DRUG INFORMATION HANDBOOK for DENTISTRY

Including Oral Medicine for Medically-Compromised Patients & Specific Oral Conditions

Senior Editors:

Richard L. Wynn, BSPharm, PhD
Timothy F. Meiller, DDS, PhD
Harold L. Crossley, DDS, PhD

17th Edition

Lexicomp™

DRUG INFORMATION HANDBOOK for DENTISTRY

Including Oral Medicine for Medically-Compromised Patients & Specific Oral Conditions

Richard L. Wynn, BSPharm, PhD
Professor of Pharmacology
Baltimore College of Dental Surgery
Dental School
University of Maryland Baltimore
Baltimore, Maryland

Timothy F. Meiller, DDS, PhD
Professor
Oncology and Diagnostic Sciences
Baltimore College of Dental Surgery
Professor of Oncology
Marlene and Stewart Greenebaum Cancer Center
University of Maryland Medical System
Baltimore, Maryland

Harold L. Crossley, DDS, PhD
Professor Emeritus
Baltimore College of Dental Surgery
Dental School
University of Maryland Baltimore
Baltimore, Maryland

Lexicomp™

NOTICE

This data is intended to serve the user as a handy reference and not as a complete drug information resource. It does not include information on every therapeutic agent available. The publication covers over 1650 commonly used drugs and is specifically designed to present important aspects of drug data in a more concise format than is typically found in medical literature or product material supplied by manufacturers.

The nature of drug information is that it is constantly evolving because of ongoing research and clinical experience and is often subject to interpretation. While great care has been taken to ensure the accuracy of the information and recommendations presented, the reader is advised that the authors, editors, reviewers, contributors, and publishers cannot be responsible for the continued currency of the information or for any errors, omissions, or the application of this information, or for any consequences arising therefrom. Therefore, the author(s) and/or the publisher shall have no liability to any person or entity with regard to claims, loss, or damage caused, or alleged to be caused, directly or indirectly, by the use of information contained herein. Because of the dynamic nature of drug information, readers are advised that decisions regarding drug therapy must be based on the independent judgment of the clinician, changing information about a drug (eg, as reflected in the literature and manufacturer's most current product information), and changing medical practices. Therefore, this data is designed to be used in conjunction with other necessary information and is not designed to be solely relied upon by any user. The user of this data hereby and forever releases the authors and publishers of this data from any and all liability of any kind that might arise out of the use of this data. The editors are not responsible for any inaccuracy of quotation or for any false or misleading implication that may arise due to the text or formulas as used or due to the quotation of revisions no longer official.

Certain of the authors, editors, and contributors have written this book in their private capacities. No official support or endorsement by any federal or state agency or pharmaceutical company is intended or inferred.

The publishers have made every effort to trace any third party copyright holders, if any, for borrowed material. If they have inadvertently overlooked any, they will be pleased to make the necessary arrangements at the first opportunity.

If you have any suggestions or questions regarding any information presented in this data, please contact our drug information pharmacists at (330) 650-6506. Book revisions are available at our website at http://www.lexi.com/home/revisions/.

This manual was produced using Lexi-Comp's Information Management System™ (LIMS) — a complete publishing service of Lexi-Comp, Inc.

Lexicomp

1100 Terex Road • Hudson, Ohio 44236
(330) 650-6506

ISBN 978-1-59195-296-1

TABLE OF CONTENTS

Part III: Sample Prescriptions

ABOUT THE EDITORS

Richard L. Wynn, BSPharm, PhD

Richard L. Wynn, PhD, is Professor of Pharmacology at the Baltimore College of Dental Surgery, Dental School, University of Maryland Baltimore. Dr Wynn has served as a dental educator, researcher, and teacher of dental pharmacology and dental hygiene pharmacology for his entire professional career. He holds a BS (pharmacy; registered pharmacist, Maryland), an MS (physiology) and a PhD (pharmacology) from the University of Maryland. Dr Wynn chaired the Department of Pharmacology at the University of Maryland Dental School from 1980 to 1995. Previously, he chaired the Department of Oral Biology at the University of Kentucky College of Dentistry.

Dr Wynn has to his credit over 350 publications including original research articles, textbooks, textbook chapters, monographs, and articles in continuing education journals. He has given close to 600 continuing education seminars to dental professionals in the U.S., Canada, and Europe. Dr Wynn has been a consultant to the drug industry for 27 years and his research laboratories have contributed to the development of new analgesics and anesthetics. He is a consultant to the Academy of General Dentistry, the American Dental Association, and a former consultant to the Council on Dental Education, Commission on Accreditation. He is a featured columnist and his drug review articles, entitled *Pharmacology Today*, appear in each issue of *General Dentistry*, a journal published by the Academy. One of his primary interests continues to be keeping dental professionals informed on all aspects of drug use in dental practice.

Timothy F. Meiller, DDS, PhD

Dr Meiller is Professor of Oncology and Diagnostic Sciences at the Baltimore College of Dental Surgery and Professor of Oncology at the Marlene and Stewart Greenebaum Cancer Center, University of Maryland Medical Systems in Baltimore. He is Director of the Oral Medicine Program in both the dental school and the cancer center. He has held his position at the Dental School for 34 years.

Dr Meiller is a Diplomate of the American Board of Oral Medicine and a graduate of Johns Hopkins University and the University of Maryland Dental and Graduate Schools, holding a DDS and a PhD in Immunology/Virology. He has over 200 publications to his credit, maintains an active general dental practice, and is a consultant to the National Institutes of Health and the Veterans Administration. He is currently engaged in ongoing investigations into cellular immune dysfunction in premalignant oral lesions, oral diseases associated with AIDS, in patients receiving therapies for cancer, and in other medically-compromised patients.

Harold L. Crossley, DDS, PhD

Dr Crossley is Professor Emeritus at the University of Maryland Dental School. A native of Rhode Island, Dr Crossley received a Bachelor of Science degree in Pharmacy from the University of Rhode Island in 1964. He later was awarded the Master of Science (1970) and Doctorate degrees (1972) in Pharmacology. The University of Maryland Dental School in Baltimore awarded Dr Crossley the DDS degree in 1980. The liaison between the classroom and his dental practice, which he mentored on a part-time basis in the Dental School Intramural Faculty Practice, produced a practical approach to understanding the pharmacology of drugs used in the dental office.

Dr Crossley has coauthored a number of articles and four books dealing with a variety of topics within the field of pharmacology. Other areas of expertise include the pharmacology of street drugs and chemical dependency. He serves on the Maryland State Dental Association's Well-Being Committee. He is an active member of Phi Kappa Phi, Omicron Kappa Upsilon Honorary Dental Society, the American College of Dentists, and International College of Dentists. He was the recipient of the 2008 Gordon Christensen Lecturer Recognition award presented by the Chicago Dental Society. He has been a consultant for the United States Drug Enforcement Administration and other law enforcement agencies since 1974. Drawing on this unique background, Dr Crossley has become nationally and internationally recognized as an expert on street drugs and chemical dependency as well as the clinical pharmacology of dental drugs.

EDITORIAL ADVISORY PANEL

Julie A. Dopheide, PharmD, BCPP
Associate Professor of Clinical Pharmacy, Psychiatry and the Behavioral Sciences
University of Southern California
Schools of Pharmacy and Medicine
Los Angeles, California

Eve Echt, MD
Medical Staff
Department of Radiology
Akron General Medical Center
Akron, Ohio

Michael S. Edwards, PharmD, MBA, BCOP
Chief, Oncology Pharmacy
Director, Oncology Pharmacy Residency Program
Walter Reed Army Medical Center
Washington, D.C.

Vicki L. Ellingrod, PharmD, BCPP
Associate Professor
University of Iowa
Iowa City, Iowa

Kelley K. Engle, BSPharm
Medical Science Pharmacist
Lexi-Comp, Inc
Hudson, Ohio

Erin Fabian, PharmD, RPh
Pharmacotherapy Specialist
Lexi-Comp, Inc
Hudson, Ohio

Elizabeth Farrington, PharmD, FCCP, FCCM, BCPS
Clinical Specialist, Pediatrics
Department of Pharmacy
University of North Carolina
Hospitals and Clinics
Chapel Hill, North Carolina

Margaret A. Fitzgerald, MS, APRN, BC, NP-C, FAANP
President
Fitzgerald Health
Education Associates, Inc.
North Andover, Massachusetts
Family Nurse Practitioner
Greater Lawrence Family Health Center
Lawrence, Massachusetts

Lawrence A. Frazee, PharmD, BCPS
Pharmacotherapy Specialist in Internal Medicine
Akron General Medical Center
Akron, Ohio

Matthew A. Fuller, PharmD, BCPS, BCPP, FASHP
Clinical Pharmacy Specialist, Psychiatry
Cleveland Department of Veterans Affairs
Medical Center
Brecksville, Ohio
Associate Clinical Professor of Psychiatry
Clinical Instructor of Psychology
Case Western Reserve University
Cleveland, Ohio
Adjunct Associate Professor of Clinical Pharmacy
University of Toledo
Toledo, Ohio

Jennifer L. Gardner, PharmD
Neonatal Clinical Pharmacy Specialist
Texas Children's Hospital
Houston, Texas

Meredith D. Girard, MD, FACP
Medical Staff
Department of Internal Medicine
Summa Health Systems
Akron, Ohio
Assistant Professor Internal Medicine
Northeast Ohio Universities College of Medicine (NEOUCOM)
Rootstown, Ohio

Morton P. Goldman, RPh, PharmD, BCPS, FCCP
Director of Pharmacotherapy Services
The Cleveland Clinic Foundation
Cleveland, Ohio

Julie A. Golembiewski, PharmD
Clinical Associate Professor
Colleges of Pharmacy and Medicine
Clinical Pharmacist, Anesthesia/Pain
University of Illinois
Chicago, Illinois

Jeffrey P. Gonzales, PharmD, BCPS
Critical Care Clinical Pharmacy Specialist
University of Maryland Medical Center
Baltimore, Maryland

Roland Grad, MDCM, MSc, CCFP, FCFP
Department of Family Medicine
McGill University
Montreal, Quebec, Canada

Larry D. Gray, PhD, ABMM
Director, Clinical Microbiology
TriHealth Laboratories
Bethesda and Good Samaritan Hospitals
Cincinnati, Ohio

Tracy Hagemann, PharmD
Associate Professor
College of Pharmacy
The University of Oklahoma
Oklahoma City, Oklahoma

Martin D. Higbee, PharmD
Associate Professor
Department of Pharmacy
Practice and Science
The University of Arizona
Tucson, Arizona

Jane Hurlburt Hodding, PharmD
Executive Director, Inpatient Pharmacy Services and Clinical Nutrition Services
Long Beach Memorial Medical Center
and Miller Children's Hospital
Long Beach, California

Sherry Luedtke, PharmD
Associate Professor and Associate Dean
Department of Pharmacy Practice
Texas Tech University
HSC School of Pharmacy
Amarillo, Texas

Vincent F. Mauro, BS, PharmD, FCCP
Professor of Clinical Pharmacy
College of Pharmacy
Adjunct Professor of Medicine
College of Medicine
The University of Toledo
Toledo, Ohio

Barrie McCombs, MD, FCFP
Medical Information Service Coordinator
The Alberta Rural Physician Action Plan
Calgary, Alberta, Canada

Timothy F. Meiller, DDS, PhD
Professor
Oncology and Diagnostic Sciences
Baltimore College of Dental Surgery
Professor of Oncology
Marlene and Stewart
Greenebaum Cancer Center
University of Maryland Medical System
Baltimore, Maryland

Geralyn M. Meny, MD
Medical Director
American Red Cross,
Penn-Jersey Region
Philadelphia, Pennsylvania

Julie Miller, PharmD
Pharmacy Clinical Specialist, Cardiology
Columbus Children's Hospital
Columbus, Ohio

Leah Millstein, MD
Assistant Professor
Division of General Internal Medicine
University of Maryland School of Medicine
Baltimore, Maryland

Kevin M. Mulieri, BS, PharmD
Pediatric Hematology/Oncology Clinical Specialist
Penn State Milton S. Hershey
Medical Center
Instructor of Pharmacology
Penn State College of Medicine
Hershey, Pennsylvania

Tom Palma, MS, RPh
Medical Science Pharmacist
Lexi-Comp, Inc
Hudson, Ohio

Susie H. Park, PharmD, BCPP
Assistant Professor of Clinical Pharmacy
University of Southern Califormia
Los Angeles, California

Alpa Patel, PharmD
Antimicrobial Clinical Pharmacist
University of Louisville Hospital
Louisville, Kentucky

Gayle Pearson, BSPharm, MSA
Drug Information Pharmacist
Peter Lougheed Centre,
Alberta Health Services
Calgary, Alberta, Canada

James A. Ponto, MS, RPh, BCNP
Chief Nuclear Pharmacist
Department of Radiology
University of Iowa, Hospitals and Clinics
Professor of Clinical Pharmacy
Department of Pharmacy
Practice and Science
University of Iowa College of Pharmacy
Iowa City, Iowa

James Reissig, PharmD
Assistant Director, Clinical Services
Akron General Medical Center
Akron, Ohio

A.J. (Fred) Remillard, PharmD
Assistant Dean,
Research and Graduate Affairs
College of Pharmacy and Nutrition
University of Saskatchewan
Saskatoon, Saskatchewan

Curtis M. Rimmermann, MD, MBA, FACC
Gus P. Karos Chair,
Clinical Cardiovascular Medicine
Department of Cardiovascular Medicine
Cleveland Clinic Foundation
Cleveland, Ohio

P. David Rogers, PharmD, PhD, FCCP
Professor and Associate Dean for Translational Research
University of Tennessee
College of Pharmacy
Memphis, Tennessee

Martha Sajatovic, MD
Professor of Psychiatry
Case Western Reserve University
Cleveland, Ohio
Department of Psychiatry
University Hospitals of Cleveland
Cleveland, Ohio

Jennifer K. Sekeres, PharmD, BCPS
Infectious Diseases Clinical Specialist
The Cleveland Clinic Foundation
Cleveland, Ohio

Todd P. Semla, MS, PharmD, BCPS, FCCP, AGSF
Clinical Pharmacy Specialist
Department of Veterans Affairs
Pharmacy Benefits
Management Services
Associate Professor, Clinical
Department of Medicine and Psychiatry
and Behavioral Health
Feinberg School of Medicine
Northwestern University
Chicago, Illinois

PREFACE TO THE SEVENTEENTH EDITION

The editors of the 17th edition of the *Drug Information Handbook for Dentistry* are extremely proud that the book remains as popular and as successful as its readers have affirmed. We thank each practitioner and student who has made the previous editions so widely accepted in the field of dentistry. In this new 17th edition, we have continued, as always, to respond to all of the comments and creative suggestions that come from our readership each year. We know that our text remains the premier companion to the daily practice of dentistry and that it complements Oral Medicine and medical reference libraries that every clinician has available in their office.

In addition to the extensive information presented, we are confident that the dental practitioners and dental hygienists who utilize the text have found it to be easy to navigate and their pharmacotherapeutics knowledge and oral medicine questions have been enhanced by its use. The complete cross-referencing of generic and brand names along with the foreign brands, makes the text the truly complete drug reference guide for dental practice.

The monographs now include over 1650 drugs and these have been updated in the 17th edition with the fields expanded in common monographs to make them easier to read and identify for all of the drugs. The fields most important to practicing dentists have been enhanced. The drugs most commonly used in dentistry have the added fields regarding specific use considerations in dentistry. Medical drugs also include dosing and dose formulation information. In addition, the adverse reaction section and the important uses and effects on dental treatment for all drugs have been updated throughout the text.

As in each previous edition, the Oral Medicine section has been updated offering a selection of prescription choices for management of common oral conditions often encountered during patient care. Stand-alone sections have now been enhanced for Antiplatelet and Anticoagulation Considerations in Dentistry, Clinical Risk Related to Drugs Prolonging QT Interval, and Osteonecrosis of the Jaw. The chapters related to pain, burning mouth, osteonecrosis as an oral complication, and others have been updated to assist in formulating a differential diagnosis. Recommended readings have been edited for most chapter subsections. Example prescriptions have been updated and remain in a stand-alone section for quicker reference. Prescribing information options are outlined and are available for easy cross reference for the dental practitioner. The subsection for Probiotics to Reduce Symptoms During Long-Term Antibiotic Therapy has been enhanced.

The alphabetical index at the back of the text continues to guide the reader through the text. The natural products section; drug synonyms; and U.S., Canadian, and Mexican brand names have all been updated. We hope that the active general dentist, the specialist, the dental hygienist, and the advanced student of dentistry remain better prepared for patient care while using this new 17th edition of the DIHD.

Richard L. Wynn

Timothy F. Meiller

Harold L. Crossley

DESCRIPTION OF SECTIONS AND FIELDS USED IN THIS HANDBOOK

The *Drug Information Handbook for Dentistry, 17th Edition* is organized into six sections: Introductory text; alphabetical listing of drug monographs; natural products; oral medicine topics; appendix; and indexes which include pharmacologic categories and alphabetical listings containing generic product names and index terms, as well as U.S., Canadian, and Mexican brand names.

INTRODUCTORY TEXT

Helpful guides to understanding the organization and format of the information in this handbook.

DRUG MONOGRAPHS

This alphabetical listing of drugs contains comprehensive monographs for medications commonly prescribed in dentistry and concise monographs for other popular drugs which dental patients may be taking. Monographs may contain the following fields:

Generic Name	U.S. adopted name
Pronunciation	Phonetic pronunciation guide
Related Information	Cross-reference(s) to pertinent information in other sections of this handbook
Related Sample Prescriptions	Cross-reference(s) to sample prescriptions.
U.S. Brand Names	Trade name(s) (manufacturer-specific) found in the United States. The symbol [DSC] appears after trade names that have been recently discontinued.
Canadian Brand Names	Trade names found in Canada.
Generic Availability (U.S.)	Indicates availability of generic products in the United States
Pharmacologic Category	Indicates one or more systematic classifications of the drug
Dental Use	Information in the **Dental Use** field indicates when a drug has an established use specific to dentistry and/or oral medicine. In some cases, these uses are considered to be unlabeled, as they are not included in the FDA-approved product labeling (see Description of Dental Use).
Use	Statements under the **Use** field reflect the approved labeling by the FDA based on accepted clinical evaluation on safety and efficacy of the drug as submitted in the New Drug Application (NDA). The "gold standard" of clinical testing of a new drug requires a randomly-selected cohort of subjects, using a double-blind and placebo controlled protocol and an acceptable method of assessment to test differences between test compound and placebo. It is assumed that by their approval of the labeling, the FDA considers the new drug "safe and effective" for treating a particular condition in a given patient population.

Unlabeled/Investigational Use	Statements under the **Unlabeled/Investigational** use field refer to other conditions, dosages, or routes of administration which are decided by the prescriber, where such uses have not been officially approved by the FDA. Such "off label" use usually occurs in response to published studies supporting a drug's effectiveness in a new use and/or alternative dosing strategy. It is important to note that individual reports do not necessarily indicate in and of themselves that the safety and effectiveness of the drug in question has been established for the new use. If an individual report is one of many studies, the clinician is encouraged to read and critically review all of the studies in order to arrive at a decision on the safety and efficacy for the "off label" use.
Local Anesthetic/ Vasoconstrictor Precautions	Specific information to prevent potential drug interactions related to anesthesia
Effects on Dental Treatment	Includes significant side effects of drug therapy which may directly or indirectly affect dental treatment or diagnosis; may also contain suggested management approaches and patient handling or care.
Effects on Bleeding	How the product affects bleeding during dental procedures
Adverse Effects	Side effects are grouped by percentage of incidence (if known) and/or body system
Dental Usual Dosage	The amount of the drug to be typically given or taken during dental treatment for children and adults
Dosage	The amount of the drug to be typically given or taken during therapy for children and adults; also includes any dosing adjustment/comments for renal impairment or hepatic failure; **Note:** For General Dosage Range: The range of dosing typically used during therapy in children and adults based upon route of administration. The information included is useful for confirming the dose is within the range but should not be used for prescribing purposes. Medications with a variety of indication-specific doses that cannot be encompassed by a range will not have a dose.
Mechanism of Action	How the drug works in the body to elicit a response
Contraindications	Information pertaining to inappropriate use of the drug as dictated by the approved labeling
Warnings/Precautions	Precautionary considerations, hazardous conditions related to use of the drug, and disease states or patient populations in which the drug should be cautiously used. Boxed warnings, when present, are clearly identified and are adapted from the FDA approved labeling. Consult the product labeling for the exact black box warning through the manufacturer's or the FDA website.
Drug Interactions	
Metabolism/Transport Effects	If a drug has demonstrated involvement with cytochrome P450 enzymes, or other metabolism or transport proteins, this field will identify the drug as an inhibitor, inducer, or substrate of the specific enzyme(s) (eg, CYP1A2 or UGT1A1). CYP450 isoenzymes are identified as substrates (minor or major), inhibitors (weak, moderate, or strong), and inducers (weak or strong).
Avoid Concomitant Use	Designates drug combinations which should not be used concomitantly, due to an unacceptable risk:benefit assessment. Frequently, the concurrent use of the agents is explicitly prohibited or contraindicated by the product labeling.

Increased Effect/Toxicity	Drug combinations that result in an increased or toxic therapeutic effect between the drug listed in the monograph and other drugs or drug classes.
Decreased Effect	Drug combinations that result in a decreased therapeutic effect between the drug listed in the monograph and other drugs or drug classes.
Ethanol/Nutrition/Herb Interactions	Information regarding potential interactions with food, nutritionals, herbal products, vitamins, or ethanol
Dietary Considerations	Includes information on how the medication should be taken relative to meals or food
Pharmacodynamics/Kinetics	
Onset of Action	The time after drug administration when therapeutic effect is observed; may also include time for peak therapeutic effect.
Duration of Action	Length of therapeutic effect.
Half-Life Elimination	The reported half-life of elimination for the parent or metabolites of the drug
Time to Peak	Describes the relative time after ingestion when concentration achieves the highest serum concentration
Pregnancy Risk Factor	Five categories established by the FDA to indicate the potential of a systemically absorbed drug for causing risk to fetus.
Lactation	Indicates if the drug listed in the monograph is present in breast milk and the manufacturers' recommendation for use while breast-feeding (where recommendation of American Academy of Pediatrics differs, notation is made).
Breast-Feeding Considerations	Information pertinent to or associated with the human use of the drug as it relates to clinical effects on the nursing infant or postpartum woman.
Product Availability	Provides availability information on products that have been approved by the FDA, but not yet available for use. Estimates for when a product may be available are included, when this information is known. May also provide any unique or critical drug availability issues.
Controlled Substance	Contains controlled substance schedule information as assigned by the United States Drug Enforcement Administration (DEA) or Canadian Controlled Substance Act (CDSA). CDSA information is only provided for drugs available in Canada and not available in the U.S.
Prescribing and Access Restrictions	Provides information on any special requirements regarding the prescribing, obtaining or dispensing of drugs, including access restrictions pertaining to drugs with REMS elements and those drugs whose access restrictions are not REMS-related.
Dosage Forms	Information with regard to form, strength, and availability of the drug in the United States. **Note:** Please consult individual product labeling for additional formulation information (eg, excipients, preservatives).
Dosage Forms: Canada	Information with regard to form, strength, and availability of products that are uniquely available in Canada, but currently not available in the United States.
Dental Comment	Pharmacology-related comments and considerations relevant to the dental professional
References	Sources and literature where the user may find additional information

NATURAL PRODUCTS: HERBAL AND DIETARY SUPPLEMENTS

This section is divided into two parts. First, is a brief introduction to popular natural products, followed by an alphabetical listing of herbal and dietary supplements commonly purchased over-the-counter which patients may be taking. Monographs may contain the following:

NATURAL PRODUCT MONOGRAPHS

Name	Common name
Related Information	Cross-reference(s) to related monographs
Pharmacologic Category	Indicates one or more systematic classifications of the drug
Reported Use	Reported uses are based on clinical efficacy in human and animal studies. These uses are not all-inclusive for each plant, but are the most widely recommended and currently accepted in the medical community.
Local Anesthetic/ Vasoconstrictor Precautions	Specific information to prevent potential interactions related to anesthesia
Effects on Bleeding	How the product affects bleeding during dental procedures
Warnings/Precautions	Cautions and hazardous conditions related to use
References	Sources used to verify included information.

ORAL MEDICINE TOPICS

This section is divided into three major parts and contains text on Oral Medicine topics. In each subsection, the systemic condition or the oral disease state is described briefly, followed by the pharmacologic considerations with which the dentist must be familiar.

I. **Dental Management and Therapeutic Considerations in Medically-Compromised Patients:** Focuses on common medical conditions and their associated drug therapies with which the dentist must be familiar. Patient profiles with commonly associated drug regimens are described.

II. **Dental Management and Therapeutic Considerations in Patients With Specific Oral Conditions:** Focuses on therapies the dentist may choose to prescribe for patients suffering from oral disease or who are in need of special care. Some overlap between these sections has resulted from systemic conditions that have oral manifestations and vice-versa. Cross-references to the descriptions and the monographs for individual drugs described elsewhere in this handbook allow for easy retrieval of information. Example prescriptions for drugs commonly used in the treatment of each condition are presented so that the clinician can evaluate alternate approaches to treatment. Seldom is there a single drug of choice.
Note: Prescriptions listed represent prototype drugs and popular prescriptions and are examples only. The pharmacologic category index is available for cross-referencing if alternatives or additional drugs are sought.

III. **Sample Prescriptions:** Examples provided for prototype drugs and popular prescriptions. Prescriptions included for the following uses: Bacterial endocarditis (prevention), prosthetic joint late infections (prevention), oral pain, bacterial infections and periodontal diseases, sinus infections treatment, antimicrobial rinses, fungal infections, viral infections, ulcerative and erosive disorders, sedation (prior to dental treatment).

APPENDIX

The appendix is broken down into various sections for easy use and offers a compilation of tables and guidelines which can often be helpful when considering patient care.

INDEXES

This section includes a pharmacologic category index with an easy-to-use classification system in alphabetical order and an alphabetical index which provides a quick reference for generic names, index terms, U.S., Canadian, and Mexican brand names. From this index, the reader can cross-reference to the monographs.

DESCRIPTION OF DENTAL USE

Unlabeled Use and Routes of Administration in Dentistry and Oral Medicine

The off-label use of a medication may involve differences in either the intended purpose or the route of administration of a particular medication. In dentistry, there are some situations which are common (clindamycin for endocarditis prophylaxis), and uncommon (application of Oralone® paste to the oral mucosa) which may be termed "unlabeled use". Depending on the degree of familiarity, the prescription of a drug for an off-label purpose may create concern on the part of healthcare professionals who are less familiar with the dental use of these medications. For example, a pharmacist may note the statement "for external use only" on the label of a tube of topical cream and question whether the drug should be applied to the oral mucosa. Usually, reinforcement of the use of a drug as well as an analysis of the likely systemic exposure/toxicity, can address these concerns.

The dentist who prescribes a drug bears the responsibility for deciding on the purpose of the prescription and the detail of the dosing regimen. These professional decisions are based on information from a variety of sources, including (but not limited to) the official labeling, sound scientific evidence, expert medical judgment, or published literature. In selected situations, these sources may justify the use of a drug in an off-label manner. Accepted professional standards indicate off-label use of a drug must be initiated in good faith, serve the best interest of the patient, and must be undertaken without fraudulent intent. Healthcare providers should recognize that the approved labeling is not intended to limit the practitioners in the exercise of his or her best professional judgment in serving the interest of patients. In addition, the purpose of labeling is not intended to impose liability for off-label use. However, it should be noted that a practitioner may be accountable for the negligent use in a civil action regardless of whether the FDA has approved the use of the drug in question. Based on these assertions, at least one medical organization (the American Academy of Pediatrics) has published in an official policy statement that the practice of medicine may actually require a practitioner to use drugs in an off-label manner in order to provide the most appropriate treatment for a given patient. Off-label use in dentistry and oral medicine is a frequently encountered issue. A discussion of the off-label use of drugs in dentistry appears in the ADA guide to Dental Therapeutics, 3rd Edition, edited by Sebastian G. Ciancio, DDS in cooperation with the ADA Council on Scientific Affairs.

CONTROLLED SUBSTANCES

Schedule I = C-I

The drugs and other substances in this schedule have no legal medical uses except research. They have a **high** potential for abuse. They include selected opiates such as heroin, opium derivatives, and hallucinogens.

Schedule II = C-II

The drugs and other substances in this schedule have legal medical uses and a **high** abuse potential which may lead to severe dependence. They include former "Class A" narcotics, amphetamines, barbiturates, and other drugs.

Schedule III = C-III

The drugs and other substances in this schedule have legal medical uses and a **lesser** degree of abuse potential which may lead to **moderate** dependence. They include former "Class B" narcotics and other drugs.

Schedule IV = C-IV

The drugs and other substances in this schedule have legal medial uses and **low** abuse potential which may lead to **moderate** dependence. They include barbiturates, benzodiazepines, propoxyphenes, and other drugs.

Schedule V = C-V

The drugs and other substances in this schedule have legal medical uses and **low** abuse potential which may lead to **moderate** dependence. They include narcotic cough preparations, diarrhea preparations, and other drugs.

Note: These are federal classifications. Your individual state may place a substance into a more restricted category. When this occurs, the more restricted category applies. Consult your state law.

PREGNANCY CATEGORIES

Pregnancy Categories (sometimes referred to as pregnancy risk factors) are a letter system currently required under the *Teratogenic Effects* subsection of the product labeling. The system was initiated in 1979. The categories are required to be part of the package insert for prescription drugs that are systemically absorbed.

The categories are defined as follows:

A Adequate and well-controlled studies in pregnant women have not shown that the drug increases the risk of fetal abnormalities.

B Animal reproduction studies show no evidence of impaired fertility or harm to the fetus; however, no adequate and well-controlled studies have been conducted in pregnant women.
or
Animal reproduction studies have shown adverse events; however, studies in pregnant women have not shown that the drug increases the risk of abnormalities.

C Animal reproduction studies have shown an adverse effect on the fetus. There are no adequate and well-controlled studies in humans and the benefits from the use of the drug in pregnant women may be acceptable, despite its potential risks.
or
Animal reproduction studies have not been conducted.

D Based on human data, the drug can cause fetal harm when administered to pregnant women, but the potential benefits from the use of the drug may be acceptable, despite its potential risks.

X Studies in animals or humans have demonstrated fetal abnormalities (or there is positive evidence of fetal risk based on reports and/or marketing experience) and the risk of using the drug in pregnant women clearly outweighs any possible benefit (for example, safer drugs or other forms of therapy are available).

The categories do not take into consideration nonteratogenic effects (that information is currently presented separately). In 2008, the Food and Drug Administration (FDA) proposed new labeling requirements which would eliminate the use of the pregnancy category system and replace it with scientific data and other information specific to the use of the drug in pregnant women. These proposed changes were suggested because the current category system may be misleading. For instance, some practitioners may believe that risk increases from category A to B to C to D to X, which is not the intent. In addition, practitioners may not be aware that some medications are categorized based on animal data, while others are based on human data. When the new labeling requirements are approved, product labeling will contain pregnancy and lactation subsections, each describing a risk summary, clinical considerations, and section for specific data.

For full descriptions of the current and proposed labeling requirements, refer to the following websites:

Labeling Requirements for Prescription Drugs and/or Insulin (Code of Federal Regulations, Title 21, Volume 4, Revised April 1, 2010). Available at: http://www.accessdata.fda.gov/scripts/cdrh/cfdocs/cfCFR/CFRSearch.cfm?fr=201.57.

Content and Format of Labeling for Human Prescription Drug and Biological Products; Requirements for Pregnancy and Lactation Labeling (Federal Register, May 29, 2008). Available at: http://frwebgate.access.gpo.gov/cgi-bin/getdoc.cgi?dbname=2008_register&docid=fr29my08-33.pdf.

FDA NAME DIFFERENTIATION PROJECT: THE USE OF TALL-MAN LETTERS

Confusion between similar drug names is an important cause of medication errors. For years, The Institute For Safe Medication Practices (ISMP), has urged generic manufacturers to use a combination of large and small letters as well as bolding (ie, chlorpro**MAZINE** and chlorpro**PAMIDE**) to help distinguish drugs with look-alike names, especially when they share similar strengths. Recently the FDA's Division of Generic Drugs began to issue recommendation letters to manufacturers suggesting this novel way to label their products to help reduce this drug name confusion. Although this project has had marginal success, the method has successfully eliminated problems with products such as diphenhydr**AMINE** and dimenhy**DRINATE**. Hospitals should also follow suit by making similar changes in their own labels, preprinted order forms, computer screens and printouts, and drug storage location labels.

Lexi-Comp, Inc. Medical Publishing will use "Tall-Man" letters for the drugs suggested by the FDA or recommended by ISMP.

The following is a list of generic and brand name product names and recommended revisions.

Drug Product	Recommended Revision
acetazolamide	aceta**ZOLAMIDE**
alprazolam	**ALPRAZ**olam
amiloride	a**MIL**oride
amlodipine	am**LODIP**ine
aripiprazole	**ARIP**iprazole
Avinza	**AVIN**za
azacitidine	aza**CITID**ine
azathioprine	aza**THIO**prine
bupropion	bu**PROP**ion
buspirone	bus**PIR**one
carbamazepine	car**BAM**azepine
carboplatin	**CARBO**platin
cefazolin	ce**FAZ**olin
cefotetan	cefo**TE**tan
cefoxitin	cef**OX**itin
ceftazidime	cef**TAZ**idime
ceftriaxone	cef**TRIAX**one
Celebrex	Cele**BREX**
Celexa	Cele**XA**
chlordiazepoxide	chlordiaze**POXIDE**
chlorpromazine	chlorpro**MAZINE**
chlorpropamide	chlorpro**PAMIDE**
cisplatin	**CIS**platin
clomiphene	clomi**PHENE**
clomipramine	clomi**PRAMINE**
clonazepam	clonaze**PAM**
clonidine	clo**NID**ine
clozapine	clo**ZAP**ine
cycloserine	cyclo**SERINE**
cyclosporine	cyclo**SPORINE**
dactinomycin	**DACTIN**omycin
daptomycin	**DAPTO**mycin
daunorubicin	**DAUNO**rubicin
dimenhydrinate	dimenhy**DRINATE**

Drug Product	Recommended Revision
diphenhydramine	diphenhydr**AMINE**
dobutamine	**DOBUT**amine
docetaxel	**DOCE**taxel
dopamine	**DOP**amine
doxorubicin	**DOXO**rubicin
duloxetine	**DUL**oxetine
ephedrine	e**PHED**rine
epinephrine	**EPINEPH**rine
fentanyl	fenta**NYL**
flavoxate	flavox**ATE**
fluoxetine	**FLU**oxetine
fluphenazine	flu**PHENAZ**ine
fluvoxamine	fluvoxa**MINE**
glipizide	glipi**ZIDE**
glyburide	gly**BURIDE**
guaifenesin	guai**FEN**esin
guanfacine	guan**FACINE**
Humalog	Huma**LOG**
Humulin	Humu**LIN**
hydralazine	hydr**ALAZINE**
hydrocodone	**HYDRO**codone
hydromorphone	**HYDRO**morphone
hydroxyzine	hydr**OXY**zine
idarubicin	**IDA**rubicin
infliximab	in**FLIX**imab
Invanz	**INV**anz
isotretinoin	**ISO**tretinoin
Klonopin	Klono**PIN**
Lamictal	La**MIC**tal
Lamisil	Lam**ISIL**
lamivudine	lami**VUD**ine
lamotrigine	lamo**TRI**gine
levetiracetam	Lev**ETIRA**cetam
levocarnitine	lev**OCARN**itine
lorazepam	**LOR**azepam
medroxyprogesterone	medroxy**PROGESTER**one
metformin	met**FORMIN**
methylprednisolone	methyl**PREDNIS**olone
methyltestosterone	methyl**TESTOSTER**one
metronidazole	metro**NIDAZOLE**
mitomycin	mito**MY**cin
mitoxantrone	Mito**XAN**trone
Nexavar	Nex**AVAR**
Nexium	Nex**IUM**
nicardipine	ni**CAR**dipine
nifedipine	**NIFE**dipine
nimodipine	ni**MOD**ipine
Novolin	Novo**LIN**
Novolog	Novo**LOG**
olanzapine	**OLANZ**apine
oxcarbazepine	**OX**carbazepine
oxycodone	oxy**CODONE**
Oxycontin	Oxy**CONTIN**

Drug Product	Recommended Revision
paclitaxel	**PACL**itaxel
paroxetine	**PAR**oxetine
pemetrexed	**PEME**trexed
pentobarbital	**PENT**obarbital
phenobarbital	**PHEN**obarbital
pralatrexate	**PRALA**trexate
prednisolone	predniso**LONE**
prednisone	predni**SONE**
Prilosec	Pri**LOSEC**
Prozac	**PRO**zac
quetiapine	**QUE**tiapine
quinidine	qui**NID**ine
quinine	qui**NINE**
rabeprazole	**RABE**prazole
Risperdal	Risper**DAL**
risperidone	risperi**DONE**
rituximab	ri**TUX**imab
romidepsin	romi**DEP**sin
romiplostim	romi**PLOS**tim
ropinirole	r**OPINIR**ole
Sandimmune	sand**IMMUNE**
Sandostatin	Sando**STATIN**
Seroquel	**SERO**quel
Sinequan	**SINE**quan
sitagliptin	sita**GLIP**tin
Solu-Cortef	Solu-**CORTEF**
Solu-Medrol	Solu-**MEDROL**
sorafenib	**SORA**fenib
sufentanil	**SUF**entanil
sulfadiazine	sulf**ADIAZINE**
sulfasalazine	sulfa**SALA**zine
sumatriptan	**SUMA**triptan
sunitinib	**SUNI**tinib
Tegretol	**TEG**retol
tiagabine	tia**GAB**ine
tizanidine	ti**ZAN**idine
tolazamide	**TOLAZ**amide
tolbutamide	**TOLBUT**amide
tramadol	tra**MAD**ol
trazodone	tra**ZOD**one
Trental	**TREN**tal
valacyclovir	val**ACY**clovir
valganciclovir	val**GAN**ciclovir
vinblastine	vin**BLAS**tine
vincristine	vin**CRIS**tine
zolmitriptan	**ZOLM**itriptan
Zyprexa	Zy**PREXA**
Zyrtec	Zyr**TEC**

"FDA and ISMP Lists of Look-Alike Drug Names with Recommended Tall Man Letter." Available at http://www.ismp.org/tools/tallmanletters.pdf. Last accessed January 6, 2011.

"Name Differentiation Project." Available at: http://www.fda.gov/Drugs/DrugSafety/MedicationErrors/ucm164587.htm. Last accessed January 6, 2011.

U.S. Pharmacopeia, "USP Quality Review: Use Caution-Avoid Confusion," March 2001, No. 76. Available at: http://www.usp.org.

PRESCRIPTION WRITING

Doctor's Name
Address
Phone Number

Patient's Name/Date

Patient's Address/Age

Rx

Drug Name/Dosage Size
Disp: Number of tablets, capsules, ounces to be dispensed (roman numerals added as precaution for abused drugs)
Sig: Direction on how drug is to be taken

Doctor's signature
State license number
DEA number (if required)

PRESCRIPTION REQUIREMENTS

1. Date
2. Full name and address of patient
3. Name and address of prescriber
4. Signature of prescriber

If Class II drug, Drug Enforcement Agency (DEA) number necessary.

If Class II and Class III narcotic, a triplicate prescription form (in the state of California) is necessary and it must be handwritten by the prescriber.

Please turn to appropriate oral medicine chapters for examples of prescriptions.

PREVENTING PRESCRIBING ERRORS

Prescribing errors account for the majority of reported medication errors and have prompted healthcare professionals to focus on the development of steps to make the prescribing process safer. Prescription legibility has been attributed to a portion of these errors and legislation has been enacted in several states to address prescription legibility. However, eliminating handwritten prescriptions and ordering medications through the use of technology [eg, computerized prescriber order entry (CPOE)] has been the primary recommendation. Whether a prescription is electronic, typed, or hand-printed, additional safe practices should be considered for implementation to maximize the safety of the prescribing process. Listed below are suggestions for safer prescribing:

- Ensure correct patient by using at least 2 patient identifiers on the prescription (eg, full name, birth date, or address). Review prescription with the patient or patient's caregiver.
- If pediatric patient, document patient's birth date or age and most recent weight. If geriatric patient, document patient's birth date or age.
- Prevent drug name confusion:
  - Use TALLman lettering (eg, buPROPion, busPIRone, predniSONE, prednisoLONE). For more information see: http://www.fda.gov/Drugs/DrugSafety/MedicationErrors/ucm164587.htm.
  - Avoid abbreviated drug names (eg, MSO_4, $MgSO_4$, MS, HCT, 6MP, MTX), as they may be misinterpreted and cause error.
  - Avoid investigational names for drugs with FDA approval (eg, FK-506, CBDCA).
  - Avoid chemical names such as 6-mercaptopurine or 6-thioguanine, as sixfold overdoses have been given when these were not recognized as chemical names. The proper names of these drugs are mercaptopurine or thioguanine.
  - Use care when prescribing drugs that look or sound similar (eg, look- alike, sound-alike drugs). Common examples include: Celebrex® vs Celexa®, hydroxyzine vs hydralazine, Zyprexa® vs Zyrtec®.
- Avoid dangerous, error-prone abbreviations (eg, regardless of letter-case: U, IU, QD, QOD, µg, cc, @). Do not use apothecary system or symbols. Additionally, text messaging abbreviations (eg, "2Day") should never be used.
  - For more information see: http://www.ismp.org/Tools/errorproneabbreviations.pdf
- Always use a leading zero for numbers less than 1 (0.5 mg is correct and .5 mg is **incorrect**) and never use a trailing zero for whole numbers (2 mg is correct and 2.0 mg is **incorrect**).
- Always use a space between a number and its units as it is easier to read. There should be no periods after the abbreviations mg or mL (10 mg is correct and 10mg is **incorrect**).
- For doses that are greater than 1,000 dosing units, use properly placed commas to prevent 10-fold errors (100,000 units is correct and 100000 units is **incorrect**).
- Do not prescribe drug dosage by the type of container in which the drug is available (eg, do not prescribe "1 amp", "2 vials", etc).
- Do not write vague or ambiguous orders which have the potential for misinterpretation by other healthcare providers. Examples of vague orders to avoid: "resume pre-op medications," "give drug per protocol," or "continue home medications."
- Review each prescription with patient (or patient's caregiver) including the medication name, indication, and directions for use.
- Take extra precautions when prescribing *high alert drugs* (drugs that can cause significant patient harm when prescribed in error). Common examples of these drugs include: Anticoagulants, chemotherapy, insulins, opiates, and sedatives.
  - For more information see: http://www.ismp.org/Tools/highalertmedications.pdf

To Err is Human: Building a Safer Health System, Kohn LT, Corrigan JM, and Donaldson MS, eds, Washington, D.C.: National Academy Press, 2000.

A Complete Outpatient Prescription[1]

A complete outpatient prescription can prevent the prescriber, the pharmacist, and/or the patient from making a mistake and can eliminate the need for further clarification. The complete outpatient prescription should contain:

- Patient's full name
- Medication indication
- Allergies
- Prescriber name and telephone or pager number
- For pediatric patients: Their birth date or age and current weight
- For geriatric patients: Their birth date or age
- Drug name, dosage form and strength
- For pediatric patients: Intended daily weight-based dose so that calculations can be checked by the pharmacist (ie, mg/kg/day or units/kg/day)
- Number or amount to be dispensed
- Complete instructions for the patient or caregiver, including the purpose of the medication, directions for use (including dose), dosing frequency, route of administration, duration of therapy, and number of refills.
- Dose should be expressed in convenient units of measure.
- When there are recognized contraindications for a prescribed drug, the prescriber should indicate knowledge of this fact to the pharmacist (ie, when prescribing a potassium salt for a patient receiving an ACE inhibitor, the prescriber should write "K serum leveling being monitored").

Upon dispensing of the final product, the pharmacist should ensure that the patient or caregiver can effectively demonstrate the appropriate administration technique. An appropriate measuring device should be provided or recommended. Household teaspoons and tablespoons should not be used to measure liquid medications due to their variability and inaccuracies in measurement; oral medication syringes are recommended.

For additional information see: http://www.ppag.org/attachments/files/111/Guidelines_Peds.pdf

[1]Levine SR, Cohen MR, Blanchard NR, et al, "Guidelines for Preventing Medication Errors in Pediatrics," *J Pediatr Pharmacol Ther*, 2001, 6:426-42.

ALPHABETICAL LISTING OF DRUGS

Abacavir (a BAK a veer)

Related Information

HIV Infection and AIDS *on page 1883*

U.S. Brand Names Ziagen®

Canadian Brand Names Ziagen®

Pharmacologic Category Antiretroviral Agent, Reverse Transcriptase Inhibitor (Nucleoside)

Use Treatment of HIV infections in combination with other antiretroviral agents

Local Anesthetic/Vasoconstrictor Precautions No information available to require special precautions

Effects on Dental Treatment No significant effects or complications reported

Effects on Bleeding No information available to require special precautions relative to altered hemostasis

Adverse Effects Hypersensitivity reactions (which may be fatal) occur in ~5% of patients. Symptoms may include anaphylaxis, fever, rash (including erythema multiforme), fatigue, diarrhea, abdominal pain; respiratory symptoms (eg, pharyngitis, dyspnea, cough, adult respiratory distress syndrome, or respiratory failure); headache, malaise, lethargy, myalgia, myolysis, arthralgia, edema, paresthesia, nausea and vomiting, mouth ulcerations, conjunctivitis, lymphadenopathy, hepatic failure, and renal failure.

Note: Rates of adverse reactions were defined during combination therapy with other antiretrovirals (lamivudine and efavirenz **or** lamivudine and zidovudine). Only reactions which occurred at a higher frequency in adults (except where noted) than in the comparator group are noted. Adverse reaction rates attributable to abacavir alone are not available.

>10%:
- Central nervous system: Headache (7% to 13%)
- Gastrointestinal: Nausea (7% to 19%, children 9%)

1% to 10%:
- Central nervous system: Depression (6%), fever/chills (6%, children 9%), anxiety (5%)
- Dermatologic: Rash (5% to 6%, children 7%)
- Endocrine & metabolic: Triglycerides increased (2% to 6%)
- Gastrointestinal: Diarrhea (7%), vomiting (children 9%), amylase increased (2%)
- Hematologic: Thrombocytopenia (1%)
- Hepatic: AST increased (6%)
- Neuromuscular & skeletal: Musculoskeletal pain (5% to 6%)
- Miscellaneous: Hypersensitivity reactions (2% to 9%; may include reactions to other components of antiretroviral regimen), infection (ENT 5%)

General Dosage Range Dosage adjustment recommended in patients with hepatic impairment

Oral:

Children 3 months to 16 years: 8 mg/kg twice daily (maximum: 300 mg twice daily)

Adults: 600 mg/day in 1-2 divided (maximum: 600 mg/day)

Mechanism of Action Nucleoside reverse transcriptase inhibitor. Abacavir is a guanosine analogue which is phosphorylated to carbovir triphosphate which interferes with HIV viral RNA-dependent DNA polymerase resulting in inhibition of viral replication.

Pharmacodynamics/Kinetics

Half-life Elimination 1.5 hours

Time to Peak 0.7-1.7 hours

Pregnancy Risk Factor C

Abacavir and Lamivudine (a BAK a veer & la MI vyoo deen)

Related Information

Abacavir *on page 24*

LamiVUDine *on page 978*

U.S. Brand Names Epzicom®

Canadian Brand Names Kivexa™

Pharmacologic Category Antiretroviral Agent, Reverse Transcriptase Inhibitor (Nucleoside)

Use Treatment of HIV infections in combination with other antiretroviral agents

Local Anesthetic/Vasoconstrictor Precautions No information available to require special precautions

Effects on Dental Treatment No significant effects or complications reported

Effects on Bleeding No information available to require special precautions relative to altered hemostasis

Adverse Effects See individual agents.

General Dosage Range Oral: *Adults:* One tablet (abacavir 600 mg and lamivudine 300 mg) once daily

Mechanism of Action Nucleoside reverse transcriptase inhibitor combination.

Abacavir is a guanosine analogue which is phosphorylated to carbovir triphosphate which interferes with HIV viral RNA-dependent DNA polymerase resulting in inhibition of viral replication.

Lamivudine is a cytosine analog. After lamivudine is triphosphorylated, the principle mode of action is inhibition of HIV reverse transcription via viral DNA chain termination; inhibits RNA-dependent DNA polymerase activities of reverse transcriptase.

Pregnancy Risk Factor C

Abacavir, Lamivudine, and Zidovudine

(a BAK a veer, la MI vyoo deen, & zye DOE vyoo deen)

Related Information

Abacavir *on page 24*
LamiVUDine *on page 978*
Zidovudine *on page 1742*

U.S. Brand Names Trizivir®

Canadian Brand Names Trizivir®

Pharmacologic Category Antiretroviral Agent, Reverse Transcriptase Inhibitor (Nucleoside)

Use Treatment of HIV infection (either alone or in combination with other antiretroviral agents) in patients whose regimen would otherwise contain the components of Trizivir®

Local Anesthetic/Vasoconstrictor Precautions No information available to require special precautions

Effects on Dental Treatment No significant effects or complications reported

Effects on Bleeding No information available to require special precautions relative to altered hemostasis

Adverse Effects Fatal hypersensitivity reactions have occurred in patients taking abacavir (in Trizivir®). If Trizivir® is to be restarted following an interruption in therapy, first evaluate the patient for previously unsuspected symptoms of hypersensitivity. Do not restart if hypersensitivity is suspected or if hypersensitivity cannot be ruled out.

The following information is based on CNA3005 study data concerning effects noted in patients receiving abacavir, lamivudine, and zidovudine. See individual agents for additional information.

>10%:
- Central nervous system: Headache (13%), malaise (12%), fatigue (12%)
- Gastrointestinal: Nausea (19%)

1% to 10%:
- Central nervous system: Fever/chills (6%), depression (6%), anxiety (5%)
- Dermatologic: Rash (5%)
- Endocrine & metabolic: Triglycerides increased (2% grade 3-4)
- Gastrointestinal: Nausea and vomiting (10%), diarrhea (7%), amylase increased (2%)
- Hematologic: Neutropenia (5%)
- Hepatic: ALT increased (6%)
- Neuromuscular & skeletal: CPK increased (7%)
- Otic: Ear infection (5%)
- Respiratory: Nose/throat infection (5%)
- Miscellaneous: Hypersensitivity (2% to 9% based on abacavir component), viral infection (5%)

Other (frequency unknown): Pancreatitis, GGT increased, fat redistribution, immune reconstitution syndrome

General Dosage Range Oral: *Adolescents ≥40 kg and Adults:* 1 tablet twice daily

Mechanism of Action The combination of abacavir, lamivudine, and zidovudine is believed to act synergistically to inhibit reverse transcriptase via DNA chain termination after incorporation of the nucleoside analogue as well as to delay the emergence of mutations conferring resistance.

Pregnancy Risk Factor C

Abatacept (ab a TA sept)

Related Information

Rheumatoid Arthritis, Osteoarthritis, and Osteoporosis *on page 1889*

U.S. Brand Names Orencia®

Canadian Brand Names Orencia®

Pharmacologic Category Antirheumatic, Disease Modifying

Use

Treatment of moderately- to severely-active adult rheumatoid arthritis (RA); may be used as monotherapy or in combination with other DMARDs

Treatment of moderately- to severely-active juvenile idiopathic arthritis (JIA); may be used as monotherapy or in combination with methotrexate

Note: Abatacept should **not** be used in combination with anakinra or TNF-blocking agents

Local Anesthetic/Vasoconstrictor Precautions No information available to require special precautions

Effects on Dental Treatment No significant effects or complications reported

Effects on Bleeding No information available to require special precautions

Adverse Effects Note: Percentages not always reported; COPD patients experienced a higher frequency of COPD-related adverse reactions (COPD exacerbation, cough, dyspnea, pneumonia, rhonchi)

>10%:

Central nervous system: Headache (≤18%)
Gastrointestinal: Nausea
Respiratory: Nasopharyngitis (12%), upper respiratory tract infection
Miscellaneous: Infection (adults 54%; children 36%), antibody formation (2% to 41%)

1% to 10%:

Cardiovascular: Hypertension (7%)
Central nervous system: Dizziness (9%), fever
Dermatologic: Rash (4%)
Gastrointestinal: Dyspepsia (6%), abdominal pain, diarrhea
Genitourinary: Urinary tract infection (6%)
Neuromuscular & skeletal: Back pain (7%), limb pain (3%)
Respiratory: Cough (8%), bronchitis, pneumonia, rhinitis, sinusitis
Miscellaneous: Infusion-related reactions (2% to 9%), herpes simplex, influenza

General Dosage Range I.V.: Repeat dose at 2 weeks and 4 weeks, then every 4 weeks thereafter

Children ≥6 years and <75 kg: 10 mg/kg/dose
Children ≥6 years and 75-100 kg: 750 mg/dose
Children ≥6 years and >100 kg: 1000 mg/dose
Adults <60 kg: 500 mg/dose
Adults 60-100 kg: 750 mg/dose
Adults >100 kg: 1000 mg/dose

Mechanism of Action Selective costimulation modulator; inhibits T-cell (T-lymphocyte) activation by binding to CD80 and CD86 on antigen presenting cells (APC), thus blocking the required CD28 interaction between APCs and T cells. Activated T lymphocytes are found in the synovium of rheumatoid arthritis patients.

Pharmacodynamics/Kinetics

Half-life Elimination 8-25 days

Pregnancy Risk Factor C

Abciximab (ab SIK si mab)

Related Information

Cardiovascular Diseases *on page 1848*

U.S. Brand Names Reopro®

Canadian Brand Names ReoPro®

Pharmacologic Category Antiplatelet Agent, Glycoprotein IIb/IIIa Inhibitor

Use Prevention of cardiac ischemic complications in patients undergoing percutaneous coronary intervention (PCI); prevention of cardiac ischemic complications in patients with unstable angina not responding to conventional therapy when PCI is scheduled within 24 hours

Note: Intended for use with aspirin and heparin, at a minimum.

Unlabeled/Investigational Use To support PCI during ST-elevation myocardial infarction (STEMI) (administered at the time of primary PCI); STEMI as an adjunct to half-dose thrombolysis (eg, tenecteplase)

Local Anesthetic/Vasoconstrictor Precautions No information available to require special precautions

Effects on Dental Treatment Key adverse event(s) related to dental treatment: Bleeding is a potential adverse effect of abciximab during dental surgery. See Effects on Bleeding.

Effects on Bleeding As with all anticoagulants, bleeding is a potential adverse effect of abciximab during dental surgery; risk is dependent on multiple variables, including the intensity of anticoagulation and patient susceptibility. Medical consult is suggested. It is unlikely that ambulatory patients presenting for dental treatment will be taking intravenous anticoagulant therapy.

Adverse Effects As with all drugs which may affect hemostasis, bleeding is associated with abciximab. Hemorrhage may occur at virtually any site. Risk is dependent on multiple variables, including the concurrent use of multiple agents which alter hemostasis and patient susceptibility.

>10%:

- Cardiovascular: Hypotension (14%), chest pain (11%)
- Gastrointestinal: Nausea (14%)
- Hematologic: Minor bleeding (4% to 17%)
- Neuromuscular & skeletal: Back pain (18%)

1% to 10%:

- Cardiovascular: Bradycardia (5%), peripheral edema (2%)
- Central nervous system: Headache (7%)
- Gastrointestinal: Vomiting (7%), abdominal pain (3%)
- Hematologic: Major bleeding (1% to 14%), thrombocytopenia: <100,000 cells/mm^3 (3% to 6%); <50,000 cells/mm^3 (0.4% to 2%)
- Local: Injection site pain (4%)

General Dosage Range I.V.: *Adults:* Bolus: 0.25 mg/kg; Infusion: 0.125 mcg/kg/minute (maximum: 10 mcg/minute)

Mechanism of Action Fab antibody fragment of the chimeric human-murine monoclonal antibody 7E3; this agent binds to platelet IIb/IIIa receptors, resulting in steric hindrance, thus inhibiting platelet aggregation

Pharmacodynamics/Kinetics

Half-life Elimination ~30 minutes

Pregnancy Risk Factor C

AbobotulinumtoxinA (aye bo BOT yoo lin num TOKS in aye)

U.S. Brand Names Dysport™

Pharmacologic Category Neuromuscular Blocker Agent, Toxin

Use Treatment of cervical dystonia in both toxin-naive and previously treated patients; temporary improvement in the appearance of moderate-severe glabellar lines associated with procerus and corrugator muscle activity

Local Anesthetic/Vasoconstrictor Precautions No information available to require special precautions

Effects on Dental Treatment Key adverse event(s) related to dental treatment: Xerostomia (normal salivary flow resumes upon discontinuation) and facial paresis.

Effects on Bleeding No information available to require special precautions

Adverse Effects

>10%:

Cervical dystonia:

- Central nervous system: Dysphonia (≤28%), fatigue (12%), headache (11%)
- Gastrointestinal: Dysphagia (15% to 39%), xerostomia (13% to 39%)
- Local: Injection site discomfort/pain (5% to 22%)
- Neuromuscular & skeletal: Weakness (11% to 56%), facial paresis (≤11%)
- Ocular: Eye disorders (≤17%, includes accommodation disorder, blurred vision, diplopia, dryness, pain, pruritus, visual acuity decreased)
- Miscellaneous: Infection (13%)

1% to 10%:

Cervical dystonia:

- Cardiovascular: Heart rate decreased
- Central nervous system: Dizziness (≤4%)
- Endocrine & metabolic: Blood glucose increased
- Neuromuscular & skeletal: Pain (7%), muscle atrophy (1%)
- Respiratory: Breathing difficulties/dyspnea (~3%; onset: ~1 week; duration: ~3 weeks)
- Miscellaneous: Antibody formation (3%)

Glabellar lines:

- Central nervous system: Headache (9%)
- Dermatologic: Contact dermatitis (2% to 3%)

Gastrointestinal: Nausea (2%)
Genitourinary: Hematuria (2%)
Local: Injection site pain/reaction (2% to 3%)
Ocular: Eyelid edema (2%), eyelid ptosis (2%)
Respiratory: Nasopharyngitis (10%), upper respiratory tract infection (3%), cough (2% to 3%), pharyngolaryngeal pain (2% to 3%), bronchitis (2% to 3%), sinusitis (2%)
Miscellaneous: Flu-like syndrome (2% to 3%)

General Dosage Range I.M.:
Adults: Cervical dystonia: Initial: 500 units/treatment; subsequent doses: 250-1000 units
Adults <65 years: Reduction of glabellar lines: 10 units (0.05 mL or 0.08 mL) into each site (total dose: 50 units)

Mechanism of Action AbobotulinumtoxinA (previously known as botulinum toxin type A) is a neurotoxin produced by *Clostridium botulinum*, spore-forming anaerobic bacillus, which appears to affect only the presynaptic membrane of the neuromuscular junction in humans, where it prevents calcium-dependent release of acetylcholine and produces a state of denervation. Muscle inactivation persists until new fibrils grow from the nerve and form junction plates on new areas of the muscle-cell walls.

Pharmacodynamics/Kinetics
Onset of Action Peak effect: Cervical dystonia: 2-4 weeks
Duration of Action Cervical dystonia: Up to 4 months

Pregnancy Risk Factor C

Acamprosate (a kam PROE sate)

U.S. Brand Names Campral®
Canadian Brand Names Campral®
Pharmacologic Category GABA Agonist/Glutamate Antagonist
Use Maintenance of alcohol abstinence
Local Anesthetic/Vasoconstrictor Precautions No information available to require special precautions
Effects on Dental Treatment Key adverse event(s) related to dental treatment: Xerostomia and changes in salivation (normal salivary flow resumes upon discontinuation) and taste perversion.
Effects on Bleeding No information available to require special precautions
Adverse Effects Note: Many adverse effects associated with treatment may be related to alcohol abstinence; reported frequency range may overlap with placebo.

>10%: Gastrointestinal: Diarrhea (10% to 17%)
1% to 10%:
Cardiovascular: Syncope, palpitation, edema (peripheral)
Central nervous system: Insomnia (6% to 9%), anxiety (5% to 8%), depression (4% to 8%), dizziness (3% to 4%), pain (2% to 4%), paresthesia (2% to 3%), headache, somnolence, amnesia, tremor, chills
Dermatologic: Pruritus (3% to 4%), rash
Endocrine & metabolic: Weight gain, libido decreased
Gastrointestinal: Anorexia (2% to 5%), flatulence (1% to 3%), nausea (3% to 4%), abdominal pain, dry mouth (1% to 3%), vomiting, dyspepsia, constipation, appetite increased, taste perversion
Genitourinary: Impotence
Neuromuscular & skeletal: Weakness (5% to 7%), back pain, myalgia, arthralgia
Ocular: Abnormal vision
Respiratory: Rhinitis, dyspnea, pharyngitis, bronchitis
Miscellaneous: Diaphoresis (2% to 3%), suicide attempt

General Dosage Range Dosage adjustment recommended in patients with renal impairment and patients <60 kg
Oral: *Adults:* 666 mg 3 times/day (maximum: 1998 mg/day)

Mechanism of Action Mechanism not fully defined. Structurally similar to gamma-amino butyric acid (GABA), acamprosate appears to increase the activity of the GABA-ergic system, and decreases activity of glutamate within the CNS, including a decrease in activity at N-methyl D-aspartate (NMDA) receptors; may also affect CNS calcium channels. Restores balance to GABA and glutamate activities which appear to be disrupted in alcohol dependence. During therapeutic use, reduces alcohol intake, but does not cause a disulfiram-like reaction following alcohol ingestion.

Pharmacodynamics/Kinetics
Half-life Elimination 20-33 hours

Pregnancy Risk Factor C

Acarbose (AY car bose)

Related Information

Endocrine Disorders and Pregnancy *on page* 1879

U.S. Brand Names Precose®

Canadian Brand Names Glucobay™

Pharmacologic Category Antidiabetic Agent, Alpha-Glucosidase Inhibitor

Use Adjunct to diet and exercise to lower blood glucose in patients with type 2 diabetes mellitus (noninsulin dependent, NIDDM)

Local Anesthetic/Vasoconstrictor Precautions No information available to require special precautions

Effects on Dental Treatment Although acarbose does not cause hypoglycemia, it is frequently used in combination and may complicate the management of hypoglecemic episodes caused by other medications. As part of its therapeutic effect, acarbose slows the absorption of complex sugars or disaccharides such as sucrose. This would delay effective treatment of hypoglycemia. Simple sugars, including glucose (dextrose), are not affected. If a patient experiences hypoglycemia, use of food items such as table sugar, candy, or cookies will NOT effectively increase blood glucose. Administration of oral glucose is required in mild-moderate hypoglycemia, and parenteral glucose is required for severe hypoglycemia.

Effects on Bleeding No information available to require special precautions

Adverse Effects >10%:

Gastrointestinal: Diarrhea (31%) and abdominal pain (19%) tend to return to pretreatment levels over time; frequency and intensity of flatulence (74%) tend to abate with time

Hepatic: Transaminases increased (≤4%)

General Dosage Range Dosage adjustment recommended in patients on concomitant therapy

Oral: *Adults:* Initial: 25 mg 1-3 times/day; Maintenance: 75-300 mg/day in 3 divided doses (maximum: ≤60 kg: 150 mg/day; >60 kg: 300 mg/day)

Mechanism of Action Competitive inhibitor of pancreatic α-amylase and intestinal brush border α-glucosidases, resulting in delayed hydrolysis of ingested complex carbohydrates and disaccharides and absorption of glucose; dose-dependent reduction in postprandial serum insulin and glucose peaks; inhibits the metabolism of sucrose to glucose and fructose

Pharmacodynamics/Kinetics

Half-life Elimination ~2 hours

Time to Peak Active drug: ~1 hour

Pregnancy Risk Factor B

Acebutolol (a se BYOO toe lole)

Related Information

Cardiovascular Diseases *on page* 1848

U.S. Brand Names Sectral®

Canadian Brand Names Apo-Acebutolol®; Mylan-Acebutolol; Mylan-Acebutolol (Type S); Novo-Acebutolol; Nu-Acebutolol; Rhotral; Sandoz-Acebutolol; Sectral®; Teva-Acebutolol

Pharmacologic Category Antiarrhythmic Agent, Class II; Beta Blocker With Intrinsic Sympathomimetic Activity

Use Treatment of hypertension; management of ventricular arrhythmias

Unlabeled/Investigational Use Treatment of chronic stable angina

Local Anesthetic/Vasoconstrictor Precautions No information available to require special precautions. Local anesthetic with vasoconstrictor can be safely used in patients medicated with acebutolol.

Effects on Dental Treatment Acebutolol is a cardioselective beta-blocker. Local anesthetic with vasoconstrictor can be safely used in patients medicated with acebutolol. Nonselective beta-blockers (ie, propranolol, nadolol) enhance the pressor response to epinephrine, resulting in hypertension and bradycardia; this has not been reported for acebutolol. Many nonsteroidal anti-inflammatory drugs, such as ibuprofen and indomethacin, can reduce the hypotensive effect of beta-blockers after 3 or more weeks of therapy with the NSAID. Short-term NSAID use (ie, 3 days) requires no special precautions in patients taking beta-blockers.

Effects on Bleeding No information available to require special precautions

Adverse Effects

>10%: Central nervous system: Fatigue (11%)

1% to 10%:

Cardiovascular: Chest pain (2%), edema (2%), bradycardia, hypotension, CHF

Central nervous system: Headache (6%), dizziness (6%), insomnia (3%), depression (2%), abnormal dreams (2%), anxiety, hyper-/hypoesthesia

Dermatologic: Rash (2%), pruritus

Gastrointestinal: Constipation (4%), diarrhea (4%), dyspepsia (4%), nausea (4%), flatulence (3%), abdominal pain, vomiting

Genitourinary: Micturition frequency (3%), dysuria, impotence, nocturia

Neuromuscular & skeletal: Myalgia (2%), back pain, joint pain

Ocular: Abnormal vision (2%), conjunctivitis, dry eyes, eye pain

Respiratory: Dyspnea (4%), rhinitis (2%), cough (1%), pharyngitis, wheezing

Potential adverse effects (based on experience with other beta-blocking agents) include agranulocytosis, allergic reactions, alopecia, catatonia, claudication, depression (reversible), disorientation, emotional lability, erythematous rash, ischemic colitis, laryngospasm, mesenteric artery thrombosis, Peyronie's disease, purpura, respiratory distress, short-term memory loss, slightly clouded sensorium, thrombocytopenia

General Dosage Range Dosage adjustment recommended in patients with renal impairment

Oral:

Adults: 200-1200 mg/day in 2 divided doses (maximum: 1200 mg/day)

Elderly: 200-800 mg/day in 2 divided doses (maximum: 800 mg/day)

Mechanism of Action Competitively blocks $beta_1$-adrenergic receptors with little or no effect on $beta_2$-receptors except at high doses; exhibits membrane stabilizing and intrinsic sympathomimetic activity

Pharmacodynamics/Kinetics

Onset of Action 1-2 hours

Duration of Action 12-24 hours

Half-life Elimination Parent drug: 3-4 hours; Metabolite: 8-13 hours

Time to Peak 2-4 hours

Pregnancy Risk Factor B

Acenocoumarol (a see no KOOM a rol)

Canadian Brand Names Sintrom®

Pharmacologic Category Anticoagulant, Coumarin Derivative

Use Prophylaxis and treatment of venous thrombosis, pulmonary embolism, and thromboembolic disorders; atrial fibrillation with risk of embolism; adjunct in the prophylaxis of coronary occlusion and transient ischemic attacks

Local Anesthetic/Vasoconstrictor Precautions No information available to require special precautions

Effects on Dental Treatment Signs of acenocoumarol overdose may first appear as bleeding from gingival tissue. See Effects on Bleeding.

Effects on Bleeding As with all anticoagulants, bleeding is a potential adverse effect of acenocoumarol during dental surgery; risk is dependent on multiple variables, including the intensity of anticoagulation and patient susceptibility. Medical consult is suggested.

Adverse Effects As with all anticoagulants, bleeding is the major adverse effect of acenocoumarol. Hemorrhage may occur at virtually any site. Risk is dependent on multiple variables, including the intensity of anticoagulation and patient susceptibility.

Frequency not defined.

Cardiovascular: Hemorrhagic shock

Central nervous system: Fever, headache, stroke (hemorrhagic)

Dermatologic: Rash, urticaria, skin necrosis

Skin necrosis/gangrene, due to paradoxical local thrombosis, is a known but rare risk of oral anticoagulant therapy. Its onset is usually within the first few days of therapy and is frequently localized to the limbs, breast, or penis. The risk of this effect is increased in patients with protein C or S deficiency.

Additional adverse reactions associated with warfarin, but likely to also occur with indanediones, include priapism and skin necrosis ("purple toe" syndrome or cutaneous gangrene).

Gastrointestinal: Gastrointestinal bleeding, melena

Genitourinary: Hematuria

Hematologic: Hemorrhage, retroperitoneal hematoma, unrecognized bleeding sites (eg, colon cancer) may be uncovered by anticoagulation. Other hematologic reactions reported with coumarin derivatives include agranulocytosis, red cell aplasia, anemia, thrombocytopenia, eosinophilia.

Hepatic: Hepatitis, hepatotoxicity, hematobilia
Ocular: Ocular hemorrhage
Respiratory: Epistaxis, hemoptysis, pulmonary hemorrhage
Miscellaneous: Hypersensitivity/allergic reactions

Dosage Note: Dosage must be individualized. The following information is based on the manufacturer's labeling in Canada. Adults:

Oral: Initial: 8-12 mg on day 1, followed by 4-8 mg on day 2. Subsequent dosage should be based on PT/INR measurements. Usual range of maintenance doses: 1-10 mg/day. Tapering of dosage is recommended prior to discontinuation.

Mechanism of Action Interferes with hepatic synthesis of vitamin K-dependent coagulation factors (II, VII, IX, X)

Contraindications Hypersensitivity to acenocoumarol, related coumarin derivatives, or any component of the formulation; hemorrhagic tendencies; hemophilia; thrombocytopenia purpura; leukemia; recent or potential surgery of the eye or CNS; major regional lumbar block anesthesia or surgery resulting in large, open surfaces; bleeding from the GI, respiratory, or GU tract; threatened abortion; aneurysm; prolonged dietary insufficiencies (vitamin K deficiency); ascorbic acid deficiency; history of bleeding diathesis; prostatectomy; continuous tube drainage of the small intestine; polyarthritis; diverticulitis; emaciation; malnutrition; cerebrovascular hemorrhage; eclampsia/pre-eclampsia; blood dyscrasias; severe uncontrolled or malignant hypertension; severe hepatic disease; pericarditis or pericardial effusion; subacute bacterial endocarditis; visceral carcinoma; following spinal puncture and other diagnostic or therapeutic procedures with potential for significant bleeding; history of warfarin-induced necrosis; an unreliable, noncompliant patient; alcoholism; patient who has a history of falls or is a significant fall risk; pregnancy

Warnings/Precautions Use care in the selection of patients appropriate for this treatment. Use with caution in trauma, acute infection (antibiotics and fever may alter response to acenocoumarol), renal insufficiency, moderate-severe hypertension, polycythemia vera, vasculitis, open wound, active TB, history of PUD, anaphylactic disorders, indwelling catheters, severe diabetes, thyroid disease, and menstruating and postpartum women. Necrosis or gangrene of the skin and other tissues can occur (rarely) due to early hypercoagulability; risk is increased in patients with protein C deficiency. "Purple toe" syndrome, due to cholesterol microembolization, has been described with coumarin-type anticoagulants. Women may be at risk of developing ovarian hemorrhage at the time of ovulation. May cause hypersensitivity reactions, including anaphylaxis; cross-reactivity among coumarin anticoagulants has been described.

Hemorrhage is the most serious risk of therapy. Risk factors for bleeding include high intensity anticoagulation (INR >4), age (>65 years), variable INRs, history of GI bleeding, hypertension, cerebrovascular disease, serious heart disease, anemia, severe diabetes, malignancy, trauma, renal insufficiency, polycythemia vera, vasculitis, open wound, history of PUD, indwelling catheters, menstruating and postpartum women, drug-drug interactions and long duration of therapy. Patient must be instructed to report bleeding, accidents, or falls. Patient must also report any new or discontinued medications, herbal or alternative products used, significant changes in smoking or dietary habits. Ensure patient cooperation especially from the alcoholic, illicit drug user, demented, or psychotic patient. The elderly may be more sensitive to anticoagulant therapy. Safety and efficacy have not been established in children.

Drug Interactions

Metabolism/Transport Effects **Substrate** of CYP1A2 (major), 2C9 (major), 2C19 (minor)

Avoid Concomitant Use

Avoid concomitant use of Acenocoumarol with any of the following: Tamoxifen

Increased Effect/Toxicity

Acenocoumarol may increase the levels/effects of: Anticoagulants; Collagenase (Systemic); Deferasirox; Drotrecogin Alfa; Ethotoin; Fosphenytoin; Phenytoin

The levels/effects of Acenocoumarol may be increased by: Abiraterone; Acetaminophen; Allopurinol; Amiodarone; Androgens; Antineoplastic Agents; Antiplatelet Agents; Bicalutamide; Capecitabine; Cephalosporins; Chloral Hydrate; Chloramphenicol; Cimetidine; Cranberry; CYP1A2 Inhibitors (Moderate); CYP1A2 Inhibitors (Strong); CYP2C9 Inhibitors (Moderate); CYP2C9 Inhibitors (Strong); Deferasirox; Desvenlafaxine; Dexmethylphenidate; Disulfiram; Dronedarone; Efavirenz; Erythromycin (Ophthalmic); Esomeprazole; Ethacrynic Acid; Ethotoin; Etoposide; Exenatide; Fenugreek; Fibric Acid Derivatives; Fluconazole; Fluorouracil; Fluorouracil (Systemic); Fluorouracil (Topical); Fosphenytoin; Gefitinib; Ginkgo Biloba; Glucagon; Green Tea; Herbs (Anticoagulant/Antiplatelet Properties); HMG-CoA Reductase Inhibitors; Ifosfamide; Itraconazole; Ivermectin; Ketoconazole; Ketoconazole (Systemic); Lansoprazole; Leflunomide; Macrolide Antibiotics; Methylphenidate; MetroNIDAZOLE; MetroNIDAZOLE (Systemic); Miconazole (Topical); Milnacipran;

Neomycin; NSAID (COX-2 Inhibitor); NSAID (Nonselective); Omeprazole; Pentosan Polysulfate Sodium; Pentoxifylline; Phenytoin; Posaconazole; Propafenone; Propoxyphene; Prostacyclin Analogues; QuiNIDine; QuiNINE; Quinolone Antibiotics; Salicylates; Selective Serotonin Reuptake Inhibitors; Sulfinpyrazone [Off Market]; Sulfonamide Derivatives; Tamoxifen; Tetracycline Derivatives; Thrombolytic Agents; Thyroid Products; Toremifene; TraMADol; Tricyclic Antidepressants; Venlafaxine; Vitamin E; Voriconazole; Vorinostat; Zafirlukast

Decreased Effect

The levels/effects of Acenocoumarol may be decreased by: Aminoglutethimide; Antineoplastic Agents; Antithyroid Agents; AzaTHIOprine; Barbiturates; Bile Acid Sequestrants; Bosentan; CarBAMazepine; Coenzyme Q-10; Contraceptives (Estrogens); Contraceptives (Progestins); CYP1A2 Inducers (Strong); CYP2C9 Inducers (Highly Effective); Dicloxacillin; Efavirenz; Glutethimide; Green Tea; Griseofulvin; Mercaptopurine; Nafcillin; Peginterferon Alfa-2b; Phytonadione; Rifamycin Derivatives; St Johns Wort; Sucralfate

Ethanol/Nutrition/Herb Interactions

Ethanol: Avoid ethanol. Acute ethanol ingestion (binge drinking) decreases the metabolism of oral anticoagulants and increases PT/INR. Chronic daily ethanol use increases the metabolism of oral anticoagulants and decreases PT/INR.

Food: The anticoagulant effects of acenocoumarol may be decreased if taken with foods rich in vitamin K. Vitamin E may increase anticoagulant effect.

Herb/Nutraceutical: St John's wort may decrease oral anticoagulant levels. Alfalfa contains large amounts of vitamin K as do many enteral products. Coenzyme Q_{10} may decrease response to oral anticoagulants. Avoid cat's claw, dong quai, evening primrose, feverfew, red clover, horse chestnut, garlic, green tea, ginseng, and ginkgo (all have additional antiplatelet activity).

Dietary Considerations Foods high in vitamin K (eg, beef liver, pork liver, green tea, and leafy green vegetables) inhibit anticoagulant effect. Do not change dietary habits once stabilized on acenocoumarol therapy. A balanced diet with a consistent intake of vitamin K is essential. Avoid large amounts of alfalfa, asparagus, broccoli, Brussels sprouts, cabbage, cauliflower, green teas, kale, lettuce, spinach, turnip greens, watercress; these decrease efficacy of oral anticoagulants. It is recommended that the diet contain a CONSISTENT vitamin K content of 70-140 mcg/day. Check with healthcare provider before changing diet. Avoid using multivitamins that contain vitamin K.

Pharmacodynamics/Kinetics

Onset of Action Peak anticoagulant effect: Oral: 36-48 hours

Half-life Elimination 8-11 hours

Time to Peak 1-3 hours

Lactation Enters breast milk/not recommended (per manufacturer)

Product Availability Not available in U.S.

Dosage Forms: Canada

Tablet:

Sintrom®: 1 mg, 4 mg

Acetaminophen (a seet a MIN oh fen)

Related Information

Antiplatelet and Anticoagulation Considerations in Dentistry *on page 1867*

Cardiovascular Diseases *on page 1848*

Oral Pain *on page 1928*

Related Sample Prescriptions

Mild/Moderate Oral Pain *on page 1980*

U.S. Brand Names Acephen™ [OTC]; APAP 500 [OTC]; Aspirin Free Anacin® Extra Strength [OTC]; Cetafen® Extra [OTC]; Cetafen® [OTC]; Excedrin® Tension Headache [OTC]; Feverall® [OTC]; Genebs Extra Strength [OTC] [DSC]; Infantaire [OTC]; Little Fevers™ [OTC]; Mapap® Arthritis Pain [OTC]; Mapap® Children's [OTC]; Mapap® Extra Strength [OTC]; Mapap® Infant's [OTC]; Mapap® Junior Rapid Tabs [OTC]; Mapap® [OTC]; Nortemp Children's [OTC]; Ofirmev™; Pain & Fever Children's [OTC]; Pain Eze [OTC]; Silapap Children's [OTC]; Silapap Infant's [OTC]; Triaminic™ Children's Fever Reducer Pain Reliever [OTC]; Tylenol® 8 Hour [OTC]; Tylenol® Arthritis Pain Extended Relief [OTC]; Tylenol® Children's Meltaways [OTC]; Tylenol® Children's [OTC]; Tylenol® Extra Strength [OTC]; Tylenol® Infant's Concentrated [OTC]; Tylenol® Jr. Meltaways [OTC]; Tylenol® [OTC]; Valorin Extra [OTC]; Valorin [OTC]

Canadian Brand Names Abenol®; Apo-Acetaminophen®; Atasol®; Novo-Gesic; Pediatrix; Tempra®; Tylenol®

Generic Availability (U.S.) Yes: Excludes extended release products; injectable formulation

Pharmacologic Category Analgesic, Miscellaneous

Dental Use Treatment of postoperative pain

Use Treatment of mild-to-moderate pain and fever (analgesic/antipyretic)

I.V.: Additional indication: Management of moderate-to-severe pain when combined with opioid analgesia

Local Anesthetic/Vasoconstrictor Precautions No information available to require special precautions

Effects on Dental Treatment No significant effects or complications reported (see Dental Comment)

Effects on Bleeding No information available to require special precautions in patients medicated only with acetaminophen; however, there is information that acetaminophen may increase levels and enhance anticoagulant effects of vitamin K antagonists acenocoumarol and warfarin (Coumadin®) (see Dental Comment)

Adverse Effects

Oral, Rectal: Frequency not defined:

Dermatologic: Rash

Endocrine & metabolic: May increase chloride, uric acid, glucose; may decrease sodium, bicarbonate, calcium

Hematologic: Anemia; blood dyscrasias (neutropenia, pancytopenia, leukopenia)

Hepatic: Bilirubin increased, alkaline phosphatase increased

Renal: Ammonia increased, nephrotoxicity with chronic overdose, analgesic nephropathy

Miscellaneous: Hypersensitivity reactions (rare)

I.V.:

>10%: Gastrointestinal: Nausea (adults 34%; children ≥5%), vomiting (adults 15%; children ≥5%)

1% to 10%:

Cardiovascular: Edema (peripheral), hypervolemia, hypo/hypertension, tachycardia

Central nervous system: Headache (adults 10%; children ≥1%), insomnia (adults 7%; children ≥1%), agitation (children ≥5%), anxiety, fatigue

Dermatologic: Pruritus (children ≥5%), rash

Endocrine & metabolic: Hypoalbuminemia, hypokalemia, hypomagnesemia, hypophosphatemia

Gastrointestinal: Constipation (children ≥5%), abdominal pain, diarrhea

Hematologic: Anemia

Hepatic: Transaminases increased

Local: Infusion site pain

Neuromuscular & skeletal: Muscle spasms, pain in extremity, trismus

Ocular: Periorbital edema

Renal: Oliguria (children ≥1%)

Respiratory: Atelectasis (children ≥5%), breath sounds abnormal, dyspnea, hypoxia, pleural effusion, pulmonary edema, stridor, wheezing

Dental Usual Dosage Postoperative pain: Oral, rectal:

Children <12 years: 10-15 mg/kg/dose every 4-6 hours as needed; do **not** exceed 5 doses (2.6 g) in 24 hours; alternatively, the following age-based doses may be used

Adults: 325-650 mg every 4-6 hours or 1000 mg 3-4 times/day; do **not** exceed 4 g/day

Dosage Note: No dose adjustment required if converting between different acetaminophen formulations.

Oral, rectal:

Children <12 years: 10-15 mg/kg/dose every 4-6 hours as needed; do **not** exceed 5 doses (2.6 g) in 24 hours; alternatively, the following age-based doses may be used; see table.

Acetaminophen Dosing (Oral and Rectal Formulations)

Age	Dosage (mg)	Age	Dosage (mg)
0-3 mo	40	4-5 y	240
4-11 mo	80	6-8 y	320
1-2 y	120	9-10 y	400
2-3 y	160	11 y	480

Note: Higher rectal doses have been studied for use in preoperative pain control in children. However, specific guidelines are not available and dosing may be product dependent. The safety and efficacy of alternating acetaminophen and ibuprofen dosing has not been established.

Adults: 325-650 mg every 4-6 hours or 1000 mg 3-4 times/day; do **not** exceed 4 g/day

I.V.:

Children 2-12 years: 15 mg/kg every 6 hours **or** 12.5 mg/kg every 4 hours; maximum single dose: 15 mg/kg/dose; maximum daily dose: 75 mg/kg/day (≤3.75 g/day)

Adolescents >12 years and Adults:

<50 kg: 15 mg/kg every 6 hours or 12.5 mg/kg every 4 hours; maximum single dose: 750 mg/dose; maximum daily dose: 75 mg/kg/day (≤3.75 g/day)

≥50 kg: 650 mg every 4 hours or 1000 mg every 6 hours; maximum single dose: 1000 mg/dose; maximum daily dose: 4 g/day

Dosing interval in renal impairment:

Oral (Aronoff, 2007):

Children:

Cl_{cr} <10 mL/minute: Administer every 8 hours

Intermittent hemodialysis or peritoneal dialysis: Administer every 8 hours

CRRT: No adjustments necessary

Adults:

Cl_{cr} 10-50 mL/minute: Administer every 6 hours

Cl_{cr} <10 mL/minute: Administer every 8 hours

Intermittent hemodialysis or peritoneal dialysis: No adjustment necessary

CRRT: Administer every 8 hours

I.V.: Cl_{cr} ≤30 mL/minute: Use with caution; consider decreasing daily dose and extending dosing interval

Dosing adjustment/comments in hepatic impairment: Use with caution. Limited, low-dose therapy is usually well tolerated in hepatic disease/cirrhosis. However, cases of hepatotoxicity at daily acetaminophen dosages <4 g/day have been reported. Avoid chronic use in hepatic impairment.

Mechanism of Action Although not fully elucidated, believed to inhibit the synthesis of prostaglandins in the central nervous system and work peripherally to block pain impulse generation; produces antipyresis from inhibition of hypothalamic heat-regulating center

Contraindications Hypersensitivity to acetaminophen or any component of the formulation; severe hepatic impairment or severe active liver disease (Ofirmev™)

Warnings/Precautions Limit dose to <4 g/day. May cause severe hepatotoxicity on acute overdose; in addition, chronic daily dosing in adults has resulted in liver damage in some patients. Use with caution in patients with alcoholic liver disease; consuming ≥3 alcoholic drinks/day may increase the risk of liver damage. Use caution in patients with hepatic impairment or active liver disease. Use of intravenous formulation is contraindicated in patients with severe hepatic impairment or severe active liver disease. Use caution in patients with known G6PD deficiency; rare reports of hemolysis have occurred. Use caution in patients with chronic malnutrition and hypovolemia (intravenous formulation). Use caution in patients with severe renal impairment; consider dosing adjustments. Hypersensitivity and anaphylactic reactions have been reported; discontinue immediately if symptoms of allergic or hypersensitivity reactions occur.

OTC labeling: When used for self-medication, patients should be instructed to contact healthcare provider if used for fever lasting >3 days or for pain lasting >10 days in adults or >5 days in children.

Drug Interactions

Metabolism/Transport Effects **Substrate** (minor) of CYP1A2, 2A6, 2C9, 2D6, 2E1, 3A4; **Inhibits** CYP3A4 (weak)

Avoid Concomitant Use There are no known interactions where it is recommended to avoid concomitant use.

Increased Effect/Toxicity

Acetaminophen may increase the levels/effects of: Dasatinib; Imatinib; SORAfenib; Vitamin K Antagonists

The levels/effects of Acetaminophen may be increased by: Conivaptan; Dasatinib; Imatinib; Isoniazid; Metyrapone; Probenecid; SORAfenib

Decreased Effect

The levels/effects of Acetaminophen may be decreased by: Anticonvulsants (Hydantoin); Barbiturates; CarBAMazepine; Cholestyramine Resin; Peginterferon Alfa-2b; Tocilizumab

Ethanol/Nutrition/Herb Interactions

Ethanol: Excessive intake of ethanol may increase the risk of acetaminophen-induced hepatotoxicity. Avoid ethanol or limit to <3 drinks/day.

Food: Rate of absorption may be decreased when given with food.

Herb/Nutraceutical: St John's wort may decrease acetaminophen levels.

Dietary Considerations Some products may contain phenylalanine.

Pharmacodynamics/Kinetics

Onset of Action

Oral: <1 hour

I.V.: Analgesia: 5-10 minutes; Antipyretic: Within 30 minutes

Peak effect: I.V.: Analgesic: 1 hour

Duration of Action

I.V., Oral: Analgesia: 4-6 hours

I.V.: Antipyretic: ≥6 hours

Half-life Elimination Prolonged following toxic doses

Neonates: 7 hours (range: 4-10 hours)

Infants: ~4 hours (range: 1-7 hours)

Children: 3 hours (range: 2-5 hours)

Adolescents: ~3 hours (range: 2-4 hours)

Adults: ~2 hours (range: 2-3 hours); may be slightly prolonged in severe renal insufficiency (Cl_{cr}<30 mL/minute): 2-5.3 hours

Time to Peak Serum: Oral: Immediate release: 10-60 minutes (may be delayed in acute overdoses); I.V.: 15 minutes

Pregnancy Risk Factor C

Lactation Enters breast milk/use caution (AAP rates "compatible"; AAP 2001 update pending)

Breast-Feeding Considerations Low concentrations of acetaminophen are excreted into breast milk and can be detected in the urine of nursing infants. Adverse reactions have generally not been observed; however, a rash caused by acetaminophen exposure was reported in one breast-feeding infant.

Dosage Forms

Caplet, oral: 500 mg

Cetafen® Extra [OTC]: 500 mg

Mapap® Extra Strength [OTC]: 500 mg

Pain Eze [OTC]: 650 mg

Tylenol® [OTC]: 325 mg

Tylenol® Extra Strength [OTC]: 500 mg

Caplet, extended release, oral:

Mapap® Arthritis Pain [OTC]: 650 mg

Tylenol® 8 Hour [OTC]: 650 mg

Tylenol® Arthritis Pain Extended Relief [OTC]: 650 mg

Capsule, oral:

Mapap® Extra Strength [OTC]: 500 mg

Captab, oral: 500 mg

Elixir, oral:

Mapap® Children's [OTC]: 160 mg/5 mL (118 mL, 480 mL)

Gelcap, oral:

Mapap® [OTC]: 500 mg

Gelcap, rapid release, oral:

Tylenol® Extra Strength [OTC]: 500 mg

Geltab, oral:

Excedrin® Tension Headache [OTC]: 500 mg

Injection, solution [preservative free]:

Ofirmev™: 10 mg/mL (100 mL)

Liquid, oral:

APAP 500 [OTC]: 500 mg/5 mL (237 mL)

Silapap Children's [OTC]: 160 mg/5 mL (118 mL, 237 mL, 473 mL)

Tylenol® Extra Strength [OTC]: 500 mg/15 mL (240 mL)

Solution, oral: 160 mg/5 mL (5 mL, 10 mL, 20 mL, 118 mL, 473 mL); 80 mg/0.8 mL (15 mL)

Infantaire [OTC]: 80 mg/0.8 mL (15 mL, 30 mL)

Little Fevers™ [OTC]: 80 mg/mL (30 mL)

Mapap® [OTC]: 80 mg/0.8 mL (15 mL)

Pain & Fever Children's [OTC]: 160 mg/5 mL (118 mL, 473 mL)

Silapap Infant's [OTC]: 80 mg/0.8 mL (15 mL, 30 mL)

Suppository, rectal: 120 mg (12s, 50s, 100s); 325 mg (12s); 650 mg (12s, 50s, 100s)

Acephen™ [OTC]: 120 mg (12s, 50s, 100s); 325 mg (6s, 12s, 50s, 100s); 650 mg (12s, 50s, 100s)

Feverall® [OTC]: 80 mg (6s, 50s); 120 mg (6s, 50s); 325 mg (6s, 50s); 650 mg (50s)

Suspension, oral: 160 mg/5 mL (5 mL, 10 mL, 10.15 mL, 20 mL, 20.3 mL)
Mapap® Children's [OTC]: 160 mg/5 mL (118 mL)
Mapap® Infant's [OTC]: 80 mg/0.8 mL (15 mL, 30 mL)
Nortemp Children's [OTC]: 160 mg/5 mL (118 mL)
Tylenol® Children's [OTC]: 160 mg/5 mL (60 mL, 120 mL)
Tylenol® Infant's Concentrated [OTC]: 80 mg/0.8 mL (15 mL, 30 mL)
Syrup, oral:
Triaminic™ Children's Fever Reducer Pain Reliever [OTC]: 160 mg/5 mL (118 mL)
Tablet, oral: 325 mg, 500 mg
Aspirin Free Anacin® Extra Strength [OTC]: 500 mg
Cetafen® [OTC]: 325 mg
Mapap® [OTC]: 325 mg
Tylenol® [OTC]: 325 mg
Valorin [OTC]: 325 mg
Valorin Extra [OTC]: 500 mg
Tablet, chewable, oral: 80 mg
Mapap® Children's [OTC]: 80 mg
Tablet, orally disintegrating, oral:
Mapap® Children's [OTC]: 80 mg
Mapap® Junior Rapid Tabs [OTC]: 160 mg
Tylenol® Children's Meltaways [OTC]: 80 mg
Tylenol® Jr. Meltaways [OTC]: 160 mg

Dental Comment Hepatotoxicity caused by acetaminophen is potentiated by chronic alcohol consumption. People who are taking acetaminophen, even at therapeutic doses, and consume alcohol are at risk of developing hepatotoxicity.

Acetaminophen may increase the levels and enhance the anticoagulant effects of vitamin K antagonists acenocoumarol and warfarin (Coumadin®). Studies have reported that acetaminophen has increased the INR in warfarin treated patients with daily acetaminophen doses as low as 2 g, particularly when taking acetaminophen for >1 week (Antlitz, 1968; Boeijinga, 1982; Gebauer, 2003; Hylek, 1998; Rubin, 1984). In addition, case reports of bleeding as a result of increased INR have been published (Bagheri, 1999; Bartle, 1991). There is no known mechanism of the interaction; furthermore, some studies have failed to demonstrate this interaction (Gadisseur, 2003; Kwan, 1995; van den Bemt, 2002). In terms of risk, the data suggest that acetaminophen and warfarin could interact in some clinically significant manner but that the benefits of concomitant use of acetaminophen for pain control in dental patients taking warfarin usually outweigh the risks. An appropriate monitoring plan should be in place to identify potential negative effects and dosage adjustments may be necessary in a minority of patients. The interaction may be more likely to occur with daily acetaminophen doses of >1.3 g for >1 week.

There are no reports of acetaminophen interacting with antiplatelet drugs such as aspirin, clopidogrel (Plavix®), or prasugrel (Effient™). Also, there are no reports of acetaminophen in combination with hydrocodone, codeine, or oxycodone interacting with warfarin (Coumadin®).

References

Ahmad N, Grad HA, Haas DA, et al, "The Efficacy of Nonopioid Analgesics for Postoperative Dental Pain: A Meta-Analysis," *Anesth Prog*, 1997, 44(4):119-26.
Antlitz AM, Mead JA Jr, and Tolentino MA, "Potentiation of Oral Anticoagulant Therapy by Acetaminophen," *Curr Ther Res Clin Exp*, 1968, 10(10):501-7.
Bagheri H, Bernhard NB, and Montastruc JL, "Potentiation of the Acenocoumarol Anticoagulant Effect by Acetaminophen," *Ann Pharmacother*, 1999, 33(4):506.
Bartle WR and Blakely JA, "Potentiation of Warfarin Anticoagulation by Acetaminophen," *JAMA*, 1991, 265(10):1260.
Bell WR, "Acetaminophen and Warfarin: Undesirable Synergy," *JAMA*, 1998, 279(9):702-3.
Boeijinga JJ, Boerstra EE, Ris P, et al, "Interaction Between Paracetamol and Coumarin Anticoagulants," *Lancet*, 1982, 1(8270):506.
Dart RC, Kuffner EK, and Rumack BH, "Treatment of Pain or Fever With Paracetamol (Acetaminophen) in the Alcoholic Patient: A Systematic Review," *Am J Ther*, 2000, 7(2):123-34.
Dionne R, "Additive Analgesia Without Opioid Side Effects," *Compend Contin Educ Dent*, 2000, 21 (7):572-4, 576-7.
Gadisseur AP, Van Der Meer FJ, and Rosendaal FR, "Sustained Intake of Paracetamol (Acetaminophen) During Oral Anticoagulant Therapy With Coumarins Does Not Cause Clinically Important INR Changes: A Randomized Double-Blind Clinical Trial," *J Thromb Haemost*, 2003, 1(4):714-7.
Gebauer MG, Nyfort-Hansen K, Henschke PJ, et al, "Warfarin and Acetaminophen Interaction," *Pharmacotherapy*, 2003, 23(1):109-12.
Hylek EM, Heiman H, Skates SJ, et al, "Acetaminophen and Other Risk Factors for Excessive Warfarin Anticoagulation," *JAMA*, 1998, 279(9):657-62.
Kwan D, Bartle WR, and Walker SE, "The Effects of Acetaminophen on Pharmacokinetics and Pharmacodynamics of Warfarin," *J Clin Pharmacol*, 1999, 39(1):68-75.
Kwan D, Bartle WR, and Walker SE, "The Effects of Acute and Chronic Acetaminophen Dosing on the Pharmacodynamics and Pharmacokinetics of (R)- and (S)-Warfarin," *Clin Pharmacol Ther*, 1995, 57:212.
Lee WM, "Drug-Induced Hepatotoxicity," *N Engl J Med*, 1995, 333(17):1118-27.
Licht H, Seeff LB, and Zimmerman HJ, "Apparent Potentiation of Acetaminophen Hepatotoxicity by Alcohol," *Ann Intern Med*, 1980, 92(4):511.
McClain CJ, Price S, Barve S, et al, "Acetaminophen Hepatotoxicity: An Update," *Curr Gastroenterol Rep*, 1999, 1(1):42-9.
Rubin RN, Mentzer RL, and Budzynski AZ, "Potentiation of Anticoagulant Effect of Warfarin by Acetaminophen (Tylenol®)," *Clin Res*, 1984, 32:698a.
Schwab JM, Schluesener HJ, and Laufer S, "COX-3: Just Another COX or the Solitary Elusive Target of Paracetamol?" *Lancet*, 2003, 361(9362):981-2.

Shek KL, Chan LN, and Nutescu E, "Warfarin-Acetaminophen Drug Interaction Revisited," *Pharmacotherapy*, 1999, 19(10):1153-8.
Tanaka E, Yamazaki K, and Misawa S, "Update: The Clinical Importance of Acetaminophen Hepatotoxicity in Nonalcoholic and Alcoholic Subjects," *J Clin Pharm Ther*, 2000, 25(5):325-32.
van den Bemt PM, Geven LM, Kuitert NA, et al, "The Potential Interaction Between Oral Anticoagulants and Acetaminophen in Everyday Practice," *Pharm World Sci*, 2002, 24(5):201-4.
Wynn RL, "Update on Nonprescription Pain Relievers for Dental Pain," *Gen Dent*, 2004, 52(2):94-8.

Acetaminophen and Codeine (a seet a MIN oh fen & KOE deen)

Related Information

Acetaminophen *on page 32*
Codeine *on page 432*

Related Sample Prescriptions

Moderate/Moderately Severe Oral Pain *on page 1980*

U.S. Brand Names Capital® and Codeine; Tylenol® with Codeine No. 3; Tylenol® with Codeine No. 4

Canadian Brand Names ratio-Emtec; ratio-Lenoltec; Triatec-30; Triatec-8; Triatec-8 Strong; Tylenol Elixir with Codeine; Tylenol No. 1; Tylenol No. 1 Forte; Tylenol No. 2 with Codeine; Tylenol No. 3 with Codeine; Tylenol No. 4 with Codeine

Generic Availability (U.S.) Yes

Pharmacologic Category Analgesic, Opioid

Dental Use Treatment of postoperative pain

Use Relief of mild-to-moderate pain

Local Anesthetic/Vasoconstrictor Precautions No information available to require special precautions

Effects on Dental Treatment No significant effects or complications reported (see Dental Comment)

Effects on Bleeding No information available to require special precautions

Adverse Effects

>10%:

- Central nervous system: Dizziness, lightheadedness, sedation
- Gastrointestinal: Nausea, vomiting
- Respiratory: Dyspnea

1% to 10%:

- Central nervous system: Dysphonia, euphoria
- Dermatologic: Pruritus
- Gastrointestinal: Abdominal pain, constipation
- Miscellaneous: Histamine release

Dental Usual Dosage Postoperative pain: Adults: Analgesic: Based on codeine (30-60 mg/dose) every 4-6 hours (maximum: 4000 mg/24 hours based on acetaminophen component)

Dosage Doses should be adjusted according to severity of pain and response of the patient. Adult doses ≥60 mg codeine fail to give commensurate relief of pain but merely prolong analgesia and are associated with an appreciably increased incidence of side effects. Oral:

Children: Analgesic:

Codeine: 0.5-1 mg codeine/kg/dose every 4-6 hours

Acetaminophen: 10-15 mg/kg/dose every 4 hours up to a maximum of 2.6 g/24 hours for children <12 years; **alternatively, the following can be used:**

- 3-6 years: 5 mL 3-4 times/day as needed of elixir
- 7-12 years: 10 mL 3-4 times/day as needed of elixir
- >12 years: 15 mL every 4 hours as needed of elixir

Adults:

Antitussive: Based on codeine (15-30 mg/dose) every 4-6 hours (maximum: 360 mg/24 hours based on codeine component)

Analgesic: Based on codeine (30-60 mg/dose) every 4-6 hours (maximum: 4000 mg/24 hours based on acetaminophen component)

1-2 tablets every 4 hours to a maximum of 12 tablets/24 hours

Dosing adjustment in renal impairment: See individual agents.

Dosing adjustment in hepatic impairment: Use with caution. Limited, low-dose therapy is usually well tolerated in hepatic disease/cirrhosis; however, cases of hepatotoxicity at daily acetaminophen dosages <4 g/day have been reported. Avoid chronic use in hepatic impairment.

Mechanism of Action Inhibits the synthesis of prostaglandins in the central nervous system and peripherally blocks pain impulse generation; produces antipyresis from inhibition of hypothalamic heat-regulating center; binds to opiate receptors in the CNS, causing inhibition of ascending pain pathways, altering the perception of and response to pain; causes cough supression by direct central action in the medulla; produces generalized CNS depression. Caffeine (contained in some non-U.S. formulations) is a CNS stimulant; use with acetaminophen and codeine increases the level of analgesia provided by each agent.

Contraindications Hypersensitivity to acetaminophen, codeine, or any component of the formulation; significant respiratory depression (in unmonitored settings); acute or severe bronchial asthma; hypercapnia; paralytic ileus

Warnings/Precautions Use with caution in patients with hypersensitivity reactions to other phenanthrene-derivative opioid agonists (morphine, hydrocodone, hydromorphone, levorphanol, oxycodone, oxymorphone); tablets contain metabisulfite which may cause allergic reactions. Tolerance or drug dependence may result from extended use. Use caution in patients with two or more copies of the variant CYP2D6*2 allele; may have extensive conversion to morphine and thus increased opioid-mediated effects.

Limit total acetaminophen dose to <4 g/day. May cause severe hepatic toxicity on acute overdose; in addition, chronic daily dosing in adults has resulted in liver damage in some patients. Use with caution in patients with alcoholic liver disease; consuming 3 alcoholic drinks/day may increase the risk of liver damage. Use caution in patients with known G6PD deficiency.

This combination should be used with caution in elderly or debilitated patients, hypotension, adrenocortical insufficiency, abdominal conditions, hepatic impairment, renal impairment, respiratory disease, thyroid disorders, prostatic hyperplasia, urethral stricture, seizure disorder, CNS depression, head injury or increased intracranial pressure. Causes sedation; caution must be used in performing tasks which require alertness (eg, operating machinery or driving). Safety and efficacy in pediatric patients have not been established. Effects may be potentiated when used with other sedative drugs or ethanol.

Note: Some non-U.S. formulations (including most Canadian formulations) may contain caffeine as an additional ingredient. Caffeine may cause CNS and cardiovascular stimulation, as well as GI irritation in high doses. Use with caution in patients with a history of peptic ulcer or GERD; avoid in patients with symptomatic cardiac arrhythmias.

Drug Interactions

Metabolism/Transport Effects Acetaminophen: **Substrate** (minor) of CYP1A2, 2A6, 2C9, 2D6, 2E1, 3A4; **Inhibits** CYP3A4 (weak)

Avoid Concomitant Use There are no known interactions where it is recommended to avoid concomitant use.

Increased Effect/Toxicity

Acetaminophen and Codeine may increase the levels/effects of: Alcohol (Ethyl); Alvimopan; CNS Depressants; Dasatinib; Desmopressin; Imatinib; Selective Serotonin Reuptake Inhibitors; SORAfenib; Thiazide Diuretics; Vitamin K Antagonists

The levels/effects of Acetaminophen and Codeine may be increased by: Amphetamines; Antipsychotic Agents (Phenothiazines); Conivaptan; Dasatinib; Droperidol; Imatinib; Isoniazid; Metyrapone; Probenecid; Somatostatin Analogs; SORAfenib; Succinylcholine

Decreased Effect

Acetaminophen and Codeine may decrease the levels/effects of: Pegvisomant

The levels/effects of Acetaminophen and Codeine may be decreased by: Ammonium Chloride; Anticonvulsants (Hydantoin); Barbiturates; CarBAMazepine; Cholestyramine Resin; CYP2D6 Inhibitors (Moderate); CYP2D6 Inhibitors (Strong); Mixed Agonist / Antagonist Opioids; Peginterferon Alfa-2b; Tocilizumab

Ethanol/Nutrition/Herb Interactions Ethanol: Excessive intake of ethanol may increase the risk of acetaminophen-induced hepatotoxicity. Avoid ethanol or limit to <3 drinks/day.

Dietary Considerations May be taken with food.

Pregnancy Risk Factor C

Lactation Enters breast milk/use caution

Breast-Feeding Considerations Refer to Codeine monograph.

Controlled Substance C-III; C-V

Dosage Forms

Solution, oral [C-V]: Acetaminophen 120 mg and codeine 12 mg per 5 mL

Suspension, oral [C-V]: Acetaminophen 120 mg and codeine 12 mg per 5 mL

Capital® and Codeine [C-V]: Acetaminophen 120 mg and codeine 12 mg per 5 mL

Tablet [C-III]: Acetaminophen 300 mg and codeine 15 mg; acetaminophen 300 mg and codeine 30 mg; acetaminophen 300 mg and codeine 60 mg

Tylenol® with Codeine No. 3: Acetaminophen 300 mg and codeine 30 mg

Tylenol® with Codeine No. 4: Acetaminophen 300 mg and codeine 60 mg

Dosage Forms: Canada Note: In countries outside of the U.S., some formulations of Tylenol® with Codeine include caffeine.

Caplet:

ratio-Lenoltec No. 1, Tylenol No. 1: Acetaminophen 300 mg, codeine 8 mg, and caffeine 15 mg

Tylenol No. 1 Forte: Acetaminophen 500 mg, codeine 8 mg, and caffeine 15 mg

Solution, oral:

Tylenol Elixir with Codeine: Acetaminophen 160 mg and codeine 8 mg per 5 mL

Tablet:

ratio-Emtec, Triatec-30: Acetaminophen 300 mg and codeine 30 mg

ratio-Lenoltec No. 1: Acetaminophen 300 mg, codeine 8 mg, and caffeine 15 mg

ratio-Lenoltec No. 2, Tylenol No. 2 with Codeine: Acetaminophen 300 mg, codeine 15 mg, and caffeine 15 mg

ratio-Lenoltec No. 3, Tylenol No. 3 with Codeine: Acetaminophen 300 mg, codeine 30 mg, and caffeine 15 mg

ratio-Lenoltec No. 4, Tylenol No. 4 with Codeine: Acetaminophen 300 mg and codeine 60 mg

Triatec-8: Acetaminophen 325 mg, codeine 8 mg, and caffeine 30 mg

Triatec-8 Strong: Acetaminophen 500 mg, codeine 8 mg, and caffeine 30 mg

Dental Comment Hepatotoxicity caused by acetaminophen is potentiated by chronic alcohol consumption. People who are taking acetaminophen, even at therapeutic doses, and consume alcohol are at risk of developing hepatotoxicity.

Acetaminophen may increase the levels and enhance the anticoagulant effects of vitamin K antagonists acenocoumarol and warfarin (Coumadin®). Studies have reported that acetaminophen has increased the INR in warfarin treated patients with daily acetaminophen doses as low as 2 g, particularly when taking acetaminophen for >1 week (Antlitz, 1968; Boeijinga, 1982; Gebauer, 2003; Hylek, 1998; Rubin, 1984). In addition, case reports of bleeding as a result of increased INR have been published (Bagheri, 1999; Bartle, 1991). There is no known mechanism of the interaction; furthermore, some studies have failed to demonstrate this interaction (Gadisseur, 2003; Kwan, 1995; van den Bemt, 2002). In terms of risk, the data suggest that acetaminophen and warfarin could interact in some clinically significant manner but that the benefits of concomitant use of acetaminophen for pain control in dental patients taking warfarin usually outweigh the risks. An appropriate monitoring plan should be in place to identify potential negative effects and dosage adjustments may be necessary in a minority of patients. The interaction may be more likely to occur with daily acetaminophen doses of >1.3 g for >1 week.

There are no reports of acetaminophen interacting with antiplatelet drugs such as aspirin, clopidogrel (Plavix®), or prasugrel (Effient™). Also, there are no reports of acetaminophen in combination with hydrocodone, codeine, or oxycodone interacting with warfarin (Coumadin®).

References

Antlitz AM, Mead JA Jr, and Tolentino MA, "Potentiation of Oral Anticoagulant Therapy by Acetaminophen," *Curr Ther Res Clin Exp*, 1968, 10(10):501-7.

Bagheri H, Bernhard NB, and Montastruc JL, "Potentiation of the Acenocoumarol Anticoagulant Effect by Acetaminophen," *Ann Pharmacother*, 1999, 33(4):506.

Bartle WR and Blakely JA, "Potentiation of Warfarin Anticoagulation by Acetaminophen," *JAMA*, 1991, 265(10):1260.

Bell WR, "Acetaminophen and Warfarin: Undesirable Synergy," *JAMA*, 1998, 279(9):702-3.

Boeijinga JJ, Boerstra EE, Ris P, et al, "Interaction Between Paracetamol and Coumarin Anticoagulants," *Lancet*, 1982, 1(8270):506.

Chang DJ, Fricke JR, Bird SR, et al, "Rofecoxib Versus Codeine/Acetaminophen in Postoperative Dental Pain: A Double-Blind, Randomized, Placebo- and Active Comparator-Controlled Clinical Trial," *Clin Ther*, 2001, 23(9):1446-55.

Dionne RA, "New Approaches to Preventing and Treating Postoperative Pain," *J Am Dent Assoc*, 1992, 123(6):26-34.

Forbes JA, Butterworth GA, Burchfield WH, et al, "Evaluation of Ketorolac, Aspirin, and an Acetaminophen-Codeine Combination in Postoperative Oral Surgery Pain," *Pharmacotherapy*, 1990, 10(6 Pt 2):77S-93S.

Gadisseur AP, Van Der Meer FJ, and Rosendaal FR, "Sustained Intake of Paracetamol (Acetaminophen) During Oral Anticoagulant Therapy With Coumarins Does Not Cause Clinically Important INR Changes: A Randomized Double-Blind Clinical Trial," *J Thromb Haemost*, 2003, 1(4):714-7.

Gebauer MG, Nyfort-Hansen K, Henschke PJ, et al, "Warfarin and Acetaminophen Interaction," *Pharmacotherapy*, 2003, 23(1):109-12.

Hylek EM, Heiman H, Skates SJ, et al, "Acetaminophen and Other Risk Factors for Excessive Warfarin Anticoagulation," *JAMA*, 1998, 279(9):657-62.

Kwan D, Bartle WR, and Walker SE, "The Effects of Acute and Chronic Acetaminophen Dosing on the Pharmacodynamics and Pharmacokinetics of (R)- and (S)-Warfarin," *Clin Pharmacol Ther*, 1995, 57:212.

Mullican WS and Lacy JR, "Tramadol/Acetaminophen Combination Tablets and Codeine/Acetaminophen Combination Capsules for the Management of Chronic Pain: A Comparative Trial," *Clin Ther*, 2001, 23 (9):1429-45.

Rubin RN, Mentzer RL, and Budzynski AZ, "Potentiation of Anticoagulant Effect of Warfarin by Acetaminophen (Tylenol®)," *Clin Res*, 1984, 32:698a.

van den Bemt PM, Geven LM, Kuitert NA, et al, "The Potential Interaction Between Oral Anticoagulants and Acetaminophen in Everyday Practice," *Pharm World Sci*, 2002, 24(5):201-4.

Wynn RL, "Narcotic Analgesics for Dental Pain: Available Products, Strengths, and Formulations," *Gen Dent*, 2001, 49(2):126-8, 130, 132 passim.

Acetaminophen and Diphenhydramine

(a seet a MIN oh fen & dye fen HYE dra meen)

Related Information

Acetaminophen *on page 32*

DiphenhydrAMINE (Systemic) *on page 540*

U.S. Brand Names Excedrin PM® [OTC]; Goody's PM® [OTC]; Legatrin PM® [OTC]; Mapap PM [OTC]; Percogesic® Extra Strength [OTC]; TopCare® Pain Relief PM [OTC]; Tylenol® PM [OTC]; Tylenol® Severe Allergy [OTC]

Pharmacologic Category Analgesic, Miscellaneous

Use Aid in the relief of insomnia accompanied by minor pain

Local Anesthetic/Vasoconstrictor Precautions No information available to require special precautions

Effects on Dental Treatment Key adverse event(s) related to dental treatment: Xerostomia (normal salivary flow resumes upon discontinuation). See Dental Comment.

Effects on Bleeding No information available to require special precautions

Adverse Effects See individual agents.

General Dosage Range Oral: *Children ≥12 years and Adults:* 50 mg of diphenhydramine HCl (76 mg diphenhydramine citrate) at bedtime

Dental Comment Hepatotoxicity caused by acetaminophen is potentiated by chronic alcohol consumption. People who are taking acetaminophen, even at therapeutic doses, and consume alcohol are at risk of developing hepatotoxicity.

Acetaminophen may increase the levels and enhance the anticoagulant effects of vitamin K antagonists acenocoumarol and warfarin (Coumadin®). Studies have reported that acetaminophen has increased the INR in warfarin treated patients with daily acetaminophen doses as low as 2 g, particularly when taking acetaminophen for >1 week (Antlitz, 1968; Boeijinga, 1982; Gebauer, 2003; Hylek, 1998; Rubin, 1984). In addition, case reports of bleeding as a result of increased INR have been published (Bagheri, 1999; Bartle, 1991). There is no known mechanism of the interaction; furthermore, some studies have failed to demonstrate this interaction (Gadisseur, 2003; Kwan, 1995; van den Bemt, 2002). In terms of risk, the data suggest that acetaminophen and warfarin could interact in some clinically significant manner but that the benefits of concomitant use of acetaminophen for pain control in dental patients taking warfarin usually outweigh the risks. An appropriate monitoring plan should be in place to identify potential negative effects and dosage adjustments may be necessary in a minority of patients. The interaction may be more likely to occur with daily acetaminophen doses of >1.3 g for >1 week.

There are no reports of acetaminophen interacting with antiplatelet drugs such as aspirin, clopidogrel (Plavix®), or prasugrel (Effient™). Also, there are no reports of acetaminophen in combination with hydrocodone, codeine, or oxycodone interacting with warfarin (Coumadin®).

Acetaminophen and Phenylephrine

(a seet a MIN oh fen & fen il EF rin)

Related Information

Acetaminophen *on page 32*

Phenylephrine (Systemic) *on page 1339*

U.S. Brand Names Alka-Seltzer Plus® Sinus Formula [OTC]; Cetafen Cold® [OTC]; Contac® Cold + Flu Maximum Strength Non-Drowsy [OTC]; Excedrin® Sinus Headache [OTC]; Mapap® Sinus Congestion and Pain Daytime [OTC]; Sinus Pain & Pressure [OTC]; Sinutab® Sinus [OTC]; Sudafed PE® Pressure + Pain [OTC]; Sudafed PE® Sinus Headache [OTC] [DSC]; Tylenol® Sinus Congestion & Pain Daytime [OTC]; Vicks® DayQuil® Sinus [OTC]

Pharmacologic Category Analgesic, Miscellaneous; Decongestant

Use Temporary relief of sinus/nasal congestion and pressure, headache, and minor aches and pains

Local Anesthetic/Vasoconstrictor Precautions Use with caution since phenylephrine is a sympathomimetic amine which could interact with epinephrine to cause a pressor response.

Effects on Dental Treatment Key adverse event(s) related to dental treatment: Tachycardia, palpitations (use vasoconstrictor with caution), and xerostomia (normal salivary flow resumes upon discontinuation). See Dental Comment.

Effects on Bleeding No information available to require special precautions

Adverse Effects See individual agents.

General Dosage Range Oral: *Children ≥12 years and Adults:* Acetaminophen 325 mg and phenylephrine 5 mg/caplet: Take 2 caplets every 4 hours as needed (maximum: 12 caplets/24 hours; maximum acetaminophen: 4 g/day)

Mechanism of Action Acetaminophen inhibits the synthesis of prostaglandins in the central nervous system and peripherally blocks pain impulse generation. Phenylephrine causes vasoconstriction of the arterioles of the nasal mucosa.

Dental Comment Hepatotoxicity caused by acetaminophen is potentiated by chronic alcohol consumption. People who are taking acetaminophen, even at therapeutic doses, and consume alcohol are at risk of developing hepatotoxicity.

Acetaminophen may increase the levels and enhance the anticoagulant effects of vitamin K antagonists acenocoumarol and warfarin (Coumadin®). Studies have reported that acetaminophen has increased the INR in warfarin treated patients with daily acetaminophen doses as low as 2 g, particularly when taking acetaminophen for >1 week (Antlitz, 1968; Boeijinga, 1982; Gebauer, 2003; Hylek, 1998; Rubin, 1984). In addition, case reports of bleeding as a result of increased INR have been published (Bagheri, 1999; Bartle, 1991). There is no known mechanism of the interaction; furthermore, some studies have failed to demonstrate this interaction (Gadisseur, 2003; Kwan, 1995; van den Bemt, 2002). In terms of risk, the data suggest that acetaminophen and warfarin could interact in some clinically significant manner but that the benefits of concomitant use of acetaminophen for pain control in dental patients taking warfarin usually outweigh the risks. An appropriate monitoring plan should be in place to identify potential negative effects and dosage adjustments may be necessary in a minority of patients. The interaction may be more likely to occur with daily acetaminophen doses of >1.3 g for >1 week.

There are no reports of acetaminophen interacting with antiplatelet drugs such as aspirin, clopidogrel (Plavix®), or prasugrel (Effient™). Also, there are no reports of acetaminophen in combination with hydrocodone, codeine, or oxycodone interacting with warfarin (Coumadin®).

Acetaminophen and Phenyltoloxamine

(a seet a MIN oh fen & fen il to LOKS a meen)

Related Information

Acetaminophen *on page 32*

U.S. Brand Names Aceta-Gesic [OTC]; BP Poly 650 [DSC]; Flextra-650 [DSC]; Flextra-DS [DSC]; Lagesic™ [DSC]; Phenagesic [OTC] [DSC]; RhinoFlex™; RhinoFlex™-650; Zgesic

Pharmacologic Category Analgesic, Miscellaneous

Use Relief of mild-to-moderate pain

Local Anesthetic/Vasoconstrictor Precautions No information available to require special precautions

Effects on Dental Treatment No significant effects or complications reported (see Dental Comment)

Effects on Bleeding No information available to require special precautions

Adverse Effects Frequency not defined.

Central nervous system: Dizziness, drowsiness, lassitude
Dermatologic: Pruritus, rash
Gastrointestinal: Nausea
Ocular: Blurred vision
Miscellaneous: Diaphoresis

General Dosage Range Oral: Based on acetaminophen component:

Children <12 years: 10-15 mg/kg/dose every 4-6 hours as needed (maximum: 2.6 g/day)

Children ≥12 years and Adults: 325-650 mg every 4-6 hours as needed (maximum: 4 g/day)

Mechanism of Action Acetaminophen inhibits the synthesis of prostaglandins in the central nervous system and peripherally blocks pain impulse generation; produces antipyresis from inhibition of hypothalamic heat-regulating center. Phenyltoloxamine is an antihistamine (H_1-blocking agent) which acts primarily to inhibit secretions in the nose, mouth, and pharynx, as well as causing CNS depression.

Pregnancy Risk Factor C

Dental Comment Hepatotoxicity caused by acetaminophen is potentiated by chronic alcohol consumption. People who are taking acetaminophen, even at therapeutic doses, and consume alcohol are at risk of developing hepatotoxicity.

Acetaminophen may increase the levels and enhance the anticoagulant effects of vitamin K antagonists acenocoumarol and warfarin (Coumadin®). Studies have reported that acetaminophen has increased the INR in warfarin treated patients with daily acetaminophen doses as low as 2 g, particularly when taking acetaminophen for >1 week (Antlitz, 1968; Boeijinga, 1982; Gebauer, 2003; Hylek, 1998; Rubin, 1984). In addition, case reports of bleeding as a result of increased INR have been published (Bagheri, 1999; Bartle, 1991). There is no known mechanism of the interaction; furthermore, some studies have failed to demonstrate this interaction

(Gadisseur, 2003; Kwan, 1995; van den Bemt, 2002). In terms of risk, the data suggest that acetaminophen and warfarin could interact in some clinically significant manner but that the benefits of concomitant use of acetaminophen for pain control in dental patients taking warfarin usually outweigh the risks. An appropriate monitoring plan should be in place to identify potential negative effects and dosage adjustments may be necessary in a minority of patients. The interaction may be more likely to occur with daily acetaminophen doses of >1.3 g for >1 week.

There are no reports of acetaminophen interacting with antiplatelet drugs such as aspirin, clopidogrel (Plavix®), or prasugrel (Effient™). Also, there are no reports of acetaminophen in combination with hydrocodone, codeine, or oxycodone interacting with warfarin (Coumadin®).

Acetaminophen and Pseudoephedrine

(a seet a MIN oh fen & soo doe e FED rin)

Related Information

Acetaminophen *on page* 32

Pseudoephedrine *on page* 1429

U.S. Brand Names Ornex® Maximum Strength [OTC]; Ornex® [OTC]

Canadian Brand Names Contac® Cold and Sore Throat, Non Drowsy, Extra Strength; Dristan® N.D.; Dristan® N.D., Extra Strength; Sinutab® Non Drowsy; Sudafed® Head Cold and Sinus Extra Strength; Tylenol® Decongestant; Tylenol® Sinus

Pharmacologic Category Alpha/Beta Agonist; Analgesic, Miscellaneous

Use Temporary relief of nasal congestion, and minor aches and pains associated with colds, flu, sinusitis, or allergies

Local Anesthetic/Vasoconstrictor Precautions Use with caution since pseudoephedrine is a sympathomimetic amine which could interact with epinephrine to cause a pressor response

Effects on Dental Treatment Key adverse event(s) related to dental treatment: Pseudoephedrine: Xerostomia (normal salivary flow resumes upon discontinuation). See Dental Comment.

Effects on Bleeding No information available to require special precautions

Adverse Effects See individual agents.

General Dosage Range Oral:

Children 6-11 years: Acetaminophen 325 mg/pseudoephedrine 30 mg every 4-6 hours (maximum: 120 mg/day pseudoephedrine)

Children ≥12 years and Adults: Acetaminophen 625-1000 mg/pseudoephedrine 60 mg every 4-6 hours (maximum: 240 mg/day pseudoephedrine)

Dental Comment Hepatotoxicity caused by acetaminophen is potentiated by chronic alcohol consumption. People who are taking acetaminophen, even at therapeutic doses, and consume alcohol are at risk of developing hepatotoxicity.

Acetaminophen may increase the levels and enhance the anticoagulant effects of vitamin K antagonists acenocoumarol and warfarin (Coumadin®). Studies have reported that acetaminophen has increased the INR in warfarin treated patients with daily acetaminophen doses as low as 2 g, particularly when taking acetaminophen for >1 week (Antlitz, 1968; Boeijinga, 1982; Gebauer, 2003; Hylek, 1998; Rubin, 1984). In addition, case reports of bleeding as a result of increased INR have been published (Bagheri, 1999; Bartle, 1991). There is no known mechanism of the interaction; furthermore, some studies have failed to demonstrate this interaction (Gadisseur, 2003; Kwan, 1995; van den Bemt, 2002). In terms of risk, the data suggest that acetaminophen and warfarin could interact in some clinically significant manner but that the benefits of concomitant use of acetaminophen for pain control in dental patients taking warfarin usually outweigh the risks. An appropriate monitoring plan should be in place to identify potential negative effects and dosage adjustments may be necessary in a minority of patients. The interaction may be more likely to occur with daily acetaminophen doses of >1.3 g for >1 week.

There are no reports of acetaminophen interacting with antiplatelet drugs such as aspirin, clopidogrel (Plavix®), or prasugrel (Effient™). Also, there are no reports of acetaminophen in combination with hydrocodone, codeine, or oxycodone interacting with warfarin (Coumadin®).

Acetaminophen and Tramadol (a seet a MIN oh fen & TRA ma dole)

Related Information

Acetaminophen *on page* 32

Oral Pain *on page* 1928

TraMADol *on page* 1656

Related Sample Prescriptions

Moderate/Moderately Severe Oral Pain *on page* 1980

U.S. Brand Names Ultracet®

Canadian Brand Names Apo-Tramadol/Acet®; Tramacet

Generic Availability (U.S.) Yes

Pharmacologic Category Analgesic, Miscellaneous; Analgesic, Opioid

Dental Use Treatment of postoperative pain (≤5 days)

Use Short-term (≤5 days) management of acute pain

Local Anesthetic/Vasoconstrictor Precautions No information available to require special precautions

Effects on Dental Treatment Key adverse event(s) related to dental treatment: Xerostomia and changes in salivation (normal salivary flow resumes upon discontinuation). See Dental Comment.

Effects on Bleeding No information available to require special precautions

Adverse Effects 1% to 10%:

Central nervous system: Somnolence (6%), dizziness (3%), insomnia (2%), anxiety, confusion, euphoria, fatigue, headache, nervousness, somnolence, tremor

Dermatologic: Pruritus (2%), rash

Endocrine & metabolic: Hot flashes

Gastrointestinal: Constipation (6%), anorexia (3%), diarrhea (3%), nausea (3%), dry mouth (2%), abdominal pain, dyspepsia, flatulence, vomiting

Genitourinary: Prostatic disorder (2%)

Neuromuscular & skeletal: Weakness

Miscellaneous: Diaphoresis increased (4%)

Dental Usual Dosage Acute postoperative pain (≤5 days): Adults: Oral: Two tablets every 4-6 hours as needed for pain relief (maximum: 8 tablets/day); treatment should not exceed 5 days

Dosage Oral: Adults: Acute pain: Two tablets every 4-6 hours as needed for pain relief (maximum: 8 tablets/day); treatment should not exceed 5 days

Dosage adjustment in renal impairment: Cl_{cr} <30 mL/minute: Maximum of 2 tablets every 12 hours; treatment should not exceed 5 days

Dosage adjustment in hepatic impairment: Use is not recommended.

Mechanism of Action

Based on **acetaminophen** component: Inhibits the synthesis of prostaglandins in the central nervous system and peripherally blocks pain impulse generation; produces antipyresis from inhibition of hypothalamic heat-regulating center

Based on **tramadol** component: Binds to μ-opiate receptors in the CNS causing inhibition of ascending pain pathways, altering the perception of and response to pain; also inhibits the reuptake of norepinephrine and serotonin, which also modifies the ascending pain pathway

Contraindications Hypersensitivity to acetaminophen, tramadol, opioids, or any component of the formulation; opioid-dependent patients; acute intoxication with ethanol, hypnotics, narcotics, centrally-acting analgesics, opioids, or psychotropic drugs; hepatic dysfunction

Note: Based on Canadian product labeling: Tramadol is contraindicated during or within 14 days following MAO inhibitor therapy

Warnings/Precautions See individual agents.

Drug Interactions

Metabolism/Transport Effects

Acetaminophen: **Substrate** (minor) of CYP1A2, 2A6, 2C9, 2D6, 2E1, 3A4; **Inhibits** CYP3A4 (weak)

Tramadol: **Substrate** of CYP2D6 (major), 3A4 (major)

Avoid Concomitant Use

Avoid concomitant use of Acetaminophen and Tramadol with any of the following: Sibutramine

Increased Effect/Toxicity

Acetaminophen and Tramadol may increase the levels/effects of: Alcohol (Ethyl); Alvimopan; CNS Depressants; Dasatinib; Desmopressin; Imatinib; MAO Inhibitors; Selective Serotonin Reuptake Inhibitors; Serotonin Modulators; SORAfenib; Thiazide Diuretics; Vitamin K Antagonists

The levels/effects of Acetaminophen and Tramadol may be increased by: Amphetamines; Antipsychotic Agents (Phenothiazines); Conivaptan; CYP3A4 Inhibitors (Moderate); CYP3A4 Inhibitors (Strong); Dasatinib; Droperidol; Imatinib; Isoniazid; Metyrapone; Probenecid; Selective Serotonin Reuptake Inhibitors; Sibutramine; SORAfenib; Succinylcholine; Tricyclic Antidepressants

Decreased Effect

Acetaminophen and Tramadol may decrease the levels/effects of: Pegvisomant

The levels/effects of Acetaminophen and Tramadol may be decreased by: Ammonium Chloride; Anticonvulsants (Hydantoin); Barbiturates; CarBAMazepine; Cholestyramine Resin; CYP2D6 Inhibitors (Moderate); CYP2D6 Inhibitors (Strong); CYP3A4 Inducers (Strong); Deferasirox; Mixed Agonist / Antagonist Opioids; Peginterferon Alfa-2b; Tocilizumab

Ethanol/Nutrition/Herb Interactions

Ethanol: Avoid ethanol (increased liver toxicity with concomitant use).

Food: May delay time to peak plasma levels, however, the extent of absorption is not affected.

Herb/Nutraceutical:

Acetaminophen: Avoid St John's wort (may decrease acetaminophen levels).

Tramadol: Avoid valerian, St John's wort, kava kava, gotu kola (may increase CNS depression).

Dietary Considerations May be taken with or without food.

Pregnancy Risk Factor C

Lactation Tramadol: Enters breast milk/contraindicated

Breast-Feeding Considerations Not recommended for postdelivery analgesia in nursing mothers.

Dosage Forms

Tablet: Acetaminophen 325 mg and tramadol 37.5 mg

Ultracet®: Acetaminophen 325 mg and tramadol 37.5 mg

Dental Comment Hepatotoxicity caused by acetaminophen is potentiated by chronic alcohol consumption. People who are taking acetaminophen, even at therapeutic doses, and consume alcohol are at risk of developing hepatotoxicity.

Acetaminophen may increase the levels and enhance the anticoagulant effects of vitamin K antagonists acenocoumarol and warfarin (Coumadin®). Studies have reported that acetaminophen has increased the INR in warfarin treated patients with daily acetaminophen doses as low as 2 g, particularly when taking acetaminophen for >1 week (Antlitz, 1968; Boeijinga, 1982; Gebauer, 2003; Hylek, 1998; Rubin, 1984). In addition, case reports of bleeding as a result of increased INR have been published (Bagheri, 1999; Bartle, 1991). There is no known mechanism of the interaction; furthermore, some studies have failed to demonstrate this interaction (Gadisseur, 2003; Kwan, 1995; van den Bemt, 2002). In terms of risk, the data suggest that acetaminophen and warfarin could interact in some clinically significant manner but that the benefits of concomitant use of acetaminophen for pain control in dental patients taking warfarin usually outweigh the risks. An appropriate monitoring plan should be in place to identify potential negative effects and dosage adjustments may be necessary in a minority of patients. The interaction may be more likely to occur with daily acetaminophen doses of >1.3 g for >1 week.

There are no reports of acetaminophen interacting with antiplatelet drugs such as aspirin, clopidogrel (Plavix®), or prasugrel (Effient™). Also, there are no reports of acetaminophen in combination with hydrocodone, codeine, or oxycodone interacting with warfarin (Coumadin®).

References

Antlitz AM, Mead JA Jr, and Tolentino MA, "Potentiation of Oral Anticoagulant Therapy by Acetaminophen," *Curr Ther Res Clin Exp*, 1968, 10(10):501-7.

Bagheri H, Bernhard NB, and Montastruc JL, "Potentiation of the Acenocoumarol Anticoagulant Effect by Acetaminophen," *Ann Pharmacother*, 1999, 33(4):506.

Bartle WR and Blakely JA, "Potentiation of Warfarin Anticoagulation by Acetaminophen," *JAMA*, 1991, 265(10):1260.

Boeijinga JJ, Boerstra EE, Ris P, et al, "Interaction Between Paracetamol and Coumarin Anticoagulants," *Lancet*, 1982, 1(8270):506.

Fricke JR Jr, Hewitt DJ, Jordan DM, et al, "A Double-Blind Placebo-Controlled Comparison of Tramadol/Acetaminophen and Tramadol in Patients With Postoperative Dental Pain," *Pain*, 2004, 109(3):250-7.

Fricke JR Jr, Karim R, Jordan D, et al, "A Double-Blind, Single-Dose Comparison of the Analgesic Efficacy of Tramadol/Acetaminophen Combination Tablets, Hydrocodone/Acetaminophen Combination Tablets, and Placebo After Oral Surgery," *Clin Ther*, 2002, 24(6):953-68.

Gadisseur AP, Van Der Meer FJ, and Rosendaal FR, "Sustained Intake of Paracetamol (Acetaminophen) During Oral Anticoagulant Therapy With Coumarins Does Not Cause Clinically Important INR Changes: A Randomized Double-Blind Clinical Trial," *J Thromb Haemost*, 2003, 1(4):714-7.

Gebauer MG, Nyfort-Hansen K, Henschke PJ, et al, "Warfarin and Acetaminophen Interaction," *Pharmacotherapy*, 2003, 23(1):109-12.

Hylek EM, Heiman H, Skates SJ, et al, "Acetaminophen and Other Risk Factors for Excessive Warfarin Anticoagulation," *JAMA*, 1998, 279(9):657-62.

Kwan D, Bartle WR, and Walker SE, "The Effects of Acute and Chronic Acetaminophen Dosing on the Pharmacodynamics and Pharmacokinetics of (R)- and (S)-Warfarin," *Clin Pharmacol Ther*, 1995, 57:212.

Medve RA, Wang J, and Karim R, "Tramadol and Acetaminophen Tablets for Dental Pain," *Anesth Prog*, 2001, 48(3):79-81.

Rubin RN, Mentzer RL, and Budzynski AZ, "Potentiation of Anticoagulant Effect of Warfarin by Acetaminophen (Tylenol®)," *Clin Res*, 1984, 32:698a.
Smith AB, Ravikumar TS, Kamin M, et al, "Combination Tramadol Plus Acetaminophen for Postsurgical Pain,' *Am J Surg*, 2004, 187(4):521-7.
van den Bemt PM, Geven LM, Kuitert NA, et al, "The Potential Interaction Between Oral Anticoagulants and Acetaminophen in Everyday Practice," *Pharm World Sci*, 2002, 24(5):201-4.
Wynn RL, "NSAIDS and Cardiovascular Effects, Celecoxib for Dental Pain, and a New Analgesic - Tramadol with Acetaminophen," *Gen Dent*, 2002, 50(3):218-222.

Acetaminophen, Aspirin, and Caffeine

(a seet a MIN oh fen, AS pir in, & KAF een)

Related Information

Acetaminophen *on page 32*
Aspirin *on page 171*
Caffeine *on page 282*

U.S. Brand Names Anacin® Advanced Headache Formula [OTC]; Excedrin® Extra Strength [OTC]; Excedrin® Migraine [OTC]; Fem-Prin® [OTC]; Goody's® Extra Strength Headache Powder [OTC]; Goody's® Extra Strength Pain Relief [OTC]; Pain-Off [OTC]; Vanquish® Extra Strength Pain Reliever [OTC]

Pharmacologic Category Analgesic, Miscellaneous

Use Relief of mild-to-moderate pain; mild-to-moderate pain associated with migraine headache

Local Anesthetic/Vasoconstrictor Precautions No information available to require special precautions

Effects on Dental Treatment Key adverse event(s) related to dental treatment: Aspirin: As with all drugs which may affect hemostasis, bleeding is associated with aspirin. Hemorrhage may occur at virtually any site; risk is dependent on multiple variables including dosage, concurrent use of multiple agents which alter hemostasis, and patient susceptibility. Many adverse effects of aspirin are dose related, and are rare at low dosages. Other serious reactions are idiosyncratic, related to allergy or individual sensitivity (see Effects on Bleeding).

Effects on Bleeding Aspirin inhibits platelet aggregation which prolongs bleeding times. Inhibition is irreversible; on discontinuation of ASA, normal platelet function returns only when new platelets are released from the bone marrow. Dental practitioners should note that recommendations differ between general surgery (eg, appendectomy, hip replacement) and dental surgery. Due to concerns for increased blood loss, ASA is typically avoided (if possible) in general surgery patients for 1-2 weeks prior to surgery (exception is in patients undergoing CABG or noncardiac surgery at high risk of cardiac events - per 2008 ACCP guidelines). However, in the case of dental surgery there is no scientific evidence to warrant discontinuance of aspirin.

Reports of major bleeding related to dental surgery attributed to aspirin use have not been published. Furthermore, interruption of therapy may result in a loss of therapeutic effect. Patients taking one aspirin tablet daily as an antithrombotic who require dental surgery should be given special consideration in consultation with the physician before removal of the aspirin. In particular, aspirin should NOT be discontinued in patients with cardiac stents that have not completed their full course of dual antiplatelet therapy (aspirin, clopidogrel); patient specific situations need to be discussed with cardiologist. When feasible, postponement of dental surgery until the completion of dual antiplatelet therapy should be considered.

Adverse Effects See individual agents.

General Dosage Range Oral: *Children >12 years and Adults:* 1-2 doses every 4-6 hours as needed (maximum: 4 g/day [based on acetaminophen and aspirin component])

Pregnancy Risk Factor D

Dental Comment There is no scientific evidence to warrant discontinuance of aspirin prior to dental surgery. Patients taking one aspirin tablet daily as an antithrombotic and who require dental surgery should be given special consideration in consultation with the physician before removal of the aspirin relative to prevention of postoperative bleeding.

Hepatotoxicity caused by acetaminophen is potentiated by chronic alcohol consumption. People who are taking acetaminophen, even at therapeutic doses, and consume alcohol are at risk of developing hepatotoxicity.

Acetaminophen may increase the levels and enhance the anticoagulant effects of vitamin K antagonists acenocoumarol and warfarin (Coumadin®). Studies have reported that acetaminophen has increased the INR in warfarin treated patients with daily acetaminophen doses as low as 2 g, particularly when taking acetaminophen for >1 week (Antlitz, 1968; Boeijinga, 1982; Gebauer, 2003; Hylek, 1998; Rubin, 1984). In addition, case reports of bleeding as a result of increased INR have been published (Bagheri, 1999; Bartle, 1991). There is no known mechanism of the interaction; furthermore, some studies have failed to demonstrate this interaction (Gadisseur, 2003; Kwan, 1995; van den Bemt, 2002). In terms of risk, the data suggest that acetaminophen and warfarin could interact in some clinically significant manner but that the benefits of concomitant use of acetaminophen for pain control in dental patients taking warfarin usually outweigh the risks. An appropriate monitoring plan should be in place to identify potential negative effects and dosage adjustments may be necessary in a minority of patients. The interaction may be more likely to occur with daily acetaminophen doses of >1.3 g for >1 week.

There are no reports of acetaminophen interacting with antiplatelet drugs such as aspirin, clopidogrel (Plavix®), or prasugrel (Effient™). Also, there are no reports of acetaminophen in combination with hydrocodone, codeine, or oxycodone interacting with warfarin (Coumadin®).

Acetaminophen, Caffeine, and Dihydrocodeine

(a seet a MIN oh fen, KAF een, & dye hye droe KOE deen)

Related Information

Acetaminophen *on page* 32

Caffeine *on page* 282

U.S. Brand Names Panlor® SS [DSC]; Trezix®; ZerLor™ [DSC]

Generic Availability (U.S.) Yes: Tablet

Pharmacologic Category Analgesic Combination (Opioid)

Dental Use Relief of moderate to moderately-severe dental pain

Use Relief of moderate to moderately-severe pain

Local Anesthetic/Vasoconstrictor Precautions No information available to require special precautions

Effects on Dental Treatment No significant effects or complications reported (see Dental Comment)

Effects on Bleeding No information available to require special precautions

Adverse Effects Frequency not defined. Most common reactions with this combination include:

Central nervous system: Dizziness, drowsiness, lightheadedness, sedation

Dermatologic: Pruritus, skin reactions

Gastrointestinal: Constipation, nausea, vomiting

Dental Usual Dosage Relief of moderate-to-moderately severe dental pain: Adults: Oral:

Panlor® SS: 1 tablet every 4 hours as needed; adjust dose based on severity of pain (maximum dose: 5 tablets/24 hours)

Trezix®: 2 capsules every 4 hours as needed; adjust dose based on severity of pain (maximum dose: 10 capsules/24 hours)

Dosage Oral: Adults: Relief of pain:

Panlor® SS, ZerLor™: 1 tablet every 4 hours as needed; adjust dose based on severity of pain (maximum dose: 5 tablets/24 hours)

Trezix®: 2 capsules every 4 hours as needed; adjust dose based on severity of pain (maximum dose: 10 capsules/24 hours)

Mechanism of Action

Acetaminophen inhibits the synthesis of prostaglandins in the central nervous system and peripherally blocks pain impulse generation; produces antipyresis from inhibition of hypothalamic heat-regulating center.

Caffeine is a CNS stimulant; use with acetaminophen and dihydrocodeine increases the level of analgesia provided by each agent.

Dihydrocodeine binds to opiate receptors in the CNS, causing inhibition of ascending pain pathways, altering the perception of and response to pain; produces generalized CNS depression.

Contraindications Hypersensitivity to acetaminophen, caffeine, dihydrocodeine, codeine, or any component of the formulation; significant respiratory depression (in unmonitored settings); acute or severe bronchial asthma; hypercapnia; paralytic ileus

Warnings/Precautions Acetaminophen may cause severe hepatotoxicity in acute overdose; limit acetaminophen to <4 g/day; in addition, chronic daily dosing in adults has resulted in liver damage in some patients. Use with caution in patients with alcoholic liver disease; consuming ≥3 alcoholic drinks/day may increase the risk of liver damage. Use caution in patients with known G6PD deficiency. Caffeine may cause CNS and cardiovascular stimulation as well as GI irritation in high doses. Dihydrocodeine should be used with caution in patients with hypersensitivity reactions to other phenanthrene-derivative opioid agonists (morphine, hydrocodone, hydromorphone, levorphanol, oxycodone, oxymorphone), respiratory diseases including asthma, emphysema, COPD, history of drug abuse or severe hepatic or renal insufficiency. Use caution with MAO inhibitors.

This combination should be used with caution in elderly or debilitated patients, hypotension, adrenocortical insufficiency, thyroid disorders, prostatic hyperplasia, urethral stricture, seizure disorder, CNS depression, head injury or increased intracranial pressure. Causes sedation; caution must be used in performing tasks which require alertness (eg, operating machinery or driving). Safety and efficacy in pediatric patients have not been established.

Drug Interactions

Metabolism/Transport Effects

Acetaminophen: **Substrate** (minor) of CYP1A2, 2A6, 2C9, 2D6, 2E1, 3A4; **Inhibits** CYP3A4 (weak)

Caffeine: **Substrate** of CYP1A2 (major), 2C9 (minor), 2D6 (minor), 2E1 (minor), 3A4 (minor); **Inhibits** CYP1A2 (weak), 3A4 (moderate)

Dihydrocodeine: **Substrate** of CYP2D6 (minor)

Avoid Concomitant Use

Avoid concomitant use of Acetaminophen, Caffeine, and Dihydrocodeine with any of the following: Iobenguane I 123

Increased Effect/Toxicity

Acetaminophen, Caffeine, and Dihydrocodeine may increase the levels/effects of: Alcohol (Ethyl); Alvimopan; CNS Depressants; Dasatinib; Desmopressin; Formoterol; Imatinib; Selective Serotonin Reuptake Inhibitors; SORAfenib; Sympathomimetics; Thiazide Diuretics; Vitamin K Antagonists

The levels/effects of Acetaminophen, Caffeine, and Dihydrocodeine may be increased by: Abiraterone; Amphetamines; Antipsychotic Agents (Phenothiazines); Atomoxetine; Conivaptan; CYP1A2 Inhibitors (Moderate); CYP1A2 Inhibitors (Strong); Dasatinib; Deferasirox; Droperidol; Imatinib; Isoniazid; Metyrapone; Probenecid; Quinolone Antibiotics; SORAfenib; Succinylcholine

Decreased Effect

Acetaminophen, Caffeine, and Dihydrocodeine may decrease the levels/effects of: Adenosine; Iobenguane I 123; Pegvisomant; Regadenoson

The levels/effects of Acetaminophen, Caffeine, and Dihydrocodeine may be decreased by: Ammonium Chloride; Anticonvulsants (Hydantoin); Barbiturates; CarBAMazepine; Cholestyramine Resin; Mixed Agonist / Antagonist Opioids; Peginterferon Alfa-2b; QuiNIDine; Tocilizumab

Ethanol/Nutrition/Herb Interactions Ethanol: Excessive intake of ethanol may increase the risk of acetaminophen-induced toxicity. Ethanol may also increase CNS depression; monitor for increased effects with coadministration. Caution patients about effects.

Pregnancy Risk Factor C

Lactation Enters breast milk/not recommended

Breast-Feeding Considerations Acetaminophen and caffeine are both excreted in breast milk. Specific information for dihydrocodeine is not available; however, similar agents (eg, codeine, morphine) are excreted in breast milk.

Controlled Substance C-III

Dosage Forms

Capsule:

Trezix®: Acetaminophen 356.4 mg, caffeine 30 mg, and dihydrocodeine 16 mg

Tablet: Acetaminophen 712.8 mg, caffeine 60 mg, and dihydrocodeine bitartrate 32 mg

Dental Comment Hepatotoxicity caused by acetaminophen is potentiated by chronic alcohol consumption. People who are taking acetaminophen, even at therapeutic doses, and consume alcohol are at risk of developing hepatotoxicity.

Acetaminophen may increase the levels and enhance the anticoagulant effects of vitamin K antagonists acenocoumarol and warfarin (Coumadin®). Studies have reported that acetaminophen has increased the INR in warfarin treated patients with daily acetaminophen doses as low as 2 g, particularly when taking acetaminophen for >1 week (Antlitz, 1968; Boeijinga, 1982; Gebauer, 2003; Hylek, 1998; Rubin, 1984). In addition, case reports of bleeding as a result of increased INR have been published (Bagheri, 1999; Bartle, 1991). There is no known mechanism of the interaction; furthermore, some studies have failed to demonstrate this interaction (Gadisseur, 2003; Kwan, 1995; van den Bemt, 2002). In terms of risk, the data suggest that acetaminophen and warfarin could interact in some clinically significant manner but that the benefits of concomitant use of acetaminophen for pain control in dental patients taking warfarin usually outweigh the risks. An appropriate monitoring plan should be in place to identify potential negative effects and dosage adjustments may be necessary in a minority of patients. The interaction may be more likely to occur with daily acetaminophen doses of >1.3 g for >1 week.

There are no reports of acetaminophen interacting with antiplatelet drugs such as aspirin, clopidogrel (Plavix®), or prasugrel (Effient™). Also, there are no reports of acetaminophen in combination with hydrocodone, codeine, or oxycodone interacting with warfarin (Coumadin®).

References

Antlitz AM, Mead JA Jr, and Tolentino MA, "Potentiation of Oral Anticoagulant Therapy by Acetaminophen," *Curr Ther Res Clin Exp*, 1968, 10(10):501-7.

Bagheri H, Bernhard NB, and Montastruc JL, "Potentiation of the Acenocoumarol Anticoagulant Effect by Acetaminophen," *Ann Pharmacother*, 1999, 33(4):506.

Bartle WR and Blakely JA, "Potentiation of Warfarin Anticoagulation by Acetaminophen," *JAMA*, 1991, 265(10):1260.

Boeijinga JJ, Boerstra EE, Ris P, et al, "Interaction Between Paracetamol and Coumarin Anticoagulants," *Lancet*, 1982, 1(8270):506.

Gadisseur AP, Van Der Meer FJ, and Rosendaal FR, "Sustained Intake of Paracetamol (Acetaminophen) During Oral Anticoagulant Therapy With Coumarins Does Not Cause Clinically Important INR Changes: A Randomized Double-Blind Clinical Trial," *J Thromb Haemost*, 2003, 1(4):714-7.

Gebauer MG, Nyfort-Hansen K, Henschke PJ, et al, "Warfarin and Acetaminophen Interaction," *Pharmacotherapy*, 2003, 23(1):109-12.

Hylek EM, Heiman H, Skates SJ, et al, "Acetaminophen and Other Risk Factors for Excessive Warfarin Anticoagulation," *JAMA*, 1998, 279(9):657-62.

Kwan D, Bartle WR, and Walker SE, "The Effects of Acute and Chronic Acetaminophen Dosing on the Pharmacodynamics and Pharmacokinetics of (R)- and (S)-Warfarin," *Clin Pharmacol Ther*, 1995, 57:212.

Rubin RN, Mentzer RL, and Budzynski AZ, "Potentiation of Anticoagulant Effect of Warfarin by Acetaminophen (Tylenol®)," *Clin Res*, 1984, 32:698a.

van den Bemt PM, Geven LM, Kuitert NA, et al, "The Potential Interaction Between Oral Anticoagulants and Acetaminophen in Everyday Practice," *Pharm World Sci*, 2002, 24(5):201-4.

Acetaminophen, Chlorpheniramine, and Pseudoephedrine (a seet a MIN oh fen, klor fen IR a meen, & soo doe e FED rin)

Related Information

Acetaminophen *on page 32*

Chlorpheniramine *on page 365*

Pseudoephedrine *on page 1429*

U.S. Brand Names Drinex [OTC] [DSC]; Relief-SF®

Pharmacologic Category Alkylamine Derivative; Alpha/Beta Agonist; Analgesic, Miscellaneous; Decongestant; Histamine H_1 Antagonist; Histamine H_1 Antagonist, First Generation

Use Temporary relief of cold, allergy, or sinus symptoms

Local Anesthetic/Vasoconstrictor Precautions Use with caution since pseudoephedrine is a sympathomimetic amine which could interact with epinephrine to cause a pressor response

Effects on Dental Treatment Key adverse event(s) related to dental treatment:

Acetaminophen: See Dental Comment.

Chlorpheniramine: Significant xerostomia with prolonged use (normal salivary flow resumes upon discontinuation).

Pseudoephedrine: Xerostomia (normal salivary flow resumes upon discontinuation).

Effects on Bleeding No information available to require special precautions

Adverse Effects See individual agents.

General Dosage Range Oral: *Children ≥12 years and Adults:* Drinex: 1 tablet 3-4 times/day (maximum: 4 tablets/24 hours); Relief-SF®: 1-2 caplets every 6 hours (maximum: 8 caplets/24 hours)

Dental Comment Hepatotoxicity caused by acetaminophen is potentiated by chronic alcohol consumption. People who are taking acetaminophen, even at therapeutic doses, and consume alcohol are at risk of developing hepatotoxicity.

Acetaminophen may increase the levels and enhance the anticoagulant effects of vitamin K antagonists acenocoumarol and warfarin (Coumadin®). Studies have reported that acetaminophen has increased the INR in warfarin treated patients with daily acetaminophen doses as low as 2 g, particularly when taking acetaminophen for >1 week (Antlitz, 1968; Boeijinga, 1982; Gebauer, 2003; Hylek, 1998; Rubin, 1984). In addition, case reports of bleeding as a result of increased INR have been published (Bagheri, 1999; Bartle, 1991). There is no known mechanism of the interaction; furthermore, some studies have failed to demonstrate this interaction (Gadisseur, 2003; Kwan, 1995; van den Bemt, 2002). In terms of risk, the data suggest that acetaminophen and warfarin could interact in some clinically significant manner but that the benefits of concomitant use of acetaminophen for pain control in dental patients taking warfarin usually outweigh the risks. An appropriate monitoring plan should be in place to identify potential negative effects and dosage adjustments may be necessary in a minority of patients. The interaction may be more likely to occur with daily acetaminophen doses of >1.3 g for >1 week.

There are no reports of acetaminophen interacting with antiplatelet drugs such as aspirin, clopidogrel (Plavix®), or prasugrel (Effient™). Also, there are no reports of acetaminophen in combination with hydrocodone, codeine, or oxycodone interacting with warfarin (Coumadin®).

Acetaminophen, Dextromethorphan, and Phenylephrine

(a seet a MIN oh fen, deks troe meth OR fan, & fen il EF rin)

Related Information

Acetaminophen *on page* 32
Dextromethorphan *on page* 504
Phenylephrine (Systemic) *on page* 1339

U.S. Brand Names Alka-Seltzer Plus® Day Cold [OTC]; Comtrex® Maximum Strength, Non-Drowsy Cold & Cough Relief [OTC]; Mapap® Multi-Symptom Cold [OTC]; Theraflu® Daytime Severe Cold & Cough [OTC]; Theraflu® Warming Relief Daytime Severe Cold & Cough [OTC]; Tylenol® Cold Head Congestion Daytime [OTC]; Tylenol® Cold Multi-Symptom Daytime [OTC]; Vicks® DayQuil® Cold/Flu Multi-Symptom [OTC]

Pharmacologic Category Analgesic, Miscellaneous; Antitussive; Decongestant

Use Temporary relief of common cold and flu symptoms (eg, pain, fever, cough, congestion)

Local Anesthetic/Vasoconstrictor Precautions Use with caution since phenylephrine is a sympathomimetic amine which could interact with epinephrine to cause a pressor response.

Effects on Dental Treatment Key adverse event(s) related to dental treatment: Tachycardia, palpitations (use vasoconstrictor with caution), and xerostomia (normal salivary flow resumes upon discontinuation). See Dental Comment.

Effects on Bleeding No information available to require special precautions

Adverse Effects See individual agents.

General Dosage Range Oral: *Children ≥6 years and Adults:* Dosage varies greatly depending on product

Dental Comment Hepatotoxicity caused by acetaminophen is potentiated by chronic alcohol consumption. People who are taking acetaminophen, even at therapeutic doses, and consume alcohol are at risk of developing hepatotoxicity.

Acetaminophen may increase the levels and enhance the anticoagulant effects of vitamin K antagonists acenocoumarol and warfarin (Coumadin®). Studies have reported that acetaminophen has increased the INR in warfarin treated patients with daily acetaminophen doses as low as 2 g, particularly when taking acetaminophen for >1 week (Antlitz, 1968; Boeijinga, 1982; Gebauer, 2003; Hylek, 1998; Rubin, 1984). In addition, case reports of bleeding as a result of increased INR have been published (Bagheri, 1999; Bartle, 1991). There is no known mechanism of the interaction; furthermore, some studies have failed to demonstrate this interaction (Gadisseur, 2003; Kwan, 1995; van den Bemt, 2002). In terms of risk, the data suggest that acetaminophen and warfarin could interact in some clinically significant manner but that the benefits of concomitant use of acetaminophen for pain control in dental patients taking warfarin usually outweigh the risks. An appropriate monitoring plan should be in place to identify potential negative effects and dosage adjustments may be necessary in a minority of patients. The interaction may be more likely to occur with daily acetaminophen doses of >1.3 g for >1 week.

There are no reports of acetaminophen interacting with antiplatelet drugs such as aspirin, clopidogrel (Plavix®), or prasugrel (Effient™). Also, there are no reports of acetaminophen in combination with hydrocodone, codeine, or oxycodone interacting with warfarin (Coumadin®).

Acetaminophen, Diphenhydramine, and Phenylephrine

(a seet a MIN oh fen, dye fen HYE dra meen, & fen il EF rin)

Related Information

Acetaminophen *on page* 32
DiphenhydrAMINE (Systemic) *on page* 540
Phenylephrine (Systemic) *on page* 1339

U.S. Brand Names Benadryl® Allergy and Cold [OTC]; Benadryl® Allergy and Sinus Headache [OTC]; Benadry® Maximum Strength Severe Allergy and Sinus Headache [OTC]; Cold Control PE [OTC]; One Tab™ Allergy & Sinus [OTC]; One Tab™ Cold & Flu [OTC]; Sudafed PE® Nighttime Cold [OTC]; Sudafed PE® Severe Cold [OTC]; Theraflu® Nighttime Severe Cold & Cough [OTC]; Theraflu® Sugar-Free Nighttime Severe Cold & Cough [OTC]; Theraflu® Warming Relief ™ Flu & Sore Throat [OTC]; Theraflu® Warming Relief™ Nighttime Severe Cold & Cough [OTC]; Tylenol® Allergy Multi-Symptom Nighttime [OTC]; Tylenol® Children's Plus Cold and Allergy [OTC]

Pharmacologic Category Alpha/Beta Agonist; Analgesic, Miscellaneous; Decongestant; Ethanolamine Derivative; Histamine H_1 Antagonist; Histamine H_1 Antagonist, First Generation

Use Temporary relief of symptoms of hay fever and the common cold, including sinus/nasal congestion and pain/pressure, headache, sneezing, runny nose, itchy/watery eyes, sore throat, fever, cough, and minor aches and pains

Local Anesthetic/Vasoconstrictor Precautions Use with caution since phenylephrine is a sympathomimetic amine which could interact with epinephrine or mepivacaine and levonordefrin (Carbocaine® 2% with Neo-Cobefrin®) to cause a pressor response.

Effects on Dental Treatment Key adverse event(s) related to dental treatment:

Acetaminophen: See Dental Comment.

Diphenhydramine: Prolonged use will cause significant xerostomia (normal salivary flow resumes upon discontinuation).

Phenylephrine: Up to 10% of patients could experience tachycardia, palpitations, and xerostomia.

Effects on Bleeding No information available to require special precautions

Adverse Effects See individual agents.

General Dosage Range Oral:

Caplet:

Children 6-11 years: One caplet every 4 hours as needed (maximum: 5 doses/caplets)

Children ≥12 years and Adults: Two caplets every 4 hours as needed (maximum: 12 caplets/24 hours)

Liquid: *Children 6-11 years and 48-95 lbs:* 10 mL every 4 hours as needed (maximum: 5 doses/24 hours)

Powder for solution: *Children ≥12 years and Adults:* One packet every 4 hours as needed (maximum: 6 doses/24 hours)

Syrup: *Children ≥12 years and Adults:* 30 mL every 4 hours as needed (maximum: 6 doses/24 hours)

Mechanism of Action

Acetaminophen inhibits the synthesis of prostaglandins in the central nervous system and peripherally blocks pain impulse generation.

Diphenhydramine is an H_1-receptor antagonist.

Phenylephrine causes vasoconstriction of the arterioles of the nasal mucosa.

Dental Comment Hepatotoxicity caused by acetaminophen is potentiated by chronic alcohol consumption. People who are taking acetaminophen, even at therapeutic doses, and consume alcohol are at risk of developing hepatotoxicity.

Acetaminophen may increase the levels and enhance the anticoagulant effects of vitamin K antagonists acenocoumarol and warfarin (Coumadin®). Studies have reported that acetaminophen has increased the INR in warfarin treated patients with daily acetaminophen doses as low as 2 g, particularly when taking acetaminophen for >1 week (Antlitz, 1968; Boeijinga, 1982; Gebauer, 2003; Hylek, 1998; Rubin, 1984). In addition, case reports of bleeding as a result of increased INR have been published (Bagheri, 1999; Bartle, 1991). There is no known mechanism of the interaction; furthermore, some studies have failed to demonstrate this interaction (Gadisseur, 2003; Kwan, 1995; van den Bemt, 2002). In terms of risk, the data suggest that acetaminophen and warfarin could interact in some clinically significant manner but that the benefits of concomitant use of acetaminophen for pain control in dental patients taking warfarin usually outweigh the risks. An appropriate monitoring plan should be in place to identify potential negative effects and dosage adjustments may be necessary in a minority of patients. The interaction may be more likely to occur with daily acetaminophen doses of >1.3 g for >1 week.

There are no reports of acetaminophen interacting with antiplatelet drugs such as aspirin, clopidogrel (Plavix®), or prasugrel (Effient™). Also, there are no reports of acetaminophen in combination with hydrocodone, codeine, or oxycodone interacting with warfarin (Coumadin®).

Acetaminophen, Isometheptene, and Dichloralphenazone

(a seet a MIN oh fen, eye soe me THEP teen, & dye KLOR al FEN a zone)

Related Information

Acetaminophen *on page* 32

U.S. Brand Names Epidrin [DSC]; Midrin® [DSC]

Pharmacologic Category Analgesic, Miscellaneous

Use Relief of migraine and tension headache

Local Anesthetic/Vasoconstrictor Precautions No information available to require special precautions

Effects on Dental Treatment No significant effects or complications reported (see Dental Comment)

Effects on Bleeding No information available to require special precautions

Adverse Effects Frequency not defined.

Central nervous system: Dizziness (transient)

Dermatological: Rash

General Dosage Range Oral: *Adults:* 2 capsules initially, then 1 capsule every hour until relief; alternatively, 1-2 capsules every 4 hours (maximum: 5 capsules/12 hours or 8 capsules/day)

Controlled Substance C-IV

Dental Comment Hepatotoxicity caused by acetaminophen is potentiated by chronic alcohol consumption. People who are taking acetaminophen, even at therapeutic doses, and consume alcohol are at risk of developing hepatotoxicity.

Acetaminophen may increase the levels and enhance the anticoagulant effects of vitamin K antagonists acenocoumarol and warfarin (Coumadin®). Studies have reported that acetaminophen has increased the INR in warfarin treated patients with daily acetaminophen doses as low as 2 g, particularly when taking acetaminophen for >1 week (Antlitz, 1968; Boeijinga, 1982; Gebauer, 2003; Hylek, 1998; Rubin, 1984). In addition, case reports of bleeding as a result of increased INR have been published (Bagheri, 1999; Bartle, 1991). There is no known mechanism of the interaction; furthermore, some studies have failed to demonstrate this interaction (Gadisseur, 2003; Kwan, 1995; van den Bemt, 2002). In terms of risk, the data suggest that acetaminophen and warfarin could interact in some clinically significant manner but that the benefits of concomitant use of acetaminophen for pain control in dental patients taking warfarin usually outweigh the risks. An appropriate monitoring plan should be in place to identify potential negative effects and dosage adjustments may be necessary in a minority of patients. The interaction may be more likely to occur with daily acetaminophen doses of >1.3 g for >1 week.

There are no reports of acetaminophen interacting with antiplatelet drugs such as aspirin, clopidogrel (Plavix®), or prasugrel (Effient™). Also, there are no reports of acetaminophen in combination with hydrocodone, codeine, or oxycodone interacting with warfarin (Coumadin®).

AcetaZOLAMIDE (a set a ZOLE a mide)

U.S. Brand Names Diamox® Sequels®

Canadian Brand Names Apo-Acetazolamide®; Diamox®

Pharmacologic Category Anticonvulsant, Miscellaneous; Carbonic Anhydrase Inhibitor; Diuretic, Carbonic Anhydrase Inhibitor; Ophthalmic Agent, Antiglaucoma

Use Treatment of glaucoma (chronic simple open-angle, secondary glaucoma, preoperatively in acute angle-closure); drug-induced edema or edema due to congestive heart failure (adjunctive therapy); centrencephalic epilepsies (immediate release dosage form); prevention or amelioration of symptoms associated with acute mountain sickness

Unlabeled/Investigational Use Metabolic alkalosis; respiratory stimulant in COPD; urine alkalinization

Local Anesthetic/Vasoconstrictor Precautions No information available to require special precautions

Effects on Dental Treatment Key adverse event(s) related to dental treatment: Metallic taste (resolves upon discontinuation)

Effects on Bleeding No information available to require special precautions

Adverse Effects Frequency not defined.

Cardiovascular: Flushing

Central nervous system: Ataxia, confusion, convulsions, depression, dizziness, drowsiness, excitement, fatigue, fever, headache, malaise

Dermatologic: Allergic skin reactions, photosensitivity, Stevens-Johnson syndrome, toxic epidermal necrolysis, urticaria

Endocrine & metabolic: Electrolyte imbalance, growth retardation (children), hyperglycemia, hypoglycemia, hypokalemia, hyponatremia, metabolic acidosis

Gastrointestinal: Appetite decreased, diarrhea, melena, nausea, taste alteration, vomiting

Genitourinary: Crystalluria, glycosuria, hematuria, polyuria, renal failure

Hematologic: Agranulocytosis, aplastic anemia, leukopenia, thrombocytopenia, thrombocytopenic purpura

Hepatic: Cholestatic jaundice, fulminant hepatic necrosis, hepatic insufficiency, liver function tests abnormal

Local: Pain at injection site

Neuromuscular & skeletal: Flaccid paralysis, paresthesia

Ocular: Myopia

Otic: Hearing disturbance, tinnitus

Miscellaneous: Anaphylaxis

General Dosage Range Dosage adjustment recommended in patients with renal impairment

I.V.:

Children: 20-40 mg/kg/day divided every 6 hours **or** 5 mg/kg (150 mg/m^2) once daily (maximum: 1 g/day)

Adults: 250-500 mg/day (maximum: 1 g/day)

Oral:

Immediate release:

Children: 5-30 mg/kg/day (150-900 mg/m^2/day) divided in 1-4 doses (maximum: 1 g/day)

Adults: 250-1000 mg/day in 1-4 divided doses (maximum: 1 g/day)

Elderly: Initial: 250 mg once or twice daily

Extended release:

Adults: 500 mg every 12-24 hours (maximum 1 g/day)

Mechanism of Action Reversible inhibition of the enzyme carbonic anhydrase resulting in reduction of hydrogen ion secretion at renal tubule and an increased renal excretion of sodium, potassium, bicarbonate, and water to decrease production of aqueous humor; also inhibits carbonic anhydrase in central nervous system to retard abnormal and excessive discharge from CNS neurons

Pharmacodynamics/Kinetics

Onset of Action Capsule, extended release: 2 hours; I.V.: 2 minutes

Peak effect: Capsule, extended release: 8-12 hours; I.V.: 15 minutes; Tablet: 2-4 hours

Duration of Action Inhibition of aqueous humor secretion: Capsule, extended release: 18-24 hours; I.V.: 4-5 hours; Tablet: 8-12 hours

Pregnancy Risk Factor C

Acetic Acid, Propylene Glycol Diacetate, and Hydrocortisone

(a SEE tik AS id, PRO pa leen GLY kole dye AS e tate, & hye droe KOR ti sone)

U.S. Brand Names Acetasol® HC; VoSol® HC

Pharmacologic Category Otic Agent, Anti-infective

Use Treatment of superficial infections of the external auditory canal caused by organisms susceptible to the action of the antimicrobial, complicated by swelling

Local Anesthetic/Vasoconstrictor Precautions No information available to require special precautions

Effects on Dental Treatment No significant effects or complications reported

Effects on Bleeding No information available to require special precautions

Adverse Effects Frequency not defined: Otic: Transient burning or stinging may be noticed occasionally when the solution is first instilled into the acutely inflamed ear

General Dosage Range Otic: *Children ≥3 years and Adults:* Instill 3-5 drops in ear(s) every 4-6 hours

Acetohydroxamic Acid (a SEE toe hye droks am ik AS id)

U.S. Brand Names Lithostat®

Canadian Brand Names Lithostat®

Pharmacologic Category Urinary Tract Product

Use Adjunctive therapy in chronic urea-splitting urinary infection

Local Anesthetic/Vasoconstrictor Precautions No information available to require special precautions

Effects on Dental Treatment No significant effects or complications reported

Effects on Bleeding Has been associated with bone marrow suppression and hemolytic anemia. No information to require specific precautions related to dental procedures.

Adverse Effects Frequency not defined.

Cardiovascular: Deep vein thrombosis (rare), embolism, palpitation, phlebitis

Central nervous system: Anorexia, anxiety, depression, headache, malaise, nervousness, tremor

Dermatologic: Flushing (with ethanol consumption), rash (nonpruritic, macular)

Gastrointestinal: Nausea, vomiting

Hematologic: Hemolytic anemia (15% with laboratory evidence; ~3% severe requiring discontinuation; may be accompanied by GI symptoms or systemic complaints of malaise and/or fatigue); hyperbilirubinemia

Respiratory: Pulmonary embolism (rare)

General Dosage Range Oral:

Children: Initial: 10 mg/kg/day

Adults: 250 mg 3-4 times/day (maximum: 10-15 mg/kg/day)

Mechanism of Action Acetohydroxamic acid inhibits bacterial urease enzymes, decreasing the formation of ammonia in the urine by urea-splitting organisms. A reduction in urinary ammonia may increase the antibacterial activity of some antibiotic agents.

Pregnancy Risk Factor X

Acetylcholine (a se teel KOE leen)

U.S. Brand Names Miochol®-E

Canadian Brand Names Miochol®-E

Pharmacologic Category Cholinergic Agonist; Ophthalmic Agent, Miotic

Use Produces complete miosis in cataract surgery, keratoplasty, iridectomy, and other anterior segment surgery where rapid miosis is required

Local Anesthetic/Vasoconstrictor Precautions No information available to require special precautions

Effects on Dental Treatment No significant effects or complications reported

Effects on Bleeding No information available to require special precautions

Adverse Effects Frequency not defined.

Cardiovascular: Bradycardia, flushing, hypotension
Central nervous system: Headache
Ocular: Clouding, corneal edema, decompensation
Respiratory: Dyspnea
Miscellaneous: Diaphoresis

General Dosage Range Intraocular: *Adults:* Instill 0.5-2 mL of 1% injection (5-20 mg)

Mechanism of Action Causes contraction of the sphincter muscles of the iris, resulting in miosis and contraction of the ciliary muscle, leading to accommodation spasm

Pharmacodynamics/Kinetics

Onset of Action Rapid

Duration of Action ~10 minutes

Pregnancy Risk Factor C

Acetylcysteine (a se teel SIS teen)

U.S. Brand Names Acetadote®

Canadian Brand Names Acetylcysteine Solution; Mucomyst®; Parvolex®

Pharmacologic Category Antidote; Mucolytic Agent

Use Antidote for acute acetaminophen (APAP) poisoning; repeated supratherapeutic ingestion (RSTI) of APAP; adjunctive mucolytic therapy in patients with abnormal or viscid mucous secretions in acute and chronic bronchopulmonary diseases; pulmonary complications of surgery and cystic fibrosis; diagnostic bronchial studies

Unlabeled/Investigational Use Prevention of contrast-induced renal dysfunction (oral, I.V.); distal intestinal obstruction syndrome (DIOS, previously referred to as meconium ileus equivalent)

Local Anesthetic/Vasoconstrictor Precautions No information available to require special precautions

Effects on Dental Treatment Key adverse event(s) related to dental treatment: Stomatitis, drowsiness, fever, vomiting, nausea, bronchospasm, rhinorrhea, hemoptysis, and dizziness

Effects on Bleeding No information available to require special precautions

Adverse Effects

Inhalation: Frequency not defined.

Central nervous system: Drowsiness, chills, fever
Gastrointestinal: Vomiting, nausea, stomatitis
Local: Irritation, stickiness on face following nebulization
Respiratory: Bronchospasm, rhinorrhea, hemoptysis
Miscellaneous: Acquired sensitization (rare), clamminess, unpleasant odor during administration

Intravenous:

>10%: Miscellaneous: Anaphylactoid reaction (8% to 18%; shorter infusion periods [eg, <60 minutes] associated with increased incidence)

1% to 10%:

Cardiovascular: Flushing (1% to 8%), tachycardia (1% to 4%), edema (1% to 2%)
Dermatologic: Urticaria (6% to 8%), rash (2% to 4%), pruritus (1% to 4%)
Gastrointestinal: Vomiting (2% to 10%), nausea (1% to 6%)
Respiratory: Pharyngitis (≤1%), rhinorrhea (≤1%), rhonchi (≤1%), throat tightness (≤1%)

General Dosage Range

Inhalation:

Nebulization:

Infants: 1-2 mL of 20% solution or 2-4 mL 10% solution 3-4 times/day

Children and Adults: 1-10 mL of 20% solution or 2-20 mL of 10% solution every 2-6 hours

Direct instillation: *Adults:* 1-4 mL of 10% or 1-2 mL of 20% solution every 1-4 hours

I.V.: Acetadote®:

Children and Adults: 21-hour regimen: Consists of 3 doses; total dose delivered: 300 mg/kg

Loading dose: 150 mg/kg (maximum: 15 g) infused over 60 minutes

Second dose: 50 mg/kg (maximum: 5 g) infused over 4 hours

Third dose: 100 mg/kg (maximum: 10 g) infused over 16 hours

Oral:

Children and Adults: Acetaminophen poisoning: 72-hour regimen: Consists of 18 doses; total dose delivered: 1330 mg/kg

Loading dose: 140 mg/kg

Maintenance dose: 70 mg/kg every 4 hours

Adults: Renal protectant for radiocontrast: 600-1200 mg twice daily for 2 days

Mechanism of Action Exerts mucolytic action through its free sulfhydryl group which opens up the disulfide bonds in the mucoproteins thus lowering mucous viscosity.

In patients with APAP toxicity, acetylcysteine acts as a hepatoprotective agent by restoring hepatic glutathione, serving as a glutathione substitute, and enhancing the nontoxic sulfate conjugation of APAP.

The presumed mechanism in preventing contrast-induced nephropathy is its ability to scavenge oxygen-derived free radicals and improve endothelium-dependent vasodilation.

Pharmacodynamics/Kinetics

Onset of Action Inhalation: 5-10 minutes

Duration of Action Inhalation: >1 hour

Half-life Elimination Reduced acetylcysteine: 2 hours; Total acetylcysteine: Adults: 5.6 hours, Newborns: 11 hours

Time to Peak Plasma: Oral: 1-2 hours

Pregnancy Risk Factor B

Acrivastine and Pseudoephedrine (AK ri vas teen & soo doe e FED rin)

Related Information

Pseudoephedrine *on page 1429*

U.S. Brand Names Semprex®-D

Pharmacologic Category Alkylamine Derivative; Alpha/Beta Agonist; Decongestant; Histamine H_1 Antagonist; Histamine H_1 Antagonist, Second Generation

Use Temporary relief of nasal congestion, decongest sinus openings, running nose, itching of nose or throat, and itchy, watery eyes due to hay fever or other upper respiratory allergies

Local Anesthetic/Vasoconstrictor Precautions Use with caution since pseudoephedrine is a sympathomimetic amine which could interact with epinephrine to cause a pressor response

Effects on Dental Treatment Key adverse event(s) related to dental treatment: Pseudoephedrine: Xerostomia (normal salivary flow resumes upon discontinuation).

Effects on Bleeding No information available to require special precautions

Adverse Effects

>10%: Central nervous system: Drowsiness, headache

1% to 10%:

Cardiovascular: Tachycardia, palpitation

Central nervous system: Nervousness, dizziness, insomnia, vertigo, lightheadedness, fatigue

Gastrointestinal: Nausea, vomiting, xerostomia, diarrhea

Genitourinary: Dysuria

Neuromuscular & skeletal: Weakness

Respiratory: Pharyngitis, cough increased

Miscellaneous: Diaphoresis

General Dosage Range Oral: *Adults:* 1 capsule 3-4 times/day

Mechanism of Action Refer to Pseudoephedrine; acrivastine is an analogue of triprolidine and it is considered to be relatively less sedating than traditional antihistamines; believed to involve competitive blockade of H_1-receptor sites resulting in the inability of histamine to combine with its receptor sites and exert its usual effects on target cells

Pharmacodynamics/Kinetics

Time to Peak Acrivastine: ~1.1 hours

Pregnancy Risk Factor B

Acyclovir (Systemic) (ay SYE kloe veer)

Related Information

Systemic Viral Diseases *on page 1904*
ValACYclovir *on page 1692*
Viral Infections *on page 1947*

Related Sample Prescriptions

Herpes Simplex (Primary) *on page 1990*
Shingles (Varicella-Zoster Virus) *on page 1990*

U.S. Brand Names Zovirax®

Canadian Brand Names Apo-Acyclovir®; Gen-Acyclovir; Mylan-Acyclovir; Novo-Acyclovir; Nu-Acyclovir; ratio-Acyclovir; Teva-Acyclovir; Zovirax®

Generic Availability (U.S.) Yes

Pharmacologic Category Antiviral Agent

Dental Use Treatment of initial and prophylaxis of recurrent mucosal and cutaneous herpes simplex (HSV-1 and HSV-2) infections in immunocompromised patients

Use Treatment of genital herpes simplex virus (HSV) and HSV encephalitis

Unlabeled/Investigational Use Prevention of HSV reactivation in HIV-positive patients; prevention of HSV reactivation in hematopoietic stem cell transplant (HSCT); prevention of HSV reactivation during periods of neutropenia in patients with cancer; prevention of varicella zoster virus (VZV) reactivation in allogenic HSCT; prevention of CMV reactivation in low-risk allogeneic HSCT; treatment of disseminated HSV or VZV in immunocompromised patients with cancer; empiric treatment of suspected encephalitis in immunocompromised patients with cancer; treatment of initial and prophylaxis of recurrent mucosal and cutaneous herpes simplex (HSV-1 and HSV-2) infections in immunocompromised patients

Local Anesthetic/Vasoconstrictor Precautions No information available to require special precautions

Effects on Dental Treatment No significant effects or complications reported

Effects on Bleeding No information available to require special precautions

Adverse Effects

Oral:

>10%: Central nervous system: Malaise (≤12%)

1% to 10%:

- Central nervous system: Headache (≤2%)
- Gastrointestinal: Nausea (2% to 5%), vomiting (≤3%), diarrhea (2% to 3%)

Parenteral:

1% to 10%:

- Dermatologic: Hives (2%), itching (2%), rash (2%)
- Gastrointestinal: Nausea/vomiting (7%)
- Hepatic: Liver function tests increased (1% to 2%)
- Local: Inflammation at injection site or phlebitis (9%)
- Renal: BUN increased (5% to 10%), creatinine increased (5% to 10%), acute renal failure

Dental Usual Dosage

Mucocutaneous HSV: Adults:

Immunocompromised (unlabeled use): Oral: 400 mg 5 times a day for 7-14 days

Dosage Note: Obese patients should be dosed using ideal body weight

Genital herpes simplex virus (HSV) infection:

I.V.: Children ≥12 years and Adults (immunocompetent): Initial episode, severe: 5 mg/kg/dose every 8 hours for 5-7 days **or** 5-10 mg/kg/dose every 8 hours for 2-7 days, follow with oral therapy to complete at least 10 days of therapy (CDC, 2010)

Oral:

Children, immunocompetent:

Initial episode (unlabeled use): 40-80 mg/kg/day divided into 3-4 doses for 5-10 days (maximum: 1 g/day)

Chronic suppression (unlabeled use; limited data): 80 mg/kg/day in 3 divided doses (maximum: 1 g/day), re-evaluate after 12 months of treatment

Children, immunocompromised (unlabeled use; CDC, 2009): Initial episode:

Children <45 kg: 60 mg/kg/day divided into 3 doses for 5-14 days (maximum: 1.2 g/day)

Adolescents: 400 mg twice daily for 5-14 days

Adults:
Initial episode: 200 mg every 4 hours while awake (5 times/day) for 10 days **or** 400 mg 3 times/day for 7-10 days (CDC, 2010)
Recurrence: 200 mg every 4 hours while awake (5 times/day) for 5 days (per manufacturer's labeling; begin at earliest signs of disease)
Alternatively, the following regimens are also recommended by the CDC: 400 mg 3 times/day for 5 days; 800 mg twice daily for 5 days; 800 mg 3 times/day for 2 days (CDC, 2010)
Chronic suppression: 400 mg twice daily or 200 mg 3-5 times/day, for up to 12 months followed by re-evaluation (per manufacturer's labeling)

Herpes zoster (shingles):
Oral: Adults (immunocompetent): 800 mg every 4 hours (5 times/day) for 7-10 days
I.V.:
Children <12 years (immunocompromised): 20 mg/kg/dose every 8 hours for 7 days
Children ≥12 years and Adults (immunocompromised): 10 mg/kg/dose or 500 mg/m^2/dose every 8 hours for 7 days

HSV encephalitis: I.V.:
Children 3 months to 12 years: 20 mg/kg/dose every 8 hours for 10 days (per manufacturer's labeling); dosing for 14-21 days also reported
Children ≥12 years and Adults: 10 mg/kg/dose every 8 hours for 10 days (per manufacturer's labeling); 10-15 mg/kg/dose every 8 hours for 14-21 days also reported

Mucocutaneous HSV:
I.V.:
Children <12 years (immunocompromised): 10 mg/kg/dose every 8 hours for 7 days
Children ≥12 years and Adults (immunocompromised): 5 mg/kg/dose every 8 hours for 7 days (per manufacturer's labeling); dosing for up to 14 days also reported
Oral: Adults (immunocompromised, unlabeled use): 400 mg 5 times a day for 7-14 days

Neonatal HSV: I.V.: Neonate: Birth to 3 months: 10 mg/kg/dose every 8 hours for 10 days (manufacturer's labeling); 20 mg/kg/dose every 8 hours for 14 (skin and mucous membrane disease) to 21 days (CNS disease) (CDC, 2010)

Varicella-zoster (chickenpox): Begin treatment within the first 24 hours of rash onset:
Oral: **Note:** The CDC HIV guidelines recommended duration of therapy is 7-10 days or until no new lesions for 48 hours (for patients with mild varicella and no or moderate immune suppression).
Children ≥2 years and ≤40 kg (immunocompetent): 20 mg/kg/dose (up to 800 mg/dose) 4 times/day for 5 days
Children >40 kg and Adults (immunocompetent): 800 mg/dose 4 times a day for 5 days
I.V.:
Manufacturer's labeling (immunocompromised):
Children <12 years: 20 mg/kg/dose every 8 hours for 7 days
Children ≥12 years and Adults: 10 mg/kg/dose every 8 hours for 7 days
CDC HIV guidelines (immunocompromised):
Children <1 year: 10 mg/kg/dose every 8 hours for 7-10 days or until no new lesions for 48 hours
Children ≥1 year: 10 mg/kg/dose or 500 mg/m^2/dose every 8 hours for 7-10 days or until no new lesions for 48 hours
Adolescents and Adults: 10-15 mg/kg/dose every 8 hours for 7-10 days

Varicella-zoster acute retinal necrosis infection in HIV-exposed/-positive (unlabeled use; CDC, 2009): I.V.: Infants and Children: 10-15 mg/kg/dose every 8 hours for 10-14 days, followed by valacyclovir for 4-6 weeks

Prevention of HSV reactivation in HIV-positive patient (unlabeled use): Oral:
Children: 20 mg/kg/dose twice daily (maximum: 400 mg/dose) (CDC, 2009)
Adults: 400-800 mg 2-3 times/day (CDC, 2010)

Prevention of HSV reactivation in HSCT (unlabeled use): *CDC recommendations:* **Note:** Start at the beginning of conditioning therapy and continue until engraftment or until mucositis resolves (~30 days)
Oral: Adults: 200 mg 3 times/day
I.V.:
Children: 250 mg/m^2/dose every 8 hours or 125 mg/m^2/dose every 6 hours
Adults: 250 mg/m^2/dose every 12 hours

Prevention of VZV reactivation in allogeneic HSCT (unlabeled use): *NCCN guidelines:* Oral: Adults: 800 mg twice a day

Prevention of CMV reactivation in low-risk allogeneic HSCT (unlabeled use): *NCCN guidelines:* **Note:** Requires close monitoring (due to weak activity); not for use in patients at high risk for CMV disease: Oral: Adults: 800 mg 4 times/day

Treatment of disseminated HSV or VZV or empiric treatment of suspected encephalitis in immunocompromised patients with cancer: (unlabeled use): *NCCN guidelines:* I.V.: Adults: 10-12 mg/kg/dose every 8 hours

Treatment of episodic HSV infection in HIV-positive patient (unlabeled use): Oral: Adults: 400 mg 3 times/day for 5-10 days (CDC, 2010)

Dosing adjustment in renal impairment:

Oral:

Cl_{cr} 10-25 mL/minute/1.73 m^2: Normal dosing regimen 800 mg every 4 hours: Administer 800 mg every 8 hours

Cl_{cr} <10 mL/minute/1.73 m^2:

Normal dosing regimen 200 mg every 4 hours or 400 mg every 12 hours: Administer 200 mg every 12 hours

Normal dosing regimen 800 mg every 4 hours: Administer 800 mg every 12 hours

I.V.:

Cl_{cr} 25-50 mL/minute/1.73 m^2: Administer recommended dose every 12 hours

Cl_{cr} 10-25 mL/minute/1.73 m^2: Administer recommended dose every 24 hours

Cl_{cr} <10 mL/minute/1.73 m^2: Administer 50% of recommended dose every 24 hours

Hemodialysis: Administer dose after dialysis

Continuous ambulatory peritoneal dialysis (CAPD): Administer 50% of normal dose once daily; no supplemental dose needed

Continuous renal replacement therapy (CRRT): Drug clearance is highly dependent on the method of renal replacement, filter type, and flow rate. Appropriate dosing requires close monitoring of pharmacologic response, signs of adverse reactions due to drug accumulation, as well as drug levels in relation to target trough (if appropriate). The following are general recommendations only (based on dialysate flow/ultrafiltration rates of 1 L/hour) and should not supersede clinical judgment:

CVVH or CVVHD/CVVHDF: 5-7.5 mg/kg every 24 hours

Note: The higher dose of 7.5 mg/kg is recommended for infections with CNS involvement (Trotman, 2005).

Mechanism of Action Acyclovir is converted to acyclovir monophosphate by virus-specific thymidine kinase then further converted to acyclovir triphosphate by other cellular enzymes. Acyclovir triphosphate inhibits DNA synthesis and viral replication by competing with deoxyguanosine triphosphate for viral DNA polymerase and being incorporated into viral DNA.

Contraindications Hypersensitivity to acyclovir, valacyclovir, or any component of the formulation

Warnings/Precautions Use with caution in immunocompromised patients; thrombocytopenic purpura/hemolytic uremic syndrome (TTP/HUS) has been reported. Use caution in the elderly, pre-existing renal disease (may require dosage modification), or in those receiving other nephrotoxic drugs. Renal failure (sometimes fatal) has been reported. Maintain adequate hydration during oral or intravenous therapy. Use I.V. preparation with caution in patients with underlying neurologic abnormalities, serious hepatic or electrolyte abnormalities, or substantial hypoxia.

Varicella-zoster: Treatment should begin within 24 hours of appearance of rash; oral route not recommended for routine use in otherwise healthy children with varicella, but may be effective in patients at increased risk of moderate-to-severe infection (>12 years of age, chronic cutaneous or pulmonary disorders, long-term salicylate therapy, corticosteroid therapy).

Drug Interactions

Avoid Concomitant Use

Avoid concomitant use of Acyclovir (Systemic) with any of the following: Zoster Vaccine

Increased Effect/Toxicity

Acyclovir (Systemic) may increase the levels/effects of: Mycophenolate; Tenofovir; Zidovudine

The levels/effects of Acyclovir (Systemic) may be increased by: Mycophenolate

Decreased Effect

Acyclovir (Systemic) may decrease the levels/effects of: Zoster Vaccine

Ethanol/Nutrition/Herb Interactions Food: Does not affect absorption of oral acyclovir.

Dietary Considerations May be taken with or without food. Some products may contain sodium.

Pharmacodynamics/Kinetics

Half-life Elimination Terminal: Neonates: 4 hours; Children 1-12 years: 2-3 hours; Adults: 3 hours

Time to Peak Serum: Oral: Within 1.5-2 hours

Pregnancy Risk Factor B

Lactation Enters breast milk/use with caution (AAP rates "compatible"; AAP 2001 update pending)

Breast-Feeding Considerations Nursing mothers with herpetic lesions near or on the breast should avoid breast-feeding. Limited data suggest exposure to the nursing infant of ~0.3 mg/kg/day following oral administration of acyclovir to the mother.

Dosage Forms

Capsule, oral: 200 mg
Zovirax®: 200 mg

Injection, powder for reconstitution: 500 mg, 1000 mg

Injection, solution [preservative free]: 50 mg/mL (10 mL, 20 mL)

Suspension, oral: 200 mg/5 mL (473 mL)
Zovirax®: 200 mg/5 mL (473 mL)

Tablet, oral: 400 mg, 800 mg
Zovirax®: 400 mg, 800 mg

Acyclovir (Topical) (ay SYE kloe veer)

Related Information

Systemic Viral Diseases *on page 1904*
Viral Infections *on page 1947*

Related Sample Prescriptions

Herpes Simplex (Primary) *on page 1990*
Herpes Simplex (Recurrent) *on page 1990*

U.S. Brand Names Zovirax®

Canadian Brand Names Zovirax®

Generic Availability (U.S.) No

Pharmacologic Category Antiviral Agent, Topical

Dental Use Treatment of initial and prophylaxis of recurrent mucosal and cutaneous herpes simplex (HSV-1 and HSV-2) infections in immunocompromised patients

Use Treatment of herpes labialis (cold sores), mucocutaneous HSV in immunocompromised patients

Local Anesthetic/Vasoconstrictor Precautions No information available to require special precautions

Effects on Dental Treatment Key adverse event(s) related to dental treatment: Topical (Zovirax® cream): Dry/cracked lips and dry/flaky skin were reported in fewer than 1 in 100 patients in clinical studies.

Effects on Bleeding No information available to require special precautions

Adverse Effects

>10%: Dermatologic: Mild pain, burning, or stinging (ointment 30%)
1% to 10%: Dermatologic: Pruritus (ointment 4%), itching

Dental Usual Dosage

Herpes labialis (cold sores): Children ≥12 years and Adults: Topical: Cream: Apply 5 times/day for 4 days

Mucocutaneous HSV: Adults: Nonlife-threatening, immunocompromised: Topical: Ointment: 1/2" ribbon of ointment for a 4" square surface area every 3 hours (6 times/day) for 7 days

Dosage Topical:

Genital HSV: Adults (immunocompromised): Ointment: Initial episode: 1/2" ribbon of ointment for a 4" square surface area every 3 hours (6 times/day) for 7 days

Herpes labialis (cold sores): Children ≥12 years and Adults: Cream: Apply 5 times/day for 4 days

Mucocutaneous HSV: Ointment: Adults (non-life-threatening, immunocompromised): 1/2" ribbon of ointment for a 4" square surface area every 3 hours (6 times/day) for 7 days

Mechanism of Action Acyclovir is converted to acyclovir monophosphate by virus-specific thymidine kinase then further converted to acyclovir triphosphate by other cellular enzymes. Acyclovir triphosphate inhibits DNA synthesis and viral replication by competing with deoxyguanosine triphosphate for viral DNA polymerase and being incorporated into viral DNA.

Contraindications Hypersensitivity to acyclovir, valacyclovir, or any component of the formulation

Warnings/Precautions

Genital herpes: Physical contact should be avoided when lesions are present; transmission may also occur in the absence of symptoms. Treatment should begin with the first signs or symptoms.

Herpes labialis: For external use only to the lips and face; do not apply to eye or inside the mouth or nose. Treatment should begin with the first signs or symptoms.

Drug Interactions

Avoid Concomitant Use There are no known interactions where it is recommended to avoid concomitant use.

Increased Effect/Toxicity There are no known significant interactions involving an increase in effect.

Decreased Effect There are no known significant interactions involving a decrease in effect.

Pregnancy Risk Factor B

Breast-Feeding Considerations When administered orally, acyclovir enters breast milk. Refer to the Acyclovir (Systemic) monograph for details. The amount of acyclovir available systemically following topical application of the cream or ointment is significantly less in comparison to oral doses. Nursing mothers with herpetic lesions near or on the breast should avoid breast-feeding.

Dosage Forms

Cream, topical:

Zovirax®: 5% (2 g, 5 g)

Ointment, topical:

Zovirax®: 5% (15 g, 30 g)

Acyclovir and Hydrocortisone (ay SYE kloe veer & hye droe KOR ti sone)

Related Information

Acyclovir (Topical) *on page 58*
Hydrocortisone (Topical) *on page 868*

U.S. Brand Names Xerese™

Generic Availability (U.S.) No

Pharmacologic Category Antiviral Agent, Topical; Corticosteroid, Topical

Use Treatment of recurrent herpes labialis (cold sores)

Local Anesthetic/Vasoconstrictor Precautions No information available to require special precautions

Effects on Dental Treatment No significant effects or complications reported

Effects on Bleeding No information available to require special precautions

Adverse Effects <1%: Dermatologic: Burning, contact dermatitis, dryness, erythema, flaking, pigmentation changes, sensitization, signs/symptoms of inflammation, tingling

Dosage Topical: Herpes labialis (cold sores): Children ≥12 years and Adults: Apply 5 times/day for 5 days

Mechanism of Action See individual agents.

Contraindications There are no contraindications listed within the manufacturer's labeling.

Warnings/Precautions Treatment should begin with the first signs or symptoms. For external use only to the lips and around the mouth; do not apply to eye, inside the mouth or nose, or on the genitals. Contact healthcare provider if cold sore fails to heal in 2 weeks. Use with caution in immunocompromised patients. Use has been associated with local sensitization (irritation).

Drug Interactions

Avoid Concomitant Use There are no known interactions where it is recommended to avoid concomitant use.

Increased Effect/Toxicity There are no known significant interactions involving an increase in effect.

Decreased Effect There are no known significant interactions involving a decrease in effect.

Pregnancy Risk Factor B

Lactation Excretion in breast milk unknown/use caution

Breast-Feeding Considerations Systemic exposure of acyclovir and hydrocortisone after topical administration is minimal. See individual agents.

Adalimumab (a da LIM yoo mab)

Related Information

Rheumatoid Arthritis, Osteoarthritis, and Osteoporosis *on page 1889*

U.S. Brand Names Humira®; Humira® Pen

Canadian Brand Names Humira®

Pharmacologic Category Antirheumatic, Disease Modifying; Gastrointestinal Agent, Miscellaneous; Monoclonal Antibody; Tumor Necrosis Factor (TNF) Blocking Agent

Use

Treatment of active rheumatoid arthritis (moderate-to-severe) and active psoriatic arthritis; may be used alone or in combination with disease-modifying antirheumatic drugs (DMARDs); treatment of ankylosing spondylitis

Treatment of moderately- to severely-active Crohn's disease in patients with inadequate response to conventional treatment, or patients who have lost response to or are intolerant of infliximab

Treatment of moderate-to-severe plaque psoriasis

Treatment of moderately- to severely-active juvenile idiopathic arthritis

Local Anesthetic/Vasoconstrictor Precautions No information available to require special precautions

Effects on Dental Treatment No significant effects or complications reported

Effects on Bleeding Rare cases of pancytopenia (including aplastic anemia) have been reported with TNF-blocking agents; potentially including significant reduction in platelet counts and altered hemostasis. In patients who are under active treatment with these agents, medical consult is suggested.

Adverse Effects

>10%:

Central nervous system: Headache (12%)

Dermatologic: Rash (6% to 12%)

Local: Injection site reaction (12% to 20%; includes erythema, itching, hemorrhage, pain, swelling)

Neuromuscular & skeletal: CPK increased (15%)

Respiratory: Upper respiratory tract infection (17%), sinusitis (11%)

Miscellaneous: Antibodies to adalimumab (3% to 26%; significance unknown), positive ANA (12%)

5% to 10%:

Cardiovascular: Hypertension (5%)

Endocrine & metabolic: Hyperlipidemia (7%), hypercholesterolemia (6%)

Gastrointestinal: Nausea (9%), abdominal pain (7%)

Genitourinary: Urinary tract infection (8%)

Hepatic: Alkaline phosphatase increased (5%)

Local: Injection site reaction (8%; other than erythema, itching, hemorrhage, pain, swelling)

Neuromuscular & skeletal: Back pain (6%)

Renal: Hematuria (5%)

Miscellaneous: Accidental injury (10%), flu-like syndrome (7%)

<5%:

Cardiovascular: Arrhythmia, atrial fibrillation, chest pain, CHF, coronary artery disorder, heart arrest, MI, palpitation, pericardial effusion, pericarditis, peripheral edema, syncope, tachycardia, thrombosis (leg), vascular disorder

Central nervous system: Confusion, fever, hypertensive encephalopathy, multiple sclerosis, subdural hematoma

Dermatologic: Cellulitis, erysipelas

Endocrine & metabolic: Dehydration, menstrual disorder, parathyroid disorder

Gastrointestinal: Diverticulitis, esophagitis, gastroenteritis, gastrointestinal hemorrhage, vomiting

Genitourinary: Cystitis, pelvic pain

Hematologic: Agranulocytosis, granulocytopenia, leukopenia, pancytopenia, paraproteinemia, polycythemia

Hepatic: Cholecystitis, cholelithiasis, hepatic necrosis

Neuromuscular & skeletal: Arthralgia, arthritis, bone fracture, bone necrosis, joint disorder, muscle cramps, myasthenia, pain in extremity, paresthesia, pyogenic arthritis, synovitis, tendon disorder, tremor

Ocular: Cataract

Renal: Kidney calculus, pyelonephritis

Respiratory: Asthma, bronchospasm, dyspnea, lung function decreased, pleural effusion, pneumonia

Miscellaneous: Adenoma, allergic reactions (1%), carcinoma (including breast, gastrointestinal, skin, urogenital), healing abnormality, herpes zoster, ketosis, lupus erythematosus syndrome, lymphoma, melanoma, postsurgical infection, sepsis, tuberculosis (reactivation of latent infection; miliary, lymphatic, peritoneal and pulmonary)

General Dosage Range SubQ:

Children ≥4 years: 15 kg to <30 kg: 20 mg every other week; ≥30 kg: 40 mg every other week

Adults: Initial: 80-160 mg; Maintenance: 40 mg every other week (maximum: 40 mg every week)

Mechanism of Action Adalimumab is a recombinant monoclonal antibody that binds to human tumor necrosis factor alpha (TNF-alpha), thereby interfering with binding to TNFα receptor sites and subsequent cytokine-driven inflammatory processes. Elevated TNF levels in the synovial fluid are involved in the pathologic pain and joint destruction in immune-mediated arthritis. Adalimumab decreases signs and symptoms of psoriatic arthritis, rheumatoid arthritis, and ankylosing spondylitis. It inhibits progression of structural damage of rheumatoid and psoriatic arthritis. Reduces signs and symptoms and maintains clinical remission in Crohn's disease; reduces epidermal thickness and inflammatory cell infiltration in plaque psoriasis.

Pharmacodynamics/Kinetics

Half-life Elimination Terminal: ~2 weeks (range: 10-20 days)

Time to Peak Serum: SubQ: 131 ± 56 hours

Pregnancy Risk Factor B

Adapalene (a DAP a leen)

U.S. Brand Names Differin®

Canadian Brand Names Differin®; Differin® XP

Pharmacologic Category Acne Products; Topical Skin Product, Acne

Use Treatment of acne vulgaris

Local Anesthetic/Vasoconstrictor Precautions No information available to require special precautions

Effects on Dental Treatment No significant effects or complications reported

Effects on Bleeding No information available to require special precautions

Adverse Effects >10%: Dermatologic: Erythema, scaling, dryness, pruritus, burning, pruritus or burning immediately after application

General Dosage Range Topical: *Children >12 years and Adults:* Apply once daily at bedtime

Mechanism of Action Retinoid-like compound which is a modulator of cellular differentiation, keratinization, and inflammatory processes, all of which represent important features in the pathology of acne vulgaris

Pregnancy Risk Factor C

Adapalene and Benzoyl Peroxide (a DAP a leen & BEN zoe il peer OKS ide)

Related Information

Adapalene *on page 61*

Benzoyl Peroxide *on page 223*

U.S. Brand Names Epiduo®

Pharmacologic Category Acne Products; Topical Skin Product; Topical Skin Product, Acne

Use Topical treatment of acne vulgaris

Local Anesthetic/Vasoconstrictor Precautions No information available to require special precautions

Effects on Dental Treatment No significant effects or complications reported

Effects on Bleeding No information available to require special precautions

Adverse Effects 1% to 10%: Dermatologic: Dry skin (<1% to 10%), scaling (<1% to 9%), erythema (1% to 8%), burning (1% to 7%), stinging (1% to 7%), contact dermatitis (3%), skin irritation (1%)

General Dosage Range Topical: *Children ≥12 years and Adults:* Apply once daily

Mechanism of Action

Benzoyl peroxide releases free-radical oxygen which oxidizes bacterial proteins in the sebaceous follicles decreasing the number of anaerobic bacteria and decreasing irritating-type free fatty acids.

Adapalene is a retinoid-like compound which is a modulator of cellular differentiation, keratinization, and inflammatory processes, all of which represent important features in the pathology of acne vulgaris.

Pregnancy Risk Factor C

Adefovir (a DEF o veer)

Related Information

HIV Infection and AIDS *on page 1883*

Systemic Viral Diseases *on page 1904*

U.S. Brand Names Hepsera®

Canadian Brand Names Hepsera™

Pharmacologic Category Antiretroviral Agent, Reverse Transcriptase Inhibitor (Nucleotide)

Use Treatment of chronic hepatitis B with evidence of active viral replication (based on persistent elevation of ALT/AST or histologic evidence), including patients with lamivudine-resistant hepatitis B

Local Anesthetic/Vasoconstrictor Precautions No information available to require special precautions

Effects on Dental Treatment No significant effects or complications reported

Effects on Bleeding No information available to require special precautions

Adverse Effects

>10%:

Central nervous system: Headache (24% to 25%)

Gastrointestinal: Abdominal pain (15%), diarrhea (up to 13%)

Hepatic: Hepatitis exacerbation (up to 25% within 12 weeks of adefovir discontinuation)

Neuromuscular & skeletal: Weakness (up to 25%)

Renal: Hematuria (grade ≥3: 11%)

1% to 10%:

Dermatologic: Rash, pruritus

Endocrine & metabolic: Hypophosphatemia (<2 mg/dL: 1% and 3% in pre-/post-liver transplant patients, respectively)

Gastrointestinal: Flatulence (up to 8%), dyspepsia (5% to 9%), nausea, vomiting

Neuromuscular & skeletal: Back pain (up to 10%)

Renal: Serum creatinine increased (≥0.5 mg/dL: 2% to 3% in compensated liver disease; incidence may be higher in patients with decompensated cirrhosis or in liver transplant recipients), renal failure

Note: In liver transplant patients with baseline renal dysfunction, frequency of increased serum creatinine has been observed to be as high as 32% to 51% at 48 and 96 weeks post-transplantation, respectively; considering the concomitant use of other potentially nephrotoxic medications, baseline renal insufficiency, and predisposing comorbidities, the role of adefovir in these changes could not be established.

Respiratory: Cough (6% to 8%), rhinitis (up to 5%)

General Dosage Range Dosage adjustment recommended in patients with renal impairment

Oral: *Children ≥12 years and Adults:* 10 mg once daily

Mechanism of Action Acyclic nucleotide reverse transcriptase inhibitor (adenosine analog) which interferes with HBV viral RNA-dependent DNA polymerase resulting in inhibition of viral replication.

Pharmacodynamics/Kinetics

Half-life Elimination 7.5 hours; prolonged in renal impairment

Time to Peak 1.75 hours

Pregnancy Risk Factor C

Adenosine (a DEN oh seen)

U.S. Brand Names Adenocard® IV; Adenoscan®

Canadian Brand Names Adenocard®; Adenoscan®; Adenosine Injection, USP; PMS-Adenosine

Pharmacologic Category Antiarrhythmic Agent, Miscellaneous; Diagnostic Agent

Use

Adenocard®: Treatment of paroxysmal supraventricular tachycardia (PSVT) including that associated with accessory bypass tracts (Wolff-Parkinson-White syndrome); when clinically advisable, appropriate vagal maneuvers should be attempted prior to adenosine administration; **not effective for conversion of atrial fibrillation, atrial flutter, or ventricular tachycardia**

Adenoscan®: Pharmacologic stress agent used in myocardial perfusion thallium-201 scintigraphy

Unlabeled/Investigational Use

ACLS/PALS Guidelines (2010): Stable, narrow-complex regular tachycardias; unstable narrow-complex regular tachycardias while preparations are made for synchronized direct-current cardioversion; stable regular monomorphic, wide-complex tachycardia as a therapeutic (if SVT) and diagnostic maneuver

Adenoscan®: Acute vasodilator testing in pulmonary artery hypertension

Local Anesthetic/Vasoconstrictor Precautions No information available to require special precautions

Effects on Dental Treatment No significant effects or complications reported

Effects on Bleeding No information available to require special precautions

Adverse Effects Note: Frequency varies based on use; higher frequency of infusion-related effects, such as flushing and lightheadedness, were reported with continuous infusion (Adenoscan®).

>10%:

- Cardiovascular: Transient new arrhythmia (eg, atrial premature contractions, atrial fibrillation, PVCs) after cardioversion (55%), facial flushing (18% to 44%)
- Central nervous system: Headache (2% to 18%), dizziness/lightheadedness (2% to 12%)
- Gastrointestinal: GI discomfort (13%)
- Neuromuscular & skeletal: Discomfort of neck, throat, jaw (<1% to 15%)
- Respiratory: Chest pressure/discomfort (7% to 40%), dyspnea (12% to 28%)

1% to 10%:

- Cardiovascular: AV block (infusion 6%; third-degree <1%), ST segment depression (3%), hypotension (<1% to 2%), chest pain, palpitation
- Central nervous system: Nervousness (2%), apprehension
- Gastrointestinal: Nausea (3%)
- Neuromuscular & skeletal: Upper extremity discomfort (≤4%), numbness (≤2%), paresthesia (≤2%)
- Respiratory: Hyperventilation
- Miscellaneous: Diaphoresis

General Dosage Range I.V.:

Children <50 kg: Initial: 0.05-0.1 mg/kg/dose (maximum initial dose: 6 mg); repeat: 0.05-0.3 mg/kg/dose (maximum: 0.3 mg/kg/dose or 12 mg/dose)

Children ≥50 kg and Adults: Initial: 6 mg; if not effective, 12 mg may be given; may repeat 12 mg if needed (maximum: 12 mg/dose)

Mechanism of Action

Antiarrhythmic actions: Slows conduction time through the AV node, interrupting the re-entry pathways through the AV node, restoring normal sinus rhythm

Myocardial perfusion scintigraphy: Adenosine also causes coronary vasodilation and increases blood flow in normal coronary arteries with little to no increase in stenotic coronary arteries; thallium-201 uptake into the stenotic coronary arteries will be less than that of normal coronary arteries revealing areas of insufficient blood flow.

Pharmacodynamics/Kinetics

Onset of Action Rapid

Duration of Action Very brief

Half-life Elimination <10 seconds

Pregnancy Risk Factor C

Adenovirus (Types 4, 7) Vaccine

(ad e noh VYE rus typs for SEV en vak SEEN)

Pharmacologic Category Vaccine, Live (Viral)

Use Prevention of acute febrile respiratory disease caused by adenovirus types 4 and 7 (approved for use in military populations)

Local Anesthetic/Vasoconstrictor Precautions No information available to require special precautions

Effects on Dental Treatment No significant effects or complications reported

Effects on Bleeding No information available to require special precautions

Adverse Effects All serious adverse reactions must be reported to the U.S. Department of Health and Human Services (DHHS) Vaccine Adverse Event Reporting System (VAERS) at 1-800-822-7967 or online at https://vaers.hhs.gov/esub/index.

>10%:

- Central nervous system: Headache (7% to 30%)
- Gastrointestinal: Nausea (5% to 14%)
- Respiratory: Nasal congestion (8% to 15%), pharyngolaryngeal pain (12% to 13%), cough (10% to 12%)

1% to 10%:
Central nervous system: Fever (≤1%)
Gastrointestinal: Diarrhea (3% to 10%)
Neuromuscular & skeletal: Limb pain (4%)
Respiratory: Rhinorrhea (4%)

General Dosage Range Oral: *Adolescents ≥17 years and Adults ≤50 years:* One tablet each of type 4 and type 7 as a single vaccine dose

Mechanism of Action Nonattenuated preparation of live adenovirus types 4 and 7 designed to release the live viruses in the intestine and replicate (in the intestinal tract) to induce immunity in individuals without (or with low) existing neutralizing antibodies to adenovirus types 4 and 7.

Pharmacodynamics/Kinetics

Onset of Action Viral shedding in the stool begins at 7 days; seroconversion occurs ~26 days following vaccination

Duration of Action Viral shedding no longer detected at 28 days

Product Availability Adenovirus (Types 4, 7) tablets: FDA approved March 2011; anticipated availability is currently undetermined

Prescribing and Access Restrictions Product is approved for use in military populations

Agalsidase Alfa (aye GAL si days AL fa)

Canadian Brand Names Replagal™

Pharmacologic Category Enzyme

Use Replacement therapy for Fabry disease

Local Anesthetic/Vasoconstrictor Precautions No information available to require special precautions

Effects on Dental Treatment No significant effects or complications reported

Effects on Bleeding No information available to require special precautions

Adverse Effects Note: The most common and serious adverse reactions are infusion reactions (symptoms may include chills, dyspnea, facial flushing, fever, hypertension, nausea, rigors, tachycardia, urticaria, and vomiting).

>10%:
Cardiovascular: Flushing (24%)
Central nervous system: Fever (20%), headache (11%)
Neuromuscular & skeletal: Rigors (20%)
Miscellaneous: IgG antibody formation (55%), infusion-related reactions (13%)

1% to 10%:
Cardiovascular: Chest tightness (7%), hypertension (4%), tachycardia (4%), chest pain (2%), edema (2%), peripheral coldness (2%), peripheral edema (2%)
Central nervous system: Dizziness (9%), fatigue (9%), fatigue aggravated (7%), hypersomnia (2%), hypoesthesia (2%), panic attack (2%), pain/discomfort (7%), somnolence (2%), vertigo (2%)
Dermatologic: Acne (9%), erythema (7%), mottled skin(4%), pruritus (4%), dry skin (2%), eczema (2%), rash (2%)
Gastrointestinal: Nausea (9%), dysgeusia (6%), diarrhea (4%), vomiting (4%), abdominal pain (2%), dyspepsia (2%), gastrointestinal upset (2%), stomach cramps (2%), stomach discomfort (2%)
Neuromuscular & skeletal: Myalgia (6%), neuropathic pain (6%), tremor (4%), musculoskeletal discomfort (2%), back pain (2%), limb pain (2%), paraesthesia (2%), weakness (2%)
Ocular: Lacrimation increased (2%), periorbital edema (2%)
Respiratory: Hoarseness (6%), throat tightness (6%), cough (4%), dyspnea (4%), nasopharyngitis (4%), pharyngitis (4%), nasal congestion (2%), snoring (2%), throat irritation (2%)
Miscellaneous: Feeling hot (4%), influenza-like syndrome(2%), parosmia (2%)

General Dosage Range I.V.: *Children and Adults:* 0.2 mg/kg every 2 weeks

Mechanism of Action Agalsidase alfa is a recombinant form of the enzyme alpha-galactosidase-A, which catalyzes the hydrolysis of globotriaosylceramide (Gb-3) and other glycosphingolipids. These compounds may accumulate (over many years) within the tissues of patients with Fabry disease, leading to renal and cardiovascular complications. Agalsidase has been noted to reduce cellular levels of Gb-3 within the liver, heart, kidney, blood vessels, and in plasma.

Pharmacodynamics/Kinetics

Half-life Elimination ~1.5-2 hours

Product Availability Not available in U.S.

Agalsidase Beta (aye GAL si days BAY ta)

U.S. Brand Names Fabrazyme®
Canadian Brand Names Fabrazyme®
Pharmacologic Category Enzyme
Use Replacement therapy for Fabry disease
Local Anesthetic/Vasoconstrictor Precautions No information available to require special precautions
Effects on Dental Treatment No significant effects or complications reported
Effects on Bleeding No information available to require special precautions
Adverse Effects Note: The most common and serious adverse reactions are infusion reactions (symptoms may include fever, tachycardia, hypertension, throat tightness, dyspnea, chills, abdominal pain, pruritus, urticaria, vomiting).

>10%:
Cardiovascular: Peripheral edema (21%)
Central nervous system: Chills (43%), headache (39%), fever (6% to 36%), fatigue (25%), dizziness (21%), pain (16%)
Gastrointestinal: Vomiting (24%)
Hematologic: Anemia (14%)
Neuromuscular & skeletal: Paresthesia (31%), limb pain (19%), back pain (16%)
Respiratory: Cough (33%), nasopharyngitis (28%), nasal congestion (19%), upper respiratory tract infection (19%), pharyngolaryngeal pain (16%), lower respiratory infection (11%)
Miscellaneous: IgG antibody formation (69% to 79%)

1% to 10%:
Cardiovascular: Hypertension (5% to 10%), chest discomfort (5%), tachycardia (5%), ventricular wall thickening (5%)
Central nervous system: Hypoesthesia (9%), insomnia (9%), anxiety (8%), depression (6%)
Dermatologic: Rash (10%), excoriation (9%), pruritus (8%), contact dermatitis (5%)
Endocrine & metabolic: Bicarbonate decreased (9%)
Gastrointestinal: Abdominal discomfort (6%), toothache (6%)
Neuromuscular & skeletal: Myalgia (8%), burning sensation (6%), muscle spasms (5%), neck pain (5%)
Otic: Tinnitus (8%), hearing impairment (5%)
Renal: Creatinine increased (9%), proteinuria (5%)
Respiratory: Sinusitis (9%), bronchitis (8%), congestion (8%), dyspnea (8%), pharyngitis (6%), wheezing (6%)
Miscellaneous: Feeling cold (10%), viral infection (5% to 6%), fungal infection (5%), infusion reactions (≥5%)

Other reported severe reactions (frequency not established): Abdominal pain, arrhythmia, ataxia, bradycardia, cardiac arrest, cardiac output decreased, chest pain, face edema, flushing, hypotension, nausea, nephrotic syndrome, pallor, stroke, throat tightness, urticaria, vertigo

General Dosage Range I.V.: *Children ≥8 years and Adults:* 1 mg/kg every 2 weeks
Mechanism of Action Agalsidase beta is a recombinant form of the enzyme alpha-galactosidase-A, which is required for the hydrolysis of GL-3 and other glycosphingolipids. The compounds may accumulate (over many years) within the tissues of patients with Fabry disease, leading to renal and cardiovascular complications. In clinical trials of limited duration, agalsidase been noted to reduce tissue inclusions of a key sphingolipid (GL-3). It is believed that long-term enzyme replacement may reduce clinical manifestations of renal failure, cardiomyopathy, and stroke. However, the relationship to a reduction in clinical manifestations has not been established.
Pharmacodynamics/Kinetics
Half-life Elimination Children: 86-151 minutes; Adults: 45-119 minutes
Pregnancy Risk Factor B

Albendazole (al BEN da zole)

U.S. Brand Names Albenza®
Pharmacologic Category Anthelmintic
Use Treatment of parenchymal neurocysticercosis caused by *Taenia solium* and cystic hydatid disease of the liver, lung, and peritoneum caused by *Echinococcus granulosus*
Unlabeled/Investigational Use Albendazole has activity against *Ascaris lumbricoides* (roundworm); *Ancylostoma caninum*; *Ancylostoma duodenale* and *Necator americanus* (hookworms); cutaneous larva migrans; *Enterobius vermicularis* (pinworm); *Giardia duodenalis* (giardiasis); *Gnathostoma spinigerum*; *Gongylonema* sp; *Mansonella perstans* (filariasis); *Oesophagostomum bifurcum*; *Opisthorchis sinensis*

(liver fluke); *Trichinella spiralis* (Trichinellosis); visceral larva migrans (toxocariasis); activity has also been shown against the liver fluke *Clonorchis sinensis*, *Giardia lamblia*, *Cysticercus cellulosae*, and *Echinococcus multilocularis*. Albendazole has also been used for the treatment of intestinal microsporidiosis (*Encephalitozoon intestinalis*), disseminated microsporidiosis (*E. hellem*, *E. cuniculi*, *E. intestinalis*, *Pleistophora* sp, *Trachipleistophora* sp, *Brachiola vesicularum*), and ocular microsporidiosis (*E. hellem*, *E. cuniculi*, *Vittaforma corneae*).

Local Anesthetic/Vasoconstrictor Precautions No information available to require special precautions

Effects on Dental Treatment No significant effects or complications reported

Effects on Bleeding No information available to require special precautions

Adverse Effects

>10%:

- Central nervous system: Headache (11% neurocysticercosis; 1% hydatid)
- Hepatic: LFTs increased (16% hydatid; <1% neurocysticercosis)

1% to 10%:

- Central nervous system: Intracranial pressure increased (≤2%), dizziness (≤1%), fever (≤1%), vertigo (≤1%), meningeal signs (1%)
- Dermatologic: Alopecia (<1% to 2%)
- Gastrointestinal: Abdominal pain (≤6%), nausea/vomiting (4% to 6%)

General Dosage Range Oral:

Children and Adults <60 kg: 15 mg/kg/day in 2 divided doses (maximum: 800 mg/day)

Children and Adults ≥60 kg: 800 mg/day in 2 divided doses (maximum: 800 mg/day)

Mechanism of Action Active metabolite, albendazole sulfoxide, causes selective degeneration of cytoplasmic microtubules in intestinal and tegmental cells of intestinal helminths and larvae; glycogen is depleted, glucose uptake and cholinesterase secretion are impaired, and desecratory substances accumulate intracellulary. ATP production decreases causing energy depletion, immobilization, and worm death.

Pharmacodynamics/Kinetics

Half-life Elimination 8-12 hours

Time to Peak Serum: 2-5 hours

Pregnancy Risk Factor C

Albuterol (al BYOO ter ole)

Related Information

Respiratory Diseases *on page 1876*

U.S. Brand Names AccuNeb®; ProAir® HFA; Proventil® HFA; Ventolin® HFA; VoSpire ER®

Canadian Brand Names Airomir; Apo-Salvent®; Apo-Salvent® AEM; Apo-Salvent® CFC Free; Apo-Salvent® Sterules; Dom-Salbutamol; Med-Salbutamol; Mylan-Salbutamol Respirator Solution; Mylan-Salbutamol Sterinebs P.F.; Novo-Salbutamol HFA; Nu-Salbutamol; PHL-Salbutamol; PMS-Salbutamol; ratio-Ipra-Sal; ratio-Salbutamol; Sandoz-Salbutamol; Ventolin®; Ventolin® Diskus; Ventolin® HFA; Ventolin® I.V. Infusion; Ventolin® Nebules P.F.

Generic Availability (U.S.) Yes

Pharmacologic Category Beta$_2$-Adrenergic Agonist

Use Treatment or prevention of bronchospasm in patients with reversible obstructive airway disease; prevention of exercise-induced bronchospasm

Local Anesthetic/Vasoconstrictor Precautions No information available to require special precautions

Effects on Dental Treatment Key adverse event(s) related to dental treatment: Xerostomia (normal salivary flow resumes upon discontinuation)

Effects on Bleeding No information available to require special precautions

Adverse Effects Incidence of adverse effects is dependent upon age of patient, dose, and route of administration.

- Cardiovascular: Angina, atrial fibrillation, arrhythmias, chest discomfort, chest pain, extrasystoles, flushing, hyper-/hypotension, palpitation, supraventricular tachycardia, tachycardia
- Central nervous system: CNS stimulation, dizziness, drowsiness, headache, insomnia, irritability, lightheadedness, migraine, nervousness, nightmares, restlessness, seizure
- Dermatologic: Angioedema, rash, urticaria
- Endocrine & metabolic: Hyperglycemia, hypokalemia, lactic acidosis
- Gastrointestinal: Diarrhea, dry mouth, dyspepsia, gastroenteritis, nausea, unusual taste, vomiting
- Genitourinary: Micturition difficulty

Local: Injection: Pain, stinging
Neuromuscular & skeletal: Muscle cramps, musculoskeletal pain, tremor, weakness
Otic: Otitis media, vertigo
Respiratory: Asthma exacerbation, bronchospasm, cough, epistaxis, laryngitis, oropharyngeal drying/irritation, oropharyngeal edema, pharyngitis, rhinitis, upper respiratory inflammation, viral respiratory infection
Miscellaneous: Allergic reaction, anaphylaxis, diaphoresis, lymphadenopathy

Dosage

Oral:

Children: Bronchospasm:
- 2-6 years: 0.1-0.2 mg/kg/dose 3 times/day; maximum dose not to exceed 12 mg/day (divided doses)
- 6-12 years: 2 mg/dose 3-4 times/day; maximum dose not to exceed 24 mg/day (divided doses)
  - Extended release: 4 mg every 12 hours; maximum dose not to exceed 24 mg/day (divided doses)

Children >12 years and Adults: Bronchospasm (treatment): 2-4 mg/dose 3-4 times/day; maximum dose not to exceed 32 mg/day (divided doses)
- Extended release: 8 mg every 12 hours; maximum dose not to exceed 32 mg/day (divided doses). A 4 mg dose every 12 hours may be sufficient in some patients, such as adults of low body weight.

Elderly: Bronchospasm (treatment): 2 mg 3-4 times/day; maximum: 8 mg 4 times/day

Metered-dose inhaler (90 mcg/puff):

Children ≤4 years *(NIH Guidelines, 2007)*:
- Quick relief: 2 puffs every 4-6 hours as needed
- Exacerbation of asthma (acute, severe): 4-8 puffs every 20 minutes for 3 doses, then every 1-4 hours as needed
- Exercise-induced bronchospasm (prevention): 1-2 puffs 5 minutes prior to exercise

Children 5-11 years *(NIH Guidelines, 2007)*:
- Bronchospasm, quick relief: 2 puffs every 4-6 hours as needed
- Exacerbation of asthma (acute, severe): 4-8 puffs every 20 minutes for 3 doses, then every 1-4 hours as needed
- Exercise-induced bronchospasm (prevention): 2 puffs 5-30 minutes prior to exercise

Children ≥12 years and Adults:
- Bronchospasm, quick relief *(NIH Guidelines, 2007)*: 2 puffs every 4-6 hours as needed
- Exacerbation of asthma (acute, severe) *(NIH Guidelines, 2007)*: 4-8 puffs every 20 minutes for up to 4 hours, then every 1-4 hours as needed
- Exercise-induced bronchospasm (prevention) *(NIH Guidelines, 2007)*: 2 puffs 5-30 minutes prior to exercise

Solution for nebulization:

Children 2-12 years (AccuNeb®): Bronchospasm: 0.63-1.25 mg 3-4 times daily as needed

Children ≤4 years *(NIH Guidelines, 2007)*:
- Quick relief: 0.63-2.5 mg every 4-6 hours as needed
- Exacerbation of asthma (acute, severe): 0.15 mg/kg (minimum: 2.5 mg) every 20 minutes for 3 doses, then 0.15-0.3 mg/kg (maximum: 10 mg) every 1-4 hours as needed **or** 0.5 mg/kg/hour by continuous nebulization

Children 5-11 years *(NIH Guidelines, 2007)*:
- Quick relief: 1.25-5 mg every 4-8 hours as needed
- Exacerbation of asthma (acute, severe): 0.15 mg/kg (minimum: 2.5 mg) every 20 minutes for 3 doses, then 0.15-0.3 mg/kg (maximum: 10 mg) every 1-4 hours as needed **or** 0.5 mg/kg/hour by continuous nebulization

Children ≥12 years and Adults:
- Bronchospasm: 2.5 mg 3-4 times daily as needed
- Quick relief *(NIH Guidelines, 2007)*: 1.25-5 mg every 4-8 hours as needed
- Exacerbation of asthma (acute, severe) *(NIH Guidelines, 2007)*: 2.5-5 mg every 20 minutes for 3 doses then 2.5-10 mg every 1-4 hours as needed, **or** 10-15 mg/hour by continuous nebulization

I.V. continuous infusion: Adults (Canadian labeling; product not available in U.S.): Severe bronchospasm and status asthmaticus: Initial: 5 mcg/minute; may increase up to 10-20 mcg/minute at 15- to 30-minute intervals if needed

Dosage adjustment in renal impairment: Use with caution in patients with renal impairment. No dosage adjustment required (including patients on hemodialysis, peritoneal dialysis, or CRRT; Aronoff, 2007).

Mechanism of Action Relaxes bronchial smooth muscle by action on $beta_2$-receptors with little effect on heart rate

Contraindications Hypersensitivity to albuterol or any component of the formulation

Injection formulation (Canadian labeling; product not available in U.S.): Hypersensitivity to albuterol or any component of the formulation; tachyarrhythmias; risk of abortion during first or second trimester

Warnings/Precautions Optimize anti-inflammatory treatment before initiating maintenance treatment with albuterol. Do not use as a component of chronic therapy without an anti-inflammatory agent. Only the mildest forms of asthma (Step 1 and/or exercise-induced) would not require concurrent use based upon asthma guidelines. Patient must be instructed to seek medical attention in cases where acute symptoms are not relieved or a previous level of response is diminished. The need to increase frequency of use may indicate deterioration of asthma, and treatment must not be delayed.

Use caution in patients with cardiovascular disease (arrhythmia or hypertension or HF), convulsive disorders, diabetes, glaucoma, hyperthyroidism, or hypokalemia. Beta-agonists may cause elevation in blood pressure, heart rate, and result in CNS stimulation/excitation. $Beta_2$-agonists may increase risk of arrhythmia, increase serum glucose, or decrease serum potassium.

Immediate hypersensitivity reactions (urticaria, angioedema, rash, bronchospasm) have been reported. Do not exceed recommended dose; serious adverse events, including fatalities, have been associated with excessive use of inhaled sympathomimetics. Rarely, paradoxical bronchospasm may occur with use of inhaled bronchodilating agents; this should be distinguished from inadequate response. All patients should utilize a spacer device or valved holding chamber when using a metered-dose inhaler; in addition, face masks should be used in children <4 years of age.

Patient response may vary between inhalers that contain chlorofluorocarbons and those which are chlorofluorocarbon-free.

Drug Interactions

Avoid Concomitant Use

Avoid concomitant use of Albuterol with any of the following: Iobenguane I 123

Increased Effect/Toxicity

Albuterol may increase the levels/effects of: Loop Diuretics; Sympathomimetics

The levels/effects of Albuterol may be increased by: Atomoxetine; Cannabinoids; MAO Inhibitors; Tricyclic Antidepressants

Decreased Effect

Albuterol may decrease the levels/effects of: Iobenguane I 123

The levels/effects of Albuterol may be decreased by: Alpha-/Beta-Blockers; Beta-Blockers (Beta1 Selective); Beta-Blockers (Nonselective); Betahistine

Ethanol/Nutrition/Herb Interactions

Food: Avoid or limit caffeine (may cause CNS stimulation).

Herb/Nutraceutical: Avoid ephedra, yohimbe (may cause CNS stimulation). Avoid St John's wort (may decrease the levels/effects of albuterol).

Dietary Considerations Oral forms should be taken with water 1 hour before or 2 hours after meals.

Pharmacodynamics/Kinetics

Onset of Action Peak effect:

Nebulization/oral inhalation: 0.5-2 hours

CFC-propelled albuterol: 10 minutes

Ventolin® HFA: 25 minutes

Oral: 2-3 hours

Duration of Action Nebulization/oral inhalation: 3-4 hours; Oral: 4-6 hours

Half-life Elimination Inhalation: 3.8 hours; Oral: 3.7-5 hours

Pregnancy Risk Factor C

Lactation Excretion in breast milk unknown/use caution

Dosage Forms

Aerosol, for oral inhalation:

ProAir® HFA: 90 mcg/inhalation (8.5 g)

Proventil® HFA: 90 mcg/inhalation (6.7 g)

Ventolin® HFA: 90 mcg/inhalation (8 g, 18 g)

Solution, for nebulization: 0.5% [100 mg/20 mL] (1s); 0.083% [2.5 mg/3 mL] (25s, 30s, 60s)

Solution, for nebulization [preservative free]: 0.021% [0.63 mg/3 mL] (25s); 0.042% [1.25 mg/3 mL] (25s, 30s); 0.083% [2.5 mg/3 mL] (10s, 24s, 25s, 30s, 60s); 0.5% [2.5 mg/0.5 mL] (10s, 30s)
AccuNeb®: 0.021% [0.63 mg/3 mL] (25s); 0.042% [1.25 mg/3 mL] (25s)
Syrup, oral: 2 mg/5 mL (473 mL, 480 mL)
Tablet, oral: 2 mg, 4 mg
Tablet, extended release, oral: 4 mg, 8 mg
VoSpire ER®: 4 mg, 8 mg

Dosage Forms: Canada
Injection, solution:
Ventolin® I.V.: 1 mg/1mL (5 mL)

Alcaftadine (al KAF ta deen)

U.S. Brand Names Lastacaft™
Pharmacologic Category Histamine H_1 Antagonist; Histamine H_1 Antagonist, Second Generation; Mast Cell Stabilizer
Use Prevention of itching associated with allergic conjunctivitis
Local Anesthetic/Vasoconstrictor Precautions No information available to require special precautions
Effects on Dental Treatment No significant effects or complications reported
Effects on Bleeding No information available to require special precautions
Adverse Effects 1% to 10%:
Central nervous system: Headache (<3%)
Ocular: Ocular reactions (<4%; includes burning, pruritus, irritation, redness, stinging)
Respiratory: Nasopharyngitis (<3%)
Miscellaneous: Influenza (<3%)
General Dosage Range Ophthalmic: *Children ≥2 years and Adults:* Instill 1 drop into each eye once daily
Mechanism of Action Direct H_1-receptor antagonist and inhibitor of histamine release from mast cells
Pharmacodynamics/Kinetics
Half-life Elimination Carboxylic acid: ~2 hours
Pregnancy Risk Factor B

Alclometasone (al kloe MET a sone)

U.S. Brand Names Aclovate®
Generic Availability (U.S.) Yes
Pharmacologic Category Corticosteroid, Topical
Dental Use Treatment of inflammation of corticosteroid-responsive dermatosis (low to medium potency topical corticosteroid)
Use Treatment of inflammation of corticosteroid-responsive dermatosis (low to medium potency topical corticosteroid)
Local Anesthetic/Vasoconstrictor Precautions No information available to require special precautions
Effects on Dental Treatment No significant effects or complications reported
Effects on Bleeding No information available to require special precautions
Adverse Effects Frequency not defined.
Dermatologic: Acne, allergic dermatitis, hypopigmentation, maceration of the skin, perioral dermatitis, skin atrophy, striae, miliaria, telangiectasia
Endocrine & metabolic: HPA suppression, Cushing's syndrome, growth retardation
Local: Burning, erythema, itching, irritation, dryness, folliculitis, hypertrichosis, papular rash
Miscellaneous: Secondary infection
Dosage Note: Therapy should be discontinued when control is achieved; if no improvement is seen within 2 weeks, reassessment of diagnosis may be necessary.
Topical:
Children ≥1 year: Apply thin film to affected area 2-3 times/day; do not use for >3 weeks
Adults: Apply a thin film to the affected area 2-3 times/day
Mechanism of Action Stimulates the synthesis of enzymes needed to decrease inflammation, suppress mitotic activity, and cause vasoconstriction
Contraindications Hypersensitivity to alclometasone or any component of the formulation; viral, fungal, or tubercular skin lesions
Warnings/Precautions Systemic absorption of topical corticosteroids may cause hypothalamic-pituitary-adrenal (HPA) axis suppression (reversible) particularly in younger children. HPA axis suppression may lead to adrenal crisis. Risk is increased

when used over large surface areas, for prolonged periods, or with occlusive dressings. Adverse systemic effects including hyperglycemia, glycosuria, fluid and electrolyte changes, and HPA suppression may occur when used on large surface areas, for prolonged periods, or with an occlusive dressing. Prolonged treatment with corticosteroids has been associated with the development of Kaposi's sarcoma (case reports); if noted, discontinuation of therapy should be considered. Allergic contact dermatitis can occur, it is usually diagnosed by failure to heal rather than clinical exacerbation. Safety and efficacy have not been established in children <1 year of age. Chronic use of corticosteroids in children may interfere with growth and development. Not for the treatment of diaper dermatitis.

Drug Interactions

Avoid Concomitant Use

Avoid concomitant use of Alclometasone with any of the following: Aldesleukin

Increased Effect/Toxicity

Alclometasone may increase the levels/effects of: Deferasirox

Decreased Effect

Alclometasone may decrease the levels/effects of: Aldesleukin; Corticorelin

Pregnancy Risk Factor C

Dosage Forms

Cream, topical: 0.05% (15 g, 45 g, 60 g)

Aclovate®: 0.05% (15 g, 60 g)

Ointment, topical: 0.05% (15 g, 45 g, 60 g)

Aclovate®: 0.05% (15 g, 60 g)

Aldesleukin (al des LOO kin)

U.S. Brand Names Proleukin®

Canadian Brand Names Proleukin®

Pharmacologic Category Antineoplastic Agent, Miscellaneous; Biological Response Modulator

Use Treatment of metastatic renal cell cancer, metastatic melanoma

Unlabeled/Investigational Use Treatment of acute myeloid leukemia (AML)

Local Anesthetic/Vasoconstrictor Precautions No information available to require special precautions

Effects on Dental Treatment Key adverse event(s) related to dental treatment: Stomatitis

Effects on Bleeding Chemotherapy may result in significant myelosuppression, potentially including significant reduction in platelet counts and altered hemostasis. In patients who are under active treatment with these agents, medical consult is suggested.

Adverse Effects

>10%:

Cardiovascular: Hypotension (71%; grade 4: 3%), peripheral edema (28%), tachycardia (23%), edema (15%), vasodilation (13%), supraventricular tachycardia (12%; grade 4: 1%), cardiovascular disorder (11%; includes blood pressure changes, HF and ECG changes)

Central nervous system: Chills (52%), confusion (34%; grade 4: 1%), fever (29%; grade 4: 1%), malaise (27%), somnolence (22%), anxiety (12%), pain (12%), dizziness (11%)

Dermatologic: Rash (42%), pruritus (24%), exfoliative dermatitis (18%)

Endocrine & metabolic: Acidosis (12%; grade 4: 1%), hypomagnesemia (12%), hypocalcemia (11%)

Gastrointestinal: Diarrhea (67%; grade 4: 2%), vomiting (19% to 50%; grade 4: 1%), nausea (19% to 35%), stomatitis (22%), anorexia (20%), weight gain (16%), abdominal pain (11%)

Hematologic: Thrombocytopenia (37%; grade 4: 1%), anemia (29%), leukopenia (16%)

Hepatic: Hyperbilirubinemia (40%; grade 4: 2%), AST increased (23%; grade 4: 1%)

Neuromuscular & skeletal: Weakness (23%)

Renal: Oliguria (63%; grade 4: 6%), creatinine increased (33%; grade 4: 1%)

Respiratory: Dyspnea (43%; grade 4: 1%), lung disorder (24%; includes pulmonary congestion, rales, and rhonchi), cough (11%), respiratory disorder (11%; includes acute respiratory distress syndrome, infiltrates and pulmonary changes)

Miscellaneous: Infection (13%; grade 4: 1%)

1% to 10%:

Cardiovascular: Arrhythmia (10%), cardiac arrest (grade 4: 1%), MI (grade 4: 1%), ventricular tachycardia (grade 4: 1%)

Central nervous system: Coma (grade 4: 2%), stupor (grade 4: 1%), psychosis (grade 4: 1%)

Gastrointestinal: Abdomen enlarged (10%)
Hematologic: Coagulation disorder (grade 4: 1%)
Hepatic: Alkaline phosphatase increased (10%)
Renal: Anuria (grade 4: 5%), acute renal failure (grade 4: 1%)
Respiratory: Rhinitis (10%), apnea (grade 4: 1%)
Miscellaneous: Sepsis (grade 4: 1%)

General Dosage Range Dosage adjustment recommended in patients who develop toxicities

I.V.: *Adults:* 600,000 int. units/kg every 8 hours (maximum: 14 doses); may repeat after 9 days for a total of 28 doses/course

Mechanism of Action Aldesleukin is a human recombinant interleukin-2 product which promotes proliferation, differentiation, and recruitment of T and B cells, natural killer (NK) cells, and thymocytes; causes cytolytic activity in a subset of lymphocytes and subsequent interactions between the immune system and malignant cells; can stimulate lymphokine-activated killer (LAK) cells and tumor-infiltrating lymphocytes (TIL) cells.

Pharmacodynamics/Kinetics

Half-life Elimination I.V.: Initial: 6-13 minutes; Terminal: 80-120 minutes

Pregnancy Risk Factor C

Alefacept (a LE fa sept)

U.S. Brand Names Amevive®

Canadian Brand Names Amevive®

Pharmacologic Category Monoclonal Antibody

Use Treatment of moderate-to-severe chronic plaque psoriasis in adults who are candidates for systemic therapy or phototherapy

Local Anesthetic/Vasoconstrictor Precautions No information available to require special precautions

Effects on Dental Treatment No significant effects or complications reported

Effects on Bleeding No information available to require special precautions

Adverse Effects

≥10%:

Hematologic: Lymphopenia (up to 10% of patients required temporary discontinuation, up to 17% during a second course of therapy)
Local: Injection site reactions (up to 16% of patients; includes pain, inflammation, bleeding, edema, or other reaction)

1% to 10%:

Central nervous system: Chills (6%; primarily during intravenous administration), dizziness (≥2%)
Dermatologic: Pruritus (≥2%)
Gastrointestinal: Nausea (≥2%)
Neuromuscular & skeletal: Myalgia (≥2%)
Respiratory: Pharyngitis (≥2%), cough increased (≥2%)
Miscellaneous: Malignancies (1% vs 0.5% in placebo), antibodies to alefacept (3%; significance unknown), infection (1% requiring hospitalization)

General Dosage Range I.M.: *Adults:* 15 mg once weekly

Mechanism of Action Binds to CD2, a receptor on the surface of lymphocytes, inhibiting their interaction with leukocyte functional antigen 3 (LFA-3). Interaction between CD2 and LFA-3 is important for the activation of T lymphocytes in psoriasis. Activated T lymphocytes secrete a number of inflammatory mediators, including interferon gamma, which are involved in psoriasis. Since CD2 is primarily expressed on T lymphocytes, treatment results in a reduction in $CD4^+$ and $CD8^+$ T lymphocytes, with lesser effects on other cell populations (NK and B lymphocytes).

Pharmacodynamics/Kinetics

Half-life Elimination 270 hours (following I.V. administration)

Pregnancy Risk Factor B

Prescribing and Access Restrictions Alefacept will be distributed directly to physician offices or to a specialty pharmacy; injections are intended to be administered in the physician's office. Contact Amevive® Start Assistance Program (ASAP) at 1-800-477-6472 to initiate treatment.

Alemtuzumab (ay lem TU zoo mab)

U.S. Brand Names Campath®

Canadian Brand Names MabCampath®

Pharmacologic Category Antineoplastic Agent, Monoclonal Antibody

Use Treatment of B-cell chronic lymphocytic leukemia (B-CLL)

Unlabeled/Investigational Use Treatment of cutaneous T-cell lymphoma, peripheral T-cell lymphoma, refractory T-cell prolymphocytic leukemia, refractory or resistant autoimmune cytopenias; preconditioning regimen and prophylaxis of graft-versus-host disease (GVHD) in allogeneic stem cell transplant; immunosuppressant in solid organ transplant (induction and rejection)

Local Anesthetic/Vasoconstrictor Precautions No information available to require special precautions

Effects on Dental Treatment Key adverse event(s) related to dental treatment: Stomatitis and mucositis.

Effects on Bleeding Chemotherapy may result in significant myelosuppression, potentially including significant reduction in platelet counts and altered hemostasis. In patients who are under active treatment with these agents, medical consult is suggested.

Adverse Effects

>10%:

Cardiovascular: Hypotension (15% to 32%), peripheral edema (13%), hypertension (11% to 15%), dysrhythmia/tachycardia/SVT (10% to 14%)

Central nervous system: Fever (69% to 85%), chills (53%), fatigue (22% to 34%), headache (13% to 24%), dysthesias (15%), dizziness (12%)

Dermatologic: Rash (13% to 40%), urticaria (16% to 30%), pruritus (14% to 24%)

Gastrointestinal: Nausea (47% to 54%), vomiting (33% to 41%), anorexia (20%), diarrhea (10% to 22%), stomatitis/mucositis (14%), abdominal pain (11%)

Hematologic: Lymphopenia (grades 3/4: 97%), neutropenia (77% to 85%; grade 3/4: 42% to 70% [median onset: 31 days, median duration: 28-37 days]), anemia (76% to 80%; grade 3/4: 12% to 47% [median onset: 31 days, median duration 8 days]), thrombocytopenia (71% to 72%; grade 3/4: 13% to 52% [median onset: 9 days; median duration: 14-21 days])

Local: Injection site reaction (SubQ administration: 90%)

Neuromuscular & skeletal: Rigors (86% to 89%), skeletal pain (24%), weakness (13%), myalgia (11%)

Respiratory: Dyspnea (14% to 26%), cough (25%), bronchitis/pneumonitis (21%), pneumonia (16%), pharyngitis (12%)

Miscellaneous: Infection (43% to 74%; grades 3/4: 21% to 37%; incidence is lower if prophylactic anti-infectives are utilized), CMV viremia (55%), infusion reactions (grades 3/4: 10% to 35%), diaphoresis (19%), CMV infection (6% to 16%), sepsis (15%; grades 3/4: 3% to 10%), herpes viral infections (1% to 11%)

1% to 10%:

Cardiovascular: Chest pain (10%)

Central nervous system: Insomnia (10%), malaise (9%), anxiety (8%), depression (7%), temperature change sensation (5%), somnolence (5%)

Dermatologic: Purpura (8%), erythema (4%)

Gastrointestinal: Dyspepsia (10%), constipation (9%)

Hematologic: Neutropenic fever (10%; grades 3/4: 5% to 10%), pancytopenia/marrow hypoplasia (5% to 6%; grade 3/4: 3%), positive Coombs' test without hemolysis (2%), autoimmune thrombocytopenia (2%), autoimmune hemolytic anemia (1%)

Neuromuscular & skeletal: Back pain (10%), tremor (3% to 7%)

Respiratory: Bronchospasm (9%), epistaxis (7%), rhinitis (7%)

Miscellaneous: Moniliasis (8%)

General Dosage Range Dosage adjustment recommended in patients who develop toxicities

I.V. (infusion): *Adults:* Initial: 3 mg/day, then 10 mg/day; Maintenance: 30 mg/day 3 times/week on alternate days; Maximum dose: 30 mg/day; 90 mg/week (cumulative)

Mechanism of Action Binds to CD52, a nonmodulating antigen present on the surface of B and T lymphocytes, a majority of monocytes, macrophages, NK cells, and a subpopulation of granulocytes. After binding to $CD52^+$ cells, an antibody-dependent lysis of leukemic cells occurs.

Pharmacodynamics/Kinetics

Half-life Elimination I.V.: 11 hours (following first 30 mg dose; range: 2-32 hours); 6 days (following the last 30 mg dose; range: 1-14 days)

Pregnancy Risk Factor C

Alendronate (a LEN droe nate)

Related Information

Osteonecrosis of the Jaw *on page 1894*

Rheumatoid Arthritis, Osteoarthritis, and Osteoporosis *on page 1889*

U.S. Brand Names Fosamax®

Canadian Brand Names Alendronate-FC; Apo-Alendronate®; CO Alendronate; Dom-Alendronate; Fosamax®; Mylan-Alendronate; Novo-Alendronate; PHL-Alendronate; PMS-Alendronate; PMS-Alendronate-FC; ratio-Alendronate; Riva-Alendronate; Sandoz-Alendronate; Teva-Alendronate

Generic Availability (U.S.) Yes: Tablet

Pharmacologic Category Bisphosphonate Derivative

Use Treatment and prevention of osteoporosis in postmenopausal females; treatment of osteoporosis in males; Paget's disease of the bone in patients who are symptomatic, at risk for future complications, or with alkaline phosphatase ≥2 times the upper limit of normal; treatment of glucocorticoid-induced osteoporosis in males and females with low bone mineral density who are receiving a daily dosage ≥7.5 mg of prednisone (or equivalent)

Local Anesthetic/Vasoconstrictor Precautions No information available to require special precautions

Effects on Dental Treatment Osteonecrosis of the jaw (ONJ), generally associated with local infection and/or tooth extraction and often with delayed healing, has been reported in patients taking bisphosphonates. Symptoms included nonhealing extraction socket or an exposed jawbone. Most reported cases of bisphosphonate-associated osteonecrosis have been in cancer patients treated with intravenous bisphosphonates. However, some have occurred in patients with postmenopausal osteoporosis taking oral bisphosphonates. Dental surgery, particularly tooth extraction, may increase the risk for ONJ. Patients who develop ONJ while on bisphosphonate therapy should receive care by an oral surgeon. See Dental Comment.

Effects on Bleeding No information available to require special precautions

Adverse Effects Note: Incidence of adverse effects (mostly GI) increases significantly in patients treated for Paget's disease at 40 mg/day.

>10%: Endocrine & metabolic: Hypocalcemia (transient, mild, 18%); hypophosphatemia (transient, mild, 10%)

1% to 10%:

Central nervous system: Headache (up to 3%)

Gastrointestinal: Abdominal pain (1% to 7%), acid reflux (1% to 4%), dyspepsia (1% to 4%), nausea (1% to 4%), flatulence (up to 4%), diarrhea (1% to 3%), gastroesophageal reflux disease (1% to 3%), constipation (up to 3%), esophageal ulcer (up to 2%), abdominal distension (up to 1%), gastritis (up to 1%), vomiting (up to 1%), dysphagia (up to 1%), gastric ulcer (1%), melena (1%)

Neuromuscular & skeletal: Musculoskeletal pain (up to 6%), muscle cramps (up to 1%)

Dosage Oral: Adults: **Note:** Patients should receive supplemental calcium and vitamin D if dietary intake is inadequate.

Osteoporosis in postmenopausal females:

Prophylaxis: 5 mg once daily **or** 35 mg once weekly

Treatment: 10 mg once daily **or** 70 mg once weekly

Osteoporosis in males: 10 mg once daily **or** 70 mg once weekly

Osteoporosis secondary to glucocorticoids in males and females: Treatment: 5 mg once daily; a dose of 10 mg once daily should be used in postmenopausal females who are not receiving estrogen.

Paget's disease of bone in males and females: 40 mg once daily for 6 months

Retreatment: Relapses during the 12 months following therapy occurred in 9% of patients who responded to treatment. Specific retreatment data are not available. Following a 6-month post-treatment evaluation period, retreatment with alendronate may be considered in patients who have relapsed based on increases in serum alkaline phosphatase, which should be measured periodically. Retreatment may also be considered in those who failed to normalize their serum alkaline phosphatase.

Elderly: No dosage adjustment is necessary

Dosage adjustment in renal impairment:

Cl_{cr} 35-60 mL/minute: None necessary

Cl_{cr} <35 mL/minute: Alendronate is not recommended due to lack of experience

Dosage adjustment in hepatic impairment: None necessary

Mechanism of Action A bisphosphonate which inhibits bone resorption via actions on osteoclasts or on osteoclast precursors; decreases the rate of bone resorption, leading to an indirect increase in bone mineral density. In Paget's disease, characterized by disordered resorption and formation of bone, inhibition of resorption leads to an indirect decrease in bone formation; but the newly-formed bone has a more normal architecture.

Contraindications Hypersensitivity to alendronate, other bisphosphonates, or any component of the formulation; hypocalcemia; abnormalities of the esophagus which delay esophageal emptying such as stricture or achalasia; inability to stand or sit upright for at least 30 minutes; oral solution should not be used in patients at risk of aspiration

Warnings/Precautions Use caution in patients with renal impairment (not recommended for use in patients with Cl_{cr} <35 mL/minute); hypocalcemia must be corrected before therapy initiation; ensure adequate calcium and vitamin D intake. May cause irritation to upper gastrointestinal mucosa. Esophagitis, dysphagia, esophageal ulcers, esophageal erosions, and esophageal stricture (rare) have been reported; risk increases in patients unable to comply with dosing instructions. Use with caution in patients with dysphagia, esophageal disease, gastritis, duodenitis, or ulcers (may worsen underlying condition). Discontinue use if new or worsening symptoms develop.

Osteonecrosis of the jaw (ONJ) has been reported in patients receiving bisphosphonates. Risk factors include invasive dental procedures (eg, tooth extraction, dental implants, boney surgery); a diagnosis of cancer, with concomitant chemotherapy or corticosteroids; poor oral hygiene, ill-fitting dentures; and comorbid disorders (anemia, coagulopathy, infection, pre-existing dental disease). Most reported cases occurred after I.V. bisphosphonate therapy; however, cases have been reported following oral therapy. A dental exam and preventative dentistry should be performed prior to placing patients with risk factors on chronic bisphosphonate therapy. The manufacturer's labeling states that discontinuing bisphosphonates in patients requiring invasive dental procedures may reduce the risk of ONJ. However, other experts suggest that there is no evidence that discontinuing therapy reduces the risk of developing ONJ (Assael, 2009). The benefit/risk must be assessed by the treating physician and/or dentist/surgeon prior to any invasive dental procedure. Patients developing ONJ while on bisphosphonates should receive care by an oral surgeon.

Atypical femur fractures have been reported in patients receiving bisphosphonates for treatment/prevention of osteoporosis. The fractures include subtrochanteric femur (bone just below the hip joint) and diaphyseal femur (long segment of the thigh bone). Some patients experience prodromal pain weeks or months before the fracture occurs. It is unclear if bisphosphonate therapy is the cause for these fractures, although the majority have been reported in patients taking bisphosphonates. Patients receiving long-term (>3-5 years) therapy may be at an increased risk. Discontinue bisphosphonate therapy in patients who develop a femoral shaft fracture.

Severe (and occasionally debilitating) bone, joint, and/or muscle pain have been reported during bisphosphonate treatment. The onset of pain ranged from a single day to several months. Consider discontinuing therapy in patients who experience severe symptoms; symptoms usually resolve upon discontinuation. Some patients experienced recurrence when rechallenged with same drug or another bisphosphonate; avoid use in patients with a history of these symptoms in association with bisphosphonate therapy.

Drug Interactions

Avoid Concomitant Use There are no known interactions where it is recommended to avoid concomitant use.

Increased Effect/Toxicity

Alendronate may increase the levels/effects of: Deferasirox; Phosphate Supplements

The levels/effects of Alendronate may be increased by: Aminoglycosides; Aspirin; Nonsteroidal Anti-Inflammatory Agents

Decreased Effect

The levels/effects of Alendronate may be decreased by: Antacids; Calcium Salts; Iron Salts; Magnesium Salts; Proton Pump Inhibitors

Ethanol/Nutrition/Herb Interactions

Ethanol: Avoid ethanol (may increase risk of osteoporosis and gastric irritation).

Food: All food and beverages interfere with absorption. Coadministration with caffeine may reduce alendronate efficacy. Coadministration with dairy products may decrease alendronate absorption. Beverages (especially orange juice and coffee) and food may reduce the absorption of alendronate as much as 60%.

Dietary Considerations Ensure adequate calcium and vitamin D intake; women and men >50 years of age should consume 1200-1500 mg/day of elemental calcium and 800-1000 int. units/day of vitamin D. Wait at least 30 minutes after taking alendronate before taking any supplement. Alendronate must be taken with plain water first thing in the morning and at least 30 minutes before the first food or beverage of the day. Do not take with mineral water or with other beverages.

Pharmacodynamics/Kinetics

Half-life Elimination Exceeds 10 years

Pregnancy Risk Factor C

Lactation Excretion in breast milk unknown/use caution

Dosage Forms

Tablet, oral: 5 mg, 10 mg, 35 mg, 40 mg, 70 mg

Fosamax®: 10 mg, 70 mg

Dental Comment According to the 2008 report by the American Dental Association (ADA), the incidence of osteonecrosis of the jawbone associated with oral bisphosphonate therapy remains low. It was also stated that the benefits of using oral bisphosphonates to prevent osteoporosis significantly outweighs the small risk of developing bisphosphonate-associated osteonecrosis (Edwards, 2008). The full 26 page report can be accessed at http://www.ada.org/sections/professionalResources/pdfs/topics_osteonecrosis_bisphosphonate_report.pdf.

The ADA review stated the incidence of oral bisphosphonate-associated osteonecrosis of the jaw was one case for every 140,000 person-years exposure to oral bisphosphonates (ADA, 2006). This figure was based on information received from Merck & Co citing 170 worldwide cases for alendronate (Fosamax®). In addition, Procter & Gamble Pharmaceuticals has cited 20 cases for risedronate (Actonel®) and Roche Laboratories, Inc has cited one case for ibandronate (Boniva®).

In addition, the ADA 2008 report reiterates that the risk of osteonecrosis of the jawbone with oral bisphosphonates is minute compared to the risks with intravenous bisphosphonates therapy in cancer patients. The ADA cites an ~20% incidence in patients receiving bisphosphonates intravenously for cancer therapy. Fewer than 10% of all cases of bisphosphonate-associated osteonecrosis of the jaw occurs in patients taking the oral drugs.

Information on alendronate (Fosamax®) use in Australia and the incidence of ONJ has been reported (Mavrokokki, 2007). A survey form was sent to all of the Australian members of the Australian and New Zealand Association of Oral and Maxillofacial Surgeons requesting cases that they had identified as ONJ in 2004 and 2005. The definition of ONJ for the survey was an area of exposed bone in the jawbone that failed to heal within 6 weeks in patients taking bisphosphonates for bone disease. The frequency of ONJ in osteoporotic patients, mainly taking weekly oral alendronate, was 1 in 8470 to 1 in 2260 (0.01% to 0.04%) patients. If extractions were carried out, the calculated frequency was 1 in 1130 to 1 in 296 (0.09% to 0.34%) patients. The minimum values in these cases were determined from the survey, whereas, the maximum values were extrapolated from survey data. The median time to onset of ONJ in alendronate patients was 24 months.

A 2010 study reported the prevalence of osteonecrosis of the jaw in patients using alendronate-type drugs was 1 out of 952 patients or ~0.1% (Lo, 2010). The study's protocol involved a survey mailed out to 13,946 members of Kaiser Permanente of Northern California healthcare delivery system; 8572 patients responded to the survey. Investigators identified respondents reporting oral problems and dental symptoms. These respondents were then interviewed by telephone for presence of dental problems including exposed bone, gingival sores, moderate periodontal disease, and persistent symptoms or complications after dental procedures. Those selected were then invited for an examination or to have their dental records reviewed. The diagnosis of ONJ was made according to the 2006 American Association of Oral and Maxillofacial Surgeons criteria which required treatment with a bisphosphonate, exposed bone in the maxillofacial region lasting >8 weeks, and no radiotherapy involving the jaw. Of the 8572 respondents, 9 cases of ONJ were identified; 5 had developed ONJ spontaneously and 4 developed ONJ after tooth extraction. Specific oral bisphosphonates were not identified. When extrapolated to patient-years of bisphosphonate exposure, this prevalence rate of 0.1% equates to a frequency of 28 cases per 100,000 person-years of oral bisphosphonate treatment.

References

American Dental Association Council on Scientific Affairs, "Dental Management of Patients Receiving Oral Bisphosphonate Therapy: Expert Panel Recommendations," *J Am Dent Assoc*, 2006, 137 (8):1144-50. Available at http://jada.ada.org/cgi/content/full/137/8/1144.

Author Unknown, "Safety Update: Bone-Building Drugs: Risks Explained," *Consumer Reports on Health*, 2006, 18(5):3.

Cartsos VM, Zhu S, and Zavras AI, "Bisphosphonate Use and the Risk of Adverse Jaw Outcomes: A Medical Claims Study of 714,217 People," J Am Dent Assoc, 2008, 139(1):23-30.

Edwards BJ, Hellstein JW, Jacobsen PL, et al, "Updated Recommendations for Managing the Care of Patients Receiving Oral Bisphosphonate Therapy: An Advisory Statement From the American Dental Association Council on Scientific Affairs," *J Am Dent Assoc*, 2008, 139(12):1674-7.

Lo JC, O'Ryan FS, Gordon NP, et al, "Prevalence of Osteonecrosis of the Jaw in Patients With Oral Bisphosphonate Exposure," *J Oral Maxillofac Surg*, 2010, 68(2):243-53.

Marx RE, Sawatari Y, Fortin M, et al, "Bisphosphonate-Induced Exposed Bone (Osteonecrosis/Osteopetrosis) of the Jaws: Risk Factors, Recognition, Prevention, and Treatment," *J Oral Maxillofac Surg*, 2005, 63(11):1567-75.

Mavrokokki T, Cheng A, Stein B, et al, "Nature and Frequency of Bisphosphonate-Associated Osteonecrosis of the Jaws in Australia," *J Oral Maxillofac Surg*, 2007, 65(3):415-23.

Alendronate and Cholecalciferol (a LEN droe nate & kole e kal SI fer ole)

Related Information

Alendronate *on page 72*

Cholecalciferol *on page 375*

U.S. Brand Names Fosamax Plus D®

Canadian Brand Names Fosavance

Pharmacologic Category Bisphosphonate Derivative; Vitamin D Analog

Use Treatment of osteoporosis in postmenopausal females; increase bone mass in males with osteoporosis

Local Anesthetic/Vasoconstrictor Precautions No information available to require special precautions

Effects on Dental Treatment Osteonecrosis of the jaw (ONJ), generally associated with local infection and/or tooth extraction and often with delayed healing, has been reported in patients taking bisphosphonates. Symptoms included nonhealing extraction socket or an exposed jawbone. Most reported cases of bisphosphonate-associated osteonecrosis have been in cancer patients treated with intravenous bisphosphonates. However, some have occurred in patients with postmenopausal osteoporosis taking oral bisphosphonates. Dental surgery, particularly tooth extraction, may increase the risk for ONJ. Patients who develop ONJ while on bisphosphonate therapy should receive care by an oral surgeon. See Dental Comment.

Effects on Bleeding No information available to require special precautions

Adverse Effects See individual agents.

General Dosage Range Oral: *Adults:* One tablet (alendronate 70 mg/cholecalciferol 2800-5600 international units) once weekly

Mechanism of Action See individual agents.

Pregnancy Risk Factor C

Dental Comment See Alendronate monograph.

Alfacalcidol (Al fa CAL ce dol)

Canadian Brand Names One-Alpha®

Pharmacologic Category Vitamin D Analog

Use Management of hypocalcemia, secondary hyperparathyroidism, and osteodystrophy in patients with chronic renal failure

Local Anesthetic/Vasoconstrictor Precautions No information available to require special precautions

Effects on Dental Treatment Key adverse event(s) related to dental treatment: Xerostomia (normal salivary flow resumes upon discontinuation) or abnormal taste.

Effects on Bleeding No information available to require special precautions

Adverse Effects Frequency not defined; as associated with Hypervitaminosis D:

Cardiovascular: Cardiac arrhythmia, hypertension

Central nervous system: Headache, hyperthermia, psychosis (rare), somnolence

Dermatologic: Pruritus

Genitourinary: Nocturia

Endocrine & metabolic: Hypercalcemia, hypercholesterolemia, hyperphosphatemia, libido decreased, polydipsia

Gastrointestinal: Anorexia, constipation, nausea, pancreatitis, taste abnormal, vomiting, weight loss, xerostomia

Hepatic: ALT increased, AST increased

Neuromuscular & skeletal: Bone pain, muscle pain, weakness

Ocular: Conjunctivitis, corneal calcification, photophobia

Renal: BUN increased, polyuria

Respiratory: Rhinorrhea

General Dosage Range Individualize dosage:

Oral: *Adults:* 0.25-3 mcg/day

I.V.: *Adults:* 1-12 mcg/week (with dialysis)

Mechanism of Action Alfacalcidol is rapidly converted to the active metabolite of vitamin D (1,25-dihydroxyvitamin D_3) in the liver, effectively bypassing renal metabolic conversion; promotes intestinal absorption of calcium and phosphorous, reabsorption of calcium from the bone, and possibly renal reabsorption of calcium

Pharmacodynamics/Kinetics

Onset of Action 6 hours

Duration of Action Effect on intestinal calcium absorption levels: 1,25-$(OH)_2$ D_3: 48 hours

Half-life Elimination Renal insufficiency: 3 hours

Time to Peak Active vitamin D levels: Oral: 12 hours; I.V.: 4 hours

Product Availability Not available in the U.S.

Alfentanil (al FEN ta nil)

U.S. Brand Names Alfenta®

Canadian Brand Names Alfentanil Injection, USP; Alfenta®

Pharmacologic Category Analgesic, Opioid; Anilidopiperidine Opioid

Use Analgesic adjunct for the induction and maintenance of general anesthesia; analgesic component for monitored anesthesia care (MAC)

Local Anesthetic/Vasoconstrictor Precautions No information available to require special precautions

Effects on Dental Treatment Key adverse event(s) related to dental treatment: Orthostatic hypotension.

Erythromycin inhibits the liver metabolism of alfentanil resulting in increased sedation and prolonged respiratory depression. Clarithromycin may act similarly.

Effects on Bleeding No information available to require special precautions

Adverse Effects

>10%:
- Cardiovascular: Bradycardia, peripheral vasodilation
- Central nervous system: Drowsiness, sedation, intracranial pressure increased
- Gastrointestinal: Nausea, vomiting, constipation
- Endocrine & metabolic: Antidiuretic hormone release
- Ocular: Miosis

1% to 10%:
- Cardiovascular: Cardiac arrhythmia, orthostatic hypotension
- Central nervous system: Confusion, CNS depression
- Ocular: Blurred vision

General Dosage Range I.V.:

Anesthetic induction: *Children ≥12 years and Adults:* Initial: 130-245 mcg/kg; Maintenance: 0.5-1.5 mcg/kg/minute

Continuous infusion: *Children ≥12 years and Adults:* Initial: 50-75 mcg/kg; Maintenance: 0.5-3 mcg/kg/minute

Incremental injection: *Children ≥12 years and Adults:*
- ≤30 minutes anesthesia: Initial: 8-20 mcg/kg; Maintenance: 3-5 mcg/kg **or** 0.5-1 mcg/kg/minute (maximum: 40 mcg/kg total dose)
- ≥30 minutes anesthesia: Initial: 20-50 mcg/kg; Maintenance: 5-15 mcg/kg (maximum: 75 mcg/kg total dose)

Mechanism of Action Binds with stereospecific receptors at many sites within the CNS, increases pain threshold, alters pain perception, inhibits ascending pain pathways; is an ultra short-acting narcotic

Pharmacodynamics/Kinetics

Onset of Action Rapid

Duration of Action Dose dependent: 30-60 minutes

Half-life Elimination Newborns, premature: 5.33-8.75 hours; Children: 40-60 minutes; Adults: 83-97 minutes

Pregnancy Risk Factor C

Controlled Substance C-II

Alfuzosin (al FYOO zoe sin)

U.S. Brand Names Uroxatral®

Canadian Brand Names Apo-Alfuzosin®; Sandoz-Alfuzosin; Xatral

Pharmacologic Category $Alpha_1$ Blocker

Use Treatment of the functional symptoms of benign prostatic hyperplasia (BPH)

Local Anesthetic/Vasoconstrictor Precautions No information available to require special precautions

Effects on Dental Treatment No significant effects or complications reported

Effects on Bleeding No information available to require special precautions

Adverse Effects 1% to 10%:
- Central nervous system: Dizziness (6%), fatigue (3%), headache (3%), pain (1% to 2%)
- Gastrointestinal: Abdominal pain (1% to 2%), constipation (1% to 2%), dyspepsia (1% to 2%), nausea (1% to 2%)
- Genitourinary: Impotence (1% to 2%)
- Respiratory: Upper respiratory tract infection (3%), bronchitis (1% to 2%), pharyngitis (1% to 2%), sinusitis (1% to 2%)

General Dosage Range Oral: *Adults:* 10 mg once daily

Mechanism of Action An antagonist of $alpha_1$-adrenoreceptors in the lower urinary tract. Smooth muscle tone is mediated by the sympathetic nervous stimulation of $alpha_1$-adrenoreceptors, which are abundant in the prostate, prostatic capsule, prostatic urethra, and bladder neck. Blockade of these adrenoreceptors can cause smooth muscles in the bladder neck and prostate to relax, resulting in an improvement in urine flow rate and a reduction in BPH symptoms.

Pharmacodynamics/Kinetics

Half-life Elimination 10 hours

Time to Peak Plasma: 8 hours following a meal

Pregnancy Risk Factor B

Alglucerase (al GLOO ser ase)

U.S. Brand Names Ceredase®
Pharmacologic Category Enzyme
Use Replacement therapy for Gaucher's disease (type 1)
Local Anesthetic/Vasoconstrictor Precautions No information available to require special precautions
Effects on Dental Treatment No significant effects or complications reported
Effects on Bleeding No information available to require special precautions
Adverse Effects Frequency not defined.
Cardiovascular: Peripheral edema
Central nervous system: Chills, fatigue, fever, headache, lightheadedness
Endocrine & metabolic: Hot flashes, menstrual abnormalities
Gastrointestinal: Abdominal discomfort, diarrhea, nausea, oral ulcerations, vomiting
Local: Injection site: Abscess, burning, discomfort, pruritus, swelling
Neuromuscular & skeletal: Backache, weakness
Miscellaneous: Dysosmia; hypersensitivity reactions (abdominal cramping, angioedema, chest discomfort, flushing, hypotension, nausea, pruritus, respiratory symptoms, urticaria); IgG antibody formation (~13%)
General Dosage Range I.V.: *Children and Adults:* Initial: 30-60 units/kg every 2 weeks; Maintenance (range): 2.5 units/kg 3 times/week to 60 units/kg once weekly to every 4 weeks
Mechanism of Action Alglucerase is a modified form of glucocerebrosidase; it is prepared from human placental tissue. Glucocerebrosidase is an enzyme deficient in Gaucher's disease. It is needed to catalyze the hydrolysis of glucocerebroside to glucose and ceramide.
Pharmacodynamics/Kinetics
Half-life Elimination ~3-11 minutes
Pregnancy Risk Factor C

Aliskiren (a lis KYE ren)

Related Information
Cardiovascular Diseases *on page* 1848
U.S. Brand Names Tekturna®
Canadian Brand Names Rasilez®
Pharmacologic Category Renin Inhibitor
Use Treatment of hypertension, alone or in combination with other antihypertensive agents
Unlabeled/Investigational Use Treatment of persistent proteinuria in patients with type 2 diabetes mellitus, hypertension, and nephropathy despite administration of optimized recommended renoprotective therapy (eg, angiotensin II receptor blocker)
Local Anesthetic/Vasoconstrictor Precautions No information available to require special precautions
Effects on Dental Treatment No significant effects or complications required
Effects on Bleeding No information available to require special precautions
Adverse Effects 1% to 10%:
Dermatologic: Rash (1%)
Endocrine & metabolic: Hyperkalemia (monotherapy ≤1%; concurrent with ACE inhibitor in patients with diabetes 6%)
Gastrointestinal: Diarrhea (2%)
Hematologic: Creatine kinase increased (>300%: 1%)
Renal: BUN increased (≤7%), serum creatinine increased (≤7%)
Respiratory: Cough (1%)
General Dosage Range Oral: *Adults:* 150-300 mg once daily (maximum: 300 mg/day)
Mechanism of Action Aliskerin is a direct renin inhibitor, resulting in blockade of the conversion of angiotensinogen to angiotensin I. Angiotensin I suppression decreases the formation of angiotensin II (Ang II), a potent blood pressure-elevating peptide (via direct vasoconstriction, aldosterone release, and sodium retention). Ang II also functions within the Renin-Angiotensin-Aldosterone System (RAAS) as a negative inhibitory feedback mediator within the renal parenchyma to suppress the further release of renin. Thus, reductions in Ang II levels suppress this feedback loop, leading to further increased plasma renin concentrations (PRC) and subsequent activity (PRA). This disinhibition effect can be potentially problematic for ACE inhibitor and ARB therapy, as increased PRA could partially overcome the pharmacologic inhibition of the RAAS. As aliskiren is a direct inhibitor of renin activity, blunting of PRA despite the increased PRC (from loss of the negative feedback) may be clinically advantageous. The effect of aliskiren on bradykinin levels is unknown.

Pharmacodynamics/Kinetics

Onset of Action Maximum antihypertensive effect: Within 2 weeks

Half-life Elimination ~24 hours (range: 16-32 hours)

Time to Peak 1-3 hours

Pregnancy Risk Factor C (1st trimester); D (2nd and 3rd trimesters)

Aliskiren, Amlodipine, and Hydrochlorothiazide

(a lis KYE ren, am LOE di peen, & hye droe klor oh THYE a zide)

Related Information

Aliskiren *on page 78*
AmLODIPine *on page 113*
Hydrochlorothiazide *on page 854*

U.S. Brand Names Amturnide™

Pharmacologic Category Calcium Channel Blocker; Calcium Channel Blocker, Dihydropyridine; Diuretic, Thiazide; Renin Inhibitor

Use Treatment of hypertension (not for initial therapy)

Local Anesthetic/Vasoconstrictor Precautions No information available to require special precautions

Effects on Dental Treatment Key adverse event(s) related to dental treatment: Hydrochlorothiazide: Orthostatic hypotension.

Fewer reports of gingival hyperplasia with amlodipine than with other CCBs (usually resolves upon discontinuation); consultation with physician is suggested.

Effects on Bleeding No information available to require special precautions

Adverse Effects Also see individual agents.

1% to 10%:

- Cardiovascular: Peripheral edema (7%)
- Central nervous system: Dizziness (4%), headache (4%)
- Respiratory: Nasopharyngitis (3%)

General Dosage Range

Oral: *Adults:* Aliskiren 150-300 mg and Amlodipine 5-10 mg and Hydrochlorothiazide 12.5-25 mg once daily (maximum recommended daily dose: Aliskiren 300 mg; amlodipine 10 mg; hydrochlorothiazide 25 mg)

Mechanism of Action

Aliskiren: Direct renin inhibitor, resulting in blockade of the conversion of angiotensinogen to angiotensin I. Angiotensin I suppression decreases the formation of angiotensin II (Ang II), a potent blood pressure-elevating peptide (via direct vasoconstriction, aldosterone release, and sodium retention). Ang II also functions within the Renin-Angiotensin-Aldosterone System (RAAS) as a negative inhibitory feedback mediator within the renal parenchyma to suppress the further release of renin. Thus, reductions in Ang II levels suppress this feedback loop, leading to further increased plasma renin concentrations (PRC) and subsequent activity (PRA). This disinhibition effect can be potentially problematic for ACE inhibitor and ARB therapy, as increased PRA could partially overcome the pharmacologic inhibition of the RAAS. As aliskiren is a direct inhibitor of renin activity, blunting of PRA despite the increased PRC (from loss of the negative feedback) may be clinically advantageous. The effect of aliskiren on bradykinin levels is unknown.

Amlodipine: Inhibits calcium ion from entering the "slow channels" or select voltage-sensitive areas of vascular smooth muscle and myocardium during depolarization, producing a relaxation of coronary vascular smooth muscle and coronary vasodilation; increases myocardial oxygen delivery in patients with vasospastic angina. Amlodipine directly acts on vascular smooth muscle to produce peripheral arterial vasodilation reducing peripheral vascular resistance and blood pressure.

Hydrochlorothiazide: Inhibits sodium reabsorption in the distal tubules causing increased excretion of sodium and water as well as potassium and hydrogen ions.

Pregnancy Risk Factor D

Aliskiren and Amlodipine (a lis KYE ren & am LOE di peen)

Related Information

Aliskiren *on page 78*
AmLODIPine *on page 113*

U.S. Brand Names Tekamlo™

Pharmacologic Category Calcium Channel Blocker; Calcium Channel Blocker, Dihydropyridine; Renin Inhibitor

Use Treatment of hypertension, alone or in combination with other antihypertensive agents, including use as initial therapy in patients likely to need multiple antihypertensives for adequate control

Local Anesthetic/Vasoconstrictor Precautions No information available to require special precautions

Effects on Dental Treatment Fewer reports of gingival hyperplasia with amlodipine than with other calcium channel blockers (usually resolves upon discontinuation); consultation with physician is suggested.

Effects on Bleeding No information available to require special precautions

Adverse Effects Frequencies reported with combination product. See individual monographs for additional adverse effects reported with each agent.

1% to 10%: Cardiovascular: Peripheral edema (6% to 9%)

General Dosage Range Oral: *Adults:* Aliskiren 150-300 mg and amlodipine 5-10 mg once daily (maximum: 300 mg/day [aliskiren]; 10 mg/day [amlodipine])

Mechanism of Action

Aliskiren is a direct renin inhibitor, resulting in blockade of the conversion of angiotensinogen to angiotensin I. Angiotensin I suppression decreases the formation of angiotensin II (Ang II), a potent blood pressure-elevating peptide (via direct vasoconstriction, aldosterone release, and sodium retention).

Amlodipine inhibits calcium ion from entering the "slow channels" or select voltage-sensitive areas of vascular smooth muscle and myocardium during depolarization, producing a relaxation of coronary vascular smooth muscle and coronary vasodilation; increases myocardial oxygen delivery in patients with vasospastic angina. Amlodipine directly acts on vascular smooth muscle to produce peripheral arterial vasodilation reducing peripheral vascular resistance and blood pressure.

Pregnancy Risk Factor D

Aliskiren and Hydrochlorothiazide

(a lis KYE ren & hye droe klor oh THYE a zide)

Related Information

Aliskiren *on page 78*

Hydrochlorothiazide *on page 854*

U.S. Brand Names Tekturna HCT®

Canadian Brand Names Rasilez HCT

Pharmacologic Category Diuretic, Thiazide; Renin Inhibitor

Use Treatment of hypertension, including use as initial therapy in patients likely to need multiple antihypertensives for adequate control

Local Anesthetic/Vasoconstrictor Precautions No information available to require special precautions

Effects on Dental Treatment Key adverse event(s) related to dental treatment: Orthostatic hypotension

Effects on Bleeding No information available to require special precautions

Adverse Effects Frequencies reported with combination product. See individual monographs for additional adverse effects reported with each agent.

>10%: Renal: BUN increased (12%)

1% to 10%:

- Central nervous system: Dizziness (2%), vertigo (1%)
- Endocrine & metabolic: Hypokalemia (2%), uric acid level increased (2%), hyperkalemia (1%)
- Gastrointestinal: Diarrhea (2%)
- Hepatic: ALT increased (1%)
- Neuromuscular & skeletal: Arthralgia (1%), weakness (1%)
- Respiratory: Cough (1%)
- Miscellaneous: Flu-like syndrome (2%)

Note: Angioedema, periorbital edema, and peripheral edema have been reported with aliskiren. Severe dermatologic reactions and pancreatitis have been reported with hydrochlorothiazide.

General Dosage Range Oral: *Adults:* Aliskiren 150-300 mg and hydrochlorothiazide 12.5-25 mg once daily (maximum: 300 mg/day [aliskiren]; 25 mg/day [hydrochlorothiazide])

Mechanism of Action Aliskiren is a direct renin inhibitor, resulting in blockade of the conversion of angiotensinogen to angiotensin I. Angiotensin I suppression decreases the formation of angiotensin II (Ang II), a potent blood pressure-elevating peptide (via direct vasoconstriction, aldosterone release, and sodium retention). Hydrochlorothiazide inhibits sodium reabsorption in the distal tubules causing increased excretion of sodium and water as well as potassium and hydrogen ions.

Pregnancy Risk Factor D

Aliskiren and Valsartan (a lis KYE ren & val SAR tan)

Related Information

Aliskiren *on page 78*

Valsartan *on page 1699*

U.S. Brand Names Valturna®

Pharmacologic Category Angiotensin II Receptor Blocker; Renin Inhibitor

Use Treatment of hypertension, including use as initial therapy in patients likely to need multiple antihypertensives for adequate control

Local Anesthetic/Vasoconstrictor Precautions No information available to require special precautions

Effects on Dental Treatment Key adverse event(s) related to dental treatment: Angioedema has been reported for both aliskiren and valsartan

Effects on Bleeding No information available to require special precautions

Adverse Effects Frequencies reported with combination product. See individual monographs for additional adverse effects reported with each agent.

1% to 10%:

- Central nervous system: Fatigue (3%), vertigo (1%)
- Endocrine & metabolic: Hyperkalemia (4%)
- Respiratory: Nasopharyngitis (3%)
- Miscellaneous: Influenza (1%)

Note: Angioedema, periorbital edema, and peripheral edema have been reported with aliskiren.

General Dosage Range Oral: *Adults:* Aliskiren 150-300 mg and valsartan 160-320 mg once daily (maximum: 300 mg/day [aliskiren]; 320 mg/day [valsartan])

Mechanism of Action

Aliskiren is a direct renin inhibitor, resulting in blockade of the conversion of angiotensinogen to angiotensin I. Angiotensin I suppression decreases the formation of angiotensin II (Ang II), a potent blood pressure-elevating peptide (via direct vasoconstriction, aldosterone release, and sodium retention).

Valsartan produces direct antagonism of the angiotensin II (AT2) receptors, unlike the ACE inhibitors. It displaces angiotensin II from the AT1 receptor and produces its blood pressure-lowering effects by antagonizing AT1-induced vasoconstriction, aldosterone release, catecholamine release, arginine vasopressin release, water intake, and hypertrophic responses. This action results in more efficient blockade of the cardiovascular effects of angiotensin II and fewer side effects than the ACE inhibitors.

Pregnancy Risk Factor D

Alitretinoin (a li TRET i noyn)

U.S. Brand Names Panretin®

Canadian Brand Names Panretin®

Pharmacologic Category Antineoplastic Agent, Miscellaneous; Retinoic Acid Derivative

Use Orphan drug: Topical treatment of cutaneous lesions in AIDS-related Kaposi's sarcoma

Unlabeled/Investigational Use Cutaneous T-cell lymphomas

Local Anesthetic/Vasoconstrictor Precautions No information available to require special precautions

Effects on Dental Treatment No significant effects or complications reported

Effects on Bleeding Although significant myelosuppression with associated altered hemostasis has been reported for many chemotherapeutic agents, myelosuppression is not common with alitretinoin and no specific precautions appear to be necessary.

Adverse Effects

>10%:

- Central nervous system: Pain (0% to 34%)
- Dermatologic: Rash (25% to 77%), pruritus (8% to 11%)
- Neuromuscular & skeletal: Paresthesia (3% to 22%)

5% to 10%:

- Cardiovascular: Edema (3% to 8%)
- Dermatologic: Exfoliative dermatitis (3% to 9%), skin disorder (0% to 8%)

General Dosage Range Topical: *Adults:* Apply twice daily

Mechanism of Action Binds to retinoid receptors to inhibit growth of Kaposi's sarcoma

Pregnancy Risk Factor D

Allopurinol (al oh PURE i nole)

U.S. Brand Names Aloprim®; Zyloprim®
Canadian Brand Names Alloprin®; Apo-Allopurinol®; Novo-Purol; Zyloprim®
Pharmacologic Category Xanthine Oxidase Inhibitor
Use
Oral: Prevention of attack of gouty arthritis and nephropathy; treatment of secondary hyperuricemia which may occur during treatment of tumors or leukemia; prevention of recurrent calcium oxalate calculi
I.V.: Treatment of elevated serum and urinary uric acid levels when oral therapy is not tolerated in patients with leukemia, lymphoma, and solid tumor malignancies who are receiving cancer chemotherapy
Local Anesthetic/Vasoconstrictor Precautions No information available to require special precautions
Effects on Dental Treatment No significant effects or complications reported
Effects on Bleeding No information available to require special precautions
Adverse Effects
Dermatologic: Rash
Endocrine & metabolic: Gout (acute)
Gastrointestinal: Diarrhea, nausea
Hepatic: Alkaline phosphatase increased, liver enzymes increased
General Dosage Range Dosage adjustment recommended in patients with renal impairment
I.V.:
Children ≤10 years: Initial: 200 mg/m^2/day as a single infusion or in equally divided doses at 6-, 8-, or 12-hour intervals
Children >10 years and Adults: 200-400 mg/m^2/day as a single infusion or in equally divided doses at 6-, 8-, or 12-hour intervals (maximum: 600 mg/day)
Oral:
Children <6 years: 150 mg/day in 3 divided doses **or** 10 mg/kg/day in 2-3 divided doses **or** 200-300 mg/m^2/day in 2-4 divided doses (maximum: 800 mg/day)
Children 6-10 years: 10 mg/kg/day **or** 300 mg/day in 2-3 divided doses **or** 200-300 mg/m^2/day in 2-4 divided doses (maximum: 800 mg/day)
Children >10 years and Adults: 100-800 mg/day in 1-3 divided doses (maximum: 800 mg/day)
Elderly: Initial: 100 mg/day
Mechanism of Action Allopurinol inhibits xanthine oxidase, the enzyme responsible for the conversion of hypoxanthine to xanthine to uric acid. Allopurinol is metabolized to oxypurinol which is also an inhibitor of xanthine oxidase; allopurinol acts on purine catabolism, reducing the production of uric acid without disrupting the biosynthesis of vital purines.
Pharmacodynamics/Kinetics
Onset of Action Peak effect: 1-2 weeks
Half-life Elimination
Normal renal function: Parent drug: 1-3 hours; Oxypurinol: 18-30 hours
End-stage renal disease: Prolonged
Time to Peak Plasma: Oral: 30-120 minutes
Pregnancy Risk Factor C

Almotriptan (al moh TRIP tan)

Related Information
Temporomandibular Dysfunction (TMD) *on page 1964*
U.S. Brand Names Axert®
Canadian Brand Names Axert®
Generic Availability (U.S.) No
Pharmacologic Category Antimigraine Agent; Serotonin 5-HT$_{1B, 1D}$ Receptor Agonist
Use Acute treatment of migraine with or without aura in adults (with a history of migraine) and adolescents (with a history of migraine lasting ≥4 hours when left untreated)
Local Anesthetic/Vasoconstrictor Precautions No information available to require special precautions
Effects on Dental Treatment Key adverse effect(s) related to dental treatment: Xerostomia (normal salivary flow resumes upon discontinuation)
Effects on Bleeding No information available to require special precautions

Adverse Effects 1% to 10%:

Central nervous system: Somnolence (≤5%), dizziness (≤4%), headache (≤2%)
Gastrointestinal: Nausea (1% to 3%), vomiting (≤2%), xerostomia (1%)
Neuromuscular & skeletal: Paresthesia (≤1%)

Dosage Oral: Children ≥12 years and Adults: Migraine: Initial: 6.25-12.5 mg in a single dose; if the headache returns, repeat the dose after 2 hours (maximum daily dose: 25 mg)

Note: The safety of treating more than 4 migraines/month has not been established.

Dosage adjustment with concomitant use of an enzyme inhibitor:

Patients receiving a potent CYP3A4 inhibitor: Initial: 6.25 mg in a single dose; maximum daily dose: 12.5 mg

Patients with renal impairment and concomitant use of a potent CYP3A4 inhibitor: Avoid use

Patients with hepatic impairment and concomitant use of a potent CYP3A4 inhibitor: Avoid use

Dosage adjustment in renal impairment: Severe renal impairment (Cl_{cr} ≤30 mL/minute): Initial: 6.25 mg in a single dose; maximum daily dose: 12.5 mg

Dosage adjustment in hepatic impairment: Initial: 6.25 mg in a single dose; maximum daily dose: 12.5 mg

Mechanism of Action Selective agonist for serotonin ($5\text{-}HT_{1B}$ and $5\text{-}HT_{1D}$ receptors) in cranial arteries; causes vasoconstriction and reduces sterile inflammation associated with antidromic neuronal transmission correlating with relief of migraine

Contraindications Hypersensitivity to almotriptan or any component of the formulation; hemiplegic or basilar migraine; known or suspected ischemic heart disease (eg, angina pectoris, MI, documented silent ischemia, coronary artery vasospasm, Prinzmetal's variant angina); cerebrovascular syndromes (eg, stroke, transient ischemic attacks); peripheral vascular disease (eg, ischemic bowel disease); uncontrolled hypertension; use within 24 hours of another $5\text{-}HT_1$ agonist; use within 24 hours of ergotamine derivatives and/or ergotamine-containing medications (eg, dihydroergotamine, ergotamine)

Warnings/Precautions Almotriptan is only indicated for the treatment of acute migraine headache; not indicated for migraine prophylaxis, or the treatment of cluster headaches, hemiplegic migraine, or basilar migraine. If a patient does not respond to the first dose, the diagnosis of acute migraine should be reconsidered.

Almotriptan should not be given to patients with documented ischemic or vasospastic CAD. Patients with risk factors for CAD (eg, hypertension, hypercholesterolemia, smoker, obesity, diabetes, strong family history of CAD, menopause, male >40 years of age) should undergo adequate cardiac evaluation prior to administration; if the cardiac evaluation is "satisfactory," the first dose of almotriptan should be given in the healthcare provider's office. All patients should undergo periodic evaluation of cardiovascular status during treatment. Cardiac events (coronary artery vasospasm, transient ischemia, myocardial infarction, ventricular tachycardia/fibrillation, cardiac arrest, and death), cerebral/subarachnoid hemorrhage, stroke, peripheral vascular ischemia, and colonic ischemia have been reported with $5\text{-}HT_1$ agonist administration. Significant elevation in blood pressure, including hypertensive crisis, has also been reported on rare occasions following $5\text{-}HT_1$ agonist administration in patients with and without a history of hypertension.

Transient and permanent blindness and partial vision loss have been reported (rare) with $5\text{-}HT_1$ agonist administration. Almotriptan contains a sulfonyl group which is structurally different from a sulfonamide. Cross-reactivity in patients with sulfonamide allergy has not been evaluated; however, the manufacturer recommends that caution be exercised in this patient population. Use with caution in liver or renal dysfunction. Symptoms of agitation, confusion, hallucinations, hyper-reflexia, myoclonus, shivering, and tachycardia (serotonin syndrome) may occur with concomitant proserotonergic drugs (ie, SSRIs/SNRIs or triptans) or agents which reduce almotriptan's metabolism. Efficacy has not been demonstrated in improvement of migraine-associated symptoms (eg, phonophobia, nausea, photophobia) in patients aged 12-17 years (Linder, 2008).

Drug Interactions

Metabolism/Transport Effects Substrate (minor) of CYP2D6, 3A4

Avoid Concomitant Use

Avoid concomitant use of Almotriptan with any of the following: Ergot Derivatives; MAO Inhibitors; Sibutramine

Increased Effect/Toxicity

Almotriptan may increase the levels/effects of: Ergot Derivatives; Serotonin Modulators

The levels/effects of Almotriptan may be increased by: CYP3A4 Inhibitors (Strong); Ergot Derivatives; MAO Inhibitors; Sibutramine

Decreased Effect
The levels/effects of Almotriptan may be decreased by: Peginterferon Alfa-2b; Tocilizumab

Dietary Considerations May be taken without regard to meals.

Pharmacodynamics/Kinetics

Half-life Elimination 3-4 hours

Time to Peak Plasma: 1-3 hours

Pregnancy Risk Factor C

Lactation Excretion in breast milk unknown/use caution

Dosage Forms

Tablet, oral:
Axert®: 6.25 mg, 12.5 mg

Alosetron (a LOE se tron)

U.S. Brand Names Lotronex®

Pharmacologic Category Selective 5-HT_3 Receptor Antagonist

Use Treatment of women with severe diarrhea-predominant irritable bowel syndrome (IBS) who have failed to respond to conventional therapy

Local Anesthetic/Vasoconstrictor Precautions No information available to require special precautions

Effects on Dental Treatment No significant effects or complications reported

Effects on Bleeding No information available to require special precautions

Adverse Effects

>10%: Gastrointestinal: Constipation (dose related; 29%)

2% to 10%: Gastrointestinal: Abdominal discomfort and pain (7%), nausea (6%), gastrointestinal discomfort and pain (5%), abdominal distention (2%), hemorrhoids (2%), regurgitation and reflux (2%)

General Dosage Range Oral: *Adults:* Initial: 0.5 mg twice daily; may increase to 1 mg twice daily if needed (maximum: 2 mg/day)

Mechanism of Action Alosetron is a potent and selective antagonist of a subtype of the serotonin 5-HT_3 receptor. 5-HT_3 receptors are ligand-gated ion channels extensively distributed on enteric neurons in the human gastrointestinal tract, as well as other peripheral and central locations. Activation of these channels affect the regulation of visceral pain, colonic transit, and gastrointestinal secretions. In patients with irritable bowel syndrome, blockade of these channels may reduce pain, abdominal discomfort, urgency, and diarrhea.

Pharmacodynamics/Kinetics

Half-life Elimination 1.5 hours for alosetron

Time to Peak 1 hour after oral administration

Pregnancy Risk Factor B

Prescribing and Access Restrictions As a requirement of the REMS program, access to the medication is restricted. Physicians must enroll in the Prometheus Prescribing Program for Lotronex® (www.lotronexppl.com or 1-888-423-5227) in order to prescribe this medication. Program stickers must be affixed to all prescriptions; no phone, fax, or computerized prescriptions are permitted with this program.

Alpha$_1$-Proteinase Inhibitor (al fa won PRO tee in ase in HI bi tor)

U.S. Brand Names Aralast NP; Glassia™; Prolastin®-C; Zemaira®

Canadian Brand Names Prolastin®-C

Pharmacologic Category Antitrypsin Deficiency Agent; Blood Product Derivative

Use Replacement therapy in congenital alpha$_1$-proteinase inhibitor (alpha$_1$-antitrypsin, A_1-PI) deficiency with clinical emphysema

Local Anesthetic/Vasoconstrictor Precautions No information available to require special precautions

Effects on Dental Treatment Key adverse event(s) related to dental treatment: Pharyngitis

Effects on Bleeding No information available to require special precautions

Adverse Effects Frequency not defined. Actual incidence may vary by product.

Cardiovascular: Chest pain, peripheral edema, vasodilation

Central nervous system: Chills, dizziness, fever, headache, lightheadedness, malaise, migraine, pain, somnolence

Dermatologic: Bruising, pruritus, rash

Endocrine & metabolic: Hot flushes

Gastrointestinal: Abdominal pain, bloating, cholangitis, diarrhea, dyspepsia, nausea, sore throat

Genitourinary: Urinary tract infection

Hematologic: Hemorrhage

Hepatic: Transaminases increased
Local: Injection site reactions (including hemorrhage and pain)
Neuromuscular & skeletal: Arthralgia, back pain, musculoskeletal discomfort, paresthesia, weakness
Ocular: Vision changes
Respiratory: Asthma exacerbation, bronchitis, bronchospasm, COPD exacerbation, cough, dyspnea, pharyngitis, respiratory tract infection (lower/upper), rhinitis, sinusitis
Miscellaneous: Flu-like syndrome, infection

General Dosage Range I.V.: *Adults:* 60 mg/kg once weekly

Mechanism of Action Alpha$_1$-antitrypsin (AAT) is the principle protease inhibitor in serum. Its major physiologic role is to render proteolytic enzymes (secreted during inflammation) inactive. A decrease in AAT, as seen in congenital AAT deficiency, leads to increased elastic damage in the lung, causing emphysema.

Pharmacodynamics/Kinetics

Half-life Elimination Metabolic: ~5-6 days

Time to Peak Serum: ~1 hour; threshold levels achieved after 3 weeks

Pregnancy Risk Factor C

ALPRAZolam (al PRAY zoe lam)

Related Information

Management of the Patient With Anxiety or Depression *on page 1968*
Temporomandibular Dysfunction (TMD) *on page 1964*

Related Sample Prescriptions

Sedation (Prior to Dental Treatment) *on page 1995*

U.S. Brand Names Alprazolam Intensol™; Niravam™; Xanax XR®; Xanax®

Canadian Brand Names Alti-Alprazolam; Apo-Alpraz®; Apo-Alpraz® TS; Mylan-Alprazolam; Novo-Alprazol; Nu-Alpraz; Xanax TS™; Xanax®

Generic Availability (U.S.) Yes: Excludes oral solution

Pharmacologic Category Benzodiazepine

Dental Use Preoperative sedation

Use Treatment of anxiety disorder (GAD); panic disorder, with or without agoraphobia; anxiety associated with depression

Unlabeled/Investigational Use Anxiety in children

Local Anesthetic/Vasoconstrictor Precautions No information available to require special precautions

Effects on Dental Treatment Key adverse event(s) related to dental treatment: Significant xerostomia and changes in salivation (normal salivary flow resumes upon discontinuation)

Effects on Bleeding No information available to require special precautions

Adverse Effects

>10%:

Central nervous system: Abnormal coordination, cognitive disorder, depression, drowsiness, fatigue, irritability, lightheadedness, memory impairment, sedation, somnolence
Gastrointestinal: Appetite increased/decreased, constipation, salivation decreased, weight gain/loss, xerostomia
Genitourinary: Micturition difficulty
Neuromuscular & skeletal: Dysarthria

1% to 10%:

Cardiovascular: Hypotension
Central nervous system: Agitation, attention disturbance, confusion, depersonalization, derealization, disorientation, disinhibition, dizziness, dream abnormalities, fear, hallucinations, hypersomnia, nightmares, seizure, talkativeness
Dermatologic: Dermatitis, pruritus, rash
Endocrine & metabolic: Libido decreased/increased, menstrual disorders
Gastrointestinal: Salivation increased
Genitourinary: Incontinence
Hepatic: Bilirubin increased, jaundice, liver enzymes increased
Neuromuscular & skeletal: Arthralgia, ataxia, myalgia, paresthesia
Ocular: Diplopia
Respiratory: Allergic rhinitis, dyspnea

Dental Usual Dosage Preoperative sedation: Adults: Oral: 0.5 mg in evening at bedtime and 0.5 mg 1 hour before procedure

Dosage Oral: **Note:** Treatment >4 months should be re-evaluated to determine the patient's continued need for the drug

Children: Anxiety (unlabeled use): Immediate release: Initial: 0.005 mg/kg/dose or 0.125 mg/dose 3 times/day; increase in increments of 0.125-0.25 mg, up to a maximum of 0.02 mg/kg/dose or 0.06 mg/kg/day (0.375-3 mg/day). See "Dose Reduction" comment.

Adults:

Anxiety: Immediate release: Effective doses are 0.5-4 mg/day in divided doses; the manufacturer recommends starting at 0.25-0.5 mg 3 times/day; titrate dose upward; usual maximum: 4 mg/day. Patients requiring doses >4 mg/day should be increased cautiously. Periodic reassessment and consideration of dosage reduction is recommended.

Anxiety associated with depression: Immediate release: Average dose required: 2.5-3 mg/day in divided doses

Ethanol withdrawal (unlabeled use): Immediate release: Usual dose: 2-2.5 mg/day in divided doses

Panic disorder:

Immediate release: Initial: 0.5 mg 3 times/day; dose may be increased every 3-4 days in increments ≤1 mg/day. Mean effective dosage: 5-6 mg/day; many patients obtain relief at 2 mg/day, as much as 10 mg/day may be required

Extended release: 0.5-1 mg once daily; may increase dose every 3-4 days in increments ≤1 mg/day (range: 3-6 mg/day)

Switching from immediate release to extended release: Patients may be switched to extended release tablets by taking the total daily dose of the immediate release tablets and giving it once daily using the extended release preparation.

Preoperative sedation: 0.5 mg in evening at bedtime and 0.5 mg 1 hour before procedure

Dose reduction: Abrupt discontinuation should be avoided. Daily dose may be decreased by 0.5 mg every 3 days, however, some patients may require a slower reduction. If withdrawal symptoms occur, resume previous dose and discontinue on a less rapid schedule.

Elderly: Initial: 0.125-0.25 mg twice daily; increase by 0.125 mg/day as needed. The smallest effective dose should be used. **Note:** Elderly patients may be more sensitive to the effects of alprazolam including ataxia and oversedation. The elderly may also have impaired renal function leading to decreased clearance. Titrate gradually, if needed.

Immediate release: Initial: 0.25 mg 2-3 times/day

Extended release: Initial: 0.5 mg once daily

Dosing adjustment in renal impairment: No guidelines for adjustment; use caution

Dosing adjustment in hepatic impairment: Reduce dose by 50% to 60% or avoid in cirrhosis

Mechanism of Action Binds to stereospecific benzodiazepine receptors on the postsynaptic GABA neuron at several sites within the central nervous system, including the limbic system, reticular formation. Enhancement of the inhibitory effect of GABA on neuronal excitability results by increased neuronal membrane permeability to chloride ions. This shift in chloride ions results in hyperpolarization (a less excitable state) and stabilization.

Contraindications Hypersensitivity to alprazolam or any component of the formulation (cross-sensitivity with other benzodiazepines may exist); narrow-angle glaucoma; concurrent use with ketoconazole or itraconazole; pregnancy

Warnings/Precautions Rebound or withdrawal symptoms, including seizures, may occur 18 hours to 3 days following abrupt discontinuation or large decreases in dose (more common in patients receiving >4 mg/day or prolonged treatment). Breakthrough anxiety may occur at the end of dosing interval. Use with caution in patients receiving concurrent CYP3A4 inhibitors. Use with caution in renal impairment or predisposition to urate nephropathy. Use with caution in elderly or debilitated patients, patients with hepatic disease (including alcoholics), renal impairment, or obese patients.

Causes CNS depression (dose related) which may impair physical and mental capabilities. Patients must be cautioned about performing tasks that require mental alertness (eg, operating machinery or driving). Effects with other sedative drugs or ethanol may be potentiated. Benzodiazepines have been associated with falls and traumatic injury and should be used with extreme caution in patients who are at risk of these events. Due to increased sensitivity in the elderly, smaller doses of benzodiazepines may be safer and as effective. Avoid using doses >2 mg daily of alprazolam (Beers Criteria). Use with caution in patients with respiratory disease or impaired gag reflex.

Use caution in patients with depression, particularly if suicidal risk may be present. Episodes of mania or hypomania have occurred in depressed patients treated with alprazolam. May cause physical or psychological dependence. Acute withdrawal may be precipitated in patients after administration of flumazenil.

Benzodiazepines have been associated with anterograde amnesia. Paradoxical reactions have been reported with benzodiazepines, particularly in adolescent/pediatric or psychiatric patients. Does not have analgesic, antidepressant, or antipsychotic properties.

Drug Interactions

Metabolism/Transport Effects Substrate of CYP3A4 (major)

Avoid Concomitant Use

Avoid concomitant use of ALPRAZolam with any of the following: Indinavir; OLANZapine

Increased Effect/Toxicity

ALPRAZolam may increase the levels/effects of: Alcohol (Ethyl); CloZAPine; CNS Depressants; Methotrimeprazine

The levels/effects of ALPRAZolam may be increased by: Antifungal Agents (Azole Derivatives, Systemic); Aprepitant; Calcium Channel Blockers (Nondihydropyridine); Cimetidine; Conivaptan; Contraceptives (Estrogens); Contraceptives (Progestins); CYP3A4 Inhibitors (Moderate); CYP3A4 Inhibitors (Strong); Dasatinib; Droperidol; Fluconazole; Fosaprepitant; Grapefruit Juice; Indinavir; Isoniazid; Macrolide Antibiotics; Methotrimeprazine; Nefazodone; OLANZapine; Protease Inhibitors; Proton Pump Inhibitors; Selective Serotonin Reuptake Inhibitors

Decreased Effect

The levels/effects of ALPRAZolam may be decreased by: CarBAMazepine; CYP3A4 Inducers (Strong); Deferasirox; Rifamycin Derivatives; St Johns Wort; Theophylline Derivatives; Tocilizumab; Yohimbine

Ethanol/Nutrition/Herb Interactions

Cigarette smoking: May decrease alprazolam concentrations up to 50%.

Ethanol: May increase CNS depression; monitor for increased effects with coadministration. Caution patients about effects.

Food: Alprazolam serum concentration is unlikely to be increased by grapefruit juice because of alprazolam's high oral bioavailability. The C_{max} of the extended release formulation is increased by 25% when a high-fat meal is given 2 hours before dosing. T_{max} is decreased 30% when food is given immediately prior to dose. T_{max} is increased by 30% when food is given ≥1 hour after dose.

Herb/Nutraceutical: St John's wort may decrease alprazolam levels. Avoid valerian, St John's wort, kava kava, gotu kola (may increase CNS depression).

Dietary Considerations Extended release tablet should be taken once daily in the morning.

Pharmacodynamics/Kinetics

Onset of Action Immediate release and extended release formulations: 1 hour

Duration of Action Immediate release: 5.1 ± 1.7 hours; Extended release: 11.3 ± 4.2 hours

Half-life Elimination

Adults (healthy): 11.2 hours (immediate release range: 6.3-26.9 hours; extended release range: 10.7-15.8 hours)

Elderly: 16.3 hours (range: 9-26.9 hours)

Alcoholic liver disease: 19.7 hours (range: 5.8-65.3 hours)

Obesity: 21.8 hours (range: 9.9-40.4 hours)

Time to Peak Immediate release: 1-2 hours; Extended release: ~9 hours; decreased by 1 hour following bedtime dosing compared to morning dosing

Pregnancy Risk Factor D

Lactation Enters breast milk/not recommended (AAP rates "of concern"; AAP 2001 update pending)

Breast-Feeding Considerations In a study of eight postpartum women, peak concentrations of alprazolam were found in breast milk ~1 hour after the maternal dose and the half-life was ~14 hours. Samples were obtained over 36 hours following a single oral dose of alprazolam 0.5 mg. Metabolites were not detected in breast milk. In this study, the estimated exposure to the breast-feeding infant was ~3% of the weight-adjusted maternal dose. Drowsiness, lethargy, or weight loss in nursing infants have been observed in case reports following maternal use of some benzodiazepines.

Controlled Substance C-IV

Dosage Forms

Solution, oral:

Alprazolam Intensol™: 1 mg/mL (30 mL)

Tablet, oral: 0.25 mg, 0.5 mg, 1 mg, 2 mg

Xanax®: 0.25 mg, 0.5 mg, 1 mg, 2 mg

Tablet, extended release, oral: 0.5 mg, 1 mg, 2 mg, 3 mg
Xanax XR®: 0.5 mg, 1 mg, 2 mg, 3 mg
Tablet, orally disintegrating, oral: 0.25 mg, 0.5 mg, 1 mg, 2 mg
Niravam™: 0.25 mg, 0.5 mg, 1 mg, 2 mg

Alprostadil (al PROS ta dill)

U.S. Brand Names Caverject Impulse®; Caverject®; Edex®; Muse®; Prostin VR Pediatric®

Canadian Brand Names Caverject®; Muse® Pellet; Prostin® VR

Pharmacologic Category Prostaglandin; Vasodilator

Use

Prostin VR Pediatric®: Temporary maintenance of patency of ductus arteriosus in neonates with ductal-dependent congenital heart disease until surgery can be performed. These defects include cyanotic (eg, pulmonary atresia, pulmonary stenosis, tricuspid atresia, Fallot's tetralogy, transposition of the great vessels) and acyanotic (eg, interruption of aortic arch, coarctation of aorta, hypoplastic left ventricle) heart disease.

Caverject®: Treatment of erectile dysfunction of vasculogenic, psychogenic, or neurogenic etiology; adjunct in the diagnosis of erectile dysfunction

Edex®, Muse®: Treatment of erectile dysfunction of vasculogenic, psychogenic, or neurogenic etiology

Unlabeled/Investigational Use Investigational: Treatment of pulmonary hypertension in infants and children with congenital heart defects with left-to-right shunts

Local Anesthetic/Vasoconstrictor Precautions No information available to require special precautions

Effects on Dental Treatment No significant effects or complications reported

Effects on Bleeding No information available to require special precautions

Adverse Effects

Intraurethral:

>10%: Genitourinary: Penile pain, urethral burning

2% to 10%:

Central nervous system: Headache, dizziness, pain

Genitourinary: Vaginal itching (female partner), testicular pain, urethral bleeding (minor)

Intracavernosal injection:

>10%: Genitourinary: Penile pain

1% to 10%:

Cardiovascular: Hypertension

Central nervous system: Headache, dizziness

Genitourinary: Prolonged erection (>4 hours, 4%), penile fibrosis, penis disorder, penile rash, penile edema

Local: Injection site hematoma and/or bruising

Intravenous:

>10%:

Cardiovascular: Flushing

Central nervous system: Fever

Respiratory: Apnea

1% to 10%:

Cardiovascular: Bradycardia, hyper-/hypotension, tachycardia, cardiac arrest, edema

Central nervous system: Seizure, headache, dizziness

Endocrine & metabolic: Hypokalemia

Gastrointestinal: Diarrhea

Hematologic: Disseminated intravascular coagulation

Neuromuscular & skeletal: Back pain

Respiratory: Upper respiratory infection, flu syndrome, sinusitis, nasal congestion, cough

Miscellaneous: Sepsis, localized pain in structures other than the injection site

General Dosage Range

I.V.: *Neonates:* Initial: 0.05-0.1 mcg/kg/minute; Maintenance: 0.01-0.4 mcg/kg/minute

Intracavernous: *Adults:* Initial: 1.25-2.5 mcg; Maintenance: Increase to effective dose no more than 3 times/week with at least 24 hours between doses (maximum: 40 mcg/dose [Edex®]; 60 mcg/dose [Caverject®])

Intraurethral: *Adults:* Initial: 125-250 mcg; Maintenance: As needed (maximum: 2 doses/day)

Mechanism of Action Causes vasodilation by means of direct effect on vascular and ductus arteriosus smooth muscle; relaxes trabecular smooth muscle by dilation of cavernosal arteries when injected along the penile shaft, allowing blood flow to and entrapment in the lacunar spaces of the penis (ie, corporeal veno-occlusive mechanism)

Pharmacodynamics/Kinetics

Onset of Action Rapid

Duration of Action <1 hour

Half-life Elimination 5-10 minutes

Pregnancy Risk Factor X/C (Muse®)

Alteplase (AL te plase)

Related Information

Cardiovascular Diseases *on page 1848*

U.S. Brand Names Activase®; Cathflo® Activase®

Canadian Brand Names Activase® rt-PA; Cathflo® Activase®

Pharmacologic Category Thrombolytic Agent

Use Management of ST-elevation myocardial infarction (STEMI) for the lysis of thrombi in coronary arteries; management of acute ischemic stroke (AIS); management of acute pulmonary embolism (PE)

Recommended criteria for treatment:

STEMI: Chest pain ≥20 minutes duration, onset of chest pain within 12 hours of treatment (or within prior 12-24 hours in patients with continuing ischemic symptoms), and ST-segment elevation >0.1 mV in at least two contiguous precordial leads or two adjacent limb leads on ECG or new or presumably new left bundle branch block (LBBB)

AIS: Onset of stroke symptoms within 3 hours of treatment

Acute pulmonary embolism: Age ≤75 years: Documented massive PE (defined as acute PE with sustained hypotension [SBP <90 mm Hg for ≤15 minutes or requiring inotropic support], persistent profound bradycardia [HR <40 bpm with signs or symptoms of shock], or pulselessness); alteplase may be considered for submassive PE with clinical evidence of adverse prognosis (eg, new hemodynamic instability, worsening respiratory insufficiency, severe RV dysfunction, or major myocardial necrosis) and low risk of bleeding complications. **Note:** Not recommended for patients with low-risk PE (eg, normotensive, no RV dysfunction, normal biomarkers) or submassive acute PE with minor RV dysfunction, minor myocardial necrosis, and no clinical worsening (Jaff, 2011).

Cathflo® Activase®: Restoration of central venous catheter function

Unlabeled/Investigational Use Acute ischemic stroke presenting 3-4.5 hours after symptom onset; acute peripheral arterial occlusive disease

Local Anesthetic/Vasoconstrictor Precautions No information available to require special precautions

Effects on Dental Treatment Key adverse event(s) related to dental treatment: As with all drugs which may affect hemostasis, bleeding is the major adverse effect associated with alteplase. Hemorrhage may occur at virtually any site; risk is dependent on multiple variables, including the dosage administered, concurrent use of multiple agents which alter hemostasis, and patient predisposition. Rapid lysis of coronary artery thrombi by thrombolytic agents may be associated with reperfusion-related atrial and/or ventricular arrhythmias. See Effects on Bleeding.

Effects on Bleeding Bleeding is the major adverse effect associated with alteplase. It is unlikely that ambulatory patients presenting for dental treatment will be taking intravenous anticoagulant therapy.

Adverse Effects As with all drugs which may affect hemostasis, bleeding is the major adverse effect associated with alteplase. Hemorrhage may occur at virtually any site. Risk is dependent on multiple variables, including the dosage administered, concurrent use of multiple agents which alter hemostasis, and patient predisposition. Rapid lysis of coronary artery thrombi by thrombolytic agents may be associated with reperfusion-related atrial and/or ventricular arrhythmia. **Note:** Lowest rate of bleeding complications expected with dose used to restore catheter function.

1% to 10%:

Cardiovascular: Hypotension

Central nervous system: Fever

Dermatologic: Bruising (1%)

Gastrointestinal: GI hemorrhage (5%), nausea, vomiting

Genitourinary: GU hemorrhage (4%)

Hematologic: Bleeding (0.5% major, 7% minor: GUSTO trial)

Local: Bleeding at catheter puncture site (15.3%, accelerated administration)

Additional cardiovascular events associated **with use in STEMI:** AV block, cardiogenic shock, heart failure, cardiac arrest, recurrent ischemia/infarction, myocardial rupture, electromechanical dissociation, pericardial effusion, pericarditis, mitral regurgitation, cardiac tamponade, thromboembolism, pulmonary edema, asystole, ventricular tachycardia, bradycardia, ruptured intracranial AV malformation, seizure, hemorrhagic bursitis, cholesterol crystal embolization

Additional events associated **with use in pulmonary embolism:** Pulmonary re-embolization, pulmonary edema, pleural effusion, thromboembolism

Additional events associated **with use in stroke:** Cerebral edema, cerebral herniation, seizure, new ischemic stroke

General Dosage Range

Intracatheter:

Children <30 kg: 110% of the internal lumen volume of the catheter; retain in catheter for 0.5-2 hours; may repeat once (maximum: 2 mg/2 mL/dose)

Children ≥30 kg and Adults: 2 mg (2 mL) retain in catheter for 0.5-2 hours; may repeat once

I.V. infusion: *Adults:* Dosage varies greatly depending on indication

Mechanism of Action Initiates local fibrinolysis by binding to fibrin in a thrombus (clot) and converts entrapped plasminogen to plasmin

Pharmacodynamics/Kinetics

Duration of Action >50% present in plasma cleared ~5 minutes after infusion terminated, ~80% cleared within 10 minutes

Pregnancy Risk Factor C

Altretamine (al TRET a meen)

U.S. Brand Names Hexalen®

Canadian Brand Names Hexalen®

Pharmacologic Category Antineoplastic Agent, Miscellaneous

Use Palliative treatment of persistent or recurrent ovarian cancer

Local Anesthetic/Vasoconstrictor Precautions No information available to require special precautions

Effects on Dental Treatment No significant effects or complications reported

Effects on Bleeding Chemotherapy may result in significant myelosuppression, potentially including significant reduction in platelet counts and altered hemostasis. In patients who are under active treatment with these agents, medical consult is suggested.

Adverse Effects

>10%:

Central nervous system: Peripheral sensory neuropathy (31%; moderate-to-severe 9%), neurotoxicity (21%; may be progressive and dose limiting)

Gastrointestinal: Nausea/vomiting (33% to 70%; severe 1%), diarrhea (48%)

Hematologic: Anemia (33%), leukopenia (5% to 15%; grade 4: 1%), neutropenia

1% to 10%:

Central nervous system: Fatigue (1%), seizure (1%)

Gastrointestinal: Stomach cramps, anorexia (1%)

Hematologic: Thrombocytopenia (9%)

Hepatic: Alkaline phosphatase increased (9%)

General Dosage Range Dosage adjustment recommended in patients who develop toxicities

Oral: *Adults:* 260 mg/m^2/day in 4 divided doses for 14 or 21 days of a 28-day cycle

Mechanism of Action Although altretamine's clinical antitumor spectrum resembles that of alkylating agents, the drug has demonstrated activity in alkylator-resistant patients. The drug selectively inhibits the incorporation of radioactive thymidine and uridine into DNA and RNA, inhibiting DNA and RNA synthesis; reactive intermediates covalently bind to microsomal proteins and DNA; can spontaneously degrade to demethylated melamines and formaldehyde which are also cytotoxic.

Pharmacodynamics/Kinetics

Half-life Elimination 13 hours

Time to Peak Plasma: 0.5-3 hours

Pregnancy Risk Factor D

Aluminum Chloride (a LOO mi num KLOR ide)

Related Information

Antiplatelet and Anticoagulation Considerations in Dentistry *on page 1867*

U.S. Brand Names Hemodent™

Generic Availability (U.S.) No

Pharmacologic Category Astringent; Hemostatic Agent

Dental Use Hemostatic; gingival retraction; to control bleeding created during a dental procedure

Use Hemostatic

Local Anesthetic/Vasoconstrictor Precautions No information available to require special precautions

Effects on Dental Treatment No significant effects or complications reported

Effects on Bleeding No information available to require special precautions

Adverse Effects No data reported.

Dental Usual Dosage Control of dental bleeding: Apply retraction cord as directed

Dosage Control of bleeding: Apply retraction cord as directed

Mechanism of Action Precipitates tissue and blood proteins causing a mechanical obstruction to hemorrhage from injured blood vessels

Contraindications No data reported

Warnings/Precautions Since large amounts of astringents may cause tissue irritation and possible damage, only small amounts should be applied.

Drug Interactions

Avoid Concomitant Use There are no known interactions where it is recommended to avoid concomitant use.

Increased Effect/Toxicity There are no known significant interactions involving an increase in effect.

Decreased Effect There are no known significant interactions involving a decrease in effect.

Dosage Forms

Cord, oral, topical:

Hemodent™: 21% (7 ft)

Liquid, oral, topical:

Hemodent™: 21% (10 mL, 20 mL, 40 mL)

Aluminum Hydroxide (a LOO mi num hye DROKS ide)

U.S. Brand Names ALternaGel® [OTC]; Dermagran® [OTC]

Canadian Brand Names Amphojel®; Basaljel®

Pharmacologic Category Antacid; Antidote; Protectant, Topical

Use Treatment of hyperacidity; hyperphosphatemia; temporary protection of minor cuts, scrapes, and burns

Local Anesthetic/Vasoconstrictor Precautions No information available to require special precautions

Effects on Dental Treatment Key adverse event(s) related to dental treatment: Chalky taste. Aluminum and magnesium ions prevent GI absorption of tetracycline by forming a large ionized chelated molecule with the aluminum ion and tetracyclines in the stomach. Aluminum hydroxide prevents GI absorption of ketoconazole and itraconazole by increasing the pH in the GI tract. Any of these drugs should be administered at least 1 hour before $Al(OH)_3$.

Effects on Bleeding No information available to require special precautions

Adverse Effects Frequency not defined.

Gastrointestinal: Constipation, discoloration of feces (white speckles), fecal impaction, nausea, stomach cramps, vomiting

Endocrine & metabolic: Hypomagnesemia, hypophosphatemia

General Dosage Range

Oral:

Children: 50-150 mg/kg/day in divided doses every 4-6 hours

Adults: 300-1200 mg 3-4 times/day

Topical: *Children and Adults:* Apply to affected area as needed; reapply at least every 12 hours

Mechanism of Action Neutralizes hydrochloride in stomach to form $Al(Cl)_3$ salt + H_2O

Pregnancy Risk Factor C

Aluminum Hydroxide and Magnesium Carbonate

(a LOO mi num hye DROKS ide & mag NEE zhum KAR bun nate)

Related Information

Aluminum Hydroxide *on page 91*

U.S. Brand Names Acid Gone Extra Strength [OTC]; Acid Gone [OTC]; Gaviscon® Extra Strength [OTC]; Gaviscon® Liquid [OTC]; Genaton™ [OTC]

Pharmacologic Category Antacid

Use Temporary relief of symptoms associated with gastric acidity

Local Anesthetic/Vasoconstrictor Precautions No information available to require special precautions

Effects on Dental Treatment Key adverse event(s) related to dental treatment: Chalky taste. Aluminum and magnesium ions prevent GI absorption of tetracycline by forming a large ionized chelated molecule with the tetracyclines in the stomach. Aluminum hydroxide prevents GI absorption of ketoconazole and itraconazole by increasing the pH in the GI tract. Any of these drugs should be administered at least 1 hour before aluminum hydroxide.

Effects on Bleeding No information available to require special precautions

Adverse Effects 1% to 10%:

Endocrine & metabolic: Hypermagnesemia, aluminum intoxication (prolonged use and concomitant renal failure), hypophosphatemia

Gastrointestinal: Constipation, diarrhea

Neuromuscular & skeletal: Osteomalacia

General Dosage Range Oral: *Adults:* 15-30 mL **or** 2-4 tablets 4 times/day

Aluminum Hydroxide and Magnesium Hydroxide

(a LOO mi num hye DROKS ide & mag NEE zhum hye DROK side)

Related Information

Aluminum Hydroxide *on page 91*

Magnesium Hydroxide *on page 1049*

U.S. Brand Names Alamag [OTC]; Mag-Al Ultimate [OTC]; Mag-Al [OTC]

Canadian Brand Names Diovol®; Diovol® Ex; Gelusil® Extra Strength; Mylanta™

Pharmacologic Category Antacid

Use Antacid for symptoms related to hyperacidity associated with heartburn, hiatal hernia, upset stomach, peptic ulcer, peptic esophagitis, or gastritis

Local Anesthetic/Vasoconstrictor Precautions No information available to require special precautions

Effects on Dental Treatment Key adverse event(s) related to dental treatment: Chalky taste. Aluminum and magnesium ions prevent GI absorption of tetracycline by forming a large ionized chelated molecule with the tetracyclines in the stomach. Aluminum hydroxide prevents GI absorption of ketoconazole and itraconazole by increasing the pH in the GI tract. Any of these drugs should be administered at least 1 hour before aluminum hydroxide.

Effects on Bleeding No information available to require special precautions

Adverse Effects Frequency not defined.

Gastrointestinal: Constipation, chalky taste, cramping, fecal discoloration (white speckles), fecal impaction, nausea, vomiting

Endocrine & metabolic: Hypophosphatemia (rare), hypermagnesemia (rare)

General Dosage Range Oral: *Children ≥12 years and Adults:* 10-20 mL 4 times/day (maximum: magnesium hydroxide 4500 mg/day; aluminum hydroxide 4500 mg/day) **or** 1-2 tablets as needed (maximum: 16 tablets)

Aluminum Hydroxide and Magnesium Trisilicate

(a LOO mi num hye DROKS ide & mag NEE zhum trye SIL i kate)

Related Information

Aluminum Hydroxide *on page 91*

U.S. Brand Names Gaviscon® Tablet [OTC]

Pharmacologic Category Antacid

Use Temporary relief of hyperacidity

Local Anesthetic/Vasoconstrictor Precautions No information available to require special precautions

Effects on Dental Treatment Key adverse event(s) related to dental treatment: Chalky taste. Aluminum and magnesium ions prevent GI absorption of tetracycline by forming a large ionized chelated molecule with the tetracyclines in the stomach. Aluminum hydroxide prevents GI absorption of ketoconazole and itraconazole by increasing the pH in the GI tract. Any of these drugs should be administered at least 1 hour before aluminum hydroxide.

Effects on Bleeding No information available to require special precautions

General Dosage Range Oral: *Adults:* 2-4 tablets 4 times/day

Pregnancy Risk Factor C

Aluminum Hydroxide, Magnesium Hydroxide, and Simethicone

(a LOO mi num hye DROKS ide, mag NEE zhum hye DROKS ide, & sye METH i kone)

Related Information

Aluminum Hydroxide *on page 91*
Magnesium Hydroxide *on page 1049*
Management of Patients Undergoing Cancer Therapy *on page 1970*
Simethicone *on page 1527*

U.S. Brand Names Alamag Plus [OTC]; Aldroxicon I [OTC]; Aldroxicon II [OTC]; Almacone Double Strength® [OTC]; Almacone® [OTC]; Gelusil® [OTC]; Maalox® Advanced Maximum Strength [OTC]; Maalox® Advanced Regular Strength [OTC]; Mi-Acid Maximum Strength [OTC] [DSC]; Mi-Acid [OTC]; Mintox Plus [OTC]; Mylanta® Classic Maximum Strength Liquid [OTC]; Mylanta® Classic Regular Strength Liquid [OTC]; Rulox [OTC]

Canadian Brand Names Diovol Plus®; Gelusil®; Mylanta® Double Strength; Mylanta® Extra Strength; Mylanta® Regular Strength

Pharmacologic Category Antacid; Antiflatulent

Use Temporary relief of hyperacidity associated with gas; may also be used for indications associated with other antacids

Local Anesthetic/Vasoconstrictor Precautions No information available to require special precautions

Effects on Dental Treatment Key adverse event(s) related to dental treatment: Chalky taste. Aluminum and magnesium ions prevent GI absorption of tetracycline by forming a large ionized chelated molecule with the tetracyclines in the stomach. Aluminum hydroxide prevents GI absorption of ketoconazole and itraconazole by increasing the pH in the GI tract. Any of these drugs should be administered at least 1 hour before aluminum hydroxide.

Effects on Bleeding No information available to require special precautions

Adverse Effects

>10%: Gastrointestinal: Chalky taste, stomach cramps, constipation, bowel motility decreased, fecal impaction, hemorrhoids

1% to 10%: Gastrointestinal: Nausea, vomiting, discoloration of feces (white speckles)

General Dosage Range Oral: *Adults:* 10-20 mL or 2-4 tablets 4-6 times/day

Pregnancy Risk Factor C

Aluminum Sulfate and Calcium Acetate

(a LOO mi num SUL fate & KAL see um AS e tate)

Related Information

Calcium Acetate *on page 285*

U.S. Brand Names Domeboro® [OTC]; Gordon Boro-Packs [OTC]; Pedi-Boro® [OTC]

Pharmacologic Category Topical Skin Product

Use Astringent wet dressing for relief of inflammatory conditions of the skin; reduce weeping that may occur in dermatitis

Local Anesthetic/Vasoconstrictor Precautions No information available to require special precautions

Effects on Dental Treatment No significant effects or complications reported

Effects on Bleeding No information available to require special precautions

General Dosage Range Topical: *Adults:* Soak affected area or wet dressing in the solution 2-4 times/day

Alvimopan (al VI moe pan)

U.S. Brand Names Entereg®

Pharmacologic Category Gastrointestinal Agent, Miscellaneous; Opioid Antagonist, Peripherally-Acting

Use Accelerate the time to upper and lower GI recovery following partial large or small bowel resection surgery with primary anastomosis

Local Anesthetic/Vasoconstrictor Precautions No information available to require special precautions

Effects on Dental Treatment No significant effects or complications reported

Effects on Bleeding No information available to require special precautions

Adverse Effects 1% to 10%: **Note:** Incidence reported limited to bowel resection patients only.

Endocrine & metabolic: Hypokalemia (10%)
Gastrointestinal: Dyspepsia (7%)
Genitourinary: Urinary retention (3%)
Hematologic: Anemia (5%)
Neuromuscular & skeletal: Back pain (3%)

General Dosage Range Oral: *Adults:* Initial: 12 mg prior to surgery; Maintenance: 12 mg twice daily (maximum: 15 doses)

Mechanism of Action An opioid receptor antagonist which blocks opioid binding at the mu receptor; alvimopan has restricted ability to cross the blood-brain barrier at therapeutic doses. It selectively and competitively binds to the GI tract mu opioid receptors and antagonizes the peripheral effects of opioids on gastrointestinal motility and secretion. Does not affect opioid analgesic effects or induce opioid withdrawal symptoms.

Pharmacodynamics/Kinetics

Half-life Elimination 10-17 hours

Time to Peak Plasma: Parent drug: ~2 hours; Metabolite: 36 hours

Pregnancy Risk Factor B

Prescribing and Access Restrictions As a requirement of the REMS program, access to this medication is restricted. Only hospitals enrolled in the ENTEREG Access Support and Education (E.A.S.E.™) Program may administer this medication. Hospital staff must be educated on the need to limit to short-term (no more than 15 doses) and inpatient use. Hospitals may contact the E.A.S.E.™ program at 1-866-423-6567 (1-866-4ADOLOR).

Amantadine (a MAN ta deen)

Related Information

Respiratory Diseases *on page 1876*
Systemic Viral Diseases *on page 1904*

Canadian Brand Names Endantadine®; Mylan-Amantadine; PMS-Amantadine; Symmetrel®

Pharmacologic Category Anti-Parkinson's Agent, Dopamine Agonist; Antiviral Agent; Antiviral Agent, Adamantane

Use Prophylaxis and treatment of influenza A viral infection (per manufacturer labeling; also refer to current ACIP guidelines for recommendations during current flu season); treatment of parkinsonism; treatment of drug-induced extrapyramidal symptoms

Local Anesthetic/Vasoconstrictor Precautions No information available to require special precautions

Effects on Dental Treatment Key adverse event(s) related to dental treatment: Xerostomia (prolonged use may cause significant xerostomia; normal salivary flow resumes upon discontinuation) and orthostatic hypotension.

Effects on Bleeding No information available to require special precautions

Adverse Effects 1% to 10%:

Cardiovascular: Orthostatic hypotension, peripheral edema
Central nervous system: Agitation, anxiety, ataxia, confusion, delirium, depression, dizziness, dream abnormality, fatigue, hallucinations, headache, insomnia, irritability, lightheadedness, nervousness, somnolence
Dermatologic: Livedo reticularis
Gastrointestinal: Anorexia, constipation, diarrhea, nausea, xerostomia
Respiratory: Dry nose

General Dosage Range Dosage adjustment recommended in patients with renal impairment

Oral:

Children 1-9 years: 4.4-8.8 mg/kg/day in 2 divided doses (maximum: 150 mg/day)
Children ≥10 years and <40 kg: 5 mg/kg/day in 2 divided doses
Children ≥10 years and ≥40 kg: 100 mg twice daily (maximum: 200 mg/day)
Adults: 200-400 mg/day in 2 divided doses (maximum: 400 mg/day)
Elderly: 100-400 mg/day in 2 divided doses (maximum: 400 mg/day)

Mechanism of Action As an antiviral, blocks the uncoating of influenza A virus preventing penetration of virus into host; antiparkinsonian activity may be due to its blocking the reuptake of dopamine into presynaptic neurons or by increasing dopamine release from presynaptic fibers

Pharmacodynamics/Kinetics

Onset of Action Antidyskinetic: Within 48 hours

Half-life Elimination Normal renal function: 16 ± 6 hours (9-31 hours); Healthy, older (≥60 years) males: 29 hours (range: 20-41 hours); End-stage renal disease: 7-10 days

Time to Peak Plasma: 2-4 hours

Pregnancy Risk Factor C

Ambenonium (am be NOE nee um)

U.S. Brand Names Mytelase®

Canadian Brand Names Mytelase®

Pharmacologic Category Cholinergic Agonist

Use Treatment of myasthenia gravis

Local Anesthetic/Vasoconstrictor Precautions No information available to require special precautions

Effects on Dental Treatment No significant effects or complications reported

Effects on Bleeding No information available to require special precautions

Adverse Effects Frequency not defined.

Cardiovascular: Arrhythmias (especially bradycardia), hypotension, carbon monoxide decreased, tachycardia, AV block, nodal rhythm, ECG changes (nonspecific), cardiac arrest, syncope, flushing

Central nervous system: Convulsions, dysarthria, dysphonia, dizziness, loss of consciousness, drowsiness, headache

Dermatologic: Skin rash, thrombophlebitis (I.V.), urticaria

Gastrointestinal: Hyperperistalsis, nausea, vomiting, salivation, diarrhea, stomach cramps, dysphagia, flatulence

Genitourinary: Urinary urgency

Neuromuscular & skeletal: Weakness, fasciculations, muscle cramps, spasms, arthralgia

Ocular: Small pupils, lacrimation

Respiratory: Bronchial secretions increased, laryngospasm, bronchiolar constriction, respiratory muscle paralysis, dyspnea, respiratory depression, respiratory arrest, bronchospasm

Miscellaneous: Diaphoresis increased, anaphylaxis, allergic reactions

General Dosage Range Oral: *Adults:* 5-25 mg 3-4 times/day

Pregnancy Risk Factor C

Ambrisentan (am bri SEN tan)

U.S. Brand Names Letairis®

Canadian Brand Names Volibris®

Pharmacologic Category Endothelin Antagonist; Vasodilator

Use Treatment of pulmonary artery hypertension (PAH) World Health Organization (WHO) Group I to improve exercise ability and decrease the rate of clinical deterioration

Local Anesthetic/Vasoconstrictor Precautions No information available to require special precautions

Effects on Dental Treatment Key adverse event(s) related to dental treatment: Endothelin antagonists have caused bleeding gums; there have been no specific reports for ambrisentan

Effects on Bleeding No information available to require special precautions

Adverse Effects

>10%:

Cardiovascular: Peripheral edema (17%)

Central nervous system: Headache (15%)

1% to 10%:

Cardiovascular: Palpitation (5%), flushing (4%)

Gastrointestinal: Constipation (4%), abdominal pain (3%)

Hematologic: Hemoglobin decreased (7% to 10%)

Respiratory: Nasal congestion (6%), dyspnea (4%), nasopharyngitis (3%), sinusitis (3%)

General Dosage Range Dosage adjustment recommended in patients on concomitant therapy.

Oral: *Adults:* Initial: 5 mg once daily (maximum: 10 mg/day)

Mechanism of Action Blocks endothelin receptor subtypes ET_A and ET_B on vascular endothelium and smooth muscle. Stimulation of ET_A receptors, located primarily in pulmonary vascular smooth muscle cells is associated with vasoconstriction and cellular proliferation. Stimulation of ET_B receptors, located in both pulmonary vascular endothelial cells and smooth muscle cells is associated with vasodilation, antiproliferative effects, and endothelin clearance. Although ambrisentan blocks both ET_A and ETB receptors, the affinity is greater for the ET_A receptor (>4000 fold higher affinity).

Pharmacodynamics/Kinetics

Half-life Elimination ~9 hours

Time to Peak ~2 hours

Pregnancy Risk Factor X

Prescribing and Access Restrictions As a requirement of the REMS program, access to this medication is restricted. Ambrisentan (Letairis®) is only available through Letairis Education and Access Program (LEAP). Only prescribers and pharmacies registered with LEAP may prescribe and dispense ambrisentan. Further information may be obtained from the manufacturer, Gilead Sciences, Inc (1-866-664-5327).

Amcinonide (am SIN oh nide)

Canadian Brand Names Amcort®; Cyclocort®; ratio-Amcinonide; Taro-Amcinonide

Pharmacologic Category Corticosteroid, Topical

Use Relief of the inflammatory and pruritic manifestations of corticosteroid-responsive dermatoses (high potency corticosteroid)

Local Anesthetic/Vasoconstrictor Precautions No information available to require special precautions

Effects on Dental Treatment No significant effects or complications reported

Effects on Bleeding No information available to require special precautions

Adverse Effects Frequency not defined.

Dermatologic: Acne, hypopigmentation, allergic dermatitis, maceration of the skin, miliaria, skin atrophy, striae, telangiectasia

Endocrine & metabolic: Cushing's syndrome, growth retardation (long-term use), HPA suppression, hyperglycemia; these reactions occur more frequently with occlusive dressings

Local: Burning, dryness, folliculitis, hypertrichosis, itching, irritation

Miscellaneous: Secondary infection

General Dosage Range Topical: *Adults:* Apply in a thin film 2-3 times/day

Mechanism of Action Stimulates the synthesis of enzymes needed to decrease inflammation, suppress mitotic activity, and cause vasoconstriction

Pregnancy Risk Factor C

Amifostine (am i FOS teen)

U.S. Brand Names Ethyol®

Canadian Brand Names Ethyol®

Pharmacologic Category Adjuvant, Chemoprotective Agent (Cytoprotective); Antidote

Use Reduce the incidence of moderate-to-severe xerostomia in patients undergoing postoperative radiation treatment for head and neck cancer, where the radiation port includes a substantial portion of the parotid glands; reduce the cumulative renal toxicity associated with repeated administration of cisplatin

Unlabeled/Investigational Use Prevention of radiation proctitis in patients with rectal cancer

Local Anesthetic/Vasoconstrictor Precautions No information available to require special precautions

Effects on Dental Treatment No significant effects or complications reported

Effects on Bleeding Although significant myelosuppression with associated altered hemostasis has been reported for many chemotherapeutic agents, myelosuppression is not significant with amifostine and no specific precautions appear to be necessary.

Adverse Effects

>10%:

Cardiovascular: Hypotension (15% to 61%; grades 3/4: 3% to 8%; dose dependent)

Gastrointestinal: Nausea/vomiting (53% to 96%; grades 3/4: 8% to 30%; dose dependent)

1% to 10%: Endocrine & metabolic: Hypocalcemia (clinically significant: 1%)

General Dosage Range I.V.: *Adults:* 910 mg/m^2 once daily 30 minutes prior to cytotoxic therapy **or** 200 mg/m^2/day 15-30 minutes prior to radiation therapy

Mechanism of Action Prodrug that is dephosphorylated by alkaline phosphatase in tissues to a pharmacologically-active free thiol metabolite. The free thiol is available to bind to, and detoxify, reactive metabolites of cisplatin; and can also act as a scavenger of free radicals that may be generated (by cisplatin or radiation therapy) in tissues.

Pharmacodynamics/Kinetics

Half-life Elimination ~8-9 minutes

Pregnancy Risk Factor C

Amikacin (am i KAY sin)

Canadian Brand Names Amikacin Sulfate Injection, USP; Amikin®

Pharmacologic Category Antibiotic, Aminoglycoside

Use Treatment of serious infections (bone infections, respiratory tract infections, endocarditis, and septicemia) due to organisms resistant to gentamicin and tobramycin, including *Pseudomonas*, *Proteus*, *Serratia*, and other gram-negative bacilli; documented infection of mycobacterial organisms susceptible to amikacin

Unlabeled/Investigational Use Bacterial endophthalmitis

Local Anesthetic/Vasoconstrictor Precautions No information available to require special precautions

Effects on Dental Treatment No significant effects or complications reported

Effects on Bleeding No information available to require special precautions

Adverse Effects 1% to 10%:

Central nervous system: Neurotoxicity

Otic: Ototoxicity (auditory), ototoxicity (vestibular)

Renal: Nephrotoxicity

General Dosage Range Dosage adjustment recommended in patients with renal impairment

I.M.: *Infants, Children, and Adults:* 5-7.5 mg/kg/dose every 8 hours (maximum: 20 mg/kg/day)

I.V.:

Infants and Children: 5-7.5 mg/kg/dose every 8 hours (maximum: 20 mg/kg/day)

Adults: 5-7.5 mg/kg/dose every 8 hours **or** 15-20 mg/kg as a single daily dose (maximum: 20 mg/kg/day)

Mechanism of Action Inhibits protein synthesis in susceptible bacteria by binding to 30S ribosomal subunits

Pharmacodynamics/Kinetics

Half-life Elimination Renal function and age dependent:

Infants: Low birth weight (1-3 days): 7-9 hours; Full-term >7 days: 4-5 hours

Children: 1.6-2.5 hours

Adults: Normal renal function: 1.4-2.3 hours; Anuria/end-stage renal disease: 28-86 hours

Time to Peak Serum: I.M.: 45-120 minutes

Pregnancy Risk Factor D

AMILoride (a MIL oh ride)

Related Information

Cardiovascular Diseases *on page 1848*

Canadian Brand Names Apo-Amiloride®; Midamor

Pharmacologic Category Diuretic, Potassium-Sparing

Use Counteracts potassium loss induced by other diuretics in the treatment of hypertension or edematous conditions including CHF, hepatic cirrhosis, and hypoaldosteronism; usually used in conjunction with more potent diuretics such as thiazides or loop diuretics

Unlabeled/Investigational Use Investigational: Cystic fibrosis; reduction of lithium-induced polyuria; pediatric hypertension

Local Anesthetic/Vasoconstrictor Precautions No information available to require special precautions

Effects on Dental Treatment No significant effects or complications reported

Effects on Bleeding No information available to require special precautions

Adverse Effects 1% to 10%:

Central nervous system: Headache, fatigue, dizziness

Endocrine & metabolic: Hyperkalemia (up to 10%; risk reduced in patients receiving kaliuretic diuretics), hyperchloremic metabolic acidosis, dehydration, hyponatremia, gynecomastia

Gastrointestinal: Nausea, diarrhea, vomiting, abdominal pain, gas pain, appetite changes, constipation

Genitourinary: Impotence

Neuromuscular & skeletal: Muscle cramps, weakness
Respiratory: Cough, dyspnea

General Dosage Range Dosage adjustment recommended in patients with renal impairment

Oral:

Adults: 5-10 mg/day in 1-2 divided doses (maximum: 20 mg/day)
Elderly: Initial: 5 mg once daily or every other day

Mechanism of Action Inhibits sodium reabsorption in the distal tubule, cortical collecting tubule, and collecting duct subsequently reducing both potassium and hydrogen excretion resulting in weak natriuretic, diuretic, and antihypertensive activity; increases sodium loss; increases potassium retention; decreases calcium excretion; decreases magnesium loss

Pharmacodynamics/Kinetics

Onset of Action 2 hours
Duration of Action 24 hours
Half-life Elimination Normal renal function: 6-9 hours; End-stage renal disease: 8-144 hours
Time to Peak Serum: 6-10 hours

Pregnancy Risk Factor B

Amiloride and Hydrochlorothiazide
(a MIL oh ride & hye droe klor oh THYE a zide)

Related Information

AMILoride *on page 97*
Hydrochlorothiazide *on page 854*

Canadian Brand Names Ami-Hydro; Apo-Amilzide®; Gen-Amilazide; Moduret; Novamilor; Nu-Amilzide

Pharmacologic Category Diuretic, Combination

Use Potassium-sparing diuretic; antihypertensive

Local Anesthetic/Vasoconstrictor Precautions No information available to require special precautions

Effects on Dental Treatment No significant effects or complications reported

Effects on Bleeding No information available to require special precautions

Adverse Effects See individual agents.

General Dosage Range Dosage adjustment recommended in patients with renal impairment

Oral:

Adults: 1-2 tablets (amiloride 5 mg/HCTZ 50 mg per tablet) once daily (maximum: 2 tablets/day)
Elderly: Initial: 1/2 to 1 tablet/day (maximum: 2 tablets/day)

Pregnancy Risk Factor B

Aminocaproic Acid (a mee noe ka PROE ik AS id)

Related Information

Antiplatelet and Anticoagulation Considerations in Dentistry *on page 1867*

U.S. Brand Names Amicar®

Pharmacologic Category Antifibrinolytic Agent; Antihemophilic Agent; Hemostatic Agent; Lysine Analog

Use To enhance hemostasis when fibrinolysis contributes to bleeding (causes may include cardiac surgery, hematologic disorders, neoplastic disorders, abruption placentae, hepatic cirrhosis, and urinary fibrinolysis)

Unlabeled/Investigational Use Treatment of traumatic hyphema; control bleeding in thrombocytopenia; control oral bleeding in congenital and acquired coagulation disorders; topical treatment (mouth rinse) of bleeding associated with dental procedures in patients on oral anticoagulant therapy; prevention of perioperative bleeding associated with cardiac surgery

Local Anesthetic/Vasoconstrictor Precautions No information available to require special precautions

Effects on Dental Treatment No significant effects or complications reported (see Effects on Bleeding)

Effects on Bleeding General dental procedures and simple restorative procedures are not associated with bleeding; therefore, there is no contraindication to general dental treatment for most patients with bleeding disorders. However, after dental extractions and other dental surgeries including deep scaling, block anesthesia, and large fillings, in patients with hemophilia, antifibrinolytic drugs such as aminocaproic acid are useful in controlling bleeding. A carefully coordinated strategy between the dental and medical team may be required to ensure adequate procedures for hemostasis. As preparation for selected dental procedures aminocaproic acid may be required.

A clinical trial reported that aminocaproic acid or tranexamic acid reduces both recurrent bleeding and the amount of clotting factor replacement therapy required. In adults, the oral dose was 50-60 mg aminocaproic acid per kg every 4 hours until dental sockets were completely healed.

Extemporaneous solutions incorporating 100 mg aminocaproic acid per 5 mL of oral solution have been used as an oral rinse with some success. Use however, must be carefully considered since it may not show efficacy in all patients with either drug-induced or hereditary coagulation problems. Studies are ongoing and commercial products may be available in the future.

Adverse Effects Frequency not defined.

Cardiovascular: Arrhythmia, bradycardia, edema, hypotension, intracranial hypertension, peripheral ischemia, syncope, thrombosis

Central nervous system: Confusion, delirium, dizziness, fatigue, hallucinations, headache, malaise, seizure, stroke

Dermatologic: Rash, pruritus

Gastrointestinal: Abdominal pain, anorexia, cramps, diarrhea, GI irritation, nausea, vomiting

Genitourinary: Dry ejaculation

Hematologic: Agranulocytosis, bleeding time increased, leukopenia, thrombocytopenia

Local: Injection site necrosis, injection site pain, injectionsite reactions

Neuromuscular & skeletal: CPK increased, myalgia, myositis, myopathy, rhabdomyolysis (rare), weakness

Ophthalmic: Vision decreased, watery eyes

Otic: Tinnitus

Renal: BUN increased, intrarenal obstruction (glomerular capillary thrombosis), myoglobinuria (rare), renal failure (rare)

Respiratory: Dyspnea, nasal congestion, pulmonary embolism

Miscellaneous: Allergic reaction, anaphylactoid reaction, anaphylaxis

General Dosage Range

I.V.: *Adults:* Dosage varies greatly depending on indication

Oral: *Adults:* Initial: Loading dose: 4-5 g for first hour; Maintenance: 1 g/hour (or 1.25 g/hour using oral solution) for 8 hours or until bleeding controlled (maximum: 30 g/day)

Mechanism of Action Binds competitively to plasminogen; blocking the binding of plasminogen to fibrin and the subsequent conversion to plasmin, resulting in inhibition of fibrin degradation (fibrinolysis).

Pharmacodynamics/Kinetics

Onset of Action ~1-72 hours

Half-life Elimination ~2 hours

Time to Peak Oral: Within 2 hours

Pregnancy Risk Factor C

Aminolevulinic Acid (a MEE noh lev yoo lin ik AS id)

U.S. Brand Names Levulan® Kerastick®

Canadian Brand Names Levulan® Kerastick®

Pharmacologic Category Photosensitizing Agent, Topical; Topical Skin Product

Use Treatment of minimally to moderately thick actinic keratoses (grade 1 or 2) of the face or scalp; to be used in conjunction with blue light illumination

Unlabeled/Investigational Use Photodynamic treatment of low-risk superficial basal cell skin cancer and low-risk squamous cell skin cancer *in situ* (Bowen's disease)

Local Anesthetic/Vasoconstrictor Precautions No information available to require special precautions

Effects on Dental Treatment Key adverse event(s) related to dental treatment: Bleeding/hemorrhage (limited to application/treatment site).

Effects on Bleeding Bleeding/hemorrhage at application or treatment site.

Adverse Effects Transient stinging, burning, itching, erythema, and edema result from the photosensitizing properties of this agent. Symptoms subside between 1 minute and 24 hours after turning off the blue light illuminator. Severe stinging or burning was reported in at least 50% of patients from at least 1 lesional site during treatment.

>10%: Dermatologic: Stinging or burning (most patients; severe: ≥50%), erythema (99%), scaling/crusted skin (64% to 71%), hyper-/hypopigmentation (22% to 36%), edematous lesions (35%), itching (14% to 25%), erosion (2% to 14%), skin disorder (5% to 12%)

1% to 10%:

Central nervous system: Dysesthesia (≤2%)

Dermatologic: Vesiculation (4% to 5%), skin ulceration (2% to 4%), pustular drug eruption (≤4%)

Hematologic: Bleeding/hemorrhage (2% to 4%)

Local: Wheal/flare (2% to 7%), scabbing (≤2%), tenderness (1% to 2%), edema (≤1%), excoriation (≤1%), local pain (≤1%), oozing (≤1%)

General Dosage Range Topical: *Adults:* Apply to actinic keratoses once; may repeat after 8 weeks

Mechanism of Action Aminolevulinic acid is a metabolic precursor of the photosensitizer protoporphyrin IX (PpIX). Photosensitization following local application of aminolevulinic acid occurs through the metabolic conversion to PpIX. When exposed to light of appropriate wavelength and energy, accumulated PpIX produces a photodynamic reaction resulting in local cytotoxicity. Precancerous and cancerous cells exhibit a higher rate of porphyrin induction compared to normal cells.

Pharmacodynamics/Kinetics

Onset of Action Peak fluorescence intensity of protoporphyrin IX (PpIX): Actinic keratosis: 11 hours ± 1 hour; Perilesional skin: 12 hours ± 1 hour

Half-life Elimination Mean fluorescence clearance half-life of PpIX for lesions: 30 ± 10 hours

Pregnancy Risk Factor C

Aminophylline (am in OFF i lin)

Related Information

Respiratory Diseases *on page 1876*

Theophylline *on page 1619*

Canadian Brand Names Phyllocontin®; Phyllocontin®-350

Pharmacologic Category Theophylline Derivative

Use Treatment of symptoms and reversible airway obstruction due to asthma or other chronic lung diseases (eg, emphysema, chronic bronchitis)

Note: The National Heart, Lung, and Blood Institute Guidelines (2007) do not recommend aminophylline I.V. for the treatment of asthma exacerbations.

Unlabeled/Investigational Use Reversal of adenosine-, dipyridamole-, or regadenoson-induced adverse reactions (eg, angina, hypotension) during nuclear cardiac stress testing

Local Anesthetic/Vasoconstrictor Precautions No information available to require special precautions

Effects on Dental Treatment Prescribe erythromycin products with caution to patients taking theophylline products. Erythromycin will delay the normal metabolic inactivation of theophyllines leading to increased blood levels; this has resulted in nausea, vomiting, and CNS restlessness.

Effects on Bleeding No information available to require special precautions

Adverse Effects Frequency not defined. Adverse events observed at therapeutic serum levels:

Cardiovascular: Flutter, tachycardia

Central nervous system: Behavior alterations (children), headache, insomnia, irritability, restlessness, seizures

Dermatologic: Allergic skin reactions, exfoliative dermatitis

Gastrointestinal: Diarrhea, nausea, vomiting

Neuromuscular & skeletal: Tremor

Renal: Diuresis (transient)

General Dosage Range

I.V.:

Neonates to Adults: Loading dose: 5.7 mg/kg

Neonates ≤24 days: Maintenance: 1.27 mg/kg every 12 hours

Neonates >24 days: Maintenance: 1.9 mg/kg every 12 hours

Children 6 weeks to 1 year: Maintenance: Equivalent theophylline dose: mg/kg/hour = (0.008)(age in weeks) + 0.21

Children 1-9 years: Maintenance: 1.01 mg/kg/hour

Children 9-12 years: Maintenance: 0.89 mg/kg/hour

Adolescents 12-16 years (smokers): Maintenance: 0.89 mg/kg/hour

Adolescents 12-16 years (nonsmokers): Maintenance: 0.63 mg/kg/hour

Adolescents >16 years and Adults ≤60 years (nonsmokers): Maintenance: 0.51 mg/kg/hour (maximum: 900 mg/day)

Adults >60 years (nonsmokers): Maintenance: 0.38 mg/kg/hour (maximum: 400 mg/day)

Oral:

Children 1-15 years and <45 kg (without risk factors for impaired clearance): Initial: 15.2-17.7 mg/kg/day divided every 4-6 hours for 3 days (maximum: 380 mg), then increase to 20.3 mg/kg/day divided every 4-6 hours for 3 days (maximum: 400 mg/day); Maintenance: 25.3 mg/kg/day divided every 4-6 hours (maximum: 760 mg/day)

Children ≥45 kg and Adults: Initial: 380 mg/day divided every 6-8 hours for 3 days, then 507 mg/day divided every 6-8 hours for 3 days; Maintenance: 760 mg/day divided every 6-8 hours

Mechanism of Action Causes bronchodilatation, diuresis, CNS and cardiac stimulation, and gastric acid secretion by blocking phosphodiesterase which increases tissue concentrations of cyclic adenine monophosphate (cAMP) which in turn promote catecholamine stimulation of lipolysis, glycogenolysis, and gluconeogenesis and induce release of epinephrine from adrenal medulla cells

Pharmacodynamics/Kinetics

Half-life Elimination Theophylline: Highly variable and dependent upon age, liver function, cardiac function, lung disease, and smoking history

Premature infants, postnatal age 3-15 days: 30 hours (range: 17-43 hours)

Premature infants, postnatal age 25-57 days: 20 hours (range: 9.4-30.6 hours)

Children 1-4 yrs: 3.4 hours (range: 1.2-5.6 hours); 6-17 years: 3.7 hours (range: 1.5-5.9 hours)

Adults 16-60 years with asthma, nonsmoking, otherwise healthy: 8.7 hours (range: 6.1-12.8 hours)

Time to Peak

Oral: Immediate release tablet: 1-2 hours; Sustained release tablet (Canadian labeling; not available in U.S.): 4-5 hours

I.V.: Within 30 minutes

Pregnancy Risk Factor C

Aminosalicylic Acid (a mee noe sal i SIL ik AS id)

Related Information

Rheumatoid Arthritis, Osteoarthritis, and Osteoporosis *on page 1889*

Tuberculosis *on page 1902*

U.S. Brand Names Paser®

Pharmacologic Category Salicylate

Use Adjunctive treatment of tuberculosis used in combination with other antitubercular agents

Unlabeled/Investigational Use Crohn's disease

Local Anesthetic/Vasoconstrictor Precautions No information available to require special precautions

Effects on Dental Treatment NSAID formulations are known to reversibly decrease platelet aggregation via mechanisms different than observed with aspirin. The dentist should be aware of the potential of abnormal coagulation. Caution should also be exercised in the use of NSAIDs in patients already on anticoagulant therapy with drugs such as warfarin (Coumadin®).

Effects on Bleeding No information available to require special precautions

Adverse Effects Frequency not defined.

Cardiovascular: Pericarditis, vasculitis

Central nervous system: Encephalopathy, fever

Dermatologic: Skin eruptions

Endocrine & metabolic: Goiter (with or without myxedema), hypoglycemia

Gastrointestinal: Abdominal pain, diarrhea, nausea, vomiting

Hematologic: Agranulocytosis, anemia (hemolytic), leukopenia, thrombocytopenia

Hepatic: Hepatitis, jaundice

Ocular: Optic neuritis

Respiratory: Eosinophilic pneumonia

General Dosage Range Dosage adjustment recommended in patients with renal impairment

Oral:

Children: 200-300 mg/kg/day in 3-4 equally divided doses

Adults: 150 mg/kg/day in 2-3 equally divided doses

Mechanism of Action Aminosalicylic acid (PAS) is a highly-specific bacteriostatic agent active against *M. tuberculosis*. Structurally related to para-aminobenzoic acid (PABA) and its mechanism of action is thought to be similar to the sulfonamides, a competitive antagonism with PABA; disrupts plate biosynthesis in sensitive organisms.

Pharmacodynamics/Kinetics
Half-life Elimination Reduced with renal impairment
Time to Peak Serum: 6 hours
Pregnancy Risk Factor C

Amiodarone (a MEE oh da rone)

Related Information
Cardiovascular Diseases *on page 1848*
Clinical Risk Related to Drugs Prolonging QT Interval *on page 1872*
U.S. Brand Names Cordarone®; Pacerone®
Canadian Brand Names Apo-Amiodarone®; Cordarone®; Dom-Amiodarone; Mylan-Amiodarone; Novo-Amiodarone; PHL-Amiodarone; PMS-Amiodarone; PRO-Amiodarone; ratio-Amiodarone; ratio-Amiodarone I.V.; Riva-Amiodarone; Sandoz-Amiodarone; Teva-Amiodarone
Generic Availability (U.S.) Yes
Pharmacologic Category Antiarrhythmic Agent, Class III
Use Management of life-threatening recurrent ventricular fibrillation (VF) or hemodynamically-unstable ventricular tachycardia (VT) refractory to other antiarrhythmic agents or in patients intolerant of other agents used for these conditions
Unlabeled/Investigational Use
Cardiac arrest with persistent ventricular tachycardia (VT) or ventricular fibrillation (VF) if defibrillation, CPR, and vasopressor administration have failed (ACLS/PALS guidelines)
Control of hemodynamically-stable monomorphic VT, polymorphic VT with a normal baseline QT interval, or wide-complex tachycardia of uncertain origin (ACLS/PALS guidelines)
Control of rapid ventricular rate due to accessory pathway conduction in pre-excited atrial arrhythmias (ACLS guidelines)
Control of stable narrow-complex tachycardia (ACLS guidelines)
Heart rate control in patients with atrial fibrillation and heart failure [no accessory pathway] (ACC/AHA/ESC Practice Guidelines)
Paroxysmal supraventricular tachycardia (SVT) (not initial drug of choice)
Prevention of postoperative atrial fibrillation associated with cardiothoracic surgery
Pharmacologic adjunct to ICD therapy to suppress symptomatic ventricular tachyarrhythmias in otherwise optimally-treated patients with heart failure (ACC/AHA/ESC Practice Guidelines)
Pharmacologic conversion of atrial fibrillation to normal sinus rhythm; maintenance of normal sinus rhythm

Local Anesthetic/Vasoconstrictor Precautions Amiodarone is one of the drugs confirmed to prolong the QT interval and is accepted as having a risk of causing torsade de pointes. The risk of drug-induced torsade de pointes is extremely low when a single QT interval prolonging drug is prescribed. In terms of epinephrine, it is not known what effect vasoconstrictors in the local anesthetic regimen will have in patients with a known history of congenital prolonged QT interval or in patients taking any medication that prolongs the QT interval. Until more information is obtained, it is suggested that the clinician consult with the physician prior to the use of a vasoconstrictor in suspected patients, and that the vasoconstrictor (epinephrine, mepivacaine and levonordefrin [Carbocaine® 2% with Neo-Cobefrin®]) be used with caution.
Effects on Dental Treatment Key adverse event(s) related to dental treatment: Oral: Abnormal salivation and taste
Effects on Bleeding No information available to require special precautions
Adverse Effects In a recent meta-analysis, patients taking lower doses of amiodarone (152-330 mg daily for at least 12 months) were more likely to develop thyroid, neurologic, skin, ocular, and bradycardic abnormalities than those taking placebo (Vorperian, 1997). Pulmonary toxicity was similar in both the low dose amiodarone group and in the placebo group but there was a trend towards increased toxicity in the amiodarone group. Gastrointestinal and hepatic events were seen to a similar extent in both the low dose amiodarone group and placebo group. As the frequency of adverse events varies considerably across studies as a function of route and dose, a consolidation of adverse event rates is provided by Goldschlager, 2000.

>10%:
Cardiovascular: Hypotension (I.V. 16%, refractory in rare cases)
Central nervous system (3% to 40%): Abnormal gait/ataxia, dizziness, fatigue, headache, malaise, impaired memory, involuntary movement, insomnia, poor coordination, peripheral neuropathy, sleep disturbances, tremor
Dermatologic: Photosensitivity (10% to 75%)
Endocrine & Metabolic: Hypothyroidism (1% to 22%)
Gastrointestinal: Nausea, vomiting, anorexia, and constipation (10% to 33%)

Hepatic: AST or ALT level >2x normal (15% to 50%)
Ocular: Corneal microdeposits (>90%; causes visual disturbance in <10%)

1% to 10%:

Cardiovascular: CHF (3%), bradycardia (3% to 5%), AV block (5%), conduction abnormalities, SA node dysfunction (1% to 3%), cardiac arrhythmia, flushing, edema. Additional effects associated with I.V. administration include asystole, atrial fibrillation, cardiac arrest, electromechanical dissociation, pulseless electrical activity (PEA), ventricular tachycardia, and cardiogenic shock.
Dermatologic: Slate blue skin discoloration (<10%)
Endocrine & metabolic: Hyperthyroidism (3% to 10%; more common in iodine-deficient regions of the world), libido decreased
Gastrointestinal: Abdominal pain, abnormal salivation, abnormal taste (oral), diarrhea, nausea (I.V.)
Hematologic: Coagulation abnormalities
Hepatic: Hepatitis and cirrhosis (<3%)
Local: Phlebitis (I.V., with concentrations >3 mg/mL)
Ocular: Visual disturbances (2% to 9%), halo vision (<5% occurring especially at night), optic neuritis (1%)
Respiratory: Pulmonary toxicity has been estimated to occur at a frequency between 2% and 7% of patients (some reports indicate a frequency as high as 17%). Toxicity may present as hypersensitivity pneumonitis; pulmonary fibrosis (cough, fever, malaise); pulmonary inflammation; interstitial pneumonitis; or alveolar pneumonitis. ARDS has been reported in up to 2% of patients receiving amiodarone, and postoperatively in patients receiving oral amiodarone.
Miscellaneous: Abnormal smell (oral)

Dosage Note: Lower loading and maintenance doses are preferable in women and all patients with low body weight.

Oral:

Children: Arrhythmias (unlabeled use):

Loading dose: 10-20 mg/kg/day in 1-2 doses for 4-14 days or until adequate control of arrhythmia or prominent adverse effects occur; alternative loading dose in children <1 year: 600-800 mg/1.73 m^2/day in 1-2 divided doses/day

Maintenance dose: Dose may be reduced to 5 mg/kg/day for several weeks (or 200-400 mg/1.73 m^2/day given once daily); if no recurrence of arrhythmia, dose may be further reduced to 2.5 mg/kg/day; maintenance doses may be given 5-7 days/week

Adults:

Ventricular arrhythmias: 800-1600 mg/day in 1-2 doses for 1-3 weeks, then when adequate arrhythmia control is achieved, decrease to 600-800 mg/day in 1-2 doses for 1 month; maintenance: 400 mg/day. Lower doses are recommended for supraventricular arrhythmias.

Atrial fibrillation:

Pharmacologic cardioversion (unlabeled use): ACC/AHA/ESC Practice Guidelines: *Inpatient:* 1.2-1.8 g/day in divided doses until 10 g total, then 200-400 mg/day maintenance. *Outpatient:* 600-800 mg/day in divided doses until 10 g total, then 200-400 mg/day maintenance; although not supported by clinical evidence, a maintenance dose of 100 mg/day is commonly used especially for the elderly or patients with low body mass (Fuster, 2006; Zimetbaum, 2007). **Note:** Other regimens have been described and may be used clinically:

400 mg 3 times/day for 5-7 days, then 400 mg/day for 1 month, then 200 mg/day

or

10 mg/kg/day for 14 days, followed by 300 mg/day for 4 weeks, followed by maintenance dosage of 200 mg/day (Roy, 2000)

Prophylaxis following open heart surgery (unlabeled use): Starting in postop recovery: 400 mg twice daily for up to 7 days. Alternative regimen of amiodarone: 600 mg/day for 7 days prior to surgery, followed by 200 mg/day until hospital discharge, has also been shown to decrease the risk of postoperative atrial fibrillation. **Note:** A variety of regimens have been used in clinical trials.

I.V.:

Children:

Arrhythmias (unlabeled use, dosing based on limited data): Loading dose: 5 mg/kg over 30 minutes; may repeat up to 3 times if no response. Maintenance dose: Continuous infusion: 10-20 mg/kg/day followed by conversion to oral therapy as appropriate

Note: I.V. administration at low flow rates (potentially associated with use in pediatrics) may result in leaching of plasticizers (DEHP) from intravenous tubing. DEHP may adversely affect male reproductive tract development. Alternative means of dosing and administration (1 mg/kg aliquots) may need to be considered.

Pulseless VT or VF (PALS dosing): 5 mg/kg (maximum: 300 mg/dose) rapid I.V. bolus or I.O.; repeat up to a maximum daily dose of 15 mg/kg. (**Note:** Maximum recommended daily dose in adolescents is 2.2 g.)

Perfusing tachycardias (PALS dosing): Loading dose: 5 mg/kg (maximum: 300 mg/dose) I.V. over 20-60 minutes or I.O.; may repeat up to maximum dose of 15 mg/kg/day. (**Note:** Maximum recommended daily dose in adolescents is 2.2 g.)

Adults:

Atrial fibrillation:

Pharmacologic cardioversion (ACC/AHA/ESC Practice Guidelines) (unlabeled use): 5-7 mg/kg over 30-60 minutes, then 1.2-1.8 g/day continuous infusion until 10 g total. Maintenance: See oral dosing.

Prophylaxis following open heart surgery (unlabeled use): Starting at postop recovery, 1000 mg infused over 24 hours for 2 days has been shown to reduce the risk of postoperative atrial fibrillation. **Note:** A variety of regimens have been used in clinical trials.

Pulseless VT or VF (ACLS, 2010): I.V. push, I.O.: Initial: 300 mg; if pulseless VT or VF continues after subsequent defibrillation attempt or recurs, administer supplemental dose of 150 mg. **Note:** *Handbook of Emergency Cardiovascular Care* (AHA, 2005) recommends dilution in 20-30 mL D_5W (ACLS guidelines do not specify); however, in this setting, administering **undiluted** is preferred (Dager, 2006; Skrifvars, 2004). **Note:** Limited experience with I.O. administration of amiodarone (ACLS, 2010).

Upon return of spontaneous circulation, follow with an infusion of 1 mg/minute for 6 hours, then 0.5 mg/minute for 18 hours (mean daily doses >2.1 g/day have been associated with hypotension).

Stable VT or SVT (unlabeled use): First 24 hours: 1050 mg according to following regimen

Step 1: 150 mg (100 mL) over first 10 minutes (mix 3 mL in 100 mL D_5W)

Step 2: 360 mg (200 mL) over next 6 hours (mix 18 mL in 500 mL D_5W): 1 mg/minute

Step 3: 540 mg (300 mL) over next 18 hours: 0.5 mg/minute

Note: After the first 24 hours: 0.5 mg/minute utilizing concentration of 1-6 mg/mL

Breakthrough stable VT or SVT: 150 mg supplemental doses in 100 mL D_5W or NS over 10 minutes (mean daily doses >2.1 g/day have been associated with hypotension)

I.V. to oral therapy conversion: Use the following as a guide:

<1 week I.V. infusion: 800-1600 mg/day

1- to 3-week I.V. infusion: 600-800 mg/day

>3-week I.V. infusion: 400 mg/day

Note: Conversion from I.V. to oral therapy has not been formally evaluated. Some experts recommend a 1-2 day overlap when converting from I.V. to oral therapy especially when treating ventricular arrhythmias.

Recommendations for conversion to intravenous amiodarone after oral administration: During long-term amiodarone therapy (ie, ≥4 months), the mean plasma-elimination half-life of the active metabolite of amiodarone is 61 days. Replacement therapy may not be necessary in such patients if oral therapy is discontinued for a period <2 weeks, since any changes in serum amiodarone concentrations during this period may **not** be clinically significant.

Elderly: No specific guidelines available. Dose selection should be cautious, at low end of dosage range, and titration should be slower to evaluate response. Although not supported by clinical evidence, a maintenance dose of 100 mg/day is commonly used especially for the elderly or patients with low body mass (Fuster, 2006; Zimetbaum, 2007).

Dosing adjustment in renal impairment: No dosage adjustment necessary

Hemodialysis: Not dialyzable (0% to 5%); supplemental dose is not necessary.

Peritoneal dialysis: Not dialyzable (0% to 5%); supplemental dose is not necessary.

Dosing adjustment in hepatic impairment: Dosage adjustment is probably necessary in substantial hepatic impairment. No specific guidelines available. If hepatic enzymes exceed 3 times normal or double in a patient with an elevated baseline, consider decreasing the dose or discontinuing amiodarone.

Mechanism of Action Class III antiarrhythmic agent which inhibits adrenergic stimulation (alpha- and beta-blocking properties), affects sodium, potassium, and calcium channels, prolongs the action potential and refractory period in myocardial tissue; decreases AV conduction and sinus node function

Contraindications Hypersensitivity to amiodarone, iodine, or any component of the formulation; severe sinus-node dysfunction; second- and third-degree heart block (except in patients with a functioning artificial pacemaker); bradycardia causing syncope (except in patients with a functioning artificial pacemaker); cardiogenic shock

Warnings/Precautions **[U.S. Boxed Warning]: Only indicated for patients with life-threatening arrhythmias because of risk of toxicity. Alternative therapies should be tried first before using amiodarone. Patients should be hospitalized when amiodarone is initiated.** Currently, the 2005 ACLS guidelines recommend I.V. amiodarone as the preferred antiarrhythmic for the treatment of pulseless VT/VF, both life-threatening arrhythmias. In patients with non-life-threatening arrhythmias (eg, atrial fibrillation), amiodarone should be used only if the use of other antiarrhythmics has proven ineffective or are contraindicated.

[U.S. Boxed Warning]: Lung damage (abnormal diffusion capacity) may occur without symptoms. Monitor for pulmonary toxicity. Evaluate new respiratory symptoms; pre-existing pulmonary disease does not increase risk of developing pulmonary toxicity, but if pulmonary toxicity develops then the prognosis is worse. The lowest effective dose should be used as appropriate for the acuity/severity of the arrhythmia being treated. **[U.S. Boxed Warning]: Liver toxicity is common, but usually mild with evidence of increased liver enzymes. Severe liver toxicity can occur and has been fatal in a few cases.**

[U.S. Boxed Warning]: Amiodarone can exacerbate arrhythmias, by making them more difficult to tolerate or reverse; other types of arrhythmias have occurred, including significant heart block, sinus bradycardia new ventricular fibrillation, incessant ventricular tachycardia, increased resistance to cardioversion, and polymorphic ventricular tachycardia associated with QT_c prolongation (torsade de pointes [TdP]). Risk may be increased with concomitant use of other antiarrhythmic agents or drugs that prolong the QT_c interval. Proarrhythmic effects may be prolonged.

Monitor pacing or defibrillation thresholds in patients with implantable cardiac devices (eg, pacemakers, defibrillators). Use very cautiously and with close monitoring in patients with thyroid or liver disease. May cause hyper- or hypothyroidism. Hyperthyroidism may result in thyrotoxicosis and may aggravate or cause breakthrough arrhythmias. If any new signs of arrhythmia appear, hyperthyroidism should be considered. Thyroid function should be monitored prior to treatment and periodically thereafter.

May cause optic neuropathy and/or optic neuritis, usually resulting in visual impairment. Corneal microdeposits occur in a majority of patients, and may cause visual disturbances in some patients (blurred vision, halos); these are not generally considered a reason to discontinue treatment. Corneal refractive laser surgery is generally contraindicated in amiodarone users. Avoid excessive exposure to sunlight; may cause photosensitivity.

Amiodarone is a potent inhibitor of CYP enzymes and transport proteins (including p-glycoprotein), which may lead to increased serum concentrations/toxicity of a number of medications. Particular caution must be used when a drug with QT_c-prolonging potential relies on metabolism via these enzymes, since the effect of elevated concentrations may be additive with the effect of amiodarone. Carefully assess risk:benefit of coadministration of other drugs which may prolong QT_c interval. Patients may still be at risk for amiodarone–related drug interactions after the drug has been discontinued. The pharmacokinetics are complex (due to prolonged duration of action and half-life) and difficult to predict. Correct electrolyte disturbances, especially hypokalemia or hypomagnesemia, prior to use and throughout therapy. Use caution when initiating amiodarone in patients on warfarin. Cases of increased INR with or without bleeding have occurred in patients treated with warfarin; monitor INR closely after initiating amiodarone in these patients.

May cause hypotension and bradycardia (infusion-rate related). Caution in surgical patients; may enhance hemodynamic effect of anesthetics; associated with increased risk of adult respiratory distress syndrome (ARDS) postoperatively. May be inappropriate in the elderly due to a risk of QT_c-interval prolongation, torsade de pointes, and lack of efficacy in the elderly (Beers Criteria). Injection contains benzyl alcohol, which has been associated with "gasping syndrome" in neonates. Safety and efficacy of amiodarone in children has not been fully established.

Drug Interactions

Metabolism/Transport Effects **Substrate** of CYP1A2 (minor), CYP2C8 (major at low concentration), CYP2C19 (minor), CYP2D6 (minor), CYP3A4 (major), P-glycoprotein; **Inhibits** CYP1A2 (weak), CYP2A6 (moderate), CYP2B6 (weak), CYP2C9 (moderate), CYP2C19 (weak), CYP2D6 (moderate), CYP3A4 (moderate), P-glycoprotein

Avoid Concomitant Use

Avoid concomitant use of Amiodarone with any of the following: Agalsidase Beta; Artemether; Dronedarone; Grapefruit Juice; Lumefantrine; Nilotinib; Pimozide; Protease Inhibitors; QuiNINE; Silodosin; Tetrabenazine; Thioridazine; Tolvaptan; Topotecan; Toremifene; Vandetanib; Ziprasidone

Increased Effect/Toxicity

Amiodarone may increase the levels/effects of: Antiarrhythmic Agents (Class Ia); Beta-Blockers; Budesonide (Systemic, Oral Inhalation); Cardiac Glycosides; Colchicine; CycloSPORINE; CycloSPORINE (Systemic); CYP2A6 Substrates; CYP2C9 Substrates (High risk); CYP2D6 Substrates; CYP3A4 Substrates; Dabigatran Etexilate; Dronedarone; Eplerenone; Everolimus; FentaNYL; Fesoterodine; Flecainide; Fosphenytoin; HMG-CoA Reductase Inhibitors; Lidocaine; Lidocaine (Systemic); Lidocaine (Topical); Loratadine; Lurasidone; P-Glycoprotein Substrates; Phenytoin; Pimecrolimus; Pimozide; QTc-Prolonging Agents; QuiNINE; Rivaroxaban; Salmeterol; Saxagliptin; Silodosin; Tamoxifen; Tetrabenazine; Thioridazine; Tolvaptan; Topotecan; Toremifene; Vandetanib; Vilazodone; Vitamin K Antagonists; Ziprasidone

The levels/effects of Amiodarone may be increased by: Alfuzosin; Artemether; Azithromycin; Azithromycin (Systemic); Calcium Channel Blockers (Nondihydropyridine); Chloroquine; Cimetidine; Ciprofloxacin; Ciprofloxacin (Systemic); Conivaptan; CYP2C8 Inhibitors (Moderate); CYP2C8 Inhibitors (Strong); CYP3A4 Inhibitors (Moderate); CYP3A4 Inhibitors (Strong); Deferasirox; Eribulin; Fingolimod; Gadobutrol; Grapefruit Juice; Lumefantrine; Nilotinib; P-Glycoprotein Inhibitors; Protease Inhibitors; QuiNINE

Decreased Effect

Amiodarone may decrease the levels/effects of: Agalsidase Beta; Clopidogrel; Codeine; Sodium Iodide I131; TraMADol

The levels/effects of Amiodarone may be decreased by: Bile Acid Sequestrants; CYP2C8 Inducers (Highly Effective); CYP3A4 Inducers (Strong); Deferasirox; Etravirine; Fosphenytoin; Grapefruit Juice; Herbs (CYP3A4 Inducers); Orlistat; Peginterferon Alfa-2b; P-Glycoprotein Inducers; Phenytoin; Rifamycin Derivatives; Tocilizumab

Ethanol/Nutrition/Herb Interactions

Food: Increases the rate and extent of absorption of amiodarone. Grapefruit juice increases bioavailability of oral amiodarone by 50% and decreases the conversion of amiodarone to N-DEA (active metabolite); altered effects are possible; use should be avoided during therapy.

Herb/Nutraceutical: St John's wort may decrease amiodarone levels or enhance photosensitization. Avoid ephedra (may worsen arrhythmia). Avoid dong quai.

Dietary Considerations Take consistently with regard to meals. Amiodarone is a potential source of large amounts of inorganic iodine; ~3 mg of inorganic iodine per 100 mg of amiodarone is released into the systemic circulation. Recommended daily allowance for iodine in adults is 150 mcg.

Grapefruit juice is not recommended.

Pharmacodynamics/Kinetics

Onset of Action Oral: 2 days to 3 weeks; I.V.: May be more rapid; Peak effect: 1 week to 5 months

Duration of Action After discontinuing therapy: 7-50 days

Note: Mean onset of effect and duration after discontinuation may be shorter in children than adults

Half-life Elimination Terminal: 40-55 days (range: 26-107 days); shorter in children

Time to Peak Serum: 3-7 hours

Pregnancy Risk Factor D

Lactation Enters breast milk/not recommended (AAP rates "of concern"; AAP 2001 update pending)

Breast-Feeding Considerations Hypothyroidism may occur in nursing infants. Both amiodarone and its active metabolite are excreted in human milk. Breast-feeding may lead to significant infant exposure and potential toxicity.

Product Availability

Nexterone®: FDA approved January 2009; expected availability first quarter 2011; consult prescribing information for additional information

Nexterone® is an injection formulation that is free of polysorbate 80 and free of benzyl alcohol.

Dosage Forms

Injection, solution: 50 mg/mL (3 mL, 9 mL, 18 mL)

Tablet, oral: 200 mg, 400 mg

Cordarone®: 200 mg

Pacerone®: 100 mg, 200 mg, 400 mg

Dental Comment Amiodarone is known to prolong the QT interval. The QT interval is measured as the time and distance between the Q point of the QRS complex and the end of the T wave in the ECG tracing. After adjustment for heart rate, the QT interval is defined as prolonged if it is more than 450 msec in men and 460 msec in women. A long QT syndrome was first described in the 1950s and 60s as a congenital syndrome involving QT interval prolongation and syncope and sudden death. Some of the congenital long QT syndromes were characterized by a peculiar electrocardiographic appearance of the QRS complex involving a premature atria beat followed by a pause, then a subsequent sinus beat showing marked QT prolongation and deformity. This type of cardiac arrhythmia was originally termed "torsade de pointes" (translated from the French as "twisting of the points"). Amiodarone is considered as having a risk of causing torsade de pointes. Since it is not known what effect vasoconstrictors in the local anesthetic regimen will have in patients with a known history of congenital prolonged QT interval or in patients taking any medication that prolongs the QT interval, a medical consult is suggested.

Amitriptyline (a mee TRIP ti leen)

Related Information

Temporomandibular Dysfunction (TMD) *on page 1964*

Canadian Brand Names Apo-Amitriptyline®; Bio-Amitriptyline; Dom-Amitriptyline; Elavil; Levate®; Novo-Triptyn; PMS-Amitriptyline

Generic Availability (U.S.) Yes

Pharmacologic Category Antidepressant, Tricyclic (Tertiary Amine)

Dental Use Management of chronic neuropathic pain in temporomandibular dysfunction (TMD)

Use Relief of symptoms of depression

Unlabeled/Investigational Use Analgesic for certain chronic and neuropathic pain (including diabetic neuropathy); prophylaxis against migraine headaches; treatment of depressive disorders in children; post-traumatic stress disorder (PTSD)

Local Anesthetic/Vasoconstrictor Precautions Amitriptyline is one of the drugs confirmed to prolong the QT interval and is accepted as having a risk of causing torsade de pointes. In terms of epinephrine, it is not known what effect vasoconstrictors in the local anesthetic regimen will have in patients with a known history of congenital prolonged QT interval or in patients taking any medication that prolongs the QT interval. Until more information is obtained, it is suggested that the clinician consult with the physician prior to the use of a vasoconstrictor in suspected patients, and that the vasoconstrictor (epinephrine, mepivacaine and levonordefrin [Carbocaine® 2% with Neo-Cobefrin®]) be used with caution. See Dental Comment.

Effects on Dental Treatment Key adverse event(s) related to dental treatment: Xerostomia and changes in salivation (normal salivary flow resumes upon discontinuation), orthostatic hypotension, stomatitis, peculiar taste, and black tongue. Amitriptyline is the most anticholinergic and sedating of the antidepressants; has pronounced effects on the cardiovascular system. Long-term treatment with TCAs such as amitriptyline increases the risk of caries by reducing salivation and salivary buffer capacity. In a study by Rundergren, et al, pathological alterations were observed in the oral mucosa of 72% of 58 patients; 55% had new carious lesions after taking TCAs for a median of 5½ years. Current research is investigating the use of the salivary stimulant pilocarpine (Salagen®) to overcome the xerostomia from amitriptyline.

Effects on Bleeding No information available to require special precautions

Adverse Effects Anticholinergic effects may be pronounced; moderate to marked sedation can occur (tolerance to these effects usually occurs).

Frequency not defined.

Cardiovascular: Orthostatic hypotension, tachycardia, ECG changes (nonspecific), AV conduction changes, cardiomyopathy (rare), MI, stroke, heart block, arrhythmia, syncope, hypertension, palpitation

Central nervous system: Restlessness, dizziness, insomnia, sedation, fatigue, anxiety, cognitive function (impaired), seizure, extrapyramidal symptoms, coma, hallucinations, confusion, disorientation, coordination impaired, ataxia, headache, nightmares, hyperpyrexia

Dermatologic: Allergic rash, urticaria, photosensitivity, alopecia

Endocrine & metabolic: Syndrome of inappropriate ADH secretion

Gastrointestinal: Weight gain, xerostomia, constipation, paralytic ileus, nausea, vomiting, anorexia, stomatitis, peculiar taste, diarrhea, black tongue

Genitourinary: Urinary retention

Hematologic: Bone marrow depression, purpura, eosinophilia

Neuromuscular & skeletal: Numbness, paresthesia, peripheral neuropathy, tremor, weakness

Ocular: Blurred vision, mydriasis, ocular pressure increased
Otic: Tinnitus
Miscellaneous: Diaphoresis, withdrawal reactions (nausea, headache, malaise)

Dental Usual Dosage Chronic neuropathic pain in temporomandibular dysfunction (TMD) (unlabeled use): Adults: Oral: Initial: 25 mg at bedtime; may increase as tolerated to 100 mg/day

Dosage

Children:

Chronic pain management (unlabeled use): Oral: Initial: 0.1 mg/kg at bedtime, may advance as tolerated over 2-3 weeks to 0.5-2 mg/kg at bedtime

Depressive disorders (unlabeled use): Oral: Initial doses of 1 mg/kg/day given in 3 divided doses with increases to 1.5 mg/kg/day have been reported in a small number of children (n=9) 9-12 years of age; clinically, doses up to 3 mg/kg/day (5 mg/kg/day if monitored closely) have been proposed

Migraine prophylaxis (unlabeled use): Oral: Initial: 0.25 mg/kg/day, given at bedtime; increase dose by 0.25 mg/kg/day to maximum 1 mg/kg/day. Reported dosing ranges: 0.1-2 mg/kg/day; maximum suggested dose: 10 mg.

Adolescents: Depressive disorders: Oral: Initial: 25-50 mg/day; may administer in divided doses; increase gradually to 100 mg/day in divided doses

Adults:

Depression: Oral: 50-150 mg/day single dose at bedtime or in divided doses; dose may be gradually increased up to 300 mg/day

Chronic pain management (unlabeled use): Oral: Initial: 25 mg at bedtime; may increase as tolerated to 100 mg/day

Diabetic neuropathy (unlabeled use): Oral: 25-100 mg/day (Bril, 2011)

Migraine prophylaxis (unlabeled use): Oral: Initial: 10-25 mg at bedtime; usual dose: 150 mg; reported dosing ranges: 10-400 mg/day

Post-traumatic stress disorder (PTSD) (unlabeled use): Oral: 75-200 mg/day

Elderly: Depression: Oral: Initial: 10-25 mg at bedtime; dose should be increased in 10-25 mg increments every week if tolerated; dose range: 25-150 mg/day

Dosing interval in hepatic impairment: Use with caution and monitor plasma levels and patient response

Hemodialysis: Nondialyzable

Mechanism of Action Increases the synaptic concentration of serotonin and/or norepinephrine in the central nervous system by inhibition of their reuptake by the presynaptic neuronal membrane

Contraindications Hypersensitivity to amitriptyline or any component of the formulation (cross-sensitivity with other tricyclics may occur); use of MAO inhibitors within past 14 days; acute recovery phase following myocardial infarction; concurrent use of cisapride

Warnings/Precautions [U.S. Boxed Warning]: Antidepressants increase the risk of suicidal thinking and behavior in children, adolescents, and young adults (18-24 years of age) with major depressive disorder (MDD) and other psychiatric disorders; consider risk prior to prescribing. Short-term studies did not show an increased risk in patients >24 years of age and showed a decreased risk in patients ≥65 years. Closely monitor for clinical worsening, suicidality, or unusual changes in behavior; the patient's family or caregiver should be instructed to closely observe the patient and communicate condition with healthcare provider. Such observation would generally include at least weekly face-to-face contact with patients or their family members or caregivers during the first 4 weeks of treatment, then every other week visits for the next 4 weeks, then at 12 weeks, and as clinically indicated beyond 12 weeks. Additional contact by telephone may be appropriate between face-to-face visits. Adults treated with antidepressants should be observed similarly for clinical worsening and suicidality, especially during the initial few months of a course of drug therapy, or at times of dose changes, either increases or decreases. A medication guide should be dispensed with each prescription. **Amitriptyline is not FDA-approved for use in children <12 years of age.**

The possibility of a suicide attempt is inherent in major depression and may persist until remission occurs. Monitor for worsening of depression or suicidality, especially during initiation of therapy (generally first 1-2 months) or with dose increases or decreases. Worsening depression and severe abrupt suicidality that are not part of the presenting symptoms may require discontinuation or modification of drug therapy. The patient's family or caregiver should be alerted to monitor patients for the emergence of suicidality and associated behaviors (such as agitation, irritability, hostility, impulsivity, and hypomania) and notify healthcare provider.

May worsen psychosis in some patients or precipitate a shift to mania or hypomania in patients with bipolar disorder. Patients presenting with depressive symptoms should be screened for bipolar disorder. Monotherapy in patients with bipolar disorder should be avoided. **Amitriptyline is not FDA approved for bipolar depression.**

The degree of sedation, anticholinergic effects, orthostasis, and conduction abnormalities are high relative to other antidepressants. Amitriptyline often causes drowsiness/sedation, resulting in impaired performance of tasks requiring alertness (eg, operating machinery or driving). Sedative effects may be additive with other CNS depressants and/or ethanol. Use with caution in patients with a history of cardiovascular disease (including previous MI, stroke, tachycardia, or conduction abnormalities). Use with caution in patients with urinary retention, benign prostatic hyperplasia, narrow-angle glaucoma, xerostomia, visual problems, constipation, or a history of bowel obstruction.

TCAs may rarely cause bone marrow suppression; monitor for any signs of infection and obtain CBC if symptoms (eg, fever, sore throat) evident. May alter glucose control - use with caution in patients with diabetes. Consider discontinuing, when possible, prior to elective surgery. Therapy should not be abruptly discontinued in patients receiving high doses for prolonged periods. May lower seizure threshold - use caution in patients with a previous seizure disorder or condition predisposing to seizures such as brain damage, alcoholism, or concurrent therapy with other drugs which lower the seizure threshold. Hyperpyrexia has been observed with TCAs in combination with anticholinergics and/or neuroleptics, particularly during hot weather. May increase the risks associated with electroconvulsive therapy. Use with caution in hyperthyroid patients or those receiving thyroid supplementation. Use with caution in patients with hepatic or renal dysfunction. Use with caution in the elderly; may be inappropriate in this age group due to its potent anticholinergic and sedative properties (Beers Criteria).

Drug Interactions

Metabolism/Transport Effects Substrate of CYP1A2 (minor), 2B6 (minor), 2C9 (minor), 2C19 (minor), 2D6 (major), 3A4 (minor); **Inhibits** CYP1A2 (weak), 2C9 (weak), 2C19 (weak), 2D6 (weak), 2E1 (weak)

Avoid Concomitant Use

Avoid concomitant use of Amitriptyline with any of the following: Artemether; Cisapride; Dronedarone; Iobenguane I 123; Lumefantrine; MAO Inhibitors; Methylene Blue; Nilotinib; Pimozide; QuiNINE; Sibutramine; Tetrabenazine; Thioridazine; Toremifene; Vandetanib; Ziprasidone

Increased Effect/Toxicity

Amitriptyline may increase the levels/effects of: Alcohol (Ethyl); Alpha-/Beta-Agonists (Direct-Acting); Alpha1-Agonists; Amphetamines; Anticholinergics; Aspirin; Beta2-Agonists; Cisapride; CNS Depressants; Desmopressin; Dronedarone; Methylene Blue; NSAID (COX-2 Inhibitor); NSAID (Nonselective); Pimozide; QTc-Prolonging Agents; QuiNIDine; QuiNINE; Serotonin Modulators; Sulfonylureas; Tetrabenazine; Thioridazine; Toremifene; TraMADol; Vandetanib; Vitamin K Antagonists; Yohimbine; Ziprasidone

The levels/effects of Amitriptyline may be increased by: Abiraterone; Alfuzosin; Altretamine; Artemether; BuPROPion; Chloroquine; Cimetidine; Cinacalcet; Ciprofloxacin; Ciprofloxacin (Systemic); Conivaptan; CYP2D6 Inhibitors (Moderate); CYP2D6 Inhibitors (Strong); Dexmethylphenidate; Divalproex; DULoxetine; Gadobutrol; Lithium; Lumefantrine; MAO Inhibitors; Methylphenidate; Metoclopramide; Nilotinib; Pramlintide; Propoxyphene; Protease Inhibitors; QuiNIDine; QuiNINE; Selective Serotonin Reuptake Inhibitors; Sibutramine; Terbinafine; Terbinafine (Systemic); Valproic Acid

Decreased Effect

Amitriptyline may decrease the levels/effects of: Acetylcholinesterase Inhibitors (Central); Alpha2-Agonists; Iobenguane I 123

The levels/effects of Amitriptyline may be decreased by: Acetylcholinesterase Inhibitors (Central); Barbiturates; CarBAMazepine; Peginterferon Alfa-2b; St Johns Wort; Tocilizumab

Ethanol/Nutrition/Herb Interactions

Ethanol: May increase CNS depression; monitor for increased effects with coadministration. Caution patients about effects.

Food: Grapefruit juice may inhibit the metabolism of some TCAs and clinical toxicity may result.

Herb/Nutraceutical: St John's wort may decrease amitriptyline levels. Avoid valerian, St John's wort, kava kava, gotu kola (may increase CNS depression).

Pharmacodynamics/Kinetics

Onset of Action Migraine prophylaxis: 6 weeks, higher dosage may be required in heavy smokers because of increased metabolism; Depression: 4-6 weeks, reduce dosage to lowest effective level

Half-life Elimination Adults: 9-27 hours (average: 15 hours)

Time to Peak Serum: ~4 hours

Pregnancy Risk Factor C

Lactation Enters breast milk/not recommended (AAP rates "of concern"; AAP 2001 update pending)

Breast-Feeding Considerations Based on information from six mother/infant pairs, following maternal use of amitriptyline 75-175 mg/day, the estimated exposure to the breast-feeding infant would be 0.2% to 1.9% of the weight-adjusted maternal dose. Adverse events have not been reported in nursing infants (four cases). Infants should be monitored for signs of adverse events; routine monitoring of infant serum concentrations is not recommended.

Dosage Forms

Tablet, oral: 10 mg, 25 mg, 50 mg, 75 mg, 100 mg, 150 mg

Dental Comment Amitriptyline is known to prolong the QT interval. The QT interval is measured as the time and distance between the Q point of the QRS complex and the end of the T wave in the ECG tracing. After adjustment for heart rate, the QT interval is defined as prolonged if it is more than 450 msec in men and 460 msec in women. A long QT syndrome was first described in the 1950s and 60s as a congenital syndrome involving QT interval prolongation and syncope and sudden death. Some of the congenital long QT syndromes were characterized by a peculiar electrocardiographic appearance of the QRS complex involving a premature atria beat followed by a pause, then a subsequent sinus beat showing marked QT prolongation and deformity. This type of cardiac arrhythmia was originally termed "torsade de pointes" (translated from the French as "twisting of the points"). Amitriptyline is considered as having a risk of causing torsade de pointes. Since it is not known what effect vasoconstrictors in the local anesthetic regimen will have in patients with a known history of congenital prolonged QT interval or in patients taking any medication that prolongs the QT interval, a medical consult is suggested.

References

Boakes AJ, Laurence DR, Teoh PC, et al, "Interactions Between Sympathomimetic Amines and Antidepressant Agents in Man," *Br Med J*, 1973, 1(849):311-5.

Friedlander AH and Mahler ME, "Major Depressive Disorder. Psychopathology, Medical Management, and Dental Implications," *J Am Dent Assoc*, 2001, 132(5):629-38.

Ganzberg S, "Psychoactive Drugs," *ADA Guide to Dental Therapeutics*, 2nd ed, Chicago, IL: ADA Publishing, a Division of ADA Business Enterprises, Inc, 2000, 376-405.

Jastak JT and Yagiela JA, "Vasoconstrictors and Local Anesthesia: A Review and Rationale for Use," *J Am Dent Assoc*, 1983, 107(4):623-30.

Rundegren J, van Dijken J, Mörnstad H, et al, "Oral Conditions in Patients Receiving Long-Term Treatment With Cyclic Antidepressant Drugs," *Swed Dent J*, 1985, 9(2):55-64.

Yagiela JA, "Adverse Drug Interactions in Dental Practice: Interactions Associated With Vasoconstrictors. Part V of a Series," *J Am Dent Assoc*, 1999, 130(5):701-9.

Amitriptyline and Chlordiazepoxide

(a mee TRIP ti leen & klor dye az e POKS ide)

Related Information

Amitriptyline *on page 107*

ChlordiazePOXIDE *on page 359*

Pharmacologic Category Antidepressant, Tricyclic (Tertiary Amine); Benzodiazepine

Use Treatment of moderate-to-severe anxiety and/or agitation and depression

Local Anesthetic/Vasoconstrictor Precautions Use with caution; epinephrine or mepivacaine and levonordefrin (Carbocaine® 2% with Neo-Cobefrin®) have been shown to have an increased pressor response in combination with TCAs

Effects on Dental Treatment Key adverse event(s) related to dental treatment:

Amitriptyline: Xerostomia and changes in salivation (normal salivary flow resumes upon discontinuation), orthostatic hypotension, stomatitis, peculiar taste, and black tongue. Amitriptyline is the most anticholinergic and sedating of the antidepressants; has pronounced effects on the cardiovascular system. Long-term treatment with TCAs such as amitriptyline increases the risk of caries by reducing salivation and salivary buffer capacity. In a study by Rundergren, et al, pathological alterations were observed in the oral mucosa of 72% of 58 patients; 55% had new carious lesions after taking TCAs for a median of 5½ years. Current research is investigating the use of the salivary stimulant pilocarpine (Salagen®) to overcome the xerostomia from amitriptyline.

Chlordiazepoxide: Over 10% of patients will experience xerostomia which disappears with cessation of drug therapy.

Effects on Bleeding No information available to require special precautions

Adverse Effects See individual agents.

General Dosage Range Oral: *Adults:* 2-6 tablets (amitriptyline 12.5-25 mg/chlordiazepoxide 5-10 mg per tablet)/day (maximum: 6 tablets/day)

Mechanism of Action See individual agents.

Pregnancy Risk Factor D

Controlled Substance C-IV

Amitriptyline and Perphenazine (a mee TRIP ti leen & per FEN a zeen)

Related Information

Amitriptyline *on page 107*

Perphenazine *on page 1331*

Canadian Brand Names Etrafon®

Pharmacologic Category Antidepressant, Tricyclic (Tertiary Amine); Antipsychotic Agent, Typical, Phenothiazine

Use Treatment of patients with moderate-to-severe anxiety and depression

Unlabeled/Investigational Use Depression with psychotic features

Local Anesthetic/Vasoconstrictor Precautions

Amitriptyline: Use with caution; epinephrine or mepivacaine and levonordefrin (Carbocaine® 2% with Neo-Cobefrin®) have been shown to have an increased pressor response in combination with TCAs

Perphenazine: No information available to require special precautions

Effects on Dental Treatment Key adverse event(s) related to dental treatment:

Amitriptyline: Xerostomia and changes in salivation (normal salivary flow resumes upon discontinuation), orthostatic hypotension, stomatitis, peculiar taste, and black tongue. Amitriptyline is the most anticholinergic and sedating of the antidepressants; has pronounced effects on the cardiovascular system. Long-term treatment with TCAs such as amitriptyline increases the risk of caries by reducing salivation and salivary buffer capacity. In a study by Rundergren, et al, pathological alterations were observed in the oral mucosa of 72% of 58 patients; 55% had new carious lesions after taking TCAs for a median of 5$^{1/2}$ years. Current research is investigating the use of the salivary stimulant pilocarpine (Salagen®) to overcome the xerostomia from amitriptyline.

Perphenazine: Extrapyramidal symptoms (pseudoparkinsonism, akathisia, dystonias, tardive dyskinesia), dizziness, seizures, headache, drowsiness, paradoxical excitement, restlessness, and hyperactivity.

Tardive dyskinesia: Prevalence rate may be 40% in elderly; development of the syndrome and the irreversible nature are proportional to duration and total cumulative dose over time. Extrapyramidal reactions are more common in elderly with up to 50% developing these reactions after 60 years of age. Drug-induced Parkinson's syndrome occurs often; akathisia is the most common extrapyramidal reaction in elderly.

Increased confusion, memory loss, psychotic behavior, and agitation frequently occur as a consequence of anticholinergic effects. Antipsychotic associated sedation in nonpsychotic patients is extremely unpleasant due to feelings of depersonalization, derealization, and dysphoria.

Effects on Bleeding No information available to require special precautions

Adverse Effects Frequency not defined.

Based on **amitriptyline** component: Anticholinergic effects may be pronounced; moderate to marked sedation can occur (tolerance to these effects usually occurs).

- Cardiovascular: Orthostatic hypotension, tachycardia, ECG changes (nonspecific), AV conduction changes
- Central nervous system: Restlessness, dizziness, insomnia, sedation, fatigue, anxiety, cognitive function impaired, seizure, extrapyramidal symptoms
- Dermatologic: Allergic rash, urticaria, photosensitivity
- Gastrointestinal: Weight gain, xerostomia, constipation
- Genitourinary: Urinary retention
- Ocular: Blurred vision, mydriasis
- Miscellaneous: Diaphoresis

Based on **perphenazine** component:

- Cardiovascular: Hyper-/hypotension, orthostatic hypotension, tachycardia, bradycardia, dizziness, cardiac arrest
- Central nervous system: Extrapyramidal symptoms (pseudoparkinsonism, akathisia, dystonias, tardive dyskinesia), dizziness, cerebral edema, seizure, headache, drowsiness, paradoxical excitement, restlessness, hyperactivity, insomnia, neuroleptic malignant syndrome (NMS), impairment of temperature regulation
- Dermatologic: Sun sensitivity increased, rash, discoloration of skin (blue-gray)
- Endocrine & metabolic: Hypoglycemia, hyperglycemia, galactorrhea, lactation, breast enlargement, gynecomastia, menstrual irregularity, amenorrhea, SIADH, libido changes
- Gastrointestinal: Constipation, weight gain, vomiting, stomach pain, nausea, xerostomia, salivation, diarrhea, anorexia, ileus
- Genitourinary: Difficulty in urination, ejaculatory disturbances, incontinence, polyuria, ejaculating dysfunction, priapism
- Hematologic: Agranulocytosis, leukopenia, eosinophilia, hemolytic anemia, thrombocytopenic purpura, pancytopenia
- Hepatic: Cholestatic jaundice, hepatotoxicity

Neuromuscular & skeletal: Tremor
Ocular: Pigmentary retinopathy, blurred vision, cornea and lens changes
Respiratory: Nasal congestion
Miscellaneous: Diaphoresis

General Dosage Range Oral: *Adults:* 1 tablet (amitriptyline 10-50 mg/perphenazine 2-4 mg per tablet) 2-4 times/day

Mechanism of Action

Amitriptyline increases the synaptic concentration of serotonin and/or norepinephrine in the central nervous system by inhibition of their reuptake by the presynaptic neuronal membrane.

Perphenazine is a piperazine phenothiazine antipsychotic which blocks postsynaptic mesolimbic dopaminergic receptors in the brain; exhibits alpha-adrenergic blocking effect and depresses the release of hypothalamic and hypophyseal hormones.

Amlexanox (am LEKS an oks)

Related Information

Ulcerative, Erosive, and Painful Oral Mucosal Disorders *on page 1950*

Related Sample Prescriptions

Recurrent Aphthous Stomatitis *on page 1992*

U.S. Brand Names Aphthasol®

Generic Availability (U.S.) No

Pharmacologic Category Anti-inflammatory, Locally Applied

Dental Use Treatment of aphthous ulcers (ie, canker sores)

Use Treatment of aphthous ulcers (ie, canker sores)

Unlabeled/Investigational Use Allergic disorders

Local Anesthetic/Vasoconstrictor Precautions No information available to require special precautions

Effects on Dental Treatment Key adverse event(s) related to dental treatment: Allergic contact dermatitis and oral irritation. Discontinue therapy if rash or contact mucositis develops (see Dental Comment).

Effects on Bleeding No information available to require special precautions

Adverse Effects 1% to 2%:

Dermatologic: Allergic contact dermatitis
Gastrointestinal: Oral irritation

Dosage Topical: Administer ~1/4 inch (0.5 cm) directly on ulcers 4 times/day following oral hygiene, after meals, and at bedtime

Mechanism of Action As a benzopyrano-bipyridine carboxylic acid derivative, amlexanox has anti-inflammatory and antiallergic properties; it inhibits chemical mediatory release of the slow-reacting substance of anaphylaxis (SRS-A) and may have antagonistic effects on interleukin-3

Contraindications Hypersensitivity to amlexanox or any component of the formulation

Warnings/Precautions Discontinue therapy if rash or contact mucositis develops. Safety and efficacy have not been established in children.

Drug Interactions

Avoid Concomitant Use There are no known interactions where it is recommended to avoid concomitant use.

Increased Effect/Toxicity There are no known significant interactions involving an increase in effect.

Decreased Effect There are no known significant interactions involving a decrease in effect.

Pharmacodynamics/Kinetics

Half-life Elimination 3.5 hours

Time to Peak Serum: 2 hours

Pregnancy Risk Factor B

Lactation Excretion in breast milk unknown/use caution

Dosage Forms

Paste, oral:

Aphthasol®: 5% (3 g)

Dental Comment Treatment of canker sores with amlexanox showed a 76% median reduction in ulcer size compared to a 40% reduction with placebo. Greer, et al, reported an overall mean reduction in ulcer size of 1.82 mm^2 for patients treated with 5% amlexanox versus an average reduction of 0.52 mm^2 for the control group. Recent studies in over thousands of patients have confirmed that amlexanox accelerates the resolution of pain and healing of aphthous ulcers more significantly than vehicle and no treatment.

References

Barrons RW, "Treatment Strategies for Recurrent Oral Aphthous Ulcers," *Am J Health Syst Pharm*, 2001, 58(1):41-50.

Binnie WH, Curro FA, Khandwala A, et al, "Amlexanox Oral Paste: A Novel Treatment That Accelerates the Healing of Aphthous Ulcers," *Compend Contin Educ Dent*, 1997, 18(11):1116-8, 1120-2, 1124 passim.

Eisen D and Lynch DP, "Selecting Topical and Systemic Agents for Recurrent Aphthous Stomatitis," *Cutis*, 2001, 68(3):201-6.

Greer RO Jr, Lindenmuth JE, Juarez T, et al, "A Double-Blind Study of Topically Applied 5% Amlexanox in the Treatment of Aphthous Ulcers," *J Oral Maxillofac Surg*, 1993, 51(3):243-8.

Khandwala A, Van Inwegen RG, and Alfano MC, "5% Amlexanox Oral Paste, A New Treatment for Recurrent Minor Aphthous Ulcers: I. Clinical Demonstration of Acceleration of Healing and Resolution of Pain," *Oral Surg Oral Med Oral Pathol Oral Radiol Endod*, 1997, 83(2):222-30.

Khandwala A, Van Inwegen RG, Charney MR, et al, "5% Amlexanox Oral Paste, A New Treatment for Recurrent Minor Aphthous Ulcers: II. Pharmacokinetics and Demonstration of Clinical Safety," *Oral Surg Oral Med Oral Pathol Oral Radiol Endod*, 1997, 83(2):231-8.

AmLODIPine (am LOE di peen)

Related Information

Calcium Channel Blockers and Gingival Hyperplasia *on page 2014*

Cardiovascular Diseases *on page 1848*

U.S. Brand Names Norvasc®

Canadian Brand Names Accel-Amlodipine; Apo-Amlodipine®; CO Amlodipine; Dom-Amlodipine; GD-Amlodipine; JAMP-Amlodipine; Mint-Amlodipine; Mylan-Amlodipine; Norvasc®; PHL-Amlodipine; PMS-Amlodipine; RAN™-Amlodipine; ratio-Amlodipine; Riva-Amlodipine; Sandoz Amlodipine; Septa-Amlodipine; Teva-Amlodipine; ZYM-Amlodipine

Generic Availability (U.S.) Yes

Pharmacologic Category Calcium Channel Blocker; Calcium Channel Blocker, Dihydropyridine

Use Treatment of hypertension; treatment of symptomatic chronic stable angina, vasospastic (Prinzmetal's) angina (confirmed or suspected); prevention of hospitalization due to angina with documented CAD (limited to patients without heart failure or ejection fraction <40%)

Local Anesthetic/Vasoconstrictor Precautions No information available to require special precautions

Effects on Dental Treatment Fewer reports of gingival hyperplasia with amlodipine than with other CCBs (usually resolves upon discontinuation); consultation with physician is suggested.

Effects on Bleeding No information available to require special precautions

Adverse Effects

>10%: Cardiovascular: Peripheral edema (2% to 15% dose related; HF patients: 27% [Packer, 1996])

1% to 10%:

- Cardiovascular: Flushing (1% to 5% dose related), palpitation (1% to 5% dose related)
- Central nervous system: Dizziness (1% to 3% dose related), fatigue (5%), somnolence (1% to 2%)
- Dermatologic: Rash (1% to 2%), pruritus (1% to 2%)
- Endocrine & metabolic: Male sexual dysfunction (1% to 2%)
- Gastrointestinal: Nausea (3%), abdominal pain (1% to 2%), dyspepsia (1% to 2%)
- Neuromuscular & skeletal: Muscle cramps (1% to 2%), weakness (1% to 2%)
- Respiratory: Dyspnea (1% to 2%), pulmonary edema (HF patients: 27% [Packer, 1996])

Dosage Oral:

Children 6-17 years: Hypertension: 2.5-5 mg once daily

Adults:

- Hypertension: Initial dose: 5 mg once daily; maximum dose: 10 mg once daily. In general, titrate in 2.5 mg increments over 7-14 days. Usual dosage range (JNC 7): 2.5-10 mg once daily.
- Angina: Usual dose: 5-10 mg; most patients require 10 mg for adequate effect

Elderly: Dosing should start at the lower end of dosing range due to possible increased incidence of hepatic, renal, or cardiac impairment. Elderly patients also show decreased clearance of amlodipine.

- Hypertension: 2.5 mg once daily
- Angina: 5 mg once daily

Dosage adjustment in renal impairment: Dialysis: Hemodialysis and peritoneal dialysis do not enhance elimination. Supplemental dose is not necessary.

Dosage adjustment in hepatic impairment:

- Angina: Administer 5 mg once daily.
- Hypertension: Administer 2.5 mg once daily.

Mechanism of Action Inhibits calcium ion from entering the "slow channels" or select voltage-sensitive areas of vascular smooth muscle and myocardium during depolarization, producing a relaxation of coronary vascular smooth muscle and coronary vasodilation; increases myocardial oxygen delivery in patients with vasospastic angina. Amlodipine directly acts on vascular smooth muscle to produce peripheral arterial vasodilation reducing peripheral vascular resistance and blood pressure.

Contraindications Hypersensitivity to amlodipine or any component of the formulation

Warnings/Precautions Increased angina and/or MI has occurred with initiation or dosage titration of calcium channel blockers. Symptomatic hypotension with or without syncope can rarely occur; blood pressure must be lowered at a rate appropriate for the patient's clinical condition. Use caution in severe aortic stenosis and/or hypertrophic cardiomyopathy with outflow tract obstruction. Use caution in patients with hepatic impairment; may require lower starting dose; titrate slowly with severe hepatic impairment. The most common side effect is peripheral edema; occurs within 2-3 weeks of starting therapy. Reflex tachycardia may occur with use. Peak antihypertensive effect is delayed; dosage titration should occur after 7-14 days on a given dose. Initiate at a lower dose in the elderly.

Drug Interactions

Metabolism/Transport Effects Substrate of CYP3A4 (major); **Inhibits** CYP1A2 (moderate), 2A6 (weak), 2B6 (weak), 2C8 (weak), 2C9 (weak), 2D6 (weak), 3A4 (weak)

Avoid Concomitant Use There are no known interactions where it is recommended to avoid concomitant use.

Increased Effect/Toxicity

AmLODIPine may increase the levels/effects of: Amifostine; Antihypertensives; Calcium Channel Blockers (Nondihydropyridine); CYP1A2 Substrates; Fosphenytoin; Hypotensive Agents; Magnesium Salts; Neuromuscular-Blocking Agents (Nondepolarizing); Nitroprusside; Phenytoin; RiTUXimab; Tacrolimus; Tacrolimus (Systemic)

The levels/effects of AmLODIPine may be increased by: Alpha1-Blockers; Antifungal Agents (Azole Derivatives, Systemic); Calcium Channel Blockers (Nondihydropyridine); Conivaptan; CycloSPORINE; CycloSPORINE (Systemic); CYP3A4 Inhibitors (Moderate); CYP3A4 Inhibitors (Strong); Dasatinib; Diazoxide; Fluconazole; Grapefruit Juice; Herbs (Hypotensive Properties); Macrolide Antibiotics; Magnesium Salts; MAO Inhibitors; Pentoxifylline; Phosphodiesterase 5 Inhibitors; Prostacyclin Analogues; Protease Inhibitors

Decreased Effect

AmLODIPine may decrease the levels/effects of: Clopidogrel; QuiNIDine

The levels/effects of AmLODIPine may be decreased by: Barbiturates; Calcium Salts; CarBAMazepine; CYP3A4 Inducers (Strong); Deferasirox; Herbs (CYP3A4 Inducers); Herbs (Hypertensive Properties); Methylphenidate; Nafcillin; Rifamycin Derivatives; Tocilizumab; Yohimbine

Ethanol/Nutrition/Herb Interactions

Food: Grapefruit juice may modestly increase amlodipine levels.

Herb/Nutraceutical: St John's wort may decrease amlodipine levels. Avoid herbs with *hypertensive* properties (bayberry, blue cohosh, cayenne, ephedra, ginger, ginseng [American], kola, licorice). Avoid herbs with *hypotensive* properties (black cohosh, California poppy, coleus, garlic, goldenseal, hawthorn, mistletoe, periwinkle, quinine, shepherd's purse).

Dietary Considerations May be taken without regard to meals.

Pharmacodynamics/Kinetics

Duration of Action Antihypertensive effect: 24 hours

Half-life Elimination Terminal: 30-50 hours; increased with hepatic dysfunction

Time to Peak Plasma: 6-12 hours

Pregnancy Risk Factor C

Lactation Excretion in breast milk unknown/not recommended

Dosage Forms

Tablet, oral: 2.5 mg, 5 mg, 10 mg

Norvasc®: 2.5 mg, 5 mg, 10 mg

References

Jorgensen MG, "Prevalence of Amlodipine-Related Gingival Hyperplasia," *J Periodontol*, 1997, 68 (7):676-8.

Wynn RL, "An Update on Calcium Channel Blocker-Induced Gingival Hyperplasia," *Gen Dent*, 1995, 43 (3):218-22.

Wynn RL, "Calcium Channel Blockers and Gingival Hyperplasia," *Gen Dent*, 1991, 39(4):240-3.

Amlodipine and Atorvastatin (am LOW di peen & a TORE va sta tin)

Related Information

AmLODIPine *on page* 113

Atorvastatin *on page* 184

U.S. Brand Names Caduet®

Canadian Brand Names Caduet®

Generic Availability (U.S.) No

Pharmacologic Category Antilipemic Agent, HMG-CoA Reductase Inhibitor; Calcium Channel Blocker; Calcium Channel Blocker, Dihydropyridine

Use For use when treatment with both amlodipine and atorvastatin is appropriate:

Amlodipine: Treatment of hypertension; treatment of chronic stable angina, vasospastic (Prinzmetal's) angina (confirmed or suspected); prevention of hospitalization or to decrease coronary revascularization procedure due to angina with documented CAD (limited to patients without heart failure or ejection fraction <40%)

Atorvastatin: Treatment of dyslipidemias or primary prevention of cardiovascular disease (atherosclerotic) as detailed here:

Primary prevention of cardiovascular disease (high-risk for CVD): To reduce the risk of MI or stroke in patients without evidence of coronary heart disease who have multiple CVD risk factors or type 2 diabetes; also reduces the risk for angina or revascularization procedures in patients with multiple CVD risk factors without evidence of coronary heart disease

Secondary prevention of cardiovascular disease: To reduce the risk of MI, stroke, revascularization procedures, angina, and hospitalization for heart failure

Treatment of dyslipidemias: To reduce elevations in total cholesterol, LDL-C, apolipoprotein B, and triglycerides in patients with elevations of one or more components, and/or to increase low HDL-C as present in heterozygous familial/nonfamilial hypercholesterolemia and mixed dyslipidemia (Fredrickson type IIa and IIb hyperlipidemias); treatment of primary dysbetalipoproteinemia (Fredrickson type III), elevated serum TG levels (Fredrickson type IV), and homozygous familial hypercholesterolemia

Treatment of heterozygous familial hypercholesterolemia (HeFH) in adolescent patients (10-17 years of age, females >1 year postmenarche) having LDL-C ≥190 mg/dL or LDL-C ≥160 mg/dL with positive family history of premature cardiovascular disease (CVD) or with two or more CVD risk factors.

Local Anesthetic/Vasoconstrictor Precautions No information available to require special precautions

Effects on Dental Treatment Key adverse event(s) related to dental treatment: Fewer reports of gingival hyperplasia with amlodipine than with other calcium channel blockers (usually resolves upon discontinuation); consultation with physician is suggested.

Effects on Bleeding No information available to require special precautions

Adverse Effects See individual agents.

Dosage Oral: **Note:** Dose is individualized; combination product may be used as initial therapy or substituted for individual components in patients currently maintained on both agents separately or in patients not adequately controlled with monotherapy (using one of the agents or an agent within same pharmacologic class).

Children 10-17 years (females >1 year postmenarche): Hypertension and hyperlipidemia:

Initial therapy: Amlodipine 2.5 mg and atorvastatin 10 mg once daily; dose may be titrated after 1-2 weeks (amlodipine component) and after 2-4 weeks (atorvastatin component) to a maximum daily dose: Amlodipine 5 mg; atorvastatin 20 mg

Add-on therapy/replacement therapy: Amlodipine 2.5-5 mg and atorvastatin 10-20 mg once daily; dose may be titrated after 1-2 weeks (amlodipine component) and after 2-4 weeks (atorvastatin component) to a maximum daily dose: Amlodipine 5 mg; atorvastatin 20 mg

Adults: Hypertension, angina, and hyperlipidemia:

Initial therapy: Amlodipine 5 mg and atorvastatin 10-20 mg once daily; dose may be titrated after 1-2 weeks (amlodipine component) and after 2-4 weeks (atorvastatin component) to a maximum daily dose: Amlodipine 10 mg; atorvastatin 80 mg

Add-on therapy/replacement therapy: Amlodipine 5-10 mg and atorvastatin 10-80 mg once daily; dose may be titrated after 1-2 weeks (amlodipine component) and after 2-4 weeks (atorvastatin component) to a maximum daily dose: Amlodipine 10 mg; atorvastatin 80 mg

Elderly: Consider starting amlodipine at the lower end of dosing range due to increased incidence of hepatic, renal, or cardiac impairment. Elderly patients also show decreased clearance of amlodipine.

Dosage adjustment for atorvastatin with concomitant medications:

Cyclosporine: Atorvastatin dose should not exceed 10 mg/day

Clarithromycin, itraconazole, ritonavir plus saquinavir, or lopinavir plus ritonavir when atorvastatin dose >20 mg: Ensure that the lowest dose necessary of atorvastatin is used

Dosage adjustment in renal impairment: No dosage adjustment is necessary

Dosage adjustment in hepatic impairment: Contraindicated in patients with active liver disease

Mechanism of Action

Amlodipine: Inhibits calcium ion from entering the "slow channels" or select voltage-sensitive areas of vascular smooth muscle and myocardium during depolarization, producing a relaxation of coronary vascular smooth muscle and coronary vasodilation; increases myocardial oxygen delivery in patients with vasospastic angina. Amlodipine directly acts on vascular smooth muscle to produce peripheral arterial vasodilation reducing peripheral vascular resistance and blood pressure.

Atorvastatin: Inhibitor of 3-hydroxy-3-methylglutaryl coenzyme A (HMG-CoA) reductase, the rate limiting enzyme in cholesterol synthesis (reduces the production of mevalonic acid from HMG-CoA); this then results in a compensatory increase in the expression of LDL receptors on hepatocyte membranes and a stimulation of LDL catabolism

Contraindications Hypersensitivity to amlodipine, atorvastatin, or any component of the formulation; active liver disease; unexplained persistent elevations of serum transaminases; pregnancy; breast-feeding

Warnings/Precautions See individual agents.

Drug Interactions

Metabolism/Transport Effects

Amlodipine: **Substrate** of CYP3A4 (major); **Inhibits** CYP1A2 (moderate), 2A6 (weak), 2B6 (weak), 2C8 (weak), 2C9 (weak), 2D6 (weak), 3A4 (weak)

Atorvastatin: **Substrate** of CYP3A4 (major), P-glycoprotein; **Inhibits** CYP3A4 (weak), P-glycoprotein

Avoid Concomitant Use

Avoid concomitant use of Amlodipine and Atorvastatin with any of the following: Red Yeast Rice; Topotecan

Increased Effect/Toxicity

Amlodipine and Atorvastatin may increase the levels/effects of: Aliskiren; Amifostine; Antihypertensives; Calcium Channel Blockers (Nondihydropyridine); CYP1A2 Substrates; DAPTOmycin; Digoxin; Diltiazem; Everolimus; Fosphenytoin; Hypotensive Agents; Magnesium Salts; Midazolam; Neuromuscular-Blocking Agents (Nondepolarizing); Nitroprusside; P-Glycoprotein Substrates; Phenytoin; RiTUXimab; Rivaroxaban; Tacrolimus; Tacrolimus (Systemic); Topotecan; Trabectedin; Verapamil

The levels/effects of Amlodipine and Atorvastatin may be increased by: Alpha1-Blockers; Amiodarone; Antifungal Agents (Azole Derivatives, Systemic); Calcium Channel Blockers (Nondihydropyridine); Colchicine; Conivaptan; CycloSPORINE; CycloSPORINE (Systemic); CYP3A4 Inhibitors (Moderate); CYP3A4 Inhibitors (Strong); Danazol; Dasatinib; Diazoxide; Diltiazem; Dronedarone; Eltrombopag; Fenofibrate; Fenofibric Acid; Fluconazole; Fusidic Acid; Gemfibrozil; Grapefruit Juice; Herbs (Hypotensive Properties); Macrolide Antibiotics; Magnesium Salts; MAO Inhibitors; Nefazodone; Niacin; Niacinamide; Pentoxifylline; P-Glycoprotein Inhibitors; Phosphodiesterase 5 Inhibitors; Prostacyclin Analogues; Protease Inhibitors; QuiNINE; Red Yeast Rice; Rifamycin Derivatives; Sildenafil; Verapamil

Decreased Effect

Amlodipine and Atorvastatin may decrease the levels/effects of: Clopidogrel; Dabigatran Etexilate; QuiNIDine

The levels/effects of Amlodipine and Atorvastatin may be decreased by: Antacids; Barbiturates; Bosentan; Calcium Salts; CarBAMazepine; CYP3A4 Inducers (Strong); Deferasirox; Efavirenz; Etravirine; Fosphenytoin; Herbs (Hypertensive Properties); Methylphenidate; Nafcillin; P-Glycoprotein Inducers; Phenytoin; Rifamycin Derivatives; St Johns Wort; Tocilizumab; Yohimbine

Ethanol/Nutrition/Herb Interactions See individual agents.

Dietary Considerations May take with food if desired; may take without regard to time of day. Before initiation of therapy with atorvastatin, patients should be placed on a standard cholesterol-lowering diet for 3-6 months and the diet should be continued during drug therapy. Red yeast rice contains an estimated 2.4 mg lovastatin per 600 mg rice.

Pregnancy Risk Factor X

Lactation Excretion in breast milk unknown/contraindicated

Breast-Feeding Considerations See individual agents.

Dosage Forms

Tablet:

Caduet®:

2.5/10: Amlodipine 2.5 mg and atorvastatin 10 mg; 2.5/20: Amlodipine 2.5 mg and atorvastatin 20 mg; 2.5/40: Amlodipine 2.5 mg and atorvastatin 40 mg

5/10: Amlodipine 5 mg and atorvastatin 10 mg; 5/20: Amlodipine 5 mg and atorvastatin 20 mg; 5/40: Amlodipine 5 mg and atorvastatin 40 mg; 5/80: Amlodipine 5 mg and atorvastatin 80 mg

10/10: Amlodipine 10 mg and atorvastatin 10 mg; 10/20: Amlodipine 10 mg and atorvastatin 20 mg; 10/40: Amlodipine 10 mg and atorvastatin 40 mg; 10/80: Amlodipine 10 mg and atorvastatin 80 mg

Amlodipine and Benazepril (am LOE di peen & ben AY ze pril)

Related Information

AmLODIPine *on page 113*

Benazepril *on page 213*

U.S. Brand Names Lotrel®

Generic Availability (U.S.) Yes

Pharmacologic Category Angiotensin-Converting Enzyme (ACE) Inhibitor; Calcium Channel Blocker; Calcium Channel Blocker, Dihydropyridine

Use Treatment of hypertension

Local Anesthetic/Vasoconstrictor Precautions No information available to require special precautions

Effects on Dental Treatment Fewer reports of gingival hyperplasia with amlodipine than with other CCBs (usually resolves upon discontinuation); consultation with physician is suggested.

Effects on Bleeding No information available to require special precautions

Adverse Effects See individual agents.

Dosage Oral: **Note:** Dose is individualized; combination product may be substituted for individual components in patients currently maintained on both agents separately or in patients not adequately controlled with monotherapy (using one of the agents or an agent within same antihypertensive class).

Adults: 2.5-10 mg (amlodipine) and 10-40 mg (benazepril) once daily; maximum: Amlodipine: 10 mg/day; benazepril: 80 mg/day

Elderly: Initial dose: 2.5 mg based on amlodipine component

Dosage adjustment in renal impairment: Cl_{cr} ≤30 mL/minute: Use of combination product is not recommended.

Dosage adjustment in hepatic impairment: Initial dose: 2.5 mg based on amlodipine component

Mechanism of Action

Amlodipine is a dihydropyridine calcium channel antagonist that inhibits transmembrane influx of calcium ions into vascular smooth muscle and cardiac muscle producing relaxation of coronary vascular smooth muscle and coronary vasodilation; amlodipine directly acts on vascular smooth muscle to produce peripheral arterial vasodilation reducing peripheral vascular resistance and blood pressure.

Benazepril lowers blood pressure by suppressing the renin-angiotensin-aldosterone system; benazepril has an antihypertensive effect even in patients with low-renin hypertension.

Contraindications Hypersensitivity to amlodipine, benazepril, other ACE inhibitors, or any component of the formulation; history of angioedema, with or without previous ACE inhibitor treatment

Warnings/Precautions Used as a replacement for separate dosing of components or combination therapy when response to single agent is suboptimal. The fixed combination is not indicated for initial treatment of hypertension. See individual agents for additional warnings/precautions.

Drug Interactions

Metabolism/Transport Effects Amlodipine: **Substrate** of CYP3A4 (major); **Inhibits** CYP1A2 (moderate), 2A6 (weak), 2B6 (weak), 2C8 (weak), 2C9 (weak), 2D6 (weak), 3A4 (weak)

Avoid Concomitant Use There are no known interactions where it is recommended to avoid concomitant use.

Increased Effect/Toxicity

Amlodipine and Benazepril may increase the levels/effects of: Allopurinol; Amifostine; Antihypertensives; AzaTHIOprine; Calcium Channel Blockers (Nondihydropyridine); CycloSPORINE; CycloSPORINE (Systemic); CYP1A2 Substrates; Ferric Gluconate; Fosphenytoin; Gold Sodium Thiomalate; Hypotensive Agents; Iron Dextran Complex; Lithium; Magnesium Salts; Neuromuscular-Blocking Agents

(Nondepolarizing); Nitroprusside; Nonsteroidal Anti-Inflammatory Agents; Phenytoin; RiTUXimab; Tacrolimus; Tacrolimus (Systemic)

The levels/effects of Amlodipine and Benazepril may be increased by: Alpha1-Blockers; Angiotensin II Receptor Blockers; Antifungal Agents (Azole Derivatives, Systemic); Calcium Channel Blockers (Nondihydropyridine); Conivaptan; CycloSPORINE; CycloSPORINE (Systemic); CYP3A4 Inhibitors (Moderate); CYP3A4 Inhibitors (Strong); Dasatinib; Diazoxide; DPP-IV Inhibitors; Eplerenone; Everolimus; Fluconazole; Grapefruit Juice; Herbs (Hypotensive Properties); Loop Diuretics; Macrolide Antibiotics; Magnesium Salts; MAO Inhibitors; Pentoxifylline; Phosphodiesterase 5 Inhibitors; Potassium Salts; Potassium-Sparing Diuretics; Prostacyclin Analogues; Protease Inhibitors; Sirolimus; Temsirolimus; Thiazide Diuretics; TiZANidine; Tolvaptan; Trimethoprim

Decreased Effect

Amlodipine and Benazepril may decrease the levels/effects of: Clopidogrel; QuiNIDine

The levels/effects of Amlodipine and Benazepril may be decreased by: Antacids; Aprotinin; Barbiturates; Calcium Salts; CarBAMazepine; CYP3A4 Inducers (Strong); Deferasirox; Herbs (CYP3A4 Inducers); Herbs (Hypertensive Properties); Methylphenidate; Nafcillin; Nonsteroidal Anti-Inflammatory Agents; Rifamycin Derivatives; Salicylates; Tocilizumab; Yohimbine

Ethanol/Nutrition/Herb Interactions

Food: Grapefruit juice may modestly increase amlodipine levels.

Herb/Nutraceutical: St John's wort may decrease amlodipine levels. Avoid herbs with *hypertensive* properties (bayberry, blue cohosh, cayenne, ephedra, ginger, ginseng [American], kola, licorice). Avoid herbs with *hypotensive* properties (black cohosh, California poppy, coleus, garlic, goldenseal, hawthorn, mistletoe, periwinkle, quinine, shepherd's purse).

Pregnancy Risk Factor D

Lactation

Amlodipine: Excretion in breast milk unknown/not recommended

Benazepril: Enters breast milk

Dosage Forms

Capsule: 2.5/10: Amlodipine 2.5 mg and benazepril 10 mg; 5/10: Amlodipine 5 mg and benazepril 10 mg; 5/20: Amlodipine 5 mg and benazepril 20 mg; 5/40: Amlodipine 5 mg and benazepril hydrochloride 40 mg; 10/20: Amlodipine 10 mg and benazepril 20 mg; 10/40: Amlodipine 10 mg and benazepril hydrochloride 40 mg

Lotrel®: 2.5/10: Amlodipine 2.5 and benazepril 10 mg; 5/10: Amlodipine 5 mg and benazepril 10 mg; 5/20: Amlodipine 5 mg and benazepril 20 mg; 5/40: Amlodipine 5 mg and benazepril 40 mg; 10/20: Amlodipine 10 mg and benazepril 20 mg; 10/40: Amlodipine 10 mg and benazepril 40 mg

References

Wynn RL, "An Update on Calcium Channel Blocker-Induced Gingival Hyperplasia," *Gen Dent*, 1995, 43 (3):218-22.

Wynn RL, "Calcium Channel Blockers and Gingival Hyperplasia," *Gen Dent*, 1991, 39(4):240-3.

Amlodipine and Olmesartan (am LOE di peen & olme SAR tan)

Related Information

AmLODIPine *on page 113*

Olmesartan *on page 1243*

U.S. Brand Names Azor™

Pharmacologic Category Angiotensin II Receptor Blocker; Calcium Channel Blocker; Calcium Channel Blocker, Dihydropyridine

Use Treatment of hypertension, including initial treatment in patients who will require multiple antihypertensives for adequate control

Local Anesthetic/Vasoconstrictor Precautions No information available to require special precautions

Effects on Dental Treatment Fewer reports of gingival hyperplasia with amlodipine than with other CCBs (usually resolves upon discontinuation); consultation with physician is suggested.

Effects on Bleeding No information available to require special precautions

Adverse Effects Reactions/percentages reported with combination product; also refer to individual agents

>10%: Cardiovascular: Peripheral edema (dose related: 18% to 26%)

Frequency not defined (limited to important or life-threatening): Hypotension, nocturia, orthostatic hypotension, palpitation, pruritus, rash, urinary frequency

General Dosage Range Oral: *Adults:* Amlodipine 5-10 mg and olmesartan 20-40 mg once daily (maximum: 10 mg/day [amlodipine]; 40 mg/day [olmesartan])

Mechanism of Action
Amlodipine inhibits calcium ion from entering the "slow channels" or select voltage-sensitive areas of vascular smooth muscle and myocardium during depolarization, producing a relaxation of coronary vascular smooth muscle and coronary vasodilation; increases myocardial oxygen delivery in patients with vasospastic angina. Amlodipine directly acts on vascular smooth muscle to produce peripheral arterial vasodilation reducing peripheral vascular resistance and blood pressure.

As a selective and competitive, nonpeptide angiotensin II receptor antagonist, olmesartan blocks the vasoconstrictor and aldosterone-secreting effects of angiotensin II; olmesartan interacts reversibly at the AT1 and AT2 receptors of many tissues and has slow dissociation kinetics; its affinity for the AT1 receptor is 12,500 times greater than the AT2 receptor. Angiotensin II receptor antagonists may induce a more complete inhibition of the renin-angiotensin system than ACE inhibitors, they do not affect the response to bradykinin, and are less likely to be associated with nonrenin-angiotensin effects (eg, cough and angioedema). Olmesartan increases urinary flow rate and, in addition to being natriuretic and kaliuretic, increases excretion of chloride, magnesium, uric acid, calcium, and phosphate.

Pregnancy Risk Factor C/D (2nd and 3rd trimesters)

Amlodipine and Valsartan (am LOE di peen & val SAR tan)

Related Information
AmLODIPine *on page 113*
Valsartan *on page 1699*

U.S. Brand Names Exforge®

Generic Availability (U.S.) No

Pharmacologic Category Angiotensin II Receptor Blocker; Calcium Channel Blocker; Calcium Channel Blocker, Dihydropyridine

Use Treatment of hypertension

Local Anesthetic/Vasoconstrictor Precautions No information available to require special precautions

Effects on Dental Treatment Key adverse event(s) related to dental treatment: Fewer reports of gingival hyperplasia with amlodipine than with other calcium channel blockers (usually resolves upon discontinuation); consultation with physician is suggested.

Effects on Bleeding No information available to require special precautions

Adverse Effects Reactions/percentages reported with combination product; also refer to individual agents

>10%: Central nervous system: Headache (11%)

1% to 10%:
- Cardiovascular: Peripheral edema (5% to 8%)
- Central nervous system: Anxiety (3%), somnolence (3%), dizziness (≤2%)
- Endocrine & metabolic: Hyperkalemia (3% to 10%)
- Gastrointestinal: Abdominal pain (upper; 3%), diarrhea (3%), nausea (3%)
- Renal: BUN increased (6%)
- Respiratory: Nasopharyngitis (4%), upper respiratory tract infection (3%), cough (2%)
- Miscellaneous: Influenza (2%)

Frequency not defined, but occurred at ≥0.2% incidence (limited to important or life-threatening): Abdominal discomfort/distension, abdominal pain, arthralgia, chest pain, colitis, constipation, depression, diabetes, dyspepsia, edema (including pitting), erectile dysfunction, erythema, fever, flushing, gastritis, hematuria, hypercholesterolemia, infection, LFTs increased, lymphadenopathy, myalgia, nephrolithiasis, palpitation, paresthesia, pharyngitis, pruritus, rash, tachycardia, vomiting, weakness, xerostomia

Dosage Oral: Dose is individualized; combination product may be used as initial therapy or substituted for individual components in patients currently maintained on both agents separately or in patients not adequately controlled with monotherapy (using one of the agents or an agent within same antihypertensive class).

Adults: Hypertension:
- Initial therapy: Amlodipine 5 mg and valsartan 160 mg once daily, dose may be titrated after 1-2 weeks of therapy. Maximum recommended doses: Amlodipine 10 mg/day; valsartan 320 mg/day
- Add-on/replacement therapy: Amlodipine 5-10 mg and valsartan 160-320 mg once daily; dose may be titrated after 3-4 weeks of therapy. Maximum recommended doses: Amlodipine 10 mg/day; valsartan 320 mg/day

Elderly: Initiate amlodipine at 2.5 mg/day due to decreased clearance

Dosing adjustment in renal impairment:
Cl_{cr} >10 mL/minute: No dosage adjustment necessary
Cl_{cr} ≤10 mL/minute: Use caution; titrate slowly

Dosing adjustment in hepatic impairment: Mild-to-moderate hepatic impairment: No initial dosage adjustment required, titrate slowly. Amlodipine and valsartan exposure increased in presence of hepatic impairment.
Amlodipine: Use caution in severe hepatic impairment; lower initial doses may be required
Valsartan: Mild-to-moderate hepatic impairment: No dosage adjustment required; however, patients with mild-to-moderate chronic disease have twice the exposure as healthy volunteers.

Mechanism of Action
Amlodipine inhibits calcium ion from entering the "slow channels" or select voltage-sensitive areas of vascular smooth muscle and myocardium during depolarization, producing a relaxation of coronary vascular smooth muscle and coronary vasodilation; increases myocardial oxygen delivery in patients with vasospastic angina. Amlodipine directly acts on vascular smooth muscle to produce peripheral arterial vasodilation reducing peripheral vascular resistance and blood pressure.

Valsartan produces direct antagonism of the angiotensin II (AT2) receptors, unlike the ACE inhibitors. It displaces angiotensin II from the AT1 receptor and produces its blood pressure-lowering effects by antagonizing AT1-induced vasoconstriction, aldosterone release, catecholamine release, arginine vasopressin release, water intake, and hypertrophic responses. This action results in more efficient blockade of the cardiovascular effects of angiotensin II and fewer side effects than the ACE inhibitors.

Contraindications There are no contraindications listed within the FDA-approved labeling.

Warnings/Precautions See individual agents.

Drug Interactions

Metabolism/Transport Effects
Amlodipine: **Substrate** of CYP3A4 (major); **Inhibits** CYP1A2 (moderate), 2A6 (weak), 2B6 (weak), 2C8 (weak), 2C9 (weak), 2D6 (weak), 3A4 (weak)
Valsartan: **Substrate** of SLCO1B1; **Inhibits** CYP2C9 (weak)

Avoid Concomitant Use There are no known interactions where it is recommended to avoid concomitant use.

Increased Effect/Toxicity
Amlodipine and Valsartan may increase the levels/effects of: ACE Inhibitors; Amifostine; Antihypertensives; Calcium Channel Blockers (Nondihydropyridine); CYP1A2 Substrates; Fosphenytoin; Hypotensive Agents; Lithium; Magnesium Salts; Neuromuscular-Blocking Agents (Nondepolarizing); Nitroprusside; Nonsteroidal Anti-Inflammatory Agents; Phenytoin; Potassium-Sparing Diuretics; RiTUXimab; Tacrolimus; Tacrolimus (Systemic)

The levels/effects of Amlodipine and Valsartan may be increased by: Alpha1-Blockers; Antifungal Agents (Azole Derivatives, Systemic); Calcium Channel Blockers (Nondihydropyridine); Conivaptan; CycloSPORINE; CycloSPORINE (Systemic); CYP3A4 Inhibitors (Moderate); CYP3A4 Inhibitors (Strong); Dasatinib; Diazoxide; Eltrombopag; Eplerenone; Fluconazole; Grapefruit Juice; Herbs (Hypotensive Properties); Macrolide Antibiotics; Magnesium Salts; MAO Inhibitors; Pentoxifylline; Phosphodiesterase 5 Inhibitors; Potassium Salts; Prostacyclin Analogues; Protease Inhibitors; Tolvaptan; Trimethoprim

Decreased Effect
Amlodipine and Valsartan may decrease the levels/effects of: Clopidogrel; QuiNIDine

The levels/effects of Amlodipine and Valsartan may be decreased by: Barbiturates; Calcium Salts; CarBAMazepine; CYP3A4 Inducers (Strong); Deferasirox; Herbs (CYP3A4 Inducers); Herbs (Hypertensive Properties); Methylphenidate; Nafcillin; Nonsteroidal Anti-Inflammatory Agents; Rifamycin Derivatives; Tocilizumab; Yohimbine

Ethanol/Nutrition/Herb Interactions
Food: Decreases rate and extent of valsartan absorption by 50% and 40%, respectively.
Herb/Nutraceutical: Avoid dong quai if using for hypertension (has estrogenic activity). Avoid ephedra, yohimbe, ginseng (may worsen hypertension). Avoid garlic (may have increased antihypertensive effects).

Dietary Considerations Avoid salt substitutes which contain potassium. May be taken with or without food.

Pregnancy Risk Factor D

Lactation Excretion in breast milk unknown/not recommended

Breast-Feeding Considerations See individual agents.

Dosage Forms

Tablet:

Exforge®: 5/160: Amlodipine 5 mg and valsartan 160 mg; 5/320 mg: Amlodipine 5 mg and valsartan 320 mg; 10/160: Amlodipine 10 mg and valsartan 160 mg; 10/320: Amlodipine 10 mg and valsartan 320 mg

Amlodipine, Valsartan, and Hydrochlorothiazide

(am LOE di peen, val SAR tan, & hye droe klor oh THYE a zide)

Related Information

AmLODIPine *on page 113*
Hydrochlorothiazide *on page 854*
Valsartan *on page 1699*

U.S. Brand Names Exforge HCT®

Pharmacologic Category Angiotensin II Receptor Blocker; Calcium Channel Blocker; Calcium Channel Blocker, Dihydropyridine; Diuretic, Thiazide

Use Treatment of hypertension (not for initial therapy)

Local Anesthetic/Vasoconstrictor Precautions No information available to require special precautions

Effects on Dental Treatment Key adverse event(s) related to dental treatment: Fewer reports of gingival hyperplasia with amlodipine than with other calcium channel blockers (usually resolves upon discontinuation); consultation with physician is suggested.

Effects on Bleeding No information available to require special precautions

Adverse Effects Reactions/percentages reported with combination product; also refer to individual agents.

>10%: Renal: BUN increased (30%)

2% to 10%:

- Cardiovascular: Edema (7%)
- Central nervous system: Dizziness (8%), headache (5%), fatigue (2%)
- Endocrine & metabolic: Hypokalemia (7%), hyperkalemia (4%)
- Gastrointestinal: Dyspepsia (2%), nausea (2%)
- Neuromuscular & Skeletal: Back pain (2%), muscle spasms (2%)
- Renal: Serum creatinine increased (2%)
- Respiratory: Nasopharyngitis (2%)

General Dosage Range Oral: *Adults:* Amlodipine 5-10 mg and valsartan 160-320 mg and hydrochlorothiazide 12.5-25 mg once daily (maximum: 10 mg/day [amlodipine]; 25 mg/day [hydrochlorothiazide]; 320 mg/day [valsartan])

Mechanism of Action

Amlodipine inhibits calcium ion from entering the "slow channels" or select voltage-sensitive areas of vascular smooth muscle and myocardium during depolarization, producing a relaxation of coronary vascular smooth muscle and coronary vasodilation; increases myocardial oxygen delivery in patients with vasospastic angina. Amlodipine directly acts on vascular smooth muscle to produce peripheral arterial vasodilation reducing peripheral vascular resistance and blood pressure.

Valsartan produces direct antagonism of the angiotensin II (AT2) receptors, unlike the ACE inhibitors. It displaces angiotensin II from the AT1 receptor and produces its blood pressure-lowering effects by antagonizing AT1-induced vasoconstriction, aldosterone release, catecholamine release, arginine vasopressin release, water intake, and hypertrophic responses. This action results in more efficient blockade of the cardiovascular effects of angiotensin II and fewer side effects than the ACE inhibitors.

Hydrochlorothiazide inhibits sodium reabsorption in the distal tubules causing increased excretion of sodium and water as well as potassium and hydrogen ions.

Pregnancy Risk Factor D

Ammonia Spirit (Aromatic) (a MOE nee ah SPEAR it, air oh MAT ik)

Generic Availability (U.S.) Yes

Pharmacologic Category Respiratory Stimulant

Dental Use Emergency use in syncope

Use Respiratory and circulatory stimulant; treatment of fainting

Local Anesthetic/Vasoconstrictor Precautions No information available to require special precautions

Effects on Dental Treatment No significant effects or complications reported

Effects on Bleeding No information available to require special precautions

Adverse Effects 1% to 10%:
Gastrointestinal: Nausea, vomiting
Respiratory: Irritation to nasal mucosa, cough

Dosage Used as "smelling salts" to treat or prevent fainting

Contraindications Hypersensitivity to ammonia or any component of the formulation

Drug Interactions

Avoid Concomitant Use There are no known interactions where it is recommended to avoid concomitant use.

Increased Effect/Toxicity There are no known significant interactions involving an increase in effect.

Decreased Effect There are no known significant interactions involving a decrease in effect.

Pregnancy Risk Factor C

Dosage Forms
Solution, for inhalation: 1.7% to 2.1% (0.33 mL, 60 mL)

Ammonium Chloride (a MOE nee um KLOR ide)

Pharmacologic Category Electrolyte Supplement, Parenteral

Use Treatment of hypochloremic states or metabolic alkalosis

Local Anesthetic/Vasoconstrictor Precautions No information available to require special precautions

Effects on Dental Treatment No significant effects or complications reported

Effects on Bleeding No information available to require special precautions

Adverse Effects Frequency not defined.
Central nervous system: Coma, drowsiness, EEG abnormalities, headache, mental confusion, seizure
Dermatologic: Rash
Endocrine & metabolic: Calcium-deficient tetany, hyperchloremia, hypokalemia, metabolic acidosis, potassium may be decreased, sodium may be decreased
Gastrointestinal: Abdominal pain, gastric irritation, nausea, vomiting
Hepatic: Ammonia may be increased
Local: Pain at site of injection
Neuromuscular & skeletal: Twitching
Respiratory: Hyperventilation

Mechanism of Action Increases acidity by increasing free hydrogen ion concentration

Pregnancy Risk Factor C

Amobarbital (am oh BAR bi tal)

U.S. Brand Names Amytal®

Canadian Brand Names Amytal®

Pharmacologic Category Barbiturate; General Anesthetic; Hypnotic; Sedative

Use Hypnotic in short-term treatment of insomnia; reduce anxiety and provide sedation preoperatively

Unlabeled/Investigational Use Therapeutic or diagnostic "Amytal® Interviewing"; Wada test

Local Anesthetic/Vasoconstrictor Precautions No information available to require special precautions

Effects on Dental Treatment No significant effects or complications reported

Effects on Bleeding No information available to require special precautions

Adverse Effects Frequency not defined and is reported as barbiturate use (not specifically amobarbital).

Cardiovascular: Bradycardia, hypotension, syncope
Central nervous system: Agitation, anxiety, ataxia, confusion, CNS depression, dizziness, fever, hallucinations, headache, insomnia, nightmares, nervousness, psychiatric disturbances, somnolence, thinking abnormal
Gastrointestinal: Constipation, nausea, vomiting
Hematologic: Megaloblastic anemia (following chronic phenobarbital use)
Hepatic: Liver damage
Local: Injection site reaction
Neuromuscular & skeletal: Hyperkinesia
Respiratory: Apnea, atelectasis (postoperative), hypoventilation
Miscellaneous: Hypersensitivity reaction (including angioedema, rash, and exfoliative dermatitis)

General Dosage Range Dosage adjustment recommended in patients with hepatic or renal impairment

I.M., I.V.:

Children 6-12 years: Sedative: 65-500 mg/dose

Adults:

Hypnotic: 65-200 mg at bedtime (maximum single dose: 1000 mg)

Sedative: 30-50 mg 2-3 times/day (maximum single dose: 1000 mg)

Mechanism of Action Interferes with transmission of impulses from the thalamus to the cortex of the brain resulting in an imbalance in central inhibitory and facilitatory mechanisms

Pharmacodynamics/Kinetics

Onset of Action I.V.: Within 5 minutes

Half-life Elimination 15-40 hours (mean: 25 hours)

Pregnancy Risk Factor D

Controlled Substance C-II

Amoxapine (a MOKS a peen)

Pharmacologic Category Antidepressant, Tricyclic (Secondary Amine)

Use Treatment of depression, psychotic depression, depression accompanied by anxiety or agitation

Local Anesthetic/Vasoconstrictor Precautions Use with caution; epinephrine and levonordefrin have been shown to have an increased pressor response in combination with TCAs. Amoxapine is one of the drugs confirmed to prolong the QT interval and is accepted as having a risk of causing torsade de pointes. The risk of drug-induced torsade de pointes is extremely low when a single QT interval prolonging drug is prescribed. In terms of epinephrine, it is not known what effect vasoconstrictors in the local anesthetic regimen will have in patients with a known history of congenital prolonged QT interval or in patients taking any medication that prolongs the QT interval. Until more information is obtained, it is suggested that the clinician consult with the physician prior to the use of a vasoconstrictor in suspected patients, and that the vasoconstrictor (epinephrine, mepivacaine and levonordefrin [Carbocaine® 2% with Neo-Cobefrin®]) be used with caution.

Effects on Dental Treatment Key adverse event(s) related to dental treatment: Xerostomia and changes in salivation (normal salivary flow resumes upon discontinuation). Long-term treatment with TCAs, such as amoxapine, increases the risk of caries by reducing salivation and salivary buffer capacity.

Effects on Bleeding No information available to require special precautions

Adverse Effects

>10%:

Central nervous system: Drowsiness

Gastrointestinal: Xerostomia, constipation

1% to 10%:

Central nervous system: Anxiety, ataxia, confusion, dizziness, excitement, headache, insomnia, nervousness, restlessness

Dermatologic: Edema, skin rash

Endocrine: Prolactin levels increased

Gastrointestinal: Nausea

Neuromuscular & skeletal: Tremor, weakness

Ocular: Blurred vision

Miscellaneous: Diaphoresis

General Dosage Range Oral:

Adolescents: Initial: 25-50 mg/day as a single dose or in divided doses; Maintenance: 25-100 mg/day as a single dose at bedtime or in divided doses (maximum: 100 mg/day)

Adults: Initial: 50-75 mg/day in 2-3 divided doses; Maintenance 50-300 mg/day in 2-3 divided doses (maximum: 600 mg/day [inpatient]; 400 mg/day [outpatient])

Mechanism of Action Reduces the reuptake of serotonin and norepinephrine. The metabolite, 7-OH-amoxapine has significant dopamine receptor blocking activity similar to haloperidol.

Pharmacodynamics/Kinetics

Onset of Action Antidepressant effect: Usually occurs after 1-2 weeks, but may require 4-6 weeks

Half-life Elimination Parent drug: 11-16 hours; Active metabolite (8-hydroxy): Adults: 30 hours

Time to Peak Serum: 1-2 hours

Pregnancy Risk Factor C

Dental Comment Amoxapine is known to prolong the QT interval. The QT interval is measured as the time and distance between the Q point of the QRS complex and the end of the T wave in the ECG tracing. After adjustment for heart rate, the QT interval is defined as prolonged if it is more than 450 msec in men and 460 msec in women. A long QT syndrome was first described in the 1950s and 60s as a congenital syndrome involving QT interval prolongation and syncope and sudden death. Some of the congenital long QT syndromes were characterized by a peculiar electrocardiographic appearance of the QRS complex involving a premature atria beat followed by a pause, then a subsequent sinus beat showing marked QT prolongation and deformity. This type of cardiac arrhythmia was originally termed "torsade de pointes" (translated from the French as "twisting of the points"). Amoxapine is considered as having a risk of causing torsade de pointes. Since it is not known what effect vasoconstrictors in the local anesthetic regimen will have in patients with a known history of congenital prolonged QT interval or in patients taking any medication that prolongs the QT interval, a medical consult is suggested.

Amoxicillin (a moks i SIL in)

Related Information

Antibiotic Prophylaxis *on page* 1910
Bacterial Infections *on page* 1933
Gastrointestinal Disorders *on page* 1874
Osteonecrosis of the Jaw *on page* 1894
Periodontal Diseases *on page* 1942

Related Sample Prescriptions

Bacterial Infections and Periodontal Diseases *on page* 1983
Infective Endocarditis (Prevention) *on page* 1978
Prosthetic Joint Late Infections (Prevention) *on page* 1979
Sinus Infection Treatment *on page* 1985

U.S. Brand Names Moxatag™

Canadian Brand Names Apo-Amoxi®; Gen-Amoxicillin; Lin-Amox; Mylan-Amoxicillin; Novamoxin®; Nu-Amoxi; PHL-Amoxicillin; PMS-Amoxicillin

Generic Availability (U.S.) Yes: Excludes extended-release formulation

Pharmacologic Category Antibiotic, Penicillin

Dental Use Antibiotic for standard prophylactic regimen for dental patients who are at risk for infective endocarditis; prophylaxis in total joint replacement patients undergoing dental procedures which produce bacteremia; antibiotic used to treat orofacial infections

Use Treatment of otitis media, sinusitis, and infections caused by susceptible organisms involving the upper and lower respiratory tract, skin, and urinary tract; prophylaxis of infective endocarditis in patients undergoing surgical or dental procedures; as part of a multidrug regimen for *H. pylori* eradication

Unlabeled/Investigational Use Postexposure prophylaxis for anthrax exposure with documented susceptible organisms

Local Anesthetic/Vasoconstrictor Precautions No information available to require special precautions

Effects on Dental Treatment Prolonged use of penicillins may lead to development of oral candidiasis

Effects on Bleeding No information available to require special precautions

Adverse Effects Frequency not defined.

Central nervous system: Agitation, anxiety, behavioral changes, confusion, dizziness, headache, hyperactivity (reversible), insomnia, seizure

Dermatologic: Acute exanthematous pustulosis, erythematous maculopapular rash, erythema multiforme, exfoliative dermatitis, hypersensitivity vasculitis, mucocutaneous candidiasis, Stevens-Johnson syndrome, toxic epidermal necrolysis, urticaria

Gastrointestinal: Black hairy tongue, diarrhea, hemorrhagic colitis, nausea, pseudomembranous colitis, tooth discoloration (brown, yellow, or gray; rare), vomiting

Hematologic: Agranulocytosis, anemia, eosinophilia, hemolytic anemia, leukopenia, thrombocytopenia, thrombocytopenia purpura

Hepatic: Acute cytolytic hepatitis, ALT increased, AST increased, cholestatic jaundice, hepatic cholestasis

Renal: Crystalluria

Miscellaneous: Anaphylaxis, serum sickness-like reaction

Dental Usual Dosage Oral:

Children >3 months and <40 kg: Prophylaxis against infective endocarditis: 50 mg/kg 30-60 minutes before procedure. **Note:** American Heart Association (AHA) guidelines now recommend prophylaxis only in patients undergoing invasive procedures and in whom underlying cardiac conditions may predispose to a higher risk of adverse outcomes should infection occur. As of April 2007, routine prophylaxis for GI/GU procedures is no longer recommended by the AHA.

Adults:

Prophylaxis against infective endocarditis: 2 g 30-60 minutes before procedure. **Note:** American Heart Association (AHA) guidelines now recommend prophylaxis only in patients undergoing invasive procedures and in whom underlying cardiac conditions may predispose to a higher risk of adverse outcomes should infection occur. As of April 2007, routine prophylaxis for GI/GU procedures is no longer recommended by the AHA.

Orofacial infection: 250-500 mg every 8 hours or 500-875 mg twice daily

Prophylaxis in total joint replacement patients undergoing dental procedures which produce bacteremia: 2 g 1 hour prior to procedure

Dosage

Usual dosage range:

Children ≤3 months: Oral: 20-30 mg/kg/day divided every 12 hours

Children >3 months and <40 kg: Oral: 20-50 mg/kg/day in divided doses every 8-12 hours

Children ≥12 years: Oral: Extended-release tablet: 775 mg once daily

Adults: Oral: 250-500 mg every 8 hours or 500-875 mg twice daily

Extended-release tablet: 775 mg once daily

Indication-specific dosing:

Children >3 months and <40 kg: Oral:

Acute otitis media: 80-90 mg/kg/day divided every 12 hours

Anthrax exposure (CDC guidelines): Note: Postexposure prophylaxis only with documented susceptible organisms: 80 mg/kg/day in divided doses every 8 hours (maximum: 500 mg/dose)

Community-acquired pneumonia:

4 months to <5 years: 80-100 mg/kg/day divided every 8 hours

5-15 years: 100 mg/kg/day divided every 8 hours; **Note:** Treatment with a macrolide or doxycycline (if age >8 years) is preferred due to higher prevalence of atypical pathogens in this age group

Ear, nose, throat, genitourinary tract, or skin/skin structure infections:

Mild-to-moderate: 25 mg/kg/day in divided doses every 12 hours **or** 20 mg/kg/day in divided doses every 8 hours

Severe: 45 mg/kg/day in divided doses every 12 hours **or** 40 mg/kg/day in divided doses every 8 hours

Tonsillitis and/or pharyngitis: Children ≥12 years: Extended-release tablet: 775 mg once daily

Lower respiratory tract infections: 45 mg/kg/day in divided doses every 12 hours **or** 40 mg/kg/day in divided doses every 8 hours

Lyme disease: 25-50 mg/kg/day divided every 8 hours (maximum: 500 mg)

Prophylaxis against infective endocarditis: 50 mg/kg 1 hour before procedure. **Note:** American Heart Association (AHA) guidelines now recommend prophylaxis only in patients undergoing invasive procedures and in whom underlying cardiac conditions may predispose to a higher risk of adverse outcomes should infection occur. As of April 2007, routine prophylaxis for GI/GU procedures is no longer recommended by the AHA.

Adults: Oral:

Anthrax exposure (CDC guidelines): Note: Postexposure prophylaxis in pregnant or nursing women only with documented susceptible organisms: 500 mg every 8 hours

Chlamydial infection during pregnancy (unlabeled use): 500 mg 3 times/day for 7 days (CDC, 2010)

Ear, nose, throat, genitourinary tract, or skin/skin structure infections:

Mild-to-moderate: 500 mg every 12 hours **or** 250 mg every 8 hours

Severe: 875 mg every 12 hours **or** 500 mg every 8 hours

Tonsillitis and/or pharyngitis: Extended-release tablet: 775 mg once daily

***Helicobacter pylori* eradication:** 1000 mg twice daily; requires combination therapy with at least one other antibiotic and an acid-suppressing agent (proton pump inhibitor or H_2 blocker)

Lower respiratory tract infections: 875 mg every 12 hours **or** 500 mg every 8 hours

Lyme disease: 500 mg every 6-8 hours (depending on size of patient) for 21-30 days

Prophylaxis against infective endocarditis: 2 g 30-60 minutes before procedure. **Note:** American Heart Association (AHA) guidelines now recommend prophylaxis only in patients undergoing invasive procedures and in whom underlying cardiac conditions may predispose to a higher risk of adverse outcomes should infection occur. As of April 2007, routine prophylaxis for GI/GU procedures is no longer recommended by the AHA.

Prophylaxis in total joint replacement patients undergoing dental procedures which produce bacteremia: 2 g 1 hour prior to procedure

Dosing interval in renal impairment: Use of certain dosage forms (eg, extended-release 775 mg tablet and immediate-release 875 mg tablet) should be avoided in patients with Cl_{cr} <30 mL/minute or patients requiring hemodialysis.

Cl_{cr} 10-30 mL/minute: 250-500 mg every 12 hours

Cl_{cr} <10 mL/minute: 250-500 mg every 24 hours

Dialysis: Moderately dialyzable (20% to 50%) by hemo- or peritoneal dialysis; approximately 50 mg of amoxicillin per liter of filtrate is removed by continuous arteriovenous or venovenous hemofiltration; dose as per Cl_{cr} <10 mL/minute guidelines

Mechanism of Action Inhibits bacterial cell wall synthesis by binding to one or more of the penicillin-binding proteins (PBPs) which in turn inhibits the final transpeptidation step of peptidoglycan synthesis in bacterial cell walls, thus inhibiting cell wall biosynthesis. Bacteria eventually lyse due to ongoing activity of cell wall autolytic enzymes (autolysins and murein hydrolases) while cell wall assembly is arrested.

Contraindications Hypersensitivity to amoxicillin, penicillin, other beta-lactams, or any component of the formulation

Warnings/Precautions In patients with renal impairment, doses and/or frequency of administration should be modified in response to the degree of renal impairment; in addition, use of certain dosage forms (eg, extended release 775 mg tablet and immediate release 875 mg tablet) should be avoided in patients with Cl_{cr} <30 mL/minute or patients requiring hemodialysis. A high percentage of patients with infectious mononucleosis have developed rash during therapy with amoxicillin; ampicillin-class antibiotics not recommended in these patients. Serious and occasionally severe or fatal hypersensitivity (anaphylactoid) reactions have been reported in patients on penicillin therapy, especially with a history of beta-lactam hypersensitivity, history of sensitivity to multiple allergens, or previous IgE-mediated reactions (eg, anaphylaxis, angioedema, urticaria). Use with caution in asthmatic patients. Prolonged use may result in fungal or bacterial superinfection, including *C. difficile*-associated diarrhea (CDAD) and pseudomembranous colitis; CDAD has been observed >2 months postantibiotic treatment. Chewable tablets contain phenylalanine.

Drug Interactions

Avoid Concomitant Use

Avoid concomitant use of Amoxicillin with any of the following: BCG

Increased Effect/Toxicity

Amoxicillin may increase the levels/effects of: Methotrexate

The levels/effects of Amoxicillin may be increased by: Allopurinol; Probenecid

Decreased Effect

Amoxicillin may decrease the levels/effects of: BCG; Mycophenolate; Typhoid Vaccine

The levels/effects of Amoxicillin may be decreased by: Fusidic Acid; Tetracycline Derivatives

Dietary Considerations May be taken with food.

Moxatag™: Take within 1 hour of finishing a meal.

Pharmacodynamics/Kinetics

Half-life Elimination

Neonates, full-term: 3.7 hours

Infants and Children: 1-2 hours

Adults: Normal renal function: 0.7-1.4 hours

Cl_{cr} <10 mL/minute: 7-21 hours

Time to Peak Capsule: 2 hours; Extended-release tablet: 3.1 hours; Suspension: 1 hour

Pregnancy Risk Factor B

Lactation Enters breast milk/use caution (AAP rates "compatible"; AAP 2001 update pending)

Breast-Feeding Considerations Very small amounts of amoxicillin are excreted in breast milk. The manufacturer recommends that caution be exercised when administering amoxicillin to nursing women. Nondose-related effects could include modification of bowel flora and allergic sensitization of the infant.

Dosage Forms

Capsule, oral: 250 mg, 500 mg

Powder for suspension, oral: 125 mg/5 mL (80 mL, 100 mL, 150 mL); 200 mg/5 mL (50 mL, 75 mL, 100 mL); 250 mg/5 mL (80 mL, 100 mL, 150 mL); 400 mg/5 mL (50 mL, 75 mL, 100 mL)

Tablet, oral: 500 mg, 875 mg

Tablet, chewable, oral: 125 mg, 200 mg, 250 mg, 400 mg

Tablet, extended release, oral:

Moxatag™: 775 mg

References

ADA Division of Legal Affairs, "A Legal Perspective on Antibiotic Prophylaxis," *J Am Dent Assoc*, 2003, 134(9):1260.

American Dental Association; American Academy of Orthopedic Surgeons, "Antibiotic Prophylaxis for Dental Patients With Total Joint Replacements," *J Am Dent Assoc*, 2003, 134(7):895-9.

American Dental Association Council on Scientific Affairs, "Combating Antibiotic Resistance," *J Am Dent Assoc*, 2004, 135(4):484-7.

Dajani AS, Taubert KA, Wilson W, et al, "Prevention of Bacterial Endocarditis. Recommendations by the American Heart Association," *JAMA*, 1997, 277(22):1794-801.

Dajani AS, Taubert KA, Wilson W, et al, "Prevention of Bacterial Endocarditis: Recommendations by the American Heart Association," *J Am Dent Assoc*, 1997, 128(8):1142-51.

Wilson W, Taubert KA, Gewitz M, et al, "Prevention of Infective Endocarditis. Guidelines From the American Heart Association. A Guideline From the American Heart Association Rheumatic Fever, Endocarditis, and Kawasaki Disease Committee, Council on Cardiovascular Disease in the Young, and the Council on Clinical Cardiology, Council on Cardiovascular Surgery and Anesthesia, and the Quality of Care and Outcomes Research Interdisciplinary Working Group," *Circulation*, 2007, 115. Available at http://circ.ahajournals.org/cgi/reprint/CIRCULATIONAHA.106.183095v1; last accessed July 26, 2007.

Wynn RL, Bergman SA, Meiller TF, et al, "Antibiotics in Treating Oral-Facial Infections of Odontogenic Origin: An Update", *Gen Dent*, 2001, 49(3):238-40, 242, 244 passim.

Amoxicillin and Clavulanate Potassium

(a moks i SIL in & klav yoo LAN ate poe TASS ee um)

Related Information

Amoxicillin *on page 124*

Bacterial Infections *on page 1933*

Related Sample Prescriptions

Bacterial Infections and Periodontal Diseases *on page 1983*

Sinus Infection Treatment *on page 1985*

U.S. Brand Names Amoclan; Augmentin ES-600® [DSC]; Augmentin XR®; Augmentin®

Canadian Brand Names Amoxi-Clav; Apo-Amoxi-Clav®; Augmentin®; Clavulin®; Novo-Clavamoxin; ratio-Aclavulanate

Generic Availability (U.S.) Yes

Pharmacologic Category Antibiotic, Penicillin

Dental Use Treatment of orofacial infections when beta-lactamase-producing staphylococci and beta-lactamase-producing *Bacteroides* are present

Use Treatment of otitis media, sinusitis, and infections caused by susceptible organisms involving the lower respiratory tract, skin and skin structure, and urinary tract; spectrum same as amoxicillin with additional coverage of beta-lactamase producing *B. catarrhalis*, *H. influenzae*, *N. gonorrhoeae*, and *S. aureus* (not MRSA). The expanded coverage of this combination makes it a useful alternative when amoxicillin resistance is present and patients cannot tolerate alternative treatments.

Local Anesthetic/Vasoconstrictor Precautions No information available to require special precautions

Effects on Dental Treatment Prolonged use of penicillins may lead to development of oral candidiasis (see Dental Comment)

Effects on Bleeding No information available to require special precautions

Adverse Effects

>10%: Gastrointestinal: Diarrhea (3% to 34%; incidence varies upon dose and regimen used)

1% to 10%:

Dermatologic: Diaper rash, skin rash, urticaria
Gastrointestinal: Abdominal discomfort, loose stools, nausea, vomiting
Genitourinary: Vaginitis, vaginal mycosis
Miscellaneous: Moniliasis

Additional adverse reactions seen with **ampicillin-class antibiotics:** Agitation, agranulocytosis, alkaline phosphatase increased, anaphylaxis, anemia, angioedema, anxiety, behavioral changes, bilirubin increased, black "hairy" tongue, confusion, convulsions, crystalluria, dizziness, enterocolitis, eosinophilia, erythema multiforme, exanthematous pustulosis, exfoliative dermatitis, gastritis, glossitis, hematuria, hemolytic anemia, hemorrhagic colitis, indigestion, insomnia, hyperactivity, interstitial nephritis, leukopenia, mucocutaneous candidiasis, pruritus, pseudomembranous colitis, serum sickness-like reaction, Stevens-Johnson syndrome, stomatitis, transaminases increased, thrombocytopenia, thrombocytopenic purpura, tooth discoloration, toxic epidermal necrolysis

Dental Usual Dosage Orofacial infections: Children >40 kg and Adults: Oral: 250-500 mg every 8 hours or 875 mg every 12 hours

Dosage Note: Dose is based on the amoxicillin component; see "Augmentin® Product-Specific Considerations" table on next page.

Usual dosage range:

Infants <3 months: Oral: 30 mg/kg/day divided every 12 hours using the 125 mg/5 mL suspension
Children ≥3 months and <40 kg: Oral: 20-90 mg/kg/day divided every 8-12 hours
Children >40 kg and Adults: Oral: 250-500 mg every 8 hours or 875 mg every 12 hours

Indication-specific dosing:

Children ≥3 months and <40 kg: Oral:

Lower respiratory tract infections, severe infections, sinusitis: 45 mg/kg/day divided every 12 hours **or** 40 mg/kg/day divided every 8 hours
Mild-to-moderate infections: 25 mg/kg/day divided every 12 hours or 20 mg/kg/day divided every 8 hours
Otitis media (Augmentin ES-600®): 90 mg/kg/day divided every 12 hours for 10 days in children with severe illness and when coverage for β-lactamase-positive *H. influenzae* and *M. catarrhalis* is needed.

Children ≥16 years and Adults: Oral:

Acute bacterial sinusitis: Extended release tablet: Two 1000 mg tablets every 12 hours for 10 days
Bite wounds (animal/human): 875 mg every 12 hours **or** 500 mg every 8 hours
Chronic obstructive pulmonary disease: 875 mg every 12 hours **or** 500 mg every 8 hours
Diabetic foot: Extended release tablet: Two 1000 mg tablets every 12 hours for 7-14 days
Diverticulitis, perirectal abscess: Extended release tablet: Two 1000 mg tablets every 12 hours for 7-10 days
Erysipelas: 875 mg every 12 hours **or** 500 mg every 8 hours
Febrile neutropenia: 875 mg every 12 hours
Pneumonia:
Aspiration: 875 mg every 12 hours
Community-acquired: Extended release tablet: Two 1000 mg tablets every 12 hours for 7-10 days
Pyelonephritis (acute, uncomplicated): 875 mg every 12 hours **or** 500 mg every 8 hours
Skin abscess: 875 mg every 12 hours

Dosing interval in renal impairment:

Cl_{cr} <30 mL/minute: Do not use 875 mg tablet or extended release tablets
Cl_{cr} 10-30 mL/minute: 250-500 mg every 12 hours
Cl_{cr} <10 mL/minute: 250-500 every 24 hours

Hemodialysis: Moderately dialyzable (20% to 50%)
250-500 mg every 24 hours; administer dose during and after dialysis. Do not use extended release tablets.

Peritoneal dialysis: Moderately dialyzable (20% to 50%)
Amoxicillin: Administer 250 mg every 12 hours
Clavulanic acid: Dose for Cl_{cr} <10 mL/minute

Continuous arteriovenous or venovenous hemofiltration effects:
Amoxicillin: ~50 mg of amoxicillin/L of filtrate is removed
Clavulanic acid: Dose for Cl_{cr} <10 mL/minute

Augmentin® Product-Specific Considerations

Strength	Form	Consideration
125 mg	S	q8h dosing
	S	For adults having difficulty swallowing tablets, 125 mg/5 mL suspension may be substituted for 500 mg tablet.
200 mg	CT, S	q12h dosing
	CT	Contains phenylalanine
	S	For adults having difficulty swallowing tablets, 200 mg/5 mL suspension may be substituted for 875 mg tablet.
250 mg	S, T	q8h dosing
	T	Not for use in patients <40 kg
	S	For adults having difficulty swallowing tablets, 250 mg/5 mL suspension may be substituted for 500 mg tablet.
400 mg	CT, S	q12h dosing
	CT	Contains phenylalanine
	S	For adults having difficulty swallowing tablets, 400 mg/5 mL suspension may be substituted for 875 mg tablet.
500 mg	T	q8h or q12h dosing
600 mg	S	q12h dosing
		Not for use in adults or children ≥40 kg
		600 mg/5 mL suspension is not equivalent to or interchangeable with 200 mg/5 mL or 400 mg/5 mL due to differences in clavulanic acid.
875 mg	T	q12h dosing; not for use in Cl_{cr} <30 mL/minute
1000 mg	XR	q12h dosing
		Not for use in children <16 years of age
		Not interchangeable with two 500 mg tablets
		Not for use if Cl_{cr} <30 mL/minute or hemodialysis

Legend: CT = chewable tablet, S = suspension, T = tablet, XR = extended release.

Mechanism of Action Clavulanic acid binds and inhibits beta-lactamases that inactivate amoxicillin resulting in amoxicillin having an expanded spectrum of activity. Amoxicillin inhibits bacterial cell wall synthesis by binding to one or more of the penicillin-binding proteins (PBPs) which in turn inhibits the final transpeptidation step of peptidoglycan synthesis in bacterial cell walls, thus inhibiting cell wall biosynthesis. Bacteria eventually lyse due to ongoing activity of cell wall autolytic enzymes (autolysins and murein hydrolases) while cell wall assembly is arrested.

Contraindications Hypersensitivity to amoxicillin, clavulanic acid, penicillin, or any component of the formulation; history of cholestatic jaundice or hepatic dysfunction with amoxicillin/clavulanate potassium therapy; Augmentin XR™: severe renal impairment (Cl_{cr} <30 mL/minute) and hemodialysis patients

Warnings/Precautions Hypersensitivity reactions, including anaphylaxis (some fatal), have been reported. Prolonged use may result in fungal or bacterial superinfection, including *C. difficile*-associated diarrhea (CDAD) and pseudomembranous colitis; CDAD has been observed >2 months postantibiotic treatment. In patients with renal impairment, doses and/or frequency of administration should be modified in response to the degree of renal impairment. High percentage of patients with infectious mononucleosis have developed rash during therapy; ampicillin-class antibiotics not recommended in these patients. Incidence of diarrhea is higher than with amoxicillin alone. Due to differing content of clavulanic acid, not all formulations are interchangeable. Low incidence of cross-allergy with cephalosporins exists. Some products contain phenylalanine.

Drug Interactions

Avoid Concomitant Use

Avoid concomitant use of Amoxicillin and Clavulanate Potassium with any of the following: BCG

Increased Effect/Toxicity

Amoxicillin and Clavulanate Potassium may increase the levels/effects of: Methotrexate

The levels/effects of Amoxicillin and Clavulanate Potassium may be increased by: Allopurinol; Probenecid

Decreased Effect

Amoxicillin and Clavulanate Potassium may decrease the levels/effects of: BCG; Mycophenolate; Typhoid Vaccine

The levels/effects of Amoxicillin and Clavulanate Potassium may be decreased by: Fusidic Acid; Tetracycline Derivatives

Dietary Considerations May be taken with meals or on an empty stomach; take with meals to increase absorption and decrease GI upset; may mix with milk, formula, or juice. Extended release tablets should be taken with food. Some products may contain sodium. Some products contain phenylalanine; if you have phenylketonuria or PKU, avoid use. All dosage forms contain potassium.

Pharmacodynamics/Kinetics

Half-life Elimination Clavulanic acid: 1 hour

Time to Peak Clavulanic acid: Serum: 1 hour

Pregnancy Risk Factor B

Lactation Enters breast milk/use caution

Breast-Feeding Considerations Amoxicillin is found in breast milk. The manufacturer recommends that caution be used if administered to breast-feeding women. The use of amoxicillin/clavulanate may be safe while breast-feeding; however, the risk of adverse events in the infant may be increased when compared to the use of amoxicillin alone. The risk of adverse events may be related to maternal dose. Nondose-related effects could include modification of bowel flora and allergic sensitization of the infant.

Dosage Forms

Powder for oral suspension: 200: Amoxicillin 200 mg and clavulanate potassium 28.5 mg per 5 mL; 250: Amoxicillin 250 mg and clavulanate potassium 62.5 mg per 5 mL; 400: Amoxicillin 400 mg and clavulanate potassium 57 mg per 5 mL; 600: Amoxicillin 600 mg and clavulanate potassium 42.9 mg per 5 mL

Amoclan:

200: Amoxicillin 200 mg and clavulanate potassium 28.5 mg per 5 mL
400: Amoxicillin 400 mg and clavulanate potassium 57 mg per 5 mL
600: Amoxicillin 600 mg and clavulanate potassium 42.9 mg per 5 mL

Augmentin®:

125: Amoxicillin 125 mg and clavulanate potassium 31.25 mg per 5 mL
250: Amoxicillin 250 mg and clavulanate potassium 62.5 mg per 5 mL

Tablet: 250: Amoxicillin 250 mg and clavulanate potassium 125 mg; 500: Amoxicillin 500 mg and clavulanate potassium 125 mg; 875: Amoxicillin 875 mg and clavulanate potassium 125 mg

Augmentin®:

500: Amoxicillin 500 mg and clavulanate potassium 125 mg
875: Amoxicillin 875 mg and clavulanate potassium 125 mg

Tablet, chewable: 200: Amoxicillin 200 mg and clavulanate potassium 28.5 mg; 400: Amoxicillin 400 mg and clavulanate potassium 57 mg

Tablet, extended release: Amoxicillin 1000 mg and clavulanate acid 62.5 mg

Augmentin XR®: 1000: Amoxicillin 1000 mg and clavulanate acid 62.5 mg

Dental Comment In maxillary sinus, anterior nasal cavity, and deep neck infections, beta-lactamase-producing staphylococci and beta-lactamase-producing *Bacteroides* usually are present. In these situations, antibiotics that resist the beta-lactamase enzyme are indicated. Amoxicillin and clavulanic acid is administered orally for moderate infections. Ampicillin sodium and sulbactam sodium (Unasyn®) is administered parenterally for more severe infections.

References

American Dental Association Council on Scientific Affairs, "Combating Antibiotic Resistance," *J Am Dent Assoc*, 2004, 135(4):484-7.

Wynn RL, Bergman SA, Meiller TF, et al, "Antibiotics in Treating Oral-Facial Infections of Odontogenic Origin: An Update," *Gen Dent*, 2001, 49(3):238-40, 242, 244 passim.

Amphotericin B Cholesteryl Sulfate Complex

(am foe TER i sin bee kole LES te ril SUL fate KOM plecks)

U.S. Brand Names Amphotec®

Canadian Brand Names Amphotec®

Pharmacologic Category Antifungal Agent, Parenteral

Use Treatment of invasive aspergillosis in patients who have failed amphotericin B deoxycholate treatment, or who have renal impairment or experience unacceptable toxicity which precludes treatment with amphotericin B deoxycholate in effective doses.

Unlabeled/Investigational Use Effective in patients with serious *Candida* species infections

Local Anesthetic/Vasoconstrictor Precautions No information available to require special precautions

Effects on Dental Treatment No significant effects or complications reported

Effects on Bleeding No information available to require special precautions

Adverse Effects

>10%: Central nervous system: Chills, fever

1% to 10%:

Cardiovascular: Hypotension, tachycardia

Central nervous system: Headache
Dermatologic: Rash
Endocrine & metabolic: Hypokalemia, hypomagnesemia
Gastrointestinal: Nausea, diarrhea, abdominal pain
Hematologic: Thrombocytopenia
Hepatic: LFT change
Neuromuscular & skeletal: Rigors
Renal: Creatinine increased
Respiratory: Dyspnea

Note: Amphotericin B colloidal dispersion has an improved therapeutic index compared to conventional amphotericin B, and has been used safely in patients with amphotericin B-related nephrotoxicity; however, continued decline of renal function has occurred in some patients.

General Dosage Range I.V.: *Children and Adults:* 3-4 mg/kg/day (maximum: 7.5 mg/kg/day)

Mechanism of Action Binds to ergosterol altering cell membrane permeability in susceptible fungi and causing leakage of cell components with subsequent cell death. Proposed mechanism suggests that amphotericin causes an oxidation-dependent stimulation of macrophages (Lyman, 1992).

Pharmacodynamics/Kinetics

Half-life Elimination 28-29 hours; prolonged with higher doses

Pregnancy Risk Factor B

Amphotericin B (Conventional) (am foe TER i sin bee con VEN sha nal)

Related Information

Fungal Infections *on page 1945*

Canadian Brand Names Fungizone®

Generic Availability (U.S.) Yes

Pharmacologic Category Antifungal Agent, Parenteral

Use Treatment of severe systemic and central nervous system infections caused by susceptible fungi such as *Candida* species, *Histoplasma capsulatum*, *Cryptococcus neoformans*, *Aspergillus* species, *Blastomyces dermatitidis*, *Torulopsis glabrata*, and *Coccidioides immitis*; fungal peritonitis; irrigant for bladder fungal infections; used in fungal infection in patients with bone marrow transplantation, amebic meningoencephalitis, ocular aspergillosis (intraocular injection), candidal cystitis (bladder irrigation), chemoprophylaxis (low-dose I.V.), immunocompromised patients at risk of aspergillosis (intranasal/nebulized), refractory meningitis (intrathecal), coccidioidal arthritis (intra-articular/I.M.).

Low-dose amphotericin B has been administered after bone marrow transplantation to reduce the risk of invasive fungal disease.

Local Anesthetic/Vasoconstrictor Precautions No information available to require special precautions

Effects on Dental Treatment No significant effects or complications reported

Effects on Bleeding No information available to require special precautions

Adverse Effects

>10%:

Central nervous system: Fever, chills, headache, malaise, generalized pain
Endocrine & metabolic: Hypokalemia, hypomagnesemia
Gastrointestinal: Anorexia
Hematologic: Anemia
Renal: Nephrotoxicity

1% to 10%:

Cardiovascular: Hypotension, hypertension, flushing
Central nervous system: Delirium, arachnoiditis, pain along lumbar nerves
Gastrointestinal: Nausea, vomiting
Genitourinary: Urinary retention
Hematologic: Leukocytosis
Local: Thrombophlebitis
Neuromuscular & skeletal: Paresthesia (especially with I.T. therapy)
Renal: Renal tubular acidosis, renal failure

Dosage Premedication: For patients who experience infusion-related immediate reactions, premedicate with the following drugs 30-60 minutes prior to drug administration: NSAID (with or without diphenhydramine) **or** acetaminophen with diphenhydramine **or** hydrocortisone 50-100 mg. If the patient experiences rigors during the infusion, meperidine may be administered.

Usual dosage ranges:

Infants and Children:

Test dose: I.V.: 0.1 mg/kg/dose to a maximum of 1 mg; infuse over 30-60 minutes. Many clinicians believe a test dose is unnecessary.

Maintenance dose: 0.25-1 mg/kg/day given once daily; infuse over 2-6 hours. Once therapy has been established, amphotericin B can be administered on an every-other-day basis at 1-1.5 mg/kg/dose; cumulative dose: 1.5-2 g over 6-10 weeks.

Duration of therapy: Varies with nature of infection, usual duration is 4-12 weeks or cumulative dose of 1-4 g

Adults:

Test dose: 1 mg infused over 20-30 minutes. Many clinicians believe a test dose is unnecessary.

Maintenance dose: Usual: 0.05-1.5 mg/kg/day; 1-1.5 mg/kg over 4-6 hours every other day may be given once therapy is established; aspergillosis, rhinocerebral mucormycosis, often require 1-1.5 mg/kg/day; do not exceed 1.5 mg/kg/day

Indication-specific dosing:

Infants and Children:

Aspergillosis (HIV-exposed/-positive): I.V.: 1-1.5 mg/kg/day once daily (CDC, 2009)

Candidiasis (HIV-exposed/-positive):

Invasive: I.V.: 0.5-1.5 mg/kg/day once daily (CDC, 2009)

Esophageal: I.V.: 0.3-0.5 mg/kg/day once daily (CDC, 2009)

Oropharyngeal, refractory: I.V.: 0.3-0.5 mg/kg/day (CDC, 2009)

Coccidioidomycosis (HIV-exposed/-positive): I.V.: 0.5-1 mg/kg/day (CDC, 2009)

***Cryptococcus*, CNS disease (HIV-exposed/-positive):** I.V.: 0.7-1 mg/kg/day plus flucytosine; **Note:** Minimum 2 week induction followed by consolidation and chronic suppressive therapy; may increase amphotericin dose to 1.5 mg/kg/day if flucytosine is not tolerated.

***Cryptococcus*, Disseminated (non-CNS disease) or severe pulmonary disease (HIV-exposed/-positive):** I.V.: 0.7-1 mg/kg/day once daily with or without flucytosine

Histoplasma, CNS or severe disseminated: I.V.: 1 mg/kg/day once daily (CDC, 2009)

Adults:

Aspergillosis, disseminated: I.V.: 0.6-0.7 mg/kg/day for 3-6 months

Bone marrow transplantation (prophylaxis): I.V.: Low-dose amphotericin B 0.1-0.25 mg/kg/day has been administered after bone marrow transplantation to reduce the risk of invasive fungal disease.

Candidemia (neutropenic or non-neutropenic): I.V.: 0.5-1 mg/kg/day until 14 days after first negative blood culture and resolution of signs and symptoms (Pappas, 2009)

Candidiasis, chronic, disseminated: I.V.: 0.5-0.7 mg/kg/day for 3-6 months and resolution of radiologic lesions (Pappas, 2009)

Dematiaceous fungi: I.V.: 0.7 mg/kg/day in combination with an azole

Endocarditis: I.V.: 0.6-1 mg/kg/day (with or without flucytosine) for 6 weeks after valve replacement; **Note:** If isolates susceptible and/or clearance demonstrated, guidelines recommend step-down to fluconazole; also for long-term suppression therapy if valve replacement is not possible (Pappas, 2009)

Endophthalmitis, fungal:

Intravitreal (unlabeled use): 10 mcg in 0.1 mL (in conjunction with systemic therapy)

I.V.: 0.7-1 mg/kg/day (with or without flucytosine) for at least 4-6 weeks (Pappas, 2009)

Esophageal candidiasis: I.V.: 0.3-0.7 mg/kg/day for 14-21 days after clinical improvement (Pappas, 2009)

Histoplasmosis: Chronic, severe pulmonary or disseminated: I.V.: 0.5-1 mg/kg/day for 7 days, then 0.8 mg/kg every other day (or 3 times/week) until total dose of 10-15 mg/kg; may continue itraconazole as suppressive therapy (lifelong for immunocompromised patients)

Meningitis:

Candidal: I.V.: 0.7-1 mg/kg/day (with or without flucytosine) for at least 4 weeks; **Note:** Liposomal amphotericin favored by IDSA guidelines based on decreased risk of nephrotoxicity and potentially better CNS penetration (Pappas, 2009)

Cryptococcal or Coccidioides: I.T.: Initial: 0.01-0.05 mg as single daily dose; may increase daily in increments of 0.025-0.1 mg as tolerated (maximum: 1.5 mg/day; most patients will tolerate a maximum dose of ~0.5 mg/treatment). Once titration to a maximum tolerated dose is achieved, that dose is administered daily. Once CSF improvement noted, may decrease frequency on a weekly basis (eg, 5 times/week, then 3 times/week, then 2 times/week, then once weekly, then once every other week, then once every 2 weeks, etc) until administration occurs once every 6 weeks. Typically, concurrent oral azole therapy is maintained (Stevens, 2001). **Note:** IDSA notes that the use of I.T. amphotericin for cryptococcal meningitis is generally discouraged and rarely necessary (Perfect, 2010).

Histoplasma: I.V.: 0.5-1 mg/kg/day for 7 days, then 0.8 mg/kg every other day (or 3 times/week) for 3 months total duration; follow with fluconazole suppressive therapy for up to 12 months

Meningoencephalitis, cryptococcal (Perfect, 2010): I.V.:

HIV positive: Induction: 0.7-1 mg/kg/day (plus flucytosine 100 mg/kg/day) for 2 weeks, then change to oral fluconazole for at least 8 weeks; alternatively, amphotericin (0.7-1 mg/kg/day) may be continued uninterrupted for 4-6 weeks; maintenance: amphotericin 1 mg/kg/week for ≥1 year may be considered, but inferior to use of azoles

HIV negative: Induction: 0.7-1 mg/kg/day (plus flucytosine 100 mg/kg/day) for 2 weeks (low-risk patients), ≥4 weeks (non-low-risk, but without neurologic complication, immunosuppression, underlying disease, and negative CSF culture at 2 weeks), >6 weeks (neurologic complication or patients intolerant of flucytosine) Follow with azole consolidation/maintenance treatment.

Oropharyngeal candidiasis: I.V.: 0.3 mg/kg/day for 7-14 days (Pappas, 2009)

Osteoarticular candidiasis: I.V.: 0.5-1 mg/kg/day for several weeks, followed by fluconazole for 6-12 months (osteomyelitis) or 6 weeks (septic arthritis) (Pappas, 2009)

Penicillium marneffei: I.V.: 0.6 mg/kg/day for 2 weeks

Pneumonia: Cryptococcal (mild-to-moderate): I.V.:

HIV positive: 0.5-1 mg/kg/day

HIV negative: 0.5-0.7 mg/kg/day (plus flucytosine) for 2 weeks

Sporotrichosis: Pulmonary, meningeal, osteoarticular, or disseminated: I.V.: Total dose of 1-2 g, then change to oral itraconazole or fluconazole for suppressive therapy

Urinary tract candidiasis (Pappas, 2009):

Fungus balls: I.V.: 0.5-0.7 mg/kg/day with or without flucytosine 25 mg/kg 4 times daily

Pyelonephritis: I.V.: 0.5-0.7 mg/kg/day with or without flucytosine 25 mg/kg 4 times daily for 2 weeks

Symptomatic cystitis: I.V.: 0.3-0.6 mg/kg/day for 1-7 days

Bladder irrigation: Irrigate with 50 mcg/mL solution instilled periodically or continuously for 5-10 days or until cultures are clear for fluconazole-resistant *Candida*

Dosing adjustment in renal impairment: If renal dysfunction is due to the drug, the daily total can be decreased by 50% or the dose can be given every other day; I.V. therapy may take several months

Dialysis: Poorly dialyzed; no supplemental dosage necessary when using hemo- or peritoneal dialysis or continuous renal replacement therapy (CRRT)

Administration in dialysate: Children and Adults: 1-2 mg/L of peritoneal dialysis fluid either with or without low-dose I.V. amphotericin B (a total dose of 2-10 mg/kg given over 7-14 days). Precipitate may form in ionic dialysate solutions.

Mechanism of Action Binds to ergosterol altering cell membrane permeability in susceptible fungi and causing leakage of cell components with subsequent cell death. Proposed mechanism suggests that amphotericin causes an oxidation-dependent stimulation of macrophages (Lyman, 1992).

Contraindications Hypersensitivity to amphotericin or any component of the formulation

Warnings/Precautions Anaphylaxis has been reported with amphotericin B-containing drugs. During the initial dosing, the drug should be administered under close clinical observation. May cause nephrotoxicity; usual risk factors include underlying renal disease, concomitant nephrotoxic medications and daily and/or cumulative dose of amphotericin. Avoid use with other nephrotoxic drugs; drug-induced renal toxicity usually improves with interrupting therapy, decreasing dosage, or increasing dosing interval. However permanent impairment may occur, especially in patients receiving large cumulative dose (eg, >5 g) and in those also receiving other nephrotoxic drugs. Hydration and sodium repletion prior to administration may reduce the risk of developing nephrotoxicity. Frequent monitoring of renal function is recommended. Acute reactions (eg, fever, shaking chills, hypotension, anorexia, nausea, vomiting, headache, tachypnea) are most common 1-3 hours after starting the infusion and diminish with continued therapy. Avoid rapid infusion to prevent hypotension, hypokalemia, arrhythmias, and shock. If therapy is stopped for >7 days, restart at the lowest dose recommended and increase gradually. Leukoencephalopathy has been reported following administration of amphotericin. Total body irradiation has been reported to be a possible predisposition.

[U.S. Boxed Warning]: Should be used primarily for treatment of progressive, potentially life-threatening fungal infections, not noninvasive forms of infection. [U.S. Boxed warning]: Verify the product name and dosage if dose exceeds 1.5 mg/kg.

Drug Interactions

Avoid Concomitant Use

Avoid concomitant use of Amphotericin B (Conventional) with any of the following: Gallium Nitrate

Increased Effect/Toxicity

Amphotericin B (Conventional) may increase the levels/effects of: Aminoglycosides; Colistimethate; CycloSPORINE; CycloSPORINE (Systemic); Flucytosine; Gallium Nitrate

The levels/effects of Amphotericin B (Conventional) may be increased by: Corticosteroids (Orally Inhaled); Corticosteroids (Systemic)

Decreased Effect

Amphotericin B (Conventional) may decrease the levels/effects of: Saccharomyces boulardii

The levels/effects of Amphotericin B (Conventional) may be decreased by: Antifungal Agents (Azole Derivatives, Systemic)

Pharmacodynamics/Kinetics

Half-life Elimination Biphasic: Initial: 15-48 hours; Terminal: 15 days

Time to Peak Within 1 hour following a 4- to 6-hour dose

Pregnancy Risk Factor B

Lactation Excretion in breast milk unknown/contraindicated

Dosage Forms

Injection, powder for reconstitution: 50 mg

Amphotericin B (Lipid Complex) (am foe TER i sin bee LIP id KOM pleks)

U.S. Brand Names Abelcet®

Canadian Brand Names Abelcet®

Pharmacologic Category Antifungal Agent, Parenteral

Use Treatment of aspergillosis or any type of progressive fungal infection in patients who are refractory to or intolerant of conventional amphotericin B therapy

Unlabeled/Investigational Use Effective in patients with serious *Candida* species infections

Local Anesthetic/Vasoconstrictor Precautions No information available to require special precautions

Effects on Dental Treatment No significant effects or complications reported

Effects on Bleeding No information available to require special precautions

Adverse Effects Nephrotoxicity and infusion-related hyperpyrexia, rigor, and chilling are reduced relative to amphotericin deoxycholate.

>10%:

- Central nervous system: Chills, fever
- Renal: Serum creatinine increased
- Miscellaneous: Multiple organ failure

1% to 10%:

- Cardiovascular: Hypotension, cardiac arrest
- Central nervous system: Headache, pain
- Dermatologic: Rash
- Endocrine & metabolic: Bilirubinemia, hypokalemia, acidosis
- Gastrointestinal: Nausea, vomiting, diarrhea, gastrointestinal hemorrhage, abdominal pain
- Renal: Renal failure
- Respiratory: Respiratory failure, dyspnea, pneumonia

General Dosage Range Dosage adjustment recommended in patients who develop toxicities

I.V.: *Children and Adults:* 2.5-5 mg/kg/day as a single daily dose (maximum: 5 mg/kg/day)

Mechanism of Action Binds to ergosterol altering cell membrane permeability in susceptible fungi and causing leakage of cell components with subsequent cell death. Proposed mechanism suggests that amphotericin causes an oxidation-dependent stimulation of macrophages.

Pharmacodynamics/Kinetics

Half-life Elimination ~24 hours

Pregnancy Risk Factor B

Amphotericin B (Liposomal) (am foe TER i sin bee lye po SO mal)

U.S. Brand Names AmBisome®

Canadian Brand Names AmBisome®

Pharmacologic Category Antifungal Agent, Parenteral

Use Empirical therapy for presumed fungal infection in febrile, neutropenic patients; treatment of patients with *Aspergillus* species, *Candida* species, and/or *Cryptococcus* species infections refractory to amphotericin B desoxycholate (conventional amphotericin), or in patients where renal impairment or unacceptable toxicity precludes the use of amphotericin B desoxycholate; treatment of cryptococcal meningitis in HIV-infected patients; treatment of visceral leishmaniasis

Unlabeled/Investigational Use Treatment of systemic *Histoplasmosis* infection

Local Anesthetic/Vasoconstrictor Precautions No information available to require special precautions

Effects on Dental Treatment Key adverse event(s) related to dental treatment: Facial swelling, postural hypotension, mucositis, stomatitis, and ulcerative stomatitis (see Dental Comment)

Effects on Bleeding No information available to require special precautions

Adverse Effects Percentage of adverse reactions is dependent upon population studied and may vary with respect to premedications and underlying illness. Incidence of decreased renal function and infusion-related events are lower than rates observed with amphotericin B deoxycholate.

>10%:

Cardiovascular: Peripheral edema (15%), edema (12% to 14%), tachycardia (9% to 19%), hypotension (7% to 14%), hypertension (8% to 20%), chest pain (8% to 12%), hypervolemia (8% to 12%)

Central nervous system: Chills (29% to 48%), insomnia (17% to 22%), headache (9% to 20%), anxiety (7% to 14%), pain (14%), confusion (9% to 13%)

Dermatologic: Rash (5% to 25%), pruritus (11%)

Endocrine & metabolic: Hypokalemia (31% to 51%), hypomagnesemia (15% to 50%), hyperglycemia (8% to 23%), hypocalcemia (5% to 18%), hyponatremia (9% to 12%)

Gastrointestinal: Nausea (16% to 40%), vomiting (11% to 32%), diarrhea (11% to 30%), abdominal pain (7% to 20%), constipation (15%), anorexia (10% to 14%)

Hematologic: Anemia (27% to 48%), blood transfusion reaction (9% to 18%), leukopenia (15% to 17%), thrombocytopenia (6% to 13%)

Hepatic: Alkaline phosphatase increased (7% to 22%), bilirubinemia (≤18%), ALT increased (15%), AST increased (13%), liver function tests abnormal (not specified) (4% to 13%)

Local: Phlebitis (9% to 11%)

Neuromuscular & skeletal: Weakness (6% to 13%), back pain (12%)

Renal: Nephrotoxicity (14% to 47%), creatinine increased (18% to 40%), BUN increased (7% to 21%), hematuria (14%)

Respiratory: Dyspnea (18% to 23%), lung disorder (14% to 18%), cough (2% to 18%), epistaxis (9% to 15%), pleural effusion (13%), rhinitis (11%)

Miscellaneous: Infusion reactions (4% to 21%), sepsis (7% to 14%), infection (11% to 13%)

2% to 10%:

Cardiovascular: Arrhythmia, atrial fibrillation, bradycardia, cardiac arrest, cardiomegaly, facial swelling, flushing, postural hypotension, valvular heart disease, vascular disorder, vasodilation

Central nervous system: Agitation, abnormal thinking, coma, depression, dysesthesia, dizziness (7% to 9%), hallucinations, malaise, nervousness, seizure, somnolence

Dermatologic: Alopecia, bruising, cellulitis, dry skin, maculopapular rash, petechia, purpura, skin discoloration, skin disorder, skin ulcer, urticaria, vesiculobullous rash

Endocrine & metabolic: Acidosis, fluid overload, hypernatremia (4%), hyperchloremia, hyperkalemia, hypermagnesemia, hyperphosphatemia, hypophosphatemia, hypoproteinemia, lactate dehydrogenase increased, nonprotein nitrogen increased

Gastrointestinal: Abdomen enlarged, amylase increased, dyspepsia, dysphagia, eructation, fecal incontinence, flatulence, gastrointestinal hemorrhage (10%), hematemesis, hemorrhoids, gum/oral hemorrhage, ileus, mucositis, rectal disorder, stomatitis, ulcerative stomatitis, xerostomia

Genitourinary: Vaginal hemorrhage

Hematologic: Coagulation disorder, hemorrhage, prothrombin decreased

Hepatic: Hepatocellular damage, hepatomegaly, veno-occlusive liver disease

Local: Injection site inflammation

Neuromuscular & skeletal: Arthralgia, bone pain, dystonia, myalgia, neck pain, paresthesia, rigors, tremor

Ocular: Conjunctivitis, dry eyes, eye hemorrhage

Renal: Abnormal renal function, acute renal failure, dysuria, renal failure, toxic nephropathy, urinary incontinence

Respiratory: Asthma, atelectasis, dry nose, hemoptysis, hyperventilation, pharyngitis, pneumonia, pulmonary edema, respiratory alkalosis, respiratory insufficiency, respiratory failure, sinusitis, hypoxia (6% to 8%)

Miscellaneous: Allergic reaction, cell-mediated immunological reaction, flu-like syndrome, graft-versus-host disease, herpes simplex, hiccup, procedural complication (8% to 10%), diaphoresis (7%)

General Dosage Range I.V.: *Children and Adults:* 3-6 mg/kg/day as a single daily dose (maximum: 6 mg/kg/day)

Mechanism of Action Binds to ergosterol altering cell membrane permeability in susceptible fungi and causing leakage of cell components with subsequent cell death. Proposed mechanism suggests that amphotericin causes an oxidation-dependent stimulation of macrophages (Lyman, 1992).

Pharmacodynamics/Kinetics

Half-life Elimination Terminal: 174 hours

Pregnancy Risk Factor B

Dental Comment Amphotericin B, liposomal is a true single bilayer liposomal drug delivery system. Liposomes are closed, spherical vesicles created by mixing specific proportions of amphophilic substances such as phospholipids and cholesterol so that they arrange themselves into multiple concentric bilayer membranes when hydrated in aqueous solutions. Single bilayer liposomes are then formed by microemulsification of multilamellar vesicles using a homogenizer. Amphotericin B, liposomal consists of these unilamellar bilayer liposomes with amphotericin B intercalated within the membrane. Due to the nature and quantity of amphophilic substances used, and the lipophilic moiety in the amphotericin B molecule, the drug is an integral part of the overall structure of the amphotericin B liposomes. Amphotericin B, liposomal contains true liposomes that are <100 nm in diameter.

Ampicillin (am pi SIL in)

Related Information

Antibiotic Prophylaxis *on page 1910*

Canadian Brand Names Apo-Ampi®; Novo-Ampicillin; Nu-Ampi

Generic Availability (U.S.) Yes

Pharmacologic Category Antibiotic, Penicillin

Dental Use I.V. or I.M. administration for the prevention of infective endocarditis in patients not allergic to penicillin and unable to take oral amoxicillin; I.V. or I.M. administration for prophylaxis in total joint replacement patients not allergic to penicillin and unable to take oral medications undergoing dental procedures which produce bacteremia

Use Treatment of susceptible bacterial infections (nonbeta-lactamase-producing organisms); treatment or prophylaxis of infective endocarditis; susceptible bacterial infections caused by streptococci, pneumococci, nonpenicillinase-producing staphylococci, *Listeria*, meningococci; some strains of *H. influenzae*, *Salmonella*, *Shigella*, *E. coli*, *Enterobacter*, and *Klebsiella*

Local Anesthetic/Vasoconstrictor Precautions No information available to require special precautions

Effects on Dental Treatment Key adverse event(s) related to dental treatment: Oral candidiasis, black hairy tongue, glossitis, sore mouth or tongue, and stomatitis.

Effects on Bleeding No information available to require special precautions

Adverse Effects Frequency not defined.

Central nervous system: Fever, penicillin encephalopathy, seizure

Dermatologic: Erythema multiforme, exfoliative dermatitis, rash, urticaria

Note: Appearance of a rash should be carefully evaluated to differentiate (if possible) nonallergic ampicillin rash from hypersensitivity reaction. Incidence is higher in patients with viral infection, *Salmonella* infection, lymphocytic leukemia, or patients that have hyperuricemia.

Gastrointestinal: Black hairy tongue, diarrhea, enterocolitis, glossitis, nausea, oral candidiasis, pseudomembranous colitis, sore mouth or tongue, stomatitis, vomiting

Hematologic: Agranulocytosis, anemia, hemolytic anemia, eosinophilia, leukopenia, thrombocytopenia purpura

Hepatic: AST increased

Renal: Interstitial nephritis (rare)

Respiratory: Laryngeal stridor

Miscellaneous: Anaphylaxis, serum sickness-like reaction

Dental Usual Dosage

Infective endocarditis prophylaxis: I.M., I.V.: Dental, oral, or respiratory tract procedures:

Infants and Children: 50 mg/kg within 30-60 minutes prior to procedure in patients not allergic to penicillin and unable to take oral amoxicillin.

Adults: 2 g within 30-60 minutes prior to procedure in patients not allergic to penicillin and unable to take oral amoxicillin.

Note: Intramuscular injections should be avoided in patients who are receiving anticoagulant therapy. In these circumstances, orally administered regimens should be given whenever possible. Intravenously administered antibiotics should be used for patients who are unable to tolerate or absorb oral medications.

Note: American Heart Association (AHA) guidelines now recommend prophylaxis only in patients undergoing invasive procedures and in whom underlying cardiac conditions may predispose to a higher risk of adverse outcomes should infection occur.

Prophylaxis in total joint replacement patient: Adults: I.M., I.V.: 2 g 1 hour prior to the procedure

Dosage

Usual dosage range:

Infants and Children:

Oral: 50-100 mg/kg/day in doses divided every 6 hours (maximum: 2-4 g/day)

I.M., I.V.: 100-400 mg/kg/day in divided doses every 6 hours (maximum: 12 g/day)

Adults: Oral, I.M., I.V.: 250-500 mg every 6 hours

Indication-specific dosing:

Infants and Children:

Prophylaxis against infective endocarditis:

Dental, oral, or respiratory tract procedures: I.M., I.V.: 50 mg/kg within 30-60 minutes prior to procedure in patients not allergic to penicillin and unable to take oral amoxicillin. Intramuscular injections should be avoided in patients who are receiving anticoagulant therapy. In these circumstances, orally administered regimens should be given whenever possible. Intravenously administered antibiotics should be used for patients who are unable to tolerate or absorb oral medications.

Note: American Heart Association (AHA) guidelines now recommend prophylaxis only in patients undergoing invasive procedures and in whom underlying cardiac conditions may predispose to a higher risk of adverse outcomes should infection occur.

Genitourinary and gastrointestinal tract procedures: I.M., I.V.:

High-risk patients: 50 mg/kg (maximum: 2 g) within 30 minutes prior to procedure, followed by ampicillin 25 mg/kg (or amoxicillin 25 mg/kg orally) 6 hours later; must be used in combination with gentamicin. **Note:** As of April 2007, routine prophylaxis for GI/GU procedures is no longer recommended by the AHA.

Moderate-risk patients: 50 mg/kg within 30 minutes prior to procedure

Mild-to-moderate infections:

Oral: 50-100 mg/kg/day in doses divided every 6 hours (maximum: 2-4 g/day)

I.M., I.V.: 100-150 mg/kg/day in divided doses every 6 hours (maximum: 2-4 g/day)

Severe infections, meningitis: I.M., I.V.: 200-400 mg/kg/day in divided doses every 6 hours (maximum: 6-12 g/day)

Adults:

Actinomycosis: I.V.: 50 mg/kg/day for 4-6 weeks then oral amoxicillin

Cholangitis (acute): I.V.: 2 g every 4 hours with gentamicin

Diverticulitis: I.M., I.V.: 2 g every 6 hours with metronidazole

Endocarditis:

Infective: I.V.: 12 g/day via continuous infusion or divided every 4 hours

Prophylaxis: Dental, oral, or respiratory tract: I.M., I.V.: 2 g within 30-60 minutes prior to procedure in patients not allergic to penicillin and unable to take oral amoxicillin. Intramuscular injections should be avoided in patients who are receiving anticoagulant therapy. In these circumstances, orally administered regimens should be given whenever possible. Intravenously administered antibiotics should be used for patients who are unable to tolerate or absorb oral medications.

Note: American Heart Association (AHA) guidelines now recommend prophylaxis only in patients undergoing invasive procedures and in whom underlying cardiac conditions may predispose to a higher risk of adverse outcomes should infection occur.

Prophylaxis in total joint replacement patient: I.M., I.V.: 2 g 1 hour prior to the procedure

Genitourinary and gastrointestinal tract procedures:
High-risk patients: I.M., I.V.: 2 g within 30 minutes prior to procedure, followed by ampicillin 1 g (or amoxicillin 1 g orally) 6 hours later; must be used in combination with gentamicin. **Note:** As of April 2007, routine prophylaxis for GI/GU procedures is no longer recommended by the AHA.
Moderate-risk patients: I.M., I.V.: 2 g within 30 minutes prior to procedure
Group B strep prophylaxis (intrapartum): I.V.: 2 g initial dose, then 1 g every 4 hours until delivery
***Listeria* infections:** I.V.: 2 g every 4 hours (consider addition of aminoglycoside)
Sepsis/meningitis: I.M., I.V.: 150-250 mg/kg/day divided every 3-4 hours (range: 6-12 g/day)
Urinary tract infections (*Enterococcus* suspected): I.V.: 1-2 g every 6 hours with gentamicin

Dosing interval in renal impairment:
Cl_{cr} >50 mL/minute: Administer every 6 hours
Cl_{cr} 10-50 mL/minute: Administer every 6-12 hours
Cl_{cr} <10 mL/minute: Administer every 12-24 hours
Hemodialysis: Moderately dialyzable (20% to 50%); administer dose after dialysis
Peritoneal dialysis: Moderately dialyzable (20% to 50%)
Administer 250 mg every 12 hours
Continuous arteriovenous or venovenous hemofiltration effects: Dose as for Cl_{cr} 10-50 mL/minute; ~50 mg of ampicillin per liter of filtrate is removed

Mechanism of Action Inhibits bacterial cell wall synthesis by binding to one or more of the penicillin-binding proteins (PBPs) which in turn inhibits the final transpeptidation step of peptidoglycan synthesis in bacterial cell walls, thus inhibiting cell wall biosynthesis. Bacteria eventually lyse due to ongoing activity of cell wall autolytic enzymes (autolysins and murein hydrolases) while cell wall assembly is arrested.

Contraindications Hypersensitivity to ampicillin, any component of the formulation, or other penicillins

Warnings/Precautions Dosage adjustment may be necessary in patients with renal impairment. Serious and occasionally severe or fatal hypersensitivity (anaphylactoid) reactions have been reported in patients on penicillin therapy, especially with a history of beta-lactam hypersensitivity, history of sensitivity to multiple allergens, or previous IgE-mediated reactions (eg, anaphylaxis, angioedema, urticaria). Use with caution in asthmatic patients. High percentage of patients with infectious mononucleosis have developed rash during therapy with ampicillin; ampicillin-class antibiotics not recommended in these patients. Appearance of a rash should be carefully evaluated to differentiate a nonallergic ampicillin rash from a hypersensitivity reaction. Ampicillin rash occurs in 5% to 10% of children receiving ampicillin and is a generalized dull red, maculopapular rash, generally appearing 3-14 days after the start of therapy. It normally begins on the trunk and spreads over most of the body. It may be most intense at pressure areas, elbows, and knees. Prolonged use may result in fungal or bacterial superinfection, including *C. difficile*-associated diarrhea (CDAD) and pseudomembranous colitis; CDAD has been observed >2 months postantibiotic treatment.

Drug Interactions

Avoid Concomitant Use

Avoid concomitant use of Ampicillin with any of the following: BCG

Increased Effect/Toxicity

Ampicillin may increase the levels/effects of: Methotrexate

The levels/effects of Ampicillin may be increased by: Allopurinol; Probenecid

Decreased Effect

Ampicillin may decrease the levels/effects of: Atenolol; BCG; Mycophenolate; Typhoid Vaccine

The levels/effects of Ampicillin may be decreased by: Chloroquine; Fusidic Acid; Tetracycline Derivatives

Ethanol/Nutrition/Herb Interactions Food: Food decreases ampicillin absorption rate; may decrease ampicillin serum concentration.

Dietary Considerations Take on an empty stomach 1 hour before or 2 hours after meals. Some products may contain sodium.

Pharmacodynamics/Kinetics

Half-life Elimination
Children and Adults: 1-1.8 hours
Anuria/end-stage renal disease: 7-20 hours

Time to Peak Oral: Within 1-2 hours

Pregnancy Risk Factor B

Lactation Enters breast milk/use caution

Breast-Feeding Considerations Ampicillin is excreted in breast milk. The manufacturer recommends that caution be exercised when administering ampicillin to nursing women. Due to the low concentrations in human milk, minimal toxicity would be expected in the nursing infant. Nondose-related effects could include modification of bowel flora and allergic sensitization.

Dosage Forms

Capsule, oral: 250 mg, 500 mg

Injection, powder for reconstitution: 125 mg, 250 mg, 500 mg, 1 g, 2 g, 10 g

Powder for suspension, oral: 125 mg/5 mL (100 mL, 200 mL); 250 mg/5 mL (100 mL, 200 mL)

References

ADA Division of Legal Affairs, "A Legal Perspective on Antibiotic Prophylaxis," *J Am Dent Assoc*, 2003, 134(9):1260.

American Dental Association; American Academy of Orthopedic Surgeons, "Antibiotic Prophylaxis for Dental Patients With Total Joint Replacements," *J Am Dent Assoc*, 2003, 134(7):895-9.

American Dental Association Council on Scientific Affairs, "Combating Antibiotic Resistance," *J Am Dent Assoc*, 2004, 135(4):484-7.

Dajani AS, Taubert KA, Wilson W, et al, "Prevention of Bacterial Endocarditis. Recommendations by the American Heart Association," *JAMA*, 1997, 277(22):1794-801.

Dajani AS, Taubert KA, Wilson W, et al, "Prevention of Bacterial Endocarditis: Recommendations by the American Heart Association," *J Am Dent Assoc*, 1997, 128(8):1142-51.

Wilson W, Taubert KA, Gewitz M, et al, "Prevention of Infective Endocarditis. Guidelines From the American Heart Association. A Guideline From the American Heart Association Rheumatic Fever, Endocarditis, and Kawasaki Disease Committee, Council on Cardiovascular Disease in the Young, and the Council on Clinical Cardiology, Council on Cardiovascular Surgery and Anesthesia, and the Quality of Care and Outcomes Research Interdisciplinary Working Group," *Circulation*, 2007, 115. Available at http://circ.ahajournals.org/cgi/reprint/CIRCULATIONAHA.106.183095v1; last accessed July 26, 2007.

Wynn RL, Bergman SA, Meiller TF, et al, "Antibiotics in Treating Oral-Facial Infections of Odontogenic Origin: An Update", *Gen Dent*, 2001, 49(3):238-40, 242, 244 passim.

Ampicillin and Sulbactam (am pi SIL in & SUL bak tam)

Related Information

Ampicillin *on page 136*

Sexually-Transmitted Diseases *on page 1903*

U.S. Brand Names Unasyn®

Canadian Brand Names Unasyn®

Generic Availability (U.S.) Yes

Pharmacologic Category Antibiotic, Penicillin

Dental Use Parenteral beta-lactamase-resistant antibiotic combination to treat more severe orofacial infections where beta-lactamase-producing staphylococci and beta-lactamase-producing *Bacteroides* are present

Use Treatment of susceptible bacterial infections involved with skin and skin structure, intra-abdominal infections, gynecological infections; spectrum is that of ampicillin plus organisms producing beta-lactamases such as *S. aureus*, *H. influenzae*, *E. coli*, *Klebsiella*, *Acinetobacter*, *Enterobacter*, and anaerobes

Local Anesthetic/Vasoconstrictor Precautions No information available to require special precautions

Effects on Dental Treatment Prolonged use of penicillins may lead to development of oral candidiasis (see Dental Comment)

Effects on Bleeding No information available to require special precautions

Adverse Effects Also see Ampicillin.

>10%: Local: Pain at injection site (I.M.)

1% to 10%:

Dermatologic: Rash

Gastrointestinal: Diarrhea

Local: Pain at injection site (I.V.), thrombophlebitis

Miscellaneous: Allergic reaction (may include serum sickness, urticaria, bronchospasm, hypotension, etc)

Dental Usual Dosage Severe orofacial infections: Adults: I.M., I.V.: 1-2 g ampicillin (1.5-3 g Unasyn®) every 6 hours (maximum: 8 g ampicillin/day, 12 g Unasyn®)

Dosage Note: Unasyn® (ampicillin/sulbactam) is a combination product. Dosage recommendations for Unasyn® are based on the ampicillin component.

Usual dosage range:

Children ≥1 year: I.V.: 100-400 mg ampicillin/kg/day divided every 6 hours (maximum: 8 g ampicillin/day, 12 g Unasyn®). **Note:** The American Academy of Pediatrics recommends a dose of up to 300 mg/kg/day for severe infection in infants >1 month of age.

Adults: I.M., I.V.: 1-2 g ampicillin (1.5-3 g Unasyn®) every 6 hours (maximum: 8 g ampicillin/day, 12 g Unasyn®)

Indication-specific dosing:

Children: ≥1 year:

Epiglottitis: I.V.: 100-200 mg ampicillin/kg/day divided in 4 doses

Mild-to-moderate infections: I.V.: 100-200 mg ampicillin/kg/day (150-300 mg Unasyn®) divided every 6 hours (maximum: 8 g ampicillin/day, 12 g Unasyn®)

Peritonsillar and retropharyngeal abscess: I.V.: 50 mg ampicillin/kg/dose every 6 hours

Severe infections: I.V.: 200-400 mg ampicillin/kg/day divided every 6 hours (maximum: 8 g ampicillin/day, 12 g Unasyn®)

Adults: Doses expressed as ampicillin/sulbactam combination:

Amnionitis, cholangitis, diverticulitis, endometritis, endophthalmitis, epididymitis/orchitis, liver abscess, osteomyelitis (diabetic foot), peritonitis: I.V.: 3 g every 6 hours; **Note:** Due to high rates of *E. coli* resistance, not recommended for the treatment of community-acquired intra-abdominal infections (Solomkin, 2010)

Endocarditis: I.V.: 3 g every 6 hours with gentamicin or vancomycin for 4-6 weeks

Orbital cellulitis: I.V.: 1.5 g every 6 hours

Parapharyngeal space infections: I.V.: 3 g every 6 hours

***Pasteurella multocida* (human, canine/feline bites):** I.V.: 1.5-3 g every 6 hours

Pelvic inflammatory disease: I.V.: 3 g every 6 hours with doxycycline

Peritonitis (CAPD): Intraperitoneal:

Anuric, intermittent: 3 g every 12 hours

Anuric, continuous: Loading dose: 1.5 g; maintenance dose: 150 mg

Pneumonia:

Aspiration, community-acquired: I.V.: 1.5-3 g every 6 hours

Hospital-acquired: I.V.: 3 g every 6 hours

Urinary tract infections, pyelonephritis: I.V.: 3 g every 6 hours for 14 days

Dosing interval in renal impairment: Note: Estimation of renal function for the purpose of drug dosing should be done using the Cockcroft-Gault formula.

Cl_{cr} 15-29 mL/minute/1.73 m^2: 1.5-3 g every 12 hours

Cl_{cr} 5-14 mL/minute/1.73 m^2: 1.5-3 g every 24 hours

Intermittent hemodialysis (IHD): 1.5-3 g every 12-24 hours (administer after hemodialysis on dialysis days) (Heintz, 2009). **Note:** Dosing dependent on the assumption of 3 times/week, complete IHD sessions.

Continuous ambulatory peritoneal dialysis (CAPD): 3 g every 24 hours

Continuous renal replacement therapy (CRRT): Drug clearance is highly dependent on the method of renal replacement, filter type, and flow rate. Appropriate dosing requires close monitoring of pharmacologic response, signs of adverse reactions due to drug accumulation, as well as drug levels in relation to target trough (if appropriate). The following are general recommendations only (based on dialysate flow/ultrafiltration rates of 1-2 L/hour and minimal residual renal function) and should not supersede clinical judgment (Heintz, 2009; Trotman, 2005):

CVVH: Initial: 3 g; maintenance: 1.5-3 g every 8-12 hours

CVVHD: Initial: 3 g; maintenance: 1.5-3 g every 8 hours

CVVHDF: Initial: 3 g; maintenance: 1.5-3 g every 6-8 hours

Mechanism of Action The addition of sulbactam, a beta-lactamase inhibitor, to ampicillin extends the spectrum of ampicillin to include some beta-lactamase-producing organisms; inhibits bacterial cell wall synthesis by binding to one or more of the penicillin-binding proteins (PBPs) which in turn inhibits the final transpeptidation step of peptidoglycan synthesis in bacterial cell walls, thus inhibiting cell wall biosynthesis. Bacteria eventually lyse due to ongoing activity of cell wall autolytic enzymes (autolysins and murein hydrolases) while cell wall assembly is arrested.

Contraindications Hypersensitivity to ampicillin, sulbactam, penicillins, or any component of the formulations

Warnings/Precautions Dosage adjustment may be necessary in patients with renal impairment. Serious and occasionally severe or fatal hypersensitivity (anaphylactoid) reactions have been reported in patients on penicillin therapy, especially with a history of beta-lactam hypersensitivity, history of sensitivity to multiple allergens, or previous IgE-mediated reactions (eg, anaphylaxis, angioedema, urticaria). Use with caution in asthmatic patients. High percentage of patients with infectious mononucleosis have developed rash during therapy with ampicillin; ampicillin-class antibiotics not recommended in these patients. Appearance of a rash should be carefully evaluated to differentiate a nonallergic ampicillin rash from a hypersensitivity reaction. Prolonged use may result in fungal or bacterial superinfection, including *C. difficile*-associated diarrhea (CDAD) and pseudomembranous colitis; CDAD has been observed >2 months postantibiotic treatment.

Drug Interactions

Avoid Concomitant Use

Avoid concomitant use of Ampicillin and Sulbactam with any of the following: BCG

Increased Effect/Toxicity

Ampicillin and Sulbactam may increase the levels/effects of: Methotrexate

The levels/effects of Ampicillin and Sulbactam may be increased by: Allopurinol; Probenecid

Decreased Effect

Ampicillin and Sulbactam may decrease the levels/effects of: Atenolol; BCG; Mycophenolate; Typhoid Vaccine

The levels/effects of Ampicillin and Sulbactam may be decreased by: Chloroquine; Fusidic Acid; Tetracycline Derivatives

Dietary Considerations Some products may contain sodium.

Pharmacodynamics/Kinetics

Half-life Elimination Sulbactam: Normal renal function: 1-1.3 hours

Pregnancy Risk Factor B

Lactation Enters breast milk/use caution

Breast-Feeding Considerations Ampicillin and sulbactam are both excreted into breast milk in low concentrations. The manufacturer recommends that caution be used if administering to lactating women. Nondose-related effects could include modification of bowel flora and allergic sensitization of the infant. The maternal dose of sulbactam does not need altered in the postpartum period. Also refer to the Ampicillin monograph.

Dosage Forms

Injection, powder for reconstitution: 1.5 g [ampicillin 1 g and sulbactam 0.5 g]; 3 g [ampicillin 2 g and sulbactam 1 g]; 15 g [ampicillin 10 g and sulbactam 5 g]

Unasyn®: 1.5 g [ampicillin 1 g and sulbactam 0.5 g]; 3 g [ampicillin 2 g and sulbactam 1 g]; 15 g [ampicillin 10 g and sulbactam 5 g]; 15 g [ampicillin 10 g and sulbactam 5 g]

Dental Comment In maxillary sinus, anterior nasal cavity, and deep neck infections, beta-lactamase-producing staphylococci and beta-lactamase-producing *Bacteroides* usually are present. In these situations, antibiotics that resist the beta-lactamase enzyme should be administered. Amoxicillin and clavulanic acid is administered orally for moderate infections. Ampicillin sodium and sulbactam sodium (Unasyn®) is administered parenterally for more severe infections.

Amsacrine (AM sah kreen)

Canadian Brand Names AMSA PD

Pharmacologic Category Antineoplastic Agent

Use Refractory acute leukemia

Unlabeled/Investigational Use Acute myeloid leukemia (AML)

Local Anesthetic/Vasoconstrictor Precautions No information available to require special precautions

Effects on Dental Treatment Key adverse event(s) related to dental treatment: Oral ulcerations and stomatitis

Effects on Bleeding Chemotherapy may result in significant myelosuppression, potentially including significant reduction in platelet counts and altered hemostasis. In patients who are under active treatment with these agents, medical consult is suggested.

Adverse Effects

>10%:

Gastrointestinal: Nausea (>10%), vomiting (>10%), stomatitis (>10%), diarrhea (>10%), perirectal abscess (>10%), abdominal pain (>10%)

Hematologic: Myelosuppression, leukopenia (nadir: 11-13 days; recovery: days 17-25)

Frequency not defined:

Cardiovascular: Atrial tachyarrhythmia, atrial tachycardia, atrial fibrillation, bradycardia, cardiomyopathy (rare), cardiopulmonary arrest, CHF (rare); ECG changes (QT prolongation, nonspecific ST segment or T wave changes); ejection fraction decreased, hypotension, sinus tachycardia, tachycardia, ventricular arrhythmia, ventricular extrasystoles, ventricular fibrillation, ventricular tachyarrhythmia

Central nervous system: Confusion, dizziness, emotional lability, fever, headache, hypoesthesia, lethargy, seizure

Dermatologic: Alopecia, cutaneous inflammatory reaction, dermatologic reaction, purpura, rash (purpuric or maculopapular), urticaria

Gastrointestinal: Anorexia, dysphagia, gingivitis, gum hemorrhage, hematemesis, weight changes

Genitourinary: Orange-red discoloration of the urine

Hematologic: Anemia, granulocytopenia, hemorrhage, pancytopenia, thrombocytopenia

Hepatic: Alkaline phosphatase increased, AST increased, bilirubin increased, hepatic insufficiency, hepatitis, hepatotoxicity, jaundice, progressive liver failure

Local: Injection site inflammation, phlebitis

Neuromuscular & skeletal: Musculoskeletal pain, paresthesia, weakness

Renal: BUN increased, creatinine increased, hematuria, proteinuria, renal failure

Respiratory: Dyspnea
Miscellaneous: Allergic reaction, infection

General Dosage Range Dosage adjustment recommended in patients with hepatic or renal impairment or patients who develop toxicities

I.V.: *Adults:* Induction: 75-125 mg/m^2/day for 5 days every 3-4 weeks; Maintenance: ~50% of induction dose every 4-8 weeks

Mechanism of Action Amsacrine has been shown to inhibit DNA synthesis by binding to, and intercalating with, DNA; inhibits topoisomerase II activity.

Pharmacodynamics/Kinetics

Half-life Elimination 1.4-5 hours; Terminal: 8-9 hours

Product Availability Not available in U.S.

Amyl Nitrite (AM il NYE trite)

Pharmacologic Category Antidote; Vasodilator

Use Coronary vasodilator in angina pectoris; adjunct in treatment of cyanide poisoning; produce changes in the intensity of heart murmurs

Local Anesthetic/Vasoconstrictor Precautions No information available to require special precautions

Effects on Dental Treatment Key adverse event(s) related to dental treatment: Postural hypotension

Effects on Bleeding No information available to require special precautions

Adverse Effects Frequency not defined.

Cardiovascular: Postural hypotension, cutaneous flushing of head, neck, and clavicular area, palpitations, tachycardia, sinus tachycardia, vasodilation
Central nervous system: Headache, incoherent speech, restlessness
Dermatologic: Contact dermatitis
Gastrointestinal: Nausea, colitis, vomiting
Genitourinary: Penile erection enhanced, retarded ejaculation
Hematologic: Heinz body hemolysis/hemolytic anemia
Ocular: Increased intraocular pressure, blurred vision
Respiratory: Tracheobronchitis

General Dosage Range Nasal inhalation: *Adults:* 1-6 inhalations from 1 crushed ampul; may repeat in 3-5 minutes

Mechanism of Action Relaxes vascular smooth muscle; decreased venous ratios and arterial blood pressure; reduces left ventricular work; decreases myocardial O_2 consumption; in cyanide poisoning, amyl nitrite converts hemoglobin to methemoglobin that binds with cyanide to form cyanate hemoglobin

Pharmacodynamics/Kinetics

Onset of Action Angina: Within 30 seconds

Duration of Action 3-15 minutes

Pregnancy Risk Factor C

Anagrelide (an AG gre lide)

U.S. Brand Names Agrylin®

Canadian Brand Names Agrylin®; Dom-Anagrelide; Mylan-Anagrelide; PMS-Anagrelide; Sandoz-Anagrelide

Pharmacologic Category Phospholipase A_2 Inhibitor; Platelet Reducing Agent

Use Treatment of thrombocythemia associated with myeloproliferative disorders (eg, chronic myelogenous leukemia, essential thrombocythemia, polycythemia vera, myeloid metaplasia with myelofibrosis, or other myeloproliferative disorder)

Local Anesthetic/Vasoconstrictor Precautions No information available to require special precautions

Effects on Dental Treatment Key adverse event(s) related to dental treatment: Orthostatic hypotension

Effects on Bleeding Anagrelide causes dose-related reduction in platelet production and could affect normal clotting; hemorrhage has been reported. Medical consult is suggested for patients under active treatment with anagrelide.

Adverse Effects

>10%:

Cardiovascular: Palpitation (26%), edema (21%)
Central nervous system: Headache (44%), dizziness (15%), pain (15%)
Gastrointestinal: Diarrhea (26%), nausea (17%), abdominal pain (16%)
Neuromuscular & skeletal: Weakness (23%)
Respiratory: Dyspnea (12%)

1% to 10%:

Cardiovascular: Peripheral edema (9%), chest pain (8%), tachycardia (8%), angina, arrhythmia, HF, hypertension, postural hypotension, syncope, thrombosis, vasodilatation

Central nervous system: Fever (9%), malaise (6%), amnesia, chills, confusion, depression, insomnia, migraine, nervousness, somnolence
Dermatologic: Rash (8%), pruritus (6%), alopecia, bruising, photosensitivity, urticaria
Endocrine & skeletal: Dehydration
Gastrointestinal: Flatulence (10%), vomiting (10%), anorexia (8%), dyspepsia (5%), aphthous stomatitis, constipation, eructation, gastritis, GI distress, GI hemorrhage, melena
Genitourinary: Dysuria
Hematologic: Thrombocytopenia (9%; grades 3/4: 5%), anemia, hemorrhage
Neuromuscular & skeletal: Back pain (6%), paresthesia (6%), arthralgia, leg cramps, myalgia
Ocular: Amblyopia, diplopia, visual field abnormality
Otic: Tinnitus
Renal: Renal abnormality (2%), renal failure (1%), hematuria
Respiratory: Pharyngitis (7%), cough (6%), asthma, bronchitis, epistaxis, pneumonia, rhinitis, sinusitis
Miscellaneous: Flu-like syndrome, lymphadenopathy

General Dosage Range Dosage adjustment recommended in patients with hepatic impairment

Oral:

Children: Initial: 0.5 mg/day; Maintenance: 0.5 mg 1-4 times/day (maximum: 10 mg/day; 2.5 mg/dose)

Adults: Initial: 0.5 mg 4 times/day **or** 1 mg twice daily (maximum: 10 mg/day; 2.5 mg/dose)

Mechanism of Action Anagrelide appears to inhibit cyclic nucleotide phosphodiesterase and the release of arachidonic acid from phospholipase, possibly by inhibiting phospholipase A_2. It also causes a dose-related reduction in platelet production, which results from decreased megakaryocyte hypermaturation (disrupts the postmitotic phase of maturation).

Pharmacodynamics/Kinetics

Onset of Action Initial: Within 7-14 days; complete response (platelets ≤600,000/mm^3): 4-12 weeks

Duration of Action 6-24 hours; upon discontinuation, platelet count begins to rise within 4 days

Half-life Elimination Plasma: 1.3 hours

Time to Peak Serum: 1 hour

Pregnancy Risk Factor C

Anakinra (an a KIN ra)

Related Information

Rheumatoid Arthritis, Osteoarthritis, and Osteoporosis *on page 1889*

U.S. Brand Names Kineret®

Canadian Brand Names Kineret®

Pharmacologic Category Antirheumatic, Disease Modifying; Interleukin-1 Receptor Antagonist

Use Treatment of moderately- to severely-active rheumatoid arthritis in adult patients who have failed one or more disease-modifying antirheumatic drugs (DMARDs); may be used alone or in combination with DMARDs (other than tumor necrosis factor-blocking agents)

Local Anesthetic/Vasoconstrictor Precautions No information available to require special precautions

Effects on Dental Treatment No significant effects or complications reported

Effects on Bleeding No information available to require special precautions

Adverse Effects

>10%:
Central nervous system: Headache (12%)
Local: Injection site reaction (majority mild, typically lasting 14-28 days, characterized by erythema, ecchymosis, inflammation, and pain; up to 71%)
Miscellaneous: Infection (39% versus 37% in placebo; serious infection 2% to 3%)

1% to 10%:
Gastrointestinal: Nausea (8%), diarrhea (7%), abdominal pain (5%)
Hematologic: Neutropenia (8%; grades 3/4: 0.4%)
Respiratory: Sinusitis (7%)
Miscellaneous: Flu-like syndrome (6%)

General Dosage Range Dosage adjustment recommended in patients with renal impairment

SubQ: *Adults:* 100 mg once daily

Mechanism of Action Antagonist of the interleukin-1 (IL-1) receptor. Endogenous IL-1 is induced by inflammatory stimuli and mediates a variety of immunological responses, including degradation of cartilage (loss of proteoglycans) and stimulation of bone resorption.

Pharmacodynamics/Kinetics

Half-life Elimination Terminal: 4-6 hours

Time to Peak SubQ: 3-7 hours

Pregnancy Risk Factor B

Anastrozole (an AS troe zole)

U.S. Brand Names Arimidex®

Canadian Brand Names Arimidex®

Pharmacologic Category Antineoplastic Agent, Aromatase Inhibitor

Use First-line treatment of locally-advanced or metastatic breast cancer (hormone receptor-positive or unknown) in postmenopausal women; treatment of advanced breast cancer in postmenopausal women with disease progression following tamoxifen therapy; adjuvant treatment of early hormone receptor-positive breast cancer in postmenopausal women

Unlabeled/Investigational Use Treatment of recurrent or metastatic endometrial or uterine cancers, treatment of recurrent ovarian cancer

Local Anesthetic/Vasoconstrictor Precautions No information available to require special precautions

Effects on Dental Treatment Key adverse event(s) related to dental treatment: Xerostomia (normal salivary flow resumes upon discontinuation).

Effects on Bleeding Although significant myelosuppression with associated altered hemostasis has been reported for many chemotherapeutic agents, myelosuppression is not significant with anastrozole and no specific precautions appear to be necessary.

Adverse Effects

>10%:

Cardiovascular: Vasodilatation (25% to 36%), ischemic cardiovascular disease (4%; 17% in patients with pre-existing ischemic heart disease), hypertension (2% to 13%), angina (2%; 12% in patients with pre-existing ischemic heart disease)

Central nervous system: Mood disturbance (19%), fatigue (19%), pain (11% to 17%), headache (9% to 13%), depression (5% to 13%)

Dermatologic: Rash (6% to 11%)

Endocrine & metabolic: Hot flashes (12% to 36%)

Gastrointestinal: Nausea (11% to 19%), vomiting (8% to 13%)

Neuromuscular & skeletal: Weakness (16% to 19%), arthritis (17%), arthralgia (2% to 15%), back pain (10% to 12%), bone pain (6% to 11%), osteoporosis (11%)

Respiratory: Pharyngitis (6% to 14%), cough increased (8% to 11%)

1% to 10%:

Cardiovascular: Peripheral edema (5% to 10%), chest pain (5% to 7%), edema (7%), venous thromboembolic events (2% to 4%), ischemic cerebrovascular events (2%), MI (1%)

Central nervous system: Insomnia (2% to 10%), dizziness (6% to 8%), anxiety (2% to 6%), fever (2% to 5%), malaise (2% to 5%), confusion (2% to 5%), nervousness (2% to 5%), somnolence (2% to 5%), lethargy (1%)

Dermatologic: Alopecia (2% to 5%), pruritus (2% to 5%)

Endocrine & metabolic: Hypercholesterolemia (9%), breast pain (2% to 8%)

Gastrointestinal: Diarrhea (8% to 9%), constipation (7% to 9%), abdominal pain (7% to 9%), weight gain (2% to 9%), anorexia (5% to 7%), xerostomia (6%), dyspepsia (7%), weight loss (2% to 5%)

Genitourinary: Urinary tract infection (2% to 8%), vulvovaginitis (6%), pelvic pain (5%), vaginal bleeding (1% to 5%), vaginitis (4%), vaginal discharge (4%), vaginal hemorrhage (2% to 4%), leukorrhea (2% to 3%), vaginal dryness (2% to 5%)

Hematologic: Anemia (2% to 5%), leukopenia (2% to 5%)

Hepatic: Liver function tests increased (1% to 10%), alkaline phosphatase increased (1% to 10%), gamma GT increased (≤5%)

Local: Thrombophlebitis (2% to 5%)

Neuromuscular & skeletal: Fracture (1% to 10%), arthrosis (7%), paresthesia (5% to 7%), joint disorder (6%), myalgia (2% to 6%), neck pain (2% to 5%), carpal tunnel syndrome (3%), hypertonia (3%)

Ocular: Cataracts (6%)

Respiratory: Dyspnea (8% to 10%), sinusitis (2% to 6%), bronchitis (2% to 5%), rhinitis (2% to 5%)

Miscellaneous: Lymphedema (10%), infection (2% to 9%), flu-like syndrome (2% to 7%), diaphoresis (2% to 5%), cyst (5%), neoplasm (5%), tumor flare (3%)

General Dosage Range Oral: *Adults:* 1 mg once daily

Mechanism of Action Potent and selective nonsteroidal aromatase inhibitor. By inhibiting aromatase, the conversion of androstenedione to estrone, and testosterone to estradiol, is prevented, thereby decreasing tumor mass or delaying progression in patients with tumors responsive to hormones. Anastrozole causes an 85% decrease in estrone sulfate levels.

Pharmacodynamics/Kinetics

Onset of Action Onset of estradiol reduction: 70% reduction after 24 hours; 80% after 2 weeks therapy

Duration of Action Duration of estradiol reduction: 6 days

Half-life Elimination ~50 hours

Time to Peak Plasma: ~2 hours without food; 5 hours with food

Pregnancy Risk Factor X

Anidulafungin (ay nid yoo la FUN jin)

Related Information

Fungal Infections *on page 1945*

U.S. Brand Names Eraxis™

Canadian Brand Names Eraxis™

Pharmacologic Category Antifungal Agent, Parenteral; Echinocandin

Use Treatment of candidemia and other forms of *Candida* infections (including those of intra-abdominal, peritoneal, and esophageal locus)

Unlabeled/Investigational Use Treatment of infections due to *Aspergillus* spp.

Local Anesthetic/Vasoconstrictor Precautions No information available to require special precautions

Effects on Dental Treatment No significant effects or complications reported

Effects on Bleeding No information available to require special precautions

Adverse Effects 2% to 10%:

Endocrine & metabolic: Hypokalemia (3%)

Gastrointestinal: Diarrhea (3%)

Hepatic: Transaminase increased (<1% to 2%)

General Dosage Range I.V.: *Adults:* Loading dose: 100-200 mg as a single dose; Maintenance: 50-100 mg daily

Mechanism of Action Noncompetitive inhibitor of 1,3-beta-D-glucan synthase resulting in reduced formation of 1,3-beta-D-glucan, an essential polysaccharide comprising 30% to 60% of *Candida* cell walls (absent in mammalian cells); decreased glucan content leads to osmotic instability and cellular lysis

Pharmacodynamics/Kinetics

Half-life Elimination 27 hours

Pregnancy Risk Factor C

Anthralin (AN thra lin)

U.S. Brand Names Dritho-Creme®; Dritho-Scalp®; Zithranol®-RR

Canadian Brand Names Anthraforte®; Anthranol®; Anthrascalp®; Micanol®

Pharmacologic Category Antipsoriatic Agent; Keratolytic Agent

Use Treatment of psoriasis (quiescent or chronic psoriasis)

Local Anesthetic/Vasoconstrictor Precautions No information available to require special precautions

Effects on Dental Treatment No significant effects or complications reported

Effects on Bleeding No information available to require special precautions

Adverse Effects Frequency not defined: Dermatologic: Transient primary irritation of uninvolved skin; temporary discoloration of skin, hair, and fingernails; contact allergic reactions; erythema

General Dosage Range Topical: *Adults:* Generally, apply once a day or as directed

Mechanism of Action Reduction of the mitotic rate and proliferation of epidermal cells in psoriasis by inhibiting synthesis of nucleic protein from inhibition of DNA synthesis to affected areas

Pregnancy Risk Factor C

Anthrax Vaccine (Adsorbed) (AN thraks vak SEEN ad SORBED)

U.S. Brand Names BioThrax®

Pharmacologic Category Vaccine, Inactivated (Bacterial)

Use Immunization against *Bacillus anthracis* in persons at high risk for exposure.

ANTHRAX VACCINE (ADSORBED)

The Advisory Committee on Immunization Practices (ACIP) recommends routine vaccination (pre-exposure vaccination) for the following:

- Persons who work directly with the organism in the laboratory
- Persons who handle animals or animal products only when
  - potentially infected in research settings;
  - in areas of high incidence of enzootic anthrax; or
  - where standards and restrictions are not sufficient to prevent exposure
- Military personnel deployed to areas with high risk of exposure as recommended by the Department of Defense (DoD)
- Persons engaged in environmental investigations or remediation efforts

Routine immunization for the general population is not recommended. Routine vaccination may be offered to emergency and other responders (police and fire departments, the National Guard, etc) on a voluntary basis under the direction of a comprehensive occupational health and safety program.

The ACIP recommends postexposure prophylaxis for the following (in the absence of completing a pre-exposure, routine vaccination schedule):

- The general public, including pregnant and breast-feeding women
- Medical professionals
- Children ages 0-18 years as determined on an event-by-event basis
- Persons engaged in handling certain animals or animal products
- Persons who work directly with the organism in the laboratory (postexposure vaccination dependant upon pre-event vaccination status)
- Military personnel as recommended by the DoD
- Persons engaged in environmental investigations or remediation efforts (post-exposure vaccination dependent upon pre-event vaccination status)
- Emergency and other responders (police and fire departments, the National Guard, etc)
- Persons working in postal facilities

Local Anesthetic/Vasoconstrictor Precautions No information available to require special precautions

Effects on Dental Treatment No significant effects or complications reported

Effects on Bleeding No information available to require special precautions

Adverse Effects All serious adverse reactions must be reported to the U.S. Department of Health and Human Services (DHHS) Vaccine Adverse Event Reporting System (VAERS) 1-800-822-7967 or online at https://vaers.hhs.gov/esub/index.

Note: Percentages reported with I.M. administration; the incidence of local reactions may be increased with SubQ administration.

>10%:

Central nervous system: Headache (4% to 64%), fatigue (5% to 62%)

Local: Tenderness (10% to 61%), erythema (8% to 31%), pain (4% to 23%), edema (1% to 16%), limitation of arm motion (1% to 16%), induration (3% to 14%), warmth (1% to 11%)

Neuromuscular & skeletal: Myalgia (2% to 72%)

Respiratory: Nasopharyngitis (12% to 15%), pharyngolaryngeal pain (12%)

1% to 10%:

Dermatologic: Pruritus (≤2%), rash (≤2%)

Endocrine & metabolic: Dysmenorrhea (7%)

Gastrointestinal: Diarrhea (6% to 8%), nausea (6%)

Local: Itching (≤9%), bruising (3% to 6%), nodule (1% to 6%)

Neuromuscular & skeletal: Back pain (7% to 9%), neck pain (3%), joint sprain (≤2%), rigors (1% to 2%)

Respiratory: Sinusitis (5% to 7%), upper respiratory tract infection (2% to 3%), sinus headache (1% to 3%)

Miscellaneous: Hypersensitivity (2% to 4%), lymphadenopathy (2% to 3%), flu-like illness (2%), tender/painful axillary adenopathy (≤1%)

General Dosage Range

I.M.: *Adults ≤65 years:* 0.5 mL

SubQ: *Adults:* 0.5 mL

Mechanism of Action Active immunization against *Bacillus anthracis*. The vaccine is prepared from a cell-free filtrate of *B. anthracis*, but no dead or live bacteria. Completion of the entire vaccination series is required for full protection.

Pregnancy Risk Factor D

Prescribing and Access Restrictions Not commercially available in U.S.; presently, all anthrax vaccine lots are owned by the U.S. Department of Defense. The Center for Disease Control (CDC) does not currently recommend routine vaccination of the general public.

Antihemophilic Factor (Human) (an tee hee moe FIL ik FAK tor HYU man)

U.S. Brand Names Hemofil M; Koāte®-DVI; Monarc-M™; Monoclate-P®

Canadian Brand Names Hemofil M

Pharmacologic Category Antihemophilic Agent; Blood Product Derivative

Use Prevention and treatment of hemorrhagic episodes in patients with hemophilia A (classic hemophilia); perioperative management of hemophilia A; can be of significant therapeutic value in patients with acquired factor VIII inhibitors not exceeding 10 Bethesda units/mL

Local Anesthetic/Vasoconstrictor Precautions No information available to require special precautions

Effects on Dental Treatment No significant effects or complications reported

Effects on Bleeding Treatment of bleeding disorders depends on many factors, including severity of disease and risks of bleeding. General dental procedures and simple restorative procedures are not associated with bleeding; therefore, there is no contraindication to general dental treatment for most patients with bleeding disorders. Surgical dental procedures are also possible for hemophiliacs and other bleeding disorders, but a carefully coordinated strategy between the dental and medical team may be required to ensure adequate hemostasis. As preparation for selected dental procedures, factor replacement, tranexamic acid, or aminocaproic acid (Amicar®) may be required. Local measures to promote hemostasis (such as collagen) are commonly used. Examples of procedures which require advance consultation include block anesthesia, deep scaling, extractions, large fillings, and any oral surgery. Medical consultation is warranted.

General Dosage Range I.V.: *Children and Adults:* Dosage varies greatly depending on indication

Mechanism of Action Protein (factor VIII) in normal plasma which is necessary for clot formation and maintenance of hemostasis; activates factor X in conjunction with activated factor IX; activated factor X converts prothrombin to thrombin, which converts fibrinogen to fibrin, and with factor XIII forms a stable clot

Pharmacodynamics/Kinetics

Half-life Elimination Mean: 8-27 hours

Pregnancy Risk Factor C

Antihemophilic Factor (Recombinant)

(an tee hee moe FIL ik FAK tor ree KOM be nant)

U.S. Brand Names Advate; Helixate® FS; Kogenate® FS; Recombinate; Xyntha™

Canadian Brand Names Advate; Helixate® FS; Kogenate®; Kogenate® FS; Recombinate; ReFacto®; Xyntha®

Pharmacologic Category Antihemophilic Agent

Use Prevention and treatment of hemorrhagic episodes in patients with hemophilia A (classic hemophilia or congenital factor VIII deficiency); perioperative management of hemophilia A; prophylaxis of joint bleeding and to reduce risk of joint damage in children with hemophilia A with no pre-existing joint damage; can be of significant therapeutic value in patients with acquired factor VIII inhibitors ≤10 Bethesda units/mL

Local Anesthetic/Vasoconstrictor Precautions No information available to require special precautions

Effects on Dental Treatment Key adverse event(s) related to dental treatment: Taste perversion.

Effects on Bleeding Treatment of bleeding disorders depends on many factors, including severity of disease and risks of bleeding. General dental procedures and simple restorative procedures are not associated with bleeding; therefore, there is no contraindication to general dental treatment for most patients with bleeding disorders. Surgical dental procedures are also possible for hemophiliacs and other bleeding disorders, but a carefully coordinated strategy between the dental and medical team may be required to ensure adequate hemostasis. As preparation for selected dental procedures, factor replacement, tranexamic acid, or aminocaproic acid (Amicar®) may be required. Local measures to promote hemostasis (such as collagen) are commonly used. Examples of procedures which require advance consultation include block anesthesia, deep scaling, extractions, large fillings, and any oral surgery. Medical consultation is warranted.

Adverse Effects >1% (actual frequency may vary by product):

Central nervous system: Chills, dizziness, fever, headache, pain

Dermatologic: Pruritus, rash, urticaria

Gastrointestinal: Diarrhea, nausea, taste perversion, vomiting

Hematologic: Hemorrhage

Local: Injection site pain, injection site inflammation, infusion site reaction

Neuromuscular & skeletal: Arthralgia, weakness

Respiratory: Cough, dyspnea, nasopharyngitis, pharyngolaryngeal pain
Miscellaneous: Catheter thrombosis, factor VIII inhibitor formation

General Dosage Range I.V.: *Children and Adults:* Dosage varies greatly depending on indication

Mechanism of Action Factor VIII replacement, necessary for clot formation and maintenance of hemostasis. It activates factor X in conjunction with activated factor IX; activated factor X converts prothrombin to thrombin, which converts fibrinogen to fibrin, and with factor XIII forms a stable clot.

Pharmacodynamics/Kinetics

Half-life Elimination Mean: 8-19 hours

Pregnancy Risk Factor C

Antihemophilic Factor/von Willebrand Factor Complex (Human) (an tee hee moe FIL ik FAK tor von WILL le brand FAK tor KOM plex HYU man)

U.S. Brand Names Alphanate®; Humate-P®; Wilate®

Canadian Brand Names Humate-P®

Pharmacologic Category Antihemophilic Agent; Blood Product Derivative

Use

Factor VIII deficiency: Alphanate®, Humate-P®: Prevention and treatment of hemorrhagic episodes in patients with hemophilia A (classical hemophilia) or acquired factor VIII deficiency (Alphanate® only); **Note:** Wilate® is not approved for use in patients with hemophilia A or acquired factor VIII deficiency

von Willebrand disease (VWD):

Alphanate®: Prophylaxis with surgical and/or invasive procedures in patients with VWD when desmopressin is either ineffective or contraindicated; **Note:** Not indicated for patients with severe VWD undergoing major surgery

Humate-P®: Treatment of spontaneous or trauma-induced bleeding, as well as prevention of excessive bleeding during and after surgery in patients with severe VWD, including mild or moderate disease where use of desmopressin is known or suspected to be inadequate; **Note:** Not indicated for the prophylaxis of spontaneous bleeding episodes

Wilate®: Treatment of spontaneous and trauma-induced bleeding in patients with severe VWD, including mild or moderate disease where use of desmopressin is known or suspected to be inadequate or contraindicated; **Note:** Not indicated for prophylaxis of spontaneous bleeding or prevention of excessive bleeding during and after surgery)

Local Anesthetic/Vasoconstrictor Precautions No information available to require special precautions

Effects on Dental Treatment No significant effects or complications reported

Effects on Bleeding Treatment of bleeding disorders depends on many factors, including severity of disease and risks of bleeding. General dental procedures and simple restorative procedures are not associated with bleeding; therefore, there is no contraindication to general dental treatment for most patients with bleeding disorders. Surgical dental procedures are also possible for hemophiliacs and other bleeding disorders, but a carefully coordinated strategy between the dental and medical team may be required to ensure adequate hemostasis. As preparation for selected dental procedures, factor replacement, desmopressin acetate (Stimate®) nasal spray, tranexamic acid, or aminocaproic acid (Amicar®) may be required. Local measures to promote hemostasis (such as collagen) are commonly used. Examples of procedures which require advance consultation include block anesthesia, deep scaling, extractions, large fillings, and any oral surgery. Medical consultation is warranted.

Adverse Effects Frequency not defined.

Cardiovascular: Cardiorespiratory arrest, chest tightness, edema, femoral venous thrombosis, flushing, hypervolemia, orthostatic hypotension, shock, thromboembolic events, vasodilation
Central nervous system: Chills, dizziness, fever, headache, lethargy, pain, seizure, somnolence
Dermatologic: Itching, pruritus, rash, urticaria
Endocrine & metabolic: Parotid gland swelling
Gastrointestinal: Nausea, vomiting
Hematologic: Hematocrit decreased (moderate), hemorrhage, hemolysis, pseudothrombocytopenia (severe)
Hepatic: ALT increased
Local: Injection site stinging, phlebitis
Neuromuscular & skeletal: Extremity pain, joint pain, paresthesia, rigors
Respiratory: Cough, dyspnea, pharyngitis, pulmonary embolus (large doses)
Miscellaneous: Allergic reactions, anaphylactic reactions, factor VIII inhibitor formation, hypersensitivity reactions, von Willebrand factor inhibitor formation

General Dosage Range I.V.: *Children and Adults:* Dosage varies greatly depending on indication

Mechanism of Action Factor VIII and von Willebrand factor (VWF), obtained from pooled human plasma, are used to replace endogenous factor VIII and VWF in patients with hemophilia or VWD. Factor VIII in conjunction with activated factor IX, activates factor X which converts prothrombin to thrombin and fibrinogen to fibrin. VWF promotes platelet aggregation and adhesion to damaged vascular endothelium and acts as a stabilizing carrier protein for factor VIII. (Circulating levels of functional VWF are measured as ristocetin cofactor activity [VWF:RCo].)

Pharmacodynamics/Kinetics

Onset of Action Shortening of bleeding time: Immediate

Duration of Action VWD: Shortening of bleeding time: <6 hours postinfusion; presence of VWF multimers detected in the plasma: ≥24 hours

Half-life Elimination

Factor VIII coagulant activity (FVIII:C): Range: 8-28 hours in patients with hemophilia A

VWF:RCo: Range: 3-34 hours in patients with VWD

Pregnancy Risk Factor C

Anti-inhibitor Coagulant Complex

(an TEE in HI bi tor coe AG yoo lant KOM pleks)

U.S. Brand Names Feiba NF; Feiba VH [DSC]

Canadian Brand Names Feiba NF

Pharmacologic Category Activated Prothrombin Complex Concentrate (aPCC); Antihemophilic Agent; Blood Product Derivative

Use Hemophilia A & B patients with inhibitors who are to undergo surgery or those who are bleeding

Unlabeled/Investigational Use Acquired hemophilia with factor VIII or factor IX inhibitor titers >5 Bethesda units (BU)

Local Anesthetic/Vasoconstrictor Precautions No information available to require special precautions

Effects on Dental Treatment No significant effects or complications reported

Effects on Bleeding Treatment of bleeding disorders depends on many factors, including severity of disease and risks of bleeding. General dental procedures and simple restorative procedures are not associated with bleeding; therefore, there is no contraindication to general dental treatment for most patients with bleeding disorders. Surgical dental procedures are also possible for hemophiliacs and other bleeding disorders, but a carefully coordinated strategy between the dental and medical team may be required to ensure adequate hemostasis. As preparation for selected dental procedures, factor replacement, tranexamic acid, or aminocaproic acid (Amicar®) may be required. Local measures to promote hemostasis (such as collagen) are commonly used. Examples of procedures which require advance consultation include block anesthesia, deep scaling, extractions, large fillings, and any oral surgery. Medical consultation is warranted.

Adverse Effects Frequency not defined.

Cardiovascular: Blood pressure decreased, MI, thromboembolism

Central nervous system: Hypoesthesia (including facial)

Dermatologic: Rash, urticaria

Hematologic: DIC

Local: Injection site pain

Miscellaneous: Allergic reaction (including anaphylaxis), anamnestic response, hypersensitivity

General Dosage Range I.V.: *Children and Adults:* 50-100 units/kg every 6-12 hours (maximum: 200 units/kg/day)

Pregnancy Risk Factor C

Antipyrine and Benzocaine (an tee PYE reen & BEN zoe kane)

Related Information

Benzocaine *on page* 218

Canadian Brand Names Auralgan®

Pharmacologic Category Otic Agent, Analgesic; Otic Agent, Cerumenolytic

Use Temporary relief of pain and reduction of swelling associated with acute congestive and serous otitis media, swimmer's ear, otitis externa; facilitates ear wax removal

Local Anesthetic/Vasoconstrictor Precautions No information available to require special precautions

Effects on Dental Treatment No significant effects or complications reported

Effects on Bleeding No information available to require special precautions

General Dosage Range Otic: *Children and Adults:* Instill drops 3-4 times/day (ear wax removal) or fill ear canal every 1-2 hours (otitis media)

Mechanism of Action Antipyrine has analgesic properties; benzocaine is a local anesthetic; the glycerin base provides decreased middle ear pressure by osmosis.

Pharmacodynamics/Kinetics

Onset of Action Pain relief: ~30 minutes

Pregnancy Risk Factor C

Antithrombin (an tee THROM bin)

U.S. Brand Names Atryn®; Thrombate III®

Canadian Brand Names Thrombate III®

Pharmacologic Category Anticoagulant; Blood Product Derivative

Use Prophylaxis (ATryn®, Thrombate III®) of thromboembolic events in patients with hereditary antithrombin (AT or AT-III) deficiency undergoing surgical or obstetrical procedures (eg, childbirth); treatment (Thrombate III®) of thromboembolism in patients with hereditary AT deficiency

Local Anesthetic/Vasoconstrictor Precautions No information available to require special precautions

Effects on Dental Treatment No significant effects or complications reported

Effects on Bleeding Treatment of bleeding disorders depends on many factors, including severity of disease and risks of bleeding. General dental procedures and simple restorative procedures are not associated with bleeding; therefore, there is no contraindication to general dental treatment for most patients with bleeding disorders. Surgical dental procedures are also possible for hemophiliacs and other bleeding disorders, but a carefully coordinated strategy between the dental and medical team may be required to ensure adequate hemostasis. As preparation for selected dental procedures, factor replacement, desmopressin acetate (Stimate®) nasal spray, tranexamic acid, or aminocaproic acid (Amicar®) may be required. Local measures to promote hemostasis (such as collagen) are commonly used. Examples of procedures which require advance consultation include block anesthesia, deep scaling, extractions, large fillings, and any oral surgery. Medical consultation is warranted.

Adverse Effects 1% to 10%:

Cardiovascular: Chest pain (≤2%)
Central nervous system: Dizziness (2%)
Hematologic: Hemorrhage (≥5%), hematoma (≤2%)
Hepatic: Liver enzyme abnormalities (≤2%)
Neuromuscular & skeletal: Hemarthrosis (≤2%)
Renal: Hematuria (≤2%)
Local: Infusion site reaction (≥5%)

General Dosage Range I.V.: *Adults:* Dosage varies greatly depending on indication

Mechanism of Action Antithrombin is the primary physiologic inhibitor of *in vivo* coagulation. It is an alpha$_2$-globulin. Its principal actions are the inactivation of thrombin, plasmin, and other active serine proteases of coagulation, including factors IXa, Xa, XIa, and XIIa. The inactivation of proteases is a major step in the normal clotting process. The strong activation of clotting enzymes at the site of every bleeding injury facilitates fibrin formation and maintains normal hemostasis. Thrombosis in the circulation would be caused by active serine proteases if they were not inhibited by antithrombin after the localized clotting process.

Pharmacodynamics/Kinetics

Half-life Elimination

Plasma derived (Thrombate III®): Biologic: 2.5 days (immunologic assay); 3.8 days (functional AT assay). Half-life may be decreased following surgery, with hemorrhage, acute thrombosis, and/or during heparin administration.

Recombinant derived (Atryn®): 12-18 hours; surgery, childbirth hemorrhage, and/or concomitant heparin may shorten half-life

Pregnancy Risk Factor B (Thrombate III®); C (ATryn®)

Antithymocyte Globulin (Equine) (an te THY moe site GLOB yu lin, E kwine)

U.S. Brand Names Atgam®

Canadian Brand Names Atgam®

Pharmacologic Category Immune Globulin; Immunosuppressant Agent; Polyclonal Antibody

Use Prevention and treatment of acute renal allograft rejection; treatment of moderate-to-severe aplastic anemia in patients not considered suitable candidates for bone marrow transplantation

Unlabeled/Investigational Use Prevention and treatment of other solid organ allograft rejection; prevention or treatment of graft-versus-host disease (GVHD) following allogeneic stem cell transplantation; treatment of myelodysplastic syndrome (MDS)

Local Anesthetic/Vasoconstrictor Precautions No information available to require special precautions

Effects on Dental Treatment Key adverse event(s) related to dental treatment: Stomatitis

Effects on Bleeding No information available to require special precautions

Adverse Effects

>10%:

- Central nervous system: Chills, fever, headache
- Dermatologic: Pruritus, rash, urticaria, wheal/flare
- Hematologic: Leukopenia, thrombocytopenia
- Neuromuscular & skeletal: Arthralgia

1% to 10%:

- Cardiovascular: Bradycardia, cardiac irregularity, chest pain, edema, heart failure, hyper-/hypotension, myocarditis
- Central nervous system: Agitation, encephalitis, lethargy, lightheadedness, listlessness, seizure, viral encephalopathy
- Gastrointestinal: Diarrhea, nausea, stomatitis, vomiting
- Hepatic: Hepatosplenomegaly, liver function tests abnormal
- Local: Injection site reactions (pain, redness, swelling), phlebitis, thrombophlebitis, burning soles/palms
- Neuromuscular & skeletal: Aches, back pain, joint stiffness, myalgia
- Ocular: Periorbital edema
- Renal: Proteinuria, renal function tests abnormal
- Respiratory: Dyspnea, pleural effusion, respiratory distress
- Miscellaneous: Anaphylactic reaction, diaphoresis, lymphadenopathy, night sweats, serum sickness, viral infection

General Dosage Range I.V.:

Children: Initial: 5-25 mg/kg/day administered daily for 8-14 days; may be followed by administration every other day (maximum: 21 doses in 28 days)

Adults: Initial: 10-20 mg/kg/day administered daily; may be followed by administration every other day (maximum: 21 doses in 28 days)

Mechanism of Action Immunosuppressant involved in the elimination of antigen-reactive T lymphocytes (killer cells) in peripheral blood or alteration in the function of T-lymphocytes, which are involved in humoral immunity and partly in cell-mediated immunity; induces complete or partial hematologic response in aplastic anemia

Pharmacodynamics/Kinetics

Half-life Elimination Plasma: 1.5-12 days

Pregnancy Risk Factor C

Apomorphine (a poe MOR feen)

U.S. Brand Names Apokyn®

Pharmacologic Category Anti-Parkinson's Agent, Dopamine Agonist

Use Treatment of hypomobility, "off" episodes with Parkinson's disease

Unlabeled/Investigational Use Treatment of erectile dysfunction

Local Anesthetic/Vasoconstrictor Precautions Apomorphine is one of the drugs confirmed to prolong the QT interval and is accepted as having a risk of causing torsade de pointes. The risk of drug-induced torsade de pointes is extremely low when a single QT interval prolonging drug is prescribed. In terms of epinephrine, it is not known what effect vasoconstrictors in the local anesthetic regimen will have in patients with a known history of congenital prolonged QT interval or in patients taking any medication that prolongs the QT interval. Until more information is obtained, it is suggested that the clinician consult with the physician prior to the use of a vasoconstrictor in suspected patients, and that the vasoconstrictor (epinephrine, mepivacaine and levonordefrin [Carbocaine® 2% with Neo-Cobefrin®]) be used with caution.

Effects on Dental Treatment Key adverse event(s) related to dental treatment: Orthostatic hypotension has been reported in significant numbers of patients.

Effects on Bleeding No information available to require special precautions

Adverse Effects

>10%:

- Cardiovascular: Chest pain/pressure or angina (15%)
- Central nervous system: Drowsiness or somnolence (35%), dizziness or orthostatic hypotension (20%)
- Gastrointestinal: Nausea and/or vomiting (30%)
- Neuromuscular & skeletal: Falls (30%), dyskinesias (24% to 35%)

Respiratory: Yawning (40%), rhinorrhea (20%)

1% to 10%:

Cardiovascular: Edema (10%), vasodilation (3%), hypotension (2%), syncope (2%), CHF

Central nervous system: Hallucinations or confusion (10%), anxiety, depression, fatigue, headache, insomnia, pain

Dermatologic: Bruising

Endocrine & metabolic: Dehydration

Gastrointestinal: Constipation, diarrhea

Local: Injection site reactions

Neuromuscular & skeletal: Arthralgias, weakness

Miscellaneous: Diaphoresis increased

General Dosage Range Dosage adjustment recommended in patients with renal impairment

SubQ: *Adults:* Initial test dose: 2 mg; Starting dose: 2-3 mg/dose at time of "off" episode; Maintenance dose: 2-6 mg/dose at time of "off" episode (maximum: 20 mg/day; 6 mg/dose; 5 doses/day)

Mechanism of Action Stimulates postsynaptic D2-type receptors within the caudate putamen in the brain.

Pharmacodynamics/Kinetics

Onset of Action SubQ: Rapid

Half-life Elimination Terminal: 40 minutes

Time to Peak Plasma: Improved motor scores: 20 minutes

Pregnancy Risk Factor C

Prescribing and Access Restrictions Apokyn® is only available through a select group of specialty pharmacies and cannot be obtained through a retail pharmacy. Apokyn® may be obtained from the following specialty pharmacies: Accredo Nova Factor or PharmaCare. To obtain the medication, contact the APOKYN Call Center at 1-877-7APOKYN (1-877-727-6596).

Dental Comment Apomorphine is known to prolong the QT interval. The QT interval is measured as the time and distance between the Q point of the QRS complex and the end of the T wave in the ECG tracing. After adjustment for heart rate, the QT interval is defined as prolonged if it is more than 450 msec in men and 460 msec in women. A long QT syndrome was first described in the 1950s and 60s as a congenital syndrome involving QT interval prolongation and syncope and sudden death. Some of the congenital long QT syndromes were characterized by a peculiar electrocardiographic appearance of the QRS complex involving a premature atria beat followed by a pause, then a subsequent sinus beat showing marked QT prolongation and deformity. This type of cardiac arrhythmia was originally termed "torsade de pointes" (translated from the French as "twisting of the points"). Apomorphine is considered as having a risk of causing torsade de pointes. Since it is not known what effect vasoconstrictors in the local anesthetic regimen will have in patients with a known history of congenital prolonged QT interval or in patients taking any medication that prolongs the QT interval, a medical consult is suggested.

Apraclonidine (a pra KLOE ni deen)

U.S. Brand Names Iopidine®

Canadian Brand Names Iopidine®

Pharmacologic Category $Alpha_2$ Agonist, Ophthalmic

Use Prevention and treatment of postsurgical intraocular pressure (IOP) elevation; short-term, adjunctive therapy in patients who require additional reduction of IOP

Local Anesthetic/Vasoconstrictor Precautions No information available to require special precautions

Effects on Dental Treatment Key adverse event(s) related to dental treatment: Xerostomia (normal salivary flow resumes upon discontinuation)

Effects on Bleeding No information available to require special precautions

Adverse Effects

Ocular:

5% to 15%: Discomfort, hyperemia, pruritus

1% to 5%: Blanching, blurred vision, conjunctivitis, discharge, dry eye, foreign body sensation, lid edema, tearing

Other body systems:

1% to 10%: Gastrointestinal: Dry mouth (10%)

<3%:

Cardiovascular: Arrhythmia, chest pain, facial edema, peripheral edema

Central nervous system: Depression, dizziness, headache, insomnia, malaise, nervousness, somnolence

Dermatologic: Contact dermatitis, dermatitis

Gastrointestinal: Constipation, nausea, taste perversion

Neuromuscular & skeletal: Abnormal coordination, myalgia, paresthesia, weakness

Respiratory: Asthma, dry nose, dyspnea, parosmia, pharyngitis, rhinitis

General Dosage Range Ophthalmic: *Adults:* 0.5%: Instill 1-2 drops in the affected eye(s) 3 times/day; 1%: Instill 1 drop in operative eye 1 hour prior to and upon completion of surgery

Mechanism of Action Apraclonidine is a potent alpha-adrenergic agent similar to clonidine; relatively selective for $alpha_2$-receptors but does retain some binding to $alpha_1$-receptors; appears to result in reduction of aqueous humor formation; its penetration through the blood-brain barrier is more polar than clonidine which reduces its penetration through the blood-brain barrier and suggests that its pharmacological profile is characterized by peripheral rather than central effects.

Pharmacodynamics/Kinetics

Onset of Action 1 hour; Peak effect: Decreased intraocular pressure: 3-5 hours

Half-life Elimination Systemic: 8 hours

Pregnancy Risk Factor C

Aprepitant (ap RE pi tant)

U.S. Brand Names Emend®

Canadian Brand Names Emend®

Generic Availability (U.S.) No

Pharmacologic Category Antiemetic; Substance P/Neurokinin 1 Receptor Antagonist

Use Prevention of acute and delayed nausea and vomiting associated with moderately- and highly-emetogenic chemotherapy (in combination with other antiemetics); prevention of postoperative nausea and vomiting (PONV)

Local Anesthetic/Vasoconstrictor Precautions No information available to require special precautions

Effects on Dental Treatment Key adverse event(s) related to dental treatment: Hiccups, stomatitis, and mucous membrane disorder.

Effects on Bleeding No information available to require special precautions

Adverse Effects Note: Adverse reactions reported as part of a combination chemotherapy regimen or with general anesthesia.

>10%:

Central nervous system: Fatigue (≤18%)

Gastrointestinal: Nausea (6% to 13%), constipation (9% to 10%)

Neuromuscular & skeletal: Weakness (≤18%)

Miscellaneous: Hiccups (11%)

1% to 10%:

Cardiovascular: Hypotension (≤6%), bradycardia (≤4%)

Central nervous system: Dizziness (≤7%)

Endocrine & metabolic: Dehydration (≤6%)

Gastrointestinal: Diarrhea (≤10%), dyspepsia (≤6%), abdominal pain (≤5%), epigastric discomfort (4%), gastritis (4%), stomatitis (3%)

Hepatic: ALT increased (≤6%), AST increased (3%)

Renal: Proteinuria (7%), BUN increased (5%)

Dosage Oral: Adults:

Prevention of chemotherapy-induced nausea/vomiting: 125 mg 1 hour prior to chemotherapy on day 1, followed by 80 mg once daily on days 2 and 3 (in combination with a corticosteroid and $5\text{-}HT_3$ antagonist antiemetic)

Prevention of PONV: 40 mg within 3 hours prior to induction

Dosage adjustment in renal impairment: No dose adjustment necessary in patients with renal disease or end-stage renal disease maintained on hemodialysis.

Dosage adjustment in hepatic impairment:

Mild-to-moderate impairment (Child-Pugh classes A and B): No adjustment necessary

Severe impairment (Child-Pugh class C): Use caution; no data available

Mechanism of Action Prevents acute and delayed vomiting by inhibiting the substance P/neurokinin 1 (NK_1) receptor; augments the antiemetic activity of $5\text{-}HT_3$ receptor antagonists and corticosteroids to inhibit acute and delayed phases of chemotherapy-induced emesis.

Contraindications Hypersensitivity to aprepitant or any component of the formulation; concurrent use with cisapride or pimozide

Warnings/Precautions Use caution with agents primarily metabolized via CYP3A4; aprepitant is a 3A4 inhibitor. Effect on orally administered 3A4 substrates is greater than those administered intravenously. Chronic continuous use is not recommended; however, a single 40 mg aprepitant oral dose is not likely to alter plasma concentrations of CYP3A4 substrates. Use caution with severe hepatic impairment; has not been studied in patients with severe hepatic impairment (Child-Pugh class C). Not studied for treatment of existing nausea and vomiting. Chronic continuous administration is not recommended.

Drug Interactions

Metabolism/Transport Effects **Substrate** of CYP1A2 (minor), 2C19 (minor), 3A4 (major); **Inhibits** CYP2C9 (weak), 2C19 (weak), 3A4 (moderate); **Induces** CYP2C9 (weak), 3A4 (weak)

Avoid Concomitant Use

Avoid concomitant use of Aprepitant with any of the following: Cisapride; Pimozide; Tolvaptan

Increased Effect/Toxicity

Aprepitant may increase the levels/effects of: Benzodiazepines (metabolized by oxidation); Budesonide (Systemic, Oral Inhalation); Cisapride; Colchicine; Corticosteroids (Systemic); CYP3A4 Substrates; Diltiazem; Eplerenone; Everolimus; FentaNYL; Halofantrine; Lurasidone; Pimecrolimus; Pimozide; Ranolazine; Salmeterol; Saxagliptin; Tolvaptan; Vilazodone

The levels/effects of Aprepitant may be increased by: Antifungal Agents (Azole Derivatives, Systemic); Conivaptan; CYP3A4 Inhibitors (Moderate); CYP3A4 Inhibitors (Strong); Dasatinib; Diltiazem

Decreased Effect

Aprepitant may decrease the levels/effects of: Contraceptives (Estrogens); Contraceptives (Progestins); CYP2C9 Substrates (High risk); PARoxetine; Saxagliptin; TOLBUTamide; Warfarin

The levels/effects of Aprepitant may be decreased by: CYP3A4 Inducers (Strong); Deferasirox; Herbs (CYP3A4 Inducers); PARoxetine; Rifamycin Derivatives; Tocilizumab

Ethanol/Nutrition/Herb Interactions

Food: Aprepitant serum concentration may be increased when taken with grapefruit juice; avoid concurrent use.

Herb/Nutraceutical: Avoid St John's wort (may decrease aprepitant levels).

Dietary Considerations May be taken with or without food.

Pharmacodynamics/Kinetics

Half-life Elimination Terminal: ~9-13 hours

Time to Peak Plasma: ~3-4 hours

Pregnancy Risk Factor B

Lactation Excretion in breast milk unknown/not recommended

Dosage Forms

Capsule, oral:

Emend®: 40 mg, 80 mg, 125 mg

Combination package, oral:

Emend®: Capsule: 80 mg (2s) and Capsule: 125 mg (1s)

Aprotinin (a proe TYE nin)

Canadian Brand Names Trasylol®

Pharmacologic Category Blood Product Derivative; Hemostatic Agent

Use Prevention of perioperative blood loss in patients who are at increased risk for blood loss and blood transfusions in association with cardiopulmonary bypass in coronary artery bypass graft surgery

Local Anesthetic/Vasoconstrictor Precautions No information available to require special precautions

Effects on Dental Treatment No significant effects or complications reported

Effects on Bleeding Treatment of bleeding disorders depends on many factors, including severity of disease and risks of bleeding. This agent is not likely to be used in a setting where dental procedures are contemplated.

Adverse Effects

>10%:

Central nervous system: Fever (15%)

Gastrointestinal: Nausea (11%)

1% to 10%:

Cardiovascular: Atrial flutter (6%), ventricular extrasystoles (6%), ventricular tachycardia (1% to 5%), heart failure (1% to 5%), arrhythmia (4%), supraventricular tachycardia (4%), bradycardia (1% to 2%), thrombosis (1% to 2%), bundle branch block (1% to 2%), cardiac arrest (1% to 2%), heart block (1% to 2%), hemorrhage (1% to 2%), myocardial ischemia (1% to 2%), pericardial effusion (1% to 2%), ventricular fibrillation (1% to 2%), shock (<1% to 2%)

Central nervous system: Agitation (1% to 2%), anxiety (1% to 2%), dizziness (1% to 2%), seizure (1% to 2%)

Endocrine & metabolic: Creatine phosphokinase increase (2%), acidosis (1% to 2%), hyperglycemia (1% to 2%), hypervolemia (1% to 2%), hypokalemia
Gastrointestinal: Diarrhea (3%), dyspepsia (1% to 2%), gastrointestinal hemorrhage (1% to 2%)
Hematologic: Disseminated intravascular coagulation (DIC), leukocytosis (1% to 2%), prothrombin decreased (1% to 2%), thrombocytopenia (1% to 2%)
Hepatic: Jaundice (1% to 2%), hepatic failure (1% to 2%)
Neuromuscular & skeletal: Arthralgia (1% to 2%)
Renal: Serum creatinine increase of >0.5 mg/dL above baseline (high dose: 9%), oliguria (1% to 2%), tubular necrosis (1% to 2%), kidney failure (1%)
Respiratory: Hypoxia (2%), pulmonary hypertension (1% to 2%), pneumonia (1% to 2%), apnea (1% to 2%), cough increased (1% to 2%)
Miscellaneous: Sepsis (1% to 2%), multisystem organ failure (1% to 2%)

General Dosage Range I.V.: *Adults:* Test dose: 1 mL (1.4 mg) 10 minutes prior to loading dose; Loading dose: 1-2 million KIU (140-280 mg; 100-200 mL); Pump prime volume: 1-2 million KIU (140-280 mg, 100-200 mL); Infusion: 250,000-500,000 KIU/hour (35-70 mg/hour; 25-50 mL/hour)

Mechanism of Action Bleeding from CABG surgery is thought to result from a systemic inflammatory response induced by the procedure. Contact of blood cells with the cardiopulmonary bypass (CPB) equipment leads to deregulated activation of the coagulation and fibrinolysis systems, with concurrent upregulation of proinflammatory cytokines. Aprotinin is a broad spectrum serine protease inhibitor that attenuates the coagulation, fibrinolytic and inflammatory pathways by interfering with the chemical mediators (thrombin, plasmin, kallikrein). Additionally, it protects platelet-expressed glycoproteins from mechanical shear forces. This preserves normal hemostatic activity through protease receptor-independent mechanisms (eg, via ADP, IIb/IIIa), while blocking CPB-induced thrombin-mediated aggregation.

Pharmacodynamics/Kinetics

Half-life Elimination 2.5 hours (plasma); terminal: 10 hours

Pregnancy Risk Factor B

Prescribing and Access Restrictions Available in U.S. under an investigational new drug (IND) process. The program will provide aprotinin for the treatment of adult patients undergoing coronary artery bypass graft (CABG) surgery requiring cardiopulmonary bypass (CPB) who are at increased risk of bleeding and transfusion during CABG surgery with no acceptable therapeutic alternative. Healthcare providers using aprotinin for this situation must also ensure that the benefits outweigh the risks for their patient. Healthcare providers with patients who may qualify can access information and forms for enrollment at http://www.trasylol.com/main.htm or contact Bayer Medical Communications at (888) 842-2937.

Arformoterol (ar for MOE ter ol)

U.S. Brand Names Brovana®

Pharmacologic Category Beta$_2$-Adrenergic Agonist; Beta$_2$-Adrenergic Agonist, Long-Acting

Use Long-term maintenance treatment of bronchoconstriction in chronic obstructive pulmonary disease (COPD), including chronic bronchitis and emphysema

Local Anesthetic/Vasoconstrictor Precautions No information available to require special precautions

Effects on Dental Treatment No significant effects or complications reported

Effects on Bleeding No information available to require special precautions

Adverse Effects 2% to 10%:
Cardiovascular: Chest pain (7%), peripheral edema (3%)
Central nervous system: Pain (8%)
Dermatologic: Rash (4%)
Gastrointestinal: Diarrhea (6%)
Neuromuscular & skeletal: Back pain (6%), leg cramps (4%)
Respiratory: Dyspnea (4%), sinusitis (5%), congestive conditions (2%)
Miscellaneous: Flu-like syndrome (3%)

General Dosage Range Nebulization: *Adults:* 5 mcg twice daily (maximum: 30 mcg/day)

Mechanism of Action Arformoterol, the (R,R)-enantiomer of the racemic formoterol, is a long-acting beta$_2$-agonist that relaxes bronchial smooth muscle by selective action on beta$_2$-receptors with little effect on cardiovascular system.

Pharmacodynamics/Kinetics

Onset of Action 7-20 minutes; Peak effect: 1-3 hours

Half-life Elimination 26 hours

Time to Peak 0.5-3 hours

Pregnancy Risk Factor C

Argatroban (ar GA troh ban)

Related Information

Cardiovascular Diseases *on page 1848*

Pharmacologic Category Anticoagulant, Thrombin Inhibitor

Use Prophylaxis or treatment of thrombosis in patients with heparin-induced thrombocytopenia (HIT); adjunct to percutaneous coronary intervention (PCI) in patients who have or are at risk of thrombosis associated with HIT

Unlabeled/Investigational Use To maintain extracorporeal circuit patency (prefilter administration) of continuous renal replacement therapy (CRRT) in critically-ill patients with HIT

Local Anesthetic/Vasoconstrictor Precautions No information available to require special precautions

Effects on Dental Treatment Key adverse event(s) related to dental treatment: Bleeding is a potential adverse effect of argatroban during dental surgery; it is unlikely that ambulatory patients presenting for dental treatment will be taking intravenous anticoagulant therapy. See Effects on Bleeding.

Effects on Bleeding As with all anticoagulants, bleeding is the major adverse effect of argatroban. Hemorrhage may occur at virtually any site; risk is dependent on multiple variables including the intensity of anticoagulation and patient susceptibility. Medical consult is suggested. It is unlikely that ambulatory patients presenting for dental treatment will be receiving intravenous anticoagulant therapy.

Adverse Effects As with all anticoagulants, bleeding is the major adverse effect of argatroban. Hemorrhage may occur at virtually any site. Risk is dependent on multiple variables, including the intensity of anticoagulation and patient susceptibility.

>10%:

Cardiovascular: Chest pain (PCI related: <1% to 15%), hypotension (7% to 11%)

Gastrointestinal: Gastrointestinal bleed (major: <1% to 3%; minor: 3% to 14%)

Genitourinary: Genitourinary bleed and hematuria (major: <1%; minor: 2% to 12%)

1% to 10%:

Cardiovascular: Vasodilation (1% to 10%), cardiac arrest (6%), ventricular tachycardia (5%), bradycardia (5%), myocardial infarction (PCI: 4%), atrial fibrillation (3%), angina (2%), CABG-related bleeding (minor, 2%), myocardial ischemia (2%), cerebrovascular disorder (<1% to 2%), thrombosis (<1% to 2%)

Central nervous system: Fever (<1% to 7%), headache (5%), pain (5%), intracranial bleeding (1% to 4%)

Dermatologic: Skin reactions (bullous eruption, rash; 1% to <10%)

Gastrointestinal: Nausea (5% to 7%), diarrhea (6%), vomiting (4% to 6%), abdominal pain (3% to 4%)

Genitourinary: Urinary tract infection (5%)

Hematologic: Hemoglobin decreased (<2 g/dL), hematocrit decreased (minor: 2% to 10%; major: <1%)

Local: Bleeding at injection or access site (minor: 2% to 5%)

Neuromuscular & skeletal: Back pain (PCI related: 8%)

Renal: Abnormal renal function (3%)

Respiratory: Dyspnea (8% to 10%), cough (3% to 10%), hemoptysis (minor: <1% to 3%), pneumonia (3%)

Miscellaneous: Sepsis (6%), infection (4%)

General Dosage Range Dosage adjustment recommended in patients with hepatic impairment

I.V.:

Children: Initial dose: 0.75 mcg/kg/minute; dosage may be adjusted in increments of 0.1-0.25 mcg/kg/minute

Adults: Bolus dose: 150-350 mcg/kg during procedure; Infusion: Initial: 2 mcg/kg/minute **or** 25 mcg/kg/minute during procedure; Maintenance: 0.5-10 mcg/kg/minute (maximum: 10 mcg/kg/minute) **or** 25-40 mcg/kg/minute during procedure

Adults (critically-ill): Initial: 0.2 mcg/kg/minute; Maintenance: 0.5-1.3 mcg/kg/minute

Mechanism of Action A direct, highly-selective thrombin inhibitor. Reversibly binds to the active thrombin site of free and clot-associated thrombin. Inhibits fibrin formation; activation of coagulation factors V, VIII, and XIII; activation of protein C; and platelet aggregation.

Pharmacodynamics/Kinetics

Onset of Action Immediate

Half-life Elimination 39-51 minutes; Hepatic impairment: ≤181 minutes

Time to Peak Steady-state: 1-3 hours

Pregnancy Risk Factor B

Arginine (AR ji neen)

U.S. Brand Names R-Gene® 10

Pharmacologic Category Diagnostic Agent

Use Pituitary function test (growth hormone)

Unlabeled/Investigational Use Management of severe, uncompensated, metabolic alkalosis (pH ≥7.55) **after** optimizing therapy with sodium and potassium supplements

Local Anesthetic/Vasoconstrictor Precautions No information available to require special precautions

Effects on Dental Treatment No significant effects or complications reported

Effects on Bleeding No information available to require special precautions

Adverse Effects 1% to 10%:

Cardiovascular: Flushing (with rapid I.V. infusion)

Central nervous system: Headache

Gastrointestinal: Nausea, vomiting

Local: Venous irritation

Neuromuscular & skeletal: Numbness

General Dosage Range I.V.:

Children: 0.5 g/kg/dose as a single dose

Adults: 30 g (300 mL) as a single dose

Mechanism of Action Stimulates pituitary release of growth hormone and prolactin through origins in the hypothalamus; patients with impaired pituitary function have lower or no increase in plasma concentrations of growth hormone after administration of arginine. Arginine hydrochloride has been used for severe metabolic alkalosis due to its high chloride content. Arginine hydrochloride has been used investigationally to treat metabolic alkalosis. Arginine contains 475 mEq of hydrogen ions and 475 mEq of chloride ions/L. Arginine is metabolized by the liver to produce hydrogen ions. It may be used in patients with relative hepatic insufficiency because arginine combines with ammonia in the body to produce urea. Arginine is a precursor to nitric oxide and can produce vasodilation and inhibition of platelet aggregation.

Pharmacodynamics/Kinetics

Half-life Elimination 0.7-1.3 hours

Time to Peak Serum: Oral: ~2 hours; I.V.: 20-30 minutes

Pregnancy Risk Factor B

ARIPiprazole (ay ri PIP ray zole)

U.S. Brand Names Abilify Discmelt®; Abilify®

Canadian Brand Names Abilify®

Generic Availability (U.S.) No

Pharmacologic Category Antipsychotic Agent, Atypical

Use

Oral: Acute and maintenance treatment of schizophrenia; acute (manic and mixed episodes) and maintenance treatment of bipolar I disorder as monotherapy or as an adjunct to lithium or valproic acid; adjunctive treatment of major depressive disorder; treatment of irritability associated with autistic disorder

Injection: Agitation associated with schizophrenia or bipolar I disorder

Unlabeled/Investigational Use Depression with psychotic features; aggression (children); conduct disorder (children); Tourette syndrome (children); psychosis/agitation related to Alzheimer's dementia

Local Anesthetic/Vasoconstrictor Precautions No information available to require special precautions

Effects on Dental Treatment Key adverse event(s) related to dental treatment: Extrapyramidal symptoms (similar to placebo) (see Dental Comment); xerostomia and changes in salivation (normal salivary flow resumes upon discontinuation).

Effects on Bleeding No information available to require special precautions

Adverse Effects Unless otherwise noted, frequency of adverse reactions is shown as reported for adult patients receiving oral administration. Spectrum and incidence of adverse effects similar in children; exceptions noted when incidence much higher in children.

>10%:

Central nervous system: Headache (27%; injection 12%), agitation (19%), insomnia (18%), anxiety (17%), EPS (dose related; 5% to 16%; children 6% to 26%), akathisia (dose related; 8% to 13%; injection 2%), sedation (dose related; 5% to 11%; children 8% to 24%; injection 3% to 9%)

Gastrointestinal: Weight gain (8% to 30%; highest frequency in patients with BMI <23), nausea (15%; injection 9%), constipation (11%), vomiting (11%; children 9% to 14%; injection 3%), dyspepsia (9%)

1% to 10%:

Cardiovascular: Orthostatic hypotension (1% to 4%; injection 1% to 3%), tachycardia (injection 2%), chest pain, hypertension, peripheral edema

Central nervous system: Dizziness (10%; injection 8%), pyrexia (children 5% to 9%), restlessness (5% to 6%), fatigue (dose related; 6%; children 8% to 17%; injection 2%), lethargy (children 2% to 5%), lightheadedness (4%), pain (3%), dystonia (children 1%), hypersomnia (1%), irritability (children 1%), coordination impaired, suicidal ideation

Dermatologic: Rash (children 2%), hyperhidrosis

Endocrine & metabolic: Dysmenorrhea (children 2%)

Gastrointestinal: Salivation increased (dose related; children 4% to 9%), appetite decreased (children 4% to 7%), appetite increased (children 7%), xerostomia (5%), toothache (4%), abdominal discomfort (3%), diarrhea (children 5%), weight loss

Local: Injection site reaction (injection)

Neuromuscular & skeletal: Tremor (dose related; 5% to 6%; children 6% to 10%), extremity pain (4%), stiffness (4%), myalgia (2%), spasm (2%), arthralgia (children 1%), dyskinesia (children 1%), CPK increased, weakness

Ocular: Blurred vision (3%; children 3% to 8%)

Respiratory: Nasopharyngitis (children 6%), pharyngolaryngeal pain (3%), cough (3%), rhinorrhea (children 2%), aspiration pneumonia, dyspnea, nasal congestion

Miscellaneous: Thirst (children 1%)

Dosage Note: Oral solution may be substituted for the oral tablet on a mg-per-mg basis, up to 25 mg. Patients receiving 30 mg tablets should be given 25 mg oral solution. Orally disintegrating tablets (Abilify Discmelt®) are bioequivalent to the immediate release tablets (Abilify®).

Children: Oral: Aggression, conduct disorder, Tourette syndrome (unlabeled uses): 5-20 mg/day

Children ≥6 years: Oral: Irritability associated with autistic disorder: Initial: 2 mg daily for 7 days, followed by an increase to target dose of 5 mg daily; subsequent dose increases may be made in 5 mg increments at intervals of ≥1 week as needed, up to a maximum of 15 mg/day

Children ≥10 years: Oral: Bipolar I disorder (acute manic or mixed episodes): Initial: 2 mg daily for 2 days, followed by 5 mg daily for 2 days with a further increase to target dose of 10 mg daily as monotherapy or as adjunct to lithium or valproic acid; subsequent dose increases may be made in 5 mg increments, up to a maximum of 30 mg/day

Adolescents ≥13 years: Oral: Schizophrenia: Initial: 2 mg daily for 2 days, followed by 5 mg daily for 2 days with a further increase to target dose of 10 mg daily; subsequent dose increases may be made in 5 mg increments up to a maximum of 30 mg/day (30 mg/day not shown to be more efficacious than 10 mg/day)

Adults:

Acute agitation (schizophrenia/bipolar mania): I.M.: 9.75 mg as a single dose (range: 5.25-15 mg); repeated doses may be given at ≥2-hour intervals to a maximum of 30 mg/day. **Note:** If ongoing therapy with aripiprazole is necessary, transition to oral therapy as soon as possible.

Bipolar I disorder (acute manic or mixed episodes): Oral:

Stabilization:

Monotherapy: Initial: 15 mg once daily. May increase to 30 mg once daily if clinically indicated; safety of doses >30 mg/day has not been evaluated

Adjunct to lithium or valproic acid: Initial: 10-15 mg once daily. May increase to 30 mg once daily if clinically indicated; safety of doses >30 mg/day has not been evaluated.

Maintenance: Continue stabilization dose for up to 6 weeks; efficacy of continued treatment >6 weeks has not been established

Depression (adjunctive with antidepressants): Oral: Initial: 2-5 mg/day (range: 2-15 mg/day); dose adjustments of up to 5 mg/day may be made in intervals of ≥1 week. **Note:** Dosing based on patients already receiving antidepressant therapy.

Schizophrenia: Oral: 10-15 mg once daily; may be increased to a maximum of 30 mg once daily (efficacy at dosages above 10-15 mg has not been shown to be increased). Dosage titration should not be more frequent than every 2 weeks.

Dosage adjustment with concurrent CYP450 inducer or inhibitor therapy:

Oral:

CYP3A4 inducers (eg, carbamazepine): Aripiprazole dose should be doubled (20-30 mg/day); dose should be subsequently reduced (10-15 mg/day) if concurrent inducer agent discontinued.

CYP3A4 inhibitors (eg, ketoconazole): Aripiprazole dose should be reduced to 1/2 of the usual dose, and proportionally increased upon discontinuation of the inhibitor agent.

CYP2D6 inhibitors (eg, fluoxetine, paroxetine): Aripiprazole dose should be reduced to 1/2 of the usual dose, and proportionally increased upon discontinuation of the inhibitor agent.

Dosage adjustment in renal impairment: No dosage adjustment required

Dosage adjustment in hepatic impairment: No dosage adjustment required

Mechanism of Action Aripiprazole is a quinolinone antipsychotic which exhibits high affinity for D_2, D_3, 5-HT_{1A}, and 5-HT_{2A} receptors; moderate affinity for D_4, 5-HT_{2C}, 5-HT_7, $alpha_1$ adrenergic, and H_1 receptors. It also possesses moderate affinity for the serotonin reuptake transporter; has no affinity for muscarinic (cholinergic) receptors. Aripiprazole functions as a partial agonist at the D_2 and 5-HT_{1A} receptors, and as an antagonist at the 5-HT_{2A} receptor.

Contraindications Hypersensitivity to aripiprazole or any component of the formulation

Warnings/Precautions [U.S. Boxed Warning]: Elderly patients with dementia-related psychosis treated with antipsychotics are at an increased risk of death compared to placebo. Most deaths appeared to be either cardiovascular (eg, heart failure, sudden death) or infectious (eg, pneumonia) in nature. In addition, an increased incidence of cerebrovascular effects (eg, transient ischemic attack, cerebrovascular accidents) has been reported in studies of placebo-controlled trials of aripiprazole in elderly patients with dementia-related psychosis. Aripiprazole is not approved for the treatment of dementia-related psychosis.

[U.S. Boxed Warning]: Antidepressants increase the risk of suicidal thinking and behavior in children, adolescents, and young adults (18-24 years of age) with major depressive disorder (MDD) and other psychiatric disorders; consider risk prior to prescribing. The possibility of a suicide attempt is inherent in major depression and may persist until remission occurs. Patients treated with antidepressants should be observed for clinical worsening and suicidality, especially during the initial few months of a course of drug therapy, or at times of dose changes, either increases or decreases. Prescriptions should be written for the smallest quantity consistent with good patient care. The patient's family or caregiver should be alerted to monitor patients for the emergence of suicidality and associated behaviors; patients should be instructed to notify their healthcare provider if any of these symptoms or worsening depression or psychosis occur.

Leukopenia, neutropenia, and agranulocytosis (sometimes fatal) have been reported in clinical trials and postmarketing reports with antipsychotic use; presence of risk factors (eg, pre-existing low WBC or history of drug-induced leuko-/neutropenia) should prompt periodic blood count assessment. Discontinue therapy at first signs of blood dyscrasias or if absolute neutrophil count $<1000/mm^3$.

A medication guide concerning the use of antidepressants should be dispensed with each prescription. **Aripiprazole is not FDA approved for adjunctive treatment of depression in children.**

May cause extrapyramidal symptoms (EPS), including pseudoparkinsonism, acute dystonic reactions, akathisia, and tardive dyskinesia (risk of these reactions is very low relative to typical/conventional antipsychotics, frequencies reported are similar to placebo). Risk of dystonia (and probably other EPS) may be greater with increased doses, use of conventional antipsychotics, males, and younger patients. May be associated with neuroleptic malignant syndrome (NMS).

May be sedating, use with caution in disorders where CNS depression is a feature. May cause orthostatic hypotension (although reported rates are similar to placebo); use caution in patients at risk of this effect or those who would not tolerate transient hypotensive episodes (cerebrovascular disease, cardiovascular disease, or other medications which may predispose).

Use caution in patients with Parkinson's disease; predisposition to seizures; and severe cardiac disease. May alter cardiac conduction; life-threatening arrhythmias have occurred with therapeutic doses of antipsychotics. Esophageal dysmotility and aspiration have been associated with antipsychotic use; use caution in patients at risk of pneumonia (eg, Alzheimer's disease). May alter temperature regulation. Significant weight gain has been observed with antipsychotic therapy; incidence varies with product. Monitor waist circumference and BMI.

Atypical antipsychotics have been associated with development of hyperglycemia; in some cases, may be extreme and associated with ketoacidosis, hyperosmolar coma, or death. Reports of hyperglycemia with aripiprazole therapy have been few and specific risk associated with this agent is not known. Use caution in patients with diabetes or other disorders of glucose regulation; monitor for worsening of glucose control.

Abilify Discmelt®: Use caution in phenylketonuria; contains phenylalanine.

Drug Interactions

Metabolism/Transport Effects Substrate (major) of CYP2D6, 3A4

Avoid Concomitant Use

Avoid concomitant use of ARIPiprazole with any of the following: Metoclopramide

Increased Effect/Toxicity

ARIPiprazole may increase the levels/effects of: Alcohol (Ethyl); CNS Depressants; Methotrimeprazine; Methylphenidate

The levels/effects of ARIPiprazole may be increased by: Abiraterone; Acetylcholinesterase Inhibitors (Central); Conivaptan; CYP2D6 Inhibitors (Moderate); CYP2D6 Inhibitors (Strong); CYP3A4 Inhibitors (Moderate); CYP3A4 Inhibitors (Strong); Darunavir; Dasatinib; Droperidol; Lithium formulations; Methotrimeprazine; Methylphenidate; Metoclopramide; Tetrabenazine

Decreased Effect

ARIPiprazole may decrease the levels/effects of: Amphetamines; Anti-Parkinson's Agents (Dopamine Agonist); Quinagolide

The levels/effects of ARIPiprazole may be decreased by: CarBAMazepine; CYP3A4 Inducers (Strong); Deferasirox; Herbs (CYP3A4 Inducers); Lithium formulations; Peginterferon Alfa-2b; Tocilizumab

Ethanol/Nutrition/Herb Interactions

Ethanol: May increase CNS depression; monitor for increased effects with coadministration. Caution patients about effects.

Food: Ingestion with a high-fat meal delays time to peak plasma level.

Herb/Nutraceutical: St John's wort may decrease aripiprazole levels. Avoid kava kava, gotu kola, valerian, St John's wort (may increase CNS depression).

Dietary Considerations May be taken with or without food. Some products may contain phenylalanine.

Pharmacodynamics/Kinetics

Onset of Action Initial: 1-3 weeks

Half-life Elimination

Aripiprazole: 75 hours; dehydro-aripiprazole: 94 hours

CYP2D6 poor metabolizers: Aripiprazole: 146 hours

Time to Peak I.M.: 1-3 hours; Tablet: 3-5 hours

With high-fat meal: Aripiprazole: Delayed by 3 hours; dehydro-aripiprazole: Delayed by 12 hours

Pregnancy Risk Factor C

Lactation Excretion in breast milk unknown/not recommended

Breast-Feeding Considerations Based on limited data from case reports, small amounts of aripiprazole have been detected in breast milk.

Dosage Forms

Injection, solution:

Abilify®: 7.5 mg/mL (1.3 mL)

Solution, oral:

Abilify®: 1 mg/mL (150 mL)

Tablet, oral:

Abilify®: 2 mg, 5 mg, 10 mg, 15 mg, 20 mg, 30 mg

Tablet, orally disintegrating, oral:

Abilify Discmelt®: 10 mg, 15 mg

Dental Comment Aripiprazole works differently from the classic antipsychotics, such as chlorpromazine, in that it does not appear to block central dopaminergic receptors, but rather seems to be a stabilizer of dopamine-serotonin central systems. The risk of extrapyramidal reactions such as pseudoparkinsonism, acute dystonic reactions, akathisia, and tardive dyskinesia are low and the frequencies reported are similar to placebo. Aripiprazole may be associated with neuroleptic malignant syndrome (NMS).

Armodafinil (ar moe DAF i nil)

U.S. Brand Names Nuvigil®

Pharmacologic Category Stimulant

Use Improve wakefulness in patients with excessive daytime sleepiness associated with narcolepsy and shift work sleep disorder (SWSD); adjunctive therapy for obstructive sleep apnea/hypopnea syndrome (OSAHS)

Local Anesthetic/Vasoconstrictor Precautions Use vasoconstrictor with caution. Patients may experience heart palpitations and increased heart rate when taking armodafinil.

Effects on Dental Treatment Key adverse event(s) related to dental treatment: Xerostomia (normal salivary flow resumes upon discontinuation).

Effects on Bleeding No information available to require special precautions

Adverse Effects

>10%: Central nervous system: Headache (14% to 23%; dose-related)

1% to 10%:

Cardiovascular: Palpitation (2%), increased heart rate (1%)

Central nervous system: Dizziness (5%), insomnia (4% to 6%; dose related), anxiety (4%), depression (1% to 3%; dose related), fatigue (2%), agitation (1%), attention disturbance (1%), depressed mood (1%), migraine (1%), nervousness (1%), pain (1%), pyrexia (1%), tremor (1%)

Dermatologic: Rash (1% to 4%; dose related), contact dermatitis (1%), hyperhidrosis (1%)

Gastrointestinal: Nausea (6% to 9%; dose related), xerostomia (2% to 7%; dose related), diarrhea (4%), abdominal pain (2%), dyspepsia (2%), anorexia (1%), appetite decreased (1%), constipation (1%), loose stools (1%), vomiting (1%)

Genitourinary: Polyuria (1%)

Hepatic: GGT increased (1%)

Neuromuscular & skeletal: Paresthesia (1%)

Respiratory: Dyspnea (1%)

Miscellaneous: Flu-like syndrome (1%), thirst (1%)

General Dosage Range Dosage adjustment recommended in patients with hepatic impairment

Oral: *Adults:* 150-250 mg once daily

Mechanism of Action The exact mechanism of action of armodafinil is unknown. It is the R-enantiomer of modafinil. Armodafinil binds to the dopamine transporter and inhibits dopamine reuptake, which may result in increased extracellular dopamine levels in the brain. However, it does not appear to be a dopamine receptor agonist and also does not appear to bind to or inhibit the most common receptors or enzymes that are relevant for sleep/wake regulation.

Pharmacodynamics/Kinetics

Half-life Elimination 15 hours; Steady state: ~7 days

Time to Peak 2 hours (fasted)

Pregnancy Risk Factor C

Controlled Substance C-IV

Artemether and Lumefantrine (ar TEM e ther & loo me FAN treen)

Related Information

Clinical Risk Related to Drugs Prolonging QT Interval *on page 1872*

U.S. Brand Names Coartem®

Pharmacologic Category Antimalarial Agent

Use Treatment of acute, uncomplicated malaria infections due to *Plasmodium falciparum*, including geographical regions where chloroquine resistance has been reported

Local Anesthetic/Vasoconstrictor Precautions Artemether and lumefantrine is one of the drugs confirmed to prolong the QT interval and is accepted as having a risk of causing torsade de pointes. The risk of drug-induced torsade de pointes is extremely low when a single QT interval prolonging drug is prescribed. In terms of epinephrine, it is not known what effect vasoconstrictors in the local anesthetic regimen will have in patients with a known history of congenital prolonged QT interval or in patients taking any medication that prolongs the QT interval. Until more information is obtained, it is suggested that the clinician consult with the physician prior to the use of a vasoconstrictor in suspected patients, and that the vasoconstrictor (epinephrine, mepivacaine and levonordefrin [Carbocaine® 2% with Neo-Cobefrin®]) be used with caution.

Effects on Dental Treatment No significant effects or complications reported

Effects on Bleeding No information available to require special precautions

Adverse Effects

>10%:

Cardiovascular: Palpitation (18%)

Central nervous system: Headache (adults 56%; children 13%), dizziness (adults 39%; children 4%), fever (25% to 29%), chills (adults 23%; children 5%), sleep disturbances (22%), fatigue (adults 17%; children 3%)

Gastrointestinal: Anorexia (adults 40%; children 13%), nausea (adults 26%; children 5%), vomiting (17% to 18%), abdominal pain (adults 17%; children 8%)

Neuromuscular & skeletal: Weakness (adults 38%; children 5%), arthralgia (adults 34%; children 3%), myalgia (adults 32%; children 3%)

Respiratory: Cough (adults 6%; children 23%)

3% to 10%:

- Central nervous system: Insomnia (5%), malaise (3%), vertigo (3%)
- Dermatologic: Pruritus (4%), rash (3%)
- Gastrointestinal: Splenomegaly (9%), diarrhea (7% to 8%)
- Hematologic: Anemia (4% to 9%)
- Hepatic: Hepatomegaly (6% to 9%), AST increased (4%)
- Respiratory: Rhinitis (4%), nasopharyngitis (3% to 4%)

General Dosage Range Oral:

Children 2 months to ≤16 years:

- 5 to <15 kg: Artemether 20 mg/lumefantrine 120 mg twice daily (maximum: 6 tablets per treatment course)
- 15 to <25 kg: Artemether 40 mg/lumefantrine 240 mg twice daily (maximum: 12 tablets per treatment course)
- 25 to <35 kg: Artemether 60 mg/lumefantrine 360 mg twice daily (maximum: 18 tablets per treatment course)
- ≥35 kg: Artemether 80 mg/lumefantrine 480 mg twice daily (maximum: 24 tablets per treatment course)

Children >16 years and Adults:

- 25 to <35 kg: Artemether 60 mg/lumefantrine 360 mg twice daily (maximum: 18 tablets per treatment course)
- ≥35 kg: Artemether 80 mg/lumefantrine 480 mg twice daily (maximum: 24 tablets per treatment course)

Mechanism of Action A coformulation of artemether and lumefantrine with activity against *Plasmodium falciparum*. Artemether and major metabolite dihydroartemisinin (DHA) are rapid schizontocides with activity attributed to the endoperoxide moiety common to each substance. Artemether inhibits an essential calcium adenosine triphosphatase. The exact mechanism of lumefantrine is unknown, but it may inhibit the formation of β-hematin by complexing with hemin. Both artemether and lumefantrine inhibit nucleic acid and protein synthesis. Artemether rapidly reduces parasite biomass and lumefantrine eliminates residual parasites.

Pharmacodynamics/Kinetics

Half-life Elimination Artemether: 1-2 hours; DHA: 2 hours; Lumefantrine: 72-144 hours

Time to Peak Plasma: Artemether: ~2 hours; Lumefantrine: ~6-8 hours

Pregnancy Risk Factor C

Dental Comment Artemether and lumefantrine is known to prolong the QT interval. The QT interval is measured as the time and distance between the Q point of the QRS complex and the end of the T wave in the ECG tracing. After adjustment for heart rate, the QT interval is defined as prolonged if it is more than 450 msec in men and 460 msec in women. A long QT syndrome was first described in the 1950s and 60s as a congenital syndrome involving QT interval prolongation and syncope and sudden death. Some of the congenital long QT syndromes were characterized by a peculiar electrocardiographic appearance of the QRS complex involving a premature atria beat followed by a pause, then a subsequent sinus beat showing marked QT prolongation and deformity. This type of cardiac arrhythmia was originally termed "torsade de pointes" (translated from the French as "twisting of the points"). Artemether and lumefantrine is considered as having a risk of causing torsade de pointes. Since it is not known what effect vasoconstrictors in the local anesthetic regimen will have in patients with a known history of congenital prolonged QT interval or in patients taking any medication that prolongs the QT interval, a medical consult is suggested.

Articaine and Epinephrine (AR ti kane & ep i NEF rin)

Related Information

EPINEPHrine (Systemic, Oral Inhalation) *on page 604*

Oral Pain *on page 1928*

U.S. Brand Names Septocaine® with epinephrine 1:100,000; Septocaine® with epinephrine 1:200,000; Zorcaine™

Canadian Brand Names Astracaine® with epinephrine 1:200,000; Astracaine® with epinephrine forte 1:100,000; Septanest® N; Septanest® SP; Ultracaine® DS; Ultracaine® DS Forte; Zorcaine™

Generic Availability (U.S.) No

Pharmacologic Category Local Anesthetic

Dental Use Local, infiltrative, or conductive anesthesia in both simple and complex dental and periodontal procedures

Use Local, infiltrative, or conductive anesthesia during simple and complex dental procedures

Local Anesthetic/Vasoconstrictor Precautions No information available to require special precautions (see Dental Comment)

Effects on Dental Treatment No significant effects or complications reported

Effects on Bleeding No information available to require special precautions

Adverse Effects Adverse reactions to Septocaine™ are characteristic of those associated with other amide-type local anesthetics; adverse reactions to this group of drugs may also result from excessive plasma levels which may be due to overdosage, unintentional intravascular injection, or slow metabolic degradation.

≥1% (in controlled trial of 882 patients):
- Central nervous system: Headache (4%), paresthesia (1%)
- Gastrointestinal: Gingivitis (1%)
- Miscellaneous: Pain (body as a whole 13%), facial edema (1%)

Additional adverse reactions reported with articaine and epinephrine: Arrhythmia, myocardial depression, asthma, convulsions, allergic reactions, injection site reactions, tissue necrosis

Dental Usual Dosage Adults:

Infiltration: Injection volume of 4% solution: 0.5-2.5 mL; total dose: 20-100 mg
Nerve block: Injection volume of 4% solution: 0.5-3.4 mL; total dose: 20-136 mg
Oral surgery: Injection volume of 4% solution: 1-5.1 mL; total dose: 40-204 mg

Note: These dosages are guides only; other dosages may be used; however, do not exceed maximum recommended dose

Special populations: The clinician is reminded that these doses serve only as a guide to the amount of anesthetic required for most routine procedures. The actual volumes to be used depend upon a number of factors, such as type and extent of surgical procedure, depth of anesthesia, degree of muscular relaxation, and condition of the patient. In all cases, the smallest dose that will produce the desired result should be given. Dosages should be reduced for pediatric patients, elderly patients, and patients with cardiac and/or liver disease.

Dosage Summary of recommended volumes and concentrations for various types of anesthetic procedures; dosages (administered by submucosal injection and/or nerve block) apply to normal healthy adults:

Infiltration: Injection volume of 4% solution: 0.5-2.5 mL; total dose: 20-100 mg
Nerve block: Injection volume of 4% solution: 0.5-3.4 mL; total dose: 20-136 mg
Oral surgery: Injection volume of 4% solution: 1-5.1 mL; total dose: 40-204 mg

Note: These dosages are guides only; other dosages may be used; however, do not exceed maximum recommended dose

Special populations: The clinician is reminded that these doses serve only as a guide to the amount of anesthetic required for most routine procedures. The actual volumes to be used depend upon a number of factors, such as type and extent of surgical procedure, depth of anesthesia, degree of muscular relaxation, and condition of the patient. In all cases, the smallest dose that will produce the desired result should be given. Dosages should be reduced for pediatric patients, elderly patients, and patients with cardiac and/or liver disease.

Children <4 years: Safety and efficacy have not been established

Children 4-16 years (dosages in a clinical trial of 61 patients):
- Simple procedures: 0.76-5.65 mg/kg (0.9-5.1 mL) was administered safely to 51 patients
- Complex procedures: 0.37-7.48 mg/kg (0.7-3.9 mL) was administered safely to 10 patients
- **Note:** Approximately 13% of the pediatric patients required additional injections for complete anesthesia

Geriatric patients (dosages in a clinical trial):
- 65-75 years:
  - Simple procedures: 0.43-4.76 mg/kg (0.9-11.9 mL) was administered safely to 35 patients
  - Complex procedures: 1.05-4.27 mg/kg (1.3-6.8 mL) was administered safely to 19 patients
- ≥75 years:
  - Simple procedures: 0.78-4.76 mg/kg (1.3-11.9 mL) was administered safely to 7 patients
  - Complex procedures: 1.12-2.17 mg/kg (1.3-5.1 mL) was administered safely to 4 patients
- **Note:** Approximately 6% of the patients 65-75 years of age (none of the patients ≥75 years of age) required additional injections for complete anesthesia, compared to 11% of the patients 17-65 years of age who required additional injections.

Maximum recommended dosages:

Children (use in pediatric patients <4 years is not recommended): Not to exceed 7 mg/kg (0.175 mL/kg) **or** 3.2 mg/lb (0.0795 mL/lb) of body weight

Adults (normal, healthy): Submucosal infiltration and/or nerve block: Not to exceed 7 mg/kg (0.175 mL/kg) **or** 3.2 mg/lb (0.0795 mL/lb) of body weight

The following numbers of dental cartridges (1.7 mL) provide the indicated amounts of articaine hydrochloride 4% and epinephrine 1:100,000:

1 cartridge provides 68 mg articaine HCl (4%) and 0.017 mg vasoconstrictor (epinephrine 1:100,000)
2 cartridges provides 136 mg articaine HCl (4%) and 0.034 mg vasoconstrictor (epinephrine 1:100,000)
3 cartridges provides 204 mg articaine HCl (4%) and 0.051 mg vasoconstrictor (epinephrine 1:100,000)
4 cartridges provides 272 mg articaine HCl (4%) and 0.068 mg vasoconstrictor (epinephrine 1:100,000)
5 cartridges provides 340 mg articaine HCl (4%) and 0.085 mg vasoconstrictor (epinephrine 1:100,000)
6 cartridges provides 408 mg articaine HCl (4%) and 0.102 mg vasoconstrictor (epinephrine 1:100,000)
7 cartridges provides 476 mg articaine HCl (4%) and 0.119 mg vasoconstrictor (epinephrine 1:100,000)
8 cartridges provides 544 mg articaine HCl (4%) and 0.136 mg vasoconstrictor (epinephrine 1:100,000)

The following numbers of dental cartridges (1.7 mL) provide the indicated amounts of articaine hydrochloride 4% and epinephrine 1:200,000:

1 cartridge provides 68 mg articaine HCl (4%) and 0.0085 mg vasoconstrictor (epinephrine 1:200,000)
2 cartridges provides 136 mg articaine HCl (4%) and 0.017 mg vasoconstrictor (epinephrine 1:200,000)
3 cartridges provides 204 mg articaine HCl (4%) and 0.026 mg vasoconstrictor (epinephrine 1:200,000)
4 cartridges provides 272 mg articaine HCl (4%) and 0.034 mg vasoconstrictor (epinephrine 1:200,000)
5 cartridges provides 340 mg articaine HCl (4%) and 0.043 mg vasoconstrictor (epinephrine 1:200,000)
6 cartridges provides 408 mg articaine HCl (4%) and 0.051 mg vasoconstrictor (epinephrine 1:200,000)
7 cartridges provides 476 mg articaine HCl (4%) and 0.060 mg vasoconstrictor (epinephrine 1:200,000)
8 cartridges provides 544 mg articaine HCl (4%) and 0.068 mg vasoconstrictor (epinephrine 1:200,000)

Mechanism of Action Local anesthetics block the generation and conduction of nerve impulses, presumably by increasing the threshold for electrical excitation in the nerve, by slowing the propagation of the nerve impulse, and by reducing the rate of rise of the action potential. In general, the progression of anesthesia is related to the diameter, myelination, and conduction velocity of the affected nerve fibers. Clinically, the order of loss of nerve function is as follows: 1) pain, 2) temperature, 3) touch, 4) proprioception, and 5) skeletal muscle tone.

Contraindications Hypersensitivity to local anesthetics of the amide type or any component of the formulation

Warnings/Precautions Intravascular injections should be avoided; aspiration should be performed prior to administration; the needle must be repositioned until no return of blood can be elicited by aspiration; however, absence of blood in the syringe does not guarantee that intravascular injection has been avoided. **Accidental intravascular injection may be associated with convulsions, followed by CNS or cardiorespiratory depression and coma, ultimately progressing to respiratory arrest.** Dental practitioners and/or clinicians using local anesthetic agents should be well trained in diagnosis and management of emergencies that may arise from the use of these agents. Resuscitative equipment, oxygen, and other resuscitative drugs should be available for immediate use.

Contains epinephrine, which can cause local tissue necrosis or systemic toxicity, usual precautions for epinephrine administration should be observed. Administration of articaine HCl with epinephrine results in a three- to fivefold increase in plasma epinephrine concentrations compared to baseline; however, in healthy adults, it does not appear to be associated with marked increases in blood pressure or heart rate, except in the case of accidental intravascular injection.

Products may contain sodium metabisulfite, which may cause allergic-type reactions (including anaphylactic symptoms, and life-threatening or less severe asthmatic episodes) in certain susceptible patients. The overall prevalence of the sulfite sensitivity in the general population is unknown, and is seen more frequently in asthmatic than in nonasthmatic persons.

To avoid serious adverse effects and high plasma levels, the lowest dosage resulting in effective anesthesia should be administered. Repeated doses may cause significant increases in blood levels with each repeated dose due to the possibility of accumulation of the drug or its metabolites. Tolerance to elevated blood levels varies with patient status. Reduced dosages, commensurate with age and physical condition, should be given to debilitated patients, elderly patients, acutely-ill patients, and pediatric patients. Use caution in patients with heart block.

Local anesthetic solutions containing a vasoconstrictor should be used cautiously. Patients with peripheral vascular disease or hypertensive vascular disease may exhibit exaggerated vasoconstrictor response, possibly resulting in ischemic injury or necrosis. It should also be used cautiously in patients during or following the administration of a potent general anesthetic agent, since cardiac arrhythmias may occur under these conditions.

Systemic absorption of local anesthetics may produce CNS and cardiovascular effects. Changes in cardiac conduction, excitability, refractoriness, contractility, and peripheral vascular resistance are minimal at blood concentrations produced by therapeutic doses. However, toxic blood concentrations depress cardiac conduction and excitability, which may lead to AV block, ventricular arrhythmias, and cardiac arrest (sometimes resulting in death). In addition, myocardial contractility is depressed and peripheral vasodilation occurs, leading to decreased cardiac output and arterial blood pressure.

Careful and constant monitoring of cardiovascular and respiratory (adequacy of ventilation) vital signs and the patient's state of consciousness should be done following each local anesthetic injection; at such times, restlessness, anxiety, tinnitus, dizziness, blurred vision, tremors, depression, or drowsiness may be early warning signs of CNS toxicity. Methemoglobinemia has been reported with articaine. Treatment is primarily symptomatic and supportive. Methemoglobinemia may be treated with methylene blue, 1-2 mg/kg I.V. infused over several minutes.

In vitro studies show that ~5% to 10% of articaine is metabolized by the human liver microsomal P450 isoenzyme system; however, no studies have been performed in patient with liver dysfunction, and caution should be used in patients with severe hepatic disease. Use with caution in patients with impaired cardiovascular function, since they may be less able to compensate for function changes associated with prolonged AV conduction produced by these drugs.

Small doses of local anesthetics injected into dental blocks may produce adverse reactions similar to systemic toxicity seen in unintentional intravascular injections at larger doses. Confusion, convulsions, respiratory depression and/or respiratory arrest, and cardiovascular stimulation or depression have been reported. These reactions may be due to intra-arterial injection of the local anesthetic with retrograde flow to the cerebral circulation. Patients receiving such blocks should be observed constantly with resuscitative equipment and personnel trained in treatment of adverse reactions immediately available. Dosage recommendations should not be exceeded. Safety and efficacy have not been established in children <4 years of age.

Drug Interactions

Avoid Concomitant Use

Avoid concomitant use of Articaine and Epinephrine with any of the following: Iobenguane I 123; Lurasidone

Increased Effect/Toxicity

Articaine and Epinephrine may increase the levels/effects of: Bromocriptine; Lurasidone; Sympathomimetics

The levels/effects of Articaine and Epinephrine may be increased by: Antacids; Atomoxetine; Beta-Blockers; Cannabinoids; Carbonic Anhydrase Inhibitors; COMT Inhibitors; Inhalational Anesthetics; MAO Inhibitors; Serotonin/Norepinephrine Reuptake Inhibitors; Tricyclic Antidepressants

Decreased Effect

Articaine and Epinephrine may decrease the levels/effects of: Benzylpenicilloyl Polylysine; Iobenguane I 123

The levels/effects of Articaine and Epinephrine may be decreased by: Spironolactone

Pharmacodynamics/Kinetics

Onset of Action 1-6 minutes

Duration of Action Complete anesthesia: ~1 hour

Half-life Elimination Articaine: 1.8 hours; Articainic acid: 1.5 hours

Pregnancy Risk Factor C

Lactation Excretion in breast milk unknown/use caution

Breast-Feeding Considerations It is not known whether articaine is excreted in human milk.

Dosage Forms

Injection, solution [for dental use]:

Septocaine® with epinephrine 1:100,000: Articaine 4% and epinephrine 1:100,000 (1.7 mL)

Septocaine® with epinephrine 1:200,000: Articaine 4% and epinephrine 1:200,000 (1.7 mL)

Zorcaine™: Articaine 4% and epinephrine 1:100,000 (1.7 mL) [contains sodium metabisulfite]

Dosage Forms: Canada

Injection, solution [for dental use]:

Astracaine® with epinephrine 1:200,000: Articaine 4% and epinephrine 1:200,000 (1.8 mL)

Astracaine® Forte with epinephrine forte 1:100,000: Articaine 4% and epinephrine 1:100,000 (1.8 mL)

Septanest® N: Articaine 4% and epinephrine 1:200,000 (1.7 mL)

Septanest® SP: Articaine 4% and epinephrine 1:100,000 (1.7 mL)

Ultracaine® DS: Articaine 4% and epinephrine 1:200,000 (1.7 mL)

Ultracaine® DS Forte: Articaine 4% and epinephrine 1:100,000 (1.7 mL)

Dental Comment Septocaine™ (articaine hydrochloride 4% and epinephrine 1:100,000) is the first FDA approval in 30 years of a new local dental anesthetic providing complete pulpal anesthesia for approximately 1 hour. Chemically, articaine contains both an amide linkage and an ester linkage, making it chemically unique in the class of local anesthetics. Since it contains the ester linkage, articaine HCl is rapidly metabolized by plasma carboxyesterase to its primary metabolite, articainic acid, which is an inactive product of this metabolism. According to the manufacturer, *in vitro* studies show that the human liver microsomal P450 isoenzyme system metabolizes approximately 5% to 10% of available articaine with nearly quantitative conversion to articainic acid. The elimination half-life of articaine is about 1.8 hours, and that of articainic acid is about 1.5 hours. Articaine is excreted primarily through urine with 53% to 57% of the administered dose eliminated in the first 24 hours following submucosal administration. Articainic acid is the primary metabolite in urine. A minor metabolite, articainic acid glucuronide, is also excreted in the urine. Articaine constitutes only 2% of the total dose excreted in urine.

The anesthetic efficacy of the articaine 4% with 1:200,000 epinephrine (A/200) was compared to that of articaine 4% with 1:100,000 (A/100) using electric pulp tester to assess anesthesia using 63 subjects after either maxillary infiltration (Moore, 2006) or inferior alveolar block (Hersh, 2006).

After maxillary infiltration of 1 mL of each formula, the onset times to anesthesia were 3.1 ± 2.3 minutes for articaine 4% and 1:200,000 epinephrine (A/200), 3 ± 2.1 minutes for articaine 4% and 1:100,000 epinephrine (A/100), 3 ± 2 minutes for articaine 4% with no epinephrine (A/no). These three mean times of onset were not statistically different. Durations of anesthesia were 41.6 ± 21.1 minutes A/200, 45 ± 23.6 minutes A/100, 13.3 ± 6.8 minutes for A/no. There was no statistically significant difference between the durations elicited by the A/200 and A/100 formulations (Moore, 2006). In the second trial of the study, also using 63 subjects, the investigators administered an inferior alveolar nerve block injection of one cartridge (1.7 mL) using a standard intra-oral injection technique for inferior alveolar block anesthesia. Pulpal anesthesia was measured again using the pulp tester.

The onset times to anesthesia were 4.7 ± 2.6 minutes A/200, 4.2 ± 2.8 minutes A/100, and 4.3 ± 2.5 minutes for A/no. There were no statistically significant differences in these times to onset. Durations of anesthesia were 51.2 ± 55.9 minutes A/200, 61.8 ± 59 minutes A/100, and 49.7 ± 44.6 minutes for A/no. There were no statistically significant differences in the duration between A/200, A/100, and A/no formulations (Hersh, 2006).

Oral paresthesia: The occurrence of oral paresthesia associated with 4% solutions of prilocaine or articaine, although rare, continue to be slightly more frequent than other local anesthetics. From 1999-2008, there were 182 cases of nonsurgical paresthesia (Gaffen, 2009). Of the cases, 172 involved mandibular block injection only. Another eight cases involved mandibular block combined with at least one other type of anesthetic injection. A single case involved infiltration around tooth number 35 and the final case involved infiltration and intraligamentary injection in the maxillary anterior region.

A 2010 report, reviewed adverse events submitted voluntarily over a 10-year period involving the dental local anesthetics articaine, bupivacaine, lidocaine, mepivacaine, and prilocaine in the United States. Articaine reported incidence: One case per 4,159,848 cartridges sold. The reported incidence of paresthesia was one case for 13,800,970 cartridges of all local anesthetics sold in the U.S. (Garisto, 2010).

References

Dower JS Jr, "A Review of Paresthesia in Association With Administration of Local Anesthesia," *Dent Today*, 2003, 22(2):64-9.

Finder RL and Moore PA, "Adverse Drug Reactions to Local Anesthesia," *Dent Clin North Am*, 2002, 46 (4):747-57, x.

Gaffen AS and Haas DA, "Retrospective Review of Voluntary Reports of Nonsurgical Paresthesia in Dentistry," *J Can Dent Assoc*, 2009, 75(8):579.

Garisto GA, Gaffen AS, Lawrence HP, et al, "Occurrence of Paresthesia After Dental Local Anesthetic Administration in the United States," *J Am Dent Assoc*, 2010, 141(7):836-44.

Haas DA, "An Update on Local Anesthetics in Dentistry," *J Can Dent Assoc*, 2002, 68(9):546-51.

Hawkins JM and Moore PA, "Local Anesthesia: Advances in Agents and Techniques," *Dent Clin North Am*, 2002, 46(4):719-32, ix.

Hersh EV, Giannakopoulos H, Levin LM, et al, "The Pharmacokinetics and Cardiovascular Effects of High-Dose Articaine With 1:100,000 and 1:200,000 Epinephrine," *J Am Dent Assoc*, 2006, 137 (11):1562-71.

"Injectable Local Anesthetics," *J Am Dent Assoc*, 2003, 134(5):628-9.

Malamed SF, Gagnon S, Leblanc D, "A Comparison Between Articaine HCl and Lidocaine HCl in Pediatric Dental Patients," *Pediatr Dent*, 2000, 22(4):307-11.

Malamed SF, "Allergy and Toxic Reactions to Local Anesthetics," *Dent Today*, 2003, 22(4):114-6, 118-21.

Malamed SF, Gagnon S, Leblanc D, "Articaine Hydrochloride: A Study of the Safety of a New Amide Local Anesthetic," *J Am Dent Assoc*, 2001, 132(2):177-85.

Malamed SF, Gagnon S, Leblanc D, "Efficacy of Articaine: A New Amide Local Anesthetic," *J Am Dent Assoc*, 2000, 131(5):635-42.

Moore PA, Boynes SG, Hersh EV, et al, "The Anesthetic Efficacy of 4 Percent Articaine 1:200,000 Epinephrine: Two Controlled Clinical Trials," *J Am Dent Assoc*, 2006, 137(11):1572-81.

Schertzer ER Jr, "Articaine vs lidocaine," *J Am Dent Assoc*, 2000, 131(9):1248, 1250.

Weaver JM, "Articaine, A New Local Anesthetic for American Dentists: Will It Supersede Lidocaine?" *Anesth Prog*, 1999, 46(4):111-2.

Wynn RL, Bergman SA, and Meiller TF, "Paresthesia Associated With Local Anesthetics: A Perspective on Articaine," *Gen Dent*, 2003, 51(6):498-501.

Artificial Tears (ar ti FISH il tears)

U.S. Brand Names Akwa Tears® [OTC]; Bion® Tears [OTC]; HypoTears PF [OTC]; HypoTears [OTC]; Liquifilm® Tears [OTC]; Moisture® Eyes PM [OTC]; Moisture® Eyes [OTC]; Murine Tears® [OTC]; Murocel® [OTC]; Nature's Tears® [OTC]; Nu-Tears® II [OTC]; Nu-Tears® [OTC]; Puralube® Tears [OTC] [DSC]; Refresh Plus® [OTC]; Refresh Tears® [OTC]; Refresh® [OTC]; Soothe® [OTC]; Systane® Free [OTC]; Systane® [OTC]; Teargen® II [OTC]; Teargen® [OTC]; Tearisol® [OTC]; Tears Again® [OTC]; Tears Naturale® Free [OTC]; Tears Naturale® II [OTC]; Tears Naturale® [OTC]; Tears Plus® [OTC]; Tears Renewed® [OTC]; Ultra Tears® [OTC]; Viva-Drops® [OTC]

Canadian Brand Names Teardrops®

Pharmacologic Category Ophthalmic Agent, Miscellaneous

Use Ophthalmic lubricant; for relief of dry eyes and eye irritation

Local Anesthetic/Vasoconstrictor Precautions No information available to require special precautions

Effects on Dental Treatment No significant effects or complications reported

Effects on Bleeding No information available to require special precautions

Adverse Effects 1% to 10%: Ocular: May cause mild stinging or temporary blurred vision

General Dosage Range Ophthalmic: *Children and Adults:* 1-2 drops into eye(s) 3-4 times/day as needed

Pregnancy Risk Factor C

Ascorbic Acid (a SKOR bik AS id)

U.S. Brand Names Acerola [OTC]; Asco-Caps-1000 [OTC]; Asco-Caps-500 [OTC]; Asco-Tabs-1000 [OTC]; Ascocid® [OTC]; Ascocid®-500 [OTC]; Ascor L 500®; Ascor L NC®; C-Gel [OTC]; C-Gram [OTC]; C-Time [OTC]; Cemill 1000 [OTC]; Cemill 500 [OTC]; Chew-C [OTC]; Dull-C® [OTC]; Mild-C® [OTC]; One Gram C [OTC]; Time-C® [OTC]; Vicks® Vitamin C [OTC]; Vita-C® [OTC]

Canadian Brand Names Proflavanol C™; Revitalose C-1000®

Pharmacologic Category Vitamin, Water Soluble

Use Prevention and treatment of scurvy; acidify the urine

Unlabeled/Investigational Use Investigational: In large doses, to decrease the severity of "colds"; dietary supplementation; a 20-year study was recently completed involving 730 individuals which indicates a possible decreased risk of death by stroke when ascorbic acid at doses ≥45 mg/day was administered

Local Anesthetic/Vasoconstrictor Precautions No information available to require special precautions

Effects on Dental Treatment No significant effects or complications reported

Effects on Bleeding No information available to require special precautions

Adverse Effects 1% to 10%: Renal: Hyperoxaluria with large doses

General Dosage Range

I.M., SubQ:

Children: 100-300 mg/day in divided doses

Adults: 100-250 mg 1-2 times/day

I.V., Oral:

Children: 100-300 mg/day in divided doses (maximum: 500 mg every 6-8 hours)

Adults: 100-250 mg 1-2 times/day (maximum: 4-12 g/day in 3-4 divided doses)

Mechanism of Action Not fully understood; necessary for collagen formation and tissue repair; involved in some oxidation-reduction reactions as well as other metabolic pathways, such as synthesis of carnitine, steroids, and catecholamines and conversion of folic acid to folinic acid

Pregnancy Risk Factor A/C (dose exceeding RDA recommendation)

Asenapine (a SEN a peen)

Related Information

Clinical Risk Related to Drugs Prolonging QT Interval *on page 1872*

U.S. Brand Names Saphris®

Pharmacologic Category Antimanic Agent; Antipsychotic Agent, Atypical

Use Acute and maintenance treatment of schizophrenia; treatment of acute mania or mixed episodes associated with bipolar I disorder (as monotherapy or in combination with lithium or valproate)

Local Anesthetic/Vasoconstrictor Precautions Asenapine is one of the drugs confirmed to prolong the QT interval and is accepted as having a risk of causing torsade de pointes. The risk of drug-induced torsade de pointes is extremely low when a single QT interval prolonging drug is prescribed. In terms of epinephrine, it is not known what effect vasoconstrictors in the local anesthetic regimen will have in patients with a known history of congenital prolonged QT interval or in patients taking any medication that prolongs the QT interval. Until more information is obtained, it is suggested that the clinician consult with the physician prior to the use of a vasoconstrictor in suspected patients, and that the vasoconstrictor (epinephrine, mepivacaine and levonordefrin [Carbocaine® 2% with Neo-Cobefrin®]) be used with caution.

Effects on Dental Treatment Key adverse event(s) related to dental treatment: Xerostomia and increase in salivation (normal salivary flow resumes upon discontinuation). Abnormal taste, toothache, and edema of the tongue have been reported. Many patients may experience orthostatic hypotension with asenapine; precautions should be taken. Asenapine may cause extrapyramidal symptoms including tardive dyskinesia; risk may be greater with increased doses.

Effects on Bleeding No information available to require special precautions

Adverse Effects Actual frequency may be dependent upon dose and/or indication.

>10%:

Central nervous system: Somnolence (13% to 24%), insomnia (6% to 16%), extrapyramidal symptoms (6% to 12%), headache (12%), akathisia (4% to 11%; dose related), dizziness (3% to 11%)

Endocrine & metabolic: Hypertriglyceridemia (13% to 15%)

1% to 10%:

Cardiovascular: Peripheral edema (3%), hypertension (2% to 3%)

Central nervous system: Hypoesthesia (4% to 7%), fatigue (3% to 4%), anxiety (4%), depression (2%), irritability (1% to 2%)

Endocrine & metabolic: Cholesterol increased (8% to 9%), glucose increased (5% to 7%), hyperprolactinemia (2% to 3%)

Gastrointestinal: Constipation (4% to 7%), vomiting (4% to 7%), weight gain (2% to 5%), dyspepsia (3% to 4%), appetite increased (≤4%), salivation increased (≤4%), abnormal taste (3%), toothache (3%), abdominal discomfort (≤3%), xerostomia (1% to 3%)

Hematologic: Creatine kinase increased (6%)

Hepatic: Transaminases increased (<1% to 3%)

Neuromuscular & skeletal: Arthralgia (3%), extremity pain (2%)

Dosage Sublingual: Adults: **Note:** Safety of doses >20 mg/day has not been evaluated:

Schizophrenia:

Acute treatment: Initial: 5 mg twice daily. Daily doses >20 mg/day in clinical trials did not appear to offer any additional benefits and increased risk of adverse effects.

Maintenance treatment: Initial: 5 mg twice daily; may increase to 10 mg twice daily after 1 week based on tolerability

Bipolar disorder:

Monotherapy: Initial: 10 mg twice daily; decrease to 5 mg twice daily if dose not tolerated

Combination therapy (with lithium or valproate): 5 mg twice daily; may increase to 10 mg twice daily based on tolerability

Dosing adjustment in renal impairment: No dosage adjustment is necessary

Dosing adjustment in hepatic impairment:

Mild-to-moderate hepatic impairment (Child-Pugh class A or B): No dosage adjustment is necessary

Severe hepatic impairment (Child-Pugh class C): Use is not recommended

Mechanism of Action Asenapine is a dibenzo-oxepino pyrrole atypical antipsychotic with mixed serotonin-dopamine antagonist activity. It exhibits high affinity for $5\text{-}HT_{1A}$, $5\text{-}HT_{1B}$, $5\text{-}HT_{2A}$, $5\text{-}HT_{2B}$, $5\text{-}HT_{2C}$, $5\text{-}HT_{5\text{-}7}$, $D_{1\text{-}4}$, H_1 and, $alpha_1$- and $alpha_2$-adrenergic receptors; moderate affinity for H_2 receptors. Asenapine has no significant affinity for muscarinic receptors. The binding affinity to the D_2 receptor is 19 times lower than the $5\text{-}HT_{2A}$ affinity (Weber, 2009). The addition of serotonin antagonism to dopamine antagonism (classic neuroleptic mechanism) is thought to improve negative symptoms of psychoses and reduce the incidence of extrapyramidal side effects as compared to typical antipsychotics.

Contraindications There are no contraindications listed in the manufacturers labeling.

Warnings/Precautions [U.S. Boxed Warning]: Elderly patients with dementia-related psychosis treated with atypical antipsychotics are at an increased risk of death compared to placebo. Most deaths appeared to be either cardiovascular (eg, heart failure, sudden death) or infectious (eg, pneumonia) in nature. In addition, an increased incidence of cerebrovascular effects (eg, transient ischemic attack, cerebrovascular accidents) has been reported in studies of placebo-controlled trials of antipsychotics in elderly patients with dementia-related psychosis. Asenapine is not approved for the treatment of dementia-related psychosis.

Leukopenia, neutropenia, and agranulocytosis (sometimes fatal) have been reported in clinical trials and postmarketing reports with antipsychotic use; presence of risk factors (eg, pre-existing low WBC or history of drug-induced leuko/neutropenia) should prompt periodic blood count assessment. Discontinue therapy at first signs of blood dyscrasias or if absolute neutrophil count $<1000/mm^3$.

May be sedating; use with caution in disorders where CNS depression is a feature. Use with caution in Parkinson's disease. Use with caution in patients at risk of seizures, including those with a history of seizures, head trauma, brain damage, alcoholism, or concurrent therapy with medications which may lower seizure threshold. Use is not recommended in severe hepatic impairment; increased drug concentrations may occur. Esophageal dysmotility and aspiration have been associated with antipsychotic use; use with caution in patients at risk of aspiration pneumonia (ie, Alzheimer's disease). Elevates prolactin levels; use with caution in breast cancer or other prolactin-dependent tumors. May alter temperature regulation.

Use with caution in patients with cardiovascular diseases (eg, heart failure, history of myocardial infarction or ischemia, cerebrovascular disease, conduction abnormalities). May cause orthostatic hypotension; use with caution in patients at risk of this effect (eg, concurrent medication use which may predispose to hypotension/bradycardia or presence of hypovolemia) or in those who would not tolerate transient hypotensive episodes. May result in QT_c prolongation. Risk may be increased by conditions or concomitant medications which cause bradycardia, hypokalemia, and/or hypomagnesemia. Avoid use in combination with QT_c-prolonging drugs and in patients with congenital long QT syndrome or patients with history of cardiac arrhythmia.

May cause extrapyramidal symptoms (EPS), including pseudoparkinsonism, acute dystonic reactions, akathisia, and tardive dyskinesia. Risk of dystonia (and probably other EPS) may be greater with increased doses, use of conventional antipsychotics, males, and younger patients. Risk of neuroleptic malignant syndrome (NMS) may be increased in patients with Parkinson's disease or Lewy body dementia. May cause hyperglycemia; in some cases may be extreme and associated with ketoacidosis, hyperosmolar coma, or death. Use with caution in patients with diabetes or other disorders of glucose regulation; monitor for worsening of glucose control. Significant weight gain has been observed with antipsychotic therapy; incidence varies with product. Monitor waist circumference and BMI.

The possibility of a suicide attempt is inherent in psychotic illness or bipolar disorder; use caution in high-risk patients during initiation of therapy. Prescriptions should be written for the smallest quantity consistent with good patient care. Use caution in elderly patients.

Drug Interactions

Avoid Concomitant Use

Avoid concomitant use of Asenapine with any of the following: Artemether; Dronedarone; Lumefantrine; Metoclopramide; Nilotinib; Pimozide; QuiNINE; Tetrabenazine; Thioridazine; Toremifene; Vandetanib; Ziprasidone

Increased Effect/Toxicity

Asenapine may increase the levels/effects of: Alcohol (Ethyl); CNS Depressants; Dronedarone; Methylphenidate; PARoxetine; Pimozide; QTc-Prolonging Agents; QuiNINE; Tetrabenazine; Thioridazine; Toremifene; Vandetanib; Ziprasidone

The levels/effects of Asenapine may be increased by: Abiraterone; Acetylcholinesterase Inhibitors (Central); Alfuzosin; Artemether; Chloroquine; Ciprofloxacin; Ciprofloxacin (Systemic); Conivaptan; CYP1A2 Inhibitors (Moderate); CYP1A2 Inhibitors (Strong); Deferasirox; FluvoxaMINE; Gadobutrol; Lithium formulations; Lumefantrine; MAO Inhibitors; Methylphenidate; Metoclopramide; Nilotinib; QuiNINE; Tetrabenazine

Decreased Effect

Asenapine may decrease the levels/effects of: Amphetamines; Anti-Parkinson's Agents (Dopamine Agonist); Quinagolide

The levels/effects of Asenapine may be decreased by: CYP1A2 Inducers (Strong); Lithium formulations; Peginterferon Alfa-2b; Tocilizumab

Ethanol/Nutrition/Herb Interactions Ethanol: May increase CNS depression; monitor for increased effects with coadministration. Caution patients about effects.

Dietary Considerations Avoid eating or drinking for at least 10 minutes after administration.

Pharmacodynamics/Kinetics

Half-life Elimination Terminal: ~24 hours

Time to Peak 0.5-1.5 hours

Pregnancy Risk Factor C

Lactation Excretion in breast milk unknown/not recommended

Dosage Forms

Tablet, sublingual:

Saphris®: 5 mg, 10 mg

Dental Comment Asenapine is known to prolong the QT interval. The QT interval is measured as the time and distance between the Q point of the QRS complex and the end of the T wave in the ECG tracing. After adjustment for heart rate, the QT interval is defined as prolonged if it is more than 450 msec in men and 460 msec in women. A long QT syndrome was first described in the 1950s and 60s as a congenital syndrome involving QT interval prolongation and syncope and sudden death. Some of the congenital long QT syndromes were characterized by a peculiar electrocardiographic appearance of the QRS complex involving a premature atria beat followed by a pause, then a subsequent sinus beat showing marked QT prolongation and deformity. This type of cardiac arrhythmia was originally termed "torsade de pointes" (translated from the French as "twisting of the points"). Asenapine is considered as having a risk of causing torsade de pointes. Since it is not known what effect vasoconstrictors in the local anesthetic regimen will have in patients with a known history of congenital prolonged QT interval or in patients taking any medication that prolongs the QT interval, a medical consult is suggested.

Asparaginase (a SPEAR a ji nase)

U.S. Brand Names Elspar®

Canadian Brand Names Kidrolase®

Pharmacologic Category Antineoplastic Agent, Miscellaneous

Use Treatment (in combination with other chemotherapy) of acute lymphoblastic leukemia (ALL)

Unlabeled/Investigational Use Treatment of lymphoblastic lymphoma

Local Anesthetic/Vasoconstrictor Precautions No information available to require special precautions

Effects on Dental Treatment Key adverse event(s) related to dental treatment: Stomatitis

Effects on Bleeding Although significant myelosuppression with associated altered hemostasis has been reported for many chemotherapeutic agents, myelosuppression is not common with asparaginase and no specific precautions appear to be necessary.

Adverse Effects Note: Immediate effects: Fever, chills, nausea, and vomiting occur in 50% to 60% of patients.

>10%:

Central nervous system: Fatigue, fever, chills, depression, agitation, seizure (10% to 60%), somnolence, stupor, confusion, coma (25%)

Endocrine & metabolic: Hyperglycemia/glucose intolerance (10%)

Gastrointestinal: Nausea, vomiting (50% to 60%), anorexia, abdominal cramps (70%), acute pancreatitis (15%, may be severe in some patients)

Hematologic: Hypofibrinogenemia and depression of clotting factors V and VIII, variable decrease in factors VII and IX, severe protein C deficiency and decrease in antithrombin III (may be dose limiting or fatal)

Hepatic: Transaminases, bilirubin, and alkaline phosphatase increased (transient)

Hypersensitivity: Acute allergic reactions (fever, rash, urticaria, arthralgia, hypotension, angioedema, bronchospasm, anaphylaxis (15% to 35%); may be dose limiting in some patients, may be fatal)

Renal: Azotemia (66%)

1% to 10%:

Endocrine & metabolic: Hyperuricemia

Gastrointestinal: Stomatitis

Miscellaneous: Allergic reaction (including anaphylaxis), antibody formation/immunogenicity (~25%)

General Dosage Range

I.M.: *Children and Adults:* 6000 units/m^2/dose 3 times/week **or** 6000 units/m^2 every ~3 days

I.V.: *Children and Adults:* Dosage varies greatly depending on indication

Intradermal: *Children and Adults:* Test dose: 0.1-0.2 mL of a 20-250 units/mL concentration

Mechanism of Action Asparaginase inhibits protein synthesis by hydrolyzing asparagine to aspartic acid and ammonia. Leukemia cells, especially lymphoblasts, require exogenous asparagine; normal cells can synthesize asparagine. Asparaginase is cycle-specific for the G_1 phase.

Pharmacodynamics/Kinetics

Half-life Elimination I.M.: 39-49 hours; I.V.: 8-30 hours

Time to Peak I.M.: 14-24 hours

Pregnancy Risk Factor C

Prescribing and Access Restrictions The *Erwinia* strain of asparaginase is no longer commercially available in the U.S., although may be obtained through clinical trials or on a compassionate use basis.

Aspirin (AS pir in)

Related Information

Antiplatelet and Anticoagulation Considerations in Dentistry *on page 1867*

Cardiovascular Diseases *on page 1848*

Oral Pain *on page 1928*

Rheumatoid Arthritis, Osteoarthritis, and Osteoporosis *on page 1889*

U.S. Brand Names Ascriptin® Maximum Strength [OTC]; Ascriptin® Regular Strength [OTC]; Aspercin [OTC]; Aspergum® [OTC]; Aspir-low [OTC]; Aspirtab [OTC]; Bayer® Aspirin Extra Strength [OTC]; Bayer® Aspirin Regimen Adult Low Strength [OTC]; Bayer® Aspirin Regimen Children's [OTC]; Bayer® Aspirin Regimen Regular Strength [OTC]; Bayer® Genuine Aspirin [OTC]; Bayer® Plus Extra Strength [OTC]; Bayer® Women's Low Dose Aspirin [OTC]; Buffasal [OTC]; Bufferin® Extra Strength [OTC]; Bufferin® [OTC]; Buffinol [OTC]; Easprin®; Ecotrin® Arthritis Strength [OTC]; Ecotrin® Low Strength [OTC]; Ecotrin® [OTC]; Halfprin® [OTC]; St Joseph® Adult Aspirin [OTC]; Tri-Buffered Aspirin [OTC]; ZORprin® [DSC]

Canadian Brand Names Asaphen; Asaphen E.C.; Entrophen®; Novasen; Praxis ASA EC 81 Mg Daily Dose

Generic Availability (U.S.) Yes: Excludes gum

Pharmacologic Category Antiplatelet Agent; Salicylate

Dental Use Treatment of postoperative pain

Use Treatment of mild-to-moderate pain, inflammation, and fever; prevention and treatment of myocardial infarction (MI), acute ischemic stroke, and transient ischemic episodes; management of rheumatoid arthritis, rheumatic fever, osteoarthritis, and gout (high dose); adjunctive therapy in revascularization procedures (coronary artery bypass graft [CABG], percutaneous transluminal coronary angioplasty [PTCA], carotid endarterectomy), stent implantation

Unlabeled/Investigational Use Low doses have been used in the prevention of pre-eclampsia, complications associated with autoimmune disorders such as lupus or antiphospholipid syndrome; alternative therapy for prevention of thromboembolism associated with atrial fibrillation in patients not candidates for warfarin; pericarditis associated with MI; prosthetic valve thromboprophylaxis

Local Anesthetic/Vasoconstrictor Precautions No information available to require special precautions

Effects on Dental Treatment Key adverse event(s) related to dental treatment: As with all drugs which may affect hemostasis, bleeding is associated with aspirin. Hemorrhage may occur at virtually any site; risk is dependent on multiple variables including dosage, concurrent use of multiple agents which alter hemostasis, and patient susceptibility. Many adverse effects of aspirin are dose related, and are rare at low dosages. Other serious reactions are idiosyncratic, related to allergy or individual sensitivity (see Dental Comment).

Aspirin and clopidogrel (Plavix®) in combination is the primary prevention strategy against stent thrombosis after placement of drug-eluting metal stents in coronary patients. Premature discontinuation of this combination antiplatelet therapy strongly increases the risk of a catastrophic event of stent thrombosis leading to myocardial infarction and/or death, so says a science advisory issued in January 2007 from the American Heart Association in collaboration with the American Dental Association and other professional healthcare organizations. The advisory stresses a 12-month therapy of aspirin and Plavix® combination after placement of a drug-eluting stent in order to prevent thrombosis at the stent site. Any elective surgery should be postponed for 1 year after stent implantation, and if surgery must be performed, consideration should be given to continuing the antiplatelet therapy during the perioperative period in high-risk patients with drug-eluting stents.

This advisory was issued from a science panel made up of representatives from the American Heart Association (AHA), the American College of Cardiology, the Society for Cardiovascular Angiography and Interventions, the American College of Surgeons, the American Dental Association (ADA), and the American College of Physicians (Grines, 2007).

Effects on Bleeding Aspirin inhibits platelet aggregation which prolongs bleeding times. Inhibition is irreversible; on discontinuation of ASA, normal platelet function returns only when new platelets are released from the bone marrow. Dental practitioners should note that recommendations differ between general surgery (eg, appendectomy, hip replacement) and dental surgery. Due to concerns for increased blood loss, ASA is typically avoided (if possible) in general surgery patients for 1-2 weeks prior to surgery (exception is in patients undergoing CABG or noncardiac surgery at high risk of cardiac events - per 2008 ACCP guidelines). However, in the case of dental surgery there is no scientific evidence to warrant discontinuance of aspirin.

Reports of major bleeding related to dental surgery attributed to aspirin use have not been published. Furthermore, interruption of therapy may result in a loss of therapeutic effect. Patients taking one aspirin tablet daily as an antithrombotic who require dental surgery should be given special consideration in consultation with the physician before removal of the aspirin. In particular, aspirin should NOT be discontinued in patients with cardiac stents that have not completed their full course of dual antiplatelet therapy (aspirin, clopidogrel); patient specific situations need to be discussed with cardiologist. When feasible, postponement of dental surgery until the completion of dual antiplatelet therapy should be considered.

Adverse Effects As with all drugs which may affect hemostasis, bleeding is associated with aspirin. Hemorrhage may occur at virtually any site. Risk is dependent on multiple variables including dosage, concurrent use of multiple agents which alter hemostasis, and patient susceptibility. Many adverse effects of aspirin are dose related, and are rare at low dosages. Other serious reactions are idiosyncratic, related to allergy or individual sensitivity. Accurate estimation of frequencies is not possible. The reactions listed below have been reported for aspirin (frequency not defined).

Cardiovascular: Hypotension, tachycardia, dysrhythmias, edema

Central nervous system: Fatigue, insomnia, nervousness, agitation, confusion, dizziness, headache, lethargy, cerebral edema, hyperthermia, coma

Dermatologic: Rash, angioedema, urticaria

Endocrine & metabolic: Acidosis, hyperkalemia, dehydration, hypoglycemia (children), hyperglycemia, hypernatremia (buffered forms)

Gastrointestinal: Nausea, vomiting, dyspepsia, epigastric discomfort, heartburn, stomach pain, gastrointestinal ulceration (6% to 31%), gastric erosions, gastric erythema, duodenal ulcers

Hematologic: Anemia, disseminated intravascular coagulation (DIC), prothrombin times prolonged, coagulopathy, thrombocytopenia, hemolytic anemia, bleeding, iron deficiency anemia

Hepatic: Hepatotoxicity, transaminases increased, hepatitis (reversible)
Neuromuscular & skeletal: Rhabdomyolysis, weakness, acetabular bone destruction (OA)
Otic: Hearing loss, tinnitus
Renal: Interstitial nephritis, papillary necrosis, proteinuria, renal impairment, renal failure (including cases caused by rhabdomyolysis), BUN increased, serum creatinine increased
Respiratory: Asthma, bronchospasm, dyspnea, laryngeal edema, hyperpnea, tachypnea, respiratory alkalosis, noncardiogenic pulmonary edema
Miscellaneous: Anaphylaxis, prolonged pregnancy and labor, stillbirths, low birth weight, peripartum bleeding, Reye's syndrome

Dental Usual Dosage Postoperative pain:
Analgesic and antipyretic: Oral, rectal:
Children: 10-15 mg/kg/dose every 4-6 hours, up to a total of 4 g/day
Adults: 325-650 mg every 4-6 hours up to 4 g/day
Anti-inflammatory: Oral: Initial:
Children: 60-90 mg/kg/day in divided doses; usual maintenance: 80-100 mg/kg/day divided every 6-8 hours; monitor serum concentrations
Adults: 2.4-3.6 g/day in divided doses; usual maintenance: 3.6-5.4 g/day; monitor serum concentrations

Dosage
Children:
Analgesic and antipyretic: Oral, rectal: 10-15 mg/kg/dose every 4-6 hours, up to a total of 4 g/day
Anti-inflammatory: Oral: Initial: 60-90 mg/kg/day in divided doses; usual maintenance: 80-100 mg/kg/day divided every 6-8 hours; monitor serum concentrations
Antiplatelet effects: Adequate pediatric studies have not been performed; pediatric dosage is derived from adult studies and clinical experience and is not well established; suggested doses have ranged from 3-5 mg/kg/day to 5-10 mg/kg/day given as a single daily dose. Doses are rounded to a convenient amount (eg, 1/2 of 81 mg tablet).
Mechanical prosthetic heart valves: 6-20 mg/kg/day given as a single daily dose (used in combination with an oral anticoagulant in children who have systemic embolism despite adequate oral anticoagulation therapy (INR 2.5-3.5) and used in combination with low-dose anticoagulation (INR 2-3) and dipyridamole when full-dose oral anticoagulation is contraindicated)
Blalock-Taussig shunts: 1-5 mg/kg/day given as a single daily dose
Kawasaki disease: Oral: 80-100 mg/kg/day divided every 6 hours; monitor serum concentrations; after fever resolves: 3-5 mg/kg/day once daily; in patients without coronary artery abnormalities, give lower dose for at least 6-8 weeks or until ESR and platelet count are normal; in patients with coronary artery abnormalities, low-dose aspirin should be continued indefinitely
Antirheumatic: Oral: 60-100 mg/kg/day in divided doses every 4 hours
Adults:
Acute ischemic stroke: Oral: 150-325 mg once daily, initiated within 48 hours (in patients who are not candidates for alteplase and not receiving systemic anticoagulation)
Analgesic and antipyretic:
Oral: 325-650 mg every 4-6 hours up to 4 g/day
Rectal: 300-600 mg every 4-6 hours up to 4 g/day
Anti-inflammatory: Oral: Initial: 2.4-3.6 g/day in divided doses; usual maintenance: 3.6-5.4 g/day; monitor serum concentrations
Atrial fibrillation (in patients not candidates for warfarin or at low risk of ischemic stroke): Oral: 75-325 mg once daily (Fuster, 2006; Singer, 2008) **or** 75-100 mg once daily (Furie, 2011)
Bioprosthetic aortic valve: Oral: 50-100 mg once daily; usual dose: 81 mg once daily
Bioprosthetic mitral valve (following 3 months of anticoagulation): Oral: 50-100 mg once daily; usual dose: 81 mg once daily
CABG: Oral: 75-100 mg once daily (usual dose: 81 mg) initiated 6 hours following surgery; if bleeding prevents administration at 6 hours after CABG, initiate as soon as possible
CABG (internal mammary bypass graft): Oral: 75-162 mg once daily
Carotid artery stenting: Oral: 81-325 mg once daily beginning at least 24 hours (preferably 4 days) prior to procedure with concomitant clopidogrel
Carotid endarterectomy: Oral: 50-100 mg once daily preoperatively and daily thereafter; usual dose: 81 mg once daily
Infrainguinal arterial reconstruction/bypass: Oral: 75-100 mg once daily (begin preoperatively); usual dose: 81 mg once daily

Mechanical heart valve (with risk factors for or history of thromboembolism while receiving oral anticoagulants): Oral: 50-100 mg once daily (in addition to warfarin) (Furie, 2011; Salem, 2008); usual dose: 81 mg once daily

Mitral annular calcification (with documented stroke, TIA, or systemic embolism): Oral: 50-100 mg once daily; usual dose: 81 mg once daily

Mitral valve prolapse (with documented stroke or TIA): Oral: 50-100 mg once daily; usual dose: 81 mg once daily

Myocardial infarction (primary prevention): Oral: 75-162 mg once daily (Antman, 2004) **or** 75-100 mg (usual dose: 81 mg) once daily (Hirsh, 2008)

Non-ST-segment elevation myocardial infarction (NSTEMI): Oral: Initial: 162-325 mg; Maintenance: 75-100 mg once daily indefinitely; usual maintenance dose: 81 mg once daily

PCI: Oral: Initial: 75-325 mg (300-325 mg in aspirin naive patients) starting at least 2 hours (preferably 24 hours) before procedure; post procedure: 162-325 mg once daily (dose and duration varies with type of stent implanted); **Note:** Dose may be reduced to 75-162 mg once daily after appropriate duration based on stent-type is complete

Pericarditis associated with myocardial infarction: Oral: 162-325 mg once daily; doses as high as 650 mg every 4-6 hours may be required

Peripheral arterial disease: Oral: 75-100 mg once daily; usual dose: 81 mg once daily

Pre-eclampsia prevention (unlabeled use): Oral: 60-81 mg once daily (usual dose: 81 mg) during gestational weeks 13-26 (patient selection criteria not established)

Prosthetic valve thromboprophylaxis in pregnancy: Oral:75-100 mg once daily; usual dose: 81 mg once daily

ST-segment elevation myocardial infarction (STEMI): Oral: Initial: 162-325 mg given on presentation (patient should chew nonenteric-coated aspirin especially if not taking before presentation); for patients unable to take oral, may use rectal suppository (300 mg). Maintenance (secondary prevention): 75-162 mg once daily indefinitely

Stroke (cardioembolic, anticoagulation contraindicated): Oral: 75-325 mg once daily

Stroke/TIA (noncardioembolic, secondary prevention): Oral: 50-325 mg once daily (Adams, 2008) **or** 50-100 mg once daily; usual dose: 81 mg once daily (Hirsh, 2008)

Dosing adjustment in renal impairment: Cl_{cr} <10 mL/minute: Avoid use.
Hemodialysis: Dialyzable (50% to 100%)

Dosing adjustment in hepatic disease: Avoid use in severe liver disease.

Mechanism of Action Irreversibly inhibits cyclooxygenase-1 and 2 (COX-1 and 2) enzymes, via acetylation, which results in decreased formation of prostaglandin precursors; irreversibly inhibits formation of prostaglandin derivative, thromboxane A_2, via acetylation of platelet cyclooxygenase, thus inhibiting platelet aggregation; has antipyretic, analgesic, and anti-inflammatory properties

Contraindications Hypersensitivity to salicylates, other NSAIDs, or any component of the formulation; asthma; rhinitis; nasal polyps; inherited or acquired bleeding disorders (including factor VII and factor IX deficiency); do not use in children (<16 years of age) for viral infections (chickenpox or flu symptoms), with or without fever, due to a potential association with Reye's syndrome; pregnancy (3rd trimester especially)

Warnings/Precautions Use with caution in patients with platelet and bleeding disorders, renal dysfunction, dehydration, erosive gastritis, or peptic ulcer disease. Heavy ethanol use (>3 drinks/day) can increase bleeding risks. Avoid use in severe renal failure or in severe hepatic failure. Low-dose aspirin for cardioprotective effects is associated with a two- to fourfold increase in UGI events (eg, symptomatic or complicated ulcers); risks of these events increase with increasing aspirin dose; during the chronic phase of aspirin dosing, doses >81 mg are not recommended unless indicated (Bhatt, 2008).

Discontinue use if tinnitus or impaired hearing occurs. Caution in mild-to-moderate renal failure (only at high dosages). Patients with sensitivity to tartrazine dyes, nasal polyps, and asthma may have an increased risk of salicylate sensitivity. In the treatment of acute ischemic stroke, avoid aspirin for 24 hours following administration of alteplase; administration within 24 hours increases the risk of hemorrhagic transformation. Concurrent use of aspirin and clopidogrel is not recommended for secondary prevention of ischemic stroke or TIA in patients unable to take oral anticoagulants due to hemorrhagic risk (Furie, 2011). Surgical patients should avoid ASA if possible, for 1-2 weeks prior to surgery, to reduce the risk of excessive bleeding (except in patients with cardiac stents that have not completed their full course of dual antiplatelet therapy [aspirin, clopidogrel]; patient-specific situations need to be discussed with cardiologist; AHA/ACC/SCAI/ACS/ADA Science Advisory provides recommendations). When used concomitantly with ≤325 mg of aspirin,

NSAIDs (including selective COX-2 inhibitors) substantially increase the risk of gastrointestinal complications (eg, ulcer); concomitant gastroprotective therapy (eg, proton pump inhibitors) is recommended (Bhatt, 2008).

When used for self-medication (OTC labeling): Children and teenagers who have or are recovering from chickenpox or flu-like symptoms should not use this product. Changes in behavior (along with nausea and vomiting) may be an early sign of Reye's syndrome; patients should be instructed to contact their healthcare provider if these occur.

Drug Interactions

Metabolism/Transport Effects **Substrate** of CYP2C9 (minor)

Avoid Concomitant Use

Avoid concomitant use of Aspirin with any of the following: Influenza Virus Vaccine (Live/Attenuated); Ketorolac; Ketorolac (Systemic)

Increased Effect/Toxicity

Aspirin may increase the levels/effects of: Alendronate; Anticoagulants; Carbonic Anhydrase Inhibitors; Collagenase (Systemic); Corticosteroids (Systemic); Divalproex; Drotrecogin Alfa; Heparin; Ibritumomab; Methotrexate; PRALAtrexate; Salicylates; Sulfonylureas; Thrombolytic Agents; Tositumomab and Iodine I 131 Tositumomab; Valproic Acid; Varicella Virus-Containing Vaccines; Vitamin K Antagonists

The levels/effects of Aspirin may be increased by: Antidepressants (Tricyclic, Tertiary Amine); Antiplatelet Agents; Calcium Channel Blockers (Nondihydropyridine); Dasatinib; Ginkgo Biloba; Glucosamine; Herbs (Anticoagulant/Antiplatelet Properties); Influenza Virus Vaccine (Live/Attenuated); Ketorolac; Ketorolac (Systemic); Loop Diuretics; Nonsteroidal Anti-Inflammatory Agents; NSAID (Nonselective); Omega-3-Acid Ethyl Esters; Pentosan Polysulfate Sodium; Pentoxifylline; Prostacyclin Analogues; Selective Serotonin Reuptake Inhibitors; Serotonin/Norepinephrine Reuptake Inhibitors; Treprostinil

Decreased Effect

Aspirin may decrease the levels/effects of: ACE Inhibitors; Loop Diuretics; NSAID (Nonselective); Probenecid; Tiludronate

The levels/effects of Aspirin may be decreased by: Corticosteroids (Systemic); Nonsteroidal Anti-Inflammatory Agents; NSAID (Nonselective)

Ethanol/Nutrition/Herb Interactions

Ethanol: Avoid ethanol (may enhance gastric mucosal damage).

Food: Food may decrease the rate but not the extent of oral absorption.

- Folic acid: Hyperexcretion of folate; folic acid deficiency may result, leading to macrocytic anemia.
- Iron: With chronic aspirin use and at doses of 3-4 g/day, iron-deficiency anemia may result.
- Sodium: Hypernatremia resulting from buffered aspirin solutions or sodium salicylate containing high sodium content. Avoid or use with caution in CHF or any condition where hypernatremia would be detrimental.
- Benedictine liqueur, prunes, raisins, tea, and gherkins: Potential salicylate accumulation.
- Fresh fruits containing vitamin C: Displace drug from binding sites, resulting in increased urinary excretion of aspirin.

Herb/Nutraceutical: Avoid cat's claw, dong quai, evening primrose, feverfew, garlic, ginger, ginkgo, red clover, horse chestnut, green tea, ginseng (all have additional antiplatelet activity). Limit curry powder, paprika, licorice; may cause salicylate accumulation. These foods contain 6 mg salicylate/100 g. An ordinary American diet contains 10-200 mg/day of salicylate.

Dietary Considerations Take with food or large volume of water or milk to minimize GI upset.

Pharmacodynamics/Kinetics

Duration of Action 4-6 hours

Half-life Elimination Parent drug: 15-20 minutes; Salicylates (dose dependent): 3 hours at lower doses (300-600 mg), 5-6 hours (after 1 g), 10 hours with higher doses

Time to Peak Serum: ~1-2 hours

Lactation Enters breast milk (AAP recommends use "with caution"; AAP 2001 update pending)

Breast-Feeding Considerations Low amounts of aspirin can be found in breast milk. Milk/plasma ratios ranging from 0.03-0.3 have been reported. Peak levels in breast milk are reported to be at ~9 hours after a dose. Metabolic acidosis was reported in one infant following an aspirin dose of 3.9 g/day in the mother. The WHO considers occasional doses of aspirin to be compatible with breast-feeding, but to avoid long-term therapy and consider monitoring the infant for adverse effects. Other sources suggest avoiding aspirin while breast-feeding due to the theoretical risk of Reye's syndrome.

Dosage Forms

Caplet, oral:
- Ascriptin® Maximum Strength [OTC]: 500 mg
- Bayer® Aspirin Extra Strength [OTC]: 500 mg
- Bayer® Genuine Aspirin [OTC]: 325 mg
- Bayer® Plus Extra Strength [OTC]: 500 mg
- Bayer® Women's Low Dose Aspirin [OTC]: 81 mg

Caplet, enteric coated, oral:
- Bayer® Aspirin Regimen Regular Strength [OTC]: 325 mg

Gum, chewing, oral:
- Aspergum® [OTC]: 227 mg (12s)

Suppository, rectal: 300 mg (12s); 600 mg (12s)

Tablet, oral: 325 mg
- Ascriptin® Regular Strength [OTC]: 325 mg
- Aspercin [OTC]: 325 mg
- Aspirtab [OTC]: 325 mg
- Bayer® Genuine Aspirin [OTC]: 325 mg
- Buffasal [OTC]: 325 mg
- Bufferin® [OTC]: 325 mg
- Bufferin® Extra Strength [OTC]: 500 mg
- Buffinol [OTC]: 324 mg
- Tri-Buffered Aspirin [OTC]: 325 mg

Tablet, chewable, oral: 81 mg
- Bayer® Aspirin Regimen Children's [OTC]: 81 mg
- St Joseph® Adult Aspirin [OTC]: 81 mg

Tablet, delayed release, enteric coated, oral:
- Easprin®: 975 mg

Tablet, enteric coated, oral: 81 mg, 325 mg, 650 mg
- Aspir-low [OTC]: 81 mg
- Bayer® Aspirin Regimen Adult Low Strength [OTC]: 81 mg
- Ecotrin® [OTC]: 325 mg
- Ecotrin® Arthritis Strength [OTC]: 500 mg
- Ecotrin® Low Strength [OTC]: 81 mg
- Halfprin® [OTC]: 81 mg, 162 mg
- St Joseph® Adult Aspirin [OTC]: 81 mg

Dental Comment The Food and Drug Administration (FDA), has issued a letter updating information and considerations regarding the use of ibuprofen (400 mg doses) in patients who are taking low dose aspirin (81 mg, immediate release; not enteric coated) for cardioprotection and stroke prevention. Ibuprofen, at these doses, may interfere with aspirin's antiplatelet effect depending upon when it is administered. Patients initiated on aspirin first (for ~1 week) then ibuprofen (400 mg 3 times/day for 10 days) seem to maintain aspirin's platelet effect (Cryer, 2005). Ibuprofen has the greatest impact on aspirin if administered less than 8 hours before aspirin (Catella-Lawson, 2001).

Patients may require counseling about the appropriate timing of ibuprofen dosing in relationship to aspirin therapy. With occasional use of ibuprofen, a clinically-significant interaction with aspirin in unlikely. To avoid interference during chronic dosing, a single dose of ibuprofen should be taken 30-120 minutes after aspirin ingestion or at least 8 hours should elapse after ibuprofen dosing before giving aspirin (FDA, 2006; Catella-Lawson, 2001).

The clinical implications of the interaction are unclear. There have not been any clinical endpoint studies conducted at this time. Avoidance of this interaction is potentially important because aspirin's vascular protection could be decreased or negated.

Other nonselective NSAIDs may have potential for a similar interaction with aspirin. Such has been described with naproxen (Capone, 2005). Acetaminophen does not appear to interfere with the antiplatelet effect of aspirin. Other clinical scenarios (use of smaller ibuprofen doses, other aspirin products, other doses of aspirin) have not been evaluated.

Additional information is available at: http://www.fda.gov/Drugs/DrugSafety/PostmarketDrugSafetyInformationforPatientsandProviders/ucm125222.htm

References

Capone ML, Sciulli MG, Tacconelli S, et al, "Pharmacodynamic Interaction of Naproxen With Low-Dose Aspirin in Healthy Subjects," *J Am Coll Cardiol*, 2005, 45(8):1295-1301.

Catella-Lawson F, Reilly MP, Kapoor SC, et al, "Cyclooxygenase Inhibitors and the Antiplatelet Effects of Aspirin," *N Engl J Med*, 2001, 345(25):1809-17.

Cryer B, Verlin RG, Cooper SA, et al, "Double-Blind, Randomized, Parallel, Placebo-Controlled Study of Ibuprofen Effects on Thromboxane B2 Concentrations in Aspirin-Treated Healthy Adult Volunteers," *Clin Ther*, 2005, 27(2):185-191.

Daniel NG, Goulet J, Bergeron M, et al, "Antiplatelet Drugs: Is There a Surgical Risk?" *J Can Dent Assoc*, 2002, 68(11):683-7.
Forbes JA, Butterworth GA, Burchfield WH, et al, "Evaluation of Ketorolac, Aspirin, and an Acetaminophen-Codeine Combination in Postoperative Oral Surgery Pain," *Pharmacotherapy*, 1990, 10(6 Pt 2):77S-93S.
Grines CL, Bonow RO, Casey DE, et al, "AHA/ACC/SCAI/ACS/ADA Science Advisory, Prevention of Premature Discontinuation of Dual Antiplatelet Therapy in Patients With Coronary Artery Stents. A Science Advisory From the American Heart Association, American College of Cardiology, Society of Cardiovascular Angiography and Interventions, American College of Surgeons, and American Dental Association With Representation From The Amercian College Of Physicians," *Circulation*, 2007, 115 (6):813-8. Available at http://www.acc.org/qualityandscience/clinical/pdfs/Final_Dual_Antiplatelet_Statement_010507.pdf.
Hurlen M, Erikssen J, Smith P, et al, "Comparison of Bleeding Complications of Warfarin and Warfarin Plus Acetylsalicylic Acid: A Study in 3166 Outpatients," *J Intern Med*, 1994, 236(3):299-304.
Jeske AH, Suchko GD, ADA Council on Scientific Affairs and Division of Science, et al, "Lack of a Scientific Basis for Routine Discontinuation of Oral Anticoagulation Therapy Before Dental Treatment," *J Am Dent Assoc*, 2003, 134(11):1492-7.
Little JW, Miller CS, Henry RG, et al, "Antithrombotic Agents: Implications in Dentistry," *Oral Surg Oral Med Oral Pathol Oral Radiol Endod*, 2002, 93(5):544-51.
Schrodi J, Recio L, Fiorellini J, et al, "The Effect of Aspirin on the Periodontal Parameter Bleeding on Probing," *J Periodontol*, 2002, 73(8):871-6.
Scully C and Wolff A, "Oral Surgery in Patients on Anticoagulant Therapy," *Oral Surg Oral Med Oral Pathol Oral Radiol Endod*, 2002, 94(1):57-64.

Aspirin and Dipyridamole (AS pir in & dye peer ID a mole)

Related Information

Aspirin *on page 171*
Cardiovascular Diseases *on page 1848*
Dipyridamole *on page 548*

U.S. Brand Names Aggrenox®

Canadian Brand Names Aggrenox®

Pharmacologic Category Antiplatelet Agent

Use Reduction in the risk of stroke in patients who have had transient ischemia of the brain or ischemic stroke due to thrombosis

Unlabeled/Investigational Use Hemodialysis graft patency

Local Anesthetic/Vasoconstrictor Precautions No information available to require special precautions

Effects on Dental Treatment Key adverse event(s) related to dental treatment: As with all drugs which may affect hemostasis, bleeding is associated with aspirin. Hemorrhage may occur at virtually any site; risk is dependent on multiple variables including dosage, concurrent use of multiple agents which alter hemostasis, and patient susceptibility. Many adverse effects of aspirin are dose related, and are rare at low dosages. Other serious reactions are idiosyncratic, related to allergy or individual sensitivity (see Dental Comment).

Effects on Bleeding Aspirin inhibits platelet aggregation which prolongs bleeding times. Inhibition is irreversible; on discontinuation of ASA, normal platelet function returns only when new platelets are released from the bone marrow. Dental practitioners should note that recommendations differ between general surgery (eg, appendectomy, hip replacement) and dental surgery. Due to concerns for increased blood loss, ASA is typically avoided (if possible) in general surgery patients for 1-2 weeks prior to surgery (exception is in patients undergoing CABG or noncardiac surgery at high risk of cardiac events - per 2008 ACCP guidelines). However, in the case of dental surgery there is no scientific evidence to warrant discontinuance of aspirin.

Reports of major bleeding related to dental surgery attributed to aspirin use have not been published. Furthermore, interruption of therapy may result in a loss of therapeutic effect. Patients taking one aspirin tablet daily as an antithrombotic who require dental surgery should be given special consideration in consultation with the physician before removal of the aspirin. In particular, aspirin should NOT be discontinued in patients with cardiac stents that have not completed their full course of dual antiplatelet therapy (aspirin, clopidogrel); patient specific situations need to be discussed with cardiologist. When feasible, postponement of dental surgery until the completion of dual antiplatelet therapy should be considered.

Dipyridamole blocks platelet aggregation and may prolong bleeding time. Prior to general surgery, it may be temporarily discontinued to restore platelet function. However, routine interruption of therapy for noninvasive dental procedures is not warranted and there is no scientific evidence to warrant the discontinuance of dipyridamole prior to dental surgery. Patients taking dipyridamole as an antithrombotic who require dental surgery should be given special consideration in consultation with physician.

Adverse Effects

>10%:

Central nervous system: Headache (39%; tolerance usually develops)
Gastrointestinal: Abdominal pain (18%), dyspepsia (18%), nausea (16%), diarrhea (13%)

1% to 10%:

Cardiovascular: Cardiac failure (2%), syncope (1%)

Central nervous system: Fatigue (6%), pain (6%), amnesia (2%), malaise (2%), seizure (2%), confusion (1%), somnolence (1%)

Dermatologic: Purpura (1%)

Gastrointestinal: Vomiting (8%), GI bleeding (4%), melena (2%), rectal bleeding (2%), hemorrhoids (1%), GI hemorrhage (1%), anorexia (1%)

Hematologic: Hemorrhage (3%), anemia (2%)

Neuromuscular & skeletal: Arthralgia (6%), back pain (5%), weakness (2%), arthritis (2%), arthrosis (1%), myalgia (1%)

Respiratory: Cough (2%), epistaxis (2%), upper respiratory tract infection (1%)

General Dosage Range Oral: *Adults:* 1 capsule (200 mg dipyridamole, 25 mg aspirin) twice daily

Mechanism of Action The antithrombotic action results from additive antiplatelet effects. Dipyridamole inhibits the uptake of adenosine into platelets, endothelial cells, and erythrocytes. Aspirin inhibits platelet aggregation by irreversible inhibition of platelet cyclooxygenase and thus inhibits the generation of thromboxane A_2.

Pregnancy Risk Factor D

Dental Comment The Food and Drug Administration (FDA), has issued a letter updating information and considerations regarding the use of ibuprofen (400 mg doses) in patients who are taking low dose aspirin (81 mg, immediate release; not enteric coated) for cardioprotection and stroke prevention. Ibuprofen, at these doses, may interfere with aspirin's antiplatelet effect depending upon when it is administered. Patients initiated on aspirin first (for ~1 week) then ibuprofen (400 mg 3 times/day for 10 days) seem to maintain aspirin's platelet effect (Cryer, 2005). Ibuprofen has the greatest impact on aspirin if administered less than 8 hours before aspirin (Catella-Lawson, 2001).

Patients may require counseling about the appropriate timing of ibuprofen dosing in relationship to aspirin therapy. With occasional use of ibuprofen, a clinically-significant interaction with aspirin in unlikely. To avoid interference during chronic dosing, a single dose of ibuprofen should be taken 30-120 minutes after aspirin ingestion or at least 8 hours should elapse after ibuprofen dosing before giving aspirin (FDA, 2006; Catella-Lawson, 2001).

The clinical implications of the interaction are unclear. There have not been any clinical endpoint studies conducted at this time. Avoidance of this interaction is potentially important because aspirin's vascular protection could be decreased or negated.

Other nonselective NSAIDs may have potential for a similar interaction with aspirin. Such has been described with naproxen (Capone, 2005). Acetaminophen does not appear to interfere with the antiplatelet effect of aspirin. Other clinical scenarios (use of smaller ibuprofen doses, other aspirin products, other doses of aspirin) have not been evaluated.

Additional information is available at: http://www.fda.gov/Drugs/DrugSafety/PostmarketDrugSafetyInformationforPatientsandProviders/ucm125222.htm

Atazanavir (at a za NA veer)

Related Information

HIV Infection and AIDS *on page 1883*

U.S. Brand Names Reyataz®

Canadian Brand Names Reyataz®

Pharmacologic Category Antiretroviral Agent, Protease Inhibitor

Use Treatment of HIV-1 infections in combination with at least two other antiretroviral agents

Local Anesthetic/Vasoconstrictor Precautions No information available to require special precautions

Effects on Dental Treatment No significant effects or complications reported

Effects on Bleeding Increased bleeding has been noted with protease inhibitors in patients with hemophilia A or B. No information available to require routine special precautions relative to hemostasis in other patients.

Adverse Effects Includes data from both treatment-naive and treatment-experienced patients. Percentages listed for adults unless otherwise specified.

>10%:

Dermatologic: Rash (3% to 21%; median onset 7 weeks)

Endocrine & metabolic: Cholesterol increased (≥240 mg/dL: 6% to 25%)

Gastrointestinal: Nausea (3% to 14%), amylase increased (≤14%)

Hepatic: Bilirubin increased (≥2.6 times ULN: 35% to 49%)

Neuromuscular & skeletal: CPK increased (6% to 11%)

Respiratory: Cough (children 21%)

2% to 10%:

Cardiovascular: AV block (first degree: 6%; second degree [children] 2%)

Central nervous system: Headache (1% to 6%; children 7%), peripheral neuropathy (<1% to 4%), insomnia (<1% to 3%), depression (2%), fever (2%; children 19%), dizziness (<1% to 2%)

Endocrine & metabolic: Triglycerides increased (<1% to 8%), hyperglycemia (≥251 mg/dL: 5%)

Gastrointestinal: Lipase increased (<1% to 5%), abdominal pain (4%), vomiting (3% to 4%; children 8%), diarrhea (1% to 3%; children 8%)

Hematologic: Neutropenia (3% to 7%), hemoglobin decreased (<1% to 5%), thrombocytopenia (2%)

Hepatic: Jaundice (5% to 9%; children 13%), ALT increased (>5 times ULN: 3% to 9%; 10% to 25% in patients seropositive for hepatitis B and/or C), AST increased (>5 times ULN: 2% to 7%; 9% to 10% in patients seropositive for hepatitis B and/ or C)

Neuromuscular & skeletal: Myalgia (4%)

Respiratory: Rhinorrhea (children 6%)

General Dosage Range Dosage adjustment recommended in patients with hepatic or renal impairment or on concomitant therapy

Oral:

Children 6-17 years:

15-24 kg (antiretroviral-naive patients): Atazanavir 150 mg once daily

25-31 kg: Atazanavir 200 mg once daily

32-38 kg: Atazanavir 250 mg once daily

≥39 kg: Atazanavir 300 mg once daily

or

15-19 kg: Atazanavir 8.5 mg/kg/dose once daily (rounded to available capsule strengths)

≥20 kg: Atazanavir 7 mg/kg/dose once daily (round to available capsule strengths) (maximum: 300 mg)

Children ≥13 years (≥39 kg) and Adults: 400 mg once daily (antiretroviral-naive) **or** atazanavir 300 mg once daily

Mechanism of Action Binds to the site of HIV-1 protease activity and inhibits cleavage of viral Gag-Pol polyprotein precursors into individual functional proteins required for infectious HIV. This results in the formation of immature, noninfectious viral particles.

Pharmacodynamics/Kinetics

Half-life Elimination Unboosted therapy: 7-8 hours; Boosted therapy (with ritonavir): 9-18 hours

Time to Peak Plasma: 2-3 hours

Pregnancy Risk Factor B

Atenolol (a TEN oh lole)

Related Information

Cardiovascular Diseases *on page 1848*

U.S. Brand Names Tenormin®

Canadian Brand Names Apo-Atenol®; CO Atenolol; Dom-Atenolol; Med-Atenolol; Mylan-Atenolol; Nu-Atenol; PHL-Atenolol; PMS-Atenolol; RAN™-Atenolol; ratio-Atenolol; Riva-Atenolol; Sandoz-Atenolol; Tenormin®; Teva-Atenolol

Generic Availability (U.S.) Yes

Pharmacologic Category Beta Blocker, Beta-1 Selective

Use Treatment of hypertension, alone or in combination with other agents; management of angina pectoris; secondary prevention postmyocardial infarction

Unlabeled/Investigational Use Acute ethanol withdrawal, supraventricular and ventricular arrhythmias, and migraine headache prophylaxis

Local Anesthetic/Vasoconstrictor Precautions No information available to require special precautions

Effects on Dental Treatment Atenolol is a cardioselective beta-blocker. Local anesthetic with vasoconstrictor can be safely used in patients medicated with atenolol. Nonselective beta-blockers (ie, propranolol, nadolol) enhance the pressor response to epinephrine, resulting in hypertension and bradycardia; this has not been reported for atenolol. Many nonsteroidal anti-inflammatory drugs, such as ibuprofen and indomethacin, can reduce the hypotensive effect of beta-blockers after 3 or more weeks of therapy with the NSAID. Short-term NSAID use (ie, 3 days) requires no special precautions in patients taking beta-blockers.

Effects on Bleeding No information available to require special precautions

Adverse Effects 1% to 10%:

Cardiovascular: Persistent bradycardia, hypotension, chest pain, edema, heart failure, second- or third-degree AV block, Raynaud's phenomenon

Central nervous system: Dizziness, fatigue, insomnia, lethargy, confusion, mental impairment, depression, headache, nightmares

Gastrointestinal: Constipation, diarrhea, nausea

Genitourinary: Impotence

Miscellaneous: Cold extremities

Dosage Oral:

Children: Hypertension: 0.5-1 mg/kg/dose given daily; range of 0.5-1.5 mg/kg/day; maximum dose: 2 mg/kg/day up to 100 mg/day

Adults:

Hypertension: 25-50 mg once daily, may increase to 100 mg/day. Doses >100 mg are unlikely to produce any further benefit.

Angina pectoris: 50 mg once daily, may increase to 100 mg/day. Some patients may require 200 mg/day.

Postmyocardial infarction: 100 mg/day or 50 mg twice daily for 6-9 days post-myocardial infarction.

Dosing interval for oral atenolol in renal impairment:

Cl_{cr} 15-35 mL/minute: Administer 50 mg/day maximum.

Cl_{cr} <15 mL/minute: Administer 50 mg every other day maximum.

Hemodialysis: Moderately dialyzable (20% to 50%) via hemodialysis; administer dose postdialysis or administer 25-50 mg supplemental dose.

Peritoneal dialysis: Elimination is not enhanced; supplemental dose is not necessary.

Mechanism of Action Competitively blocks response to beta-adrenergic stimulation, selectively blocks $beta_1$-receptors with little or no effect on $beta_2$-receptors except at high doses

Contraindications Hypersensitivity to atenolol or any component of the formulation; sinus bradycardia; sinus node dysfunction; heart block greater than first-degree (except in patients with a functioning artificial pacemaker); cardiogenic shock; uncompensated cardiac failure; pulmonary edema; pregnancy

Warnings/Precautions Consider pre-existing conditions such as sick sinus syndrome before initiating. Administer cautiously in compensated heart failure and monitor for a worsening of the condition (efficacy of atenolol in heart failure has not been established). **[U.S. Boxed Warning]: Beta-blocker therapy should not be withdrawn abruptly (particularly in patients with CAD), but gradually tapered to avoid acute tachycardia, hypertension, and/or ischemia.** Use caution with concurrent use of beta-blockers and either verapamil or diltiazem; bradycardia or heart block can occur. Beta-blockers should be avoided in patients with bronchospastic disease (asthma). Atenolol, with B_1 selectivity, has been used cautiously in bronchospastic disease with close monitoring. Use cautiously in peripheral arterial disease, especially if severe disease is present. Use cautiously in patients with diabetes - may mask hypoglycemic symptoms. Use cautiously in the renally impaired (dosage adjustment required). Use care with anesthetic agents which decrease myocardial function. Caution in myasthenia gravis or psychiatric disease (may cause CNS depression). Adequate alpha-blockade is required prior to use of any beta-blocker for patients with untreated pheochromocytoma. May induce or exacerbate psoriasis. Use caution with history of severe anaphylaxis to allergens; patients taking beta-blockers may become more sensitive to repeated challenges. Treatment of anaphylaxis (eg, epinephrine) in patients taking beta-blockers may be ineffective or promote undesirable effects.

Drug Interactions

Avoid Concomitant Use

Avoid concomitant use of Atenolol with any of the following: Methacholine

Increased Effect/Toxicity

Atenolol may increase the levels/effects of: Alpha-/Beta-Agonists (Direct-Acting); Alpha1-Blockers; Alpha2-Agonists; Amifostine; Antihypertensives; Bupivacaine; Cardiac Glycosides; Fingolimod; Hypotensive Agents; Insulin; Lidocaine; Lidocaine (Systemic); Lidocaine (Topical); Mepivacaine; Methacholine; Midodrine; RiTUXimab; Sulfonylureas

The levels/effects of Atenolol may be increased by: Acetylcholinesterase Inhibitors; Amiodarone; Anilidopiperidine Opioids; Calcium Channel Blockers (Nondihydropyridine); Diazoxide; Dipyridamole; Disopyramide; Dronedarone; Glycopyrrolate; Herbs (Hypotensive Properties); MAO Inhibitors; Pentoxifylline; Phosphodiesterase 5 Inhibitors; Prostacyclin Analogues; Reserpine

Decreased Effect

Atenolol may decrease the levels/effects of: Beta2-Agonists; Theophylline Derivatives

The levels/effects of Atenolol may be decreased by: Ampicillin; Herbs (Hypertensive Properties); Methylphenidate; Nonsteroidal Anti-Inflammatory Agents; Yohimbine

Ethanol/Nutrition/Herb Interactions

Food: Atenolol serum concentrations may be decreased if taken with food.

Herb/Nutraceutical: Avoid dong quai if using for hypertension (has estrogenic activity). Avoid ephedra, yohimbe, ginseng (may worsen hypertension). Avoid garlic (may have increased antihypertensive effect).

Dietary Considerations May be taken without regard to meals.

Pharmacodynamics/Kinetics

Onset of Action Peak effect: Oral: 2-4 hours

Duration of Action Normal renal function: 12-24 hours

Half-life Elimination Beta:

Neonates: ≤35 hours; Mean: 16 hours

Children: 4.6 hours; children >10 years may have prolonged half-life (>5 hours) compared to children 5-10 years (<5 hours)

Adults: Normal renal function: 6-7 hours, prolonged with renal impairment; End-stage renal disease: 15-35 hours

Time to Peak Plasma: Oral: 2-4 hours

Pregnancy Risk Factor D

Lactation Enters breast milk/use caution (AAP recommends "use with caution"; AAP 2001 update pending)

Breast-Feeding Considerations Atenolol is excreted in breast milk and has been detected in the serum and urine of nursing infants. Peak concentrations in breast milk have been reported to occur between 2-8 hours after the maternal dose and in some cases are higher than the peak maternal serum concentration. Although most studies have not reported adverse events in nursing infants, avoiding maternal use while nursing infants with renal dysfunction or infants <44 weeks postconceptual age has been suggested. Beta-blockers with less distribution into breast milk may be preferred. The manufacturer recommends that caution be exercised when administering atenolol to nursing women.

Dosage Forms

Tablet, oral: 25 mg, 50 mg, 100 mg

Tenormin®: 25 mg, 50 mg, 100 mg

References

Foster CA and Aston SJ, "Propranolol-Epinephrine Interaction: A Potential Disaster," *Plast Reconstr Surg*, 1983, 72(1):74-8.

Wong DG, Spence JD, Lamki L, et al, "Effect of Nonsteroidal Anti-inflammatory Drugs on Control of Hypertension of Beta-Blockers and Diuretics," *Lancet*, 1986, 1(8488):997-1001.

Wynn RL, "Dental Nonsteroidal Anti-inflammatory Drugs and Prostaglandin-Based Drug Interactions-Part Two," *Gen Dent*, 1992, 40(2):104, 106, 108.

Wynn RL, "Epinephrine Interactions With Beta-Blockers," *Gen Dent*, 1994, 42(1):16, 18.

Atenolol and Chlorthalidone (a TEN oh lole & klor THAL i done)

Related Information

Atenolol *on page 179*

Chlorthalidone *on page 373*

U.S. Brand Names Tenoretic®

Canadian Brand Names Apo-Atenidone®; Novo-Atenolthalidone; Tenoretic®; Teva-Atenolol Chlorthalidone

Pharmacologic Category Beta Blocker, Beta-1 Selective; Diuretic, Thiazide

Use Treatment of hypertension with a cardioselective beta-blocker and a diuretic

Local Anesthetic/Vasoconstrictor Precautions No information available to require special precautions

Effects on Dental Treatment Atenolol is a cardioselective beta-blocker. Local anesthetic with vasoconstrictor can be safely used in patients medicated with atenolol. Nonselective beta-blockers (ie, propranolol, nadolol) enhance the pressor response to epinephrine, resulting in hypertension and bradycardia; this has not been reported for atenolol. Many nonsteroidal anti-inflammatory drugs, such as ibuprofen and indomethacin, can reduce the hypotensive effect of beta-blockers after 3 or more weeks of therapy with the NSAID. Short-term NSAID use (ie, 3 days) requires no special precautions in patients taking beta-blockers.

Effects on Bleeding No information available to require special precautions

Adverse Effects See individual agents.

General Dosage Range Dosage adjustment recommended in patients with renal impairment

Oral: *Adults:* Initial: 50 mg (atenolol) and 25 mg (chlorthalidone) once daily; Maintenance: 50-100 mg (atenolol) and 25 mg (chlorthalidone) once daily (maximum: Atenolol 100 mg/day; chlorthalidone 25 mg/day)

Pregnancy Risk Factor D

Atomoxetine (AT oh mox e teen)

U.S. Brand Names Strattera®

Canadian Brand Names Strattera®

Generic Availability (U.S.) No

Pharmacologic Category Norepinephrine Reuptake Inhibitor, Selective

Use Treatment of attention deficit/hyperactivity disorder (ADHD)

Local Anesthetic/Vasoconstrictor Precautions Use vasoconstrictor with caution. Atomoxetine may increase heart rate or blood pressure in the presence of pressor agents. Pressor agents include the vasoconstrictors epinephrine or mepivacaine and levonordefrin (Carbocaine® 2% with Neo-Cobefrin®)

Effects on Dental Treatment Key adverse event(s) related to dental treatment: Xerostomia (normal salivary flow resumes upon discontinuation)

Effects on Bleeding No information available to require special precautions

Adverse Effects Percentages as reported in children and adults; some adverse reactions may be increased in "poor metabolizers" (CYP2D6).

>10%:

Central nervous system: Headache (2% to 19%), insomnia (2% to 15%), somnolence (4% to 11%)

Gastrointestinal: Xerostomia (21%), nausea (7% to 21%), abdominal pain (7% to 18%), appetite decreased (11% to 16%), vomiting (3% to 11%)

1% to 10%:

Cardiovascular: Systolic blood pressure increased (4% to 5%), diastolic pressure increased (≤4%), palpitation (3%), flushing (≥2%), tachycardia (≤2%), orthostatic hypotension (<2%)

Central nervous system: Fatigue/lethargy (6% to 9%), dizziness (5% to 6%), irritability (≤6%), chills (3%), sleep disturbance (3%), mood swings (1% to 2%)

Dermatologic: Hyperhidrosis (4%), rash (2%)

Endocrine & metabolic: Hot flashes (8%), dysmenorrhea (6%), libido decreased (4%), menstruation disturbance (2%), orgasm abnormal (2%)

Gastrointestinal: Constipation (1% to 9%), dyspepsia (4%), anorexia (<3%), weight loss (2% to 3%)

Genitourinary: Erectile disturbance (9%), urinary hesitation/retention (7%), dysuria (3%), ejaculatory disturbance (3%), prostatitis (2%)

Neuromuscular & skeletal: Paresthesia (3% adults; postmarketing observation in children), tremor (2%)

Ocular: Mydriasis (≥2%)

Respiratory: Sinus headache (3%)

Miscellaneous: Jittery feeling (2%)

Dosage Oral: **Note:** Atomoxetine may be discontinued without the need for tapering dose.

Children ≥6 years and ≤70 kg: ADHD: Initial: 0.5 mg/kg/day, increase after minimum of 3 days to ~1.2 mg/kg/day; may administer as either a single daily dose or 2 evenly divided doses in morning and late afternoon/early evening. Maximum daily dose: 1.4 mg/kg or 100 mg, whichever is less.

Dosage adjustment in patients receiving strong CYP2D6 inhibitors (eg, paroxetine, fluoxetine, quinidine) or patients known to be CYP2D6 poor metabolizers: Do not exceed 1.2 mg/kg/day; dose adjustments should occur only after 4 weeks.

Children ≥6 years and >70 kg and Adults: ADHD: Initial: 40 mg/day, increased after minimum of 3 days to ~80 mg/day; may administer as either a single daily dose or two evenly divided doses in morning and late afternoon/early evening. May increase to 100 mg/day in 2-4 additional weeks to achieve optimal response.

Dosage adjustment in patients receiving strong CYP2D6 inhibitors (eg, paroxetine, fluoxetine, quinidine) or patients known to be CYP2D6 poor metabolizers: Do not exceed 80 mg/day; dose adjustments should occur only after 4 weeks.

Elderly: Use has not been evaluated in the elderly

Dosage adjustment in renal impairment: No adjustment needed

Dosage adjustment in hepatic impairment:

Moderate hepatic insufficiency (Child-Pugh class B): All doses should be reduced to 50% of normal

Severe hepatic insufficiency (Child-Pugh class C): All doses should be reduced to 25% of normal

Mechanism of Action Selectively inhibits the reuptake of norepinephrine (Ki 4.5nM) with little to no activity at the other neuronal reuptake pumps or receptor sites.

Contraindications Hypersensitivity to atomoxetine or any component of the formulation; use with or within 14 days of MAO inhibitors; narrow-angle glaucoma; current or past history of pheochromocytoma

Warnings/Precautions [U.S. Boxed Warning]: Use caution in pediatric patients; may be an increased risk of suicidal ideation. Closely monitor for clinical worsening, suicidality, or unusual changes in behavior; especially during the initial few months of a course of drug therapy, or at times of dose changes, either increases or decreases. The child's family or caregiver should be instructed to closely observe the patient and communicate condition with healthcare provider. New or worsening symptoms of hostility or aggressive behaviors have been associated with atomoxetine, particularly with the initiation of therapy. Use caution in patients with a history of psychotic illness or bipolar disorder; therapy may induce mixed/manic disorder or psychotic symptoms. Atomoxetine is not approved for major depressive disorder. Patients presenting with depressive symptoms should be screened for bipolar disorder. Recommended to be used as part of a comprehensive treatment program for attention deficit disorders. Atomoxetine does not worsen anxiety in patients with existing anxiety disorders or tics related to Tourette's disorder.

Use caution with hepatic disease (dosage adjustments necessary in hepatic impairment). Use may be associated with rare but severe hepatotoxicity; discontinue and do not restart if signs or symptoms of hepatotoxic reaction (eg, jaundice, pruritus, flu-like symptoms) or laboratory evidence of liver disease are noted. Use caution in patients who are poor metabolizers of CYP2D6 metabolized drugs ("poor metabolizers"), bioavailability increases.

Orthostasis can occur; use caution in patients predisposed to hypotension or those with abrupt changes in heart rate or blood pressure. CNS stimulant use has been associated with serious cardiovascular events including sudden death in patients with pre-existing structural cardiac abnormalities or other serious heart problems (sudden death in children and adolescents; sudden death, stroke, and MI in adults). These products should be avoided in patients with known serious structural cardiac abnormalities, cardiomyopathy, serious heart rhythm abnormalities, or other serious cardiac problems that could increase the risk of sudden death that these conditions alone carry. Patients should be carefully evaluated for cardiac disease prior to initiation of therapy. May cause increased heart rate or blood pressure; use caution with hypertension or other cardiovascular disease. Use caution with renal impairment. May cause urinary retention/hesitancy; use caution in patients with history of urinary retention or bladder outlet obstruction. Priapism has been associated with use (rarely). Allergic reactions (including angioneurotic edema, urticaria, and rash) may occur (rare).

Growth should be monitored during treatment. Height and weight gain may be reduced during the first 9-12 months of treatment, but should recover by 3 years of therapy. Safety and efficacy have not been evaluated in pediatric patients <6 years of age.

Drug Interactions

Metabolism/Transport Effects Substrate of CYP2C19 (minor), 2D6 (major)

Avoid Concomitant Use

Avoid concomitant use of Atomoxetine with any of the following: Iobenguane I 123; MAO Inhibitors

Increased Effect/Toxicity

Atomoxetine may increase the levels/effects of: Alcohol (Ethyl); Beta2-Agonists; CNS Depressants; Methotrimeprazine; Sympathomimetics

The levels/effects of Atomoxetine may be increased by: Abiraterone; CYP2D6 Inhibitors (Moderate); CYP2D6 Inhibitors (Strong); Darunavir; Droperidol; MAO Inhibitors; Methotrimeprazine

Decreased Effect

Atomoxetine may decrease the levels/effects of: Iobenguane I 123

The levels/effects of Atomoxetine may be decreased by: Peginterferon Alfa-2b

Ethanol/Nutrition/Herb Interactions Ethanol: May increase CNS depression; monitor for increased effects with coadministration. Caution patients about effects.

Dietary Considerations May be taken with or without food.

Pharmacodynamics/Kinetics

Half-life Elimination Atomoxetine: 5 hours (up to 24 hours in poor metabolizers); Active metabolites: 4-hydroxyatomoxetine: 6-8 hours; N-desmethylatomoxetine: 6-8 hours (34-40 hours in poor metabolizers)

Time to Peak Plasma: 1-2 hours

Pregnancy Risk Factor C

Lactation Excretion in breast milk unknown/use caution

Dosage Forms

Capsule, oral:

Strattera®: 10 mg, 18 mg, 25 mg, 40 mg, 60 mg, 80 mg, 100 mg

Atorvastatin (a TORE va sta tin)

Related Information

Cardiovascular Diseases *on page 1848*

U.S. Brand Names Lipitor®

Canadian Brand Names Apo-Atorvastatin®; CO Atorvastatin; GD-Atorvastatin; Lipitor®; Novo-Atorvastatin; PMS-Atorvastatin; RAN™-Atorvastatin; Sandoz-Atorvastatin

Generic Availability (U.S.) No

Pharmacologic Category Antilipemic Agent, HMG-CoA Reductase Inhibitor

Use Treatment of dyslipidemias or primary prevention of cardiovascular disease (atherosclerotic) as detailed below:

Primary prevention of cardiovascular disease (high-risk for CVD): To reduce the risk of MI or stroke in patients without evidence of heart disease who have multiple CVD risk factors or type 2 diabetes. Treatment reduces the risk for angina or revascularization procedures in patients with multiple risk factors.

Secondary prevention of cardiovascular disease: To reduce the risk of nonfatal MI, nonfatal stroke, revascularization procedures, hospitalization for heart failure, and angina in patients with evidence of coronary heart disease.

Treatment of dyslipidemias: To reduce elevations in total cholesterol (C), LDL-C, apolipoprotein B, and triglycerides in patients with elevations of one or more components, and/or to increase low HDL-C as present in Fredrickson type IIa, IIb, III, and IV hyperlipidemias, heterozygous familial and nonfamilial hypercholesterolemia, and homozygous familial hypercholesterolemia

Treatment of heterozygous familial hypercholesterolemia (HeFH) in adolescent patients (10-17 years of age, females >1 year postmenarche) having LDL-C ≥190 mg/dL or LDL-C ≥160 mg/dL with positive family history of premature cardiovascular disease (CVD) or with two or more CVD risk factors.

Unlabeled/Investigational Use Secondary prevention in patients who have experienced a noncardioembolic stroke/TIA or following an ACS event regardless of baseline LDL-C using intensive lipid-lowering therapy

Local Anesthetic/Vasoconstrictor Precautions No information available to require special precautions

Effects on Dental Treatment No significant effects or complications reported

Effects on Bleeding No information available to require special precautions

Adverse Effects

>10%:

- Gastrointestinal: Diarrhea (5% to 14%)
- Neuromuscular & skeletal: Arthralgia (4% to 12%)
- Respiratory: Nasopharyngitis (4% to 13%)

2% to 10%:

- Central nervous system: Insomnia (1% to 5%)
- Gastrointestinal: Nausea (4% to 7%), dyspepsia (3% to 6%)
- Genitourinary: Urinary tract infection (4% to 8%)
- Hepatic: Transaminases increased (2% to 3% with 80 mg/day dosing)
- Neuromuscular & skeletal: Limb pain (3% to 9%), myalgia (3% to 8%), muscle spasms (2% to 5%), musculoskeletal pain (2% to 5%)
- Respiratory: Pharyngolaryngeal pain (1% to 4%)

Additional class-related events or case reports (not necessarily reported with atorvastatin therapy): Cataracts, cirrhosis, dermatomyositis, eosinophilia, erectile dysfunction, extraocular muscle movement impaired, fulminant hepatic necrosis, gynecomastia, hemolytic anemia, interstitial lung disease, ophthalmoplegia, peripheral nerve palsy, polymyalgia rheumatica, positive ANA, renal failure (secondary to rhabdomyolysis), systemic lupus erythematosus-like syndrome, thyroid dysfunction, tremor, vasculitis, vertigo

Dosage Oral:

Primary prevention: Note: Doses should be individualized according to the baseline LDL-cholesterol concentrations, the recommended goal of therapy, and patient response; adjustments should be made at intervals of 2-4 weeks (4 weeks for children)

Children 10-17 years (females >1 year postmenarche): HeFH: 10 mg once daily (maximum: 20 mg/day)

Adults:

Hypercholesterolemia (heterozygous familial and nonfamilial) and mixed hyperlipidemia (Fredrickson types IIa and IIb): Initial: 10-20 mg once daily; patients requiring >45% reduction in LDL-C may be started at 40 mg once daily; range: 10-80 mg once daily

Homozygous familial hypercholesterolemia: 10-80 mg once daily

Secondary prevention:

Clinically-evident coronary heart disease: Initial: 80 mg once daily; adjust based on patient tolerability and recommended goal LDL-C (LaRosa, 2005)

Intensive lipid-lowering after an ACS event regardless of baseline LDL (unlabeled use): Initial: 80 mg once daily; adjust based on patient tolerability and recommended goal LDL-C (Cannon, 2004; Pederson, 2005; Schwartz, 2001). **Note:** Currently, the ACC/AHA guidelines for UA/NSTEMI do not specify which statin to use (Anderson, 2007).

Noncardioembolic stroke/TIA (unlabeled use): Initial: 80 mg once daily; adjust based on patient tolerability and recommended goal LDL-C (Adams, 2008; Amarenco, 2006)

Dosage adjustment for atorvastatin with concomitant medications:

Cyclosporine: Atorvastatin dose should not exceed 10 mg/day

Clarithromycin, itraconazole, ritonavir plus saquinavir, or lopinavir plus ritonavir when atorvastatin dose >20 mg: Ensure that the lowest dose necessary of atorvastatin is used.

Dosing adjustment in renal impairment: No dosage adjustment is necessary.

Dosing adjustment in hepatic impairment: Contraindicated in active liver disease or in patients with unexplained persistent elevations of serum transaminases.

Mechanism of Action Inhibitor of 3-hydroxy-3-methylglutaryl coenzyme A (HMG-CoA) reductase, the rate-limiting enzyme in cholesterol synthesis (reduces the production of mevalonic acid from HMG-CoA); this then results in a compensatory increase in the expression of LDL receptors on hepatocyte membranes and a stimulation of LDL catabolism

Contraindications Hypersensitivity to atorvastatin or any component of the formulation; active liver disease; unexplained persistent elevations of serum transaminases; pregnancy; breast-feeding

Warnings/Precautions Secondary causes of hyperlipidemia should be ruled out prior to therapy. Atorvastatin has not been studied when the primary lipid abnormality is chylomicron elevation (Fredrickson types I and V). Liver function must be monitored by periodic laboratory assessment. May cause hepatic dysfunction. Use with caution in patients who consume large amounts of ethanol or have a history of liver disease; use is contraindicated in patients with active liver disease or unexplained persistent elevations of serum transaminases. Monitoring is recommended. Patients with a history of hemorrhagic stroke may be at increased risk for another hemorrhagic stroke with use.

Rhabdomyolysis with acute renal failure has occurred. Risk is dose related and is increased with concurrent use of lipid-lowering agents which may cause rhabdomyolysis (fibric acid derivatives or niacin at doses ≥1 g/day) or during concurrent use with potent CYP3A4 inhibitors (including amiodarone, clarithromycin, cyclosporine, erythromycin, itraconazole, ketoconazole, nefazodone, grapefruit juice in large quantities, verapamil, or protease inhibitors such as indinavir, nelfinavir, or ritonavir). Ensure patient is on the lowest effective atorvastatin dose. If concurrent use of clarithromycin or combination protease inhibitors (eg, lopinavir/ritonavir or ritonavir/saquinavir) is warranted consider dose adjustment of atorvastatin. Monitor closely if used with other drugs associated with myopathy. Weigh the risk versus benefit when combining any of these drugs with atorvastatin. Discontinue in any patient experiencing an acute or serious condition predisposing to renal failure secondary to rhabdomyolysis. Based upon current evidence, HMG-CoA reductase inhibitor therapy should be continued in the perioperative period unless risk outweighs cardioprotective benefit. Use with caution in patients with advanced age, these patients are predisposed to myopathy. Safety and efficacy have not been established in patients <10 years of age or in premenarcheal girls.

Drug Interactions

Metabolism/Transport Effects **Substrate** of CYP3A4 (major), P-glycoprotein; **Inhibits** CYP3A4 (weak), P-glycoprotein

Avoid Concomitant Use

Avoid concomitant use of Atorvastatin with any of the following: Red Yeast Rice; Silodosin; Topotecan

Increased Effect/Toxicity

Atorvastatin may increase the levels/effects of: Aliskiren; DAPTOmycin; Digoxin; Diltiazem; Everolimus; Midazolam; P-Glycoprotein Substrates; Rivaroxaban; Silodosin; Topotecan; Trabectedin; Verapamil

The levels/effects of Atorvastatin may be increased by: Amiodarone; Antifungal Agents (Azole Derivatives, Systemic); Colchicine; Conivaptan; CycloSPORINE; CycloSPORINE (Systemic); CYP3A4 Inhibitors (Moderate); CYP3A4 Inhibitors (Strong); Danazol; Dasatinib; Diltiazem; Dronedarone; Eltrombopag; Fenofibrate; Fenofibric Acid; Fluconazole; Fusidic Acid; Gemfibrozil; Grapefruit Juice; Macrolide

Antibiotics; Nefazodone; Niacin; Niacinamide; P-Glycoprotein Inhibitors; Protease Inhibitors; QuiNINE; Red Yeast Rice; Rifamycin Derivatives; Sildenafil; Verapamil

Decreased Effect

Atorvastatin may decrease the levels/effects of: Dabigatran Etexilate

The levels/effects of Atorvastatin may be decreased by: Antacids; Bosentan; CYP3A4 Inducers (Strong); Deferasirox; Efavirenz; Etravirine; Fosphenytoin; P-Glycoprotein Inducers; Phenytoin; Rifamycin Derivatives; St Johns Wort; Tocilizumab

Ethanol/Nutrition/Herb Interactions

Ethanol: Avoid excessive ethanol consumption (due to potential hepatic effects).

Food: Atorvastatin serum concentrations may be increased by grapefruit juice; avoid concurrent intake of large quantities (>1 quart/day). Red yeast rice contains an estimated 2.4 mg lovastatin per 600 mg rice.

Herb/Nutraceutical: St John's wort may decrease atorvastatin levels.

Dietary Considerations May take with food if desired; may take without regard to time of day. Before initiation of therapy, patients should be placed on a standard cholesterol-lowering diet for 3-6 months and the diet should be continued during drug therapy. Red yeast rice contains an estimated 2.4 mg lovastatin per 600 mg rice. Atorvastatin serum concentration may be increased when taken with grapefruit juice; avoid concurrent intake of large quantities (>1 quart/day).

Pharmacodynamics/Kinetics

Onset of Action Initial changes: 3-5 days; Maximal reduction in plasma cholesterol and triglycerides: 2 weeks

Half-life Elimination Parent drug: 14 hours; Equipotent metabolites: 20-30 hours

Time to Peak Serum: 1-2 hours

Pregnancy Risk Factor X

Lactation Excretion in breast milk unknown/contraindicated

Dosage Forms

Tablet, oral:

Lipitor®: 10 mg, 20 mg, 40 mg, 80 mg

References

Siedlik PH, Olson, SC, Yang BB, et al, "Erythromycin Coadministration Increases Plasma Atorvastatin Concentrations," *J Clin Pharmacol*, 1999, 39(5):501-4.

Atovaquone (a TOE va kwone)

Related Information

Systemic Viral Diseases *on page 1904*

U.S. Brand Names Mepron®

Canadian Brand Names Mepron®

Pharmacologic Category Antiprotozoal

Use Acute oral treatment of mild-to-moderate *Pneumocystis jirovecii* pneumonia (PCP) in patients who are intolerant to co-trimoxazole; prophylaxis of PCP in patients who are intolerant to co-trimoxazole

Unlabeled/Investigational Use Treatment of babesiosis; treatment/suppression of *Toxoplasma gondii* encephalitis; primary prophylaxis of HIV-infected persons at high risk for developing *Toxoplasma gondii* encephalitis

Local Anesthetic/Vasoconstrictor Precautions No information available to require special precautions

Effects on Dental Treatment Key adverse event(s) related to dental treatment: Oral moniliasis

Effects on Bleeding No information available to require special precautions

Adverse Effects Note: Adverse reaction statistics have been compiled from studies including patients with advanced HIV disease; consequently, it is difficult to distinguish reactions attributed to atovaquone from those caused by the underlying disease or a combination thereof.

>10%:

Central nervous system: Fever (14% to 40%), headache (16% to 31%), insomnia (10% to 19%), depression, pain

Dermatologic: Rash (22% to 46%), pruritus (5% to ≥10%)

Gastrointestinal: Diarrhea (19% to 42%), nausea (21% to 32%), vomiting (14% to 22%), abdominal pain (4% to 21%)

Neuromuscular & skeletal: Weakness (8% to 31%), myalgia

Respiratory: Cough (14% to 25%), rhinitis (5% to 24%), dyspnea (15% to 21%), sinusitis (7% to ≥10%)

Miscellaneous: Infection (18% to 22%), diaphoresis, flu-like syndrome

1% to 10%:

Cardiovascular: Hypotension (≤1%)

Central nervous system: Dizziness (3% to 8%), anxiety (≤7%)

Endocrine & metabolic: Hyponatremia (7% to 10%), hyperglycemia (≤9%), hypoglycemia (≤1%)
Gastrointestinal: Amylase increased (7% to 8%), anorexia (≤7%), dyspepsia (≤5%), constipation (≤3%), taste perversion (≤3%)
Hematologic: Anemia (4% to 6%), neutropenia (3% to 5%)
Hepatic: Liver enzymes increased (4% to 8%)
Renal: BUN increased (≤1%), creatinine increased (≤1%)
Respiratory: Bronchospasm (2% to 4%)
Miscellaneous: Oral moniliasis (5% to 10%)

General Dosage Range Oral: *Children 13-16 years and Adults:* 1500 mg/day in 1-2 divided doses

Mechanism of Action Inhibits electron transport in mitochondria resulting in the inhibition of key metabolic enzymes responsible for the synthesis of nucleic acids and ATP

Pharmacodynamics/Kinetics

Half-life Elimination 1.5-4 days

Pregnancy Risk Factor C

Atovaquone and Proguanil (a TOE va kwone & pro GWA nil)

Related Information

Atovaquone *on page 186*

U.S. Brand Names Malarone®

Canadian Brand Names Malarone®; Malarone® Pediatric

Pharmacologic Category Antimalarial Agent

Use Prevention or treatment of acute, uncomplicated *P. falciparum* malaria

Local Anesthetic/Vasoconstrictor Precautions No information available to require special precautions

Effects on Dental Treatment No significant effects or complications reported

Effects on Bleeding No information available to require special precautions

Adverse Effects The following adverse reactions were reported in patients being treated for malaria. When used for prophylaxis, reactions are similar to those seen with placebo.

>10%:

Gastrointestinal: Abdominal pain (17%), nausea (12%), vomiting (children 10% to 13%, adults 12%)
Hepatic: Transaminase increases (ALT 27%, AST 17%; increased LFT values typically normalized after ~4 weeks)

1% to 10%:

Central nervous system: Headache (10%), dizziness (5%)
Dermatologic: Pruritus (children 6%)
Gastrointestinal: Diarrhea (children 6%, adults 8%), anorexia (5%)
Neuromuscular & skeletal: Weakness (8%)

General Dosage Range Oral:

Children 5-8 kg: Treatment: 125 mg/50 mg as a single daily dose
Children 9-10 kg: Treatment: 187.5 mg/75 mg as a single daily dose
Children 11-20 kg: Prophylaxis: 62.5 mg/25 mg; Treatment: 250 mg/100 mg as a single daily dose
Children 21-30 kg: Prophylaxis: 125 mg/50 mg; Treatment: 500 mg/200 mg as a single daily dose
Children 31-40 kg: Prophylaxis: 187.5 mg/75 mg; Treatment: 750 mg/300 mg as a single daily dose
Children >40 kg and Adults: Prophylaxis: 250 mg/100 mg; Treatment: 1 g/400 mg as a single daily dose

Mechanism of Action

Atovaquone: Selectively inhibits parasite mitochondrial electron transport.
Proguanil: The metabolite cycloguanil inhibits dihydrofolate reductase, disrupting deoxythymidylate synthesis. Together, atovaquone/cycloguanil affect the erythrocytic and exoerythrocytic stages of development.

Pharmacodynamics/Kinetics

Half-life Elimination Proguanil: 12-21 hours

Time to Peak Proguanil: Plasma: 2-4 hours

Pregnancy Risk Factor C

Atropine (A troe peen)

Related Information

Dentin Hypersensitivity, Acid Erosion, High Caries Index, and Xerostomia *on page 1955*

U.S. Brand Names AtroPen®; Atropine Care™; Isopto® Atropine; Sal-Tropine™

Canadian Brand Names Dioptic's Atropine Solution; Isopto® Atropine

Generic Availability (U.S.) Yes: Excludes tablet

Pharmacologic Category Anticholinergic Agent; Anticholinergic Agent, Ophthalmic; Antidote; Antispasmodic Agent, Gastrointestinal; Ophthalmic Agent, Mydriatic

Dental Use Reduction of salivation and bronchial secretions

Use

Injection: Preoperative medication to inhibit salivation and secretions; treatment of symptomatic sinus bradycardia, AV block (nodal level); antidote for acetylcholinesterase inhibitor poisoning (carbamate insecticides, nerve agents, organophosphate insecticides); adjuvant use with anticholinesterases (eg, edrophonium, neostigmine) to decrease their side effects during reversal of neuromuscular blockade

Note: Use is no longer recommended in the management of asystole or pulseless electrical activity (PEA) (ACLS, 2010).

Ophthalmic: Produce mydriasis and cycloplegia for examination of the retina and optic disc and accurate measurement of refractive errors; uveitis

Oral: Inhibit salivation and secretions

Local Anesthetic/Vasoconstrictor Precautions No information available to require special precautions

Effects on Dental Treatment Key adverse event(s) related to dental treatment: Xerostomia and changes in salivation (normal salivary flow resumes upon discontinuation), dry throat, and nasal dryness

Effects on Bleeding No information available to require special precautions

Adverse Effects Severity and frequency of adverse reactions are dose related and vary greatly; listed reactions are limited to significant and/or life-threatening.

Cardiovascular: Arrhythmia, flushing, hypotension, palpitation, tachycardia

Central nervous system: Ataxia, coma, delirium, disorientation, dizziness, drowsiness, excitement, fever, hallucinations, headache, insomnia, nervousness

Dermatologic: Anhidrosis, urticaria, rash, scarlatiniform rash

Gastrointestinal: Bloating, constipation, delayed gastric emptying, loss of taste, nausea, paralytic ileus, vomiting, xerostomia, dry throat, nasal dryness

Genitourinary: Urinary hesitancy, urinary retention

Neuromuscular & skeletal: Weakness

Ocular: Angle-closure glaucoma, blurred vision, cycloplegia, dry eyes, mydriasis, ocular tension increased

Respiratory: Dyspnea, laryngospasm, pulmonary edema

Miscellaneous: Anaphylaxis

Dental Usual Dosage Inhibit salivation and secretions (preanesthesia): Adults (doses <0.5 mg have been associated with paradoxical bradycardia):

I.M., I.V., SubQ: 0.4-0.6 mg 30-60 minutes preop and repeat every 4-6 hours as needed

Oral: 0.4 mg; may repeat in 4 hours if necessary; 0.4 mg initial dose may be exceeded in certain cases and may repeat in 4 hours if necessary (see Dental Comment)

Dosage

Neonates, Infants, and Children: Doses <0.1 mg have been associated with paradoxical bradycardia.

Inhibit salivation and secretions (preanesthesia): Oral, I.M., I.V., SubQ:

<5 kg: 0.02 mg/kg/dose 30-60 minutes preop then every 4-6 hours as needed. Use of a minimum dosage of 0.1 mg in neonates <5 kg will result in dosages >0.02 mg/kg. There is no documented minimum dosage in this age group.

>5 kg: 0.01-0.02 mg/kg/dose to a maximum 0.4 mg/dose 30-60 minutes preop; minimum dose: 0.1 mg

Alternate dosing:

3-7 kg (7-16 lb): 0.1 mg

8-11 kg (17-24 lb): 0.15 mg

11-18 kg (24-40 lb): 0.2 mg

18-29 kg (40-65 lb): 0.3 mg

>30 kg (>65 lb): 0.4 mg

Bradycardia:

I.V., I.O.: 0.02 mg/kg, minimum dose 0.1 mg, maximum single dose: 0.5 mg; may repeat once in 3-5 minutes to a maximum total dose of 0.04 mg/kg or 1 mg (PALS, 2010). When treating bradycardia in neonates, reserve use for those patients unresponsive to improved oxygenation and epinephrine.

Intratracheal: 0.04-0.06 mg/kg; may repeat once if needed (PALS, 2010)

Infants and Children: Nerve agent toxicity management: See **Note** under adult dosing.

Prehospital ("in the field"): I.M.:

Birth to <2 years: Mild-to-moderate symptoms: 0.05 mg/kg; severe symptoms: 0.1 mg/kg

2-10 years: Mild-to-moderate symptoms: 1 mg; severe symptoms: 2 mg

>10 years: Mild-to-moderate symptoms: 2 mg; severe symptoms: 4 mg

Hospital/emergency department: I.M.:

Birth to <2 years: Mild-to-moderate symptoms: 0.05 mg/kg I.M. **or** 0.02 mg/kg I.V.; severe symptoms: 0.1 mg/kg I.M. **or** 0.02 mg/kg I.V.

2-10 years: Mild-to-moderate symptoms: 1 mg; severe symptoms: 2 mg

>10 years: Mild-to-moderate symptoms: 2 mg; severe symptoms: 4 mg

Note: Pralidoxime is a component of the management of nerve agent toxicity; consult Pralidoxime for specific route and dose. For prehospital ("in the field") management, repeat atropine I.M. (children: 0.05-0.1 mg/kg) at 5-10 minute intervals until secretions have diminished and breathing is comfortable or airway resistance has returned to near normal. For hospital management, repeat atropine I.M. (infants 1 mg; all others: 2 mg) at 5-10 minute intervals until secretions have diminished and breathing is comfortable or airway resistance has returned to near normal.

Children: Organophosphate or carbamate poisoning:

I.V.: 0.03-0.05 mg/kg every 10-20 minutes until atropine effect, then every 1-4 hours for at least 24 hours

I.M. (AtroPen®): Mild symptoms: Administer dose listed below as soon as exposure is known or suspected. If severe symptoms develop after first dose, 2 additional doses should be repeated in 10 minutes; do not administer more than 3 doses. Severe symptoms: Immediately administer 3 doses as follows:

<6.8 kg (15 lb): Use of **AtroPen® formulation not recommended;** administer atropine 0.05 mg/kg

6.8-18 kg (15-40 lb): 0.5 mg/dose

18-41 kg (40-90 lb): 1 mg/dose

>41 kg (>90 lb): 2 mg/dose

Adults (doses <0.5 mg have been associated with paradoxical bradycardia):

Inhibit salivation and secretions (preanesthesia):

I.M., I.V., SubQ: 0.4-0.6 mg 30-60 minutes preop and repeat every 4-6 hours as needed

Oral: 0.4 mg; may repeat in 4 hours if necessary; 0.4 mg initial dose may be exceeded in certain cases and may repeat in 4 hours if necessary

Bradycardia: **Note:** Atropine may be ineffective in heart transplant recipients: I.V.: 0.5 mg every 3-5 minutes, not to exceed a total of 3 mg or 0.04 mg/kg (ACLS, 2010)

Neuromuscular blockade reversal: I.V.: 25-30 mcg/kg 30-60 seconds before neostigmine or 7-10 mcg/kg 30-60 seconds before edrophonium

Organophosphate or carbamate poisoning: **Note:** The dose of atropine required varies considerably with the severity of poisoning. Total amount of atropine used in carbamate poisoning is usually less. Severely poisoned patients may exhibit significant tolerance to atropine; ≥2 times the suggested doses may be needed. Titrate to pulmonary status (decreased bronchial secretions). Once patient is stable for a period of time, the dose/dosing frequency may be decreased. If atropinization occurs after 1-2 mg of atropine then re-evaluate working diagnosis.

I.V.: Initial: 1-5 mg; doses should be doubled every 5 minutes until signs of muscarinic excess abate (clearing of bronchial secretions, bronchospasm, and adequate oxygenation). Overly aggressive dosing may cause anticholinergic toxicity (eg, delirium, hyperthermia, and muscle twitching).

I.V. Infusion: 0.5-1 mg/hour or 10% to 20% of loading dose/hour

I.M. (AtroPen®): Mild symptoms: Administer 2 mg as soon as exposure is known or suspected. If severe symptoms develop after first dose, 2 additional doses should be repeated in 10 minutes; do not administer more than 3 doses. Severe symptoms: Immediately administer three 2 mg doses.

Nerve agent toxicity management: I.M.: See **Note**. Prehospital ("in the field") or hospital/emergency department: Mild-to-moderate symptoms: 2-4 mg; severe symptoms: 6 mg

Note: Pralidoxime is a component of the management of nerve agent toxicity; consult Pralidoxime for specific route and dose. For prehospital ("in the field") management, repeat atropine I.M. (2 mg) at 5-10 minute intervals until secretions have diminished and breathing is comfortable or airway resistance has returned to near normal. For hospital management, repeat atropine I.M. (2 mg) at 5-10 minute intervals until secretions have diminished and breathing is comfortable or airway resistance has returned to near normal.

Mydriasis, cycloplegia (preprocedure): Ophthalmic (1% solution): Instill 1-2 drops 1 hour before procedure.

Uveitis: Ophthalmic:

1% solution: Instill 1-2 drops 4 times/day

Ointment: Apply a small amount in the conjunctival sac up to 3 times/day; compress the lacrimal sac by digital pressure for 1-3 minutes after instillation

Elderly, frail patients: Nerve agent toxicity management (unlabeled use): I.M.: See **Note** under adult dosing.

Prehospital ("in the field"): Mild-to-moderate symptoms: 1 mg; severe symptoms: 2-4 mg

Hospital/emergency department: Mild-to-moderate symptoms: 1 mg; severe symptoms: 2 mg

Mechanism of Action Blocks the action of acetylcholine at parasympathetic sites in smooth muscle, secretory glands, and the CNS; increases cardiac output, dries secretions. Atropine reverses the muscarinic effects of cholinergic poisoning. The primary goal in cholinergic poisonings is reversal of bronchorrhea and bronchoconstriction. Atropine has no effect on the nicotinic receptors responsible for muscle weakness, fasciculations, and paralysis.

Contraindications Hypersensitivity to atropine or any component of the formulation; narrow-angle glaucoma; adhesions between the iris and lens; tachycardia; obstructive GI disease; paralytic ileus; intestinal atony of the elderly or debilitated patient; severe ulcerative colitis; toxic megacolon complicating ulcerative colitis; hepatic disease; obstructive uropathy; renal disease; myasthenia gravis (unless used to treat side effects of acetylcholinesterase inhibitor); asthma; thyrotoxicosis; Mobitz type II block

Warnings/Precautions Use with caution in children with spastic paralysis; use with caution in elderly patients. Low doses cause a paradoxical decrease in heart rates. Heat prostration may occur in hot weather. Use with caution in patients with autonomic neuropathy, prostatic hyperplasia, hyperthyroidism, HF, cardiac arrhythmias, chronic lung disease, biliary tract disease; anticholinergic agents are generally not well tolerated in the elderly and their use should be avoided when possible. Atropine is rarely used except as a preoperative agent or in the acute treatment of bradyarrhythmias. In heart transplant recipients, atropine will likely be ineffective in treatment of bradycardia due to lack of vagal innervation of the transplanted heart; cholinergic reinnervation may occur over time (years), so atropine may be used cautiously; however, some may experience paradoxical slowing of the heart rate and high-degree AV block upon administration (ACLS, 2010: Bernheim, 2004).

Avoid relying on atropine for effective treatment of type II second-degree or third-degree AV block (with or without a new wide QRS complex). Asystole or bradycardic pulseless electrical activity (PEA): Although no evidence exists for significant detrimental effects, routine use is unlikely to have a therapeutic benefit and is no longer recommended (ACLS, 2010).

AtroPen®: There are no absolute contraindications for the use of atropine in severe organophosphate poisonings, however in mild poisonings, use caution in those patients where the use of atropine would be otherwise contraindicated. Formulation for use by trained personnel only.

Drug Interactions

Avoid Concomitant Use There are no known interactions where it is recommended to avoid concomitant use.

Increased Effect/Toxicity

Atropine may increase the levels/effects of: AbobotulinumtoxinA; Anticholinergics; Cannabinoids; OnabotulinumtoxinA; Potassium Chloride; RimabotulinumtoxinB

The levels/effects of Atropine may be increased by: Pramlintide

Decreased Effect

Atropine may decrease the levels/effects of: Acetylcholinesterase Inhibitors (Central); Secretin

The levels/effects of Atropine may be decreased by: Acetylcholinesterase Inhibitors (Central)

Pharmacodynamics/Kinetics

Onset of Action I.V.: Rapid

Half-life Elimination 2-3 hours

Pregnancy Risk Factor B/C (manufacturer specific)

Lactation Enters breast milk/use caution (AAP rates "compatible"; AAP 2001 update pending)

Breast-Feeding Considerations Trace amounts of atropine are excreted into breast milk. Anticholinergic agents may suppress lactation.

Prescribing and Access Restrictions The AtroPen® formulation is available for use primarily by the Department of Defense.

Dosage Forms

Injection, solution: 0.05 mg/mL (5 mL); 0.1 mg/mL (5 mL, 10 mL); 0.4 mg/mL (1 mL, 20 mL); 1 mg/mL (1 mL)

AtroPen®: 0.25 mg/0.3 mL (0.3 mL); 0.5 mg/0.7 mL (0.7 mL); 1 mg/0.7 mL (0.7 mL); 2 mg/0.7 mL (0.7 mL)

Injection, solution [preservative free]: 0.4 mg/0.5 mL (0.5 mL); 0.4 mg/mL (1 mL); 1 mg/mL (1 mL)

Ointment, ophthalmic: 1% (3.5 g)

Solution, ophthalmic: 1% (2 mL, 5 mL, 15 mL)

Atropine Care™: 1% (2 mL)

Isopto® Atropine: 1% (5 mL, 15 mL)

Tablet, oral:

Sal-Tropine™: 0.4 mg

Dental Comment The possibility of the need for an initial dose in excess of 0.4 mg has been confirmed by the American Dental Association in its recommendation on the use of this medication to reduce salivation during dental procedures.

Attapulgite (at a PULL gite)

Related Information

Management of Patients Undergoing Cancer Therapy *on page 1970*

Ulcerative, Erosive, and Painful Oral Mucosal Disorders *on page 1950*

Canadian Brand Names Kaopectate® Children's [OTC]; Kaopectate® Extra Strength [OTC]; Kaopectate® [OTC]

Pharmacologic Category Antidiarrheal

Use Symptomatic treatment of diarrhea and cramps

Local Anesthetic/Vasoconstrictor Precautions No information available to require special precautions

Effects on Dental Treatment No significant effects or complications reported

Effects on Bleeding No information available to require special precautions

General Dosage Range Oral:

Children 3-6 years: 300 mg/dose (maximum dose: 2100 mg/day)

Children 6-12 years: 600-750 mg/dose (maximum dose: 4500 mg/day)

Children >12 years and Adults: 1200-1500 mg/dose (maximum dose: 8400 mg/day)

Mechanism of Action Nonselectively absorbs excess intestinal fluid, thereby reducing stool liquidity. May interfere with absorption of nutrients and other drugs as well.

Product Availability Not available in U.S.

Auranofin (au RANE oh fin)

Related Information

Rheumatoid Arthritis, Osteoarthritis, and Osteoporosis *on page 1889*

U.S. Brand Names Ridaura®

Canadian Brand Names Ridaura®

Pharmacologic Category Gold Compound

Use Management of active stage of classic or definite rheumatoid arthritis in patients who do not respond to or tolerate other agents; psoriatic arthritis; adjunctive or alternative therapy for pemphigus

Local Anesthetic/Vasoconstrictor Precautions No information available to require special precautions

Effects on Dental Treatment Key adverse event(s) related to dental treatment: Glossitis and stomatitis.

Effects on Bleeding May be associated (rarely) with thrombocytopenia. No information available to require routine special precautions.

Adverse Effects

>10%:

Dermatologic: Rash (24%), pruritus (17%)

Gastrointestinal: Diarrhea/loose stools (47%), abdominal pain (14%), stomatitis (13%)

Ocular: Conjunctivitis

Renal: Proteinuria

1% to 10%:

Dermatologic: Alopecia, urticaria

Gastrointestinal: Anorexia, constipation, dyspepsia, dysgeusia, flatulence, glossitis

Hematologic: Anemia, eosinophilia, leukopenia, thrombocytopenia

Hepatic: Transaminases increased

Renal: Hematuria, proteinuria

General Dosage Range Dosage adjustment recommended in patients with renal impairment

Oral:

Children: Initial: 0.1 mg/kg/day; Maintenance: 0.1-0.2 mg/kg/day in 1-2 divided doses (maximum: 0.2 mg/kg/day)

Adults: Initial: 6 mg/day; Maintenance: 6-9 mg/day (maximum: 9 mg/day)

Mechanism of Action The exact mechanism of action of gold is unknown; gold is taken up by macrophages which results in inhibition of phagocytosis and lysosomal membrane stabilization; other actions observed are decreased serum rheumatoid factor and alterations in immunoglobulins. Additionally, complement activation is decreased, prostaglandin synthesis is inhibited, and lysosomal enzyme activity is decreased.

Pharmacodynamics/Kinetics

Onset of Action Delayed; therapeutic response may require as long as 3-4 months

Duration of Action Prolonged

Half-life Elimination Single or multiple dosing dependent: 21-31 days

Time to Peak Serum: ~2 hours

Pregnancy Risk Factor C

AzaCITIDine (ay za SYE ti deen)

U.S. Brand Names Vidaza®

Pharmacologic Category Antineoplastic Agent, DNA Methylation Inhibitor

Use Treatment of myelodysplastic syndrome (MDS)

Unlabeled/Investigational Use Treatment of acute myelogenous leukemia (AML)

Local Anesthetic/Vasoconstrictor Precautions No information available to require special precautions

Effects on Dental Treatment Key adverse event(s) related to dental treatment: Mucositis, gingival bleeding, oral mucosal petechiae, stomatitis, oral hemorrhage, and tongue ulceration.

Effects on Bleeding Chemotherapy may result in significant myelosuppression, potentially including significant reduction in platelet counts and altered hemostasis. In patients who are under active treatment with these agents, medical consult is suggested.

Adverse Effects

>10%:

Cardiovascular: Peripheral edema (7% to 19%), chest pain (16%), pallor (16%), pitting edema (15%)

Central nervous system: Fever (30% to 52%), fatigue (13% to 36%), headache (22%), dizziness (19%), anxiety (5% to 13%), depression (12%), insomnia (9% to 11%), malaise (11%), pain (11%)

Dermatologic: Bruising (19% to 31%), petechiae (11% to 24%), erythema (7% to 17%), skin lesion (15%), rash (10% to 14%), pruritus (12%)

Endocrine & metabolic: Hypokalemia (6% to 13%)

Gastrointestinal: Nausea (48% to 71%), vomiting (27% to 54%), diarrhea (36%), constipation (34% to 50%), anorexia (13% to 21%), weight loss (16%), abdominal pain (11% to 16%), abdominal tenderness (12%)

Hematologic: Thrombocytopenia (66% to 70%; grades 3/4: 58%), anemia (51% to 70%; grades 3/4: 14%), neutropenia (32% to 66%; grades 3/4: 61%), leukopenia (18% to 48%; grades 3/4: 15%), febrile neutropenia (14% to 16%; grades 3/4: 13%), myelosuppression (nadir: days 10-17; recovery: days 28-31)

Local: Injection site reactions (14% to 29%): Erythema (35% to 43%; more common with I.V. administration), pain (19% to 23%; more common with I.V. administration), bruising (5% to 14%)

Neuromuscular & skeletal: Weakness (29%), rigors (26%), arthralgia (22%), limb pain (20%), back pain (19%), myalgia (16%)

Respiratory: Cough (11% to 30%), dyspnea (5% to 29%), pharyngitis (20%), epistaxis (16%), nasopharyngitis (15%), upper respiratory tract infection (9% to 13%), pneumonia (11%), crackles (11%)

Miscellaneous: Diaphoresis (11%)

5% to 10%:

Cardiovascular: Cardiac murmur (10%), hypertension (≤9%), tachycardia (9%), hypotension (7%), syncope (6%), chest wall pain (5%)

Central nervous system: Lethargy (7% to 8%), hypoesthesia (5%), postprocedural pain (5%)

Dermatologic: Cellulitis (8%), urticaria (6%), dry skin (5%), skin nodule (5%)

Gastrointestinal: Gingival bleeding (10%), oral mucosal petechiae (8%), stomatitis (8%), weight loss (≤8%), dyspepsia (6% to 7%), hemorrhoids (7%), abdominal distension (6%), loose stools (6%), dysphagia (5%), oral hemorrhage (5%), tongue ulceration (5%)
Genitourinary: Dysuria (8%), urinary tract infection (8% to 9%)
Hematologic: Hematoma (9%), postprocedural hemorrhage (6%)
Local: Injection site reactions: Pruritus (7%), hematoma (6%), rash (6%), granuloma (5%), induration (5%), pigmentation change (5%), swelling (5%)
Neuromuscular & skeletal: Muscle cramps (6%)
Renal: Hematuria (≤6%)
Respiratory: Rhinorrhea (10%), rales (9%), wheezing (9%), breath sounds decreased (8%), pharyngolaryngeal pain (6%), pleural effusion (6%), postnasal drip (6%), rhinitis (6%), rhonchi (6%), nasal congestion (6%), atelectasis (5%), sinusitis (5%)
Miscellaneous: Lymphadenopathy (10%), herpes simplex (9%), night sweats (9%), transfusion reaction (7%), mouth hemorrhage (5%)

General Dosage Range Dosage adjustment recommended in patients who develop toxicities

I.V., SubQ: *Adults:* 75-100 mg/m^2/day for 7 days/28-day treatment cycle

Mechanism of Action Antineoplastic effects may be a result of azacitidine's ability to promote hypomethylation of DNA leading to direct toxicity of abnormal hematopoietic cells in the bone marrow.

Pharmacodynamics/Kinetics

Half-life Elimination I.V., SubQ: ~4 hours

Time to Peak SubQ: 30 minutes

Pregnancy Risk Factor D

AzaTHIOprine (ay za THYE oh preen)

U.S. Brand Names Azasan®; Imuran®

Canadian Brand Names Apo-Azathioprine®; Imuran®; Mylan-Azathioprine; Teva-Azathioprine

Generic Availability (U.S.) Yes

Pharmacologic Category Immunosuppressant Agent

Dental Use Adjunct with prednisone for managing severe erosive lichen planus, major aphthous stomatitis, erythema multiforme, and benign mucous membrane pemphigoid

Use Adjunctive therapy in prevention of rejection of kidney transplants; management of active rheumatoid arthritis (RA)

Unlabeled/Investigational Use Adjunct in prevention of rejection of solid organ (nonrenal) transplants; steroid-sparing agent for corticosteroid-dependent Crohn's disease (CD) and ulcerative colitis (UC); maintenance of remission in CD; fistulizing CD; dermatomyositis/polymyositis; erythema multiforme; pemphigus vulgaris

Local Anesthetic/Vasoconstrictor Precautions No information available to require special precautions

Effects on Dental Treatment No significant effects or complications reported

Effects on Bleeding May be associated (rarely) with thrombocytopenia. No information available to require routine special precautions.

Adverse Effects Frequency not always defined; dependent upon dose, duration, indication, and concomitant therapy.

Central nervous system: Fever, malaise
Gastrointestinal: Nausea/vomiting (RA: 12%), diarrhea
Hematologic: Leukopenia (renal transplant: >50%; RA: 28%), thrombocytopenia
Hepatic: Alkaline phosphatase increased, bilirubin increased, hepatotoxicity, transaminases increased
Neuromuscular & skeletal: Myalgia
Miscellaneous: Infection (renal transplant: 20%; RA: <1%; includes bacterial, fungal, protozoal, viral); neoplasia (other than lymphoma: 3%)

Dental Usual Dosage Adjunctive management of severe recurrent aphthous stomatitis (unlabeled use): Adults: Oral: 50 mg once daily in conjunction with prednisone

Dosage Note: Patients with intermediate TPMT activity may be at risk for increased myelosuppression; those with low or absent TPMT activity receiving conventional azathioprine doses are at risk for developing severe, life-threatening myelotoxicity. Dosage reductions are recommended for patients with reduced TPMT activity.

I.V. dose is equivalent to oral dose (dosing should be transitioned from I.V. to oral as soon as tolerated):

Children (unlabeled) and Adults:

Renal transplantation (treatment usually started the day of transplant, however, has been initiated [rarely] 1-3 days prior to transplant): Oral, I.V.: Initial: 3-5 mg/kg/day usually given as a single daily dose, then 1-3 mg/kg/day maintenance

Rheumatoid arthritis: Oral:

Initial: 1 mg/kg/day given once daily or divided twice daily for 6-8 weeks; increase by 0.5 mg/kg every 4 weeks until response or up to 2.5 mg/kg/day; an adequate trial should be a minimum of 12 weeks

Maintenance dose: Reduce dose by 0.5 mg/kg every 4 weeks until lowest effective dose is reached; optimum duration of therapy not specified; may be discontinued abruptly

Adults: Oral:

Adjunctive management of severe recurrent aphthous stomatitis (unlabeled use): 50 mg once daily in conjunction with prednisone

Adjunctive management of dermatomyositis/polymyositis (unlabeled use): 50 mg/day in conjunction with prednisone; increase by 50 mg/week to total dose of 2-3 mg/kg/day (Briemberg, 2003); **Note:** Onset of beneficial effects may take 3-6 months; however, may be preferred over methotrexate in patients with pulmonary or hepatic toxicity.

Reduction of steroid use in CD or UC, maintenance of remission in CD or fistulizing disease (unlabeled uses): Initial: 50 mg once daily; may increase by 25 mg/day every 1-2 weeks as tolerated to target dose of 2-3 mg/kg/day

Dosage adjustment for concomitant use with allopurinol: Reduce azathioprine dose to one-third or one-fourth the usual dose when used concurrently with allopurinol. Patients with low or absent TPMT activity may require further dose reductions or discontinuation.

Dosage adjustment for toxicity:

Rapid WBC count decrease, persistently low WBC count, or serious infection: Reduce dose or temporarily withhold treatment

Severe toxicity in renal transplantation: May require discontinuation

Hepatic veno-occlusive disease: Permanently discontinue

Dosing adjustment in renal impairment: Although dosage reductions are recommended, specific guidelines are not available in the FDA-approved labeling; the following guidelines have been used by some clinicians (Aronoff, 2007):

Cl_{cr} >50 mL/minute: No adjustment recommended

Cl_{cr} 10-50 mL/minute: Administer 75% of normal dose

Cl_{cr} <10 mL/minute: Administer 50% of normal dose

Hemodialysis (dialyzable; ~45% removed in 8 hours): Children: Administer 50% of normal dose; Adults: Supplement: 0.25 mg/kg

CAPD: Children: Administer 50% of normal dose; Adults: Unknown

CRRT: Children and Adults: Administer 75% of normal dose

Mechanism of Action Azathioprine is an imidazolyl derivative of mercaptopurine; antagonizes purine metabolism and may inhibit synthesis of DNA, RNA, and proteins; may also interfere with cellular metabolism and inhibit mitosis. The 6-thioguanine nucleotides appear to mediate the majority of azathioprine's immunosuppressive and toxic effects.

Contraindications Hypersensitivity to azathioprine or any component of the formulation; pregnancy (in patients with rheumatoid arthritis); patients with rheumatoid arthritis and a history of treatment with alkylating agents (eg, cyclophosphamide, chlorambucil, melphalan) may have a prohibitive risk of neoplasia with azathioprine treatment

Warnings/Precautions [U.S. Boxed Warning]: Chronic immunosuppression increases the risk of neoplasia and serious infections. Azathioprine has mutagenic potential to both men and women. Dose-related, delayed hematologic toxicities (leukopenia, thrombocytopenia, macrocytic anemia, pancytopenia) may occur; may be more severe with renal transplants undergoing rejection; dosage modification for hematologic toxicity may be necessary. Use with caution in patients with liver disease or renal impairment; monitor hematologic function closely. Azathioprine is metabolized to mercaptopurine; concomitant use may result in profound myelosuppression and should be avoided. Patients with genetic deficiency of thiopurine methyltransferase (TPMT) or concurrent therapy with drugs which may inhibit TPMT may be sensitive to myelosuppressive effects. Patients with intermediate TPMT activity may be at risk for increased myelosuppression; those with low or absent TPMT activity are at risk for developing severe myelotoxicity. TPMT genotyping or phenotyping may assist in identifying patients at risk for developing toxicity. TPMT testing does not substitute for CBC monitoring. Xanthine oxidase inhibitors may increase risk for hematologic toxicity; reduce azathioprine dose when used concurrently with allopurinol; patients with low or absent TPMT activity may require further dose reductions or discontinuation.

Hepatotoxicity (transaminase, bilirubin, and alkaline phosphatase elevations) may occur, usually in renal transplant patients and generally within 6 months of transplant; normally reversible with discontinuation; monitor liver function periodically. Rarely, hepatic veno-occlusive disease (VOD) has been reported; discontinue if hepatic VOD is suspected. Gastrointestinal toxicity may occur within the first several weeks of therapy and is reversible. Symptoms may include severe nausea, vomiting, diarrhea, rash, fever, malaise, myalgia, hypotension, and liver enzyme abnormalities. **[U.S. Boxed Warning]: Should be prescribed by physicians familiar with the risks, including hematologic toxicities and mutagenic potential.** Immune response to vaccines may be diminished. Hazardous agent - use appropriate precautions for handling and disposal.

Drug Interactions

Avoid Concomitant Use

Avoid concomitant use of AzaTHIOprine with any of the following: BCG; Febuxostat; Mercaptopurine; Natalizumab; Pimecrolimus; Roflumilast; Tacrolimus (Topical)

Increased Effect/Toxicity

AzaTHIOprine may increase the levels/effects of: Leflunomide; Mercaptopurine; Natalizumab; Vaccines (Live)

The levels/effects of AzaTHIOprine may be increased by: 5-ASA Derivatives; ACE Inhibitors; Allopurinol; Denosumab; Febuxostat; Pimecrolimus; Ribavirin; Roflumilast; Sulfamethoxazole; Tacrolimus (Topical); Trastuzumab; Trimethoprim

Decreased Effect

AzaTHIOprine may decrease the levels/effects of: BCG; Sipuleucel-T; Vaccines (Inactivated); Vitamin K Antagonists

The levels/effects of AzaTHIOprine may be decreased by: Echinacea

Ethanol/Nutrition/Herb Interactions Herb/Nutraceutical: Avoid cat's claw, echinacea (have immunostimulant properties).

Dietary Considerations May be taken with food.

Pharmacodynamics/Kinetics

Half-life Elimination Parent drug: 12 minutes; mercaptopurine: 0.7-3 hours; End-stage renal disease: Slightly prolonged

Time to Peak Plasma: 1-2 hours (including metabolites)

Pregnancy Risk Factor D

Lactation Enters breast milk/not recommended

Breast-Feeding Considerations Due to risk of immunosuppression and serious adverse effects in the nursing infant, breast-feeding is not recommended.

Dosage Forms

Injection, powder for reconstitution: 100 mg

Tablet, oral: 50 mg

Azasan®: 75 mg, 100 mg

Imuran®: 50 mg

References

Beissert S, Werfel T, Frieling U, et al, "A Comparison of Oral Methylprednisolone Plus Azathioprine or Mycophenolate Mofetil for the Treatment of Pemphigus," *Arch Dermatol*, 2006, 142(11):1447-54.

Jones RR, "Azathioprine Therapy in the Management of Persistent Erythema Multiforme," *Br J Dermatol*, 1981, 105(4):465-7.

Azelaic Acid (a zeh LAY ik AS id)

U.S. Brand Names Azelex®; Finacea®; Finacea® Plus™

Canadian Brand Names Finacea®

Pharmacologic Category Topical Skin Product, Acne

Use Topical treatment of inflammatory papules and pustules of mild-to-moderate rosacea; mild-to-moderate inflammatory acne vulgaris

Finacea®: Not FDA-approved for the treatment of acne

Local Anesthetic/Vasoconstrictor Precautions No information available to require special precautions

Effects on Dental Treatment No significant effects or complications reported

Effects on Bleeding No information available to require special precautions

Adverse Effects

>5%: Dermatologic: Pruritus (1% to 6%), burning/stinging/itching (1% to 6%)

1% to 5%:

Dermatologic: Acne (<1% to 1%), edema, erythema, rash, peeling, dermatitis, contact dermatitis, irritation, scaling/dry skin/xerosis

Neuromuscular & skeletal: Paresthesia

General Dosage Range Topical: *Children ≥12 years and Adults:* Massage gently into affected areas twice daily.

Mechanism of Action Azelaic acid is a dietary constituent normally found in whole grain cereals; can be formed endogenously. Exact mechanism is not known. *In vitro*, azelaic acid possesses antimicrobial activity against *Propionibacterium acnes* and *Staphylococcus epidermidis*. May decrease microcomedo formation.

Pharmacodynamics/Kinetics

Half-life Elimination Topical: Healthy subjects: 12 hours

Pregnancy Risk Factor B

Azelastine (Nasal) (a ZEL as teen)

U.S. Brand Names Astelin®; Astepro®

Canadian Brand Names Astelin®

Pharmacologic Category Histamine H_1 Antagonist; Histamine H_1 Antagonist, Second Generation

Use Treatment of the symptoms of seasonal allergic rhinitis such as rhinorrhea, sneezing, and nasal pruritus; treatment of the symptoms of vasomotor rhinitis

Local Anesthetic/Vasoconstrictor Precautions No information available to require special precautions

Effects on Dental Treatment Key adverse event(s) related to dental treatment: Bitter taste, xerostomia (normal salivary flow resumes upon discontinuation), aphthous stomatitis, glossitis, and burning sensation in throat. Chronic use of antihistamines will inhibit salivary flow, particularly in elderly patients. May contribute to periodontal disease and oral discomfort.

Effects on Bleeding No information available to require special precautions

Adverse Effects Note: Adverse reactions may be dose-, indication-, or product-dependent:

>10%:
- Central nervous system: Headache (Astelin® 8% to 15%; Astepro® 1% to 3%), somnolence (<1% to 12%)
- Gastrointestinal: Bitter taste (Astelin® 8% to 20%; Astepro® 6% to 7%)
- Respiratory: Cold symptoms/rhinitis (2% to 17%), cough (11%)

2% to 10%:
- Central nervous system: Dysesthesia (8%), dizziness (2%), fatigue (2%)
- Gastrointestinal: Nausea (3%), weight gain (2%), xerostomia (3%)
- Neuromuscular & skeletal: Myalgia (≤2%)
- Ocular: Conjunctivitis (<2% to 5%)
- Respiratory: Asthma (5%), nasal burning (4%), pharyngitis (4%), paroxysmal sneezing (3%), sinusitis (3%), epistaxis (2% to 3%)

<2%:
- Cardiovascular: Flushing, hypertension, tachycardia
- Central nervous system: Abnormal thinking, anxiety, depersonalization, depression, drowsiness, fever, hypoesthesia, malaise, nervousness, sleep disorder, vertigo
- Dermatologic: Contact dermatitis, eczema, furunculosis, hair and follicle infection, skin laceration
- Endocrine & metabolic: Amenorrhea, breast pain
- Gastrointestinal: Abdominal pain, aphthous stomatitis, appetite increased, constipation, diarrhea, gastroenteritis, glossitis, loss of taste, ulcerative stomatitis, toothache, vomiting
- Genitourinary: Albuminuria, hematuria, polyuria
- Hepatic: ALT increased
- Neuromuscular & skeletal: Back pain, extremity pain, hyperkinesia, rheumatoid arthritis, temporomandibular dislocation
- Ocular: Eye pain, watery eyes
- Respiratory: Bronchitis, bronchospasm, laryngitis, nasal congestion, nocturnal dyspnea, postnasal drip, sinus hypersecretion, throat burning
- Miscellaneous: Allergic reactions, viral infection

General Dosage Range Intranasal:

Children 5-11 years: 1 spray in each nostril twice daily

Children ≥12 years and Adults: 1-2 sprays in each nostril twice daily

Mechanism of Action Competes with histamine for H_1-receptor sites on effector cells and inhibits the release of histamine and other mediators involved in the allergic response; when used intranasally, reduces hyper-reactivity of the airways; increases the motility of bronchial epithelial cilia, improving mucociliary transport

Pharmacodynamics/Kinetics

Onset of Action Peak effect: 3 hours

Duration of Action 12 hours

Half-life Elimination Azelastine: 22-25 hours; Desmethylazelastine: 52-57 hours

Time to Peak Serum: 2-4 hours

Pregnancy Risk Factor C

Azilsartan (ay zil SAR tan)

U.S. Brand Names Edarbi™

Pharmacologic Category Angiotensin II Receptor Blocker

Use Treatment of hypertension; may be used alone or in combination with other antihypertensives

Local Anesthetic/Vasoconstrictor Precautions No information available to require special precautions

Effects on Dental Treatment Key adverse event(s) related to dental treatment: Orthostatic hypotension

Effects on Bleeding No information available to require special precautions

Adverse Effects

Cardiovascular: Hypotension, orthostatic hypotension
Central nervous system: Dizziness, fatigue
Gastrointestinal: Diarrhea (2%), nausea
Hematologic: Hemoglobin decreased, hematocrit decreased, RBC decreased
Neuromuscular & skeletal: Muscle spasm, weakness
Renal: Serum creatinine increased
Respiratory: Cough

General Dosage Range Oral: *Adults:* 40-80 mg once daily

Mechanism of Action Angiotensin II (which is formed by enzymatic conversion from angiotensin I) is the primary pressor agent of the renin-angiotensin system. Effects of angiotensin II include vasoconstriction, stimulation of aldosterone synthesis/release, cardiac stimulation, and renal sodium reabsorption. Azilsartan inhibits angiotensin II's vasoconstrictor and aldosterone-secreting effects by selectively blocking the binding of angiotensin II to the AT_1 receptor in vascular smooth muscle and adrenal gland tissues (azilsartan has a stronger affinity for the AT_1 receptor than the AT_2 receptor). The action is independent of the angiotensin II synthesis pathways. Azilsartan does not inhibit ACE (kininase II), therefore it does not affect the response to bradykinin (the clinical relevance of this is unknown) and does not bind to or inhibit other receptors or ion channels of importance in cardiovascular regulation.

Pharmacodynamics/Kinetics

Half-life Elimination ~11 hours

Time to Peak Serum: 1.5-3 hours

Pregnancy Risk Factor C (1st trimester); D (2nd and 3rd trimesters)

Azithromycin (Systemic) (az ith roe MYE sin)

Related Information

Antibiotic Prophylaxis *on page 1910*
Bacterial Infections *on page 1933*
Clinical Risk Related to Drugs Prolonging QT Interval *on page 1872*
Periodontal Diseases *on page 1942*
Sexually-Transmitted Diseases *on page 1903*

Related Sample Prescriptions

Bacterial Infections and Periodontal Diseases *on page 1983*
Infective Endocarditis (Prevention) *on page 1978*
Sinus Infection Treatment *on page 1985*

U.S. Brand Names Zithromax®; Zithromax® TRI-PAK™; Zithromax® Z-PAK®; Zmax®

Canadian Brand Names Apo-Azithromycin®; CO Azithromycin; Dom-Azithromycin; Mylan-Azithromycin; Novo-Azithromycin; PHL-Azithromycin; PMS-Azithromycin; PRO-Azithromycin; ratio-Azithromycin; Riva-Azithromycin; Sandoz-Azithromycin; Zithromax®

Generic Availability (U.S.) Yes: Excludes extended release microspheres

Pharmacologic Category Antibiotic, Macrolide

Dental Use Alternate oral antibiotic for prevention of infective endocarditis in individuals allergic to penicillins or ampicillin, when amoxicillin cannot be used; alternate antibiotic in the treatment of common orofacial infections caused by aerobic gram-positive cocci and susceptible anaerobes

Use Oral, I.V.: Treatment of acute otitis media due to *H. influenzae*, *M. catarrhalis*, or *S. pneumoniae*; pharyngitis/tonsillitis due to *S. pyogenes*; treatment of mild-to-moderate upper and lower respiratory tract infections, infections of the skin and skin structure, community-acquired pneumonia, pelvic inflammatory disease (PID), sexually-transmitted diseases (urethritis/cervicitis), pharyngitis/tonsillitis, and genital ulcer disease (chancroid) due to susceptible strains of *Chlamydophila pneumoniae*, *C. trachomatis*, *M. catarrhalis*, *H. influenzae*, *S. aureus*, *S. pneumoniae*, *Mycoplasma genitalium*, *Mycoplasma pneumoniae*, and *C. psittaci*; acute bacterial exacerbations of chronic obstructive pulmonary disease (COPD) due to *H. influenzae, M. catarrhalis,* or *S. pneumoniae*; acute bacterial sinusitis

Unlabeled/Investigational Use Prevention of (or to delay onset of) or treatment of MAC in patients with advanced HIV infection; prophylaxis of infective endocarditis in patients who are allergic to penicillin and undergoing surgical or dental procedures; pertussis

Local Anesthetic/Vasoconstrictor Precautions No information available to require special precautions

Effects on Dental Treatment No significant effects or complications reported

Effects on Bleeding No information available to require special precautions

Adverse Effects

>10%: Gastrointestinal: Diarrhea (4% to 9%; high single-dose regimens 12% to 14%), nausea (≤7%; high single-dose regimens 18%)

2% to 10%:

Dermatologic: Pruritus, rash

Gastrointestinal: Abdominal pain, anorexia, cramping, vomiting (especially with high single-dose regimens)

Genitourinary: Vaginitis

Local: (with I.V. administration): Injection site pain, inflammation

Dental Usual Dosage

Prophylaxis against infective endocarditis (unlabeled use): Oral:

Children: 15 mg/kg 30-60 minutes before procedure (maximum: 500 mg). **Note:** American Heart Association (AHA) guidelines now recommend prophylaxis only in patients undergoing invasive procedures and in whom underlying cardiac conditions may predispose to a higher risk of adverse outcomes should infection occur. As of April 2007, routine prophylaxis for GI/GU procedures is no longer recommended by the AHA.

Adolescents ≥16 years and Adults: 500 mg 30-60 minutes prior to the procedure. **Note:** American Heart Association (AHA) guidelines now recommend prophylaxis only in patients undergoing invasive procedures and in whom underlying cardiac conditions may predispose to a higher risk of adverse outcomes should infection occur. As of April 2007, routine prophylaxis for GI/GU procedures is no longer recommended by the AHA.

Bacterial sinusitis: Oral:

Children ≥6 months: 10 mg/kg once daily for 3 days (maximum: 500 mg/day)

Adolescents ≥16 years and Adults: 500 mg/day for a total of 3 days

Extended release suspension (Zmax®): 2 g as a single dose

Orofacial infections: Adolescents ≥16 years and Adults: Oral: 500 mg/day, then 250 mg days 2-5

Treatment of periodontal disease: 500 mg once daily for 4-7 days

Dosage Note: Extended release suspension (Zmax®) is not interchangeable with immediate release formulations. Use should be limited to approved indications. All doses are expressed as immediate release azithromycin unless otherwise specified.

Usual dosage range:

Children ≥6 months: Oral: 5-12 mg/kg given once daily (maximum: 500 mg/day) **or** 30 mg/kg as a single dose (maximum: 1500 mg)

Extended release suspension (Zmax®): 60 mg/kg as a single dose; **Note:** Extended release suspension (Zmax®): Dose in mL is equal to the weight in lbs for patients <75 lbs (34 kg). Pediatric patients ≥75 lbs should receive the adult dose.

Adolescents ≥16 years and Adults:

Oral: 250-600 mg once daily **or** 1-2 g as a single dose

Extended release suspension (Zmax®): 2 g as a single dose

I.V.: 250-500 mg once daily

Indication-specific dosing:

Children: Oral:

Bacterial sinusitis: 10 mg/kg once daily for 3 days (maximum: 500 mg/day)

Cat scratch disease (unlabeled use): <45.5 kg: 10 mg/kg as a single dose, then 5 mg/kg once daily for 4 days

Community-acquired pneumonia: 10 mg/kg on day 1 (maximum: 500 mg/day) followed by 5 mg/kg/day once daily on days 2-5 (maximum: 250 mg/day)

Extended release suspension (Zmax®):

<75 lbs (34 kg): 60 mg/kg as a single dose; dose in mL is equal to the weight in lbs for patients <75 lbs (34 kg)

≥75 lbs (34 kg): Refer to adult dose

Disseminated *M. avium* (unlabeled use; CDC, 2009):

Treatment: 10-12 mg/kg/day (maximum: 500 mg)

Primary prophylaxis: 20 mg/kg (maximum: 1200 mg) once weekly (preferred) or alternatively, 5 mg/kg/day once daily (maximum: 250 mg/day)

Secondary prophylaxis: 5 mg/kg/day once daily (maximum: 250 mg/day) in combination with ethambutol, with or without rifabutin

Otitis media:

1-day regimen: 30 mg/kg as a single dose (maximum: 1500 mg)

3-day regimen: 10 mg/kg once daily for 3 days (maximum: 500 mg/day)

5-day regimen: 10 mg/kg on day 1 (maximum: 500 mg/day) followed by 5 mg/kg/day once daily on days 2-5 (maximum: 250 mg/day)

Pertussis (CDC, 2005):

Children <6 months: 10 mg/kg/day for 5 days

Children ≥6 months: 10 mg/kg on day 1 (maximum: 500 mg/day) followed by 5 mg/kg/day once daily on days 2-5 (maximum: 250 mg/day)

Pharyngitis, tonsillitis: Children ≥2 years: 12 mg/kg/day once daily for 5 days (maximum: 500 mg/day)

Prophylaxis against infective endocarditis (unlabeled use): 15 mg/kg 30-60 minutes before procedure (maximum: 500 mg). **Note:** American Heart Association (AHA) guidelines now recommend prophylaxis only in patients undergoing invasive procedures and in whom underlying cardiac conditions may predispose to a higher risk of adverse outcomes should infection occur. As of April 2007, routine prophylaxis for GI/GU procedures is no longer recommended by the AHA.

Uncomplicated chlamydial urethritis or cervicitis (unlabeled use): Children ≥45 kg: 1 g as a single dose (CDC, 2010)

Adolescents ≥16 years and Adults:

Bacterial sinusitis: Oral: 500 mg/day for a total of 3 days

Extended release suspension (Zmax®): 2 g as a single dose

Cat scratch disease (unlabeled use): Oral: >45.5 kg: 500 mg as a single dose, then 250 mg once daily for 4 days

Chancroid due to *H. ducreyi*: Oral: 1 g as a single dose (CDC, 2010)

Community-acquired pneumonia:

Oral: Extended release suspension (Zmax®): 2 g as a single dose

I.V.: 500 mg as a single dose for at least 2 days, follow I.V. therapy by the oral route with a single daily dose of 500 mg to complete a 7- to 10-day course of therapy.

Disseminated *M. avium* complex disease in patients with advanced HIV infection (unlabeled use): Oral:

Prophylaxis: 1200 mg once weekly (may be combined with rifabutin)

Treatment: 600 mg daily (in combination with ethambutol 15 mg/kg)

Gonococcal infection, uncomplicated (cervix, pharynx, rectum, urethra): Oral: 1 g as a single dose (in combination with a cephalosporin) (CDC, 2010)

Note: Monotherapy with azithromycin (1 g and 2 g) have been associated with resistance and/or treatment failure; use in combination with a cephalosporin (CDC, 2010). However, a single 2 g azithromycin dose is still an FDA-approved dose for gonococcal urethritis and cervicitis and also may be appropriate for treatment of a gonococcal infection in pregnant women who cannot tolerate a cephalosporin (CDC, 2010).

Granuloma inguinale (donovanosis): Oral: 1 g once a week for at least 3 weeks (and until lesions have healed) (CDC, 2010)

Mild-to-moderate respiratory tract, skin, and soft tissue infections: Oral: 500 mg in a single loading dose on day 1 followed by 250 mg/day as a single dose on days 2-5

Alternative regimen: Bacterial exacerbation of COPD: 500 mg/day for a total of 3 days

Pelvic inflammatory disease (PID): I.V.: 500 mg as a single dose for 1-2 days, follow I.V. therapy by the oral route with a single daily dose of 250 mg to complete a 7-day course of therapy

Pertussis (CDC, 2005): Oral: 500 mg on day 1 followed by 250 mg/day on days 2-5 (maximum: 500 mg/day)

Prophylaxis against infective endocarditis (unlabeled use): Oral: 500 mg 30-60 minutes prior to the procedure. **Note:** American Heart Association (AHA) guidelines now recommend prophylaxis only in patients undergoing invasive procedures and in whom underlying cardiac conditions may predispose to a higher risk of adverse outcomes should infection occur. As of April 2007, routine prophylaxis for GI/GU procedures is no longer recommended by the AHA.

Prophylaxis against sexually-transmitted diseases following sexual assault: Oral: 1 g as a single dose (in combination with a cephalosporin and metronidazole) (CDC, 2010)

Urethritis/cervicitis: Oral: *Due to C. trachomatis or M. genitalium*: 1 g as a single dose

Dosage adjustment in renal impairment: Use caution in patients with GFR <10 mL/minute

Dosage adjustment in hepatic impairment: Use with caution due to potential for hepatotoxicity (rare). Specific guidelines for dosing in hepatic impairment have not been established.

Mechanism of Action Inhibits RNA-dependent protein synthesis at the chain elongation step; binds to the 50S ribosomal subunit resulting in blockage of transpeptidation

Contraindications Hypersensitivity to azithromycin, other macrolide (eg, azalide or ketolide) antibiotics, or any component of the formulation

Warnings/Precautions Use with caution in patients with pre-existing liver disease; hepatic impairment, including hepatocellular and/or cholestatic hepatitis, with or without jaundice, has been observed. Discontinue if symptoms of malaise, nausea, vomiting, abdominal colic, and fever. Allergic reactions have been reported (rare); reappearance of allergic reaction may occur without further azithromycin exposure. May mask or delay symptoms of incubating gonorrhea or syphilis, so appropriate culture and susceptibility tests should be performed prior to initiating azithromycin. Prolonged use may result in fungal or bacterial superinfection, including *C. difficile*-associated diarrhea (CDAD) and pseudomembranous colitis; CDAD has been observed >2 months postantibiotic treatment. Use caution with renal dysfunction. Prolongation of the QT_c interval has been reported with macrolide antibiotics; use caution in patients at risk of prolonged cardiac repolarization. Use with caution in patients with myasthenia gravis. Safety and efficacy of systemically-administered azithromycin (oral, intravenous) have not been established in children <6 months of age with acute otitis media, acute bacterial sinusitis, or community-acquired pneumonia, or in children <2 years of age with pharyngitis/tonsillitis.

Oral suspensions (immediate release and extended release) are not interchangeable.

Drug Interactions

Metabolism/Transport Effects Substrate of CYP3A4 (minor); **Inhibits** CYP3A4 (weak)

Avoid Concomitant Use

Avoid concomitant use of Azithromycin (Systemic) with any of the following: Artemether; BCG; Dronedarone; Lumefantrine; Nilotinib; Pimozide; QuiNINE; Tetrabenazine; Thioridazine; Toremifene; Vandetanib; Ziprasidone

Increased Effect/Toxicity

Azithromycin (Systemic) may increase the levels/effects of: Amiodarone; Cardiac Glycosides; CycloSPORINE; CycloSPORINE (Systemic); Dronedarone; Pimozide; QTc-Prolonging Agents; QuiNINE; Tacrolimus; Tacrolimus (Systemic); Tacrolimus (Topical); Tetrabenazine; Thioridazine; Toremifene; Vandetanib; Vitamin K Antagonists; Ziprasidone

The levels/effects of Azithromycin (Systemic) may be increased by: Alfuzosin; Artemether; Chloroquine; Ciprofloxacin; Ciprofloxacin (Systemic); Conivaptan; Gadobutrol; Lumefantrine; Nelfinavir; Nilotinib; QuiNINE

Decreased Effect

Azithromycin (Systemic) may decrease the levels/effects of: BCG; Typhoid Vaccine

The levels/effects of Azithromycin (Systemic) may be decreased by: Tocilizumab

Ethanol/Nutrition/Herb Interactions Food: Rate and extent of GI absorption may be altered depending upon the formulation. Azithromycin suspension, not tablet form, has significantly increased absorption (46%) with food.

Dietary Considerations

Some products may contain sodium and/or sucrose.

Oral suspension, immediate release, may be administered with or without food.

Oral suspension, extended release, should be taken on an empty stomach (at least 1 hour before or 2 hours following a meal).

Tablet may be administered with food to decrease GI effects.

Pharmacodynamics/Kinetics

Half-life Elimination Terminal: Oral, I.V.: Immediate release: 68-72 hours; Extended release: 59 hours

Time to Peak Oral: Serum: Immediate release: 2-3 hours; Extended release: 5 hours

Pregnancy Risk Factor B

Lactation Enters breast milk/use caution

Breast-Feeding Considerations Azithromycin is excreted in low amounts into breast milk. The manufacturer recommends that caution be exercised when administering azithromycin to breast-feeding women. Nondose-related effects could include modification of bowel flora.

Dosage Forms

Injection, powder for reconstitution: 500 mg

Zithromax®: 500 mg

Microspheres for suspension, extended release, oral:

Zmax®: 2 g/bottle (60 mL)

Powder for suspension, oral: 100 mg/5 mL (15 mL); 200 mg/5 mL (15 mL, 22.5 mL, 30 mL); 1 g/packet (3s, 10s)

Zithromax®: 100 mg/5 mL (15 mL); 200 mg/5 mL (15 mL, 22.5 mL, 30 mL); 1 g/packet (3s, 10s)

Tablet, oral: 250 mg, 500 mg, 600 mg

Zithromax®: 250 mg, 500 mg, 600 mg

Zithromax® TRI-PAK™: 500 mg

Zithromax® Z-PAK®: 250 mg

References

ADA Division of Legal Affairs, "A Legal Perspective on Antibiotic Prophylaxis," *J Am Dent Assoc*, 2003, 134(9):1260.

American Dental Association Council on Scientific Affairs, "Combating Antibiotic Resistance," *J Am Dent Assoc*, 2004, 135(4):484-7.

Cotter CJ and Bierne JC, "Azithromycin for Odontogenic Infection," *J Oral Maxillofac Surg*, 2003, 61 (10):1238.

Dajani AS, Taubert KA, Wilson W, et al, "Prevention of Bacterial Endocarditis. Recommendations by the American Heart Association," *JAMA*, 1997, 277(22):1794-801.

Dajani AS, Taubert KA, Wilson W, et al, "Prevention of Bacterial Endocarditis: Recommendations by the American Heart Association," *J Am Dent Assoc*, 1997, 128(8):1142-51.

Moore PA, "Dental Therapeutic Indications for the Newer Long-Acting Macrolide Antibiotics," *J Am Dent Assoc*, 1999, 130(9):1341-3.

Williams JD, Maskell JP, Shain H, et al, "Comparative *In Vitro* Activity of Azithromycin, Macrolides (Erythromycin, Clarithromycin and Spiramycin) and Streptogramin RP 59500 Against Oral Organisms," *J Antimicrob Chemother*, 1992, 30(1):27-37.

Wilson W, Taubert KA, Gewitz M, et al, "Prevention of Infective Endocarditis. Guidelines From the American Heart Association. A Guideline From the American Heart Association Rheumatic Fever, Endocarditis, and Kawasaki Disease Committee, Council on Cardiovascular Disease in the Young, and the Council on Clinical Cardiology, Council on Cardiovascular Surgery and Anesthesia, and the Quality of Care and Outcomes Research Interdisciplinary Working Group," *Circulation*, 2007, 115. Available at http://circ.ahajournals.org/cgi/reprint/CIRCULATIONAHA.106.183095v1; accessed August 6, 2007.

Wynn RL, "New Erythromycins," *Gen Dent*, 1996, 44(4):304-7.

Wynn RL, Bergman SA, Meiller TF, et al, "Antibiotics in Treating Oral-Facial Infections of Odontogenic Origin: An Update," *Gen Dent*, 2001, 49(3):238-40, 242, 244 passim.

Aztreonam (AZ tree oh nam)

U.S. Brand Names Azactam®; Cayston®

Canadian Brand Names Azactam®

Pharmacologic Category Antibiotic, Miscellaneous

Use

Injection: Treatment of patients with urinary tract infections, lower respiratory tract infections, septicemia, skin/skin structure infections, intra-abdominal infections, and gynecological infections caused by susceptible gram-negative bacilli

Inhalation: Improve respiratory symptoms in cystic fibrosis (CF) patients with *Pseudomonas aeruginosa*

Local Anesthetic/Vasoconstrictor Precautions No information available to require special precautions

Effects on Dental Treatment No significant effects or complications reported

Effects on Bleeding No information available to require special precautions

Adverse Effects

Injection: Adults: 1% to 10%:

Dermatologic: Rash

Gastrointestinal: Diarrhea, nausea, vomiting

Local: Thrombophlebitis, pain at injection site

Inhalation:

>10%:

Central nervous system: Pyrexia (13%; more often observed in children)

Respiratory: Cough (54%), nasal congestion (16%), pharyngeal pain (12%), wheezing (16%)

1% to 10%:

Cardiovascular: Chest discomfort (8%)

Dermatologic: Rash (2%)

Gastrointestinal: Abdominal pain (7%), vomiting (6%)

Respiratory: Bronchospasm (3%)

General Dosage Range Dosage adjustment recommended in patients with renal impairment

I.M.:

Children >1 month: 30-50 mg/kg/dose every 6-8 hours (maximum: 8 g/day)

Adults: 500 mg to 1 g every 8-12 hours

I.V.:

Children >1 month: 30-50 mg/kg/dose every 6-8 hours (maximum: 8 g/day)

Adults: 1-2 g every 6-12 hours (maximum: 8 g/day)

Oral inhalation: *Children ≥7 years and Adults:* 75 mg 3 times/day

Mechanism of Action Inhibits bacterial cell wall synthesis by binding to one or more of the penicillin-binding proteins (PBPs) which in turn inhibits the final transpeptidation step of peptidoglycan synthesis in bacterial cell walls, thus inhibiting cell wall biosynthesis. Bacteria eventually lyse due to ongoing activity of cell wall autolytic enzymes (autolysins and murein hydrolases) while cell wall assembly is arrested. Monobactam structure makes cross-allergenicity with beta-lactams unlikely.

Pharmacodynamics/Kinetics

Half-life Elimination Injection:

Children 2 months to 12 years: 1.7 hours

Adults: Normal renal function: 1.7-2.9 hours

End-stage renal disease: 6-8 hours

Time to Peak I.M., I.V. push: Within 60 minutes; I.V. infusion: 1.5 hours

Pregnancy Risk Factor B

Prescribing and Access Restrictions Cayston® (aztreonam inhalation solution) is only available through a select group of specialty pharmacies and cannot be obtained through a retail pharmacy. Because Cayston® may only be used with the Altera® Nebulizer System, it can only be obtained from the following specialty pharmacies: Cystic Fibrosis Services, Inc; IV Solutions; Foundation Care; and Pharmaceutical Specialties, Inc. This network of specialty pharmacies ensures proper access to both the drug and device. To obtain the medication and proper nebulizer, contact the Cayston Access Program at 1-877-7CAYSTON (1-877-722-9786) or at www.cayston.com.

Bacitracin (bas i TRAY sin)

U.S. Brand Names Baci-Rx [DSC]; Baciguent® [OTC]; BACiiM™

Canadian Brand Names Baciguent®; Baciject®

Pharmacologic Category Antibiotic, Miscellaneous; Antibiotic, Ophthalmic; Antibiotic, Topical

Use Treatment of susceptible bacterial infections mainly; has activity against gram-positive bacilli; due to toxicity risks, systemic and irrigant uses of bacitracin should be limited to situations where less toxic alternatives would not be effective

Unlabeled/Investigational Use Oral administration: Successful in antibiotic-associated colitis; has been used for enteric eradication of vancomycin-resistant enterococci (VRE)

Local Anesthetic/Vasoconstrictor Precautions No information available to require special precautions

Effects on Dental Treatment No significant effects or complications reported

Effects on Bleeding No information available to require special precautions

Adverse Effects

1% to 10%:

Cardiovascular: Hypotension, edema of the face/lips, chest tightness

Central nervous system: Pain

Dermatologic: Rash, itching

Gastrointestinal: Anorexia, nausea, vomiting, diarrhea, rectal itching

Hematologic: Blood dyscrasias

Miscellaneous: Diaphoresis

<1%: Rare cases of anaphylaxis have been reported in association with topical and intraoperative exposures.

General Dosage Range

I.M.:

Infants ≤2.5 kg: 900 units/kg/day in 2-3 divided doses

Infants >2.5 kg: 1000 units/kg/day in 2-3 divided doses

Children: 800-1200 units/kg/day divided every 8 hours

Irrigation: *Children and Adults:* 50-100 units/mL in solution for irrigation, apply 1-5 times/day or as needed

Ophthalmic: *Children and Adults:* Instill 1/4" to 1/2" ribbon every 3-4 hours (acute infections) or 2-3 times/day (mild-to-moderate infections)

Oral: *Adults:* 25,000 units 4 times/day

Topical: *Children and Adults:* Apply 1-5 times/day

Mechanism of Action Inhibits bacterial cell wall synthesis by preventing transfer of mucopeptides into the growing cell wall

Pharmacodynamics/Kinetics

Duration of Action 6-8 hours

Time to Peak Serum: I.M.: 1-2 hours

Bacitracin and Polymyxin B (bas i TRAY sin & pol i MIKS in bee)

Related Information

Bacitracin *on page* 202

Polymyxin B *on page* 1370

U.S. Brand Names AK-Poly-Bac™; Polysporin® [OTC]

Canadian Brand Names LID-Pack®; Optimyxin®

Pharmacologic Category Antibiotic, Ophthalmic; Antibiotic, Topical

Use Treatment of superficial infections caused by susceptible organisms

Local Anesthetic/Vasoconstrictor Precautions No information available to require special precautions

Effects on Dental Treatment No significant effects or complications reported

Effects on Bleeding No information available to require special precautions

Adverse Effects 1% to 10%: Local: Rash, itching, burning, anaphylactoid reactions, swelling, conjunctival erythema

General Dosage Range

Ophthalmic: *Children and Adults:* Instill 1/2" ribbon in the affected eye(s) every 3-4 hours (acute infections) **or** 2-3 times/day (mild-to-moderate infections)

Topical: *Children and Adults:* Apply to affected area 1-4 times/day

Mechanism of Action See individual agents.

Pregnancy Risk Factor C

Bacitracin, Neomycin, and Polymyxin B
(bas i TRAY sin, nee oh MYE sin, & pol i MIKS in bee)

Related Information

Bacitracin *on page* 202

Neomycin *on page* 1197

Polymyxin B *on page* 1370

U.S. Brand Names Neosporin® Neo To Go® [OTC]; Neosporin® Topical [OTC]

Pharmacologic Category Antibiotic, Ophthalmic; Antibiotic, Topical

Use Helps prevent infection in minor cuts, scrapes, and burns; short-term treatment of superficial external ocular infections caused by susceptible organisms

Local Anesthetic/Vasoconstrictor Precautions No information available to require special precautions

Effects on Dental Treatment No significant effects or complications reported

Effects on Bleeding No information available to require special precautions

Adverse Effects Frequency not defined.

Dermatologic: Reddening, allergic contact dermatitis

Local: Itching, failure to heal, swelling, irritation

Ophthalmic: Conjunctival edema

Miscellaneous: Anaphylaxis

General Dosage Range

Ophthalmic: *Children and Adults:* Instill 1/2" every 3-4 hours

Topical: *Children and Adults:* Apply 1-3 times/day

Mechanism of Action See individual agents.

Pregnancy Risk Factor C

Bacitracin, Neomycin, Polymyxin B, and Hydrocortisone
(bas i TRAY sin, nee oh MYE sin, pol i MIKS in bee, & hye droe KOR ti sone)

Related Information

Bacitracin *on page* 202

Hydrocortisone (Topical) *on page* 868

Neomycin *on page* 1197

Polymyxin B *on page* 1370

U.S. Brand Names Cortisporin® Ointment

Canadian Brand Names Cortisporin® Topical Ointment

Pharmacologic Category Antibiotic, Ophthalmic; Antibiotic, Topical; Corticosteroid, Ophthalmic; Corticosteroid, Topical

Use Prevention and treatment of susceptible inflammatory conditions where bacterial infection (or risk of infection) is present

Local Anesthetic/Vasoconstrictor Precautions No information available to require special precautions

Effects on Dental Treatment No significant effects or complications reported

Effects on Bleeding No information available to require special precautions

Adverse Effects Frequency not defined. For additional information, see individual agents.

Ophthalmic ointment:

Dermatologic: Delayed wound healing, rash

Ocular: Cataracts, corneal thinning, glaucoma, irritation, keratitis (bacterial), intraocular pressure increase, optic nerve damage, scleral thinning

Miscellaneous: Hypersensitivity (including anaphylaxis), secondary infection, sensitization to kanamycin, paromomycin, streptomycin, and gentamicin

Topical ointment:

Dermatologic: Acneiform eruptions, allergic contact dermatitis, burning skin, dryness, folliculitis, hypertrichosis, hypopigmentation, irritation, maceration of skin, miliaria, ocular hypertension, perioral dermatitis, pruritus, skin atrophy, striae

Otic: Ototoxicity

Renal: Nephrotoxicity

Miscellaneous: Hypersensitivity (including anaphylaxis), secondary infection, sensitization to karamycin, paromycin, streptomycin, and gentamicin

General Dosage Range

Ophthalmic: *Children and Adults:* Instill 1/2 inch every 3-4 hours

Topical: *Children and Adults:* Apply sparingly 2-4 times/day

Mechanism of Action See individual agents.

Pregnancy Risk Factor C

Bacitracin, Neomycin, Polymyxin B, and Pramoxine

(bas i TRAY sin, nee oh MYE sin, pol i MIKS in bee, & pra MOKS een)

Related Information

Bacitracin *on page 202*

Neomycin *on page 1197*

Polymyxin B *on page 1370*

Pramoxine *on page 1384*

U.S. Brand Names Neosporin® + Pain Relief Ointment [OTC]; Tri Biozene [OTC]

Pharmacologic Category Antibiotic, Topical

Use Prevention and treatment of susceptible superficial topical infections and provide temporary relief of pain or discomfort

Local Anesthetic/Vasoconstrictor Precautions No information available to require special precautions

Effects on Dental Treatment No significant effects or complications reported

Effects on Bleeding No information available to require special precautions

General Dosage Range Topical: *Children ≥2 years and Adults:* Apply 1-3 times/day to infected areas

Baclofen (BAK loe fen)

U.S. Brand Names Gablofen®; Lioresal®

Canadian Brand Names Apo-Baclofen®; Dom-Baclofen; Lioresal®; Liotec; Med-Baclofen; Mylan-Baclofen; Novo-Baclofen; Nu-Baclo; PHL-Baclofen; PMS-Baclofen; ratio-Baclofen; Riva-Baclofen

Pharmacologic Category Skeletal Muscle Relaxant

Use Treatment of reversible spasticity associated with multiple sclerosis or spinal cord lesions

Orphan drug: Intrathecal: Treatment of intractable spasticity caused by spinal cord injury, multiple sclerosis, and other spinal disease (spinal ischemia or tumor, transverse myelitis, cervical spondylosis, degenerative myelopathy)

Unlabeled/Investigational Use Intractable hiccups, intractable pain relief, bladder spasticity, trigeminal neuralgia, cerebral palsy, short-term treatment of spasticity in children with cerebral palsy, Huntington's chorea

Local Anesthetic/Vasoconstrictor Precautions No information available to require special precautions

Effects on Dental Treatment No significant effects or complications reported

Effects on Bleeding No information available to require special precautions

Adverse Effects

>10%:

Central nervous system: Drowsiness, vertigo, psychiatric disturbances, insomnia, slurred speech, ataxia, hypotonia

Neuromuscular & skeletal: Weakness

1% to 10%:
- Cardiovascular: Hypotension
- Central nervous system: Fatigue, confusion, headache
- Dermatologic: Rash
- Gastrointestinal: Nausea, constipation
- Genitourinary: Polyuria

General Dosage Range

Intrathecal:

Children: Test dose: 25-100 mcg; Initial infusion: Infuse at a 24-hourly rate dosed at twice the test dose

Adults: Test dose: 50-100 mcg; Initial infusion: Infuse at a 24-hourly rate dosed at twice the test dose

Oral:

Adults: Initial: 5 mg 3 times/day; Maintenance: Up to 80 mg/day in 2-3 divided doses

Elderly: Initial: 5 mg 2-3 times/day, increasing gradually as needed

Mechanism of Action Inhibits the transmission of both monosynaptic and polysynaptic reflexes at the spinal cord level, possibly by hyperpolarization of primary afferent fiber terminals, with resultant relief of muscle spasticity

Pharmacodynamics/Kinetics

Onset of Action 3-4 days; Peak effect: 5-10 days

Half-life Elimination 3.5 hours

Time to Peak Serum: Oral: Within 2-3 hours

Pregnancy Risk Factor C

Balanced Salt Solution (BAL anced salt soe LOO shun)

U.S. Brand Names AquaLase™; BSS Plus®; BSS®; Navstel®

Canadian Brand Names BSS Plus®; BSS®; Eye-Stream®

Pharmacologic Category Irrigating Solution; Ophthalmic Agent, Miscellaneous

Use

Irrigation solution for ophthalmic surgery:
- AquaLase™, BSS®: Intraocular or extraocular irrigating solution
- BSS Plus®, Navstel®: Intraocular irrigating solution

Irrigation solution for eyes, ears, nose, or throat

Local Anesthetic/Vasoconstrictor Precautions No information available to require special precautions

Effects on Dental Treatment No significant effects or complications reported

Effects on Bleeding No information available to require special precautions

Adverse Effects

>10%: Ocular: Intraocular pressure increased (11% to 12%), cataract (7% to 11%)

1% to 10%:
- Central nervous system: Headache (3%)
- Ocular: Discomfort (3% to 5%), dry eyes (3% to 5%), macular edema (4%), conjunctival hyperemia (3% to 4%), posterior capsule opacification (2% to 3%), iritis (1% to 3%), retinal hemorrhage (1% to 3%), blurred vision (1% to 2%)

General Dosage Range Irrigation: *Children and Adults:* Based on standard for each surgical procedure

Pregnancy Risk Factor C

Balsalazide (bal SAL a zide)

U.S. Brand Names Colazal®

Pharmacologic Category 5-Aminosalicylic Acid Derivative; Anti-inflammatory Agent

Use Treatment of mild-to-moderate active ulcerative colitis

Local Anesthetic/Vasoconstrictor Precautions No information available to require special precautions

Effects on Dental Treatment No significant effects or complications reported

Effects on Bleeding No information available to require special precautions

Adverse Effects

>10%:
- Central nervous system: Headache (children 15%; adults 8%)
- Gastrointestinal: Abdominal pain (children 12% to 13%; adults 6%)

1% to 10%:
- Central nervous system: Insomnia (adults 2%), fatigue (children 4%; adults 2%), fever (children 6%; adults 2%)
- Endocrine & metabolic: Dysmenorrhea (children 3%)

Gastrointestinal: Diarrhea (children 9%; adults 5%), ulcerative colitis exacerbation (children 6%; adults 1%), nausea (children 4%; adults 5%), vomiting (children 10%; adults 4%), hematochezia (children 4%), stomatitis (children 3%), anorexia (adults 2%), dyspepsia (adults 2%), flatulence (adults 2%), cramps (adults 1%), constipation (adults 1%), xerostomia (adults 1%)
Genitourinary: Urinary tract infection (adults 1%)
Neuromuscular & skeletal: Arthralgia (adults 4%), back pain (adults 2%), myalgia (adults 1%)
Respiratory: Respiratory infection (adults 4%), cough (children 3%; adults 2%), pharyngitis (children 6%; adults 2%), pharyngolaryngeal pain (children 3%), rhinitis (adults 2%)
Miscellaneous: Flu-like syndrome (children 4%; adults 1%)

General Dosage Range Oral:
Children ≥5 years: 750 mg **or** 2.25 g 3 times/day
Adults: 2.25 g 3 times/day

Mechanism of Action Balsalazide is a prodrug, converted by bacterial azoreduction to 5-aminosalicylic acid (mesalamine, active), 4-aminobenzoyl-β-alanine (inert), and their metabolites. 5-aminosalicylic acid may decrease inflammation by blocking the production of arachidonic acid metabolites topically in the colon mucosa.

Pharmacodynamics/Kinetics
Onset of Action Delayed; may require several days to weeks
Half-life Elimination Primary effect is topical (colonic mucosa); systemic half-life not determined
Time to Peak Balsalazide: 1-2 hours

Pregnancy Risk Factor B

Barium (BA ree um)

U.S. Brand Names Bar-Test™; Cat-Pak™; E-Z Cat® Dry; E-Z-Cat®; E-Z-Disk™; Entero VU™ 24%; Esopho-Cat®; Liquid Polibar Plus®; Liquid Polibar®; Readi-Cat®; Readi-Cat® 2; Varibar® Honey; Varibar® Nectar; Varibar® Pudding; Varibar® Thin Honey; VoLumen®

Pharmacologic Category Radiopaque Agents

Use Diagnostic aid for computed tomography or x-ray examinations of the GI tract

Local Anesthetic/Vasoconstrictor Precautions No information available to require special precautions

Effects on Dental Treatment No significant effects or complications reported

Effects on Bleeding No information available to require special precautions

Basiliximab (ba si LIK si mab)

U.S. Brand Names Simulect®

Canadian Brand Names Simulect®

Pharmacologic Category Immunosuppressant Agent; Monoclonal Antibody

Use Prophylaxis of acute organ rejection in renal transplantation (in combination with cyclosporine and corticosteroids)

Unlabeled/Investigational Use Treatment of refractory acute graft-versus-host disease (GVHD); prevention of liver or cardiac transplant rejection

Local Anesthetic/Vasoconstrictor Precautions No information available to require special precautions

Effects on Dental Treatment Key adverse event(s) related to dental treatment: Facial edema and ulcerative stomatitis. Causes gingival hypertrophy (GH) similar to that caused by cyclosporine; early reports indicate that frequency/incidence of basiliximab-induced GH not as high as cyclosporine-induced GH.

Effects on Bleeding No information available to require special precautions

Adverse Effects Administration of basiliximab did not appear to increase the incidence or severity of adverse effects in clinical trials. Adverse events were reported in 96% of both the placebo and basiliximab groups.

>10%:
Cardiovascular: Hypertension, peripheral edema
Central nervous system: Fever, headache, insomnia, pain
Dermatologic: Acne, wound complications
Endocrine & metabolic: Hypercholesterolemia, hyperglycemia, hyper-/hypokalemia, hyperuricemia, hypophosphatemia
Gastrointestinal: Abdominal pain, constipation, diarrhea, dyspepsia, nausea, vomiting
Genitourinary: Urinary tract infection
Hematologic: Anemia
Neuromuscular & skeletal: Tremor

Respiratory: Dyspnea, infection (upper respiratory)
Miscellaneous: Viral infection

3% to 10%:

Cardiovascular: Abnormal heart sounds, angina, arrhythmia, atrial fibrillation, chest pain, generalized edema, heart failure, hypotension, tachycardia
Central nervous system: Agitation, anxiety, depression, dizziness, fatigue, hypoesthesia, malaise
Dermatologic: Cyst, hypertrichosis, pruritus, rash, skin disorder, skin ulceration
Endocrine & metabolic: Acidosis, dehydration, diabetes mellitus, fluid overload, glucocorticoids increased, hyper-/hypocalcemia, hyperlipemia, hypertriglyceridemia, hypoglycemia, hypomagnesemia, hyponatremia, hypoproteinemia
Gastrointestinal: Abdomen enlarged, esophagitis, flatulence, gastroenteritis, GI hemorrhage, gingival hyperplasia, melena, moniliasis, stomatitis (including ulcerative), weight gain
Genitourinary: Bladder disorder, dysuria, genital edema (male), impotence, ureteral disorder, urinary frequency, urinary retention
Hematologic: Hematoma, hemorrhage, leukopenia, polycythemia, purpura, thrombocytopenia, thrombosis
Neuromuscular & skeletal: Arthralgia, arthropathy, back pain, cramps, fracture, hernia, leg pain, myalgia, neuropathy, paresthesia, rigors, weakness
Ocular: Abnormal vision, cataract, conjunctivitis
Renal: Albuminuria, hematuria, nonprotein nitrogen increased, oliguria, renal function abnormal, renal tubular necrosis
Respiratory: Bronchitis, bronchospasm, cough, pharyngitis, pneumonia, pulmonary edema, sinusitis, rhinitis
Miscellaneous: Accidental trauma, cytomegalovirus (CMV) infection, herpes infection (simplex and zoster), infection, sepsis

General Dosage Range I.V.:

Children <35 kg: 10 mg within 2 hours prior to transplant surgery, followed by a second 10 mg dose 4 days after transplantation

Children ≥35 kg and Adults: 20 mg within 2 hours prior to transplant surgery, followed by a second 20 mg dose 4 days after transplantation

Mechanism of Action Chimeric (murine/human) immunosuppressant monoclonal antibody which blocks the alpha-chain of the interleukin-2 (IL-2) receptor complex; this receptor is expressed on activated T lymphocytes and is a critical pathway for activating cell-mediated allograft rejection

Pharmacodynamics/Kinetics

Duration of Action Mean: 36 days (determined by IL-2R alpha saturation)

Half-life Elimination Children 1-11 years: 9.5 days; Adolescents 12-16 years: 9.1 days; Adults: Mean: 7.2 days

Pregnancy Risk Factor B

BCG (bee see jee)

U.S. Brand Names BCG Vaccine; TheraCys®; TICE® BCG

Canadian Brand Names ImmuCyst®; Oncotice™; Pacis™

Pharmacologic Category Biological Response Modulator; Vaccine, Live (Bacterial)

Use

BCG intravesical: Treatment and prophylaxis of carcinoma *in situ* of the bladder; prophylaxis of primary or recurrent superficial papillary tumors following transurethral resection

BCG vaccine: Immunization against *Mycobacterium tuberculosis* in persons not previously infected and who are at high risk for exposure

BCG vaccine is not routinely administered for the prevention of *M. tuberculosis* in the United States. The Advisory Committee on Immunization Practices (ACIP) recommends vaccination be considered for the following:

- Children with a negative tuberculin skin test who are continually exposed to (and cannot be separated from) adults who are untreated or ineffectively treated for TB disease when the child cannot be given long-term treatment for infection **or** if the adult has TB caused by strains resistant to isoniazid and rifampin.
- Healthcare workers with a high percentage of patients with *M. tuberculosis* strains resistant to both isoniazid and rifampin, if there is ongoing transmission of the resistant strains and subsequent infection is likely, or if comprehensive infection-control precautions have not been successful. In addition, healthcare workers should be counseled on the risks and benefits of vaccination and treatment of latent TB infection

Local Anesthetic/Vasoconstrictor Precautions No information available to require special precautions

Effects on Dental Treatment No significant effects or complications reported

Effects on Bleeding No information available to require special precautions

Adverse Effects All serious adverse reactions must be reported to the U.S. Department of Health and Human Services (DHHS) Vaccine Adverse Event Reporting System (VAERS) 1-800-822-7967 or online at https://vaers.hhs.gov/esub/index.

Adverse reactions associated with **intravesicular administration**:

>10%:

Central nervous system: Malaise (7% to 40%), fever (17% to 38%), chills (9% to 34%), pain (17%)

Gastrointestinal: Nausea/vomiting (3% to 16%), anorexia/weight loss (2% to 11%)

Genitourinary: Dysuria (52% to 60%), bladder irritation (50% to 60%), urinary urgency/frequency (6% to 50%), hematuria (26% to 39%), cystitis (6% to 29%), urinary tract infection (2% to 18%)

Hematological: Anemia (≤21%)

Miscellaneous: Flu-like syndrome (24% to 33%)

1% to 10%:

Central nervous system: Fatigue (7%), headache/dizziness (2% to 5%)

Dermatologic: Rash (≤5%)

Gastrointestinal: Diarrhea (6%), abdominal pain (2% to 5%), constipation (≤5%)

Genitourinary: Genital pain (10%), hemorrhagic cystitis (9%), bladder cramps/pain (8%), urinary incontinence (2% to 6%), bladder spasm (5%), contracted bladder (≤5%), nocturia (5%), urinary debris (2% to 5%), genital inflammation/abscess (2%)

Hematological: Leukopenia (≤5%), coagulopathy (≤5%), thrombocytopenia (<5%)

Neuromuscular & skeletal: Arthralgia/myalgia (3% to 7%), cramps/pain (4% to 6%), rigors (3%)

Renal: Renal toxicity (10%)

Respiratory: Pulmonary infection (<5%)

Miscellaneous: Infection (3% to 5%), diaphoresis (3%), allergy (2%)

<1%: Abscesses, conjunctivitis, disseminated sepsis, epididymitis, granulomatous chorioretinitis, hepatitis, hepatic granuloma, iritis, keratitis, *M. bovis* infection (lung, liver, bone, bone marrow, kidney, lymph nodes, prostate), orchitis, pneumonitis, prostatitis, skin ulceration, urethritis, urinary obstruction, uveitis

Adverse reactions associated with **BCG vaccination**: Axillary lymphadenopathy, cervical lymphadenopathy, disseminated BCG infection (BCG osteomyelitis; may occur from 4 months to 2 years after vaccination), local reactions (induration, itching, lesions, lymphadenitis, pustule, tenderness, ulceration). Local reactions may persist for up to 3 months; more severe manifestations may occur up to 5 months after vaccination and persist for several weeks.

General Dosage Range

Percutaneous:

Children <1 month: 0.2-0.3 mL (half-strength dilution)

Children >1 month and Adults: 0.2-0.3 mL (full-strength dilution)

Intravesicular: *Adults:*

TheraCys®: 1 dose instilled into bladder (for 2 hours) once weekly for 6 weeks followed by 1 treatment at 3, 6, 12, 18, and 24 months after initial treatment

TICE® BCG: 1 dose instilled into bladder (for 2 hours) once weekly for 6 weeks (may repeat cycle 1 time), followed by once monthly for 6-12 months

Mechanism of Action BCG live is an attenuated strain of bacillus Calmette-Guérin (*Mycobacterium bovis*) used as a biological response modifier. BCG live, when used intravesicularly for treatment of bladder carcinoma *in situ*, is thought to cause a local, chronic inflammatory response involving macrophage and leukocyte infiltration of the bladder. By a mechanism not fully understood, this local inflammatory response leads to destruction of superficial tumor cells of the urothelium. BCG is active immunotherapy which stimulates the host's immune mechanism to reject the tumor. Evidence of systemic immune response is also commonly seen, manifested by a positive PPD tuberculin skin test reaction, however, its relationship to clinical efficacy is not well-established.

Pregnancy Risk Factor C

Becaplermin (be KAP ler min)

U.S. Brand Names Regranex®

Canadian Brand Names Regranex®

Pharmacologic Category Growth Factor, Platelet-Derived; Topical Skin Product

Use Adjunctive treatment of diabetic neuropathic ulcers occurring on the lower limbs and feet that extend into subcutaneous tissue (or beyond) and have adequate blood supply

Local Anesthetic/Vasoconstrictor Precautions No information available to require special precautions

Effects on Dental Treatment No significant effects or complications reported

Effects on Bleeding No information available to require special precautions

Adverse Effects 1% to 10%: Dermatologic: Erythematous rash (2%)

General Dosage Range Topical: *Adults:* Apply once daily; to determine the length of gel to apply to the ulcer, measure the greatest length of the ulcer by the greatest width of the ulcer. Tube size and unit of measure will determine the formula used in the calculation. Recalculate amount of gel needed every 1-2 weeks, depending on the rate of change in ulcer area.

Centimeters: 15 g tube: [ulcer length (cm) x width (cm)] divided by 4 = length of gel (cm); 2 g tube: [ulcer length (cm) x width (cm)] divided by 2 = length of gel (cm)

Inches: 15 g tube: [length (in) x width (in)] x 0.6 = length of gel (in); 2 g tube: [length (in) x width (in)] x 1.3 = length of gel (in)

Mechanism of Action Recombinant B-isoform homodimer of human platelet-derived growth factor (rPDGF-BB) which enhances formation of new granulation tissue, induces fibroblast proliferation and differentiation to promote wound healing; also promotes angiogenesis.

Pharmacodynamics/Kinetics

Onset of Action Complete healing: 15% of patients within 8 weeks, 25% at 10 weeks

Pregnancy Risk Factor C

Beclomethasone (Oral Inhalation) (be kloe METH a sone)

Related Information

Respiratory Diseases *on page 1876*

U.S. Brand Names QVAR®

Canadian Brand Names QVAR®; Vanceril® AEM

Generic Availability (U.S.) No

Pharmacologic Category Corticosteroid, Inhalant (Oral)

Use Oral inhalation: Maintenance and prophylactic treatment of asthma; includes those who require corticosteroids and those who may benefit from a dose reduction/elimination of systemically-administered corticosteroids. Not for relief of acute bronchospasm.

Local Anesthetic/Vasoconstrictor Precautions No information available to require special precautions

Effects on Dental Treatment Key adverse event(s) related to dental treatment: Oral candidiasis, xerostomia (normal salivary flow resumes upon discontinuation), nasal dryness, and dry throat. Localized infections with *Candida albicans* or *Aspergillus niger* occur frequently in the mouth and pharynx with repetitive use of an oral inhaler; may require treatment with appropriate antifungal therapy or discontinuance of inhaler use.

Effects on Bleeding No information available to require special precautions

Adverse Effects Frequency not defined.

Central nervous system: Agitation, depression, dizziness, dysphonia, headache, lightheadedness, mental disturbances

Dermatologic: Acneiform lesions, angioedema, atrophy, bruising, pruritus, purpura, striae, rash, urticaria

Endocrine & metabolic: Cushingoid features, growth velocity reduction in children and adolescents, HPA function suppression, weight gain

Gastrointestinal: Dry/irritated nose, throat and mouth, hoarseness, localized *Candida* or *Aspergillus* infection, loss of smell, loss of taste, nausea, unpleasant smell, unpleasant taste, vomiting

Ocular: Cataracts, glaucoma, intraocular pressure increased

Respiratory: Cough, paradoxical bronchospasm, pharyngitis, sinusitis, wheezing

Miscellaneous: Anaphylactic/anaphylactoid reactions, death (due to adrenal insufficiency, reported during and after transfer from systemic corticosteroids to aerosol in asthmatic patients), immediate and delayed hypersensitivity reactions

Dosage Nasal inhalation and oral inhalation dosage forms are not to be used interchangeably.

Inhalation, oral: Asthma (doses should be titrated to the lowest effective dose once asthma is controlled) (QVAR®):

Children 5-11 years: Initial: 40 mcg twice daily; maximum dose: 80 mcg twice daily

Children ≥12 years and Adults:

Patients previously on bronchodilators only: Initial dose 40-80 mcg twice daily; maximum dose: 320 mcg twice day

Patients previously on inhaled corticosteroids: Initial dose 40-160 mcg twice daily; maximum dose: 320 mcg twice daily

NIH Asthma Guidelines (NIH, 2007): HFA formulation (eg, QVAR®): Administer in divided doses:
Children 5-11 years:
"Low" dose: 80-160 mcg/day
"Medium" dose: >160-320 mcg/day
"High" dose: >320 mcg/day
Children ≥12 years and Adults:
"Low" dose: 80-240 mcg/day
"Medium" dose: >240-480 mcg/day
"High" dose: >480 mcg/day

Mechanism of Action Controls the rate of protein synthesis; depresses the migration of polymorphonuclear leukocytes, fibroblasts; reverses capillary permeability and lysosomal stabilization at the cellular level to prevent or control inflammation

Contraindications Hypersensitivity to beclomethasone or any component of the formulation; status asthmaticus

Warnings/Precautions May cause hypercorticism or suppression of hypothalamic-pituitary-adrenal (HPA) axis, particularly in younger children or in patients receiving high doses for prolonged periods. HPA axis suppression may lead to adrenal crisis. Withdrawal and discontinuation of a corticosteroid should be done slowly and carefully. Particular care is required when patients are transferred from systemic corticosteroids to inhaled products due to possible adrenal insufficiency or withdrawal from steroids, including an increase in allergic symptoms. Patients receiving >20 mg per day of prednisone (or equivalent) may be most susceptible. Fatalities have occurred due to adrenal insufficiency in asthmatic patients during and after transfer from systemic corticosteroids to aerosol steroids; aerosol steroids do **not** provide the systemic steroid needed to treat patients having trauma, surgery, or infections.

Bronchospasm may occur with wheezing after inhalation; if this occurs, stop steroid and treat with a fast-acting bronchodilator. Supplemental steroids (oral or parenteral) may be needed during stress or severe asthma attacks. Not to be used in status asthmaticus or for the relief of acute bronchospasm. Corticosteroid use may cause psychiatric disturbances, including depression, euphoria, insomnia, mood swings, and personality changes. Pre-existing psychiatric conditions may be exacerbated by corticosteroid use. Prolonged use of corticosteroids may also increase the incidence of secondary infection, mask acute infection (including fungal infections), prolong or exacerbate viral infections, or limit response to vaccines. Exposure to chickenpox should be avoided; corticosteroids should not be used to treat ocular herpes simplex. Corticosteroids should not be used for cerebral malaria. Close observation is required in patients with latent tuberculosis and/or TB reactivity; restrict use in active TB (only in conjunction with antituberculosis treatment). Prolonged treatment with corticosteroids has been associated with the development of Kaposi's sarcoma (case reports); if noted, discontinuation of therapy should be considered.

Use with caution in patients with thyroid disease, hepatic impairment, renal impairment, cardiovascular disease, diabetes, glaucoma, cataracts, myasthenia gravis, patients at risk for osteoporosis, patients at risk for seizures, or GI diseases (diverticulitis, peptic ulcer, ulcerative colitis) due to perforation risk. Use caution following acute MI (corticosteroids have been associated with myocardial rupture). Because of the risk of adverse effects, systemic corticosteroids should be used cautiously in the elderly in the smallest possible effective dose for the shortest duration.

Orally-inhaled corticosteroids may cause a reduction in growth velocity in pediatric patients (~1 centimeter per year [range: 0.3-1.8 cm per year] and related to dose and duration of exposure). To minimize the systemic effects of orally-inhaled corticosteroids, each patient should be titrated to the lowest effective dose. Growth should be routinely monitored in pediatric patients. Safety and efficacy have not been established in children <5 years of age. There have been reports of systemic corticosteroid withdrawal symptoms (eg, joint/muscle pain, lassitude, depression) when withdrawing oral inhalation therapy.

Drug Interactions

Avoid Concomitant Use

Avoid concomitant use of Beclomethasone (Oral Inhalation) with any of the following: Aldesleukin; BCG; Natalizumab; Pimecrolimus; Roflumilast; Tacrolimus (Topical)

Increased Effect/Toxicity

Beclomethasone (Oral Inhalation) may increase the levels/effects of: Amphotericin B; Deferasirox; Leflunomide; Loop Diuretics; Natalizumab; Thiazide Diuretics

The levels/effects of Beclomethasone (Oral Inhalation) may be increased by: Denosumab; Pimecrolimus; Roflumilast; Tacrolimus (Topical); Trastuzumab

Decreased Effect

Beclomethasone (Oral Inhalation) may decrease the levels/effects of: Aldesleukin; Antidiabetic Agents; BCG; Corticorelin; Sipuleucel-T; Vaccines (Inactivated)

The levels/effects of Beclomethasone (Oral Inhalation) may be decreased by: Echinacea

Pharmacodynamics/Kinetics

Onset of Action Therapeutic effect: 1-4 weeks

Half-life Elimination BDP: 0.5 hours; 17-BMP: 3 hours

Time to Peak Plasma: Oral inhalation: BDP: 0.5 hours; 17-BMP: 0.7 hours

Pregnancy Risk Factor C

Lactation Excretion in breast milk unknown/use caution

Breast-Feeding Considerations Other corticosteroids have been found in breast milk; however, information for beclomethasone is not available.

Dosage Forms

Aerosol, for oral inhalation:

QVAR®: 40 mcg/inhalation (8.7 g); 80 mcg/inhalation (8.7 g)

Beclomethasone (Nasal) (be kloe METH a sone)

U.S. Brand Names Beconase AQ®

Canadian Brand Names Apo-Beclomethasone®; Gen-Beclo; Nu-Beclomethasone; Rivanase AQ

Generic Availability (U.S.) No

Pharmacologic Category Corticosteroid, Nasal

Use Symptomatic treatment of seasonal or perennial rhinitis; prevent recurrence of nasal polyps following surgery.

Local Anesthetic/Vasoconstrictor Precautions No information available to require special precautions

Effects on Dental Treatment No significant effects or complications reported

Effects on Bleeding No information available to require special precautions

Adverse Effects Frequency not defined.

Central nervous system: Headache, lightheadedness

Dermatologic: Angioedema, rash, urticaria

Endocrine & metabolic: Growth velocity reduction in children and adolescents, HPA function suppression (dose related), weight gain

Gastrointestinal: Dry/irritated nose, throat and mouth, hoarseness, localized *Candida* or *Aspergillus* infection, loss of smell, loss of taste, nausea, unpleasant smell, unpleasant taste, vomiting

Local: Burning, epistaxis, localized *Candida* infection, nasal septum perforation (rare), nasal stuffiness, nosebleeds, rhinorrhea, sneezing, transient irritation, ulceration of nasal mucosa (rare)

Ocular: Cataracts (rare), glaucoma (rare), intraocular pressure increased (rare), tearing

Respiratory: Cough, paradoxical bronchospasm (rare), pharyngitis, sinusitis, wheezing

Miscellaneous: Anaphylactic/anaphylactoid reactions, immediate and delayed hypersensitivity reactions

Dosage Nasal inhalation and oral inhalation dosage forms are not to be used interchangeably.

Inhalation, nasal: Rhinitis, nasal polyps (Beconase® AQ): Children ≥6 years and Adults: 1-2 inhalations each nostril twice daily; total dose 168-336 mcg/day

Mechanism of Action Controls the rate of protein synthesis; depresses the migration of polymorphonuclear leukocytes, fibroblasts; reverses capillary permeability and lysosomal stabilization at the cellular level to prevent or control inflammation

Contraindications Hypersensitivity to beclomethasone or any component of the formulation; status asthmaticus

Warnings/Precautions May cause hypercorticism or suppression of hypothalamic-pituitary-adrenal (HPA) axis, particularly in younger children or in patients receiving high doses for prolonged periods. HPA axis suppression may lead to adrenal crisis. Withdrawal and discontinuation of a corticosteroid should be done slowly and carefully. Particular care is required when patients are transferred from systemic corticosteroids to inhaled products due to possible adrenal insufficiency or withdrawal from steroids, including an increase in allergic symptoms. Patients receiving >20 mg per day of prednisone (or equivalent) may be most susceptible. Fatalities have occurred due to adrenal insufficiency in asthmatic patients during and after transfer from systemic corticosteroids to aerosol steroids; aerosol steroids do not provide the systemic steroid needed to treat patients having trauma, surgery, or infections.

Avoid nasal corticosteroid use in patients with recent nasal septal ulcers, nasal surgery or nasal trauma until healing has occurred.

Intranasal corticosteroids may cause a reduction in growth velocity in pediatric patients (~1 centimeter per year [range: 0.3-1.8 cm per year] and related to dose and duration of exposure). To minimize the systemic effects of intranasal corticosteroids, each patient should be titrated to the lowest effective dose. Growth should be routinely monitored in pediatric patients. Safety and efficacy have not been established in children <5 years of age. There have been reports of systemic corticosteroid withdrawal symptoms (eg, joint/muscle pain, lassitude, depression) when withdrawing oral inhalation therapy.

Drug Interactions

Avoid Concomitant Use There are no known interactions where it is recommended to avoid concomitant use.

Increased Effect/Toxicity

Beclomethasone (Nasal) may increase the levels/effects of: Deferasirox

Decreased Effect

Beclomethasone (Nasal) may decrease the levels/effects of: Corticorelin

Pharmacodynamics/Kinetics

Half-life Elimination BDP: 0.5 hours; 17-BMP: 3 hours

Pregnancy Risk Factor C

Lactation Excretion in breast milk unknown/use caution

Breast-Feeding Considerations Other corticosteroids have been found in breast milk; however, information for beclomethasone is not available. Inhaled corticosteroids are recommended for the treatment of asthma (most information available using budesonide) while breast-feeding.

Dosage Forms

Suspension, intranasal:

Beconase AQ®: 42 mcg/inhalation (25 g)

Belimumab (be LIM yoo mab)

U.S. Brand Names Benlysta®

Pharmacologic Category Monoclonal Antibody

Use Treatment of autoantibody-positive (antinuclear antibody [ANA] and/or anti-double-stranded DNA [anti-ds-DNA]) systemic lupus erythematosus (SLE) in addition to standard therapy

Local Anesthetic/Vasoconstrictor Precautions No information available to require special precautions

Effects on Dental Treatment No significant effects or complications reported

Effects on Bleeding No information available to require special precautions

Adverse Effects

>10%: Gastrointestinal: Nausea (15%), diarrhea (12%)

≥3% to 10%:

Central nervous system: Fever (10%), insomnia (7%), migraine (5%), depression (5%), anxiety (4%)

Gastrointestinal: Viral gastroenteritis (3%)

Genitourinary: Cystitis (4%)

Hematologic: Leukopenia (4%)

Neuromuscular & skeletal: Pain in extremity (6%)

Respiratory: Bronchitis (9%), nasopharyngitis (9%), pharyngitis (5%)

General Dosage Range I.V.: *Adults:* 10 mg/kg every 2 weeks for 3 doses; Maintenance: 10 mg/kg every 4 weeks

Mechanism of Action Belimumab is an IgG1λ monoclonal antibody that prevents the survival of B lymphocytes by blocking the binding of soluble human B lymphocyte stimulator protein (BLyS) to receptors on B lymphocytes. This reduces the activity of B-cell mediated immunity and the autoimmune response.

Pharmacodynamics/Kinetics

Onset of Action B cells: 8 weeks; Clinical improvement (SLE Responder Index and flare reduction): 16 weeks (Navarra, 2011)

Half-life Elimination 19.4 days

Pregnancy Risk Factor C

Belladonna and Opium (bel a DON a & OH pee um)

Related Information

Opium Tincture *on page 1255*

Pharmacologic Category Analgesic Combination (Opioid); Antispasmodic Agent, Urinary

Use Relief of moderate-to-severe pain associated with ureteral spasms not responsive to nonopioid analgesics and to space intervals between injections of opiates

Local Anesthetic/Vasoconstrictor Precautions No information available to require special precautions

Effects on Dental Treatment Key adverse event(s) related to dental treatment: Xerostomia and changes in salivation (normal salivary flow resumes upon discontinuation), and dry throat and nose.

Effects on Bleeding No information available to require special precautions

Adverse Effects Frequency not defined.

Cardiovascular: Palpitation
Central nervous system: Dizziness, drowsiness
Dermatologic: Pruritus, urticaria
Gastrointestinal: Constipation, nausea, vomiting, xerostomia
Genitourinary: Urinary retention
Ocular: Blurred vision, photophobia

General Dosage Range Rectal: *Children >12 years and Adults:* 1 suppository 1-2 times/day (maximum: 4 doses/day)

Mechanism of Action The pharmacologically active agents present in the belladonna component are atropine and scopolamine. Atropine blocks the action of acetylcholine at parasympathetic sites in smooth muscle, secretory glands, and the CNS causing a relaxation of smooth muscle and drying of secretions. The principle agent in opium is morphine. Morphine binds to opiate receptors in the CNS, causing inhibition of ascending pain pathways, altering the perception of and response to pain.

Pregnancy Risk Factor C

Controlled Substance C-II

Benazepril (ben AY ze pril)

Related Information

Cardiovascular Diseases *on page 1848*

U.S. Brand Names Lotensin®

Canadian Brand Names Apo-Benazepril®; Lotensin®

Generic Availability (U.S.) Yes

Pharmacologic Category Angiotensin-Converting Enzyme (ACE) Inhibitor

Use Treatment of hypertension, either alone or in combination with other antihypertensive agents

Local Anesthetic/Vasoconstrictor Precautions No information available to require special precautions

Effects on Dental Treatment No significant effects or complications reported

Effects on Bleeding No information available to require special precautions

Adverse Effects

1% to 10%:

Cardiovascular: Postural dizziness (2%)
Central nervous system: Headache (6%), dizziness (4%), somnolence (2%)
Renal: Serum creatinine increased (2%), worsening of renal function may occur in patients with bilateral renal artery stenosis or hypovolemia
Respiratory: Cough (1% to 10%)

Eosinophilic pneumonitis, anaphylaxis, renal insufficiency, and renal failure have been reported with other ACE inhibitors. In addition, a syndrome including fever, myalgia, arthralgia, interstitial nephritis, vasculitis, rash, eosinophilia, and elevated ESR has been reported to be associated with ACE inhibitors.

Dosage Oral: Hypertension:

Children ≥6 years: Initial: 0.2 mg/kg/day (up to 10 mg/day) as monotherapy; dosing range: 0.1-0.6 mg/kg/day (maximum dose: 40 mg/day)

Adults: Initial: 10 mg/day in patients not receiving a diuretic; 20-80 mg/day as a single dose or 2 divided doses; the need for twice-daily dosing should be assessed by monitoring peak (2-6 hours after dosing) and trough responses.

Note: Patients taking diuretics should have them discontinued 2-3 days prior to starting benazepril. If they cannot be discontinued, then initial dose should be 5 mg; restart after blood pressure is stabilized if needed.

Elderly: Oral: Initial: 5-10 mg/day in single or divided doses; usual range: 20-40 mg/day; adjust for renal function; also see **Note** in adult dosing.

Dosing interval in renal impairment: Cl_{cr} <30 mL/minute:

Children: Use is not recommended.

Adults: Administer 5 mg/day initially; maximum daily dose: 40 mg.

Hemodialysis: Moderately dialyzable (20% to 50%); administer dose postdialysis or administer 25% to 35% supplemental dose.

Peritoneal dialysis: Supplemental dose is not necessary.

Mechanism of Action Competitive inhibition of angiotensin I being converted to angiotensin II, a potent vasoconstrictor, through the angiotensin I-converting enzyme (ACE) activity, with resultant lower levels of angiotensin II which causes an increase in plasma renin activity and a reduction in aldosterone secretion

Contraindications Hypersensitivity to benazepril or any component of the formulation; patients with a history of angioedema (with or without prior ACE inhibitor therapy)

Warnings/Precautions Anaphylactic reactions may occur rarely with ACE inhibitors. At any time during treatment (especially following first dose) angioedema may occur rarely with ACE inhibitors. It may involve the head and neck (potentially compromising airway) or the intestine (presenting with abdominal pain). African-Americans and patients with idiopathic or hereditary angioedema may be at an increased risk. Prolonged frequent monitoring may be required especially if tongue, glottis, or larynx are involved as they are associated with airway obstruction. Patients with a history of airway surgery may have a higher risk of airway obstruction. Aggressive early and appropriate management is critical. Contraindicated in patients with history of angioedema with or without prior ACE inhibitor therapy. Hypersensitivity reactions may be seen during hemodialysis (eg, CVVHD) with high-flux dialysis membranes (eg, AN69), and rarely, during low density lipoprotein apheresis with dextran sulfate cellulose. Rare cases of anaphylactoid reactions have been reported in patients undergoing sensitization treatment with hymenoptera (bee, wasp) venom while receiving ACE inhibitors.

Symptomatic hypotension with or without syncope can occur with ACE inhibitors (usually with the first several doses); effects are most often observed in volume depleted patients; close monitoring of patient is required especially with initial dosing and dosing increases; blood pressure must be lowered at a rate appropriate for the patient's clinical condition. Initiation of therapy in patients with ischemic heart disease or cerebrovascular disease warrants close observation due to the potential consequences posed by falling blood pressure (eg, MI, stroke). **[U.S. Boxed Warning]: Based on human data, ACEIs can cause injury and death to the developing fetus when used in the second and third trimesters. ACEIs should be discontinued as soon as possible once pregnancy is detected.** Use with caution in hypertrophic cardiomyopathy with outflow tract obstruction, severe aortic stenosis, or before, during, or immediately after major surgery.

Hyperkalemia may occur with ACE inhibitors; risk factors include renal dysfunction, diabetes mellitus, concomitant use of potassium-sparing diuretics, potassium supplements and/or potassium containing salts. Use cautiously, if at all, with these agents and monitor potassium closely. Cough may occur with ACE inhibitors. Other causes of cough should be considered (eg, pulmonary congestion in patients with heart failure) and excluded prior to discontinuation. Use with caution in patients with diabetes receiving insulin or oral antidiabetic agents; may be at increased risk for episodes of hypoglycemia.

May be associated with deterioration of renal function and/or increases in serum creatinine, particularly in patients with low renal blood flow (eg, renal artery stenosis, heart failure) whose glomerular filtration rate (GFR) is dependent on efferent arteriolar vasoconstriction by angiotensin II; deterioration may result in oliguria, acute renal failure, and progressive azotemia. Small increases in serum creatinine may occur following initiation; consider discontinuation only in patients with progressive and/or significant deterioration in renal function. Use with caution in patients with unstented unilateral/bilateral renal artery stenosis. When unstented bilateral renal artery stenosis is present, use is generally avoided due to the elevated risk of deterioration in renal function unless possible benefits outweigh risks. Concurrent use of angiotensin receptor blockers may increase the risk of clinically-significant adverse events (eg, renal dysfunction, hyperkalemia).

Rare toxicities associated with ACE inhibitors include cholestatic jaundice (which may progress to fulminant hepatic necrosis), agranulocytosis, neutropenia, or leukopenia with myeloid hypoplasia. Patients with collagen vascular diseases (especially with concomitant renal impairment) or renal impairment alone may be at increased risk for hematologic toxicity; periodically monitor CBC with differential in these patients.

Drug Interactions

Avoid Concomitant Use There are no known interactions where it is recommended to avoid concomitant use.

Increased Effect/Toxicity

Benazepril may increase the levels/effects of: Allopurinol; Amifostine; Antihypertensives; AzaTHIOprine; CycloSPORINE; CycloSPORINE (Systemic); Ferric Gluconate; Gold Sodium Thiomalate; Hypotensive Agents; Iron Dextran Complex; Lithium; Nonsteroidal Anti-Inflammatory Agents; RiTUXimab

The levels/effects of Benazepril may be increased by: Angiotensin II Receptor Blockers; Diazoxide; DPP-IV Inhibitors; Eplerenone; Everolimus; Herbs (Hypotensive Properties); Loop Diuretics; MAO Inhibitors; Pentoxifylline; Phosphodiesterase 5 Inhibitors; Potassium Salts; Potassium-Sparing Diuretics; Prostacyclin Analogues; Sirolimus; Temsirolimus; Thiazide Diuretics; TiZANidine; Tolvaptan; Trimethoprim

Decreased Effect

The levels/effects of Benazepril may be decreased by: Antacids; Aprotinin; Herbs (Hypertensive Properties); Methylphenidate; Nonsteroidal Anti-Inflammatory Agents; Salicylates; Yohimbine

Ethanol/Nutrition/Herb Interactions Herb/Nutraceutical: Avoid bayberry, blue cohosh, cayenne, ephedra, ginger, ginseng (American), kola, licorice (may worsen hypertension). Avoid black cohosh, California poppy, coleus, golden seal, hawthorn, mistletoe, periwinkle, quinine, shepherd's purse (may have increased antihypertensive effect).

Pharmacodynamics/Kinetics

Onset of Action

Reduction in plasma angiotensin-converting enzyme (ACE) activity: Peak effect: 1-2 hours after 2-20 mg dose

Reduction in blood pressure: Peak effect: Single dose: 2-4 hours; Continuous therapy: 2 weeks

Duration of Action Reduction in plasma angiotensin-converting enzyme (ACE) activity: >90% inhibition for 24 hours after 5-20 mg dose

Half-life Elimination Benazeprilat: Effective: 10-11 hours; Terminal: Children: 5 hours, Adults: 22 hours

Time to Peak Parent drug: 0.5-1 hour

Pregnancy Risk Factor D

Lactation Enters breast milk

Breast-Feeding Considerations Small amounts of benazepril and benazeprilat are found in breast milk.

Dosage Forms

Tablet, oral: 5 mg, 10 mg, 20 mg, 40 mg

Lotensin®: 5 mg, 10 mg, 20 mg, 40 mg

Benazepril and Hydrochlorothiazide

(ben AY ze pril & hye droe klor oh THYE a zide)

Related Information

Benazepril *on page 213*

Hydrochlorothiazide *on page 854*

U.S. Brand Names Lotensin HCT®

Pharmacologic Category Angiotensin-Converting Enzyme (ACE) Inhibitor; Diuretic, Thiazide

Use Treatment of hypertension

Local Anesthetic/Vasoconstrictor Precautions No information available to require special precautions

Effects on Dental Treatment No significant effects or complications reported

Effects on Bleeding No information available to require special precautions

Adverse Effects See individual agents.

General Dosage Range Oral: *Adults:* Benazepril 5-20 mg and hydrochlorothiazide 6.25-25 mg daily

Mechanism of Action Benazepril is a competitive inhibitor of angiotensin-converting enzyme (ACE); prevents conversion of angiotensin I to angiotensin II, a potent vasoconstrictor. This results in lower levels of angiotensin II which causes an increase in plasma renin activity and a reduction in aldosterone secretion. Hydrochlorothiazide inhibits sodium reabsorption in the distal tubules causing increased excretion of sodium and water as well as potassium and hydrogen ions.

Pregnancy Risk Factor D

Bendamustine (ben da MUS teen)

U.S. Brand Names Treanda®

Pharmacologic Category Antineoplastic Agent; Antineoplastic Agent, Alkylating Agent; Antineoplastic Agent, Alkylating Agent (Nitrogen Mustard)

Use Treatment of chronic lymphocytic leukemia (CLL); treatment of progressed indolent B-cell non-Hodgkin's lymphoma (NHL)

Unlabeled/Investigational Use Treatment of mantle cell lymphoma; salvage therapy for relapsed multiple myeloma; first-line therapy for follicular lymphoma; treatment of Waldenstrom's macroglobulinemia

Local Anesthetic/Vasoconstrictor Precautions No information available to require special precautions

Effects on Dental Treatment Key adverse event(s) related to dental treatment: Stomatitis, xerostomia (normal salivary flow resumes upon discontinuation).

Effects on Bleeding Chemotherapy may result in significant myelosuppression, potentially including significant reduction in platelet counts and altered hemostasis. In patients who are under active treatment with these agents, medical consult is suggested.

Adverse Effects

>10%:

Cardiovascular: Peripheral edema (≤13%)

Central nervous system: Fatigue (9% to 57%), fever (24% to 34%), headache (≤21%), chills (6% to 14%), dizziness (≤14%), insomnia (≤13%)

Dermatologic: Rash (8% to 16%; grades 3/4: ≤3%)

Endocrine & metabolic: Dehydration (≤14%)

Gastrointestinal: Nausea (20% to 75%), vomiting (16% to 40%), diarrhea (9% to 37%), constipation (≤29%), anorexia (≤23%), weight loss (7% to 18%), stomatitis (≤15%), abdominal pain (5% to 13%), appetite loss (≤13%), dyspepsia (≤11%)

Hematologic: Myelosuppression (nadir: in week 3), lymphopenia (68% to 99%; grades 3/4: 47% to 94%), leukopenia (61% to 94%; grades 3/4: 28% to 56%), anemia (88% to 89%; grades 3/4: 11% to 13%), thrombocytopenia (77% to 86%; grades 3/4: 11% to 25%), neutropenia (75% to 86%; grades 3/4: 43% to 60%)

Hepatic: Bilirubin increased (≤34%; grades 3/4: 3%)

Neuromuscular & skeletal: Back pain (≤14%), weakness (8% to 11%)

Respiratory: Cough (4% to 22%), dyspnea (≤16%)

1% to 10%:

Cardiovascular: Tachycardia (≤7%), hypotension (≤6%), chest pain (≤6%), hypertension aggravated (≤3%)

Central nervous system: Anxiety (≤8%), depression (≤6%), pain (≤6%)

Dermatologic: Pruritus (5% to 6%), dry skin (≤5%)

Endocrine & metabolic: Hypokalemia (≤9%), hyperuricemia (≤7%; grades 3/4: 2%), hyperglycemia (grades 3/4: ≤3%), hypocalcemia (grades 3/4: ≤2%), hyponatremia (grades 3/4: ≤2%)

Gastrointestinal: Gastroesophageal reflux disease (≤10%), xerostomia (9%), taste alteration (≤7%), oral candidiasis (≤6%), abdominal distention (≤5%)

Genitourinary: Urinary tract infection (≤10%)

Hematologic: Febrile neutropenia (3% to 6%)

Hepatic: ALT increased (grades 3/4: ≤3%), AST increased (grades 3/4: ≤1%)

Local: Infusion site pain (≤6%), catheter site pain (≤5%)

Neuromuscular & skeletal: Arthralgia (≤6%), bone pain (≤5%), limb pain (≤5%)

Renal: Creatinine increased (grades 3/4: ≤2%)

Respiratory: Upper respiratory infection (10%), sinusitis (≤9%), pharyngolaryngeal pain (≤8%), pneumonia (≤8%), nasopharyngitis (6% to 7%), wheezing (≤5%), nasal congestion (≤5%)

Miscellaneous: Herpes infection (3% to 10%), infection (≤6%; grades 3/4: 2%), hypersensitivity (≤5%; grades 3/4: 1%), diaphoresis (≤5%), night sweats (≤5%)

General Dosage Range Dosage adjustment recommended in patients who develop toxicities

I.V.: *Adults:* 100 mg/m^2 on days 1 and 2 of a 28-day treatment cycle **or** 120 mg/m^2 on days 1 and 2 of a 21-day treatment cycle

Mechanism of Action Bendamustine is an alkylating agent (nitrogen mustard derivative) with a benzimidazole ring (purine analog) which demonstrates only partial cross-resistance (*in vitro*) with other alkylating agents. It leads to cell death via single and double strand DNA cross-linking. Bendamustine is active against quiescent and dividing cells. The primary cytotoxic activity is due to bendamustine (as compared to metabolites).

Pharmacodynamics/Kinetics

Half-life Elimination Bendamustine: ~40 minutes; M3: ~3 hours; M4: ~30 minutes

Time to Peak At end of infusion

Pregnancy Risk Factor D

Bentoquatam (BEN toe kwa tam)

U.S. Brand Names Ivy Block® [OTC]

Pharmacologic Category Topical Skin Product

Use Skin protectant for the prevention of allergic contact dermatitis to poison oak, ivy, and sumac

Local Anesthetic/Vasoconstrictor Precautions No information available to require special precautions

Effects on Dental Treatment No significant effects or complications reported

Effects on Bleeding No information available to require special precautions

General Dosage Range Topical: *Children >6 years and Adults:* Apply to skin 15 minutes prior to potential exposure to poison ivy, poison oak, or poison sumac, and reapply every 4 hours

Mechanism of Action An organoclay substance which is capable of absorbing or binding to urushiol, the active principle in poison oak, ivy, and sumac. Bentoquatam serves as a barrier, blocking urushiol skin contact/absorption.

Benzalkonium Chloride and Isopropyl Alcohol

(benz al KOE nee um KLOR ide & eye so PRO pil AL koe hol)

Related Information

Viral Infections *on page* 1947

Related Sample Prescriptions

Herpes Simplex (Recurrent) *on page* 1990

U.S. Brand Names Viroxyn® [OTC]

Generic Availability (U.S.) No

Pharmacologic Category Antiseptic, Topical

Dental Use Topical: Germicidal for the treatment of cold sores/fever blisters

Local Anesthetic/Vasoconstrictor Precautions No information available to require special precautions

Effects on Dental Treatment No significant effects or complications reported (see Dental Comment)

Effects on Bleeding No information available to require special precautions

Adverse Effects Frequency not defined

Ocular: Irritation (following inadvertent contact)

Respiratory: Vapors may cause cough, dyspnea

Dosage Topical: One single application treatment to affected area. Secondary events (new viral load in the initial lesion, which may occur 12-72 hours after initial symptoms) or additional sore presentations will require additional treatment with a new vial. See Dental Comment for application instructions.

Manufacturer states medication should not be used >3 times/day; however, instructions indicate that a single application is generally effective if instructions are followed.

Mechanism of Action Germicidal due to disruption of the viral capsid coat by the quaternary ammonium benzalkonium chloride ingredient.

Contraindications Hypersensitivity to benzalkonium chloride, isopropyl alcohol, or any component of the formulation

Warnings/Precautions For topical use only; ingestion may lead to gastric irritation or distress. Avoid contact with eyes; flush with eye bath if inadvertent contact occurs. Avoid use of anionic cleansers or acidic products for at least 1 hour following application (active ingredient will be neutralized). Avoid the use of soap, toothpaste, cleansers, or drinks containing citric acid (including lemonade and orange juice). Should not be used >3 times/day. Avoid use in pregnant or lactating women. Avoid use in children <2 years of age. Formulation in isopropyl alcohol is flammable; avoid use near sparks, flames, or high temperatures.

Drug Interactions

Avoid Concomitant Use There are no known interactions where it is recommended to avoid concomitant use.

Increased Effect/Toxicity There are no known significant interactions involving an increase in effect.

Decreased Effect There are no known significant interactions involving a decrease in effect.

Dosage Forms

Solution, topical:

Viroxyn® [OTC]: Benzalkonium 0.13% in isopropyl alcohol

Dental Comment Use this product according to the following directions from the manufacturer. 1) Prior to treatment, clean area to be treated of all other preparations (ointments, treatments, lipstick). Do not use soap or other cleansers. A dry wipe may be sufficient, or you may use water or alcohol if necessary. 2) Remove cap from vial and replace on the other end over the clear plastic tube. Hold vial between thumb and index finger, applicator end up. Pinch vial in the center at top of cap until the inner ampoule of medication breaks. 3) Hold white applicator down and allow medication to saturate the swab. If necessary, pinch vial gently until a drop of medication just appears. 4) Place the applicator against the area of skin to be treated so that the tip of the applicator is held flat against the skin. The key is to massage medication into the sore and the surrounding area by rubbing. Do not rub so hard that you cause damage to the skin. For best results, the patient should massage drug into the sore by rubbing. The rubbing should proceed for about 10 minutes or until all the drug has been massaged into the sore. The application may sting. This is normal and should subside quickly. For best results, medication must penetrate the subepidermal layers of the skin to site of infection. The ingredients facilitate penetration, but mechanical action is critical. Simply dabbing the drug onto the sore is not likely to give best results. 5) If treating at prodrome (tingling sensation before lesion erupts), a more vigorous rubbing is easily tolerated and gives best results. If the lesion has progressed to vesicle or ulcerated lesion, the patient may prefer to rub less vigorously but for a longer time period. 6) Keep applicator saturated at all times. If necessary, pause and hold vial so as to allow medication to flow into applicator. When finished recap vial. Dispose of immediately. Do not disassemble. Store at room temperature. Flammable; do not expose to high heat or flame. Keep out of reach of children.

Benzocaine (BEN zoe kane)

Related Information

Management of Patients Undergoing Cancer Therapy *on page 1970*
Oral Pain *on page 1928*

Related Sample Prescriptions

Recurrent Aphthous Stomatitis *on page 1992*

U.S. Brand Names Americaine® Hemorrhoidal [OTC]; Anbesol® Baby [OTC]; Anbesol® Cold Sore Therapy [OTC]; Anbesol® Jr. [OTC]; Anbesol® Maximum Strength [OTC]; Anbesol® [OTC]; Benzodent® [OTC]; Bi-Zets [OTC]; Boil-Ease® Pain Relieving [OTC]; Cepacol® Fizzlers™ [OTC]; Cepacol® Sore Throat Pain Relief [OTC]; Cepacol® Sore Throat Plus Coating Relief [OTC]; Chiggerex® Plus [OTC]; ChiggerTox® [OTC]; Cylex® [OTC] [DSC]; Dent's Extra Strength Toothache Gum [OTC]; Dentapaine [OTC]; Dermoplast® Antibacterial [OTC]; Dermoplast® Pain Relieving [OTC]; Detane® [OTC]; Foille® [OTC]; HDA® Toothache [OTC]; Hurricaine® [OTC]; Ivy-Rid® [OTC]; Kank-A® Soft Brush [OTC]; Lanacane® Maximum Strength [OTC]; Lanacane® [OTC]; Little Teethers® [OTC]; Medicone® Hemorrhoidal [OTC]; Mycinettes® [OTC]; Orabase® with Benzocaine [OTC]; Orajel® Baby Daytime and Nighttime [OTC]; Orajel® Baby Teething Nighttime [OTC]; Orajel® Baby Teething [OTC]; Orajel® Cold Sore [OTC]; Orajel® Denture Plus [OTC]; Orajel® Maximum Strength [OTC]; Orajel® Medicated Mouth Sore [OTC]; Orajel® Medicated Toothache [OTC]; Orajel® Mouth Sore [OTC]; Orajel® Multi-Action Cold Sore [OTC]; Orajel® PM Maximum Strength [OTC]; Orajel® Ultra Mouth Sore [OTC]; Orajel® [OTC]; Outgro® [OTC]; Red Cross™ Canker Sore [OTC]; Rid-A-Pain Dental [OTC]; Sepasoothe® [OTC]; Skeeter Stik® [OTC]; Sore Throat Relief [OTC]; Sting-Kill® [OTC]; Tanac® [OTC]; Thorets [OTC]; Trocaine® [OTC]; Zilactin® Tooth & Gum Pain [OTC]; Zilactin®-B [OTC]

Canadian Brand Names Anbesol® Baby; Zilactin Baby®; Zilactin-B®

Generic Availability (U.S.) Yes: Lozenge, liquid

Pharmacologic Category Local Anesthetic

Dental Use Ester-type topical local anesthetic for temporary relief of pain associated with toothache, minor sore throat pain, and canker sore

Use Temporary relief of pain associated with pruritic dermatosis, pruritus, minor burns, acute congestive, bee stings, and insect bites; mouth and gum irritations (toothache, minor sore throat pain, canker sores, dentures, orthodontia, teething, mucositis, stomatitis); sunburn; hemorrhoids; anesthetic lubricant for passage of catheters and endoscopic tubes

Local Anesthetic/Vasoconstrictor Precautions No information available to require special precautions

Effects on Dental Treatment No significant effects or complications reported (see Dental Comment).

Effects on Bleeding No information available to require special precautions

Adverse Effects Frequency not defined.

Hematologic: Methemoglobinemia

Local: Burning, contact dermatitis, edema, erythema, pruritus, rash, stinging, tenderness, urticaria

Miscellaneous: Hypersensitivity

Dental Usual Dosage Relief of pain (toothache, minor sore throat pain, and canker sore): Children ≥2 years and Adults: Topical (oral): 10% to 20%: Apply thin layer to affected area up to 4 times daily

Dosage Note: These are general dosing guidelines; refer to specific product labeling for dosing instructions.

Children ≥4 months: Topical (oral): Teething pain: 7.5% to 10%: Apply to affected gum area up to 4 times daily

Children ≥2 years and Adults:
Topical:
Bee stings, insect bites, minor burns, sunburn: 5% to 20%: Apply to affected area 3-4 times a day as needed. In cases of bee stings, remove stinger before treatment.
Lubricant for passage of catheters and instruments: 20%: Apply evenly to exterior of instrument prior to use.
Topical (oral): Mouth and gum irritation: 10% to 20%: Apply thin layer to affected area up to 4 times daily
Children ≥5 years and Adults: Oral: Sore throat: Allow 1 lozenge (10-15 mg) to dissolve slowly in mouth; may repeat every 2 hours as needed
Children ≥12 years and Adults: Rectal: Hemorrhoids: 5% to 20%: Apply externally to affected area up to 6 times daily

Mechanism of Action Ester local anesthetic blocks both the initiation and conduction of nerve impulses by decreasing the neuronal membrane's permeability to sodium ions, which results in inhibition of depolarization with resultant blockade of conduction

Contraindications Hypersensitivity to benzocaine, other ester-type local anesthetics, or any component of the formulation; secondary bacterial infection of area; ophthalmic use

Warnings/Precautions Methemoglobinemia has been reported following topical use (rare), particularly with higher concentration (14% to 20%) spray formulations applied to the mouth or mucous membranes. When applied as a spray to the mouth or throat, multiple sprays (or sprays of longer than indicated duration) are not recommended. Use caution with breathing problems (asthma, bronchitis, emphysema, in smokers), inflamed/damaged mucosa, heart disease, and hemoglobin or enzyme abnormalities (glucose-6-phosphate dehydrogenase deficiency, hemoglobin-M disease, NADH-methemoglobin reductase deficiency, pyruvate-kinase deficiency). Alternatives to benzocaine sprays, such as topical lidocaine preparations, should be considered for patients at higher risk of this reaction. Due to the heightened risk of methemoglobinemia, not recommended for use in patients <2 years of age unless under the advice and supervision by a healthcare professional.

The classical clinical finding of methemoglobinemia is chocolate brown-colored arterial blood. However, suspected cases should be confirmed by co-oximetry, which yields a direct and accurate measure of methemoglobin levels. Standard pulse oximetry readings or arterial blood gas values are not reliable. Clinically significant methemoglobinemia requires immediate treatment.

When topical anesthetics are used prior to cosmetic or medical procedures, the lowest amount of anesthetic necessary for pain relief should be applied. High systemic levels and toxic effects (eg, methemoglobinemia, irregular heart beats, respiratory depression, seizures, death) have been reported in patients who (without supervision of a trained professional) have applied topical anesthetics in large amounts (or to large areas of the skin), left these products on for prolonged periods of time, or have used wraps/dressings to cover the skin following application.

When used for self-medication (OTC), notify healthcare provider if condition worsens or does not improve within 7 days, or if swelling, rash, or fever develops. Do not use on open wounds. Avoid contact with the eyes.

Drug Interactions

Avoid Concomitant Use There are no known interactions where it is recommended to avoid concomitant use.

Increased Effect/Toxicity There are no known significant interactions involving an increase in effect.

Decreased Effect There are no known significant interactions involving a decrease in effect.

Dietary Considerations Some products may contain sodium.

Pregnancy Risk Factor C

Lactation Excretion in breast milk unknown/use caution

Dosage Forms

Aerosol, oral:
Hurricaine® [OTC]: 20% (60 mL)

Aerosol, topical:
Dermoplast® Antibacterial [OTC]: 20% (82.5 mL)
Dermoplast® Pain Relieving [OTC]: 20% (60 mL, 82.5 mL)
Ivy-Rid® [OTC]: 2% (85 g)
Lanacane® Maximum Strength [OTC]: 20% (120 mL)

Combination package, oral:
Orajel® Baby Daytime and Nighttime [OTC]: gel, oral (Daytime Regular formula): benzocaine 7.5% (5.3 g) [1 tube] and gel, oral (Nighttime formula): benzocaine 10% (5.3 g) [1 tube]

Cream, oral:
- Benzodent® [OTC]: 20% (7.5 g, 30 g)
- Orajel® PM Maximum Strength [OTC]: 20% (5.3 g, 7 g)

Cream, topical:
- Lanacane® [OTC]: 6% (28 g, 60 g)
- Lanacane® Maximum Strength [OTC]: 20% (28 g)

Gel, oral: 20% (15 g)
- Anbesol® [OTC]: 10% (7.1 g)
- Anbesol® Baby [OTC]: 7.5% (7.1 g)
- Anbesol® Jr. [OTC]: 10% (7.1 g)
- Anbesol® Maximum Strength [OTC]: 20% (7.1 g, 10 g)
- Dentapaine [OTC]: 20% (11 g)
- HDA® Toothache [OTC]: 6.5% (15 mL)
- Hurricaine® [OTC]: 20% (30 g); 20% (5.25 g, 30 g)
- Kank-A® Soft Brush [OTC]: 20% (2 g)
- Little Teethers® [OTC]: 7.5% (9.4 g)
- Orabase® with Benzocaine [OTC]: 20% (7 g)
- Orajel® [OTC]: 10% (5.3 g, 7 g, 9.4 g)
- Orajel® Baby Teething [OTC]: 7.5% (11.9 g); 7.5% (9.4 g)
- Orajel® Baby Teething Nighttime [OTC]: 10% (5.3 g)
- Orajel® Denture Plus [OTC]: 15% (9 g)
- Orajel® Maximum Strength [OTC]: 20% (5.4 g, 7 g, 9.4 g, 11.9 g)
- Orajel® Mouth Sore [OTC]: 20% (5.3 g, 9.4 g, 11.9 g)
- Orajel® Multi-Action Cold Sore [OTC]: 20% (9.4 g)
- Orajel® Ultra Mouth Sore [OTC]: 15% (9.4 g)
- Zilactin®-B [OTC]: 10% (7.5 g)

Gel, topical:
- Detane® [OTC]: 7.5% (15 g)

Liquid, oral: 20% (15 mL)
- Anbesol® [OTC]: 10% (9.3 mL)
- Anbesol® Maximum Strength [OTC]: 20% (9.3 mL)
- Hurricaine® [OTC]: 20% (30 mL)
- Orajel® Baby Teething [OTC]: 7.5% (13.3 mL)
- Orajel® Maximum Strength [OTC]: 20% (13.5 mL)
- Rid-A-Pain Dental [OTC]: 6.3% (30 mL)
- Tanac® [OTC]: 10% (13 mL)

Liquid, topical:
- ChiggerTox® [OTC]: 2% (30 mL)
- Outgro® [OTC]: 20% (9.3 mL)
- Skeeter Stik® [OTC]: 5% (14 mL)

Lozenge, oral: 6 mg (18s)
- Bi-Zets [OTC]: 15 mg (10s)
- Cepacol® Sore Throat Pain Relief [OTC]: 15 mg (16s, 18s)
- Cepacol® Sore Throat Plus Coating Relief [OTC]: 15 mg (18s)
- Mycinettes® [OTC]: 15 mg (12s)
- Sepasoothe® [OTC]: 10 mg (6s, 24s, 100s, 250s, 500s)
- Sore Throat Relief [OTC]: 10 mg (100s, 250s, 500s)
- Thorets [OTC]: 18 mg (300s)
- Trocaine® [OTC]: 10 mg (50s, 300s)

Ointment, oral:
- Anbesol® Cold Sore Therapy [OTC]: 20% (7.1 g)
- Red Cross™ Canker Sore [OTC]: 20% (7.5 g)

Ointment, rectal:
- Americaine® Hemorrhoidal [OTC]: 20% (30 g)
- Medicone® Hemorrhoidal [OTC]: 20% (28.4 g)

Ointment, topical:
- Boil-Ease® Pain Relieving [OTC]: 20% (30 g)
- Chiggerex® Plus [OTC]: 6% (50 g)
- Foille® [OTC]: 5% (3.5 g, 14 g, 28 g)

Pad, topical:
- Sting-Kill® [OTC]: 20% (8s)

Paste, oral:
- Orabase® with Benzocaine [OTC]: 20% (6 g)

Solution, oral:
- Hurricaine® [OTC]: 20% (30 mL)

Swab, oral:
Hurricaine® [OTC]: 20% (8s, 72s)
Orajel® Baby Teething [OTC]: 7.5% (12s)
Orajel® Cold Sore [OTC]: 20% (12s)
Orajel® Medicated Mouth Sore [OTC]: 20% (8s, 12s)
Orajel® Medicated Toothache [OTC]: 20% (8s, 12s)
Zilactin® Tooth & Gum Pain [OTC]: 20% (8s)

Swab, topical:
Boil-Ease® Pain Relieving [OTC]: 20% (12s)
Sting-Kill® [OTC]: 20% (5s)

Tablet, orally dissolving, oral:
Cepacol® Fizzlers™ [OTC]: 6 mg (12s)

Wax, oral:
Dent's Extra Strength Toothache Gum [OTC]: 20% (1 g)

Dental Comment Health Canada has issued a reminder to healthcare professionals that benzocaine sprays must be used judiciously to minimize the risk of methemoglobinemia. Almost all reported cases have been associated with higher concentration (14% to 20% benzocaine) spray products used in the mouth and on other mucous membranes. Alternatives to benzocaine sprays, such as topical lidocaine preparations, should be considered for patients at higher risk of this reaction.

Benzocaine, Butamben, and Tetracaine

(BEN zoe kane, byoo TAM ben, & TET ra kane)

Related Information
Benzocaine *on page* 218
Tetracaine (Topical) *on page* 1610

U.S. Brand Names Cetacaine®; Exactacain™

Generic Availability (U.S.) No

Pharmacologic Category Local Anesthetic

Dental Use Topical anesthetic for accessible mucous membranes

Use Topical anesthetic to control pain in surgical or endoscopic procedures; anesthetic for accessible mucous membranes except for the eyes

Local Anesthetic/Vasoconstrictor Precautions No information available to require special precautions

Effects on Dental Treatment Key adverse event(s) related to dental treatment: A patient history of allergy to ester-type local anesthetics contraindicates the use of this product (see Dental Comment).

Effects on Bleeding No information available to require special precautions

Adverse Effects Frequency not defined. Also see individual monographs for Benzocaine and Tetracaine (Topical).
Dermatologic: Contact dermatitis (eg, erythema, pruritus, vesiculation, oozing); dehydration of the epithelium; escharotic effect
Miscellaneous: Hypersensitivity/anaphylaxis reaction (rare)

Dental Usual Dosage Topical anesthetic (Exactacain™): Adults: 3 metered sprays (maximum dose: 6 metered sprays); each metered spray delivers 9.3 mg benzocaine, 1.3 mg butamben, 1.3 mg tetracaine

Dosage Topical anesthetic: **Note:** Decrease dose in the acutely-ill patient.
Children: Dose has not been established; dose reduction is suggested
Adults:
Cetacaine®:
Aerosol: Apply for ≤1 second; use of sprays >2 seconds is contraindicated
Gel: Apply ~1/2 inch (13 mm) x 3/16 inch (5 mm); application of >1 inch (26 cm) x 3/16 inch (5 mm) is contraindicated
Liquid: Apply 6-7 drops (0.2 mL); application of >12-14 drops (0.4 mL) is contraindicated
Exactacain™: 3 metered sprays (use of >6 metered sprays is contraindicated)
Elderly: Dose reduction is suggested

Mechanism of Action Reversible blockage of initiation and conduction of nerve impulses by deceasing the neuronal membrane's permeability to sodium ions

Contraindications Hypersensitivity to benzocaine, butamben, tetracaine, or any component of the formulation; ophthalmic use; cholinesterase deficiencies; large areas of denuded or inflamed tissue; administration in excess of product labeling

Warnings/Precautions For topical use only. Methemoglobinemia has been reported following topical benzocaine use (rare), particularly with higher concentration (14% to 20%) spray formulations applied to the mouth or mucous membranes. The classical clinical finding of methemoglobinemia is chocolate brown-colored arterial blood. However, suspected cases should be confirmed by co-oximetry, which yields a direct and accurate measure of methemoglobin levels.

Standard pulse oximetry readings or arterial blood gas values are not reliable. Clinically-significant methemoglobinemia requires immediate treatment.

Use caution with breathing problems (asthma, bronchitis, emphysema, in smokers), inflamed/damaged mucosa, heart disease, children <6 months of age, and hemoglobin or enzyme abnormalities (glucose-6-phosphate dehydrogenase deficiency, hemoglobin-M disease, NADH-methemoglobin reductase deficiency, pyruvate-kinase deficiency). Alternatives to benzocaine sprays, such as topical lidocaine preparations, should be considered for patients at higher risk of this reaction.

When topical anesthetics are used prior to cosmetic or medical procedures, the lowest amount of anesthetic necessary for pain relief should be applied. High systemic levels and toxic effects (eg, methhemoglobinemia, irregular heart beats, respiratory depression, seizures, death) have been reported in patients who (without supervision of a trained professional) have applied topical anesthetics in large amounts (or to large areas of the skin), left these products on for prolonged periods of time, or have used wraps/dressings to cover the skin following application.

Use caution in debilitated, elderly, acutely ill, and very young patients; dose adjustment is suggested. Do not use under dentures or cotton rolls; retention of active ingredients may cause escharotic effect.

Drug Interactions

Avoid Concomitant Use There are no known interactions where it is recommended to avoid concomitant use.

Increased Effect/Toxicity There are no known significant interactions involving an increase in effect.

Decreased Effect There are no known significant interactions involving a decrease in effect.

Pharmacodynamics/Kinetics

Onset of Action ~30 seconds

Duration of Action 30-60 minutes

Dosage Forms

Aerosol, topical [spray]:

Cetacaine®: Benzocaine 14%, butamben 2%, and tetracaine 2% (56 g)

Exactacain™: Benzocaine 14%, butamben 2%, and tetracaine 2% (60 g)

Gel, topical:

Cetacaine®: Benzocaine 14%, butamben 2%, and tetracaine 2% (29 g)

Liquid, topical:

Cetacaine®: Benzocaine 14%, butamben 2%, and tetracaine 2% (56 g)

Dental Comment Manufacturer indication for use is suppression of gag reflex for gastroenterological procedures.

Health Canada has issued a reminder to healthcare professionals that benzocaine sprays must be used judiciously to minimize the risk of methemoglobinemia. Almost all reported cases have been associated with higher concentration (14% to 20% benzocaine) spray products used in the mouth and on other mucous membranes. Alternatives to benzocaine sprays, such as topical lidocaine preparations, should be considered for patients at higher risk of this reaction.

Benzoin (BEN zoin)

U.S. Brand Names Benz-Protect Swabs™ [OTC]; Sprayzoin™ [OTC]

Pharmacologic Category Antibiotic, Topical; Topical Skin Product

Use Protective application for irritations of the skin; sometimes used in boiling water as steam inhalants for its expectorant and soothing action

Local Anesthetic/Vasoconstrictor Precautions No information available to require special precautions

Effects on Dental Treatment No significant effects or complications reported

Effects on Bleeding No information available to require special precautions

General Dosage Range Topical: *Children and Adults:* Apply 1-2 times/day

Benzonatate (ben ZOE na tate)

Related Information

Management of Patients Undergoing Cancer Therapy *on page 1970*

U.S. Brand Names Tessalon®; Zonatuss™

Canadian Brand Names Tessalon®

Generic Availability (U.S.) Yes: Capsule (softgel)

Pharmacologic Category Antitussive

Use Symptomatic relief of nonproductive cough

Local Anesthetic/Vasoconstrictor Precautions No information available to require special precautions

Effects on Dental Treatment No significant effects or complications reported

Effects on Bleeding No information available to require special precautions

Adverse Effects 1% to 10%:

Central nervous system: Sedation, headache, dizziness
Dermatologic: Rash
Gastrointestinal: GI upset
Neuromuscular & skeletal: Chest numbness
Ocular: Burning sensation in eyes
Respiratory: Nasal congestion

Dosage Children >10 years and Adults: Oral: 100 mg 3 times/day or every 4 hours up to 600 mg/day

Mechanism of Action Tetracaine congener with antitussive properties; suppresses cough by topical anesthetic action on the respiratory stretch receptors

Contraindications Hypersensitivity to benzonatate, related compounds (such as tetracaine), or any component of the formulation

Drug Interactions

Avoid Concomitant Use There are no known interactions where it is recommended to avoid concomitant use.

Increased Effect/Toxicity There are no known significant interactions involving an increase in effect.

Decreased Effect There are no known significant interactions involving a decrease in effect.

Pharmacodynamics/Kinetics

Onset of Action Therapeutic: 15-20 minutes

Duration of Action 3-8 hours

Pregnancy Risk Factor C

Lactation Excretion in breast milk unknown/use caution

Dosage Forms

Capsule, oral:
Zonatuss™: 150 mg

Capsule, softgel, oral: 100 mg, 200 mg
Tessalon®: 100 mg, 200 mg

Benzoyl Peroxide (BEN zoe il peer OKS ide)

U.S. Brand Names 10 Benzagel®; 5 Benzagel®; Acne Clear Maximum Strength [OTC]; Benzac® AC; Benzac® W; BenzaShave®; BenzEFoam™; Benziq™; BPO; Brevoxyl®-4 [DSC]; Brevoxyl®-8 [DSC]; Clearskin [OTC]; Clinac® BPO; Desquam-X® 10 [OTC]; Desquam-X® 5 [OTC]; Inova™; Levoclen® Acne Wash Kit; Levoclen™-4; Levoclen™-8; Neutrogena® Clear Pore™ [OTC]; Neutrogena® On The Spot® Acne Treatment [OTC]; OXY® Chill Factor® [OTC]; OXY® [OTC]; Pacnex™; Palmer's® Skin Success Invisible Acne [OTC]; PanOxyl® Aqua Gel [OTC]; PanOxyl® Bar [OTC]; Triaz®; Zapzyt® [OTC]; ZoDerm®; ZoDerm® Hydrating Wash™; ZoDerm® Redi-Pads™

Canadian Brand Names Acetoxyl®; Benoxyl®; Benzac AC®; Benzac W® Gel; Benzac W® Wash; Desquam-X®; Oxyderm™; PanOxyl®; Solugel®

Pharmacologic Category Acne Products; Topical Skin Product; Topical Skin Product, Acne

Use Treatment of mild-to-moderate acne vulgaris and acne rosacea

Local Anesthetic/Vasoconstrictor Precautions No information available to require special precautions

Effects on Dental Treatment No significant effects or complications reported

Effects on Bleeding No information available to require special precautions

Adverse Effects 1% to 10%: Dermatologic: Irritation, contact dermatitis, dryness, erythema, peeling, stinging

General Dosage Range Topical: *Adolescents and Adults:*

Cleanser: Wash once or twice daily
Topical formulations: Apply sparingly once daily; gradually increase to 2-3 times/day if needed

Mechanism of Action Releases free-radical oxygen which oxidizes bacterial proteins in the sebaceous follicles decreasing the number of anaerobic bacteria and decreasing irritating-type free fatty acids

Pregnancy Risk Factor C

Benzoyl Peroxide and Hydrocortisone

(BEN zoe il peer OKS ide & hye droe KOR ti sone)

Related Information

Benzoyl Peroxide *on page* 223

Hydrocortisone (Topical) *on page* 868

U.S. Brand Names Vanoxide-HC®

Canadian Brand Names Vanoxide-HC®

Pharmacologic Category Acne Products; Topical Skin Product; Topical Skin Product, Acne

Use Treatment of acne vulgaris and oily skin

Local Anesthetic/Vasoconstrictor Precautions No information available to require special precautions

Effects on Dental Treatment No significant effects or complications reported

Effects on Bleeding No information available to require special precautions

Adverse Effects See individual agents.

General Dosage Range Topical: *Adolescents and Adults:* Apply thin film 1-3 times/day

Pregnancy Risk Factor C

Benzphetamine (benz FET a meen)

U.S. Brand Names Didrex®

Pharmacologic Category Anorexiant; Sympathomimetic

Use Short-term (few weeks) adjunct to caloric restriction in exogenous obesity

Pharmacotherapy for weight loss is recommended only for obese patients with a body mass index ≥30 kg/m^2, or ≥27 kg/m^2 in the presence of other risk factors such as hypertension, diabetes, and/or dyslipidemia or a high waist circumference; therapy should be used in conjunction with a comprehensive weight management program.

Local Anesthetic/Vasoconstrictor Precautions Use with caution since amphetamines have actions similar to epinephrine and norepinephrine

Effects on Dental Treatment Key adverse event(s) related to dental treatment: Xerostomia (normal salivary flow resumes upon discontinuation) and metallic taste.

Effects on Bleeding No information available to require special precautions

Adverse Effects Frequency not defined.

Cardiovascular: Cardiomyopathy/ischemic events (with chronic amphetamine use), hypertension, palpitation, tachycardia

Central nervous system: Depression (with withdrawal), dizziness, headache, insomnia, psychosis (rare), restlessness

Dermatologic: Skin reactions, urticaria

Endocrine & metabolic: Libido changes

Gastrointestinal: Diarrhea, nausea, unpleasant taste, xerostomia

Neuromuscular & skeletal: Tremor

Miscellaneous: Diaphoresis, overstimulation

General Dosage Range Oral: *Children ≥12 years and Adults:* Initial: 25-50 mg once daily; Maintenance: 25-50 mg 1-3 times/day (maximum: 150 mg/day)

Mechanism of Action Benzphetamine is a sympathomimetic amine with pharmacologic properties similar to the amphetamines. The mechanism of action in reducing appetite appears to be secondary to CNS effects, including stimulation of the hypothalamus to release norepinephrine.

Pregnancy Risk Factor X

Controlled Substance C-III

Benztropine (BENZ troe peen)

U.S. Brand Names Cogentin®

Canadian Brand Names Apo-Benztropine®

Pharmacologic Category Anti-Parkinson's Agent, Anticholinergic; Anticholinergic Agent

Use Adjunctive treatment of Parkinson's disease; treatment of drug-induced extrapyramidal symptoms (except tardive dyskinesia)

Local Anesthetic/Vasoconstrictor Precautions No information available to require special precautions

Effects on Dental Treatment Key adverse event(s) related to dental treatment: Xerostomia and changes in salivation (normal salivary flow resumes upon discontinuation), dry throat, and nasal dryness (very prevalent).

Effects on Bleeding No information available to require special precautions

Adverse Effects Frequency not defined.

Cardiovascular: Tachycardia

Central nervous system: Confusion, disorientation, memory impairment, toxic psychosis, visual hallucinations

Dermatologic: Rash

Endocrine & metabolic: Heat stroke, hyperthermia

Gastrointestinal: Constipation, dry throat, ileus, nasal dryness, nausea, vomiting, xerostomia

Genitourinary: Urinary retention, dysuria

Ocular: Blurred vision, mydriasis

Miscellaneous: Fever

General Dosage Range

I.M., I.V.:

Children >3 years: 0.02-0.05 mg/kg 1-2 times/day

Adults: 1-4 mg/dose 1-2 times/day

Oral:

Children >3 years: 0.02-0.05 mg/kg 1-2 times/day

Adults: 0.5-8 mg/day in 1-2 divided doses

Elderly: Initial: 0.5 mg 1-2 times/day (maximum: 4 mg/day)

Mechanism of Action Possesses both anticholinergic and antihistaminic effects. *In vitro* anticholinergic activity approximates that of atropine; *in vivo* it is only about half as active as atropine. Animal data suggest its antihistaminic activity and duration of action approach that of pyrilamine maleate. May also inhibit the reuptake and storage of dopamine, thereby prolonging the action of dopamine.

Pharmacodynamics/Kinetics

Onset of Action Oral: Within 1 hour; Parenteral: Within 15 minutes

Duration of Action 6-48 hours

Pregnancy Risk Factor C

Benzydamine (ben ZID a meen)

Canadian Brand Names Apo-Benzydamine®; Dom-Benzydamine; Novo-Benzydamine; PMS-Benzydamine; ratio-Benzydamine; Sun-Benz®; Tantum®

Pharmacologic Category Local Anesthetic, Oral

Dental Use Symptomatic treatment of pain associated with acute pharyngitis; treatment of pain associated with radiation-induced oropharyngeal mucositis

Use Symptomatic treatment of pain associated with acute pharyngitis; treatment of pain associated with radiation-induced oropharyngeal mucositis

Local Anesthetic/Vasoconstrictor Precautions No information available to require special precautions

Effects on Dental Treatment Key adverse event(s) related to dental treatment: Numbness, burning/stinging sensation, and xerostomia (normal salivary flow resumes upon discontinuation).

Effects on Bleeding No information available to require special precautions

Adverse Effects

Central nervous system: Drowsiness, headache

Gastrointestinal: Nausea and/or vomiting (2%), xerostomia

Local: Numbness (10%), burning/stinging sensation (8%)

Respiratory: Cough, pharyngeal irritation

Dental Usual Dosage

Acute pharyngitis: Adults: Oral rinse: Gargle with 15 mL every 1½-3 hours until symptoms resolve. Patient should expel solution from mouth following use; solution should not be swallowed.

Radiation-associated mucositis: Adults: Oral rinse: 15 mL as a gargle or rinse 3-4 times/day; contact between the liquid and the oral mucosa should be maintained for at least 30 seconds, followed by expulsion from the mouth.

Dosage Oral rinse: Adults:

Acute pharyngitis: Gargle with 15 mL of undiluted solution every 1½-3 hours until symptoms resolve. Patient should expel solution from mouth following use; solution should not be swallowed.

Mucositis: 15 mL of undiluted solution as a gargle or rinse 3-4 times/day; contact should be maintained for at least 30 seconds, followed by expulsion from the mouth

Dosage adjustment in renal impairment: No adjustment required.

Mechanism of Action Local anesthetic and anti-inflammatory, reduces local pain and inflammation. Does not interfere with arachidonic acid metabolism.

Contraindications Hypersensitivity to benzydamine or any component of the formulation

Warnings/Precautions May cause local irritation and/or burning sensation in patients with altered mucosal integrity. Dilution (1:1 in warm water) may attenuate this effect. Use caution in renal impairment.

Drug Interactions

Metabolism/Transport Effects Substrate (minor) of CYP1A2, 2C19, 2D6, 3A4

Avoid Concomitant Use There are no known interactions where it is recommended to avoid concomitant use.

Increased Effect/Toxicity There are no known significant interactions involving an increase in effect.

Decreased Effect There are no known significant interactions involving a decrease in effect.

Lactation Excretion in breast milk unknown/use caution

Product Availability Not available in U.S.

Dosage Forms: Canada

Oral rinse: 0.15% (100 mL, 250 mL)

Benzylpenicilloyl Polylysine (BEN zil pen i SIL oyl pol i LIE seen)

U.S. Brand Names Pre-Pen®

Pharmacologic Category Diagnostic Agent

Use Adjunct in assessing the risk of administering penicillin (penicillin G or benzylpenicillin) in patients suspected of clinical penicillin hypersensitivity

Unlabeled/Investigational Use Adjunct in assessment of hypersensitivity to other beta-lactam antibiotics (penicillins and cephalosporins) to determine the safety of penicillin administration in patients with a history of reaction to cephalosporins

Local Anesthetic/Vasoconstrictor Precautions No information available to require special precautions

Effects on Dental Treatment No significant effects or complications reported

Effects on Bleeding No information available to require special precautions

Adverse Effects Frequency not defined.

Cardiovascular: Hypotension
Dermatologic: Angioneurotic edema, pruritus, erythema, urticaria
Local: Inflammation (intense; at skin test site), wheal (locally)
Respiratory: Dyspnea
Miscellaneous: Systemic allergic reactions (including anaphylaxis; rare)

General Dosage Range

Intradermal: *Children and Adults:* Inject a volume of skin test solution sufficient to raise a small intradermal bleb ~3 mm in diameter, in duplicate

Puncture test (first step): *Children and Adults:* Apply a small drop of solution to make a single shallow puncture of the epidermis

Mechanism of Action Benzylpenicilloyl polylysine, a conjugate of the benzylpenicilloyl structural group (hapten) and the poly-l-lysine carrier (protein), is an antigen which reacts with benzylpenicilloyl IgE antibodies to elicit the release of chemical mediators, thereby producing type I (immediate or accelerated) urticarial reactions in patients hypersensitive to penicillins.

Pregnancy Risk Factor C

Bepotastine (be poe TAS teen)

U.S. Brand Names Bepreve™

Pharmacologic Category Histamine H_1 Antagonist; Histamine H_1 Antagonist, Second Generation; Mast Cell Stabilizer

Use Treatment of itching associated with allergic conjunctivitis

Local Anesthetic/Vasoconstrictor Precautions No information available to require special precautions

Effects on Dental Treatment Key adverse event(s) related to dental treatment: Taste abnormalities reported in ≤25% of patients

Effects on Bleeding No information available to require special precautions

Adverse Effects

Central nervous system: Headache
Gastrointestinal: Taste abnormality
Ocular: Irritation
Respiratory: Nasopharyngitis

General Dosage Range Ophthalmic: *Children ≥2 years and Adults:* Instill 1 drop into the affected eye(s) twice daily

Mechanism of Action Direct H_1-receptor antagonist and inhibits release of histamine from mast cells

Pregnancy Risk Factor C

Beractant (ber AKT ant)

U.S. Brand Names Survanta®
Canadian Brand Names Survanta®
Pharmacologic Category Lung Surfactant
Use Prevention and treatment of respiratory distress syndrome (RDS) in premature infants

Prophylactic therapy: Body weight <1250 g in infants at risk for developing, or with evidence of, surfactant deficiency (administer within 15 minutes of birth)
Rescue therapy: Treatment of infants with RDS confirmed by x-ray and requiring mechanical ventilation (administer as soon as possible - within 8 hours of age)

Local Anesthetic/Vasoconstrictor Precautions No information available to require special precautions
Effects on Dental Treatment No significant effects or complications reported
Effects on Bleeding No information available to require special precautions
Adverse Effects During the dosing procedure:
>10%: Cardiovascular: Transient bradycardia
1% to 10%: Respiratory: Oxygen desaturation

General Dosage Range Intratracheal: *Premature infants:* Administer 100 mg phospholipids (4 mL/kg); may repeat if needed, no more frequently than every 6 hours to a maximum of 4 doses/48 hours for prophylactic treatment (maximum: 4 doses/24 hours for rescue treatment)
Mechanism of Action Replaces deficient or ineffective endogenous lung surfactant in neonates with respiratory distress syndrome (RDS) or in neonates at risk of developing RDS. Surfactant prevents the alveoli from collapsing during expiration by lowering surface tension between air and alveolar surfaces.

Besifloxacin (be si FLOX a sin)

U.S. Brand Names Besivance™
Pharmacologic Category Antibiotic, Ophthalmic; Antibiotic, Quinolone
Use Treatment of bacterial conjunctivitis
Local Anesthetic/Vasoconstrictor Precautions No information available to require special precautions
Effects on Dental Treatment No significant effects or complications reported
Effects on Bleeding No information available to require special precautions
Adverse Effects 1% to 2%:
Central nervous system: Headache
Ocular: Conjunctival redness (2%), blurred vision, irritation, pain, pruritus

General Dosage Range Ophthalmic: *Children ≥1 year and Adults:* 1 drop into affected eye(s) 3 times/day (4-12 hours apart)
Mechanism of Action Inhibits both DNA gyrase and topoisomerase IV. DNA gyrase is an essential bacterial enzyme required for DNA replication, transcription, and repair. Topoisomerase IV is an essential bacterial enzyme required for decatenation during cell division. Inhibition effect is bactericidal.
Pharmacodynamics/Kinetics
Half-life Elimination ~7 hours
Pregnancy Risk Factor C

Beta-Carotene (BAY ta KARE oh teen)

U.S. Brand Names A-Caro-25 [OTC]; B-Caro-T™ [OTC]; Lumitene™ [OTC]
Pharmacologic Category Vitamin, Fat Soluble
Unlabeled/Investigational Use Prophylaxis and treatment of polymorphous light eruption; prophylaxis against photosensitivity reactions in erythropoietic protoporphyria
Local Anesthetic/Vasoconstrictor Precautions No information available to require special precautions
Effects on Dental Treatment No significant effects or complications reported
Effects on Bleeding No information available to require special precautions
Adverse Effects >10%: Dermatologic: Carotenodermia (yellowing of palms, hands, or soles of feet, and to a lesser extent the face)
General Dosage Range Oral:
Children <14 years (unlabeled use): 30-150 mg/day
Adults (unlabeled use): 30-300 mg/day

Mechanism of Action The exact mechanism of action in erythropoietic protoporphyria has not as yet been elucidated; although patient must become carotenemic before effects are observed, there appears to be more than a simple internal light screen responsible for the drug's action. A protective effect was achieved when beta-carotene was added to blood samples. The concentrations of solutions used were similar to those achieved in treated patients. Topically applied beta-carotene is considerably less effective than systemic therapy.

Pregnancy Risk Factor C

Betaine (BAY ta een)

U.S. Brand Names Cystadane®

Canadian Brand Names Cystadane®

Pharmacologic Category Homocystinuria, Treatment Agent

Use Treatment of homocystinuria (eg, deficiencies or defects in cystathionine beta-synthase [CBS], 5,10-methylene tetrahydrofolate reductase [MTHFR], and cobalamin cofactor metabolism [CBL])

Local Anesthetic/Vasoconstrictor Precautions No information available to require special precautions

Effects on Dental Treatment No significant effects or complications reported

Effects on Bleeding No information available to require special precautions

Adverse Effects

Frequency not defined: Gastrointestinal: Diarrhea, dysgeusia, GI distress, nausea

Postmarketing and/or case reports: Alopecia, anorexia, agitation, cerebral edema (associated with hypermethioninemia), dental disorders, depression, hives, glossitis, irritability, personality disorder, sleep disturbances, skin odor abnormalities, urinary incontinence, vomiting

General Dosage Range Oral:

Children <3 years: Initial: 100 mg/kg/day, then increase weekly by 50 mg/kg increments, as needed

Children ≥3 years and Adults: 3 g twice daily (maximum: 20 g/day)

Mechanism of Action Betaine acts as a methyl group donor in the remethylation of homocysteine to methionine. Homocystinuria is an inborn error of metabolism in which elevated plasma homocysteine levels can lead to mental retardation, ocular abnormalities, osteoporosis, premature atherosclerosis and thromboembolic disease. Remethylation is one of the two divergent pathways in the metabolism of homocysteine. The second pathway involves transulfuration of homocysteine to produce cysteine. A number of enzymes and cofactors are also involved in these pathways.

Pregnancy Risk Factor C

Prescribing and Access Restrictions Cystadane® may be obtained by contacting Accredo Health Group Inc at 1-888-454-8860.

Betamethasone (bay ta METH a sone)

Related Information

Respiratory Diseases *on page 1876*

Related Sample Prescriptions

Recurrent Aphthous Stomatitis *on page 1992*

U.S. Brand Names Beta-Val® [DSC]; Celestone®; Celestone® Soluspan®; Diprolene®; Diprolene® AF; Luxíq®

Canadian Brand Names Betaderm; Betaject™; Betnesol®; Betnovate®; Celestone® Soluspan®; Diprolene® Glycol; Diprosone®; Ectosone; Prevex® B; Taro-Sone; Topilene®; Topisone®; Valisone® Scalp Lotion

Generic Availability (U.S.) Yes: Excludes aerosol, solution

Pharmacologic Category Corticosteroid, Systemic; Corticosteroid, Topical

Dental Use Treatment of a variety of oral diseases of allergic, inflammatory, or autoimmune origin

Use Inflammatory dermatoses such as seborrheic or atopic dermatitis, neurodermatitis, anogenital pruritus, psoriasis, inflammatory phase of xerosis

Unlabeled/Investigational Use Accelerate fetal lung maturation in patients with preterm labor

Local Anesthetic/Vasoconstrictor Precautions No information available to require special precautions

Effects on Dental Treatment No significant effects or complications reported

Effects on Bleeding No information available to require special precautions

Adverse Effects

Systemic:

Cardiovascular: Congestive heart failure, edema, hyper-/hypotension

Central nervous system: Dizziness, headache, insomnia, intracranial pressure increased, lightheadedness, nervousness, pseudotumor cerebri, seizure, vertigo

Dermatologic: Ecchymoses, facial erythema, fragile skin, hirsutism, hyper-/hypopigmentation, perioral dermatitis (oral), petechiae, striae, wound healing impaired
Endocrine & metabolic: Amenorrhea, Cushing's syndrome, diabetes mellitus, growth suppression, hyperglycemia, hypokalemia, menstrual irregularities, pituitary-adrenal axis suppression, protein catabolism, sodium retention, water retention
Local: Injection site reactions (intra-articular use), sterile abscess
Neuromuscular & skeletal: Arthralgia, muscle atrophy, fractures, muscle weakness, myopathy, osteoporosis, necrosis (femoral and humeral heads)
Ocular: Cataracts, glaucoma, intraocular pressure increased
Miscellaneous: Anaphylactoid reaction, diaphoresis, hypersensitivity, secondary infection

Topical:

Dermatologic: Acneiform eruptions, allergic dermatitis, burning, dry skin, erythema, folliculitis, hypertrichosis, irritation, miliaria, pruritus, skin atrophy, striae, vesiculation
Endocrine and metabolic effects have occasionally been reported with topical use.

Dental Usual Dosage Allergic or inflammatory diseases: Topical: Gel: Apply small quantity with Q-tip to affected area 3-4 times/day

Dosage Base dosage on severity of disease and patient response

Children: Use lowest dose listed as initial dose for adrenocortical insufficiency (physiologic replacement)
- I.M.: ≤12 years: 0.0175-0.125 mg base/kg/day divided every 6-12 hours **or** 0.5-7.5 mg base/m^2/day divided every 6-12 hours
- Oral: ≤12 years: 0.0175-0.25 mg/kg/day divided every 6-8 hours **or** 0.5-7.5 mg/m^2/day divided every 6-8 hours
- Topical:
  - ≤12 years: Use is not recommended.
  - ≥13 years: Use minimal amount for shortest period of time to avoid HPA axis suppression
    - Gel, augmented formulation: Apply once or twice daily; rub in gently. **Note:** Do not exceed 2 weeks of treatment or 50 g/week.
    - Lotion: Apply a few drops twice daily
      - Augmented formulation: Apply a few drops once or twice daily; rub in gently. **Note:** Do not exceed 2 weeks of treatment or 50 mL/week.
    - Cream/ointment: Apply once or twice daily.
      - Augmented formulation: Apply once or twice daily. **Note:** Do not exceed 2 weeks of treatment or 45 g/week.

Adolescents and Adults:
- Oral: 2.4-4.8 mg/day in 2-4 doses; range: 0.6-7.2 mg/day
- I.M.: Betamethasone sodium phosphate and betamethasone acetate: 0.6-9 mg/day (generally, 1/3 to 1/2 of oral dose) divided every 12-24 hours

Adults:
- Intrabursal, intra-articular, intradermal: 0.25-2 mL
- Intralesional: Rheumatoid arthritis/osteoarthritis:
  - Very large joints: 1-2 mL
  - Large joints: 1 mL
  - Medium joints: 0.5-1 mL
  - Small joints: 0.25-0.5 mL
- Topical:
  - Foam: Apply to the scalp twice daily, once in the morning and once at night
  - Gel, augmented formulation: Apply once or twice daily; rub in gently. **Note:** Do not exceed 2 weeks of treatment or 50 g/week.
  - Lotion: Apply a few drops twice daily
    - Augmented formulation: Apply a few drops once or twice daily; rub in gently. **Note:** Do not exceed 2 weeks of treatment or 50 mL/week.
  - Cream/ointment: Apply once or twice daily
    - Augmented formulation: Apply once or twice daily. **Note:** Do not exceed 2 weeks of treatment or 45 g/week.

Dosing adjustment in hepatic impairment: Adjustments may be necessary in patients with liver failure because betamethasone is extensively metabolized in the liver

Mechanism of Action Controls the rate of protein synthesis; depresses the migration of polymorphonuclear leukocytes, fibroblasts; reverses capillary permeability and lysosomal stabilization at the cellular level to prevent or control inflammation

Contraindications Hypersensitivity to betamethasone, other corticosteroids, or any component of the formulation; systemic fungal infections; I.M. administration contraindicated in idiopathic thrombocytopenia purpura

Warnings/Precautions Very high potency topical products are not for treatment of rosacea, perioral dermatitis; not for use on face, groin, or axillae; not for use in a diapered area. Avoid concurrent use of other corticosteroids.

May cause hypercorticism or suppression of hypothalamic-pituitary-adrenal (HPA) axis, particularly in younger children or in patients receiving high doses for prolonged periods. HPA axis suppression may lead to adrenal crisis. Withdrawal and discontinuation of a corticosteroid should be done slowly and carefully. Particular care is required when patients are transferred from systemic corticosteroids to inhaled products due to possible adrenal insufficiency or withdrawal from steroids, including an increase in allergic symptoms. Patients receiving >20 mg per day of prednisone (or equivalent) may be most susceptible. Fatalities have occurred due to adrenal insufficiency in asthmatic patients during and after transfer from systemic corticosteroids to aerosol steroids; aerosol steroids do not provide the systemic steroid needed to treat patients having trauma, surgery, or infections. In stressful situations, HPA axis-suppressed patients should receive adequate supplementation with natural glucocorticoids (hydrocortisone or cortisone) rather than betamethasone (due to lack of mineralocorticoid activity).

Acute myopathy has been reported with high dose corticosteroids, usually in patients with neuromuscular transmission disorders; may involve ocular and/or respiratory muscles; monitor creatine kinase; recovery may be delayed. Corticosteroid use may cause psychiatric disturbances, including depression, euphoria, insomnia, mood swings, and personality changes. Pre-existing psychiatric conditions may be exacerbated by corticosteroid use. Prolonged use of corticosteroids may also increase the incidence of secondary infection, mask acute infection (including fungal infections), prolong or exacerbate viral infections, or limit response to vaccines. Exposure to chickenpox should be avoided; corticosteroids should not be used to treat ocular herpes simplex. Corticosteroids should not be used for cerebral malaria or viral hepatitis. Close observation is required in patients with latent tuberculosis and/or TB reactivity; restrict use in active TB (only in conjunction with antituberculosis treatment). Prolonged treatment with corticosteroids has been associated with the development of Kaposi's sarcoma (case reports); if noted, discontinuation of therapy should be considered. High-dose corticosteroids should not be used to manage acute head injury.

Use with caution in patients with thyroid disease, hepatic impairment, renal impairment, cardiovascular disease, diabetes, glaucoma, cataracts, myasthenia gravis, patients at risk for osteoporosis, patients at risk for seizures, or GI diseases (diverticulitis, peptic ulcer, ulcerative colitis) due to perforation risk. Use caution following acute MI (corticosteroids have been associated with myocardial rupture). Because of the risk of adverse effects, systemic corticosteroids should be used cautiously in the elderly in the smallest possible effective dose for the shortest duration. Do not use occlusive dressings on weeping or exudative lesions and general caution with occlusive dressings should be observed; adverse effects may be increased. Discontinue if skin irritation or contact dermatitis should occur; do not use in patients with decreased skin circulation. Withdraw therapy with gradual tapering of dose. May affect growth velocity; growth should be routinely monitored in pediatric patients. Topical use in patients ≤12 years of age is not recommended.

Drug Interactions

Metabolism/Transport Effects Inhibits CYP3A4 (weak)

Avoid Concomitant Use

Avoid concomitant use of Betamethasone with any of the following: Aldesleukin; BCG; Natalizumab; Pimecrolimus; Roflumilast; Tacrolimus (Topical)

Increased Effect/Toxicity

Betamethasone may increase the levels/effects of: Acetylcholinesterase Inhibitors; Amphotericin B; Deferasirox; Leflunomide; Loop Diuretics; Natalizumab; NSAID (COX-2 Inhibitor); NSAID (Nonselective); Thiazide Diuretics; Vaccines (Live); Warfarin

The levels/effects of Betamethasone may be increased by: Antifungal Agents (Azole Derivatives, Systemic); Aprepitant; Calcium Channel Blockers (Nondihydropyridine); Denosumab; Estrogen Derivatives; Fluconazole; Fosaprepitant; Macrolide Antibiotics; Neuromuscular-Blocking Agents (Nondepolarizing); Pimecrolimus; Quinolone Antibiotics; Roflumilast; Salicylates; Tacrolimus (Topical); Trastuzumab

Decreased Effect

Betamethasone may decrease the levels/effects of: Aldesleukin; Antidiabetic Agents; BCG; Calcitriol; Corticorelin; Isoniazid; Salicylates; Sipuleucel-T; Vaccines (Inactivated)

The levels/effects of Betamethasone may be decreased by: Aminoglutethimide; Antacids; Barbiturates; Bile Acid Sequestrants; Echinacea; Mitotane; Primidone; Rifamycin Derivatives

Ethanol/Nutrition/Herb Interactions

Ethanol: Avoid ethanol (may enhance gastric mucosal irritation).

Food: Betamethasone interferes with calcium absorption.

Herb/Nutraceutical: Avoid cat's claw, echinacea (have immunostimulant properties).

Dietary Considerations May be taken with food to decrease GI distress.

Pharmacodynamics/Kinetics

Half-life Elimination 6.5 hours

Time to Peak Serum: I.V.: 10-36 minutes

Pregnancy Risk Factor C

Lactation Excretion in breast milk unknown/use caution

Breast-Feeding Considerations Corticosteroids are excreted in human milk. The onset of milk secretion after birth may be delayed and the volume of milk produced may be decreased by antenatal betamethasone therapy; this affect was seen when delivery occurred 3-9 days after the betamethasone dose in women between 28 and 34 weeks gestation. Antenatal betamethasone therapy did not affect milk production when birth occurred <3 days or >10 days of treatment. It is not known if systemic absorption following topical administration results in detectable quantities in human milk. Use with caution while breast-feeding; do not apply to nipples.

Dosage Forms

Aerosol, topical:

Luxíq®: 0.12% (50 g, 100 g)

Cream, topical: 0.05% (15 g, 45 g, 50 g); 0.1% (15 g, 45 g)

Diprolene® AF: 0.05% (15 g, 50 g)

Gel, topical: 0.05% (15 g, 50 g)

Injection, suspension: Betamethasone sodium phosphate 3 mg and betamethasone acetate 3 mg per 1 mL (5 mL)

Celestone® Soluspan®: Betamethasone sodium phosphate 3 mg and betamethasone acetate 3 mg per 1 mL (5 mL)

Lotion, topical: 0.05% (30 mL, 60 mL); 0.1% (60 mL)

Diprolene®: 0.05% (30 mL, 60 mL)

Ointment, topical: 0.05% (15 g, 45 g, 50 g); 0.1% (15 g, 45 g)

Diprolene®: 0.05% (15 g, 50 g)

Solution, oral:

Celestone®: 0.6 mg/5 mL (118 mL)

Betamethasone and Clotrimazole (bay ta METH a sone & kloe TRIM a zole)

Related Information

Betamethasone *on page* 228

Clotrimazole (Topical) *on page* 426

U.S. Brand Names Lotrisone®

Canadian Brand Names Lotriderm®

Generic Availability (U.S.) Yes

Pharmacologic Category Antifungal Agent, Topical; Corticosteroid, Topical

Dental Use Treatment of a variety of oral diseases of allergic, inflammatory, or autoimmune origin

Use Topical treatment of various dermal fungal infections (including tinea pedis, cruris, and corpora in patients ≥17 years of age)

Local Anesthetic/Vasoconstrictor Precautions No information available to require special precautions

Effects on Dental Treatment No significant effects or complications reported

Effects on Bleeding No information available to require special precautions

Adverse Effects Also see individual agents. 1% to 10%:

Dermatologic: Dry skin (2%)

Local: Burning (2%)

Neuromuscular & skeletal: Paresthesia (2%)

Other reactions reported with topical corticosteroid use: Acneiform eruption dermatitis, bruising, folliculitis, hypertrichosis, hypopigmentation, striae, telangiectasia

Dental Usual Dosage Allergic or inflammatory diseases: Children ≥17 years and Adults: Topical: Apply to affected area twice daily, morning and evening

Dosage

Children <17 years: Do not use

Children ≥17 years and Adults:

Allergic or inflammatory diseases: Topical: Apply to affected area twice daily, morning and evening

Tinea corporis, tinea cruris: Topical: Massage into affected area twice daily, morning and evening; do not use for longer than 2 weeks; re-evaluate after 1 week if no clinical improvement; do not exceed 45 g cream/week or 45 mL lotion/week

Tinea pedis: Topical: Massage into affected area twice daily, morning and evening; do not use for longer than 4 weeks; re-evaluate after 2 weeks if no clinical improvement; do not exceed 45 g cream/week or 45 mL lotion/week

Elderly: Use with caution; skin atrophy and skin ulceration (rare) have been reported in patients with thinning skin; do not use for diaper dermatitis or under occlusive dressings

Mechanism of Action Betamethasone dipropionate is a corticosteroid which controls the rate of protein synthesis; depresses the migration of polymorphonuclear leukocytes, fibroblasts; reverses capillary permeability and lysosomal stabilization at the cellular level to prevent or control inflammation. Clotrimazole is an antifungal agent that binds to phospholipids in the fungal cell membrane altering cell wall permeability resulting in loss of essential intracellular elements.

Contraindications Hypersensitivity to betamethasone, clotrimazole, other corticosteroids or imidazoles, or any component of the formulation

Warnings/Precautions For topical use only; discontinue use if irritation occurs. Systemic absorption of topical corticosteroids may cause hypothalamic-pituitary-adrenal (HPA) axis suppression (reversible) particularly in younger children. HPA axis suppression may lead to adrenal crisis. Risk is increased when used over large surface areas, for prolonged periods, or with occlusive dressings. Adverse systemic effects including hyperglycemia, glycosuria, fluid and electrolyte changes, and HPA suppression may occur when used on large surface areas, for prolonged periods, or with an occlusive dressing. Prolonged treatment with corticosteroids has been associated with the development of Kaposi's sarcoma (case reports); if noted, discontinuation of therapy should be considered. Use with caution in the elderly. Not for use in pediatric patients <17 years of age. Do not use for diaper dermatitis.

Drug Interactions

Metabolism/Transport Effects

Betamethasone: **Inhibits** CYP3A4 (weak)

Clotrimazole: **Inhibits** CYP1A2 (weak), 2A6 (weak), 2B6 (weak), 2C8/9 (weak), 2C19 (weak), 2D6 (weak), 2E1 (weak), 3A4 (moderate)

Avoid Concomitant Use

Avoid concomitant use of Betamethasone and Clotrimazole with any of the following: Aldesleukin; BCG; Natalizumab; Pimecrolimus; Roflumilast; Tacrolimus (Topical); Tolvaptan

Increased Effect/Toxicity

Betamethasone and Clotrimazole may increase the levels/effects of: Acetylcholinesterase Inhibitors; Amphotericin B; Budesonide (Systemic, Oral Inhalation); Colchicine; CYP3A4 Substrates; Deferasirox; Eplerenone; Everolimus; FentaNYL; Halofantrine; Leflunomide; Loop Diuretics; Lurasidone; Natalizumab; NSAID (COX-2 Inhibitor); NSAID (Nonselective); Ranolazine; Salmeterol; Tacrolimus; Tacrolimus (Systemic); Thiazide Diuretics; Tolvaptan; Vaccines (Live); Vilazodone; Warfarin

The levels/effects of Betamethasone and Clotrimazole may be increased by: Antifungal Agents (Azole Derivatives, Systemic); Aprepitant; Calcium Channel Blockers (Nondihydropyridine); Denosumab; Estrogen Derivatives; Fluconazole; Fosaprepitant; Macrolide Antibiotics; Neuromuscular-Blocking Agents (Nondepolarizing); Pimecrolimus; Quinolone Antibiotics; Roflumilast; Salicylates; Tacrolimus (Topical); Trastuzumab

Decreased Effect

Betamethasone and Clotrimazole may decrease the levels/effects of: Aldesleukin; Antidiabetic Agents; BCG; Calcitriol; Corticorelin; Isoniazid; Saccharomyces boulardii; Salicylates; Sipuleucel-T; Vaccines (Inactivated)

The levels/effects of Betamethasone and Clotrimazole may be decreased by: Aminoglutethimide; Antacids; Barbiturates; Bile Acid Sequestrants; Echinacea; Mitotane; Primidone; Rifamycin Derivatives

Pregnancy Risk Factor C

Lactation Excretion in breast milk unknown/use caution

Breast-Feeding Considerations Betamethasone: Systemic corticosteroids are excreted in human milk. The extent of topical absorption is variable. Use with caution while breast-feeding; do not apply to nipples.

Dosage Forms

Cream: Betamethasone 0.05% and clotrimazole 1% (15 g, 45 g)

Lotrisone®: Betamethasone 0.05% and clotrimazole 1% (15 g, 45 g)

Lotion: Betamethasone 0.05% and clotrimazole 1% (30 mL)

Lotrisone®: Betamethasone 0.05% and clotrimazole 1% (30 mL)

Betaxolol (Systemic) (be TAKS oh lol)

Related Information

Cardiovascular Diseases *on page 1848*

U.S. Brand Names Kerlone®

Canadian Brand Names Sandoz-Betaxolol

Pharmacologic Category Beta Blocker, Beta-1 Selective

Use Management of hypertension

Unlabeled/Investigational Use Treatment of coronary artery disease

Local Anesthetic/Vasoconstrictor Precautions No information available to require special precautions

Effects on Dental Treatment Betaxolol is a cardioselective beta-blocker. Local anesthetic with vasoconstrictor can be safely used in patients medicated with betaxolol. Nonselective beta-blockers (ie, propranolol, nadolol) enhance the pressor response to epinephrine, resulting in hypertension and bradycardia; this has not been reported for betaxolol. Many nonsteroidal anti-inflammatory drugs, such as ibuprofen and indomethacin, can reduce the hypotensive effect of beta-blockers after 3 or more weeks of therapy with the NSAID. Short-term NSAID use (ie, 3 days) requires no special precautions in patients taking beta-blockers.

Effects on Bleeding No information available to require special precautions

Adverse Effects 2% to 10%:

Cardiovascular: Bradycardia (6% to 8%; symptomatic bradycardia: <1% to 2%; dose-dependent), chest pain (2% to 7%), palpitation (2%), edema (≤2%; similar to placebo)

Central nervous system: Fatigue (3% to 10%), insomnia (1% to 5%), lethargy (3%)

Gastrointestinal: Nausea (2% to 6%), dyspepsia (4% to 5%), diarrhea (2%)

Neuromuscular & skeletal: Arthralgia (3% to 5%), paresthesia (2%)

Respiratory: Dyspnea (2%), pharyngitis (2%)

Miscellaneous: Antinuclear antibody positive (5%), cold extremities (2%)

General Dosage Range Dosage adjustment recommended in patients with renal impairment

Oral:

Adults: 5-20 mg/day

Elderly: Initial dose: 5 mg/day

Mechanism of Action Competitively blocks $beta_1$-receptors, with little or no effect on $beta_2$-receptors

Pharmacodynamics/Kinetics

Onset of Action 1-1.5 hours

Half-life Elimination 14-22 hours; prolonged in hepatic disease and/or chronic renal failure

Time to Peak 1.5-6 hours

Pregnancy Risk Factor C

Bethanechol (be THAN e kole)

U.S. Brand Names Urecholine®

Canadian Brand Names Duvoid®; PMS-Bethanechol

Pharmacologic Category Cholinergic Agonist

Use Treatment of acute postoperative and postpartum nonobstructive (functional) urinary retention; treatment of neurogenic atony of the urinary bladder with retention

Unlabeled/Investigational Use Gastroesophageal reflux

Local Anesthetic/Vasoconstrictor Precautions No information available to require special precautions

Effects on Dental Treatment This is a cholinergic agent similar to pilocarpine; expect to see salivation and sweating in patients.

Effects on Bleeding No information available to require special precautions

Adverse Effects Frequency not defined.

Cardiovascular: Hypotension, tachycardia, flushed skin

Central nervous system: Headache, malaise, seizure

Gastrointestinal: Abdominal cramps, belching, borborygmi, colicky pain, diarrhea, nausea, vomiting, salivation

Genitourinary: Urinary urgency

Ocular: Lacrimation, miosis

Respiratory: Asthmatic attacks, bronchial constriction

Miscellaneous: Diaphoresis

General Dosage Range Oral: *Adults:* 10-100 mg 2-4 times/day

Mechanism of Action Due to stimulation of the parasympathetic nervous system, bethanechol increases bladder muscle tone causing contractions which initiate urination. Bethanechol also stimulates gastric motility, increases gastric tone and may restore peristalsis.

Pharmacodynamics/Kinetics

Onset of Action 30-90 minutes

Duration of Action Up to 6 hours

Pregnancy Risk Factor C

Bevacizumab (be vuh SIZ uh mab)

U.S. Brand Names Avastin®

Canadian Brand Names Avastin®

Pharmacologic Category Antineoplastic Agent, Monoclonal Antibody; Vascular Endothelial Growth Factor (VEGF) Inhibitor

Use Treatment of metastatic colorectal cancer; treatment of unresectable, locally advanced, recurrent or metastatic nonsquamous, nonsmall cell lung cancer; treatment of metastatic HER-2 negative breast cancer (who have not received chemotherapy for metastatic disease); treatment of progressive glioblastoma; treatment of metastatic renal cell cancer (not an approved use in Canada)

Note: For the treatment of metastatic breast cancer, effectiveness is based on improvement in progression-free survival; not indicated for the treatment of breast cancer with metastatic disease that has progressed following anthracycline and taxane treatment. For the treatment of glioblastoma, effectiveness is based on improvement in objective response rate.

Unlabeled/Investigational Use Treatment of recurrent ovarian cancer, recurrent cervical cancer, soft tissue sarcomas (angiosarcoma or hemangiopericytoma/solitary fibrous tumor), age-related macular degeneration (AMD)

Local Anesthetic/Vasoconstrictor Precautions No information available to require special precautions

Effects on Dental Treatment Key adverse event(s) related to dental treatment: Xerostomia (normal salivary flow resumes upon discontinuation), stomatitis, taste disorder, and gingival bleeding.

Effects on Bleeding Chemotherapy may result in significant myelosuppression, potentially including significant reduction in platelet counts and altered hemostasis. In patients who are under active treatment with these agents, medical consult is suggested.

Adverse Effects Percentages reported as monotherapy and as part of combination chemotherapy regimens. Some studies only reported hematologic toxicities grades ≥4 and nonhematologic toxicities grades ≥3.

>10%:

- Cardiovascular: Hypertension (23% to 67%; grades 3/4: 5% to 18%), thromboembolic event (≤21%; grades 3/4: 15%; venous thrombus/embolus: 8%; grades 3/4: 5% to 7%; arterial thrombosis 6%; grades 3/4: 3%), hypotension (7% to 15%)
- Central nervous system: Pain (31% to 62%), headache (24% to 37%; grades 3/4: 2% to 4%), dizziness (19% to 26%), fatigue (≤45%; grades 3/4: 4% to 19%), sensory neuropathy (grades 3/4: 1% to 17%; in combination with paclitaxel: 24%)
- Dermatologic: Alopecia (6% to 32%), dry skin (7% to 20%), exfoliative dermatitis (3% to 19%), skin discoloration (2% to 16%)
- Endocrine & metabolic: Hypokalemia (12% to 16%)
- Gastrointestinal: Abdominal pain (50% to 61%; grades 3/4: 8%), vomiting (47% to 52%; grades 3/4: 6% to 11%), anorexia (35% to 43%), constipation (29% to 40%), diarrhea (grades 3/4: 1% to 34%), stomatitis (25% to 32%), gastrointestinal hemorrhage (19% to 24%), dyspepsia (17% to 24%), taste disorder (14% to 21%), flatulence (11% to 19%), weight loss (9% to 20%), nausea (grades 3/4: 4% to 12%)
- Hematologic: Hemorrhage (≤40%; grades 3/4: 1% to 5%), leukopenia (grades 3/4: 37%), neutropenia (grade 4: 6% to 27%)
- Neuromuscular & skeletal: Weakness (57% to 74%), myalgia (8% to 19%), back pain (≤12%)
- Ocular: Tearing increased (6% to 18%)
- Renal: Proteinuria (4% to 36%; grades 3/4: ≤7%; median onset: 5.6 months; median time to resolution: 6.1 months)
- Respiratory: Upper respiratory infection (40% to 47%), epistaxis (16% to 35%), dyspnea (25% to 26%), rhinitis
- Miscellaneous: Infection (≤55%; serious: 9% to 14%; pneumonia, catheter, or wound infections)

1% to 10%:

Cardiovascular: DVT (6% to 9%; grades 3/4: 9%), HF (grades 3/4: 1% to 4%), syncope (grades 3/4: 3%), intra-abdominal venous thrombosis (grades 3/4: 3%), cardio-/cerebrovascular arterial thrombotic event (2% to 4%), left ventricular dysfunction (grades 3/4: 1%)

Central nervous system: Confusion (1% to 6%), abnormal gait (1% to 5%); CNS hemorrhage (1% to 5%; grades 3/4: 1%), reversible posterior leukoencephalopathy syndrome ([RPLS] ≤1%)

Dermatologic: Nail disorder (2% to 8%), skin ulcer (≤6%), rash desquamation (grades 3/4: 3%), wound dehiscence (1% to 6%), acne (≤1%)

Endocrine & metabolic: Dehydration (grades 3/4: 3% to 10%), hyponatremia (grades 3/4: 4%)

Gastrointestinal: Xerostomia (4% to 7%), colitis (1% to 6%), ileus (grades 3/4: 4% to 5%), gingival bleeding (2% to 4%), fistula (1%), gastrointestinal perforation (≤4%), gastroesophageal reflux (≤2%), gingivitis (≤2%), mouth ulceration (≤2%), tooth abscess (≤2%), intra-abdominal abscess (1%), gastritis (≤1%), gingival pain (≤1%)

Genitourinary: Polyuria/urgency (3% to 6%), vaginal hemorrhage (4%)

Hematologic: Neutropenic fever/infection (5%; grades 3 and/or 4: 4% to 5%), thrombocytopenia (5%)

Hepatic: Bilirubinemia (1% to 6%)

Neuromuscular & skeletal: Bone pain (grades 3/4: 4%), neuropathy (other than sensory: grades 3/4: 1% to 5%)

Ocular: Blurred vision (≤2%)

Otic: Tinnitus (≤2%), deafness (≤1%)

Respiratory: Voice alteration (5% to 9%), pneumonitis/pulmonary infiltrates (grades 3/4: 5%), hemoptysis (nonsquamous histology 2%), pulmonary embolism (≤1%)

Miscellaneous: Infusion reactions (<3%)

General Dosage Range I.V.: *Adults:* 5 or 10 mg/kg every 2 weeks **or** 15 mg/kg every 3 weeks

Mechanism of Action Bevacizumab is a recombinant, humanized monoclonal antibody which binds to, and neutralizes, vascular endothelial growth factor (VEGF), preventing its association with endothelial receptors, Flt-1 and KDR. VEGF binding initiates angiogenesis (endothelial proliferation and the formation of new blood vessels). The inhibition of microvascular growth is believed to retard the growth of all tissues (including metastatic tissue).

Pharmacodynamics/Kinetics

Half-life Elimination ~20 days (range: 11-50 days)

Pregnancy Risk Factor C

Bexarotene (Systemic) (beks AIR oh teen)

U.S. Brand Names Targretin®

Canadian Brand Names Targretin®

Pharmacologic Category Antineoplastic Agent, Miscellaneous

Use Treatment of cutaneous manifestations of cutaneous T-cell lymphoma in patients who are refractory to at least one prior systemic therapy

Local Anesthetic/Vasoconstrictor Precautions No information available to require special precautions

Effects on Dental Treatment Key adverse event(s) related to dental treatment: Xerostomia (normal salivary flow resumes upon discontinuation) and gingivitis.

Effects on Bleeding Chemotherapy may result in significant myelosuppression, potentially including significant reduction in platelet counts and altered hemostasis. In patients who are under active treatment with these agents, medical consult is suggested.

Adverse Effects First percentage is at a dose of 300 mg/m^2/day; the second percentage is at a dose >300 mg/m^2/day.

>10%:

Cardiovascular: Peripheral edema (13% to 11%)

Central nervous system: Headache (30% to 42%), chills (10% to 13%)

Dermatologic: Rash (17% to 23%), exfoliative dermatitis (10% to 28%)

Endocrine & metabolic: Hyperlipidemia (about 79% in both dosing ranges), hypercholesteremia (32% to 62%), hypothyroidism (29% to 53%)

Hematologic: Leukopenia (17% to 47%)

Neuromuscular & skeletal: Weakness (20% to 45%)

Miscellaneous: Infection (13% to 23%)

<10%:
- Cardiovascular: Hemorrhage, hypertension, angina pectoris, right heart failure, tachycardia, cerebrovascular accident
- Central nervous system: Fever (5% to 17%), insomnia (5% to 11%), subdural hematoma, syncope, depression, agitation, ataxia, confusion, dizziness, hyperesthesia
- Dermatologic: Dry skin (about 10% for both dosing ranges), alopecia (4% to 11%), skin ulceration, acne, skin nodule, maculopapular rash, serous drainage, vesicular bullous rash, cheilitis
- Endocrine & metabolic: Hypoproteinemia, hyperglycemia, weight loss/gain, breast pain
- Gastrointestinal: Abdominal pain (11% to 4%), nausea (16% to 8%), diarrhea (7% to 42%), vomiting (4% to 13%), anorexia (2% to 23%), constipation, xerostomia, flatulence, colitis, dyspepsia, gastroenteritis, gingivitis, melena, pancreatitis, serum amylase increased
- Genitourinary: Albuminuria, hematuria, urinary incontinence, urinary tract infection, urinary urgency, dysuria, kidney function abnormality
- Hematologic: Hypochromic anemia (4% to 13%), anemia (6% to 25%), eosinophilia, thrombocythemia, coagulation time increased, lymphocytosis, thrombocytopenia
- Hepatic: LDH increase (7% to 13%), hepatic failure
- Neuromuscular & skeletal: Back pain (2% to 11%), arthralgia, myalgia, bone pain, myasthenia, arthrosis, neuropathy
- Ocular: Dry eyes, conjunctivitis, blepharitis, corneal lesion, visual field defects, keratitis
- Otic: Ear pain, otitis externa
- Renal: Creatinine increased
- Respiratory: Pharyngitis, rhinitis, dyspnea, pleural effusion, bronchitis, cough increased, lung edema, hemoptysis, hypoxia
- Miscellaneous: Flu-like syndrome (4% to 13%), bacterial infection (1% to 13%)

General Dosage Range Oral: *Adults:* 300-400 mg/m^2 once daily

Mechanism of Action The exact mechanism is unknown. Binds and activates retinoid X receptor subtypes. Once activated, these receptors function as transcription factors that regulate the expression of genes which control cellular differentiation and proliferation. Bexarotene inhibits the growth *in vitro* of some tumor cell lines of hematopoietic and squamous cell origin.

Pharmacodynamics/Kinetics

Half-life Elimination ~7 hours

Time to Peak ~2 hours

Pregnancy Risk Factor X

Bexarotene (Topical) (beks AIR oh teen)

U.S. Brand Names Targretin®

Canadian Brand Names Targretin®

Pharmacologic Category Antineoplastic Agent, Miscellaneous

Use Treatment of cutaneous lesions in patients with refractory cutaneous T-cell lymphoma (stage 1A and 1B) or who have not tolerated other therapies

Local Anesthetic/Vasoconstrictor Precautions No information available to require special precautions

Effects on Dental Treatment No significant effects or complications reported

Effects on Bleeding No information available to require special precautions

Adverse Effects
- Cardiovascular: Edema (10%)
- Central nervous system: Headache (14%), weakness (6%), pain (30%)
- Dermatologic: Rash (14% to 72%), pruritus (6% to 40%), contact dermatitis (14%), exfoliative dermatitis (6%)
- Endocrine & metabolic: Hyperlipidemia (10%)
- Hematologic: Leukopenia (6%), lymphadenopathy (6%)
- Neuromuscular & skeletal: Paresthesia (6%)
- Respiratory: Cough (6%), pharyngitis (6%)
- Miscellaneous: Diaphoresis (6%), infection (18%)

General Dosage Range Topical: *Adults:* Initial: Apply once every other day for first week; Maintenance: Apply 1-4 times/day

Mechanism of Action The exact mechanism is unknown. Binds and activates retinoid X receptor subtypes. Once activated, these receptors function as transcription factors that regulate the expression of genes which control cellular differentiation and proliferation.

Pregnancy Risk Factor X

Bicalutamide (bye ka LOO ta mide)

U.S. Brand Names Casodex®

Canadian Brand Names Apo-Bicalutamide®; Casodex®; CO Bicalutamide; Dom-Bicalutamide; JAMP-Bicalutamide; Mylan-Bicalutamide; Novo-Bicalutamide; PHL-Bicalutamide; PMS-Bicalutamide; PRO-Bicalutamide; ratio-Bicalutamide; Sandoz-Bicalutamide

Pharmacologic Category Antineoplastic Agent, Antiandrogen

Use Treatment of metastatic prostate cancer (in combination with an LHRH agonist)

Unlabeled/Investigational Use Monotherapy for locally-advanced prostate cancer

Local Anesthetic/Vasoconstrictor Precautions No information available to require special precautions

Effects on Dental Treatment Key adverse event(s) related to dental treatment: Xerostomia (normal salivary flow resumes upon discontinuation).

Effects on Bleeding Although significant myelosuppression with associated altered hemostasis has been reported for many chemotherapeutic agents, myelosuppression is not common with bicalutamide and no specific precautions appear to be necessary.

Adverse Effects Adverse reaction percentages reported as part of combination regimen with an LHRH analogue unless otherwise noted.

>10%:

- Cardiovascular: Peripheral edema (13%)
- Central nervous system: Pain (35%)
- Endocrine & metabolic: Hot flashes (53%), breast pain (6%; monotherapy [150 mg]: 39% to 85%), gynecomastia (9%; monotherapy [150 mg]: 38% to 73%)
- Gastrointestinal: Constipation (22%), nausea (15%), diarrhea (12%), abdominal pain (11%)
- Genitourinary: Pelvic pain (21%), hematuria (12%), nocturia (12%)
- Hematologic: Anemia (11%)
- Neuromuscular & skeletal: Back pain (25%), weakness (22%)
- Respiratory: Dyspnea (13%)
- Miscellaneous: Infection (18%)

≥2% to 10%:

- Cardiovascular: Chest pain (8%), hypertension (8%), angina pectoris (2% to <5%), cardiac arrest (2% to <5%), CHF (2% to <5%), edema (2% to <5%), MI (2% to <5%), coronary artery disorder (2% to <5%), syncope (2% to <5%)
- Central nervous system: Dizziness (10%), headache (7%), insomnia (7%), anxiety (5%), depression (4%), chills (2% to <5%), confusion (2% to <5%), fever (2% to <5%), nervousness (2% to <5%), somnolence (2% to <5%)
- Dermatologic: Rash (9%), alopecia (2% to <5%), dry skin (2% to <5%), pruritus (2% to <5%), skin carcinoma (2% to <5%)
- Endocrine & metabolic: Hyperglycemia (6%), dehydration (2% to <5%), gout (2% to <5%), hypercholesterolemia (2% to <5%), libido decreased (2% to <5%)
- Gastrointestinal: Dyspepsia (7%), weight loss (7%), anorexia (6%), flatulence (6%), vomiting (6%), weight gain (5%), dysphagia (2% to <5%), gastrointestinal carcinoma (2% to <5%), melena (2% to <5%), periodontal abscess (2% to <5%), rectal hemorrhage (2% to <5%), xerostomia (2% to <5%)
- Genitourinary: Urinary tract infection (9%), impotence (7%), polyuria (6%), urinary retention (5%), urinary impairment (5%), urinary incontinence (4%), dysuria (2% to <5%), urinary urgency (2% to <5%)
- Hepatic: LFTs increased (7%), alkaline phosphatase increased (5%)
- Neuromuscular & skeletal: Bone pain (9%), paresthesia (8%), myasthenia (7%), arthritis (5%), pathological fracture (4%), hypertonia (2% to <5%), leg cramps (2% to <5%), myalgia (2% to <5%), neck pain (2% to <5%), neuropathy (2% to <5%)
- Ocular: Cataract (2% to <5%)
- Renal: BUN increased (2% to <5%), creatinine increased (2% to <5%), hydronephrosis (2% to <5%)
- Respiratory: Cough (8%), pharyngitis (8%), bronchitis (6%), pneumonia (4%), rhinitis (4%), asthma (2% to <5%), epistaxis (2% to <5%), sinusitis (2% to <5%)
- Miscellaneous: Flu-like syndrome (7%), diaphoresis (6%), cyst (2% to <5%), hernia (2% to <5%), herpes zoster (2% to <5%), sepsis (2% to <5%)

General Dosage Range Oral: *Adults:* 50 mg once daily

Mechanism of Action Androgen receptor inhibitor; pure nonsteroidal antiandrogen that binds to androgen receptors; specifically a competitive inhibitor for the binding of dihydrotestosterone and testosterone; prevents testosterone stimulation of cell growth in prostate cancer

Pharmacodynamics/Kinetics

Half-life Elimination Active enantiomer: ~6 days, ~10 days in severe liver disease

Time to Peak Active enantiomer: ~31 hours

Pregnancy Risk Factor X

Bimatoprost (bi MAT oh prost)

U.S. Brand Names Latisse®; Lumigan®

Canadian Brand Names Lumigan®; Lumigan® RC

Pharmacologic Category Ophthalmic Agent, Antiglaucoma; Ophthalmic Agent, Miscellaneous; Prostaglandin, Ophthalmic

Use Reduction of intraocular pressure (IOP) in patients with open-angle glaucoma or ocular hypertension; hypotrichosis treatment of the eyelashes

Local Anesthetic/Vasoconstrictor Precautions No information available to require special precautions

Effects on Dental Treatment No significant effects or complications reported

Effects on Bleeding No information available to require special precautions

Adverse Effects Adverse reactions and percentages are for Lumigan® unless noted:

>10%: Ocular: Conjunctival hyperemia (25% to 45%; Latisse®: <4%), growth of eyelashes, ocular pruritus (Latisse®: <4%)

1% to 10%:

Central nervous system: Headache (1% to 5%)

Dermatologic: Skin hyperpigmentation (Latisse®: <4%), abnormal hair growth

Hepatic: Liver function tests abnormal (1% to 5%)

Neuromuscular & skeletal: Weakness (1% to 5%)

Ocular: Dryness (Latisse®: <4%), erythema of the eyelid (Latisse®: <4%), irritation (Latisse®: <4%), allergic conjunctivitis, asthenopia, blepharitis, burning, cataract, conjunctival edema, conjunctival hemorrhage, discharge, eyelash darkening, foreign body sensation, iris pigmentation increased (may be delayed), pain, photophobia, pigmentation of periocular skin, superficial punctate keratitis, tearing, visual disturbance

Miscellaneous: Infections (10%; primarily colds and upper respiratory tract infections)

General Dosage Range

Ophthalmic: *Adults:* Instill 1 drop into affected eye(s) once daily

Ophthalmic, topical: *Adults:* Place 1 drop on applicator and apply evenly along the skin of the upper eyelid at base of eyelashes once daily

Mechanism of Action As a synthetic analog of prostaglandin with ocular hypotensive activity, bimatoprost decreases intraocular pressure by increasing the outflow of aqueous humor. Bimatoprost may increase the percent and duration of hairs in the growth phase, resulting in eyelash growth..

Pharmacodynamics/Kinetics

Onset of Action Reduction of IOP: ~4 hours; Peak effect: Maximum reduction of IOP: ~8-12 hours

Half-life Elimination I.V.: ≤45 minutes

Time to Peak ≤10 minutes

Pregnancy Risk Factor C

Bisacodyl (bis a KOE dil)

U.S. Brand Names Alophen® [OTC]; Bisac-Evac™ [OTC]; Biscolax™ [OTC]; Correctol® Tablets [OTC]; Dacodyl™ [OTC]; Doxidan® [OTC]; Dulcolax® [OTC]; ex-lax® Ultra [OTC]; Femilax™ [OTC]; Fleet® Bisacodyl [OTC]; Fleet® Stimulant Laxative [OTC]; Veracolate® [OTC]

Canadian Brand Names Apo-Bisacodyl®; Carter's Little Pills®; Dulcolax®; Gentlax®

Pharmacologic Category Laxative, Stimulant

Use Treatment of constipation; colonic evacuation prior to procedures or examination

Local Anesthetic/Vasoconstrictor Precautions No information available to require special precautions

Effects on Dental Treatment No significant effects or complications reported

Effects on Bleeding No information available to require special precautions

General Dosage Range

Oral:

Children >6 years: 5-10 mg (0.3 mg/kg) once daily

Adults: 5-15 mg as a single dose (maximum: 30 mg)

Rectal:
Children <2 years: 5 mg as a single dose
Children ≥2 years and Adults: 10 mg as a single dose

Mechanism of Action Stimulates peristalsis by directly irritating the smooth muscle of the intestine, possibly the colonic intramural plexus; alters water and electrolyte secretion producing net intestinal fluid accumulation and laxation

Pharmacodynamics/Kinetics
Onset of Action Oral: 6-10 hours; Rectal: 0.25-1 hour

Pregnancy Risk Factor C

Bismuth (BIZ muth)

Related Information
Gastrointestinal Disorders *on page 1874*

U.S. Brand Names Bismatrol Maximum Strength [OTC]; Bismatrol [OTC]; Diotame [OTC]; Kao-Tin [OTC]; Kaopectate® Extra Strength [OTC]; Kaopectate® [OTC]; Maalox® Total Relief® [OTC] [DSC]; Peptic Relief [OTC]; Pepto Relief [OTC]; Pepto-Bismol® Maximum Strength [OTC]; Pepto-Bismol® [OTC]

Pharmacologic Category Antidiarrheal

Use Subsalicylate formulation: Symptomatic treatment of mild, nonspecific diarrhea; control of traveler's diarrhea (enterotoxigenic *Escherichia coli*); as part of a multidrug regimen for *H. pylori* eradication to reduce the risk of duodenal ulcer recurrence

Local Anesthetic/Vasoconstrictor Precautions No information available to require special precautions

Effects on Dental Treatment Key adverse event(s) related to dental treatment: Darkening of tongue.

Effects on Bleeding No information available to require special precautions

Adverse Effects Frequency not defined; subsalicylate formulation:
Central nervous system: Anxiety, confusion, headache, mental depression, slurred speech
Gastrointestinal: Discoloration of the tongue (darkening), grayish black stools, impaction may occur in infants and debilitated patients
Neuromuscular & skeletal: Muscle spasms, weakness
Otic: Hearing loss, tinnitus

General Dosage Range Oral:
Subsalicylate based on 262 mg/5 mL liquid or 262 mg tablet (diarrhea):
Children 3-6 years: 1/3 tablet **or** 5 mL every 30 minutes to 1 hour as needed (maximum: 8 doses/day)
Children 6-9 years: 2/3 tablet **or** 10 mL every 30 minutes to 1 hour as needed (maximum: 8 doses/day)
Children 9-12 years: 1 tablet **or** 15 mL every 30 minutes to 1 hour as needed (maximum: 8 doses/day)
Subsalicylate based on 262 mg/15 mL liquid or 262 mg tablet:
Children >12 years: Diarrhea: 2 tablets **or** 30 mL every 30 minutes to 1 hour as needed (maximum: 8 doses/day)
Adults:
Diarrhea: 2 tablets **or** 30 mL every 30 minutes to 1 hour as needed (maximum: 8 doses/day)
H. pylori eradication: 524 mg 4 times/day

Mechanism of Action Bismuth subsalicylate exhibits both antisecretory and antimicrobial action. This agent may provide some anti-inflammatory action as well. The salicylate moiety provides antisecretory effect and the bismuth exhibits antimicrobial directly against bacterial and viral gastrointestinal pathogens.

Pharmacodynamics/Kinetics
Half-life Elimination Terminal: Bismuth: Highly variable

Pregnancy Risk Factor C/D (3rd trimester)

Bismuth, Metronidazole, and Tetracycline
(BIZ muth, me troe NI da zole, & tet ra SYE kleen)

Related Information
Bismuth *on page 239*
MetroNIDAZOLE (Systemic) *on page 1126*
Tetracycline *on page 1611*

U.S. Brand Names Helidac®; Pylera™

Pharmacologic Category Antibiotic, Miscellaneous; Antibiotic, Tetracycline Derivative; Antidiarrheal

Use As part of a multidrug regimen for *H. pylori* eradication to reduce the risk of duodenal ulcer recurrence in combination with an H_2 agonist (Helidac®) or omeprazole (Pylera™)

Local Anesthetic/Vasoconstrictor Precautions No information available to require special precautions

Effects on Dental Treatment Tetracyclines are not recommended for use during pregnancy since they can cause enamel hypoplasia and permanent teeth discoloration; long-term use associated with oral candidiasis.

Effects on Bleeding No information available to require special precautions

Adverse Effects Also see individual agents.

Helidac® (includes studies with/without concomitant acid-suppression therapy):

>10%: Gastrointestinal: Nausea (12%)

1% to 10%:

Central nervous system: Dizziness (2%), headache (2%), insomnia (1%), pain (1%)

Gastrointestinal: Abdominal pain (7%), diarrhea (7%), melena (3%), anorexia (2%), constipation (2%), dyspepsia (2%), tongue discoloration (2%), vomiting (2%), abnormal stools (1%), anal discomfort (1%), duodenal ulcer (1%), flatulence (1%), GI hemorrhage (1%), taste perversion (1%)

Neuromuscular & skeletal: Weakness (2%), paresthesia (1%)

Respiratory: Upper respiratory infection (2%), sinusitis (1%)

Pylera™ (with concomitant omeprazole):

>10%: Gastrointestinal: Abnormal stools (16%)

1% to 10%:

Cardiovascular: Chest pain (1%), palpitation (1%)

Central nervous system: Headache (8%), dizziness (3%), pain (2%), anxiety (1%)

Dermatologic: Maculopapular rash (1%)

Gastrointestional: Abdominal pain (9%), diarrhea (9%), dyspepsia (9%), nausea (8%), taste perversion (5%), gastritis (1%), gastroenteritis (1%), vomiting (1%), xerostomia (1%)

Genitourinary: Vaginitis (4%), urine abnormality (2%)

Hepatic: ALT increased (2%), AST increased (1%)

Neuromuscular & skeletal: Weakness (4%), back pain (2%)

Respiratory: Pharyngitis (2%), rhinitis (1%)

Miscellaneous: Flu-like syndrome (5%), infection (1% to 2%)

General Dosage Range Oral: *Adults:*

Helidac®: 2 bismuth subsalicylate 262.4 mg tablets, 1 metronidazole 250 mg tablet, and 1 tetracycline 500 mg capsule 4 times/day at meals and bedtime

Pylera™: 3 capsules 4 times/day after meals and at bedtime

Mechanism of Action Bismuth, metronidazole, and tetracycline individually have demonstrated *in vitro* activity against most susceptible strains of *H. pylori* isolated from patients with duodenal ulcers. Resistance to metronidazole is increasing in the U.S.; an alternative regimen, not containing metronidazole, if *H. pylori* is not eradicated follow therapy.

Pregnancy Risk Factor D

Bisoprolol (bis OH proe lol)

Related Information

Cardiovascular Diseases *on page 1848*

U.S. Brand Names Zebeta®

Canadian Brand Names Apo-Bisoprolol®; Novo-Bisoprolol; PHL-Bisoprolol; PMS-Bisoprolol; PRO-Bisoprolol; Sandoz-Bisoprolol; ZYM-Bisoprolol

Pharmacologic Category Beta Blocker, Beta-1 Selective

Use Treatment of hypertension, alone or in combination with other agents

Unlabeled/Investigational Use Chronic stable angina, supraventricular arrhythmias, PVCs, heart failure (HF)

Local Anesthetic/Vasoconstrictor Precautions No information available to require special precautions

Effects on Dental Treatment Bisoprolol is a cardioselective beta-blocker. Local anesthetic with vasoconstrictor can be safely used in patients medicated with bisoprolol. Nonselective beta-blockers (ie, propranolol, nadolol) enhance the pressor response to epinephrine, resulting in hypertension and bradycardia; this has not been reported for bisoprolol. Many nonsteroidal anti-inflammatory drugs, such as ibuprofen and indomethacin, can reduce the hypotensive effect of beta-blockers after 3 or more weeks of therapy with the NSAID. Short-term NSAID use (ie, 3 days) requires no special precautions in patients taking beta-blockers.

Effects on Bleeding No information available to require special precautions

Adverse Effects 1% to 10%:
- Cardiovascular: Chest pain (1% to 2%)
- Central nervous system: Fatigue (dose related; 6% to 8%), insomnia (2% to 3%), hypoesthesia (1% to 2%)
- Gastrointestinal: Diarrhea (dose related; 3% to 4%), nausea (2%), vomiting (1% to 2%)
- Neuromuscular & skeletal: Arthralgia, asthenia (dose related; ≤2%)
- Respiratory: Upper respiratory infection (5%), rhinitis (3% to 4%), sinusitis (dose related; 2%), dyspnea (1% to 2%)

General Dosage Range Dosage adjustment recommended in patients with renal impairment

Oral:

Adults: Initial: 2.5-5 mg once daily; Maintenance: 2.5-20 mg once daily

Elderly: Initial: 2.5 mg/day

Mechanism of Action Selective inhibitor of beta$_1$-adrenergic receptors; competitively blocks beta$_1$-receptors, with little or no effect on beta$_2$-receptors at doses ≤20 mg

Pharmacodynamics/Kinetics

Onset of Action 1-2 hours

Half-life Elimination Normal renal function: 9-12 hours; Cl_{cr} <40 mL/minute: 27-36 hours; Hepatic cirrhosis: 8-22 hours

Time to Peak 2-4 hours

Pregnancy Risk Factor C

Bisoprolol and Hydrochlorothiazide

(bis OH proe lol & hye droe klor oh THYE a zide)

Related Information

Bisoprolol *on page 240*

Hydrochlorothiazide *on page 854*

U.S. Brand Names Ziac®

Canadian Brand Names Ziac®

Pharmacologic Category Beta Blocker, Beta-1 Selective; Diuretic, Thiazide

Use Treatment of hypertension

Unlabeled/Investigational Use Treatment of hypertension in the pediatric patient

Local Anesthetic/Vasoconstrictor Precautions No information available to require special precautions

Effects on Dental Treatment Bisoprolol is a cardioselective beta-blocker. Local anesthetic with vasoconstrictor can be safely used in patients medicated with bisoprolol. Nonselective beta-blockers (ie, propranolol, nadolol) enhance the pressor response to epinephrine, resulting in hypertension and bradycardia; this has not been reported for bisoprolol. Many nonsteroidal anti-inflammatory drugs, such as ibuprofen and indomethacin, can reduce the hypotensive effect of beta-blockers after 3 or more weeks of therapy with the NSAID. Short-term NSAID use (ie, 3 days) requires no special precautions in patients taking beta-blockers.

Effects on Bleeding No information available to require special precautions

Adverse Effects See individual agents.

General Dosage Range Oral: *Adults:* Initial: Bisoprolol 2.5 mg and hydrochlorothiazide 6.25 mg once daily; Maintenance: Bisoprolol 2.5-20 mg and hydrochlorothiazide 6.25-12.5 mg once daily; Maximum dose (manufacturer recommended): Bisoprolol 20 mg and hydrochlorothiazide 12.5 mg once daily

Mechanism of Action See individual agents.

Pregnancy Risk Factor C

Bivalirudin (bye VAL i roo din)

Related Information

Cardiovascular Diseases *on page 1848*

U.S. Brand Names Angiomax®

Canadian Brand Names Angiomax®

Pharmacologic Category Anticoagulant, Thrombin Inhibitor

Use Anticoagulant used in conjunction with aspirin for patients with unstable angina undergoing percutaneous transluminal coronary angioplasty (PTCA) or percutaneous coronary intervention (PCI) with provisional glycoprotein IIb/IIIa inhibitor; anticoagulant used in conjunction with aspirin for patients undergoing PCI with (or at risk of) heparin-induced thrombocytopenia (HIT) / thrombosis syndrome (HITTS)

Unlabeled/Investigational Use Heparin-induced thrombocytopenia (HIT); ST-elevation myocardial infarction (STEMI) undergoing primary PCI

Local Anesthetic/Vasoconstrictor Precautions No information available to require special precautions

Effects on Dental Treatment Key adverse event(s) related to dental treatment: Bleeding is the major adverse effect of bivalirudin. Additional adverse effects are often related to idiosyncratic reactions, the frequency is difficult to estimate. Adverse reactions reported were generally less than those seen with heparin. See Effects on Bleeding.

Effects on Bleeding As with all anticoagulants, bleeding is the major adverse effect of bivalirudin. Hemorrhage may occur at virtually any site; risk is dependent on multiple variables including the intensity of anticoagulation and patient susceptibility. Medical consult is suggested. It is unlikely that ambulatory patients presenting for dental treatment will be receiving intravenous anticoagulant therapy.

Adverse Effects As with all anticoagulants, bleeding is the major adverse effect of bivalirudin. Hemorrhage may occur at virtually any site. Risk is dependent on multiple variables, including the intensity of anticoagulation, concurrent use of a glycoprotein IIb/IIIa inhibitor, and patient susceptibility. Additional adverse effects are often related to idiosyncratic reactions, and the frequency is difficult to estimate. Adverse reactions reported were generally less than those seen with heparin.

>10%:

- Cardiovascular: Hypotension (≤12%)
- Central nervous system: Pain (≤15%), headache (≤12%)
- Gastrointestinal: Nausea (≤15%)
- Hematologic: Minor hemorrhage (REPLACE-2 study: Protocol defined: 14%, compared to 26% with heparin; TIMI defined: 1%, compared to 3% with heparin)
- Neuromuscular & skeletal: Back pain (9% to 42%)

1% to 10%:

- Cardiovascular: Hypertension (6%), bradycardia (5%), angina (≤5%)
- Central nervous system: Insomnia (7%), anxiety (6%), fever (5%), nervousness (5%)
- Gastrointestinal: Vomiting (≤6%), dyspepsia (5%), abdominal pain (5%)
- Genitourinary: Urinary retention (4%)
- Hematologic: Major hemorrhage (Protocol defined: 2% to 4%, compared to 4% to 9% with heparin; REPLACE-2 Study: TIMI defined: 0.6%, compared to 0.9% with heparin), transfusion required (1% to 2%, compared to 2% to 6% with heparin)
- Local: Injection site pain (≤8%)
- Neuromuscular & skeletal: Pelvic pain (6%)

General Dosage Range Dosage adjustment recommend in patients with renal impairment

I.V.: *Adults:* Bolus: 0.75 mg/kg; may repeat at 0.3 mg/kg if necessary; Infusion: 1.75 mg/kg/hour for duration of procedure and up to 4 hours postprocedure if needed; after 4 hours may continue 0.2 mg/kg/minute for up to 20 hours if needed

Mechanism of Action Bivalirudin acts as a specific and reversible direct thrombin inhibitor; it binds to the catalytic and anionic exosite of both circulating and clot-bound thrombin. Catalytic binding site occupation functionally inhibits coagulant effects by preventing thrombin-mediated cleavage of fibrinogen to fibrin monomers, and activation of factors V, VIII, and XIII. Shows linear dose- and concentration-dependent prolongation of ACT, aPTT, PT, and TT.

Pharmacodynamics/Kinetics

Onset of Action Immediate

Duration of Action Coagulation times return to baseline ~1 hour following discontinuation of infusion

Half-life Elimination Normal renal function (Cl_{cr} ≥90 mL/minute): 25 minutes; Severe renal impairment (Cl_{cr} 10-29 mL/minute): 57 minutes; Dialysis-dependent patients (off dialysis): 3.5 hours

Pregnancy Risk Factor B

Bleomycin (blee oh MYE sin)

Canadian Brand Names Blenoxane®; Bleomycin Injection, USP

Pharmacologic Category Antineoplastic Agent, Antibiotic

Use Treatment of squamous cell carcinomas of the head and neck, penis, cervix, or vulva, testicular carcinoma, Hodgkin's lymphoma, and non-Hodgkin's lymphoma; sclerosing agent for malignant pleural effusion

Unlabeled/Investigational Use Treatment of ovarian germ cell tumors

Local Anesthetic/Vasoconstrictor Precautions No information available to require special precautions

Effects on Dental Treatment Key adverse event(s) related to dental treatment: Stomatitis and mucositis.

Effects on Bleeding Although significant myelosuppression with associated altered hemostasis has been reported for many chemotherapeutic agents, myelosuppression is not common with bleomycin and no specific precautions appear to be necessary.

Adverse Effects

>10%:

Dermatologic: Pain at the tumor site, phlebitis. About 50% of patients develop erythema, rash, striae, induration, hyperkeratosis, vesiculation, and peeling of the skin, particularly on the palmar and plantar surfaces of the hands and feet. Hyperpigmentation (50%), alopecia, nailbed changes may also occur. These effects appear dose related and reversible with discontinuation.

Gastrointestinal: Stomatitis and mucositis (30%), anorexia, weight loss

Respiratory: Tachypnea, rales, acute or chronic interstitial pneumonitis, and pulmonary fibrosis (5% to 10%); hypoxia and death (1%). Symptoms include cough, dyspnea, and bilateral pulmonary infiltrates. The pathogenesis is not certain, but may be due to damage of pulmonary, vascular, or connective tissue. Response to steroid therapy is variable and somewhat controversial.

Miscellaneous: Acute febrile reactions (25% to 50%)

1% to 10%:

Dermatologic: Skin thickening, diffuse scleroderma, onycholysis, pruritus

Miscellaneous: Anaphylactoid-like reactions (characterized by hypotension, confusion, fever, chills, and wheezing; onset may be immediate or delayed for several hours); idiosyncratic reactions (1% in lymphoma patients)

General Dosage Range Dosage adjustment recommended in patients with renal impairment

I.V.: *Adults:* Dosage varies greatly depending on indication

Intrapleural: *Adults:* 60 units as a single instillation

Mechanism of Action Inhibits synthesis of DNA; binds to DNA leading to single- and double-strand breaks; also inhibits (to a lesser degree) RNA and protein synthesis

Pharmacodynamics/Kinetics

Half-life Elimination Biphasic: Renal function dependent:

Normal renal function: Initial: 1.3 hours; Terminal: 9 hours

End-stage renal disease: Initial: 2 hours; Terminal: 30 hours

Time to Peak Serum: I.M.: Within 30 minutes

Pregnancy Risk Factor D

Bortezomib (bore TEZ oh mib)

U.S. Brand Names Velcade®

Canadian Brand Names Velcade®

Pharmacologic Category Antineoplastic Agent; Proteasome Inhibitor

Use Treatment of multiple myeloma; treatment of relapsed or refractory mantle cell lymphoma

Unlabeled/Investigational Use Treatment of Waldenström's macroglobulinemia, peripheral T-cell lymphoma, cutaneous T-Cell lymphomas (mycosis fungoides), systemic light-chain amyloidosis

Local Anesthetic/Vasoconstrictor Precautions No information available to require special precautions

Effects on Dental Treatment Key adverse event(s) related to dental treatment: Abnormal taste and stomatitis.

Effects on Bleeding Chemotherapy may result in significant myelosuppression, potentially including significant reduction in platelet counts and altered hemostasis. In patients who are under active treatment with these agents, medical consult is suggested.

Adverse Effects

>10%:

Cardiovascular: Edema (11% to 23%), cardiac disorder (treatment emergent: 15%), hypotension (13%; grades 3/4: 3%)

Central nervous system: Psychiatric disturbance (≤35%), fever (34%), dysesthesia (22%), headache (22%), insomnia (20%), dizziness (17%; excludes vertigo)

Dermatologic: Rash (18%)

Gastrointestinal: Nausea (55%), diarrhea (52%), constipation (41%), anorexia (36%), vomiting (33%), abdominal pain (15%), abnormal taste, dyspepsia

Hematologic: Thrombocytopenia (36%; grade 4: 5%; nadir: day 11; recovery: by day 21), anemia (29%; grade 4: <1%), neutropenia (17%; grade 4: 3%; nadir: day 11; recovery: by day 21)

Neuromuscular & skeletal: Weakness (64%; grades 3/4: 16%), peripheral neuropathy (39%; grade 3: 11%; grade 4: <1%), paresthesia (22%), arthralgia (17%), limb pain (15%), bone pain (14%), back pain (13%), myalgia (12%), muscle cramps (11%), rigors (≤11%)

Respiratory: Dyspnea (21%), cough (20%), respiratory tract infection (12% to 15%), nasopharyngitis (12%), pneumonia (12%)

Miscellaneous: Herpesvirus infections (12%)

1% to 10%:

Cardiovascular: Heart failure (5%; includes acute pulmonary edema, cardiac failure, congestive cardiac failure, cardiogenic shock, pulmonary edema)

Central nervous system: Anxiety (10%)

Endocrine & metabolic: Dehydration (10%), hypercalcemia (grade 4: 2%)

Hematologic: Bleeding events (≥grade 3: 4%)

Local: Injection site irritation (5%)

Frequency not defined (including postmarketing and/or case reports; limited to important or life-threatening): Acute diffuse infiltrative pulmonary disease, acute respiratory distress syndrome, alkaline phosphatase increased, amyloidosis, anaphylaxis, angina, angioedema, ascites, aspergillosis, atelectasis, atrial fibrillation, atrial flutter, AV block, bacteremia, bradycardia, cardiac amyloidosis, blurred vision, bronchitis, cardiac arrest, cardiac tamponade, cardiopulmonary arrest, cerebral hemorrhage, cerebrovascular accident, cholestasis, coma, confusion, conjunctival infection/irritation, cranial palsy, deep venous thrombosis, diplopia, disseminated intravascular coagulation (DIC), duodenitis (hemorrhagic), DVT, dysautonomia, dysphagia, encephalopathy, embolism, epistaxis, fecal impaction, fracture, gastritis (hemorrhagic), gastroenteritis, GGT increased, glomerular nephritis, hearing impairment, hematemesis, hematuria, hemoptysis, hemorrhagic cystitis, hepatic failure, hepatic hemorrhage, hepatitis, hepatocellular damage, herpes meningoencephalitis, hyperbilirubinemia, hyper-/hypoglycemia, hyper-/hypokalemia, hyper-/hyponatremia, hypersensitivity, hyperuricemia, hypocalcemia, hypoxia, ileus, immune complex hypersensitivity, inappropriate ADH secretion, injection site reaction, interstitial pneumonia, intestinal obstruction, intestinal perforation, intracerebral hemorrhage, ischemic colitis, ischemic stroke, laryngeal edema, left ventricular ejection fraction decreased, leukocytoclastic vasculitis, leukopenia, listeriosis, lymphopenia, melena, mental status change, MI, myocardial ischemia, neuralgia, neutropenic fever, ophthalmic herpes, oral candidiasis, pancreatitis, paralytic ileus, pericardial effusion, pericarditis, peritonitis, pleural effusion, pneumonitis, portal vein thrombosis, proliferative glomerular nephritis, pruritus, psychosis, pulmonary embolism, pulmonary hypertension, pulmonary infiltrate, QT_c prolongation, renal calculus, renal failure, respiratory failure, respiratory insufficiency, reversible posterior leukoencephalopathy syndrome (RPLS), seizure, septic shock, sepsis, sinus arrest, spinal cord compression, Stevens-Johnson syndrome, stomatitis, stroke (hemorrhagic), subarachnoid hemorrhage, subdural hematoma, suicidal ideation, Sweet's syndrome (acute febrile neutrophilic dermatosis), syncope, tachycardia, torsade de pointes, toxic epidermal necrolysis, toxoplasmosis, transaminases increased, transient ischemic attack, tumor lysis syndrome, urinary incontinence, urinary retention, urinary tract infection, urticaria, ventricular tachycardia

General Dosage Range Dosage adjustment recommended in patients with hepatic impairment or who develop toxicities.

I.V.: *Adults:* Dosage varies greatly depending on indication

Mechanism of Action Bortezomib inhibits proteasomes, enzyme complexes which regulate protein homeostasis within the cell. Specifically, it reversibly inhibits chymotrypsin-like activity at the 26S proteasome, leading to activation of signaling cascades, cell-cycle arrest, and apoptosis.

Pharmacodynamics/Kinetics

Half-life Elimination Single dose: 9-15 hours; multiple dosing: 1 mg/m^2: 40-193 hours; 1.3 mg/m^2: 76-108 hour

Pregnancy Risk Factor D

Bosentan (boe SEN tan)

U.S. Brand Names Tracleer®

Canadian Brand Names Tracleer®

Pharmacologic Category Endothelin Antagonist; Vasodilator

Use Treatment of pulmonary artery hypertension (PAH) (WHO Group I) in patients with World Health Organization (WHO) Class II, III, or IV symptoms to improve exercise capacity and decrease the rate of clinical deterioration

Local Anesthetic/Vasoconstrictor Precautions No information available to require special precautions

Effects on Dental Treatment Key adverse event(s) related to dental treatment: Endothelin antagonists have caused bleeding gums; there have been no specific reports for bosentan

Effects on Bleeding No information available to require special precautions

Adverse Effects

>10%:

Cardiovascular: Edema (11%)

Central nervous system: Headache (15%)

Endocrine & metabolic: Spermatogenesis inhibition (25%)

Hematologic: Hemoglobin decreased (≥1 g/dL in up to 57%; <11 g/dL: 3% to 6%; typically in first 6 weeks of therapy)

Hepatic: Transaminases increased (>3 times upper limit of normal; up to 12%; dose-related)

Respiratory: Respiratory tract infection (22%)

1% to 10%:

Cardiovascular: Chest pain (5%), syncope (5%), flushing (4%), hypotension (4%), palpitation (4%)

Dermatologic: Pruritus (2%)

Hematologic: Anemia (3%)

Hepatic: Abnormal hepatic function (4%)

Neuromuscular & skeletal: Arthralgia (4%)

Respiratory: Sinusitis (4%)

General Dosage Range Dosage adjustment recommended in patients with hepatic impairment or on concomitant therapy

Oral:

Children >12 years and Adults <40 kg: Initial: 62.5 mg twice daily; Maintenance: 62.5 mg twice daily

Children >12 years and Adults ≥40 kg: Initial: 62.5 mg twice daily; Maintenance: 125 mg twice daily

Mechanism of Action Blocks endothelin receptors on vascular endothelium and smooth muscle. Stimulation of these receptors is associated with vasoconstriction. Although bosentan blocks both ET_A and ET_B receptors, the affinity is higher for the A subtype.

Pharmacodynamics/Kinetics

Half-life Elimination 5 hours; prolonged with heart failure, possibly with PAH

Time to Peak Plasma: 3-5 hours

Pregnancy Risk Factor X

Prescribing and Access Restrictions As a requirement of the REMS program, access to this medication is restricted. Bosentan (Tracleer®) is only available through Tracleer® Access Program (T.A.P.). Only prescribers and pharmacies registered with T.A.P. may prescribe and dispense bosentan. Further information may be obtained from the manufacturer, Actelion Pharmaceuticals (1-866-228-3546).

Brimonidine (bri MOE ni deen)

U.S. Brand Names Alphagan® P

Canadian Brand Names Alphagan®; Apo-Brimonidine P®; Apo-Brimonidine®; PMS-Brimonidine Tartrate; ratio-Brimonidine; Sandoz-Brimonidine

Pharmacologic Category $Alpha_2$ Agonist, Ophthalmic; Ophthalmic Agent, Antiglaucoma

Use Lowering of intraocular pressure (IOP) in patients with open-angle glaucoma or ocular hypertension

Local Anesthetic/Vasoconstrictor Precautions No information available to require special precautions

Effects on Dental Treatment Key adverse event(s) related to dental treatment: Xerostomia (normal salivary flow resumes upon discontinuation).

Effects on Bleeding No information available to require special precautions

Adverse Effects Actual frequency of adverse reactions may be formulation dependent; percentages reported with Alphagan® P:

>10%:

Central nervous system: Somnolence (adults 1% to 4%; children 25% to 83%)

Ocular: Allergic conjunctivitis, conjunctival hyperemia, eye pruritus

1% to 10% (unless otherwise noted 1% to 4%):

Cardiovascular: Hypertension (5% to 9%), hypotension

Central nervous system: Alertness decreased (children), dizziness, fatigue, headache, insomnia

Dermatologic: Rash

Endocrine & metabolic: Hypercholesterolemia

Gastrointestinal: Xerostomia (5% to 9%), dyspepsia

Neuromuscular & skeletal: Weakness
Ocular: Burning sensation (5% to 9%), conjunctival folliculosis (5% to 9%), ocular allergic reaction (5% to 9%), visual disturbance (5% to 9%), blepharitis, blepharoconjunctivitis, blurred vision, cataract, conjunctival edema, conjunctival hemorrhage, conjunctivitis, dry eye, epiphora, eye discharge, eyelid disorder, eyelid edema, eyelid erythema, follicular conjunctivitis, foreign body sensation, irritation, keratitis, pain, photophobia, stinging, superficial punctate keratopathy, visual acuity worsened, visual field defect, vitreous detachment, vitreous floaters, watery eyes
Respiratory: Bronchitis, cough, dyspnea, pharyngitis, rhinitis, sinus infection, sinusitis
Miscellaneous: Allergic reaction, flu-like syndrome, infection

General Dosage Range Ophthalmic: *Children ≥2 years and Adults:* Instill 1 drop in affected eye(s) 3 times/day

Mechanism of Action Selective agonism for alpha$_2$-receptors; causes reduction of aqueous humor formation and increased uveoscleral outflow

Pharmacodynamics/Kinetics

Onset of Action Peak effect: 2 hours

Half-life Elimination ~2 hours

Time to Peak Plasma: 0.5-2.5 hours

Pregnancy Risk Factor B

Brinzolamide (brin ZOH la mide)

U.S. Brand Names Azopt®

Canadian Brand Names Azopt®

Pharmacologic Category Carbonic Anhydrase Inhibitor; Ophthalmic Agent, Antiglaucoma

Use Lowers intraocular pressure in patients with ocular hypertension or open-angle glaucoma

Local Anesthetic/Vasoconstrictor Precautions No information available to require special precautions

Effects on Dental Treatment Key adverse event(s) related to dental treatment: Taste disturbances.

Effects on Bleeding No information available to require special precautions

Adverse Effects 1% to 10%:
Dermatologic: Dermatitis (1% to 5%)
Gastrointestinal: Taste disturbances (5% to 10%)
Ocular: Blurred vision (5% to 10%), blepharitis (1% to 5%), dry eye (1% to 5%), foreign body sensation (1% to 5%), eye discharge (1% to 5%), eye pain (1% to 5%), itching of eye (1% to 5%)
Respiratory: Rhinitis (1% to 5%)

General Dosage Range Ophthalmic: *Adults:* Instill 1 drop in affected eye(s) 3 times/day

Mechanism of Action Brinzolamide inhibits carbonic anhydrase, leading to decreased aqueous humor secretion. This results in a reduction of intraocular pressure.

Pharmacodynamics/Kinetics

Onset of Action Peak effect: 2 hours

Duration of Action 8-12 hours

Pregnancy Risk Factor C

Brinzolamide and Timolol (brin ZOH la mide & TIM oh lol)

Related Information
Brinzolamide *on page 246*
Timolol (Ophthalmic) *on page 1633*

Canadian Brand Names Azarga™

Pharmacologic Category Beta-Adrenergic Blocker, Nonselective; Carbonic Anhydrase Inhibitor; Ophthalmic Agent, Antiglaucoma

Use Treatment of elevated intraocular pressure in patients with ocular hypertension or open-angle glaucoma

Local Anesthetic/Vasoconstrictor Precautions No information available to require special precautions

Effects on Dental Treatment Key adverse event(s) related to dental treatment: Taste perversion has been reported.

Effects on Bleeding No information available to require special precautions

Adverse Effects Percentages as reported with combination product. Also see individual agents.

1% to 10%:

Gastrointestinal: Taste perversion (2%)

Ocular: Blurred vision (6%), eye irritation (4%), eye pain (3%), foreign body sensation in eyes (1%)

General Dosage Range Ophthalmic: *Adults:* Instill 1 drop twice daily

Mechanism of Action

Brinzolamide inhibits carbonic anhydrase, leading to decreased aqueous humor secretion. This results in a reduction of intraocular pressure.

Timolol: Blocks both $beta_1$- and $beta_2$-adrenergic receptors, reduces intraocular pressure by reducing aqueous humor production or possibly outflow.

Product Availability Not available in U.S.

Bromazepam (broe MA ze pam)

Canadian Brand Names Apo-Bromazepam®; Lectopam®; Mylan-Bromazepam; Novo-Bromazepam; Nu-Bromazepam; PRO-Doc Limitee Bromazepam

Pharmacologic Category Benzodiazepine

Use Short-term, symptomatic treatment of anxiety

Local Anesthetic/Vasoconstrictor Precautions No information available to require special precautions

Effects on Dental Treatment Key adverse event(s) related to dental treatment: Xerostomia (normal salivary flow resumes upon discontinuation).

Effects on Bleeding No information available to require special precautions

Adverse Effects Frequency not defined.

Cardiovascular: Cardiac arrest, hypotension, palpitation, tachycardia

Central nervous system: Anterograde amnesia, ataxia, confusion, depression, dizziness, drowsiness, euphoria, headache, lethargy, physical and psychological dependence, seizure. In addition, paradoxical reactions (including aggression, agitation, excitation, hallucinations, nightmares, release of hostility, restlessness, and psychosis) are known to occur with benzodiazepines.

Dermatologic: Pruritus, rash

Endocrine & metabolic: Hyperglycemia, hypoglycemia, libido changes

Gastrointestinal: Gastritis (rare), nausea, vomiting, xerostomia

Genitourinary: Incontinence

Hematologic: Hemoglobin decreased, hematocrit decreased, WBCs increased/decreased

Hepatic: Transaminases increased, alkaline phosphatase increased, bilirubin increased

Neuromuscular & skeletal: Weakness, muscle spasm

Ocular: Blurred vision, diplopia

Respiratory: Respiratory depression

Miscellaneous: Allergic reactions including anaphylaxis have been reported with benzodiazepines

General Dosage Range Oral:

Adults: Initial: 6-18 mg/day in divided doses; Maintenance: 6-30 mg/day in divided doses

Elderly: Initial: 3 mg/day in divided doses

Mechanism of Action Binds to stereospecific benzodiazepine receptors on the postsynaptic GABA neuron at several sites within the central nervous system, including the limbic system, reticular formation. Enhancement of the inhibitory effect of GABA on neuronal excitability results by increased neuronal membrane permeability to chloride ions. This shift in chloride ions results in hyperpolarization (a less excitable state) and stabilization.

Pharmacodynamics/Kinetics

Half-life Elimination 20 hours

Time to Peak Serum: ≤2 hours (may be delayed by food)

Product Availability Not available in U.S.

Bromfenac (BROME fen ak)

U.S. Brand Names Bromday™; Xibrom® [DSC]

Pharmacologic Category Nonsteroidal Anti-inflammatory Drug (NSAID), Ophthalmic

Use Treatment of postoperative inflammation and reduction in ocular pain following cataract removal

Local Anesthetic/Vasoconstrictor Precautions No information available to require special precautions

Effects on Dental Treatment The dentist should be aware of the potential of abnormal coagulation. Caution should also be exercised in the use of NSAIDs in patients already on anticoagulant therapy with drugs such as warfarin (Coumadin®). See Effects on Bleeding.

Effects on Bleeding Nonselective NSAIDs are known to reversibly decrease platelet aggregation via mechanisms different than observed with aspirin. Platelet function is restored as the drug is eliminated from the body. Dental professionals should be aware that recommendations differ between dental and general surgery. NSAIDs should be avoided (if possible) in general surgery patients for 3-5 half-lives of the drug (usually 1-3 days) prior to surgery to reduce the risk of excessive bleeding. However, there is no scientific evidence to warrant discontinuance of NSAIDs prior to dental surgery. In medically complicated patients or extensive oral surgery, the decision to interrupt therapy must be based on the risk to benefit in an individual patient and a medical consult is suggested. Routine interruption of NSAID therapy for most dental procedures is not warranted. If therapy is continued without interruption, the clinician should anticipate the potential for slower clotting times.

Adverse Effects 2% to 7%:

Central nervous system: Headache

Ocular: Abnormal sensation, conjunctival hyperemia, iritis, irritation (burning/stinging), pain, pruritus, redness

General Dosage Range Ophthalmic: *Adults:*

Bromday™: Instill 1 drop into affected eye(s) once daily

Xibrom®: Instill 1 drop into affected eye(s) twice daily

Mechanism of Action Inhibits prostaglandin synthesis by decreasing the activity of the enzyme, cyclooxygenase, which results in decreased formation of prostaglandin precursors.

Pharmacodynamics/Kinetics

Half-life Elimination 0.5-4 hours (following oral administration)

Pregnancy Risk Factor C

Bromocriptine (broe moe KRIP teen)

U.S. Brand Names Cycloset®; Parlodel®; Parlodel® SnapTabs®

Canadian Brand Names Apo-Bromocriptine®; Dom-Bromocriptine; PMS-Bromocriptine

Pharmacologic Category Anti-Parkinson's Agent, Dopamine Agonist; Antidiabetic Agent, Dopamine Agonist; Ergot Derivative

Use Treatment of hyperprolactinemia associated with amenorrhea with or without galactorrhea, infertility, or hypogonadism; treatment of prolactin-secreting adenomas; treatment of acromegaly; treatment of Parkinson's disease

Cycloset®: Management of type 2 diabetes mellitus (noninsulin dependent, NIDDM) as an adjunct to diet and exercise

Unlabeled/Investigational Use Neuroleptic malignant syndrome

Local Anesthetic/Vasoconstrictor Precautions No information available to require special precautions

Effects on Dental Treatment Key adverse event(s) related to dental treatment: Orthostatic hypotension.

Effects on Bleeding No information available to require special precautions

Adverse Effects Note: Frequency of adverse effects may vary by dose and/or indication.

>10%:

- Central nervous system: Dizziness, fatigue, headache
- Gastrointestinal: Constipation, nausea
- Neuromuscular & skeletal: Weakness
- Respiratory: Rhinitis

1% to 10%:

- Cardiovascular: Hypotension (including postural/orthostatic), Raynaud's syndrome exacerbation, syncope
- Central nervous system: Drowsiness, fatigue, lightheadedness, somnolence
- Endocrine & metabolic: Hypoglycemia (4%; in combination with sulfonylureas or other antidiabetic agents: 7% to 9%)
- Gastrointestinal: Abdominal cramps, anorexia, diarrhea, dyspepsia, GI bleeding, vomiting, xerostomia
- Neuromuscular & skeletal: Digital vasospasm
- Ocular: Amblyopia
- Respiratory: Nasal congestion, sinusitis
- Miscellaneous: Infection, flu-like syndrome

General Dosage Range Oral:

Children 11-15 years: Initial: 1.25-2.5 mg daily; Maintenance: 2.5-10 mg/day

Children ≥16 years: Initial: 1.25-2.5 mg daily; Maintenance: 2.5-15 mg/day

Adults: Dosage varies greatly depending on indication

Mechanism of Action Semisynthetic ergot alkaloid derivative and a dopamine receptor agonist which activates postsynaptic dopamine receptors in the tuberoinfundibular (inhibiting pituitary prolactin secretion) and nigrostriatal pathways (enhancing coordinated motor control).

In the treatment of type 2 diabetes mellitus, the mechanism of action is unknown; however, bromocriptine is believed to affect circadian rhythms which are mediated, in part, by dopaminergic activity, and are believed to play a role in obesity and insulin resistance. It is postulated that bromocriptine (when administered during the morning and released into the systemic circulation in a rapid, "pulse-like" dose) may reset hypothalamic circadian activities which have been altered by obesity, thereby resulting in the reversal of insulin resistance and decreases in glucose production, without increasing serum insulin concentrations.

Pharmacodynamics/Kinetics

Onset of Action Parlodel®: Prolactin decreasing effect: 1-2 hours

Half-life Elimination Cycloset®: ~6 hours; Parlodel®: Biphasic: Terminal: 15 hours (range 8-20 hours)

Time to Peak Serum: Parlodel®: 1-3 hours; Cycloset®: 53 minutes

Pregnancy Risk Factor B

Brompheniramine (brome fen IR a meen)

U.S. Brand Names Bidhist [DSC]; Bromax; Lodrane® 24 [DSC]; LoHist-12; Respa®-BR [DSC]; TanaCof-XR [DSC]

Pharmacologic Category Alkylamine Derivative; Histamine H_1 Antagonist; Histamine H_1 Antagonist, First Generation

Use Symptomatic relief of perennial and seasonal allergic rhinitis, vasomotor rhinitis, and other respiratory allergies

Local Anesthetic/Vasoconstrictor Precautions No information available to require special precautions

Effects on Dental Treatment Key adverse event(s) related to dental treatment: Xerostomia (normal salivary flow resumes upon discontinuation). Chronic use of antihistamines will inhibit salivary flow, particularly in elderly patients; this may contribute to periodontal disease and oral discomfort.

Effects on Bleeding No information available to require special precautions

Adverse Effects Frequency not defined.

Cardiovascular: Angina, blood pressure increased, chest tightness, circulatory collapse, extrasystoles, hypotension, palpitation, tachycardia

Central nervous system: Anxiety, chills, confusion, coordination impaired, dizziness, drowsiness, euphoria, excitation, fatigue, headache, hysteria, insomnia, irritability, nervousness, neuritis, restlessness, sedation, seizure, stimulation, tension, vertigo

Dermatologic: Photosensitivity, rash, urticaria

Endocrine & metabolic: Early menses

Gastrointestinal: Abdominal cramps, anorexia, constipation, diarrhea, dry throat, epigastric distress, heartburn, nausea, vomiting, xerostomia

Genitourinary: Dysuria, polyuria, urinary retention

Hematologic: Agranulocytosis, hemolytic anemia, hypoplastic anemia, thrombocytopenia

Neuromuscular & skeletal: Paresthesia, tremor, weakness

Ocular: Blurred vision, diplopia, mydriasis

Otic: Labyrinthitis (acute), tinnitus

Respiratory: Dry nose, nasal congestion, thickening of bronchial secretions, wheezing

Miscellaneous: Anaphylactic shock, diaphoresis

General Dosage Range Oral:

Children 6-12 years:

Lodrane® 24: One capsule once daily

LoHist-12: One tablet every 12 hours (maximum: 2 tablets/day)

Children >12 years and Adults:

Bromax, Respa®-BR: One tablet twice daily

Lodrane® 24: 1-2 capsules once daily

LoHist-12: 1-2 tablets every 12 hours (maximum: 4 tablets/day)

Mechanism of Action Competes with histamine for H_1-receptor sites on effector cells

Pregnancy Risk Factor C

Brompheniramine and Pseudoephedrine
(brome fen IR a meen & soo doe e FED rin)

Related Information
Brompheniramine *on page* 249
Pseudoephedrine *on page* 1429

U.S. Brand Names Bromaline® [OTC]; Brotapp [OTC]

Pharmacologic Category Alkylamine Derivative; Alpha/Beta Agonist; Decongestant; Histamine H_1 Antagonist; Histamine H_1 Antagonist, First Generation

Use Temporary relief of symptoms associated with seasonal and perennial allergic rhinitis, the common cold, or sinusitis

Local Anesthetic/Vasoconstrictor Precautions Use with caution since pseudoephedrine is a sympathomimetic amine which could interact with epinephrine to cause a pressor response

Effects on Dental Treatment Key adverse event(s) related to dental treatment:
Brompheniramine: Prolonged use may decrease salivary flow.
Pseudoephedrine: Xerostomia (normal salivary flow resumes upon discontinuation).

Effects on Bleeding No information available to require special precautions

Adverse Effects Frequency not defined.
Cardiovascular: Arrhythmias, flushing, hypertension, pallor, palpitation, tachycardia
Central nervous system: Convulsions, CNS stimulation, dizziness, excitability (children; rare), giddiness, hallucinations, headache, insomnia, irritability, lassitude, nervousness, sedation
Gastrointestinal: Anorexia, diarrhea, dyspepsia, nausea, vomiting, xerostomia
Neuromuscular skeletal: Tremors, weakness
Ocular: Diplopia
Renal: Dysuria, polyuria, urinary retention (with BPH)
Respiratory: Respiratory difficulty

General Dosage Range
Oral: Liquid:
Children 6-11 years: Brompheniramine 2 mg/pseudoephedrine 30 mg every 6 hours (maximum: 4 doses/day)
Children ≥12 years and Adults: Brompheniramine 4 mg/pseudoephedrine 60 mg every 6 hours (maximum: 4 doses/day)

Mechanism of Action Brompheniramine maleate is an antihistamine with H_1-receptor activity; pseudoephedrine, a sympathomimetic amine and isomer of ephedrine, acts as a decongestant in respiratory tract mucous membranes with less vasoconstrictor action than ephedrine in normotensive individuals.

Pharmacodynamics/Kinetics
Time to Peak Brompheniramine (syrup): 5 hours

Pregnancy Risk Factor C

Budesonide (Systemic, Oral Inhalation) (byoo DES oh nide)

U.S. Brand Names Entocort® EC; Pulmicort Flexhaler®; Pulmicort Respules®

Canadian Brand Names Entocort®; Pulmicort®

Generic Availability (U.S.) Yes: Suspension for nebulization

Pharmacologic Category Corticosteroid, Inhalant (Oral); Corticosteroid, Systemic

Use
Nebulization: Maintenance and prophylactic treatment of asthma
Oral capsule: Treatment of active Crohn's disease (mild-to-moderate) involving the ileum and/or ascending colon; maintenance of remission (for up to 3 months) of Crohn's disease (mild-to-moderate) involving the ileum and/or ascending colon
Oral inhalation: Maintenance and prophylactic treatment of asthma; includes patients who require oral corticosteroids and those who may benefit from systemic dose reduction/elimination

Local Anesthetic/Vasoconstrictor Precautions No information available to require special precautions

Effects on Dental Treatment Key adverse event(s) related to dental treatment: Xerostomia (normal salivary flow resumes upon discontinuation), dry throat, abnormal taste, and herpes simplex. Localized infections with *Candida albicans* or *Aspergillus niger* have occurred frequently in the mouth and pharynx with repetitive use of oral inhaler of corticosteroids. These infections may require treatment with appropriate antifungal therapy or discontinuance of treatment with corticosteroid inhaler.

Effects on Bleeding No information available to require special precautions

Adverse Effects Reaction severity varies by dose and duration; not all adverse reactions have been reported with each dosage form.

>10%:

Central nervous system: Headache (≤21%)

Gastrointestinal: Nausea (≤11%)

Respiratory: Respiratory infection, rhinitis

Miscellaneous: Symptoms of HPA axis suppression and/or hypercorticism may occur in >10% of patients following administration of dosage forms which result in higher systemic exposure (ie, oral capsule), but may be less frequent than rates observed with comparator drugs (prednisolone). These symptoms may be rare (<1%) following administration via methods which result in lower exposures (topical).

1% to 10%:

Cardiovascular: Chest pain, edema, flushing, hypertension, palpitation, syncope, tachycardia

Central nervous system: Amnesia, dizziness, dysphonia, emotional lability, fatigue, fever, insomnia, malaise, migraine, nervousness, pain, sleep disorder, somnolence, vertigo

Dermatologic: Acne, alopecia, bruising, contact dermatitis, eczema, hirsutism, pruritus, pustular rash, rash, striae

Endocrine & metabolic: Adrenal insufficiency, hypokalemia, menstrual disorder

Gastrointestinal: Abdominal pain, anorexia, diarrhea, dyspepsia, flatulence, gastroenteritis (including viral), glossitis, intestinal obstruction, oral candidiasis, taste perversion, tongue edema, vomiting, weight gain, xerostomia

Genitourinary: Dysuria, hematuria, nocturia, pyuria

Hematologic: Cervical lymphadenopathy, leukocytosis, purpura

Hepatic: Alkaline phosphatase increased

Neuromuscular & skeletal: Arthralgia, back pain, fracture, hyperkinesis, hypertonia, myalgia, neck pain, paresthesia, weakness

Ocular: Conjunctivitis, eye infection

Otic: Earache, ear infection, external ear infection

Respiratory: Bronchitis, bronchospasm, cough, epistaxis, hoarseness, nasal congestion, nasal irritation, pharyngitis, sinusitis, stridor, throat irritation

Miscellaneous: Abscess, allergic reaction, C-reactive protein increased, erythrocyte sedimentation rate increased, fat distribution (moon face, buffalo hump); flu-like syndrome, herpes simplex, infection, moniliasis, viral infection, voice alteration

Dosage

Nebulization: Children 12 months to 8 years: Asthma: Pulmicort Respules®: Titrate to lowest effective dose once patient is stable; start at 0.25 mg/day or use as follows:

Previous therapy of bronchodilators alone: 0.5 mg/day administered as a single dose or divided twice daily (maximum daily dose: 0.5 mg)

Previous therapy of inhaled corticosteroids: 0.5 mg/day administered as a single dose or divided twice daily (maximum daily dose: 1 mg)

Previous therapy of oral corticosteroids: 1 mg/day administered as a single dose or divided twice daily (maximum daily dose: 1 mg)

NIH Asthma Guidelines (NIH, 2007):

Children 0-4 years:

"Low" dose: 0.25-0.5 mg/day

"Medium" dose: >0.5-1 mg/day

"High" dose: >1 mg/day

Children 5-11 years:

"Low" dose: 0.5 mg/day

"Medium" dose: 1 mg/day

"High" dose: 2 mg/day

Oral inhalation: Asthma:

Children ≥6 years:

Pulmicort Flexhaler™: Initial: 180 mcg twice daily (some patients may be initiated at 360 mcg twice daily); maximum: 360 mcg twice daily

NIH Asthma Guidelines (NIH, 2007) (administer in divided doses twice daily):

Children 5-11 years:

"Low" dose: 180-400 mcg/day

"Medium" dose: >400-800 mcg/day

"High" dose: >800 mcg/day

Children ≥12 years: Refer to adult dosing.

Pulmicort® Turbuhaler®: [CAN, not available in the U.S.]: Initial (during periods of severe asthma or when switching from oral corticosteroid therapy): 200-400 mcg daily in 2 divided doses; Maintenance: Individualized, lowest effective dose.

Adults:

Pulmicort Flexhaler™: Initial: 360 mcg twice daily (selected patients may be initiated at 180 mcg twice daily); maximum: 720 mcg twice daily

NIH Asthma Guidelines (NIH, 2007) (administer in divided doses twice daily):

"Low" dose: 180-600 mcg/day

"Medium" dose: >600-1200 mcg/day

"High" dose: >1200 mcg/day

Pulmicort® Turbuhaler® [CAN, not available in the U.S.]: Initial (during periods of severe asthma or when switching from oral corticosteroid therapy): 400-2400 mcg daily in 2-4 divided doses; Maintenance: 200-400 mcg twice daily (higher doses may be needed for short periods of time). **Note:** Patients taking 400 mcg/day may take as a single daily dose

Oral: Crohn's disease (active): Adults: 9 mg once daily in the morning for up to 8 weeks; recurring episodes may be treated with a repeat 8-week course of treatment

Note: Patients receiving CYP3A4 inhibitors should be monitored closely for signs and symptoms of hypercorticism; dosage reduction may be required. If switching from oral prednisolone, prednisolone dosage should be tapered while budesonide (Entocort™ EC) treatment is initiated.

Maintenance of remission: Following treatment of active disease (control of symptoms with CDAI <150), treatment may be continued at a dosage of 6 mg once daily for up to 3 months. If symptom control is maintained for 3 months, tapering of the dosage to complete cessation is recommended. Continued dosing beyond 3 months has not been demonstrated to result in substantial benefit.

Dosage adjustment in hepatic impairment: Monitor closely for signs and symptoms of hypercorticism; dosage reduction may be required.

Mechanism of Action Controls the rate of protein synthesis; depresses the migration of polymorphonuclear leukocytes, fibroblasts; reverses capillary permeability and lysosomal stabilization at the cellular level to prevent or control inflammation. Has potent glucocorticoid activity and weak mineralocorticoid activity.

Contraindications Hypersensitivity to budesonide or any component of the formulation; primary treatment of status asthmaticus, acute episodes of asthma; not for relief of acute bronchospasm

Canadian labeling: Additional contraindications (not in U.S. labeling): Moderate-to-severe bronchiectasis, pulmonary tuberculosis (active or quiescent), untreated respiratory infection (bacterial, fungal, or viral)

Warnings/Precautions May cause hypercorticism or suppression of hypothalamic-pituitary-adrenal (HPA) axis, particularly in younger children or in patients receiving high doses for prolonged periods. HPA axis suppression may lead to adrenal crisis. Withdrawal and discontinuation of a corticosteroid should be done slowly and carefully. Particular care is required when patients are transferred from systemic corticosteroids to inhaled products due to possible adrenal insufficiency or withdrawal from steroids, including an increase in allergic symptoms. Patients receiving >20 mg per day of prednisone (or equivalent) may be most susceptible. Fatalities have occurred due to adrenal insufficiency in asthmatic patients during and after transfer from systemic corticosteroids to aerosol steroids; aerosol steroids do not provide the systemic steroid needed to treat patients having trauma, surgery, or infections. Do not use this product to transfer patients directly from oral corticosteroid therapy.

Bronchospasm may occur with wheezing after inhalation; if this occurs stop steroid and treat with a fast-acting bronchodilator (eg, albuterol). Supplemental steroids (oral or parenteral) may be needed during stress or severe asthma attacks. Not to be used in status asthmaticus or for the relief of acute bronchospasm. Acute myopathy has been reported with high-dose corticosteroids, usually in patients with neuromuscular transmission disorders; may involve ocular and/or respiratory muscles; monitor creatine kinase; recovery may be delayed. Corticosteroid use may cause psychiatric disturbances, including depression, euphoria, insomnia, mood swings, and personality changes. Pre-existing psychiatric conditions may be exacerbated by corticosteroid use. Prolonged use of corticosteroids may also increase the incidence of secondary infection, mask acute infection (including fungal infections), prolong or exacerbate viral infections, or limit response to vaccines. Exposure to chickenpox should be avoided; corticosteroids should not be used to treat ocular herpes simplex. Corticosteroids should not be used for cerebral malaria or viral hepatitis. Close observation is required in patients with latent tuberculosis and/or TB reactivity; restrict use in active TB (only in conjunction with antituberculosis treatment). *Candida albicans* infections may occur in the mouth and pharynx; rinsing (and spitting) with water after inhaler use may decrease risk. Prolonged treatment with corticosteroids has been associated with the development of Kaposi's sarcoma (case reports); if noted, discontinuation of therapy should be considered.

Use with caution in patients with thyroid disease, hepatic impairment, renal impairment, cardiovascular disease, diabetes, glaucoma, cataracts, myasthenia gravis, patients at risk for osteoporosis, patients at risk for seizures, or GI diseases (diverticulitis, peptic ulcer, ulcerative colitis) due to perforation risk. Use caution following acute MI (corticosteroids have been associated with myocardial rupture). Because of the risk of adverse effects, systemic corticosteroids should be used cautiously in the elderly in the smallest possible effective dose for the shortest duration.

Orally-inhaled corticosteroids may cause a reduction in growth velocity in pediatric patients (~1 centimeter per year [range: 0.3-1.8 cm per year] and related to dose and duration of exposure). To minimize the systemic effects of orally-inhaled corticosteroids, each patient should be titrated to the lowest effective dose. Growth should be routinely monitored in pediatric patients. Withdraw systemic therapy with gradual tapering of dose. There have been reports of systemic corticosteroid withdrawal symptoms (eg, joint/muscle pain, lassitude, depression) when withdrawing oral inhalation therapy. Pulmicort Flexhaler™ contains lactose; very rare anaphylactic reactions have been reported in patients with severe milk protein allergy.

Drug Interactions

Metabolism/Transport Effects **Substrate** of CYP3A4 (major)

Avoid Concomitant Use

Avoid concomitant use of Budesonide (Systemic, Oral Inhalation) with any of the following: Aldesleukin; BCG; Grapefruit Juice; Natalizumab; Pimecrolimus; Roflumilast; Tacrolimus (Topical)

Increased Effect/Toxicity

Budesonide (Systemic, Oral Inhalation) may increase the levels/effects of: Amphotericin B; Deferasirox; Leflunomide; Loop Diuretics; Natalizumab; Thiazide Diuretics

The levels/effects of Budesonide (Systemic, Oral Inhalation) may be increased by: CYP3A4 Inhibitors (Moderate); CYP3A4 Inhibitors (Strong); Dasatinib; Denosumab; Grapefruit Juice; Pimecrolimus; Roflumilast; Tacrolimus (Topical); Trastuzumab

Decreased Effect

Budesonide (Systemic, Oral Inhalation) may decrease the levels/effects of: Aldesleukin; Antidiabetic Agents; BCG; Corticorelin; Sipuleucel-T; Vaccines (Inactivated)

The levels/effects of Budesonide (Systemic, Oral Inhalation) may be decreased by: Antacids; Bile Acid Sequestrants; Echinacea; Tocilizumab

Ethanol/Nutrition/Herb Interactions Food: Grapefruit juice may double systemic exposure of orally-administered budesonide. Administration of capsules with a high-fat meal delays peak concentration, but does not alter the extent of absorption.

Dietary Considerations Avoid grapefruit juice when using oral capsules.

Pharmacodynamics/Kinetics

Onset of Action Pulmicort Respules®: 2-8 days; Inhalation: 24 hours

Peak effect: Pulmicort Respules®: 4-6 weeks; Inhalation: 1-2 weeks

Half-life Elimination 2-3.6 hours

Time to Peak Capsule: 0.5-10 hours (variable in Crohn's disease); Pulmicort Respules®: 10-30 minutes; Inhalation: 1-2 hours

Pregnancy Risk Factor C (capsule)/B (inhalation)

Lactation Enters breast milk/use caution

Breast-Feeding Considerations Following use of the powder for oral inhalation, ~0.3% to 1% of the maternal dose was found in breast milk. The maximum concentration appeared within 45 minutes of dosing. Plasma budesonide levels obtained from infants ~90 minutes after breast-feeding (~140 minutes after maternal dose) were below the limit of quantification. Concentrations of budesonide in breast milk are expected to be higher following administration of oral capsules than after an inhaled dose.

Dosage Forms

Capsule, enteric coated, oral:

Entocort® EC: 3 mg

Powder, for oral inhalation:

Pulmicort Flexhaler®: 90 mcg/inhalation (165 mg); 180 mcg/inhalation (225 mg)

Suspension, for nebulization: 0.25 mg/2 mL (30s); 0.5 mg/2 mL (30s)

Pulmicort Respules®: 0.25 mg/2 mL (30s); 0.5 mg/2 mL (30s); 1 mg/2 mL (30s)

Dosage Forms: Canada

Powder for oral inhalation:

Pulmicort Turbuhaler®: 100 mcg/inhalation, 200 mcg/inhalation, 400 mcg/inhalation

Budesonide (Nasal) (byoo DES oh nide)

U.S. Brand Names Rhinocort Aqua®

Canadian Brand Names Gen-Budesonide AQ; Mylan-Budesonide AQ; Rhinocort® Aqua™; Rhinocort® Turbuhaler®

Generic Availability (U.S.) No

Pharmacologic Category Corticosteroid, Nasal

Use Management of symptoms of seasonal or perennial rhinitis

Canadian labeling: Additional use (not in U.S. labeling): Prevention and treatment of nasal polyps

Local Anesthetic/Vasoconstrictor Precautions No information available to require special precautions

Effects on Dental Treatment No significant effects or complications reported

Effects on Bleeding No information available to require special precautions

Adverse Effects 1% to 10%:

Respiratory: Epistaxis (8%), pharyngitis (4%), bronchospasm (2%), coughing (2%), nasal irritation (2%)

Miscellaneous: Although reported at higher rates with systemic administration, symptoms of HPA axis suppression and/or hypercorticism may occur rarely (<1%) following administration via methods which result in lower exposures (nasal).

Dosage Nasal inhalation:

U.S. labeling (Rhinocort® Aqua®): Rhinitis: Children ≥6 years and Adults: 64 mcg/day as a single 32 mcg spray in each nostril. Some patients who do not achieve adequate control may benefit from increased dosage. A reduced dosage may be effective after initial control is achieved.

Maximum dose: Children <12 years: 128 mcg/day; Adults: 256 mcg/day

Canadian labeling:

Rhinocort® Aqua®: Children ≥6 years and Adults:

Nasal polyps: 256 mcg/day administered as a single 64 mcg spray in each nostril twice daily

Rhinitis: Initial: 256 mcg/day administered as two 64 mcg sprays in each nostril once daily or a single 64 mcg spray in each nostril twice daily; Maintenance: Individualize, lowest effective dose

Maximum dose: 256 mcg/day

Rhinocort® Turbuhaler®: Children ≥6 years and Adults:

Nasal polyps: 100 mcg into each nostril twice daily (maximum: 400 mcg/day)

Rhinitis: Initial: 200 mcg into each nostril once daily; Maintenance: Individualize, lowest effective dose (maximum: 400 mcg/day)

Mechanism of Action Controls the rate of protein synthesis; depresses the migration of polymorphonuclear leukocytes, fibroblasts; reverses capillary permeability and lysosomal stabilization at the cellular level to prevent or control inflammation. Has potent glucocorticoid activity and weak mineralocorticoid activity.

Contraindications Hypersensitivity to budesonide or any component of the formulation

Canadian labeling: Additional contraindications (not in U.S. labeling): Pulmonary tuberculosis (active or quiescent), untreated respiratory infection (bacterial, fungal, or viral); use in patients <6 years of age

Warnings/Precautions May delay wound healing; avoid nasal corticosteroid use in patients with recent nasal septal ulcers, nasal surgery or nasal trauma until healing has occurred. Localized *Candida albicans* infections of the nose and/or pharynx may occur (rarely). Prolonged use of corticosteroids may also increase the incidence of secondary infection, mask acute infection (including fungal infections), prolong or exacerbate viral infections, or limit response to vaccines. Exposure to chickenpox should be avoided. Close observation is required in patients with latent tuberculosis and/or TB reactivity restrict use in active TB (only in conjunction with antituberculosis treatment).

Intranasal corticosteroids may cause a reduction in growth velocity in pediatric patients (~1 centimeter per year [range 0.3-1.8 cm per year] and related to dose and duration of exposure). To minimize the systemic effects of orally-inhaled and intranasal corticosteroids, each patient should be titrated to the lowest effective dose. Growth should be routinely monitored in pediatric patients.

Drug Interactions

Metabolism/Transport Effects **Substrate** of CYP3A4 (major)

Avoid Concomitant Use There are no known interactions where it is recommended to avoid concomitant use.

Increased Effect/Toxicity

Budesonide (Nasal) may increase the levels/effects of: Deferasirox

The levels/effects of Budesonide (Nasal) may be increased by: CYP3A4 Inhibitors (Strong)

Decreased Effect

Budesonide (Nasal) may decrease the levels/effects of: Corticorelin

The levels/effects of Budesonide (Nasal) may be decreased by: Tocilizumab

Pharmacodynamics/Kinetics

Onset of Action Rhinocort® Aqua®: ~10 hours

Peak effect: Rhinocort® Aqua®: ~2 weeks

Half-life Elimination 2-3.6 hours

Time to Peak Nasal: 1 hour

Pregnancy Risk Factor B

Lactation Enters breast milk/use caution

Breast-Feeding Considerations Following use of the powder for oral inhalation, ~0.3% to 1% of the maternal dose was found in breast milk. The maximum concentration appeared within 45 minutes of dosing. Plasma budesonide levels obtained from infants ~90 minutes after breast-feeding (~140 minutes after maternal dose) were below the limit of quantification. Concentrations of budesonide in breast milk are expected to be higher following administration of oral capsules than after an inhaled dose.

Dosage Forms

Suspension, intranasal:

Rhinocort Aqua®: 32 mcg/inhalation (8.6 g)

Dosage Forms: Canada

Powder for nasal inhalation:

Rhinocort® Turbuhaler®: 100 mcg/inhalation

Suspension, intranasal [spray]:

Rhinocort® Aqua®: 64 mcg/inhalation

Bumetanide (byoo MET a nide)

Related Information

Cardiovascular Diseases *on page 1848*

Canadian Brand Names Burinex®

Pharmacologic Category Diuretic, Loop

Use Management of edema secondary to heart failure or hepatic or renal disease (including nephrotic syndrome)

Unlabeled/Investigational Use Treatment of hypertension

Local Anesthetic/Vasoconstrictor Precautions No information available to require special precautions

Effects on Dental Treatment No significant effects or complications reported

Effects on Bleeding No information available to require special precautions

Adverse Effects

>10%:

Endocrine & metabolic: Hyperuricemia (18%), hypochloremia (15%), hypokalemia (15%)

Renal: Azotemia (11%)

1% to 10%:

Central nervous system: Dizziness (1%)

Endocrine & metabolic: Hyponatremia (9%), hyperglycemia (7%), phosphorus altered (5%), CO_2 content altered (4%), bicarbonate altered (3%), calcium altered (2%)

Neuromuscular & skeletal: Muscle cramps (1%)

Renal: Serum creatinine increased (7%)

Miscellaneous: LDH altered (1%)

General Dosage Range

I.M., I.V.:

Infants and children: 0.015-0.1 mg/kg/dose every 6-24 hours (maximum: 10 mg/day)

Adults: 0.5-1 mg/dose; may repeat in 2-3 hours for up to 2 doses (maximum: 10 mg/day)

Oral:

Infants and children: 0.015-0.1 mg/kg/dose every 6-24 hours (maximum: 10 mg/day)

Adults: 0.5-2 mg 1-2 times/day; may repeat in 4-5 hours for up to 2 doses (maximum: 10 mg/day)

Mechanism of Action Inhibits reabsorption of sodium and chloride in the ascending loop of Henle and proximal renal tubule, interfering with the chloride-binding cotransport system, thus causing increased excretion of water, sodium, chloride, magnesium, phosphate, and calcium; it does not appear to act on the distal tubule

Pharmacodynamics/Kinetics

Onset of Action Oral, I.M.: 0.5-1 hour; I.V.: 2-3 minutes

Peak effect: Oral: 1-2 hours; I.V.: 15-30 minutes

Duration of Action 4-6 hours

Half-life Elimination Neonates: ~6 hours; Infants (1 month): ~2.4 hours; Adults: 1-1.5 hours

Pregnancy Risk Factor C

Bupivacaine (byoo PIV a kane)

Related Information

Oral Pain *on page 1928*

U.S. Brand Names Bupivacaine Spinal; Marcaine®; Marcaine® Spinal; Sensorcaine®; Sensorcaine®-MPF; Sensorcaine®-MPF Spinal

Canadian Brand Names Marcaine®; Sensorcaine®

Pharmacologic Category Local Anesthetic

Use Local or regional anesthesia; spinal anesthesia; diagnostic and therapeutic procedures; obstetrical procedures (only 0.25% and 0.5% concentrations)

0.25%: Local infiltration, peripheral nerve block, sympathetic block, caudal or epidural block

0.5%: Peripheral nerve block, caudal and epidural block

0.75% **(not for obstetrical anesthesia)**: Retrobulbar block, epidural block. **Note:** Reserve for surgical procedures where a high degree of muscle relaxation and prolonged effect are necessary

Local Anesthetic/Vasoconstrictor Precautions No information available to require special precautions

Effects on Dental Treatment No significant effects or complications reported

Effects on Bleeding No information available to require special precautions

Adverse Effects Note: Incidence of adverse reactions is difficult to define. Most effects are dose related, and are often due to accelerated absorption from the injection site, unintentional intravascular injection, or slow metabolic degradation. The development of any central nervous system symptoms may be an early indication of more significant toxicity (seizure).

Cardiovascular: Hypotension, bradycardia, palpitation, heart block, ventricular arrhythmia, cardiac arrest

Central nervous system: Restlessness, anxiety, dizziness, seizure (0.1%); rare symptoms (usually associated with unintentional subarachnoid injection during high spinal anesthesia) include persistent anesthesia, paresthesia, paralysis, headache, septic meningitis, and cranial nerve palsies

Gastrointestinal: Nausea, vomiting; rare symptoms (usually associated with unintentional subarachnoid injection during high spinal anesthesia) include fecal incontinence and loss of sphincter control

Genitourinary: Rare symptoms (usually associated with unintentional subarachnoid injection during high spinal anesthesia) include urinary incontinence, loss of perineal sensation, and loss of sexual function

Neuromuscular & skeletal: Chondrolysis (continuous intra-articular administration), weakness

Ocular: Blurred vision, pupillary constriction

Otic: Tinnitus

Respiratory: Apnea, hypoventilation (usually associated with unintentional subarachnoid injection during high spinal anesthesia)

Miscellaneous: Allergic reactions (urticaria, pruritus, angioedema), anaphylactoid reactions

General Dosage Range

Caudal block: *Children >12 years and Adults:* 15-30 mL of 0.25% or 0.5%

Epidural block: *Children >12 years and Adults:* 10-20 mL of 0.25% or 0.5% in 3-5 mL increments **or** 10-20 mL of 0.75% if high degree of muscle relaxation and prolonged effects needed

Infiltration (local): *Children >12 years and Adults:* 0.25% (maximum: 175 mg)

Nerve block: *Children >12 years and Adults:*

Peripheral: 5 mL of 0.25% or 0.5% (maximum: 400 mg/day)

Sympathetic: 20-50 mL of 0.25%

Retrobulbar anesthesia: *Children >12 years and Adults:* 2-4 mL of 0.75%

Spinal: *Adults:* Preservative free solution of 0.75% bupivacaine in 8.25% dextrose:

Cesarean section: 1-1.4 mL

Lower abdominal procedures: 1.6 mL

Lower extremity and perineal procedures: 1 mL

Normal vaginal delivery: 0.8 mL (higher doses may be required in some patients)

Mechanism of Action Blocks both the initiation and conduction of nerve impulses by decreasing the neuronal membrane's permeability to sodium ions, which results in inhibition of depolarization with resultant blockade of conduction

Pharmacodynamics/Kinetics

Onset of Action Anesthesia (route and dose dependent): 1-17 minutes

Duration of Action Route and dose dependent: 2-9 hours

Half-life Elimination Age dependent: Neonates: 8.1 hours; Adults: 2.7 hours

Time to Peak Plasma: Caudal, epidural, or peripheral nerve block: 30-45 minutes

Pregnancy Risk Factor C

Bupivacaine and Epinephrine (byoo PIV a kane & ep i NEF rin)

Related Information

Bupivacaine *on page 256*

EPINEPHrine (Systemic, Oral Inhalation) *on page 604*

Oral Pain *on page 1928*

U.S. Brand Names Marcaine® with Epinephrine; Sensorcaine® with Epinephrine; Sensorcaine®-MPF with Epinephrine; Vivacaine™

Canadian Brand Names Sensorcaine® with Epinephrine

Generic Availability (U.S.) Yes

Pharmacologic Category Local Anesthetic

Dental Use Local anesthesia

Use Local anesthetic (injectable) for peripheral nerve block, infiltration, sympathetic block, caudal or epidural block, retrobulbar block

Local Anesthetic/Vasoconstrictor Precautions No information available to require special precautions

Effects on Dental Treatment It is common to misinterpret psychogenic responses to local anesthetic injection as an allergic reaction. Intraoral injections are perceived by many patients as a stressful procedure in dentistry. Common symptoms to this stress are diaphoresis, palpitations, and hyperventilation. Patients may exhibit hypersensitivity to bisulfites contained in local anesthetic solution to prevent oxidation of epinephrine. In general, patients reacting to bisulfites have a history of asthma and their airways are hyper-reactive to asthmatic syndrome.

Degree of adverse effects in the CNS and cardiovascular system is directly related to the blood levels of bupivacaine: Bradycardia, hypersensitivity reactions (rare; may be manifest as dermatologic reactions and edema at injection site), asthmatic syndromes.

High blood levels: Anxiety, restlessness, disorientation, confusion, dizziness, tremors, seizures, CNS depression (resulting in somnolence, unconsciousness and possible respiratory arrest), nausea, and vomiting.

Effects on Bleeding No information available to require special precautions

Adverse Effects See individual agents.

Dental Usual Dosage

Infiltration and nerve block in maxillary and mandibular area: Children >12 years and Adults: 9 mg (1.8 mL) of bupivacaine as a 0.5% solution with epinephrine 1:200,000 per injection site. A second dose may be administered if necessary to produce adequate anesthesia after allowing up to 10 minutes for onset. Up to a maximum of 90 mg of bupivacaine hydrochloride per dental appointment. The effective anesthetic dose varies with procedure, intensity of anesthesia needed, duration of anesthesia required, and physical condition of the patient; always use the lowest effective dose along with careful aspiration.

The following numbers of dental carpules (1.8 mL) provide the indicated amounts of bupivacaine hydrochloride 0.5% and vasoconstrictor (epinephrine 1:200,000). See table.

# of Cartridges (1.8 mL)	mg Bupivacaine (0.5%)	mg Vasoconstrictor (Epinephrine 1:200,000)
1	9	0.009
2	18	0.018
3	27	0.027
4	36	0.036
5	45	0.045
6	54	0.054
7	63	0.063
8	72	0.072
9	81	0.081
10	90	0.090

Note: Adult and children doses of bupivacaine hydrochloride with epinephrine cited from USP Dispensing Information (USP DI), 17th ed, The United States Pharmacopeial Convention, Inc, Rockville, MD, 1997, 134.

Dosage Dose varies with procedure, depth of anesthesia, vascularity of tissues, duration of anesthesia, and condition of patient. Do not use solutions containing preservatives for caudal or epidural block.

Children >12 years and Adults:

Caudal block (preservative free): 15-30 mL of 0.25% or 0.5%

Epidural block (other than caudal block, preservative free): 10-20 mL of 0.25% or 0.5%. Administer in 3-5 mL increments, allowing sufficient time to detect toxic manifestations of inadvertent I.V. or I.T. administration.

Surgical procedures requiring a high degree of muscle relaxation and prolonged effects only: 10-20 mL of 0.75% (**Note:** Not to be used in obstetrical cases)

Local anesthesia: Infiltration: 0.25% infiltrated locally (maximum: 175 mg of bupivacaine)

Peripheral nerve block: 5 mL of 0.25% or 0.5% (maximum: 400 mg/day of bupivacaine)

Retrobulbar anesthesia: 2-4 mL of 0.75%

Sympathetic nerve block: 20-50 mL of 0.25%

Infiltration and nerve block in maxillary and mandibular area: 9 mg (1.8 mL) of bupivacaine as a 0.5% solution with epinephrine 1:200,000 per injection site. A second dose may be administered if necessary to produce adequate anesthesia after allowing up to 10 minutes for onset. Up to a maximum of 90 mg of bupivacaine hydrochloride per dental appointment. The effective anesthetic dose varies with procedure, intensity of anesthesia needed, duration of anesthesia required, and physical condition of the patient; always use the lowest effective dose along with careful aspiration.

Note: Adult and children doses of bupivacaine hydrochloride with epinephrine cited from USP Dispensing Information (USP DI), 17th ed, The United States Pharmacopeial Convention, Inc, Rockville, MD, 1997, 134.

Mechanism of Action Local anesthetics bind selectively to the intracellular surface of sodium channels to block influx of sodium into the axon. As a result, depolarization necessary for action potential propagation and subsequent nerve function is prevented. The block at the sodium channel is reversible. When drug diffuses away from the axon, sodium channel function is restored and nerve propagation returns.

Epinephrine prolongs the duration of the anesthetic actions of bupivacaine by causing vasoconstriction (alpha-adrenergic receptor agonist) of the vasculature surrounding the nerve axons. This prevents the diffusion of bupivacaine away from the nerves resulting in a longer retention in the axon

Contraindications Hypersensitivity to bupivacaine, epinephrine, amide-type local anesthetics, or any component of the formulation

Warnings/Precautions Some commercially available formulations contain sodium metabisulfite, which may cause allergic-type reactions. Do not use solutions containing preservatives for caudal or epidural block. Intravascular injections should be avoided. Local anesthetics have been associated with rare occurrences of sudden respiratory arrest. Convulsions due to systemic toxicity leading to cardiac arrest have also been reported, presumably following unintentional intravascular injection. **[U.S. Boxed Warning]: The 0.75% is not recommended for obstetrical anesthesia.** A test dose is recommended prior to epidural administration and all reinforcing doses with continuous catheter technique. Use caution with cardiovascular dysfunction, hepatic impairment, or patients with compromised blood supply.

Use caution in debilitated, elderly, or acutely ill patients; dose reduction may be required. Dental practitioners and/or clinicians using local anesthetic agents should be well trained in diagnosis and management of emergencies that may arise from the use of these agents. Resuscitative equipment, oxygen, and other resuscitative drugs should be available for immediate use. Not recommended for use in children <12 years of age.

Continuous intra-articular infusion of local anesthetics after arthroscopic or other surgical procedures is **not** an approved use; chondrolysis (primarily shoulder joint) has occurred following infusion, with some requiring arthroplasty or shoulder replacement.

Drug Interactions

Metabolism/Transport Effects Bupivacaine: **Substrate** (minor) of CYP1A2, 2C19, 2D6, 3A4

Avoid Concomitant Use

Avoid concomitant use of Bupivacaine and Epinephrine with any of the following: Iobenguane I 123; Lurasidone

Increased Effect/Toxicity

Bupivacaine and Epinephrine may increase the levels/effects of: Bromocriptine; Lurasidone; Sympathomimetics

The levels/effects of Bupivacaine and Epinephrine may be increased by: Antacids; Atomoxetine; Beta-Blockers; Cannabinoids; Carbonic Anhydrase Inhibitors; COMT Inhibitors; Conivaptan; Inhalational Anesthetics; MAO Inhibitors; Serotonin/Norepinephrine Reuptake Inhibitors; Tricyclic Antidepressants

Decreased Effect

Bupivacaine and Epinephrine may decrease the levels/effects of: Benzylpenicilloyl Polylysine; Iobenguane I 123

The levels/effects of Bupivacaine and Epinephrine may be decreased by: Peginterferon Alfa-2b; Spironolactone; Tocilizumab

Pregnancy Risk Factor C

Lactation Enters breast milk/not recommended

Dosage Forms

Injection, solution [preservative free]: Bupivacaine 0.25% and epinephrine 1:200,000 (10 mL, 30 mL); bupivacaine 0.5% and epinephrine 1:200,000 (10 mL, 30 mL)

Marcaine® with Epinephrine: Bupivacaine 0.25% and epinephrine 1:200,000 (10 mL, 30 mL); bupivacaine 0.5% and epinephrine 1:200,000 (10 mL, 30 mL)

Sensorcaine® MPF with Epinephrine: Bupivacaine 0.25% and epinephrine 1:200,000 (10 mL, 30 mL); bupivacaine 0.5% and epinephrine 1:200,000 (10 mL, 30 mL); bupivacaine 0.75% and epinephrine 1:200,000 (30 mL)

Injection, solution: Bupivacaine 0.25% and epinephrine 1:200,000 (50 mL); bupivacaine 0.5% and epinephrine 1:200,000 (50 mL)

Marcaine® with Epinephrine, Sensorcaine® with Epinephrine: Bupivacaine 0.25% and epinephrine 1:200,000 (50 mL); bupivacaine 0.5% and epinephrine 1:200,000 (50 mL)

Injection, solution [for dental use]:

Marcaine® with Epinephrine, Vivacaine™: Bupivacaine 0.5% and epinephrine 1:200,000 (1.8 mL)

Dental Comment Oral paresthesia: The occurrence of oral paresthesia associated with 4% solutions of prilocaine or articaine, although rare, continue to be slightly more frequent than other local anesthetics. From 1999-2008, there were 182 cases of nonsurgical paresthesia (Gaffen, 2009). Of the cases, 172 involved mandibular block injection only. Another eight cases involved mandibular block combined with at least one other type of anesthetic injection. A single case involved infiltration around tooth number 35 and the final case involved infiltration and intraligamentary injection in the maxillary anterior region.

A 2010 report, reviewed adverse events submitted voluntarily over a 10-year period involving the dental local anesthetics articaine, bupivacaine, lidocaine, mepivacaine, and prilocaine in the United States. Bupivacaine reported incidence: One case per 124,286,050 cartridges sold. The reported incidence of paresthesia was one case for 13,800,970 cartridges of all local anesthetics sold in the U.S. (Garisto, 2010).

References

Ayoub ST and Coleman AE, "A Review of Local Anesthetics," *Gen Dent*, 1992, 40(4):285-7, 289-90.

Budenz AW, "Local Anesthetics in Dentistry: Then and Now," *J Calif Dent Assoc*, 2003, 31(5):388-96.

Dower JS Jr, "A Review of Paresthesia in Association With Administration of Local Anesthesia," *Dent Today*, 2003, 22(2):64-9.

Finder RL and Moore PA, "Adverse Drug Reactions to Local Anesthesia," *Dent Clin North Am*, 2002, 46 (4):747-57, x.

Gaffen AS and Haas DA, "Retrospective Review of Voluntary Reports of Nonsurgical Paresthesia in Dentistry," *J Can Dent Assoc*, 2009, 75(8):579.

Garisto GA, Gaffen AS, Lawrence HP, et al, "Occurrence of Paresthesia After Dental Local Anesthetic Administration in the United States," *J Am Dent Assoc*, 2010, 141(7):836-44.

Haas DA, "An Update on Local Anesthetics in Dentistry," *J Can Dent Assoc*, 2002, 68(9):546-51.

Hawkins JM and Moore PA, "Local Anesthesia: Advances in Agents and Techniques," *Dent Clin North Am*, 2002, 46(4):719-32, ix.
"Injectable Local Anesthetics," *J Am Dent Assoc*, 2003, 134(5):628-9.
Jastak JT and Yagiela JA, "Vasoconstrictors and Local Anesthesia: A Review and Rationale for Use," *J Am Dent Assoc*, 1983, 107(4):623-30.
MacKenzie TA and Young ER, "Local Anesthetic Update," *Anesth Prog*, 1993, 40(2):29-34.
Malamed SF, "Allergy and Toxic Reactions to Local Anesthetics," *Dent Today*, 2003, 22(4):114-6, 118-21.
Wahl MJ, Schmitt MM, Overton DA, et al, "Injection Pain of Bupivacaine With Epinephrine vs. Prilocaine Plain," *J Am Dent Assoc*, 2002, 133(12):1652-6.
Wynn RL, "Epinephrine Interactions With Beta-Blockers," *Gen Dent*, 1994, 42(1):16, 18.
Yagiela JA, "Local Anesthetics," *Anesth Prog*, 1991, 38(4-5):128-41.

Buprenorphine (byoo pre NOR feen)

U.S. Brand Names Buprenex®; Butrans™; Subutex®
Canadian Brand Names Buprenex®; Subutex®
Generic Availability (U.S.) Yes: Excludes patch
Pharmacologic Category Analgesic, Opioid; Analgesic, Opioid Partial Agonist
Use
Injection: Management of moderate-to-severe pain
Sublingual tablet: Treatment of opioid dependence
Transdermal patch: Management of moderate-to-severe chronic pain in patients requiring an around-the-clock opioid analgesic for an extended period of time
Unlabeled/Investigational Use Injection: Management of opioid withdrawal in heroin-dependent hospitalized patients
Local Anesthetic/Vasoconstrictor Precautions No information available to require special precautions
Effects on Dental Treatment No significant effects or complications reported
Effects on Bleeding No information available to require special precautions
Adverse Effects

Injection:
>10%: Central nervous system: Sedation
1% to 10%:
Cardiovascular: Hypotension
Central nervous system: Respiratory depression, dizziness, headache
Gastrointestinal: Vomiting, nausea
Ocular: Miosis
Otic: Vertigo
Miscellaneous: Diaphoresis

Tablet:
>10%:
Central nervous system: Headache (30%), pain (24%), insomnia (21% to 25%), anxiety (12%), depression (11%)
Gastrointestinal: Nausea (10% to 14%), abdominal pain (12%), constipation (8% to 11%)
Neuromuscular & skeletal: Back pain (14%), weakness (14%)
Respiratory: Rhinitis (11%)
Miscellaneous: Withdrawal syndrome (19%; placebo 37%), infection (12% to 20%), diaphoresis (12% to 13%)
1% to 10%:
Central nervous system: Chills (6%), nervousness (6%), somnolence (5%), dizziness (4%), fever (3%)
Gastrointestinal: Vomiting (5% to 8%), diarrhea (5%), dyspepsia (3%)
Ocular: Lacrimation (5%)
Respiratory: Cough (4%), pharyngitis (4%)
Miscellaneous: Flu-like syndrome (6%)

Transdermal patch:
>10%:
Central nervous system: Headache (16%), dizziness (16%), somnolence (14%),
Gastrointestinal: Nausea (23%), constipation (14%), vomiting (11%)
Local: Application site pruritus (15%)
1% to 10%:
Cardiovascular: Peripheral edema (7%), chest pain, hypertension
Central nervous system: Fatigue (5%), insomnia (3%), hypoesthesia (2%), anxiety, depression, fever, migraine
Dermatologic: Pruritus (4%), rash (2%)
Gastrointestinal: Xerostomia (7%), diarrhea (3%), abdominal discomfort (2%), anorexia (2%), upper abdominal pain
Genitourinary: Urinary tract infection (3%)
Local: Application site erythema (7%); application site rash (6%), application site irritation

Neuromuscular & skeletal: Pain in extremity (3%), back pain (3%), joint swelling (3%), paresthesia (2%), tremor (2%), muscles spasms, musculoskeletal pain, myalgia, neck pain, weakness

Respiratory: Dyspnea (3%), bronchitis, cough, nasopharyngitis, pharyngolaryngeal pain, sinusitis, upper respiratory tract infection

Miscellaneous: Hyperhydrosis (4%), fall (4%), flu-like syndrome

Dosage

I.M., I.V.: Acute pain (moderate-to-severe): **Note: Long-term use is not recommended.** The following recommendations are guidelines and do not represent the maximum doses that may be required in all patients. Doses should be titrated to pain relief/prevention. In high-risk patients (eg, elderly, debilitated, presence of respiratory disease) and/or concurrent CNS depressant use, reduce dose by one-half. Buprenorphine has an analgesic ceiling.

Children 2-12 years: I.M., slow I.V.: 2-6 mcg/kg every 4-6 hours

Children ≥13 years and Adults:

I.M.: Initial: Opiate-naive: 0.3 mg every 6-8 hours as needed; initial dose (up to 0.3 mg) may be repeated once in 30-60 minutes after the initial dose if needed; usual dosage range: 0.15-0.6 mg every 4-8 hours as needed

Slow I.V.: Initial: Opiate-naive: 0.3 mg every 6-8 hours as needed; initial dose (up to 0.3 mg) may be repeated once in 30-60 minutes after the initial dose if needed

Adults: I.V. infusion: Opiate withdrawal in heroin-dependent hospitalized patients (unlabeled): 0.3-0.9 mg (diluted in 50-100 mL of NS) over 20-30 minutes every 6-12 hours (Welsh, 2002)

Sublingual tablet: Children ≥16 years and Adults: Opioid dependence: **Note:** The combination product, buprenorphine and naloxone, is preferred therapy over buprenorphine monotherapy for induction treatment (and stabilization/maintenance treatment) for short-acting opioid dependence (U.S. Department of Health and Human Services, 2005).

Manufacturer's labeling:

Induction: Day 1: 8 mg; Day 2 and subsequent induction days: 16 mg; usual induction dosage range: 12-16 mg/day (induction usually accomplished over 3-4 days). Treatment should begin at least 4 hours after last use of heroin or other short-acting opioids, preferably when first signs of withdrawal appear. Titrating dose to clinical effectiveness should be done as rapidly as possible to prevent undue withdrawal symptoms and patient drop-out during the induction period. There is little controlled experience with induction in patients on methadone or other long-acting opioids; consult expert physician experienced with this procedure.

Maintenance: Target dose: 16 mg/day; in some patients 12 mg/day may be effective; patients should be switched to the buprenorphine/naloxone combination product for maintenance and unsupervised therapy

Transdermal patch: Adults: Chronic pain (moderate-to-severe):

Opioid-naive patients: Initial: 5 mcg/hour applied once every 7 days

Opioid-experienced patients (conversion from other opioids to buprenorphine): Taper the current around-the-clock opioid for up to 7 days to ≤30 mg/day of oral morphine or equivalent before initiating therapy. Short-acting analgesics as needed may be continued until analgesia with transdermal buprenorphine is attained. There is a potential for buprenorphine to precipitate withdrawal in patients already receiving opioids.

Patients who were receiving daily dose of <30 mg of oral morphine equivalents: Initial: 5 mcg/hour applied once every 7 days

Patients who were receiving daily dose of 30-80 mg of oral morphine equivalents: Initial: 10 mcg/hour applied once every 7 days

Dose titration (opioid-naive or opioid-experienced patients): May increase dose, based on patient's supplemental short-acting analgesic requirements, with a minimum titration interval of 72 hours (maximum dose: 20 mcg/hour applied once every 7 days; risk for QT_c prolongation increases with doses ≥20 mcg/hour patch).

Discontinuation of therapy: Taper dose gradually to prevent withdrawal; consider initiating immediate-release opioids, if needed.

Elderly:

I.M., slow I.V.: 0.15 mg every 6 hours; elderly patients are more likely to suffer from confusion and drowsiness compared to younger patients

Transdermal patch: Chronic pain (moderate-to-severe): No specific dosage adjustments required; use caution due to potential for increased risk of adverse events. Refer to adult dosing.

Dosage adjustment in hepatic impairment:

Injection, sublingual tablet: Use caution due to extensive hepatic metabolism; dosage adjustments recommended although no specific recommendations are provided by the manufacturer.

Transdermal patch:

Mild-to-moderate impairment: Initial: 5 mcg/hour applied once every 7 days

Severe impairment: Not studied; consider alternative therapy with more flexibility for dosing adjustments

Mechanism of Action Buprenorphine exerts its analgesic effect via high affinity binding to μ opiate receptors in the CNS; displays partial mu agonist and weak kappa antagonist activity

Contraindications Hypersensitivity to buprenorphine or any component of the formulation

Transdermal patch: Additional contraindications: Significant respiratory depression; severe asthma; known or suspected paralytic ileus; management of mild, acute, or intermittent pain; management of pain requiring short-term opioid analgesia; management of postoperative pain

Warnings/Precautions An opioid-containing analgesic regimen should be tailored to each patient's needs and based upon the type of pain being treated (acute versus chronic), the route of administration, degree of tolerance for opioids (naive versus chronic user), age, weight, and medical condition. The optimal analgesic dose varies widely among patients. Doses should be titrated to pain relief/prevention.

May cause CNS depression, which may impair physical or mental abilities. Effects with other sedative drugs or ethanol may be potentiated. Elderly may be more sensitive to CNS depressant and constipating effects. May cause respiratory depression - use caution in patients with respiratory disease or pre-existing respiratory depression. Hypersensitivity reactions, including bronchospasm, angioneurotic edema, and anaphylactic shock, have also been reported. Potential for drug dependency exists, abrupt cessation may precipitate withdrawal. Use caution in elderly, debilitated, pediatric patients, depression or suicidal tendencies. Tolerance, psychological and physical dependence may occur with prolonged use. Partial antagonist activity may precipitate acute narcotic withdrawal in opioid-dependent individuals.

Hepatitis has been reported with buprenorphine use; hepatic events ranged from transient, asymptomatic transaminase elevations to hepatic failure; in many cases, patients had preexisting hepatic dysfunction. Monitor liver function tests in patients at increased risk for hepatotoxicity (eg, history of alcohol abuse, pre-existing hepatic dysfunction, I.V. drug abusers) prior to and during therapy. Use with caution in patients with hepatic impairment; dosage adjustments are recommended in hepatic impairment.

Use with caution in patients with pulmonary or renal function impairment. Also use caution in patients with head injury or increased ICP, biliary tract dysfunction, patients with history of hyperthyroidism, morbid obesity, adrenal insufficiency, prostatic hyperplasia, urinary stricture, CNS depression, toxic psychosis, pancreatitis, alcoholism, delirium tremens, or kyphoscoliosis. May cause hypotension; use with caution in patients with hypovolemia, cardiovascular disease (including acute MI), or drugs which may exaggerate hypotensive effects (including phenothiazines or general anesthetics). May obscure diagnosis or clinical course of patients with acute abdominal conditions. Opioid therapy may lower seizure threshold; use caution in patients with a history of seizure disorders.

Transdermal patch: **[U.S. Boxed Warning]: Do not exceed one 20 mcg/hour transdermal patch due to the risk of QT_c-interval prolongation.** Avoid using in patients with history of long QT syndrome or in patients with predisposing factors increasing the risk of QT abnormalities (eg, concurrent medications such as antiarrhythmics, hypokalemia, unstable heart failure, unstable atrial fibrillation). **[U.S. Boxed Warning]: Healthcare provider should be alert to problems of abuse, misuse, and diversion.**

Sublingual tablets, which are used for induction treatment of opioid dependence, should not be started until effects of withdrawal are evident.

Drug Interactions

Metabolism/Transport Effects Substrate of CYP3A4 (major); **Inhibits** CYP1A2 (weak), 2A6 (weak), 2C19 (weak), 2D6 (weak)

Avoid Concomitant Use

Avoid concomitant use of Buprenorphine with any of the following: Atazanavir; MAO Inhibitors

Increased Effect/Toxicity

Buprenorphine may increase the levels/effects of: Alcohol (Ethyl); Alvimopan; CNS Depressants; Desmopressin; MAO Inhibitors; Selective Serotonin Reuptake Inhibitors; Thiazide Diuretics

The levels/effects of Buprenorphine may be increased by: Amphetamines; Antipsychotic Agents (Phenothiazines); Atazanavir; Conivaptan; CYP3A4 Inhibitors (Moderate); CYP3A4 Inhibitors (Strong); Dasatinib; Droperidol; Succinylcholine

Decreased Effect

Buprenorphine may decrease the levels/effects of: Analgesics (Opioid); Atazanavir; Pegvisomant

The levels/effects of Buprenorphine may be decreased by: Ammonium Chloride; CYP3A4 Inducers (Strong); Deferasirox; Efavirenz; Herbs (CYP3A4 Inducers); Mixed Agonist / Antagonist Opioids; Tocilizumab

Ethanol/Nutrition/Herb Interactions

Ethanol: May increase CNS depression; monitor for increased effects with coadministration. Caution patients about effect.

Herb/Nutraceutical: Avoid valerian, St John's wort, kava kava, gotu kola (may increase CNS depression).

Pharmacodynamics/Kinetics

Onset of Action Analgesic: I.M: Within 15 minutes; Peak effect: I.M.: ~1 hour; Transdermal patch: Steady state achieved by day 3

Duration of Action I.M.: ≥6 hours

Half-life Elimination I.V.: 2.2-3 hours; Apparent terminal half-life: Sublingual tablet: ~37 hours; Transdermal patch: ~26 hours. **Note:** Extended elimination half-life for sublingual administration may be due to depot effect (Kuhlman, 1996).

Time to Peak Plasma: Sublingual: 30 minutes to 1 hour (Kuhlman, 1996)

Pregnancy Risk Factor C

Lactation Enters breast milk/not recommended

Controlled Substance C-III

Prescribing and Access Restrictions Prescribing of tablets for opioid dependence is limited to physicians who have met the qualification criteria and have received a DEA number specific to prescribing this product. Tablets will be available through pharmacies and wholesalers which normally provide controlled substances.

Dosage Forms

Injection, solution: 0.3 mg/mL (1 mL)

Buprenex®: 0.3 mg/mL (1 mL)

Patch, transdermal:

Butrans™: 5 mcg/hour (4s); 10 mcg/hour (4s); 20 mcg/hour (4s)

Tablet, sublingual: 2 mg, 8 mg

Subutex®: 2 mg, 8 mg

Buprenorphine and Naloxone (byoo pre NOR feen & nal OKS one)

Related Information

Buprenorphine *on page 260*

Naloxone *on page 1179*

U.S. Brand Names Suboxone®

Pharmacologic Category Analgesic, Opioid; Analgesic, Opioid Partial Agonist

Use Maintenance treatment for opioid dependence

Local Anesthetic/Vasoconstrictor Precautions No information available to require special precautions

Effects on Dental Treatment No significant effects or complications reported

Effects on Bleeding No information available to require special precautions

Adverse Effects Also see individual agents.

>10%:

Central nervous system: Headache (36%), pain (22%)

Gastrointestinal: Vomiting (8%), erythema (oral mucosa; film), glossodynia (film), oral hypoesthesia (film)

Miscellaneous: Withdrawal syndrome (25%; placebo 37%), diaphoresis (14%)

1% to 10%:

Cardiovascular: Vasodilation (9%)

Gastrointestinal: Vomiting (7%)

General Dosage Range Sublingual: *Children ≥16 years and Adults:* 4-24 mg/day (target dose: 16 mg/day)

Mechanism of Action See individual agents.

Pharmacodynamics/Kinetics

Half-life Elimination Film: Buprenorphine: 24-42 hours; Naloxone: 2-12 hours

Pregnancy Risk Factor C

Controlled Substance C-III

Prescribing and Access Restrictions Prescribing of tablets for opioid dependence is limited to physicians who have met the qualification criteria and have received a DEA number specific to prescribing this product. Tablets will be available through pharmacies and wholesalers which normally provide controlled substances.

BuPROPion (byoo PROE pee on)

U.S. Brand Names Aplenzin™; Budeprion SR®; Budeprion XL®; Buproban®; Wellbutrin SR®; Wellbutrin XL®; Wellbutrin®; Zyban®

Canadian Brand Names Bupropion SR®; Novo-Bupropion SR; PMS-Bupropion SR; ratio-Bupropion SR; Sandoz-Bupropion SR; Wellbutrin® SR; Wellbutrin® XL; Zyban®

Generic Availability (U.S.) Yes: Excludes bupropion hydrobromide tablet, sustained release hydrochloride tablet

Pharmacologic Category Antidepressant, Dopamine-Reuptake Inhibitor; Smoking Cessation Aid

Use Treatment of major depressive disorder, including seasonal affective disorder (SAD); adjunct in smoking cessation

Unlabeled/Investigational Use Attention-deficit/hyperactivity disorder (ADHD); depression associated with bipolar disorder

Local Anesthetic/Vasoconstrictor Precautions Part of the mechanism of bupropion is to block reuptake of norepinephrine along with dopamine. Because of the potential for norepinephrine elevation within CNS synapses, it is suggested that vasoconstrictor be administered with caution and to monitor vital signs in dental patients taking antidepressants that affect norepinephrine in this way.

Effects on Dental Treatment Key adverse event(s) related to dental treatment: Abnormal taste, significant xerostomia (normal salivary flow resumes with discontinuation).

Effects on Bleeding No information available to require special precautions

Adverse Effects Frequencies, when reported, reflect highest incidence reported with sustained release product.

>10%:

- Cardiovascular: Tachycardia (11%)
- Central nervous system: Headache (25% to 34%), insomnia (11% to 20%), dizziness (6% to 11%)
- Gastrointestinal: Xerostomia (17% to 26%), weight loss (14% to 23%), nausea (1% to 18%)
- Respiratory: Pharyngitis (3% to 13%)

1% to 10%:

- Cardiovascular: Palpitation (2% to 6%), arrhythmias (5%), chest pain (3% to 4%), hypertension (2% to 4%; may be severe), flushing (1% to 4%), hypotension (3%)
- Central nervous system: Agitation (2% to 9%), confusion (8%), anxiety (5% to 7%), hostility (6%), nervousness (3% to 5%), sleep disturbance (4%), sensory disturbance (4%), migraine (1% to 4%), abnormal dreams (3%), irritability (2% to 3%), somnolence (2% to 3%), pain (2% to 3%), memory decreased (≤3%), fever (1% to 2%), CNS stimulation (1% to 2%), depression
- Dermatologic: Rash (1% to 5%), pruritus (2% to 4%), urticaria (1% to 2%)
- Endocrine & metabolic: Menstrual complaints (2% to 5%), hot flashes (1% to 3%), libido decreased (3%)
- Gastrointestinal: Constipation (5% to 10%), abdominal pain (2% to 9%), diarrhea (5% to 7%), flatulence (6%), anorexia (3% to 5%), appetite increased (4%), taste perversion (2% to 4%), vomiting (2% to 4%), dyspepsia (3%), dysphagia (≤2%)
- Genitourinary: Polyuria (2% to 5%), urinary urgency (≤2%), vaginal hemorrhage (≤2%), UTI (≤1%)
- Neuromuscular & skeletal: Tremor (3% to 6%), myalgia (2% to 6%), weakness (2% to 4%), arthralgia (1% to 4%), arthritis (2%), akathisia (≤2%), paresthesia (1% to 2%), twitching (1% to 2%), neck pain
- Ocular: Blurred vision (2% to 3%), amblyopia (2%)
- Otic: Tinnitus (3% to 6%), auditory disturbance (5%)
- Respiratory: Upper respiratory infection (9%), cough increased (1% to 4%), sinusitis (1% to 5%)
- Miscellaneous: Infection (8% to 9%), diaphoresis (5% to 6%), allergic reaction (including anaphylaxis, pruritus, urticaria)

Dosage Oral:

Children and Adolescents: ADHD (unlabeled use): Hydrochloride salt: 1.4-6 mg/kg/day

Adults:

Depression:

Immediate release hydrochloride salt: 100 mg 3 times/day; begin at 100 mg twice daily; may increase to a maximum dose of 450 mg/day

Sustained release hydrochloride salt: Initial: 150 mg/day in the morning; may increase to 150 mg twice daily by day 4 if tolerated; target dose: 300 mg/day given as 150 mg twice daily; maximum dose: 400 mg/day given as 200 mg twice daily

Extended release:

Hydrochloride salt: Initial: 150 mg/day in the morning; may increase as early as day 4 of dosing to 300 mg/day; maximum dose: 450 mg/day

Hydrobromide salt (Aplenzin™): Target dose: 348 mg/day in the morning. Patients not previously on bupropion: Initial: 174 mg/day in the morning; may increase as early as day 4 of dosing to 348 mg/day; maximum dose: 522 mg/day. **Note:** 174 mg strength currently not available; 348 mg tablet cannot be split.

Switching from hydrochloride salt formulation (eg, Wellbutrin® immediate release, SR®, XL®) to hydrobromide salt formulation (Aplenzin™): **Note:** Patients being treated twice daily with bupropion hydrochloride would be switched to the equivalent once daily dose of bupropion hydrobromide.

Bupropion hydrochloride 150 mg is equivalent to bupropion hydrobromide 174 mg

Bupropion hydrochloride 300 mg is equivalent to bupropion hydrobromide 348 mg

Bupropion hydrochloride 450 mg is equivalent to bupropion hydrobromide 522 mg

SAD (Wellbutrin XL®): Initial: 150 mg/day in the morning; if tolerated, may increase after 1 week to 300 mg/day

Note: Prophylactic treatment should be reserved for those patients with frequent depressive episodes and/or significant impairment. Initiate treatment in the Autumn prior to symptom onset, and discontinue in early Spring with dose tapering to 150 mg/day for 2 weeks

Smoking cessation (Zyban®): Initiate with 150 mg once daily for 3 days; increase to 150 mg twice daily; treatment should continue for 7-12 weeks

Note: Therapy should begin at least 1 week before target quit date. Target quit dates are generally in the second week of treatment. If patient successfully quits smoking after 7-12 weeks, may consider ongoing maintenance therapy based on individual patient risk:benefit. Efficacy of maintenance therapy (300 mg/day) has been demonstrated for up to 6 months. Conversely, if significant progress has not been made by the seventh week of therapy, success is unlikely and treatment discontinuation should be considered.

Elderly: Depression: Hydrochloride salt: 50-100 mg/day, increase by 50-100 mg every 3-4 days as tolerated; there is evidence that the elderly respond at 150 mg/day in divided doses, but some may require a higher dose. **Note:** Patients with Alzheimer's dementia-related depression may require a lower starting dosage of 37.5 mg once or twice daily (100 mg/day sustained release), increased as needed up to 300 mg/day in divided doses (300 mg/day for sustained release)

Dosing conversion between hydrochloride salt (eg, Wellbutrin®) immediate, sustained, and extended release products: Convert using same total daily dose (up to the maximum recommended dose for a given dosage form), but adjust frequency as indicated for sustained (twice daily) or extended (once daily) release products.

Dosing adjustment/comments in renal impairment: Use with caution and consider a reduction in dosing frequency; limited pharmacokinetic information suggests elimination of bupropion and/or the active metabolites may be reduced.

Moderate-to-severe renal impairment: Bupropion exposure was approximately twofold higher compared to normal subjects following a 150 mg single dose administration.

End-stage renal failure: Per the manufacturer, the elimination of hydroxybupropion and threohydrobupropion are reduced in patients with end-stage renal failure.

Dosing adjustment in hepatic impairment:

Note: The mean AUC increased by ~1.5-fold for hydroxybupropion and ~2.5-fold for erythro/threohydrobupropion; median T_{max} was observed 19 hours later for hydroxybupropion, 31 hours later for erythro/threohydrobupropion; mean half-life for hydroxybupropion increased fivefold, and increased twofold for erythro/threohydrobupropion in patients with severe hepatic cirrhosis compared to healthy volunteers.

Mild-to-moderate hepatic impairment: Use with caution and/or reduced dose/frequency

Severe hepatic cirrhosis: Use with extreme caution; maximum dose:

Aplenzin™: 174 mg every other day

Wellbutrin®: 75 mg/day

Wellbutrin SR®: 100 mg/day or 150 mg every other day

Wellbutrin XL®: 150 mg every other day

Zyban®: 150 mg every other day

Mechanism of Action Aminoketone antidepressant structurally different from all other marketed antidepressants; like other antidepressants the mechanism of bupropion's activity is not fully understood. Bupropion is a relatively weak inhibitor of the neuronal uptake of norepinephrine and dopamine, and does not inhibit monoamine oxidase or the reuptake of serotonin. Metabolite inhibits the reuptake of norepinephrine. The primary mechanism of action is thought to be dopaminergic and/or noradrenergic.

Contraindications Hypersensitivity to bupropion or any component of the formulation; seizure disorder; history of anorexia/bulimia; use of MAO inhibitors within 14 days; patients undergoing abrupt discontinuation of ethanol or sedatives (including benzodiazepines); patients receiving other dosage forms of bupropion

Warnings/Precautions [U.S. Boxed Warning]: Use in treating psychiatric disorders: Antidepressants increase the risk of suicidal thinking and behavior in children, adolescents, and young adults (18-24 years of age) with major depressive disorder (MDD) and other psychiatric disorders; consider risk prior to prescribing. Short-term studies did not show an increased risk in patients >24 years of age and showed a decreased risk in patients ≥65 years. All patients must be closely monitored for clinical worsening, suicidality, or unusual changes in behavior, especially during the initiation of therapy (generally first 1-2 months) or following an increase or decrease in dosage. The patient's family or caregiver should be instructed to closely observe the patient and communicate condition with healthcare provider. A medication guide should be dispensed with each prescription. **Bupropion is not FDA approved for use in children.**

[U.S. Boxed Warning]: Use in smoking cessation: Serious neuropsychiatric events, including depression, suicidal thoughts, and suicide, have been reported with use; some cases may have been complicated by symptoms of nicotine withdrawal following smoking cessation. Smoking cessation (with or without treatment) is associated with nicotine withdrawal symptoms and the exacerbation of underlying psychiatric illness; however, some of the behavioral disturbances were reported in treated patients who continued to smoke. These neuropsychiatric symptoms (eg, mood disturbances, psychosis, hostility) have occurred in patients with and without pre-existing psychiatric disease; many cases resolved following therapy discontinuation although in some cases, symptoms persisted. Monitor all patients for behavioral changes and psychiatric symptoms (eg, agitation, depression, suicidal behavior, suicidal ideation); inform patients to discontinue treatment and contact their healthcare provider immediately if they experience any behavioral and/or mood changes.

The possibility of a suicide attempt is inherent in major depression and may persist until remission occurs. Use caution in high-risk patients. Worsening depression and severe abrupt suicidality that are not part of the presenting symptoms may require discontinuation or modification of drug therapy. The patient's family or caregiver should be alerted to monitor patients for the emergence of suicidality and associated behaviors (such as agitation, irritability, hostility, impulsivity, and hypomania) and notify the healthcare provider.

May worsen psychosis in some patients or precipitate a shift to mania or hypomania in patients with bipolar disorder. Patients presenting with depressive symptoms should be screened for bipolar disorder. Monotherapy in patients with bipolar disorder should be avoided. **Bupropion is not FDA approved for bipolar depression.**

The risk of seizures is dose-dependent and increased in patients with a history of seizures, anorexia/bulimia, head trauma, CNS tumor, severe hepatic cirrhosis, abrupt discontinuation of sedative-hypnotics or ethanol, medications which lower seizure threshold (antipsychotics, antidepressants, theophyllines, systemic steroids), stimulants, or hypoglycemic agents. Risk of seizures may also be increased by chewing, crushing, or dividing long-acting products. Risk may be reduced by limiting the daily dose to bupropion hydrochloride ≤450 mg or bupropion hydrobromide 522 mg. Gradually increase dose incrementally to reduce risk. Discontinue and do not restart in patients experiencing a seizure.

May cause CNS stimulation (restlessness, anxiety, insomnia) or anorexia. May increase the risks associated with electroconvulsive therapy. Consider discontinuing, when possible, prior to elective surgery. May cause weight loss; use caution in patients where weight loss is not desirable. The incidence of sexual dysfunction with bupropion is generally lower than with SSRIs.

Use caution in patients with cardiovascular disease, history of hypertension, or coronary artery disease; treatment-emergent hypertension (including some severe cases) has been reported, both with bupropion alone and in combination with nicotine transdermal systems. All children diagnosed with ADHD who may be candidates for stimulant medications should have a thorough cardiovascular assessment to identify risk factors for sudden cardiac death prior to initiation of drug therapy. Use with caution in patients with hepatic or renal dysfunction and in elderly patients; reduced dose and/or frequency may be recommended. Elderly patients may be at greater risk of accumulation during chronic dosing. May cause motor or cognitive impairment in some patients; use with caution if tasks requiring alertness such as operating machinery or driving are undertaken. Arthralgia, myalgia, and fever with rash and other symptoms suggestive of delayed hypersensitivity resembling serum sickness have been reported.

Extended release tablet: Insoluble tablet shell may remain intact and be visible in the stool.

Drug Interactions

Metabolism/Transport Effects Substrate of CYP1A2 (minor), 2A6 (minor), 2B6 (major), 2C9 (minor), 2D6 (minor), 2E1 (minor), 3A4 (minor); **Inhibits** CYP2D6 (strong)

Avoid Concomitant Use

Avoid concomitant use of BuPROPion with any of the following: MAO Inhibitors; Tamoxifen; Thioridazine

Increased Effect/Toxicity

BuPROPion may increase the levels/effects of: Alcohol (Ethyl); Atomoxetine; CNS Depressants; CYP2D6 Substrates; Fesoterodine; Methotrimeprazine; Nebivolol; Tamoxifen; Tetrabenazine; Thioridazine; Tricyclic Antidepressants

The levels/effects of BuPROPion may be increased by: Conivaptan; CYP2B6 Inhibitors (Moderate); CYP2B6 Inhibitors (Strong); Droperidol; MAO Inhibitors; Methotrimeprazine; Quazepam

Decreased Effect

BuPROPion may decrease the levels/effects of: Codeine; TraMADol

The levels/effects of BuPROPion may be decreased by: CYP2B6 Inducers (Strong); Lopinavir; Peginterferon Alfa-2b; Ritonavir; Tocilizumab

Ethanol/Nutrition/Herb Interactions

Ethanol: May increase CNS depression; monitor for increased effects with coadministration. Caution patients about effects.

Herb/Nutraceutical: Avoid valerian, St John's wort, SAMe, gotu kola, kava kava (may increase CNS depression).

Pharmacodynamics/Kinetics

Half-life Elimination

Distribution: 3-4 hours

Elimination: 21 ± 9 hours; Metabolites: Hydroxybupropion: 20 ± 5 hours; Erythrohydrobupropion: 33 ± 10 hours; Threohydrobupropion: 37 ± 13 hours

Extended release (Aplenzin™): 21 ± 7 hours; Metabolites: Hydroxybupropion: 24 ± 5 hours; Erythrohydrobupropion: 31 ± 8 hours; Threohydrobupropion: 51 ± 9 hours

Time to Peak

Bupropion: Immediate release: Within 2 hours; Sustained release: Within 3 hours; Extended release: ~5 hours

Metabolite: Hydroxybupropion: Immediate release: ~3 hours; Extended release, sustained release: ~6-7 hours

Pregnancy Risk Factor C

Lactation Enters breast milk/not recommended (AAP rates "of concern"; AAP 2001 update pending)

Breast-Feeding Considerations Bupropion and its metabolites are excreted into breast milk, although neither bupropion nor its metabolites have been detected in the plasma of breast-fed infants. Adverse events have not been reported in older breast-fed infants; however, a seizure was noted in one 6-month old infant (a causal effect could not be confirmed). Breast-feeding is not recommended by the manufacturer.

Dosage Forms

Tablet, oral: 75 mg, 100 mg

Wellbutrin®: 75 mg, 100 mg

Tablet, extended release, oral: 100 mg, 150 mg, 200 mg, 300 mg

Aplenzin™: 174 mg, 348 mg, 522 mg

Budeprion SR®: 100 mg, 150 mg

Budeprion XL®: 150 mg, 300 mg

Buproban®: 150 mg

Wellbutrin XL®: 150 mg, 300 mg

Tablet, sustained release, oral:

Wellbutrin SR®: 100 mg, 150 mg, 200 mg

Zyban®: 150 mg

References

Tonstad S and Johnston JA, "Does Bupropion Have Advantages Over Other Medical Therapies in the Cessation of Smoking?" *Expert Opin Pharmacother*, 2004, 5(4):727-34.

Buserelin (BYOO se rel in)

Canadian Brand Names Suprefact®; Suprefact® Depot

Pharmacologic Category Gonadotropin Releasing Hormone Agonist

Use Palliative treatment in patients with hormone-dependent advanced prostate cancer (stage D); treatment of endometriosis in women who do not require surgical intervention as first-line therapy (length of therapy is usually 6 months, but no longer than 9 months)

Unlabeled/Investigational Use Diagnostic test for hypogonadotropic hypogonadism in males with delayed puberty

Local Anesthetic/Vasoconstrictor Precautions Buserelin may cause hypertension and palpitations. Monitor blood pressure prior to dental procedures if using local anesthesia with vasoconstrictor. There have been no reports of any direct interaction with buserelin and vasoconstrictor.

Effects on Dental Treatment No significant effects or complications reported

Effects on Bleeding No information available to require special precautions

Adverse Effects Note: Adverse reaction profile differs based on population/medication and route of administration.

Depot:

>10%:

Endocrine & metabolic: Hot flushes (14% to 23%)

Genitourinary: Impotence (2% to 23%)

Neuromuscular & skeletal: Weakness (<1% to 14%)

1% to 10%:

Cardiovascular: Hypertension (2% to 9%), palpitation (5%), edema (1%)

Central nervous system: Dizziness (5%), insomnia (<1% to 5%), depression (2%), pain (2%)

Endocrine & metabolic: Libido decreased (2% to 5%)

Gastrointestinal: Appetite increased (5%), nausea (5%)

Local: Injection site reaction (1% to 5%)

Neuromuscular & skeletal: Arthralgia (5%), myalgia (5%)

SubQ or intranasal:

>10%:

Central nervous system: Headache (20% to 29%)

Endocrine & metabolic: Libido decreased (12% to 85%), hot flushes (66% to 72%), vaginal dryness (29%), menorrhagia (24%)

Genitourinary: Impotence (75% to 80%)

Local: Injection site reaction: (8% to 12%)

1% to 10%:

Cardiovascular: Edema (1% to 5%), palpitation (1% to 5%)

Central nervous system: Dizziness (9%), depression (8%), emotional lability (7%), anxiety (1% to 5%), hostility (1% to 5%), insomnia (1% to 5%), migraine (1% to 5%), nervousness (1% to 5%), pain (1% to 5%), malaise, sleep disorder

Dermatologic: Acne (5%), dry skin (1% to 5%), purpura (1% to 5%), skin disorder (1% to 5%), flare reaction (1% to 2%), pruritus

Endocrine & metabolic: Breast pain (1% to 5%), hirsutism (1% to 5%), menstrual disorder (1% to 5%), gynecomastia (1% to 2%), premenstrual syndrome

Gastrointestinal: Nausea (5% to 7%), constipation (1% to 5%), diarrhea (1% to 5%), gastrointestinal fullness (1% to 5%), taste perversion (1% to 5%), weight loss/gain (1% to 5%), xerostomia (1% to 2%), flatulence, sore throat, vomiting

Genitourinary: Dyspareunia (1% to 5%), vaginitis (1% to 5%), leukorrhea, pelvic pain, vaginal discharge, vaginal discomfort

Neuromuscular & skeletal: Weakness (7%), arthralgia (1% to 5%), myalgia (1% to 5%), neck rigidity (1% to 5%), paresthesia (1% to 5%), back pain

Respiratory: Upper respiratory infection (1% to 5%), rhinitis (1% to 5%), dry nose (1% to 2%)

Miscellaneous: Diaphoresis (1% to 2%), infection

General Dosage Range

Intranasal: *Adults:* 400 mcg (200 mcg into each nostril) 3 times/day

SubQ: *Adults:*

Implants: 6.3 mg every 8 weeks **or** 9.45 mg every 12 weeks

Injection: Initial: 500 mcg every 8 hours for 7 days; maintenance: 200 mcg once daily

Mechanism of Action Synthetic peptide analog of Gonadotropin hormone releasing hormone (GnRH) with substitutions at positions 6 and 10; altered peptide structure results in a significantly magnified GnRH agonist effect with an extended duration of activity. Following an initial rise in the pituitary gonadotropins luteinizing hormone (LH) and follicle-stimulating hormone (FSH), chronic administration of buserelin results in a sustained suppression of LH and FSH and an interference with the production of ovarian and testicular steroids. Eventually, a decline in gonadal steroids to castration levels is observed.

Pharmacodynamics/Kinetics

Half-life Elimination 70-80 minutes; Depot implants: 20-30 Days

Time to Peak Depot: <1 day

Product Availability Not available in U.S.

BusPIRone (byoo SPYE rone)

Related Information

Management of the Patient With Anxiety or Depression *on page 1968*

Canadian Brand Names Apo-Buspirone®; BuSpar®; Buspirex; Bustab®; CO Buspirone; Dom-Buspirone; Gen-Buspirone; Lin-Buspirone; Mylan-Buspirone; Novo-Buspirone; Nu-Buspirone; PMS-Buspirone; ratio-Buspirone; Riva-Buspirone

Generic Availability (U.S.) Yes

Pharmacologic Category Antianxiety Agent, Miscellaneous

Use Management of generalized anxiety disorder (GAD)

Unlabeled/Investigational Use Management of aggression in mental retardation and secondary mental disorders; major depression; potential augmenting agent for antidepressants; premenstrual syndrome

Local Anesthetic/Vasoconstrictor Precautions No information available to require special precautions

Effects on Dental Treatment Key adverse event(s) related to dental treatment: Xerostomia (normal salivary flow resumes upon discontinuation).

Effects on Bleeding No information available to require special precautions

Adverse Effects

>10%: Central nervous system: Dizziness (12%)

1% to 10%:

Cardiovascular: Chest pain (≥1%)

Central nervous system: Drowsiness (10%), headache (6%), nervousness (5%), lightheadedness (3%), anger/hostility (2%), confusion (2%), excitement (2%), dream disturbance (≥1%)

Dermatologic: Rash (1%)

Gastrointestinal: Nausea (8%), diarrhea (2%)

Neuromuscular & skeletal: Numbness (2%), weakness (2%), musculoskeletal pain (1%), paresthesia (1%), incoordination (1%), tremor (1%)

Ocular: Blurred vision (2%)

Otic: Tinnitus (≥1%)

Respiratory: Nasal congestion (≥1%), sore throat (≥1%)

Miscellaneous: Diaphoresis (1%)

Dosage Oral:

Generalized anxiety disorder:

Children ≥6 years and Adolescents: Initial: 5 mg daily; increase in increments of 5 mg/day at weekly intervals as needed, to a maximum dose of 60 mg/day divided into 2-3 doses

Adults: 15 mg/day (7.5 mg twice daily); may increase in increments of 5 mg/day every 2-3 days to a maximum of 60 mg/day; target dose for most people is 20-30 mg/day (10-15 mg twice daily)

Elderly: Initial: 5 mg twice daily, increase by 5 mg/day every 2-3 days as needed up to 20-30 mg/day; maximum daily dose: 60 mg/day.

Dosing adjustment in renal impairment: Patients with impaired renal function demonstrated increased plasma levels and a prolonged half-life of buspirone. Use in patients with severe renal impairment not recommended.

Dosing adjustment in hepatic impairment: Patients with impaired hepatic function demonstrated increased plasma levels and a prolonged half-life of buspirone. Use in patients with severe hepatic impairment not recommended.

Mechanism of Action The mechanism of action of buspirone is unknown. Buspirone has a high affinity for serotonin $5\text{-}HT_{1A}$ and $5\text{-}HT_2$ receptors, without affecting benzodiazepine-GABA receptors. Buspirone has moderate affinity for dopamine D_2 receptors.

Contraindications Hypersensitivity to buspirone or any component of the formulation

Warnings/Precautions Use in severe hepatic or renal impairment is not recommended; does not prevent or treat withdrawal from benzodiazepines. Low potential for cognitive or motor impairment. Use with MAO inhibitors may result in hypertensive reactions. Restlessness syndrome has been reported in small number of patients; monitor for signs of any dopamine-related movement disorders. Buspirone does not exhibit cross-tolerance with benzodiazepines or other sedative/hypnotic agents. If substituting buspirone for any of these agents, gradually withdraw the drug(s) prior to initiating buspirone. Safety and efficacy of buspirone have not been established in children <6 years of age; no long-term safety/efficacy data available in children.

Drug Interactions

Metabolism/Transport Effects Substrate of CYP2D6 (minor), 3A4 (major)

Avoid Concomitant Use

Avoid concomitant use of BusPIRone with any of the following: MAO Inhibitors; Sibutramine

Increased Effect/Toxicity

BusPIRone may increase the levels/effects of: Alcohol (Ethyl); Antidepressants (Serotonin Reuptake Inhibitor/Antagonist); CNS Depressants; MAO Inhibitors; Methotrimeprazine; Selective Serotonin Reuptake Inhibitors; Serotonin Modulators

The levels/effects of BusPIRone may be increased by: Antifungal Agents (Azole Derivatives, Systemic); Calcium Channel Blockers (Nondihydropyridine); Conivaptan; CYP3A4 Inhibitors (Moderate); CYP3A4 Inhibitors (Strong); Dasatinib; Droperidol; Grapefruit Juice; Macrolide Antibiotics; Methotrimeprazine; Selective Serotonin Reuptake Inhibitors; Sibutramine

Decreased Effect

The levels/effects of BusPIRone may be decreased by: CYP3A4 Inducers (Strong); Deferasirox; Peginterferon Alfa-2b; Rifamycin Derivatives; Tocilizumab; Yohimbine

Ethanol/Nutrition/Herb Interactions

Ethanol: May increase CNS depression; monitor for increased effects with coadministration. Caution patients about effects.

Food: Food may decrease the absorption of buspirone, but it may also decrease the first-pass metabolism, thereby increasing the bioavailability of buspirone. Grapefruit juice may cause increased buspirone concentrations; avoid intake of large quantities of grapefruit juice.

Herb/Nutraceutical: St John's wort may decrease buspirone levels or increase CNS depression. Avoid valerian, gotu kola, kava kava (may increase CNS depression).

Dietary Considerations Avoid large quantities of grapefruit juice.

Pharmacodynamics/Kinetics

Half-life Elimination 2-3 hours

Time to Peak Serum: 40-90 minutes

Pregnancy Risk Factor B

Lactation Excretion in breast milk unknown/not recommended

Dosage Forms

Tablet, oral: 5 mg, 7.5 mg, 10 mg, 15 mg, 30 mg

Busulfan (byoo SUL fan)

U.S. Brand Names Busulfex®; Myleran®

Canadian Brand Names Busulfex®; Myleran®

Pharmacologic Category Antineoplastic Agent, Alkylating Agent

Use

Oral: Chronic myelogenous leukemia (CML); conditioning regimens for bone marrow transplantation

I.V.: Combination therapy with cyclophosphamide as a conditioning regimen prior to allogeneic hematopoietic progenitor cell transplantation for chronic myelogenous leukemia

Unlabeled/Investigational Use Oral: Bone marrow disorders, such as polycythemia vera and myeloid metaplasia; thrombocytosis

Local Anesthetic/Vasoconstrictor Precautions No information available to require special precautions

Effects on Dental Treatment Key adverse event(s) related to dental treatment: Xerostomia (normal salivary flow resumes upon discontinuation), mucositis/stomatitis.

Effects on Bleeding Chemotherapy may result in significant myelosuppression, potentially including significant reduction in platelet counts and altered hemostasis. In patients who are under active treatment with these agents, medical consult is suggested.

Adverse Effects

I.V.:

>10%:

Cardiovascular: Tachycardia (44%), hypertension (36%; grades 3/4: 7%), edema (28% to 79%), thrombosis (33%), chest pain (26%), vasodilation (25%), hypotension (11%; grades 3/4: 3%)

Central nervous system: Insomnia (84%), fever (80%), anxiety (72% to 75%), headache (69%), chills (46%), pain (44%), dizziness (30%), depression (23%), confusion (11%)

Dermatologic: Rash (57%), pruritus (28%), alopecia (2% to 15%)

Endocrine & metabolic: Hypomagnesemia (77%), hyperglycemia (66%; grades 3/4: 15%), hypokalemia (64%), hypocalcemia (49%), hypophosphatemia (17%)
Gastrointestinal: Nausea (98%), mucositis/stomatitis (97%; grades 3/4: 26%), vomiting (43% to 95%), anorexia (85%), diarrhea (84%; grades 3/4: 5%), abdominal pain (72%), dyspepsia (44%), constipation (38%), xerostomia (26%), rectal disorder (25%), abdominal fullness (23%)
Hematologic: Myelosuppression (≤100%), neutropenia (100%; median recovery: 13 days), thrombocytopenia (98%; median onset: 5-6 days), lymphopenia (children: 79%), anemia (69%)
Hepatic: Hyperbilirubinemia (49%; grades 3/4: 30%), ALT increased (31%; grades 3/4: 7%), veno-occlusive disease (adults: 8% to 12%; children: 21%), jaundice (12%)
Local: Injection site inflammation (25%), injection site pain (15%)
Neuromuscular & skeletal: Weakness (51%), back pain (23%), myalgia (16%), arthralgia (13%)
Renal: Creatinine increased (21%), oliguria (15%)
Respiratory: Rhinitis (44%), lung disorder (34%), cough (28%), epistaxis (25%), dyspnea (25%), pneumonia (children: 21%), hiccup (18%), pharyngitis (18%)
Miscellaneous: Infection (51%), allergic reaction (26%)

1% to 10%:

Cardiovascular: Arrhythmia (5%), cardiomegaly (5%), atrial fibrillation (2%), ECG abnormal (2%), heart block (2%), heart failure (grade 3/4: 2%), pericardial effusion (2%), tamponade (children with thalassemia: 2%), ventricular extrasystoles (2%), hypervolemia
Central nervous system: Lethargy (7%), hallucination (5%), agitation (2%), delirium (2%), encephalopathy (2%), seizure (2%), somnolence (2%), cerebral hemorrhage (1%)
Dermatologic: Vesicular rash (10%), vesiculobullous rash (10%), skin discoloration (8%), maculopapular rash (8%), acne (7%), exfoliative dermatitis (5%), erythema nodosum (2%)
Endocrine & metabolic: Hyponatremia (2%)
Gastrointestinal: Ileus (8%), weight gain (8%), hematemesis (2%), pancreatitis (2%)
Hematologic: Prothrombin time increased (2%)
Hepatic: Hepatomegaly (6%)
Renal: Hematuria (8%), dysuria (7%), hemorrhagic cystitis (grade 3/4: 7%), BUN increased (3%)
Respiratory: Asthma (8%), alveolar hemorrhage (5%), hyperventilation (5%), hemoptysis (3%), pleural effusion (3%), sinusitis (3%), atelectasis (2%), hypoxia (2%)

Oral: Frequency not defined:

Central nervous system: Seizure
Dermatologic: Hyperpigmentation of skin (busulfan tan 5% to 10%), alopecia, rash, urticaria
Endocrine & metabolic: Amenorrhea, ovarian suppression
Hematologic: Myelosuppression (anemia, leukopenia, thrombocytopenia), pancytopenia

General Dosage Range

I.V.:

Children ≤12 kg: **BMT:** 1.1 mg/kg (ideal body weight) every 6 hours for 16 doses
Children >12 kg: **BMT:** 0.8 mg/kg (ideal body weight) every 6 hours for 16 doses
Adults: **BMT:** 0.8 mg/kg (ideal body weight or actual body weight, whichever is lower) every 6 hours for 16 doses

Oral:

Children: Induction: 0.06-0.12 mg/kg/day **or** 1.8-4.6 mg/m^2/day; Maintenance: Titrate to maintain leukocyte counts above 40,000/mm^3; **BMT:** 1 mg/kg (ideal body weight) every 6 hours for 16 doses
Adults: Induction: 60 mcg/kg/day or 1.8 mg/m^2/day; usual range: 4-12 mg/day; Maintenance: 1-4 mg/day to 2 mg/week; **BMT:** 1 mg/kg (ideal body weight) every 6 hours for 16 doses

Mechanism of Action Busulfan is an alkylating agent which reacts with the N-7 position of guanosine and interferes with DNA replication and transcription of RNA. Busulfan has a more marked effect on myeloid cells than on lymphoid cells and is also very toxic to hematopoietic stem cells. Busulfan exhibits little immunosuppressive activity. Interferes with the normal function of DNA by alkylation and cross-linking the strands of DNA.

Pharmacodynamics/Kinetics

Duration of Action 28 days
Half-life Elimination After first dose: 3.4 hours; After last dose: 2.3 hours
Time to Peak Serum: Oral: Within 4 hours; I.V.: Within 5 minutes

Pregnancy Risk Factor D

Butabarbital (byoo ta BAR bi tal)

U.S. Brand Names Butisol Sodium®

Pharmacologic Category Barbiturate

Use Sedative; hypnotic

Local Anesthetic/Vasoconstrictor Precautions No information available to require special precautions

Effects on Dental Treatment No significant effects or complications reported

Effects on Bleeding No information available to require special precautions

Adverse Effects

1% to 3%: Central nervous system: Somnolence

Frequency not defined, postmarketing, and/or case reports: Agranulocytosis, anaphylaxis, angioedema, complex sleep-related activities, dependence, exfoliative dermatitis, fever, headache, hypersensitivity reactions, liver damage, megaloblastic anemia, rash, respiratory depression, Stevens-Johnson syndrome, thrombocytopenia, thrombophlebitis

General Dosage Range Oral:

Children: 2-6 mg/kg preoperatively (maximum: 100 mg)

Adults: 15-30 mg 3-4 times/day **or** 50-100 mg as a single dose

Mechanism of Action Interferes with transmission of impulses from the thalamus to the cortex of the brain resulting in an imbalance in central inhibitory and facilitatory mechanisms

Pharmacodynamics/Kinetics

Onset of Action 45-60 minutes

Duration of Action 6-8 hours

Half-life Elimination ~100 hours

Pregnancy Risk Factor D

Controlled Substance C-III

Butalbital, Acetaminophen, and Caffeine

(byoo TAL bi tal, a seet a MIN oh fen, & KAF een)

Related Information

Acetaminophen *on page* 32

Caffeine *on page* 282

U.S. Brand Names Alagesic LQ; Alagesic [DSC]; Anolor 300; Dolgic® Plus; Esgic-Plus™; Esgic®; Fioricet®; Margesic; Orbivan™; Repan®; Zebutal®

Pharmacologic Category Barbiturate

Use Relief of the symptomatic complex of tension or muscle contraction headache

Local Anesthetic/Vasoconstrictor Precautions No information available to require special precautions

Effects on Dental Treatment No significant effects or complications reported (see Dental Comment)

Effects on Bleeding No information available to require special precautions

Adverse Effects Note: Specific percentages not reported.

Frequently observed:

Central nervous system: Dizziness, drowsiness, lightheadedness, sedation

Gastrointestinal: Abdominal pain, nausea, vomiting

Respiratory: Dyspnea

Miscellaneous: Intoxicated feeling

General Dosage Range Oral: *Adults:* 1-2 tablets/capsules or 15-30 mL every 4 hours (maximum: 6 tablets/capsules daily; 180 mL/day)

Mechanism of Action

Butalbital is a short- to intermediate-acting barbiturate. Barbiturates depress the sensory cortex, decrease motor activity, alter cerebellar function, and produce drowsiness, sedation, hypnosis, and dose-dependent respiratory depression.

Acetaminophen inhibits the synthesis of prostaglandins in the central nervous system and peripherally blocks pain impulse generation; produces antipyresis from inhibition of hypothalamic heat-regulating center

Caffeine increases levels of 3'5' cyclic AMP by inhibiting phosphodiesterase; CNS stimulant which increases medullary respiratory center sensitivity to carbon dioxide, stimulates central inspiratory drive, and improves skeletal muscle contraction (diaphragmatic contractility)

Pharmacodynamics/Kinetics

Half-life Elimination Butalbital: 35 hours

Pregnancy Risk Factor C

Dental Comment Hepatotoxicity caused by acetaminophen is potentiated by chronic alcohol consumption. People who are taking acetaminophen, even at therapeutic doses, and consume alcohol are at risk of developing hepatotoxicity.

Acetaminophen may increase the levels and enhance the anticoagulant effects of vitamin K antagonists acenocoumarol and warfarin (Coumadin®). Studies have reported that acetaminophen has increased the INR in warfarin treated patients with daily acetaminophen doses as low as 2 g, particularly when taking acetaminophen for >1 week (Antlitz, 1968; Boeijinga, 1982; Gebauer, 2003; Hylek, 1998; Rubin, 1984). In addition, case reports of bleeding as a result of increased INR have been published (Bagheri, 1999; Bartle, 1991). There is no known mechanism of the interaction; furthermore, some studies have failed to demonstrate this interaction (Gadisseur, 2003; Kwan, 1995; van den Bemt, 2002). In terms of risk, the data suggest that acetaminophen and warfarin could interact in some clinically significant manner but that the benefits of concomitant use of acetaminophen for pain control in dental patients taking warfarin usually outweigh the risks. An appropriate monitoring plan should be in place to identify potential negative effects and dosage adjustments may be necessary in a minority of patients. The interaction may be more likely to occur with daily acetaminophen doses of >1.3 g for >1 week.

There are no reports of acetaminophen interacting with antiplatelet drugs such as aspirin, clopidogrel (Plavix®), or prasugrel (Effient™). Also, there are no reports of acetaminophen in combination with hydrocodone, codeine, or oxycodone interacting with warfarin (Coumadin®).

Butalbital, Acetaminophen, Caffeine, and Codeine

(byoo TAL bi tal, a seet a MIN oh fen, KAF een, & KOE deen)

Related Information

Acetaminophen *on page* 32

Caffeine *on page* 282

Codeine *on page* 432

U.S. Brand Names Fioricet® with Codeine

Generic Availability (U.S.) Yes

Pharmacologic Category Analgesic Combination (Opioid); Barbiturate

Use Relief of symptoms of complex tension (muscle contraction) headache

Local Anesthetic/Vasoconstrictor Precautions No information available to require special precautions

Effects on Dental Treatment Key adverse event(s) related to dental treatment: Xerostomia (normal salivary flow resumes upon discontinuation). See Dental Comment.

Effects on Bleeding No information available to require special precautions

Adverse Effects Frequency not defined.

Cardiovascular: Syncope, tachycardia

Central nervous system: Agitation, depression, dizziness, drowsiness, euphoria, excitement, fatigue, fever, headache, high energy, intoxicated feeling, lightheadedness, mental confusion, sedation, seizure, sluggishness

Dermatologic: Hyperhidrosis, pruritus

Endocrine & metabolic: Hot flashes

Gastrointestinal: Abdominal pain, constipation, dysphagia, flatulence, heartburn, nausea, vomiting, xerostomia

Neuromuscular & skeletal: Leg pain, muscle fatigue, numbness, paresthesia, shaky feeling

Ocular: Heavy eyelids

Otic: Earache, tinnitus

Renal: Diuresis

Respiratory: Dyspnea, nasal congestion

Miscellaneous: Allergic reaction

Note: Potential reactions associated with components of Fioricet® with Codeine include agranulocytosis, cardiac stimulation, dependence, erythema multiforme, hyperglycemia, irritability, nephrotoxicity, rash, thrombocytopenia, toxic epidermal necrolysis, tremor

Dosage Oral: Adults: 1-2 capsules every 4 hours. Total daily dosage should not exceed 6 capsules.

Dosing adjustment/comments in hepatic impairment: Use with caution. Limited, low-dose therapy usually well tolerated in hepatic disease/cirrhosis. However, cases of hepatotoxicity at daily acetaminophen dosages <4 g/day have been reported. Avoid chronic use in hepatic impairment.

Mechanism of Action Combination product for the treatment of tension headache. Contains codeine (narcotic analgesic), butalbital (barbiturate), caffeine (CNS stimulant), and acetaminophen (nonopiate, nonsalicylate analgesic).

Contraindications Hypersensitivity to butalbital, codeine, caffeine, acetaminophen, or any component of the formulation; porphyria

Warnings/Precautions May cause CNS depression, which may impair physical or mental abilities; patients must be cautioned about performing tasks which require mental alertness (eg, operating machinery or driving). Limit acetaminophen to <4 g/day. Use with caution in patients with alcoholic liver disease; consuming ≥3 alcoholic drinks/day may increase the risk of liver damage. Effects may be potentiated when used with other sedative drugs or ethanol. May cause severe hepatic toxicity in acute overdose. In addition, chronic daily dosing in adults has resulted in liver damage in some patients. Use with caution in patients with hypersensitivity reactions to other phenanthrene-derivative opioid agonists (eg, morphine, hydrocodone, oxycodone). Use caution with Addison's disease, known G6PD deficiency, severe renal or hepatic impairment. Use caution in patients with head injury or other intracranial lesions, acute abdominal conditions, urethral stricture of BPH, thyroid dysfunction, or in patients with respiratory diseases. Use caution in patients with two or more copies of the variant CYP2D6*2 allele; may have extensive conversion from codeine to morphine and thus increased opioid-mediated effects. Elderly (not recommended for use) and/or debilitated patients may be more susceptible to CNS depressants, as well as constipating effects of narcotics. Tolerance or drug dependence may result from extended use. Caffeine may cause CNS and cardiovascular stimulation, as well as GI irritation in high doses. Use with caution in patients with a history of peptic ulcer or GERD; avoid in patients with symptomatic cardiac arrhythmias. Safety and efficacy in pediatric patients have not been established.

Drug Interactions

Metabolism/Transport Effects

Acetaminophen: **Substrate** (minor) of CYP1A2, 2A6, 2C9, 2D6, 2E1, 3A4; **Inhibits** CYP3A4 (weak)

Caffeine: **Substrate** of CYP1A2 (major), 2C9 (minor), 2D6 (minor), 2E1 (minor), 3A4 (minor); **Inhibits** CYP1A2 (weak), 3A4 (moderate)

Codeine: **Substrate** of CYP2D6 (major), 3A4 (minor); **Inhibits** CYP2D6 (weak)

Avoid Concomitant Use

Avoid concomitant use of Butalbital, Acetaminophen, Caffeine, and Codeine with any of the following: Iobenguane I 123; Voriconazole

Increased Effect/Toxicity

Butalbital, Acetaminophen, Caffeine, and Codeine may increase the levels/effects of: Alcohol (Ethyl); Alvimopan; CNS Depressants; Dasatinib; Desmopressin; Formoterol; Imatinib; Meperidine; QuiNIDine; Selective Serotonin Reuptake Inhibitors; SORAfenib; Sympathomimetics; Thiazide Diuretics; Vitamin K Antagonists

The levels/effects of Butalbital, Acetaminophen, Caffeine, and Codeine may be increased by: Abiraterone; Amphetamines; Antipsychotic Agents (Phenothiazines); Atomoxetine; Chloramphenicol; Conivaptan; CYP1A2 Inhibitors (Moderate); CYP1A2 Inhibitors (Strong); Dasatinib; Deferasirox; Divalproex; Droperidol; Felbamate; Imatinib; Isoniazid; Metyrapone; Primidone; Probenecid; Quinolone Antibiotics; Somatostatin Analogs; SORAfenib; Succinylcholine; Valproic Acid

Decreased Effect

Butalbital, Acetaminophen, Caffeine, and Codeine may decrease the levels/effects of: Acetaminophen; Adenosine; Beta-Blockers; Calcium Channel Blockers; Chloramphenicol; Contraceptives (Estrogens); Contraceptives (Progestins); Corticosteroids (Systemic); CycloSPORINE; CycloSPORINE (Systemic); Disopyramide; Divalproex; Doxycycline; Etoposide; Etoposide Phosphate; Felbamate; Fosphenytoin; Griseofulvin; Iobenguane I 123; LamoTRIgine; Methadone; Pegvisomant; Phenytoin; Propafenone; QuiNIDine; Regadenoson; Teniposide; Theophylline Derivatives; Tricyclic Antidepressants; Valproic Acid; Vitamin K Antagonists; Voriconazole

The levels/effects of Butalbital, Acetaminophen, Caffeine, and Codeine may be decreased by: Ammonium Chloride; Anticonvulsants (Hydantoin); Barbiturates; CarBAMazepine; Cholestyramine Resin; CYP2D6 Inhibitors (Moderate); CYP2D6 Inhibitors (Strong); Mixed Agonist / Antagonist Opioids; Peginterferon Alfa-2b; Pyridoxine; Rifamycin Derivatives; Tocilizumab

Ethanol/Nutrition/Herb Interactions Ethanol: Avoid ethanol (may increase CNS depression).

Pregnancy Risk Factor C (per manufacturer)

Lactation Enters breast milk/not recommended

Breast-Feeding Considerations Refer to individual agents. Information specific to butalbital is not available. Discontinuation of breast-feeding or discontinuation of the drug should be considered.

Controlled Substance C-III

Dosage Forms

Capsule: Butalbital 50 mg, acetaminophen 325 mg, caffeine 40 mg, and codeine 30 mg

Fioricet® with Codeine: Butalbital 50 mg, acetaminophen 325 mg, caffeine 40 mg, and codeine 30 mg

Dental Comment Hepatotoxicity caused by acetaminophen is potentiated by chronic alcohol consumption. People who are taking acetaminophen, even at therapeutic doses, and consume alcohol are at risk of developing hepatotoxicity.

Acetaminophen may increase the levels and enhance the anticoagulant effects of vitamin K antagonists acenocoumarol and warfarin (Coumadin®). Studies have reported that acetaminophen has increased the INR in warfarin treated patients with daily acetaminophen doses as low as 2 g, particularly when taking acetaminophen for >1 week (Antlitz, 1968; Boeijinga, 1982; Gebauer, 2003; Hylek, 1998; Rubin, 1984). In addition, case reports of bleeding as a result of increased INR have been published (Bagheri, 1999; Bartle, 1991). There is no known mechanism of the interaction; furthermore, some studies have failed to demonstrate this interaction (Gadisseur, 2003; Kwan, 1995; van den Bemt, 2002). In terms of risk, the data suggest that acetaminophen and warfarin could interact in some clinically significant manner but that the benefits of concomitant use of acetaminophen for pain control in dental patients taking warfarin usually outweigh the risks. An appropriate monitoring plan should be in place to identify potential negative effects and dosage adjustments may be necessary in a minority of patients. The interaction may be more likely to occur with daily acetaminophen doses of >1.3 g for >1 week.

There are no reports of acetaminophen interacting with antiplatelet drugs such as aspirin, clopidogrel (Plavix®), or prasugrel (Effient™). Also, there are no reports of acetaminophen in combination with hydrocodone, codeine, or oxycodone interacting with warfarin (Coumadin®).

References

Antlitz AM, Mead JA Jr, and Tolentino MA, "Potentiation of Oral Anticoagulant Therapy by Acetaminophen," *Curr Ther Res Clin Exp*, 1968, 10(10):501-7.

Bagheri H, Bernhard NB, and Montastruc JL, "Potentiation of the Acenocoumarol Anticoagulant Effect by Acetaminophen," *Ann Pharmacother*, 1999, 33(4):506.

Bartle WR and Blakely JA, "Potentiation of Warfarin Anticoagulation by Acetaminophen," *JAMA*, 1991, 265(10):1260.

Boeijinga JJ, Boerstra EE, Ris P, et al, "Interaction Between Paracetamol and Coumarin Anticoagulants," *Lancet*, 1982, 1(8270):506.

Gadisseur AP, Van Der Meer FJ, and Rosendaal FR, "Sustained Intake of Paracetamol (Acetaminophen) During Oral Anticoagulant Therapy With Coumarins Does Not Cause Clinically Important INR Changes: A Randomized Double-Blind Clinical Trial," *J Thromb Haemost*, 2003, 1(4):714-7.

Gebauer MG, Nyfort-Hansen K, Henschke PJ, et al, "Warfarin and Acetaminophen Interaction," *Pharmacotherapy*, 2003, 23(1):109-12.

Hylek EM, Heiman H, Skates SJ, et al, "Acetaminophen and Other Risk Factors for Excessive Warfarin Anticoagulation," *JAMA*, 1998, 279(9):657-62.

Kwan D, Bartle WR, and Walker SE, "The Effects of Acute and Chronic Acetaminophen Dosing on the Pharmacodynamics and Pharmacokinetics of (R)- and (S)-Warfarin," *Clin Pharmacol Ther*, 1995, 57:212.

Rubin RN, Mentzer RL, and Budzynski AZ, "Potentiation of Anticoagulant Effect of Warfarin by Acetaminophen (Tylenol®)," *Clin Res*, 1984, 32:698a.

van den Bemt PM, Geven LM, Kuitert NA, et al, "The Potential Interaction Between Oral Anticoagulants and Acetaminophen in Everyday Practice," *Pharm World Sci*, 2002, 24(5):201-4.

Butalbital and Acetaminophen (byoo TAL bi tal & a seet a MIN oh fen)

Related Information

Acetaminophen *on page 32*

PHENobarbital *on page 1333*

U.S. Brand Names Bupap; Cephadyn; Phrenilin®; Phrenilin® Forte; Promacet; Sedapap®

Pharmacologic Category Analgesic, Miscellaneous; Barbiturate

Use Relief of the symptomatic complex of tension or muscle contraction headache

Local Anesthetic/Vasoconstrictor Precautions No information available to require special precautions

Effects on Dental Treatment No significant effects or complications reported (see Dental Comment)

Effects on Bleeding No information available to require special precautions

Adverse Effects

Frequently observed:

- Central nervous system: Dizziness, drowsiness, lightheadedness, sedation
- Gastrointestinal: Abdominal pain, nausea, vomiting
- Respiratory: Dyspnea
- Miscellaneous: Intoxicated feeling

Infrequently observed:

- Cardiovascular: Tachycardia
- Central nervous system: Agitation, confusion, depression, euphoria, excitement, faintness, fever, headache, seizure
- Dermatologic: Hyperhidrosis, pruritus
- Endocrine & metabolic: Hot spells
- Gastrointestinal: Constipation, dysphagia, heartburn, flatulence, xerostomia
- Neuromuscular & skeletal: Leg pain, muscle fatigue, numbness, paresthesia
- Ocular: Heavy eyelids
- Otic: Earache, tinnitus

Renal: Diuresis
Respiratory: Nasal congestion
Miscellaneous: Allergic reaction, high energy, shaky feeling, sluggishness

General Dosage Range Oral: *Adults:* 1 tablet/capsule every 4 hours as needed (maximum: 6 doses/day) **or** Phrenilin®: 1-2 tablets every 4 hours as needed (maximum: 6 tablets/day)

Mechanism of Action

Butalbital is a short- to intermediate-acting barbiturate. Barbiturates depress the sensory cortex, decrease motor activity, alter cerebellar function, and produce drowsiness, sedation, hypnosis, and dose-dependent respiratory depression.

Acetaminophen inhibits the synthesis of prostaglandins in the central nervous system and peripherally blocks pain impulse generation; produces antipyresis from inhibition of hypothalamic heat-regulating center.

Pharmacodynamics/Kinetics

Half-life Elimination Butalbital: 35 hours

Pregnancy Risk Factor C

Dental Comment Hepatotoxicity caused by acetaminophen is potentiated by chronic alcohol consumption. People who are taking acetaminophen, even at therapeutic doses, and consume alcohol are at risk of developing hepatotoxicity.

Acetaminophen may increase the levels and enhance the anticoagulant effects of vitamin K antagonists acenocoumarol and warfarin (Coumadin®). Studies have reported that acetaminophen has increased the INR in warfarin treated patients with daily acetaminophen doses as low as 2 g, particularly when taking acetaminophen for >1 week (Antlitz, 1968; Boeijinga, 1982; Gebauer, 2003; Hylek, 1998; Rubin, 1984). In addition, case reports of bleeding as a result of increased INR have been published (Bagheri, 1999; Bartle, 1991). There is no known mechanism of the interaction; furthermore, some studies have failed to demonstrate this interaction (Gadisseur, 2003; Kwan, 1995; van den Bemt, 2002). In terms of risk, the data suggest that acetaminophen and warfarin could interact in some clinically significant manner but that the benefits of concomitant use of acetaminophen for pain control in dental patients taking warfarin usually outweigh the risks. An appropriate monitoring plan should be in place to identify potential negative effects and dosage adjustments may be necessary in a minority of patients. The interaction may be more likely to occur with daily acetaminophen doses of >1.3 g for >1 week.

There are no reports of acetaminophen interacting with antiplatelet drugs such as aspirin, clopidogrel (Plavix®), or prasugrel (Effient™). Also, there are no reports of acetaminophen in combination with hydrocodone, codeine, or oxycodone interacting with warfarin (Coumadin®).

Butalbital, Aspirin, and Caffeine (byoo TAL bi tal, AS pir in, & KAF een)

Related Information

Aspirin *on page 171*
Caffeine *on page 282*

U.S. Brand Names Fiorinal®

Canadian Brand Names Fiorinal®

Pharmacologic Category Barbiturate

Use Relief of the symptomatic complex of tension or muscle contraction headache

Local Anesthetic/Vasoconstrictor Precautions No information available to require special precautions

Effects on Dental Treatment Key adverse event(s) related to dental treatment: Aspirin: As with all drugs which may affect hemostasis, bleeding is associated with aspirin. Hemorrhage may occur at virtually any site; risk is dependent on multiple variables including dosage, concurrent use of multiple agents which alter hemostasis, and patient susceptibility. Many adverse effects of aspirin are dose related, and are rare at low dosages. Other serious reactions are idiosyncratic, related to allergy or individual sensitivity (see Effects on Bleeding).

Effects on Bleeding Aspirin inhibits platelet aggregation which prolongs bleeding times. Inhibition is irreversible; on discontinuation of ASA, normal platelet function returns only when new platelets are released from the bone marrow. Dental practitioners should note that recommendations differ between general surgery (eg, appendectomy, hip replacement) and dental surgery. Due to concerns for increased blood loss, ASA is typically avoided (if possible) in general surgery patients for 1-2 weeks prior to surgery (exception is in patients undergoing CABG or noncardiac surgery at high risk of cardiac events - per 2008 ACCP guidelines). However, in the case of dental surgery there is no scientific evidence to warrant discontinuance of aspirin.

Reports of major bleeding related to dental surgery attributed to aspirin use have not been published. Furthermore, interruption of therapy may result in a loss of therapeutic effect. Patients taking one aspirin tablet daily as an antithrombotic who require dental surgery should be given special consideration in consultation with the physician before removal of the aspirin. In particular, aspirin should NOT be discontinued in patients with cardiac stents that have not completed their full course of dual antiplatelet therapy (aspirin, clopidogrel); patient specific situations need to be discussed with cardiologist. When feasible, postponement of dental surgery until the completion of dual antiplatelet therapy should be considered.

Adverse Effects

>10%:

Central nervous system: Dizziness, lightheadedness, drowsiness, "hangover" effect

Gastrointestinal: Heartburn, stomach pain, dyspepsia, epigastric discomfort, nausea

1% to 10%:

Central nervous system: Confusion, mental depression, unusual excitement, nervousness, faint feeling, headache, insomnia, nightmares, fatigue

Dermatologic: Skin rash

Gastrointestinal: Constipation, vomiting, gastrointestinal ulceration

Hematologic: Hemolytic anemia

Neuromuscular & skeletal: Weakness

Respiratory: Troubled breathing

Miscellaneous: Anaphylactic shock

General Dosage Range Oral: *Adults:* 1-2 tablets/capsules every 4 hours (maximum: 6 tablets/capsules daily)

Pregnancy Risk Factor C/D (prolonged use or high doses at term)

Controlled Substance C-III

Dental Comment There is no scientific evidence to warrant discontinuance of aspirin prior to dental surgery. Patients taking one aspirin tablet daily as an antithrombotic and who require dental surgery should be given special consideration in consultation with the physician before removal of the aspirin relative to prevention of postoperative bleeding.

Butalbital, Aspirin, Caffeine, and Codeine

(byoo TAL bi tal, AS pir in, KAF een, & KOE deen)

Related Information

Aspirin *on page 171*

Caffeine *on page 282*

Codeine *on page 432*

U.S. Brand Names Ascomp® with Codeine; Fiorinal® with Codeine

Canadian Brand Names Fiorinal®-C 1/2; Fiorinal®-C 1/4; Tecnal C 1/2; Tecnal C 1/4

Pharmacologic Category Analgesic Combination (Opioid); Barbiturate

Use Relief of symptoms of complex tension (muscle contraction) headache

Local Anesthetic/Vasoconstrictor Precautions No information available to require special precautions

Effects on Dental Treatment Key adverse event(s) related to dental treatment: Aspirin: As with all drugs which may affect hemostasis, bleeding is associated with aspirin. Hemorrhage may occur at virtually any site; risk is dependent on multiple variables including dosage, concurrent use of multiple agents which alter hemostasis, and patient susceptibility. Many adverse effects of aspirin are dose related, and are rare at low dosages. Other serious reactions are idiosyncratic, related to allergy or individual sensitivity (see Effects on Bleeding).

Effects on Bleeding Aspirin inhibits platelet aggregation which prolongs bleeding times. Inhibition is irreversible; on discontinuation of ASA, normal platelet function returns only when new platelets are released from the bone marrow. Dental practitioners should note that recommendations differ between general surgery (eg, appendectomy, hip replacement) and dental surgery. Due to concerns for increased blood loss, ASA is typically avoided (if possible) in general surgery patients for 1-2 weeks prior to surgery (exception is in patients undergoing CABG or noncardiac surgery at high risk of cardiac events - per 2008 ACCP guidelines). However, in the case of dental surgery there is no scientific evidence to warrant discontinuance of aspirin.

Reports of major bleeding related to dental surgery attributed to aspirin use have not been published. Furthermore, interruption of therapy may result in a loss of therapeutic effect. Patients taking one aspirin tablet daily as an antithrombotic who require dental surgery should be given special consideration in consultation with the physician before removal of the aspirin. In particular, aspirin should NOT be discontinued in patients with cardiac stents that have not completed their full course of dual antiplatelet therapy (aspirin, clopidogrel); patient specific situations need to be discussed with cardiologist. When feasible, postponement of dental surgery until the completion of dual antiplatelet therapy should be considered.

Adverse Effects

1% to 10%:

Central nervous system: Dizziness/lightheadedness (3%), drowsiness (2%), intoxicated feeling (1%)

Gastrointestinal: Abdominal pain/nausea (4%)

Note: Potential reactions associated with components of Fiorinal® with Codeine include acute airway obstruction, anemia, bleeding time prolonged, cardiac stimulation, dependence, hemolytic anemia, hepatitis, hyperglycemia, irritability, nephrotoxicity, occult blood loss, peptic ulcer, pruritus, renal toxicity (high doses, prolonged therapy) thrombocytopenia, tremor, urate excretion impaired

General Dosage Range Oral: *Adults:* 1-2 capsules every 4 hours as needed (maximum: 6 capsules/day)

Mechanism of Action Butalbital is a short-to-intermediate acting barbiturate; aspirin inhibits prostaglandin synthesis and has analgesic, antipyretic and anti-inflammatory actions; caffeine is a CNS stimulant; codeine is a narcotic analgesic and antitussive which produced generalized CNS depression. The combination product is for the treatment of tension headache; however, the role of each component in the relief of symptoms is not completely understood.

Pregnancy Risk Factor C (per manufacturer)

Controlled Substance C-III

Dental Comment There is no scientific evidence to warrant discontinuance of aspirin prior to dental surgery. Patients taking one aspirin tablet daily as an antithrombotic and who require dental surgery should be given special consideration in consultation with the physician before removal of the aspirin relative to prevention of postoperative bleeding.

Butenafine (byoo TEN a feen)

U.S. Brand Names Lotrimin® ultra™ [OTC]; Mentax®

Pharmacologic Category Antifungal Agent, Topical

Use Topical treatment of tinea pedis (athlete's foot), tinea cruris (jock itch), tinea corporis (ringworm), and tinea versicolor

Local Anesthetic/Vasoconstrictor Precautions No information available to require special precautions

Effects on Dental Treatment No significant effects or complications reported

Effects on Bleeding No information available to require special precautions

Adverse Effects >1%: Dermatologic: Burning, contact dermatitis, erythema, irritation, pruritus, stinging

General Dosage Range Topical: *Children >12 years and Adults:* Apply to affected area once or twice daily

Mechanism of Action Butenafine exerts fungicidal activity against dermatophytes (eg trichophyton, epidermophyton) by blocking squalene epoxidation, resulting in inhibition of ergosterol synthesis and subsequent weakening of fungal cell membranes.

Pharmacodynamics/Kinetics

Half-life Elimination Biphasic: Alpha: 35 hours; Beta: >150 hours

Time to Peak Serum: 6-15 hours

Pregnancy Risk Factor C

Butoconazole (byoo toe KOE na zole)

U.S. Brand Names Gynazole-1®

Canadian Brand Names Femstat® One; Gynazole-1®

Pharmacologic Category Antifungal Agent, Vaginal

Use Local treatment of vulvovaginal candidiasis

Local Anesthetic/Vasoconstrictor Precautions No information available to require special precautions

Effects on Dental Treatment No significant effects or complications reported

Effects on Bleeding No information available to require special precautions

Adverse Effects Frequency not defined.

Gastrointestinal: Abdominal pain or cramping

Genitourinary: Pelvic pain; vulvar/vaginal burning, itching, soreness, and swelling

General Dosage Range Intravaginal: *Adults:* Insert 1 applicatorful at bedtime

Mechanism of Action Increases cell membrane permeability in susceptible fungi (*Candida*)

Pharmacodynamics/Kinetics
Time to Peak 12-24 hours
Pregnancy Risk Factor C (use only in 2nd or 3rd trimester)

Butorphanol (byoo TOR fa nole)

Canadian Brand Names Apo-Butorphanol®; PMS-Butorphanol
Pharmacologic Category Analgesic, Opioid
Use
Parenteral: Management of moderate-to-severe pain; preoperative medication; supplement to balanced anesthesia; management of pain during labor
Nasal spray: Management of moderate-to-severe pain, including migraine headache pain
Local Anesthetic/Vasoconstrictor Precautions No information available to require special precautions
Effects on Dental Treatment Key adverse event(s) related to dental treatment: Xerostomia (normal salivary flow resumes upon discontinuation) and unpleasant aftertaste.
Effects on Bleeding No information available to require special precautions
Adverse Effects
>10%:
Central nervous system: Somnolence (43%), dizziness (19%), insomnia (nasal spray 11%)
Gastrointestinal: Nausea/vomiting (13%)
Respiratory: Nasal congestion (nasal spray 13%)
1% to 10%:
Cardiovascular: Palpitation, vasodilation
Central nervous system: Anxiety, confusion, headache, lethargy, lightheadedness
Dermatologic: Pruritus
Gastrointestinal: Anorexia, constipation, stomach pain, unpleasant aftertaste, xerostomia
Neuromuscular & skeletal: Tremor, paresthesia, weakness
Ocular: Blurred vision
Otic: Ear pain, tinnitus
Respiratory: Bronchitis, cough, dyspnea, epistaxis, nasal irritation, pharyngitis, rhinitis, sinus congestion, sinusitis, upper respiratory infection
Miscellaneous: Diaphoresis increased
General Dosage Range Dosage adjustment recommended in patients with hepatic or renal impairment
I.M.:
Adults: Initial: 2 mg, may repeat every 3-4 hours as needed; Usual range: 1-4 mg every 3-4 hours as needed **or** 2 mg prior to surgery
Elderly: Initial: 1/2 of the recommended dose, repeated dosing generally should be at least 6 hours apart
I.V.:
Adults: Initial: 1 mg, may repeat every 3-4 hours as needed; Usual range: 0.5-2 mg every 3-4 hours as needed **or** 2 mg and/or an incremental dose of 0.5-1 mg (up to 0.06 mg/kg) as supplement to surgery
Elderly: Initial: 1/2 of the recommended dose, repeated dosing generally should be at least 6 hours apart
Intranasal:
Adults: Initial: 1 spray (~1 mg) in 1 nostril, may repeat in 60-90 minutes, then repeat initial dose sequence in 3-4 hours after last dose as needed; may use initial dose of 1 spray in each nostril (2 mg) in patients who will remain recumbent
Elderly: Initial: Should not exceed 1 mg, may repeat after 90-120 minutes
Mechanism of Action Mixed narcotic agonist-antagonist with central analgesic actions; binds to opiate receptors in the CNS, causing inhibition of ascending pain pathways, altering the perception of and response to pain; produces generalized CNS depression
Pharmacodynamics/Kinetics
Onset of Action I.M.: 5-10 minutes; I.V.: <10 minutes; Nasal: Within 15 minutes
Peak effect: I.M.: 0.5-1 hour; I.V.: 4-5 minutes
Duration of Action I.M., I.V.: 3-4 hours; Nasal: 4-5 hours
Half-life Elimination 2.5-4 hours
Pregnancy Risk Factor C
Controlled Substance C-IV

C1 Inhibitor (Human) (cee won in HIB i ter HYU man)

U.S. Brand Names Berinert®; Cinryze™

Pharmacologic Category Blood Product Derivative

Use

Berinert®: Treatment of acute abdominal or facial attacks of hereditary angioedema (HAE)

Cinryze™: Routine prophylaxis against angioedema attacks in patients with HAE or inherited C1 inhibitor deficiency

Local Anesthetic/Vasoconstrictor Precautions No information available to require special precautions

Effects on Dental Treatment No significant effects or complications reported

Effects on Bleeding C1 inhibitor plays a role in the regulation of the complement and intrinsic coagulation pathway; consider potential risk of thrombosis.

Adverse Effects

>10%: Central nervous system: Headache (≤12%)

1% to 10%:

- Dermatologic: Pruritus, rash
- Gastrointestinal: Abdominal pain, abnormal taste
- Neuromuscular & skeletal: Back pain, extremity pain
- Respiratory: Bronchitis, nasopharyngitis, sinusitis, upper respiratory tract infection
- Miscellaneous: Limb injury

General Dosage Range Oral: *Adolescents and Adults:* 1000 units every 3-4 days **or** 20 units/kg

Mechanism of Action C1 inhibitor, one of the serine proteinase inhibitors found in human blood, plays a role in regulating the complement and intrinsic coagulation (contact system) pathway, and is also involved in the fibrinolytic and kinin pathways. C1 inhibitor therapy in patients with C1 inhibitor deficiency, such as HAE, is believed to suppress contact system activation via inactivation of plasma kallikrein and factor XIIa, thus preventing bradykinin production. Unregulated bradykinin production is thought to contribute to the increased vascular permeability and angioedema observed in HAE.

Pharmacodynamics/Kinetics

Onset of Action Increased plasma C1 inhibitor levels observed ~1 hour or less

Half-life Elimination

Berinert®: 22 hours (range: 17-24 hours)

Cinryze™: 56 hours (range: 11-108 hours)

Time to Peak ~4 hours

Pregnancy Risk Factor C

Prescribing and Access Restrictions Assistance with procurement and reimbursement of Cinryze™ is available for healthcare providers and patients through the CINRYZE*Solutions*® program (telephone: 1-877-945-1000) or at http://www.-cinryze.com/Cinryze_Solutions/Default.aspx

Cabazitaxel (ca baz i TAKS el)

U.S. Brand Names Jevtana®

Pharmacologic Category Antineoplastic Agent, Antimicrotubular; Antineoplastic Agent, Taxane Derivative

Use Treatment of hormone-refractory metastatic prostate cancer (in patients previously treated with a docetaxel-containing regimen)

Local Anesthetic/Vasoconstrictor Precautions No information available to require special precautions

Effects on Dental Treatment Key adverse event(s) related to dental treatment: Taste alteration

Effects on Bleeding Chemotherapy may result in significant myelosuppression, potentially including significant reduction in platelet counts and altered hemostasis. In patients who are under active treatment with these agents, medical consult is suggested.

Adverse Effects Note: Adverse reactions reported for combination therapy with prednisone.

>10%:

- Central nervous system: Fatigue (37%), fever (12%)
- Gastrointestinal: Diarrhea (47%; grades 3/4: 6%), nausea (34%), vomiting (22%), constipation (20%), abdominal pain (17%), anorexia (16%), taste alteration (11%)
- Hematologic: Anemia (98%; grades 3/4: 11%), leukopenia (96%; grades 3/4: 69%), neutropenia (94%; grades 3/4: 82%; nadir: 12 days [range: 4-17 days]), thrombocytopenia (48%; grades 3/4: 4%)
- Neuromuscular & skeletal: Weakness (20%), back pain (16%), peripheral neuropathy (13%; grades 3/4: <1%), arthralgia (11%)
- Renal: Hematuria (17%)
- Respiratory: Dyspnea (12%), cough (11%)

1% to 10%:

Cardiovascular: Peripheral edema (9%), arrhythmia (5%), hypotension (5%)
Central nervous system: Dizziness (8%), headache (8%), pain (5%)
Dermatologic: Alopecia (10%)
Endocrine & metabolic: Dehydration (5%)
Gastrointestinal: Dyspepsia (10%), weight loss (9%), mucosal inflammation (6%)
Genitourinary: Urinary tract infection (8%), dysuria (7%)
Hematologic: Neutropenic fever (grades 3/4: 7%)
Hepatic: ALT increased (grades 3/4: ≤1%), AST increased (grades 3/4: ≤1%), bilirubin increased (grades 3/4: ≤1%)
Neuromuscular & skeletal: Muscle spasm (7%)

General Dosage Range Dosage adjustment recommended in patients with hepatic impairment or who develop toxicities

I.V.: *Adults:* 25 mg/m^2 once every 3 weeks

Mechanism of Action Cabazitaxel is a taxane derivative which is a microtubule inhibitor; it binds to tubulin promoting assembly into microtubules and inhibiting disassembly which stabilizes microtubules. This inhibits microtubule depolymerization and cell division, arresting the cell cycle and inhibiting tumor proliferation. Unlike other taxanes, cabazitaxel has a poor affinity for multidrug resistance (MDR) proteins, therefore conferring activity in resistant tumors.

Pharmacodynamics/Kinetics

Half-life Elimination Terminal: 95 hours

Pregnancy Risk Factor D

Cabergoline (ca BER goe leen)

Canadian Brand Names CO Cabergoline; Dostinex®

Pharmacologic Category Ergot Derivative

Use Treatment of hyperprolactinemic disorders, either idiopathic or due to pituitary adenomas

Local Anesthetic/Vasoconstrictor Precautions No information available to require special precautions

Effects on Dental Treatment Key adverse event(s) related to dental treatment: Xerostomia (normal salivary flow resumes upon discontinuation), throat irritation, and toothache.

Effects on Bleeding No information available to require special precautions

Adverse Effects

>10%:

Central nervous system: Headache (26%), dizziness (15% to 17%)
Gastrointestinal: Nausea (27% to 29%)

1% to 10%:

Cardiovascular: Postural hypotension (4%), hypotension (1%), dependent edema (1%), edema (peripheral 1%), palpitation (1%), syncope (1%)
Central nervous system: Fatigue (5% to 7%), vertigo (1% to 4%), depression (3%), somnolence (2% to 5%), nervousness (1% to 2%), anxiety (1%), insomnia (1%), concentration impaired (1%), malaise (1%)
Dermatologic: Acne (1%), pruritus (1%)
Endocrine: Hot flashes (1% to 3%), breast pain (1% to 2%), dysmenorrhea (1%)
Gastrointestinal: Constipation (7% to 10%), abdominal pain (5%), dyspepsia (2% to 5%), vomiting (2% to 4%), xerostomia (2%), diarrhea (2%), flatulence (2%), anorexia (1%), throat irritation (1%), toothache (1%)
Neuromuscular & skeletal: Weakness (6% to 9%), pain (2%), paresthesia (1% to 2%), arthralgia (1%)
Ocular: Abnormal vision (1%), periorbital edema (1%)
Respiratory: Rhinitis (1%)
Miscellaneous: Flu-like syndrome (1%)

General Dosage Range Oral: *Adults:* Initial: 0.25 mg twice weekly; Maintenance: Up to 1 mg twice weekly

Mechanism of Action Cabergoline is a long acting dopamine receptor agonist with a high affinity for D_2 receptors; prolactin secretion by the anterior pituitary is predominantly under hypothalamic inhibitory control exerted through the release of dopamine. It is a potent 5-HT_{2B}-receptor agonist, which may contribute to observed fibrotic/valvulopathic events.

Pharmacodynamics/Kinetics

Half-life Elimination 63-69 hours

Time to Peak 2-3 hours

Pregnancy Risk Factor B

Caffeine (KAF een)

U.S. Brand Names Cafcit®; Enerjets [OTC]; No Doz® Maximum Strength [OTC]; Vivarin® [OTC]

Pharmacologic Category Stimulant

Use

Caffeine citrate: Treatment of idiopathic apnea of prematurity

Caffeine and sodium benzoate: Treatment of acute respiratory depression (not a preferred agent)

Caffeine [OTC labeling]: Restore mental alertness or wakefulness when experiencing fatigue

Unlabeled/Investigational Use Caffeine and sodium benzoate: Treatment of spinal puncture headache; CNS stimulant; diuretic; augmentation of seizure induction during electroconvulsive therapy (ECT)

Local Anesthetic/Vasoconstrictor Precautions No information available to require special precautions

Effects on Dental Treatment No significant effects or complications reported

Effects on Bleeding No information available to require special precautions

Adverse Effects Frequency not specified; primarily serum-concentration related.

Cardiovascular: Angina, arrhythmia (ventricular), chest pain, flushing, palpitation, sinus tachycardia, tachycardia (supraventricular), vasodilation

Central nervous system: Agitation, delirium, dizziness, hallucinations, headache, insomnia, irritability, psychosis, restlessness

Dermatologic: Urticaria

Gastrointestinal: Esophageal sphincter tone decreased, gastritis

Neuromuscular & skeletal: Fasciculations

Ocular: Intraocular pressure increased (>180 mg caffeine), miosis

Renal: Diuresis

General Dosage Range

I.M. (caffeine and sodium benzoate):

Children: 8 mg/kg every 4 hours as needed

Adults: 250 mg as a single dose; may repeat as needed (maximum: 500 mg/dose; 2500 mg/day)

I.V.:

Neonates (caffeine citrate): Loading dose: 10-20 mg/kg; Maintenance: 5 mg/kg once daily

Children (caffeine and sodium benzoate): 8 mg/kg every 4 hours as needed

Adults (caffeine and sodium benzoate): 250 mg as a single dose; may repeat as needed (maximum: 500 mg/dose; 2500 mg/day) **or** 300-2000 mg (electroconvulsive therapy)

Oral:

Neonates (caffeine citrate): Loading dose: 10-20 mg/kg; Maintenance: 5 mg/kg once daily

Children ≥12 years and Adults: 100-200 mg every 3-4 hours as needed (OTC labeling)

SubQ (caffeine and sodium benzoate): *Children:* 8 mg/kg every 4 hours as needed

Mechanism of Action Increases levels of 3'5' cyclic AMP by inhibiting phosphodiesterase; CNS stimulant which increases medullary respiratory center sensitivity to carbon dioxide, stimulates central inspiratory drive, and improves skeletal muscle contraction (diaphragmatic contractility); prevention of apnea may occur by competitive inhibition of adenosine

Pharmacodynamics/Kinetics

Half-life Elimination

Neonates: 72-96 hours (range: 40-230 hours)

Children >9 months and Adults: 5 hours

Time to Peak Serum: Oral: Within 30 minutes to 2 hours

Pregnancy Risk Factor C

Calcipotriene (kal si POE try een)

U.S. Brand Names Calcitrene™; Dovonex®

Canadian Brand Names Dovonex®

Pharmacologic Category Topical Skin Product; Vitamin D Analog

Use Treatment of plaque psoriasis; chronic, moderate-to-severe psoriasis of the scalp

Unlabeled/Investigational Use Vitiligo

Local Anesthetic/Vasoconstrictor Precautions No information available to require special precautions

Effects on Dental Treatment No significant effects or complications reported
Effects on Bleeding No information available to require special precautions
Adverse Effects Frequency may vary with site of application.
>10%: Dermatologic: Burning, itching, rash, skin irritation, stinging, tingling
1% to 10%: Dermatologic: Dermatitis, dry skin, erythema, peeling, pruritus, worsening of psoriasis
General Dosage Range Topical: *Adults:* Cream, solution: Apply a thin film to affected area 2 times/day; Ointment: Apply a thin film to affected area 1-2 times/day
Mechanism of Action Synthetic vitamin D_3 analog which regulates skin cell production and proliferation
Pharmacodynamics/Kinetics
Onset of Action Improvement begins after 2 weeks; marked improvement seen after 8 weeks
Pregnancy Risk Factor C

Calcitonin (kal si TOE nin)

Related Information
Rheumatoid Arthritis, Osteoarthritis, and Osteoporosis *on page 1889*
U.S. Brand Names Fortical®; Miacalcin®
Canadian Brand Names Apo-Calcitonin®; Calcimar®; Caltine®; Miacalcin® NS; PRO-Calcitonin; Sandoz-Calcitonin
Pharmacologic Category Antidote; Hormone
Use Treatment of Paget's disease of bone (osteitis deformans); adjunctive therapy for hypercalcemia; treatment of osteoporosis in women >5 years postmenopause
Local Anesthetic/Vasoconstrictor Precautions No information available to require special precautions
Effects on Dental Treatment No significant effects or complications reported
Effects on Bleeding No information available to require special precautions
Adverse Effects Unless otherwise noted, frequencies reported are with nasal spray.
>10%: Respiratory: Rhinitis (≤12%, including ulcerative)
1% to 10%:
Cardiovascular: Flushing (nasal spray: <1%; injection: 2% to 5%), angina (1% to 3%), hypertension (1% to 3%)
Central nervous system: Depression (1% to 3%), dizziness (1% to 3%), fatigue (1% to 3%)
Dermatologic: Erythematous rash (1% to 3%)
Gastrointestinal: Nausea (injection: 10%; nasal spray: 2%), abdominal pain (1% to 3%), constipation (1% to 3%), diarrhea (1% to 3%), dyspepsia (1% to 3%)
Genitourinary: Cystitis (1% to 3%)
Local: Injection site reactions (injection: 10%)
Neuromuscular & skeletal: Back pain (5%), arthrosis (1% to 3%), myalgia (1% to 3%), paresthesia (1% to 3%)
Ocular: Conjunctivitis (1% to 3%), lacrimation abnormality (1% to 3%)
Respiratory: Nasal ulcerations (3%), bronchospasm (1% to 3%), sinusitis (1% to 3%), upper respiratory tract infection (1% to 3%)
Miscellaneous: Flu-like syndrome (1% to 3%), infection (1% to 3%), lymphadenopathy (1% to 3%)
General Dosage Range
I.M., SubQ: *Adults:* Paget's disease/osteoporosis: 50-100 units every 1-3 days; Hypercalcemia: 4-8 units/kg every 12 hours (maximum: 8 units/kg every 6 hours)
Intranasal: *Adults:* 200 units (1 spray) in one nostril daily
Mechanism of Action Peptide sequence similar to human calcitonin; functionally antagonizes the effects of parathyroid hormone. Directly inhibits osteoclastic bone resorption; promotes the renal excretion of calcium, phosphate, sodium, magnesium, and potassium by decreasing tubular reabsorption; increases the jejunal secretion of water, sodium, potassium, and chloride
Pharmacodynamics/Kinetics
Onset of Action
Hypercalcemia: I.M., SubQ: ~2 hours
Paget's disease: Within a few months; may take up to 1 year for neurologic symptom improvement
Duration of Action Hypercalcemia: I.M., SubQ: 6-8 hours
Half-life Elimination Terminal: I.M. 58 minutes; SubQ 59-64 minutes; Nasal: ~18 minutes
Time to Peak Plasma: SubQ ~23 minutes; Nasal: ~13 minutes
Pregnancy Risk Factor C

Calcitriol (kal si TRYE ole)

U.S. Brand Names Calcijex®; Rocaltrol®; Vectical™

Canadian Brand Names Calcijex®; Rocaltrol®

Pharmacologic Category Vitamin D Analog

Use

Oral, injection: Management of hypocalcemia in patients on chronic renal dialysis; management of secondary hyperparathyroidism in patients with chronic kidney disease (CKD); management of hypocalcemia in hypoparathyroidism and pseudohypoparathyroidism

Topical: Management of mild-to-moderate plaque psoriasis

Unlabeled/Investigational Use Decrease severity of psoriatic lesions in psoriatic vulgaris; vitamin D-dependent rickets

Local Anesthetic/Vasoconstrictor Precautions No information available to require special precautions

Effects on Dental Treatment Key adverse event(s) related to dental treatment: Metallic taste and xerostomia (normal salivary flow resumes upon discontinuation).

Effects on Bleeding No information available to require special precautions

Adverse Effects

Oral, I.V.: Frequency not defined.

Cardiovascular: Cardiac arrhythmia, hypertension

Central nervous system: Apathy, headache, hypothermia, psychosis, sensory disturbances, somnolence

Dermatologic: Erythema multiforme, pruritus

Endocrine & metabolic: Dehydration, growth suppression, hypercalcemia, hypercholesterolemia, hypermagnesemia, hyperphosphatemia, libido decreased, polydipsia

Gastrointestinal: Abdominal pain, anorexia, constipation, metallic taste, nausea, pancreatitis, stomach ache, vomiting, weight loss, xerostomia

Genitourinary: Nocturia, urinary tract infection

Hepatic: ALT increased, AST increased

Local: Injection site pain (mild)

Neuromuscular & skeletal: Bone pain, myalgia, dystrophy, soft tissue calcification, weakness

Ocular: Conjunctivitis, photophobia

Renal: Albuminuria, BUN increased, creatinine increased, hypercalciuria, nephrocalcinosis, polyuria

Respiratory: Rhinorrhea

Miscellaneous: Allergic reaction

Topical:

>10%: Endocrine: Hypercalcemia (≤24%)

1% to 10%:

Dermatologic: Skin discomfort (3%), pruritus (1% to 3%)

Genitourinary: Urine abnormality (4%)

Renal: Hypercalciuria (3%)

General Dosage Range Dosage adjustment recommended in patients who develop toxicities

I.V.: *Adults:* 0.5-4 mcg 3 times/week

Oral:

Children: 0.25-0.2 mcg/day **or** 0.01-0.015 mcg/kg/day (maximum: 0.5 mcg/day)

Adults: 0.25 mcg every other day to 2 mcg once daily

Topical: *Adults:* Apply to affected areas twice daily (maximum: 200 g/week)

Mechanism of Action Calcitriol is a potent active metabolite of vitamin D. Vitamin D promotes absorption of calcium in the intestines and retention at the kidneys thereby increasing calcium levels in the serum; decreases excessive serum phosphatase levels, parathyroid hormone levels, and decreases bone resorption; increases renal tubule phosphate resorption

The mechanism by which calcitriol is beneficial in the treatment of psoriasis has not been established.

Pharmacodynamics/Kinetics

Onset of Action Oral: ~2-6 hours

Duration of Action Oral, I.V.: 3-5 days

Half-life Elimination Children ~27 hours; Normal adults: 5-8 hours; Hemodialysis: 16-22 hours

Time to Peak Oral: 3-6 hours; Hemodialysis: 8-12 hours

Pregnancy Risk Factor C

Calcium Acetate (KAL see um AS e tate)

Related Information

Rheumatoid Arthritis, Osteoarthritis, and Osteoporosis *on page 1889*

U.S. Brand Names Eliphos™; PhosLo®

Canadian Brand Names PhosLo®

Pharmacologic Category Antidote; Calcium Salt; Phosphate Binder

Use Control of hyperphosphatemia in end-stage renal failure; does not promote aluminum absorption

Local Anesthetic/Vasoconstrictor Precautions No information available to require special precautions

Effects on Dental Treatment No significant effects or complications reported

Effects on Bleeding No information available to require special precautions

Adverse Effects 1% to 10%:

Endocrine & metabolic: Hypercalcemia

Gastrointestinal: Nausea, vomiting

General Dosage Range Oral:

Children 0-6 months: Adequate intake:: 200 mg/day

Children 7-12 months: Adequate intake:: 260 mg/day

Children 1-3 years: RDA: 700 mg/day

Children 4-8 years: RDA: 1000 mg/day

Children 9-18 years: RDA 1300 mg/day

Adults: Initial: 1334 mg with each meal; Maintenance: 2001-2668 mg with each meal

Adults 19-50 years: RDA: 1000 mg/day

Adults ≥51 years, females: RDA: 1200 mg/day

Adults 51-70 years, males: RDA: 1000 mg/day

Adults >70 years, males: RDA: 1200 mg/day

Mechanism of Action Combines with dietary phosphate to form insoluble calcium phosphate which is excreted in feces

Pregnancy Risk Factor C

Product Availability

Phoslyra™ (calcium acetate) 667 mg/5 mL oral solution: FDA approved April 2011; expected availability undetermined

Phoslyra™ is a phosphate binder approved to reduce serum phosphorus in patients with end-stage renal disease.

Calcium and Vitamin D (KAL see um & VYE ta min dee)

U.S. Brand Names Cal-CYUM [OTC]; Caltrate® 600+D [OTC]; Caltrate® 600+Soy™ [OTC]; Caltrate® ColonHealth™ [OTC]; Chew-Cal [OTC]; Citracal® Maximum [OTC]; Citracal® Petites [OTC]; Citracal® Regular [OTC]; Liqua-Cal [OTC]; Os-Cal® 500+D [OTC]; Oysco 500+D [OTC]; Oysco D [OTC]; Oyst-Cal-D 500 [OTC]; Oyst-Cal-D [OTC]

Generic Availability (U.S.) Yes

Pharmacologic Category Calcium Salt; Electrolyte Supplement, Oral; Vitamin, Fat Soluble

Use Dietary supplement, antacid

Local Anesthetic/Vasoconstrictor Precautions No information available to require special precautions

Effects on Dental Treatment No significant effects or complications reported

Effects on Bleeding No information available to require special precautions

Adverse Effects Frequency not defined; also see individual agents

Central nervous system: Headache

Endocrine & metabolic: Hypercalcemia, hypercalciuria

Gastrointestinal: Gastrointestinal discomfort

Dosage Oral: Adults: Refer to individual monographs for dietary reference intake.

Dosage adjustment in renal impairment: Use caution in severe renal impairment

Contraindications Hypersensitivity to any component of the formulation; hypophosphatemia, hypercalcemia, evidence of vitamin D toxicity; history of kidney stones

Warnings/Precautions Constipation, bloating, and gas are common with calcium supplements. Use with caution patients with respiratory failure, renal impairment or respiratory acidosis. Use with caution in patients with renal failure to avoid hypercalcemia; frequent monitoring of serum calcium and phosphorus is necessary. Use caution when administering calcium supplements to patients with a history of kidney stones. Hypercalcemia and hypercalciuria are most likely to occur in hypoparathyroid patients receiving high doses of vitamin D. Calcium absorption is impaired in achlorhydria; common in elderly, use an alternate salt (eg, citrate) and administer with food. Calcium administration interferes with absorption of some minerals and drugs; use with caution. Taking calcium (≤500 mg) with food improves absorption.

Some products may contain soy, tartrazine, or phenylalanine, or may be derived from shellfish.

Drug Interactions

Avoid Concomitant Use

Avoid concomitant use of Calcium Carbonate and Vitamin D with any of the following: Calcium Acetate

Increased Effect/Toxicity

Calcium Carbonate and Vitamin D may increase the levels/effects of: Alpha-/Beta-Agonists; Amphetamines; Calcium Acetate; Calcium Polystyrene Sulfonate; Dexmethylphenidate; Methylphenidate; QuiNIDine; Sodium Polystyrene Sulfonate

The levels/effects of Calcium Carbonate and Vitamin D may be increased by: Thiazide Diuretics

Decreased Effect

Calcium Carbonate and Vitamin D may decrease the levels/effects of: ACE Inhibitors; Allopurinol; Anticonvulsants (Hydantoin); Antipsychotic Agents (Phenothiazines); Atazanavir; Bisacodyl; Bisphosphonate Derivatives; Calcium Channel Blockers; Cefditoren; Cefpodoxime; Cefuroxime; Chloroquine; Corticosteroids (Oral); Dabigatran Etexilate; Dasatinib; Delavirdine; DOBUTamine; Eltrombopag; Erlotinib; Estramustine; Gabapentin; HMG-CoA Reductase Inhibitors; Iron Salts; Isoniazid; Itraconazole; Ketoconazole; Ketoconazole (Systemic); Mesalamine; Methenamine; Mycophenolate; Penicillamine; Phosphate Supplements; Protease Inhibitors; Quinolone Antibiotics; Tetracycline Derivatives; Thyroid Products; Trientine

The levels/effects of Calcium Carbonate and Vitamin D may be decreased by: Trientine

Ethanol/Nutrition/Herb Interactions

Ethanol: Avoid ethanol (may increase risk of osteoporosis).

Food: Food may increase calcium absorption. Calcium may decrease iron absorption. Bran, foods high in oxalates, or whole grain cereals may decrease calcium absorption.

Dietary Considerations Take (preferably with food) 2 hours before or after other medications to minimize GI upset. Some products may contain phenylalanine (avoid use in phenylketonurics).

Breast-Feeding Considerations Available evidence suggests safe use during lactation.

Dosage Forms

Caplet, oral:

Citracal® Maximum [OTC]: Calcium 315 mg and vitamin D 250 int. units

Capsule, softgel, oral: Calcium 500 mg and vitamin D 500 int. units; calcium 600 mg and vitamin D 100 int. units; calcium 600 mg and vitamin D 200 int. units

Liqua-Cal [OTC]: Calcium 600 mg and vitamin D 200 int. units

Tablet, oral: Calcium 250 mg and vitamin D 125 int. units; calcium 500 mg and vitamin D 125 int. units; calcium 500 mg and vitamin D 200 int. units; calcium 600 mg and vitamin D 125 int. units; calcium 600 mg and vitamin D 200 int. units

Caltrate® 600+D [OTC]: Calcium 600 mg and vitamin D 200 int. units

Caltrate® 600+Soy™ [OTC]: Calcium 600 mg and vitamin D 200 int. units

Caltrate® ColonHealth™ [OTC]: Calcium 600 mg and vitamin D 200 int. units

Citracal® Petites [OTC]: Calcium 200 mg and vitamin D 250 int. units

Citracal® Regular [OTC]: Calcium 250 mg and vitamin D 200 int. units

Oysco D [OTC]: Calcium 250 mg and vitamin D 125 int. units

Oysco 500+D [OTC]: Calcium 500 mg and vitamin D 200 int. units

Oyst-Cal-D [OTC]: Calcium 250 mg and vitamin D 125 int. units

Oyst-Cal-D 500 [OTC]: Calcium 500 mg and vitamin D 200 int. units

Tablet, chewable: Calcium 500 mg and vitamin D 100 int. units; calcium 600 mg and vitamin D 400 int. units

Os-Cal® 500+D [OTC]: Calcium 500 mg and vitamin D 400 int. units

Wafer, chewable:

Cal-CYUM [OTC]: Calcium 519 mg and vitamin D 150 int. units (50s)

Chew-Cal [OTC]: Calcium 333 mg and vitamin D 40 int. units (100s, 250s)

Calcium Carbonate (KAL see um KAR bun ate)

Related Information

Rheumatoid Arthritis, Osteoarthritis, and Osteoporosis *on page 1889*

U.S. Brand Names Alcalak [OTC]; Alka-Mints® [OTC]; Cal-Gest [OTC]; Cal-Mint [OTC]; Calcarb 600 [OTC] [DSC]; Calci-Chew® [OTC]; Calci-Mix® [OTC]; Caltrate® 600 [OTC]; Children's Pepto [OTC]; Chooz® [OTC]; Florical® [OTC]; Maalox®

Children's [OTC]; Maalox® Regular Strength [OTC]; Nephro-Calci® [OTC]; Nutralox® [OTC]; Oysco 500 [OTC]; Oystercal™ 500 [OTC]; Rolaids® Extra Strength [OTC]; Super Calcium 600 [OTC]; Titralac™ [OTC]; Tums® E-X [OTC]; Tums® Extra Strength Sugar Free [OTC]; Tums® Quickpak [OTC]; Tums® Smoothies™ [OTC]; Tums® Ultra [OTC]; Tums® [OTC]

Canadian Brand Names Apo-Cal®; Calcite-500; Caltrate®; Caltrate® Select; Os-Cal®

Pharmacologic Category Antacid; Antidote; Calcium Salt; Electrolyte Supplement, Oral

Use As an antacid; treatment and prevention of calcium deficiency or hyperphosphatemia (eg, osteoporosis, osteomalacia, mild/moderate renal insufficiency, hypoparathyroidism, postmenopausal osteoporosis, rickets); has been used to bind phosphate

Local Anesthetic/Vasoconstrictor Precautions No information available to require special precautions

Effects on Dental Treatment Key adverse event(s) related to dental treatment: Xerostomia (normal salivary flow resumes upon discontinuation).

Effects on Bleeding No information available to require special precautions

Adverse Effects Well tolerated

1% to 10%:

Central nervous system: Headache

Endocrine & metabolic: Hypophosphatemia, hypercalcemia

Gastrointestinal: Constipation, laxative effect, acid rebound, nausea, vomiting, anorexia, abdominal pain, xerostomia, flatulence

Miscellaneous: Milk-alkali syndrome with very high, chronic dosing and/or renal failure (headache, nausea, irritability, weakness, alkalosis, hypercalcemia, renal impairment)

General Dosage Range Oral:

Neonates: 50-150 mg/kg/day in 4-6 divided doses (maximum: 1 g/day)

Children <2 years: 45-65 mg/kg/day in 4 divided doses

Children 2-5 years (24-47 lbs): Antacid: 161 mg (elemental calcium) as needed (maximum: 483 mg/day); Hypocalcemia: 45-65 mg/kg/day in 4 divided doses

Children 6-11 years (48-95 lbs): Antacid: 322 mg (elemental calcium) as needed (maximum: 966 mg/day); Hypocalcemia: 45-65 mg/kg/day in 4 divided doses

Children >11 years: 45-65 mg/kg/day in 4 divided doses

Adults ≤51 years: Antacid: 1-2 tablets or 5-10 mL every 2 hours (maximum: 7000 mg/day); Hypocalcemia/dietary: 500-2000 mg/day in 2-4 divided doses

Adults >51 years: Antacid: 1-2 tablets or 5-10 mL every 2 hours (maximum: 7000 mg/day); Hypocalcemia/dietary: 500-2000 mg/day in 2-4 divided doses; Osteoporosis: 1200 mg/day

Mechanism of Action As dietary supplement, used to prevent or treat negative calcium balance; in osteoporosis, it helps to prevent or decrease the rate of bone loss. The calcium in calcium salts moderates nerve and muscle performance and allows normal cardiac function. Also used to treat hyperphosphatemia in patients with advanced renal insufficiency by combining with dietary phosphate to form insoluble calcium phosphate, which is excreted in feces. Calcium salts as antacids neutralize gastric acidity resulting in increased gastric and duodenal bulb pH; they additionally inhibit proteolytic activity of peptic if the pH is increased >4 and increase lower esophageal sphincter tone.

Calcium Carbonate and Magnesium Hydroxide

(KAL see um KAR bun ate & mag NEE zhum hye DROKS ide)

Related Information

Calcium Carbonate *on page* 286

Magnesium Hydroxide *on page* 1049

U.S. Brand Names Mi-Acid™ Double Strength [OTC]; Mylanta® Gelcaps® [OTC]; Mylanta® Supreme [OTC]; Mylanta® Ultra [OTC]; Rolaids® Extra Strength [OTC]; Rolaids® [OTC]

Pharmacologic Category Antacid

Use Hyperacidity

Local Anesthetic/Vasoconstrictor Precautions No information available to require special precautions

Effects on Dental Treatment No significant effects or complications reported

Effects on Bleeding No information available to require special precautions

General Dosage Range Oral: *Adults:* 2-4 tablets between meals and at bedtime

Calcium Carbonate and Simethicone

(KAL see um KAR bun ate & sye METH i kone)

Related Information

Calcium Carbonate *on page* 286

Simethicone *on page* 1527

U.S. Brand Names Gas Ban™ [OTC]; Maalox® Advanced Maximum Strength [OTC]; Maalox® Junior Plus Antigas [OTC]; Titralac® Plus [OTC]

Pharmacologic Category Antacid; Antiflatulent

Use Relief of acid indigestion, heartburn, bloating, pressure, and discomfort of gas

Local Anesthetic/Vasoconstrictor Precautions No information available to require special precautions

Effects on Dental Treatment Do not give tetracyclines concomitantly.

Effects on Bleeding No information available to require special precautions

Adverse Effects Frequency not defined: Gastrointestinal: Constipation

General Dosage Range Oral:

Children 6-11 years: Maalox® Junior Plus Antigas: Two tablets as symptoms occur or as directed by healthcare provider (maximum: 6 tablets/24 hours)

Children ≥12 years; Maalox® Advanced Maximum Strength: 1-2 tablets as symptoms occur or as directed by healthcare provider (maximum: 8 tablets/24 hours)

Adults: Maalox® Advanced Maximum Strength: 1-2 tablets as symptoms occur or as directed by healthcare provider (maximum: 8 tablets/24 hours); Titralac® Plus: Two tablets every 2-3 hours as needed (maximum: 19 tablets/24 hours)

Pregnancy Risk Factor C

Calcium Chloride (KAL see um KLOR ide)

Pharmacologic Category Calcium Salt; Electrolyte Supplement, Parenteral

Use Treatment of acute symptomatic hypocalcemia; cardiac disturbances of hyperkalemia or hypocalcemia; emergent treatment of hypocalcemic tetany; treatment of severe hypermagnesemia

Unlabeled/Investigational Use Calcium channel blocker overdose; beta-blocker overdose; severe hyperkalemia (K+ >6.5 mEq/L with toxic ECG changes) [ACLS guidelines]; malignant arrhythmias (including cardiac arrest) associated with hypermagnesemia [ACLS guidelines]

Local Anesthetic/Vasoconstrictor Precautions No information available to require special precautions

Effects on Dental Treatment No significant effects or complications reported

Effects on Bleeding No information available to require special precautions

Adverse Effects Frequency not defined. I.V.:

Cardiovascular: Arrhythmia, bradycardia, cardiac arrest, hypotension, syncope, vasodilation

Endocrine & metabolic: Hypercalcemia

Gastrointestinal: Irritation, chalky taste

Hepatic: Serum amylase increased

Neuromuscular & skeletal: Tingling sensation

Renal: Renal calculi

Miscellaneous: Hot flashes

Postmarketing and/or case reports: Calcinosis cutis

General Dosage Range I.V.:

Neonates: 20 mg/kg or 40-60 mg/kg/dose every 6-8 hours **or** 32 mg for each 100 mL of citrated blood infused

Infants and Children: 10-20 mg/kg **or** 35-50 mg/kg every 6-8 hours **or** 32 mg for each 100 mL of citrated blood infused

Adults: 500-1000 mg; repeat as appropriate **or** 20-50 mg/kg/hour **or** 200-500 mg per 500 mL of citrated blood

Mechanism of Action Moderates nerve and muscle performance via action potential excitation threshold regulation

Pregnancy Risk Factor C

Calcium Citrate (KAL see um SIT rate)

Related Information

Rheumatoid Arthritis, Osteoarthritis, and Osteoporosis *on page* 1889

U.S. Brand Names Cal-C-Caps [OTC]; Cal-Cee [OTC]; Cal-Citrate™ 225 [OTC]; Calcitrate [OTC]

Canadian Brand Names Osteocit®

Pharmacologic Category Calcium Salt

Use Antacid; treatment and prevention of calcium deficiency or hyperphosphatemia (eg, osteoporosis, osteomalacia, mild/moderate renal insufficiency, hypoparathyroidism, postmenopausal osteoporosis, rickets)

Local Anesthetic/Vasoconstrictor Precautions No information available to require special precautions

Effects on Dental Treatment No significant effects or complications reported

Effects on Bleeding No information available to require special precautions

Adverse Effects Frequency not defined:

Mild hypercalcemia (calcium: >10.5 mg/dL) may be asymptomatic or manifest itself as constipation, anorexia, nausea, and vomiting

More severe hypercalcemia (calcium: >12 mg/dL) is associated with confusion, delirium, stupor, and coma

Central nervous system: Headache

Endocrine & metabolic: Hypophosphatemia, hypercalcemia

Gastrointestinal: Nausea, anorexia, vomiting, abdominal pain, constipation

Miscellaneous: Thirst

General Dosage Range Oral:

Children 0-6 months: RDA: 210 mg/day

Children 7-12 months: RDA: 270 mg/day

Children 1-3 years: RDA: 500 mg/day

Children 4-8 years: RDA: 800 mg/day

Children 9-18 years: RDA: 1300 mg/day

Adults: 500-2000 mg divided 2-4 times/day

Mechanism of Action Moderates nerve and muscle performance via action potential excitation threshold regulation

Pregnancy Risk Factor C

Calcium Glubionate (KAL see um gloo BYE oh nate)

Related Information

Rheumatoid Arthritis, Osteoarthritis, and Osteoporosis *on page 1889*

U.S. Brand Names Calcionate [OTC]

Pharmacologic Category Calcium Salt

Use Dietary supplement

Local Anesthetic/Vasoconstrictor Precautions No information available to require special precautions

Effects on Dental Treatment No significant effects or complications reported

Effects on Bleeding No information available to require special precautions

Adverse Effects Frequency not defined; symptoms reported with hypercalcemia:

Gastrointestinal: Abdominal pain, anorexia, constipation, nausea, thirst, vomiting, xerostomia

Genitourinary: Polyuria

General Dosage Range Oral:

Children 0-6 months: RDA: 210 mg/day

Children 7-12 months: RDA: 270 mg/day

Children 1-3 years: RDA: 500 mg/day

Children 4-8 years: RDA: 800 mg/day

Children 9-18 years: RDA: 1300 mg/day

Adults 19-50 years: RDA: 1000 mg/day

Adults ≥51 years: RDA: 1200 mg/day

Mechanism of Action As dietary supplement, used to prevent or treat negative calcium balance. The calcium in calcium salts moderates nerve and muscle performance and allows normal cardiac function.

Calcium Gluconate (KAL see um GLOO koe nate)

Related Information

Rheumatoid Arthritis, Osteoarthritis, and Osteoporosis *on page 1889*

U.S. Brand Names Cal-G [OTC]; Cal-GLU™ [OTC]

Pharmacologic Category Calcium Salt; Electrolyte Supplement, Oral; Electrolyte Supplement, Parenteral

Use Treatment and prevention of hypocalcemia; treatment of tetany, cardiac disturbances of hyperkalemia, cardiac resuscitation when epinephrine fails to improve myocardial contractions, hypocalcemia; calcium supplementation; hydrofluoric acid (HF) burns

Unlabeled/Investigational Use Calcium channel blocker overdose

Local Anesthetic/Vasoconstrictor Precautions No information available to require special precautions

Effects on Dental Treatment No significant effects or complications reported

Effects on Bleeding No information available to require special precautions

Adverse Effects Frequency not defined.

I.V.:

Cardiovascular: Arrhythmia, bradycardia, cardiac arrest, hypotension, vasodilation, and syncope may occur following rapid I.V. injection

Central nervous system: Sense of oppression

Gastrointestinal: Chalky taste

Local: Abscess and necrosis following I.M. administration

Neuromuscular & skeletal: Tingling sensation

Miscellaneous: Heat waves

Oral: Gastrointestinal: Constipation

General Dosage Range

I.V.: *Neonates, Children, and Adults:* Dosage varies greatly depending on indication

Oral:

Children: 200-500 mg/kg/day (calcium gluconate salt containing 0.465 mEq [9.3 mg]/mL elemental calcium) divided every 6 hours

Adults: 500 mg to 2 g 2-4 times/day (calcium gluconate salt containing 0.465 mEq [9.3 mg]/mL elemental calcium)

Mechanism of Action As dietary supplement, used to prevent or treat negative calcium balance; in osteoporosis, it helps to prevent or decrease the rate of bone loss. The calcium in calcium salts moderates nerve and muscle performance and allows normal cardiac function.

Pregnancy Risk Factor C

Calcium Lactate (KAL see um LAK tate)

Related Information

Rheumatoid Arthritis, Osteoarthritis, and Osteoporosis *on page 1889*

Pharmacologic Category Calcium Salt

Use Adjunct in prevention of postmenopausal osteoporosis; treatment and prevention of calcium depletion

Local Anesthetic/Vasoconstrictor Precautions No information available to require special precautions

Effects on Dental Treatment No significant effects or complications reported

Effects on Bleeding No information available to require special precautions

General Dosage Range Oral:

Children 0-6 months: RDA: 210 mg/day

Children 7-12 months: RDA: 270 mg/day

Children 1-3 years: RDA: 500 mg/day

Children 4-8 years: RDA: 800 mg/day

Children 9-18 years: RDA: 1300 mg/day

Adults 19-50 years: RDA: 1000 mg/day

Adults ≥51 years: RDA: 1200 mg/day

Mechanism of Action As dietary supplement, used to prevent or treat negative calcium balance; in osteoporosis, it helps to prevent or decrease the rate of bone loss. The calcium in calcium salts moderates nerve and muscle performance and allows normal cardiac function.

Pregnancy Risk Factor C

Calcium Phosphate (Tribasic) (KAL see um FOS fate tri BAY sik)

Related Information

Rheumatoid Arthritis, Osteoarthritis, and Osteoporosis *on page 1889*

U.S. Brand Names Posture® [OTC]

Pharmacologic Category Calcium Salt

Use Dietary supplement

Local Anesthetic/Vasoconstrictor Precautions No information available to require special precautions

Effects on Dental Treatment No significant effects or complications reported

Effects on Bleeding No information available to require special precautions

General Dosage Range Oral:

Children 0-6 months: RDA: 210 mg/day

Children 7-12 months: RDA: 270 mg/day

Children 1-3 years: RDA: 500 mg/day

Children 4-8 years: RDA: 800 mg/day

Children 9-18 years: RDA: 1300 mg/day

Adults: 2 tablets daily

Mechanism of Action As dietary supplement, used to prevent or treat negative calcium balance; in osteoporosis, it helps to prevent or decrease the rate of bone loss. The calcium in calcium salts moderates nerve and muscle performance and allows normal cardiac function.

Calfactant (kaf AKT ant)

U.S. Brand Names Infasurf®

Pharmacologic Category Lung Surfactant

Use Prevention of respiratory distress syndrome (RDS) in premature infants at high risk for RDS and for the treatment ("rescue") of premature infants who develop RDS

Prophylaxis: Therapy at birth with calfactant is indicated for premature infants <29 weeks of gestational age at significant risk for RDS. Should be administered as soon as possible, preferably within 30 minutes after birth.

Treatment: For infants ≤72 hours of age with RDS (confirmed by clinical and radiologic findings) and requiring endotracheal intubation.

Local Anesthetic/Vasoconstrictor Precautions No information available to require special precautions

Effects on Dental Treatment No significant effects or complications reported

Effects on Bleeding No information available to require special precautions

Adverse Effects

Cardiovascular: Bradycardia (34%), cyanosis (65%)

Respiratory: Airway obstruction (39%), reflux (21%), requirement for manual ventilation (16%), reintubation (1% to 10%)

General Dosage Range Intratracheal: *Premature infants:* 3 mL/kg (body weight at birth) every 12 hours for a total of 3 doses

Mechanism of Action Endogenous lung surfactant is essential for effective ventilation because it modifies alveolar surface tension, thereby stabilizing the alveoli. Lung surfactant deficiency is the cause of respiratory distress syndrome (RDS) in premature infants and lung surfactant restores surface activity to the lungs of these infants.

Camphor and Phenol (KAM for & FEE nole)

Related Information

Phenol *on page 1336*

U.S. Brand Names Campho-Phenique® [OTC]

Pharmacologic Category Topical Skin Product

Use Relief of pain and itching associated with minor burns, sunburn, minor cuts, insect bites, minor skin irritation; temporary relief of pain from cold sores

Local Anesthetic/Vasoconstrictor Precautions No information available to require special precautions

Effects on Dental Treatment No significant effects or complications reported

Effects on Bleeding No information available to require special precautions

General Dosage Range Topical: *Adults:* Apply 1-3 times/day

Pregnancy Risk Factor C

Canakinumab (can a KIN ue mab)

U.S. Brand Names Ilaris®

Pharmacologic Category Interleukin-1 Beta Inhibitor; Interleukin-1 Inhibitor; Monoclonal Antibody

Use Treatment of cryopyrin-associated periodic syndromes (CAPS), including familial cold autoinflammatory syndrome (FCAS) and Muckle-Wells syndrome (MWS)

Local Anesthetic/Vasoconstrictor Precautions No information available to require special precautions

Effects on Dental Treatment No significant effects or complications reported

Effects on Bleeding No information available to require special precautions

Adverse Effects

>10%:

Central nervous system: Headache (14%), vertigo (9% to 14%)

Gastrointestinal: Diarrhea (20%), nausea (14%), gastroenteritis (11%), weight gain (11%)

Neuromuscular and skeletal: Musculoskeletal pain (11%)

Respiratory: Nasopharyngitis (34%), rhinitis (17%), bronchitis (11%), pharyngitis (11%)

Miscellaneous: Influenza (17%)

1% to 10%: Local: Injection site reactions (7% to 9%)

General Dosage Range SubQ:
Children ≥4 years and 15-40 kg: 2-3 mg/kg every 8 weeks
Children ≥4 years and Adults >40 kg: 150 mg every 8 weeks

Mechanism of Action Canakinumab reduces inflammation by binding to interleukin-1 beta (IL-1β) (no binding to IL-1 alpha or IL-1 receptor antagonist) and preventing interaction with cell surface receptors. Cryopyrin-associated periodic syndromes (CAPS) refers to rare genetic syndromes caused by mutations in the nucleotide-binding domain, leucine rich family (NLR), pyrin domain containing 3 (NLRP-3) gene or the cold-induced autoinflammatory syndrome-1 (CIAS1) gene. Cryopyrin, a protein encoded by this gene, regulates IL-1β activation. Deficiency of cryopyrin results in excessive inflammation.

Pharmacodynamics/Kinetics
Half-life Elimination 26 days
Time to Peak Serum: Children: 2-7 days; Adults: ~7 days

Pregnancy Risk Factor C

Candesartan (kan de SAR tan)

Related Information
Cardiovascular Diseases *on page* 1848

U.S. Brand Names Atacand®

Canadian Brand Names Atacand®

Generic Availability (U.S.) No

Pharmacologic Category Angiotensin II Receptor Blocker

Use Alone or in combination with other antihypertensive agents in treating essential hypertension; treatment of heart failure (NYHA class II-IV)

Local Anesthetic/Vasoconstrictor Precautions No information available to require special precautions

Effects on Dental Treatment No significant effects or complications reported

Effects on Bleeding No information available to require special precautions

Adverse Effects
Cardiovascular: Angina, hypotension (CHF 19%), MI, palpitation, tachycardia
Central nervous system: Dizziness, lightheadedness, drowsiness, headache, vertigo, anxiety, depression, somnolence, fever
Dermatologic: Angioedema, rash
Endocrine & metabolic: Hyperglycemia, hyperkalemia (CHF <1% to 6%), hypertriglyceridemia, hyperuricemia
Gastrointestinal: Dyspepsia, gastroenteritis
Genitourinary: Hematuria
Neuromuscular & skeletal: Back pain, CPK increased, myalgia, paresthesia, weakness
Renal: Serum creatinine increased (up to 13% in patients with CHF with drug discontinuation required in 6%)
Respiratory: Dyspnea, epistaxis, pharyngitis, rhinitis, upper respiratory tract infection
Miscellaneous: Diaphoresis increased

Dosage Adults: Oral:
Hypertension: Usual dose is 4-32 mg once daily; dosage must be individualized. Blood pressure response is dose related over the range of 2-32 mg. The usual recommended starting dose of 16 mg once daily when it is used as monotherapy in patients who are not volume depleted. It can be administered once or twice daily with total daily doses ranging from 8-32 mg. Larger doses do not appear to have a greater effect and there is relatively little experience with such doses.
Congestive heart failure: Initial: 4 mg once daily; double the dose at 2-week intervals, as tolerated; target dose: 32 mg
Note: In selected cases, concurrent therapy with an ACE inhibitor may provide additional benefit.
Elderly: No initial dosage adjustment is necessary for elderly patients (although higher concentrations (C_{max}) and AUC were observed in these populations), for patients with mildly impaired renal function, or for patients with mildly impaired hepatic function.
Dosage adjustment in hepatic impairment:
Mild hepatic impairment: No initial dosage adjustment required
Moderate hepatic impairment: Consider initiation at lower dosages (AUC increased by 145%).
Severe hepatic impairment and/or cholestasis: Contraindicated

Mechanism of Action Candesartan is an angiotensin receptor antagonist. Angiotensin II acts as a vasoconstrictor. In addition to causing direct vasoconstriction, angiotensin II also stimulates the release of aldosterone. Once aldosterone is released, sodium as well as water are reabsorbed. The end result is an elevation in blood pressure. Candesartan binds to the AT1 angiotensin II receptor. This binding prevents angiotensin II from binding to the receptor thereby blocking the vasoconstriction and the aldosterone secreting effects of angiotensin II.

Contraindications Hypersensitivity to candesartan or any component of the formulation; severe hepatic impairment and/or cholestasis; pregnancy; breast-feeding

Warnings/Precautions [U.S. Boxed Warning]: Based on human data, drugs that act on the angiotensin system can cause injury and death to the developing fetus when used in the second and third trimesters. Angiotensin receptor blockers should be discontinued as soon as possible once pregnancy is detected. May cause hyperkalemia; avoid potassium supplementation unless specifically required by healthcare provider. Avoid use or use a smaller dose in patients who are volume depleted; correct depletion first. May be associated with deterioration of renal function and/or increases in serum creatinine, particularly in patients with low renal blood flow (eg, renal artery stenosis, heart failure) whose glomerular filtration rate (GFR) is dependent on efferent arteriolar vasoconstriction by angiotensin II. Use with caution in unstented unilateral/bilateral renal artery stenosis, pre-existing renal insufficiency, or significant aortic/mitral stenosis. Use with caution in patients with moderate hepatic impairment. Contraindicated with severe hepatic impairment and/or cholestasis. Use caution when initiating in heart failure; may need to adjust dose, and/or concurrent diuretic therapy, because of candesartan-induced hypotension. Hypotension may occur during major surgery and anesthesia; use cautiously before, during, and immediately after such interventions. Although concurrent therapy with an ACE inhibitor may be rational in select patients, concurrent use of ACE inhibitors may increase the risk of clinically-significant adverse events (eg, renal dysfunction, hyperkalemia).

Drug Interactions

Metabolism/Transport Effects Substrate of CYP2C9 (minor); **Inhibits** CYP2C8 (weak), 2C9 (weak)

Avoid Concomitant Use There are no known interactions where it is recommended to avoid concomitant use.

Increased Effect/Toxicity

Candesartan may increase the levels/effects of: ACE Inhibitors; Amifostine; Antihypertensives; Hypotensive Agents; Lithium; Nonsteroidal Anti-Inflammatory Agents; Potassium-Sparing Diuretics; RiTUXimab

The levels/effects of Candesartan may be increased by: Diazoxide; Eplerenone; Herbs (Hypotensive Properties); MAO Inhibitors; Pentoxifylline; Phosphodiesterase 5 Inhibitors; Potassium Salts; Prostacyclin Analogues; Tolvaptan; Trimethoprim

Decreased Effect

The levels/effects of Candesartan may be decreased by: Herbs (Hypertensive Properties); Methylphenidate; Nonsteroidal Anti-Inflammatory Agents; Yohimbine

Ethanol/Nutrition/Herb Interactions Herb/Nutraceutical: Avoid dong quai if using for hypertension (has estrogenic activity). Avoid ephedra, yohimbe, ginseng (may worsen hypertension). Avoid garlic (may have increased antihypertensive effect).

Pharmacodynamics/Kinetics

Onset of Action 2-3 hours; Peak effect: 6-8 hours

Duration of Action >24 hours

Half-life Elimination Dose dependent: 5-9 hours

Time to Peak 3-4 hours

Pregnancy Risk Factor C (1st trimester); D (2nd and 3rd trimesters)

Lactation Enters breast milk/contraindicated

Dosage Forms

Tablet, oral:

Atacand®: 4 mg, 8 mg, 16 mg, 32 mg

Candesartan and Hydrochlorothiazide

(kan de SAR tan & hye droe klor oh THYE a zide)

Related Information

Candesartan *on page* 292

Hydrochlorothiazide *on page* 854

U.S. Brand Names Atacand HCT®

Canadian Brand Names Atacand® Plus

Pharmacologic Category Angiotensin II Receptor Blocker; Diuretic, Thiazide

Use Treatment of hypertension; combination product should not be used for initial therapy

Local Anesthetic/Vasoconstrictor Precautions No information available to require special precautions

Effects on Dental Treatment No significant effects or complications reported

Effects on Bleeding No information available to require special precautions

Adverse Effects Reactions which follow have been reported with the combination product; see individual drug agents for additional adverse reactions that may be expected from each agent.

1% to 10%:

- Central nervous system: Dizziness (3%), headache (3%, placebo 5%)
- Neuromuscular & skeletal: Back pain (3%)
- Respiratory: Upper respiratory tract infection (4%)
- Miscellaneous: Flu-like syndrome (2%)

General Dosage Range Oral: *Adults:* Candesartan 16-32 mg/day in 1-2 divided doses and hydrochlorothiazide 12.5-25 mg once daily

Mechanism of Action

Candesartan: Candesartan is an angiotensin receptor antagonist. Angiotensin II acts as a vasoconstrictor. In addition to causing direct vasoconstriction, angiotensin II also stimulates the release of aldosterone. Once aldosterone is released, sodium as well as water are reabsorbed. The end result is an elevation in blood pressure. Candesartan binds to the AT1 angiotensin II receptor. This binding prevents angiotensin II from binding to the receptor, thereby blocking the vasoconstriction and the aldosterone-secreting effects of angiotensin II.

Hydrochlorothiazide: Inhibits sodium reabsorption in the distal tubules causing increased excretion of sodium and water as well as potassium and hydrogen ions

Pregnancy Risk Factor C/D (2nd and 3rd trimesters)

Cantharidin (kan THAR e din)

Canadian Brand Names Canthacur®; Cantharone®

Pharmacologic Category Keratolytic Agent

Use Removal of ordinary and periungual warts

Local Anesthetic/Vasoconstrictor Precautions No information available to require special precautions

Effects on Dental Treatment No significant effects or complications reported

Effects on Bleeding No information available to require special precautions

Adverse Effects 1% to 10%:

- Cardiovascular: Syncope
- Central nervous system: Delirium, ataxia
- Dermatologic: Dermal irritation, dermal burns, acantholysis
- Gastrointestinal: GI hemorrhage, rectal bleeding, dysphagia
- Genitourinary: Priapism
- Hepatic: Fatty degeneration
- Neuromuscular & skeletal: Hyper-reflexia
- Ocular: Conjunctivitis, iritis, keratitis
- Renal: Proteinuria, hematuria
- Respiratory: Burning of oropharynx

General Dosage Range Topical: *Children and Adults:* Apply directly to lesion, cover with nonporous tape, remove tape in 24 hours, reapply if necessary

Pregnancy Risk Factor C

Capecitabine (ka pe SITE a been)

Related Information

Fluorouracil (Systemic) *on page 754*

U.S. Brand Names Xeloda®

Canadian Brand Names Xeloda®

Pharmacologic Category Antineoplastic Agent, Antimetabolite; Antineoplastic Agent, Antimetabolite (Pyrimidine Analog)

Use Treatment of metastatic colorectal cancer; adjuvant therapy of Dukes' C colon cancer; treatment of metastatic breast cancer

Unlabeled/Investigational Use Treatment of gastric cancer, pancreatic cancer, esophageal cancer, ovarian cancer, metastatic renal cell cancer, neuroendocrine tumors, metastatic CNS lesions

Local Anesthetic/Vasoconstrictor Precautions No information available to require special precautions

Effects on Dental Treatment Key adverse event(s) related to dental treatment: Stomatitis, abnormal taste, and taste disturbance.

Effects on Bleeding Chemotherapy may result in significant myelosuppression, potentially including significant reduction in platelet counts and altered hemostasis. In patients who are under active treatment with these agents, medical consult is suggested.

Adverse Effects Frequency listed derived from monotherapy trials.

>10%:

Cardiovascular: Edema (9% to 15%)

Central nervous system: Fatigue (16% to 42%), fever (7% to 18%), pain (12%)

Dermatologic: Palmar-plantar erythrodysesthesia (hand-and-foot syndrome) (54% to 60%; grade 3: 11% to 17%; may be dose limiting), dermatitis (27% to 37%)

Gastrointestinal: Diarrhea (47% to 57%; may be dose limiting; grade 3: 12% to 13%; grade 4: 2% to 3%), nausea (34% to 53%), vomiting (15% to 37%), abdominal pain (7% to 35%), stomatitis (22% to 25%), appetite decreased (26%), anorexia (9% to 23%), constipation (9% to 15%)

Hematologic: Lymphopenia (94%; grade 4: 14%), anemia (72% to 80%; grade 4: <1% to 1%), neutropenia (2% to 26%; grade 4: 2%), thrombocytopenia (24%; grade 4: 1%)

Hepatic: Bilirubin increased (22% to 48%; grades 3/4: 11% to 23%)

Neuromuscular & skeletal: Paresthesia (21%)

Ocular: Eye irritation (13% to 15%)

Respiratory: Dyspnea (14%)

5% to 10%:

Cardiovascular: Venous thrombosis (8%), chest pain (6%)

Central nervous system: Headache (5% to 10%), lethargy (10%), dizziness (6% to 8%), insomnia (7% to 8%), mood alteration (5%), depression (5%)

Dermatologic: Nail disorder (7%), rash (7%), skin discoloration (7%), alopecia (6%), erythema (6%)

Endocrine & metabolic: Dehydration (7%)

Gastrointestinal: Motility disorder (10%), oral discomfort (10%), dyspepsia (6% to 8%), upper GI inflammatory disorders (colorectal cancer: 8%), hemorrhage (6%), ileus (6%), taste perversion (colorectal cancer: 6%)

Neuromuscular & skeletal: Back pain (10%), weakness (10%), neuropathy (10%), myalgia (9%), arthralgia (8%), limb pain (6%)

Ocular: Abnormal vision (colorectal cancer: 5%), conjunctivitis (5%)

Respiratory: Cough (7%)

Miscellaneous: Viral infection (colorectal cancer: 5%)

General Dosage Range Dosage adjustment recommended in patients with renal impairment or who develop toxicities

Oral: *Adults:* 1250 mg/m^2 twice daily for 2 weeks, every 21 days

Mechanism of Action Capecitabine is a prodrug of fluorouracil. It undergoes hydrolysis in the liver and tissues to form fluorouracil which is the active moiety. Fluorouracil is a fluorinated pyrimidine antimetabolite that inhibits thymidylate synthetase, blocking the methylation of deoxyuridylic acid to thymidylic acid, interfering with DNA, and to a lesser degree, RNA synthesis. Fluorouracil appears to be phase specific for the G_1 and S phases of the cell cycle.

Pharmacodynamics/Kinetics

Half-life Elimination 0.5-1 hour

Time to Peak 1.5 hours; Fluorouracil: 2 hours

Pregnancy Risk Factor D

Capreomycin (kap ree oh MYE sin)

Related Information

Tuberculosis *on page 1902*

U.S. Brand Names Capastat® Sulfate

Pharmacologic Category Antibiotic, Miscellaneous; Antitubercular Agent

Use Treatment of tuberculosis in conjunction with at least one other antituberculosis agent

Local Anesthetic/Vasoconstrictor Precautions No information available to require special precautions

Effects on Dental Treatment No significant effects or complications reported

Effects on Bleeding No information available to require special precautions

Adverse Effects

>10%:

Otic: Ototoxicity (subclinical hearing loss: 11%; clinical loss: 3%)

Renal: Nephrotoxicity (36%, increased BUN)

1% to 10%: Hematologic: Eosinophilia (dose related, mild)

General Dosage Range Dosage adjustment recommended in patients with renal impairment

I.M., I.V.: *Adults:* 1 g/day (maximum: 20 mg/kg/day) for 60-120 days, followed by 1 g 2-3 times/week

Mechanism of Action Capreomycin is a cyclic polypeptide antimicrobial. It is administered as a mixture of capreomycin IA and capreomycin IB. The mechanism of action of capreomycin is not well understood. Mycobacterial species that have become resistant to other agents are usually still sensitive to the action of capreomycin. However, significant cross-resistance with viomycin, kanamycin, and neomycin occurs.

Pharmacodynamics/Kinetics

Half-life Elimination Normal renal function: 4-6 hours; Cl_{cr} 100-110 mL/minute: 5-6 hours; Cl_{cr} 50-80 mL/minute: 7-10 hours; Cl_{cr} 20-40 mL/minute: 12-20 hours; Cl_{cr} 10 mL/minute: 29 hours; Cl_{cr} 0 mL/minute: 55 hours

Time to Peak Serum: I.M.: 1-2 hours

Pregnancy Risk Factor C

Capsaicin (kap SAY sin)

Related Information

Cayenne *on page 1774*

Ulcerative, Erosive, and Painful Oral Mucosal Disorders *on page 1950*

U.S. Brand Names Capzasin-HP® [OTC]; Capzasin-P® [OTC]; DiabetAid® Pain and Tingling Relief [OTC]; Qutenza™; Salonpas® Hot [OTC]; Zostrix® Diabetic Foot Pain [OTC]; Zostrix® Neuropathy [OTC] [DSC]; Zostrix® [OTC]; Zostrix®-HP [OTC]

Canadian Brand Names Zostrix®; Zostrix® H.P.

Generic Availability (U.S.) Yes: Cream

Pharmacologic Category Analgesic, Topical; Topical Skin Product; Transient Receptor Potential Vanilloid 1 (TRPV1) Agonist

Dental Use Potential use as topical agent in burning mouth syndrome and oral mucositis

Use

Topical patch (Qutenza™): Management of postherpetic neuralgia (PHN)

OTC labeling: Temporary treatment of minor pain associated with muscles and joints due to backache, strains, sprains, bruises, cramps or arthritis; temporary relief of pain associated with diabetic neuropathy

Unlabeled/Investigational Use Diabetic neuropathy; treatment of pain associated with psoriasis and intractable pruritus. Potential use as topical agent in burning mouth syndrome and oral mucositis.

Local Anesthetic/Vasoconstrictor Precautions No information available to require special precautions

Effects on Dental Treatment No significant effects or complications reported

Effects on Bleeding No information available to require special precautions

Adverse Effects Topical patch (Qutenza™, capsaicin 8%):

>10%: Local: Erythema (63%), pain (42%)

1% to 10%:

- Cardiovascular: Hypertension (2%; transient)
- Dermatologic: Pruritus (2%)
- Gastrointestinal: Nausea (5%), vomiting (3%)
- Local: Pruritus (6%), papules (6%), edema (4%), dryness (2%), swelling (2%)
- Respiratory: Nasopharyngitis (4%), sinusitis (3%), bronchitis (2%)

Dental Usual Dosage Topical: Apply cream or gel to affected area 3-4 times/day

Dosage Topical:

Children ≥12 years and Adults: Pain relief: OTC labeling: Patch (Salonpas®-Hot): Apply patch to affected area up to 3-4 times/day for 7 days. Patch may remain in place for up to 8 hours.

Adults:

Pain relief: OTC labeling: Topical products (cream, gel, liquid, lotion): Apply to affected area 3-4 times/day; efficacy may be decreased if used less than 3 times/day; best results seen after 2-4 weeks of continuous use

Postherpetic neuralgia: Patch (Qutenza™ [capsaicin 8%]): Apply patch to most painful area for 60 minutes. Up to 4 patches may be applied in a single application. Treatment may be repeated ≥3 months as needed for return of pain (do not apply more frequently than every 3 months). Area should be pretreated with a topical anesthetic prior to patch application.

Diabetic neuropathy (unlabeled use): Cream (0.075%): Apply 4 times/day (Bril, 2011)

Mechanism of Action Capsaicin, a transient receptor potential vanilloid 1 receptor (TRPV1) agonist, activates TRPV1 ligand-gated cation channels on nociceptive nerve fibers, resulting in depolarization, initiation of action potential, and pain signal transmission to the spinal cord; capsaicin exposure results in subsequent desensitization of the sensory axons and inhibition of pain transmission initiation. In arthritis, capsaicin induces release of substance P, the principal chemomediator of pain impulses from the periphery to the CNS, from peripheral sensory neurons; after repeated application, capsaicin depletes the neuron of substance P and prevents reaccumulation. The functional link between substance P and the capsaicin receptor, TRPV1, is not well understood.

Contraindications There are no contraindications listed in the manufacturer's labeling.

Warnings/Precautions

Topical high-concentration capsaicin patch (Qutenza™): Do not apply to face, scalp, or allow contact with eyes or mucous membranes. If an unintended area of skin is inadvertently exposed, the cleansing gel should be used. Post-application pain should be treated with local cooling methods and/or analgesics (opioids may be necessary). Avoid rapid removal of patches to decrease risk of aerosolization of capsaicin; inhalation of airborne capsaicin may result in coughing or sneezing; if shortness of breath occurs, medical care is required; remove patches gently and slowly to decrease risk of aerosolization. Use with caution in patients with uncontrolled hypertension, or a history of cardiovascular or cerebrovascular events; transient increases in blood pressure due to treatment-related pain have occurred during and after application of patch.

Topical OTC products: Apply externally; avoid contact with eyes or mucous membranes. Should not be applied to broken or irritated skin. Treated area should not be exposed to heat or direct sunlight. Affected area should not be bandaged. Transient burning may occur and generally disappears after several days; discontinue use if severe burning develops. Stop use and consult a healthcare provider if redness or irritation develops, symptoms get worse, or symptoms resolve and then recur.

Drug Interactions

Metabolism/Transport Effects Substrate of CYP2E1 (minor)

Avoid Concomitant Use There are no known interactions where it is recommended to avoid concomitant use.

Increased Effect/Toxicity There are no known significant interactions involving an increase in effect.

Decreased Effect There are no known significant interactions involving a decrease in effect.

Pharmacodynamics/Kinetics

Half-life Elimination Half-life elimination: Topical patch (capsaicin 8%): 1.64 hours (Babbar, 2009)

Pregnancy Risk Factor B (Qutenza™)

Lactation Excretion in breast milk unknown/use caution

Breast-Feeding Considerations When using the topical high concentration (capsaicin 8%) patch, Qutenza™, the manufacturer recommends not breast-feeding on the day of treatment after the patch has been applied to reduce any potential infant exposure.

Dosage Forms

Cream, topical: 0.025% (60 g); 0.075% (60 g)
- Capzasin-HP® [OTC]: 0.1% (42.5 g)
- Capzasin-P® [OTC]: 0.035% (42.5 g)
- Zostrix® [OTC]: 0.025% (60 g)
- Zostrix® Diabetic Foot Pain [OTC]: 0.075% (60 g)
- Zostrix®-HP [OTC]: 0.075% (60 g)

Gel, topical:
- Capzasin-P® [OTC]: 0.025% (42.5 g)

Liquid, topical:
- Capzasin-P® [OTC]: 0.15% (29.5 mL)

Lotion, topical:
- DiabetAid® Pain and Tingling Relief [OTC]: 0.025% (120 mL)

Patch, topical:
- Qutenza™: 8% (1s, 2s)
- Salonpas® Hot [OTC]: 0.025% (1s)

References

Buchanan J and Zakrzewska J, "Burning Mouth Syndrome," *Clin Evid (online)*, March 14, 2008. Available at http://www.ncbi.nlm.nih.gov/pmc/articles/PMC2907957/pdf/2008-1301.pdf.

Mínguez Serra MP, Salort Llorca C, Silvestre Donat FJ, "Pharmacological Treatment of Burning Mouth Syndrome: A Review and Update," *Med Oral Patol Oral Cir Bucal*, 2007, 12(4):E299-304.

Captopril (KAP toe pril)

Related Information

Cardiovascular Diseases *on page 1848*

Canadian Brand Names Alti-Captopril; Apo-Capto®; Capoten®; Gen-Captopril; Mylan-Captopril; Novo-Captopril; Nu-Capto; PMS-Captopril

Generic Availability (U.S.) Yes

Pharmacologic Category Angiotensin-Converting Enzyme (ACE) Inhibitor

Use Management of hypertension; treatment of heart failure, left ventricular dysfunction after myocardial infarction, diabetic nephropathy

Unlabeled/Investigational Use To delay the progression of nephropathy and reduce risks of cardiovascular events in hypertensive patients with type 1 or 2 diabetes mellitus; treatment of hypertensive crisis, rheumatoid arthritis; diagnosis of anatomic renal artery stenosis, hypertension secondary to scleroderma renal crisis; diagnosis of aldosteronism, idiopathic edema, Bartter's syndrome, postmyocardial infarction for prevention of ventricular failure; increase circulation in Raynaud's phenomenon, hypertension secondary to Takayasu's disease

Local Anesthetic/Vasoconstrictor Precautions No information available to require special precautions

Effects on Dental Treatment Key adverse event(s) related to dental treatment: Loss or diminished perception of taste and orthostatic hypotension.

Effects on Bleeding No information available to require special precautions

Adverse Effects

Frequency not defined:

Cardiovascular: Angioedema, cardiac arrest, cerebrovascular insufficiency, rhythm disturbances, orthostatic hypotension, syncope, flushing, pallor, angina, MI, Raynaud's syndrome, CHF

Central nervous system: Ataxia, confusion, depression, nervousness, somnolence

Dermatologic: Bullous pemphigus, erythema multiforme, Stevens-Johnson syndrome, exfoliative dermatitis

Endocrine & metabolic: Alkaline phosphatase increased, bilirubin increased, gynecomastia

Gastrointestinal: Pancreatitis, glossitis, dyspepsia

Genitourinary: Urinary frequency, impotence

Hematologic: Anemia, thrombocytopenia, pancytopenia, agranulocytosis, anemia

Hepatic: Jaundice, hepatitis, hepatic necrosis (rare), cholestasis, hyponatremia (symptomatic), transaminases increased

Neuromuscular & skeletal: Asthenia, myalgia, myasthenia

Ocular: Blurred vision

Renal: Renal insufficiency, renal failure, nephrotic syndrome, polyuria, oliguria

Respiratory: Bronchospasm, eosinophilic pneumonitis, rhinitis

Miscellaneous: Anaphylactoid reactions

1% to 10%:

Cardiovascular: Hypotension (1% to 3%), tachycardia (1%), chest pain (1%), palpitation (1%)

Dermatologic: Rash (maculopapular or urticarial) (4% to 7%), pruritus (2%); in patients with rash, a positive ANA and/or eosinophilia has been noted in 7% to 10%.

Endocrine & metabolic: Hyperkalemia (1% to 11%)

Hematologic: Neutropenia may occur in up to 4% of patients with renal insufficiency or collagen-vascular disease.

Renal: Proteinuria (1%), serum creatinine increased, worsening of renal function (may occur in patients with bilateral renal artery stenosis or hypovolemia)

Respiratory: Cough (<1% to 2%)

Miscellaneous: Hypersensitivity reactions (rash, pruritus, fever, arthralgia, and eosinophilia) have occurred in 4% to 7% of patients (depending on dose and renal function); dysgeusia - loss of taste or diminished perception (2% to 4%)

Dosage Note: Titrate dose according to patient's response; use lowest effective dose. Oral:

Infants: Initial: 0.15-0.3 mg/kg/dose; titrate dose upward to maximum of 6 mg/kg/day in 1-4 divided doses; usual required dose: 2.5-6 mg/kg/day

Children: Initial: 0.5 mg/kg/dose; titrate upward to maximum of 6 mg/kg/day in 2-4 divided doses

Older Children: Initial: 6.25-12.5 mg/dose every 12-24 hours; titrate upward to maximum of 6 mg/kg/day

Adolescents: Initial: 12.5-25 mg/dose given every 8-12 hours; increase by 25 mg/dose to maximum of 450 mg/day

Adults:

Acute hypertension (urgency/emergency): 12.5-25 mg, may repeat as needed (may be given sublingually, but no therapeutic advantage demonstrated)

Heart failure:

Initial dose: 6.25-12.5 mg 3 times/day in conjunction with cardiac glycoside and diuretic therapy; initial dose depends upon patient's fluid/electrolyte status

Target dose: 50 mg 3 times/day

Hypertension:

Initial dose: 12.5-25 mg 2-3 times/day; may increase by 12.5-25 mg/dose at 1- to 2-week intervals up to 50 mg 3 times/day; maximum dose: 150 mg 3 times/day; add diuretic before further dosage increases

Usual dose range (JNC 7): 25-100 mg/day in 2 divided doses

LV dysfunction after MI: Initial dose: 6.25 mg followed by 12.5 mg 3 times/day; then increase to 25 mg 3 times/day during next several days and then gradually increase over next several weeks to target dose of 50 mg 3 times/day (some dose schedules are more aggressive to achieve an increased goal dose within the first few days of initiation.)

Diabetic nephropathy: 25 mg 3 times/day; other antihypertensives often given concurrently

Dosing adjustment in renal impairment:

Cl_{cr} 10-50 mL/minute: Administer at 75% of normal dose.

Cl_{cr} <10 mL/minute: Administer at 50% of normal dose.

Note: Smaller dosages given every 8-12 hours are indicated in patients with renal dysfunction; renal function and leukocyte count should be carefully monitored during therapy.

Hemodialysis: Moderately dialyzable (20% to 50%); administer dose postdialysis or administer 25% to 35% supplemental dose.

Peritoneal dialysis: Supplemental dose is not necessary.

Mechanism of Action Competitive inhibitor of angiotensin-converting enzyme (ACE); prevents conversion of angiotensin I to angiotensin II, a potent vasoconstrictor; results in lower levels of angiotensin II which causes an increase in plasma renin activity and a reduction in aldosterone secretion

Contraindications Hypersensitivity to captopril, any other ACE inhibitor, or any component of the formulation; angioedema related to previous treatment with an ACE inhibitor

Warnings/Precautions Anaphylactic reactions may occur rarely with ACE inhibitors. At any time during treatment (especially following first dose) angioedema may occur rarely with ACE inhibitors; may involve the head and neck (potentially compromising airway) or the intestine (presenting with abdominal pain). African-Americans and patients with idiopathic or hereditary angioedema may be at an increased risk. Prolonged frequent monitoring may be required especially if tongue, glottis, or larynx are involved as they are associated with airway obstruction. Patients with a history of airway surgery may have a higher risk of airway obstruction. Aggressive early and appropriate management is critical. Use in patients with previous angioedema associated with ACE inhibitor therapy is contraindicated. Severe anaphylactoid reactions may be seen during hemodialysis (eg, CVVHD) with high-flux dialysis membranes (eg, AN69), and rarely, during low density lipoprotein apheresis with dextran sulfate cellulose. Rare cases of anaphylactoid reactions have been reported in patients undergoing sensitization treatment with hymenoptera (bee, wasp) venom while receiving ACE inhibitors.

Symptomatic hypotension with or without syncope can occur with ACE inhibitors (usually with the first several doses); effects are most often observed in volume depleted patients; close monitoring of patient is required especially with initial dosing and dosing increases; blood pressure must be lowered at a rate appropriate for the patient's clinical condition. Initiation of therapy in patients with ischemic heart disease or cerebrovascular disease warrants close observation due to the potential consequences posed by falling blood pressure (eg, MI, stroke). Use with caution in hypertrophic cardiomyopathy with outflow tract obstruction, severe aortic stenosis, or before, during, or immediately after major surgery. **[U.S. Boxed Warning]: Based on human data, ACEIs can cause injury and death to the developing fetus when used in the second and third trimesters. ACEIs should be discontinued as soon as possible once pregnancy is detected.**

Hyperkalemia may occur with ACE inhibitors; risk factors include renal dysfunction, diabetes mellitus, concomitant use of potassium-sparing diuretics, potassium supplements and/or potassium containing salts. Use cautiously, if at all, with these agents and monitor potassium closely. Cough may occur with ACE inhibitors. Other causes of cough should be considered (eg, pulmonary congestion in patients with heart failure) and excluded prior to discontinuation.

May be associated with deterioration of renal function and/or increases in serum creatinine, particularly in patients with low renal blood flow (eg, renal artery stenosis, heart failure) whose glomerular filtration rate (GFR) is dependent on efferent arteriolar vasoconstriction by angiotensin II; deterioration may result in oliguria, acute renal failure, and progressive azotemia. Small increases in serum creatinine may occur following initiation; consider discontinuation only in patients with progressive and/or significant deterioration in renal function. Use with caution in patients with unstented unilateral/bilateral renal artery stenosis. When unstented bilateral renal artery stenosis is present, use is generally avoided due to the elevated risk of deterioration in renal function unless possible benefits outweigh risks. Concurrent use of angiotensin receptor blockers may increase the risk of clinically-significant adverse events (eg, renal dysfunction, hyperkalemia).

Rare toxicities associated with ACE inhibitors include cholestatic jaundice (which may progress to fulminant hepatic necrosis), agranulocytosis, neutropenia, or leukopenia with myeloid hypoplasia. Patients with collagen vascular diseases (especially with concomitant renal impairment) or renal impairment alone may be at increased risk for hematologic toxicity; closely monitor CBC with differential for the first 3 months of therapy and periodically thereafter in these patients.

Drug Interactions

Metabolism/Transport Effects Substrate of CYP2D6 (major)

Avoid Concomitant Use There are no known interactions where it is recommended to avoid concomitant use.

Increased Effect/Toxicity

Captopril may increase the levels/effects of: Allopurinol; Amifostine; Antihypertensives; AzaTHIOprine; CycloSPORINE; CycloSPORINE (Systemic); Ferric Gluconate; Gold Sodium Thiomalate; Hypotensive Agents; Iron Dextran Complex; Lithium; Nonsteroidal Anti-Inflammatory Agents; RiTUXimab

The levels/effects of Captopril may be increased by: Abiraterone; Angiotensin II Receptor Blockers; CYP2D6 Inhibitors (Moderate); CYP2D6 Inhibitors (Strong); Darunavir; Diazoxide; DPP-IV Inhibitors; Eplerenone; Everolimus; Herbs (Hypotensive Properties); Loop Diuretics; MAO Inhibitors; Pentoxifylline; Phosphodiesterase 5 Inhibitors; Potassium Salts; Potassium-Sparing Diuretics; Prostacyclin Analogues; Sirolimus; Temsirolimus; Thiazide Diuretics; TiZANidine; Tolvaptan; Trimethoprim

Decreased Effect

The levels/effects of Captopril may be decreased by: Antacids; Aprotinin; Herbs (Hypertensive Properties); Methylphenidate; Nonsteroidal Anti-Inflammatory Agents; Peginterferon Alfa-2b; Salicylates; Yohimbine

Ethanol/Nutrition/Herb Interactions

Food: Captopril serum concentrations may be decreased if taken with food. Long-term use of captopril may result in a zinc deficiency which can result in a decrease in taste perception.

Herb/Nutraceutical: Avoid bayberry, blue cohosh, cayenne, ephedra, ginger, ginseng (American), kola, licorice (may worsen hypertension). Avoid black cohosh, california poppy, coleus, golden seal, hawthorn, mistletoe, periwinkle, quinine, shepherd's purse (may have increased antihypertensive effect).

Dietary Considerations Should be taken at least 1 hour before or 2 hours after eating.

Pharmacodynamics/Kinetics

Onset of Action Peak effect: Blood pressure reduction: 1-1.5 hours after dose

Duration of Action Dose related, may require several weeks of therapy before full hypotensive effect

Half-life Elimination Renal and cardiac function dependent: Adults: Healthy volunteers: 1.9 hours; Heart failure: 2.06 hours; Anuria: 20-40 hours

Time to Peak 1 hour

Pregnancy Risk Factor C (1st trimester); D (2nd and 3rd trimesters)

Lactation Enters breast milk/not recommended (AAP rates "compatible"; AAP 2001 update pending)

Breast-Feeding Considerations Captopril is excreted in breast milk. Breast-feeding is not recommended by the manufacturer.

Dosage Forms

Tablet, oral: 12.5 mg, 25 mg, 50 mg, 100 mg

Captopril and Hydrochlorothiazide

(KAP toe pril & hye droe klor oh THYE a zide)

Related Information

Captopril *on page 297*

Hydrochlorothiazide *on page 854*

Pharmacologic Category Angiotensin-Converting Enzyme (ACE) Inhibitor; Diuretic, Thiazide

Use Management of hypertension

Local Anesthetic/Vasoconstrictor Precautions No information available to require special precautions

Effects on Dental Treatment No significant effects or complications reported

Effects on Bleeding No information available to require special precautions

Adverse Effects See individual agents.

General Dosage Range Oral: *Adults:* Captopril 25-150 mg and hydrochlorothiazide 15-50 mg once daily

Mechanism of Action Captopril is a competitive inhibitor of angiotensin-converting enzyme (ACE); prevents conversion of angiotensin I to angiotensin II, a potent vasoconstrictor. This results in lower levels of angiotensin II which causes an increase in plasma renin activity and a reduction in aldosterone secretion. Hydrochlorothiazide inhibits sodium reabsorption in the distal tubules causing increased excretion of sodium and water as well as potassium and hydrogen ions.

Pregnancy Risk Factor C/D (2nd and 3rd trimesters)

Carbachol (KAR ba kole)

U.S. Brand Names Isopto® Carbachol; Miostat®

Canadian Brand Names Isopto® Carbachol; Miostat®

Pharmacologic Category Cholinergic Agonist; Ophthalmic Agent, Antiglaucoma; Ophthalmic Agent, Miotic

Use Lowers intraocular pressure in the treatment of glaucoma; cause miosis during surgery

Local Anesthetic/Vasoconstrictor Precautions No information available to require special precautions

Effects on Dental Treatment Key adverse event(s) related to dental treatment: Increased salivation.

Effects on Bleeding No information available to require special precautions

Adverse Effects Frequency not defined.

Cardiovascular: Arrhythmia, flushing, hypotension, syncope

Central nervous system: Headache

Gastrointestinal: Abdominal cramps, diarrhea, epigastric distress, salivation, vomiting

Genitourinary: Urinary bladder tightness

Ocular: Bullous keratopathy, burning (transient), ciliary spasm, conjunctival injection, corneal clouding, irritation, postoperative iritis (following cataract extraction), retinal detachment, stinging (transient)

Respiratory: Asthma

Miscellaneous: Diaphoresis

General Dosage Range Ophthalmic: *Adults:* Instill 1-2 drops up to 3 times/day **or** 0.5 mL as a single dose

Mechanism of Action Synthetic direct-acting cholinergic agent that causes miosis by stimulating muscarinic receptors in the eye

Pharmacodynamics/Kinetics

Onset of Action

Ophthalmic instillation: Miosis: 10-20 minutes

Intraocular administration: Miosis: 2-5 minutes

Duration of Action

Ophthalmic instillation: Reduction in intraocular pressure: 4-8 hours

Intraocular administration: 24 hours

Pregnancy Risk Factor C

CarBAMazepine (kar ba MAZ e peen)

Related Information

Temporomandibular Dysfunction (TMD) *on page 1964*

U.S. Brand Names Carbatrol®; Epitol®; Equetro®; TEGretol®; TEGretol®-XR

Canadian Brand Names Apo-Carbamazepine®; Carbamazepine; Dom-Carbamazepine; Mapezine®; Mylan-Carbamazepine CR; Nu-Carbamazepine; PMS-Carbamazepine; Sandoz-Carbamazepine; Taro-Carbamazepine Chewable; Tegretol®; Teva-Carbamazepine

Generic Availability (U.S.) Yes: Excludes capsule (extended release)

Pharmacologic Category Anticonvulsant, Miscellaneous

Dental Use Pain relief of trigeminal or glossopharyngeal neuralgia

Use

Carbatrol®, Tegretol®, Tegretol®-XR: Partial seizures with complex symptomatology (psychomotor, temporal lobe), generalized tonic-clonic seizures (grand mal), mixed seizure patterns, trigeminal neuralgia

Equetro®: Acute manic and mixed episodes associated with bipolar 1 disorder

Unlabeled/Investigational Use Treatment of restless leg syndrome and post-traumatic stress disorders

Local Anesthetic/Vasoconstrictor Precautions No information available to require special precautions

Effects on Dental Treatment Key adverse event(s) related to dental treatment: Xerostomia (normal salivary flow resumes upon discontinuation).

Effects on Bleeding No information available to require special precautions

Adverse Effects Frequency not defined, unless otherwise specified.

Cardiovascular: Arrhythmias, AV block, bradycardia, chest pain (bipolar use), CHF, edema, hyper-/hypotension, lymphadenopathy, syncope, thromboembolism, thrombophlebitis

Central nervous system: Amnesia (bipolar use), anxiety (bipolar use), aseptic meningitis (case report), ataxia (bipolar use 15%), confusion, depression (bipolar use), dizziness (bipolar use 44%), fatigue, headache (bipolar use 22%), sedation, slurred speech, somnolence (bipolar use 32%)

Dermatologic: Alopecia, alterations in skin pigmentation, erythema multiforme, exfoliative dermatitis, photosensitivity reaction, pruritus (bipolar use 8%), purpura, rash, Stevens-Johnson syndrome, toxic epidermal necrolysis, urticaria

Endocrine & metabolic: Chills, fever, hyponatremia, syndrome of inappropriate ADH secretion (SIADH)

Gastrointestinal: Abdominal pain, anorexia, constipation, diarrhea, dyspepsia (bipolar use), gastric distress, nausea (bipolar use 29%), pancreatitis, vomiting (bipolar use 18%), xerostomia (bipolar use)

Genitourinary: Azotemia, impotence, renal failure, urinary frequency, urinary retention

Hematologic: Acute intermittent porphyria, agranulocytosis, aplastic anemia, bone marrow suppression, eosinophilia, leukocytosis, leukopenia, pancytopenia, thrombocytopenia

Hepatic: Abnormal liver function tests, hepatic failure, hepatitis, jaundice

Neuromuscular & skeletal: Back pain, pain (bipolar use 12%), peripheral neuritis, weakness

Ocular: Blurred vision, conjunctivitis, lens opacities, nystagmus

Otic: Hyperacusis, tinnitus

Miscellaneous: Diaphoresis, hypersensitivity (including multiorgan reactions, may include disorders mimicking lymphoma, eosinophilia, hepatosplenomegaly, vasculitis); infection (bipolar use 12%)

Dental Usual Dosage Trigeminal or glossopharyngeal neuralgia: Oral:

Adults: Initial: 200 mg/day in 2 divided doses (tablets, extended release tablets, or extended release capsules) or 4 divided doses (oral suspension) with food, gradually increasing in increments of 200 mg/day as needed

Maintenance: Usual: 400-800 mg daily in 2 divided doses (tablets, extended release tablets, or extended release capsules) or 4 divided doses (oral suspension); maximum dose: 1200 mg/day

Dosage Dosage must be adjusted according to patient's response and serum concentrations. Administer tablets (chewable or conventional) in 2-3 divided doses daily and suspension in 4 divided doses daily. Oral:

Epilepsy:

Children:

<6 years: Initial: 10-20 mg/kg/day divided twice or 3 times daily as tablets or 4 times/day as suspension; increase dose every week until optimal response and therapeutic levels are achieved

Maintenance dose: Divide into 3-4 doses daily (tablets or suspension); maximum recommended dose: 35 mg/kg/day

6-12 years: Initial: 200 mg/day in 2 divided doses (tablets or extended release tablets) or 4 divided doses (oral suspension); increase by up to 100 mg/day at weekly intervals using a twice daily regimen of extended release tablets or 3-4 times daily regimen of other formulations until optimal response and therapeutic levels are achieved

Maintenance: Usual: 400-800 mg/day; maximum recommended dose: 1000 mg/day

Note: Children <12 years who receive ≥400 mg/day of carbamazepine may be converted to extended release capsules (Carbatrol®) using the same total daily dosage divided twice daily

Children >12 years and Adults: Initial: 400 mg/day in 2 divided doses (tablets or extended release tablets) or 4 divided doses (oral suspension); increase by up to 200 mg/day at weekly intervals using a twice daily regimen of extended release tablets or capsules, or a 3-4 times/day regimen of other formulations until optimal response and therapeutic levels are achieved; usual dose: 800-1200 mg/day

Maximum recommended doses:

Children 12-15 years: 1000 mg/day

Children >15 years: 1200 mg/day

Adults: 1600 mg/day; however, some patients have required up to 1.6-2.4 g/day

Trigeminal or glossopharyngeal neuralgia: Adults: Initial: 200 mg/day in 2 divided doses (tablets, extended release tablets, or extended release capsules) or 4 divided doses (oral suspension) with food, gradually increasing in increments of 200 mg/day as needed

Maintenance: Usual: 400-800 mg daily in 2 divided doses (tablets, extended release tablets, or extended release capsules) or 4 divided doses (oral suspension); maximum dose: 1200 mg/day

Bipolar disorder: Adults: Initial: 400 mg/day in 2 divided doses (tablets, extended release tablets, or extended release capsules) or 4 divided doses (oral suspension), may adjust by 200 mg/day increments; maximum dose: 1600 mg/day.

Note: Equetro® is the only formulation specifically approved by the FDA for the management of bipolar disorder.

Dosing adjustment in renal impairment: Dosage adjustments are not required or recommended in the manufacturer's labeling; however, the following guidelines have been used by some clinicians (Aronoff, 2007):

Children and Adults:

GFR <10 mL/minute: Administer 75% of dose

Hemodialysis, peritoneal dialysis: Administer 75% of dose

Continuous renal replacement therapy (CRRT):

Children: Administer 75% of dose

Adults: No dosage adjustment recommended

Dosing adjustment in hepatic impairment: Use with caution in hepatic impairment; metabolized primarily in the liver

Mechanism of Action In addition to anticonvulsant effects, carbamazepine has anticholinergic, antineuralgic, antidiuretic, muscle relaxant, antimanic, antidepressive, and antiarrhythmic properties; may depress activity in the nucleus ventralis of the thalamus or decrease synaptic transmission or decrease summation of temporal stimulation leading to neural discharge by limiting influx of sodium ions across cell membrane or other unknown mechanisms; stimulates the release of ADH and potentiates its action in promoting reabsorption of water; chemically related to tricyclic antidepressants

Contraindications Hypersensitivity to carbamazepine, tricyclic antidepressants, or any component of the formulation; bone marrow depression; with or within 14 days of MAO inhibitor use; concurrent use of nefazodone

Warnings/Precautions **[U.S. Boxed Warning]: Potentially fatal blood cell abnormalities have been reported.** Patients with a previous history of adverse hematologic reaction to any drug may be at increased risk.

Antiepileptics are associated with an increased risk of suicidal behavior/thoughts with use (regardless of indication); patients should be monitored for signs/symptoms of depression, suicidal tendencies, and other unusual behavior changes during therapy and instructed to inform their healthcare provider immediately if symptoms occur.

Administer carbamazepine with caution to patients with history of cardiac damage, ECG abnormalities (or at risk for ECG abnormalities), hepatic or renal disease. When used to treat bipolar disorder, the smallest effective dose is suggested to reduce the risk for overdose/suicide; high-risk patients should be monitored for suicidal ideations. Prescription should be written for the smallest quantity consistent with good patient care. May activate latent psychosis and/or cause confusion or agitation; elderly patients may be at an increased risk for psychiatric effects. Potentially serious, sometimes fatal multiorgan hypersensitivity reactions have been reported with some antiepileptic drugs; monitor for signs and symptoms of possible disparate manifestations associated with lymphatic, hepatic, renal, and/or hematologic organ systems; gradual discontinuation and conversion to alternate therapy may be required.

Carbamazepine is not effective in absence, myoclonic, or akinetic seizures; exacerbation of certain seizure types have been seen after initiation of carbamazepine therapy in children with mixed seizure disorders. Abrupt discontinuation is not recommended in patients being treated for seizures. Dizziness or drowsiness may occur; caution should be used when performing tasks which require alertness until the effects are known. Effects with other sedative drugs or ethanol may be potentiated. Carbamazepine has a high potential for drug interactions; use caution in patients taking strong CYP3A4 inducers or inhibitors or medications significantly metabolized via CYP1A2, 2B6, 2C9, 2C19, and 3A4. Coadministration of carbamazepine and nefazodone may lead to insufficient plasma levels of nefazodone; combination is contraindicated. Carbamazepine has mild anticholinergic activity; use with caution in patients with increased intraocular pressure, or sensitivity to anticholinergic effects. Severe dermatologic reactions, including toxic epidermal necrolysis and Stevens-Johnson syndrome, although rarely reported, have resulted in fatalities. **[U.S. Boxed Warning]: Use caution and screen for the genetic susceptibility genotype (*HLA-B*1502* allele) in Asian patients. Patients with a positive result should not be started on carbamazepine.** Discontinue if there are any signs of hypersensitivity. Elderly patients may have an increased risk of SIADH-like syndrome.

Administration of the suspension will yield higher peak and lower trough serum levels than an equal dose of the tablet form; consider a lower starting dose given more frequently (same total daily dose) when using the suspension.

Drug Interactions

Metabolism/Transport Effects **Substrate** of CYP2C8 (minor), 3A4 (major); **Induces** CYP1A2 (strong), 2B6 (strong), 2C8 (strong), 2C9 (strong), 2C19 (strong), 3A4 (strong), P-glycoprotein

Avoid Concomitant Use

Avoid concomitant use of CarBAMazepine with any of the following: Dabigatran Etexilate; Dronedarone; Etravirine; Everolimus; Lurasidone; MAO Inhibitors; Nefazodone; Nilotinib; Pazopanib; Praziquantel; Ranolazine; Roflumilast; RomiDEPsin; Tolvaptan; Vandetanib; Voriconazole

Increased Effect/Toxicity

CarBAMazepine may increase the levels/effects of: Adenosine; Alcohol (Ethyl); ClomiPRAMINE; CNS Depressants; Desmopressin; Fosphenytoin; Lithium; MAO Inhibitors; Methotrimeprazine; Phenytoin

The levels/effects of CarBAMazepine may be increased by: Allopurinol; Antifungal Agents (Azole Derivatives, Systemic); Calcium Channel Blockers (Nondihydropyridine); Carbonic Anhydrase Inhibitors; Cimetidine; Conivaptan; CYP3A4 Inhibitors (Moderate); CYP3A4 Inhibitors (Strong); Danazol; Darunavir; Dasatinib; Droperidol; Fluconazole; Grapefruit Juice; Isoniazid; LamoTRIgine; Macrolide Antibiotics; Methotrimeprazine; Nefazodone; Propoxyphene; Protease Inhibitors; QuiNINE; Selective Serotonin Reuptake Inhibitors; Thiazide Diuretics; Zolpidem

Decreased Effect

CarBAMazepine may decrease the levels/effects of: Acetaminophen; ARIPiprazole; Bendamustine; Benzodiazepines (metabolized by oxidation); Calcium Channel Blockers (Dihydropyridine); Calcium Channel Blockers (Nondihydropyridine); Caspofungin; CloZAPine; Contraceptives (Estrogens); Contraceptives (Progestins); CycloSPORINE; CycloSPORINE (Systemic); CYP1A2 Substrates; CYP2B6 Substrates; CYP2C19 Substrates; CYP2C8 Substrates (High risk); CYP2C9 Substrates (High risk); CYP3A4 Substrates; Dabigatran Etexilate; Divalproex; Doxycycline; Dronedarone; Etravirine; Everolimus; Exemestane; Felbamate; Flunarizine; Fosphenytoin; Gefitinib; GuanFACINE; Haloperidol; Imatinib; Irinotecan; Ixabepilone; Lacosamide; LamoTRIgine; Lopinavir; Lurasidone; Maraviroc; Mebendazole; Methadone; Nefazodone; Nilotinib; Paliperidone; Pazopanib; P-Glycoprotein Substrates; Phenytoin; Praziquantel; Protease Inhibitors; QuiNINE; Ranolazine; RisperiDONE; Roflumilast; RomiDEPsin; Rufinamide; Saxagliptin; Selective Serotonin Reuptake Inhibitors; SORAfenib; Tadalafil; Temsirolimus; Theophylline Derivatives; Thyroid Products; Tolvaptan; Topiramate; Treprostinil; Tricyclic Antidepressants; Ulipristal; Valproic Acid; Vandetanib; Vecuronium; Vitamin K Antagonists; Voriconazole; Ziprasidone; Zolpidem

The levels/effects of CarBAMazepine may be decreased by: CYP3A4 Inducers (Strong); Deferasirox; Divalproex; Felbamate; Fosphenytoin; Herbs (CYP3A4 Inducers); Ketorolac; Ketorolac (Systemic); Mefloquine; Methylfolate; Phenytoin; Rufinamide; Theophylline Derivatives; Tocilizumab; Valproic Acid

Ethanol/Nutrition/Herb Interactions

Ethanol: May increase CNS depression; monitor for increased effects with coadministration. Caution patients about effects.

Food: Carbamazepine serum levels may be increased if taken with food. Carbamazepine serum concentration may be increased if taken with grapefruit juice; avoid concurrent use.

Herb/Nutraceutical: Avoid evening primrose (seizure threshold decreased). Avoid valerian, St John's wort, kava kava, gotu kola (may increase CNS depression).

Dietary Considerations Drug may cause GI upset, take with large amount of water or food to decrease GI upset. May need to split doses to avoid GI upset.

Pharmacodynamics/Kinetics

Half-life Elimination Half-life is variable because of autoinduction which is usually complete 3-5 weeks after initiation of a fixed carbamazepine regimen.

Carbamazepine: Initial: 25-65 hours; Extended release: 35-40 hours; Multiple doses: Children: 8-14 hours; Adults: 12-17 hours

Epoxide metabolite: Initial: 25-43 hours

Time to Peak Unpredictable:

Immediate release: Suspension: 1.5 hour; tablet: 4-5 hours

Extended release: Carbatrol®, Equetro®: 12-26 hours (single dose), 4-8 hours (multiple doses); Tegretol®-XR: 3-12 hours

Pregnancy Risk Factor D

Lactation Enters breast milk/not recommended (AAP rates "compatible"; AAP 2001 update pending)

Breast-Feeding Considerations Carbamazepine and its metabolites are found in breast milk. The manufacturer does not recommend use while breast-feeding.

Dosage Forms

Capsule, extended release, oral:

Carbatrol®: 100 mg, 200 mg, 300 mg

Equetro®: 100 mg, 200 mg, 300 mg

Suspension, oral: 100 mg/5 mL (5 mL, 10 mL, 450 mL)

TEGretol®: 100 mg/5 mL (450 mL)

Tablet, oral: 200 mg, 400 mg

Epitol®: 200 mg

TEGretol®: 200 mg

Tablet, chewable, oral: 100 mg

TEGretol®: 100 mg

Tablet, extended release, oral: 200 mg, 400 mg

TEGretol®-XR: 100 mg, 200 mg, 400 mg

Carbamide Peroxide (KAR ba mide per OKS ide)

U.S. Brand Names Auraphene B® [OTC]; Auro® [OTC]; Cankaid® [OTC]; Debrox® [OTC]; E-R-O® [OTC]; Gly-Oxide® [OTC]; Murine® Ear Wax Removal Kit [OTC]; Murine® Ear [OTC]; Otix® [OTC]

Generic Availability (U.S.) Yes

Pharmacologic Category Anti-inflammatory, Locally Applied; Otic Agent, Cerumenolytic

Dental Use Relief of minor inflammation of gums, oral mucosal surfaces, and lips (including canker sores and dental irritation)

Use Relief of minor inflammation of gums, oral mucosal surfaces, and lips including canker sores and dental irritation; emulsify and disperse ear wax

Local Anesthetic/Vasoconstrictor Precautions No information available to require special precautions

Effects on Dental Treatment No significant effects or complications reported

Effects on Bleeding No information available to require special precautions

Adverse Effects Frequency not defined.

Dermatologic: Rash

Local: Irritation, redness

Miscellaneous: Superinfection

Dental Usual Dosage Minor inflammation of gums, oral mucosal surfaces and lips: Children and Adults: Topical: Oral solution (should not be used for >7 days): Apply several drops undiluted on affected area 4 times/day after meals and at bedtime; expectorate after 2-3 minutes **or** place 10 drops onto tongue, mix with saliva, swish for several minutes, expectorate

Dosage Children and Adults:

Oral: Inflammation/dental irritation: Solution (should not be used for >7 days): Oral preparation should not be used in children <2 years of age; apply several drops undiluted on affected area 4 times/day after meals and at bedtime; expectorate after 2-3 minutes **or** place 10 drops onto tongue, mix with saliva, swish for several minutes, expectorate

Otic:

Children <12 years: Tilt head sideways and individualize the dose according to patient size; 3 drops (range: 1-5 drops) twice daily for up to 4 days, tip of applicator should not enter ear canal; keep drops in ear for several minutes by keeping head tilted and placing cotton in ear

Children ≥12 years and Adults: Tilt head sideways and instill 5-10 drops twice daily up to 4 days, tip of applicator should not enter ear canal; keep drops in ear for several minutes by keeping head tilted and placing cotton in ear

Mechanism of Action Carbamide peroxide releases hydrogen peroxide which serves as a source of nascent oxygen upon contact with catalase; deodorant action is probably due to inhibition of odor-causing bacteria; softens impacted cerumen due to its foaming action

Contraindications Hypersensitivity to carbamide peroxide or any component of the formulation; otic preparation should not be used in patients with a perforated tympanic membrane; ear drainage, ear pain, or rash in the ear

Warnings/Precautions

Oral: With prolonged use of oral carbamide peroxide, there is a potential for overgrowth of opportunistic organisms, damage to periodontal tissues, and delayed wound healing; should not be used for longer than 7 days. Not for OTC use in children <2 years of age.

Otic: Do not use if ear drainage or discharge, ear pain, irritation, or rash in ear. Should not be used for longer than 4 days. Not for OTC use in children <12 years of age.

Drug Interactions

Avoid Concomitant Use There are no known interactions where it is recommended to avoid concomitant use.

Increased Effect/Toxicity There are no known significant interactions involving an increase in effect.

Decreased Effect There are no known significant interactions involving a decrease in effect.

Pharmacodynamics/Kinetics

Onset of Action ~24 hours

Dosage Forms

Liquid, oral: 10% (60 mL)
- Cankaid® [OTC]: 10% (15 mL)
- Gly-Oxide® [OTC]: 10% (15 mL, 60 mL)

Solution, otic: 6.5% (15 mL)
- Auraphene B® [OTC]: 6.5% (15 mL)
- Auro® [OTC]: 6.5% (22.2 mL)
- Debrox® [OTC]: 6.5% (15 mL, 30 mL)
- E-R-O® [OTC]: 6.5% (15 mL)
- Murine® Ear [OTC]: 6.5% (15 mL)
- Murine® Ear Wax Removal Kit [OTC]: 6.5% (15 mL)
- Otix® [OTC]: 6.5% (15 mL)

Carbetapentane and Chlorpheniramine

(kar bay ta PEN tane & klor fen IR a meen)

Related Information

Chlorpheniramine *on page 365*

U.S. Brand Names C-Tanna 12 [DSC]; Tannic-12 S [DSC]; Tussi-12 S™; Tussi-12®; Tussizone-12 RF™

Pharmacologic Category Alkylamine Derivative; Antitussive; Histamine H_1 Antagonist; Histamine H_1 Antagonist, First Generation

Use Symptomatic relief of cough associated with upper respiratory tract conditions, such as the common cold, bronchitis, bronchial asthma

Local Anesthetic/Vasoconstrictor Precautions No information available to require special precautions

Effects on Dental Treatment Key adverse event(s) related to dental treatment: Dry mucous membranes. Chronic use of antihistamines will inhibit salivary flow, particularly in elderly patients; this may contribute to periodontal disease and oral discomfort.

Effects on Bleeding No information available to require special precautions

Adverse Effects Frequency not defined.

Central nervous system: Drowsiness, excitation (children), sedation

Gastrointestinal: GI motility decreased, dry mucous membranes

General Dosage Range Oral:

Children 2-6 years: Carbetapentane 15-30 mg and chlorpheniramine 2-4 mg every 12 hours

Children >6 years: Carbetapentane 30-60 mg and chlorpheniramine 4-8 mg every 12 hours

Adults: Carbetapentane 60-120 mg and chlorpheniramine 5-10 mg every 12 hours

Mechanism of Action Carbetapentane is a nonopioid cough suppressant; chlorpheniramine is an H_1-receptor antagonist

Pregnancy Risk Factor C

Carbetapentane, Phenylephrine, and Pyrilamine

(kar bay ta PEN tane, fen il EF rin, & peer Il a meen)

Related Information

Phenylephrine (Systemic) *on page 1339*

U.S. Brand Names C-Tanna 12D [DSC]; Tussi-12® D [DSC]; Tussi-12® DS [DSC]

Pharmacologic Category Alpha/Beta Agonist; Antitussive; Decongestant; Ethylenediamine Derivative; Histamine H_1 Antagonist; Histamine H_1 Antagonist, First Generation

Use Symptomatic relief of cough associated with respiratory tract conditions such as the common cold, bronchial asthma, acute and chronic bronchitis

Local Anesthetic/Vasoconstrictor Precautions Use with caution since phenylephrine is a sympathomimetic amine which could interact with epinephrine to cause a pressor response

Effects on Dental Treatment Key adverse event(s) related to dental treatment: Tachycardia, palpitations (use vasoconstrictor with caution), and xerostomia (normal salivary flow resumes upon discontinuation).

Effects on Bleeding No information available to require special precautions

Adverse Effects Frequency not defined.

Central nervous system: Drowsiness, sedation

Gastrointestinal: Xerostomia

General Dosage Range Oral:

Children 2-6 years: Tussi-12® DS: 2.5-5 mL every 12 hours

Children 6-11 years: Tussi-12® D: 1/2 to 1 tablet every 12 hours; Tussi-12® DS: 5-10 mL every 12 hours

Children ≥12 years and Adults: Tussi-12® D: 1-2 tablets every 12 hours

Mechanism of Action

Carbetapentane is a nonopioid cough suppressant

Phenylephrine hydrochloride is a sympathomimetic agent (primarily alpha), decongestant.

Pyrilamine is an H_1-receptor antagonist.

Pregnancy Risk Factor C

Carbidopa (kar bi DOE pa)

U.S. Brand Names Lodosyn®

Pharmacologic Category Anti-Parkinson's Agent, Decarboxylase Inhibitor

Use Given with levodopa in the treatment of parkinsonism to enable a lower dosage of levodopa to be used and a more rapid response to be obtained and to decrease side effects; for details of administration and dosage, see Levodopa; has no effect without levodopa

Local Anesthetic/Vasoconstrictor Precautions No information available to require special precautions

Effects on Dental Treatment Key adverse event(s) related to dental treatment: Orthostatic hypotension. Dopaminergic therapy in Parkinson's disease includes the use of carbidopa in combination with levodopa. Carbidopa/levodopa combination is associated with orthostatic hypotension. Patients medicated with this drug combination should be carefully assisted from the chair and observed for signs of orthostatic hypotension.

Effects on Bleeding No information available to require special precautions

Adverse Effects Adverse reactions are associated with concomitant administration with levodopa

>10%: Central nervous system: Anxiety, confusion, nervousness, mental depression

1% to 10%:

Cardiovascular: Orthostatic hypotension, palpitation, cardiac arrhythmia

Central nervous system: Memory loss, insomnia, fatigue, hallucinations, ataxia, dystonic movements

Gastrointestinal: Nausea, vomiting, GI bleeding

Ocular: Blurred vision

General Dosage Range Oral: *Adults:* 70-100 mg/day (maximum: 200 mg/day)

Mechanism of Action Carbidopa is a peripheral decarboxylase inhibitor with little or no pharmacological activity when given alone in usual doses. It inhibits the peripheral decarboxylation of levodopa to dopamine; and as it does not cross the blood-brain barrier, unlike levodopa, effective brain concentrations of dopamine are produced with lower doses of levodopa. At the same time, reduced peripheral formation of dopamine reduces peripheral side-effects, notably nausea and vomiting, and cardiac arrhythmias, although the dyskinesias and adverse mental effects associated with levodopa therapy tend to develop earlier.

Pharmacodynamics/Kinetics

Half-life Elimination 1-2 hours

Pregnancy Risk Factor C

Carbidopa and Levodopa (kar bi DOE pa & lee voe DOE pa)

Related Information

Carbidopa *on page 307*

U.S. Brand Names Parcopa®; Sinemet®; Sinemet® CR

Canadian Brand Names Apo-Levocarb®; Apo-Levocarb® CR; Dom-Levo-Carbidopa; Duodopa™; Endo®-Levodopa/Carbidopa; Levocarb CR; Novo-Levocarbidopa; Nu-Levocarb; PRO-Levocarb; Sinemet®; Sinemet® CR

Pharmacologic Category Anti-Parkinson's Agent, Decarboxylase Inhibitor; Anti-Parkinson's Agent, Dopamine Precursor

Use Idiopathic Parkinson's disease; postencephalitic parkinsonism; symptomatic parkinsonism

Duodopa™ intestinal gel: Canadian labeling (not available in U.S.): Treatment of advanced levodopa-responsive Parkinson's disease in which severe motor symptoms are not controlled by other Parkinson's agents

Unlabeled/Investigational Use Restless leg syndrome

Local Anesthetic/Vasoconstrictor Precautions No information available to require special precautions

Effects on Dental Treatment Key adverse event(s) related to dental treatment: Xerostomia (normal salivary flow resumes upon discontinuation) and taste alterations. Dopaminergic therapy in Parkinson's disease (ie, treatment with levodopa and carbidopa combination) is associated with orthostatic hypotension. Patients medicated with this drug combination should be carefully assisted from the chair and observed for signs of orthostatic hypotension.

Effects on Bleeding No information available to require special precautions

Adverse Effects Frequency not defined.

Cardiovascular: Arrhythmia, chest pain, edema, flushing, hypotension, hypertension, MI, orthostatic hypotension, palpitation, phlebitis, syncope

Central nervous system: Agitation, anxiety, ataxia, confusion, delusions, dementia, depression (with or without suicidal tendencies), disorientation, dizziness, dreams abnormal, EPS, euphoria, faintness, falling, fatigue, gait abnormalities, headache, hallucinations, impulse control symptoms, insomnia, malaise, memory impairment, mental acuity decreased, nervousness, neuroleptic malignant syndrome, nightmares, on-off phenomena, paranoid ideation, pathological gambling, psychosis, seizure (causal relationship not established), somnolence

Dermatologic: Alopecia, malignant melanoma, rash

Endocrine & metabolic: Hot flashes, hyperglycemia, hypokalemia, libido increased (including hypersexuality), uric acid increased

Gastrointestinal: Abdominal pain, abdominal distress, anorexia, bruxism, constipation, diarrhea, discoloration of saliva, duodenal ulcer, dyspepsia, dysphagia, flatulence, GI bleeding, heartburn, nausea, sialorrhea, taste alterations, tongue burning sensation, weight gain/loss, vomiting, xerostomia

Genitourinary: Discoloration of urine, glycosuria, urinary frequency, priapism, proteinuria, urinary incontinence, urinary retention, urinary tract infection

Hematologic: Agranulocytosis, anemia, Coombs' test abnormal, hematocrit decreased, hemoglobin decreased, hemolytic anemia, leukopenia

Hepatic: Alkaline phosphatase abnormal, ALT abnormal, AST abnormal, bilirubin abnormal, LDH abnormal

Neuromuscular & skeletal: Back pain, dyskinesias (including choreiform, dystonic and other involuntary movements), leg pain, muscle cramps, muscle twitching, numbness, paresthesia, peripheral neuropathy, shoulder pain, tremor increased, trismus, weakness

Ocular: Blepharospasm, blurred vision, diplopia, Horner's syndrome reactivation, mydriasis, oculogyric crises (may be associated with acute dystonic reactions)

Renal: Difficult urination

Respiratory: Cough, dyspnea, hoarseness, pharyngeal pain, upper respiratory infection

Miscellaneous: Discoloration of sweat, diaphoresis increased, hiccups, hypersensitivity reactions (angioedema, pruritus, urticaria, bullous lesions [including pemphigus-like reactions], Henoch-Schönlein purpura)

General Dosage Range Oral: *Adults:* Immediate release: Initial: Carbidopa 25 mg/levodopa 100 mg 3 times/day (maximum: 8 tablets of any strength/day **or** 200 mg of carbidopa and 2000 mg of levodopa); Controlled release: *Adults:* Initial: Carbidopa 50 mg/levodopa 200 mg 2 times/day, at intervals not <6 hours (maximum: 8 tablets/day)

Mechanism of Action Parkinson's symptoms are due to a lack of striatal dopamine; levodopa circulates in the plasma to the blood-brain-barrier (BBB), where it crosses, to be converted by striatal enzymes to dopamine; carbidopa inhibits the peripheral plasma breakdown of levodopa by inhibiting its decarboxylation, and thereby increases available levodopa at the BBB

Pharmacodynamics/Kinetics

Half-life Elimination Immediate release: Levodopa (in presence of carbidopa): 1.5 hours; Half-life may be prolonged with controlled release formulations due to continuous absorption.

Time to Peak Immediate release: 0.5 hours; Controlled release: 2 hours; Intestinal gel: therapeutic plasma levels reached 10-30 minutes following morning bolus dose

Pregnancy Risk Factor C

Prescribing and Access Restrictions Duodopa™ intestinal gel (Canadian labeling; product not available in U.S.): In Canada, the Duodopa™ Education Program is a risk mitigation program established to provide safe and effective use of Duodopa™ in advanced Parkinson's patients. The program involves:

- Education of prescribing neurologists and other healthcare providers on suitable candidates for treatment, surgical procedures (PEG tube placement), and follow-up care including infusion device education.
- Distribution of educational materials to patients and caregivers describing Duodopa™ intestinal gel and its proper use, PEG tube placement, and complications associated with the mode of administration and/or PEG tube placement.

Carbinoxamine (kar bi NOKS a meen)

U.S. Brand Names Palgic®

Pharmacologic Category Ethanolamine Derivative; Histamine H_1 Antagonist; Histamine H_1 Antagonist, First Generation

Use Seasonal and perennial allergic rhinitis; vasomotor rhinitis; urticaria; decrease severity of other allergic reactions

Local Anesthetic/Vasoconstrictor Precautions No information available to require special precautions

Effects on Dental Treatment Key adverse event(s) related to dental treatment: Xerostomia (normal salivary flow resumes upon discontinuation).

Effects on Bleeding No information available to require special precautions

Adverse Effects Frequency not defined.

Cardiovascular: Extrasystoles, hypotension, palpitation, tachycardia

Central nervous system: Chills, confusion, coordination impaired (most frequent), dizziness (most frequent), euphoria, excitability (children), fatigue, headache, insomnia, irritability, nervousness, neuritis, restlessness, sedation (most frequent), seizure, sleepiness (most frequent), vertigo

Dermatologic: Photosensitivity, rash, urticaria

Endocrine & metabolic: Early menses

Gastrointestinal: Anorexia, constipation, diarrhea, epigastric distress (most frequent), heartburn, nausea, vomiting, xerostomia

Genitourinary: Difficult urination, urinary frequency, urinary retention

Hematologic: Agranulocytosis, hemolytic anemia, thrombocytopenia

Neuromuscular & skeletal: Paresthesia, tremor, weakness

Ocular: Blurred vision, diplopia

Renal: Polyuria

Respiratory: Bronchial secretions thickening (most frequent), chest tightness, nasal congestion, nasopharyngeal dryness, wheezing

Miscellaneous: Hypersensitivity reactions (including anaphylactic shock), diaphoresis

General Dosage Range Oral:

Children >3-6 years: 2-5 mg 3-4 times/day

Children >6 years: 4-6 mg 3-4 times/day

Adults: 4-8 mg 3-4 times/day

Mechanism of Action Carbinoxamine competes with histamine for H_1-receptor sites on effector cells in the gastrointestinal tract, blood vessels, and respiratory tract.

Pharmacodynamics/Kinetics

Half-life Elimination 10-20 hours

Pregnancy Risk Factor C

CARBOplatin (KAR boe pla tin)

Canadian Brand Names Paraplatin-AQ

Pharmacologic Category Antineoplastic Agent, Alkylating Agent; Antineoplastic Agent, Platinum Analog

Use Treatment of advanced ovarian cancer

Unlabeled/Investigational Use Treatment of bladder cancer, breast cancer (metastatic), central nervous system tumors, cervical cancer (recurrent or metastatic), endometrial cancer, esophageal cancer, head and neck cancer, Hodgkin's lymphoma (relapsed or refractory), malignant pleural mesothelioma, melanoma (advanced or metastatic), merkel cell carcinoma, neuroendocrine tumors (adrenal gland and carcinoid tumors), non-Hodgkin's lymphomas (relapsed or refractory), nonsmall cell lung cancer, prostate cancer, sarcomas (Ewing's sarcoma and osteosarcoma), small-cell lung cancer, testicular cancer, thymic malignancies, unknown primary adenocarcinoma, and as a conditioning regimen prior to hematopoietic stem cell transplantation

Local Anesthetic/Vasoconstrictor Precautions No information available to require special precautions

Effects on Dental Treatment Key adverse event(s) related to dental treatment: Stomatitis, mucositis, and taste dysgeusia.

Effects on Bleeding Chemotherapy may result in significant myelosuppression, potentially including significant reduction in platelet counts and altered hemostasis. In patients who are under active treatment with these agents, medical consult is suggested.

Adverse Effects Percentages reported with single-agent therapy.

>10%:

Central nervous system: Pain (23%)

Endocrine & metabolic: Hyponatremia (29% to 47%), hypomagnesemia (29% to 43%), hypocalcemia (22% to 31%), hypokalemia (20% to 28%)

Gastrointestinal: Vomiting (65% to 81%), abdominal pain (17%), nausea (without vomiting: 10% to 15%)

Hematologic: Myelosuppression (dose related and dose limiting; nadir at ~21 days; recovery by ~28 days), anemia (71% to 90%; grades 3/4: 21%), leukopenia (85%; grades 3/4: 15% to 26%), neutropenia (67%; grades 3/4: 16% to 21%), thrombocytopenia (62%; grades 3/4: 25% to 35%)

Hepatic: Alkaline phosphatase increased (24% to 37%), AST increased (15% to 19%)

Neuromuscular & skeletal: Weakness (11%)

Renal: Creatinine clearance decreased (27%), BUN increased (14% to 22%)

Miscellaneous: Hypersensitivity/allergic reaction (2% to 16%)

1% to 10%:

Central nervous system: Neurotoxicity (5%)

Dermatologic: Alopecia (2% to 3%)

Gastrointestinal: Constipation (6%), diarrhea (6%), stomatitis/mucositis (1%), taste dysgeusia (1%)

Hematologic: Bleeding (5%), hemorrhagic complications (5%)

Hepatic: Bilirubin increased (5%)

Neuromuscular & skeletal: Peripheral neuropathy (4% to 6%)

Ocular: Visual disturbance (1%)

Otic: Ototoxicity (1%)

Renal: Creatinine increased (6% to 10%)

Miscellaneous: Infection (5%)

General Dosage Range Dosage adjustment recommended in renal impairment or who develop toxicities

I.V.: *Adults:* 300-360 mg/m^2 every 4 weeks **or** AUC of 4-6 (using Calvert formula)

Mechanism of Action Carboplatin is a platinum compound alkylating agent which covalently binds to DNA; interferes with the function of DNA by producing interstrand DNA cross-links

Pharmacodynamics/Kinetics

Half-life Elimination Cl_{cr} >60 mL/minute: Carboplatin: 2.6-5.9 hours (based on a dose of 300-500 mg/m^2); Platinum (from carboplatin): ≥5 days

Pregnancy Risk Factor D

Carboprost Tromethamine (KAR boe prost tro METH a meen)

U.S. Brand Names Hemabate®

Canadian Brand Names Hemabate®

Pharmacologic Category Abortifacient; Prostaglandin

Use Termination of pregnancy; treatment of refractory postpartum uterine bleeding

Unlabeled/Investigational Use Investigational: Hemorrhagic cystitis

Local Anesthetic/Vasoconstrictor Precautions No information available to require special precautions

Effects on Dental Treatment No significant effects or complications reported

Effects on Bleeding No information available to require special precautions

Adverse Effects Frequency not defined. Effects due to increased smooth muscle contractility are most common.

Cardiovascular: Chest pain, flushing, hypertension, syncope, palpitation, tachycardia, tightness of chest

Central nervous system: Anxiety, chills/shivering, dizziness, drowsiness, dystonia, faintness, headache, lethargy, lightheadedness, nervousness, sleep disturbance, temperature elevation (may be drug induced or due to postabortion endometritis), vasovagal syndrome, vertigo

Dermatologic: Rash

Endocrine & metabolic: Breast tenderness, dysmenorrhea-like pain, endometritis, hot flashes, thyroid storm

Gastrointestinal: Choking sensation, diarrhea (~2/3 patients), dry throat, epigastric pain, gagging/retching, hematemesis, nausea (~1/3 patients), taste alteration, thirst, throat fullness, vomiting (~2/3 patients), xerostomia

Genitourinary: Perforated uterus, posterior cervical perforation, urinary tract infection, uterine bleeding (excessive), uterine rupture, uterine sacculation

Local: Injection site pain

Neuromuscular & skeletal: Backache, leg cramps, muscular pain, paresthesia, torticollis, weakness

Ocular: Blurred vision, eye pain, eyelid twitching

Otic: Tinnitus

Respiratory: Asthma, cough, bronchospasm, dyspnea, epistaxis, hyperventilation, pulmonary edema, respiratory distress, upper respiratory tract infection, wheezing

Miscellaneous: Diaphoresis, hiccups, retained placental fragment, septic shock

General Dosage Range I.M.: *Adults (females):* Abortion: 250 mcg at 1.5- to 3.5-hour intervals, a 500 mcg dose may be given if uterine response is not adequate after several 250 mcg doses (maximum total dose: 12 mg); Postpartum bleeding: 250 mcg; may repeat if needed (maximum total dose: 2 mg [8 doses])

Mechanism of Action Carboprost tromethamine is a prostaglandin similar to prostaglandin F_2 alpha (dinoprost) except for the addition of a methyl group at the C-15 position. This substitution produces longer duration of activity than dinoprost; carboprost stimulates uterine contractility which usually results in expulsion of the products of conception and is used to induce abortion between 13-20 weeks of pregnancy. Hemostasis at the placentation site is achieved through the myometrial contractions produced by carboprost.

Pregnancy Risk Factor C

Carboxymethylcellulose (kar boks ee meth il SEL yoo lose)

U.S. Brand Names Optive™ [OTC]; Refresh Liquigel™ [OTC]; Refresh Plus® [OTC]; Refresh Tears® [OTC]; Tears Again® Gel Drops™ [OTC]; Tears Again® Night & Day™ [OTC]; Theratears® [OTC]

Canadian Brand Names Celluvisc™; Refresh Plus®; Refresh Tears®

Pharmacologic Category Ophthalmic Agent, Miscellaneous

Use Artificial tear substitute

Local Anesthetic/Vasoconstrictor Precautions No information available to require special precautions

Effects on Dental Treatment No significant effects or complications reported

Effects on Bleeding No information available to require special precautions

General Dosage Range Ophthalmic: *Adults:* Instill 1-2 drops into eye(s) 3-4 times/day

Carisoprodol (kar eye soe PROE dole)

U.S. Brand Names Soma®

Generic Availability (U.S.) Yes

Pharmacologic Category Skeletal Muscle Relaxant

Dental Use Treatment of muscle spasms and pain associated with acute temporomandibular joint (TMJ) pain

Use Short-term (2-3 weeks) treatment of acute musculoskeletal pain

Local Anesthetic/Vasoconstrictor Precautions No information available to require special precautions

Effects on Dental Treatment No significant effects or complications reported

Effects on Bleeding No information available to require special precautions

Adverse Effects

>10%: Central nervous system: Drowsiness (13% to 17%)

1% to 10%: Central nervous system: Dizziness (7% to 8%), headache (3% to 5%)

Dental Usual Dosage Treatment of muscle spasms and pain associated with acute TMJ pain: Adults: Oral: 250-350 mg 3 times/day and at bedtime

Dosage Note: Carisoprodol should only be used for short periods (2-3 weeks) due to lack of evidence of effectiveness with prolonged use.

Oral: Children ≥16 years and Adults: 250-350 mg 3 times/day and at bedtime

Dosing adjustment in renal impairment: Use in renal impairment has not been studied; use with caution

Dialysis: Removed by hemo- and peritoneal dialysis

Dosing adjustment in hepatic impairment: Use in hepatic impairment has not been studied; use with caution

Mechanism of Action Precise mechanism is not yet clear, but many effects have been ascribed to its central depressant actions. In animals, carisoprodol blocks interneuronal activity and depresses polysynaptic neuron transmission in the spinal cord and reticular formation of the brain. It is also metabolized to meprobamate, which has anxiolytic and sedative effects.

Contraindications Hypersensitivity to carisoprodol, meprobamate, or any component of the formulation; acute intermittent porphyria

Warnings/Precautions Can cause CNS depression, which may impair physical or mental abilities. Patients must be cautioned about performing tasks which require mental alertness (eg, operating machinery or driving); postmarketing reports of motor vehicle accidents have been associated with use. Effects with other CNS-depressant drugs or ethanol may be potentiated. Use with caution in patients with hepatic/renal dysfunction. Tolerance or drug dependence may result from extended use. Limit use to 2-3 weeks; use caution in patients who may be prone to addiction. May precipitate withdrawal after abrupt cessation of prolonged use.

Idiosyncratic reactions and/or severe allergic reactions may occur. Idiosyncratic reactions occur following the initial dose and may include severe weakness, transient quadriplegia, euphoria, or vision loss (temporary). Has been associated (rarely) with seizures in patients with and without seizure history. Carisoprodol should be used with caution in patients who are poor CYP2C19 metabolizers; poor metabolizers have been shown to have a fourfold increase in exposure to carisoprodol and a 50% reduced exposure to the metabolite meprobamate compared to normal metabolizers. This class of medication is poorly tolerated by the elderly due to anticholinergic effects, sedation, and weakness. Efficacy is questionable at dosages tolerated by elderly patients (Beers Criteria).

Drug Interactions

Metabolism/Transport Effects **Substrate** of CYP2C19 (major)

Avoid Concomitant Use There are no known interactions where it is recommended to avoid concomitant use.

Increased Effect/Toxicity

Carisoprodol may increase the levels/effects of: Alcohol (Ethyl); CNS Depressants; Methotrimeprazine

The levels/effects of Carisoprodol may be increased by: CYP2C19 Inhibitors (Moderate); CYP2C19 Inhibitors (Strong); Droperidol; Methotrimeprazine

Decreased Effect

The levels/effects of Carisoprodol may be decreased by: CYP2C19 Inducers (Strong)

Ethanol/Nutrition/Herb Interactions Ethanol: May increase CNS depression; monitor for increased effects with coadministration. Caution patients about effects.

Dietary Considerations May be taken with or without food.

Pharmacodynamics/Kinetics

Onset of Action ~30 minutes

Duration of Action 4-6 hours

Half-life Elimination ~2 hours; Meprobamate: 10 hours

Time to Peak 1.5-2 hours

Pregnancy Risk Factor C

Lactation Enters breast milk/use caution

Breast-Feeding Considerations Carisoprodol levels in breast milk may be 2-4 times that of maternal plasma levels. The estimated dose to the infant was reported as 6.9% of the weight adjusted maternal dose in one case report and ~4% of the weight-adjusted maternal dose in another. In both cases, breast milk production was decreased requiring supplemental formula or cessation of breast-feeding. Other than slight sedation reported in one infant, no symptoms of withdrawal or other adverse events were noted in these 2 cases. Effects on long-term development are not known.

Dosage Forms

Tablet, oral: 350 mg

Soma®: 250 mg, 350 mg

Carisoprodol and Aspirin (kar eye soe PROE dole & AS pir in)

Related Information

Aspirin *on page 171*

Carisoprodol *on page 311*

U.S. Brand Names Soma® Compound

Generic Availability (U.S.) Yes

Pharmacologic Category Skeletal Muscle Relaxant

Dental Use Treatment of muscle spasms and pain associated with acute temporomandibular joint pain (TMJ)

Use Relief of discomfort associated with acute, painful skeletal muscle conditions

Local Anesthetic/Vasoconstrictor Precautions No information available to require special precautions

Effects on Dental Treatment Key adverse event(s) related to dental treatment: Aspirin: As with all drugs which may affect hemostasis, bleeding is associated with aspirin. Hemorrhage may occur at virtually any site; risk is dependent on multiple variables including dosage, concurrent use of multiple agents which alter hemostasis, and patient susceptibility. Many adverse effects of aspirin are dose related, and are rare at low dosages. Other serious reactions are idiosyncratic, related to allergy or individual sensitivity (see Effects on Bleeding).

Effects on Bleeding Aspirin inhibits platelet aggregation which prolongs bleeding times. Inhibition is irreversible; on discontinuation of ASA, normal platelet function returns only when new platelets are released from the bone marrow. Dental practitioners should note that recommendations differ between general surgery (eg, appendectomy, hip replacement) and dental surgery. Due to concerns for increased blood loss, ASA is typically avoided (if possible) in general surgery patients for 1-2 weeks prior to surgery (exception is in patients undergoing CABG or noncardiac surgery at high risk of cardiac events – per 2008 ACCP guidelines). However, in the case of dental surgery there is no scientific evidence to warrant discontinuance of aspirin.

Reports of major bleeding related to dental surgery attributed to aspirin use have not been published. Furthermore, interruption of therapy may result in a loss of therapeutic effect. Patients taking one aspirin tablet daily as an antithrombotic who require dental surgery should be given special consideration in consultation with the physician before removal of the aspirin. In particular, aspirin should NOT be discontinued in patients with cardiac stents that have not completed their full course of dual antiplatelet therapy (aspirin, clopidogrel); patient specific situations need to be discussed with cardiologist. When feasible, postponement of dental surgery until the completion of dual antiplatelet therapy should be considered.

Adverse Effects See individual agents.

Dental Usual Dosage Treatment of muscle spasms and pain associated with acute TMJ pain: Adults: Oral: 1-2 tablets 4 times/day

Dosage Oral:

Children ≥16 years and Adults: Acute skeletal muscle pain: 1-2 tablets 4 times/day for 2-3 weeks (maximum: 8 tablets/24 hours)

Elderly: Avoid use in the elderly due to risk of orthostatic hypotension and CNS depression

Dosing adjustment in renal impairment: Use in renal impairment has not been studied; use with caution

Dosing adjustment in hepatic impairment: Use in hepatic impairment has not been studied; use with caution

Mechanism of Action See individual agents.

Contraindications Hypersensitivity to a carbamate (eg, meprobamate); serious gastrointestinal complications (eg, bleeding, perforations, obstruction) due to aspirin use; aspirin-induced asthma; acute intermittent porphyria

Warnings/Precautions Can cause CNS depression, which may impair physical or mental abilities. Patients must be cautioned about performing tasks which require mental alertness (eg, operating machinery or driving); postmarketing reports of motor vehicle accidents have been associated with use. Sedative effects may be potentiated when used with other CNS-depressant drugs or ethanol. Serious GI effects (eg, bleeding, perforation, and intestinal obstruction) may occur (possibly fatal) with aspirin use. Idiosyncratic reactions may occur (rarely) following initial dosing and may include severe weakness, transient quadriplegia, euphoria, or temporary vision loss. Use with caution in patients with a history of GI bleeding from ulcers; history of poor baseline health; geriatric patients; patients taking high doses of aspirin; patients taking concurrent anticoagulants, NSAIDs, or large amounts of ethanol.

Patients with sensitivity to tartrazine dyes, nasal polyps, and asthma may have an increased risk of salicylate sensitivity. Carisoprodol has been associated (rarely) with seizures in patients with and without seizure history. Idiosyncratic reactions may occur (rarely) following initial dosing and may include severe weakness, transient quadriplegia, euphoria, or temporary vision loss. Use with caution in patients with a history of drug abuse or acute alcoholism; potential for drug dependency exists. Tolerance, psychological and physical dependence may occur with prolonged use. Abrupt discontinuation following prolonged use may lead to withdrawal symptoms; use >3 weeks not recommended.

Use with caution in patients with hepatic or renal impairment; not studied. Abrupt discontinuation following prolonged use may lead to withdrawal symptoms; use >3 weeks not recommended. Aspirin should be avoided (if possible) in surgical patients for 1-2 weeks prior to surgery, to reduce the risk of excessive bleeding. Carisoprodol should be used with caution in patients with reduced function alleles of CYP2C19; poor metabolizers have been shown to have a fourfold increase in exposure to carisoprodol and a 50% reduced exposure to the metabolite meprobamate compared to normal metabolizers. Avoid or use with caution in the elderly (>65 years of age); may be more sensitive to anticholinergic effects, sedation, and weakness. Efficacy is questionable at dosages tolerated by elderly patients (Beers Criteria).

Drug Interactions

Metabolism/Transport Effects

Carisoprodol: **Substrate** of CYP2C19 (major)
Aspirin: **Substrate** of CYP2C9 (minor)

Avoid Concomitant Use

Avoid concomitant use of Carisoprodol and Aspirin with any of the following: Influenza Virus Vaccine (Live/Attenuated); Ketorolac; Ketorolac (Systemic)

Increased Effect/Toxicity

Carisoprodol and Aspirin may increase the levels/effects of: Alcohol (Ethyl); Alendronate; Anticoagulants; Carbonic Anhydrase Inhibitors; CNS Depressants; Collagenase (Systemic); Corticosteroids (Systemic); Divalproex; Drotrecogin Alfa; Heparin; Ibritumomab; Methotrexate; Methotrimeprazine; PRALAtrexate; Salicylates; Sulfonylureas; Thrombolytic Agents; Tositumomab and Iodine I 131 Tositumomab; Valproic Acid; Varicella Virus-Containing Vaccines; Vitamin K Antagonists

The levels/effects of Carisoprodol and Aspirin may be increased by: Antidepressants (Tricyclic, Tertiary Amine); Antiplatelet Agents; Calcium Channel Blockers (Nondihydropyridine); CYP2C19 Inhibitors (Moderate); CYP2C19 Inhibitors (Strong); Dasatinib; Droperidol; Ginkgo Biloba; Glucosamine; Herbs (Anticoagulant/Antiplatelet Properties); Influenza Virus Vaccine (Live/Attenuated); Ketorolac; Ketorolac (Systemic); Loop Diuretics; Methotrimeprazine; Nonsteroidal Anti-Inflammatory Agents; NSAID (Nonselective); Omega-3-Acid Ethyl Esters; Pentosan Polysulfate Sodium; Pentoxifylline; Prostacyclin Analogues; Selective Serotonin Reuptake Inhibitors; Serotonin/Norepinephrine Reuptake Inhibitors; Treprostinil

Decreased Effect

Carisoprodol and Aspirin may decrease the levels/effects of: ACE Inhibitors; Loop Diuretics; NSAID (Nonselective); Probenecid; Tiludronate

The levels/effects of Carisoprodol and Aspirin may be decreased by: Corticosteroids (Systemic); CYP2C19 Inducers (Strong); Nonsteroidal Anti-Inflammatory Agents; NSAID (Nonselective)

Ethanol/Nutrition/Herb Interactions Ethanol: May increase CNS depression; monitor for increased effects with coadministration. Caution patients about effects.

Pregnancy Risk Factor D

Lactation Enters breast milk/not recommended

Breast-Feeding Considerations See individual agents.

Dosage Forms

Tablet: Carisoprodol 200 mg and aspirin 325 mg
Soma® Compound: Carisoprodol 200 mg and aspirin 325 mg

Dental Comment There is no scientific evidence to warrant discontinuance of aspirin prior to dental surgery. Patients taking one aspirin tablet daily as an antithrombotic and who require dental surgery should be given special consideration in consultation with the physician before removal of the aspirin relative to prevention of postoperative bleeding.

Carisoprodol, Aspirin, and Codeine

(kar eye soe PROE dole, AS pir in, and KOE deen)

Related Information

Aspirin *on page* 171
Carisoprodol *on page* 311
Codeine *on page* 432

Generic Availability (U.S.) Yes

Pharmacologic Category Skeletal Muscle Relaxant

Dental Use Treatment of muscle spasms and pain associated with acute temporomandibular joint pain (TMJ)

Use Skeletal muscle relaxant

Local Anesthetic/Vasoconstrictor Precautions No information available to require special precautions

Effects on Dental Treatment Key adverse event(s) related to dental treatment: Aspirin: As with all drugs which may affect hemostasis, bleeding is associated with aspirin. Hemorrhage may occur at virtually any site; risk is dependent on multiple variables including dosage, concurrent use of multiple agents which alter hemostasis, and patient susceptibility. Many adverse effects of aspirin are dose related, and are rare at low dosages. Other serious reactions are idiosyncratic, related to allergy or individual sensitivity (see Effects on Bleeding).

Effects on Bleeding Aspirin inhibits platelet aggregation which prolongs bleeding times. Inhibition is irreversible; on discontinuation of ASA, normal platelet function returns only when new platelets are released from the bone marrow. Dental practitioners should note that recommendations differ between general surgery (eg, appendectomy, hip replacement) and dental surgery. Due to concerns for increased blood loss, ASA is typically avoided (if possible) in general surgery patients for 1-2 weeks prior to surgery (exception is in patients undergoing CABG or noncardiac surgery at high risk of cardiac events - per 2008 ACCP guidelines). However, in the case of dental surgery there is no scientific evidence to warrant discontinuance of aspirin.

Reports of major bleeding related to dental surgery attributed to aspirin use have not been published. Furthermore, interruption of therapy may result in a loss of therapeutic effect. Patients taking one aspirin tablet daily as an antithrombotic who require dental surgery should be given special consideration in consultation with the physician before removal of the aspirin. In particular, aspirin should NOT be discontinued in patients with cardiac stents that have not completed their full course of dual antiplatelet therapy (aspirin, clopidogrel); patient specific situations need to be discussed with cardiologist. When feasible, postponement of dental surgery until the completion of dual antiplatelet therapy should be considered.

Adverse Effects See individual agents.

Dental Usual Dosage Treatment of muscle spasms and pain associated with acute TMJ pain: Adults: Oral: 1 or 2 tablets 4 times/day

Dosage Oral:

Adults: 1 or 2 tablets 4 times/day (maximum: 8 tablets/day); treatment should be temporary (2-3 weeks)

Elderly: Avoid or use with caution in the elderly (>65 years of age); adverse effects (eg, orthostatic hypotension and CNS depression) may be potentiated.

Mechanism of Action See individual agents.

Contraindications Hypersensitivity to a carbamate (eg, meprobamate); serious gastrointestinal complications (eg, bleeding, perforations, obstruction) due to aspirin use; aspirin-induced asthma; acute intermittent porphyria

Warnings/Precautions Use with caution in patients with hypersensitivity reactions to other phenanthrene-derivative opioid agonists (hydrocodone, hydromorphone, levorphanol, oxycodone, oxymorphone); hepatic or renal dysfunction; cardiovascular disease; biliary tract impairment; gastrointestinal disease; respiratory disease. May obscure diagnosis or clinical course of patients with acute abdominal conditions. May cause CNS depression, which may impair physical or mental abilities; patients must be cautioned about performing tasks which require mental alertness (eg, operating machinery or driving). May cause hypotension; use with caution in patients with hypovolemia, cardiovascular disease (including acute MI), or drugs which may exaggerate hypotensive effects (including phenothiazines or general anesthetics). Carisoprodol has been associated (rarely) with seizures in patients with and without seizure history.

Patients with sensitivity to tartrazine dyes, nasal polyps, and asthma may have an increased risk of salicylate sensitivity. Effects with other sedatives or ethanol may be potentiated. Use caution with concomitant use of aspirin, NSAIDs, warfarin, or other drugs that affect coagulation; the risk of bleeding may be potentiated. Use caution in patients with two or more copies of the variant CYP2D6*2 allele. Use with caution in elderly patients; adverse effects may be potentiated. Safety and efficacy have not been established in children <16 years of age. Tolerance or drug dependence may result from extended use; abrupt discontinuation may lead to withdrawal symptoms. Limit use to 2-3 weeks; use caution in patients who may be prone to addiction. Aspirin products should be avoided (if possible) for 1-2 weeks prior to surgery.

Drug Interactions

Metabolism/Transport Effects

Carisoprodol: **Substrate** of CYP2C19 (major)

Aspirin: **Substrate** of CYP2C9 (minor)

Avoid Concomitant Use

Avoid concomitant use of Carisoprodol, Aspirin, and Codeine with any of the following: Influenza Virus Vaccine (Live/Attenuated); Ketorolac; Ketorolac (Systemic)

Increased Effect/Toxicity

Carisoprodol, Aspirin, and Codeine may increase the levels/effects of: Alcohol (Ethyl); Alendronate; Alvimopan; Anticoagulants; Carbonic Anhydrase Inhibitors; CNS Depressants; Collagenase (Systemic); Corticosteroids (Systemic); Desmopressin; Divalproex; Drotrecogin Alfa; Heparin; Ibritumomab; Methotrexate; PRALAtrexate; Salicylates; Selective Serotonin Reuptake Inhibitors; Sulfonylureas; Thiazide Diuretics; Thrombolytic Agents; Tositumomab and Iodine I 131 Tositumomab; Valproic Acid; Varicella Virus-Containing Vaccines; Vitamin K Antagonists

The levels/effects of Carisoprodol, Aspirin, and Codeine may be increased by: Amphetamines; Antidepressants (Tricyclic, Tertiary Amine); Antiplatelet Agents; Antipsychotic Agents (Phenothiazines); Calcium Channel Blockers (Nondihydropyridine); CYP2C19 Inhibitors (Moderate); CYP2C19 Inhibitors (Strong); Dasatinib; Droperidol; Ginkgo Biloba; Glucosamine; Herbs (Anticoagulant/Antiplatelet Properties); Influenza Virus Vaccine (Live/Attenuated); Ketorolac; Ketorolac (Systemic); Loop Diuretics; NSAID (Nonselective); Omega-3-Acid Ethyl Esters; Pentosan Polysulfate Sodium; Pentoxifylline; Prostacyclin Analogues; Selective Serotonin Reuptake Inhibitors; Serotonin/Norepinephrine Reuptake Inhibitors; Somatostatin Analogs; Succinylcholine; Treprostinil

Decreased Effect

Carisoprodol, Aspirin, and Codeine may decrease the levels/effects of: ACE Inhibitors; Loop Diuretics; NSAID (Nonselective); Pegvisomant; Probenecid; Tiludronate

The levels/effects of Carisoprodol, Aspirin, and Codeine may be decreased by: Ammonium Chloride; Corticosteroids (Systemic); CYP2C19 Inducers (Strong); CYP2D6 Inhibitors (Moderate); CYP2D6 Inhibitors (Strong); Mixed Agonist/Antagonist Opioids; NSAID (Nonselective)

Ethanol/Nutrition/Herb Interactions

Ethanol: May increase CNS depression; monitor for increased effects with coadministration. Caution patients about effects.

Herb/Nutraceutical: St John's wort may decrease codeine levels. Avoid valerian, St John's wort, kava kava, gotu kola (may increase CNS depression). Avoid cat's claw, dong quai, evening primrose, feverfew, garlic, ginger, ginkgo, red clover, horse chestnut, green tea, ginseng (all have additional antiplatelet activity). Limit curry powder, paprika, licorice; may cause salicylate accumulation (these foods contain 6 mg salicylate/100 g; an ordinary American diet contains 10-200 mg/day of salicylate).

Pregnancy Risk Factor D

Lactation Enters breast milk/not recommended

Breast-Feeding Considerations Refer to Codeine monograph.

Controlled Substance C-III

Dosage Forms

Tablet: Carisoprodol 200 mg, aspirin 325 mg, and codeine 16 mg

Dental Comment There is no scientific evidence to warrant discontinuance of aspirin prior to dental surgery. Patients taking one aspirin tablet daily as an antithrombotic and who require dental surgery should be given special consideration in consultation with the physician before removal of the aspirin relative to prevention of postoperative bleeding.

Carmustine (kar MUS teen)

U.S. Brand Names BiCNU®; Gliadel®

Canadian Brand Names BiCNU®; Gliadel Wafer®

Pharmacologic Category Antineoplastic Agent; Antineoplastic Agent, Alkylating Agent; Antineoplastic Agent, Alkylating Agent (Nitrosourea)

Use

Injection: Treatment of brain tumors (glioblastoma, brainstem glioma, medulloblastoma, astrocytoma, ependymoma, and metastatic brain tumors), multiple myeloma, Hodgkin's disease (relapsed or refractory), non-Hodgkin's lymphomas (relapsed or refractory)

Wafer (implant): Adjunct to surgery in patients with recurrent glioblastoma multiforme; adjunct to surgery and radiation in patients with high-grade malignant glioma

Unlabeled/Investigational Use Treatment of metastatic melanoma

Local Anesthetic/Vasoconstrictor Precautions No information available to require special precautions

Effects on Dental Treatment Key adverse event(s) related to dental treatment: Stomatitis.

Effects on Bleeding Chemotherapy may result in significant myelosuppression, potentially including significant reduction in platelet counts and altered hemostasis.

In patients who are under active treatment with these agents, medical consult is suggested.

Adverse Effects

>10%:

Cardiovascular: Hypotension (with high-dose I.V. therapy, due to the alcohol content of the diluent)

Central nervous system: Ataxia, dizziness

Postoperatively: Seizure (wafer 5% to 54%), brain edema (wafer 4% to 23%)

Dermatologic: Burning (with skin contact), hyperpigmentation of skin (with skin contact)

Gastrointestinal: Severe nausea and vomiting, usually begins within 2-4 hours of drug administration and lasts for 4-6 hours; dose related. Patients should receive a prophylactic antiemetic regimen.

Hematologic: Myelosuppression (cumulative, dose related, delayed, and dose limiting), thrombocytopenia (onset: 28 days; recovery: 35-42 days), leukopenia (onset: 35-42 days; recovery: 42-56 days)

Hepatic: Reversible increases in bilirubin, alkaline phosphatase, and AST occur in 20% to 25% of patients

Local: Pain and burning at injection site, phlebitis

Neuromuscular & skeletal: Weakness (wafer 22%)

Ocular: Ocular toxicities (transient conjunctival flushing and blurred vision), retinal hemorrhages

Respiratory: Interstitial fibrosis occurs in up to 50% of patients receiving a cumulative dose >1400 mg/m^2, or bone marrow transplantation doses; may be delayed up to 3 years; rare in patients receiving lower doses. A history of lung disease or concomitant bleomycin therapy may increase the risk of this reaction. Patients with forced vital capacity (FVC) or carbon monoxide diffusing capacity of the lungs (DLCO) <70% of predicted are at higher risk.

Miscellaneous: Disease progression/performance deterioration (wafer 82%)

1% to 10%:

Cardiovascular: Chest pain, deep thrombophlebitis (wafer), facial edema (wafer), peripheral edema (wafer)

Central nervous system: Wafer: Amnesia, anxiety, aphasia, ataxia, brain abscess, confusion, convulsion, CSF leaks, depression, diplopia, dizziness, facial paralysis, headache, hemiplegia, hydrocephalus, hypoesthesia, insomnia, intracranial hypertension, meningitis, somnolence, speech disorder, stupor

Dermatologic: Facial flushing, probably due to the alcohol diluent; alopecia, rash (wafer), wound healing abnormal (wafer)

Gastrointestinal: Abdominal pain, anorexia, constipation, diarrhea, stomatitis

Hematologic: Anemia, hemorrhage (wafer)

Local: Abscess (wafer)

Neuromuscular & skeletal: Back pain

General Dosage Range Dosage adjustment recommended in patients with renal impairment

I.V.: *Adults:* 150-200 mg/m^2 every 6-8 weeks **or** 75-100 mg/m^2/day for 2 days every 6-8 weeks

Implantation: *Adults:* Up to 8 wafers may be placed in the resection cavity (total dose: 62.6 mg)

Mechanism of Action Interferes with the normal function of DNA and RNA by alkylation and cross-linking the strands of DNA and RNA, and by possible protein modification; may also inhibit enzyme processes by carbamylation of amino acids in protein

Pharmacodynamics/Kinetics

Half-life Elimination Biphasic: Initial: 1.4 minutes; Secondary: 20 minutes (active metabolites: plasma half-life of 67 hours)

Pregnancy Risk Factor D

Carteolol (Ophthalmic) (KAR tee oh lole)

Pharmacologic Category Ophthalmic Agent, Antiglaucoma

Use Treatment of chronic open-angle glaucoma and intraocular hypertension

Local Anesthetic/Vasoconstrictor Precautions No information available to require special precautions

Effects on Dental Treatment No significant effects or complications reported

Effects on Bleeding No information available to require special precautions

Adverse Effects

>10%: Ocular: Conjunctival hyperemia

1% to 10%: Ocular: Anisocoria, corneal punctate keratitis, corneal sensitivity decreased, corneal staining, eye pain, vision disturbances

General Dosage Range Ophthalmic: *Adults:* Instill 1 drop in affected eye(s) twice daily

Mechanism of Action Blocks both beta$_1$- and beta$_2$-receptors and has mild intrinsic sympathomimetic activity; reduces intraocular pressure by decreasing aqueous humor production

Pregnancy Risk Factor C

Carvedilol (KAR ve dil ole)

Related Information

Cardiovascular Diseases *on page 1848*

U.S. Brand Names Coreg CR®; Coreg®

Canadian Brand Names Apo-Carvedilol®; Coreg®; Dom-Carvedilol; Mylan-Carvedilol; Novo-Carvedilol; PHL-Carvedilol; PMS-Carvedilol; RAN™-Carvedilol; ratio-Carvedilol; ZYM-Carvedilol

Generic Availability (U.S.) Yes: Tablet

Pharmacologic Category Beta Blocker With Alpha-Blocking Activity

Use Mild-to-severe heart failure of ischemic or cardiomyopathic origin (usually in addition to standard therapy); left ventricular dysfunction following myocardial infarction (MI) (clinically stable with LVEF ≤40%); management of hypertension

Unlabeled/Investigational Use Angina pectoris

Local Anesthetic/Vasoconstrictor Precautions No information available to require special precautions

Effects on Dental Treatment Key adverse event(s) related to dental treatment: Postural hypotension. Periodontitis has been reported in product labeling for carvedilol; no other reports have confirmed this effect; any possible mechanism for this effect is unknown. Many nonsteroidal anti-inflammatory drugs, such as ibuprofen and indomethacin, can reduce the hypotensive effect of beta-blockers after 3 or more weeks of therapy with the NSAID. Short-term NSAID use (ie, 3 days) requires no special precautions in patients taking beta-blockers.

Effects on Bleeding No information available to require special precautions

Adverse Effects Note: Frequency ranges include data from hypertension and heart failure trials. Higher rates of adverse reactions have generally been noted in patients with heart failure. However, the frequency of adverse effects associated with placebo is also increased in this population.

>10%:

- Cardiovascular: Hypotension (9% to 20%)
- Central nervous system: Dizziness (2% to 32%), fatigue (4% to 24%)
- Endocrine & metabolic: Hyperglycemia (5% to 12%)
- Gastrointestinal: Diarrhea (1% to 12%), weight gain (10% to 12%)
- Neuromuscular & skeletal: Weakness (7% to 11%)

1% to 10%:

- Cardiovascular: Bradycardia (2% to 10%), syncope (3% to 8%), peripheral edema (1% to 7%), generalized edema (5% to 6%), angina (1% to 6%), dependent edema (≤4%), AV block, cerebrovascular accident, hypertension, hyper-/hypovolemia, postural hypotension, palpitation
- Central nervous system: Headache (5% to 8%), depression, fever, hypoesthesia, hypotonia, insomnia, malaise, somnolence, vertigo
- Endocrine & metabolic: Hypercholesterolemia (1% to 4%), hypertriglyceridemia (1%), diabetes mellitus, gout, hyperkalemia, hyperuricemia, hypoglycemia, hyponatremia
- Gastrointestinal: Nausea (2% to 9%), vomiting (1% to 6%), abdominal pain, melena, periodontitis, weight loss
- Genitourinary: Impotence
- Hematologic: Anemia, prothrombin decreased, purpura, thrombocytopenia
- Hepatic: Alkaline phosphatase increased (1% to 3%), GGT increased, transaminases increased
- Neuromuscular & skeletal: Back pain (2% to 7%), arthralgia (1% to 6%), arthritis, muscle cramps, paresthesia
- Ocular: Blurred vision (1% to 5%)
- Renal: BUN increased (≤6%), nonprotein nitrogen increased (6%), albuminuria, creatinine increased, glycosuria, hematuria, renal insufficiency
- Respiratory: Cough (5% to 8%), nasopharyngitis (4%), rales (4%), dyspnea (>3%), pulmonary edema (>3%), rhinitis (2%), nasal congestion (1%), sinus congestion (1%)
- Miscellaneous: Injury (3% to 6%), allergy, flu-like syndrome, sudden death

Dosage Oral: Adults: Reduce dosage if heart rate drops to <55 beats/minute.

Hypertension:

Immediate release: 6.25 mg twice daily; if tolerated, dose should be maintained for 1-2 weeks, then increased to 12.5 mg twice daily. If necessary, dosage may be increased to a maximum of 25 mg twice daily after 1-2 weeks.

Extended release: Initial: 20 mg once daily, if tolerated, dose should be maintained for 1-2 weeks then increased to 40 mg once daily if necessary; maximum dose: 80 mg once daily

Heart failure:

Immediate release: 3.125 mg twice daily for 2 weeks; if this dose is tolerated, may increase to 6.25 mg twice daily. Double the dose every 2 weeks to the highest dose tolerated by patient. (Prior to initiating therapy, other heart failure medications should be stabilized and fluid retention minimized.)

Maximum recommended dose:

Mild-to-moderate heart failure:

<85 kg: 25 mg twice daily

>85 kg: 50 mg twice daily

Severe heart failure: 25 mg twice daily

Extended release: Initial: 10 mg once daily for 2 weeks; if the dose is tolerated, increase dose to 20 mg, 40 mg, and 80 mg over successive intervals of at least 2 weeks. Maintain on lower dose if higher dose is not tolerated.

Left ventricular dysfunction following MI: **Note**: Should be initiated only after patient is hemodynamically stable and fluid retention has been minimized.

Immediate release: Initial 3.125-6.25 mg twice daily; increase dosage incrementally (ie, from 6.25-12.5 mg twice daily) at intervals of 3-10 days, based on tolerance, to a target dose of 25 mg twice daily.

Extended release: Initial: 10-20 mg once daily; increase dosage incrementally at intervals of 3-10 days, based on tolerance, to a target dose of 80 mg once daily.

Angina pectoris (unlabeled use): Immediate release: 25-50 mg twice daily

Conversion from immediate release to extended release (Coreg CR®):

Current dose immediate release tablets 3.125 mg twice daily: Convert to extended release capsules 10 mg once daily

Current dose immediate release tablets 6.25 mg twice daily: Convert to extended release capsules 20 mg once daily

Current dose immediate release tablets 12.5 mg twice daily: Convert to extended release capsules 40 mg once daily

Current dose immediate release tablets 25 mg twice daily: Convert to extended release capsules 80 mg once daily

Dosing adjustment in renal impairment: None necessary

Dosing adjustment in hepatic impairment: Use is contraindicated in severe liver dysfunction.

Mechanism of Action As a racemic mixture, carvedilol has nonselective beta-adrenoreceptor and alpha-adrenergic blocking activity. No intrinsic sympathomimetic activity has been documented. Associated effects in hypertensive patients include reduction of cardiac output, exercise- or beta-agonist-induced tachycardia, reduction of reflex orthostatic tachycardia, vasodilation, decreased peripheral vascular resistance (especially in standing position), decreased renal vascular resistance, reduced plasma renin activity, and increased levels of atrial natriuretic peptide. In CHF, associated effects include decreased pulmonary capillary wedge pressure, decreased pulmonary artery pressure, decreased heart rate, decreased systemic vascular resistance, increased stroke volume index, and decreased right arterial pressure (RAP).

Contraindications Serious hypersensitivity to carvedilol or any component of the formulation; decompensated cardiac failure requiring intravenous inotropic therapy; bronchial asthma or related bronchospastic conditions; second- or third-degree AV block, sick sinus syndrome, and severe bradycardia (except in patients with a functioning artificial pacemaker); cardiogenic shock; severe hepatic impairment

Warnings/Precautions Consider pre-existing conditions such as sick sinus syndrome before initiating. Heart failure patients may experience a worsening of renal function (rare); risk factors include ischemic heart disease, diffuse vascular disease, underlying renal dysfunction, and systolic BP <100 mm Hg. Initiate cautiously and monitor for possible deterioration in patient status (eg, symptoms of HF). Worsening heart failure or fluid retention may occur during upward titration; dose reduction or temporary discontinuation may be necessary. Adjustment of other medications (ACE inhibitors and/or diuretics) may also be required.

Symptomatic hypotension with or without syncope may occur with carvedilol (usually within the first 30 days of therapy); close monitoring of patient is required especially with initial dosing and dosing increases; blood pressure must be lowered at a rate appropriate for the patient's clinical condition. Initiation with a low dose, gradual up-titration, and administration with food may help to decrease the occurrence of hypotension or syncope. Patients should be advised to avoid driving or other hazardous tasks during initiation of therapy due to the risk of syncope. Beta-blocker therapy should not be withdrawn abruptly (particularly in patients with CAD), but gradually tapered to avoid acute tachycardia, hypertension, and/or ischemia.

In general, patients with bronchospastic disease should not receive beta-blockers; if used at all, should be used cautiously with close monitoring. May precipitate or aggravate symptoms of arterial insufficiency in patients with PVD and Raynaud's disease; use with caution and monitor for progression of arterial obstruction. Use caution with concurrent use of verapamil or diltiazem; bradycardia or heart block can occur. Use cautiously in patients with diabetes because it can mask prominent hypoglycemic symptoms. In patients with heart failure and diabetes, use of carvedilol may worsen hyperglycemia; may require adjustment of antidiabetic agents. May mask signs of hyperthyroidism (eg, tachycardia); if hyperthyroidism is suspected, carefully manage and monitor; abrupt withdrawal may exacerbate symptoms of hyperthyroidism or precipitate thyroid storm. May induce or exacerbate psoriasis. Use with caution in patients with myasthenia gravis or psychiatric disease (may cause CNS depression). Use with caution in patients with mild-to-moderate hepatic impairment; use is contraindicated in patients with severe impairment. Manufacturer recommends discontinuation of therapy if liver injury occurs (confirmed by laboratory testing). Adequate alpha-blockade is required prior to use of any beta-blocker for patients with untreated pheochromocytoma. Use caution with history of severe anaphylaxis to allergens; patients taking beta-blockers may become more sensitive to repeated challenges. Treatment of anaphylaxis (eg, epinephrine) in patients taking beta-blockers may be ineffective or promote undesirable effects. Use care with anesthetic agents that decrease myocardial function.

Intraoperative floppy iris syndrome has been observed in cataract surgery patients who were on or were previously treated with $alpha_1$-blockers; causality has not been established and there appears to be no benefit in discontinuing alpha-blocker therapy prior to surgery. Instruct patients to inform ophthalmologist of carvedilol use when considering eye surgery.

Drug Interactions

Metabolism/Transport Effects Substrate of CYP1A2 (minor), CYP2C9 (major), CYP2D6 (major), CYP2E1 (minor), CYP3A4 (minor), P-glycoprotein; **Inhibits** P-glycoprotein

Avoid Concomitant Use

Avoid concomitant use of Carvedilol with any of the following: Methacholine; Topotecan

Increased Effect/Toxicity

Carvedilol may increase the levels/effects of: Alpha-/Beta-Agonists (Direct-Acting); Alpha1-Blockers; Alpha2-Agonists; Amifostine; Antihypertensives; Antipsychotic Agents (Phenothiazines); Bupivacaine; Cardiac Glycosides; Colchicine; CycloSPORINE; CycloSPORINE (Systemic); Dabigatran Etexilate; Digoxin; Everolimus; Fingolimod; Hypotensive Agents; Insulin; Lidocaine; Lidocaine (Systemic); Lidocaine (Topical); Mepivacaine; Methacholine; Midodrine; P-Glycoprotein Substrates; RiTUXimab; Rivaroxaban; Sulfonylureas; Topotecan

The levels/effects of Carvedilol may be increased by: Abiraterone; Acetylcholinesterase Inhibitors; Aminoquinolines (Antimalarial); Amiodarone; Anilidopiperidine Opioids; Antipsychotic Agents (Phenothiazines); Calcium Channel Blockers (Nondihydropyridine); Cimetidine; Conivaptan; CYP2C9 Inhibitors (Moderate); CYP2C9 Inhibitors (Strong); CYP2D6 Inhibitors (Moderate); CYP2D6 Inhibitors (Strong); Darunavir; Diazoxide; Dipyridamole; Disopyramide; Dronedarone; Herbs (Hypotensive Properties); MAO Inhibitors; Pentoxifylline; P-Glycoprotein Inhibitors; Phosphodiesterase 5 Inhibitors; Propafenone; Propoxyphene; Prostacyclin Analogues; QuiNIDine; Reserpine; Selective Serotonin Reuptake Inhibitors

Decreased Effect

Carvedilol may decrease the levels/effects of: Beta2-Agonists; Theophylline Derivatives

The levels/effects of Carvedilol may be decreased by: Barbiturates; Herbs (Hypertensive Properties); Methylphenidate; Nonsteroidal Anti-Inflammatory Agents; Peginterferon Alfa-2b; P-Glycoprotein Inducers; Rifamycin Derivatives; Tocilizumab; Yohimbine

Ethanol/Nutrition/Herb Interactions

Food: Food decreases rate but not extent of absorption. Administration with food minimizes risks of orthostatic hypotension.

Herb/Nutraceutical: Avoid herbs with hypertensive properties (bayberry, blue cohosh, cayenne, ephedra, ginger, ginseng [American], kola, licorice); may diminish the antihypertensive effect of carvedilol. Avoid herbs with hypotensive properties (black cohosh, California poppy, coleus, golden seal, hawthorn, mistletoe, periwinkle, quinine, shepherd's purse); may enhance the hypotensive effect of carvedilol.

Dietary Considerations Should be taken with food to minimize the risk of orthostatic hypotension.

Pharmacodynamics/Kinetics

Onset of Action 1-2 hours; Peak antihypertensive effect: ~1-2 hours

Half-life Elimination 7-10 hours

Time to Peak Extended release: 5 hours

Pregnancy Risk Factor C

Lactation Excretion in breast milk unknown/not recommended

Breast-Feeding Considerations It is not known if carvedilol is excreted into human milk. The manufacturer suggests that a decision should be made to either discontinue nursing or discontinue the medication.

Dosage Forms

Capsule, extended release, oral:
Coreg CR®: 10 mg, 20 mg, 40 mg, 80 mg

Tablet, oral: 3.125 mg, 6.25 mg, 12.5 mg, 25 mg
Coreg®: 3.125 mg, 6.25 mg, 12.5 mg, 25 mg

References

Foster CA and Aston SJ, "Propranolol-Epinephrine Interaction: A Potential Disaster," *Plast Reconstr Surg*, 1983, 72(1):74-8.
Wong DG, Spence JD, Lamki L, et al, "Effect of Nonsteroidal Anti-inflammatory Drugs on Control of Hypertension of Beta-Blockers and Diuretics," *Lancet*, 1986, 1(8488):997-1001.
Wynn RL, "Dental Nonsteroidal Anti-inflammatory Drugs and Prostaglandin-Based Drug Interactions, Part Two," *Gen Dent*, 1992, 40(2):104, 106, 108.
Wynn RL, "Epinephrine Interactions With Beta-Blockers," *Gen Dent*, 1994, 42(1):16, 18.

Caspofungin (kas poe FUN jin)

Related Information

Fungal Infections *on page 1945*

U.S. Brand Names Cancidas®

Canadian Brand Names Cancidas®

Pharmacologic Category Antifungal Agent, Parenteral; Echinocandin

Use Treatment of invasive *Aspergillus* infections in patients who are refractory or intolerant of other therapy; treatment of candidemia and other *Candida* infections (intra-abdominal abscesses, esophageal, peritonitis, pleural space); empirical treatment for presumed fungal infections in febrile neutropenic patient

Local Anesthetic/Vasoconstrictor Precautions No information available to require special precautions

Effects on Dental Treatment No significant effects or complications reported

Effects on Bleeding No information available to require special precautions

Adverse Effects

>10%:
- Cardiovascular: Hypotension (3% to 20%), peripheral edema (6% to 11%), tachycardia (4% to 11%)
- Central nervous system: Fever (6% to 30%), chills (9% to 23%), headache (5% to 15%)
- Dermatologic: Rash (4% to 23%)
- Endocrine & metabolic: Hypokalemia (5% to 23%)
- Gastrointestinal: Diarrhea (6% to 27%), vomiting (6% to 17%), nausea (4% to 15%)
- Hematologic: Hemoglobin decreased (18% to 21%), hematocrit decreased (13% to 18%), WBC decreased (12%), anemia (2% to 11%)
- Hepatic: Serum alkaline phosphatase increased (9% to 22%), transaminases increased (2% to 18%), bilirubin increased (5% to 13%)
- Local: Phlebitis/thrombophlebitis (18%)
- Renal: Serum creatinine increased (3% to 11%)
- Respiratory: Respiratory failure (2% to 20%), cough (6% to 11%), pneumonia (4% to 11%)
- Miscellaneous: Infusion reactions (20% to 35%), septic shock (11% to 14%)

5% to 10%:
- Cardiovascular: Hypertension (5% to 6%; children 9% to 10%)
- Dermatologic: Erythema (4% to 9%), pruritus (6% to 7%)
- Endocrine & metabolic: Hypomagnesemia (7%), hyperglycemia (6%)
- Gastrointestinal: Mucosal inflammation (4% to 10%), abdominal pain (4% to 9%)
- Hepatic: Albumin decreased (7%)
- Local: Infection (1% to 9%, central line)
- Renal: Hematuria (10%), blood urea nitrogen increased (4% to 9%)
- Respiratory: Dyspnea (9%), pleural effusion (9%), respiratory distress (≤8%), rales (7%)
- Miscellaneous: Sepsis (5% to 7%)

General Dosage Range Dosage adjustment recommended in patients with hepatic impairment or on concomitant therapy

I.V.:

Children 3 months to 17 years: 70 mg/m^2 on day 1, subsequent dosing: 50-70 mg/m^2 once daily (maximum dose: 70 mg/day)

Adults: Initial: 70 mg on day 1; Subsequent dose: 50-70 mg once daily

Mechanism of Action Inhibits synthesis of β(1,3)-D-glucan, an essential component of the cell wall of susceptible fungi. Highest activity in regions of active cell growth. Mammalian cells do not require β(1,3)-D-glucan, limiting potential toxicity.

Pharmacodynamics/Kinetics

Half-life Elimination Beta (distribution): 9-11 hours; Terminal: 40-50 hours

Pregnancy Risk Factor C

Castor Oil (KAS tor oyl)

Pharmacologic Category Laxative, Miscellaneous

Use Preparation for rectal or bowel examination or surgery; rarely used to relieve constipation; also applied to skin as emollient and protectant

Local Anesthetic/Vasoconstrictor Precautions No information available to require special precautions

Effects on Dental Treatment No significant effects or complications reported

Effects on Bleeding No information available to require special precautions

Adverse Effects Frequency not defined.

Cardiovascular: Hypotension

Central nervous system: Dizziness

Endocrine & metabolic: Electrolyte disturbance

Gastrointestinal: Abdominal cramps, diarrhea, nausea

Genitourinary: Pelvic congestion

General Dosage Range Oral:

Children 2-11 years: 5-15 mL as a single dose

Children ≥12 years and Adults: 15-60 mL as a single dose

Mechanism of Action Acts primarily in the small intestine; hydrolyzed to ricinoleic acid which reduces net absorption of fluid and electrolytes and stimulates peristalsis

Pharmacodynamics/Kinetics

Onset of Action 2-6 hours

Cefaclor (SEF a klor)

Related Information

Bacterial Infections *on page 1933*

U.S. Brand Names Raniclor™

Canadian Brand Names Apo-Cefaclor®; Ceclor®; Novo-Cefaclor; Nu-Cefaclor; PMS-Cefaclor

Generic Availability (U.S.) Yes: Excludes chewable tablet

Pharmacologic Category Antibiotic, Cephalosporin (Second Generation)

Dental Use Alternative antibiotic for treatment of orofacial infections in patients allergic to penicillins; susceptible bacteria including aerobic gram-positive bacteria and anaerobes

Use Treatment of susceptible bacterial infections including otitis media, lower respiratory tract infections, acute exacerbations of chronic bronchitis, pharyngitis and tonsillitis, urinary tract infections, skin and skin structure infections

Local Anesthetic/Vasoconstrictor Precautions No information available to require special precautions

Effects on Dental Treatment No significant effects or complications reported (see Dental Comment)

Effects on Bleeding No information available to require special precautions

Adverse Effects

1% to 10%:

Dermatologic: Rash (maculopapular, erythematous, or morbilliform) (1% to 2%)

Gastrointestinal: Diarrhea (3%)

Genitourinary: Vaginitis (2%)

Hematologic: Eosinophilia (2%)

Hepatic: Transaminases increased (3%)

Miscellaneous: Moniliasis (2%)

Reactions reported with other cephalosporins: Fever, abdominal pain, superinfection, renal dysfunction, toxic nephropathy, hemorrhage, cholestasis

Dental Usual Dosage Orofacial infections: Adults: Oral: Dosing range: 250-500 mg every 8 hours

Dosage

Usual dosage range:

Children >1 month: Oral: 20-40 mg/kg/day divided every 8-12 hours (maximum dose: 1 g/day)

Adults: Oral: 250-500 mg every 8 hours

Indication-specific dosing:

Children: Oral:

Otitis media: 40 mg/kg/day divided every 12 hours

Pharyngitis: 20 mg/kg/day divided every 12 hours

Dosing adjustment in renal impairment:

Cl_{cr} 10-50 mL/minute: Administer 50% to 100% of dose

Cl_{cr} <10 mL/minute: Administer 50% of dose

Hemodialysis: Moderately dialyzable (20% to 50%)

Mechanism of Action Inhibits bacterial cell wall synthesis by binding to one or more of the penicillin-binding proteins (PBPs) which in turn inhibits the final transpeptidation step of peptidoglycan synthesis in bacterial cell walls, thus inhibiting cell wall biosynthesis. Bacteria eventually lyse due to ongoing activity of cell wall autolytic enzymes (autolysins and murein hydrolases) while cell wall assembly is arrested.

Contraindications Hypersensitivity to cefaclor, any component of the formulation, or other cephalosporins

Warnings/Precautions Modify dosage in patients with severe renal impairment. Prolonged use may result in fungal or bacterial superinfection, including *C. difficile*-associated diarrhea (CDAD) and pseudomembranous colitis; CDAD has been observed >2 months postantibiotic treatment. Use with caution in patients with a history of penicillin allergy, especially IgE-mediated reactions (eg, anaphylaxis, urticaria). Beta-lactamase-negative, ampicillin-resistant (BLNAR) strains of *H. influenzae* should be considered resistant to cefaclor. Extended release tablets are not approved for use in children <16 years of age. Some products may contain phenylalanine.

Drug Interactions

Avoid Concomitant Use

Avoid concomitant use of Cefaclor with any of the following: BCG

Increased Effect/Toxicity

The levels/effects of Cefaclor may be increased by: Probenecid

Decreased Effect

Cefaclor may decrease the levels/effects of: BCG; Typhoid Vaccine

Ethanol/Nutrition/Herb Interactions Food: Cefaclor serum levels may be decreased slightly if taken with food. The bioavailability of cefaclor extended release tablets is decreased 23% and the maximum concentration is decreased 67% when taken on an empty stomach.

Dietary Considerations Capsule, chewable tablet, and suspension may be taken with or without food. Some products may contain phenylalanine.

Pharmacodynamics/Kinetics

Half-life Elimination 0.5-1 hour; prolonged with renal impairment

Time to Peak Capsule: 60 minutes; Suspension: 45 minutes

Pregnancy Risk Factor B

Lactation Enters breast milk/use caution

Breast-Feeding Considerations Small amounts of cefaclor are excreted in breast milk. The manufacturer recommends that caution be exercised when administering cefaclor to nursing women. Nondose-related effects could include modification of bowel flora.

Dosage Forms

Capsule, oral: 250 mg, 500 mg

Powder for suspension, oral: 125 mg/5 mL (75 mL, 150 mL); 250 mg/5 mL (75 mL, 150 mL); 375 mg/5 mL (50 mL, 100 mL)

Tablet, chewable, oral:

Raniclor™: 250 mg, 375 mg

Tablet, extended release, oral: 500 mg

Dental Comment Patients allergic to penicillins can use a cephalosporin; the incidence of cross-reactivity between penicillins and cephalosporins is 1% when the allergic reaction to penicillin is delayed. Cefaclor is effective against anaerobic bacteria, but the sensitivity of alpha-hemolytic *Streptococcus* varies; approximately 10% of strains are resistant. Nearly 70% are intermediately sensitive. If the patient has a history of immediate reaction to penicillin, the incidence of cross-reactivity is 20%; cephalosporins are contraindicated in these patients.

Cefadroxil (sef a DROKS il)

Related Information

Bacterial Infections *on page 1933*

Canadian Brand Names Apo-Cefadroxil®; Novo-Cefadroxil; PRO-Cefadroxil

Generic Availability (U.S.) Yes

Pharmacologic Category Antibiotic, Cephalosporin (First Generation)

Dental Use Alternative antibiotic for treatment of orofacial infections in patients allergic to penicillins; susceptible bacteria including aerobic gram-positive bacteria and anaerobes

Use Treatment of susceptible bacterial infections, including those caused by group A beta-hemolytic *Streptococcus*

Local Anesthetic/Vasoconstrictor Precautions No information available to require special precautions

Effects on Dental Treatment No significant effects or complications reported

Effects on Bleeding No information available to require special precautions

Adverse Effects

1% to 10%: Gastrointestinal: Diarrhea

Reactions reported with other cephalosporins: Toxic epidermal necrolysis, abdominal pain, superinfection, renal dysfunction, toxic nephropathy, aplastic anemia, hemolytic anemia, hemorrhage, prothrombin time prolonged, BUN increased, creatinine increased, eosinophilia, pancytopenia, seizure

Dental Usual Dosage Orofacial infections: Oral: Adults: Dosage range: 250-500 mg every 8 hours

Dosage

Usual dosage range: Oral:

Children: 30 mg/kg/day divided twice daily up to a maximum of 2 g/day

Adults: 1-2 g/day in 2 divided doses

Indication-specific dosing: Orofacial infections: Adults: 250-500 mg every 8 hours

Dosing interval in renal impairment:

Cl_{cr} 10-25 mL/minute: Administer every 24 hours

Cl_{cr} <10 mL/minute: Administer every 36 hours

Mechanism of Action Inhibits bacterial cell wall synthesis by binding to one or more of the penicillin-binding proteins (PBPs) which in turn inhibits the final transpeptidation step of peptidoglycan synthesis in bacterial cell walls, thus inhibiting cell wall biosynthesis. Bacteria eventually lyse due to ongoing activity of cell wall autolytic enzymes (autolysins and murein hydrolases) while cell wall assembly is arrested.

Contraindications Hypersensitivity to cefadroxil, any component of the formulation, or other cephalosporins

Warnings/Precautions Modify dosage in patients with severe renal impairment. Use with caution in patients with a history of penicillin allergy, especially IgE-mediated reactions (eg, anaphylaxis, angioedema, urticaria). Prolonged use may result in fungal or bacterial superinfection, including *C. difficile*-associated diarrhea (CDAD) and pseudomembranous colitis; CDAD has been observed >2 months postantibiotic treatment.

Drug Interactions

Avoid Concomitant Use

Avoid concomitant use of Cefadroxil with any of the following: BCG

Increased Effect/Toxicity

The levels/effects of Cefadroxil may be increased by: Probenecid

Decreased Effect

Cefadroxil may decrease the levels/effects of: BCG; Typhoid Vaccine

Ethanol/Nutrition/Herb Interactions Food: Concomitant administration with food, infant formula, or cow's milk does **not** significantly affect absorption.

Pharmacodynamics/Kinetics

Half-life Elimination 1-2 hours; Renal failure: 20-24 hours

Time to Peak Serum: 70-90 minutes

Pregnancy Risk Factor B

Lactation Enters breast milk (small amounts)/use caution (AAP rates "compatible"; AAP 2001 update pending)

Breast-Feeding Considerations Very small amounts of cefadroxil are excreted in breast milk. The manufacturer recommends that caution be exercised when administering cefadroxil to nursing women. Nondose-related effects could include modification of bowel flora.

Dosage Forms

Capsule, oral: 500 mg

Powder for suspension, oral: 250 mg/5 mL (50 mL, 100 mL); 500 mg/5 mL (75 mL, 100 mL)

Tablet, oral: 1 g

References

ADA Division of Legal Affairs, "A Legal Perspective on Antibiotic Prophylaxis," *J Am Dent Assoc*, 2003, 134(9):1260.

"Advisory Statement. Antibiotic Prophylaxis for Dental Patients With Total Joint Replacements. American Dental Association; American Academy of Orthopedic Surgeons," *J Am Dent Assoc*, 1997, 128 (7):1004-8.

American Dental Association Council on Scientific Affairs, "Combating Antibiotic Resistance," *J Am Dent Assoc*, 2004, 135(4):484-7.

Dajani AS, Taubert KA, Wilson W, et al, "Prevention of Bacterial Endocarditis. Recommendations by the American Heart Association," *JAMA*, 1997, 277(22):1794-801.

Dajani AS, Taubert KA, Wilson W, et al, "Prevention of Bacterial Endocarditis: Recommendations by the American Heart Association," *J Am Dent Assoc*, 1997, 128(8):1142-51.

Donowitz GR and Mandell GL, "Drug Therapy. Beta-Lactam Antibiotics (1)," *N Engl J Med*, 1988, 318 (7):419-26.

Donowitz GR and Mandell GL, "Drug Therapy. Beta-Lactam Antibiotics (2)," *N Engl J Med*, 1988, 318 (8):490-500.

Gustaferro CA and Steckelberg JM, "Cephalosporin Antimicrobial Agents and Related Compounds," *Mayo Clin Proc*, 1991, 66(10):1064-73.

Wilson W, Taubert KA, Gewitz M, et al, "Prevention of Infective Endocarditis. Guidelines From the American Heart Association. A Guideline From the American Heart Association Rheumatic Fever, Endocarditis, and Kawasaki Disease Committee, Council on Cardiovascular Disease in the Young, and the Council on Clinical Cardiology, Council on Cardiovascular Surgery and Anesthesia, and the Quality of Care and Outcomes Research Interdisciplinary Working Group," *Circulation*, 2007, 115. Available at http://circ.ahajournals.org/cgi/reprint/CIRCULATIONAHA.106.183095v1; last accessed July 26, 2007.

CeFAZolin (sef A zoe lin)

Related Information

Antibiotic Prophylaxis *on page 1910*

Generic Availability (U.S.) Yes

Pharmacologic Category Antibiotic, Cephalosporin (First Generation)

Dental Use Alternative antibiotic for prevention of infective endocarditis when parenteral administration is needed. Individuals allergic to amoxicillin (penicillins) may receive cefazolin provided they have not had an immediate, local, or systemic IgE-mediated anaphylactic allergic reaction to penicillin. Alternate antibiotic for premedication in patients not allergic to penicillin who may be at potential increased risk of hematogenous total joint infection when parenteral administration is needed.

Use Treatment of respiratory tract, skin, genital, urinary tract, biliary tract, bone and joint infections, and septicemia due to susceptible gram-positive cocci (except *Enterococcus*); some gram-negative bacilli including *E. coli*, *Proteus*, and *Klebsiella* may be susceptible; surgical prophylaxis

Unlabeled/Investigational Use Prophylaxis against infective endocarditis

Local Anesthetic/Vasoconstrictor Precautions No information available to require special precautions

Effects on Dental Treatment No significant effects or complications reported

Effects on Bleeding No information available to require special precautions

Adverse Effects Frequency not defined.

Central nervous system: Fever, seizure

Dermatologic: Rash, pruritus, Stevens-Johnson syndrome

Gastrointestinal: Diarrhea, nausea, vomiting, abdominal cramps, anorexia, pseudomembranous colitis, oral candidiasis

Genitourinary: Vaginitis

Hepatic: Transaminases increased, hepatitis

Hematologic: Eosinophilia, neutropenia, leukopenia, thrombocytopenia, thrombocytosis

Local: Pain at injection site, phlebitis

Renal: BUN increased, serum creatinine increased, renal failure

Miscellaneous: Anaphylaxis

Reactions reported with other cephalosporins: Toxic epidermal necrolysis, abdominal pain, cholestasis, superinfection, toxic nephropathy, aplastic anemia, hemolytic anemia, hemorrhage, prothrombin time prolonged, pancytopenia

Dental Usual Dosage

Infective endocarditis prophylaxis (unlabeled use): I.M., I.V.:

Infants and Children: 50 mg/kg 30-60 minutes before procedure; maximum dose: 1 g

Adults: 1 g 30-60 minutes before procedure.

Note: Intramuscular injections should be avoided in patients who are receiving anticoagulant therapy. In these circumstances, orally administered regimens should be given whenever possible. Intravenously administered antibiotics should be used for patients who are unable to tolerate or absorb oral medications.

Note: American Heart Association (AHA) guidelines now recommend prophylaxis only in patients undergoing invasive procedures and in whom underlying cardiac conditions may predispose to a higher risk of adverse outcomes should infection occur. As of April 2007, routine prophylaxis for GI/GU procedures is no longer recommended by the AHA.

Prophylaxis in total joint replacement patient: I.M., I.V.: Adults: 1 g 1 hour prior to the procedure

Dosage

Usual dosage range: I.M., I.V.:

Children >1 month: 25-100 mg/kg/day divided every 6-8 hours; maximum: 6 g/day

Adults: 250 mg to 1.5 g every 6-12 (usually 8) hours, depending on severity of infection; maximum dose: 12 g/day

Indication-specific dosing:

Infants and Children: I.M., I.V.:

Prophylaxis against infective endocarditis (unlabeled use): 50 mg/kg 30-60 minutes before procedure; maximum dose: 1 g. Intramuscular injections should be avoided in patients who are receiving anticoagulant therapy. In these circumstances, orally administered regimens should be given whenever possible. Intravenously administered antibiotics should be used for patients who are unable to tolerate or absorb oral medications.

Note: American Heart Association (AHA) guidelines now recommend prophylaxis only in patients undergoing invasive procedures and in whom underlying cardiac conditions may predispose to a higher risk of adverse outcomes should infection occur. As of April 2007, routine prophylaxis for GI/GU procedures is no longer recommended by the AHA.

Adults: I.M., I.V.:

Cholecystitis, mild-to-moderate: I.V.: 1-2 g every 8 hours for 4-7 days (provided source controlled)

Endocarditis due to MSSA (without prosthesis) (unlabeled use): I.V.: 2 g every 8 hours; **Note:** Recommended for penicillin-allergic (nonanaphylactoid) patients (Baddour, 2005)

Intra-abdominal infection, complicated, community-acquired, mild-to-moderate (in combination with metronidazole): I.V.: 1-2 g every 8 hours for 4-7 days (provided source controlled)

Prophylaxis against infective endocarditis (unlabeled use): 1 g 30-60 minutes before procedure. Intramuscular injections should be avoided in patients who are receiving anticoagulant therapy. In these circumstances, orally administered regimens should be given whenever possible. Intravenously administered antibiotics should be used for patients who are unable to tolerate or absorb oral medications.

Note: American Heart Association (AHA) guidelines now recommend prophylaxis only in patients undergoing invasive procedures and in whom underlying cardiac conditions may predispose to a higher risk of adverse outcomes should infection occur. As of April 2007, routine prophylaxis for GI/GU procedures is no longer recommended by the AHA.

Moderate-to-severe infections: 500 mg to 1 g every 6-8 hours

Mild infection with gram-positive cocci: 250-500 mg every 8 hours

Perioperative prophylaxis: 1-2 g within 60 minutes prior to surgery (may repeat in 2-5 hours intraoperatively); followed by 500 mg to 1 g every 6-8 hours for 24 hours postoperatively

Cardiothoracic surgery: 1 g within 60 minutes prior to incision, followed by 1 g at sternotomy and 1 g after cardiopulmonary bypass; may continue 1 g every 6 hours for 24-48 hours postoperatively (Eagle, 2004)

Cholecystectomy: 1-2 g every 8 hours, discontinue within 24 hours unless infection outside gallbladder suspected

Total joint replacement: 1 g 1 hour prior to the procedure

Pneumococcal pneumonia: 500 mg every 12 hours

Severe infection: 1-1.5 g every 6 hours

UTI (uncomplicated): 1 g every 12 hours

Dosing adjustment in renal impairment:

Cl_{cr} 35-54 mL/minute: Administer full dose in intervals of ≥8 hours

Cl_{cr} 11-34 mL/minute: Administer 1/2 usual dose every 12 hours

Cl_{cr} ≤10 mL/minute: Administer 1/2 usual dose every 18-24 hours

Hemodialysis: Moderately dialyzable (20% to 50%); administer dose postdialysis or administer supplemental dose of 0.5-1 g after dialysis

Continuous ambulatory peritoneal dialysis (CAPD): Administer 0.5 g every 12 hours

Continuous renal replacement therapy (CRRT): Drug clearance is highly dependent on the method of renal replacement, filter type, and flow rate. Appropriate dosing requires close monitoring of pharmacologic response, signs of adverse reactions due to drug accumulation, as well as drug levels in relation to target trough (if appropriate). The following are general recommendations only (based on dialysate flow/ultrafiltration rates of 1 L/hour) and should not supersede clinical judgment:
CVVH: 1-2 g every 12 hours
CVVHD/CVVHDF: 2 g every 12 hours

Mechanism of Action Inhibits bacterial cell wall synthesis by binding to one or more of the penicillin-binding proteins (PBPs) which in turn inhibits the final transpeptidation step of peptidoglycan synthesis in bacterial cell walls, thus inhibiting cell wall biosynthesis. Bacteria eventually lyse due to ongoing activity of cell wall autolytic enzymes (autolysins and murein hydrolases) while cell wall assembly is arrested.

Contraindications Hypersensitivity to cefazolin sodium, any component of the formulation, or other cephalosporins

Warnings/Precautions Modify dosage in patients with severe renal impairment. Use with caution in patients with a history of penicillin allergy, especially IgE-mediated reactions (eg, anaphylaxis, angioedema, urticaria). Prolonged use may result in fungal or bacterial superinfection, including *C. difficile*-associated diarrhea (CDAD) and pseudomembranous colitis; CDAD has been observed >2 months postantibiotic treatment. May be associated with increased INR, especially in nutritionally-deficient patients, prolonged treatment, hepatic or renal disease. Use with caution in patients with a history of seizure disorder; high levels, particularly in the presence of renal impairment, may increase risk of seizures.

Drug Interactions

Avoid Concomitant Use

Avoid concomitant use of CeFAZolin with any of the following: BCG

Increased Effect/Toxicity

CeFAZolin may increase the levels/effects of: Fosphenytoin; Phenytoin; Vitamin K Antagonists

The levels/effects of CeFAZolin may be increased by: Probenecid

Decreased Effect

CeFAZolin may decrease the levels/effects of: BCG; Typhoid Vaccine

Dietary Considerations Some products may contain sodium.

Pharmacodynamics/Kinetics

Half-life Elimination 90-150 minutes; prolonged with renal impairment

Time to Peak Serum: I.M.: 0.5-2 hours

Pregnancy Risk Factor B

Lactation Enters breast milk (small amounts)/use caution (AAP rates "compatible"; AAP 2001 update pending)

Breast-Feeding Considerations Small amounts of cefazolin are excreted in breast milk. The manufacturer recommends that caution be exercised when administering cefazolin to nursing women. Nondose-related effects could include modification of bowel flora.

Dosage Forms

Infusion, premixed iso-osmotic dextrose solution: 1 g (50 mL)

Injection, powder for reconstitution: 500 mg, 1 g, 10 g, 20 g, 100 g, 300 g

References

ADA Division of Legal Affairs, "A Legal Perspective on Antibiotic Prophylaxis," *J Am Dent Assoc*, 2003, 134(9):1260.

"Advisory Statement. Antibiotic Prophylaxis for Dental Patients With Total Joint Replacements. American Dental Association; American Academy of Orthopedic Surgeons," *J Am Dent Assoc*, 1997, 128 (7):1004-8.

American Dental Association; American Academy of Orthopedic Surgeons, "Antibiotic Prophylaxis for Dental Patients With Total Joint Replacements," *J Am Dent Assoc*, 2003, 134(7):895-9.

American Dental Association Council on Scientific Affairs, "Combating Antibiotic Resistance," *J Am Dent Assoc*, 2004, 135(4):484-7.

Dajani AS, Taubert KA, Wilson W, et al, "Prevention of Bacterial Endocarditis. Recommendations by the American Heart Association," *JAMA*, 1997, 277(22):1794-801.

Dajani AS, Taubert KA, Wilson W, et al, "Prevention of Bacterial Endocarditis: Recommendations by the American Heart Association," *J Am Dent Assoc*, 1997, 128(8):1142-51.

Donowitz GR and Mandell GL, "Drug Therapy. Beta-Lactam Antibiotics (1)," *N Engl J Med*, 1988, 318 (7):419-26.

Donowitz GR and Mandell GL, "Drug Therapy. Beta-Lactam Antibiotics (2)," *N Engl J Med*, 1988, 318 (8):490-500.

Gustaferro CA and Steckelberg JM, "Cephalosporin Antimicrobial Agents and Related Compounds," *Mayo Clin Proc*, 1991, 66(10):1064-73.

Wilson W, Taubert KA, Gewitz M, et al, "Prevention of Infective Endocarditis. Guidelines From the American Heart Association. A Guideline From the American Heart Association Rheumatic Fever, Endocarditis, and Kawasaki Disease Committee, Council on Cardiovascular Disease in the Young, and the Council on Clinical Cardiology, Council on Cardiovascular Surgery and Anesthesia, and the Quality of Care and Outcomes Research Interdisciplinary Working Group," *Circulation*, 2007, 115. Available at http://circ.ahajournals.org/cgi/reprint/CIRCULATIONAHA.106.183095v1; last accessed July 26, 2007.

Cefdinir (SEF di ner)

U.S. Brand Names Omnicef®
Canadian Brand Names Omnicef®
Pharmacologic Category Antibiotic, Cephalosporin (Third Generation)
Use Treatment of community-acquired pneumonia, acute exacerbations of chronic bronchitis, acute bacterial otitis media, acute maxillary sinusitis, pharyngitis/tonsillitis, and uncomplicated skin and skin structure infections.
Local Anesthetic/Vasoconstrictor Precautions No information available to require special precautions
Effects on Dental Treatment No significant effects or complications reported
Effects on Bleeding No information available to require special precautions
Adverse Effects
>10%: Gastrointestinal: Diarrhea (8% to 15%)
1% to 10%:
Central nervous system: Headache (2%)
Dermatologic: Rash (≤3%)
Endocrine & metabolic: Bicarbonate decreased (≤1%), hyperglycemia (≤1%), hyperphosphatemia (≤1%)
Gastrointestinal: Nausea (≤3%), abdominal pain (≤1%), vomiting (≤1%)
Genitourinary: Vaginal moniliasis (≤4%), urine leukocytes increased (≤2%), urine pH increased (≤1%), urine specific gravity increased (≤1%), vaginitis (≤1%)
Hematologic: Lymphocytes increased (≤2%), eosinophils increased (1%), lymphocytes decreased (1%), platelets increased (≤1%), PMN changes (≤1%), WBC decreased/increased (≤1%)
Hepatic: Alkaline phosphatase increased (≤1%), ALT increased (≤1%)
Renal: Proteinuria (1% to 2%), microhematuria (≤1%), glycosuria (≤1%)
Miscellaneous: GGT increased (≤1%), lactate dehydrogenase increased (≤1%)
Additional reactions reported with other cephalosporins: Agranulocytosis, angioedema, aplastic anemia, asterixis, encephalopathy, hemorrhage, interstitial nephritis, neuromuscular excitability, PT prolonged, seizure, superinfection, and toxic nephropathy
General Dosage Range Dosage adjustment recommended in patients with renal impairment
Oral:
Children 6 months to 12 years: 14 mg/kg/day in 1-2 divided doses (maximum: 600 mg/day)
Children >12 years and Adults: 600 mg/day in 1-2 divided doses
Mechanism of Action Inhibits bacterial cell wall synthesis by binding to one or more of the penicillin-binding proteins (PBPs) which in turn inhibits the final transpeptidation step of peptidoglycan synthesis in bacterial cell walls, thus inhibiting cell wall biosynthesis. Bacteria eventually lyse due to ongoing activity of cell wall autolytic enzymes (autolysins and murein hydrolases) while cell wall assembly is arrested.
Pharmacodynamics/Kinetics
Half-life Elimination ~100 minutes
Time to Peak 3 hours
Pregnancy Risk Factor B

Cefditoren (sef de TOR en)

Related Information
Bacterial Infections *on page* 1933
U.S. Brand Names Spectracef®
Generic Availability (U.S.) Yes
Pharmacologic Category Antibiotic, Cephalosporin (Third Generation)
Dental Use Bactericidal antibiotic for infections due to susceptible organisms
Use Treatment of acute bacterial exacerbation of chronic bronchitis or community-acquired pneumonia (due to susceptible organisms including *Haemophilus influenzae*, *Haemophilus parainfluenzae*, *Streptococcus pneumoniae*-penicillin susceptible only, *Moraxella catarrhalis*); pharyngitis or tonsillitis (*Streptococcus pyogenes*); and uncomplicated skin and skin-structure infections (*Staphylococcus aureus* - not MRSA, *Streptococcus pyogenes*)
Local Anesthetic/Vasoconstrictor Precautions No information available to require special precautions
Effects on Dental Treatment No significant effects or complications reported
Effects on Bleeding No information available to require special precautions

Adverse Effects

>10%: Gastrointestinal: Diarrhea (11% to 15%)

1% to 10%:

Central nervous system: Headache (2% to 3%)

Endocrine & metabolic: Glucose increased (1% to 2%)

Gastrointestinal: Nausea (4% to 6%), abdominal pain (2%), dyspepsia (1% to 2%), vomiting (1%)

Genitourinary: Vaginal moniliasis (3% to 6%)

Hematologic: Hematocrit decreased (2%)

Renal: Hematuria (3%), urinary white blood cells increased (2%)

Reactions reported with other cephalosporins: Anaphylaxis, aplastic anemia, cholestasis, hemorrhage, hemolytic anemia, renal dysfunction, reversible hyperactivity, serum sickness-like reaction, toxic nephropathy

Dental Usual Dosage Dental infections (unlabeled use): Children ≥12 years and Adults: Oral: 400 mg twice daily for 10 days

Dosage

Usual dosage range:

Children ≥12 years and Adults: Oral: 200-400 mg twice daily

Indication-specific dosing:

Children ≥12 years and Adults: Oral:

Acute bacterial exacerbation of chronic bronchitis: 400 mg twice daily for 10 days

Dental infections (unlabeled use): 400 mg twice daily for 10 days

Community-acquired pneumonia: 400 mg twice daily for 14 days

Pharyngitis, tonsillitis, uncomplicated skin and skin structure infections: 200 mg twice daily for 10 days

Dosage adjustment in renal impairment:

Cl_{cr} 30-49 mL/minute/1.73 m^2: Maximum dose: 200 mg twice daily

Cl_{cr} <30 mL/minute/1.73 m^2: Maximum dose: 200 mg once daily

End-stage renal disease: Appropriate dosing not established

Dosage adjustment in hepatic impairment:

Mild-to-moderate impairment: Adjustment not required

Severe impairment (Child-Pugh Class C): Specific guidelines not available

Mechanism of Action Inhibits bacterial cell wall synthesis by binding to one or more of the penicillin-binding proteins (PBPs) which in turn inhibits the final transpeptidation step of peptidoglycan synthesis in bacterial cell walls, thus inhibiting cell wall biosynthesis. Bacteria eventually lyse due to ongoing activity of cell wall autolytic enzymes (autolysins and murein hydrolases) while cell wall assembly is arrested.

Contraindications Hypersensitivity to cefditoren, any component of the formulation, other cephalosporins, or milk protein; carnitine deficiency

Warnings/Precautions Use with caution in patients with a history of penicillin allergy, especially IgE-mediated reactions (eg, anaphylaxis, urticaria). Prolonged use may result in fungal or bacterial superinfection, including *C. difficile*-associated diarrhea (CDAD) and pseudomembranous colitis; CDAD has been observed >2 months postantibiotic treatment. Caution in individuals with seizure disorders; high levels, particularly in the presence of renal impairment, may increase risk of seizures. Use caution in patients with renal or hepatic impairment; modify dosage in patients with severe renal impairment. Cefditoren causes renal excretion of carnitine; do not use in patients with carnitine deficiency; not for long-term therapy due to the possible development of carnitine deficiency over time. May prolong prothrombin time; use with caution in patients with a history of bleeding disorder. Cefditoren tablets contain sodium caseinate, which may cause hypersensitivity reactions in patients with milk protein hypersensitivity; this does not affect patients with lactose intolerance.

Drug Interactions

Avoid Concomitant Use There are no known interactions where it is recommended to avoid concomitant use.

Increased Effect/Toxicity

The levels/effects of Cefditoren may be increased by: Probenecid

Decreased Effect

The levels/effects of Cefditoren may be decreased by: Antacids; H2-Antagonists; Proton Pump Inhibitors

Ethanol/Nutrition/Herb Interactions Food: Moderate- to high-fat meals increase bioavailability and maximum plasma concentration.

Dietary Considerations Cefditoren should be taken with meals. Plasma carnitine levels are decreased during therapy (39% with 200 mg dosing, 63% with 400 mg dosing); normal concentrations return within 7-10 days after treatment is discontinued.

Pharmacodynamics/Kinetics

Half-life Elimination 1.6 ± 0.4 hours

Time to Peak 1.5-3 hours

Pregnancy Risk Factor B

Lactation Excretion in breast milk unknown/use caution

Breast-Feeding Considerations It is not known whether cefditoren is excreted in human milk. The manufacturer recommends caution when using cefditoren during breast-feeding. Other cephalosporins are considered safe during breast-feeding. If cefditoren reaches the breast milk, the limited oral absorption may minimize the effect on the nursing infant. Nondose-related effects could include modification of bowel flora.

Dosage Forms

Tablet, oral: 200 mg, 400 mg

Spectracef®: 200 mg, 400 mg

Cefepime (SEF e pim)

U.S. Brand Names Maxipime®

Canadian Brand Names Maxipime®

Pharmacologic Category Antibiotic, Cephalosporin (Fourth Generation)

Use Treatment of uncomplicated and complicated urinary tract infections, including pyelonephritis caused by *Escherichia coli, Klebsiella pneumoniae*, or *Proteus mirabilis*; monotherapy for febrile neutropenia; uncomplicated skin and skin structure infections caused by *Streptococcus pyogenes* or methicillin-susceptible staphylococci; moderate-to-severe pneumonia caused by *Streptococcus pneumoniae, Pseudomonas aeruginosa, Klebsiella pneumoniae*, or *Enterobacter* species; complicated intra-abdominal infections (in combination with metronidazole) caused by *E. coli, P. aeruginosa, K. pneumoniae, Enterobacter* species, or *Bacteroides fragilis* against methicillin-susceptible staphylococci, *Enterobacter* sp, and many other gram-negative bacilli.

Children 2 months to 16 years: Empiric therapy of febrile neutropenia patients, uncomplicated skin/soft tissue infections, pneumonia, and uncomplicated/complicated urinary tract infections, including pyelonephritis.

Unlabeled/Investigational Use Brain abscess (postneurosurgical prevention); malignant otitis externa; septic lateral/cavernous sinus thrombosis

Local Anesthetic/Vasoconstrictor Precautions No information available to require special precautions

Effects on Dental Treatment No significant effects or complications reported

Effects on Bleeding No information available to require special precautions

Adverse Effects

>10%: Hematologic: Positive Coombs' test without hemolysis (16%)

1% to 10%:

Central nervous system: Fever (1%), headache (1%)

Dermatologic: Rash (1% to 4%), pruritus (1%)

Endocrine & metabolic: Hypophosphatemia (3%)

Gastrointestinal: Diarrhea (≤3%), nausea (≤2%), vomiting (≤1%)

Hematologic: Eosinophils (2%)

Hepatic: ALT increased (3%), AST increased (2%), PTT abnormal (2%), PT abnormal (1%)

Local: Inflammation, phlebitis, and pain (1%)

Reactions reported with other cephalosporins: Aplastic anemia, erythema multiforme, hemolytic anemia, hemorrhage, pancytopenia, PT prolonged, renal dysfunction, Stevens-Johnson syndrome, superinfection, toxic epidermal necrolysis, toxic nephropathy, vaginitis

General Dosage Range Dosage adjustment recommended in patients with renal impairment

I.M.:

Children ≥2 months: 50 mg/kg/dose every 12 hours

Adults: 500-1000 mg every 12 hours

I.V.:

Children ≥2 months: 50 mg/kg/dose every 8-12 hours

Adults: 1-2 g every 8-12 hours

Mechanism of Action Inhibits bacterial cell wall synthesis by binding to one or more of the penicillin-binding proteins (PBPs) which in turn inhibits the final transpeptidation step of peptidoglycan synthesis in bacterial cell walls, thus inhibiting cell wall biosynthesis. Bacteria eventually lyse due to ongoing activity of cell wall autolytic enzymes (autolysis and murein hydrolases) while cell wall assembly is arrested.

Pharmacodynamics/Kinetics
Half-life Elimination 2 hours
Time to Peak I.M.: 1-2 hours; I.V.: 0.5 hours
Pregnancy Risk Factor B

Cefixime (sef IKS eem)

Related Information
Sexually-Transmitted Diseases *on page 1903*
U.S. Brand Names Suprax®
Canadian Brand Names Suprax®
Pharmacologic Category Antibiotic, Cephalosporin (Third Generation)
Use Treatment of urinary tract infections, otitis media, respiratory infections due to susceptible organisms including *S. pneumoniae* and *S. pyogenes*, *H. influenzae*, and many Enterobacteriaceae; uncomplicated cervical/urethral gonorrhea due to *N. gonorrhoeae*
Local Anesthetic/Vasoconstrictor Precautions No information available to require special precautions
Effects on Dental Treatment No significant effects or complications reported
Effects on Bleeding No information available to require special precautions
Adverse Effects
>10%: Gastrointestinal: Diarrhea (16%)
2% to 10%: Gastrointestinal: Abdominal pain, nausea, dyspepsia, flatulence, loose stools
Reactions reported with other cephalosporins: Interstitial nephritis, aplastic anemia, hemolytic anemia, hemorrhage, pancytopenia, agranulocytosis, colitis, superinfection
General Dosage Range Dosage adjustment recommended in patients with renal impairment
Oral:
Children ≥6 months to 12 years and ≤50 kg: 8-20 mg/kg/day divided every 12-24 hours (maximum: 400 mg/day)
Children >12 years or >50 kg and Adults: 400 mg/day divided every 12-24 hours **or** 20-30 mg/kg/day in 2 divided doses
Mechanism of Action Inhibits bacterial cell wall synthesis by binding to one or more of the penicillin-binding proteins (PBPs); which in turn inhibits the final transpeptidation step of peptidoglycan synthesis in bacterial cell walls, thus inhibiting cell wall biosynthesis. Bacteria eventually lyse due to ongoing activity of cell wall autolytic enzymes (autolysins and murein hydrolases) while cell wall assembly is arrested.
Pharmacodynamics/Kinetics
Half-life Elimination Normal renal function: 3-4 hours; Renal failure: Up to 11.5 hours
Time to Peak Serum: 2-6 hours; delayed with food
Pregnancy Risk Factor B

Cefotaxime (sef oh TAKS eem)

Related Information
Sexually-Transmitted Diseases *on page 1903*
U.S. Brand Names Claforan®
Canadian Brand Names Claforan®
Pharmacologic Category Antibiotic, Cephalosporin (Third Generation)
Use Treatment of susceptible infection in respiratory tract, skin and skin structure, bone and joint, urinary tract, gynecologic as well as septicemia, and documented or suspected meningitis. Active against most gram-negative bacilli (not *Pseudomonas*) and gram-positive cocci (not enterococcus). Active against many penicillin-resistant pneumococci.
Local Anesthetic/Vasoconstrictor Precautions No information available to require special precautions
Effects on Dental Treatment No significant effects or complications reported
Effects on Bleeding No information available to require special precautions
Adverse Effects
1% to 10%:
Dermatologic: Rash, pruritus
Gastrointestinal: Diarrhea, nausea, vomiting, colitis
Local: Pain at injection site

Reactions reported with other cephalosporins: Agranulocytosis, aplastic anemia, cholestasis, hemolytic anemia, hemorrhage, nephropathy, pancytopenia, renal dysfunction, seizure, superinfection.

General Dosage Range Dosage adjustment recommended in patients with hepatic or renal impairment

I.M.:

Children 1 month to 12 years and <50 kg: 50-200 mg/kg/day in divided doses every 6-8 hours (maximum: 12 g/day)

Children >12 years and ≥50 kg and Adults: 1-2 g every 8-12 hours **or** as a single dose

I.V.:

Children 1 month to 12 years and <50 kg: 50-200 mg/kg/day in divided doses every 6-8 hours (maximum: 12 g/day)

Children >12 years and ≥50 kg and Adults: 1-2 g every 4-12 hours

Mechanism of Action Inhibits bacterial cell wall synthesis by binding to one or more of the penicillin-binding proteins (PBPs) which in turn inhibits the final transpeptidation step of peptidoglycan synthesis in bacterial cell walls, thus inhibiting cell wall biosynthesis. Bacteria eventually lyse due to ongoing activity of cell wall autolytic enzymes (autolysins and murein hydrolases) while cell wall assembly is arrested.

Pharmacodynamics/Kinetics

Half-life Elimination

Cefotaxime: Premature neonates <1 week: 5-6 hours; Full-term neonates <1 week: 2-3.4 hours; Adults: 1-1.5 hours, prolonged with renal and/or hepatic impairment

Desacetylcefotaxime: 1.5-1.9 hours; prolonged with renal impairment

Time to Peak Serum: I.M.: Within 30 minutes

Pregnancy Risk Factor B

CefoTEtan (SEF oh tee tan)

Generic Availability (U.S.) Yes

Pharmacologic Category Antibiotic, Cephalosporin (Second Generation)

Use Surgical prophylaxis; intra-abdominal infections and other mixed infections; respiratory tract, skin and skin structure, bone and joint, urinary tract and gynecologic as well as septicemia; active against gram-negative enteric bacilli including *E. coli*, *Klebsiella*, and *Proteus*; less active against staphylococci and streptococci than first generation cephalosporins, but active against anaerobes including *Bacteroides fragilis*

Local Anesthetic/Vasoconstrictor Precautions No information available to require special precautions

Effects on Dental Treatment No significant effects or complications reported

Effects on Bleeding Although cefotetan contains the methyltetrazolethiol side chain, bleeding has not been a significant problem.

Adverse Effects

1% to 10%:

Gastrointestinal: Diarrhea (1%)

Hepatic: Transaminases increased (1%)

Miscellaneous: Hypersensitivity reactions (1%)

Reactions reported with other cephalosporins: Seizure, Stevens-Johnson syndrome, toxic epidermal necrolysis, renal dysfunction, toxic nephropathy, cholestasis, aplastic anemia, hemolytic anemia, hemorrhage, pancytopenia, agranulocytosis, colitis, superinfection

Dosage

Usual dosage range:

Children (unlabeled use): I.M., I.V.: 20-40 mg/kg/dose every 12 hours (maximum: 6 g/day)

Adults: I.M., I.V.: 1-6 g/day in divided doses every 12 hours

Indication-specific dosing:

Children (unlabeled use):

Preoperative prophylaxis: I.M., I.V.: 40 mg/kg 30-60 minutes prior to surgery

Adolescents and Adults:

Pelvic inflammatory disease: I.V.: 2 g every 12 hours; used in combination with doxycycline

Adults:

Orbital cellulitis, odontogenic infections: I.V.: 2 g every 12 hours

Preoperative prophylaxis: I.M., I.V.: 1-2 g 30-60 minutes prior to surgery; when used for cesarean section, dose should be given as soon as umbilical cord is clamped

Susceptible infections: I.M., I.V.: 1-6 g/day in divided doses every 12 hours; usual dose: 1-2 g every 12 hours for 5-10 days; 1-2 g may be given every 24 hours for urinary tract infection; **Note:** Due to high rates of *B. fragilis* group resistance, not recommended for the treatment of community-acquired intra-abdominal infections (Solomkin, 2010)

Urinary tract infection: I.M., I.V.: 1-2 g may be given every 24 hours

Dosing interval in renal impairment:

Cl_{cr} 10-30 mL/minute: Administer every 24 hours

Cl_{cr} <10 mL/minute: Administer every 48 hours

Hemodialysis: Dialyzable (5% to 20%); administer 1/4 the usual dose every 24 hours on days between dialysis; administer 1/2 the usual dose on the day of dialysis.

Continuous arteriovenous or venovenous hemodiafiltration effects: Administer 750 mg every 12 hours

Mechanism of Action Inhibits bacterial cell wall synthesis by binding to one or more of the penicillin-binding proteins (PBPs) which in turn inhibits the final transpeptidation step of peptidoglycan synthesis in bacterial cell walls, thus inhibiting cell wall biosynthesis. Bacteria eventually lyse due to ongoing activity of cell wall autolytic enzymes (autolysins and murein hydrolases) while cell wall assembly is arrested.

Contraindications Hypersensitivity to cefotetan, any component of the formulation, or other cephalosporins; previous cephalosporin-associated hemolytic anemia

Warnings/Precautions Modify dosage in patients with severe renal impairment. Although cefotetan contains the methyltetrazolethiol side chain, bleeding has not been a significant problem. Use with caution in patients with a history of penicillin allergy, especially IgE-mediated reactions (eg, anaphylaxis, urticaria). Cefotetan has been associated with a higher risk of hemolytic anemia relative to other cephalosporins (approximately threefold); monitor carefully during use and consider cephalosporin-associated immune anemia in patients who have received cefotetan within 2-3 weeks (either as treatment or prophylaxis). Prolonged use may result in fungal or bacterial superinfection, including *C. difficile*-associated diarrhea (CDAD) and pseudomembranous colitis; CDAD has been observed >2 months postantibiotic treatment. May be associated with increased INR, especially in nutritionally-deficient patients, prolonged treatment, hepatic or renal disease.

Drug Interactions

Avoid Concomitant Use

Avoid concomitant use of CefoTEtan with any of the following: BCG

Increased Effect/Toxicity

CefoTEtan may increase the levels/effects of: Alcohol (Ethyl); Vitamin K Antagonists

The levels/effects of CefoTEtan may be increased by: Probenecid

Decreased Effect

CefoTEtan may decrease the levels/effects of: BCG; Typhoid Vaccine

Ethanol/Nutrition/Herb Interactions Ethanol: Avoid ethanol (may cause a disulfiram-like reaction).

Dietary Considerations Some products may contain sodium.

Pharmacodynamics/Kinetics

Half-life Elimination 3-5 hours

Time to Peak Serum: I.M.: 1.5-3 hours

Pregnancy Risk Factor B

Lactation Enters breast milk (small amounts)/use caution

Breast-Feeding Considerations Very small amounts of cefotetan are excreted in human milk. The manufacturer recommends caution when giving cefotetan to a breast-feeding mother. Nondose-related effects could include modification of bowel flora.

Dosage Forms

Injection, powder for reconstitution: 1 g, 2 g, 10 g

CefOXitin (se FOKS i tin)

Related Information

Sexually-Transmitted Diseases *on page 1903*

U.S. Brand Names Mefoxin®

Canadian Brand Names Apo-Cefoxitin®

Generic Availability (U.S.) Yes: Excludes infusion

Pharmacologic Category Antibiotic, Cephalosporin (Second Generation)

Use Less active against staphylococci and streptococci than first generation cephalosporins, but active against anaerobes including *Bacteroides fragilis*; active against gram-negative enteric bacilli including *E. coli*, *Klebsiella*, and *Proteus*; used predominantly for respiratory tract, skin, bone and joint, urinary tract and gynecologic as well as septicemia; surgical prophylaxis; intra-abdominal infections and other mixed infections; indicated for bacterial *Eikenella corrodens* infections

Local Anesthetic/Vasoconstrictor Precautions No information available to require special precautions

Effects on Dental Treatment No significant effects or complications reported

Effects on Bleeding No information available to require special precautions

Adverse Effects

1% to 10%: Gastrointestinal: Diarrhea

Reactions reported with other cephalosporins: Agranulocytosis, aplastic anemia, cholestasis, colitis, erythema multiforme, hemolytic anemia, hemorrhage, pancytopenia, renal dysfunction, serum-sickness reactions, seizure, Stevens-Johnson syndrome, superinfection, toxic nephropathy, vaginitis

Dosage

Usual dosage range:

Infants >3 months and Children: I.M., I.V.: 80-160 mg/kg/day in divided doses every 4-6 hours (maximum dose: 12 g/day)

Adults: I.M., I.V.: 1-2 g every 6-8 hours (maximum dose: 12 g/day)

Note: I.M. injection is painful

Indication-specific dosing:

Infants >3 months and Children:

Mild-to-moderate infection: I.M., I.V.: 80-100 mg/kg/day in divided doses every 4-6 hours

Perioperative prophylaxis: I.V.: 30-40 mg/kg 30-60 minutes prior to surgery followed by 30-40 mg/kg/dose every 6 hours for no more than 24 hours after surgery depending on the procedure

Severe infection: I.M., I.V.: 100-160 mg/kg/day in divided doses every 4-6 hours

Adolescents and Adults:

Perioperative prophylaxis: I.M., I.V.: 1-2 g 30-60 minutes prior to surgery (may repeat in 2-5 hours intraoperatively) followed by 1-2 g every 6-8 hours for no more than 24 hours after surgery depending on the procedure

Adults:

Amnionitis, endomyometritis: I.M., I.V.: 2 g every 6-8 hours

Aspiration pneumonia, empyema, orbital cellulitis, parapharyngeal space, human bites: I.M., I.V.: 2 g every 8 hours

Intra-abdominal infection, complicated, community acquired, mild-to-moderate: I.V.: 2 g every 6 hours for 4-7 days (provided source controlled)

Liver abscess: I.V.: 1 g every 4 hours

Mycobacterium species, not MTB or MAI: I.V.: 12 g/day with amikacin

Pelvic inflammatory disease:

Inpatients: I.V.: 2 g every 6 hours **plus** doxycycline 100 mg I.V. or 100 mg orally every 12 hours until improved, followed by doxycycline 100 mg orally twice daily to complete 14 days

Outpatients: I.M.: 2 g **plus** probenecid 1 g orally as a single dose, followed by doxycycline 100 mg orally twice daily for 14 days

Dosing interval in renal impairment:

Cl_{cr} 30-50 mL/minute: Administer 1-2 g every 8-12 hours

Cl_{cr} 10-29 mL/minute: Administer 1-2 g every 12-24 hours

Cl_{cr} 5-9 mL/minute: Administer 0.5-1 g every 12-24 hours

Cl_{cr} <5 mL/minute: Administer 0.5-1 g every 24-48 hours

Hemodialysis: Moderately dialyzable (20% to 50%); administer a loading dose of 1-2 g after each hemodialysis; maintenance dose as noted above based on Cl_{cr}

Continuous arteriovenous or venovenous hemodiafiltration effects: Dose as for Cl_{cr} 10-50 mL/minute

Mechanism of Action Inhibits bacterial cell wall synthesis by binding to one or more of the penicillin-binding proteins (PBPs) which in turn inhibits the final transpeptidation step of peptidoglycan synthesis in bacterial cell walls, thus inhibiting cell wall biosynthesis. Bacteria eventually lyse due to ongoing activity of cell wall autolytic enzymes (autolysins and murein hydrolases) while cell wall assembly is arrested.

Contraindications Hypersensitivity to cefoxitin, any component of the formulation, or other cephalosporins

Warnings/Precautions Modify dosage in patients with severe renal impairment. Prolonged use may result in superinfection. Use with caution in patients with a history of penicillin allergy, especially IgE-mediated reactions (eg, anaphylaxis, urticaria). Prolonged use may result in fungal or bacterial superinfection, including *C. difficile*-associated diarrhea (CDAD) and pseudomembranous colitis; CDAD has been observed >2 months postantibiotic treatment.

Drug Interactions

Avoid Concomitant Use

Avoid concomitant use of CefOXitin with any of the following: BCG

Increased Effect/Toxicity

CefOXitin may increase the levels/effects of: Vitamin K Antagonists

The levels/effects of CefOXitin may be increased by: Probenecid

Decreased Effect

CefOXitin may decrease the levels/effects of: BCG; Typhoid Vaccine

Dietary Considerations Some products may contain sodium.

Pharmacodynamics/Kinetics

Half-life Elimination 45-60 minutes; significantly prolonged with renal impairment

Time to Peak Serum: I.M.: 20-30 minutes

Pregnancy Risk Factor B

Lactation Enters breast milk/use caution (AAP rates "compatible"; AAP 2001 update pending)

Breast-Feeding Considerations Very small amounts of cefoxitin are excreted in breast milk. The manufacturer recommends that caution be exercised when administering cefoxitin to nursing women. Nondose-related effects could include modification of bowel flora. Cefoxitin pharmacokinetics may be altered immediately postpartum.

Dosage Forms

Infusion, premixed iso-osmotic dextrose solution:

Mefoxin®: 1 g (50 mL); 2 g (50 mL)

Injection, powder for reconstitution: 1 g, 2 g, 10 g

Cefpodoxime (sef pode OKS eem)

Pharmacologic Category Antibiotic, Cephalosporin (Third Generation)

Use Treatment of susceptible acute, community-acquired pneumonia caused by *S. pneumoniae* or nonbeta-lactamase producing *H. influenzae*; acute uncomplicated gonorrhea caused by *N. gonorrhoeae*; uncomplicated skin and skin structure infections caused by *S. aureus* or *S. pyogenes*; acute otitis media caused by *S. pneumoniae*, *H. influenzae*, or *M. catarrhalis*; pharyngitis or tonsillitis; and uncomplicated urinary tract infections caused by *E. coli*, *Klebsiella*, and *Proteus*

Local Anesthetic/Vasoconstrictor Precautions No information available to require special precautions

Effects on Dental Treatment No significant effects or complications reported

Effects on Bleeding No information available to require special precautions

Adverse Effects

>10%:

Dermatologic: Diaper rash (12%)

Gastrointestinal: Diarrhea in infants and toddlers (15%)

1% to 10%:

Central nervous system: Headache (1%)

Dermatologic: Rash (1%)

Gastrointestinal: Diarrhea (7%), nausea (4%), abdominal pain (2%), vomiting (1% to 2%)

Genitourinary: Vaginal infection (3%)

Reactions reported with other cephalosporins: Seizure, Stevens-Johnson syndrome, toxic epidermal necrolysis, erythema multiforme, urticaria, serum-sickness reactions, renal dysfunction, interstitial nephritis toxic nephropathy, cholestasis, aplastic anemia, hemolytic anemia, hemorrhage, pancytopenia, agranulocytosis, colitis, vaginitis, superinfection

General Dosage Range Dosage adjustment recommended in patients with renal impairment

Oral:

Children 2 months to 12 years: 10 mg/kg/day divided every 12 hours (maximum: 400 mg/day)

Children ≥12 years and Adults: 100-400 mg every 12 hours **or** 200 mg as a single dose

Mechanism of Action Inhibits bacterial cell wall synthesis by binding to one or more of the penicillin-binding proteins (PBPs) which in turn inhibits the final transpeptidation step of peptidoglycan synthesis in bacterial cell walls, thus inhibiting cell wall biosynthesis. Bacteria eventually lyse due to ongoing activity of cell wall autolytic enzymes (autolysins and murein hydrolases) while cell wall assembly is arrested.

Pharmacodynamics/Kinetics

Half-life Elimination 2.2 hours; prolonged with renal impairment

Time to Peak Within 1 hour

Pregnancy Risk Factor B

Cefprozil (sef PROE zil)

Canadian Brand Names Apo-Cefprozil®; Cefzil®; Mint-Cefprozil; RAN™-Cefprozil; Sandoz-Cefprozil

Generic Availability (U.S.) Yes

Pharmacologic Category Antibiotic, Cephalosporin (Second Generation)

Use Treatment of otitis media and infections involving the respiratory tract and skin and skin structure; active against methicillin-sensitive staphylococci, many streptococci, and various gram-negative bacilli including *E. coli*, some *Klebsiella*, *P. mirabilis*, *H. influenzae*, and *Moraxella*.

Local Anesthetic/Vasoconstrictor Precautions No information available to require special precautions

Effects on Dental Treatment No significant effects or complications reported

Effects on Bleeding No information available to require special precautions

Adverse Effects

1% to 10%:

Central nervous system: Dizziness (1%)

Dermatologic: Diaper rash (2%)

Gastrointestinal: Diarrhea (3%), nausea (4%), vomiting (1%), abdominal pain (1%)

Genitourinary: Vaginitis, genital pruritus (2%)

Hepatic: Transaminases increased (2%)

Miscellaneous: Superinfection

Reactions reported with other cephalosporins: Seizure, toxic epidermal necrolysis, renal dysfunction, interstitial nephritis, toxic nephropathy, aplastic anemia, hemolytic anemia, hemorrhage, pancytopenia, agranulocytosis, colitis, vaginitis, superinfection

Dosage

Usual dosage range:

Infants and Children >6 months to 12 years: Oral: 7.5-15 mg/kg/day divided every 12 hours

Children >12 years and Adults: Oral: 250-500 mg every 12 hours or 500 mg every 24 hours

Indication-specific dosing:

Infants and Children >6 months to 12 years: Oral:

Otitis media: 15 mg/kg every 12 hours for 10 days

Children 2-12 years: Oral:

Pharyngitis/tonsillitis: 7.5-15 mg/kg/day divided every 12 hours for 10 days (administer for >10 days if due to *S. pyogenes*); maximum: 1 g/day

Uncomplicated skin and skin structure infections: 20 mg/kg every 24 hours for 10 days; maximum: 1 g/day

Children >12 years and Adults: Oral:

Pharyngitis/tonsillitis: 500 mg every 24 hours for 10 days

Secondary bacterial infection of acute bronchitis or acute bacterial exacerbation of chronic bronchitis: 500 mg every 12 hours for 10 days

Uncomplicated skin and skin structure infections: 250 mg every 12 hours or 500 mg every 12-24 hours for 10 days

Dosing adjustment in renal impairment: Cl_{cr} <30 mL/minute: Reduce dose by 50%

Hemodialysis: Reduced by hemodialysis; administer dose after the completion of hemodialysis

Mechanism of Action Inhibits bacterial cell wall synthesis by binding to one or more of the penicillin-binding proteins (PBPs) which in turn inhibits the final transpeptidation step of peptidoglycan synthesis in bacterial cell walls, thus inhibiting cell wall biosynthesis. Bacteria eventually lyse due to ongoing activity of cell wall autolytic enzymes (autolysins and murein hydrolases) while cell wall assembly is arrested.

Contraindications Hypersensitivity to cefprozil, any component of the formulation, or other cephalosporins

Warnings/Precautions Modify dosage in patients with severe renal impairment. Use with caution in patients with a history of penicillin allergy, especially IgE-mediated reactions (eg, anaphylaxis, urticaria). Prolonged use may result in fungal or bacterial superinfection, including *C. difficile*-associated diarrhea (CDAD) and pseudomembranous colitis; CDAD has been observed >2 months postantibiotic treatment. Some products may contain phenylalanine.

Drug Interactions

Avoid Concomitant Use

Avoid concomitant use of Cefprozil with any of the following: BCG

Increased Effect/Toxicity

The levels/effects of Cefprozil may be increased by: Probenecid

Decreased Effect

Cefprozil may decrease the levels/effects of: BCG; Typhoid Vaccine

Ethanol/Nutrition/Herb Interactions Food: Food delays cefprozil absorption.

Dietary Considerations May be taken with food. Oral suspension may contain phenylalanine; consult product labeling.

Pharmacodynamics/Kinetics

Half-life Elimination Normal renal function: 1.3 hours

Time to Peak Serum: Fasting: 1.5 hours

Pregnancy Risk Factor B

Lactation Enters breast milk/use caution (AAP rates "compatible"; AAP 2001 update pending)

Breast-Feeding Considerations Small amounts of cefprozil are excreted in breast milk. The manufacturer recommends that caution be exercised when administering cefprozil to nursing women. Nondose-related effects could include modification of bowel flora.

Dosage Forms

Powder for suspension, oral: 125 mg/5 mL (50 mL, 75 mL, 100 mL); 250 mg/5 mL (50 mL, 75 mL, 100 mL)

Tablet, oral: 250 mg, 500 mg

Ceftaroline Fosamil (sef TAR oh leen FOS a mil)

U.S. Brand Names Teflaro™

Pharmacologic Category Antibiotic, Cephalosporin (Fifth Generation)

Use Treatment of acute bacterial skin and skin structure infections (ABSSSI) caused by susceptible isolates of *Staphylococcus aureus* (including methicillin-susceptible and –resistant isolates), *Streptococcus pyogenes, Streptococcus agalactiae, Escherichia coli, Klebsiella pneumoniae*, and *Klebsiella oxytoca,* and community-acquired pneumonia (CAP) caused by *Streptococcus pneumoniae* (including cases with concurrent bacteremia), *Staphylococcus aureus* (methicillin-susceptible isolates only), *Haemophilus influenzae, Klebsiella pneumoniae, Klebsiella oxytoca,* and *Escherichia coli*

Local Anesthetic/Vasoconstrictor Precautions No information available to require special precautions

Effects on Dental Treatment No significant effects or complications reported

Effects on Bleeding No information available to require special precautions

Adverse Effects

>10%: Hematologic: Positive Coombs' test without hemolysis (~11%)

2% to 10%:

Central nervous system: Headache (3% to 5%), insomnia (3% to 4%)

Dermatologic: Pruritus (3% to 4%), rash (3%)

Endocrine & metabolic: Hypokalemia (2%)

Gastrointestinal: Diarrhea (5%), nausea (4%), constipation (2%), vomiting (2%)

Hepatic: Transaminases increased (2%)

Local: Phlebitis (2%)

General Dosage Range Dosage adjustment recommended in patients with renal impairment.

I.V.: *Adults:* 600 mg every 12 hours

Mechanism of Action Inhibits bacterial cell wall synthesis by binding to penicillin-binding proteins (PBPs) 1 through 3. This action blocks the final transpeptidation step of peptidoglycan synthesis in bacterial cell walls and inhibits cell wall biosynthesis.Bacteria eventually lyse due to ongoing activity of cell wall autolytic enzymes (autolysis and murein hydrolases) while cell wall assembly is arrested. Ceftaroline has a strong affinity for PBP2a, a modified PBP in MRSA, and PBP2x in *S. pneumoniae*, contributing to its spectrum of activity against these bacteria.

Pharmacodynamics/Kinetics

Half-life Elimination Normal renal function: 2.4 hours; Moderate renal impairment (Cl_{cr} 30-50 ml/minute): 4.5 hours

Time to Peak 1 hour

Pregnancy Risk Factor B

CefTAZidime (SEF tay zi deem)

U.S. Brand Names Fortaz®; Tazicef®

Canadian Brand Names Fortaz®

Pharmacologic Category Antibiotic, Cephalosporin (Third Generation)

Use Treatment of documented susceptible *Pseudomonas aeruginosa* infection and infections due to other susceptible aerobic gram-negative organisms; empiric therapy of a febrile, granulocytopenic patient

Unlabeled/Investigational Use Bacterial endophthalmitis
Local Anesthetic/Vasoconstrictor Precautions No information available to require special precautions
Effects on Dental Treatment No significant effects or complications reported
Effects on Bleeding No information available to require special precautions
Adverse Effects
1% to 10%:
Gastrointestinal: Diarrhea (1%)
Local: Pain at injection site (1%)
Miscellaneous: Hypersensitivity reactions (2%)
Reactions reported with other cephalosporins: Seizure, urticaria, serum-sickness reactions, renal dysfunction, interstitial nephritis, toxic nephropathy, BUN increased, creatinine increased, cholestasis, aplastic anemia, hemolytic anemia, pancytopenia, agranulocytosis, colitis, prolonged PT, hemorrhage, superinfection
General Dosage Range Dosage adjustment recommended in patients with renal impairment
I.M.: *Adults:* 500 mg to 2 g every 8-12 hours
I.V.:
Children 1 month to 12 years: 30-50 mg/kg every 8 hours (maximum: 6 g/day)
Children ≥12 years and Adults: 500 mg to 2 g every 8-12 hours (maximum: 6 g/day)
Mechanism of Action Inhibits bacterial cell wall synthesis by binding to one or more of the penicillin-binding proteins (PBPs) which in turn inhibits the final transpeptidation step of peptidoglycan synthesis in bacterial cell walls, thus inhibiting cell wall biosynthesis. Bacteria eventually lyse due to ongoing activity of cell wall autolytic enzymes (autolysins and murein hydrolases) while cell wall assembly is arrested.
Pharmacodynamics/Kinetics
Half-life Elimination 1-2 hours, prolonged with renal impairment; Neonates <23 days: 2.2-4.7 hours
Time to Peak Serum: I.M.: ~1 hour
Pregnancy Risk Factor B

Ceftibuten (sef TYE byoo ten)

Related Information
Bacterial Infections *on page 1933*
U.S. Brand Names Cedax®
Generic Availability (U.S.) No
Pharmacologic Category Antibiotic, Cephalosporin (Third Generation)
Use Treatment of acute exacerbations of chronic bronchitis, acute bacterial otitis media, and pharyngitis/tonsillitis
Local Anesthetic/Vasoconstrictor Precautions No information available to require special precautions
Effects on Dental Treatment No significant effects or complications reported
Effects on Bleeding No information available to require special precautions
Adverse Effects
1% to 10%:
Central nervous system: Headache (≤3%), dizziness (≤1%)
Gastrointestinal: Nausea (≤4%), diarrhea (3% to 4%), dyspepsia (≤2%), loose stools (≤2%), abdominal pain (1% to 2%), vomiting (1% to 2%)
Hematologic: Eosinophils increased (3%), hemoglobin decreased (1% to 2%), platelets increased (≤1%)
Hepatic: ALT increased (≤1%), bilirubin increased (≤1%)
Renal: BUN increased (2% to 4%)
Additional reactions reported with other cephalosporins: Allergic reaction, agranulocytosis, angioedema, aplastic anemia, anaphylaxis, asterixis, cholestasis, drug fever, encephalopathy, erythema multiforme, hemolytic anemia, hemorrhage, interstitial nephritis, neuromuscular excitability, neutropenia, pancytopenia, prolonged PT, renal dysfunction, seizure, superinfection, toxic nephropathy
Dosage
Usual dosage range:
Children 6 months to <12 years: Oral: 9 mg/kg/day for 10 days (maximum dose: 400 mg/day)
Children ≥12 years and Adults: Oral: 400 mg once daily for 10 days
Dosage adjustment in renal impairment:
Cl_{cr} ≥50 mL//minute: No adjustment needed
Cl_{cr} 30-49 mL//minute: Administer 4.5 mg/kg or 200 mg every 24 hours
Cl_{cr} 5-29 mL/minute: Administer 2.25 mg/kg or 100 mg every 24 hours.

Hemodialysis: Administer 400 mg or 9 mg/kg (maximum: 400 mg) after each hemodialysis session

Mechanism of Action Inhibits bacterial cell wall synthesis by binding to one or more of the penicillin-binding proteins (PBPs) which in turn inhibits the final transpeptidation step of peptidoglycan synthesis in bacterial cell walls, thus inhibiting cell wall biosynthesis. Bacteria eventually lyse due to ongoing activity of cell wall autolytic enzymes (autolysins and murein hydrolases) while cell wall assembly is arrested.

Contraindications Hypersensitivity to ceftibuten, any component of the formulation, or other cephalosporins

Warnings/Precautions Modify dosage in patients with moderate-to-severe renal impairment. Prolonged use may result in fungal or bacterial superinfection, including *C. difficile*-associated diarrhea (CDAD) and pseudomembranous colitis; CDAD has been observed >2 months postantibiotic treatment. Use with caution in patients with a history of colitis and other gastrointestinal diseases. Use with caution in patients with a history of penicillin allergy, especially IgE-mediated reactions (eg, anaphylaxis, urticaria). Oral suspension formulation contains sucrose.

Drug Interactions

Avoid Concomitant Use

Avoid concomitant use of Ceftibuten with any of the following: BCG

Increased Effect/Toxicity

The levels/effects of Ceftibuten may be increased by: Probenecid

Decreased Effect

Ceftibuten may decrease the levels/effects of: BCG; Typhoid Vaccine

Dietary Considerations

Capsule: Take without regard to food.

Suspension: Take 2 hours before or 1 hour after meals.

Pharmacodynamics/Kinetics

Half-life Elimination 2 hours; Cl_{cr} 30-49 mL/minute: 7 hours; Cl_{cr} 5-29 mL/minute: 13 hours; Cl_{cr} <5 mL/minute: 22 hours

Time to Peak 2-3 hours

Pregnancy Risk Factor B

Lactation Excretion in breast milk unknown/use caution

Breast-Feeding Considerations Ceftibuten was not detectable in milk after a single 200 mg dose (limit of detection: 1 mcg/mL). It is not known if it would be detectable after a 400 mg dose or multiple doses. The manufacturer recommends that caution be exercised when administering ceftibuten to nursing women. If ceftibuten does reach the human milk, nondose-related effects could include modification of bowel flora.

Dosage Forms

Capsule, oral:

Cedax®: 400 mg

Powder for suspension, oral:

Cedax®: 90 mg/5 mL (60 mL, 90 mL, 120 mL); 180 mg/5 mL (30 mL, 60 mL)

CefTRIAXone (sef trye AKS one)

Related Information

Antibiotic Prophylaxis *on page 1910*

Sexually-Transmitted Diseases *on page 1903*

U.S. Brand Names Rocephin®

Canadian Brand Names Ceftriaxone for Injection; Ceftriaxone Sodium for Injection BP; Rocephin®

Pharmacologic Category Antibiotic, Cephalosporin (Third Generation)

Use Treatment of lower respiratory tract infections, acute bacterial otitis media, skin and skin structure infections, bone and joint infections, intra-abdominal and urinary tract infections, pelvic inflammatory disease (PID), uncomplicated gonorrhea, bacterial septicemia, and meningitis; used in surgical prophylaxis

Unlabeled/Investigational Use Treatment of chancroid, epididymitis, complicated gonococcal infections; sexually-transmitted diseases (STD); periorbital or buccal cellulitis; salmonellosis or shigellosis; atypical community-acquired pneumonia; epiglottitis, Lyme disease; used in chemoprophylaxis for high-risk contacts and persons with invasive meningococcal disease; sexual assault; typhoid fever, Whipple's disease

Local Anesthetic/Vasoconstrictor Precautions No information available to require special precautions

Effects on Dental Treatment No significant effects or complications reported

Effects on Bleeding No information available to require special precautions

Adverse Effects

>10%: Local: Induration (I.M. 5% to 17%), warmth (I.M.), tightness (I.M.)

1% to 10%:

Dermatologic: Rash (2%)

Gastrointestinal: Diarrhea (3%)

Hematologic: Eosinophilia (6%), thrombocytosis (5%), leukopenia (2%)

Hepatic: Transaminases increased (3%)

Local: Tenderness at injection site (I.V. 1%), pain

Renal: BUN increased (1%)

Reactions reported with other cephalosporins: Angioedema, allergic reaction, aplastic anemia, asterixis, cholestasis, encephalopathy, hemorrhage, hepatic dysfunction, hyperactivity (reversible), hypertonia, interstitial nephritis, LDH increased, neuromuscular excitability, pancytopenia, paresthesia, renal dysfunction, superinfection, toxic nephropathy

General Dosage Range Dosage adjustment recommended in patients with hepatic and renal impairment

I.M.:

Children: 50-100 mg/kg/day divided every 12-24 hours (maximum: 4 g/day) **or** 125 mg or 50 mg/kg as a single dose

Adults: 1-2 g every 12-24 hours **or** 125-250 mg as a single dose

I.V.:

Children: 50-100 mg/kg/day divided every 12-24 hours (maximum: 4 g/day)

Adults: 1-2 g every 12-24 hours

Mechanism of Action Inhibits bacterial cell wall synthesis by binding to one or more of the penicillin-binding proteins (PBPs) which in turn inhibits the final transpeptidation step of peptidoglycan synthesis in bacterial cell walls, thus inhibiting cell wall biosynthesis. Bacteria eventually lyse due to ongoing activity of cell wall autolytic enzymes (autolysins and murein hydrolases) while cell wall assembly is arrested.

Pharmacodynamics/Kinetics

Half-life Elimination Normal renal and hepatic function: 5-9 hours; Renal impairment (mild-to-severe): 12-16 hours

Time to Peak Serum: I.M.: 2-3 hours

Pregnancy Risk Factor B

Cefuroxime (se fyoor OKS eem)

Related Information

Bacterial Infections *on page 1933*

U.S. Brand Names Ceftin®; Zinacef®

Canadian Brand Names Apo-Cefuroxime®; Ceftin®; Cefuroxime For Injection; PRO-Cefuroxime; ratio-Cefuroxime

Generic Availability (U.S.) Yes

Pharmacologic Category Antibiotic, Cephalosporin (Second Generation)

Use Treatment of infections caused by staphylococci, group B streptococci, *H. influenzae* (type A and B), *E. coli*, *Enterobacter*, *Salmonella*, and *Klebsiella*; treatment of susceptible infections of the upper and lower respiratory tract, otitis media, urinary tract, uncomplicated skin and soft tissue, bone and joint, sepsis, uncomplicated gonorrhea, and early Lyme disease; surgical prophylaxis

Local Anesthetic/Vasoconstrictor Precautions No information available to require special precautions

Effects on Dental Treatment No significant effects or complications reported

Effects on Bleeding No information available to require special precautions

Adverse Effects

>10%: Gastrointestinal: Diarrhea (4% to 11%, duration-dependent)

1% to 10%:

Dermatologic: Diaper rash (3%)

Endocrine & metabolic: Alkaline phosphatase increased (2%), lactate dehydrogenase increased (1%)

Gastrointestinal: Nausea/vomiting (3% to 7%)

Genitourinary: Vaginitis (≤5%)

Hematologic: Eosinophilia (7%), hemoglobin and hematocrit decreased (10%)

Hepatic: Transaminases increased (2% to 4%)

Local: Thrombophlebitis (2%)

Reactions reported with other cephalosporins: Agranulocytosis, aplastic anemia, asterixis, encephalopathy, hemorrhage, neuromuscular excitability, serum-sickness reactions, superinfection, toxic nephropathy

Dosage Note: Cefuroxime axetil film-coated tablets and oral suspension are not bioequivalent and are not substitutable on a mg/mg basis

Usual dosage range:

Children 3 months to 12 years:

Oral: 20-30 mg/kg/day in 2 divided doses

I.M., I.V.: 75-150 mg/kg/day divided every 8 hours (maximum dose: 6 g/day)

Children ≥13 years and Adults:

Oral: 250-500 mg twice daily

I.M., I.V.: 750 mg to 1.5 g every 6-8 hours or 100-150 mg/kg/day in divided doses every 6-8 hours (maximum: 6 g/day)

Indication-specific dosing:

Children ≥3 months to 12 years:

Acute bacterial maxillary sinusitis, acute otitis media, and impetigo:

Oral: Suspension: 30 mg/kg/day in 2 divided doses for 10 days (maximum dose: 1 g/day); tablet: 250 mg twice daily for 10 days

I.M., I.V.: 75-150 mg/kg/day divided every 8 hours (maximum dose: 6 g/day)

Epiglottitis: Oral: 150 mg/kg/day in 3 divided doses for 7-10 days

Pharyngitis/tonsillitis:

Oral: Suspension: 20 mg/kg/day (maximum: 500 mg/day) in 2 divided doses for 10 days; tablet: 125 mg every 12 hours for 10 days

I.M., I.V.: 75-150 mg/kg day divided every 8 hours (maximum: 6 g/day)

Children ≥13 years and Adults (all oral doses listed are for tablet formulation):

Bronchitis (acute and exacerbations of chronic bronchitis):

Oral: 250-500 mg every 12 hours for 10 days

I.V.: 500-750 mg every 8 hours (complete therapy with oral dosing)

Cellulitis, orbital: I.V.: 1.5 g every 8 hours

Gonorrhea:

Disseminated: I.M., I.V.: 750 mg every 8 hours

Uncomplicated:

Oral: 1 g as a single dose

I.M.: 1.5 g as single dose (administer in 2 different sites with probenecid)

Lyme disease (early): Oral: 500 mg twice daily for 20 days

Pharyngitis/tonsillitis and sinusitis: Oral: 250 mg twice daily for 10 days

Pneumonia (uncomplicated): I.V.: 750 mg every 8 hours

Severe or complicated infections: I.M., I.V.: 1.5 g every 8 hours (up to 1.5 g every 6 hours in life-threatening infections)

Skin/skin structure infection (uncomplicated):

Oral: 250-500 mg every 12 hours for 10 days

I.M., I.V.: 750 mg every 8 hours

Surgical prophylaxis: I.V.: 1.5 g 30 minutes to 1 hour prior to procedure (if procedure is prolonged can give 750 mg every 8 hours I.M.)

Open heart: I.V.: 1.5 g every 12 hours to a total of 6 g

Urinary tract infection (uncomplicated):

Oral: 125-250 mg every 12 hours for 7-10 days

I.M., I.V.: 750 mg every 8 hours

Adults:

Cholecystitis, mild-to-moderate: I.V.: 1.5 g every 8 hours for 4-7 days (provided source controlled)

Intra-abdominal infection, complicated, community-acquired, mild-to-moderate (in combination with metronidazole): I.V.: 1.5 g every 8 hours for 4-7 days (provided source controlled)

Surgical prophylaxis:

Cholecystectomy: I.V.: 1.5 g every 8 hours, discontinue within 24 hours unless infection outside gallbladder suspected

Dosing adjustment in renal impairment:

Cl_{cr} 10-20 mL/minute: Administer every 12 hours

Cl_{cr} <10 mL/minute: Administer every 24 hours

Hemodialysis: Dialyzable (25%)

Peritoneal dialysis: Dose every 24 hours

Continuous renal replacement therapy (CRRT): 1 g every 12 hours

Mechanism of Action Inhibits bacterial cell wall synthesis by binding to one or more of the penicillin-binding proteins (PBPs) which in turn inhibits the final transpeptidation step of peptidoglycan synthesis in bacterial cell walls, thus inhibiting cell wall biosynthesis. Bacteria eventually lyse due to ongoing activity of cell wall autolytic enzymes (autolysins and murein hydrolases) while cell wall assembly is arrested.

Contraindications Hypersensitivity to cefuroxime, any component of the formulation, or other cephalosporins

Warnings/Precautions Modify dosage in patients with severe renal impairment. Use with caution in patients with a history of penicillin allergy, especially IgE-mediated reactions (eg, anaphylaxis, urticaria). Prolonged use may result in fungal or bacterial superinfection, including *C. difficile*-associated diarrhea (CDAD) and pseudomembranous colitis; CDAD has been observed >2 months postantibiotic treatment. May be associated with increased INR, especially in nutritionally-deficient patients, prolonged treatment, hepatic or renal disease. Tablets and oral suspension are not bioequivalent (do not substitute on a mg-per-mg basis). Some products may contain phenylalanine.

Drug Interactions

Avoid Concomitant Use

Avoid concomitant use of Cefuroxime with any of the following: BCG

Increased Effect/Toxicity

The levels/effects of Cefuroxime may be increased by: Probenecid

Decreased Effect

Cefuroxime may decrease the levels/effects of: BCG; Typhoid Vaccine

The levels/effects of Cefuroxime may be decreased by: Antacids; H2-Antagonists

Ethanol/Nutrition/Herb Interactions Food: Bioavailability is increased with food; cefuroxime serum levels may be increased if taken with food or dairy products.

Dietary Considerations Some products may contain phenylalanine and/or sodium.

Oral suspension: May be taken with food.

Pharmacodynamics/Kinetics

Half-life Elimination Children 1-2 hours; Adults: 1-2 hours; prolonged with renal impairment

Time to Peak Serum: I.M.: ~15-60 minutes; I.V.: 2-3 minutes; Oral: Children: 3-4 hours; Adults: 2-3 hours

Pregnancy Risk Factor B

Lactation Enters breast milk/use caution

Breast-Feeding Considerations Cefuroxime is excreted in breast milk. Manufacturer recommendations vary; caution is recommended if cefuroxime I.V. is given to a nursing woman and it is recommended to consider discontinuing nursing temporarily during treatment following oral cefuroxime. Nondose-related effects could include modification of bowel flora.

Dosage Forms

Infusion, premixed iso-osmotic solution:

Zinacef®: 750 mg (50 mL); 1.5 g (50 mL)

Injection, powder for reconstitution: 750 mg, 1.5 g, 7.5 g, 75 g

Zinacef®: 750 mg, 1.5 g, 7.5 g

Powder for suspension, oral: 125 mg/5 mL (100 mL); 250 mg/5 mL (50 mL, 100 mL)

Ceftin®: 125 mg/5 mL (100 mL); 250 mg/5 mL (50 mL, 100 mL)

Tablet, oral: 250 mg, 500 mg

Ceftin®: 250 mg, 500 mg

Celecoxib (se le KOKS ib)

Related Information

Oral Pain *on page 1928*

Rheumatoid Arthritis, Osteoarthritis, and Osteoporosis *on page 1889*

U.S. Brand Names CeleBREX®

Canadian Brand Names Celebrex®

Generic Availability (U.S.) No

Pharmacologic Category Nonsteroidal Anti-inflammatory Drug (NSAID), COX-2 Selective

Dental Use Management of acute dental pain

Use Relief of the signs and symptoms of osteoarthritis, ankylosing spondylitis, juvenile idiopathic arthritis (JIA), and rheumatoid arthritis; management of acute pain; treatment of primary dysmenorrhea

Local Anesthetic/Vasoconstrictor Precautions No information available to require special precautions

Effects on Dental Treatment Key adverse event(s) related to dental treatment: Stomatitis, abnormal taste, xerostomia (normal salivary flow resumes upon discontinuation), and tooth disorder.

Effects on Bleeding Nonselective NSAIDs are known to reversibly decrease platelet aggregation via mechanisms different than observed with aspirin. Celecoxib selectively inhibits only the COX-2 enzyme, and does not inhibit COX-1, which is involved in platelet aggregation. According to the manufacturer, celecoxib, at single doses up to 800 mg and multiple doses of 600 mg twice daily, had no effect on platelet aggregation or bleeding time. Comparative NSAIDs (naproxen 500 mg twice daily, ibuprofen 800 mg 3 times daily, or diclofenac 75 mg twice daily) significantly reduced platelet aggregation and prolonged the bleeding times. See Dental Comment.

Adverse Effects

≥2%

Cardiovascular: Peripheral edema

Central nervous system: Dizziness, fever, headache, insomnia

Dermatologic: Rash

Gastrointestinal: Abdominal pain, diarrhea, dyspepsia, flatulence, nausea, vomiting

Neuromuscular & skeletal: Arthralgia, back pain

Respiratory: Cough, nasopharyngitis, pharyngitis, rhinitis, sinusitis, upper respiratory tract infection

0.1% to 1.9%:

Cardiovascular: Angina, aortic valve incompetence, chest pain, coronary artery disorder, edema, facial edema, hypertension (aggravated), MI, palpitation, sinus bradycardia, tachycardia, ventricular hypertrophy

Central nervous system: Anxiety, depression, fatigue, hypoesthesia, migraine, nervousness, pain, somnolence, vertigo

Dermatologic: Alopecia, bruising, cellulitis, dermatitis, dry skin, photosensitivity, pruritus, rash (erythematous), rash (maculopapular), urticaria

Endocrine & metabolic: Hot flashes, hypercholesterolemia, hyperglycemia, hypokalemia, ovarian cyst, testosterone decreased

Gastrointestinal: Anorexia, appetite increased, constipation, diverticulitis, dysphagia, eructation, esophagitis, gastritis, gastroenteritis, gastroesophageal reflux, gastrointestinal ulcer, hemorrhoids, hiatal hernia, melena, stomatitis, tenesmus, weight gain, xerostomia

Genitourinary: Cystitis, dysuria, urinary frequency

Hematologic: Anemia, thrombocythemia

Hepatic: Alkaline phosphatase increased, transaminases increased

Neuromuscular & skeletal: Arthrosis, CPK increased, hypertonia, leg cramps, myalgia, paresthesia, synovitis, tendonitis

Ocular: Conjunctival hemorrhage, vitreous floaters

Otic: Deafness, labyrinthitis, tinnitus

Renal: Albuminuria, BUN increased, creatinine increased, hematuria, nonprotein nitrogen increased, renal calculi

Respiratory: Bronchitis, bronchospasm, dyspnea, epistaxis, laryngitis, pneumonia

Miscellaneous: Allergic reactions, allergy aggravated, cyst, diaphoresis, flu-like syndrome

Dental Usual Dosage Acute dental pain: Adults: Oral: 400 mg, followed by an additional 200 mg if needed on day 1; maintenance dose: 200 mg twice daily as needed

Dosage Note: Use the lowest effective dose for the shortest duration of time, consistent with individual patient treatment goals. Oral:

Children ≥2 years: Juvenile idiopathic arthritis (JIA):

≥10 kg to ≤25 kg: 50 mg twice daily

>25 kg: 100 mg twice daily

Adults:

Acute pain or primary dysmenorrhea: Initial dose: 400 mg, followed by an additional 200 mg if needed on day 1; maintenance dose: 200 mg twice daily as needed.

Canadian labeling: Recommended maximum dose for treatment of acute pain: 400 mg/day up to 7 days

Ankylosing spondylitis: 200 mg/day as a single dose or in divided doses twice daily; if no effect after 6 weeks, may increase to 400 mg/day. If no response following 6 weeks of treatment with 400 mg/day, consider discontinuation and alternative treatment.

Canadian labeling: Recommended maximum dose: 200 mg/day

Osteoarthritis: 200 mg/day as a single dose or in divided doses twice daily

Rheumatoid arthritis: 100-200 mg twice daily

Elderly: No specific adjustment based on age is recommended. However, the AUC in elderly patients may be increased by 50% as compared to younger subjects. Initiate at the lowest recommended dose in patients weighing <50 kg.

*Dosing adjustment in poor CYP2C9 metabolizers (eg, CYP2C9*3/*3):* Consider reducing initial dose by 50%; consider alternative treatment in patients with JIA who are poor CYP2C9 metabolizers.

Canadian labeling: Recommended maximum dose: 100 mg/day

Dosing adjustment in renal impairment:

Advanced renal disease: Use is not recommended, however, if celecoxib treatment cannot be avoided, monitor renal function closely

Severe renal insufficiency: Use is not recommended.
Canadian labeling: Cl_{cr} <30 mL/minute: Use is contraindicated.
Abnormal renal function tests (persistent or worsening): Discontinue use

Dosing adjustment in hepatic impairment:
Moderate hepatic impairment (Child-Pugh class B): Reduce dose by 50%
Severe hepatic impairment (Child-Pugh class C): Use is not recommended
Canadian labeling: Use is contraindicated.
Abnormal liver function tests (persistent or worsening): Discontinue use

Mechanism of Action Inhibits prostaglandin synthesis by decreasing the activity of the enzyme, cyclooxygenase-2 (COX-2), which results in decreased formation of prostaglandin precursors; has antipyretic, analgesic, and anti-inflammatory properties. Celecoxib does not inhibit cyclooxygenase-1 (COX-1) at therapeutic concentrations.

Contraindications Hypersensitivity to celecoxib, sulfonamides, aspirin, other NSAIDs, or any component of the formulation; perioperative pain in the setting of coronary artery bypass graft (CABG) surgery

Canadian labeling: Additional contraindications (not in U.S. labeling): Pregnancy (third trimester); women who are breast-feeding; severe, uncontrolled heart failure; active gastrointestinal ulcer (gastric, duodenal, peptic) or bleeding; inflammatory bowel disease; cerebrovascular bleeding; severe liver impairment or active hepatic disease; severe renal impairment (Cl_{cr} <30 mL/minute) or deteriorating renal disease; known hyperkalemia; use in children

Warnings/Precautions **[U.S. Boxed Warning]: NSAIDs are associated with an increased risk of serious (and potentially fatal) adverse cardiovascular thrombotic events, including MI and stroke.** Risk may be increased with duration of use or pre-existing cardiovascular risk factors or disease. Carefully evaluate individual cardiovascular risk profiles prior to prescribing. New-onset or exacerbation of hypertension may occur (NSAIDS may impair response to thiazide or loop diuretics); may contribute to cardiovascular events; monitor blood pressure; use with caution in patients with hypertension. May cause sodium and fluid retention; use with caution in patients with edema, cerebrovascular disease, or ischemic heart disease. Avoid use in heart failure. Long-term cardiovascular risk in children has not been evaluated.

[U.S. Boxed Warning]: Celecoxib is contraindicated for treatment of perioperative pain in the setting of coronary artery bypass graft (CABG) surgery. Risk of MI and stroke may be increased with use following CABG surgery.

[U.S. Boxed Warning]: NSAIDs may increase risk of serious gastrointestinal ulceration, bleeding, and perforation (may be fatal). These events may occur at any time during therapy and without warning. Use caution with a history of GI disease (bleeding or ulcers), concurrent therapy with aspirin, anticoagulants and/or corticosteroids, smoking, use of alcohol, the elderly or debilitated patients. When used concomitantly with ≤325 mg of aspirin, a substantial increase in the risk of gastrointestinal complications (eg, ulcer) occurs; concomitant gastroprotective therapy (eg, proton pump inhibitors) is recommended (Bhatt, 2008).

Use the lowest effective dose for the shortest duration of time, consistent with individual patient goals, to reduce risk of cardiovascular or GI adverse events. Alternate therapies should be considered for patients at high risk.

NSAIDs may cause serious skin adverse events including exfoliative dermatitis, Stevens-Johnson syndrome (SJS), and toxic epidermal necrolysis (TEN); may occur without warning and in patients without prior known sulfa allergy. Anaphylactoid reactions may occur, even without prior exposure; patients with "aspirin triad" (bronchial asthma, aspirin intolerance, rhinitis) may be at increased risk. Do not use in patients who experience bronchospasm, asthma, rhinitis, or urticaria with NSAID or aspirin therapy. Use with caution in other forms of asthma.

Use with caution in patients with decreased hepatic (dosage adjustments are recommended for moderate hepatic impairment; not recommended for patients with severe hepatic impairment) or renal function. Transaminase elevations have been reported with use; closely monitor patients with any abnormal LFT. Severe hepatic reactions (eg, fulminant hepatitis, liver failure) have occurred with NSAID use, rarely; discontinue if signs or symptoms of liver disease develop, if systemic manifestations occur, or with persistent or worsening abnormal hepatic function tests. NSAID use may compromise existing renal function; dose-dependent decreases in prostaglandin synthesis may result from NSAID use, causing a reduction in renal blood flow which may cause renal decompensation (usually reversible). Patients with impaired renal function, dehydration, heart failure, liver dysfunction, those taking diuretics, ACE inhibitors, angiotensin II receptor blockers, and the elderly are at greater risk for renal toxicity. Rehydrate patient before starting therapy; monitor renal function closely. Not recommended for use in patients with advanced renal disease or severe renal insufficiency; discontinue use with persistent or worsening abnormal renal function tests. Long-term NSAID use may result in renal papillary necrosis. Should not be considered a treatment or replacement of corticosteroid-dependent diseases.

Anaphylactoid reactions may occur, even with no prior exposure to celecoxib. Use with caution in patients with known or suspected deficiency of cytochrome P450 isoenzyme 2C9; poor metabolizers may have higher plasma levels due to reduced metabolism; consider reduced initial doses. Alternate therapies should be considered in patients with JIA who are poor metabolizers of CYP2C9.

Anemia may occur with use; monitor hemoglobin or hematocrit in patients on long-term treatment. Celecoxib does not affect PT, PTT or platelet counts; does not inhibit platelet aggregation at approved doses.

When used for juvenile idiopathic arthritis (JIA), celecoxib is not FDA-approved in children <2 years of age or in children <10 kg. Use caution with systemic onset JIA (may be at risk for disseminated intravascular coagulation). Safety and efficacy have not been established for use in children for indications other than JIA.

Drug Interactions

Metabolism/Transport Effects **Substrate** of CYP2C9 (major), 3A4 (minor); **Inhibits** CYP2C8 (moderate), 2D6 (weak)

Avoid Concomitant Use

Avoid concomitant use of Celecoxib with any of the following: Ketorolac; Ketorolac (Systemic); Thioridazine

Increased Effect/Toxicity

Celecoxib may increase the levels/effects of: Aminoglycosides; Anticoagulants; Antiplatelet Agents; Bisphosphonate Derivatives; CycloSPORINE; CycloSPORINE (Systemic); CYP2C8 Substrates (High risk); CYP2D6 Substrates; Deferasirox; Desmopressin; Digoxin; Eplerenone; Fesoterodine; Haloperidol; Lithium; Methotrexate; Nebivolol; Nonsteroidal Anti-Inflammatory Agents; Potassium-Sparing Diuretics; PRALAtrexate; Quinolone Antibiotics; Tamoxifen; Thioridazine; Thrombolytic Agents; Vancomycin; Vitamin K Antagonists

The levels/effects of Celecoxib may be increased by: ACE Inhibitors; Angiotensin II Receptor Blockers; Antidepressants (Tricyclic, Tertiary Amine); Conivaptan; Corticosteroids (Systemic); CYP2C9 Inhibitors (Moderate); CYP2C9 Inhibitors (Strong); Herbs (Anticoagulant/Antiplatelet Properties); Ketorolac; Ketorolac (Systemic); Probenecid; Selective Serotonin Reuptake Inhibitors; Treprostinil

Decreased Effect

Celecoxib may decrease the levels/effects of: ACE Inhibitors; Angiotensin II Receptor Blockers; Antiplatelet Agents; Beta-Blockers; Codeine; Eplerenone; HydrALAZINE; Loop Diuretics; Potassium-Sparing Diuretics; Thiazide Diuretics; TraMADol

The levels/effects of Celecoxib may be decreased by: Bile Acid Sequestrants; CYP2C9 Inducers (Highly Effective); Peginterferon Alfa-2b; Tocilizumab

Ethanol/Nutrition/Herb Interactions

Ethanol: Avoid ethanol (increased GI irritation).

Food: Peak concentrations are delayed and AUC is increased by 10% to 20% when taken with a high-fat meal.

Herb/Nutraceutical: Avoid concomitant use with herbs possessing anticoagulation/antiplatelet properties, including alfalfa, anise, bilberry, bladderwrack, bromelain, cat's claw, celery, chamomile, coleus, cordyceps, dong quai, evening primrose, fenugreek, feverfew, garlic, ginger, ginkgo biloba, ginseng (American, Panax, Siberian), grapeseed, green tea, guggul, horse chestnuts, horseradish, licorice, prickly ash, red clover, reishi, SAMe (S-adenosylmethionine), sweet clover, turmeric, white willow.

Dietary Considerations May be taken without regard to meals.

Pharmacodynamics/Kinetics

Half-life Elimination ~11 hours (fasted)

Time to Peak ~3 hours

Pregnancy Risk Factor C (prior to 30 weeks gestation)/D (≥30 weeks gestation)

Lactation Enters breast milk/use caution

Breast-Feeding Considerations Small amounts of celecoxib are found in breast milk. The manufacturer recommends that caution be exercised when administering celecoxib to nursing women.

Dosage Forms

Capsule, oral:

CeleBREX®: 50 mg, 100 mg, 200 mg, 400 mg

Dental Comment The product labeling for **all** prescription nonsteroidal anti-inflammatory agents (NSAIDs) now include boxed warnings regarding an increased risk of cardiovascular (CV) events and gastrointestinal (GI) bleeding associated with their use and a contraindication for use in patients who have recently undergone coronary artery bypass graft (CABG) surgery. Medication guides are also now required for these products. Manufacturers of over-the-counter products are to include warnings about potential skin reactions, which are already included in prescription labeling.

The FDA encourages physicians to consider this information in risk-to-benefit evaluations while considering the use of the COX-2 selective celecoxib (CeleBREX®) in patients. Similar COX-2 selective drugs, including rofecoxib (Vioxx®) and valdecoxib (Bextra®), were pulled from the market due to increased risks of adverse CV events associated with their use. In addition, the FDA advises an evaluation of alternative therapy. If physicians determine that continued use is appropriate for individual patients, the lowest effective dose of celecoxib should be prescribed.

The association between selective COX-2 inhibitors and increased cardiovascular risk has been noted previously and prompted by publication of a meta-analysis entitled "Risk of Cardiovascular Events Associated With Selective COX-2 Inhibitors" in the August 22, 2001, edition of the *Journal of the American Medical Association (JAMA)*. The researchers re-evaluated four previously published trials, assessing cardiovascular events in patients receiving either celecoxib or rofecoxib. They found an association between the use of COX-2 inhibitors and cardiovascular events (including MI and ischemic stroke). The annualized MI rate was found to be significantly higher in patients receiving celecoxib or rofecoxib than in the control (placebo) group from a recent meta-analysis of primary prevention trials. Although cause and effect cannot be established (these trials were originally designed to assess GI effects, not cardiovascular ones), the authors believe the available data raise a cautionary flag concerning the risk of cardiovascular events with the use of COX-2 inhibitors.

Cross-reactivity, including bronchospasm, is a concern with aspirin and other NSAIDs, in aspirin-sensitive patients. The manufacturer suggests that celecoxib should not be administered to patients with this type of aspirin sensitivity and should be used with caution in patients with pre-existing asthma.

The manufacturer studied the effect of celecoxib on the anticoagulant effect of warfarin and found no alteration of anticoagulant effect, as determined by prothrombin time, in patients taking 2-5 mg daily. However, the manufacturer has issued a caution when using celecoxib with warfarin since those patients are at increased risk of bleeding complications.

References

Dionne R, "COX-2 Inhibitors: Better Than Ibuprofen for Dental Pain?" *Compend Contin Educ Dent*, 1999, 20(6):518-20, 522-4.

Doyle G, Jayawardena S, Ashraf E, et al, "Efficacy and Tolerability of Nonprescription Ibuprofen Versus Celecoxib for Dental Pain," *J Clin Pharmacol*, 2002, 42(8):912-9.

Everts B, Wahrborg P, and Hedner T, "COX-2 Specific Inhibitors - The Emergence of a New Class of Analgesic and Anti-inflammatory Drugs," *Clin Rheumatol*, 2000, 19(5):331-43.

Jeske AH, "Selecting New Drugs for Pain Control: Evidence-Based Decisions or Clinical Impressions?" *J Am Dent Assoc*, 2002, 133(8):1052-6.

Jouzeau JY, Terlain B, Abid A, et al, "Cyclo-oxygenase Isoenzymes. How Recent Findings Affect Thinking About Nonsteroidal Anti-inflammatory Drugs," *Drugs*, 1997, 53(4):563-82.

Kaplan-Machlis B and Klostermeyer BS, "The Cyclo-oxygenase-2 Inhibitors: Safety and Effectiveness," *Ann Pharmacother*, 1999, 33(9):979-88.

Karim A, et al, "Celecoxib, A Specific COX-2 Inhibitor, Lacks Significant Drug-Drug Interactions With Methotrexate or Warfarin," *Arthritis Rheum*, 1998, 41(9 Suppl):315:1698.

Kellstein D, Ott D, Jayawardene S, et al, "Analgesic Efficacy of a Single Dose of Lumiracoxib Compared With Rofecoxib, Celecoxib and Placebo in the Treatment of Post-Operative Dental Pain," *Int J Clin Pract*, 2004, 58(3):244-50.

Kurumbail RG, Stevens AM, Gierse JK, et al, "Structural Basis for Selective Inhibition of Cyclo-oxygenase-2 By Anti-inflammatory Agents," *Nature*, 1996, 384(6610):644-8.

Malmstrom K, Daniels S, Kotey P, et al, "Comparison of Rofecoxib and Celecoxib, Two Cyclooxygenase-2 Inhibitors, in Postoperative Dental Pain: A Randomized Placebo- and Active-Comparator-Controlled Clinical Trial," *Clin Ther*, 1999, 21(10):1653-63.

Moore PA and Hersh EV, "Celecoxib and Rofecoxib. The Role of COX-2 Inhibitors in Dental Practice," *J Am Dent Assoc*, 2001, 132(4):451-6.

Needleman P and Isakson PC, "The Discovery and Function of COX-2," *J Rheumatol*, 1997, 24(S49):6-8.

Simon LS, et al, "Preliminary Study of the Safety and Efficacy of SC-58635, A Novel Cyclo-oxygenase 2 Inhibitor: Efficacy and Safety in Two Placebo-Controlled Trials in Osteoarthritis and Rheumatoid Arthritis, and Studies of Gastrointestinal and Platelet Effects," *Arthritis Rheum*, 1998, 41:1591-1602.

Wynn RL, "The New COX-2 Inhibitors: Rofecoxib (Vioxx®) and Celecoxib (Celebrex™)," *Gen Dent*, 2000, 48(1):16-20.

Cellulose (Oxidized/Regenerated)

(SEL yoo lose, OKS i dyzed re JEN er aye ted)

Related Information

Antiplatelet and Anticoagulation Considerations in Dentistry *on page 1867*

U.S. Brand Names Surgicel®; Surgicel® Fibrillar; Surgicel® NuKnit

Generic Availability (U.S.) No

Pharmacologic Category Hemostatic Agent

Dental Use To control bleeding created during a dental procedure

Use Hemostatic; temporary packing for the control of capillary, venous, or small arterial hemorrhage

Local Anesthetic/Vasoconstrictor Precautions No information available to require special precautions

Effects on Dental Treatment No significant effects or complications reported

Effects on Bleeding Due to hemostatic effects may be used to control bleeding in dental procedures.

Adverse Effects Frequency not defined.

Central nervous system: Headache

Respiratory: Nasal burning or stinging, sneezing (rhinological procedures)

Miscellaneous: Encapsulation of fluid, foreign body reactions (with or without) infection

Dental Usual Dosage Control bleeding created during a dental procedure: Topical: Minimal amounts of the fabric strip are laid on the bleeding site or held firmly against the tissues until hemostasis occurs; remove excess material

Dosage Minimal amounts of the fabric strip are laid on the bleeding site or held firmly against the tissues until hemostasis occurs; remove excess material

Mechanism of Action Cellulose, oxidized regenerated is saturated with blood at the bleeding site and swells into a brownish or black gelatinous mass which aids in the formation of a clot. When used in small amounts, it is absorbed from the sites of implantation with little or no tissue reaction. In addition to providing hemostasis, oxidized regenerated cellulose also has been shown *in vitro* to have bactericidal properties.

Contraindications Hypersensitivity to any component of the formulation; implantation into bone defects; hemorrhage from large arteries; nonhemorrhagic oozing; use as an adhesion product

Warnings/Precautions Pain, numbness, or paralysis have been reported if used near a bony or neural space and left inside patient; use minimum amount necessary to achieve hemostasis. Remove as much of agent as possible after hemostasis is achieved. Do not leave in a contaminated or infected space. Always remove completely following hemostasis if applied in proximity to foramina in bone, areas of bony confine, the spinal cord or optic nerve and chasm; product may swell and exert unwanted pressure. The material should not be moistened before insertion since the hemostatic effect is greater when applied dry. The material should not be impregnated with anti-infective agents. Its hemostatic effect is not enhanced by the addition of thrombin.

Drug Interactions

Avoid Concomitant Use There are no known interactions where it is recommended to avoid concomitant use.

Increased Effect/Toxicity There are no known significant interactions involving an increase in effect.

Decreased Effect There are no known significant interactions involving a decrease in effect.

Pregnancy Risk Factor No data reported

Dosage Forms

Fabric, fibrous:

Surgicel® Fibrillar:

1" x 2" (10s)
2" x 4" (10s)
4" x 4" (10s)

Fabric, knitted:

Surgicel® NuKnit:

1" x 1" (24s)
1" x 3½" (10s)
3" x 4" (24s)
6" x 9" (10s)

Fabric, sheer weave:

Surgicel®:

½" x 2" (24s)
2" x 3" (24s)
2" x 14" (24s)
4" x 8" (24s)

Cephalexin (sef a LEKS in)

Related Information

Antibiotic Prophylaxis *on page* 1910

Bacterial Infections *on page* 1933

Related Sample Prescriptions

Bacterial Infections and Periodontal Diseases *on page* 1983

Infective Endocarditis (Prevention) *on page* 1978

Prosthetic Joint Late Infections (Prevention) *on page* 1979

U.S. Brand Names Keflex®

Canadian Brand Names Apo-Cephalex®; Dom-Cephalexin; Keflex®; Keftab®; Novo-Lexin; Nu-Cephalex; PMS-Cephalexin

Generic Availability (U.S.) Yes

Pharmacologic Category Antibiotic, Cephalosporin (First Generation)

Dental Use Prophylaxis in total joint replacement patients undergoing dental procedures which produce bacteremia; alternative oral antibiotic for prevention of infective endocarditis in individuals allergic to penicillins or ampicillin

Note: Individuals allergic to amoxicillin (penicillins) may receive cephalexin provided they have not had an immediate, local, or systemic IgE-mediated anaphylactic allergic reaction to penicillin.

Use Treatment of susceptible bacterial infections including respiratory tract infections, otitis media, skin and skin structure infections, bone infections, and genitourinary tract infections, including acute prostatitis; alternative therapy for acute infective endocarditis prophylaxis

Local Anesthetic/Vasoconstrictor Precautions No information available to require special precautions

Effects on Dental Treatment No significant effects or complications reported (see Dental Comment)

Effects on Bleeding No information available to require special precautions

Adverse Effects Frequency not defined.

Central nervous system: Agitation, confusion, dizziness, fatigue, hallucinations, headache

Dermatologic: Angioedema, erythema multiforme (rare), rash, Stevens-Johnson syndrome (rare), toxic epidermal necrolysis (rare), urticaria

Gastrointestinal: Abdominal pain, diarrhea, dyspepsia, gastritis, nausea (rare), pseudomembranous colitis, vomiting (rare)

Genitourinary: Genital pruritus, genital moniliasis, vaginitis, vaginal discharge

Hematologic: Eosinophilia, hemolytic anemia, neutropenia, thrombocytopenia

Hepatic: ALT increased, AST increased, cholestatic jaundice (rare), transient hepatitis (rare)

Neuromuscular & skeletal: Arthralgia, arthritis, joint disorder

Renal: Interstitial nephritis (rare)

Miscellaneous: Allergic reactions, anaphylaxis

Dental Usual Dosage

Prophylaxis against infective endocarditis (dental, oral, or respiratory tract procedures): Oral:

Children >1 year: 50 mg/kg 30-60 minutes prior to procedure; maximum: 2 g

Children >15 years and Adults: 2 g 30-60 minutes prior to procedure

Note: American Heart Association (AHA) guidelines now recommend prophylaxis only in patients undergoing invasive procedures and in whom underlying cardiac conditions may predispose to a higher risk of adverse outcomes should infection occur.

Prophylaxis in total joint replacement patients undergoing dental procedures which produce bacteremia: Oral: Adults: 2 g 1 hour prior to procedure

Dosage

Usual dosage range:

Children >1 year: Oral: 25-100 mg/kg/day every 6-8 hours (maximum: 4 g/day)

Adults: Oral: 250-1000 mg every 6 hours; maximum: 4 g/day

Indication-specific dosing:

Children >1 year: Oral:

Furunculosis: 25-50 mg/kg/day in 4 divided doses

Impetigo: 25 mg/kg/day in 4 divided doses

Otitis media: 75-100 mg/kg/day in 4 divided doses

Prophylaxis against infective endocarditis (dental, oral, or respiratory tract procedures): 50 mg/kg 30-60 minutes prior to procedure (maximum: 2 g). **Note:** American Heart Association (AHA) guidelines now recommend prophylaxis only in patients undergoing invasive procedures and in whom underlying cardiac conditions may predispose to a higher risk of adverse outcomes should infection occur.

Severe infections: 50-100 mg/kg/day in divided doses every 6-8 hours

Skin abscess: 50 mg/kg/day in 4 divided doses (maximum: 4 g)

Streptococcal pharyngitis, skin and skin structure infections: 25-50 mg/kg/day divided every 12 hours

Children >15 years and Adults: Oral:

Cellulitis and mastitis: 500 mg every 6 hours

Furunculosis/skin abscess: 250 mg 4 times/day

Prophylaxis against infective endocarditis (dental, oral, or respiratory tract procedures): 2 g 30-60 minutes prior to procedure. **Note:** American Heart Association (AHA) guidelines now recommend prophylaxis only in patients undergoing invasive procedures and in whom underlying cardiac conditions may predispose to a higher risk of adverse outcomes should infection occur.

Prophylaxis in total joint replacement patients undergoing dental procedures which produce bacteremia: 2 g 1 hour prior to procedure

Streptococcal pharyngitis, skin and skin structure infections: 500 mg every 12 hours

Uncomplicated cystitis: 500 mg every 12 hours for 7-14 days

Dosing adjustment in renal impairment: Adults:

Cl_{cr} 10-50 mL/minute: 500 mg every 8-12 hours

Cl_{cr} <10: 250-500 mg every 12-24 hours

Hemodialysis: 250 mg every 12-24 hours; moderately dialyzable (20% to 50%); give dose after dialysis session

Mechanism of Action Inhibits bacterial cell wall synthesis by binding to one or more of the penicillin-binding proteins (PBPs) which in turn inhibits the final transpeptidation step of peptidoglycan synthesis in bacterial cell walls, thus inhibiting cell wall biosynthesis. Bacteria eventually lyse due to ongoing activity of cell wall autolytic enzymes (autolysins and murein hydrolases) while cell wall assembly is arrested.

Contraindications Hypersensitivity to cephalexin, any component of the formulation, or other cephalosporins

Warnings/Precautions Modify dosage in patients with severe renal impairment. Use with caution in patients with a history of penicillin allergy, especially IgE-mediated reactions (eg, anaphylaxis, urticaria). Prolonged use may result in fungal or bacterial superinfection, including *C. difficile*-associated diarrhea (CDAD) and pseudomembranous colitis; CDAD has been observed >2 months postantibiotic treatment. May be associated with increased INR, especially in nutritionally-deficient patients, prolonged treatment, hepatic or renal disease.

Drug Interactions

Avoid Concomitant Use

Avoid concomitant use of Cephalexin with any of the following: BCG

Increased Effect/Toxicity

Cephalexin may increase the levels/effects of: MetFORMIN

The levels/effects of Cephalexin may be increased by: Probenecid

Decreased Effect

Cephalexin may decrease the levels/effects of: BCG; Typhoid Vaccine

Ethanol/Nutrition/Herb Interactions Food: Peak antibiotic serum concentration is lowered and delayed, but total drug absorbed is not affected. Cephalexin serum levels may be decreased if taken with food.

Dietary Considerations Take without regard to food. If GI distress, take with food.

Pharmacodynamics/Kinetics

Half-life Elimination Adults: 0.5-1.2 hours; prolonged with renal impairment

Time to Peak Serum: ~1 hour

Pregnancy Risk Factor B

Lactation Enters breast milk (small amounts)/use caution

Breast-Feeding Considerations Small amounts of cephalexin are excreted in breast milk. The manufacturer recommends that caution be exercised when administering cephalexin to nursing women. Maximum milk concentration occurs ~4 hours after a single oral dose and gradually disappears by 8 hours after administration. Nondose-related effects could include modification of bowel flora.

Dosage Forms

Capsule, oral: 250 mg, 500 mg

Keflex®: 250 mg, 500 mg, 750 mg

Powder for suspension, oral: 125 mg/5 mL (100 mL, 200 mL); 250 mg/5 mL (100 mL, 200 mL)

Tablet, oral: 250 mg, 500 mg

Dental Comment Cephalexin is effective against anaerobic bacteria, but the sensitivity of alpha-hemolytic *Streptococcus* vary; approximately 10% of strains are resistant. Nearly 70% are intermediately sensitive. Patients allergic to penicillins can use a cephalosporin; the incidence of cross-reactivity between penicillins and cephalosporins is 1% when the allergic reaction to penicillin is delayed. If the patient has a history of immediate reaction to penicillin, the incidence of cross-reactivity is 20%; cephalosporins are contraindicated in these patients.

References

ADA Division of Legal Affairs, "A Legal Perspective on Antibiotic Prophylaxis," *J Am Dent Assoc*, 2003, 134(9):1260.

"Advisory Statement. Antibiotic Prophylaxis for Dental Patients With Total Joint Replacements. American Dental Association; American Academy of Orthopedic Surgeons," *J Am Dent Assoc*, 1997, 128 (7):1004-8.

American Dental Association; American Academy of Orthopedic Surgeons, "Antibiotic Prophylaxis for Dental Patients With Total Joint Replacements," *J Am Dent Assoc*, 2003, 134(7):895-9.

American Dental Association Council on Scientific Affairs, "Combating Antibiotic Resistance," *J Am Dent Assoc*, 2004, 135(4):484-7.

Dajani AS, Taubert KA, Wilson W, et al, "Prevention of Bacterial Endocarditis. Recommendations by the American Heart Association," *JAMA*, 1997, 277(22):1794-801.

Dajani AS, Taubert KA, Wilson W, et al, "Prevention of Bacterial Endocarditis: Recommendations by the American Heart Association," *J Am Dent Assoc*, 1997, 128(8):1142-51.

Saxon A, Beall GN, Rohr AS, et al, "Immediate Hypersensitivity Reactions to Beta-Lactam Antibiotics," *Ann Intern Med*, 1987, 107(2):204-15.
Wilson W, Taubert KA, Gewitz M, et al, "Prevention of Infective Endocarditis. Guidelines From the American Heart Association. A Guideline From the American Heart Association Rheumatic Fever, Endocarditis, and Kawasaki Disease Committee, Council on Cardiovascular Disease in the Young, and the Council on Clinical Cardiology, Council on Cardiovascular Surgery and Anesthesia, and the Quality of Care and Outcomes Research Interdisciplinary Working Group," *Circulation*, 2007, 115. Available at http://circ.ahajournals.org/cgi/reprint/CIRCULATIONAHA.106.183095v1; last accessed July 26, 2007.
Wynn RL, Bergman SA, Meiller TF, et al, "Antibiotics in Treating Oral-Facial Infections of Odontogenic Origin: An Update," *Gen Dent*, 2001, 49(3):238-40, 242, 244 passim.

Certolizumab Pegol (cer to LIZ u mab PEG ol)

Related Information
Rheumatoid Arthritis, Osteoarthritis, and Osteoporosis *on page* 1889
U.S. Brand Names Cimzia®
Canadian Brand Names Cimzia®
Pharmacologic Category Antirheumatic, Disease Modifying; Gastrointestinal Agent, Miscellaneous; Tumor Necrosis Factor (TNF) Blocking Agent
Use Treatment of moderately- to severely-active Crohn's disease in patients who have inadequate response to conventional therapy; moderately- to severely-active rheumatoid arthritis (as monotherapy or in combination with nonbiological disease-modifying antirheumatic drugs [DMARDS])
Local Anesthetic/Vasoconstrictor Precautions No information available to require special precautions
Effects on Dental Treatment Key adverse event(s) related to dental treatment: Aphthous ulcers reported in <1% of patients.
Effects on Bleeding No information available to require special precautions
Adverse Effects
>10%:
Central nervous system: Headache (5% to 18%)
Gastrointestinal: Nausea (≤11%)
Respiratory: Upper respiratory infection (6% to 20%), nasopharyngitis (4% to 13%)
Miscellaneous: Infection (14% to 38%; serious: 3%)
1% to 10%:
Cardiovascular: Hypertension (≤5%)
Central nervous system: Dizziness (≤6%), fever (≤5%), fatigue (≤3%)
Dermatologic: Rash (9%)
Gastrointestinal: Abdominal pain (≤6%), vomiting (5%)
Genitourinary: Urinary tract infection (≤8%)
Local: Injection site reactions (includes bleeding, burning, erythema, inflammation, pain, rash: ≤7%; incidence higher with placebo)
Neuromuscular & skeletal: Arthralgia (6% to 7%), back pain (≤4%)
Respiratory: Cough (≤6%), bronchitis (≤3%), pharyngitis (≤3%)
Miscellaneous: Antibody formation (7% to 8%), positive ANA (≤4%)
General Dosage Range SubQ: Adults: Initial: 400 mg, repeat dose 2 and 4 weeks after initial dose; Maintenance: 400 mg every 4 weeks **or** 200 mg every other week
Mechanism of Action Certolizumab pegol is a pegylated humanized antibody Fab' fragment of tumor necrosis factor alpha (TNF-alpha) monoclonal antibody. Certolizumab pegol binds to and selectively neutralizes human TNF-alpha activity. (Elevated levels of TNF-alpha have a role in the inflammatory process associated with Crohn's disease and in joint destruction associated with rheumatoid arthritis.) Since it is not a complete antibody (lacks Fc region), it does not induce complement activation, antibody-dependent cell-mediated cytotoxicity, or apoptosis. Pegylation of certolizumab allows for delayed elimination and therefore an extended half-life.
Pharmacodynamics/Kinetics
Half-life Elimination ~14 days
Time to Peak Plasma: 54-171 hours
Pregnancy Risk Factor B

Cetirizine (se TI ra zeen)

U.S. Brand Names All Day Allergy [OTC]; ZyrTEC® Allergy [OTC]; ZyrTEC® Children's Allergy [OTC]; ZyrTEC® Children's Hives Relief [OTC]
Canadian Brand Names Apo-Cetirizine®; PMS-Cetirizine; Reactine™
Generic Availability (U.S.) Yes
Pharmacologic Category Histamine H_1 Antagonist; Histamine H_1 Antagonist, Second Generation; Piperazine Derivative
Use Perennial and seasonal allergic rhinitis and other allergic symptoms including urticaria; chronic idiopathic urticaria
Local Anesthetic/Vasoconstrictor Precautions No information available to require special precautions

Effects on Dental Treatment Key adverse event(s) related to dental treatment: Xerostomia and increased salivation (normal salivary flow resumes upon discontinuation).

Effects on Bleeding No information available to require special precautions

Adverse Effects

>10%: Central nervous system: Headache (children 11% to 14%, placebo 12%), somnolence (adults 14%, children 2% to 4%)

2% to 10%:

Central nervous system: Insomnia (children 9%, adults <2%), fatigue (adults 6%), malaise (4%), dizziness (adults 2%)

Gastrointestinal: Abdominal pain (children 4% to 6%), dry mouth (adults 5%), diarrhea (children 2% to 3%), nausea (children 2% to 3%, placebo 2%), vomiting (children 2% to 3%)

Respiratory: Epistaxis (children 2% to 4%, placebo 3%), pharyngitis (children 3% to 6%, placebo 3%), bronchospasm (children 2% to 3%, placebo 2%)

Dosage Oral:

Children:

6-12 months: Chronic urticaria, perennial allergic rhinitis: 2.5 mg once daily

12 months to <2 years: Chronic urticaria, perennial allergic rhinitis: 2.5 mg once daily; may increase to 2.5 mg every 12 hours if needed

2-5 years: Chronic urticaria, perennial or seasonal allergic rhinitis: Initial: 2.5 mg once daily; may be increased to 2.5 mg every 12 hours **or** 5 mg once daily

Children ≥6 years and Adults: Chronic urticaria, perennial or seasonal allergic rhinitis: 5-10 mg once daily, depending upon symptom severity

Elderly: Initial: 5 mg once daily; may increase to 10 mg/day. **Note:** Manufacturer recommends 5 mg/day in patients ≥77 years of age.

Dosage adjustment in renal/hepatic impairment:

Children <6 years: Cetirizine use not recommended

Children 6-11 years: <2.5 mg once daily

Children ≥12 and Adults:

Cl_{cr} 11-31 mL/minute, hemodialysis, or hepatic impairment: Administer 5 mg once daily

Cl_{cr} <11 mL/minute, not on dialysis: Cetirizine use not recommended

Mechanism of Action Competes with histamine for H_1-receptor sites on effector cells in the gastrointestinal tract, blood vessels, and respiratory tract

Contraindications Hypersensitivity to cetirizine, hydroxyzine, or any component of the formulation

Warnings/Precautions Cetirizine should be used cautiously in patients with hepatic or renal dysfunction; dosage adjustment recommended. Use with caution in the elderly; may be more sensitive to adverse effects. May cause drowsiness; use caution performing tasks which require alertness (eg, operating machinery or driving). Effects may be potentiated when used with other sedative drugs or ethanol.

Drug Interactions

Metabolism/Transport Effects **Substrate** of CYP3A4 (minor), P-glycoprotein

Avoid Concomitant Use There are no known interactions where it is recommended to avoid concomitant use.

Increased Effect/Toxicity

Cetirizine may increase the levels/effects of: Alcohol (Ethyl); Anticholinergics; CNS Depressants

The levels/effects of Cetirizine may be increased by: Conivaptan; Droperidol; P-Glycoprotein Inhibitors; Pramlintide

Decreased Effect

Cetirizine may decrease the levels/effects of: Acetylcholinesterase Inhibitors (Central); Benzylpenicilloyl Polylysine; Betahistine

The levels/effects of Cetirizine may be decreased by: Acetylcholinesterase Inhibitors (Central); Amphetamines; P-Glycoprotein Inducers; Tocilizumab

Ethanol/Nutrition/Herb Interactions Ethanol: May increase CNS depression; monitor for increased effects with coadministration. Caution patients about effects.

Dietary Considerations May be taken with or without food.

Pharmacodynamics/Kinetics

Onset of Action 15-30 minutes

Half-life Elimination 8 hours

Time to Peak Serum: 1 hour

Pregnancy Risk Factor B

Lactation Enters breast milk/not recommended

Dosage Forms

Capsule, liquid gel, oral:

ZyrTEC® Allergy [OTC]: 10 mg

Syrup, oral: 5 mg/5 mL (5 mL, 118 mL, 120 mL, 473 mL, 480 mL)
ZyrTEC® Children's Allergy [OTC]: 5 mg/5 mL (118 mL)
ZyrTEC® Children's Hives Relief [OTC]: 5 mg/5 mL (118 mL)
Tablet, oral: 5 mg, 10 mg
All Day Allergy [OTC]: 10 mg
ZyrTEC® Allergy [OTC]: 10 mg
Tablet, chewable, oral: 5 mg, 10 mg
All Day Allergy [OTC]: 5 mg
ZyrTEC® Children's Allergy [OTC]: 5 mg, 10 mg

Cetirizine and Pseudoephedrine (se TI ra zeen & soo doe e FED rin)

Related Information
Cetirizine *on page* 350
Pseudoephedrine *on page* 1429
U.S. Brand Names ZyrTEC-D® Allergy & Congestion [OTC]
Canadian Brand Names Reactine® Allergy and Sinus
Pharmacologic Category Alpha/Beta Agonist; Decongestant; Histamine H_1 Antagonist; Histamine H_1 Antagonist, Second Generation; Piperazine Derivative
Use Treatment of symptoms of seasonal or perennial allergic rhinitis
Local Anesthetic/Vasoconstrictor Precautions Use with caution since pseudoephedrine is a sympathomimetic amine which could interact with epinephrine to cause a pressor response
Effects on Dental Treatment Key adverse event(s) related to dental treatment: Pseudoephedrine: Xerostomia (normal salivary flow resumes upon discontinuation).
Effects on Bleeding No information available to require special precautions
Adverse Effects Percentages reported with combination product. Additional adverse effects reported; refer to individual agents.

1% to 10%:
Central nervous system: Insomnia (4%), fatigue (2%), somnolence (2%), dizziness (1%)
Gastrointestinal: Xerostomia (4%)
Respiratory: Pharyngitis (2%), epistaxis (1%)

General Dosage Range Dosage adjustment recommended in patients with hepatic or renal impairment
Oral: *Children ≥12 years:* 1 tablet twice daily (maximum: 2 tablets/day)
Mechanism of Action Cetirizine is an antihistamine; exhibits selective inhibition of H_1 receptors. Pseudoephedrine is a sympathomimetic and exerts a decongestant action on nasal mucosa.
Pharmacodynamics/Kinetics
Half-life Elimination Cetirizine: 7.9 hours; Pseudoephedrine: 6 hours
Time to Peak Cetirizine: 2.2 hours; Pseudoephedrine: 4.4 hours
Pregnancy Risk Factor C

Cetrorelix (set roe REL iks)

U.S. Brand Names Cetrotide®
Canadian Brand Names Cetrotide®
Pharmacologic Category Gonadotropin Releasing Hormone Antagonist
Use Inhibits premature luteinizing hormone (LH) surges in women undergoing controlled ovarian stimulation
Local Anesthetic/Vasoconstrictor Precautions No information available to require special precautions
Effects on Dental Treatment No significant effects or complications reported
Effects on Bleeding No information available to require special precautions
Adverse Effects 1% to 10%:
Central nervous system: Headache (1%)
Endocrine & metabolic: Ovarian hyperstimulation syndrome, WHO grade II or III (4%)
Gastrointestinal: Nausea (1%)
Hepatic: ALT, AST, GGT, and alkaline phosphatase increased (1% to 2%)

General Dosage Range SubQ: *Adults (females):* 0.25 mg once daily **or** 3 mg as a single dose
Mechanism of Action Competes with naturally-occurring GnRH for binding on receptors of the pituitary. This delays luteinizing hormone surge, preventing ovulation until the follicles are of adequate size.
Pharmacodynamics/Kinetics
Onset of Action 0.25 mg dose: 2 hours; 3 mg dose: 1 hour
Duration of Action 3 mg dose (single dose): 4 days

Half-life Elimination 0.25 mg dose: 5 hours; 0.25 mg multiple doses: 20.6 hours; 3 mg dose: 62.8 hours

Time to Peak 0.25 mg dose: 1 hour; 3 mg dose: 1.5 hours

Pregnancy Risk Factor X

Cetuximab (se TUK see mab)

U.S. Brand Names Erbitux®

Canadian Brand Names Erbitux®

Pharmacologic Category Antineoplastic Agent, Monoclonal Antibody; Epidermal Growth Factor Receptor (EGFR) Inhibitor

Use Treatment of metastatic colorectal cancer; treatment of squamous cell cancer of the head and neck

Note: Subset analyses (retrospective) in metastatic colorectal cancer trials have not shown a benefit with EGFR inhibitor treatment in patients whose tumors have codon 12 or 13 *KRAS* mutations; use is not recommended in these patients.

Unlabeled/Investigational Use Treatment of EGFR-expressing advanced non-small cell lung cancer (NSCLC)

Local Anesthetic/Vasoconstrictor Precautions No information available to require special precautions

Effects on Dental Treatment No significant effects or complications reported

Effects on Bleeding Although significant myelosuppression with associated altered hemostasis has been reported for many chemotherapeutic agents, myelosuppression is not common with cetuximab and no specific precautions appear to be necessary.

Adverse Effects Except where noted, percentages reported for cetuximab monotherapy.

>10%:

- Central nervous system: Fatigue (89%), pain (17% to 51%), headache (26% to 33%), insomnia (10% to 30%), fever (27% to 30%), confusion (15%), anxiety (14%), chills/rigors (13%), depression (7% to 13%)
- Dermatologic: Acneiform rash (76% to 90%; grades 3/4: 1% to 17%; onset: ≤14 days), rash (89%), dry skin (49%), pruritus (11% to 40%), nail changes/disorder (16% to 21%)
- Endocrine & metabolic: Hypomagnesemia (55%; grades 3/4: 6% to 17%)
- Gastrointestinal: Abdominal pain (26% to 59%), constipation (26% to 46%), diarrhea (25% to 39%), vomiting (25% to 37%), nausea (mild-to-moderate 29%), weight loss (7% to 27%), anorexia (23%), stomatitis (10% to 25%), xerostomia (11%)
- Neuromuscular & skeletal: Weakness (45% to 48%), bone pain (15%)
- Respiratory: Dyspnea (17% to 48%), cough (11% to 29%)
- Miscellaneous: Infection (13% to 35%), infusion reaction (15% to 21%; grades 3/4: 2% to 5%; 90% of severe reactions occurred with first infusion)

1% to 10%:

- Cardiovascular: Peripheral edema (10%), cardiopulmonary arrest (2%; with radiation therapy)
- Dermatologic: Alopecia (4%), skin disorder (4%)
- Endocrine & metabolic: Dehydration (2% to 10%)
- Gastrointestinal: Dyspepsia (6%)
- Hematologic: Anemia (9%)
- Hepatic: Alkaline phosphatase increased (5% to 10%), transaminases increased (5% to 10%)
- Neuromuscular & skeletal: Back pain (10%)
- Ocular: Conjunctivitis (7%)
- Renal: Renal failure (1%)
- Respiratory: Pulmonary embolus (1%)
- Miscellaneous: Sepsis (1% to 4%)

General Dosage Range Dosage adjustment recommended in patients who develop toxicities

I.V.: *Adults:* Loading dose: 400 mg/m^2; Maintenance: 250 mg/m^2 weekly

Mechanism of Action Recombinant human/mouse chimeric monoclonal antibody which binds specifically to the epidermal growth factor receptor (EGFR, HER1, c-ErbB-1) and competitively inhibits the binding of epidermal growth factor (EGF) and other ligands. Binding to the EGFR blocks phosphorylation and activation of receptor-associated kinases, resulting in inhibition of cell growth, induction of apoptosis, and decreased matrix metalloproteinase and vascular endothelial growth factor production. EGFR signal transduction results in *KRAS* wild-type activation; cells with *KRAS* mutations appear to be unaffected by EGFR inhibition.

Pharmacodynamics/Kinetics
Half-life Elimination ~112 hours (range: 63-230 hours)
Pregnancy Risk Factor C

Cetylpyridinium (SEE til peer i DI nee um)

U.S. Brand Names Cepacol® [OTC]; DiabetAid Therapeutic Gingivitis Mouth Rinse [OTC]
Generic Availability (U.S.) No
Pharmacologic Category Antiseptic, Oral Mouthwash
Dental Use Antiseptic to aid in the prevention and reduction of plaque and gingivitis, and to freshen breath
Use Antiseptic to aid in the prevention and reduction of plaque and gingivitis, and to freshen breath
Local Anesthetic/Vasoconstrictor Precautions No information available to require special precautions
Effects on Dental Treatment Key adverse event(s) related to dental treatment: Tooth and tongue staining and oral irritation.
Effects on Bleeding No information available to require special precautions
Adverse Effects Frequency not defined: Gastrointestinal: Tooth and tongue staining, oral irritation
Dental Usual Dosage Prevention and reduction of plaque and gingivitis, and to freshen breath: Children ≥6 years and Adults: Oral (OTC labeling): Rinse or gargle as directed; may be used before or after brushing (2-3 times/day)
Dosage Children ≥6 years and Adults: Oral (OTC labeling): Rinse or gargle to freshen mouth; may be used before or after brushing
Contraindications Hypersensitivity to cetylpyridinium or any component of the formulation
Warnings/Precautions Not labeled for OTC use in children <6 years of age.
Drug Interactions
Avoid Concomitant Use There are no known interactions where it is recommended to avoid concomitant use.
Increased Effect/Toxicity There are no known significant interactions involving an increase in effect.
Decreased Effect There are no known significant interactions involving a decrease in effect.
Pregnancy Risk Factor C
Dosage Forms
Liquid, oral:
Cepacol® [OTC]: 0.05% (360 mL, 720 mL)
DiabetAid Therapeutic Gingivitis Mouth Rinse [OTC]: 0.1% (480 mL)

Cetylpyridinium and Benzocaine (SEE til peer i DI nee um & BEN zoe kane)

Related Information
Benzocaine *on page 218*
Cetylpyridinium *on page 354*
Canadian Brand Names Cepacol®; Kank-A®
Pharmacologic Category Local Anesthetic
Dental Use Antiseptic/anesthetic for oral cavity
Use Symptomatic relief of sore throat
Local Anesthetic/Vasoconstrictor Precautions No information available to require special precautions
Effects on Dental Treatment No significant effects or complications reported
Effects on Bleeding No information available to require special precautions
Dosage Antiseptic/anesthetic: Oral: Dissolve in mouth as needed for sore throat
Drug Interactions
Avoid Concomitant Use There are no known interactions where it is recommended to avoid concomitant use.
Increased Effect/Toxicity There are no known significant interactions involving an increase in effect.
Decreased Effect There are no known significant interactions involving a decrease in effect.
Pregnancy Risk Factor C
Product Availability Not available in U.S.

Cevimeline (se vi ME leen)

Related Information

Dentin Hypersensitivity, Acid Erosion, High Caries Index, and Xerostomia *on page 1955*

Management of Patients Undergoing Cancer Therapy *on page 1970*

U.S. Brand Names Evoxac®

Canadian Brand Names Evoxac®

Generic Availability (U.S.) No

Pharmacologic Category Cholinergic Agonist

Dental Use Treatment of symptoms of dry mouth in patients with Sjögren's syndrome

Use Treatment of symptoms of dry mouth in patients with Sjögren's syndrome

Local Anesthetic/Vasoconstrictor Precautions No information available to require special precautions

Effects on Dental Treatment Key adverse event(s) related to dental treatment: Excessive salivation, salivary gland pain, xerostomia (normal salivary flow resumes upon discontinuation), ulcerative stomatitis, and tooth disorder.

Effects on Bleeding No information available to require special precautions

Adverse Effects

>10%:

Central nervous system: Headache (14%; placebo 20%)

Gastrointestinal: Nausea (14%), diarrhea (10%)

Respiratory: Rhinitis (11%), sinusitis (12%), upper respiratory infection (11%)

Miscellaneous: Diaphoresis increased (19%)

1% to 10%:

Cardiovascular: Peripheral edema, chest pain, edema, palpitation

Central nervous system: Dizziness (4%), fatigue (3%), pain (3%), insomnia (2%), anxiety (1%), fever, depression, migraine, hypoesthesia, vertigo

Dermatologic: Rash (4%; placebo 6%), pruritus, skin disorder, erythematous rash

Endocrine & metabolic: Hot flashes (2%)

Gastrointestinal: Dyspepsia (8%; placebo 9%), abdominal pain (8%), vomiting (5%), excessive salivation (2%), constipation, salivary gland pain, dry mouth, sialoadenitis, gastroesophageal reflux, flatulence, ulcerative stomatitis, eructation, amylase increased, anorexia, tooth disorder

Genitourinary: Urinary tract infection (6%), vaginitis, cystitis

Hematologic: Anemia

Local: Abscess

Neuromuscular & skeletal: Back pain (5%), arthralgia (4%), skeletal pain (3%), rigors (1%), hypertonia, tremor, myalgia, hyporeflexia, leg cramps

Ocular: Conjunctivitis (4%), abnormal vision, eye pain, eye abnormality, xerophthalmia

Otic: Earache, otitis media

Respiratory: Coughing (6%), bronchitis (4%), pneumonia, epistaxis

Miscellaneous: Flu-like syndrome, infection, fungal infection, allergy, hiccups

Dental Usual Dosage Dry mouth (in Sjögren's syndrome): Adults: Oral: 30 mg 3 times/day

Dosage Adults: Oral: 30 mg 3 times/day

Elderly: No specific dosage adjustment is recommended; however, use caution when initiating due to potential for increased sensitivity

Dosage adjustment in renal/hepatic impairment: Not studied; no specific dosage adjustment is recommended

Mechanism of Action Binds to muscarinic (cholinergic) receptors, causing an increase in secretion of exocrine glands (including salivary glands)

Contraindications Hypersensitivity to cevimeline or any component of the formulation; uncontrolled asthma; narrow-angle glaucoma; acute iritis; other conditions where miosis is undesirable

Warnings/Precautions May alter cardiac conduction and/or heart rate; use caution in patients with significant cardiovascular disease, including angina, myocardial infarction, or conduction disturbances. Cevimeline has the potential to increase bronchial smooth muscle tone, airway resistance, and bronchial secretions; use with caution in patients with controlled asthma, COPD, or chronic bronchitis. May cause decreased visual acuity (particularly at night and in patients with central lens changes) and impaired depth perception. Patients should be cautioned about driving at night or performing hazardous activities in reduced lighting. May cause a variety of parasympathomimetic effects, which may be particularly dangerous in elderly patients; excessive sweating may lead to dehydration in some patients.

Use with caution in patients with a history of biliary stones or nephrolithiasis; cevimeline may induce smooth muscle spasms, precipitating cholangitis, cholecystitis, biliary obstruction, renal colic, or ureteral reflux in susceptible patients. Patients with a known or suspected deficiency of CYP2D6 may be at higher risk of adverse effects.

Drug Interactions

Metabolism/Transport Effects Substrate (minor) of CYP2D6, CYP3A4

Avoid Concomitant Use There are no known interactions where it is recommended to avoid concomitant use.

Increased Effect/Toxicity

The levels/effects of Cevimeline may be increased by: Acetylcholinesterase Inhibitors; Conivaptan

Decreased Effect

The levels/effects of Cevimeline may be decreased by: Peginterferon Alfa-2b; Tocilizumab

Dietary Considerations Take with or without food.

Pharmacodynamics/Kinetics

Half-life Elimination 5 hours

Time to Peak 1.5-2 hours

Pregnancy Risk Factor C

Lactation Excretion in breast milk unknown/not recommended

Dosage Forms

Capsule, oral:

Evoxac®: 30 mg

Charcoal, Activated (CHAR kole AK tiv ay ted)

U.S. Brand Names Actidose® with Sorbitol [OTC]; Actidose®-Aqua [OTC]; Char-Caps [OTC]; Charcoal Plus® DS [OTC]; CharcoCaps® [OTC]; EZ-Char® [OTC]; Kerr Insta-Char® [OTC]; Requa® Activated Charcoal [OTC]

Canadian Brand Names Charcadole®; Charcadole® TFS; Charcadole®, Aqueous

Pharmacologic Category Antidote

Use Emergency treatment in poisoning by drugs and chemicals; aids the elimination of certain drugs and improves decontamination of excessive ingestions of sustained-release products or in the presence of bezoars; repetitive doses have proven useful to enhance the elimination of certain drugs (eg, carbamazepine, dapsone, phenobarbital, quinine, or theophylline); repetitive doses for gastric dialysis in uremia to adsorb various waste products; dietary supplement (digestive aid)

Local Anesthetic/Vasoconstrictor Precautions No information available to require special precautions

Effects on Dental Treatment No significant effects or complications reported

Effects on Bleeding No information available to require special precautions

Adverse Effects Frequency not defined.

Endocrine & metabolic: Hypernatremia, hypokalemia, and hypermagnesemia may occur with coadministration of cathartics

Gastrointestinal: Vomiting (incidence may increase with sorbitol), diarrhea (with sorbitol), constipation, swelling of abdomen, bowel obstruction, appendicitis

Respiratory: Aspiration (both gastric contents and charcoal)

Miscellaneous: Fecal discoloration (black)

General Dosage Range Oral:

Children <1 year: 10-25 g **or** 0.5-1 g/kg as a single dose; additional doses can be given as 0.25 g/kg/hour or equivalent

Children 1-12 years: 25-50 g **or** 0.5-1 g/kg as a single dose; additional doses can be given as 0.25 g/kg/hour or equivalent

Children >12 years: 25-100 g **or** 1 g/kg as a single dose; additional doses can be given as 12.5 g/hour (0.25 g/kg/hour) or equivalent

Adults: Acute poisoning: 25-100 mg as a single dose; additional doses can be given as 12.5 g/hour or equivalent; Dietary supplement: 500-520 mg after meals, may repeat in 2 hours (maximum: 10 g/day)

Mechanism of Action Adsorbs toxic substances or irritants, thus inhibiting GI absorption; adsorbs intestinal gas; the addition of sorbitol results in hyperosmotic laxative action causing catharsis

Pregnancy Risk Factor C

Chloral Hydrate (KLOR al HYE drate)

Related Information

Management of the Patient With Anxiety or Depression *on page 1968*

U.S. Brand Names Somnote®

Canadian Brand Names PMS-Chloral Hydrate

Generic Availability (U.S.) Yes: Syrup and suppositories

Pharmacologic Category Hypnotic, Nonbenzodiazepine

Dental Use Short-term sedative/hypnotic for dental procedures

Use Short-term sedative and hypnotic (<2 weeks); sedative/hypnotic for diagnostic procedures; sedative prior to EEG evaluations

Local Anesthetic/Vasoconstrictor Precautions No information available to require special precautions

Effects on Dental Treatment No significant effects or complications reported

Effects on Bleeding No information available to require special precautions

Adverse Effects Frequency not defined.

Central nervous system: Ataxia, disorientation, sedation, excitement (paradoxical), dizziness, fever, headache, confusion, lightheadedness, nightmares, hallucinations, drowsiness, "hangover" effect

Dermatologic: Rash, urticaria

Gastrointestinal: Gastric irritation, nausea, vomiting, diarrhea, flatulence

Hematologic: Leukopenia, eosinophilia, acute intermittent porphyria

Miscellaneous: Physical and psychological dependence may occur with prolonged use of large doses

Dental Usual Dosage

Conscious sedation: Children: Oral: 50-75 mg/kg/dose 30-60 minutes prior to procedure; may repeat 30 minutes after initial dose if needed, to a total maximum dose of 120 mg/kg or 1 g total

Hypnotic: Adults: Oral, rectal: 500-1000 mg at bedtime or 30 minutes prior to procedure, not to exceed 2 g/24 hours

Sedation, anxiety: Oral, rectal:

Children: 5-15 mg/kg/dose every 8 hours (maximum: 500 mg/dose)

Adults: 250 mg 3 times/day

Dosage

Children:

Sedation or anxiety: Oral, rectal: 5-15 mg/kg/dose every 8 hours (maximum: 500 mg/dose)

Prior to EEG: Oral, rectal: 20-25 mg/kg/dose, 30-60 minutes prior to EEG; may repeat in 30 minutes to maximum of 100 mg/kg or 2 g total

Hypnotic: Oral, rectal: 20-40 mg/kg/dose up to a maximum of 50 mg/kg/24 hours or 1 g/dose or 2 g/24 hours

Conscious sedation: Oral: 50-75 mg/kg/dose 30-60 minutes prior to procedure; may repeat 30 minutes after initial dose if needed, to a total maximum dose of 120 mg/kg or 1 g total

Adults: Oral, rectal:

Sedation, anxiety: 250 mg 3 times/day

Hypnotic: 500-1000 mg at bedtime or 30 minutes prior to procedure, not to exceed 2 g/24 hours

Discontinuation: Withdraw gradually over 2 weeks if patient has been maintained on high doses for prolonged period of time. Do not stop drug abruptly; sudden withdrawal may result in delirium.

Dosing adjustment/comments in renal impairment: Cl_{cr} <50 mL/minute: Avoid use

Hemodialysis: Dialyzable (50% to 100%); supplemental dose is not necessary

Dosing adjustment/comments in hepatic impairment: Avoid use in patients with severe hepatic impairment

Mechanism of Action Central nervous system depressant effects are due to its active metabolite trichloroethanol, mechanism unknown

Contraindications Hypersensitivity to chloral hydrate or any component of the formulation; hepatic or renal impairment; gastritis or ulcers; severe cardiac disease

Warnings/Precautions Hazardous agent - use appropriate precautions for handling and disposal. Use with caution in patients with porphyria. Use with caution in neonates. Drug may accumulate with repeated use; prolonged use in neonates associated with hyperbilirubinemia. Tolerance to hypnotic effect develops, therefore, not recommended for use >2 weeks. Taper dosage to avoid withdrawal with prolonged use. Trichloroethanol (TCE), a metabolite of chloral hydrate, is a carcinogen in mice; there is no data in humans. Chloral hydrate is considered a second line hypnotic agent in the elderly. Recent interpretive guidelines from the Centers for Medicare and Medicaid Services (CMS) discourage the use of chloral hydrate in residents of long-term care facilities.

Drug Interactions

Avoid Concomitant Use There are no known interactions where it is recommended to avoid concomitant use.

Increased Effect/Toxicity

Chloral Hydrate may increase the levels/effects of: Alcohol (Ethyl); CNS Depressants; Methotrimeprazine; Vitamin K Antagonists

The levels/effects of Chloral Hydrate may be increased by: Droperidol; Methotrimeprazine

Decreased Effect

The levels/effects of Chloral Hydrate may be decreased by: Flumazenil

Ethanol/Nutrition/Herb Interactions

Ethanol: May increase CNS depression; monitor for increased effects with coadministration. Caution patients about effects.

Herb/Nutraceutical: Avoid valerian, St John's wort, kava kava, gotu kola (may increase CNS depression).

Pharmacodynamics/Kinetics

Onset of Action Time to sleep: 0.5-1 hour

Duration of Action 4-8 hours

Half-life Elimination Active metabolite: 8-11 hours

Pregnancy Risk Factor C

Lactation Enters breast milk/compatible

Controlled Substance C-IV

Dosage Forms

Capsule, oral:

Somnote®: 500 mg

Suppository, rectal: 500 mg (25s)

Syrup, oral: 500 mg/5 mL (5 mL, 473 mL, 480 mL)

Chlorambucil (klor AM byoo sil)

U.S. Brand Names Leukeran®

Canadian Brand Names Leukeran®

Pharmacologic Category Antineoplastic Agent, Alkylating Agent

Use Management of chronic lymphocytic leukemia (CLL), Hodgkin's lymphoma, non-Hodgkin's lymphoma (NHL)

Unlabeled/Investigational Use Treatment of nephrotic syndrome, Waldenström's macroglobulinemia

Local Anesthetic/Vasoconstrictor Precautions No information available to require special precautions

Effects on Dental Treatment Key adverse event(s) related to dental treatment: Stomatitis.

Effects on Bleeding Chemotherapy may result in significant myelosuppression, potentially including significant reduction in platelet counts and altered hemostasis. In patients who are under active treatment with these agents, medical consult is suggested.

Adverse Effects Frequency not always defined.

Central nervous system: Agitation (rare), ataxia (rare), confusion (rare), drug fever, focal/generalized seizure (rare), hallucinations (rare)

Dermatologic: Angioneurotic edema, erythema multiforme (rare), rash, skin hypersensitivity, Stevens-Johnson syndrome (rare), toxic epidermal necrolysis (rare), urticaria

Endocrine & metabolic: Amenorrhea, infertility, SIADH (rare)

Gastrointestinal: Diarrhea (infrequent), nausea (infrequent), oral ulceration (infrequent), vomiting (infrequent)

Genitourinary: Azoospermia, cystitis (sterile)

Hematologic: Neutropenia (25%; dose- and duration-related; onset: 3 weeks; recovery: 10 days after last dose), bone marrow failure (irreversible), bone marrow suppression, anemia, leukemia (secondary), leukopenia, lymphopenia, pancytopenia, thrombocytopenia

Hepatic: Hepatotoxicity, jaundice

Neuromuscular & skeletal: Flaccid paresis (rare), muscular twitching (rare), myoclonia (rare), peripheral neuropathy, tremor (rare)

Respiratory: Interstitial pneumonia, pulmonary fibrosis

Miscellaneous: Allergic reactions, malignancies (secondary)

General Dosage Range Dosage adjustment recommended in patients with renal impairment or who develop toxicities

Oral:

Adults: 0.1-0.2 mg/kg/day for 3-6 weeks **or** 0.4 mg/kg biweekly or monthly (may increase by 0.1 mg/kg/dose) **or** 0.03-0.1 mg/kg/day

Elderly: Usual dose: 2-4 mg/day

Mechanism of Action Interferes with DNA replication and RNA transcription by alkylation and cross-linking the strands of DNA

Pharmacodynamics/Kinetics
Half-life Elimination ~1.5 hours; Phenylacetic acid mustard: ~1.8 hours
Time to Peak Within 1 hour; Phenylacetic acid mustard: 1.2-2.6 hours
Pregnancy Risk Factor D

Chloramphenicol (klor am FEN i kole)

Canadian Brand Names Chloromycetin®; Chloromycetin® Succinate; Diochloram®; Pentamycetin®
Pharmacologic Category Antibiotic, Miscellaneous
Use Treatment of serious infections due to organisms resistant to other less toxic antibiotics or when its penetrability into the site of infection is clinically superior to other antibiotics to which the organism is sensitive; useful in infections caused by *Bacteroides*, *H. influenzae*, *Neisseria meningitidis*, *Salmonella*, and *Rickettsia*; active against many vancomycin-resistant enterococci
Local Anesthetic/Vasoconstrictor Precautions No information available to require special precautions
Effects on Dental Treatment Key adverse event(s) related to dental treatment: Glossitis and stomatitis.
Effects on Bleeding Rare serious bone marrow suppression may occur which could alter hemostasis. In the absence of this effect (which would have other corresponding symptoms), no information is available to require routine special precautions.
Adverse Effects Frequency not defined.
Central nervous system: Confusion, delirium, depression, fever, headache
Dermatologic: Angioedema, rash, urticaria
Gastrointestinal: Diarrhea, enterocolitis, glossitis, nausea, stomatitis, vomiting
Hematologic: Aplastic anemia, bone marrow suppression, granulocytopenia, hypoplastic anemia, pancytopenia, thrombocytopenia
Ocular: Optic neuritis
Miscellaneous: Anaphylaxis, hypersensitivity reactions, Gray syndrome
General Dosage Range I.V.:
Neonates: Loading dose: 20 mg/kg, followed by maintenance dose based on postnatal age:
≤7 days: 25 mg/kg/day once every 24 hours
>7 days, ≤2000 g: 25 mg/kg/day once every 24 hours
>7 days, >2000 g: 50 mg/kg/day divided every 12 hours
Infants >30 days, Children, and Adults: 50-100 mg/kg/day divided every 6 hours (maximum: 4 g/day)
Mechanism of Action Reversibly binds to 50S ribosomal subunits of susceptible organisms preventing amino acids from being transferred to growing peptide chains thus inhibiting protein synthesis
Pharmacodynamics/Kinetics
Half-life Elimination
Normal renal function:
Chloramphenicol: Adults: ~4 hours; Children 4-6 hours; Infants: Significantly prolonged
Chloramphenicol succinate: Adults: ~3 hours
End-stage renal disease: Chloramphenicol: 3-7 hours
Hepatic disease: Prolonged

ChlordiazePOXIDE (klor dye az e POKS ide)

Canadian Brand Names Apo-Chlordiazepoxide®
Pharmacologic Category Benzodiazepine
Use Management of anxiety disorder or for the short-term relief of symptoms of anxiety; withdrawal symptoms of acute alcoholism; preoperative apprehension and anxiety
Local Anesthetic/Vasoconstrictor Precautions No information available to require special precautions
Effects on Dental Treatment Key adverse event(s) related to dental treatment: Xerostomia (normal salivary flow resumes upon discontinuation).
Effects on Bleeding No information available to require special precautions
Adverse Effects
>10%:
Central nervous system: Drowsiness, fatigue, ataxia, lightheadedness, memory impairment, dysarthria, irritability
Dermatologic: Rash
Endocrine & metabolic: Libido decreased, menstrual disorders

Gastrointestinal: Xerostomia, salivation decreased, appetite increased or decreased, weight gain/loss
Genitourinary: Micturition difficulties

1% to 10%:
Cardiovascular: Hypotension
Central nervous system: Confusion, dizziness, disinhibition, akathisia
Dermatologic: Dermatitis
Endocrine & metabolic: Libido increased
Gastrointestinal: Salivation increased
Genitourinary: Sexual dysfunction, incontinence
Neuromuscular & skeletal: Rigidity, tremor, muscle cramps
Otic: Tinnitus
Respiratory: Nasal congestion

General Dosage Range Dosage adjustment recommended in patients with renal impairment

I.M.:
Children >6 years: 0.5 mg/kg/day divided every 6-8 hours
Adults: Initial: 50-100 mg followed by 25-50 mg 3-4 times/day as needed **or** 50-100 mg prior to surgery (maximum: 300 mg/day)

I.V.: *Adults:* Initial: 50-100 mg followed by 25-50 mg 3-4 times/day as needed **or** 50-100 mg to start, may repeat in 2-4 hours as needed (maximum: 300 mg/day)

Oral:
Children >6 years: 0.5 mg/kg/day divided every 6-8 hours
Adults: 15-100 mg/day in 3-4 divided doses **or** 50-100 mg to start, may repeat in 2-4 hours as needed (maximum: 300 mg/day)
Elderly: Anxiety: 5 mg 2-4 times/day

Mechanism of Action Binds to stereospecific benzodiazepine receptors on the postsynaptic GABA neuron at several sites within the central nervous system, including the limbic system, reticular formation. Enhancement of the inhibitory effect of GABA on neuronal excitability results by increased neuronal membrane permeability to chloride ions. This shift in chloride ions results in hyperpolarization (a less excitable state) and stabilization.

Pharmacodynamics/Kinetics

Half-life Elimination 6.6-25 hours; End-stage renal disease: 5-30 hours; Cirrhosis: 30-63 hours

Time to Peak Serum: Oral: Within 2 hours; I.M.: Results in lower peak plasma levels than oral

Controlled Substance C-IV

Chlorhexidine Gluconate (klor HEKS i deen GLOO koe nate)

Related Information
Bacterial Infections *on page 1933*
Dentin Hypersensitivity, Acid Erosion, High Caries Index, and Xerostomia *on page 1955*
Management of Patients Undergoing Cancer Therapy *on page 1970*
Osteonecrosis of the Jaw *on page 1894*
Periodontal Diseases *on page 1942*
Ulcerative, Erosive, and Painful Oral Mucosal Disorders *on page 1950*

Related Sample Prescriptions
Antimicrobial Oral Rinses *on page 1987*

U.S. Brand Names Avagard™ [OTC]; Bactoshield® CHG [OTC]; Betasept® [OTC]; ChloraPrep® Frepp® [OTC]; ChloraPrep® Sepp® [OTC]; ChloraPrep® [OTC]; Chlorascrub™ Maxi [OTC]; Chlorascrub™ [OTC]; Dyna-Hex® [OTC]; Hibiclens® [OTC]; Hibistat® [OTC]; Operand® Chlorhexidine Gluconate [OTC]; Peridex®; PerioChip®; PerioGard® [OTC]

Canadian Brand Names Hibidil® 1:2000; ORO-Clense; Peridex® Oral Rinse

Generic Availability (U.S.) Yes: Oral liquid

Pharmacologic Category Antibiotic, Oral Rinse; Antibiotic, Topical

Dental Use
Antibacterial dental rinse; chlorhexidine is active against gram-positive and gram-negative organisms, facultative anaerobes, aerobes, and yeast
Chip, for periodontal pocket insertion: Indicated as an adjunct to scaling and root planing procedures for reduction of pocket depth in patients with adult periodontitis; may be used as part of a periodontal maintenance program

Use Skin cleanser for line placement, skin wounds, preoperative skin preparation; germicidal hand rinse; antibacterial dental rinse. Chlorhexidine is active against gram-positive and gram-negative organisms, facultative anaerobes, aerobes, and yeast. Chip, for periodontal pocket insertion: Reduces pocket depth in patients with adult periodontitis

Orphan drug: Peridex®: Oral mucositis with cytoreductive therapy when used for patients undergoing bone marrow transplant

Local Anesthetic/Vasoconstrictor Precautions No information available to require special precautions

Effects on Dental Treatment Key adverse event(s) related to dental treatment: Increased tartar on teeth, altered taste perception, staining of oral surfaces (mucosa, teeth, dorsum of tongue), and oral/tongue irritation. Staining may be visible as soon as 1 week after therapy begins and is more pronounced when there is a heavy accumulation of unremoved plaque and when teeth fillings have rough surfaces. Stain does not have a clinically adverse effect but because removal may not be possible, patient with frontal restoration should be advised of the potential permanency of the stain.

Effects on Bleeding No information available to require special precautions

Adverse Effects

Oral:

>10%: Tartar on teeth increased, taste changes. Staining of oral surfaces (mucosa, teeth, dorsum of tongue) may be visible as soon as 1 week after therapy begins and is more pronounced when there is a heavy accumulation of unremoved plaque and when teeth fillings have rough surfaces. Stain does not have a clinically adverse effect but because removal may not be possible, patient with frontal restoration should be advised of the potential permanency of the stain.

1% to 10%: Gastrointestinal: Tongue irritation, oral irritation

Topical: Skin erythema and roughness, dryness, sensitization, allergic reactions

Dental Usual Dosage Adults:

Oral rinse (Peridex®, PerioGard®):

Floss and brush teeth, completely rinse toothpaste from mouth and swish 15 mL (one capful) undiluted oral rinse around in mouth for 30 seconds, then expectorate. Caution patient not to swallow the medicine and instruct not to eat for 2-3 hours after treatment (cap on bottle measures 15 mL).

Treatment of gingivitis: Oral prophylaxis: Swish for 30 seconds with 15 mL chlorhexidine, then expectorate; repeat twice daily (morning and evening). Patient should have a re-evaluation followed by a dental prophylaxis every 6 months.

Periodontal chip: One chip is inserted into a periodontal pocket with a probing pocket depth ≥5 mm. Up to 8 chips may be inserted in a single visit. Treatment is recommended every 3 months in pockets with a remaining depth ≥5 mm. If dislodgment occurs 7 days or more after placement, the subject is considered to have had the full course of treatment. If dislodgment occurs within 48 hours, a new chip should be inserted. The chip biodegrades completely and does not need to be removed. Patients should avoid dental floss at the site of PerioChip® insertion for 10 days after placement because flossing might dislodge the chip.

Insertion of periodontal chip: Pocket should be isolated and surrounding area dried prior to chip insertion. The chip should be grasped using forceps with the rounded edges away from the forceps. The chip should be inserted into the periodontal pocket to its maximum depth. It may be maneuvered into position using the tips of the forceps or a flat instrument.

Dosage Adults:

Oral rinse (Peridex®, PerioGard®):

Floss and brush teeth, completely rinse toothpaste from mouth and swish 15 mL (one capful) undiluted oral rinse around in mouth for 30 seconds, then expectorate. Caution patient not to swallow the medicine and instruct not to eat for 2-3 hours after treatment (cap on bottle measures 15 mL).

Treatment of gingivitis: Oral prophylaxis: Swish for 30 seconds with 15 mL chlorhexidine, then expectorate; repeat twice daily (morning and evening). Patient should have a re-evaluation followed by a dental prophylaxis every 6 months.

Periodontal chip: One chip is inserted into a periodontal pocket with a probing pocket depth ≥5 mm. Up to 8 chips may be inserted in a single visit. Treatment is recommended every 3 months in pockets with a remaining depth ≥5 mm. If dislodgment occurs 7 days or more after placement, the subject is considered to have had the full course of treatment. If dislodgment occurs within 48 hours, a new chip should be inserted. The chip biodegrades completely and does not need to be removed. Patients should avoid dental floss at the site of PerioChip® insertion for 10 days after placement because flossing might dislodge the chip.

Insertion of periodontal chip: Pocket should be isolated and surrounding area dried prior to chip insertion. The chip should be grasped using forceps with the rounded edges away from the forceps. The chip should be inserted into the periodontal pocket to its maximum depth. It may be maneuvered into position using the tips of the forceps or a flat instrument.

Cleanser:

Surgical scrub: Scrub 3 minutes and rinse thoroughly, wash for an additional 3 minutes

Hand sanitizer (Avagard™): Dispense 1 pumpful in palm of one hand; dip fingertips of opposite hand into solution and work it under nails. Spread remainder evenly over hand and just above elbow, covering all surfaces. Repeat on other hand. Dispense another pumpful in each hand and reapply to each hand up to the wrist. Allow to dry before gloving.

Hand wash: Wash for 15 seconds and rinse

Hand rinse: Rub 15 seconds and rinse

Mechanism of Action The bactericidal effect of chlorhexidine is a result of the binding of this cationic molecule to negatively charged bacterial cell walls and extramicrobial complexes. At low concentrations, this causes an alteration of bacterial cell osmotic equilibrium and leakage of potassium and phosphorous resulting in a bacteriostatic effect. At high concentrations of chlorhexidine, the cytoplasmic contents of the bacterial cell precipitate and result in cell death.

Contraindications Hypersensitivity to chlorhexidine gluconate or any component of the formulation

Warnings/Precautions

Oral: Staining of oral surfaces (mucosa, teeth, tooth restorations, dorsum of tongue) may occur; may be visible as soon as 1 week after therapy begins and is more pronounced when there is a heavy accumulation of unremoved plaque and when teeth fillings have rough surfaces. Stain does not have a clinically adverse effect, but because removal may not be possible, patient with frontal restoration should be advised of the potential permanency of the stain.

Topical: For topical use only. Avoid application over large surfaces or into open wounds. Keep out of eyes and ears. May stain fabric. There have been case reports of anaphylaxis following chlorhexidine disinfection. Not for preoperative preparation of face or head; avoid contact with meninges (do not use on lumbar puncture sites). Solutions may be flammable (contain isopropyl alcohol); avoid exposure to open flame and/or ignition source (eg, electrocautery) until completely dry; avoid application to hairy areas which may significantly delay drying time. Avoid use in children <2 months of age due to increased absorption and/or irritation.

Drug Interactions

Avoid Concomitant Use There are no known interactions where it is recommended to avoid concomitant use.

Increased Effect/Toxicity There are no known significant interactions involving an increase in effect.

Decreased Effect There are no known significant interactions involving a decrease in effect.

Pharmacodynamics/Kinetics

Duration of Action Avagard™: Topical hand sanitizer: Duration of antimicrobial protection: 6 hours

Time to Peak Peridex®, PerioGard®: Plasma: Detectable levels not present after 12 hours

Pregnancy Risk Factor B

Dosage Forms

Chip, for periodontal pocket insertion:
PerioChip®: 2.5 mg (20s)

Liquid, oral: 0.12% (15 mL, 473 mL, 475 mL, 480 mL)
Peridex®: 0.12% (118 mL, 473 mL, 1920 mL)
PerioGard® [OTC]: 0.12% (480 mL)

Liquid, topical:
Betasept® [OTC]: 4% (118 mL, 237 mL, 473 mL, 946 mL, 3840 mL)
Dyna-Hex® [OTC]: 2% (120 mL, 480 mL, 960 mL, 3840 mL); 4% (120 mL, 240 mL, 480 mL, 960 mL, 3840 mL)
Hibiclens® [OTC]: 4% (15 mL, 118 mL, 236 mL, 473 mL, 946 mL, 3840 mL)
Operand® Chlorhexidine Gluconate [OTC]: 2% (118 mL); 4% (118 mL, 237 mL, 472 mL, 946 mL, 3785 mL)

Lotion, topical:
Avagard™ [OTC]: 1% (500 mL)

Solution, topical:
Bactoshield® CHG [OTC]: 2% (120 mL, 480 mL, 750 mL, 960 mL, 3840 mL); 4% (120 mL, 473 mL, 960 mL, 3840 mL)

Sponge, topical:
ChloraPrep® [OTC]: 2% (25s); 2% (25s); 2% (25s); 2% (25s); 2% (25s); 2% (25s); 2% (25s); 2% (25s)
ChloraPrep® Frepp® [OTC]: 2% (20s)
ChloraPrep® Sepp® [OTC]: 2% (200s)

Sponge/Brush, topical:
Bactoshield® CHG [OTC]: 4% (300s)

Swab, topical:
Chlorascrub™ [OTC]: 3.15% (100s)

Swabsticks, topical:
ChloraPrep® [OTC]: 2% (48s, 120s)
Chlorascrub™ [OTC]: 3.15% (50s)
Chlorascrub™ Maxi [OTC]: 3.15% (30s)

Wipe, topical:
Hibistat® [OTC]: 0.5% (50s)

References

al-Tannir MA and Goodman HS, "A Review of Chlorhexidine and Its Use in Special Populations," *Spec Care Dentist*, 1994, 14(3):116-22.
Ercan E, Ozekinci T, Atakul F, et al, "Antibacterial Activity of 2% Chlorhexidine Gluconate and 5.25% Sodium Hypochlorite in Infected Root Canal: *In Vivo* Study," *J Endod*, 2004, 30(2):84-7.
Johnson BT, "Uses of Chlorhexidine in Dentistry," *Gen Dent*, 1995, 43(2):126-32, 134-40.
Noiri Y, Okami Y, Narimatsu M, et al, "Effects of Chlorhexidine, Minocycline, and Metronidazole on Porphyromonas Gingivalis Strain 381 in Biofilms," *J Periodontol*, 2003, 74(11):1647-51.
Reddy MS, Jeffcoat MK, Geurs NC, et al, "Efficacy of Controlled-Release Subgingival Chlorhexidine to Enhance Periodontal Regeneration," *J Periodontol*, 2003, 74(4):411-9.
Soskolne WA, Proskin HM, and Stabholz A, "Probing Depth Changes Following 2 Years of Periodontal Maintenance Therapy Including Adjunctive Controlled Release of Chlorhexidine," *J Periodontol*, 2003, 74(4):420-7.

Chlorophyll (KLOR oh fil)

U.S. Brand Names Nullo® [OTC]

Pharmacologic Category Gastrointestinal Agent, Miscellaneous

Use Control fecal odors in colostomy or ileostomy

Local Anesthetic/Vasoconstrictor Precautions No information available to require special precautions

Effects on Dental Treatment No significant effects or complications reported

Effects on Bleeding No information available to require special precautions

Adverse Effects Frequency not defined: Gastrointestinal: Diarrhea, green stools, abdominal cramping

General Dosage Range

Oral: *Children >12 years and Adults:* 100-200 mg/day in divided doses (maximum: 300 mg/day)

Ostomy: *Children >12 years and Adults:* Place 1-2 tablets in empty pouch each time it is reused or changed

Chloroprocaine (klor oh PROE kane)

Related Information

Oral Pain *on page 1928*

U.S. Brand Names Nesacaine®; Nesacaine®-MPF

Canadian Brand Names Nesacaine®-CE

Pharmacologic Category Local Anesthetic

Use Infiltration anesthesia, peripheral nerve block, epidural anesthesia

Local Anesthetic/Vasoconstrictor Precautions No information available to require special precautions

Effects on Dental Treatment No significant effects or complications reported

Effects on Bleeding No information available to require special precautions

Adverse Effects Frequency not always defined.
Cardiovascular: Bradycardia, cardiac arrest, hypotension, ventricular arrhythmia
Central nervous system: Anxiety, dizziness, restlessness, tinnitus, unconsciousness
Dermatologic: Angioneurotic edema, erythema, pruritus, urticaria
Neuromuscular & skeletal: Chondrolysis (continuous intra-articular administration)
Ocular: Blurred vision
Respiratory: Respiratory arrest
Miscellaneous: Allergic reactions, anaphylactoid reactions

General Dosage Range

Caudal block: *Adults:* Preservative-free: 2% or 3%: 15-25 mL; may repeat at 40-60 minute intervals

Infiltration and peripheral nerve block:

Children >3 years: Infiltration: Concentrations of 0.5-1% (maximum without epinephrine: 11 mg/kg); Nerve block: Concentrations of 1% to 1.5% (maximum without epinephrine: 11 mg/kg)

Adults: Dosage varies greatly depending on indication

Lumbar epidural block: *Adults:* Preservative-free: 2% or 3%: 2-2.5 mL per segment; Usual total volume: 15-25 mL, may repeat with doses that are 2-6 mL less than total initial dose every 40-50 minutes

Mechanism of Action Chloroprocaine HCl is benzoic acid, 4-amino-2-chloro-2-(diethylamino) ethyl ester monohydrochloride. Chloroprocaine is an ester-type local anesthetic, which stabilizes the neuronal membranes and prevents initiation and transmission of nerve impulses thereby affecting local anesthetic actions. Local anesthetics including chloroprocaine, reversibly prevent generation and conduction of electrical impulses in neurons by decreasing the transient increase in permeability to sodium. The differential sensitivity generally depends on the size of the fiber; small fibers are more sensitive than larger fibers and require a longer period for recovery. Sensory pain fibers are usually blocked first, followed by fibers that transmit sensations of temperature, touch, and deep pressure. High concentrations block sympathetic somatic sensory and somatic motor fibers. The spread of anesthesia depends upon the distribution of the solution. This is primarily dependent on the volume of drug injected.

Pharmacodynamics/Kinetics

Onset of Action 6-12 minutes

Duration of Action 30-60 minutes

Half-life Elimination *In vitro,* plasma: Adults: 21 seconds; Neonates: 43 seconds

Pregnancy Risk Factor C

Chloroquine (KLOR oh kwin)

Related Information

Clinical Risk Related to Drugs Prolonging QT Interval *on page* 1872

U.S. Brand Names Aralen®

Canadian Brand Names Aralen®; Novo-Chloroquine

Pharmacologic Category Aminoquinoline (Antimalarial)

Use Suppression/chemoprophylaxis or treatment of acute malaria due to susceptible *Plasmodium malariae, P. vivax, P. ovale, P. falciparum*; extraintestinal amebiasis

Unlabeled/Investigational Use Rheumatoid arthritis; discoid lupus erythematosus

Local Anesthetic/Vasoconstrictor Precautions No information available to require special precautions

Effects on Dental Treatment Key adverse event(s) related to dental treatment: Stomatitis.

Effects on Bleeding Rare hematologic toxicity may result in thrombocytopenia. No information available to require routine special precautions.

Adverse Effects Frequency not defined.

Cardiovascular: Cardiomyopathy, ECG changes (rare; including prolonged QRS and QT_c intervals), hypotension (rare), torsade de pointes (rare)

Central nervous system: Agitation, anxiety, confusion, delirium, depression, hallucinations, headache, insomnia, personality changes, polyneuritis, psychosis,

Dermatologic: Alopecia, erythema multiforme (rare), exfoliative dermatitis (rare), hair bleaching, lichen planus eruptions, photosensitivity, pleomorphic skin eruptions, pruritus, skin/mucosal pigmentary changes (blue-black), Stevens-Johnson syndrome (rare), toxic epidermal necrolysis (rare), urticaria

Gastrointestinal: Abdominal cramps, anorexia, diarrhea, nausea, vomiting

Hematologic: Rare cases of agranulocytosis (reversible), aplastic anemia, neutropenia, pancytopenia, thrombocytopenia

Hepatic: Hepatitis, liver enzymes increased

Neuromuscular & skeletal: Depression of deep tendon reflexes, myopathy, neuromyopathy, proximal muscle atrophy

Ocular: Accommodation disturbances, blurred vision, corneal opacities (reversible), nyctalopia, retinopathy (including irreversible changes in some patients long-term or high-dose therapy), visual field defects

Otic: Hearing reduced (risk increased in patients with pre-existing auditory damage), nerve deafness, tinnitus

Miscellaneous: Anaphylaxis, angioedema

General Dosage Range Dosage adjustment recommended in patients with renal impairment

Oral: *Children and Adults:* Dosage varies greatly depending on indication

Mechanism of Action Binds to and inhibits DNA and RNA polymerase; interferes with metabolism and hemoglobin utilization by parasites; inhibits prostaglandin effects; chloroquine concentrates within parasite acid vesicles and raises internal pH resulting in inhibition of parasite growth; may involve aggregates of ferriprotoporphyrin IX acting as chloroquine receptors causing membrane damage; may also interfere with nucleoprotein synthesis

Pharmacodynamics/Kinetics

Duration of Action Small amounts may be present in urine months following discontinuation of therapy

Half-life Elimination 3-5 days

Time to Peak Serum: 1-2 hours

Chlorothiazide (klor oh THYE a zide)

Related Information
Cardiovascular Diseases *on page* 1848

U.S. Brand Names Diuril®; Sodium Diuril®

Canadian Brand Names Diuril®

Pharmacologic Category Diuretic, Thiazide

Use Management of mild-to-moderate hypertension; adjunctive treatment of edema

Local Anesthetic/Vasoconstrictor Precautions No information available to require special precautions

Effects on Dental Treatment Key adverse event(s) related to dental treatment: Orthostatic hypotension.

Effects on Bleeding No information available to require special precautions

Adverse Effects Frequency not defined.

Cardiovascular: Hypotension, orthostatic hypotension, necrotizing angiitis

Central nervous system: Dizziness, fever, headache, restlessness, vertigo

Dermatologic: Alopecia, erythema multiforme, exfoliative dermatitis, photosensitivity, purpura, rash, Stevens-Johnson syndrome, toxic epidermal necrolysis, urticaria

Endocrine & metabolic: Cholesterol increased, hyperglycemia, hyperuricemia, hypochloremic alkalosis, hypokalemia, hyponatremia, hypomagnesemia, triglycerides increased

Gastrointestinal: Abdominal cramping, anorexia, constipation, diarrhea, gastric irritation, nausea, pancreatitis, sialadenitis, vomiting

Genitourinary: Impotence

Hematologic: Agranulocytosis, aplastic anemia, hemolytic anemia, leukopenia, thrombocytopenia

Hepatic: Jaundice

Neuromuscular & skeletal: Muscle spasm, paresthesia, weakness

Ocular: Blurred vision, xanthopsia

Renal: Glycosuria, hematuria (I.V.), interstitial nephritis, renal failure, renal dysfunction

Respiratory: Pneumonitis, pulmonary edema, respiratory distress

Miscellaneous: Anaphylactic reactions, systemic lupus erythematosus

General Dosage Range

I.V.: *Adults:* 250-1000 mg once or twice daily (maximum: 1000 mg/day)

Oral:

Children <6 months: 10-30 mg/kg/day in 2 divided doses (maximum: 375 mg/day)

Children ≥6 months: 10-20 mg/kg/day in 1-2 divided doses (maximum: 375 mg/day)

Adults: 250-2000 mg/day in 1-2 divided doses (maximum: 1000 mg/day [CHF])

Mechanism of Action Inhibits sodium and chloride reabsorption in the distal tubules causing increased excretion of sodium, chloride, and water resulting in diuresis. Loss of potassium, hydrogen ions, magnesium, phosphate, and bicarbonate also occurs.

Pharmacodynamics/Kinetics

Onset of Action Diuresis: Oral: 2 hours; I.V.: 15 minutes

Duration of Action Diuretic action: Oral: 6-12 hours; I.V.: ~2 hours

Half-life Elimination 1-2 hours

Time to Peak Oral: ~4 hours; I.V.: 30 minutes

Pregnancy Risk Factor C

Chlorpheniramine (klor fen IR a meen)

Related Information
Bacterial Infections *on page* 1933

Related Sample Prescriptions
Sinus Infection Treatment *on page* 1985

U.S. Brand Names Ahist™; Aller-Chlor® [OTC]; Chlor Hist [OTC]; Chlor-Trimeton® Allergy [OTC]; Chlorphen [OTC]; Diabetic Tussin® for Children Allergy Relief [OTC]; Ed Chlorped [DSC]; Ed-Chlor-Tan [DSC]; Ed-Chlortan; P-Tann [DSC]; Teldrin® HBP [OTC]

Canadian Brand Names Chlor-Tripolon®; Novo-Pheniram

Generic Availability (U.S.) Yes: Syrup, tablet

Pharmacologic Category Alkylamine Derivative; Histamine H_1 Antagonist; Histamine H_1 Antagonist, First Generation

Dental Use Treatment of histamine-induced allergic symptoms

Use Perennial and seasonal allergic rhinitis and other allergic symptoms including urticaria

Local Anesthetic/Vasoconstrictor Precautions No information available to require special precautions

Effects on Dental Treatment Key adverse event(s) related to dental treatment: Xerostomia (normal salivary flow resumes upon discontinuation). Chronic use of antihistamines will inhibit salivary flow, particularly in elderly patients; this may contribute to periodontal disease and oral discomfort.

Effects on Bleeding No information available to require special precautions

Adverse Effects

>10%:

Central nervous system: Slight to moderate drowsiness

Respiratory: Thickening of bronchial secretions

1% to 10%:

Central nervous system: Headache, excitability, fatigue, nervousness, dizziness

Gastrointestinal: Nausea, xerostomia, diarrhea, abdominal pain, appetite increase, weight gain

Genitourinary: Urinary retention

Neuromuscular & skeletal: Arthralgia, weakness

Ocular: Diplopia

Renal: Polyuria

Respiratory: Pharyngitis

Dosage Oral:

Children: 0.35 mg/kg/day in divided doses every 4-6 hours

2-6 years: 1 mg every 4-6 hours, not to exceed 6 mg in 24 hours

6-12 years: 2 mg every 4-6 hours, not to exceed 12 mg/day or sustained release 8 mg at bedtime

Children >12 years and Adults: 4 mg every 4-6 hours, not to exceed 24 mg/day or sustained release 8-12 mg every 8-12 hours, not to exceed 24 mg/day

Elderly: 4 mg once or twice daily. **Note:** Duration of action may be 36 hours or more when serum concentrations are low.

Hemodialysis: Supplemental dose is not necessary

Mechanism of Action Competes with histamine for H_1-receptor sites on effector cells in the gastrointestinal tract, blood vessels, and respiratory tract

Contraindications Hypersensitivity to chlorpheniramine maleate or any component of the formulation; narrow-angle glaucoma; bladder neck obstruction; symptomatic prostate hypertrophy; during acute asthmatic attacks; stenosing peptic ulcer; pyloroduodenal obstruction. Avoid use in premature and term newborns due to possible association with SIDS.

Warnings/Precautions Causes sedation, caution must be used in performing tasks which require alertness (eg, operating machinery or driving). Sedative effects of CNS depressants or ethanol are potentiated. Use with caution in patients with urinary tract obstruction, symptomatic prostatic hyperplasia, thyroid dysfunction, increased intraocular pressure, and cardiovascular disease (including hypertension and ischemic heart disease). May be inappropriate for use in elderly due to potent anticholinergic effects; nonanticholinergic antihistamines preferred for treating allergic reactions (Beers Criteria). Antihistamines may cause excitation in young children. Not for OTC use in children <2 years of age.

Drug Interactions

Metabolism/Transport Effects **Substrate** of CYP2D6 (minor), 3A4 (major); **Inhibits** CYP2D6 (weak)

Avoid Concomitant Use There are no known interactions where it is recommended to avoid concomitant use.

Increased Effect/Toxicity

Chlorpheniramine may increase the levels/effects of: Alcohol (Ethyl); Anticholinergics; CNS Depressants

The levels/effects of Chlorpheniramine may be increased by: Conivaptan; CYP3A4 Inhibitors (Moderate); CYP3A4 Inhibitors (Strong); Dasatinib; Droperidol; Pramlintide

Decreased Effect

Chlorpheniramine may decrease the levels/effects of: Acetylcholinesterase Inhibitors (Central); Benzylpenicilloyl Polylysine; Betahistine

The levels/effects of Chlorpheniramine may be decreased by: Acetylcholinesterase Inhibitors (Central); Amphetamines; Peginterferon Alfa-2b; Tocilizumab

Ethanol/Nutrition/Herb Interactions Ethanol: May increase CNS depression; monitor for increased effects with coadministration. Caution patients about effects.

Dietary Considerations May be taken with food or water.

Pharmacodynamics/Kinetics

Half-life Elimination Serum: 20-24 hours

Pregnancy Risk Factor C

Lactation Excretion in breast milk unknown/not recommended

Dosage Forms

Syrup, oral:

Aller-Chlor® [OTC]: 2 mg/5 mL (118 mL)

Diabetic Tussin® for Children Allergy Relief [OTC]: 2 mg/5 mL (118 mL)

Tablet, oral: 4 mg

Aller-Chlor® [OTC]: 4 mg

Chlor Hist [OTC]: 4 mg

Chlor-Trimeton® Allergy [OTC]: 4 mg

Chlorphen [OTC]: 4 mg

Ed-Chlortan: 4 mg

Teldrin® HBP [OTC]: 4 mg

Tablet, extended release, oral:

Chlor-Trimeton® Allergy [OTC]: 12 mg

Tablet, long acting, oral:

Ahist™: 12 mg

Chlorpheniramine and Acetaminophen

(klor fen IR a meen & a seet a MIN oh fen)

Related Information

Acetaminophen *on page* 32

Chlorpheniramine *on page* 365

U.S. Brand Names Coricidin HBP® Cold and Flu [OTC]

Pharmacologic Category Alkylamine Derivative; Analgesic, Miscellaneous; Histamine H_1 Antagonist; Histamine H_1 Antagonist, First Generation

Use Symptomatic relief of congestion, headache, aches and pains of colds and flu

Local Anesthetic/Vasoconstrictor Precautions No information available to require special precautions

Effects on Dental Treatment Key adverse event(s) related to dental treatment: Chronic use of antihistamines will inhibit salivary flow, particularly in elderly patients; this may contribute to periodontal disease and oral discomfort. See Dental Comment.

Effects on Bleeding No information available to require special precautions

Adverse Effects See individual agents.

General Dosage Range Oral: *Adults:* 2 tablets every 4 hours

Dental Comment Hepatotoxicity caused by acetaminophen is potentiated by chronic alcohol consumption. People who are taking acetaminophen, even at therapeutic doses, and consume alcohol are at risk of developing hepatotoxicity.

Acetaminophen may increase the levels and enhance the anticoagulant effects of vitamin K antagonists acenocoumarol and warfarin (Coumadin®). Studies have reported that acetaminophen has increased the INR in warfarin treated patients with daily acetaminophen doses as low as 2 g, particularly when taking acetaminophen for >1 week (Antlitz, 1968; Boeijinga, 1982; Gebauer, 2003; Hylek, 1998; Rubin, 1984). In addition, case reports of bleeding as a result of increased INR have been published (Bagheri, 1999; Bartle, 1991). There is no known mechanism of the interaction; furthermore, some studies have failed to demonstrate this interaction (Gadisseur, 2003; Kwan, 1995; van den Bemt, 2002). In terms of risk, the data suggest that acetaminophen and warfarin could interact in some clinically significant manner but that the benefits of concomitant use of acetaminophen for pain control in dental patients taking warfarin usually outweigh the risks. An appropriate monitoring plan should be in place to identify potential negative effects and dosage adjustments may be necessary in a minority of patients. The interaction may be more likely to occur with daily acetaminophen doses of >1.3 g for >1 week.

There are no reports of acetaminophen interacting with antiplatelet drugs such as aspirin, clopidogrel (Plavix®), or prasugrel (Effient™). Also, there are no reports of acetaminophen in combination with hydrocodone, codeine, or oxycodone interacting with warfarin (Coumadin®).

Chlorpheniramine and Phenylephrine (klor fen IR a meen & fen il EF rin)

Related Information

Chlorpheniramine *on page* 365

Phenylephrine (Systemic) *on page* 1339

U.S. Brand Names Actifed® Cold & Allergy [OTC] *[reformulation]*; C-Phen [DSC]; Ceron [DSC]; Dallergy Drops [DSC]; Dallergy®-JR [DSC]; Dec-Chlorphen [DSC]; Ed A-Hist™ [DSC]; Ed ChlorPed D; NoHist [DSC]; PD-Hist-D; Phenabid® [DSC]; R-Tanna; R-Tanna Pediatric; Rynatan®; Rynatan® Pediatric; Sildec PE [DSC]; Sudafed PE® Sinus & Allergy [OTC] [DSC]; Sudafed PE® Sinus + Allergy [OTC]; Tannate Pediatric [DSC]; Triaminic® Cold and Allergy [OTC]

Pharmacologic Category Alkylamine Derivative; Alpha/Beta Agonist; Decongestant; Histamine H_1 Antagonist; Histamine H_1 Antagonist, First Generation

Use Temporary relief of upper respiratory conditions such as nasal congestion, runny nose, and sneezing due to the common cold, hay fever, or allergic or vasomotor rhinitis

Local Anesthetic/Vasoconstrictor Precautions Use with caution since phenylephrine is a sympathomimetic amine which could interact with epinephrine to cause a pressor response

Effects on Dental Treatment Key adverse event(s) related to dental treatment:

Chlorpheniramine: Prolonged use will cause significant xerostomia (normal salivary flow resumes upon discontinuation).

Phenylephrine: Up to 10% of patients could experience tachycardia, palpitations, and xerostomia (prolonged use worsens); use vasoconstrictor with caution.

Effects on Bleeding No information available to require special precautions

Adverse Effects See individual agents.

General Dosage Range Oral: *Children ≥2 years and Adults:* Dosage varies greatly depending on product

Pregnancy Risk Factor C

Chlorpheniramine and Pseudoephedrine

(klor fen IR a meen & soo doe e FED rin)

Related Information

Chlorpheniramine *on page* 365

Pseudoephedrine *on page* 1429

U.S. Brand Names Dicel® Chewable [OTC]; Dicel® Suspension; LoHist-D; Neutrahist Pediatric [OTC] [DSC]; Suclor™ [DSC]; SudaHist® [DSC]; Sudal® 12 [DSC]

Canadian Brand Names Triaminic® Cold & Allergy

Pharmacologic Category Alkylamine Derivative; Alpha/Beta Agonist; Decongestant; Histamine H_1 Antagonist; Histamine H_1 Antagonist, First Generation

Use Relief of nasal congestion associated with the common cold, hay fever, and other allergies, sinusitis, eustachian tube blockage, and vasomotor and allergic rhinitis

Local Anesthetic/Vasoconstrictor Precautions Use with caution since pseudoephedrine is a sympathomimetic amine which could interact with epinephrine to cause a pressor response

Effects on Dental Treatment Key adverse event(s) related to dental treatment:

Chlorpheniramine: Prolonged use will cause significant xerostomia (normal salivary flow resumes upon discontinuation).

Pseudoephedrine: Xerostomia (prolonged use worsens; normal salivary flow resumes upon discontinuation).

Effects on Bleeding No information available to require special precautions

Adverse Effects See individual agents.

General Dosage Range Oral:

Immediate release: *Children ≥2 years and Adults:* Dosage varies greatly depending on product

Sustained release: *Children ≥12 years and Adults:* Deconamine® SR: Chlorpheniramine maleate 8 mg and pseudoephedrine hydrochloride 120 mg every 12 hours

Mechanism of Action

Chlorpheniramine competes with histamine for H_1-receptor sites on effector cells in the gastrointestinal tract, blood vessels, and respiratory tract.

Pseudoephedrine is a sympathomimetic amine and isomer of ephedrine; acts as a decongestant in respiratory tract mucous membranes with less vasoconstrictor action than ephedrine in normotensive individuals.

Pregnancy Risk Factor C

Chlorpheniramine, Ephedrine, Phenylephrine, and Carbetapentane

(klor fen IR a meen, e FED rin, fen il EF rin, & kar bay ta PEN tane)

Related Information

Chlorpheniramine *on page* 365

EPHEDrine (Systemic) *on page* 603

Phenylephrine (Systemic) *on page* 1339

U.S. Brand Names Quad Tann® [DSC]; Rynatuss®; Tetra Tannate Pediatric [DSC]

Pharmacologic Category Alkylamine Derivative; Alpha/Beta Agonist; Antitussive; Decongestant; Histamine H_1 Antagonist; Histamine H_1 Antagonist, First Generation

Use Symptomatic relief of cough with a decongestant and an antihistamine

Local Anesthetic/Vasoconstrictor Precautions
Ephedrine: Use vasoconstrictor with caution since ephedrine may enhance cardiostimulation and vasopressor effects of sympathomimetics
Phenylephrine: Use with caution since phenylephrine is a sympathomimetic amine which could interact with epinephrine to cause a pressor response

Effects on Dental Treatment Key adverse event(s) related to dental treatment:
Chlorpheniramine: Prolonged use will cause significant xerostomia (normal salivary flow resumes upon discontinuation).
Ephedrine: No significant effects or complications reported.
Phenylephrine: Up to 10% of patients could experience tachycardia, palpitations, and xerostomia; use vasoconstrictor with caution.

Effects on Bleeding No information available to require special precautions

General Dosage Range Oral:
Children 2-6 years: 2.5-5 mL every 12 hours
Children >6 years: 5-10 mL every 12 hours
Adults: 1-2 tablets every 12 hours

Pregnancy Risk Factor C

Chlorpheniramine, Phenylephrine, and Dextromethorphan (klor fen IR a meen, fen il EF rin, & deks troe meth OR fan)

Related Information
Chlorpheniramine *on page 365*
Dextromethorphan *on page 504*
Phenylephrine (Systemic) *on page 1339*

U.S. Brand Names Ceron-DM [DSC]; Corfen DM [DSC]; De-Chlor DM [DSC]; De-Chlor DR [DSC]; Donatussin DM; Ed A-Hist DM [DSC]; Father John's® Plus [OTC]; Neo DM [DSC]; NoHist-DMX [DSC]; PD-Cof [DSC]; PE-Hist DM [DSC]; Sildec PE-DM [DSC]

Pharmacologic Category Alkylamine Derivative; Alpha/Beta Agonist; Antitussive; Decongestant; Histamine H_1 Antagonist; Histamine H_1 Antagonist, First Generation

Use Temporary relief of cough and upper respiratory symptoms associated with allergies or the common cold

Local Anesthetic/Vasoconstrictor Precautions
Chlorpheniramine, Dextromethorphan: No information available to require special precautions
Phenylephrine: Use with caution since phenylephrine is a sympathomimetic amine which could interact with epinephrine to cause a pressor response

Effects on Dental Treatment Key adverse event(s) related to dental treatment:
Chlorpheniramine: Prolonged use will cause significant xerostomia (normal salivary flow resumes upon discontinuation).
Dextromethorphan: No significant effects or complications reported
Phenylephrine: Up to 10% of patients could experience tachycardia, palpitations, and xerostomia (prolonged use worsens); use vasoconstrictor with caution.

Effects on Bleeding No information available to require special precautions

Adverse Effects See individual agents.

General Dosage Range Oral: *Children ≥6 years and Adults:* Dosage varies greatly depending on product

Pregnancy Risk Factor C

Chlorpheniramine, Phenylephrine, and Methscopolamine
(klor fen IR a meen, fen il EF rin, & meth skoe POL a meen)

Related Information
Chlorpheniramine *on page 365*
Methscopolamine *on page 1106*
Phenylephrine (Systemic) *on page 1339*

U.S. Brand Names aerohist plus™ [DSC]; aeroKid™; AH-Chew® [DSC]; AH-Chew™ Ultra [DSC]; Chlor-Mes [DSC]; Chlor-Mes-D [DSC]; Dallergy® [DSC]; Dehistine [DSC]; DryMax; Duradryl®; Histatab PH [DSC]; OMNIhist® II L.A. [DSC]; Ralix [DSC]; Rescon®; Triall™ [DSC]

Pharmacologic Category Alkylamine Derivative; Alpha/Beta Agonist; Anticholinergic Agent; Decongestant; Histamine H_1 Antagonist; Histamine H_1 Antagonist, First Generation

Use Treatment of upper respiratory symptoms such as respiratory congestion, allergic rhinitis, vasomotor rhinitis, sinusitis, and allergic skin reactions of urticaria and angioedema

Local Anesthetic/Vasoconstrictor Precautions Use with caution since phenylephrine is a sympathomimetic amine which could interact with epinephrine to cause a pressor response

Effects on Dental Treatment Key adverse event(s) related to dental treatment:
Chlorpheniramine: Significant xerostomia with prolonged use (normal salivary flow resumes upon discontinuation).
Methscopolamine: Anticholinergic side effects can cause a reduction of saliva production or secretion contributes to discomfort and dental disease (ie, caries, oral candidiasis and periodontal disease).
Phenylephrine: Tachycardia, palpitations, and xerostomia; use vasoconstrictor with caution.

Effects on Bleeding No information available to require special precautions

Adverse Effects Frequency not defined.
Cardiovascular: Arrhythmias, bradycardia, cardiovascular collapse, flushing, hypotension, pallor, palpitation, tachycardia
Central nervous system: Anxiety, convulsions, CNS depression, dizziness, drowsiness, excitability, fear, giddiness, hallucinations, headache, insomnia, irritability, lassitude, restlessness, tenseness, tremor
Gastrointestinal: Constipation, dysphagia, gastric irritation, nausea, xerostomia
Genitourinary: Dysuria, urinary retention
Neuromuscular & skeletal: Weakness
Ocular: Blurred vision, mydriasis
Respiratory: Dry nose, dry throat, respiratory difficulty

General Dosage Range Oral: *Children ≥6 years and Adults:* Dosage varies greatly depending on product

Mechanism of Action
Chlorpheniramine maleate: Antihistamine
Phenylephrine hydrochloride: Sympathomimetic agent (primarily alpha), decongestant
Methscopolamine nitrate: Derivative of scopolamine, antisecretory effects

Pregnancy Risk Factor C

Chlorpheniramine, Phenylephrine, and Phenyltoloxamine

(klor fen IR a meen, fen il EF rin, & fen il tole LOKS a meen)

Related Information
Chlorpheniramine *on page* 365
Phenylephrine (Systemic) *on page* 1339

U.S. Brand Names Chlorex-A [DSC]; Nalex®-A; NoHist-A; Rhinacon A

Pharmacologic Category Alkylamine Derivative; Alpha/Beta Agonist; Decongestant; Ethanolamine Derivative; Histamine H_1 Antagonist; Histamine H_1 Antagonist, First Generation

Use Symptomatic relief of rhinitis and nasal congestion due to colds or allergy

Local Anesthetic/Vasoconstrictor Precautions Use with caution since phenylephrine is a sympathomimetic amine which could interact with epinephrine to cause a pressor response

Effects on Dental Treatment Key adverse event(s) related to dental treatment:
Chlorpheniramine: Prolonged use will cause significant xerostomia (normal salivary flow resumes upon discontinuation).
Phenylephrine: Up to 10% of patients could experience tachycardia, palpitations, and xerostomia; use vasoconstrictor with caution.

Effects on Bleeding No information available to require special precautions

Adverse Effects Frequency not defined.
Cardiovascular: Hypotension, palpitation
Central nervous system: Headache, dizziness, sedation, excitation (children), nervousness, seizure
Dermatologic: Urticaria, drug rash
Gastrointestinal: Dry mouth, anorexia, nausea, vomiting, diarrhea, constipation, GI upset
Genitourinary: Urinary frequency, urinary retention
Hematologic: Agranulocytosis, leukopenia, thrombocytopenia
Ocular: Blurred vision
Respiratory: Dry nose/throat, thickening of bronchial secretions, wheezing, stuffy nose, tightness of chest

General Dosage Range Oral:
Children 2-6 years: Nalex®-A: 1.25-2.5 mL every 4-6 hours
Children 6-12 years: Nalex®-A: 5 mL every 4-6 hours **or** one-half tablet 2-3 times/day
Children >12 years and Adults: Nalex®-A: 10 mL every 4-6 hours **or** 1 tablet 2-3 times/day

Pregnancy Risk Factor C

Chlorpheniramine, Pseudoephedrine, and Codeine

(klor fen IR a meen, soo doe e FED rin, & KOE deen)

Related Information

Chlorpheniramine *on page 365*

Codeine *on page 432*

Pseudoephedrine *on page 1429*

U.S. Brand Names Phenylhistine DH

Pharmacologic Category Alkylamine Derivative; Alpha/Beta Agonist; Analgesic, Opioid; Antitussive; Decongestant; Histamine H_1 Antagonist; Histamine H_1 Antagonist, First Generation

Use Temporary relief of cough associated with minor throat or bronchial irritation or nasal congestion due to common cold, allergic rhinitis, or sinusitis

Local Anesthetic/Vasoconstrictor Precautions Use with caution since pseudoephedrine is a sympathomimetic amine which could interact with epinephrine to cause a pressor response

Effects on Dental Treatment Key adverse event(s) related to dental treatment:

Chlorpheniramine: Significant xerostomia with prolonged use (normal salivary flow resumes upon discontinuation).

Pseudoephedrine: Xerostomia (normal salivary flow resumes upon discontinuation).

Effects on Bleeding No information available to require special precautions

Adverse Effects See individual agents.

General Dosage Range Oral:

Children 6-11 years: 5 mL every 4 hours (maximum: 20 mL/24 hours)

Children ≥12 years and Adults: 10 mL every 4 hours (maximum: 40 mL/24 hours)

Pregnancy Risk Factor C

Controlled Substance C-V

Chlorpheniramine, Pyrilamine, and Phenylephrine

(klor fen IR a meen, pye RIL a meen, & fen il EF rin)

Related Information

Chlorpheniramine *on page 365*

Phenylephrine (Systemic) *on page 1339*

U.S. Brand Names Conal [DSC]; MyHist-PD; Nalex A 12; Poly Hist Forte® [DSC]; Poly Hist PD [DSC]; Pyrichlor PE™; Ru-Hist Forte; Triplex™ AD [DSC]

Pharmacologic Category Alkylamine Derivative; Alpha/Beta Agonist; Decongestant; Ethylenediamine Derivative; Histamine H_1 Antagonist; Histamine H_1 Antagonist, First Generation

Use Symptomatic relief of rhinitis and nasal congestion due to colds or allergy

Local Anesthetic/Vasoconstrictor Precautions Use with caution since phenylephrine is a sympathomimetic amine which could interact with epinephrine or mepivacaine and levonordefrin (Carbocaine® 2% with Neo-Cobefrin®) to cause a pressor response.

Effects on Dental Treatment Key adverse event(s) related to dental treatment:

Chlorpheniramine and pyrilamine: Prolonged use will cause significant xerostomia (normal salivary flow resumes upon discontinuation).

Phenylephrine: Up to 10% of patients could experience tachycardia, palpitations, and xerostomia.

Effects on Bleeding No information available to require special precautions

Adverse Effects Frequency not defined.

Cardiovascular: Hyper-/hypotension, palpitation

Central nervous system: Dizziness, excitation (children), headache, nervousness, sedation, seizure

Dermatologic: Drug rash, urticaria

Gastrointestinal: Anorexia, constipation, diarrhea, dry mouth, GI upset, nausea, vomiting

Genitourinary: Urinary frequency, urinary retention

Hematologic: Agranulocytosis, leukopenia, thrombocytopenia

Ocular: Blurred vision

Respiratory: Dry nose/throat, stuffy nose, thickening of bronchial secretions, tightness of chest, wheezing

General Dosage Range Oral: *Children ≥2 years and Adults:* Dosage varies greatly depending on product

Pregnancy Risk Factor C

ChlorproMAZINE (klor PROE ma zeen)

Related Information

Clinical Risk Related to Drugs Prolonging QT Interval *on page* 1872

Canadian Brand Names Largactil®; Novo-Chlorpromazine

Pharmacologic Category Antimanic Agent; Antipsychotic Agent, Typical, Phenothiazine

Use Management of psychotic disorders (control of mania, treatment of schizophrenia); control of nausea and vomiting; relief of restlessness and apprehension before surgery; acute intermittent porphyria; adjunct in the treatment of tetanus; intractable hiccups; combativeness and/or explosive hyperexcitable behavior in children 1-12 years of age and in short-term treatment of hyperactive children

Unlabeled/Investigational Use Behavioral symptoms associated with dementia (elderly); psychosis/agitation related to Alzheimer's dementia

Local Anesthetic/Vasoconstrictor Precautions Most pharmacology textbooks state that in presence of phenothiazines, systemic doses of epinephrine paradoxically decrease the blood pressure. This is the so called "epinephrine reversal" phenomenon. This has never been observed when epinephrine is given by infiltration as part of the anesthesia procedure. Chlorpromazine is one of the drugs confirmed to prolong the QT interval and is accepted as having a risk of causing torsade de pointes. The risk of drug-induced torsade de pointes is extremely low when a single QT interval prolonging drug is prescribed. In terms of epinephrine, it is not known what effect vasoconstrictors in the local anesthetic regimen will have in patients with a known history of congenital prolonged QT interval or in patients taking any medication that prolongs the QT interval. Until more information is obtained, it is suggested that the clinician consult with the physician prior to the use of a vasoconstrictor in suspected patients, and that the vasoconstrictor (epinephrine, mepivacaine and levonordefrin [Carbocaine® 2% with Neo-Cobefrin®]) be used with caution.

Effects on Dental Treatment Key adverse event(s) related to dental treatment:

Xerostomia (normal salivary flow resumes upon discontinuation).

Significant hypotension may occur, especially when the drug is administered parenterally. Orthostatic hypotension is due to alpha-receptor blockade; elderly are at greater risk.

Tardive dyskinesia: Prevalence rate may be 40% in elderly; development of the syndrome and the irreversible nature are proportional to duration and total cumulative dose over time. Extrapyramidal reactions are more common in elderly with up to 50% developing these reactions after 60 years of age. Drug-induced Parkinson's syndrome occurs often; akathisia is the most common extrapyramidal reaction in elderly.

Increased confusion, memory loss, psychotic behavior, and agitation frequently occur as a consequence of anticholinergic effects. Antipsychotic-associated sedation in nonpsychotic patients is extremely unpleasant due to feelings of depersonalization, derealization, and dysphoria.

Effects on Bleeding No information available to require special precautions

Adverse Effects Frequency not defined.

Cardiovascular: Postural hypotension, tachycardia, dizziness, nonspecific QT changes

Central nervous system: Drowsiness, dystonias, akathisia, pseudoparkinsonism, tardive dyskinesia, neuroleptic malignant syndrome, seizure

Dermatologic: Photosensitivity, dermatitis, skin pigmentation (slate gray)

Endocrine & metabolic: Lactation, breast engorgement, false-positive pregnancy test, amenorrhea, gynecomastia, hyper- or hypoglycemia

Gastrointestinal: Xerostomia, constipation, nausea

Genitourinary: Urinary retention, ejaculatory disorder, impotence

Hematologic: Agranulocytosis, eosinophilia, leukopenia, hemolytic anemia, aplastic anemia, thrombocytopenic purpura

Hepatic: Jaundice

Ocular: Blurred vision, corneal and lenticular changes, epithelial keratopathy, pigmentary retinopathy

General Dosage Range

I.M., I.V.:

Children ≥6 months: 0.5-1 mg/kg every 6-8 hours (maximum: <5 years [<22.7 kg]: 40 mg/day; 5-12 years [22.7-45.5 kg]: 75 mg/day)

Adults: Initial: 25 mg; may repeat (25-50 mg) in 1-4 hours; Usual dose: 300-800 mg/day (maximum: 400 mg every 4-6 hours)

Oral:

Children ≥6 months: 0.5-1 mg/ kg every 4-6 hours as needed

Adults: Dosage varies greatly depending on indication

Mechanism of Action Chlorpromazine is an aliphatic phenothiazine antipsychotic which blocks postsynaptic mesolimbic dopaminergic receptors in the brain; exhibits a strong alpha-adrenergic blocking effect and depresses the release of hypothalamic and hypophyseal hormones; believed to depress the reticular activating system, thus affecting basal metabolism, body temperature, wakefulness, vasomotor tone, and emesis

Pharmacodynamics/Kinetics

Onset of Action I.M.: 15 minutes; Oral: 30-60 minutes

Half-life Elimination Biphasic: Initial: 2 hours; Terminal: 30 hours

Dental Comment Chlorpromazine is known to prolong the QT interval. The QT interval is measured as the time and distance between the Q point of the QRS complex and the end of the T wave in the ECG tracing. After adjustment for heart rate, the QT interval is defined as prolonged if it is more than 450 msec in men and 460 msec in women. A long QT syndrome was first described in the 1950s and 60s as a congenital syndrome involving QT interval prolongation and syncope and sudden death. Some of the congenital long QT syndromes were characterized by a peculiar electrocardiographic appearance of the QRS complex involving a premature atria beat followed by a pause, then a subsequent sinus beat showing marked QT prolongation and deformity. This type of cardiac arrhythmia was originally termed "torsade de pointes" (translated from the French as "twisting of the points"). Chlorpromazine is considered as having a risk of causing torsade de pointes. Since it is not known what effect vasoconstrictors in the local anesthetic regimen will have in patients with a known history of congenital prolonged QT interval or in patients taking any medication that prolongs the QT interval, a medical consult is suggested.

ChlorproPAMIDE (klor PROE pa mide)

Related Information

Endocrine Disorders and Pregnancy *on page 1879*

Canadian Brand Names Apo-Chlorpropamide®; Novo-Propamide

Pharmacologic Category Antidiabetic Agent, Sulfonylurea

Use Management of blood sugar in type 2 diabetes mellitus (noninsulin dependent, NIDDM)

Unlabeled/Investigational Use Neurogenic diabetes insipidus

Local Anesthetic/Vasoconstrictor Precautions No information available to require special precautions

Effects on Dental Treatment Chlorpropamide-dependent patients with diabetes (noninsulin dependent, Type 2) should be appointed for dental treatment in morning in order to minimize chance of stress-induced hypoglycemia.

Effects on Bleeding No information available to require special precautions

Adverse Effects Frequency not defined.

Central nervous system: Dizziness, headache

Dermatologic: Erythema multiforme, exfoliative dermatitis, maculopapular eruptions, photosensitivity, pruritus, urticaria

Endocrine & metabolic: Disulfiram-like reactions, hypoglycemia, SIADH

Gastrointestinal: Anorexia, diarrhea, hunger, nausea, proctocolitis, vomiting

Hematologic: Agranulocytosis, aplastic anemia, eosinophilia, hemolytic anemia, leukopenia, pancytopenia, porphyria cutanea tarda, thrombocytopenia

Hepatic: Cholestatic jaundice, hepatic porphyria, hepatitis, liver failure

General Dosage Range Oral:

Adults: Initial: 250 mg/day; Maintenance: 100-500 mg/day (maximum: 750 mg/day)

Elderly: Initial: 100-125 mg/day

Mechanism of Action Stimulates insulin release from the pancreatic beta cells; reduces glucose output from the liver; insulin sensitivity is increased at peripheral target sites

Pharmacodynamics/Kinetics

Onset of Action 1 hour; Peak effect: 3-6 hours

Duration of Action 24 hours

Half-life Elimination ~36 hours, prolonged in elderly or with renal impairment; End-stage renal disease: 50-200 hours

Time to Peak Serum: 2-4 hours

Pregnancy Risk Factor C

Chlorthalidone (klor THAL i done)

Related Information

Cardiovascular Diseases *on page 1848*

U.S. Brand Names Thalitone®

Canadian Brand Names Apo-Chlorthalidone®

Pharmacologic Category Diuretic, Thiazide

Use Management of mild-to-moderate hypertension when used alone or in combination with other agents; treatment of edema associated with heart failure or nephrotic syndrome. Recent studies have found chlorthalidone effective in the treatment of isolated systolic hypertension in the elderly.

Unlabeled/Investigational Use Pediatric hypertension

Local Anesthetic/Vasoconstrictor Precautions No information available to require special precautions

Effects on Dental Treatment No significant effects or complications reported

Effects on Bleeding No information available to require special precautions

Adverse Effects 1% to 10%:

Dermatologic: Photosensitivity

Endocrine & metabolic: Hypokalemia

Gastrointestinal: Anorexia, epigastric distress

General Dosage Range Oral:

Adults: 12.5-100 mg/day **or** 100 mg 3 times/week (maximum: 200 mg/day)

Elderly: Initial: 12.5-25 mg/day or every other day

Mechanism of Action Sulfonamide-derived diuretic that inhibits sodium and chloride reabsorption in the cortical-diluting segment of the ascending loop of Henle

Pharmacodynamics/Kinetics

Onset of Action Peak effect: 2-6 hours

Duration of Action 24-72 hours

Half-life Elimination 40-60 hours; may be prolonged with renal impairment; Anuria: 81 hours

Pregnancy Risk Factor B

Chlorzoxazone (klor ZOKS a zone)

Related Information

Temporomandibular Dysfunction (TMD) *on page 1964*

U.S. Brand Names Parafon Forte® DSC

Canadian Brand Names Parafon Forte®; Strifon Forte®

Generic Availability (U.S.) Yes

Pharmacologic Category Skeletal Muscle Relaxant

Dental Use Treatment of muscle spasm and pain associated with acute temporomandibular joint pain (TMJ)

Use Symptomatic treatment of muscle spasm and pain associated with acute musculoskeletal conditions

Local Anesthetic/Vasoconstrictor Precautions No information available to require special precautions

Effects on Dental Treatment No significant effects or complications reported

Effects on Bleeding No information available to require special precautions

Adverse Effects Frequency not defined.

Central nervous system: Dizziness, drowsiness lightheadedness, paradoxical stimulation, malaise

Dermatologic: Rash, petechiae, ecchymoses (rare), angioneurotic edema

Gastrointestinal: Nausea, vomiting, stomach cramps

Genitourinary: Urine discoloration

Hepatic: Liver dysfunction

Miscellaneous: Anaphylaxis (very rare)

Dental Usual Dosage Treatment of muscle spasm and pain associated with acute TMJ pain: Oral:

Children: 20 mg/kg/day or 600 mg/m^2/day in 3-4 divided doses

Adults: 250-500 mg 3-4 times/day up to 750 mg 3-4 times/day

Dosage Oral:

Children: 20 mg/kg/day or 600 mg/m^2/day in 3-4 divided doses

Adults: 250-500 mg 3-4 times/day up to 750 mg 3-4 times/day

Mechanism of Action Acts on the spinal cord and subcortical levels by depressing polysynaptic reflexes

Contraindications Hypersensitivity to chlorzoxazone or any component of the formulation; impaired liver function

Warnings/Precautions This class of medication is poorly tolerated by the elderly due to anticholinergic effects, sedation, and weakness. Efficacy is questionable at dosages tolerated by elderly patients (Beers Criteria).

Drug Interactions

Metabolism/Transport Effects Substrate of CYP1A2 (minor), 2A6 (minor), 2D6 (minor), 2E1 (major), 3A4 (minor); **Inhibits** CYP2E1 (weak), 3A4 (weak)

Avoid Concomitant Use There are no known interactions where it is recommended to avoid concomitant use.

Increased Effect/Toxicity

Chlorzoxazone may increase the levels/effects of: Alcohol (Ethyl); CNS Depressants; Methotrimeprazine

The levels/effects of Chlorzoxazone may be increased by: Conivaptan; Disulfiram; Droperidol; Isoniazid; Methotrimeprazine

Decreased Effect

The levels/effects of Chlorzoxazone may be decreased by: Peginterferon Alfa-2b; Tocilizumab

Ethanol/Nutrition/Herb Interactions Ethanol: May increase CNS depression; monitor for increased effects with coadministration. Caution patients about effects.

Pharmacodynamics/Kinetics

Onset of Action ~1 hour

Duration of Action 6-12 hours

Pregnancy Risk Factor C

Lactation Excretion in breast milk unknown/not recommended

Dosage Forms

Caplet, oral:

Parafon Forte® DSC: 500 mg

Tablet, oral: 500 mg

Cholecalciferol (kole e kal SI fer ole)

U.S. Brand Names Bio-D-Mulsion Forte® [OTC]; Bio-D-Mulsion® [OTC]; D-3 [OTC]; D3-50™ [OTC]; D3-5™ [OTC]; DDrops®; DDrops® Baby [OTC]; DDrops® Kids [OTC]; DDrops® [OTC]; Delta® D3 [OTC]; Enfamil® D-Vi-Sol™ [OTC]; Maximum D3® [OTC]; Vitamin D3 [OTC]

Canadian Brand Names D-Vi-Sol®

Pharmacologic Category Vitamin D Analog

Use Dietary supplement, treatment of vitamin D deficiency, or prophylaxis of deficiency

Local Anesthetic/Vasoconstrictor Precautions No information available to require special precautions

Effects on Dental Treatment Key adverse event(s) related to dental treatment: Metallic taste and xerostomia (normal salivary flow resumes upon discontinuation).

Effects on Bleeding No information available to require special precautions

Adverse Effects Frequency not defined: Endocrine & metabolic: Hypervitaminosis D (signs and symptoms include hypercalcemia, resulting in headache, nausea, vomiting, lethargy, confusion, sluggishness, abdominal pain, bone pain, polyuria, polydipsia, weakness, cardiac arrhythmias [eg, QT shortening, sinus tachycardia], soft tissue calcification, calciuria, and nephrocalcinosis)

General Dosage Range Oral: *Adults:* 200-1000 units/day

Pharmacodynamics/Kinetics

Half-life Elimination 14 hours

Time to Peak 11 hours

Pregnancy Risk Factor C

Cholestyramine Resin (koe LES teer a meen REZ in)

Related Information

Cardiovascular Diseases *on page* 1848

U.S. Brand Names Prevalite®; Questran®; Questran® Light

Canadian Brand Names Novo-Cholamine; Novo-Cholamine Light; Olestyr; PMS-Cholestyramine; Questran®; Questran® Light Sugar Free; ZYM-Cholestyramine-Light; ZYM-Cholestyramine-Regular

Pharmacologic Category Antilipemic Agent, Bile Acid Sequestrant

Use Adjunct in the management of primary hypercholesterolemia; pruritus associated with elevated levels of bile acids; diarrhea associated with excess fecal bile acids; binding toxicologic agents; pseudomembraneous colitis

Local Anesthetic/Vasoconstrictor Precautions No information available to require special precautions

Effects on Dental Treatment No significant effects or complications reported

Effects on Bleeding Although chronic use at high dosages may be associated with bleeding problems, there is no information available to require routine special precautions in patients receiving this medication. The possibility of delayed coagulation should be anticipated.

Adverse Effects

>10%: Gastrointestinal: Constipation, heartburn, nausea, vomiting, stomach pain

1% to 10%:

Central nervous system: Headache

Gastrointestinal: Belching, bloating, diarrhea

General Dosage Range Oral:

Children: 240 mg/kg/day in 3 divided doses

Adults: 4-24 g/day in 1-6 divided doses

Mechanism of Action Forms a nonabsorbable complex with bile acids in the intestine, releasing chloride ions in the process; inhibits enterohepatic reuptake of intestinal bile salts and thereby increases the fecal loss of bile salt-bound low density lipoprotein cholesterol

Pharmacodynamics/Kinetics

Onset of Action Peak effect: 21 days

Pregnancy Risk Factor C

Choline Magnesium Trisalicylate

(KOE leen mag NEE zhum trye sa LIS i late)

Related Information

Rheumatoid Arthritis, Osteoarthritis, and Osteoporosis *on page* 1889

Temporomandibular Dysfunction (TMD) *on page* 1964

Generic Availability (U.S.) Yes

Pharmacologic Category Salicylate

Use Management of osteoarthritis, rheumatoid arthritis, and other arthritis; acute painful shoulder

Local Anesthetic/Vasoconstrictor Precautions No information available to require special precautions

Effects on Dental Treatment The dentist should be aware of the potential of abnormal coagulation. Caution should also be exercised in the use of NSAIDs in patients already on anticoagulant therapy with drugs such as warfarin (Coumadin®). See Effects on Bleeding.

Effects on Bleeding Nonacetylated salicylate formulations are known to reversibly decrease platelet aggregation via mechanisms different than observed with aspirin. Platelet function is restored as the drug is eliminated from the body. The dentist should be aware of the potential of abnormal coagulation. Caution should also be exercised in the use of NSAIDs in patients already on anticoagulant therapy with drugs such as warfarin (Coumadin®).

With respect to surgery, dental practitioners should note that recommendations differ between general surgery (eg, appendectomy, hip replacement) and dental surgery. NSAIDs should be avoided (if possible) in general surgery patients for 3-5 half-lives of the drug (usually 1-3 days) prior to surgery to reduce the risk of excessive bleeding. However, there is no scientific evidence to warrant discontinuance of NSAIDs prior to dental surgery. In medically complicated patients or extensive oral surgery, the decision to interrupt therapy must be based on the risk to benefit in an individual patient and a medical consult is suggested. Routine interruption of NSAID therapy for most dental procedures is not warranted. If therapy is continued without interruption, the clinician should anticipate the potential for slower clotting times.

Adverse Effects

<20%:

Gastrointestinal: Nausea, vomiting, diarrhea, heartburn, dyspepsia, epigastric pain, constipation

Otic: Tinnitus

<2%:

Central nervous system: Headache, lightheadedness, dizziness, drowsiness, lethargy

Otic: Hearing impairment

Dosage Oral (based on total salicylate content):

Children <37 kg: 50 mg/kg/day given in 2 divided doses; 2250 mg/day for heavier children

Adults: 500 mg to 1.5 g 2-3 times/day **or** 3 g at bedtime; usual maintenance dose: 1-4.5 g/day

Elderly: 750 mg 3 times/day

Dosing adjustment/comments in renal impairment: Avoid use in severe renal impairment

Mechanism of Action Weakly inhibits cyclooxygenase enzymes, which results in decreased formation of prostaglandin precursors; antipyretic, analgesic, and anti-inflammatory properties.

Other proposed mechanisms not fully elucidated (and possibly contributing to the anti-inflammatory effect to varying degrees) include inhibiting chemotaxis, altering lymphocyte activity, inhibiting neutrophil aggregation/activation, and decreasing proinflammatory cytokine levels.

Contraindications Hypersensitivity to salicylates, other nonacetylated salicylates, other NSAIDs, or any component of the formulation; bleeding disorders; pregnancy (3rd trimester)

Warnings/Precautions Salicylate salts may not inhibit platelet aggregation and, therefore, should not be substituted for aspirin in the prophylaxis of thrombosis. Use with caution in patients with impaired hepatic or renal function, dehydration, erosive gastritis, asthma, or peptic ulcer. Children and teenagers who have or are recovering from chickenpox or flu-like symptoms should not use this product. Changes in behavior (along with nausea and vomiting) may be an early sign of Reye's syndrome; patients should be instructed to contact their healthcare provider if these occur.

Elderly are a high-risk population for adverse effects from NSAIDs. As many as 60% of elderly can develop peptic ulceration and/or hemorrhage asymptomatically. Use lowest effective dose for shortest period possible. Tinnitus or impaired hearing may indicate toxicity. Tinnitus may be a difficult and unreliable indication of toxicity due to age-related hearing loss or eighth cranial nerve damage. CNS adverse effects may be observed in the elderly at lower doses than younger adults.

Drug Interactions

Avoid Concomitant Use

Avoid concomitant use of Choline Magnesium Trisalicylate with any of the following: Influenza Virus Vaccine (Live/Attenuated)

Increased Effect/Toxicity

Choline Magnesium Trisalicylate may increase the levels/effects of: Anticoagulants; Carbonic Anhydrase Inhibitors; Corticosteroids (Systemic); Divalproex; Drotrecogin Alfa; Methotrexate; PRALAtrexate; Salicylates; Sulfonylureas; Thrombolytic Agents; Valproic Acid; Varicella Virus-Containing Vaccines; Vitamin K Antagonists

The levels/effects of Choline Magnesium Trisalicylate may be increased by: Antiplatelet Agents; Calcium Channel Blockers (Nondihydropyridine); Ginkgo Biloba; Herbs (Anticoagulant/Antiplatelet Properties); Influenza Virus Vaccine (Live/Attenuated); Loop Diuretics; Treprostinil

Decreased Effect

Choline Magnesium Trisalicylate may decrease the levels/effects of: ACE Inhibitors; Loop Diuretics; Probenecid

The levels/effects of Choline Magnesium Trisalicylate may be decreased by: Corticosteroids (Systemic)

Ethanol/Nutrition/Herb Interactions

Ethanol: Avoid ethanol (may enhance gastric mucosal irritation).

Food: May decrease the rate but not the extent of oral absorption.

Herb/Nutraceutical: Avoid cat's claw, dong quai, evening primrose, feverfew, garlic, ginger, ginkgo, red clover, horse chestnut, green tea, ginseng (all have additional antiplatelet activity). Limit curry powder, paprika, licorice, Benedictine liqueur, prunes, raisins, tea, and gherkins; may cause salicylate accumulation. These foods contain 6 mg salicylate/100 g.

Dietary Considerations Take with food or large volume of water or milk to minimize GI upset. Liquid may be mixed with fruit juice just before drinking. Hypermagnesemia resulting from magnesium salicylate; avoid or use with caution in renal insufficiency.

Pharmacodynamics/Kinetics

Onset of Action Peak effect: ~2 hours

Half-life Elimination Dose dependent: Low dose: 2-3 hours; High dose: 30 hours

Time to Peak Serum: ~2 hours

Pregnancy Risk Factor C/D (3rd trimester)

Lactation Enters breast milk/use caution

Breast-Feeding Considerations Excreted in breast milk; peak levels occur 9-12 hours after dose. Use caution if used during breast-feeding.

Dosage Forms

Liquid, oral: 500 mg/5 mL (240 mL)

Chorionic Gonadotropin (Human)

(kor ee ON ik goe NAD oh troe pin, HYU man)

Related Information

Chorionic Gonadotropin (Recombinant) *on page 378*

U.S. Brand Names Novarel®; Pregnyl®

Canadian Brand Names Chorionic Gonadotropin for Injection; Pregnyl®

Pharmacologic Category Gonadotropin; Ovulation Stimulator

Use Induces ovulation and pregnancy in anovulatory, infertile females; treatment of hypogonadotropic hypogonadism, prepubertal cryptorchidism; spermatogenesis induction with follitropin alfa

Local Anesthetic/Vasoconstrictor Precautions No information available to require special precautions

Effects on Dental Treatment No significant effects or complications reported

Effects on Bleeding No information available to require special precautions

Adverse Effects Frequency not always defined.

Cardiovascular: Edema

Central nervous system: Depression, fatigue, headache, irritability, restlessness

Endocrine & metabolic: Gynecomastia, precocious puberty

Local: Injection site reaction, pain at injection site

Miscellaneous: Hypersensitivity reaction (local or systemic)

General Dosage Range I.M.:

Children: Dosage varies greatly depending on indication

Adults (females): 5000-10,000 units 1 day following last dose of menotropins

Adults (males): 1000-2000 units 2-3 times/week

Mechanism of Action Luteinizing hormone obtained from the urine of pregnant women. Stimulates production of gonadal steroid hormones by causing production of androgen by the testes; as a substitute for luteinizing hormone (LH) to stimulate ovulation

Pharmacodynamics/Kinetics

Half-life Elimination Biphasic: Initial: 11 hours; Terminal: 23 hours

Pregnancy Risk Factor X

Chorionic Gonadotropin (Recombinant)

(kor ee ON ik goe NAD oh troe pin ree KOM be nant)

Related Information

Chorionic Gonadotropin (Human) *on page 377*

U.S. Brand Names Ovidrel®

Canadian Brand Names Ovidrel®

Pharmacologic Category Gonadotropin; Ovulation Stimulator

Use As part of an assisted reproductive technology (ART) program, induces ovulation in infertile females who have been pretreated with follicle stimulating hormones (FSH); induces ovulation and pregnancy in infertile females when the cause of infertility is functional

Local Anesthetic/Vasoconstrictor Precautions No information available to require special precautions

Effects on Dental Treatment No significant effects or complications reported

Effects on Bleeding No information available to require special precautions

Adverse Effects

2% to 10%:

Endocrine & metabolic: Ovarian cyst (3%), ovarian hyperstimulation (<2% to 3%)

Gastrointestinal: Abdominal pain (3% to 4%), nausea (3%), vomiting (3%)

Local: Injection site: Pain (8%), bruising (3% to 5%), reaction (<2% to 3%), inflammation (<2% to 2%)

Miscellaneous: Postoperative pain (5%)

<2%:

Cardiovascular: Cardiac arrhythmia, heart murmur

Central nervous system: Dizziness, emotional lability, fever, headache, insomnia, malaise

Dermatologic: Pruritus, rash

Endocrine & metabolic: Breast pain, hot flashes, hyperglycemia, intermenstrual bleeding, vaginal hemorrhage

Gastrointestinal: Abdominal enlargement, diarrhea, flatulence

Genitourinary: Cervical carcinoma, cervical lesion, dysuria, genital herpes, genital moniliasis, leukorrhea, urinary incontinence, urinary tract infection, vaginal discomfort, vaginal hemorrhage, vaginitis

Hematologic: Leukocytosis

Neuromuscular & skeletal: Back pain, paresthesia

Renal: Albuminuria

Respiratory: Cough, pharyngitis, upper respiratory tract infection

Miscellaneous: Ectopic pregnancy, hiccups

In addition, the following have been reported with menotropin therapy: Adnexal torsion, hemoperitoneum, mild-to-moderate ovarian enlargement, pulmonary and vascular complications. Ovarian neoplasms have also been reported (rare) with multiple drug regimens used for ovarian induction (relationship not established).

General Dosage Range SubQ: *Adults (female):* 250 mcg given 1 day following last dose of follicle stimulating agent
Mechanism of Action Luteinizing hormone analogue produced by recombinant DNA techniques; stimulates late follicular maturation and intitates rupture of the ovarian follicle once follicular development has occurred
Pharmacodynamics/Kinetics
Half-life Elimination Initial: 4 hours; Terminal: 29 hours
Time to Peak 12-24 hours
Pregnancy Risk Factor X

Ciclesonide (Oral Inhalation) (sye KLES oh nide)

U.S. Brand Names Alvesco®
Canadian Brand Names Alvesco®
Generic Availability (U.S.) No
Pharmacologic Category Corticosteroid, Inhalant (Oral)
Use Prophylactic management of bronchial asthma
Local Anesthetic/Vasoconstrictor Precautions No information available to require special precautions
Effects on Dental Treatment No significant effects or complications reported
Effects on Bleeding No information available to require special precautions
Adverse Effects
>10%:
Central nervous system: Headache (≤11%)
Respiratory: Nasopharyngitis (≤11%)
1% to 10%:
Cardiovascular: Facial edema (≥3%)
Central nervous system: Dizziness (≥3%), fatigue (≥3%), dysphonia (1%)
Dermatologic: Urticaria (≥3%)
Gastrointestinal: Gastroenteritis (≥3%), oral candidiasis (≥3%)
Neuromuscular & skeletal: Arthralgia (≤4%), musculoskeletal chest pain (≥3%), back pain (≥3%), extremity pain (≥3%)
Ocular: Conjunctivitis (≥3%)
Otic: Ear pain (2%)
Respiratory: Upper respiratory infection (≤9%), epistaxis (≤8%), nasal congestion (≤6%), sinusitis (≤6%), pharyngolaryngeal pain (≤ 5%), hoarseness (≥3%), pneumonia (≥3%), paradoxical bronchospasm (2%)
Miscellaneous: Influenza (≥3%)
Dosage Oral inhalation (Alvesco®):
Asthma: **Note:** Titrate to the lowest effective dose once asthma stability is achieved:
U.S. labeling: Children ≥12 years and Adults:
Prior therapy with bronchodilators alone: Initial: 80 mcg twice daily (maximum dose: 320 mcg/day)
Prior therapy with inhaled corticosteroids: Initial: 80 mcg twice daily (maximum dose: 640 mcg/day)
Prior therapy with oral corticosteroids: Initial: 320 mcg twice daily (maximum dose: 640 mcg/day)
Canadian labeling:
Children 6-11 years: Initial: 100-200 mcg once daily; maintenance: 100-200 mcg/day (1-2 puffs once daily)
Children ≥12 years and Adults: Initial: 400 mcg once daily; maintenance: 100-800 mcg/day (1-2 puffs once or twice daily)

Conversion from oral to inhaled steroid: Initiation of oral inhalation therapy should begin in patients who have previously been stabilized on oral corticosteroids (OCS). A gradual dose reduction of OCS should begin ~7-10 days after starting inhaled therapy. U.S. labeling recommends reducing prednisone dose no more rapidly than ≤2.5 mg/day on a weekly basis. The Canadian labeling recommends decreasing the daily dose of prednisone by 1 mg (or equivalent of other OCS) every 7 days in closely monitored patients, and every 10 days in patients whom close monitoring is not possible. In the presence of withdrawal symptoms, resume previous OCS dose for 1 week before attempting further dose reductions.
Mechanism of Action Ciclesonide is a nonhalogenated, glucocorticoid prodrug that is hydrolyzed to the pharmacologically active metabolite des-ciclesonide following administration. Des-ciclesonide has a high affinity for the glucocorticoid receptor and exhibits anti-inflammatory activity. The mechanism of action for corticosteroids is believed to be a combination of three important properties – anti-inflammatory activity, immunosuppressive properties, and antiproliferative actions.
Contraindications Hypersensitivity to ciclesonide or any component of the formulation; primary treatment of acute asthma or status asthmaticus; moderate-to-severe bronchiectasis

Canadian labeling: Additional contraindications (not in U.S. labeling): Untreated fungal, bacterial, or tuberculosis infections of the respiratory tract; moderate-to-severe bronchiectasis

Warnings/Precautions May cause hypercorticism or suppression of hypothalamic-pituitary-adrenal (HPA) axis, particularly in younger children or in patients receiving high doses for prolonged periods. HPA axis suppression may lead to adrenal crisis. Withdrawal and discontinuation of a corticosteroid should be done slowly and carefully. Particular care is required when patients are transferred from systemic corticosteroids to inhaled products due to possible adrenal insufficiency or withdrawal from steroids, including an increase in allergic symptoms. Patients receiving >20 mg per day of prednisone (or equivalent) may be most susceptible. Fatalities have occurred due to adrenal insufficiency in asthmatic patients during and after transfer from systemic corticosteroids to aerosol steroids; aerosol steroids do **not** provide the systemic steroid needed to treat patients having trauma, surgery, or infections.

Bronchospasm may occur with wheezing after inhalation; if this occurs stop steroid and treat with a fast-acting bronchodilator. Supplemental steroids (oral or parenteral) may be needed during stress or severe asthma attacks. Not to be used in status asthmaticus or for the relief of acute bronchospasm. Oropharyngeal thrush due to candida albicans infection may occur with use. Prolonged use of corticosteroids may also increase the incidence of secondary infection, mask acute infection (including fungal infections), prolong or exacerbate viral infections, or limit response to vaccines. Exposure to chickenpox and measles should be avoided; corticosteroids should not be used to treat ocular herpes simplex. Close observation is required in patients with latent tuberculosis and/or TB reactivity; restrict use in active TB (only in conjunction with antituberculosis treatment). Use in patients with TB is contraindicated in the Canadian labeling. Prolonged treatment with corticosteroids has been associated with the development of Kaposi's sarcoma (case reports); if noted, discontinuation of therapy should be considered.

Use with caution in patients with thyroid disease, severe hepatic impairment, glaucoma, cataracts, patients at risk for osteoporosis, and patients at risk for seizures.

Orally inhaled corticosteroids may cause a reduction in growth velocity in pediatric patients (~1 cm per year [range: 0.3-1.8 cm per year] and related to dose and duration of exposure). To minimize the systemic effects of orally inhaled corticosteroids, each patient should be titrated to the lowest effective dose. Growth should be routinely monitored in pediatric patients.

Drug Interactions

Metabolism/Transport Effects Substrate of CYP3A4 (major), 2D6 (minor)

Avoid Concomitant Use

Avoid concomitant use of Ciclesonide (Oral Inhalation) with any of the following: Aldesleukin

Increased Effect/Toxicity

Ciclesonide (Oral Inhalation) may increase the levels/effects of: Deferasirox

The levels/effects of Ciclesonide (Oral Inhalation) may be increased by: CYP3A4 Inhibitors (Moderate); Dasatinib

Decreased Effect

Ciclesonide (Oral Inhalation) may decrease the levels/effects of: Aldesleukin; Corticorelin

The levels/effects of Ciclesonide (Oral Inhalation) may be decreased by: Tocilizumab

Pharmacodynamics/Kinetics

Half-life Elimination ~5-7 hours

Time to Peak ~1 hour (active metabolite)

Pregnancy Risk Factor C

Lactation Excretion in breast milk unknown/use caution

Dosage Forms

Aerosol, for oral inhalation:

Alvesco®: 80 mcg/inhalation (6.1 g); 160 mcg/inhalation (6.1 g)

Dosage Forms: Canada

Aerosol for oral inhalation:

Alvesco®: 50 mcg/inhalation; 100 mcg/inhalation; 200 mcg/inhalation

Ciclesonide (Nasal) (sye KLES oh nide)

U.S. Brand Names Omnaris™

Canadian Brand Names Omnaris™

Pharmacologic Category Corticosteroid, Nasal

Use Management of seasonal and perennial allergic rhinitis

Local Anesthetic/Vasoconstrictor Precautions No information available to require special precautions

Effects on Dental Treatment No significant effects or complications reported

Effects on Bleeding No information available to require special precautions

Adverse Effects

>10%:

Central nervous system: Headache (≤11%)

Respiratory: Nasopharyngitis (≤11%)

1% to 10%:

Central nervous system: Dysphonia (1%)

Respiratory: Upper respiratory infection (≤9%), epistaxis (≤8%), nasal congestion (≤6%), sinusitis (≤6%), pharyngolaryngeal pain (≤5%), hoarseness (≥3%), pneumonia (≥3%), paradoxical bronchospasm (2%)

Miscellaneous: Influenza (≥3%)

General Dosage Range Intranasal: *Children ≥6 years and Adults:* 2 sprays (50 mcg/spray) per nostril once daily (maximum: 200 mcg/day)

Pharmacodynamics/Kinetics

Onset of Action 24-48 hours; further improvement observed over 1-2 weeks in seasonal allergic rhinitis or 5 weeks in perennial allergic rhinitis

Pregnancy Risk Factor C

Ciclopirox (sye kloe PEER oks)

U.S. Brand Names Loprox®; Penlac®

Canadian Brand Names Loprox®; Penlac®; Stieprox®

Pharmacologic Category Antifungal Agent, Topical

Use

Cream/suspension: Treatment of tinea pedis (athlete's foot), tinea cruris (jock itch), tinea corporis (ringworm), cutaneous candidiasis, and tinea versicolor (pityriasis)

Gel: Treatment of tinea pedis (athlete's foot), tinea corporis (ringworm); seborrheic dermatitis of the scalp

Lacquer (solution): Topical treatment of mild-to-moderate onychomycosis of the fingernails and toenails due to *Trichophyton rubrum* (not involving the lunula) and the immediately-adjacent skin

Shampoo: Treatment of seborrheic dermatitis of the scalp

Local Anesthetic/Vasoconstrictor Precautions No information available to require special precautions

Effects on Dental Treatment No significant effects or complications reported

Effects on Bleeding No information available to require special precautions

Adverse Effects

Central nervous system: Headache

Dermatologic: Alopecia, dry skin, erythema, facial edema, hair discoloration (rare; shampoo formulation in light-haired individuals), nail disorder (shape or color change with lacquer), pruritus, rash

Local: Burning sensation (gel: 34%; ≤1% with other forms), irritation, redness, or pain

General Dosage Range Topical:

Cream/suspension: *Children >10 years and Adults:* Apply twice daily

Gel: *Children >16 years and Adults:* Apply twice daily

Lacquer: *Children ≥12 years and Adults:* Apply to adjacent skin and affected nails daily; remove with alcohol every 7 days

Shampoo: *Children >16 years and Adults:* Apply 5-10 mL to wet hair, lather, and leave in place ~3 minutes, rinse; repeat twice weekly (allow minimum of 3 days between applications)

Mechanism of Action Inhibiting transport of essential elements in the fungal cell disrupting the synthesis of DNA, RNA, and protein

Pharmacodynamics/Kinetics

Half-life Elimination Biologic: 1.7 hours (suspension); elimination: 5.5 hours (gel)

Pregnancy Risk Factor B

Cidofovir (si DOF o veer)

Related Information

Systemic Viral Diseases *on page 1904*

U.S. Brand Names Vistide®

Pharmacologic Category Antiviral Agent

Use Treatment of cytomegalovirus (CMV) retinitis in patients with acquired immunodeficiency syndrome (AIDS). **Note:** Should be administered with probenecid.

Local Anesthetic/Vasoconstrictor Precautions No information available to require special precautions

Effects on Dental Treatment Key adverse event(s) related to dental treatment: Stomatitis and abnormal taste.

Effects on Bleeding No information available to require special precautions relative to altered hemostasis.

Adverse Effects

>10%:

Central nervous system: Chills, fever, headache, pain
Dermatologic: Alopecia, rash
Gastrointestinal: Nausea, vomiting, diarrhea, anorexia
Hematologic: Anemia, neutropenia
Neuromuscular & skeletal: Weakness
Ocular: Intraocular pressure decreased, iritis, ocular hypotony, uveitis
Renal: Creatinine increased, proteinuria, renal toxicity
Respiratory: Cough, dyspnea
Miscellaneous: Infection, oral moniliasis, serum bicarbonate decreased

1% to 10%:

Renal: Fanconi syndrome
Respiratory: Pneumonia

Frequency not defined (limited to important or life-threatening reactions):

Cardiovascular: Cardiomyopathy, cardiovascular disorder, CHF, edema, postural hypotension, shock, syncope, tachycardia
Central nervous system: Agitation, amnesia, anxiety, confusion, convulsion, dizziness, hallucinations, insomnia, malaise, vertigo
Dermatologic: Photosensitivity reaction, skin discoloration, urticaria
Endocrine & metabolic: Adrenal cortex insufficiency
Gastrointestinal: Abdominal pain, aphthous stomatitis, colitis, constipation, dysphagia, fecal incontinence, gastritis, GI hemorrhage, gingivitis, melena, proctitis, splenomegaly, stomatitis, tongue discoloration
Genitourinary: Urinary incontinence
Hematologic: Hypochromic anemia, leukocytosis, leukopenia, lymphadenopathy, lymphoma-like reaction, pancytopenia, thrombocytopenia, thrombocytopenic purpura
Hepatic: Hepatomegaly, hepatosplenomegaly, jaundice, liver function tests abnormal, liver damage, liver necrosis
Local: Injection site reaction
Neuromuscular & skeletal: Tremor
Ocular: Amblyopia, blindness, cataract, conjunctivitis, corneal lesion, diplopia, vision abnormal
Otic: Hearing loss
Miscellaneous: Allergic reaction, sepsis

General Dosage Range Dosage adjustment recommended in patients with renal impairment

I.V.: *Adults:* Induction: 5 mg/kg once weekly for 2 consecutive weeks; Maintenance: 5 mg/kg once every 2 weeks

Mechanism of Action Cidofovir is converted to cidofovir diphosphate which is the active intracellular metabolite; cidofovir diphosphate suppresses CMV replication by selective inhibition of viral DNA synthesis. Incorporation of cidofovir into growing viral DNA chain results in reductions in the rate of viral DNA synthesis.

Pharmacodynamics/Kinetics

Half-life Elimination Plasma: ~2.6 hours

Pregnancy Risk Factor C

Cilazapril (sye LAY za pril)

Canadian Brand Names Apo-Cilazapril®; CO Cilazapril; Inhibace®; Mylan-Cilazapril; Novo-Cilazapril; PHL-Cilazapril; PMS-Cilazapril

Pharmacologic Category Angiotensin-Converting Enzyme (ACE) Inhibitor

Use Management of hypertension; treatment of heart failure

Local Anesthetic/Vasoconstrictor Precautions No information available to require special precautions

Effects on Dental Treatment Key adverse event(s) related to dental treatment: Orthostatic hypotension.

Effects on Bleeding No information available to require special precautions

Adverse Effects 1% to 10%:

Cardiovascular: Palpitation (up to 1%), hypotension (symptomatic, up to 1% in CHF patients), orthostatic hypotension (2%)
Central nervous system: Headache (3% to 5%), dizziness (3% to 8%), fatigue (2% to 3%)

Gastrointestinal: Nausea (1% to 3%)
Neuromuscular & skeletal: Weakness (0.3% to 2%)
Renal: Serum creatinine increased
Respiratory: Cough (2% in hypertension, up to 7.5% in CHF patients)

General Dosage Range Dosage adjustment recommended in patients with hepatic or renal impairment

Oral:

Adults: Initial: 0.5-5 mg once daily (maximum: 2.5 mg/day [CHF]; 10 mg/day [HTN])

Elderly: Initial: 1.25 mg once daily

Mechanism of Action Competitive inhibitor of angiotensin-converting enzyme (ACE); prevents conversion of angiotensin I to angiotensin II, a potent vasoconstrictor; results in lower levels of angiotensin II which causes an increase in plasma renin activity and a reduction in aldosterone secretion.

Pharmacodynamics/Kinetics

Onset of Action Antihypertensive: ~1 hour

Duration of Action Therapeutic effect: 24 hours

Half-life Elimination Cilazaprilat: Terminal: 36-49 hours

Time to Peak 3-7 hours

Product Availability Not available in U.S.

Cilazapril and Hydrochlorothiazide

(sye LAY za pril & hye droe klor oh THYE a zide)

Related Information

Cilazapril *on page 382*
Hydrochlorothiazide *on page 854*

Canadian Brand Names Apo-Cilazapril®/Hctz; Inhibace® Plus; Novo-Cilazapril/HCTZ

Pharmacologic Category Angiotensin-Converting Enzyme (ACE) Inhibitor; Diuretic, Thiazide

Use Treatment of mild-to-moderate hypertension in patients who have been stabilized on the individual agents given in the same proportions; not indicated for initial treatment of hypertension

Local Anesthetic/Vasoconstrictor Precautions No information available to require special precautions

Effects on Dental Treatment Key adverse event(s) related to dental treatment: Orthostatic hypotension.

Effects on Bleeding No information available to require special precautions

Adverse Effects 1% to 10%:

Cardiovascular: Palpitation (1%)
Central nervous system: Dizziness (4%), fatigue (3%), somnolence (1%)
Gastrointestinal: Nausea (1%)
Genitourinary: Polyuria (1%)
Hematologic: Transient neutropenia (1%)
Hepatic: Transaminases increased (≤1%)
Respiratory: Cough (3%)

General Dosage Range Oral: *Adults:* 1 tablet (cilazapril 5 mg/hydrochlorothiazide 12.5 mg) once daily

Product Availability Not available in U.S.

Cilostazol (sil OH sta zol)

U.S. Brand Names Pletal®

Pharmacologic Category Antiplatelet Agent; Phosphodiesterase Enzyme Inhibitor

Use Symptomatic management of peripheral vascular disease, primarily intermittent claudication

Unlabeled/Investigational Use Adjunct with aspirin and clopidogrel for prevention of stent thrombosis and restenosis after coronary stent placement

Local Anesthetic/Vasoconstrictor Precautions No information available to require special precautions

Effects on Dental Treatment No significant effects or complications reported

Effects on Bleeding Cilostazol decreases platelet aggregation but does not increase bleeding times. Prior to elective general surgery, it may be temporarily discontinued (usually for 4 days) to restore platelet function. However, routine interruption of therapy for noninvasive dental procedures is not warranted and there is no scientific evidence to warrant the discontinuance of cilostazol prior to dental surgery.

Adverse Effects
>10%:
Central nervous system: Headache (27% to 34%)
Gastrointestinal: Abnormal stools (12% to 15%), diarrhea (12% to 19%)
Respiratory: Rhinitis (7% to 12%)
Miscellaneous: Infection (10% to 14%)
2% to 10%:
Cardiovascular: Peripheral edema (7% to 9%), palpitation (5% to 10%), tachycardia (4%)
Central nervous system: Dizziness (9% to 10%), vertigo (up to 3%)
Gastrointestinal: Dyspepsia (6%), nausea (6% to 7%), abdominal pain (4% to 5%), flatulence (2% to 3%)
Neuromuscular & skeletal: Back pain (6% to 7%), myalgia (2% to 3%)
Respiratory: Pharyngitis (7% to 10%), cough (3% to 4%)

General Dosage Range Dosage adjustment recommended in patients on concomitant therapy

Oral: *Adults:* 100 mg twice daily

Mechanism of Action Cilostazol and its metabolites are inhibitors of phosphodiesterase III. As a result, cyclic AMP is increased leading to reversible inhibition of platelet aggregation, vasodilation, and inhibition of vascular smooth muscle cell proliferation.

Pharmacodynamics/Kinetics

Onset of Action 2-4 weeks; may require up to 12 weeks

Half-life Elimination 11-13 hours

Pregnancy Risk Factor C

Cimetidine (sye MET i deen)

Related Information
Gastrointestinal Disorders *on page 1874*

U.S. Brand Names Tagamet HB 200® [OTC]

Canadian Brand Names Apo-Cimetidine®; Dom-Cimetidine; Mylan-Cimetidine; Novo-Cimetidine; Nu-Cimet; PMS-Cimetidine; Tagamet® HB

Pharmacologic Category Histamine H_2 Antagonist

Use Short-term treatment of active duodenal ulcers and benign gastric ulcers; maintenance therapy of duodenal ulcer; treatment of gastric hypersecretory states; treatment of gastroesophageal reflux disease (GERD)

OTC labeling: Prevention or relief of heartburn, acid indigestion, or sour stomach

Unlabeled/Investigational Use Part of a multidrug regimen for *H. pylori* eradication to reduce the risk of duodenal ulcer recurrence

Local Anesthetic/Vasoconstrictor Precautions No information available to require special precautions

Effects on Dental Treatment No significant effects or complications reported

Effects on Bleeding No information available to require special precautions

Adverse Effects
1% to 10%:
Central nervous system: Headache (2% to 4%), dizziness (1%), somnolence (1%), agitation
Endocrine & metabolic: Gynecomastia (<1% to 4%)
Gastrointestinal: Diarrhea (1%)
Frequency not defined:
Cardiovascular: AV block, bradycardia, hypotension, tachycardia, vasculitis
Central nervous system: Confusion, fever
Dermatologic: Alopecia, erythema multiforme, exfoliative dermatitis, Stevens-Johnson syndrome, toxic epidermal necrolysis, rash
Endocrine & metabolic: Edema of the breasts, sexual ability decreased
Gastrointestinal: Nausea, pancreatitis, vomiting
Hematologic: Agranulocytosis, aplastic anemia, hemolytic anemia (immune-based), neutropenia, pancytopenia, thrombocytopenia
Hepatic: ALT increased, AST increased, hepatic fibrosis (case report)
Neuromuscular & skeletal: Arthralgia, myalgia, polymyositis
Renal: Creatinine increased, interstitial nephritis
Miscellaneous: Anaphylaxis, pneumonia (causal relationship not established)

General Dosage Range Dosage adjustment recommended in patients with renal impaiment

Oral:
Children <12 years: 20-40 mg/kg/day divided every 6 hours
Children ≥12 years: 20-40 mg/kg/day divided every 6 hours **or** 200 mg 1-2 times/day [OTC]

Adults: 300-600 mg 4 times/day **or** 400-800 mg 1-2 times/day **or** 200 mg 1-2 times/day [OTC]

Mechanism of Action Competitive inhibition of histamine at H_2 receptors of the gastric parietal cells resulting in reduced gastric acid secretion, gastric volume and hydrogen ion concentration reduced

Pharmacodynamics/Kinetics

Onset of Action 1 hour

Duration of Action 80% reduction in gastric acid secretion for 4-5 hours after 300 mg dose

Half-life Elimination Neonates: 3.6 hours; Children: 1.4 hours; Adults: 2 hours

Time to Peak Serum: Oral: 1-2 hours

Pregnancy Risk Factor B

Cinacalcet (sin a KAL cet)

U.S. Brand Names Sensipar®

Canadian Brand Names Sensipar®

Pharmacologic Category Calcimimetic

Use Treatment of secondary hyperparathyroidism in patients with chronic kidney disease (CKD) on dialysis; treatment of hypercalcemia in patients with parathyroid carcinoma; treatment of severe hypercalcemia in patients with primary hyperparathyroidism who are unable to undergo parathyroidectomy

Local Anesthetic/Vasoconstrictor Precautions No information available to require special precautions

Effects on Dental Treatment No significant effects or complications reported

Effects on Bleeding No information available to require special precautions

Adverse Effects

>10%:

Central nervous system: Fatigue (12% to 21%), headache (≤21%), depression (10% to 18%)

Endocrine & metabolic: Hypocalcemia (≤66%), dehydration (≤24%), hypercalcemia (12% to 21%)

Gastrointestinal: Nausea (31% to 66%), vomiting (27% to 52%), diarrhea (≤21%), anorexia (6% to 21%), constipation (10% to 18%)

Hematologic: Anemia (6% to 17%)

Neuromuscular & skeletal: Parasthesia (14% to 29%), fracture (12% to 21%), weakness (7% to 17%), arthralgia (6% to 17%), myalgia (≤15%), limb pain (10% to 12%)

Respiratory: Upper respiratory infection (10% to 12%)

1% to 10%:

Cardiovascular: Hypertension (≤7%)

Central nervous system: Dizziness (≤10%), seizure (1%)

Endocrine & metabolic: Testosterone decreased

Neuromuscular & skeletal: Chest pain (noncardiac; ≤6%)

General Dosage Range Dosage adjustment recommended in patients on concomitant therapy or who develop toxicities

Oral: *Adults:* Initial: 30 mg once or twice daily; Maintenance: Increase dose incrementally every 2-4 weeks to normalize calcium levels or maintain iPTH level (maximum: 360 mg/day [parathyroid cancer, primary hyperparathyroidism]; 180 mg/day [secondary hyperparathyroidism])

Mechanism of Action Increases the sensitivity of the calcium-sensing receptor on the parathyroid gland thereby, concomitantly lowering parathyroid hormone (PTH), serum calcium, and serum phosphorus levels, preventing progressive bone disease and adverse events associated with mineral metabolism disorders.

Pharmacodynamics/Kinetics

Half-life Elimination Terminal: 30-40 hours; moderate hepatic impairment: 65 hours; severe hepatic impairment: 84 hours

Time to Peak ~2-6 hours

Pregnancy Risk Factor C

Ciprofloxacin (Systemic) (sip roe FLOKS a sin)

Related Information

Periodontal Diseases *on page 1942*

Sexually-Transmitted Diseases *on page 1903*

Related Sample Prescriptions

Bacterial Infections and Periodontal Diseases *on page 1983*

U.S. Brand Names Cipro®; Cipro® I.V.; Cipro® XR; Proquin® XR

Canadian Brand Names Apo-Ciproflox®; Cipro®; Cipro® XL; CO Ciprofloxacin; Dom-Ciprofloxacin; Mint-Ciprofloxacin; Mylan-Ciprofloxacin; Novo-Ciprofloxacin; PHL-Ciprofloxacin; PMS-Ciprofloxacin; PRO-Ciprofloxacin; RAN™-Ciprofloxacin; ratio-Ciprofloxacin; Riva-Ciprofloxacin; Sandoz-Ciprofloxacin; Taro-Ciprofloxacin

Generic Availability (U.S.) Yes: Excludes suspension

Pharmacologic Category Antibiotic, Quinolone

Dental Use Useful as a single agent or in combination with metronidazole in the treatment of periodontitis associated with the presence of *Actinobacillus actinomycetemcomitans* (AA), as well as enteric rods/pseudomonads

Use

Children: Complicated urinary tract infections and pyelonephritis due to *E. coli*. **Note:** Although effective, ciprofloxacin is not the drug of first choice in children.

Children and Adults: To reduce incidence or progression of disease following exposure to aerolized *Bacillus anthracis*.

Adults: Treatment of the following infections when caused by susceptible bacteria: Urinary tract infections; acute uncomplicated cystitis in females; chronic bacterial prostatitis; lower respiratory tract infections (including acute exacerbations of chronic bronchitis); acute sinusitis; skin and skin structure infections; bone and joint infections; complicated intra-abdominal infections (in combination with metronidazole); infectious diarrhea; typhoid fever due to *Salmonella typhi* (eradication of chronic typhoid carrier state has not been proven); uncomplicated cervical and urethra gonorrhea (due to *N. gonorrhoeae*); nosocomial pneumonia; empirical therapy for febrile neutropenic patients (in combination with piperacillin)

Note: As of April 2007, the CDC no longer recommends the use of fluoroquinolones for the treatment of gonococcal disease.

Unlabeled/Investigational Use Acute pulmonary exacerbations in cystic fibrosis (children); cutaneous/gastrointestinal/oropharyngeal anthrax (treatment, children and adults); disseminated gonococcal infection (adults); chancroid (adults); prophylaxis to *Neisseria meningitidis* following close contact with an infected person; empirical therapy (oral) for febrile neutropenia in low-risk cancer patients; HACEK group endocarditis; infectious diarrhea (children); periodontitis

Local Anesthetic/Vasoconstrictor Precautions No information available to require special precautions

Effects on Dental Treatment No significant effects or complications reported

Effects on Bleeding No information available to require special precautions

Adverse Effects 1% to 10%:

Central nervous system: Neurologic events (children 2%, includes dizziness, insomnia, nervousness, somnolence); fever (children 2%); headache (I.V. administration); restlessness (I.V. administration)

Dermatologic: Rash (children 2%, adults 1%)

Gastrointestinal: Nausea (3%); diarrhea (children 5%, adults 2%); vomiting (children 5%, adults 1%); abdominal pain (children 3%, adults <1%); dyspepsia (children 3%)

Hepatic: ALT increased, AST increased (adults 1%)

Local: Injection site reactions (I.V. administration)

Respiratory: Rhinitis (children 3%)

Dental Usual Dosage Treatment of periodontitis: Adults: Oral: 500 mg every 12 hours for 8-10 days

Dosage Note: Extended release tablets and immediate release formulations are not interchangeable. Unless otherwise specified, oral dosing reflects the use of immediate release formulations.

Usual dosage ranges:

Children (see Warnings/Precautions):

Oral: 20-30 mg/kg/day in 2 divided doses; maximum dose: 1.5 g/day

I.V.: 20-30 mg/kg/day divided every 12 hours; maximum dose: 800 mg/day

Adults:

Oral: 250-750 mg every 12 hours

I.V.: 200-400 mg every 12 hours

Indication-specific dosing:

Children:

Anthrax:

Inhalational (postexposure prophylaxis):

Oral: 15 mg/kg/dose every 12 hours for 60 days; maximum: 500 mg/dose

I.V.: 10 mg/kg/dose every 12 hours for 60 days; do **not** exceed 400 mg/dose (800 mg/day)

Cutaneous (treatment, CDC guidelines): Oral: 10-15 mg/kg every 12 hours for 60 days (maximum: 1 g/day); amoxicillin 80 mg/kg/day divided every 8 hours is an option for completion of treatment after clinical improvement. **Note:** In the presence of systemic involvement, extensive edema, lesions on head/neck, refer to I.V. dosing for treatment of inhalational/gastrointestinal/oropharyngeal anthrax.

Inhalational/gastrointestinal/oropharyngeal (treatment, CDC guidelines): I.V.: Initial: 10-15 mg/kg every 12 hours for 60 days (maximum: 500 mg/dose); switch to oral therapy when clinically appropriate; refer to adult dosing for notes on combined therapy and duration

Cystic fibrosis (unlabeled use):

Oral: 40 mg/kg/day divided every 12 hours administered following 1 week of I.V. therapy has been reported in a clinical trial; total duration of therapy: 10-21 days

I.V.: 30 mg/kg/day divided every 8 hours for 1 week, followed by oral therapy, has been reported in a clinical trial

Urinary tract infection (complicated) or pyelonephritis:

Oral: 20-30 mg/kg/day in 2 divided doses (every 12 hours) for 10-21 days; maximum: 1.5 g/day

I.V.: 6-10 mg/kg every 8 hours for 10-21 days (maximum: 400 mg/dose)

Adults:

Anthrax:

Inhalational (postexposure prophylaxis):

Oral: 500 mg every 12 hours for 60 days

I.V.: 400 mg every 12 hours for 60 days

Cutaneous (treatment, CDC guidelines): Oral: Immediate release formulation: 500 mg every 12 hours for 60 days. **Note:** In the presence of systemic involvement, extensive edema, lesions on head/neck, refer to I.V. dosing for treatment of inhalational/gastrointestinal/oropharyngeal anthrax

Inhalational/gastrointestinal/oropharyngeal (treatment, CDC guidelines): I.V.: 400 mg every 12 hours. **Note:** Initial treatment should include two or more agents predicted to be effective (per CDC recommendations). Continue combined therapy for 60 days.

Bone/joint infections:

Oral: 500-750 mg twice daily for 4-6 weeks

I.V.: Mild-to-moderate: 400 mg every 12 hours for 4-6 weeks; Severe/complicated: 400 mg every 8 hours for 4-6 weeks

Chancroid (unlabeled use): Oral: 500 mg twice daily for 3 days (CDC, 2010)

Endocarditis due to HACEK organisms (AHA guidelines, unlabeled use): **Note:** Not first-line option; use only if intolerant of beta-lactam therapy:

Oral: 500 mg every 12 hours for 4 weeks

I.V.: 400 mg every 12 hours for 4 weeks

Febrile neutropenia: I.V.: 400 mg every 8 hours for 7-14 days (combination therapy generally recommended)

Gonococcal infections:

Urethral/cervical gonococcal infections: Oral: 250-500 mg as a single dose (CDC recommends concomitant doxycycline or azithromycin due to possible coinfection with *Chlamydia*; **Note:** As of April 2007, the CDC no longer recommends the use of fluoroquinolones for the treatment of uncomplicated gonococcal disease.

Disseminated gonococcal infection (CDC guidelines): Oral: 500 mg twice daily to complete 7 days of therapy (initial treatment with ceftriaxone 1 g I.M./I.V. daily for 24-48 hours after improvement begins); **Note:** As of April 2007, the CDC no longer recommends the use of fluoroquinolones for the treatment of more serious gonococcal disease, unless no other options exist and susceptibility can be confirmed via culture.

Granuloma inguinale (donovanosis) (unlabeled use): Oral: 750 mg twice daily for at least 3 weeks (and until lesions have healed) (CDC, 2010)

Infectious diarrhea: Oral:

Salmonella: 500 mg twice daily for 5-7 days

Shigella: 500 mg twice daily for 3 days

Traveler's diarrhea: Mild: 750 mg for one dose; Severe: 500 mg twice daily for 3 days

Vibrio cholerae: 1 g for one dose

Intra-abdominal, complicated, community-acquired (in combination with metronidazole): **Note:** Avoid using in settings where *E. coli* susceptibility to fluoroquinolones is <90%:

Oral: 500 mg every 12 hours for 7-14 days

I.V.: 400 mg every 12 hours for 7-14 days; **Note:** 2010 IDSA guidelines recommend treatment duration of 4-7 days (provided source controlled)

Lower respiratory tract, skin/skin structure infections:

Oral: 500-750 mg twice daily for 7-14 days

I.V.: Mild-to-moderate: 400 mg every 12 hours for 7-14 days; Severe/complicated: 400 mg every 8 hours for 7-14 days

Nosocomial pneumonia: I.V.: 400 mg every 8 hours for 10-14 days

Periodontitis (unlabeled use): Oral: 500 mg every 12 hours for 8-10 days

Prostatitis (chronic, bacterial): Oral: 500 mg every 12 hours for 28 days

Sinusitis (acute): Oral: 500 mg every 12 hours for 10 days
Typhoid fever: Oral: 500 mg every 12 hours for 10 days
Urinary tract infection:
Acute uncomplicated, cystitis:
Oral:
Immediate release formulation: 250 mg every 12 hours for 3 days
Extended release formulation (Cipro® XR, Proquin® XR): 500 mg every 24 hours for 3 days
I.V.: 200 mg every 12 hours for 7-14 days
Complicated (including pyelonephritis):
Oral:
Immediate release formulation: 500 mg every 12 hours for 7-14 days
Extended release formulation (Cipro® XR): 1000 mg every 24 hours for 7-14 days
I.V.: 400 mg every 12 hours for 7-14 days
Elderly: No adjustment needed in patients with normal renal function

Dosing adjustment in renal impairment: Adults:
Cl_{cr} 30-50 mL/minute: Oral: 250-500 mg every 12 hours
Cl_{cr} <30 mL/minute: Acute uncomplicated pyelonephritis or complicated UTI: Oral: Extended release formulation: 500 mg every 24 hours
Cl_{cr} 5-29 mL/minute:
Oral: 250-500 mg every 18 hours
I.V.: 200-400 mg every 18-24 hours
Dialysis: Only small amounts of ciprofloxacin are removed by hemo- or peritoneal dialysis (<10%); usual dose: Oral: 250-500 mg every 24 hours following dialysis
Continuous renal replacement therapy (CRRT): I.V.:
CVVH: 200 mg every 12 hours
CVVHD or CVVHDF: 200-400 mg every 12 hours

Mechanism of Action Inhibits DNA-gyrase in susceptible organisms; inhibits relaxation of supercoiled DNA and promotes breakage of double-stranded DNA

Contraindications Hypersensitivity to ciprofloxacin, any component of the formulation, or other quinolones; concurrent administration of tizanidine

Warnings/Precautions **[U.S. Boxed Warning]: There have been reports of tendon inflammation and/or rupture with quinolone antibiotics; risk may be increased with concurrent corticosteroids, organ transplant recipients, and in patients >60 years of age.** Rupture of the Achilles tendon sometimes requiring surgical repair has been reported most frequently; but other tendon sites (eg, rotator cuff, biceps) have also been reported. Strenuous physical activity, rheumatoid arthritis, and renal impairment may be an independent risk factor for tendonitis. Discontinue at first sign of tendon inflammation or pain. May occur even after discontinuation of therapy. Use with caution in patients with rheumatoid arthritis; may increase risk of tendon rupture. CNS stimulation may occur (tremor, restlessness, confusion, and very rarely hallucinations or seizures). Use with caution in patients with known or suspected CNS disorder. Potential for seizures, although very rare, may be increased with concomitant NSAID therapy. Use with caution in individuals at risk of seizures. Fluoroquinolones may prolong QT_c interval; avoid use in patients with a history of QT_c prolongation, uncorrected hypokalemia, hypomagnesemia, or concurrent administration of other medications known to prolong the QT interval (including Class Ia and Class III antiarrhythmics, cisapride, erythromycin, antipsychotics, and tricyclic antidepressants). Prolonged use may result in fungal or bacterial superinfection, including *C. difficile*-associated diarrhea (CDAD) and pseudomembranous colitis; CDAD has been observed >2 months postantibiotic treatment. Rarely crystalluria has occurred; urine alkalinity may increase the risk. Ensure adequate hydration during therapy. Adverse effects, including those related to joints and/or surrounding tissues, are increased in pediatric patients and therefore, ciprofloxacin should not be considered as drug of choice in children (exception is anthrax treatment). Rare cases of peripheral neuropathy may occur.

Fluoroquinolones have been associated with the development of serious, and sometimes fatal, hypoglycemia, most often in elderly diabetics but also in patients without diabetes. This occurred most frequently with gatifloxacin (no longer available systemically), but may occur at a lower frequency with other quinolones.

Severe hypersensitivity reactions, including anaphylaxis, have occurred with quinolone therapy. Reactions may present as typical allergic symptoms after a single dose, or may manifest as severe idiosyncratic dermatologic, vascular, pulmonary, renal, hepatic, and/or hematologic events, usually after multiple doses. Prompt discontinuation of drug should occur if skin rash or other symptoms arise. **[U.S. Boxed Warning]: Quinolones may exacerbate myasthenia gravis; avoid use (rare, potentially life-threatening weakness of respiratory muscles may occur).** Use caution in renal impairment. Avoid excessive sunlight and take precautions to limit exposure (eg, loose fitting clothing, sunscreen); may cause moderate-to-severe phototoxicity reactions. Discontinue use if photosensitivity occurs. Since ciprofloxacin is ineffective in the treatment of syphilis and may mask symptoms, all patients should be tested for syphilis at the time of gonorrheal diagnosis and 3 months later. Hemolytic reactions may (rarely) occur with quinolone use in patients with latent or actual G6PD deficiency.

Ciprofloxacin is a potent inhibitor of CYP1A2. Coadministration of drugs which depend on this pathway may lead to substantial increases in serum concentrations and adverse effects.

Drug Interactions

Metabolism/Transport Effects Substrate of P-glycoprotein; **Inhibits** CYP1A2 (strong), 3A4 (weak)

Avoid Concomitant Use

Avoid concomitant use of Ciprofloxacin (Systemic) with any of the following: BCG; TiZANidine

Increased Effect/Toxicity

Ciprofloxacin (Systemic) may increase the levels/effects of: Bendamustine; Caffeine; Corticosteroids (Systemic); CYP1A2 Substrates; Erlotinib; Methotrexate; Pentoxifylline; QTc-Prolonging Agents; ROPINIRole; Ropivacaine; Sulfonylureas; Theophylline Derivatives; TiZANidine; Vitamin K Antagonists

The levels/effects of Ciprofloxacin (Systemic) may be increased by: Insulin; Nonsteroidal Anti-Inflammatory Agents; P-Glycoprotein Inhibitors; Probenecid

Decreased Effect

Ciprofloxacin (Systemic) may decrease the levels/effects of: BCG; Fosphenytoin; Mycophenolate; Phenytoin; Sulfonylureas; Typhoid Vaccine

The levels/effects of Ciprofloxacin (Systemic) may be decreased by: Antacids; Calcium Salts; Didanosine; Iron Salts; Lanthanum; Magnesium Salts; P-Glycoprotein Inducers; Quinapril; Sevelamer; Sucralfate; Zinc Salts

Ethanol/Nutrition/Herb Interactions

Food: Food decreases rate, but not extent, of absorption. Ciprofloxacin serum levels may be decreased if taken with dairy products or calcium-fortified juices. Ciprofloxacin may increase serum caffeine levels if taken with caffeine.

Enteral feedings may decrease plasma concentrations of ciprofloxacin probably by >30% inhibition of absorption. Ciprofloxacin should not be administered with enteral feedings. The feeding would need to be discontinued for 1-2 hours prior to and after ciprofloxacin administration. Nasogastric administration produces a greater loss of ciprofloxacin bioavailability than does nasoduodenal administration.

Herb/Nutraceutical: Avoid dong quai, St John's wort (may also cause photosensitization).

Dietary Considerations Food: Drug may cause GI upset; take without regard to meals (manufacturer prefers that immediate release tablet is taken 2 hours after meals). Extended release tablet may be taken with meals that contain dairy products (calcium content <800 mg), but not with dairy products alone.

Dairy products, calcium-fortified juices, oral multivitamins, and mineral supplements: Absorption of ciprofloxacin is decreased by divalent and trivalent cations. The manufacturer states that the usual dietary intake of calcium (including meals which include dairy products) has not been shown to interfere with ciprofloxacin absorption. Immediate release ciprofloxacin and Cipro® XR may be taken 2 hours before or 6 hours after, and Proquin® XR may be taken 4 hours before or 6 hours after, any of these products.

Caffeine: Patients consuming regular large quantities of caffeinated beverages may need to restrict caffeine intake if excessive cardiac or CNS stimulation occurs.

Pharmacodynamics/Kinetics

Half-life Elimination Children: 2.5 hours; Adults: Normal renal function: 3-5 hours

Time to Peak Oral:

Immediate release tablet: 0.5-2 hours

Extended release tablet: Cipro® XR: 1-2.5 hours; Proquin® XR: 3.5-8.7 hours

Pregnancy Risk Factor C

Lactation Enters breast milk/not recommended (AAP rates "compatible"; AAP 2001 update pending)

Breast-Feeding Considerations Ciprofloxacin is excreted in breast milk. Breast-feeding is not recommended by the manufacturer. Due to the low concentrations in human milk, minimal toxicity would be expected in the nursing infant and infant serum levels were undetectable in one report. Nondose-related effects could include modification of bowel flora. There has been a single case report of perforated pseudomembranous colitis in a breast-feeding infant whose mother was taking ciprofloxacin.

Dosage Forms

Infusion, premixed in D_5W: 200 mg (100 mL); 400 mg (200 mL)
Cipro® I.V.: 200 mg (100 mL); 400 mg (200 mL)
Infusion, premixed in D_5W [preservative free]: 200 mg (100 mL); 400 mg (200 mL)
Injection, solution: 10 mg/mL (20 mL, 40 mL, 120 mL)
Injection, solution [preservative free]: 10 mg/mL (20 mL)
Microcapsules for suspension, oral:
Cipro®: 250 mg/5 mL (100 mL); 500 mg/5 mL (100 mL)
Tablet, oral: 100 mg, 250 mg, 500 mg, 750 mg
Cipro®: 250 mg, 500 mg
Tablet, extended release, oral: 500 mg, 1000 mg
Cipro® XR: 500 mg, 1000 mg
Proquin® XR: 500 mg

References

Rams TE and Slots J, "Antibiotics in Periodontal Therapy: An Update," *Compendium*, 1992, 13(12):1130, 1132, 1134.
Wynn RL, Bergman SA, Meiller TF, et al, "Antibiotics in Treating Oral-Facial Infections of Odontogenic Origin: An Update," *Gen Dent*, 2001, 49(3):238-40, 242, 244 passim.

Ciprofloxacin and Dexamethasone
(sip roe FLOKS a sin & deks a METH a sone)

U.S. Brand Names Ciprodex®
Canadian Brand Names Ciprodex®
Pharmacologic Category Antibiotic, Otic; Antibiotic/Corticosteroid, Otic; Corticosteroid, Otic
Use Treatment of acute otitis media in pediatric patients with tympanostomy tubes or acute otitis externa in children and adults
Local Anesthetic/Vasoconstrictor Precautions No information available to require special precautions
Effects on Dental Treatment No significant effects or complications reported
Effects on Bleeding No information available to require special precautions
Adverse Effects 1% to 10%: Otic: Discomfort (3%), pain (<1% to 2%), pruritus (1%)
General Dosage Range Otic: *Children and Adults:* Instill 4 drops into affected ear(s) twice daily
Mechanism of Action Ciprofloxacin is a quinolone antibiotic; dexamethasone is a corticosteroid used to decrease inflammation accompanying bacterial infections
Pharmacodynamics/Kinetics
Time to Peak Plasma: Otic: Ciprofloxacin: 15 minutes to 2 hours
Pregnancy Risk Factor C

Ciprofloxacin and Hydrocortisone
(sip roe FLOKS a sin & hye droe KOR ti sone)

U.S. Brand Names Cipro® HC
Canadian Brand Names Cipro® HC
Pharmacologic Category Antibiotic/Corticosteroid, Otic
Use Treatment of acute otitis externa, sometimes known as "swimmer's ear"
Local Anesthetic/Vasoconstrictor Precautions No information available to require special precautions
Effects on Dental Treatment No significant effects or complications reported
Effects on Bleeding No information available to require special precautions
General Dosage Range Otic: *Children >1 year and Adults:* 3 drops into affected ear(s) twice daily
Pregnancy Risk Factor C

Cisapride (SIS a pride)

U.S. Brand Names Propulsid®
Pharmacologic Category Gastrointestinal Agent, Prokinetic
Use Treatment of nocturnal symptoms of gastroesophageal reflux disease (GERD); has demonstrated effectiveness for gastroparesis, refractory constipation, and non-ulcer dyspepsia
Local Anesthetic/Vasoconstrictor Precautions Cisapride is one of the drugs confirmed to prolong the QT interval and is accepted as having a risk of causing torsade de pointes. The risk of drug-induced torsade de pointes is extremely low when a single QT interval prolonging drug is prescribed. In terms of epinephrine, it is not known what effect vasoconstrictors in the local anesthetic regimen will have in patients with a known history of congenital prolonged QT interval or in patients taking any medication that prolongs the QT interval. Until more information is obtained, it is suggested that the clinician consult with the physician prior to the

use of a vasoconstrictor in suspected patients, and that the vasoconstrictor (epinephrine, mepivacaine and levonordefrin [Carbocaine® 2% with Neo-Cobefrin®]) be used with caution.

Effects on Dental Treatment Key adverse event(s) related to dental treatment: Xerostomia (normal salivary flow resumes upon discontinuation).

Effects on Bleeding No information available to require special precautions

Adverse Effects

>5%:

Central nervous system: Headache

Dermatologic: Rash

Gastrointestinal: Diarrhea, GI cramping, dyspepsia, flatulence, nausea, xerostomia

Respiratory: Rhinitis

<5%:

Cardiovascular: Tachycardia

Central nervous system: Extrapyramidal effects, somnolence, fatigue, seizure, insomnia, anxiety

Hematologic: Thrombocytopenia, increased LFTs, pancytopenia, leukopenia, granulocytopenia, aplastic anemia

Respiratory: Sinusitis, cough, upper respiratory tract infection, increased incidence of viral infection

General Dosage Range

Oral:

Children: 0.15-0.3 mg/kg 3-4 times/day (maximum: 10 mg/dose)

Adults: Initial: 5-10 mg 4 times/day, may increase to 20 mg 4 times/day if needed

Mechanism of Action Enhances the release of acetylcholine at the myenteric plexus. *In vitro* studies have shown cisapride to have serotonin-4 receptor agonistic properties which may increase gastrointestinal motility and cardiac rate; increases lower esophageal sphincter pressure and lower esophageal peristalsis; accelerates gastric emptying of both liquids and solids.

Pharmacodynamics/Kinetics

Onset of Action 0.5-1 hour

Half-life Elimination 6-12 hours

Pregnancy Risk Factor C

Prescribing and Access Restrictions In U.S., available via limited-access protocol only. Call 877-795-4247 for more information.

Dental Comment Cisapride is known to prolong the QT interval. The QT interval is measured as the time and distance between the Q point of the QRS complex and the end of the T wave in the ECG tracing. After adjustment for heart rate, the QT interval is defined as prolonged if it is more than 450 msec in men and 460 msec in women. A long QT syndrome was first described in the 1950s and 60s as a congenital syndrome involving QT interval prolongation and syncope and sudden death. Some of the congenital long QT syndromes were characterized by a peculiar electrocardiographic appearance of the QRS complex involving a premature atria beat followed by a pause, then a subsequent sinus beat showing marked QT prolongation and deformity. This type of cardiac arrhythmia was originally termed "torsade de pointes" (translated from the French as "twisting of the points"). Cisapride is considered as having a risk of causing torsade de pointes. Since it is not known what effect vasoconstrictors in the local anesthetic regimen will have in patients with a known history of congenital prolonged QT interval or in patients taking any medication that prolongs the QT interval, a medical consult is suggested.

CISplatin (SIS pla tin)

Pharmacologic Category Antineoplastic Agent, Alkylating Agent; Antineoplastic Agent, Platinum Analog

Use Treatment of advanced bladder cancer, metastatic testicular cancer, and metastatic ovarian cancer

Unlabeled/Investigational Use Treatment of head and neck cancer, breast cancer, gastric cancer, esophageal cancer, cervical cancer, prostate cancer, non-small cell lung cancer, small cell lung cancer; Hodgkin's and non-Hodgkin's lymphoma; neuroblastoma; sarcomas, myeloma, melanoma, mesothelioma, hepatoblastoma, and osteosarcoma

Local Anesthetic/Vasoconstrictor Precautions No information available to require special precautions

Effects on Dental Treatment No significant effects or complications reported

Effects on Bleeding Chemotherapy may result in significant myelosuppression, potentially including significant reduction in platelet counts and altered hemostasis. In patients who are under active treatment with these agents, medical consult is suggested.

Adverse Effects
>10%:
Central nervous system: Neurotoxicity: Peripheral neuropathy is dose- and duration-dependent.
Gastrointestinal: Nausea and vomiting (76% to 100%)
Hematologic: Myelosuppression (25% to 30%; nadir: day 18-23; recovery: by day 39; mild with moderate doses, mild-to-moderate with high-dose therapy)
Hepatic: Liver enzymes increased
Renal: Nephrotoxicity (acute renal failure and chronic renal insufficiency)
Otic: Ototoxicity (10% to 30%; manifested as high frequency hearing loss; ototoxicity is especially pronounced in children)
1% to 10%: Local: Tissue irritation

General Dosage Range Dosage adjustment recommended in patients with renal impairment
I.V.: *Adults:* 50-70 mg/m^2 every 3-4 weeks **or** 75-100 mg/m^2/day every 4 weeks **or** 20 mg/m^2/day for 5 days every 3 weeks

Mechanism of Action Inhibits DNA synthesis by the formation of DNA cross-links; denatures the double helix; covalently binds to DNA bases and disrupts DNA function; may also bind to proteins; the *cis*-isomer is 14 times more cytotoxic than the *trans*-isomer; both forms cross-link DNA but cis-platinum is less easily recognized by cell enzymes and, therefore, not repaired. Cisplatin can also bind two adjacent guanines on the same strand of DNA producing intrastrand cross-linking and breakage.

Pharmacodynamics/Kinetics
Half-life Elimination Initial: 20-30 minutes; Beta: 60 minutes; Terminal: ~24 hours; Secondary half-life: 44-73 hours

Pregnancy Risk Factor D

Citalopram (sye TAL oh pram)

Related Information
Escitalopram *on page 625*

U.S. Brand Names CeleXA®

Canadian Brand Names Apo-Citalopram®; Celexa®; Citalopram-Odan; CO Citalopram; CTP 30; Dom-Citalopram; JAMP-Citalopram; Mint-Citalopram; Mylan-Citalopram; NG-Citalopram; Novo-Citalopram; PHL-Citalopram; PMS-Citalopram; RAN™-Citalo; ratio-Citalopram; Riva-Citalopram; Sandoz-Citalopram; Septa-Citalopram; Teva-Citalopram

Generic Availability (U.S.) Yes

Pharmacologic Category Antidepressant, Selective Serotonin Reuptake Inhibitor

Use Treatment of depression

Unlabeled/Investigational Use Treatment of mild dementia-associated agitation in nonpsychotic patients; smoking cessation; ethanol abuse; obsessive-compulsive disorder (OCD) in children; diabetic neuropathy

Local Anesthetic/Vasoconstrictor Precautions Although caution should be used in patients taking tricyclic antidepressants, no interactions have been reported with vasoconstrictors and citalopram, a nontricyclic antidepressant which acts to increase serotonin; no precautions appear to be needed

Effects on Dental Treatment Key adverse event(s) related to dental treatment: Xerostomia (normal salivary flow resumes upon discontinuation). Premarketing trials reported abnormal taste. See Effects on Bleeding and Dental Comment.

Effects on Bleeding May impair platelet aggregation resulting in increased risk of bleeding events, particularly if used concomitantly with aspirin, NSAIDs, warfarin, or other anticoagulants. Bleeding related to SSRI use has been reported to range from relatively minor bruising and epistaxis to life-threatening hemorrhage. Routine interruption of therapy for most dental procedures is not warranted. In medically complicated patients or extensive oral surgery, the decision to interrupt therapy must be based on the risk to benefit in an individual patient and a medical consult is suggested. If therapy is continued without interruption, the clinician should anticipate the potential for a prolonged bleeding time.

Adverse Effects
>10%:
Central nervous system: Somnolence (18%; dose related), insomnia (15%; dose related)
Gastrointestinal: Nausea (21%), xerostomia (20%)
Miscellaneous: Diaphoresis (11%; dose related)

1% to 10%:

Cardiovascular: Heart rate decreased, postural hypotension, tachycardia

Central nervous system: Fatigue (5%; dose related), anorexia (4%), anxiety (4%), agitation (3%), fever (2%), yawning (2%; dose related), amnesia, apathy, concentration impaired, confusion, depression, migraine, suicide attempt

Dermatologic: Rash, pruritus

Endocrine & metabolic: Libido decreased (1% to 4%), dysmenorrhea (3%), amenorrhea, sexual dysfunction

Gastrointestinal: Diarrhea (8%), dyspepsia (5%), vomiting (4%), abdominal pain (3%), flatulence, salivation increased, taste perversion, weight gain/loss

Genitourinary: Ejaculation disorder (6%), impotence (3%; dose related), polyuria

Neuromuscular & skeletal: Tremor (8%), arthralgia (2%), myalgia (2%), paresthesia

Ocular: Abnormal accommodation

Respiratory: Rhinitis (5%), upper respiratory tract infection (5%), sinusitis (3%), cough

Dosage Oral:

Children and Adolescents: Obsessive-compulsive disorder (unlabeled use): 10-40 mg/day

Adults: Depression: Initial: 20 mg/day, generally with an increase to 40 mg/day; doses of more than 40 mg are not usually necessary. Should a dose increase be necessary, it should occur in 20 mg increments at intervals of no less than 1 week. Maximum dose: 60 mg/day; reduce dosage in elderly or those with hepatic impairment.

Elderly:

Depression: Initial: 20 mg once daily; increase dose to 40 mg/day in nonresponsive patients

Alzheimer's dementia-related depression (unlabeled use): Initial: 5-10 mg/day; may increase at multi-week intervals to maximum of 40 mg/day

Dosage adjustment in renal impairment:

Mild-to-moderate impairment: No dosage adjustment needed

Severe impairment: Cl_{cr} <20 mL/minute: Use with caution

Dosage adjustment in hepatic impairment: 20 mg once daily; increase dose to 40 mg/day in nonresponsive patients

Mechanism of Action A racemic bicyclic phthalane derivative, citalopram selectively inhibits serotonin reuptake in the presynaptic neurons and has minimal effects on norepinephrine or dopamine. Uptake inhibition of serotonin is primarily due to the *S*-enantiomer of citalopram. Displays little to no affinity for serotonin, dopamine, adrenergic, histamine, GABA, or muscarinic receptor subtypes.

Contraindications Hypersensitivity to citalopram or any component of the formulation; concomitant use with MAO inhibitors or within 2 weeks of discontinuing MAO inhibitors; concomitant use with pimozide

Warnings/Precautions [U.S. Boxed Warning]: Antidepressants increase the risk of suicidal thinking and behavior in children, adolescents, and young adults (18-24 years of age) with major depressive disorder (MDD) and other psychiatric disorders; consider risk prior to prescribing. Short-term studies did not show an increased risk in patients >24 years of age and showed a decreased risk in patients ≥65 years. Closely monitor patients for clinical worsening, suicidality, or unusual changes in behavior, particularly during the initial 1-2 months of therapy or during periods of dosage adjustments (increases or decreases); the patient's family or caregiver should be instructed to closely observe the patient and communicate condition with healthcare provider. A medication guide concerning the use of antidepressants should be dispensed with each prescription. **Citalopram is not FDA approved for use in children.**

The possibility of a suicide attempt is inherent in major depression and may persist until remission occurs. Use caution in high-risk patients. Worsening depression and severe abrupt suicidality that are not part of the presenting symptoms may require discontinuation or modification of drug therapy. The patient's family or caregiver should be alerted to monitor patients for the emergence of suicidality and associated behaviors (such as agitation, irritability, hostility, impulsivity, and hypomania) and call healthcare provider.

May worsen psychosis in some patients or precipitate a shift to mania or hypomania in patients with bipolar disorder. Patients presenting with depressive symptoms should be screened for bipolar disorder. Monotherapy in patients with bipolar disorder should be avoided. **Citalopram is not FDA approved for the treatment of bipolar depression.**

Serotonin syndrome and neuroleptic malignant syndrome (NMS)-like reactions have occurred with serotonin/norepinephrine reuptake inhibitors (SNRIs) and selective serotonin reuptake inhibitors (SSRIs) when used alone, and particularly when used in combination with serotonergic agents (eg, triptans) or antidopaminergic agents (eg, antipsychotics). Concurrent use with MAO inhibitors is contraindicated. May increase the risks associated with electroconvulsive therapy. Has a low potential to impair cognitive or motor performance; caution operating hazardous machinery or driving.

Use with caution in patients with hepatic or renal dysfunction, in elderly patients, concomitant CNS depressants, and pregnancy (high doses of citalopram have been associated with teratogenicity in animals). Use caution with concomitant use of aspirin, NSAIDs, warfarin, or other drugs that affect coagulation; the risk of bleeding may be potentiated. May cause hyponatremia/SIADH (elderly at increased risk); volume depletion and diuretics may increase risk. May cause or exacerbate sexual dysfunction. Upon discontinuation of citalopram therapy, gradually taper dose. If intolerable symptoms occur following a decrease in dosage or upon discontinuation of therapy, then resuming the previous dose with a more gradual taper should be considered.

Drug Interactions

Metabolism/Transport Effects Substrate of CYP2C19 (major), 2D6 (minor), 3A4 (major); **Inhibits** CYP1A2 (weak), 2B6 (weak), 2C19 (weak), 2D6 (weak)

Avoid Concomitant Use

Avoid concomitant use of Citalopram with any of the following: Artemether; Dronedarone; Iobenguane I 123; Lumefantrine; MAO Inhibitors; Methylene Blue; Nilotinib; Pimozide; QuiNINE; Sibutramine; Tetrabenazine; Thioridazine; Toremifene; Tryptophan; Vandetanib; Ziprasidone

Increased Effect/Toxicity

Citalopram may increase the levels/effects of: Alcohol (Ethyl); Alpha-/Beta-Blockers; Anticoagulants; Antidepressants (Serotonin Reuptake Inhibitor/Antagonist); Antiplatelet Agents; Aspirin; BusPIRone; CarBAMazepine; CloZAPine; CNS Depressants; Collagenase (Systemic); Desmopressin; Dextromethorphan; Dronedarone; Drotrecogin Alfa; Haloperidol; Ibritumomab; Lithium; Methadone; Methylene Blue; Mexiletine; NSAID (COX-2 Inhibitor); NSAID (Nonselective); Pimozide; QTc-Prolonging Agents; QuiNINE; RisperiDONE; Salicylates; Serotonin Modulators; Tetrabenazine; Thioridazine; Thrombolytic Agents; Toremifene; Tositumomab and Iodine I 131 Tositumomab; TraMADol; Tricyclic Antidepressants; Vandetanib; Vitamin K Antagonists; Ziprasidone

The levels/effects of Citalopram may be increased by: Alfuzosin; Analgesics (Opioid); Artemether; BusPIRone; Chloroquine; Cimetidine; Ciprofloxacin; Ciprofloxacin (Systemic); Conivaptan; CYP2C19 Inhibitors (Moderate); CYP2C19 Inhibitors (Strong); CYP3A4 Inhibitors (Moderate); CYP3A4 Inhibitors (Strong); Fluconazole; Gadobutrol; Glucosamine; Herbs (Anticoagulant/Antiplatelet Properties); Lumefantrine; Macrolide Antibiotics; MAO Inhibitors; Metoclopramide; Nilotinib; Omega-3-Acid Ethyl Esters; Pentosan Polysulfate Sodium; Pentoxifylline; Prostacyclin Analogues; QuiNINE; Sibutramine; TraMADol; Tryptophan

Decreased Effect

Citalopram may decrease the levels/effects of: Iobenguane I 123

The levels/effects of Citalopram may be decreased by: CarBAMazepine; CYP2C19 Inducers (Strong); CYP3A4 Inducers (Strong); Cyproheptadine; Deferasirox; Peginterferon Alfa-2b; Tocilizumab

Ethanol/Nutrition/Herb Interactions

Ethanol: May increase CNS depression; monitor for increased effects with coadministration. Caution patients about effects.

Herb/Nutraceutical: Avoid valerian, St John's wort, SAMe, kava kava, and gotu kola (may increase CNS depression).

Dietary Considerations May be taken without regard to food.

Pharmacodynamics/Kinetics

Onset of Action Depression: The onset of action is within a week; however, individual response varies greatly and full response may not be seen until 8-12 weeks after initiation of treatment.

Half-life Elimination 24-48 hours (average: 35 hours); doubled with hepatic impairment

Time to Peak Serum: 1-6 hours, average within 4 hours

Pregnancy Risk Factor C

Lactation Enters breast milk/consider risk:benefit

Breast-Feeding Considerations Citalopram and its metabolites are excreted in human milk. According to the manufacturer, the decision to continue or discontinue breast-feeding during therapy should take into account the risk of exposure to the infant and the benefits of treatment to the mother. Excessive somnolence, decreased feeding, colic, irritability, restlessness, and weight loss have been reported in breast-fed infants. The long-term effects on development and behavior have not been studied; therefore, citalopram should be prescribed to a mother who is breast-feeding only when the benefits outweigh the potential risks.

Dosage Forms

Solution, oral: 10 mg/5 mL (240 mL)

Tablet, oral: 10 mg, 20 mg, 40 mg

CeleXA®: 10 mg, 20 mg, 40 mg

Dental Comment Problems with SSRI-induced bruxism have been reported and may preclude their use; clinicians attempting to evaluate any patient with bruxism or involuntary muscle movement, who is simultaneously being treated with an SSRI drug, should be aware of the potential association.

Citric Acid, Magnesium Carbonate, and Glucono-Delta-Lactone (SI trik AS id, mag NEE see um KAR bo nate, and GLOO kon o DEL ta LAK tone)

U.S. Brand Names Renacidin®

Pharmacologic Category Genitourinary Irrigant; Urinary Tract Product

Use Prevention of formation of calcifications of indwelling urinary tract catheters; treatment of renal and bladder calculi of the apatite or struvite type

Local Anesthetic/Vasoconstrictor Precautions No information available to require special precautions

Effects on Dental Treatment No significant effects or complications reported

Effects on Bleeding No information available to require special precautions

Adverse Effects

>10%:

Central nervous system: Fever (20% to 40%)

Genitourinary: Urothelial ulceration with or without edema (13%)

Miscellaneous: Transient flank pain

1% to 10%:

Endocrine & metabolic: Hypermagnesemia, hyperphosphatemia

Genitourinary: Urinary tract infection, dysuria, hematuria, bladder irritability

Neuromuscular & skeletal: Back pain

Renal: Creatinine increased

General Dosage Range Irrigation: *Adults:* 30-60 mL into catheter 2-3 times/day **or** 30 mL into bladder, retained for 30-60 minutes then drained 4-6 times **or** 60-120 mL/hour

Mechanism of Action Magnesium from the irrigating solution is exchanged for calcium in the stone matrix. The magnesium stones are soluble and are able to dissolve in the acidic pH of the solution.

Pregnancy Risk Factor C

Citric Acid, Sodium Citrate, and Potassium Citrate (SIT rik AS id, SOW dee um SIT rate, & poe TASS ee um SIT rate)

Related Information

Potassium Citrate *on page 1378*

U.S. Brand Names Cytra-3; Tricitrates

Pharmacologic Category Alkalinizing Agent, Oral

Use Conditions where long-term maintenance of an alkaline urine is desirable as in control and dissolution of uric acid and cystine calculi of the urinary tract

Local Anesthetic/Vasoconstrictor Precautions No information available to require special precautions

Effects on Dental Treatment No significant effects or complications reported

Effects on Bleeding No information available to require special precautions

Adverse Effects Frequency not defined.

Cardiovascular: Cardiac abnormalities

Endocrine & metabolic: Metabolic alkalosis, calcium levels, hyperkalemia, hypernatremia

Gastrointestinal: Diarrhea

Neuromuscular & skeletal: Tetany

General Dosage Range Oral:

Children: 5-15 mL after meals and at bedtime

Adults: 15-30 mL after meals and at bedtime

Pregnancy Risk Factor Not established

Cladribine (KLA dri been)

U.S. Brand Names Leustatin®

Canadian Brand Names Leustatin®

Pharmacologic Category Antineoplastic Agent, Antimetabolite; Antineoplastic Agent, Antimetabolite (Purine Analog)

Use Treatment of hairy cell leukemia

Unlabeled/Investigational Use Treatment of chronic lymphocytic leukemia (CLL), chronic myelogenous leukemia (CML), non-Hodgkin's lymphomas, progressive multiple sclerosis

Local Anesthetic/Vasoconstrictor Precautions No information available to require special precautions

Effects on Dental Treatment No significant effects or complications reported

Effects on Bleeding Chemotherapy may result in significant myelosuppression, potentially including significant reduction in platelet counts and altered hemostasis. In patients who are under active treatment with these agents, medical consult is suggested.

Adverse Effects

>10%:

Central nervous system: Fever (69%; ≥104°F: 11%), fatigue (11% to 45%), headache (7% to 22%)
Dermatologic: Rash (10% to 27%)
Gastrointestinal: Nausea (28%), appetite decreased (17%), vomiting (13%)
Hematologic: Myelosuppression, common, dose limiting (nadir: 5-10 days, recovery: 4-8 weeks); neutropenia (70%); anemia (37%); thrombocytopenia (12%)
Local: Injection site reactions (9% to 19%)
Respiratory: Abnormal breath sounds (11%)
Miscellaneous: Infection (28%)

1% to 10%:

Cardiovascular: Edema (6%), tachycardia (6%), thrombosis (2%)
Central nervous system: Dizziness (9%), chills (9%), insomnia (7%), malaise (5% to 7%), pain (6%)
Dermatologic: Purpura (10%), petechiae (8%), pruritus (6%), erythema (6%)
Gastrointestinal: Diarrhea (10%), constipation (9%), abdominal pain (6%)
Local: Phlebitis (2%)
Neuromuscular & skeletal: Weakness (9%), myalgia (7%), arthralgia (5%)
Respiratory: Cough (7% to 10%), abnormal chest sounds (9%), dyspnea (7%), epistaxis (5%)
Miscellaneous: Diaphoresis (9%)

General Dosage Range Dosage adjustment recommended in patients with renal impairment

I.V.: *Adults:* Continuous infusion: 0.09 mg/kg/day days 1-7 every 28-35 days

Mechanism of Action A purine nucleoside analogue; prodrug which is activated via phosphorylation by deoxycytidine kinase to a 5'-triphosphate derivative. This active form incorporates into DNA to result in the breakage of DNA strand and shutdown of DNA synthesis. This also results in a depletion of nicotinamide adenine dinucleotide and adenosine triphosphate (ATP). Cladribine is cell-cycle nonspecific.

Pharmacodynamics/Kinetics

Half-life Elimination Biphasic: Alpha: 25 minutes; Beta: 6.7 hours; Terminal, mean: Normal renal function: 5.4 hours

Pregnancy Risk Factor D

Clarithromycin (kla RITH roe mye sin)

Related Information

Antibiotic Prophylaxis *on page 1910*
Bacterial Infections *on page 1933*
Cardiovascular Diseases *on page 1848*
Clinical Risk Related to Drugs Prolonging QT Interval *on page 1872*
Gastrointestinal Disorders *on page 1874*
Respiratory Diseases *on page 1876*

U.S. Brand Names Biaxin®; Biaxin® XL

Canadian Brand Names Apo-Clarithromycin®; Biaxin®; Biaxin® XL; Dom-Clarithromycin; Mylan-Clarithromycin; PMS-Clarithromycin; RAN™-Clarithromycin; ratio-Clarithromycin; Riva-Clarithromycin; Sandoz-Clarithromycin

Generic Availability (U.S.) Yes

Pharmacologic Category Antibiotic, Macrolide

Dental Use Alternate oral antibiotic for prevention of infective endocarditis in individuals allergic to penicillins or ampicillin, when amoxicillin cannot be used; alternate antibiotic in the treatment of common orofacial infections caused by aerobic gram-positive cocci and susceptible anaerobes

Use

Children:

Acute otitis media (*H. influenzae*, *M. catarrhalis*, or *S. pneumoniae*)
Community-acquired pneumonia due to susceptible *Mycoplasma pneumoniae*, *S. pneumoniae*, or *Chlamydia pneumoniae* (TWAR)

Pharyngitis/tonsillitis due to susceptible *S. pyogenes*, acute maxillary sinusitis due to susceptible *H. influenzae, S. pneumoniae,* or *Moraxella catarrhalis*, uncomplicated skin/skin structure infections due to susceptible *S. aureus, S. pyogenes,* and mycobacterial infections

Prevention of disseminated mycobacterial infections due to MAC disease in patients with advanced HIV infection

Adults:

Pharyngitis/tonsillitis due to susceptible *S. pyogenes*

Acute maxillary sinusitis due to susceptible *H. influenzae, M. catarrhalis,* or *S. pneumoniae*

Acute exacerbation of chronic bronchitis due to susceptible *H. influenzae, H. parainfluenzae, M. catarrhalis*, or *S. pneumoniae*

Community-acquired pneumonia due to susceptible *H. influenzae, H. parainfluenzae, Mycoplasma pneumoniae, S. pneumoniae,* or *Chlamydia pneumoniae* (TWAR), *Moraxella catarrhalis*

Uncomplicated skin/skin structure infections due to susceptible *S. aureus, S. pyogenes*

Disseminated mycobacterial infections due to *M. avium* or *M. intracellulare*

Prevention of disseminated mycobacterial infections due to *M. avium* complex (MAC) disease (eg, patients with advanced HIV infection)

Duodenal ulcer disease due to *H. pylori* in regimens with other drugs including amoxicillin and lansoprazole or omeprazole, ranitidine bismuth citrate, bismuth subsalicylate, tetracycline, and/or an H_2 antagonist

Unlabeled/Investigational Use Pertussis (CDC guidelines); alternate antibiotic for prophylaxis of infective endocarditis in patients who are allergic to penicillin and undergoing surgical or dental procedures (ACC/AHA guidelines)

Local Anesthetic/Vasoconstrictor Precautions Clarithromycin is one of the drugs confirmed to prolong the QT interval and is accepted as having a risk of causing torsade de pointes. In terms of epinephrine, it is not known what effect vasoconstrictors in the local anesthetic regimen will have in patients with a known history of congenital prolonged QT interval or in patients taking any medication that prolongs the QT interval. Until more information is obtained, it is suggested that the clinician consult with the physician prior to the use of a vasoconstrictor in suspected patients, and that the vasoconstrictor (epinephrine, mepivacaine and levonordefrin [Carbocaine® 2% with Neo-Cobefrin®]) be used with caution. See Dental Comment.

Effects on Dental Treatment Key adverse event(s) related to dental treatment: Abnormal taste.

Effects on Bleeding No information available to require special precautions

Adverse Effects 1% to 10%:

Central nervous system: Headache (adults and children 2%)

Dermatologic: Rash (children 3%)

Gastrointestinal: Abnormal taste (adults 3% to 7%), diarrhea (adults 3% to 6%; children 6%), vomiting (children 6%), nausea (adults 3%), abdominal pain (adults 2%; children 3%), dyspepsia (adults 2%)

Hepatic: Prothrombin time increased (adults 1%)

Renal: BUN increased (4%)

Dental Usual Dosage Prophylaxis against infective endocarditis (unlabeled use): Oral:

Children: 15 mg/kg 30-60 minutes before procedure

Adults: 500 mg 30-60 minutes prior to procedure

Note: American Heart Association (AHA) guidelines now recommend prophylaxis only in patients undergoing invasive procedures and in whom underlying cardiac conditions may predispose to a higher risk of adverse outcomes should infection occur. As of April 2007, routine prophylaxis for GI/GU procedures is no longer recommended by the AHA.

Dosage

Usual dosage range:

Children ≥6 months: Oral: 7.5 mg/kg every 12 hours (maximum: 500 mg/dose) for 10 days

Adults: Oral: 250-500 mg every 12 hours **or** 1000 mg (two 500 mg extended release tablets) once daily for 7-14 days

Indication-specific dosing:

Children: Oral:

Community-acquired pneumonia, sinusitis, bronchitis, skin infections: 15 mg/kg/day divided every 12 hours for 10 days

Mycobacterial infection (prevention and treatment):

Manufacturer's recommendation: 7.5 mg/kg/dose (maximum: 500 mg/dose) twice daily. **Note:** Safety of clarithromycin for MAC not studied in children <20 months.

HIV-exposed/-positive (unlabeled use; CDC, 2009):

Primary prophylaxis: 7.5 mg/kg/dose (maximum: 500 mg/dose) twice daily

Secondary prophylaxis: 7.5 mg/kg/dose (maximum: 500 mg/dose) twice daily, plus ethambutol, with or without rifabutin

Treatment: 7.5-15 mg/kg/dose (maximum: 500 mg/dose) twice daily plus ethambutol, plus rifabutin (for severe disease)

Pertussis (unlabeled use; CDC, 2005):

Children 1-5 months: 15 mg/kg/day divided every 12 hours for 7 days

Children ≥6 months: 15 mg/kg/day divided every 12 hours for 7 days (maximum: 1 g/day)

Prophylaxis against infective endocarditis (unlabeled use): 15 mg/kg 30-60 minutes before procedure. **Note:** American Heart Association (AHA) guidelines now recommend prophylaxis only in patients undergoing invasive procedures and in whom underlying cardiac conditions may predispose to a higher risk of adverse outcomes should infection occur. As of April 2007, routine prophylaxis for GI/GU procedures is no longer recommended by the AHA.

Adults: Oral:

Acute exacerbation of chronic bronchitis:

M. catarrhalis and *S. pneumoniae*: 250 mg every 12 hours for 7-14 days **or** 1000 mg (two 500 mg extended release tablets) once daily for 7 days

H. influenzae: 500 mg every 12 hours for 7-14 days **or** 1000 mg (two 500 mg extended release tablets) once daily for 7 days

H. parainfluenzae: 500 mg every 12 hours for 7 days **or** 1000 mg (two 500 mg extended release tablets) once daily for 7 days

Acute maxillary sinusitis: 500 mg every 12 hours **or** 1000 mg (two 500 mg extended release tablets) once daily for 14 days

Mycobacterial infection (prevention and treatment): 500 mg twice daily (use with other antimycobacterial drugs, eg, ethambutol or rifampin)

Peptic ulcer disease: Eradication of *Helicobacter pylori*: Dual or triple combination regimens with bismuth subsalicylate, amoxicillin, an H_2-receptor antagonist, or proton-pump inhibitor: 500 mg every 8-12 hours for 10-14 days

Pertussis (unlabeled use; CDC, 2005): 500 mg twice daily for 7 days

Pharyngitis, tonsillitis: 250 mg every 12 hours for 10 days

Pneumonia:

C. pneumoniae, *M. pneumoniae*, and *S. pneumoniae*: 250 mg every 12 hours for 7-14 days **or** 1000 mg (two 500 mg extended release tablets) once daily for 7 days

H. influenzae: 250 mg every 12 hours for 7 days **or** 1000 mg (two 500 mg extended release tablets) once daily for 7 days

H. parainfluenzae and *M. catarrhalis*: 1000 mg (two 500 mg extended release tablets) once daily for 7 days

Prophylaxis against infective endocarditis (unlabeled use): 500 mg 30-60 minutes prior to procedure. **Note:** American Heart Association (AHA) guidelines now recommend prophylaxis only in patients undergoing invasive procedures and in whom underlying cardiac conditions may predispose to a higher risk of adverse outcomes should infection occur. As of April 2007, routine prophylaxis for GI/GU procedures is no longer recommended by the AHA.

Skin and skin structure infection, uncomplicated: 250 mg every 12 hours for 7-14 days

Elderly: Pharmacokinetics are similar to those in younger adults; may have age-related reductions in renal function; monitor and adjust dose if necessary

Dosing adjustment in renal impairment:

Cl_{cr} <30 mL/minute: Half the normal dose or double the dosing interval

Hemodialysis: Administer after HD session is completed.

In combination with ritonavir:

Cl_{cr} 30-60 mL/minute: Decrease clarithromycin dose by 50%

Cl_{cr} <30 mL/minute: Decrease clarithromycin dose by 75%

Dosing adjustment in hepatic impairment: No dosing adjustment is needed as long as renal function is normal

Mechanism of Action Exerts its antibacterial action by binding to 50S ribosomal subunit resulting in inhibition of protein synthesis. The 14-OH metabolite of clarithromycin is twice as active as the parent compound against certain organisms.

Contraindications Hypersensitivity to clarithromycin, erythromycin, or any macrolide antibiotic; use with ergot derivatives, pimozide, cisapride

Warnings/Precautions Dosage adjustment required with severe renal impairment; decreased dosage or prolonged dosing interval may be appropriate. Use with caution in patients with myasthenia gravis. Colchicine toxicity (including fatalities) has been reported with concomitant use. Prolonged use may result in fungal or bacterial superinfection, including *C. difficile*-associated diarrhea (CDAD) and pseudomembranous colitis; CDAD has been observed >2 months postantibiotic treatment. Macrolides (including clarithromycin) have been associated with rare QT prolongation and ventricular arrhythmias, including torsade de pointes. Use caution in patients with coronary artery disease. Avoid use of extended release tablets (Biaxin® XL) in patients with known stricture/narrowing of the GI tract.

Drug Interactions

Metabolism/Transport Effects Substrate of CYP3A4 (major); **Inhibits** CYP1A2 (weak), CYP3A4 (strong), P-glycoprotein

Avoid Concomitant Use

Avoid concomitant use of Clarithromycin with any of the following: Alfuzosin; Artemether; BCG; Cisapride; Conivaptan; Dihydroergotamine; Disopyramide; Dronedarone; Eplerenone; Ergotamine; Everolimus; Fluticasone (Oral Inhalation); Halofantrine; Lumefantrine; Lurasidone; Nilotinib; Nisoldipine; Pimozide; QuiNINE; Ranolazine; Rivaroxaban; RomiDEPsin; Salmeterol; Silodosin; Tamsulosin; Tetrabenazine; Thioridazine; Tolvaptan; Topotecan; Toremifene; Vandetanib; Ziprasidone

Increased Effect/Toxicity

Clarithromycin may increase the levels/effects of: Alfentanil; Alfuzosin; Almotriptan; Alosetron; Antifungal Agents (Azole Derivatives, Systemic); Antineoplastic Agents (Vinca Alkaloids); Benzodiazepines (metabolized by oxidation); Bortezomib; Brinzolamide; Budesonide (Nasal); Budesonide (Systemic, Oral Inhalation); BusPIRone; Calcium Channel Blockers; CarBAMazepine; Cardiac Glycosides; Ciclesonide; Cilostazol; Cisapride; CloZAPine; Colchicine; Conivaptan; Corticosteroids (Orally Inhaled); Corticosteroids (Systemic); CycloSPORINE; CycloSPORINE (Systemic); CYP3A4 Substrates; Dabigatran Etexilate; Dienogest; Dihydroergotamine; Disopyramide; Dronedarone; Dutasteride; Eletriptan; Eplerenone; Ergot Derivatives; Ergotamine; Everolimus; FentaNYL; Fesoterodine; Fluticasone (Nasal); Fluticasone (Oral Inhalation); GlipiZIDE; GlyBURIDE; GuanFACINE; Halofantrine; HMG-CoA Reductase Inhibitors; Ixabepilone; Lumefantrine; Lurasidone; Maraviroc; MethylPREDNISolone; Nilotinib; Nisoldipine; Paricalcitol; Pazopanib; P-Glycoprotein Substrates; Phosphodiesterase 5 Inhibitors; Pimecrolimus; Pimozide; Protease Inhibitors; QTc-Prolonging Agents; QuiNIDine; QuiNINE; Ranolazine; Repaglinide; Rifamycin Derivatives; Rivaroxaban; RomiDEPsin; Salmeterol; Saxagliptin; Selective Serotonin Reuptake Inhibitors; Silodosin; Sirolimus; SORAfenib; Tacrolimus; Tacrolimus (Systemic); Tacrolimus (Topical); Tadalafil; Tamsulosin; Temsirolimus; Tetrabenazine; Theophylline Derivatives; Thioridazine; Tolvaptan; Topotecan; Toremifene; Vandetanib; Vilazodone; Vitamin K Antagonists; Zidovudine; Ziprasidone; Zopiclone

The levels/effects of Clarithromycin may be increased by: Alfuzosin; Antifungal Agents (Azole Derivatives, Systemic); Artemether; Chloroquine; Ciprofloxacin; Ciprofloxacin (Systemic); CYP3A4 Inhibitors (Moderate); CYP3A4 Inhibitors (Strong); Gadobutrol; Lumefantrine; Nilotinib; Protease Inhibitors; QuiNINE

Decreased Effect

Clarithromycin may decrease the levels/effects of: BCG; Clopidogrel; Prasugrel; Typhoid Vaccine; Zidovudine

The levels/effects of Clarithromycin may be decreased by: CYP3A4 Inducers (Strong); Deferasirox; Etravirine; Herbs (CYP3A4 Inducers); Protease Inhibitors; Tocilizumab

Ethanol/Nutrition/Herb Interactions

Food: Immediate release: Food delays rate, but not extent of absorption; Extended release: Food increases clarithromycin AUC by ~30% relative to fasting conditions.

Herb/Nutraceutical: St John's wort may decrease clarithromycin levels.

Dietary Considerations Clarithromycin immediate release tablets and oral suspension may be given with or without meals, and may be taken with milk. Extended release tablets should be taken with food.

Pharmacodynamics/Kinetics

Half-life Elimination Immediate release: Clarithromycin: 3-7 hours; 14-OH-clarithromycin: 5-9 hours

Time to Peak Immediate release: 2-4 hours

Pregnancy Risk Factor C

Lactation Excretion in breast milk unknown/use caution

Breast-Feeding Considerations It is not known if clarithromycin is excreted in human breast milk. The manufacturer recommends that caution be exercised when administering clarithromycin to breast-feeding women.

Other macrolides are considered compatible with breast-feeding and clarithromycin is used therapeutically in infants. Nondose-related effects could include modification of bowel flora.

Dosage Forms

Granules for suspension, oral: 125 mg/5 mL (50 mL, 100 mL); 250 mg/5 mL (50 mL, 100 mL)

Biaxin®: 125 mg/5 mL (50 mL, 100 mL); 250 mg/5 mL (50 mL, 100 mL)

Tablet, oral: 250 mg, 500 mg
Biaxin®: 250 mg, 500 mg
Tablet, extended release, oral: 500 mg
Biaxin® XL: 500 mg

Dental Comment The FDA issued a special alert in December 2005 stating that short-term therapy with clarithromycin in patients with stable coronary artery disease may cause significantly higher cardiovascular mortality. The use of 500 mg clarithromycin daily for 14 days in patients with the above condition resulted in significantly higher all-cause mortality compared to patients taking placebo. This information is provided to the dental practitioner on the possible association between short-term use of clarithromycin for infections and increases in mortality in patients with a history of stable coronary artery disease.

Clarithromycin is known to prolong the QT interval. The QT interval is measured as the time and distance between the Q point of the QRS complex and the end of the T wave in the ECG tracing. After adjustment for heart rate, the QT interval is defined as prolonged if it is more than 450 msec in men and 460 msec in women. A long QT syndrome was first described in the 1950s and 60s as a congenital syndrome involving QT interval prolongation and syncope and sudden death. Some of the congenital long QT syndromes were characterized by a peculiar electrocardiographic appearance of the QRS complex involving a premature atria beat followed by a pause, then a subsequent sinus beat showing marked QT prolongation and deformity. This type of cardiac arrhythmia was originally termed "torsade de pointes" (translated from the French as "twisting of the points"). Clarithromycin is considered as having a risk of causing torsade de pointes. Since it is not known what effect vasoconstrictors in the local anesthetic regimen will have in patients with a known history of congenital prolonged QT interval or in patients taking any medication that prolongs the QT interval, a medical consult is suggested.

References

ADA Division of Legal Affairs, "A Legal Perspective on Antibiotic Prophylaxis," *J Am Dent Assoc*, 2003, 134(9):1260.

American Dental Association Council on Scientific Affairs, "Combating Antibiotic Resistance," *J Am Dent Assoc*, 2004, 135(4):484-7.

Amsden GW, "Erythromycin, Clarithromycin, and Azithromycin: Are the Differences Real?" *Clin Ther*, 1996, 18(1):56-72.

Dajani AS, Taubert KA, Wilson W, et al, "Prevention of Bacterial Endocarditis. Recommendations by the American Heart Association," *JAMA*, 1997, 277(22):1794-801.

Dajani AS, Taubert KA, Wilson W, et al, "Prevention of Bacterial Endocarditis: Recommendations by the American Heart Association," *J Am Dent Assoc*, 1997, 128(8):1142-51.

Moore PA, "Dental Therapeutic Indications for the Newer Long-Acting Macrolide Antibiotics," *J Am Dent Assoc*, 1999, 130(9):1341-3.

"Pimozide (Orap) Contraindicated With Clarithromycin (Biaxin®) and Other Macrolide Antibiotics," *FDA Medical Bulletin*, October 1996, 26 (3).

Wilson W, Taubert KA, Gewitz M, et al, "Prevention of Infective Endocarditis. Guidelines From the American Heart Association. A Guideline From the American Heart Association Rheumatic Fever, Endocarditis, and Kawasaki Disease Committee, Council on Cardiovascular Disease in the Young, and the Council on Clinical Cardiology, Council on Cardiovascular Surgery and Anesthesia, and the Quality of Care and Outcomes Research Interdisciplinary Working Group," *Circulation*, 2007, 115. Available at http://circ.ahajournals.org/cgi/reprint/CIRCULATIONAHA.106.183095v1; last accessed July 26, 2007.

Wynn RL, "New Erythromycins," *Gen Dent*, 1996, 44(4):304-7.

Wynn RL, Bergman SA, Meiller TF, et al, "Antibiotics in Treating Oral-Facial Infections of Odontogenic Origin: An Update," *Gen Dent*, 2001, 49(3):238-40, 242, 244 passim.

Clemastine (KLEM as teen)

U.S. Brand Names Tavist® Allergy [OTC]

Pharmacologic Category Ethanolamine Derivative; Histamine H_1 Antagonist; Histamine H_1 Antagonist, First Generation

Use Perennial and seasonal allergic rhinitis and other allergic symptoms including urticaria

Local Anesthetic/Vasoconstrictor Precautions No information available to require special precautions

Effects on Dental Treatment Key adverse event(s) related to dental treatment: Xerostomia (normal salivary flow resumes upon discontinuation).

Effects on Bleeding No information available to require special precautions

Adverse Effects Frequency not defined.

Cardiovascular: Palpitation, hypotension, tachycardia

Central nervous system: Dyscoordination, sedation, somnolence slight to moderate, sleepiness, confusion, restlessness, nervousness, insomnia, irritability, fatigue, headache, dizziness increased

Dermatologic: Rash, photosensitivity

Gastrointestinal: Diarrhea, nausea, xerostomia, epigastric distress, vomiting, constipation

Genitourinary: Urinary frequency, difficult urination, urinary retention

Hematologic: Hemolytic anemia, thrombocytopenia, agranulocytosis

Ocular: Blurred vision

Otic: Tinnitus
Respiratory: Thickening of bronchial secretions
Miscellaneous: Anaphylaxis

General Dosage Range Oral:

Children <6 years: 0.05 mg/kg/day (base) **or** 0.335-0.67 mg/day (fumarate) in 2-3 divided doses (maximum: 1.34 mg/day [fumarate] or 1 mg/day [base])

Children 6-12 years: 0.67-1.34 mg fumarate (0.5-1 mg base) twice daily (maximum: 4.02 mg/day [3 mg base])

Children ≥12 years and Adults: 1.34-2.68 mg fumarate (1-2 mg base) 2-3 times/day (maximum: 8.04 mg/day [6 mg base])

Mechanism of Action Competes with histamine for H_1-receptor sites on effector cells in the gastrointestinal tract, blood vessels, and respiratory tract

Pharmacodynamics/Kinetics

Onset of Action Peak effect: Therapeutic: 5-7 hours

Duration of Action 8-16 hours

Pregnancy Risk Factor B

Clevidipine (klev ID i peen)

Related Information

Calcium Channel Blockers and Gingival Hyperplasia *on page 2014*

U.S. Brand Names Cleviprex™

Pharmacologic Category Calcium Channel Blocker; Calcium Channel Blocker, Dihydropyridine

Use Management of hypertension

Local Anesthetic/Vasoconstrictor Precautions No information available to require special precautions

Effects on Dental Treatment Key adverse event(s) related to dental treatment: Although other calcium channel blockers (eg, nifedipine, diltiazem) have been associated with gingival hyperplasia, there are no reports that clevidipine has caused this adverse effect.

Effects on Bleeding No information available to require special precautions

Adverse Effects

>10%:
Central nervous system: Fever (19%), insomnia (12%)
Gastrointestinal: Nausea (5% to 21%)

1% to 10%:
Central nervous system: Headache (6%)
Gastrointestinal: Vomiting (3%)
Hematologic: Postprocedural hemorrhage (3%)
Renal: Acute renal failure (9%)
Respiratory: Pneumonia (3%), respiratory failure (3%)

General Dosage Range I.V.: *Adults:* Initial: 1-2 mg/hour; Usual maintenance: 4-6 mg/hour; Maximum: 21 mg/hour (1000 mL/24 hours)

Mechanism of Action Dihydropyridine calcium channel blocker with potent arterial vasodilating activity. Inhibits calcium ion influx through the L-type calcium channels during depolarization in arterial smooth muscle, producing a decrease in mean arterial pressure (MAP) by reducing systemic vascular resistance.

Pharmacodynamics/Kinetics

Onset of Action 2-4 minutes after start of infusion

Duration of Action I.V.: 5-15 minutes

Half-life Elimination Biphasic: Initial: 1 minute (predominant); Terminal: 15 minutes

Pregnancy Risk Factor C

Clidinium and Chlordiazepoxide (kli DI nee um & klor dye az e POKS ide)

Related Information

ChlordiazePOXIDE *on page 359*

U.S. Brand Names Librax® *[original formulation]*

Canadian Brand Names Apo-Chlorax®; Librax®

Pharmacologic Category Antispasmodic Agent, Gastrointestinal; Benzodiazepine

Use Adjunct treatment of peptic ulcer; treatment of irritable bowel syndrome

Local Anesthetic/Vasoconstrictor Precautions No information available to require special precautions

Effects on Dental Treatment Key adverse event(s) related to dental treatment: Xerostomia and changes in salivation (normal salivary flow resumes upon discontinuation).

Effects on Bleeding No information available to require special precautions

Adverse Effects 1% to 10%:

Central nervous system: Drowsiness, ataxia, confusion, anticholinergic side effects
Gastrointestinal: Dry mouth, constipation, nausea

General Dosage Range Oral: *Adults:* 1-2 capsules 3-4 times/day

Pregnancy Risk Factor D

Clindamycin (Systemic) (klin da MYE sin)

Related Information

Antibiotic Prophylaxis *on page 1910*
Bacterial Infections *on page 1933*
Periodontal Diseases *on page 1942*
Sexually-Transmitted Diseases *on page 1903*

Related Sample Prescriptions

Bacterial Infections and Periodontal Diseases *on page 1983*
Infective Endocarditis (Prevention) *on page 1978*
Prosthetic Joint Late Infections (Prevention) *on page 1979*

U.S. Brand Names Cleocin HCl®; Cleocin Pediatric®; Cleocin Phosphate®

Canadian Brand Names Alti-Clindamycin; Apo-Clindamycin®; Clindamycin Injection, USP; Clindamycine; Gen-Clindamycin; Mylan-Clindamycin; Novo-Clindamycin; NV-Clindamycin; PMS-Clindamycin; ratio-Clindamycin; Riva-Clindamycin; Teva-Clindamycin

Generic Availability (U.S.) Yes

Pharmacologic Category Antibiotic, Lincosamide

Dental Use Alternate oral antibiotic for prevention of infective endocarditis in individuals allergic to penicillins or ampicillin, when amoxicillin cannot be used; alternate I.M. or I.V. antibiotic for prevention of infective endocarditis in patients allergic to penicillins or ampicillin and unable to take oral medication; alternate oral antibiotic for prophylaxis for dental patients with total joint replacement who are allergic to penicillin; alternate I.V. antibiotic for prophylaxis for dental patients with total joint replacement who are allergic to penicillin and unable to take oral medications; alternate antibiotic in the treatment of common orofacial infections caused by aerobic gram-positive cocci and susceptible anaerobes; treatment of periodontal disease

Use Treatment of susceptible bacterial infections, mainly those caused by anaerobes, streptococci, pneumococci, and staphylococci; pelvic inflammatory disease (I.V.)

Unlabeled/Investigational Use May be useful in PCP; alternate treatment for toxoplasmosis; bacterial vaginosis (oral); alternate treatment for MRSA infections; alternate antibiotic for prophylaxis of infective endocarditis in patients who are allergic to penicillin and undergoing surgical or dental procedures (ACC/AHA guidelines)

Local Anesthetic/Vasoconstrictor Precautions No information available to require special precautions

Effects on Dental Treatment No significant effects or complications reported

Effects on Bleeding No information available to require special precautions

Adverse Effects Frequency not defined.

Cardiovascular: Cardiac arrest (rare; I.V. administration), hypotension (rare; I.V. administration)
Dermatologic: Erythema multiforme (rare), exfoliative dermatitis (rare), pruritus, rash, Stevens-Johnson syndrome (rare), urticaria
Gastrointestinal: Abdominal pain, diarrhea, esophagitis, nausea, pseudomembranous colitis, vomiting
Genitourinary: Vaginitis
Hematologic: Agranulocytosis, eosinophilia (transient), neutropenia (transient), thrombocytopenia
Hepatic: Jaundice, liver function test abnormalities
Local: Induration/pain/sterile abscess (I.M.), thrombophlebitis (I.V.)
Neuromuscular & skeletal: Polyarthritis (rare)
Renal: Renal dysfunction (rare)
Miscellaneous: Anaphylactoid reactions (rare)

Dental Usual Dosage

Orofacial infection:
- Children:
  - Oral: 10-20 mg/kg/day in 3-4 equally divided doses
  - I.V.: 15-25 mg/kg/day in 3-4 equally divided doses
- Adults:
  - Oral: 150-450 mg/dose for 7 days; maximum dose: 1.8 g/day
  - I.V.: 600-900 mg every 8 hours

Treatment of periodontal disease: Oral: 300 mg every 8 hours for 8 days

Infective endocarditis prophylaxis:
Children:
Oral: 20 mg/kg 30-60 minutes before procedure
I.M., I.V.: 20 mg/kg 30-60 minutes before procedure. **Note:** Intramuscular injections should be avoided in patients who are receiving anticoagulant therapy. In these circumstances, orally administered regimens should be given whenever possible. Intravenously administered antibiotics should be used for patients who are unable to tolerate or absorb oral medications.
Adults:
Oral: 600 mg 30-60 minutes before procedure
I.M., I.V.: 600 mg 30-60 minutes before procedure. **Note:** Intramuscular injections should be avoided in patients who are receiving anticoagulant therapy. In these circumstances, orally administered regimens should be given whenever possible. Intravenously administered antibiotics should be used for patients who are unable to tolerate or absorb oral medications.
Prophylaxis in total joint replacement patients undergoing dental procedures which produce bacteremia:
Adults:
Oral: 600 mg 1 hour prior to procedure
I.V.: 600 mg 1 hour prior to procedure (for patients unable to take oral medication)

Dosage

Usual dosage ranges:
Infants and Children:
Oral: 8-20 mg/kg/day as hydrochloride; 8-25 mg/kg/day as palmitate in 3-4 divided doses (minimum dose of palmitate: 37.5 mg 3 times/day)
I.M., I.V.:
<1 month: 15-20 mg/kg/day in 3-4 divided doses
>1 month: 20-40 mg/kg/day in 3-4 divided doses
Adults:
Oral: 150-450 mg/dose every 6-8 hours; maximum dose: 1.8 g/day
I.M., I.V.: 1.2-2.7 g/day in 2-4 divided doses; maximum dose: 4.8 g/day

Indication-specific dosing:
Children:
Anthrax (unlabeled use): I.V.: 7.5 mg/kg every 6 hours
Babesiosis (unlabeled use): Oral: 20-40 mg/kg/day divided every 8 hours for 7-10 days plus quinine (*Medical Letter*, 2007)
Cellulitis due to MRSA (unlabeled use): Oral: 10-13 mg/kg/dose every 6-8 hours for 5-10 days (maximum: 40 mg/kg/day) (Liu, 2011)
Complicated skin/soft tissue infection due to MRSA (unlabeled use): I.V., Oral: 10-13 mg/kg/dose every 6-8 hours for 7-14 days (maximum: 40 mg/kg/day) (Liu, 2011)
Orofacial infections:
Oral: 10-20 mg/kg/day in 3-4 equally divided doses
I.V.: 15-25 mg/kg/day in 3-4 equally divided doses
Osteomyelitis due to MRSA (unlabeled use): I.V., Oral: 10-13 mg/kg/dose every 6-8 hours for a minimum of 4-6 weeks (maximum: 40 mg/kg/day) (Liu, 2011)
Pneumonia due to MRSA (unlabeled use): I.V., Oral: 10-13 mg/kg/dose every 6-8 hours for 7-21 days (maximum: 40 mg/kg/day) (Liu, 2011)
Prophylaxis against infective endocarditis (unlabeled use):
Oral: 20 mg/kg 30-60 minutes before procedure (Wilson, 2007)
I.M., I.V.: 20 mg/kg 30-60 minutes before procedure. Intramuscular injections should be avoided in patients who are receiving anticoagulant therapy. In these circumstances, orally administered regimens should be given whenever possible. Intravenously administered antibiotics should be used for patients who are unable to tolerate or absorb oral medications. (Wilson, 2007)
Note: American Heart Association (AHA) guidelines now recommend prophylaxis only in patients undergoing invasive procedures and in whom underlying cardiac conditions may predispose to a higher risk of adverse outcomes should infection occur. As of April 2007, routine prophylaxis for GI/GU procedures is no longer recommended by the AHA.
Septic arthritis due to MRSA (unlabeled use): I.V., Oral: 10-13 mg/kg/dose every 6-8 hours for minimum of 3-4 weeks (maximum: 40 mg/kg/day) (Liu, 2011)
Toxoplasmosis (HIV-exposed/-positive; secondary prevention [unlabeled use]): Oral: 20-30 mg/kg/day divided every 6-8 hours (plus pyrimethamine and leucovorin calcium) (CDC, 2009)
Adults:
Amnionitis: I.V.: 450-900 mg every 8 hours
Anthrax (unlabeled use): I.V.: 900 mg every 8 hours with ciprofloxacin or doxycycline

Babesiosis (unlabeled use):
Oral: 600 mg 3 times/day for 7-10 days with quinine (*Medical Letter*, 2007)
I.V.: 1.2 g twice daily for 7-10 days with quinine (*Medical Letter*, 2007)

Bacterial vaginosis (unlabeled use): Oral: 300 mg twice daily for 7 days (CDC, 2010)

Bite wounds (canine): Oral: 300 mg 4 times/day with a fluoroquinolone

Cellulitis due to MRSA (unlabeled use): Oral: 300-450 mg 3 times/day for 5-10 days (Liu, 2011)

Complicated skin/soft tissue infection due to MRSA (unlabeled use): I.V., Oral: 600 mg 3 times/day for 7-14 days (Liu, 2011)

Gangrenous pyomyositis: I.V.: 900 mg every 8 hours with penicillin G

Group B streptococcus (neonatal prophylaxis): I.V.: 900 mg every 8 hours until delivery

Orofacial/parapharyngeal space infections:
Oral: 150-450 mg every 6 hours for 7 days, maximum 1.8 g/day
I.V.: 600-900 mg every 8 hours

Osteomyelitis due to MRSA (unlabeled use): I.V., Oral: 600 mg 3 times/day for a minimum of 8 weeks (some experts combine with rifampin) (Liu, 2011)

Pelvic inflammatory disease: I.V.: 900 mg every 8 hours with gentamicin (conventional or single daily dosing); 24 hours after clinical improvement may convert to oral doxycycline 100 mg twice daily **or** clindamycin 450 mg 4 times/day to complete 14 days of total therapy. Avoid doxycycline if tubo-ovarian abscess is present. (CDC, 2010)

***Pneumocystis jiroveci* pneumonia (unlabeled use):**
I.V.: 600-900 mg every 6-8 hours with primaquine for 21 days (CDC, 2009)
Oral: 300-450 mg every 6-8 hours with primaquine for 21 days (CDC,2009)

Pneumonia due to MRSA (unlabeled use): I.V., Oral: 600 mg 3 times/day for 7-21 days (Liu, 2011)

Prophylaxis against infective endocarditis (unlabeled use):
Oral: 600 mg 30-60 minutes before procedure (Wilson, 2007)
I.M., I.V.: 600 mg 30-60 minutes before procedure. Intramuscular injections should be avoided in patients who are receiving anticoagulant therapy. In these circumstances, orally administered regimens should be given whenever possible. Intravenously administered antibiotics should be used for patients who are unable to tolerate or absorb oral medications. (Wilson, 2007)

Note: American Heart Association (AHA) guidelines now recommend prophylaxis only in patients undergoing invasive procedures and in whom underlying cardiac conditions may predispose to a higher risk of adverse outcomes should infection occur. As of April 2007, routine prophylaxis for GI/GU procedures is no longer recommended by the AHA.

Prophylaxis in total joint replacement patients undergoing dental procedures which produce bacteremia (unlabeled use):
Oral: 600 mg 1 hour prior to procedure (ADA, 2003)
I.V.: 600 mg 1 hour prior to procedure (for patients unable to take oral medication) (ADA, 2003)

Septic arthritis due to MRSA (unlabeled use): I.V., Oral: 600 mg 3 times/day for 3-4 weeks (Liu, 2011)

Toxic shock syndrome: I.V.: 900 mg every 8 hours with penicillin G or ceftriaxone

Toxoplasmosis (HIV-exposed/positive; secondary prevention [unlabeled use]): Oral: 600 mg every 8 hours (with pyrimethamine and leucovorin calcium) (CDC, 2009)

Dosing adjustment in renal impairment: No adjustment required.

Dosing adjustment in hepatic impairment: No adjustment required. Use caution with severe hepatic impairment.

Mechanism of Action Reversibly binds to 50S ribosomal subunits preventing peptide bond formation thus inhibiting bacterial protein synthesis; bacteriostatic or bactericidal depending on drug concentration, infection site, and organism

Contraindications Hypersensitivity to clindamycin, lincomycin, or any component of the formulation

Warnings/Precautions Dosage adjustment may be necessary in patients with severe hepatic dysfunction. **[U.S. Boxed Warning]: Can cause severe and possibly fatal colitis.** Prolonged use may result in fungal or bacterial superinfection, including *C. difficile*-associated diarrhea (CDAD) and pseudomembranous colitis; CDAD has been observed >2 months postantibiotic treatment. Use with caution in patients with a history of gastrointestinal disease. Discontinue drug if significant diarrhea, abdominal cramps, or passage of blood and mucus occurs. Some dosage forms contain benzyl alcohol or tartrazine. Use caution in atopic patients. Not appropriate for use in the treatment of meningitis due to inadequate penetration into the CSF.

Drug Interactions

Avoid Concomitant Use

Avoid concomitant use of Clindamycin (Systemic) with any of the following: BCG; Erythromycin; Erythromycin (Systemic)

Increased Effect/Toxicity

Clindamycin (Systemic) may increase the levels/effects of: Neuromuscular-Blocking Agents

Decreased Effect

Clindamycin (Systemic) may decrease the levels/effects of: BCG; Erythromycin (Systemic); Typhoid Vaccine

The levels/effects of Clindamycin (Systemic) may be decreased by: Erythromycin; Kaolin

Ethanol/Nutrition/Herb Interactions

Food: Peak concentrations may be delayed with food.

Herb/Nutraceutical: St John's wort may decrease clindamycin levels.

Dietary Considerations May be taken with food.

Pharmacodynamics/Kinetics

Half-life Elimination Neonates: Premature: 8.7 hours; Full-term: 3.6 hours; Children: ~2 hours; Adults: ~2-3 hours; Elderly 4 hours (range: 3.4-5.1 hours)

Time to Peak Serum: Oral: Within 60 minutes; I.M.: 1-3 hours

Pregnancy Risk Factor B

Lactation Enters breast milk/not recommended (AAP rates "compatible"; AAP 2001 update pending)

Breast-Feeding Considerations Small amounts of clindamycin transfer to human milk. The manufacturer does not recommend the use of clindamycin during breast-feeding. Nondose-related effects could include modification of bowel flora. There has been one published case of bloody stools in a nursing infant, but a causal relationship was not proven.

Dosage Forms

Capsule, oral: 75 mg, 150 mg, 300 mg

Cleocin HCl®: 75 mg, 150 mg, 300 mg

Granules for solution, oral: 75 mg/5 mL (100 mL)

Cleocin Pediatric®: 75 mg/5 mL (100 mL)

Infusion, premixed in D_5W:

Cleocin Phosphate®: 300 mg (50 mL); 600 mg (50 mL); 900 mg (50 mL)

Injection, solution: 150 mg/mL (2 mL, 4 mL, 6 mL, 60 mL)

Cleocin Phosphate®: 150 mg/mL (2 mL, 4 mL, 6 mL, 60 mL)

Dental Comment Clindamycin has not been shown to interfere with oral contraceptive activity; however, it reduces GI microflora, thus, oral contraceptive users should be advised to use additional methods of birth control. About 1% of clindamycin users develop pseudomembranous colitis. Symptoms may occur 2-9 days after initiation of therapy; however, it has never occurred with the 1-dose regimen of clindamycin used to prevent bacterial endocarditis.

References

ADA Division of Legal Affairs, "A Legal Perspective on Antibiotic Prophylaxis," *J Am Dent Assoc*, 2003, 134(9):1260.

"Advisory Statement. Antibiotic Prophylaxis for Dental Patients With Total Joint Replacements. American Dental Association; American Academy of Orthopedic Surgeons," *J Am Dent Assoc*, 1997, 128 (7):1004-8.

American Dental Association; American Academy of Orthopedic Surgeons, "Antibiotic Prophylaxis for Dental Patients With Total Joint Replacements," *J Am Dent Assoc*, 2003, 134(7):895-9.

American Dental Association Council on Scientific Affairs, "Combating Antibiotic Resistance," *J Am Dent Assoc*, 2004, 135(4):484-7.

Dajani AS, Taubert KA, Wilson W, et al, "Prevention of Bacterial Endocarditis. Recommendations by the American Heart Association," *JAMA*, 1997, 277(22):1794-801.

Dajani AS, Taubert KA, Wilson W, et al, "Prevention of Bacterial Endocarditis: Recommendations by the American Heart Association," *J Am Dent Assoc*, 1997, 128(8):1142-51.

Sandor GK, Low DE, Judd PL, et al, "Antimicrobial Treatment Options in the Management of Odontogenic Infections," *J Can Dent Assoc*, 1998, 64(7):508-14.

Wilson W, Taubert KA, Gewitz M, et al, "Prevention of Infective Endocarditis. Guidelines From the American Heart Association. A Guideline From the American Heart Association Rheumatic Fever, Endocarditis, and Kawasaki Disease Committee, Council on Cardiovascular Disease in the Young, and the Council on Clinical Cardiology, Council on Cardiovascular Surgery and Anesthesia, and the Quality of Care and Outcomes Research Interdisciplinary Working Group," *Circulation*, 2007, 115. Available at http://circ.ahajournals.org/cgi/reprint/CIRCULATIONAHA.106.183095v1; last accessed July 26, 2007.

Wynn RL and Bergman SA, "Antibiotics and Their Use in the Treatment of Orofacial Infections, Part I and Part II," *Gen Dent*, 1994, 42(5):398-402, 498-502.

Wynn RL, Bergman SA, Meiller TF, et al, "Antibiotics in Treating Oral-Facial Infections of Odontogenic Origin: An Update," *Gen Dent*, 2001, 49(3):238-40, 242, 244 passim.

Wynn RL, "Clindamycin: An Often Forgotten but Important Antibiotic," *AGD Impact*, 1994, 22:10.

Clindamycin (Topical) (klin da MYE sin)

U.S. Brand Names Cleocin T®; Cleocin®; Cleocin® Vaginal Ovule; Clindagel®; ClindaMax®; ClindaReach®; Clindesse®; Evoclin®

Canadian Brand Names Clinda-T; Clindasol™; Clindets; Dalacin® C; Dalacin® T; Dalacin® Vaginal; Taro-Clindamycin

Pharmacologic Category Antibiotic, Lincosamide; Topical Skin Product, Acne

Use Treatment of bacterial vaginosis (vaginal cream, vaginal suppository); topically in treatment of severe acne

Local Anesthetic/Vasoconstrictor Precautions No information available to require special precautions

Effects on Dental Treatment No significant effects or complications reported

Effects on Bleeding No information available to require special precautions

Adverse Effects

Topical:

>10%: Dermatologic: Dryness, burning, itching, scaliness, erythema, or peeling of skin (lotion, solution); oiliness (gel, lotion)

1% to 10%: Central nervous system: Headache (3%)

Vaginal:

>10%: Genitourinary: Vaginal candidiasis (≤13%), vulvovaginal pruritus (from *Candida albicans*)

1% to 10%:

Dermatologic: Pruritus (≤1%)

Genitourinary: Vulvovaginal disorder (3% to 7%), vulvovaginitis (4% to 6%), vaginal pain (≤2%), trichomonal vaginitis (1%)

Miscellaneous: Fungal infection (1% to 2%)

General Dosage Range

Intravaginal: *Adults:* Insert 1 ovule or applicatorful once daily **or** 1 applicatorful as a single dose (Clindesse®)

Topical: *Children ≥12 years and Adults:* Apply once or twice daily

Mechanism of Action Reversibly binds to 50S ribosomal subunits preventing peptide bond formation thus inhibiting bacterial protein synthesis; bacteriostatic or bactericidal depending on drug concentration, infection site, and organism

Pharmacodynamics/Kinetics

Half-life Elimination Vaginal cream: 1.5-2.6 hours following repeated dosing; Vaginal suppository: 11 hours (range: 4-35 hours, limited by absorption rate)

Time to Peak Vaginal cream: ~10-14 hours (range: 4-24 hours); Vaginal suppository: ~5 hours (range: 1-10 hours)

Pregnancy Risk Factor B

Clindamycin and Benzoyl Peroxide

(klin da MYE sin & BEN zoe il peer OKS ide)

Related Information

Benzoyl Peroxide *on page 223*

Clindamycin (Topical) *on page 405*

U.S. Brand Names Acanya®; BenzaClin®; Duac® CS [DSC]

Canadian Brand Names BenzaClin®; Clindoxyl

Pharmacologic Category Acne Products; Topical Skin Product; Topical Skin Product, Acne

Use Topical treatment of acne vulgaris

Local Anesthetic/Vasoconstrictor Precautions No information available to require special precautions

Effects on Dental Treatment No significant effects or complications reported

Effects on Bleeding No information available to require special precautions

Adverse Effects

>10%: Dermatologic: Erythema (<1% to 26%), scaling (≤1% to 18%), peeling (2% to 17%), dry skin (1% to 15%), itching (<1% to 15%)

1% to 10%: Dermatologic: Burning (≤1% to 8%), stinging (≤1% to 6%), pruritus (2%), sunburn (1%)

General Dosage Range Topical: *Children ≥12 years and Adults:* Apply once daily (Acanya®, Duac® CS) **or** twice daily (BenzaClin®) to affected areas

Mechanism of Action Clindamycin and benzoyl peroxide have activity against *Propionibacterium acnes in vitro*. This organism has been associated with acne vulgaris. Benzoyl peroxide releases free-radical oxygen which oxidizes bacterial proteins in the sebaceous follicles decreasing the number of anaerobic bacteria and decreasing irritating-type free fatty acids. Clindamycin reversibly binds to 50S ribosomal subunits preventing peptide bond formation thus inhibiting bacterial protein synthesis; bacteriostatic or bactericidal depending on drug concentration, infection site, and organism.

Pregnancy Risk Factor C

Clindamycin and Tretinoin (klin da MYE sin & TRET i noyn)

Related Information

Clindamycin (Topical) *on page 405*

Tretinoin (Topical) *on page 1668*

U.S. Brand Names Veltin™; Ziana™

Pharmacologic Category Acne Products; Retinoic Acid Derivative; Topical Skin Product; Topical Skin Product, Acne

Use Treatment of acne vulgaris

Local Anesthetic/Vasoconstrictor Precautions No information available to require special precautions

Effects on Dental Treatment No significant effects or complications reported

Effects on Bleeding No information available to require special precautions

General Dosage Range Topical: *Children ≥12 years and Adults:* Apply pea-size amount to entire face once daily at bedtime

Mechanism of Action Clindamycin reversibly binds to 50S ribosomal subunits preventing peptide chain elongation thus inhibiting bacterial protein synthesis. Clindamycin exhibits *in vitro* activity against *Propionibacterium acnes*, an organism associated with acne vulgaris. Topical tretinoin is believed to decrease follicular epithelial cells cohesiveness and increase follicular epithelial cell turnover resulting in decreased microcomedo formation and increased expulsion of comedones.

Pregnancy Risk Factor C

Clobazam (KLOE ba zam)

Canadian Brand Names Apo-Clobazam®; Clobazam-10; Dom-Clobazam; Frisium®; Novo-Clobazam; PMS-Clobazam

Pharmacologic Category Benzodiazepine

Use Adjunctive treatment of epilepsy

Unlabeled/Investigational Use Monotherapy for epilepsy or intermittent seizures

Local Anesthetic/Vasoconstrictor Precautions No information available to require special precautions

Effects on Dental Treatment Key adverse event(s) related to dental treatment: Xerostomia (normal salivary flow resumes upon discontinuation). Paradoxical reactions (including excitation, agitation, hallucinations, and psychosis) are known to occur with benzodiazepines.

Effects on Bleeding No information available to require special precautions

Adverse Effects

Central nervous system: Drowsiness (17%), ataxia (4%), dizziness (2%), nervousness (2%), behavior disorder (1%), hostility (1%), anterograde amnesia, confusion, disorientation, headache, lethargy, sedation, slurred speech; paradoxical reactions (including aggression, agitation, anxiety, delusions, difficulty falling asleep, excitation, hallucinations, irritability, nightmares, rage, restlessness, psychosis, and suicidal tendencies)

Dermatologic: Rash, Stevens-Johnson syndrome, toxic epidermal necrolysis, urticaria

Endocrine: Libido decreased

Gastrointestinal: Weight gain (2%), constipation, nausea, xerostomia

Hematologic: Decreased WBCs and other hematologic abnormalities have been rarely associated with benzodiazepines

Neuromuscular & skeletal: Gait instability, muscle spasm, muscle weakness, tremor

Ocular: Blurred vision (1%), double vision, nystagmus

General Dosage Range Dosage adjustment recommended in patients with hepatic or renal impairment

Oral:

Children <2 years: 0.5-1 mg/kg/day

Children 2-16 years: Initial: 5 mg/day; Maintenance: Up to 40 mg/day

Adults: Initial: 5-15 mg/day; Maintenance: Up to 80 mg/day

Mechanism of Action Clobazam is a 1,5 benzodiazepine which binds to stereospecific benzodiazepine receptors on the postsynaptic GABA neuron at several sites within the central nervous system, including the limbic system, reticular formation. Enhancement of the inhibitory effect of GABA on neuronal excitability results by increased neuronal membrane permeability to chloride ions. This shift in chloride ions results in hyperpolarization (a less excitable state) and stabilization.

Pharmacodynamics/Kinetics

Half-life Elimination 18 hours; N-desmethyl (active): 42 hours

Time to Peak 15 minutes to 4 hours

Product Availability Not available in U.S.

Clobetasol (kloe BAY ta sol)

Related Information

Ulcerative, Erosive, and Painful Oral Mucosal Disorders *on page 1950*

Related Sample Prescriptions

Erosive Lichen Planus, Other Biopsy-Proven Desquamative Oral Diseases, and Major Aphthae *on page 1992*

Recurrent Aphthous Stomatitis *on page 1992*

U.S. Brand Names Clobex®; Cormax®; Olux-E™; Olux®; Olux®/Olux-E™ CP [DSC]; Temovate E®; Temovate®

Canadian Brand Names Clobex®; Dermovate®; Gen-Clobetasol; Mylan-Clobetasol Cream; Mylan-Clobetasol Ointment; Mylan-Clobetasol Scalp Application; Novo-Clobetasol; PMS-Clobetasol; ratio-Clobetasol; Taro-Clobetasol

Generic Availability (U.S.) Yes: Excludes lotion, shampoo, spray

Pharmacologic Category Corticosteroid, Topical

Dental Use Short-term relief of oral mucosal inflammation

Use Short-term relief of inflammation of moderate-to-severe corticosteroid-responsive dermatoses (very high potency topical corticosteroid)

Local Anesthetic/Vasoconstrictor Precautions No information available to require special precautions

Effects on Dental Treatment No significant effects or complications reported

Effects on Bleeding No information available to require special precautions

Adverse Effects Frequency not defined; may depend upon formulation used, length of application, surface area covered, and the use of occlusive dressings.

Endocrine & metabolic: Adrenal suppression, Cushing's syndrome, hyperglycemia

Local: Application site: Burning, cracking/fissuring of the skin, dryness, erythema, folliculitis, irritation, numbness, pruritus, skin atrophy, stinging, telangiectasia

Renal: Glucosuria

Effects reported with other high-potency topical steroids: Acneiform eruptions, allergic contact dermatitis, hypertrichosis, hypopigmentation, maceration of the skin, miliaria, perioral dermatitis, secondary infection

Dental Usual Dosage Oral mucosal inflammation: Children ≥12 years and Adults: Cream: Apply twice daily for up to 2 weeks (maximum dose: 50 g/week); discontinue application when control is achieved; if no improvement is seen, reassessment of diagnosis may be necessary

Dosage Topical: Discontinue when control achieved; if improvement not seen within 2 weeks, reassessment of diagnosis may be necessary.

Children <12 years: Use is not recommended

Children ≥12 years and Adults:

- Oral mucosal inflammation, dental (unlabeled use): Cream: Apply twice daily for up to 2 weeks (maximum dose: 50 g/week); discontinue application when control is achieved; if no improvement is seen, reassessment of diagnosis may be necessary
- Steroid-responsive dermatoses:
  - Cream, emollient cream, gel, ointment: Apply twice daily for up to 2 weeks (maximum dose: 50 g/week)
  - Foam (Olux-E™): Apply to affected area twice daily for up to 2 weeks (maximum dose: 50 g/week); do not apply to face or intertriginous areas
- Steroid-responsive dermatoses: Foam (Olux®), solution: Apply to affected scalp twice daily for up to 2 weeks (maximum dose: 50 g/week or 50 mL/week)
- Mild-to-moderate plaque-type psoriasis of nonscalp areas: Foam (Olux®): Apply to affected area twice daily for up to 2 weeks (maximum dose: 50 g/week); do not apply to face or intertriginous areas

Children ≥16 years and Adults: Moderate-to-severe plaque-type psoriasis: Emollient cream, lotion: Apply twice daily for up to 2 weeks, has been used for up to 4 weeks when application is <10% of body surface area; use with caution (maximum dose: 50 g/week)

Children ≥18 years and Adults:

- Moderate-to-severe plaque-type psoriasis: Spray: Apply by spraying directly onto affected area twice daily; should be gently rubbed into skin. Should be used for not longer than 4 weeks; treatment beyond 2 weeks should be limited to localized lesions which have not improved sufficiently. Total dose should not exceed 50 g/week or 59 mL/week.
- Scalp psoriasis: Shampoo: Apply thin film to dry scalp once daily; leave in place for 15 minutes, then add water, lather; rinse thoroughly
- Steroid-responsive dermatoses: Lotion: Apply twice daily for up to 2 weeks (maximum dose: 50 g/week)

Mechanism of Action Stimulates the synthesis of enzymes needed to decrease inflammation, suppress mitotic activity, and cause vasoconstriction

Contraindications Hypersensitivity to clobetasol or any component of the formulation; viral, fungal, or tubercular skin lesions

Warnings/Precautions Systemic absorption of topical corticosteroids may cause hypothalamic-pituitary-adrenal (HPA) axis suppression (reversible) particularly in younger children. HPA axis suppression may lead to adrenal crisis. Risk is increased when used over large surface areas, for prolonged periods, or with occlusive dressings. Allergic contact dermatitis can occur, it is usually diagnosed by failure to heal rather than clinical exacerbation. Prolonged treatment with corticosteroids has been associated with the development of Kaposi's sarcoma (case reports); if noted, discontinuation of therapy should be considered. Adverse systemic effects including hyperglycemia, glycosuria, fluid and electrolyte changes, and HPA suppression may occur when used on large surface areas, for prolonged periods, or with an occlusive dressing. Use in children <12 years of age is not recommended. Do not use on the face, axillae, or groin.

Drug Interactions

Avoid Concomitant Use

Avoid concomitant use of Clobetasol with any of the following: Aldesleukin

Increased Effect/Toxicity

Clobetasol may increase the levels/effects of: Deferasirox

Decreased Effect

Clobetasol may decrease the levels/effects of: Aldesleukin; Corticorelin

Pregnancy Risk Factor C

Lactation Excretion in breast milk unknown/use caution

Breast-Feeding Considerations It is not known if topical application will result in detectable quantities in breast milk.

Dosage Forms

Aerosol, topical: 0.05% (50 g, 100 g)
Olux-E™: 0.05% (50 g, 100 g)
Olux®: 0.05% (50 g, 100 g)

Cream, topical: 0.05% (15 g, 30 g, 45 g, 60 g)
Temovate E®: 0.05% (60 g)

Gel, topical: 0.05% (15 g, 30 g, 60 g)
Temovate®: 0.05% (60 g)

Lotion, topical:
Clobex®: 0.05% (30 mL, 59 mL, 118 mL)

Ointment, topical: 0.05% (15 g, 30 g, 45 g, 60 g)
Cormax®: 0.05% (15 g, 45 g)
Temovate®: 0.05% (15 g, 30 g)

Shampoo, topical:
Clobex®: 0.05% (118 mL)

Solution, topical: 0.05% (25 mL, 50 mL)
Clobex®: 0.05% (59 mL, 125 mL)
Cormax®: 0.05% (25 mL, 50 mL)
Temovate®: 0.05% (50 mL)

Clocortolone (kloe KOR toe lone)

U.S. Brand Names Cloderm®

Canadian Brand Names Cloderm®

Pharmacologic Category Corticosteroid, Topical

Use Inflammation of corticosteroid-responsive dermatoses (intermediate-potency topical corticosteroid)

Local Anesthetic/Vasoconstrictor Precautions No information available to require special precautions

Effects on Dental Treatment No significant effects or complications reported

Effects on Bleeding No information available to require special precautions

Adverse Effects 1% to 10%:

Dermatologic: Itching, erythema

Local: Burning, dryness, irritation, papular rash

General Dosage Range Topical: *Adults:* Apply sparingly to affected area 1-4 times/day

Mechanism of Action Stimulates the synthesis of enzymes needed to decrease inflammation, suppress mitotic activity, and cause vasoconstriction

Pregnancy Risk Factor C

Clodronate (KLOE droh nate)

Related Information

Osteonecrosis of the Jaw *on page 1894*

Canadian Brand Names Bonefos®; Clasteon®

Pharmacologic Category Bisphosphonate Derivative

Use Management of hypercalcemia of malignancy; management of osteolysis due to bone metastases of malignancy

Local Anesthetic/Vasoconstrictor Precautions No information available to require special precautions

Effects on Dental Treatment Osteonecrosis of the jaw (ONJ), generally associated with local infection and/or tooth extraction and often with delayed healing, has been reported in patients taking bisphosphonates. Symptoms included nonhealing extraction socket or an exposed jawbone. Most reported cases of bisphosphonate-associated osteonecrosis have been in cancer patients treated with intravenous bisphosphonates. However, some have occurred in patients with postmenopausal osteoporosis taking oral bisphosphonates. Dental surgery, particularly tooth extraction, may increase the risk for ONJ. Patients who develop ONJ while on bisphosphonate therapy should receive care by an oral surgeon. See Dental Comment.

Effects on Bleeding No information available to require special precautions

Adverse Effects

>10%: Hepatic: Transaminases increased (≤18%; >2 x ULN: 2%)

1% to 10%:

- Endocrine & metabolic: Hypocalcemia (≤3%)
- Gastrointestinal: GI disturbances (≤10%; includes anorexia, diarrhea, gastric pain, nausea, vomiting)
- Renal: Serum creatinine increased (1%), BUN increased

General Dosage Range Dosage adjustment recommended in patients with renal impairment

I.V.: *Adults:* 1500 mg as single dose (Clasteon®) **or** 300 mg/day (Clasteon®, Bonefos®); Maximum therapy: 10 days (Clasteon®); 7 days (Bonefos®)

Oral: *Adults:* 1600-2400 mg/day in 1-2 divided doses (maximum: 3200 mg/day)

Mechanism of Action A bisphosphonate which lowers serum calcium by inhibition of bone resorption via actions on osteoclasts or on osteoclast precursors.

Pharmacodynamics/Kinetics

Onset of Action Calcium-lowering effects: I.V.: Within 48 hours

Duration of Action Calcium-lowering effects: 5 days to 3 weeks following discontinuation

Half-life Elimination Terminal: Oral: ~6 hours; I.V.: 13 hours (serum); prolonged in bone tissue

Time to Peak Plasma: Oral: 30 minutes

Product Availability Not available in U.S.

Dental Comment The American Association of Oral and Maxillofacial Surgeons position paper on bisphosphonate-related osteonecrosis of the jaws, 2009 update, stated that I.V. bisphosphonate exposure in the setting of managing malignancy remains the major risk factor for the development of ONJ. After reviewing case series, case-controlled studies, and cohort studies, the estimates of the cumulative incidence of I.V. bisphosphonate-associated ONJ ranges from 0.8% to 12%.

Two reports have attempted to assess more accurately the percent of cancer patients developing ONJ after bisphosphonate treatment. Maerevoet et al, reported that among 194 patients treated with Zometa® every 3-4 weeks, nine developed ONJ. Before receiving Zometa®, six had received Aredia® 90 mg every 3-4 weeks. The median duration of treatment with Aredia® was 39 months and for Zometa® 18 months. The incidence of ONJ in these patients was calculated to be 4.6%. Durie et al, described the results of a survey by the International Myeloma Foundation in 2004 to assess the risk factors of ONJ. Out of 1203 respondents, 904 had myeloma and 299 had breast cancer. Of the myeloma patients, 62 developed ONJ and 54 had suspicious findings. Of the breast cancer patients, 13 had ONJ and 23 had suspicious findings. The total number of cases of either ONJ or suspicious findings was 152. ONJ developed in 10% of 211 patients receiving Zometa® compared to 4% of 413 receiving Aredia®. The mean time to onset of ONJ among patients taking Zometa® was 18 months; the mean time to onset after Aredia® was 6 years. It should be noted that an early report by authors from Novartis Pharmaceuticals Corporation stressed that Aredia® and Zometa® had been used in 2.5 million patients world wide and reports of ONJ during their extensive use had been rare (Tarassoff, 2003). In addition, these authors stated that review of the reported cases revealed multiple risk factors for avascular necrosis. McMahon et al, followed up with a report that, along with other factors, bisphosphonates are additional stressors of bone health that can tip the balance to osteonecrosis. They suggested that the prevention of ONJ should be stressed such as the elimination of chronic dental infections prior to chemotherapy and bisphosphonate use in cancer patients.

Clofarabine (klo FARE a been)

U.S. Brand Names Clolar®

Pharmacologic Category Antineoplastic Agent, Antimetabolite (Purine Analog)

Use Treatment of relapsed or refractory acute lymphoblastic leukemia (ALL)

Unlabeled/Investigational Use Relapsed and refractory acute myeloid leukemia (AML) and myelodysplastic syndrome (MDS)

Local Anesthetic/Vasoconstrictor Precautions No information available to require special precautions

Effects on Dental Treatment Key adverse event(s) related to dental treatment: Mucosal inflammation and gingival bleeding.

Effects on Bleeding Chemotherapy may result in significant myelosuppression, potentially including significant reduction in platelet counts and altered hemostasis. In patients who are under active treatment with these agents, medical consult is suggested.

Adverse Effects

>10%:

- Cardiovascular: Tachycardia (35%), hypotension (29%), flushing (19%), hypertension (13%), edema (12%)
- Central nervous system: Headache (43%), fever (39%), chills (34%), fatigue (34%), anxiety (21%), pain (15%)
- Dermatologic: Pruritus (43%), rash (38%), petechiae (26%), palmar-plantar erythrodysesthesia syndrome (16%), erythema (11%)
- Gastrointestinal: Vomiting (78%; grades 3/4: 9%), nausea (73%; grades 3/4: 15%), diarrhea (56%), abdominal pain (8% to 35%), anorexia (30%), mucosal inflammation (16%), gingival bleeding (14%), oral candidiasis (11%)
- Genitourinary: Hematuria (13%)
- Hematologic: Leukopenia (grades 3/4: 88%), anemia (83%; grades 3/4: 75%), lymphopenia (grades 3/4: 82%), thrombocytopenia (81%; grades 3/4: 80%), neutropenia (grades 3/4: 10% to 64%), febrile neutropenia (55%; grade 4: 3%)
- Hepatic: ALT increased (81%; grades 3/4: 43% to 44%), AST increased (74%; grades 3/4: 36%), bilirubin increased (45%; grades 3/4: 13%)
- Neuromuscular & skeletal: Limb pain (30%), myalgia (14%)
- Renal: Creatinine increased (50%; grades 3/4: 8%)
- Respiratory: Epistaxis (27%), dyspnea (13%), pleural effusion (12%)
- Miscellaneous: Infection (83%; includes bacterial, fungal, and viral), catheter-related infection (12%)

1% to 10%:

- Cardiovascular: Pericardial effusion (8%)
- Central nervous system: Irritability (10%), lethargy (10%), somnolence (10%), agitation (5%), mental status change
- Dermatologic: Cellulitis (8%), pruritic rash (8%)
- Gastrointestinal: Proctalgia (8%), clostridium colitis (7%), stomatitis (7%), mouth hemorrhage (5%), oral mucosal petechiae (5%), cecitis (1% to 4%), pancreatitis (1% to 4%)
- Hepatic: Jaundice (8%)
- Neuromuscular & skeletal: Back pain (10%), bone pain (10%), weakness (10%), arthralgia (9%)
- Respiratory: Pneumonia (10%), respiratory distress (10%), tachypnea (9%), upper respiratory tract infection (5%), pulmonary edema (1% to 4%)
- Miscellaneous: Herpes simplex (10%), sepsis (10%), bacteremia (9%), candidiasis (7%), herpes zoster (7%), septic shock (7%), staphylococcus bacteremia (6%), tumor lysis syndrome (grade 3: 6%), capillary leak syndrome (4%), hypersensitivity (1% to 4%), SIRS (2%)

General Dosage Range Dosage adjustment recommended in patients who develop toxicities

I.V.: *Children >1 year and Adults ≤21 years:* 52 mg/m^2/day days 1 through 5; repeat every 2-6 weeks

Mechanism of Action Clofarabine, a purine (deoxyadenosine) nucleoside analog, is metabolized to clofarabine 5'-triphosphate. Clofarabine 5'-triphosphate decreases cell replication and repair as well as causing cell death. To decrease cell replication and repair, clofarabine 5'-triphosphate competes with deoxyadenosine triphosphate for the enzymes ribonucleotide reductase and DNA polymerase. Cell replication is decreased when clofarabine 5'-triphosphate inhibits ribonucleotide reductase from reacting with deoxyadenosine triphosphate to produce deoxynucleotide triphosphate which is needed for DNA synthesis. Cell replication is also decreased when clofarabine 5'-triphosphate competes with DNA polymerase for incorporation into the DNA chain; when done during the repair process, cell repair is affected. To cause cell death, clofarabine 5'-triphosphate alters the mitochondrial membrane by releasing proteins, an inducing factor and cytochrome C.

Pharmacodynamics/Kinetics

Half-life Elimination ~5.2 hours

Pregnancy Risk Factor D

ClomiPHENE (KLOE mi feen)

U.S. Brand Names Clomid®; Serophene®

Canadian Brand Names Clomid®; Milophene®; Serophene®

Pharmacologic Category Ovulation Stimulator; Selective Estrogen Receptor Modulator (SERM)

Use Treatment of ovulatory failure in patients desiring pregnancy

Local Anesthetic/Vasoconstrictor Precautions No information available to require special precautions

Effects on Dental Treatment No significant effects or complications reported

Effects on Bleeding No information available to require special precautions

Adverse Effects

>10%: Endocrine & metabolic: Ovarian enlargement (14%)

1% to 10%:

- Central nervous system: Headache (1%)
- Endocrine & metabolic: Hot flashes (10%), breast discomfort (2%), abnormal uterine bleeding (1%)
- Gastrointestinal: Distention/bloating/discomfort (6%), nausea (2%), vomiting (2%)
- Ocular: Visual symptoms (2%, includes blurring of vision, diplopia, floaters, lights, phosphenes, photophobia, scotomata, waves)

General Dosage Range Oral: *Adults (females):* First course: 50 mg/day for 5 days; Second course (if needed): 100 mg/day for 5 days

Mechanism of Action Clomiphene is a racemic mixture consisting of zuclomiphene (~38%) and enclomiphene (~62%), each with distinct pharmacologic properties. Enclomiphene is much less potent in inducing ovulation; however, it is more rapidly absorbed and metabolized, allowing the more potent activity of zuclomiphene to predominate. Zuclomiphene acts at the level of the hypothalamus, occupying cell surface and intracellular estrogen receptors (ERs) for longer durations than estrogen. This interferes with receptor recycling, effectively depleting hypothalamic ERs and inhibiting normal estrogenic negative feedback. Impairment of the feedback signal results in increased pulsatile GnRH secretion from the hypothalamus and subsequent pituitary gonadotropin (FSH, LH) release, causing growth of the ovarian follicle, followed by follicular rupture.

Pharmacodynamics/Kinetics

Onset of Action Ovulation: 5-10 days following course of treatment

Duration of Action Effects are cumulative; ovulation may occur in the cycle following the last treatment

Half-life Elimination 5-7 days

Time to Peak ~6 hours

Pregnancy Risk Factor X

ClomiPRAMINE (kloe MI pra meen)

U.S. Brand Names Anafranil®

Canadian Brand Names Anafranil®; Apo-Clomipramine®; CO Clomipramine; Gen-Clomipramine

Pharmacologic Category Antidepressant, Tricyclic (Tertiary Amine)

Use Treatment of obsessive-compulsive disorder (OCD)

Unlabeled/Investigational Use Depression, panic attacks, chronic pain

Local Anesthetic/Vasoconstrictor Precautions Use with caution; epinephrine and levonordefrin have been shown to have an increased pressor response in combination with TCAs. Clomipramine is one of the drugs confirmed to prolong the QT interval and is accepted as having a risk of causing torsade de pointes. The risk of drug-induced torsade de pointes is extremely low when a single QT interval prolonging drug is prescribed. In terms of epinephrine, it is not known what effect vasoconstrictors in the local anesthetic regimen will have in patients with a known history of congenital prolonged QT interval or in patients taking any medication that prolongs the QT interval. Until more information is obtained, it is suggested that the clinician consult with the physician prior to the use of a vasoconstrictor in suspected patients, and that the vasoconstrictor (epinephrine, mepivacaine and levonordefrin [Carbocaine® 2% with Neo-Cobefrin®]) be used with caution.

Effects on Dental Treatment Key adverse event(s) related to dental treatment: Xerostomia and changes in salivation (normal salivary flow resumes upon discontinuation). Long-term treatment with TCAs, such as clomipramine, increases the risk of caries by reducing salivation and salivary buffer capacity.

Effects on Bleeding No information available to require special precautions

Adverse Effects Data shown for children reflects both children and adolescents studied in clinical trials.

>10%:

Central nervous system: Dizziness (54%), somnolence (54%), drowsiness, headache (52%; children 28%), fatigue (39%), insomnia (25%; children 11%), malaise, nervousness (18%; children 4%)

Endocrine & metabolic: Libido changes (21%), hot flushes (5%)

Gastrointestinal: Xerostomia (84%, children 63%) constipation (47%; children 22%), nausea (33%; children 9%), dyspepsia (22%; children 13%), weight gain (18%; children 2%), diarrhea (13%; children 7%), anorexia (12%; children 22%), abdominal pain (11%), appetite increased (11%)

Genitourinary: Ejaculation failure (42%), impotence (20%), micturition disorder (14%; children 4%)

Neuromuscular & skeletal: Tremor (54%), myoclonus (13%; children 2%), myalgia (13%)

Ocular: Abnormal vision (18%; children 7%)

Respiratory: Pharyngitis (14%), rhinitis (12%)

Miscellaneous: Diaphoresis increased (29%; children 9%)

1% to 10%:

Cardiovascular: Flushing (8%), postural hypotension (6%), palpitation (4%), tachycardia (4%; children 2%), chest pain (4%), edema (2%)

Central nervous system: Anxiety (9%), memory impairment (9%), twitching (7%), depression (5%), concentration impaired (5%), fever (4%), hypertonia (4%), abnormal dreaming (3%), agitation (3%), confusion (3%), migraine (3%), pain (3%), psychosomatic disorder (3%), speech disorder (3%), yawning (3%), aggressiveness (children 2%), chills (2%), depersonalization (2%), emotional lability (2%), irritability (2%), panic reaction (1%)

Dermatologic: Rash (8%), pruritus (6%), purpura (3%), dermatitis (2%), acne (2%), dry skin (2%), urticaria (1%)

Endocrine & metabolic: Amenorrhea (1%), breast enlargement (2%), breast pain (1%), hot flashes (5%), lactation (nonpuerperal) (4%)

Gastrointestinal: Taste disturbance (8%), vomiting (7%), flatulence (6%), tooth disorder (5%), dysphagia (2%), esophagitis (1%)

Genitourinary: UTI (2% to 6%), micturition frequency (5%), dysuria (2%), leucorrhea (2%), vaginitis (2%), urinary retention (2%)

Neuromuscular & skeletal: Paresthesia (9%), back pain (6%), arthralgia (3%), paresis (children 2%), weakness (1%)

Ocular: Lacrimation abnormal (3%), mydriasis (2%), conjunctivitis (1%)

Otic: Tinnitus (6%)

Respiratory: Sinusitis (6%), coughing (6%), bronchospasm (2%; children 7%), epistaxis (2%)

General Dosage Range Oral:

Children ≥10 years: Initial: 25 mg/day; Maintenance: Up to 3 mg/kg/day (maximum: 200 mg/day)

Adults: Initial: 25 mg/day; Maintenance: Up to 250 mg/day

Mechanism of Action Clomipramine appears to affect serotonin uptake while its active metabolite, desmethylclomipramine, affects norepinephrine uptake

Pharmacodynamics/Kinetics

Half-life Elimination Clomipramine: Mean: 32 hours (range: 19-37 hours); DMI: Mean: 69 hours (range: 54-77 hours)

Time to Peak 2-6 hours

Pregnancy Risk Factor C

Dental Comment Clomipramine is known to prolong the QT interval. The QT interval is measured as the time and distance between the Q point of the QRS complex and the end of the T wave in the ECG tracing. After adjustment for heart rate, the QT interval is defined as prolonged if it is more than 450 msec in men and 460 msec in women. A long QT syndrome was first described in the 1950s and 60s as a congenital syndrome involving QT interval prolongation and syncope and sudden death. Some of the congenital long QT syndromes were characterized by a peculiar electrocardiographic appearance of the QRS complex involving a premature atria beat followed by a pause, then a subsequent sinus beat showing marked QT prolongation and deformity. This type of cardiac arrhythmia was originally termed "torsade de pointes" (translated from the French as "twisting of the points"). Clomipramine is considered as having a risk of causing torsade de pointes. Since it is not known what effect vasoconstrictors in the local anesthetic regimen will have in patients with a known history of congenital prolonged QT interval or in patients taking any medication that prolongs the QT interval, a medical consult is suggested.

ClonazePAM (kloe NA ze pam)

U.S. Brand Names KlonoPIN®

Canadian Brand Names Alti-Clonazepam; Apo-Clonazepam®; Clonapam; CO Clonazepam; Gen-Clonazepam; Klonopin®; Mylan-Clonazepam; Novo-Clonazepam; Nu-Clonazepam; PMS-Clonazepam; PRO-Clonazepam; Rho®-Clonazepam; Rivotril®; Sandoz-Clonazepam; ZYM-Clonazepam

Generic Availability (U.S.) Yes

Pharmacologic Category Benzodiazepine

Dental Use Burning mouth syndrome

Use Alone or as an adjunct in the treatment of petit mal variant (Lennox-Gastaut), akinetic, and myoclonic seizures; petit mal (absence) seizures unresponsive to succimides; panic disorder with or without agoraphobia

Unlabeled/Investigational Use Restless legs syndrome; neuralgia; multifocal tic disorder; parkinsonian dysarthria; bipolar disorder; adjunct therapy for schizophrenia; burning mouth syndrome

Local Anesthetic/Vasoconstrictor Precautions No information available to require special precautions

Effects on Dental Treatment Key adverse event(s) related to dental treatment: Xerostomia and changes in salivation (normal salivary flow resumes upon discontinuation), gum soreness, and coated tongue.

Effects on Bleeding No information available to require special precautions

Adverse Effects Reactions reported in patients with seizure and/or panic disorder. Frequency not always defined.

Cardiovascular: Edema (ankle or facial), palpitation

Central nervous system: Amnesia, ataxia (seizure disorder ~30%; panic disorder 5%), behavior problems (seizure disorder ~25%), coma, confusion, depression, dizziness, drowsiness (seizure disorder ~50%), emotional lability, fatigue, fever, hallucinations, headache, hypotonia, hysteria, insomnia, intellectual ability reduced, memory disturbance, nervousness; paradoxical reactions (including aggressive behavior, agitation, anxiety, excitability, hostility, irritability, nervousness, nightmares, sleep disturbance, vivid dreams); psychosis, slurred speech, somnolence (panic disorder 37%), suicidal attempt, suicide ideation, vertigo

Dermatologic: Hair loss, hirsutism, skin rash

Endocrine & metabolic: Dysmenorrhea, libido increased/decreased

Gastrointestinal: Abdominal pain, anorexia, appetite increased/decreased, coated tongue, constipation, dehydration, diarrhea, gastritis, gum soreness, nausea, weight changes (loss/gain), xerostomia

Genitourinary: Colpitis, dysuria, ejaculation delayed, enuresis, impotence, micturition frequency, nocturia, urinary retention, urinary tract infection

Hematologic: Anemia, eosinophilia, leukopenia, thrombocytopenia

Hepatic: Alkaline phosphatase increased (transient), hepatomegaly, serum transaminases increased (transient)

Neuromuscular & skeletal: Choreiform movements, coordination abnormal, dysarthria, muscle pain, muscle weakness, myalgia, tremor

Ocular: Blurred vision, eye movements abnormal, diplopia, nystagmus

Respiratory: Chest congestion, cough, bronchitis, hypersecretions, pharyngitis, respiratory depression, respiratory tract infection, rhinitis, rhinorrhea, shortness of breath, sinusitis

Miscellaneous: Allergic reaction, aphonia, dysdiadochokinesis, encopresis, "glassy-eyed" appearance, hemiparesis, lymphadenopathy

Dental Usual Dosage Burning mouth syndrome (unlabeled use): Adults: Oral: 0.25-3 mg/day in 2 divided doses, in morning and evening

Dosage Oral:

Children <10 years or 30 kg: Seizure disorders:

Initial daily dose: 0.01-0.03 mg/kg/day (maximum: 0.05 mg/kg/day) given in 2-3 divided doses; increase by no more than 0.5 mg every third day until seizures are controlled or adverse effects seen

Usual maintenance dose: 0.1-0.2 mg/kg/day divided 3 times/day, not to exceed 0.2 mg/kg/day

Adults:

Burning mouth syndrome (unlabeled use): 0.25-3 mg/day in 2 divided doses, in morning and evening

Seizure disorders:

Initial daily dose not to exceed 1.5 mg given in 3 divided doses; may increase by 0.5-1 mg every third day until seizures are controlled or adverse effects seen (maximum: 20 mg/day)

Usual maintenance dose: 0.05-0.2 mg/kg; do not exceed 20 mg/day

Panic disorder: 0.25 mg twice daily; increase in increments of 0.125-0.25 mg twice daily every 3 days; target dose: 1 mg/day (maximum: 4 mg/day)

Discontinuation of treatment: To discontinue, treatment should be withdrawn gradually. Decrease dose by 0.125 mg twice daily every 3 days until medication is completely withdrawn.

Elderly: Initiate with low doses and observe closely

Hemodialysis: Supplemental dose is not necessary

Mechanism of Action The exact mechanism is unknown, but believed to be related to its ability to enhance the activity of GABA; suppresses the spike-and-wave discharge in absence seizures by depressing nerve transmission in the motor cortex

Contraindications Hypersensitivity to clonazepam or any component of the formulation (cross-sensitivity with other benzodiazepines may exist); significant liver disease; narrow-angle glaucoma; pregnancy

Warnings/Precautions Antiepileptics are associated with an increased risk of suicidal behavior/thoughts with use (regardless of indication); patients should be monitored for signs/symptoms of depression, suicidal tendencies, and other unusual behavior changes during therapy and instructed to inform their healthcare provider immediately if symptoms occur.

Use with caution in elderly or debilitated patients, patients with hepatic disease (including alcoholics), or renal impairment. Use with caution in patients with respiratory disease or impaired gag reflex or ability to protect the airway from secretions (salivation may be increased). Worsening of seizures may occur when added to patients with multiple seizure types. Concurrent use with valproic acid may result in absence status. Monitoring of CBC and liver function tests has been recommended during prolonged therapy.

Causes CNS depression (dose related) resulting in sedation, dizziness, confusion, or ataxia which may impair physical and mental capabilities. Patients must be cautioned about performing tasks which require mental alertness (eg, operating machinery or driving). Use with caution in patients receiving other CNS depressants or psychoactive agents. Effects with other sedative drugs or ethanol may be potentiated. Benzodiazepines have been associated with falls and traumatic injury and should be used with extreme caution in patients who are at risk of these events (especially the elderly).

Use caution in patients with depression, particularly if suicidal risk may be present. Use with caution in patients with a history of drug dependence. Benzodiazepines have been associated with dependence and acute withdrawal symptoms, including seizures, on discontinuation or reduction in dose. Acute withdrawal, including seizures, may be precipitated in patients after administration of flumazenil to patients receiving long-term benzodiazepine therapy.

Benzodiazepines have been associated with anterograde amnesia. Paradoxical reactions, including hyperactive or aggressive behavior, have been reported with benzodiazepines, particularly in adolescent/pediatric or psychiatric patients. Does not have analgesic, antidepressant, or antipsychotic properties.

Drug Interactions

Metabolism/Transport Effects **Substrate** of CYP3A4 (major)

Avoid Concomitant Use

Avoid concomitant use of ClonazePAM with any of the following: OLANZapine

Increased Effect/Toxicity

ClonazePAM may increase the levels/effects of: Alcohol (Ethyl); CloZAPine; CNS Depressants; Fosphenytoin; Methotrimeprazine; Phenytoin

The levels/effects of ClonazePAM may be increased by: Antifungal Agents (Azole Derivatives, Systemic); Aprepitant; Calcium Channel Blockers (Nondihydropyridine); Cimetidine; Conivaptan; Contraceptives (Estrogens); Contraceptives (Progestins); CYP3A4 Inhibitors (Moderate); CYP3A4 Inhibitors (Strong); Dasatinib; Droperidol; Fluconazole; Fosaprepitant; Grapefruit Juice; Isoniazid; Macrolide Antibiotics; Methotrimeprazine; Nefazodone; OLANZapine; Proton Pump Inhibitors; Selective Serotonin Reuptake Inhibitors

Decreased Effect

The levels/effects of ClonazePAM may be decreased by: CarBAMazepine; CYP3A4 Inducers (Strong); Deferasirox; Rifamycin Derivatives; St Johns Wort; Theophylline Derivatives; Tocilizumab; Yohimbine

Ethanol/Nutrition/Herb Interactions

Ethanol: May increase CNS depression; monitor for increased effects with coadministration. Caution patients about effects.

Food: Clonazepam serum concentration is unlikely to be increased by grapefruit juice because of clonazepam's high oral bioavailability.

Herb/Nutraceutical: St John's wort may decrease clonazepam levels. Avoid valerian, St John's wort, kava kava, gotu kola (may increase CNS depression).

Pharmacodynamics/Kinetics

Onset of Action 20-60 minutes

Duration of Action Infants and young children: 6-8 hours; Adults: ≤12 hours

Half-life Elimination Children: 22-33 hours; Adults: 19-50 hours

Time to Peak Serum: 1-3 hours; Steady-state: 5-7 days

Pregnancy Risk Factor D

Lactation Enters breast milk/not recommended

Breast-Feeding Considerations Clonazepam enters breast milk. Drowsiness, lethargy, or weight loss in nursing infants have been observed in case reports following maternal use of some benzodiazepines.

Controlled Substance C-IV

Dosage Forms

Tablet, oral: 0.5 mg, 1 mg, 2 mg

KlonoPIN®: 0.5 mg, 1 mg, 2 mg

Tablet, orally disintegrating, oral: 0.125 mg, 0.25 mg, 0.5 mg, 1 mg, 2 mg

References

Buchanan J and Zakrzewska J, "Burning Mouth Syndrome," *Clin Evid (online)*, March 14, 2008. Available at http://www.ncbi.nlm.nih.gov/pmc/articles/PMC2907957/pdf/2008-1301.pdf.

Mínguez Serra MP, Salort Llorca C, Silvestre Donat FJ, "Pharmacological Treatment of Burning Mouth Syndrome: A Review and Update," *Med Oral Patol Oral Cir Bucal*, 2007, 12(4):E299-304.

CloNIDine (KLON i deen)

Related Information

Cardiovascular Diseases *on page 1848*

U.S. Brand Names Catapres-TTS®-1; Catapres-TTS®-2; Catapres-TTS®-3; Catapres®; Duraclon®; Kapvay™; Nexiclon™ XR

Canadian Brand Names Apo-Clonidine®; Carapres®; Dixarit®; Dom-Clonidine; Novo-Clonidine; Nu-Clonidine

Generic Availability (U.S.) Yes: Excludes extended release tablets, oral suspension

Pharmacologic Category Alpha$_2$-Adrenergic Agonist

Use

Oral:

Immediate release: Management of hypertension (monotherapy or as adjunctive therapy)

Extended release:

Kapvay™: Treatment of attention-deficit/hyperactivity disorder (ADHD) (monotherapy or as adjunctive therapy)

Nexiclon™ XR: Management of hypertension (monotherapy or as adjunctive therapy)

Epidural (Duraclon®): For continuous epidural administration as adjunctive therapy with opioids for treatment of severe cancer pain in patients tolerant to or unresponsive to opioids alone; epidural clonidine is generally more effective for neuropathic pain and less effective (or possibly ineffective) for somatic or visceral pain

Transdermal patch: Management of hypertension (monotherapy or as adjunctive therapy)

Unlabeled/Investigational Use Heroin or nicotine withdrawal; severe pain; dysmenorrhea; vasomotor symptoms associated with menopause; ethanol dependence; prophylaxis of migraines; glaucoma; diabetes-associated diarrhea; impulse control disorder, clozapine-induced sialorrhea; aid in the diagnosis of growth hormone deficiency

Local Anesthetic/Vasoconstrictor Precautions No information available to require special precautions

Effects on Dental Treatment Key adverse event(s) related to dental treatment: Significant xerostomia (normal salivary flow resumes upon discontinuation), orthostatic hypotension, and abnormal taste.

Effects on Bleeding No information available to require special precautions

Adverse Effects Frequency not always defined.

Oral, Transdermal: Incidence of adverse events may be less with transdermal compared to oral due to the lower peak/trough ratio.

Cardiovascular: Bradycardia (≤4%), palpitation (1%), tachycardia (1%), arrhythmia, atrioventricular block, chest pain, CHF, ECG abnormalities, flushing, orthostatic hypotension, pallor, Raynaud's phenomenon, syncope

Central nervous system: Drowsiness (12% to 38%), headache (1% to 29%), fatigue (4% to 16%), dizziness (2% to 16%), sedation (3% to 10%), insomnia (≤6%), lethargy (3%), nervousness (1% to 3%), mental depression (1%), aggression, agitation, anxiety, behavioral changes, CVA, delirium, delusional perception, fever, hallucinations (visual and auditory), irritability, malaise, nightmares, restlessness, vivid dreams

Dermatologic: Transient localized skin reactions characterized by pruritus and erythema (transdermal 15% to 50%), contact dermatitis (transdermal 8% to 34%), vesiculation (transdermal 7%), allergic contact sensitization (transdermal 5%), hyperpigmentation (transdermal 5%), burning (transdermal 3%), edema (3%), excoriation (transdermal 3%) blanching (transdermal 1%), generalized macular rash (1%), papules (transdermal 1%), throbbing (transdermal 1%), alopecia, angioedema, hives, localized hypopigmentation (transdermal), rash, urticaria

Endocrine & metabolic: Sexual dysfunction (3%), gynecomastia (1%), creatine phosphokinase increased (transient; oral), hyperglycemia (transient; oral), libido decreased

Gastrointestinal: Xerostomia (≤40%), constipation (2% to 10%), anorexia (1%), taste perversion (1%), weight gain (<1%), abdominal pain (oral), diarrhea, nausea, parotid gland pain (oral), parotitis (oral), pseudo-obstruction (oral), throat pain, vomiting

Genitourinary: Erectile dysfunction (2% to 3%), nocturia (1%), dysuria, enuresis, urinary retention

Hematologic: Thrombocytopenia (oral)

Hepatic: Liver function test (mild transient abnormalities; ≤1%), hepatitis

Neuromuscular & skeletal: Weakness (10%), arthralgia (1%), myalgia (1%), leg cramps (<1%), numbness (localized, transdermal), pain in extremities, paresthesia, tremor

Ocular: Accommodation disorder, blurred vision, burning eyes, dry eyes, lacrimation decreased, lacrimation increased

Otic: Ear pain, otitis media

Renal: Pollakiuria

Respiratory: Asthma, epistaxis, nasal congestion, nasal dryness, nasopharyngitis, respiratory tract infection, rhinorrhea

Miscellaneous: Withdrawal syndrome (1%), flu-like syndrome, thirst

Epidural: Note: The following adverse events occurred more often than placebo in cancer patients with intractable pain being treated with concurrent epidural morphine.

>10%:

Cardiovascular: Hypotension (45%), postural hypotension (32%)

Central nervous system: Confusion (13%), dizziness (13%)

Gastrointestinal: Xerostomia (13%)

1% to 10%:

Cardiovascular: Chest pain (5%)

Central nervous system: Hallucinations (5%)

Gastrointestinal: Nausea/vomiting (8%)

Otic: Tinnitus (5%)

Miscellaneous: Diaphoresis (5%)

Dosage Note: Dosing is expressed as the salt (clonidine hydrochloride) unless otherwise noted. Formulations of clonidine (immediate release versus extended release) are not interchangeable on a mg:mg basis due to different pharmacokinetic profiles. This includes commercially available oral suspension (Nexiclon™ XR) which is an extended release preparation and should not be used interchangeably with any extemporaneously prepared clonidine oral suspension.

Children:

Oral:

Hypertension (unlabeled use): Children ≥12 years: Immediate release: Initial: 0.2 mg/day in 2 divided doses; increase gradually, if needed, in 0.1 mg/day increments at weekly intervals; maximum: 2.4 mg/day (rarely required) (NHBPEP, Fourth Report)

Severe hypertension (unlabeled use): Children: Immediate release: 0.05-0.1 mg/dose; may repeat up to a maximum total dose of 0.8 mg (NHBPEP, Fourth Report)

Clonidine tolerance test (test of growth hormone release from pituitary) (unlabeled use):
0.15 mg/m^2 as a single dose (Lanes, 1982)
or
5 mcg/kg as a single dose; maximum dose: 250 mcg (Richmond, 2008)

ADHD: **Note:** May be used alone or as an adjunct to stimulants.
Immediate release (unlabeled indication; Pliszka, 2007):
Children ≤45 kg: Initial: 0.05 mg at bedtime; sequentially increase every 3-7 days by 0.05 mg increments as twice daily, then 3 times daily, then 4 times daily; maximum daily dose: 0.2 mg/day for patients weighing 27-40.5 kg; 0.3 mg/day for patients weighing 40.5-45 kg. When discontinuing therapy, taper gradually over 1-2 weeks.
Children >45 kg: Initial: 0.1 mg at bedtime; sequentially increase every 3-7 days by 0.1 mg increments as twice daily, then 3 times daily, then 4 times daily; maximum daily dose: 0.4 mg/day. When discontinuing therapy, taper gradually over 1-2 weeks.
Extended release (Kapvay™): Children ≥6 years: Initial: 0.1 mg at bedtime; increase in 0.1 mg/day increments every 7 days until desired response, doses should be administered twice daily (either split equally or with the higher split dosage given at bedtime); maximum: 0.4 mg/day. **Note:** Maintenance treatment for >5 weeks has not been evaluated. When discontinuing therapy, taper daily dose by ≤0.1 mg every 3-7 days.

Epidural infusion: Pain management: Reserved for cancer patients with severe intractable pain, unresponsive to other opioid analgesics: Initial: 0.5 mcg/kg/**hour**; adjust with caution, based on clinical effect

Adults:
Oral:
Hypertension:
Immediate release: Initial dose: 0.1 mg twice daily (maximum recommended dose: 2.4 mg/day); usual dose range (JNC 7): 0.1-0.8 mg/day in 2 divided doses
Extended release (Nexiclon™ XR): Initial: 0.17 mg clonidine base once daily at bedtime; may increase increments of 0.09 mg/day every 7 days; maintenance: usual dose range: 0.17-0.52 mg clonidine base once daily; maximum: 0.52 mg/day clonidine base
Conversion between immediate release clonidine hydrochloride and extended release (Nexiclon™ XR) clonidine base:
Current dose immediate release tablets 0.05 mg twice daily: Convert to extended release tablet of 0.09 mg clonidine base once daily
Current dose immediate release tablets 0.1 mg twice daily: Convert to extended release tablet of 0.17 mg clonidine base once daily
Current dose immediate release tablets 0.2 mg twice daily: Convert to extended release tablet of 0.34 mg clonidine base once daily
Current dose immediate release tablets 0.3 mg twice daily: convert to extended release tablets of 0.52 mg clonidine base once daily

Acute hypertension (urgency) (unlabeled use): Initial 0.1-0.2 mg; may be followed by additional doses of 0.1 mg every hour, if necessary, to a maximum total dose of 0.7 mg (Atkin, 1992; Jaker, 1989)
Unlabeled route of administration: Sublingual: Initial: 0.1-0.2 mg; followed by 0.05-0.1 mg every hour until blood pressure controlled or a cumulative dose of 0.7 mg is reached (Cunningham, 1994; Matuschka, 1999)

Nicotine withdrawal symptoms (unlabeled use): Initial: 0.1 mg twice daily; titrate by 0.1 mg/day every 7 days if needed; dosage range used in clinical trials: 0.15-0.75 mg/day; duration of therapy ranged from 3-10 weeks in clinical trials (Fiore, 2008)

Transdermal:
Hypertension: Initial: 0.1 mg/24 hour patch applied once every 7 days and increase by 0.1 mg at 1- to 2-week intervals (dosages >0.6 mg/24 hours do not improve efficacy); usual dose range (JNC 7): 0.1-0.3 mg/24 hour patch applied once every 7 days
Nicotine withdrawal symptoms (unlabeled use): Initial: 0.1 mg/24 hour patch applied once every 7 days and increase by 0.1 mg at 1-week intervals if necessary; dosage range used in clinical trials: 0.1-0.2 mg/24 hour patch applied once every 7 days; duration of therapy ranged from 3-10 weeks in clinical trials (Fiore, 2008)

Note: If transitioning from oral to transdermal therapy, overlap oral regimen for 1-2 days; transdermal route takes 2-3 days to achieve therapeutic effects.
Conversion from oral to transdermal:
Day 1: Place Catapres-TTS® 1; administer 100% of oral dose.
Day 2: Administer 50% of oral dose.
Day 3: Administer 25% of oral dose.
Day 4: Patch remains, no further oral supplement necessary.

Epidural infusion: Pain management: Reserved for cancer patients with severe intractable pain, unresponsive to other opioid analgesics: Starting dose: 30 mcg/hour; titrate as required for relief of pain or presence of side effects; experience with doses >40 mcg/hour is limited; should be considered an adjunct to opioid therapy

Elderly: Oral: Hypertension:

Immediate release: Initial: 0.1 mg once daily at bedtime, increase gradually as needed

Extended release (Nexiclon™ XR): No specific recommendations are provided by the manufacturer although a lower initial dose is recommended.

Dosing adjustment in renal impairment: Bradycardia, sedation, and hypotension may be more likely to occur in patients with renal failure; may consider using doses at the lower end of the dosing range and monitor closely

Not dialyzable (0% to 5%) via hemodialysis; supplemental dose is not necessary; unclear how much is removed via peritoneal dialysis. Oral antihypertensive drugs given preferentially at night may reduce the nocturnal surge of blood pressure and minimize the intradialytic hypotension that may occur when taken the morning before a dialysis session (K/DOQI, 2005).

Oral: Extended release (Nexiclon™ XR):

Moderate-to-severe impairment (not on dialysis): No dosage adjustment recommended; titrate slowly

End-stage kidney disease (on maintenance dialysis): Initial: 0.09 mg clonidine base/day; titrate slowly

Mechanism of Action Stimulates alpha$_2$-adrenoceptors in the brain stem, thus activating an inhibitory neuron, resulting in reduced sympathetic outflow from the CNS, producing a decrease in peripheral resistance, renal vascular resistance, heart rate, and blood pressure; epidural clonidine may produce pain relief at spinal presynaptic and postjunctional alpha$_2$-adrenoceptors by preventing pain signal transmission; pain relief occurs only for the body regions innervated by the spinal segments where analgesic concentrations of clonidine exist. For the treatment of ADHD, the mechanism of action is unknown; it has been proposed that postsynaptic alpha$_2$-agonist stimulation regulates subcortical activity in the prefrontal cortex, the area of the brain responsible for emotions, attentions, and behaviors and causes reduced hyperactivity, impulsiveness, and distractibility.

Contraindications Hypersensitivity to clonidine hydrochloride or any component of the formulation

Epidural administration: Injection site infection; concurrent anticoagulant therapy; bleeding diathesis; administration above the C4 dermatome

Warnings/Precautions May cause CNS depression, which may impair physical or mental abilities; patients must be cautioned about performing tasks which require mental alertness (eg, operating machinery or driving). Sedating effects may be potentiated when used with other CNS-depressant drugs or ethanol. Use with caution in patients with severe coronary insufficiency; conduction disturbances; recent MI, CVA, or chronic renal insufficiency. May cause dose dependent reductions in heart rate; use with caution in patients with preexisting bradycardia or those predisposed to developing bradycardia. Caution in sinus node dysfunction. Use with caution in patients concurrently receiving agents known to reduce SA node function and/or AV nodal conduction (eg, digoxin, diltiazem, metoprolol, verapamil). May cause significant xerostomia. Clonidine may cause eye dryness in patients who wear contact lenses.

[U.S. Boxed Warning]: Must dilute concentrated epidural injectable (500 mcg/mL) solution prior to use. Epidural clonidine is not recommended for perioperative, obstetrical, or postpartum pain due to risk of hemodynamic instability. Clonidine injection should be administered via a continuous epidural infusion device. Monitor closely for catheter-related infection such as meningitis or epidural abscess. Epidural clonidine is not recommended for use in patients with severe cardiovascular disease or hemodynamic instability; may lead to cardiovascular instability (hypotension, bradycardia). Symptomatic hypotension may occur with use; in all patients, use epidural clonidine with caution due to the potential for severe hypotension especially in women and those of low body weight. Most hypotensive episodes occur within the first 4 days of initiation; however, episodes may occur throughout the duration of therapy.

Gradual withdrawal is needed (taper oral immediate release or epidural dose gradually over 2-4 days to avoid rebound hypertension) if drug needs to be stopped. Patients should be instructed about abrupt discontinuation (causes rapid increase in BP and symptoms of sympathetic overactivity). In patients on both a beta-blocker and clonidine where withdrawal of clonidine is necessary, withdraw the beta-blocker first and several days before clonidine withdrawal, then slowly decrease clonidine. In children and adolescents, extended release formulation (Kapvay™) should be tapered in decrements of no more than 0.1 mg every 3-7 days. Discontinue oral immediate release formulations within 4 hours of surgery then restart as soon as possible afterwards. Discontinue oral extended release formulations up to 28 hours prior to surgery, then restart the following day.

Oral formulations of clonidine (immediate release versus extended release) are not interchangeable on a mg:mg basis due to different pharmacokinetic profiles. This includes commercially available oral suspension (Nexiclon™ XR) which is an extended release preparation and should not be used interchangeably with any extemporaneously prepared clonidine oral suspension.

Transdermal patch may contain conducting metal (eg, aluminum); remove patch prior to MRI. Due to the potential for altered electrical conductivity, remove transdermal patch before cardioversion or defibrillation. Localized contact sensitization to the transdermal system has been reported; in these patients, allergic reactions (eg, generalized rash, urticaria, angioedema) have also occurred following subsequent substitution of oral therapy.

Clonidine may be inappropriate for use in the elderly due to CNS adverse events and orthostatic hypotension (Beers Criteria). In pediatric patients, epidural clonidine should be reserved for cancer patients with severe intractable pain, unresponsive to other analgesics or epidural or spinal opioids. Use oral formulations with caution in pediatric patients since children commonly have gastrointestinal illnesses with vomiting and are susceptible to hypertensive episodes due to abrupt inability to take oral medication.

Drug Interactions

Avoid Concomitant Use

Avoid concomitant use of CloNIDine with any of the following: Iobenguane I 123

Increased Effect/Toxicity

CloNIDine may increase the levels/effects of: Amifostine; Antihypertensives; Hypotensive Agents; RiTUXimab

The levels/effects of CloNIDine may be increased by: Beta-Blockers; Diazoxide; Herbs (Hypotensive Properties); MAO Inhibitors; Methylphenidate; Pentoxifylline; Phosphodiesterase 5 Inhibitors; Prostacyclin Analogues

Decreased Effect

CloNIDine may decrease the levels/effects of: Iobenguane I 123

The levels/effects of CloNIDine may be decreased by: Antidepressants (Alpha2-Antagonist); Herbs (Hypertensive Properties); Serotonin/Norepinephrine Reuptake Inhibitors; Tricyclic Antidepressants; Yohimbine

Ethanol/Nutrition/Herb Interactions

Ethanol: Avoid ethanol (may increase CNS depression). *In vitro* studies have shown high concentrations of alcohol may increase the rate of release of Nexiclon™ XR.

Herb/Nutraceutical: Avoid dong quai if using for hypertension (has estrogenic activity). Avoid ephedra, yohimbe, ginseng (may worsen hypertension). Avoid valerian, St John's wort, kava kava, gotu kola (may increase CNS depression).

Pharmacodynamics/Kinetics

Onset of Action Oral: 0.5-1 hour; Transdermal: Initial application: 2-3 days

Duration of Action 6-10 hours

Half-life Elimination Adults: Normal renal function: 12-16 hours; Renal impairment: Up to 41 hours

Epidural administration: CSF half-life elimination: 0.8-1.8 hours

Time to Peak Oral: Immediate release: 3-5 hours; Extended release: 7-8 hours

Pregnancy Risk Factor C

Lactation Enters breast milk/not recommended

Breast-Feeding Considerations Enters breast milk with concentrations approximately twice maternal serum concentrations

Dosage Forms

Injection, solution [preservative free]: 100 mcg/mL (10 mL); 500 mcg/mL (10 mL)
Duraclon®: 100 mcg/mL (10 mL); 500 mcg/mL (10 mL)

Patch, transdermal: 0.1 mg/24 hours (4s); 0.2 mg/24 hours (4s); 0.3 mg/24 hours (4s)
Catapres-TTS®-1: 0.1 mg/24 hours (4s)
Catapres-TTS®-2: 0.2 mg/24 hours (4s)
Catapres-TTS®-3: 0.3 mg/24 hours (4s)

Suspension, extended release, oral:
Nexiclon™ XR: 0.09 mg/mL (118 mL)

Tablet, oral: 0.1 mg, 0.2 mg, 0.3 mg
Catapres®: 0.1 mg, 0.2 mg, 0.3 mg

Tablet, extended release, oral:
Kapvay™: 0.1 mg
Nexiclon™ XR: 0.17 mg

Clonidine and Chlorthalidone (KLON i deen & klor THAL i done)

Related Information

Chlorthalidone *on page 373*

CloNIDine *on page 416*

U.S. Brand Names Clorpres®

Pharmacologic Category Alpha$_2$-Adrenergic Agonist; Diuretic, Thiazide

Use Management of mild-to-moderate hypertension

Local Anesthetic/Vasoconstrictor Precautions No information available to require special precautions

Effects on Dental Treatment Key adverse event(s) related to dental treatment: Clonidine: Significant xerostomia (normal salivary flow resumes upon discontinuation), orthostatic hypotension, and abnormal taste.

Effects on Bleeding No information available to require special precautions

Adverse Effects See individual agents.

General Dosage Range Oral: *Adults:* 1 tablet (clonidine 0.1-0.3 mg/chlorthalidone 15 mg/tablet) 1-2 times/day (maximum: clonidine 0.6 mg; chlorthalidone 30 mg)

Pregnancy Risk Factor C

Clopidogrel (kloh PID oh grel)

Related Information

Antiplatelet and Anticoagulation Considerations in Dentistry *on page 1867*

Cardiovascular Diseases *on page 1848*

U.S. Brand Names Plavix®

Canadian Brand Names Plavix®

Generic Availability (U.S.) No

Pharmacologic Category Antiplatelet Agent; Antiplatelet Agent, Thienopyridine

Use Reduces rate of atherothrombotic events (myocardial infarction, stroke, vascular deaths) in patients with recent MI or stroke, or established peripheral arterial disease; reduces rate of atherothrombotic events in patients with unstable angina (UA) or non-ST-segment elevation (NSTEMI) managed medically or with percutaneous coronary intervention (PCI) (with or without stent) or CABG; reduces rate of death and atherothrombotic events in patients with ST-segment elevation MI (STEMI) managed medically

Unlabeled/Investigational Use In patients with allergy or major gastrointestinal intolerance to aspirin, initial treatment of acute coronary syndromes (ACS) or prevention of coronary artery bypass graft closure (saphenous vein)

Local Anesthetic/Vasoconstrictor Precautions No information available to require special precautions

Effects on Dental Treatment Aspirin and clopidogrel (Plavix®) in combination is the primary prevention strategy against stent thrombosis after placement of drug-eluting metal stents in coronary patients. Premature discontinuation of this combination antiplatelet therapy strongly increases the risk of a catastrophic event of stent thrombosis leading to myocardial infarction and/or death, so says a science advisory issued in January 2007 from the American Heart Association in collaboration with the American Dental Association and other professional healthcare organizations. The advisory stresses a 12-month therapy of aspirin and Plavix® combination after placement of a drug-eluting stent in order to prevent thrombosis at the stent site. Any elective surgery should be postponed for 1 year after stent implantation, and if surgery must be performed, consideration should be given to continuing the antiplatelet therapy during the perioperative period in high-risk patients with drug-eluting stents.

This advisory was issued from a science panel made up of representatives from the American Heart Association (AHA), the American College of Cardiology, the Society for Cardiovascular Angiography and Interventions, the American College of Surgeons, the American Dental Association (ADA), and the American College of Physicians (Grines, 2007).

Effects on Bleeding Clopidogrel blocks platelet aggregation and may prolong bleeding time. Inhibition is irreversible; on discontinuation of clopidogrel, normal platelet function returns only when new platelets are released from the bone marrow. Dental practitioners should note that recommendations differ between general surgery (eg, appendectomy, hip replacement) and dental surgery. Prior to elective general surgery, it may be temporarily discontinued (usually for 5-10 days) to restore platelet function. However, routine interruption of therapy for noninvasive dental procedures is NOT warranted and there is no scientific evidence to warrant the discontinuance of clopidogrel prior to dental surgery. In particular, clopidogrel should

NOT be discontinued in patients with cardiac stents that have not completed their full course of dual antiplatelet therapy (aspirin, clopidogrel/ticlopidine); patient specific situations need to be discussed with cardiologist. When feasible, postponement of dental surgery until the completion of dual antiplatelet therapy should be considered.

Adverse Effects As with all drugs which may affect hemostasis, bleeding is associated with clopidogrel. Hemorrhage may occur at virtually any site. Risk is dependent on multiple variables, including the concurrent use of multiple agents which alter hemostasis and patient susceptibility.

3% to 10%:

Dermatologic: Rash (4%), pruritus (3%)

Hematologic: Bleeding (major 4%; minor 5%), purpura/bruising (5%), epistaxis (3%)

1% to 3%:

Gastrointestinal: GI hemorrhage (2%)

Hematologic: Hematoma

Dosage Oral: Adults:

Recent MI, recent stroke, or established arterial disease: 75 mg once daily

Acute coronary syndrome (ACS):

Unstable angina, non-ST-segment elevation myocardial infarction (UA/NSTEMI): Initial: 300 mg loading dose, followed by 75 mg once daily for at least 1 month and ideally up to 12 months (in combination with aspirin 75-162 mg once daily indefinitely) (Wright, 2011).

ST-segment elevation myocardial infarction (STEMI): 75 mg once daily (in combination with aspirin 162-325 mg initially followed by 81-162 mg/day). **Note:** CLARITY-TIMI 28 used a 300 mg loading dose (with thrombolysis) demonstrating an improvement in patency rate of the infarct related artery and reduction in ischemic complications. The duration of therapy was <28 days (usually until hospital discharge) unless nonprimary percutaneous coronary intervention (PCI) was performed (Sabatine, 2005).

The American College of Chest Physicians (Goodman, 2008) recommends:

Patients ≤75 years: Initial: 300 mg loading dose, followed by 75 mg once daily for up to 28 days (in combination with aspirin)

Patients >75 years: 75 mg once daily for up to 28 days (with or without thrombolysis)

Percutaneous coronary intervention (PCI) for UA/NSTEMI or STEMI: Loading dose: 300-600 mg (600 mg may be preferred for early invasive strategy with UA/NSTEMI) given as early as possible before or at the time of PCI followed by 75 mg once daily; may consider a maintenance dose of 150 mg once daily for 6 days then 75 mg once daily thereafter in patients not at high risk for bleeding (CURRENT-OASIS 7 Investigators, 2010; Wright, 2011). **Note:** If an initial loading dose of 300 mg was given prior to PCI, a supplemental loading dose of 300 mg (total loading dose of 600 mg) may be administered (Kushner, 2009). For patients with UA/NSTEMI, it has been recommended that the loading dose be given at least 2 hours (or 24 hours in patients unable to take aspirin) prior to PCI (*Chest* guidelines, 2008).

Duration of clopidogrel (in combination with aspirin) after stent placement: **Premature interruption of therapy may result in stent thrombosis with subsequent fatal and nonfatal MI.** With STEMI, clopidogrel for at least 12 months regardless of stent type (ie, either bare metal or drug eluting stent) is recommended (Kushner, 2009). With UA/NSTEMI, at least 12 months of clopidogrel is recommended in patients receiving a drug eluting stent (DES) unless the risk of bleeding outweighs the benefits. For bare metal stent (BMS) placement, at least 1 month and ideally up to 12 months duration is recommended unless the risk of bleeding outweighs the benefits then a minimum of 2 weeks is recommended (Wright, 2011). In either setting, a duration >15 months may be considered in patients with DES placement (Kushner, 2009; Wright 2011). For patients without ongoing ACS, clopidogrel should be continued for at least 1 month (for BMS) or at least 12 months (for DES) (Becker, 2008).

CYP2C19 poor metabolizers (ie, *CYP2C19*2* or **3* carriers): An appropriate regimen for this patient population has not been established in clinical outcome trials; however, a higher dose regimen of 600 mg loading dose followed by 150 mg once daily has demonstrated an increase in antiplatelet response in this patient population.

Prevention of coronary artery bypass graft closure (saphenous vein) [*Chest* guidelines, 2008]: Aspirin-allergic patients (unlabeled use): Loading dose: 300 mg administered 6 hours following procedure; maintenance: 75 mg/day

Dosing adjustment in renal impairment and elderly: None necessary

Dosing adjustment in hepatic impairment: Use with caution; experience is limited. **Note:** Inhibition of ADP-induced platelet aggregation and mean bleeding time prolongation were similar in patients with severe hepatic impairment compared to healthy subjects after repeated doses of 75 mg once daily for 10 days.

Mechanism of Action Clopidogrel requires *in vivo* biotransformation to an active thiol metabolite. The active metabolite irreversibly blocks the $P2Y_{12}$ component of ADP receptors on the platelet surface, which prevents activation of the GPIIb/IIIa receptor complex, thereby reducing platelet aggregation. Platelets blocked by clopidogrel are affected for the remainder of their lifespan (~7-10 days).

Contraindications Hypersensitivity to clopidogrel or any component of the formulation; active pathological bleeding such as peptic ulcer or intracranial hemorrhage

Canadian labeling: Additional contraindications (not in U.S. labeling): Significant liver impairment or cholestatic jaundice

Warnings/Precautions [U.S. Boxed Warning]: Patients with one or more copies of the variant *CYP2C19*2* and/or *CYP2C19*3* alleles (and potentially other reduced-function variants) may have reduced conversion of clopidogrel to its active thiol metabolite. Lower active metabolite exposure may result in reduced platelet inhibition and, thus, a higher rate of cardiovascular events following MI or stent thrombosis following PCI. Although evidence is insufficient to recommend routine genetic testing, tests are available to determine CYP2C19 genotype and may be used to determine therapeutic strategy; alternative treatment or treatment strategies may be considered if patient is identified as a CYP2C19 poor metabolizer. Genetic testing may be considered prior to initiating clopidogrel in patients at moderate or high risk for poor outcomes (eg, PCI in patients with extensive and/or very complex disease). The optimal dose for CYP2C19 poor metabolizers has yet to be determined. After initiation of clopidogrel, functional testing (eg, VerifyNow® P2Y12 assay) may also be done to determine clopidogrel responsiveness (Holmes, 2010).

Use with caution in patients who may be at risk of increased bleeding, including patients with PUD, trauma, or surgery. In patients with coronary stents, premature interruption of therapy may result in stent thrombosis with subsequent fatal and nonfatal MI. Duration of therapy, in general, is determined by the type of stent placed (bare metal or drug eluting) and whether an ACS event was ongoing at the time of placement. Consider discontinuing 5 days before elective surgery (except in patients with cardiac stents that have not completed their full course of dual antiplatelet therapy; patient-specific situations need to be discussed with cardiologist; AHA/ACC/SCAI/ACS/ADA Science Advisory provides recommendations). Use caution in concurrent treatment with anticoagulants (eg, heparin, warfarin) or other antiplatelet drugs; bleeding risk is increased. Concurrent use with drugs known to inhibit CYP2C19 (eg, proton pump inhibitors) may reduce levels of active metabolite and subsequently reduce clinical efficacy and increase the risk of cardiovascular events; if possible, avoid concurrent use of moderate-to-strong CYP2C19 inhibitors. In patients requiring antacid therapy, consider use of an acid-reducing agent lacking (eg, ranitidine) or with less CYP2C19 inhibition. If a PPI is necessary, the use of pantoprazole, a weak CYP2C19 inhibitor, has been shown to have less of an effect on the pharmacologic activity of clopidogrel. Of the PPIs, lansoprazole exhibits the most potent CYP2C19 inhibitory effects (Li, 2004).Use with caution in patients with severe liver or renal disease (experience is limited). Cases of TTP (usually occurring within the first 2 weeks of therapy), resulting in some fatalities, have been reported; urgent plasmapheresis is required. Use in patients with severe hepatic impairment or cholestatic jaundice is contraindicated in the Canadian labeling. Cases of TTP (usually occurring within the first 2 weeks of therapy), resulting in some fatalities, have been reported; urgent plasmapheresis is required. Concurrent use of aspirin and clopidogrel is not recommended for secondary prevention of ischemic stroke or TIA in patients unable to take oral anticoagulants due to hemorrhagic risk (Furie, 2011)

Drug Interactions

Metabolism/Transport Effects Substrate of CYP2C19, 3A4, 1A2 (minor); **Inhibits** CYP2B6 (moderate), 2C9 (weak)

Avoid Concomitant Use

Avoid concomitant use of Clopidogrel with any of the following: CYP2C19 Inhibitors (Moderate); CYP2C19 Inhibitors (Strong); Omeprazole

Increased Effect/Toxicity

Clopidogrel may increase the levels/effects of: Anticoagulants; Antiplatelet Agents; Collagenase (Systemic); CYP2B6 Substrates; Drotrecogin Alfa; Ibritumomab; Salicylates; Thrombolytic Agents; Tositumomab and Iodine I 131 Tositumomab; Warfarin

The levels/effects of Clopidogrel may be increased by: Dasatinib; Glucosamine; Herbs (Anticoagulant/Antiplatelet Properties); Nonsteroidal Anti-Inflammatory Agents; Omega-3-Acid Ethyl Esters; Pentosan Polysulfate Sodium; Pentoxifylline; Prostacyclin Analogues; Rifamycin Derivatives

Decreased Effect

The levels/effects of Clopidogrel may be decreased by: Amiodarone; Calcium Channel Blockers; CYP2C19 Inhibitors (Moderate); CYP2C19 Inhibitors (Strong); Dexlansoprazole; Esomeprazole; Lansoprazole; Macrolide Antibiotics; Nonsteroidal Anti-Inflammatory Agents; Omeprazole; Pantoprazole; RABEprazole

Ethanol/Nutrition/Herb Interactions Herb/Nutraceutical: Avoid alfalfa, anise, bilberry, bladderwrack, bromelain, cat's claw, chamomile, coleus, cordyceps, dong quai, evening primrose oil, fenugreek, feverfew, garlic, ginger, ginkgo biloba, ginseng (American), ginseng (Panax), ginseng (Siberian), grape seed, green tea, guggul, horse chestnut seed, horseradish, licorice, prickly ash, red clover, reishi, SAMe (S-adenosylmethionine), sweet clover, turmeric, white willow (all have additional antiplatelet activity).

Dietary Considerations May be taken without regard to meals.

Pharmacodynamics/Kinetics

Onset of Action

Onset of action: Inhibition of platelet aggregation (IPA): Dose-dependent:
- 300-600 mg loading dose: Detected within 2 hours
- 50-100 mg/day: Detected by the second day of treatment

Peak effect: Time to maximal IPA: Dose-dependent: **Note:** Degree of IPA based on adenosine diphosphate (ADP) concentration used during light aggregometry:
- 300-600 mg loading dose:
  - ADP 5 µmol/L: 20% to 30% IPA at 6 hours post administration (Montelescot, 2006)
  - ADP 20 µmol/L: 30% to 37% IPA at 6 hours post administration (Montelescot, 2006)
- 50-100 mg/day: ADP 5 µmol/L: 50% to 60% IPA at 5-7 days (Herbert, 1993)

Half-life Elimination Parent drug: ~6 hours; Active metabolite: ~30 minutes

Time to Peak Serum: ~0.75 hours

Pregnancy Risk Factor B

Lactation Excretion in breast milk unknown/not recommended

Dosage Forms

Tablet, oral:

Plavix®: 75 mg, 300 mg

Dental Comment There is no scientific evidence to warrant the discontinuance of clopidogrel prior to dental surgery. Patients taking one clopidogrel tablet daily as an antithrombotic and who require dental surgery should be given special consideration in consultation with physician.

References

Daniel NG, Goulet J, Bergeron M, et al, "Antiplatelet Drugs: Is There a Surgical Risk?" *J Can Dent Assoc*, 2002, 68(11):683-7.

Grines CL, Bonow RO, Casey DE, et al, "AHA/ACC/SCAI/ACS/ADA Science Advisory, Prevention of Premature Discontinuation of Dual Antiplatelet Therapy in Patients With Coronary Artery Stents. A Science Advisory From the American Heart Association, American College of Cardiology, Society of Cardiovascular Angiography and Interventions, American College of Surgeons, and American Dental Association With Representation From The Amercian College Of Physicians," *Circulation*, 2007, 115 (6):813-8. Available at http://www.acc.org/qualityandscience/clinical/pdfs/Final_Dual_Antiplatelet_-Statement_010507.pdf.

Jeske AH, Suchko GD, ADA Council on Scientific Affairs and Division of Science, et al, "Lack of a Scientific Basis for Routine Discontinuation of Oral Anticoagulation Therapy Before Dental Treatment," *J Am Dent Assoc*, 2003, 134(11):1492-7.

Little JW, Miller CS, Henry RG, et al, "Antithrombotic Agents: Implications in Dentistry," *Oral Surg Oral Med Oral Pathol Oral Radiol Endod*, 2002, 93(5):544-51.

Scully C and Wolff A, "Oral Surgery in Patients on Anticoagulant Therapy," *Oral Surg Oral Med Oral Pathol Oral Radiol Endod*, 2002, 94(1):57-64.

Wynn RL, "Clopidogrel (Plavix): Dental Considerations of an Antiplatelet Drug," *Gen Dent*, 2001, 49 (6):564-8.

Clorazepate (klor AZ e pate)

U.S. Brand Names Tranxene® T-Tab®

Canadian Brand Names Apo-Clorazepate®; Novo-Clopate

Pharmacologic Category Benzodiazepine

Use Treatment of generalized anxiety disorder; management of ethanol withdrawal; adjunct anticonvulsant in management of partial seizures

Local Anesthetic/Vasoconstrictor Precautions No information available to require special precautions

Effects on Dental Treatment Key adverse event(s) related to dental treatment: Xerostomia (normal salivary flow resumes upon discontinuation). Many patients will experience drowsiness; orthostatic hypotension is possible. It is suggested that narcotic analgesics not be given for pain control to patients taking clorazepate due to enhanced sedation.

Effects on Bleeding No information available to require special precautions

Adverse Effects Frequency not defined.

Cardiovascular: Hypotension

Central nervous system: Drowsiness, fatigue, ataxia, lightheadedness, memory impairment, insomnia, anxiety, headache, depression, slurred speech, confusion, nervousness, dizziness, irritability

Dermatologic: Rash

Endocrine & metabolic: Libido decreased

Gastrointestinal: Xerostomia, constipation, diarrhea, nausea, salivation decreased, vomiting, appetite increased or decreased

Hepatic: Jaundice, transaminase increased

Neuromuscular & skeletal: Dysarthria, tremor

Ocular: Blurred vision, diplopia

General Dosage Range Oral:

Children 9-12 years: Initial: 3.75-7.5 mg twice daily; Maintenance: Up to 60 mg/day in 2-3 divided doses

Children >12 years: Initial: Up to 7.5 mg 2-3 times/day; Maintenance: Up to 90 mg/day

Adults: Initial: 7.5-15 mg 2-4 times/day; Maintenance: Up to 90 mg/day

Elderly: Anxiety: 7.5 mg 1-2 times/day

Mechanism of Action Binds to stereospecific benzodiazepine receptors on the postsynaptic GABA neuron at several sites within the central nervous system, including the limbic system, reticular formation. Enhancement of the inhibitory effect of GABA on neuronal excitability results by increased neuronal membrane permeability to chloride ions. This shift in chloride ions results in hyperpolarization (a less excitable state) and stabilization.

Pharmacodynamics/Kinetics

Onset of Action 1-2 hours

Duration of Action Variable, 8-24 hours

Half-life Elimination Adults: Nordiazepam: 40-50 hours; Oxazepam: 6-8 hours

Time to Peak Serum: ~1 hour

Controlled Substance C-IV

Clotrimazole (Oral) (kloe TRIM a zole)

Related Information

Fungal Infections *on page 1945*

Related Sample Prescriptions

Topical Fungal Infections *on page 1988*

Generic Availability (U.S.) Yes

Pharmacologic Category Antifungal Agent, Oral Nonabsorbed

Dental Use Treatment of susceptible fungal infections, including oropharyngeal candidiasis; limited data suggest that clotrimazole troches may be effective for prophylaxis against oropharyngeal candidiasis in neutropenic patients

Use Treatment of susceptible fungal infections, including oropharyngeal candidiasis; limited data suggest that clotrimazole troches may be effective for prophylaxis against oropharyngeal candidiasis in neutropenic patients

Local Anesthetic/Vasoconstrictor Precautions No information available to require special precautions

Effects on Dental Treatment No significant effects or complications reported

Effects on Bleeding No information available to require special precautions

Adverse Effects

>10%: Hepatic: Abnormal liver function tests

Frequency not defined:

Dermatologic: Pruritus

Gastrointestinal: Nausea, vomiting

Dental Usual Dosage Oropharyngeal candidiasis: Children >3 years and Adults: Oral:

Prophylaxis: 10 mg troche dissolved 3 times/day for the duration of chemotherapy or until steroids are reduced to maintenance levels

Treatment: 10 mg troche dissolved slowly 5 times/day for 14 consecutive days

Dosage Oral: Children >3 years and Adults:

Prophylaxis: 10 mg troche dissolved 3 times/day for the duration of chemotherapy or until steroids are reduced to maintenance levels

Treatment: 10 mg troche dissolved slowly 5 times/day for 14 consecutive days

Mechanism of Action Binds to phospholipids in the fungal cell membrane altering cell wall permeability resulting in loss of essential intracellular elements

Contraindications Hypersensitivity to clotrimazole or any component of the formulation

Warnings/Precautions Clotrimazole should not be used for treatment of systemic fungal infection. Safety and effectiveness of clotrimazole lozenges (troches) in children <3 years of age have not been established.

Drug Interactions

Metabolism/Transport Effects **Inhibits** CYP1A2 (weak), 2A6 (weak), 2B6 (weak), 2C8 (weak), 2C9 (weak), 2C19 (weak), 2D6 (weak), 2E1 (weak), 3A4 (moderate)

Avoid Concomitant Use

Avoid concomitant use of Clotrimazole (Oral) with any of the following: Tolvaptan

Increased Effect/Toxicity

Clotrimazole (Oral) may increase the levels/effects of: Budesonide (Systemic, Oral Inhalation); Colchicine; CYP3A4 Substrates; Eplerenone; Everolimus; FentaNYL; Halofantrine; Lurasidone; Pimecrolimus; Ranolazine; Salmeterol; Saxagliptin; Tacrolimus; Tacrolimus (Systemic); Tolvaptan; Vilazodone

Decreased Effect

Clotrimazole (Oral) may decrease the levels/effects of: Saccharomyces boulardii

Pregnancy Risk Factor C

Lactation Excretion in breast milk unknown

Dosage Forms

Troche, oral: 10 mg

Clotrimazole (Topical) (kloe TRIM a zole)

U.S. Brand Names Anti-Fungal™ [OTC]; Cruex® [OTC]; Gyne-Lotrimin® 3 [OTC]; Gyne-Lotrimin® 7 [OTC]; Lotrimin® AF Athlete's Foot [OTC]; Lotrimin® AF for Her [OTC]; Lotrimin® AF Jock Itch [OTC]

Canadian Brand Names Canesten® Topical; Canesten® Vaginal; Clotrimaderm; Trivagizole-3®

Generic Availability (U.S.) Yes: Cream, solution

Pharmacologic Category Antifungal Agent, Topical; Antifungal Agent, Vaginal

Use Treatment of susceptible fungal infections, including dermatophytoses, superficial mycoses, and cutaneous candidiasis, as well as vulvovaginal candidiasis

Local Anesthetic/Vasoconstrictor Precautions No information available to require special precautions

Effects on Dental Treatment No significant effects or complications reported

Effects on Bleeding No information available to require special precautions

Adverse Effects Vaginal: 1% to 10%: Genitourinary: Vulvar/vaginal burning

Dental Usual Dosage Cutaneous candidiasis: Children >3 years and Adults: Topical (cream, solution): Apply twice daily; if no improvement occurs after 4 weeks of therapy, re-evaluate diagnosis.

Dosage

Children >3 years and Adults: Topical (cream, solution): Apply twice daily; if no improvement occurs after 4 weeks of therapy, re-evaluate diagnosis

Children >12 years and Adults:

Vaginal: Cream:

1%: Insert 1 applicatorful vaginal cream daily (preferably at bedtime) for 7 consecutive days

2%: Insert 1 applicatorful vaginal cream daily (preferably at bedtime) for 3 consecutive days

Topical (cream, solution): Apply to affected area twice daily (morning and evening) for 7 consecutive days

Mechanism of Action Binds to phospholipids in the fungal cell membrane altering cell wall permeability resulting in loss of essential intracellular elements

Contraindications Hypersensitivity to clotrimazole or any component of the formulation

Warnings/Precautions Avoid contact with eyes.

Drug Interactions

Avoid Concomitant Use There are no known interactions where it is recommended to avoid concomitant use.

Increased Effect/Toxicity There are no known significant interactions involving an increase in effect.

Decreased Effect There are no known significant interactions involving a decrease in effect.

Pharmacodynamics/Kinetics

Time to Peak Serum: Vaginal cream: ~24 hours

Pregnancy Risk Factor B

Lactation Excretion in breast milk unknown/use caution

Breast-Feeding Considerations Following topical and vaginal administration, clotrimazole is poorly absorbed systemically.

Dosage Forms

Cream, topical: 1% (15 g, 30 g, 45 g)
- Anti-Fungal™ [OTC]: 1% (113 g)
- Cruex® [OTC]: 1% (15 g)
- Lotrimin® AF Athlete's Foot [OTC]: 1% (12 g)
- Lotrimin® AF for Her [OTC]: 1% (24 g)
- Lotrimin® AF Jock Itch [OTC]: 1% (12 g)

Cream, vaginal: 1% (45 g); 2% (21 g)
- Gyne-Lotrimin® 7 [OTC]: 1% (45 g)
- Gyne-Lotrimin® 3 [OTC]: 2% (21 g)

Solution, topical: 1% (10 mL, 30 mL)

Cloxacillin (kloks a SIL in)

Canadian Brand Names Apo-Cloxi®; Cloxacillin; Novo-Cloxin; Nu-Cloxi

Pharmacologic Category Antibiotic, Penicillin

Dental Use Treatment of susceptible orofacial infections (notably penicillinase-producing staphylococci)

Use Treatment of bacterial infections including endocarditis, pneumonia, bone and joint infections, skin and soft-tissue infections, and sepsis that are caused by susceptible strains of penicillinase-producing staphylococci. **Note:** Exhibits good activity against *Staphylococcus aureus*; has activity against many streptococci, but is less active than penicillin and is generally not used in clinical practice to treat streptococcal infections.

Local Anesthetic/Vasoconstrictor Precautions No information available to require special precautions

Effects on Dental Treatment Key adverse event(s) related to dental treatment: Prolonged use of penicillins may lead to development of oral candidiasis.

Effects on Bleeding No information available to require special precautions

Adverse Effects Frequency not defined.

Cardiovascular: Hypotension

Central nervous system: Confusion, fever, lethargy, seizure (high doses and/or renal failure)

Dermatologic: Pruritus, rash, urticaria

Gastrointestinal: Abdominal pain, black or hairy tongue, diarrhea, flatulence, nausea, oral candidiasis, pseudomembranous colitis, stomatitis, vomiting

Hematologic: Agranulocytosis, bone marrow depression, eosinophilia, granulocytopenia, hemolytic anemia, leukopenia, neutropenia, thrombocytopenia

Hepatic: Alkaline phosphatase increased, ALT increased, AST increased, hepatotoxicity

Local: Thrombophlebitis

Neuromuscular & skeletal: Arthralgia, myalgia, myoclonus

Renal: Hematuria, interstitial nephritis, proteinuria, renal insufficiency, renal tubular damage

Respiratory: Bronchospasm, laryngeal edema, laryngospasm, sneezing, wheezing

Miscellaneous: Anaphylaxis, angioedema, allergic reaction, serum sickness-like reaction

Dental Usual Dosage Susceptible orofacial infections: Children >20 kg and Adults: Oral: 250-500 mg every 6 hours

Dosage Note: Dose and duration of therapy can vary depending on infecting organism, severity of infection, and clinical response of patient. Treat severe staphylococcal infections for at least 14 days; endocarditis and osteomyelitis require an extended duration of therapy for 4-6 weeks. The intravenous route should be used for severe infections.

Usual dosage range:

Oral:
- Children ≤20 kg: 25-50 mg/kg/day in divided doses every 6 hours
- Children >20 kg and Adults: 250-500 mg every 6 hours (manufacturer recommended maximum adult dose: 6 g/day)

I.M., I.V.:
- Children ≤20 kg: 25-50 mg/kg/day in divided doses every 6 hours; up to 200 mg/kg/day has been used in some studies for severe infections (Nunn, 2007; St. John, 1981)
- Children >20 kg and Adults: 250-500 mg every 6 hours (manufacturer recommended maximum adult dose: 6 g/day)

Indication-specific dosing: Dosing recommendations of World Health Organization unless otherwise noted:

Arthritis (septic), methicillin-sensitive *Staphylococcus aureus* (MSSA) (unlabeled dosing):

Children 2 months to 5 years: I.M., I.V.: 25-50 mg/kg (maximum: 2 g) every 4-6 hours given with ceftriaxone until clinical improvement, **followed by** oral therapy: 12.5 mg/kg (maximum: 500 mg) every 6 hours; total duration of therapy 2-3 weeks

Children >5 years: I.M., I.V.: 25-50 mg/kg (maximum: 2 g) every 4-6 hours (maximum daily dose: 12 g/day) until clinical improvement, **followed by** oral therapy: 25 mg/kg (maximum: 500 mg) every 6 hours; total duration of therapy 2-3 weeks

Adults: I.M., I.V.: 2 g every 6 hours for 2-3 weeks; **Note:** Oral therapy of 1 g every 6 hours may be used to complete therapy if parenteral therapy is discontinued prior to 2-3 week duration

Endocarditis (MSSA) (unlabeled dosing): I.V.:

Children: 50 mg/kg (maximum: 2 g) every 4 hours for 6 weeks; give with gentamicin for initial 7 days

Adults:

Native valve: 2 g every 4 hours for 6 weeks; may give with gentamicin for initial 5 days (Choudri, 2000)

Prosthetic valve: 2 g every 4 hours for 6 weeks; give with gentamicin for 2 weeks and rifampin for 6 weeks (Choudri, 2000)

Uncomplicated endocarditis in I.V. drug users: 2 g every 4 hours for 4 weeks and gentamicin for initial 5 days **or** 2 g every 4 hours and gentamicin both given for 2 weeks total (Choudri, 2000)

Osteomyelitis (MSSA) (unlabeled dosing):

Children 2 months to 5 years: I.M., I.V.: 25-50 mg/kg (maximum: 2 g) every 4-6 hours given with ceftriaxone until clinical improvement, **followed by** oral therapy: 12.5 mg/kg (maximum: 500 mg) every 6 hours; total duration of therapy 3-4 weeks

Children >5 years: I.M., I.V.: 25-50 mg/kg (maximum: 2 g) every 4-6 hours (maximum daily dose: 12 g/day) until clinical improvement, **followed by** oral therapy: 25 mg/kg (maximum: 500 mg) every 6 hours; total duration of therapy 3-4 weeks

Adults: I.M., I.V.: 2 g every 6 hours for 4-6 weeks (preferred) **or** for a minimum of 14 days, **followed by** 1 g every 6 hours orally to complete 4-6 weeks of therapy

Pneumonia (MSSA) (unlabeled dosing):

Children 2 months to 5 years: Oral: 25-50 mg/kg (maximum: 2 g) every 6 hours for at least 3 weeks with gentamicin

Children >5 years: I.M., I.V.: 50 mg/kg (maximum: 2 g) every 6 hours for 10-14 days

Adults: I.M., I.V.: 1-2 g every 6 hours for 10-14 days

Dosage adjustment in renal impairment: No dosage adjustment necessary

Mechanism of Action Inhibits bacterial cell wall synthesis by binding to one or more of the penicillin-binding proteins (PBPs) which in turn inhibit the final transpeptidation step of peptidoglycan synthesis in bacterial cell walls, thus inhibiting cell wall biosynthesis. Bacteria eventually lyse due to ongoing activity of cell wall autolytic enzymes (autolysins and murein hydrolases) while cell wall assembly is arrested.

Contraindications Hypersensitivity to cloxacillin, other penicillins, cephalosporins, or any component of the formulation

Warnings/Precautions Serious and occasionally severe or fatal hypersensitivity (anaphylactoid) reactions have been reported in patients on penicillin therapy, especially with a history of beta-lactam hypersensitivity, history of sensitivity to multiple allergens, or previous IgE-mediated reactions (eg, anaphylaxis, angioedema, urticaria). Use with caution in renal impairment as the rate of elimination is decreased. Use with caution in asthmatic patients. Prolonged use may result in fungal or bacterial superinfection, including *C. difficile*-associated diarrhea (CDAD) and pseudomembranous colitis; CDAD has been observed >2 months postantibiotic treatment. Use with caution in patients with a history of seizure disorders, particularly in the presence of renal impairment as increased serum levels may increase risk for seizures. Penicillin transport across the blood-brain barrier may be enhanced by inflamed meninges or during cardiopulmonary bypass increasing the risk of myoclonia, seizures, or reduced consciousness especially in patients with renal failure. Penicillin use has been associated with hematologic disorders (eg, agranulocytosis, neutropenia, thrombocytopenia) believed to be a hypersensitivity phenomena. Reactions are most often reversible upon discontinuing therapy. Renal clearance may be reduced in neonates; more frequent evaluation of clinical status and serum levels as well as more frequent dosage adjustments may be necessary with this patient population.

Drug Interactions

Avoid Concomitant Use

Avoid concomitant use of Cloxacillin with any of the following: BCG

Increased Effect/Toxicity

Cloxacillin may increase the levels/effects of: Methotrexate

The levels/effects of Cloxacillin may be increased by: Probenecid

Decreased Effect

Cloxacillin may decrease the levels/effects of: BCG; Mycophenolate; Typhoid Vaccine

The levels/effects of Cloxacillin may be decreased by: Fusidic Acid; Tetracycline Derivatives

Ethanol/Nutrition/Herb Interactions Food: Decreases cloxacillin absorption; serum levels are reduced by ~50%.

Dietary Considerations Should be taken 1 hour before or 2 hours after meals with water.

Pharmacodynamics/Kinetics

Half-life Elimination 0.5-1.5 hours; prolonged with renal impairment and in neonates

Time to Peak Serum: ~1 hour

Lactation Enters breast milk/use caution

Product Availability Not available in U.S.

Dosage Forms: Canada

Capsule: 250 mg, 500 mg

Injection, powder for reconstitution: 250 mg, 500 mg, 1000 mg, 2000 mg

Powder for suspension, oral: 125 mg/5 mL

CloZAPine (KLOE za peen)

U.S. Brand Names Clozaril®; FazaClo®

Canadian Brand Names Apo-Clozapine®; Clozaril®; Gen-Clozapine; PMS-Clozapine

Pharmacologic Category Antipsychotic Agent, Atypical

Use Treatment-refractory schizophrenia; to reduce risk of recurrent suicidal behavior in schizophrenia or schizoaffective disorder

Unlabeled/Investigational Use Schizoaffective disorder, bipolar disorder, childhood psychosis, severe obsessive-compulsive disorder; psychosis/agitation related to Alzheimer's dementia

Local Anesthetic/Vasoconstrictor Precautions Most pharmacology textbooks state that in presence of phenothiazines, systemic doses of epinephrine paradoxically decrease the blood pressure. This is the so called "epinephrine reversal" phenomenon. This has never been observed when epinephrine is given by infiltration as part of the local anesthesia procedure.

Effects on Dental Treatment Key adverse event(s) related to dental treatment: Sialorrhea and xerostomia (normal salivary flow resumes upon discontinuation). Many patients may experience orthostatic hypotension with clozapine; precautions should be taken; do not use atropine-like drugs for xerostomia in patients taking clozapine due to significant potentiation.

Effects on Bleeding No information available to require special precautions

Adverse Effects

>10%:

Cardiovascular: Tachycardia (25%)

Central nervous system: Drowsiness (39% to 46%), dizziness (19% to 27%), insomnia (2% to 20%)

Gastrointestinal: Sialorrhea (31% to 48%), weight gain (4% to 31%), constipation (14% to 25%), nausea/vomiting (3% to 17%)

1% to 10%:

Cardiovascular: Hypotension (9%), syncope (6%), hypertension (4%), angina (1%), ECG changes (1%)

Central nervous system: Headache (7%), agitation (4%), akinesia (4%), nightmares (4%), restlessness (4%), akathisia (3%), confusion (3%), seizure (3%), anxiety (1%), ataxia (1%), depression (1%), lethargy (1%), myoclonic jerks (1%), slurred speech (1%)

Dermatologic: Rash (2%)

Gastrointestinal: Abdominal discomfort/heartburn (4% to 14%), xerostomia (6%), diarrhea (2%), anorexia (1%), throat discomfort (1%)

Genitourinary: Urinary abnormalities (eg, abnormal ejaculation, retention, urgency, incontinence; 1% to 2%)

Hematologic: Agranulocytosis (1%), eosinophilia (1%), leukocytosis, leukopenia

Hepatic: Liver function tests abnormal (1%)

Neuromuscular & skeletal: Tremor (6%), hypokinesia (4%), rigidity (3%), hyperkinesia (1%), weakness (1%), pain (1%), spasm (1%)
Ocular: Visual disturbances (5%)
Respiratory: Dyspnea (1%), nasal congestion (1%)
Miscellaneous: Diaphoresis (6%), tongue numbness (1%)

General Dosage Range Dosage adjustment recommended in patients who develop toxicities

Oral: *Adults:* Initial: 12.5 mg once or twice daily; Maintenance: 12.5-900 mg/day (maximum: 900 mg/day)

Mechanism of Action Clozapine (dibenzodiazepine antipsychotic) exhibits weak antagonism of D_1, D_2, D_3, and D_5 dopamine receptor subtypes, but shows high affinity for D_4; in addition, it blocks the serotonin ($5HT_2$), alpha-adrenergic, histamine H_1, and cholinergic receptors

Pharmacodynamics/Kinetics

Half-life Elimination Steady state: 12 hours (range: 4-66 hours)

Time to Peak 2.5 hours (range: 1-6 hours)

Pregnancy Risk Factor B

Prescribing and Access Restrictions

U.S.: Clozaril® is deemed to have an approved REMS program. As a requirement of the REMS program, access to this medication is restricted. Patient-specific registration is required to dispense clozapine. Monitoring systems for individual clozapine manufacturers are independent. If a patient is switched from one brand/manufacturer of clozapine to another, the patient must be entered into a new registry (must be completed by the prescriber and delivered to the dispensing pharmacy). Healthcare providers, including pharmacists dispensing clozapine, should verify the patient's hematological status and qualification to receive clozapine with all existing registries. The manufacturer of Clozaril® requests that healthcare providers submit all WBC/ANC values following discontinuation of therapy to the Clozaril National Registry for all nonrechallengable patients until WBC is ≥3500/mm^3 and ANC is ≥2000/mm^3.

Canada: Distribution of clozapine is available only through the Clozaril Support and Assistance Network (CSAN). Details regarding CSAN are available to Canadian practitioners at (800-267-2726).

Coal Tar (KOLE tar)

U.S. Brand Names Balnetar® [OTC]; Betatar Gel® [OTC]; Cutar® [OTC]; Denorex® Therapeutic Protection 2-in-1 Shampoo + Conditioner [OTC]; Denorex® Therapeutic Protection [OTC]; DHS® Tar [OTC]; DHS™ Tar Gel [OTC]; Exorex® Penetrating Emulsion #2 [OTC]; Exorex® Penetrating Emulsion [OTC]; ionil-T® Plus [OTC]; ionil-T® [OTC]; MG217® Medicated Tar Extra Strength [OTC]; MG217® Medicated Tar Intensive Strength [OTC]; MG217® Medicated Tar [OTC]; Neutrogena® T/Gel® Extra Strength [OTC]; Neutrogena® T/Gel® Stubborn Itch Control [OTC]; Neutrogena® T/Gel® [OTC]; Oxipor® VHC [OTC]; Pentrax® [OTC]; Scytera™ [OTC]; Tera-Gel™ [OTC]; Thera-Gel [OTC]; Zetar® [OTC]

Canadian Brand Names Balnetar®; Estar®; Targel®

Pharmacologic Category Topical Skin Product

Use Topically for controlling dandruff, seborrheic dermatitis, or psoriasis

Local Anesthetic/Vasoconstrictor Precautions No information available to require special precautions

Effects on Dental Treatment No significant effects or complications reported

Effects on Bleeding No information available to require special precautions

Adverse Effects Frequency not defined: Dermatologic: Dermatitis, folliculitis. irritation, photosensitivity

General Dosage Range Topical: *Adults:*
Bath: Add 60-90 mL (5-20%) or 15-25 mL (30%) to bath water, soak 5-20 minutes, use once daily to every 3 days
Scalp: Apply to lesions 3-12 hours before each shampoo
Shampoo: Rub into wet hair, rinse, repeat leaving on 5 minutes; apply twice weekly for 2 weeks then once weekly
Skin: Apply to affected areas 1-4 times/day, decrease to 2-3 times/week once condition controlled
Soap: Use on affected areas instead of regular soap

Pregnancy Risk Factor C

Coal Tar and Salicylic Acid (KOLE tar & sal i SIL ik AS id)

Related Information

Coal Tar *on page* 430

Salicylic Acid *on page* 1504

U.S. Brand Names Tarsum® [OTC]; X-Seb T® Pearl [OTC]; X-Seb T® Plus [OTC]

Canadian Brand Names Sebcur/T®

Pharmacologic Category Topical Skin Product

Use Seborrheal dermatitis, dandruff, psoriasis

Local Anesthetic/Vasoconstrictor Precautions No information available to require special precautions

Effects on Dental Treatment No significant effects or complications reported

Effects on Bleeding No information available to require special precautions

General Dosage Range Topical:

Gel: *Adults:* Apply to plaques, leave on up to 1 hour then rinse

Shampoo: *Adults:* Apply to wet hair, massage into scalp then rinse

Pregnancy Risk Factor C

Cocaine (koe KANE)

Pharmacologic Category Local Anesthetic

Use Topical anesthesia for mucous membranes

Local Anesthetic/Vasoconstrictor Precautions Although plain local anesthetic is not contraindicated, vasoconstrictor is absolutely contraindicated in any patient under the influence of or within 2 hours of cocaine use

Effects on Dental Treatment Key adverse event(s) related to dental treatment: Loss of taste perception. See Dental Comment.

Effects on Bleeding No information available to require special precautions

Adverse Effects

>10%:

Central nervous system: CNS stimulation

Gastrointestinal: Loss of taste perception

Respiratory: Rhinitis, nasal congestion

Miscellaneous: Loss of smell

1% to 10%:

Cardiovascular: Heart rate decreased with low doses, tachycardia with moderate doses, hypertension, cardiomyopathy, cardiac arrhythmia, myocarditis, QRS prolongation, Raynaud's phenomenon, cerebral vasculitis, thrombosis, fibrillation (atrial), flutter (atrial), sinus bradycardia, CHF, pulmonary hypertension, sinus tachycardia, tachycardia (supraventricular), arrhythmia (ventricular), vasoconstriction

Central nervous system: Fever, nervousness, restlessness, euphoria, excitation, headache, psychosis, hallucinations, agitation, seizure, slurred speech, hyperthermia, dystonic reactions, cerebral vascular accident, vasculitis, clonic-tonic reactions, paranoia, sympathetic storm

Dermatologic: Skin infarction, pruritus, madarosis

Gastrointestinal: Nausea, anorexia, colonic ischemia, spontaneous bowel perforation

Genitourinary: Priapism, uterine rupture

Hematologic: Thrombocytopenia

Neuromuscular & skeletal: Chorea (extrapyramidal), paresthesia, tremor, fasciculations

Ocular: Mydriasis (peak effect at 45 minutes; may last up to 12 hours), sloughing of the corneal epithelium, ulceration of the cornea, iritis, mydriasis, chemosis

Renal: Myoglobinuria, necrotizing vasculitis

Respiratory: Tachypnea, nasal mucosa damage (when snorting), hyposmia, bronchiolitis obliterans organizing pneumonia

Miscellaneous: "Washed-out" syndrome

General Dosage Range Topical: *Adults:* Do not exceed 1 mg/kg (1% to 10% concentration)

Mechanism of Action Ester local anesthetic blocks both the initiation and conduction of nerve impulses by decreasing the neuronal membrane's permeability to sodium ions, which results in inhibition of depolarization with resultant blockade of conduction; interferes with the uptake of norepinephrine by adrenergic nerve terminals producing vasoconstriction

Pharmacodynamics/Kinetics

Onset of Action ~1 minute; Peak effect: ~5 minutes

Duration of Action Dose dependent: ≥30 minutes; cocaine metabolites may appear in urine of neonates up to 5 days after birth due to maternal cocaine use shortly before birth

Half-life Elimination 75 minutes

Pregnancy Risk Factor C/X (nonmedicinal use)

Controlled Substance C-II

Dental Comment The cocaine user, regardless of how the cocaine was administered, presents a potential life-threatening situation in the dental operatory. A patient under the influence of cocaine could be compared to a car going 100 mph. Blood pressure is elevated, heart rate is likely increased, and the use of a local anesthetic with epinephrine may result in a medical emergency. Such patients can be identified by their jitteriness, irritability, talkativeness, tremors, and short, abrupt speech patterns. These same signs and symptoms may also be seen in a normal dental patient with preoperative dental anxiety; therefore, the dentist must be particularly alert in order to identify the potential cocaine abuser. If cocaine use is suspected, the patient should never be given a local anesthetic with vasoconstrictor, for fear of exacerbating the cocaine-induced sympathetic response. Life-threatening episodes of cardiac arrhythmias and hypertensive crises have been reported when local anesthetic with vasoconstrictor was administered to a patient under the influence of cocaine. No local anesthetic, used by any dentist, can interfere with, nor test positive by cocaine in any urine testing screen. Therefore, the dentist does not need to be concerned with any false drug-use accusations associated with dental anesthesia.

Codeine (KOE deen)

Related Information

Oral Pain *on page* 1928

Canadian Brand Names Codeine Contin®

Generic Availability (U.S.) Yes

Pharmacologic Category Analgesic, Opioid; Antitussive

Dental Use Treatment of postoperative pain

Use Treatment of mild-to-moderate pain; antitussive in lower doses

Local Anesthetic/Vasoconstrictor Precautions No information available to require special precautions

Effects on Dental Treatment No significant effects or complications reported (see Dental Comment)

Effects on Bleeding No information available to require special precautions

Adverse Effects

>10%:
- Central nervous system: Drowsiness
- Gastrointestinal: Constipation

1% to 10%:
- Cardiovascular: Hypotension, tachycardia or bradycardia
- Central nervous system: Confusion, dizziness, false feeling of well being, headache, lightheadedness, malaise, paradoxical CNS stimulation, restlessness
- Dermatologic: Rash, urticaria
- Gastrointestinal: Anorexia, nausea, vomiting, xerostomia
- Genitourinary: Ureteral spasm, urination decreased
- Hepatic: LFTs increased
- Local: Burning at injection site
- Neuromuscular & skeletal: Weakness
- Ocular: Blurred vision
- Respiratory: Dyspnea
- Miscellaneous: Histamine release

Frequency not defined: ALT increased, AST increased

Dental Usual Dosage Postoperative pain: Adults: Oral: 30 mg every 4-6 hours as needed; patients with prior opiate exposure may require higher initial doses. Usual range: 15-120 mg every 4-6 hours as needed

Dosage Note: These are guidelines and do not represent the maximum doses that may be required in all patients. Doses should be titrated to pain relief/prevention. Doses >1.5 mg/kg body weight are not recommended.

Analgesic:

Children: Oral, I.M., SubQ: 0.5-1 mg/kg/dose every 4-6 hours as needed; maximum: 60 mg/dose

Adults:

Oral: 30 mg every 4-6 hours as needed; patients with prior opiate exposure may require higher initial doses. Usual range: 15-120 mg every 4-6 hours as needed.

Note: The American Pain Society recommends an initial dose of 30-60 mg for adults with moderate pain.

Oral, controlled release formulation (Codeine Contin®, not available in U.S.): 50-300 mg every 12 hours. **Note:** A patient's codeine requirement should be established using prompt release formulations; conversion to long acting products may be considered when chronic, continuous treatment is required. Higher dosages should be reserved for use only in opioid-tolerant patients.

I.M., SubQ: 30 mg every 4-6 hours as needed; patients with prior opiate exposure may require higher initial doses. Usual range: 15-120 mg every 4-6 hours as needed; more frequent dosing may be needed

Antitussive: Oral (for nonproductive cough):

Children: 1-1.5 mg/kg/day in divided doses every 4-6 hours as needed: Alternative dose according to age:

2-6 years: 2.5-5 mg every 4-6 hours as needed; maximum: 30 mg/day

6-12 years: 5-10 mg every 4-6 hours as needed; maximum: 60 mg/day

Adults: 10-20 mg/dose every 4-6 hours as needed; maximum: 120 mg/day

Dosing adjustment in renal impairment:

Cl_{cr} 10-50 mL/minute: Administer 75% of dose

Cl_{cr} <10 mL/minute: Administer 50% of dose

Dosing adjustment in hepatic impairment: Probably necessary in hepatic insufficiency

Mechanism of Action Binds to opiate receptors in the CNS, causing inhibition of ascending pain pathways, altering the perception of and response to pain; causes cough supression by direct central action in the medulla; produces generalized CNS depression

Contraindications Hypersensitivity to codeine or any component of the formulation; pregnancy (prolonged use or high doses at term)

Warnings/Precautions Use with caution in patients with hypersensitivity reactions to other phenanthrene-derivative opioid agonists (morphine, hydrocodone, hydromorphone, levorphanol, oxycodone, oxymorphone); respiratory diseases including asthma, emphysema, COPD, adrenal insufficiency, biliary tract impairment, CNS depression/coma, head trauma, morbid obesity, prostatic hyperplasia, urinary stricture, thyroid dysfunction, or severe liver or renal insufficiency; some preparations contain sulfites which may cause allergic reactions; tolerance or drug dependence may result from extended use. May obscure diagnosis or clinical course of patients with acute abdominal conditions. May cause CNS depression, which may impair physical or mental abilities; patients must be cautioned about performing tasks which require mental alertness (eg, operating machinery or driving). May cause hypotension; use with caution in patients with hypovolemia, cardiovascular disease (including acute MI), or drugs which may exaggerate hypotensive effects (including phenothiazines or general anesthetics). Use caution in patients with two or more copies of the variant CYP2D6*2 allele; may have extensive conversion to morphine and thus increased opioid-mediated effects.

Not recommended for use for cough control in patients with a productive cough; not recommended as an antitussive for children <2 years of age; the elderly and debilitated patients may be particularly susceptible to adverse effects of narcotics

Not approved for I.V. administration (although this route has been used clinically). If given intravenously, must be given slowly and the patient should be lying down. Rapid intravenous administration of narcotics may increase the incidence of serious adverse effects, in part due to limited opportunity to assess response prior to administration of the full dose. Access to respiratory support should be immediately available.

Concurrent use of agonist/antagonist analgesics may precipitate withdrawal symptoms and/or reduced analgesic efficacy in patients following prolonged therapy with mu opioid agonists. Abrupt discontinuation following prolonged use may also lead to withdrawal symptoms.

Drug Interactions

Metabolism/Transport Effects **Substrate** of CYP2D6 (major), 3A4 (minor); **Inhibits** CYP2D6 (weak)

Avoid Concomitant Use There are no known interactions where it is recommended to avoid concomitant use.

Increased Effect/Toxicity

Codeine may increase the levels/effects of: Alcohol (Ethyl); Alvimopan; CNS Depressants; Desmopressin; Selective Serotonin Reuptake Inhibitors; Thiazide Diuretics

The levels/effects of Codeine may be increased by: Amphetamines; Antipsychotic Agents (Phenothiazines); Droperidol; Somatostatin Analogs; Succinylcholine

Decreased Effect
Codeine may decrease the levels/effects of: Pegvisomant

The levels/effects of Codeine may be decreased by: Ammonium Chloride; CYP2D6 Inhibitors (Moderate); CYP2D6 Inhibitors (Strong); Mixed Agonist/Antagonist Opioids

Ethanol/Nutrition/Herb Interactions
Ethanol: May increase CNS depression; monitor for increased effects with coadministration. Caution patients about effects.
Herb/Nutraceutical: St John's wort may decrease codeine levels. Avoid valerian, St John's wort, kava kava, gotu kola (may increase CNS depression).

Pharmacodynamics/Kinetics
Onset of Action Oral: 0.5-1 hour; I.M.: 10-30 minutes; Peak effect: Oral: 1-1.5 hours; I.M.: 0.5-1 hour
Duration of Action 4-6 hours
Half-life Elimination 2.5-3.5 hours

Pregnancy Risk Factor C

Lactation Enters breast milk/use caution (AAP rates "compatible"; AAP 2001 update pending)

Breast-Feeding Considerations Codeine and its metabolite (morphine) are found in breast milk and can be detected in the serum of nursing infants. The relative dose to a nursing infant has been calculated to be ~1% of the weight-adjusted maternal dose. Higher levels of morphine may be found in the breast milk of lactating mothers who are "ultra-rapid metabolizers" of codeine; patients with two or more copies of the variant CYP2D6*2 allele may have extensive conversion to morphine and thus increased opioid-mediated effects. In one case, excessively high serum concentrations of morphine were reported in a breast-fed infant following maternal use of acetaminophen with codeine. The mother was later found to be an "ultra-rapid metabolizer" of codeine; symptoms in the infant included feeding difficulty and lethargy, followed by death. Caution should be used since most persons are not aware if they have the genotype resulting in "ultra-rapid metabolizer" status. When codeine is used in breast-feeding women, it is recommended to use the lowest dose for the shortest duration of time and observe the infant for increased sleepiness, difficulty in feeding or breathing, or limpness.

Controlled Substance C-II

Dosage Forms
Powder, for prescription compounding: USP: 100% (10 g, 25 g)
Tablet, oral: 15 mg, 30 mg, 60 mg

Dosage Forms: Canada
Tablet, controlled release:
Codeine Contin®: 50 mg, 100 mg, 150 mg, 200 mg

Dental Comment It is recommended that codeine not be used as the sole entity for analgesia because of moderate efficacy along with relatively high incidence of nausea, sedation, and constipation. In addition, codeine has some narcotic addiction liability. Codeine in combination with acetaminophen or aspirin is recommended. Maximum effective analgesic dose of codeine is 60 mg (1 grain). Beyond 60 mg increases respiratory depression only. Sodium thiosulfate is an effective chemical antidote for codeine poisoning.

References
Desjardins PJ, Cooper SA, Gallegos TL, et al, "The Relative Analgesic Efficacy of Propiram Fumarate, Codeine, Aspirin, and Placebo in Postimpaction Dental Pain," *J Clin Pharmacol*, 1984, 24(1):35-42.
Forbes JA, Keller CK, Smith JW, et al, "Analgesic Effect of Naproxen Sodium, Codeine, a Naproxen-Codeine Combination and Aspirin on the Postoperative Pain of Oral Surgery," *Pharmacotherapy*, 1986, 6(5):211-8.

Colchicine (KOL chi seen)

U.S. Brand Names Colcrys®

Pharmacologic Category Colchicine

Use Prevention and treatment of acute gout flares; treatment of familial Mediterranean fever (FMF)

Unlabeled/Investigational Use Primary biliary cirrhosis; pericarditis

Local Anesthetic/Vasoconstrictor Precautions No information available to require special precautions

Effects on Dental Treatment No significant effects or complications reported

Effects on Bleeding No information available to require special precautions

Adverse Effects
>10%: Gastrointestinal: Gastrointestinal disorders including abdominal pain, cramping, nausea, vomiting (up to 26%), diarrhea (up to 23%)
1% to 10%: Respiratory: Pharyngolaryngeal pain (3%)

General Dosage Range Dosage adjustment recommended in patients with renal impairment or on concomitant therapy

Oral:

Children 4-6 years: 0.3-1.8 mg/day in 1-2 divided doses
Children 6-12 years: 0.9-1.8 mg/day in 1-2 divided doses
Children 12-16 years: 1.2-2.4 mg/day in 1-2 divided doses
Children >16 years and Adults: 0.6-2.4 mg/day in 1-2 divided doses **or** Initial: 1.2 mg; repeat with 0.6 mg in 1 hour (maximum total therapy: 1.8 mg)

Mechanism of Action Disrupts cytoskeletal functions by inhibiting β-tubulin polymerization into microtubules, preventing activation, degranulation, and migration of neutrophils associated with mediating some gout symptoms. In familial Mediterranean fever, may interfere with intracellular assembly of the inflammasome complex present in neutrophils and monocytes that mediate activation of interleukin-1β.

Pharmacodynamics/Kinetics

Onset of Action Oral: Pain relief: ~18-24 hours

Half-life Elimination 27-31 hours (multiple oral doses; young, healthy volunteers)

Time to Peak Serum: Oral: 0.5-3 hours

Pregnancy Risk Factor C

Colchicine and Probenecid (KOL chi seen & proe BEN e sid)

Related Information

Colchicine *on page 434*
Probenecid *on page 1404*

Pharmacologic Category Anti-inflammatory Agent; Antigout Agent; Uricosuric Agent

Use Treatment of chronic gouty arthritis when complicated by frequent, recurrent acute attacks of gout

Local Anesthetic/Vasoconstrictor Precautions No information available to require special precautions

Effects on Dental Treatment No significant effects or complications reported

Effects on Bleeding No information available to require special precautions

Adverse Effects 1% to 10%:

Cardiovascular: Flushing
Central nervous system: Headache, dizziness
Dermatologic: Rash, alopecia
Gastrointestinal: Anorexia, nausea, vomiting, diarrhea, abdominal pain
Hematologic: Anemia, leukopenia, aplastic anemia, agranulocytosis
Hepatic: Hepatic necrosis, hepatotoxicity
Neuromuscular & skeletal: Peripheral neuritis, myopathy
Renal: Nephrotic syndrome, uric acid stones, polyuria
Miscellaneous: Hypersensitivity reactions

General Dosage Range Dosage adjustment recommended in patients with renal impairment

Oral: *Adults:* Initial: 1 tablet daily; Maintenance: 1 tablet twice daily

Pregnancy Risk Factor C

Colesevelam (koh le SEV a lam)

Related Information

Cardiovascular Diseases *on page 1848*

U.S. Brand Names Welchol®

Canadian Brand Names Welchol®

Generic Availability (U.S.) No

Pharmacologic Category Antilipemic Agent, Bile Acid Sequestrant

Use Management of elevated LDL in primary hypercholesterolemia (Fredrickson type IIa) when used alone or in combination with an HMG-CoA reductase inhibitor; management of heterozygous familial hypercholesterolemia (heFH) in adolescent patients (males and postmenarchal females 10-17 years of age) when used alone or in combination with an HMG-CoA reductase inhibitor, in patients who after an adequate trial of dietary therapy have LDL-C ≥190 mg/dL or LDL-C ≥160 mg/dL with positive family history of premature cardiovascular disease (CVD) or with two or more CVD risk factors; improve glycemic control in type 2 diabetes mellitus (noninsulin dependent, NIDDM) in conjunction with diet, exercise, and insulin or oral antidiabetic agents

Local Anesthetic/Vasoconstrictor Precautions No information available to require special precautions

Effects on Dental Treatment No significant effects or complications reported

Effects on Bleeding No information available to require special precautions

Adverse Effects

>10%: Gastrointestinal: Constipation (11%)

2% to 10%:

Gastrointestinal: Dyspepsia (8%)

Neuromuscular & skeletal: Weakness (4%), myalgia (2%)

Respiratory: Pharyngitis (3%)

Incidence less than or equal to placebo: Infection, headache, pain, back pain, abdominal pain, flu syndrome, flatulence, diarrhea, nausea, sinusitis, rhinitis, cough

Dosage Oral:

Children 10-17 years (males and postmenarchal females) and Adults:

Once-daily dosing: 3.75 g (oral suspension or 6 tablets)

Twice-daily dosing: 1.875 g (oral suspension or 3 tablets)

Note: Due to large tablet size, oral suspension is recommended in pediatric patients.

Elderly: No recommendations made

Dosage adjustment in renal impairment: No recommendations made

Dosage adjustment in hepatic impairment: No recommendations made

Mechanism of Action Colesevelam binds bile acids including glycocholic acid in the intestine, impeding their reabsorption. Increases the fecal loss of bile salt-bound LDL-C

Contraindications History of bowel obstruction; serum triglyceride concentration >500 mg/dL; history of hypertriglyceridemia-induced pancreatitis

Warnings/Precautions Use with caution in treating patients with serum triglyceride concentrations >300 mg/dL (may cause increased concentrations) or in patients susceptible to fat-soluble vitamin deficiencies. Discontinue if triglyceride concentrations exceed 500 mg/dL or hypertriglyceridemia-induced pancreatitis occurs. Use in patients with gastroparesis, other severe GI motility disorders, or a history of major GI tract surgery is not recommended due to constipating effects of colesevelam. Patients with dysphagia or swallowing disorders should use the oral suspension form of colesevelam due to large tablet size and risk for esophageal obstruction.

Minimal effects are seen on HDL-C and triglyceride levels. Secondary causes of hypercholesterolemia should be excluded before initiation. Colesevelam has not been studied in Fredrickson Type I, III, IV, or V dyslipidemias. Colesevelam is not indicated for the management of type 1 diabetes, particularly in the acute management (eg, DKA). It is also not indicated in type 2 diabetes mellitus as monotherapy and must be used as an adjunct to diet, exercise, and glycemic control with insulin or oral antidiabetic agents. Combination with dipeptidyl peptidase 4 inhibitors or thiazolidinediones has not been studied extensively.

Some products may contain phenylalanine.

Drug Interactions

Avoid Concomitant Use There are no known interactions where it is recommended to avoid concomitant use.

Increased Effect/Toxicity There are no known significant interactions involving an increase in effect.

Decreased Effect

Colesevelam may decrease the levels/effects of: Amiodarone; Antidiabetic Agents (Thiazolidinedione); Chenodiol; Contraceptives (Estrogens); Contraceptives (Progestins); Corticosteroids (Oral); Ethinyl Estradiol; Ezetimibe; GlyBURIDE; Leflunomide; Loop Diuretics; Methotrexate; Niacin; Nonsteroidal Anti-Inflammatory Agents; Norethindrone; Phenytoin; Pravastatin; Propranolol; Raloxifene; Tetracycline Derivatives; Thiazide Diuretics; Thyroid Products; Ursodiol; Vitamin D Analogs; Vitamin K Antagonists

Dietary Considerations Should be taken with meal(s) and a liquid. Follow dietary guidelines. Some products may contain phenylalanine.

Pharmacodynamics/Kinetics

Onset of Action Peak effect: Therapeutic: ~2 weeks

Half-life Elimination 0.05% was excreted in the urine after 1 month of chronic dosing

Pregnancy Risk Factor B

Lactation Excretion in breast milk unknown

Dosage Forms

Granules for suspension, oral:

Welchol®: 3.75 g/packet (30s)

Tablet, oral:

Welchol®: 625 mg

References

Davidson MH, Dillon MA, Gordon B, et al, "Colesevelam Hydrochloride (Cholestagel): A New, Potent Bile Acid Sequestrant Associated With a Low Incidence of Gastrointestinal Side Effects," *Arch Intern Med*, 1999, 159(16):1893-900.

"Executive Summary of The Third Report of The National Cholesterol Education Program (NCEP) Expert Panel on Detection, Evaluation, And Treatment of High Blood Cholesterol In Adults (Adult Treatment Panel III)," *JAMA*, 2001, 285(19):2486-97.

Steinmetz KL, "Colesevelam Hydrochloride," *Am J Health Syst Pharm*, 2002, 59:932-9.

Colestipol (koe LES ti pole)

Related Information

Cardiovascular Diseases *on page 1848*

U.S. Brand Names Colestid®; Colestid® Flavored

Canadian Brand Names Colestid®

Pharmacologic Category Antilipemic Agent, Bile Acid Sequestrant

Use Adjunct in management of primary hypercholesterolemia; regression of arteriolosclerosis; relief of pruritus associated with elevated levels of bile acids; possibly used to decrease plasma half-life of digoxin in toxicity

Local Anesthetic/Vasoconstrictor Precautions No information available to require special precautions

Effects on Dental Treatment No significant effects or complications reported

Effects on Bleeding Although chronic use at high dosages may be associated with bleeding problems, there is no information available to require routine special precautions in patients receiving this medication. The possibility of delayed coagulation should be anticipated.

Adverse Effects

>10%: Gastrointestinal: Constipation

1% to 10%:

Central nervous system: Headache, dizziness, anxiety, vertigo, drowsiness, fatigue

Gastrointestinal: Abdominal pain and distention, belching, flatulence, nausea, vomiting, diarrhea

General Dosage Range Oral: *Adults:* Granules: Initial: 5 g 1-2 times/day; Maintenance: 5-30 g/day in 1-4 divided doses; Tablets: Initial: 2 g 1-2 times/day; Maintenance: 2-16 g/day

Mechanism of Action Binds with bile acids to form an insoluble complex that is eliminated in feces; it thereby increases the fecal loss of bile acid-bound low density lipoprotein cholesterol

Pregnancy Risk Factor C

Colistimethate (koe lis ti METH ate)

U.S. Brand Names Coly-Mycin® M

Canadian Brand Names Coly-Mycin® M

Pharmacologic Category Antibiotic, Miscellaneous

Use Treatment of infections due to sensitive strains of certain gram-negative bacilli which are resistant to other antibacterials or in patients allergic to other antibacterials

Unlabeled/Investigational Use Used as nebulized inhalation in the prevention of *Pseudomonas aeruginosa* respiratory tract infections in immunocompromised patients, and used as nebulized inhalation adjunct agent for the treatment of *P. aeruginosa* infections in patients with cystic fibrosis and other seriously ill or chronically ill patients

Local Anesthetic/Vasoconstrictor Precautions No information available to require special precautions

Effects on Dental Treatment No significant effects or complications reported

Effects on Bleeding No information available to require special precautions

Adverse Effects Frequency not defined.

Central nervous system: Dizziness, fever, headache, slurred speech, vertigo

Dermatologic: Pruritus, rash, urticaria

gastrointestinal: GI upset

Neuromuscular & skeletal: Paresthesia (extremities, oral); weakness (lower limb)

Renal: BUN increased, creatinine increased, nephrotoxicity, proteinuria, urine output decreased

Respiratory: Apnea, respiratory arrest

General Dosage Range Dosage adjustment recommended in patients with renal impairment

I.M., I.V.: *Children and Adults:* 2.5-5 mg/kg/day in 2-4 divided doses

Mechanism of Action Hydrolyzed to colistin, which acts as a cationic detergent which damages the bacterial cytoplasmic membrane causing leaking of intracellular substances and cell death

Pharmacodynamics/Kinetics

Half-life Elimination I.M., I.V.: 2-3 hours; Anuria: ≤2-3 days

Time to Peak I.V.: 10 minutes

Pregnancy Risk Factor C

Collagen (Absorbable) (KOL la jen, ab SORB able)

Related Information

Antiplatelet and Anticoagulation Considerations in Dentistry *on page 1867*

U.S. Brand Names CollaCote®; CollaPlug®; CollaTape®

Generic Availability (U.S.) Yes

Pharmacologic Category Hemostatic Agent

Dental Use Control of bleeding created during dental surgery

Use Hemostatic

Local Anesthetic/Vasoconstrictor Precautions No information available to require special precautions

Effects on Dental Treatment No significant effects or complications reported

Effects on Bleeding General dental procedures and simple restorative procedures are not associated with bleeding; therefore, there is no contraindication with these general dental procedures for most patients with bleeding disorders. However, after dental extractions and other dental surgeries including deep scaling, block anesthesia, and large fillings, in patients with hemophilia, drugs such as collagen may be useful in controlling bleeding. A carefully coordinated strategy between the dental and medical team may be required to ensure adequate procedures for hemostasis.

Adverse Effects No data reported.

Dental Usual Dosage Control of bleeding: Children and Adults: Topical: A sufficiently large dressing should be selected so as to completely cover the oral wound

Dosage Children and Adults: A sufficiently large dressing should be selected so as to completely cover the oral wound

Mechanism of Action The highly porous sponge structure absorbs blood and wound exudate. The collagen component causes aggregation of platelets which bind to collagen fibrils. The aggregated platelets degranulate, releasing coagulation factors that promote the formation of fibrin.

Contraindications No data reported

Warnings/Precautions Should not be used on infected or contaminated wounds

Drug Interactions

Avoid Concomitant Use There are no known interactions where it is recommended to avoid concomitant use.

Increased Effect/Toxicity There are no known significant interactions involving an increase in effect.

Decreased Effect There are no known significant interactions involving a decrease in effect.

Lactation Compatible

Dosage Forms

Wound dressing:

Generics:

3/8" x 3/4"

3/4" x 1 1/2"

1" x 3"

Brands:

CollaCote®, CollaPlug®, CollaTape®:

3/8" x 3/4"

3/4" x 1 1/2"

1" x 3"

Collagenase (Systemic) (KOL la je nase)

U.S. Brand Names Xiaflex™

Pharmacologic Category Enzyme

Use Treatment of Dupuytren's contracture with a palpable cord

Adverse Effects

>10%:

Dermatologic: Bruising (70%), pruritus (15%)

Hematologic: Lymphadenopathy (13%)

Local: Injection site hemorrhage (38%), injection site reaction (24% to 35%; includes erythema, inflammation, irritation, pain, swelling, tenderness)

Miscellaneous: Antibody formation (≥86%), peripheral edema (primarily as swelling of injected hand: 73%), pain in extremity (35%), neutralizing antibodies (10% to 21% to AUX-I and AUX-II, respectively)

1% to 10%:

Dermatologic: laceration (9%), erythema (6%)

Miscellaneous: Lymph node pain (8%), axillary pain (6%)

General Dosage Range Intralesional: *Adults:* 0.58 mg per cord

Mechanism of Action Collagenase clostridium histolyticum contains two forms of microbial collagenase (Collagenase AUX-1 and Collagenase AUX-II) isolated and purified from the fermentation of *Clostridium histolyticum* bacteria; collagenase lyses collagen, leading to enzymatic disruption of contracted Dupuytren's cord (comprised primarily of collagen)

Pregnancy Risk Factor B

Collagenase (Topical) (KOL la je nase)

U.S. Brand Names Santyl®

Pharmacologic Category Enzyme, Topical Debridement

Use Promotes debridement of necrotic tissue in dermal ulcers and severe burns

Local Anesthetic/Vasoconstrictor Precautions No information available to require special precautions

Effects on Dental Treatment No significant effects or complications reported

Effects on Bleeding No information available to require special precautions

Adverse Effects Frequency not defined.

Local: Irritation, pain and burning may occur at site of application

General Dosage Range Topical: *Children and Adults:* Apply once daily

Mechanism of Action Collagenase is an enzyme derived from the fermentation of *Clostridium histolyticum* and differs from other proteolytic enzymes in that its enzymatic action has a high specificity for native and denatured collagen. Collagenase will not attack collagen in healthy tissue or newly formed granulation tissue. In addition, it does not act on fat, fibrin, keratin, or muscle.

Pregnancy Risk Factor C

Collagen Hemostat (KOL la jen HEE moe stat)

Related Information

Antiplatelet and Anticoagulation Considerations in Dentistry *on page* 1867

U.S. Brand Names Avitene®; Avitene® Flour; Avitene® Ultrafoam™; EndoAvitene®; Helistat®; Helitene®; Instat™ MCH; SyringeAvitene™

Generic Availability (U.S.) No

Pharmacologic Category Hemostatic Agent

Dental Use Adjunct to hemostasis when control of bleeding by ligature is ineffective or impractical

Use Adjunct to hemostasis when control of bleeding by ligature is ineffective or impractical

Local Anesthetic/Vasoconstrictor Precautions No information available to require special precautions

Effects on Dental Treatment No significant effects or complications reported

Effects on Bleeding General dental procedures and simple restorative procedures are not associated with bleeding; therefore, there is no contraindication with these general dental procedures for most patients with bleeding disorders. However, after dental extractions and other dental surgeries including deep scaling, block anesthesia, and large fillings, in patients with hemophilia, drugs such as collagen may be useful in controlling bleeding. A carefully coordinated strategy between the dental and medical team may be required to ensure adequate procedures for hemostasis.

Adverse Effects Frequency not defined.

Miscellaneous: Adhesion formation, allergic reaction, edema, foreign body reaction, hematoma, inflammation, potentiation of infection

Dental Usual Dosage Hemostasis: Adults: Topical: Apply dry directly to source of bleeding; remove excess material after ~10-15 minutes

Dosage Apply dry directly to source of bleeding; remove excess material after ~10-15 minutes

Mechanism of Action Collagen hemostat is an absorbable topical hemostatic agent prepared from purified bovine corium collagen and shredded into fibrils. Physically, microfibrillar collagen hemostat yields a large surface area. Chemically, it is collagen with hydrochloric acid noncovalently bound to some of the available amino groups in the collagen molecules. When in contact with a bleeding surface, collagen hemostat attracts platelets which adhere to its fibrils and undergo the ▶

release phenomenon. This triggers aggregation of the platelets into thrombi in the interstices of the fibrous mass, initiating the formation of a physiologic platelet plug.

Contraindications Hypersensitivity to any component of the formulation; products of bovine origin; closure of skin incisions, contaminated wounds; application to bone surfaces to which prosthetic materials are attached with methylmethacrylate adhesives

Warnings/Precautions Pain, numbness, or paralysis have been reported if used near a bony or neural space and left inside patient; use minimum amount necessary to achieve hemostasis. Remove as much of agent as possible after hemostasis is achieved. Do not leave in a contaminated or infected space. Fragments of MCH may pass through filters of blood scavenging systems; avoid reintroduction of blood from operative sites treated with MCH. Not intended to treat systemic coagulation disorders. Not for use when origin of bleeding is unknown.

Drug Interactions

Avoid Concomitant Use There are no known interactions where it is recommended to avoid concomitant use.

Increased Effect/Toxicity There are no known significant interactions involving an increase in effect.

Decreased Effect There are no known significant interactions involving a decrease in effect.

Pharmacodynamics/Kinetics

Onset of Action Hemostasis: 2-5 minutes

Dosage Forms

Powder, topical:
- Avitene® Flour: (0.5 g, 1 g, 5 g)
- Helitene®: (0.5 g, 1 g)
- Instat™ MCH: (0.5 g, 1 g)
- SyringeAvitene™: (1 g)

Sheet, topical:
- Avitene®: (1s, 6s)
- EndoAvitene®: (6s)

Sponge:
- Avitene® Ultrafoam™: (6s)

Sponge, topical:
- Helistat®: (10s, 18s)

Conivaptan (koe NYE vap tan)

U.S. Brand Names Vaprisol®

Pharmacologic Category Vasopressin Antagonist

Use Treatment of euvolemic and hypervolemic hyponatremia in hospitalized patients

Local Anesthetic/Vasoconstrictor Precautions No information available to require special precautions

Effects on Dental Treatment Key adverse event(s) related to dental treatment: Dry mouth, oral candidiasis, orthostatic hypotension.

Effects on Bleeding No information available to require special precautions

Adverse Effects

>10%:
- Cardiovascular: Orthostatic hypotension (6% to 14%)
- Central nervous system: Fever (5% to 11%)
- Endocrine & metabolic: Hypokalemia (10% to 22%)
- Local: Injection site reactions including pain, erythema, phlebitis, swelling (63% to 73%)

1% to 10%:
- Cardiovascular: Hypertension (6% to 8%), hypotension (5% to 8%), peripheral edema (3% to 8%), phlebitis (5%), atrial fibrillation (2% to 5%), ECG abnormality (≤5%)
- Central nervous system: Headache (8% to 10%), insomnia (4% to 5%), confusion (≤5%), pain (2%)
- Dermatologic: Pruritus (1% to 5%), erythema (3%)
- Endocrine & metabolic: Hyponatremia (6% to 8%), hypomagnesemia (2% to 5%), hyper-/hypoglycemia (3%)
- Gastrointestinal: Constipation (6% to 8%), vomiting (5% to 7%), diarrhea (≤7%), nausea (3% to 5%), dry mouth (4%), dehydration (2%), oral candidiasis (2%)
- Genitourinary: Urinary tract infection (4% to 5%)
- Hematologic: Anemia (5% to 6%)
- Renal: Polyuria (5% to 6%), hematuria (2%)
- Respiratory: Pneumonia (2% to 5%), pharyngolaryngeal pain (1% to 5%)
- Miscellaneous: Thirst (3% to 6%)

General Dosage Range Dosage adjustment recommended in patients with hepatic or renal impairment

I.V.: *Adults:* Loading dose: 20 mg bolus, followed by 20 mg as continuous infusion over 24 hours; Maintenance: 20-40 mg/day as a continuous infusion over 24 hours (maximum therapy: 4 days)

Mechanism of Action Conivaptan is an arginine vasopressin (AVP) receptor antagonist with affinity for AVP receptor subtypes V_{1A} and V_2. The antidiuretic action of AVP is mediated through activation of the V_2 receptor, which functions to regulate water and electrolyte balance at the level of the collecting ducts in the kidney. Serum levels of AVP are commonly elevated in euvolemic or hypervolemic hyponatremia, which results in the dilution of serum sodium and the relative hyponatremic state. Antagonism of the V_2 receptor by conivaptan promotes the excretion of free water (without loss of serum electrolytes) resulting in net fluid loss, increased urine output, decreased urine osmolality, and subsequent restoration of normal serum sodium concentrations.

Pharmacodynamics/Kinetics

Half-life Elimination ~5-8 hours

Pregnancy Risk Factor C

Copper (KOP er)

Pharmacologic Category Trace Element, Parenteral

Use Supplement to intravenous solutions given for total parenteral nutrition (TPN) to maintain copper serum levels and to prevent depletion of endogenous stores and subsequent deficiency symptoms

Local Anesthetic/Vasoconstrictor Precautions No information available to require special precautions

Effects on Dental Treatment No significant effects or complications reported

Effects on Bleeding No information available to require special precautions

General Dosage Range I.V. (as a parenteral nutrition component):

Infants and Children: 20 mcg/kg/day

Adults: 0.3-1.5 mg/day

Mechanism of Action Copper is an essential nutrient which serves as a cofactor for serum ceruloplasmin, an oxidase necessary for proper formation of the iron carrier protein, transferrin. It also helps maintain normal rates of red and white blood cell formation and helps prevent development of deficiency symptoms: Leukopenia, neutropenia, anemia, depressed ceruloplasmin levels, impaired transferring formation, secondary iron deficiency and osteoporosis.

Pregnancy Risk Factor C

Corticorelin (kor ti koe REL in)

U.S. Brand Names Acthrel®

Pharmacologic Category Diagnostic Agent, ACTH-Dependent Hypercortisolism

Use Diagnostic test used in adrenocorticotropic hormone (ACTH)-dependent Cushing's syndrome to differentiate between pituitary and ectopic production of ACTH

Local Anesthetic/Vasoconstrictor Precautions No information available to require special precautions

Effects on Dental Treatment No significant effects or complications reported

Effects on Bleeding No information available to require special precautions

Adverse Effects

>10%: Cardiovascular: Flushing (face, neck and upper chest, 16%)

1% to 10%:

Gastrointestinal: Metallic taste (transient, 5%)

Respiratory: Dyspnea (urge to inspire, 6%)

General Dosage Range I.V.: *Adults:* 1 mcg/kg

Mechanism of Action Stimulates adrenocorticotropic hormone (ACTH) release from anterior pituitary. ACTH stimulates the adrenal cortex to produce cortisol.

Pharmacodynamics/Kinetics

Onset of Action I.V.: Plasma ACTH level increases 2 minutes after injection; plasma cortisol level increases within 10 minutes after injection

Duration of Action I.V.: Plasma ACTH and cortisol levels remain elevated for up to 2 hours

Time to Peak Plasma: ACTH: 15-60 minutes; cortisol: 30-120 minutes; both levels show a dose-dependent, biphasic response with a second lower peak 2-3 hours after injection

Pregnancy Risk Factor C

Corticotropin (kor ti koe TROE pin)

U.S. Brand Names H.P. Acthar®

Pharmacologic Category Corticosteroid, Systemic

Use Acute exacerbations of multiple sclerosis; infantile spasms; adjunctive therapy for exacerbations/acute episodes of rheumatic disorders (psoriatic arthritis, rheumatoid arthritis, juvenile idiopathic arthritis [JIA], ankylosing spondylitis); exacerbations or maintenance therapy for collagen diseases (systemic lupus erythematosus, systemic dermatomyositis); severe erythema multiforme; Stevens-Johnson syndrome; serum sickness; severe acute/chronic allergic and inflammatory ophthalmic disease (keratitis, iritis, iridocyclitis, diffuse posterior uveitis and choroiditis, optic neuritis, chorioretinitis, anterior segment inflammation); symptomatic sarcoidosis; to induce diuresis for remission of proteinuria in patients with nephrotic syndrome without idiopathic uremia or due to lupus erythematosus

Local Anesthetic/Vasoconstrictor Precautions No information available to require special precautions

Effects on Dental Treatment No significant effects or complications reported

Effects on Bleeding No information available to require special precautions

Adverse Effects

Adverse events associated with cortisol elevation; frequency not defined:

- Cardiovascular: Blood pressure increased
- Central nervous system: Behavioral changes, mood changes
- Endocrine & metabolic: Fluid retention, glucose intolerance
- Gastrointestinal: Appetite increased, weight gain

Adverse events in children <2 years of age observed with doses of 75 units/m^2 twice daily (frequency increased and additional adverse events observed with 150 units/m^2 once-daily dosing):

>10%:

- Cardiovascular: Hypertension (11%)
- Central nervous system: Seizure (12%)
- Miscellaneous: Infection (20%)

1% to 10%:

- Cardiovascular: Cardiac hypertrophy (3%)
- Central nervous system: Irritability (7%), pyrexia (5%)
- Endocrine & metabolic: Cushingoid syndrome (3%)
- Gastrointestinal: Appetite decreased (3%), diarrhea (3%), vomiting (3%), weight gain (1%)
- Respiratory: Nasal congestion (1%)

General Dosage Range

I.M.:

Children <2 years: 75 units/m^2/dose twice daily (infantile spasms) followed by gradual downward titration of dose

Children >2 years: 40-80 units every 24-72 hours

Adults: 80-120 units/day for 2-3 weeks (MS) **or** 40-80 units every 24-72 hours (indications other than MS)

SubQ:

Children >2 years: 40-80 units every 24-72 hours

Adults: 80-120 units/day for 2-3 weeks (MS) **or** 40-80 units every 24-72 hours (indications other than MS)

Mechanism of Action Stimulates the adrenal cortex to secrete adrenal steroids (including hydrocortisone, cortisone), androgenic substances, and a small amount of aldosterone

Pharmacodynamics/Kinetics

Half-life Elimination ACTH: 15 minutes

Prescribing and Access Restrictions H.P. Acthar® Gel is only available through specialty pharmacy distribution and not through traditional distribution sources (eg, wholesalers, retail pharmacies). Hospitals wishing to acquire H.P. Acthar® Gel should contact CuraScipt Specialty Distribution (1-877-599-7748).

After treatment is initiated, discharge or outpatient prescriptions should be submitted to the Acthar Support and Access Program (A.S.A.P.) in order to ensure an uninterrupted supply of the medication. The Acthar Referral/Prescription form is available online at http://www.acthar.com/files/Acthar-Prescription-Referral-Form.-pdf.

Additional information is available for the A.S.A.P. at http://www.acthar.com/health-care-professionals/physician-patient-referrals or by calling 1-888-435-2284.

Cortisone (KOR ti sone)

Related Information

Respiratory Diseases *on page 1876*

Triamcinolone (Systemic) *on page 1669*

Pharmacologic Category Corticosteroid, Systemic

Use Management of adrenocortical insufficiency

Local Anesthetic/Vasoconstrictor Precautions No information available to require special precautions

Effects on Dental Treatment A compromised immune response may occur if patient has been taking systemic cortisone. The need for corticosteroid coverage in these patients should be considered before any dental treatment; consult with physician.

Effects on Bleeding No information available to require special precautions

Adverse Effects

>10%:

- Central nervous system: Insomnia, nervousness
- Gastrointestinal: Increased appetite, indigestion

1% to 10%:

- Dermatologic: Hirsutism
- Endocrine & metabolic: Diabetes mellitus
- Neuromuscular & skeletal: Arthralgia
- Ocular: Cataracts, glaucoma
- Respiratory: Epistaxis

General Dosage Range Oral:

Children: 0.5-10 mg/kg/day **or** 20-300 mg/m^2/day divided every 6-8 hours

Adults: 25-300 mg /day divided every 12-24 hours

Mechanism of Action Decreases inflammation by suppression of migration of polymorphonuclear leukocytes and reversal of increased capillary permeability

Pharmacodynamics/Kinetics

Onset of Action Peak effect: Oral: ~2 hours; I.M.: 20-48 hours

Duration of Action 30-36 hours

Half-life Elimination 0.5-2 hours; End-stage renal disease: 3.5 hours

Cosyntropin (koe sin TROE pin)

U.S. Brand Names Cortrosyn®

Canadian Brand Names Cortrosyn®

Pharmacologic Category Diagnostic Agent

Use Diagnostic test to differentiate primary adrenal from secondary (pituitary) adrenocortical insufficiency

Local Anesthetic/Vasoconstrictor Precautions No information available to require special precautions

Effects on Dental Treatment No significant effects or complications reported

Effects on Bleeding No information available to require special precautions

Adverse Effects Frequency not defined.

- Cardiovascular: Bradycardia, hypertension, peripheral edema, tachycardia
- Dermatologic: Rash
- Local: Whealing with redness at the injection site
- Miscellaneous: Anaphylaxis, hypersensitivity reaction

General Dosage Range I.M., I.V.:

Children ≤2 years: 0.125 mg

Children >2 years and Adults: 0.25 mg

Mechanism of Action Stimulates the adrenal cortex to secrete adrenal steroids (including hydrocortisone, cortisone), androgenic substances, and a small amount of aldosterone

Pharmacodynamics/Kinetics

Time to Peak Serum: I.M., IVP: ~1 hour; plasma cortisol levels rise in healthy individuals within 5 minutes

Pregnancy Risk Factor C

Cromolyn (Systemic, Oral Inhalation) (KROE moe lin)

Related Information

Respiratory Diseases *on page 1876*

U.S. Brand Names Gastrocrom®

Canadian Brand Names Nalcrom®; Nu-Cromolyn; PMS-Sodium Cromoglycate

Pharmacologic Category Mast Cell Stabilizer

Use

Inhalation: May be used as an adjunct in the prophylaxis of allergic disorders, including asthma; prevention of exercise-induced bronchospasm

Oral: Systemic mastocytosis

Unlabeled/Investigational Use Oral: Food allergy, treatment of inflammatory bowel disease

Local Anesthetic/Vasoconstrictor Precautions No information available to require special precautions

Effects on Dental Treatment Key adverse event(s) related to dental treatment:

Inhalation: Unpleasant taste.

Systemic: Glossitis, stomatitis, and unpleasant taste.

Effects on Bleeding No information available to require special precautions

Adverse Effects Frequency not defined.

Cardiovascular: Angioedema, chest pain, edema, flushing, palpitation, premature ventricular contractions, tachycardia

Central nervous system: Anxiety, behavior changes, convulsions, depression, dizziness, fatigue, hallucinations, headache, irritability, insomnia, lethargy, migraine, nervousness, hypoesthesia, postprandial lightheadedness, psychosis

Dermatologic: Erythema, photosensitivity, pruritus, purpura, rash, urticaria

Gastrointestinal: Abdominal pain, constipation, diarrhea, dyspepsia, dysphagia, esophagospasm, flatulence, glossitis, nausea, stomatitis, vomiting

Genitourinary: Dysuria, urinary frequency

Hematologic: Neutropenia, pancytopenia, polycythemia

Hepatic: Liver function test abnormal

Local: Burning

Neuromuscular & skeletal: Arthralgia, leg stiffness, leg weakness, myalgia, paresthesia

Otic: Tinnitus

Respiratory: Dyspnea, pharyngitis

Miscellaneous: Lupus erythematosus

General Dosage Range

Inhalation: Nebulization: *Children ≥2 years and Adults:* Initial: 20 mg 4 times/day; Maintenance: 20 mg 3-4 times/day **or** 20 mg prior to exercise or allergen exposure

Oral:

Children 2-12 years: 100 mg 4 times/day (maximum: 40 mg/kg/day)

Children >12 years and Adults: 200 mg 4 times/day (maximum: 40 mg/kg/day)

Mechanism of Action Prevents the mast cell release of histamine, leukotrienes, and slow-reacting substance of anaphylaxis by inhibiting degranulation after contact with antigens

Pharmacodynamics/Kinetics

Onset of Action Response to treatment: Oral: May occur within 2-6 weeks

Half-life Elimination 80-90 minutes

Time to Peak Serum: Inhalation: ~15 minutes

Pregnancy Risk Factor B

Crotamiton (kroe TAM i tonn)

U.S. Brand Names Eurax®

Pharmacologic Category Scabicidal Agent

Use Treatment of scabies (*Sarcoptes scabiei*) and symptomatic treatment of pruritus

Local Anesthetic/Vasoconstrictor Precautions No information available to require special precautions

Effects on Dental Treatment No significant effects or complications reported

Effects on Bleeding No information available to require special precautions

Adverse Effects Frequency not defined. Topical:

Dermatologic: Contact dermatitis, pruritus, rash

Local: Local irritation

Miscellaneous: Allergic sensitivity reactions, warm sensation

General Dosage Range Topical: *Children and Adults:* Pruritus: Massage into affected areas as needed; Scabies: Apply a thin layer from the neck to the toes, repeat in 24 hours; take a cleansing bath 48 hours after final application, may repeat after 7-10 days

Mechanism of Action Crotamiton has scabicidal activity against *Sarcoptes scabiei*; mechanism of action unknown

Pregnancy Risk Factor C

Cyanocobalamin (sye an oh koe BAL a min)

U.S. Brand Names CaloMist™; Ener-B® [OTC]; Nascobal®; Twelve Resin-K [OTC]

Generic Availability (U.S.) Yes: Excludes nasal spray

Pharmacologic Category Vitamin, Water Soluble

Use Treatment of pernicious anemia; vitamin B_{12} deficiency due to dietary deficiencies or malabsorption diseases, inadequate secretion of intrinsic factor, and inadequate utilization of B_{12} (eg, during neoplastic treatment); increased B_{12} requirements due to pregnancy, thyrotoxicosis, hemorrhage, malignancy, liver or kidney disease

CaloMist™: Maintenance of vitamin B_{12} concentrations after initial correction in patients with B_{12} deficiency without CNS involvement

Local Anesthetic/Vasoconstrictor Precautions No information available to require special precautions

Effects on Dental Treatment No significant effects or complications reported

Effects on Bleeding No information available to require special precautions

Adverse Effects Frequency not defined.

Cardiovascular: CHF, peripheral vascular disorder, peripheral vascular thrombosis

Central nervous system: Anxiety, dizziness, headache, hypoesthesia, incoordination, pain, nervousness

Dermatologic: Itching, urticaria, exanthema (transient)

Gastrointestinal: Diarrhea, dyspepsia, glossitis, nausea, sore throat, vomiting

Hematologic: Polycythemia vera

Neuromuscular & skeletal: Abnormal gait, arthritis, back pain, myalgia, paresthesia, weakness

Respiratory: Dyspnea, pulmonary edema, rhinitis

Miscellaneous: Anaphylaxis (parenteral) and infection

Dosage

Adequate intake:

Children:

0-6 months: 0.4 mcg/day

7-12 months: 0.5 mcg/day

Recommended intake:

Children:

1-3 years: 0.9 mcg/day

4-8 years: 1.2 mcg/day

9-13 years: 1.8 mcg/day

Children >14 years and Adults: 2.4 mcg/day

Pregnancy: 2.6 mcg/day

Lactation: 2.8 mcg/day

Vitamin B_{12} deficiency:

I.M., deep SubQ:

Children (dosage not well established): 0.2 mcg/kg for 2 days, followed by 1000 mcg/day for 2-7 days, followed by 100 mcg/week for one month; for malabsorptive causes of B_{12} deficiency, monthly maintenance doses of 100 mcg have been recommended **or** as an alternative 100 mcg/day for 10-15 days, then once or twice weekly for several months

Adults: Initial: 30 mcg/day for 5-10 days; maintenance: 100-200 mcg/month

Intranasal: Adults:

Nascobal®: 500 mcg in one nostril once weekly

CaloMist™: Maintenance therapy (following correction of vitamin B_{12} deficiency): 25 mcg in each nostril daily (50 mcg/day). If inadequate response, 25 mcg in each nostril twice daily (100 mcg/day).

Oral: Adults: 250 mcg/day

Pernicious anemia: I.M., deep SubQ (administer concomitantly with folic acid if needed, 1 mg/day for 1 month):

Children: 30-50 mcg/day for 2 or more weeks (to a total dose of 1000-5000 mcg), then follow with 100 mcg/month as maintenance dosage

Adults: 100 mcg/day for 6-7 days; if improvement, administer same dose on alternate days for 7 doses, then every 3-4 days for 2-3 weeks; once hematologic values have returned to normal, maintenance dosage: 100 mcg/month. **Note:** Alternative dosing of 1000 mcg/day for 5 days (followed by 500-1000 mcg/month) has been used.

Hematologic remission (without evidence of nervous system involvement): Adults:

Intranasal (Nascobal®): 500 mcg in one nostril once weekly

Oral: 1000-2000 mcg/day

I.M., SubQ: 100-1000 mcg/month

Schilling test: Adults: I.M.: 1000 mcg

Mechanism of Action Coenzyme for various metabolic functions, including fat and carbohydrate metabolism and protein synthesis, used in cell replication and hematopoiesis

Contraindications Hypersensitivity to cyanocobalamin, cobalt, or any component of the formulation

Warnings/Precautions I.M./SubQ routes are used to treat pernicious anemia; oral and intranasal administration are not indicated until hematologic remission and no signs of nervous system involvement. Treatment of severe vitamin B_{12} megaloblastic anemia may result in thrombocytosis and severe hypokalemia, sometimes fatal, due to intracellular potassium shift upon anemia resolution. Vitamin B_{12} deficiency masks signs of polycythemia vera; use caution in other conditions where folic acid or vitamin B_{12} administration alone might mask true diagnosis, despite hematologic response. Vitamin B_{12} deficiency for >3 months results in irreversible degenerative CNS lesions; neurologic manifestations will not be prevented with folic acid unless vitamin B_{12} is also given. Spinal cord degeneration might also occur when folic acid used as a substitute for vitamin B_{12} in anemia prevention. Use caution in Leber's disease patients; B_{12} treatment may result in rapid optic atrophy. Some parenteral products contain aluminum; use caution in patients with impaired renal function and neonates. Some products contain benzyl alcohol which has been associated with "gasping syndrome" in neonates. Avoid intravenous route; anaphylactic shock has occurred. Intradermal test dose of vitamin B_{12} is recommended for any patient suspected of cyanocobalamin sensitivity prior to intranasal or injectable administration. Efficacy of intranasal products in patients with nasal pathology or with other concomitant intranasal therapy has not been determined.

Drug Interactions

Avoid Concomitant Use There are no known interactions where it is recommended to avoid concomitant use.

Increased Effect/Toxicity There are no known significant interactions involving an increase in effect.

Decreased Effect

The levels/effects of Cyanocobalamin may be decreased by: Chloramphenicol; Colchicine

Ethanol/Nutrition/Herb Interactions Ethanol: Heavy consumption >2 weeks may impair vitamin B_{12} absorption.

Dietary Considerations Strict vegetarian diets (eg, without eggs or dairy products) may result in vitamin B_{12} deficiency.

Pregnancy Risk Factor A/C (dose exceeding RDA recommendation); C (intranasal)

Lactation Enters breast milk/compatible

Breast-Feeding Considerations Vegetarian diets which contain no animal products do not supply any vitamin B_{12}. Deficiency recognized in infants of vegetarian mothers who were breast-fed; consider supplementation during breast-feeding.

Dosage Forms

Injection, solution: 1000 mcg/mL (1 mL, 10 mL, 30 mL)

Lozenge, oral: 50 mcg (100s); 100 mcg (100s); 250 mcg (100s, 250s); 500 mcg (100s, 250s)

Lozenge, sublingual: 500 mcg (100s)

Solution, intranasal:

CaloMist™: 25 mcg/spray (10.7 mL)

Nascobal®: 500 mcg/spray (2.3 mL)

Tablet, for buccal application/oral/sublingual:

Twelve Resin-K [OTC]: 1000 mcg

Tablet, oral: 50 mcg, 100 mcg, 250 mcg, 500 mcg, 1000 mcg

Ener-B® [OTC]: 100 mcg, 500 mcg, 1000 mcg

Tablet, sublingual: 1000 mcg, 2500 mcg, 5000 mcg

Tablet, timed release, oral: 1000 mcg

Ener-B® [OTC]: 1500 mcg

Cyclizine (SYE kli zeen)

U.S. Brand Names Bonine® for Kids [OTC]; Marezine® [OTC]

Pharmacologic Category Histamine H_1 Antagonist; Histamine H_1 Antagonist, First Generation; Piperazine Derivative

Use Prevention and treatment of nausea, vomiting, and vertigo associated with motion sickness

Local Anesthetic/Vasoconstrictor Precautions No information available to require special precautions

Effects on Dental Treatment Key adverse event(s) related to dental treatment: Xerostomia (normal salivary flow resumes upon discontinuation).

Effects on Bleeding No information available to require special precautions

Adverse Effects

>10%:

Central nervous system: Drowsiness

Gastrointestinal: Xerostomia

1% to 10%:
- Central nervous system: Headache
- Dermatologic: Dermatitis
- Gastrointestinal: Nausea
- Genitourinary: Urinary retention
- Ocular: Diplopia
- Renal: Polyuria

General Dosage Range Oral:
Children 6-12 years: 25 mg up to 3 times/day (maximum: 75 mg/day)
Adults: 50 mg prior to departure; may repeat in 4-6 hours if needed (maximum: 200 mg/day)

Mechanism of Action Cyclizine is a piperazine derivative with properties of histamines. The precise mechanism of action in inhibiting the symptoms of motion sickness is not known. It may have effects directly on the labyrinthine apparatus and central actions on the labyrinthine apparatus and on the chemoreceptor trigger zone. Cyclizine exerts a central anticholinergic action.

Pregnancy Risk Factor B

Cyclobenzaprine (sye kloe BEN za preen)

Related Information
Temporomandibular Dysfunction (TMD) *on page 1964*

U.S. Brand Names Amrix®; Fexmid®; Flexeril®

Canadian Brand Names Apo-Cyclobenzaprine®; Dom-Cyclobenzaprine; Flexeril®; Flexitec; Gen-Cyclobenzaprine; Mylan-Cyclobenzaprine; Novo-Cycloprine; Nu-Cyclobenzaprine; PHL-Cyclobenzaprine; PMS-Cyclobenzaprine; ratio-Cyclobenzaprine; Riva-Cycloprine

Generic Availability (U.S.) Yes: Excludes capsule

Pharmacologic Category Skeletal Muscle Relaxant

Dental Use Treatment of muscle spasm associated with acute temporomandibular joint pain (TMJ)

Use Treatment of muscle spasm associated with acute, painful musculoskeletal conditions

Unlabeled/Investigational Use Treatment of muscle spasm associated with acute temporomandibular joint pain (TMJ)

Local Anesthetic/Vasoconstrictor Precautions No information available to require special precautions

Effects on Dental Treatment Key adverse event(s) related to dental treatment: Xerostomia and changes in salivation (normal salivary flow resumes upon discontinuation).

Effects on Bleeding No information available to require special precautions

Adverse Effects

>10%:
- Central nervous system: Drowsiness (29% to 39%), dizziness (1% to 11%)
- Gastrointestinal: Xerostomia (21% to 32%)

1% to 10%:
- Central nervous system: Fatigue (1% to 6%), headache (1% to 5%), confusion (1% to 3%), irritability (1% to 3%), mental acuity decreased (1% to 3%), nervousness (1% to 3%), somnolence (1% to 2%)
- Gastrointestinal: Dyspepsia (≤4%), abdominal pain (1% to 3%), constipation (1% to 3%), diarrhea (1% to 3%), nausea (1% to 3%), unpleasant taste (1% to 3%)
- Neuromuscular & skeletal: Weakness (1% to 3%)
- Ocular: Blurred vision (1% to 3%)
- Respiratory: Pharyngitis (1% to 3%), upper respiratory infection (1% to 3%)

Dental Usual Dosage Treatment of muscle spasm associated with acute TMJ pain (**Note:** Do not use longer than 2-3 weeks): Oral:
Adults: Initial: 5 mg 3 times/day; may increase to 7.5-10 mg 3 times/day if needed
Elderly: 5 mg 3 times/day; plasma concentration and incidence of adverse effects are increased in the elderly; dose should be titrated slowly

Dosage Oral: Muscle spasm: **Note:** Do not use longer than 2-3 weeks
Capsule, extended release:
- Adults: Usual: 15 mg once daily; some patients may require up to 30 mg once daily
- Elderly: Use not recommended

Tablet, immediate release:
- Children ≥15 years and Adults: Initial: 5 mg 3 times/day; may increase up to 10 mg 3 times/day if needed
- Elderly: Initial: 5 mg; titrate dose slowly and consider less frequent dosing

Dosage adjustment in hepatic impairment:
Capsule, extended release: Mild-to-severe impairment: Use not recommended.
Tablet, immediate release:
Mild impairment: Initial: 5 mg; use with caution; titrate slowly and consider less frequent dosing
Moderate-to-severe impairment: Use not recommended

Mechanism of Action Centrally-acting skeletal muscle relaxant pharmacologically related to tricyclic antidepressants; reduces tonic somatic motor activity influencing both alpha and gamma motor neurons

Contraindications Hypersensitivity to cyclobenzaprine or any component of the formulation; during or within 14 days of MAO inhibitors; hyperthyroidism; congestive heart failure; arrhythmias; heart block or conduction disturbances; acute recovery phase of MI

Warnings/Precautions May cause CNS depression, which may impair physical or mental abilities; patients must be cautioned about performing tasks which require mental alertness (eg, operating machinery or driving). Cyclobenzaprine shares the toxic potentials of the tricyclic antidepressants (including arrhythmias, tachycardia, and conduction time prolongation) and the usual precautions of tricyclic antidepressant therapy should be observed; use with caution in patients with urinary hesitancy or retention, angle-closure glaucoma or increased intraocular pressure, hepatic impairment, or in the elderly. This class of medication is poorly tolerated by the elderly due to anticholinergic effects, sedation, and weakness; efficacy is questionable at dosages tolerated by elderly patients (Beers Criteria). Extended release capsules not recommended for use in mild-to-severe hepatic impairment or in the elderly. Do not use concomitantly or within 14 days after MAO inhibitors; combination may cause hypertensive crisis, severe convulsions. Effects may be potentiated when used with other CNS depressants or ethanol.

Drug Interactions

Metabolism/Transport Effects Substrate of CYP1A2 (major), 2D6 (minor), 3A4 (minor)

Avoid Concomitant Use

Avoid concomitant use of Cyclobenzaprine with any of the following: MAO Inhibitors

Increased Effect/Toxicity

Cyclobenzaprine may increase the levels/effects of: Alcohol (Ethyl); Anticholinergics; CNS Depressants; MAO Inhibitors; Methotrimeprazine

The levels/effects of Cyclobenzaprine may be increased by: Abiraterone; Conivaptan; CYP1A2 Inhibitors (Moderate); CYP1A2 Inhibitors (Strong); Deferasirox; Methotrimeprazine; Pramlintide

Decreased Effect

Cyclobenzaprine may decrease the levels/effects of: Acetylcholinesterase Inhibitors (Central)

The levels/effects of Cyclobenzaprine may be decreased by: Acetylcholinesterase Inhibitors (Central); Peginterferon Alfa-2b; Tocilizumab

Ethanol/Nutrition/Herb Interactions
Ethanol: May increase CNS depression; monitor for increased effects with coadministration. Caution patients about effects.
Food: Food increases bioavailability (peak plasma concentrations increased by 35% and area under the curve by 20%) of the extended release capsule.
Herb/Nutraceutical: Avoid valerian, kava kava, gotu kola (may increase CNS depression).

Pharmacodynamics/Kinetics

Half-life Elimination Range: 8-37 hours; Immediate release tablet: 18 hours; Extended release capsule: 32-33 hours

Time to Peak Extended release capsule: 7-8 hours

Pregnancy Risk Factor B

Lactation Excretion in breast milk unknown/use caution

Dosage Forms

Capsule, extended release, oral:
Amrix®: 15 mg, 30 mg

Tablet, oral: 5 mg, 10 mg
Fexmid®: 7.5 mg
Flexeril®: 5 mg, 10 mg

Cyclopentolate (sye kloe PEN toe late)

U.S. Brand Names AK-Pentolate™; Cyclogyl®; Cylate™
Canadian Brand Names Cyclogyl®; Diopentolate®
Pharmacologic Category Anticholinergic Agent, Ophthalmic

Use Diagnostic procedures requiring mydriasis and cycloplegia

Local Anesthetic/Vasoconstrictor Precautions No information available to require special precautions

Effects on Dental Treatment No significant effects or complications reported

Effects on Bleeding No information available to require special precautions

Adverse Effects 1% to 10%:

Cardiovascular: Tachycardia

Central nervous system: Ataxia, hallucinations, hyperactivity, incoherent speech, psychosis, restlessness, seizure

Dermatologic: Burning sensation

Ocular: Intraocular pressure increased, loss of visual accommodation

Miscellaneous: Allergic reaction

General Dosage Range Ophthalmic:

Children: Instill 1 drop of 0.5%, 1%, or 2% in eye followed by 1 drop of 0.5% or 1% in 5 minutes, if necessary

Adults: Instill 1 drop of 1% followed by another drop in 5 minutes; 2% solution in heavily pigmented iris

Mechanism of Action Prevents the muscle of the ciliary body and the sphincter muscle of the iris from responding to cholinergic stimulation, causing mydriasis and cycloplegia

Pharmacodynamics/Kinetics

Onset of Action Peak effect: Cycloplegia: 25-75 minutes; Mydriasis: 30-60 minutes

Duration of Action ≤24 hours

Pregnancy Risk Factor C

Cyclopentolate and Phenylephrine (sye kloe PEN toe late & fen il EF rin)

Related Information

Cyclopentolate *on page 448*

U.S. Brand Names Cyclomydril®

Pharmacologic Category Ophthalmic Agent, Antiglaucoma

Use Induce mydriasis greater than that produced with cyclopentolate HCl alone

Local Anesthetic/Vasoconstrictor Precautions No information available to require special precautions

Effects on Dental Treatment No significant effects or complications reported

Effects on Bleeding No information available to require special precautions

General Dosage Range Ophthalmic: *Neonates, Children, and Adults:* Instill 1 drop into eyes every 5-10 minutes, for up to 3 doses

Pregnancy Risk Factor C

Cyclophosphamide (sye kloe FOS fa mide)

Canadian Brand Names Procytox®

Generic Availability (U.S.) Yes

Pharmacologic Category Antineoplastic Agent, Alkylating Agent

Dental Use Treatment of Wegener's granulomatosis, systemic lupus erythematosus

Use

Oncology-related uses: Treatment of Hodgkin's lymphoma, non-Hodgkin's lymphoma (including Burkitt's lymphoma), chronic lymphocytic leukemia (CLL), chronic myelocytic leukemia (CML), acute myelocytic leukemia (AML), acute lymphocytic leukemia (ALL), mycosis fungoides, multiple myeloma, neuroblastoma, retinoblastoma; breast cancer; ovarian adenocarcinoma

Nononcology uses: Treatment of refractory nephrotic syndrome in children

Unlabeled/Investigational Use

Oncology-related uses: Ewing's sarcoma, rhabdomyosarcoma, Wilms tumor, ovarian germ cell tumors, small cell lung cancer, testicular cancer, pheochromocytoma, bone marrow transplantation conditioning regimen

Nononcology uses: Severe rheumatoid disorders, Wegener's granulomatosis, myasthenia gravis, multiple sclerosis, systemic lupus erythematosus, lupus nephritis, autoimmune hemolytic anemia, idiopathic thrombocytic purpura (ITP), and antibody-induced pure red cell aplasia; juvenile idiopathic arthritis (JIA)

Local Anesthetic/Vasoconstrictor Precautions No information available to require special precautions

Effects on Dental Treatment Key adverse event(s) related to dental treatment: Mucositis and stomatitis.

Effects on Bleeding Chemotherapy may result in significant myelosuppression, potentially including significant reduction in platelet counts and altered hemostasis. In patients who are under active treatment with these agents, medical consult is suggested.

Adverse Effects

>10%:

Dermatologic: Alopecia (40% to 60%) but hair will usually regrow although it may be a different color and/or texture. Hair loss usually begins 3-6 weeks after the start of therapy.

Endocrine & metabolic: Fertility: May cause sterility; interferes with oogenesis and spermatogenesis; may be irreversible in some patients; gonadal suppression (amenorrhea)

Gastrointestinal: Nausea and vomiting (usually beginning 6-10 hours after administration; severe with high-dose therapy); anorexia, diarrhea, mucositis, and stomatitis are also seen

Genitourinary: Severe, potentially fatal, acute hemorrhagic cystitis or urinary fibrosis (7% to 40%)

Hematologic: Anemia, leukopenia (dose-related; recovery: 7-10 days after cessation), thrombocytopenia

1% to 10%:

Cardiovascular: Facial flushing

Central nervous system: Headache

Dermatologic: Skin rash

Respiratory: Nasal congestion occurs when I.V. doses are administered too rapidly; patients experience runny eyes, rhinorrhea, sinus congestion, and sneezing during or immediately after the infusion.

Dosage Details concerns dosing in combination regimens should also be consulted.

Children: Oral:

Malignancy: Usual range (in the manufacturer's labeling): 1-5 mg/kg/day (initial and maintenance dosing)

Nephrotic syndrome: 2.5-3 mg/kg/day every day for 60-90 days (when refractory or intolerant to corticosteroid treatment)

Children and Adults: I.V.:

Single doses: 400-1800 mg/m^2 (30-50 mg/kg) per treatment course (1-5 days) which can be repeated at 2-4 week intervals

Continuous daily doses: 60-120 mg/m^2 (1-2.5 mg/kg) per day

Autologous BMT (unlabeled use): IVPB: 50 mg/kg/dose x 4 days **or** 60 mg/kg/dose for 2 days; total dose is usually divided over 2-4 days

JIA/vasculitis (unlabeled use): 10 mg/kg every 2 weeks

SLE (unlabeled use): 500 mg/m^2 every month; may increase up to a maximum dose of 1 g/m^2 every month (Austin, 1986)

Adults: Oral:

Malignancy: Usual range (in the manufacturer's labeling): 1-5 mg/kg/day (initial and maintenance dosing)

Breast cancer (unlabeled dosing; combination chemotherapy):

CEF: 75 mg/m^2/day days 1-14 every 28 days (Levine, 1998)

CMF: 100 mg/m^2/day days 1-14 every 28 days (Bonadonna, 1995; Levine, 1998)

Nephrotic syndrome (refractory; unlabeled use): 2.5-3 mg/kg/day every day for 60-90 days (when refractory or intolerant to corticosteroid treatment)

Dosing adjustment in renal impairment: The FDA-approved labeling states there is insufficient evidence to recommend dosage adjustment and therefore, does not contain renal dosing adjustment guidelines. The following guidelines have been used by some clinicians (Aronoff, 2007): Children and Adults:

Cl_{cr} <10 mL/minute: Administer 75% of normal dose

Hemodialysis effects: Moderately dialyzable (20% to 50%)

Administer 50% of dose posthemodialysis

Continuous ambulatory peritoneal dialysis (CAPD): Administer 75% of normal dose

Continuous renal replacement therapy (CRRT): Administer 100% of normal dose

Dosing adjustment in hepatic impairment: The pharmacokinetics of cyclophosphamide are not significantly altered in the presence of hepatic insufficiency. The FDA-approved labeling does not contain hepatic dosing adjustment guidelines. The following guidelines have been used by some clinicians (Floyd, 2006):

Serum bilirubin 3.1-5 mg/dL or transaminases >3 times ULN: Administer 75% of dose

Serum bilirubin >5 mg/mL: Avoid use

Mechanism of Action Cyclophosphamide is an alkylating agent that prevents cell division by cross-linking DNA strands and decreasing DNA synthesis. It is a cell cycle phase nonspecific agent. Cyclophosphamide also possesses potent immunosuppressive activity. Cyclophosphamide is a prodrug that must be metabolized to active metabolites in the liver.

Contraindications Hypersensitivity to cyclophosphamide or any component of the formulation; severely depressed bone marrow function

Warnings/Precautions Hazardous agent - use appropriate precautions for handling and disposal. Dosage adjustment may be needed for renal or hepatic failure. Hemorrhagic cystitis may occur; increased hydration and frequent voiding is recommended. Immunosuppression may occur; monitor for infections. May cause cardiotoxicity (HF, usually with higher doses); may potentiate the cardiotoxicity of anthracyclines. May impair fertility; interferes with oogenesis and spermatogenesis. Secondary malignancies (usually delayed) have been reported

Drug Interactions

Metabolism/Transport Effects **Substrate** of CYP2A6 (minor), 2B6 (major), 2C9 (minor), 2C19 (minor), 3A4 (minor); **Inhibits** CYP3A4 (weak); **Induces** CYP2B6 (weak), 2C8 (weak), 2C9 (weak)

Avoid Concomitant Use

Avoid concomitant use of Cyclophosphamide with any of the following: BCG; Belimumab; Etanercept; Natalizumab; Pimecrolimus; Roflumilast; Tacrolimus (Topical); Vaccines (Live)

Increased Effect/Toxicity

Cyclophosphamide may increase the levels/effects of: Leflunomide; Natalizumab; Succinylcholine; Vaccines (Live); Vitamin K Antagonists

The levels/effects of Cyclophosphamide may be increased by: Allopurinol; Belimumab; Conivaptan; CYP2B6 Inhibitors (Moderate); CYP2B6 Inhibitors (Strong); Denosumab; Etanercept; Pentostatin; Pimecrolimus; Quazepam; Roflumilast; Tacrolimus (Topical); Trastuzumab

Decreased Effect

Cyclophosphamide may decrease the levels/effects of: BCG; Cardiac Glycosides; Sipuleucel-T; Vaccines (Inactivated); Vaccines (Live); Vitamin K Antagonists

The levels/effects of Cyclophosphamide may be decreased by: CYP2B6 Inducers (Strong); Echinacea; Tocilizumab

Ethanol/Nutrition/Herb Interactions Herb/Nutraceutical: Avoid black cohosh, dong quai in estrogen-dependent tumors.

Dietary Considerations Tablets should be administered during or after meals.

Pharmacodynamics/Kinetics

Half-life Elimination 3-12 hours

Time to Peak Serum: Oral: ~1 hour

Pregnancy Risk Factor D

Lactation Enters breast milk/contraindicated

Dosage Forms

Injection, powder for reconstitution: 500 mg, 1 g, 2 g

Tablet, oral: 25 mg, 50 mg

CycloSERINE (sye kloe SER een)

Related Information

Tuberculosis *on page* 1902

U.S. Brand Names Seromycin®

Pharmacologic Category Antibiotic, Miscellaneous; Antitubercular Agent

Use Adjunctive treatment in pulmonary or extrapulmonary tuberculosis

Unlabeled/Investigational Use Treatment of Gaucher's disease

Local Anesthetic/Vasoconstrictor Precautions No information available to require special precautions

Effects on Dental Treatment No significant effects or complications reported

Effects on Bleeding No information available to require special precautions

Adverse Effects Frequency not defined.

Cardiovascular: Cardiac arrhythmia

Central nervous system: Drowsiness, headache, dizziness, vertigo, seizure, confusion, psychosis, paresis, coma

Dermatologic: Rash

Endocrine & metabolic: Vitamin B_{12} deficiency

Hematologic: Folate deficiency

Hepatic: Liver enzymes increased

Neuromuscular & skeletal: Tremor

General Dosage Range Dosage adjustment recommended in patients with renal impairment

Oral:

Children: 10-20 mg/kg/day in 2 divided doses (maximum: 1000 mg/day)

Adults: Initial: 250 mg every 12 hours for 14 days; Maintenance: 500-1000 mg/day in 2 divided doses

Mechanism of Action Inhibits bacterial cell wall synthesis by competing with amino acid (D-alanine) for incorporation into the bacterial cell wall; bacteriostatic or bactericidal

Pharmacodynamics/Kinetics

Half-life Elimination Normal renal function: 10 hours

Time to Peak Serum: 3-4 hours

Pregnancy Risk Factor C

CycloSPORINE (Systemic) (SYE kloe spor een)

U.S. Brand Names Gengraf®; Neoral®; SandIMMUNE®

Canadian Brand Names Apo-Cyclosporine®; Neoral®; Rhoxal-cyclosporine; Sandimmune® I.V.; Sandoz-Cyclosporine

Generic Availability (U.S.) Yes

Pharmacologic Category Calcineurin Inhibitor; Immunosuppressant Agent

Dental Use Used as an immunosuppressive agent

Use Prophylaxis of organ rejection in kidney, liver, and heart transplants, has been used with azathioprine and/or corticosteroids; severe, active rheumatoid arthritis (RA) not responsive to methotrexate alone; severe, recalcitrant plaque psoriasis in nonimmunocompromised adults unresponsive to or unable to tolerate other systemic therapy

Unlabeled/Investigational Use Allogenic stem cell transplants for prevention and treatment of graft-versus-host disease; also used in some cases of severe autoimmune disease (eg, SLE) that are resistant to corticosteroids and other therapy; focal segmental glomerulosclerosis; severe ulcerative colitis

Local Anesthetic/Vasoconstrictor Precautions No information available to require special precautions

Effects on Dental Treatment Key adverse event(s) related to dental treatment: Mouth sores, swallowing difficulty, gingivitis, gum hyperplasia, xerostomia (normal salivary flow resumes upon discontinuation), abnormal taste, tongue disorder, tooth disorder, and gingival bleeding.

Effects on Bleeding No information available to require special precautions

Adverse Effects Adverse reactions reported with systemic use, including rheumatoid arthritis, psoriasis, and transplantation (kidney, liver, and heart). Percentages noted include the highest frequency regardless of indication/dosage. Frequencies may vary for specific conditions or formulation.

>10%:

- Cardiovascular: Hypertension (8% to 53%), edema (5% to 14%)
- Central nervous system: Headache (2% to 25%)
- Dermatologic: Hirsutism (21% to 45%), hypertrichosis (5% to 19%)
- Endocrine & metabolic: Triglycerides increased (15%), female reproductive disorder (9% to 11%)
- Gastrointestinal: Nausea (23%), diarrhea (3% to 13%), gum hyperplasia (2% to 16%), abdominal discomfort (<1% to 15%), dyspepsia (2% to 12%)
- Neuromuscular & skeletal: Tremor (7% to 55%), paresthesia (1% to 11%), leg cramps/muscle contractions (2% to 12%)
- Renal: Renal dysfunction/nephropathy (10% to 38%), creatinine increased (16% to ≥50%)
- Respiratory: Upper respiratory infection (1% to 14%)
- Miscellaneous: Infection (3% to 25%)

Kidney, liver, and heart transplant only (≤2% unless otherwise noted):

- Cardiovascular: Flushes (<1% to 4%), MI
- Central nervous system: Convulsions (1% to 5%), anxiety, confusion, fever, lethargy
- Dermatologic: Acne (1% to 6%), brittle fingernails, hair breaking, pruritus
- Endocrine & metabolic: Gynecomastia (<1% to 4%), hyperglycemia
- Gastrointestinal: Nausea (2% to 10%), vomiting (2% to 10%), diarrhea (3% to 8%), abdominal discomfort (<1% to 7%), cramps (0% to 4%), anorexia, constipation, gastritis, mouth sores, pancreatitis, swallowing difficulty, upper GI bleed, weight loss
- Hematologic: Leukopenia (<1% to 6%), anemia, thrombocytopenia
- Hepatic: Hepatotoxicity (<1% to 7%)
- Neuromuscular & skeletal: Paresthesia (1% to 3%), joint pain, muscle pain, tingling, weakness
- Ocular: Conjunctivitis, visual disturbance
- Otic: Hearing loss, tinnitus
- Renal: Hematuria
- Respiratory: Sinusitis (<1% to 7%)
- Miscellaneous: Lymphoma (<1% to 6%), allergic reactions, hiccups, night sweats

Rheumatoid arthritis only (1% to <3% unless otherwise noted):

Cardiovascular: Hypertension (8%), edema (5%), chest pain (4%), arrhythmia (2%), abnormal heart sounds, cardiac failure, MI, peripheral ischemia

Central nervous system: Dizziness (8%), pain (6%), insomnia (4%), depression (3%), migraine (2%), anxiety, hypoesthesia, emotional lability, impaired concentration, malaise, nervousness, paranoia, somnolence, vertigo

Dermatologic: Purpura (3%), abnormal pigmentation, angioedema, cellulitis, dermatitis, dry skin, eczema, folliculitis, nail disorder, pruritus, skin disorder, urticaria

Endocrine & metabolic: Menstrual disorder (3%), breast fibroadenosis, breast pain, diabetes mellitus, goiter, hot flashes, hyperkalemia, hyperuricemia, hypoglycemia, libido increased/decreased

Gastrointestinal: Vomiting (9%), flatulence (5%), gingivitis (4%), gum hyperplasia (2%), constipation, dry mouth, dysphagia, enanthema, eructation, esophagitis, gastric ulcer, gastritis, gastroenteritis, gingival bleeding, glossitis, peptic ulcer, salivary gland enlargement, taste perversion, tongue disorder, tooth disorder, weight loss/gain

Genitourinary: Leukorrhea (1%), abnormal urine, micturition urgency, nocturia, polyuria, pyelonephritis, urinary incontinence, uterine hemorrhage

Hematologic: Anemia, leukopenia

Hepatic: Bilirubinemia

Neuromuscular & skeletal: Paresthesia (8%), tremor (8%), leg cramps/muscle contractions (2%), arthralgia, bone fracture, joint dislocation, myalgia, neuropathy, stiffness, synovial cyst, tendon disorder, weakness

Ocular: Abnormal vision, cataract, conjunctivitis, eye pain

Otic: Tinnitus, deafness, vestibular disorder

Renal: BUN increased, hematuria, renal abscess

Respiratory: Cough (5%), dyspnea (5%), sinusitis (4%), abnormal chest sounds, bronchospasm, epistaxis

Miscellaneous: Infection (9%), abscess, allergy, bacterial infection, carcinoma, fungal infection, herpes simplex, herpes zoster, lymphadenopathy, moniliasis, diaphoresis increased, tonsillitis, viral infection

Psoriasis only (1% to <3% unless otherwise noted):

Cardiovascular: Chest pain, flushes

Central nervous system: Psychiatric events (4% to 5%), pain (3% to 4%), dizziness, fever, insomnia, nervousness, vertigo

Dermatologic: Hypertrichosis (5% to 7%), acne, dry skin, folliculitis, keratosis, pruritus, rash, skin malignancies

Endocrine & metabolic: Hot flashes

Gastrointestinal: Nausea (5% to 6%), diarrhea (5% to 6%), gum hyperplasia (4% to 6%), abdominal discomfort (3% to 6%), dyspepsia (2% to 3%), abdominal distention, appetite increased, constipation, gingival bleeding

Genitourinary: Micturition increased

Hematologic: Bleeding disorder, clotting disorder, platelet disorder, red blood cell disorder

Hepatic: Hyperbilirubinemia

Neuromuscular & skeletal: Paresthesia (5% to 7%), arthralgia (1% to 6%)

Ocular: Abnormal vision

Respiratory: Bronchospasm (5%), cough (5%), dyspnea (5%), rhinitis (5%), respiratory infection

Miscellaneous: Flu-like syndrome (8% to 10%)

Dental Usual Dosage Note: Neoral®/Genraf® and Sandimmune® are not bioequivalent and cannot be used interchangeably.

Autoimmune diseases: Adults: 1-3 mg/kg/day

Dosage Neoral®/Genraf® and Sandimmune® are not bioequivalent and cannot be used interchangeably.

Children: Transplant: Refer to adult dosing; children may require, and are able to tolerate, larger doses than adults.

Adults:

Newly-transplanted patients: Adjunct therapy with corticosteroids is recommended. Initial dose should be given 4-12 hours prior to transplant or may be given postoperatively; adjust initial dose to achieve desired plasma concentration

Oral: Dose is dependent upon type of transplant and formulation:

Cyclosporine (modified):

Renal: 9 ± 3 mg/kg/day, divided twice daily

Liver: 8 ± 4 mg/kg/day, divided twice daily

Heart: 7 ± 3 mg/kg/day, divided twice daily

Cyclosporine (non-modified): Initial doses of 10-14 mg/kg/day have been used for renal transplants (the manufacturer's labeling includes dosing from initial clinical trials of 15 mg/kg/day [range: 14-18 mg/kg/day]; however, this higher dosing level is rarely used any longer). Continue initial dose daily for 1-2 weeks; taper by 5% per week to a maintenance dose of 5-10 mg/kg/day; some renal transplant patients may be dosed as low as 3 mg/kg/day

Note: When using the non-modified formulation, cyclosporine levels may increase in liver transplant patients when the T-tube is closed; dose may need decreased

I.V.: Cyclosporine (non-modified): Manufacturer's labeling: Initial dose: 5-6 mg/kg/day or one-third of the oral dose as a single dose, infused over 2-6 hours; use should be limited to patients unable to take capsules or oral solution; patients should be switched to an oral dosage form as soon as possible

Note: Many transplant centers administer cyclosporine as "divided dose" infusions (in 2-3 doses/day) or as a continuous (24-hour) infusion; dosages range from 3-7.5 mg/kg/day. Specific institutional protocols should be consulted.

Conversion to cyclosporine (modified) from cyclosporine (non-modified): Start with daily dose previously used and adjust to obtain preconversion cyclosporine trough concentration. Plasma concentrations should be monitored every 4-7 days and dose adjusted as necessary, until desired trough level is obtained. When transferring patients with previously poor absorption of cyclosporine (non-modified), monitor trough levels at least twice weekly (especially if initial dose exceeds 10 mg/kg/day); high plasma levels are likely to occur.

Rheumatoid arthritis: Oral: Cyclosporine (modified): Initial dose: 2.5 mg/kg/day, divided twice daily; salicylates, NSAIDs, and oral glucocorticoids may be continued (refer to Drug Interactions); dose may be increased by 0.5-0.75 mg/kg/day if insufficient response is seen after 8 weeks of treatment; additional dosage increases may be made again at 12 weeks (maximum dose: 4 mg/kg/day). Discontinue if no benefit is seen by 16 weeks of therapy.

Note: Increase the frequency of blood pressure monitoring after each alteration in dosage of cyclosporine. Cyclosporine dosage should be decreased by 25% to 50% in patients with no history of hypertension who develop sustained hypertension during therapy and, if hypertension persists, treatment with cyclosporine should be discontinued.

Psoriasis: Oral: Cyclosporine (modified): Initial dose: 2.5 mg/kg/day, divided twice daily; dose may be increased by 0.5 mg/kg/day if insufficient response is seen after 4 weeks of treatment. Additional dosage increases may be made every 2 weeks if needed (maximum dose: 4 mg/kg/day). Discontinue if no benefit is seen by 6 weeks of therapy. Once patients are adequately controlled, the dose should be decreased to the lowest effective dose. Doses lower than 2.5 mg/kg/day may be effective. Treatment longer than 1 year is not recommended.

Note: Increase the frequency of blood pressure monitoring after each alteration in dosage of cyclosporine. Cyclosporine dosage should be decreased by 25% to 50% in patients with no history of hypertension who develop sustained hypertension during therapy and, if hypertension persists, treatment with cyclosporine should be discontinued.

Focal segmental glomerulosclerosis (unlabeled use): Oral: Initial: 3.5-5 mg/kg/day divided every 12 hours (in combination with oral prednisone) (Braun, 2008; Cattran, 1999)

Lupus nephritis (unlabeled use): Oral: Initial: 4 mg/kg/day for 1 month (reduce dose if trough concentrations >200 ng/mL); reduce dose by 0.5 mg/kg every 2 weeks to a maintenance dose of 2.5-3 mg/kg/day (Moroni, 2006)

Severe ulcerative colitis (steroid-refractory) (unlabeled use):

I.V.: Cyclosporine (non-modified): 2-4 mg/kg/day, infused continuously over 24 hours. (Lichtiger, 1994; Van Assche, 2003). **Note:** Some studies suggest no therapeutic difference between low-dose (2 mg/kg) and high-dose (4 mg/kg) cyclosporine regimens (Van Assche, 2003).

Oral: Cyclosporine (modified): 2.3-3 mg/kg every 12 hours (Weber 2006; De Saussure 2005)

Note: Patients responsive to I.V. therapy should be switched to oral therapy when possible.

Dosage adjustment in renal impairment: For severe psoriasis:

Serum creatinine levels ≥25% above pretreatment levels: Take another sample within 2 weeks; if the level remains ≥25% above pretreatment levels, decrease dosage of cyclosporine (modified) by 25% to 50%. If two dosage adjustments do not reverse the increase in serum creatinine levels, treatment should be discontinued.

Serum creatinine levels ≥50% above pretreatment levels: Decrease cyclosporine dosage by 25% to 50%. If two dosage adjustments do not reverse the increase in serum creatinine levels, treatment should be discontinued.

Hemodialysis: Supplemental dose is not necessary.

Peritoneal dialysis: Supplemental dose is not necessary.

Dosage adjustment in hepatic impairment: Probably necessary; monitor levels closely

Mechanism of Action Inhibition of production and release of interleukin II and inhibits interleukin II-induced activation of resting T-lymphocytes.

Contraindications Hypersensitivity to cyclosporine or any component of the formulation. I.V. cyclosporine is contraindicated in hypersensitivity to polyoxyethylated castor oil (Cremophor® EL).

Rheumatoid arthritis and psoriasis: Abnormal renal function, uncontrolled hypertension, malignancies. Concomitant treatment with PUVA or UVB therapy, methotrexate, other immunosuppressive agents, coal tar, or radiation therapy are also contraindications for use in patients with psoriasis.

Warnings/Precautions Hazardous agent - use appropriate precautions for handling and disposal. **[U.S. Boxed Warning]: Renal impairment, including structural kidney damage has occurred (when used at high doses); monitor renal function closely.** Elevations in serum creatinine and BUN generally respond to dosage reductions. Use caution with other potentially nephrotoxic drugs (eg, acyclovir, aminoglycoside antibiotics, amphotericin B, ciprofloxacin). **[U.S. Boxed Warning]: Increased risk of lymphomas and other malignancies, particularly those of the skin;** risk is related to intensity/duration of therapy and the use of >1 immunosuppressive agent; all patients should avoid excessive sun/UV light exposure. **[U.S. Boxed Warning]: Increased risk of infection; fatal infections have been reported.** Latent viral infections may be activated (including BK virus which is associated with nephropathy) and result in serious adverse effects. **[U.S. Boxed Warning]: May cause hypertension.** Use caution when changing dosage forms. **[U.S. Boxed Warning]: Cyclosporine (modified) has increased bioavailability as compared to cyclosporine (non-modified) and cannot be used interchangeably without close monitoring.** Monitor cyclosporine concentrations closely following the addition, modification, or deletion of other medications; live, attenuated vaccines may be less effective; use should be avoided. Increased hepatic enzymes and bilirubin have occurred (when used at high doses); improvement usually seen with dosage reduction.

Transplant patients: To be used initially with corticosteroids. May cause significant hyperkalemia and hyperuricemia, seizures (particularly if used with high dose corticosteroids), and encephalopathy. Other neurotoxic events (eg, optic disc edema including papilledema and visual impairment) have been reported rarely. Make dose adjustments based on cyclosporine blood concentrations. **[U.S. Boxed Warning]: Adjustment of dose should only be made under the direct supervision of an experienced physician.** Anaphylaxis has been reported with I.V. use; reserve for patients who cannot take oral form. **[U.S. Boxed Warning]: Risk of skin cancer may be increased in transplant patients.** Due to the increased risk for nephrotoxicity in renal transplantation, avoid using standard doses of cyclosporine in combination with everolimus; reduced cyclosporine doses are recommended; monitor cyclosporine concentrations closely. Cyclosporine and everolimus combination therapy may increase the risk for proteinuria. Cyclosporine combined with either everolimus or sirolimus may increase the risk for thrombotic microangiopathy/thrombotic thrombocytopenic purpura/hemolytic uremic syndrome (TMA/TTP/HUS).

Psoriasis: Patients should avoid excessive sun exposure; safety and efficacy in children <18 years of age have not been established. **[U.S. Boxed Warning]: Risk of skin cancer may be increased with a history of PUVA and possibly methotrexate or other immunosuppressants, UVB, coal tar, or radiation.**

Rheumatoid arthritis: Safety and efficacy for use in juvenile idiopathic arthritis (JIA) have not been established. If receiving other immunosuppressive agents, radiation or UV therapy, concurrent use of cyclosporine is not recommended.

Products may contain corn oil, ethanol, or propylene glycol; injection also contains Cremophor® EL (polyoxyethylated castor oil), which has been associated with rare anaphylactic reactions.

Drug Interactions

Metabolism/Transport Effects **Substrate** of CYP3A4 (major), P-glycoprotein; **Inhibits** CYP2C9 (weak), CYP3A4 (moderate), P-glycoprotein

Avoid Concomitant Use

Avoid concomitant use of CycloSPORINE (Systemic) with any of the following: Aliskiren; BCG; Bosentan; Dronedarone; Natalizumab; Pimecrolimus; Pitavastatin; Roflumilast; Silodosin; Sitaxentan; Tacrolimus; Tacrolimus (Systemic); Tacrolimus (Topical); Tolvaptan; Topotecan; Vaccines (Live)

Increased Effect/Toxicity

CycloSPORINE (Systemic) may increase the levels/effects of: Aliskiren; Ambrisentan; Bosentan; Budesonide (Systemic, Oral Inhalation); Calcium Channel Blockers (Dihydropyridine); Calcium Channel Blockers (Nondihydropyridine); Cardiac Glycosides; Caspofungin; Colchicine; CYP3A4 Substrates; Dabigatran Etexilate; Dexamethasone; Dexamethasone (Systemic); DOXOrubicin; Dronedarone; Eplerenone; Etoposide; Etoposide Phosphate; Everolimus; Ezetimibe; FentaNYL;

Fibric Acid Derivatives; Halofantrine; HMG-CoA Reductase Inhibitors; Imipenem; Leflunomide; Lurasidone; Methotrexate; MethylPREDNISolone; Minoxidil; Minoxidil (Systemic); Minoxidil (Topical); Natalizumab; P-Glycoprotein Substrates; Pitavastatin; PrednisoLONE; PrednisoLONE (Systemic); PredniSONE; Protease Inhibitors; Ranolazine; Repaglinide; Rivaroxaban; Salmeterol; Saxagliptin; Silodosin; Sirolimus; Sitaxentan; Tacrolimus; Tacrolimus (Systemic); Tacrolimus (Topical); Tolvaptan; Topotecan; Vaccines (Live); Vilazodone

The levels/effects of CycloSPORINE (Systemic) may be increased by: ACE Inhibitors; Aminoglycosides; Amiodarone; Amphotericin B; Androgens; Antifungal Agents (Azole Derivatives, Systemic); Bromocriptine; Calcium Channel Blockers (Nondihydropyridine); Carvedilol; Conivaptan; CYP3A4 Inhibitors (Moderate); CYP3A4 Inhibitors (Strong); Dasatinib; Denosumab; Dexamethasone; Dexamethasone (Systemic); Ezetimibe; Fluconazole; GlyBURIDE; Grapefruit Juice; Imatinib; Imipenem; Macrolide Antibiotics; Melphalan; Methotrexate; MethylPREDNISolone; Metoclopramide; MetroNIDAZOLE; MetroNIDAZOLE (Systemic); Nonsteroidal Anti-Inflammatory Agents; Norfloxacin; Omeprazole; P-Glycoprotein Inhibitors; Pimecrolimus; PrednisoLONE; PrednisoLONE (Systemic); PredniSONE; Protease Inhibitors; Pyrazinamide; Quinupristin; Roflumilast; Sirolimus; Sulfonamide Derivatives; Tacrolimus; Tacrolimus (Systemic); Tacrolimus (Topical); Temsirolimus; Trastuzumab

Decreased Effect

CycloSPORINE (Systemic) may decrease the levels/effects of: BCG; GlyBURIDE; Mycophenolate; Sipuleucel-T; Vaccines (Inactivated); Vaccines (Live)

The levels/effects of CycloSPORINE (Systemic) may be decreased by: Armodafinil; Ascorbic Acid; Barbiturates; Bosentan; CarBAMazepine; CYP3A4 Inducers (Strong); Deferasirox; Dexamethasone; Dexamethasone (Systemic); Echinacea; Efavirenz; Fibric Acid Derivatives; Fosphenytoin; Griseofulvin; Imipenem; MethylPREDNISolone; Modafinil; Nafcillin; Orlistat; P-Glycoprotein Inducers; Phenytoin; PrednisoLONE; PrednisoLONE (Systemic); PredniSONE; Probucol; Rifamycin Derivatives; Somatostatin Analogs; St Johns Wort; Sulfinpyrazone [Off Market]; Sulfonamide Derivatives; Terbinafine; Tocilizumab; Vitamin E

Ethanol/Nutrition/Herb Interactions

Food: Grapefruit juice increases cyclosporine serum concentrations.

Herb/Nutraceutical: Avoid St John's wort; as an enzyme inducer, it may increase the metabolism of and decrease plasma levels of cyclosporine; organ rejection and graft loss have been reported. Avoid cat's claw, echinacea (have immunostimulant properties).

Dietary Considerations Administer this medication consistently with relation to time of day and meals. Avoid grapefruit juice with oral cyclosporine use.

Pharmacodynamics/Kinetics

Half-life Elimination Oral: May be prolonged with hepatic impairment and shorter in pediatric patients due to the higher metabolism rate

Cyclosporine (non-modified): Biphasic: Alpha: 1.4 hours; Terminal: 19 hours (range: 10-27 hours)

Cyclosporine (modified): Biphasic: Terminal: 8.4 hours (range: 5-18 hours)

Time to Peak Serum: Oral:

Cyclosporine (non-modified): 2-6 hours; some patients have a second peak at 5-6 hours

Cyclosporine (modified): Renal transplant: 1.5-2 hours

Pregnancy Risk Factor C

Lactation Enters breast milk/not recommended

Dosage Forms

Capsule, oral: 25 mg, 100 mg
Gengraf®: 25 mg, 100 mg

Capsule, softgel, oral: 25 mg, 50 mg, 100 mg
Neoral®: 25 mg, 100 mg
SandIMMUNE®: 25 mg, 100 mg

Injection, solution: 50 mg/mL (5 mL)
SandIMMUNE®: 50 mg/mL (5 mL)

Injection, solution [preservative free]: 50 mg/mL (5 mL)

Solution, oral: 100 mg/mL (50 mL)
Gengraf®: 100 mg/mL (50 mL)
Neoral®: 100 mg/mL (50 mL)
SandIMMUNE®: 100 mg/mL (50 mL)

References

Ferrari SL, Goffin E, Mourad M, et al, "The Interaction Between Clarithromycin and Cyclosporine in Kidney Transplant Recipients," *Transplantation*, 1994, 58(6):725-7.

Harnett JD, Parfrey PS, Paul MD, et al, "Erythromycin-Cyclosporine Interaction in Renal Transplant Recipients," *Transplantation*, 1987, 43(2):316-8.

CycloSPORINE (Ophthalmic) (SYE kloe spor een)

U.S. Brand Names Restasis®

Pharmacologic Category Immunosuppressant Agent

Use Increase tear production when suppressed tear production is presumed to be due to keratoconjunctivitis sicca-associated ocular inflammation (in patients not already using topical anti-inflammatory drugs or punctal plugs)

Local Anesthetic/Vasoconstrictor Precautions No information available to require special precautions

Effects on Dental Treatment No significant effects or complications reported

Effects on Bleeding No information available to require special precautions

Adverse Effects

>10%: Ocular: Burning (17%)

1% to 10%: Ocular: Hyperemia (conjunctival 5%), eye pain, pruritus, stinging

General Dosage Range Ophthalmic (Restasis®): *Children ≥16 years and Adults:* Instill 1 drop in each eye every 12 hours

Pregnancy Risk Factor C

Cyproheptadine (si proe HEP ta deen)

Pharmacologic Category Histamine H_1 Antagonist; Histamine H_1 Antagonist, First Generation; Piperidine Derivative

Use Perennial and seasonal allergic rhinitis and other allergic symptoms including urticaria

Unlabeled/Investigational Use Migraine headache prophylaxis, pruritus, spasticity associated with spinal cord damage

Local Anesthetic/Vasoconstrictor Precautions No information available to require special precautions

Effects on Dental Treatment Key adverse event(s) related to dental treatment: Xerostomia (normal salivary flow resumes upon discontinuation)

Effects on Bleeding No information available to require special precautions

Adverse Effects Frequency not defined.

Cardiovascular: Extrasystoles, hypotension, palpitation, tachycardia

Central nervous system: Confusion, coordination disturbed, dizziness, excitation, euphoria, faintness, hallucinations, headache, hysteria, insomnia, irritability, nervousness, neuritis, restlessness, sedation, seizure, sleepiness, tremor, vertigo

Dermatologic: Angioedema, photosensitivity, rash, urticaria

Gastrointestinal: Abdominal pain, anorexia, appetite increased, constipation, diarrhea, nausea, vomiting, xerostomia

Genitourinary: Difficult urination, urinary frequency, urinary retention

Hematologic: Agranulocytosis, hemolytic anemia, leukopenia, thrombocytopenia

Hepatic: Cholestasis, hepatic failure, hepatitis, jaundice

Neuromuscular & skeletal: Paresthesia

Ocular: Blurred vision, diplopia

Otic: Labyrinthitis (acute), tinnitus

Respiratory: Bronchial secretions (thickening), nasal congestion, pharyngitis

Miscellaneous: Allergic reactions, anaphylactic shock, chills, diaphoresis, fatigue

General Dosage Range

Oral:

Children 2-6 years: 2 mg every 8-12 hours (not to exceed 12 mg/day)

Children 7-14 years: 4 mg every 8-12 hours (not to exceed 16 mg/day)

Adults: 4-20 mg/day divided every 8 hours (not to exceed 0.5 mg/kg/day)

Mechanism of Action A potent antihistamine and serotonin antagonist, competes with histamine for H_1-receptor sites on effector cells in the gastrointestinal tract, blood vessels, and respiratory tract

Pharmacodynamics/Kinetics

Time to Peak Plasma: 6-9 hours (Hintze, 1975)

Pregnancy Risk Factor B

Cysteamine (sis TEE a meen)

U.S. Brand Names Cystagon®

Pharmacologic Category Anticystine Agent; Urinary Tract Product

Use Treatment of nephropathic cystinosis

Local Anesthetic/Vasoconstrictor Precautions No information available to require special precautions

Effects on Dental Treatment No significant effects or complications reported

Effects on Bleeding No information available to require special precautions

Adverse Effects

>5%:

Central nervous system: Fever (22%), lethargy (11%)
Dermatologic: Rash (7%)
Gastrointestinal: Vomiting (35%), anorexia (31%), diarrhea (16%)

<5%:

Cardiovascular: Hypertension
Central nervous system: Abnormal thinking, ataxia, confusion, depression, dizziness, emotional lability, encephalopathy, hallucinations, headache, impaired cognition, jitteriness, nervousness, nightmares, seizure, somnolence
Dermatologic: Urticaria
Endocrine & metabolic: Dehydration
Gastrointestinal: Abdominal pain, bad breath, constipation, duodenal ulceration, duodenitis, dyspepsia, gastroenteritis, gastrointestinal bleeding, gastrointestinal ulcers, nausea
Hematologic: Anemia, leukopenia
Hepatic: Abnormal LFTs
Neuromuscular & skeletal: Hyperkinesia, tremor
Otic: Hearing decreased

General Dosage Range Oral:

Children <12 years: Initial: 1/4 to 1/6 of maintenance dose; Maintenance: 1.3 g/m^2/day **or** 60 mg/kg/day in 4 divided doses (maximum dose: 1.95 g/m^2/day; 90 mg/kg/day)

Children ≥12 years and Adults >110 lbs: Initial: 1/4 to 1/6 of maintenance dose; Maintenance: 2 g/day in 4 divided doses (maximum: 1.95 g/m^2/day; 90 mg/kg/day)

Mechanism of Action Reacts with cystine within the lysosome to convert it to cysteine and to a cysteine-cysteamine mixed disulfide, both of which can then exit the lysosome in patients with cystinosis, an inherited defect of lysosomal transport

Pharmacodynamics/Kinetics

Onset of Action 1-1.8 hours

Duration of Action 6 hours

Time to Peak 1.4 hours

Pregnancy Risk Factor C

Cysteine (SIS te een)

U.S. Brand Names Cysteine-500

Pharmacologic Category Nutritional Supplement

Use Supplement to crystalline amino acid solutions, in particular the specialized pediatric formulas (eg, Aminosyn® PF, TrophAmine®) to meet the intravenous amino acid nutritional requirements of infants receiving parenteral nutrition (PN)

Local Anesthetic/Vasoconstrictor Precautions No information available to require special precautions

Effects on Dental Treatment No significant effects or complications reported

Effects on Bleeding No information available to require special precautions

Adverse Effects Frequency not defined.

Central nervous system: Fever
Endocrine & metabolic: Metabolic acidosis
Gastrointestinal: Nausea
Renal: Azotemia, BUN increased

General Dosage Range I.V.: *Neonates and Infants ≤2 years:* Added as a fixed ratio to crystalline amino acid solution: 40 mg cysteine per g of amino acids; dosage will vary with the daily amino acid dosage; individual doses of cysteine of 0.8-1 mmol/kg/day have also been added directly to the daily PN solution

Mechanism of Action Cysteine is a sulfur-containing amino acid synthesized from methionine via the transulfuration pathway. It is a precursor of the tripeptide glutathione and also of taurine. Newborn infants have a relative deficiency of the enzyme necessary to affect this conversion. Cysteine may be considered an essential amino acid in infants.

Cytarabine (sye TARE a been)

Canadian Brand Names Cytosar®

Pharmacologic Category Antineoplastic Agent, Antimetabolite; Antineoplastic Agent, Antimetabolite (Pyrimidine Analog)

Use Remission induction in acute myeloid leukemia (AML), treatment of acute lymphocytic leukemia (ALL) and chronic myelocytic leukemia (CML; blast phase); prophylaxis and treatment of meningeal leukemia

Unlabeled/Investigational Use Postinduction, postremission consolidation, and salvage treatment of AML; treatment of primary central nervous system (CNS) lymphoma; treatment of relapsed or refractory Hodgkin's lymphoma; treatment of non-Hodgkin's lymphomas (NHL)

Local Anesthetic/Vasoconstrictor Precautions No information available to require special precautions

Effects on Dental Treatment Key adverse event(s) related to dental treatment: Mucositis

Effects on Bleeding Chemotherapy may result in significant myelosuppression, potentially including significant reduction in platelet counts and altered hemostasis. In patients who are under active treatment with these agents, medical consult is suggested.

Adverse Effects Note: Frequency not defined.

Frequent:

Central nervous system: Fever

Dermatologic: Rash

Gastrointestinal: Anal inflammation, anal ulceration, anorexia, diarrhea, mucositis, nausea, vomiting

Hematologic: Myelosuppression, neutropenia (onset: 1-7 days; nadir [biphasic]: 7-9 days and at 15-24 days; recovery [biphasic]: 9-12 and at 24-34 days), thrombocytopenia (onset: 5 days; nadir: 12-15 days; recovery 15-25 days), anemia, bleeding, leukopenia, megaloblastosis, reticulocytes decreased

Hepatic: Hepatic dysfunction, transaminases increased (acute)

Local: Thrombophlebitis

Less frequent:

Cardiovascular: Chest pain, pericarditis

Central nervous system: Dizziness, headache, neural toxicity, neuritis

Dermatologic: Alopecia, pruritus, skin freckling, skin ulceration, urticaria

Gastrointestinal: Abdominal pain, bowel necrosis, esophageal ulceration, esophagitis, pancreatitis, sore throat

Genitourinary: Urinary retention

Hepatic: Jaundice

Local: Injection site cellulitis

Ocular: Conjunctivitis

Renal: Renal dysfunction

Respiratory: Dyspnea

Miscellaneous: Allergic edema, anaphylaxis, sepsis

Infrequent and/or case reports: Acute respiratory distress syndrome, amylase increased, angina, aseptic meningitis, cardiopulmonary arrest (acute), cerebral dysfunction, cytarabine syndrome (bone pain, chest pain, conjunctivitis, fever, maculopapular rash, malaise, myalgia); exanthematous pustulosis, hyperuricemia, injection site inflammation (SubQ injection), injection site pain (SubQ injection), interstitial pneumonitis, lipase increased, pancreatitis, paralysis (intrathecal and I.V. combination therapy), reversible posterior leukoencephalopathy syndrome (RPLS), rhabdomyolysis, toxic megacolon, veno-occlusive liver disease

Adverse events associated with high-dose cytarabine (CNS, gastrointestinal, ocular, and pulmonary toxicities are more common with high-dose regimens):

Cardiovascular: Cardiomegaly, cardiomyopathy (in combination with cyclophosphamide)

Central nervous system: Coma, neurotoxicity (dose-related, cerebellar toxicity may occur in patients receiving high-dose cytarabine [>36-48 g/m^2/cycle]; incidence may up to 55% in patients with renal impairment), personality change, somnolence

Dermatologic: Alopecia (complete), desquamation, rash (severe)

Gastrointestinal: Gastrointestinal ulcer, peritonitis, pneumatosis cystoides intestinalis

Hepatic: Hyperbilirubinemia, liver abscess, liver damage, necrotizing colitis

Neuromuscular & skeletal: Peripheral neuropathy (motor and sensory)

Ocular: Corneal toxicity, hemorrhagic conjunctivitis

Respiratory: Pulmonary edema, syndrome of sudden respiratory distress

Miscellaneous: Sepsis

Adverse events associated with intrathecal cytarabine administration:

Central nervous system: Accessory nerve paralysis, fever, necrotizing leukoencephalopathy (with concurrent cranial irradiation, I.T. methotrexate, and I.T. hydrocortisone), neurotoxicity, paraplegia

Gastrointestinal: Dysphagia, nausea, vomiting

Ocular: Blindness (with concurrent systemic chemotherapy and cranial irradiation), diplopia

Respiratory: Cough, hoarseness

Miscellaneous: Aphonia

General Dosage Range Dosage adjustment recommended in patients with hepatic or renal impairment

I.T.:

Children <1 year: 15-20 mg/dose
Children 1-2 years: 16-30 mg/dose
Children 2-3 years: 20-50 mg/dose
Children ≥3 years: 20-70 mg/dose
Adults: 40-100 mg/dose

I.V.: *Children and Adults:* Induction: 100-200 mg/m^2/day for 7 days

Mechanism of Action Inhibits DNA synthesis. Cytosine gains entry into cells by a carrier process, and then must be converted to its active compound, aracytidine triphosphate. Cytosine is a pyrimidine analog and is incorporated into DNA; however, the primary action is inhibition of DNA polymerase resulting in decreased DNA synthesis and repair. The degree of cytotoxicity correlates linearly with incorporation into DNA; therefore, incorporation into the DNA is responsible for drug activity and toxicity. Cytarabine is specific for the S phase of the cell cycle (blocks progression from the G_1 to the S phase).

Pharmacodynamics/Kinetics

Half-life Elimination I.V.: Initial: 7-20 minutes; Terminal: 1-3 hours; I.T.: 2-6 hours

Time to Peak I.M., SubQ: 20-60 minutes

Pregnancy Risk Factor D

Cytarabine (Liposomal) (sye TARE a been lip po SOE mal)

U.S. Brand Names DepoCyt®

Canadian Brand Names DepoCyt®

Pharmacologic Category Antineoplastic Agent, Antimetabolite (Pyrimidine Antagonist)

Use Treatment of lymphomatous meningitis

Local Anesthetic/Vasoconstrictor Precautions No information available to require special precautions

Effects on Dental Treatment No significant effects or complications reported

Effects on Bleeding Chemotherapy may result in significant myelosuppression, potentially including significant reduction in platelet counts and altered hemostasis. In patients who are under active treatment with these agents, medical consult is suggested.

Adverse Effects

>10%:

Cardiovascular: Peripheral edema (11%)
Central nervous system: Chemical arachnoiditis (without dexamethasone premedication: 100%; with dexamethasone premedication: 33% to 42%; grade 4: 19% to 30%; onset: ≤5 days); headache (56%), confusion (33%), fever (32%), fatigue (25%), seizure (20% to 22%), dizziness (18%), lethargy (16%), insomnia (14%), memory impairment (14%), pain (14%)
Endocrine & metabolic: Dehydration (13%)
Gastrointestinal: Nausea (46%), vomiting (44%), constipation (25%), diarrhea (12%), appetite decreased (11%)
Genitourinary: Urinary tract infection (14%)
Hematologic: Anemia (12%), thrombocytopenia (3% to 11%)
Neuromuscular & skeletal: Weakness (40%), back pain (24%), abnormal gait (23%), limb pain (15%), neck pain (14%), arthralgia (11%), neck stiffness (11%)
Ocular: Blurred vision (11%)

1% to 10%:

Cardiovascular: Tachycardia (9%), hypotension (8%), hypertension (6%), syncope (3%), edema (2%)
Central nervous system: Agitation (10%), hypoesthesia (10%), depression (8%), anxiety (7%), sensory neuropathy (3%)
Dermatologic: Pruritus (2%)
Endocrine & metabolic: Hypokalemia (7%), hyponatremia (7%), hyperglycemia (6%)
Gastrointestinal: Abdominal pain (9%), dysphagia (8%), anorexia (5%), hemorrhoids (3%), mucosal inflammation (3%)
Genitourinary: Incontinence (7%), urinary retention (5%)
Hematologic: Neutropenia (10%), contusion (2%)
Neuromuscular & skeletal: Muscle weakness (10%), tremor (9%), peripheral neuropathy (4%), abnormal reflexes (3%)
Otic: Hypoacusis (6%)
Respiratory: Dyspnea (10%), cough (7%), pneumonia (6%)
Miscellaneous: Diaphoresis (2%)

General Dosage Range Dosage adjustment recommended in patients who develop toxicities

I.T.: *Adults:* Induction: 50 mg every 14 days for a total of 2 doses (weeks 1 and 3); Consolidation: 50 mg every 14 days for 3 doses (weeks 5, 7, and 9), followed by 50 mg at week 13; Maintenance: 50 mg every 28 days for 4 doses (weeks 17, 21, 25, and 29)

Mechanism of Action Cytarabine liposomal is a sustained-release formulation of the active ingredient cytarabine, an antimetabolite which acts through inhibition of DNA synthesis and is cell cycle-specific for the S phase of cell division. Cytarabine is converted intracellularly to its active metabolite cytarabine-5'-triphosphate (ara-CTP). Ara-CTP also appears to be incorporated into DNA and RNA; however, the primary action is inhibition of DNA polymerase, resulting in decreased DNA synthesis and repair. The liposomal formulation allows for gradual release, resulting in prolonged exposure.

Pharmacodynamics/Kinetics

Half-life Elimination CSF: 6-82 hours

Time to Peak CSF: Intrathecal: <1 hour

Pregnancy Risk Factor D

Dabigatran Etexilate (da BIG a tran ett EX ill ate)

Related Information

Cardiovascular Diseases *on page 1848*

U.S. Brand Names Pradaxa®

Canadian Brand Names Pradax™

Pharmacologic Category Anticoagulant, Thrombin Inhibitor

Use Prevention of stroke and systemic embolism in patients with nonvalvular atrial fibrillation

2011 ACCF/AHA/HRS atrial fibrillation guidelines: Not recommended for patients with coexisting prosthetic heart valve or hemodynamically significant valve disease, severe renal failure (Cl_{cr} <15 mL/minute), or advanced liver disease (impaired baseline clotting function)

Canadian labeling: Additional uses (not in U.S. labeling): Postoperative thromboprophylaxis in patients who have undergone total hip or knee replacement procedures

Local Anesthetic/Vasoconstrictor Precautions No information available to require special precautions

Effects on Dental Treatment Dabigatran etexilate is converted *in vivo* to the active dabigatran, a specific, reversible, direct thrombin inhibitor. It causes bleeding by preventing thrombin-mediated effects, and by inhibiting thrombin-induced platelet aggregation.

Effects on Bleeding Dabigatran etexilate is converted *in vivo* to the active dabigatran, a specific, reversible, direct thrombin inhibitor. It causes bleeding by preventing thrombin-mediated effects and by inhibiting thrombin-induced platelet aggregation. There is no scientific evidence to warrant discontinuation of dabigatran etexilate prior to dental surgery. Product labeling states that discontinuation for invasive procedures places the patient at increased risk of stroke.

Adverse Effects Adverse reactions listed below are reflective of both the U.S. and Canadian product information. **Important:** No specific antidote exists for dabigatran reversal. Therapy for severe hemorrhage may include transfusions of fresh frozen plasma, packed red blood cells, or surgical intervention when appropriate (Wann, 2011).

>10%:

Gastrointestinal: Dyspepsia (11%; includes abdominal discomfort/pain, epigastric discomfort)

Hematologic: Bleeding (8% to 33%; major: ≤6%)

1% to 10%:

Gastrointestinal: GI hemorrhage (≤6%), gastritis-like symptoms (eg, GERD, esophagitis, erosive gastritis, GI ulcer)

Hematologic: Anemia (1% to 4%), hematoma (1% to 2%), hemoglobin decreased (1% to 2%), hemorrhage (postprocedural or wound: 1% to 2%)

Hepatic: ALT increased (≥3 x ULN: 2% to 3%)

Renal: Hematuria (1%)

Miscellaneous: Wound secretion (5%), postprocedural discharge (1%)

General Dosage Range Dosage adjustment recommended in patients with renal impairment

Oral: *Adults:* 150 mg twice daily

Mechanism of Action Prodrug lacking anticoagulant activity that is converted *in vivo* to the active dabigatran, a specific, reversible, direct thrombin inhibitor that inhibits both free and fibrin-bound thrombin. Inhibits coagulation by preventing thrombin-mediated effects, including cleavage of fibrinogen to fibrin monomers, activation of factors V, VIII, XI, and XIII, and inhibition of thrombin-induced platelet aggregation.

Pharmacodynamics/Kinetics

Half-life Elimination 12-17 hours; Elderly: 14-17 hours; Mild-to-moderate renal impairment: 15-18 hours; Severe renal impairment: 28 hours (Stangier, 2010)

Time to Peak Plasma: Dabigatran: 1 hour; delayed 2 hours by food (no effect on bioavailability)

Pregnancy Risk Factor C

Dacarbazine (da KAR ba zeen)

Canadian Brand Names Dacarbazine for Injection

Pharmacologic Category Antineoplastic Agent, Alkylating Agent (Triazene)

Use Treatment of malignant melanoma, Hodgkin's disease

Unlabeled/Investigational Use Treatment of soft-tissue sarcomas, islet cell tumors, pheochromocytoma, medullary carcinoma of the thyroid

Local Anesthetic/Vasoconstrictor Precautions No information available to require special precautions

Effects on Dental Treatment Key adverse event(s) related to dental treatment: Metallic taste.

Effects on Bleeding Chemotherapy may result in significant myelosuppression, potentially including significant reduction in platelet counts and altered hemostasis. In patients who are under active treatment with these agents, medical consult is suggested.

Adverse Effects Frequency not always defined.

Dermatologic: Alopecia

Gastrointestinal: Nausea and vomiting (>90%), anorexia

Hematologic: Myelosuppression (onset: 5-7 days; nadir: 7-10 days; recovery: 21-28 days), leukopenia, thrombocytopenia

Local: Pain on infusion

General Dosage Range Dosage adjustment recommended in patients with renal impairment

I.V.:

Children: 375 mg/m^2 on days 1 and 15, repeat every 28 days

Adults: 375 mg/m^2 days 1 and 15 every 4 weeks **or** 250 mg/m^2 days 1-5 every 3 weeks

Mechanism of Action Dacarbazine is an alkylating agent. It is converted to the active alkylating metabolite MTIC [(methyl-triazene-1-yl)-imidazole-4-carboxamide]. The cytotoxic effects of MTIC are manifested through alkylation of DNA at the O^6, N^7 guanine positions which appears to attack cross-links strands of DNA resulting in the inhibition of DNA, RNA, and protein synthesis.

Pharmacodynamics/Kinetics

Half-life Elimination Biphasic: Initial: 20-40 minutes, Terminal: 5 hours; Patients with renal and hepatic dysfunction: Initial: 55 minutes, Terminal: 7.2 hours

Pregnancy Risk Factor C

Daclizumab (dac KLYE zue mab)

U.S. Brand Names Zenapax® [DSC]

Canadian Brand Names Zenapax®

Pharmacologic Category Immunosuppressant Agent; Monoclonal Antibody

Use Prophylaxis of acute rejection in renal transplantation (in combination with cyclosporine and corticosteroids)

Unlabeled/Investigational Use Treatment of refractory acute graft-versus-host disease; prevention of cardiac transplant rejection

Local Anesthetic/Vasoconstrictor Precautions No information available to require special precautions

Effects on Dental Treatment No significant effects or complications reported

Effects on Bleeding No information available to require special precautions

Adverse Effects Adverse effects reported during clinical trial use of daclizumab may be related to the patient population, transplant procedure, and concurrent transplant medications; incidences reported with daclizumab were similar to those reported with placebo. Diarrhea, fever, postoperative pain, pruritus, respiratory tract infection, urinary tract infection, hypertension (aggravated), and vomiting occurred more often in children than adults.

≥5%:

Cardiovascular: Chest pain, edema (including peripheral), hyper-/hypotension, tachycardia, thrombosis

Central nervous system: Dizziness, fatigue, fever, headache, insomnia, pain, post-traumatic pain

Dermatologic: Acne, cellulitis, wound healing impaired

Endocrine & metabolic: Hyperglycemia (32%)

Gastrointestinal: Abdominal distention, abdominal pain, constipation, diarrhea, dyspepsia, epigastric pain, nausea, pyrosis, vomiting

Genitourinary: Dysuria

Hematologic: Bleeding

Neuromuscular & skeletal: Back pain, musculoskeletal pain, tremor

Renal: Oliguria, renal tubular necrosis

Respiratory: Cough, dyspnea, pulmonary edema

Miscellaneous: Anti-daclizumab antibody formation (children 34%; adults 14%), malignancy (2% to 6%), lymphocele, wound infection

≥2% to <5%:

Central nervous system: Anxiety, depression, shivering

Dermatologic: Hirsutism, pruritus, rash

Endocrine & metabolic: Dehydration, diabetes mellitus, fluid overload

Gastrointestinal: Flatulence, gastritis, hemorrhoids

Genitourinary: Urinary retention, urinary tract bleeding

Local: Injection site reaction

Neuromuscular & skeletal: Arthralgia, leg cramps, myalgia, neuropathy, weakness

Ocular: Vision blurred

Renal: Hydronephrosis, renal damage, renal insufficiency

Respiratory: Abnormal breath sounds, atelectasis, congestion, hypoxia, pharyngitis, pleural effusion, rales, rhinitis

Miscellaneous: Diaphoresis, night sweats

General Dosage Range I.V.: *Children and Adults:* 1 mg/kg within 24 hours before transplantation (day 0), then every 14 days for 4 additional doses

Mechanism of Action Daclizumab is a chimeric (90% human, 10% murine) monoclonal IgG antibody produced by recombinant DNA technology. Daclizumab inhibits immune reactions by binding and blocking the alpha-chain of the Tac subunit of the interleukin-2 receptor (CD25) complex located on the surface of activated lymphocytes.

Pharmacodynamics/Kinetics

Half-life Elimination Estimated: Adults: Terminal: ~20 days (range: 11-38 days); Children: ~13 days

Pregnancy Risk Factor C

Product Availability Zenapax®: Due to diminishing market demand, the manufacturer of daclizumab has discontinued production; it is anticipated that available supplies will be depleted in January 2010; all remaining lots will expire in 2011.

DACTINomycin (dak ti noe MYE sin)

U.S. Brand Names Cosmegen®

Canadian Brand Names Cosmegen®

Pharmacologic Category Antineoplastic Agent, Antibiotic

Use Treatment of Wilms' tumor, childhood rhabdomyosarcoma, Ewing's sarcoma, metastatic testicular tumors (nonseminomatous), gestational trophoblastic neoplasm; regional perfusion (palliative or adjunctive) of locally recurrent or locoregional solid tumors (sarcomas, carcinomas and adenocarcinomas)

Unlabeled/Investigational Use Treatment of ovarian cancer (germ cell or stromal tumors), osteosarcoma, soft tissue sarcoma (other than rhabdomyosarcoma)

Local Anesthetic/Vasoconstrictor Precautions No information available to require special precautions

Effects on Dental Treatment Key adverse event(s) related to dental treatment: Stomatitis and mucositis

Effects on Bleeding Chemotherapy may result in significant myelosuppression, potentially including significant reduction in platelet counts and altered hemostasis. In patients who are under active treatment with these agents, medical consult is suggested.

Adverse Effects Frequency not defined.

Central nervous system: Fatigue, fever, lethargy, malaise

Dermatologic: Acne, alopecia (reversible), cheilitis; increased pigmentation, sloughing, or erythema of previously irradiated skin; skin eruptions

Endocrine & metabolic: Growth retardation, hyperuricemia, hypocalcemia

Gastrointestinal: Abdominal pain, anorexia, diarrhea, dysphagia, esophagitis, GI ulceration, mucositis, nausea, pharyngitis, proctitis, stomatitis, vomiting

Hematologic: Agranulocytosis, anemia, aplastic anemia, febrile neutropenia, leukopenia, myelosuppression (onset: 7 days, nadir: 14-21 days, recovery: 21-28 days), neutropenia, pancytopenia, reticulocytopenia, thrombocytopenia, thrombocytopenia (immune mediated)
Hepatic: Ascites, bilirubin increased, hepatic failure, hepatitis, hepatomegaly, hepatopathy thrombocytopenia syndrome, hepatotoxicity, liver function test abnormality, veno-occlusive liver disease
Local: Erythema, edema, epidermolysis, pain, tissue necrosis, and ulceration (following extravasation)
Neuromuscular & skeletal: Myalgia
Renal: Renal function abnormality
Respiratory: Pneumonitis
Miscellaneous: Anaphylactoid reaction, infection

General Dosage Range

I.V.:

Children >6 months: 15 mcg/kg/day **or** 400-600 mcg/m²/day for 5 days every 3-6 weeks

Adults: 12-15 mcg/kg/day **or** 400-600 mcg/m²/day for 5 days every 3-6 weeks **or** 1000 mcg/m² on day 1 **or** 500 mcg/dose days 1 and 2

Regional perfusion: *Adults:* Lower extremity or pelvis: 50 mcg/kg; Upper extremity: 35 mcg/kg

Mechanism of Action Binds to the guanine portion of DNA intercalating between guanine and cytosine base pairs inhibiting DNA and RNA synthesis and protein synthesis

Pharmacodynamics/Kinetics

Half-life Elimination ~36 hours; Children: Range: 14-43 hours

Pregnancy Risk Factor D

Dalfampridine (dal FAM pri deen)

U.S. Brand Names Ampyra™

Pharmacologic Category Potassium Channel Blocker

Use Treatment to improve walking in multiple sclerosis (MS) patients

Local Anesthetic/Vasoconstrictor Precautions No information available to require special precautions

Effects on Dental Treatment No significant effects or complications reported

Effects on Bleeding No information available to require special precautions

Adverse Effects

>10%: Genitourinary: Urinary tract infection (12%)

1% to 10%:

Central nervous system: Insomnia (9%), dizziness (7%), headache (7%), multiple sclerosis relapse (4%), seizures (up to 4%; dose-dependent)
Gastrointestinal: Nausea (7%), constipation (3%), dyspepsia (2%)
Neuromuscular & skeletal: Weakness (7%), back pain (5%), balance disorder (5%), paresthesia (4%)
Respiratory: Nasopharyngitis (4%), pharyngolaryngeal pain (2%)

General Dosage Range Oral: Extended release: *Adults:* 10 mg every 12 hours

Mechanism of Action Nonspecific potassium channel blocker which improves conduction in focally demyelinated axons by delaying repolarization and prolonging the duration of action potentials. Enhanced neuronal conduction is thought to strengthen skeletal muscle fiber twitch activity, thereby, improving peripheral motor neurologic function.

Pharmacodynamics/Kinetics

Half-life Elimination 5-7 hours; prolonged in severe renal impairment (~3 times longer)

Pregnancy Risk Factor C

Dalteparin (dal TE pa rin)

Related Information

Cardiovascular Diseases *on page 1848*

U.S. Brand Names Fragmin®

Canadian Brand Names Fragmin®

Pharmacologic Category Low Molecular Weight Heparin

Use Prevention of deep vein thrombosis which may lead to pulmonary embolism, in patients requiring abdominal surgery who are at risk for thromboembolism complications (eg, patients >40 years of age, obesity, patients with malignancy, history of deep vein thrombosis or pulmonary embolism, and surgical procedures requiring general anesthesia and lasting >30 minutes); prevention of DVT in patients undergoing hip-replacement surgery; patients immobile during an acute illness; acute treatment of unstable angina or non-Q-wave myocardial infarction; prevention of ischemic complications in patients on concurrent aspirin therapy; in patients with cancer, extended treatment (6 months) of acute symptomatic venous thromboembolism (DVT and/or PE) to reduce the recurrence of venous thromboembolism

Unlabeled/Investigational Use Active treatment of deep vein thrombosis (noncancer patients)

Local Anesthetic/Vasoconstrictor Precautions No information available to require special precautions

Effects on Dental Treatment Key adverse event(s) related to dental treatment: Bleeding is the major adverse effect of dalteparin. Adverse reactions reported were generally less than those seen with heparin. See Effects on Bleeding.

Effects on Bleeding As with all anticoagulants, bleeding is the major adverse effect of dalteparin. Hemorrhage may occur at virtually any site; risk is dependent on multiple variables including the intensity of anticoagulation and patient susceptibility. At the recommended doses, LMWHs do not significantly influence platelet aggregation or affect global clotting time (ie, PT or aPTT). Medical consult is suggested.

Adverse Effects Note: As with all anticoagulants, bleeding is the major adverse effect of dalteparin. Hemorrhage may occur at virtually any site. Risk is dependent on multiple variables.

>10%:
- Hematologic: Bleeding (3% to 14%)

1% to 10%:
- Hematologic: Wound hematoma (up to 3%)
- Hepatic: AST >3 times upper limit of normal (5% to 9%), ALT >3 times upper limit of normal (4% to 10%)
- Local: Pain at injection site (up to 12%), injection site hematoma (up to 7%)

General Dosage Range SubQ: *Adults:* Prophylaxis: 2500-5000 int. units daily; Treatment: 120 int. units/kg every 12 hours (maximum: 10,000 int. units/dose) **or** ~150-200 int. units/kg (maximum: 18,000 int. units/dose) once daily

Mechanism of Action Low molecular weight heparin analog with a molecular weight of 4000-6000 daltons; the commercial product contains 3% to 15% heparin with a molecular weight <3000 daltons, 65% to 78% with a molecular weight of 3000-8000 daltons and 14% to 26% with a molecular weight >8000 daltons; while dalteparin has been shown to inhibit both factor Xa and factor IIa (thrombin), the antithrombotic effect of dalteparin is characterized by a higher ratio of antifactor Xa to antifactor IIa activity (ratio = 4)

Pharmacodynamics/Kinetics

Onset of Action 1-2 hours

Duration of Action >12 hours

Half-life Elimination Route dependent: 2-5 hours

Time to Peak Serum: 4 hours

Pregnancy Risk Factor B

Danaparoid (da NAP a roid)

Canadian Brand Names Orgaran®

Pharmacologic Category Anticoagulant; Heparinoid

Use Prevention of postoperative deep vein thrombosis following elective hip replacement surgery

Unlabeled/Investigational Use Systemic anticoagulation for patients with heparin-induced thrombocytopenia: Factor Xa inhibition is used to monitor degree of anticoagulation if necessary

Local Anesthetic/Vasoconstrictor Precautions No information available to require special precautions

Effects on Dental Treatment Key adverse event(s) related to dental treatment: Bleeding is the major adverse effect of danaparoid. See Effects on Bleeding.

Effects on Bleeding As with all anticoagulants, bleeding is the major adverse effect of danaparoid. Hemorrhage may occur at virtually any site; risk is dependent on multiple variables including the intensity of anticoagulation and patient susceptibility. At the recommended doses, LMWHs do not significantly influence platelet aggregation or affect global clotting time (ie, PT or aPTT). Medical consult is suggested.

Adverse Effects As with all anticoagulants, bleeding is the major adverse effect of danaparoid. Hemorrhage may occur at virtually any site. Risk is dependent on multiple variables.

>10%:
- Central nervous system: Fever (22%)
- Gastrointestinal: Nausea (4% to 14%), constipation (4% to 11%)

1% to 10%:

Cardiovascular: Peripheral edema (3%), edema (3%)

Central nervous system: Insomnia (3%), headache (3%), asthenia (2%), dizziness (2%), pain (9%)

Dermatologic: Rash (2% to 5%), pruritus (4%)

Gastrointestinal: Vomiting (3%)

Genitourinary: Urinary tract infection (3% to 4%), urinary retention (2%)

Hematologic: Anemia (2%)

Local: Injection site pain (8% to 14%), injection site hematoma (5%)

Neuromuscular & skeletal: Joint disorder (3%)

Miscellaneous: Infection (2%)

General Dosage Range Dosage adjustment recommended in patients with renal impairment

SubQ: *Adults:* 750 anti-Xa units every 12 hours

Mechanism of Action Prevents fibrin formation in coagulation pathway via thrombin generation inhibition by anti-Xa and anti-IIa effects.

Pharmacodynamics/Kinetics

Onset of Action Peak effect: SubQ: Maximum antifactor Xa and antithrombin (antifactor IIa) activities occur in 2-5 hours

Half-life Elimination Plasma: Mean: Terminal: ~24 hours

Pregnancy Risk Factor B

Product Availability Not available in U.S.

Danazol (DA na zole)

Canadian Brand Names Cyclomen®

Pharmacologic Category Androgen

Use Treatment of endometriosis, fibrocystic breast disease, and hereditary angioedema

Local Anesthetic/Vasoconstrictor Precautions No information available to require special precautions

Effects on Dental Treatment No significant effects or complications reported

Effects on Bleeding Although thromboembolism, thrombotic, and thrombophlebitic events have been reported (including life-threatening or fatal strokes), there is no information available to require special precautions related to dental procedures.

Adverse Effects Frequency not defined.

Cardiovascular: Benign intracranial hypertension (rare), edema, flushing, hypertension

Central nervous system: Anxiety (rare), chills (rare), convulsions (rare), depression, dizziness, emotional lability, fainting, fever (rare), Guillain-Barré syndrome, headache, nervousness, sleep disorders, tremor

Dermatologic: Acne, hair loss, mild hirsutism, maculopapular rash, papular rash, petechial rash, pruritus, purpuric rash, seborrhea, Stevens-Johnson syndrome (rare), photosensitivity (rare), urticaria, vesicular rash

Endocrine & metabolic: Amenorrhea (which may continue post therapy), breast size reduction, clitoris hypertrophy, glucose intolerance, HDL decreased, LDL increased, libido changes, nipple discharge, menstrual disturbances (spotting, altered timing of cycle), semen abnormalities (changes in volume, viscosity, sperm count/motility), spermatogenesis reduction

Gastrointestinal: Appetite changes (rare), bleeding gums (rare), constipation, gastroenteritis, nausea, pancreatitis (rare), vomiting, weight gain

Genitourinary: Vaginal dryness, vaginal irritation, pelvic pain

Hematologic: Eosinophilia, erythrocytosis (reversible), leukocytosis, leukopenia, platelet count increased, polycythemia, RBC increased, thrombocytopenia

Hepatic: Cholestatic jaundice, hepatic adenoma, jaundice, liver enzymes (elevated), malignant tumors (after prolonged use), peliosis hepatis

Neuromuscular & skeletal: Back pain, carpal tunnel syndrome (rare), extremity pain, joint lockup, joint pain, joint swelling, muscle cramps, neck pain, paresthesia, spasms, weakness

Ocular: Cataracts (rare), visual disturbances

Renal: Hematuria

Respiratory: Nasal congestion (rare)

Miscellaneous: Voice change (hoarseness, sore throat, instability, deepening of pitch), diaphoresis

General Dosage Range Oral:

Adults (females): 100-800 mg/day in 2 divided doses

Adults (females/males): Hereditary angioedema: Initial: 200 mg 2-3 times/day; after favorable response decrease dosage by 50% or less

Mechanism of Action Suppresses pituitary output of follicle-stimulating hormone and luteinizing hormone that causes regression and atrophy of normal and ectopic endometrial tissue; decreases rate of growth of abnormal breast tissue; reduces attacks associated with hereditary angioedema by increasing levels of C4 component of complement

Pharmacodynamics/Kinetics

Onset of Action Therapeutic: ~4 weeks

Half-life Elimination Variable: 4.5 hours

Time to Peak Serum: Within 2 hours

Pregnancy Risk Factor X

Dantrolene (DAN troe leen)

U.S. Brand Names Dantrium®; Revonto™

Canadian Brand Names Dantrium®

Pharmacologic Category Skeletal Muscle Relaxant

Use Treatment of spasticity associated with upper motor neuron disorders (eg, spinal cord injury, stroke, cerebral palsy, or multiple sclerosis); management of malignant hyperthermia; prevention of malignant hyperthermia in susceptible individuals (preoperative/postoperative administration)

Unlabeled/Investigational Use Neuroleptic malignant syndrome (NMS)

Local Anesthetic/Vasoconstrictor Precautions No information available to require special precautions

Effects on Dental Treatment No significant effects or complications reported

Effects on Bleeding No information available to require special precautions

Adverse Effects Frequency not defined.

Cardiovascular: Blood pressure (altered), heart failure, tachycardia

Central nervous system: Chills, confusion, dizziness, drowsiness, fatigue, fever, headache, insomnia, lightheadedness, malaise, mental depression, nervousness, seizure, speech disturbance

Dermatologic: Eczematoid eruption, hair growth (abnormal), pruritus, rash, urticaria

Gastrointestinal: Abdominal cramps, anorexia, constipation, diarrhea, dysphagia, gastric irritation, gastrointestinal hemorrhage, nausea, taste change, vomiting

Genitourinary: Crystalluria, difficult erection, difficult urination, nocturia, polyuria, urinary frequency, urinary incontinence, urinary retention

Hematologic: Anemia (aplastic), leukopenia, thrombocytopenia

Hepatic: Hepatitis

Local: Injection site reaction (pain, erythema, swelling), thrombophlebitis, tissue necrosis

Neuromuscular & skeletal: Back pain, muscle weakness, myalgia

Ocular: Blurred vision, diplopia, tearing (excessive)

Renal: Hematuria

Respiratory: Feeling of suffocation, pleural effusion (associated with pericarditis), pulmonary edema, respiratory depression

Miscellaneous: Anaphylaxis, diaphoresis, lymphocytic lymphoma, sialorrhea

General Dosage Range

I.V.: *Children and Adults:* 1-2.5 mg/kg; may repeat up to cumulative dose of 10 mg/kg **or** 2.5 mg/kg as a single dose

Oral:

Children: 4-8 mg/kg/day in 4 divided doses **or** 0.5-2 mg/kg/dose 1-3 times/day (maximum: 400 mg/day)

Adults: 4-8 mg/kg/day in 4 divided doses **or** 25-100 mg 1-3 times/day (maximum: 400 mg/day)

Mechanism of Action Acts directly on skeletal muscle by interfering with release of calcium ion from the sarcoplasmic reticulum; prevents or reduces the increase in myoplasmic calcium ion concentration that activates the acute catabolic processes associated with malignant hyperthermia

Pharmacodynamics/Kinetics

Half-life Elimination 4-8 hours

Pregnancy Risk Factor C

Dapsone (Systemic) (DAP sone)

Related Information

HIV Infection and AIDS *on page 1883*

Generic Availability (U.S.) Yes

Pharmacologic Category Antibiotic, Miscellaneous

Dental Use Pemphigus vulgaris (oral), aphthous ulcers (severe), bullous systemic lupus erythematosus; all in consultation with patient's physician as significant monitoring required

Use Treatment of leprosy and dermatitis herpetiformis (infections caused by *Mycobacterium leprae*)

Unlabeled/Investigational Use Prophylaxis of toxoplasmosis in severely-immunocompromised patients; alternative agent for *Pneumocystis jiroveci* pneumonia (PCP) prophylaxis (monotherapy) and treatment (in combination with trimethoprim); pemphigus vulgaris (oral), aphthous ulcers (severe), bullous systemic lupus erythematosus; all in consultation with patient's physician as significant monitoring required

Local Anesthetic/Vasoconstrictor Precautions No information available to require special precautions

Effects on Dental Treatment No significant effects or complications reported

Effects on Bleeding No information available to require special precautions

Adverse Effects Frequency not always defined.

>10%: Hematologic: Reticulocyte increase (2% to 12%), hemolysis (>10%; dose related; seen in patients with and without G6PD deficiency), hemoglobin decrease (>10%; 1-2 g/dL; almost all patients), methemoglobinemia (>10%), red cell life span shortened (>10%), Agranulocytosis, anemia, leukopenia, pure red cell aplasia (case report)

Cardiovascular: Tachycardia

Central nervous system: Fever, headache, insomnia, psychosis, vertigo

Dermatologic: Bullous and exfoliative dermatitis, erythema nodosum, exfoliative dermatitis, morbilliform and scarlatiniform reactions, phototoxicity, Stevens-Johnson syndrome, toxic epidural necrolysis, urticaria

Endocrine & metabolic: Hypoalbuminemia (without proteinuria), male infertility

Gastrointestinal: Abdominal pain, nausea, pancreatitis, vomiting

Hepatic: Cholestatic jaundice, hepatitis

Neuromuscular & skeletal: Drug-induced lupus erythematosus, lower motor neuron toxicity (prolonged therapy), peripheral neuropathy (rare, nonleprosy patients)

Ocular: Blurred vision

Otic: Tinnitus

Renal: Albuminuria, nephrotic syndrome, renal papillary necrosis

Respiratory: Interstitial pneumonitis, pulmonary eosinophilia

Miscellaneous: Infectious mononucleosis-like syndrome (rash, fever, lymphadenopathy, hepatic dysfunction)

Dental Usual Dosage Oral: Adults:

Aphthous ulcers, severe (unlabeled use): 50 mg once daily

Bullous systemic lupus erythematosus (unlabeled use): 100 mg once daily

Dosage Oral:

Aphthous ulcers, severe (unlabeled use): Adults: 50 mg once daily

Bullous systemic lupus erythematosus (unlabeled use): Adults: 100 mg once daily

Leprosy:

Children: 1-2 mg/kg/24 hours, up to a maximum of 100 mg/day, in combination with other antileprosy agents; duration of therapy is variable

Adults: 100 mg/day, in combination with other antileprosy agents; duration of therapy is variable

Dermatitis herpetiformis: Adults: Start at 50 mg/day, increase to 300 mg/day, or higher to achieve full control, reduce dosage to minimum level as soon as possible

Pneumocystis jiroveci pneumonia, alternative therapy (unlabeled use):

Prophylaxis (primary or secondary):

Infants and Children: 2 mg/kg/day once daily (maximum dose: 100 mg/day) or 4 mg/kg/dose once weekly (maximum dose: 200 mg) (CDC, 2009)

Adolescents and Adults: 100 mg/day once daily or divided in 2 doses as monotherapy **or** 50 mg daily in combination with weekly pyrimethamine and leucovorin (CDC, 2009)

Treatment:

Infants and Children: 2 mg/kg/day once daily (maximum dose: 100 mg/day) in combination with trimethoprim for 21 days

Adolescents and Adults: 100 mg/day once daily in combination with trimethoprim for 21 days

Dosing adjustment in renal impairment: No specific guidelines are available

Mechanism of Action Competitive antagonist of para-aminobenzoic acid (PABA) and prevents normal bacterial utilization of PABA for the synthesis of folic acid

Contraindications Hypersensitivity to dapsone or any component of the formulation

Warnings/Precautions Use with caution in patients with severe anemia, G6PD, methemoglobin reductase deficiency or hemoglobin M deficiency; hypersensitivity to other sulfonamides; aplastic anemia, agranulocytosis and other severe blood dyscrasias have resulted in death; monitor carefully; serious dermatologic reactions (including toxic epidermal necrolysis) are rare but potential occurrences; sulfone reactions may also occur as potentially fatal hypersensitivity reactions; these, but not leprosy reactional states, require drug discontinuation. Motor loss and muscle weakness have been reported with use. Prolonged use may result in fungal or bacterial superinfection, including *C. difficile*-associated diarrhea and pseudomembranous colitis.

Drug Interactions

Metabolism/Transport Effects Substrate of CYP2C8 (minor), 2C9 (major), 2C19 (minor), 2E1 (minor), 3A4 (major)

Avoid Concomitant Use

Avoid concomitant use of Dapsone (Systemic) with any of the following: BCG

Increased Effect/Toxicity

Dapsone (Systemic) may increase the levels/effects of: Antimalarial Agents; Trimethoprim

The levels/effects of Dapsone (Systemic) may be increased by: Antimalarial Agents; Conivaptan; CYP2C9 Inhibitors (Moderate); CYP2C9 Inhibitors (Strong); CYP3A4 Inhibitors (Moderate); CYP3A4 Inhibitors (Strong); Dasatinib; Probenecid; Trimethoprim

Decreased Effect

Dapsone (Systemic) may decrease the levels/effects of: BCG; Typhoid Vaccine

The levels/effects of Dapsone (Systemic) may be decreased by: CYP2C9 Inducers (Highly Effective); CYP3A4 Inducers (Strong); Deferasirox; Herbs (CYP3A4 Inducers); Peginterferon Alfa-2b; Rifamycin Derivatives; Tocilizumab

Ethanol/Nutrition/Herb Interactions Herb/Nutraceutical: St John's wort may decrease dapsone levels.

Dietary Considerations Do not give with antacids, alkaline foods, or drugs.

Pharmacodynamics/Kinetics

Half-life Elimination 30 hours (range: 10-50 hours)

Pregnancy Risk Factor C

Lactation Enters breast milk/not recommended (AAP rates "compatible"; AAP 2001 update pending)

Breast-Feeding Considerations Dapsone is excreted in breast milk and can be detected in the serum of nursing infants. Hemolytic anemia has been reported in a breast-fed infant. Breast-feeding is not recommended by the manufacturer due to the potential for carcinogenicity observed in animal studies and the potential for hemolysis in the neonate, especially if there is a family history of G6PD deficiency.

Dosage Forms

Tablet, oral: 25 mg, 100 mg

References

Fabbri P, Cardinali C, Giomi B, et al, "Cutaneous Lupus Erythematosus: Diagnosis and Management," *Am J Clin Dermatol*, 2003, 4(7):449-65.

Werth VP, Fivenson D, Pandya AG, et al, "Multicenter Randomized, Double-Blind, Placebo, Controlled Clinical Trial of Dapsone as a Glucocorticoid-Sparing Agent in Maintenance-Phase Pemphigus Vulgaris," *Arch Dermatol*, 2008, 144(1):25-32.

Dapsone (Topical) (DAP sone)

U.S. Brand Names Aczone®

Pharmacologic Category Topical Skin Product, Acne

Use Topical treatment of acne vulgaris

Local Anesthetic/Vasoconstrictor Precautions No information available to require special precautions

Effects on Dental Treatment No significant effects or complications reported

Effects on Bleeding No information available to require special precautions

Adverse Effects Frequency not always defined.

Cardiovascular: Facial edema

Central nervous system: Depression, psychosis, suicide attempt, tonic-clonic movement

Gastrointestinal: Abdominal pain, pancreatitis, vomiting

Respiratory: Sinusitis (2%)

General Dosage Range Topical: *Children ≥12 years and Adults:* Apply pea-sized amount (approximately) in thin layer to affected areas twice daily

Pregnancy Risk Factor C

DAPTOmycin (DAP toe mye sin)

U.S. Brand Names Cubicin®

Canadian Brand Names Cubicin®

Pharmacologic Category Antibiotic, Cyclic Lipopeptide

Use Treatment of complicated skin and skin structure infections caused by susceptible aerobic gram-positive organisms; *Staphylococcus aureus* bacteremia, including right-sided native valve infective endocarditis caused by MSSA or MRSA

Unlabeled/Investigational Use Treatment of severe infections caused by MRSA or VRE

Local Anesthetic/Vasoconstrictor Precautions No information available to require special precautions

Effects on Dental Treatment No significant effects or complications reported

Effects on Bleeding No information available to require special precautions

Adverse Effects

>10%:

Gastrointestinal: Diarrhea (5% to 12%), vomiting (3% to 12%), constipation (6% to 11%)

Hematologic: Anemia (2% to 13%)

1% to 10%:

Cardiovascular: Peripheral edema (7%), chest pain (7%), hypertension (1% to 6%), hypotension (2% to 5%)

Central nervous system: Insomnia (5% to 9%), headache (5% to7%), fever (2% to 7%), dizziness (2% to 6%), anxiety (5%)

Dermatologic: Rash (4% to 7%), pruritus (3% to 6%), erythema (5%)

Endocrine & metabolic: Hypokalemia (9%), hyperkalemia (5%), hyperphosphatemia (3%)

Gastrointestinal: Nausea (6% to 10%), abdominal pain (6%), dyspepsia (1% to 4%), loose stool (4%), GI hemorrhage (2%)

Genitourinary: Urinary tract infection (2% to 7%)

Hematologic: INR increased (2%), eosinophilia (2%)

Hepatic: Transaminases increased (2% to 3%), alkaline phosphatase increased (2%)

Local: Injection site reaction (3% to 6%)

Neuromuscular & skeletal: CPK increased (3% to 9%), limb pain (2% to 9%), back pain (7%), weakness (5%), arthralgia (1% to 3%)

Renal: Renal failure (2% to 3%)

Respiratory: Pharyngolaryngeal pain (8%), pleural effusion (6%), cough (3%), pneumonia (3%), dyspnea (2% to 3%)

Miscellaneous: Osteomyelitis (6%), bacteremia (5%), diaphoresis (5%), sepsis (5%), infection (fungal, 2% to 3%)

General Dosage Range Dosage adjustment recommended in patients with renal impairment

I.V.: *Adults:* 4-6 mg/kg once daily

Mechanism of Action Daptomycin binds to components of the cell membrane of susceptible organisms and causes rapid depolarization, inhibiting intracellular synthesis of DNA, RNA, and protein. Daptomycin is bactericidal in a concentration-dependent manner.

Pharmacodynamics/Kinetics

Half-life Elimination 8-9 hours (up to 28 hours in renal impairment)

Pregnancy Risk Factor B

Darbepoetin Alfa (dar be POE e tin AL fa)

U.S. Brand Names Aranesp®; Aranesp® SingleJect®

Canadian Brand Names Aranesp®

Pharmacologic Category Colony Stimulating Factor; Growth Factor; Recombinant Human Erythropoietin

Use Treatment of anemia (elevate or maintain red blood cell level and decrease the need for transfusions) associated with chronic renal failure (including patients on dialysis and not on dialysis); treatment of anemia due to concurrent chemotherapy in patients with metastatic cancer (nonmyeloid malignancies)

Note: Darbepoetin is **not** indicated for use in cancer patients under the following conditions:

- receiving hormonal therapy, therapeutic biologic products, or radiation therapy unless also receiving concurrent myelosuppressive chemotherapy
- receiving myelosuppressive therapy when the expected outcome is curative

Unlabeled/Investigational Use Treatment of symptomatic anemia in myelodysplastic syndrome (MDS)

Local Anesthetic/Vasoconstrictor Precautions No information available to require special precautions

Effects on Dental Treatment No significant effects or complications reported

Effects on Bleeding Although ESAs have been associated with thromboembolic events, there is no information available to require special precautions for dental procedures.

Adverse Effects

>10%:

Cardiovascular: Edema (21%), hypertension (4% to 20%), hypotension (20%)

Central nervous system: Fatigue (9% to 33%), fever (4% to 19%), headache (12% to 15%), dizziness (7% to 14%)

Gastrointestinal: Diarrhea (14% to 22%), constipation (5% to 18%), vomiting (2% to 14%), nausea (11%)

Neuromuscular & skeletal: Muscle spasm (17%), arthralgia (9% to 13%)

Respiratory: Upper respiratory infection (15%)

Miscellaneous: Infection (24%)

1% to 10%:

Cardiovascular: Peripheral edema (10%), arrhythmia/arrest (8%), angina/chest pain (7% to 8%), fluid overload (6%), thrombosis (6%), CHF (5%), MI (2%)

Central nervous system: Stroke (2% to 5%), seizure (≤1%), TIA (≤1%)

Dermatologic: Rash (7%), pruritus (6%)

Endocrine & metabolic: Dehydration (3% to 5%)

Gastrointestinal: Abdominal pain (10%)

Local: Vascular access hemorrhage (7%), injection site pain (6%), vascular access infection (6%), vascular access thrombosis (6%)

Neuromuscular & skeletal: Limb pain (8%), myalgia (8%), back pain (7%), weakness (5%)

Respiratory: Dyspnea (2% to 10%), cough (9%), bronchitis (5%), pneumonia (3%), pulmonary embolism (1%)

Miscellaneous: Flu-like syndrome (6%)

General Dosage Range

I.V.:

Children 1-18 years: 6.25-200 mcg/week

Adults: 0.45 mcg/kg once weekly **or** 0.75 mcg/kg once every 2 weeks

SubQ:

Children 1-18 years: 6.25-200 mcg/week

Adults: 0.45-4.5 mcg/kg/week **or** 0.75 mcg/kg once every 2 weeks **or** 500 mcg once every 3 weeks

Mechanism of Action Induces erythropoiesis by stimulating the division and differentiation of committed erythroid progenitor cells; induces the release of reticulocytes from the bone marrow into the bloodstream, where they mature to erythrocytes. There is a dose response relationship with this effect. This results in an increase in reticulocyte counts followed by a rise in hematocrit and hemoglobin levels. When administered SubQ or I.V., darbepoetin's half-life is ~3 times that of epoetin alfa concentrations.

Pharmacodynamics/Kinetics

Onset of Action Increased hemoglobin levels not generally observed until 2-6 weeks after initiating treatment

Half-life Elimination Note: Darbepoetin half-life is approximately threefold longer than epoetin alfa following I.V. administration

CRF: Adults:

I.V.: 21 hours

SubQ: Nondialysis patients: 70 hours (range: 35-139 hours); Dialysis patients: 46 hours (range: 12-89 hours)

Cancer: Adults: SubQ: 74 hours (range: 24-144 hours); Children: 49 hours

Time to Peak SubQ:

CRF: Adults: 48 hours (range: 12-72 hours; independent of dialysis); Children: 36 hours (range: 10-58 hours)

Cancer: Adults: 71-90 hours (range: 28-123 hours); Children: 71 hours (range: 21-143 hours)

Pregnancy Risk Factor C

Prescribing and Access Restrictions As a requirement of the REMS program, access to this medication is restricted. Healthcare providers and hospitals must be enrolled in the ESA APPRISE (Assisting Providers and Cancer Patients with Risk Information for the Safe use of ESAs) Oncology Program (866-284-8089; http://www.esa-apprise.com) to prescribe or dispense ESAs (ie, darbepoetin alfa, epoetin alfa) to patients with cancer.

Darifenacin (dar i FEN a sin)

U.S. Brand Names Enablex®

Canadian Brand Names Enablex®

Pharmacologic Category Anticholinergic Agent

Use Management of symptoms of bladder overactivity (urge incontinence, urgency, and frequency)

Local Anesthetic/Vasoconstrictor Precautions No information available to require special precautions

Effects on Dental Treatment Key adverse event(s) related to dental treatment: Xerostomia (normal salivary flow resumes upon discontinuation). Prolonged xerostomia may contribute to discomfort and dental disease (eg, caries, periodontal disease, and oral candidiasis).

Effects on Bleeding No information available to require special precautions

Adverse Effects

>10%: Gastrointestinal: Xerostomia (19% to 35%), constipation (15% to 21%)

1% to 10%:

Cardiovascular: Hypertension (≥1%), peripheral edema (≥1%)

Central nervous system: Headache (7%), dizziness (<2%), pain (≥1%)

Dermatological: Dry skin (≥1%), pruritus (≥1%), rash (≥1%)

Gastrointestinal: Dyspepsia (3% to 8%), abdominal pain (2% to 4%), nausea (2% to 4%), vomiting (≥1%), weight gain (≥1%)

Genitourinary: Urinary tract infection (4% to 5%), vaginitis (≥1%), urinary retention (acute)

Neuromuscular & skeletal: Weakness (<3%), arthralgia (≥1%), back pain (≥1%)

Ocular: Dry eyes (2%), abnormal vision (≥1%)

Respiratory: Bronchitis (≥1%), pharyngitis (≥1%), rhinitis (≥1%), sinusitis (≥1%)

Miscellaneous: Flu-like syndrome (1% to 3%)

General Dosage Range Dosage adjustment recommended in patients with hepatic impairment or on concomitant therapy

Oral: *Adults:* Initial: 7.5 mg once daily; Maintenance: 7.5-15 mg once daily

Mechanism of Action Selective antagonist of the M3 muscarinic (cholinergic) receptor subtype. Blockade of the receptor limits bladder contractions, reducing the symptoms of bladder irritability/overactivity (urge incontinence, urgency and frequency).

Pharmacodynamics/Kinetics

Half-life Elimination ~13-19 hours

Time to Peak Plasma: ~7 hours

Pregnancy Risk Factor C

Darunavir (dar OO na veer)

Related Information

HIV Infection and AIDS *on page 1883*

U.S. Brand Names Prezista®

Canadian Brand Names Prezista®

Pharmacologic Category Antiretroviral Agent, Protease Inhibitor

Use Treatment of HIV-1 infections in combination with ritonavir and other antiretroviral agents

Local Anesthetic/Vasoconstrictor Precautions No information available to require special precautions

Effects on Dental Treatment No significant effects or complications reported

Effects on Bleeding Increased bleeding has been noted with protease inhibitors in patients with hemophilia A or B. No information available to require routine special precautions relative to hemostasis in other patients.

Adverse Effects As a class, protease inhibitors potentially cause dyslipidemias which includes elevated cholesterol and triglycerides and a redistribution of body fat centrally to cause increased abdominal girth, buffalo hump, facial atrophy, and breast enlargement. These agents also cause hyperglycemia. Frequency of adverse events is reported for darunavir/ritonavir. See also Ritonavir monograph.

>10%:

Endocrine & metabolic: Hypercholesterolemia (grade 2: 16% to 25%; grade 3: 1% to 10%), LDL increased (grade 2: 14%; grade 3: 5% to 8%)

Gastrointestinal: Vomiting (children 13%; adults 2% to 5%), diarrhea (8% to 14%)

2% to 10%:

Central nervous system: Headache (children 9%; adults 3% to 6%), fatigue (children 3%; adults ≤2%)

Dermatologic: Rash (5% to 10%)

Endocrine & metabolic: Hyperglycemia (grade 2: 7% to 10%; grade 3: ≤1%; grade 4: <1%), triglycerides increased (grade 2: 3% to 10%; grade 3: 1% to 7%; grade 4: ≤3%), diabetes mellitus (2%)

Gastrointestinal: Abdominal pain (children 10%; adults 5% to 6%), nausea (3% to 7%), amylase increased (grade 2: 5% to 6%; grade 3: 3% to 7%), lipase increased (grade 2: 2% to 3%; grade 3: ≤2%; grade 4: <1%), abdominal distention (2%), anorexia (2%), dyspepsia (2%)

Hepatic: ALT increased (grade 2: 7%, grade 3: 2% to 3%; grade 4: ≤1%), AST increased (grade 2: 6%; grade 3: 2% to 4%; grade 4: <1%), alkaline phosphatase (grade 2: ≤2%; grade 3: <1%)

Neuromuscular & skeletal: Weakness (≤3%)

General Dosage Range Dosage adjustment recommended in patients on concomitant therapy or who develop toxicities.

Oral:

Children ≥6 years and ≥20 kg to <30 kg: Darunavir: 375 mg twice daily; Ritonavir: 50 mg twice daily

Children ≥6 years and ≥30 kg to <40 kg: Darunavir: 450 mg twice daily; Ritonavir: 60 mg twice daily

Children ≥6 years and ≥40 kg: Darunavir: 600 mg twice daily; Ritonavir: 100 mg twice daily

Adults: Darunavir: 600 mg twice daily; Ritonavir: 100 mg twice daily **or** Darunavir: 800 mg once daily; Ritonavir: 100 mg once daily

Mechanism of Action Binds to the site of HIV-1 protease activity and inhibits cleavage of viral Gag-Pol polyprotein precursors into individual functional proteins required for infectious HIV. This results in the formation of immature, noninfectious viral particles.

Pharmacodynamics/Kinetics

Half-life Elimination ~15 hours

Pregnancy Risk Factor C

Dasatinib (da SA ti nib)

Related Information

Clinical Risk Related to Drugs Prolonging QT Interval *on page* 1872

U.S. Brand Names Sprycel®

Canadian Brand Names Sprycel®

Pharmacologic Category Antineoplastic Agent, Tyrosine Kinase Inhibitor

Use Treatment of chronic myelogenous leukemia (CML) in chronic, accelerated or blast (myeloid or lymphoid) phase resistant or intolerant to prior therapy (including imatinib); treatment of newly-diagnosed Philadelphia chromosome-positive (Ph+) CML in chronic phase; treatment of Philadelphia chromosome-positive (Ph+) acute lymphoblastic leukemia (ALL) resistant or intolerant to prior therapy

Unlabeled/Investigational Use Post-stem cell transplant (allogeneic) follow-up treatment of CML; treatment of gastrointestinal stromal tumor (GIST)

Local Anesthetic/Vasoconstrictor Precautions Dasatinib is one of the drugs confirmed to prolong the QT interval and is accepted as having a risk of causing torsade de pointes. The risk of drug-induced torsade de pointes is extremely low when a single QT interval prolonging drug is prescribed. In terms of epinephrine, it is not known what effect vasoconstrictors in the local anesthetic regimen will have in patients with a known history of congenital prolonged QT interval or in patients taking any medication that prolongs the QT interval. Until more information is obtained, it is suggested that the clinician consult with the physician prior to the use of a vasoconstrictor in suspected patients, and that the vasoconstrictor (epinephrine, mepivacaine and levonordefrin [Carbocaine® 2% with Neo-Cobefrin®]) be used with caution.

Effects on Dental Treatment Key adverse event(s) related to dental treatment: Mucositis/stomatitis, taste perversion.

Effects on Bleeding Chemotherapy may result in significant myelosuppression, potentially including significant reduction in platelet counts and altered hemostasis. In patients who are under active treatment with these agents, medical consult is suggested.

Adverse Effects

≥10%:

Cardiovascular: Fluid retention (21% to 35%; grades 3/4: 1% to 8%), superficial edema (3% to 19%; grades 3/4: ≤1%)

Central nervous system: Headache (12% to 33%), fatigue (8% to 24%), fever (5% to 18%)

Dermatologic: Rash (11% to 21%; includes drug eruption, erythema, erythema multiforme, erythematous rash, erythrosis, exfoliative rash, follicular rash, heat rash, macular rash, maculopapular rash, milia, papular rash, pruritic rash, pustular rash, skin exfoliation, skin irritation, urticaria vesiculosa, vesicular rash)

Endocrine & metabolic: Hypophosphatemia (grades 3/4: 5% to 18%), hypokalemia (grades 3/4: ≤15%), hypocalcemia (grades 3/4: <1% to 12%)

Gastrointestinal: Diarrhea (18% to 31%; grades 3/4: ≤5%), nausea (9% to 24%), vomiting (5% to 16%), abdominal pain (3% to 12%)

Hematologic: Thrombocytopenia (grades 3/4: 19% to 85%), neutropenia (grades 3/4: 22% to 79%), anemia (grades 3/4: 11% to 74%), hemorrhage (6% to 26%; grades 3/4: 1% to 9%), neutropenic fever (grades 3/4: 1% to 12%)
Neuromuscular & skeletal: Musculoskeletal pain (≤19%), myalgia (3% to 13%), arthralgia (≤12%)
Respiratory: Pleural effusion (12% to 24%; grades 3/4: ≤11%), dyspnea (3% to 20%; grades 3/4: 2% to 3%)
Miscellaneous: Infection (9% to 12%, includes bacterial, fungal, viral)

1% to <10%:

Cardiovascular: Generalized edema (≤1%), pericardial effusion (≤3%; grades 3/4: ≤1%), CHF/cardiac dysfunction (≤4%; includes cardiac failure, cardiomyopathy, diastolic dysfunction, ejection fraction decreased, left ventricular dysfunction, ventricular failure); arrhythmia, chest pain, flushing, hypertension, palpitation
Central nervous system: CNS bleeding (≤3%; grades 3/4: ≤3%), chills, depression, dizziness, insomnia, pain, somnolence
Dermatologic: Acne, alopecia, dermatitis, dry skin, eczema, hyperhydrosis, pruritus, urticaria
Gastrointestinal: Gastrointestinal bleeding (2% to 9%; grades 3/4: 1% to 7%), abdominal distention, anorexia, colitis (including neutropenic colitis), constipation, dyspepsia, enterocolitis, gastritis, mucositis/stomatitis, oral soft tissue disorder, taste alteration, weight loss/gain
Hematologic: Contusion, pancytopenia
Hepatic: Bilirubin increased (grades 3/4: ≤6%), ALT increased (grades 3/4: ≤5%), AST increased (grades 3/4: ≤4%)
Neuromuscular & skeletal: Muscle inflammation (4%), muscle weakness, neuropathy, peripheral neuropathy, weakness
Ocular: Visual disorder (blurred vision, acuity reduced, visual disturbance), xerophthalmia
Otic: Tinnitus
Renal: Serum creatinine increased (grades 3/4: ≤8%)
Respiratory: Pulmonary edema (≤4%; grades 3/4: ≤3%), cough, lung infiltration, pneumonia (bacterial, viral or fungal), pneumonitis, pulmonary hypertension, upper respiratory tract infection/inflammation
Miscellaneous: Herpes virus infection

General Dosage Range Dosage adjustment recommended in patients on concomitant therapy or who develop toxicities

Oral: *Adults:* 100-180 mg once daily

Mechanism of Action BCR-ABL tyrosine kinase inhibitor; targets most imatinib-resistant BCR-ABL mutations (except the T315I and F317V mutants) by distinctly binding to active and inactive ABL-kinase. Kinase inhibition halts proliferation of leukemia cells. Also inhibits SRC family (including SRC, LKC, YES, FYN); c-KIT, EPHA2 and platelet derived growth factor receptor (PDGFRβ)

Pharmacodynamics/Kinetics

Half-life Elimination Terminal: 3-5 hours

Time to Peak 0.5-6 hours

Pregnancy Risk Factor D

Dental Comment Dasatinib is known to prolong the QT interval. The QT interval is measured as the time and distance between the Q point of the QRS complex and the end of the T wave in the ECG tracing. After adjustment for heart rate, the QT interval is defined as prolonged if it is more than 450 msec in men and 460 msec in women. A long QT syndrome was first described in the 1950s and 60s as a congenital syndrome involving QT interval prolongation and syncope and sudden death. Some of the congenital long QT syndromes were characterized by a peculiar electrocardiographic appearance of the QRS complex involving a premature atria beat followed by a pause, then a subsequent sinus beat showing marked QT prolongation and deformity. This type of cardiac arrhythmia was originally termed "torsade de pointes" (translated from the French as "twisting of the points"). Dasatinib is considered as having a risk of causing torsade de pointes. Since it is not known what effect vasoconstrictors in the local anesthetic regimen will have in patients with a known history of congenital prolonged QT interval or in patients taking any medication that prolongs the QT interval, a medical consult is suggested.

DAUNOrubicin Citrate (Liposomal)

(daw noe ROO bi sin SI trate lip po SOE mal)

U.S. Brand Names DaunoXome®

Pharmacologic Category Antineoplastic Agent, Anthracycline

Use First-line treatment of advanced HIV-associated Kaposi's sarcoma (KS)

Local Anesthetic/Vasoconstrictor Precautions No information available to require special precautions

Effects on Dental Treatment Key adverse event(s) related to dental treatment: Stomatitis.

Effects on Bleeding Chemotherapy may result in significant myelosuppression, potentially including significant reduction in platelet counts and altered hemostasis. In patients who are under active treatment with these agents, medical consult is suggested.

Adverse Effects

>10%:

Cardiovascular: Edema (11%)

Central nervous system: Fatigue (49%), fever (47%), headache (25%), neutropenic fever (17%)

Gastrointestinal: Nausea (54%), diarrhea (38%), abdominal pain (23%), anorexia (23%), vomiting (23%)

Hematologic: Myelosuppression (onset: 7 days; nadir: 14 days; recovery 21 days), neutropenia (up to 55%; grade 4: 15%), anemia (up to 55%; grade 4: 2%), thrombocytopenia (up to 12%; grade 4: 1%)

Neuromuscular & skeletal: Rigors (19%), back pain (16%), neuropathy (13%)

Respiratory: Cough (28%), dyspnea (26%), rhinitis (12%)

Miscellaneous: Opportunistic infections (40%), allergic reactions (24%), diaphoresis (14%), infusion-related reactions (14%; includes back pain, flushing, chest tightness)

1% to 10%:

Cardiovascular: Chest pain (10%), hypertension (≤5%), palpitation (≤5%), syncope (≤5%), tachycardia (≤5%), LVEF decreased (3%), CHF/cardiomyopathy

Central nervous system: Depression (10%), malaise (10%), dizziness (8%), insomnia (6%), abnormal thinking (≤5%), amnesia (≤5%), anxiety (≤5%), ataxia (≤5%), confusion (≤5%), emotional lability (≤5%), hallucination (≤5%), meningitis (≤5%), seizure (≤5%), somnolence (≤5%)

Dermatologic: Alopecia (8%), pruritus (7%), dry skin (≤5%), folliculitis (≤5%), seborrhea (≤5%)

Endocrine & metabolic: Dehydration (≤5%), hot flashes (≤5%)

Gastrointestinal: Stomatitis (10%), constipation (7%), tenesmus (5%), appetite increased (≤5%), dental caries (≤5%), dysphagia (≤5%), gastrointestinal hemorrhage (≤5%), gastritis (≤5%), gingival bleeding (≤5%), hemorrhoids (≤5%), melena (≤5%), splenomegaly (≤5%), taste perversion (≤5%), xerostomia (≤5%)

Genitourinary: Dysuria (≤5%), nocturia (≤5%), polyuria (≤5%)

Hepatic: Hepatomegaly (≤5%)

Local: Injection site inflammation (≤5%)

Neuromuscular & skeletal: Arthralgia (7%), myalgia (7%), gait abnormal (≤5%), hyperkinesia (≤5%), hypertonia (≤5%), tremor (≤5%)

Ocular: Abnormal vision (5%) conjunctivitis (≤5%), eye pain (≤5%)

Otic: Deafness (≤5%), earache (≤5%), tinnitus (≤5%)

Respiratory: Sinusitis (8%), hemoptysis (≤5%), pulmonary infiltrate (≤5%), sputum increased (≤5%)

Miscellaneous: Flu-like syndrome (5%), hiccups (≤5%), lymphadenopathy (≤5%), thirst (≤5%)

General Dosage Range Dosage adjustment recommended in patients with hepatic or renal impairment

I.V.: *Adults:* 40 mg/m^2 every 2 weeks

Mechanism of Action Liposomes have been shown to penetrate solid tumors more effectively, possibly because of their small size and longer circulation time. Once in tissues, daunorubicin is released. Daunorubicin inhibits DNA and RNA synthesis by intercalation between DNA base pairs and by steric obstruction; and intercalates at points of local uncoiling of the double helix. Although the exact mechanism is unclear, it appears that direct binding to DNA (intercalation) and inhibition of DNA repair (topoisomerase II inhibition) result in blockade of DNA and RNA synthesis and fragmentation of DNA.

Pharmacodynamics/Kinetics

Half-life Elimination Distribution: 4.4 hours; Terminal: 3-5 hours

Pregnancy Risk Factor D

DAUNOrubicin Hydrochloride (daw noe ROO bi sin hye droe KLOR ide)

U.S. Brand Names Cerubidine®

Canadian Brand Names Cerubidine®

Pharmacologic Category Antineoplastic Agent, Anthracycline

Use Treatment of acute lymphocytic leukemia (ALL) and acute myeloid leukemia (AML)

Local Anesthetic/Vasoconstrictor Precautions No information available to require special precautions

Effects on Dental Treatment Key adverse event(s) related to dental treatment: Stomatitis and discoloration of saliva.

Effects on Bleeding Chemotherapy may result in significant myelosuppression, potentially including significant reduction in platelet counts and altered hemostasis. In patients who are under active treatment with these agents, medical consult is suggested.

Adverse Effects

>10%:

Cardiovascular: Transient ECG abnormalities (supraventricular tachycardia, S-T wave changes, atrial or ventricular extrasystoles); generally asymptomatic and self-limiting. CHF, dose related, may be delayed for 7-8 years after treatment.

Dermatologic: Alopecia(reversible), radiation recall

Gastrointestinal: Mild nausea or vomiting, stomatitis

Genitourinary: Discoloration of urine (red)

Hematologic: Myelosuppression (onset: 7 days; nadir: 10-14 days; recovery: 21-28 days), primarily leukopenia; thrombocytopenia and anemia

1% to 10%:

Dermatologic: Skin "flare" at injection site; discoloration of saliva, sweat, or tears

Endocrine & metabolic: Hyperuricemia

Gastrointestinal: Abdominal pain, GI ulceration, diarrhea

General Dosage Range Dosage adjustment recommended in patients with hepatic or renal impairment

I.V.:

Children <2 years or BSA <0.5 m²: 1 mg/kg/dose per protocol with frequency dependent on regimen employed (maximum cumulative dose: 10 mg/kg)

Children ≥2 years and BSA ≥0.5 m²: 25 mg/m² on day 1 every week for 4 cycles **or** 30-60 mg/m²/day for 3 days (maximum cumulative dose: 300 mg/m²)

Adults <60 years: 30-60 mg/m²/day for 2-3 days (maximum cumulative dose: 550 mg/m²; 400 mg/m² with chest irradiation)

Adults ≥60 years: 30 mg/m²/day for 2-3 days (maximum cumulative dose: 550 mg/m²; 400 mg/m² with chest irradiation)

Mechanism of Action Inhibition of DNA and RNA synthesis by intercalation between DNA base pairs and by steric obstruction. Daunomycin intercalates at points of local uncoiling of the double helix. Although the exact mechanism is unclear, it appears that direct binding to DNA (intercalation) and inhibition of DNA repair (topoisomerase II inhibition) result in blockade of DNA and RNA synthesis and fragmentation of DNA.

Pharmacodynamics/Kinetics

Half-life Elimination Distribution: 2 minutes; Elimination: 14-20 hours; Terminal: 18.5 hours; Daunorubicinol plasma half-life: 24-48 hours

Pregnancy Risk Factor D

Decitabine (de SYE ta been)

U.S. Brand Names Dacogen™

Pharmacologic Category Antineoplastic Agent, DNA Methylation Inhibitor

Use Treatment of myelodysplastic syndrome (MDS)

Unlabeled/Investigational Use Treatment of acute myelogenous leukemia (AML), sickle cell anemia

Local Anesthetic/Vasoconstrictor Precautions No information available to require special precautions

Effects on Dental Treatment Key adverse event(s) related to dental treatment: Oral mucosal petechiae, stomatitis, gingival bleeding, tongue ulceration, oral candidiasis, lip ulceration, mucosal inflammation, gingival pain have been reported.

Effects on Bleeding Chemotherapy may result in significant myelosuppression, potentially including significant reduction in platelet counts and altered hemostasis. In patients who are under active treatment with these agents, medical consult is suggested.

Adverse Effects

>10%:

Cardiovascular: Peripheral edema (25% to 27%), pallor (23%), edema (5% to 18%), cardiac murmur (16%), hypotension (6% to 11%)

Central nervous system: Fever (6% to 53%), fatigue (46%), headache (23% to 28%), insomnia (14% to 28%), dizziness (18% to 21%), chills (16%), pain (5% to 13%), confusion (8% to 12%), lethargy (12%), anxiety (9% to 11%), hypoesthesia (11%)

Dermatologic: Petechiae (12% to 39%), bruising (9% to 22%), rash (11% to 19%), erythema (5% to 14%), cellulitis (9% to 12%), lesions (5% to 11%), pruritus (9% to 11%)

Endocrine & metabolic: Hyperglycemia (6% to 33%), hypoalbuminemia (7% to 24%), hypomagnesemia (5% to 24%), hypokalemia (12% to 22%), hyperkalemia (13%), hyponatremia (19%)
Gastrointestinal: Nausea (40% to 42%), constipation (30% to 35%), diarrhea (28% to 34%), vomiting (16% to 25%), anorexia/appetite decreased (8% to 23%), abdominal pain (5% to 14%), oral mucosal petechiae (13%), stomatitis (11% to 12%), dyspepsia (10% to 12%)
Hematologic: Neutropenia (38% to 90%; grades 3/4: 37% to 87%; recovery 28-50 days), thrombocytopenia (27% to 89%; grades 3/4: 24% to 85%), anemia (31% to 82%; grades 3/4: 22%), febrile neutropenia (20% to 29%; grades 3/4: 23%), leukopenia (6% to 28%; grades 3/4: 22%), lymphadenopathy (12%)
Hepatic: Hyperbilirubinemia (6% to 14%), alkaline phosphatase increased (11%)
Local: Tenderness (11%)
Neuromuscular & skeletal: Rigors (22%), arthralgia (17% to 20%), limb pain (18% to 19%), back pain (17% to 18%), weakness (15%)
Respiratory: Cough (27% to 40%), dyspnea (29%), pneumonia (20% to 22%), pharyngitis (16%), lung crackles (14%), epistaxis (13%)

5% to 10%:
Cardiovascular: Tachycardia (8%), chest pain/discomfort (6% to 7%), facial edema (6%), hypertension (6%), heart failure (5%)
Central nervous system: Depression (9%), malaise (5%)
Dermatologic: Alopecia (8%), dry skin (8%), urticaria (6%)
Endocrine & metabolic: Hyperuricemia (10%), LDH increased (8%), bicarbonate increased (6%), dehydration (6% to 8%), hypochloremia (6%), bicarbonate decreased (5%), hypoproteinemia (5%)
Gastrointestinal: Mucosal inflammation (9%), weight loss (9%), gingival bleeding (8%), hemorrhoids (8%), loose stools (7%), tongue ulceration (7%), dysphagia (5% to 6%), oral candidiasis (6%), toothache (6%), abdominal distension (5%), gastroesophageal reflux (5%), glossodynia (5%), lip ulceration (5%), oral pain (5%), tooth abscess (5%)
Genitourinary: Urinary tract infection (7%), dysuria (6%), polyuria (5%)
Hematologic: Bacteremia (5% to 8%), hematoma (5%), pancytopenia (5%), thrombocythemia (5%)
Hepatic: Ascites (10%), AST increased (10%), hypobilirubinemia (5%)
Local: Catheter infection (8%), catheter site erythema (5%), catheter site pain (5%), injection site swelling (5%)
Neuromuscular & skeletal: Myalgia (5% to 9%), falling (8%), chest wall pain (7%), muscle spasm (7%), bone pain (6%), musculoskeletal pain/discomfort (5% to 6%), crepitation (5%)
Ocular: Blurred vision (6%)
Otic: Ear pain (6%)
Respiratory: Breath sounds abnormal (5% to 10%), hypoxia (10%), upper respiratory tract infection (10%), pharyngolaryngeal pain (8%), rales (8%), pulmonary edema (6%), sinusitis (5% to 6%), pleural effusion (5%), postnasal drip (5%), sinus congestion (5%)
Miscellaneous: Candidal infection (10%), staphylococcal infection (7%), transfusion reaction (7%), night sweats (5%)

General Dosage Range Dosage adjustment recommended in patients who develop toxicities

I.V.: *Adults:* 15 mg/m^2 every 8 hours for 3 days every 6 weeks **or** 20 mg/m^2 daily for 5 days every 28 days

Mechanism of Action After phosphorylation, decitabine is incorporated into DNA and inhibits DNA methyltransferase causing hypomethylation and subsequent cell death (within the S-phase of the cell cycle).

Pharmacodynamics/Kinetics

Half-life Elimination ~30-35 minutes

Time to Peak At end of infusion

Pregnancy Risk Factor D

Deferasirox (de FER a sir ox)

U.S. Brand Names Exjade®

Canadian Brand Names Exjade®

Pharmacologic Category Antidote; Chelating Agent

Use Treatment of chronic iron overload due to blood transfusions (transfusional hemosiderosis)

Local Anesthetic/Vasoconstrictor Precautions No information available to require special precautions

Effects on Dental Treatment No significant effects or complications reported

Effects on Bleeding Rare thrombocytopenia has been reported; however, there is no information available to require routine precautions relative to altered hemostasis.

Adverse Effects

>10%:

Central nervous system: Fever (19%), headache (16%)

Dermatologic: Rash (dose related; 8% to 11%)

Gastrointestinal: Abdominal pain (dose related; 21% to 28%), diarrhea (dose related; 12% to 20%), nausea (dose related; 11% to 23%), vomiting (dose related; 10% to 21%)

Renal: Serum creatinine increased (dose related; 7% to 38%), proteinuria (19%)

Respiratory: Cough (14%), nasopharyngitis (13%), pharyngolaryngeal pain (11%)

Miscellaneous: Influenza (11%)

1% to 10%:

Central nervous system: Fatigue (6%)

Dermatologic: Urticaria (4%)

Hepatic: ALT increased (2% to 8%), transaminitis (4%)

Neuromuscular & skeletal: Arthralgia (7%), back pain (6%)

Otic: Ear infection (5%)

Respiratory: Respiratory tract infection (10%), bronchitis (9%), pharyngitis (8%), acute tonsillitis (6%), rhinitis (6%)

General Dosage Range Dosage adjustment recommended in patients with renal impairment or on concomitant therapy

Oral: *Children ≥2 years and Adults:* Initial: 20 mg/kg once daily; Maintenance: 20-30 mg/kg once daily (maximum dose: 40 mg/kg/day)

Mechanism of Action Selectively binds iron, forming a complex which is excreted primarily through the feces.

Pharmacodynamics/Kinetics

Half-life Elimination 8-16 hours

Time to Peak ~1.5-4 hours

Pregnancy Risk Factor C

Prescribing and Access Restrictions Deferasirox (Exjade®) is only available through a restricted distribution program called EPASS™ Complete Care. Prescribers must enroll patients in this program in order to obtain the medication. For patient enrollment, contact 1-888-90-EPASS (1-888-903-7277).

Deferoxamine (de fer OKS a meen)

U.S. Brand Names Desferal®

Canadian Brand Names Desferal®; PMS-Deferoxamine

Pharmacologic Category Antidote; Chelating Agent

Use Adjunct in the treatment of acute iron intoxication; treatment of chronic iron overload secondary to multiple transfusions

Canadian labeling (unlabeled use in the U.S.): Diagnosis of aluminum overload; treatment of chronic aluminum overload in patients with end-stage renal failure undergoing maintenance dialysis

Unlabeled/Investigational Use Diagnosis or treatment of aluminum induced toxicity associated with chronic kidney disease (CKD)

Local Anesthetic/Vasoconstrictor Precautions No information available to require special precautions

Effects on Dental Treatment No significant effects or complications reported

Effects on Bleeding No information available to require special precautions

Adverse Effects Frequency not defined.

Cardiovascular: Flushing, hypotension, shock, tachycardia

Central nervous system: Dizziness, encephalopathy (aluminum toxicity/dialysis-related), fever, headache, seizure

Dermatologic: Angioedema, rash, urticaria

Endocrine & metabolic: Growth retardation (children), hyperparathyroidism (aggravated), hypocalcemia

Gastrointestinal: Abdominal discomfort, abdominal pain, diarrhea, nausea, vomiting

Genitourinary: Dysuria, urine discoloration (reddish color)

Hematologic: Leukopenia, thrombocytopenia

Hepatic: Hepatic dysfunction, transaminases increased

Local: Injection site: Burning, crust, edema, erythema, eschar, induration, infiltration, irritation, pain, pruritus, swelling, vesicles, wheal formation

Neuromuscular & skeletal: Arthralgia, metaphyseal dysplasia (children <3 years; dose related), muscle spasms, myalgia, neuropathy (peripheral, sensory, motor, or mixed), paresthesia

Ocular: Blurred vision, cataract, corneal opacities, dyschromatopsia, loss of vision, night blindness, optic neuritis, peripheral vision impaired, retinal pigment abnormalities, scotoma, visual acuity decreased, visual field defects

Otic: Hearing loss, tinnitus
Renal: Acute renal failure, renal tubular disorders, serum creatinine increased
Respiratory: Acute respiratory distress syndrome (dyspnea, cyanosis, and/or interstitial infiltrates), asthma
Miscellaneous: Anaphylaxis (with or without shock), hypersensitivity reaction, infections (*Yersinia*, mucormycosis)

General Dosage Range Dosage adjustment recommended in patients with renal impairment

I.M.:
Children ≥3 years: Maximum: 6 g/24 hours
Adults: Initial: 1000 mg, followed by 500 mg every 4 hours for 2 doses; Maintenance: 500 mg every 4-12 hours **or** 500-1000 mg once daily (maximum: 6 g/day)

I.V.:
Children ≥3 years: 15 mg/kg/hour (maximum: 6 g/24 hours)
Adults: Initial: 1000 mg, followed by 500 mg every 4 hours for 2 doses; Maintenance: 500 mg every 4-12 hours **or** 2000 mg with each unit of blood (maximum: 6 g/day)

SubQ:
Children ≥3 years: 20-40 mg/kg/day (maximum: 1000-2000 mg/day)
Adults: 1-2 g once daily **or** 20-40 mg/kg/day

Mechanism of Action Complexes with trivalent ions (ferric ions) to form ferrioxamine, which are removed by the kidneys, slows accumulation of hepatic iron and retards or eliminates progression of hepatic fibrosis. Also known to inhibit DNA synthesis *in vitro*.

Pharmacodynamics/Kinetics
Half-life Elimination 14 hours (plasma half-life: 20-30 minutes)

Pregnancy Risk Factor C

Degarelix (deg a REL ix)

U.S. Brand Names Firmagon®

Canadian Brand Names Firmagon®

Pharmacologic Category Antineoplastic Agent, Gonadotropin-Releasing Hormone Antagonist; Gonadotropin Releasing Hormone Antagonist

Use Treatment of advanced prostate cancer

Local Anesthetic/Vasoconstrictor Precautions Degarelix may prolong QT interval; it is suggested that the clinician consult with the physician prior to use of vasoconstrictor in suspected patients; use vasoconstrictor (epinephrine, mepivacaine and levonordefrin [Carbocaine® 2% with Neo-Cobefrin®]) with caution.

Effects on Dental Treatment No significant effects or complications reported

Effects on Bleeding No information available to require special precautions

Adverse Effects
>10%:
Endocrine & metabolic: Hot flashes (26%)
Local: Injections site reactions (35%, grade 3: ≤2%; pain 28%, erythema 17%, swelling 6%, induration 4%, nodule 3%)

1% to 10%:
Cardiovascular: Hypertension (6%)
Central nervous system: Chills (5%), dizziness (1% to 5%), fever (1% to 5%), headache (1% to 5%), insomnia (1% to 5%), fatigue (3%)
Dermatologic: Hyperhydrosis
Endocrine & metabolic: Hypercholesterolemia (3%), gynecomastia, testicular atrophy
Gastrointestinal: Weight gain (9%), constipation (5%), nausea (1% to 5%), diarrhea
Genitourinary: Urinary tract infection (5%), erectile dysfunction
Hepatic: ALT increased (10%; grade 3: <1%), AST increased (5%; grade 3: <1%), GGT increased
Neuromuscular & skeletal: Back pain (6%), arthralgia (5%), weakness (1% to 5%)
Miscellaneous: Antidegarelix antibody formation (10%), night sweats (1% to 5%)

General Dosage Range SubQ: *Adults:* Loading dose: 240 mg; Maintenance dose: 80 mg every 28 days

Mechanism of Action Gonadotropin-releasing hormone (GnRH) antagonist which reversibly binds to GnRH receptors in the anterior pituitary gland, blocking the receptor and decreasing secretion of luteinizing hormone (LH) and follicle stimulation hormone (FSH), resulting in rapid androgen deprivation by decreasing testosterone production, thereby decreasing testosterone levels. Testosterone levels do not exhibit an initial surge, or flare, as is typical with GnRH agonists.

Pharmacodynamics/Kinetics

Onset of Action Rapid; ~96% of patients had testosterone levels ≤50 ng/dL within 3 days (Klotz, 2008)

Half-life Elimination Loading dose: SubQ: ~53 days

Time to Peak Plasma: Loading dose: SubQ: Within 2 days

Pregnancy Risk Factor X

Dental Comment Degarelix is known to prolong the QT interval. The QT interval is measured as the time and distance between the Q point of the QRS complex and the end of the T wave in the ECG tracing. After adjustment for heart rate, the QT interval is defined as prolonged if it is more than 450 msec in men and 460 msec in women. A long QT syndrome was first described in the 1950s and 60s as a congenital syndrome involving QT interval prolongation and syncope and sudden death. Some of the congenital long QT syndromes were characterized by a peculiar electrocardiographic appearance of the QRS complex involving a premature atria beat followed by a pause, then a subsequent sinus beat showing marked QT prolongation and deformity. This type of cardiac arrhythmia was originally termed "torsade de pointes" (translated from the French as "twisting of the points"). Degarelix is considered as having a risk of causing torsade de pointes. Since it is not known what effect vasoconstrictors in the local anesthetic regimen will have in patients with a known history of congenital prolonged QT interval or in patients taking any medication that prolongs the QT interval, a medical consult is suggested.

Delavirdine (de la VIR deen)

Related Information

HIV Infection and AIDS *on page 1883*

U.S. Brand Names Rescriptor®

Canadian Brand Names Rescriptor®

Pharmacologic Category Antiretroviral Agent, Reverse Transcriptase Inhibitor (Non-nucleoside)

Use Treatment of HIV-1 infection in combination with at least two additional antiretroviral agents

Local Anesthetic/Vasoconstrictor Precautions No information available to require special precautions

Effects on Dental Treatment No significant effects or complications reported

Effects on Bleeding No information available to require special precautions relative to altered hemostasis.

Adverse Effects

Frequency of adverse reactions reported from occurrence in clinical trials with delavirdine when used as part of combination antiretroviral therapy.

>10%:

Central nervous system: Headache (19% to 20%), depressive symptoms (10% to 15%), fever (4% to 12%)

Dermatologic: Rash (16% to 32%)

Gastrointestinal: Nausea (20% to 25%), vomiting (3% to 11%)

1% to 10%:

Central nervous system: Anxiety (6% to 8%)

Endocrine & metabolic: Transaminases increased (2% to 5%), amylase increased (3%), bilirubin increased (2%)

Gastrointestinal: Diarrhea, vomiting, abdominal pain (4% to 6%)

Hematologic: Prothrombin time increased (2%), hemoglobin decreased (1% to 3%)

Respiratory: Bronchitis (6% to 8%)

Frequency not defined (limited to important or life threatening): Abscess, adenopathy, alkaline phosphatase increased, allergic reaction, angioedema, anorexia, arrhythmia, bloody stool, bone pain, bruising, cardiac insufficiency, cardiac rate abnormal, cardiomyopathy, chest congestion, cognitive impairment, colitis, confusion, conjunctivitis, dermal leukocytoclastic vasculitis, desquamation, diverticulitis, dyspnea, emotional lability, eosinophilia, erythema multiforme, fecal incontinence, fungal dermatitis, gamma glutamyl transpeptidase increased, gastroenteritis, gastrointestinal bleeding, granulocytosis, gum hemorrhage, hallucination, hematuria, hepatomegaly, hyperglycemia, hyperkalemia, hypertension, hypertriglyceridemia, hyperuricemia, hypocalcemia, hyponatremia, hypophosphatemia, infection, jaundice, kidney pain, leukopenia, lipase increased, menstrual irregularities, moniliasis (oral/vaginal), pancreatitis, pancytopenia, paralysis, peripheral vascular disorder, pneumonia, postural hypotension, purpura, redistribution of body fat, renal calculi, serum creatinine increased, spleen disorder, Stevens-Johnson syndrome, tetany, thrombocytopenia, urinary tract infection, vertigo

General Dosage Range Oral: *Children ≥16 years and Adults:* 400 mg 3 times/day

Mechanism of Action Delavirdine binds directly to reverse transcriptase, blocking RNA-dependent and DNA-dependent DNA polymerase activities

Pharmacodynamics/Kinetics
Half-life Elimination 5.8 hours (range: 2-11 hours)
Time to Peak Plasma: 1 hour
Pregnancy Risk Factor C

Delmopinol (del MOE pi nol)

U.S. Brand Names Decapinol®
Generic Availability (U.S.) No
Pharmacologic Category Antibacterial, Oral Rinse
Dental Use Treatment of gingivitis; used to decrease the adhesion of oral plaque
Local Anesthetic/Vasoconstrictor Precautions No information available to require special precautions
Effects on Dental Treatment No significant effects or complications reported
Dental Usual Dosage Treatment of gingivitis; used to decrease the adhesion of oral plaque: Adults: Oral: Rinse mouth with 10 mL for 1 minute twice daily (after brushing and flossing)
Mechanism of Action Reduces adhesion of plaque-causing bacteria, reducing the formation of new plaque and promoting the removal of deposits with normal mechanical disruption (brushing and flossing). Ultimately causes a reduction in both plaque and gingivitis. Decapinol® is regulated as a medical device because the primary mode of action is to serve as a physical barrier without chemical activity.
Contraindications Hypersensitivity to delmopinol or any component of the formulation
Warnings/Precautions Not for ingestion, patients should be instructed not to swallow solution. May cause transient anesthetic effects, dry mouth, or changes in taste following use. Light staining may occur, which may be removed by brushing the teeth. Patients should be instructed to avoid eating or drinking for 30 minutes following use. Should be used as an adjunct to normal mechanical hygiene. Avoid use in pregnant women (lack of data). Not recommended for use in children <12 years of age.

Note: Preliminary monograph: A decision to market this product within the U.S. is pending. At the time of publication, it is not possible to determine when this product will be available in the U.S. market.

Pregnancy Risk Factor
The manufacturer does not recommend use in pregnant women.
Lactation Excretion unknown/not recommended
References
Hase JC, Attstrom R, Edwardsson S, et al, "6-Month Use of 0.2% Delmopinol Hydrochloride in Comparison With 0.2% Chlorhexidine Digluconate and Placebo (I). Effect on Plaque Formation and Gingivitis," *J Clin Periodontol*, 1998, 25(9):746-53.
Klinge B, Matsson L, Attstrom R, et al, "Effect of Local Application of Delmopinol Hydrochloride on Developing and Early Established Supragingival Plaque in Humans," *J Clin Periodontol*, 1996, 23 (6):543-7.
Lang NP, Hase JC, Grassi M, et al, "Plaque Formation and Gingivitis After Supervised Mouthrinsing With 0.2% Delmopinol Hydrochloride, 0.2% Chlorhexidine Digluconate and Placebo for 6 Months," *Oral Dis*, 1998, 4(2):105-13.

Demeclocycline (dem e kloe SYE kleen)

Pharmacologic Category Antibiotic, Tetracycline Derivative
Use Treatment of susceptible bacterial infections (acne, gonorrhea, pertussis, and urinary tract infections) caused by both gram-negative and gram-positive organisms
Unlabeled/Investigational Use Treatment of chronic syndrome of inappropriate secretion of antidiuretic hormone (SIADH)
Local Anesthetic/Vasoconstrictor Precautions No information available to require special precautions
Effects on Dental Treatment Tetracyclines are not recommended for use during pregnancy or in children ≤8 years of age since they have been reported to cause enamel hypoplasia and permanent teeth discoloration. Tetracyclines should only be used in these patients if other agents are contraindicated or alternative antimicrobials will not eradicate the organism. Long-term use associated with oral candidiasis.
Effects on Bleeding No information available to require special precautions
Adverse Effects Frequency not defined.
Cardiovascular: Pericarditis
Central nervous system: Bulging fontanels (infants), dizziness, headache, pseudotumor cerebri (adults)
Dermatologic: Angioneurotic edema, erythema multiforme, erythematous rash, maculopapular rash, photosensitivity, pigmentation of skin, Stevens-Johnson syndrome (rare), urticaria
Endocrine & metabolic: Discoloration of thyroid gland (brown/black), nephrogenic diabetes insipidus

Gastrointestinal: Anorexia, diarrhea, dysphagia, enterocolitis, esophageal ulcerations, glossitis, nausea, pancreatitis, vomiting
Genitourinary: Balanitis
Hematologic: Eosinophilia, neutropenia, hemolytic anemia, thrombocytopenia
Hepatic: Hepatitis (rare), hepatotoxicity (rare), liver enzymes increased, liver failure (rare)
Neuromuscular & skeletal: Myasthenic syndrome, polyarthralgia, tooth discoloration (children <8 years, rarely in adults)
Ocular: Visual disturbances
Otic: Tinnitus
Renal: Acute renal failure
Respiratory: Pulmonary infiltrates
Miscellaneous: Anaphylaxis, anaphylactoid purpura, lupus-like syndrome, systemic lupus erythematosus exacerbation

General Dosage Range Oral:
Children ≥8 years: 8-12 mg/kg/day divided every 6-12 hours
Adults: 600 mg/day in 2 or 4 divided doses

Mechanism of Action Inhibits protein synthesis by binding with the 30S and possibly the 50S ribosomal subunit(s) of susceptible bacteria; may also cause alterations in the cytoplasmic membrane; inhibits the action of ADH in patients with chronic SIADH

Pharmacodynamics/Kinetics
Onset of Action SIADH: Several days
Half-life Elimination 10-17 hours
Time to Peak Serum: 3-6 hours

Pregnancy Risk Factor D

Denileukin Diftitox (de ni LOO kin DIF ti toks)

U.S. Brand Names ONTAK®

Pharmacologic Category Antineoplastic Agent, Miscellaneous

Use Treatment of persistent or recurrent cutaneous T-cell lymphoma (CTCL) whose malignant cells express the CD25 component of the IL-2 receptor

Unlabeled/Investigational Use Treatment of CTCL types mycosis fungoides (MF) and Sézary syndrome (SS); peripheral T-cell lymphoma (second-line treatment)

Local Anesthetic/Vasoconstrictor Precautions No information available to require special precautions

Effects on Dental Treatment No significant effects or complications reported

Effects on Bleeding No information available to require special precautions

Adverse Effects
>10%:
Cardiovascular: Capillary leak syndrome (33%; serious: 11%), peripheral edema (20% to 26%), vasodilation (22%), hypotension (7% to 16%), chest pain (4% to 13%), tachycardia (12%), thrombosis-related events (7% to 11%)
Central nervous system: Fever (49% to 64%), fatigue (44% to 47%), headache (26% to 29%), dizziness (11% to 13%), pain (11% to 13%)
Dermatologic: Rash (20% to 24%), pruritus (16% to 18%)
Endocrine & metabolic: Hypoalbuminemia (14% to 17%)
Gastrointestinal: Nausea (47% to 60%), vomiting (13% to 35%), diarrhea (22%), anorexia (9% to 20%), taste disturbance (11% to 13%)
Hematologic: Lymphopenia (70%; 24% had lymphopenia at baseline)
Hepatic: ALT increased (84%), AST increased (84%)
Neuromuscular & skeletal: Rigors (42% to 47%), myalgia (18% to 20%), weakness (18%), back pain (16% to 18%), arthralgia (13% to 16%)
Respiratory: Cough (18% to 20%), upper respiratory infection (13%), dyspnea (11% to 13%)
Miscellaneous: Antibody formation (76% to 100%) neutralizing antibodies (45% to 97%), flu-like syndrome (≤85%), infusion reaction (71%; serious: 8%), infection (48%)
1% to 10%:
Cardiovascular: Arrhythmia (6%), hypertension (6%)
Hematologic: Leukopenia (grades 3/4: 3% to 6%), neutropenia (grades 3/4: 3%), thrombocytopenia (grades 3/4: 3%)
Local: Injection site reaction (8%)
Ocular: Visual changes (serious: 4%; includes loss of visual acuity)
Renal: Serum creatinine increased (3% to 10%), proteinuria/casts/hematuria (6%)

General Dosage Range Dosage adjustment recommended in patients who develop toxicities
I.V.: *Adults:* 9 or 18 mcg/kg/day days 1-5 every 21 days

Mechanism of Action Denileukin diftitox is a fusion protein (a combination of amino acid sequences from diphtheria toxin and interleukin-2) which selectively delivers the cytotoxic activity of diphtheria toxin to targeted cells. It interacts with the high-affinity IL-2 receptor on the surface of malignant cells to inhibit intracellular protein synthesis, rapidly leading to cell death.

Pharmacodynamics/Kinetics

Half-life Elimination Distribution: 2-5 minutes; Terminal: 70-80 minutes

Denosumab (den OH sue mab)

Related Information

Osteonecrosis of the Jaw *on page* 1894

U.S. Brand Names Prolia™; Xgeva™

Canadian Brand Names Prolia™

Generic Availability (U.S.) No

Pharmacologic Category Monoclonal Antibody

Use Treatment of osteoporosis in postmenopausal women at high risk for fracture; prevention of skeletal-related events (eg, fracture, spinal cord compression, bone pain requiring radiation therapy) in patients with bone metastases from solid tumors

Unlabeled/Investigational Use Prevention of bone loss due to androgen deprivation therapy in nonmetastatic prostate cancer; prevention of bone loss due to aromatase inhibitor therapy in breast cancer; treatment of bone destruction caused by rheumatoid arthritis

Local Anesthetic/Vasoconstrictor Precautions No information available to require special precautions

Effects on Dental Treatment Cases of osteonecrosis of the jaw bone (ONJ) have been associated with denosumab exposure. ONJ presents clinically as exposed necrotic bone of at least 8 weeks duration with or without the presence of pain, infection, or previous trauma in a patient who has not received radiation to the jaws. Since ONJ is also associated with bisphosphonate exposure, and osteoclasts are the common targets of bisphosphonates and denosumab, osteoclastic inhibition may play a central role in ONJ associated with these two classes of drugs. Patients developing ONJ while on denosumab therapy should receive care by an oral surgeon. See Warnings/Precautions and Dental Comment.

Effects on Bleeding No information available to require special precautions

Adverse Effects A postmarketing safety program for Prolia™ is available to collect information on adverse events; more information is available at http://www.-proliasafety.com. To report adverse events for either Prolia™ or Xgeva™, prescribers may also call Amgen at 800-772-6436 or FDA at 800-332-1088. **Note:** Adverse events and frequencies occurred in patients with osteoporosis unless otherwise noted as occurring in patients with cancer.

>10%:

- Central nervous system: Fatigue (cancer patients: 45%), headache (cancer patients: 13%)
- Dermatologic: Dermatitis (11%), eczema (11%), rash (3% to 11%)
- Endocrine & metabolic: Hypophosphatemia (cancer patients: 32%; grade 3: 15%), hypocalcemia (2%; cancer patients: 18%; grade 3: 3%)
- Gastrointestinal: Nausea (cancer patients: 31%), diarrhea (cancer patients: 20%)
- Neuromuscular & skeletal: Limb pain (12%), weakness (cancer patients: 45%; osteoporosis: 2%)
- Respiratory: Dyspnea (cancer patients: 21%), cough (cancer patients: 15%)

1% to 10%:

- Cardiovascular: Peripheral edema (5%), angina (3%)
- Endocrine & metabolic: Hypercholesterolemia (7%)
- Gastrointestinal: Flatulence (2%)
- Neuromuscular & skeletal: Sciatica (5%), bone pain (4%), myalgia (3%), osteonecrosis of the jaw ([ONJ] cancer patients: 2%)
- Respiratory: Upper respiratory tract infection (5%)
- Miscellaneous: New malignancies (5%), infections (nonfatal, serious; 4%)

Dosage SubQ: Adults:

Prevention of skeletal-related events in bone metastases from solid tumors (Xgeva™): 120 mg every 4 weeks

Treatment of osteoporosis in postmenopausal females (Prolia™): 60 mg as a single dose, once every 6 months

Prevention of androgen-induced bone loss in nonmetastatic prostate cancer (unlabeled use): 60 mg as a single dose, once every 6 months (Smith, 2009)

Prevention of aromatase inhibitor-induced bone loss in breast cancer (unlabeled use): 60 mg as a single dose, once every 6 months for 4 doses (Ellis, 2008)

Dosage adjustment in renal impairment: Dose adjustment is not needed; monitor patients with severe impairment (Cl_{cr} <30 mL/minute or on dialysis) due to increased risk of hypocalcemia.

Mechanism of Action Denosumab is a monoclonal antibody with affinity for nuclear factor-kappa ligand (RANKL). Osteoblasts secrete RANKL; RANKL activates osteoclast precursors and subsequent osteolysis which promotes release of bone-derived growth factors, such as insulin-like growth factor-1 (IGF1) and transforming growth factor-beta (TGF-beta), and increases serum calcium levels. Denosumab binds to RANKL, blocks the interaction between RANKL and RANK (a receptor located on osteoclast surfaces), and prevents osteoclast formation, leading to decreased bone resorption and increased bone mass in osteoporosis. In solid tumors with bony metastases, RANKL inhibition decreases osteoclastic activity leading to decreased skeletal related events and tumor-induced bone destruction.

Contraindications

Prolia™: Hypocalcemia

Xgeva™: There are no contraindications listed in the manufacturer's labeling.

Warnings/Precautions Denosumab may cause or exacerbate hypocalcemia. Monitor calcium levels; correct pre-existing hypocalcemia prior to therapy. Use caution in patients with a history of hypoparathyroidism, thyroid surgery, parathyroid surgery, malabsorption syndromes, excision of small intestine, severe renal impairment or other conditions which would predispose the patient to hypocalcemia; monitor closely during therapy. Ensure adequate calcium and vitamin D intake; supplement with calcium and vitamin D; magnesium supplementation may also be necessary. Incidence of infections may be increased, including serious skin infections, abdominal, urinary, ear, or periodontal infections. Endocarditis has also been reported following use. Patients should be advised to contact healthcare provider if signs or symptoms of severe infection or cellulitis develop. Use with caution in patients with impaired immune systems or using concomitant immunosuppressive therapy; may be at increased risk for serious infections. Evaluate the need for continued treatment with serious infection. Osteonecrosis of the jaw (ONJ) has been reported in patients receiving denosumab. Risk factors include invasive dental procedures (eg, tooth extraction, dental implants, boney surgery); a diagnosis of cancer, concomitant chemotherapy or corticosteroids, poor oral hygiene, ill-fitting dentures; and comorbid disorders (anemia, coagulopathy, infection, pre-existing dental disease). Patients should maintain good oral hygiene during treatment. A dental exam and preventative dentistry should be performed prior to therapy. The benefit/risk must be assessed by the treating physician and/or dentist/surgeon prior to any invasive dental procedure; avoid invasive procedures in patients with bone metastases receiving therapy for prevention of skeletal-related events. Patients developing ONJ while on denosumab therapy should receive care by a dentist or oral surgeon; extensive dental surgery to treat ONJ may exacerbate ONJ.

Postmenopausal osteoporosis: For use in women at high risk for fracture which is defined as a history of osteoporotic fracture or multiple risk factors for fracture. May also be used in women who failed or did not tolerate other therapies.

Bone metastases: Denosumab is not indicated for the prevention of skeletal-related events in patients with multiple myeloma. In trials of with multiple myeloma patients, denosumab was noninferior to zoledronic acid in delaying time to first skeletal-related event and mortality was increased in a subset of the denosumab-treated group.

Denosumab therapy results in significant suppression of bone turnover; the long term effects of treatment are not known but may contribute to adverse outcomes such as ONJ, atypical fractures, or delayed fracture healing; monitor. Use with caution in patients with renal impairment (Cl_{cr} <30 mL/minute) or patients on dialysis; risk of hypocalcemia is increased. Dose adjustment is not needed. Dermatitis, eczema, and rash (which are not necessarily specific to the injection site) have been reported. Consider discontinuing use if symptoms occur. Packaging may contain natural latex rubber. Safety and efficacy have not been established in children; use may impair bone growth in children with open growth plates or inhibit eruption of dentition.

Drug Interactions

Avoid Concomitant Use There are no known interactions where it is recommended to avoid concomitant use.

Increased Effect/Toxicity

Denosumab may increase the levels/effects of: Immunosuppressants

Decreased Effect There are no known significant interactions involving a decrease in effect.

Ethanol/Nutrition/Herb Interactions Ethanol: Avoid ethanol (may increase risk of osteoporosis).

Dietary Considerations Ensure adequate calcium and vitamin D intake. Calcium 1000 mg/day and vitamin D ≥400 units/day is recommended in product labeling (Prolia™).

Women and men >50 years of age should consume elemental calcium 1200-1500 mg/day and vitamin D 800-1000 int. units/day (National Osteoporosis Foundation Guidelines, 2010).

Pharmacodynamics/Kinetics

Onset of Action Decreases markers of bone resorption by ~85% within 3 days; maximal reductions observed within 1 month

Duration of Action Markers of bone resorption return to baseline within 12 months of discontinuing therapy

Half-life Elimination ~25-28 days

Time to Peak Serum: 10 days (range 3-21 days)

Pregnancy Risk Factor C

Lactation Excretion unknown/not recommended

Breast-Feeding Considerations According to the manufacturer, the decision to continue or discontinue breast-feeding during therapy should take into account the risk of exposure to the infant and the benefits of treatment to the mother. In animal studies, mammary gland development was impaired following exposure to denosumab during pregnancy, resulting in impaired lactation postpartum.

Dosage Forms

Injection, solution [preservative free]:

Prolia™: 60 mg/mL (1 mL)

Xgeva™: 70 mg/mL (1.7 mL)

Dental Comment In head-to-head comparison trials of denosumab and zoledronate (a bisphosphonate) for the treatment of bone metastasis in patients with cancer, 20 cases of ONJ were detected out of a total of 1026 subjects (2.0%) exposed to denosumab. There were 14 cases of ONJ observed out of a total of 1020 subjects (1.4%) exposed to zoledronate (Kyrgidis, 2010). The case of a 60-year old male cancer patient who developed ONJ after treatment with denosumab has been published (Taylor, 2010). In that report, the patient participated in a trial for a phase 3 study of denosumab. The patient had never been prescribed a bisphosphonate medication before treatment with denosumab. Clinical and radiological features of the lesion were diagnostic of probable ONJ. After discontinuation of the denosumab, the patient was treated with antibiotics and chlorhexidine rinses for a week. The necrotic bone sequestered 12 months later, and 15 months after initial presentation, the mucosa had healed with no further symptoms. Another case reported the development of ONJ in a 65-year old women being treated for giant cell tumor with denosumab. Although the patient was medically compromised and on multiple medications, the authors proposed that a common thread in ONJ development is inhibition of osteoclastic activity, mediated in this case by denosumab.

References

Kyrgidis A and Toulis KA, "Denosumab-Related Osteonecrosis of the Jaws," *Osteoporos Int*, 2010, [epub ahead of print].

Taylor KH, Middlefell LS, and Mizen KD, "Osteonecrosis of the Jaws Induced by Anti-RANK Ligand Therapy," *Br J Oral Maxillofac Surg*, 2010, 48(3):221-3.

Desipramine (des IP ra meen)

U.S. Brand Names Norpramin®

Canadian Brand Names Alti-Desipramine; Apo-Desipramine®; Norpramin®; Nu-Desipramine; PMS-Desipramine

Pharmacologic Category Antidepressant, Tricyclic (Secondary Amine)

Use Treatment of depression

Unlabeled/Investigational Use Analgesic adjunct in chronic pain; peripheral neuropathies (including diabetic neuropathy); substance-related disorders (eg, cocaine withdrawal); attention-deficit/hyperactivity disorder (ADHD); depression in children ≤12 years of age

Local Anesthetic/Vasoconstrictor Precautions Use with caution; epinephrine and levonordefrin have been shown to have an increased pressor response in combination with TCAs. Desipramine is one of the drugs confirmed to prolong the QT interval and is accepted as having a risk of causing torsade de pointes. The risk of drug-induced torsade de pointes is extremely low when a single QT interval prolonging drug is prescribed. In terms of epinephrine, it is not known what effect vasoconstrictors in the local anesthetic regimen will have in patients with a known history of congenital prolonged QT interval or in patients taking any medication that prolongs the QT interval. Until more information is obtained, it is suggested that the clinician consult with the physician prior to the use of a vasoconstrictor in suspected patients, and that the vasoconstrictor (epinephrine, mepivacaine and levonordefrin [Carbocaine® 2% with Neo-Cobefrin®]) be used with caution.

Effects on Dental Treatment Key adverse event(s) related to dental treatment: Xerostomia and changes in salivation (normal salivary flow resumes upon discontinuation), unpleasant taste, stomatitis, and black tongue. Long-term treatment with TCAs increases the risk of caries by reducing salivation and salivary buffer capacity.

Effects on Bleeding No information available to require special precautions

Adverse Effects Frequency not defined.

Cardiovascular: Arrhythmias, edema, flushing, heart block, hyper-/hypotension, MI, palpitation, stroke, tachycardia

Central nervous system: Agitation, anxiety, ataxia, confusion, delirium, disorientation, dizziness, drowsiness, drug fever, exacerbation of psychosis, extrapyramidal symptoms, fatigue, hallucinations, headache, hypomania, incoordination, insomnia, nervousness, parkinsonian syndrome, restlessness, seizure

Dermatologic: Alopecia, itching, petechiae, photosensitivity, skin rash, urticaria

Endocrine & metabolic: Breast enlargement, galactorrhea, hyper-/hypoglycemia, impotence, libido changes, SIADH

Gastrointestinal: Abdominal cramps, anorexia, black tongue, constipation, decreased lower esophageal sphincter tone may cause GE reflux, diarrhea, heartburn, nausea, paralytic ileus, stomatitis, unpleasant taste, vomiting, weight gain/loss, xerostomia

Genitourinary: Difficult urination, polyuria, sexual dysfunction, testicular edema, urinary retention

Hematologic: Agranulocytosis, eosinophilia, purpura, thrombocytopenia

Hepatic: Cholestatic jaundice, hepatitis, liver enzymes increased

Neuromuscular & skeletal: Fine muscle tremor, numbness, paresthesia of extremities, peripheral neuropathy, tingling, weakness

Ocular: Blurred vision, disturbances of accommodation, intraocular pressure increased, mydriasis

Otic: Tinnitus

Miscellaneous: Allergic reaction, diaphoresis (excessive)

General Dosage Range Oral:

Adolescents: Initial: 25-50 mg once daily; Maintenance: 25-100 mg/day in single or divided doses (maximum: 150 mg/day)

Adults: Initial: 75 mg/day in divided doses; Maintenance: 75-200 mg/day in single or divided doses (maximum: 300 mg/day)

Elderly: Initial: 10-25 mg/day; Maintenance: 75-150 mg/day

Mechanism of Action Traditionally believed to increase the synaptic concentration of norepinephrine (and to a lesser extent, serotonin) in the central nervous system by inhibition of its reuptake by the presynaptic neuronal membrane. However, additional receptor effects have been found including desensitization of adenyl cyclase, down regulation of beta-adrenergic receptors, and down regulation of serotonin receptors.

Pharmacodynamics/Kinetics

Onset of Action 1-3 weeks; Maximum antidepressant effect: >2 weeks

Half-life Elimination Adults: 7-60 hours

Time to Peak Plasma: 4-6 hours

Dental Comment Desipramine is known to prolong the QT interval. The QT interval is measured as the time and distance between the Q point of the QRS complex and the end of the T wave in the ECG tracing. After adjustment for heart rate, the QT interval is defined as prolonged if it is more than 450 msec in men and 460 msec in women. A long QT syndrome was first described in the 1950s and 60s as a congenital syndrome involving QT interval prolongation and syncope and sudden death. Some of the congenital long QT syndromes were characterized by a peculiar electrocardiographic appearance of the QRS complex involving a premature atria beat followed by a pause, then a subsequent sinus beat showing marked QT prolongation and deformity. This type of cardiac arrhythmia was originally termed "torsade de pointes" (translated from the French as "twisting of the points"). Desipramine is considered as having a risk of causing torsade de pointes. Since it is not known what effect vasoconstrictors in the local anesthetic regimen will have in patients with a known history of congenital prolonged QT interval or in patients taking any medication that prolongs the QT interval, a medical consult is suggested.

Desirudin (des i ROO din)

Related Information

Cardiovascular Diseases *on page 1848*

U.S. Brand Names Iprivask®

Pharmacologic Category Anticoagulant, Thrombin Inhibitor

Use Prophylaxis of deep vein thrombosis (DVT) in patients undergoing surgery for hip replacement

Local Anesthetic/Vasoconstrictor Precautions No information available to require special precautions
Effects on Dental Treatment No significant effects or complications reported
Effects on Bleeding As with all anticoagulants, bleeding is the major adverse effect of desirudin during dental surgery. Hemorrhage may occur at virtually any site; risk is dependent on multiple variables, including the intensity of anticoagulation and patient susceptibility. Medical consult is suggested. It is unlikely that ambulatory patients presenting for dental treatment will be taking intravenous anticoagulant therapy.
Adverse Effects As with all anticoagulants, bleeding is the major adverse effect. Hemorrhage may occur at any site.

2% to 10%:
- Gastrointestinal: Nausea (2%)
- Hematologic: Hematoma (6%), hemorrhage (major, <1% to 3%; may include cases of intracranial, retroperitoneal, intraocular, intraspinal, or prosthetic joint hemorrhage), anemia (3%)
- Local: Injection site mass (4%), deep thrombophlebitis (2%)
- Miscellaneous: Wound secretion (4%)

General Dosage Range Dosage adjustment recommended in patients with renal impairment
SubQ: *Adults:* 15 mg every 12 hours
Mechanism of Action Desirudin is a direct, highly selective thrombin inhibitor. Reversibly binds to the active thrombin site of free and clot-associated thrombin. Inhibits fibrin formation, activation of coagulation factors V, VII, and XIII, and thrombin-induced platelet aggregation resulting in a dose-dependent prolongation of the activated partial thromboplastin time (aPTT).
Pharmacodynamics/Kinetics
Half-life Elimination ~2 hours; Prolonged with renal impairment (Cl_{cr} <31 mL/minute/1.73 m^2: Up to 12 hours)
Time to Peak Plasma: 1-3 hours
Pregnancy Risk Factor C

Desloratadine (des lor AT a deen)

U.S. Brand Names Clarinex®
Canadian Brand Names Aerius®; Aerius® Kids
Generic Availability (U.S.) No
Pharmacologic Category Histamine H_1 Antagonist; Histamine H_1 Antagonist, Second Generation; Piperidine Derivative
Use Relief of nasal and non-nasal symptoms of seasonal allergic rhinitis (SAR) and perennial allergic rhinitis (PAR); treatment of chronic idiopathic urticaria (CIU)
Local Anesthetic/Vasoconstrictor Precautions No information available to require special precautions
Effects on Dental Treatment Key adverse event(s) related to dental treatment: Xerostomia (normal salivary flow resumes upon discontinuation)
Effects on Bleeding No information available to require special precautions
Adverse Effects

>10%: Central nervous system: Headache (14%)

1% to 10%:
- Central nervous system: Fatigue (2% to 5%), somnolence (2%), dizziness (4%)
- Endocrine & metabolic: Dysmenorrhea (2%)
- Gastrointestinal: Xerostomia (3%), nausea (5%), dyspepsia (3%)
- Neuromuscular & skeletal: Myalgia (2% to 3%)
- Respiratory: Pharyngitis (3% to 4%)

Dosage Oral:

Children:
- 6-11 months: 1 mg once daily
- 12 months to 5 years: 1.25 mg once daily
- 6-11 years: 2.5 mg once daily

Children ≥12 years and Adults: 5 mg once daily

Dosage adjustment in renal/hepatic impairment:
- Children: Not established
- Adults: 5 mg every other day

Mechanism of Action Desloratadine, a major metabolite of loratadine, is a long-acting tricyclic antihistamine with selective peripheral histamine H_1 receptor antagonistic activity and additional anti-inflammatory properties.
Contraindications Hypersensitivity to desloratadine, loratadine, or any component of the formulation

Warnings/Precautions Dose should be adjusted in patients with liver or renal impairment. Use with caution in patients known to be slow metabolizers of desloratadine (incidence of side effects may be increased). Some products may contain phenylalanine. Safety and efficacy have not been established for children <6 months of age.

Drug Interactions

Metabolism/Transport Effects Substrate of P-glycoprotein

Avoid Concomitant Use There are no known interactions where it is recommended to avoid concomitant use.

Increased Effect/Toxicity

Desloratadine may increase the levels/effects of: Alcohol (Ethyl); Anticholinergics; CNS Depressants

The levels/effects of Desloratadine may be increased by: Droperidol; P-Glycoprotein Inhibitors; Pramlintide

Decreased Effect

Desloratadine may decrease the levels/effects of: Acetylcholinesterase Inhibitors (Central); Benzylpenicilloyl Polylysine; Betahistine

The levels/effects of Desloratadine may be decreased by: Acetylcholinesterase Inhibitors (Central); Amphetamines; P-Glycoprotein Inducers

Ethanol/Nutrition/Herb Interactions

Ethanol: May increase CNS depression; monitor for increased effects with coadministration. Caution patients about effects.

Food: Does not affect bioavailability.

Dietary Considerations May be taken with or without food. Some products may contain phenylalanine.

Pharmacodynamics/Kinetics

Half-life Elimination 27 hours

Time to Peak 3 hours

Pregnancy Risk Factor C

Lactation Enters breast milk/not recommended

Dosage Forms

Syrup, oral:

Clarinex®: 0.5 mg/mL (480 mL)

Tablet, oral:

Clarinex®: 5 mg

Tablet, orally disintegrating, oral:

Clarinex®: 2.5 mg, 5 mg

Desloratadine and Pseudoephedrine

(des lor AT a deen & soo doe e FED rin)

Related Information

Desloratadine *on page 487*

Pseudoephedrine *on page 1429*

U.S. Brand Names Clarinex-D® 12 Hour; Clarinex-D® 24 Hour

Pharmacologic Category Alpha/Beta Agonist; Decongestant; Histamine H_1 Antagonist; Histamine H_1 Antagonist, Second Generation; Piperidine Derivative

Use Relief of symptoms of seasonal allergic rhinitis, in children ≥12 years of age and adults

Local Anesthetic/Vasoconstrictor Precautions No information available to require special precautions

Effects on Dental Treatment Key adverse event(s) related to dental treatment: Pseudoephedrine: Xerostomia (normal salivary flow resumes upon discontinuation).

Effects on Bleeding No information available to require special precautions

Adverse Effects See also individual agents. Percentages as reported with the combination products:

1% to 10%:

Central nervous system: Insomnia (5% to 10%), headache (6% to 8%), fatigue (3% to 4%), somnolence (3%), dizziness (2% to 3%), hyperactivity (2%), nervousness (2%)

Gastrointestinal: Xerostomia (8%), anorexia (2%), nausea (2%)

Respiratory: Pharyngitis (3%)

Miscellaneous: Infection (2%)

General Dosage Range Dosage adjustment recommended in patients with renal impairment

Oral: *Children ≥12 years and Adults:* 12 hour: 1 tablet twice daily; 24 hour: 1 tablet once daily

Mechanism of Action
Desloratadine, a major metabolite of loratadine, is a long-acting tricyclic antihistamine with selective peripheral histamine H_1 receptor antagonistic activity and additional anti-inflammatory properties.
Pseudoephedrine directly stimulates alpha-adrenergic receptors of respiratory mucosa causing vasoconstriction; directly stimulates beta-adrenergic receptors causing bronchial relaxation, increased heart rate and contractility.

Pharmacodynamics/Kinetics
Onset of Action Antihistaminic activity: 1 hour
Time to Peak Desloratadine: 4-7 hours; Pseudoephedrine: 6-9 hours

Pregnancy Risk Factor C

Desmopressin (des moe PRES in)

U.S. Brand Names DDAVP®; Stimate®

Canadian Brand Names Apo-Desmopressin®; DDAVP®; DDAVP® Melt; Minirin®; Novo-Desmopressin; Octostim®; PMS-Desmopressin

Pharmacologic Category Antihemophilic Agent; Hemostatic Agent; Vasopressin Analog, Synthetic

Use
Injection: Treatment of diabetes insipidus; maintenance of hemostasis and control of bleeding in hemophilia A with factor VIII coagulant activity levels >5% and mild-to-moderate classic von Willebrand's disease (type 1) with factor VIII coagulant activity levels >5%
Nasal solutions (DDAVP® Nasal Spray and DDAVP® Rhinal Tube): Treatment of central diabetes insipidus
Nasal spray (Stimate®): Maintenance of hemostasis and control of bleeding in hemophilia A with factor VIII coagulant activity levels >5% and mild-to-moderate classic von Willebrand's disease (type 1) with factor VIII coagulant activity levels >5%
Tablet: Treatment of central diabetes insipidus, temporary polyuria and polydipsia following pituitary surgery or head trauma, primary nocturnal enuresis

Unlabeled/Investigational Use Uremic bleeding associated with acute or chronic renal failure; prevention of surgical bleeding in patients with uremia

Local Anesthetic/Vasoconstrictor Precautions No information available to require special precautions

Effects on Dental Treatment No significant effects or complications reported

Effects on Bleeding General dental procedures and simple restorative procedures are not associated with bleeding; therefore, there is no contraindication to general dental treatment for most patients with bleeding disorders. However, after dental extractions and other dental surgeries including deep scaling, block anesthesia, and large fillings, in patients with hemophilia, antifibrinolytic drugs are useful in controlling bleeding. A carefully coordinated strategy between the dental and medical team may be required to ensure adequate procedures for hemostasis. Although desmopressin is medically useful for maintenance of hemostasis and control of bleeding, there is no information available for its use in the hemophiliac dental patient. As preparation for selected dental procedures, tranexamic acid or aminocaproic acid may be appropriate.

Adverse Effects Frequency may not be defined (may be dose or route related).
Cardiovascular: Blood pressure increased/decreased (I.V.), facial flushing
Central nervous system: Headache (2% to 5%), dizziness (intranasal; ≤3%), chills (intranasal; 2%)
Dermatologic: Rash
Endocrine & metabolic: Hyponatremia, water intoxication
Gastrointestinal: Abdominal pain (intranasal; 2%), gastrointestinal disorder (intranasal; ≤2%), nausea (intranasal; ≤2%), abdominal cramps, sore throat
Hepatic: Transient increases in liver transaminases (associated primarily with tablets)
Local: Injection: Burning pain, erythema, and swelling at the injection site
Neuromuscular & Skeletal: Weakness (intranasal; ≤2%)
Ocular: Conjunctivitis (intranasal; ≤2%), eye edema (intranasal; ≤2%), lacrimation disorder (intranasal; ≤2%)
Respiratory: Rhinitis (intranasal; 3% to 8%), epistaxis (intranasal; ≤3%), nostril pain (intranasal; ≤2%), cough, nasal congestion, upper respiratory infection

General Dosage Range
I.V.:
Children ≥3 months: 0.3 mcg/kg as a single dose, may repeat dose if needed
Adults: 2-4 mcg/day in 2 divided doses **or** 1/10 of the intranasal maintenance dose **or** 0.3 mcg/kg as a single dose

Intranasal:

Children 3-11 months: Initial: 5 mcg/day (0.05 mL/day) in 1-2 divided doses; Maintenance: 5-30 mcg/day (0.05-0.3 mL/day) in 1-2 divided doses

Children 12 months to 12 years: Initial: 5 mcg/day (0.05 mL/day) in 1-2 divided doses; Maintenance: 5-30 mcg/day (0.05-0.3 mL/day) in 1-2 divided doses **or** 150 mcg (1 spray of high concentration) as a single dose

Children >12 years and Adults <50 kg: 10-40 mcg/day (0.1-0.4 mL) in 1-3 divided doses **or** 150 mcg (1 spray of high concentration spray) as a single dose

Children >12 years and Adults ≥50 kg: 10-40 mcg/day in 1-3 divided doses **or** 300 mcg (1 spray each nostril of high concentration spray) as a single dose

Oral:

Children 4-5 years: Initial: 0.05 mg twice daily; Maintenance: 0.1-1.2 mg/day in 2-3 divided doses

Children ≥6 years: Initial: 0.05 mg twice daily **or** 0.2 mg at bedtime; Maintenance: 0.1-1.2 mg/day in 2-3 divided doses **or** 0.2-0.6 mg at bedtime

Adults: 0.2-0.6 mg at bedtime **or** 0.1-1.2 mg/day in 2-3 divided doses

SubQ: *Adults:* 2-4 mcg/day in 2 divided doses **or** 1/10 of the intranasal maintenance dose

Mechanism of Action In a dose dependent manner, desmopressin increases cyclic adenosine monophosphate (cAMP) in renal tubular cells which increases water permeability resulting in decreased urine volume and increased urine osmolality; increases plasma levels of von Willebrand factor, factor VIII, and t-PA contributing to a shortened activated partial thromboplastin time (aPTT) and bleeding time.

Pharmacodynamics/Kinetics

Onset of Action

Intranasal: Antidiuretic: 15-30 minutes; Increased factor VIII and von Willebrand factor (vWF) activity (dose related): 30 minutes

Peak effect: Antidiuretic: 1 hour; Increased factor VIII and vWF activity: 1.5 hours

I.V. infusion: Increased factor VIII and vWF activity: 30 minutes (dose related)

Peak effect: 1.5-2 hours

Oral tablet: Antidiuretic: ~1 hour

Peak effect: 4-7 hours

Duration of Action Intranasal, I.V. infusion, Oral tablet: ~6-14 hours

Half-life Elimination Intranasal: ~3.5 hours; I.V. infusion: 3 hours; Oral tablet: 2-3 hours

Renal impairment: ≤9 hours

Pregnancy Risk Factor B

Desonide (DES oh nide)

U.S. Brand Names Desonate®; DesOwen®; LoKara™; Verdeso™

Canadian Brand Names Desocort®; PMS-Desonide

Pharmacologic Category Corticosteroid, Topical

Use Treatment of inflammatory and pruritic manifestations of corticosteroid responsive dermatosis (low-to-medium potency corticosteroid); mild-to-moderate atopic dermatitis

Local Anesthetic/Vasoconstrictor Precautions No information available to require special precautions

Effects on Dental Treatment No significant effects or complications reported

Effects on Bleeding No information available to require special precautions

General Dosage Range Topical:

Children ≥3 months: Aerosol, gel: Apply 2 times/day sparingly

Adults: Apply 2-3 times/day sparingly

Mechanism of Action Stimulates the synthesis of enzymes needed to decrease inflammation, suppress mitotic activity, and cause vasoconstriction

Pregnancy Risk Factor C

Desoximetasone (des oks i MET a sone)

U.S. Brand Names Topicort®; Topicort®-LP

Canadian Brand Names Taro-Desoximetasone; Topicort®

Generic Availability (U.S.) Yes

Pharmacologic Category Corticosteroid, Topical

Dental Use Short-term relief of inflammation of moderate-to-severe corticosteroid-responsive dermatosis (intermediate- to high-potency topical corticosteroid)

Use Relieves inflammation and pruritic symptoms of corticosteroid-responsive dermatosis (intermediate- to high-potency topical corticosteroid)

Local Anesthetic/Vasoconstrictor Precautions No information available to require special precautions

Effects on Dental Treatment No significant effects or complications reported

Effects on Bleeding No information available to require special precautions

Dosage Desoximetasone is a potent fluorinated topical corticosteroid. Therapy should be discontinued when control is achieved; if no improvement is seen, reassessment of diagnosis may be necessary.

Cream, gel: Children and Adults: Apply a thin film to affected area twice daily

Ointment: Children ≥10 years and Adults: Apply a thin film to affected area twice daily

Mechanism of Action Stimulates the synthesis of enzymes needed to decrease inflammation, suppress mitotic activity, and cause vasoconstriction

Contraindications Hypersensitivity to desoximetasone or any component of the formulation; topical fungal infections; tuberculosis of skin herpes simplex

Warnings/Precautions Systemic absorption of topical corticosteroids may cause hypothalamic-pituitary-adrenal (HPA) axis suppression (reversible) particularly in younger children. HPA axis suppression may lead to adrenal crisis. Risk is increased when used over large surface areas, for prolonged periods, or with occlusive dressings. Prolonged treatment with corticosteroids has been associated with the development of Kaposi's sarcoma (case reports); if noted, discontinuation of therapy should be considered. Adverse systemic effects including hyperglycemia, glycosuria, fluid and electrolyte changes, and HPA suppression may occur when used on large surface areas, for prolonged periods, or with an occlusive dressing. Chronic use of corticosteroids in children may interfere with growth and development. Safety and efficacy of desoximetasone ointment have not been established in children <10 years of age.

Drug Interactions

Avoid Concomitant Use

Avoid concomitant use of Desoximetasone with any of the following: Aldesleukin

Increased Effect/Toxicity

Desoximetasone may increase the levels/effects of: Deferasirox

Decreased Effect

Desoximetasone may decrease the levels/effects of: Aldesleukin; Corticorelin

Pharmacodynamics/Kinetics

Half-life Elimination Emollient cream: 15-17 hours

Pregnancy Risk Factor C

Lactation Excretion in breast milk unknown/use caution

Dosage Forms

Cream, topical: 0.05% (15 g, 60 g); 0.25% (15 g, 60 g)

Topicort®: 0.25% (15 g, 60 g)

Topicort®-LP: 0.05% (15 g, 60 g)

Gel, topical: 0.05% (15 g, 60 g)

Topicort®: 0.05% (15 g, 60 g)

Ointment, topical: 0.25% (15 g, 60 g)

Topicort®: 0.25% (15 g, 60 g)

Desvenlafaxine (des ven la FAX een)

U.S. Brand Names Pristiq®

Canadian Brand Names Pristiq®

Pharmacologic Category Antidepressant, Serotonin/Norepinephrine Reuptake Inhibitor

Use Treatment of major depressive disorder

Local Anesthetic/Vasoconstrictor Precautions Part of the mechanism of desvenlafaxine is to block reuptake of norepinephrine along with dopamine. Because of the potential for norepinephrine elevation within CNS synapses, it is suggested that vasoconstrictor be administered with caution and to monitor vital signs in dental patients taking antidepressants that affect norepinephrine in this way. This is particularly important in patients taking desvenlafaxine, which has been noted to cause a sustained increase in blood pressure or heart rate. Dose-related increase in systolic and diastolic blood pressure have also been reported.

Effects on Dental Treatment Key adverse event(s) related to dental treatment: Significant xerostomia (normal salivary flow resumes upon discontinuation). See Effects on Bleeding.

Effects on Bleeding May impair platelet aggregation resulting in increased risk of bleeding events, particularly if used concomitantly with aspirin, NSAIDs, warfarin, or other anticoagulants. Bleeding related to SSRI use has been reported to range from relatively minor bruising and epistaxis to life-threatening hemorrhage. Routine interruption of therapy for most dental procedures is not warranted. In medically complicated patients or extensive oral surgery, the decision to interrupt therapy must be based on the risk to benefit in an individual patient and a medical consult is suggested. If therapy is continued without interruption, the clinician should anticipate the potential for a prolonged bleeding time.

Adverse Effects Reported for 50-100 mg/day.

>10%:

Central nervous system: Dizziness (10% to 13%), insomnia (9% to 12%)

Gastrointestinal: Nausea (22% to 26%), xerostomia (11% to 17%), diarrhea (9% to 11%)

Miscellaneous: Diaphoresis (10% to 11%)

1% to 10%:

Cardiovascular: Palpitation (≤3%), orthostatic hypotension (<2%; elderly 8%), syncope (<2%), hypertension (dose related; ≤1% of patients taking 50-100 mg daily had sustained diastolic BP ≥90 mm Hg)

Central nervous system: Somnolence (≤9%), fatigue (7%), anxiety (3% to 5%), abnormal dreams (2% to 3%), irritability (2%), vertigo (1% to 2%), feeling jittery (≤2%), depersonalization (<2%), extrapyramidal symptoms (<2%), hypomania (<2%), seizures (<2%), concentration decreased (≤1%)

Dermatologic: Rash (1%)

Endocrine & metabolic: Libido decreased (males 4% to 5%), cholesterol (increased by ≥50 mg/dL and ≥261 mg/dL: 3% to 4%), anorgasmia (females 1%; males ≤3%), hot flushes (1%), low density lipoprotein cholesterol (increased by ≥50 mg/dL and ≥190 mg/dL: ≤1%), sexual dysfunction (males ≤1%)

Gastrointestinal: Constipation (9%), anorexia (5% to 8%), vomiting (≤4%), weight loss (≤2%), weight gain (<2%)

Genitourinary: Urinary hesitancy (≤1%)

Hepatic: Liver function tests abnormal (<2%)

Neuromuscular & skeletal: Tremor (≤3%), paresthesia (2%), weakness (≤2%), stiffness (<2%)

Ocular: Blurred vision (3% to 4%), mydriasis (2%)

Otic: Tinnitus (≤2%)

Renal: Proteinuria (6% to 8%)

Respiratory: Epistaxis (<2%)

Miscellaneous: Ejaculation retarded (1% to 5%), erectile dysfunction (3% to 6%), hypersensitivity reaction (<2%), yawning (1%), ejaculation failure (≤1%)

Class-wide adverse effects: Gastrointestinal hemorrhage, hallucinations, photosensitivity

General Dosage Range Dosage adjustment recommended in patients with hepatic or renal impairment

Oral: *Adults:* Initial: 50 mg once daily

Mechanism of Action Desvenlafaxine is a potent and selective serotonin and norepinephrine reuptake inhibitor.

Pharmacodynamics/Kinetics

Half-life Elimination ~11 hours; prolonged in renal failure

Time to Peak Serum: ~7.5 hours

Pregnancy Risk Factor C

Dexamethasone (Systemic) (deks a METH a sone)

Related Information

Respiratory Diseases *on page 1876*

Ulcerative, Erosive, and Painful Oral Mucosal Disorders *on page 1950*

Related Sample Prescriptions

Erosive Lichen Planus, Other Biopsy-Proven Desquamative Oral Diseases, and Major Aphthae *on page 1992*

Recurrent Aphthous Stomatitis *on page 1992*

U.S. Brand Names Baycadron™; Dexamethasone Intensol™; DexPak® 10 Day TaperPak®; DexPak® 13 Day TaperPak®; DexPak® 6 Day TaperPak®

Canadian Brand Names Apo-Dexamethasone®; Dexasone®

Generic Availability (U.S.) Yes

Pharmacologic Category Anti-inflammatory Agent; Antiemetic; Corticosteroid, Systemic

Dental Use Treatment of a variety of oral diseases of allergic, inflammatory or autoimmune origin; aphthous stomatitis (systemic dexamethasone used topically); lichen planus (erosive) and other oral vesiculoerosive diseases

Use Primarily as an anti-inflammatory or immunosuppressant agent in the treatment of a variety of diseases including those of allergic, dermatologic, endocrine, hematologic, inflammatory, neoplastic, nervous system, renal, respiratory, rheumatic, and autoimmune origin; may be used in management of cerebral edema, chronic swelling, as a diagnostic agent, diagnosis of Cushing's syndrome, antiemetic

Unlabeled/Investigational Use

Dexamethasone suppression test: General indicator consistent with depression and/or suicide

Accelerate fetal lung maturation in patients with preterm labor

Local Anesthetic/Vasoconstrictor Precautions No information available to require special precautions

Effects on Dental Treatment No significant effects or complications reported

Effects on Bleeding No information available to require special precautions

Adverse Effects Frequency not defined.

Cardiovascular: Arrhythmia, bradycardia, cardiac arrest, cardiomyopathy, CHF, circulatory collapse, edema, hypertension, myocardial rupture (post-MI), syncope, thromboembolism, vasculitis

Central nervous system: Depression, emotional instability, euphoria, headache, intracranial pressure increased, insomnia, malaise, mood swings, neuritis, personality changes, pseudotumor cerebri (usually following discontinuation), psychic disorders, seizure, vertigo

Dermatologic: Acne, allergic dermatitis, alopecia, angioedema, bruising, dry skin, erythema, fragile skin, hirsutism, hyper-/hypopigmentation, hypertrichosis, perianal pruritus (following I.V. injection), petechiae, rash, skin atrophy, skin test reaction impaired, striae, urticaria, wound healing impaired

Endocrine & metabolic: Adrenal suppression, carbohydrate tolerance decreased, Cushing's syndrome, diabetes mellitus, glucose intolerance decreased, growth suppression (children), hyperglycemia, hypokalemic alkalosis, menstrual irregularities, negative nitrogen balance, pituitary-adrenal axis suppression, protein catabolism, sodium retention

Gastrointestinal: Abdominal distention, appetite increased, gastrointestinal hemorrhage, gastrointestinal perforation, nausea, pancreatitis, peptic ulcer, ulcerative esophagitis, weight gain

Genitourinary: Altered (increased or decreased) spermatogenesis

Hepatic: Hepatomegaly, transaminases increased

Local: Postinjection flare (intra-articular use), thrombophlebitis

Neuromuscular & skeletal: Arthropathy, aseptic necrosis (femoral and humoral heads), fractures, muscle mass loss, myopathy (particularly in conjunction with neuromuscular disease or neuromuscular-blocking agents), neuropathy, osteoporosis, parasthesia, tendon rupture, vertebral compression fractures, weakness

Ocular: Cataracts, exophthalmos, glaucoma, intraocular pressure increased

Renal: Glucosuria

Respiratory: Pulmonary edema

Miscellaneous: Abnormal fat deposition, anaphylactoid reaction, anaphylaxis, avascular necrosis, diaphoresis, hiccups, hypersensitivity, impaired wound healing, infections, Kaposi's sarcoma, moon face, secondary malignancy

Dental Usual Dosage

Erosive lichen planus and major aphthae: Oral: For 3 days, rinse with 1 tablespoonful (15 mL) 4 times/day and swallow; then for 3 days, rinse with 1 teaspoonful (5 mL) 4 times/day and swallow; then for 3 days, rinse with 1 teaspoonful (5 mL) 4 times/day and swallow every other time. Then for 3 days rinse with 1 teaspoonful (5 mL) 4 times/day and expectorate. Continue the rinse and expectorate mode for 2 minutes, but discontinue medication when mouth becomes completely comfortable.

Recurrent aphthous stomatitis: Rinse with 1 teaspoonful for 2 minutes 4 times/day and expectorate

Dosage Refer to individual protocols.

Children:

Antiemetic (prior to chemotherapy): Refer to individual protocols and emetogenic potential: I.V.: 10 mg/m^2/dose every 12-24 hours on days of chemotherapy for severely emetogenic chemotherapy courses

Anti-inflammatory immunosuppressant: Oral, I.M., I.V.: 0.08-0.3 mg/kg/day **or** 2.5-10 mg/m^2/day in divided doses every 6-12 hours

Extubation or airway edema: Oral, I.M., I.V.: 0.5-2 mg/kg/day in divided doses every 6 hours beginning 24 hours prior to extubation and continuing for 4-6 doses afterwards

Cerebral edema: I.V.: Loading dose: 1-2 mg/kg/dose as a single dose; maintenance: 1-1.5 mg/kg/day (maximum: 16 mg/day) in divided doses every 4-6 hours, taper off over 1-6 weeks

Bacterial meningitis: Infants and Children >6 weeks: I.V.: 0.15 mg/kg/dose every 6 hours for the first 2-4 days of antibiotic treatment; start dexamethasone 10-20 minutes before or with the first dose of antibiotic

Physiologic replacement: Oral, I.M., I.V.: 0.03-0.15 mg/kg/day **or** 0.6-0.75 mg/m^2/day in divided doses every 6-12 hours

Adults:
Antiemetic:
Prophylaxis: Oral, I.V.: 10-20 mg 15-30 minutes before treatment on each treatment day
Continuous infusion regimen: Oral or I.V.: 10 mg every 12 hours on each treatment day
Mildly emetogenic therapy: Oral, I.M., I.V.: 4 mg every 4-6 hours
Delayed nausea/vomiting: Oral: 4-10 mg 1-2 times/day for 2-4 days **or**
8 mg every 12 hours for 2 days; then
4 mg every 12 hours for 2 days **or**
20 mg 1 hour before chemotherapy; then
10 mg 12 hours after chemotherapy; then
8 mg every 12 hours for 4 doses; then
4 mg every 12 hours for 4 doses
Anti-inflammatory:
Oral, I.M., I.V. (injections should be given as sodium phosphate): 0.75-9 mg/day in divided doses every 6-12 hours
Intra-articular, intralesional, or soft tissue (as sodium phosphate): 0.4-6 mg/day
Multiple myeloma: Oral, I.V.: 40 mg/day, days 1 to 4, 9 to 12, and 17 to 20, repeated every 4 weeks (alone or as part of a regimen)
Cerebral edema: I.V. 10 mg stat, 4 mg I.M./I.V. every 6 hours until response is maximized, then switch to oral regimen, then taper off if appropriate; dosage may be reduced after 2-4 days and gradually discontinued over 5-7 days
Extubation or airway edema: Oral, I.M., I.V. (injections should be given as sodium phosphate): 0.5-2 mg/kg/day in divided doses every 6 hours beginning 24 hours prior to extubation and continuing for 4-6 doses afterwards
Dexamethasone suppression test (depression/suicide indicator) (unlabeled use): Oral: 1 mg at 11 PM, draw blood at 8 AM the following day for plasma cortisol determination
Cushing's syndrome, diagnostic: Oral: 1 mg at 11 PM, draw blood at 8 AM; greater accuracy for Cushing's syndrome may be achieved by the following:
Dexamethasone 0.5 mg by mouth every 6 hours for 48 hours (with 24-hour urine collection for 17-hydroxycorticosteroid excretion)
Differentiation of Cushing's syndrome due to ACTH excess from Cushing's due to other causes: Oral: Dexamethasone 2 mg every 6 hours for 48 hours (with 24-hour urine collection for 17-hydroxycorticosteroid excretion)
Multiple sclerosis (acute exacerbation): 30 mg/day for 1 week, followed by 4-12 mg/day for 1 month
Physiological replacement: Oral, I.M., I.V. (should be given as sodium phosphate): 0.03-0.15 mg/kg/day **or** 0.6-0.75 mg/m^2/day in divided doses every 6-12 hours
Treatment of shock:
Addisonian crisis/shock (ie, adrenal insufficiency/responsive to steroid therapy): I.V. (given as sodium phosphate): 4-10 mg as a single dose, which may be repeated if necessary
Unresponsive shock (ie, unresponsive to steroid therapy): I.V. (given as sodium phosphate): 1-6 mg/kg as a single I.V. dose or up to 40 mg initially followed by repeat doses every 2-6 hours while shock persists
Hemodialysis: Supplemental dose is not necessary
Peritoneal dialysis: Supplemental dose is not necessary

Mechanism of Action Decreases inflammation by suppression of neutrophil migration, decreased production of inflammatory mediators, and reversal of increased capillary permeability; suppresses normal immune response. Dexamethasone's mechanism of antiemetic activity is unknown.

Contraindications Hypersensitivity to dexamethasone or any component of the formulation; systemic fungal infections, cerebral malaria

Warnings/Precautions Use with caution in patients with thyroid disease, hepatic impairment, renal impairment, cardiovascular disease, diabetes, glaucoma, cataracts, myasthenia gravis, patients at risk for osteoporosis, patients at risk for seizures, or GI diseases (diverticulitis, peptic ulcer, ulcerative colitis) due to perforation risk. Use caution following acute MI (corticosteroids have been associated with myocardial rupture). Because of the risk of adverse effects, systemic corticosteroids should be used cautiously in the elderly in the smallest possible effective dose for the shortest duration. May affect growth velocity; growth should be routinely monitored in pediatric patients. Withdraw therapy with gradual tapering of dose.

May cause hypercorticism or suppression of hypothalamic-pituitary-adrenal (HPA) axis, particularly in younger children or in patients receiving high doses for prolonged periods. HPA axis suppression may lead to adrenal crisis. Withdrawal and discontinuation of a corticosteroid should be done slowly and carefully. Particular care is required when patients are transferred from systemic corticosteroids to inhaled products due to possible adrenal insufficiency or withdrawal from steroids, including an increase in allergic symptoms. Patients receiving >20 mg per day of prednisone (or equivalent) may be most susceptible. Fatalities have occurred due to adrenal insufficiency in asthmatic patients during and after transfer from systemic corticosteroids to aerosol steroids; aerosol steroids do not provide the systemic steroid needed to treat patients having trauma, surgery, or infections. Dexamethasone does not provide adequate mineralocorticoid activity in adrenal insufficiency (may be employed as a single dose while cortisol assays are performed). The lowest possible dose should be used during treatment; discontinuation and/or dose reductions should be gradual.

Acute myopathy has been reported with high dose corticosteroids, usually in patients with neuromuscular transmission disorders; may involve ocular and/or respiratory muscles; monitor creatine kinase; recovery may be delayed. Corticosteroid use may cause psychiatric disturbances, including depression, euphoria, insomnia, mood swings, and personality changes. Pre-existing psychiatric conditions may be exacerbated by corticosteroid use. Prolonged use of corticosteroids may also increase the incidence of secondary infection, mask acute infection (including fungal infections), prolong or exacerbate viral infections, or limit response to vaccines. Exposure to chickenpox should be avoided; corticosteroids should not be used to treat ocular herpes simplex. Corticosteroids should not be used for cerebral malaria or viral hepatitis. Close observation is required in patients with latent tuberculosis and/or TB reactivity; restrict use in active TB (only in conjunction with antituberculosis treatment). Prolonged treatment with corticosteroids has been associated with the development of Kaposi's sarcoma (case reports); if noted, discontinuation of therapy should be considered. High-dose corticosteroids should not be used to manage acute head injury.

Drug Interactions

Metabolism/Transport Effects Substrate of CYP3A4 (major), P-glycoprotein; **Induces** CYP2A6 (weak), CYP2B6 (weak), CYP2C8 (weak), CYP2C9 (weak), CYP3A4 (strong), P-glycoprotein

Avoid Concomitant Use

Avoid concomitant use of Dexamethasone (Systemic) with any of the following: Aldesleukin; BCG; Dabigatran Etexilate; Dronedarone; Everolimus; Lurasidone; Natalizumab; Nilotinib; Nisoldipine; Pazopanib; Pimecrolimus; Praziquantel; Ranolazine; Roflumilast; RomiDEPsin; Tacrolimus (Topical); Tolvaptan; Vandetanib

Increased Effect/Toxicity

Dexamethasone (Systemic) may increase the levels/effects of: Acetylcholinesterase Inhibitors; Amphotericin B; CycloSPORINE; CycloSPORINE (Systemic); Deferasirox; Leflunomide; Lenalidomide; Loop Diuretics; Natalizumab; NSAID (COX-2 Inhibitor); NSAID (Nonselective); Thalidomide; Thiazide Diuretics; Vaccines (Live); Warfarin

The levels/effects of Dexamethasone (Systemic) may be increased by: Antifungal Agents (Azole Derivatives, Systemic); Aprepitant; Asparaginase; Calcium Channel Blockers (Nondihydropyridine); Conivaptan; CycloSPORINE; CycloSPORINE (Systemic); CYP3A4 Inhibitors (Moderate); CYP3A4 Inhibitors (Strong); Dasatinib; Denosumab; Estrogen Derivatives; Fluconazole; Fosaprepitant; Macrolide Antibiotics; Neuromuscular-Blocking Agents (Nondepolarizing); P-Glycoprotein Inhibitors; Pimecrolimus; Quinolone Antibiotics; Roflumilast; Salicylates; Tacrolimus (Topical); Trastuzumab

Decreased Effect

Dexamethasone (Systemic) may decrease the levels/effects of: Aldesleukin; Antidiabetic Agents; BCG; Calcitriol; Caspofungin; Corticorelin; CycloSPORINE; CycloSPORINE (Systemic); CYP3A4 Substrates; Dabigatran Etexilate; Dronedarone; Everolimus; Exemestane; Gefitinib; GuanFACINE; Imatinib; Isoniazid; Ixabepilone; Lurasidone; Maraviroc; NIFEdipine; Nilotinib; Nisoldipine; Pazopanib; P-Glycoprotein Substrates; Praziquantel; Ranolazine; RomiDEPsin; Salicylates; Sipuleucel-T; SORAfenib; Tadalafil; Tolvaptan; Ulipristal; Vaccines (Inactivated); Vandetanib

The levels/effects of Dexamethasone (Systemic) may be decreased by: Aminoglutethimide; Antacids; Barbiturates; Bile Acid Sequestrants; CYP3A4 Inducers (Strong); Echinacea; Herbs (CYP3A4 Inducers); Mitotane; P-Glycoprotein Inducers; Primidone; Rifamycin Derivatives; Tocilizumab

Ethanol/Nutrition/Herb Interactions

Ethanol: Avoid ethanol (may enhance gastric mucosal irritation).

Food: Dexamethasone interferes with calcium absorption. Limit caffeine.

Herb/Nutraceutical: Avoid cat's claw, echinacea (have immunostimulant properties).

Dietary Considerations May be taken with meals to decrease GI upset. May need diet with increased potassium, pyridoxine, vitamin C, vitamin D, folate, calcium, and phosphorus.

Pharmacodynamics/Kinetics

Onset of Action Acetate: Prompt

Duration of Action Metabolic effect: 72 hours; acetate is a long-acting repository preparation

Half-life Elimination Normal renal function: 1.8-3.5 hours; Biological half-life: 36-54 hours

Time to Peak Serum: Oral: 1-2 hours; I.M.: ~8 hours

Pregnancy Risk Factor C

Lactation Excretion in breast milk unknown/use caution

Breast-Feeding Considerations Corticosteroids are excreted in human milk; information specific to dexamethasone has not been located.

Dosage Forms

Elixir, oral: 0.5 mg/5 mL (237 mL)
 Baycadron™: 0.5 mg/5 mL (237 mL)

Injection, solution: 4 mg/mL (1 mL, 5 mL, 30 mL); 10 mg/mL (1 mL, 10 mL)

Injection, solution [preservative free]: 10 mg/mL (1 mL)

Solution, oral: 0.5 mg/5 mL (240 mL, 500 mL)
 Dexamethasone Intensol™: 1 mg/mL (30 mL)

Tablet, oral: 0.5 mg, 0.75 mg, 1 mg, 1.5 mg, 2 mg, 4 mg, 6 mg
 DexPak® 6 Day TaperPak®: 1.5 mg
 DexPak® 10 Day TaperPak®: 1.5 mg
 DexPak® 13 Day TaperPak®: 1.5 mg

Dexbrompheniramine and Pseudoephedrine

(deks brom fen EER a meen & soo doe e FED rin)

Related Information
 Pseudoephedrine *on page 1429*

Canadian Brand Names Drixoral®

Pharmacologic Category Alkylamine Derivative; Alpha/Beta Agonist; Decongestant; Histamine H_1 Antagonist; Histamine H_1 Antagonist, First Generation

Use Relief of symptoms of upper respiratory mucosal congestion in seasonal and perennial nasal allergies, acute rhinitis, rhinosinusitis, and eustachian tube blockage

Local Anesthetic/Vasoconstrictor Precautions Use with caution since pseudoephedrine is a sympathomimetic amine which could interact with epinephrine to cause a pressor response

Effects on Dental Treatment Key adverse event(s) related to dental treatment: Pseudoephedrine: Xerostomia (normal salivary flow resumes upon discontinuation)

Effects on Bleeding No information available to require special precautions

General Dosage Range Oral: *Children >12 years and Adults:* 1 tablet every 8-12 hours

Pregnancy Risk Factor B

Dexchlorpheniramine (deks klor fen EER a meen)

Pharmacologic Category Alkylamine Derivative; Histamine H_1 Antagonist; Histamine H_1 Antagonist, First Generation

Use Perennial and seasonal allergic rhinitis and other allergic symptoms including urticaria

Local Anesthetic/Vasoconstrictor Precautions No information available to require special precautions

Effects on Dental Treatment Key adverse event(s) related to dental treatment: Significant xerostomia (normal salivary flow resumes upon discontinuation)

Effects on Bleeding No information available to require special precautions

Adverse Effects

>10%:
 Central nervous system: Slight to moderate drowsiness
 Respiratory: Thickening of bronchial secretions

1% to 10%:
 Central nervous system: Headache, fatigue, nervousness, dizziness
 Gastrointestinal: Appetite increase, weight gain, nausea, diarrhea, abdominal pain, xerostomia
 Neuromuscular & skeletal: Arthralgia
 Respiratory: Pharyngitis

General Dosage Range Oral:

Regular release:
 Children 2-5 years: 0.5 mg every 4-6 hours
 Children 6-11 years: 1 mg every 4-6 hours
 Adults: 2 mg every 4-6 hours

Timed release:
Children 6-11 years: 4 mg at bedtime
Adults: 4-6 mg at bedtime **or** every 8-10 hours

Mechanism of Action Competes with histamine for H_1-receptor sites on effector cells in the gastrointestinal tract, blood vessels, and respiratory tract. Dexchlorpheniramine is the predominant active isomer of chlorpheniramine and is approximately twice as active as the racemic compound.

Pharmacodynamics/Kinetics
Onset of Action ~1 hour
Duration of Action 3-6 hours

Pregnancy Risk Factor B

Dexlansoprazole (deks lan SOE pra zole)

Related Information
Gastrointestinal Disorders *on page* 1874

U.S. Brand Names Dexilant™

Canadian Brand Names Dexilant™

Pharmacologic Category Proton Pump Inhibitor; Substituted Benzimidazole

Use Short-term (4 weeks) treatment of heartburn associated with nonerosive GERD; short-term (up to 8 weeks) treatment of all grades of erosive esophagitis; to maintain healing of erosive esophagitis for up to 6 months

Local Anesthetic/Vasoconstrictor Precautions No information available to require special precautions

Effects on Dental Treatment Key adverse event(s) related to dental treatment: Xerostomia (normal salivary flow resumes upon discontinuation) and taste alteration has been reported in <2% of patients.

Effects on Bleeding No information available to require special precautions

Adverse Effects 2% to 10%:
Gastrointestinal: Diarrhea (5%), abdominal pain (4%), nausea (3%), flatulence (1% to 3%), vomiting (1% to 2%)
Respiratory: Upper respiratory tract infection (2% to 3%)

General Dosage Range Dosage adjustment recommended in patients with hepatic impairment
Oral: *Adults:* 30-60 mg once daily

Mechanism of Action Proton pump inhibitor; decreases acid secretion in gastric parietal cells through inhibition of (H+, K+)-ATPase enzyme system, blocking the final step in gastric acid production

Pharmacodynamics/Kinetics
Half-life Elimination ~1-2 hours
Time to Peak Serum: **Note:** Two distinct peaks secondary to dual release formulation:
Peak 1: 1-2 hours
Peak 2: 4-5 hours

Pregnancy Risk Factor B

Dexmedetomidine (deks MED e toe mi deen)

U.S. Brand Names Precedex®

Canadian Brand Names Precedex®

Pharmacologic Category $Alpha_2$-Adrenergic Agonist; Sedative

Use Sedation of initially intubated and mechanically ventilated patients during treatment in an intensive care setting; sedation prior to and/or during surgical or other procedures of nonintubated patients

Unlabeled/Investigational Use Unlabeled uses include premedication prior to anesthesia induction with thiopental; relief of pain and reduction of opioid dose following laparoscopic tubal ligation; as an adjunct anesthetic in ophthalmic surgery; treatment of shivering; premedication to attenuate the cardiostimulatory and postanesthetic delirium of ketamine; use in children

Local Anesthetic/Vasoconstrictor Precautions No information available to require special precautions

Effects on Dental Treatment Key adverse event(s) related to dental treatment: Xerostomia and changes in salivation (normal salivary flow resumes upon discontinuation)

Effects on Bleeding No information available to require special precautions

Adverse Effects
>10%:
Cardiovascular: Hypotension (24% to 54%), bradycardia (5% to 14%)
Respiratory: Respiratory depression (37%; placebo 32%)

1% to 10%:
Cardiovascular: Atrial fibrillation (4% to 5%), hypovolemia (3%)
Endocrine & metabolic: Hypocalcemia (1%)
Gastrointestinal: Nausea (3% to 9%), xerostomia (3% to 4%)
Renal: Urine output decreased (1%)
Respiratory: Pleural effusion (2%), wheezing (≤1%)

General Dosage Range I.V.: *Adults:* Loading infusion: 0.5-1 mcg/kg; Maintenance infusion: 0.2-1 mcg/kg/**hour**

Mechanism of Action Selective alpha$_2$-adrenoceptor agonist with anesthetic and sedative properties thought to be due to activation of G-proteins by apha$_{2a}$-adrenoceptors in the brainstem resulting in inhibition of norepinephrine release; peripheral alpha$_{2b}$-adrenoceptors are activated at high doses or with rapid I.V. administration resulting in vasoconstriction.

Pharmacodynamics/Kinetics
Onset of Action I.V. Bolus: 5-10 minutes; Peak effect: 15-30 minutes
Duration of Action Dose dependent: 60-120 minutes
Half-life Elimination ~6 minutes; Terminal: ~2 hours

Pregnancy Risk Factor C

Dexmethylphenidate (dex meth il FEN i date)

U.S. Brand Names Focalin®; Focalin® XR
Pharmacologic Category Central Nervous System Stimulant
Use Treatment of attention-deficit/hyperactivity disorder (ADHD)
Local Anesthetic/Vasoconstrictor Precautions No information available to require special precautions
Effects on Dental Treatment Key adverse event(s) related to dental treatment: Xerostomia (normal salivary flow resumes upon discontinuation).
Effects on Bleeding No information available to require special precautions
Adverse Effects Actual frequency may be dependent upon dose and/or formulation.

>10%:
Central nervous system: Headache (25% to 39%), insomnia (children 5% to 17%), restlessness (adults 12%), anxiety (5% to 11%)
Gastrointestinal: Appetite decreased (children 30%), xerostomia (adults 7% to 20%), abdominal pain (children 15%)

1% to 10%:
Central nervous system: Dizziness (adults 6%), fever (children 5%), irritability (children ≤5%), depression (children ≤3%), mood swings (children ≤3%)
Dermatologic: Pruritus (children ≤3%)
Gastrointestinal: Nausea (children 9%), dyspepsia (5% to 9%), vomiting (children 2% to 9%), anorexia (children 5% to 7%), pharyngolaryngeal pain (adults 4% to 7%)
Respiratory: Nasal congestion (children ≤5%)

Frequency not defined: Ocular: Accommodation difficulties, blurred vision
Also refer to Methylphenidate for adverse effects seen with other methylphenidate products.

General Dosage Range Oral:
Extended release:
Children ≥6 years: Initial: 5 mg once daily; Maintenance: Up to 30 mg/day
Adults: Initial: 10 mg once daily; Maintenance: Up to 40 mg/day
Immediate release: *Children ≥6 years and Adults:* Initial: 2.5 mg twice daily; Maintenance: Up to 20 mg/day in 2 divided doses (at least 4 hours apart)

Mechanism of Action Dexmethylphenidate is the more active, *d-threo*-enantiomer, of racemic methylphenidate. It is a CNS stimulant; blocks the reuptake of norepinephrine and dopamine, and increases their release into the extraneuronal space.

Pharmacodynamics/Kinetics
Onset of Action Extended release: ≥0.5 hours
Duration of Action Extended release: 12 hours
Half-life Elimination Immediate release: Adults: 2-4.5 hours; children: 2-3 hours
Time to Peak Fasting:
Immediate release: 1-1.5 hours
Extended release: First peak: 1.5 hours (range: 1-4 hours); Second peak: 6.5 hours (range: 4.5-7 hours)

Pregnancy Risk Factor C
Controlled Substance C-II

Dexpanthenol (deks PAN the nole)

Pharmacologic Category Gastrointestinal Agent, Stimulant; Topical Skin Product

Use Prophylactic use to minimize paralytic ileus; treatment of postoperative distention; topical to relieve itching and to aid healing of minor dermatoses

Local Anesthetic/Vasoconstrictor Precautions No information available to require special precautions

Effects on Dental Treatment No significant effects or complications reported

Effects on Bleeding No information available to require special precautions

Adverse Effects Frequency not defined.

Cardiovascular: Slight drop in blood pressure
Central nervous system: Agitation
Dermatologic: Dermatitis, irritation, itching, urticaria
Gastrointestinal: Diarrhea, hyperperistalsis, vomiting
Neuromuscular & skeletal: Paresthesia
Respiratory: Dyspnea
Miscellaneous: Allergic reactions

General Dosage Range I.M.: *Adults:* Initial: 250-500 mg; repeat in 2 hours, followed by doses every 6 hours if needed

Mechanism of Action A pantothenic acid B vitamin analog that is converted to coenzyme A internally; coenzyme A is essential to normal fatty acid synthesis, amino acid synthesis and acetylation of choline in the production of the neurotransmitter, acetylcholine

Pregnancy Risk Factor C

Dexrazoxane (deks ray ZOKS ane)

U.S. Brand Names Totect®; Zinecard®

Canadian Brand Names Zinecard®

Pharmacologic Category Antidote; Cardioprotectant

Use

Zinecard®: Reduction of the incidence and severity of cardiomyopathy associated with doxorubicin administration in women with metastatic breast cancer who have received a cumulative doxorubicin dose of 300 mg/m^2 and who would benefit from continuing therapy with doxorubicin. (Not recommended for use with initial doxorubicin therapy.)

Totect®: Treatment of anthracycline-induced extravasation.

Unlabeled/Investigational Use Reduction of the incidence and severity of cardiomyopathy associated with doxorubicin administration (cumulative doses >300 mg/m^2) in patients with malignancies other than metastatic breast cancer who would benefit from continuing therapy with doxorubicin; reduction of the incidence and severity of cardiomyopathy associated with continued epirubicin administration for advanced breast cancer

Local Anesthetic/Vasoconstrictor Precautions No information available to require special precautions

Effects on Dental Treatment No significant effects or complications reported

Effects on Bleeding Chemotherapy may result in significant myelosuppression, potentially including significant reduction in platelet counts and altered hemostasis. In patients who are under active treatment with these agents, medical consult is suggested.

Adverse Effects Note: Most adverse reactions are thought to be attributed to chemotherapy, except for increased myelosuppression, pain at injection site, and phlebitis.

Prevention of doxorubicin cardiomyopathy (reactions listed are those which were greater in the dexrazoxane arm in a comparison of chemotherapy plus dexrazoxane vs chemotherapy alone):

Central nervous system: Fatigue/malaise, fever
Dermatologic: Alopecia, streaking/erythema
Endocrine & metabolic: Serum calcium decreased, serum triglycerides increased
Gastrointestinal: Serum amylase increased
Hematologic: Granulocytopenia, hemorrhage, leukopenia, myelosuppression, neutropenia, thrombocytopenia
Local: Extravasation, injection site pain, phlebitis
Neuromuscular & skeletal: Neurotoxicity
Miscellaneous: Infection, sepsis

Anthracycline extravasation:

Cardiovascular: Peripheral edema
Central nervous system: Depression, dizziness, fatigue, fever, headache, insomnia
Dermatologic: Alopecia
Endocrine & metabolic: Hypercalcemia, hyponatremia
Gastrointestinal: Abdominal pain, anorexia, constipation, diarrhea, nausea, vomiting

Hematologic: Anemia, leukopenia, neutropenia, neutropenic fever, thrombocytopenia
Hepatic: Alkaline phosphatase increased, ALT increased, AST increased, bilirubin increased, LDH increased
Local: Injection site pain/discomfort, phlebitis
Renal: Creatinine increased
Respiratory: Cough, dyspnea, pneumonia
Miscellaneous: Infection

General Dosage Range Dosage adjustment recommended in patients with renal impairment

I.V.: *Adults:* A 10:1 ratio of dexrazoxane:doxorubicin (500 mg/m^2 dexrazoxane: 50 mg/m^2 doxorubicin) **or** 1000 mg/m^2 on days 1 and 2 (maximum dose: 2000 mg), followed by 500 mg/m^2 on day 3 (maximum dose: 1000 mg)

Mechanism of Action Derivative of ethylenediaminetetraacetic acid (EDTA); potent intracellular chelating agent. The mechanism of cardioprotectant activity is not fully understood. Appears to be converted intracellularly to a ring-opened chelating agent that interferes with iron-mediated oxygen free radical generation thought to be responsible, in part, for anthracycline-induced cardiomyopathy. In the management of anthracycline-induced extravasation, dexrazoxane may act by reversibly inhibiting topoisomerase II, protecting tissue from anthracycline cytotoxicity, thereby decreasing tissue damage.

Pharmacodynamics/Kinetics

Half-life Elimination 2-2.5 hours

Pregnancy Risk Factor C (Zinecard®) / D (Totect®)

Dextran (DEKS tran)

U.S. Brand Names LMD®

Pharmacologic Category Plasma Volume Expander

Use Blood volume expander used in treatment of shock or impending shock when blood or blood products are not available; dextran 40 is also used as a priming fluid in cardiopulmonary bypass and for prophylaxis of venous thrombosis and pulmonary embolism in surgical procedures associated with a high risk of thromboembolic complications

Local Anesthetic/Vasoconstrictor Precautions No information available to require special precautions

Effects on Dental Treatment No significant effects or complications reported

Effects on Bleeding No information available to require special precautions, although caution in patients with active hemorrhage is recommended.

General Dosage Range I.V.:

Dextran 40:

Children: Total dose should not exceed 20 mL/kg during first 24 hours

Adults: 500-1000 mL at a rate of 20-40 mL/minute (maximum: 20 mL/kg/day for first 24 hours); 10 mL/kg/day thereafter (5 days total therapy) **or** 50-100 g on the day of surgery, then 50 g (4 mL/minute) every 2-3 days during the period of risk

Dextran 70:

Children: Total dose should not exceed 20 mL/kg during first 24 hours

Adults: 500-1000 mL at a rate of 20-40 mL/minute (maximum: 20 mL/kg/day for first 24 hours)

Mechanism of Action Produces plasma volume expansion by virtue of its highly colloidal starch structure, similar to albumin

Pharmacodynamics/Kinetics

Onset of Action Minutes to 1 hour (depending upon the molecular weight polysaccharide administered)

Pregnancy Risk Factor C

Dextroamphetamine (deks troe am FET a meen)

U.S. Brand Names Dexedrine® Spansule®; ProCentra®

Canadian Brand Names Dexedrine®

Pharmacologic Category Stimulant

Use Narcolepsy; attention-deficit/hyperactivity disorder (ADHD)

Unlabeled/Investigational Use Depression

Local Anesthetic/Vasoconstrictor Precautions Use vasoconstrictor with caution in patients taking dextroamphetamine. Amphetamines enhance the sympathomimetic response of epinephrine and norepinephrine leading to potential hypertension and cardiotoxicity.

Effects on Dental Treatment Key adverse event(s) related to dental treatment: Xerostomia (normal salivary flow resumes upon discontinuation). Up to 10% of patients taking dextroamphetamines may present with hypertension. Monitor blood pressure prior to using local anesthetic with vasoconstrictors.

Effects on Bleeding No information available to require special precautions

Adverse Effects Frequency not defined.

Cardiovascular: Cardiomyopathy, hypertension, palpitation, tachycardia

Central nervous system: Aggression, dizziness, dyskinesia, dysphoria, euphoria, exacerbation of motor and phonic tics, headache, insomnia, mania, overstimulation, psychosis, restlessness, Tourette's syndrome

Dermatologic: Urticaria

Endocrine & metabolic: Libido changes

Gastrointestinal: Anorexia, constipation, diarrhea, unpleasant taste, weight loss, xerostomia

Genitourinary: Impotence

Neuromuscular & skeletal: Tremor

Ocular: Accommodation abnormalities, blurred vision

General Dosage Range Oral:

Children 3-5 years: Initial: 2.5 mg once daily; Maintenance: 0.1-0.5 mg/kg once daily (maximum: 40 mg/day)

Children 6-12 years: Initial: 5 mg once or twice daily; Maintenance: 5-20 mg (0.1-0.5 mg/kg) once daily (maximum: 40 mg [ADHD]: 60 mg [narcolepsy])

Children >12 years: Initial: 5-10 mg/day in 1-2 divided doses; Maximum: Up to 40 mg/day [ADHD] or 60 mg/day [narcolepsy]

Adults: Initial: 10 mg once daily; Maximum: Up to 60 mg/day

Mechanism of Action Amphetamines are noncatecholamine, sympathomimetic amines that promote release of catecholamines (primarily dopamine and norepinephrine) from their storage sites in the presynaptic nerve terminals. A less significant mechanism may include their ability to block the reuptake of catecholamines by competitive inhibition.

Pharmacodynamics/Kinetics

Onset of Action 1-1.5 hours

Half-life Elimination Adults: 10-13 hours

Time to Peak Serum: Immediate release: ~3 hours; sustained release: ~8 hours

Pregnancy Risk Factor C

Controlled Substance C-II

Dextroamphetamine and Amphetamine

(deks troe am FET a meen & am FET a meen)

Related Information

Dextroamphetamine *on page 500*

U.S. Brand Names Adderall XR®; Adderall®

Canadian Brand Names Adderall XR®

Generic Availability (U.S.) Yes

Pharmacologic Category Stimulant

Use Attention-deficit/hyperactivity disorder (ADHD); narcolepsy

Local Anesthetic/Vasoconstrictor Precautions Use vasoconstrictor with caution in patients taking dextroamphetamine. Amphetamines enhance the sympathomimetic response of epinephrine and norepinephrine leading to potential hypertension and cardiotoxicity.

Effects on Dental Treatment Key adverse event(s) related to dental treatment: Tooth disorder; up to 10% of patients taking dextroamphetamines may present with hypertension. Monitor blood pressure prior to using local anesthetic with vasoconstrictors.

Effects on Bleeding No information available to require special precautions

Adverse Effects

As reported with Adderall XR®:

>10%:

Central nervous system: Insomnia (12% to 27%), headache (up to 26% in adults)

Gastrointestinal: Appetite decreased (22% to 36%), abdominal pain (11% to 14%), dry mouth (2% to 35%), weight loss (4% to 11%)

1% to 10%:

Cardiovascular: Tachycardia (up to 6% in adults), palpitation (2% to 4%)

Central nervous system: Emotional lability (2% to 9%), agitation (up to 8% in adults), anxiety (8%), dizziness (2% to 7%), nervousness (6%), fever (5%), somnolence (2% to 4%)

Dermatologic: Photosensitization (2% to 4%)

Endocrine & metabolic: Dysmenorrhea (2% to 4%), impotence (2% to 4%), libido decreased (2% to 4%)

Gastrointestinal: Nausea (2% to 8%), vomiting (2% to 7%), diarrhea (2% to 6%), constipation (2% to 4%), dyspepsia (2% to 4%), tooth disorder (2% to 4%)
Genitourinary: Urinary tract infection (5%)
Neuromuscular & skeletal: Twitching (2% to 4%), weakness (2% to 6%)
Respiratory: Dyspnea (2% to 4%)
Miscellaneous: Diaphoresis (2% to 4%), infection (2% to 4%), speech disorder (2% to 4%)

Adverse reactions reported with other amphetamines include: Adverse reactions reported with other amphetamines include: Anaphylaxis, angioedema, anorexia, cardiomyopathy, depression, dyskinesia, dysphoria, euphoria, exacerbation of motor and phonic tics, exacerbation of Tourette's syndrome, hypertension, MI, overstimulation, psychosis, rash, restlessness, seizure, stroke, taste disturbance, tremor, urticaria

Dosage Oral: **Note:** Use lowest effective individualized dose; administer first dose as soon as awake

ADHD:

Children: <3 years: Not recommended

Children: 3-5 years (Adderall®): Initial 2.5 mg/day given every morning; increase daily dose in 2.5 mg increments at weekly intervals until optimal response is obtained (maximum dose: 40 mg/day given in 1-3 divided doses); use intervals of 4-6 hours between additional doses

Children: ≥6 years:

Adderall®: Initial: 5 mg 1-2 times/day; increase daily dose in 5 mg increments at weekly intervals until optimal response is obtained (usual maximum dose: 40 mg/day given in 1-3 divided doses); use intervals of 4-6 hours between additional doses

Adderall XR®: 5-10 mg once daily in the morning; if needed, may increase daily dose in 5-10 mg increments at weekly intervals (maximum dose: 30 mg/day)

Adolescents 13-17 years (Adderall XR®): 10 mg once daily in the morning; maybe increased to 20 mg/day after 1 week if symptoms are not controlled; higher doses (up to 60 mg/day) have been evaluated; however, there is not adequate evidence that higher doses afford additional benefit.

Adults (Adderall XR®): Initial: 20 mg once daily in the morning; higher doses (up to 60 mg once daily) have been evaluated; however, there is not adequate evidence that higher doses afforded additional benefit

Narcolepsy (Adderall®):

Children: 6-12 years: Initial: 5 mg/day; increase daily dose in 5 mg at weekly intervals until optimal response is obtained (maximum dose: 60 mg/day given in 1-3 divided doses with intervals of 4-6 hours between doses)

Children >12 years and Adults: Initial: 10 mg/day; increase daily dose in 10 mg increments at weekly intervals until optimal response is obtained (maximum dose: 60 mg/day given in 1-3 divided doses with intervals of 4-6 hours between doses)

Mechanism of Action Amphetamines are noncatecholamine, sympathomimetic amines that promote release of catecholamines (primarily dopamine and norepinephrine) from their storage sites in the presynaptic nerve terminals. A less significant mechanism may include their ability to block the reuptake of catecholamines by competitive inhibition.

Contraindications Hypersensitivity to dextroamphetamine, amphetamine, or any component of the formulation; advanced arteriosclerosis; symptomatic cardiovascular disease; moderate-to-severe hypertension; hyperthyroidism; hypersensitivity or idiosyncrasy to the sympathomimetic amines; glaucoma; agitated states; patients with a history of drug abuse; with or within 14 days following MAO inhibitor (hypertensive crisis)

Warnings/Precautions [U.S. Boxed Warning]: Use has been associated with serious cardiovascular events including sudden death in patients with preexisting structural cardiac abnormalities or other serious heart problems (sudden death in children and adolescents; sudden death, stroke and MI in adults. These products should be avoided in the patients with known serious structural cardiac abnormalities, cardiomyopathy, serious heart rhythm abnormalities, or other serious cardiac problems that could increase the risk of sudden death that these conditions alone carry. Patients should be carefully evaluated for cardiac disease prior to initiation of therapy. Use with caution in patients with hypertension and other cardiovascular conditions that might be exacerbated by increases in blood pressure or heart rate. Amphetamines may impair the ability to engage in potentially hazardous activities. May cause visual disturbances.

Use with caution in patients with psychiatric or seizure disorders. May exacerbate symptoms of behavior and thought disorder in psychotic patients. Stimulants may unmask tics in individuals with coexisting Tourette's syndrome. **[U.S. Boxed Warning]: Potential for drug dependency exists; prolonged use may lead to drug dependency.** Use is contraindicated in patients with history of ethanol or drug abuse. Prescriptions should be written for the smallest quantity consistent with good patient care to minimize possibility of overdose. Abrupt discontinuation following high doses or for prolonged periods may result in symptoms for withdrawal.

May be inappropriate for use in the elderly due to CNS stimulant adverse effects (Beers Criteria). Safety and efficacy have not been established in children <3 years of age. Appetite suppression may occur; monitor weight during therapy, particularly in children. Use of stimulants has been associated with suppression of growth; monitor growth rate during treatment.

Drug Interactions

Metabolism/Transport Effects Amphetamine: **Inhibits** CYP2D6 (weak)

Avoid Concomitant Use

Avoid concomitant use of Dextroamphetamine and Amphetamine with any of the following: Iobenguane I 123; MAO Inhibitors

Increased Effect/Toxicity

Dextroamphetamine and Amphetamine may increase the levels/effects of: Analgesics (Opioid); Sympathomimetics

The levels/effects of Dextroamphetamine and Amphetamine may be increased by: Alkalinizing Agents; Antacids; Atomoxetine; Cannabinoids; Carbonic Anhydrase Inhibitors; MAO Inhibitors; Proton Pump Inhibitors; Tricyclic Antidepressants

Decreased Effect

Dextroamphetamine and Amphetamine may decrease the levels/effects of: Antihistamines; Ethosuximide; Iobenguane I 123; PHENobarbital; Phenytoin

The levels/effects of Dextroamphetamine and Amphetamine may be decreased by: Ammonium Chloride; Antipsychotics; Gastrointestinal Acidifying Agents; Lithium; Methenamine; Peginterferon Alfa-2b

Ethanol/Nutrition/Herb Interactions

Ethanol: Avoid ethanol (may increase CNS depression).

Food: Dextroamphetamine serum levels may be altered if taken with acidic food, juices, or vitamin C. Avoid caffeine.

Herb/Nutraceutical: Avoid ephedra (may cause hypertension or arrhythmias).

Pharmacodynamics/Kinetics

Onset of Action 30-60 minutes

Duration of Action 4-6 hours

Half-life Elimination

Children 6-12 years: d-amphetamine: 9 hours; l-amphetamine: 11 hours

Adolescents 13-17 years: d-amphetamine: 11 hours; l-amphetamine: 13-14 hours

Adults: d-amphetamine: 10 hours; l-amphetamine: 13 hours

Time to Peak T_{max}: Adderall®: 3 hours; Adderall XR®: 7 hours

Pregnancy Risk Factor C

Lactation Enters breast milk/contraindicated

Controlled Substance C-II

Dosage Forms

Capsule, extended release:

5 mg [dextroamphetamine sulfate 1.25 mg, dextroamphetamine saccharate 1.25 mg, amphetamine aspartate monohydrate 1.25 mg, amphetamine sulfate 1.25 mg]

10 mg [dextroamphetamine sulfate 2.5 mg, dextroamphetamine saccharate 2.5 mg, amphetamine aspartate monohydrate 2.5 mg, amphetamine sulfate 2.5 mg]

15 mg [dextroamphetamine sulfate 3.75 mg, dextroamphetamine saccharate 3.75 mg, amphetamine aspartate monohydrate 3.75 mg, amphetamine sulfate 3.75 mg]

20 mg [dextroamphetamine sulfate 5 mg, dextroamphetamine saccharate 5 mg, amphetamine aspartate monohydrate 5 mg, amphetamine sulfate 5 mg]

25 mg [dextroamphetamine sulfate 6.25 mg, dextroamphetamine saccharate 6.25 mg, amphetamine aspartate monohydrate 6.25 mg, amphetamine sulfate 6.25 mg]

30 mg [dextroamphetamine sulfate 7.5 mg, dextroamphetamine saccharate 7.5 mg, amphetamine aspartate monohydrate 7.5 mg, amphetamine sulfate 7.5 mg]

Adderall XR®:

5 mg [dextroamphetamine 1.25 mg, dextroamphetamine saccharate 1.25 mg, amphetamine aspartate monohydrate 1.25 mg, amphetamine sulfate 1.25 mg]

10 mg [dextroamphetamine sulfate 2.5 mg, dextroamphetamine saccharate 2.5 mg, amphetamine aspartate monohydrate 2.5 mg, amphetamine sulfate 2.5 mg]

15 mg [dextroamphetamine sulfate 3.75 mg, dextroamphetamine saccharate 3.75 mg, amphetamine aspartate monohydrate 3.75 mg, amphetamine sulfate 3.75 mg]

20 mg [dextroamphetamine sulfate 5 mg, dextroamphetamine saccharate 5 mg, amphetamine aspartate monohydrate 5 mg, amphetamine sulfate 5 mg]
25 mg [dextroamphetamine sulfate 6.25 mg, dextroamphetamine saccharate 6.25 mg, amphetamine aspartate monohydrate 6.25 mg, amphetamine sulfate 6.25 mg]
30 mg [dextroamphetamine sulfate 7.5 mg, dextroamphetamine saccharate 7.5 mg, amphetamine aspartate monohydrate 7.5 mg, amphetamine sulfate 7.5 mg]

Tablet: 5 mg, 7.5 mg, 10 mg, 12.5 mg, 15 mg, 20 mg, 30 mg
5 mg [dextroamphetamine sulfate 1.25 mg, dextroamphetamine saccharate 1.25 mg, amphetamine aspartate monohydrate 1.25 mg, amphetamine sulfate 1.25 mg]
7.5 mg [dextroamphetamine sulfate 1.875 mg, dextroamphetamine saccharate 1.875 mg, amphetamine aspartate monohydrate 1.875 mg, amphetamine sulfate 1.875 mg]
10 mg [dextroamphetamine sulfate 2.5 mg, dextroamphetamine saccharate 2.5 mg, amphetamine aspartate monohydrate 2.5 mg, amphetamine sulfate 2.5 mg]
12.5 mg [dextroamphetamine sulfate 3.125 mg, dextroamphetamine saccharate 3.125 mg, amphetamine aspartate monohydrate 3.125 mg, amphetamine sulfate 3.125 mg]
15 mg [dextroamphetamine sulfate 3.75 mg, dextroamphetamine saccharate 3.75 mg, amphetamine aspartate monohydrate 3.75 mg, amphetamine sulfate 3.75 mg]
20 mg [dextroamphetamine sulfate 5 mg, dextroamphetamine saccharate 5 mg, amphetamine aspartate monohydrate 5 mg, amphetamine sulfate 5 mg]
30 mg [dextroamphetamine sulfate 7.5 mg, dextroamphetamine saccharate 7.5 mg, amphetamine aspartate monohydrate 7.5 mg, amphetamine sulfate 7.5 mg]

Adderall®:
5 mg [dextroamphetamine sulfate 1.25 mg, dextroamphetamine saccharate 1.25 mg, amphetamine aspartate monohydrate 1.25 mg, amphetamine sulfate 1.25 mg]
7.5 mg [dextroamphetamine 1.875 mg, dextroamphetamine saccharate 1.875 mg, amphetamine aspartate monohydrate 1.875 mg, amphetamine sulfate 1.875 mg]
10 mg [dextroamphetamine sulfate 2.5 mg, dextroamphetamine saccharate 2.5 mg, amphetamine aspartate monohydrate 2.5 mg, amphetamine sulfate 2.5 mg]
12.5 mg [dextroamphetamine sulfate 3.125 mg, dextroamphetamine saccharate 3.125 mg, amphetamine aspartate monohydrate 3.125 mg, amphetamine sulfate 3.125 mg]
15 mg [dextroamphetamine sulfate 3.75 mg, dextroamphetamine saccharate 3.75 mg, amphetamine aspartate monohydrate 3.75 mg, amphetamine sulfate 3.75 mg]
20 mg [dextroamphetamine sulfate 5 mg, dextroamphetamine saccharate 5 mg, amphetamine aspartate monohydrate 5 mg, amphetamine sulfate 5 mg]
30 mg [dextroamphetamine sulfate 7.5 mg, dextroamphetamine saccharate 7.5 mg, amphetamine aspartate monohydrate 7.5 mg, amphetamine sulfate 7.5 mg]

Dextromethorphan (deks troe meth OR fan)

U.S. Brand Names Creo-Terpin® [OTC]; Creomulsion® Adult Formula [OTC]; Creomulsion® for Children [OTC]; Delsym® [OTC]; Father John's® [OTC]; Hold® DM [OTC]; Nycoff [OTC]; PediaCare® Children's Long-Acting Cough [OTC]; Robafen Cough [OTC]; Robitussin® Children's Cough Long-Acting [OTC]; Robitussin® Cough Long Acting [OTC]; Robitussin® CoughGels™ Long-Acting [OTC]; Scot-Tussin® Diabetes [OTC]; Silphen-DM [OTC]; Triaminic Thin Strips® Children's Long Acting Cough [OTC]; Triaminic® Children's Cough Long Acting [OTC]; Trocal® [OTC]; Vicks® 44® Cough Relief [OTC]; Vicks® DayQuil® Cough [OTC]

Pharmacologic Category Antitussive; N-Methyl-D-Aspartate Receptor Antagonist

Use Symptomatic relief of coughs caused by the common cold or inhaled irritants

Unlabeled/Investigational Use *N*-methyl-D-aspartate (NMDA) antagonist

Local Anesthetic/Vasoconstrictor Precautions No information available to require special precautions

Effects on Dental Treatment No significant effects or complications reported

Effects on Bleeding No information available to require special precautions

General Dosage Range Oral:

Extended release:

Children 4-6 years: 15 mg twice daily (maximum: 30 mg/day)

Children 6-12 years: 30 mg twice daily (maximum: 60 mg/day)

Children >12 years and Adults: 60 mg twice daily (maximum: 120 mg/day)

Immediate release:

Children 4-6 years: 2.5-7.5 mg every 4-8 hours (maximum: 30 mg/day)

Children 6-12 years: 5-10 mg every 4 hours **or** 15 mg every 6-8 hours (maximum: 60 mg/day)

Children >12 years and Adults: 10-20 mg every 4 hours **or** 30 mg every 6-8 hours (maximum: 120 mg/day)

Mechanism of Action Decreases the sensitivity of cough receptors and interrupts cough impulse transmission by depressing the medullary cough center through sigma receptor stimulation; structurally related to codeine

Pharmacodynamics/Kinetics

Onset of Action Antitussive: 15-30 minutes

Duration of Action ≤6 hours

Half-life Elimination Dextromethorphan: Extensive metabolizers: 2-4 hours; poor metabolizers: 24 hours

Time to Peak 2-3 hours

Dextromethorphan and Chlorpheniramine

(deks troe meth OR fan & klor fen IR a meen)

Related Information

Chlorpheniramine *on page 365*

Dextromethorphan *on page 504*

U.S. Brand Names Coricidin® HBP Cough & Cold [OTC]; Dimetapp® Children's Long Acting Cough Plus Cold [OTC]; Robitussin® Children's Cough & Cold Long-Acting [OTC]; Robitussin® Cough & Cold Long-Acting [OTC]; Scot-Tussin® DM Maximum Strength [OTC]; Triaminic® Children's Softchews® Cough & Runny Nose [OTC]

Pharmacologic Category Alkylamine Derivative; Antitussive; Histamine H_1 Antagonist; Histamine H_1 Antagonist, First Generation

Use Symptomatic relief of runny nose, sneezing, itchy/watery eyes, cough, and other upper respiratory symptoms associated with hay fever, common cold, or upper respiratory allergies

Local Anesthetic/Vasoconstrictor Precautions No information available to require special precautions

Effects on Dental Treatment Key adverse event(s) related to dental treatment: Chlorpheniramine: Prolonged use will cause significant xerostomia (normal salivary flow resumes upon discontinuation).

Effects on Bleeding No information available to require special precautions

Adverse Effects See individual agents.

General Dosage Range Oral:

Children 6-11 years: Dextromethorphan 10-15 mg and chlorpheniramine 2 mg every 4-6 hours as needed (maximum: 60 mg dextromethorphan and 10 mg chlorpheniramine/24 hours)

Children ≥12 years and Adults: Dextromethorphan 30 mg and chlorpheniramine 4 mg every 6 hours as needed (maximum: 120 mg dextromethorphan and 16 mg chlorpheniramine/24 hours)

Mechanism of Action

Chlorpheniramine maleate: Antihistamine with H_1-receptor activity

Dextromethorphan: A non-narcotic antitussive, increases cough threshold by its activity on the medulla oblongata

Dextromethorphan and Phenylephrine

(deks troe meth OR fan & fen il EF rin)

Related Information

Dextromethorphan *on page 504*

Phenylephrine (Systemic) *on page 1339*

U.S. Brand Names PediaCare® Children's Multi-Symptom Cold [OTC]; Safetussin® CD [OTC]; Sudafed PE® Children's Cold & Cough [OTC]; Triaminic Thin Strips® Children's Day Time Cold & Cough [OTC]; Triaminic® Day Time Cold & Cough [OTC]

Pharmacologic Category Antitussive; Decongestant

Use Temporary relief of symptoms of hay fever, the common cold, and upper respiratory allergies including sinus/nasal congestion, minor bronchial/throat irritation, and cough

Local Anesthetic/Vasoconstrictor Precautions Use with caution since phenylephrine is a sympathomimetic amine which could interact with epinephrine to cause a pressor response

Effects on Dental Treatment No significant effects or complications reported

Effects on Bleeding No information available to require special precautions

Adverse Effects See individual agents.

General Dosage Range Oral:

Children ≥4-12 years: Dosage varies greatly depending on product

Children ≥12 years and Adults: Safetussin® CD: 10 mL every 6 hours as needed (maximum: 40 mL/24 hours)

Mechanism of Action See individual agents.

Dextromethorphan and Quinidine (deks troe meth OR fan & KWIN i deen)

Related Information

Dextromethorphan *on page* 504

QuiNIDine *on page* 1447

U.S. Brand Names Nuedexta™

Canadian Brand Names Nuedexta™

Pharmacologic Category Antiarrhythmic Agent, Class Ia; N-Methyl-D-Aspartate Receptor Antagonist

Use Treatment of pseudobulbar affect (PBA)

Local Anesthetic/Vasoconstrictor Precautions See individual agents

Effects on Dental Treatment See individual agents

Effects on Bleeding See individual agents

Adverse Effects Also refer to individual agents.

>10%: Gastrointestinal: Diarrhea (13%)

1% to 10%:

- Cardiovascular: Peripheral edema (5%)
- Central nervous system: Dizziness (10%)
- Gastrointestinal: Vomiting (5%), flatulence (3%)
- Genitourinary: Urinary tract infection (4%)
- Hepatic: GGT increased (3%)
- Neuromuscular & skeletal: Weakness (5%)
- Respiratory: Cough (5%)
- Miscellaneous: Influenza (4%)

General Dosage Range

Oral: *Adults:* Initial: Once capsule once daily for 7 days; Maintenance: One capsule twice daily

Mechanism of Action Dextromethorphan may relieve the symptoms of PBA by binding to sigma-1 receptors in the brain which may be involved in behavior, however the exact mechanism of action is not known. Quinidine is used to block the rapid metabolism of dextromethorphan, thereby increasing serum concentrations. The dose of quinidine in this combination product provides serum concentrations 1% to 3% of those needed to treat cardiac arrhythmias.

Pharmacodynamics/Kinetics

Half-life Elimination Dextromethorphan: 13 hours in extensive metabolizers; Quinidine: 7 hours in extensive metabolizers

Time to Peak Dextromethorphan: 3-4 hours; Quinidine: 1-2 hours

Pregnancy Risk Factor C

Dental Comment See individual agents

Dextrose (DEKS trose)

U.S. Brand Names BD™ Glucose [OTC]; Dex4® [OTC]; Enfamil® Glucose [OTC]; GlucoBurst® [OTC]; Glutol™ [OTC]; Glutose 15™ [OTC]; Glutose 45™ [OTC]; Insta-Glucose® [OTC]; Similac® Glucose [OTC]

Pharmacologic Category Antidote, Hypoglycemia; Intravenous Nutritional Therapy

Use

Oral: Treatment of hypoglycemia

5% and 10% solutions: Peripheral infusion to provide calories and fluid replacement

25% (hypertonic) solution: Treatment of acute symptomatic episodes of hypoglycemia in infants and children to restore depressed blood glucose levels; adjunctive treatment of hyperkalemia when combined with insulin

50% (hypertonic) solution: Treatment of insulin-induced hypoglycemia (hyperinsulinemia or insulin shock) and adjunctive treatment of hyperkalemia in adolescents and adults

≥10% solutions: Infusion after admixture with amino acids for nutritional support

Local Anesthetic/Vasoconstrictor Precautions No information available to require special precautions

Effects on Dental Treatment No significant effects or complications reported

Effects on Bleeding No information available to require special precautions

Adverse Effects Frequency not defined. **Note:** Most adverse effects are associated with excessive dosage or rate of infusion.

Cardiovascular: Edema, dehydration, hyper-/hypovolemia, phlebitis, venous thrombosis

Central nervous system: Fever, hyperosmolar syndrome, mental confusion, unconsciousness

Endocrine & metabolic: Acidosis, hyperglycemia, hypokalemia, hypophosphatemia, hypomagnesemia

Genitourinary: Ketonuria, glycosuria, polyuria

Gastrointestinal: Diarrhea (oral), nausea, polydipsia

Local: Pain, tissue necrosis, vein irritation

Respiratory: Pulmonary edema, tachypnea

General Dosage Range

I.V.:

Infants ≤6 months: 0.25-1 g/kg/dose (maximum: 25 g/dose)

Children >6 months to 12 years: 0.5-1 g/kg/dose (maximum: 25 g/dose)

Adolescents and and Adults: 10-50 g/dose

Oral: *Children >2 years and and Adults:* 10-20 g as a single dose, may repeat if needed

Mechanism of Action Dextrose, a monosaccharide, is a source of calories and fluid for patients unable to obtain an adequate oral intake; may decrease body protein and nitrogen losses; promotes glycogen deposition in the liver. When used in the treatment of hyperkalemia (combined with insulin), dextrose stimulates the uptake of potassium by cells, especially in muscle tissue, lowering serum potassium.

Pharmacodynamics/Kinetics

Onset of Action

Treatment of hypoglycemia: Oral: 10 minutes

Treatment of hyperkalemia: Maximum effect: I.V.: 30 minutes

Time to Peak Oral: 40 minutes

Pregnancy Risk Factor C/A (oral)

Diatrizoate Meglumine (dye a tri ZOE ate MEG loo meen)

U.S. Brand Names Cystografin®; Cystografin® Dilute

Pharmacologic Category Iodinated Contrast Media; Radiological/Contrast Media, Ionic (High Osmolality)

Use

Solution for instillation: Retrograde cystourethrography; retrograde or ascending pyelography

Solution for injection: Arthrography, cerebral angiography, direct cholangiography, discography, drip infusion pyelography, excretory urography, peripheral arteriography, splenoportography, venography; contrast enhancement of computed tomographic head and body imaging

Local Anesthetic/Vasoconstrictor Precautions No information available to require special precautions

Effects on Dental Treatment No significant effects or complications reported

Effects on Bleeding No information available to require special precautions

Adverse Effects

<10%:

Cardiovascular: Flushing (49%)

Gastrointestinal: Taste perversion (11%)

Local: Injection site reaction (12%)

Renal: Nephrosis (excretory urography: 23%)

1% to 10%:

Cardiovascular: Edema, hypertension

Central nervous system: Dizziness (5%), agitation, chills, fever, headache

Dermatologic: Urticaria (1%)

Gastrointestinal: Nausea (6%), vomiting (3%)

Local: Extravasation

Neuromuscular & skeletal: Parasthesia (6%)

Renal: Hematuria (retrograde GU procedures), urinary tract infections (retrograde GU procedures)

Respiratory: Cough (2%), rhinitis (1%), sneezing

Miscellaneous: Allergic reaction, diaphoresis

Pregnancy Risk Factor C

Diatrizoate Meglumine and Diatrizoate Sodium

(dye a tri ZOE ate MEG loo meen & dye a tri ZOE ate SOW dee um)

Related Information

Diatrizoate Meglumine *on page* 507
Diatrizoate Sodium *on page* 508

U.S. Brand Names Gastrografin®; MD-76®R; MD-Gastroview®

Pharmacologic Category Iodinated Contrast Media; Radiological/Contrast Media, Ionic (High Osmolality)

Use

Oral/rectal: Examination of GI tract; adjunct to contrast enhancement in computed tomography of the torso

Injection: Angiocardiography, aortography, central venography, cerebral angiography, cholangiography, digital arteriography, excretory urography, nephrotomography, peripheral angiography, peripheral arteriography, renal arteriography, renal venography, splenoportography, visceral arteriography; contrast enhancement of computed tomographic imaging

Local Anesthetic/Vasoconstrictor Precautions No information available to require special precautions

Effects on Dental Treatment No significant effects or complications reported

Effects on Bleeding No information available to require special precautions

Adverse Effects Frequency not defined.

Cardiovascular: Tachyarrhythmia
Dermatologic: Urticaria
Gastrointestinal: Diarrhea, nausea, vomiting
Respiratory: Dyspnea, hypoxia
Miscellaneous: Anaphylaxis

General Dosage Range

Oral:

Children <5 years: 30 mL, dilute 1:1 (if <10 kg or debilitated, dilute 1:3)
Children 5-10 years: 60 mL, dilute 1:1 (if <10 kg or debilitated, dilute 1:3)
Adults: 30-90 mL **or** 25-77 mL in 1000 mL tap water

Rectal:

Children <5 years: Dilute 1:5 in tap water
Children ≥5 years: Dilute 90 mL in 500 mL tap water
Adults: Dilute 240 mL in 1000 mL tap water

Pregnancy Risk Factor B/C (manufacturer dependent)

Diatrizoate Meglumine and Iodipamide Meglumine

(dye a tri ZOE ate MEG loo meen & eye oh DI pa mide MEG loo meen)

Related Information

Diatrizoate Meglumine *on page* 507
Iodipamide Meglumine *on page* 934

U.S. Brand Names Sinografin®

Pharmacologic Category Iodinated Contrast Media; Radiological/Contrast Media, Ionic (Low Osmolality)

Use Hysterosalpingography

Local Anesthetic/Vasoconstrictor Precautions No information available to require special precautions

Effects on Dental Treatment No significant effects or complications reported

Effects on Bleeding No information available to require special precautions

Adverse Effects Frequency not defined.

Cardiovascular: Bradycardia (rare), cardiac arrest (rare), hypotension, syncope
Central nervous system: Chills, dizziness, fever
Gastrointestinal: Abdominal pain, abdominal tenderness, nausea, vomiting
Miscellaneous: Anaphylactoid reactions, hypersensitivity reactions (including sweating, flushing, pruritus, urticaria, rash, arthralgia, respiratory distress, and circulatory collapse)

General Dosage Range Intrauterine: *Adults:* Usual dose: 3-4 mL; Total dosage range: 1.5-10 mL

Diatrizoate Sodium (dye a tri ZOE ate SOW dee um)

U.S. Brand Names Hypaque™ Sodium

Pharmacologic Category Iodinated Contrast Media; Radiological/Contrast Media, Ionic (High Osmolality)

Use Radiographic examination of GI tract

Local Anesthetic/Vasoconstrictor Precautions No information available to require special precautions

Effects on Dental Treatment No significant effects or complications reported

Effects on Bleeding No information available to require special precautions

Adverse Effects Frequency not defined.

Dermatologic: Urticaria

Gastrointestinal: Diarrhea, nausea, vomiting

Hematologic: Eosinophilia

Miscellaneous: Anaphylactic reaction

General Dosage Range

Oral:

Infants and Children: 20% to 40% solution: 30-75 mL

Adults: 25% to 40% solution: 90-180 mL

Rectal: Enema:

Infants and Children: 10% to 15% solution: 100-500 mL depending on weight of patient

Adults: 15% to 25% solution: 500-1000 mL

Mechanism of Action When administered orally or given as an enema, the medium produces excellent opacification and delineation of the upper and lower gastrointestinal tract; however, because of dilution, contrast in the small bowel may be unsatisfactory.

Pregnancy Risk Factor C

Diazepam (dye AZ e pam)

Related Information

Management of the Patient With Anxiety or Depression *on page 1968*

Temporomandibular Dysfunction (TMD) *on page 1964*

Related Sample Prescriptions

Sedation (Prior to Dental Treatment) *on page 1995*

U.S. Brand Names Diastat®; Diastat® AcuDial™; Diazepam Intensol™; Valium®

Canadian Brand Names Apo-Diazepam®; Diastat®; Diastat® Rectal Delivery System; Diazemuls®; Novo-Dipam; Valium®

Generic Availability (U.S.) Yes

Pharmacologic Category Benzodiazepine

Dental Use Oral medication for preoperative dental anxiety; sedative component in I.V. conscious sedation in oral surgery patients; skeletal muscle relaxant

Use Management of anxiety disorders, ethanol withdrawal symptoms; skeletal muscle relaxant; treatment of convulsive disorders; preoperative or preprocedural sedation and amnesia

Rectal gel: Management of selected, refractory epilepsy patients on stable regimens of antiepileptic drugs requiring intermittent use of diazepam to control episodes of increased seizure activity

Unlabeled/Investigational Use Panic disorders; short-term treatment of spasticity in children with cerebral palsy

Local Anesthetic/Vasoconstrictor Precautions No information available to require special precautions

Effects on Dental Treatment Key adverse event(s) related to dental treatment: Xerostomia and changes in salivation (normal salivary flow resumes upon discontinuation).

Effects on Bleeding No information available to require special precautions

Adverse Effects Frequency not defined. Adverse reactions may vary by route of administration.

Cardiovascular: Hypotension, vasodilatation

Central nervous system: Amnesia, ataxia, confusion, depression, drowsiness, fatigue, headache, slurred speech, paradoxical reactions (eg, aggressiveness, agitation, anxiety, delusions, hallucinations, inappropriate behavior, increased muscle spasms, insomnia, irritability, psychoses, rage, restlessness, sleep disturbances, stimulation), vertigo

Dermatologic: Rash

Endocrine & metabolic: Libido changes

Gastrointestinal: Constipation, diarrhea, nausea, salivation changes (dry mouth or hypersalivation)

Genitourinary: Incontinence, urinary retention

Hepatic: Jaundice

Local: Phlebitis, pain with injection

Neuromuscular & skeletal: Dysarthria, tremor, weakness

Ocular: Blurred vision, diplopia

Respiratory: Apnea, asthma, respiratory rate decreased

Dental Usual Dosage

Anxiety/sedation/skeletal muscle relaxant: Adults:

Oral: 2-10 mg 2-4 times/day

I.M., I.V.: 2-10 mg, may repeat in 3-4 hours if needed

Anxiety: Elderly: Oral: Initial: 1-2 mg 1-2 times/day; increase gradually as needed, rarely need to use >10 mg/day (watch for hypotension and excessive sedation)

Skeletal muscle relaxant: Elderly: Oral: Initial: 2-5 mg 2-4 times/day

Dosage Oral absorption is more reliable than I.M.

Children:

Conscious sedation for procedures: Oral: 0.2-0.3 mg/kg (maximum: 10 mg) 45-60 minutes prior to procedure

Muscle spasm associated with tetanus: I.V., I.M.:

Infants >30 days: 1-2 mg/dose every 3-4 hours as needed

Children ≥5 years: 5-10 mg/dose every 3-4 hours as needed

Sedation/muscle relaxant/anxiety:

Oral: 0.12-0.8 mg/kg/day in divided doses every 6-8 hours

I.M., I.V.: 0.04-0.3 mg/kg/dose every 2-4 hours to a maximum of 0.6 mg/kg within an 8-hour period if needed

Spasticity in cerebral palsy (unlabeled use): Oral: Dose should be individualized:

Children ≤5 years: <8.5 kg: 0.5-1 mg at bedtime; 8.5-15 kg: 1-2 mg at bedtime (Mathew, 2005)

Children 5-16 years: 1.25 mg 3 times daily to 5 mg 4 times daily (Engle, 1966)

Status epilepticus:

I.V.: Infants >30 days and Children: 0.1-0.3 mg/kg given over ≤5 mg/minute; may repeat dose after 5-10 minutes; maximum: 10 mg/dose (Hegenbarth, 2008)

Rectal gel: 0.5 mg/kg, then 0.25 mg/kg in 10 minutes if needed

Anticonvulsant (acute treatment): Rectal gel:

Children <2 years: Safety and efficacy have not been studied

Children 2-5 years: 0.5 mg/kg

Children 6-11 years: 0.3 mg/kg

Children ≥12 years: 0.2 mg/kg

Note: Dosage should be rounded upward to the next available dose, 2.5, 5, 7.5, 10, 12.5, 15, 17.5, and 20 mg/dose; dose may be repeated in 4-12 hours if needed; do not use for more than 5 episodes per month or more than one episode every 5 days

Adolescents: Conscious sedation for procedures:

Oral: 10 mg

I.V.: 5 mg, may repeat with 1/2 dose if needed

Adults:

Acute ethanol withdrawal: Oral: 10 mg 3-4 times during first 24 hours, then decrease to 5 mg 3-4 times/day as needed

Anticonvulsant (acute treatment): Rectal gel: 0.2 mg/kg

Note: Dosage should be rounded upward to the next available dose, 2.5, 5, 7.5, 10, 12.5, 15, 17.5, and 20 mg/dose; dose may be repeated in 4-12 hours if needed; do not use for more than 5 episodes per month or more than one episode every 5 days.

Anxiety (symptoms/disorders):

Oral: 2-10 mg 2-4 times/day

I.M., I.V.: 2-10 mg, may repeat in 3-4 hours if needed

Muscle spasm: I.V., I.M.: Initial: 5-10 mg; then 5-10 mg in 3-4 hours, if necessary. Larger doses may be required if associated with tetanus.

Sedation in the ICU patient: I.V.: 0.03-0.1 mg/kg every 30 minutes to 6 hours

Skeletal muscle relaxant (adjunct therapy): Oral: 2-10 mg 3-4 times/day

Status epilepticus:

I.V.: 5-10 mg every 5-10 minutes given over ≤5 mg/minute; maximum dose: 30 mg

Rectal gel: Premonitory/out-of-hospital treatment: 10 mg once; may repeat once if necessary

Rapid tranquilization of agitated patient (administer every 30-60 minutes): Oral: 5-10 mg; average total dose for tranquilization: 20-60 mg

Elderly/debilitated patients:

Oral: 2-2.5 mg 1-2 times/day initially; increase gradually as needed and tolerated

Rectal gel: Due to the increased half-life in elderly and debilitated patients, consider reducing dose.

Dosing adjustment in renal impairment: No dose adjustment recommended; decrease dose if administered for prolonged periods.

I.V.: Risk of propylene glycol toxicity; monitor closely if using for prolonged periods or at high doses

Hemodialysis: Not dialyzable (0% to 5%); supplemental dose is not necessary

Dosing adjustment in hepatic impairment: Use with caution

Mechanism of Action Binds to stereospecific benzodiazepine receptors on the postsynaptic GABA neuron at several sites within the central nervous system, including the limbic system, reticular formation. Enhancement of the inhibitory effect of GABA on neuronal excitability results by increased neuronal membrane permeability to chloride ions. This shift in chloride ions results in hyperpolarization (a less excitable state) and stabilization.

Contraindications Hypersensitivity to diazepam or any component of the formulation (cross-sensitivity with other benzodiazepines may exist); myasthenia gravis; severe respiratory insufficiency; severe hepatic insufficiency; sleep apnea syndrome; acute narrow-angle glaucoma; not for use in children <6 months of age (oral)

Warnings/Precautions Withdrawal has also been associated with an increase in the seizure frequency. Use with caution with drugs which may decrease diazepam metabolism. Use with caution in debilitated patients, obese patients, patients with hepatic disease (including alcoholics), or renal impairment. Active metabolites with extended half-lives may lead to delayed accumulation and adverse effects. Use with caution in patients with respiratory disease or impaired gag reflex.

Acute hypotension, muscle weakness, apnea, and cardiac arrest have occurred with parenteral administration. Acute effects may be more prevalent in patients receiving concurrent barbiturates, narcotics, or ethanol. Appropriate resuscitative equipment and qualified personnel should be available during administration and monitoring. Avoid use of the injection in patients with shock, coma, or acute ethanol intoxication. Intra-arterial injection or extravasation of the parenteral formulation should be avoided. Parenteral formulation contains propylene glycol, which has been associated with toxicity when administered in high dosages. Administration of rectal gel should only be performed by individuals trained to recognize characteristic seizure activity and monitor response.

Causes CNS depression (dose-related) resulting in sedation, dizziness, confusion, or ataxia which may impair physical and mental capabilities. Patients must be cautioned about performing tasks which require mental alertness (eg, operating machinery or driving). Use with caution in patients receiving other CNS depressants or psychoactive agents. Effects with other sedative drugs or ethanol may be potentiated. The dosage of narcotics should be reduced by approximately 1/3 when diazepam is added. Benzodiazepines have been associated with falls and traumatic injury and should be used with extreme caution in patients who are at risk of these events (especially the elderly). Benzodiazepines with long half-lives may produce prolonged sedation and increase the risk of falls and fracture. Short- or intermediate-acting benzodiazepines are preferred in elderly patients (Beers Criteria).

Use with caution in patients taking strong CYP3A4 inhibitors, moderate or strong CYP3A4 and CYP2C19 inducers and major CYP3A4 substrates.

Use caution in patients with depression or anxiety associated with depression, particularly if suicidal risk may be present. Use with caution in patients with a history of drug dependence. Benzodiazepines have been associated with dependence and acute withdrawal symptoms on discontinuation or reduction in dose. Acute withdrawal, including seizures, may be precipitated in patients after administration of flumazenil to patients receiving long-term benzodiazepine therapy.

Diazepam has been associated with anterograde amnesia. Psychiatric and paradoxical reactions, including hyperactive or aggressive behavior, have been reported with benzodiazepines, particularly in adolescent/pediatric or elderly patients. Does not have analgesic, antidepressant, or antipsychotic properties.

Rectal gel: Safety and efficacy have not been established in children <2 years of age.

Oral: Safety and efficacy have not been established in children <6 months of age.

Injection: Safety and efficacy have not been established in children <30 days of age. Solution for injection may contain sodium benzoate, benzyl alcohol, or benzoic acid. Large amounts have been associated with "gasping syndrome" in neonates.

Drug Interactions

Metabolism/Transport Effects **Substrate** of CYP1A2 (minor), 2B6 (minor), 2C9 (minor), 2C19 (major), 3A4 (major); **Inhibits** CYP2C19 (weak), 3A4 (weak)

Avoid Concomitant Use

Avoid concomitant use of Diazepam with any of the following: OLANZapine

Increased Effect/Toxicity

Diazepam may increase the levels/effects of: Alcohol (Ethyl); CloZAPine; CNS Depressants; Fosphenytoin; Methotrimeprazine; Phenytoin

The levels/effects of Diazepam may be increased by: Antifungal Agents (Azole Derivatives, Systemic); Aprepitant; Calcium Channel Blockers (Nondihydropyridine); Cimetidine; Conivaptan; Contraceptives (Estrogens); Contraceptives (Progestins); CYP2C19 Inhibitors (Moderate); CYP2C19 Inhibitors (Strong); CYP3A4

Inhibitors (Moderate); CYP3A4 Inhibitors (Strong); Dasatinib; Disulfiram; Droperidol; Fluconazole; Fosamprenavir; Fosaprepitant; Grapefruit Juice; Isoniazid; Macrolide Antibiotics; Methotrimeprazine; Nefazodone; OLANZapine; Proton Pump Inhibitors; Ritonavir; Saquinavir; Selective Serotonin Reuptake Inhibitors

Decreased Effect

The levels/effects of Diazepam may be decreased by: CarBAMazepine; CYP2C19 Inducers (Strong); CYP3A4 Inducers (Strong); Deferasirox; Rifamycin Derivatives; St Johns Wort; Theophylline Derivatives; Tocilizumab; Yohimbine

Ethanol/Nutrition/Herb Interactions

Ethanol: May increase CNS depression; monitor for increased effects with coadministration. Caution patients about effects.

Food: Diazepam serum concentrations may be increased if taken with food. Grapefruit juice may increase diazepam serum concentrations; avoid concurrent use.

Herb/Nutraceutical: St John's wort may decrease diazepam levels. Avoid valerian, St John's wort, kava kava, gotu kola (may increase CNS depression).

Pharmacodynamics/Kinetics

Onset of Action I.V.: Status epilepticus: Almost immediate

Duration of Action I.V.: Status epilepticus: 20-30 minutes

Half-life Elimination Parent drug: Adults: 20-50 hours; increased half-life in neonates, elderly, and those with severe hepatic disorders; Active major metabolite (desmethyldiazepam): 50-100 hours; may be prolonged in neonates

Pregnancy Risk Factor D

Lactation Enters breast milk/not recommended (AAP rates "of concern"; AAP 2001 update pending)

Breast-Feeding Considerations Diazepam and N-desmethyldiazepam can be found in breast milk; the oxazepam metabolite has also been detected in the urine of a nursing infant. Drowsiness, lethargy, or weight loss in nursing infants have been observed in case reports following maternal use of some benzodiazepines, including diazepam.

Controlled Substance C-IV

Dosage Forms

Gel, rectal: 10 mg (2 mL); 20 mg (4 mL); 5 mg/mL (0.5 mL)
Diastat®: 5 mg/mL (0.5 mL)
Diastat® AcuDial™: 10 mg (2 mL); 20 mg (4 mL)

Injection, solution: 5 mg/mL (2 mL, 10 mL)

Solution, oral: 5 mg/5 mL (5 mL, 500 mL)
Diazepam Intensol™: 5 mg/mL (30 mL)

Tablet, oral: 2 mg, 5 mg, 10 mg
Valium®: 2 mg, 5 mg, 10 mg

Diazoxide (dye az OKS ide)

U.S. Brand Names Proglycem®

Canadian Brand Names Proglycem®

Pharmacologic Category Antihypoglycemic Agent; Vasodilator, Direct-Acting

Use Hypoglycemia related to islet cell adenoma, carcinoma, hyperplasia, or adenomatosis; nesidioblastosis; leucine sensitivity; extrapancreatic malignancy

Local Anesthetic/Vasoconstrictor Precautions No information available to require special precautions

Effects on Dental Treatment No significant effects or complications reported

Effects on Bleeding No information available to require special precautions

Adverse Effects Frequency not defined.

Cardiovascular: Hypotension, palpitation, tachycardia

Central nervous system: Anxiety, dizziness, fever, headache, insomnia, malaise, polyneuritis

Dermatologic: Hirsutism, pruritus, purpura, rash, scalp hair loss

Endocrine & metabolic: Breast lump enlargement, diabetic ketoacidosis, fluid retention, galactorrhea, gout, hyperglycemia, hyperosmolar nonketotic coma, sodium retention

Gastrointestinal: Abdominal pain, anorexia, diarrhea, ileus, nausea, pancreatitis, pancreatic necrosis, taste loss (transient), vomiting

Hematologic: Bleeding (excessive), eosinophilia, hemoglobin/hematocrit decreased, neutropenia (transient), thrombocytopenia

Hepatic: Alkaline phosphatase increased, AST increased

Neuromuscular & skeletal: Weakness

Ocular: Blurred vision, cataracts (transient), diplopia, lacrimation, ring scotoma, subconjunctival hemorrhage

Renal: Albuminuria, azotemia, creatinine clearance decreased, glucosuria, hematuria, nephrotic syndrome (reversible), uric acid increased, urinary output decreased

Miscellaneous: Abnormal facial features (children with chronic use), IgG decreased, lymphadenopathy

General Dosage Range Oral:

Infants: 8-15 mg/kg/day in divided doses every 8-12 hours

Children and Adults: 3-8 mg/kg/day in divided doses every 8-12 hours

Mechanism of Action Activates potassium channels. Inhibits insulin release from the pancreas

Pharmacodynamics/Kinetics

Onset of Action Hyperglycemic: Oral: ~1 hour

Duration of Action Hyperglycemic: Oral: Normal renal function: 8 hours

Half-life Elimination Oral: Children: 9-24 hours; Adults: 24-36 hours

Pregnancy Risk Factor C

Dibucaine (DYE byoo kane)

U.S. Brand Names Nupercainal® [OTC]

Generic Availability (U.S.) Yes

Pharmacologic Category Local Anesthetic

Dental Use Amide derivative local anesthetic for minor skin conditions

Use Fast, temporary relief of pain and itching due to hemorrhoids, minor burns

Local Anesthetic/Vasoconstrictor Precautions No information available to require special precautions

Effects on Dental Treatment No significant effects or complications reported

Effects on Bleeding No information available to require special precautions

Adverse Effects 1% to 10%:

Dermatologic: Angioedema, contact dermatitis

Local: Burning

Dental Usual Dosage Local pain (local anesthetic): Children and Adults: Topical: Apply gently to the affected areas; no more than 30 g for adults or 7.5 g for children should be used in any 24-hour period

Dosage Children and Adults: Topical: Apply gently to the affected areas; no more than 30 g for adults or 7.5 g for children should be used in any 24-hour period

Mechanism of Action Local anesthetics bind selectively to the intracellular surface of sodium channels to block influx of sodium into the axon. As a result, depolarization necessary for action potential propagation and subsequent nerve function is prevented. The block at the sodium channel is reversible. When drug diffuses away from the axon, sodium channel function is restored and nerve propagation returns.

Contraindications Hypersensitivity to amide-type anesthetics, ophthalmic use

Warnings/Precautions When topical anesthetics are used prior to cosmetic or medical procedures, the lowest amount of anesthetic necessary for pain relief should be applied. High systemic levels and toxic effects (eg, methhemoglobinemia, irregular heart beats, respiratory depression, seizures, death) have been reported in patients who (without supervision of a trained professional) have applied topical anesthetics in large amounts (or to large areas of the skin), left these products on for prolonged periods of time, or have used wraps/dressings to cover the skin following application.

Drug Interactions

Avoid Concomitant Use There are no known interactions where it is recommended to avoid concomitant use.

Increased Effect/Toxicity There are no known significant interactions involving an increase in effect.

Decreased Effect There are no known significant interactions involving a decrease in effect.

Pharmacodynamics/Kinetics

Onset of Action ~15 minutes

Duration of Action 2-4 hours

Breast-Feeding Considerations No data reported; however, topical administration is probably compatible.

Dosage Forms

Ointment, topical: 1% [10 mg/g] (30 g, 454 g)

Nupercainal® [OTC]: 1% [10 mg/g] (30 g, 60 g)

Diclofenac (Systemic) (dye KLOE fen ak)

Related Information

Rheumatoid Arthritis, Osteoarthritis, and Osteoporosis *on page 1889*

Temporomandibular Dysfunction (TMD) *on page 1964*

U.S. Brand Names Cambia™; Cataflam®; Voltaren®-XR; Zipsor™

Canadian Brand Names Apo-Diclo Rapide®; Apo-Diclo®; Apo-Diclo® SR®; Cataflam®; Diclofenac ECT; Diclofenac Sodium; Diclofenac Sodium SR; Diclofenac SR; Dom-Diclofenac; Dom-Diclofenac SR; Novo-Difenac ECT; Novo-Difenac K; Novo-Difenac Suppositories; Novo-Difenac-SR; Nu-Diclo; Nu-Diclo-SR; Pennsaid®; PMS-Diclofenac; PMS-Diclofenac SR; PMS-Diclofenac-K; PRO-Diclo-Rapide; Sandoz-Diclofenac; Sandoz-Diclofenac Rapide; Sandoz-Diclofenac SR; Voltaren Rapide®; Voltaren SR®; Voltaren®

Generic Availability (U.S.) Yes: Excludes capsule, oral solution

Pharmacologic Category Nonsteroidal Anti-inflammatory Drug (NSAID); Nonsteroidal Anti-inflammatory Drug (NSAID), Oral

Dental Use Immediate-release tablets: Acute treatment of mild-to-moderate pain

Use

Capsule: Relief of mild-to-moderate acute pain

Immediate-release tablet: Ankylosing spondylitis; primary dysmenorrhea; acute and chronic treatment of rheumatoid arthritis, osteoarthritis

Delayed-release tablet: Acute and chronic treatment of rheumatoid arthritis, osteoarthritis, ankylosing spondylitis

Extended-release tablet: Chronic treatment of osteoarthritis, rheumatoid arthritis

Oral solution: Treatment of acute migraine with or without aura

Suppository (CAN; not available in U.S.): Symptomatic treatment of rheumatoid arthritis and osteoarthritis (including degenerative joint disease of hip)

Unlabeled/Investigational Use Juvenile idiopathic arthritis (JIA)

Local Anesthetic/Vasoconstrictor Precautions No information available to require special precautions

Effects on Dental Treatment The dentist should be aware of the potential of abnormal coagulation. Caution should also be exercised in the use of NSAIDs in patients already on anticoagulant therapy with drugs such as warfarin (Coumadin®). See Effects on Bleeding.

Effects on Bleeding Nonselective NSAIDs are known to reversibly decrease platelet aggregation via mechanisms different than observed with aspirin. Platelet function is restored as the drug is eliminated from the body. Dental professionals should be aware that recommendations differ between dental and general surgery. NSAIDs should be avoided (if possible) in general surgery patients for 3-5 half-lives of the drug (usually 1-3 days) prior to surgery to reduce the risk of excessive bleeding. However, there is no scientific evidence to warrant discontinuance of NSAIDs prior to dental surgery. In medically complicated patients or extensive oral surgery, the decision to interrupt therapy must be based on the risk to benefit in an individual patient and a medical consult is suggested. Routine interruption of NSAID therapy for most dental procedures is not warranted. If therapy is continued without interruption, the clinician should anticipate the potential for slower clotting times.

Adverse Effects

Oral:

1% to 10%:

Cardiovascular: Edema

Central nervous system: Dizziness, headache

Dermatologic: Pruritus, rash

Endocrine & metabolic: Fluid retention

Gastrointestinal: Abdominal distension, abdominal pain, constipation, diarrhea, dyspepsia, flatulence, GI perforation, heartburn, nausea, peptic ulcer/GI bleed, vomiting

Hematologic: Anemia, bleeding time increased

Hepatic: Liver enzyme abnormalities (>3 x ULN; ≤4%)

Otic: Tinnitus

Renal: Renal function abnormal

Miscellaneous: Diaphoresis increased

Rectal suppository (CAN; not available in U.S.): Also refer to adverse reactions associated with oral formulations.

Dental Usual Dosage Pain: Adults: Oral: Starting dose: 50 mg 3 times/day; maximum dose: 150 mg/day

Dosage Adults:

Oral:

Analgesia:

Immediate release tablet: Starting dose: 50 mg 3 times/day (maximum dose: 150 mg/day); may administer 100 mg loading dose, followed by 50 mg every 8 hours (maximum dose day 1: 200 mg/day; maximum dose day 2 and thereafter: 150 mg/day)

Immediate release capsule: 25 mg 4 times/day

Primary dysmenorrhea: Immediate release tablet: Starting dose: 50 mg 3 times/day (maximum dose: 150 mg/day); may administer 100 mg loading dose, followed by 50 mg every 8 hours (maximum dose day 1: 200 mg/day; maximum dose day 2 and thereafter: 150 mg/day)

Rheumatoid arthritis: Immediate or delayed release tablet: 150-200 mg/day in 2-4 divided doses; Extended release tablet: 100-200 mg/day

Canadian labeling: 150 mg/day in 3 divided doses (75-150 mg/day of slow release tablet)

Osteoarthritis: Immediate or delayed release tablet: 100-150 mg/day in 2-3 divided doses; Extended release tablet: 100 mg/day

Canadian labeling: 150 mg/day in 3 divided doses (75-150 mg/day of slow release tablet)

Ankylosing spondylitis: Delayed release tablet: 100-125 mg/day in 4-5 divided doses

Migraine: Oral solution: 50 mg (one packet) as a single dose at the time of migraine onset; safety and efficacy of a second dose have not been established

Rectal suppository (not available in U.S.):

Osteoarthritis: *Canadian labeling:* Insert 50 mg or 100 mg suppository rectally as single dose to substitute for final (third) oral daily dose; maximum combined dose (rectal and oral): 150 mg/day

Rheumatoid arthritis: *Canadian labeling:* Insert 50 mg or 100 mg suppository rectally as single dose to substitute for final (third) oral daily dose (maximum combined dose [rectal and oral]: 150 mg/day

Dosage adjustment in renal impairment: Not recommended in patients with advanced renal disease or significant renal impairment

Dosage adjustment in hepatic impairment: May require dosage adjustment; use oral solution only if benefits outweigh risks

Elderly: No specific dosing recommendations; elderly may demonstrate adverse effects at lower doses than younger adults, and >60% may develop asymptomatic peptic ulceration with or without hemorrhage; monitor renal function

Mechanism of Action Reversibly inhibits cyclooxygenase-1 and 2 (COX-1 and 2) enzymes, which results in decreased formation of prostaglandin precursors; has antipyretic, analgesic, and anti-inflammatory properties

Other proposed mechanisms not fully elucidated (and possibly contributing to the anti-inflammatory effect to varying degrees), include inhibiting chemotaxis, altering lymphocyte activity, inhibiting neutrophil aggregation/activation, and decreasing proinflammatory cytokine levels.

Contraindications Hypersensitivity to diclofenac or any component of the formulation; hypersensitivity to bovine protein (capsule formulation only); patients who exhibit asthma, urticaria, or other allergic-type reactions after taking aspirin or other NSAIDs; perioperative pain in the setting of coronary artery bypass graft (CABG) surgery

Canadian labeling: Additional contraindications (not in U.S. labeling): Uncontrolled heart failure, active gastric/duodenal/peptic ulcer; active GI bleed or perforation; regional ulcer, gastritis, or ulcerative colitis; cerebrovascular bleeding or other bleeding disorders; inflammatory bowel disease; severe hepatic impairment; active hepatic disease; severe renal impairment (Cl_{cr} <30 mL/minute) or deteriorating renal disease; known hyperkalemia; patients <16 years of age; breast-feeding; pregnancy (third trimester); use of diclofenac suppository if recent history of bleeding or inflammatory lesions of rectum/anus

Warnings/Precautions [U.S. Boxed Warning]: NSAIDs are associated with an increased risk of adverse cardiovascular thrombotic events, including MI and stroke. Risk may be increased with duration of use or pre-existing cardiovascular risk factors or disease. Carefully evaluate individual cardiovascular risk profiles prior to prescribing. May cause new-onset hypertension or worsening of existing hypertension. Monitor blood pressure closely. Use caution with fluid retention. Avoid use in heart failure. Concurrent administration of ibuprofen, and potentially other nonselective NSAIDs, may interfere with aspirin's cardioprotective effect. **[U.S. Boxed Warning]: Use is contraindicated for treatment of perioperative pain in the setting of coronary artery bypass graft (CABG) surgery.** Risk of MI and stroke may be increased with use following CABG surgery.

NSAID use may compromise existing renal function; dose-dependent decreases in prostaglandin synthesis may result from NSAID use, reducing renal blood flow which may cause renal decompensation. NSAID use may increase the risk for hyperkalemia. Patients with impaired renal function, dehydration, heart failure, liver dysfunction, those taking diuretics and ACEI, and the elderly are at greater risk of renal toxicity and hyperkalemia. Rehydrate patient before starting therapy; monitor renal function closely. Not recommended for use in patients with advanced renal disease. Long-term NSAID use may result in renal papillary necrosis while persistent urinary symptoms (eg, dysuria, bladder pain), cystitis, or hematuria may occur anytime after initiating NSAID therapy. Discontinue therapy with symptom onset and evaluate for origin.

[U.S. Boxed Warning]: NSAIDs may increase risk of gastrointestinal irritation, inflammation, ulceration, bleeding, and perforation. These events may occur at any time during therapy and without warning. Use caution with a history of GI disease (bleeding or ulcers), concurrent therapy with aspirin, anticoagulants and/or corticosteroids, smoking, use of alcohol, the elderly or debilitated patients. When used concomitantly with ≤325 mg of aspirin, a substantial increase in the risk of gastrointestinal complications (eg, ulcer) occurs; concomitant gastroprotective therapy (eg, proton pump inhibitors) is recommended (Bhatt, 2008).

Use the lowest effective dose for the shortest duration of time, consistent with individual patient goals, to reduce risk of cardiovascular or GI adverse events. Alternate therapies should be considered for patients at high risk.

NSAIDs may cause photosensitivity or serious skin adverse events including exfoliative dermatitis, Stevens-Johnson syndrome (SJS), and toxic epidermal necrolysis (TEN); discontinue use at first sign of skin rash or hypersensitivity. Anaphylactoid reactions may occur, even without prior exposure; patients with "aspirin triad" (bronchial asthma, aspirin intolerance, rhinitis) may be at increased risk. Do not use in patients who experience bronchospasm, asthma, rhinitis, or urticaria with NSAID or aspirin therapy. Use caution in other forms of asthma. Platelet adhesion and aggregation may be decreased; may prolong bleeding time; patients with coagulation disorders or who are receiving anticoagulants should be monitored closely. Anemia may occur; patients on long-term NSAID therapy should be monitored for anemia. Rarely, NSAID use may cause severe blood dyscrasias (eg, agranulocytosis, aplastic anemia, thrombocytopenia).

Use with caution in patients with impaired hepatic function. Closely monitor patients with any abnormal LFT. Diclofenac can cause transaminase elevations; initiate monitoring 4-8 weeks into therapy. Rarely, severe hepatic reactions (eg, fulminant hepatitis, liver failure) have occurred; discontinue all formulations if signs or symptoms of liver disease develop, or if systemic manifestations occur. Use with caution in hepatic porphyria (may trigger attack).

NSAIDS may cause drowsiness, dizziness, blurred vision, and other neurologic effects which may impair physical or mental abilities; patients must be cautioned about performing tasks which require mental alertness (eg, operating machinery or driving). Discontinue use with blurred or diminished vision and perform ophthalmologic exam. Monitor vision with long-term therapy. The elderly are at increased risk for adverse effects (especially peptic ulceration, CNS effects, and renal toxicity) from NSAIDs even at low doses. May increase the risk of aseptic meningitis, especially in patients with systemic lupus erythematosus (SLE) and mixed connective tissue disorders.

Withhold for at least 4-6 half-lives prior to surgical or dental procedures. Safety and efficacy have not been established in children.

Capsule: Contains gelatin; use is contraindicated in patients with history of hypersensitivity to bovine protein.

Oral solution: Only indicated for the acute treatment of migraine; not indicated for migraine prophylaxis or cluster headache. Not bioequivalent to other forms of diclofenac (even same dose); do not interchange products. Contains phenylalanine.

Drug Interactions

Metabolism/Transport Effects **Substrate** (minor) of CYP1A2, 2B6, 2C8, 2C9, 2C19, 2D6, 3A4; **Inhibits** CYP1A2 (moderate), 2C9 (weak), 2E1 (weak), 3A4 (weak)

Avoid Concomitant Use

Avoid concomitant use of Diclofenac (Systemic) with any of the following: Ketorolac; Ketorolac (Systemic)

Increased Effect/Toxicity

Diclofenac (Systemic) may increase the levels/effects of: Aminoglycosides; Anticoagulants; Antiplatelet Agents; Bisphosphonate Derivatives; Collagenase (Systemic); CycloSPORINE; CycloSPORINE (Systemic); CYP1A2 Substrates; Deferasirox; Desmopressin; Digoxin; Drotrecogin Alfa; Eplerenone; Haloperidol; Ibritumomab; Lithium; Methotrexate; Nonsteroidal Anti-Inflammatory Agents; PEMEtrexed; Potassium-Sparing Diuretics; PRALAtrexate; Quinolone Antibiotics; Salicylates; Thrombolytic Agents; Tositumomab and Iodine I 131 Tositumomab; Vancomycin; Vitamin K Antagonists

The levels/effects of Diclofenac (Systemic) may be increased by: ACE Inhibitors; Angiotensin II Receptor Blockers; Antidepressants (Tricyclic, Tertiary Amine); Conivaptan; Corticosteroids (Systemic); Dasatinib; Glucosamine; Herbs

(Anticoagulant/Antiplatelet Properties); Ketorolac; Ketorolac (Systemic); Nonsteroidal Anti-Inflammatory Agents; Omega-3-Acid Ethyl Esters; Pentosan Polysulfate Sodium; Pentoxifylline; Probenecid; Prostacyclin Analogues; Selective Serotonin Reuptake Inhibitors; Serotonin/Norepinephrine Reuptake Inhibitors; Treprostinil; Voriconazole

Decreased Effect

Diclofenac (Systemic) may decrease the levels/effects of: ACE Inhibitors; Angiotensin II Receptor Blockers; Antiplatelet Agents; Beta-Blockers; Eplerenone; HydrALAZINE; Loop Diuretics; Potassium-Sparing Diuretics; Salicylates; Thiazide Diuretics

The levels/effects of Diclofenac (Systemic) may be decreased by: Bile Acid Sequestrants; Nonsteroidal Anti-Inflammatory Agents; Peginterferon Alfa-2b; Salicylates; Tocilizumab

Ethanol/Nutrition/Herb Interactions

Ethanol: Avoid ethanol (may enhance gastric mucosal irritation).

Herb/Nutraceutical: Avoid alfalfa, anise, bilberry, bladderwrack, bromelain, cat's claw, celery, chamomile, coleus, cordyceps, dong quai, evening primrose, fenugreek, feverfew, garlic, ginger, ginkgo biloba, grapeseed, green tea, ginseng (Siberian), guggul, horse chestnut, horseradish, licorice, prickly ash, red clover, reishi, SAMe (s-adenosylmethionine), sweet clover, turmeric, white willow (all have additional antiplatelet activity).

Dietary Considerations Oral formulations may be taken with food to decrease GI distress. Food may reduce effectiveness of oral solution. Some products may contain phenylalanine.

Diclofenac potassium = Cataflam®; potassium content: 5.8 mg (0.15 mEq) per 50 mg tablet

Pharmacodynamics/Kinetics

Onset of Action

Cataflam® is more rapid than sodium salt (Voltaren®) because it dissolves in the stomach instead of the duodenum

Suppository: more rapid onset, but slower rate of absorption when compared to enteric coated tablet

Half-life Elimination ~2 hours

Time to Peak Serum: Cambia™: ~0.25 hours; Cataflam®: ~1 hour; Voltaren®: ~2 hours; Voltaren® XR ~5 hours; Zipsor™: ~0.5 hour; Suppository: ≤1 hour. **Note:** Suppository: C_{max}: Approximately two-thirds of that observed with enteric coated tablet (equivalent 50 mg dose).

Pregnancy Risk Factor C (oral)/D (≥30 weeks gestation [oral])

Lactation Excreted in breast milk/not recommended

Breast-Feeding Considerations Low concentrations of diclofenac can be found in breast milk. Breast-feeding is not recommended by the manufacturer. Use while breast-feeding is contraindicated in Canadian labeling.

Dosage Forms

Capsule, liquid filled, oral:

Zipsor™: 25 mg

Powder for solution, oral:

Cambia™: 50 mg/packet (1s)

Tablet, oral: 50 mg

Cataflam®: 50 mg

Tablet, delayed release, enteric coated, oral: 25 mg, 50 mg, 75 mg

Tablet, extended release, oral: 100 mg

Voltaren®-XR: 100 mg

Dosage Forms: Canada

Suppository:

Voltaren®: 50 mg, 100mg

References

Kubitzek F, Ziegler G, Gold MS, et al, "Analgesic Efficacy of Low-Dose Diclofenac Versus Paracetamol and Placebo in Postoperative Dental Pain," *J Orofac Pain*, 2003, 17(3):237-44.

Diclofenac (Topical) (dye KLOE fen ak)

U.S. Brand Names Flector®; Pennsaid®; Solaraze®; Voltaren® Gel

Canadian Brand Names Voltaren® Emulgel™

Pharmacologic Category Nonsteroidal Anti-inflammatory Drug (NSAID); Nonsteroidal Anti-inflammatory Drug (NSAID), Topical

Use

Topical gel 1%: Relief of osteoarthritis pain in joints amenable to topical therapy (eg, ankle, elbow, foot, hand, knee, wrist)

Canadian labeling (not in U.S. labeling): Relief of pain associated with acute, localized joint/muscle injuries (eg, sports injuries, strains) in patients ≥16 years of age

Topical gel 3%: Actinic keratosis (AK) in conjunction with sun avoidance

Topical patch: Acute pain due to minor strains, sprains, and contusions

Topical solution: Relief of osteoarthritis pain of the knee

Local Anesthetic/Vasoconstrictor Precautions No information available to require special precautions

Effects on Dental Treatment No significant effects or complications reported

Effects on Bleeding No information available to require special precautions

Adverse Effects

Topical gel:

>10%: Local: Application site reactions (incidence increased with 3% gel): Pruritus (≤52%), rash (35% to 46%), contact dermatitis (4% to 33%), dry skin (≤27%), pain (15% to 26%), exfoliation (3% gel; 6% to 24%), paresthesia (≤20%)

1% to 10% (reported for 3% gel):

- Cardiovascular: Chest pain, hypertension
- Central nervous system: Headache, pain
- Dermatologic: Pruritus, rash, skin ulcer
- Endocrine & metabolic: Hypercholesterolemia, hyperglycemia
- Gastrointestinal: Abdominal pain, diarrhea, dyspepsia
- Genitourinary: Hematuria
- Hepatic: Liver enzymes increased
- Local: Alopecia, edema, photosensitivity
- Neuromuscular and skeletal: Arthralgia, arthrosis, back pain, CPK increased, hypokinesia, myalgia, neck pain, weakness
- Ocular: Conjunctivitis
- Respiratory: Asthma, dyspnea, pneumonia, sinusitis
- Miscellaneous: Flu-like syndrome

Topical solution:

>10%: Dermatologic: Dry skin (application site 32%; nonapplication site 2%)

1% to 10%:

- Cardiovascular: Edema (3%)
- Dermatologic: Contact dermatitis (2% to 9%), rash (3%), bruising (2%), pruritus (application site4%; nonapplication site 2%)
- Gastrointestinal: Dyspepsia (8%), abdominal pain (6%), diarrhea (4%), flatulence (4%), nausea (4%), constipation (3%), halitosis (1%)
- Neuromuscular & skeletal: Paresthesia (2%)
- Respiratory: Sinusitis (1%)
- Miscellaneous: Infection (3%)

Transdermal patch:

1% to 10%:

- Central nervous system: Dizziness, hypoesthesia
- Dermatologic: Dermatitis (2%), dermal allergic reaction
- Gastrointestinal: Nausea (3%), dysgeusia (2%), abdominal pain, constipation, diarrhea, gastritis, vomiting, xerostomia
- Local: Application site dryness, irritation, erythema, atrophy, discoloration, hyperhidrosis, and vesicles, edema, itching
- Neuromuscular & skeletal: Hyperkinesia

General Dosage Range Topical: *Adults:*

1% gel: Apply 2-4 g to affected joint 4 times/day (maximum: 16 g/day single joint of lower extremity, 8 g/day single joint of upper extremity); Maximum total body dose of 1% gel should not exceed 32 g per day.

3% gel: Apply to lesion area twice daily

Patch: Apply 1 patch twice daily

Solution: Apply 40 drops to each affected knee 4 times/day

Pharmacodynamics/Kinetics

Half-life Elimination Patch: ~12 hours

Time to Peak Serum: Flector®: 10-20 hours; Pennsaid®: 5-17 hours; Solaraze® Gel: ~5 hours; Voltaren® Gel: 10-14 hours

Pregnancy Risk Factor B (topical gel 3%); C (topical gel 1%, topical solution, topical patch) D (topical solution ≥30 weeks gestation)

Diclofenac and Misoprostol (dye KLOE fen ak & mye soe PROST ole)

Related Information

Diclofenac (Systemic) *on page* 513
Misoprostol *on page* 1146
Rheumatoid Arthritis, Osteoarthritis, and Osteoporosis *on page* 1889

U.S. Brand Names Arthrotec®

Canadian Brand Names Arthrotec®

Pharmacologic Category Nonsteroidal Anti-inflammatory Drug (NSAID), Oral; Prostaglandin

Use Treatment of osteoarthritis and rheumatoid arthritis in patients at high risk for NSAID-induced gastric and duodenal ulceration

Local Anesthetic/Vasoconstrictor Precautions No information available to require special precautions

Effects on Dental Treatment The dentist should be aware of the potential of abnormal coagulation. Caution should also be exercised in the use of NSAIDs in patients already on anticoagulant therapy with drugs such as warfarin (Coumadin®). See Effects on Bleeding.

Effects on Bleeding Nonselective NSAIDs are known to reversibly decrease platelet aggregation via mechanisms different than observed with aspirin. Platelet function is restored as the drug is eliminated from the body. Dental professionals should be aware that recommendations differ between dental and general surgery. NSAIDs should be avoided (if possible) in general surgery patients for 3-5 half-lives of the drug (usually 1-3 days) prior to surgery to reduce the risk of excessive bleeding. However, there is no scientific evidence to warrant discontinuance of NSAIDs prior to dental surgery. In medically complicated patients or extensive oral surgery, the decision to interrupt therapy must be based on the risk to benefit in an individual patient and a medical consult is suggested. Routine interruption of NSAID therapy for most dental procedures is not warranted. If therapy is continued without interruption, the clinician should anticipate the potential for slower clotting times.

Adverse Effects Percentages reported with combination product. Also see individual agents.

>10%: Gastrointestinal: Abdominal pain (21%), diarrhea (19%), dyspepsia (14%), nausea (11%)

1% to 10%: Gastrointestinal: Flatulence (9%)

General Dosage Range Oral: *Adults:* Arthrotec® 50: One tablet 2-4 times/day; Arthrotec® 75: One tablet twice daily

Mechanism of Action See individual agents.

Pregnancy Risk Factor X

Dicloxacillin (dye kloks a SIL in)

Related Information

Bacterial Infections *on page* 1933

Canadian Brand Names Dycill®; Pathocil®

Generic Availability (U.S.) Yes

Pharmacologic Category Antibiotic, Penicillin

Dental Use Treatment of susceptible orofacial infections (notably penicillinase-producing staphylococci)

Use Treatment of systemic infections such as pneumonia, skin and soft tissue infections, and osteomyelitis caused by penicillinase-producing staphylococci

Local Anesthetic/Vasoconstrictor Precautions No information available to require special precautions

Effects on Dental Treatment Key adverse event(s) related to dental treatment: Prolonged use of penicillins may lead to development of oral candidiasis.

Effects on Bleeding No information available to require special precautions

Adverse Effects 1% to 10%: Gastrointestinal: Nausea, diarrhea, abdominal pain

Dental Usual Dosage Susceptible orofacial infections: Children >40 kg and Adults: 125-250 mg every 6 hours

Dosage

Usual dosage range:

Newborns: Use not recommended
Children <40 kg: Oral: 12.5-100 mg/kg/day divided every 6 hours
Children >40 kg: Oral: 125-250 mg every 6 hours
Adults: Oral: 125-1000 mg every 6 hours

Indication-specific dosing:

Children: Oral:
Furunculosis: 25-50 mg/kg/day divided every 6 hours
Osteomyelitis: 50-100 mg/kg/day in divided doses every 6 hours

Adults: Oral:

Erysipelas, furunculosis, mastitis, otitis externa, septic bursitis, skin abscess: 500 mg every 6 hours

Impetigo: 250 mg every 6 hours

Prosthetic joint (long-term suppression therapy): 250 mg twice daily

***Staphylococcus aureus*, methicillin susceptible infection if no I.V. access:** 500-1000 mg every 6-8 hours

Dosage adjustment in renal impairment: Not necessary

Hemodialysis: Not dialyzable (0% to 5%); supplemental dosage not necessary

Peritoneal dialysis: Supplemental dosage not necessary

Continuous arteriovenous or venovenous hemofiltration: Supplemental dosage not necessary

Mechanism of Action Inhibits bacterial cell wall synthesis by binding to one or more of the penicillin-binding proteins (PBPs) which in turn inhibits the final transpeptidation step of peptidoglycan synthesis in bacterial cell walls, thus inhibiting cell wall biosynthesis. Bacteria eventually lyse due to ongoing activity of cell wall autolytic enzymes (autolysins and murein hydrolases) while cell wall assembly is arrested.

Contraindications Hypersensitivity to dicloxacillin, penicillin, or any component of the formulation

Warnings/Precautions Monitor PT if patient concurrently on warfarin. Use with caution in neonates; elimination of drug is slow. Serious and occasionally severe or fatal hypersensitivity (anaphylactoid) reactions have been reported in patients on penicillin therapy, especially with a history of beta-lactam hypersensitivity, history of sensitivity to multiple allergens, or previous IgE-mediated reactions (eg, anaphylaxis, angioedema, urticaria). Use with caution in asthmatic patients. Prolonged use may result in fungal or bacterial superinfection, including *C. difficile*-associated diarrhea and pseudomembranous colitis.

Drug Interactions

Metabolism/Transport Effects Induces CYP3A4 (weak)

Avoid Concomitant Use

Avoid concomitant use of Dicloxacillin with any of the following: BCG

Increased Effect/Toxicity

Dicloxacillin may increase the levels/effects of: Methotrexate

The levels/effects of Dicloxacillin may be increased by: Probenecid

Decreased Effect

Dicloxacillin may decrease the levels/effects of: BCG; Mycophenolate; Saxagliptin; Typhoid Vaccine; Vitamin K Antagonists

The levels/effects of Dicloxacillin may be decreased by: Fusidic Acid; Tetracycline Derivatives

Ethanol/Nutrition/Herb Interactions Food: Decreases drug absorption rate; decreases drug serum concentration.

Dietary Considerations Administer on an empty stomach 1 hour before or 2 hours after meals. Some products may contain sodium.

Pharmacodynamics/Kinetics

Half-life Elimination 0.6-0.8 hour; slightly prolonged with renal impairment

Time to Peak Serum: 0.5-2 hours

Pregnancy Risk Factor B

Lactation Excretion in breast milk unknown/use caution

Breast-Feeding Considerations It is not known if dicloxacillin crosses into human milk. The manufacturer recommends that caution be exercised when administering dicloxacillin to nursing women. Other penicillins distribute into human milk and are considered safe for use during breast-feeding. Nondose-related effects could include modification of bowel flora.

Dosage Forms

Capsule, oral: 250 mg, 500 mg

Dicyclomine (dye SYE kloe meen)

U.S. Brand Names Bentyl®

Canadian Brand Names Bentylol®; Formulex®; Lomine; Riva-Dicyclomine

Pharmacologic Category Anticholinergic Agent

Use Treatment of functional bowel/irritable bowel syndrome

Unlabeled/Investigational Use Urinary incontinence

Local Anesthetic/Vasoconstrictor Precautions No information available to require special precautions

Effects on Dental Treatment Key adverse event(s) related to dental treatment: Xerostomia and changes in salivation (normal salivary flow resumes upon discontinuation)

Effects on Bleeding No information available to require special precautions

Adverse Effects Adverse reactions are included here that have been reported for pharmacologically similar drugs with anticholinergic/antispasmodic action.

Cardiovascular: Syncope, tachycardia, palpitation
Central nervous system: Dizziness (29%), lightheadedness (11%), drowsiness (9%), tingling, headache, nervousness (6%), numbness, mental confusion and/or excitement, dyskinesia, lethargy, speech disturbance, insomnia
Dermatologic: Rash, urticaria, itching, and other dermal manifestations
Endocrine & metabolic: Suppression of lactation
Gastrointestinal: Xerostomia (33%), nausea (14%), vomiting, constipation, bloated feeling, abdominal pain, taste loss, anorexia
Genitourinary: Urinary hesitancy, urinary retention, impotence
Local: Irritation (injection), focal coagulation necrosis (injection)
Neuromuscular & skeletal: Weakness (7%)
Ocular: Blurred vision (27%), diplopia, mydriasis, cycloplegia, increased ocular tension
Respiratory: Dyspnea, apnea, asphyxia, nasal stuffiness or congestion, sneezing, throat congestion
Miscellaneous: Anaphylaxis, diaphoresis decreased, severe allergic reaction

General Dosage Range

I.M.: *Adults:* 80 mg/day in 4 divided doses

Oral:

Adults: Initial: 20 mg 4 times/day; Maintenance: Up to 160 mg/day in 4 divided doses

Elderly: Initial: 10-20 mg 4 times/day

Mechanism of Action Blocks the action of acetylcholine at parasympathetic sites in smooth muscle, secretory glands and the CNS

Pharmacodynamics/Kinetics

Onset of Action 1-2 hours

Duration of Action ≤4 hours

Half-life Elimination Initial: 1.8 hours; Terminal: 9-10 hours

Pregnancy Risk Factor B

Didanosine (dye DAN oh seen)

Related Information

HIV Infection and AIDS *on page* 1883

U.S. Brand Names Videx®; Videx® EC

Canadian Brand Names Videx®; Videx® EC

Pharmacologic Category Antiretroviral Agent, Reverse Transcriptase Inhibitor (Nucleoside)

Use Treatment of HIV infection; always to be used in combination with at least two other antiretroviral agents

Local Anesthetic/Vasoconstrictor Precautions No information available to require special precautions

Effects on Dental Treatment Key adverse event(s) related to dental treatment: Xerostomia (normal salivary flow resumes upon discontinuation).

Effects on Bleeding No information available to require special precautions relative to effects on hemostasis.

Adverse Effects As reported in monotherapy studies; risk of toxicity may increase when combined with other agents.

>10%:

Gastrointestinal: Diarrhea (19% to 28%), amylase increased (15% to 17%), abdominal pain (7% to 13%)
Neuromuscular & skeletal: Peripheral neuropathy (17% to 20%)

1% to 10%:

Dermatologic: Rash/pruritus (7% to 9%)
Endocrine & metabolic: Uric acid increased (2% to 3%)
Gastrointestinal: Pancreatitis (1% to 7% dose dependent); patients >65 years of age had a higher frequency of pancreatitis than younger patients patients (10% vs 5% in younger patients)
Hepatic: AST increased (7% to 9%), ALT increased (6% to 9%), alkaline phosphatase increased (1% to 4%)

General Dosage Range Dosage adjustment recommended in patients with renal impairment

Oral:

Delayed release:

Children ≥6 years and 20 kg to <25 kg: 200 mg once daily

Children ≥6 years and 25 kg to <60 kg and Adults <60 kg: 250 mg once daily

Children and Adults ≥60 kg: 400 mg once daily

Pediatric powder for oral solution (Videx®):

Infants 2 weeks to 8 months: 100 mg/m^2 twice daily

Children >8 months to 18 years: 120 mg/m^2 twice daily

Adolescents and Adults <60 kg: 125 mg twice daily **or** 250 mg once daily

Adolescents and Adults ≥60 kg: 200 mg twice daily **or** 400 mg once daily

Mechanism of Action Didanosine, a purine nucleoside (adenosine) analog and the deamination product of dideoxyadenosine (ddA), inhibits HIV replication *in vitro* in both T cells and monocytes. Didanosine is converted within the cell to the mono-, di-, and triphosphates of ddA. These ddA triphosphates act as substrate and inhibitor of HIV reverse transcriptase substrate and inhibitor of HIV reverse transcriptase thereby blocking viral DNA synthesis and suppressing HIV replication.

Pharmacodynamics/Kinetics

Half-life Elimination

Children and Adolescents: 0.8 hour

Adults: Normal renal function: 1.5 hours; however, active metabolite, ddATP, has an intracellular half-life >12 hours *in vitro*; Renal impairment: 2.5-5 hours

Time to Peak Delayed release capsules: 2 hours; Powder for suspension: 0.25-1.5 hours

Pregnancy Risk Factor B

Diethylene Triamine Penta-Acetic Acid

(dye ETH i leen TRYE a meen PEN ta a SEE tik AS id)

U.S. Brand Names Ca-DTPA; Zn-DTPA

Pharmacologic Category Antidote

Use Treatment of known or suspected internal contamination with plutonium, americium, or curium

Local Anesthetic/Vasoconstrictor Precautions No information available to require special precautions

Effects on Dental Treatment Key adverse event(s) related to dental treatment: Metallic taste

Effects on Bleeding No information available to require special precautions

Adverse Effects Frequency not defined.

Cardiovascular: Chest pain

Central nervous system: Headache, lightheadedness

Dermatologic: Dermatitis

Gastrointestinal: Diarrhea, metallic taste, nausea

Local: Injection site reactions

Neuromuscular & skeletal: Pelvic pain

Respiratory: Cough and/or wheezing (using Ca-DTPA following nebulization in patients with asthma)

Miscellaneous: Allergic reaction, magnesium depletion, manganese depletion, metalloproteinases, zinc depletion

General Dosage Range I.V.:

Children <12 years: Initial: Ca-DTPA: 14 mg/kg/day (maximum dose: 1 g/day); Maintenance: Zn-DTPA: 14 mg/kg/day (maximum: 1 g/day)

Children ≥12s years and Adults: Ca-DTPA: 1 g/day; Zn-DTPA: 1 g/day

Mechanism of Action Ca-DTPA and Zn-DTPA form chelates with metal ions. The radioactive chelates are then excreted in the urine. Treatment is most effective when radiocontaminants are in circulation or interstitial fluids. Radiocontaminants eventually sequester in liver and bone, therefore, effectiveness of treatment decreases with time after exposure.

Pharmacodynamics/Kinetics

Half-life Elimination Ca-DTPA, Zn-DTPA: May be increased by renal impairment

Pregnancy Risk Factor C (Ca-DTPA)/B (Zn-DTPA)

Diethylpropion (dye eth il PROE pee on)

Canadian Brand Names Tenuate®; Tenuate® Dospan®

Pharmacologic Category Anorexiant; Sympathomimetic

Use Short-term (few weeks) adjunct in the management of exogenous obesity

Pharmacotherapy for weight loss is recommended only for obese patients with a body mass index ≥30 kg/m^2, or ≥27 kg/m^2 in the presence of other risk factors such as hypertension, diabetes, and/or dyslipidemia or a high waist circumference; therapy should be used in conjunction with a comprehensive weight management program.

Local Anesthetic/Vasoconstrictor Precautions Use vasoconstrictor with caution in patients taking diethylpropion. Amphetamine-like drugs such as diethylpropion enhance the sympathomimetic response of epinephrine and norepinephrine leading to potential hypertension and cardiotoxicity.

Effects on Dental Treatment Key adverse event(s) related to dental treatment: Xerostomia and changes in salivation (normal salivary flow resumes upon discontinuation), and metallic taste (the use of local anesthetic without vasoconstrictor is recommended in these patients).

Effects on Bleeding No information available to require special precautions

Adverse Effects Frequency not defined.

Cardiovascular: Arrhythmia, ECG changes, hypertension, palpitation, precordial pain, pulmonary hypertension, tachycardia, valvulopathy

Central nervous system: Anxiety, CVA, depression, dizziness, drowsiness, dysphoria, euphoria, headache, insomnia, jitteriness, malaise, nervousness, overstimulation, psychosis, restlessness, seizure

Dermatologic: Alopecia, ecchymosis, erythema, rash, urticaria

Endocrine & metabolic: Libido changes, gynecomastia, menstrual irregularities

Gastrointestinal: Abdominal discomfort, constipation, diarrhea, nausea, unpleasant taste, vomiting, xerostomia

Genitourinary: Dysuria, impotence, polyuria

Hematologic: Bone marrow depression, agranulocytosis, leukopenia

Neuromuscular & skeletal: Dyskinesia, muscle pain, tremor

Ocular: Blurred vision, mydriasis

Respiratory: Dyspnea

Miscellaneous: Diaphoresis, tachyphylaxis

General Dosage Range Oral:

Controlled release: *Children >16 years and Adults:* 75 mg at midmorning

Immediate release: *Children >16 years and Adults:* 25 mg 3 times/day

Mechanism of Action Diethylpropion s a sympathomimetic amine with pharmacologic properties similar to the amphetamines. It is also structurally similar to bupropion. The mechanism of action in reducing appetite appears to be secondary to CNS effects, including stimulation of the hypothalamus to release norepinephrine

Pharmacodynamics/Kinetics

Half-life Elimination Aminoketone metabolites: ~4-6 hours

Pregnancy Risk Factor B

Controlled Substance C-IV

Difenoxin and Atropine (dye fen OKS in & A troe peen)

Related Information

Atropine *on page 188*

U.S. Brand Names Motofen®

Pharmacologic Category Antidiarrheal

Use Treatment of diarrhea

Local Anesthetic/Vasoconstrictor Precautions No information available to require special precautions

Effects on Dental Treatment Key adverse event(s) related to dental treatment: Xerostomia (normal salivary flow resumes upon discontinuation)

Effects on Bleeding No information available to require special precautions

Adverse Effects 1% to 10%:

Central nervous system: Dizziness, drowsiness, lightheadedness, headache

Gastrointestinal: Nausea, vomiting, xerostomia, epigastric distress

General Dosage Range Oral: *Adults:* 2 tablets (each tablet contains difenoxin hydrochloride 1 mg and atropine sulfate 0.025 mg) initially, then 1 tablet after each loose stool (maximum: 8 tablets/day)

Pharmacodynamics/Kinetics

Time to Peak Plasma: Within 40-60 minutes

Pregnancy Risk Factor C

Controlled Substance C-IV

Diflorasone (dye FLOR a sone)

U.S. Brand Names ApexiCon® E; ApexiCon™

Pharmacologic Category Corticosteroid, Topical

Use Relieves inflammation and pruritic symptoms of corticosteroid-responsive dermatosis (high to very high potency topical corticosteroid)

Local Anesthetic/Vasoconstrictor Precautions No information available to require special precautions

Effects on Dental Treatment No significant effects or complications reported

Effects on Bleeding No information available to require special precautions

General Dosage Range Topical: *Adults:* Cream: Apply 2-4 times/day; Ointment: Apply 1-3 times/day

Mechanism of Action Decreases inflammation by suppression of migration of polymorphonuclear leukocytes and reversal of increased capillary permeability

Pregnancy Risk Factor C

Diflunisal (dye FLOO ni sal)

Related Information

Oral Pain *on page 1928*

Rheumatoid Arthritis, Osteoarthritis, and Osteoporosis *on page 1889*

Temporomandibular Dysfunction (TMD) *on page 1964*

Related Sample Prescriptions

Mild/Moderate Oral Pain *on page 1980*

Canadian Brand Names Apo-Diflunisal®; Novo-Diflunisal; Nu-Diflunisal

Generic Availability (U.S.) Yes

Pharmacologic Category Nonsteroidal Anti-inflammatory Drug (NSAID), Oral

Dental Use Treatment of postoperative pain

Use Management of inflammatory disorders usually including rheumatoid arthritis and osteoarthritis; can be used as an analgesic for treatment of mild-to-moderate pain

Local Anesthetic/Vasoconstrictor Precautions No information available to require special precautions

Effects on Dental Treatment The dentist should be aware of the potential of abnormal coagulation. Caution should also be exercised in the use of NSAIDs in patients already on anticoagulant therapy with drugs such as warfarin (Coumadin®). See Effects on Bleeding.

Effects on Bleeding Nonselective NSAIDs are known to reversibly decrease platelet aggregation via mechanisms different than observed with aspirin. Platelet function is restored as the drug is eliminated from the body. Dental professionals should be aware that recommendations differ between dental and general surgery. NSAIDs should be avoided (if possible) in general surgery patients for 3-5 half-lives of the drug (usually 1-3 days) prior to surgery to reduce the risk of excessive bleeding. However, there is no scientific evidence to warrant discontinuance of NSAIDs prior to dental surgery. In medically complicated patients or extensive oral surgery, the decision to interrupt therapy must be based on the risk to benefit in an individual patient and a medical consult is suggested. Routine interruption of NSAID therapy for most dental procedures is not warranted. If therapy is continued without interruption, the clinician should anticipate the potential for slower clotting times.

Adverse Effects 1% to 10%:

Central nervous system: Headache (3% to 9%), dizziness (1% to 3%), insomnia (1% to 3%), somnolence (1% to 3%), fatigue (1% to 3%)

Dermatologic: Rash (3% to 9%)

Gastrointestinal: Nausea (3% to 9%), dyspepsia (3% to 9%), GI pain (3% to 9%), diarrhea (3% to 9%), constipation (1% to 3%), flatulence (1% to 3%), vomiting (1% to 3%), GI ulceration

Otic: Tinnitus (1% to 3%)

Dental Usual Dosage Mild-to-moderate pain: Adults: Oral: Initial: 500-1000 mg followed by 250-500 mg every 8-12 hours; maximum daily dose: 1.5 g

Dosage Adults: Oral:

Mild-to-moderate pain: Initial: 500-1000 mg followed by 250-500 mg every 8-12 hours; maximum daily dose: 1.5 g

Arthritis: 500-1000 mg/day in 2 divided doses; maximum daily dose: 1.5 g

Dosing adjustment in renal impairment: Use with caution; Cl_{cr} <50 mL/minute: Administer 50% of normal dose (Aronoff, 1998)

Hemodialysis: No supplement required

CAPD: No supplement require

CAVH: Dose for GFR 10-50

Mechanism of Action Reversibly inhibits cyclooxygenase-1 and 2 (COX-1 and 2) enzymes, which results in decreased formation of prostaglandin precursors; has antipyretic, analgesic, and anti-inflammatory properties.

Other proposed mechanisms not fully elucidated (and possibly contributing to the anti-inflammatory effect to varying degrees) include inhibiting chemotaxis, altering lymphocyte activity, inhibiting neutrophil aggregation/activation, and decreasing proinflammatory cytokine levels.

Contraindications Hypersensitivity to diflunisal, aspirin, other NSAIDs, or any component of the formulation; perioperative pain in the setting of coronary artery bypass graft (CABG) surgery

Warnings/Precautions [U.S. Boxed Warning]: NSAIDs are associated with an increased risk of adverse cardiovascular thrombotic events, including MI and stroke. Risk may be increased with duration of use or pre-existing cardiovascular risk factors or disease. Carefully evaluate individual cardiovascular risk profiles prior to prescribing. May cause new-onset hypertension or worsening of existing hypertension. Use caution with fluid retention. Avoid use in heart failure. Concurrent administration of ibuprofen, and potentially other nonselective NSAIDs, may interfere with aspirin's cardioprotective effect. **[U.S. Boxed Warning]: Use is contraindicated for treatment of perioperative pain in the setting of coronary artery bypass graft (CABG) surgery.** Risk of MI and stroke may be increased with use following CABG surgery.

[U.S. Boxed Warning]: NSAIDs may increase risk of gastrointestinal irritation, inflammation, ulceration, bleeding, and perforation. Use caution with a history of GI disease (bleeding or ulcers), concurrent therapy with aspirin, anticoagulants and/or corticosteroids, smoking, use of alcohol, the elderly or debilitated patients. When used concomitantly with ≤325 mg of aspirin, a substantial increase in the risk of gastrointestinal complications (eg, ulcer) occurs; concomitant gastroprotective therapy (eg, proton pump inhibitors) is recommended (Bhatt, 2008).

Platelet adhesion and aggregation may be decreased; may prolong bleeding time; patients with coagulation disorders or who are receiving anticoagulants should be monitored closely. Anemia may occur; patients on long-term NSAID therapy should be monitored for anemia. Rarely, NSAID use may cause severe blood dyscrasias (eg, agranulocytosis, aplastic anemia, thrombocytopenia).

NSAID use may compromise existing renal function; dose-dependent decreases in prostaglandin synthesis may result from NSAID use, reducing renal blood flow which may cause renal decompensation. NSAID use may increase the risk for hyperkalemia. Patients with impaired renal function, dehydration, heart failure, liver dysfunction, those taking diuretics, and ACE inhibitors, and the elderly are at greater risk of renal toxicity and hyperkalemia. Rehydrate patient before starting therapy; monitor renal function closely. Not recommended for use in patients with advanced renal disease. Long-term NSAID use may result in renal papillary necrosis. Use with caution in patients with decreased hepatic function.

NSAIDS may cause drowsiness, dizziness, blurred vision and other neurologic effects which may impair physical or mental abilities; patients must be cautioned about performing tasks which require mental alertness (eg, operating machinery or driving). Discontinue use with blurred or diminished vision and perform ophthalmologic exam. Monitor vision with long-term therapy.

Use the lowest effective dose for the shortest duration of time, consistent with individual patient goals, to reduce risk of cardiovascular or GI adverse events.

NSAIDs may cause serious skin adverse events including exfoliative dermatitis, Stevens-Johnson syndrome (SJS), and toxic epidermal necrolysis (TEN); discontinue use at first sign of skin rash or hypersensitivity. Do not use in patients who experience bronchospasm, asthma, rhinitis, or urticaria with NSAID or aspirin therapy. Use caution in other forms of asthma.

A hypersensitivity syndrome has been reported; monitor for constitutional symptoms and cutaneous findings; other organ dysfunction may be involved.

Diflunisal is a derivative of acetylsalicylic acid and therefore may be associated with Reye's syndrome. Withhold for at least 4-6 half-lives prior to surgical or dental procedures.

Drug Interactions

Avoid Concomitant Use

Avoid concomitant use of Diflunisal with any of the following: Ketorolac; Ketorolac (Systemic)

Increased Effect/Toxicity

Diflunisal may increase the levels/effects of: Aminoglycosides; Anticoagulants; Antiplatelet Agents; Bisphosphonate Derivatives; Collagenase (Systemic); CycloSPORINE; CycloSPORINE (Systemic); Deferasirox; Desmopressin; Digoxin; Drotrecogin Alfa; Eplerenone; Haloperidol; Ibritumomab; Lithium; Methotrexate; Nonsteroidal Anti-Inflammatory Agents; PEMEtrexed; Potassium-Sparing Diuretics; PRALAtrexate; Quinolone Antibiotics; Salicylates; Thrombolytic Agents; Tositumomab and Iodine I 131 Tositumomab; Vancomycin; Vitamin K Antagonists

The levels/effects of Diflunisal may be increased by: ACE Inhibitors; Angiotensin II Receptor Blockers; Antidepressants (Tricyclic, Tertiary Amine); Corticosteroids (Systemic); Dasatinib; Glucosamine; Herbs (Anticoagulant/Antiplatelet Properties); Ketorolac; Ketorolac (Systemic); Nonsteroidal Anti-Inflammatory Agents; Omega-3-Acid Ethyl Esters; Pentosan Polysulfate Sodium; Pentoxifylline; Probenecid; Prostacyclin Analogues; Selective Serotonin Reuptake Inhibitors; Serotonin/Norepinephrine Reuptake Inhibitors; Treprostinil

Decreased Effect

Diflunisal may decrease the levels/effects of: ACE Inhibitors; Angiotensin II Receptor Blockers; Antiplatelet Agents; Beta-Blockers; Eplerenone; HydrALAZINE; Loop Diuretics; Potassium-Sparing Diuretics; Salicylates; Thiazide Diuretics

The levels/effects of Diflunisal may be decreased by: Bile Acid Sequestrants; Nonsteroidal Anti-Inflammatory Agents; Salicylates

Ethanol/Nutrition/Herb Interactions

Ethanol: Avoid ethanol (may enhance gastric mucosal irritation).

Herb/Nutraceutical: Avoid alfalfa, anise, bilberry, bladderwrack, bromelain, cat's claw, celery, chamomile, coleus, cordyceps, dong quai, evening primrose, fenugreek, feverfew, garlic, ginger, ginkgo biloba, ginseng (American, Panax, Siberian), grapeseed, green tea, guggul, horse chestnut seed, horseradish, licorice, prickly ash, red clover, reishi, SAMe (S-adenosylmethionine), sweet clover, turmeric, white willow (all have additional antiplatelet activity).

Dietary Considerations Should be taken with food to decrease GI upset.

Pharmacodynamics/Kinetics

Onset of Action Analgesic: ~1 hour; maximal effect: 2-3 hours

Duration of Action 8-12 hours

Half-life Elimination 8-12 hours; prolonged with renal impairment

Time to Peak Serum: 2-3 hours

Pregnancy Risk Factor C

Lactation Enters breast milk/not recommended

Breast-Feeding Considerations Diflunisal is excreted into breast milk at levels of 2% to 7% of those in maternal plasma. Breast-feeding is not recommended by the manufacturer.

Dosage Forms

Tablet, oral: 500 mg

Dental Comment The advantage of diflunisal as a pain reliever is its 12-hour duration of effect. In many cases, this long effect will ensure a full night sleep during the postoperative pain period.

References

Ahmad N, Grad HA, Haas DA, et al, "The Efficacy of Nonopioid Analgesics for Postoperative Dental Pain: A Meta-Analysis," *Anesth Prog*, 1997, 44(4):119-26.

Brooks PM and Day RO, "Nonsteroidal Anti-inflammatory Drugs - Differences and Similarities," *N Engl J Med*, 1991, 324(24):1716-25.

Dionne R, "Additive Analgesia Without Opioid Side Effects," *Compend Contin Educ Dent*, 2000, 21 (7):572-4, 576-7.

Dionne RA, "New Approaches to Preventing and Treating Postoperative Pain," *J Am Dent Assoc*, 1992, 123(6):26-34.

Dionne RA and Berthold CW, "Therapeutic Uses of Nonsteroidal Anti-inflammatory Drugs in Dentistry," *Crit Rev Oral Biol Med*, 2001, 12(4):315-30.

Forbes JA, Calderazzo JP, Bowser MW, et al, "A 12-Hour Evaluation of the Analgesic Efficacy of Diflunisal, Aspirin, and Placebo in Postoperative Dental Pain," *J Clin Pharmacol*, 1982, 22(2-3):89-96.

Gobetti JP, "Controlling Dental Pain," *J Am Dent Assoc*, 1992, 123(6):47-52.

Nguyen AM, Graham DY, Gage T, et al, "Nonsteroidal Anti-inflammatory Drug Use in Dentistry: Gastrointestinal Implications," *Gen Dent*, 1999, 47(6):590-6.

Selcuk E, Gomel M, Bellibas SE, et al, "Comparison of the Analgesic Effects of Diflunisal and Paracetamol in the Treatment of Postoperative Dental Pain," *Int J Clin Pharmacol Res*, 1996, 16(2-3):57-65.

Difluprednate (dye floo PRED nate)

U.S. Brand Names Durezol®

Pharmacologic Category Corticosteroid, Ophthalmic

Use Treatment of inflammation and pain following ocular surgery

Local Anesthetic/Vasoconstrictor Precautions No information available to require special precautions

Effects on Dental Treatment No significant effects or complications reported

Effects on Bleeding No information available to require special precautions

Adverse Effects

5% to 15%: Ocular: Anterior chamber cells/flare, blepharitis, ciliary and conjunctival hyperemia, conjunctival/corneal edema, pain, photophobia, posterior capsule opacification

1% to 5%: Ocular: Inflammation, iritis, punctuate keratitis, visual acuity reduced

General Dosage Range Ophthalmic: *Adults:* Instill 1 drop in affected eye(s) 2-4 times/day

Mechanism of Action Corticosteroids inhibit the inflammatory response including edema, capillary dilation, leukocyte migration, and scar formation. Difluprednate penetrates cells readily to induce the production of lipocortins. These proteins modulate the activity of prostaglandins and leukotrienes.

Pregnancy Risk Factor C

Digoxin (di JOKS in)

Related Information

Cardiovascular Diseases *on page 1848*

U.S. Brand Names Lanoxin®

Canadian Brand Names Apo-Digoxin®; Digoxin CSD; Lanoxin®; Pediatric Digoxin CSD; PMS-Digoxin; Toloxin®

Generic Availability (U.S.) Yes

Pharmacologic Category Antiarrhythmic Agent, Miscellaneous; Cardiac Glycoside

Use Treatment of mild-to-moderate (or stage C as recommended by the ACCF/AHA) heart failure (HF); atrial fibrillation (rate-control)

Note: In treatment of atrial fibrillation (AF), use is not considered first-line unless AF coexistent with heart failure or in sedentary patients (Fuster, 2006).

Unlabeled/Investigational Use Fetal tachycardia with or without hydrops; to slow ventricular rate in supraventricular tachyarrhythmias such as supraventricular tachycardia (SVT) excluding atrioventricular reciprocating tachycardia (AVRT)

Local Anesthetic/Vasoconstrictor Precautions Use vasoconstrictor with caution due to risk of cardiac arrhythmias with digoxin

Effects on Dental Treatment Sensitive gag reflex may cause difficulty in taking a dental impression.

Effects on Bleeding No information available to require special precautions

Adverse Effects Incidence not always reported.

Cardiovascular: Accelerated junctional rhythm, asystole, atrial tachycardia with or without block, AV dissociation, first-, second- (Wenckebach), or third-degree heart block, facial edema, PR prolongation, PVCs (especially bigeminy or trigeminy), ST segment depression, ventricular tachycardia or ventricular fibrillation

Central nervous system: Dizziness (6%), mental disturbances (5%), headache (4%), apathy, anxiety, confusion, delirium, depression, fever, hallucinations

Dermatologic: Rash (erythematous, maculopapular [most common], papular, scarlatiniform, vesicular or bullous), pruritus, urticaria, angioneurotic edema

Gastrointestinal: Nausea (4%), vomiting (2%), diarrhea (4%), abdominal pain, anorexia

Neuromuscular & skeletal: Weakness

Ocular: Visual disturbances (blurred or yellow vision)

Respiratory: Laryngeal edema

Children are more likely to experience cardiac arrhythmia as a sign of excessive dosing. The most common are conduction disturbances or tachyarrhythmia (atrial tachycardia with or without block) and junctional tachycardia. Ventricular tachyarrhythmias are less common. In infants, sinus bradycardia may be a sign of digoxin toxicity. Any arrhythmia seen in a child on digoxin should be considered as digoxin toxicity. The gastrointestinal and central nervous system symptoms are not frequently seen in children.

Dosage

Children: When changing from oral (tablets or liquid) or I.M. to I.V. therapy, dosage should be reduced by 20% to 25%. Refer to the following: See table.

Dosage Recommendations for Digoxin[1]

Age	Total Digitalizing Dose[2,3] (mcg/kg)		Daily Maintenance Dose[3,4] (mcg/kg)	
	Oral	I.V. or I.M.[5]	Oral	I.V. or I.M.[5]
Preterm infant	20-30	15-25	5-7.5	4-6
Full-term infant	25-35	20-30	6-10	5-8
1 mo - 2 y	35-60	30-50	10-15	7.5-12
2-5 y	30-40	25-35	7.5-10	6-9
5-10 y	20-35	15-30	5-10	4-8
>10 y	10-15	8-12	2.5-5	2-3

[1]**Heart failure:** A lower serum digoxin concentration may be adequate to treat heart failure (compared to cardiac arrhythmias); consider doses at the lower end of the recommended range for treatment of heart failure; a digitalizing dose (loading dose) may not be necessary when treating heart failure (Ross, 2001).

[2]**Do not give full total digitalizing dose (TDD) at once.** Give one-half of the total digitalizing dose (TDD) in the initial dose, then give one-quarter of the TDD in each of two subsequent doses at 6- to 8-hour intervals. Obtain ECG 6 hours after each dose to assess potential toxicity.

[3]Based on lean body weight and normal renal function for age. Decrease dose in patients with decreased renal function; digitalizing dose often not recommended in infants and children.

[4]Divided every 12 hours in infants and children <10 years of age. Given once daily to children >10 years of age and adults.

[5]I.M. not preferred due to severe injection site pain. If I.M. route is necessary, administer as deep injection followed by massage of injection site.

Adults:

Atrial fibrillation (rate control) in patients with heart failure: Loading dose: I.V.: 0.25 mg every 2 hours, up to 1.5 mg within 24 hours; for nonacute situations, may administer 0.5 mg orally once daily for 2 days followed by oral maintenance dose. Maintenance dose: I.V., Oral: 0.125-0.375 mg once daily (Fuster, 2006)

Heart failure: Daily maintenance dose (**Note:** Loading dose not recommended): Oral: 0.125-0.25 mg once daily; higher daily doses (up to 0.5 mg/day) are rarely necessary. If patient is >70 years of age, has impaired renal function, or has a low lean body mass, low doses (eg, 0.125 mg daily or every other day) should be used (Hunt, 2009).

Supraventricular tachyarrhythmias (rate control):

Initial: Total digitalizing dose:

Oral: 0.75-1.5 mg

I.V., I.M.: 0.5-1 mg (**Note:** I.M. not preferred due to severe injection site pain.)

Give 1/2 (one-half) of the total digitalizing dose (TDD) as the initial dose, then give 1/4 (one-quarter) of the TDD in each of 2 subsequent doses at 6- to 8-hour intervals. Obtain ECG 6 hours after each dose to assess potential toxicity.

Daily maintenance dose:

Oral: 0.125-0.5 mg once daily

I.V., I.M.: 0.1-0.4 mg once daily (**Note:** I.M. not preferred due to severe injection site pain.)

Elderly: Dose is based on lean body weight and normal renal function for age. Decrease dose in patients with decreased renal function (see dosing adjustment in renal impairment).

Heart failure: If patient is >70 years, low doses (eg, 0.125 mg daily or every other day) should be used (Hunt, 2009).

Dosing adjustment/interval in renal impairment:

Loading dose: If loading dose necessary, reduce dose by 50% in ESRD

Maintenance dose:

Cl_{cr} 10-50 mL/minute: Administer 25% to 75% of dose or every 36 hours

Cl_{cr} <10 mL/minute: Administer 10% to 25% of dose or every 48 hours

Hemodialysis: Not dialyzable (0% to 5%)

Mechanism of Action

Heart failure: Inhibition of the sodium/potassium ATPase pump in myocardial cells results in a transient increase of intracellular sodium, which in turn promotes calcium influx via the sodium-calcium exchange pump leading to increased contractility.

Supraventricular arrhythmias: Direct suppression of the AV node conduction to increase effective refractory period and decrease conduction velocity - positive inotropic effect, enhanced vagal tone, and decreased ventricular rate to fast atrial arrhythmias. Atrial fibrillation may decrease sensitivity and increase tolerance to higher serum digoxin concentrations.

Contraindications Hypersensitivity to digoxin (rare) or other forms of digitalis, or any component of the formulation; ventricular fibrillation

Warnings/Precautions Watch for proarrhythmic effects (especially with digoxin toxicity). Withdrawal in clinically stable patients with HF may lead to recurrence of HF symptoms. During an episode of atrial fibrillation or flutter in patients with an accessory bypass tract (eg, Wolff-Parkinson-White syndrome), use has been associated with increased anterograde conduction down the accessory pathway leading to ventricular fibrillation; avoid use in such patients. Avoid use in patients with second- or third-degree heart block (except in patients with a functioning artificial pacemaker); incomplete AV block (eg, Stokes-Adams attack) may progress to complete block with digoxin administration. HF patients with preserved left ventricular function including patients with restrictive cardiomyopathy, constrictive pericarditis, and amyloid heart disease may be susceptible to digoxin toxicity; avoid use unless used to control ventricular response with atrial fibrillation. Digoxin should not be used in patients with low EF, sinus rhythm, and no HF symptoms since the risk of harm may be greater than clinical benefit. Avoid use in patients with hypertrophic cardiomyopathy (HCM) and outflow tract obstruction unless used to control ventricular response with atrial fibrillation; outflow obstruction may worsen due to the positive inotropic effects of digoxin.

Use with caution in patients with hyperthyroidism, hypothyroidism, recent acute MI (within 6 months), sinus nodal disease (eg, sick sinus syndrome). Reduce dose with renal impairment and when amiodarone, propafenone, quinidine, or verapamil are added to a patient on digoxin; use with caution in patients taking strong inducers or inhibitors of P-glycoprotein (eg, cyclosporine). Avoid rapid I.V. administration of calcium in digitalized patients; may produce serious arrhythmias.

Atrial arrhythmias associated with hypermetabolic states are very difficult to treat; treat underlying condition first; if digoxin is used, ensure digoxin toxicity does not occur. Patients with beri beri heart disease may fail to adequately respond to digoxin therapy; treat underlying thiamine deficiency concomitantly. Correct electrolyte disturbances, especially hypokalemia or hypomagnesemia, prior to use and throughout therapy; toxicity may occur despite therapeutic digoxin concentrations. Hypercalcemia may increase the risk of digoxin toxicity; maintain normocalcemia. It is not necessary to routinely reduce or hold digoxin therapy prior to elective electrical cardioversion for atrial fibrillation; however, exclusion of digoxin toxicity (eg, clinical and ECG signs) is necessary prior to cardioversion. If signs of digoxin excess exist, withhold digoxin and delay cardioversion until toxicity subsides; usually >24 hours. Use with caution in the elderly; may develop exaggerated serum/tissue concentrations due to age-related alterations in clearance and pharmacodynamics differences; dosage reduction may be necessary; in general, avoid doses >0.125 mg/day (Beers Criteria).

Drug Interactions

Metabolism/Transport Effects **Substrate** of CYP3A4 (minor), P-glycoprotein

Avoid Concomitant Use There are no known interactions where it is recommended to avoid concomitant use.

Increased Effect/Toxicity

Digoxin may increase the levels/effects of: Adenosine; Colchicine; Dronedarone; Midodrine

The levels/effects of Digoxin may be increased by: Aminoquinolines (Antimalarial); Amiodarone; Atorvastatin; Beta-Blockers; Calcium Channel Blockers (Nondihydropyridine); Calcium Polystyrene Sulfonate; Carvedilol; Conivaptan; CycloSPORINE; CycloSPORINE (Systemic); Dronedarone; Etravirine; Glycopyrrolate; Itraconazole; Macrolide Antibiotics; Milnacipran; Nefazodone; Neuromuscular-Blocking Agents; Nonsteroidal Anti-Inflammatory Agents; Paricalcitol; P-Glycoprotein Inhibitors; Posaconazole; Potassium-Sparing Diuretics; Propafenone; Protease Inhibitors; QuiNIDine; QuiNINE; Ranolazine; Reserpine; SitaGLIPtin; Sodium Polystyrene Sulfonate; Spironolactone; Telmisartan; Tolvaptan; Vitamin D Analogs

Decreased Effect

Digoxin may decrease the levels/effects of: Antineoplastic Agents (Anthracycline)

The levels/effects of Digoxin may be decreased by: 5-ASA Derivatives; Acarbose; Aminoglycosides; Antineoplastic Agents; Antineoplastic Agents (Anthracycline); Bile Acid Sequestrants; Kaolin; Penicillamine; P-Glycoprotein Inducers; Potassium-Sparing Diuretics; St Johns Wort; Sucralfate; Tocilizumab

Ethanol/Nutrition/Herb Interactions

Food: Digoxin peak serum concentrations may be decreased if taken with food. Meals containing increased fiber (bran) or foods high in pectin may decrease oral absorption of digoxin.

Herb/Nutraceutical: Avoid ephedra (risk of cardiac stimulation). Avoid natural licorice (causes sodium and water retention and increases potassium loss).

Dietary Considerations Maintain adequate amounts of potassium in diet to decrease risk of hypokalemia (hypokalemia may increase risk of digoxin toxicity).

Pharmacodynamics/Kinetics

Onset of Action

Heart rate control: Oral: 1-2 hours; I.V.: 5-60 minutes

Peak effect: Heart rate control: Oral: 2-8 hours; I.V.: 1-6 hours; **Note:** In patients with atrial fibrillation, median time to ventricular rate control in one study was 6 hours (range: 3-15 hours) (Siu, 2009)

Duration of Action Adults: 3-4 days

Half-life Elimination

Age, renal and cardiac function dependent:

Neonates: Premature: 61-170 hours; Full-term: 35-45 hours

Infants: 18-25 hours

Children: 18-36 hours

Adults: 36-48 hours

Adults, anephric: 3.5-5 days

Parent drug: 38 hours; Metabolites: Digoxigenin: 4 hours; Monodigitoxoside: 3-12 hours

Time to Peak Serum: Oral: 1-3 hours

Pregnancy Risk Factor C

Lactation Enters breast milk/use caution (AAP rates "compatible"; AAP 2001 update pending)

Breast-Feeding Considerations Digoxin is excreted into breast milk and similar concentrations are found within mother's serum and milk. The manufacturer recommends that caution be used in nursing women.

Dosage Forms

Injection, solution: 250 mcg/mL (1 mL, 2 mL)

Lanoxin®: 100 mcg/mL (1 mL); 250 mcg/mL (2 mL)

Solution, oral: 50 mcg/mL (2.5 mL, 5 mL, 60 mL)

Tablet, oral: 125 mcg, 250 mcg

Lanoxin®: 125 mcg, 250 mcg

Dosage Forms: Canada

Tablet, oral:

Apo-Digoxin®: 62.5 mcg, 125 mcg, 250 mcg

Digoxin Immune Fab (di JOKS in i MYUN fab)

U.S. Brand Names Digibind® [DSC]; DigiFab®

Canadian Brand Names Digibind®

Pharmacologic Category Antidote

Use Treatment of life-threatening or potentially life-threatening digoxin intoxication, including:

- acute digoxin ingestion (ie, >10 mg in adults or >4 mg in children)
- chronic ingestions leading to steady-state digoxin concentrations >6 ng/mL in adults or >4 ng/mL in children
- manifestations of digoxin toxicity due to overdose (life-threatening ventricular arrhythmias, progressive bradycardia, second- or third-degree heart block not responsive to atropine, serum potassium >5 mEq/L in adults or >6 mEq in children)

Local Anesthetic/Vasoconstrictor Precautions No information available to require special precautions

Effects on Dental Treatment No significant effects or complications reported

Effects on Bleeding No information available to require special precautions

Adverse Effects Frequency not defined.

Cardiovascular: Effects (due to withdrawal of digitalis) include exacerbation of heart failure, rapid ventricular response in patients with atrial fibrillation; postural hypotension

Endocrine & metabolic: Hypokalemia

Local: Phlebitis

Miscellaneous: Allergic reactions, serum sickness

General Dosage Range I.V.:

Acute ingestion of known amount: *Children and Adults:* Dose (vials) = Total body load (mg) / (0.5 mg digitalis bound/vial)

Based on steady-state digoxin concentration:

Infants and Children ≤20 kg: Dose (mg) = [(serum digoxin concentration [ng/mL] x weight [kg]) / 100] x (mg/vial)

Note: Digibind® 38 mg/vial or DigiFab™ 40 mg/vial

Adults: Dose (vials) = (serum digoxin concentration [ng/mL] x weight [kg]) / 100

Amount ingested and blood level unknown:

Children ≤20 kg: Acute toxicity: 20 vials total in 2 divided doses; Chronic toxicity: 1 vial may be sufficient

Children >20 kg and Adults: Acute toxicity: 20 vials total in 2 divided doses; Chronic toxicity: 6 vials

Mechanism of Action Digoxin immune antigen-binding fragments (Fab) are specific antibodies for the treatment of digitalis intoxication in carefully selected patients; binds with molecules of digoxin or digitoxin and then is excreted by the kidneys and removed from the body

Pharmacodynamics/Kinetics

Onset of Action I.V.: Improvement in 2-30 minutes for toxicity

Half-life Elimination 15-20 hours; prolonged with renal impairment

Pregnancy Risk Factor C

Dihydrocodeine, Aspirin, and Caffeine

(dye hye droe KOE deen, AS pir in, & KAF een)

Related Information

Aspirin *on page 171*
Caffeine *on page 282*
Codeine *on page 432*
Oral Pain *on page 1928*

U.S. Brand Names Synalgos®-DC

Generic Availability (U.S.) No

Pharmacologic Category Analgesic, Opioid

Dental Use Management of postoperative pain

Use Management of mild-to-moderate pain that requires relaxation

Local Anesthetic/Vasoconstrictor Precautions No information available to require special precautions

Effects on Dental Treatment Key adverse event(s) related to dental treatment: Dihydrocodeine: nausea, followed by sedation and constipation. Elderly are a high-risk population for adverse effects from nonsteroidal anti-inflammatory agents. As many as 60% of elderly patients with GI complications from NSAIDs can develop peptic ulceration and/or hemorrhage asymptomatically. Concomitant disease and drug use contribute to the risk of GI adverse effects. Use lowest effective dose for shortest period possible. Consider renal function decline with age.

Aspirin: As with all drugs which may affect hemostasis, bleeding is associated with aspirin. Hemorrhage may occur at virtually any site; risk is dependent on multiple variables including dosage, concurrent use of multiple agents which alter hemostasis, and patient susceptibility. Many adverse effects of aspirin are dose related, and are rare at low dosages. Other serious reactions are idiosyncratic, related to allergy or individual sensitivity (see Effects on Bleeding).

Effects on Bleeding Aspirin inhibits platelet aggregation which prolongs bleeding times. Inhibition is irreversible; on discontinuation of ASA, normal platelet function returns only when new platelets are released from the bone marrow. Dental practitioners should note that recommendations differ between general surgery (eg, appendectomy, hip replacement) and dental surgery. Due to concerns for increased blood loss, ASA is typically avoided (if possible) in general surgery patients for 1-2 weeks prior to surgery (exception is in patients undergoing CABG or noncardiac surgery at high risk of cardiac events – per 2008 ACCP guidelines). However, in the case of dental surgery there is no scientific evidence to warrant discontinuance of aspirin.

Adverse Effects

>10%:

Central nervous system: Lightheadedness, dizziness, drowsiness, sedation
Dermatologic: Pruritus, skin reactions
Gastrointestinal: Nausea, vomiting, constipation

1% to 10%:

Cardiovascular: Hypotension, palpitation, bradycardia, peripheral vasodilation
Central nervous system: Increased intracranial pressure
Endocrine & metabolic: Antidiuretic hormone release
Gastrointestinal: Biliary tract spasm
Genitourinary: Urinary tract spasm
Ocular: Miosis
Respiratory: Respiratory depression
Miscellaneous: Histamine release, physical and psychological dependence with prolonged use

Dental Usual Dosage Management of postoperative pain: Oral:

Adults: 1-2 capsules every 4-6 hours as needed for pain
Elderly: Initial dosing should be cautious (low end of adult dosing range)

Dosage
Adults: Oral: 1-2 capsules every 4-6 hours as needed for pain
Elderly: Initial dosing should be cautious (low end of adult dosing range)

Mechanism of Action Binds to opiate receptors in the CNS, causing inhibition of ascending pain pathways, altering the perception of and response to pain; causes cough suppression by direct central action in the medulla; produces generalized CNS depression

Contraindications Hypersensitivity to dihydrocodeine or any component of the formulation; pregnancy (prolonged use or high doses at term)

Warnings/Precautions May cause CNS depression, which may impair physical or mental abilities; patients must be cautioned about performing tasks which require mental alertness (eg, operating machinery or driving). Discontinue use if tinnitus or impaired hearing occurs. Use with caution in patients with hypersensitivity reactions to other phenanthrene-derivative opioid agonists (morphine, hydrocodone, hydromorphone, levorphanol, oxycodone, oxymorphone); patients with sensitivity to tartrazine dyes, nasal polyps, and asthma may have an increased risk of salicylate sensitivity; respiratory diseases including asthma, emphysema, COPD, adrenal insufficiency, biliary tract impairment, CNS depression, coma, head trauma, prostatic hyperplasia, urinary stricture, thyroid dysfunction bleeding disorders, GI disease, or severe liver or renal insufficiency; may obscure diagnosis or clinical course of patients with acute abdominal conditions; heavy ethanol use (>3 drinks/day) can increase bleeding risks; ASA should be avoided (if possible) in surgical patients for 1-2 weeks prior to surgery; some preparations contain sulfites which may cause allergic reactions; dextromethorphan has equivalent antitussive activity but has much lower toxicity in accidental overdose; tolerance of drug dependence may result from extended use

Drug Interactions

Metabolism/Transport Effects **Substrate** of CYP2D6 (minor) based on dihydrocodeine

Avoid Concomitant Use

Avoid concomitant use of Dihydrocodeine, Aspirin, and Caffeine with any of the following: Influenza Virus Vaccine (Live/Attenuated); Iobenguane I 123; Ketorolac; Ketorolac (Systemic)

Increased Effect/Toxicity

Dihydrocodeine, Aspirin, and Caffeine may increase the levels/effects of: Alcohol (Ethyl); Alendronate; Alvimopan; Anticoagulants; Carbonic Anhydrase Inhibitors; CNS Depressants; Collagenase (Systemic); Corticosteroids (Systemic); Desmopressin; Divalproex; Drotrecogin Alfa; Formoterol; Heparin; Ibritumomab; Methotrexate; PRALAtrexate; Salicylates; Selective Serotonin Reuptake Inhibitors; Sulfonylureas; Sympathomimetics; Thiazide Diuretics; Thrombolytic Agents; Tositumomab and Iodine I 131 Tositumomab; Valproic Acid; Varicella Virus-Containing Vaccines; Vitamin K Antagonists

The levels/effects of Dihydrocodeine, Aspirin, and Caffeine may be increased by: Abiraterone; Amphetamines; Antidepressants (Tricyclic, Tertiary Amine); Antiplatelet Agents; Antipsychotic Agents (Phenothiazines); Atomoxetine; Calcium Channel Blockers (Nondihydropyridine); Conivaptan; CYP1A2 Inhibitors (Moderate); CYP1A2 Inhibitors (Strong); Dasatinib; Deferasirox; Droperidol; Ginkgo Biloba; Glucosamine; Herbs (Anticoagulant/Antiplatelet Properties); Influenza Virus Vaccine (Live/Attenuated); Ketorolac; Ketorolac (Systemic); Loop Diuretics; Nonsteroidal Anti-Inflammatory Agents; NSAID (Nonselective); Omega-3-Acid Ethyl Esters; Pentosan Polysulfate Sodium; Pentoxifylline; Prostacyclin Analogues; Quinolone Antibiotics; Selective Serotonin Reuptake Inhibitors; Serotonin/Norepinephrine Reuptake Inhibitors; Succinylcholine; Treprostinil

Decreased Effect

Dihydrocodeine, Aspirin, and Caffeine may decrease the levels/effects of: ACE Inhibitors; Adenosine; Iobenguane I 123; Loop Diuretics; NSAID (Nonselective); Pegvisomant; Probenecid; Regadenoson; Tiludronate

The levels/effects of Dihydrocodeine, Aspirin, and Caffeine may be decreased by: Ammonium Chloride; Corticosteroids (Systemic); Mixed Agonist / Antagonist Opioids; Nonsteroidal Anti-Inflammatory Agents; NSAID (Nonselective); Peginterferon Alfa-2b; QuiNIDine; Tocilizumab

Ethanol/Nutrition/Herb Interactions Ethanol: May increase CNS depression; monitor for increased effects with coadministration. Caution patients about effects.

Pharmacodynamics/Kinetics

Onset of Action 10-30 minutes

Duration of Action 4-6 hours

Half-life Elimination Serum: 3.8 hours

Time to Peak Serum: 30-60 minutes

Pregnancy Risk Factor B/D (prolonged use or high doses at term)

Lactation Excretion in breast milk unknown/use caution

Breast-Feeding Considerations

Acetaminophen: May be taken while breast-feeding.

Aspirin: Use cautiously due to potential adverse effects in nursing infants.

Dihydrocodeine: No data reported.

Controlled Substance C-III

Dosage Forms

Capsule, oral:

Synalgos®-DC: Dihydrocodeine 16 mg, aspirin 356.4 mg, and caffeine 30 mg

Dental Comment There is no scientific evidence to warrant discontinuance of aspirin prior to dental surgery. Patients taking one aspirin tablet daily as an antithrombotic and who require dental surgery should be given special consideration in consultation with the physician before removal of the aspirin relative to prevention of postoperative bleeding.

Dihydrocodeine, Chlorpheniramine, and Phenylephrine

(dye hye droe KOE deen, klor fen IR a meen, & fen il EF rin)

Related Information

Chlorpheniramine *on page* 365

Codeine *on page* 432

Phenylephrine (Systemic) *on page* 1339

U.S. Brand Names Coldcough PD; DiHydro-PE [OTC]; Novahistine DH; Tusscough DHC™

Pharmacologic Category Alkylamine Derivative; Alpha/Beta Agonist; Analgesic, Opioid; Antitussive; Decongestant; Histamine H_1 Antagonist; Histamine H_1 Antagonist, First Generation

Use Symptomatic relief of cough and congestion associated with the upper respiratory tract

Local Anesthetic/Vasoconstrictor Precautions No information available to require special precautions

Effects on Dental Treatment Key adverse event(s) related to dental treatment:

Chlorpheniramine: Prolonged use will cause significant xerostomia (normal salivary flow resumes upon discontinuation).

Phenylephrine: Up to 10% of patients could experience tachycardia, palpitations, and xerostomia; use vasoconstrictor with caution.

Effects on Bleeding No information available to require special precautions

Adverse Effects See individual agents.

General Dosage Range

Oral:

Children 2-6 years: Novahistine DH: 1.25-2.5 mL every 4-6 hours as needed (maximum: 10 mL/day)

Children 6-12 years: Novahistine DH: 2.5-5 mL every 4-6 hours as needed (maximum: 20 mL/day)

Children >12 years and Adults: Novahistine DH: 5-10 mL every 4-6 hours as needed (maximum: 40 mL/day)

Mechanism of Action

Dihydrocodeine: Binds to opiate receptors in the CNS; suppresses cough in medullary center; produces generalized CNS depression

Chlorpheniramine: Competes with histamine for H_1-receptor sites on effector cells in the gastrointestinal tract, blood vessels, and respiratory tract

Phenylephrine: Potent, direct-acting alpha-adrenergic stimulator with weak beta-adrenergic activity; causes vasoconstriction of the arterioles of the nasal mucosa and conjunctiva

Pregnancy Risk Factor C

Controlled Substance C-III; C-V

Dihydrocodeine, Pseudoephedrine, and Guaifenesin

(dye hye droe KOE deen, soo doe e FED rin, & gwye FEN e sin)

Related Information

Codeine *on page* 432

GuaiFENesin *on page* 835

Pseudoephedrine *on page* 1429

U.S. Brand Names DiHydro-GP; Pancof®-EXP

Pharmacologic Category Antitussive/Decongestant/Expectorant

Use Temporary relief of cough and congestion associated with upper respiratory tract infections and allergies

Local Anesthetic/Vasoconstrictor Precautions Use with caution since pseudoephedrine is a sympathomimetic amine which could interact with epinephrine to cause a pressor response

Effects on Dental Treatment No significant effects or complications reported

Effects on Bleeding No information available to require special precautions

Adverse Effects Refer to individual agents.

General Dosage Range Oral:

Children 2-6 years: 1.25-2.5 mL every 4-6 hours as needed

Children 6-12 years: 2.5-5 mL every 4-6 hours as needed

Children ≥12 years and Adults: 5-10 mL every 4-6 hours as needed

Mechanism of Action

Dihydrocodeine is an antitussive and analgesic chemically related to codeine. Codeine binds to opiate receptors in the CNS, causing inhibition of ascending pain pathways, altering the perception of and response to pain; causes cough supression by direct central action in the medulla; produces generalized CNS depression.

Pseudoephedrine directly stimulates alpha-adrenergic receptors of respiratory mucosa causing vasoconstriction; directly stimulates beta-adrenergic receptors causing bronchial relaxation, increased heart rate and contractility.

Guaifenesin is thought to act as an expectorant by irritating the gastric mucosa and stimulating respiratory tract secretions, thereby increasing respiratory fluid volumes and decreasing phlegm viscosity.

Pregnancy Risk Factor C

Dihydroergotamine (dye hye droe er GOT a meen)

U.S. Brand Names D.H.E. 45®; Migranal®

Canadian Brand Names Migranal®

Pharmacologic Category Antimigraine Agent; Ergot Derivative

Use Treatment of migraine headache with or without aura; injection also indicated for treatment of cluster headaches

Unlabeled/Investigational Use Adjunct for DVT prophylaxis for hip surgery, for orthostatic hypotension, xerostomia secondary to antidepressant use, and pelvic congestion with pain

Local Anesthetic/Vasoconstrictor Precautions No information available to require special precautions

Effects on Dental Treatment Key adverse event(s) related to dental treatment: Rhinitis and abnormal taste.

Effects on Bleeding Rare but significant events related to hemorrhage (cerebral hemorrhage, subarachnoid hemorrhage, and stroke) have occurred following use of the injection. However, there is no information related to special precautions associated with bleeding related to dental procedures.

Adverse Effects

>10%: Nasal spray: Respiratory: Rhinitis (26%)

1% to 10%: Nasal spray:

- Central nervous system: Dizziness (4%), somnolence (3%)
- Endocrine & metabolic: Hot flashes (1%)
- Gastrointestinal: Nausea (10%), taste disturbance (8%), vomiting (4%), diarrhea (2%)
- Local: Application site reaction (6%)
- Neuromuscular & skeletal: Weakness (1%), stiffness (1%)
- Respiratory: Pharyngitis (3%)

General Dosage Range

I.M., SubQ: *Adults:* 1 mg initially, may repeat hourly up to 3 mg total (maximum: 6 mg/week)

I.V.: *Adults:* 1 mg initially, may repeat hourly up to 2 mg total (maximum: 6 mg/week)

Intranasal: *Adults:* 1 spray (0.5 mg) in each nostril initially, may repeat after 15 minutes up to 4 sprays total (maximum: 6 sprays/24 hours; 8 sprays/week)

Mechanism of Action Ergot alkaloid alpha-adrenergic blocker directly stimulates vascular smooth muscle to vasoconstrict peripheral and cerebral vessels; also has effects on serotonin receptors

Pharmacodynamics/Kinetics

Onset of Action I.M.: 15-30 minutes

Duration of Action I.M.: 3-4 hours

Half-life Elimination ~9-10 hours

Time to Peak Serum: I.M.: 24 minutes; I.V.: 1-2 minutes; Intranasal: 30-60 minutes; SubQ 15-45 minutes

Pregnancy Risk Factor X

Diltiazem (dil TYE a zem)

Related Information

Calcium Channel Blockers and Gingival Hyperplasia *on page 2014*
Cardiovascular Diseases *on page 1848*

U.S. Brand Names Cardizem®; Cardizem® CD; Cardizem® LA; Cartia XT®; Dilacor XR®; Dilt-CD; Dilt-XR; Diltia XT®; Diltzac; Matzim™ LA; Taztia XT®; Tiazac®

Canadian Brand Names Apo-Diltiaz CD®; Apo-Diltiaz SR®; Apo-Diltiaz TZ®; Apo-Diltiaz®; Apo-Diltiaz® Injectable; Cardizem® CD; Diltiazem HCl ER®; Diltiazem Hydrochloride Injection; Diltiazem TZ; Diltiazem-CD; Med-Diltiazem; Nu-Diltiaz; Nu-Diltiaz-CD; PMS-Diltiazem CD; ratio-Diltiazem CD; Sandoz-Diltiazem CD; Sandoz-Diltiazem T; Teva-Diltiazem; Teva-Diltiazem CD; Tiazac®; Tiazac® XC

Generic Availability (U.S.) Yes

Pharmacologic Category Antiarrhythmic Agent, Class IV; Calcium Channel Blocker; Calcium Channel Blocker, Nondihydropyridine

Use

Oral: Essential hypertension; chronic stable angina or angina from coronary artery spasm

Injection: Control of rapid ventricular rate in patients with atrial fibrillation or atrial flutter; conversion of paroxysmal supraventricular tachycardia (PSVT)

Unlabeled/Investigational Use

ACLS guidelines: Injection: Stable narrow-complex tachycardia uncontrolled or unconverted by adenosine or vagal maneuvers or if SVT is recurrent

Pediatric hypertension

Local Anesthetic/Vasoconstrictor Precautions No information available to require special precautions

Effects on Dental Treatment Key adverse event(s) related to dental treatment: Diltiazem has been reported to cause >10% incidence of gingival hyperplasia; usually disappears with discontinuation (consultation with physician is suggested).

Effects on Bleeding No information available to require special precautions

Adverse Effects Note: Frequencies represent ranges for various dosage forms. Patients with impaired ventricular function and/or conduction abnormalities may have higher incidence of adverse reactions.

>10%:
- Cardiovascular: Edema (2% to 15%)
- Central nervous system: Headache (5% to 12%)

2% to 10%:
- Cardiovascular: AV block (first degree 2% to 8%), edema (lower limb 2% to 8%), pain (6%), bradycardia (2% to 6%), hypotension (<2% to 4%), vasodilation (2% to 3%), extrasystoles (2%), flushing (1% to 2%), palpitation (1% to 2%)
- Central nervous system: Dizziness (3% to 10%), nervousness (2%)
- Dermatologic: Rash (1% to 4%)
- Endocrine & metabolic: Gout (1% to 2%)
- Gastrointestinal: Dyspepsia (1% to 6%), constipation (<2% to 4%), vomiting (2%), diarrhea (1% to 2%)
- Local: Injection site reactions: Burning, itching (4%)
- Neuromuscular & skeletal: Weakness (1% to 4%), myalgia (2%)
- Respiratory: Rhinitis (<2% to 10%), pharyngitis (2% to 6%), dyspnea (1% to 6%), bronchitis (1% to 4%), cough (≤3), sinus congestion (1% to 2%)

Dosage

Children (unlabeled use): Minimal information available; some centers use the following: Oral: Hypertension: Immediate release tablets: Initial: 1.5-2 mg/kg/day divided in 3 doses/day (maximum dose 6 mg/kg/day up to 360 mg/day) (Flynn, 2000)

Adults:

Oral:

Angina:

Capsule, extended release:

Dilacor XR®, Dilt-XR, Diltia XT®: Initial: 120 mg once daily; titrate over 7-14 days; usual dose range: 120-320 mg/day: maximum: 480 mg/day

Cardizem® CD, Cartia XT®, Dilt-CD: Initial: 120-180 mg once daily; titrate over 7-14 days; usual dose range: 120-320 mg/day; maximum: 480 mg/day

Tiazac®, Taztia XT®: Initial: 120-180 mg once daily; titrate over 7-14 days; usual dose range: 120-320 mg/day; maximum: 540 mg/day

Tablet, extended release (Cardizem® LA, Tiazac® XC [CAN; not available in U.S.]): 180 mg once daily; may increase at 7- to 14-day intervals; usual dose range: 120-320 mg/day; maximum: 360 mg/day

Tablet, immediate release (Cardizem®): Usual starting dose: 30 mg 4 times/day; titrate dose gradually at 1- to 2-day intervals; usual dose range: 120-320 mg/day

Hypertension:

Capsule, extended release (once-daily dosing):

Cardizem® CD, Cartia XT®, Dilt-CD: Initial: 180-240 mg once daily; dose adjustment may be made after 14 days; usual dose range (JNC 7): 180-420 mg/day; maximum: 480 mg/day

Dilacor® XR, Diltia XT®, Dilt-XR: Initial: 180-240 mg once daily; dose adjustment may be made after 14 days; usual dose range (JNC 7): 180-420 mg/day; maximum: 540 mg/day

Tiazac®, Taztia XT®: Initial: 120-240 mg once daily; dose adjustment may be made after 14 days; usual dose range (JNC 7): 180-420 mg/day; maximum: 540 mg/day

Capsule, extended release (twice-daily dosing): Initial: 60-120 mg twice daily; dose adjustment may be made after 14 days; usual range: 240-360 mg/day

Note: Diltiazem is available as a generic intended for either once- or twice-daily dosing, depending on the formulation; verify appropriate extended release capsule formulation is administered.

Tablet, extended release (Cardizem® LA, Tiazac® XC [CAN; not available in U.S.]): Initial: 180-240 mg once daily; dose adjustment may be made after 14 days; usual dose range (JNC 7): 120-540 mg/day

Note: Elderly: Patients ≥60 years may respond to a lower initial dose (ie, 120 mg once daily using extended release capsule)

I.V.: *Atrial fibrillation, atrial flutter, PSVT:*

Initial bolus dose: 0.25 mg/kg actual body weight over 2 minutes (average adult dose: 20 mg); ACLS guideline recommends 15-20 mg

Repeat bolus dose (may be administered after 15 minutes if the response is inadequate): 0.35 mg/kg actual body weight over 2 minutes (average adult dose: 25 mg); ACLS guideline recommends 20-25 mg

Continuous infusion (infusions >24 hours or infusion rates >15 mg/hour are not recommended): Initial infusion rate of 10 mg/hour; rate may be increased in 5 mg/hour increments up to 15 mg/hour as needed; some patients may respond to an initial rate of 5 mg/hour.

If diltiazem injection is administered by continuous infusion for >24 hours, the possibility of decreased diltiazem clearance, prolonged elimination half-life, and increased diltiazem and/or diltiazem metabolite plasma concentrations should be considered.

Conversion from I.V. diltiazem to oral diltiazem:

Oral dose (mg/day) is approximately equal to [rate (mg/hour) x 3 + 3] x 10.

3 mg/hour = 120 mg/day
5 mg/hour = 180 mg/day
7 mg/hour = 240 mg/day
11 mg/hour = 360 mg/day

Dosing adjustment in renal impairment: Use with caution; no dosing adjustments recommended

Dialysis: Not removed by hemo- or peritoneal dialysis; supplemental dose is not necessary.

Dosing adjustment in hepatic impairment: Use with caution; no specific dosing recommendations available; extensively metabolized by the liver; half-life is increased in patients with cirrhosis

Mechanism of Action Nondihydropyridine calcium channel blocker which inhibits calcium ion from entering the "slow channels" or select voltage-sensitive areas of vascular smooth muscle and myocardium during depolarization, producing a relaxation of coronary vascular smooth muscle and coronary vasodilation; increases myocardial oxygen delivery in patients with vasospastic angina

Contraindications

Oral: Hypersensitivity to diltiazem or any component of the formulation; sick sinus syndrome (except in patients with a functioning artificial pacemaker); second- or third-degree AV block (except in patients with a functioning artificial pacemaker); severe hypotension (systolic <90 mm Hg); acute MI and pulmonary congestion

Intravenous (I.V.): Hypersensitivity to diltiazem or any component of the formulation; sick sinus syndrome (except in patients with a functioning artificial pacemaker); second- or third-degree AV block (except in patients with a functioning artificial pacemaker); severe hypotension (systolic <90 mm Hg); cardiogenic shock; administration concomitantly or within a few hours of the administration of I.V. beta-blockers; atrial fibrillation or flutter associated with accessory bypass tract (eg, Wolff-Parkinson-White syndrome); ventricular tachycardia (with wide-complex tachycardia, must determine whether origin is supraventricular or ventricular)

Canadian labeling: Additional contraindications (not in U.S. labeling): I.V. and Oral: Pregnancy; use in women of childbearing potential

Warnings/Precautions Can cause first-, second-, and third-degree AV block or sinus bradycardia and risk increases with agents known to slow cardiac conduction. The most common side effect is peripheral edema; occurs within 2-3 weeks of starting therapy. Symptomatic hypotension with or without syncope can rarely occur; blood pressure must be lowered at a rate appropriate for the patient's clinical condition. Use caution when using diltiazem together with a beta-blocker; may result in conduction disturbances, hypotension, and worsened LV function. Simultaneous administration of I.V. diltiazem and an I.V. beta-blocker or administration within a few hours of each other may result in asystole and is contraindicated. Use with other agents known to either reduce SA node function and/or AV nodal conduction (eg, digoxin) or reduce sympathetic outflow (eg, clonidine) may increase the risk of serious bradycardia. Use caution in left ventricular dysfunction (may exacerbate condition). Avoid use of diltiazem in patients with heart failure and reduced ejection fraction (Hunt, 2009). Use with caution with hypertrophic obstructive cardiomyopathy; routine use is currently not recommended due to insufficient evidence (Maron, 2003). Use with caution in hepatic or renal dysfunction. Transient dermatologic reactions have been observed with use; if reaction persists, discontinue. May (rarely) progress to erythema multiforme or exfoliative dermatitis.

Drug Interactions

Metabolism/Transport Effects Substrate of CYP2C9 (minor), 2D6 (minor), 3A4 (major), P-glycoprotein; **Inhibits** CYP2C9 (weak), 2D6 (weak), 3A4 (moderate)

Avoid Concomitant Use

Avoid concomitant use of Diltiazem with any of the following: Tolvaptan

Increased Effect/Toxicity

Diltiazem may increase the levels/effects of: Alfentanil; Amifostine; Amiodarone; Antihypertensives; Aprepitant; Atorvastatin; Benzodiazepines (metabolized by oxidation); Beta-Blockers; Budesonide (Systemic, Oral Inhalation); BusPIRone; Calcium Channel Blockers (Dihydropyridine); CarBAMazepine; Cardiac Glycosides; Colchicine; Corticosteroids (Systemic); CycloSPORINE; CycloSPORINE (Systemic); CYP3A4 Substrates; Dronedarone; Eletriptan; Eplerenone; Everolimus; Fingolimod; Fosaprepitant; Fosphenytoin; Halofantrine; Hypotensive Agents; Lithium; Lovastatin; Lurasidone; Magnesium Salts; Midodrine; Neuromuscular-Blocking Agents (Nondepolarizing); Nitroprusside; Phenytoin; Pimecrolimus; QuiNIDine; Ranolazine; Red Yeast Rice; RiTUXimab; Salicylates; Salmeterol; Saxagliptin; Simvastatin; Tacrolimus; Tacrolimus (Systemic); Tacrolimus (Topical); Tolvaptan; Vilazodone

The levels/effects of Diltiazem may be increased by: Alpha1-Blockers; Anilidopiperidine Opioids; Antifungal Agents (Azole Derivatives, Systemic); Aprepitant; Atorvastatin; Calcium Channel Blockers (Dihydropyridine); Cimetidine; Conivaptan; CycloSPORINE; CycloSPORINE (Systemic); CYP3A4 Inhibitors (Moderate); CYP3A4 Inhibitors (Strong); Dasatinib; Diazoxide; Dronedarone; Fluconazole; Fosaprepitant; Grapefruit Juice; Herbs (Hypotensive Properties); Lovastatin; Macrolide Antibiotics; Magnesium Salts; MAO Inhibitors; Pentoxifylline; P-Glycoprotein Inhibitors; Phosphodiesterase 5 Inhibitors; Prostacyclin Analogues; Protease Inhibitors; Simvastatin

Decreased Effect

Diltiazem may decrease the levels/effects of: Clopidogrel

The levels/effects of Diltiazem may be decreased by: Barbiturates; Calcium Salts; CarBAMazepine; Colestipol; CYP3A4 Inducers (Strong); Deferasirox; Herbs (CYP3A4 Inducers); Herbs (Hypertensive Properties); Methylphenidate; Nafcillin; Peginterferon Alfa-2b; P-Glycoprotein Inducers; Rifamycin Derivatives; Tocilizumab; Yohimbine

Ethanol/Nutrition/Herb Interactions

Ethanol: Avoid ethanol (may increase risk of hypotension or vasodilation).

Food: Diltiazem serum levels may be elevated if taken with food. Serum concentrations were not altered by grapefruit juice in small clinical trials.

Herb/Nutraceutical: St John's wort may decrease diltiazem levels. Avoid bayberry, blue cohosh, cayenne, ephedra, ginger, ginseng (American), kola, licorice, yohimbe (may worsen hypertension). Avoid black cohosh, California poppy, coleus, garlic, golden seal, hawthorn, mistletoe, periwinkle, quinine, shepherd's purse (may have increased antihypertensive effect).

Pharmacodynamics/Kinetics

Onset of Action Oral: Immediate release tablet: 30-60 minutes; I.V.: 3 minutes

Duration of Action I.V.: Bolus: 1-3 hours; Continuous infusion (after discontinuation): 0.5-10 hours

Half-life Elimination Immediate release tablet: 3-4.5 hours, may be prolonged with renal impairment; Extended release tablet: 6-9 hours; Extended release capsules: 5-10 hours; I.V.: single dose: ~3.4 hours; continuous infusion: 4-5 hours

Time to Peak Serum: Immediate release tablet: 2-4 hours; Extended release tablet: 11-18 hours; Extended release capsule: 10-14 hours

Pregnancy Risk Factor C

Lactation Enters breast milk/not recommended (AAP considers "compatible"; AAP 2001 update pending)

Breast-Feeding Considerations Diltiazem is excreted into breastmilk in concentrations similar to those in the maternal plasma.

Dosage Forms

Capsule, extended release, oral: 60 mg, 90 mg, 120 mg, 180 mg, 240 mg, 300 mg, 360 mg, 420 mg
- Cardizem® CD: 120 mg, 180 mg, 240 mg, 300 mg, 360 mg
- Cartia XT®: 120 mg, 180 mg, 240 mg, 300 mg
- Dilacor XR®: 240 mg
- Dilt-CD: 120 mg, 180 mg, 240 mg, 300 mg
- Dilt-XR: 120 mg, 180 mg, 240 mg
- Diltia XT®: 120 mg, 180 mg, 240 mg
- Diltzac: 120 mg, 180 mg, 240 mg, 300 mg, 360 mg
- Taztia XT®: 120 mg, 180 mg, 240 mg, 300 mg, 360 mg
- Tiazac®: 120 mg, 180 mg, 240 mg, 300 mg, 360 mg, 420 mg

Injection, powder for reconstitution: 100 mg

Injection, solution: 5 mg/mL (5 mL, 10 mL, 25 mL)

Tablet, oral: 30 mg, 60 mg, 90 mg, 120 mg
- Cardizem®: 30 mg, 60 mg, 90 mg, 120 mg

Tablet, extended release, oral:
- Cardizem® LA: 120 mg, 180 mg, 240 mg, 300 mg, 360 mg, 420 mg
- Matzim™ LA: 180 mg, 240 mg, 300 mg, 360 mg, 420 mg

Dosage Forms: Canada

Tablet, extended release:
- Tiazac® XC: 120 mg, 180 mg, 240 mg, 300 mg, 360 mg

DimenhyDRINATE (dye men HYE dri nate)

U.S. Brand Names Dramamine® [OTC]; Driminate [OTC]; TripTone® [OTC]

Canadian Brand Names Apo-Dimenhydrinate®; Children's Motion Sickness Liquid; Dimenhydrinate Injection; Dinate®; Gravol®; Nauseatol; Novo-Dimenate; PMS-Dimenhydrinate; Sandoz-Dimenhydrinate

Pharmacologic Category Ethanolamine Derivative; Histamine H_1 Antagonist; Histamine H_1 Antagonist, First Generation

Use Treatment and prevention of nausea, vertigo, and vomiting associated with motion sickness

Local Anesthetic/Vasoconstrictor Precautions No information available to require special precautions

Effects on Dental Treatment Key adverse event(s) related to dental treatment: Significant xerostomia (normal salivary flow resumes upon discontinuation).

Effects on Bleeding No information available to require special precautions

Adverse Effects Frequency not defined.
- Cardiovascular: Tachycardia
- Central nervous system: Dizziness, drowsiness, excitation, headache, insomnia, lassitude, nervousness, restlessness
- Dermatologic: Rash
- Gastrointestinal: Anorexia, epigastric distress, nausea, xerostomia
- Genitourinary: Dysuria
- Ocular: Blurred vision
- Respiratory: Thickening of bronchial secretions

General Dosage Range

Oral:
- *Children 2-5 years:* 12.5-25 mg every 6-8 hours (maximum: 75 mg/day)
- *Children 6-12 years:* 25-50 mg every 6-8 hours (maximum: 150 mg/day)

I.M.:
- *Children:* 1.25 mg/kg **or** 37.5 mg/m^2 4 times/day (maximum: 300 mg/day)
- *Adults:* 50-100 mg every 4 hours

I.V.: *Adults:* 50-100 mg every 4 hours

Mechanism of Action Competes with histamine for H_1-receptor sites on effector cells in the gastrointestinal tract, blood vessels, and respiratory tract; blocks chemoreceptor trigger zone, diminishes vestibular stimulation, and depresses labyrinthine function through its central anticholinergic activity

Pharmacodynamics/Kinetics

Onset of Action Oral: ~15-30 minutes

Pregnancy Risk Factor B

Dimercaprol (dye mer KAP role)

U.S. Brand Names BAL in Oil®
Pharmacologic Category Antidote
Use Antidote to gold, arsenic (except arsine), or acute mercury poisoning (except nonalkyl mercury); adjunct to edetate CALCIUM disodium in lead poisoning
Local Anesthetic/Vasoconstrictor Precautions No information available to require special precautions
Effects on Dental Treatment No significant effects or complications reported
Effects on Bleeding No information available to require special precautions
Adverse Effects Frequency not always defined.
Cardiovascular: Chest pain, hypertension (dose related), tachycardia (dose related)
Central nervous system: Anxiety, fever (children ~30%), headache, nervousness
Dermatologic: Abscess
Gastrointestinal: Abdominal pain, burning sensation (lips, mouth, throat), nausea, salivation, throat irritation/pain, vomiting
Genitourinary: Burning sensation (penis)
Hematologic: Leukopenia (polymorphonuclear)
Local: Injection site pain
Neuromuscular & skeletal: Paresthesias (hand), weakness
Ocular: Blepharospasm, conjunctivitis, lacrimation
Renal: Acute renal insufficiency
Respiratory: Rhinorrhea, throat constriction
Miscellaneous: Diaphoresis
General Dosage Range I.M.: *Children and Adults:* Dosage varies greatly depending on indication
Mechanism of Action Sulfhydryl group combines with ions of various heavy metals to form relatively stable, nontoxic, soluble chelates which are excreted in urine
Pharmacodynamics/Kinetics
Time to Peak Serum: 0.5-1 hour
Pregnancy Risk Factor C

Dinoprostone (dye noe PROST one)

U.S. Brand Names Cervidil®; Prepidil®; Prostin E2®
Canadian Brand Names Cervidil®; Prepidil®; Prostin E_2®
Pharmacologic Category Abortifacient; Prostaglandin
Use
Endocervical gel: Promote cervical ripening in patients at or near term in whom there is a medical or obstetrical indication for the induction of labor
Suppositories: Terminate pregnancy from 12th through 20th week of gestation; evacuate uterus in cases of missed abortion or intrauterine fetal death up to 28 weeks of gestation; manage benign hydatidiform mole (nonmetastatic gestational trophoblastic disease)
Vaginal insert: Initiation and/or continuation of cervical ripening in patients at or near term in whom there is a medical or obstetrical indication for the induction of labor
Local Anesthetic/Vasoconstrictor Precautions No information available to require special precautions
Effects on Dental Treatment No significant effects or complications reported
Effects on Bleeding No information available to require special precautions
Adverse Effects
Endocervical gel: 1% to 10%:
Central nervous system: Fever (1%)
Gastrointestinal: GI upset (6%)
Genitourinary: Abnormal uterine contractions (7%), warm feeling in vagina (2%)
Neuromuscular & skeletal: Back pain (3%)

Suppository: Frequency not defined:
Cardiovascular: Arrhythmia, chest pain, chest tightness, hypotension, syncope
Central nervous system: Chills, dizziness, fever, headache, shivering, tension
Dermatologic: Rash, skin discoloration
Endocrine & metabolic: Breast tenderness, endometritis, hot flashes
Gastrointestinal: Dehydration, diarrhea, nausea, vomiting
Genitourinary: uterine rupture, urinary retention, vaginal pain, vaginismus, vaginitis, vulvitis
Neuromuscular & skeletal: Arthralgia, backache, joint inflammation/pain (new or exacerbated), leg cramps (nocturnal), muscle cramp/pain, myalgia, paresthesia, stiff neck, tremor, weakness
Ocular: Blurred vision, eye pain
Otic: Hearing impairment

Respiratory: Cough, dyspnea, laryngitis, pharyngitis, wheezing
Miscellaneous: Diaphoresis

Vaginal insert: 1% to 10%: Genitourinary: Uterine hyperstimulation *without* fetal distress (2% to 5%), uterine hyperstimulation *with* fetal distress (3%)

General Dosage Range

Endocervical: *Children (females of reproductive age) and Adults (females):* 0.5 mg; may repeat every 6 hours if needed. Maximum cumulative dose: 1.5 mg/24 hours

Intravaginal: *Children (females of reproductive age) and Adults (females):* Insert: 10 mg; remove at onset of active labor or after 12 hours; Suppository: 20 mg every 3-5 hours until abortion occurs

Mechanism of Action A synthetic prostaglandin E_2 abortifacient that stimulates uterine contractions similar to those seen during natural labor. Prostaglandin E_2 plays a role in cervical ripening, which allows the fetus to pass through the birth canal.

Pharmacodynamics/Kinetics

Onset of Action Uterine contractions: Vaginal suppository: Within 10 minutes

Duration of Action Vaginal insert: 0.3 mg/hour over 12 hours; Vaginal suppository: Up to 2-3 hours

Half-life Elimination 2.5-5 minutes

Time to Peak Endocervical gel: 30-45 minutes

Pregnancy Risk Factor C

DiphenhydrAMINE (Systemic) (dye fen HYE dra meen)

Related Information

Management of Patients Undergoing Cancer Therapy *on page 1970*
Ulcerative, Erosive, and Painful Oral Mucosal Disorders *on page 1950*
Viral Infections *on page 1947*

Related Sample Prescriptions

Recurrent Aphthous Stomatitis *on page 1992*

U.S. Brand Names Aler-Cap [OTC]; Aler-Dryl [OTC]; Aler-Tab [OTC]; AllerMax® [OTC]; Altaryl [OTC]; Anti-Hist [OTC]; Banophen™ [OTC]; Benadryl® Allergy Quick Dissolve [OTC]; Benadryl® Allergy [OTC]; Benadryl® Children's Allergy FastMelt® [OTC]; Benadryl® Children's Allergy Perfect Measure™ [OTC]; Benadryl® Children's Allergy [OTC]; Benadryl® Children's Dye Free Allergy [OTC]; Benadryl® Dye-Free Allergy [OTC]; Compoz® [OTC]; Diphen [OTC]; Diphenhist® [OTC]; Genahist™ [OTC] [DSC]; Histaprin [OTC]; Nytol® Quick Caps [OTC]; Nytol® Quick Gels [OTC]; PediaCare® Children's Allergy [OTC]; PediaCare® Children's NightTime Cough [OTC]; Siladryl Allergy [OTC]; Silphen [OTC]; Simply Sleep® [OTC]; Sleep-ettes D [OTC]; Sleep-Tabs [OTC]; Sleepinal® [OTC]; Sominex® Maximum Strength [OTC]; Sominex® [OTC]; Theraflu® Thin Strips® Multi Symptom [OTC]; Triaminic Thin Strips® Children's Cough & Runny Nose [OTC]; Twilite® [OTC]; Unisom® SleepGels® Maximum Strength [OTC]; Unisom® SleepMelts™ [OTC]

Canadian Brand Names Allerdryl®; Allernix; Benadryl®; Nytol®; Nytol® Extra Strength; PMS-Diphenhydramine; Simply Sleep®; Sominex®

Generic Availability (U.S.) Yes: Excludes orally-disintegrating tablet, strip

Pharmacologic Category Ethanolamine Derivative; Histamine H_1 Antagonist; Histamine H_1 Antagonist, First Generation

Dental Use Symptomatic relief of nasal mucosal congestion; symptomatic relief of oral erosions (systemic diphenhydramine used topically) including aphthous stomatitis

Use Symptomatic relief of allergic symptoms caused by histamine release including nasal allergies and allergic dermatosis; adjunct to epinephrine in the treatment of anaphylaxis; nighttime sleep aid; prevention or treatment of motion sickness; antitussive; management of Parkinsonian syndrome including drug-induced extrapyramidal symptoms

Local Anesthetic/Vasoconstrictor Precautions No information available to require special precautions

Effects on Dental Treatment Key adverse event(s) related to dental treatment: Xerostomia (normal salivary flow resumes upon discontinuation) and dry mucous membranes. Chronic use of antihistamines will inhibit salivary flow, particularly in elderly patients; may contribute to periodontal disease and oral discomfort. See Dental Comment.

Effects on Bleeding No information available to require special precautions

Adverse Effects Frequency not defined.

Cardiovascular: Chest tightness, extrasystoles, hypotension, palpitation, tachycardia

Central nervous system: Chills, confusion, convulsion, disturbed coordination, dizziness, euphoria, excitation, fatigue, headache, insomnia, irritability, nervousness, paradoxical excitement, restlessness, sedation, sleepiness, vertigo
Endocrine & metabolic: Menstrual irregularities (early menses)
Gastrointestinal: Anorexia, constipation, diarrhea, dry mucous membranes, epigastric distress, nausea, throat tightness, vomiting, xerostomia
Genitourinary: Difficult urination, urinary frequency, urinary retention
Hematologic: Agranulocytosis, hemolytic anemia, thrombocytopenia
Neuromuscular & skeletal: Neuritis, paresthesia, tremor
Ocular: Blurred vision, diplopia
Otic: Labyrinthitis (acute), tinnitus
Respiratory: Nasal stuffiness, thickening of bronchial secretions, wheezing
Miscellaneous: Anaphylactic shock, diaphoresis

Dental Usual Dosage

Symptomatic relief of nasal mucosal congestion: Adults: Oral: 25-50 mg every 6-8 hours

Symptomatic relief of oral erosions (used topically): Adults: Rinse with 1-2 teaspoonfuls every 2 hours and expectorate

Dosage Note: Dosages are expressed as the hydrochloride salt.

Children:
- Allergic reactions or motion sickness: Oral, I.M., I.V.: 5 mg/kg/day or 150 mg/m²/day in divided doses every 6-8 hours, not to exceed 300 mg/day
  - Alternate dosing by age: Oral:
    - 2 to <6 years: 6.25 mg every 4-6 hours; maximum: 37.5 mg/day
    - 6 to <12 years: 12.5-25 mg every 4-6 hours; maximum: 150 mg/day
    - ≥12 years: 25-50 mg every 4-6 hours; maximum: 300 mg/day
- Night-time sleep aid: Oral: Children ≥12 years: 50 mg at bedtime
- Antitussive: Oral:
  - 2 to <6 years: 6.25 mg every 4 hours; maximum: 37.5 mg/day
  - 6 to <12 years: 12.5 mg every 4 hours; maximum: 75 mg/day
  - ≥12 years: 25 mg every 4 hours; maximum: 150 mg/day
- Treatment of dystonic reactions: I.M., I.V.: 0.5-1 mg/kg/dose

Adults:
- Allergic reactions or motion sickness: Oral: 25-50 mg every 6-8 hours
- Antitussive: Oral: 25 mg every 4 hours; maximum: 150 mg/24 hours
- Night-time sleep aid: Oral: 50 mg at bedtime
- Allergic reactions or motion sickness: I.M., I.V.: 10-50 mg per dose; single doses up to 100 mg may be used if needed; not to exceed 400 mg/day
- Dystonic reaction: I.M., I.V.: 50 mg in a single dose; may repeat in 20-30 minutes if necessary

Elderly: Initial: 25 mg 2-3 times/day increasing as needed

Mechanism of Action Competes with histamine for H_1-receptor sites on effector cells in the gastrointestinal tract, blood vessels, and respiratory tract; anticholinergic and sedative effects are also seen

Contraindications Hypersensitivity to diphenhydramine or any component of the formulation; acute asthma; neonates or premature infants; breast-feeding; use as a local anesthetic (injection)

Warnings/Precautions Causes sedation, caution must be used in performing tasks which require alertness (eg, operating machinery or driving). Sedative effects of CNS depressants or ethanol are potentiated. Should not be used as a hypnotic in the elderly; may cause excessive sedation and confusion; may be inappropriate in this age group when used as an antihistamine due to potent anticholinergic effects (nonanticholinergic antihistamines preferred); when used for emergency allergic reactions, use the smallest effective dose (Beers Criteria). Antihistamines may cause excitation in young children. Use with caution in patients with angle-closure glaucoma, pyloroduodenal obstruction (including stenotic peptic ulcer), urinary tract obstruction (including bladder neck obstruction and symptomatic prostatic hyperplasia), asthma, hyperthyroidism, increased intraocular pressure, and cardiovascular disease (including hypertension and tachycardia). Some preparations contain soy protein; avoid use in patients with soy protein or peanut allergies. Some products may contain phenylalanine.

Self-medication (OTC use): Do not use with other products containing diphenhydramine, even ones used on the skin. Oral products are not for OTC use in children <6 years of age.

Drug Interactions

Metabolism/Transport Effects **Inhibits** CYP2D6 (moderate)

Avoid Concomitant Use There are no known interactions where it is recommended to avoid concomitant use.

Increased Effect/Toxicity

DiphenhydrAMINE (Systemic) may increase the levels/effects of: Alcohol (Ethyl); Anticholinergics; CNS Depressants; CYP2D6 Substrates; Fesoterodine; Nebivolol; Tamoxifen

The levels/effects of DiphenhydrAMINE (Systemic) may be increased by: Droperidol; Pramlintide

Decreased Effect

DiphenhydrAMINE (Systemic) may decrease the levels/effects of: Acetylcholinesterase Inhibitors (Central); Benzylpenicilloyl Polylysine; Betahistine; Codeine; TraMADol

The levels/effects of DiphenhydrAMINE (Systemic) may be decreased by: Acetylcholinesterase Inhibitors (Central); Amphetamines

Ethanol/Nutrition/Herb Interactions

Ethanol: May increase CNS depression; monitor for increased effects with coadministration. Caution patients about effects.

Herb/Nutraceutical: Avoid valerian, St John's wort, kava kava, gotu kola (may increase CNS depression).

Dietary Considerations Some products may contain sodium and/or phenylalanine.

Pharmacodynamics/Kinetics

Onset of Action Maximum sedative effect: 1-3 hours

Duration of Action 4-7 hours

Half-life Elimination 2-10 hours; Elderly: 13.5 hours

Time to Peak Serum: 2-4 hours

Pregnancy Risk Factor B

Lactation Enters breast milk/contraindicated

Breast-Feeding Considerations Infants may be more sensitive to the effects of antihistamines. Use while breast-feeding is contraindicated by the manufacturer.

Dosage Forms

Caplet, oral:

Aler-Dryl [OTC]: 50 mg
AllerMax® [OTC]: 50 mg
Anti-Hist [OTC]: 25 mg
Compoz® [OTC]: 50 mg
Histaprin [OTC]: 25 mg
Nytol® Quick Caps [OTC]: 25 mg
Simply Sleep® [OTC]: 25 mg
Sleep-ettes D [OTC]: 50 mg
Sominex® Maximum Strength [OTC]: 50 mg
Twilite® [OTC]: 50 mg

Capsule, oral: 25 mg, 50 mg

Aler-Cap [OTC]: 25 mg
Banophen™ [OTC]: 25 mg
Benadryl® Allergy [OTC]: 25 mg
Diphen [OTC]: 25 mg
Diphenhist® [OTC]: 25 mg
Sleepinal® [OTC]: 50 mg

Capsule, softgel, oral:

Benadryl® Dye-Free Allergy [OTC]: 25 mg
Compoz® [OTC]: 50 mg
Nytol® Quick Gels [OTC]: 50 mg
Unisom® SleepGels® Maximum Strength [OTC]: 50 mg

Captab, oral:

Diphenhist® [OTC]: 25 mg

Elixir, oral:

Altaryl [OTC]: 12.5 mg/5 mL (120 mL, 480 mL, 3840 mL)
Banophen™ [OTC]: 12.5 mg/5 mL (120 mL, 480 mL)

Injection, solution: 50 mg/mL (1 mL, 10 mL)

Injection, solution [preservative free]: 50 mg/mL (1 mL)

Liquid, oral:

AllerMax® [OTC]: 12.5 mg/5 mL (120 mL)
Benadryl® Children's Allergy [OTC]: 12.5 mg/5 mL (118 mL, 236 mL)
Benadryl® Children's Allergy Perfect Measure™ [OTC]: 12.5 mg/5 mL (5 mL)
Benadryl® Children's Dye Free Allergy [OTC]: 12.5 mg/5 mL (118 mL)
Siladryl Allergy [OTC]: 12.5 mg/5 mL (118 mL, 237 mL, 473 mL)

Solution, oral: 12.5 mg/5 mL (5 mL, 10 mL, 20 mL)

Diphenhist® [OTC]: 12.5 mg/5 mL (120 mL, 480 mL)

Strip, orally disintegrating, oral:
Benadryl® Allergy Quick Dissolve [OTC]: 25 mg (10s)
Theraflu® Thin Strips® Multi Symptom [OTC]: 25 mg (12s, 24s)
Triaminic Thin Strips® Children's Cough & Runny Nose [OTC]: 12.5 mg (14s)
Syrup, oral:
PediaCare® Children's Allergy [OTC]: 12.5 mg/5 mL (118 mL)
PediaCare® Children's NightTime Cough [OTC]: 12.5 mg/5 mL (118 mL)
Silphen [OTC]: 12.5 mg/5 mL (118 mL, 237 mL, 473 mL)
Tablet, oral: 25 mg, 50 mg
Aler-Tab [OTC]: 25 mg
Banophen™ [OTC]: 25 mg
Benadryl® Allergy [OTC]: 25 mg
Sleep-Tabs [OTC]: 25 mg
Sominex® [OTC]: 25 mg
Tablet, orally dissolving, oral:
Benadryl® Children's Allergy FastMelt® [OTC]: 12.5 mg
Unisom® SleepMelts™ [OTC]: 25 mg

Dental Comment 25-50 mg of diphenhydramine orally every 4-6 hours can be used to treat mild dermatologic manifestations of allergic reactions to penicillin and other antibiotics. Diphenhydramine is not recommended as local anesthetic for either infiltration route or nerve block since the vehicle has caused local necrosis upon injection. A 50:50 mixture of diphenhydramine liquid (12.5 mg/5 mL) in Kaopectate® or Maalox® is used as a local application for recurrent aphthous ulcers; swish 1 tablespoonful for 2 minutes 4 times/day.

DiphenhydrAMINE (Topical) (dye fen HYE dra meen)

U.S. Brand Names Banophen™ Anti-Itch [OTC]; Benadryl® Extra Strength Itch Stopping [OTC]; Benadryl® Itch Relief Extra Strength [OTC]; Benadryl® Itch Stopping Extra Strength [OTC]; Benadryl® Itch Stopping [OTC]; Dermamycin® [OTC]; Diphenhist® [OTC]

Canadian Brand Names Benadryl® Cream; Benadryl® Itch Relief Stick; Benadryl® Spray

Generic Availability (U.S.) Yes: Excludes gel, liquid stick, spray

Pharmacologic Category Ethanolamine Derivative; Histamine H_1 Antagonist; Histamine H_1 Antagonist, First Generation; Topical Skin Product

Use Topically for relief of pain and itching associated with insect bites, minor cuts and burns, or rashes due to poison ivy, poison oak, and poison sumac

Local Anesthetic/Vasoconstrictor Precautions No information available to require special precautions

Effects on Dental Treatment No significant effects or complications reported

Effects on Bleeding No information available to require special precautions

Adverse Effects Frequency not defined.
Dermatologic: Photosensitivity, rash, urticaria

Dosage
Children:
Relief of pain and itching: Topical: Children ≥2 years: Apply 1% or 2% to affected area up to 3-4 times/day
Adults:
Relief of pain and itching: Topical: Apply 1% or 2% to affected area up to 3-4 times/day

Contraindications Hypersensitivity to diphenhydramine or any component of the formulation; neonates or premature infants; breast-feeding

Warnings/Precautions Self-medication (OTC use): Topical products should not be used on large areas of the body, or on chicken pox or measles. Healthcare provider should be contacted if topical use is needed for >7 days. Topical products are not for OTC use in children <2 years of age. Do not use with other products containing diphenhydramine.

Drug Interactions
Metabolism/Transport Effects Inhibits CYP2D6 (moderate)
Avoid Concomitant Use There are no known interactions where it is recommended to avoid concomitant use.
Increased Effect/Toxicity
DiphenhydrAMINE (Topical) may increase the levels/effects of: Alcohol (Ethyl); Anticholinergics; CNS Depressants

The levels/effects of DiphenhydrAMINE (Topical) may be increased by: Droperidol; Pramlintide
Decreased Effect
DiphenhydrAMINE (Topical) may decrease the levels/effects of: Acetylcholinesterase Inhibitors (Central); Benzylpenicilloyl Polylysine; Betahistine

The levels/effects of DiphenhydrAMINE (Topical) may be decreased by: Acetylcholinesterase Inhibitors (Central); Amphetamines

Dosage Forms

Cream, topical: 2% (30 g)
Banophen™ Anti-Itch [OTC]: 2% (28.4 g)
Benadryl® Itch Stopping [OTC]: 1% (14.2 g, 28.3 g)
Benadryl® Itch Stopping Extra Strength [OTC]: 2% (14.2 g, 28.3 g)
Dermamycin® [OTC]: 2% (28 g)
Diphenhist® [OTC]: 2% (28.4 g)

Gel, topical:
Benadryl® Extra Strength Itch Stopping [OTC]: 2% (120 mL)

Liquid, topical:
Benadryl® Itch Relief Extra Strength [OTC]: 2% (14 mL)
Benadryl® Itch Stopping Extra Strength [OTC]: 2% (59 mL)
Dermamycin® [OTC]: 2% (60 mL)

Diphenhydramine and Phenylephrine

(dye fen HYE dra meen & fen il EF rin)

Related Information

DiphenhydrAMINE (Systemic) *on page 540*
Phenylephrine (Systemic) *on page 1339*

U.S. Brand Names Aldex® CT; Benadryl-D® Allergy & Sinus [OTC]; Benadryl-D® Children's Allergy & Sinus [OTC]; Dimetapp® Children's Nighttime Cold & Congestion [OTC]; Robitussin® Night Time Cough & Cold [OTC]; Triaminic® Children's Night Time Cold & Cough [OTC]; Triaminic® Children's Thin Strips® Night Time Cold & Cough [OTC]

Pharmacologic Category Alpha/Beta Agonist; Decongestant; Ethanolamine Derivative; Histamine H_1 Antagonist; Histamine H_1 Antagonist, First Generation

Use Temporary relief of symptoms of allergic rhinitis, sinusitis, and other upper respiratory conditions, including sinus/nasal congestion, sneezing, stuffy/runny nose, itchy/watery eyes, and cough

Local Anesthetic/Vasoconstrictor Precautions Use with caution since phenylephrine is a sympathomimetic amine which could interact with epinephrine or mepivacaine and levonordefrin (Carbocaine® 2% with Neo-Cobefrin®) to cause a pressor response.

Effects on Dental Treatment Key adverse event(s) related to dental treatment:
Diphenhydramine: Prolonged use will cause significant xerostomia (normal salivary flow resumes upon discontinuation).
Phenylephrine: Up to 10% of patients could experience tachycardia, palpitations, and xerostomia.

Effects on Bleeding No information available to require special precautions

Adverse Effects Frequency not defined.
Cardiovascular: Chest tightness, extrasystoles, hypotension, palpitation, tachycardia
Central nervous system: Chills, confusion, coordination impaired, dizziness, drowsiness, euphoria, excitation, fatigue, headache, insomnia, irritability, nervousness, neuritis, restlessness, sedation, seizure, vertigo
Dermatologic: Photosensitivity, rash, urticaria
Endocrine & metabolic: Early menses
Gastrointestinal: Anorexia, constipation, diarrhea, dry mucous membranes, epigastric distress, nausea, vomiting, xerostomia
Genitourinary: Dysuria, polyuria, urinary retention
Hematologic: Agranulocytosis, hemolytic anemia, thrombocytopenia
Neuromuscular & skeletal: Paresthesia, tremor
Ocular: Blurred vision, diplopia
Otic: Labyrinthitis, tinnitus
Respiratory: Bronchial secretions (thickening), nasal congestion, throat tightness, wheezing
Miscellaneous: Anaphylaxis, diaphoresis

General Dosage Range Oral:
Children 6-11 years: Aldex® CT: 1/2 to 1 tablet every 6 hours; OTC labeling: 5-10 mL or 1 strip every 4 hours as needed (maximum: 6 doses/24 hours)
Children ≥12 years and Adults: Aldex® CT: 1-2 tablets every 6 hours; OTC labeling: 10-20 mL every 4 hours as needed or 1 tablet every 4 hours as needed (maximum: 6 doses/24 hours)

Mechanism of Action
Diphenhydramine is an H_1-receptor antagonist.
Phenylephrine is a potent, direct-acting alpha-adrenergic stimulator.

Pregnancy Risk Factor C

Diphenoxylate and Atropine (dye fen OKS i late & A troe peen)

Related Information

Atropine *on page* 188

U.S. Brand Names Lomotil®

Canadian Brand Names Lomotil®

Pharmacologic Category Antidiarrheal

Use Treatment of diarrhea

Local Anesthetic/Vasoconstrictor Precautions No information available to require special precautions

Effects on Dental Treatment Key adverse event(s) related to dental treatment: Significant xerostomia (normal salivary flow resumes upon discontinuation).

Effects on Bleeding No information available to require special precautions

Adverse Effects Frequency not defined.

Cardiovascular: Tachycardia

Central nervous system: Confusion, depression, dizziness, drowsiness, euphoria, flushing, headache, hyperthermia, lethargy, malaise, restlessness, sedation

Dermatologic: Angioneurotic edema, dry skin, pruritus, urticaria

Gastrointestinal: Abdominal discomfort, anorexia, gum swelling, nausea, pancreatitis, paralytic ileus, toxic megacolon, vomiting, xerostomia

Genitourinary: Urinary retention

Neuromuscular & skeletal: Numbness

Miscellaneous: Anaphylaxis

General Dosage Range Oral:

Children 2-12 years: Initial: Diphenoxylate 0.3-0.4 mg/kg/day in 4 divided doses (maximum: 10 mg/day); Maintenance: Reduce as needed, may be as low as 25% of the initial daily dose

Adults: Initial: Diphenoxylate 5 mg 4 times/day (maximum: 20 mg/day); Maintenance: Reduce as needed, may be as low as 5 mg/day

Mechanism of Action Diphenoxylate inhibits excessive GI motility and GI propulsion; commercial preparations contain a subtherapeutic amount of atropine to discourage abuse

Pharmacodynamics/Kinetics

Onset of Action Diphenoxylate: Antidiarrheal: 45-60 minutes

Duration of Action Diphenoxylate: Antidiarrheal: 3-4 hours

Half-life Elimination Diphenoxylate: 2.5 hours; Diphenoxylic acid: 12-14 hours

Time to Peak Diphenoxylate: Serum: 2 hours

Pregnancy Risk Factor C

Controlled Substance C-V

Diphtheria and Tetanus Toxoids, Acellular Pertussis, and Poliovirus Vaccine

(dif THEER ee a & TET a nus TOKS oyds, ay CEL yoo lar per TUS sis & POE lee oh VYE rus vak SEEN)

U.S. Brand Names Kinrix®

Pharmacologic Category Vaccine, Inactivated (Bacterial); Vaccine, Inactivated (Viral)

Use Active immunization against diphtheria, tetanus, pertussis, and poliomyelitis, used as the 5th dose in the DTaP series and the 4th dose in the IPV series

The Advisory Committee on Immunization Practices (ACIP) recommends routine vaccination for use as the fifth dose in the DTaP series and the fourth dose in the IPV series in children who received DTaP (Infanrix®) and/or DTaP-Hepatitis B-IPV (Pediarix®) as the first 3 doses and DTaP (Infanrix®) as the fourth dose. Whenever feasible, the same manufacturer should be used to provide the pertussis component; however, vaccination should not be deferred if a specific brand is not known or is not available.

Local Anesthetic/Vasoconstrictor Precautions No information available to require special precautions

Effects on Dental Treatment No significant effects or complications reported

Effects on Bleeding No information available to require special precautions

Adverse Effects All serious adverse reactions must be reported to the U.S. Department of Health and Human Services (DHHS) Vaccine Adverse Event Reporting System (VAERS) 1-800-822-7967 or online at https://vaers.hhs.gov/esub/index.

Adverse events reported within 4 days of vaccination: >10%:

Central nervous system: Drowsiness (19%, grade 3: 1%), fever (≥99.5°F: 16%, >100.4: 7%, >104: <1%)

Gastrointestinal: Loss of appetite (16%; grade 3: 1%)

Local: Injection site: Pain (57%; grade 3: 2%), redness (37%; ≥50 mm: 18%, ≥110 mm: 3%), arm circumference increase (36%, >20 mm: 7%, >30 mm: 2%), swelling (26%; ≥50 mm: 10%, ≥110 mm: 1%)

General Dosage Range I.M.: *Children 4-6 years:* 0.5 mL

Mechanism of Action Promotes active immunity to diphtheria, tetanus, pertussis, and poliovirus (types 1, 2 and 3) by inducing production of specific antibodies and antitoxins.

Pharmacodynamics/Kinetics

Onset of Action Immune response observed to all components ~1 month following vaccination

Pregnancy Risk Factor C

Diphtheria and Tetanus Toxoids, Acellular Pertussis, Hepatitis B (Recombinant), Poliovirus (Inactivated), and *Haemophilus influenzae* B Conjugate (Adsorbed) Vaccine

(dif THEER ee a & TET a nus TOKS oyds, ay CEL yoo lar per TUS sis, hep a TYE tis bee ree KOM be nant, POE lee oh VYE rus in ak ti VAY ted, & hem OF fi lus in floo EN za bee KON joo gate ad SORBED vak SEEN)

Canadian Brand Names Infanrix Hexa™

Pharmacologic Category Vaccine, Inactivated (Bacterial, Viral)

Use Active primary immunization against diphtheria, tetanus, pertussis, hepatitis B, poliomyelitis and disease caused by *Haemophilus influenzae* type b in infants and children 6 weeks to 2 years of age; booster immunization (at 18 months) in infants who previously received a full primary vaccination course of each component of the vaccine

Local Anesthetic/Vasoconstrictor Precautions No information available to require special precautions

Effects on Dental Treatment No significant effects or complications reported

Effects on Bleeding No information available to require special precautions

Adverse Effects **All serious adverse reactions may be reported to local provincial/territorial health agencies or to the Vaccine Safety Section at Public Health Agency of Canada (1-866-844-0018).**

Frequency not always defined.

>10%:

Central nervous system: Irritability (83%), sleeping increased (63%), fever ≥38°C (100.4°F) (56%), sleeping decreased (51%), crying abnormal (43%), fatigue, restlessness

Local: Injection Site: Redness (49%), pain (43%), swelling (36%)

Gastrointestinal: Loss of appetite (49%), diarrhea (36%), vomiting (25%)

1% to 10%:

Central nervous system: Fever >39.5°C (103.1°F), nervousness

Local: Injection site: Induration

General Dosage Range I.M.: *Children 6 weeks to 2 years:* Primary immunization: 0.5 mL every 8 weeks for a total of 3 doses; booster dose: 0.5 mL

Mechanism of Action Promotes active immunity to diphtheria, tetanus, pertussis, hepatitis B, poliovirus (types 1, 2 and 3), and *Haemophilus influenzae* type B by inducing production of specific antibodies and antitoxins.

Pharmacodynamics/Kinetics

Onset of Action Immune response observed to all components 1 month following the 3-dose series

Product Availability Not available in U.S.

Diphtheria and Tetanus Toxoids, Acellular Pertussis, Poliovirus and *Haemophilus* b Conjugate Vaccine

(dif THEER ee a & TET a nus TOKS oyds ay CEL yoo lar per TUS sis POE lee oh VYE rus & hem OF fi lus in floo EN za bee KON joo gate vak SEEN)

U.S. Brand Names Pentacel®

Canadian Brand Names Pediacel®; Pentacel®

Pharmacologic Category Vaccine, Inactivated (Bacterial); Vaccine, Inactivated (Viral)

Use Active immunization against diphtheria, tetanus, pertussis, poliomyelitis, and invasive disease caused by *H. influenzae* type b in children 6 weeks through 4 years of age

Advisory Committee on Immunization Practices (ACIP) recommends that Pentacel® (DTaP-IPV/Hib) may be used to provide the recommended DTaP, IPV, and Hib immunization in children <5 years of age. Whenever feasible, the same manufacturer should be used to provide the pertussis component; however, vaccination should not be deferred if a specific brand is not known or is not available. The Hib component in Pentacel® contains a tetanus toxoid conjugate. A Hib vaccine containing the PRP-OMP conjugate (PedvaxHIB®) may provide a more rapid seroconversion following the first dose and may be preferable to use in certain populations (eg, American Indian or Alaska Native children).

Local Anesthetic/Vasoconstrictor Precautions No information available to require special precautions

Effects on Dental Treatment No significant effects or complications reported

Effects on Bleeding No information available to require special precautions

Adverse Effects All serious adverse reactions must be reported to the U.S. Department of Health and Human Services (DHHS) Vaccine Adverse Event Reporting System (VAERS) 1-800-822-7967 or online at https://vaers.hhs.gov/esub/index. In Canada, adverse reactions may be reported to local provincial/territorial health agencies or to the Vaccine Safety Section at Public Health Agency of Canada (1-866-844-0018).

>10%:

Central nervous system: Fussiness/irritability (54% to 77%; >3 hours 4% to 5%), inconsolable crying (36% to 60%; >3 hours ≤2%), lethargy/decreased activity (24% to 46%; severe ≤3%), fever ≥38°C (6% to 16%)

Local: Injection site reactions: Tenderness (39% to 56%; severe 1% to 5%), arm circumference increase >5 mm (34%; >40 mm <1%), redness >5 mm (7% to 17%)

1% to 10%: Local: Injection site reaction: Swelling >5 mm (5% to 10%)

General Dosage Range I.M.: *Children 6 weeks to ≤4 years:* 0.5 mL

Pregnancy Risk Factor C

Diphtheria, Tetanus Toxoids, Acellular Pertussis, Hepatitis B (Recombinant), and Poliovirus Vaccine

(dif THEER ee a, TET a nus TOKS oyds, ay CEL yoo lar per TUS sis, hep a TYE tis bee ree KOM be nant, & POE lee oh VYE rus vak SEEN)

Related Information

Hepatitis B Vaccine (Recombinant) *on page* 848
Poliovirus Vaccine (Inactivated) *on page* 1367
Tetanus Toxoid (Adsorbed) *on page* 1607

U.S. Brand Names Pediarix®

Canadian Brand Names Pediarix®

Pharmacologic Category Vaccine, Inactivated (Bacterial); Vaccine, Inactivated (Viral)

Use Combination vaccine for the active immunization against diphtheria, tetanus, pertussis, hepatitis B virus (all known subtypes), and poliomyelitis (caused by poliovirus types 1, 2, and 3)

The Advisory Committee on Immunization Practices (ACIP) recommends Pediarix® for the following:

- Primary vaccination for DTaP, Hep B, and IPV in children at 2, 4, and 6 months of age.
- To complete the primary vaccination series in children who have received DTaP (Infanrix®) and who are scheduled to receive the other components of the vaccine. Whenever feasible, the same manufacturer should be used to provide the pertussis component; however, vaccination should not be deferred if a specific brand is not known or is not available. HepB and IPV from different manufacturers are interchangeable.

Local Anesthetic/Vasoconstrictor Precautions No information available to require special precautions

Effects on Dental Treatment No significant effects or complications reported

Effects on Bleeding No information available to require special precautions

Adverse Effects All serious adverse reactions must be reported to the U.S. Department of Health and Human Services (DHHS) Vaccine Adverse Event Reporting System (VAERS) 1-800-822-7967 or online at https://vaers.hhs.gov/esub/index. In Canada, adverse reactions may be reported to local provincial/territorial health agencies or to the Vaccine Safety Section at Public Health Agency of Canada (1-866-844-0018).

Adverse events reported within 4 days of vaccination at 2-, 4-, and 6 months of age in patients given Pediarix® concomitantly with Hib conjugate vaccine and PCV7 vaccine.

>10%:

Central nervous system: Irritability/fussiness (61% to 65%; grade 3: 3% to 4%), drowsiness (41% to 57%), fever ≥100.4°F (28% to 39%)

Gastrointestinal: Loss of appetite (26% to 31%; grade 3: <1%)

Local: Injection site: Redness (25% to 40%; >20 mm: 1% to 3%), pain (31% to 36%; grade 3: 2% to 3%), swelling (17% to 29%; >20 mm: 2% to 3%)

1% to 10%: Central nervous system: Fever >103.1°F (≤1%)

Additional and postmarketing events: Anaphylactic/anaphylactoid reaction, angioedema, anorexia, apnea, arthus-type hypersensitivity reactions, brachial neuritis, bulging fontanelle, consciousness depressed, cough, cranial mononeuropathy, crying, cyanosis, demyelinating disease, diarrhea, dyspnea, encephalitis, erythema, fatigue, febrile convulsion, Guillain-Barré syndrome, hypersensitivity reaction, hypotonia, hypotonic-hyporesposnive episode, injection site reactions (cellulitis, induration, itching, nodule, warmth, vesicles), insomnia, lethargy, limb pain, limb swelling, liver function test abnormalities, nervousness, pallor, peripheral mononeuropathy, petechiae, rash, restlessness, screaming, seizure, SIDS, somnolence, upper respiratory tract infection, urticaria, vomiting

General Dosage Range I.M.: *Children 6 weeks to <7 years:* 0.5 mL/dose for a total of 3 doses

Mechanism of Action Promotes active immunity to diphtheria, tetanus, pertussis, hepatitis B and poliovirus (types 1, 2 and 3) by inducing production of specific antibodies and antitoxins.

Pharmacodynamics/Kinetics

Onset of Action Immune response observed to all components 1 month following the 3-dose series.

Pregnancy Risk Factor C

Dipivefrin (dye PI ve frin)

Canadian Brand Names Ophtho-Dipivefrin™; PMS-Dipivefrin; Propine®

Pharmacologic Category Alpha/Beta Agonist; Ophthalmic Agent, Antiglaucoma; Ophthalmic Agent, Vasoconstrictor

Use Reduces elevated intraocular pressure in chronic open-angle glaucoma; also used to treat ocular hypertension, low tension, and secondary glaucomas

Local Anesthetic/Vasoconstrictor Precautions No information available to require special precautions

Effects on Dental Treatment No significant effects or complications reported

Effects on Bleeding No information available to require special precautions

Adverse Effects 1% to 10%:

Central nervous system: Headache

Local: Burning, stinging

Ocular: Blepharoconjunctivitis, blurred vision, bulbar conjunctival follicles, cystoid macular edema, ocular congestion, ocular pain, mydriasis, photophobia

General Dosage Range Ophthalmic: *Adults:* Instill 1 drop every 12 hours

Mechanism of Action Dipivefrin is a prodrug of epinephrine which is the active agent that stimulates alpha- and/or beta-adrenergic receptors increasing aqueous humor outflow

Pharmacodynamics/Kinetics

Onset of Action

Ocular pressure: ~30 minutes

Mydriasis: ~30 minutes

Duration of Action

Ocular pressure effect: ≥12 hours

Mydriasis: Several hours

Pregnancy Risk Factor B

Dipyridamole (dye peer ID a mole)

U.S. Brand Names Persantine®

Canadian Brand Names Apo-Dipyridamole FC®; Dipyridamole For Injection; Persantine®

Pharmacologic Category Antiplatelet Agent; Vasodilator

Use

Oral: Used with warfarin to decrease thrombosis in patients after artificial heart valve replacement

I.V.: Diagnostic agent in CAD

Unlabeled/Investigational Use Stroke prevention (in combination with aspirin)

Local Anesthetic/Vasoconstrictor Precautions No information available to require special precautions

Effects on Dental Treatment No significant effects or complications reported

Effects on Bleeding Dipyridamole blocks platelet aggregation and may prolong bleeding time. Prior to general surgery, it may be temporarily discontinued to restore platelet function. However, routine interruption of therapy for noninvasive dental procedures is not warranted and there is no scientific evidence to warrant the discontinuance of dipyridamole prior to dental surgery. Patients taking dipyridamole as an antithrombotic who require dental surgery should be given special consideration in consultation with physician.

Adverse Effects

Oral:

>10%: Dizziness (14%)

1% to 10%:

Central nervous system: Headache (2%)

Dermatologic: Rash (2%)

Gastrointestinal: Abdominal distress (6%)

Frequency not defined: Diarrhea, vomiting, flushing, pruritus, angina pectoris, liver dysfunction

I.V.:

>10%:

Cardiovascular: Exacerbation of angina pectoris (20%)

Central nervous system: Dizziness (12%), headache (12%)

1% to 10%:

Cardiovascular: Hypotension (5%), hypertension (2%), blood pressure lability (2%), ECG abnormalities (ST-T changes, extrasystoles; 5% to 8%), pain (3%), tachycardia (3%)

Central nervous system: Flushing (3%), fatigue (1%)

Gastrointestinal: Nausea (5%)

Neuromuscular & skeletal: Paresthesia (1%)

Respiratory: Dyspnea (3%)

General Dosage Range

I.V.: *Adults:* 0.14 mg/kg/minute for 4 minutes (maximum: 60 mg)

Oral: *Children ≥12 years and Adults:* 75-100 mg 4 times/day

Mechanism of Action Inhibits the activity of adenosine deaminase and phosphodiesterase, which causes an accumulation of adenosine, adenine nucleotides, and cyclic AMP; these mediators then inhibit platelet aggregation and may cause vasodilation; may also stimulate release of prostacyclin or PGD_2; causes coronary vasodilation

Pharmacodynamics/Kinetics

Half-life Elimination Terminal: 10-12 hours

Time to Peak Serum: 2-2.5 hours

Pregnancy Risk Factor B

Disopyramide (dye soe PEER a mide)

Related Information

Cardiovascular Diseases *on page 1848*

Clinical Risk Related to Drugs Prolonging QT Interval *on page 1872*

U.S. Brand Names Norpace®; Norpace® CR

Canadian Brand Names Norpace®; Rythmodan®; Rythmodan®-LA

Pharmacologic Category Antiarrhythmic Agent, Class Ia

Use Suppression and prevention of unifocal and multifocal atrial and premature, ventricular premature complexes, coupled ventricular tachycardia; effective in the conversion of atrial fibrillation, atrial flutter, and paroxysmal atrial tachycardia to normal sinus rhythm and prevention of the recurrence of these arrhythmias after conversion by other methods

Unlabeled/Investigational Use Hypertrophic obstructive cardiomyopathy (HOCM)

Local Anesthetic/Vasoconstrictor Precautions Disopyramide is one of the drugs confirmed to prolong the QT interval and is accepted as having a risk of causing torsade de pointes. The risk of drug-induced torsade de pointes is extremely low when a single QT interval prolonging drug is prescribed. In terms of epinephrine, it is not known what effect vasoconstrictors in the local anesthetic regimen will have in patients with a known history of congenital prolonged QT interval or in patients taking any medication that prolongs the QT interval. Until more information is obtained, it is suggested that the clinician consult with the physician prior to the use of a vasoconstrictor in suspected patients, and that the vasoconstrictor (epinephrine, mepivacaine and levonordefrin [Carbocaine® 2% with Neo-Cobefrin®]) be used with caution.

Effects on Dental Treatment Key adverse event(s) related to dental treatment: Xerostomia (normal salivary flow resumes upon discontinuation).

Effects on Bleeding No information available to require special precautions

Adverse Effects The most common adverse effects are related to cholinergic blockade. The most serious adverse effects of disopyramide are hypotension and CHF.

>10%:
- Gastrointestinal: Xerostomia (32%), constipation (11%)
- Genitourinary: Urinary hesitancy (14% to 23%)

1% to 10%:
- Cardiovascular: CHF, hypotension, cardiac conduction disturbance, edema, syncope, chest pain
- Central nervous system: Fatigue, headache, malaise, dizziness, nervousness
- Dermatologic: Rash, generalized dermatoses, pruritus
- Endocrine & metabolic: Cholesterol increased, hypokalemia, triglycerides increased
- Gastrointestinal: Dry throat, nausea, abdominal distension, flatulence, abdominal bloating, anorexia, diarrhea, vomiting, weight gain
- Genitourinary: Urinary retention, urinary frequency, urinary urgency, impotence (1% to 3%)
- Neuromuscular & skeletal: Muscle weakness, muscular pain
- Ocular: Blurred vision, dry eyes
- Respiratory: Dyspnea

General Dosage Range Dosage adjustment recommended in patients with hepatic or renal impairment

Oral:

Controlled release:
- *Adults <50 kg:* 200 mg every 12 hours
- *Adults ≥50 kg:* 300 mg every 12 hours

Immediate release:
- *Children <1 year:* 10-30 mg/kg/day in 4 divided doses
- *Children 1-4 years:* 10-20 mg/kg/day in 4 divided doses
- *Children 4-12 years:* 10-15 mg/kg/day in 4 divided doses
- *Children 12-18 years:* 6-15 mg/kg/day in 4 divided doses
- *Adults <50 kg:* 100 mg every 6 hours
- *Adults ≥50 kg:* Initial: 150 mg every 6 hours; Maintenance: 150-400 mg every 6 hours

Mechanism of Action Class Ia antiarrhythmic: Decreases myocardial excitability and conduction velocity; reduces disparity in refractory between normal and infarcted myocardium; possesses anticholinergic, peripheral vasoconstrictive, and negative inotropic effects

Pharmacodynamics/Kinetics

Onset of Action 0.5-3.5 hours

Duration of Action 1.5-8.5 hours

Half-life Elimination Adults: 4-10 hours; prolonged with hepatic or renal impairment

Time to Peak Within 2 hours

Pregnancy Risk Factor C

Dental Comment Disopyramide is known to prolong the QT interval. The QT interval is measured as the time and distance between the Q point of the QRS complex and the end of the T wave in the ECG tracing. After adjustment for heart rate, the QT interval is defined as prolonged if it is more than 450 msec in men and 460 msec in women. A long QT syndrome was first described in the 1950s and 60s as a congenital syndrome involving QT interval prolongation and syncope and sudden death. Some of the congenital long QT syndromes were characterized by a peculiar electrocardiographic appearance of the QRS complex involving a premature atria beat followed by a pause, then a subsequent sinus beat showing marked QT prolongation and deformity. This type of cardiac arrhythmia was originally termed "torsade de pointes" (translated from the French as "twisting of the points"). Disopyramide is considered as having a risk of causing torsade de pointes. Since it is not known what effect vasoconstrictors in the local anesthetic regimen will have in patients with a known history of congenital prolonged QT interval or in patients taking any medication that prolongs the QT interval, a medical consult is suggested.

Disulfiram (dye SUL fi ram)

U.S. Brand Names Antabuse®

Pharmacologic Category Aldehyde Dehydrogenase Inhibitor

Use Management of chronic alcoholism

Local Anesthetic/Vasoconstrictor Precautions No information available to require special precautions

Effects on Dental Treatment No significant effects or complications reported

Effects on Bleeding No information available to require special precautions

Adverse Effects Frequency not defined.

Central nervous system: Drowsiness, headache, fatigue, psychosis
Dermatologic: Rash, acneiform eruptions, allergic dermatitis
Gastrointestinal: Metallic or garlic-like aftertaste
Genitourinary: Impotence
Hepatic: Hepatitis (cholestatic and fulminant), hepatic failure (multiple case reports)
Neuromuscular & skeletal: Peripheral neuritis, polyneuritis, peripheral neuropathy
Ocular: Optic neuritis

General Dosage Range Oral: *Adults:* Initial: 500 mg once daily; Maintenance: 125-500 mg once daily (maximum: 500 mg/day)

Mechanism of Action Disulfiram is a thiuram derivative which interferes with aldehyde dehydrogenase. When taken concomitantly with alcohol, there is an increase in serum acetaldehyde levels. High acetaldehyde causes uncomfortable symptoms including flushing, nausea, thirst, palpitations, chest pain, vertigo, and hypotension. This reaction is the basis for disulfiram use in postwithdrawal long-term care of alcoholism.

Pharmacodynamics/Kinetics

Onset of Action Full effect: 12 hours

Duration of Action ~1-2 weeks after last dose

Pregnancy Risk Factor C

Divalproex (dye VAL proe ex)

U.S. Brand Names Depakote®; Depakote® ER; Depakote® Sprinkle

Canadian Brand Names Apo-Divalproex®; Dom-Divalproex; Epival®; Mylan-Divalproex; Novo-Divalproex; Nu-Divalproex; PHL-Divalproex; PMS-Divalproex

Generic Availability (U.S.) Yes

Pharmacologic Category Anticonvulsant, Miscellaneous; Antimanic Agent; Histone Deacetylase Inhibitor

Use Monotherapy and adjunctive therapy in the treatment of patients with complex partial seizures; monotherapy and adjunctive therapy of simple and complex absence seizures; adjunctive therapy in patients with multiple seizure types that include absence seizures

Depakote®, Depakote® ER: Mania associated with bipolar disorder; migraine prophylaxis

Unlabeled/Investigational Use Diabetic neuropathy

Local Anesthetic/Vasoconstrictor Precautions No information available to require special precautions

Effects on Dental Treatment Key adverse event(s) related to dental treatment: Periodontal abscess and taste perversion.

Effects on Bleeding Has been associated with dose-related thrombocytopenia. Normal coagulation may generally be expected unless thrombocytopenia is present and severe.

Adverse Effects

>10%:

Central nervous system: Headache (≤31%), somnolence (≤30%), dizziness (12% to 25%), insomnia (>1% to 15%), nervousness (>1% to 11%), pain (1% to 11%)
Dermatologic: Alopecia (>1% to 24%)
Gastrointestinal: Nausea (15% to 48%), vomiting (7% to 27%), diarrhea (7% to 23%), abdominal pain (7% to 23%), dyspepsia (7% to 23%), anorexia (>1% to 12%)
Hematologic: Thrombocytopenia (1% to 24%; dose related)
Neuromuscular & skeletal: Tremor (≤57%), weakness (6% to 27%)
Ocular: Diplopia (>1% to 16%), amblyopia/blurred vision (≤12%)
Miscellaneous: Infection (≤20%), flu-like syndrome (12%)

1% to 10%:

Cardiovascular: Peripheral edema (>1% to 8%), chest pain (>1% to <5%), edema (>1% to <5%), facial edema (>1% to <5%), hypertension (>1% to <5%), hypotension (>1% to <5%), palpitation (>1% to <5%), postural hypotension (>1% to <5%), tachycardia (>1% to <5%), vasodilation(>1% to <5%), arrhythmia
Central nervous system: Ataxia (>1% to 8%), amnesia (>1% to 7%), emotional lability (>1% to 6%), fever (>1% to 6%), abnormal thinking (≤6%), depression (>1% to 5%), abnormal dreams (>1% to <5%), agitation (>1% to <5%), anxiety (>1% to <5%), catatonia (>1% to <5%), chills (>1% to <5%), confusion (>1% to <5%), coordination abnormal (>1% to <5%), hallucination (>1% to <5%), malaise (>1% to <5%), personality disorder (>1% to <5%), speech disorder (>1% to <5%),

tardive dyskinesia (>1% to <5%), vertigo (>1% to <5%), euphoria (1%), hypoesthesia (1%)

Dermatologic: Rash (>1% to 6%), bruising (>1% to 5%), discoid lupus erythematosus (>1% to <5%), dry skin (>1% to <5%), furunculosis (>1% to <5%), petechia (>1% to <5%), pruritus (>1% to <5), seborrhea (>1% to <5%)

Endocrine & metabolic: Amenorrhea (>1% to <5%), dysmenorrhea (>1% to <5%), metrorrhagia (>1% to <5%), hypoproteinemia

Gastrointestinal: Weight gain (4% to 9%), weight loss (6%); appetite increased (≤6%), constipation (>1% to 5%), xerostomia (>1% to 5%), eructation (>1% to <5%), fecal incontinence (>1% to <5%), flatulence (>1% to <5%), gastroenteritis (>1% to <5%), glossitis (>1% to <5%), hematemesis (>1% to <5%), pancreatitis (>1% to <5%), periodontal abscess (>1% to <5%), stomatitis (>1% to <5%), taste perversion (>1% to <5%), dysphagia, gum hemorrhage, mouth ulceration

Genitourinary: Cystitis (>1% to 5%), dysuria (>1% to 5%), urinary frequency (>1% to <5%), urinary incontinence (>1% to <5%), vaginal hemorrhage (>1% to 5%), vaginitis (>1% to <5%)

Hepatic: ALT increased (>1% to <5%), AST increased (>1% to <5%)

Local: Injection site pain (3%), injection site reaction (2%), injection site inflammation (1%)

Neuromuscular & skeletal: Back pain (≤8%), abnormal gait (>1% to <5%), arthralgia (>1% to <5%), arthrosis (>1% to <5%), dysarthria (>1% to <5%), hypertonia (>1% to <5%), hypokinesia (>1% to <5%), leg cramps (>1% to <5%), myalgia (>1% to <5%), myasthenia (>1% to <5%), neck pain (>1% to <5%), neck rigidity (>1% to <5%), paresthesia (>1% to <5%), reflex increased (>1% to <5%), twitching (>1% to <5%)

Ocular: Nystagmus (1% to 8%), dry eyes (>1% to 5%), eye pain (>1% to 5%), abnormal vision (>1% to <5%), conjunctivitis (>1% to <5%)

Otic: Tinnitus (1% to 7%), ear pain (>1% to 5%), deafness (>1% to <5%), otitis media (>1% to <5%)

Respiratory: Pharyngitis (2% to 8%), bronchitis (5%), rhinitis (>1% to 5%), dyspnea (1% to 5%), cough (>1% to <5%), epistaxis (>1% to <5%), pneumonia (>1% to <5%), sinusitis (>1% to <5%)

Miscellaneous: Diaphoresis (1%), hiccups

Dosage Oral: Equivalent oral dosages of divalproex and valproic acid deliver the same quantities of valproate ion.

Seizure disorders: **Note:** Administer doses >250 mg/day in divided doses.

Simple and complex absence seizures: Children and Adults: Initial: 15 mg/kg/day; increase by 5-10 mg/kg/day at weekly intervals until therapeutic levels are achieved; maximum: 60 mg/kg/day. Larger maintenance doses may be required in younger children.

Complex partial seizures: Children ≥10 years and Adults: Initial: 10-15 mg/kg/day; increase by 5-10 mg/kg/day at weekly intervals until therapeutic levels are achieved; maximum: 60 mg/kg/day. Larger maintenance doses may be required in younger children.

Note: Regular release and delayed release formulations are usually given in 2-4 divided doses/day; extended release formulation (Depakote® ER) is usually given once daily. Conversion to Depakote® ER from a stable dose of Depakote® may require an increase in the total daily dose between 8% and 20% to maintain similar serum concentrations. Depakote® ER is not recommended for use in children <10 years of age.

Mania: Adults:

Depakote® tablet: Initial: 750 mg/day in divided doses; dose should be adjusted as rapidly as possible to desired clinical effect; maximum recommended dosage: 60 mg/kg/day

Depakote® ER: Initial: 25 mg/kg/day given once daily; dose should be adjusted as rapidly as possible to desired clinical effect; maximum recommended dose: 60 mg/kg/day.

Migraine prophylaxis: Children ≥16 years and Adults:

Depakote® tablet: 250 mg twice daily; adjust dose based on patient response, up to 1000 mg/day

Depakote® ER: 500 mg once daily for 7 days, then increase to 1000 mg once daily; adjust dose based on patient response; usual dosage range: 500-1000 mg/day

Diabetic neuropathy (unlabeled use): Adults: 500-1200 mg/day (Bril, 2011)

Elderly: Elimination is decreased in the elderly. Studies of elderly patients with dementia show a high incidence of somnolence. In some patients, this was associated with weight loss. Starting doses should be lower and increases should be slow, with careful monitoring of nutritional intake and dehydration. Safety and efficacy for use in patients >65 years have not been studied for migraine prophylaxis.

Dosing adjustment in renal impairment: A 27% reduction in clearance of unbound valproate is seen in patients with Cl_{cr} <10 mL/minute. Hemodialysis reduces valproate concentrations by 20%, therefore no dose adjustment is needed in patients with renal failure. Protein binding is reduced, monitoring only total valproate concentrations may be misleading.

Dosing adjustment/comments in hepatic impairment: Reduce dose. Clearance is decreased with liver impairment. Hepatic disease is also associated with decreased albumin concentrations and 2- to 2.6-fold increase in the unbound fraction. Free concentrations of valproate may be elevated while total concentrations appear normal. Use is contraindicated in severe impairment.

Mechanism of Action Causes increased availability of gamma-aminobutyric acid (GABA), an inhibitory neurotransmitter, to brain neurons or may enhance the action of GABA or mimic its action at postsynaptic receptor sites

Contraindications Hypersensitivity to divalproex, derivatives, or any component of the formulation; hepatic disease or significant impairment; urea cycle disorders

Warnings/Precautions [U.S. Boxed Warning]: Hepatic failure resulting in fatalities has occurred in patients; children <2 years of age are at considerable risk. Other risk factors include organic brain disease, mental retardation with severe seizure disorders, congenital metabolic disorders, and patients on multiple anticonvulsants. Hepatotoxicity has usually been reported within 6 months of therapy initiation. Monitor patients closely for appearance of malaise, weakness, facial edema, anorexia, jaundice, and vomiting; discontinue immediately with signs/symptom of significant or suspected impairment. Liver function tests should be performed at baseline and at regular intervals after initiation of therapy, especially within the first 6 months. Hepatic dysfunction may progress despite discontinuing treatment. Should only be used as monotherapy in children <2 years of age and patients at high risk for hepatotoxicity. Contraindicated with severe impairment.

[U.S. Boxed Warning]: Cases of life-threatening pancreatitis, occurring at the start of therapy or following years of use, have been reported in adults and children. Some cases have been hemorrhagic with rapid progression of initial symptoms to death. Promptly evaluate symptoms of abdominal pain, nausea, vomiting, and/or anorexia; should generally be discontinued if pancreatitis is diagnosed.

[U.S. Boxed Warning]: May cause teratogenic effects such as neural tube defects (eg, spina bifida). Use in women of childbearing potential requires that benefits of use in mother be weighed against the potential risk to fetus, especially when used for conditions not associated with permanent injury or risk of death (eg, migraine).

May cause severe thrombocytopenia, inhibition of platelet aggregation, and bleeding. Tremors may indicate overdosage; use with caution in patients receiving other anticonvulsants. Hypersensitivity reactions affecting multiple organs have been reported in association with divalproex use; may include dermatologic and/or hematologic changes (eosinophilia, neutropenia, thrombocytopenia) or symptoms of organ dysfunction.

Hyperammonemia and/or encephalopathy, sometimes fatal, have been reported following the initiation of divalproex therapy and may be present with normal transaminase levels. Ammonia levels should be measured in patients who develop unexplained lethargy and vomiting, changes in mental status, or in patients who present with hypothermia (unintentional drop in core body temperature to <35°C/95°F). Discontinue therapy if ammonia levels are increased and evaluate for possible urea cycle disorder (UCD); contraindicated in patients with UCD. Evaluation of UCD should be considered for the following patients prior to the start of therapy: History of unexplained encephalopathy or coma; encephalopathy associated with protein load; pregnancy or postpartum encephalopathy; unexplained mental retardation; history of elevated plasma ammonia or glutamine; history of cyclical vomiting and lethargy; episodic extreme irritability, ataxia; low BUN or protein avoidance; family history of UCD or unexplained infant deaths (particularly male); or signs or symptoms of UCD (hyperammonemia, encephalopathy, respiratory alkalosis). Hypothermia has been reported with divalproex therapy; may or may not be associated with hyperammonemia; may also occur with concomitant topiramate therapy.

In vitro studies have suggested divalproex stimulates the replication of HIV and CMV viruses under experimental conditions. The clinical consequence of this is unknown, but should be considered when monitoring affected patients.

Antiepileptics are associated with an increased risk of suicidal behavior/thoughts with use (regardless of indication); patients should be monitored for signs/symptoms of depression, suicidal tendencies, and other unusual behavior changes during therapy and instructed to inform their healthcare provider immediately if symptoms occur.

Anticonvulsants should not be discontinued abruptly because of the possibility of increasing seizure frequency; divalproex should be withdrawn gradually to minimize the potential of increased seizure frequency, unless safety concerns require a more rapid withdrawal. Concomitant use with carbapenem antibiotics may reduce valproic acid levels to subtherapeutic levels; monitor levels frequently and consider alternate therapy if levels drop significantly or lack of seizure control occurs. Concomitant use with clonazepam may induce absence status. Patients treated for bipolar disorder should be monitored closely for clinical worsening or suicidality; prescriptions should be written for the smallest quantity consistent with good patient care.

CNS depression may occur with divalproex use. Patients must be cautioned about performing tasks which require mental alertness (operating machinery or driving). Effects with other sedative drugs or ethanol may be potentiated. Use with caution in the elderly.

Drug Interactions

Metabolism/Transport Effects For divalproex: **Substrate** (minor) of CYP2A6, 2B6, 2C9, 2C19, 2E1; **Inhibits** CYP2C9 (weak), 2C19 (weak), 2D6 (weak), 3A4 (weak); **Induces** CYP2A6 (weak)

Avoid Concomitant Use There are no known interactions where it is recommended to avoid concomitant use.

Increased Effect/Toxicity

Divalproex may increase the levels/effects of: Barbiturates; Ethosuximide; LamoTRIgine; LORazepam; Paliperidone; Primidone; RisperiDONE; Rufinamide; Temozolomide; Tricyclic Antidepressants; Vorinostat; Zidovudine

The levels/effects of Divalproex may be increased by: ChlorproMAZINE; Felbamate; GuanFACINE; Salicylates; Topiramate

Decreased Effect

Divalproex may decrease the levels/effects of: CarBAMazepine; Fosphenytoin; OXcarbazepine; Phenytoin

The levels/effects of Divalproex may be decreased by: Barbiturates; CarBAMazepine; Carbapenems; Ethosuximide; Fosphenytoin; Methylfolate; Phenytoin; Primidone; Protease Inhibitors; Rifampin

Ethanol/Nutrition/Herb Interactions

Ethanol: Avoid ethanol (may increase CNS depression).

Food: Food may delay but does not affect the extent of absorption. Valproic acid serum concentrations may be decreased if taken with food. Milk has no effect on absorption.

Herb/Nutraceutical: Avoid evening primrose (seizure threshold decreased).

Dietary Considerations Divalproex may cause GI upset; take with large amount of water or food to decrease GI upset. May need to split doses to avoid GI upset.

Depakote® Sprinkle capsule contents may be mixed with semisolid food (eg, applesauce or pudding) in patients having difficulty swallowing; particles should be swallowed and not chewed.

Pharmacodynamics/Kinetics

Half-life Elimination Increased in neonates and with liver disease; Children >2 months: 7-13 hours; Adults: 9-16 hours

Time to Peak Serum: Depakote® tablet: ~4 hours; Depakote® ER: 4-17 hours

Pregnancy Risk Factor D

Lactation Enters breast milk/not recommended (AAP considers "compatible"; AAP 2001 update pending)

Breast-Feeding Considerations Breast milk concentrations of valproic acid have been reported as 1% to 10% of maternal concentration. The weight-adjusted dose to the infant has been calculated to be ~4%.

Dosage Forms

Capsule, sprinkle, oral: 125 mg

Depakote® Sprinkle: 125 mg

Tablet, delayed release, oral: 125 mg, 250 mg, 500 mg

Depakote®: 125 mg, 250 mg, 500 mg

Tablet, extended release, oral: 250 mg, 500 mg

Depakote® ER: 250 mg, 500 mg

DOBUTamine (doe BYOO ta meen)

Related Information

Cardiovascular Diseases *on page 1848*

Canadian Brand Names Dobutamine Injection, USP; Dobutrex®

Pharmacologic Category Adrenergic Agonist Agent

Use Short-term management of patients with cardiac decompensation

Unlabeled/Investigational Use Positive inotropic agent for use in myocardial dysfunction related to sepsis; stress echocardiography

Local Anesthetic/Vasoconstrictor Precautions No information available to require special precautions

Effects on Dental Treatment No significant effects or complications reported

Effects on Bleeding No information available to require special precautions

Adverse Effects Incidence of adverse events is not always reported.

Cardiovascular: Increased heart rate, increased blood pressure, increased ventricular ectopic activity, hypotension, premature ventricular beats (5%, dose related), anginal pain (1% to 3%), nonspecific chest pain (1% to 3%), palpitation (1% to 3%)

Central nervous system: Fever (1% to 3%), headache (1% to 3%), paresthesia

Endocrine & metabolic: Slight decrease in serum potassium

Gastrointestinal: Nausea (1% to 3%)

Hematologic: Thrombocytopenia (isolated cases)

Local: Phlebitis, local inflammatory changes and pain from infiltration, cutaneous necrosis (isolated cases)

Neuromuscular & skeletal: Mild leg cramps

Respiratory: Dyspnea (1% to 3%)

General Dosage Range I.V.: *Children and Adults:* 2.5-20 mcg/kg/minute (maximum: 40 mcg/kg/minute)

Mechanism of Action Stimulates $beta_1$-adrenergic receptors, causing increased contractility and heart rate, with little effect on $beta_2$- or alpha-receptors

Pharmacodynamics/Kinetics

Onset of Action I.V.: 1-10 minutes; Peak effect: 10-20 minutes

Half-life Elimination 2 minutes

Pregnancy Risk Factor B

DOCEtaxel (doe se TAKS el)

U.S. Brand Names Taxotere®

Canadian Brand Names Taxotere®

Pharmacologic Category Antineoplastic Agent, Antimicrotubular; Antineoplastic Agent, Natural Source (Plant) Derivative; Antineoplastic Agent, Taxane Derivative

Use Treatment of breast cancer (locally advanced/metastatic or adjuvant treatment of operable node-positive); locally-advanced or metastatic nonsmall cell lung cancer (NSCLC); hormone refractory, metastatic prostate cancer; advanced gastric adenocarcinoma; locally-advanced squamous cell head and neck cancer

Unlabeled/Investigational Use Treatment of bladder cancer (metastatic), ovarian cancer, cervical cancer (relapsed), esophageal cancer, small cell lung cancer (relapsed), soft tissue sarcoma, Ewing's sarcoma, osteosarcoma, and unknown-primary adenocarcinoma

Local Anesthetic/Vasoconstrictor Precautions No information available to require special precautions

Effects on Dental Treatment Key adverse event(s) related to dental treatment: Mucositis, stomatitis, and taste perversion.

Effects on Bleeding Chemotherapy may result in significant myelosuppression, potentially including significant reduction in platelet counts and altered hemostasis. In patients who are under active treatment with these agents, medical consult is suggested.

Adverse Effects Percentages reported for docetaxel monotherapy; frequency may vary depending on diagnosis, dose, liver function, prior treatment, and premedication. The incidence of adverse events was usually higher in patients with elevated liver function tests.

>10%:

Cardiovascular: Fluid retention (13% to 60%; dose dependent)

Central nervous system: Neurosensory events (20% to 58%; including neuropathy), fever (31% to 35%), neuromotor events (16%)

Dermatologic: Alopecia (56% to 76%), cutaneous events (20% to 48%), nail disorder (11% to 41%)

Gastrointestinal: Stomatitis (19% to 53%; severe 1% to 8%), diarrhea (23% to 43%; severe: 5% to 6%), nausea (34% to 42%), vomiting (22% to 23%)

Hematologic: Neutropenia (84% to 99%; grade 4: 75% to 86%; nadir (median): 7 days, duration (severe neutropenia): 7 days; dose dependent), leukopenia (84% to 99%; grade 4: 32% to 44%), anemia (65% to 94%; dose dependent; grades 3/4: 8% to 9%), thrombocytopenia (8% to 14%; grade 4: 1%; dose dependent), febrile neutropenia (6% to 12%; dose dependent)

Hepatic: Transaminases increased (4% to 19%)

Neuromuscular & skeletal: Weakness (53% to 66%; severe 13% to 18%), myalgia (3% to 23%)
Respiratory: Pulmonary events (41%)
Miscellaneous: Infection (1% to 34%; dose dependent), hypersensitivity (1% to 21%; with premedication 15%)

1% to 10%:

Cardiovascular: Left ventricular ejection fraction decreased (prostate cancer: 10%; metastatic breast cancer: 8%), hypotension (3%)
Gastrointestinal: Taste perversion (6%)
Hepatic: Bilirubin increased (9%), alkaline phosphatase increased (4% to 7%)
Local: Infusion-site reactions (4%, including hyperpigmentation, inflammation, redness, dryness, phlebitis, extravasation, swelling of the vein)
Neuromuscular and skeletal: Arthralgia (3% to 9%)
Ocular: Epiphora associated with canalicular stenosis (≤77% with weekly administration; ≤1% with every 3-week administration)

General Dosage Range Dosage adjustment recommended in patients with hepatic impairment, on concomitant therapy, or who develop toxicities.

I.V.: *Adults:* 60-100 mg/m^2 every 3 weeks

Mechanism of Action Docetaxel promotes the assembly of microtubules from tubulin dimers, and inhibits the depolymerization of tubulin which stabilizes microtubules in the cell. This results in inhibition of DNA, RNA, and protein synthesis. Most activity occurs during the M phase of the cell cycle.

Pharmacodynamics/Kinetics

Half-life Elimination Terminal: ~11 hours

Pregnancy Risk Factor D

Product Availability Docefrez™: FDA approved May 2011; expected availability undetermined

Docosanol (doe KOE san ole)

Related Information

Viral Infections *on page 1947*

Related Sample Prescriptions

Herpes Simplex (Recurrent) *on page 1990*

U.S. Brand Names Abreva® [OTC]

Generic Availability (U.S.) No

Pharmacologic Category Antiviral Agent, Topical

Dental Use Treatment of herpes simplex of the face or lips

Use Treatment of herpes simplex of the face or lips

Local Anesthetic/Vasoconstrictor Precautions No information available to require special precautions

Effects on Dental Treatment No significant effects or complications reported (see Dental Comment)

Effects on Bleeding No information available to require special precautions

Adverse Effects Limited information; headache reported (frequency similar to placebo)

Dental Usual Dosage Herpes simplex (face/lips): Children ≥12 years and Adults: Topical: Apply 5 times/day to affected area of face or lips. Start at first sign of cold sore or fever blister and continue until healed.

Dosage Children ≥12 years and Adults: Topical: Apply 5 times/day to affected area of face or lips. Start at first sign of cold sore or fever blister and continue until healed.

Mechanism of Action Prevents viral entry and replication at the cellular level

Contraindications Hypersensitivity to docosanol or any component of the formulation

Warnings/Precautions For external use only. Do not apply to inside of mouth or around eyes. Not for use in children <12 years of age.

Drug Interactions

Avoid Concomitant Use There are no known interactions where it is recommended to avoid concomitant use.

Increased Effect/Toxicity There are no known significant interactions involving an increase in effect.

Decreased Effect There are no known significant interactions involving a decrease in effect.

Dosage Forms

Cream, topical:

Abreva® [OTC]: 10% (2 g)

Dental Comment Wash hands before and after applying cream. Begin treatment at first tingle of cold sore or fever blister. Rub into area gently, but completely. Do not apply directly to inside of mouth or around eyes. Contact healthcare provider if sore gets worse or does not heal within 10 days. Do not share this product with others, may spread infection. Notify healthcare professional if pregnant or breast-feeding.

Docusate (DOK yoo sate)

U.S. Brand Names Colace® [OTC]; Correctol® [OTC]; Diocto [OTC]; Docu-Soft [OTC]; DocuSoft S™ [OTC]; Dok™ [OTC]; DSS® [OTC]; Dulcolax® Stool Softener [OTC]; Dulcolax® [OTC]; Enemeez® Plus [OTC]; Enemeez® [OTC]; Fleet® Pedia-Lax™ Liquid Stool Softener [OTC]; Fleet® Sof-lax® [OTC]; Kaopectate® Stool Softener [OTC]; Phillips'® Liquid-Gels® [OTC]; Phillips'® Stool Softener Laxative [OTC]; Silace [OTC]

Canadian Brand Names Apo-Docusate-Sodium®; Colace®; Colax-C®; Novo-Docusate Calcium; Novo-Docusate Sodium; PMS-Docusate Calcium; PMS-Docusate Sodium; Regulex®; Selax®; Soflax™

Pharmacologic Category Stool Softener

Use Stool softener in patients who should avoid straining during defecation and constipation associated with hard, dry stools; prophylaxis for straining (Valsalva) following myocardial infarction. A safe agent to be used in elderly; some evidence that doses <200 mg are ineffective; stool softeners are unnecessary if stool is well hydrated or "mushy" and soft; shown to be ineffective used long-term.

Unlabeled/Investigational Use Ceruminolytic

Local Anesthetic/Vasoconstrictor Precautions No information available to require special precautions

Effects on Dental Treatment Key adverse event(s) related to dental treatment: Throat irritation.

Effects on Bleeding No information available to require special precautions

Adverse Effects 1% to 10%:

Gastrointestinal: Intestinal obstruction, diarrhea, abdominal cramping

Miscellaneous: Throat irritation

General Dosage Range

Oral:

Children <3 years: 10-40 mg/day in 1-4 divided doses

Children 3-6 years: 20-60 mg/day in 1-4 divided doses

Children 6-12 years: 40-150 mg/day in 1-4 divided doses

Adolescents and Adults: 50-500 mg/day in 1-4 divided doses

Rectal: *Older children and Adults:* Add 50-100 mg to enema fluid

Mechanism of Action Reduces surface tension of the oil-water interface of the stool resulting in enhanced incorporation of water and fat allowing for stool softening

Pharmacodynamics/Kinetics

Onset of Action 12-72 hours

Pregnancy Risk Factor C

Dofetilide (doe FET il ide)

Related Information

Clinical Risk Related to Drugs Prolonging QT Interval *on page* 1872

U.S. Brand Names Tikosyn®

Canadian Brand Names Tikosyn®

Pharmacologic Category Antiarrhythmic Agent, Class III

Use Maintenance of normal sinus rhythm in patients with chronic atrial fibrillation/atrial flutter of longer than 1-week duration who have been converted to normal sinus rhythm; conversion of atrial fibrillation and atrial flutter to normal sinus rhythm

Local Anesthetic/Vasoconstrictor Precautions Dofetilide is one of the drugs confirmed to prolong the QT interval and is accepted as having a risk of causing torsade de pointes. The risk of drug-induced torsade de pointes is extremely low when a single QT interval prolonging drug is prescribed. In terms of epinephrine, it is not known what effect vasoconstrictors in the local anesthetic regimen will have in patients with a known history of congenital prolonged QT interval or in patients taking any medication that prolongs the QT interval. Until more information is obtained, it is suggested that the clinician consult with the physician prior to the use of a vasoconstrictor in suspected patients, and that the vasoconstrictor (epinephrine, mepivacaine and levonordefrin [Carbocaine® 2% with Neo-Cobefrin®]) be used with caution.

Effects on Dental Treatment No significant effects or complications reported

Effects on Bleeding No information available to require special precautions

Adverse Effects

Supraventricular arrhythmia patients (incidence > placebo)

>10%: Central nervous system: Headache (11%)

2% to 10%:

Central nervous system: Dizziness (8%), insomnia (4%)

Cardiovascular: Ventricular tachycardia (2.6% to 3.7%), chest pain (10%), torsade de pointes (3.3% in CHF patients and 0.9% in patients with a recent MI; up to 10.5% in patients receiving doses in excess of those recommended). Torsade de pointes occurs most frequently within the first 3 days of therapy.

Dermatologic: Rash (3%)

Gastrointestinal: Nausea (5%), diarrhea (3%), abdominal pain (3%)

Neuromuscular & skeletal: Back pain (3%)

Respiratory: Respiratory tract infection (7%), dyspnea (6%)

Miscellaneous: Flu syndrome (4%)

<2%:

Central nervous system: CVA, facial paralysis, flaccid paralysis, migraine, paralysis

Cardiovascular: AV block (0.4% to 1.5%), ventricular fibrillation (0% to 0.4%), bundle branch block, heart block, edema, heart arrest, myocardial infarct, sudden death, syncope

Dermatologic: Angioedema

Gastrointestinal: Liver damage

Neuromuscular & skeletal: Paresthesia

Respiratory: Cough

>2% (incidence ≤ placebo): Anxiety, pain, angina, atrial fibrillation, hypertension, palpitation, supraventricular tachycardia, peripheral edema, urinary tract infection, weakness, arthralgia, diaphoresis

General Dosage Range Dosage adjustment recommended in patients with renal impairment

Oral: *Adults:* Initial: 500 mcg twice daily; Maintenance: 125-500 mcg twice daily **or** 125 mcg once daily

Mechanism of Action Vaughan Williams Class III antiarrhythmic activity. Blockade of the cardiac ion channel carrying the rapid component of the delayed rectifier potassium current. Dofetilide has no effect on sodium channels, adrenergic alpha-receptors, or adrenergic beta-receptors. It increases the monophasic action potential duration due to delayed repolarization. The increase in the QT interval is a function of prolongation of both effective and functional refractory periods in the His-Purkinje system and the ventricles. Changes in cardiac conduction velocity and sinus node function have not been observed in patients with or without structural heart disease. PR and QRS width remain the same in patients with pre-existing heart block and or sick sinus syndrome.

Pharmacodynamics/Kinetics

Half-life Elimination 10 hours

Time to Peak Serum: Fasting: 2-3 hours

Pregnancy Risk Factor C

Prescribing and Access Restrictions Tikosyn® is deemed to have an approved REMS program. As a requirement of the REMS program, access to this medication is restricted. Tikosyn® is only available to prescribers and hospitals that have confirmed their participation in a designated Tikosyn® Education Program. The program provides comprehensive education about the importance of in-hospital treatment initiation and individualized dosing.

T.I.P.S. is the Tikosyn® In Pharmacy System designated to allow retail pharmacies to stock and dispense Tikosyn® once they have been enrolled. A participating pharmacy must confirm receipt of the T.I.P.S. program materials and educate its pharmacy staff about the procedures required to fill an outpatient prescription for Tikosyn®. The T.I.P.S. enrollment form is available at www.tikosyn.com. Tikosyn® is only available from a special mail order pharmacy, and enrolled retail pharmacies. Pharmacists must verify that the hospital/prescriber is a confirmed participant before Tikosyn® is provided. For participant verification, the pharmacist may call 1-800-788-7353 or use the web site located at www.tikosynlist.com. Further details and directions on the program are provided at www.tikosyn.com.

Dofetilide therapy must be initiated/adjusted in a hospital setting with proper monitoring under the guidance of experienced personnel.

Dental Comment Dofetilide is known to prolong the QT interval. The QT interval is measured as the time and distance between the Q point of the QRS complex and the end of the T wave in the ECG tracing. After adjustment for heart rate, the QT interval is defined as prolonged if it is more than 450 msec in men and 460 msec in women. A long QT syndrome was first described in the 1950s and 60s as a congenital syndrome involving QT interval prolongation and syncope and sudden death. Some of the congenital long QT syndromes were characterized by a peculiar electrocardiographic appearance of the QRS complex involving a premature atria beat followed by a pause, then a subsequent sinus beat showing marked QT prolongation and deformity. This type of cardiac arrhythmia was originally termed "torsade de pointes" (translated from the French as "twisting of the points"). Dofetilide is considered as having a risk of causing torsade de pointes. Since it is not known what effect vasoconstrictors in the local anesthetic regimen will have in patients with a known history of congenital prolonged QT interval or in patients taking any medication that prolongs the QT interval, a medical consult is suggested.

Dolasetron (dol A se tron)

U.S. Brand Names Anzemet®

Canadian Brand Names Anzemet®

Pharmacologic Category Antiemetic; Selective 5-HT_3 Receptor Antagonist

Use

U.S. labeling:

Injection: Prevention and treatment of postoperative nausea and vomiting

Oral: Prevention of nausea and vomiting associated with emetogenic cancer chemotherapy (initial and repeat courses); prevention of postoperative nausea and vomiting

Canadian labeling: Oral: Prevention of nausea and vomiting associated with emetogenic cancer chemotherapy (initial and repeat courses)

Local Anesthetic/Vasoconstrictor Precautions Dolasetron is one of the drugs confirmed to prolong the QT interval and is accepted as having a risk of causing torsade de pointes. The risk of drug-induced torsade de pointes is extremely low when a single QT interval prolonging drug is prescribed. In terms of epinephrine, it is not known what effect vasoconstrictors in the local anesthetic regimen will have in patients with a known history of congenital prolonged QT interval or in patients taking any medication that prolongs the QT interval. Until more information is obtained, it is suggested that the clinician consult with the physician prior to the use of a vasoconstrictor in suspected patients, and that the vasoconstrictor (epinephrine, mepivacaine and levonordefrin [Carbocaine® 2% with Neo-Cobefrin®]) be used with caution.

Effects on Dental Treatment Key adverse event(s) related to dental treatment: Taste alterations.

Effects on Bleeding No information available to require special precautions

Adverse Effects Adverse events may vary according to indication

>10%:

Central nervous system: Headache (7% to 24%)

Gastrointestinal: Diarrhea (2% to 12%)

1% to 10%:

Cardiovascular: Bradycardia (4% to 5%), hypertension (≤3%), tachycardia (2% to 3%)

Central nervous system: Dizziness (1% to 6%), fatigue (3% to 6%), fever (4%), pain (≤2%), chills/shivering (1% to 2%)

Gastrointestinal: Dyspepsia (≤3%), abdominal pain (≤3%)

Hepatic: Abnormal hepatic function (4%)

Renal: Oliguria (3%)

General Dosage Range

I.V.:

Children 2-16 years: 0.35 mg/kg as a single dose (maximum: 12.5 mg)

Adults: 12.5 mg or 100 mg as a single dose

Oral:

Children 2-16 years: 1.2-1.8 mg/kg as a single dose (maximum: 100 mg/dose)

Adults: 100 mg as single dose

Mechanism of Action Selective serotonin receptor (5-HT_3) antagonist, blocking serotonin both peripherally (primary site of action) and centrally at the chemoreceptor trigger zone

Pharmacodynamics/Kinetics

Half-life Elimination Dolasetron: ≤10 minutes; hydrodolasetron: Adults: 6-8 hours; Children: 4-6 hours; Severe renal impairment: 11 hours; Severe hepatic impairment: 11 hours

Time to Peak Hydrodolasetron: I.V.: 0.6 hours; Oral: ~1 hour

Pregnancy Risk Factor B

Dental Comment Dolasetron is known to prolong the QT interval. The QT interval is measured as the time and distance between the Q point of the QRS complex and the end of the T wave in the ECG tracing. After adjustment for heart rate, the QT interval is defined as prolonged if it is more than 450 msec in men and 460 msec in women. A long QT syndrome was first described in the 1950s and 60s as a congenital syndrome involving QT interval prolongation and syncope and sudden death. Some of the congenital long QT syndromes were characterized by a peculiar electrocardiographic appearance of the QRS complex involving a premature atria beat followed by a pause, then a subsequent sinus beat showing marked QT prolongation and deformity. This type of cardiac arrhythmia was originally termed "torsade de pointes" (translated from the French as "twisting of the points"). Dolasetron is considered as having a risk of causing torsade de pointes. Since it is not known what effect vasoconstrictors in the local anesthetic regimen will have in patients with a known history of congenital prolonged QT interval or in patients taking any medication that prolongs the QT interval, a medical consult is suggested.

Donepezil (doh NEP e zil)

U.S. Brand Names Aricept®; Aricept® ODT

Canadian Brand Names Aricept®; Aricept® RDT

Generic Availability (U.S.) Yes

Pharmacologic Category Acetylcholinesterase Inhibitor (Central)

Use Treatment of mild, moderate, or severe dementia of the Alzheimer's type

Unlabeled/Investigational Use Behavioral syndromes in dementia; mild-to-moderate dementia associated with Parkinson's disease; Lewy body dementia

Local Anesthetic/Vasoconstrictor Precautions No information available to require special precautions

Effects on Dental Treatment No significant effects or complications reported

Effects on Bleeding No information available to require special precautions

Adverse Effects

>10%:

Central nervous system: Insomnia (2% to 14%)

Gastrointestinal: Nausea (3% to 19%; dose related), diarrhea (5% to 15%; dose related)

Miscellaneous: Accident (7% to 13%), infection (11%)

1% to 10%:

Cardiovascular: Hypertension (3%), chest pain (2%), hemorrhage (2%), syncope (2%), hypotension, atrial fibrillation, bradycardia, ECG abnormal, edema, heart failure, hot flashes, peripheral edema, vasodilation

Central nervous system: Headache (3% to 10%), pain (3% to 9%), fatigue (1% to 8%), dizziness (2% to 8%), abnormal dreams (3%), hostility (3%), nervousness (1% to 3%), hallucinations (3%), depression (2% to 3%), confusion (2%), emotional lability (2%), personality disorder (2%), fever (2%), somnolence (2%), abnormal crying, aggression, agitation, anxiety, aphasia, delusions, irritability, restlessness, seizure, vertigo

Dermatologic: Bruising (4% to 5%), eczema (3%), pruritus, rash, skin ulcer, urticaria

Endocrine & metabolic: Dehydration (1% to 2%), hyperlipemia (2%), libido increased

Gastrointestinal: Anorexia (2% to 8%), vomiting (3% to 9%; dose related), weight loss (3% to 5%; dose related), abdominal pain, bloating, constipation, dyspepsia, epigastric pain, fecal incontinence, gastroenteritis, GI bleeding, toothache

Genitourinary: Urinary frequency (2%), urinary incontinence (1% to 3%), cystitis, hematuria, glycosuria, nocturia, UTI

Hematologic: Contusion (≤2%), anemia

Hepatic: Alkaline phosphatase increased

Neuromuscular & skeletal: Muscle cramps (3% to 8%), back pain (3%), CPK increased (3%), arthritis (1% to 2%), ataxia, bone fracture, gait abnormal, lactate dehydrogenase increased, paresthesia, tremor, weakness (1% to 2%)

Ocular: Blurred vision, cataract, eye irritation

Respiratory: Bronchitis, cough increased, dyspnea, pharyngitis, pneumonia, sore throat

Miscellaneous: Diaphoresis, fungal infection, flu symptoms, wandering

Dosage Oral:

Adults: Alzheimer's dementia:

Mild-to-moderate: Initial: 5 mg once daily; may increase to 10 mg once daily after 4-6 weeks; effective dosage range in clinical studies: 5-10 mg/day

Moderate-to-severe: Initial: 5 mg once daily; may increase to 10 mg once daily after 4-6 weeks; may increase further to 23 mg once daily after ≥3 months; effective dosage range in clinical studies: 10-23 mg/day

Elderly: Refer to adult dosing. **Note:** The Canadian labeling recommends a maximum dose of 5 mg once daily in elderly women of low body weight.

Mechanism of Action Alzheimer's disease is characterized by cholinergic deficiency in the cortex and basal forebrain, which contributes to cognitive deficits. Donepezil reversibly and noncompetitively inhibits centrally-active acetylcholinesterase, the enzyme responsible for hydrolysis of acetylcholine. This appears to result in increased concentrations of acetylcholine available for synaptic transmission in the central nervous system.

Contraindications Hypersensitivity to donepezil, piperidine derivatives, or any component of the formulation

Warnings/Precautions Cholinesterase inhibitors may have vagotonic effects which may cause bradycardia and/or heart block with or without a history of cardiac disease; syncopal episodes have been associated with donepezil. Alzheimer's treatment guidelines consider bradycardia to be a relative contraindication for use of centrally-active cholinesterase inhibitors. Use with caution with sick sinus syndrome or other supraventricular cardiac conduction abnormalities, COPD, or asthma. Use with caution in patients with a history of seizure disorder; cholinomimetics may potentially cause generalized seizures, although seizure activity may also result from Alzheimer's disease. Use with caution in patients at risk of ulcer disease (eg, previous history or NSAID use), or in patients with bladder outlet obstruction. May cause dose-related diarrhea, nausea, and/or vomiting, which usually resolves in 1-3 weeks. May cause anorexia and/or weight loss (dose-related). May exaggerate neuromuscular blockade effects of depolarizing neuromuscular-blocking agents (eg, succinylcholine).

Drug Interactions

Metabolism/Transport Effects Substrate (minor) of CYP2D6, 3A4

Avoid Concomitant Use There are no known interactions where it is recommended to avoid concomitant use.

Increased Effect/Toxicity

Donepezil may increase the levels/effects of: Antipsychotics; Beta-Blockers; Cholinergic Agonists; Succinylcholine

The levels/effects of Donepezil may be increased by: Conivaptan; Corticosteroids (Systemic)

Decreased Effect

Donepezil may decrease the levels/effects of: Anticholinergics; Neuromuscular-Blocking Agents (Nondepolarizing)

The levels/effects of Donepezil may be decreased by: Anticholinergics; Peginterferon Alfa-2b; Tocilizumab

Ethanol/Nutrition/Herb Interactions Herb/Nutraceutical: St John's wort may decrease donepezil levels. Ginkgo biloba may increase adverse effects/toxicity of acetylcholinesterase inhibitors.

Dietary Considerations May take with or without food.

Pharmacodynamics/Kinetics

Half-life Elimination 70 hours; time to steady-state: 15 days

Time to Peak Plasma: Tablet, 10 mg: 3 hours; Tablet, 23 mg: ~8 hours; **Note:** Peak plasma concentrations almost twofold higher for the 23 mg tablet compared to the 10 mg tablet

Pregnancy Risk Factor C

Lactation Excretion in breast milk unknown/not recommended

Dosage Forms

Tablet, oral: 5 mg, 10 mg

Aricept®: 5 mg, 10 mg, 23 mg

Tablet, orally disintegrating, oral: 5 mg, 10 mg

Aricept® ODT: 5 mg, 10 mg

Doripenem (dore i PEN em)

U.S. Brand Names Doribax®

Canadian Brand Names Doribax®

Pharmacologic Category Antibiotic, Carbapenem

Use Treatment of complicated intra-abdominal infections and complicated urinary tract infections (including pyelonephritis) due to susceptible gram-positive, gram-negative (including *Pseudomonas aeruginosa*), and anaerobic bacteria

Unlabeled/Investigational Use Treatment of nosocomial pneumonia

Local Anesthetic/Vasoconstrictor Precautions No information available to require special precautions

Effects on Dental Treatment Prolonged use of doripenem may lead to development of oral candidiasis.

Effects on Bleeding No information available to require special precautions

Adverse Effects

>10%:

Central nervous system: Headache (4% to 16%)

Gastrointestinal: Nausea (4% to 12%), diarrhea (6% to 11%)

1% to 10%:
Dermatologic: Rash (1% to 5%; includes allergic/bullous dermatitis, erythema, macular/papular eruptions, urticaria, and erythema multiforme), pruritus (≤3%)
Gastrointestinal: Oral candidiasis (1%)
Hematologic: Anemia (2% to 10%)
Hepatic: Transaminases increased (1% to 2%)
Local: Phlebitis (4% to 8%)
Renal: Renal impairment/failure (≤1%)
Miscellaneous: Vulvomycotic infection (1% to 2%)

General Dosage Range Dosage adjustment recommended in patients with renal impairment

I.V.: *Adults:* 500 mg every 8 hours

Mechanism of Action Inhibits bacterial cell wall synthesis by binding to several of the penicillin-binding proteins, which in turn inhibits the final transpeptidation step of peptidoglycan synthesis in bacterial cell walls, thus inhibiting cell wall biosynthesis; bacteria eventually lyse due to ongoing activity of cell wall autolytic enzymes (autolysins and murein hydrolases) while cell wall assembly is arrested.

Pharmacodynamics/Kinetics

Half-life Elimination ~1 hour

Pregnancy Risk Factor B

Dornase Alfa (DOOR nase AL fa)

U.S. Brand Names Pulmozyme®

Canadian Brand Names Pulmozyme®

Pharmacologic Category Enzyme; Mucolytic Agent

Use Management of cystic fibrosis patients to reduce the frequency of respiratory infections that require parenteral antibiotics in patients with FVC ≥40% of predicted; in conjunction with standard therapies, to improve pulmonary function in patients with cystic fibrosis

Local Anesthetic/Vasoconstrictor Precautions No information available to require special precautions

Effects on Dental Treatment Key adverse event(s) related to dental treatment: Pharyngitis

Effects on Bleeding No information available to require special precautions

Adverse Effects Adverse events were similar in children using the PARI BABY™ nebulizer (facemask as opposed to mouthpiece) with the addition of cough (45% in children 3 months to <5 years; 30% in children 5 to ≤10 years).

>10%:
Cardiovascular: Chest pain (18% to 25%)
Central nervous system: Fever (32% in patients with FVC <40%)
Dermatologic: Rash (3% to 12%)
Respiratory: Pharyngitis (32% to 40%), rhinitis (30% in patients with FVC <40%); FVC decrease ≥10% of predicted (22% in patients with FVC <40%), dyspnea (17% in patients with FVC <40%)
Miscellaneous: Voice alteration (12% to 18%)

1% to 10%:
Gastrointestinal: Dyspepsia (≤3%)
Ocular: Conjunctivitis (1% to 5%)
Respiratory: Laryngitis (3% to 4%)
Miscellaneous: Dornase alfa serum antibodies (2% to 4%)

Postmarketing and/or case reports: Headache, urticaria

General Dosage Range Inhalation: *Children ≥3 months and Adults:* 2.5 mg once daily

Mechanism of Action The hallmark of cystic fibrosis lung disease is the presence of abundant, purulent airway secretions composed primarily of highly polymerized DNA. The principal source of this DNA is the nuclei of degenerating neutrophils, which is present in large concentrations in infected lung secretions. The presence of this DNA produces a viscous mucous that may contribute to the decreased mucociliary transport and persistent infections that are commonly seen in this population. Dornase alfa is a deoxyribonuclease (DNA) enzyme produced by recombinant gene technology. Dornase selectively cleaves DNA, thus reducing mucous viscosity and as a result, airflow in the lung is improved and the risk of bacterial infection may be decreased.

Pharmacodynamics/Kinetics

Onset of Action Nebulization: Enzyme levels are measured in sputum in ~15 minutes

Duration of Action Rapidly declines

Pregnancy Risk Factor B

Dorzolamide (dor ZOLE a mide)

U.S. Brand Names Trusopt®
Canadian Brand Names Trusopt®
Pharmacologic Category Carbonic Anhydrase Inhibitor; Ophthalmic Agent, Antiglaucoma
Use Treatment of elevated intraocular pressure in patients with ocular hypertension or open-angle glaucoma
Local Anesthetic/Vasoconstrictor Precautions No information available to require special precautions
Effects on Dental Treatment No significant effects or complications reported
Effects on Bleeding No information available to require special precautions
Adverse Effects
>10%:
Gastrointestinal: Bitter taste following administration (25%)
Ocular: Burning, stinging or discomfort immediately following administration (33%); superficial punctate keratitis (10% to 15%); signs and symptoms of ocular allergic reaction (10%)
1% to 5%: Ocular: Blurred vision, conjunctivitis, dryness, lid reactions, photophobia, redness, tearing
General Dosage Range Ophthalmic: *Children and Adults:* Instill 1 drop into affected eye(s) 3 times/day
Mechanism of Action Reversible inhibition of the enzyme carbonic anhydrase resulting in reduction of hydrogen ion secretion at renal tubule and an increased renal excretion of sodium, potassium, bicarbonate, and water to decrease production of aqueous humor; also inhibits carbonic anhydrase in central nervous system to retard abnormal and excessive discharge from CNS neurons
Pharmacodynamics/Kinetics
Onset of Action Peak effect: 2 hours
Duration of Action 8-12 hours
Half-life Elimination Terminal RBC: 147 days; washes out of RBCs nonlinearly, resulting in a rapid decline of drug concentration initially, followed by a slower elimination phase with a half-life of about 4 months
Pregnancy Risk Factor C

Dorzolamide and Timolol (dor ZOLE a mide & TYE moe lole)

Related Information
Dorzolamide *on page* 563
Timolol (Ophthalmic) *on page* 1633
U.S. Brand Names Cosopt®
Canadian Brand Names Apo-Dorzo-Timop; Cosopt®; Sandoz-Dorzolamide/Timolol
Pharmacologic Category Beta-Adrenergic Blocker, Nonselective; Carbonic Anhydrase Inhibitor; Ophthalmic Agent, Antiglaucoma
Use Treatment of elevated intraocular pressure in patients with ocular hypertension or open-angle glaucoma
Local Anesthetic/Vasoconstrictor Precautions No information available to require special precautions
Effects on Dental Treatment Key adverse event(s) related to dental treatment: Taste perversion.
Effects on Bleeding No information available to require special precautions
Adverse Effects Percentages as reported with combination product. Also see individual agents.

>5%:
Gastrointestinal: Taste perversion (≤30%)
Ocular: Burning/stinging (≤30%), blurred vision (5% to 15%), conjunctival hyperemia (5% to 15%), itching (5% to 15%), superficial punctuate keratitis (5% to 15%)
1% to 5%:
Cardiovascular: Hypertension
Central nervous system: Dizziness, headache
Gastrointestinal: Abdominal pain, dyspepsia, nausea
Genitourinary: Urinary tract infection
Neuromuscular & skeletal: Back pain

Ocular: Blepharitis, cloudy vision, conjunctival discharge, conjunctival edema, conjunctival follicles, conjunctivitis, corneal erosion, corneal staining, cortical lens opacity, dryness, eye debris, eye/eyelid discharge, eye/eyelid pain, eyelid edema, eyelid erythema, eyelid exudate/scales, foreign body sensation, glaucomatous cupping, lens nucleus discoloration, lens opacity, post-subcapsular cataract, tearing, visual field defect, vitreous detachment

Respiratory: Bronchitis, cough, pharyngitis, sinusitis, upper respiratory infection

Miscellaneous: Flu

General Dosage Range Ophthalmic: *Children ≥2 years and Adults:* Instill 1 drop into affected eye(s) twice daily

Mechanism of Action

Dorzolamide: Inhibits carbonic anhydrase in the ciliary processes of the eye resulting decreased bicarbonate ion formation which decreases sodium and fluid transport, thus decreasing aqueous humor secretion and reduces intraocular pressure.

Timolol: Blocks both $beta_1$- and $beta_2$-adrenergic receptors, reduces intraocular pressure by reducing aqueous humor production or possibly outflow

Pregnancy Risk Factor C

Doxapram (DOKS a pram)

U.S. Brand Names Dopram®

Pharmacologic Category Respiratory Stimulant; Stimulant

Use Respiratory and CNS stimulant for respiratory depression secondary to anesthesia, drug-induced CNS depression; acute hypercapnia secondary to COPD

Local Anesthetic/Vasoconstrictor Precautions No information available to require special precautions

Effects on Dental Treatment No significant effects or complications reported

Effects on Bleeding No information available to require special precautions

Adverse Effects Frequency not defined.

Cardiovascular: Arrhythmia, blood pressure increased, chest pain, chest tightness, flushing, heart rate changes, T waves lowered, ventricular tachycardia, ventricular fibrillation

Central nervous system: Apprehension, Babinski turns positive, disorientation, dizziness, hallucinations, headache, hyperactivity, pyrexia, seizure

Dermatologic: Burning sensation, pruritus

Gastrointestinal: Defecation urge, diarrhea, nausea, vomiting

Genitourinary: Spontaneous voiding, urinary retention

Hematologic: Hematocrit decreased, hemoglobin decreased, hemolysis, red blood cell count decreased

Local: Phlebitis

Neuromuscular & skeletal: Clonus, deep tendon reflexes increase, fasciculations, involuntary muscle movement, muscle spasm, paresthesia

Ocular: Pupillary dilatation

Renal: Albuminuria, BUN increased

Respiratory: Bronchospasm, cough, dyspnea, hiccups, hyperventilation, laryngospasm, rebound hypoventilation, tachypnea

Miscellaneous: Diaphoresis

General Dosage Range I.V.: *Adults:* 0.5-1 mg/kg every 5 minutes until response (maximum total dose: 2 mg/kg) **or** 1-5 mg/minute until response; should not be continued >2 hours (maximum total dose: 4 mg/kg; 3 g/day)

Mechanism of Action Stimulates respiration through action on respiratory center in medulla or indirectly on peripheral carotid chemoreceptors

Pharmacodynamics/Kinetics

Onset of Action Respiratory stimulation: I.V.: 20-40 seconds; Peak effect: 1-2 minutes

Duration of Action 5-12 minutes

Half-life Elimination Serum: Adults: Mean: 3.4 hours

Pregnancy Risk Factor B

Doxazosin (doks AY zoe sin)

Related Information

Cardiovascular Diseases *on page 1848*

U.S. Brand Names Cardura®; Cardura® XL

Canadian Brand Names Alti-Doxazosin; Apo-Doxazosin®; Cardura-1™; Cardura-2™; Cardura-4™; Gen-Doxazosin; Mylan-Doxazosin; Novo-Doxazosin

Generic Availability (U.S.) Yes: Excludes extended release tablet

Pharmacologic Category $Alpha_1$ Blocker

Use

Immediate release formulation: Treatment of hypertension as monotherapy or in conjunction with diuretics, ACE inhibitors, beta-blockers, or calcium antagonists

Immediate release and extended release formulations: Treatment of urinary outflow obstruction and/or obstructive and irritative symptoms associated with benign prostatic hyperplasia (BPH)

Unlabeled/Investigational Use Pediatric hypertension

Local Anesthetic/Vasoconstrictor Precautions No information available to require special precautions

Effects on Dental Treatment Key adverse event(s) related to dental treatment: Xerostomia (normal salivary flow resumes upon discontinuation) and orthostatic hypotension

Effects on Bleeding No information available to require special precautions

Adverse Effects Note: Type and frequency of adverse reactions reflect combined data from BPH and hypertension trials and immediate release and extended release products.

>10%: Central nervous system: Dizziness (5% to 19%), headache (5% to 14%)

1% to 10%:

Cardiovascular: Orthostatic hypotension (dose related; 0.3% up to 2%), edema (3% to 4%), hypotension (1% to 2%), palpitation (1% to 2%), chest pain (1% to 2%), arrhythmia (1%), syncope (2%), flushing (1%)

Central nervous system: Fatigue (8% to 12%), somnolence (1% to 5%), nervousness (2%), pain (2%), vertigo (2% to 4%), insomnia (1%), anxiety (1%), paresthesia (1%), movement disorder (1%), ataxia (1%), hypertonia (1%), depression (1%)

Dermatologic: Rash (1%), pruritus (1%)

Endocrine & metabolic: Sexual dysfunction (2%)

Gastrointestinal: Abdominal pain (2%), diarrhea (2%), dyspepsia (1% to 2%), nausea (1% to 3%), xerostomia (1% to 2%), constipation (1%), flatulence (1%)

Genitourinary: Urinary tract infection (1%), impotence (1%), polyuria (2%), incontinence (1%)

Neuromuscular & skeletal: Back pain (2% to 3%), weakness (1% to 7%), arthritis (1%), muscle weakness (1%), myalgia (≤1%), muscle cramps (1%)

Ocular: Abnormal vision (1% to 2%), conjunctivitis (1%)

Otic: Tinnitus (1%)

Respiratory: Respiratory tract infection (5%), rhinitis (3%), dyspnea (1% to 3%), respiratory disorder (1%), epistaxis (1%)

Miscellaneous: Diaphoresis increased (1%), flu-like syndrome (1%)

Dosage Oral:

Children (unlabeled use): Hypertension: Immediate release: Initial: 1 mg once daily; maximum: 4 mg/day

Adults:

Immediate release: 1 mg once daily in morning or evening; may be increased to 2 mg once daily. Thereafter titrate upwards, if needed, over several weeks, balancing therapeutic benefit with doxazosin-induced postural hypotension.

BPH: Goal: 4-8 mg/day; maximum dose: 8 mg/day

Hypertension: Maximum dose: 16 mg/day

Reinitiation of therapy: If therapy is discontinued for several days, restart at 1 mg dose and titrate as before

Extended release: BPH: 4 mg once daily with breakfast; titrate based on response and tolerability every 3-4 weeks to maximum recommended dose of 8 mg/day

Reinitiation of therapy: If therapy is discontinued for several days, restart at 4 mg dose and titrate as before.

Conversion to extended release from immediate release: Omit final evening dose of immediate release prior to starting morning dosing with extended release product; initiate extended release product using 4 mg once daily

Dosing adjustment in hepatic impairment: Use with caution in mild-to-moderate hepatic dysfunction. Do not use with severe impairment.

Mechanism of Action

Hypertension: Competitively inhibits postsynaptic alpha$_1$-adrenergic receptors which results in vasodilation of veins and arterioles and a decrease in total peripheral resistance and blood pressure; ~50% as potent on a weight by weight basis as prazosin.

BPH: Competitively inhibits postsynaptic alpha$_1$-adrenergic receptors in prostatic stromal and bladder neck tissues. This reduces the sympathetic tone-induced urethral stricture causing BPH symptoms.

Contraindications Hypersensitivity to quinazolines (prazosin, terazosin), doxazosin, or any component of the formulation

Warnings/Precautions Can cause significant orthostatic hypotension and syncope, especially with first dose; anticipate a similar effect if therapy is interrupted for a few days, if dosage is rapidly increased, or if another antihypertensive drug (particularly vasodilators) or a PDE-5 inhibitor is introduced. Discontinue if symptoms of angina occur or worsen. Patients should be cautioned about performing hazardous tasks when starting new therapy or adjusting dosage upward. Prostate cancer should be ruled out before starting for BPH. Use with caution in mild-to-moderate hepatic impairment; not recommended in severe dysfunction. Intraoperative floppy iris syndrome has been observed in cataract surgery patients who were on or were previously treated with alpha$_1$-blockers. Causality has not been established and there appears to be no benefit in discontinuing alpha-blocker therapy prior to surgery. May be inappropriate in the elderly due to potential for dry mouth, hypotension, and urinary problems (Beers Criteria).

The extended release formulation consists of drug within a nondeformable matrix; following drug release/absorption, the matrix/shell is expelled in the stool. The use of nondeformable products in patients with known stricture/narrowing of the GI tract has been associated with symptoms of obstruction. Use caution in patients with increased GI retention (eg, chronic constipation) as doxazosin exposure may be increased. Extended release formulation is not indicated for use in women or for the treatment of hypertension.

Drug Interactions

Avoid Concomitant Use

Avoid concomitant use of Doxazosin with any of the following: Alpha1-Blockers

Increased Effect/Toxicity

Doxazosin may increase the levels/effects of: Alpha1-Blockers; Amifostine; Antihypertensives; Calcium Channel Blockers; Hypotensive Agents; RiTUXimab

The levels/effects of Doxazosin may be increased by: Beta-Blockers; Diazoxide; Herbs (Hypotensive Properties); MAO Inhibitors; Pentoxifylline; Phosphodiesterase 5 Inhibitors; Prostacyclin Analogues

Decreased Effect

The levels/effects of Doxazosin may be decreased by: Herbs (Hypertensive Properties); Methylphenidate; Yohimbine

Ethanol/Nutrition/Herb Interactions Herb/Nutraceutical: Avoid dong quai if using for hypertension (has estrogenic activity). Avoid ephedra, yohimbe, ginseng (may worsen hypertension). Avoid saw palmetto when used for BPH (due to limited experience with this combination). Avoid garlic (may have increased antihypertensive effect).

Dietary Considerations Cardura® XL: Take with morning meal.

Pharmacodynamics/Kinetics

Duration of Action >24 hours

Half-life Elimination Immediate release: ~22 hours; Extended release: 15-19 hours

Time to Peak Serum: Immediate release: 2-3 hours; Extended release: 8-9 hours

Pregnancy Risk Factor C

Lactation Excretion in breast milk unknown/use caution

Breast-Feeding Considerations The extended release formulation is not indicated for use in women.

Dosage Forms

Tablet, oral: 1 mg, 2 mg, 4 mg, 8 mg

Cardura®: 1 mg, 2 mg, 4 mg, 8 mg

Tablet, extended release, oral:

Cardura® XL: 4 mg, 8 mg

Doxepin (Systemic) (DOKS e pin)

Related Information

Management of the Patient With Anxiety or Depression *on page 1968*

U.S. Brand Names Silenor®

Canadian Brand Names Apo-Doxepin®; Doxepine; Novo-Doxepin; Sinequan®

Generic Availability (U.S.) Yes: Excludes tablet

Pharmacologic Category Antidepressant, Tricyclic (Tertiary Amine)

Use Depression; treatment of insomnia (with difficulty of sleep maintenance)

Unlabeled/Investigational Use Analgesic for certain chronic and neuropathic pain; anxiety

Local Anesthetic/Vasoconstrictor Precautions Doxepin is one of the drugs confirmed to prolong the QT interval and is accepted as having a risk of causing torsade de pointes. In terms of epinephrine, it is not known what effect vasoconstrictors in the local anesthetic regimen will have in patients with a known history of congenital prolonged QT interval or in patients taking any medication that prolongs the QT interval. Until more information is obtained, it is suggested that the clinician consult with the physician prior to the use of a vasoconstrictor in suspected patients, and that the vasoconstrictor (epinephrine, mepivacaine and levonordefrin [Carbocaine® 2% with Neo-Cobefrin®]) be used with caution. See Dental Comment.

Effects on Dental Treatment Key adverse event(s) related to dental treatment: Xerostomia and changes in salivation (normal salivary flow resumes upon discontinuation)

Oral: Aphthous stomatitis, unpleasant taste, trouble with gums

Long-term treatment with TCAs increases the risk of caries by reducing salivation and salivary buffer capacity.

Effects on Bleeding No information available to require special precautions

Adverse Effects Actual frequency may be dependent on diagnosis.

Cardiovascular: Flushing, hypertension (<3%), hypotension, tachycardia

Central nervous system: Ataxia, chills, confusion, disorientation, dizziness, drowsiness, fatigue, hallucinations, headache, seizure, somnolence/sedation (6% to 9%)

Dermatologic: Alopecia, photosensitivity, pruritus, rash

Endocrine & metabolic: Blood sugar increased/decreased, breast enlargement, galactorrhea, gynecomastia, libido increased/decreased, SIADH

Gastrointestinal: Anorexia, aphthous stomatitis, constipation, diarrhea, gastroenteritis (≤2%), indigestion, nausea (2%), trouble with gums, unpleasant taste, vomiting, weight gain, xerostomia; lower esophageal sphincter tone decrease may cause GE reflux

Genitourinary: Testicular edema, urinary retention

Hematologic: Agranulocytosis, eosinophilia, leukopenia, purpura, thrombocytopenia, purpura

Hepatic: Jaundice

Neuromuscular & skeletal: Extrapyramidal symptoms, numbness, paresthesia, tardive dyskinesia, tremor, weakness

Ocular: Blurred vision

Otic: Tinnitus

Respiratory: Asthma exacerbation, nasopharyngitis/upper respiratory tract infection (≤4%)

Miscellaneous: Allergic reactions, diaphoresis (excessive)

Dosage Oral:

Depression or anxiety (entire daily dose may be given at bedtime):

Adults: Initial: 25-150 mg/day at bedtime or in 2-3 divided doses; may gradually increase up to 300 mg/day; single dose should not exceed 150 mg; select patients may respond to 25-50 mg/day

Elderly: Initial: 10-25 mg at bedtime; increase by 10-25 mg every 3 days for inpatients and weekly for outpatients if tolerated. Rarely does the maximum dose required exceed 75 mg/day; a single bedtime dose is recommended.

Insomnia (Silenor®):

Adults: 3-6 mg once daily 30 minutes prior to bedtime; maximum dose: 6 mg/day

Elderly: 3 mg once daily; increase to 6 mg once daily if clinically needed

Dosing adjustment in hepatic impairment: Use a lower dose and adjust gradually

Silenor®: Initial: 3 mg once daily

Mechanism of Action Increases the synaptic concentration of serotonin and norepinephrine in the central nervous system by inhibition of their reuptake by the presynaptic neuronal membrane; antagonizes the histamine (H_1) receptor for sleep maintenance

Contraindications Hypersensitivity to doxepin, drugs from similar chemical class, or any component of the formulation; narrow-angle glaucoma; urinary retention; use of MAO inhibitors within 14 days

Warnings/Precautions [U.S. Boxed Warning]: Antidepressants increase the risk of suicidal thinking and behavior in children, adolescents, and young adults (18-24 years of age) with major depressive disorder (MDD) and other psychiatric disorders; consider risk prior to prescribing. Short-term studies did not show an increased risk in patients >24 years of age and showed a decreased risk in patients ≥65 years. Closely monitor for clinical worsening, suicidality, or unusual changes in behavior; the patient's family or caregiver should be instructed to closely observe the patient and communicate condition with healthcare provider. A medication guide should be dispensed with each prescription. **Doxepin is approved for treatment of depression in adolescents.**

The possibility of a suicide attempt is inherent in major depression and may persist until remission occurs. Monitor for worsening of depression or suicidality, especially during initiation of therapy (generally first 1-2 months) or with dose increases or decreases. Use caution in high-risk patients. Worsening depression and severe abrupt suicidality that are not part of the presenting symptoms may require discontinuation or modification of drug therapy. The patient's family or caregiver should be alerted to monitor patients for the emergence of suicidality and associated behaviors (such as agitation, irritability, hostility, impulsivity, and hypomania) and call healthcare provider.

Risk of suicidal behavior may be increased regardless of doxepin dose; antidepressant doses of doxepin are 10- to 100-fold higher than doses for insomnia.

May worsen psychosis in some patients or precipitate a shift to mania or hypomania in patients with bipolar disorder. Patients presenting with depressive symptoms should be screened for bipolar disorder. Monotherapy in patients with bipolar disorder should be avoided. **Doxepin is not FDA approved for the treatment of bipolar depression.**

Should only be used for insomnia after evaluation of potential causes of sleep disturbance. Failure of sleep disturbance to resolve after 7-10 days may indicate psychiatric or medical illness. An increased risk for hazardous sleep-related activities has been noted; discontinue use with any sleep-related episodes. The risks of sedative and anticholinergic effects are high relative to other antidepressant agents. Doxepin frequently causes sedation, which may result in impaired performance of tasks requiring alertness (eg, operating machinery or driving). Sedative effects may be additive with other CNS depressants and/or ethanol. Also use caution in patients with benign prostatic hyperplasia, xerostomia, visual problems, constipation, or history of bowel obstruction.

May cause orthostatic hypotension or conduction disturbances (risks are moderate relative to other antidepressants). Use with caution in patients with a history of cardiovascular disease (including previous MI, stroke, tachycardia, or conduction abnormalities). Use with caution in patients with respiratory compromise or sleep apnea; use is generally not recommended with severe sleep apnea. Consider discontinuation, when possible, prior to elective surgery. Therapy should not be abruptly discontinued in patients receiving high doses for prolonged periods.

Use caution in patients with a previous seizure disorder or condition predisposing to seizures such as brain damage, alcoholism, or concurrent therapy with other drugs which lower the seizure threshold. Use with caution in hyperthyroid patients or those receiving thyroid supplementation. Use with caution in patients with hepatic or renal dysfunction. Use as an antidepressant in the elderly may be inappropriate due to potent anticholinergic and sedating effects (Beers Criteria).

Drug Interactions

Metabolism/Transport Effects Substrate (major) of CYP1A2, 2D6, 3A4

Avoid Concomitant Use

Avoid concomitant use of Doxepin (Systemic) with any of the following: Artemether; Dronedarone; Iobenguane I 123; Lumefantrine; MAO Inhibitors; Methylene Blue; Nilotinib; Pimozide; QuiNINE; Sibutramine; Tetrabenazine; Thioridazine; Toremifene; Vandetanib; Ziprasidone

Increased Effect/Toxicity

Doxepin (Systemic) may increase the levels/effects of: Alcohol (Ethyl); Alpha-/Beta-Agonists (Direct-Acting); Alpha1-Agonists; Amphetamines; Anticholinergics; Aspirin; Beta2-Agonists; CNS Depressants; Desmopressin; Dronedarone; Methylene Blue; NSAID (COX-2 Inhibitor); NSAID (Nonselective); Pimozide; QTc-Prolonging Agents; QuiNIDine; QuiNINE; Serotonin Modulators; Sulfonylureas; Tetrabenazine; Thioridazine; Toremifene; TraMADol; Vandetanib; Vitamin K Antagonists; Yohimbine; Ziprasidone

The levels/effects of Doxepin (Systemic) may be increased by: Abiraterone; Alfuzosin; Altretamine; Artemether; BuPROPion; Chloroquine; Cimetidine; Cinacalcet; Ciprofloxacin; Ciprofloxacin (Systemic); Conivaptan; CYP2D6 Inhibitors (Moderate); CYP2D6 Inhibitors (Strong); Dexmethylphenidate; Divalproex; DULoxetine; Gadobutrol; Lithium; Lumefantrine; MAO Inhibitors; Methylphenidate; Metoclopramide; Nilotinib; Pramlintide; Propoxyphene; Protease Inhibitors; QuiNIDine; QuiNINE; Selective Serotonin Reuptake Inhibitors; Sibutramine; Terbinafine; Terbinafine (Systemic); Valproic Acid

Decreased Effect

Doxepin (Systemic) may decrease the levels/effects of: Acetylcholinesterase Inhibitors (Central); Alpha2-Agonists; Iobenguane I 123

The levels/effects of Doxepin (Systemic) may be decreased by: Acetylcholinesterase Inhibitors (Central); Barbiturates; CarBAMazepine; Peginterferon Alfa-2b; St Johns Wort; Tocilizumab

Ethanol/Nutrition/Herb Interactions

Ethanol: May increase CNS depression; monitor for increased effects with coadministration. Caution patients about effects.

Food: A high-fat meal increases the bioavailability of Silenor® and delays the peak plasma concentration by ~3 hours

Herb/Nutraceutical: Avoid valerian, St John's wort, SAMe, kava kava (may increase risk of serotonin syndrome and/or excessive sedation).

Pharmacodynamics/Kinetics

Onset of Action Peak effect: Antidepressant: Usually >2 weeks; Anxiolytic: May occur sooner

Half-life Elimination Adults: Doxepin: ~15 hours; N-desmethyldoxepin: 31 hours

Time to Peak Serum: Hypnotic: 3.5 hours

Pregnancy Risk Factor C

Lactation Enters breast milk/use caution (AAP rates "of concern"; AAP 2001 update pending)

Breast-Feeding Considerations Drowsiness and apnea have been reported in a nursing infant following maternal use of doxepin for depression.

Dosage Forms

Capsule, oral: 10 mg, 25 mg, 50 mg, 75 mg, 100 mg, 150 mg

Solution, oral: 10 mg/mL (118 mL, 120 mL)

Tablet, oral:

Silenor®: 3 mg, 6 mg

Dental Comment Doxepin is known to prolong the QT interval. The QT interval is measured as the time and distance between the Q point of the QRS complex and the end of the T wave in the ECG tracing. After adjustment for heart rate, the QT interval is defined as prolonged if it is more than 450 msec in men and 460 msec in women. A long QT syndrome was first described in the 1950s and 60s as a congenital syndrome involving QT interval prolongation and syncope and sudden death. Some of the congenital long QT syndromes were characterized by a peculiar electrocardiographic appearance of the QRS complex involving a premature atria beat followed by a pause, then a subsequent sinus beat showing marked QT prolongation and deformity. This type of cardiac arrhythmia was originally termed "torsade de pointes" (translated from the French as "twisting of the points"). Doxepin is considered as having a risk of causing torsade de pointes. Since it is not known what effect vasoconstrictors in the local anesthetic regimen will have in patients with a known history of congenital prolonged QT interval or in patients taking any medication that prolongs the QT interval, a medical consult is suggested.

References

Friedlander AH and Mahler ME, "Major Depressive Disorder. Psychopathology, Medical Management and Dental Implications," *J Am Dent Assoc*, 2001, 132(5):629-38.

Ganzberg S, "Psychoactive Drugs," *ADA Guide to Dental Therapeutics*, 2nd ed, Chicago, IL: ADA Publishing, a Division of ADA Business Enterprises, Inc, 2000, 376-405.

Jastak JT and Yagiela JA, "Vasoconstrictors and Local Anesthesia: A Review and Rationale for Use," *J Am Dent Assoc*, 1983, 107(4):623-30.

Rundegren J, van Dijken J, Mörnstad H, et al, "Oral Conditions in Patients Receiving Long-Term Treatment With Cyclic Antidepressant Drugs," *Swed Dent J*, 1985, 9(2):55-64.

Yagiela JA, "Adverse Drug Interactions in Dental Practice: Interactions Associated With Vasoconstrictors. Part V of a Series," *J Am Dent Assoc*, 1999, 130(5):701-9.

Doxepin (Topical) (DOKS e pin)

U.S. Brand Names Prudoxin™; Zonalon®

Canadian Brand Names Zonalon®

Generic Availability (U.S.) No

Pharmacologic Category Topical Skin Product

Dental Use Cream: Treatment of burning mouth syndrome and neuropathic pain

Use Short-term (<8 days) management of moderate pruritus in adults with atopic dermatitis or lichen simplex chronicus

Unlabeled/Investigational Use Cream: Treatment of burning mouth syndrome and neuropathic pain

Local Anesthetic/Vasoconstrictor Precautions No information available to require special precautions

Effects on Dental Treatment Key adverse event(s) related to dental treatment: Xerostomia and changes in salivation (normal salivary flow resumes upon discontinuation)

Topical: Taste alteration

Long-term treatment with TCAs increases the risk of caries by reducing salivation and salivary buffer capacity.

Effects on Bleeding No information available to require special precautions

Adverse Effects

>10%:

Central nervous system: Drowsiness (22%)

Dermatologic: Stinging/burning (23%)

1% to 10%:

Cardiovascular: Edema: (1%)

Central nervous system: Dizziness (2%), emotional changes (2%)

Gastrointestinal: Xerostomia (10%), taste alteration (2%)

Dental Usual Dosage Treatment of burning mouth syndrome and neuropathic pain (unlabeled uses): Adults: Oral: Topical: Cream: Apply 3-4 times daily

Dosage

Oral: Topical: Burning mouth syndrome (unlabeled use): Cream: Apply 3-4 times daily

Topical: Pruritus: Adults and Elderly: Apply a thin film 4 times/day with at least 3- to 4-hour interval between applications; not recommended for use >8 days. **Note:** Low-dose (25-50 mg) oral administration has also been used to treat pruritus, but systemic effects are increased.

Contraindications Hypersensitivity to doxepin, drugs from similar chemical class, or any component of the formulation; narrow-angle glaucoma; urinary retention; use of MAO inhibitors within 14 days; use in a patient during acute recovery phase of MI

Warnings/Precautions Cream formulation is for external use only (not for ophthalmic, vaginal, or oral use). Do not use occlusive dressings. Use for >8 days may increase risk of contact sensitization. Doxepin is significantly absorbed following topical administration; plasma levels may be similar to those achieved with oral administration. Systemic absorption may be significant. The risks of sedative and anticholinergic effects caused by doxepin are high relative to other antidepressant agents. Doxepin frequently causes sedation, which may result in impaired performance of tasks requiring alertness (eg, operating machinery or driving). Sedative effects may be additive with other CNS depressants and/or ethanol. Also use caution in patients with benign prostatic hyperplasia, xerostomia, visual problems, constipation, or history of bowel obstruction.

May cause orthostatic hypotension or conduction disturbances. Use with caution in patients with a history of cardiovascular disease (including previous MI, stroke, tachycardia, or conduction abnormalities). Consider discontinuation, when possible, prior to elective surgery. Use caution in patients with a previous seizure disorder or condition predisposing to seizures such as brain damage, alcoholism, or concurrent therapy with other drugs which lower the seizure threshold. Use with caution in hyperthyroid patients or those receiving thyroid supplementation. Use with caution in patients with hepatic or renal dysfunction.

Drug Interactions

Metabolism/Transport Effects Substrate (major) of CYP1A2, 2D6, 3A4

Avoid Concomitant Use

Avoid concomitant use of Doxepin (Topical) with any of the following: Artemether; Dronedarone; Iobenguane I 123; Lumefantrine; MAO Inhibitors; Methylene Blue; Nilotinib; Pimozide; QuiNINE; Sibutramine; Tetrabenazine; Thioridazine; Toremifene; Vandetanib; Ziprasidone

Increased Effect/Toxicity

Doxepin (Topical) may increase the levels/effects of: Alcohol (Ethyl); Alpha-/Beta-Agonists (Direct-Acting); Alpha1-Agonists; Amphetamines; Anticholinergics; Aspirin; Beta2-Agonists; CNS Depressants; Desmopressin; Dronedarone; Methylene Blue; NSAID (COX-2 Inhibitor); NSAID (Nonselective); Pimozide; QTc-Prolonging Agents; QuiNIDine; QuiNINE; Serotonin Modulators; Sulfonylureas; Tetrabenazine; Thioridazine; Toremifene; TraMADol; Vandetanib; Vitamin K Antagonists; Yohimbine; Ziprasidone

The levels/effects of Doxepin (Topical) may be increased by: Abiraterone; Alfuzosin; Altretamine; Artemether; BuPROPion; Chloroquine; Cimetidine; Cinacalcet; Ciprofloxacin; Ciprofloxacin (Systemic); Conivaptan; CYP2D6 Inhibitors (Moderate); CYP2D6 Inhibitors (Strong); Dexmethylphenidate; Divalproex; DULoxetine; Gadobutrol; Lithium; Lumefantrine; MAO Inhibitors; Methylphenidate; Metoclopramide; Nilotinib; Pramlintide; Propoxyphene; Protease Inhibitors; QuiNIDine; QuiNINE; Selective Serotonin Reuptake Inhibitors; Sibutramine; Terbinafine; Terbinafine (Systemic); Valproic Acid

Decreased Effect

Doxepin (Topical) may decrease the levels/effects of: Acetylcholinesterase Inhibitors (Central); Alpha2-Agonists; Iobenguane I 123

The levels/effects of Doxepin (Topical) may be decreased by: Acetylcholinesterase Inhibitors (Central); Barbiturates; CarBAMazepine; Peginterferon Alfa-2b; St Johns Wort; Tocilizumab

Pregnancy Risk Factor B

Lactation Enters breast milk/not recommended (AAP rates "of concern"; AAP 2001 update pending)

Breast-Feeding Considerations Drowsiness and apnea have been reported in a nursing infant following maternal use of oral doxepin. Following topical application, plasma levels may be similar to those achieved with oral administration.

Dosage Forms

Cream, topical:

Prudoxin™: 5% (45 g)

Zonalon®: 5% (30 g, 45 g)

References

Buchanan J and Zakrzewska J, "Burning Mouth Syndrome," *Clin Evid (online)*, March 14, 2008. Available at http://www.ncbi.nlm.nih.gov/pmc/articles/PMC2907957/pdf/2008-1301.pdf.

Mínguez Serra MP, Salort Llorca C, Silvestre Donat FJ, "Pharmacological Treatment of Burning Mouth Syndrome: A Review and Update," *Med Oral Patol Oral Cir Bucal*, 2007, 12(4):E299-304.

Doxercalciferol (doks er kal si fe FEER ole)

U.S. Brand Names Hectorol®

Canadian Brand Names Hectorol®

Pharmacologic Category Vitamin D Analog

Use Treatment of secondary hyperparathyroidism in patients with chronic kidney disease

Local Anesthetic/Vasoconstrictor Precautions No information available to require special precautions

Effects on Dental Treatment No significant effects or complications reported

Effects on Bleeding No information available to require special precautions

Adverse Effects Note: As reported in dialysis patients.

>10%:

- Cardiovascular: Edema (34%)
- Central nervous system: Headache (28%), malaise (28%), dizziness (12%)
- Gastrointestinal: Nausea/vomiting (21%)
- Respiratory: Dyspnea (12%)

1% to 10%:

- Cardiovascular: Bradycardia (7%)
- Central nervous system: Sleep disorder (3%)
- Dermatologic: Pruritus (8%)
- Endocrine & metabolic: Hypercalcemia (I.V. ~1%), hyperphosphatemia (I.V. 2% to 4%)
- Gastrointestinal: Anorexia (5%), dyspepsia (5%), weight gain (5%)
- Neuromuscular & skeletal: Arthralgia (5%)
- Miscellaneous: Abscess (3%)

General Dosage Range

I.V.: *Adults:* Initial: 4 mcg 3 times/week after dialysis; Maintenance: Up to 18 mcg/week

Oral:

Adults (dialysis patients): Initial: 10 mcg 3 times/week at dialysis; Maintenance: Up to 60 mcg/week

Adults (predialysis patients): Initial: 1 mcg/day; Maintenance: Up to 3.5 mcg/day

Mechanism of Action Doxercalciferol is metabolized to the active form of vitamin D. The active form of vitamin D controls the intestinal absorption of dietary calcium, the tubular reabsorption of calcium by the kidneys, and in conjunction with PTH, the mobilization of calcium from the skeleton.

Pharmacodynamics/Kinetics

Half-life Elimination Active metabolite: 32-37 hours; up to 96 hours

Pregnancy Risk Factor B

DOXOrubicin (doks oh ROO bi sin)

Related Information

DOXOrubicin (Liposomal) *on page* 572

U.S. Brand Names Adriamycin®

Canadian Brand Names Adriamycin®

Pharmacologic Category Antineoplastic Agent, Anthracycline

Use Treatment of acute lymphocytic leukemia (ALL), acute myeloid leukemia (AML), Hodgkin's disease, malignant lymphoma, soft tissue and bone sarcomas, thyroid cancer, small cell lung cancer, breast cancer, gastric cancer, ovarian cancer, bladder cancer, neuroblastoma, and Wilms' tumor

Unlabeled/Investigational Use Treatment of multiple myeloma, endometrial carcinoma, uterine sarcoma, head and neck cancer, liver cancer, kidney cancer

Local Anesthetic/Vasoconstrictor Precautions No information available to require special precautions

Effects on Dental Treatment Key adverse event(s) related to dental treatment: Stomatitis and mucositis.

Effects on Bleeding Chemotherapy may result in significant myelosuppression, potentially including significant reduction in platelet counts and altered hemostasis.

In patients who are under active treatment with these agents, medical consult is suggested.

Adverse Effects Frequency not defined.

Cardiovascular:

Acute cardiotoxicity: Atrioventricular block, bradycardia, bundle branch block, ECG abnormalities, extrasystoles (atrial or ventricular), sinus tachycardia, ST-T wave changes, supraventricular tachycardia, tachyarrhythmia, ventricular tachycardia

Delayed cardiotoxicity: LVEF decreased, CHF (manifestations include ascites, cardiomegaly, dyspnea, edema, gallop rhythm, hepatomegaly, oliguria, pleural effusion, pulmonary edema, tachycardia); myocarditis, pericarditis

Central nervous system: Malaise

Dermatologic: Alopecia, itching, photosensitivity, radiation recall, rash; discoloration of saliva, sweat, or tears

Endocrine & metabolic: Amenorrhea, dehydration, infertility (may be temporary), hyperuricemia

Gastrointestinal: Abdominal pain, anorexia, colon necrosis, diarrhea, GI ulceration, mucositis, nausea, vomiting

Genitourinary: Discoloration of urine

Hematologic: Leukopenia/neutropenia (75%; nadir: 10-14 days; recovery: by day 21); thrombocytopenia and anemia

Local: Skin "flare" at injection site, urticaria

Neuromuscular & skeletal: Weakness

General Dosage Range

Dosage adjustment recommended in patients with hepatic impairment or who develop toxicities

I.V.: *Children and Adults:* Dosage varies greatly depending on indication

Mechanism of Action Inhibition of DNA and RNA synthesis by intercalation between DNA base pairs by inhibition of topoisomerase II and by steric obstruction. Doxorubicin intercalates at points of local uncoiling of the double helix. Although the exact mechanism is unclear, it appears that direct binding to DNA (intercalation) and inhibition of DNA repair (topoisomerase II inhibition) result in blockade of DNA and RNA synthesis and fragmentation of DNA. Doxorubicin is also a powerful iron chelator; the iron-doxorubicin complex can bind DNA and cell membranes and produce free radicals that immediately cleave the DNA and cell membranes.

Pharmacodynamics/Kinetics

Half-life Elimination

Distribution: 5-10 minutes

Elimination: Doxorubicin: 1-3 hours; Metabolites: 3-3.5 hours

Terminal: 17-48 hours

Male: 54 hours; Female: 35 hours

Pregnancy Risk Factor D

DOXOrubicin (Liposomal) (doks oh ROO bi sin lip pah SOW mal)

Related Information

DOXOrubicin *on page 571*

U.S. Brand Names Doxil®

Canadian Brand Names Caelyx®; Myocet™

Pharmacologic Category Antineoplastic Agent, Anthracycline

Use Treatment of ovarian cancer, multiple myeloma, and AIDS-related Kaposi's sarcoma

Unlabeled/Investigational Use Treatment of metastatic breast cancer, Hodgkin's lymphoma, cutaneous T-cell lymphomas (mycosis fungoides and Sézary syndrome), advanced soft tissue sarcomas; recurrent or metastatic cervical cancer, advanced or metastatic uterine sarcoma

Local Anesthetic/Vasoconstrictor Precautions No information available to require special precautions

Effects on Dental Treatment Key adverse event(s) related to dental treatment: Xerostomia (normal salivary flow resumes upon discontinuation), mucositis, gingivitis, glossitis, mouth ulceration, taste perversion, and stomatitis.

Effects on Bleeding Chemotherapy may result in significant myelosuppression, potentially including significant reduction in platelet counts and altered hemostasis. In patients who are under active treatment with these agents, medical consult is suggested.

Adverse Effects

>10%:

Cardiovascular: Peripheral edema (≤11%)

Central nervous system: Fever (8% to 21%), headache (≤11%), pain (≤21%)

Dermatologic: Palmar-plantar erythrodysesthesia/hand-foot syndrome (≤51% in ovarian cancer [grades 3/4: 24%]; 3% in Kaposi's sarcoma), rash (≤29% in ovarian cancer, ≤5% in Kaposi's sarcoma), alopecia (9% to 19%)
Gastrointestinal: Nausea (17% to 46%), stomatitis (5% to 41%), vomiting (8% to 33%), constipation (≤30%), diarrhea (5% to 21%), anorexia (≤20%), mucositis (≤14%), dyspepsia (≤12%), intestinal obstruction (≤11%)
Hematologic: Myelosuppression (onset: 7 days; nadir: 10-14 days; recovery: 21-28 days), thrombocytopenia (13% to 65%; grades 3/4: 1%), neutropenia (12% to 62%; grade 4: 4%), leukopenia (36%), anemia (6% to 74%; grade 4: <1%)
Neuromuscular & skeletal: Weakness (7% to 40%), back pain (≤12%)
Respiratory: Pharyngitis (≤16%), dyspnea (≤15%)
Miscellaneous: Infection (≤12%)

1% to 10%:
Cardiovascular: Cardiac arrest, chest pain, deep thrombophlebitis, edema, hypotension, pallor, tachycardia, vasodilation
Central nervous system: Agitation, anxiety, chills, confusion, depression, dizziness, emotional lability, insomnia, somnolence, vertigo
Dermatologic: Acne, bruising, dry skin (6%), exfoliative dermatitis, fungal dermatitis, furunculosis, maculopapular rash, pruritus, skin discoloration, vesiculobullous rash
Endocrine & metabolic: Dehydration, hypercalcemia, hyperglycemia, hypokalemia, hyponatremia
Gastrointestinal: Abdomen enlarged, anorexia, ascites, cachexia, dyspepsia, dysphagia, esophagitis, flatulence, gingivitis, glossitis, ileus, mouth ulceration, oral moniliasis, rectal bleeding, taste perversion, weight loss, xerostomia
Genitourinary: Cystitis, dysuria, leukorrhea, pelvic pain, polyuria, urinary incontinence, urinary tract infection, urinary urgency, vaginal bleeding, vaginal moniliasis
Hematologic: Hemolysis, prothrombin time increased
Hepatic: ALT increased, alkaline phosphatase increased, hyperbilirubinemia
Local: Thrombophlebitis
Neuromuscular & skeletal: Arthralgia, hypertonia, myalgia, neuralgia, neuritis (peripheral), neuropathy, paresthesia (≤10%), pathological fracture
Ocular: Conjunctivitis, dry eyes, retinitis
Otic: Ear pain
Renal: Albuminuria, hematuria
Respiratory: Apnea, cough (≤10%), epistaxis, pleural effusion, pneumonia, rhinitis, sinusitis
Miscellaneous: Allergic reaction; infusion-related reactions (7%; includes bronchospasm, chest tightness, chills, dyspnea, facial edema, flushing, headache, herpes simplex/zoster, hypotension, pruritus); moniliasis, diaphoresis

General Dosage Range Dosage adjustment recommended in patients with hepatic impairment or who develop toxicities

I.V.: *Adults:* 20-30 mg/m^2 every 3 weeks **or** 50 mg/m^2/dose every 4 weeks

Mechanism of Action Doxorubicin inhibits DNA and RNA synthesis by intercalating between DNA base pairs causing steric obstruction and inhibits topoisomerase-II at the point of DNA cleavage. Doxorubicin is also a powerful iron chelator. The iron-doxorubicin complex can bind DNA and cell membranes, producing free hydroxyl (OH) radicals that cleave DNA and cell membranes. Active throughout entire cell cycle. Doxorubicin liposomal is a pegylated formulation which protects the liposomes, and thereby increases blood circulation time.

Pharmacodynamics/Kinetics

Half-life Elimination Terminal: Distribution: 4.7-5.2 hours, Elimination: 44-55 hours

Pregnancy Risk Factor D

Doxycycline (doks i SYE kleen)

Related Information

Periodontal Diseases *on page 1942*
Sexually-Transmitted Diseases *on page 1903*

Related Sample Prescriptions

Bacterial Infections and Periodontal Diseases *on page 1983*

U.S. Brand Names Adoxa®; Adoxa® Pak™ 1/150; Adoxa® Pak™ 1/75; Alodox™; Doryx®; Doxy 100™; Monodox®; Ocudox™; Oracea®; Oraxyl™; Periostat®; Vibramycin®

Canadian Brand Names Apo-Doxy Tabs®; Apo-Doxy®; Dom-Doxycycline; Doxycin; Doxytab; Novo-Doxylin; Nu-Doxycycline; Periostat®; PHL-Doxycycline; PMS-Doxycycline; Vibra-Tabs®; Vibramycin®

Generic Availability (U.S.) Yes: Excludes capsule (variable release), syrup

Pharmacologic Category Antibiotic, Tetracycline Derivative

Dental Use Treatment of periodontitis associated with presence of *Actinobacillus actinomycetemcomitans* (AA); adjunct to scaling and root planing to promote attachment level gain and to reduce pocket depth in adult periodontitis (systemic levels are subinhibitory against bacteria)

Use Principally in the treatment of infections caused by susceptible *Rickettsia*, *Chlamydia*, and *Mycoplasma*; alternative to mefloquine for malaria prophylaxis; treatment for syphilis, uncomplicated *Neisseria gonorrhoeae*, *Listeria*, *Actinomyces israelii*, and *Clostridium* infections in penicillin-allergic patients; used for community-acquired pneumonia and other common infections due to susceptible organisms; anthrax due to *Bacillus anthracis,* including inhalational anthrax (postexposure); treatment of infections caused by uncommon susceptible gram-negative and gram-positive organisms including *Borrelia recurrentis*, *Ureaplasma urealyticum*, *Haemophilus ducreyi*, *Yersinia pestis*, *Francisella tularensis*, *Vibrio cholerae*, *Campylobacter fetus*, *Brucella* spp, *Bartonella bacilliformis*, and *Klebsiella granulomatis,* Q fever, Lyme disease; treatment of inflammatory lesions associated with rosacea; intestinal amebiasis; severe acne

Unlabeled/Investigational Use Sclerosing agent for pleural effusion injection; vancomycin-resistant enterococci (VRE); alternate treatment for MRSA infections; treatment of periodontitis (refractory); localized juvenile periodontitis (LIP)

Local Anesthetic/Vasoconstrictor Precautions No information available to require special precautions

Effects on Dental Treatment Key adverse event(s) related to dental treatment: Glossitis and tooth discoloration (children). Opportunistic "superinfection" with *Candida albicans*; tetracyclines are not recommended for use during pregnancy or in children ≤8 years of age since they have been reported to cause enamel hypoplasia and permanent teeth discoloration. The use of tetracyclines should only be used in these patients if other agents are contraindicated or alternative antimicrobials will not eradicate the organism.

Effects on Bleeding No information available to require special precautions

Adverse Effects Frequency not defined.

Cardiovascular: Intracranial hypertension, pericarditis

Dermatologic: Angioneurotic edema, erythema multiforme, exfoliative dermatitis (rare), photosensitivity, rash, skin hyperpigmentation, Stevens-Johnson syndrome, toxic epidermal necrolysis, urticaria

Endocrine & metabolic: Brown/black discoloration of thyroid gland (no dysfunction reported), hypoglycemia

Gastrointestinal: Anorexia, diarrhea, dysphagia, enterocolitis, esophagitis (rare), esophageal ulcerations (rare), glossitis, inflammatory lesions in anogenital region, nausea, oral (mucosal) pigmentation, pseudomembranous colitis, tooth discoloration (children), vomiting

Hematologic: Eosinophilia, hemolytic anemia, neutropenia, thrombocytopenia

Hepatic: Hepatotoxicity (rare)

Renal: BUN increased (dose related)

Miscellaneous: Anaphylactoid purpura, anaphylaxis, bulging fontanels (infants), serum sickness, SLE exacerbation

Note: Adverse effects in clinical trials occurring at a frequency more than 1% greater than placebo:

Periostat®: Diarrhea, dyspepsia, joint pain, menstrual cramp, nausea, dyspepsia, pain

Oracea®: Abdominal distention, abdominal pain, anxiety, AST increased, back pain, fungal infection, hyperglycemia, influenza, LDH increased, nasal congestion, nasopharyngitis, pain, sinus headache, sinusitis, xerostomia

Dental Usual Dosage Adults: Oral: Treatment of periodontitis (refractory): 100-200 mg once daily for 21 days. **Note:** A specific formulation (Periostat®) containing a subantimicrobial dosage is also available for use as an adjunct to scaling and root planing. In addition, doxycycline gel (Atridox™) is available for subgingival application (see Doxycycline Hyclate Periodontal Extended-Release Liquid monograph).

Dosage

Usual dosage range:

Children >8 years (≤45 kg): Oral, I.V.: 2-5 mg/kg/day in 1-2 divided doses, not to exceed 200 mg/day

Children >8 years (>45 kg) and Adults: Oral, I.V.: 100-200 mg/day in 1-2 divided doses

Indication-specific dosing:

Children:

Anthrax: Doxycycline should be used in children if antibiotic susceptibility testing, exhaustion of drug supplies, or allergic reaction preclude use of penicillin or ciprofloxacin. For treatment, the consensus recommendation does not include a loading dose for doxycycline.

Inhalational (postexposure prophylaxis) (ACIP, 2010): Oral, I.V. (use oral route when possible):

≤8 years: 2.2 mg/kg every 12 hours for 60 days
>8 years and ≤45 kg: 2.2 mg/kg every 12 hours for 60 days
>8 years and >45 kg: 100 mg every 12 hours for 60 days

Cutaneous (treatment): Oral: See dosing for "Inhalational (postexposure prophylaxis)"

Note: In the presence of systemic involvement, extensive edema, and/or lesions on head/neck, doxycycline should initially be administered I.V.

Inhalational/gastrointestinal/oropharyngeal (treatment): I.V.: Refer to dosing for inhalational anthrax (postexposure prophylaxis); switch to oral therapy when clinically appropriate

Note: Initial treatment should include two or more agents predicted to be effective (CDC, 2001). Agents suggested for use in conjunction with doxycycline or ciprofloxacin include rifampin, vancomycin, imipenem, penicillin, ampicillin, chloramphenicol, clindamycin, and clarithromycin. May switch to oral antimicrobial therapy when clinically appropriate. Continue combined therapy for 60 days

Cellulitis (purulent) due to community-acquired MRSA (unlabeled use): Oral: Children >8 years and ≤45 kg: 2 mg/kg/dose every 12 hours for 5-10 days (Liu, 2011)

Localized juvenile periodontitis (LIP) (unlabeled use): 50-100 mg/day

Q fever: Oral, I.V.: 2.2 mg/kg twice/day for 15-21 days (CDC, 2009). Some clinicians may recommend trimethoprim/sulfamethoxazole for children <8 years of age (Hartzell, 2008). **Note:** Use of tetracyclines should be avoided during tooth development (children ≤8 years of age) unless other drugs are unlikely to be effective or are contraindicated.

Tickborne rickettsial disease: Oral, I.V.: Children ≤8 years: 2.2 mg/kg (maximum dose: 100 mg) every 12 hours for 5-7 days; severe or complicated disease may require longer treatment; human granulocytotropic anaplasmosis (HGA) should be treated for 10-14 days. **Note:** The American Academy of Pediatrics Committee on Infectious Diseases identifies doxycycline as the drug of choice in children of any age.

Tularemia: I.V. (may transition to oral if clinically indicated) (Dennis, 2001):

Children <45 kg: 2.2 mg/kg every 12 hours for 14-21 days
Children ≥45 kg: 100 mg every 12 hours for 14-21 days

Children ≥8 years:

Lyme disease: Oral (Halperin, 2007; Wormser, 2006):

Prevention: 4 mg/kg (maximum: 200 mg) administered as a single dose; **Note:** Initiate within 72 hours of tick removal

Treatment (early lyme disease without neurologic manifestations): 1-2 mg/kg twice daily for 10-21 days (maximum: 100 mg/dose)

Treatment (meningitis and other early neurologic manifestations): 4-8 mg/kg/day in 2 divided doses for 10-28 days (maximum: 200 mg/dose)

Malaria prophylaxis: Oral: 2 mg/kg/day (maximum: 100 mg/day). Start 1-2 days prior to travel to endemic area; continue daily during travel and for 4 weeks after leaving endemic area

Children >8 years (and >45 kg) and Adults:

Cellulitis (purulent) due to community-acquired MRSA (unlabeled use): Oral: 100 mg twice daily for 5-10 days (Liu, 2011)

Chlamydial infections, uncomplicated: Oral: 100 mg twice daily for 7 days

Tickborne rickettsial disease: Oral, I.V.: 100 mg twice daily for 5-7 days; severe or complicated disease may require longer treatment; human granulocytotropic anaplasmosis (HGA) should be treated for 10-14 days. **Note:** The American Academy of Pediatrics Committee on Infectious Diseases identifies doxycycline as the drug of choice in children of any age.

Adults:

Anthrax:

Inhalational (postexposure prophylaxis): Oral, I.V. (use oral route when possible): 100 mg every 12 hours for 60 days (ACIP, 2010)

Cutaneous (treatment): Oral: 100 mg every 12 hours for 60 days. **Note:** In the presence of systemic involvement, extensive edema, lesions on head/neck, refer to I.V. dosing for treatment of inhalational/gastrointestinal/oropharyngeal anthrax

Inhalational/gastrointestinal/oropharyngeal (treatment): I.V.: Initial: 100 mg every 12 hours; switch to oral therapy when clinically appropriate; some recommend initial loading dose of 200 mg, followed by 100 mg every 8-12 hours (Franz, 1997). **Note:** Initial treatment should include two or more agents predicted to be effective (CDC, 2001). Agents suggested for use in conjunction with doxycycline or ciprofloxacin include rifampin, vancomycin, imipenem, penicillin, ampicillin, chloramphenicol, clindamycin, and clarithromycin. May switch to oral antimicrobial therapy when clinically appropriate. Continue combined therapy for 60 days

Brucellosis: Oral: 100 mg twice daily for 6 weeks with rifampin or streptomycin

Community-acquired pneumonia, bronchitis: Oral, I.V.: 100 mg twice daily (Ailani, 1999; Mandell, 2007)

Epididymitis: Oral: 100 mg twice daily for 10 days (in combination with ceftriaxone) (CDC, 2010)

Gonococcal infection, uncomplicated (cervix, pharynx, rectum, urethra): Oral: 100 mg twice daily for 7 days (in combination with a cephalosporin) (CDC, 2010)

Alternatively, the manufacturer recommends a single-visit dose in nonanorectal infections in men: 300 mg initially, repeat dose in 1 hour (total dose: 600 mg)

Granuloma inguinale (donovanosis): Oral: 100 mg twice daily for at least 3 weeks (and until lesions have healed) (CDC, 2010)

Lyme disease: Oral (Halperin, 2007; Wormser, 2006):

Prevention: Initiate within 72 hours of tick removal: 200 mg administered as a single dose

Treatment (early lyme disease without neurologic manifestations): 100 mg twice daily for 10-21 days

Treatment (meningitis or other early neurologic manifestations): 100-200 mg twice daily for 14 days (range: 10-28 days)

Lymphogranuloma venereum: Oral: 100 mg twice daily for 21 days (CDC, 2010)

Malaria prophylaxis: 100 mg/day. Start 1-2 days prior to travel to endemic area; continue daily during travel and for 4 weeks after leaving endemic area

Nongonococcal urethritis: Oral: 100 mg twice daily for 7 days (CDC, 2010)

Pelvic inflammatory disease:

Treatment, inpatient: Oral, I.V.: 100 mg twice daily (in combination with cefoxitin or cefotetan); may transition to oral doxycycline (add clindamycin or metronidazole if tubo-ovarian abscess present) to complete 14 days of treatment (CDC, 2010)

Treatment, outpatient: Oral: 100 mg twice daily for 14 days (with or without metronidazole); preceded by a single I.M. dose of cefoxitin (plus oral probenecid) or ceftriaxone (CDC, 2010)

Periodontitis: Oral (Periostat®): 20 mg twice daily as an adjunct following scaling and root planing

Periodontitis, refractory (unlabeled use): Oral: 100-200 mg daily

Proctitis: Oral: 100 mg twice daily for 7 days (in combination with ceftriaxone) (CDC, 2010)

Q fever: Oral: 100 mg every 12 hours for 15-21days (CDC, 2009)

Rosacea (Oracea®): Oral: 40 mg once daily in the morning

Sclerosing agent for pleural effusion (unlabeled use): Intrapleural: 500 mg as a single dose in 100 mL NS (Porcel, 2006); may require a repeat dose (Kvale, 2007)

Syphilis:

Primary/secondary syphilis: Oral: 100 mg twice daily for 14 days (CDC, 2010)

Latent syphilis: Oral: 100 mg twice daily for 28 days (CDC, 2010)

Tularemia: I.V. (may transition to oral if clinically appropriate): Initial: 100 mg every 12 hours for 14-21 days (Dennis, 2001)

Vibrio cholerae: Oral: 300 mg as a single dose (WHO, 2004)

***Yersinia pestis* (plague):** Oral, I.V.: 200 mg initially then 100 mg twice daily **or** 200 mg once daily for 10 days (Daya, 2005; Inglesby, 2000)

Dosing adjustment in renal impairment: No adjustment necessary

Dialysis: Not dialyzable; 0% to 5% by hemo- and peritoneal methods or by continuous arteriovenous or venovenous hemofiltration: No supplemental dosage necessary

Mechanism of Action Inhibits protein synthesis by binding with the 30S and possibly the 50S ribosomal subunit(s) of susceptible bacteria; may also cause alterations in the cytoplasmic membrane

Periostat® capsules (proposed mechanism): Has been shown to inhibit collagenase activity *in vitro*. Also has been noted to reduce elevated collagenase activity in the gingival crevicular fluid of patients with periodontal disease. Systemic levels do not reach inhibitory concentrations against bacteria.

Contraindications Hypersensitivity to doxycycline, tetracycline or any component of the formulation

Warnings/Precautions Photosensitivity reaction may occur with this drug; avoid prolonged exposure to sunlight or tanning equipment. Antianabolic effects of tetracyclines can increase BUN (dose-related). Autoimmune syndromes have been reported. Hepatotoxicity rarely occurs; if symptomatic, conduct LFT and discontinue drug. Pseudotumor cerebri has been (rarely) reported with tetracycline use; usually resolves with discontinuation. Prolonged use may result in fungal or bacterial superinfection, including *C. difficile*-associated diarrhea (CDAD) and pseudomembranous colitis; CDAD has been observed >2 months postantibiotic treatment. May cause tissue hyperpigmentation, enamel hypoplasia, or permanent tooth discoloration; use of tetracyclines should be avoided during tooth development (children ≤8 years of age) unless other drugs are not likely to be effective or are contraindicated. However, recommended in treatment of anthrax exposure and tickborne rickettsial diseases. Do not use during pregnancy. In addition to affecting tooth development, tetracycline use has been associated with retardation of skeletal development and reduced bone growth.

Additional specific warnings: Oracea®: Should not be used for the treatment or prophylaxis of bacterial infections, since the lower dose of drug per capsule may be subefficacious and promote resistance. Syrup contains sodium metabisulfite. Effectiveness of products intended for use in periodontitis has not been established in patients with coexistent oral candidiasis; use with caution in patients with a history or predisposition to oral candidiasis.

Drug Interactions

Metabolism/Transport Effects Inhibits CYP3A4 (moderate)

Avoid Concomitant Use

Avoid concomitant use of Doxycycline with any of the following: BCG; Retinoic Acid Derivatives

Increased Effect/Toxicity

Doxycycline may increase the levels/effects of: Neuromuscular-Blocking Agents; Retinoic Acid Derivatives; Vitamin K Antagonists

Decreased Effect

Doxycycline may decrease the levels/effects of: BCG; Penicillins; Typhoid Vaccine

The levels/effects of Doxycycline may be decreased by: Antacids; Barbiturates; Bile Acid Sequestrants; Bismuth; Bismuth Subsalicylate; Calcium Salts; CarBAMazepine; Fosphenytoin; Iron Salts; Magnesium Salts; Phenytoin; Quinapril; Sucralfate

Ethanol/Nutrition/Herb Interactions

Ethanol: Chronic ethanol ingestion may reduce the serum concentration of doxycycline.

Food: Doxycycline serum levels may be slightly decreased if taken with food or milk. Administration with iron or calcium may decrease doxycycline absorption. May decrease absorption of calcium, iron, magnesium, zinc, and amino acids.

Herb/Nutraceutical: St John's wort may decrease doxycycline levels. Avoid dong quai, St John's wort (may also cause photosensitization).

Dietary Considerations

Tetracyclines (in general): Take with food if gastric irritation occurs. While administration with food may decrease GI absorption of doxycycline by up to 20%, administration on an empty stomach is not recommended due to GI intolerance. Of currently available tetracyclines, doxycycline has the least affinity for calcium.

Oracea®: Take on an empty stomach 1 hour before or 2 hours after meals.

Some products may contain sodium.

Pharmacodynamics/Kinetics

Half-life Elimination 12-15 hours (usually increases to 22-24 hours with multiple doses); End-stage renal disease: 18-25 hours; Oracea®: 21 hours

Time to Peak Serum: 1.5-4 hours

Pregnancy Risk Factor D

Lactation Enters breast milk/not recommended

Breast-Feeding Considerations Tetracyclines, including doxycycline, are excreted in breast milk and therefore, breast-feeding is not recommended by the manufacturer.

Doxycycline is less bound to the calcium in maternal milk which may lead to increased absorption compared to other tetracyclines. Only minimal amounts of doxycycline are excreted in human milk and the relative amount of tooth staining has been reported to be lower when compared to other tetracycline analogs. Nondose-related effects could include modification of bowel flora.

Dosage Forms

Capsule, oral: 50 mg, 100 mg
Adoxa®: 150 mg
Monodox®: 50 mg, 75 mg, 100 mg
Ocudox™: 50 mg
Oraxyl™: 20 mg
Vibramycin®: 100 mg

Capsule, variable release, oral:
Oracea®: 40 mg [30 mg (immediate release) and 10 mg (delayed release)]

Injection, powder for reconstitution: 100 mg
Doxy 100™: 100 mg

Powder for suspension, oral:
Vibramycin®: 25 mg/5 mL (60 mL)

Syrup, oral:
Vibramycin®: 50 mg/5 mL (473 mL)

Tablet, oral: 20 mg, 50 mg, 75 mg, 100 mg, 150 mg
Adoxa®: 50 mg
Adoxa® Pak™ 1/150: 150 mg
Adoxa® Pak™ 1/75: 75 mg
Alodox™: 20 mg
Periostat®: 20 mg

Tablet, delayed release coated beads, oral: 75 mg, 100 mg

Tablet, delayed release coated pellets, oral:
Doryx®: 75 mg, 100 mg, 150 mg

Doxycycline Hyclate Periodontal Extended-Release Liquid (doks i SYE kleen HI klayt per ee oh DON tal ik STEN did ri LES LIK wid)

Related Information

Doxycycline *on page 573*
Periodontal Diseases *on page 1942*

U.S. Brand Names Atridox®

Canadian Brand Names Atridox®

Generic Availability (U.S.) No

Pharmacologic Category Antibiotic, Tetracycline Derivative

Dental Use Treatment of chronic adult periodontitis for gain in clinical attachment, reduction in probing depth, and reduction in bleeding upon probing

Use Used exclusively in dental applications

Local Anesthetic/Vasoconstrictor Precautions No information available to require special precautions

Effects on Dental Treatment Key adverse event(s) related to dental treatment: Discoloration of teeth (in children), gum discomfort, toothache, periodontal abscess, tooth sensitivity, broken tooth, tooth mobility, endodontic abscess, and jaw pain

Mechanical oral hygiene procedures (ie, tooth brushing, flossing) should be avoided in any treated area for 7 days.

Effects reported in clinical trials were similar in incidence between doxycycline-containing product and vehicle alone; comparable to standard therapies including scaling and root planing or oral hygiene. Although there is no known relationship between doxycycline and hypertension, unspecified essential hypertension was noted in 1.6% of the doxycycline gel group, as compared to 0.2% in the vehicle group (allergic reactions to the vehicle were also reported in two patients).

Effects on Bleeding No information available to require special precautions

Adverse Effects

>10%: Discoloration of teeth in children

Doxycycline periodontal gel (Atridox®): The adverse effects reported in clinical trials were similar in incidence between doxycycline-containing product and vehicle alone. In addition, these effects were comparable to standard therapies including scaling and root planning or oral hygiene. Events associated with application reported with an incidence >1% included: gum discomfort (18%), toothache (14%), periodontal abscess (10%), tooth sensitivity (8%), broken tooth (5%), tooth mobility (2%), endodontic abscess (2%) and jaw pain (1%). Systemic adverse events included headache (27%), muscle aches (7%), diarrhea (3%), upset stomach (4%), and nausea (2%). Although there is no known relationship between doxycycline and hypertension, unspecified essential hypertension was noted in 1.6% of the doxycycline gel group, as compared to 0.2% in the vehicle group. Allergic reactions to the vehicle were also reported in two patients.

Dental Usual Dosage Oral, subgingival: Dose depends on size, shape and number of pockets treated. Application may be repeated four months after initial treatment. The delivery system consists of 2 separate syringes in a single pouch. Syringe A contains 450 mg of a bioabsorbable polymer gel; syringe B contains doxycycline hyclate 50 mg. To prepare for instillation, couple syringe A to syringe B. Inject contents of syringe A (purple stripe) into syringe B, then push contents back into syringe A. Repeat this mixing cycle at a rate of one cycle per second for 100 cycles. If syringes are stored prior to use (a maximum of 3 days), repeat mixing cycle 10 times before use. After appropriate mixing, contents should be in syringe A. Holding syringes vertically, with syringe A at the bottom, pull back on the syringe A plunger, allowing contents to flow down barrel for several seconds. Uncouple syringes and attach enclosed blunt cannula to syringe A. Local anesthesia is not required for placement. Cannula tip may be bent to resemble periodontal probe and used to explore pocket. Express product from syringe until pocket is filled. To separate tip from formulation, turn tip towards the tooth and press against tooth surface to achieve separation. An appropriate dental instrument may be used to pack gel into the pocket. Pockets may be covered with either Coe-pak™ or Octyldent™ dental adhesive.

Dosage Adults: Subgingival application: Dose depends on size, shape and number of pockets treated. Contains 50 mg doxycycline hyclate per 500 mg of formulation in each final blended syringe product. Application may be repeated four months after initial treatment.

Atridox® subgingival controlled-release product: The delivery system consists of 2 separate syringes in a single pouch. Syringe A contains 450 mg of a bioabsorbable polymer gel; syringe B contains doxycycline hyclate 50 mg. To prepare for instillation, couple syringe A to syringe B. Inject contents of syringe A (purple stripe) into syringe B, then push contents back into syringe A. Repeat this mixing cycle at a rate of one cycle per second for 100 cycles. If syringes are stored prior to use (a maximum of 3 days), repeat mixing cycle 10 times before use. After appropriate mixing, contents should be in syringe A. Holding syringes vertically, with syringe A at the bottom, pull back on the syringe A plunger, allowing contents to flow down barrel for several seconds. Uncouple syringes and attach enclosed blunt cannula to syringe A. Local anesthesia is not required for placement. Cannula tip may be bent to resemble periodontal probe and used to explore pocket. Express product from syringe until pocket is filled. To separate tip from formulation, turn tip towards the tooth and press against tooth surface to achieve separation. An appropriate dental instrument may be used to pack gel into the pocket. Pockets may be covered with either Coe-Pak™ or Octyldent™ dental adhesive.

Mechanism of Action Inhibits protein synthesis by binding with the 30S and possibly the 50S ribosomal subunit(s) of susceptible bacteria; may also cause alterations in the cytoplasmic membrane

Doxycycline inhibits collagenase *in vitro* and has been shown to inhibit collagenase in the gingival crevicular fluid in adults with periodontitis

Contraindications Hypersensitivity to doxycycline, tetracycline or any component of the formulation; children <8 years of age; severe hepatic dysfunction; pregnancy

Warnings/Precautions Photosensitivity reaction may occur with this drug; avoid prolonged exposure to sunlight or tanning equipment. Prolonged use may result in fungal or bacterial superinfection, including *C. difficile*-associated diarrhea (CDAD) and pseudomembranous colitis; CDAD has been observed >2 months postantibiotic treatment. May cause tissue hyperpigmentation, enamel hypoplasia, or permanent tooth discoloration; use of tetracyclines should be avoided during tooth development (children ≤8 years of age) unless other drugs are not likely to be effective or are contraindicated. However, recommended in treatment of anthrax exposure. Do not use during pregnancy. In addition to affecting tooth development, tetracycline use has been associated with retardation of skeletal development and reduced bone growth.

Additional specific warnings for doxycycline gel (Atridox®) for subgingival application: This product has not been evaluated or tested in immunocompromised patients, in patients with oral candidiasis, or in conditions characterized by severe periodontal defects with little remaining periodontium. May result in overgrowth of nonsusceptible organisms, including fungi. Effects of treatment >6 months have not been evaluated. Has not been evaluated for use in regeneration of alveolar bone

Drug Interactions

Avoid Concomitant Use There are no known interactions where it is recommended to avoid concomitant use.

Increased Effect/Toxicity There are no known significant interactions involving an increase in effect.

Decreased Effect There are no known significant interactions involving a decrease in effect.

Dietary Considerations May be taken with food, milk, or water.

Pregnancy Risk Factor D

Dosage Forms
Liquid, subgingival:
Atridox®: 10% (4 units, 6 units)

Doxylamine (dox IL a meen)

U.S. Brand Names Aldex® AN
Canadian Brand Names Unisom®-2
Pharmacologic Category Ethanolamine Derivative; Histamine H_1 Antagonist; Histamine H_1 Antagonist, First Generation
Use Treatment of short-term insomnia
Local Anesthetic/Vasoconstrictor Precautions No information available to require special precautions
Effects on Dental Treatment Key adverse event(s) related to dental treatment: Dry mucous membranes and significant xerostomia (normal salivary flow resumes upon discontinuation)
Effects on Bleeding No information available to require special precautions
Adverse Effects Frequency not defined.
Cardiovascular: Palpitation, tachycardia
Central nervous system: Dizziness, disorientation, drowsiness, headache, paradoxical CNS stimulation, vertigo
Gastrointestinal: Anorexia, dry mucous membranes, diarrhea, constipation, epigastric pain, xerostomia
Genitourinary: Dysuria, urinary retention
Ocular: Blurred vision, diplopia
General Dosage Range Oral: *Adults:* 1 tablet 30 minutes before bedtime
Mechanism of Action Doxylamine competes with histamine for H_1-receptor sites on effector cells; blocks chemoreceptor trigger zone, diminishes vestibular stimulation, and depresses labyrinthine function through its central anticholinergic activity.
Pharmacodynamics/Kinetics
Half-life Elimination 10-12 hours
Pregnancy Risk Factor B

Dronabinol (droe NAB i nol)

U.S. Brand Names Marinol®
Canadian Brand Names Marinol®
Pharmacologic Category Antiemetic; Appetite Stimulant
Use Chemotherapy-associated nausea and vomiting refractory to other antiemetic(s); AIDS-related anorexia
Unlabeled/Investigational Use Cancer-related anorexia
Local Anesthetic/Vasoconstrictor Precautions No information available to require special precautions
Effects on Dental Treatment Key adverse event(s) related to dental treatment: Xerostomia (normal salivary flow resumes upon discontinuation) and orthostatic hypotension
Effects on Bleeding No information available to require special precautions
Adverse Effects Frequency not always specified.
>1%:
Cardiovascular: Palpitations, tachycardia, vasodilation/facial flushing
Central nervous system: Euphoria (8% to 24%, dose related), abnormal thinking (3% to 10%), dizziness (3% to 10%), paranoia (3% to 10%), somnolence (3% to 10%), amnesia, anxiety, ataxia, confusion, depersonalization, hallucination
Gastrointestinal: Abdominal pain (3% to 10%), nausea (3% to 10%), vomiting (3% to 10%)
Neuromuscular & skeletal: Weakness
General Dosage Range Oral:
Children: Initial: 5 mg/m^2 as a single dose; Maintenance: 5 mg/m^2/dose every 2-4 hours for a total of 4-6 doses/day (maximum: 15 mg/m^2/dose)
Adults: Initial: 5 mg/m^2 as a single dose; Maintenance: 5 mg/m^2/dose every 2-4 hours for a total of 4-6 doses/day (maximum: 15 mg/m^2/dose) **or** Initial: 2.5 mg twice daily; Maintenance: Titrate up to 20 mg/day in 2 divided doses
Mechanism of Action Unknown, may inhibit endorphins in the brain's emetic center, suppress prostaglandin synthesis, and/or inhibit medullary activity through an unspecified cortical action. Some pharmacologic effects appear to involve sympathimometic activity; tachyphylaxis to some effect (eg, tachycardia) may occur, but appetite-stimulating effects do not appear to wane over time. Antiemetic activity may be due to effect on cannabinoid receptors (CB1) within the central nervous system.

Pharmacodynamics/Kinetics

Onset of Action Within 1 hour; Peak effect: 2-4 hours

Duration of Action 24 hours (appetite stimulation)

Half-life Elimination Dronabinol: 25-36 hours (terminal); Dronabinol metabolites: 44-59 hours

Time to Peak Serum: 0.5-4 hours

Pregnancy Risk Factor C

Controlled Substance C-III

Dronedarone (droe NE da rone)

U.S. Brand Names Multaq®

Canadian Brand Names Multaq®

Pharmacologic Category Antiarrhythmic Agent, Class III

Use To reduce the risk of hospitalization related to paroxysmal or persistent atrial fibrillation (AF) or atrial flutter (AFL) in patients with a recent episode of AF/AFL and associated cardiovascular risk factors (eg, age >70 years, hypertension, diabetes, prior cerebrovascular accident, left atrial diameter ≥50 mm or left ventricular ejection fraction <40%), who are in normal sinus rhythm or will be cardioverted

Local Anesthetic/Vasoconstrictor Precautions Dronedarone is one of the drugs confirmed to prolong the QT interval and is accepted as having a risk of causing torsade de pointes. The risk of drug-induced torsade de pointes is extremely low when a single QT interval prolonging drug is prescribed. In terms of epinephrine, it is not known what effect vasoconstrictors in the local anesthetic regimen will have in patients with a known history of congenital prolonged QT interval or in patients taking any medication that prolongs the QT interval. Until more information is obtained, it is suggested that the clinician consult with the physician prior to the use of a vasoconstrictor in suspected patients, and that the vasoconstrictor (epinephrine, mepivacaine and levonordefrin [Carbocaine® 2% with Neo-Cobefrin®]) be used with caution.

Effects on Dental Treatment No significant effects or complications reported (see Dental Comment)

Effects on Bleeding No information available to require special precautions

Adverse Effects

>10%:

Cardiovascular: QT_c (Bazett) prolongation (28% [placebo: 19%]; defined as >450 msec in males or >470 msec in females)

Renal: Serum creatinine increased ≥10% (51%; occurred 5 days after initiation)

1% to 10%:

Cardiovascular: Bradycardia (3%)

Dermatologic: Allergic dermatitis (≤5%), dermatitis (≤5%), eczema (≤5%), pruritus (≤5%), rash (≤5%; described as generalized, macular, maculopapular, erythematous)

Gastrointestinal: Diarrhea (9%), nausea (5%), abdominal pain (4%), dyspepsia (2%), vomiting (2%)

Neuromuscular & skeletal: Weakness (7%)

General Dosage Range Oral: *Adults:* 400 mg twice daily

Mechanism of Action A noniodinated antiarrhythmic agent structurally related to amiodarone exhibiting properties of all 4 antiarrhythmic classes. Dronedarone inhibits sodium (I_{Na}) and potassium (I_{kr}, I_{kS}, I_{k1}, and $I_{k\text{-}ACh}$) channels resulting in prolongation of the action potential and refractory period in myocardial tissue without reverse-use dependent effects; decreases AV conduction and sinus node function through inhibition of calcium ($I_{Ca\text{-}L}$) channels and beta$_1$-receptor blocking activity. Similar to amiodarone, dronedarone also inhibits alpha$_1$-receptor mediated increases in blood pressure.

Pharmacodynamics/Kinetics

Half-life Elimination 13-19 hours

Time to Peak Plasma: 3-6 hours

Pregnancy Risk Factor X

Dental Comment Dronedarone is known to prolong the QT interval. The QT interval is measured as the time and distance between the Q point of the QRS complex and the end of the T wave in the ECG tracing. After adjustment for heart rate, the QT interval is defined as prolonged if it is more than 450 msec in men and 460 msec in women. A long QT syndrome was first described in the 1950s and 60s as a congenital syndrome involving QT interval prolongation and syncope and sudden death. Some of the congenital long QT syndromes were characterized by a peculiar electrocardiographic appearance of the QRS complex involving a premature atria beat followed by a pause, then a subsequent sinus beat showing marked QT prolongation and deformity. This type of cardiac arrhythmia was originally termed "torsade de pointes" (translated from the French as "twisting of the points").

Dronedarone is considered as having a risk of causing torsade de pointes. Since it is not known what effect vasoconstrictors in the local anesthetic regimen will have in patients with a known history of congenital prolonged QT interval or in patients taking any medication that prolongs the QT interval, a medical consult is suggested.

Droperidol (droe PER i dole)

Related Information

Clinical Risk Related to Drugs Prolonging QT Interval *on page 1872*

Canadian Brand Names Droperidol Injection, USP

Pharmacologic Category Antiemetic; Antipsychotic Agent, Typical

Use Prevention and/or treatment of nausea and vomiting from surgical and diagnostic procedures

Local Anesthetic/Vasoconstrictor Precautions Manufacturer's information states that droperidol may block vasopressor activity of epinephrine. This has not been observed during use of epinephrine as a vasoconstrictor in local anesthesia. Droperidol is one of the drugs confirmed to prolong the QT interval and is accepted as having a risk of causing torsade de pointes. The risk of drug-induced torsade de pointes is extremely low when a single QT interval prolonging drug is prescribed. In terms of epinephrine, it is not known what effect vasoconstrictors in the local anesthetic regimen will have in patients with a known history of congenital prolonged QT interval or in patients taking any medication that prolongs the QT interval. Until more information is obtained, it is suggested that the clinician consult with the physician prior to the use of a vasoconstrictor in suspected patients, and that the vasoconstrictor (epinephrine, mepivacaine and levonordefrin [Carbocaine® 2% with Neo-Cobefrin®]) be used with caution.

Effects on Dental Treatment Key adverse event(s) related to dental treatment: Orthostatic hypotension

Effects on Bleeding No information available to require special precautions

Adverse Effects Frequency not defined.

Cardiovascular: Cardiac arrest, hypertension, hypotension (especially orthostatic), QT_c prolongation (dose dependent), tachycardia, torsade de pointes, ventricular tachycardia

Central nervous system: Anxiety, chills, depression (postoperative, transient), dizziness, drowsiness (postoperative) increased, dysphoria, extrapyramidal symptoms (akathisia, dystonia, oculogyric crisis), hallucinations (postoperative), hyperactivity, neuroleptic malignant syndrome (NMS) (rare), restlessness

Respiratory: Bronchospasm, laryngospasm

Miscellaneous: Anaphylaxis, shivering

General Dosage Range I.M., I.V.:

Children 2-12 years: Maximum: 0.1 mg/kg; additional doses may be repeated

Adults: Maximum initial dose: 2.5 mg; additional doses of 1.25 mg may be administered

Mechanism of Action Droperidol is a butyrophenone antipsychotic; antiemetic effect is a result of blockade of dopamine stimulation of the chemoreceptor trigger zone. Other effects include alpha-adrenergic blockade, peripheral vascular dilation, and reduction of the pressor effect of epinephrine resulting in hypotension and decreased peripheral vascular resistance; may also reduce pulmonary artery pressure

Pharmacodynamics/Kinetics

Onset of Action 3-10 minutes; Peak effect: Within 30 minutes

Duration of Action 2-4 hours, may extend to 12 hours

Half-life Elimination ~2.3 hours

Pregnancy Risk Factor C

Dental Comment Droperidol is known to prolong the QT interval. The QT interval is measured as the time and distance between the Q point of the QRS complex and the end of the T wave in the ECG tracing. After adjustment for heart rate, the QT interval is defined as prolonged if it is more than 450 msec in men and 460 msec in women. A long QT syndrome was first described in the 1950s and 60s as a congenital syndrome involving QT interval prolongation and syncope and sudden death. Some of the congenital long QT syndromes were characterized by a peculiar electrocardiographic appearance of the QRS complex involving a premature atria beat followed by a pause, then a subsequent sinus beat showing marked QT prolongation and deformity. This type of cardiac arrhythmia was originally termed "torsade de pointes" (translated from the French as "twisting of the points"). Droperidol is considered as having a risk of causing torsade de pointes. Since it is not known what effect vasoconstrictors in the local anesthetic regimen will have in patients with a known history of congenital prolonged QT interval or in patients taking any medication that prolongs the QT interval, a medical consult is suggested.

Drospirenone and Estradiol (droh SPYE re none & es tra DYE ole)

U.S. Brand Names Angeliq®

Canadian Brand Names Angeliq®

Pharmacologic Category Estrogen and Progestin Combination

Use Treatment of moderate-to-severe vasomotor symptoms associated with menopause; treatment of vulvar and vaginal atrophy associated with menopause

Local Anesthetic/Vasoconstrictor Precautions No information available to require special precautions

Effects on Dental Treatment When prescribing antibiotics, patient must be warned to use additional methods of birth control if on oral contraceptives.

Effects on Bleeding No information available to require special precautions related to hemostasis in dental procedures.

Adverse Effects

>10%:

Endocrine & metabolic: Breast pain (19%)

Gastrointestinal: Abdominal pain (11%)

Respiratory: Upper respiratory tract infection (19%)

1% to 10%:

Cardiovascular: Peripheral edema (2%)

Central nervous system: Headache (10%), pain (8%)

Gastrointestinal: Abdomen enlarged (7%)

Genitourinary: Vaginal hemorrhage (9%), endometrial disorder (2%), leukorrhea (1%)

Neuromuscular & skeletal: Back pain (7%)

Respiratory: Flu-like syndrome (7%), sinusitis (5%)

Additional adverse effects reported with estrogens and/or progestins: Abdominal cramps, acne, abnormal uterine bleeding, aggravation of porphyria, amenorrhea, anaphylactoid reactions, anaphylaxis, antifactor Xa decreased, antithrombin III decreased, appetite changes, bloating, breast enlargement, breast tenderness, cerebral embolism, cerebral thrombosis, chloasma, cholestatic jaundice, cholecystitis, cholelithiasis, chorea, contact lens intolerance, corneal curvature steepening, cystitis-like syndrome, decreased carbohydrate tolerance, depression, dementia, dizziness, dysmenorrhea; factors VII, VIII, IX, X, XII, VII-X complex, and II-VII-X complex increased; endometrial hyperplasia, erythema multiforme, erythema nodosum, galactorrhea, hemorrhagic eruption, fatigue, fibrinogen increased, impaired glucose tolerance, HDL-cholesterol increased, hirsutism, hypertension, gallbladder disease, insomnia, LDL-cholesterol decreased, libido changes, melasma, migraine, mood disturbances, nausea, nervousness, optic neuritis, pancreatitis, platelet aggregability and platelet count increased, premenstrual-like syndrome, PT and PTT accelerated, pulmonary embolism, pyrexia, retinal thrombosis, scalp hair loss, somnolence, stroke, thrombophlebitis, thyroid-binding globulin increased, total thyroid hormone (T_4) increased, triglycerides increased, urticaria, uterine leiomyomata size increased, vaginal candidiasis, vomiting, weight gain/loss

General Dosage Range Oral: *Adults (females):* 1 tablet daily

Mechanism of Action

Drospirenone is a synthetic progestin and spironolactone analog with antimineralocorticoid and antiandrogenic activity. Counteracts estrogen effects causing endometrial thinning.

Estrogens are responsible for the development and maintenance of the female reproductive system and secondary sexual characteristics. Estradiol is the principal intracellular human estrogen and is more potent than estrone and estriol at the receptor level; it is the primary estrogen secreted prior to menopause. Following menopause, estrone and estrone sulfate are more highly produced. Estrogens modulate the pituitary secretion of gonadotropins, luteinizing hormone, and follicle-stimulating hormone through a negative feedback system; estrogen replacement reduces elevated levels of these hormones in postmenopausal women.

Pharmacodynamics/Kinetics

Time to Peak Drospirenone: 1 hour; Estradiol: 6-8 hours

Drotrecogin Alfa (dro TRE coe jin AL fa)

U.S. Brand Names Xigris®

Canadian Brand Names Xigris®

Pharmacologic Category Protein C (Activated)

Use Reduction of mortality from severe sepsis (associated with organ dysfunction) in adults at high risk of death (eg, APACHE II score ≥25)

Unlabeled/Investigational Use Purpura fulminans

Local Anesthetic/Vasoconstrictor Precautions No information available to require special precautions

Effects on Dental Treatment Key adverse event(s) related to dental treatment: As with all drugs which may affect hemostasis, bleeding is the major adverse effect associated with drotrecogin alfa. Hemorrhage may occur at virtually any site; risk is dependent on multiple variables, including the dosage administered, concurrent use of multiple agents which alter hemostasis, and patient predisposition.

Effects on Bleeding Associated with increased bleeding risk. Unlikely to be used in a setting where dental procedures are considered.

Adverse Effects As with all drugs which may affect hemostasis, bleeding is the major adverse effect associated with drotrecogin alfa. Hemorrhage may occur at virtually any site. Risk is dependent on multiple variables, including the dosage administered, concurrent use of multiple agents which alter hemostasis, and patient predisposition.

>10%:
- Dermatologic: Bruising
- Gastrointestinal: Gastrointestinal bleeding

1% to 10%: Hematologic: Bleeding (serious 2.4% during infusion vs 3.5% during 28-day study period; individual events listed as <1%)

General Dosage Range I.V.: *Adults:* 24 mcg/kg/**hour** for 96 hours

Mechanism of Action Inhibits factors Va and VIIIa, limiting thrombotic effects. Additional *in vitro* data suggest inhibition of plasminogen activator inhibitor-1 (PAF-1) resulting in profibrinolytic activity, inhibition of macrophage production of tumor necrosis factor, blocking of leukocyte adhesion, and limitation of thrombin-induced inflammatory responses. Relative contribution of effects on the reduction of mortality from sepsis is not completely understood.

Pharmacodynamics/Kinetics

Duration of Action Plasma nondetectable within 2 hours of discontinuation

Half-life Elimination 1.6 hours

Pregnancy Risk Factor C

DULoxetine (doo LOX e teen)

U.S. Brand Names Cymbalta®

Canadian Brand Names Cymbalta®

Pharmacologic Category Antidepressant, Serotonin/Norepinephrine Reuptake Inhibitor

Use Acute and maintenance treatment of major depressive disorder (MDD); treatment of generalized anxiety disorder (GAD); management of diabetic peripheral neuropathic pain (DPNP); management of fibromyalgia (FM); chronic musculoskeletal pain

Unlabeled/Investigational Use Treatment of stress incontinence

Local Anesthetic/Vasoconstrictor Precautions Although duloxetine is not a tricyclic antidepressant, it does block norepinephrine reuptake within the CNS synapses as part of its mechanism. It has been suggested that vasoconstrictors be administered with caution and to monitor vital signs in dental patients taking antidepressants that affect norepinephrine in this way.

Effects on Dental Treatment Key adverse event(s) related to dental treatment: Xerostomia and changes in salivation (normal salivary flow resumes upon discontinuation). See Effects on Bleeding.

Effects on Bleeding May impair platelet aggregation resulting in increased risk of bleeding events, particularly if used concomitantly with aspirin, NSAIDs, warfarin, or other anticoagulants. Bleeding related to SSRI use has been reported to range from relatively minor bruising and epistaxis to life-threatening hemorrhage. Routine interruption of therapy for most dental procedures is not warranted. In medically complicated patients or extensive oral surgery, the decision to interrupt therapy must be based on the risk to benefit in an individual patient and a medical consult is suggested. If therapy is continued without interruption, the clinician should anticipate the potential for a prolonged bleeding time.

Adverse Effects

>10%:
- Central nervous system: Headache (13% to 14%), somnolence (10% to 12%; dose related), fatigue (10 to 11%)
- Gastrointestinal: Nausea (23% to 25%), xerostomia (11% to 15%; dose related)

1% to 10%:
- Cardiovascular: Palpitation (1% to 2%)
- Central nervous system: Dizziness (10%), insomnia (10%; dose related), agitation (3% to 5%), anxiety (3%), dreams abnormal (1% to 2%), yawning (1% to 2%), hypoesthesia (≥1%), lethargy (≥1%), vertigo (≥1%), chills (1%), sleep disorder (1%)

Dermatologic: Hyperhydrosis (6% to 7%)
Endocrine & metabolic: Libido decreased (2% to 4%), hot flushes (1% to 3%), orgasm abnormality (1% to 3%)
Gastrointestinal: Constipation (10%; dose related), diarrhea (9% to 10%), appetite decreased (7% to 9%; dose related), abdominal pain (4% to 6%), vomiting (3% to 5%), dyspepsia (2%), weight loss (2%), flatulence (≥1%), taste abnormal (≥1%), weight gain (≥1%)
Genitourinary: Erectile dysfunction (4% to 5%), ejaculation delayed (3%; dose related), ejaculatory dysfunction (2%)
Hepatic: ALT >3x ULN (1%)
Neuromuscular & skeletal: Muscle spasms (3%), tremor (2% to 3%; dose related), musculoskeletal pain (≥1%), paresthesia (≥1%), rigors (≥1%)
Ocular: Blurred vision (1% to 3%)
Respiratory: Nasopharyngitis (5%), cough (3%)
Miscellaneous: Influenza (3%)

General Dosage Range Oral:
Adults: 30-60 mg/day in 1-2 divided doses (maximum: 120 mg/day)
Elderly: Initial: 20 mg 1-2 times/day

Mechanism of Action Duloxetine is a potent inhibitor of neuronal serotonin and norepinephrine reuptake and a weak inhibitor of dopamine reuptake. Duloxetine has no significant activity for muscarinic cholinergic, H_1-histaminergic, or alpha$_2$-adrenergic receptors. Duloxetine does not possess MAO-inhibitory activity.

Pharmacodynamics/Kinetics
Half-life Elimination 12 hours (range: 8-17 hours)
Time to Peak 6 hours; 10 hours when ingested with food

Pregnancy Risk Factor C

Dutasteride (doo TAS teer ide)

U.S. Brand Names Avodart®
Canadian Brand Names Avodart®
Pharmacologic Category 5 Alpha-Reductase Inhibitor
Use Treatment of symptomatic benign prostatic hyperplasia (BPH) as monotherapy or combination therapy with tamsulosin
Unlabeled/Investigational Use Treatment of male patterned baldness; prostate cancer prevention (to reduce the incidence)
Local Anesthetic/Vasoconstrictor Precautions No information available to require special precautions
Effects on Dental Treatment No significant effects or complications reported
Effects on Bleeding No information available to require special precautions

Adverse Effects
1% to 10%: Endocrine & metabolic: Impotence (1% to 5%), libido decreased (≤3%), ejaculation disorders (≤1%), gynecomastia (including breast tenderness, breast enlargement; ≤1%)
Frequency not defined: Endocrine & metabolic: TSH increased
Note: Frequency of adverse events (except gynecomastia) tends to decrease with continued use (>6 months).

General Dosage Range Oral: *Adults (males):* 0.5 mg once daily

Mechanism of Action Dutasteride is a 4-azo analog of testosterone and is a competitive, selective inhibitor of both reproductive tissues (type 2) and skin and hepatic (type 1) 5α-reductase. This results in inhibition of the conversion of testosterone to dihydrotestosterone and markedly suppresses serum dihydrotestosterone levels.

Pharmacodynamics/Kinetics
Half-life Elimination Terminal: ~5 weeks
Time to Peak 2-3 hours

Pregnancy Risk Factor X

Dutasteride and Tamsulosin (doo TAS teer ide & tam SOO loe sin)

Related Information
Dutasteride *on page 585*
Tamsulosin *on page 1583*

U.S. Brand Names Jalyn™
Pharmacologic Category 5 Alpha-Reductase Inhibitor; Alpha$_1$ Blocker
Use Treatment of symptomatic benign prostatic hyperplasia (BPH)
Local Anesthetic/Vasoconstrictor Precautions No information available to require special precautions

Effects on Dental Treatment Key adverse event(s) related to dental treatment: Tamsulosin: Orthostatic hypotension has been reported; monitor patient for dizziness while rising from dental chair.

Effects on Bleeding No information available to require special precautions

Adverse Effects Frequencies reported for when products used in combination. See individual monographs for additional adverse effects reported with each agent.

1% to 10%:

Central nervous system: Dizziness (2%)

Endocrine & metabolic: Libido decreased (5%), breast enlargement/tenderness (3%)

Genitourinary: Abnormal ejaculation (10%), impotence (8%)

General Dosage Range Oral: *Adults (males):* 1 capsule (0.5 mg dutasteride/0.4 mg tamsulosin) once daily

Mechanism of Action Dutasteride is a 4-azo analog of testosterone and is a competitive, selective inhibitor of both reproductive tissues (type 2) and skin and hepatic (type 1) 5α-reductase. This results in inhibition of the conversion of testosterone to dihydrotestosterone and markedly suppresses serum dihydrotestosterone levels.

Tamsulosin is an antagonist of $alpha_{1A}$-adrenoreceptors in the prostate. Smooth muscle tone in the prostate is mediated by $alpha_{1A}$-adrenoreceptors; blocking them leads to relaxation of smooth muscle in the bladder neck and prostate, causing an improvement of urine flow and decreased symptoms of BPH. Approximately 75% of the $alpha_1$-receptors in the prostate are of the $alpha_{1A}$subtype.

Pregnancy Risk Factor X

Dyclonine (DYE kloe neen)

U.S. Brand Names Sucrets® Children's [OTC]; Sucrets® Maximum Strength [OTC]; Sucrets® Regular Strength [OTC]

Pharmacologic Category Local Anesthetic, Oral

Use Temporary relief of pain associated with oral mucosa

Local Anesthetic/Vasoconstrictor Precautions No information available to require special precautions

Effects on Dental Treatment No significant effects or complications reported

Effects on Bleeding No information available to require special precautions

Adverse Effects

Local: Irritation, numbness, pain, stinging

Miscellaneous: Allergic reactions, cold/heat sensation

General Dosage Range Oral: Lozenge: *Children ≥2 years and Adults:* One lozenge every 2 hours as needed (maximum: 10 lozenges/day)

Dyphylline (DYE fi lin)

U.S. Brand Names Dylix; Lufyllin®

Pharmacologic Category Theophylline Derivative

Use Bronchodilator in reversible airway obstruction due to asthma, chronic bronchitis, or emphysema

Local Anesthetic/Vasoconstrictor Precautions No information available to require special precautions

Effects on Dental Treatment Do not prescribe any erythromycin product to patients taking theophylline products. Erythromycin will delay the normal metabolic inactivation of theophyllines leading to increased blood levels; this has resulted in nausea, vomiting and CNS restlessness.

Effects on Bleeding No information available to require special precautions

Adverse Effects Frequency not defined. Reactions reported with other xanthine derivatives and may be dose related.

Cardiovascular: Circulatory failure, extrasystoles, flushing, hypotension, palpitation, tachycardia, ventricular arrhythmias

Central nervous system: Agitation, convulsion, fever, headache, hyperexcitability, insomnia, irritability, restlessness

Endocrine & metabolic: ADH syndrome, dehydration, hyperglycemia

Gastrointestinal: Diarrhea, epigastric pain, hematemesis, nausea, vomiting

Neuromuscular & skeletal: Muscle twitching

Renal: Albuminuria, diuresis, hematuria

Respiratory: Respiratory arrest, tachypnea

General Dosage Range Dosage adjustment recommended in patients with renal impairment

Oral: *Adults:* Up to 15 mg/kg 4 times/day

Mechanism of Action Causes bronchodilatation, through phosphodiesterase inhibition which increases concentrations of cyclic adenine monophosphate (cAMP) and produces relaxation of bronchial smooth muscle.

Pharmacodynamics/Kinetics

Half-life Elimination ~2 hours

Time to Peak ~45 minutes

Pregnancy Risk Factor C

Ecallantide (e KAL lan tide)

U.S. Brand Names Kalbitor®

Pharmacologic Category Kallikrein Inhibitor

Use Treatment of acute attacks of hereditary angioedema (HAE)

Local Anesthetic/Vasoconstrictor Precautions No information available to require special precautions

Effects on Dental Treatment No significant effects or complications reported

Effects on Bleeding No information available to require special precautions

Adverse Effects

>10%:

Central nervous system: Headache (8% to 16%), fatigue (12%)

Gastrointestinal: Nausea (5% to 13%), diarrhea (4% to 11%)

1% to 10%:

Central nervous system: Fever (4% to 5%)

Dermatologic: Pruritus (5%), rash (3%), urticaria (2%)

Gastrointestinal: Vomiting (6%), upper abdominal pain (5%)

Local: Injection site reactions (3% to 7%; includes bruising, erythema, irritation, pain, pruritus, urticaria)

Respiratory: Upper respiratory infection (8%), nasopharyngitis (3% to 6%)

Miscellaneous: Antibody formation (5% to 7%), anaphylaxis (4%)

General Dosage Range SubQ: *Children ≥16 years and Adults:* 30 mg; may repeat once (maximum: 60 mg/24 hours)

Mechanism of Action Ecallantide is a recombinant protein which inhibits the conversion of high molecular weight kininogen to bradykinin by selectively and reversibly inhibiting plasma kallikrein. Unregulated bradykinin production is thought to contribute to the increased vascular permeability and angioedema observed in HAE.

Pharmacodynamics/Kinetics

Onset of Action 30 minutes to 4 hours

Half-life Elimination 1.5-2.5 hours

Time to Peak ~2-3 hours

Pregnancy Risk Factor C

Echothiophate Iodide (ek oh THYE oh fate EYE oh dide)

U.S. Brand Names Phospholine Iodide®

Pharmacologic Category Acetylcholinesterase Inhibitor; Ophthalmic Agent, Antiglaucoma; Ophthalmic Agent, Miotic

Use Used as miotic in treatment of chronic, open-angle glaucoma; may be useful in specific cases of angle-closure glaucoma (postiridectomy or where surgery refused/contraindicated); postcataract surgery-related glaucoma; accommodative esotropia

Local Anesthetic/Vasoconstrictor Precautions No information available to require special precautions

Effects on Dental Treatment No significant effects or complications reported

Effects on Bleeding No information available to require special precautions

Adverse Effects Frequency not defined.

Cardiovascular: Bradycardia, cardiac irregularities, flushing, hypotension

Gastrointestinal: Diarrhea, nausea, vomiting

Neurologic & skeletal: Muscle weakness

Ocular: Blurred vision, browache, burning eyes, ciliary redness, conjunctival redness/thickening, intraocular pressure increases (paradoxical), iris cysts, lacrimation, lid muscle twitching, miosis, myopia, latent iritis or uveitis activation, lens opacities, retinal detachment, stinging

Respiratory: Dyspnea

Miscellaneous: Diaphoresis, nasolacrimal canal obstruction

General Dosage Range Ophthalmic:

Children: Diagnosis: Instill 1 drop of (0.125%) into both eyes at bedtime for 2-3 weeks; Treatment: Instill 1 drop of 0.06% once daily **or** 0.125% every other day (maximum: 0.125% daily)

Adults: Initial: 1 drop (0.03%) twice daily; Maintenance: 1 dose daily or every other day

Mechanism of Action Long-acting inhibition of cholinesterase enhances activity of endogenous acetylcholine. Reduced degradation of acetylcholine leads to continuous stimulation of the ciliary muscle producing miosis; other effects include potentiation of accommodation and facilitation of aqueous humor outflow, with attendant reduction in intraocular pressure.

Pharmacodynamics/Kinetics

Onset of Action Miosis: 10-30 minutes; Intraocular pressure decrease: 4-8 hours

Peak effect: Intraocular pressure decrease: 24 hours

Duration of Action Miosis: 1-4 weeks

Pregnancy Risk Factor C

Econazole (e KONE a zole)

Pharmacologic Category Antifungal Agent, Topical

Use Topical treatment of tinea pedis (athlete's foot), tinea cruris (jock itch), tinea corporis (ringworm), tinea versicolor, and cutaneous candidiasis

Local Anesthetic/Vasoconstrictor Precautions No information available to require special precautions

Effects on Dental Treatment No significant effects or complications reported

Effects on Bleeding No information available to require special precautions

Adverse Effects 1% to 10%: Dermatologic: Burning (3%), erythema (3%), itching (3%), stinging (3%)

General Dosage Range Topical: *Children and Adults:* Apply sufficient quantity once or twice daily

Mechanism of Action Alters fungal cell wall membrane permeability; may interfere with RNA and protein synthesis, and lipid metabolism

Pregnancy Risk Factor C

Eculizumab (e kue LIZ oo mab)

U.S. Brand Names Soliris®

Canadian Brand Names Soliris®

Pharmacologic Category Monoclonal Antibody; Monoclonal Antibody, Complement Inhibitor

Use Treatment of paroxysmal nocturnal hemoglobinuria (PNH) to reduce hemolysis

Local Anesthetic/Vasoconstrictor Precautions No information available to require special precautions

Effects on Dental Treatment No significant effects or complications reported

Effects on Bleeding Although significant myelosuppression with associated altered hemostasis has been reported for many chemotherapeutic agents, myelosuppression is not common with eculizumab and no specific precautions appear to be necessary.

Adverse Effects

>10%:

- Central nervous system: Headache (44%; serious: 2%; usually occurs within 48 hours of each of the first 2 induction doses), fatigue (12%)
- Gastrointestinal: Nausea (16%), abdominal pain, diarrhea, vomiting
- Genitourinary: Urinary tract infection
- Neuromuscular & skeletal: Back pain (19%), arthralgia
- Respiratory: Nasopharyngitis (23%), cough (12%)

1% to 10%:

- Central nervous system: Fever (serious: 2%)
- Gastrointestinal: Constipation (7%)
- Hematologic: Anemia (serious: 2%)
- Neuromuscular & skeletal: Limb pain (7%), myalgia (7%)
- Respiratory: Respiratory tract infection (7%), sinusitis (7%)
- Miscellaneous: Herpes infections (7%), flu-like syndrome (5%), viral infection (serious: 2%), meningococcal infection (1%)

General Dosage Range I.V.: *Adults:* 600 mg once weekly for 4 weeks, followed by 900 mg 1 week later; Maintenance: 900 mg every 2 weeks

Mechanism of Action Eculizumab is a humanized monoclonal IgG antibody that binds to complement protein C5, preventing cleavage into C5a and C5b. Blocking the formation of C5b inhibits the subsequent formation of terminal complex C5b-9 or membrane attack complex (MAC). Terminal complement-mediated intravascular hemolysis is a key clinical feature of paroxysmal nocturnal hemoglobinuria. Blocking the formation of MAC results in stabilization of hemoglobin and a reduction in the need for RBC transfusions.

Pharmacodynamics/Kinetics
Onset of Action PNH: Reduced hemolysis: ≤1 week
Half-life Elimination ~11 days (range: ~8-15 days)
Pregnancy Risk Factor C
Prescribing and Access Restrictions Patients and providers must enroll with Soliris® OneSource™ (1-888-765-4747) program prior to treatment initiation.

Edetate CALCIUM Disodium (ED e tate KAL see um dye SOW dee um)

U.S. Brand Names Calcium Disodium Versenate®
Pharmacologic Category Chelating Agent
Use Treatment of symptomatic acute and chronic lead poisoning or for symptomatic patients with high blood lead levels
Unlabeled/Investigational Use Possibly useful in poisoning by zinc, manganese, and certain heavy radioisotopes
Local Anesthetic/Vasoconstrictor Precautions No information available to require special precautions
Effects on Dental Treatment No significant effects or complications reported
Effects on Bleeding No information available to require special precautions
Adverse Effects Frequency not defined.
Cardiovascular: Arrhythmia, ECG changes, hypotension
Central nervous system: Chills, fatigue, fever, headache, malaise
Dermatologic: Cheilosis, dermatitis, rash
Endocrine & metabolic: Hypercalcemia
Gastrointestinal: Anorexia, GI upset, nausea, thirst (excessive), vomiting
Hematologic: Anemia, bone marrow suppression (transient)
Hepatic: Alkaline phosphatase decreased, liver function test increased (mild)
Local: Thrombophlebitis (I.V. infusion when concentration >5 mg/mL), pain at injection site (I.M. injection)
Neuromuscular & skeletal: Arthralgia, myalgia, numbness, tremor
Ocular: Lacrimation
Renal: Glucosuria, nephrotoxicity, renal tubular necrosis, microscopic hematuria, proteinuria, urinary frequency/urgency
Respiratory: Nasal congestion, sneezing
Miscellaneous: Iron, magnesium, and/or zinc deficiency (with chronic therapy)
General Dosage Range Dosage adjustment recommended in patients with renal impairment
I.M., I.V.: *Children and Adults:* 1000-1500 mg/m^2/day (25-75 mg/kg/day)
Mechanism of Action Calcium is displaced by divalent and trivalent heavy metals, forming a nonionizing soluble complex that is excreted in urine
Pharmacodynamics/Kinetics
Onset of Action Chelation of lead: I.V.: 1 hour
Half-life Elimination 20-60 minutes
Pregnancy Risk Factor B

Edrophonium (ed roe FOE nee um)

U.S. Brand Names Enlon®
Canadian Brand Names Enlon®; Tensilon®
Pharmacologic Category Acetylcholinesterase Inhibitor; Antidote; Diagnostic Agent
Use Diagnosis of myasthenia gravis; differentiation of cholinergic crises from myasthenia crises; reversal of nondepolarizing neuromuscular blockers
Local Anesthetic/Vasoconstrictor Precautions No information available to require special precautions
Effects on Dental Treatment No significant effects or complications reported
Effects on Bleeding No information available to require special precautions
Adverse Effects Frequency not defined.
Cardiovascular: Arrhythmias (especially bradycardia), AV block, carbon monoxide decreased, cardiac arrest, ECG changes (nonspecific), flushing, hypotension, nodal rhythm, syncope, tachycardia
Central nervous system: Convulsions, dizziness, drowsiness, dysarthria, dysphonia, headache, loss of consciousness
Dermatologic: Skin rash, thrombophlebitis (I.V.), urticaria
Gastrointestinal: Diarrhea, dysphagia, flatulence, hyperperistalsis, nausea, salivation, stomach cramps, vomiting
Genitourinary: Urinary urgency
Neuromuscular & skeletal: Arthralgias, fasciculations, muscle cramps, spasms, weakness

Ocular: Lacrimation, small pupils
Respiratory: Bronchiolar constriction, bronchospasm, dyspnea, bronchial secretions increased, laryngospasm, respiratory arrest, respiratory depression, respiratory muscle paralysis
Miscellaneous: Allergic reactions, anaphylaxis, diaphoresis increased

General Dosage Range

I.M.:

Infants: 0.5-1 mg
Children ≤34 kg: 1 mg
Children >34 kg: 5 mg
Adults: 10 mg, followed by 2 mg if no response

I.V.:

Infants: 0.1 mg, followed by 0.4 mg if no response (maximum total dose: 0.5 mg)
Children ≤34 kg: 0.04 mg/kg as single dose or followed by 0.16 mg/kg if no response **or** 1 mg, followed by 1mg every 30-45 seconds if no response (maximum total dose: 5 mg)
Children >34 kg: 0.04 mg/kg as single dose or followed by 0.16 mg/kg if no response **or** 2 mg, followed by 1 mg every 30-45 seconds if no response (maximum total dose: 10 mg)
Adults: 2 mg test dose, followed by 8 mg if no response **or** 1-10 mg as a single dose **or** 10 mg every 5-10 minutes up to 40 mg **or** 1 mg; may repeat after 1 minute

Mechanism of Action Inhibits destruction of acetylcholine by acetylcholinesterase. This facilitates transmission of impulses across myoneural junction and results in increased cholinergic responses such as miosis, increased tonus of intestinal and skeletal muscles, bronchial and ureteral constriction, bradycardia, and increased salivary and sweat gland secretions.

Pharmacodynamics/Kinetics

Onset of Action I.M.: 2-10 minutes; I.V.: 30-60 seconds
Duration of Action I.M.: 5-30 minutes: I.V.: 10 minutes
Half-life Elimination Adults: 1.2-2.4 hours; Anephric patients: 2.4-4.4 hours

Pregnancy Risk Factor C

Edrophonium and Atropine (ed roe FOE nee um & A troe peen)

Related Information

Atropine *on page* 188
Edrophonium *on page* 589

U.S. Brand Names Enlon-Plus®

Pharmacologic Category Acetylcholinesterase Inhibitor; Anticholinergic Agent; Antidote

Use Reversal of nondepolarizing neuromuscular blockers; adjunct treatment of respiratory depression caused by curare overdose

Local Anesthetic/Vasoconstrictor Precautions Bradyarrhythmias, tachycardia, and premature ventricular contractions have been reported; use vasoconstrictor with caution

Effects on Dental Treatment No significant effects or complications reported

Effects on Bleeding No information available to require special precautions

Adverse Effects See individual agents.

General Dosage Range I.V.: *Adults:* 0.05-0.1 mL/kg (0.5-1 mg/kg of edrophonium and 0.007-0.014 mg/kg of atropine)

Mechanism of Action

Edrophonium: Inhibits destruction of acetylcholine by acetylcholinesterase. This facilitates transmission of impulses across myoneural junction and results in increased cholinergic response.

Atropine: Minimizes or prevents the muscarinic cholinergic effects caused by edrophonium (eg, bradycardia, bronchocontriction, and increased secretions).

Pharmacodynamics/Kinetics

Onset of Action Edrophonium: Antagonism of nondepolarizing muscle relaxants: 3 minutes; Atropine: Heart rate: Immediate
Duration of Action Edrophonium: Antagonism of nondepolarizing muscle relaxants: 70 minutes; Atropine: Heart rate: 170 minutes
Half-life Elimination Edrophonium: Adults: 1.2-2.4 hours; Anephric patients: 2.4-4.4 hours
Time to Peak Edrophonium: Antagonism of nondepolarizing muscle relaxants: 1.2 minutes; Atropine: Heart rate: 2-16 minutes

Pregnancy Risk Factor C

Efavirenz (e FAV e renz)

Related Information

HIV Infection and AIDS *on page 1883*

U.S. Brand Names Sustiva®

Canadian Brand Names Sustiva®

Pharmacologic Category Antiretroviral Agent, Reverse Transcriptase Inhibitor (Non-nucleoside)

Use Treatment of HIV-1 infections in combination with at least two other antiretroviral agents

Local Anesthetic/Vasoconstrictor Precautions No information available to require special precautions

Effects on Dental Treatment Key adverse event(s) related to dental treatment: Abnormal taste

Effects on Bleeding No information available to require special precautions related to hemostasis.

Adverse Effects Unless otherwise noted, frequency of adverse events is as reported in adults receiving combination antiretroviral therapy.

>10%:

Central nervous system: Dizziness (2% to 28%; children 16%), fever (children 21%), depression (up to 19%; severe: 1% to 2%), insomnia (up to 16%), anxiety (2% to 13%), pain (1% to 13%; children 14%), headache (2% to 8%; children 11%)

Dermatologic: Rash (5% to 26%, grade 3/4: <1%; children up to 46%, grade 3/4: 2% to 4%)

Endocrine & metabolic: HDL increased (25% to 35%), total cholesterol increased (20% to 40%), triglycerides increased (≥751 mg/dL: 6% to 11%)

Gastrointestinal: Diarrhea (3% to 14%; children: up to 39%), nausea (2% to 12%; children 12%), vomiting (3% to 6%; children 12%)

Respiratory: Cough (children 16%)

1% to 10%:

Central nervous system: Impaired concentration (up to 8%), somnolence (up to 7%), fatigue (up to 8%), abnormal dreams (1% to 6%), nervousness (2% to 7%), hallucinations (1%)

Dermatologic: Pruritus (up to 9%)

Endocrine & metabolic: Hyperglycemia (>250 mg/dL: 2% to 5%)

Gastrointestinal: Dyspepsia (up to 4%), abdominal pain (2% to 3%), anorexia (up to 2%), amylase increased (grade 3/4: up to 6%)

Hematologic: Neutropenia (grade 3/4: 2% to 10%)

Hepatic: Transaminases increased (grade 3/4: 2% to 8%, incidence higher with hepatitis B and/or C coinfection)

General Dosage Range Dosage adjustment recommended in patients on concomitant therapy

Oral:

Children ≥3 years and 10 kg to <15 kg: 200 mg once daily
Children ≥3 years and 15 kg to <20 kg: 250 mg once daily
Children ≥3 years and 20 kg to <25 kg: 300 mg once daily
Children ≥3 years and 25 kg to <32.5 kg: 350 mg once daily
Children ≥3 years and 32.5 kg to <40 kg: 400 mg once daily
Children ≥3 years and ≥40 kg and Adults: 600 mg once daily

Mechanism of Action As a non-nucleoside reverse transcriptase inhibitor, efavirenz has activity against HIV-1 by binding to reverse transcriptase. It consequently blocks the RNA-dependent and DNA-dependent DNA polymerase activities including HIV-1 replication. It does not require intracellular phosphorylation for antiviral activity.

Pharmacodynamics/Kinetics

Half-life Elimination Single dose: 52-76 hours; Multiple doses: 40-55 hours

Time to Peak 3-5 hours

Pregnancy Risk Factor D

Prescribing and Access Restrictions Efavirenz oral solution is available only through an expanded access (compassionate use) program. Enrollment information may be obtained by calling 877-372-7097.

Efavirenz, Emtricitabine, and Tenofovir

(e FAV e renz, em trye SYE ta been, & te NOE fo veer)

Related Information

Efavirenz *on page 591*
Emtricitabine *on page 595*
HIV Infection and AIDS *on page 1883*
Tenofovir *on page 1600*

U.S. Brand Names Atripla®

Canadian Brand Names Atripla®

Pharmacologic Category Antiretroviral Agent, Reverse Transcriptase Inhibitor (Non-nucleoside); Antiretroviral Agent, Reverse Transcriptase Inhibitor (Nucleoside); Antiretroviral Agent, Reverse Transcriptase Inhibitor (Nucleotide)

Use Treatment of HIV infection

Local Anesthetic/Vasoconstrictor Precautions No information available to require special precautions

Effects on Dental Treatment Key adverse event(s) related to dental treatment: Efavirenz alone has caused xerostomia (normal salivary flow resumes upon discontinuation) and abnormal taste (see individual monographs). No significant effects or complications reported with combination drug.

Effects on Bleeding No information available to require special precautions related to hemostasis.

Adverse Effects The complete adverse reaction profile of combination therapy has not been established. **See individual agents.** The following adverse effects were noted in clinical trials with combination therapy:

>10%: Endocrine & metabolic: Hypercholesterolemia (22%)

1% to 10%:

Central nervous system: Depression (9%), fatigue (9%), dizziness (8%), headache (6%), anxiety (5%), insomnia (5%), somnolence (4%), abnormal dreams

Dermatologic: Rash (7%)

Endocrine & metabolic: Triglycerides increased (4%), hyperglycemia (2%)

Gastrointestinal: Nausea (9%), diarrhea (9%), serum amylase increased (8%), vomiting (2%)

Hematologic: Neutropenia (3%)

Hepatic: AST increased (3%), ALT increased (2%), alkaline phosphatase increased (1%)

Neuromuscular & skeletal: Creatine increased (9%)

Renal: Hematuria (3%)

Respiratory: Sinusitis (8%), upper respiratory infection (8%), nasopharyngitis (5%)

General Dosage Range Oral: *Adults:* 1 tablet (efavirenz 600 mg/emtricitabine 200 mg/tenofovir 300 mg) once daily

Mechanism of Action See individual agents.

Pregnancy Risk Factor D

Eflornithine (ee FLOR ni theen)

U.S. Brand Names Vaniqa®

Canadian Brand Names Vaniqa®

Pharmacologic Category Antiprotozoal; Topical Skin Product

Use Cream: Females ≥12 years: Reduce unwanted hair from face and adjacent areas under the chin

Orphan status: Injection: Treatment of meningoencephalitic stage of *Trypanosoma brucei gambiense* infection (sleeping sickness)

Local Anesthetic/Vasoconstrictor Precautions No information available to require special precautions

Effects on Dental Treatment No significant effects or complications reported

Effects on Bleeding No information available to require special precautions

Adverse Effects

Injection:

>10%: Hematologic (reversible): Anemia (55%), leukopenia (37%), thrombocytopenia (14%)

1% to 10%:

Central nervous system: Seizure (may be due to the disease) (8%), dizziness

Dermatologic: Alopecia

Gastrointestinal: Vomiting, diarrhea

Hematologic: Eosinophilia

Otic: Hearing impairment

Topical:
>10%: Dermatologic: Acne (11% to 21%), pseudofolliculitis barbae (5% to 15%)
1% to 10%:
Central nervous system: Headache (4% to 5%), dizziness (1%), vertigo (0.3% to 1%)
Dermatologic: Pruritus (3% to 4%), burning skin (2% to 4%), tingling skin (1% to 4%), dry skin (2% to 3%), rash (1% to 3%), facial edema (0.3% to 3%), alopecia (1% to 2%), skin irritation (1% to 2%), erythema (0% to 2%), ingrown hair (0.3% to 2%), folliculitis (0% to 1%)
Gastrointestinal: Dyspepsia (2%), anorexia (0.7% to 2%)

General Dosage Range Dosage adjustment recommended in patients with renal impairment
I.V.: *Adults:* 100 mg/kg/dose every 6 hours
Topical: *Children and Adults:* Apply thin layer to affected areas twice daily

Mechanism of Action Eflornithine exerts antitumor and antiprotozoal effects through specific, irreversible ("suicide") inhibition of the enzyme ornithine decarboxylase (ODC). ODC is the rate-limiting enzyme in the biosynthesis of putrescine, spermine, and spermidine, the major polyamines in nucleated cells. Polyamines are necessary for the synthesis of DNA, RNA, and proteins and are, therefore, necessary for cell growth and differentiation. Although many microorganisms and higher plants are able to produce polyamines from alternate biochemical pathways, all mammalian cells depend on ornithine decarboxylase to produce polyamines. Eflornithine inhibits ODC and rapidly depletes animal cells of putrescine and spermidine; the concentration of spermine remains the same or may even increase. Rapidly dividing cells appear to be most susceptible to the effects of eflornithine. Topically, the inhibition of ODC in the skin leads to a decreased rate of hair growth.

Pharmacodynamics/Kinetics
Half-life Elimination I.V.: 3-3.5 hours; Topical: 8 hours

Pregnancy Risk Factor C

Eletriptan (el e TRIP tan)

Related Information
Temporomandibular Dysfunction (TMD) *on page* 1964

U.S. Brand Names Relpax®

Canadian Brand Names Relpax®

Pharmacologic Category Antimigraine Agent; Serotonin 5-$HT_{1B, 1D}$ Receptor Agonist

Use Acute treatment of migraine, with or without aura

Local Anesthetic/Vasoconstrictor Precautions No information available to require special precautions

Effects on Dental Treatment Key adverse event(s) related to dental treatment: Xerostomia (normal salivary flow resumes upon discontinuation)

Effects on Bleeding No information available to require special precautions

Adverse Effects 1% to 10%:
Cardiovascular: Chest pain/tightness (1% to 4%; placebo 1%), palpitation
Central nervous system: Dizziness (3% to 7%; placebo 3%), somnolence (3% to 7%; placebo 4%), headache (3% to 4%; placebo 3%), chills, pain, vertigo
Gastrointestinal: Nausea (4% to 8%; placebo 5%), xerostomia (2% to 4%, placebo 2%), dysphagia (1% to 2%), abdominal pain/discomfort (1% to 2%; placebo 1%), dyspepsia (1% to 2%; placebo 1%)
Neuromuscular & skeletal: Weakness (4% to 10%), paresthesia (3% to 4%), back pain, hypertonia, hypoesthesia
Respiratory: Pharyngitis
Miscellaneous: Diaphoresis

General Dosage Range Oral: *Adults:* 20-40 mg as a single dose, may repeat (maximum: 80 mg/day)

Mechanism of Action Selective agonist for serotonin (5-HT_{1B} and 5-HT_{1D} receptors) in cranial arteries; causes vasoconstriction and reduces sterile inflammation associated with antidromic neuronal transmission correlating with relief of migraine

Pharmacodynamics/Kinetics
Half-life Elimination ~4 hours (Elderly: 4.4-5.7 hours); Metabolite: ~13 hours
Time to Peak Plasma: 1.5-2 hours

Pregnancy Risk Factor C

Eltrombopag (el TROM boe pag)

U.S. Brand Names Promacta®

Canadian Brand Names Revolade™

Pharmacologic Category Colony Stimulating Factor; Thrombopoietic Agent

Use Treatment of thrombocytopenia in patients with chronic immune (idiopathic) thrombocytopenic purpura (ITP) at risk for bleeding who have had insufficient response to corticosteroids, immune globulin, or splenectomy

Local Anesthetic/Vasoconstrictor Precautions No information available to require special precautions

Effects on Dental Treatment Key adverse event(s) related to dental treatment: Risk of bleeding in soft tissues upon discontinuation of therapy due to rebound thrombocytopenia; monitor for at least 4 weeks after discontinuation of treatment.

Effects on Bleeding Eltrombopag is used in the management of severe thrombocytopenia. Thromboembolism may occur with excess increases in platelet levels during therapy. Risk of bleeding is increased with discontinuation of therapy due to rebound thrombocytopenia.

Medical consultation is warranted. Treatment of bleeding disorders depends on many factors, including severity of disease and risks of bleeding. General dental procedures and simple restorative procedures are not associated with bleeding; therefore, there is generally no contraindication to general dental treatment for most patients with bleeding disorders. Surgical dental procedures are also possible for hemophiliacs and other bleeding disorders, but a carefully coordinated strategy between the dental and medical team may be required to ensure adequate hemostasis. Examples of procedures which require advance consultation include block anesthesia, deep scaling, extractions, large fillings, and any oral surgery.

Adverse Effects

>10%: Hepatic: Liver function tests abnormal (11%)

1% to 10%:

- Central nervous system: Headache (10%), fatigue (4%)
- Dermatologic: Rash (3%), alopecia (2%)
- Gastrointestinal: Diarrhea (9%), nausea (4% to 9%), vomiting (6%), xerostomia (2%)
- Genitourinary: Urinary tract infection (5%)
- Hematologic: Myelofibrosis (Extension study: Grade ≤1: 93%; grade 2: 7%), rebound thrombocytopenia (8%)
- Hepatic: Hyperbilirubinemia (6%), ALT increased (5% to 6%), AST increased (4%), alkaline phosphatase increased (2%)
- Neuromuscular & skeletal: Myalgia (5%), back pain (3%), paresthesia (3%)
- Ocular: Cataract (4% to 7%)
- Respiratory: Upper respiratory infection (7%), oropharyngeal pain (4%), pharyngitis (4%)
- Miscellaneous: Influenza (3%)

General Dosage Range Dosage adjustment recommended in patients with hepatic impairment, of East-Asian ethnicity, or who develop toxicities

Oral: *Adults:* 50 mg once daily (maximum: 75 mg/day)

Mechanism of Action Thrombopoietin (TPO) nonpeptide agonist which increases platelet counts by binding to and activating the human TPO receptor. Activates intracellular signal transduction pathways to increase proliferation and differentiation of marrow progenitor cells. Does not induce platelet aggregation or activation.

Pharmacodynamics/Kinetics

Onset of Action Platelet count increase: Within 1-2 weeks; Peak platelet count increase: 14-16 days

Duration of Action Platelets return to baseline: 1-2 weeks after last dose

Half-life Elimination

~21-32 hours in healthy individuals; ~26-35 hours in patients with ITP

Time to Peak 2-6 hours

Pregnancy Risk Factor C

Prescribing and Access Restrictions As a requirement of the REMS program, access to this medication is restricted. Eltrombopag is approved for marketing under a Food and Drug Administration (FDA) approved, risk management, and restricted distribution program called Promacta® Cares™ (1-877-977-6622). Patients, prescribers, and pharmacies must be enrolled in the program.

Emedastine (em e DAS teen)

U.S. Brand Names Emadine®

Pharmacologic Category Histamine H_1 Antagonist; Histamine H_1 Antagonist, Second Generation

Use Treatment of allergic conjunctivitis

Local Anesthetic/Vasoconstrictor Precautions No information available to require special precautions

Effects on Dental Treatment No significant effects or complications reported

Effects on Bleeding No information available to require special precautions

Adverse Effects
>10%: Central nervous system: Headache (11%)
1% to 10%:
Cardiovascular: Hyperemia
Central nervous system: Abnormal dreams
Dermatologic: Dermatitis, keratitis, pruritus
Gastrointestinal: Taste (unpleasant)
Neuromuscular & skeletal: Weakness
Ocular: Blurred vision, corneal infiltrates, corneal staining, dry eyes, transient burning or stinging
Respiratory: Rhinitis, sinusitis
Miscellaneous: Tearing

General Dosage Range Ophthalmic: *Children ≥3 years and Adults:* Instill 1 drop in affected eye up to 4 times/day

Mechanism of Action Selective histamine H_1-receptor antagonist for topical ophthalmic use

Pharmacodynamics/Kinetics
Half-life Elimination Oral: Plasma: 3-4 hours

Pregnancy Risk Factor B

Emtricitabine (em trye SYE ta been)

Related Information
HIV Infection and AIDS *on page 1883*

U.S. Brand Names Emtriva®

Canadian Brand Names Emtriva®

Pharmacologic Category Antiretroviral Agent, Reverse Transcriptase Inhibitor (Nucleoside)

Use Treatment of HIV infection in combination with at least two other antiretroviral agents

Local Anesthetic/Vasoconstrictor Precautions No information available to require special precautions

Effects on Dental Treatment No significant effects or complications reported

Effects on Bleeding No information available to require special precautions related to hemostasis.

Adverse Effects Clinical trials were conducted in patients receiving other antiretroviral agents, and it is not possible to correlate frequency of adverse events with emtricitabine alone. The range of frequencies of adverse events is generally comparable to comparator groups, with the exception of hyperpigmentation, which occurred more frequently in patients receiving emtricitabine. Unless otherwise noted, percentages are as reported in adults.

>10%:
Central nervous system: Dizziness (4% to 25%), headache (6% to 22%), fever (children 18%), insomnia (5% to 16%), abnormal dreams (2% to 11%)
Dermatologic: Hyperpigmentation (children 32%; adults 2% to 4%; primarily of palms and/or soles but may include tongue, arms, lip and nails; generally mild and nonprogressive without associated local reactions such as pruritus or rash); rash (17% to 30%; includes pruritus, maculopapular rash, vesiculobullous rash, pustular rash, and allergic reaction)
Gastrointestinal: Diarrhea (children 20%; adults 9% to 23%), vomiting (children 23%; adults 9%), nausea (13% to 18%), abdominal pain (8% to 14%), gastroenteritis (children 11%)
Neuromuscular & skeletal: Weakness (12% to 16%), CPK increased (grades 3/4: 11% to 12%)
Otic: Otitis media (children 23%)
Respiratory: Cough (children 28%; adults 14%), rhinitis (children 20%; adults 12% to 18%), pneumonia (children 15%)
Miscellaneous: Infection (children 44%)
1% to 10%:
Central nervous system: Depression (6% to 9%), neuropathy/neuritis (4%)
Endocrine & metabolic: Serum triglycerides increased (grades 3/4: 4% to 10%), disordered glucose homeostasis (grades 3/4: 2% to 3%), serum amylase increased (grades 3/4: children 9%; adults 2% to 5%), serum lipase increased (grades 3/4: ≤1%)
Gastrointestinal: Dyspepsia (4% to 8%), serum amylase increased (grades 3/4: 8%)
Genitourinary: Hematuria (grades 3/4: 3%)
Hematologic: Anemia (children: 7%), neutropenia (grades 3/4: children 2%; adults 5%)

Hepatic: Transaminases increased (grades 3/4: 2% to 6%), alkaline phosphatase increased (>550 units/L: 1%), bilirubin increased (grades 3/4: 1%)
Neuromuscular & skeletal: Creatinine kinase increased (grades 3/4: 9%), myalgia (4% to 6%), paresthesia (5% to 6%), arthralgia (3% to 5%)
Respiratory: Upper respiratory tract infection (8%), sinusitis (8%), pharyngitis (5%)

General Dosage Range Dosage adjustment recommended in patients with renal impairment

Oral:

Capsule: *Children 3 months to 17 years and >33 kg and Adults:* 200 mg once daily
Solution:
Children <3 months: 3 mg/kg/day
Children 3 months to 17 years: 6 mg/kg once daily (maximum: 240 mg/day)
Adults: 240 mg once daily

Mechanism of Action Nucleoside reverse transcriptase inhibitor; emtricitabine is a cytosine analogue which is phosphorylated intracellularly to emtricitabine 5'-triphosphate which interferes with HIV viral RNA dependent DNA polymerase resulting in inhibition of viral replication.

Pharmacodynamics/Kinetics

Half-life Elimination Normal renal function: Adults: 10 hours; children: 5-18 hours

Time to Peak Plasma: 1-2 hours

Pregnancy Risk Factor B

Emtricitabine and Tenofovir (em trye SYE ta been & te NOE fo veer)

Related Information

Emtricitabine *on page* 595
HIV Infection and AIDS *on page* 1883
Tenofovir *on page* 1600

U.S. Brand Names Truvada®

Canadian Brand Names Truvada®

Pharmacologic Category Antiretroviral Agent, Reverse Transcriptase Inhibitor (Nucleoside); Antiretroviral Agent, Reverse Transcriptase Inhibitor (Nucleotide)

Use Treatment of HIV infection in combination with other antiretroviral agents

Unlabeled/Investigational Use Treatment of hepatitis B in patients with antiviral-resistant HBV or coinfection with HIV; pre-exposure prophylaxis (PrEP) for prevention of HIV infection in men who have sex with men who are at high risk for acquiring HIV

Local Anesthetic/Vasoconstrictor Precautions No information available to require special precautions

Effects on Dental Treatment No significant effects or complications reported

Effects on Bleeding No information available to require special precautions related to hemostasis.

Adverse Effects The adverse reaction profile of combination therapy has not been established. See individual agents.

General Dosage Range Dosage adjustment recommended in patients with renal impairment

Oral: *Adults:* 1 tablet (emtricitabine 200 mg and tenofovir 300 mg) once daily

Mechanism of Action Nucleoside and nucleotide reverse transcriptase inhibitor combination; emtricitabine is a cytosine analogue while tenofovir disoproxil fumarate (TDF) is an analog of adenosine 5'-monophosphate. Each drug interferes with HIV viral RNA dependent DNA polymerase resulting in inhibition of viral replication.

Pregnancy Risk Factor B

Enalapril (e NAL a pril)

Related Information

Cardiovascular Diseases *on page* 1848

U.S. Brand Names Vasotec®

Canadian Brand Names Apo-Enalapril®; CO Enalapril; Mylan-Enalapril; Novo-Enalapril; PMS-Enalapril; PRO-Enalapril; RAN™-Enalapril; ratio-Enalapril; Riva-Enalapril; Sandoz-Enalapril; Sig-Enalapril; Taro-Enalapril; Vasotec®; Vasotec® I.V.

Generic Availability (U.S.) Yes

Pharmacologic Category Angiotensin-Converting Enzyme (ACE) Inhibitor

Use Treatment of hypertension; treatment of symptomatic heart failure; treatment of asymptomatic left ventricular dysfunction

Unlabeled/Investigational Use

Unlabeled: To delay the progression of nephropathy and reduce risks of cardiovascular events in hypertensive patients with type 1 or 2 diabetes mellitus; hypertensive crisis, diabetic nephropathy, hypertension secondary to scleroderma renal crisis, diagnosis of aldosteronism, idiopathic edema, Bartter's syndrome, postmyocardial infarction for prevention of ventricular failure

Investigational: Severe congestive heart failure in infants, neonatal hypertension, acute cardiogenic pulmonary edema (enalaprilat)

Local Anesthetic/Vasoconstrictor Precautions No information available to require special precautions

Effects on Dental Treatment Key adverse event(s) related to dental treatment: Abnormal taste and orthostatic hypotension

Effects on Bleeding No information available to require special precautions

Adverse Effects Note: Frequency ranges include data from hypertension and heart failure trials. Higher rates of adverse reactions have generally been noted in patients with CHF. However, the frequency of adverse effects associated with placebo is also increased in this population.

1% to 10%:

Cardiovascular: Hypotension (0.9% to 7%), chest pain (2%), syncope (0.5% to 2%), orthostasis (2%), orthostatic hypotension (2%)

Central nervous system: Headache (2% to 5%), dizziness (4% to 8%), fatigue (2% to 3%)

Dermatologic: Rash (2%)

Gastrointestinal: Abnormal taste, abdominal pain, vomiting, nausea, diarrhea, anorexia, constipation

Neuromuscular & skeletal: Weakness

Renal: Serum creatinine increased (0.2% to 20%), worsening of renal function (in patients with bilateral renal artery stenosis or hypovolemia)

Respiratory (1% to 2%): Bronchitis, cough, dyspnea

Dosage Use lower listed initial dose in patients with hyponatremia, hypovolemia, severe congestive heart failure, decreased renal function, or in those receiving diuretics.

Oral: **Enalapril**: Children 1 month to 17 years: Hypertension: Initial: 0.08 mg/kg/day (up to 5 mg) in 1-2 divided doses; adjust dosage based on patient response; doses >0.58 mg/kg (40 mg) have not been evaluated in pediatric patients

Investigational: Congestive heart failure: Initial oral doses of **enalapril**: 0.1 mg/kg/day increasing as needed over 2 weeks to 0.5 mg/kg/day have been used in infants

Investigational: Neonatal hypertension: I.V. doses of **enalaprilat**: 5-10 mcg/kg/dose administered every 8-24 hours have been used; monitor patients carefully; select patients may require higher doses

Adults:

Oral: **Enalapril:**

Asymptomatic left ventricular dysfunction: 2.5 mg twice daily, titrated as tolerated to 20 mg/day

Heart failure: Initial: 2.5 mg once or twice daily (usual range: 5-40 mg/day in 2 divided doses); titrate slowly at 1- to 2-week intervals. Target dose: 10-20 mg twice daily (ACC/AHA 2009 Heart Failure Guidelines)

Hypertension: 2.5-5 mg/day then increase as required, usually at 1- to 2-week intervals; usual dose range (JNC 7): 2.5-40 mg/day in 1-2 divided doses. **Note:** Initiate with 2.5 mg if patient is taking a diuretic which cannot be discontinued. May add a diuretic if blood pressure cannot be controlled with enalapril alone.

I.V.: **Enalaprilat:**

Heart failure: Avoid I.V. administration in patients with unstable heart failure or those suffering acute myocardial infarction.

Hypertension: 1.25 mg/dose, given over 5 minutes every 6 hours; doses as high as 5 mg/dose every 6 hours have been tolerated for up to 36 hours. **Note:** If patients are concomitantly receiving diuretic therapy, begin with 0.625 mg I.V. over 5 minutes; if the effect is not adequate after 1 hour, repeat the dose and administer 1.25 mg at 6-hour intervals thereafter; if adequate, administer 0.625 mg I.V. every 6 hours.

Conversion from I.V. to oral therapy if not concurrently on diuretics: 5 mg once daily; subsequent titration as needed; if concurrently receiving diuretics and responding to 0.625 mg I.V. every 6 hours, initiate with 2.5 mg/day.

Dosing adjustment in renal impairment:

Oral: Enalapril:

Cl_{cr} 30-80 mL/minute: Administer 5 mg/day titrated upwards to maximum of 40 mg.

Cl_{cr} <30 mL/minute: Administer 2.5 mg day; titrated upward until blood pressure is controlled.

For heart failure patients with sodium <130 mEq/L or serum creatinine >1.6 mg/dL, initiate dosage with 2.5 mg/day, increasing to twice daily as needed. Increase further in increments of 2.5 mg/dose at >4-day intervals to a maximum daily dose of 40 mg.

I.V.: Enalaprilat:

Cl_{cr} >30 mL/minute: Initiate with 1.25 mg every 6 hours and increase dose based on response.

Cl_{cr} <30 mL/minute: Initiate with 0.625 mg every 6 hours and increase dose based on response.

Hemodialysis: Moderately dialyzable (20% to 50%); administer dose postdialysis (eg, 0.625 mg I.V. every 6 hours) or administer 20% to 25% supplemental dose following dialysis; Clearance: 62 mL/minute.

Peritoneal dialysis: Supplemental dose is not necessary, although some removal of drug occurs.

Dosing adjustment in hepatic impairment: Hydrolysis of enalapril to enalaprilat may be delayed and/or impaired in patients with severe hepatic impairment, but the pharmacodynamic effects of the drug do not appear to be significantly altered; no dosage adjustment.

Mechanism of Action Competitive inhibitor of angiotensin-converting enzyme (ACE); prevents conversion of angiotensin I to angiotensin II, a potent vasoconstrictor; results in lower levels of angiotensin II which causes an increase in plasma renin activity and a reduction in aldosterone secretion

Contraindications Hypersensitivity to enalapril or enalaprilat; angioedema related to previous treatment with an ACE inhibitor; patients with idiopathic or hereditary angioedema

Warnings/Precautions Anaphylactic reactions may occur rarely with ACE inhibitors. At any time during treatment (especially following first dose) angioedema may occur rarely with ACE inhibitors; it may involve the head and neck (potentially compromising airway) or the intestine (presenting with abdominal pain). African-Americans may be at an increased risk. Prolonged frequent monitoring may be required especially if tongue, glottis, or larynx are involved as they are associated with airway obstruction. Patients with a history of airway surgery may have a higher risk of airway obstruction. Aggressive early and appropriate management is critical. Use in patients with idiopathic or hereditary angioedema or previous angioedema associated with ACE inhibitor therapy is contraindicated. Severe anaphylactoid reactions may be seen during hemodialysis (eg, CVVHD) with high-flux dialysis membranes (eg, AN69), and rarely, during low density lipoprotein apheresis with dextran sulfate cellulose. Rare cases of anaphylactoid reactions have been reported in patients undergoing sensitization treatment with hymenoptera (bee, wasp) venom while receiving ACE inhibitors.

Symptomatic hypotension with or without syncope can occur with ACE inhibitors (usually with the first several doses); effects are most often observed in volume depleted patients; correct volume depletion prior to initiation; close monitoring of patient is required especially with initial dosing and dosing increases; blood pressure must be lowered at a rate appropriate for the patient's clinical condition. Initiation of therapy in patients with ischemic heart disease or cerebrovascular disease warrants close observation due to the potential consequences posed by falling blood pressure (eg, MI, stroke). Use with caution in hypertrophic cardiomyopathy with outflow tract obstruction, severe aortic stenosis, or before, during, or immediately after major surgery. **[U.S. Boxed Warning]: Based on human data, ACEIs can cause injury and death to the developing fetus when used in the second and third trimesters. ACEIs should be discontinued as soon as possible once pregnancy is detected.** Injection contains benzyl alcohol which has been associated with "gasping syndrome" in neonates.

Hyperkalemia may occur with ACE inhibitors; risk factors include renal dysfunction, diabetes mellitus, concomitant use of potassium-sparing diuretics, potassium supplements, and/or potassium-containing salts. Use cautiously, if at all, with these agents and monitor potassium closely. Cough may occur with ACE inhibitors. Other causes of cough should be considered (eg, pulmonary congestion in patients with heart failure) and excluded prior to discontinuation.

May be associated with deterioration of renal function and/or increases in serum creatinine, particularly in patients with low renal blood flow (eg, renal artery stenosis, heart failure) whose glomerular filtration rate (GFR) is dependent on efferent arteriolar vasoconstriction by angiotensin II; deterioration may result in oliguria, acute renal failure, and progressive azotemia. Small increases in serum creatinine may occur following initiation; consider discontinuation only in patients with progressive and/or significant deterioration in renal function. Use with caution in patients with unstented unilateral/bilateral renal artery stenosis. When unstented bilateral renal artery stenosis is present, use is generally avoided due to the elevated risk of deterioration in renal function unless possible benefits outweigh risks. Concurrent use of angiotensin receptor blockers may increase the risk of clinically-significant adverse events (eg, renal dysfunction, hyperkalemia).

Rare toxicities associated with ACE inhibitors include cholestatic jaundice (which may progress to fulminant hepatic necrosis), agranulocytosis, neutropenia or leukopenia with myeloid hypoplasia. Patients with collagen vascular diseases (especially with concomitant renal impairment) or renal impairment alone may be at increased risk for hematologic toxicity; periodically monitor CBC with differential in these patients.

Drug Interactions

Metabolism/Transport Effects Substrate of CYP3A4 (minor)

Avoid Concomitant Use There are no known interactions where it is recommended to avoid concomitant use.

Increased Effect/Toxicity

Enalapril may increase the levels/effects of: Allopurinol; Amifostine; Antihypertensives; AzaTHIOprine; CycloSPORINE; CycloSPORINE (Systemic); Ferric Gluconate; Gold Sodium Thiomalate; Hypotensive Agents; Iron Dextran Complex; Lithium; Nonsteroidal Anti-Inflammatory Agents; RiTUXimab

The levels/effects of Enalapril may be increased by: Angiotensin II Receptor Blockers; Conivaptan; Diazoxide; DPP-IV Inhibitors; Eplerenone; Everolimus; Herbs (Hypotensive Properties); Loop Diuretics; MAO Inhibitors; Pentoxifylline; Phosphodiesterase 5 Inhibitors; Potassium Salts; Potassium-Sparing Diuretics; Prostacyclin Analogues; Sirolimus; Temsirolimus; Thiazide Diuretics; TiZANidine; Tolvaptan; Trimethoprim

Decreased Effect

The levels/effects of Enalapril may be decreased by: Antacids; Aprotinin; CYP3A4 Inducers (Strong); Deferasirox; Herbs (CYP3A4 Inducers); Herbs (Hypertensive Properties); Methylphenidate; Nonsteroidal Anti-Inflammatory Agents; Salicylates; Tocilizumab; Yohimbine

Ethanol/Nutrition/Herb Interactions Herb/Nutraceutical: Avoid bayberry, blue cohosh, cayenne, ephedra, ginger, ginseng (American), kola, licorice (may worsen hypertension). Avoid black cohosh, california poppy, coleus, golden seal, hawthorn, mistletoe, periwinkle, quinine, shepherd's purse (may have increased antihypertensive effect).

Dietary Considerations Limit salt substitutes or potassium-rich diet.

Pharmacodynamics/Kinetics

Onset of Action Oral: ~1 hour, I.V.: ≤15 minutes; Peak effect: Oral: 4-6 hours, I.V.: 1-4 hours

Duration of Action Oral: 12-24 hours; I.V.: ~6 hours

Half-life Elimination

Enalapril: Adults: Healthy: 2 hours; Congestive heart failure: 3.4-5.8 hours
Enalaprilat: Infants 6 weeks to 8 months of age: 6-10 hours; Adults: 35-38 hours

Time to Peak Serum: Oral: Enalapril: 0.5-1.5 hours; Enalaprilat (active): 3-4.5 hours

Pregnancy Risk Factor C (1st trimester); D (2nd and 3rd trimesters)

Lactation Enters breast milk/not recommended (AAP rates "compatible"; AAP 2001 update pending)

Breast-Feeding Considerations Enalapril and enalaprilat are excreted in breast milk. Breast-feeding is not recommended by the manufacturer.

Dosage Forms

Injection, solution: 1.25 mg/mL (1 mL, 2 mL)
Tablet, oral: 2.5 mg, 5 mg, 10 mg, 20 mg
Vasotec®: 2.5 mg, 5 mg, 10 mg, 20 mg

Enalapril and Felodipine (e NAL a pril & fe LOE di peen)

Related Information

Enalapril *on page* 596
Felodipine *on page* 710

U.S. Brand Names Lexxel® [DSC]

Canadian Brand Names Lexxel®

Pharmacologic Category Angiotensin-Converting Enzyme (ACE) Inhibitor; Calcium Channel Blocker; Calcium Channel Blocker, Dihydropyridine

Use Treatment of hypertension, however, not indicated for initial treatment of hypertension; replacement therapy in patients receiving separate dosage forms (for patient convenience); when monotherapy with one component fails to achieve desired antihypertensive effect, or when dose-limiting adverse effects limit upward titration of monotherapy

Local Anesthetic/Vasoconstrictor Precautions No information available to require special precautions

Effects on Dental Treatment Key adverse event(s) related to dental treatment: Gingival hyperplasia (fewer reports with felodipine than with other CCBs); resolves upon discontinuation (consultation with physician is suggested).

Effects on Bleeding No information available to require special precautions

Adverse Effects See individual agents.

General Dosage Range Dosage adjustment recommended in patients with renal impairment

Oral:

Adults: Enalapril 5-20 mg and felodipine 2.5-10 mg once daily

Elderly: Initial: Felodipine 2.5 mg daily

Mechanism of Action See individual agents.

Pregnancy Risk Factor C/D (2nd and 3rd trimesters)

Enalapril and Hydrochlorothiazide

(e NAL a pril & hye droe klor oh THYE a zide)

Related Information

Enalapril *on page* 596

Hydrochlorothiazide *on page* 854

U.S. Brand Names Vaseretic®

Canadian Brand Names Vaseretic®

Pharmacologic Category Angiotensin-Converting Enzyme (ACE) Inhibitor; Diuretic, Thiazide

Use Treatment of hypertension

Local Anesthetic/Vasoconstrictor Precautions No information available to require special precautions

Effects on Dental Treatment No significant effects or complications reported

Effects on Bleeding No information available to require special precautions

Adverse Effects See individual agents.

General Dosage Range Oral: *Adults:* Enalapril 5-10 mg and hydrochlorothiazide 12.5-25 mg once daily (maximum: 40 mg/day [enalapril]; 50 mg/day [hydrochlorothiazide])

Pregnancy Risk Factor C/D (2nd and 3rd trimesters)

Enfuvirtide (en FYOO vir tide)

Related Information

HIV Infection and AIDS *on page* 1883

U.S. Brand Names Fuzeon®

Canadian Brand Names Fuzeon®

Pharmacologic Category Antiretroviral Agent, Fusion Protein Inhibitor

Use Treatment of HIV-1 infection in combination with other antiretroviral agents in treatment-experienced patients with evidence of HIV-1 replication despite ongoing antiretroviral therapy

Local Anesthetic/Vasoconstrictor Precautions No information available to require special precautions

Effects on Dental Treatment Key adverse event(s) related to dental treatment: Xerostomia (normal salivary flow resumes upon discontinuation) and taste disturbance

Effects on Bleeding No information available to require special precautions related to hemostasis.

Adverse Effects

>10%:

- Gastrointestinal: Diarrhea (32%), nausea (23%)
- Local: Injection site infection (children 11%), injection site reactions (98%; may include pain, erythema, induration, pruritus, ecchymosis, nodule or cyst formation)

1% to 10%:

- Dermatologic: Folliculitis (2%)
- Gastrointestinal: Weight loss (7%), abdominal pain (4%), appetite decreased (3%), pancreatitis (3%), anorexia (2%), xerostomia (2%)
- Hematologic: Eosinophilia (2% to 9%)
- Hepatic: Transaminases increased (4%, grade 4: 1%)
- Local: Injection site infection (adults 2%)
- Neuromuscular & skeletal: CPK increased (3% to 7%), limb pain (3%), myalgia (3%)
- Ocular: Conjunctivitis (2%)
- Respiratory: Sinusitis (6%), cough (4%), pneumonia (3%)
- Miscellaneous: Infections (4% to 6%), herpes simplex (4%), flu-like syndrome (2%)

General Dosage Range Dosage adjustment recommended in patients with renal impairment

SubQ:

Children 6-16 years: 2 mg/kg twice daily (maximum: 90 mg/dose)

Adolescents ≥16 years and Adults: 90 mg twice daily

Mechanism of Action Binds to the first heptad-repeat (HR1) in the gp41 subunit of the viral envelope glycoprotein. Inhibits the fusion of HIV-1 virus with CD4 cells by blocking the conformational change in gp41 required for membrane fusion and entry into CD4 cells

Pharmacodynamics/Kinetics

Half-life Elimination 3.8 hours

Time to Peak 4-8 hours

Pregnancy Risk Factor B

Enoxaparin (ee noks a PA rin)

Related Information

Cardiovascular Diseases *on page 1848*

U.S. Brand Names Lovenox®

Canadian Brand Names Enoxaparin Injection; Lovenox®; Lovenox® HP

Pharmacologic Category Low Molecular Weight Heparin

Use

Acute coronary syndromes: Unstable angina (UA), non-ST-elevation (NSTEMI), and ST-elevation myocardial infarction (STEMI)

DVT prophylaxis: Following hip or knee replacement surgery, abdominal surgery, or in medical patients with severely-restricted mobility during acute illness who are at risk for thromboembolic complications

DVT treatment (acute): Inpatient treatment (patients with and without pulmonary embolism) and outpatient treatment (patients without pulmonary embolism)

Note: High-risk patients include those with one or more of the following risk factors: >40 years of age, obesity, general anesthesia lasting >30 minutes, malignancy, history of deep vein thrombosis or pulmonary embolism

Unlabeled/Investigational Use Prophylaxis and treatment of thromboembolism in children; anticoagulant bridge therapy during temporary interruption of vitamin K antagonist therapy in patients at high risk for thromboembolism; DVT prophylaxis following moderate-risk general surgery, major gynecologic surgery and following higher-risk general surgery for cancer; management of venous thromboembolism (VTE) during pregnancy (Hirsh, 2008)

Local Anesthetic/Vasoconstrictor Precautions No information available to require special precautions

Effects on Dental Treatment Key adverse event(s) related to dental treatment: Bleeding is the major adverse effect of enoxaparin. See Effects on Bleeding.

Effects on Bleeding As with all anticoagulants, bleeding is the major adverse effect of enoxaparin. Hemorrhage may occur at virtually any site; risk is dependent on multiple variables including the intensity of anticoagulation and patient susceptibility. At the recommended doses, enoxaparin does not significantly influence platelet aggregation or affect global clotting time (ie, PT or aPTT). Medical consult is suggested.

Adverse Effects As with all anticoagulants, bleeding is the major adverse effect of enoxaparin. Hemorrhage may occur at virtually any site. Risk is dependent on multiple variables. At the recommended doses, single injections of enoxaparin do not significantly influence platelet aggregation or affect global clotting time (ie, PT or aPTT).

1% to 10%:

Central nervous system: Fever (5% to 8%), confusion, pain

Dermatologic: Erythema, bruising

Gastrointestinal: Nausea (3%), diarrhea

Hematologic: Hemorrhage (major, <1% to 4%; includes cases of intracranial, retroperitoneal, or intraocular hemorrhage; incidence varies with indication/population), thrombocytopenia (moderate 1%; severe 0.1% - see **"Note"**), anemia (<2%)

Hepatic: ALT increased, AST increased

Local: Injection site hematoma (9%), local reactions (irritation, pain, ecchymosis, erythema)

Renal: Hematuria (<2%)

Note: Thrombocytopenia with thrombosis: Cases of heparin-induced thrombocytopenia (some complicated by organ infarction, limb ischemia, or death) have been reported.

General Dosage Range Dosage adjustment recommended in patients with renal impairment

SubQ: *Adults:* Prophylaxis: 30 mg every 12 hours **or** 40 mg once daily; Treatment: 1 mg/kg every 12 hours **or** 1.5 mg/kg once daily

STEMI indication only:

<75 years: 30 mg I.V. bolus plus 1 mg/kg SubQ every 12 hours

≥75 years: 0.75 mg/kg SubQ every 12 hours

Mechanism of Action Standard heparin consists of components with molecular weights ranging from 4000-30,000 daltons with a mean of 16,000 daltons. Heparin acts as an anticoagulant by enhancing the inhibition rate of clotting proteases by antithrombin III impairing normal hemostasis and inhibition of factor Xa. Low molecular weight heparins have a small effect on the activated partial thromboplastin time and strongly inhibit factor Xa. Enoxaparin is derived from porcine heparin that undergoes benzylation followed by alkaline depolymerization. The average molecular weight of enoxaparin is 4500 daltons which is distributed as (≤20%) 2000 daltons (≥68%) 2000-8000 daltons, and (≤15%) >8000 daltons. Enoxaparin has a higher ratio of antifactor Xa to antifactor IIa activity than unfractionated heparin.

Pharmacodynamics/Kinetics

Onset of Action Peak effect: SubQ: Antifactor Xa and antithrombin (antifactor IIa): 3-5 hours

Duration of Action 40 mg dose: Antifactor Xa activity: ~12 hours

Half-life Elimination Plasma: 2-4 times longer than standard heparin, independent of dose; based on anti-Xa activity: 4.5-7 hours

Pregnancy Risk Factor B

Entacapone (en TA ka pone)

U.S. Brand Names Comtan®

Canadian Brand Names Comtan®

Pharmacologic Category Anti-Parkinson's Agent, COMT Inhibitor

Use Adjunct to levodopa/carbidopa therapy in patients with idiopathic Parkinson's disease who experience "wearing-off" symptoms at the end of a dosing interval

Local Anesthetic/Vasoconstrictor Precautions No information available to require special precautions

Effects on Dental Treatment Key adverse event(s) related to dental treatment: Orthostatic hypotension and abnormal taste. Dopaminergic therapy in Parkinson's disease (ie, treatment with levodopa) is associated with orthostatic hypotension. Entacapone enhances levodopa bioavailability and may increase the occurrence of hypotension/syncope in the dental patient. The patient should be carefully assisted from the chair and observed for signs of orthostatic hypotension.

Effects on Bleeding No information available to require special precautions

Adverse Effects

>10%:

Gastrointestinal: Nausea (14%)

Neuromuscular & skeletal: Dyskinesia (25%), placebo (15%)

1% to 10%:

Cardiovascular: Orthostatic hypotension (4%), syncope (1%)

Central nervous system: Dizziness (8%), fatigue (6%), hallucinations (4%), anxiety (2%), somnolence (2%), agitation (1%)

Dermatologic: Purpura (2%)

Gastrointestinal: Diarrhea (10%), abdominal pain (8%), constipation (6%), vomiting (4%), dry mouth (3%), dyspepsia (2%), flatulence (2%), gastritis (1%), taste perversion (1%)

Genitourinary: Brown-orange urine discoloration (10%)

Neuromuscular & skeletal: Hyperkinesia (10%), hypokinesia (9%), back pain (4%), weakness (2%)

Respiratory: Dyspnea (3%)

Miscellaneous: Diaphoresis increased (2%), bacterial infection (1%)

General Dosage Range Oral: *Adults:* 200 mg with each dose of levodopa/carbidopa (maximum: 1600 mg/day)

Mechanism of Action Entacapone is a reversible and selective inhibitor of catechol-O-methyltransferase (COMT). When entacapone is taken with levodopa, the pharmacokinetics are altered, resulting in more sustained levodopa serum levels compared to levodopa taken alone. The resulting levels of levodopa provide for increased concentrations available for absorption across the blood-brain barrier, thereby providing for increased CNS levels of dopamine, the active metabolite of levodopa.

Pharmacodynamics/Kinetics

Onset of Action Rapid; Peak effect: 1 hour

Half-life Elimination B phase: 0.4-0.7 hours; Y phase: 2.4 hours

Time to Peak Serum: 1 hour

Pregnancy Risk Factor C

Entecavir (en TE ka veer)

Related Information

HIV Infection and AIDS *on page* 1883

Systemic Viral Diseases *on page* 1904

U.S. Brand Names Baraclude®

Canadian Brand Names Baraclude®

Pharmacologic Category Antiretroviral Agent, Reverse Transcriptase Inhibitor (Nucleoside)

Use Treatment of chronic hepatitis B infection, with compensated or decompensated liver disease, in adults with evidence of active viral replication and either evidence of persistent transaminase elevations or histologically-active disease

Local Anesthetic/Vasoconstrictor Precautions No information available to require special precautions

Effects on Dental Treatment No significant effects or complications reported

Effects on Bleeding No information available to require special precautions related to hemostasis.

Adverse Effects

>10%:

Cardiovascular: Peripheral edema (16% with decompensated liver disease)

Central nervous system: Pyrexia (14% with decompensated liver disease)

Hepatic: Ascites (15% with decompensated liver disease), ALT increased (>5 x ULN: 11% to 12%; post-treatment flare [lamivudine refractory]: >10 x ULN and >2 x baseline: 12%)

1% to 10%:

Central nervous system: Headache (2% to 4%), fatigue (1% to 3%), dizziness

Endocrine & metabolic: Hyperglycemia (2% to 3%), blood bicarbonate decreased (2% with decompensated liver disease)

Gastrointestinal: Lipase increased (7%), amylase increased (2% to 3%), diarrhea (≤1%), dyspepsia (≤1%), nausea

Hepatic: Hepatic encephalopathy (10% with decompensated liver disease), bilirubin increased (2% to 3%), ALT increased (>10 x ULN and >2 x baseline: 2%; post-treatment flare [nucleoside-naive]: >10 x ULN and >2 x baseline: 2% to 8%)

Renal: Hematuria (9%), glycosuria (4%), creatinine increased (1% to 2%)

Respiratory: Upper respiratory tract infection (10% with decompensated liver disease)

General Dosage Range Dosage adjustment recommended in patients with renal impairment.

Oral: *Adolescents ≥16 years and Adults:* 0.5-1 mg once daily

Mechanism of Action Entecavir is intracellularly phosphorylated to guanosine triphosphate which competes with natural substrates to effectively inhibit hepatitis B viral polymerase; enzyme inhibition blocks reverse transcriptase activity thereby reducing viral DNA synthesis.

Pharmacodynamics/Kinetics

Half-life Elimination Terminal: ~5-6 days; accumulation: ~24 hours

Time to Peak 0.5-1.5 hours

Pregnancy Risk Factor C

EPHEDrine (Systemic) (e FED rin)

Pharmacologic Category Alpha/Beta Agonist

Use Treatment of nasal congestion, idiopathic orthostatic hypotension, anesthesia-induced hypotension

Unlabeled/Investigational Use Postoperative nausea and vomiting (PONV)

Local Anesthetic/Vasoconstrictor Precautions Use vasoconstrictor with caution since ephedrine may enhance cardiostimulation and vasopressor effects of sympathomimetics such as epinephrine

Effects on Dental Treatment Key adverse event(s) related to dental treatment: Xerostomia (normal salivary flow resumes upon discontinuation)

Effects on Bleeding No information available to require special precautions

Adverse Effects Frequency not defined.

Cardiovascular: Arrhythmias, chest pain, elevation or depression of blood pressure, hypertension, palpitation, tachycardia, unusual pallor

Central nervous system: Agitation, anxiety, apprehension, CNS stimulating effects, dizziness, excitation, fear, headache hyperactivity, insomnia, irritability, nervousness, restlessness, tension
Gastrointestinal: Anorexia, GI upset, nausea, vomiting, xerostomia
Genitourinary: Painful urination
Neuromuscular & skeletal: Trembling, tremor (more common in the elderly), weakness
Respiratory: Dyspnea
Miscellaneous: Diaphoresis increased

General Dosage Range

I.V.:

Children: 0.2-0.3 mg/kg/dose every 4-6 hours

Adults: 5-25 mg/dose; repeat after 5-10 minutes as needed, then every 3-4 hours (maximum: 150 mg/day)

Oral: *Children ≥12 years and Adults:* 12.5-50 mg every 4 hours as needed (maximum: 150 mg/day)

Mechanism of Action Releases tissue stores of norepinephrine and thereby produces an alpha- and beta-adrenergic stimulation; longer-acting and less potent than epinephrine

Pharmacodynamics/Kinetics

Duration of Action Oral: 3-6 hours

Half-life Elimination 2.5-3.6 hours

Pregnancy Risk Factor C

Epinastine (ep i NAS teen)

U.S. Brand Names Elestat®

Pharmacologic Category Histamine H_1 Antagonist; Histamine H_1 Antagonist, Second Generation

Use Treatment of allergic conjunctivitis

Local Anesthetic/Vasoconstrictor Precautions No information available to require special precautions

Effects on Dental Treatment No significant effects or complications reported

Effects on Bleeding No information available to require special precautions

Adverse Effects 1% to 10%:

Central nervous system: Headache (1% to 3%)
Ocular: Burning sensation, folliculosis, hyperemia, pruritus
Respiratory: Cough (1% to 3%), pharyngitis (1% to 3%), rhinitis (1% to 3%), sinusitis (1% to 3%)
Miscellaneous: Infection (10%; defined as cold symptoms and upper respiratory infection)

General Dosage Range Ophthalmic: *Children ≥3 years and Adults:* Instill 1 drop into each eye twice daily

Mechanism of Action Selective H_1-receptor antagonist; inhibits release of histamine from the mast cell

Pharmacodynamics/Kinetics

Onset of Action 3-5 minutes

Duration of Action 8 hours

Half-life Elimination 12 hours

Pregnancy Risk Factor C

EPINEPHrine (Systemic, Oral Inhalation) (ep i NEF rin)

U.S. Brand Names Adrenaclick™ [DSC]; Adrenalin®; EpiPen 2-Pak®; EpiPen Jr 2-Pak®; EpiPen®; EpiPen® Jr.; Primatene® Mist [OTC]; S2® [OTC]; Twinject®

Canadian Brand Names Adrenalin®; Epi E-Z Pen®; EpiPen®; EpiPen® Jr; Twinject®

Generic Availability (U.S.) Yes: Solution for injection

Pharmacologic Category Alpha/Beta Agonist

Dental Use Emergency drug for treatment of anaphylactic reactions; used as vasoconstrictor to prolong local anesthesia

Use Treatment of bronchospasms, bronchial asthma, viral croup, anaphylactic reactions, cardiac arrest; added to local anesthetics to decrease systemic absorption of intraspinal and local anesthetics and increase duration of action; decrease superficial hemorrhage

Unlabeled/Investigational Use ACLS guidelines: Ventricular fibrillation (VF) or pulseless ventricular tachycardia (VT) unresponsive to initial defibrillatory shocks; pulseless electrical activity; asystole; hypotension/shock unresponsive to volume resuscitation; symptomatic bradycardia unresponsive to atropine or pacing; inotropic support

Local Anesthetic/Vasoconstrictor Precautions No information available to require special precautions

Effects on Dental Treatment Key adverse event(s) related to dental treatment: Xerostomia (normal salivary flow resumes upon discontinuation) and dry throat.

Effects on Bleeding No information available to require special precautions

Adverse Effects Frequency not defined.

Cardiovascular: Angina, cardiac arrhythmia, chest pain, flushing, hypertension, pallor, palpitation, sudden death, tachycardia (parenteral), vasoconstriction, ventricular ectopy

Central nervous system: Anxiety (transient), apprehensiveness, cerebral hemorrhage, dizziness, headache, insomnia, lightheadedness, nervousness, restlessness

Gastrointestinal: Dry throat, loss of appetite, nausea, vomiting, xerostomia

Genitourinary: Acute urinary retention in patients with bladder outflow obstruction

Neuromuscular & skeletal: Tremor, weakness

Ocular: Allergic lid reaction, burning, eye pain, ocular irritation, precipitation of or exacerbation of narrow-angle glaucoma, transient stinging

Respiratory: Dyspnea, pulmonary edema

Miscellaneous: Diaphoresis

Dental Usual Dosage Hypersensitivity reaction:

Infants and Children:

SubQ, I.V.: 0.01 mg/kg every 20 minutes; larger doses or continuous infusion may be needed for some anaphylactic reactions

SubQ, I.M.:

15-30 kg: Twinject®: 0.15 mg (for self-administration following severe allergic reactions to insect stings, food, etc)

>30 kg: Refer to adult dosing

I.M.:

<30 kg: EpiPen® Jr: 0.15 mg (for self-administration following severe allergic reactions to insect stings, food, etc)

>30 kg: Refer to adult dosing

Adults:

I.M., SubQ: 0.3-0.5 mg (1:1000) every 15-20 minutes if condition requires (I.M route is preferred)

>30 kg: Twinject®: 0.3 mg (for self-administration following severe allergic reactions to insect stings, food, etc)

I.M.: >30 kg: EpiPen®: 0.3 mg (for self-administration following severe allergic reactions to insect stings, food, etc)

I.V.: 0.1 mg (1:10,000) over 5 minutes. May infuse at 1-4 mcg/minute to prevent the need to repeat injections frequently.

Dosage

Neonates: Cardiac arrest (Neonatal resuscitation guidelines, 2010):

I.V.: 0.01-0.03 mg/kg (0.1-0.3 mL/kg of **1:10,000** solution) every 3-5 minutes until return of spontaneous circulation

Intratracheal: Although I.V. route is preferred, may administer 0.05-0.1 mg/kg (0.5-1 mL/kg of **1:10,000** solution) every 3-5 minutes until I.V. access established or return of spontaneous circulation

Infants and Children:

Asystole/pulseless arrest, pulseless VT/VF (after failed defibrillation attempts) (PALS, 2010):

I.V., I.O.: 0.01 mg/kg (0.1 mL/kg of **1:10,000** solution) (maximum single dose: 1 mg) every 3-5 minutes until return of spontaneous circulation

Intratracheal: 0.1 mg/kg (0.1 mL/kg of **1:1000** solution) (maximum single dose: 2.5 mg) every 3-5 minutes until I.V./I.O. access established or return of spontaneous circulation

Postresuscitation infusion to maintain cardiac output or stabilize: I.V., I.O.: 0.1-1 mcg/kg/minute; doses <0.3 mcg/kg/minute generally produce beta-adrenergic effects and higher doses (>0.3 mcg/kg/minute) generally produce alpha-adrenergic vasoconstriction; titrate dosage to desired effect

Bradycardia (symptomatic; unresponsive to atropine or pacing):

I.V., I.O.: 0.01 mg/kg (0.1 mL/kg of **1:10,000** solution) (maximum single dose: 1 mg) every 3-5 minutes as needed

Intratracheal: 0.1 mg/kg or (0.1 mL/kg of **1:1000** solution) (maximum single dose: 2.5 mg) every 3-5 minutes as needed until I.V./I.O. access established

Continuous infusion: I.V., I.O.: 0.1-1 mcg/kg/minute; doses <0.3 mcg/kg/minute generally produce beta-adrenergic effects and higher doses (>0.3 mcg/kg/minute) generally produce alpha-adrenergic vasoconstriction; titrate dosage to desired effect

Bronchodilator:

SubQ: 0.01 mg/kg (0.01 mL/kg of **1:1000** solution) (maximum single dose: 0.5 mg) every 20 minutes for 3 doses

Nebulization: S2® (racepinephrine, OTC labeling):

Children <4 years: Jet nebulizer: Croup: 0.05 mL/kg (maximum dose: 0.5 mL); dilute in 3 mL of NS. Administer over ~15 minutes; do not administer more frequently than every 2 hours

Children ≥4 years: Refer to adult dosing.

Inhalation: Children ≥4 years: Primatene® Mist: Refer to adult dosing.

Hypersensitivity reaction: **Note:** SubQ administration results in slower absorption and is less reliable. I.M. administration in the anterolateral aspect of the middle third of the thigh is preferred in the setting of anaphylaxis (ACLS guidelines, 2010; Kemp, 2008).

I.M., SubQ: 0.01 mg/kg (0.01 mL/kg of **1:1000** solution) (maximum single dose: 0.3 mg) every 5-15 minutes; larger I.M. or SubQ doses, use of I.V. route, or continuous infusion may be needed for severe anaphylactic reactions (Kemp, 2008; Lieberman, 2010). If clinician deems appropriate, the 5-minute interval between injections may be shortened to allow for more frequent administration (Lieberman, 2010).

Self-administration following severe allergic reactions (eg, insect stings, food): **Note:** World Health Organization (WHO) and Anaphylaxis Canada recommend the availability of 1 dose for every 10-20 minutes of travel time to a medical emergency facility:

EpiPen® Jr: I.M., SubQ: Children 15-29 kg: 0.15 mg; if anaphylactic symptoms persist, dose may be repeated in 5-15 minutes using an additional EpiPen® Jr

EpiPen®: I.M., SubQ: Children ≥30 kg: 0.3 mg; if anaphylactic symptoms persist, dose may be repeated in 5-15 minutes using an additional EpiPen®

Twinject®: I.M. SubQ:

Children 15-29 kg: 0.15 mg; if anaphylactic symptoms persist, dose may be repeated in 5-15 minutes using the same device after partial disassembly

Children ≥30 kg: 0.3 mg; if anaphylactic symptoms persist, dose may be repeated in 5-15 minutes using the same device after partial disassembly

Alternate auto-injector dose: I.M. (Sicherer, 2007):

Children 10-25 kg: 0.15 mg

Children >25 kg: 0.3 mg

Hypotension/shock, fluid-resistant (unlabeled use): Continuous I.V. infusion: 0.1-1 mcg/kg/minute; doses up to 5 mcg/kg/minute may rarely be necessary (Hegenbarth, 2008)

Adults:

Asystole/pulseless arrest, pulseless VT/VF (ACLS, 2010):

I.V., I.O.: 1 mg every 3-5 minutes until return of spontaneous circulation; if this approach fails, higher doses of epinephrine (up to 0.2 mg/kg) have been used for treatment of specific problems (eg, beta-blocker or calcium channel blocker overdose)

Intratracheal: 2-2.5 mg every 3-5 minutes until I.V./I.O. access established or return of spontaneous circulation; dilute in 5-10 mL NS or sterile water. **Note:** Absorption may be greater with sterile water (Naganobu, 2000).

Bradycardia (symptomatic; unresponsive to atropine or pacing): I.V. infusion: 2-10 mcg/minute **or** 0.1-0.5 mcg/kg/minute (7-35 mcg/minute in a 70 kg patient); titrate to desired effect (ACLS, 2010)

Bronchodilator:

SubQ: 0.3-0.5 mg (**1:1000** solution) every 20 minutes for 3 doses

Nebulization: S2® (racepinephrine, OTC labeling):

Hand-bulb nebulizer: Add 0.5 mL (~10 drops) to nebulizer; 1-3 inhalations up to every 3 hours if needed

Jet nebulizer: Add 0.5 mL (~10 drops) to nebulizer and dilute with 3 mL of NS; administer over ~15 minutes every 3-4 hours as needed

Inhalation: Primatene® Mist (OTC labeling): One inhalation, wait at least 1 minute; if not relieved, may use once more. Do not use again for at least 3 hours.

Hypersensitivity reaction: **Note:** SubQ administration results in slower absorption and is less reliable. I.M. administration in the anterolateral aspect of the middle third of the thigh is preferred in the setting of anaphylaxis (ACLS guidelines, 2010; Kemp, 2008).

I.M., SubQ: 0.2-0.5 mg (**1:1000** solution) every 5-15 minutes in the absence of clinical improvement (ACLS, 2010; Kemp, 2008; Lieberman, 2010). If clinician deems appropriate, the 5-minute interval between injections may be shortened to allow for more frequent administration (Lieberman, 2010).

I.V.: 0.1 mg (**1:10,000** solution) over 5 minutes; may infuse at 1-4 mcg/minute to prevent the need to repeat injections frequently **or** may initiate with an infusion at 5-15 mcg/minute (with crystalloid administration) (ACLS, 2010; Brown, 2004). In general, I.V. administration should only be done in patients who are profoundly hypotensive or are in cardiopulmonary arrest refractory to volume resuscitation and several epinephrine injections (Lieberman, 2010).

Self-administration following severe allergic reactions (eg, insect stings, food): **Note:** The World Health Organization (WHO) and Anaphylaxis Canada recommend the availability of one dose for every 10-20 minutes of travel time to a medical emergency facility. More than 2 doses should only be administered under direct medical supervision.

Twinject®: I.M., SubQ: 0.3 mg; if anaphylactic symptoms persist, dose may be repeated in 5-15 minutes using the same device after partial disassembly

EpiPen®: I.M., SubQ: 0.3 mg; if anaphylactic symptoms persist, dose may be repeated in 5-15 minutes using an additional EpiPen®

Hypotension/shock, severe and fluid resistant (unlabeled use): I.V. infusion: Initial: 0.1-0.5 mcg/kg/minute (7-35 mcg/minute in a 70 kg patient); titrate to desired response (ACLS, 2010)

Mechanism of Action Stimulates alpha-, beta$_1$-, and beta$_2$-adrenergic receptors resulting in relaxation of smooth muscle of the bronchial tree, cardiac stimulation (increasing myocardial oxygen consumption), and dilation of skeletal muscle vasculature; small doses can cause vasodilation via beta$_2$-vascular receptors; large doses may produce constriction of skeletal and vascular smooth muscle

Contraindications There are no absolute contraindications to the use of injectable epinephrine (including EpiPen®, EpiPen® Jr, and Twinject®) in a life-threatening situation.

Oral inhalation: Concurrent use or within 2 weeks of MAO inhibitors

Injectable solution: Per the manufacturer, contraindicated in narrow-angle glaucoma; shock; during general anesthesia with halogenated hydrocarbons or cyclopropane (currently not available in U.S.); individuals with organic brain damage; with local anesthesia of the digits; during labor; heart failure; coronary insufficiency

Warnings/Precautions Use with caution in elderly patients, patients with diabetes mellitus, cardiovascular diseases (eg, coronary artery disease, hypertension), thyroid disease, cerebrovascular disease, Parkinson's disease, or patients taking tricyclic antidepressants. Some products contain sulfites as preservatives; the presence of sulfites in some products (eg, EpiPen® and Twinject®) should not deter administration during a serious allergic or other emergency situation even if the patient is sulfite-sensitive. Accidental injection into digits, hands, or feet may result in local reactions, including injection site pallor, coldness and hypoesthesia or injury, resulting in bruising, bleeding, discoloration, erythema or skeletal injury; patient should seek immediate medical attention if this occurs. Rapid I.V. administration may cause death from cerebrovascular hemorrhage or cardiac arrhythmias; however, rapid I.V. administration during pulseless arrest is necessary.

Oral inhalation: Use with caution in patients with prostate enlargement or urinary retention; may cause temporary worsening of symptoms.

Self medication (OTC use): Oral inhalation: Prior to self-medication, patients should contact healthcare provider. The product should only be used in persons with a diagnosis of asthma. If symptoms are not relieved in 20 minutes or become worse do not continue to use the product - seek immediate medical assistance. The product should not be used more frequently or at higher doses than recommended unless directed by a healthcare provider. This product should not be used in patients who have required hospitalization for asthma or if a patient is taking prescription medication for asthma. Do not use if you have taken a MAO inhibitor (certain drugs used for depression, Parkinson's disease, or other conditions) within 2 weeks.

Drug Interactions

Avoid Concomitant Use

Avoid concomitant use of EPINEPHrine (Systemic, Oral Inhalation) with any of the following: Iobenguane I 123; Lurasidone

Increased Effect/Toxicity

EPINEPHrine (Systemic, Oral Inhalation) may increase the levels/effects of: Bromocriptine; Lurasidone; Sympathomimetics

The levels/effects of EPINEPHrine (Systemic, Oral Inhalation) may be increased by: Antacids; Atomoxetine; Beta-Blockers; Cannabinoids; Carbonic Anhydrase Inhibitors; COMT Inhibitors; Inhalational Anesthetics; MAO Inhibitors; Serotonin/Norepinephrine Reuptake Inhibitors; Tricyclic Antidepressants

Decreased Effect

EPINEPHrine (Systemic, Oral Inhalation) may decrease the levels/effects of: Benzylpenicilloyl Polylysine; Iobenguane I 123

The levels/effects of EPINEPHrine (Systemic, Oral Inhalation) may be decreased by: Spironolactone

Ethanol/Nutrition/Herb Interactions Herb/Nutraceutical: Avoid ephedra, yohimbe (may cause CNS stimulation).

Pharmacodynamics/Kinetics

Onset of Action Bronchodilation: SubQ: ~5-10 minutes; Inhalation: ~1 minute

Pregnancy Risk Factor C

Lactation Excretion in breast milk unknown

Dosage Forms

Aerosol, for oral inhalation:

Primatene® Mist [OTC]: 0.22 mg/inhalation (15 mL)

Injection, solution: 0.1 mg/mL (10 mL); 0.15 mg/0.15 mL (1.1 mL); 0.3 mg/0.3 mL (1.1 mL); 1 mg/mL (1 mL, 30 mL)

Adrenalin®: 1 mg/mL (1 mL, 30 mL)

EpiPen 2-Pak®: 0.3 mg/0.3 mL (2 mL)

EpiPen Jr 2-Pak®: 0.15 mg/0.3 mL (2 mL)

EpiPen®: 0.3 mg/0.3 mL (2 mL)

EpiPen® Jr.: 0.15 mg/0.3 mL (2 mL)

Twinject®: 0.15 mg/0.15 mL (1.1 mL); 0.3 mg/0.3 mL (1.1 mL)

Injection, solution [preservative free]: 1 mg/mL (1 mL)

Solution, for oral inhalation [preservative free]:

S2® [OTC]: 2.25% (0.5 mL)

References

"2005 American Heart Association Guidelines for Cardiopulmonary Resuscitation and Emergency Cardiovascular Care," *Circulation*, 2005, 112(24 Suppl): 1-211.

Cydulka R, Davison R, Grammer L, et al, "The Use of Epinephrine in the Treatment of Older Adult Asthmatics," *Ann Emerg Med*, 1988, 17(4):322-6.

Davis C and Wax P, "Subcutaneous Epinephrine O.D. in a Child Resulting in Dysrhythmias and Myocardial Ischemia," *Vet Hum Toxicol*, 1994, 36:367.

Illi A, Sundberg S, Ojala-Karlsson P, et al, "The Effect of Entacapone on the Disposition and Hemodynamic Effects of Intravenous Isoproterenol and Epinephrine," *Clin Pharmacol Ther*, 1995, 58(2):221-7.

Klein JS, Rich MR, and Yunginger JW, "Myocardial Ischemia Without Coronary Artery Disease After Epinephrine Overdose for Insect Sting Reaction," *J Allergy Clin Immunol*, 1995, 95(2):371.

Kuracheck SC and Rockoff MA, "Inadvertent Intravenous Administration of Racemic Epinephrine," *JAMA*, 1984, 253(10):1441-2.

Murphy FT, Manown TJ, Knutson SW, et al, "Epinephrine-Induced Lactic Acidosis in the Setting of Status Asthmaticus," *South Med J*, 1995, 88(5):577-9.

National Asthma Education and Prevention Program, "Expert Panel Report 2: Guidelines for the Diagnosis and Management of Asthma," Bethesda, MD, National Institutes of Health, 1997. NIH publication 97-4051.

Nicholson KE and Rogers JE, "Cocaine and Adrenaline Paste: A Fatal Combination?" *BMJ*, 1995, 311 (6999):250-1.

Riou B, Barriot P, Rimailho A, et al, "Treatment of Severe Chloroquine Poisoning," *N Engl J Med*, 1988, 318(1):1-6.

Scalzo A, Keith G, and Thompson M, "Fatal Outcome After Massive Epinephrine Overdose by Intravenous Injection of an OTC Asthma Inhaler," *Clin Toxicol*, 1995, 33(5):501-2.

Stiell IG, Hebert PC, Wells GA, et al, "Vasopressin Versus Epinephrine for Inhospital Cardiac Arrest: A Randomised Controlled Trial," *Lancet*, 2001, 358(9276):105-9.

Waisman Y, Klein BL, Boenning DA, et al, "Prospective Randomized Double-Blind Study Comparing L-Epinephrine and Racemic Epinephrine Aerosols in the Treatment of Laryngotracheitis (Croup)," *Pediatrics*, 1992, 89(2):302-6.

Wenzel V, Krismer AC, Arntz HR, et al, "A Comparison of Vasopressin and Epinephrine for Out-of-Hospital Cardiopulmonary Resuscitation. European Resuscitation Council Vasopressor during Cardiopulmonary Resuscitation Study Group," *N Engl J Med*, 2004, 350(2):105-13.

Epinephrine and Chlorpheniramine (ep i NEF rin & klor fen IR a meen)

Related Information

Chlorpheniramine *on page 365*

EPINEPHrine (Systemic, Oral Inhalation) *on page 604*

U.S. Brand Names Ana-Kit®

Pharmacologic Category Antidote

Use Anaphylaxis emergency treatment of insect bites or stings by the sensitive patient that may occur within minutes of insect sting or exposure to an allergic substance

Local Anesthetic/Vasoconstrictor Precautions No information available to require special precautions

Effects on Dental Treatment No significant effects or complications reported

Effects on Bleeding No information available to require special precautions

General Dosage Range

I.M., SubQ: Epinephrine (1:1000):

Children <2 years: 0.05-0.1 mL

Children 2-6 years: 0.15 mL

Children 6-12 years: 0.2 mL

Children >12 years and Adults: 0.3 mL

Oral: Chlorpheniramine (2 mg/tablet):
Children <6 years: 1 tablet
Children 6-12 years: 2 tablets
Children >12 years and Adults: 4 tablets

Epinephrine (Racemic) and Aluminum Potassium Sulfate

(ep i NEF rin, ra SEE mik and a LOO mi num poe TASS ee um SUL fate)

Related Information
EPINEPHrine (Systemic, Oral Inhalation) *on page 604*

U.S. Brand Names Van R Gingibraid®

Generic Availability (U.S.) No

Pharmacologic Category Adrenergic Agonist Agent; Alpha/Beta Agonist; Astringent; Vasoconstrictor

Dental Use Gingival retraction

Local Anesthetic/Vasoconstrictor Precautions No information available to require special precautions

Effects on Dental Treatment Key adverse event(s) related to dental treatment: Tissue retraction around base of the tooth (therapeutic effect).

Effects on Bleeding No information available to require special precautions

Adverse Effects No data reported.

Dental Usual Dosage Gingival retraction: Adults: Pass the impregnated yarn around the neck of the tooth and place into gingival sulcus; normal tissue moisture, water, or gingival retraction solutions activate impregnated yarn. Limit use to one quadrant of the mouth at a time; recommended use is for 3-8 minutes in the mouth.

Mechanism of Action Epinephrine stimulates $alpha_1$ adrenergic receptors to cause vasoconstriction in blood vessels in gingiva; aluminum potassium sulfate, precipitates tissue and blood proteins

Contraindications Hypersensitivity to epinephrine or any component of the formulation; cardiovascular disease, hyperthyroidism, or diabetes; do not apply to areas of heavy or deep bleeding or over exposed bone

Warnings/Precautions Caution should be exercised whenever using gingival retraction cords with epinephrine since it delivers vasoconstrictor doses of racemic epinephrine to patients; the general medical history should be thoroughly evaluated before using in any patient

Dosage Forms

Yarn, saturated in solution of racemic epinephrine 8% and aluminum potassium sulfate 7% (Van R Gingibraid®):
Type "0e": 0.20 ± 0.10 mg epinephrine/inch; Type "1e": 0.40 ± 0.20 mg epinephrine/inch; Type "2e": 0.60 ± 0.20 mg epinephrine/inch

Epirubicin (ep i ROO bi sin)

U.S. Brand Names Ellence®

Canadian Brand Names Ellence®; Pharmorubicin®

Pharmacologic Category Antineoplastic Agent, Anthracycline

Use Adjuvant therapy for primary breast cancer

Unlabeled/Investigational Use Treatment of esophageal cancer, gastric cancer, soft tissue sarcoma, uterine sarcoma

Local Anesthetic/Vasoconstrictor Precautions No information available to require special precautions

Effects on Dental Treatment Key adverse event(s) related to dental treatment: Mucositis

Effects on Bleeding Chemotherapy may result in significant myelosuppression, potentially including significant reduction in platelet counts and altered hemostasis. In patients who are under active treatment with these agents, medical consult is suggested.

Adverse Effects Percentages reported as part of combination chemotherapy regimens.

>10%:
Central nervous system: Lethargy (1% to 46%)
Dermatologic: Alopecia (69% to 96%)
Endocrine & metabolic: Amenorrhea (69% to 72%), hot flashes (5% to 39%)
Gastrointestinal: Nausea/vomiting (83% to 92%; grades 3/4: 22% to 25%), mucositis (9% to 59%; grades 3/4: ≤9%), diarrhea (7% to 25%)
Hematologic: Leukopenia (50% to 80%; grades 3/4: 2% to 59%), neutropenia (54% to 80%; grades 3/4: 11% to 67%; nadir: 10-14 days; recovery: 21 days), anemia (13% to 72%; grades 3/4: ≤6%), thrombocytopenia (5% to 49%; grades 3/4: ≤5%)
Local: Injection site reactions (3% to 20%; grades 3/4: <1%)

Ocular: Conjunctivitis (1% to 15%)
Miscellaneous: Infection (15% to 22%; grades 3/4: ≤2%)

1% to 10%:

Cardiovascular: LVEF decreased (asymptomatic; delayed: 1% to 2%), HF (0.4% to 1.5%)
Central nervous system: Fever (1% to 5%)
Dermatologic: Rash (1% to 9%), skin changes (1% to 5%)
Gastrointestinal: Anorexia (2% to 3%)
Hematologic: Neutropenic fever (grades 3/4: ≤6%)

General Dosage Range Dosage adjustment recommended in patients with hepatic or renal impairment or who develop toxicities

I.V.: *Adults:* 100 mg/m² on day 1 every 3 weeks **or** 60 mg/m² on days 1 and 8 every 4 weeks

Mechanism of Action Epirubicin is an anthracycline antineoplastic agent; known to inhibit DNA and RNA synthesis by steric obstruction after intercalating between DNA base pairs; active throughout entire cell cycle. Intercalation triggers DNA cleavage by topoisomerase II, resulting in cytocidal activity. Also inhibits DNA helicase, and generates cytotoxic free radicals.

Pharmacodynamics/Kinetics

Half-life Elimination Triphasic; Mean terminal: 33 hours

Pregnancy Risk Factor D

Eplerenone (e PLER en one)

Related Information

Cardiovascular Diseases *on page 1848*

U.S. Brand Names Inspra™

Pharmacologic Category Diuretic, Potassium-Sparing; Selective Aldosterone Blocker

Use Treatment of hypertension (may be used alone or in combination with other antihypertensive agents); treatment of heart failure (HF) following acute MI

Local Anesthetic/Vasoconstrictor Precautions No information available to require special precautions

Effects on Dental Treatment No significant effects or complications reported

Effects on Bleeding No information available to require special precautions

Adverse Effects

>10%: Endocrine & metabolic: Hyperkalemia ([HF post-MI: K >5.5 mEq/L: 16%; K ≥6 mEq/L: 6%] [HTN: K >5.5 mEq/L at doses ≤100 mg: ≤1%; doses >100 mg: 9%]), hypertriglyceridemia (1% to 15%, dose related)

1% to 10%:

Central nervous system: Dizziness (3%), fatigue (2%)
Endocrine & metabolic: Hyponatremia (2%, dose related), breast pain (males <1% to 1%), gynecomastia (males <1% to 1%), hypercholesterolemia (<1% to 1%)
Gastrointestinal: Diarrhea (2%), abdominal pain (1%)
Genitourinary: Abnormal vaginal bleeding (<1% to 2%)
Renal: Creatinine increased (HF post-MI: 6%), albuminuria (1%)
Respiratory: Cough (2%)
Miscellaneous: Flu-like syndrome (2%)

General Dosage Range Dosage adjustment recommended in patients on concomitant therapy or based on potassium concentrations

Oral: *Adults:* Initial: 25-50 mg once daily; Maintenance: 50 mg once or twice daily (maximum: 100 mg/day)

Mechanism of Action Aldosterone, a mineralocorticoid, increases blood pressure primarily by inducing sodium and water retention. Overexpression of aldosterone is thought to contribute to myocardial fibrosis (especially following myocardial infarction) and vascular fibrosis. Mineralocorticoid receptors are located in the kidney, heart, blood vessels, and brain. Eplerenone selectively blocks mineralocorticoid receptors reducing blood pressure in a dose-dependent manner and appears to prevent myocardial and vascular fibrosis.

Pharmacodynamics/Kinetics

Half-life Elimination 4-6 hours

Time to Peak Plasma: ~1.5 hours; may take up to 4 weeks for full antihypertensive effect

Pregnancy Risk Factor B

Epoetin Alfa (e POE e tin AL fa)

U.S. Brand Names Epogen®; Procrit®

Canadian Brand Names Eprex®

Pharmacologic Category Colony Stimulating Factor

Use Treatment of anemia (elevate or maintain red blood cell level and decrease the need for transfusions) associated with HIV (zidovudine) therapy, chronic renal failure (including patients on dialysis and not on dialysis); reduction of allogeneic blood transfusion for elective, noncardiac, nonvascular surgery; treatment of anemia due to concurrent chemotherapy in patients with metastatic cancer (nonmyeloid malignancies) receiving chemotherapy for a minimum of 2 months

Note: Erythropoietin is **not** indicated for use in cancer patients under the following conditions:

- receiving hormonal therapy, therapeutic biologic products, or radiation therapy unless also receiving concurrent myelosuppressive chemotherapy
- receiving myelosuppressive therapy when the expected outcome is curative
- anemia due to other factors (eg, iron deficiency, folate deficiency, or gastrointestinal bleed)

Not intended for patients who require immediate correction of severe anemia or as a substitute for emergency transfusion.

Unlabeled/Investigational Use Treatment of anemia associated with critical illness; anemia of prematurity; symptomatic anemia in myelodysplastic syndrome (MDS)

Local Anesthetic/Vasoconstrictor Precautions No information available to require special precautions

Effects on Dental Treatment No significant effects or complications reported

Effects on Bleeding Although ESAs have been associated with thromboembolic events, there is no information available to require special precautions for dental procedures.

Adverse Effects

>10%:

Cardiovascular: Hypertension (5% to 24%), thrombotic/vascular events (coronary artery bypass graft surgery: 23%), edema (6% to 17%), deep vein thrombosis (≤11%)

Central nervous system: Fever (29% to 51%), dizziness (5% to 21%), insomnia (13% to 21%), headache (10% to 19%)

Dermatologic: Pruritus (14% to 22%), skin pain (4% to 18%), rash (≤16%)

Gastrointestinal: Nausea (11% to 58%), constipation (42% to 53%), vomiting (8% to 29%), diarrhea (6% to 21%), dyspepsia (7% to 11%)

Genitourinary: Urinary tract infection (3% to 12%)

Local: Injection site reaction (<10% to 29%)

Neuromuscular & skeletal: Arthralgia (≤11%), paresthesia (≤11%)

Respiratory: Cough (≤18%), congestion (≤15%), dyspnea (13% to 14%), upper respiratory infection (≤11%)

1% to 10%:

Central nervous system: Seizure (1% to 3%)

Local: Clotted vascular access (7%)

General Dosage Range

I.V.:

Children: Initial: 50 units/kg 3 times/week; Maintenance: 50-400 units/kg 1-3 times/week **or** 600 units/kg once weekly (maximum: 40,000 units)

Adults: Initial: 50-100 units/kg 3 times/week; Maintenance: 75-150 units/kg/week **or** 100-300 units/kg 3 times/week

SubQ:

Children: Initial: 50 units/kg 3 times/week; Maintenance: 50-400 units/kg 1-3 times/week

Adults: Dosage varies greatly depending on indication

Mechanism of Action Induces erythropoiesis by stimulating the division and differentiation of committed erythroid progenitor cells; induces the release of reticulocytes from the bone marrow into the bloodstream, where they mature to erythrocytes. There is a dose response relationship with this effect. This results in an increase in reticulocyte counts followed by a rise in hematocrit and hemoglobin levels.

Pharmacodynamics/Kinetics

Onset of Action Several days; Peak effect: Hemoglobin level: 2-6 weeks

Half-life Elimination Cancer: SubQ: 16-67 hours; Chronic renal failure: I.V.: 4-13 hours

Time to Peak Serum: Chronic renal failure: SubQ: 5-24 hours

Pregnancy Risk Factor C

Prescribing and Access Restrictions As a requirement of the REMS program, access to this medication is restricted. Healthcare providers and hospitals must be enrolled in the ESA APPRISE (Assisting Providers and Cancer Patients with Risk Information for the Safe use of ESAs) Oncology Program (866-284-8089; http://www.esa-apprise.com) to prescribe or dispense ESAs (ie, epoetin alfa, darbepoetin alfa) to patients with cancer.

Epoprostenol (e poe PROST en ole)

U.S. Brand Names Flolan®; Veletri®

Canadian Brand Names Flolan®

Pharmacologic Category Prostacyclin; Prostaglandin; Vasodilator

Use Treatment of idiopathic pulmonary arterial hypertension (IPAH); pulmonary hypertension associated with the scleroderma spectrum of disease (SSD) in NYHA Class III and Class IV patients who do not respond adequately to conventional therapy

Unlabeled/Investigational Use Acute vasodilator testing in pulmonary arterial hypertension (PAH)

Inhalation: Intraoperative treatment of pulmonary hypertension in patients undergoing cardiac surgery with cardiopulmonary bypass; post-cardiothoracic surgery pulmonary hypertension, right ventricular dysfunction, or refractory hypoxemia

Local Anesthetic/Vasoconstrictor Precautions No information available to require special precautions

Effects on Dental Treatment No significant effects or complications reported. Epoprostenol is an inhibitor of platelet aggregation and may enhance the risk of bleeding with other antiplatelet agents (such as aspirin and/or NSAIDs).

Effects on Bleeding Epoprostenol is an inhibitor of platelet aggregation and may prolong bleeding times.

Adverse Effects Note: Adverse events reported during dose initiation and escalation include flushing (58%), headache (49%), nausea/vomiting (32%), hypotension (16%), anxiety/nervousness/agitation (11%), chest pain (11%), dizziness, abdominal pain, bradycardia, musculoskeletal pain, dyspnea, back pain, diaphoresis, dyspepsia, hypoesthesia/paresthesia, and tachycardia are also reported. The following adverse events have been reported during chronic administration for IPAH. Although some may be related to the underlying disease state, anxiety, diarrhea, flu-like syndrome, flushing, headache, jaw pain, nausea, nervousness, and vomiting are clearly contributed to epoprostenol.

>10%:

- Cardiovascular: Chest pain (52% to 67%), palpitation (63%), tachycardia (35% to 43%), flushing (23% to 42%), arrhythmia (27%), bradycardia (15%), hypotension (13%)
- Central nervous system: Dizziness (83%), headache (46% to 83%), chills/fever/sepsis/flu-like syndrome (13% to 25%), anxiety/nervousness/tremor (7% to 21%), depression/depression psychotic (13%)
- Dermatologic: Skin ulcer (39%), eczema/rash/urticaria (25%)
- Gastrointestinal: Nausea/vomiting (41% to 67%), anorexia (66%), diarrhea (37% to 50%), weight loss (27%)
- Hematologic: Hemorrhage (11% to 19%)
- Hepatic: Ascites (23%)
- Local: Injection site reactions: Infection (21%), pain (13%)
- Neuromuscular & skeletal: Weakness (87% to 100%), pain/neck pain/arthralgia (84%), jaw pain (54% to 75%), arthritis (52%), myalgia (44%), musculoskeletal pain (35%; predominantly involving legs and feet), back pain (13%), hypoesthesia/hyperparesthesia/paresthesia (5% to 12%)
- Respiratory: Dyspnea (90%)
- Miscellaneous: Diaphoresis (41%)

1% to 10%:

- Cardiovascular: Supraventricular tachycardia (8%), cerebrovascular accident (4%), MI (4%)
- Central nervous system: Insomnia (9%), seizure (4%), somnolence (4%)
- Dermatologic: Rash (10%), pruritus (4%)
- Endocrine & metabolic: Hypokalemia (6%), hyperkalemia (4%)
- Gastrointestinal: Abdominal pain (14%), constipation (4% to 6%), weight gain (6%), flatulence (5%), abdominal enlargement (4%)
- Genitourinary: Urinary tract infection (7%)
- Hematologic: Thrombocytopenia (4%)
- Ocular: Amblyopia (8%), vision abnormality (4%)
- Renal: Hematuria (5%)
- Respiratory: Epistaxis (4% to 9%), pleural effusion (4% to 7%), pharyngitis (5%), pneumonia (5%), pneumothorax (4%), pulmonary edema (4%)

General Dosage Range I.V.: *Adults:* Initial: 1-2 ng/kg/minute; increase dose in increments of 1-2 ng/kg/minute every 15 minutes until response

Mechanism of Action Epoprostenol is also known as prostacyclin and PGI_2. It is a strong vasodilator of all vascular beds. In addition, it is a potent endogenous inhibitor of platelet aggregation. The reduction in platelet aggregation results from epoprostenol's activation of intracellular adenylate cyclase and the resultant increase in cyclic adenosine monophosphate concentrations within the platelets. Additionally, it is capable of decreasing thrombogenesis and platelet clumping in the lungs by inhibiting platelet aggregation.

Pharmacodynamics/Kinetics

Half-life Elimination 6 minutes

Pregnancy Risk Factor B

Prescribing and Access Restrictions Orders for epoprostenol are distributed by two sources in the United States. Information on orders or reimbursement assistance may be obtained from either Accredo Health, Inc (1-800-935-6526) or TheraCom, Inc (1-877-356-5264).

Eprosartan (ep roe SAR tan)

Related Information

Cardiovascular Diseases *on page 1848*

U.S. Brand Names Teveten®

Canadian Brand Names Teveten®

Generic Availability (U.S.) No

Pharmacologic Category Angiotensin II Receptor Blocker

Use Treatment of hypertension; may be used alone or in combination with other antihypertensives

Local Anesthetic/Vasoconstrictor Precautions No information available to require special precautions

Effects on Dental Treatment No significant effects or complications reported

Effects on Bleeding No information available to require special precautions

Adverse Effects 1% to 10%:

Central nervous system: Fatigue (2%), depression (1%)

Endocrine & metabolic: Hypertriglyceridemia (1%)

Gastrointestinal: Abdominal pain (2%)

Genitourinary: Urinary tract infection (1%)

Respiratory: Upper respiratory tract infection (8%), rhinitis (4%), pharyngitis (4%), cough (4%)

Miscellaneous: Viral infection (2%), injury (2%)

Dosage Adults: Oral: Dosage must be individualized; can administer once or twice daily with total daily doses of 400-800 mg. Usual starting dose is 600 mg once daily as monotherapy in patients who are euvolemic. Limited clinical experience with doses >800 mg.

Dosage adjustment in renal impairment: No starting dosage adjustment is necessary; however, carefully monitor the patient

Dosage adjustment in hepatic impairment: No starting dosage adjustment is necessary; however, carefully monitor the patient

Elderly: No starting dosage adjustment is necessary; however, carefully monitor the patient

Mechanism of Action Angiotensin II is formed from angiotensin I in a reaction catalyzed by angiotensin-converting enzyme (ACE, kininase II). Angiotensin II is the principal pressor agent of the renin-angiotensin system, with effects that include vasoconstriction, stimulation of synthesis and release of aldosterone, cardiac stimulation, and renal reabsorption of sodium. Eprosartan blocks the vasoconstrictor and aldosterone-secreting effects of angiotensin II by selectively blocking the binding of angiotensin II to the AT1 receptor in many tissues, such as vascular smooth muscle and the adrenal gland. Its action is therefore independent of the pathways for angiotensin II synthesis. Blockade of the renin-angiotensin system with ACE inhibitors, which inhibit the biosynthesis of angiotensin II from angiotensin I, is widely used in the treatment of hypertension. ACE inhibitors also inhibit the degradation of bradykinin, a reaction also catalyzed by ACE. Because eprosartan does not inhibit ACE (kininase II), it does not affect the response to bradykinin. Whether this difference has clinical relevance is not yet known. Eprosartan does not bind to or block other hormone receptors or ion channels known to be important in cardiovascular regulation.

Contraindications Hypersensitivity to eprosartan or any component of the formulation

Warnings/Precautions [U.S. Boxed Warning]: Based on human data, drugs that act on the angiotensin system can cause injury and death to the developing fetus when used in the second and third trimesters. Angiotensin receptor blockers should be discontinued as soon as possible once pregnancy is detected. May cause hyperkalemia; avoid potassium supplementation unless specifically required by healthcare provider. Avoid use or use a smaller dose in patients who are volume depleted; correct depletion first. May be associated with deterioration of renal function and/or increases in serum creatinine, particularly in patients with low renal blood flow (eg, renal artery stenosis, heart failure) whose glomerular filtration rate (GFR) is dependent on efferent arteriolar vasoconstriction by angiotensin II. Use with caution in unstented unilateral/bilateral renal artery stenosis. When unstented bilateral renal artery stenosis is present, use is generally avoided due to the elevated risk of deterioration in renal function unless possible benefits outweigh risks. Use with caution in pre-existing renal insufficiency; significant aortic/mitral stenosis. Concurrent use of ACE inhibitors may increase the risk of clinically-significant adverse events (eg, renal dysfunction, hyperkalemia).

Drug Interactions

Metabolism/Transport Effects Inhibits CYP2C9 (weak)

Avoid Concomitant Use There are no known interactions where it is recommended to avoid concomitant use.

Increased Effect/Toxicity

Eprosartan may increase the levels/effects of: ACE Inhibitors; Amifostine; Antihypertensives; Hypotensive Agents; Lithium; Nonsteroidal Anti-Inflammatory Agents; Potassium-Sparing Diuretics; RiTUXimab

The levels/effects of Eprosartan may be increased by: Diazoxide; Eplerenone; Herbs (Hypotensive Properties); MAO Inhibitors; Pentoxifylline; Phosphodiesterase 5 Inhibitors; Potassium Salts; Prostacyclin Analogues; Tolvaptan; Trimethoprim

Decreased Effect

The levels/effects of Eprosartan may be decreased by: Herbs (Hypertensive Properties); Methylphenidate; Nonsteroidal Anti-Inflammatory Agents; Yohimbine

Ethanol/Nutrition/Herb Interactions Herb/Nutraceutical: Avoid dong quai if using for hypertension (has estrogenic activity). Avoid ephedra, yohimbe, ginseng (may worsen hypertension). Avoid garlic (may have increased antihypertensive effect).

Pharmacodynamics/Kinetics

Half-life Elimination Terminal: 5-9 hours

Time to Peak Serum: Fasting: 1-2 hours

Pregnancy Risk Factor C (1st trimester); D (2nd and 3rd trimesters)

Lactation Not recommended

Dosage Forms

Tablet, oral:

Teveten®: 400 mg, 600 mg

Eprosartan and Hydrochlorothiazide

(ep roe SAR tan & hye droe klor oh THYE a zide)

Related Information

Eprosartan *on page 613*

Hydrochlorothiazide *on page 854*

U.S. Brand Names Teveten® HCT

Canadian Brand Names Teveten® HCT; Teveten® Plus

Pharmacologic Category Angiotensin II Receptor Blocker; Diuretic, Thiazide

Use Treatment of hypertension (not indicated for initial treatment)

Local Anesthetic/Vasoconstrictor Precautions No information available to require special precautions

Effects on Dental Treatment No significant effects or complications reported

Effects on Bleeding No information available to require special precautions

Adverse Effects Percentages reported with combination product; other reactions have been reported (see individual agents for additional information).

1% to 10%:

Central nervous system: Dizziness (4%), headache (3%), fatigue (2%)
Hematologic: Neutrophil count decreased (1%)
Neuromuscular & skeletal: Back pain (3%)
Renal: BUN increased (1%)

General Dosage Range Oral: *Adults:* Eprosartan 600 mg and hydrochlorothiazide 12.5-25 mg once daily

Mechanism of Action Hydrochlorothiazide inhibits sodium reabsorption in the distal tubules causing increased excretion of sodium and water as well as potassium and hydrogen ions. **Eprosartan** blocks the vasoconstrictor and aldosterone-secreting effects of angiotensin II by selectively blocking the binding of angiotensin II to the AT1 receptor in many tissues, such as vascular smooth muscle and the adrenal gland.

Pregnancy Risk Factor C/D (2nd and 3rd trimesters)

Eptifibatide (ep TIF i ba tide)

Related Information

Cardiovascular Diseases *on page* 1848

U.S. Brand Names Integrilin®

Canadian Brand Names Integrilin®

Pharmacologic Category Antiplatelet Agent, Glycoprotein IIb/IIIa Inhibitor

Use Treatment of patients with acute coronary syndrome (unstable angina/non-Q wave myocardial infarction [UA/NQMI]), including patients who are to be managed medically and those undergoing percutaneous coronary intervention (PCI including angioplasty, intracoronary stenting)

Unlabeled/Investigational Use To support PCI during ST-elevation myocardial infarction (administered at the time of primary PCI)

Local Anesthetic/Vasoconstrictor Precautions No information available to require special precautions

Effects on Dental Treatment Key adverse event(s) related to dental treatment: Bleeding; patients weighing <70 kg may have an increased risk of major bleeding. See Effects on Bleeding.

Effects on Bleeding As with all anticoagulants, bleeding is a potential adverse effect of eptifibatide during dental surgery; risk is dependent on multiple variables, including the intensity of anticoagulation and patient susceptibility. It is unlikely that ambulatory patients presenting for dental treatment will be receiving intravenous anticoagulant therapy.

Adverse Effects Bleeding is the major drug-related adverse effect. Access site is often primary source of bleeding complications. Incidence of bleeding is also related to heparin intensity. Patients weighing <70 kg may have an increased risk of major bleeding.

>10%: Hematologic: Bleeding (major: 1% to 11%; minor: 3% to 14%; transfusion required: 2% to 13%)

1% to 10%:
- Cardiovascular: Hypotension (up to 7%)
- Hematologic: Thrombocytopenia (1% to 3%)
- Local: Injection site reaction

General Dosage Range Dosage adjustment recommended in patients with renal impairment

I.V.: *Adults:* Bolus: 180 mcg/kg (maximum: 22.6 mg), repeat once for PCI; Infusion: 2 mcg/kg/minute (maximum: 15 mg/hour)

Mechanism of Action Eptifibatide is a cyclic heptapeptide which blocks the platelet glycoprotein IIb/IIIa receptor, the binding site for fibrinogen, von Willebrand factor, and other ligands. Inhibition of binding at this final common receptor reversibly blocks platelet aggregation and prevents thrombosis.

Pharmacodynamics/Kinetics

Onset of Action Within 1 hour

Duration of Action Platelet function restored ~4 hours following discontinuation

Half-life Elimination 2.5 hours

Pregnancy Risk Factor B

Ergocalciferol (er goe kal SIF e role)

U.S. Brand Names Calciferol™ [OTC]; Drisdol®; Drisdol® [OTC]

Canadian Brand Names Drisdol®; Ostoforte®

Pharmacologic Category Vitamin D Analog

Use Treatment of refractory rickets, hypophosphatemia, hypoparathyroidism; dietary supplement

Unlabeled/Investigational Use Prevention and treatment of vitamin D deficiency in patients with chronic kidney disease (CKD)

Local Anesthetic/Vasoconstrictor Precautions No information available to require special precautions

Effects on Dental Treatment Key adverse event(s) related to dental treatment: Metallic taste and xerostomia (normal salivary flow resumes upon discontinuation).

Effects on Bleeding No information available to require special precautions

Adverse Effects Frequency not defined: Endocrine & metabolic: Hypervitaminosis D (signs and symptoms include hypercalcemia, resulting in headache, nausea, vomiting, lethargy, confusion, sluggishness, abdominal pain, bone pain, polyuria, polydipsia, weakness, cardiac arrhythmias [eg, QT shortening, sinus tachycardia], soft tissue calcification, calciuria, and nephrocalcinosis)

General Dosage Range Oral: *Children and Adults:* Dosage varies greatly depending on indication

Mechanism of Action Stimulates calcium and phosphate absorption from the small intestine, promotes secretion of calcium from bone to blood; promotes renal tubule phosphate resorption

Pharmacodynamics/Kinetics

Onset of Action Peak effect: ~1 month following daily doses

Pregnancy Risk Factor C (manufacturer); A/C (dose exceeding RDA recommendation; per expert analysis)

Ergoloid Mesylates (ER goe loid MES i lates)

Canadian Brand Names Hydergine®

Pharmacologic Category Ergot Derivative

Use Treatment of cerebrovascular insufficiency in primary progressive dementia, Alzheimer's dementia, and senile onset

Local Anesthetic/Vasoconstrictor Precautions No information available to require special precautions

Effects on Dental Treatment Key adverse event(s) related to dental treatment: Orthostatic hypotension.

Effects on Bleeding No information available to require special precautions

Adverse Effects Adverse effects are minimal; most common include transient nausea, gastrointestinal disturbances and sublingual irritation with SL tablets; other common side effects include:

Cardiovascular: Bradycardia, orthostatic hypotension
Dermatologic: Flushing, skin rash
Ocular: Blurred vision
Respiratory: Nasal congestion

General Dosage Range Oral: *Adults:* Initial: 1 mg 3 times/day; Maintenance: 3-12 mg/day in 3 divided doses

Mechanism of Action Ergoloid mesylates do not have the vasoconstrictor effects of the natural ergot alkaloids; exact mechanism in dementia is unknown; originally classed as peripheral and cerebral vasodilator, now considered a "metabolic enhancer"; there is no specific evidence which clearly establishes the mechanism by which ergoloid mesylate preparations produce mental effects, nor is there conclusive evidence that the drug particularly affects cerebral arteriosclerosis or cerebrovascular insufficiency

Pharmacodynamics/Kinetics

Half-life Elimination Serum: 3.5 hours

Time to Peak Serum: ~1 hour

Pregnancy Risk Factor C

Ergotamine (er GOT a meen)

U.S. Brand Names Ergomar®

Pharmacologic Category Antimigraine Agent; Ergot Derivative

Use Abort or prevent vascular headaches, such as migraine, migraine variants, or so-called "histaminic cephalalgia"

Local Anesthetic/Vasoconstrictor Precautions No information available to require special precautions

Effects on Dental Treatment No significant effects or complications reported

Effects on Bleeding Rare but significant events related to hemorrhage (cerebral hemorrhage, subarachnoid hemorrhage, and stroke) have occurred following injection of some agents in this class. However, there is no information related to special precautions associated with bleeding related to dental procedures.

Adverse Effects Frequency not defined.

Cardiovascular: Absence of pulse, bradycardia, cardiac valvular fibrosis, cyanosis, edema, ECG changes, gangrene, hypertension, ischemia, precordial distress and pain, tachycardia, vasospasm
Central nervous system: Vertigo
Dermatologic: Itching
Gastrointestinal: Nausea, vomiting
Genitourinary: Retroperitoneal fibrosis
Neuromuscular & skeletal: Muscle pain, numbness, paresthesia, weakness
Respiratory: Pleuropulmonary fibrosis
Miscellaneous: Cold extremities

General Dosage Range

Sublingual: *Adults:* 1 tablet initially, then 1 tablet every 30 minutes if needed (maximum: 3 tablets/day; 5 tablets/week)

Mechanism of Action Has partial agonist and/or antagonist activity against tryptaminergic, dopaminergic and alpha-adrenergic receptors depending upon their site; is a highly active uterine stimulant; it causes constriction of peripheral and cranial blood vessels and produces depression of central vasomotor centers

Pharmacodynamics/Kinetics

Half-life Elimination 2 hours

Time to Peak Serum: 0.5-3 hours

Pregnancy Risk Factor X

Ergotamine and Caffeine (er GOT a meen & KAF een)

Related Information

Caffeine *on page 282*

Ergotamine *on page 616*

U.S. Brand Names Cafergot®; Migergot

Canadian Brand Names Cafergor®

Pharmacologic Category Antimigraine Agent; Ergot Derivative; Stimulant

Use Abort or prevent vascular headaches, such as migraine, migraine variants, or so-called "histaminic cephalalgia"

Local Anesthetic/Vasoconstrictor Precautions No information available to require special precautions

Effects on Dental Treatment No significant effects or complications reported

Effects on Bleeding Rare but significant events related to hemorrhage (cerebral hemorrhage, subarachnoid hemorrhage, and stroke) have occurred following injection of some agents in this class. However, there is no information related to special precautions associated with bleeding related to dental procedures.

Adverse Effects Frequency not defined.

Cardiovascular: Absence of pulse, bradycardia, cardiac valvular fibrosis, cyanosis, edema, ECG changes, gangrene, hypertension, ischemia, precordial distress and pain, tachycardia, vasospasm

Central nervous system: Vertigo

Dermatologic: Itching

Gastrointestinal: Anal or rectal ulcer (with overuse of suppository), nausea, vomiting

Genitourinary: Retroperitoneal fibrosis

Neuromuscular & skeletal: Muscle pain, numbness, paresthesia, weakness

Respiratory: Pleuropulmonary fibrosis

Miscellaneous: Cold extremities

General Dosage Range

Oral: *Adults:* 2 tablets initially, then 1 tablet every 30 minutes as needed (maximum: 6 tablets/attack; 10 tablets/week)

Rectal: *Adults:* 1 suppository initially; may repeat after 1 hour if needed (maximum: 2 doses/attack; 5 doses/week)

Mechanism of Action Has partial agonist and/or antagonist activity against tryptaminergic, dopaminergic and alpha-adrenergic receptors depending upon their site; is a highly active uterine stimulant; it causes constriction of peripheral and cranial blood vessels and produces depression of central vasomotor centers

Pharmacodynamics/Kinetics

Half-life Elimination 2 hours

Time to Peak Serum: Ergotamine: 0.5-3 hours

Pregnancy Risk Factor X

Eribulin (er i BUE lin)

U.S. Brand Names Halaven™

Pharmacologic Category Antineoplastic Agent, Antimicrotubular

Use Treatment of metastatic breast cancer in patients who have received at least 2 prior chemotherapy regimens

Local Anesthetic/Vasoconstrictor Precautions No information available to require special precautions

Effects on Dental Treatment Key adverse event(s) related to dental treatment: Xerostomia (normal salivary flow resumes upon discontinuation), stomatitis, mucosal inflammation, or taste alteration.

Effects on Bleeding Chemotherapy may result in significant myelosuppression, potentially including significant reduction in platelet counts and altered hemostasis. In patients who are under active treatment with these agents, medical consult is suggested.

Adverse Effects

>10%:

Central nervous system: Central nervous system: Fatigue (54%), fever (21%), headache (19%)

Dermatologic: Alopecia (45%)

Gastrointestinal: Nausea (35%), stomatitis (5% to 18%), constipation (25%), weight loss (21%), anorexia (20%), diarrhea (18%), vomiting (18%)

Hematologic: Neutropenia (82%; grades 3: 28%; grade 4: 29%; nadir: 13 days; recovery: 8 days), anemia (58%; grades 3/4: 2%)

Hepatic: ALT increased (18%)

Neuromuscular & skeletal: Weakness (54%), peripheral neuropathy (35%; grades 3/4: ≤8%), arthralgia/myalgia (22%), back pain (16%), bone pain (12%), limb pain (11%)

Respiratory: Dyspnea (16%), cough (14%)

1% to 10%:

Cardiovascular: Peripheral edema

Central nervous system: Depression, dizziness, insomnia

Dermatologic: Rash

Endocrine & metabolic: Hypokalemia

Gastrointestinal: Mucosal inflammation (9%), abdominal pain, dyspepsia, taste alteration, xerostomia

Genitourinary: Urinary tract infection (10%)

Hematologic: Neutropenic fever (5%), thrombocytopenia (grades 3/4: 1%)

Neuromuscular & skeletal: Muscle spasm

Ocular: Lacrimation increased

Respiratory: Upper respiratory infection

General Dosage Range Dosage adjustment recommended in patients with renal or hepatic impairment or who develop toxicities

I.V.: *Adults:* 1.4 mg/m^2/dose days 1 and 8 every 3 weeks

Mechanism of Action Eribulin is a non-taxane microtubule inhibitor which is a halichondrin B analog. It inhibits the growth phase of the microtubule by inhibiting formation of mitotic spindles causing mitotic blockage and arresting the cell cycle at the G_2/M phase; suppresses microtubule polymerization yet does not affect depolymerization.

Pharmacodynamics/Kinetics

Half-life Elimination ~40 hours

Pregnancy Risk Factor D

Erlotinib (er LOE tye nib)

U.S. Brand Names Tarceva®

Canadian Brand Names Tarceva®

Pharmacologic Category Antineoplastic Agent, Tyrosine Kinase Inhibitor; Epidermal Growth Factor Receptor (EGFR) Inhibitor

Use Treatment of locally advanced or metastatic nonsmall cell lung cancer (NSCLC) refractory to at least 1 prior chemotherapy regimen (as monotherapy); maintenance treatment of locally advanced or metastatic NCSLC which has not progressed after 4-6 cycles of first line platinum-based chemotherapy; locally advanced, unresectable or metastatic pancreatic cancer (first-line therapy in combination with gemcitabine)

Unlabeled/Investigational Use First-line treatment of NSCLC with known EGFR mutation; treatment of head and neck cancer

Local Anesthetic/Vasoconstrictor Precautions No information available to require special precautions

Effects on Dental Treatment Key adverse event(s) related to dental treatment: Xerostomia (normal salivary flow resumes upon discontinuation), mucositis, abnormal taste, and stomatitis.

Effects on Bleeding Although significant myelosuppression with associated altered hemostasis has been reported for many chemotherapeutic agents, myelosuppression is not common with erlotinib and no specific precautions appear to necessary.

Adverse Effects

Adverse reactions reported with monotherapy:

>10%:

Central nervous system: Fatigue (9% to 52%)

Dermatologic: Rash (49% to 75%; grade 3: 6% to 8%; grade 4: <1%; median onset: 8 days), pruritus (7% to 13%), dry skin (4% to 12%)

Gastrointestinal: Diarrhea (20% to 54%; grade 3: 2% to 6%; grade 4: <1%; median onset: 12 days), anorexia (9% to 52%), nausea (33%), vomiting (23%), stomatitis (17%), abdominal pain (11%)

Ocular: Conjunctivitis (12%), keratoconjunctivitis sicca (12%)

Respiratory: Dyspnea (41%), cough (33%)

Miscellaneous: Infection (24%)
1% to 10%:
Dermatologic: Acne (6%), dermatitis acneiform (5%), paronychia (4%)
Gastrointestinal: Weight loss (4%)
Hepatic: ALT increased (grade 2: 2% to 4%; grade 3: 1%), hyperbilirubinemia (grade 2: 4%; grade 3: <1%)
Respiratory: Pneumonitis/pulmonary infiltrate (3%), pulmonary fibrosis (3%)

Adverse reactions reported with combination (erlotinib plus gemcitabine) therapy:
Cardiovascular: Edema (37%), thrombotic events (grades 3/4: 11%), deep venous thrombosis (4%), cerebrovascular accident (2%; including cerebral hemorrhage), MI/myocardial ischemia (2%), arrhythmia, syncope
Central nervous system: Fatigue (79%), fever (36%), depression (19%), dizziness (15%), headache (15%), anxiety (13%)
Dermatologic: Rash (69%), alopecia (14%)
Gastrointestinal: Nausea (60%), anorexia (52%), diarrhea (48%), abdominal pain (46%), vomiting (42%), weight loss (39%), stomatitis (22%), dyspepsia (17%), flatulence (13%), ileus, pancreatitis
Hematologic: Hemolytic anemia, microangiopathic hemolytic anemia with thrombocytopenia (1%)
Hepatic: ALT increased (grade 2: 31%, grade 3: 13%, grade 4: <1%), AST increased (grade 2: 24%, grade 3: 10%, grade 4 <1%), hyperbilirubinemia (grade 2: 17%, grade 3: 10%, grade 4: <1%)
Neuromuscular & skeletal: Bone pain (25%), myalgia (21%), neuropathy (13%), rigors (12%)
Renal: Renal insufficiency
Respiratory: Dyspnea (24%), cough (16%), interstitial lung disease (ILD)-like events (3%)
Miscellaneous: Infection (39%)

General Dosage Range Dosage adjustment recommended in patients with hepatic impairment, on concomitant therapy, who smoke, or who develop toxicities
Oral: *Adults:* 100-150 mg/day

Mechanism of Action The mechanism of erlotinib's antitumor action is not fully characterized. It is known to inhibit overall epidermal growth factor receptor (HER1/EGFR) - tyrosine kinase. Active competitive inhibition of adenosine triphosphate inhibits downstream signal transduction of ligand dependent HER1/EGFR activation.

Pharmacodynamics/Kinetics
Half-life Elimination 24-36 hours
Time to Peak Plasma: 1-7 hours

Pregnancy Risk Factor D

Ertapenem (er ta PEN em)

U.S. Brand Names INVanz®
Canadian Brand Names Invanz®
Pharmacologic Category Antibiotic, Carbapenem

Use Treatment of the following moderate-severe infections: Complicated intra-abdominal infections, complicated skin and skin structure infections (including diabetic foot infections without osteomyelitis), complicated UTI (including pyelonephritis), acute pelvic infections (including postpartum endomyometritis, septic abortion, post surgical gynecologic infections), and community-acquired pneumonia. Prophylaxis of surgical site infection following elective colorectal surgery. Antibacterial coverage includes aerobic gram-positive organisms, aerobic gram-negative organisms, anaerobic organisms.

Note: Methicillin-resistant *Staphylococcus*, *Enterococcus* spp, penicillin-resistant strains of *Streptococcus pneumoniae*, beta-lactamase-positive strains of *Haemophilus influenzae* are **resistant** to ertapenem, as are most *Pseudomonas aeruginosa*.

Local Anesthetic/Vasoconstrictor Precautions No information available to require special precautions

Effects on Dental Treatment Key adverse event(s) related to dental treatment: Oral candidiasis

Effects on Bleeding No information available to require special precautions

Adverse Effects Note: Percentages reported in adults.
1% to 10%:
Cardiovascular: Edema (3%), chest pain (1% to 2%), hypertension (1% to 2%), hypotension (1% to 2%), tachycardia (1% to 2%)

Central nervous system: Headache (6% to 7%); altered mental status (eg, agitation, confusion, disorientation, decreased mental acuity, changed mental status, somnolence, stupor) (3% to 5%); fever (2% to 5%), insomnia (3%), dizziness (2%), fatigue (1%), anxiety (1%)
Dermatologic: Rash (2% to 3%), pruritus (1% to 2%), erythema (1% to 2%)
Endocrine & metabolic: Hypokalemia (2%), hyperglycemia (1% to 2%), hyperkalemia (≤1%)
Gastrointestinal: Diarrhea (9% to 10%), nausea (6% to 9%), abdominal pain (4%), vomiting (4%), constipation (3% to 4%), acid regurgitation (1% to 2%), dyspepsia (1%), oral candidiasis (≤1%)
Genitourinary: Urine WBCs increased (2% to 3%), urine RBCs increased (1% to 3%), vaginitis (1% to 3%)
Hematologic: Thrombocytosis (4% to 7%), hematocrit/hemoglobin decreased (3% to 5%), eosinophils increased (1% to 2%), leukopenia (1% to 2%), neutrophils decreased (1% to 2%), thrombocytopenia (1%), prothrombin time increased (≤1%)
Hepatic: Hepatic enzyme increased (7% to 9%), alkaline phosphatase increase (4% to 7%), albumin decreased (1% to 2%), bilirubin (total) increased (1% to 2%)
Local: Infused vein complications (5% to 7%), phlebitis/thrombophlebitis (2%), extravasation (1% to 2%)
Neuromuscular & skeletal: Weakness (1%), leg pain (≤1%)
Renal: Serum creatinine increased (1%)
Respiratory: Dyspnea (1% to 3%), cough (1% to 2%), pharyngitis (1%), rales/rhonchi (1%), respiratory distress (≤1%)

General Dosage Range Dosage adjustment recommended in patients with renal impairment

I.M., I.V.:

Children 3 months to 12 years: 15 mg/kg twice daily (maximum: 1 g/day)
Adolescents ≥13 years and Adults: 1 g once daily or as single dose

Mechanism of Action Inhibits bacterial cell wall synthesis by binding to one or more of the penicillin-binding proteins; which in turn inhibits the final transpeptidation step of peptidoglycan synthesis in bacterial cell walls, thus inhibiting cell wall biosynthesis. Bacteria eventually lyse due to ongoing activity of cell wall autolytic enzymes (autolysins and murein hydrolases) while cell wall assembly is arrested.

Pharmacodynamics/Kinetics

Half-life Elimination

Children 3 months to 12 years: ~2.5 hours
Children ≥13 years and Adults: ~4 hours

Time to Peak I.M.: ~2.3 hours

Pregnancy Risk Factor B

Erythromycin (Systemic) (er ith roe MYE sin)

Related Information

Bacterial Infections *on page 1933*
Cardiovascular Diseases *on page 1848*
Clinical Risk Related to Drugs Prolonging QT Interval *on page 1872*
Respiratory Diseases *on page 1876*

Related Sample Prescriptions

Bacterial Infections and Periodontal Diseases *on page 1983*

U.S. Brand Names E.E.S.®; Ery-Tab®; EryPed®; Erythro-RX; Erythrocin®; Erythrocin® Lactobionate-I.V.; PCE®

Canadian Brand Names Apo-Erythro Base®; Apo-Erythro E-C®; Apo-Erythro-ES®; Apo-Erythro-S®; EES®; Erybid™; Eryc®; Novo-Rythro Estolate; Novo-Rythro Ethylsuccinate; Nu-Erythromycin-S; PCE®

Generic Availability (U.S.) Yes: Capsule, tablet (as base, ethylsuccinate, and stearate)

Pharmacologic Category Antibiotic, Macrolide

Dental Use Alternative to penicillin VK for treatment of orofacial infections

Use Treatment of susceptible bacterial infections including *S. pyogenes*, some *S. pneumoniae*, some *S. aureus*, *M. pneumoniae*, *Legionella pneumophila*, diphtheria, pertussis, *Chlamydia*, erythrasma, *N. gonorrhoeae*, *E. histolytica*, syphilis and nongonococcal urethritis, and *Campylobacter* gastroenteritis; used in conjunction with neomycin for decontaminating the bowel

Unlabeled/Investigational Use Treatment of gastroparesis, chancroid; preoperative gut sterilization

Local Anesthetic/Vasoconstrictor Precautions Erythromycin is one of the drugs confirmed to prolong the QT interval and is accepted as having a risk of causing torsade de pointes. In terms of epinephrine, it is not known what effect vasoconstrictors in the local anesthetic regimen will have in patients with a known history of congenital prolonged QT interval or in patients taking any medication that prolongs the QT interval. Until more information is obtained, it is suggested that the clinician consult with the physician prior to the use of a vasoconstrictor in suspected patients, and that the vasoconstrictor (epinephrine, mepivacaine and levonordefrin [Carbocaine® 2% with Neo-Cobefrin®]) be used with caution. See Dental Comment.

Effects on Dental Treatment Key adverse event(s) related to dental treatment: Oral candidiasis.

Effects on Bleeding No information available to require special precautions

Adverse Effects Frequency not defined. Incidence may vary with formulation.

Cardiovascular: QT_c prolongation, torsade de pointes, ventricular arrhythmia, ventricular tachycardia

Central nervous system: Seizure

Dermatitis: Pruritus, rash

Gastrointestinal: Abdominal pain, anorexia, diarrhea, infantile hypertrophic pyloric stenosis, nausea, oral candidiasis, pancreatitis, pseudomembranous colitis, vomiting

Hepatic: Cholestatic jaundice (most common with estolate), hepatitis, liver function tests abnormal

Local: Phlebitis at the injection site, thrombophlebitis

Neuromuscular & skeletal: Weakness

Otic: Hearing loss

Miscellaneous: Allergic reactions, anaphylaxis, hypersensitivity reactions, urticaria

Dental Usual Dosage Treatment of orofacial infections: Adults: Oral:

Base: 250-500 mg every 6-12 hours

Ethylsuccinate: 400-800 mg every 6-12 hours

Dosage Note: Due to differences in absorption, 400 mg erythromycin ethylsuccinate produces the same serum levels as 250 mg erythromycin base or stearate.

Usual dosage range:

Infants and Children:

Oral:

Base: 30-50 mg/kg/day in 2-4 divided doses; maximum: 2 g/day

Ethylsuccinate: 30-50 mg/kg/day in 2-4 divided doses; maximum: 3.2 g/day

Stearate: 30-50 mg/kg/day in 2-4 divided doses; maximum: 2 g/day

I.V.: Lactobionate: 15-50 mg/kg/day divided every 6 hours, not to exceed 4 g/day

Adults:

Oral:

Base: 250-500 mg every 6-12 hours; maximum 4 g/day

Ethylsuccinate: 400-800 mg every 6-12 hours; maximum: 4 g/day

I.V.: Lactobionate: 15-20 mg/kg/day divided every 6 hours or 500 mg to 1 g every 6 hours, or given as a continuous infusion over 24 hours; maximum: 4 g/24 hours

Indication-specific dosing:

Neonates:

Conjunctivitis, neonatal *(C. trachomatis):* Oral: 50 mg/kg/day (base or ethylsuccinate) in 4 divided doses for 14 days

Infants:

Pneumonia *(C. trachomatis):* Oral: 50 mg/kg/day (base or ethylsuccinate) in 4 divided doses for 14 days (CDC, 2010)

Children:

***Bartonella sp* infections (bacillary angiomatosis [BA], peliosis hepatis [PH]) (unlabeled use):** Oral: 40 mg/kg/day (ethylsuccinate) in 4 divided doses (maximum: 2 g/day) for 3 months (BA) or 4 months (PH)

Chlamydial infection *(C. trachomatis):* Children <45 kg: Oral: 50 mg/kg/day (base or ethylsuccinate) in 4 divided doses for 14 days (CDC, 2010)

Mild/moderate infection: Oral: 30-50 mg/kg/day in divided doses every 6-12 hours

Pertussis: Oral: 40-50 mg/kg/day in 4 divided doses for 14 days; maximum 2 g/day (not preferred agent for infants <1 month due to IHPS)

Pharyngitis, tonsillitis (streptococcal): Oral: 20 mg (base)/kg/day or 40 mg (ethylsuccinate)/kg/day in 2 divided doses for 10 days. **Note:** No longer preferred therapy due to increased organism resistance.

Preop bowel preparation: Oral: 20 mg (base)/kg at 1, 2, and 11 PM on the day before surgery combined with mechanical cleansing of the large intestine and oral neomycin

Severe infection: I.V.: 15-50 mg/kg/day; maximum: 4 g/day

Adults:

***Bartonella sp* infections (bacillary angiomatosis [BA], peliosis hepatis [PH]) (unlabeled use):** Oral: 500 mg (base) 4 times/day for 3 months (BA) or 4 months (PH)

Chancroid (unlabeled use): Oral: 500 mg (base) 3 times/day for 7 days; **Note:** Not a preferred agent; isolates with intermediate resistance have been documented (CDC, 2010)

Gastrointestinal prokinetic (unlabeled use): I.V.: 200 mg initially followed by 250 mg (base) orally 3 times/day 30 minutes before meals. Lower dosages have been used in some trials.

Granuloma inguinale (donovanosis) (unlabeled use): Oral: 500 mg (base) 4 times/day for 21 days (CDC, 2010)

Legionnaires' disease: Oral: 1.6-4 g (ethylsuccinate)/day or 1-4 g (base)/day in divided doses for 21 days. **Note:** No longer preferred therapy and only used in nonhospitalized patients.

Lymphogranuloma venereum: Oral: 500 mg (base) 4 times/day for 21 days; **Note:** Preferred therapy for pregnant or lactating women (CDC, 2010)

Nongonococcal urethritis (including coinfection with *C. trachomatis*): Oral: 500 mg (base) 4 times/day for 7 days or 800 mg (ethylsuccinate) 4 times/day for 7 days. **Note:** May use 250 mg (base) or 400 mg (ethylsuccinate) 4 times/day for 14 days if gastrointestinal intolerance.

Pertussis: Oral: 500 mg (base) every 6 hours for 14 days

Preop bowel preparation: Oral: 1 g erythromycin base at 1, 2, and 11 PM on the day before surgery combined with mechanical cleansing of the large intestine and oral neomycin

Dosage adjustment in renal impairment: Dialysis: Slightly dialyzable (5% to 20%); no supplemental dosage necessary in hemo- or peritoneal dialysis or in continuous arteriovenous or venovenous hemofiltration

Mechanism of Action Inhibits RNA-dependent protein synthesis at the chain elongation step; binds to the 50S ribosomal subunit resulting in blockage of transpeptidation

Contraindications Hypersensitivity to erythromycin, any macrolide antibiotics, or any component of the formulation

Concomitant use with pimozide or cisapride

Warnings/Precautions Use caution with hepatic impairment with or without jaundice has occurred, it may be accompanied by malaise, nausea, vomiting, abdominal colic, and fever; discontinue use if these occur. Use caution with other medication relying on CYP3A4 metabolism; high potential for drug interactions exists. Prolonged use may result in fungal or bacterial superinfection, including *C. difficile*-associated diarrhea (CDAD) and pseudomembranous colitis; CDAD has been observed >2 months postantibiotic treatment. Use in infants has been associated with infantile hypertrophic pyloric stenosis (IHPS). Macrolides have been associated with rare QT_c prolongation and ventricular arrhythmias, including torsade de pointes. Use caution in elderly patients, as risk of adverse events may be increased. Use caution in myasthenia gravis patients; erythromycin may aggravate muscular weakness.

Drug Interactions

Metabolism/Transport Effects **Substrate** of CYP2B6 (minor), CYP3A4 (major), P-glycoprotein; **Inhibits** CYP1A2 (weak), CYP3A4 (moderate), P-glycoprotein

Avoid Concomitant Use

Avoid concomitant use of Erythromycin (Systemic) with any of the following: Artemether; BCG; Cisapride; Disopyramide; Dronedarone; Lincosamide Antibiotics; Lumefantrine; Nilotinib; Pimozide; QuiNINE; Silodosin; Tetrabenazine; Thioridazine; Tolvaptan; Topotecan; Toremifene; Vandetanib; Ziprasidone

Increased Effect/Toxicity

Erythromycin (Systemic) may increase the levels/effects of: Alfentanil; Antifungal Agents (Azole Derivatives, Systemic); Antineoplastic Agents (Vinca Alkaloids); Benzodiazepines (metabolized by oxidation); Budesonide (Systemic, Oral Inhalation); BusPIRone; Calcium Channel Blockers; CarBAMazepine; Cardiac Glycosides; Cilostazol; Cisapride; CloZAPine; Colchicine; Corticosteroids (Systemic); CycloSPORINE; CycloSPORINE (Systemic); CYP3A4 Substrates; Dabigatran Etexilate; Disopyramide; Dronedarone; Eletriptan; Eplerenone; Ergot Derivatives; Everolimus; FentaNYL; Fexofenadine; HMG-CoA Reductase Inhibitors; Lurasidone; P-Glycoprotein Substrates; Phosphodiesterase 5 Inhibitors; Pimecrolimus; Pimozide; QTc-Prolonging Agents; QuiNIDine; QuiNINE; Repaglinide; Rifamycin Derivatives; Rivaroxaban; Salmeterol; Saxagliptin; Selective Serotonin Reuptake Inhibitors; Silodosin; Sirolimus; Tacrolimus; Tacrolimus (Systemic); Tacrolimus (Topical); Temsirolimus; Tetrabenazine; Theophylline Derivatives; Thioridazine; Tolvaptan; Topotecan; Toremifene; Vandetanib; Vitamin K Antagonists; Ziprasidone; Zopiclone

The levels/effects of Erythromycin (Systemic) may be increased by: Alfuzosin; Antifungal Agents (Azole Derivatives, Systemic); Artemether; Chloroquine; Ciprofloxacin; Ciprofloxacin (Systemic); Conivaptan; CYP3A4 Inhibitors (Moderate);

CYP3A4 Inhibitors (Strong); Gadobutrol; Lumefantrine; Nilotinib; P-Glycoprotein Inhibitors; QuiNINE

Decreased Effect

Erythromycin (Systemic) may decrease the levels/effects of: BCG; Clopidogrel; Typhoid Vaccine; Zafirlukast

The levels/effects of Erythromycin (Systemic) may be decreased by: CYP3A4 Inducers (Strong); Deferasirox; Etravirine; Herbs (CYP3A4 Inducers); Lincosamide Antibiotics; P-Glycoprotein Inducers; Tocilizumab

Ethanol/Nutrition/Herb Interactions

Ethanol: Avoid ethanol (may decrease absorption of erythromycin or enhance ethanol effects).

Food: Erythromycin serum levels may be altered if taken with food (formulation-dependent).

Herb/Nutraceutical: St John's wort may decrease erythromycin levels.

Dietary Considerations Drug may cause GI upset; may take with food. Some products may contain sodium.

Pharmacodynamics/Kinetics

Half-life Elimination Peak: 1.5-2 hours; End-stage renal disease: 5-6 hours

Time to Peak Serum: Base: 4 hours; Ethylsuccinate: 0.5-2.5 hours; delayed with food due to differences in absorption

Pregnancy Risk Factor B

Lactation Enters breast milk/use caution (AAP considers "compatible"; AAP 2001 update pending)

Breast-Feeding Considerations Erythromycin is excreted in breast milk; therefore, the manufacturer recommends that caution be exercised when administering erythromycin to breast-feeding women.

Due to the low concentrations in human milk, minimal toxicity would be expected in the nursing infant. One case report and a cohort study raise the possibility for a connection with pyloric stenosis in neonates exposed to erythromycin via breast milk and an alternative antibiotic may be preferred for breast-feeding mothers of infants in this age group. Nondose-related effects could include modification of bowel flora.

Dosage Forms

Capsule, delayed release, enteric coated pellets, oral: 250 mg

Granules for suspension, oral:

E.E.S.®: 200 mg/5 mL (100 mL, 200 mL)

Injection, powder for reconstitution:

Erythrocin® Lactobionate-I.V.: 500 mg

Powder, for prescription compounding:

Erythro-RX: USP: 100% (50 g)

Powder for suspension, oral:

EryPed®: 200 mg/5 mL (100 mL); 400 mg/5 mL (100 mL)

Tablet, oral: 250 mg, 400 mg, 500 mg

E.E.S.®: 400 mg

Erythrocin®: 250 mg, 500 mg

Tablet, delayed release, enteric coated, oral:

Ery-Tab®: 250 mg, 333 mg, 500 mg

Tablet, polymer coated particles, oral:

PCE®: 333 mg, 500 mg

Dental Comment Erythromycin is known to prolong the QT interval. The QT interval is measured as the time and distance between the Q point of the QRS complex and the end of the T wave in the ECG tracing. After adjustment for heart rate, the QT interval is defined as prolonged if it is more than 450 msec in men and 460 msec in women. A long QT syndrome was first described in the 1950s and 60s as a congenital syndrome involving QT interval prolongation and syncope and sudden death. Some of the congenital long QT syndromes were characterized by a peculiar electrocardiographic appearance of the QRS complex involving a premature atria beat followed by a pause, then a subsequent sinus beat showing marked QT prolongation and deformity. This type of cardiac arrhythmia was originally termed "torsade de pointes" (translated from the French as "twisting of the points"). Erythromycin is considered as having a risk of causing torsade de pointes. Since it is not known what effect vasoconstrictors in the local anesthetic regimen will have in patients with a known history of congenital prolonged QT interval or in patients taking any medication that prolongs the QT interval, a medical consult is suggested.

Many patients cannot tolerate erythromycin because of abdominal pain and nausea; the mechanism of this adverse effect appears to be the motilin agonistic properties of erythromycin in the GI tract. For these patients, clindamycin is indicated as the alternative antibiotic for treatment of orofacial infections.

HMG-CoA reductase inhibitors, also known as the statins, effectively decrease the hepatic cholesterol biosynthesis resulting in the reduction of blood LDL-cholesterol concentrations. The AUC of atorvastatin (Lipitor®) was increased 33% by erythromycin administration. Combination of erythromycin and lovastatin (Mevacor®) has been associated with rhabdomyolysis (Ayanian, et al). The mechanism of erythromycin is inhibiting the CYP3A4 metabolism of atorvastatin, lovastatin, and cerivastatin. Simvastatin (Zocor®) would likely be affected in a similar manner by the coadministration of erythromycin. Clarithromycin (Biaxin®) may exert a similar effect as erythromycin on atorvastatin, lovastatin, cerivastatin, and simvastatin.

References

American Dental Association Council on Scientific Affairs, "Combating Antibiotic Resistance," *J Am Dent Assoc*, 2004, 135(4):484-7.

Wynn RL and Bergman SA, "Antibiotics and Their Use in the Treatment of Orofacial Infections, Part I and Part II," *Gen Dent*, 1994, 42(5):398-402, 498-502.

Wynn RL, "Current Concepts of the Erythromycins," *Gen Dent*, 1991, 39(6):408, 410-1.

Erythromycin and Benzoyl Peroxide

(er ith roe MYE sin & BEN zoe il per OKS ide)

Related Information

Benzoyl Peroxide *on page 223*

U.S. Brand Names Benzamycin®; Benzamycin® Pak

Pharmacologic Category Acne Products; Topical Skin Product, Acne

Use Topical control of acne vulgaris

Local Anesthetic/Vasoconstrictor Precautions No information available to require special precautions

Effects on Dental Treatment No significant effects or complications reported

Effects on Bleeding No information available to require special precautions

General Dosage Range Topical: *Adolescents ≥12 years and Adults:* Apply twice daily

Pregnancy Risk Factor C

Erythromycin and Sulfisoxazole (er ith roe MYE sin & sul fi SOKS a zole)

Related Information

Erythromycin (Systemic) *on page 620*

U.S. Brand Names E.S.P.®

Canadian Brand Names Pediazole®

Pharmacologic Category Antibiotic, Macrolide; Antibiotic, Macrolide Combination; Antibiotic, Sulfonamide Derivative

Use Treatment of susceptible bacterial infections of the upper and lower respiratory tract, otitis media in children caused by susceptible strains of *Haemophilus influenzae*, and many other infections in patients allergic to penicillin

Local Anesthetic/Vasoconstrictor Precautions No information available to require special precautions

Effects on Dental Treatment Key adverse event(s) related to dental treatment: Oral candidiasis.

Effects on Bleeding No information available to require special precautions

Adverse Effects Frequency not defined.

Cardiovascular: Ventricular arrhythmia,

Central nervous system: Headache, fever

Dermatologic: Rash, Stevens-Johnson syndrome, toxic epidermal necrolysis

Gastrointestinal: Abdominal pain, cramping, nausea, vomiting, oral candidiasis, hypertrophic pyloric stenosis, diarrhea, pseudomembranous colitis

Hematologic: Agranulocytosis, aplastic anemia, eosinophilia

Hepatic: Hepatic necrosis, cholestatic jaundice

Local: Phlebitis at the injection site, thrombophlebitis

Renal: Toxic nephrosis, crystalluria

Miscellaneous: Hypersensitivity reactions

General Dosage Range Dosage adjustment recommended in patients with renal impaiment

Oral:

Children ≥2 months: 50 mg/kg/day erythromycin and 150 mg/kg/day sulfisoxazole in divided doses every 6 hours

Adults: 400 mg erythromycin and 1200 mg sulfisoxazole every 6 hours

Mechanism of Action Erythromycin inhibits bacterial protein synthesis; sulfisoxazole competitively inhibits bacterial synthesis of folic acid from para-aminobenzoic acid

Pregnancy Risk Factor C

Escitalopram (es sye TAL oh pram)

Related Information

Citalopram *on page 392*

Clinical Risk Related to Drugs Prolonging QT Interval *on page 1872*

U.S. Brand Names Lexapro®

Canadian Brand Names Cipralex®

Generic Availability (U.S.) No

Pharmacologic Category Antidepressant, Selective Serotonin Reuptake Inhibitor

Use Treatment of major depressive disorder; generalized anxiety disorders (GAD)

Unlabeled/Investigational Use Treatment of mild dementia-associated agitation in nonpsychotic patients

Local Anesthetic/Vasoconstrictor Precautions Although caution should be used in patients taking tricyclic antidepressants, no interactions have been reported with vasoconstrictors and escitalopram, a nontricyclic antidepressant which acts to increase serotonin; no precautions appear to be needed

Effects on Dental Treatment Key adverse event(s) related to dental treatment: Xerostomia (normal salivary flow resumes upon discontinuation) and toothache. See Effects on Bleeding.

Effects on Bleeding May impair platelet aggregation resulting in increased risk of bleeding events, particularly if used concomitantly with aspirin, NSAIDs, warfarin, or other anticoagulants. Bleeding related to SSRI use has been reported to range from relatively minor bruising and epistaxis to life-threatening hemorrhage. Routine interruption of therapy for most dental procedures is not warranted. In medically complicated patients or extensive oral surgery, the decision to interrupt therapy must be based on the risk to benefit in an individual patient and a medical consult is suggested. If therapy is continued without interruption, the clinician should anticipate the potential for a prolonged bleeding time.

Adverse Effects

>10%:

Central nervous system: Headache (24%), somnolence (6% to 13%), insomnia (9% to 12%)

Gastrointestinal: Nausea (15% to 18%)

Genitourinary: Ejaculation disorder (9% to 14%)

1% to 10%:

Central nervous system: Fatigue (5% to 8%), dizziness (5%), abnormal dreaming (3%), lethargy (3%), yawning (2%)

Endocrine & metabolic: Libido decreased (3% to 7%), anorgasmia (2% to 6%), menstrual disorder (2%)

Gastrointestinal: Xerostomia (6% to 9%), diarrhea (8%), constipation (3% to 5%), appetite decreased (3%), indigestion (3%), vomiting (3%), abdominal pain (2%), flatulence (2%), toothache (2%)

Genitourinary: Impotence (2% to 3%)

Neuromuscular & skeletal: Neck/shoulder pain (3%), paresthesia (2%)

Respiratory: Rhinitis (5%), sinusitis (3%)

Miscellaneous: Diaphoresis (4% to 5%), flu-like syndrome (5%)

Dosage Oral:

Children ≥12 years: Major depressive disorder: Initial: 10 mg once daily; dose may be increased to 20 mg once daily after at least 3 weeks

Adults: Major depressive disorder, generalized anxiety disorder: Initial: 10 mg once daily; dose may be increased to 20 mg once daily after at least 1 week

Elderly: 10 mg once daily

Dosage adjustment in renal impairment:

Mild-to-moderate impairment: No dosage adjustment needed

Severe impairment: Cl_{cr} <20 mL/minute: Use with caution

Dosage adjustment in hepatic impairment: 10 mg once daily

Mechanism of Action Escitalopram is the S-enantiomer of the racemic derivative citalopram, which selectively inhibits the reuptake of serotonin with little to no effect on norepinephrine or dopamine reuptake. It has no or very low affinity for $5\text{-HT}_{1\text{-}7}$, alpha- and beta-adrenergic, $D_{1\text{-}5}$, $H_{1\text{-}3}$, $M_{1\text{-}5}$, and benzodiazepine receptors. Escitalopram does not bind to or has low affinity for Na^+, K^+, Cl^-, and Ca^{++} ion channels.

Contraindications Hypersensitivity to escitalopram, citalopram, or any component of the formulation; concomitant use with pimozide; concomitant use or within 2 weeks of MAO inhibitors

Warnings/Precautions [U.S. Boxed Warning]: Antidepressants increase the risk of suicidal thinking and behavior in children, adolescents, and young adults (18-24 years of age) with major depressive disorder (MDD) and other psychiatric disorders; consider risk prior to prescribing. Short-term studies did not show an increased risk in patients >24 years of age and showed a decreased risk in patients ≥65 years. Closely monitor patients for clinical worsening, suicidality, or unusual changes in behavior, particularly during the initial 1-2 months of therapy or during periods of dosage adjustments (increases or decreases); the patient's family or caregiver should be instructed to closely observe the patient and communicate condition with healthcare provider. A medication guide concerning the use of antidepressants should be dispensed with each prescription. **Escitalopram is not FDA approved for use in children <12 years of age.**

The possibility of a suicide attempt is inherent in major depression and may persist until remission occurs. Use caution in high-risk patients. Worsening depression and severe abrupt suicidality that are not part of the presenting symptoms may require discontinuation or modification of drug therapy. The patient's family or caregiver should be alerted to monitor patients for the emergence of suicidality and associated behaviors (such as agitation, irritability, hostility, impulsivity, and hypomania) and call healthcare provider.

May worsen psychosis in some patients or precipitate a shift to mania or hypomania in patients with bipolar disorder. Patients presenting with depressive symptoms should be screened for bipolar disorder. Monotherapy in patients with bipolar disorder should be avoided. Escitalopram is not FDA approved for the treatment of bipolar depression. Escitalopram is not FDA approved for the treatment of bipolar depression.

Serotonin syndrome and neuroleptic malignant syndrome (NMS)-like reactions have occurred with serotonin/norepinephrine reuptake inhibitors (SNRIs) and selective serotonin reuptake inhibitors (SSRIs) when used alone, and particularly when used in combination with serotonergic agents (eg, triptans) or antidopaminergic agents (eg, antipsychotics). Concurrent use or within 2 weeks of an MAO inhibitor is contraindicated. May increase the risks associated with electroconvulsive therapy. Has a low potential to impair cognitive or motor performance; caution operating hazardous machinery or driving.

Use caution with a previous seizure disorder or condition predisposing to seizures such as brain damage, alcoholism, or concurrent therapy with other drugs which lower the seizure threshold. May cause hyponatremia/SIADH (elderly at increased risk); volume depletion (diuretics may increase risk) may occur. May cause or exacerbate sexual dysfunction. Use caution with severe renal impairment or liver impairment; concomitant CNS depressants; pregnancy (high doses of citalopram have been associated with teratogenicity in animals). Use caution with concomitant use of aspirin, NSAIDs, warfarin, or other drugs that affect coagulation; the risk of bleeding may be potentiated.

Upon discontinuation of escitalopram therapy, gradually taper dose. If intolerable symptoms occur following a decrease in dosage or upon discontinuation of therapy, then resuming the previous dose with a more gradual taper should be considered.

Safety and efficacy have not been established in children <12 years of age with major depressive disorder or in children <18 years with generalized anxiety disorder.

Drug Interactions

Metabolism/Transport Effects **Substrate** (major) of CYP2C19, 3A4; **Inhibits** CYP2D6 (weak)

Avoid Concomitant Use

Avoid concomitant use of Escitalopram with any of the following: Artemether; Dronedarone; Iobenguane I 123; Lumefantrine; MAO Inhibitors; Methylene Blue; Nilotinib; Pimozide; QuiNINE; Sibutramine; Tetrabenazine; Thioridazine; Toremifene; Tryptophan; Vandetanib; Ziprasidone

Increased Effect/Toxicity

Escitalopram may increase the levels/effects of: Alcohol (Ethyl); Alpha-/Beta-Blockers; Anticoagulants; Antidepressants (Serotonin Reuptake Inhibitor/Antagonist); Antiplatelet Agents; Aspirin; BusPIRone; CarBAMazepine; CloZAPine; CNS Depressants; Collagenase (Systemic); Desmopressin; Dextromethorphan; Dronedarone; Drotrecogin Alfa; Haloperidol; Ibritumomab; Lithium; Methadone; Methylene Blue; Mexiletine; NSAID (COX-2 Inhibitor); NSAID (Nonselective); Pimozide; QTc-Prolonging Agents; QuiNINE; RisperiDONE; Salicylates; Serotonin Modulators; Tetrabenazine; Thioridazine; Thrombolytic Agents; Toremifene; Tositumomab and Iodine I 131 Tositumomab; TraMADol; Tricyclic Antidepressants; Vandetanib; Vitamin K Antagonists; Ziprasidone

The levels/effects of Escitalopram may be increased by: Alfuzosin; Analgesics (Opioid); Artemether; BusPIRone; Chloroquine; Cimetidine; Ciprofloxacin; Ciprofloxacin (Systemic); Conivaptan; CYP2C19 Inhibitors (Moderate); CYP2C19 Inhibitors (Strong); CYP3A4 Inhibitors (Moderate); CYP3A4 Inhibitors (Strong); Gadobutrol; Glucosamine; Herbs (Anticoagulant/Antiplatelet Properties); Lumefantrine; Macrolide Antibiotics; MAO Inhibitors; Metoclopramide; Nilotinib; Omega-3-Acid Ethyl Esters; Pentosan Polysulfate Sodium; Pentoxifylline; Prostacyclin Analogues; QuiNINE; Sibutramine; TraMADol; Tryptophan

Decreased Effect

Escitalopram may decrease the levels/effects of: Iobenguane I 123

The levels/effects of Escitalopram may be decreased by: CarBAMazepine; CYP2C19 Inducers (Strong); CYP3A4 Inducers (Strong); Cyproheptadine; Deferasirox; Tocilizumab

Ethanol/Nutrition/Herb Interactions

Ethanol: May increase CNS depression; monitor for increased effects with coadministration. Caution patients about effects.

Herb/Nutraceutical: Avoid valerian, St John's wort, SAMe, kava kava, and gotu kola (may increase CNS depression).

Dietary Considerations May be taken with or without food.

Pharmacodynamics/Kinetics

Onset of Action Depression: The onset of action is within a week; however, individual response varies greatly and full response may not be seen until 8-12 weeks after initiation of treatment.

Half-life Elimination Escitalopram: 27-32 hours; S-DCT: 59 hours

Time to Peak Escitalopram: ~5 hours; S-DCT: 14 hours

Pregnancy Risk Factor C

Lactation Enters breast milk/consider risk:benefit

Breast-Feeding Considerations Escitalopram and its metabolite are excreted into breast milk. Limited data is available concerning the effects escitalopram may have in the nursing infant and the long-term effects on development and behavior have not been studied. According to the manufacturer, the decision to continue or discontinue breast-feeding during therapy should take into account the risk of exposure to the infant and the benefits of treatment to the mother. Escitalopram is the S-enantiomer of the racemic derivative citalopram; also refer to the Citalopram monograph.

Dosage Forms

Solution, oral:

Lexapro®: 1 mg/mL (240 mL)

Tablet, oral:

Lexapro®: 5 mg, 10 mg, 20 mg

Dosage Forms: Canada

Tablet:

Cipralex®: 10 mg, 20 mg

Esmolol (ES moe lol)

U.S. Brand Names Brevibloc

Canadian Brand Names Brevibloc®

Pharmacologic Category Antiarrhythmic Agent, Class II; Beta Blocker, Beta-1 Selective

Use Treatment of supraventricular tachycardia (SVT) and atrial fibrillation/flutter (control ventricular rate); treatment of intraoperative and postoperative tachycardia and/or hypertension; treatment of noncompensatory sinus tachycardia

Unlabeled/Investigational Use In children, for SVT and postoperative hypertension

Local Anesthetic/Vasoconstrictor Precautions No information available to require special precautions

Effects on Dental Treatment Esmolol is a cardioselective beta-blocker. Local anesthetic with vasoconstrictor can be safely used in patients medicated with esmolol. Nonselective beta-blockers (ie, propranolol, nadolol) enhance the pressor response to epinephrine, resulting in hypertension and bradycardia; this has not been reported for esmolol. Many nonsteroidal anti-inflammatory drugs, such as ibuprofen and indomethacin, can reduce the hypotensive effect of beta-blockers after 3 or more weeks of therapy with the NSAID. Short-term NSAID use (ie, 3 days) requires no special precautions in patients taking beta-blockers.

Effects on Bleeding No information available to require special precautions

Adverse Effects

>10%:

Cardiovascular: Asymptomatic hypotension (dose related: 25% to 38%), symptomatic hypotension (dose related: 12%)

Miscellaneous: Diaphoresis (10%)

1% to 10%:

Cardiovascular: Peripheral ischemia (1%)

Central nervous system: Dizziness (3%), somnolence (3%), confusion (2%), headache (2%), agitation (2%), fatigue (1%)

Gastrointestinal: Nausea (7%), vomiting (1%)

Local: Pain on injection (8%), infusion site reaction

General Dosage Range I.V.: *Adults:* Bolus: 80 mg **or** 500 mcg/kg; Infusion: 50-200 mcg/kg/minute (maximum: 300 mcg/kg/minute)

Mechanism of Action Class II antiarrhythmic: Competitively blocks response to $beta_1$-adrenergic stimulation with little or no effect of $beta_2$-receptors except at high doses, no intrinsic sympathomimetic activity, no membrane stabilizing activity

Pharmacodynamics/Kinetics

Onset of Action Beta-blockade: I.V.: 2-10 minutes (quickest when loading doses are administered)

Duration of Action Hemodynamic effects: 10-30 minutes; prolonged following higher cumulative doses, extended duration of use

Half-life Elimination Adults: Esmolol: 9 minutes; Acid metabolite: 3.7 hours; elimination of metabolite decreases with end-stage renal disease

Pregnancy Risk Factor C

Esomeprazole (es oh ME pray zol)

Related Information

Gastrointestinal Disorders *on page 1874*

Omeprazole *on page 1247*

U.S. Brand Names NexIUM®; NexIUM® I.V.

Canadian Brand Names Nexium®

Generic Availability (U.S.) No

Pharmacologic Category Proton Pump Inhibitor; Substituted Benzimidazole

Use

Oral: Short-term (4-8 weeks) treatment of erosive esophagitis; maintaining symptom resolution and healing of erosive esophagitis; treatment of symptomatic gastroesophageal reflux disease (GERD); as part of a multidrug regimen for *Helicobacter pylori* eradication in patients with duodenal ulcer disease (active or history of within the past 5 years); prevention of gastric ulcers in patients at risk (age ≥60 years and/or history of gastric ulcer) associated with continuous NSAID therapy; long-term treatment of pathological hypersecretory conditions including Zollinger-Ellison syndrome

Canadian labeling: Additional use (not in U.S. labeling): Oral: Treatment of nonerosive reflux disease (NERD)

I.V.: Short-term (≤10 days) treatment of gastroesophageal reflux disease (GERD) when oral therapy is not possible or appropriate

Unlabeled/Investigational Use I.V.: Prevention of recurrent peptic ulcer bleeding postendoscopy

Local Anesthetic/Vasoconstrictor Precautions No information available to require special precautions

Effects on Dental Treatment Key adverse event(s) related to dental treatment: Xerostomia (normal salivary flow resumes upon discontinuation)

Effects on Bleeding No information available to require special precautions

Adverse Effects Unless otherwise specified, percentages represent adverse reactions identified in clinical trials evaluating the oral formulation.

>10%: Central nervous system: Headache (I.V. 11%; oral ≤8%)

1% to 10%:

Cardiovascular: Hypertension (≤3%), chest pain (>1%)

Central nervous system: Pain (4%), dizziness (oral >1%; I.V. 3%), anxiety (2%), insomnia (2%), pyrexia (2%), fatigue (>1%)

Dermatologic: Rash (>1%), pruritus (I.V. ≤1%)

Endocrine & metabolic: Hypercholesterolemia (2%)

Gastrointestinal: Flatulence (oral ≤5%; I.V. 10%), diarrhea (oral ≤7%; I.V. 4%), abdominal pain (oral ≤6%; I.V. 6%), nausea (oral 5%; I.V. 6%), dyspepsia (oral >1%; I.V. 6%), gastritis (≤6%), constipation (oral 2%; I.V. 3%), vomiting (≤3%), benign GI neoplasm (>1%), dyspepsia (>1%), duodenitis (>1%), epigastric pain (>1%), esophageal disorder (>1%), gastroenteritis (>1%), GI mucosal discoloration (>1%), serum gastrin increased (>1%), tooth disorder (>1%), xerostomia (1%)

Genitourinary: Urinary tract infection (4%)

Hematologic: Anemia (>1%)

Hepatic: Transaminases increased (>1%)

Local: Injection site reaction (I.V. 2%)

Neuromuscular & skeletal: Arthralgia (3%), back pain (>1%), fracture (>1%), arthropathy (1%), myalgia (1%)

Respiratory: Respiratory infection (oral ≤9%; I.V. 1%), bronchitis (4%), sinusitis (oral ≤4%; I.V. 2%), coughing (>1%), rhinitis (>1%), dyspnea (1%)

Miscellaneous: Accident/injury (≤8%), viral infection (4%), allergy (2%), ear infection (2%), hernia (>1%), flu-like syndrome (1%)

Dosage

Oral:

Children 1-11 years: **Note:** Safety and efficacy of doses >1 mg/kg/day and/or therapy beyond 8 weeks have not been established.

Symptomatic GERD: 10 mg once daily for up to 8 weeks

Erosive esophagitis (healing):

<20 kg: 10 mg once daily for 8 weeks

≥20 kg: 10-20 mg once daily for 8 weeks

Nonerosive reflux disease (NERD) (Canadian labeling): 10 mg once daily for up to 8 weeks

Adolescents 12-17 years:

GERD: 20-40 mg once daily for up to 8 weeks

NERD (Canadian labeling): 20 mg once daily for 2-4 weeks; lack of symptom control after 4 weeks warrants further evaluation

Adults:

Erosive esophagitis (healing): Initial: 20-40 mg once daily for 4-8 weeks; if incomplete healing, may continue for an additional 4-8 weeks; maintenance: 20 mg once daily (controlled studies did not extend beyond 6 months)

NERD (Canadian labeling): Initial: 20 mg once daily for 2-4 weeks; lack of symptom control after 4 weeks warrants further evaluation; maintenance (in patients with successful initial therapy): 20 mg once daily as needed

Symptomatic GERD: 20 mg once daily for 4 weeks; may continue an additional 4 weeks if symptoms persist

Helicobacter pylori eradication:

Manufacturer labeling: 40 mg once daily administered with amoxicillin 1000 mg *and* clarithromycin 500 mg twice daily for 10 days

American College of Gastroenterology guidelines (Chey, 2007):

Nonpenicillin allergy: 40 mg once daily administered with amoxicillin 1000 mg *and* clarithromycin 500 mg twice daily for 10-14 days

Penicillin allergy: 40 mg once daily administered with clarithromycin 500 mg *and* metronidazole 500 mg twice daily for 10-14 days **or** 40 mg once daily administered with bismuth subsalicylate 525 mg *and* metronidazole 250 mg *plus* tetracycline 500 mg 4 times/day for 10-14 days

Canadian labeling: 20 mg twice daily for 7 days; requires combination therapy

Prevention of NSAID-induced gastric ulcers: 20-40 mg once daily for up to 6 months

Treatment of NSAID-induced gastric ulcers (Canadian labeling): 20 mg once daily for 4-8 weeks.

Pathological hypersecretory conditions (Zollinger-Ellison syndrome): 40 mg twice daily; adjust regimen to individual patient needs; doses up to 240 mg/day have been administered

I.V.:

Treatment of GERD (short-term): **Note:** Indicated only in cases where oral therapy is inappropriate or not possible; safety/efficacy ≥10 days has not been established.

Children 1-11 months: 0.5 mg/kg once daily

Children 1-17 years: <55 kg: 10 mg once daily; ≥55 kg: 20 mg once daily

Adults: 20 mg or 40 mg once daily

Prevention of recurrent peptic ulcer bleeding postendoscopy (unlabeled use; Sung, 2009): Adults: 80 mg over 30 minutes, followed by 8 mg/hour infusion for 72 hours, then 40 mg *orally* once daily for 27 additional days

Elderly: No dosage adjustment needed.

Dosage adjustment in renal impairment: No dosage adjustment needed

Dosage adjustment in hepatic impairment:

Safety and efficacy not established in children with hepatic impairment.

Mild-to-moderate hepatic impairment (Child-Pugh class A or B): No dosage adjustment needed

Severe hepatic impairment (Child-Pugh class C): Dose should not exceed 20 mg/day

Mechanism of Action Proton pump inhibitor suppresses gastric acid secretion by inhibition of the H^+/K^+-ATPase in the gastric parietal cell. Esomeprazole is the S-isomer of omeprazole.

Contraindications Hypersensitivity to esomeprazole, substituted benzimidazoles (eg, omeprazole, lansoprazole), or any component of the formulation

Warnings/Precautions Use of proton pump inhibitors may increase the risk of gastrointestinal infections (eg, *Salmonella, Campylobacter*). Relief of symptoms does not preclude the presence of a gastric malignancy. Atrophic gastritis (by biopsy) has been noted with long-term omeprazole therapy; this may also occur with esomeprazole. No reports of enterochromaffin-like (ECL) cell carcinoids, dysplasia, or neoplasia have occurred. Severe liver dysfunction may require dosage reductions. Safety and efficacy of I.V. therapy >10 days have not been established; transition from I.V. to oral therapy as soon possible. Bioavailability may be increased in Asian populations, the elderly, and patients with hepatic dysfunction. Decreased *H. pylori* eradication rates have been observed with short-term (≤7 days) combination therapy. The American College of Gastroenterology recommends 10-14 days of therapy (triple or quadruple) for eradication of *H. pylori* (Chey, 2007). Proton pump inhibitors may diminish the therapeutic effect of clopidogrel, thought to be due to reduced formation of the active metabolite of clopidogrel; an increase in the risk of cardiovascular events may occur. The manufacturer of clopidogrel recommends avoidance of concomitant administration of another PPI (ie, omeprazole); similar recommendations with esomeprazole would appear prudent.

Increased incidence of osteoporosis-related bone fractures of the hip, spine, or wrist may occur with proton pump inhibitor therapy. Patients on high-dose or long-term therapy should be monitored. Use the lowest effective dose for the shortest duration of time, use vitamin D and calcium supplementation, and follow appropriate guidelines to reduce risk of fractures in patients at risk.

Drug Interactions

Metabolism/Transport Effects **Substrate** of CYP2C19 (major), 3A4 (major); **Inhibits** CYP2C19 (moderate)

Avoid Concomitant Use

Avoid concomitant use of Esomeprazole with any of the following: Delavirdine; Erlotinib; Nelfinavir; Posaconazole

Increased Effect/Toxicity

Esomeprazole may increase the levels/effects of: Amphetamines; Benzodiazepines (metabolized by oxidation); Cilostazol; CYP2C19 Substrates; Dexmethylphenidate; Methotrexate; Methylphenidate; Raltegravir; Saquinavir; Tacrolimus; Tacrolimus (Systemic); Vitamin K Antagonists; Voriconazole

The levels/effects of Esomeprazole may be increased by: Conivaptan; Fluconazole; Ketoconazole; Ketoconazole (Systemic)

Decreased Effect

Esomeprazole may decrease the levels/effects of: Atazanavir; Bisphosphonate Derivatives; Cefditoren; Clopidogrel; Dabigatran Etexilate; Dasatinib; Delavirdine; Erlotinib; Gefitinib; Indinavir; Iron Salts; Itraconazole; Ketoconazole; Ketoconazole (Systemic); Mesalamine; Mycophenolate; Nelfinavir; Posaconazole

The levels/effects of Esomeprazole may be decreased by: CYP2C19 Inducers (Strong); Tipranavir; Tocilizumab

Ethanol/Nutrition/Herb Interactions Food: Absorption is decreased by 43% to 53% when taken with food.

Dietary Considerations Take at least 1 hour before meals; best if taken before breakfast. The contents of the capsule may be mixed in applesauce or water; pellets also remain intact when exposed to orange juice, apple juice, and yogurt.

Pharmacodynamics/Kinetics

Half-life Elimination ~1-1.5 hours

Time to Peak Oral: 1.5-2 hours

Pregnancy Risk Factor B

Lactation Excretion in breast milk unknown/not recommended

Breast-Feeding Considerations Esomeprazole excretion into breast milk has not been studied. However, omeprazole is excreted in breast milk, and therefore considered likely that esomeprazole is similarly excreted; breast-feeding is not recommended.

Dosage Forms

Capsule, delayed release, oral:
NexIUM®: 20 mg, 40 mg

Granules for suspension, delayed release, oral:
NexIUM®: 10 mg/packet (30s); 20 mg/packet (30s); 40 mg/packet (30s)

Injection, powder for reconstitution:
NexIUM® I.V.: 20 mg, 40 mg

Dosage Forms: Canada Note: Strength expressed as base.

Granules, for oral suspension, delayed release, as magnesium:
Nexium®: 10 mg/packet (28s)

Tablet, extended release, as magnesium:
Nexium®: 20 mg, 40 mg

Estazolam (es TA zoe lam)

Pharmacologic Category Benzodiazepine

Use Short-term management of insomnia

Local Anesthetic/Vasoconstrictor Precautions No information available to require special precautions

Effects on Dental Treatment Key adverse event(s) related to dental treatment: Significant xerostomia (normal salivary flow resumes upon discontinuation)

Effects on Bleeding No information available to require special precautions

Adverse Effects

>10%:

Central nervous system: Somnolence

Neuromuscular & skeletal: Weakness

1% to 10%:

Cardiovascular: Flushing, palpitation

Central nervous system: Anxiety, confusion, dizziness, hypokinesia, abnormal coordination, hangover effect, agitation, amnesia, apathy, emotional lability, euphoria, hostility, seizure, sleep disorder, stupor, twitch

Dermatologic: Dermatitis, pruritus, rash, urticaria

Gastrointestinal: Xerostomia, constipation, appetite increased/decreased, flatulence, gastritis, perverse taste

Genitourinary: Frequent urination, menstrual cramps, urinary hesitancy, urinary frequency, vaginal discharge/itching

Neuromuscular & skeletal: Paresthesia

Ocular: Photophobia, eye pain, eye swelling

Respiratory: Cough, dyspnea, asthma, rhinitis, sinusitis

Miscellaneous: Diaphoresis

General Dosage Range Oral:

Adults: 0.5-2 mg at bedtime

Elderly: Initial: 0.5 mg at bedtime in small or debilitated patients

Mechanism of Action Binds to stereospecific benzodiazepine receptors on the postsynaptic GABA neuron at several sites within the central nervous system, including the limbic system, reticular formation. Enhancement of the inhibitory effect of GABA on neuronal excitability results by increased neuronal membrane permeability to chloride ions. This shift in chloride ions results in hyperpolarization (a less excitable state) and stabilization.

Pharmacodynamics/Kinetics

Onset of Action ~1 hour

Duration of Action Variable

Half-life Elimination 10-24 hours (no significant changes in elderly)

Time to Peak Serum: 0.5-1.6 hours

Pregnancy Risk Factor X

Controlled Substance C-IV

Estradiol (Systemic) (es tra DYE ole)

Related Information

Endocrine Disorders and Pregnancy *on page 1879*

Rheumatoid Arthritis, Osteoarthritis, and Osteoporosis *on page 1889*

U.S. Brand Names Alora®; Climara®; Delestrogen®; Depo®-Estradiol; Divigel®; Elestrin®; Estrace®; Estraderm®; Estrasorb®; EstroGel®; Evamist™; Femring®; Femtrace®; Menostar®; Vivelle-Dot®

Canadian Brand Names Climara®; Depo®-Estradiol; Estraderm®; Estradot®; EstroGel®; Menostar®; Oesclim®; Sandoz-Estradiol Derm 100; Sandoz-Estradiol Derm 50; Sandoz-Estradiol Derm 75

Pharmacologic Category Estrogen Derivative

Use Treatment of moderate-to-severe vasomotor symptoms associated with menopause; treatment of moderate-to-severe vulvar and vaginal atrophy associated with menopause; hypoestrogenism (due to hypogonadism, castration, or primary ovarian failure); advanced prostatic cancer (palliation); metastatic breast cancer (palliation) in men and postmenopausal women; postmenopausal osteoporosis (prophylaxis)

Local Anesthetic/Vasoconstrictor Precautions No information available to require special precautions

Effects on Dental Treatment No significant effects or complications reported

Effects on Bleeding No information available to require special precautions

Adverse Effects Frequency not defined. Some adverse reactions observed with estrogen and/or progestin combination therapy.

Cardiovascular: Chest pain, DVT, edema, hypertension, MI, stroke, syncope, TIA, vasodilation, venous thromboembolism

Central nervous system: Anxiety, dementia, dizziness, epilepsy exacerbation, headache, insomnia, irritability, mental depression, migraine, mood disturbances, nervousness

Dermatologic: Angioedema, chloasma, dermatitis, erythema multiforme, erythema nodosum, hemorrhagic eruption, hirsutism, loss of scalp hair, melasma, rash, pruritus, urticaria

Endocrine & metabolic: Breast cancer, breast enlargement, breast pain, breast tenderness, carbohydrate intolerance, fibrocystic breast changes, fluid retention, galactorrhea, hot flashes, hypocalcemia, libido changes, nipple discharge, nipple pain
Gastrointestinal: Abdominal cramps, abdominal pain, bloating, cholecystitis, cholelithiasis, constipation, diarrhea, dyspepsia, flatulence, gallbladder disease, gastritis, nausea, pancreatitis, vomiting, weight gain/loss
Genitourinary: Alterations in frequency and flow of bleeding patterns, breakthrough bleeding, cervical ectropion changes, cervical secretion changes, cystitis, dysmenorrhea, endometrial cancer, endometrial hyperplasia, genital eruption, menorrhagia, metrorrhagia, ovarian cancer, ovarian cyst, Pap smear suspicious, spotting, uterine leiomyomata size increased, leukorrhea, uterine cancer, uterine enlargement, uterine pain, urinary incontinence, urogenital pruritus, vaginal candidiasis, vaginal discharge, vaginal moniliasis, vaginitis
Hematologic: Aggravation of porphyria
Hepatic: Cholestatic jaundice, hepatic hemangioma enlargement
Local: Thrombophlebitis
Gel, spray: Application site reaction
Transdermal patches: Erythema, irritation
Neuromuscular & skeletal: Arthralgia, back pain, chorea, leg cramps, myalgia, muscle cramps, skeletal pain, weakness
Ocular: Blindness, contact lens intolerance, corneal curvature steepening, retinal vascular thrombosis
Respiratory: Asthma exacerbation, pulmonary thromboembolism
Miscellaneous: Anaphylactoid/anaphylactic reactions, hypersensitivity reactions

General Dosage Range

I.M.:

Cypionate:

Adults (females): Hypoestrogenism: 1.5-2 mg monthly
Adults (females): Menopause: 1-5 mg every 3-4 weeks

Valerate:

Adults (females): Menopause: 10-20 mg every 4 weeks
Adults (males): Prostate cancer: 30 mg or more every 1-2 weeks

Oral:

Adults (females):

Estrace®: Breast cancer: 10 mg 3 times/day; Hypoestrogenism: 1-2 mg/day; Menopause: 0.5-2 mg/day
Femtrace®: Menopause: 0.45-1.8 mg/day

Adults (males): Estrace®: Prostate cancer: 1-2 mg 3 times/day; Breast cancer: 10 mg 3 times/day

Intravaginal: *Adults (females):* (Femring®): 0.05-0.1 mg, leave in place for 3 months

Topical: *Adults (females):*

Emulsion (Estrasorb®): 3.48 g applied once daily in the morning
Gel: 1.25 g/day (EstroGel®) or 0.87 g/day (Elestrin®) or 0.25-1 g/day (Divigel®) applied at the same time each day
Spray (Evamist™): 1 spray (1.53 mg) per day; dosing range: 1-3 sprays/day

Transdermal: *Adults (females):*

Alora®, Estraderm®, Vivelle-Dot®: Apply twice weekly continuously or cyclically (3 weeks on, 1 week off)
Climara®: Apply once weekly continuously or cyclically (3 weeks on, 1 week off)
Menostar®: Apply once weekly continuously

Mechanism of Action Estrogens are responsible for the development and maintenance of the female reproductive system and secondary sexual characteristics. Estradiol is the principle intracellular human estrogen and is more potent than estrone and estriol at the receptor level; it is the primary estrogen secreted prior to menopause. Following menopause, estrone and estrone sulfate are more highly produced. Estrogens modulate the pituitary secretion of gonadotropins, luteinizing hormone, and follicle-stimulating hormone through a negative feedback system; estrogen replacement reduces elevated levels of these hormones in postmenopausal women.

Pharmacodynamics/Kinetics

Half-life Elimination Femtrace®: 21-26 hours

Time to Peak Plasma: Oral: Femtrace®: 0.4-0.75 hours

Pregnancy Risk Factor X

Estradiol and Dienogest (es tra DYE ole & dye EN oh jest)

Related Information

Estradiol (Systemic) *on page 631*

U.S. Brand Names Natazia™

Pharmacologic Category Contraceptive; Estrogen and Progestin Combination

Use Prevention of pregnancy

Unlabeled/Investigational Use Treatment of hypermenorrhea (menorrhagia); pain associated with endometriosis; dysmenorrhea; dysfunctional uterine bleeding

Local Anesthetic/Vasoconstrictor Precautions No information available to require special precautions

Effects on Dental Treatment No significant effects or complications reported

Effects on Bleeding No information available to require special precautions

Adverse Effects

>10%: Central nervous system: Headache (13%, including migraine)

1% to 10%:

Dermatologic: Acne (4%)

Endocrine & metabolic: Metrorrhagia and irregular menstruation (8%), breast pain/discomfort/tenderness (7%)

Gastrointestinal: Nausea or vomiting (7%), weight gain (3%)

Frequency not defined: DVT, focal nodular hyperplasia of the liver, MI, ruptured ovarian cyst, uterine leiomyoma

The following reactions have been associated with oral contraceptive use:

Increased risk or evidence of association with use:

Cardiovascular: Arterial thromboembolism, cerebral hemorrhage, cerebral thrombosis, hypertension, mesenteric thrombosis, MI, venous thrombosis (with or without embolism)

Gastrointestinal: Gallbladder disease

Hepatic: Hepatic adenomas, liver tumors (benign)

Local: Thrombophlebitis

Ocular: Retinal thrombosis

Respiratory: Pulmonary embolism

Adverse reactions considered drug related:

Cardiovascular: Edema, varicose vein aggravation

Central nervous system: Depression, migraine, mood changes

Dermatologic: Chloasma, melasma, rash (allergic)

Endocrine & metabolic: Amenorrhea, breakthrough bleeding, breast changes (enlargement, pain, secretion, tenderness), fluid retention, infertility (temporary), lactation decreased (with use immediately postpartum), menstrual flow changes, spotting

Gastrointestinal: Abdominal bloating, abdominal cramps, abdominal pain, appetite changes, nausea, weight changes, vomiting

Genitourinary: Cervical ectropion, cervical secretion, vaginal candidiasis, vaginitis

Hematologic: Folate decreased, porphyria exacerbation

Hepatic: Cholestatic jaundice

Neuromuscular & skeletal: Chorea exacerbation

Ocular: Contact lens intolerance, corneal curvature changes (steepening)

Miscellaneous: Anaphylactic/anaphylactoid reactions (including angioedema, circulatory collapse, respiratory collapse, urticaria), SLE exacerbation

General Dosage Range Oral: *Children and Adults (females, postmenarche):* 1 tablet daily

Mechanism of Action Combination hormonal contraceptives inhibit ovulation and may also cause changes in the cervical mucus, rendering it unfavorable for sperm penetration even if ovulation occurs. The four-phasic formulation provides the estrogen in decreasing concentrations and the progestin in increasing concentrations over the 28-day cycle.

Pharmacodynamics/Kinetics

Half-life Elimination Estradiol: ~14 hours; Dienogest: ~11 hours

Time to Peak

Estradiol: ~6 hours; Dienogest: ~1 hour

Pregnancy Risk Factor X

Estradiol and Norethindrone (es tra DYE ole & nor eth IN drone)

Related Information

Endocrine Disorders and Pregnancy *on page 1879*

Estradiol (Systemic) *on page 631*

Norethindrone *on page 1226*

U.S. Brand Names Activella®; CombiPatch®; Mimvey™

Canadian Brand Names Estalis-Sequi®; Estalis®

Pharmacologic Category Estrogen and Progestin Combination

Use Women with an intact uterus:

Tablet: Treatment of moderate-to-severe vasomotor symptoms associated with menopause; treatment of vulvar and vaginal atrophy; prophylaxis for postmenopausal osteoporosis

Transdermal patch: Treatment of moderate-to-severe vasomotor symptoms associated with menopause; treatment of vulvar and vaginal atrophy; treatment of hypoestrogenism due to hypogonadism, castration, or primary ovarian failure

Local Anesthetic/Vasoconstrictor Precautions No information available to require special precautions

Effects on Dental Treatment No significant effects or complications reported

Effects on Bleeding No information available to require special precautions related to hemostasis in dental procedures.

Adverse Effects Frequency not defined.

Cardiovascular: Altered blood pressure, cardiovascular accident, edema, MI, stroke, venous thromboembolism, thrombophlebitis

Central nervous system: Dementia, dizziness, emotional lability, fatigue, headache, insomnia, irritability, mental depression, migraine, mood changes, nervousness, seizure

Dermatologic: Chloasma, erythema multiforme, erythema nodosum, hemorrhagic eruption, hirsutism, itching, loss of scalp hair, melasma, pruritus, seborrhea, skin rash

Endocrine & metabolic: Breast cancer, breast enlargement, breast tenderness, breast pain, fibrocystic breast changes, galactorrhea, hypocalcemia, libido changes, nipple discharge, triglycerides increased

Gastrointestinal: Abdominal pain, bloating, changes in appetite, cramps, flatulence, gallbladder disease, gastroenteritis, nausea, pancreatitis, vomiting, weight gain/loss

Genitourinary: Alterations in frequency and flow of menses, changes in cervical secretions, cystitis-like syndrome, endometrial cancer, endometrial hyperplasia, endometrial thickening, endometriosis exacerbation, genital moniliasis, ovarian cancer, ovarian cyst, postmenopausal bleeding, premenstrual-like syndrome, size of uterine leiomyomata increased, uterine fibroid, vaginal candidiasis, vaginal hemorrhage, vaginitis

Hematologic: Aggravation of porphyria

Hepatic: Cholestatic jaundice

Local: Application site reaction (transdermal patch)

Neuromuscular & skeletal: Arthralgia, back pain, chorea, extremity pain, leg cramps, myalgia, weakness

Ocular: Contact lens intolerance, corneal curvature steepening, retinal vascular thrombosis

Respiratory: Asthma exacerbation, nasopharyngitis, pharyngitis, pulmonary thromboembolism, rhinitis, sinusitis, upper respiratory tract infection

Miscellaneous: Allergic reactions, carbohydrate intolerance, flu-like syndrome, viral infection

General Dosage Range

Oral: *Adults (females):* 1 tablet daily

Transdermal: *Adults (females):* Apply 1 patch twice weekly

Pharmacodynamics/Kinetics

Half-life Elimination Activella®: Estradiol: 12-14 hours; Norethindrone: 8-11 hours

Time to Peak Activella®: Estradiol: 5-8 hours

Estradiol and Norgestimate (es tra DYE ole & nor JES ti mate)

Related Information

Endocrine Disorders and Pregnancy *on page 1879*

Estradiol (Systemic) *on page 631*

U.S. Brand Names Prefest™

Pharmacologic Category Estrogen and Progestin Combination

Use Women with an intact uterus: Treatment of moderate-to-severe vasomotor symptoms associated with menopause; treatment of atrophic vaginitis; prevention of osteoporosis

Local Anesthetic/Vasoconstrictor Precautions No information available to require special precautions

Effects on Dental Treatment No significant effects or complications reported

Effects on Bleeding No information available to require special precautions related to hemostasis in dental procedures.

Adverse Effects

>10%:

Central nervous system: Headache (23%)
Endocrine & metabolic: Breast pain (16%)
Gastrointestinal: Abdominal pain (12%)
Neuromuscular & skeletal: Back pain (12%)
Respiratory: Upper respiratory tract infection (21%)
Miscellaneous: Flu-like syndrome (11%)

1% to 10%:

Central nervous system: Fatigue (6%), pain (6%), depression (5%), dizziness (5%)
Endocrine & metabolic: Vaginal bleeding (9%), dysmenorrhea (8%), vaginitis (7%)
Gastrointestinal: Nausea (6%), flatulence (5%)
Neuromuscular & skeletal: Arthralgia (9%), myalgia (5%)
Respiratory: Sinusitis (8%), pharyngitis (7%), cough (5%)
Miscellaneous: Viral infection (6%)

Additional adverse effects associated with **estrogens and progestins**; frequency not defined:

Cardiovascular: Edema, hypertension, MI, stroke, venous thrombosis
Central nervous system: Anxiety, epilepsy exacerbation, insomnia, irritability, migraine, mood disturbances, nervousness, pyrexia, somnolence
Dermatologic: Acne, chloasma, erythema multiforme, erythema nodosum, hemorrhagic eruptions, hirsutism, itching, melasma, pruritus, rash, scalp hair loss, urticaria
Endocrine & metabolic: Amenorrhea, breast cancer, breast discharge, breast enlargement, Breast tenderness, carbohydrate tolerance decreased, endometrial cancer, endometrial hyperplasia, fibrocystic breast changes, galactorrhea, hypocalcemia, libido changes, ovarian cancer, triglycerides increased
Gastrointestinal: Abdominal cramps, appetite changes, bloating, gallbladder disease, pancreatitis, vomiting, weight gain/loss
Genitourinary: Abnormal withdrawal bleeding/flow, breakthrough bleeding, cervical secretion changes, cystitis syndrome, uterine leiomyomata size increased, vaginal candidiasis, vaginal bleeding/spotting
Hematologic: Anemia, porphyria
Hepatic: Cholestatic jaundice
Local: Thrombophlebitis
Neuromuscular & skeletal: Chorea
Ocular: Contact lens intolerance, corneal curvature steepening, neuro-ocular lesions
Respiratory: Asthma exacerbation, pulmonary embolism
Miscellaneous: Anaphylaxis

General Dosage Range Oral: *Adults (females):* 1 tablet of estradiol 1 mg once daily for 3 days, followed by 1 tablet of estradiol 1 mg and norgestimate 0.09 mg once daily for 3 days; repeat sequence continuously

Mechanism of Action Estrogens are responsible for the development and maintenance of the female reproductive system and secondary sexual characteristics. Estradiol is the principle intracellular human estrogen and is more potent than estrone and estriol at the receptor level; it is the primary estrogen secreted prior to menopause. Following menopause, estrone and estrone sulfate are more highly produced. Estrogens modulate the pituitary secretion of gonadotropins, luteinizing hormone, and follicle-stimulating hormone through a negative feedback system; estrogen replacement reduces elevated levels of these hormones in postmenopausal women.

Progestins inhibit gonadotropin production which then prevents follicular maturation and ovulation. In women with adequate estrogen, progestins transform a proliferative endometrium into a secretory endometrium; when administered with estradiol, reduces the incidence of endometrial hyperplasia and risk of adenocarcinoma.

Pharmacodynamics/Kinetics

Half-life Elimination Norgestimate: 17-deacetylnorgestimate: 37 hours

Pregnancy Risk Factor X

Estramustine (es tra MUS teen)

U.S. Brand Names Emcyt®

Canadian Brand Names Emcyt®

Pharmacologic Category Antineoplastic Agent, Alkylating Agent; Antineoplastic Agent, Hormone; Antineoplastic Agent, Hormone (Estrogen/Nitrogen Mustard)

Use Palliative treatment of progressive or metastatic prostate cancer

Local Anesthetic/Vasoconstrictor Precautions No information available to require special precautions

Effects on Dental Treatment No significant effects or complications reported

Effects on Bleeding Although significant myelosuppression with associated altered hemostasis has been reported for many chemotherapeutic agents, myelosuppression is not common with estramustine and no specific precautions appear to necessary.

Adverse Effects

>10%:

Cardiovascular: Edema (20%)

Endocrine & metabolic: Gynecomastia (75%), breast tenderness (71%), libido decreased

Gastrointestinal: Nausea (16%), diarrhea (13%), gastrointestinal upset (12%)

Hepatic: LDH increased (2% to 33%), AST increased (2% to 33%)

Respiratory: Dyspnea (12%)

1% to 10%:

Cardiovascular: CHF (3%), MI (3%), cerebrovascular accident (2%), chest pain (1%), flushing (1%)

Central nervous system: Lethargy (4%), insomnia (3%), emotional lability (2%), anxiety (1%), headache (1%)

Dermatologic: Bruising (3%), dry skin (2%), pruritus (2%), hair thinning (1%), rash (1%), skin peeling (1%)

Gastrointestinal: Anorexia (4%), flatulence (2%), burning throat (1%), gastrointestinal bleeding (1%), thirst (1%), vomiting (1%)

Hematologic: Leukopenia (4%), thrombocytopenia (1%)

Hepatic: Bilirubin increased (1% to 2%)

Local: Thrombophlebitis (3%)

Neuromuscular & skeletal: Leg cramps (9%)

Ocular: Tearing (1%)

Respiratory: Pulmonary embolism (2%), upper respiratory discharge (1%), hoarseness (1%)

General Dosage Range Oral: *Adults (males):* 14 mg/kg/day (range: 10-16 mg/kg/day) in 3 or 4 divided doses

Mechanism of Action Combines the effects of estradiol and nitrogen mustard. It appears to bind to microtubule proteins, preventing normal tubulin function. The antitumor effect may be due solely to an estrogenic effect. Estramustine causes a marked decrease in plasma testosterone and an increase in estrogen levels.

Pharmacodynamics/Kinetics

Half-life Elimination Terminal: 15-24 hours

Time to Peak Serum: 2-3 hours

Estrogens (Conjugated A/Synthetic)

(ES troe jenz, KON joo gate ed, aye, sin THET ik)

Related Information

Endocrine Disorders and Pregnancy *on page 1879*

U.S. Brand Names Cenestin®

Canadian Brand Names Cenestin

Pharmacologic Category Estrogen Derivative

Use Treatment of moderate-to-severe vasomotor symptoms of menopause; treatment of vulvar and vaginal atrophy

Local Anesthetic/Vasoconstrictor Precautions No information available to require special precautions

Effects on Dental Treatment No significant effects or complications reported

Effects on Bleeding No information available to require special precautions related to hemostasis in dental procedures.

Adverse Effects

>10%:

Central nervous system: Headache (11% to 68%), dizziness (11%), pain (11%)

Endocrine & metabolic: Breast pain (29%), endometrial thickening (19%), metrorrhagia (14%)

Gastrointestinal: Abdominal pain (9% to 28%), nausea (9% to 18%)

Neuromuscular & skeletal: Paresthesia (8% to 33%), back pain (14%)

Respiratory: Upper respiratory tract infection (13%)

Miscellaneous: Infection (2% to 14%)

1% to 10%:

Central nervous system: Anxiety (6%), fever (1%)

Gastrointestinal: Dyspepsia (10%), vomiting (7%), constipation (6%), diarrhea (6%), weight gain (6%)

Genitourinary: Vaginitis (8%)

Neuromuscular & skeletal: Leg cramps (10%), hypertonia (6%)

Respiratory: Rhinitis (6% to 8%), cough (6%)

In addition, the following have been reported with estrogen and/or progestin therapy:
Cardiovascular: Edema, hypertension, MI, stroke, venous thromboembolism
Central nervous system: Epilepsy exacerbation, irritability, mental depression, migraine, mood disturbances, nervousness
Dermatologic: Angioedema, chloasma, erythema multiforme, erythema nodosum, hemorrhagic eruption, hirsutism, melasma, pruritus, rash, scalp hair loss, urticaria
Endocrine & metabolic: Breast cancer, breast enlargement, breast tenderness, glucose tolerance impaired, HDL-cholesterol increased, hyper-/hypocalcemia, LDL-cholesterol decreased, libido changes, serum triglycerides/phospholipids increased, thyroid-binding globulin increased, total thyroid hormone (T_4) increased
Gastrointestinal: Abdominal cramps, bloating, cholecystitis, cholelithiasis, gallbladder disease, pancreatitis, weight gain/loss
Genitourinary: Alterations in frequency and flow of menses, cervical secretion changes, endometrial cancer, endometrial hyperplasia, uterine leiomyomata size increased, vaginal candidiasis
Hematologic: Aggravation of porphyria, antithrombin III and antifactor Xa decreased, fibrinogen levels increased, platelet aggregability and platelet count increased; prothrombin and factors VII, VIII, IX, X increased
Hepatic: Cholestatic jaundice, hepatic hemangiomas enlarged
Neuromuscular & skeletal: Arthralgias, chorea, leg cramps
Local: Thrombophlebitis
Ocular: Contact lens intolerance, retinal vascular thrombosis, corneal curvature steepening
Respiratory: Asthma exacerbation, pulmonary thromboembolism
Miscellaneous: Anaphylactoid/anaphylactic reactions, carbohydrate intolerance

General Dosage Range Oral: *Adults (females):* 0.3-1.25 mg once daily

Mechanism of Action Conjugated A/synthetic estrogens contain a mixture of 9 synthetic estrogen substances, including sodium estrone sulfate, sodium equilin sulfate, sodium 17 alpha-dihydroequilin, sodium 17 alpha-estradiol and sodium 17 beta-dihydroequilin. Estrogens are responsible for the development and maintenance of the female reproductive system and secondary sexual characteristics. Estradiol is the principle intracellular human estrogen and is more potent than estrone and estriol at the receptor level; it is the primary estrogen secreted prior to menopause. Following menopause, estrone and estrone sulfate are more highly produced. Estrogens modulate the pituitary secretion of gonadotropins, luteinizing hormone, and follicle-stimulating hormone through a negative feedback system; estrogen replacement reduces elevated levels of these hormones in postmenopausal women.

Estrogens (Conjugated B/Synthetic)

(ES troe jenz, KON joo gate ed, bee, sin THET ik)

U.S. Brand Names Enjuvia™

Pharmacologic Category Estrogen Derivative

Use Treatment of moderate-to-severe vasomotor symptoms of menopause; treatment of vulvar and vaginal atrophy associated with menopause; treatment of moderate-to-severe vaginal dryness and pain with intercourse associated with menopause

Local Anesthetic/Vasoconstrictor Precautions No information available to require special precautions

Effects on Dental Treatment No significant effects or complications reported

Effects on Bleeding No information available to require special precautions related to hemostasis in dental procedures.

Adverse Effects

>10%:
Central nervous system: Headache (15% to 25%), pain (10% to 19%)
Endocrine & metabolic: Breast pain (up to 14%)
Gastrointestinal: Abdominal pain (4% to 15%), nausea (7% to 12%)

1% to 10%:
Central nervous system: Dizziness (1% to 7%)
Endocrine & metabolic: Dysmenorrhea (1% to 8%)
Gastrointestinal: Flatulence (4% to 7%)
Genitourinary: Vaginitis (2% to 7%)
Neuromuscular & skeletal: Paresthesia (up to 6%)
Respiratory: Bronchitis (up to 7%), rhinitis (4% to 7%), sinusitis (3% to 7%)
Miscellaneous: Flu-like syndrome (4% to 7%)

In addition, the following have been reported with estrogen and/or progestin therapy:
Cardiovascular: Edema, hypertension, MI, stroke, venous thromboembolism
Central nervous system: Epilepsy exacerbation, irritability, mental depression, migraine, mood disturbances, nervousness

Dermatologic: Angioedema, chloasma, erythema multiforme, erythema nodosum, hemorrhagic eruption, hirsutism, loss of scalp hair, melasma, pruritus, rash, urticaria

Endocrine & metabolic: Breast cancer, breast enlargement, breast tenderness, HDL-cholesterol increased, hyper-/hypocalcemia, impaired glucose tolerance, LDL-cholesterol decreased, libido (changes in), serum triglycerides/phospholipids increased, thyroid-binding globulin increased, total thyroid hormone (T_4) increased

Gastrointestinal: Abdominal cramps, bloating, cholecystitis, cholelithiasis, gallbladder disease, pancreatitis, weight gain/loss

Genitourinary: Alterations in frequency and flow of menses, changes in cervical secretions, endometrial cancer, endometrial hyperplasia, increased size of uterine leiomyomata, vaginal candidiasis

Hematologic: Aggravation of porphyria; antithrombin III and antifactor Xa decreased; fibrinogen levels increased; platelet aggregability and platelet count increased; prothrombin and factors VII, VIII, IX, X increased

Hepatic: Cholestatic jaundice, hepatic hemangiomas enlarged

Local: Thrombophlebitis

Neuromuscular & skeletal: Arthralgias, chorea, leg cramps

Ocular: Contact lens intolerance, corneal curvature steepening, retinal vascular thrombosis

Respiratory: Asthma exacerbation, pulmonary thromboembolism

Miscellaneous: Anaphylactoid/anaphylactic reactions, carbohydrate intolerance

General Dosage Range Oral: *Adults (females):* 0.3-1.25 mg once daily

Mechanism of Action Conjugated B/synthetic estrogens contain a mixture of 10 synthetic estrogen substances, including sodium estrone sulfate, sodium equilin sulfate, sodium 17-alpha-dihydroequilin, sodium 17-alpha-estradiol, and sodium 17-beta-dihydroequilin. Estrogens are responsible for the development and maintenance of the female reproductive system and secondary sexual characteristics. Estradiol is the principle intracellular human estrogen and is more potent than estrone and estriol at the receptor level; it is the primary estrogen secreted prior to menopause. Following menopause, estrone and estrone sulfate are more highly produced. Estrogens modulate the pituitary secretion of gonadotropins, luteinizing hormone, and follicle-stimulating hormone through a negative feedback system; estrogen replacement reduces elevated levels of these hormones in postmenopausal women.

Pharmacodynamics/Kinetics

Half-life Elimination Conjugated estrone: 8-20 hours; conjugated equilin: 5-17 hours

Estrogens (Conjugated/Equine, Systemic)

(ES troe jenz KON joo gate ed, EE kwine)

Related Information

Endocrine Disorders and Pregnancy *on page 1879*

U.S. Brand Names Premarin®

Canadian Brand Names C.E.S.®; Premarin®

Generic Availability (U.S.) No

Pharmacologic Category Estrogen Derivative

Use Treatment of moderate-to-severe vasomotor symptoms associated with menopause; treatment of vulvar and vaginal atrophy; hypoestrogenism (due to hypogonadism, castration, or primary ovarian failure); prostatic cancer (palliation); breast cancer (palliation); osteoporosis (prophylaxis, postmenopausal women at significant risk only); abnormal uterine bleeding; moderate-to-severe dyspareunia (pain during intercourse) due to vaginal/vulvar atrophy of menopause

Unlabeled/Investigational Use Uremic bleeding

Local Anesthetic/Vasoconstrictor Precautions No information available to require special precautions

Effects on Dental Treatment No significant effects or complications reported

Effects on Bleeding No information available to require special precautions

Adverse Effects

Note: Percentages reported in postmenopausal women following oral use.

>10%:

Central nervous system: Headache (26% to 32%; placebo 28%)

Endocrine & metabolic: Breast pain (7% to 12%; placebo 9%)

Gastrointestinal: Abdominal pain (15% to 17%)

Genitourinary: Vaginal hemorrhage (2% to 14%)

Neuromuscular & skeletal: Back pain (13% to 14%)

1% to 10%:

Central nervous system: Nervousness (2% to 5%)
Dermatologic: Pruritus (4% to 5%)
Gastrointestinal: Flatulence (6% to 7%)
Genitourinary: Vaginitis (5% to 7%), leukorrhea (4% to 7%), vaginal moniliasis (5% to 6%)
Neuromuscular & skeletal: Weakness (7% to 8%), leg cramps (3% to 7%)

Additional adverse reactions reported with injection or vaginal cream; frequency not defined:

Genitourinary: Cystis-like syndrome, genital pruritus, vulvovaginal discomfort
Local: injection site: Edema, pain, phlebitis

In addition, the following have been reported with estrogen and/or progestin therapy:
Cardiovascular: DVT, edema, hypertension, MI, stroke, superficial venous thrombosis
Central nervous system: Dementia, dizziness, epilepsy exacerbation, headache, irritability, mental depression, migraine, mood disturbances, nervousness
Dermatologic: Angioedema, chloasma, erythema multiforme, erythema nodosum, hemorrhagic eruption, hirsutism, loss of scalp hair, melasma, pruritus, rash, urticaria
Endocrine & metabolic: Breast cancer, breast discharge, breast enlargement, breast tenderness, dysmenorrhea, fibrocystic breast changes, galactorrhea, glucose intolerance, HDL-cholesterol increased, hyper-/hypocalcemia, LDL-cholesterol decreased, libido (changes in), ovarian cancer, serum triglycerides/phospholipids increased, thyroid-binding globulin increased, total thyroid hormone (T_4) increased
Gastrointestinal: Abdominal cramps, bloating, cholecystitis, cholelithiasis, gallbladder disease, ischemic colitis, nausea, pancreatitis, vomiting, weight gain/loss
Genitourinary: Abnormal uterine bleeding/spotting, changes in cervical ectropion, changes in cervical secretions, endometrial cancer, endometrial hyperplasia, increased size of uterine leiomyomata, vaginal candidiasis
Hematologic: Aggravation of porphyria, antithrombin III and antifactor Xa decreased; factors II, II-VII-X complex, VII, VIII, VII-X complex, IX, X, and XII increased; increased beta-thromboglobulin, fibrinogen levels, plasminogen/plasminogen activity, platelet aggregability, platelet count, and prothrombin
Hepatic: Cholestatic jaundice, hepatic hemangiomas enlarged
Neuromuscular & skeletal: Arthralgias, chorea, leg cramps
Local: Thrombophlebitis
Ocular: Contact lens intolerance, corneal curvature steepening, retinal vascular thrombosis
Respiratory: Asthma exacerbation, pulmonary thromboembolism
Miscellaneous: Anaphylactoid/anaphylactic reactions, benign meningioma growth potentiation

Dosage Adults:

Male: Androgen-dependent prostate cancer palliation: Oral: 1.25-2.5 mg 3 times/day

Female:

Prevention of postmenopausal osteoporosis: Oral: Initial: 0.3 mg/day cyclically* or daily, depending on medical assessment of patient. Dose may be adjusted based on bone mineral density and clinical response. The lowest effective dose should be used.

Moderate-to-severe vasomotor symptoms associated with menopause: Oral: Initial: 0.3 mg/day, cyclically* or daily, depending on medical assessment of patient. The lowest dose that will control symptoms should be used. Medication should be discontinued as soon as possible.

Vulvar and vaginal atrophy:

Oral: Initial: 0.3 mg/day; the lowest dose that will control symptoms should be used. May be given cyclically* or daily, depending on medical assessment of patient. Medication should be discontinued as soon as possible.

Abnormal uterine bleeding:

Acute/heavy bleeding:

Oral (unlabeled route): 1.25 mg, may repeat every 4 hours for 24 hours, followed by 1.25 mg once daily for 7-10 days

I.M., I.V.: 25 mg, may repeat in 6-12 hours if needed

Note: Treatment should be followed by a low-dose oral contraceptive; medroxyprogesterone acetate along with or following estrogen therapy can also be given

Nonacute/lesser bleeding: Oral (unlabeled route): 1.25 mg once daily for 7-10 days

Female hypogonadism: Oral: 0.3-0.625 mg/day given cyclically*; dose may be titrated in 6- to 12-month intervals; progestin treatment should be added to maintain bone mineral density once skeletal maturity is achieved.

Female castration, primary ovarian failure: Oral: 1.25 mg/day given cyclically*; adjust according to severity of symptoms and patient response. For maintenance, adjust to the lowest effective dose.

***Cyclic administration:** Either 3 weeks on, 1 week off **or** 25 days on, 5 days off

Male and Female:

Breast cancer palliation, metastatic disease in selected patients: Oral: 10 mg 3 times/day for at least 3 months

Uremic bleeding (unlabeled use): I.V.: 0.6 mg/kg/day for 5 days

Elderly: Refer to adult dosing; a higher incidence of stroke and invasive breast cancer was observed in women >75 years in a WHI substudy.

Mechanism of Action Conjugated estrogens contain a mixture of estrone sulfate, equilin sulfate, 17 alpha-dihydroequilin, 17 alpha-estradiol and 17 beta-dihydroequilin. Estrogens are responsible for the development and maintenance of the female reproductive system and secondary sexual characteristics. Estradiol is the principle intracellular human estrogen and is more potent than estrone and estriol at the receptor level; it is the primary estrogen secreted prior to menopause. Following menopause, estrone and estrone sulfate are more highly produced. Estrogens modulate the pituitary secretion of gonadotropins, luteinizing hormone, and follicle-stimulating hormone through a negative feedback system; estrogen replacement reduces elevated levels of these hormones in postmenopausal women.

Contraindications Hypersensitivity to estrogens or any component of the formulation; undiagnosed abnormal vaginal bleeding; history of or current thrombophlebitis or venous thromboembolic disorders (including DVT, PE); active or recent (within 1 year) arterial thromboembolic disease (eg, stroke, MI); carcinoma of the breast (except in appropriately selected patients being treated for metastatic disease); estrogen-dependent tumor; hepatic dysfunction or disease; pregnancy

Warnings/Precautions

Cardiovascular-related considerations: **[U.S. Boxed Warning]: Estrogens with or without progestin should not be used to prevent cardiovascular disease.** Use caution with cardiovascular disease or dysfunction. May increase the risks of hypertension, myocardial infarction (MI), stroke, pulmonary emboli (PE), and deep vein thrombosis; incidence of these effects was shown to be significantly increased in postmenopausal women using conjugated estrogens (CE) alone or in combination with medroxyprogesterone acetate (MPA). Nonfatal MI, PE, and thrombophlebitis have also been reported in males taking high doses of CE (eg, for prostate cancer). Estrogen compounds are generally associated with lipid effects such as increased HDL-cholesterol and decreased LDL-cholesterol. Triglycerides may also be increased; use with caution in patients with familial defects of lipoprotein metabolism. Whenever possible, estrogens should be discontinued at least 4 weeks prior to and for 2 weeks following elective surgery associated with an increased risk of thromboembolism or during periods of prolonged immobilization.

Neurological considerations: **[U.S. Boxed Warning]: The risk of dementia may be increased in postmenopausal women;** increased incidence was observed in women ≥65 years of age taking CE alone or in combination with MPA.

Cancer-related considerations: **[U.S. Boxed Warning]: Adequate diagnostic measures, including endometrial sampling, if indicated, should be performed to rule out malignancy in all cases of undiagnosed abnormal vaginal bleeding. Unopposed estrogens may increase the risk of endometrial carcinoma in postmenopausal women with an intact uterus.** Risk appears to be associated with long-term use The use of a progestin should be considered when administering estrogens to postmenopausal women with an intact uterus. Estrogens may exacerbate endometriosis. Malignant transformation of residual endometrial implants has been reported posthysterectomy with estrogen only therapy. Consider adding a progestin in women with residual endometriosis posthysterectomy. Presentation of irregular, unresolving vaginal bleeding warrants further evaluation including endometrial sampling, if indicated, to rule out malignancy. Estrogens may increase the risk of breast cancer. An increased risk of invasive breast cancer was observed in postmenopausal women using CE in combination with MPA; a smaller increase in risk was seen with estrogen therapy alone in observational studies. An increase in abnormal mammograms has also been reported with estrogen and progestin therapy. Estrogen use may lead to severe hypercalcemia in patients with breast cancer and bone metastases; discontinue estrogen if hypercalcemia occurs.

Estrogens may cause retinal vascular thrombosis; discontinue permanently if papilledema or retinal vascular lesions are observed on examination. Use with caution in patients with diseases which may be exacerbated by fluid retention, including asthma, epilepsy, migraine, diabetes, heart failure, or renal dysfunction. Use with caution in patients with a history of severe hypocalcemia, SLE, hepatic hemangiomas, porphyria, endometriosis, and gallbladder disease. Use caution with history of cholestatic jaundice associated with past estrogen use or pregnancy. May be inappropriate for use in the elderly due to potential of increased risk of breast and endometrial cancers and lack of proven cardioprotection (Beers Criteria). Prior to puberty, estrogens may cause premature closure of the epiphyses, premature breast development in girls or gynecomastia in boys. Vaginal bleeding and vaginal cornification may also be induced in girls.

[U.S. Boxed Warning]: Estrogens with or without progestin should be used for shortest duration possible at the lowest effective dose consistent with treatment goals. Before prescribing estrogen therapy to postmenopausal women, the risks and benefits must be weighed for each patient. Women should be informed of these risks and benefits, as well as possible effects of progestin when added to estrogen therapy. Estrogens with or without progestin should be used for shortest duration possible consistent with treatment goals. Conduct periodic risk:benefit assessments.

Drug Interactions

Metabolism/Transport Effects

Based on estradiol and estrone: **Substrate** of CYP1A2 (major), 2A6 (minor), 2B6 (minor), 2C9 (minor), 2C19 (minor), 2D6 (minor), 2E1 (minor), 3A4 (major); Inhibits CYP1A2 (weak), 2C8 (weak); Induces CYP3A4 (weak)

Avoid Concomitant Use

Avoid concomitant use of Estrogens (Conjugated/Equine, Systemic) with any of the following: Anastrozole

Increased Effect/Toxicity

Estrogens (Conjugated/Equine, Systemic) may increase the levels/effects of: Corticosteroids (Systemic); ROPINIRole; Tipranavir

The levels/effects of Estrogens (Conjugated/Equine, Systemic) may be increased by: Ascorbic Acid; Conivaptan; Herbs (Estrogenic Properties)

Decreased Effect

Estrogens (Conjugated/Equine, Systemic) may decrease the levels/effects of: Anastrozole; Chenodiol; Saxagliptin; Somatropin; Thyroid Products; Ursodiol

The levels/effects of Estrogens (Conjugated/Equine, Systemic) may be decreased by: CYP1A2 Inducers (Strong); CYP3A4 Inducers (Strong); Deferasirox; Herbs (CYP3A4 Inducers); Peginterferon Alfa-2b; Tipranavir; Tocilizumab

Ethanol/Nutrition/Herb Interactions

Ethanol: Avoid ethanol (routine use increases estrogen plasma concentrations and risk of breast cancer). Ethanol may also increase the risk of osteoporosis.

Food: Folic acid absorption may be decreased.

Herb/Nutraceutical: St John's wort may decrease levels. Herbs with estrogenic properties may enhance the adverse/toxic effect of estrogen derivatives; examples include alfalfa, black cohosh, bloodroot, hops, kudzu, licorice, red clover, saw palmetto, soybean, thyme, wild yam, yucca.

Dietary Considerations Ensure adequate calcium and vitamin D intake when used for the prevention of osteoporosis. Powder for reconstitution for injection (25 mg) contains lactose 200 mg.

Pharmacodynamics/Kinetics

Half-life Elimination Total estrone: 27 hours

Time to Peak Total estrone: 7 hours

Lactation Enters breast milk/use caution

Breast-Feeding Considerations Estrogen has been shown to decrease the quantity and quality of human milk. Use only if clearly needed. Monitor the growth of the infant closely.

Dosage Forms

Injection, powder for reconstitution:

Premarin®: 25 mg

Tablet, oral:

Premarin®: 0.3 mg, 0.45 mg, 0.625 mg, 0.9 mg, 1.25 mg

Estrogens (Conjugated/Equine) and Medroxyprogesterone

(ES troe jenz KON joo gate ed/EE kwine & me DROKS ee proe JES te rone)

Related Information

Endocrine Disorders and Pregnancy *on page* 1879

Estrogens (Conjugated/Equine, Systemic) *on page* 638

MedroxyPROGESTERone *on page* 1061

U.S. Brand Names Premphase®; Prempro®

Canadian Brand Names Premphase®; Premplus®; Prempro®

Pharmacologic Category Estrogen and Progestin Combination

Use Women with an intact uterus: Treatment of moderate-to-severe vasomotor symptoms associated with menopause; treatment of moderate-to-severe vulvar and vaginal atrophy due to menopause; postmenopausal osteoporosis (prophylaxis)

Local Anesthetic/Vasoconstrictor Precautions No information available to require special precautions

Effects on Dental Treatment No significant effects or complications reported

Effects on Bleeding No information available to require special precautions related to hemostasis in dental procedures.

Adverse Effects

>10%:

Central nervous system: Headache (28% to 37%), pain (11% to 13%), depression (6% to 11%)
Endocrine & metabolic: Breast pain (32% to 38%), dysmenorrhea (5% to 13%)
Gastrointestinal: Abdominal pain (16% to 23%), nausea (9% to 11%)
Neuromuscular & skeletal: Back pain (13% to 16%)
Respiratory: Pharyngitis (11% to 13%)
Miscellaneous: Infection (16% to 18%), flu-like syndrome (10% to 13%)

1% to 10%:

Cardiovascular: Peripheral edema (3% to 4%)
Central nervous system: Dizziness (3% to 5%)
Dermatologic: Pruritus (5% to 10%), rash (4% to 6%)
Endocrine & metabolic: Leukorrhea (5% to 9%)
Gastrointestinal: Flatulence (8% to 9%), diarrhea (5% to 6%), dyspepsia (5% to 6%)
Genitourinary: Vaginitis (5% to 7%), cervical changes (4% to 5%), pelvic pain (4 to 5%), vaginal hemorrhage (1% to 3%)
Neuromuscular & skeletal: Weakness (6% to 10%), arthralgia (7% to 9%), leg cramps (3% to 5%), hypertonia (3% to 4%)
Respiratory: Sinusitis (7% to 8%), rhinitis (6% to 8%)

General Dosage Range Oral: *Adults (females):* Prempro®: Conjugated estrogen 0.3-0.625 mg/mPA 1.5-5 mg once daily **or** Premphase®: One 0.625 mg tablet daily on days 1 through 14 and 1 conjugated estrogen 0.625 mg/mPA 5 mg tablet daily on days 15 through 28

Mechanism of Action

Conjugated estrogens contain a mixture of estrone sulfate, equilin sulfate, 17 alpha-dihydroequilin, 17 alpha-estradiol, and 17 beta-dihydroequilin. Estrogens are responsible for the development and maintenance of the female reproductive system and secondary sexual characteristics. Estradiol is the principle intracellular human estrogen and is more potent than estrone and estriol at the receptor level; it is the primary estrogen secreted prior to menopause. Following menopause, estrone and estrone sulfate are more highly produced. Estrogens modulate the pituitary secretion of gonadotropins, luteinizing hormone, and follicle-stimulating hormone through a negative feedback system; estrogen replacement reduces elevated levels of these hormones in postmenopausal women.

MPA inhibits gonadotropin production which then prevents follicular maturation and ovulation. In women with adequate estrogen, MPA transforms a proliferative endometrium into a secretory endometrium; when administered with conjugated estrogens, reduces the incidence of endometrial hyperplasia and risk of adenocarcinoma.

Estrogens (Esterified) (ES troe jenz, es TER i fied)

Related Information

Endocrine Disorders and Pregnancy *on page 1879*

U.S. Brand Names Menest®

Canadian Brand Names Estragyn; Estratab®; Menest®

Pharmacologic Category Estrogen Derivative

Use Treatment of moderate-to-severe vasomotor symptoms associated with menopause; treatment of moderate-to-severe vulvar and vaginal atrophy associated with menopause; hypoestrogenism (due to hypogonadism, castration, or primary ovarian failure); advanced prostatic cancer (palliation), metastatic breast cancer (palliation) in men and postmenopausal women

Local Anesthetic/Vasoconstrictor Precautions No information available to require special precautions

Effects on Dental Treatment No significant effects or complications reported

Effects on Bleeding No information available to require special precautions related to hemostasis in dental procedures.

Adverse Effects Frequency not defined.

Cardiovascular: Edema, hypertension, MI, stroke, venous thromboembolism

Central nervous system: Dementia exacerbation, dizziness, epilepsy exacerbation, headache, irritability, mental depression, migraine, mood disturbances, nervousness

Dermatologic: Angioedema, chloasma, erythema multiforme, erythema nodosum, hemorrhagic eruption, hirsutism, pruritus, loss of scalp hair, melasma, rash, urticaria

Endocrine & metabolic: Breast cancer, breast enlargement, breast tenderness, carbohydrate intolerance, fibrocystic breast changes, galactorrhea, hypocalcemia, libido (changes in), nipple discharge, premenstrual like syndrome

Gastrointestinal: Abdominal cramps, bloating, gallbladder disease, nausea, pancreatitis, vomiting, weight gain/loss

Genitourinary: Alterations in frequency and flow of menstrual patterns, breakthrough bleeding, changes in cervical secretions, cervical ectropion changes, cystitis-like syndrome, dysmenorrhea, endometrial hyperplasia, endometrial cancer, increased size of uterine leiomyomata, ovarian cancer, vaginal candidiasis, vaginitis

Hematologic: Aggravation of porphyria

Hepatic: Cholestatic jaundice, hemangioma enlargement

Local: Thrombophlebitis

Neuromuscular & skeletal: Arthralgia, chorea, leg cramps

Ocular: Contact lens intolerance, corneal curvature steepening, retinal vascular thrombosis

Respiratory: Asthma exacerbation, pulmonary embolism

Miscellaneous: Anaphylactoid/anaphylactic reactions

General Dosage Range

Oral:

Adults (females): Hypogonadism: 2.5-7.5 mg/day for 20 days followed by a 10-day rest, repeat until response; Castration or ovarian failure: 1.25 mg/day, cyclically; Menopause 0.3-1.25 mg/day given cyclically; Breast cancer: 10 mg 3 times/day

Adults (males): Breast cancer: 10 mg 3 times/day; Prostate cancer: 1.25-2.5 mg 3 times/day

Mechanism of Action Esterified estrogens contain a mixture of estrogenic substances; the principle component is estrone. Preparations contain 75% to 85% sodium estrone sulfate and 6% to 15% sodium equilin sulfate such that the total is not <90%. Estrogens are responsible for the development and maintenance of the female reproductive system and secondary sexual characteristics. Estradiol is the principle intracellular human estrogen and is more potent than estrone and estriol at the receptor level; it is the primary estrogen secreted prior to menopause. In males and following menopause in females, estrone and estrone sulfate are more highly produced. Estrogens modulate the pituitary secretion of gonadotropins, luteinizing hormone, and follicle-stimulating hormone through a negative feedback system; estrogen replacement reduces elevated levels of these hormones.

Estrogens (Esterified) and Methyltestosterone

(ES troe jenz es TER i fied & meth il tes TOS te rone)

Related Information

Endocrine Disorders and Pregnancy *on page 1879*

Estrogens (Esterified) *on page 642*

MethylTESTOSTERone *on page 1119*

U.S. Brand Names Covaryx®; Covaryx® H.S.; EEMT™; EEMT™ HS; Estratest® H.S. [DSC]; Estratest® [DSC]

Pharmacologic Category Estrogen and Progestin Combination

Use Treatment of moderate-to-severe vasomotor symptoms associated with menopause not improved by estrogens alone

Local Anesthetic/Vasoconstrictor Precautions No information available to require special precautions

Effects on Dental Treatment No significant effects or complications reported

Effects on Bleeding No information available to require special precautions related to hemostasis in dental procedures.

Adverse Effects Refer to the Estrogens (Esterified) and the Testosterone monographs.

General Dosage Range Oral: *Adults (females):* Usual dosage range (based on esterified estrogen component): 0.625-1.25 mg every day for 3 weeks and then discontinued for 1 week off

Mechanism of Action

Conjugated estrogens: Activate estrogen receptors (DNA protein complex) located in estrogen-responsive tissues. Once activated, regulate transcription of certain genes leading to observed effects.

Testosterone: Increases synthesis of DNA, RNA, and various proteins in target tissues

Pregnancy Risk Factor X

Estropipate (ES troe pih pate)

Related Information

Endocrine Disorders and Pregnancy *on page 1879*

Canadian Brand Names Ogen®

Pharmacologic Category Estrogen Derivative

Use Treatment of moderate-to-severe vasomotor symptoms associated with menopause; treatment of vulvar and vaginal atrophy; hypoestrogenism (due to hypogonadism, castration, or primary ovarian failure); osteoporosis (prophylaxis, in women at significant risk only)

Local Anesthetic/Vasoconstrictor Precautions No information available to require special precautions

Effects on Dental Treatment No significant effects or complications reported

Effects on Bleeding No information available to require special precautions related to hemostasis in dental procedures.

Adverse Effects Frequency not defined.

Cardiovascular: Edema, hypertension, venous thromboembolism

Central nervous system: Dizziness, headache, mental depression, migraine

Dermatologic: Chloasma, erythema multiforme, erythema nodosum, hemorrhagic eruption, hirsutism, loss of scalp hair, melasma

Endocrine & metabolic: Breast enlargement, breast tenderness, libido (changes in), increased thyroid-binding globulin, increased total thyroid hormone (T_4), increased serum triglycerides/phospholipids, increased HDL-cholesterol, decreased LDL-cholesterol, impaired glucose tolerance, hypercalcemia

Gastrointestinal: Abdominal cramps, bloating, cholecystitis, cholelithiasis, gallbladder disease, nausea, pancreatitis, vomiting, weight gain/loss

Genitourinary: Alterations in frequency and flow of menses, changes in cervical secretions, endometrial cancer, increased size of uterine leiomyomata, vaginal candidiasis

Hematologic: Antithrombin III decreased; antifactor Xa decreased; fibrinogen levels increased; platelet aggregability increased; platelet count increased; porphyria aggravation; prothrombin and factors VII, VIII, IX, X increased

Hepatic: Cholestatic jaundice

Neuromuscular & skeletal: Chorea

Ocular: Ocular: Contact lens intolerance, corneal curvature steepening

Respiratory: Pulmonary thromboembolism

Miscellaneous: Carbohydrate intolerance

General Dosage Range Dosage adjustment recommended in patients with hepatic impairment

Oral: *Adults (females):* 0.75-6 mg once daily or cyclically [menopause] **or** 1.5-9 mg for the first 3 weeks, followed by a rest period of 8-10 days [hypoestrogenism] **or** 0.75 mg for 25 days of a 31 day cycle [osteoporosis]

Mechanism of Action Estrogens are responsible for the development and maintenance of the female reproductive system and secondary sexual characteristics. Estradiol is the principle intracellular human estrogen and is more potent than estrone and estriol at the receptor level; it is the primary estrogen secreted prior to menopause. In males and following menopause in females, estrone and estrone sulfate are more highly produced. Estrogens modulate the pituitary secretion of gonadotropins, luteinizing hormone, and follicle-stimulating hormone through a negative feedback system; estrogen replacement reduces elevated levels of these hormones. Estropipate is prepared from purified crystalline estrone that has been solubilized as the sulfate and stabilized with piperazine.

Pregnancy Risk Factor X

Eszopiclone (es zoe PIK lone)

U.S. Brand Names Lunesta®

Generic Availability (U.S.) No

Pharmacologic Category Hypnotic, Nonbenzodiazepine

Use Treatment of insomnia

Local Anesthetic/Vasoconstrictor Precautions No information available to require special precautions

Effects on Dental Treatment Key adverse event(s) related to dental treatment: Unpleasant taste and xerostomia (normal salivary flow resumes upon discontinuation).

Effects on Bleeding No information available to require special precautions

Adverse Effects

>10%:

Central nervous system: Headache (15% to 21%)

Gastrointestinal: Unpleasant taste (8% to 34%)

1% to 10%:

Cardiovascular: Chest pain, peripheral edema

Central nervous system: Somnolence (8% to 10%), dizziness (5% to 7%), pain (4% to 5%), nervousness (up to 5%), depression (1% to 4%), confusion (up to 3%), hallucinations (1% to 3%), anxiety (1% to 3%), abnormal dreams (1% to 3%), migraine

Dermatologic: Rash (3% to 4%), pruritus (1% to 4%)

Endocrine & metabolic: Libido decreased (up to 3%), dysmenorrhea (up to 3%), gynecomastia (males up to 3%)

Gastrointestinal: Xerostomia (3% to 7%), dyspepsia (2% to 6%), nausea (4% to 5%), diarrhea (2% to 4%), vomiting (up to 3%)

Genitourinary: Urinary tract infection (up to 3%)

Neuromuscular & skeletal: Neuralgia (up to 3%)

Miscellaneous: Infection (5% to 10%), viral infection (3%), accidental injury (up to 3%)

Dosage Oral:

Adults: Insomnia: Initial: 2 mg immediately before bedtime (maximum dose: 3 mg)

Concurrent use with strong CYP3A4 inhibitor: 1 mg immediately before bedtime; if needed, dose may be increased to 2 mg

Elderly:

Difficulty **falling** asleep: Initial: 1 mg immediately before bedtime; maximum dose: 2 mg

Difficulty **staying** asleep: 2 mg immediately before bedtime

Dosage adjustment in renal impairment: None required

Dosage adjustment in hepatic impairment:

Mild-to-moderate: Use with caution; dosage adjustment unnecessary

Severe: Initial dose: 1 mg; maximum dose: 2 mg

Mechanism of Action May interact with GABA-receptor complexes at binding domains located close to or allosterically coupled to benzodiazepine receptors.

Contraindications There are no contraindications listed within the manufacturer's labeling.

Warnings/Precautions Symptomatic treatment of insomnia should be initiated only after careful evaluation of potential causes of sleep disturbance. Tolerance did not develop over 6 months of use. Use with caution in patients with depression or a history of drug dependence. Abrupt discontinuance may lead to withdrawal symptoms. Use with caution in patients receiving other CNS depressants or psychoactive medications. Hypnotics/sedatives have been associated with abnormal thinking and behavior changes including decreased inhibition, aggression, bizarre behavior, agitation, hallucinations, and depersonalization. These changes may occur unpredictably and may indicate previously unrecognized psychiatric disorders; evaluate appropriately. Amnesia may occur. May impair physical and mental capabilities. Postmarketing studies have indicated that the use of hypnotic/sedative agents for sleep has been associated with hypersensitivity reactions including anaphylaxis as well as angioedema. An increased risk for hazardous sleep-related activities such as sleep-driving (as well as cooking and eating food and making phone calls while asleep) has also been noted. Use caution in patients with respiratory compromise, hepatic dysfunction, elderly or those taking strong CYP3A4 inhibitors. Because of the rapid onset of action, administer immediately prior to bedtime or after the patient has gone to bed and is having difficulty falling asleep.

Drug Interactions

Metabolism/Transport Effects Substrate of CYP2E1 (minor), 3A4 (major)

Avoid Concomitant Use There are no known interactions where it is recommended to avoid concomitant use.

Increased Effect/Toxicity

Eszopiclone may increase the levels/effects of: Alcohol (Ethyl); CNS Depressants; Methotrimeprazine

The levels/effects of Eszopiclone may be increased by: Antifungal Agents (Azole Derivatives, Systemic); Conivaptan; CYP3A4 Inhibitors (Moderate); CYP3A4 Inhibitors (Strong); Dasatinib; Droperidol; Methotrimeprazine

Decreased Effect

The levels/effects of Eszopiclone may be decreased by: CYP3A4 Inducers (Strong); Deferasirox; Flumazenil; Herbs (CYP3A4 Inducers); Tocilizumab

Ethanol/Nutrition/Herb Interactions

Ethanol: Ethanol: May increase CNS depression; monitor for increased effects with coadministration. Caution patients about effects.

Food: Onset of action may be reduced if taken with or immediately after a heavy meal.
Herb/Nutraceutical: Avoid valerian, St John's wort, kava kava, gotu kola (may increase CNS depression).

Dietary Considerations Avoid taking after a heavy meal; may delay onset.

Pharmacodynamics/Kinetics

Half-life Elimination ~6 hours; Elderly (≥65 years): ~9 hours

Time to Peak ~1 hour

Pregnancy Risk Factor C

Lactation Excretion in breast milk unknown/use caution

Controlled Substance C-IV

Dosage Forms

Tablet, oral:
Lunesta®: 1 mg, 2 mg, 3 mg

Etanercept (et a NER sept)

Related Information

Rheumatoid Arthritis, Osteoarthritis, and Osteoporosis *on page 1889*

U.S. Brand Names Enbrel®; Enbrel® SureClick®

Canadian Brand Names Enbrel®

Generic Availability (U.S.) No

Pharmacologic Category Antirheumatic, Disease Modifying; Tumor Necrosis Factor (TNF) Blocking Agent

Use Treatment of moderately- to severely-active rheumatoid arthritis (RA); moderately- to severely-active polyarticular juvenile idiopathic arthritis (JIA); psoriatic arthritis; active ankylosing spondylitis (AS); moderate-to-severe chronic plaque psoriasis

Local Anesthetic/Vasoconstrictor Precautions No information available to require special precautions

Effects on Dental Treatment No significant effects or complications reported

Effects on Bleeding No information available to require special precautions

Adverse Effects Percentages reported for adults except where specified.

>10%:
- Central nervous system: Headache (17%; children 19%)
- Gastrointestinal: Abdominal pain (5%; children 19%), vomiting (3%; children 13%)
- Local: Injection site reaction (14% to 37%; erythema, itching, pain or swelling)
- Respiratory: Respiratory tract infection (upper; 12% to 29%), rhinitis (12%)
- Miscellaneous: Infection (35%; children 62%), positive ANA (11%), positive anti-double-stranded DNA antibodies (15% by RIA, 3% by *Crithidia luciliae* assay)

≥3% to 10%:
- Central nervous system: Dizziness (7%)
- Dermatologic: Rash (5%)
- Gastrointestinal: Nausea (children 9%), dyspepsia (4%)
- Neuromuscular & skeletal: Weakness (5%)
- Respiratory: Pharyngitis (7%), cough (6%), respiratory disorder (5%), sinusitis (3%)

Dosage SubQ:

Children 2-17 years: Juvenile idiopathic arthritis:
- Once-weekly dosing: 0.8 mg/kg (maximum: 50 mg/dose) once weekly
- Twice-weekly dosing: 0.4 mg/kg (maximum: 25 mg/dose) twice weekly (individual doses should be separated by 72-96 hours)

Adults:
- Rheumatoid arthritis, psoriatic arthritis, ankylosing spondylitis:
  - Once-weekly dosing: 50 mg once weekly
  - Twice weekly dosing: 25 mg given twice weekly (individual doses should be separated by 72-96 hours)
- Plaque psoriasis:
  - Initial: 50 mg twice weekly, 72-96 hours apart; maintain initial dose for 3 months (starting doses of 25 or 50 mg once weekly have also been used successfully)
  - Maintenance dose: 50 mg once weekly

Elderly: Refer to adult dosing. Although greater sensitivity of some elderly patients cannot be ruled out, no overall differences in safety or effectiveness were observed.

Mechanism of Action Etanercept is a recombinant DNA-derived protein composed of tumor necrosis factor receptor (TNFR) linked to the Fc portion of human IgG1. Etanercept binds tumor necrosis factor (TNF) and blocks its interaction with cell surface receptors. TNF plays an important role in the inflammatory processes and the resulting joint pathology of rheumatoid arthritis (RA), polyarticular-course juvenile idiopathic arthritis (JIA), ankylosing spondylitis (AS), and plaque psoriasis.

Contraindications Hypersensitivity to etanercept or any component of the formulation; patients with sepsis (mortality may be increased)

Warnings/Precautions [U.S. Boxed Warning]: Serious and potentially fatal infections have been reported including bacterial, mycobacterial, viral, and invasive fungal infections; usually in patients taking concomitant immunosuppressive medication; infection may be disseminated, rather than localized, upon presentation. Cases of unrecognized invasive fungal infections (eg, histoplasmosis, blastomycosis, coccidioidomycosis, listeriosis, candidiasis, aspergillosis, pneumocystosis) have also been reported with anti-TNF agent use. Discontinue administration if patient develops a serious infection or sepsis. Caution should be exercised when considering the use in patients with chronic infection, history of recurrent infection, or predisposition to infection (eg, poorly-controlled diabetes or residence/travel from areas of endemic mycoses). Do not give to patients with an active chronic or localized infection. Patients should be educated about the symptoms of infection and closely monitored for signs and symptoms while undergoing treatment. **[U.S. Boxed Warning]: Tuberculosis (disseminated or extrapulmonary) has been reported in patients receiving etanercept; both reactivation of latent infection and new infections have been reported.** Patients should be evaluated for tuberculosis risk factors and for latent tuberculosis infection with a tuberculin skin test prior to starting therapy. Treatment of latent tuberculosis should be initiated before etanercept therapy; consider antituberculosis treatment if adequate course of treatment cannot be confirmed in patients with a history of latent or active tuberculosis or with risk factors despite negative skin test. Some patients who tested negative prior to therapy have developed active infection; monitor for signs and symptoms of tuberculosis in all patients. Rare reactivation of hepatitis B has occurred in chronic carriers of the virus; evaluate prior to initiation and during treatment in patients at risk for hepatitis B infection. Patients should be brought up to date with all immunizations before initiating therapy. Live vaccines should not be given concurrently with etanercept. Patients with a significant exposure to varicella virus should temporarily discontinue etanercept. Treatment with varicella zoster immune globulin should be considered.

[U.S. Boxed Warning]: Lymphoma and other malignancies have been reported in children and adolescent patients receiving TNF-blocking agents, including etanercept. Half of the malignancies reported in children were lymphomas (Hodgkin's and non-Hodgkin's) while other cases varied and included malignancies not typically observed in this population. The impact of etanercept on the development and course of malignancy is not fully defined. Compared to the general population, an increased risk of lymphoma has been noted in clinical trials; however, rheumatoid arthritis alone has been previously associated with an increased rate of lymphoma. Lymphomas and other malignancies were also observed (at rates higher than expected for the general population) in adult patients receiving etanercept. Etanercept is not recommended for use in patients with Wegener's granulomatosis who are receiving immunosuppressive therapy. Treatment may result in the formation of autoimmune antibodies; cases of autoimmune disease have not been described. Non-neutralizing antibodies to etanercept may also be formed. Rarely, a reversible lupus-like syndrome has occurred.

Allergic reactions may occur; if an anaphylactic reaction or other serious allergic reaction occurs, administration should be discontinued immediately and appropriate therapy initiated. Use with caution in patients with pre-existing or recent onset CNS demyelinating disorders; rare cases of new onset or exacerbation of CNS demyelinating disorders have occurred; may present with mental status changes and some may be associated with permanent disability. Optic neuritis, transverse myelitis, multiple sclerosis, and new onset or exacerbation of seizures have been reported. Use with caution in patients with heart failure or decreased left ventricular function; worsening and new-onset heart failure has been reported. Use caution in patients with a history of significant hematologic abnormalities; has been associated with pancytopenia and aplastic anemia (rare). Discontinue if significant hematologic abnormalities are confirmed. Use with caution in patients with moderate to severe alcoholic hepatitis. Compared to placebo, the mortality rate in patients treated with etanercept was similar at one month but significantly higher after 6 months

Due to a higher incidence of serious infections, concomitant use with anakinra is not recommended. Some dosage forms may contain dry natural rubber (latex). Some dosage forms may contain benzyl alcohol which has been associated with "gasping syndrome" in neonates.

Drug Interactions

Avoid Concomitant Use

Avoid concomitant use of Etanercept with any of the following: Abatacept; Anakinra; BCG; Belimumab; Canakinumab; Certolizumab Pegol; Cyclophosphamide; Natalizumab; Pimecrolimus; Rilonacept; Roflumilast; Tacrolimus (Topical); Vaccines (Live)

Increased Effect/Toxicity

Etanercept may increase the levels/effects of: Abatacept; Anakinra; Belimumab; Canakinumab; Certolizumab Pegol; Cyclophosphamide; Leflunomide; Natalizumab; Rilonacept; Vaccines (Live)

The levels/effects of Etanercept may be increased by: Denosumab; Pimecrolimus; Roflumilast; Tacrolimus (Topical); Trastuzumab

Decreased Effect

Etanercept may decrease the levels/effects of: BCG; Sipuleucel-T; Vaccines (Inactivated); Vaccines (Live)

The levels/effects of Etanercept may be decreased by: Echinacea

Ethanol/Nutrition/Herb Interactions Herb/Nutraceutical: Echinacea may decrease the therapeutic effects of etanercept (avoid concurrent use).

Pharmacodynamics/Kinetics

Onset of Action ~2-3 weeks; RA: 1-2 weeks

Half-life Elimination RA: SubQ: 72-132 hour

Time to Peak RA: SubQ: 35-103 hours

Pregnancy Risk Factor B

Lactation Excretion in breast milk unknown/not recommended

Breast-Feeding Considerations It is not known whether etanercept is excreted in human milk. Because many drugs and immunoglobulins are excreted in human milk and the potential for serious adverse reactions exists, a decision should be made whether to discontinue nursing or to discontinue the drug, taking into account the importance of the drug to the mother.

Dosage Forms

Injection, powder for reconstitution:

Enbrel®: 25 mg

Injection, solution [preservative free]:

Enbrel®: 50 mg/mL (0.51 mL, 0.98 mL)

Enbrel® SureClick®: 50 mg/mL (0.98 mL)

Ethacrynic Acid (eth a KRIN ik AS id)

Related Information

Cardiovascular Diseases *on page 1848*

U.S. Brand Names Edecrin®; Sodium Edecrin®

Canadian Brand Names Edecrin®

Pharmacologic Category Diuretic, Loop

Use Management of edema associated with congestive heart failure; hepatic cirrhosis or renal disease; short-term management of ascites due to malignancy, idiopathic edema, and lymphedema

Local Anesthetic/Vasoconstrictor Precautions No information available to require special precautions

Effects on Dental Treatment No significant effects or complications reported

Effects on Bleeding No information available to require special precautions

Adverse Effects Frequency not defined.

Central nervous system: Headache, fatigue, apprehension, confusion, fever, chills, encephalopathy (patients with pre-existing liver disease); vertigo

Dermatologic: Skin rash, Henoch-Schönlein purpura (in patient with rheumatic heart disease)

Endocrine & metabolic: Hyponatremia, hyperglycemia, variations in phosphorus, CO_2 content, bicarbonate, and calcium; reversible hyperuricemia, gout, hyperglycemia, hypoglycemia (occurred in two uremic patients who received doses above those recommended)

Gastrointestinal: Anorexia, malaise, abdominal discomfort or pain, dysphagia, nausea, vomiting, diarrhea, gastrointestinal bleeding, acute pancreatitis (rare)

Genitourinary: Hematuria

Hepatic: Jaundice, abnormal liver function tests

Hematology: Agranulocytosis, severe neutropenia, thrombocytopenia

Local: Thrombophlebitis (with intravenous use), local irritation and pain

Ocular: Blurred vision

Otic: Tinnitus, temporary or permanent deafness

Renal: Serum creatinine increased

General Dosage Range

I.V.: *Adults:* 0.5-1 mg/kg/dose (maximum: 100 mg/dose)

Oral:

Children: 1-3 mg/kg/day

Adults: 50-400 mg/day in 1-2 divided doses

Elderly: Initial: 25-50 mg/day

Mechanism of Action Inhibits reabsorption of sodium and chloride in the ascending loop of Henle and distal renal tubule, interfering with the chloride-binding cotransport system, thus causing increased excretion of water, sodium, chloride, magnesium, and calcium

Pharmacodynamics/Kinetics

Onset of Action Diuresis: Oral: ~30 minutes; I.V.: 5 minutes; Peak effect: Oral: 2 hours; I.V.: 30 minutes

Duration of Action Oral: 12 hours; I.V.: 2 hours

Half-life Elimination Normal renal function: 2-4 hours

Pregnancy Risk Factor B

Ethambutol (e THAM byoo tole)

Related Information

Tuberculosis *on page 1902*

U.S. Brand Names Myambutol®

Canadian Brand Names Etibi®

Pharmacologic Category Antitubercular Agent

Use Treatment of pulmonary tuberculosis in conjunction with other antituberculosis agents

Unlabeled/Investigational Use Other mycobacterial diseases in conjunction with other antimycobacterial agents

Local Anesthetic/Vasoconstrictor Precautions No information available to require special precautions

Effects on Dental Treatment No significant effects or complications reported

Effects on Bleeding No information available to require special precautions

Adverse Effects Frequency not defined.

Cardiovascular: Myocarditis, pericarditis

Central nervous system: Confusion, disorientation, dizziness, fever, hallucinations, headache, malaise

Dermatologic: Dermatitis, erythema multiforme, exfoliative dermatitis, pruritus, rash

Endocrine & metabolic: Acute gout or hyperuricemia

Gastrointestinal: Abdominal pain, anorexia, GI upset, nausea, vomiting

Hematologic: Eosinophilia, leukopenia, lymphadenopathy, neutropenia, thrombocytopenia

Hepatic: Hepatitis, hepatotoxicity (possibly related to concurrent therapy), LFTs abnormal

Neuromuscular & skeletal: Arthralgia, peripheral neuritis

Ocular: Optic neuritis; symptoms may include decreased acuity, scotoma, color blindness, or visual defects (usually reversible with discontinuation, irreversible blindness has been described)

Renal: Nephritis

Respiratory: Infiltrates (with or without eosinophilia), pneumonitis

Miscellaneous: Anaphylaxis, anaphylactoid reaction; hypersensitivity syndrome (cutaneous reactions, eosinophilia, and organ-specific inflammation)

General Dosage Range Dosage adjustment recommended in patients with renal impairment

Oral:

Children: 15-20 mg/kg/day (maximum: 1 g/day) **or** 50 mg/kg twice weekly (maximum: 2.5 g/dose)

Adults: Daily therapy: 1.5-2.5 g/kg/day (maximum dose: 1.5-2.5 g); 3 times/week DOT: 25-30 mg/kg/dose (maximum dose: 2.4 g/dose); Twice weekly DOT: 50 mg/kg/dose (maximum dose: 4 g/dose)

Mechanism of Action Inhibits arabinosyl transferase resulting in impaired mycobacterial cell wall synthesis

Pharmacodynamics/Kinetics

Half-life Elimination 2.5-3.6 hours; End-stage renal disease: 7-15 hours

Time to Peak Serum: 2-4 hours

Pregnancy Risk Factor C

Ethanolamine Oleate (ETH a nol a meen OH lee ate)

U.S. Brand Names Ethamolin®

Pharmacologic Category Sclerosing Agent

Use Orphan drug: Sclerosing agent used for bleeding esophageal varices

Local Anesthetic/Vasoconstrictor Precautions No information available to require special precautions

Effects on Dental Treatment No significant effects or complications reported

Effects on Bleeding No information available to require special precautions

Adverse Effects 1% to 10%:
Central nervous system: Pyrexia (1.8%)
Gastrointestinal: Esophageal ulcer (2%), esophageal stricture (1.3%)
Respiratory: Pleural effusion (2%), pneumonia (1.2%)
Miscellaneous: Retrosternal pain (1.6%)

General Dosage Range Injection: *Adults:* 1.5-5 mL per varix (maximum: 20 mL total)

Mechanism of Action Derived from oleic acid and similar in physical properties to sodium morrhuate; however, the exact mechanism of the hemostatic effect used in endoscopic injection sclerotherapy is not known. Intravenously injected ethanolamine oleate produces a sterile inflammatory response resulting in fibrosis and occlusion of the vein; a dose-related extravascular inflammatory reaction occurs when the drug diffuses through the venous wall. Autopsy results indicate that variceal obliteration occurs secondary to mural necrosis and fibrosis. Thrombosis appears to be a transient reaction.

Pregnancy Risk Factor C

Ethinyl Estradiol and Desogestrel

(ETH in il es tra DYE ole & des oh JES trel)

U.S. Brand Names Apri®; Azurette™; Caziant®; Cesia® [DSC]; Cyclessa®; Desogen®; Emoquette™; Kariva®; Mircette®; Ortho-Cept®; Reclipsen®; Solia® [DSC]; Velivet™

Canadian Brand Names Cyclessa®; Linessa®; Marvelon®; Ortho-Cept®

Generic Availability (U.S.) Yes

Pharmacologic Category Contraceptive; Estrogen and Progestin Combination

Use Prevention of pregnancy

Unlabeled/Investigational Use Treatment of hypermenorrhea (menorrhagia); pain associated with endometriosis; dysmenorrhea; dysfunctional uterine bleeding

Local Anesthetic/Vasoconstrictor Precautions No information available to require special precautions

Effects on Dental Treatment When prescribing antibiotics, patient must be warned to use additional methods of birth control if on oral contraceptives.

Effects on Bleeding No information available to require special precautions

Adverse Effects The following reactions have been associated with oral contraceptive use:

Increased risk or evidence of association with use:
Cardiovascular: Arterial thromboembolism, cerebral hemorrhage, cerebral thrombosis, hypertension, mesenteric thrombosis, MI, venous thrombosis (with or without embolism)
Gastrointestinal: Gallbladder disease
Hepatic: Hepatic adenomas, liver tumors (benign)
Local: Thrombophlebitis
Ocular: Retinal thrombosis
Respiratory: Pulmonary embolism

Adverse reactions considered drug related:
Cardiovascular: Edema, varicose vein aggravation
Central nervous system: Depression, migraine, mood changes
Dermatologic: Chloasma, melasma, rash (allergic)
Endocrine & metabolic: Amenorrhea, breakthrough bleeding, breast changes (enlargement, pain, secretion, tenderness), fluid retention, infertility (temporary), lactation decreased (with use immediately postpartum), menstrual flow changes, spotting
Gastrointestinal: Abdominal bloating, abdominal cramps, abdominal pain, appetite changes, nausea, weight changes, vomiting
Genitourinary: Cervical ectropion, cervical secretion, vaginal candidiasis, vaginitis
Hematologic: Folate decreased, porphyria exacerbation
Hepatic: Cholestatic jaundice
Neuromuscular & skeletal: Chorea exacerbation
Ocular: Contact lens intolerance, corneal curvature changes (steepening)
Miscellaneous: Anaphylactic/anaphylactoid reactions (including angioedema, circulatory collapse, respiratory collapse, urticaria), SLE exacerbation

Adverse reactions in which association is not confirmed or denied: Acne, Budd-Chiari syndrome, cataracts, colitis, cystitis-like syndrome, dizziness, dysmenorrhea, erythema multiforme, erythema nodosum, headache, hemolytic uremic syndrome, hemorrhagic eruption, hirsutism, libido changes, nervousness, optic neuritis (with or without partial or complete loss of vision), pancreatitis, premenstrual syndrome, renal function impaired, scalp hair loss

Dosage Oral: Adults: Females: Contraception:

Schedule 1 (Sunday starter): Dose begins on first Sunday after onset of menstruation; if the menstrual period starts on Sunday, take first tablet that very same day. **With a Sunday start, an additional method of contraception should be used until after the first 7 days of consecutive administration.**

For 21-tablet package: Dosage is 1 tablet daily for 21 consecutive days, followed by 7 days off of the medication; a new course begins on the 8th day after the last tablet is taken.

For 28-tablet package: Dosage is 1 tablet daily without interruption.

Schedule 2 (Day 1 starter): Dose starts on first day of menstrual cycle taking 1 tablet daily.

For 21-tablet package: Dosage is 1 tablet daily for 21 consecutive days, followed by 7 days off of the medication; a new course begins on the 8th day after the last tablet is taken.

For 28-tablet package: Dosage is 1 tablet daily without interruption.

If all doses have been taken on schedule and one menstrual period is missed, continue dosing cycle. If two consecutive menstrual periods are missed, pregnancy test is required before new dosing cycle is started.

Missed doses **monophasic formulations** (refer to package insert for complete information):

One dose missed: Take as soon as remembered or take 2 tablets next day

Two consecutive doses missed in the first 2 weeks: Take 2 tablets as soon as remembered or 2 tablets next 2 days. **An additional method of contraception should be used for 7 days after missed dose.**

Two consecutive doses missed in week 3 or three consecutive doses missed at any time:

Schedule 1 (Sunday starter): Continue to take 1 tablet daily until Sunday, then discard the rest of the pack, and a new pack is started that same day.

Schedule 2 (Day 1 starter): Current pack should be discarded, and a new pack started that same day. **An additional method of contraception should be used for 7 days after missed dose.**

Missed doses **biphasic/triphasic formulations** (refer to package insert for complete information):

One dose missed: Take as soon as remembered or take 2 tablets next day.

Two consecutive doses missed in week 1 or week 2 of the pack: Take 2 tablets as soon as remembered and 2 tablets the next day. Resume taking 1 tablet daily until the pack is empty. **An additional method of contraception should be used for 7 days after a missed dose.**

Two consecutive doses missed in week 3 of the pack; **an additional method of contraception must be used for 7 days after a missed dose**:

Schedule 1 (Sunday starter): Take 1 tablet every day until Sunday. Discard the remaining pack and start a new pack of pills on the same day.

Schedule 2 (Day 1 starter): Discard the remaining pack and start a new pack the same day.

Three or more consecutive doses missed; **an additional method of contraception must be used for 7 days after a missed dose**:

Schedule 1 (Sunday starter): Take 1 tablet every day until Sunday; on Sunday, discard the pack and start a new pack.

Schedule 2 (Day 1 starter): Discard the remaining pack and begin new pack of tablets starting on the same day.

Dosage adjustment in renal impairment: Specific guidelines not available; use with caution and monitor blood pressure closely. Consider other forms of contraception.

Dosage adjustment in hepatic impairment: Contraindicated in patients with hepatic impairment

Mechanism of Action Combination hormonal contraceptives inhibit ovulation via a negative feedback mechanism on the hypothalamus, which alters the normal pattern of gonadotropin secretion of a follicle-stimulating hormone (FSH) and luteinizing hormone by the anterior pituitary. The follicular phase FSH and midcycle surge of gonadotropins are inhibited. In addition, combination hormonal contraceptives produce alterations in the genital tract, including changes in the cervical mucus, rendering it unfavorable for sperm penetration even if ovulation occurs. Changes in the endometrium may also occur, producing an unfavorable environment for nidation. Combination hormonal contraceptive drugs may alter the tubal transport of the ova through the fallopian tubes. Progestational agents may also alter sperm fertility.

Contraindications Hypersensitivity to ethinyl estradiol, etonogestrel, desogestrel, or any component of the formulation; history of or current thrombophlebitis or venous thromboembolic disorders (including DVT, PE); active or recent (within 1 year) arterial thromboembolic disease (eg, stroke, MI); cerebral vascular disease, coronary artery disease, valvular heart disease with complications, severe hypertension;

diabetes mellitus with vascular involvement; severe headache with focal neurological symptoms; known or suspected breast carcinoma, endometrial cancer, estrogen-dependent neoplasms, undiagnosed abnormal genital bleeding; hepatic dysfunction or tumor, cholestatic jaundice of pregnancy, jaundice with prior combination hormonal contraceptive use; major surgery with prolonged immobilization; heavy smoking (≥15 cigarettes/day) in patients >35 years of age; pregnancy

Warnings/Precautions Combination hormonal contraceptives do not protect against HIV infection or other sexually-transmitted diseases. **[U.S. Boxed Warning]: The risk of cardiovascular side effects increases in women who smoke cigarettes, especially those who are >35 years of age; women who use combination hormonal contraceptives should be strongly advised not to smoke.** Combination hormonal contraceptives may lead to increased risk of myocardial infarction, use with caution in patients with risk factors for coronary artery disease. May increase the risk of thromboembolism. Whenever possible, combination hormonal contraceptives should be discontinued at least 4 weeks prior to and for 2 weeks following elective surgery associated with an increased risk of thromboembolism or during periods of prolonged immobilization. Combination hormonal contraceptives may have a dose-related risk of vascular disease, hypertension, and gallbladder disease. Women with hypertension or renal disease should be encouraged to use another form of contraception. The use of combination hormonal contraceptives has been associated with a slight increase in frequency of breast cancer, however, studies are not consistent. Combination hormonal contraceptives may cause glucose intolerance or effect serum triglyceride and lipoprotein levels. Retinal thrombosis has been reported (rarely). Use caution in conditions that may be aggravated by fluid retention, depression, or history of migraine. Not for use prior to menarche.

The minimum dosage combination of estrogen/progestin that will effectively treat the individual patient should be used. New patients should be started on products containing ≤0.035 mg of estrogen per tablet.

Drug Interactions

Metabolism/Transport Effects

Ethinyl estradiol: **Substrate** of CYP2C9 (minor), 3A4 (major), 3A5-7 (minor); **Inhibits** CYP1A2 (weak), 2B6 (weak), 2C8 (weak), 2C19 (weak), 3A4 (weak)

Desogestrel: **Substrate** of CYP2C19 (major)

Avoid Concomitant Use

Avoid concomitant use of Ethinyl Estradiol and Desogestrel with any of the following: Anastrozole; Griseofulvin

Increased Effect/Toxicity

Ethinyl Estradiol and Desogestrel may increase the levels/effects of: Benzodiazepines (metabolized by oxidation); Corticosteroids (Systemic); CYP1A2 Substrates; ROPINIRole; Selegiline; Theophylline Derivatives; Tipranavir; TiZANidine; Tranexamic Acid; Voriconazole

The levels/effects of Ethinyl Estradiol and Desogestrel may be increased by: Ascorbic Acid; Conivaptan; Herbs (Estrogenic Properties); Herbs (Progestogenic Properties); Voriconazole

Decreased Effect

Ethinyl Estradiol and Desogestrel may decrease the levels/effects of: Anastrozole; Chenodiol; LamoTRIgine; Protease Inhibitors; Thyroid Products; Ursodiol; Vitamin K Antagonists

The levels/effects of Ethinyl Estradiol and Desogestrel may be decreased by: Acitretin; Aminoglutethimide; Aprepitant; Armodafinil; Artemether; Barbiturates; Bile Acid Sequestrants; Bosentan; CarBAMazepine; Colesevelam; CYP3A4 Inducers (Strong); Deferasirox; Felbamate; Fosaprepitant; Fosphenytoin; Griseofulvin; LamoTRIgine; Modafinil; Mycophenolate; Nafcillin; OXcarbazepine; Phenytoin; Protease Inhibitors; Retinoic Acid Derivatives; Rifamycin Derivatives; Rufinamide; St Johns Wort; Tipranavir; Tocilizumab; Topiramate

Ethanol/Nutrition/Herb Interactions

Food: CNS effects of caffeine may be enhanced if combination hormonal contraceptives are used concurrently with caffeine. Grapefruit juice increases ethinyl estradiol concentrations and would be expected to increase progesterone serum levels as well; clinical implications are unclear.

Herb/Nutraceutical: St John's wort may decrease levels. Herbs with estrogenic properties may enhance the adverse/toxic effect of estrogen derivatives; examples include alfalfa, black cohosh, bloodroot, hops, kudzu, licorice, red clover, saw palmetto, soybean, thyme, wild yam, yucca. Herbs with progestogenic properties may enhance the adverse/toxic effect of progestins; examples include bloodroot, chasteberry, damiana, oregano, yucca.

Dietary Considerations Should be taken at same time each day.

Pharmacodynamics/Kinetics

Half-life Elimination Etonogestrel: ~38 hours; Ethinyl estradiol: ~26 hours

Pregnancy Risk Factor X

Lactation Enters breast milk/not recommended

Breast-Feeding Considerations Jaundice and breast enlargement in the nursing infant have been reported following the use of combination hormonal contraceptives. May decrease the quality and quantity of breast milk; a nonhormonal form of contraception is recommended.

Dosage Forms

Tablet, low-dose formulations:

Azurette™:
- Day 1-21: Ethinyl estradiol 0.02 mg and desogestrel 0.15 mg [21 white tablets]
- Day 22-23: 2 inactive green tablets
- Day 24-28: Ethinyl estradiol 0.01 mg [5 blue tablets] (28s)

Kariva®:
- Day 1-21: Ethinyl estradiol 0.02 mg and desogestrel 0.15 mg [21 white tablets]
- Day 22-23: 2 inactive light green tablets
- Day 24-28: Ethinyl estradiol 0.01 mg [5 light blue tablets] (28s)

Mircette®:
- Day 1-21: Ethinyl estradiol 0.02 mg and desogestrel 0.15 mg [21 white tablets]
- Day 22-23: 2 inactive green tablets
- Day 24-28: Ethinyl estradiol 0.01 mg [5 yellow tablets] (28s)

Tablet, monophasic formulations:

Apri® 28: Ethinyl estradiol 0.03 mg and desogestrel 0.15 mg (28s) [21 rose tablets and 7 white inactive tablets]

Desogen®, Reclipsen®: Ethinyl estradiol 0.03 mg and desogestrel 0.15 mg (28s) [21 white tablets and 7 green inactive tablets]

Emoquette™: Ethinyl estradiol 0.03 mg and desogestrel 0.15 mg (28s) [21 white tablets and 7 light green inactive tablets]

Ortho-Cept® 28: Ethinyl estradiol 0.03 mg and desogestrel 0.15 mg (28s) [21 light orange tablets and 7 green inactive tablets]

Tablet, triphasic formulations:

Caziant®:
- Day 1-7: Ethinyl estradiol 0.025 mg and desogestrel 0.1 mg [7 white tablets]
- Day 8-14: Ethinyl estradiol 0.025 mg and desogestrel 0.125 mg [7 light blue tablets]
- Day 15-21: Ethinyl estradiol 0.025 mg and desogestrel 0.15 mg [7 blue tablets]
- Day 22-28: 7 green inactive tablets (28s)

Cyclessa®:
- Day 1-7: Ethinyl estradiol 0.025 mg and desogestrel 0.1 mg [7 light yellow tablets]
- Day 8-14: Ethinyl estradiol 0.025 mg and desogestrel 0.125 mg [7 orange tablets]
- Day 15-21: Ethinyl estradiol 0.025 mg and desogestrel 0.15 mg [7 red tablets]
- Day 22-28: 7 green inactive tablets (28s)

Velivet™:
- Day 1-7: Ethinyl estradiol 0.025 mg and desogestrel 0.1 mg [7 beige tablets]
- Day 8-14: Ethinyl estradiol 0.025 mg and desogestrel 0.125 mg [7 orange tablets]
- Day 15-21: Ethinyl estradiol 0.025 mg and desogestrel 0.15 mg [7 pink tablets]
- Day 22-28: 7 white inactive tablets (28s)

Ethinyl Estradiol and Drospirenone

(ETH in il es tra DYE ole & droh SPYE re none)

Related Information

Endocrine Disorders and Pregnancy *on page 1879*

U.S. Brand Names Gianvi™; Loryna™; Ocella™; Yasmin®; Yaz®; Zarah®

Canadian Brand Names Yasmin®; Yaz®

Generic Availability (U.S.) Yes

Pharmacologic Category Contraceptive; Estrogen and Progestin Combination

Use Females: Prevention of pregnancy; treatment of premenstrual dysphoric disorder (PMDD); treatment of acne

Unlabeled/Investigational Use Treatment of hypermenorrhea (menorrhagia); pain associated with endometriosis; dysmenorrhea; dysfunctional uterine bleeding

Local Anesthetic/Vasoconstrictor Precautions No information available to require special precautions

Effects on Dental Treatment When prescribing antibiotics, patient must be warned to use additional methods of birth control if on oral contraceptives.

Effects on Bleeding No information available to require special precautions

Adverse Effects The following reactions have been associated with oral contraceptive use:

Increased risk or evidence of association with use:

Cardiovascular: Arterial thromboembolism, cerebral hemorrhage, cerebral thrombosis, hypertension, mesenteric thrombosis, MI

Gastrointestinal: Gallbladder disease

Hepatic: Hepatic adenomas, liver tumors (benign)

Local: Thrombophlebitis

Ocular: Retinal thrombosis

Respiratory: Pulmonary embolism

Adverse reactions considered drug related:

Cardiovascular: Edema, varicose vein aggravation

Central nervous system: Depression, migraine

Dermatologic: Melasma, rash (allergic)

Endocrine & metabolic: Amenorrhea, breakthrough bleeding, breast changes (enlargement, pain, secretion, tenderness), carbohydrate tolerance decreased, infertility (temporary), lactation decreased (with use immediately postpartum), menstrual flow changes, spotting

Gastrointestinal: Abdominal bloating, abdominal cramps, nausea, weight changes, vomiting

Genitourinary: Cervical ectropion, cervical secretion/erosion, vaginal candidiasis

Hematologic: Folate decreased, porphyria exacerbation

Hepatic: Cholestatic jaundice

Neuromuscular & skeletal: Chorea exacerbation

Ocular: Contact lens intolerance, corneal curvature changes (steepening)

Miscellaneous: Anaphylactic/anaphylactoid reactions (including angioedema, circulatory collapse, respiratory collapse, urticaria), SLE exacerbation

Adverse reactions in which association is not confirmed or denied: Acne, appetite changes, Budd-Chiari syndrome, cataracts, colitis, cystitis-like syndrome, dizziness, dysmenorrhea, erythema multiforme, erythema nodosum, headache, hemolytic uremic syndrome, hemorrhagic eruption, hirsutism, libido changes, nervousness, optic neuritis (with or without partial or complete loss of vision), pancreatitis, premenstrual syndrome, porphyria, renal function impaired, scalp hair loss, vaginitis

Dosage Oral:

Children ≥14 years and Adults: Females: Acne (Yaz®): Refer to dosing for contraception

Adults: Females: Contraception (Yasmin®, Yaz®), PMDD (Yaz®): Dosage is 1 tablet daily for 28 consecutive days. Dosing may be started on the first day of menstrual period (Day 1 starter) or on the first Sunday after the onset of the menstrual period (Sunday starter). **An additional method of contraception should be used until after the first 7 days of consecutive administration.**

Day 1 starter: Dose starts on first day of menstrual cycle taking 1 tablet daily.

Sunday starter: Dose begins on first Sunday after onset of menstruation; if the menstrual period starts on Sunday, take first tablet that very same day.

Switching from a different contraceptive:

Oral contraceptive: Start on the same day that a new pack of the previous oral contraceptive would have been taken

Transdermal patch, vaginal ring, injection: Start on the day the next dose would have been due

IUD or implant: Start on the day of removal

Use after childbirth (in women who are not breast-feeding) or after second trimester abortion: Therapy may be started ≥4 weeks postpartum. Pregnancy should be ruled out prior to treatment if menstrual periods have not restarted and an additional method of contraception (nonhormonal) should be used until after the first 7 days of consecutive administration.

Missed doses:

If all doses have been taken on schedule and one menstrual period is missed, continue dosing cycle. If two consecutive menstrual periods are missed, pregnancy test is required before new dosing cycle is started.

If doses have been missed during the first 3 weeks and the menstrual period is missed, pregnancy should be ruled out prior to continuing treatment.

Missed doses (monophasic formulations) (refer to package insert for complete information):

One dose missed: Take as soon as remembered or take 2 tablets next day

Two consecutive doses missed in the first 2 weeks: Take 2 tablets as soon as remembered or 2 tablets next 2 days. **An additional method of contraception should be used for 7 days after missed dose.**

Two consecutive doses missed in week 3 or three consecutive doses missed at any time: **An additional method of contraception must be used for 7 days after a missed dose.**

Day 1 starter: Current pack should be discarded, and a new pack should be started that same day.

Sunday starter: Continue dose of 1 tablet daily until Sunday, then discard the rest of the pack, and a new pack should be started that same day.

Any number of doses missed in week 4: Continue taking one pill each day until pack is empty; no back-up method of contraception is needed

Dosage adjustment in renal impairment: Contraindicated in patients with renal dysfunction

Dosage adjustment in hepatic impairment: Contraindicated in patients with hepatic dysfunction

Mechanism of Action Combination oral contraceptives inhibit ovulation via a negative feedback mechanism on the hypothalamus, which alters the normal pattern of gonadotropin secretion of a follicle-stimulating hormone (FSH) and luteinizing hormone by the anterior pituitary. The follicular phase FSH and midcycle surge of gonadotropins are inhibited. In addition, oral contraceptives produce alterations in the genital tract, including changes in the cervical mucus, rendering it unfavorable for sperm penetration even if ovulation occurs. Changes in the endometrium may also occur, producing an unfavorable environment for nidation. Oral contraceptive drugs may alter the tubal transport of the ova through the fallopian tubes. Progestational agents may also alter sperm fertility. Drospirenone is a spironolactone analogue with antimineralocorticoid and antiandrogenic activity.

Contraindications Adrenal insufficiency, breast cancer or other estrogen- or progestin-dependent neoplasms (current or a history of), hepatic tumors or disease, pregnancy, renal impairment, undiagnosed abnormal uterine bleeding. Use is also contraindicated in women at high risk of arterial or venous thrombotic diseases including: Cerebrovascular disease, coronary artery disease, diabetes mellitus with vascular disease, DVT or PE (current or history of), hypercoagulopathies (inherited or acquired), headaches with focal neurological symptoms, hypertension (uncontrolled), migraine headaches if >35 years of age, thrombogenic valvular or rhythm diseases of the heart (eg, subacute bacterial endocarditis with valvular disease or atrial fibrillation), women >35 years of age who smoke.

Warnings/Precautions Oral contraceptives do not protect against HIV infection or other sexually-transmitted diseases. **[U.S. Boxed Warning]: The risk of cardiovascular side effects is increased in women who smoke cigarettes; risk increases with age (especially women >35 years of age) and the number of cigarettes smoked; women who use combination hormonal contraceptives should be strongly advised not to smoke.** Oral contraceptives may lead to increased risk of stroke or myocardial infarction, use with caution in patients with risk factors for cardiovascular disease. Contraceptives may increase the risk of thromboembolism; discontinue if an arterial or venous thrombotic event occurs. Risk may be greater with contraceptives containing drospirenone. Whenever possible, combination hormonal contraceptives should be discontinued at least 4 weeks prior to and for 2 weeks following elective surgery associated with an increased risk of thromboembolism or during periods of prolonged immobilization. Oral contraceptives may have a dose-related risk of vascular disease, hypertension, and gallbladder disease. Women with hypertension should be encouraged to use another form of contraception. The use of combination hormonal contraceptives has been associated with a slight increase in frequency of breast cancer, however, studies are not consistent. Combination hormonal contraceptives may cause glucose intolerance or effect serum triglyceride and lipoprotein levels. Estrogens may cause retinal vascular thrombosis; discontinue if migraine, loss of vision, proptosis, diplopia or other visual disturbances occur; discontinue permanently if papilledema or retinal vascular lesions are observed on examination. Use with caution in patients with conditions that may be aggravated by fluid retention, depression, or patients with history of migraine. Evaluate new, recurrent, severe or persistent headaches. Not for use prior to menarche. Estrogens may induce or exacerbate symptoms in women with hereditary angioedema. Use caution with a history of chloasma gravidarum; women with a tendency to chloasma should avoid sun and ultraviolet radiation exposure during therapy. Cholestasis may occur in women with a history of pregnancy-related or previous oral contraceptive-related cholestasis. Combination hormonal contraceptives may effect serum triglyceride and lipoprotein levels. Use with caution in patients with familial defects of lipoprotein metabolism; consider an alternate form of contraception in women with uncontrolled dyslipidemias.

The minimum dosage combination of estrogen/progestin that will effectively treat the individual patient should be used. Unscheduled bleeding/spotting may especially occur within the first 3 months of use. Development of irregular, unresolving vaginal bleeding following previously regular cycles warrants further evaluation including endometrial sampling, if indicated, to rule out malignancy.

Acne use: For use only in females ≥14 years who have reached menarche, who also desire combination hormonal contraceptive therapy, are unresponsive to topical treatments, and have no contraindications to combination hormonal contraceptive use.

PMDD use: For use only in females who desire combination hormonal contraceptive therapy; use for more than 3 menstrual cycles has not been evaluated. Has not been evaluated for the treatment of premenstrual syndrome

Drospirenone has antimineralocorticoid activity that may lead to hyperkalemia in patients with renal insufficiency, hepatic dysfunction, or adrenal insufficiency. Use caution with medications that may increase serum potassium.

Drug Interactions

Metabolism/Transport Effects

Ethinyl estradiol: **Substrate** of CYP2C9 (minor), 3A4 (major), 3A5-7 (minor); **Inhibits** CYP1A2 (weak), 2B6 (weak), 2C8 (weak), 2C19 (weak), 3A4 (weak)

Drospirenone: **Substrate** of CYP3A4 (minor); **Inhibits** CYP1A2 (weak), 2C9 (weak), 2C19 (weak), 3A4 (weak)

Avoid Concomitant Use

Avoid concomitant use of Ethinyl Estradiol and Drospirenone with any of the following: Anastrozole; Griseofulvin; Tacrolimus

Increased Effect/Toxicity

Ethinyl Estradiol and Drospirenone may increase the levels/effects of: ACE Inhibitors; Amifostine; Ammonium Chloride; Antihypertensives; Benzodiazepines (metabolized by oxidation); Cardiac Glycosides; Corticosteroids (Systemic); CYP1A2 Substrates; Hypotensive Agents; Potassium-Sparing Diuretics; RiTUXimab; ROPINIRole; Selegiline; Tacrolimus; Theophylline Derivatives; Tipranavir; TiZANidine; Tranexamic Acid; Voriconazole

The levels/effects of Ethinyl Estradiol and Drospirenone may be increased by: Angiotensin II Receptor Blockers; Ascorbic Acid; Conivaptan; Diazoxide; Eplerenone; Herbs (Estrogenic Properties); Herbs (Hypotensive Properties); Herbs (Progestogenic Properties); MAO Inhibitors; Nonsteroidal Anti-Inflammatory Agents; Pentoxifylline; Phosphodiesterase 5 Inhibitors; Potassium Salts; Prostacyclin Analogues; Tolvaptan; Voriconazole

Decreased Effect

Ethinyl Estradiol and Drospirenone may decrease the levels/effects of: Anastrozole; Cardiac Glycosides; Chenodiol; LamoTRIgine; Protease Inhibitors; QuiNIDine; Thyroid Products; Ursodiol; Vitamin K Antagonists

The levels/effects of Ethinyl Estradiol and Drospirenone may be decreased by: Acitretin; Aminoglutethimide; Aprepitant; Armodafinil; Artemether; Barbiturates; Bile Acid Sequestrants; Bosentan; CarBAMazepine; Colesevelam; CYP3A4 Inducers (Strong); Deferasirox; Felbamate; Fosaprepitant; Fosphenytoin; Griseofulvin; Herbs (Hypertensive Properties); LamoTRIgine; Methylphenidate; Modafinil; Mycophenolate; Nafcillin; Nonsteroidal Anti-Inflammatory Agents; OXcarbazepine; Phenytoin; Protease Inhibitors; Retinoic Acid Derivatives; Rifamycin Derivatives; Rufinamide; St Johns Wort; Tipranavir; Tocilizumab; Topiramate; Yohimbine

Ethanol/Nutrition/Herb Interactions

Food: CNS effects of caffeine may be enhanced if oral contraceptives are used concurrently with caffeine. Grapefruit juice increases ethinyl estradiol plasma concentrations; clinical implications are unclear.

Herb/Nutraceutical: St John's wort may decrease levels. Herbs with estrogenic properties may enhance the adverse/toxic effect of estrogen derivatives; examples include alfalfa, black cohosh, bloodroot, hops, kudzu, licorice, red clover, saw palmetto, soybean, thyme, wild yam, yucca. Herbs with progestogenic properties may enhance the adverse/toxic effect of progestins; examples include bloodroot, chasteberry, damiana, oregano, yucca.

Dietary Considerations

Should be taken at the same time each day; may be taken with or without a meal

Pharmacodynamics/Kinetics

Half-life Elimination

Terminal: Drospirenone: ~30 hours; Ethinyl estradiol: ~24 hours

Time to Peak

1-3 hours

Pregnancy Risk Factor X

Lactation Enters breast milk/not recommended

Breast-Feeding Considerations The amount of drospirenone excreted in breast milk is ~0.02%, resulting in a maximum of ~3 mcg/day drospirenone to the infant. Jaundice and breast enlargement in the nursing infant have been reported following the use of other oral contraceptives. In addition, may decrease the quality and quantity of breast milk. Other forms of contraception are recommended while breast-feeding.

Dosage Forms

Tablet, oral:

Gianvi™: Ethinyl estradiol 0.03 mg and drospirenone 3 mg (28s) [24 light pink active tablets and 4 white inactive tablets]

Loryna™: Ethinyl estradiol 0.02 mg and drospirenone 3 mg (28s) [24 peach active tablets and 4 white inactive tablets]

Ocella™, Yasmin®: Ethinyl estradiol 0.03 mg and drospirenone 3 mg (28s) [21 yellow active tablets and 7 white inactive tablets]

Yaz®: Ethinyl estradiol 0.02 mg and drospirenone 3 mg (28s) [24 light pink active tablets and 4 white inactive tablets]

Zarah®: Ethinyl estradiol 0.03 mg and drospirenone 3 mg (28s) [21 blue active tablets and 7 peach inactive tablets]

Ethinyl Estradiol and Ethynodiol Diacetate

(ETH in il es tra DYE ole & e thye noe DYE ole dye AS e tate)

U.S. Brand Names Kelnor™; Zovia®

Canadian Brand Names Demulen® 30

Generic Availability (U.S.) Yes

Pharmacologic Category Contraceptive; Estrogen and Progestin Combination

Use Prevention of pregnancy

Unlabeled/Investigational Use Treatment of hypermenorrhea (menorrhagia); pain associated with endometriosis; dysmenorrhea; dysfunctional uterine bleeding

Local Anesthetic/Vasoconstrictor Precautions No information available to require special precautions

Effects on Dental Treatment When prescribing antibiotics, patient must be warned to use additional methods of birth control if on oral contraceptives.

Effects on Bleeding No information available to require special precautions

Adverse Effects Frequency not defined.

Cardiovascular: Arterial thromboembolism, cerebral hemorrhage, cerebral thrombosis, edema, hypertension, mesenteric thrombosis, MI

Central nervous system: Depression, dizziness, headache, migraine, nervousness, premenstrual syndrome, stroke

Dermatologic: Acne, erythema multiforme, erythema nodosum, hirsutism, loss of scalp hair, melasma (may persist), rash (allergic)

Endocrine & metabolic: Amenorrhea, breakthrough bleeding, breast enlargement, breast secretion, breast tenderness, carbohydrate intolerance, lactation decreased (postpartum), glucose tolerance decreased, libido changes, menstrual flow changes, sex hormone-binding globulins (SHBG) increased, spotting, temporary infertility (following discontinuation), thyroid-binding globulin increased, triglycerides increased

Gastrointestinal: Abdominal cramps, appetite changes, bloating, cholestasis, colitis, gallbladder disease, jaundice, nausea, vomiting, weight gain/loss

Genitourinary: Cervical erosion changes, cervical secretion changes, cystitis-like syndrome, vaginal candidiasis, vaginitis

Hematologic: Antithrombin III decreased, folate levels decreased, hemolytic uremic syndrome, norepinephrine induced platelet aggregability increased, porphyria, prothrombin increased; factors VII, VIII, IX, and X increased

Hepatic: Benign liver tumors, Budd-Chiari syndrome, cholestatic jaundice, hepatic adenomas

Local: Thrombophlebitis

Ocular: Cataracts, change in corneal curvature (steepening), contact lens intolerance, optic neuritis, retinal thrombosis

Renal: Impaired renal function

Respiratory: Pulmonary thromboembolism

Miscellaneous: Hemorrhagic eruption

Dosage Oral: Adults: Females: Contraception:

Schedule 1 (Sunday starter): Dose begins on first Sunday after onset of menstruation; if the menstrual period starts on Sunday, take first tablet that very same day. **With a Sunday start, an additional method of contraception should be used until after the first 7 days of consecutive administration.**

For 21-tablet package: 1 tablet/day for 21 consecutive days, followed by 7 days off of the medication; a new course begins on the 8th day after the last tablet is taken.

For 28-tablet package: 1 tablet/day without interruption.

Schedule 2 (Day 1 starter): Dose starts on first day of menstrual cycle taking 1 tablet daily.

For 21-tablet package: 1 tablet/day for 21 consecutive days, followed by 7 days off of the medication; a new course begins on the 8th day after the last tablet is taken.

For 28-tablet package: 1 tablet/day without interruption.

If all doses have been taken on schedule and one menstrual period is missed, continue dosing cycle. If two consecutive menstrual periods are missed, pregnancy test is required before new dosing cycle is started.

Missed doses **monophasic formulations** (refer to package insert for complete information):

One dose missed: Take as soon as remembered or take 2 tablets next day

Two consecutive doses missed in the first 2 weeks: Take 2 tablets as soon as remembered or 2 tablets next 2 days. **An additional method of contraception should be used for 7 days after missed dose.**

Two consecutive doses missed in week 3 or three consecutive doses missed at any time: **An additional method of contraception should be used for 7 days after missed dose:**

Schedule 1 (Sunday starter): Continue dose of 1 tablet daily until Sunday, then discard the rest of the pack, and a new pack should be started that same day.

Schedule 2 (Day 1 starter): Current package should be discarded, and a new pack should be started that same day.

Dosage adjustment in renal impairment: Specific guidelines not available; use with caution and monitor blood pressure closely. Consider other forms of contraception.

Dosage adjustment in hepatic impairment: Contraindicated in patients with hepatic impairment

Mechanism of Action Combination hormonal contraceptives inhibit ovulation via a negative feedback mechanism on the hypothalamus, which alters the normal pattern of gonadotropin secretion of a follicle-stimulating hormone (FSH) and luteinizing hormone by the anterior pituitary. The follicular phase FSH and midcycle surge of gonadotropins are inhibited. In addition, combination hormonal contraceptives produce alterations in the genital tract, including changes in the cervical mucus, rendering it unfavorable for sperm penetration even if ovulation occurs. Changes in the endometrium may also occur, producing an unfavorable environment for nidation. Combination hormonal contraceptive drugs may alter the tubal transport of the ova through the fallopian tubes. Progestational agents may also alter sperm fertility.

Contraindications Hypersensitivity to ethinyl estradiol, ethynodiol diacetate, or any component of the formulation; history of or current thrombophlebitis or venous thromboembolic disorders (including DVT, PE); active or recent (within 1 year) arterial thromboembolic disease (eg, stroke, MI); cerebral vascular disease, coronary artery disease, valvular heart disease with complications, severe hypertension; diabetes mellitus with vascular involvement; severe headache with focal neurological symptoms; known or suspected breast carcinoma, endometrial cancer, estrogen-dependent neoplasms, undiagnosed abnormal genital bleeding; hepatic dysfunction or tumor, cholestatic jaundice of pregnancy, jaundice with prior combination hormonal contraceptive use; major surgery with prolonged immobilization; heavy smoking (≥15 cigarettes/day) in patients >35 years of age; pregnancy

Warnings/Precautions Combination hormonal contraceptives do not protect against HIV infection or other sexually-transmitted diseases. **[U.S. Boxed Warning]: The risk of cardiovascular side effects increases in women who smoke cigarettes, especially those who are >35 years of age; women who use combination hormonal contraceptives should be strongly advised not to smoke.** Combination hormonal contraceptives may lead to increased risk of myocardial infarction, use with caution in patients with risk factors for coronary artery disease. May increase the risk of thromboembolism. Whenever possible, combination hormonal contraceptives should be discontinued at least 4 weeks prior to and for 2 weeks following elective surgery associated with an increased risk of thromboembolism or during periods of prolonged immobilization. Combination hormonal contraceptives may have a dose-related risk of vascular disease, hypertension, and gallbladder disease. Women with hypertension or renal disease should be encouraged to use a nonhormonal form of contraception. The use of combination hormonal contraceptives has been associated with a slight increase in frequency of breast cancer, however, studies are not consistent. Combination hormonal contraceptives may cause glucose intolerance or effect serum triglyceride and lipoprotein levels. Retinal thrombosis has been reported (rarely). Use caution with conditions that may be aggravated by fluid retention, depression, or history of migraine. Not for use prior to menarche.

The minimum dosage combination of estrogen/progestin that will effectively treat the individual patient should be used. New patients should be started on products containing ≤0.035 mg of estrogen per tablet.

Drug Interactions

Metabolism/Transport Effects Ethinyl estradiol: **Substrate** of CYP2C9 (minor), 3A4 (major), 3A5-7 (minor); **Inhibits** CYP1A2 (weak), 2B6 (weak), 2C8 (weak), 2C19 (weak), 3A4 (weak)

Avoid Concomitant Use

Avoid concomitant use of Ethinyl Estradiol and Ethynodiol Diacetate with any of the following: Anastrozole; Griseofulvin

Increased Effect/Toxicity

Ethinyl Estradiol and Ethynodiol Diacetate may increase the levels/effects of: Benzodiazepines (metabolized by oxidation); Corticosteroids (Systemic); CYP1A2 Substrates; ROPINIRole; Selegiline; Theophylline Derivatives; Tipranavir; TiZANidine; Tranexamic Acid; Voriconazole

The levels/effects of Ethinyl Estradiol and Ethynodiol Diacetate may be increased by: Ascorbic Acid; Conivaptan; Herbs (Estrogenic Properties); Herbs (Progestogenic Properties); Voriconazole

Decreased Effect

Ethinyl Estradiol and Ethynodiol Diacetate may decrease the levels/effects of: Anastrozole; Chenodiol; LamoTRIgine; Protease Inhibitors; Thyroid Products; Ursodiol; Vitamin K Antagonists

The levels/effects of Ethinyl Estradiol and Ethynodiol Diacetate may be decreased by: Acitretin; Aminoglutethimide; Aprepitant; Armodafinil; Artemether; Barbiturates; Bile Acid Sequestrants; Bosentan; CarBAMazepine; Colesevelam; CYP3A4 Inducers (Strong); Deferasirox; Felbamate; Fosaprepitant; Fosphenytoin; Griseofulvin; LamoTRIgine; Modafinil; Mycophenolate; Nafcillin; OXcarbazepine; Phenytoin; Protease Inhibitors; Retinoic Acid Derivatives; Rifamycin Derivatives; Rufinamide; St Johns Wort; Tipranavir; Tocilizumab; Topiramate

Ethanol/Nutrition/Herb Interactions

Food: CNS effects of caffeine may be enhanced if combination hormonal contraceptives are used concurrently with caffeine. Grapefruit juice increases ethinyl estradiol concentrations and would be expected to increase progesterone serum levels as well; clinical implications are unclear.

Herb/Nutraceutical: St John's wort may decrease levels. Herbs with estrogenic properties may enhance the adverse/toxic effect of estrogen derivatives; examples include alfalfa, black cohosh, bloodroot, hops, kudzu, licorice, red clover, saw palmetto, soybean, thyme, wild yam, yucca. Herbs with progestogenic properties may enhance the adverse/toxic effect of progestins; examples include bloodroot, chasteberry, damiana, oregano, yucca.

Dietary Considerations Should be taken with food at same time each day.

Pharmacodynamics/Kinetics

Half-life Elimination

Ethynodiol diacetate (converted to norethindrone) Terminal: 5-14 hours

Pregnancy Risk Factor X

Lactation Enters breast milk/not recommended

Breast-Feeding Considerations Jaundice and breast enlargement in the nursing infant have been reported following the use of combination hormonal contraceptives. May decrease the quality and quantity of breast milk; a nonhormonal form of contraception is recommended.

Dosage Forms

Tablet, monophasic formulations:

Kelnor™ 1/35: Ethinyl estradiol 0.035 mg and ethynodiol diacetate 1 mg [21 light yellow tablets and 7 white inactive tablets] (28s)

Zovia® 1/35-28: Ethinyl estradiol 0.035 mg and ethynodiol diacetate 1 mg [21 light pink tablets and 7 white inactive tablets] (28s)

Zovia® 1/50-28: Ethinyl estradiol 0.05 mg and ethynodiol diacetate 1 mg [21 pink tablets and 7 white inactive tablets] (28s)

Ethinyl Estradiol and Etonogestrel

(ETH in il es tra DYE ole & et oh noe JES trel)

Related Information

Endocrine Disorders and Pregnancy *on page* 1879

Etonogestrel *on page* 694

U.S. Brand Names NuvaRing®

Canadian Brand Names NuvaRing®

Generic Availability (U.S.) No

Pharmacologic Category Contraceptive; Estrogen and Progestin Combination

Use Prevention of pregnancy

Unlabeled/Investigational Use Treatment of hypermenorrhea (menorrhagia); pain associated with endometriosis; dysmenorrhea; dysfunctional uterine bleeding

Local Anesthetic/Vasoconstrictor Precautions No information available to require special precautions

Effects on Dental Treatment When prescribing antibiotics, patient must be warned to use additional methods of birth control if on oral contraceptives.

Effects on Bleeding No information available to require special precautions

Adverse Effects

The most common adverse reactions associated with NuvaRing® (5% to 14%): Headache, nausea, sinusitis, upper respiratory tract infection, vaginal secretion, vaginitis, and weight gain. The following reactions have been associated with combination hormonal contraceptive use:

Increased risk or evidence of association with use:

Cardiovascular: Arterial thromboembolism, cerebral hemorrhage, cerebral thrombosis, hypertension, mesenteric thrombosis, MI, venous thrombosis (with or without embolism)

Gastrointestinal: Gallbladder disease

Hepatic: Hepatic adenomas, liver tumors (benign)

Local: Thrombophlebitis

Ocular: Retinal thrombosis

Respiratory: Pulmonary embolism

Adverse reactions considered drug related:

Cardiovascular: Edema, varicose vein aggravation

Central nervous system: Depression, migraine, mood changes

Dermatologic: Chloasma, melasma, rash (allergic)

Endocrine & metabolic: Amenorrhea, breakthrough bleeding, breast changes (enlargement, pain, secretion, tenderness), fluid retention, infertility (temporary), lactation decreased (with use immediately postpartum), menstrual flow changes, spotting

Gastrointestinal: Abdominal bloating, abdominal cramps, abdominal pain, appetite changes, nausea, weight changes, vomiting

Genitourinary: Cervical ectropion, cervical secretion, vaginal candidiasis, vaginitis

Hematologic: Folate decreased, porphyria exacerbation

Hepatic: Cholestatic jaundice

Neuromuscular & skeletal: Chorea exacerbation

Ocular: Contact lens intolerance, corneal curvature changes (steepening)

Miscellaneous: Anaphylactic/anaphylactoid reactions (including angioedema, circulatory collapse, respiratory collapse, urticaria), SLE exacerbation

Adverse reactions in which association is not confirmed or denied: Acne, Budd-Chiari syndrome, cataracts, colitis, cystitis-like syndrome, dizziness, dysmenorrhea, erythema multiforme, erythema nodosum, headache, hemolytic uremic syndrome, hemorrhagic eruption, hirsutism, libido changes, nervousness, optic neuritis (with or without partial or complete loss of vision), pancreatitis, premenstrual syndrome, renal function impaired, scalp hair loss

Dosage Vaginal: Adults: Females: Contraception: One ring, inserted vaginally and left in place for 3 consecutive weeks, then removed for 1 week. A new ring is inserted 7 days after the last was removed (even if bleeding is not complete) and should be inserted at approximately the same time of day the ring was removed the previous week.

Initial treatment should begin as follows (pregnancy should always be ruled out first):

No hormonal contraceptive use in the past month: Insert ring on the first day of menstrual cycle ("Day 1"). May also insert on days 2-5 even if bleeding is not complete, however, **a spermicide or barrier method of contraception should be used for the following 7 days.***

Switching from combination oral contraceptive: Ring can be inserted on any day within 7 days after the last **active** tablet in the cycle was taken and no later than the first day a new cycle of tablets would begin. Additional forms of contraception are not needed.

Switching from progestin-only contraceptive: **A spermicide or barrier method of contraception should be used for the following 7 days with any of the following.***

If previously using a progestin-only mini-pill, insert the ring on any day of the month; do not skip days between the last pill and insertion of the ring.

If previously using an implant, insert the ring on the same day of implant removal.

If previously using a progestin-containing IUD, insert the ring on day of IUD removal.

If previously using a progestin injection, insert the ring on the day the next injection would be given.

Following complete 1st trimester abortion: Insert ring within the first 5 days of abortion. If not inserted within 5 days, follow instructions for "No hormonal contraceptive use within the past month" and instruct patient to use a non-hormonal contraceptive in the interim.

Following delivery or 2nd trimester abortion: Insert ring 4 weeks postpartum (in women who are not breast-feeding) or following 2nd trimester abortion. **A spermicide or barrier method of contraception should be used for the following 7 days.***

If the ring is accidentally removed from the vagina at anytime during the 3-week period of use, it may be rinsed with cool or lukewarm water (not hot) and reinserted as soon as possible. If the ring is not reinserted within 3 hours, contraceptive effectiveness will be decreased. **A spermicide or barrier method of contraception should be used until the ring has been in place for 7 consecutive days.***

If the ring has been removed for longer than 1 week, pregnancy must be ruled out prior to restarting therapy. **A spermicide or barrier method of contraception should be used for the following 7 days.***

If the ring has been left in place for >3 weeks, a new ring should be inserted following a 1-week (ring-free) interval. Protection continues during week 4, however, if the ring is left in place >4 weeks, pregnancy must be ruled out prior to insertion and **a spermicide or barrier method of contraception should be used for the following 7 days.***

Disconnected ring: In the event the ring disconnects at the weld joint, discard and replace with a new ring.

***Note:** Diaphragms may interfere with proper ring placement, and therefore, are not recommended for use as an additional form of contraception.

Dosage adjustment in renal impairment: Specific guidelines not available; use with caution and monitor blood pressure closely. Consider other forms of contraception.

Dosage adjustment in hepatic impairment: Contraindicated in patients with hepatic impairment

Mechanism of Action Combination hormonal contraceptives inhibit ovulation via a negative feedback mechanism on the hypothalamus, which alters the normal pattern of gonadotropin secretion of a follicle-stimulating hormone (FSH) and luteinizing hormone by the anterior pituitary. The follicular phase FSH and midcycle surge of gonadotropins are inhibited. In addition, combination hormonal contraceptives produce alterations in the genital tract, including changes in the cervical mucus, rendering it unfavorable for sperm penetration even if ovulation occurs. Changes in the endometrium may also occur, producing an unfavorable environment for nidation. Combination hormonal contraceptive drugs may alter the tubal transport of the ova through the fallopian tubes. Progestational agents may also alter sperm fertility.

Contraindications Hypersensitivity to ethinyl estradiol, etonogestrel, or any component of the formulation; history of or current thrombophlebitis or venous thromboembolic disorders (including DVT, PE); active or recent (within 1 year) arterial thromboembolic disease (eg, stroke, MI); major surgery with prolonged immobilization, cerebral vascular disease, coronary artery disease, valvular heart disease with complications, severe hypertension; diabetes mellitus with vascular involvement; severe headache with focal neurological symptoms; known or suspected breast carcinoma or personal history of breast cancer, endometrial cancer, estrogen-dependent neoplasms, undiagnosed abnormal genital bleeding; active liver disease or tumor, cholestatic jaundice of pregnancy, jaundice with prior combination hormonal contraceptive use; heavy smoking (≥15 cigarettes/day) in patients >35 years of age; pregnancy

Warnings/Precautions Combination hormonal contraceptive agents do not protect against HIV infection or other sexually-transmitted diseases. **[U.S. Boxed Warning]: The risk of cardiovascular side effects increases in women who smoke cigarettes, especially those who are >35 years of age; women who use combination hormonal contraceptives should be strongly advised not to smoke.** May lead to increased risk of myocardial infarction, use with caution in patients with risk factors for coronary artery disease. May increase the risk of thromboembolism. Whenever possible, combination hormonal contraceptives should be discontinued at least 4 weeks prior to and for 2 weeks following elective surgery associated with an increased risk of thromboembolism or during periods of prolonged immobilization. May have a dose-related risk of vascular disease, hypertension, and gallbladder disease. Women with hypertension or renal disease should be encouraged to use another form of contraception. The use of combination hormonal contraceptives has been associated with a slight increase in frequency of breast cancer, however, studies are not consistent. Combination hormonal contraceptives may effect serum triglyceride and lipoprotein levels. May have adverse effects on glucose tolerance; use caution in women with diabetes. Retinal thrombosis has been reported (rarely); discontinue permanently if loss of vision occurs, or if papilledema or retinal vascular lesions are observed on examination. Use caution with conditions that may be aggravated by fluid retention, depression, or history of migraine. Combination hormonal contraceptives may be poorly metabolized in women with hepatic impairment. Not for use prior to menarche.

Vaginally-administered combination hormonal contraceptive agents may have a similar adverse effects associated with oral contraceptive products. In order to reduce some of the possible risks, the minimum dosage combination of estrogen/progestin that will effectively treat the individual patient should be used. May not be appropriate for use in women with conditions that make the vagina susceptible to irritation or ulceration. Ensure proper vaginal placement of the ring to avoid inadvertent urinary bladder insertion.

Drug Interactions

Metabolism/Transport Effects

Ethinyl estradiol: **Substrate** of CYP2C9 (minor), 3A4 (major), 3A5-7 (minor); **Inhibits** CYP1A2 (weak), 2B6 (weak), 2C8 (weak), 2C19 (weak), 3A4 (weak)

Etonogestrel: **Substrate** of CYP3A4 (minor)

Avoid Concomitant Use

Avoid concomitant use of Ethinyl Estradiol and Etonogestrel with any of the following: Anastrozole; Griseofulvin

Increased Effect/Toxicity

Ethinyl Estradiol and Etonogestrel may increase the levels/effects of: Benzodiazepines (metabolized by oxidation); Corticosteroids (Systemic); CYP1A2 Substrates; ROPINIRole; Selegiline; Theophylline Derivatives; Tipranavir; TiZANidine; Tranexamic Acid; Voriconazole

The levels/effects of Ethinyl Estradiol and Etonogestrel may be increased by: Ascorbic Acid; Conivaptan; Herbs (Estrogenic Properties); Herbs (Progestogenic Properties); Voriconazole

Decreased Effect

Ethinyl Estradiol and Etonogestrel may decrease the levels/effects of: Anastrozole; Chenodiol; LamoTRIgine; Protease Inhibitors; Thyroid Products; Ursodiol; Vitamin K Antagonists

The levels/effects of Ethinyl Estradiol and Etonogestrel may be decreased by: Acitretin; Aminoglutethimide; Aprepitant; Armodafinil; Artemether; Barbiturates; Bile Acid Sequestrants; Bosentan; CarBAMazepine; Colesevelam; CYP3A4 Inducers (Strong); Deferasirox; Efavirenz; Felbamate; Fosaprepitant; Fosphenytoin; Griseofulvin; LamoTRIgine; Modafinil; Mycophenolate; Nafcillin; OXcarbazepine; Phenytoin; Protease Inhibitors; Retinoic Acid Derivatives; Rifamycin Derivatives; Rufinamide; St Johns Wort; Tipranavir; Tocilizumab; Topiramate

Ethanol/Nutrition/Herb Interactions

Food: CNS effects of caffeine may be enhanced if combination hormonal contraceptives are used concurrently with caffeine. Grapefruit juice increases ethinyl estradiol concentrations and would be expected to increase progesterone serum levels as well; clinical implications are unclear.

Herb/Nutraceutical: St John's wort may decrease levels. Herbs with estrogenic properties may enhance the adverse/toxic effect of estrogen derivatives; examples include alfalfa, black cohosh, bloodroot, hops, kudzu, licorice, red clover, saw palmetto, soybean, thyme, wild yam, yucca. Herbs with progestogenic properties may enhance the adverse/toxic effect of progestins; examples include bloodroot, chasteberry, damiana, oregano, yucca.

Pharmacodynamics/Kinetics

Duration of Action

Serum levels (contraceptive effectiveness) decrease after 3 weeks of continuous use

Half-life Elimination Ethinyl estradiol: 45 hours; Etonogestrel: 29 hours

Time to Peak Vaginal: Ethinyl estradiol: 60 hours; Etonogestrel: 200 hours

Pregnancy Risk Factor X

Lactation Enters breast milk/not recommended

Breast-Feeding Considerations Jaundice and breast enlargement in the nursing infant have been reported following the use of combination hormonal contraceptives. May decrease the quality and quantity of breast milk; alternative form of contraception is recommended.

Dosage Forms

Ring, vaginal:

NuvaRing®: Ethinyl estradiol 0.015 mg/day and etonogestrel 0.12 mg/day (1s) [3-week duration]

Ethinyl Estradiol and Levonorgestrel

(ETH in il es tra DYE ole & LEE voe nor jes trel)

Related Information

Levonorgestrel *on page 1003*

U.S. Brand Names Aviane™; Enpresse®; Introvale™; Jolessa™; Lessina®; Levora®; LoSeasonique®; Lutera®; Lybrel®; Nordette® 28; Portia®; Quasense®; Seasonale®; Seasonique®; Sronyx®; Trivora®

Canadian Brand Names Alesse®; Aviane®; Min-Ovral®; Seasonale®; Triphasil®; Triquilar®

Generic Availability (U.S.) Yes

Pharmacologic Category Contraceptive; Estrogen and Progestin Combination

Use Prevention of pregnancy; postcoital contraception

Unlabeled/Investigational Use Treatment of hypermenorrhea (menorrhagia); pain associated with endometriosis; dysmenorrhea; dysfunctional uterine bleeding

Local Anesthetic/Vasoconstrictor Precautions No information available to require special precautions

Effects on Dental Treatment When prescribing antibiotics, patient must be warned to use additional methods of birth control if on oral contraceptives.

Effects on Bleeding No information available to require special precautions

Adverse Effects The following reactions have been associated with oral contraceptive use:

Increased risk or evidence of association with use:

Cardiovascular: Arterial thromboembolism, cerebral hemorrhage, cerebral thrombosis, hypertension, mesenteric thrombosis, MI, venous thrombosis (with or without embolism)

Gastrointestinal: Gallbladder disease

Hepatic: Hepatic adenomas, liver tumors (benign)

Local: Thrombophlebitis

Ocular: Retinal thrombosis

Respiratory: Pulmonary embolism

Adverse reactions considered drug related:

Cardiovascular: Edema, varicose vein aggravation

Central nervous system: Depression, migraine, mood changes

Dermatologic: Chloasma, melasma, rash (allergic)

Endocrine & metabolic: Amenorrhea, breakthrough bleeding, breast changes (enlargement, pain, secretion, tenderness), carbohydrate tolerance decreased, fluid retention, infertility (temporary), lactation decreased (with use immediately postpartum), menstrual flow changes, spotting

Gastrointestinal: Abdominal bloating, abdominal cramps, abdominal pain, appetite changes, nausea, weight changes, vomiting

Genitourinary: Cervical ectropion, cervical secretion/erosion, endocervical hyperplasia, fibroid enlargement, vaginal candidiasis, vaginitis

Hematologic: Folate decreased, porphyria exacerbation

Hepatic: Cholestatic jaundice, focal nodular hyperplasia

Neuromuscular & skeletal: Chorea exacerbation

Ocular: Contact lens intolerance, corneal curvature changes (steepening)

Respiratory: Rhinitis

Miscellaneous: Anaphylactic/anaphylactoid reactions (including angioedema, circulatory collapse, respiratory collapse, urticaria), SLE exacerbation

Adverse reactions in which association is not confirmed or denied: Acne, auditory disturbances, Budd-Chiari syndrome, cataracts, cervical smear abnormal, colitis, cystitis-like syndrome, dizziness, dysmenorrhea, erythema multiforme, erythema nodosum, headache, hemolytic uremic syndrome, hemorrhagic eruption, hirsutism, libido changes, nervousness, optic neuritis (with or without partial or complete loss of vision), pancreatitis, premenstrual syndrome, renal function impaired, scalp hair loss

Dosage Oral: Adults: Females:

Contraception, 28-day cycle:

Schedule 1 (Sunday starter): Dose begins on first Sunday after onset of menstruation; if the menstrual period starts on Sunday, take first tablet that very same day. With a Sunday start, an additional method of contraception should be used until after the first 7 days of consecutive administration:

For 21-tablet package: 1 tablet/day for 21 consecutive days, followed by 7 days off of the medication; a new course begins on the 8th day after the last tablet is taken

For 28-tablet package: 1 tablet/day without interruption

Schedule 2 (Day 1 starter): Dose starts on first day of menstrual cycle taking 1 tablet/day:

For 21-tablet package: 1 tablet/day for 21 consecutive days, followed by 7 days off of the medication; a new course begins on the 8th day after the last tablet is taken

For 28-tablet package: 1 tablet/day without interruption

If all doses have been taken on schedule and one menstrual period is missed, continue dosing cycle. If two consecutive menstrual periods are missed, pregnancy test is required before new dosing cycle is started.

Missed doses **monophasic formulations** (refer to package insert for complete information):

One dose missed: Take as soon as remembered or take 2 tablets next day

Two consecutive doses missed in the first 2 weeks: Take 2 tablets as soon as remembered or 2 tablets next 2 days. An additional method of contraception should be used for 7 days after missed dose.

Two consecutive doses missed in week 3 or three consecutive doses missed at any time: An additional method of contraception must be used for 7 days after a missed dose:

Schedule 1 (Sunday starter): Continue dose of 1 tablet daily until Sunday, then discard the rest of the pack, and a new pack should be started that same day.

Schedule 2 (Day 1 starter): Current pack should be discarded, and a new pack should be started that same day.

Missed doses **biphasic/triphasic formulations** (refer to package insert for complete information):

One dose missed: Take as soon as remembered or take 2 tablets next day.

Two consecutive doses missed in week 1 or week 2 of the pack: Take 2 tablets as soon as remembered and 2 tablets the next day. Resume taking 1 tablet daily until the pack is empty. An additional method of contraception should be used for 7 days after a missed dose.

Two consecutive doses missed in week 3 of the pack: An additional method of contraception must be used for 7 days after a missed dose.

Schedule 1 (Sunday starter): Take 1 tablet every day until Sunday. Discard the remaining pack and start a new pack of pills on the same day.

Schedule 2 (Day 1 starter): Discard the remaining pack and start a new pack the same day.

Three or more consecutive doses missed: An additional method of contraception must be used for 7 days after a missed dose.

Schedule 1 (Sunday starter): Take 1 tablet every day until Sunday; on Sunday, discard the pack and start a new pack.

Schedule 2 (Day 1 starter): Discard the remaining pack and begin new pack of tablets starting on the same day.

Contraception, 91-day cycle (extended cycle regimen): Dose begins on first Sunday after onset of menstruation; if the menstrual period starts on Sunday, take first tablet that very same day. An additional method of contraception should be used until after the first 7 days of consecutive administration:

Seasonale®: One active tablet/day for 84 consecutive days, followed by 1 inactive tablet/day for 7 days; if all doses have been taken on schedule and one menstrual period is missed, pregnancy should be ruled out prior to continuing therapy.

Seasonique®, LoSeasonique®: One active tablet/day for 84 consecutive days, followed by 1 low dose estrogen tablet/day for 7 days; if all doses have been taken on schedule and one menstrual period is missed, pregnancy should be ruled out prior to continuing therapy.

Missed doses:

One dose missed: Take as soon as remembered or take 2 tablets the next day

Two consecutive doses missed: Take 2 tablets as soon as remembered or 2 tablets the next 2 days. An additional nonhormonal method of contraception should be used for 7 consecutive days after the missed dose.

Three or more consecutive doses missed: Do not take the missed doses; continue taking 1 tablet/day until pack is complete. Bleeding may occur during the following week. An additional nonhormonal method of contraception should be used for 7 consecutive days after the missed dose.

Any number of pills during week 13: Throw away the missed pills and keep taking scheduled pills until the pack is finished. A back-up method of contraception is not needed

Contraception, continuous use (extended cycle regimen): Lybrel®: Take one tablet daily, at the same time each day, without a tablet-free interval. Therapy should be initiated as follows:

No previous contraception: Begin on the first day of menstrual cycle. Back-up contraception is not needed.

Previously taking a 21-day or 28-day combination hormonal contraceptive: Begin on day 1 of the withdrawal bleed (at the latest, 7 days after the last active tablet). Back-up contraception is not needed.

Previously using a progestin-only pill: Begin the day after taking a progestin only pill. Back-up contraception is needed for the first 7 days of therapy.

Previously using contraceptive implant: Begin the day of implant removal. Back-up contraception is needed for the first 7 days of therapy.

Previously using contraceptive injection: Begin when the next injection is due. Back-up contraception is needed for the first 7 days of therapy.

Missed doses:

One dose missed: Take as soon as remembered then take the next tablet at the regular time (2 tablets in 1 day). An additional nonhormonal method of contraception should also be used for 7 consecutive days.

Two consecutive doses missed: If remembered the day of the second missed tablet, take 2 tablets as soon as remembered, then 1 tablet the next day. If remembered the day after the second tablet is missed, take 2 tablets the day remembered, then 2 tablets the next day. An additional nonhormonal method of contraception should also be used for 7 consecutive days.

Three or more consecutive doses missed: Take 1 tablet daily and contact healthcare provider; do not take the missed pills. An additional nonhormonal method of contraception should also be used for 7 consecutive days.

Dosage adjustment in renal impairment: Specific guidelines not available; use with caution and monitor blood pressure closely. Consider other forms of contraception.

Dosage adjustment in hepatic impairment: Contraindicated in patients with hepatic impairment

Mechanism of Action Combination hormonal contraceptives inhibit ovulation via a negative feedback mechanism on the hypothalamus, which alters the normal pattern of gonadotropin secretion of a follicle-stimulating hormone (FSH) and luteinizing hormone by the anterior pituitary. The follicular phase FSH and midcycle surge of gonadotropins are inhibited. In addition, combination hormonal contraceptives produce alterations in the genital tract, including changes in the cervical mucus, rendering it unfavorable for sperm penetration even if ovulation occurs. Changes in the endometrium may also occur, producing an unfavorable environment for nidation. Combination hormonal contraceptive drugs may alter the tubal transport of the ova through the fallopian tubes. Progestational agents may also alter sperm fertility.

Contraindications Hypersensitivity to ethinyl estradiol, levonorgestrel, or any component of the formulation; history of or current thrombophlebitis or venous thromboembolic disorders (including DVT, PE); active or recent (within 1 year) arterial thromboembolic disease (eg, stroke, MI); cerebral vascular disease, coronary artery disease, valvular heart disease with complications, severe/uncontrolled hypertension, thrombogenic rhythm disorders, hereditary or acquired thrombophilias; diabetes mellitus with vascular involvement; severe headache with focal neurological symptoms or migraine headaches with or without aura if >35 years of age; known or suspected breast carcinoma, endometrial cancer, estrogen- or progestin-dependent neoplasms, undiagnosed abnormal genital bleeding; hepatic dysfunction or tumor, cholestatic jaundice of pregnancy, jaundice with prior combination hormonal contraceptive use; major surgery with prolonged immobilization; heavy smoking (≥15 cigarettes/day) in patients >35 years of age; pregnancy

Canadian-labeling: Additional contraindication: Ocular lesions due to ophthalmic vascular disease including partial or complete loss of vision or defect in visual fields; severe dyslipoproteinemia; hereditary or acquired predisposition for venous or arterial thrombosis

Warnings/Precautions Combination hormonal contraceptives do not protect against HIV infection or other sexually-transmitted diseases. **[U.S. Boxed Warning]: The risk of cardiovascular side effects increases in women who smoke cigarettes, especially those who are >35 years of age; women who use combination hormonal contraceptives should be strongly advised not to smoke.** Use with caution in patients with risk factors for coronary artery disease; may lead to increased risk of myocardial infarction. May have a dose-related risk of vascular disease and hypertension; women with hypertension should be encouraged to use a nonhormonal form of contraception. May increase the risk of thromboembolism. Whenever possible, combination hormonal contraceptives should be discontinued at least 4 weeks prior to and for 2 weeks following elective surgery associated with an increased risk of thromboembolism or during periods of prolonged immobilization. Combination hormonal contraceptives may have a dose-related risk of gallbladder disease and may worsen existing gallbladder disease. Women with renal disease should be encouraged to use another form of contraception. May have adverse effects on glucose tolerance; use caution in women with diabetes. Combination hormonal contraceptives may affect serum triglyceride and lipoprotein levels. Triglycerides may also be increased; use with caution in patients with familial defects of lipoprotein metabolism. The use of combination hormonal contraceptives has been associated with a slight increase in frequency of breast cancer, however, studies are not consistent. Retinal thrombosis has been reported (rarely); discontinue permanently if papilledema or retinal vascular lesions are observed on examination or if loss of vision or other visual disturbances occur. Use caution with conditions that may be aggravated by fluid retention, depression, or history of migraine. Evaluate new, recurrent, severe or persistent headaches. Use with migraine headaches with or without aura if >35 years of age is contraindicated. Not for use prior to menarche.

Presentation of irregular, unresolving vaginal bleeding warrants further evaluation including endometrial sampling, if indicated, to rule out malignancy; evaluate hypothalamic-pituitary-function in women with persistent (≥6 months) amenorrhea (especially associated with breast secretion) following discontinuation of therapy. Discontinue use with the onset of sudden enlargement, pain, or tenderness of fibroids (leiomyomata). Extremely rare hepatic adenomas and focal nodular hyperplasia resulting in fatal intra-abdominal hemorrhage have been reported in association with long-term oral contraceptive use; presentation of an abdominal mass, acute abdominal pain, or intra-abdominal bleeding warrants further evaluation to rule out source.

The minimum dosage combination of estrogen/progestin that will effectively treat the individual patient should be used. New patients should be started on products containing ≤0.035 mg of estrogen per tablet. Extended cycle regimen contraceptives provide more hormonal exposure per year than conventional monthly contraceptives.

Drug Interactions

Metabolism/Transport Effects

Ethinyl estradiol: **Substrate** of CYP2C9 (minor), 3A4 (major), 3A5-7 (minor); **Inhibits** CYP1A2 (weak), 2B6 (weak), 2C8 (weak), 2C19 (weak), 3A4 (weak)

Levonorgestrel: **Substrate** of CYP3A4 (major)

Avoid Concomitant Use

Avoid concomitant use of Ethinyl Estradiol and Levonorgestrel with any of the following: Anastrozole; Griseofulvin

Increased Effect/Toxicity

Ethinyl Estradiol and Levonorgestrel may increase the levels/effects of: Benzodiazepines (metabolized by oxidation); Corticosteroids (Systemic); CYP1A2 Substrates; ROPINIRole; Selegiline; Theophylline Derivatives; Tipranavir; TiZANidine; Tranexamic Acid; Voriconazole

The levels/effects of Ethinyl Estradiol and Levonorgestrel may be increased by: Ascorbic Acid; Conivaptan; Herbs (Estrogenic Properties); Herbs (Progestogenic Properties); Voriconazole

Decreased Effect

Ethinyl Estradiol and Levonorgestrel may decrease the levels/effects of: Anastrozole; Chenodiol; LamoTRIgine; Protease Inhibitors; Thyroid Products; Ursodiol; Vitamin K Antagonists

The levels/effects of Ethinyl Estradiol and Levonorgestrel may be decreased by: Acitretin; Aminoglutethimide; Aprepitant; Armodafinil; Artemether; Barbiturates; Bile Acid Sequestrants; Bosentan; CarBAMazepine; Colesevelam; CYP3A4 Inducers (Strong); Deferasirox; Felbamate; Fosaprepitant; Fosphenytoin; Griseofulvin; LamoTRIgine; Modafinil; Mycophenolate; Nafcillin; OXcarbazepine; Phenytoin; Protease Inhibitors; Retinoic Acid Derivatives; Rifamycin Derivatives; Rufinamide; St Johns Wort; Tipranavir; Tocilizumab; Topiramate

Ethanol/Nutrition/Herb Interactions

Food: CNS effects of caffeine may be enhanced if combination hormonal contraceptives are used concurrently with caffeine. Grapefruit juice increases ethinyl estradiol plasma concentrations and would be expected to increase progesterone serum levels as well; clinical implications are unclear.

Herb/Nutraceutical: St John's wort may decrease levels. Herbs with estrogenic properties may enhance the adverse/toxic effect of estrogen derivatives; examples include alfalfa, black cohosh, bloodroot, hops, kudzu, licorice, red clover, saw palmetto, soybean, thyme, wild yam, yucca. Herbs with progestogenic properties may enhance the adverse/toxic effect of progestins; examples include bloodroot, chasteberry, damiana, oregano, yucca. Impaired folate metabolism and reduced serum levels of cyanocobalamin have been reported with oral contraceptive use; increased dietary intake or supplementation may be necessary.

Dietary Considerations Should be taken at the same time each day.

Pharmacodynamics/Kinetics

Half-life Elimination Ethinyl estradiol: 12-23 hours; Levonorgestrel: 22-49 hours

Pregnancy Risk Factor X

Lactation Enters breast milk/not recommended

Breast-Feeding Considerations Jaundice and breast enlargement in the nursing infant have been reported following the use of combination hormonal contraceptives. May decrease the quality and quantity of breast milk; alternative form of contraception is recommended.

Dosage Forms

Tablet, oral [low-dose formulation]:

Aviane™: Ethinyl estradiol 0.02 mg and levonorgestrel 0.1 mg (28s) [21 orange tablets and 7 light green inactive tablets]

Lutera®, Sronyx®: Ethinyl estradiol 0.02 mg and levonorgestrel 0.1 mg (28s) [21 white tablets and 7 peach inactive tablets]

Tablet, oral [monophasic formulation]:

Levora®: Ethinyl estradiol 0.03 mg and levonorgestrel 0.15 mg (28s) [21 white tablets and 7 peach inactive tablets]

Nordette® 28: Ethinyl estradiol 0.03 mg and levonorgestrel 0.15 mg (28s) [21 light orange tablets and 7 pink inactive tablets]

Portia® 28: Ethinyl estradiol 0.03 mg and levonorgestrel 0.15 mg (28s) [21 pink tablets and 7 white inactive tablets]

Tablet, oral [extended cycle regimen]:

Introvale™: Ethinyl estradiol 0.03 mg and levonorgestrel 0.15 mg (91s) [84 peach tablets and 7 white inactive tablets]

Jolessa™, Seasonale®: Ethinyl estradiol 0.03 mg and levonorgestrel 0.15 mg (91s) [84 pink tablets and 7 white inactive tablets]

LoSeasonique®: Ethinyl estradiol 0.02 mg and levonorgestrel 0.1 mg (91s) [84 orange tablets] and ethinyl estradiol 0.01 mg [7 yellow tablets]

Quasense®: Ethinyl estradiol 0.03 mg and levonorgestrel 0.15 mg] (91s) [84 white tablets and 7 peach inactive tablets]

Seasonique®: Ethinyl estradiol 0.03 mg and levonorgestrel 0.15 mg (91s) [84 light blue-green tablets] and ethinyl estradiol 0.01 mg [7 yellow tablets]

Tablet, oral [noncyclic regimen]:

Lybrel®: Ethinyl estradiol 0.02 mg and levonorgestrel 0.09 mg (28s) [28 yellow tablets]

Tablet, oral [triphasic formulation]:

Enpresse®:

- Day 1-6: Ethinyl estradiol 0.03 mg and levonorgestrel 0.05 mg [6 pink tablets]
- Day 7-11: Ethinyl estradiol 0.04 mg and levonorgestrel 0.075 mg [5 white tablets]
- Day 12-21: Ethinyl estradiol 0.03 mg and levonorgestrel 0.125 mg [10 orange tablets]
- Day 22-28: 7 light green inactive tablets (28s)

Trivora®:

- Day 1-6: Ethinyl estradiol 0.03 mg and levonorgestrel 0.05 mg [6 blue tablets]
- Day 7-11: Ethinyl estradiol 0.04 mg and levonorgestrel 0.075 mg [5 white tablets]
- Day 12-21: Ethinyl estradiol 0.03 mg and levonorgestrel 0.125 mg [10 pink tablets]
- Day 22-28: 7 peach inactive tablets (28s)

Ethinyl Estradiol and Norelgestromin

(ETH in il es tra DYE ole & nor el JES troe min)

U.S. Brand Names Ortho Evra®

Canadian Brand Names Evra®

Pharmacologic Category Contraceptive; Estrogen and Progestin Combination

Use Prevention of pregnancy

Local Anesthetic/Vasoconstrictor Precautions No information available to require special precautions

Effects on Dental Treatment When prescribing antibiotics, patient must be warned to use additional methods of birth control if on oral contraceptives.

Effects on Bleeding No information available to require special precautions

Adverse Effects The following reactions have been reported with the contraceptive patch. Adverse reactions associated with oral combination hormonal contraceptive agents are also likely to appear with the topical contraceptive patch (frequency difficult to anticipate).

>10%:

- Central nervous system: Headache (21%)
- Endocrine & metabolic: Breast symptoms (22%; including discomfort, engorgement, pain)
- Gastrointestinal: Nausea (17%)
- Miscellaneous: Application site disorder (17%)

1% to 10%:

- Cardiovascular: Blood pressure increased (<2.5%)
- Central nervous system: Anxiety/mood disorders (6%), dizziness (3%), fatigue (3%), migraine (3%), insomnia (<2.5%), malaise (<2.5%)

Dermatologic: Acne (3%), pruritus (3%), chloasma (<2.5%), contact dermatitis (<2.5%), erythema (<2.5%), skin irritation (<2.5%)
Endocrine & metabolic: Dysmenorrhea (8%), menstrual disorders (6%), weight gain (3%), fluid retention (<2.5%), galactorrhea (<2.5%), libido changes (<2.5%)
Gastrointestinal: Abdominal pain (8%), vomiting (5%), diarrhea (4%), vaginal yeast infection (4%), abdominal distension (<2.5%)
Genitourinary: Vaginal bleeding (6%), genital discharge (<2.5%), uterine spasm (<2.5%), vaginal discharge (<2.5%), vulvovaginal dryness (<2.5%)
Hepatic: Cholecystitis (<2.5%), lipid disorders (<2.5%)
Neuromuscular & skeletal: Muscle spasms (<2.5%)
Respiratory: Pulmonary embolism (<2.5%)
Miscellaneous: Premenstrual syndrome (<2.5%)

Dosage Topical: Adults: Females:

Contraception: Apply one patch each week for 3 weeks (21 total days); followed by one week that is patch-free. Each patch should be applied on the same day each week ("patch change day") and only one patch should be worn at a time. No more than 7 days should pass during the patch-free interval.

Schedule 1 (Sunday starter): Dose begins on first Sunday after onset of menstruation; if the menstrual period starts on Sunday, apply one patch that very same day. **With a Sunday start, an additional method of contraception (nonhormonal) must be used until after the first 7 days of consecutive administration.** Each patch change will then occur on Sunday.

Schedule 2 (Day 1 starter): Dose starts on first day of menstrual cycle, applying one patch during the first 24 hours of menstrual cycle. No back-up method of contraception is needed as long as the patch is applied on the first day of cycle. Each patch change will then occur on that same day of the week.

Additional dosing considerations:

No bleeding during patch-free week/missed menstrual period: If patch has been applied as directed, continue treatment on usual "patch change day". If used correctly, no bleeding during patch-free week does not necessarily indicate pregnancy. However, if no withdrawal bleeding occurs for 2 consecutive cycles, pregnancy should be ruled out. If patch has not been applied as directed, and one menstrual period is missed, pregnancy should be ruled out prior to continuing treatment.

If a patch becomes partially or completely detached for <24 hours: Try to reapply to same place, or replace with a new patch immediately. Do not reapply if patch is no longer sticky, if it is sticking to itself or another surface, or if it has material sticking to it.

If a patch becomes partially or completely detached for >24 hours (or time period is unknown): Apply a new patch and use this day of the week as the new "patch change day" from this point on. **An additional method of contraception (nonhormonal) should be used until after the first 7 days of consecutive administration.**

Switching from oral contraceptives: Apply first patch on the first day of withdrawal bleeding. If there is no bleeding within 5 days of taking the last active tablet, pregnancy must first be ruled out. If patch is applied later than the first day of bleeding, **an additional method of contraception (nonhormonal) should be used until after the first 7 days of consecutive administration**

Use after childbirth: Therapy should not be started <4 weeks after childbirth. Pregnancy should be ruled out prior to treatment if menstrual periods have not restarted. **An additional method of contraception (nonhormonal) should be used until after the first 7 days of consecutive administration.**

Use after abortion or miscarriage: Therapy may be started immediately if abortion/miscarriage occur within the first trimester. If therapy is not started within 5 days, follow instructions for first time use. If abortion/miscarriage occur during the second trimester, therapy should not be started for at least 4 weeks. Follow directions for use after childbirth.

Dosage adjustment in renal impairment: Specific guidelines not available; use with caution and monitor blood pressure closely. Consider other forms of contraception.

Dosage adjustment in hepatic impairment: Contraindicated in patients with hepatic impairment

Mechanism of Action Combination hormonal contraceptives inhibit ovulation via a negative feedback mechanism on the hypothalamus, which alters the normal pattern of gonadotropin secretion of a follicle-stimulating hormone (FSH) and luteinizing hormone by the anterior pituitary. The follicular phase FSH and midcycle surge of gonadotropins are inhibited. In addition, combination hormonal contraceptives produce alterations in the genital tract, including changes in the cervical mucus, rendering it unfavorable for sperm penetration even if ovulation occurs. Changes in the endometrium may also occur, producing an unfavorable environment for nidation. Combination hormonal contraceptive drugs may alter the tubal transport of the ova through the fallopian tubes. Progestational agents may also alter sperm fertility.

Contraindications Hypersensitivity to ethinyl estradiol, norelgestromin, or any component of the formulation; history of or current thrombophlebitis or venous thromboembolic disorders (including DVT, PE); active or recent (within 1 year) arterial thromboembolic disease (eg, stroke, MI); cerebral vascular disease, coronary artery disease, valvular heart disease with complications, persistent blood pressure values of ≥160/100 mm Hg; diabetes mellitus with vascular involvement; known or suspected breast carcinoma, endometrial cancer, estrogen-dependent neoplasms; undiagnosed abnormal genital bleeding; hepatic dysfunction or tumor, cholestatic jaundice of pregnancy, jaundice with prior combination hormonal contraceptive use; major surgery with prolonged immobilization; pregnancy

Warnings/Precautions Combination hormonal contraceptives do not protect against HIV infection or other sexually-transmitted diseases. **[U.S. Boxed Warning]: The risk of cardiovascular side effects is increased in women who smoke cigarettes; risk increases with age (especially women >35 years of age) and the number of cigarettes smoked; women who use combination hormonal contraceptives should be strongly advised not to smoke. Avoid use in patients >35 years of age who smoke.** Combination hormonal contraceptives may lead to increased risk of myocardial infarction, use with caution in patients with risk factors for coronary artery disease. All combination hormonal contraceptives may increase the risk of thromboembolism. **[U.S. Boxed Warning]: The risk of venous thromboembolism (VTE) may be further increased with use of the contraceptive patch due to increased estrogen exposure in comparison to oral contraceptives.** Whenever possible, combination hormonal contraceptives should be discontinued at least 4 weeks prior to and for 2 weeks following elective surgery associated with an increased risk of thromboembolism or during periods of prolonged immobilization. Combination hormonal contraceptives may have a dose-related risk of vascular disease, hypertension, and gallbladder disease. Cholestasis may occur in women with a history of pregnancy-related or previous oral contraceptive-related cholestasis. Women with hypertension or renal disease should be encouraged to use a nonhormonal form of contraception. The use of combination hormonal contraceptives has been associated with a slight increase in frequency of breast cancer; however, studies are not consistent. Use is contraindicated in women with breast cancer (current or history of). Combination hormonal contraceptives may cause glucose intolerance or affect serum triglyceride and lipoprotein levels. Estrogens may cause retinal vascular thrombosis; discontinue if migraine, loss of vision, proptosis, diplopia or other visual disturbances occur; discontinue permanently if papilledema or retinal vascular lesions are observed on examination. Use caution with conditions that may be aggravated by fluid retention, depression, or history of migraine. Presentation of irregular, unresolving vaginal bleeding warrants further evaluation including endometrial sampling, if indicated, to rule out malignancy. Extremely rare adenomas and focal nodular hyperplasia resulting in fatal intra-abdominal hemorrhage have been reported in association with long-term oral contraceptive use. The minimum dosage combination of estrogen/progestin that will effectively treat the individual patient should be used. Not for use prior to menarche.

The combination hormonal contraceptive patch may have adverse effects similar to those associated with oral contraceptive products. Risk of complications increases with other risk factors such as hypertension, hyperlipidemias, obesity and diabetes. The topical patch may be less effective in patients weighing ≥90 kg (198 lb) and an increased incidence of pregnancy has been reported in this population; consider another form of contraception.

Drug Interactions

Metabolism/Transport Effects

Ethinyl estradiol: **Substrate** of CYP2C9 (minor), 3A4 (major), 3A5-7 (minor); **Inhibits** CYP1A2 (weak), 2B6 (weak), 2C8 (weak), 2C19 (weak), 3A4 (weak)

Norelgestromin: **Substrate** of CYP3A4 (minor)

Avoid Concomitant Use

Avoid concomitant use of Ethinyl Estradiol and Norelgestromin with any of the following: Anastrozole; Griseofulvin

Increased Effect/Toxicity

Ethinyl Estradiol and Norelgestromin may increase the levels/effects of: Benzodiazepines (metabolized by oxidation); Corticosteroids (Systemic); CYP1A2 Substrates; ROPINIRole; Selegiline; Theophylline Derivatives; Tipranavir; TiZANidine; Tranexamic Acid; Voriconazole

The levels/effects of Ethinyl Estradiol and Norelgestromin may be increased by: Ascorbic Acid; Conivaptan; Herbs (Estrogenic Properties); Herbs (Progestogenic Properties); Voriconazole

Decreased Effect

Ethinyl Estradiol and Norelgestromin may decrease the levels/effects of: Anastrozole; Chenodiol; LamoTRIgine; Protease Inhibitors; Thyroid Products; Ursodiol; Vitamin K Antagonists

The levels/effects of Ethinyl Estradiol and Norelgestromin may be decreased by: Acitretin; Aminoglutethimide; Aprepitant; Armodafinil; Artemether; Barbiturates; Bile Acid Sequestrants; Bosentan; CarBAMazepine; Colesevelam; CYP3A4 Inducers (Strong); Deferasirox; Felbamate; Fosaprepitant; Fosphenytoin; Griseofulvin; LamoTRIgine; Modafinil; Mycophenolate; Nafcillin; OXcarbazepine; Phenytoin; Protease Inhibitors; Retinoic Acid Derivatives; Rifamycin Derivatives; Rufinamide; St Johns Wort; Tipranavir; Tocilizumab; Topiramate

Ethanol/Nutrition/Herb Interactions

Food: CNS effects of caffeine may be enhanced if combination hormonal contraceptives are used concurrently with caffeine. Grapefruit juice increases ethinyl estradiol concentrations and would be expected to increase progesterone serum levels as well; clinical implications are unclear.

Herb/Nutraceutical: St John's wort may decrease levels. Herbs with estrogenic properties may enhance the adverse/toxic effect of estrogen derivatives; examples include alfalfa, black cohosh, bloodroot, hops, kudzu, licorice, red clover, saw palmetto, soybean, thyme, wild yam, yucca. Herbs with progestogenic properties may enhance the adverse/toxic effect of progestins; examples include bloodroot, chasteberry, damiana, oregano, yucca.

Pharmacodynamics/Kinetics

Half-life Elimination Topical: Ethinyl estradiol: ~17 hours; Norelgestromin: ~28 hours

Pregnancy Risk Factor X

Lactation Enters breast milk/not recommended

Breast-Feeding Considerations Jaundice and breast enlargement in the nursing infant have been reported following the use of combination hormonal contraceptives. May decrease the quality and quantity of breast milk; a nonhormonal form of contraception is recommended.

Dosage Forms

Patch, transdermal:

Ortho Evra®: Ethinyl estradiol 0.75 mg and norelgestromin 6 mg [releases ethinyl estradiol 20 mcg and norelgestromin 150 mcg per day] (1s, 3s)

Dosage Forms: Canada

Patch, transdermal:

Evra®: Ethinyl estradiol 0.6 mg and norelgestromin 6 mg (1s, 3s)

Ethinyl Estradiol and Norethindrone

(ETH in il es tra DYE ole & nor eth IN drone)

Related Information

Endocrine Disorders and Pregnancy *on page* 1879

Norethindrone *on page* 1226

U.S. Brand Names Aranelle®; Balziva™; Brevicon®; Estrostep® Fe; Femcon® Fe; femhrt®; femhrt® Lo; Generess™ Fe; Jinteli™; Junel® 1.5/30; Junel® 1/20; Junel® Fe 1.5/30; Junel® Fe 1/20; Leena®; Lo Loestrin™ Fe; Loestrin® 21 1.5/30; Loestrin® 21 1/20; Loestrin® 24 Fe; Loestrin® Fe 1.5/30; Loestrin® Fe 1/20; Microgestin® 1.5/30; Microgestin® 1/20; Microgestin® Fe 1.5/30; Microgestin® Fe 1/20; Modicon®; Necon® 0.5/35; Necon® 1/35; Necon® 10/11; Necon® 7/7/7; Norinyl® 1+35; Nortrel® 0.5/35; Nortrel® 1/35; Nortrel® 7/7/7; Ortho-Novum® 1/35; Ortho-Novum® 7/7/7; Ovcon® 35; Ovcon® 50; Tilia™ Fe; Tri-Legest™ Fe; Tri-Norinyl®; Zenchent™; Zeosa™

Canadian Brand Names Brevicon® 0.5/35; Brevicon® 1/35; FemHRT®; Loestrin™ 1.5/30; Minestrin™ 1/20; Ortho® 0.5/35; Ortho® 1/35; Ortho® 7/7/7; Select™ 1/35; Synphasic®

Generic Availability (U.S.) Yes

Pharmacologic Category Contraceptive; Estrogen and Progestin Combination

Use Prevention of pregnancy; treatment of acne; moderate-to-severe vasomotor symptoms associated with menopause; prevention of osteoporosis (in women at significant risk only)

Unlabeled/Investigational Use Treatment of hypermenorrhea (menorrhagia); pain associated with endometriosis, dysmenorrhea; dysfunctional uterine bleeding

Local Anesthetic/Vasoconstrictor Precautions No information available to require special precautions

Effects on Dental Treatment When prescribing antibiotics, patient must be warned to use additional methods of birth control if on oral contraceptives.

Effects on Bleeding No information available to require special precautions

Adverse Effects The following reactions have been associated with oral contraceptive use:

Increased risk or evidence of association with use:

Cardiovascular: Arterial thromboembolism, cerebral hemorrhage, cerebral thrombosis, hypertension, mesenteric thrombosis, MI, venous thrombosis (with or without embolism)
Gastrointestinal: Gallbladder disease
Hepatic: Hepatic adenomas, liver tumors (benign)
Local: Thrombophlebitis
Ocular: Retinal thrombosis
Renal: Impaired renal function
Respiratory: Pulmonary embolism

Adverse reactions considered drug related:

Cardiovascular: Edema, varicose vein aggravation
Central nervous system: Depression, migraine, mood changes
Dermatologic: Chloasma, melasma, rash (allergic)
Endocrine & metabolic: Amenorrhea, breakthrough bleeding, breast changes (enlargement, pain, secretion, tenderness), fluid retention, infertility (temporary), lactation decreased (with use immediately postpartum), menstrual flow changes, spotting
Gastrointestinal: Abdominal bloating, abdominal cramps, abdominal pain, appetite changes, nausea, weight changes, vomiting
Genitourinary: Cervical ectropion, cervical secretion, vaginal candidiasis, vaginitis
Hematologic: Folate decreased, porphyria exacerbation
Hepatic: Cholestatic jaundice
Neuromuscular & skeletal: Chorea exacerbation
Ocular: Contact lens intolerance, corneal curvature changes (steepening)
Miscellaneous: Anaphylactic/anaphylactoid reactions (including angioedema, circulatory collapse, respiratory collapse, urticaria), SLE exacerbation

Adverse reactions in which association is not confirmed or denied: Acne, Budd-Chiari syndrome, cataracts, colitis, cystitis-like syndrome, dizziness, dysmenorrhea, erythema multiforme, erythema nodosum, headache, hemolytic uremic syndrome, hemorrhagic eruption, hirsutism, libido changes, nervousness, optic neuritis (with or without partial or complete loss of vision), pancreatitis, premenstrual syndrome, renal function impaired, scalp hair loss

The following have been associated with femhrt® and in general, are similar to placebo. Also refer to adverse reactions observed with oral contraceptives for additional reactions observed with estrogen/progestin therapy:

>10%: Central nervous system: Headache (15% to 18%)

1% to 10%:

Central nervous system: Depression (4% to 6%), nervousness (2% to 5%)
Endocrine & metabolic: Breast pain (8% to 9%)
Gastrointestinal: Abdominal pain (8% to 10%), nausea/vomiting (5% to 7%), diarrhea (4% to 6%), dyspepsia (3% to 5%)
Genitourinary: Urinary tract infection (4% to 6%), vaginitis (5%)
Respiratory: Sinusitis (8% to 9%)

Dosage Oral:

Adolescents ≥15 years and Adults: Females: Acne: Estrostep® Fe: Refer to dosing for contraception

Adults: Females:

Moderate-to-severe vasomotor symptoms associated with menopause: Initial: femhrt® 0.5/2.5: 1 tablet daily; patient should be re-evaluated at 3- to 6-month intervals to determine if treatment is still necessary; patient should be maintained at the lowest effective dose

Prevention of osteoporosis: Initial: femhrt® 0.5/2.5: 1 tablet daily; patient should be maintained on the lowest effective dose

Contraception:

Schedule 1 (Sunday starter): Dose begins on first Sunday after onset of menstruation; if the menstrual period starts on Sunday, take first tablet that very same day. This schedule is not preferred for Lo Loestrin Fe. With a Sunday start, an additional method of contraception should be used until after the first 7 days of consecutive administration (all products).

For 21-tablet package: Dosage is 1 tablet daily for 21 consecutive days, followed by 7 days off of the medication; a new course begins on the 8th day after the last tablet is taken.

For 28-tablet package: Dosage is 1 tablet daily without interruption.

Schedule 2 (Day 1 starter): Dose starts on first day of menstrual cycle taking 1 tablet daily.

For 21-tablet package: Dosage is 1 tablet daily for 21 consecutive days, followed by 7 days off of the medication; a new course begins on the 8th day after the last tablet is taken.

For 28-tablet package: Dosage is 1 tablet daily without interruption.

If all doses have been taken on schedule and one menstrual period is missed, continue dosing cycle. If two consecutive menstrual periods are missed, pregnancy test is required before new dosing cycle is started.

Missed doses **monophasic formulations** (refer to package insert for complete information):

One dose missed: Take as soon as remembered. Take the next tablet at your regular time. You may take 2 tablets in 1 day.

Two consecutive doses missed in the first 2 weeks: Take 2 tablets as soon as remembered and 2 tablets the next day. An additional method of contraception should be used for 7 days after missed dose.

Two consecutive doses missed in week 3 (all products) or in week 4 (Lo Loestrin Fe), or three consecutive doses missed at any time (all products): An additional method of contraception must be used for 7 days after a missed dose.

Schedule 1 (Sunday starter): Continue dose of 1 tablet daily until Sunday, then discard the rest of the pack, and a new pack should be started that same day.

Schedule 2 (Day 1 starter): Current pack should be discarded, and a new pack should be started that same day.

Missed doses **biphasic/triphasic formulations** (refer to package insert for complete information):

One dose missed: Take the next tablet at your regular time. You may take 2 tablets in 1 day.

Two consecutive doses missed in week 1 or week 2 of the pack: Take 2 tablets as soon as remembered and 2 tablets the next day. Resume taking 1 tablet daily until the pack is empty. An additional method of contraception should be used for 7 days after a missed dose.

Two consecutive doses missed in week 3 of the pack: An additional method of contraception must be used for 7 days after a missed dose.

Schedule 1 (Sunday Starter): Take 1 tablet every day until Sunday. Discard the remaining pack and start a new pack of pills on the same day.

Schedule 2 (Day 1 starter): Discard the remaining pack and start a new pack the same day.

Three or more consecutive doses missed: An additional method of contraception must be used for 7 days after a missed dose.

Schedule 1 (Sunday Starter): Take 1 tablet every day until Sunday; on Sunday, discard the pack and start a new pack.

Schedule 2 (Day 1 Starter): Discard the remaining pack and begin new pack of tablets starting on the same day.

Switching from a different contraceptive:

Oral contraceptive: Start on the same day that a new pack of the previous oral contraceptive would have been taken.

Transdermal patch, vaginal ring, injection: Start on the day the next dose would have been due.

IUD or implant: Start on the day of removal. A backup method of contraception may be required following IUD removal.

Use after childbirth (in women who are not breast-feeding) or after second trimester abortion: Therapy may be started ≥4 weeks postpartum. Pregnancy should be ruled out prior to treatment if menstrual periods have not restarted and an additional method of contraception (nonhormonal) should be used until after the first 7 days of consecutive administration.

Dosage adjustment in renal impairment: Specific guidelines not available; use with caution and monitor blood pressure closely. Consider other forms of contraception.

Dosage adjustment in hepatic impairment: Contraindicated in patients with hepatic impairment.

Mechanism of Action Combination oral contraceptives inhibit ovulation via a negative feedback mechanism on the hypothalamus, which alters the normal pattern of gonadotropin secretion of a follicle-stimulating hormone (FSH) and luteinizing hormone by the anterior pituitary. The follicular phase FSH and midcycle surge of gonadotropins are inhibited. In addition, combination hormonal contraceptives produce alterations in the genital tract, including changes in the cervical mucus, rendering it unfavorable for sperm penetration even if ovulation occurs. Changes in the endometrium may also occur, producing an unfavorable environment for nidation. Combination hormonal contraceptive drugs may alter the tubal transport of the ova through the fallopian tubes. Progestational agents may also alter sperm fertility.

In postmenopausal women, exogenous estrogen is used to replace decreased endogenous production. The addition of progestin reduces the incidence of endometrial hyperplasia and risk of endometrial cancer in women with an intact uterus.

Contraindications Hypersensitivity to ethinyl estradiol, norethindrone, norethindrone acetate, or any component of the formulation; breast cancer or other estrogen- or progestin-dependent neoplasms (current or a history of), hepatic tumors or disease, pregnancy, undiagnosed abnormal uterine bleeding. Use is also contraindicated in women at high risk of arterial or venous thrombotic diseases including: Cerebrovascular disease, coronary artery disease, diabetes mellitus with vascular disease, DVT or PE (current or history of), hypercoagulopathies (inherited or acquired), headaches with focal neurological symptoms, hypertension (uncontrolled), migraine headaches if >35 years of age, thrombogenic valvular or rhythm diseases of the heart (eg, subacute bacterial endocarditis with valvular disease or atrial fibrillation), women >35 years of age who smoke.

Warnings/Precautions [U.S. Boxed Warning]: Estrogens with or without progestin should not be used to prevent cardiovascular disease. Use caution with cardiovascular disease or dysfunction. May increase the risks of hypertension, myocardial infarction (MI), stroke, pulmonary emboli (PE), and deep vein thrombosis; incidence of these effects was shown to be significantly increased in postmenopausal women using conjugated equine estrogens (CEE) in combination with medroxyprogesterone acetate (MPA). Nonfatal MI, PE, and thrombophlebitis have also been reported in males taking high doses of CEE (eg, for prostate cancer). When used for contraception, use with caution in patients with risk factors for cardiovascular disease; may also lead to increased risk of cerebrovascular events (stroke). May have a dose-related risk of vascular disease and hypertension; women with hypertension should be encouraged to use another form of contraception. Monitor women with well-controlled hypertension and discontinue if blood pressure rises significantly. Use is contraindicated with uncontrolled hypertension. Combination hormonal contraceptives may effect serum triglyceride and lipoprotein levels. Estrogen compounds are generally associated with lipid effects such as increased HDL-cholesterol and decreased LDL-cholesterol. Progestins may be associated with decreased HDL-cholesterol. Triglycerides may also be increased; use with caution in patients with familial defects of lipoprotein metabolism.

[U.S. Boxed Warning]: The risk of cardiovascular side effects increases in women who smoke cigarettes, the risk is increased in women who are >35 years of age and the number of cigarettes smoked. Use is contraindicated in women >35 years of age who smoke; all women who use combination hormonal contraceptives should be strongly advised not to smoke.

[U.S. Boxed Warning]: Estrogens with or without progestin should be used for shortest duration possible at the lowest effective dose consistent with treatment goals. Before prescribing estrogen therapy to postmenopausal women, the risks and benefits must be weighed for each patient. Women should be informed of these risks and benefits, as well as possible effects of progestin when added to estrogen therapy. Estrogens with or without progestin should be used for shortest duration possible consistent with treatment goals. Conduct periodic risk:benefit assessments.

[U.S. Boxed Warning]: The risk of dementia may be increased in postmenopausal women; increased incidence was observed in women ≥65 years of age taking CEE alone or in combination with MPA.

Estrogens may increase the risk of breast cancer. The use of combination hormonal contraceptives has been associated with a slight increase in frequency of breast cancer, however studies are not consistent. Use for contraception is contraindicated in women with breast cancer (current or history of). An increased risk of invasive breast cancer was observed in postmenopausal women using CEE in combination with MPA; a smaller increase in risk was seen with estrogen therapy alone in observational studies. An increase in abnormal mammograms has also been reported with estrogen and progestin therapy in postmenopausal women. Estrogen use may lead to severe hypercalcemia in postmenopausal patients with breast cancer and bone metastases; discontinue estrogen if hypercalcemia occurs. Unopposed estrogens may increase the risk of endometrial carcinoma in postmenopausal women with an intact uterus. Risk appears to be associated with long-term use. The use of a progestin should be considered when administering estrogens to postmenopausal women with an intact uterus. Adequate diagnostic measures, including endometrial sampling (if indicated), should be performed to rule out malignancy in all cases of undiagnosed abnormal vaginal bleeding. Postmenopausal estrogen therapy and combined estrogen/progesterone therapy may increase the risk of ovarian cancer; however, the absolute risk to an individual woman is small. Although results from various studies are not consistent, risk does not appear to be significantly associated with the duration, route, or dose of therapy. In one study, the risk decreased after 2 years following discontinuation of therapy. Estrogens may exacerbate endometriosis. Malignant transformation of residual endometrial implants has been reported posthysterectomy with estrogen only therapy. Consider adding a progestin in women with residual endometriosis posthysterectomy.

Extremely rare hepatic adenomas and focal nodular hyperplasia resulting in fatal intra-abdominal hemorrhage have been reported in association with long-term oral contraceptive use. Presentation of an abdominal mass, acute abdominal pain, or intra-abdominal bleeding warrants further evaluation to rule out source. Steroid hormones may be poorly metabolized in patients with hepatic dysfunction. Discontinue if jaundice develops or if acute or chronic hepatic disturbances occur. Use is contraindicated with hepatic disease. Cholestasis may occur in women with a history of pregnancy-related or previous estrogen-related cholestasis.

Estrogens may cause retinal vascular thrombosis; discontinue if papilledema or retinal vascular lesions are observed on examination or if loss of vision, proptosis, diplopia or other visual disturbances occur. Estrogens may induce or exacerbate symptoms in women with hereditary angioedema. Use caution in women with diabetes; may have adverse effects on glucose tolerance. Use caution with a history of chloasma gravidarum; women with a tendency to chloasma should avoid sun and ultraviolet radiation exposure during therapy. Use with caution in patients with a history of migraine. Evaluate new, recurrent, severe, or persistent headaches. Use of combination oral contraceptives is contraindicated in women with headaches with focal neurological symptoms or migraine headaches if >35 years of age. Use with caution in patients with depression, porphyria, SLE, and in patients with diseases which may be exacerbated by fluid retention, including asthma, epilepsy, or renal dysfunction (women with renal disease should be encouraged to use a nonhormonal form of contraception). Use with caution in patients with gallbladder disease; may have a dose-related risk of gallbladder disease. Use with caution in patients with severe hypocalcemia.

Combination hormonal contraceptives are not for use prior to menarche. Unscheduled bleeding/spotting may occur within the first 3 months of combination oral contraceptive use. Presentation of irregular, unresolving vaginal bleeding following previously regular cycles warrants further evaluation including endometrial sampling, if indicated, to rule out malignancy. Whenever possible, discontinue at least 4 weeks prior to and for 2 weeks following elective surgery associated with an increased risk of thromboembolism or during periods of prolonged immobilization. When used for acne, use only in females ≥15 years, who also desire combination hormonal contraceptive therapy, are unresponsive to topical treatments, have no contraindications to combination hormonal contraceptive use, and plan to stay on therapy for ≥6 months. When used solely for the prevention of osteoporosis in women at significant risk, nonestrogen treatment options should be considered.

The minimum dosage combination of estrogen/progestin that will effectively treat the individual patient should be used. New patients should be started on products containing ≤0.035 mg of estrogen per tablet. Safety and efficacy have not been established for Lo Loestrin Fe in women with a BMI >35 kg/m^2. Combination hormonal contraceptives do not protect against HIV infection or other sexually-transmitted diseases.

Drug Interactions

Metabolism/Transport Effects

Ethinyl estradiol: **Substrate** of CYP2C9 (minor), 3A4 (major), 3A5-7 (minor); **Inhibits** CYP1A2 (weak), 2B6 (weak), 2C8 (weak), 2C19 (weak), 3A4 (weak)

Norethindrone: **Substrate** of CYP3A4 (major); Induces CYP2C19 (weak)

Avoid Concomitant Use

Avoid concomitant use of Ethinyl Estradiol and Norethindrone with any of the following: Anastrozole; Griseofulvin

Increased Effect/Toxicity

Ethinyl Estradiol and Norethindrone may increase the levels/effects of: Benzodiazepines (metabolized by oxidation); Corticosteroids (Systemic); CYP1A2 Substrates; ROPINIRole; Selegiline; Theophylline Derivatives; Tipranavir; TiZANidine; Tranexamic Acid; Voriconazole

The levels/effects of Ethinyl Estradiol and Norethindrone may be increased by: Ascorbic Acid; Conivaptan; Herbs (Estrogenic Properties); Herbs (Progestogenic Properties); Voriconazole

Decreased Effect

Ethinyl Estradiol and Norethindrone may decrease the levels/effects of: Anastrozole; Chenodiol; LamoTRIgine; Protease Inhibitors; Thyroid Products; Ursodiol; Vitamin K Antagonists

The levels/effects of Ethinyl Estradiol and Norethindrone may be decreased by: Acitretin; Aminoglutethimide; Aprepitant; Armodafinil; Artemether; Barbiturates; Bile Acid Sequestrants; Bosentan; CarBAMazepine; Colesevelam; CYP3A4 Inducers (Strong); Darunavir; Deferasirox; Felbamate; Fosaprepitant; Fosphenytoin; Griseofulvin; LamoTRIgine; Modafinil; Mycophenolate; Nafcillin; OXcarbazepine; Phenytoin; Protease Inhibitors; Retinoic Acid Derivatives; Rifamycin Derivatives; Rufinamide; St Johns Wort; Tipranavir; Tocilizumab; Topiramate

Ethanol/Nutrition/Herb Interactions

Ethanol: Routine use increases estrogen level and risk of breast cancer; avoid ethanol. Ethanol may also increase the risk of osteoporosis.

Food: CNS effects of caffeine may be enhanced if combination hormonal contraceptives are used concurrently with caffeine. Grapefruit juice increases ethinyl estradiol concentrations and would be expected to increase progesterone serum levels as well; clinical implications are unclear. Norethindrone absorption is increased by 27% following administration with food.

Herb/Nutraceutical: St John's wort may decrease levels. Herbs with estrogenic properties may enhance the adverse/toxic effect of estrogen derivatives; examples include alfalfa, black cohosh, bloodroot, hops, kudzu, licorice, red clover, saw palmetto, soybean, thyme, wild yam, yucca. Herbs with progestogenic properties may enhance the adverse/toxic effect of progestins; examples include bloodroot, chasteberry, damiana, oregano, yucca.

Dietary Considerations Should be taken at same time each day. May be taken without regard to meals. Ensure adequate calcium and vitamin D intake when used for the prevention of osteoporosis.

Pharmacodynamics/Kinetics

Half-life Elimination Ethinyl estradiol: 19-24 hours

Pregnancy Risk Factor X

Lactation Enters breast milk/not recommended

Breast-Feeding Considerations Jaundice and breast enlargement in the nursing infant have been reported following the use of combination hormonal contraceptives. May decrease the quality and quantity of breast milk; alternative form of contraception is recommended.

Dosage Forms

Tablet, oral:

femhrt® 1/5: Ethinyl estradiol 0.005 mg and norethindrone acetate 1 mg (28s, 90s) [white tablets]

femhrt® Lo 0.5/2.5: Ethinyl estradiol 0.0025 mg and norethindrone acetate 0.5 mg (28s, 90s) [white tablets]

Jinteli™: Ethinyl estradiol 0.005 mg and norethindrone acetate 1 mg (28s, 90s) [white tablets]

Tablet, oral, monophasic formulations:

Balziva™: Ethinyl estradiol 0.035 mg and norethindrone 0.4 mg (28s) [21 light peach tablets and 7 white inactive tablets]

Brevicon®: Ethinyl estradiol 0.035 mg and norethindrone 0.5 mg (28s) [21 blue tablets and 7 orange inactive tablets]

Junel® 1/20: Ethinyl estradiol 0.02 mg and norethindrone acetate 1 mg (21s) [yellow tablets]

Junel® 1.5/30, Loestrin® 21 1.5/30: Ethinyl estradiol 0.03 mg and norethindrone acetate 1.5 mg (21s) [pink tablets]

Junel® Fe 1/20: Ethinyl estradiol 0.02 mg and norethindrone acetate 1 mg [21 yellow tablets] and ferrous fumarate 75 mg [7 brown tablets] (28s)

Junel® Fe 1.5/30, Loestrin® Fe 21 1.5/30: Ethinyl estradiol 0.03 mg and norethindrone acetate 1.5 mg [21 pink tablets] and ferrous fumarate 75 mg [7 brown tablets] (28s)

Loestrin® 21 1/20: Ethinyl estradiol 0.02 mg and norethindrone acetate 1 mg (21s) [light yellow tablets]

Lo Loestrin Fe: Ethinyl estradiol 0.01 mg and norethindrone acetate 1mg [24 blue tablets] and ethinyl estradiol 0.01 mg [2 white tablets] and ferrous fumarate 75 mg [2 brown tablets] (28s)

Loestrin® 24 Fe: Ethinyl estradiol 0.02 mg and norethindrone acetate 1 mg [24 white tablets] and ferrous fumarate 75 mg [4 brown tablets] (28s)

Loestrin® Fe 1/20: Ethinyl estradiol 0.02 mg and norethindrone acetate 1 mg [21 light yellow tablets] and ferrous fumarate 75 mg [7 brown tablets] (28s)

Loestrin® Fe 1.5/30: Ethinyl estradiol 0.03 mg and norethindrone acetate 1.5 mg [21 pink tablets] and ferrous fumarate 75 mg [7 brown tablets] (28s)

Microgestin® 1/20: Ethinyl estradiol 0.02 mg and norethindrone acetate 1 mg (21s) [white tablets]

Microgestin® 1.5/30: Ethinyl estradiol 0.03 mg and norethindrone acetate 1.5 mg (21s) [green tablets]

Microgestin® Fe 1/20: Ethinyl estradiol 0.02 mg and norethindrone acetate 1 mg [21 white tablets] and ferrous fumarate 75 mg [7 brown tablets] (28s)

Microgestin® Fe 1.5/30: Ethinyl estradiol 0.03 mg and norethindrone acetate 1.5 mg [21 green tablets] and ferrous fumarate 75 mg [7 brown tablets] (28s)
Modicon®: Ethinyl estradiol 0.035 mg and norethindrone 0.5 mg (28s) [21 white tablets and 7 green inactive tablets]
Necon® 0.5/35, Nortrel® 0.5/35: Ethinyl estradiol 0.035 mg and norethindrone 0.5 mg (28s) [21 light yellow tablets and 7 white inactive tablets]
Necon® 1/35: Ethinyl estradiol 0.035 mg and norethindrone 1 mg (28s) [21 dark yellow tablets and 7 white inactive tablets]
Norinyl® 1+35: Ethinyl estradiol 0.035 mg and norethindrone 1 mg (28s) [21 yellow-green tablets and 7 orange inactive tablets]
Nortrel® 1/35:
Ethinyl estradiol 0.035 mg and norethindrone 1 mg (21s) [yellow tablets]
Ethinyl estradiol 0.035 mg and norethindrone 1 mg (28s) [21 yellow tablets and 7 white inactive tablets]
Ortho-Novum® 1/35: Ethinyl estradiol 0.035 mg and norethindrone 1 mg (28s) [21 peach tablets and 7 green inactive tablets]
Ovcon® 35: Ethinyl estradiol 0.035 mg and norethindrone 0.4 mg (28s) [21 light peach tablets and 7 green inactive tablets]
Ovcon® 50: Ethinyl estradiol 0.05 mg and norethindrone 1 mg (28s) [21 yellow tablets and 7 green inactive tablets]
Zenchent™: Ethinyl estradiol 0.035 mg and norethindrone 0.4 mg (28s) [21 orange tablets and 7 white inactive tablets]

Tablet, chewable, oral, monophasic formulations:
Femcon® Fe: Ethinyl estradiol 0.035 mg and norethindrone 0.4 mg [21 white tablets] and ferrous fumarate 75 mg [7 brown tablets] (28s)
Generess™ Fe: Ethinyl estradiol 0.025 mg and norethindrone 0.8 mg [24 light green tablets] and ferrous fumarate 75 mg [4 brown tablets] (28s)
Zeosa™: Ethinyl estradiol 0.035 mg and norethindrone 0.4 mg [21 light yellow tablets] and ferrous fumarate 75 mg [7 brown tablets] (28s)

Tablet, oral, biphasic formulations:
Necon® 10/11:
Day 1-10: Ethinyl estradiol 0.035 mg and norethindrone 0.5 mg [10 light yellow tablets]
Day 11-21: Ethinyl estradiol 0.035 mg and norethindrone 1 mg [11 dark yellow tablets]
Day 22-28: 7 white inactive tablets (28s)

Tablet, oral, triphasic formulations:
Aranelle®:
Day 1-7: Ethinyl estradiol 0.035 mg and norethindrone 0.5 mg [7 light yellow tablets]
Day 8-16: Ethinyl estradiol 0.035 mg and norethindrone 1 mg [9 white tablets]
Day 17-21: Ethinyl estradiol 0.035 mg and norethindrone 0.5 mg [5 light yellow tablets]
Day 22-28: 7 peach inactive tablets (28s)
Estrostep® Fe, Tilia™ Fe::
Day 1-5: Ethinyl estradiol 0.02 mg and norethindrone acetate 1 mg [5 white triangular tablets]
Day 6-12: Ethinyl estradiol 0.03 mg and norethindrone acetate 1 mg [7 white square tablets]
Day 13-21: Ethinyl estradiol 0.035 mg and norethindrone acetate 1 mg [9 white round tablets]
Day 22-28: Ferrous fumarate 75 mg [7 brown tablets] (28s)
Leena®:
Day 1-7: Ethinyl estradiol 0.035 mg and norethindrone 0.5 mg [7 light blue tablets]
Day 8-16: Ethinyl estradiol 0.035 mg and norethindrone 1 mg [9 light yellow-green tablets]
Day 17-21: Ethinyl estradiol 0.035 mg and norethindrone 0.5 mg [5 light blue tablets]
Day 22-28: 7 orange inactive tablets (28s)
Necon® 7/7/7, Ortho-Novum® 7/7/7:
Day 1-7: Ethinyl estradiol 0.035 mg and norethindrone 0.5 mg [7 white tablets]
Day 8-14: Ethinyl estradiol 0.035 mg and norethindrone 0.75 mg [7 light peach tablets]
Day 15-21: Ethinyl estradiol 0.035 mg and norethindrone 1 mg [7 peach tablets]
Day 22-28: 7 green inactive tablets (28s)

Nortrel® 7/7/7:
- Day 1-7: Ethinyl estradiol 0.035 mg and norethindrone 0.5 mg [7 light yellow tablets]
- Day 8-14: Ethinyl estradiol 0.035 mg and norethindrone 0.75 mg [7 blue tablets]
- Day 15-21: Ethinyl estradiol 0.035 mg and norethindrone 1 mg [7 peach tablets]
- Day 22-28: 7 white inactive tablets (28s)

Tri-Legest™ Fe:
- Day 1-5: Ethinyl estradiol 0.02 mg and norethindrone acetate 1 mg [5 light pink tablets]
- Day 6-12: Ethinyl estradiol 0.03 mg and norethindrone acetate 1 mg [7 light yellow tablets]
- Day 13-21: Ethinyl estradiol 0.035 mg and norethindrone acetate 1 mg [9 light blue tablets]
- Day 22-28: Ferrous fumarate 75 mg [7 brown tablets] (28s)

Tri-Norinyl®:
- Day 1-7: Ethinyl estradiol 0.035 mg and norethindrone 0.5 mg [7 blue tablets]
- Day 8-16: Ethinyl estradiol 0.035 mg and norethindrone 1 mg [9 yellow-green tablets]
- Day 17-21: Ethinyl estradiol 0.035 mg and norethindrone 0.5 mg [5 blue tablets]
- Day 22-28: 7 orange inactive tablets (28s)

Ethinyl Estradiol and Norgestimate

(ETH in il es tra DYE ole & nor JES ti mate)

Related Information

Endocrine Disorders and Pregnancy *on page 1879*

U.S. Brand Names MonoNessa®; Ortho Tri-Cyclen®; Ortho Tri-Cyclen® Lo; Ortho-Cyclen®; Sprintec®; Tri-Sprintec®; TriNessa®

Canadian Brand Names Cyclen®; Tri-Cyclen®; Tri-Cyclen® Lo

Generic Availability (U.S.) Yes

Pharmacologic Category Contraceptive; Estrogen and Progestin Combination

Use Prevention of pregnancy; treatment of acne

Unlabeled/Investigational Use Treatment of hypermenorrhea (menorrhagia); pain associated with endometriosis; dysmenorrhea; dysfunctional uterine bleeding

Local Anesthetic/Vasoconstrictor Precautions No information available to require special precautions

Effects on Dental Treatment When prescribing antibiotics, patient must be warned to use additional methods of birth control if on oral contraceptives.

Effects on Bleeding No information available to require special precautions

Adverse Effects The following reactions have been associated with oral contraceptive use:

Increased risk or evidence of association with use:
- Cardiovascular: Arterial thromboembolism, cerebral hemorrhage, cerebral thrombosis, hypertension, mesenteric thrombosis, MI, venous thrombosis (with or without embolism)
- Gastrointestinal: Gallbladder disease
- Hepatic: Hepatic adenomas, liver tumors (benign)
- Local: Thrombophlebitis
- Ocular: Retinal thrombosis
- Respiratory: Pulmonary embolism

Adverse reactions considered drug related:
- Cardiovascular: Edema, varicose vein aggravation
- Central nervous system: Depression, migraine, mood changes
- Dermatologic: Chloasma, melasma, rash (allergic)
- Endocrine & metabolic: Amenorrhea, breakthrough bleeding, breast changes (enlargement, pain, secretion, tenderness), fluid retention, infertility (temporary), lactation decreased (with use immediately postpartum), menstrual flow changes, spotting
- Gastrointestinal: Abdominal bloating, abdominal cramps, abdominal pain, appetite changes, nausea, weight changes, vomiting
- Genitourinary: Cervical ectropion, cervical secretion, vaginal candidiasis, vaginitis
- Hematologic: Folate decreased, porphyria exacerbation
- Hepatic: Cholestatic jaundice
- Neuromuscular & skeletal: Chorea exacerbation
- Ocular: Contact lens intolerance, corneal curvature changes (steepening)
- Miscellaneous: Anaphylactic/anaphylactoid reactions (including angioedema, circulatory collapse, respiratory collapse, urticaria), SLE exacerbation

Adverse reactions in which association is not confirmed or denied: Acne, Budd-Chiari syndrome, cataracts, colitis, cystitis-like syndrome, dizziness, dysmenorrhea, erythema multiforme, erythema nodosum, headache, hemolytic uremic syndrome, hemorrhagic eruption, hirsutism, libido changes, nervousness, optic neuritis (with or without partial or complete loss of vision), pancreatitis, premenstrual syndrome, renal function impaired, scalp hair loss

Dosage Oral:

Children ≥15 years and Adults: Females: Acne (Ortho Tri-Cyclen®): Refer to dosing for contraception

Adults: Females:

Contraception:

Schedule 1 (Sunday starter): Dose begins on first Sunday after onset of menstruation; if the menstrual period starts on Sunday, take first tablet that very same day. **With a Sunday start, an additional method of contraception should be used until after the first 7 days of consecutive administration.**

For 21-tablet package: Dosage is 1 tablet daily for 21 consecutive days, followed by 7 days off of the medication; a new course begins on the 8th day after the last tablet is taken.

For 28-tablet package: Dosage is 1 tablet daily without interruption.

Schedule 2 (Day 1 starter): Dose starts on first day of menstrual cycle taking 1 tablet daily.

For 21-tablet package: Dosage is 1 tablet daily for 21 consecutive days, followed by 7 days off of the medication; a new course begins on the 8th day after the last tablet is taken.

For 28-tablet package: Dosage is 1 tablet daily without interruption.

If all doses have been taken on schedule and one menstrual period is missed, continue dosing cycle. If two consecutive menstrual periods are missed, pregnancy test is required before new dosing cycle is started.

Missed doses **monophasic formulations** (refer to package insert for complete information):

One dose missed: Take as soon as remembered or take 2 tablets next day

Two consecutive doses missed in the first 2 weeks: Take 2 tablets as soon as remembered or 2 tablets next 2 days. **An additional method of contraception should be used for 7 days after missed dose.**

Two consecutive doses missed in week 3 or three consecutive doses missed at any time: **An additional method of contraception must be used for 7 days after a missed dose:**

Schedule 1 (Sunday starter): Continue dose of 1 tablet daily until Sunday, then discard the rest of the pack, and a new pack should be started that same day.

Schedule 2 (Day 1 starter): Current pack should be discarded, and a new pack should be started that same day.

Missed doses **biphasic/triphasic formulations** (refer to package insert for complete information):

One dose missed: Take as soon as remembered or take 2 tablets next day.

Two consecutive doses missed in week 1 or week 2 of the pack: Take 2 tablets as soon as remembered and 2 tablets the next day. Resume taking 1 tablet daily until the pack is empty. **An additional method of contraception must be used for 7 days after a missed dose.**

Two consecutive doses missed in week 3 of the pack. **An additional method of contraception must be used for 7 days after a missed dose.**

Schedule 1 (Sunday starter): Take 1 tablet every day until Sunday. Discard the remaining pack and start a new pack of pills on the same day.

Schedule 2 (Day 1 starter): Discard the remaining pack and start a new pack the same day.

Three or more consecutive doses missed. **An additional method of contraception must be used for 7 days after a missed dose.**

Schedule 1 (Sunday starter): Take 1 tablet every day until Sunday; on Sunday, discard the pack and start a new pack.

Schedule 2 (Day 1 starter): Discard the remaining pack and begin new pack of tablets starting on the same day.

Dosage adjustment in renal impairment: Specific guidelines not available; use with caution and monitor blood pressure closely. Consider other forms of contraception.

Dosage adjustment in hepatic impairment: Contraindicated in patients with hepatic impairment.

Mechanism of Action Combination hormonal contraceptives inhibit ovulation via a negative feedback mechanism on the hypothalamus, which alters the normal pattern of gonadotropin secretion of a follicle-stimulating hormone (FSH) and luteinizing hormone by the anterior pituitary. The follicular phase FSH and midcycle surge of gonadotropins are inhibited. In addition, combination hormonal contraceptives produce alterations in the genital tract, including changes in the cervical mucus, rendering it unfavorable for sperm penetration even if ovulation occurs. Changes in the endometrium may also occur, producing an unfavorable environment for nidation. Combination hormonal contraceptive drugs may alter the tubal transport of the ova through the fallopian tubes. Progestational agents may also alter sperm fertility.

Contraindications Hypersensitivity to ethinyl estradiol, norgestimate, or any component of the formulation; history of or current thrombophlebitis or venous thromboembolic disorders (including DVT, PE); active or recent (within 1 year) arterial thromboembolic disease (eg, stroke, MI); cerebral vascular disease, coronary artery disease, valvular heart disease with complications, severe hypertension; diabetes with vascular involvement; severe headache with focal neurological symptoms; known or suspected breast carcinoma, endometrial cancer, estrogen-dependent neoplasms, undiagnosed abnormal genital bleeding; hepatic dysfunction or tumor, cholestatic jaundice of pregnancy, jaundice with prior combination hormonal contraceptive use; major surgery with prolonged immobilization; heavy smoking (≥15 cigarettes/day) in patients >35 years of age; pregnancy

Warnings/Precautions Combination hormonal contraceptives do not protect against HIV infection or other sexually-transmitted diseases. **[U.S. Boxed Warning]: The risk of cardiovascular side effects increases in women who smoke cigarettes, especially those who are >35 years of age; women who use combination hormonal contraceptives should be strongly advised not to smoke.** Combination hormonal contraceptives may lead to increased risk of myocardial infarction, use with caution in patients with risk factors for coronary artery disease. May increase the risk of thromboembolism. Whenever possible, combination hormonal contraceptives should be discontinued at least 4 weeks prior to and for 2 weeks following elective surgery associated with an increased risk of thromboembolism or during periods of prolonged immobilization. Combination hormonal contraceptives may have a dose-related risk of vascular disease, hypertension, and gallbladder disease. Women with hypertension or renal disease should be encouraged to use a nonhormonal form of contraception. The use of combination hormonal contraceptives has been associated with a slight increase in frequency of breast cancer, however, studies are not consistent. Combination hormonal contraceptives may cause glucose intolerance or effect serum triglyceride and lipoprotein levels. Retinal thrombosis has been reported (rarely). Use caution with conditions that may be aggravated by fluid retention, depression, or history of migraine. Not for use prior to menarche.

The minimum dosage combination of estrogen/progestin that will effectively treat the individual patient should be used. New patients should be started on products containing ≤0.035 mg of estrogen per tablet.

Acne: For use only in females ≥15 years, who also desire combination hormonal contraceptive therapy, are unresponsive to topical treatments, and have no contraindications to combination hormonal contraceptive use.

Drug Interactions

Metabolism/Transport Effects Ethinyl estradiol: **Substrate** of CYP2C9 (minor), 3A4 (major), 3A5-7 (minor); **Inhibits** CYP1A2 (weak), 2B6 (weak), 2C8 (weak), 2C19 (weak), 3A4 (weak)

Avoid Concomitant Use

Avoid concomitant use of Ethinyl Estradiol and Norgestimate with any of the following: Anastrozole; Griseofulvin

Increased Effect/Toxicity

Ethinyl Estradiol and Norgestimate may increase the levels/effects of: Benzodiazepines (metabolized by oxidation); Corticosteroids (Systemic); CYP1A2 Substrates; ROPINIRole; Selegiline; Theophylline Derivatives; Tipranavir; TiZANidine; Tranexamic Acid; Voriconazole

The levels/effects of Ethinyl Estradiol and Norgestimate may be increased by: Ascorbic Acid; Conivaptan; Herbs (Estrogenic Properties); Herbs (Progestogenic Properties); Voriconazole

Decreased Effect

Ethinyl Estradiol and Norgestimate may decrease the levels/effects of: Anastrozole; Chenodiol; LamoTRIgine; Protease Inhibitors; Thyroid Products; Ursodiol; Vitamin K Antagonists

The levels/effects of Ethinyl Estradiol and Norgestimate may be decreased by: Acitretin; Aminoglutethimide; Aprepitant; Armodafinil; Artemether; Barbiturates; Bile Acid Sequestrants; Bosentan; CarBAMazepine; Colesevelam; CYP3A4 Inducers (Strong); Deferasirox; Efavirenz; Felbamate; Fosaprepitant; Fosphenytoin; Griseofulvin; LamoTRIgine; Modafinil; Mycophenolate; Nafcillin; OXcarbazepine; Phenytoin; Protease Inhibitors; Retinoic Acid Derivatives; Rifamycin Derivatives; Rufinamide; St Johns Wort; Tipranavir; Tocilizumab; Topiramate

Ethanol/Nutrition/Herb Interactions

Food: CNS effects of caffeine may be enhanced if combination hormonal contraceptives are used concurrently with caffeine. Grapefruit juice increases ethinyl estradiol concentrations and would be expected to increase progesterone serum levels as well; clinical implications are unclear.

Herb/Nutraceutical: St John's wort may decrease levels. Herbs with estrogenic properties may enhance the adverse/toxic effect of estrogen derivatives; examples include alfalfa, black cohosh, bloodroot, hops, kudzu, licorice, red clover, saw palmetto, soybean, thyme, wild yam, yucca. Herbs with progestogenic properties may enhance the adverse/toxic effect of progestins; examples include bloodroot, chasteberry, damiana, oregano, yucca.

Dietary Considerations Should be taken at same time each day.

Pharmacodynamics/Kinetics

Half-life Elimination EE: 10-16 hours; NGMN: 18-25 hours; NG: 38-45 hours

Time to Peak EE and NGM: ~2 hours

Pregnancy Risk Factor X

Lactation Enters breast milk/not recommended

Breast-Feeding Considerations Jaundice and breast enlargement in the nursing infant have been reported following the use of combination hormonal contraceptives. May decrease the quality and quantity of breast milk; a nonhormonal form of contraception is recommended.

Dosage Forms

Tablet, monophasic formulations:

MonoNessa®, Ortho-Cyclen®: Ethinyl estradiol 0.035 mg and norgestimate 0.25 mg (28s) [21 blue tablets and 7 green inactive tablets]

Sprintec®: Ethinyl estradiol 0.035 mg and norgestimate 0.25 mg (28s) [21 blue tablets and 7 white inactive tablets]

Tablet, triphasic formulations:

Ortho Tri-Cyclen®, TriNessa®:

Day 1-7: Ethinyl estradiol 0.035 mg and norgestimate 0.18 mg [7 white tablets]

Day 8-14: Ethinyl estradiol 0.035 mg and norgestimate 0.215 mg [7 light blue tablets]

Day 15-21: Ethinyl estradiol 0.035 mg and norgestimate 0.25 mg [7 blue tablets]

Day 22-28: 7 green inactive tablets (28s)

Tri-Sprintec®:

Day 1-7: Ethinyl estradiol 0.035 mg and norgestimate 0.18 mg [7 gray tablets]

Day 8-14: Ethinyl estradiol 0.035 mg and norgestimate 0.215 mg [7 light blue tablets]

Day 15-21: Ethinyl estradiol 0.035 mg and norgestimate 0.25 mg [7 blue tablets]

Day 22-28: 7 white inactive tablets (28s)

Ortho Tri-Cyclen® Lo:

Day 1-7: Ethinyl estradiol 0.025 mg and norgestimate 0.18 mg [7 white tablets]

Day 8-14: Ethinyl estradiol 0.025 mg and norgestimate 0.215 mg [7 light blue tablets]

Day 15-21: Ethinyl estradiol 0.025 mg and norgestimate 0.25 mg [7 dark blue tablets]

Day 22-28: 7 green inactive tablets (28s)

Ethinyl Estradiol and Norgestrel (ETH in il es tra DYE ole & nor JES trel)

U.S. Brand Names Cryselle® 28; Lo/Ovral®-28; Low-Ogestrel®; Ogestrel®

Canadian Brand Names Lo-Femenal 21; Ovral®

Generic Availability (U.S.) Yes

Pharmacologic Category Contraceptive; Estrogen and Progestin Combination

Use Prevention of pregnancy; postcoital contraceptive or "morning after" pill

Unlabeled/Investigational Use Treatment of hypermenorrhea (menorrhagia); pain associated with endometriosis; dysmenorrhea; dysfunctional uterine bleeding

Local Anesthetic/Vasoconstrictor Precautions No information available to require special precautions

Effects on Dental Treatment When prescribing antibiotics, patient must be warned to use additional methods of birth control if on oral contraceptives.

Effects on Bleeding No information available to require special precautions

Adverse Effects Frequency not defined.

Cardiovascular: Arterial thromboembolism, cerebral hemorrhage, cerebral thrombosis, edema, hypertension, mesenteric thrombosis, MI

Central nervous system: Depression, dizziness, headache, migraine, nervousness, premenstrual syndrome, stroke

Dermatologic: Acne, erythema multiforme, erythema nodosum, hirsutism, loss of scalp hair, melasma (may persist), rash (allergic)

Endocrine & metabolic: Amenorrhea, breakthrough bleeding, breast enlargement, breast secretion, breast tenderness, carbohydrate intolerance, lactation decreased (postpartum), glucose tolerance decreased, libido changes, menstrual flow changes, sex hormone-binding globulins (SHBG) increased, spotting, temporary infertility (following discontinuation), thyroid-binding globulin increased, triglycerides increased

Gastrointestinal: Abdominal cramps, appetite changes, bloating, cholestasis, colitis, gallbladder disease, jaundice, nausea, vomiting, weight gain/loss

Genitourinary: Cervical erosion changes, cervical secretion changes, cystitis-like syndrome, vaginal candidiasis, vaginitis

Hematologic: Antithrombin III decreased, folate levels decreased, hemolytic uremic syndrome, norepinephrine induced platelet aggregability increased, porphyria, prothrombin increased; factors VII, VIII, IX, and X

Hepatic: Benign liver tumors, Budd-Chiari syndrome, cholestatic jaundice, hepatic adenomas

Local: Thrombophlebitis

Ocular: Cataracts, change in corneal curvature (steepening), contact lens intolerance, optic neuritis, retinal thrombosis

Renal: Impaired renal function

Respiratory: Pulmonary thromboembolism

Miscellaneous: Hemorrhagic eruption

Dosage Oral: Adults: Females:

Contraception:

Schedule 1 (Sunday starter): Dose begins on first Sunday after onset of menstruation; if the menstrual period starts on Sunday, take first tablet that very same day. **With a Sunday start, an additional method of contraception should be used until after the first 7 days of consecutive administration.**

For 21-tablet package: Dosage is 1 tablet daily for 21 consecutive days, followed by 7 days off of the medication; a new course begins on the 8th day after the last tablet is taken.

For 28-tablet package: Dosage is 1 tablet daily without interruption.

Schedule 2 (Day 1 starter): Dose starts on first day of menstrual cycle taking 1 tablet daily.

For 21-tablet package: Dosage is 1 tablet daily for 21 consecutive days, followed by 7 days off of the medication; a new course begins on the 8th day after the last tablet is taken.

For 28-tablet package: Dosage is 1 tablet daily without interruption.

If all doses have been taken on schedule and one menstrual period is missed, continue dosing cycle. If two consecutive menstrual periods are missed, pregnancy test is required before new dosing cycle is started.

Missed doses **monophasic formulations** (refer to package insert for complete information):

One dose missed: Take as soon as remembered or take 2 tablets next day

Two consecutive doses missed in the first 2 weeks: Take 2 tablets as soon as remembered or 2 tablets next 2 days. **An additional method of contraception should be used for 7 days after missed dose.**

Two consecutive doses missed in week 3 or three consecutive doses missed at any time:

Schedule 1 (Sunday starter): Continue to take 1 tablet daily until Sunday, then discard the rest of the pack, and a new pack is started that same day.

Schedule 2 (Day 1 starter): Current pack should be discarded, and a new pack started that same day. **An additional method of contraception should be used for 7 days after missed dose.**

Postcoital contraception:

Ethinyl estradiol 0.03 mg and norgestrel 0.3 mg formulation: 4 tablets within 72 hours of unprotected intercourse and 4 tablets 12 hours after first dose

Ethinyl estradiol 0.05 mg and norgestrel 0.5 mg formulation: 2 tablets within 72 hours of unprotected intercourse and 2 tablets 12 hours after first dose

Dosage adjustment in renal impairment: Specific guidelines not available; use with caution and monitor blood pressure closely. Consider other forms of contraception.

Dosage adjustment in hepatic impairment: Contraindicated in patients with hepatic impairment.

Mechanism of Action Combination hormonal contraceptives inhibit ovulation via a negative feedback mechanism on the hypothalamus, which alters the normal pattern of gonadotropin secretion of a follicle-stimulating hormone (FSH) and luteinizing hormone by the anterior pituitary. The follicular phase FSH and midcycle surge of gonadotropins are inhibited. In addition, combination hormonal contraceptives produce alterations in the genital tract, including changes in the cervical mucus, rendering it unfavorable for sperm penetration even if ovulation occurs. Changes in the endometrium may also occur, producing an unfavorable environment for nidation. Combination hormonal contraceptive drugs may alter the tubal transport of the ova through the fallopian tubes. Progestational agents may also alter sperm fertility.

Contraindications Hypersensitivity to ethinyl estradiol, norgestrel, or any component of the formulation; history of or current thrombophlebitis or venous thromboembolic disorders (including DVT, PE); active or recent (within 1 year) arterial thromboembolic disease (eg, stroke, MI); cerebral vascular disease, coronary artery disease, valvular heart disease with complications, severe hypertension; diabetes mellitus with vascular involvement; severe headache with focal neurological symptoms; known or suspected breast carcinoma, endometrial cancer, estrogen-dependent neoplasms, undiagnosed abnormal genital bleeding; hepatic dysfunction or tumor, cholestatic jaundice of pregnancy, jaundice with prior combination hormonal contraceptive use; major surgery with prolonged immobilization; heavy smoking (≥15 cigarettes/day) in patients >35 years of age; pregnancy

Warnings/Precautions Combination hormonal contraceptives do not protect against HIV infection or other sexually-transmitted diseases. **[U.S. Boxed Warning]: The risk of cardiovascular side effects increases in women who smoke cigarettes, especially those who are >35 years of age; women who use combination hormonal contraceptives should be strongly advised not to smoke.** Combination hormonal contraceptives may lead to increased risk of myocardial infarction, use with caution in patients with risk factors for coronary artery disease. May increase the risk of thromboembolism. Whenever possible, combination hormonal contraceptives should be discontinued at least 4 weeks prior to and for 2 weeks following elective surgery associated with an increased risk of thromboembolism or during periods of prolonged immobilization. Combination hormonal contraceptives may have a dose-related risk of vascular disease, hypertension, and gallbladder disease. Women with hypertension or renal disease should be encouraged to use another form of contraception. The use of combination hormonal contraceptives has been associated with a slight increase in frequency of breast cancer, however, studies are not consistent. Combination hormonal contraceptives may cause glucose intolerance or effect serum triglyceride and lipoprotein levels. Retinal thrombosis has been reported (rarely). Use caution with conditions that may be aggravated by fluid retention, depression, or history of migraine. Not for use prior to menarche.

The minimum dosage combination of estrogen/progestin that will effectively treat the individual patient should be used. New patients should be started on products containing ≤0.035 mg of estrogen per tablet.

Drug Interactions

Metabolism/Transport Effects

Ethinyl estradiol: **Substrate** of CYP2C9 (minor), 3A4 (major), 3A5-7 (minor); **Inhibits** CYP1A2 (weak), 2B6 (weak), 2C8 (weak), 2C19 (weak), 3A4 (weak)

Norgestrel: **Substrate** of CYP3A4 (major)

Avoid Concomitant Use

Avoid concomitant use of Ethinyl Estradiol and Norgestrel with any of the following: Anastrozole; Griseofulvin

Increased Effect/Toxicity

Ethinyl Estradiol and Norgestrel may increase the levels/effects of: Benzodiazepines (metabolized by oxidation); Corticosteroids (Systemic); CYP1A2 Substrates; ROPINIRole; Selegiline; Theophylline Derivatives; Tipranavir; TiZANidine; Tranexamic Acid; Voriconazole

The levels/effects of Ethinyl Estradiol and Norgestrel may be increased by: Ascorbic Acid; Conivaptan; Herbs (Estrogenic Properties); Herbs (Progestogenic Properties); Voriconazole

Decreased Effect

Ethinyl Estradiol and Norgestrel may decrease the levels/effects of: Anastrozole; Chenodiol; LamoTRIgine; Protease Inhibitors; Thyroid Products; Ursodiol; Vitamin K Antagonists

The levels/effects of Ethinyl Estradiol and Norgestrel may be decreased by: Acitretin; Aminoglutethimide; Aprepitant; Armodafinil; Artemether; Barbiturates; Bile Acid Sequestrants; Bosentan; CarBAMazepine; Colesevelam; CYP3A4 Inducers (Strong); Deferasirox; Felbamate; Fosaprepitant; Fosphenytoin; Griseofulvin; LamoTRIgine; Modafinil; Mycophenolate; Nafcillin; OXcarbazepine; Phenytoin; Protease Inhibitors; Retinoic Acid Derivatives; Rifamycin Derivatives; Rufinamide; St Johns Wort; Tipranavir; Tocilizumab; Topiramate

Ethanol/Nutrition/Herb Interactions

Food: CNS effects of caffeine may be enhanced if combination hormonal contraceptives are used concurrently with caffeine. Grapefruit juice increases ethinyl estradiol concentrations and would be expected to increase progesterone serum levels as well; clinical implications are unclear.

Herb/Nutraceutical: St John's wort may decrease levels. Herbs with estrogenic properties may enhance the adverse/toxic effect of estrogen derivatives; examples include alfalfa, black cohosh, bloodroot, hops, kudzu, licorice, red clover, saw palmetto, soybean, thyme, wild yam, yucca. Herbs with progestogenic properties may enhance the adverse/toxic effect of progestins; examples include bloodroot, chasteberry, damiana, oregano, yucca.

Dietary Considerations Should be taken at same time each day.

Pregnancy Risk Factor X

Lactation Enters breast milk/not recommended

Breast-Feeding Considerations Jaundice and breast enlargement in the nursing infant have been reported following the use of combination hormonal contraceptives. May decrease the quality and quantity of breast milk; a nonhormonal form of contraception is recommended.

Dosage Forms

Tablet, monophasic formulations: Ethinyl estradiol 0.03 mg and norgestrel 0.3 mg [21 white tablets and 7 pink inactive tablets] (28s)

Cryselle® 28: Ethinyl estradiol 0.03 mg and norgestrel 0.3 mg [21 white tablets and 7 light green inactive tablets] (28s)

Low-Ogestrel®: Ethinyl estradiol 0.03 mg and norgestrel 0.3 mg [21 white tablets and 7 peach inactive tablets] (28s)

Lo/Ovral®-28: Ethinyl estradiol 0.03 mg and norgestrel 0.3 mg [21 white tablets and 7 pink inactive tablets] (28s)

Ogestrel®: Ethinyl estradiol 0.05 mg and norgestrel 0.5 mg [21 white tablets and 7 peach inactive tablets] (28s)

Ethinyl Estradiol, Drospirenone, and Levomefolate

(ETH in il es tra DYE ole, droh SPYE re none, & lee voe me FOE late)

U.S. Brand Names Beyaz™; Safyral™

Pharmacologic Category Contraceptive; Estrogen and Progestin Combination

Use Females: Prevention of pregnancy; treatment of premenstrual dysphoric disorder (PMDD); treatment of acne; folate supplementation

Unlabeled/Investigational Use Treatment of hypermenorrhea (menorrhagia); pain associated with endometriosis; dysmenorrhea; dysfunctional uterine bleeding

Local Anesthetic/Vasoconstrictor Precautions No information available to require special precautions

Effects on Dental Treatment When prescribing antibiotics, patient must be warned to use additional methods of birth control if on oral contraceptives.

Effects on Bleeding No information available to require special precautions

Adverse Effects Note: Percentages reported with Beyaz™

>10%:

Central nervous system: Headache/migraine (6% to 13%)

Endocrine & metabolic: Menstrual irregularities (4% to 25%, including menorrhagia, metrorrhagia, spotting, vaginal hemorrhage), breast pain/tenderness (3% to 11%)

Gastrointestinal: Nausea/vomiting (4% to 16%)

1% to 10%:

Central nervous system: Fatigue (4%), irritability (3%), affect lability (2%)

Endocrine & metabolic: Libido decreased (3%)

Gastrointestinal: Weight gain (3%)

Frequency not defined: Cervical dysplasia, cervix carcinoma stage 0

For additional adverse events and postmarketing reports, refer to the Ethinyl Estradiol and Drospirenone (Yasmin®, Yaz®) monograph.

Dosage Oral:

Children ≥14 years and Adults: Females: Acne (Beyaz™): Refer to dosing for contraception

Adults: Females: PMDD (Beyaz™): Refer to dosing for contraception

Adults: Females: Contraception (Beyaz™, Safyral™): Dosage is 1 tablet daily

Beyaz™: One pink tablet daily for 24 consecutive days, then one light orange tablet daily on days 25-28

Safyral™: One orange tablet daily for 21 consecutive days, then one light orange tablet daily on days 22-28

Dose should be taken at the same time each day, either after the evening meal or at bedtime. Dosing may be started on the first day of menstrual period (Day 1 starter) or on the first Sunday after the onset of the menstrual period (Sunday starter).

Day 1 starter: Dose starts on first day of menstrual cycle taking 1 tablet daily. If first dose is taken later than the first day of the menstrual cycle, **an additional method of contraception should be used until after the first 7 days of consecutive administration.**

Sunday starter: Dose begins on first Sunday after onset of menstruation; if the menstrual period starts on Sunday, take first tablet that very same day. **With a Sunday start, an additional method of contraception should be used until after the first 7 days of consecutive administration.**

Switching from a different contraceptive:

Oral contraceptive: Start on the same day that a new pack of the previous oral contraceptive would have been taken

Transdermal patch, vaginal ring, injection: Start on the day the next dose would have been due

IUD or implant: Start on the day of removal

Use after childbirth (in women who are not breast-feeding) or after second trimester abortion: Therapy may be started ≥4 weeks postpartum. Pregnancy should be ruled out prior to treatment if menstrual periods have not restarted and an additional method of contraception (nonhormonal) should be used until after the first 7 days of consecutive administration.

Missed doses:

If all doses have been taken on schedule and one menstrual period is missed, continue dosing cycle. If two consecutive menstrual periods are missed, rule out pregnancy and discontinue if pregnancy is confirmed.

If doses have been missed during the first 3 weeks or if active tablets (pink tablets) were started later than as directed and the menstrual period is missed, pregnancy should be ruled out prior to continuing treatment.

Missed doses (monophasic formulations) (refer to package insert for complete information):

One dose missed: Take as soon as remembered or take 2 tablets next day

Two consecutive doses missed in the first 2 weeks: Take 2 tablets as soon as remembered or 2 tablets next 2 days. **An additional method of contraception should be used for 7 days after missed dose.**

Two consecutive doses missed in week 3 or three consecutive doses missed at any time: **An additional method of contraception must be used for 7 days after a missed dose.**

Day 1 starter: Current pack should be discarded, and a new pack should be started that same day.

Sunday starter: Continue dose of 1 tablet daily until Sunday, then discard the rest of the pack, and a new pack should be started that same day.

Any number of doses missed in week 4: Throw away the pills that were missed. Continue taking one pill each day until pack is empty; no back-up method of contraception is needed

Dosage adjustment in renal impairment: Contraindicated in patients with renal dysfunction

Dosage adjustment in hepatic impairment: Contraindicated in patients with hepatic disease. Exposure to drospirenone is ~3 times higher with moderate liver impairment; information not available for severe impairment.

Mechanism of Action Combination oral contraceptives inhibit ovulation via a negative feedback mechanism on the hypothalamus, which alters the normal pattern of gonadotropin secretion of a follicle-stimulating hormone (FSH) and luteinizing hormone by the anterior pituitary. The follicular phase FSH and midcycle surge of gonadotropins are inhibited. In addition, oral contraceptives produce alterations in the genital tract, including changes in the cervical mucus, rendering it unfavorable for sperm penetration even if ovulation occurs. Changes in the endometrium may also occur, producing an unfavorable environment for nidation. Oral contraceptive drugs may alter the tubal transport of the ova through the fallopian tubes. Progestational agents may also alter sperm fertility. Drospirenone is a spironolactone analogue with antimineralocorticoid and antiandrogenic activity.

Contraindications Adrenal insufficiency, breast cancer or other estrogen- or progestin-dependent neoplasms (current or a history of), hepatic tumors or disease, pregnancy, renal impairment, undiagnosed abnormal uterine bleeding. Use is also contraindicated in women at high risk of arterial or venous thrombotic diseases including: Cerebrovascular disease, coronary artery disease, diabetes mellitus with vascular disease, DVT or PE (current or history of), hypercoagulopathies (inherited or acquired), headaches with focal neurological symptoms, hypertension (uncontrolled), migraine headaches if >35 years of age, thrombogenic valvular or rhythm diseases of the heart (eg, subacute bacterial endocarditis with valvular disease or atrial fibrillation), women >35 years of age who smoke.

Warnings/Precautions [U.S. Boxed Warning]: The risk of cardiovascular side effects is increased in women who smoke cigarettes; risk increases with age (especially women >35 years of age) and the number of cigarettes smoked; women who use combination hormonal contraceptives should be strongly advised not to smoke. Use with caution in patients with risk factors for coronary artery disease; may lead to increased risk of myocardial infarction or stroke. May have a dose-related risk of vascular disease and hypertension; women with hypertension should be encouraged to use another form of contraception. Monitor women with well-controlled hypertension and discontinue if blood pressure rises significantly. Use is contraindicated with uncontrolled hypertension or hypertension with vascular disease. Contraceptives may increase the risk of thromboembolism. Discontinue if an arterial or deep venous thrombotic event occurs. Risk may be greater with contraceptives containing drospirenone. Estrogens may induce or exacerbate symptoms of angioedema in women with hereditary angioedema.

Steroid hormones are poorly metabolized in patients with hepatic dysfunction. Discontinue if jaundice develops or if acute or chronic hepatic disturbances occur. Use is contraindicated with hepatic disease. Cholestasis may occur in women with a history of pregnancy related or previous oral contraceptive related cholestasis. Drospirenone has antimineralocorticoid activity that may lead to hyperkalemia in patients with renal insufficiency, hepatic dysfunction, or adrenal insufficiency; use caution with medications that may increase serum potassium. Combination hormonal contraceptives may effect serum triglyceride and lipoprotein levels. Estrogen compounds are generally associated with lipid effects such as increased HDL-cholesterol and decreased LDL-cholesterol. Progestins may be associated with decreased HDL-cholesterol. Triglycerides may also be increased; use with caution in patients with familial defects of lipoprotein metabolism. Combination hormonal contraceptives may have adverse effects on glucose tolerance; use caution in women with diabetes. Use may have a dose-related risk of gallbladder disease.

The use of combination hormonal contraceptives has been associated with a slight increase in frequency of breast cancer; however, studies are not consistent. Use is contraindicated in women with breast cancer (current or history of). Extremely rare adenomas and focal nodular hyperplasia resulting in fatal intra-abdominal hemorrhage have been reported in association with long-term oral contraceptive use. Presentation of an abdominal mass, acute abdominal pain, or intra-abdominal bleeding warrants further evaluation to rule out source.

Estrogens may cause retinal vascular thrombosis; discontinue if migraine, loss of vision, proptosis, diplopia or other visual disturbances occur; discontinue permanently if papilledema or retinal vascular lesions are observed on examination. Use with caution in patients with a history of migraine. Evaluate new, recurrent, severe, or persistent headaches. Use is contraindicated in women with headaches with focal neurological symptoms or migraine headaches if > 35 years of age. Use with caution in patients with diseases which may be exacerbated by fluid retention, including asthma, epilepsy, diabetes or renal dysfunction; use with caution in patients with depression. Use caution with a history of chloasma gravidarum; women with a tendency to chloasma should avoid sun and ultraviolet radiation exposure during therapy.

Unscheduled bleeding /spotting may occur within the first 3 months of use. Presentation of irregular, unresolving vaginal bleeding following previously regular cycles warrants further evaluation including endometrial sampling, if indicated, to rule out malignancy. Inform patients that oral contraceptives do not protect against HIV infection or other sexually-transmitted diseases. The minimum dosage combination of estrogen/progestin that will effectively treat the individual patient should be used. Not for use prior to menarche. Whenever possible, should be discontinued at least 4 weeks prior to and for 2 weeks following elective surgery associated with an increased risk of thromboembolism or during periods of prolonged immobilization.

Acne use: For use only in females ≥14 years of age who have reached menarche, who also desire combination hormonal contraceptive therapy.

PMDD use: For use only in females who desire combination hormonal contraceptive therapy; use for more than 3 menstrual cycles has not been evaluated. Has not been evaluated for the treatment of premenstrual syndrome.

Drug Interactions

Avoid Concomitant Use

Avoid concomitant use of Ethinyl Estradiol, Drospirenone, and Levomefolate with any of the following: Anastrozole; Griseofulvin; Raltitrexed; Tacrolimus

Increased Effect/Toxicity

Ethinyl Estradiol, Drospirenone, and Levomefolate may increase the levels/effects of: ACE Inhibitors; Amifostine; Ammonium Chloride; Antihypertensives; Benzodiazepines (metabolized by oxidation); Cardiac Glycosides; Corticosteroids (Systemic); CYP1A2 Substrates; Hypotensive Agents; Potassium-Sparing Diuretics; RiTUXimab; ROPINIRole; Selegiline; Tacrolimus; Theophylline Derivatives; Tipranavir; TiZANidine; Tranexamic Acid; Voriconazole

The levels/effects of Ethinyl Estradiol, Drospirenone, and Levomefolate may be increased by: Angiotensin II Receptor Blockers; Ascorbic Acid; Conivaptan; Diazoxide; Eplerenone; Herbs (Estrogenic Properties); Herbs (Hypotensive Properties); Herbs (Progestogenic Properties); MAO Inhibitors; Nonsteroidal Anti-Inflammatory Agents; Pentoxifylline; Phosphodiesterase 5 Inhibitors; Potassium Salts; Prostacyclin Analogues; Tolvaptan; Voriconazole

Decreased Effect

Ethinyl Estradiol, Drospirenone, and Levomefolate may decrease the levels/effects of: Anastrozole; Cardiac Glycosides; Chenodiol; Fosphenytoin; LamoTRIgine; PHENobarbital; Phenytoin; Primidone; Protease Inhibitors; QuiNIDine; Raltitrexed; Thyroid Products; Ursodiol; Vitamin K Antagonists

The levels/effects of Ethinyl Estradiol, Drospirenone, and Levomefolate may be decreased by: Acitretin; Aminoglutethimide; Aprepitant; Armodafinil; Artemether; Barbiturates; Bile Acid Sequestrants; Bosentan; CarBAMazepine; Colesevelam; CYP3A4 Inducers (Strong); Deferasirox; Felbamate; Fosaprepitant; Fosphenytoin; Griseofulvin; Herbs (Hypertensive Properties); LamoTRIgine; Methylphenidate; Modafinil; Mycophenolate; Nafcillin; Nonsteroidal Anti-Inflammatory Agents; OXcarbazepine; Phenytoin; Protease Inhibitors; Retinoic Acid Derivatives; Rifamycin Derivatives; Rufinamide; St Johns Wort; Tipranavir; Tocilizumab; Topiramate; Yohimbine

Ethanol/Nutrition/Herb Interactions

Food: CNS effects of caffeine may be enhanced if oral contraceptives are used concurrently with caffeine. Grapefruit juice increases ethinyl estradiol plasma concentrations; clinical implications are unclear. Food decreases the maximum plasma concentrations of drospirenone and ethinyl estradiol by ~40%.

Herb/Nutraceutical: St John's wort may decrease levels. Herbs with estrogenic properties may enhance the adverse/toxic effect of estrogen derivatives; examples include alfalfa, black cohosh, bloodroot, hops, kudzu, licorice, red clover, saw palmetto, soybean, thyme, wild yam, yucca. Herbs with progestogenic properties may enhance the adverse/toxic effect of progestins; examples include bloodroot, chasteberry, damiana, oregano, yucca.

Dietary Considerations Should be taken at the same time each day; may be taken with or without a meal. Consider other sources of folic acid and ensure supplementation continues once therapy is discontinued. The RDA for folate in women 14–50 years of age is 400 mcg/day of dietary folate equivalents. The USPSTF recommends that all women of reproductive potential should take a supplement containing folic acid 400-800 mcg/day in order to decrease the risk of neural tube defects.

Pharmacodynamics/Kinetics

Half-life Elimination Terminal: Drospirenone: ~31 hours; Ethinyl estradiol: ~24 hours; levomefolate calcium: ~4-5 hours

Time to Peak Drospirenone, ethinyl estradiol: 1-2 hours; Levomefolate calcium: 0.5-1.5 hours

Lactation Enters breast milk/not recommended

Breast-Feeding Considerations The amount of drospirenone excreted in breast milk is ~0.02%, resulting in a maximum of ~3 mcg/day drospirenone to the infant. Jaundice and breast enlargement in the nursing infant have been reported following the use of other oral contraceptives. In addition, may decrease the quality and quantity of breast milk. Other forms of contraception are recommended while breast-feeding.

Dosage Forms

Tablet, oral:

Beyaz™: Ethinyl estradiol 0.02 mg, drospirenone 3 mg, and levomefolate calcium 0.451 mg [24 pink tablets] and levomefolate calcium 0.451 mg [4 light orange tablets] (28s)

Safyral™: Ethinyl estradiol 0.03 mg, drospirenone 3 mg, and levomefolate calcium 0.451 mg [21 orange tablets] and levomefolate calcium 0.451 mg [7 light orange tablets] (28s)

Ethionamide (e thye on AM ide)

Related Information

Tuberculosis *on page* 1902

U.S. Brand Names Trecator®

Canadian Brand Names Trecator®

Pharmacologic Category Antitubercular Agent

Use Treatment of tuberculosis and other mycobacterial diseases, in conjunction with other antituberculosis agents, when first-line agents have failed or resistance has been demonstrated

Local Anesthetic/Vasoconstrictor Precautions No information available to require special precautions

Effects on Dental Treatment Key adverse event(s) related to dental treatment: Postural hypotension, metallic taste, and stomatitis.

Effects on Bleeding No information available to require special precautions

Adverse Effects Frequency not defined.

Cardiovascular: Postural hypotension

Central nervous system: Depression, dizziness, drowsiness, headache, psychiatric disturbances, restlessness, seizure

Dermatologic: Acne, alopecia, photosensitivity, purpura, rash

Endocrine & metabolic: Gynecomastia, hypoglycemia, hypothyroidism or goiter, pellagra-like syndrome

Gastrointestinal: Abdominal pain, anorexia, diarrhea, excessive salivation, metallic taste, nausea, stomatitis, vomiting, weight loss

Genitourinary: Impotence

Hematologic: Thrombocytopenia

Hepatic: Hepatitis, jaundice, liver function tests increased

Neuromuscular & skeletal: Peripheral neuritis, weakness (common)

Ocular: Blurred vision, diplopia, optic neuritis

Respiratory: Olfactory disturbances

Miscellaneous: Hypersensitivity reaction

General Dosage Range Dosage adjustment recommended in patients with renal impairment

Oral:

Children: 15-20 mg/kg/day in 2-3 divided doses (maximum: 1 g/day)

Adults: 250-750 mg/day in 1-4 divided doses (maximum: 1 g/day)

Mechanism of Action Inhibits peptide synthesis

Pharmacodynamics/Kinetics

Half-life Elimination 2-3 hours

Time to Peak Serum: 1 hour

Pregnancy Risk Factor C

Ethosuximide (eth oh SUKS i mide)

U.S. Brand Names Zarontin®

Canadian Brand Names Zarontin®

Pharmacologic Category Anticonvulsant, Succinimide

Use Management of absence (petit mal) seizures

Local Anesthetic/Vasoconstrictor Precautions No information available to require special precautions

Effects on Dental Treatment No significant effects or complications reported

Effects on Bleeding No information available to require special precautions

Adverse Effects Frequency not defined.

Central nervous system: Aggressiveness, ataxia, concentration impaired, dizziness, drowsiness, euphoria, fatigue, headache, hyperactivity, inability to concentrate, irritability, lethargy, mental depression (with cases of overt suicidal intentions), night terrors, paranoid psychosis, sleep disturbance

Dermatologic: Hirsutism, pruritus, rash, Stevens-Johnson syndrome, urticaria

Endocrine & metabolic: Libido increased

Gastrointestinal: Abdominal pain, anorexia, cramps, diarrhea, epigastric pain, gastric upset, gum hypertrophy, nausea, tongue swelling, vomiting, weight loss

Genitourinary: Hematuria (microscopic), vaginal bleeding

Hematologic: Agranulocytosis, eosinophilia, leukopenia, pancytopenia

Ocular: Myopia

Miscellaneous: Allergic reaction, hiccups, systemic lupus erythematosus

General Dosage Range Oral:
Children 3-6 years: Initial: 250 mg/day; Maintenance: 20 mg/kg/day (maximum: 1.5 g/day in divided doses)
Children ≥6 years: Initial: 500 mg/day; Maintenance: 20 mg/kg/day (maximum: 1.5 g/day in divided doses)
Adults: Initial: 500 mg/day (maximum: 1.5 g/day in divided doses)

Mechanism of Action Increases the seizure threshold and suppresses paroxysmal spike-and-wave pattern in absence seizures; depresses nerve transmission in the motor cortex

Pharmacodynamics/Kinetics
Half-life Elimination Serum: Children: 30 hours; Adults: 50-60 hours
Time to Peak Serum: Capsule: ~2-4 hours; Syrup: <2-4 hours

Ethotoin (ETH oh toyn)

U.S. Brand Names Peganone®
Pharmacologic Category Anticonvulsant, Hydantoin
Use Generalized tonic-clonic or complex-partial seizures
Local Anesthetic/Vasoconstrictor Precautions No information available to require special precautions
Effects on Dental Treatment No significant effects or complications reported
Effects on Bleeding No information available to require special precautions
Adverse Effects Frequency not defined.
Cardiovascular: Chest pain
Central nervous system: Ataxia, dizziness, fatigue, fever, headache, insomnia
Dermatologic: Skin rash, Stevens-Johnson syndrome
Gastrointestinal: Diarrhea, gingival hyperplasia, nausea, vomiting
Hematologic: Blood dyscrasias
Neuromuscular & skeletal: Numbness
Ocular: Diplopia, nystagmus
Miscellaneous: Lymphadenopathy, systemic lupus erythematosus (SLE)-like syndrome

General Dosage Range Oral:
Children ≥1 year: Maximum initial dose: 750 mg/day; usual maintenance dose: 0.5-1 g/day; maximum dose: 3 g/day
Adults: Initial dose: ≤1 g/day; usual maintenance dose: 2-3 g/day

Mechanism of Action Stabilizes the seizure threshold and prevents the spread of seizure activity
Pharmacodynamics/Kinetics
Half-life Elimination 3-9 hours
Pregnancy Risk Factor D

Ethyl Chloride (ETH il KLOR ide)

U.S. Brand Names Gebauer's Ethyl Chloride®
Pharmacologic Category Local Anesthetic
Use Local anesthetic in minor operative procedures and to relieve pain caused by insect stings and burns, and irritation caused by myofascial and visceral pain syndromes
Local Anesthetic/Vasoconstrictor Precautions No information available to require special precautions
Effects on Dental Treatment Key adverse event(s) related to dental treatment: Mucous membrane irritation. See Dental Comment.
Effects on Bleeding No information available to require special precautions
Adverse Effects 1% to 10%: Mucous membrane irritation, freezing may alter skin pigment
General Dosage Range Topical: *Adults:* Dosage varies greatly depending on indication
Pregnancy Risk Factor C
Dental Comment Spray for a few seconds to the point of frost formation when the tissue becomes white; avoid prolonged spraying of skin beyond this point

Ethyl Chloride and Dichlorotetrafluoroethane
(ETH il KLOR ide & dye klor oh te tra floo or oh ETH ane)

Related Information
Ethyl Chloride *on page 688*
U.S. Brand Names Fluro-Ethyl® [DSC]
Pharmacologic Category Local Anesthetic

Use Topical refrigerant anesthetic to control pain associated with minor surgical procedures, dermabrasion, injections, contusions, and minor strains

Local Anesthetic/Vasoconstrictor Precautions No information available to require special precautions

Effects on Dental Treatment No significant effects or complications reported

Effects on Bleeding No information available to require special precautions

General Dosage Range Topical: *Adults:* Apply as a fine mist approximately 2" to 4" from site of application

Pregnancy Risk Factor C

Etidronate (e ti DROE nate)

Related Information

Osteonecrosis of the Jaw *on page* 1894

U.S. Brand Names Didronel®

Canadian Brand Names Co-Etidronate; Mylan-Etidronate

Pharmacologic Category Bisphosphonate Derivative

Use Symptomatic treatment of Paget's disease; prevention and treatment of heterotopic ossification due to spinal cord injury or after total hip replacement

Local Anesthetic/Vasoconstrictor Precautions No information available to require special precautions

Effects on Dental Treatment Key adverse event(s) related to dental treatment: Abnormal taste.

Osteonecrosis of the jaw (ONJ), generally associated with local infection and/or tooth extraction and often with delayed healing, has been reported in patients taking bisphosphonates. Symptoms included nonhealing extraction socket or an exposed jawbone. Most reported cases of bisphosphonate-associated osteonecrosis have been in cancer patients treated with intravenous bisphosphonates. However, some have occurred in patients with postmenopausal osteoporosis taking oral bisphosphonates. Dental surgery, particularly tooth extraction, may increase the risk for ONJ. Patients who develop ONJ while on bisphosphonate therapy should receive care by an oral surgeon. See Dental Comment.

Effects on Bleeding No information available to require special precautions

Adverse Effects Frequency not defined.

Gastrointestinal: Diarrhea, nausea

Neuromuscular & skeletal: Bone pain

General Dosage Range Oral: *Adults:* 5-20 mg/kg/day

Mechanism of Action Decreases bone resorption by inhibiting osteocystic osteolysis; decreases mineral release and matrix or collagen breakdown in bone

Pharmacodynamics/Kinetics

Onset of Action 1-3 months

Duration of Action Can persist for 12 months without continuous therapy

Half-life Elimination 1-6 hours

Pregnancy Risk Factor C

Dental Comment According to the 2008 report by the American Dental Association (ADA), the incidence of osteonecrosis of the jawbone associated with oral bisphosphonate therapy remains low. It was also stated that the benefits of using oral bisphosphonates to prevent osteoporosis significantly outweighs the small risk of developing bisphosphonate-associated osteonecrosis (Edwards, 2008). The full 26 page report can be accessed at http://www.ada.org/sections/professionalResources/pdfs/topics_osteonecrosis_bisphosphonate_report.pdf.

The ADA review stated the incidence of oral bisphosphonate-associated osteonecrosis of the jaw was one case for every 140,000 person-years exposure to oral bisphosphonates (ADA, 2006). This figure was based on information received from Merck & Co citing 170 worldwide cases for alendronate (Fosamax®). In addition, Procter & Gamble Pharmaceuticals has cited 20 cases for risedronate (Actonel®) and Roche Laboratories, Inc has cited one case for ibandronate (Boniva®).

In addition, the ADA 2008 report reiterates that the risk of osteonecrosis of the jawbone with oral bisphosphonates is minute compared to the risks with intravenous bisphosphonates therapy in cancer patients. The ADA cites an ~20% incidence in patients receiving bisphosphonates intravenously for cancer therapy. Fewer than 10% of all cases of bisphosphonate-associated osteonecrosis of the jaw occurs in patients taking the oral drugs.

Information on alendronate (Fosamax®) use in Australia and the incidence of ONJ has been reported (Mavrokokki, 2007). A survey form was sent to all of the Australian members of the Australian and New Zealand Association of Oral and Maxillofacial Surgeons requesting cases that they had identified as ONJ in 2004 and 2005. The definition of ONJ for the survey was an area of exposed bone in the jawbone that failed to heal within 6 weeks in patients taking bisphosphonates for bone disease. The frequency of ONJ in osteoporotic patients, mainly taking weekly oral alendronate, was 1 in 8470 to 1 in 2260 (0.01% to 0.04%) patients. If extractions were carried out, the calculated frequency was 1 in 1130 to 1 in 296 (0.09% to 0.34%) patients. The minimum values in these cases were determined from the survey, whereas, the maximum values were extrapolated from survey data. The median time to onset of ONJ in alendronate patients was 24 months.

A 2010 study reported the prevalence of osteonecrosis of the jaw in patients using alendronate-type drugs was 1 out of 952 patients or ~0.1% (Lo, 2010). The study's protocol involved a survey mailed out to 13,946 members of Kaiser Permanente of Northern California healthcare delivery system; 8572 patients responded to the survey. Investigators identified respondents reporting oral problems and dental symptoms. These respondents were then interviewed by telephone for presence of dental problems including exposed bone, gingival sores, moderate periodontal disease, and persistent symptoms or complications after dental procedures. Those selected were then invited for an examination or to have their dental records reviewed. The diagnosis of ONJ was made according to the 2006 American Association of Oral and Maxillofacial Surgeons criteria which required treatment with a bisphosphonate, exposed bone in the maxillofacial region lasting >8 weeks, and no radiotherapy involving the jaw. Of the 8572 respondents, 9 cases of ONJ were identified; 5 had developed ONJ spontaneously and 4 developed ONJ after tooth extraction. Specific oral bisphosphonates were not identified. When extrapolated to patient-years of bisphosphonate exposure, this prevalence rate of 0.1% equates to a frequency of 28 cases per 100,000 person-years of oral bisphosphonate treatment.

Etidronate and Calcium Carbonate

(e ti DROE nate & KAL see um KAR bun ate)

Related Information

Calcium Carbonate *on page* 286

Etidronate *on page* 689

Canadian Brand Names CO Etidrocal; Didrocal®; Mylan-Eti-Cal Carepac; Novo-Etidronatecal

Pharmacologic Category Bisphosphonate Derivative; Calcium Salt

Use Treatment and prevention of postmenopausal osteoporosis; prevention of corticosteroid-induced osteoporosis

Local Anesthetic/Vasoconstrictor Precautions No information available to require special precautions

Effects on Dental Treatment Osteonecrosis of the jaw (ONJ), generally associated with local infection and/or tooth extraction and often with delayed healing, has been reported in patients taking bisphosphonates. Symptoms included nonhealing extraction socket or an exposed jawbone. Most reported cases of bisphosphonate-associated osteonecrosis have been in cancer patients treated with intravenous bisphosphonates. However, some have occurred in patients with postmenopausal osteoporosis taking oral bisphosphonates. Dental surgery, particularly tooth extraction, may increase the risk for ONJ. Patients who develop ONJ while on bisphosphonate therapy should receive care by an oral surgeon. See Dental Comment.

Effects on Bleeding No information available to require special precautions

Adverse Effects >10%:

Central nervous system: Dizziness (16%), headache (13%)

Gastrointestinal: Diarrhea (37%), nausea (18%), flatulence (17%), constipation (13%), dyspepsia (12%), vomiting (11%)

General Dosage Range Oral: *Adults:* Etidronate disodium 400 mg once daily for 14 days, followed by calcium carbonate 1250 mg (500 mg elemental calcium) once daily for 76 days

Mechanism of Action See individual agents.

Product Availability Not available in U.S.

Dental Comment See Etidronate monograph.

Etodolac (ee toe DOE lak)

Related Information

Oral Pain *on page* 1928

Rheumatoid Arthritis, Osteoarthritis, and Osteoporosis *on page* 1889

Temporomandibular Dysfunction (TMD) *on page* 1964

Canadian Brand Names Apo-Etodolac®; Utradol™

Generic Availability (U.S.) Yes

Pharmacologic Category Nonsteroidal Anti-inflammatory Drug (NSAID), Oral

Dental Use Management of postoperative pain

Use Acute and long-term use in the management of signs and symptoms of osteoarthritis; rheumatoid arthritis and juvenile idiopathic arthritis (JIA); management of acute pain

Local Anesthetic/Vasoconstrictor Precautions No information available to require special precautions

Effects on Dental Treatment The dentist should be aware of the potential of abnormal coagulation. Caution should also be exercised in the use of NSAIDs in patients already on anticoagulant therapy with drugs such as warfarin (Coumadin®). See Effects on Bleeding.

Effects on Bleeding Nonselective NSAIDs are known to reversibly decrease platelet aggregation via mechanisms different than observed with aspirin. Platelet function is restored as the drug is eliminated from the body. Dental professionals should be aware that recommendations differ between dental and general surgery. NSAIDs should be avoided (if possible) in general surgery patients for 3-5 half-lives of the drug (usually 1-3 days) prior to surgery to reduce the risk of excessive bleeding. However, there is no scientific evidence to warrant discontinuance of NSAIDs prior to dental surgery. In medically complicated patients or extensive oral surgery, the decision to interrupt therapy must be based on the risk to benefit in an individual patient and a medical consult is suggested. Routine interruption of NSAID therapy for most dental procedures is not warranted. If therapy is continued without interruption, the clinician should anticipate the potential for slower clotting times.

Adverse Effects 1% to 10%:

Central nervous system: Dizziness (3% to 9%), chills/fever (1% to 3%), depression (1% to 3%), nervousness (1% to 3%)

Dermatologic: Rash (1% to 3%), pruritus (1% to 3%)

Gastrointestinal: Dyspepsia (10%), abdominal cramps (3% to 9%), diarrhea (3% to 9%), flatulence (3% to 9%), nausea (3% to 9%), vomiting (1% to 3%), constipation (1% to 3%), melena (1% to 3%), gastritis (1% to 3%)

Genitourinary: Dysuria (1% to 3%)

Neuromuscular & skeletal: Weakness (3% to 9%)

Ocular: Blurred vision (1% to 3%)

Otic: Tinnitus (1% to 3%)

Renal: Polyuria (1% to 3%)

Dental Usual Dosage Acute pain: Adults: Oral: Immediate release formulation: 200-400 mg every 6-8 hours, as needed, not to exceed total daily doses of 1000 mg

Dosage Note: For chronic conditions, response is usually observed within 2 weeks.

Children 6-16 years: Oral: Juvenile idiopathic arthritis (JIA): Extended release formulation:

20-30 kg: 400 mg once daily

31-45 kg: 600 mg once daily

46-60 kg: 800 mg once daily

>60 kg: 1000 mg once daily

Adults: Oral:

Acute pain: Immediate release formulation: 200-400 mg every 6-8 hours, as needed, not to exceed total daily doses of 1000 mg

Rheumatoid arthritis, osteoarthritis:

Immediate release formulation: 400 mg 2 times/day **or** 300 mg 2-3 times/day **or** 500 mg 2 times/day (doses >1000 mg/day have not been evaluated)

Extended release formulation: 400-1000 mg once daily

Elderly: Refer to adult dosing; in patients ≥65 years, no dosage adjustment required based on pharmacokinetics. The elderly are more sensitive to antiprostaglandin effects and may need dosage adjustments.

Dosage adjustment in renal impairment:

Mild-to-moderate: No adjustment required

Severe: Use not recommended; use with caution

Hemodialysis: Not removed

Dosage adjustment in hepatic impairment: No adjustment required.

Mechanism of Action Reversibly inhibits cyclooxygenase-1 and 2 (COX-1 and 2) enzymes, which results in decreased formation of prostaglandin precursors; has antipyretic, analgesic, and anti-inflammatory properties

Other proposed mechanisms not fully elucidated (and possibly contributing to the anti-inflammatory effect to varying degrees), include inhibiting chemotaxis, altering lymphocyte activity, inhibiting neutrophil aggregation/activation, and decreasing proinflammatory cytokine levels.

Contraindications Hypersensitivity to etodolac, aspirin, other NSAIDs, or any component of the formulation; perioperative pain in the setting of coronary artery bypass graft (CABG) surgery

Warnings/Precautions [U.S. Boxed Warning]: NSAIDs are associated with an increased risk of adverse cardiovascular thrombotic events, including MI and stroke. Risk may be increased with duration of use or pre-existing cardiovascular risk factors or disease. Carefully evaluate individual cardiovascular risk profiles prior to prescribing. May cause new-onset hypertension or worsening of existing hypertension. Use caution with fluid retention. Avoid use in heart failure. Concurrent administration of ibuprofen, and potentially other nonselective NSAIDs, may interfere with aspirin's cardioprotective effect. **[U.S. Boxed Warning]: Use is contraindicated for treatment of perioperative pain in the setting of coronary artery bypass graft (CABG) surgery**. Risk of MI and stroke may be increased with use following CABG surgery.

[U.S. Boxed Warning]: NSAIDs may increase risk of gastrointestinal irritation, inflammation, ulceration, bleeding, and perforation. These events may occur at any time during therapy and without warning. Use caution with a history of GI disease (bleeding or ulcers), concurrent therapy with aspirin, anticoagulants and/or corticosteroids, smoking, use of alcohol, the elderly or debilitated patients. When used concomitantly with ≤325 mg of aspirin, a substantial increase in the risk of gastrointestinal complications (eg, ulcer) occurs; concomitant gastroprotective therapy (eg, proton pump inhibitors) is recommended (Bhatt, 2008).

Platelet adhesion and aggregation may be decreased; may prolong bleeding time; patients with coagulation disorders or who are receiving anticoagulants should be monitored closely. Anemia may occur; patients on long-term NSAID therapy should be monitored for anemia. Rarely, NSAID use may cause severe blood dyscrasias (eg, agranulocytosis, aplastic anemia, thrombocytopenia).

NSAID use may compromise existing renal function; dose-dependent decreases in prostaglandin synthesis may result from NSAID use, reducing renal blood flow which may cause renal decompensation. NSAID use may increase the risk for hyperkalemia. Patients with impaired renal function, dehydration, heart failure, liver dysfunction, those taking diuretics and ACE inhibitors, and the elderly are at greater risk for renal toxicity and hyperkalemia. Rehydrate patient before starting therapy; monitor renal function closely. Not recommended for use in patients with advanced renal disease. Long-term NSAID use may result in renal papillary necrosis.

Use the lowest effective dose for the shortest duration of time, consistent with individual patient goals, to reduce risk of cardiovascular or GI adverse events. Alternate therapies should be considered for patients at high risk.

NSAIDs may cause serious skin adverse events including exfoliative dermatitis, Stevens-Johnson syndrome (SJS), and toxic epidermal necrolysis (TEN); discontinue use at first sign of skin rash or hypersensitivity. Anaphylactoid reactions may occur, even without prior exposure; patients with "aspirin triad" (bronchial asthma, aspirin intolerance, rhinitis) may be at increased risk. Do not use in patients who experience bronchospasm, asthma, rhinitis, or urticaria with NSAID or aspirin therapy. Use caution in other forms of asthma.

Use with caution in patients with decreased hepatic function. Closely monitor patients with any abnormal LFT. Severe hepatic reactions (eg, fulminant hepatitis, liver failure) have occurred with NSAID use, rarely; discontinue if signs or symptoms of liver disease develop, or if systemic manifestations occur.

NSAIDS may cause drowsiness, dizziness, blurred vision and other neurologic effects which may impair physical or mental abilities; patients must be cautioned about performing tasks which require mental alertness (eg, operating machinery or driving). Discontinue use with blurred or diminished vision and perform ophthalmologic exam. Monitor vision with long-term therapy. The elderly are at increased risk for adverse effects (especially peptic ulceration, CNS effects, renal toxicity) from NSAIDs even at low doses.

Withhold for at least 4-6 half-lives prior to surgical or dental procedures.

Use of extended release product consisting of a nondeformable matrix should be avoided in patients with stricture/narrowing of the GI tract; symptoms of obstruction have been associated with nondeformable products.

Drug Interactions

Avoid Concomitant Use

Avoid concomitant use of Etodolac with any of the following: Ketorolac; Ketorolac (Systemic)

Increased Effect/Toxicity

Etodolac may increase the levels/effects of: Aminoglycosides; Anticoagulants; Antiplatelet Agents; Bisphosphonate Derivatives; Collagenase (Systemic); CycloSPORINE; CycloSPORINE (Systemic); Deferasirox; Desmopressin; Digoxin; Drotrecogin Alfa; Eplerenone; Haloperidol; Ibritumomab; Lithium; Methotrexate; Nonsteroidal Anti-Inflammatory Agents; PEMEtrexed; Potassium-Sparing

Diuretics; PRALAtrexate; Quinolone Antibiotics; Salicylates; Thrombolytic Agents; Tositumomab and Iodine I 131 Tositumomab; Vancomycin; Vitamin K Antagonists

The levels/effects of Etodolac may be increased by: ACE Inhibitors; Angiotensin II Receptor Blockers; Antidepressants (Tricyclic, Tertiary Amine); Corticosteroids (Systemic); Dasatinib; Glucosamine; Herbs (Anticoagulant/Antiplatelet Properties); Ketorolac; Ketorolac (Systemic); Nonsteroidal Anti-Inflammatory Agents; Omega-3-Acid Ethyl Esters; Pentosan Polysulfate Sodium; Pentoxifylline; Probenecid; Prostacyclin Analogues; Selective Serotonin Reuptake Inhibitors; Serotonin/Norepinephrine Reuptake Inhibitors; Treprostinil

Decreased Effect

Etodolac may decrease the levels/effects of: ACE Inhibitors; Angiotensin II Receptor Blockers; Antiplatelet Agents; Beta-Blockers; Eplerenone; HydrALAZINE; Loop Diuretics; Potassium-Sparing Diuretics; Salicylates; Thiazide Diuretics

The levels/effects of Etodolac may be decreased by: Bile Acid Sequestrants; Nonsteroidal Anti-Inflammatory Agents; Salicylates

Ethanol/Nutrition/Herb Interactions

Ethanol: Avoid ethanol (may enhance gastric mucosal irritation).

Food: Etodolac peak serum levels may be decreased if taken with food.

Herb/Nutraceutical: Avoid alfalfa, anise, bilberry, bladderwrack, bromelain, cat's claw, celery, chamomile, coleus, cordyceps, dong quai, evening primrose, fenugreek, feverfew, garlic, ginger, ginkgo biloba, ginseng (American, Panax, Siberian), grapeseed, green tea, guggul, horse chestnut seed, horseradish, licorice, prickly ash, red clover, reishi, SAMe (S-adenosylmethionine), sweet clover, turmeric, white willow (all have additional antiplatelet activity).

Dietary Considerations May be taken with food to decrease GI upset.

Pharmacodynamics/Kinetics

Onset of Action Analgesic: 2-4 hours; Maximum anti-inflammatory effect: A few days

Half-life Elimination Terminal: Adults: 5-8 hours; Extended release: Children (6-16 years): 12 hours

Time to Peak Immediate release: Adults: 1-2 hours; Extended release: 5-7 hours, increased 1.4-3.8 hours with food

Pregnancy Risk Factor C

Lactation Excretion in breast milk unknown/not recommended

Breast-Feeding Considerations It is not known if etodolac is excreted into breast milk. Use of etodolac while breast-feeding is not recommended by the manufacturer.

Dosage Forms

Capsule, oral: 200 mg, 300 mg

Tablet, oral: 400 mg, 500 mg

Tablet, extended release, oral: 400 mg, 500 mg, 600 mg

References

Brooks PM and Day RO, "Nonsteroidal Anti-inflammatory Drugs - Differences and Similarities," *N Engl J Med*, 1991, 324(24):1716-25.

Tucker PW, Smith JR, and Adams DF, "A Comparison of 2 Analgesic Regimens for the Control of Postoperative Periodontal Discomfort," *J Periodontol*, 1996, 67(2):125-9.

Etomidate (e TOM i date)

U.S. Brand Names Amidate®

Canadian Brand Names Amidate®

Pharmacologic Category General Anesthetic

Use Induction and maintenance of general anesthesia

Unlabeled/Investigational Use Sedation for diagnosis of seizure foci

Local Anesthetic/Vasoconstrictor Precautions No information available to require special precautions

Effects on Dental Treatment Key adverse event(s) related to dental treatment: Hiccups.

Effects on Bleeding No information available to require special precautions

Adverse Effects

>10%:

Endocrine & metabolic: Adrenal suppression

Gastrointestinal: Nausea, vomiting on emergence from anesthesia

Local: Pain at injection site (30% to 80%)

Neuromuscular & skeletal: Myoclonus (33%), transient skeletal movements, uncontrolled eye movements

1% to 10%: Hiccups

General Dosage Range I.V.: *Children >10 years and Adults:* Induction: 0.2-0.6 mg/kg; Maintenance: 5-20 mcg/kg/minute

Mechanism of Action Ultrashort-acting nonbarbiturate hypnotic (benzylimidazole) used for the induction of anesthesia; chemically, it is a carboxylated imidazole which produces a rapid induction of anesthesia with minimal cardiovascular effects; produces EEG burst suppression at high doses

Pharmacodynamics/Kinetics

Onset of Action 30-60 seconds; Peak effect: 1 minute

Duration of Action 3-5 minutes; terminated by redistribution

Half-life Elimination Terminal: 2.6 hours

Pregnancy Risk Factor C

Etonogestrel (e toe noe JES trel)

U.S. Brand Names Implanon™

Pharmacologic Category Contraceptive; Progestin

Use Prevention of pregnancy; for use in women who request long-acting (up to 3 years) contraception

Local Anesthetic/Vasoconstrictor Precautions No information available to require special precautions

Effects on Dental Treatment Key adverse event(s) related to dental treatment: Until more is known about the mechanism of interaction, use caution in prescribing antibiotics to female patients taking progestin-only contraceptives.

Effects on Bleeding No information available to require special precautions

Adverse Effects

>10%:

Central nervous system: Headache (25%)

Dermatologic: Acne (14%)

Endocrine & metabolic: Infrequent menstrual bleeding (<3 episodes/90 days: 34%), amenorrhea (no bleeding in 90 days: 22%), prolonged menstrual bleeding (lasting >14 days: 18%), breast pain (13%), menstrual bleeding irregularities requiring discontinuation (11%)

Gastrointestinal: Weight gain (14%), abdominal pain (11%)

Genitourinary: Vaginitis (15%)

Respiratory: Upper respiratory tract infection (13%), pharyngitis (11%)

5% to 10%:

Central nervous system: Dizziness (7%), emotional lability (7%), depression (6%), nervousness (6%), pain (6%)

Endocrine & metabolic: Dysmenorrhea (7%), frequent menstrual bleeding (>5 episodes/90 days: 7%)

Gastrointestinal: Nausea (6%)

Genitourinary: Leukorrhea (10%)

Local: Insertion site pain (5%)

Neuromuscular & skeletal: Back pain (7%)

Respiratory: Sinusitis (6%)

Miscellaneous: Flu-like syndrome (8%)

General Dosage Range Subdermal: *Children and Adults (females, postmenarche):* Implant 1 rod for up to 3 years

Mechanism of Action Etonogestrel is the active metabolite of desogestrel. It prevents pregnancy by suppressing ovulation, increasing the viscosity of cervical mucous, and inhibiting endometrial proliferation.

Pharmacodynamics/Kinetics

Onset of Action Serum levels sufficient to inhibit ovulation: ≤8 hours of implant

Duration of Action Implant: Each rod maintains etonogestrel levels sufficient to inhibit ovulation for 3 years

Half-life Elimination ~25 hours

Prescribing and Access Restrictions Only healthcare providers who have undergone training in the insertion and removal procedures will be able to order Implanon™. Materials related to the insertion and removal of Implanon™ are available from the manufacturer (877-467-5266).

Etoposide (e toe POE side)

U.S. Brand Names Toposar®

Pharmacologic Category Antineoplastic Agent, Podophyllotoxin Derivative; Antineoplastic Agent, Topoisomerase II Inhibitor

Use Treatment of refractory testicular tumors (injectable formulation); treatment of small cell lung cancer

Unlabeled/Investigational Use Treatment of acute lymphocytic leukemia (ALL), refractory acute myeloid leukemia (AML), recurrent or metastatic breast cancer, central nervous system tumors, Ewing's sarcoma, gestational trophoblastic disease, Hodgkin's lymphoma, merkel cell cancer, refractory multiple myeloma, neuroblastoma, neuroendocrine tumors (adrenal gland and carcinoid tumors), non-Hodgkin's lymphomas, nonsmall-cell lung cancer (NSCLC), osteosarcoma, ovarian cancer, prostate cancer, retinoblastoma, metastatic soft tissue sarcoma, thymic malignancies, unknown-primary adenocarcinoma, Wilms' tumor; conditioning regimen for hematopoietic cell transplantation

Local Anesthetic/Vasoconstrictor Precautions No information available to require special precautions

Effects on Dental Treatment Key adverse event(s) related to dental treatment: Mucositis (especially at high doses) and stomatitis.

Effects on Bleeding Chemotherapy may result in significant myelosuppression, potentially including significant reduction in platelet counts and altered hemostasis. In patients who are under active treatment with these agents, medical consult is suggested.

Adverse Effects Note: The following may occur with higher doses used in stem cell transplantation: Alopecia, ethanol intoxication, hepatitis, hypotension (infusion-related), metabolic acidosis, mucositis, nausea and vomiting (severe), secondary malignancy, skin lesions (resembling Stevens-Johnson syndrome).

>10%:
- Dermatologic: Alopecia (8% to 66%)
- Gastrointestinal: Nausea/vomiting (31% to 43%), anorexia (10% to 13%), diarrhea (1% to 13%)
- Hematologic: Leukopenia (60% to 91%; grade 4: 3% to 17%; nadir: 7-14 days; recovery: by day 20), thrombocytopenia (22% to 41%; grades 3/4: 1% to 20%; nadir 9-16 days; recovery: by day 20), anemia (≤33%)

1% to 10%:
- Cardiovascular: Hypotension (1% to 2%; due to rapid infusion)
- Gastrointestinal: Stomatitis (1% to 6%), abdominal pain (up to 2%)
- Hepatic: Hepatic toxicity (up to 3%)
- Neuromuscular & skeletal: Peripheral neuropathy (1% to 2%)
- Miscellaneous: Anaphylactic-like reaction (I.V. infusion 1% to 2%; oral capsules <1%; including chills, fever, tachycardia, bronchospasm, dyspnea)

General Dosage Range Dosage adjustment recommended in patients with hepatic or renal impairment

I.V., oral: *Adults:* Dosage varies greatly depending on indication

Mechanism of Action Etoposide has been shown to delay transit of cells through the S phase and arrest cells in late S or early G_2 phase. The drug may inhibit mitochondrial transport at the NADH dehydrogenase level or inhibit uptake of nucleosides into HeLa cells. It is a topoisomerase II inhibitor and appears to cause DNA strand breaks. Etoposide does not inhibit microtubular assembly.

Pharmacodynamics/Kinetics

Half-life Elimination Terminal: I.V.: 4-11 hours; Children: Normal renal/hepatic function: 6-8 hours

Pregnancy Risk Factor D

Etoposide Phosphate (e toe POE side FOS fate)

Related Information

Etoposide *on page* 694

U.S. Brand Names Etopophos®

Pharmacologic Category Antineoplastic Agent, Podophyllotoxin Derivative; Antineoplastic Agent, Topoisomerase II Inhibitor

Use Treatment of refractory testicular tumors; treatment of small cell lung cancer

Local Anesthetic/Vasoconstrictor Precautions No information available to require special precautions

Effects on Dental Treatment Key adverse event(s) related to dental treatment: Mucositis (especially at high doses), stomatitis, and taste perversion.

Effects on Bleeding Chemotherapy may result in significant myelosuppression, potentially including significant reduction in platelet counts and altered hemostasis. In patients who are under active treatment with these agents, medical consult is suggested.

Adverse Effects Note: Also see adverse reactions for **etoposide;** etoposide phosphate is converted to etoposide, adverse reactions experienced with etoposide would also be expected with etoposide phosphate.

>10%:
- Central nervous system: Chills/fever (24%)
- Dermatologic: Alopecia (33% to 44%)
- Gastrointestinal: Nausea/vomiting (37%), anorexia (16%), mucositis (11%)

Hematologic: Leukopenia (91%; grade 4: 17%; nadir: day 15-22; recovery: usually by day 21), neutropenia (88%; grade 4: 37%; nadir: day 12-19; recovery: usually by day 21), anemia (72%; grades 3/4: 19%), thrombocytopenia (23%; grade 4: 9%; nadir: day 10-15; recovery: usually by day 21)
Neuromuscular & skeletal: Weakness/malaise (39%)

1% to 10%:

Cardiovascular: Hypotension (1% to 5%), hypertension (3%), facial flushing (2%)
Central nervous system: Dizziness (5%)
Dermatologic: Skin rash (3%)
Gastrointestinal: Constipation (8%), abdominal pain (7%), diarrhea (6%), taste perversion (6%)
Local: Extravasation/phlebitis (5%; including swelling, pain, cellulitis, necrosis, and/or skin necrosis at site of infiltration)
Miscellaneous: Anaphylactic-type reactions (3%; including chills, diaphoresis, fever, rigor, tachycardia, bronchospasm, dyspnea, pruritus)

General Dosage Range Dosage adjustment recommended in patients with hepatic or renal impairment

I.V.: *Adults:* Dosage varies greatly depending on indication

Mechanism of Action Etoposide phosphate is converted *in vivo* to the active moiety, etoposide, by dephosphorylation. Etoposide inhibits mitotic activity; inhibits cells from entering prophase; inhibits DNA synthesis. Initially thought to be mitotic inhibitors similar to podophyllotoxin, but actually have no effect on microtubule assembly. However, later shown to induce DNA strand breakage and inhibition of topoisomerase II (an enzyme which breaks and repairs DNA); etoposide acts in late S or early G2 phases.

Pharmacodynamics/Kinetics

Half-life Elimination Terminal: 4-11 hours; Children: Normal renal/hepatic function: 6-8 hours

Pregnancy Risk Factor D

Etravirine (et ra VIR een)

Related Information

HIV Infection and AIDS *on page 1883*

U.S. Brand Names Intelence®

Canadian Brand Names Intelence™

Pharmacologic Category Antiretroviral Agent, Reverse Transcriptase Inhibitor (Non-nucleoside)

Use Treatment of HIV-1 infection in combination with at least two additional antiretroviral agents in treatment-experienced patients exhibiting viral replication with documented non-nucleoside reverse transcriptase inhibitor (NNRTI) resistance

Local Anesthetic/Vasoconstrictor Precautions No information available to require special precautions

Effects on Dental Treatment Key adverse event(s) related to dental treatment: Stomatitis has been reported.

Effects on Bleeding No information available to require special precautions related to hemostasis.

Adverse Effects

>10%:

Dermatologic: Rash (≥ grade 2: 10%)
Endocrine & metabolic: Cholesterol (total) increased (≤300 mg/dL: 20%; >300 mg/dL: 8%), hyperglycemia (≤250 mg/dL: 15%; 251-500 mg/dL: 4%), LDL increased (≤190 mg/dL: 13%)
Gastrointestinal: Nausea

2% to 10%:

Endocrine & metabolic: Triglycerides increased (≤750 mg/dL: 9%; >750 mg/dL: 4% to 6%)
Hepatic: ALT increased (≤5 x ULN: 6%; >5 x ULN: 3%), AST increased (≤5 x ULN: 6%; >5 x ULN: 3%)
Neuromuscular & skeletal: Peripheral neuropathy (≥ grade 2: 4%)
Renal: Creatinine increased (≤1.8 x ULN: 6%; >1.8 x ULN: 2%)

General Dosage Range Oral: *Adults:* 200 mg twice daily

Mechanism of Action As a non-nucleoside reverse transcriptase inhibitor, etravirine has activity against HIV-1 by binding to reverse transcriptase. It consequently blocks the RNA-dependent and DNA-dependent DNA polymerase activities, including HIV-1 replication. It does not require intracellular phosphorylation for antiviral activity.

Pharmacodynamics/Kinetics

Half-life Elimination 41 hours (± 20 hours)

Time to Peak 2.5-4 hours

Pregnancy Risk Factor B

Everolimus (e ver OH li mus)

U.S. Brand Names Afinitor®; Zortress®

Pharmacologic Category Antineoplastic Agent, mTOR Kinase Inhibitor; Immunosuppressant Agent; mTOR Kinase Inhibitor

Use Treatment of advanced renal cell cancer (RCC), after sunitinib or sorafenib failure (Afinitor®); treatment of subependymal giant cell astrocytoma (SEGA) associated with tuberous sclerosis, in patients who are not candidates for curative surgical resection (Afinitor®); prophylaxis of organ rejection in patients at low-moderate immunologic risk receiving renal transplants (Zortress®)

Unlabeled/Investigational Use Prophylaxis of organ rejection in heart transplant recipients; treatment of advanced pancreatic neuroendocrine tumors; treatment of relapsed or refractory Waldenström's macroglobulinemia (WM)

Local Anesthetic/Vasoconstrictor Precautions No information available to require special precautions

Effects on Dental Treatment Key adverse event(s) related to dental treatment: High incidence of mouth ulcers, mucositis, and stomatitis; xerostomia and taste alterations have been observed (normal salivary flow resumes upon discontinuation)

Effects on Bleeding No information available to require special precautions

Adverse Effects

>10%:

Cardiovascular: Peripheral edema (RCC: 25%; renal transplantation: 45%; SEGA: 4%), hypertension (RCC, SEGA: 4%; renal transplant: 30%)

Central nervous system: Fever (19% to 32%), fatigue (RCC: 31%; renal transplant: 9%; SEGA: 7%), seizure (SEGA: 29%), headache (18% to 19%), personality change (SEGA: 18%), insomnia (9% to 17%), dizziness (7% to 14%)

Dermatologic: Rash (18% to 29%), acneiform dermatitis (SEGA: 25%; RCC: 3%), cellulitis (SEGA: 21%), dry skin (13% to 18%), contact dermatitis (14%), excoriation (14%), pruritus (14%), acne (11%)

Endocrine & metabolic: Hypercholesterolemia (RCC: 77%; grade 3: 4%; SEGA: 68%; renal transplant: 17%), hypertriglyceridemia (RCC: 73%; grade 3: <1%; SEGA: 11% to 43%; renal transplant: <10%), hyperglycemia (RCC: 57%; grade 3: 15%; grade 4: <1%; SEGA: 25%; renal transplant: 12%), hypoglycemia (SEGA: 32%), hypophosphatemia (RCC: 37%; grade 3: 6%; renal transplant: 13%), hyperlipidemia (renal transplant: 21%), hyperkalemia (renal transplant: 18%), hypocalcemia (17%), dyslipidemia (renal transplant: 15%), hypomagnesemia (renal transplant: 14%), hypokalemia (renal transplant: 12%)

Gastrointestinal: Stomatitis (SEGA: 86%; grade 3: 4%; RCC: 44%; grade 3: 4%; grade 4: <1%; renal transplant: 8%), constipation (renal transplant: 38%; SEGA: 11%), diarrhea (RCC: 30%; grade 3: 1%; SEGA: 25%; renal transplantation: 19%), nausea (26% to 29%: grade 3: 1%), anorexia (25%), vomiting (15% to 21%; grade 3: 2%), mucosal inflammation (19%; grade 3: 1%), gastroenteritis (SEGA: 18%), abdominal pain (3% to 13%)

Genitourinary: Urinary tract infection (renal transplant: 22%; RCC: 5%), dysuria (renal transplant: 11%)

Hematologic: Anemia (RCC: 92%; grade 3: 12%; grade 4: 1%; SEGA: 39%; renal transplant: 26%), lymphocytopenia (51%; grade 3: 16%; grade 4: 2%), leukopenia (SEGA: 54%; RCC: 26%; renal transplant: 3%), thrombocytopenia (21% to 23%; grade 3: 1%; renal transplant <10%), neutropenia (14%; grade 4: <4%)

Hepatic: AST increased (25% to 89%; grade 3: <4%; grade 4: <1%), ALT increased (21% to 46%; grade 3: 1%)

Neuromuscular & skeletal: Weakness (33%), limb pain (10% to 12%), back pain (renal transplant: 11%)

Otic: Otitis (SEGA: 14% to 36%)

Renal: Creatinine increased (RCC: 50%; grade 3: 1%; renal transplant: 18%; SEGA: 11%), hematuria (renal transplant: 12%)

Respiratory: Upper respiratory infection (SEGA: 82%; renal transplant: 16%), sinusitis (3% to 39%), cough (RCC: 30%; SEGA: 21%; renal transplant: 7%), dyspnea (24%; grade 3: 6%; grade 4: 1%), epistaxis (≤18%), nasal congestion (14%), pneumonitis (includes alveolitis, interstitial lung disease, lung infiltrate, pulmonary alveolar hemorrhage, pulmonary toxicity; 14%; grade 3: 4%), rhinitis (14%), pharyngitis (SEGA: 4% to 11%)

Miscellaneous: Infection (RCC: All infections: 37%; grade 3: 7%; grade 4: 3%; renal transplant: 62%)

1% to 10%:

Cardiovascular: Chest pain (5%), tachycardia (3%), heart failure (1%), angina, atrial fibrillation, chest discomfort, deep vein thrombosis, edema (generalized), hypotension, palpitation, syncope

Central nervous system: Chills (4%), agitation, anxiety, depression, hallucination, hemiparesis, hypesthesia, malaise, somnolence
Dermatologic: Nail disorder (5%), palmar-plantar erythrodysesthesia syndrome ([hand-foot syndrome] 5%), erythema 4%, onychoclasis (4%), pityriasis rosea (4%), skin lesions (4%), alopecia, hirsutism, incision complications, hyperhydrosis, hypertrichosis
Endocrine & metabolic: Diabetes mellitus (exacerbation: 2%; new-onset: <9%), acidosis, cushingoid syndrome, dehydration, gout, hypercalcemia, hyperparathyroidism, hyperphosphatemia, hyperuricemia, hypoglycemia, hyponatremia, iron deficiency, vitamin B_{12} deficiency
Gastrointestinal: Taste alteration (10%), weight loss (9%), xerostomia (8%), gastritis (7%), hemorrhoids (5%), dyspepsia (4%), dysphagia (4%), abdominal distention, epigastric discomfort, flatulence, gastroesophageal reflux, gingival hypertrophy, hematemesis, ileus, peritonitis
Genitourinary: Bladder spasm, erectile dysfunction, ovarian cysts, pollakiuria, polyuria, pyuria, scrotal edema, urinary retention, urinary urgency
Hematologic: Hemorrhage (3%), leukocytosis, lymphadenopathy, thrombocythemia
Hepatic: Bilirubin increased (3%; grade 3: <1%; grade 4: <1%)
Neuromuscular & skeletal: Tremor (8%), paresthesia (5%), jaw pain (3%), arthralgia, joint swelling, muscle spasm, musculoskeletal pain, myalgia, osteonecrosis, osteopenia, osteoporosis, spondylitis
Ocular: Eyelid edema (4%), ocular hyperemia (4%), conjunctivitis (2%), blurred vision, cataract
Renal: Renal failure (3%), BUN increased, hydronephrosis, interstitial nephritis, proteinuria, renal artery thrombosis, renal impairment
Respiratory: Pleural effusion (7%), nasopharyngitis (6%), pneumonia (6%), bronchitis (4%), pharyngolaryngeal pain (4%), rhinorrhea (3%), atelectasis, nasal congestion, pulmonary edema, sinus congestion, wheezing
Miscellaneous: BK virus infection, candidiasis, night sweats

General Dosage Range Dosage adjustment recommended in patients with hepatic impairment, on concomitant therapy, or who develop toxicities

Oral: *Children ≥3 years and Adults:* Dosage varies greatly depending on indication

Mechanism of Action Everolimus is a macrolide immunosuppressant and an m-TOR inhibitor which has antiproliferative and antiangiogenic properties. Reduces protein synthesis and cell proliferation by binding to the FK binding protein-12 (FKBP-12), an intracellular protein, to form a complex that inhibits activation of mTOR (mammalian target of rapamycin) serine-threonine kinase activity. Also reduces angiogenesis by inhibiting vascular endothelial growth factor (VEGF) and hypoxia-inducible factor (HIF-1) expression.

Pharmacodynamics/Kinetics

Half-life Elimination ~30 hours

Time to Peak 1-2 hours

Pregnancy Risk Factor D (Afinitor®) / C (Zortress®)

Exemestane (ex e MES tane)

U.S. Brand Names Aromasin®

Canadian Brand Names Aromasin®

Pharmacologic Category Antineoplastic Agent, Aromatase Inactivator

Use Treatment of advanced breast cancer in postmenopausal women whose disease has progressed following tamoxifen therapy; adjuvant treatment of postmenopausal estrogen receptor-positive early breast cancer following 2-3 years of tamoxifen (for a total of 5 years of adjuvant therapy)

Local Anesthetic/Vasoconstrictor Precautions No information available to require special precautions

Effects on Dental Treatment No significant effects or complications reported

Effects on Bleeding Although significant myelosuppression with associated altered hemostasis has been reported for many chemotherapeutic agents, myelosuppression is not common with exemestane and no specific precautions appear to necessary.

Adverse Effects

>10%:

Cardiovascular: Hypertension (5% to 15%)
Central nervous system: Fatigue (8% to 22%), insomnia (11% to 14%), pain (13%), headache (7% to 13%), depression (6% to 13%)
Dermatological: Hyperhidrosis (4% to 18%), alopecia (15%)
Endocrine & metabolic: Hot flashes (13% to 33%)
Gastrointestinal: Nausea (9% to 18%), abdominal pain (6% to 11%)
Hepatic: Alkaline phosphatase increased (14% to 15%)

Neuromuscular & skeletal: Arthralgia (15% to 29%)

1% to 10%:

Cardiovascular: Edema (6% to 7%); cardiac ischemic events (2%: MI, angina, myocardial ischemia); chest pain

Central nervous system: Dizziness (8% to 10%), anxiety (4% to 10%), fever (5%), confusion, hypoesthesia

Dermatologic: Dermatitis (8%), itching, rash

Endocrine & metabolic: Weight gain (8%)

Gastrointestinal: Diarrhea (4% to 10%), vomiting (7%), anorexia (6%), constipation (5%), appetite increased (3%), dyspepsia

Genitourinary: Urinary tract infection (2% to 5%)

Hepatic: Bilirubin increased (5% to 7%)

Neuromuscular & skeletal: Back pain (9%), limb pain (9%), myalgia (6%), osteoarthritis (6%), weakness (6%), osteoporosis (5%), pathological fracture (4%), paresthesia (3%), carpal tunnel syndrome (2%), cramps (2%)

Ocular: Visual disturbances (5%)

Renal: Creatinine increased (6%)

Respiratory: Dyspnea (10%), cough (6%), bronchitis, pharyngitis, rhinitis, sinusitis, upper respiratory infection

Miscellaneous: Flu-like syndrome (6%), lymphedema, infection

A dose-dependent decrease in sex hormone-binding globulin has been observed with daily doses of daily doses ≥2.5 mg. Serum luteinizing hormone and follicle-stimulating hormone levels have increased with this medicine.

General Dosage Range Dosage adjustment recommended in patients on concomitant therapy

Oral: *Adults (postmenopausal females):* 25 mg once daily

Mechanism of Action Exemestane is an irreversible, steroidal aromatase inactivator. It is structurally related to androstenedione, and is converted to an intermediate that irreversibly blocks the active site of the aromatase enzyme, leading to inactivation ("suicide inhibition") and thus preventing conversion of androgens to estrogens in peripheral tissues. In postmenopausal breast cancers where growth is estrogen-dependent, this medicine will lower circulating estrogens.

Pharmacodynamics/Kinetics

Half-life Elimination 24 hours

Time to Peak Women with breast cancer: 1.2 hours

Pregnancy Risk Factor D

Exenatide (ex EN a tide)

U.S. Brand Names Byetta®

Pharmacologic Category Antidiabetic Agent, Glucagon-Like Peptide-1 (GLP-1) Receptor Agonist

Use Treatment of type 2 diabetes mellitus (noninsulin dependent, NIDDM) to improve glycemic control

Local Anesthetic/Vasoconstrictor Precautions No information available to require special precautions

Effects on Dental Treatment No significant effects or complications reported

Effects on Bleeding No information available to require special precautions

Adverse Effects Percentages as reported for combination therapy (sulfonylurea and/or metformin; thiazolidinedione and/or metformin) unless otherwise noted:

>10%:

Endocrine & metabolic: Hypoglycemia (monotherapy 4% to 5%; combination therapy: sulfonylurea - 14% to 36%; metformin - similar to placebo; thiazolidinedione - 11%)

Gastrointestinal: Nausea (monotherapy 8%; combination therapy 40% to 44%; dose-dependent), vomiting (monotherapy 4%; combination therapy 13%), diarrhea (monotherapy <2%; combination therapy 6% to 13%)

Miscellaneous: Anti-exenatide antibodies (low titers 38%, high titers 6%)

1% to 10%:

Central nervous system: Dizziness (monotherapy <2%; combination therapy 9%), headache (9%)

Dermatologic: Hyperhidrosis (3%)

Endocrine & metabolic: Appetite decreased (<2%)

Gastrointestinal: Dyspepsia (monotherapy 3%; combination therapy 6% to 7%), GERD (3%)

Neuromuscular & skeletal: Weakness (4%)

Miscellaneous: Feeling jittery (9%)

General Dosage Range SubQ: *Adults:* Initial: 5 mcg twice daily; Maintenance: 5-10 mcg twice daily

Mechanism of Action Exenatide is an analog of the hormone incretin (glucagon-like peptide 1 or GLP-1) which increases glucose-dependent insulin secretion, decreases inappropriate glucagon secretion, increases B-cell growth/replication, slows gastric emptying, and decreases food intake. Exenatide administration results in decreases in hemoglobin A_{1c} by approximately 0.5% to 1%.

Pharmacodynamics/Kinetics

Half-life Elimination 2.4 hours

Time to Peak SubQ: 2.1 hours

Pregnancy Risk Factor C

Ezetimibe (ez ET i mibe)

Related Information

Cardiovascular Diseases *on page 1848*

U.S. Brand Names Zetia®

Canadian Brand Names Ezetrol®

Generic Availability (U.S.) No

Pharmacologic Category Antilipemic Agent, 2-Azetidinone

Use Use in combination with dietary therapy for the treatment of primary hypercholesterolemia (as monotherapy or in combination with HMG-CoA reductase inhibitors); homozygous sitosterolemia; homozygous familial hypercholesterolemia (in combination with atorvastatin or simvastatin); mixed hyperlipidemia (in combination with fenofibrate)

Local Anesthetic/Vasoconstrictor Precautions No information available to require special precautions

Effects on Dental Treatment No significant effects or complications reported

Effects on Bleeding No information available to require special precautions

Adverse Effects 1% to 10%:

Central nervous system: Fatigue (2%)

Gastrointestinal: Diarrhea (4%)

Hepatic: Transaminases increased (with HMG-CoA reductase inhibitors) (≥3 x ULN, 1%)

Neuromuscular & skeletal: Arthralgia (3%), pain in extremity (3%)

Respiratory: Upper respiratory tract infection (4%), sinusitis (3%)

Miscellaneous: Influenza (2%)

Dosage Oral:

Children ≥10 years and Adults: 10 mg/day

Elderly: Refer to adult dosing

Dosage adjustment in renal impairment: AUC increased with severe impairment (Cl_{cr} <30 mL/minute); no dosing adjustment recommended

Dosage adjustment in hepatic impairment: AUC increased with hepatic impairment

Mild impairment (Child-Pugh class A): No dosing adjustment necessary

Moderate-to-severe impairment (Child-Pugh classes B and C): Use of ezetimibe not recommended

Mechanism of Action Inhibits absorption of cholesterol at the brush border of the small intestine via the sterol transporter, Niemann-Pick C1-Like1 (NPC1L1). This leads to a decreased delivery of cholesterol to the liver, reduction of hepatic cholesterol stores and an increased clearance of cholesterol from the blood; decreases total C, LDL-cholesterol (LDL-C), ApoB, and triglycerides (TG) while increasing HDL-cholesterol (HDL-C).

Contraindications Hypersensitivity to ezetimibe or any component of the formulation; concomitant use with an HMG-CoA reductase inhibitor in patients with active hepatic disease, unexplained persistent elevations in serum transaminases; pregnancy; breast-feeding

Warnings/Precautions Secondary causes of hyperlipidemia should be ruled out prior to therapy. Use caution with severe renal (Cl_{cr} <30 mL/minute) or mild hepatic impairment (Child-Pugh class A); not recommended for use with moderate or severe hepatic impairment (Child-Pugh classes B and C). Concurrent use of ezetimibe and fibric acid derivatives may increase the risk of cholelithiasis.

Drug Interactions

Metabolism/Transport Effects Substrate of SLCO1B1

Avoid Concomitant Use There are no known interactions where it is recommended to avoid concomitant use.

Increased Effect/Toxicity

Ezetimibe may increase the levels/effects of: CycloSPORINE; CycloSPORINE (Systemic)

The levels/effects of Ezetimibe may be increased by: CycloSPORINE; CycloSPORINE (Systemic); Eltrombopag; Fibric Acid Derivatives

Decreased Effect

The levels/effects of Ezetimibe may be decreased by: Bile Acid Sequestrants

Ethanol/Nutrition/Herb Interactions Food: Ezetimibe did not cause meaningful reductions in fat-soluble vitamin concentrations during a 2-week clinical trial. Effects of long-term therapy have not been evaluated.

Dietary Considerations May be taken without regard to meals. Before initiation of therapy, patients should be placed on a standard cholesterol-lowering diet for 6 weeks and the diet should be continued during drug therapy.

Pharmacodynamics/Kinetics

Half-life Elimination 22 hours (ezetimibe and metabolite)

Time to Peak Plasma: 4-12 hours

Pregnancy Risk Factor C

Lactation Excretion in breast milk unknown/not recommended

Dosage Forms

Tablet, oral:

Zetia®: 10 mg

Ezetimibe and Simvastatin (ez ET i mibe & SIM va stat in)

Related Information

Ezetimibe *on page 700*

Simvastatin *on page 1527*

U.S. Brand Names Vytorin®

Pharmacologic Category Antilipemic Agent, 2-Azetidinone; Antilipemic Agent, HMG-CoA Reductase Inhibitor

Use Used in combination with dietary modification for the treatment of primary hypercholesterolemia and homozygous familial hypercholesterolemia

Local Anesthetic/Vasoconstrictor Precautions No information available to require special precautions

Effects on Dental Treatment No significant effects or complications reported

Effects on Bleeding No information available to require special precautions

Adverse Effects Percentages refer to combination Vytorin®. Also see individual agents.

1% to 10%:

Central nervous system: Headache (6%)

Gastrointestinal: Diarrhea (3%)

Hepatic: ALT increased (4%)

Neuromuscular & skeletal: Myalgia (4%), pain in extremity (2%)

Respiratory: Upper respiratory infection (4%)

Miscellaneous: Influenza (2%)

General Dosage Range Dosage adjustment recommended in patients with renal impairment or on concomitant therapy

Oral: *Adults:* Ezetimibe 10 mg and simvastatin 10-80 mg once daily

Mechanism of Action

Ezetimibe: Inhibits absorption of cholesterol at the brush border of the small intestine, leading to a decreased delivery of cholesterol to the liver. Ezetimibe inhibits the enzyme Niemann-Pick C1-Like1 (NPC1L1), a sterol transporter.

Simvastatin: A methylated derivative of lovastatin that acts by competitively inhibiting 3-hydroxy-3-methylglutaryl-coenzyme A (HMG-CoA) reductase, the enzyme that catalyzes the rate-limiting step in cholesterol biosynthesis.

Pregnancy Risk Factor X

Factor VIIa (Recombinant) (FAK ter SEV en aye ree KOM be nant)

U.S. Brand Names NovoSeven® RT

Canadian Brand Names Niastase®; Niastase® RT

Pharmacologic Category Antihemophilic Agent

Use Treatment of bleeding episodes and prevention of bleeding in surgical interventions in patients with either hemophilia A or B with inhibitors to factor VIII or factor IX, acquired hemophilia, or congenital factor VII deficiency

Unlabeled/Investigational Use Reduction of hematoma growth in patients with acute intracerebral hemorrhage, warfarin-related intracerebral hemorrhage

Local Anesthetic/Vasoconstrictor Precautions No information available to require special precautions

Effects on Dental Treatment No significant effects or complications reported

Effects on Bleeding Treatment of bleeding disorders depends on many factors, including severity of disease and risks of bleeding. General dental procedures and simple restorative procedures are not associated with bleeding; therefore, there is no contraindication to general dental treatment for most patients with bleeding disorders. Surgical dental procedures are also possible for hemophiliacs and other bleeding disorders, but a carefully coordinated strategy between the dental and medical team may be required to ensure adequate hemostasis. As preparation for selected dental procedures, factor replacement, tranexamic acid, or aminocaproic acid (Amicar®) may be required. Local measures to promote hemostasis (such as collagen) are commonly used. Examples of procedures which require advance consultation include block anesthesia, deep scaling, extractions, large fillings, and any oral surgery. Medical consultation is warranted.

Adverse Effects 1% to 10%:

Cardiovascular: Hypertension (2%), bradycardia (1%), edema (1%), hypotension (1%)
Central nervous system: Fever (4%), headache (1%), pain (1%)
Dermatologic: Pruritus (1%), purpura (1%), rash (1%)
Gastrointestinal: Vomiting (1%)
Hematologic: Plasma fibrinogen decreased (2%), disseminated intravascular coagulation (1%), fibrinolysis increased (1%), prothrombin decreased (1%)
Local: Injection site reaction (1%)
Neuromuscular & skeletal: Arthrosis (1%)
Renal: Abnormal renal function (1%)
Respiratory: Pneumonia (1%)
Miscellaneous: Allergic reactions (1%)

General Dosage Range I.V.: *Children and Adults:* Dosage varies greatly depending on indication

Mechanism of Action Recombinant factor VIIa, a vitamin K-dependent glycoprotein, promotes hemostasis by activating the extrinsic pathway of the coagulation cascade. It replaces deficient activated coagulation factor VII, which complexes with tissue factor and may activate coagulation factor X to Xa and factor IX to IXa. When complexed with other factors, coagulation factor Xa converts prothrombin to thrombin, a key step in the formation of a fibrin-platelet hemostatic plug.

Pharmacodynamics/Kinetics

Half-life Elimination 2.3 hours (range: 1.7-2.7)

Pregnancy Risk Factor C

Factor IX (FAK ter nyne)

U.S. Brand Names AlphaNine® SD; BeneFix®; Mononine®

Canadian Brand Names BeneFix®; Immunine® VH; Mononine®

Pharmacologic Category Antihemophilic Agent; Blood Product Derivative

Use Prevention and control of bleeding in patients with factor IX deficiency (hemophilia B or Christmas disease)

Local Anesthetic/Vasoconstrictor Precautions No information available to require special precautions

Effects on Dental Treatment No significant effects or complications reported

Effects on Bleeding Treatment of bleeding disorders depends on many factors, including severity of disease and risks of bleeding. General dental procedures and simple restorative procedures are not associated with bleeding; therefore, there is no contraindication to general dental treatment for most patients with bleeding disorders. Surgical dental procedures are also possible for hemophiliacs and other bleeding disorders, but a carefully coordinated strategy between the dental and medical team may be required to ensure adequate hemostasis. As preparation for selected dental procedures, factor replacement, tranexamic acid, or aminocaproic acid (Amicar®) may be required. Local measures to promote hemostasis (such as collagen) are commonly used. Examples of procedures which require advance consultation include block anesthesia, deep scaling, extractions, large fillings, and any oral surgery. Medical consultation is warranted.

Adverse Effects Frequency not defined.

Cardiovascular: Cyanosis, flushing, hypotension, chest tightness, thrombosis
Central nervous system: Chills, dizziness, drowsiness, fever (including transient fever following rapid administration), headache, lethargy, lightheadedness, somnolence
Dermatologic: Angioedema, photosensitivity reaction, rash, urticaria
Gastrointestinal: Abnormal taste, diarrhea, nausea, vomiting
Hematologic: Disseminated intravascular coagulation (DIC)
Hepatic: Alkaline phosphatase increased, ALT increased, AST increased
Local: Injection site reactions: Cellulitis, discomfort, pain, phlebitis, stinging
Neuromuscular & skeletal: Neck tightness, paresthesia, rigors
Ocular: Visual disturbance
Respiratory: Allergic rhinitis, asthma, cough, dyspnea, hypoxia, laryngeal edema, lung disorder

Miscellaneous: Allergic reaction, anaphylaxis, burning sensation in jaw/skull, factor IX inhibitor development, hypersensitivity reaction

Postmarketing and/or case reports: HAV seroconversion, inadequate response/recovery, nephrotic syndrome (associated with immune tolerance induction), parvovirus B19 seroconversion, renal infarction

General Dosage Range I.V.: *Children and Adults:* Dosage varies greatly depending on indication

Mechanism of Action Replaces deficient clotting factor IX. Hemophilia B, or Christmas disease, is an X-linked inherited disorder of blood coagulation characterized by insufficient or abnormal synthesis of the clotting protein factor IX. Factor IX is a vitamin K-dependent coagulation factor which is synthesized in the liver. Factor IX is activated by factor XIa in the intrinsic coagulation pathway. Activated factor IX (IXa), in combination with factor VII:C activates factor X to Xa, resulting ultimately in the conversion of prothrombin to thrombin and the formation of a fibrin clot. The infusion of exogenous factor IX to replace the deficiency present in hemophilia B temporarily restores hemostasis.

Pharmacodynamics/Kinetics

Half-life Elimination IX component: Adults: 21-31 hours; children: 14-28 hours

Pregnancy Risk Factor C

Factor IX Complex (Human) (FAK ter nyne KOM pleks HYU man)

U.S. Brand Names Bebulin® VH; Profilnine® SD

Pharmacologic Category Antihemophilic Agent; Blood Product Derivative; Prothrombin Complex Concentrate (PCC)

Use Animal reproduction studies have not been conducted. There are no adequate and well-controlled studies in pregnant women.

Unlabeled/Investigational Use Emergent correction of warfarin-induced coagulopathy (with clinically significant bleeding); **Note:** Products contain low or nontherapeutic levels of factor VII component; use of fresh frozen plasma (FFP) should be considered

Local Anesthetic/Vasoconstrictor Precautions No information available to require special precautions

Effects on Dental Treatment No significant effects or complications reported

Effects on Bleeding Treatment of bleeding disorders depends on many factors, including severity of disease and risks of bleeding. General dental procedures and simple restorative procedures are not associated with bleeding; therefore, there is no contraindication to general dental treatment for most patients with bleeding disorders. Surgical dental procedures are also possible for hemophiliacs and other bleeding disorders, but a carefully coordinated strategy between the dental and medical team may be required to ensure adequate hemostasis. As preparation for selected dental procedures, factor replacement, tranexamic acid, or aminocaproic acid (Amicar®) may be required. Local measures to promote hemostasis (such as collagen) are commonly used. Examples of procedures which require advance consultation include block anesthesia, deep scaling, extractions, large fillings, and any oral surgery. Medical consultation is warranted.

Adverse Effects Frequency not defined.

Cardiovascular: Flushing, thrombosis (sometimes fatal)

Central nervous system: Chills, fever, headache, lethargy, somnolence

Dermatologic: Rash, urticaria

Gastrointestinal: Nausea, vomiting

Hematologic: DIC

Neuromuscular & skeletal: Paresthesia

Respiratory: Dyspnea

Miscellaneous: Anaphylactic shock, clotting factor antibodies (development of), heparin-induced thrombocytopenia (with products containing heparin)

General Dosage Range I.V.: *Children and Adults:* Dosage varies greatly depending on indication

Mechanism of Action Replaces deficient clotting factor including factor X; hemophilia B, or Christmas disease, is an X-linked recessively inherited disorder of blood coagulation characterized by insufficient or abnormal synthesis of the clotting protein factor IX. Factor IX is a vitamin K-dependent coagulation factor which is synthesized in the liver. Factor IX is activated by factor XIa in the intrinsic coagulation pathway. Activated factor IX (IXa), in combination with factor VII:C, activates factor X to Xa, resulting ultimately in the conversion of prothrombin to thrombin and the formation of a fibrin clot. The infusion of exogenous factor IX to replace the deficiency present in hemophilia B temporarily restores hemostasis.

Pharmacodynamics/Kinetics

Half-life Elimination IX component: ~24 hours

Pregnancy Risk Factor C

Factor XIII Concentrate (Human)

(FAK ter THIR teen KON cen trate HYU man)

Pharmacologic Category Antihemophilic Agent; Blood Product Derivative

Use Prophylaxis against bleeding episodes in congenital factor XIII deficiency

Local Anesthetic/Vasoconstrictor Precautions No information available to require special precautions

Effects on Dental Treatment No significant effects or complications reported

Effects on Bleeding Treatment of bleeding disorders depends on many factors, including severity of disease and risks of bleeding. General dental procedures and simple restorative procedures are not associated with bleeding; therefore, there is no contraindication to general dental treatment for most patients with bleeding disorders. Surgical dental procedures are also possible for hemophiliacs and other bleeding disorders, but a carefully coordinated strategy between the dental and medical team may be required to ensure adequate hemostasis. As preparation for selected dental procedures, factor replacement, tranexamic acid, or aminocaproic acid (Amicar®) may be required. Local measures to promote hemostasis (such as collagen) are commonly used. Examples of procedures which require advance consultation include block anesthesia, deep scaling, extractions, large fillings, and any oral surgery. Medical consultation is warranted.

Adverse Effects >1%:

Central nervous system: Chills, fever, headache
Dermatologic: Bruising, erythema, pruritus, rash
Gastrointestinal: Abdominal pain, diarrhea, vomiting
Hematologic: Hematoma, thrombin-antithrombin levels increased
Hepatic: Liver function tests (increased)
Neuromuscular & skeletal: Arthralgia
Respiratory: Epistaxis, upper respiratory tract infection
Miscellaneous: Allergy, flu-like syndrome

General Dosage Range I.V.: *Children and Adults:* Initial: 40 units/kg; Maintenance: Varies depending on desired factor XIII trough levels

Mechanism of Action Factor XIII (FXIII) is an endogenous plasma glycoprotein found in platelets, monocytes and macrophages that is converted to activated factor XIII (FXIIIa) in the presence of calcium ions. Once activated, FXIIIa cross-links fibrin and cross-links plasmin inhibitor to protect and strengthen the hemostatic platelet plug.

Pharmacodynamics/Kinetics

Duration of Action Plasma levels of FXIII: ~28 days

Half-life Elimination Children (<16): 5.7 days; Adults: 7.1 days

Time to Peak 1.7 hours postinfusion

Pregnancy Risk Factor C

Product Availability

Corifact™: FDA approved February 2011; availability expected in April 2011

Corifact™ is a human plasma-derived factor XIII replacement product approved to prevent bleeding in individuals with congenital factor XIII deficiency.

Famciclovir (fam SYE kloe veer)

Related Information

Systemic Viral Diseases *on page 1904*
Viral Infections *on page 1947*

Related Sample Prescriptions

Herpes Simplex (Recurrent) *on page 1990*
Shingles (Varicella-Zoster Virus) *on page 1990*

U.S. Brand Names Famvir®

Canadian Brand Names Apo-Famciclovir®; CO Famciclovir; Famvir®; PMS-Famciclovir; Sandoz-Famciclovir

Generic Availability (U.S.) Yes

Pharmacologic Category Antiviral Agent

Dental Use Management of acute herpes zoster (shingles); treatment of recurrent herpes labialis in immunocompetent patients

Use Treatment of acute herpes zoster (shingles); treatment and suppression of recurrent episodes of genital herpes in immunocompetent patients; treatment of herpes labialis (cold sores) in immunocompetent patients; treatment of recurrent mucocutaneous/genital herpes simplex in HIV-infected patients

Local Anesthetic/Vasoconstrictor Precautions No information available to require special precautions

Effects on Dental Treatment No significant effects or complications reported

Effects on Bleeding No information available to require special precautions

Adverse Effects Note: Frequencies vary with dose and duration. Single-dose treatment (herpes labialis) was associated only with headache (10%), diarrhea (2%), fatigue (1%), and dysmenorrhea (1%).

>10%:
Central nervous system: Headache (14% to 39%)
Gastrointestinal: Nausea (3% to 13%)

1% to 10%:
Central nervous system: Fatigue (1% to 5%), migraine (1% to 3%)
Dermatologic: Pruritus (≤4%), rash (≤3%)
Endocrine & metabolic: Dysmenorrhea (≤8%)
Gastrointestinal: Diarrhea (5% to 9%), abdominal pain (≤8%), flatulence (1% to 5%), vomiting (1% to 5%)
Hematologic: Neutropenia (3%)
Hepatic: Transaminases increased (2% to 3%), bilirubin increased (2%)
Neuromuscular & skeletal: Paresthesia (≤3%)

Dosage Adults: Oral:

Acute herpes zoster: 500 mg every 8 hours for 7 days (**Note:** Initiate therapy within 72 hours of rash onset.)

Genital herpes simplex virus (HSV) infection in immunocompetent patients:
Initial episode: 250 mg 3 times/day for 7-10 days (CDC, 2010)
Recurrence: 1000 mg twice daily for 1 day (**Note:** Initiate therapy within 6 hours of symptoms/lesions)
Alternatively, the following regimens are also recommended: 125 mg twice daily for 5 days or 500 mg as a single dose, followed by 250 mg twice daily for 2 days (CDC, 2010)
Suppressive therapy: 250 mg twice daily for up to 1 year; **Note:** Duration not established, but efficacy/safety have been demonstrated for 1 year (CDC, 2010)

Recurrent herpes labialis (cold sores): 1500 mg as a single dose; initiate therapy at first sign or symptom such as tingling, burning, or itching (initiated within 1 hour in clinical studies)

Recurrent mucocutaneous/genital HSV infection in HIV patients: 500 mg twice daily for 7 days or 5-10 days (CDC, 2010)

Prevention of HSV reactivation in HIV patients: 500 mg twice daily (CDC, 2010)

Dosing interval in renal impairment:

Herpes zoster:
Cl_{cr} 40-59 mL/minute: Administer 500 mg every 12 hours
Cl_{cr} 20-39 mL/minute: Administer 500 mg every 24 hours
Cl_{cr} <20 mL/minute: Administer 250 mg every 24 hours
Hemodialysis: Administer 250 mg after each dialysis session.

Recurrent genital herpes: Treatment (single day regimen):
Cl_{cr} 40-59 mL/minute: Administer 500 mg every 12 hours for 1 day
Cl_{cr} 20-39 mL/minute: Administer 500 mg as a single dose
Cl_{cr} <20 mL/minute: Administer 250 mg as a single dose
Hemodialysis: Administer 250 mg as a single dose after dialysis session.

Recurrent genital herpes: Suppression:
Cl_{cr} 20-39 mL/minute: Administer 125 mg every 12 hours
Cl_{cr} <20 mL/minute: Administer 125 mg every 24 hours
Hemodialysis: Administer 125 mg after each dialysis session.

Recurrent herpes labialis: Treatment (single dose regimen):
Cl_{cr} 40-59 mL/minute: Administer 750 mg as a single dose
Cl_{cr} 20-39 mL/minute: Administer 500 mg as a single dose
Cl_{cr} <20 mL/minute: Administer 250 mg as a single dose
Hemodialysis: Administer 250 mg as a single dose after dialysis session.

Recurrent orolabial or genital herpes in HIV-infected patients:
Cl_{cr} 20-39 mL/minute: Administer 500 mg every 24 hours
Cl_{cr} <20 mL/minute: Administer 250 mg every 24 hours
Hemodialysis: Administer 250 mg after each dialysis session.

Mechanism of Action Famciclovir undergoes rapid biotransformation to the active compound, penciclovir (prodrug), which is phosphorylated by viral thymidine kinase in HSV-1, HSV-2, and VZV-infected cells to a monophosphate form; this is then converted to penciclovir triphosphate and competes with deoxyguanosine triphosphate to inhibit HSV-2 polymerase, therefore, herpes viral DNA synthesis/replication is selectively inhibited.

Contraindications Hypersensitivity to famciclovir, penciclovir, or any component of the formulation

Warnings/Precautions Has not been studied in immunocompromised patients or patients with ophthalmic, disseminated zoster, or with initial episode of genital herpes. Dosage adjustment is required in patients with renal insufficiency. Tablets contain lactose; do not use with galactose intolerance, severe lactase deficiency, or glucose-galactose malabsorption syndromes.

Drug Interactions

Avoid Concomitant Use

Avoid concomitant use of Famciclovir with any of the following: Zoster Vaccine

Increased Effect/Toxicity There are no known significant interactions involving an increase in effect.

Decreased Effect

Famciclovir may decrease the levels/effects of: Zoster Vaccine

Ethanol/Nutrition/Herb Interactions Food: Rate of absorption and/or conversion to penciclovir and peak concentration are reduced with food, but bioavailability is not affected.

Dietary Considerations May be taken without regard to meals.

Pharmacodynamics/Kinetics

Half-life Elimination Penciclovir: 2-4 hours; Prolonged in renal impairment: Cl_{cr} 20-39 mL/minute: 5-8 hours, Cl_{cr} <20 mL/minute: 3-24 hours

Time to Peak Penciclovir: 0.9 hours; C_{max} and T_{max} are decreased and prolonged with noncompensated hepatic impairment

Pregnancy Risk Factor B

Lactation Excretion in breast milk unknown/not recommended

Breast-Feeding Considerations There is no specific data describing the excretion of famciclovir in breast milk. Breast-feeding is not recommended by the manufacturer unless the potential benefits outweigh any possible risk. If herpes lesions are on breast, breast-feeding should be avoided in order to avoid transmission to infant.

Dosage Forms

Tablet, oral: 125 mg, 250 mg, 500 mg

Famvir®: 125 mg, 250 mg, 500 mg

Famotidine (fa MOE ti deen)

Related Information

Gastrointestinal Disorders *on page 1874*

U.S. Brand Names Heartburn Relief Maximum Strength [OTC]; Heartburn Relief [OTC]; Pepcid®; Pepcid® AC Maximum Strength [OTC]; Pepcid® AC [OTC]

Canadian Brand Names Acid Control; Apo-Famotidine®; Apo-Famotidine® Injectable; Famotidine Omega; Mylan-Famotidine; Novo-Famotidine; Nu-Famotidine; Pepcid®; Pepcid® AC; Pepcid® I.V.; Ulcidine

Generic Availability (U.S.) Yes: Infusion, Injection, oral suspension, tablet

Pharmacologic Category Histamine H_2 Antagonist

Use Maintenance therapy and treatment of duodenal ulcer; treatment of gastroesophageal reflux disease (GERD), active benign gastric ulcer; pathological hypersecretory conditions

OTC labeling: Relief of heartburn, acid indigestion, and sour stomach

Unlabeled/Investigational Use Part of a multidrug regimen for *H. pylori* eradication to reduce the risk of duodenal ulcer recurrence; stress ulcer prophylaxis in critically-ill patients; symptomatic relief in gastritis

Local Anesthetic/Vasoconstrictor Precautions No information available to require special precautions

Effects on Dental Treatment No significant effects or complications reported

Effects on Bleeding No information available to require special precautions

Adverse Effects

Note: Agitation and vomiting have been reported in up to 14% of pediatric patients <1 year of age.

1% to 10%:

Central nervous system: Headache (5%), dizziness (1%)

Gastrointestinal: Diarrhea (2%), constipation (1%)

Dosage

Children: Treatment duration and dose should be individualized

Peptic ulcer: 1-16 years:

Oral: 0.5 mg/kg/day at bedtime or divided twice daily (maximum dose: 40 mg/day); doses of up to 1 mg/kg/day have been used in clinical studies

I.V.: 0.25 mg/kg every 12 hours (maximum dose: 40 mg/day); doses of up to 0.5 mg/kg have been used in clinical studies

GERD: Oral:

<3 months: 0.5 mg/kg once daily

3-12 months: 0.5 mg/kg twice daily

1-16 years: 1 mg/kg/day divided twice daily (maximum dose: 40 mg twice daily); doses of up to 2 mg/kg/day have been used in clinical studies

Children ≥12 years and Adults: Heartburn, indigestion, sour stomach: OTC labeling: Oral: 10-20 mg every 12 hours; dose may be taken 15-60 minutes before eating foods known to cause heartburn

Adults:

Duodenal ulcer: Oral: Acute therapy: 40 mg/day at bedtime (or 20 mg twice daily) for 4-8 weeks; maintenance therapy: 20 mg/day at bedtime

Helicobacter pylori eradication (unlabeled use): Oral: 40 mg once daily; requires combination therapy with antibiotics

Gastric ulcer: Oral: Acute therapy: 40 mg/day at bedtime

Hypersecretory conditions: Oral: Initial: 20 mg every 6 hours, may increase in increments up to 160 mg every 6 hours

GERD: Oral: 20 mg twice daily for 6 weeks

Esophagitis and accompanying symptoms due to GERD: Oral: 20 mg or 40 mg twice daily for up to 12 weeks

Patients unable to take oral medication: I.V.: 20 mg every 12 hours

Dosing adjustment in renal impairment: Cl_{cr} <50 mL/minute: Manufacturer recommendation: Administer 50% of dose **or** increase the dosing interval to every 36-48 hours (to limit potential CNS adverse effects).

Mechanism of Action Competitive inhibition of histamine at H_2 receptors of the gastric parietal cells, which inhibits gastric acid secretion

Contraindications Hypersensitivity to famotidine, other H_2 antagonists, or any component of the formulation

Warnings/Precautions Modify dose in patients with moderate-to-severe renal impairment. Relief of symptoms does not preclude the presence of a gastric malignancy. Reversible confusional states, usually clearing within 3-4 days after discontinuation, have been linked to use. Increased age (>50 years) and renal or hepatic impairment are thought to be associated. Multidose vials for injection contain benzyl alcohol.

OTC labeling: When used for self-medication, patients should be instructed not to use if they have difficulty swallowing, are vomiting blood, or have bloody or black stools. Not for use with other acid reducers.

Drug Interactions

Avoid Concomitant Use

Avoid concomitant use of Famotidine with any of the following: Delavirdine; Erlotinib

Increased Effect/Toxicity

Famotidine may increase the levels/effects of: Dexmethylphenidate; Methylphenidate; Saquinavir

Decreased Effect

Famotidine may decrease the levels/effects of: Atazanavir; Cefditoren; Cefpodoxime; Cefuroxime; Dasatinib; Delavirdine; Erlotinib; Fosamprenavir; Gefitinib; Indinavir; Iron Salts; Itraconazole; Ketoconazole; Ketoconazole (Systemic); Mesalamine; Nelfinavir; Posaconazole

Ethanol/Nutrition/Herb Interactions

Ethanol: Avoid ethanol (may cause gastric mucosal irritation).

Food: Famotidine bioavailability may be increased if taken with food.

Dietary Considerations May be taken without regard to meals.

Pharmacodynamics/Kinetics

Onset of Action Antisecretory effect: Oral: Within 1 hour; I.V.: Within 30 minutes

Peak effect: Antisecretory effect: Oral: Within 1-3 hours (dose-dependent)

Duration of Action Antisecretory effect: I.V., Oral: 10-12 hours

Half-life Elimination

Infants: 0-3 months: ~8-10.5 hours; >3-12 months: ~4.5 hours

Children: 3.4 hours

Adults: 2.5-3.5 hours; prolonged with renal impairment; Oliguria: >20 hours

Time to Peak Serum: Oral: ~1-3 hours

Pregnancy Risk Factor B

Lactation Enters breast milk/not recommended

Breast-Feeding Considerations Famotidine is excreted into breast milk with peak concentrations occurring ~6 hours after the maternal dose. According to the manufacturer, the decision to continue or discontinue breast-feeding during therapy should take into account the risk of exposure to the infant and the benefits of treatment to the mother.

Dosage Forms

Infusion, premixed in NS [preservative free]: 20 mg (50 mL)

Injection, solution: 10 mg/mL (4 mL, 20 mL, 50 mL)

Injection, solution [preservative free]: 10 mg/mL (2 mL)

Powder for suspension, oral: 40 mg/5 mL (50 mL)

Pepcid®: 40 mg/5 mL (50 mL)

Tablet, oral: 10 mg, 20 mg, 40 mg
Heartburn Relief [OTC]: 10 mg
Heartburn Relief Maximum Strength [OTC]: 20 mg
Pepcid®: 20 mg, 40 mg
Pepcid® AC [OTC]: 10 mg
Pepcid® AC Maximum Strength [OTC]: 20 mg
Tablet, chewable, oral:
Pepcid® AC Maximum Strength [OTC]: 20 mg

Famotidine, Calcium Carbonate, and Magnesium Hydroxide (fa MOE ti deen, KAL see um KAR bun ate, & mag NEE zhum hye DROKS ide)

Related Information
Calcium Carbonate *on page 286*
Famotidine *on page 706*
Magnesium Hydroxide *on page 1049*

U.S. Brand Names Pepcid® Complete® [OTC]; Tums® Dual Action [OTC]

Canadian Brand Names Pepcid® Complete® [OTC]

Pharmacologic Category Antacid; Histamine H_2 Antagonist

Use Relief of heartburn due to acid indigestion

Local Anesthetic/Vasoconstrictor Precautions No information available to require special precautions

Effects on Dental Treatment No significant effects or complications reported

Effects on Bleeding No information available to require special precautions

Adverse Effects See individual agents.

General Dosage Range Oral: *Children ≥12 years and Adults:* 1 tablet (famotidine 10 mg/calcium carbonate 800 mg/magnesium hydroxide 165 mg) as needed (maximum: 2 tablets/day)

Mechanism of Action
Famotidine: H_2 antagonist
Calcium carbonate: Antacid
Magnesium hydroxide: Antacid

Fat Emulsion (fat e MUL shun)

U.S. Brand Names Intralipid®; Liposyn® II [DSC]; Liposyn® III

Canadian Brand Names Intralipid®; Liposyn® II

Pharmacologic Category Caloric Agent

Use Source of calories and essential fatty acids for patients requiring parenteral nutrition of extended duration; prevention and treatment of essential fatty acid deficiency (EFAD)

Unlabeled/Investigational Use Local anesthetic-induced cardiac arrest unresponsive to conventional resuscitation

Local Anesthetic/Vasoconstrictor Precautions No information available to require special precautions

Effects on Dental Treatment No significant effects or complications reported

Effects on Bleeding No information available to require special precautions

Adverse Effects <1%: Allergic reactions, back pain, brown pigment deposition in the reticuloendothelial system ("intravenous fat pigment"), chest pain, cholestasis, cyanosis, diaphoresis, dizziness, dyspnea, flushing, headache, hepatomegaly, hypercoagulability, hyperlipidemia, infusion site irritation, jaundice, leucopenia, liver function tests increased, nausea, pancreatitis, overloading syndrome (focal seizures, fever, leukocytosis, hepatomegaly, splenomegaly, shock), thrombocytopenia, vomiting

General Dosage Range I.V.:
Premature infants: Initial: 0.25-0.5 g/kg/day; Maintenance: Up to 3 g/kg/day (≤1 g/kg/day if on phototherapy)
Infants and Children: Initial: 0.5-1 g/kg/day; Maintenance: Up to 3 g/kg/day
Adults: Initial: 1 g/kg/day; Maintenance: Up to 2.5-3 g/kg/day **or** 500 mL twice weekly

Mechanism of Action Fat emulsion is metabolized and utilized as an energy source; provides the essential fatty acids, linoleic acid, and alpha linolenic acid necessary for normal structure and function of cell membranes; in local anesthetic toxicity, lipid emulsion probably extracts lipophilic local anesthesia from cardiac muscle

Pharmacodynamics/Kinetics
Half-life Elimination 0.5-1 hour

Pregnancy Risk Factor C

Febuxostat (feb UX oh stat)

U.S. Brand Names Uloric®

Canadian Brand Names Uloric®

Pharmacologic Category Xanthine Oxidase Inhibitor

Use Chronic management of hyperuricemia in patients with gout

Local Anesthetic/Vasoconstrictor Precautions No information available to require special precautions

Effects on Dental Treatment Key adverse event(s) related to dental treatment: Xerostomia (normal salivary flow resumes upon discontinuation) and taste alteration has been reported in <1% of patients.

Effects on Bleeding No information available to require special precautions

Adverse Effects 1% to 10%:

Dermatologic: Rash (1% to 2%)

Hepatic: Liver function abnormalities (5% to 7%)

Neuromuscular & skeletal: Arthralgia (1%)

General Dosage Range Oral: *Adults:* 40-80 mg once daily

Mechanism of Action Selectively inhibits xanthine oxidase, the enzyme responsible for the conversion of hypoxanthine to xanthine to uric acid thereby decreasing uric acid. At therapeutic concentration does not inhibit other enzymes involved in purine and pyrimidine synthesis.

Pharmacodynamics/Kinetics

Half-life Elimination ~5-8 hours

Time to Peak Plasma: 1-1.5 hours

Pregnancy Risk Factor C

Felbamate (FEL ba mate)

U.S. Brand Names Felbatol®

Pharmacologic Category Anticonvulsant, Miscellaneous

Use Not as a first-line antiepileptic treatment; only in those patients who respond inadequately to alternative treatments and whose epilepsy is so severe that a substantial risk of aplastic anemia and/or liver failure is deemed acceptable in light of the benefits conferred by its use. Patient must be fully advised of risk and provide signed written informed consent. Felbamate can be used as either monotherapy or adjunctive therapy in the treatment of partial seizures (with and without generalization) and in adults with epilepsy. Used as adjunctive therapy in the treatment of partial and generalized seizures associated with Lennox-Gastaut syndrome in children.

Local Anesthetic/Vasoconstrictor Precautions No information available to require special precautions

Effects on Dental Treatment Key adverse event(s) related to dental treatment: Xerostomia (normal salivary flow resumes upon discontinuation) and abnormal taste.

Effects on Bleeding Has been associated with rare aplastic anemia. No information available to require routine special precautions.

Adverse Effects

>10%:

Central nervous system: Somnolence (children 48%; adults 19%), headache (children 7%; adults 7% to 37%), fever (children 23%; adults 3%), dizziness (18%), insomnia (9% to 18%), fatigue (7% to 17%), nervousness (7% to 16%)

Dermatologic: Purpura (children 13%)

Gastrointestinal: Anorexia (children 55%; adults 19%), vomiting (children 39%; adults 9% to 17%), nausea (children 7%; adults 34%), constipation (7% to 13%), dyspepsia (7% to 12%)

Respiratory: Upper respiratory infection (children 45%; adults 5% to 9%)

1% to 10%:

Cardiovascular: Chest pain (3%), facial edema (3%), palpitation (≥1%), tachycardia (≥1%)

Central nervous system: Nervousness (7% to 16%), abnormal thinking (7%), emotional lability (children 7%), ataxia (4% to 7%), depression (5%), anxiety (5%), stupor (3%), malaise (≥1%), agitation (≥1%), psychological disturbances (≥1%), aggressive reaction (≥1%), euphoria (≤1%), hallucination (≤1%), migraine (≤1%), suicide attempt (≤1%)

Dermatologic: Skin rash (children 10%; adults 3% to 4%), acne (3%), pruritus (≥1%), bullous eruption (≤1%), urticaria (≤1%)

Endocrine and metabolic: Hypophosphatemia (≤1% to 3%), intramenstrual bleeding (3%), hypokalemia (≤1%), hyponatremia (≤1%)

Gastrointestinal: Hiccup (children 10%), weight loss (3% to 7%), taste perversion (6%), diarrhea (5%), abdominal pain (5%), xerostomia (3%), weight gain (≥1%), appetite increased (≤1%), esophagitis (≤1%)
Genitourinary: Urinary tract infection (3%)
Hematologic: Leukopenia (1% to 7%), granulocytopenia (≤1%), lymphadenopathy (≤1%), leukocytosis (≤1%), thrombocytopenia (≤1%)
Hepatic: Liver function tests increased (1% to 4%), alkaline phosphatase increased (≤1%)
Neuromuscular & skeletal: Abnormal gait (children 10%; adults 5%), pain (children 7%), tremor (6%), paresthesia (4%), myalgia (3%), weakness (≥1%), dystonia (≤1%)
Ocular: Miosis (7%), diplopia (3% to 6%), abnormal vision (5%)
Otic: Otitis media (children 10%; adults 3%)
Respiratory: Pharyngitis (children 10%; adults 3%), cough (children 7%), rhinitis (7%), sinusitis (4%)
Miscellaneous: Flu-like syndrome (≥1%), lymphadenopathy (≥1%)

General Dosage Range Dosage adjustment recommended in patients with renal impairment or on concomitant therapy

Oral:

Children 2-14 years: Initial: 15 mg/kg/day in divided doses 3 or 4 times/day; Maintenance: Up to 45 mg/kg/day in divided doses 3 or 4 times/day (maximum: 3600 mg/day)

Children >14 years and Adults: Initial: 1200 mg/day in divided doses 3 or 4 times/day; Maintenance: Up to 3600 mg/day in divided doses 3 or 4 times/day.

Mechanism of Action Mechanism of action is unknown but has properties in common with other marketed anticonvulsants; has weak inhibitory effects on GABA-receptor binding, benzodiazepine receptor binding, and is devoid of activity at the MK-801 receptor binding site of the NMDA receptor-ionophore complex.

Pharmacodynamics/Kinetics

Half-life Elimination 20-23 hours (average); prolonged in renal dysfunction

Time to Peak Serum: 3-5 hours

Pregnancy Risk Factor C

Prescribing and Access Restrictions A patient "informed consent" form should be completed and signed by the patient and physician. Copies are available from MEDA Pharmaceuticals by calling 800-526-3840.

Felodipine (fe LOE di peen)

Related Information

Calcium Channel Blockers and Gingival Hyperplasia *on page 2014*
Cardiovascular Diseases *on page 1848*

Canadian Brand Names Plendil®; Renedil®

Pharmacologic Category Calcium Channel Blocker; Calcium Channel Blocker, Dihydropyridine

Use Treatment of hypertension

Unlabeled/Investigational Use Pediatric hypertension

Local Anesthetic/Vasoconstrictor Precautions No information available to require special precautions

Effects on Dental Treatment Key adverse event(s) related to dental treatment: Gingival hyperplasia (fewer reports than other CCBs, resolves upon discontinuation, consultation with physician is suggested).

Effects on Bleeding No information available to require special precautions

Adverse Effects

>10%: Central nervous system: Headache (11% to 15%)
2% to 10%: Cardiovascular: Peripheral edema (2% to 17%), tachycardia (0.4% to 2.5%), flushing (4% to 7%)

General Dosage Range Dosage adjustment recommended in patients with hepatic impairment

Oral:

Adults: Initial: 2.5-10 mg once daily; Maintenance: 2.5-20 mg once daily (maximum: 20 mg/day)

Elderly: Initial: 2.5 mg/day

Mechanism of Action Inhibits calcium ions from entering the "slow channels" or select voltage-sensitive areas of vascular smooth muscle and myocardium during depolarization, producing a relaxation of coronary vascular smooth muscle and coronary vasodilation; increases myocardial oxygen delivery in patients with vasospastic angina

Pharmacodynamics/Kinetics

Onset of Action Antihypertensive: 2-5 hours

Duration of Action Antihypertensive effect: 24 hours

Half-life Elimination Immediate release: 11-16 hours

Pregnancy Risk Factor C

Fenofibrate (fen oh FYE brate)

Related Information

Cardiovascular Diseases *on page 1848*

U.S. Brand Names Antara®; Fenoglide®; Lipofen®; Lofibra®; TriCor®; Triglide®

Canadian Brand Names Apo-Feno-Micro®; Apo-Feno-Super®; Apo-Fenofibrate®; Dom-Fenofibrate Micro; Feno-Micro-200; Fenofibrate Micro; Fenofibrate-S; Fenomax; Lipidil EZ®; Lipidil Micro®; Lipidil Supra®; Mylan-Fenofibrate Micro; Novo-Fenofibrate; Novo-Fenofibrate Micronized; Novo-Fenofibrate-S; Nu-Fenofibrate; PHL-Fenofibrate Micro; PHL-Fenofibrate Supra; PMS-Fenofibrate Micro; PRO-Feno-Super; ratio-Fenofibrate MC; Riva-Fenofibrate Micro; Sandoz-Fenofibrate S

Generic Availability (U.S.) Yes: Micronized capsule and tablet

Pharmacologic Category Antilipemic Agent, Fibric Acid

Use Adjunct to dietary therapy for the treatment of adults with elevations of serum triglyceride levels (types IV and V hyperlipidemia); adjunct to dietary therapy for the reduction of low density lipoprotein cholesterol (LDL-C), total cholesterol (total-C), triglycerides, and apolipoprotein B (apo B), and to increase high density lipoprotein cholesterol (HDL-C) in adult patients with primary hypercholesterolemia or mixed dyslipidemia (Fredrickson types IIa and IIb)

Local Anesthetic/Vasoconstrictor Precautions No information available to require special precautions

Effects on Dental Treatment Key adverse event(s) related to dental treatment: Dry mouth and tooth disorder.

Effects on Bleeding No information available to require special precautions

Adverse Effects

>10%: Hepatic: Liver function tests increased (dose related; 3% to 13%)

1% to 10%:

- Central nervous system: Headache (3%)
- Gastrointestinal: Abdominal pain (5%), constipation (2%), nausea (2%)
- Neuromuscular & skeletal: Back pain (3%), CPK increased (3%)
- Respiratory: Respiratory disorder (6%), rhinitis (2%)

Dosage Oral:

Adults:

Hypertriglyceridemia: Initial:

- Antara® (micronized): 43-130 mg/day; maximum dose: 130 mg/day
- Fenoglide®: 40-120 mg/day; maximum dose: 120 mg/day
- Lipidil EZ® [CAN; not available in U.S.]: 145 mg/day; maximum dose: 145 mg/day
- Lipidil Micro® [CAN; not available in U.S.]: 200 mg/day; maximum dose: 200 mg/day
- Lipidil Supra® [CAN; not available in U.S.]: 160 mg/day; maximum dose: 200 mg/day
- Lipofen®: 50-150 mg/day; maximum dose: 150 mg/day
- Lofibra® (micronized): 67-200 mg/day with meals; maximum dose: 200 mg/day
- Lofibra® (tablets): 54-160 mg/day; maximum dose: 160 mg/day
- TriCor®: 48-145 mg/day; maximum dose: 145 mg/day
- Triglide®: 50-160 mg/day; maximum dose: 160 mg/day

Hypercholesterolemia or mixed hyperlipidemia:

- Antara® (micronized): 130 mg/day
- Fenoglide®: 120 mg/day
- Lipidil EZ® [CAN; not available in U.S.]: 145 mg/day; maximum dose: 145 mg/day
- Lipidil Micro® [CAN; not available in U.S.]: 200 mg/day; maximum dose: 200 mg/day
- Lipidil Supra® [CAN; not available in U.S.]: 160 mg/day; maximum dose: 200 mg/day
- Lipofen®: 150 mg/day
- Lofibra® (micronized): 200 mg/day
- Lofibra® (tablets): 160 mg/day
- TriCor®: 145 mg/day
- Triglide®: 160 mg/day

Elderly: Initial:
- Antara® (micronized): 43 mg/day
- Fenoglide®: Adjust dosage based on creatinine clearance
- Lipidil EZ® [CAN; not available in U.S.]: 48 mg/day
- Lipidil Micro® [CAN; not available in U.S.]: Adjust dosage based on creatinine clearance
- Lipidil Supra® [CAN; not available in U.S.]: Adjust dosage based on creatinine clearance
- Lipofen®: 50 mg/day
- Lofibra® (micronized): 67 mg/day
- Lofibra® (tablets): 54 mg/day
- TriCor®: Adjust dosage based on creatinine clearance
- Triglide®: 50 mg/day

Dosage adjustment/interval in renal impairment: Monitor renal function and lipid panel before adjusting. Decrease dose or increase dosing interval for patients with renal failure: **Note:** Use in severe renal impairment is contraindicated (see specific product labeling):
- Antara® (micronized): 43 mg/day
- Fenoglide®: Cl_{cr} 31-80 mL/minute: 40 mg/day
- Lipidil EZ® [CAN; not available in U.S.]: Cl_{cr} ≥20-50 mL/minute: 48 mg/day
- Lipidil Micro® [CAN; not available in U.S.]: Cl_{cr} ≥20-100 mL/minute: 67 mg/day; **Note:** Lipidil Micro® 67 mg capsules are discontinued in Canada. Micronized formulation at this dosage strength is available through other manufacturers in Canada.
- Lipidil Supra® [CAN; not available in U.S.]: Cl_{cr} ≥20-100 mL/minute: 100 mg/day
- Lipofen®: 50 mg/day
- Lofibra® (micronized): 67 mg/day
- Lofibra® (tablets): 54 mg/day
- TriCor®: Cl_{cr} 31-80 mL/minute: 48 mg/day
- Triglide®: 50 mg/day

Mechanism of Action Fenofibric acid, an agonist for the nuclear transcription factor peroxisome proliferator-activated receptor-alpha (PPAR-alpha), downregulates apoprotein C-III (an inhibitor of lipoprotein lipase) and upregulates the synthesis of apolipoprotein A-I, fatty acid transport protein, and lipoprotein lipase resulting in an increase in VLDL catabolism, fatty acid oxidation, and elimination of triglyceride-rich particles; as a result of a decrease in VLDL levels, total plasma triglycerides are reduced by 30% to 60%; modest increase in HDL occurs in some hypertriglyceridemic patients.

Contraindications Hypersensitivity to fenofibrate or any component of the formulation; hepatic dysfunction including primary biliary cirrhosis and unexplained persistent liver function abnormalities; severe renal dysfunction; pre-existing gallbladder disease; breast-feeding (only Fenoglide®)

Canadian labeling: Additional contraindications (not in U.S. labeling): Pregnancy; breast-feeding; known photoallergy or phototoxic reaction during treatment with fibrates or ketoprofen; allergy to soya lecithin or peanut or arachis oil

Warnings/Precautions Secondary causes of hyperlipidemia should be ruled out prior to therapy. Hepatic transaminases can become significantly elevated (dose-related); hepatocellular, chronic active, and cholestatic hepatitis have been reported. Regular monitoring of liver function tests is required. Increases in serum creatinine (>2 mg/dL) have been observed with use; monitor renal function in patients with renal impairment and consider monitoring patients with increased risk for developing renal impairment. May cause cholelithiasis. Use with caution in patient taking oral anticoagulants (eg, warfarin); adjustments in anticoagulation therapy may be required. Use caution with HMG-CoA reductase inhibitors (may lead to myopathy, rhabdomyolysis). In combination with HMG-CoA reductase inhibitors, fenofibrate is generally regarded as safer than gemfibrozil due to limited pharmacokinetic interaction with statins. Therapy should be withdrawn if an adequate response is not obtained after 2-3 months of therapy at the maximal daily dose. The occurrence of pancreatitis may represent a failure of efficacy in patients with severely elevated triglycerides. May cause mild-to-moderate decreases in hemoglobin, hematocrit, and WBC upon initiation of therapy which usually stabilizes with long-term therapy. Agranulocytosis and thrombocytopenia have rarely been reported. Periodic monitoring of blood counts is recommended during the first year of therapy.

Rare hypersensitivity reactions may occur. Use has been associated with pulmonary embolism (PE) and deep vein thrombosis (DVT). Use with caution in patients with risk factors for VTE. Dose adjustment is required for renal impairment and may be required for elderly patients.

Drug Interactions

Metabolism/Transport Effects **Substrate** of CYP3A4 (minor); **Inhibits** CYP2A6 (weak), 2C8 (weak), 2C9 (weak), 2C19 (weak)

Avoid Concomitant Use There are no known interactions where it is recommended to avoid concomitant use.

Increased Effect/Toxicity

Fenofibrate may increase the levels/effects of: Colchicine; Ezetimibe; HMG-CoA Reductase Inhibitors; Sulfonylureas; Vitamin K Antagonists; Warfarin

The levels/effects of Fenofibrate may be increased by: Conivaptan; CycloSPORINE; CycloSPORINE (Systemic)

Decreased Effect

Fenofibrate may decrease the levels/effects of: Chenodiol; CycloSPORINE; CycloSPORINE (Systemic); Ursodiol

The levels/effects of Fenofibrate may be decreased by: Bile Acid Sequestrants; Tocilizumab

Dietary Considerations

Fenoglide®, Lofibra® (capsules [micronized] and tablets), Lipofen®: Take with meals.

Antara®, TriCor®, Triglide®: May be taken with or without food.

Canadian products [not available in U.S.]:

Lipidil Micro®, Lipidil Supra®: Take with meals.

Lipidil EZ®: May be taken with or without food.

Pharmacodynamics/Kinetics

Half-life Elimination Half-life elimination: Fenofibric acid: Mean: 20 hours (range: 10-35 hours)

Time to Peak 3-8 hours

Pregnancy Risk Factor C

Lactation Excretion in breast milk unknown/not recommended

Breast-Feeding Considerations Tumor formation was observed in animal studies; nursing is not recommended if the medication cannot be discontinued.

Dosage Forms

Capsule, oral: 67 mg, 134 mg, 200 mg

Antara®: 43 mg, 130 mg

Lipofen®: 50 mg, 150 mg

Lofibra®: 67 mg, 134 mg, 200 mg

Tablet, oral: 54 mg, 160 mg

Fenoglide®: 40 mg, 120 mg

Lofibra®: 54 mg, 160 mg

TriCor®: 48 mg, 145 mg

Triglide®: 50 mg, 160 mg

Fenofibric Acid (fen oh FYE brik AS id)

U.S. Brand Names Fibricor™; TriLipix®

Generic Availability (U.S.) Yes

Pharmacologic Category Antilipemic Agent, Fibric Acid

Use Adjunct to dietary therapy for the treatment of severely elevated serum triglyceride levels; adjunct to dietary therapy for the reduction of low density lipoprotein cholesterol (LDL-C), total cholesterol (total-C), triglycerides, and apolipoprotein B (apo B) and to increase high density lipoprotein cholesterol (HDL-C) in patients with primary hypercholesterolemia or mixed dyslipidemia

TriLipix™ is also indicated as adjunct to dietary therapy concomitantly with a statin to reduce triglyceride levels and increase HDL-C levels in patients with mixed dyslipidemia and coronary heart disease (CHD) or at risk for CHD

Local Anesthetic/Vasoconstrictor Precautions No information available to require special precautions

Effects on Dental Treatment No significant effects or complications reported

Effects on Bleeding No information available to require special precautions

Adverse Effects Adverse reactions and frequency reported as observed during monotherapy and concurrent administration with a statin (HMG-CoA reductase inhibitor).

>10%: Central nervous system: Headache (12% to 13%)

1% to 10%:

Central nervous system: Dizziness (3% to 4%), pain (1% to 4%), fatigue (2% to 3%)

Gastrointestinal: Nausea (4% to 6%), dyspepsia (3% to 5%), diarrhea (3% to 4%), constipation (3%)

Hepatic: ALT increased (monotherapy: 1%; coadministered with statin: 3%)

Neuromuscular & skeletal: Back pain (4% to 6%), pain in extremities (3% to 5%), arthralgia (4%), myalgia (3% to 4%), muscle spasm (2% to 3%)

Respiratory: Nasopharyngitis (4% to 5%), upper respiratory infection (4% to 5%), sinusitis (3% to 4%)

Additional adverse reactions when fenofibric acid coadministered with a statin (frequency not defined): AST increased, bronchitis, cough, CPK increased, hepatic enzymes increased, hypertension, influenza, insomnia, musculoskeletal pain, pharyngolaryngeal pain, urinary tract infection

Dosage Oral:

Adults:

Mixed dyslipidemia (coadministered with a statin): TriLipix™: 135 mg once daily (maximum: 135 mg/day)

Hypertriglyceridemia:

Fibricor™: Initial: 35-105 mg once daily; Maintenance: Individualize according to patient response (maximum: 105 mg/day)

TriLipix™: Initial: 45-135 mg once daily; Maintenance: Individualize according to patient response (maximum: 135 mg/day)

Primary hypercholesterolemia or mixed dyslipidemia:

Fibricor™: 105 mg once daily (maximum: 105 mg/day)

TriLipix™: 135 mg once daily (maximum: 135 mg/day)

Elderly: Dosage based on renal function

Dosage adjustment/interval in renal impairment:

Mild-to-moderate impairment (Cl_{cr} 30-80 mL/minute): Initial: Fibricor™: 35 mg once daily or TriLipix™: 45 mg once daily; only increase once effects on lipids and renal function evaluated

Severe impairment (Cl_{cr} <30 mL/minute; with or without dialysis): Contraindicated

Mechanism of Action Fenofibric acid, an agonist for the nuclear transcription factor peroxisome proliferator-activated receptor-alpha (PPAR-alpha), downregulates apoprotein C-III (an inhibitor of lipoprotein lipase) and upregulates the synthesis of apolipoprotein A-I, fatty acid transport protein, and lipoprotein lipase resulting in an increase in VLDL catabolism, fatty acid oxidation, and elimination of triglyceride-rich particles; as a result of a decrease in VLDL levels, total plasma triglycerides are reduced by 30% to 60%; modest increased in HDL occurs in some hypertriglyceridemia patients.

Contraindications Hypersensitivity to fenofibric acid, choline fenofibrate, fenofibrate, or any component of the formulation; hepatic dysfunction including primary biliary cirrhosis and unexplained persistent liver function abnormalities; severe renal dysfunction (including patients on dialysis); pre-existing gallbladder disease; breast-feeding

Warnings/Precautions Secondary causes of hyperlipidemia should be ruled out prior to therapy. Has been associated with rare myositis or rhabdomyolysis; patients should be monitored closely. Risk increased in the elderly, patients with diabetes mellitus, renal failure, or hypothyroidism. Patients should be instructed to report unexplained muscle pain, tenderness, weakness, or brown urine. Hepatic transaminases can become significantly elevated (dose-related); hepatocellular, chronic active, and cholestatic hepatitis have been reported. Regular monitoring of liver function tests is required. Increases in serum creatinine (>2 mg/dL) have been observed with use; monitor renal function in patients with renal impairment and consider monitoring patients with increased risk for developing renal impairment. May cause cholelithiasis discontinue if gallstones found upon gallbladder studies. Use caution with oral anticoagulants; adjustments in therapy may be required.

Use caution with HMG-CoA reductase inhibitors (may lead to myopathy, rhabdomyolysis). In combination with HMG-CoA reductase inhibitors, fenofibric acid derivatives are generally regarded as safer than gemfibrozil due to limited pharmacokinetic interaction. Therapy should be withdrawn if an adequate response is not obtained after 2-3 months of therapy at the maximal daily dose. The occurrence of pancreatitis may represent a failure of efficacy in patients with severely elevated triglycerides. May cause mild-to-moderate decreases in hemoglobin, hematocrit, and WBC upon initiation of therapy, which usually stabilizes with long-term therapy. Rare hypersensitivity reactions may occur. Use has been associated with pulmonary embolism (PE) and deep vein thrombosis (DVT). Use with caution in patients with risk factors for VTE. Dose adjustment is required for renal impairment and elderly patients.

Drug Interactions

Avoid Concomitant Use There are no known interactions where it is recommended to avoid concomitant use.

Increased Effect/Toxicity

Fenofibric Acid may increase the levels/effects of: Carvedilol; Colchicine; CYP2C9 Substrates (High risk); Ezetimibe; HMG-CoA Reductase Inhibitors; Sulfonylureas; Vitamin K Antagonists; Warfarin

The levels/effects of Fenofibric Acid may be increased by: CycloSPORINE; CycloSPORINE (Systemic)

Decreased Effect

Fenofibric Acid may decrease the levels/effects of: Chenodiol; CycloSPORINE; CycloSPORINE (Systemic); Ursodiol

The levels/effects of Fenofibric Acid may be decreased by: Bile Acid Sequestrants

Dietary Considerations May be taken with or without food. Patients should follow appropriate lipid-lowering diet.

Pharmacodynamics/Kinetics

Half-life Elimination ~20 hours

Time to Peak Fibricor™: ~2.5 hours; TriLipix™: 4-5 hours

Pregnancy Risk Factor C

Lactation Excretion in breast milk unknown/contraindicated

Dosage Forms

Capsule, delayed release, oral:

TriLipix®: 45 mg, 135 mg

Tablet, oral: 35 mg, 105 mg

Fibricor™: 35 mg, 105 mg

Fenoldopam (fe NOL doe pam)

U.S. Brand Names Corlopam®

Canadian Brand Names Corlopam®

Pharmacologic Category Dopamine Agonist

Use Treatment of severe hypertension (up to 48 hours in adults), including in patients with renal compromise; short-term (up to 4 hours) blood pressure reduction in pediatric patients

Local Anesthetic/Vasoconstrictor Precautions No information available to require special precautions

Effects on Dental Treatment Key adverse event(s) related to dental treatment: Xerostomia and changes in salivation (normal salivary flow resumes upon discontinuation).

Effects on Bleeding No information available to require special precautions

Adverse Effects Frequency not always defined.

Cardiovascular: Angina, asymptomatic T wave flattening on ECG, chest pain, edema, facial flushing (>5%), fibrillation (atrial), flutter (atrial), hypotension (>5%), tachycardia

Central nervous system: Dizziness, headache (>5%)

Endocrine & metabolic: Hypokalemia

Gastrointestinal: Abdominal pain/fullness, diarrhea, nausea (>5%), vomiting, xerostomia

Local: Injection site reactions

Ocular: Intraocular pressure increased, blurred vision

Hepatic: Increases in portal pressure in cirrhotic patients

General Dosage Range I.V.:

Children: Initial: 0.2 mcg/kg/minute, may increase to 0.3-0.5 mcg/kg/minute every 20-30 minutes (maximum: 0.8 mcg/kg/minute)

Adults: Initial: 0.1-0.3 mcg/kg/minute, may increase in increments of 0.05-0.1 mcg/kg/minute every 15 minutes (maximum: 1.6 mcg/kg/minute)

Mechanism of Action A selective postsynaptic dopamine agonist (D_1-receptors) which exerts hypotensive effects by decreasing peripheral vasculature resistance with increased renal blood flow, diuresis, and natriuresis; 6 times as potent as dopamine in producing renal vasodilitation; has minimal adrenergic effects

Pharmacodynamics/Kinetics

Onset of Action I.V.: 10 minutes

Duration of Action I.V.: 1 hour

Half-life Elimination I.V.: Children: 3-5 minutes; Adults: ~5 minutes

Pregnancy Risk Factor B

Fenoprofen (fen oh PROE fen)

Related Information

Rheumatoid Arthritis, Osteoarthritis, and Osteoporosis *on page* 1889

Temporomandibular Dysfunction (TMD) *on page* 1964

U.S. Brand Names Nalfon®

Canadian Brand Names Nalfon®

Generic Availability (U.S.) Yes: Tablet

Pharmacologic Category Nonsteroidal Anti-inflammatory Drug (NSAID), Oral

Use Symptomatic treatment of acute and chronic rheumatoid arthritis and osteoarthritis; relief of mild-to-moderate pain

Local Anesthetic/Vasoconstrictor Precautions No information available to require special precautions

Effects on Dental Treatment The dentist should be aware of the potential of abnormal coagulation. Caution should also be exercised in the use of NSAIDs in patients already on anticoagulant therapy with drugs such as warfarin (Coumadin®). See Effects on Bleeding.

Effects on Bleeding Nonselective NSAIDs are known to reversibly decrease platelet aggregation via mechanisms different than observed with aspirin. Platelet function is restored as the drug is eliminated from the body. Dental professionals should be aware that recommendations differ between dental and general medical surgery. NSAIDs should be avoided (if possible) in general medical surgery patients for 3-5 half-lives of the drug (usually 1-3 days) prior to surgery to reduce the risk of excessive bleeding. However, there is no scientific evidence to warrant discontinuance of NSAIDs prior to dental surgery. In medically complicated patients or extensive oral surgery, the decision to interrupt therapy must be based on the risk to benefit in an individual patient and a medical consult is suggested. Routine interruption of NSAID therapy for most dental procedures is not warranted. If therapy is continued without interruption, the clinician should anticipate the potential for slower clotting times.

Adverse Effects 1% to 10%:

Cardiovascular: Peripheral edema (5%), palpitation (3%)

Central nervous system: Headache (9%), somnolence (9%), dizziness (7%), nervousness (6%), fatigue (2%), confusion (1%)

Dermatologic: Itching (4%), rash (4%)

Gastrointestinal: Dyspepsia (10%), nausea (8%), constipation (7%), vomiting (3%), abdominal pain (2%)

Neuromuscular & skeletal: Weakness (5%), tremor (2%)

Ocular: Blurred vision (2%)

Otic: Tinnitus (5%), hearing decreased (2%)

Respiratory: Dyspnea (3%), nasopharyngitis (1%)

Miscellaneous: Diaphoresis (5%)

Dosage Adults: Oral:

Rheumatoid arthritis, osteoarthritis: 300-600 mg 3-4 times/day; maximum dose: 3.2 g/day

Mild-to-moderate pain: 200 mg every 4-6 hours as needed; maximum dose: 3.2 g/day

Dosage adjustment in renal impairment: Not recommended in patients with advanced renal disease

Mechanism of Action Reversibly inhibits cyclooxygenase-1 and 2 (COX-1 and 2) enzymes, which results in decreased formation of prostaglandin precursors; has antipyretic, analgesic, and anti-inflammatory properties

Other proposed mechanisms not fully elucidated (and possibly contributing to the anti-inflammatory effect to varying degrees), include inhibiting chemotaxis, altering lymphocyte activity, inhibiting neutrophil aggregation/activation, and decreasing proinflammatory cytokine levels.

Contraindications Hypersensitivity to fenoprofen, aspirin, or other NSAIDs, or any component of the formulation; perioperative pain in the setting of coronary artery bypass graft (CABG) surgery; significant renal dysfunction

Warnings/Precautions **[U.S. Boxed Warning]: NSAIDs are associated with an increased risk of adverse cardiovascular thrombotic events, including MI and stroke.** Risk may be increased with duration of use or pre-existing cardiovascular risk factors or disease. Carefully evaluate individual cardiovascular risk profiles prior to prescribing. May cause new-onset hypertension or worsening of existing hypertension. Use caution with fluid retention. Avoid use in heart failure. Concurrent administration of ibuprofen, and potentially other nonselective NSAIDs, may interfere with aspirin's cardioprotective effect. **[U.S. Boxed Warning]: Use is contraindicated for treatment of perioperative pain in the setting of coronary artery bypass graft (CABG) surgery.** Risk of MI and stroke may be increased with use following CABG surgery.

NSAID use may compromise existing renal function; dose-dependent decreases in prostaglandin synthesis may result from NSAID use, reducing renal blood flow which may cause renal decompensation. NSAID use may increase the risk for hyperkalemia. Patients with impaired renal function, dehydration, heart failure, liver dysfunction, those taking diuretics, and ACE inhibitors, and the elderly are at greater risk of renal toxicity and hyperkalemia. Rehydrate patient before starting therapy; monitor renal function closely. Not recommended for use in patients with advanced renal disease. Long-term NSAID use may result in renal papillary necrosis.

[U.S. Boxed Warning]: NSAIDs may increase risk of gastrointestinal irritation, inflammation, ulceration, bleeding, and perforation. These events may occur at any time during therapy and without warning. Use caution with a history of GI disease (bleeding or ulcers), concurrent therapy with aspirin, anticoagulants and/or corticosteroids, smoking, use of alcohol, the elderly or debilitated patients. When used concomitantly with ≤325 mg of aspirin, a substantial increase in the risk of gastrointestinal complications (eg, ulcer) occurs; concomitant gastroprotective therapy (eg, proton pump inhibitors) is recommended (Bhatt, 2008).

Platelet adhesion and aggregation may be decreased; may prolong bleeding time; patients with coagulation disorders or who are receiving anticoagulants should be monitored closely. Anemia may occur; patients on long-term NSAID therapy should be monitored for anemia. Rarely, NSAID use has been associated with potentially severe blood dyscrasias (eg, agranulocytosis, thrombocytopenia, aplastic anemia).

Use the lowest effective dose for the shortest duration of time, consistent with individual patient goals, to reduce risk of cardiovascular or GI adverse events. Alternate therapies should be considered for patients at high risk.

NSAIDs may cause serious skin adverse events including exfoliative dermatitis, Stevens-Johnson syndrome (SJS), and toxic epidermal necrolysis (TEN); discontinue use at first sign of skin rash or hypersensitivity. Anaphylactoid reactions may occur, even without prior exposure; patients with "aspirin triad" (bronchial asthma, aspirin intolerance, rhinitis) may be at increased risk. Do not use in patients who experience bronchospasm, asthma, rhinitis, or urticaria with NSAID or aspirin therapy. Use caution in other forms of asthma.

Use with caution in patients with decreased hepatic function. Closely monitor patients with any abnormal LFT. Severe hepatic reactions (eg, fulminant hepatitis, liver failure) have occurred with NSAID use, rarely; discontinue if signs or symptoms of liver disease develop, or if systemic manifestations occur.

NSAIDS may cause drowsiness, dizziness, blurred vision and other neurologic effects which may impair physical or mental abilities; patients must be cautioned about performing tasks which require mental alertness (eg, operating machinery or driving). Discontinue use with blurred or diminished vision and perform ophthalmologic exam. Monitor vision with long-term therapy. The elderly are at increased risk for adverse effects (especially peptic ulceration, CNS effects, renal toxicity) from NSAIDs even at low doses.

Withhold for at least 4-6 half-lives prior to surgical or dental procedures.

Drug Interactions

Avoid Concomitant Use

Avoid concomitant use of Fenoprofen with any of the following: Ketorolac; Ketorolac (Systemic)

Increased Effect/Toxicity

Fenoprofen may increase the levels/effects of: Aminoglycosides; Anticoagulants; Antiplatelet Agents; Bisphosphonate Derivatives; Collagenase (Systemic); CycloSPORINE; CycloSPORINE (Systemic); Deferasirox; Desmopressin; Digoxin; Drotrecogin Alfa; Eplerenone; Haloperidol; Ibritumomab; Lithium; Methotrexate; Nonsteroidal Anti-Inflammatory Agents; PEMEtrexed; Potassium-Sparing Diuretics; PRALAtrexate; Quinolone Antibiotics; Salicylates; Thrombolytic Agents; Tositumomab and Iodine I 131 Tositumomab; Vancomycin; Vitamin K Antagonists

The levels/effects of Fenoprofen may be increased by: ACE Inhibitors; Angiotensin II Receptor Blockers; Antidepressants (Tricyclic, Tertiary Amine); Corticosteroids (Systemic); Dasatinib; Glucosamine; Herbs (Anticoagulant/Antiplatelet Properties); Ketorolac; Ketorolac (Systemic); Nonsteroidal Anti-Inflammatory Agents; Omega-3-Acid Ethyl Esters; Pentosan Polysulfate Sodium; Pentoxifylline; Probenecid; Prostacyclin Analogues; Selective Serotonin Reuptake Inhibitors; Serotonin/Norepinephrine Reuptake Inhibitors; Treprostinil

Decreased Effect

Fenoprofen may decrease the levels/effects of: ACE Inhibitors; Angiotensin II Receptor Blockers; Antiplatelet Agents; Beta-Blockers; Eplerenone; HydrALAZINE; Loop Diuretics; Potassium-Sparing Diuretics; Salicylates; Thiazide Diuretics

The levels/effects of Fenoprofen may be decreased by: Bile Acid Sequestrants; Nonsteroidal Anti-Inflammatory Agents; Salicylates

Ethanol/Nutrition/Herb Interactions

Ethanol: Avoid ethanol (may enhance gastric mucosal irritation).

Food: Fenoprofen peak serum levels may be decreased if taken with food; total amount absorbed is not affected.

Herb/Nutraceutical: Avoid alfalfa, anise, bilberry, bladderwrack, bromelain, cat's claw, celery, chamomile, coleus, cordyceps, dong quai, evening primrose, fenugreek, feverfew, garlic, ginger, ginkgo biloba, ginseng (American, Panax, Siberian), grapeseed, green tea, guggul, horse chestnut seed, horseradish, licorice, prickly ash, red clover, reishi, SAMe (S-adenosylmethionine), sweet clover, turmeric, white willow (all have additional antiplatelet activity).

Dietary Considerations May be taken with food to decrease GI distress.

Pharmacodynamics/Kinetics

Onset of Action A few days; full benefit: up to 2-3 weeks

Half-life Elimination 2.5-3 hours

Time to Peak Serum: ~2 hours

Pregnancy Risk Factor C

Lactation Enters breast milk/not recommended

Breast-Feeding Considerations Very low levels of fenoprofen are found in breast milk. Breast-feeding is not recommended by the manufacturer.

Dosage Forms

Capsule, oral:

Nalfon®: 200 mg

Tablet, oral: 600 mg

FentaNYL (FEN ta nil)

U.S. Brand Names Abstral®; Actiq®; Duragesic®; Fentora®; Onsolis™; Sublimaze® [DSC]

Canadian Brand Names Actiq®; Duragesic®; Duragesic® MAT; Fentanyl Citrate Injection, USP; Novo-Fentanyl; PMS-Fentanyl MTX; RAN™-Fentanyl Matrix Patch; RAN™-Fentanyl Transdermal System; ratio-Fentanyl

Generic Availability (U.S.) Yes: Excludes buccal film, buccal tablet, sublingual tablet

Pharmacologic Category Analgesic, Opioid; Anilidopiperidine Opioid; General Anesthetic

Dental Use Adjunct in preoperative intravenous conscious sedation in patients undergoing dental surgery

Use

Injection: Relief of pain, preoperative medication, adjunct to general or regional anesthesia

Iontophoretic transdermal system (Ionsys™): Short-term, in-hospital management of acute postoperative pain

Transdermal patch (eg, Duragesic®): Management of persistent moderate-to-severe chronic pain

Transmucosal lozenge (eg, Actiq®), buccal tablet (Fentora®), buccal film (Onsolis™), sublingual tablet (Abstral®): Management of breakthrough cancer pain in opioid-tolerant patients

Local Anesthetic/Vasoconstrictor Precautions No information available to require special precautions

Effects on Dental Treatment Key adverse event(s) related to dental treatment: Xerostomia, changes in salivation (normal salivary flow resumes upon discontinuation), and orthostatic hypotension. Actiq® may contribute to dental caries due to sugar content of oral lozenge; advise patients to maintain good oral hygiene. See Dental Comment.

Effects on Bleeding No information available to require special precautions

Adverse Effects

>10%:

Cardiovascular: Bradycardia, edema

Central nervous system: CNS depression, confusion, dizziness, drowsiness, fatigue, headache, sedation

Endocrine & metabolic: Dehydration

Gastrointestinal: Constipation, nausea, vomiting, xerostomia

Local: Application-site reaction erythema

Neuromuscular & skeletal: Chest wall rigidity (high dose I.V.), muscle rigidity, weakness

Ocular: Miosis

Respiratory: Dyspnea, respiratory depression

Miscellaneous: Diaphoresis

1% to 10%:

Cardiovascular: Cardiac arrhythmia, chest pain, DVT, flushing, hyper-/hypotension, orthostatic hypotension, pallor, palpitation, peripheral edema, syncope, tachycardia, vasodilation

Central nervous system: Abnormal dreams, abnormal thinking, agitation, amnesia, anxiety, attention disturbance, DVT, depression, dysphoria, euphoria, fever, hallucinations, hypoesthesia, insomnia, lethargy, malaise, mental status change, migraine, nervousness, paranoid reaction, somnolence, stupor, vertigo

Dermatologic: Alopecia, bruising, cellulitis, erythema, hyperhidrosis, papules, pruritus, rash
Endocrine & metabolic: Breast pain, hot flashes, hyper-/hypocalcemia, hyper-/hypoglycemia, hypoalbuminemia, hypokalemia, hypomagnesemia
Gastrointestinal: Abdominal pain, abnormal taste, anorexia, appetite decreased, biliary tract spasm, diarrhea, dyspepsia, dysphagia (buccal tablet/film), flatulence, GI hemorrhage, gingival pain (buccal tablet), gingivitis (lozenge), glossitis (lozenge), ileus, intestinal obstruction (buccal film), periodontal abscess (lozenge/buccal tablet), stomatitis (lozenge/buccal tablet/sublingual tablet), tongue disorder (sublingual tablet), ulceration (gingival, lip, mouth; transmucosal use), weight loss
Genitourinary: Dysuria, erectile dysfunction, urinary incontinence, urinary retention, vaginitis, vaginal hemorrhage
Hematologic: Anemia, leukopenia, neutropenia, thrombocytopenia
Hepatic: Ascites, jaundice
Local: Application site pain, application site irritation
Neuromuscular & skeletal: Abnormal coordination, abnormal gait, arthralgia, back pain, myalgia, neuropathy, paresthesia, rigors, tremor
Ocular: Blurred vision, diplopia
Renal: Renal failure
Respiratory: Apnea, asthma, bronchitis, cough, epistaxis, hemoptysis, hypoventilation, hypoxia, nasopharyngitis, pharyngolaryngeal pain, pharyngitis, pneumonia, rhinitis, sinusitis, upper respiratory infection, wheezing
Miscellaneous: Flu-like syndrome, hiccups, hypersensitivity, lymphadenopathy, night sweats, parosmia, speech disorder, withdrawal syndrome

Dental Usual Dosage Surgery: Adults:
Premedication: I.M., slow I.V.: 25-100 mcg/dose 30-60 minutes prior to surgery
Adjunct to regional anesthesia: Slow I.V.: 25-100 mcg/dose over 1-2 minutes. **Note:** An I.V. should be in place with regional anesthesia so the I.M. route is rarely used but still maintained as an option in the package labeling.

Dosage Note: These are guidelines and do not represent the maximum doses that may be required in all patients. Doses and dosage intervals should be titrated to pain relief/prevention. Monitor vital signs routinely. Single I.M. doses have a duration of 1-2 hours, single I.V. doses last 0.5-1 hour.

Minor procedures/analgesia (unlabeled use): I.V.:
Children 1-12 years: 0.5-2 mcg/kg/dose given 3 minutes prior to procedure; may repeat every 1-2 hours
Children >12 years: 0.5-2 mcg/kg/dose (maximum: 50 mcg/dose) given 3 minutes prior to procedure; may repeat in 5 minutes if necessary; if more than 2 doses are needed, repeat with a maximum of 25 mcg/dose up to 5 times

Surgery:
Children ≥2 years: Adjunct to anesthesia (induction and maintenance): Slow I.V.: 2-3 mcg/kg/dose every 1-2 hours as needed
Adults:
Premedication: I.M., slow I.V.: 50-100 mcg/dose 30-60 minutes prior to surgery
Adjunct to regional anesthesia: Slow I.V.: 25-100 mcg/dose over 1-2 minutes. **Note:** An I.V. should be in place with regional anesthesia so the I.M. route is rarely used but still maintained as an option in the package labeling.
Adjunct to general anesthesia: Slow I.V.:
Low dose: 0.5-2 mcg/kg/dose depending on the indication
Moderate dose: Initial: 2-20 mcg/kg/dose; Maintenance (bolus or infusion): 1-2 mcg/kg/**hour**. Discontinuing fentanyl infusion 30-60 minutes prior to the end of surgery will usually allow adequate ventilation upon emergence from anesthesia. For "fast-tracking" and early extubation following major surgery, total fentanyl doses are limited to 10-15 mcg/kg.
High dose: 20-50 mcg/kg/dose; **Note:** High-dose fentanyl as an adjunct to general anesthesia is rarely used, but is still described in the manufacturer's label.

Pain management:
Children (unlabeled use): I.V.: 0.5-2 mcg/kg/dose given every 1-2 hours as needed; continuous infusion: 0.5-2 mcg/kg/**hour**; titrate to desired effects
Patient-controlled analgesia (PCA) (unlabeled use; American Pain Society, 2008): Children <50 kg: **Note:** Opiate-naive: Consider lower end of dosing range:
Usual concentration: 10 mcg/mL
Demand dose: 0.5-1 mcg/kg/dose
Lockout interval: 6-8 minutes
Usual basal rate: 0-0.5 mcg/kg/**hour**

Adults:

I.V. (unlabeled use): Bolus at start of infusion: 1-2 mcg/kg **or** 25-100 mcg/dose; continuous infusion rate: 1-2 mcg/kg/**hour or** 25-200 mcg/hour

Severe pain: I.M, I.V. (unlabeled): 50-100 mcg/dose every 1-2 hours as needed; patients with prior opiate exposure may tolerate higher initial doses

Patient-controlled analgesia (PCA) (unlabeled use): I.V.:

Usual concentration: 10 mcg/mL

Demand dose: Usual: 20 mcg; range: 10-50 mcg

Lockout interval: 5-8 minutes

Usual basal rate: ≤50 mcg/hour

Critically-ill patients (unlabeled dose): Slow I.V.: 25-100 mcg (based on ~70 kg patient) **or** 0.35-1.5 mcg/kg every 30-60 minutes as needed. **Note:** More frequent dosing may be needed (eg, mechanically-ventilated patients).

Continuous infusion: 50-700 mcg/hour (based on ~70 kg patient) **or** 0.7-10 mcg/kg/**hour**

Intrathecal (I.T.) (unlabeled use; American Pain Society, 2008): **Must be preservative-free.** Doses must be adjusted for age, injection site, and patient's medical condition and degree of opioid tolerance.

Single dose: 5-25 mcg/dose; may provide adequate relief for up to 6 hours

Continuous infusion: Not recommended in acute pain management due to risk of excessive accumulation. For chronic cancer pain, infusion of very small doses may be practical (American Pain Society, 2008).

Epidural (unlabeled use; American Pain Society, 2008): **Must be preservative-free.** Doses must be adjusted for age, injection site, and patient's medical condition and degree of opioid tolerance

Single dose: 25-100 mcg/dose; may provide adequate relief for up to 8 hours

Continuous infusion: 25-100 mcg/hour

Breakthrough cancer pain: For patients who are tolerant to and currently receiving opioid therapy for persistent cancer pain; dosing should be individually titrated to provide adequate analgesia with minimal side effects. Dose titration should be done if patient requires more than 1 dose/breakthrough pain episode for several consecutive episodes. Patients experiencing >4 breakthrough pain episodes/day should have the dose of their long-term opioid re-evaluated.

Children ≥16 years and Adults: Lozenge: Initial dose: 200 mcg; the second dose may be started 15 minutes after completion of the first dose if pain unrelieved. A maximum of 1 additional dose can be given per pain episode; must wait at least 4 hours before treating another episode. Consumption should be limited to ≤4 units/day. Additional requirements suggest need for improved baseline therapy.

Adults:

Buccal film (Onsolis™): Initial dose: 200 mcg for all patients **Note:** Patients previously using another transmucosal product should be initiated at doses of 200 mcg; do **not** switch patients using any other fentanyl product on a mcg-per-mcg basis.

Dose titration: If titration required, increase dose in 200 mcg increments once per episode using multiples of the 200 mcg film; do not redose within a single episode of breakthrough pain and separate single doses by ≥2 hours. During titration, do not exceed 4 simultaneous applications of the 200 mcg films (800 mcg). If >800 mcg required, treat next episode with one 1200 mcg film (maximum dose: 1200 mcg). Once maintenance dose is determined, all other unused films should be disposed of and that strength (using a single film) should be used. During any pain episode, if adequate relief is not achieved after 30 minutes following buccal film application, a rescue medication (as determined by healthcare provider) may be used.

Maintenance: Determined dose applied as a single film once per episode and separated by ≥2 hours (dose range: 200-1200 mcg); limit to 4 applications/day. Consider increasing the around-the-clock opioid therapy in patients experiencing >4 breakthrough pain episodes/day.

Buccal tablet (Fentora®): Initial dose: 100 mcg; a second 100 mcg dose, if needed, may be started 30 minutes after the start of the first dose. **Note:** For patients previously using the transmucosal lozenge (Actiq®), the initial dose should be selected using the conversions listed below (maximum: 2 doses per breakthrough pain episode every 4 hours).

Dose titration, if required, should be done using multiples of the 100 mcg tablets. Patient can take two 100 mcg tablets (one on each side of mouth). If that dose is not successful, can use four 100 mcg tablets (two on each side of mouth). If titration requires >400 mcg/dose, then use 200 mcg tablets.

Conversion from lozenge to buccal tablet (Fentora®):
Lozenge dose 200-400 mcg, then buccal tablet 100 mcg
Lozenge dose 600-800 mcg, then buccal tablet 200 mcg
Lozenge dose 1200-1600 mcg, then buccal tablet 400 mcg

Note: Four 100 mcg buccal tablets deliver approximately 12% and 13% higher values of C_{max} and AUC, respectively, compared to one 400 mcg buccal tablet. To prevent confusion, patient should only have one strength available at a time. Using more than four buccal tablets at a time has not been studied.

Sublingual tablet (Abstral®): Initial dose: 100 mcg for all patients; if pain is unrelieved, a second dose may be given 30 minutes after administration of the first dose. A maximum of 2 doses can be given per breakthrough pain episode; must wait at least 2 hours before treating another episode. **Note:** Patients previously using another fentanyl product should be initiated at a dose of 100 mcg; do not convert patients from other fentanyl products to Abstral® on a mcg-per-mcg basis.

Dose titration: If titration required, increase in 100 mcg increments (up to 400 mcg) over consecutive breakthrough episodes. If titration requires >400 mcg/dose, increase in increments of 200 mcg, starting with 600 mcg dose. During titration, patients may use multiples of 100 mcg and/or 200 mcg tablets for any single dose; do not exceed 4 tablets at one time; safety and efficacy of doses >800 mcg have not been evaluated.

Maintenance dose: Once maintenance dose for breakthrough pain episode has been determined, use only 1 tablet in the appropriate strength per episode (if pain is unrelieved a second dose may be given after 30 minutes; maximum of 2 doses/episode of breakthrough pain); separate treatment of subsequent episodes by ≥2 hours; limit treatment to ≤4 breakthrough episodes/day. Consider increasing the around-the-clock long-acting opioid therapy in patients experiencing >4 breakthrough pain episodes/day; if long-acting opioid therapy dose altered, re-evaluate and retitrate Abstral® dose as needed.

Elderly >65 years: Transmucosal lozenge (eg, Actiq®): In clinical trials, patients who were >65 years of age were titrated to a mean dose that was 200 mcg less than that of younger patients.

Chronic pain management: Children ≥2 years and Adults (opioid-tolerant patients):
Transdermal patch (Duragesic®):

Initial: To convert patients from oral or parenteral opioids to transdermal patch, a 24-hour analgesic requirement should be calculated (based on prior opiate use). Using the tables, the appropriate initial dose can be determined. The initial fentanyl dosage may be approximated from the 24-hour morphine dosage equivalent and titrated to minimize adverse effects and provide analgesia. With the initial application, the absorption of transdermal fentanyl requires several hours to reach plateau; therefore transdermal fentanyl is inappropriate for management of acute pain. Change patch every 72 hours.

Conversion from continuous infusion of fentanyl: In patients who have adequate pain relief with a fentanyl infusion, fentanyl may be converted to transdermal dosing at a rate equivalent to the intravenous rate. A two-step taper of the infusion to be completed over 12 hours has been recommended (Kornick, 2001) after the patch is applied. The infusion is decreased to 50% of the original rate six hours after the application of the first patch, and subsequently discontinued twelve hours after application.

Titration: Short-acting agents may be required until analgesic efficacy is established and/or as supplements for "breakthrough" pain. The amount of supplemental doses should be closely monitored. Appropriate dosage increases may be based on daily supplemental dosage using the ratio of 45 mg/24 hours of oral morphine to a 12.5 mcg/hour increase in fentanyl dosage.

Frequency of adjustment: The dosage should not be titrated more frequently than every 3 days after the initial dose or every 6 days thereafter. Patients should wear a consistent fentanyl dosage through two applications (6 days) before dosage increase based on supplemental opiate dosages can be estimated. **Note:** Upon discontinuation, ~17 hours are required for a 50% decrease in fentanyl levels.

Frequency of application: The majority of patients may be controlled on every 72-hour administration; however, a small number of patients require every 48-hour administration.

Dose conversion guidelines for transdermal fentanyl (see tables below and on next page).

Note: U.S. and Canadian dose conversion guidelines differ. Consult appropriate table.

U.S. Labeling: Dose Conversion Guidelines: Recommended Initial Duragesic® Dose Based Upon Daily Oral Morphine Dose[1,2]

Oral 24-Hour Morphine (mg/day)	Duragesic® Dose[3] (mcg/h)
60-134	25
135-224	50
225-314	75
315-404	100
405-494	125
495-584	150
585-674	175
675-764	200
765-854	225
855-944	250
945-1034	275
1035-1124	300

[1]The table should NOT be used to convert from transdermal fentanyl (Duragesic®) to other opioid analgesics. Rather, following removal of the patch, titrate the dose of the new opioid until adequate analgesia is achieved.

[2]Recommendations are based on U.S. product labeling for Duragesic®.

[3]Pediatric patients initiating therapy on a 25 mcg/hour Duragesic® system should be opioid-tolerant and receiving at least 60 mg oral morphine equivalents per day.

U.S. Labeling: Dose Conversion Guidelines[1,2]

Current Analgesic	Daily Dosage (mg/day)			
Morphine (I.M./I.V.)	10-22	23-37	38-52	53-67
Oxycodone (oral)	30-67	67.5-112	112.5-157	157.5-202
Oxycodone (I.M./I.V.)	15-33	33.1-56	56.1-78	78.1-101
Codeine (oral)	150-447	448-747	748-1047	1048-1347
Hydromorphone (oral)	8-17	17.1-28	28.1-39	39.1-51
Hydromorphone (I.V.)	1.5-3.4	3.5-5.6	5.7-7.9	8-10
Meperidine (I.M.)	75-165	166-278	279-390	391-503
Methadone (oral)	20-44	45-74	75-104	105-134
Methadone (I.M.)	10-22	23-37	38-52	53-67
Fentanyl transdermal recommended dose (mcg/h)	**25 mcg/h**	**50 mcg/h**	**75 mcg/h**	**100 mcg/h**

[1]The table should NOT be used to convert from transdermal fentanyl (Duragesic®) to other opioid analgesics. Rather, following removal of the patch, titrate the dose of the new opioid until adequate analgesia is achieved.

[2]Recommendations are based on U.S. product labeling for Duragesic®.

Transdermal patch (Duragesic® MAT [Canada; not available in U.S.]): Adults:

Canadian Labeling: Dose Conversion Guidelines (Adults): Recommended Initial Duragesic® MAT Dose Based Upon Daily Oral Morphine Dose[1,2]

Oral 24-Hour Morphine (Current Dose in mg/day)	Duragesic® MAT Dose (Initial Dose in mcg/h)
45-59	12
60-134	25
135-179	37
180-224	50
225-269	62
270-314	75
315-359	87
360-404	100
405-494	125
495-584	150
585-674	175
675-764	200
765-854	225
855-944	250
945-1034	275
1035-1124	300

[1]The table should NOT be used to convert from transdermal fentanyl (Duragesic® MAT) to other opioid analgesics. Rather, following removal of the patch, titrate the dose of the new opioid until adequate analgesia is achieved.

[2]Recommendations are based on Canadian product labeling for Duragesic® MAT.

Note: The 12 mcg/hour dose included in this table is to be used for incremental dose adjustment and is generally not recommended for initial dosing, except for patients in whom lower starting doses are deemed clinically appropriate.

Canadian Labeling: Dose Conversion Guidelines (Adults)[1,2]

Current Analgesic	Daily Dosage (mg/day)						
Morphine[3] (I.M./I.V.)	20-44	45-60	61-75	76-90	n/a[4]	n/a[4]	n/a[4]
Oxycodone (oral)	30-66	67-90	91-112	113-134	135-157	158-179	180-202
Codeine (oral)	150-447	448-597	598-747	748-897	898-1047	1048-1197	1198-1347
Hydromorphone (oral)	8-16	17-22	23-28	29-33	34-39	40-45	46-51
Hydromorphone (I.V.)	4-8.4	8.5-11.4	11.5-14.4	14.5-16.5	16.6-19.5	19.6-22.5	22.6-25.5
Fentanyl transdermal recommended dose (mcg/h)	**25 mcg/h**	**37 mcg/h**	**50 mcg/h**	**62 mcg/h**	**75 mcg/h**	**87 mcg/h**	**100 mcg/h**

[1]The table should NOT be used to convert from transdermal fentanyl (Duragesic® MAT) to other opioid analgesics. Rather, following removal of the patch, titrate the dose of the new opioid until adequate analgesia is achieved.

[2]Recommendations are based on Canadian product labeling for Duragesic® MAT.

[3]Morphine dose conversion based upon I.M to oral dose ratio of 1:3.

[4]Insufficient data available to provide specific dosing recommendations. Use caution; adjust dose conservatively.

Dosing adjustment in hepatic impairment: Actiq®: Although fentanyl kinetics may be altered in hepatic disease, Actiq® can be used successfully in the management of breakthrough cancer pain. Doses should be titrated to reach clinical effect with careful monitoring of patients with severe hepatic disease.

Mechanism of Action Binds with stereospecific receptors at many sites within the CNS, increases pain threshold, alters pain reception, inhibits ascending pain pathways

Contraindications Hypersensitivity to fentanyl or any component of the formulation

Transdermal system: Severe respiratory disease or depression including acute asthma (unless patient is mechanically ventilated); paralytic ileus; patients requiring short-term therapy, management of intermittent pain

Transmucosal buccal tablets (Fentora®), buccal films (Onsolis™), lozenges (eg, Actiq®), sublingual tablets (Abstral®), and/or transdermal patches (eg, Duragesic®): Contraindicated in the management of acute or postoperative pain (including headache, migraine, dental pain, or use in emergency room), and in patients who are not opioid tolerant

Warnings/Precautions An opioid-containing analgesic regimen should be tailored to each patient's needs and based upon the type of pain being treated (acute versus chronic), the route of administration, degree of tolerance for opioids (naive versus chronic user), age, weight, and medical condition. The optimal analgesic dose varies widely among patients. Doses should be titrated to pain relief/prevention. May cause CNS depression, which may impair physical or mental abilities; patients must be cautioned about performing tasks which require mental alertness (eg, operating machinery or driving). When using with other CNS depressants, reduce dose of one or both agents. Fentanyl shares the toxic potentials of opiate agonists, and precautions of opiate agonist therapy should be observed; use with caution in patients with bradycardia or bradyarrhythmias; rapid I.V. infusion may result in skeletal muscle and chest wall rigidity leading to respiratory distress and/or apnea, bronchoconstriction, laryngospasm; inject slowly over 3-5 minutes. **[U.S. Boxed Warning]: Healthcare provider should be alert to problems of abuse, misuse, and diversion.** Tolerance or drug dependence may result from extended use. The elderly may be particularly susceptible to the CNS depressant and constipating effects of narcotics. Use extreme caution in patients with COPD or other chronic respiratory conditions. Use caution with head injuries, morbid obesity, renal impairment, or hepatic dysfunction. **[U.S. Boxed Warning]: Use with strong or moderate CYP3A4 inhibitors may result in increased effects and potentially fatal respiratory depression.** Use is not recommended with MAO inhibitors or within 14 days of MAO inhibitor use; severe and unpredictable adverse effects may result. Concurrent use of agonist/antagonist analgesics may precipitate withdrawal symptoms and/or reduced analgesic efficacy in patients following prolonged therapy with mu opioid agonists. Abrupt discontinuation following prolonged use may also lead to withdrawal symptoms. Safety and efficacy have not been established in children <16 years of age for the lozenge and <18 years of age for the buccal tablet.

[U.S. Boxed Warning]: Safety and efficacy of the transdermal patch have been limited to children ≥2 years of age who are opioid-tolerant. [U.S. Boxed Warning]: Buccal film (Onsolis™), sublingual tablet (Abstral®): Not indicated for use in opioid-tolerant cancer patients <18 years of age. [U.S. Boxed Warning]: Buccal film, buccal tablet, sublingual tablet, and lozenge preparations contain an amount of medication that can be fatal to children. Keep all units out of the reach of children and discard any open units properly. Patients and caregivers should be counseled on the dangers to children including the risk of exposure to partially-consumed units.

[U.S. Boxed Warning] Abstral®, Actiq®, Duragesic®, Fentora®, Onsolis™: May cause potentially life-threatening hypoventilation, respiratory depression, and/or death; Abstral®, Actiq®, Duragesic®, Fentora®, or Onsolis™ should only be prescribed for opioid-tolerant patients. Risk of respiratory depression increased in elderly patients, debilitated patients, and patients with conditions associated with hypoxia or hypercapnia; usually occurs after administration of initial dose in non-tolerant patients or when given with other drugs that depress respiratory function.

Transmucosal: Lozenge (eg, Actiq®), buccal tablet (Fentora®), buccal film (Onsolis™), sublingual tablet (Abstral®): **[U.S. Boxed Warning]: Should be used only for the care of opioid-tolerant cancer patients with breakthrough pain and is intended for use by specialists who are knowledgeable in treating cancer pain.** Not approved for use in management of acute or postoperative pain.

Transmucosal: Buccal film (eg, Onsolis™): **[U.S. Boxed Warning]: Available only through the FOCUS Program, a restricted distribution program with prescriber, pharmacy, and patient required enrollment. [U.S. Boxed Warning]: Onsolis™ is contraindicated in the management of acute or postoperative pain, including headache/migraine. [U.S. Boxed Warning]: Due to higher bioavailability of fentanyl in the buccal film formulation, do not substitute Onsolis™ on a mcg-per-mcg basis for any other fentanyl product. Serious adverse events, including death, may occur when used inappropriately**

(improper dose or patient selection). All patients must begin therapy with a 200 mcg dose and titrate, if needed. During therapy, patients must wait at least 2 hours before taking another dose.

Transmucosal: Buccal tablet (Fentora®): **[U.S. Boxed Warning]: Due to the higher bioavailability of fentanyl in Fentora®, when converting patients from oral transmucosal fentanyl citrate (OTFC, Actiq®) to Fentora®, do not substitute Fentora®): on a mcg-per-mcg basis for any other fentanyl product. [U.S. Boxed Warning]: Fentora® is contraindicated in the management of acute or postoperative pain, including headache/migraine. Serious adverse events, including death, have been reported when used inappropriately (improper dose or patient selection). [U.S. Boxed Warning]: Patients using Fentora® who experience breakthrough pain may only take one additional dose using the same strength and must wait four hours before taking another dose.**

Transmucosal: Lozenge (Actiq®): **[U.S. Boxed Warning]: The substitution of Actiq® for any other fentanyl product may result in a fatal overdose. Do not convert patients on a mcg-per-mcg basis to Actiq® from other fentanyl products. Do not substitute Actiq® for any other fentanyl product. [U.S. Boxed Warning]: Patients using fentanyl lozenges who experience breakthrough pain may only take 1 additional dose using the same strength and must wait 4 hours before taking another dose.**

Transmucosal: Sublingual tablet (Abstral®): **[U.S. Boxed Warning]: Available only through the ABSTRAL REMS program. Prescribers who prescribe to out-patients, outpatients, pharmacies, and distributors are required to enroll in the program. [U.S. Boxed Warning]: Abstral® is contraindicated in opioid nontolerant patients. [U.S. Boxed Warning]: Due to differing pharmacokinetics of fentanyl in the sublingual tablet formulation, do not substitute Abstral® on a mcg-per-mcg basis for any other fentanyl product. Serious adverse events, including death, may occur when used inappropriately (improper dose or patient selection). All patients must begin therapy with a 100 mcg dose. During therapy, patients must wait at least 2 hours before treating another episode of breakthrough pain.**

Transdermal patches (eg, Duragesic®): **[U.S. Boxed Warning]: Indicated for the management of persistent moderate-to-severe pain when around the clock pain control is needed for an extended time period. Should only be used in patients who are already receiving opioid therapy, are opioid tolerant, and who require a total daily dose equivalent to 25 mcg/hour transdermal patch. Contraindicated in patients who are not opioid tolerant, in the management of short-term analgesia, or in the management of postoperative pain. Should be applied only to intact skin. Use of a patch that has been cut, damaged, or altered in any way may result in overdosage.** Serum fentanyl concentrations may increase approximately one-third for patients with a body temperature of 40°C secondary to a temperature-dependent increase in fentanyl release from the patch and increased skin permeability. **[U.S. Boxed Warning]: Avoid exposure of application site and surrounding area to direct external heat sources.** Patients who experience fever or increase in core temperature should be monitored closely. Patients who experience adverse reactions should be monitored for at least 24 hours after removal of the patch. Transdermal patch may contain conducting metal (eg, aluminum); remove patch prior to MRI.

Drug Interactions

Metabolism/Transport Effects Substrate of CYP3A4 (major); **Inhibits** CYP3A4 (weak)

Avoid Concomitant Use

Avoid concomitant use of FentaNYL with any of the following: MAO Inhibitors

Increased Effect/Toxicity

FentaNYL may increase the levels/effects of: Alcohol (Ethyl); Alvimopan; Beta-Blockers; Calcium Channel Blockers (Nondihydropyridine); CNS Depressants; Desmopressin; MAO Inhibitors; Selective Serotonin Reuptake Inhibitors; Thiazide Diuretics

The levels/effects of FentaNYL may be increased by: Amphetamines; Antipsychotic Agents (Phenothiazines); CYP3A4 Inhibitors (Moderate); CYP3A4 Inhibitors (Strong); Dasatinib; Droperidol; MAO Inhibitors; Succinylcholine

Decreased Effect

FentaNYL may decrease the levels/effects of: Pegvisomant

The levels/effects of FentaNYL may be decreased by: Ammonium Chloride; Mixed Agonist / Antagonist Opioids; Rifamycin Derivatives; Tocilizumab

Ethanol/Nutrition/Herb Interactions

Ethanol: May increase CNS depression; monitor for increased effects with coadministration. Caution patients about effects.

Food: Fentanyl concentrations may be increased by grapefruit juice; avoid concurrent intake of large quantities (>1 quart/day).

Herb/Nutraceutical: St John's wort may decrease fentanyl levels. Avoid valerian, St John's wort, kava kava, gotu kola (may increase CNS depression).

Dietary Considerations Transmucosal lozenge contains 2 g sugar per unit.

Pharmacodynamics/Kinetics

Onset of Action Analgesic: I.M.: 7-8 minutes; I.V.: Almost immediate; Transdermal (initial placement): 6 hours; Transmucosal: 5-15 minutes

Peak effect: Analgesic: Transdermal (initial placement): 12 hours; Transmucosal: 15-30 minutes

Duration of Action I.M.: 1-2 hours; I.V.: 0.5-1 hour; Transdermal (removal of patch/no replacement): 12 hours; Transmucosal: Related to blood level; respiratory depressant effect may last longer than analgesic effect

Half-life Elimination

I.V.: 2-4 hours

Transdermal patch: 17 hours (13-22 hours, half-life is influenced by absorption rate)

Transmucosal: Lozenge: 7 hours; Buccal film: ~14 hours; Buccal tablet: 100-200 mcg: 3-4 hours, 400-800 mcg: 11-12 hours; Sublingual tablet: 100-200 mcg: 5-7 hours; 400-800 mcg: 10-14 hours

Time to Peak

Buccal film: 0.75-4 hours (median: 1 hour)

Buccal tablet: 20-240 minutes (median: 47 minutes)

Lozenge: 20-480 minutes (median: 20-40 minutes)

Sublingual tablet: 15-240 minutes (median: 30-60 minutes)

Transdermal patch: 24-72 hours, after several sequential 72-hour applications, steady state serum concentrations are reached

Pregnancy Risk Factor C

Lactation Enters breast milk/not recommended (AAP rates "compatible"; AAP 2001 update pending)

Breast-Feeding Considerations Fentanyl is excreted in low concentrations into breast milk. Breast-feeding is considered acceptable following single doses to the mother; however, limited information is available when used long-term. **Note:** Transdermal patch, transmucosal lozenge, sublingual tablet, buccal tablet (Fentora®), and buccal film (Onsolis™) are not recommended in nursing women due to potential for sedation and/or respiratory depression. Symptoms of opioid withdrawal may occur in infants following the cessation of breast-feeding.

Controlled Substance C-II

Prescribing and Access Restrictions As a requirement of the REMS program, access is restricted.

Abstral® (fentanyl sublingual tablet) is only available through the ABSTRAL REMS (Risk Evaluation and Mitigation Strategy) program. For outpatient use, enrollment in the ABSTRAL REMS program is required for prescribers, outpatient pharmacies, and patients. For inpatient use, enrollment in the ABSTRAL REMS program is required for inpatient pharmacies; patient and prescriber enrollment is not required for inpatient use. Distributors must also be enrolled in the program. Further information may be obtained by calling the ABSTRAL REMS program at 1-888-227-8725 or online at www.abstralrems.com

Onsolis™ (fentanyl buccal film) is only available through the restricted distribution program (FOCUS™). Enrollment in the FOCUS™ program is required for prescribers, pharmacies, and patients. Further information may be obtained from the manufacturer, Meda Pharmaceuticals, Inc (1-877-466-7654).

Dosage Forms

Film, for buccal application:

Onsolis™: 200 mcg (30s); 400 mcg (30s); 600 mcg (30s); 800 mcg (30s); 1200 mcg (30s)

Injection, solution [preservative free]: 0.05 mg/mL (2 mL, 5 mL, 10 mL, 20 mL, 30 mL, 50 mL)

Lozenge, oral: 200 mcg (30s); 400 mcg (30s); 600 mcg (30s); 800 mcg (30s); 1200 mcg (30s); 1600 mcg (30s)

Actiq®: 200 mcg (30s); 400 mcg (30s); 600 mcg (30s); 800 mcg (30s); 1200 mcg (30s); 1600 mcg (30s)

Patch, transdermal: 12.5 mcg/hr (5s); 25 mcg/hr (5s); 50 mcg/hr (5s); 75 mcg/hr (5s); 100 mcg/hr (5s)

Duragesic®: 12.5 mcg/hr (5s); 25 mcg/hr (5s); 50 mcg/hr (5s); 75 mcg/hr (5s); 100 mcg/hr (5s)

Powder, for prescription compounding: USP: 100% (1 g)

Tablet, for buccal application:

Fentora®: 100 mcg (28s); 200 mcg (28s); 400 mcg (28s); 600 mcg (28s); 800 mcg (28s)

Tablet, sublingual:
Abstral®: 100 mcg (12s, 32s); 200 mcg (12s, 32s); 300 mcg (12s, 32s); 400 mcg (12s, 32s); 600 mcg (32s); 800 mcg (32s)

Dosage Forms: Canada

Patch, transdermal, as base: 12 mcg/hr (5s); 25 mcg/hr (5s); 50 mcg/hr (5s); 75 mcg/hr (5s); 100 mcg/hr (5s)
Duragesic® MAT: 12 mcg/hr (5s); 25 mcg/hr (5s); 50 mcg/hr (5s); 75 mcg/hr (5s); 100 mcg/hr (5s)

Dental Comment Transdermal fentanyl should not be used as a pain reliever in dentistry due to danger of hypoventilation

Actiq® is a solid formulation of fentanyl with a high sugar content of 2 g hydrated dextrates per unit. Frequent use of Actiq® could result in significant dental problems including risk of dental decay. Dry mouth caused by fentanyl could add to the risk of caries. Oral adverse reactions reported in clinical trials have included tooth caries, gum hemorrhage, mouth ulcerations, oral moniliasis, dry mouth, and cheilitis.

Sedation: There is a subsequent slow release from muscle and fat which results in a terminal half-life that is beyond that of morphine. Fentanyl does not induce the release of histamine; therefore, fentanyl is preferable in patients with a predisposition to bronchospasm. Fentanyl is a good choice for use in cardiac patients because it lacks direct myocardial depression. The incidence of nausea is less than that reported with morphine or meperidine. The clinician should wait 2 to 3 minutes between doses to allow time for observation of the clinical effects of each administered dose.

References

Dionne RA, Yagiela JA, Moore PA, et al, "Comparing Efficacy and Safety of Four Intravenous Sedation Regimens in Dental Outpatients," *Am Dent Assoc*, 2001, 132(6):740-51.

Ferric Gluconate (FER ik GLOO koe nate)

U.S. Brand Names Ferrlecit®; Nulecit™

Canadian Brand Names Ferrlecit®

Pharmacologic Category Iron Salt

Use Repletion of total body iron content in patients with iron-deficiency anemia who are undergoing hemodialysis in conjunction with erythropoietin therapy

Unlabeled/Investigational Use Cancer-/chemotherapy-associated anemia

Local Anesthetic/Vasoconstrictor Precautions No information available to require special precautions

Effects on Dental Treatment Key adverse event(s) related to dental treatment: Xerostomia (normal salivary flow resumes upon discontinuation). Do not prescribe tetracyclines simultaneously with iron since GI tract absorption of both tetracycline and iron may be inhibited.

Effects on Bleeding No information available to require special precautions

Adverse Effects Frequency not defined.

Cardiovascular: Angina, bradycardia, chest pain, edema, hyper-/hypotension, hypervolemia, MI, pulmonary edema, syncope, tachycardia, thrombosis, vasodilation
Central nervous system: Agitation, chills, dizziness, fatigue, fever, headache, insomnia, malaise, pain, somnolence
Dermatologic: Pruritus, rash
Endocrine & metabolic: Hyper-/hypokalemia, hypoglycemia
Gastrointestinal: Abdominal pain, anorexia, diarrhea, dyspepsia, epigastric pain, eructation, flatulence, melena, nausea, vomiting
Genitourinary: Urinary tract infection
Hematologic: Abnormal erythrocytes, leukocytosis, lymphadenopathy
Local: Injection site reactions, injection site pain
Neuromuscular & skeletal: Arthralgia, back pain, cramps, groin pain, leg cramps, myalgia, paresthesia, rigors, weakness
Ocular: Blurred vision, conjunctivitis
Respiratory: Cough, dyspnea, pneumonia, rhinitis, upper respiratory infection
Miscellaneous: Carcinoma, diaphoresis increased, flu-like syndrome, hypersensitivity reactions, infection, sepsis

General Dosage Range I.V.:

Children ≥6 years: 1.5 msg/kg of elemental iron at 8 sequential dialysis sessions (maximum: 125 mg/dose)
Adults: 125 mg of elemental iron at ~8 sequential dialysis treatments to make a cumulative dose of 1 g

Mechanism of Action Supplies a source to elemental iron necessary to the function of hemoglobin, myoglobin and specific enzyme systems; allows transport of oxygen via hemoglobin

Pharmacodynamics/Kinetics
Half-life Elimination Bound: 1 hour
Pregnancy Risk Factor B

Ferric Hexacyanoferrate (FER ik hex a SYE an oh fer ate)

U.S. Brand Names Radiogardase®
Pharmacologic Category Antidote
Use Treatment of known or suspected internal contamination with radioactive cesium and/or radioactive or nonradioactive thallium
Local Anesthetic/Vasoconstrictor Precautions No information available to require special precautions
Effects on Dental Treatment No significant effects or complications reported
Effects on Bleeding No information available to require special precautions
Adverse Effects
>10%: Gastrointestinal: Constipation (24%)
1% to 10%: Endocrine & metabolic: Hypokalemia (7%)
Frequency not defined: Gastrointestinal: Gastric distress, fecal discoloration (blue)
General Dosage Range Oral:
Children 2-12 years: 1 g 3 times/day
Children >12 years and Adults: 1-3 g 3 times/day
Mechanism of Action Binds to cesium and thallium isotopes in the gastrointestinal tract following their ingestion or excretion in the bile; reduces their gastrointestinal reabsorption (enterohepatic circulation)
Pharmacodynamics/Kinetics
Half-life Elimination
Cesium-137: Effective: Adults: 80 days, decreased by 69% with ferric hexacyanoferrate; adolescents: 62 days, decreased by 46% with ferric hexacyanoferrate; children: 42 days, decreased by 43% with ferric hexacyanoferrate
Nonradioactive thallium: Biological: 8-10 days; with ferric hexacyanoferrate: 3 days
Pregnancy Risk Factor C

Ferrous Fumarate (FER us FYOO ma rate)

U.S. Brand Names Femiron® [OTC]; Ferretts® [OTC]; Ferro-Sequels® [OTC]; Ferrocite™ [OTC]; Hemocyte® [OTC]; Ircon® [OTC]
Canadian Brand Names Palafer®
Pharmacologic Category Iron Salt
Use Prevention and treatment of iron-deficiency anemias
Local Anesthetic/Vasoconstrictor Precautions No information available to require special precautions
Effects on Dental Treatment Key adverse event(s) related to dental treatment: Staining of teeth. Do not prescribe tetracyclines simultaneously with iron since GI tract absorption of both tetracycline and iron may be inhibited.
Effects on Bleeding No information available to require special precautions
Adverse Effects
>10%: Gastrointestinal: Constipation, dark stools, nausea, stomach cramping, vomiting
1% to 10%:
Gastrointestinal: Diarrhea, heartburn, staining of teeth
Genitourinary: Discoloration of urine
General Dosage Range Oral:
Children: 1-6 mg elemental iron/kg/day in 1-3 divided doses
Adults: 60 mg elemental iron 2-4 times/day
Mechanism of Action Replaces iron found in hemoglobin, myoglobin, and enzymes; allows the transportation of oxygen via hemoglobin
Pharmacodynamics/Kinetics
Onset of Action Hematologic response: Oral, parenteral iron salts: ~3-10 days
Peak effect: Reticulocytosis: 5-10 days; hemoglobin values increase within 2-4 weeks

Ferrous Gluconate (FER us GLOO koe nate)

U.S. Brand Names Ferate [OTC]; Fergon® [OTC]
Canadian Brand Names Apo-Ferrous Gluconate®; Novo-Ferrogluc
Pharmacologic Category Iron Salt
Use Prevention and treatment of iron-deficiency anemias
Local Anesthetic/Vasoconstrictor Precautions No information available to require special precautions

Effects on Dental Treatment Key adverse event(s) related to dental treatment: Staining of teeth. Do not prescribe tetracyclines simultaneously with iron since GI tract absorption of both tetracycline and iron may be inhibited.

Effects on Bleeding No information available to require special precautions

Adverse Effects

>10%: Gastrointestinal: Constipation, dark stools, nausea, stomach cramping, vomiting

1% to 10%:

Gastrointestinal: Diarrhea, heartburn, staining of teeth

Genitourinary: Discoloration of urine

General Dosage Range Oral:

Children: 1-6 mg Fe/kg/day in 1-3 divided doses

Adults: 60 mg 1-4 times/day

Mechanism of Action Replaces iron found in hemoglobin, myoglobin, and enzymes; allows the transportation of oxygen via hemoglobin

Pharmacodynamics/Kinetics

Onset of Action Hematologic response: Oral: 3-10 days; peak reticulocytosis occurs in 5-10 days, and hemoglobin values increase in ~2-4 weeks

Ferrous Sulfate (FER us SUL fate)

U.S. Brand Names Feosol® [OTC]; Fer-In-Sol® [OTC]; Fer-iron [OTC]; MyKidz Iron 10™ [OTC]; Slow FE® [OTC]

Canadian Brand Names Apo-Ferrous Sulfate®; Fer-In-Sol®; Ferodan™

Pharmacologic Category Iron Salt

Use Prevention and treatment of iron-deficiency anemias

Local Anesthetic/Vasoconstrictor Precautions No information available to require special precautions

Effects on Dental Treatment Do not prescribe tetracyclines simultaneously with iron since GI tract absorption of both tetracycline and iron may be inhibited. Liquid preparations may temporarily stain the teeth.

Effects on Bleeding No information available to require special precautions

Adverse Effects

>10%: Gastrointestinal: Constipation, dark stools, epigastric pain, GI irritation, nausea, stomach cramping, vomiting

1% to 10%:

Gastrointestinal: Diarrhea, heartburn

Genitourinary: Discoloration of urine

Miscellaneous: Liquid preparations may temporarily stain the teeth

General Dosage Range Oral:

Extended release: *Adults:* 250 mg 1-2 times/day

Immediate release:

Children: 1-6 mg Fe/kg/day in 1-3 divided doses (maximum: 15 mg/day [prophylaxis dosing])

Adults: 300 mg 1-4 times/day

Mechanism of Action Replaces iron, found in hemoglobin, myoglobin, and other enzymes; allows the transportation of oxygen via hemoglobin

Pharmacodynamics/Kinetics

Onset of Action Hematologic response: Oral: ~3-10 days

Peak effect: Reticulocytosis: 5-10 days; hemoglobin increases within 2-4 weeks

Ferumoxides (fer yoo MOX ides)

Pharmacologic Category Radiological/Contrast Media, Nonionic (Low Osmolality); Radiological/Contrast Media, Paramagnetic Agent

Use For I.V. administration as an adjunct to MRI (in adult patients) to enhance the T2 weighted images used in the detection and evaluation of lesions of the liver

Local Anesthetic/Vasoconstrictor Precautions No information available to require special precautions

Effects on Dental Treatment No significant effects or complications reported

Effects on Bleeding No information available to require special precautions

General Dosage Range I.V.: *Adults:* 0.56 mg of iron (0.05 mL/kg body weight) as a single dose

Pregnancy Risk Factor C

Ferumoxytol (fer ue MOX i tol)

U.S. Brand Names Feraheme®

Pharmacologic Category Iron Salt

Use Treatment of iron-deficiency anemia in chronic kidney disease

Local Anesthetic/Vasoconstrictor Precautions No information available to require special precautions

Effects on Dental Treatment No significant effects or complications reported

Effects on Bleeding No information available to require special precautions

Adverse Effects 1% to 10%:

Cardiovascular: Hypotension (≤3%), edema (2%), peripheral edema (2%), chest pain (1%), hypertension (1%)

Central nervous system: Dizziness (3%), headache (2%), fever (1%)

Dermatologic: Pruritus (1%), rash (1%)

Gastrointestinal: Diarrhea (4%), nausea (3%), constipation (2%), vomiting (2%), abdominal pain (1%)

Neuromuscular & skeletal: Back pain (1%), muscle spasms (1%)

Respiratory: Cough (1%), dyspnea (1%)

Miscellaneous: Hypersensitivity reactions (≤4%; serious reactions: <1%)

General Dosage Range I.V.: *Adults:* 510 mg (17 mL) as a single dose; repeat once 3-8 days later

Mechanism of Action Superparamagnetic iron oxide coated with a low molecular weight semisynthetic carbohydrate; iron-carbohydrate complex enters the reticuloendothelial system macrophages of the liver, spleen, and bone marrow where the iron is released from the complex. The released iron is either transported into storage pools or is transported via plasma transferrin for incorporation into hemoglobin.

Pharmacodynamics/Kinetics

Half-life Elimination ~15 hours; ferumoxytol is not removed by hemodialysis

Pregnancy Risk Factor C

Fesoterodine (fes oh TER oh deen)

U.S. Brand Names Toviaz™

Pharmacologic Category Anticholinergic Agent

Use Treatment of patients with an overactive bladder with symptoms of urinary frequency, urgency, or urge incontinence.

Local Anesthetic/Vasoconstrictor Precautions No information available to require special precautions

Effects on Dental Treatment Key adverse event(s) related to dental treatment: Prolonged use will cause significant xerostomia (normal salivary flow resumes upon discontinuation).

Effects on Bleeding No information available to require special precautions

Adverse Effects

>10%: Gastrointestinal: Xerostomia (19% to 35%; dose related)

1% to 10%:

Central nervous system: Insomnia (1%)

Dermatological: Rash (1%)

Gastrointestinal: Constipation (4% to 6%), dyspepsia (2%), nausea (1% to 2%), abdominal pain (1%)

Genitourinary: Urinary tract infection (3% to 4%), dysuria (1% to 2%), urinary retention (1%)

Hepatic: ALT increased (1%), GGT increased (1%)

Neuromuscular & skeletal: Back pain (1% to 2%)

Ocular: Dry eyes (1% to 4%)

Respiratory: Upper respiratory tract infection (2% to 3%), cough (1% to 2%), dry throat (1% to 2%)

Miscellaneous: Peripheral edema (1%)

General Dosage Range Dosage adjustment recommended in patients with renal impairment or on concomitant therapy

Oral: *Adults:* 4-8 mg once daily

Mechanism of Action Fesoterodine acts as a prodrug and is converted to an active metabolite, 5-hydroxymethyl tolterodine (5-HMT); 5-HMT is responsible for fesoterodine's antimuscarinic activity and acts as a competitive antagonist of muscarinic receptors.

Urinary bladder contractions are mediated by muscarinic receptors; fesoterodine inhibits the receptors in the bladder preventing symptoms of urgency and frequency.

Pharmacodynamics/Kinetics

Half-life Elimination ~7 hours

Time to Peak Plasma: 5-HMT: ~5 hours; C_{max} higher in poor CYP2D6 metabolizers

Pregnancy Risk Factor C

Fexofenadine (feks oh FEN a deen)

U.S. Brand Names Allegra®; Allegra® Allergy 12 Hour [OTC]; Allegra® Allergy 24 Hour [OTC]; Allegra® Children's Allergy ODT [OTC]; Allegra® Children's Allergy [OTC]; Allegra® ODT [DSC]

Canadian Brand Names Allegra®

Generic Availability (U.S.) Yes: Excludes orally disintegrating tablet and suspension

Pharmacologic Category Histamine H_1 Antagonist; Histamine H_1 Antagonist, Second Generation; Piperidine Derivative

Use Relief of symptoms associated with seasonal allergic rhinitis; treatment of chronic idiopathic urticaria

OTC labeling: Relief of symptoms associated with allergic rhinitis

Local Anesthetic/Vasoconstrictor Precautions No information available to require special precautions

Effects on Dental Treatment No significant effects or complications reported

Effects on Bleeding No information available to require special precautions

Adverse Effects

>10%:

- Central nervous system: Headache (5% to 11%)
- Gastrointestinal: Vomiting (children 6 months to 5 years: 4% to 12%)

1% to 10%:

- Central nervous system: Fatigue (1% to 3%), somnolence (1% to 3%), dizziness (2%), fever (2%), pain (2%), drowsiness (1%)
- Endocrine & metabolic: Dysmenorrhea (2%)
- Gastrointestinal: Diarrhea (3% to 4%), nausea (2%), dyspepsia (1% to 2%)
- Neuromuscular & skeletal: Myalgia (3%), back pain (2% to 3%), pain in extremities (2%)
- Otic: Otitis media (2% to 4%)
- Respiratory: Upper respiratory tract infection (3% to 4%), cough (2% to 4%), rhinorrhea (1% to 2%)
- Miscellaneous: Viral infection (3%)

Dosage Oral:

Chronic idiopathic urticaria: Children 6 months to <2 years: 15 mg twice daily

Chronic idiopathic urticaria, seasonal allergic rhinitis:

- Children 2-11 years: 30 mg twice daily
- Children ≥12 years and Adults: 60 mg twice daily **or** 180 mg once daily
- Elderly: Starting dose: Use caution; adjust dose for renal impairment

Allergic rhinitis (OTC labeling):

- Children 2-11 years: 30 mg twice daily
- Children ≥12 years and Adults: 60 mg twice daily **or** 180 mg once daily

Dosing adjustment in renal impairment: Cl_{cr} <80 mL/minute:

- Children 6 months to <2 years: Initial: 15 mg once daily
- Children 2-11 years: Initial: 30 mg once daily
- Children ≥12 years and Adults: Initial: 60 mg once daily

Hemodialysis: Not effectively removed by hemodialysis

Mechanism of Action Fexofenadine is an active metabolite of terfenadine and like terfenadine it competes with histamine for H_1-receptor sites on effector cells in the gastrointestinal tract, blood vessels and respiratory tract; it appears that fexofenadine does not cross the blood brain barrier to any appreciable degree, resulting in a reduced potential for sedation

Contraindications Hypersensitivity to fexofenadine or any component of the formulation

Warnings/Precautions Use with caution in patients with renal impairment; dosage adjustment recommended. Safety and efficacy in children <6 months of age have not been established; orally disintegrating tablet not recommended for use in children <6 years of age. Orally disintegrating tablet contains phenylalanine.

Drug Interactions

Metabolism/Transport Effects Substrate of CYP3A4 (minor), P-glycoprotein, SLCO1B1; **Inhibits** CYP2D6 (weak)

Avoid Concomitant Use There are no known interactions where it is recommended to avoid concomitant use.

Increased Effect/Toxicity

Fexofenadine may increase the levels/effects of: Alcohol (Ethyl); Anticholinergics; CNS Depressants

The levels/effects of Fexofenadine may be increased by: Conivaptan; Droperidol; Eltrombopag; Erythromycin; Erythromycin (Systemic); Itraconazole; Ketoconazole; Ketoconazole (Systemic); P-Glycoprotein Inhibitors; Pramlintide; Verapamil

Decreased Effect

Fexofenadine may decrease the levels/effects of: Acetylcholinesterase Inhibitors (Central); Benzylpenicilloyl Polylysine; Betahistine

The levels/effects of Fexofenadine may be decreased by: Acetylcholinesterase Inhibitors (Central); Amphetamines; Antacids; Grapefruit Juice; P-Glycoprotein Inducers; Rifampin; Tocilizumab

Ethanol/Nutrition/Herb Interactions

Ethanol: May increase CNS depression; monitor for increased effects with coadministration. Caution patients about effects.

Food: Fruit juice (apple, grapefruit, orange) may decrease bioavailability of fexofenadine by ~36%.

Herb/Nutraceutical: St John's wort may decrease fexofenadine levels.

Dietary Considerations Some products may contain phenylalanine and/or sodium. Take suspension and tablets with water only; do not administer with fruit juices.

Pharmacodynamics/Kinetics

Onset of Action 60 minutes

Duration of Action Antihistaminic effect: ≥12 hours

Half-life Elimination 14.4 hours (31% to 72% longer in renal impairment)

Time to Peak Serum: ODT: 2 hours (4 hours with high-fat meal); Tablet: ~2.6 hours; Suspension: ~1 hour

Pregnancy Risk Factor C

Lactation Excretion in breast milk unknown/use caution (AAP rates "compatible"; AAP 2001 update pending)

Dosage Forms

Suspension, oral:

Allegra®: 6 mg/mL (300 mL)

Allegra® Children's Allergy [OTC]: 6 mg/mL (120 mL)

Tablet, oral: 30 mg, 60 mg, 180 mg

Allegra® Allergy 12 Hour [OTC]: 60 mg

Allegra® Allergy 24 Hour [OTC]: 180 mg

Allegra® Children's Allergy [OTC]: 30 mg

Tablet, orally disintegrating, oral:

Allegra® Children's Allergy ODT [OTC]: 30 mg

Fexofenadine and Pseudoephedrine

(feks oh FEN a deen & soo doe e FED rin)

Related Information

Fexofenadine *on page 731*

Pseudoephedrine *on page 1429*

U.S. Brand Names Allegra-D® 12 Hour; Allegra-D® 24 Hour

Canadian Brand Names Allegra-D®

Pharmacologic Category Alpha/Beta Agonist; Decongestant; Histamine H_1 Antagonist; Histamine H_1 Antagonist, Second Generation; Piperidine Derivative

Use Relief of symptoms associated with seasonal allergic rhinitis in adults and children ≥12 years of age

Local Anesthetic/Vasoconstrictor Precautions Use with caution since pseudoephedrine is a sympathomimetic amine which could interact with epinephrine to cause a pressor response

Effects on Dental Treatment Key adverse event(s) related to dental treatment: Pseudoephedrine: Xerostomia (normal salivary flow resumes upon discontinuation).

Effects on Bleeding No information available to require special precautions

Adverse Effects See individual agents.

General Dosage Range Dosage adjustment recommended in patients with renal impairment

Oral: *Children ≥12 years and Adults:* 1 tablet (fexofenadine 60 mg/pseudoephedrine 120 mg) twice daily **or** 1 tablet (fexofenadine 180 mg/pseudoephedrine 240 mg) once daily

Pregnancy Risk Factor C

Fibrinogen Concentrate (Human) (fi BRIN o gin KON suhn trate HYU man)

U.S. Brand Names RiaSTAP®

Pharmacologic Category Blood Product Derivative

Use Treatment of acute bleeding episodes in patients with congenital fibrinogen deficiency (afibrinogenemia and hypofibrinogenemia)

Local Anesthetic/Vasoconstrictor Precautions No information available to require special precautions

Effects on Dental Treatment No significant effects or complications reported

Effects on Bleeding Fibrinogen concentrate is used in patients with congenital fibrinogen deficiency; it promotes blood clotting; there is the potential risk of thrombosis with use

General Dosage Range I.V.: *Children and Adults:* When baseline fibrinogen level is known: Dose (mg/kg) = [Target level (mg/dL) - measured level (mg/dL)] **divided by** 1.7 (mg/dL per mg/kg body weight) **or** when baseline fibrinogen level is not known: 70 mg/kg

Mechanism of Action Fibrinogen (coagulation factor I), a protein found in normal plasma, is required to clot blood. Fibrinogen concentrate made from pooled human plasma replaces this protein which is missing or reduced in patients with a congenital fibrinogen deficiency.

Pharmacodynamics/Kinetics

Half-life Elimination 61-97 hours (range: 56-117 hours); may be decreased in children <16 years of age

Pregnancy Risk Factor C

Fibrin Sealant (FI brin SEEL ent)

Related Information

Antiplatelet and Anticoagulation Considerations in Dentistry *on page* 1867

U.S. Brand Names Artiss; Evicel™; TachoSil®; Tisseel

Canadian Brand Names Tisseel

Pharmacologic Category Blood Product Derivative; Hemostatic Agent

Use

Artiss: Aid in adhering autologous skin grafts in burn patients (not indicated for hemostasis)

Evicel™: Adjunct to hemostasis in surgery when control of bleeding by conventional surgical techniques is ineffective or impractical

TachoSil®: Adjunct to hemostasis in cardiovascular surgery when control of bleeding by conventional surgical technique is ineffective or impractical

Tisseel: Adjunct to hemostasis in cardiopulmonary bypass surgery (including fully heparinized patients) and splenic injury (due to blunt or penetrating trauma to the abdomen) when the control of bleeding by conventional surgical techniques is ineffective or impractical; adjunctive sealant for closure of colostomies

Local Anesthetic/Vasoconstrictor Precautions No information available to require special precautions

Effects on Dental Treatment No significant effects or complications reported

Effects on Bleeding No information available to require special precautions

Adverse Effects May be related to aprotinin contained in some products. Frequency may vary by product.

1% to 10%:

- Cardiovascular: Bradycardia (≤10%)
- Central nervous system: Fever (6%)
- Dermatologic: Pruritus (≤1%)
- Local: Skin graft failure (Artiss: 4%)

General Dosage Range Topical: *Children >6 months and Adults:* Dosage varies greatly depending on product

Mechanism of Action Formation of a biodegradable adhesive is done by duplicating the last step of the coagulation cascade, the formation of fibrin from fibrinogen. Fibrinogen is the main component of the sealant solution. The solution also contains thrombin, which transforms fibrinogen from the sealer protein solution into fibrin, and fibrinolysis inhibitor (aprotinin), which prevents the premature degradation of fibrin. When mixed as directed, a viscous solution forms that sets into an elastic coagulum.

Pharmacodynamics/Kinetics

Onset of Action Artiss: Full adherence achieved: ~2 hours

Time to hemostasis: Evicel™: 4-10 minutes; TachoSil®: 6 minutes; Tisseel: 5 minutes

Pregnancy Risk Factor C

Filgrastim (fil GRA stim)

U.S. Brand Names Neupogen®

Canadian Brand Names Neupogen®

Pharmacologic Category Colony Stimulating Factor

Use

Cancer patients (nonmyeloid malignancies) receiving myelosuppressive chemotherapy to decrease the incidence of infection (febrile neutropenia) in regimens associated with a high incidence of neutropenia with fever

Acute myelogenous leukemia (AML) following induction or consolidation chemotherapy to shorten time to neutrophil recovery and reduce the duration of fever

Cancer patients (nonmyeloid malignancies) receiving bone marrow transplant to shorten the duration of neutropenia and neutropenia-related events (eg, neutropenic fever)

Peripheral stem cell transplantation to mobilize hematopoietic progenitor cells for leukapheresis collection

Severe chronic neutropenia (SCN; chronic administration) to reduce the incidence and duration of neutropenic complications (fever, infections, oropharyngeal ulcers) in symptomatic patients with congenital, cyclic, or idiopathic neutropenia

Unlabeled/Investigational Use Treatment of anemia in myelodysplastic syndrome; mobilization of hematopoietic stem cells (HSC) for collection and subsequent autologous transplantation (in combination with plerixafor) in patients with non-Hodgkin's lymphoma (NHL) and multiple myeloma (MM); treatment of neutropenia in HIV-infected patients receiving zidovudine; hepatitis C treatment-associated neutropenia

Local Anesthetic/Vasoconstrictor Precautions No information available to require special precautions

Effects on Dental Treatment No significant effects or complications reported

Effects on Bleeding No information available to require special precautions. Medical consultation may be considered to confirm adequate platelet counts.

Adverse Effects

>10%:

- Central nervous system: Fever (12%)
- Dermatologic: Petechiae (≤17%), rash (≤12%)
- Endocrine & metabolic: LDH increased, uric acid increased
- Gastrointestinal: Splenomegaly (severe chronic neutropenia: 30%; rare in other patients)
- Hepatic: Alkaline phosphatase increased (21%)
- Neuromuscular & skeletal: Bone/skeletal pain (22% to 33%; dose related), commonly in the lower back, posterior iliac crest, and sternum
- Respiratory: Epistaxis (9% to 15%)

1% to 10%:

- Cardiovascular: Hyper-/hypotension (4%), myocardial infarction/arrhythmias (3%)
- Central nervous system: Headache (7%)
- Gastrointestinal: Nausea (10%), vomiting (7%), peritonitis (≤2%)
- Hematologic: Leukocytosis (2%)
- Miscellaneous: Transfusion reaction (≤10%)

General Dosage Range

I.V.: *Children and Adults:* 5-10 mcg/kg/day

SubQ: *Children and Adults:* 5-10 mcg/kg/day **or** 6 mcg/kg twice daily

Mechanism of Action Stimulates the production, maturation, and activation of neutrophils; filgrastim activates neutrophils to increase both their migration and cytotoxicity.

Pharmacodynamics/Kinetics

Onset of Action ~24 hours; plateaus in 3-5 days

Duration of Action Neutrophil counts generally return to baseline within 4 days

Half-life Elimination 1.8-3.5 hours

Time to Peak Serum: SubQ: 2-8 hours

Pregnancy Risk Factor C

Finasteride (fi NAS teer ide)

U.S. Brand Names Propecia®; Proscar®

Canadian Brand Names CO Finasteride; JAMP-Finasteride; Mylan-Finasteride; Novo-Finasteride; PMS-Finasteride; Propecia®; Proscar®; ratio-Finasteride; Sandoz-Finasteride

Pharmacologic Category 5 Alpha-Reductase Inhibitor

Use

Propecia®: Treatment of male pattern hair loss in **men only**. Safety and efficacy were demonstrated in men between 18-41 years of age.

Proscar®: Treatment of symptomatic benign prostatic hyperplasia (BPH); can be used in combination with an alpha-blocker, doxazosin

Unlabeled/Investigational Use Prostate cancer prevention (to reduce the incidence); treatment of female hirsutism

Local Anesthetic/Vasoconstrictor Precautions No information available to require special precautions

Effects on Dental Treatment No significant effects or complications reported

Effects on Bleeding No information available to require special precautions

Adverse Effects Note: "Combination therapy" refers to finasteride and doxazosin.

>10%:

Endocrine & metabolic: Impotence (5% to 19%; combination therapy 23%), libido decreased (2% to 10%; combination therapy 12%)

Neuromuscular & skeletal: Weakness (5%; combination therapy 17%)

1% to 10%:

Cardiovascular: Postural hypotension (9%; combination therapy 18%), edema (1%; combination therapy 3%)

Central nervous system: Dizziness (7%; combination therapy 23%), somnolence (2%; combination therapy 3%)

Dermatologic: Rash (1%)

Genitourinary: Ejaculation disturbances (<1% to 7%; combination therapy 14%), decreased volume of ejaculate (2% to 4%)

Endocrine & metabolic: Gynecomastia (1% to 2%), breast tenderness (≤1%)

Respiratory: Dyspnea (1%; combination therapy 2%), rhinitis (1%; combination therapy 2%)

General Dosage Range Oral: *Adults:* 1 mg or 5 mg once daily

Mechanism of Action Finasteride is a competitive inhibitor of both tissue and hepatic 5-alpha reductase. This results in inhibition of the conversion of testosterone to dihydrotestosterone and markedly suppresses serum dihydrotestosterone levels

Pharmacodynamics/Kinetics

Onset of Action BPH: 6 months; Male pattern hair loss: ≥3 months of daily use.

Duration of Action

After a single oral dose as small as 0.5 mg: 65% depression of plasma dihydrotestosterone levels persists 5-7 days

After 6 months of treatment with 5 mg/day: Circulating dihydrotestosterone levels are reduced to castrate levels without significant effects on circulating testosterone; levels return to normal within 14 days of discontinuation of treatment

Half-life Elimination 6 hours (range: 3-16 hours); Elderly: 8 hours (range: 6-15 hours)

Time to Peak Serum: 1-2 hours

Pregnancy Risk Factor X

Fingolimod (fin GOL i mod)

U.S. Brand Names Gilenya™

Canadian Brand Names Gilenya®

Pharmacologic Category Sphingosine 1-Phosphate (S1P) Receptor Modulator

Use Treatment of relapsing forms of multiple sclerosis (MS) to reduce the frequency of clinical exacerbations and delay disability progression

Local Anesthetic/Vasoconstrictor Precautions No information available to require special precautions

Effects on Dental Treatment Key adverse event(s) related to dental treatment: Increased blood pressure may occur with fingolimod; assess and plan treatment according to patient's blood pressure. Fingolimod causes immune suppression; medical consult needed prior to dental surgery.

Effects on Bleeding No information available to require special precautions

Adverse Effects

>10%:

Central nervous system: Headache (25%)

Gastrointestinal: Diarrhea (12%)

Hepatic: ALT increased (14%), AST increased (14%)

Neuromuscular & skeletal: Back pain (12%)

Miscellaneous: Flu-like syndrome (13%)

1% to 10%:

Cardiovascular: Hypertension (6%), bradycardia (4%)

Central nervous system: Depression (8%), dizziness (7%), migraine (5%)

Dermatologic: Alopecia (4%), eczema (3%), pruritus (3%)

Endocrine & metabolic: Triglycerides increased (3%)

Gastrointestinal: Gastroenteritis (5%), weight loss (5%)

Hematologic: Lymphopenia (4%), leukopenia (3%)

Hepatic: GGT increased (5%)

Neuromuscular & skeletal: Paresthesia (5%), weakness (3%)

Ocular: Blurred vision (4%), eye pain (3%)

Respiratory: Cough (10%), bronchitis (8%), dyspnea (8%), sinusitis (7%)

Miscellaneous: Herpes infection (9%), tinea infection (4%)

General Dosage Range Oral: *Adults:* 0.5 mg once daily

Mechanism of Action Fingolimod-phosphate, active metabolite of fingolimod, binds to sphingosine 1-phosphate receptors 1, 3, 4, and 5. The amount of lymphocytes available to the central nervous system are decreased which reduces central inflammation.

Pharmacodynamics/Kinetics

Half-life Elimination 6-9 days

Time to Peak Plasma: 12-16 hours

Pregnancy Risk Factor C

Flavocoxid (fla vo KOKS id)

U.S. Brand Names Limbrel 250™; Limbrel 500™; Limbrel™ [DSC]

Pharmacologic Category Anti-inflammatory Agent; Nutritional Supplement

Use Clinical dietary management of the metabolic processes of osteoarthritis

Local Anesthetic/Vasoconstrictor Precautions No information available to require special precautions

Effects on Dental Treatment No significant effects or complications reported. May enhance risk of bleeding associated with NSAIDs.

Effects on Bleeding May alter platelet aggregation due to inhibition of cyclooxygenase (COX).

Adverse Effects ≥2%:

Cardiovascular: Hypertension, varicose veins

Dermatologic: Psoriasis

Gastrointestinal: Occult stools (statistically similar to placebo)

Neuromuscular & skeletal: Fluid on the knee

General Dosage Range Oral: *Adults:* 250-500 mg every 12 hours

Mechanism of Action Exerts anti-inflammatory properties through nonspecific inhibition of cyclooxygenase (COX) and lipoxygenase (5-LOX) pathways; may also possess general analgesic and antioxidant/anticytokine properties

Pharmacodynamics/Kinetics

Onset of Action 1-2 hours

FlavoxATE (fla VOKS ate)

Canadian Brand Names Apo-Flavoxate®; Urispas®

Pharmacologic Category Antispasmodic Agent, Urinary

Use Antispasmodic to provide symptomatic relief of dysuria, nocturia, suprapubic pain, urgency, and incontinence due to detrusor instability and hyper-reflexia in elderly with cystitis, urethritis, urethrocystitis, urethrotrigonitis, and prostatitis

Local Anesthetic/Vasoconstrictor Precautions No information available to require special precautions

Effects on Dental Treatment Key adverse event(s) related to dental treatment: Xerostomia and changes in salivation (normal salivary flow resumes upon discontinuation), and dry throat.

Effects on Bleeding No information available to require special precautions

Adverse Effects Frequency not defined.

Cardiovascular: Palpitations, tachycardia

Central nervous system: Confusion (especially in the elderly), drowsiness, fatigue, headache, hyperpyrexia, nervousness, vertigo

Dermatologic: Rash, urticaria

Gastrointestinal: Constipation, dry throat, nausea, vomiting, xerostomia

Genitourinary: Dysuria

Hematologic: Leukopenia

Ocular: Blurred vision, intraocular pressure increased

General Dosage Range Oral: *Children >12 years and Adults:* 100-200 mg 3-4 times/day

Mechanism of Action Synthetic antispasmodic with similar actions to that of propantheline; it exerts a direct relaxant effect on smooth muscles via phosphodiesterase inhibition, providing relief to a variety of smooth muscle spasms; it is especially useful for the treatment of bladder spasticity, whereby it produces an increase in urinary capacity

Pharmacodynamics/Kinetics

Onset of Action 55-60 minutes

Pregnancy Risk Factor B

Flecainide (fle KAY nide)

Related Information

Cardiovascular Diseases *on page* 1848

U.S. Brand Names Tambocor™

Canadian Brand Names Apo-Flecainide®; Tambocor™

Pharmacologic Category Antiarrhythmic Agent, Class Ic

Use Prevention and suppression of documented life-threatening ventricular arrhythmias (eg, sustained ventricular tachycardia); controlling symptomatic, disabling supraventricular tachycardias in patients without structural heart disease in whom other agents fail

Local Anesthetic/Vasoconstrictor Precautions Flecainide is one of the drugs confirmed to prolong the QT interval and is accepted as having a risk of causing torsade de pointes. The risk of drug-induced torsade de pointes is extremely low when a single QT interval prolonging drug is prescribed. In terms of epinephrine, it is not known what effect vasoconstrictors in the local anesthetic regimen will have in patients with a known history of congenital prolonged QT interval or in patients taking any medication that prolongs the QT interval. Until more information is obtained, it is suggested that the clinician consult with the physician prior to the use of a vasoconstrictor in suspected patients, and that the vasoconstrictor (epinephrine, mepivacaine and levonordefrin [Carbocaine® 2% with Neo-Cobefrin®]) be used with caution.

Effects on Dental Treatment No significant effects or complications reported

Effects on Bleeding No information available to require special precautions

Adverse Effects

>10%:

- Central nervous system: Dizziness (19% to 30%)
- Ocular: Visual disturbances (16%)
- Respiratory: Dyspnea (~10%)

1% to 10%:

- Cardiovascular: Palpitation (6%), chest pain (5%), edema (3.5%), tachycardia (1% to 3%), proarrhythmic (4% to 12%), sinus node dysfunction (1.2%)
- Central nervous system: Headache (4% to 10%), fatigue (8%), nervousness (5%) additional symptoms occurring at a frequency between 1% and 3%: fever, malaise, hypoesthesia, paresis, ataxia, vertigo, syncope, somnolence, tinnitus, anxiety, insomnia, depression
- Dermatologic: Rash (1% to 3%)
- Gastrointestinal: Nausea (9%), constipation (1%), abdominal pain (3%), anorexia (1% to 3%), diarrhea (0.7% to 3%)
- Neuromuscular & skeletal: Tremor (5%), weakness (5%), paresthesia (1%)
- Ocular: Diplopia (1% to 3%), blurred vision

General Dosage Range Dosage adjustment recommended in patients with renal impairment

Oral:

Children: Initial: 3 mg/kg/day **or** 50-100 mg/m^2/day in 3 divided doses; Maintenance: 3-6 mg/kg/day **or** 100-150 mg/m^2/day in 3 divided doses (maximum: 11 mg/kg/day; 200 mg/m^2/day)

Adults: Initial: 50-100 mg every 12 hours; Maintenance: 100-400 mg/day in 2 divided doses (maximum: 400 mg/day)

Mechanism of Action Class Ic antiarrhythmic; slows conduction in cardiac tissue by altering transport of ions across cell membranes; causes slight prolongation of refractory periods; decreases the rate of rise of the action potential without affecting its duration; increases electrical stimulation threshold of ventricle, His-Purkinje system; possesses local anesthetic and moderate negative inotropic effects

Pharmacodynamics/Kinetics

Half-life Elimination Infants: 11-12 hours; Children: 8 hours; Adults: 7-22 hours, increased with congestive heart failure or renal dysfunction; End-stage renal disease: 19-26 hours

Time to Peak Serum: ~1.5-3 hours

Pregnancy Risk Factor C

Dental Comment Flecainide is known to prolong the QT interval. The QT interval is measured as the time and distance between the Q point of the QRS complex and the end of the T wave in the ECG tracing. After adjustment for heart rate, the QT interval is defined as prolonged if it is more than 450 msec in men and 460 msec in women. A long QT syndrome was first described in the 1950s and 60s as a congenital syndrome involving QT interval prolongation and syncope and sudden death. Some of the congenital long QT syndromes were characterized by a peculiar electrocardiographic appearance of the QRS complex involving a premature atria beat followed by a pause, then a subsequent sinus beat showing marked QT prolongation and deformity. This type of cardiac arrhythmia was originally termed "torsade de pointes" (translated from the French as "twisting of the points"). Flecainide is considered as having a risk of causing torsade de pointes. Since it is not known what effect vasoconstrictors in the local anesthetic regimen will have in patients with a known history of congenital prolonged QT interval or in patients taking any medication that prolongs the QT interval, a medical consult is suggested.

Floctafenine (flok ta FEN een)

Canadian Brand Names Apo-Floctafenine®

Pharmacologic Category Nonsteroidal Anti-inflammatory Drug (NSAID), Oral

Use Short-term management of acute, mild-to-moderate pain

Local Anesthetic/Vasoconstrictor Precautions No information available to require special precautions

Effects on Dental Treatment Key adverse event(s) related to dental treatment: Xerostomia and changes in salivation (normal salivary flow resumes upon discontinuation), bitter taste. See Effects on Bleeding.

Effects on Bleeding Nonselective NSAIDs are known to reversibly decrease platelet aggregation via mechanisms different than observed with aspirin. Platelet function is restored as the drug is eliminated from the body. Dental professionals should be aware that recommendations differ between dental and general medical surgery. NSAIDs should be avoided (if possible) in general medical surgery patients for 3-5 half-lives of the drug (usually 1-3 days) prior to surgery to reduce the risk of excessive bleeding. However, there is no scientific evidence to warrant discontinuance of NSAIDs prior to dental surgery. In medically complicated patients or extensive oral surgery, the decision to interrupt therapy must be based on the risk to benefit in an individual patient and a medical consult is suggested. Routine interruption of NSAID therapy for most dental procedures is not warranted. If therapy is continued without interruption, the clinician should anticipate the potential for slower clotting times.

Adverse Effects Frequency not defined.

Cardiovascular: Edema, flushing, tachycardia

Central nervous system: Depression, dizziness, drowsiness, fatigue, headache, insomnia, irritability, malaise, nervousness, vertigo

Dermatologic: Angioedema, pruritus, rash, urticaria

Endocrine & metabolic: Fluid retention, hyperkalemia

Gastrointestinal: Abdominal pain, bitter taste, constipation, diarrhea, dyspepsia, flatulence, gastrointestinal bleeding, gastrointestinal ulcer, gross bleeding with perforation, heartburn, nausea, vomiting, xerostomia

Hematologic: Agranulocytosis, aplastic anemia, bleeding, leukopenia, neutropenia, thrombocytopenia

Hepatic: Hepatotoxicity, liver enzymes increased

Ocular: Blurred and/or diminished vision

Otic: Tinnitus

Renal: Burning micturition, cystitis, dysuria, hematuria, interstitial nephritis, polyuria, reversible acute renal insufficiency with or without oliguria/anuria, strong smelling urine, urethritis

Respiratory: Asthmatic-type dyspnea

Miscellaneous: Anaphylaxis, diaphoresis, thirst

General Dosage Range Dosage adjustment recommended in patients with renal impairment

Oral: *Adults:* 200-400 mg every 6-8 hours as needed (maximum: 1200 mg/day)

Mechanism of Action Reversibly inhibits cyclooxygenase-1 and 2 (COX-1 and 2) enzymes, which results in decreased formation of prostaglandin precursors; has antipyretic, analgesic, and anti-inflammatory properties

Other proposed mechanisms not fully elucidated (and possibly contributing to the anti-inflammatory effect to varying degrees), include inhibiting chemotaxis, altering lymphocyte activity, inhibiting neutrophil aggregation/activation, and decreasing proinflammatory cytokine levels.

Pharmacodynamics/Kinetics

Duration of Action 6-8 hours

Half-life Elimination Initial phase (distribution): 1 hour; second phase (elimination): 8 hours

Time to Peak 1-2 hours

Product Availability Not available in U.S.

Floxuridine (floks YOOR i deen)

Canadian Brand Names FUDR®

Pharmacologic Category Antineoplastic Agent, Antimetabolite (Pyrimidine Analog)

Use Management of hepatic metastases of colorectal and gastric cancers

Local Anesthetic/Vasoconstrictor Precautions No information available to require special precautions

Effects on Dental Treatment Key adverse event(s) related to dental treatment: Stomatitis.

Effects on Bleeding Chemotherapy may result in significant myelosuppression, potentially including significant reduction in platelet counts and altered hemostasis. In patients who are under active treatment with these agents, medical consult is suggested.

Adverse Effects

>10%:

Gastrointestinal: Stomatitis, diarrhea; may be dose limiting

Hematologic: Myelosuppression, may be dose limiting; leukopenia, thrombocytopenia, anemia

Onset: 4-7 days

Nadir: 5-9 days

Recovery: 21 days

1% to 10%:

Dermatologic: Alopecia, photosensitivity, hyperpigmentation of the skin, localized erythema, dermatitis

Gastrointestinal: Anorexia

Hepatic: Biliary sclerosis, cholecystitis, jaundice

General Dosage Range Dosage adjustment recommended in patients with hepatic impairment

Intra-arterial: *Adults:* 0.1-0.6 mg/kg/day

Mechanism of Action Mechanism of action and pharmacokinetics are very similar to fluorouracil; floxuridine is the deoxyribonucleotide of fluorouracil. Floxuridine is a fluorinated pyrimidine antagonist which inhibits DNA and RNA synthesis and methylation of deoxyuridylic acid to thymidylic acid.

Pregnancy Risk Factor D

Fluconazole (floo KOE na zole)

Related Information

Clinical Risk Related to Drugs Prolonging QT Interval *on page* 1872

Fungal Infections *on page* 1945

Related Sample Prescriptions

Systemic Fungal Infections *on page* 1988

U.S. Brand Names Diflucan®

Canadian Brand Names Apo-Fluconazole®; CanesOral®; CO Fluconazole; Diflucan®; Dom-Fluconazole; Fluconazole Injection; Fluconazole Omega; Mylan-Fluconazole; Novo-Fluconazole; PHL-Fluconazole; PMS-Fluconazole; PRO-Fluconazole; Riva-Fluconazole; Taro-Fluconazole; ZYM-Fluconazole

Generic Availability (U.S.) Yes

Pharmacologic Category Antifungal Agent, Oral; Antifungal Agent, Parenteral

Dental Use Treatment of susceptible fungal infections in the oral cavity including candidiasis, oral thrush, and chronic mucocutaneous candidiasis treatment of esophageal and oropharyngeal candidiasis caused by *Candida* species; treatment of severe, chronic mucocutaneous candidiasis caused by *Candida* species

Use Treatment of candidiasis (vaginal, oropharyngeal, esophageal, urinary tract infections, peritonitis, pneumonia, and systemic infections); cryptococcal meningitis; antifungal prophylaxis in allogeneic bone marrow transplant recipients

Unlabeled/Investigational Use Cryptococcal pneumonia; candidal intertrigo

Local Anesthetic/Vasoconstrictor Precautions No information available to require special precautions

Effects on Dental Treatment Key adverse event(s) related to dental treatment: Abnormal taste.

Effects on Bleeding No information available to require special precautions

Adverse Effects Frequency not always defined.

Cardiovascular: Angioedema, pallor, QT prolongation (rare, case reports), torsade de pointes (rare, case reports)

Central nervous system: Headache (2% to 13%), dizziness (1%), seizure

Dermatologic: Rash (2%), alopecia, toxic epidermal necrolysis, Stevens-Johnson syndrome

Endocrine & metabolic: Hypercholesterolemia, hypertriglyceridemia, hypokalemia

Gastrointestinal: Nausea (2% to 7%), abdominal pain (2% to 6%), vomiting (2% to 5%), diarrhea (2% to 3%), dyspepsia (1%), taste perversion (1%)

Hematologic: Agranulocytosis, leukopenia, neutropenia, thrombocytopenia

Hepatic: Alkaline phosphatase increased, ALT increased, AST increased, cholestasis, hepatic failure (rare), hepatitis, jaundice

Respiratory: Dyspnea
Miscellaneous: Anaphylactic reactions (rare)

Dental Usual Dosage Candidiasis: Adults:

Usual dosage range: 200-400 mg/day; duration and dosage depends on severity of infection

Oropharyngeal (long-term suppression): 200 mg/day; chronic therapy is recommended in immunocompromised patients with history of oropharyngeal candidiasis (OPC)

Dosage The daily dose of fluconazole is the same for oral and I.V. administration

Usual dosage ranges:

Neonates: First 2 weeks of life, especially premature neonates: Same dose as older children every 72 hours

Children: Loading dose: 6-12 mg/kg; maintenance: 3-12 mg/kg/day; duration and dosage depends on severity of infection

Adults: 150 mg once **or** 200-800 mg/day; duration and dosage depends on severity of infection

Indication-specific dosing:

Children:

Candidiasis:

Oropharyngeal:

Manufacturer's recommendation: Loading dose: 6 mg/kg; maintenance: 3 mg/kg/day once daily for 2 weeks

HIV-exposed/-positive: 3-6 mg/kg/day once daily (maximum: 400 mg/day) (CDC, 2009)

Esophageal:

Manufacturer's recommendation: Loading dose: 6 mg/kg; maintenance: 3-12 mg/kg/day once daily for 21 days and at least 2 weeks following resolution of symptoms

HIV-exposed/-positive: Loading dose: 6 mg/kg once on day 1; maintenance: 3-6 mg/kg/day once daily (maximum: 400 mg/day) (CDC, 2009)

Relapse suppression (HIV-exposed/-positive): 3-6 mg/kg/day once daily (maximum: 200 mg/day) (CDC, 2009)

Invasive disease (independent of HIV status): 5-6 mg/kg every 12 hours for 28 days (maximum: 600 mg/day) (CDC, 2009)

Coccidioidomycosis (CDC, 2009):

Meningeal and disseminated disease (HIV-exposed/-positive): 5-6 mg/kg/dose every 12 hours (maximum: 800 mg/day)

Relapse suppression (HIV-exposed/-positive): 6 mg/kg/day once daily (maximum: 400 mg/day)

Histoplasmosis, relapse suppression (HIV-exposed/-positive): 3-6 mg/kg/day once daily (maximum: 200 mg/day) (CDC, 2009)

Cryptococcal disease (CDC, 2009):

Meningitis (consolidation): Loading dose: 12 mg/kg once on day 1; maintenance: 6-12 mg/kg/day once daily for a minimum of 8 weeks (maximum: 800 mg/day)

Disseminated (non-CNS) or severe pulmonary disease: Loading dose: 12 mg/kg once on day 1; maintenance: 6-12 mg/kg/day once daily (maximum: 600 mg/day)

Relapse suppression (HIV-exposed/-positive): 6 mg/kg/day once daily (maximum: 200 mg/day)

Adults:

Candidiasis (Pappas, 2009):

Candidemia (neutropenic and non-neutropenic): Loading dose: 800 mg on first day, then 400 mg/day for 14 days after first negative blood culture and resolution of signs/symptoms; **Note:** Not recommended for neutropenic patients with recent azole exposure and critical illness

Chronic, disseminated: 400 mg/day until calcification or lesion resolution

CNS candidemia: 400-800 mg/day until CSF/radiological abnormalities resolved; **Note:** Recommended as alternative therapy in patients intolerant of amphotericin B

Oropharyngeal: 100-200 mg/day for 7-14 days for uncomplicated, moderate-to-severe disease; chronic therapy of 100 mg 3 times weekly is recommended in immunocompromised patients with history of oropharyngeal candidiasis (OPC)

Osteoarticular: 400 mg/day for 6-12 months (osteomyelitis) or 6 weeks (septic arthritis)

Esophageal: 200-400 mg/day for 14-21 days

Prophylaxis:

Solid organ: 200-400 mg/day for 7-14 days

Neutropenic patients: 400 mg/day for duration of neutropenia

Urinary tract:
Fungus balls: 200-400 mg/day
Pyelonephritis: 200-400 mg/day for 2 weeks
Symptomatic cystitis: 200 mg/day for 2 weeks
Vaginal:
Uncomplicated: 150 mg as a single dose
Complicated: 150 mg every 72 hours for 3 doses
Recurrent: 150 mg daily for 10-14 days, followed by 150 mg once weekly for 6 months

Candidal intertrigo (unlabeled use; Coldiron, 1991; Nozickova, 1998; Stengel, 1994): 50 mg/day **or** 150 mg once weekly

Coccidiomycosis (unlabeled use; Galgiani, 2005): 400-800 mg/day; doses of 800-1000 mg/day have been used for meningeal disease; usual duration of therapy ranges from 3-6 months for primary uncomplicated infections and up to 1 year for pulmonary (chronic and diffuse) infection

Endocarditis, prosthetic valve, early (unlabeled use; Pappas, 2009): 400-800 mg/day for 6 weeks after valve replacement (as step-down in stable, culture-negative patients); long-term suppression in absence of valve replacement: 400-800 mg/day

Endophthalmitis (Pappas, 2009): 400-800 mg/day for 4-6 weeks until examination indicates resolution

Meningitis, cryptococcal (Perfect, 2010):
Induction therapy: Typically consists of an amphotericin product and flucytosine for 2-6 weeks
Consolidation therapy: Fluconazole 400-800 mg/day for 8 weeks
Maintenance therapy: 200 mg/day for 6-12 months (post-transplant patients; non-HIV infected patients) **or** ≥1 year (HIV-infected patients may require lifelong therapy; CDC, 2009)

Pericarditis or myocarditis (Pappas, 2009): 400-800 mg/day

Pneumonia, cryptococcal (mild-to-moderate) (unlabeled use; Perfect, 2010): 400 mg/day for 6-12 months (HIV-infected patients may require lifelong therapy; CDC, 2009)

Dosing adjustment/interval in renal impairment:
No adjustment for vaginal candidiasis single-dose therapy
For multiple dosing, administer usual load then adjust daily doses as follows:
Cl_{cr} ≤50 mL/minute (no dialysis): Administer 50% of recommended dose or administer every 48 hours.
Hemodialysis: 50% is removed by hemodialysis; administer 100% of daily dose (according to indication) after each dialysis treatment.

Continuous renal replacement therapy (CRRT): Drug clearance is highly dependent on the method of renal replacement, filter type, and flow rate. Appropriate dosing requires close monitoring of pharmacologic response, signs of adverse reactions due to drug accumulation, as well as drug levels in relation to target trough (if appropriate). The following are general recommendations only (based on dialysate flow/ultrafiltration rates of 1 L/hour) and should not supersede clinical judgment:
CVVH: 200-400 mg every 24 hours
CVVHD/CVVHDF: 400-800 mg every 24 hours
Note: Higher daily doses of 400 mg (CVVH) and 800 mg (CVVHD/CVVHDF) should be considered when treating resistant organisms and/or when employing combined ultrafiltration and dialysis flow rates of ≥2 L/hour for CVVHD/CVVHDF (Trotman, 2005).

Mechanism of Action Interferes with fungal cytochrome P450 activity (lanosterol 14-α-demethylase), decreasing ergosterol synthesis (principal sterol in fungal cell membrane) and inhibiting cell membrane formation

Contraindications Hypersensitivity to fluconazole or any component of the formulation (cross-reaction with other azole antifungal agents may occur, but has not been established; use caution); concomitant administration with cisapride or terfenadine

Warnings/Precautions Should be used with caution in patients with renal and hepatic dysfunction or previous hepatotoxicity from other azole derivatives. Patients who develop abnormal liver function tests during fluconazole therapy should be monitored closely and discontinued if symptoms consistent with liver disease develop. Rare exfoliative skin disorders have been observed; monitor closely if rash develops and discontinue if lesions progress. The manufacturer reports rare cases of QT_c prolongation and torsade de pointes associated with fluconazole use and advises caution in patients with concomitant medications or conditions which are arrhythmogenic. However, given the limited number of cases and the presence of multiple confounding variables, the likelihood that fluconazole causes conduction abnormalities appears remote.

Drug Interactions

Metabolism/Transport Effects Inhibits CYP1A2 (weak), 2C9 (strong), 2C19 (strong), 3A4 (moderate)

Avoid Concomitant Use

Avoid concomitant use of Fluconazole with any of the following: Artemether; Cisapride; Clopidogrel; Conivaptan; Dofetilide; Dronedarone; Lumefantrine; Nilotinib; Pimozide; QuiNIDine; QuiNINE; Ranolazine; Tetrabenazine; Thioridazine; Tolvaptan; Toremifene; Vandetanib; Voriconazole; Ziprasidone

Increased Effect/Toxicity

Fluconazole may increase the levels/effects of: Alfentanil; Aprepitant; Benzodiazepines (metabolized by oxidation); Bosentan; Budesonide (Systemic, Oral Inhalation); BusPIRone; Busulfan; Calcium Channel Blockers; CarBAMazepine; Carvedilol; Cilostazol; Cinacalcet; Cisapride; Citalopram; Colchicine; Conivaptan; Corticosteroids (Systemic); CycloSPORINE; CycloSPORINE (Systemic); CYP2C19 Substrates; CYP2C9 Substrates (High risk); CYP3A4 Substrates; DOCEtaxel; Dofetilide; Dronedarone; Eletriptan; Eplerenone; Erlotinib; Eszopiclone; Etravirine; Everolimus; FentaNYL; Fosaprepitant; Fosphenytoin; Gefitinib; HMG-CoA Reductase Inhibitors; Imatinib; Irbesartan; Irinotecan; Losartan; Lurasidone; Macrolide Antibiotics; Methadone; Phenytoin; Phosphodiesterase 5 Inhibitors; Pimecrolimus; Pimozide; Protease Inhibitors; Proton Pump Inhibitors; QTc-Prolonging Agents; QuiNIDine; QuiNINE; Ramelteon; Ranolazine; Repaglinide; Rifamycin Derivatives; Salmeterol; Saxagliptin; Sirolimus; Solifenacin; Sulfonylureas; SUNItinib; Tacrolimus; Tacrolimus (Systemic); Tacrolimus (Topical); Temsirolimus; Tetrabenazine; Thioridazine; Tolterodine; Tolvaptan; Toremifene; Vandetanib; Vilazodone; Vitamin K Antagonists; Voriconazole; Zidovudine; Ziprasidone; Zolpidem

The levels/effects of Fluconazole may be increased by: Alfuzosin; Artemether; Chloroquine; Ciprofloxacin; Ciprofloxacin (Systemic); Etravirine; Gadobutrol; Grapefruit Juice; Lumefantrine; Macrolide Antibiotics; Nilotinib; Protease Inhibitors; QuiNINE

Decreased Effect

Fluconazole may decrease the levels/effects of: Amphotericin B; Clopidogrel; Saccharomyces boulardii

The levels/effects of Fluconazole may be decreased by: Didanosine; Etravirine; Fosphenytoin; Phenytoin; Rifamycin Derivatives; Sucralfate

Dietary Considerations Take without regard to meals.

Pharmacodynamics/Kinetics

Half-life Elimination Normal renal function: ~30 hours

Time to Peak Oral: 1-2 hours

Pregnancy Risk Factor C

Lactation Enters breast milk/not recommended (AAP rates "compatible"; AAP 2001 update pending)

Breast-Feeding Considerations Fluconazole is found in breast milk at concentration similar to plasma.

Dosage Forms

Infusion, premixed iso-osmotic dextrose solution: 200 mg (100 mL); 400 mg (200 mL)
Diflucan®: 400 mg (200 mL)

Infusion, premixed iso-osmotic sodium chloride solution: 100 mg (50 mL); 200 mg (100 mL); 400 mg (200 mL)
Diflucan®: 200 mg (100 mL); 400 mg (200 mL)

Infusion, premixed iso-osmotic sodium chloride solution [preservative free]: 200 mg (100 mL); 400 mg (200 mL)

Powder for suspension, oral: 10 mg/mL (35 mL); 40 mg/mL (35 mL)
Diflucan®: 10 mg/mL (35 mL); 40 mg/mL (35 mL)

Tablet, oral: 50 mg, 100 mg, 150 mg, 200 mg
Diflucan®: 50 mg, 100 mg, 150 mg, 200 mg

Flucytosine (floo SYE toe seen)

U.S. Brand Names Ancobon®

Canadian Brand Names Ancobon®

Pharmacologic Category Antifungal Agent, Oral

Use Adjunctive treatment of systemic fungal infections (eg, septicemia, endocarditis, UTI, meningitis, or pulmonary) caused by susceptible strains of *Candida* or *Cryptococcus*

Local Anesthetic/Vasoconstrictor Precautions No information available to require special precautions

Effects on Dental Treatment No significant effects or complications reported

Effects on Bleeding No information available to require special precautions

Adverse Effects Frequency not defined.

Cardiovascular: Cardiac arrest, myocardial toxicity, ventricular dysfunction, chest pain

Central nervous system: Ataxia, confusion, dizziness, drowsiness, fatigue, hallucinations, headache, parkinsonism, psychosis, pyrexia, sedation, seizure, vertigo

Dermatologic: Rash, photosensitivity, pruritus, toxic epidermal necrolysis, urticaria

Endocrine & metabolic: Hypoglycemia, hypokalemia

Gastrointestinal: Abdominal pain, diarrhea, dry mouth, duodenal ulcer, hemorrhage, loss of appetite, nausea, ulcerative colitis, vomiting

Hematologic: Agranulocytosis, anemia, aplastic anemia, eosinophilia, leukopenia, pancytopenia, thrombocytopenia

Hepatic: Acute hepatic injury, bilirubin increased, hepatic dysfunction, jaundice, liver enzymes increased

Neuromuscular & skeletal: Paresthesia, peripheral neuropathy, weakness

Otic: Hearing loss

Renal: Azotemia, BUN increased, crystalluria, renal failure, serum creatinine increased

Respiratory: Dyspnea, respiratory arrest

Miscellaneous: Allergic reaction

General Dosage Range Dosage adjustment recommended in patients with renal impairment

Oral: *Adults:* 50-150 mg/kg/day in divided doses every 6 hours

Mechanism of Action Penetrates fungal cells and is converted to fluorouracil which competes with uracil interfering with fungal RNA and protein synthesis

Pharmacodynamics/Kinetics

Half-life Elimination Normal renal function: 2-5 hours; Anuria: 85 hours (range: 30-250); End stage renal disease: 75-200 hours

Time to Peak Serum: ~1-2 hours

Pregnancy Risk Factor C

Fludarabine (floo DARE a been)

U.S. Brand Names Fludara®; Oforta™

Canadian Brand Names Fludara®

Pharmacologic Category Antineoplastic Agent, Antimetabolite (Purine Analog)

Use Treatment of progressive or refractory B-cell chronic lymphocytic leukemia (CLL)

Canadian labeling: Second-line treatment of chronic lymphocytic leukemia (CLL); second-line treatment of low-grade, refractory non-Hodgkin's lymphoma (NHL)

Unlabeled/Investigational Use Treatment of non-Hodgkin's lymphomas (NHL); acute myeloid leukemia (AML), either refractory or in poor risk patients; relapsed acute lymphocytic leukemia (ALL) or AML in pediatric patients; Waldenström's macroglobulinemia (WM); reduced-intensity conditioning regimens prior to allogeneic hematopoietic stem cell transplantation (generally administered in combination with busulfan or cyclophosphamide and antithymocyte globulin or lymphocyte immune globulin, or in combination with melphalan and alemtuzumab)

Local Anesthetic/Vasoconstrictor Precautions No information available to require special precautions

Effects on Dental Treatment Key adverse event(s) related to dental treatment: Stomatitis.

Effects on Bleeding Chemotherapy may result in significant myelosuppression, potentially including significant reduction in platelet counts and altered hemostasis. In patients who are under active treatment with these agents, medical consult is suggested.

Adverse Effects

>10%:

Cardiovascular: Edema (8% to 19%)

Central nervous system: Fever (11% to 69%), fatigue (10% to 38%), pain (5% to 22%), chills (11% to 19%)

Dermatologic: Rash (4% to 15%)

Gastrointestinal: Nausea/vomiting (1% to 36%), anorexia (≤34%), diarrhea (5% to 15%), gastrointestinal bleeding (3% to 13%)

Genitourinary: Urinary tract infection (2% to 15%)

Hematologic: Myelosuppression (nadir: 10-14 days; recovery: 5-7 weeks; dose-limiting toxicity), anemia (14% to 60%), neutropenia (grade 4: 37% to 59%; nadir: ~13 days), thrombocytopenia (17% to 55%; nadir: ~16 days)

Neuromuscular & skeletal: Weakness (9% to 65%), myalgia (4% to 16%), paresthesia (4% to 12%)

Ocular: Visual disturbance (3% to 15%)

Respiratory: Cough (≤44%), pneumonia (3% to 22%), dyspnea (1% to 22%), upper respiratory infection (2% to 16%), rhinitis (≤11%)
Miscellaneous: Infection (12% to 44%), diaphoresis (≤14%)
1% to 10%:
Cardiovascular: Peripheral edema (≤7%), angina (≤6%), chest pain (≤5%), CHF (≤3%), arrhythmia (≤3%), cerebrovascular accident (≤3%), MI (≤3%), supraventricular tachycardia (≤3%), deep vein thrombosis (1% to 3%), phlebitis (1% to 3%), aneurysm (≤1%), transient ischemic attack (≤1%)
Central nervous system: Headache (≤9%), malaise (6% to 8%), sleep disorder (1% to 3%), cerebellar syndrome (≤1%), depression (≤1%), mentation impaired (≤1%)
Dermatologic: Alopecia (≤3%), pruritus (1% to 3%), seborrhea (≤1%)
Endocrine & metabolic: Hyperglycemia (1% to 6%), LDH increased (≤6%), dehydration (≤1%)
Gastrointestinal: Abdominal pain (≤10%), stomatitis (≤9%), weight loss (≤6%), esophagitis (≤3%), constipation (1% to 3%), mucositis (≤2%), dysphagia (≤1%)
Genitourinary: Dysuria (3% to 4%), hesitancy (≤3%)
Hematologic: Hemorrhage (≤1%), myelodysplastic syndrome/acute myeloid leukemia (usually associated with prior or concurrent treatment with other anticancer agents)
Hepatic: Cholelithiasis (≤3%), liver function tests abnormal (1% to 3%), liver failure (≤1%)
Neuromuscular & skeletal: Back pain (≤9%), osteoporosis (≤2%), arthralgia (≤1%)
Otic: Hearing loss (2% to 6%)
Renal: Hematuria (2% to 3%), renal failure (≤1%), renal function test abnormal (≤1%), proteinuria (≤1%)
Respiratory: Bronchitis (≤9%), pharyngitis (≤9%), allergic pneumonitis (≤6%), hemoptysis (1% to 6%), sinusitis (≤5%), epistaxis (≤1%), hypoxia (≤1%)
Miscellaneous: Flu-like syndrome (5% to 8%), herpes simplex infection (≤8%), anaphylaxis (≤1%), tumor lysis syndrome (1%)

General Dosage Range Dosage adjustment recommended in patients with renal impairment or who develop toxicities.
Oral: *Adults:* 40 mg/m^2/day for 5 days every 28 days
I.V.: *Adults:* 25 mg/m^2/day for 5 days every 28 days

Mechanism of Action Fludarabine inhibits DNA synthesis by inhibition of DNA polymerase and ribonucleotide reductase; also inhibits DNA primase and DNA ligase I

Pharmacodynamics/Kinetics
Half-life Elimination 2-fluoro-ara-A: ~20 hours
Time to Peak Oral: 1-2 hours

Pregnancy Risk Factor D

Fludrocortisone (floo droe KOR ti sone)

Canadian Brand Names Florinef®
Generic Availability (U.S.) Yes
Pharmacologic Category Corticosteroid, Systemic
Use Partial replacement therapy for primary and secondary adrenocortical insufficiency in Addison's disease; treatment of salt-losing adrenogenital syndrome
Local Anesthetic/Vasoconstrictor Precautions No information available to require special precautions
Effects on Dental Treatment No significant effects or complications reported
Effects on Bleeding No information available to require special precautions
Adverse Effects Frequency not defined.
Cardiovascular: CHF, edema, hypertension
Central nervous system: Dizziness, headache, seizures
Dermatologic: Acne, bruising, rash
Endocrine & metabolic: HPA suppression, hyperglycemia, hypokalemic alkalosis, suppression of growth
Gastrointestinal: Peptic ulcer
Neuromuscular & skeletal: Muscle weakness
Ocular: Cataracts
Miscellaneous: Anaphylaxis (generalized), diaphoresis

Dosage Oral:
Infants and Children: 0.05-0.1 mg/day
Adults: 0.1-0.2 mg/day with ranges of 0.1 mg 3 times/week to 0.2 mg/day
Addison's disease: Initial: 0.1 mg/day; if transient hypertension develops, reduce the dose to 0.05 mg/day. Preferred administration with cortisone (10-37.5 mg/day) or hydrocortisone (10-30 mg/day).
Salt-losing adrenogenital syndrome: 0.1-0.2 mg/day

Mechanism of Action Promotes increased reabsorption of sodium and loss of potassium from renal distal tubules

Contraindications Hypersensitivity to fludrocortisone or any component of the formulation; systemic fungal infections

Warnings/Precautions May cause hypercorticism or suppression of hypothalamic-pituitary-adrenal (HPA) axis, particularly in younger children or in patients receiving high doses for prolonged periods. HPA axis suppression may lead to adrenal crisis. Withdrawal and discontinuation of a corticosteroid should be done slowly and carefully. Fludrocortisone is primarily a mineralocorticoid agonist, but may also inhibit the HPA axis. May increase risk of infection and/or limit response to vaccinations; close observation is required in patients with latent tuberculosis and/or TB reactivity. Restrict use in active TB (only in conjunction with antituberculosis treatment). Use with caution in patients with sodium retention and potassium loss, hepatic impairment, myocardial infarction, osteoporosis, and/or renal impairment. Use with caution in the elderly. Withdraw therapy with gradual tapering of dose.

Drug Interactions

Avoid Concomitant Use

Avoid concomitant use of Fludrocortisone with any of the following: Aldesleukin; BCG; Natalizumab; Pimecrolimus; Roflumilast; Tacrolimus (Topical)

Increased Effect/Toxicity

Fludrocortisone may increase the levels/effects of: Acetylcholinesterase Inhibitors; Amphotericin B; Deferasirox; Leflunomide; Loop Diuretics; Natalizumab; NSAID (COX-2 Inhibitor); NSAID (Nonselective); Thiazide Diuretics; Vaccines (Live); Warfarin

The levels/effects of Fludrocortisone may be increased by: Antifungal Agents (Azole Derivatives, Systemic); Aprepitant; Calcium Channel Blockers (Nondihydropyridine); Denosumab; Estrogen Derivatives; Fluconazole; Fosaprepitant; Macrolide Antibiotics; Neuromuscular-Blocking Agents (Nondepolarizing); Pimecrolimus; Quinolone Antibiotics; Roflumilast; Salicylates; Tacrolimus (Topical); Trastuzumab

Decreased Effect

Fludrocortisone may decrease the levels/effects of: Aldesleukin; Antidiabetic Agents; BCG; Calcitriol; Corticorelin; Isoniazid; Salicylates; Sipuleucel-T; Vaccines (Inactivated)

The levels/effects of Fludrocortisone may be decreased by: Aminoglutethimide; Antacids; Barbiturates; Bile Acid Sequestrants; Echinacea; Mitotane; Primidone; Rifamycin Derivatives

Dietary Considerations Systemic use of mineralocorticoids/corticosteroids may require a diet with increased potassium, vitamins A, B_6, C, D, folate, calcium, zinc, and phosphorus, and decreased sodium. With fludrocortisone, a decrease in dietary sodium is often not required as the increased retention of sodium is usually the desired therapeutic effect.

Pharmacodynamics/Kinetics

Half-life Elimination Plasma: 30-35 minutes; Biological: 18-36 hours

Time to Peak Serum: ~1.7 hours

Pregnancy Risk Factor C

Lactation Excretion in breast milk unknown/use caution

Breast-Feeding Considerations Corticosteroids are excreted in human milk; information specific to fludrocortisone has not been located.

Dosage Forms

Tablet, oral: 0.1 mg

Flumazenil (FLOO may ze nil)

U.S. Brand Names Romazicon®

Canadian Brand Names Anexate®; Flumazenil Injection; Flumazenil Injection, USP; Romazicon®

Generic Availability (U.S.) Yes

Pharmacologic Category Antidote

Use Benzodiazepine antagonist; reverses sedative effects of benzodiazepines used in conscious sedation and general anesthesia; treatment of benzodiazepine overdose

Local Anesthetic/Vasoconstrictor Precautions No information available to require special precautions

Effects on Dental Treatment Key adverse event(s) related to dental treatment: Xerostomia (normal salivary flow resumes upon discontinuation).

Effects on Bleeding No information available to require special precautions

Adverse Effects

>10%: Gastrointestinal: Vomiting, nausea

1% to 10%:

Cardiovascular: Vasodilation (1% to 3%), palpitation

Central nervous system: Dizziness (10%), agitation (3% to 9%), emotional lability (1% to 3%), fatigue (1% to 3%), headache (1% to 3%)

Gastrointestinal: Xerostomia

Local: Pain at injection site (3% to 9%)

Neuromuscular & skeletal: Tremor, weakness, paresthesia (1% to 3%)

Ocular: Abnormal vision, blurred vision (3% to 9%)

Respiratory: Dyspnea, hyperventilation (3% to 9%)

Miscellaneous: Diaphoresis

Dosage

Children and Adults: I.V.: See table.

Flumazenil

Pediatric Dosage	
Pediatric dosage for **reversal of conscious sedation and general anesthesia:**	
Initial dose	0.01 mg/kg over 15 seconds (maximum: 0.2 mg)
Repeat doses (maximum: 4 doses)	0.005-0.01 mg/kg (maximum: 0.2 mg) repeated at 1-minute intervals
Maximum total cumulative dose	1 mg or 0.05 mg/kg (whichever is lower)
Adult Dosage	
Adult dosage for **reversal of conscious sedation and general anesthesia:**	
Initial dose	0.2 mg intravenously over 15 seconds
Repeat doses (maximum: 4 doses)	If desired level of consciousness is not obtained, 0.2 mg may be repeated at 1-minute intervals.
Maximum total cumulative dose	1 mg (usual dose: 0.6-1 mg) **In the event of resedation:** Repeat doses may be given at 20-minute intervals with maximum of 1 mg/dose and 3 mg/hour.
Adult dosage for **suspected benzodiazepine overdose:**	
Initial dose	0.2 mg intravenously over 30 seconds; if the desired level of consciousness is not obtained, 0.3 mg can be given over 30 seconds
Repeat doses	0.5 mg over 30 seconds repeated at 1-minute intervals
Maximum total cumulative dose	3 mg (usual dose: 1-3 mg) Patients with a partial response at 3 mg may require additional titration up to a total dose of 5 mg. If a patient has not responded 5 minutes after cumulative dose of 5 mg, the major cause of sedation is not likely due to benzodiazepines. **In the event of resedation:** May repeat doses at 20-minute intervals with maximum of 1 mg/dose and 3 mg/hour.

Resedation: Repeated doses may be given at 20-minute intervals as needed; repeat treatment doses of 1 mg (at a rate of 0.5 mg/minute) should be given at any time and no more than 3 mg should be given in any hour. After intoxication with high doses of benzodiazepines, the duration of a single dose of flumazenil is not expected to exceed 1 hour; if desired, the period of wakefulness may be prolonged with repeated low intravenous doses of flumazenil, or by an infusion of 0.1-0.4 mg/hour. Most patients with benzodiazepine overdose will respond to a cumulative dose of 1-3 mg and doses >3 mg do not reliably produce additional effects. Rarely, patients with a partial response at 3 mg may require additional titration up to a total dose of 5 mg. **If a patient has not responded 5 minutes after receiving a cumulative dose of 5 mg, the major cause of sedation is not likely to be due to benzodiazepines.**

Elderly: No differences in safety or efficacy have been reported. However, increased sensitivity may occur in some elderly patients.

Dosing in renal impairment: Not significantly affected by renal failure (Cl_{cr} <10 mL/minute) or hemodialysis beginning 1 hour after drug administration

Dosing in hepatic impairment: Use caution with initial and/or repeat doses in patients with liver disease

Mechanism of Action Competitively inhibits the activity at the benzodiazepine receptor site on the GABA/benzodiazepine receptor complex. Flumazenil does not antagonize the CNS effect of drugs affecting GABA-ergic neurons by means other than the benzodiazepine receptor (ethanol, barbiturates, general anesthetics) and does not reverse the effects of opioids

Contraindications Hypersensitivity to flumazenil, benzodiazepines, or any component of the formulation; patients given benzodiazepines for control of potentially life-threatening conditions (eg, control of intracranial pressure or status epilepticus); patients who are showing signs of serious cyclic-antidepressant overdosage

Warnings/Precautions **[U.S. Boxed Warning]: Benzodiazepine reversal may result in seizures in some patients.** Patients who may develop seizures include patients on benzodiazepines for long-term sedation, tricyclic antidepressant overdose patients, concurrent major sedative-hypnotic drug withdrawal, recent therapy with repeated doses of parenteral benzodiazepines, myoclonic jerking or seizure activity prior to flumazenil administration. Flumazenil may not reliably reverse respiratory depression/hypoventilation. Flumazenil is not a substitute for evaluation of oxygenation; establishing an airway and assisting ventilation, as necessary, is always the initial step in overdose management. Resedation occurs more frequently in patients where a large single dose or cumulative dose of a benzodiazepine is administered along with a neuromuscular-blocking agent and multiple anesthetic agents. Flumazenil should be used with caution in the intensive care unit because of increased risk of unrecognized benzodiazepine dependence in such settings. Should not be used to diagnose benzodiazepine-induced sedation. Reverse neuromuscular blockade before considering use. Flumazenil does not antagonize the CNS effects of other GABA agonists (such as ethanol, barbiturates, or general anesthetics); nor does it reverse narcotics. Flumazenil does not consistently reverse amnesia; patient may not recall verbal instructions after procedure.

Use with caution in patients with a history of panic disorder; may provoke panic attacks. Use caution in drug and ethanol-dependent patients; these patients may also be dependent on benzodiazepines. Not recommended for treatment of benzodiazepine dependence. Use with caution in head injury patients. Use caution in patients with mixed drug overdoses; toxic effects of other drugs taken may emerge once benzodiazepine effects are reversed. Use caution in hepatic dysfunction and in patients relying on a benzodiazepine for seizure control. Safety and efficacy have not been established in children <1 year of age.

Drug Interactions

Avoid Concomitant Use There are no known interactions where it is recommended to avoid concomitant use.

Increased Effect/Toxicity There are no known significant interactions involving an increase in effect.

Decreased Effect

Flumazenil may decrease the levels/effects of: Hypnotics (Nonbenzodiazepine)

Pharmacodynamics/Kinetics

Onset of Action 1-3 minutes; 80% response within 3 minutes; Peak effect: 6-10 minutes

Duration of Action Resedation: ~1 hour; duration related to dose given and benzodiazepine plasma concentrations; reversal effects of flumazenil may wear off before effects of benzodiazepine

Half-life Elimination Adults: Alpha: 7-15 minutes; Terminal: 41-79 minutes; Moderate hepatic dysfunction: 1.3 hours; Severe hepatic impairment: 2.4 hours

Pregnancy Risk Factor C

Lactation Excretion in breast milk unknown/use caution

Dosage Forms

Injection, solution: 0.1 mg/mL (5 mL, 10 mL)

Romazicon®: 0.1 mg/mL (5 mL, 10 mL)

Dental Comment **Sedation:** Patients should be monitored for at least 1 hour following administration of flumazenil to ensure full recovery. Flumazenil should only be used in an emergency situation and not as a means of hastening recovery from conscious sedation. When used to hasten recovery, emergence can be sudden and unpleasant. Flumazenil should be used with caution in patients routinely taking benzodiazepines for other therapeutic uses, withdrawal symptoms will be induced.

Flunarizine (floo NAR i zeen)

Canadian Brand Names Apo-Flunarizine®; Novo-Flunarizine; Sibelium®

Pharmacologic Category Calcium Channel Antagonist

Use Prophylaxis of classic (with aura) or common (without aura) migraine; symptomatic treatment of vestibular vertigo (due to a diagnosed functional disorder of the vestibular system)

Local Anesthetic/Vasoconstrictor Precautions No information available to require special precautions

Effects on Dental Treatment Key adverse event(s) related to dental treatment: Xerostomia and changes in salivation (normal salivary flow resumes upon discontinuation).

Effects on Bleeding No information available to require special precautions

Adverse Effects Frequency not defined.

Central nervous system: Anxiety, dizziness, drowsiness, fatigue, insomnia, vertigo
Dermatologic: Rash
Endocrine & metabolic: Galactorrhea, prolactin levels increased
Gastrointestinal: Appetite increased, epigastric pain, heartburn, nausea, vomiting, weight gain, xerostomia
Neuromuscular & skeletal: Asthenia/weakness, muscle ache

General Dosage Range Oral:

Adults <65 years: 5-10 mg once daily
Elderly ≥65 years: 2.5-5 mg once daily

Mechanism of Action Flunarizine is a selective calcium channel antagonist that prevents cellular calcium overload by reducing transmembrane calcium influx; also has antihistamine properties.

Pharmacodynamics/Kinetics

Half-life Elimination ~19 days
Time to Peak 2-4 hours

Product Availability Not available in U.S.

Flunisolide (Oral Inhalation) (floo NISS oh lide)

Related Information

Respiratory Diseases *on page* 1876

U.S. Brand Names AeroBid® [DSC]; AeroBid®-M [DSC]

Canadian Brand Names Alti-Flunisolide; Apo-Flunisolide®; PMS-Flunisolide

Pharmacologic Category Corticosteroid, Inhalant (Oral)

Use Steroid-dependent asthma

Local Anesthetic/Vasoconstrictor Precautions No information available to require special precautions

Effects on Dental Treatment Key adverse event(s) related to dental treatment: *Candida* infections of the pharynx, sore throat, bitter taste, palpitations, dizziness, headache, nervousness, GI irritation, sneezing, coughing, upper respiratory tract infection, bronchitis, increased susceptibility to infections, xerostomia (normal salivary flow resumes upon discontinuation), dry throat, loss of taste, and diaphoresis.

Effects on Bleeding No information available to require special precautions

Adverse Effects

>10%:

Central nervous system: Headache (25%)
Gastrointestinal: Nausea (25%), vomiting (25%), sore throat (20%), aftertaste (8% to 17%)
Respiratory: Upper respiratory infection (25%), cold symptoms (15%)

1% to 10%:

Cardiovascular: Chest pain, chest tightness, edema, hypertension, palpitation, peripheral edema, tachycardia
Central nervous system: Anxiety, chills, dizziness, depression, fatigue, faintness, fever, hyper-/hypoactivity, insomnia, malaise, moodiness, nervousness, shakiness, vertigo
Dermatologic: Acne, eczema, hives, pruritus, rash, urticaria
Endocrine & metabolic: Menstrual disturbances
Gastrointestinal: Appetite decreased/increased, constipation, diarrhea, dyspepsia, dry throat, flatulence, glossitis, heartburn, loss of taste, mouth discomfort, oral candidiasis, stomach upset, throat irritation, weight gain
Neuromuscular & skeletal: Numbness, weakness
Ocular: Blurred vision, discomfort
Respiratory: Bronchitis, chest congestion, cough increased, dyspnea, epistaxis, hoarseness, laryngitis, pharyngitis, pleurisy, pneumonia, sinusitis, wheezing
Miscellaneous: Diaphoresis, flu-like syndrome, infection, lymphadenopathy

General Dosage Range Oral inhalation:

Children 6-15 years: 2 inhalations twice daily (maximum: 4 inhalations/day)
Children ≥16 years and Adults: 2 inhalations twice daily (maximum: 8 inhalations/day)

Mechanism of Action Decreases inflammation by suppression of migration of polymorphonuclear leukocytes and reversal of increased capillary permeability; does not depress hypothalamus

Pharmacodynamics/Kinetics

Half-life Elimination 1.8 hours

Pregnancy Risk Factor C

Flunisolide (Nasal) (floo NISS oh lide)

Canadian Brand Names Apo-Flunisolide®; Nasalide®; Rhinalar®

Pharmacologic Category Corticosteroid, Nasal

Use Seasonal or perennial rhinitis

Local Anesthetic/Vasoconstrictor Precautions No information available to require special precautions

Effects on Dental Treatment Key adverse event(s) related to dental treatment: *Candida* infections of the nose, atrophic rhinitis, sneezing, nasal congestion, nasal dryness and burning, increased susceptibility to infections, dry throat, epistaxis

Effects on Bleeding No information available to require special precautions

Adverse Effects

>10%: Respiratory: Nasal congestion (15%), nasal burning/stinging (13%)

1% to 10%:

Respiratory: Nasal dryness, nasal irritation, rhinitis, sneezing

Miscellaneous: Loss of smell

General Dosage Range Intranasal:

Children 6-14 years: 1-2 sprays 2-3 times/day (maximum: 4 sprays/day in each nostril)

Children ≥15 years and Adults: 2 sprays twice daily (maximum: 8 sprays/day in each nostril)

Mechanism of Action Decreases inflammation by suppression of migration of polymorphonuclear leukocytes and reversal of increased capillary permeability; does not depress hypothalamus

Pregnancy Risk Factor C

Fluocinolone (Topical) (floo oh SIN oh lone)

U.S. Brand Names Capex®; Derma-Smoothe/FS®

Canadian Brand Names Capex®; Derma-Smoothe/FS®; Synalar®

Generic Availability (U.S.) Yes: Excludes oil, shampoo

Pharmacologic Category Corticosteroid, Topical

Dental Use Relief of inflammatory and pruritic manifestations (low, medium, high potency topical corticosteroid)

Use Relief of susceptible inflammatory dermatosis [low, medium corticosteroid]; dermatitis or psoriasis of the scalp; atopic dermatitis in adults and children ≥3 months of age

Local Anesthetic/Vasoconstrictor Precautions No information available to require special precautions

Effects on Dental Treatment No significant effects or complications reported

Effects on Bleeding No information available to require special precautions

Adverse Effects Frequency not defined.

Cardiovascular: Intracranial hypertension (rare)

Central nervous system: Telangiectasia

Dermatologic: Acneiform eruptions, allergic contact dermatitis, atopic dermatitis (secondary), burning, dryness, erythema, folliculitis, irritation, itching, hypertrichosis, hypopigmentation, keratosis pilaris, miliaria, papules, perioral dermatitis, pustules, shiny skin, skin atrophy, striae

Endocrine & metabolic: Cushing's syndrome, HPA axis suppression

Otic: Ear infection

Miscellaneous: Herpes simplex, secondary infection

Dental Usual Dosage Inflammatory and pruritic manifestations: Adults: Topical: Apply to oral lesion 4 times/day, after meals and at bedtime

Dosage Topical:

Atopic dermatitis (Derma-Smoothe/FS® body oil):

Children ≥3 months: Moisten skin; apply a thin film to affected area twice daily; do not use for longer than 4 weeks

Adults: Apply a thin film to affected area 3 times/day

Corticosteroid-responsive dermatoses: Children and Adults: Cream, ointment, solution: Apply a thin layer to affected area 2-4 times/day; may use occlusive dressings to manage psoriasis or recalcitrant conditions

Inflammatory and pruritic manifestations (dental use): Adults: Apply to oral lesion 4 times/day, after meals and at bedtime

Scalp psoriasis (Derma-Smoothe/FS® scalp oil): Adults: Massage thoroughly into wet or dampened hair/scalp; cover with shower cap. Leave on overnight (or for at least 4 hours). Remove by washing hair with shampoo and rinsing thoroughly.

Seborrheic dermatitis of the scalp (Capex®): Adults: Apply no more than 1 ounce to scalp once daily; work into lather and allow to remain on scalp for ~5 minutes. Remove from hair and scalp by rinsing thoroughly with water.

Mechanism of Action A synthetic fluorinated corticosteroid of low-to-moderate potency. The mechanism of action for all topical corticosteroids is not well defined, however, is believed to be a combination of anti-inflammatory, antipruritic, and vasoconstrictive properties.

Contraindications Hypersensitivity to fluocinolone or any component of the formulation; TB of skin, herpes (including varicella)

Warnings/Precautions Adverse systemic effects may occur when used on large areas of the body, denuded areas, for prolonged periods of time, or with an occlusive dressing. Infants and children may be more susceptible to systemic toxicity from equivalent doses due to larger skin surface to body mass ratio. Infants and small children may be more susceptible to adrenal axis suppression from topical corticosteroid therapy. Allergic contact dermatitis can occur, it is usually diagnosed by failure to heal rather than clinical exacerbation.

Topical: Not for oral, ophthalmic, or intravaginal use; do not apply to the face, axillae, groin, or diaper area unless directed by hea lthcare provider. Safety and efficacy of Derma-Smoothe/FS® body oil have not been established in children <3 months of age. Derma-Smoothe/FS® and contains peanut oil; use caution in peanut-sensitive individuals.

Drug Interactions

Avoid Concomitant Use

Avoid concomitant use of Fluocinolone (Topical) with any of the following: Aldesleukin

Increased Effect/Toxicity

Fluocinolone (Topical) may increase the levels/effects of: Deferasirox

Decreased Effect

Fluocinolone (Topical) may decrease the levels/effects of: Aldesleukin; Corticorelin

Pregnancy Risk Factor C

Lactation Excretion in breast milk unknown/use caution

Breast-Feeding Considerations Systemic corticosteroids are excreted in human milk. It is not known if sufficient quantities of fluocinolone are absorbed following topical administration to produce detectable amounts in breast milk. Hypertension in the nursing infant has been reported following corticosteroid ointment applied to the nipples. Use with caution.

Dosage Forms

Cream, topical: 0.01% (15 g, 60 g); 0.025% (15 g, 60 g)

Oil, topical:

Derma-Smoothe/FS®: 0.01% (120 mL)

Ointment, topical: 0.025% (15 g, 60 g)

Shampoo, topical:

Capex®: 0.01% (120 mL)

Solution, topical: 0.01% (60 mL)

Fluocinolone, Hydroquinone, and Tretinoin

(floo oh SIN oh lone, HYE droe kwin one, & TRET i noyn)

Related Information

Fluocinolone (Topical) *on page 749*
Hydroquinone *on page 872*
Tretinoin (Topical) *on page 1668*

U.S. Brand Names Tri-Luma™

Pharmacologic Category Corticosteroid, Topical; Depigmenting Agent; Retinoic Acid Derivative

Use Short-term treatment of moderate-to-severe melasma of the face

Local Anesthetic/Vasoconstrictor Precautions No information available to require special precautions

Effects on Dental Treatment Key adverse event(s) related to dental treatment: Xerostomia (normal salivary flow resumes upon discontinuation).

Effects on Bleeding No information available to require special precautions

Adverse Effects

>10%:

Dermatologic: Erythema (41%), desquamation (38%), burning (18%), dry skin (14%), pruritus (11%)

1% to 10%:

Cardiovascular: Telangiectasia (3%)

Central nervous system: Paresthesia (3%), hyperesthesia (2%)

Dermatologic: Acne (5%), pigmentation change (2%), irritation (2%), papules (1%), rash (1%), rosacea (1%), vesicles (1%)

Gastrointestinal: Xerostomia (1%)

General Dosage Range Topical: *Adults:* Apply a thin film 30 minutes prior to bedtime daily

Mechanism of Action Not clearly defined. Hydroquinone may interrupt melanin synthesis (tyrosine-tyrosinase pathway); reduces hyperpigmentation.

Pregnancy Risk Factor C

Fluocinonide (floo oh SIN oh nide)

Related Information

Ulcerative, Erosive, and Painful Oral Mucosal Disorders *on page* 1950

Related Sample Prescriptions

Mild Lichen Planus *on page* 1992

Recurrent Aphthous Stomatitis *on page* 1992

U.S. Brand Names Vanos™

Canadian Brand Names Lidemol®; Lidex®; Lyderm®; Tiamol®; Topactin; Topsyn®

Generic Availability (U.S.) Yes

Pharmacologic Category Corticosteroid, Topical

Dental Use Relief of inflammatory and pruritic manifestations (high potency topical corticosteroid)

Use Anti-inflammatory, antipruritic; treatment of plaque-type psoriasis (up to 10% of body surface area) [high-potency topical corticosteroid]

Local Anesthetic/Vasoconstrictor Precautions No information available to require special precautions

Effects on Dental Treatment No significant effects or complications reported

Effects on Bleeding No information available to require special precautions

Adverse Effects Frequency not defined.

Cardiovascular: Intracranial hypertension

Dermatologic: Acne, allergic dermatitis, contact dermatitis, dry skin, folliculitis, hypertrichosis, hypopigmentation, maceration of the skin, miliaria, perioral dermatitis, pruritus, skin atrophy, striae, telangiectasia

Endocrine & metabolic: Cushing's syndrome, growth retardation, HPA suppression, hyperglycemia

Local: Burning, irritation

Renal: Glycosuria

Miscellaneous: Secondary infection

Dental Usual Dosage Pruritus and inflammation: Children and Adults: Topical (0.05% cream): Apply thin layer to affected area 2-4 times/day depending on the severity of the condition. Therapy should be discontinued when control is achieved; if no improvement is seen, reassessment of diagnosis may be necessary.

Dosage

Children and Adults: Pruritus and inflammation: Topical (0.05% cream): Apply thin layer to affected area 2-4 times/day depending on the severity of the condition. Therapy should be discontinued when control is achieved; if no improvement is seen, reassessment of diagnosis may be necessary.

Children ≥12 years and Adults: Plaque-type psoriasis (Vanos™): Topical (0.1% cream): Apply a thin layer once or twice daily to affected areas (limited to <10% of body surface area). **Note:** Not recommended for use >2 consecutive weeks or >60 g/week total exposure. Discontinue when control is achieved.

Mechanism of Action Fluorinated topical corticosteroid considered to be of high potency. The mechanism of action for all topical corticosteroids is not well defined, however, is felt to be a combination of three important properties: anti-inflammatory activity, immunosuppressive properties, and antiproliferative actions.

Contraindications Hypersensitivity to fluocinonide or any component of the formulation; viral, fungal, or tubercular skin lesions, herpes simplex

Warnings/Precautions Systemic absorption of topical corticosteroids may cause hypothalamic-pituitary-adrenal (HPA) axis suppression (reversible) particularly in younger children. HPA axis suppression may lead to adrenal crisis. Risk is increased when used over large surface areas, for prolonged periods, or with occlusive dressings. Allergic contact dermatitis can occur, it is usually diagnosed by failure to heal rather than clinical exacerbation. Prolonged treatment with corticosteroids has been associated with the development of Kaposi's sarcoma (case reports); if noted, discontinuation of therapy should be considered. Adverse systemic effects including hyperglycemia, glycosuria, fluid and electrolyte changes, and HPA suppression may occur when used on large surface areas, for prolonged periods, or with an occlusive dressing. Lower-strength cream (0.05%) may be used cautiously on face or opposing skin surfaces that may rub or touch (eg, skin folds of the groin, axilla, and breasts); higher-strength (0.1%) should not be used on the face, groin, or axillae. Use of the 0.1% cream for >2 weeks or in patients <12 years of age is not recommended. Chronic use of corticosteroids in children may interfere with growth and development.

Drug Interactions

Avoid Concomitant Use

Avoid concomitant use of Fluocinonide with any of the following: Aldesleukin

Increased Effect/Toxicity

Fluocinonide may increase the levels/effects of: Deferasirox

Decreased Effect

Fluocinonide may decrease the levels/effects of: Aldesleukin; Corticorelin

Pregnancy Risk Factor C

Dosage Forms

Cream, topical:

Vanos™: 0.1% (30 g, 60 g)

Cream, anhydrous, emollient, topical: 0.05% (15 g, 30 g, 60 g, 120 g)

Cream, aqueous, emollient, topical: 0.05% (15 g, 30 g, 60 g)

Gel, topical: 0.05% (15 g, 30 g, 60 g)

Ointment, topical: 0.05% (15 g, 30 g, 60 g)

Solution, topical: 0.05% (20 mL, 60 mL)

Fluoride (FLOR ide)

Related Information

Dentin Hypersensitivity, Acid Erosion, High Caries Index, and Xerostomia *on page 1955*

Management of Patients Undergoing Cancer Therapy *on page 1970*

U.S. Brand Names Act® Kids [OTC]; Act® Restoring™ [OTC]; Act® Total Care™ [OTC]; Act® [OTC]; CaviRinse™; Clinpro™ 5000; ControlRx™; ControlRx™ Multi; Denta 5000 Plus™; DentaGel™; Epiflur™; Fluor-A-Day®; Fluorabon™; Fluorinse®; Fluoritab; Flura-Drops®; Gel-Kam® Rinse; Gel-Kam® [OTC]; Just For Kids™ [OTC]; Lozi-Flur™; NeutraCare®; NeutraGard® Advanced; Omni Gel™ [OTC]; Ortho-Wash™; PerioMed™; Phos-Flur®; Phos-Flur® Rinse [OTC]; PreviDent®; PreviDent® 5000 Booster; PreviDent® 5000 Dry Mouth; PreviDent® 5000 Plus®; PreviDent® 5000 Sensitive; StanGard® Perio; Stop®

Canadian Brand Names Fluor-A-Day

Generic Availability (U.S.) Yes: Excludes lozenge, gel drops

Pharmacologic Category Nutritional Supplement

Dental Use Prevention of dental caries

Use Prevention of dental caries

Local Anesthetic/Vasoconstrictor Precautions No information available to require special precautions

Effects on Dental Treatment Key adverse event(s) related to dental treatment: Products containing stannous fluoride may stain teeth. See Dental Comment.

Effects on Bleeding No information available to require special precautions

Dosage Oral:

The recommended daily dose of oral fluoride supplement (mg), based on fluoride ion content (ppm) in drinking water (2.2 mg of sodium fluoride is equivalent to 1 mg of fluoride ion): See table.

Fluoride Ion

Fluoride Content of Drinking Water	Daily Dose, Oral (mg)
<0.3 ppm	
Birth - 6 mo	None
6 mo - 3 y	0.25
3-6 y	0.5
6-16 y	1
0.3-0.6 ppm	
Birth - 6 mo	None
6 mo - 3 y	None
3-6 y	0.25
6-16 y	0.5

Adapted from Recommended Dosage Schedule of The American Dental Association, The American Academy of Pediatric Dentistry, and The American Academy of Pediatrics.

Cream: Children ≥6 years and Adults: Brush teeth with cream once daily regardless of fluoride content of drinking water

Dental rinse or gel:

Children 6-12 years: 5-10 mL rinse or apply to teeth and spit daily after brushing

Adults: 10 mL rinse or apply to teeth and spit daily after brushing

PreviDent® rinse: Children >6 years and Adults: Once weekly, rinse 10 mL vigorously around and between teeth for 1 minute, then spit; this should be done preferably at bedtime, after thoroughly brushing teeth; for maximum benefit, do not eat, drink, or rinse mouth for at least 30 minutes after treatment; do not swallow

Fluorinse®: Children >6 years and Adults: Once weekly, vigorously swish 5-10 mL in mouth for 1 minute, then spit

Lozenge (Lozi-Flur™): Adults: One lozenge daily regardless of fluoride content of drinking water

Mechanism of Action Promotes remineralization of decalcified enamel; inhibits the cariogenic microbial process in dental plaque; increases tooth resistance to acid dissolution

Contraindications Hypersensitivity to fluoride, tartrazine, or any component of the formulation; when fluoride content of drinking water exceeds 0.7 ppm; low sodium or sodium-free diets; do not use 1 mg tablets in children <3 years of age or when drinking water fluoride content is ≥0.3 ppm; do not use 1 mg/5 mL rinse (as supplement) in children <6 years of age

Warnings/Precautions Prolonged ingestion with excessive doses may result in dental fluorosis and osseous changes; do **not** exceed recommended dosage. Some products contain tartrazine.

Drug Interactions

Avoid Concomitant Use There are no known interactions where it is recommended to avoid concomitant use.

Increased Effect/Toxicity There are no known significant interactions involving an increase in effect.

Decreased Effect There are no known significant interactions involving a decrease in effect.

Dietary Considerations Do not administer with milk; do **not** allow eating or drinking for 30 minutes after use.

Pregnancy Risk Factor C

Dosage Forms

Cream, oral: 1.1% (51 g)
- Denta 5000 Plus™: 1.1% (51 g)
- PreviDent® 5000 Plus®: 1.1% (51 g)

Gel, oral:
- PreviDent® 5000 Booster: 1.1% (100 mL, 106 mL)
- PreviDent® 5000 Dry Mouth: 1.1% (100 mL)
- PreviDent® 5000 Sensitive: 1.1% (100 mL)

Gel, topical: 1.1% (56 g)
- DentaGel™: 1.1% (56 g)
- Gel-Kam® [OTC]: 0.4% (129 g)
- Just For Kids™ [OTC]: 0.4% (122 g)
- NeutraCare®: 1.1% (60 g)
- NeutraGard® Advanced: 1.1% (60 g)
- Omni Gel™ [OTC]: 0.4% (122 g); 0.4% (122 g)
- Phos-Flur®: 1.1% (51 g)
- PreviDent®: 1.1% (56 g)
- Stop®: 0.4% (120 g)

Liquid, oral:
- Fluoritab: 0.125 mg/drop

Lozenge, oral:
- Lozi-Flur™: 2.21 mg (90s)

Paste, oral:
- Clinpro™ 5000: 1.1% (113 g)
- ControlRx™: 1.1% (57 g)
- ControlRx™ Multi: 1.1% (57 g)

Solution, oral: 1.1 mg/mL (50 mL); 0.2% (473 mL); 0.63% (300 mL)
- Act® [OTC]: 0.05% (532 mL)
- Act® Kids [OTC]: 0.05% (500 mL, 532 mL)
- Act® Restoring™ [OTC]: 0.02% (1000 mL); 0.05% (532 mL)
- Act® Total Care™ [OTC]: 0.02% (1000 mL); 0.05% (88 mL, 532 mL)
- CaviRinse™: 0.2% (240 mL)
- Fluor-A-Day®: 0.278 mg/drop (30 mL)
- Fluorabon™: 0.55 mg/0.6 mL (60 mL)
- Fluorinse®: 0.2% (480 mL)
- Flura-Drops®: 0.55 mg/drop (24 mL)
- Gel-Kam® Rinse: 0.63% (300 mL)
- OrthoWash™: 0.044% (480 mL)
- PerioMed™: 0.63% (284 mL)
- Phos-Flur® Rinse [OTC]: 0.044% (473 mL, 500 mL)
- PreviDent®: 0.2% (473 mL)

StanGard® Perio: 0.63% (284 mL)

Tablet, chewable, oral: 0.55 mg, 1.1 mg, 2.2 mg

Epiflur™: 0.55 mg, 1.1 mg, 2.2 mg

Fluor-A-Day®: 0.56 mg, 1.1 mg, 2.2 mg

Fluoritab: 1.1 mg, 2.2 mg

Dental Comment Neutral pH fluoride preparations are preferred in patients with oral mucositis to reduce tissue irritation; long-term use of acidulated fluorides has been associated with enamel demineralization and damage to porcelain crowns

References

Wynn RL, "Fluoride: After 50 Years, a Clearer Picture of Its Mechanism," *Gen Dent*, 2002, 50(2):118-22, 124, 126.

Fluorometholone (flure oh METH oh lone)

U.S. Brand Names Flarex®; FML Forte®; FML®

Canadian Brand Names Flarex®; FML Forte®; FML®; PMS-Fluorometholone

Pharmacologic Category Corticosteroid, Ophthalmic

Use Treatment of steroid-responsive inflammatory conditions of the eye

Local Anesthetic/Vasoconstrictor Precautions No information available to require special precautions

Effects on Dental Treatment No significant effects or complications reported

Effects on Bleeding No information available to require special precautions

Adverse Effects Frequency not defined.

Gastrointestinal: Taste perversion

Ocular: Anterior uveitis, bleb formation increased, blurred vision, burning, cataract formation, conjunctival hyperemia, conjunctivitis, corneal ulcers, delayed wound healing, glaucoma, glaucoma with optic nerve damage, intraocular pressure increased, irritation, keratitis, mydriasis, perforation of the globe, ptosis, secondary ocular infection (bacterial, fungal, viral), stinging, visual acuity and field defects

Miscellaneous: Allergic reaction, systemic hypercorticoidism (rare)

General Dosage Range Ophthalmic:

Ointment: *Children >2 years and Adults:* Apply small amount (~1/2" ribbon) every 4 hours (initial: 24-48 hours) **or** 1-3 times/day

Suspension:

Children >2 years: Instill 1 drop every 4 hours (initial: 24-48 hours) **or** 1 drop 2-4 times/day

Adults: Instill 2 drops (initial: 24-48 hours) **or** 1-2 drops 2-4 times/day

Mechanism of Action Decreases inflammation by suppression of migration of polymorphonuclear leukocytes and reversal of increased capillary permeability

Pregnancy Risk Factor C

Fluorouracil (Systemic) (flure oh YOOR a sil)

Related Information

Capecitabine *on page* 294

U.S. Brand Names Adrucil®

Pharmacologic Category Antineoplastic Agent, Antimetabolite (Pyrimidine Analog)

Use Treatment of carcinomas of the breast, colon, rectum, pancreas, or stomach

Unlabeled/Investigational Use Treatment of head and neck cancer, esophageal cancer, anal cancer, cervical cancer, bladder cancer, renal cell cancer, and unknown primary cancer

Local Anesthetic/Vasoconstrictor Precautions No information available to require special precautions

Effects on Dental Treatment Key adverse event(s) related to dental treatment: Stomatitis.

Effects on Bleeding Chemotherapy may result in significant myelosuppression, potentially including significant reduction in platelet counts and altered hemostasis. In patients who are under active treatment with these agents, medical consult is suggested.

Adverse Effects Toxicity depends on duration of treatment

Cardiovascular: Angina, arrhythmia, heart failure, MI, myocardial ischemia, vasospasm, ventricular ectopy

Central nervous system: Acute cerebellar syndrome, confusion, disorientation, euphoria, headache, nystagmus, stroke

Dermatologic: Alopecia, dermatitis, dry skin, fissuring, palmar-plantar erythrodysesthesia syndrome, pruritic maculopapular rash, photosensitivity, Stevens-Johnson syndrome, toxic epidermal necrolysis, vein pigmentations

Gastrointestinal: Anorexia, bleeding, diarrhea, esophagopharyngitis, mesenteric ischemia (acute), nausea, sloughing, stomatitis, ulceration, vomiting

Hematologic: Myelosuppression (nadir: 9-14 days; recovery by day 30), agranulocytosis, anemia, leukopenia, pancytopenia, thrombocytopenia
Local: Thrombophlebitis
Ocular: Lacrimation, lacrimal duct stenosis, photophobia, visual changes
Respiratory: Epistaxis
Miscellaneous: Anaphylaxis, generalized allergic reactions, nail loss

General Dosage Range Dosage adjustment recommended in patients with hepatic or renal impairment

I.V.: *Adults:* Dosage varies greatly depending on indication

Mechanism of Action A pyrimidine antimetabolite that interferes with DNA synthesis by blocking the methylation of deoxyuridylic acid; fluorouracil inhibits thymidylate synthetase (TS), or is incorporated into RNA. The reduced folate cofactor is required for tight binding to occur between the 5-FdUMP and TS.

Pharmacodynamics/Kinetics

Duration of Action ~3 weeks

Half-life Elimination Biphasic: Initial: 6-20 minutes; two metabolites, FdUMP and FUTP, have prolonged half-lives depending on the type of tissue

Pregnancy Risk Factor D

FLUoxetine (floo OKS e teen)

Related Information

Clinical Risk Related to Drugs Prolonging QT Interval *on page 1872*
Management of the Patient With Anxiety or Depression *on page 1968*

U.S. Brand Names PROzac®; PROzac® Weekly™; Sarafem®; Selfemra® [DSC]

Canadian Brand Names Apo-Fluoxetine®; CO Fluoxetine; Dom-Fluoxetine; Fluoxetine; FXT 40; Gen-Fluoxetine; Mylan-Fluoxetine; Novo-Fluoxetine; Nu-Fluoxetine; PHL-Fluoxetine; PMS-Fluoxetine; PRO-Fluoxetine; Prozac®; ratio-Fluoxetine; Riva-Fluoxetine; Sandoz-Fluoxetine; Teva-Fluoxetine; ZYM-Fluoxetine

Generic Availability (U.S.) Yes

Pharmacologic Category Antidepressant, Selective Serotonin Reuptake Inhibitor

Use Treatment of major depressive disorder (MDD); treatment of binge-eating and vomiting in patients with moderate-to-severe bulimia nervosa; obsessive-compulsive disorder (OCD); premenstrual dysphoric disorder (PMDD); panic disorder with or without agoraphobia; in combination with olanzapine for treatment-resistant or bipolar I depression

Unlabeled/Investigational Use Selective mutism; treatment of mild dementia-associated agitation in nonpsychotic patients; post-traumatic stress disorder (PTSD); social anxiety disorder; chronic neuropathic pain, fibromyalgia; Raynaud's phenomenon

Local Anesthetic/Vasoconstrictor Precautions Although caution should be used in patients taking tricyclic antidepressants, no interactions have been reported with vasoconstrictors and fluoxetine, a nontricyclic antidepressant which acts to increase serotonin; no precautions appear to be needed. Fluoxetine is one of the drugs confirmed to prolong the QT interval and is accepted as having a risk of causing torsade de pointes. The risk of drug-induced torsade de pointes is extremely low when a single QT interval prolonging drug is prescribed. In terms of epinephrine, it is not known what effect vasoconstrictors in the local anesthetic regimen will have in patients with a known history of congenital prolonged QT interval or in patients taking any medication that prolongs the QT interval. Until more information is obtained, it is suggested that the clinician consult with the physician prior to the use of a vasoconstrictor in suspected patients, and that the vasoconstrictor (epinephrine, mepivacaine and levonordefrin [Carbocaine® 2% with Neo-Cobefrin®]) be used with caution.

Effects on Dental Treatment Key adverse event(s) related to dental treatment: Xerostomia (normal salivary flow resumes upon discontinuation) and taste perversion. Problems with SSRI-induced bruxism have been reported and may preclude their use. Clinicians attempting to evaluate any patient with bruxism or involuntary muscle movement, who is simultaneously being treated with an SSRI drug, should be aware of this potential association. See Effects on Bleeding.

Effects on Bleeding May impair platelet aggregation resulting in increased risk of bleeding events, particularly if used concomitantly with aspirin, NSAIDs, warfarin, or other anticoagulants. Bleeding related to SSRI use has been reported to range from relatively minor bruising and epistaxis to life-threatening hemorrhage. Routine interruption of therapy for most dental procedures is not warranted. In medically complicated patients or extensive oral surgery, the decision to interrupt therapy must be based on the risk to benefit in an individual patient and a medical consult is suggested. If therapy is continued without interruption, the clinician should anticipate the potential for a prolonged bleeding time.

Adverse Effects Percentages listed for adverse effects as reported in placebo-controlled trials and were generally similar in adults and children; actual frequency may be dependent upon diagnosis and in some cases the range presented may be lower than or equal to placebo for a particular disorder.

>10%:

Central nervous system: Insomnia (10% to 33%), headache (21%), somnolence (5% to 17%), anxiety (6% to 15%), nervousness (8% to 14%)

Endocrine & metabolic: Libido decreased (1% to 11%)

Gastrointestinal: Nausea (12% to 29%), diarrhea (8% to 18%), anorexia (4% to 17%), xerostomia (4% to 12%)

Neuromuscular & skeletal: Weakness (7% to 21%), tremor (3% to 13%)

Respiratory: Pharyngitis (3% to 11%), yawn (≤11%)

1% to 10%:

Cardiovascular: Vasodilation (1% to 5%), chest pain, hemorrhage, hypertension, palpitation

Central nervous system: Dizziness (9%), abnormal dreams (1% to 5%), abnormal thinking (2%), agitation, amnesia, chills, confusion, emotional lability, sleep disorder

Dermatologic: Rash (2% to 6%), pruritus (4%)

Endocrine & metabolic: Ejaculation abnormal (≤7%), impotence (≤7%), menorrhagia (≥2%)

Gastrointestinal: Dyspepsia (6% to 10%), constipation (5%), flatulence (3%), vomiting (3%), thirst (≥2%), weight loss (2%), appetite increased, taste perversion, weight gain

Genitourinary: Urinary frequency

Neuromuscular & skeletal: Hyperkinesia (≥2%)

Ocular: Vision abnormal (2%)

Otic: Ear pain, tinnitus

Respiratory: Sinusitis (1% to 6%)

Miscellaneous: Flu-like syndrome (3% to 10%), diaphoresis (2% to 8%), epistaxis (≥2%)

Dosage Oral: **Note:** Upon discontinuation of fluoxetine therapy, gradually taper dose. If intolerable symptoms occur following a dose reduction, consider resuming the previously prescribed dose and/or decrease dose at a more gradual rate.

Children:

Depression: 8-18 years: 10-20 mg/day; lower-weight children can be started at 10 mg/day, may increase to 20 mg/day after 1 week if needed

Obsessive-compulsive disorder: 7-17 years: Initial: 10 mg/day; may increase after 2 weeks if inadequate clinical response to 20 mg/day; further increases may be considered after several weeks to recommended range of 20-30 mg/day (lower weight children) or 20-60 mg/day (adolescents and higher weight children)

Selective mutism (unlabeled use): 5-18 years: Initial: 5-10 mg/day; titrate upwards as needed (usual maximum dose: 60 mg/day)

Adults: 20 mg/day in the morning; may increase after several weeks by 20 mg/day increments; maximum: 80 mg/day; doses >20 mg may be given once daily or divided twice daily. **Note:** Lower doses of 5-10 mg/day have been used for initial treatment.

Indication-specific dosing:

Bulimia nervosa: 60 mg/day

Depression: Initial: 20 mg/day; may increase after several weeks if inadequate response (maximum: 80 mg/day). Patients maintained on Prozac® 20 mg/day may be changed to Prozac® Weekly™ 90 mg/week, starting dose 7 days after the last 20 mg/day dose

Depression associated with bipolar disorder (in combination with olanzapine): Initial: 20 mg in the evening; adjust as tolerated to usual range of 20-50 mg/day. See **"Note"**.

Fibromyalgia (unlabeled use): Range: 20-80 mg/day (Arnold, 2002)

Obsessive-compulsive disorder: Initial: 20 mg/day; may increase after several weeks if inadequate response; recommended range: 20-60 mg/day (maximum: 80 mg/day)

Panic disorder: Initial: 10 mg/day; after 1 week, increase to 20 mg/day; may increase after several weeks; doses >60 mg/day have not been evaluated

Post-traumatic stress disorder (PTSD) (unlabeled use): 20-40 mg/day

Premenstrual dysphoric disorder (Sarafem®): 20 mg/day continuously, **or** 20 mg/day starting 14 days prior to menstruation and through first full day of menses (repeat with each cycle)

Raynaud's phenomena (unlabeled use): 20 mg/day (Coleiro, 2001)

Social anxiety disorder (unlabeled use): Target dose: 40 mg/day; range 30-60 mg/day (Davidson, 2004)

Treatment-resistant depression (in combination with olanzapine): Initial: 20 mg in the evening; adjust as tolerated to usual range of 20-50 mg/day. See **"Note."**

Note: When using individual components of fluoxetine with olanzapine rather than fixed dose combination product (Symbyax®), approximate dosage correspondence is as follows:

Olanzapine 2.5 mg + fluoxetine 20 mg = Symbyax® 3/25
Olanzapine 5 mg + fluoxetine 20 mg = Symbyax® 6/25
Olanzapine 12.5 mg + fluoxetine 20 mg = Symbyax® 12/25
Olanzapine 5 mg + fluoxetine 50 mg = Symbyax® 6/50
Olanzapine 12.5 mg + fluoxetine 50 mg = Symbyax® 12/50

Elderly: Depression: Some patients may require an initial dose of 10 mg/day with dosage increases of 10 and 20 mg every several weeks as tolerated; should not be taken at night unless patient experiences sedation

Dosing adjustment in renal impairment:

Single dose studies: Pharmacokinetics of fluoxetine and norfluoxetine were similar among subjects with all levels of impaired renal function, including anephric patients on chronic hemodialysis

Chronic administration: Additional accumulation of fluoxetine or norfluoxetine may occur in patients with severely impaired renal function

Hemodialysis: Not removed by hemodialysis; use of lower dose or less frequent dosing is not usually necessary.

Dosing adjustment in hepatic impairment: Elimination half-life of fluoxetine is prolonged in patients with hepatic impairment; a lower or less frequent dose of fluoxetine should be used in these patients

Cirrhosis patients: Administer a lower dose or less frequent dosing interval

Compensated cirrhosis without ascites: Administer 50% of normal dose

Mechanism of Action Inhibits CNS neuron serotonin reuptake; minimal or no effect on reuptake of norepinephrine or dopamine; does not significantly bind to alpha-adrenergic, histamine, or cholinergic receptors

Contraindications Hypersensitivity to fluoxetine or any component of the formulation; patients currently receiving MAO inhibitors, pimozide, or thioridazine

Note: MAO inhibitor therapy must be stopped for 14 days before fluoxetine is initiated. Treatment with MAO inhibitors or thioridazine should not be initiated until 5 weeks after the discontinuation of fluoxetine.

Warnings/Precautions [U.S. Boxed Warning]: Antidepressants increase the risk of suicidal thinking and behavior in children, adolescents, and young adults (18-24 years of age) with major depressive disorder (MDD) and other psychiatric disorders; consider risk prior to prescribing. Short-term studies did not show an increased risk in patients >24 years of age and showed a decreased risk in patients ≥65 years. Closely monitor patients for clinical worsening, suicidality, or unusual changes in behavior, particularly during the initial 1-2 months of therapy or during periods of dosage adjustments (increases or decreases); the patient's family or caregiver should be instructed to closely observe the patient and communicate condition with healthcare provider. A medication guide concerning the use of antidepressants should be dispensed with each prescription. **Fluoxetine is FDA approved for the treatment of OCD in children ≥7 years of age and MDD in children ≥8 years of age.**

The possibility of a suicide attempt is inherent in major depression and may persist until remission occurs. Use caution in high-risk patients. Worsening depression and severe abrupt suicidality that are not part of the presenting symptoms may require discontinuation or modification of drug therapy. The patient's family or caregiver should be alerted to monitor patients for the emergence of suicidality and associated behaviors (such as agitation, irritability, hostility, impulsivity, and hypomania) and call healthcare provider.

May worsen psychosis in some patients or precipitate a shift to mania or hypomania in patients with bipolar disorder. Patients presenting with depressive symptoms should be screened for bipolar disorder. Monotherapy in patients with bipolar disorder should be avoided. **Fluoxetine monotherapy is not FDA approved for the treatment of bipolar depression.** May cause insomnia, anxiety, nervousness, or anorexia. Use with caution in patients where weight loss is undesirable. May impair cognitive or motor performance; caution operating hazardous machinery or driving.

Serotonin syndrome and neuroleptic malignant syndrome (NMS)-like reactions have occurred with serotonin/norepinephrine reuptake inhibitors (SNRIs) and selective serotonin reuptake inhibitors (SSRIs) when used alone, and particularly when used in combination with serotonergic agents (eg, triptans) or antidopaminergic agents (eg, antipsychotics). Concurrent use with MAO inhibitors is contraindicated. Fluoxetine may elevate plasma levels of thioridazine or pimozide and increase the risk of QT_c interval prolongation. This may lead to serious ventricular arrhythmias, such as torsade de pointes-type arrhythmias, and sudden death. Fluoxetine use has been associated with occurrences of significant rash and allergic events, including vasculitis, lupus-like syndrome, laryngospasm, anaphylactoid reactions, and pulmonary inflammatory disease. Discontinue if underlying cause of rash cannot be identified.

Use caution in patients with a previous seizure disorder or condition predisposing to seizures such as brain damage, alcoholism, or concurrent therapy with other drugs which lower the seizure threshold. Use with caution in patients with hepatic or severe renal dysfunction and in elderly patients. Fluoxetine (daily) may be inappropriate for use in the elderly due to risk of agitation, sleep disturbances, and excessive CNS stimulation, attributed to this drug's long half-life (Beers Criteria). May cause hyponatremia/SIADH (elderly at increased risk); volume depletion (diuretics may increase risk). May increase the risks associated with electroconvulsive treatment. Use caution with concomitant use of NSAIDs, ASA, or other drugs that affect coagulation; the risk of bleeding may be potentiated. Use caution with history of MI or unstable heart disease; use in these patients is limited. May alter glycemic control in patients with diabetes. Due to the long half-life of fluoxetine and its metabolites, the effects and interactions noted may persist for prolonged periods following discontinuation. May cause or exacerbate sexual dysfunction. Discontinuation symptoms (eg, dysphoric mood, irritability, agitation, confusion, anxiety, insomnia, hypomania) may occur upon abrupt discontinuation. Taper dose when discontinuing therapy.

Drug Interactions

Metabolism/Transport Effects Substrate of CYP1A2 (minor), 2B6 (minor), 2C9 (major), 2C19 (minor), 2D6 (major), 2E1 (minor), 3A4 (minor); **Inhibits** CYP1A2 (moderate), 2B6 (weak), 2C9 (weak), 2C19 (moderate), 2D6 (strong), 3A4 (weak)

Avoid Concomitant Use

Avoid concomitant use of FLUoxetine with any of the following: Artemether; Clopidogrel; Dronedarone; Iobenguane I 123; Lumefantrine; MAO Inhibitors; Methylene Blue; Nilotinib; Pimozide; QuiNINE; Sibutramine; Tamoxifen; Tetrabenazine; Thioridazine; Toremifene; Tryptophan; Vandetanib; Ziprasidone

Increased Effect/Toxicity

FLUoxetine may increase the levels/effects of: Alcohol (Ethyl); Alpha-/Beta-Blockers; Anticoagulants; Antidepressants (Serotonin Reuptake Inhibitor/Antagonist); Antiplatelet Agents; Aspirin; Atomoxetine; Benzodiazepines (metabolized by oxidation); Beta-Blockers; BusPIRone; CarBAMazepine; CloZAPine; CNS Depressants; Collagenase (Systemic); CYP1A2 Substrates; CYP2C19 Substrates; CYP2D6 Substrates; Desmopressin; Dextromethorphan; Dronedarone; Drotrecogin Alfa; Fesoterodine; Fosphenytoin; Galantamine; Haloperidol; Ibritumomab; Lithium; Methadone; Methylene Blue; Mexiletine; NSAID (COX-2 Inhibitor); NSAID (Nonselective); Phenytoin; Pimozide; Propafenone; QTc-Prolonging Agents; QuiNIDine; QuiNINE; RisperiDONE; Salicylates; Serotonin Modulators; Tamoxifen; Tetrabenazine; Thioridazine; Thrombolytic Agents; Toremifene; Tositumomab and Iodine I 131 Tositumomab; TraMADol; Tricyclic Antidepressants; Vandetanib; Vitamin K Antagonists; Ziprasidone

The levels/effects of FLUoxetine may be increased by: Abiraterone; Alfuzosin; Analgesics (Opioid); Artemether; BusPIRone; Chloroquine; Cimetidine; Ciprofloxacin; Ciprofloxacin (Systemic); Conivaptan; CYP2C9 Inhibitors (Moderate); CYP2C9 Inhibitors (Strong); CYP2D6 Inhibitors (Moderate); CYP2D6 Inhibitors (Strong); Darunavir; Gadobutrol; Glucosamine; Herbs (Anticoagulant/Antiplatelet Properties); Lumefantrine; Macrolide Antibiotics; MAO Inhibitors; Metoclopramide; Nilotinib; Omega-3-Acid Ethyl Esters; Pentosan Polysulfate Sodium; Pentoxifylline; Prostacyclin Analogues; QuiNINE; Sibutramine; TraMADol; Tryptophan

Decreased Effect

FLUoxetine may decrease the levels/effects of: Clopidogrel; Iobenguane I 123

The levels/effects of FLUoxetine may be decreased by: CarBAMazepine; CYP2C9 Inducers (Highly Effective); Cyproheptadine; Peginterferon Alfa-2b; Tocilizumab

Ethanol/Nutrition/Herb Interactions

Ethanol: May increase CNS depression; monitor for increased effects with coadministration. Caution patients about effects.

Herb/Nutraceutical: Avoid valerian, St John's wort, kava kava, gotu kola (may increase CNS depression).

Dietary Considerations May be taken without regard to meals.

Pharmacodynamics/Kinetics

Onset of Action Depression: The onset of action is within a week; however, individual response varies greatly and full response may not be seen until 8-12 weeks after initiation of treatment.

Half-life Elimination Adults: Parent drug: 1-3 days (acute), 4-6 days (chronic), 7.6 days (cirrhosis); Metabolite (norfluoxetine): 9.3 days (range: 4-16 days), 12 days (cirrhosis)

Time to Peak Serum: 6-8 hours

Pregnancy Risk Factor C

Lactation Enters breast milk/not recommended (AAP rates "of concern"; AAP 2001 update pending)

Breast-Feeding Considerations Fluoxetine and its metabolite are excreted into breast milk and can be detected in the serum of breast-feeding infants. Concentrations in breast milk are variable. Colic, irritability, slow weight gain, and feeding and sleep disorders have been reported in nursing infants. Breast-feeding is not recommended by the manufacturer.

Because the long-term effects on development and behavior have not been studied and adverse effects have been noted in some infants exposed, one should prescribe fluoxetine to a mother who is breast-feeding only when the benefits outweigh the potential risks.

Dosage Forms

Capsule, oral: 10 mg, 20 mg, 40 mg
PROzac®: 10 mg, 20 mg, 40 mg

Capsule, delayed release, enteric coated pellets, oral: 90 mg
PROzac® Weekly™: 90 mg

Solution, oral: 20 mg/5 mL (5 mL, 120 mL)

Tablet, oral: 10 mg, 20 mg
Sarafem®: 10 mg, 15 mg, 20 mg

Dental Comment Fluoxetine is known to prolong the QT interval. The QT interval is measured as the time and distance between the Q point of the QRS complex and the end of the T wave in the ECG tracing. After adjustment for heart rate, the QT interval is defined as prolonged if it is more than 450 msec in men and 460 msec in women. A long QT syndrome was first described in the 1950s and 60s as a congenital syndrome involving QT interval prolongation and syncope and sudden death. Some of the congenital long QT syndromes were characterized by a peculiar electrocardiographic appearance of the QRS complex involving a premature atria beat followed by a pause, then a subsequent sinus beat showing marked QT prolongation and deformity. This type of cardiac arrhythmia was originally termed "torsade de pointes" (translated from the French as "twisting of the points"). Fluoxetine is considered as having a risk of causing torsade de pointes. Since it is not known what effect vasoconstrictors in the local anesthetic regimen will have in patients with a known history of congenital prolonged QT interval or in patients taking any medication that prolongs the QT interval, a medical consult is suggested.

References

Friedlander AH and Mahler ME, "Major Depressive Disorder. Psychopathology, Medical Management, and Dental Implications," *J Am Dent Assoc*, 2001, 132(5):629-38.
Gerber PE and Lynd LD, "Selective Serotonin Reuptake Inhibitor-induced Movement Disorders," *Ann Pharmacother*, 1998, 32(6):692-8.
Wynn RL, "New Antidepressant Medications," *Gen Dent*, 1997, 45(1):24-8.

Fluoxymesterone (floo oks i MES te rone)

U.S. Brand Names Androxy™

Pharmacologic Category Androgen

Use Replacement of endogenous testicular hormone; in females, palliative treatment of breast cancer

Unlabeled/Investigational Use Stimulation of erythropoiesis, angioneurotic edema

Local Anesthetic/Vasoconstrictor Precautions No information available to require special precautions

Effects on Dental Treatment No significant effects or complications reported

Effects on Bleeding No information available to require special precautions

Adverse Effects

>10%:
- Male: Priapism
- Female: Menstrual problems (amenorrhea), virilism, breast soreness
- Cardiovascular: Edema
- Dermatologic: Acne

1% to 10%:
- Male: Prostatic carcinoma, hirsutism (increase in pubic hair growth), impotence, testicular atrophy
- Cardiovascular: Edema
- Gastrointestinal: GI irritation, nausea, vomiting
- Genitourinary: Prostatic hyperplasia
- Hepatic: Hepatic dysfunction

General Dosage Range Oral:
Adults (females): 10-40 mg/day in divided doses
Adults (males): 2.5-20 mg/day

Mechanism of Action Synthetic androgenic anabolic hormone responsible for the normal growth and development of male sex hormones and development of male sex organs and maintenance of secondary sex characteristics; synthetic testosterone derivative with significant androgen activity; stimulates RNA polymerase activity resulting in an increase in protein production; increases bone development; halogenated derivative of testosterone with up to 5 times the activity of methyltestosterone

Pharmacodynamics/Kinetics
Half-life Elimination 10-100 minutes

Pregnancy Risk Factor X

Controlled Substance C-III

FluPHENAZine (floo FEN a zeen)

Canadian Brand Names Apo-Fluphenazine Decanoate®; Apo-Fluphenazine®; Modecate®; Modecate® Concentrate; PMS-Fluphenazine Decanoate

Pharmacologic Category Antipsychotic Agent, Typical, Phenothiazine

Use Management of manifestations of psychotic disorders and schizophrenia; depot formulation may offer improved outcome in individuals with psychosis who are nonadherent with oral antipsychotics

Unlabeled/Investigational Use Psychosis/agitation related to Alzheimer's dementia

Local Anesthetic/Vasoconstrictor Precautions Most pharmacology textbooks state that in the presence of phenothiazines, systemic doses of epinephrine paradoxically decrease the blood pressure. This is the so called "epinephrine reversal" phenomenon. This has never been observed when epinephrine is given by infiltration as part of the anesthesia procedure.

Effects on Dental Treatment Key adverse event(s) related to dental treatment: Xerostomia and increased salivation (normal salivary flow resumes upon discontinuation). Orthostatic hypotension and nasal congestion are possible and since the drug is a dopamine antagonist, extrapyramidal symptoms of the TMJ are a possibility.

Effects on Bleeding No information available to require special precautions

Adverse Effects Frequency not defined.
Cardiovascular: Hyper-/hypotension, tachycardia, fluctuations in blood pressure, arrhythmia, edema
Central nervous system: Parkinsonian symptoms, akathisia, dystonias, tardive dyskinesia, dizziness, hyper-reflexia, headache, cerebral edema, drowsiness, lethargy, restlessness, excitement, bizarre dreams, EEG changes, depression, seizure, NMS, altered central temperature regulation
Dermatologic: Dermatitis, eczema, erythema, itching, photosensitivity, rash, seborrhea, skin pigmentation, urticaria
Endocrine & metabolic: Menstrual cycle changes, breast pain, amenorrhea, galactorrhea, gynecomastia, libido changes, prolactin increased, SIADH
Gastrointestinal: Weight gain, appetite loss, salivation, xerostomia, constipation, paralytic ileus, laryngeal edema
Genitourinary: Ejaculatory disturbances, impotence, polyuria, bladder paralysis, enuresis
Hematologic: Agranulocytosis, leukopenia, thrombocytopenia, nonthrombocytopenic purpura, eosinophilia, pancytopenia
Hepatic: Cholestatic jaundice, hepatotoxicity
Neuromuscular & skeletal: Trembling of fingers, SLE, facial hemispasm
Ocular: Pigmentary retinopathy, cornea and lens changes, blurred vision, glaucoma
Respiratory: Nasal congestion, asthma

General Dosage Range
I.M. (hydrochloride): *Adults:* Initial: 1.25 mg as a single dose; Maintenance: 2.5-10 mg/day in divided doses every 6-8 hours
I.M., SubQ (Depot): *Adults:* Initial: 6.25-25 mg every 2-4 weeks (maximum: 100 mg)
Oral: *Adults:* 1-20 mg/day in divided doses every 6-8 hours (maximum: 40 mg/day)

Mechanism of Action Fluphenazine is a piperazine phenothiazine antipsychotic which blocks postsynaptic mesolimbic dopaminergic D_1 and D_2 receptors in the brain; depresses the release of hypothalamic and hypophyseal hormones; believed to depress the reticular activating system, thus affecting basal metabolism, body temperature, wakefulness, vasomotor tone, and emesis

Pharmacodynamics/Kinetics
Onset of Action Decanoate: 24-72 hours; Peak effect: Neuroleptic: Decanoate: 48-96 hours

Duration of Action Hydrochloride salt: 6-8 hours; Decanoate: ~4 weeks
Half-life Elimination Derivative dependent: Hydrochloride: ~14-16.4 hours; Decanoate: ~14 days
Time to Peak Serum: Hydrochloride: Oral: 2 hours; Decanoate: 8-10 hours

Flurandrenolide (flure an DREN oh lide)

U.S. Brand Names Cordran®; Cordran® SP
Canadian Brand Names Cordran®
Pharmacologic Category Corticosteroid, Topical
Use Inflammation of corticosteroid-responsive dermatoses [medium potency topical corticosteroid]
Local Anesthetic/Vasoconstrictor Precautions No information available to require special precautions
Effects on Dental Treatment No significant effects or complications reported
Effects on Bleeding No information available to require special precautions
Adverse Effects Frequency not defined.
Cardiovascular: Intracranial hypertension
Dermatologic: Acne, acneiform eruptions, allergic contact dermatitis, dry skin, folliculitis, hyperpigmentation, hypertrichosis, itching, maceration of the skin, miliaria, perioral dermatitis, skin atrophy, striae
Endocrine & metabolic: Cushing's syndrome, growth retardation, HPA suppression
Local: Burning, irritation
Miscellaneous: Secondary infection
General Dosage Range Topical:
Children: Apply 1-2 times/day
Adults: Apply 2-3 times/day
Mechanism of Action Decreases inflammation by suppression of migration of polymorphonuclear leukocytes and reversal of increased capillary permeability
Pregnancy Risk Factor C

Flurazepam (flure AZ e pam)

Canadian Brand Names Apo-Flurazepam®; Dalmane®; Som Pam
Generic Availability (U.S.) Yes
Pharmacologic Category Hypnotic, Benzodiazepine
Use Short-term treatment of insomnia
Local Anesthetic/Vasoconstrictor Precautions No information available to require special precautions
Effects on Dental Treatment Key adverse event(s) related to dental treatment: Xerostomia and changes in salivation (normal salivary flow resumes upon discontinuation), and bitter taste.
Effects on Bleeding No information available to require special precautions
Adverse Effects Frequency not defined.
Cardiovascular: Chest pain, flushing, hypotension, palpitation
Central nervous system: Apprehension, ataxia, confusion, depression, dizziness, drowsiness, euphoria, faintness, falling, hallucinations, hangover effect, headache, irritability, lightheadedness, memory impairment, nervousness, paradoxical reactions, restlessness, slurred speech, staggering, talkativeness
Dermatologic: Pruritus, rash
Gastrointestinal: Appetite increased/decreased, bitter taste, constipation, diarrhea, GI pain, heartburn, nausea, salivation increased/excessive, upset stomach, vomiting, weight gain/loss, xerostomia
Hematologic: Granulocytopenia, leukopenia
Hepatic: Alkaline phosphatase increased, ALT increased, AST increased, cholestatic jaundice, total bilirubin increased
Neuromuscular & skeletal: Body/joint pain, dysarthria, reflex slowing, weakness
Ocular: Blurred vision, burning eyes, difficulty focusing
Respiratory: Apnea, dyspnea
Miscellaneous: Diaphoresis, drug dependence
Postmarketing and/or case reports: Anaphylaxis, angioedema, complex sleep-related behavior (sleep-driving, cooking or eating food, making phone calls)
Dosage Oral: Insomnia:
Children:
<15 years: Dose not established
≥15 years: 15 mg at bedtime
Adults: 15-30 mg at bedtime
Elderly: 15 mg at bedtime; avoid use if possible

Mechanism of Action Binds to stereospecific benzodiazepine receptors on the postsynaptic GABA neuron at several sites within the central nervous system, including the limbic system, reticular formation. Enhancement of the inhibitory effect of GABA on neuronal excitability results by increased neuronal membrane permeability to chloride ions. This shift in chloride ions results in hyperpolarization (a less excitable state) and stabilization.

Contraindications Hypersensitivity to flurazepam or any component of the formulation (cross-sensitivity with other benzodiazepines may exist); narrow-angle glaucoma; pregnancy

Warnings/Precautions Use with caution in elderly or debilitated patients, patients with hepatic disease (including alcoholics), or renal impairment. Use with caution in patients with respiratory disease or impaired gag reflex. Avoid use in patients with sleep apnea.

Causes CNS depression (dose related); patients must be cautioned about performing tasks which require mental alertness (eg, operating machinery or driving). Use with caution in patients receiving other CNS depressants or psychoactive agents. Benzodiazepines have been associated with falls and traumatic injury and should be used with extreme caution in patients who are at risk of these events. Benzodiazepines with long half-lives may produce prolonged sedation and increase the risk of falls and fracture. Short- or medium-acting benzodiazepines are preferred in elderly patients (Beers Criteria).

Use caution in patients with depression, particularly if suicidal risk may be present. Use with caution in patients with a history of drug dependence. Benzodiazepines have been associated with dependence and acute withdrawal symptoms on discontinuation or reduction in dose (may occur after as little as 10 days of use).

As a hypnotic, should be used only after evaluation of potential causes of sleep disturbance. Failure of sleep disturbance to resolve after 7-10 days may indicate psychiatric or medical illness. A worsening of insomnia or the emergence of new abnormalities of thought or behavior may represent unrecognized psychiatric or medical illness and requires immediate and careful evaluation. Postmarketing studies have indicated that the use of hypnotic/sedative agents for sleep has been associated with hypersensitivity reactions including anaphylaxis as well as angioedema. An increased risk for hazardous sleep-related activities such as sleep-driving; cooking and eating food, and making phone calls while asleep have also been noted.

Benzodiazepines have been associated with anterograde amnesia. Paradoxical reactions have been reported, particularly in adolescent/pediatric or psychiatric patients. Does not have analgesic, antidepressant, or antipsychotic properties.

Drug Interactions

Metabolism/Transport Effects **Substrate** of CYP3A4 (major); **Inhibits** CYP2E1 (weak)

Avoid Concomitant Use

Avoid concomitant use of Flurazepam with any of the following: OLANZapine

Increased Effect/Toxicity

Flurazepam may increase the levels/effects of: Alcohol (Ethyl); CloZAPine; CNS Depressants; Fosphenytoin; Methotrimeprazine; Phenytoin

The levels/effects of Flurazepam may be increased by: Antifungal Agents (Azole Derivatives, Systemic); Aprepitant; Calcium Channel Blockers (Nondihydropyridine); Cimetidine; Conivaptan; Contraceptives (Estrogens); Contraceptives (Progestins); CYP3A4 Inhibitors (Moderate); CYP3A4 Inhibitors (Strong); Dasatinib; Droperidol; Fluconazole; Fosamprenavir; Fosaprepitant; Grapefruit Juice; Isoniazid; Macrolide Antibiotics; Methotrimeprazine; Nefazodone; OLANZapine; Proton Pump Inhibitors; Ritonavir; Saquinavir; Selective Serotonin Reuptake Inhibitors

Decreased Effect

The levels/effects of Flurazepam may be decreased by: CarBAMazepine; CYP3A4 Inducers (Strong); Deferasirox; Rifamycin Derivatives; St Johns Wort; Theophylline Derivatives; Tocilizumab; Yohimbine

Ethanol/Nutrition/Herb Interactions

Ethanol: May increase CNS depression; monitor for increased effects with coadministration. Caution patients about effects.

Food: Serum levels and response to flurazepam may be increased by grapefruit juice, but unlikely because of flurazepam's high oral bioavailability.

Herb/Nutraceutical: Avoid valerian, St John's wort, kava kava, gotu kola (may increase CNS depression).

Pharmacodynamics/Kinetics

Onset of Action Hypnotic: 15-20 minutes; Peak effect: 3-6 hours

Duration of Action 7-8 hours

Half-life Elimination
Flurazepam: 2.3 hours
N-desalkylflurazepam:
Adults: Single dose: 74-90 hours; Multiple doses: 111-113 hours
Elderly (61-85 years): Single dose: 120-160 hours; Multiple doses: 126-158 hours

Time to Peak N-desalkylflurazepam: 10.6 hours (range: 7.6-13.6 hours); N-hydroxyethylflurazepam: ~1 hour

Lactation Excretion in breast milk unknown

Breast-Feeding Considerations Drowsiness, lethargy, or weight loss in nursing infants have been observed in case reports following maternal use of some benzodiazepines.

Controlled Substance C-IV

Dosage Forms
Capsule, oral: 15 mg, 30 mg

Flurbiprofen (Systemic) (flure BI proe fen)

Related Information
Rheumatoid Arthritis, Osteoarthritis, and Osteoporosis *on page 1889*
Temporomandibular Dysfunction (TMD) *on page 1964*

Canadian Brand Names Alti-Flurbiprofen; Ansaid®; Apo-Flurbiprofen®; Froben-SR®; Froben®; Novo-Flurprofen; Nu-Flurprofen

Generic Availability (U.S.) Yes

Pharmacologic Category Nonsteroidal Anti-inflammatory Drug (NSAID), Oral

Dental Use Management of postoperative pain

Use Treatment of rheumatoid arthritis and osteoarthritis

Unlabeled/Investigational Use Management of postoperative pain

Local Anesthetic/Vasoconstrictor Precautions No information available to require special precautions

Effects on Dental Treatment The dentist should be aware of the potential of abnormal coagulation. Caution should also be exercised in the use of NSAIDs in patients already on anticoagulant therapy with drugs such as warfarin (Coumadin®). See Effects on Bleeding.

Effects on Bleeding Nonselective NSAIDs are known to reversibly decrease platelet aggregation via mechanisms different than observed with aspirin. Platelet function is restored as the drug is eliminated from the body. Dental professionals should be aware that recommendations differ between dental and general surgery. NSAIDs should be avoided (if possible) in general surgery patients for 3-5 half-lives of the drug (usually 1-3 days) prior to surgery to reduce the risk of excessive bleeding. However, there is no scientific evidence to warrant discontinuance of NSAIDs prior to dental surgery. In medically complicated patients or extensive oral surgery, the decision to interrupt therapy must be based on the risk to benefit in an individual patient and a medical consult is suggested. Routine interruption of NSAID therapy for most dental procedures is not warranted. If therapy is continued without interruption, the clinician should anticipate the potential for slower clotting times.

Adverse Effects >1%:
Cardiovascular: Edema
Central nervous system: Amnesia, anxiety, depression, dizziness, headache, insomnia, malaise, nervousness, somnolence, vertigo
Dermatologic: Rash
Gastrointestinal: Abdominal pain, constipation, diarrhea, dyspepsia, flatulence, GI bleeding, nausea, vomiting, weight changes
Hepatic: Liver enzymes increased
Neuromuscular & skeletal: Reflexes increased, tremor, weakness
Ocular: Vision changes
Otic: Tinnitus
Respiratory: Rhinitis

Dental Usual Dosage Management of postoperative pain: Adults: Oral: 100 mg every 12 hours

Dosage Oral:
Rheumatoid arthritis and osteoarthritis: 200-300 mg/day in 2, 3, or 4 divided doses; do not administer more than 100 mg for any single dose; maximum: 300 mg/day
Dental: Management of postoperative pain (unlabeled use): 100 mg every 12 hours
Dosage adjustment in renal impairment: Not recommended in patients with advanced renal disease.

Mechanism of Action Reversibly inhibits cyclooxygenase-1 and 2 (COX-1 and 2) enzymes, which results in decreased formation of prostaglandin precursors; has antipyretic, analgesic, and anti-inflammatory properties

Other proposed mechanisms not fully elucidated (and possibly contributing to the anti-inflammatory effect to varying degrees), include inhibiting chemotaxis, altering lymphocyte activity, inhibiting neutrophil aggregation/activation, and decreasing proinflammatory cytokine levels.

Contraindications Hypersensitivity to flurbiprofen, aspirin, other NSAIDs, or any component of the formulation; perioperative pain in the setting of coronary artery bypass (CABG) surgery

Warnings/Precautions **[U.S. Boxed Warning]: NSAIDs are associated with an increased risk of adverse cardiovascular thrombotic events, including MI and stroke.** Risk may be increased with duration of use or pre-existing cardiovascular risk factors or disease. Carefully evaluate individual cardiovascular risk profiles prior to prescribing. May cause new-onset hypertension or worsening of existing hypertension. Use caution with fluid retention. Avoid use in heart failure. Concurrent administration of ibuprofen, and potentially other nonselective NSAIDs, may interfere with aspirin's cardioprotective effect. **[U.S. Boxed Warning]: Use is contraindicated for treatment of perioperative pain in the setting of coronary artery bypass graft (CABG) surgery.** Risk of MI and stroke may be increased with use following CABG surgery.

Platelet adhesion and aggregation may be decreased; may prolong bleeding time; patients with coagulation disorders or who are receiving anticoagulants should be monitored closely. Anemia may occur; patients on long-term NSAID therapy should be monitored for anemia. NSAID use may compromise existing renal function; dose-dependent decreases in prostaglandin synthesis may result from NSAID use, reducing renal blood flow which may cause renal decompensation. Patients with impaired renal function, dehydration, heart failure, liver dysfunction, those taking diuretics, and ACE inhibitors, and the elderly are at greater risk of renal toxicity. Rehydrate patient before starting therapy; monitor renal function closely. Not recommended for use in patients with advanced renal disease. Long-term NSAID use may result in renal papillary necrosis.

[U.S. Boxed Warning]: NSAIDs may increase risk of gastrointestinal irritation, inflammation, ulceration, bleeding, and perforation. These events may occur at any time during therapy and without warning. Use caution with a history of GI disease (bleeding or ulcers), concurrent therapy with aspirin, anticoagulants and/or corticosteroids, smoking, use of alcohol, the elderly, or debilitated patients. When used concomitantly with ≤325 mg of aspirin, a substantial increase in the risk of gastrointestinal complications (eg, ulcer) occurs; concomitant gastroprotective therapy (eg, proton pump inhibitors) is recommended (Bhatt, 2008).

Use the lowest effective dose for the shortest duration of time, consistent with individual patient goals, to reduce risk of cardiovascular or GI adverse events. Alternate therapies should be considered for patients at high risk.

NSAIDs may cause serious skin adverse events including exfoliative dermatitis, Stevens-Johnson syndrome (SJS), and toxic epidermal necrolysis (TEN); discontinue use at first sign of skin rash or hypersensitivity. Anaphylactoid reactions may occur, even without prior exposure; patients with "aspirin triad" (bronchial asthma, aspirin intolerance, rhinitis) may be at increased risk. Do not use in patients who experience bronchospasm, asthma, rhinitis, or urticaria with NSAID or aspirin therapy. Use caution in other forms of asthma.

Use with caution in patients with decreased hepatic function. Closely monitor patients with any abnormal LFT. Severe hepatic reactions (eg, fulminant hepatitis, liver failure) have occurred with NSAID use, rarely; discontinue if signs or symptoms of liver disease develop, or if systemic manifestations occur.

The elderly are at increased risk for adverse effects (especially peptic ulceration, CNS effects, renal toxicity) from NSAIDs even at low doses.

Withhold for at least 4-6 half-lives prior to surgical or dental procedures. Safety and efficacy have not been established in children.

Drug Interactions

Metabolism/Transport Effects **Substrate** of CYP2C9 (minor); **Inhibits** CYP2C9 (strong)

Avoid Concomitant Use

Avoid concomitant use of Flurbiprofen (Systemic) with any of the following: Ketorolac; Ketorolac (Systemic)

Increased Effect/Toxicity

Flurbiprofen (Systemic) may increase the levels/effects of: Aminoglycosides; Anticoagulants; Antiplatelet Agents; Bisphosphonate Derivatives; Collagenase (Systemic); CycloSPORINE; CycloSPORINE (Systemic); Deferasirox; Desmopressin; Digoxin; Drotrecogin Alfa; Eplerenone; Haloperidol; Ibritumomab; Lithium; Methotrexate; Nonsteroidal Anti-Inflammatory Agents; PEMEtrexed; Potassium-Sparing

Diuretics; PRALAtrexate; Quinolone Antibiotics; Salicylates; Thrombolytic Agents; Tositumomab and Iodine I 131 Tositumomab; Vancomycin; Vitamin K Antagonists

The levels/effects of Flurbiprofen (Systemic) may be increased by: ACE Inhibitors; Angiotensin II Receptor Blockers; Antidepressants (Tricyclic, Tertiary Amine); Corticosteroids (Systemic); Dasatinib; Glucosamine; Herbs (Anticoagulant/Antiplatelet Properties); Ketorolac; Ketorolac (Systemic); Nonsteroidal Anti-Inflammatory Agents; Omega-3-Acid Ethyl Esters; Pentosan Polysulfate Sodium; Pentoxifylline; Probenecid; Prostacyclin Analogues; Selective Serotonin Reuptake Inhibitors; Serotonin/Norepinephrine Reuptake Inhibitors; Treprostinil

Decreased Effect

Flurbiprofen (Systemic) may decrease the levels/effects of: ACE Inhibitors; Angiotensin II Receptor Blockers; Antiplatelet Agents; Beta-Blockers; Eplerenone; HydrALAZINE; Loop Diuretics; Potassium-Sparing Diuretics; Salicylates; Thiazide Diuretics

The levels/effects of Flurbiprofen (Systemic) may be decreased by: Bile Acid Sequestrants; Nonsteroidal Anti-Inflammatory Agents; Salicylates

Ethanol/Nutrition/Herb Interactions

Ethanol: Avoid ethanol (may enhance gastric mucosal irritation).

Food: Food may decrease the rate but not the extent of absorption.

Herb/Nutraceutical: Avoid alfalfa, anise, bilberry, bladderwrack, bromelain, cat's claw, celery, chamomile, coleus, cordyceps, dong quai, evening primrose, fenugreek, feverfew, garlic, ginger, ginkgo biloba, ginseng (American, Panax, Siberian), grapeseed, green tea, guggul, horse chestnut seed, horseradish, licorice, prickly ash, red clover, reishi, SAMe (S-adenosylmethionine), sweet clover, turmeric, white willow (all have additional antiplatelet activity).

Dietary Considerations May be taken with food, milk, or antacid to decrease GI effects.

Pharmacodynamics/Kinetics

Onset of Action ~1-2 hours

Half-life Elimination 5.7 hours

Time to Peak 1.5 hours

Pregnancy Risk Factor C

Lactation Enters breast milk/not recommended

Breast-Feeding Considerations Low levels of flurbiprofen are found in breast milk. Breast-feeding is not recommended by the manufacturer. The pharmacokinetics of flurbiprofen immediately postpartum are similar to healthy volunteers.

Dosage Forms

Tablet, oral: 50 mg, 100 mg

References

Ahmad N, Grad HA, Haas DA, et al, "The Efficacy of Nonopioid Analgesics for Postoperative Dental Pain: A Meta-Analysis," *Anesth Prog*, 1997, 44(4):119-26.

Bragger U, Muhle T, Fourmousis I, et al, "Effect of the NSAID Flurbiprofen on Remodeling After Periodontal Surgery," *J Periodontal Res*, 1997, 32(7):575-82.

Cooper SA and Kupperman A, "The Analgesic Efficacy of Flurbiprofen Compared to Acetaminophen With Codeine," *J Clin Dent*, 1991, 2(3):70-4.

Dionne R, "Additive Analgesia Without Opioid Side Effects," *Compend Contin Educ Dent*, 2000, 21 (7):572-4, 576-7.

Dionne RA, "Suppression of Dental Pain by the Preoperative Administration of Flurbiprofen," *Am J Med*, 1986, 80(3A):41-9.

Dionne RA and Berthold CW, "Therapeutic Uses of Nonsteroidal Anti-inflammatory Drugs in Dentistry," *Crit Rev Oral Biol Med*, 2001, 12(4):315-30.

Dionne RA, Snyder J, and Hargreaves KM, "Analgesic Efficacy of Flurbiprofen in Comparison With Acetaminophen, Acetaminophen Plus Codeine, and Placebo After Impacted Third Molar Removal," *J Oral Maxillofac Surg*, 1994, 52(9):919-24.

Doroschak AM, Bowles WR, and Hargreaves KM, "Evaluation of the Combination of Flurbiprofen and Tramadol for Management of Endodontic Pain," *J Endod*, 1999, 25(10):660-3.

Forbes JA, Yorio CC, Selinger LR, et al, "An Evaluation of Flurbiprofen, Aspirin, and Placebo in Postoperative Oral Surgery Pain," *Pharmacotherapy*, 1989, 9(2):66-73.

Gallardo F and Rossi E, "Analgesic Efficacy of Flurbiprofen as Compared to Acetaminophen and Placebo After Periodontal Surgery," *J Periodontol*, 1990, 61(4):224-7.

Jeffcoat MK, Reddy MS, Haigh S, et al, "A Comparison of Topical Ketorolac, Systemic Flurbiprofen, and Placebo for the Inhibition of Bone Loss in Adult Periodontitis," *J Periodontol*, 1995, 66(5):329-38.

Jeffcoat MK, Reddy MS, Wang IC, et al, "The Effect of Systemic Flurbiprofen on Bone Supporting Dental Implants," *J Am Dent Assoc*, 1995, 126(3):305-11.

Malmberg AB and Yaksh TL, "Antinociception Produced by Spinal Delivery of the S and R Enantiomers of Flurbiprofen in the Formalin Test," *Eur J Pharmacol*, 1994, 256(2):205-9.

Nguyen AM, Graham DY, Gage T, et al, "Nonsteroidal Anti-inflammatory Drug Use in Dentistry: Gastrointestinal Implications," *Gen Dent*, 1999, 47(6):590-6.

Flutamide (FLOO ta mide)

Canadian Brand Names Apo-Flutamide®; Euflex®; Eulexin®; Novo-Flutamide

Pharmacologic Category Antineoplastic Agent, Antiandrogen

Use Treatment of metastatic prostatic carcinoma in combination therapy with LHRH agonist analogues

Unlabeled/Investigational Use Female hirsutism

Local Anesthetic/Vasoconstrictor Precautions No information available to require special precautions

Effects on Dental Treatment No significant effects or complications reported

Effects on Bleeding Although significant myelosuppression with associated altered hemostasis has been reported for many chemotherapeutic agents, myelosuppression is not common with flutamide and no specific precautions appear to necessary.

Adverse Effects

>10%:

Endocrine & metabolic: Gynecomastia, hot flashes, breast tenderness, galactorrhea (9% to 42%), impotence, libido decreased, tumor flare

Gastrointestinal: Nausea, vomiting (11% to 12%)

Hepatic: AST increased (transient; mild), LDH increased (transient; mild)

1% to 10%:

Cardiovascular: Hypertension (1%), edema

Central nervous system: Drowsiness, confusion, depression, anxiety, nervousness, headache, dizziness, insomnia

Dermatologic: Ecchymosis, photosensitivity, pruritus

Gastrointestinal: Anorexia, appetite increased, constipation, indigestion, upset stomach (4% to 6%); diarrhea

Hematologic: Anemia (6%), leukopenia (3%), thrombocytopenia (1%)

Neuromuscular & skeletal: Weakness (1%)

Miscellaneous: Herpes zoster

General Dosage Range Oral: *Adults:* 250 mg 3 times/day

Mechanism of Action Nonsteroidal antiandrogen that inhibits androgen uptake or inhibits binding of androgen in target tissues

Pharmacodynamics/Kinetics

Half-life Elimination 5-6 hours (2-hydroxyflutamide)

Pregnancy Risk Factor D

Fluticasone (Oral Inhalation) (floo TIK a sone)

Related Information

Respiratory Diseases *on page* 1876

U.S. Brand Names Flovent® Diskus®; Flovent® HFA

Canadian Brand Names Flovent® Diskus®; Flovent® HFA

Generic Availability (U.S.) No

Pharmacologic Category Corticosteroid, Inhalant (Oral)

Use Maintenance treatment of asthma as prophylactic therapy; also indicated for patients requiring oral corticosteroid therapy for asthma to assist in total discontinuation or reduction of total oral dose

Local Anesthetic/Vasoconstrictor Precautions No information available to require special precautions

Effects on Dental Treatment Localized infections with *Candida albicans* or *Aspergillus niger* have occurred frequently in the mouth and pharynx with repetitive use of oral inhaler of corticosteroids. These infections may require treatment with appropriate antifungal therapy or discontinuance of treatment with corticosteroid inhaler.

Effects on Bleeding No information available to require special precautions

Adverse Effects

>10%:

Central nervous system: Headache (2% to 14%)

Respiratory: Upper respiratory tract infection (14% to 21%), throat irritation (3% to 22%)

3% to 10%:

Central nervous system: Fever (1% to 7%)

Gastrointestinal: Oral candidiasis (≤9%), nausea/vomiting (1% to 8%), gastrointestinal infection (including viral; 1% to 5%), gastrointestinal discomfort/pain (1% to 4%)

Neuromuscular & skeletal: Musculoskeletal pain (2% to 5%), muscle injury (1% to 5%)

Respiratory: Sinusitis/sinus infection (4% to 10%), lower respiratory tract infections/pneumonia (1% to 7%; COPD diagnosis and age >65 years increase risk), cough (1% to 6%), bronchitis (≤8%), hoarseness/dysphonia (2% to 6%), upper respiratory tract inflammation (≤5%), viral respiratory infection (1% to 5%), rhinitis (1% to 4%)

Miscellaneous: Viral infection (≤5%)

1% to 3%:

Cardiovascular: Chest symptoms, edema, palpitation

Central nervous system: Cranial nerve paralysis, dizziness, fatigue, malaise, migraine, mood disorders, pain, sleep disorder

Dermatologic: Acne, dermatitis/dermatosis, eczema, folliculitis, photodermatitis, infection (fungal, viral), pruritus, rash, urticaria

Endocrine & metabolic: Fluid disturbance, goiter, uric acid metabolism disturbance
Gastrointestinal: Abdominal discomfort/pain, appetite changes, dental discomfort/pain, diarrhea, dyspepsia, gastroenteritis, hyposalivation, oral discomfort/pain, oral erythema/rash, oral ulcerations, oropharyngeal plaques, tooth decay, weight gain
Genitourinary: Reproductive organ infections (bacterial), urinary tract infection
Hematologic: Hematoma
Hepatic: Cholecystitis
Neuromuscular & skeletal: Arthralgia, articular rheumatism, muscle cramps/spasms, muscle pain, muscle stiffness/tightness/rigidity, musculoskeletal inflammation
Ocular: Blepharoconjunctivitis, conjunctivitis, keratitis
Otic: Otitis
Respiratory: Epistaxis, hoarseness/dysphonia, laryngitis, nasal sinus disorder, pharyngitis/throat infection, rhinorrhea/postnasal drip, throat constriction
Miscellaneous: Infection (bacterial, fungal); injuries (including muscle, soft tissue); polyps (ear, nose, throat); tonsillitis

Dosage Inhalation, oral: Asthma:
Children:
Flovent® HFA:
Children 4-11 years: 88 mcg twice daily
Children ≥12 years: Refer to adult dosing.
NIH Asthma Guidelines (NIH, 2007) (administer in divided doses twice daily):
"Low" dose:
0-4 years: 176 mcg/day
5-11 years: 88-176 mcg/day
≥12 years: 88-264 mcg/day
"Medium" dose:
0-4 years: >176-352 mcg/day
5-11 years: >176-352 mcg/day
≥12 years: >264-440 mcg/day
"High" dose:
0-4 years: >352 mcg/day
5-11 years: >352 mcg/day
≥12 years: >440 mcg/day
Flovent® Diskus® *(U.S. labeling)*:
Children 4-11 years: Usual starting dose: 50 mcg twice daily; may increase to 100 mcg twice daily in patients not adequately controlled after 2 weeks of therapy. Higher starting doses may be considered in patients with poorer asthma control or those requiring high ranges of inhaled corticosteroids. Titrate to the lowest effective dose once asthma stability is achieved (maximum dose: 100 mcg twice daily)
Children >11 years: Refer to adult dosing.
Flovent® Diskus® *(Canadian labeling)*:
Children 4-16 years: Usual starting dose: 50-100 mcg twice daily; may increase to 200 mcg twice daily in patients not adequately controlled; titrate to the lowest effective dose once asthma stability is achieved
Children ≥16 years: Refer to adult dosing.

Adults: **Note:** Titrate to the lowest effective dose once asthma stability is achieved
Flovent® HFA: Manufacturers labeling: Dosing based on previous therapy
Bronchodilator alone: Recommended starting dose: 88 mcg twice daily; highest recommended dose: 440 mcg twice daily
Inhaled corticosteroids: Recommended starting dose: 88-220 mcg twice daily; highest recommended dose: 440 mcg twice daily; a higher starting dose may be considered in patients previously requiring higher doses of inhaled corticosteroids
Oral corticosteroids: Recommended starting dose: 440 mcg twice daily
Highest recommended dose: 880 mcg twice daily; starting dose is patient dependent. In patients on chronic oral corticosteroids therapy, reduce prednisone dose no faster than 2.5-5 mg/day on a weekly basis; begin taper after 1 week of fluticasone therapy.
NIH Asthma Guidelines (NIH, 2007) (administer in divided doses twice daily):
"Low" dose: 88-264 mcg/day
"Medium" dose: >264-440 mcg/day
"High" dose: >440 mcg/day
Flovent® Diskus® *(U.S. labeling)*: **Note:** May increase dose after 2 weeks of therapy in patients not adequately controlled. Higher starting doses may be considered in patients with poorer asthma control or those requiring high ranges of inhaled corticosteroids. Titrate to the lowest effective dose once asthma stability is achieved.

Bronchodilator alone: Recommended starting dose: 100 mcg twice daily; maximum recommended dose: 500 mcg twice daily
Inhaled corticosteroids: Recommended starting dose: 100-250 mcg twice daily; maximum recommended dose: 500 mcg twice daily
Oral corticosteroids: Recommended starting dose: 500-1000 mcg twice daily; maximum recommended dose: 1000 mcg twice daily. Starting dose is patient dependent. In patients on chronic oral corticosteroids therapy, reduce prednisone dose no faster than 2.5 mg/day on a weekly basis; begin taper after 1 week of fluticasone therapy.

Flovent® Diskus® *(Canadian labeling)*:
Mild asthma: 100-250 mcg twice daily
Moderate asthma: 250-500 mcg twice daily
Severe asthma: 500 mcg twice daily; may increase to 1000 mcg twice daily in very severe patients requiring high doses of corticosteroids

Elderly: No differences in safety have been observed in the elderly when compared to younger patients. Based on current data, no dosage adjustment is needed based on age.

Dosage adjustment in hepatic impairment: Fluticasone is primarily cleared in the liver. Fluticasone plasma levels may be increased in patients with hepatic impairment, use with caution; monitor.

Mechanism of Action Fluticasone belongs to a group of corticosteroids which utilizes a fluorocarbothioate ester linkage at the 17 carbon position; extremely potent vasoconstrictive and anti-inflammatory activity. The effectiveness of inhaled fluticasone is due to its direct local effect.

Contraindications Hypersensitivity to fluticasone or any component of the formulation; primary treatment of status asthmaticus or acute bronchospasm

Warnings/Precautions May cause hypercorticism or suppression of hypothalamic-pituitary-adrenal (HPA) axis, particularly in younger children or in patients receiving high doses for prolonged periods. HPA axis suppression may lead to adrenal crisis. Withdrawal and discontinuation of a corticosteroid should be done slowly and carefully. Particular care is required when patients are transferred from systemic corticosteroids to inhaled products due to possible adrenal insufficiency or withdrawal from steroids, including an increase in allergic symptoms. Patients receiving ≥20 mg per day of prednisone (or equivalent) may be most susceptible. Concurrent use of ritonavir (and potentially other strong inhibitors of CYP3A4) may increase fluticasone levels and effects on HPA suppression. Fatalities have occurred due to adrenal insufficiency in asthmatic patients during and after transfer from systemic corticosteroids to aerosol steroids; aerosol steroids do **not** provide the systemic steroid needed to treat patients having trauma, surgery, or infections.

Bronchospasm may occur with wheezing after inhalation; if this occurs, stop steroid and treat with a fast-acting bronchodilator. Supplemental steroids (oral or parenteral) may be needed during stress or severe asthma attacks. Corticosteroid use may cause psychiatric disturbances, including depression, euphoria, insomnia, mood swings, and personality changes. Pre-existing psychiatric conditions may be exacerbated by corticosteroid use. Prolonged use of corticosteroids may also increase the incidence of secondary infection, mask acute infection (including fungal infections), prolong or exacerbate viral infections, or limit response to vaccines. Exposure to chickenpox should be avoided; corticosteroids should not be used to treat ocular herpes simplex. Corticosteroids should not be used for cerebral malaria. Close observation is required in patients with latent tuberculosis and/or TB reactivity; restrict use in active TB (only in conjunction with antituberculosis treatment). Rare cases of vasculitis (Churg-Strauss syndrome) or other eosinophilic conditions can occur. Prolonged treatment with corticosteroids has been associated with the development of Kaposi's sarcoma (case reports); if noted, discontinuation of therapy should be considered.

Use with caution in patients with thyroid disease, hepatic impairment, renal impairment, cardiovascular disease, diabetes, glaucoma, cataracts, myasthenia gravis, patients at risk for osteoporosis, patients at risk for seizures, or GI diseases (diverticulitis, peptic ulcer, ulcerative colitis) due to perforation risk. Use caution following acute MI (corticosteroids have been associated with myocardial rupture). Because of the risk of adverse effects, systemic corticosteroids should be used cautiously in the elderly in the smallest possible effective dose for the shortest duration.

Orally-inhaled corticosteroids may cause a reduction in growth velocity in pediatric patients (~1 centimeter per year [range: 0.3-1.8 cm per year] and related to dose and duration of exposure). To minimize the systemic effects of orally-inhaled corticosteroids, each patient should be titrated to the lowest effective dose. Growth should be routinely monitored in pediatric patients.

Not to be used in status asthmaticus or for the relief of acute bronchospasm. Flovent® Diskus® contains lactose; very rare anaphylactic reactions have been reported in patients with severe milk protein allergy. There have been reports of systemic corticosteroid withdrawal symptoms (eg, joint/muscle pain, lassitude, depression) when withdrawing oral inhalation therapy. Local yeast infections (eg, oral pharyngeal candidiasis) may occur. Lower respiratory tract infections, including pneumonia, have been reported in patients with COPD with an even higher incidence in the elderly.

Drug Interactions

Metabolism/Transport Effects Substrate of CYP3A4 (major)

Avoid Concomitant Use

Avoid concomitant use of Fluticasone (Oral Inhalation) with any of the following: Aldesleukin; BCG; CYP3A4 Inhibitors (Strong); Natalizumab; Pimecrolimus; Roflumilast; Tacrolimus (Topical)

Increased Effect/Toxicity

Fluticasone (Oral Inhalation) may increase the levels/effects of: Amphotericin B; Deferasirox; Leflunomide; Loop Diuretics; Natalizumab; Thiazide Diuretics

The levels/effects of Fluticasone (Oral Inhalation) may be increased by: CYP3A4 Inhibitors (Moderate); CYP3A4 Inhibitors (Strong); Dasatinib; Denosumab; Pimecrolimus; Roflumilast; Tacrolimus (Topical); Trastuzumab

Decreased Effect

Fluticasone (Oral Inhalation) may decrease the levels/effects of: Aldesleukin; Antidiabetic Agents; BCG; Corticorelin; Sipuleucel-T; Vaccines (Inactivated)

The levels/effects of Fluticasone (Oral Inhalation) may be decreased by: Echinacea; Tocilizumab

Ethanol/Nutrition/Herb Interactions Herb/Nutraceutical: In theory, St John's wort may decrease serum levels of fluticasone by inducing CYP3A4 isoenzymes.

Dietary Considerations Flovent® Diskus® contains lactose; very rare anaphylactic reactions have been reported in patients with severe milk protein allergy.

Pharmacodynamics/Kinetics

Onset of Action Maximal benefit may take 1-2 weeks or longer

Pregnancy Risk Factor C

Lactation Excretion in breast milk unknown/use caution

Breast-Feeding Considerations Systemic corticosteroids are excreted in human milk. It is not known if sufficient quantities of fluticasone are absorbed following inhalation to produce detectable amounts in breast milk. The use of inhaled corticosteroids is not considered a contraindication to breast feeding.

Dosage Forms

Aerosol, for oral inhalation:

Flovent® HFA: 44 mcg/inhalation (10.6 g); 110 mcg/inhalation (12 g); 220 mcg/inhalation (12 g)

Powder, for oral inhalation:

Flovent® Diskus®: 50 mcg (60s); 100 mcg (60s); 250 mcg (60s)

Dosage Forms: Canada

Powder, for oral inhalation [prefilled blister pack]:

Flovent® Diskus®: 50 mcg (28s, 60s); 100 mcg (28s, 60s); 250 mcg (28s, 60s); 500 mcg (28s, 60s)

Fluticasone (Nasal) (floo TIK a sone)

U.S. Brand Names Flonase®; Veramyst®

Canadian Brand Names Apo-Fluticasone®; Avamys®; Flonase®; ratio-Fluticasone

Pharmacologic Category Corticosteroid, Nasal

Use

Flonase®: Management of seasonal and perennial allergic rhinitis and nonallergic rhinitis

Veramyst®, Avamys® [CAN]: Management of seasonal and perennial allergic rhinitis

Local Anesthetic/Vasoconstrictor Precautions No information available to require special precautions

Effects on Dental Treatment No significant effects or complications reported

Effects on Bleeding No information available to require special precautions

Adverse Effects

>10%: Central nervous system: Headache (7% to 16%)

1% to 10%:

Central nervous system: Dizziness (1% to 3%), fever (1% to 5%)

Gastrointestinal: Nausea/vomiting (3% to 5%), abdominal pain (1% to 3%), diarrhea (1% to 3%)

Neuromuscular & skeletal: Back pain (1%)
Respiratory: Pharyngitis (6% to 8%), epistaxis (4% to 7%), asthma symptoms (3% to 7%), cough (3% to 4%), pharyngolaryngeal pain (2% to 4%), blood in nasal mucous (1% to 3%), bronchitis (1% to 3%), runny nose (1% to 3%), nasal ulcer (1%)
Miscellaneous: Aches and pains (1% to 3%), flu-like syndrome (1% to 3%)

General Dosage Range Intranasal:
Propionate (Flonase®):
Children ≥4 years: Initial: 1 spray (50 mcg/spray) per nostril once daily; Maintenance: 1-2 sprays (100 mcg) per nostril once daily (maximum: 2 sprays in each nostril [200 mcg]/day)
Adults: Initial: 2 sprays (50 mcg/spray) per nostril once daily; Maintenance: 1-2 sprays per nostril once daily
Furoate (Veramyst®):
Children 2-11 years: Initial: 1 spray (27.5 mcg/spray) per nostril once daily; Maintenance 1-2 sprays per nostril once daily (55-110 mcg/day) (maximum: 2 sprays in each nostril [110 mcg]/day)
Children ≥12 years and Adults: Initial: 2 sprays (27.5 mcg/spray) per nostril once daily; Maintenance 1-2 sprays per nostril once daily (55-110 mcg/day) (maximum: 2 sprays in each nostril [110 mcg]/day)

Mechanism of Action Fluticasone belongs to a group of corticosteroids which utilizes a fluorocarbothioate ester linkage at the 17 carbon position; extremely potent vasoconstrictive and anti-inflammatory activity

Pharmacodynamics/Kinetics
Onset of Action Maximal benefit may take several days

Pregnancy Risk Factor C

Fluticasone and Salmeterol (floo TIK a sone & sal ME te role)

Related Information
Fluticasone (Oral Inhalation) *on page 766*
Salmeterol *on page 1506*

U.S. Brand Names Advair Diskus®; Advair® HFA

Canadian Brand Names Advair Diskus®; Advair®

Generic Availability (U.S.) No

Pharmacologic Category $Beta_2$-Adrenergic Agonist; $Beta_2$-Adrenergic Agonist, Long-Acting; Corticosteroid, Inhalant (Oral)

Use Maintenance treatment of asthma; maintenance treatment of COPD

Local Anesthetic/Vasoconstrictor Precautions No information available to require special precautions

Effects on Dental Treatment Localized infections with *Candida albicans* or *Aspergillus niger* have occurred frequently in the mouth and pharynx with repetitive use of oral inhaler of corticosteroids. These infections may require treatment with appropriate antifungal therapy or discontinuance of treatment with corticosteroid inhaler.

Effects on Bleeding No information available to require special precautions

Adverse Effects Percentages reported in patients with asthma; also see individual agents:
>10%:
Central nervous system: Headache (12% to 21%)
Respiratory: Upper respiratory tract infection (16% to 27%), pharyngitis (9% to 13%)
>3% to 10%:
Central nervous system: Dizziness (1% to 4%)
Endocrine & metabolic: Menstruation symptoms (3% to 5%)
Gastrointestinal: Nausea/vomiting (3% to 6%), diarrhea (2% to 4%), pain/discomfort (1% to 4%), oral candidiasis (1% to 4%), gastrointestinal infections (including viral, ≤4%)
Neuromuscular & skeletal: Musculoskeletal pain (2% to 7%), muscle pain (≤4%)
Respiratory: Throat irritation (7% to 9%), bronchitis (2% to 8%), upper respiratory tract inflammation (4% to 7%), lower respiratory tract infections/pneumonia (1% to 7%; COPD diagnosis and age >65 years increase risk), cough (3% to 6%), sinusitis (4% to 5%), hoarseness/dysphonia (1% to 5%), viral respiratory tract infection (3% to 5%)
1% to 3%:
Cardiovascular: Arrhythmia, chest symptoms, fluid retention, MI, palpitation, syncope, tachycardia
Central nervous system: Compressed nerve syndromes, hypnagogic effects, migraine, pain, sleep disorders, tremor

Dermatologic: Dermatitis, dermatosis, eczema, hives, skin flakiness, urticaria, viral skin infection

Endocrine & metabolic: Hypothyroidism

Gastrointestinal: Constipation, dental discomfort/pain, gastrointestinal infection, hemorrhoids, oral discomfort/pain, oral erythema/rash, oral ulcerations, unusual taste, weight gain

Genitourinary: Urinary tract infection

Hematologic: Contusions/hematomas

Hepatic: Abnormal liver function tests

Neuromuscular & skeletal: Arthralgia, articular rheumatism, bone/cartilage disorders, bone pain, cramps, fractures, muscle injuries (≤3%), muscle spasm, muscle stiffness, tightness/rigidity

Ocular: Conjunctivitis, edema, eye redness, keratitis, xerophthalmia

Respiratory: Blood in nasal mucosa, congestion, ear/nose/throat infection, epistaxis, laryngitis, lower respiratory hemorrhage, nasal irritation, rhinitis, rhinorrhea/postnasal drip, sneezing

Miscellaneous: Allergies/allergic reactions, bacterial infection, burns, candidiasis (≤3%), diaphoresis, sweat/sebum disorders, viral infection, wounds and lacerations

Dosage Oral inhalation: **Note:** Do not use to transfer patients from systemic corticosteroid therapy.

COPD: Adults:

Advair Diskus®: Fluticasone 250 mcg/salmeterol 50 mcg twice daily, 12 hours apart. **Note:** This is the maximum dose.

Advair Diskus® [Canadian labeling; not in approved U.S. labeling]: Fluticasone 250 mcg/salmeterol 50 mcg **or** fluticasone 500 mcg/salmeterol 50 mcg twice daily, 12 hours apart.

Maximum dose: Fluticasone 500 mcg/salmeterol 50 mcg per inhalation (2 inhalations/day)

Asthma:

Children 4-11 years: Advair Diskus®: Fluticasone 100 mcg/salmeterol 50 mcg twice daily, 12 hours apart. **Note:** This is the maximum dose.

Children ≥12 years and Adults:

Advair Diskus®: One inhalation twice daily, morning and evening, 12 hours apart

Maximum dose: Fluticasone 500 mcg/salmeterol 50 mcg per inhalation (2 inhalations/day)

Advair® HFA: Two inhalations twice daily, morning and evening, 12 hours apart

Maximum dose: Fluticasone 230 mcg/salmeterol 21 mcg per inhalation (4 inhalations/day)

Advair® 125 or Advair® 250 [Canadian labeling; not in approved U.S. labeling]: Two inhalations twice daily, morning and evening, 12 hours apart

Maximum dose: Fluticasone 250 mcg/salmeterol 25 mcg per inhalation (4 inhalations/day)

Note: Initial dose prescribed should be based upon previous dose of inhaled-steroid asthma therapy. Dose should be increased after 2 weeks if adequate response is not achieved. Patients should be titrated to lowest effective dose once stable. Each suggestion below specifies the product strength to use; remember to **use 1 inhalation for Diskus® and 2 inhalations for HFA.**

Patients not currently on inhaled corticosteroids:

Advair Diskus®: Fluticasone 100 mcg/salmeterol 50 mcg **or** fluticasone 250 mcg/salmeterol 50 mcg

Advair® HFA: Fluticasone 45 mcg/salmeterol 21 mcg **or** fluticasone 115 mcg/salmeterol 21 mcg

Patients currently using inhaled beclomethasone dipropionate:

≤160 mcg/day: Fluticasone 100 mcg/salmeterol 50 mcg **or** Advair® HFA: Fluticasone 45 mcg/salmeterol 21 mcg

320 mcg/day: Fluticasone 250 mcg/salmeterol 50 mcg **or** Advair® HFA: Fluticasone 115 mcg/salmeterol 21 mcg

640 mcg/day: Fluticasone 500 mcg/salmeterol 50 mcg **or** Advair® HFA: Fluticasone 230 mcg/salmeterol 21 mcg

Patients currently using inhaled budesonide:

≤400 mcg/day: Fluticasone 100 mcg/salmeterol 50 mcg **or** Advair® HFA: Fluticasone 45 mcg/salmeterol 21 mcg

800-1200 mcg/day: Fluticasone 250 mcg/salmeterol 50 mcg **or** Advair® HFA: Fluticasone 115 mcg/salmeterol 21 mcg

1600 mcg/day: Fluticasone 500 mcg/salmeterol 50 mcg **or** Advair® HFA: Fluticasone 230 mcg/salmeterol 21 mcg

Patients currently using inhaled flunisolide CFC aerosol:
≤1000 mcg/day: Fluticasone 100 mcg/salmeterol 50 mcg **or** Advair® HFA: Fluticasone 45 mcg/salmeterol 21 mcg
1250-2000 mcg/day: Fluticasone 250 mcg/salmeterol 50 mcg **or** Advair® HFA: Fluticasone 115 mcg/salmeterol 21 mcg
Patients currently using inhaled flunisolide HFA inhalation aerosol:
≤320 mcg/day: Fluticasone 100 mcg/salmeterol 50 mcg **or** Advair® HFA: Fluticasone 45 mcg/salmeterol 21 mcg
640 mcg/day: Fluticasone 250 mcg/salmeterol 50 mcg **or** Advair® HFA: Fluticasone 115 mcg/salmeterol 21 mcg
Patients currently using inhaled fluticasone HFA aerosol:
≤176 mcg/day: Fluticasone 100 mcg/salmeterol 50 mcg **or** Advair® HFA: Fluticasone 45 mcg/salmeterol 21 mcg
440 mcg/day: Fluticasone 250 mcg/salmeterol 50 mcg **or** Advair® HFA: Fluticasone 115 mcg/salmeterol 21 mcg
660-880 mcg/day: Fluticasone 500 mcg/salmeterol 50 mcg **or** Advair® HFA: Fluticasone 230 mcg/salmeterol 21 mcg
Patients currently using inhaled fluticasone propionate powder:
≤200 mcg/day: Fluticasone 100 mcg/salmeterol 50 mcg **or** Advair® HFA: Fluticasone 45 mcg/salmeterol 21 mcg
500 mcg/day: Fluticasone 250 mcg/salmeterol 50 mcg **or** Advair® HFA: Fluticasone 115 mcg/salmeterol 21 mcg
1000 mcg/day: Fluticasone 500 mcg/salmeterol 50 mcg **or** Advair® HFA: Fluticasone 230 mcg/salmeterol 21 mcg
Patients currently using inhaled mometasone furoate powder:
220 mcg/day: Fluticasone 100 mcg/salmeterol 50 mcg **or** Advair® HFA: Fluticasone 45 mcg/salmeterol 21 mcg
440 mcg/day: Fluticasone 250 mcg/salmeterol 50 mcg **or** Advair® HFA: Fluticasone 115 mcg/salmeterol 21 mcg
880 mcg/day: Fluticasone 500 mcg/salmeterol 50 mcg **or** Advair® HFA: Fluticasone 230 mcg/salmeterol 21 mcg
Patients currently using inhaled triamcinolone acetonide:
≤1000 mcg/day: Fluticasone 100 mcg/salmeterol 50 mcg **or** Advair® HFA: Fluticasone 45 mcg/salmeterol 21 mcg
1100-1600 mcg/day: Fluticasone 250 mcg/salmeterol 50 mcg **or** Advair® HFA: Fluticasone 115 mcg/salmeterol 21 mcg

Elderly: No differences in safety or effectiveness have been seen in studies of patients ≥65 years of age. However, increased sensitivity may be seen in the elderly. Use with caution in patients with concomitant cardiovascular disease.

Dosage adjustment in renal impairment: Specific guidelines are not available

Dosage adjustment in hepatic impairment: No dosage adjustment required; manufacturer suggests close monitoring of patients with hepatic impairment.

Mechanism of Action Combination of fluticasone (corticosteroid) and salmeterol (long-acting $beta_2$-agonist) designed to improve pulmonary function and control over what is produced by either agent when used alone. Because fluticasone and salmeterol act locally in the lung, plasma levels do not predict therapeutic effect.

Fluticasone: The mechanism of action for all topical corticosteroids is believed to be a combination of three important properties: Anti-inflammatory activity, immunosuppressive properties, and antiproliferative actions. Fluticasone has extremely potent vasoconstrictive and anti-inflammatory activity.

Salmeterol: Relaxes bronchial smooth muscle by selective action on $beta_2$-receptors with little effect on heart rate

Contraindications Hypersensitivity to fluticasone, salmeterol, or any component of the formulation; status asthmaticus; acute episodes of asthma or COPD; severe hypersensitivity to milk proteins (Advair Diskus®)

Warnings/Precautions See individual agents.

Drug Interactions

Metabolism/Transport Effects Fluticasone: **Substrate** of CYP3A4 (major); Salmeterol: **Substrate** of CYP3A4 (major)

Avoid Concomitant Use

Avoid concomitant use of Fluticasone and Salmeterol with any of the following: Aldesleukin; BCG; CYP3A4 Inhibitors (Strong); Iobenguane I 123; Natalizumab; Pimecrolimus; Roflumilast; Tacrolimus (Topical)

Increased Effect/Toxicity

Fluticasone and Salmeterol may increase the levels/effects of: Amphotericin B; Deferasirox; Leflunomide; Loop Diuretics; Natalizumab; Sympathomimetics; Thiazide Diuretics

The levels/effects of Fluticasone and Salmeterol may be increased by: Atomoxetine; Cannabinoids; CYP3A4 Inhibitors (Moderate); CYP3A4 Inhibitors (Strong); Dasatinib; Denosumab; MAO Inhibitors; Pimecrolimus; Roflumilast; Tacrolimus (Topical); Trastuzumab; Tricyclic Antidepressants

Decreased Effect

Fluticasone and Salmeterol may decrease the levels/effects of: Aldesleukin; Antidiabetic Agents; BCG; Corticorelin; Iobenguane I 123; Sipuleucel-T; Vaccines (Inactivated)

The levels/effects of Fluticasone and Salmeterol may be decreased by: Alpha-/Beta-Blockers; Beta-Blockers (Beta1 Selective); Beta-Blockers (Nonselective); Betahistine; Echinacea; Tocilizumab

Dietary Considerations Advair Diskus® powder for oral inhalation contains lactose; very rare anaphylactic reactions have been reported in patients with severe milk protein allergy.

Pregnancy Risk Factor C

Lactation

Fluticasone: Excretion in breast milk unknown/use caution

Salmeterol: Enters breast milk/use caution

Dosage Forms

Aerosol, for oral inhalation:

Advair® HFA:

45/21: Fluticasone propionate 45 mcg and salmeterol 21 mcg (8 g, 12 g) [chlorofluorocarbon free]

115/21: Fluticasone propionate 115 mcg and salmeterol 21 mcg (8 g, 12 g) [chlorofluorocarbon free]

230/21: Fluticasone propionate 230 mcg and salmeterol 21 mcg (8 g, 12 g) [chlorofluorocarbon free]

Powder, for oral inhalation:

Advair Diskus®:

100/50: Fluticasone propionate 100 mcg and salmeterol 50 mcg (14s, 60s)

250/50: Fluticasone propionate 250 mcg and salmeterol 50 mcg (60s)

500/50: Fluticasone propionate 500 mcg and salmeterol 50 mcg (60s)

Dosage Forms: Canada

Aerosol, for oral inhalation:

Advair®: 125/25: Fluticasone propionate 125 mcg and salmeterol 25 mcg (12 g); 250/25: Fluticasone propionate 250 mcg and salmeterol 25 mcg (12 g)

Fluvastatin (FLOO va sta tin)

Related Information

Cardiovascular Diseases *on page* 1848

U.S. Brand Names Lescol®; Lescol® XL

Canadian Brand Names Lescol®; Lescol® XL

Pharmacologic Category Antilipemic Agent, HMG-CoA Reductase Inhibitor

Use To be used as a component of multiple risk factor intervention in patients at risk for atherosclerosis vascular disease due to hypercholesterolemia

Adjunct to dietary therapy to reduce elevated total cholesterol (total-C), LDL-C, triglyceride, and apolipoprotein B (apo-B) levels and to increase HDL-C in primary hypercholesterolemia and mixed dyslipidemia (Fredrickson types IIa and IIb); to slow the progression of coronary atherosclerosis in patients with coronary heart disease; reduce risk of coronary revascularization procedures in patients with coronary heart disease

Local Anesthetic/Vasoconstrictor Precautions No information available to require special precautions

Effects on Dental Treatment No significant effects or complications reported

Effects on Bleeding No information available to require special precautions

Adverse Effects As reported with fluvastatin capsules; in general, adverse reactions reported with fluvastatin extended release tablet were similar, but the incidence was less.

1% to 10%:

Central nervous system: Headache (9%), fatigue (3%), insomnia (3%)

Gastrointestinal: Dyspepsia (8%), diarrhea (5%), abdominal pain (5%), nausea (3%)

Genitourinary: Urinary tract infection (2%)

Neuromuscular & skeletal: Myalgia (5%)

Respiratory: Sinusitis (3%), bronchitis (2%)

General Dosage Range Oral:
Extended release: *Children 10-16 years (females 1 year postmenarche) and Adults:* 80 mg once daily
Immediate release:
Adolescents 10-16 years (females 1 year postmenarche): Initial: 20 mg once daily; Maintenance: Up to 80 mg/day in 2 divided doses
Adults: Initial: 20-40 mg once daily; Maintenance: Up to 80 mg/day in 2 divided doses

Mechanism of Action Acts by competitively inhibiting 3-hydroxyl-3-methylglutaryl-coenzyme A (HMG-CoA) reductase, the enzyme that catalyzes the reduction of HMG-CoA to mevalonate; this is an early rate-limiting step in cholesterol biosynthesis. HDL is increased while total, LDL, and VLDL cholesterols; apolipoprotein B; and plasma triglycerides are decreased.

Pharmacodynamics/Kinetics
Onset of Action Peak effect: Maximal LDL-C reductions achieved within 4 weeks
Half-life Elimination Capsule: <3 hours; Extended release tablet: 9 hours
Time to Peak Capsule: 1 hour; Extended release tablet: 3 hours

Pregnancy Risk Factor X

FluvoxaMINE (floo VOKS a meen)

Related Information
Management of the Patient With Anxiety or Depression *on page* 1968

U.S. Brand Names Luvox® CR

Canadian Brand Names Alti-Fluvoxamine; Apo-Fluvoxamine®; Luvox®; Novo-Fluvoxamine; Nu-Fluvoxamine; PMS-Fluvoxamine; Rhoxal-fluvoxamine; Riva-Fluvox; Sandoz-Fluvoxamine

Generic Availability (U.S.) Yes: Excludes extended release capsule

Pharmacologic Category Antidepressant, Selective Serotonin Reuptake Inhibitor

Use Treatment of obsessive-compulsive disorder (OCD); treatment of social anxiety disorder

Unlabeled/Investigational Use Treatment of major depression; panic disorder; anxiety disorders in children; treatment of mild dementia-associated agitation in nonpsychotic patients; post-traumatic stress disorder (PTSD)

Local Anesthetic/Vasoconstrictor Precautions Although caution should be used in patients taking tricyclic antidepressants, no interactions have been reported with vasoconstrictors and fluvoxamine, a nontricyclic antidepressant which acts to increase serotonin; no precautions appear to be needed

Effects on Dental Treatment Key adverse event(s) related to dental treatment: Xerostomia (normal salivary flow resumes upon discontinuation) and abnormal taste. Problems with SSRI-induced bruxism have been reported and may preclude their use; clinicians attempting to evaluate any patient with bruxism or involuntary muscle movement, who is simultaneously being treated with an SSRI drug, should be aware of the potential association. See Effects on Bleeding and Dental Comment.

Effects on Bleeding May impair platelet aggregation resulting in increased risk of bleeding events, particularly if used concomitantly with aspirin, NSAIDs, warfarin, or other anticoagulants. Bleeding related to SSRI use has been reported to range from relatively minor bruising and epistaxis to life-threatening hemorrhage. Routine interruption of therapy for most dental procedures is not warranted. In medically complicated patients or extensive oral surgery, the decision to interrupt therapy must be based on the risk to benefit in an individual patient and a medical consult is suggested. If therapy is continued without interruption, the clinician should anticipate the potential for a prolonged bleeding time.

Adverse Effects Frequency varies by dosage form and indication. Adverse reactions reported as a composite of all indications.

>10%:
Central nervous system: Headache (22% to 35%), insomnia (21% to 35%), somnolence (22% to 27%), dizziness (11% to 15%), nervousness (10% to 12%)
Gastrointestinal: Nausea (34% to 40%), diarrhea (11% to 18%), xerostomia (10% to 14%), anorexia (6% to 14%)
Genitourinary: Ejaculation abnormal (8% to 11%)
Neuromuscular & skeletal: Weakness (14% to 26%)

1% to 10%:
Cardiovascular: Chest pain (3%), palpitation (3%), vasodilation (2% to 3%), hypertension (1% to 2%), edema (≤1%), hypotension (≤1%), syncope (≤1%), tachycardia (≤1%)
Central nervous system: Pain (10%), anxiety (5% to 8%), abnormal dreams (3%), abnormal thinking (3%), agitation (2% to 3%), apathy (≥1% to 3%), chills (2%), CNS stimulation (2%), depression (2%), neurosis (2%), amnesia, malaise, manic reaction, psychotic reaction

Dermatologic: Bruising (4%), acne (2%)
Endocrine & metabolic: Libido decreased (2% to 10%; incidence higher in males), anorgasmia (2% to 5%), sexual function abnormal (2% to 4%), menorrhagia (3%)
Gastrointestinal: Dyspepsia (8% to 10%), constipation (4% to 10%), vomiting (4% to 6%), abdominal pain (5%), flatulence (4%), taste perversion (2% to 3%), tooth disorder (2% to 3%), dysphagia (2%), gingivitis (2%), weight loss (≤1% to 2%), weight gain
Genitourinary: Polyuria (2% to 3%), impotence (2%), urinary tract infection (2%), urinary retention (1%)
Hepatic: Liver function tests abnormal (≥1% to 2%)
Neuromuscular & skeletal: Tremor (5% to 8%), myalgia (5%), paresthesia (3%), hypertonia (2%), twitching (2%), hyper-/hypokinesia, myoclonus
Ocular: Amblyopia (2% to 3%)
Respiratory: Upper respiratory infection (9%), pharyngitis (6%), yawn (2% to 5%), laryngitis (3%), bronchitis (2%), dyspnea (2%), epistaxis (2%), cough increased, sinusitis
Miscellaneous: Diaphoresis (6% to 7%), flu-like syndrome (3%), viral infection (2%)

Dosage Oral:

Obsessive-compulsive disorder:

Children 8-17 years: Immediate release: Initial: 25 mg once daily at bedtime; may be increased in 25 mg increments at 4- to 7-day intervals, as tolerated, to maximum therapeutic benefit; usual dose range: 50-200 mg/day. **Note:** When total daily dose exceeds 50 mg, the dose should be given in 2 divided doses with larger portion administered at bedtime.

Maximum: Children: 8-11 years: 200 mg/day, adolescents: 300 mg/day; lower doses may be effective in female versus male patients

Adults:

Immediate release: Initial: 50 mg once daily at bedtime; may be increased in 50 mg increments at 4- to 7-day intervals, as tolerated; usual dose range: 100-300 mg/day; maximum dose: 300 mg/day. **Note:** When total daily dose exceeds 100 mg, the dose should be given in 2 divided doses with larger portion administered at bedtime.

Extended release: Initial: 100 mg once daily at bedtime; may be increased in 50 mg increments at intervals of at least 1 week; usual dosage range: 100-300 mg/day; maximum dose: 300 mg/day

Social anxiety disorder: Adults: Extended release: Initial: 100 mg once daily at bedtime; may be increased in 50 mg increments at intervals of at least 1 week; usual dosage range: 100-300 mg/day; maximum dose: 300 mg/day

Post-traumatic stress disorder (PTSD) (unlabeled use): Adults: Immediate release: 75 mg twice daily

Elderly: Reduce dose, titrate slowly

Dosage adjustment in hepatic impairment: Reduce dose, titrate slowly

Mechanism of Action Inhibits CNS neuron serotonin uptake; minimal or no effect on reuptake of norepinephrine or dopamine; does not significantly bind to alpha-adrenergic, histamine or cholinergic receptors

Contraindications Hypersensitivity to fluvoxamine or any component of the formulation; concurrent use with alosetron, pimozide, thioridazine, or tizanidine; use with or within 14 days of MAO inhibitors

Warnings/Precautions [U.S. Boxed Warning]: Antidepressants increase the risk of suicidal thinking and behavior in children, adolescents, and young adults (18-24 years of age) with major depressive disorder (MDD) and other psychiatric disorders; consider risk prior to prescribing. Short-term studies did not show an increased risk in patients >24 years of age and showed a decreased risk in patients ≥65 years. Closely monitor patients for clinical worsening, suicidality, or unusual changes in behavior, particularly during the initial 1-2 months of therapy or during periods of dosage adjustments (increases or decreases); the patient's family or caregiver should be instructed to closely observe the patient and communicate condition with healthcare provider. A medication guide concerning the use of antidepressants should be dispensed with each prescription. **Fluvoxamine is FDA approved for the treatment of OCD in children ≥8 years of age; extended release capsules are not FDA approved for use in children.**

The possibility of a suicide attempt is inherent in major depression and may persist until remission occurs. Use caution in high-risk patients. Worsening depression and severe abrupt suicidality that are not part of the presenting symptoms may require discontinuation or modification of drug therapy. The patient's family or caregiver should be alerted to monitor patients for the emergence of suicidality and associated behaviors (such as agitation, irritability, hostility, impulsivity, and hypomania) and call healthcare provider.

May worsen psychosis in some patients or precipitate a shift to mania or hypomania in patients with bipolar disorder. Patients presenting with depressive symptoms should be screened for bipolar disorder. Monotherapy in patients with bipolar disorder should be avoided. **Fluvoxamine is not FDA approved for the treatment of bipolar depression.**

Serotonin syndrome and neuroleptic malignant syndrome (NMS)-like reactions have occurred with serotonin/norepinephrine reuptake inhibitors (SNRIs) and selective serotonin reuptake inhibitors (SSRIs) when used alone, and particularly when used in combination with serotonergic agents (eg, triptans) or antidopaminergic agents (eg, antipsychotics). Concurrent use with MAO inhibitors is contraindicated. Fluvoxamine has a low potential to impair cognitive or motor performance; caution operating hazardous machinery or driving. Use caution in patients with a previous seizure disorder or condition predisposing to seizures such as brain damage, alcoholism, or concurrent therapy with other drugs which lower the seizure threshold. Fluvoxamine may significantly increase alosetron concentrations; concurrent use **contraindicated.** Potential for QT_c prolongation and arrhythmia with thioridazine and pimozide; concurrent use of fluvoxamine with either of these agents is **contraindicated.** Concomitant use with tizanidine may cause a significant decrease in blood pressure and increase in drowsiness; concurrent use is **contraindicated.** Fluvoxamine levels may be lower in patients who smoke.

May increase the risks associated with electroconvulsive therapy. Use with caution in patients with hepatic dysfunction and in elderly patients. May cause hyponatremia/SIADH (elderly at increased risk); volume depletion (diuretics may increase risk). Use with caution in patients at risk of bleeding or receiving concurrent anticoagulant therapy, although not consistently noted, fluvoxamine may cause impairment in platelet function. May cause or exacerbate sexual dysfunction.

Drug Interactions

Metabolism/Transport Effects Substrate (major) of CYP1A2, 2D6; **Inhibits** CYP1A2 (strong), 2B6 (weak), 2C9 (weak), 2C19 (strong), 2D6 (weak), 3A4 (weak)

Avoid Concomitant Use

Avoid concomitant use of FluvoxaMINE with any of the following: Alosetron; Clopidogrel; Iobenguane I 123; MAO Inhibitors; Methylene Blue; Pimozide; Ramelteon; Sibutramine; Thioridazine; TiZANidine; Tryptophan

Increased Effect/Toxicity

FluvoxaMINE may increase the levels/effects of: Alcohol (Ethyl); Alosetron; Anticoagulants; Antidepressants (Serotonin Reuptake Inhibitor/Antagonist); Antiplatelet Agents; Asenapine; Aspirin; Bendamustine; Benzodiazepines (metabolized by oxidation); Bromazepam; BusPIRone; CarBAMazepine; CloZAPine; CNS Depressants; Collagenase (Systemic); CYP1A2 Substrates; CYP2C19 Substrates; Desmopressin; Drotrecogin Alfa; DULoxetine; Erlotinib; Fosphenytoin; Haloperidol; Ibritumomab; Lithium; Methadone; Methotrimeprazine; Methylene Blue; Mexiletine; NSAID (COX-2 Inhibitor); NSAID (Nonselective); OLANZapine; Phenytoin; Pimozide; Propafenone; Propranolol; QuiNIDine; Ramelteon; Roflumilast; Ropivacaine; Salicylates; Serotonin Modulators; Theophylline Derivatives; Thioridazine; Thrombolytic Agents; TiZANidine; Tositumomab and Iodine I 131 Tositumomab; TraMADol; Tricyclic Antidepressants; Vitamin K Antagonists

The levels/effects of FluvoxaMINE may be increased by: Abiraterone; Analgesics (Opioid); BusPIRone; Cimetidine; CYP1A2 Inhibitors (Moderate); CYP1A2 Inhibitors (Strong); CYP2D6 Inhibitors (Moderate); CYP2D6 Inhibitors (Strong); Darunavir; Dasatinib; Deferasirox; Droperidol; Glucosamine; Herbs (Anticoagulant/Antiplatelet Properties); MAO Inhibitors; Methotrimeprazine; Metoclopramide; Omega-3-Acid Ethyl Esters; Pentosan Polysulfate Sodium; Pentoxifylline; Prostacyclin Analogues; Sibutramine; TraMADol; Tryptophan

Decreased Effect

FluvoxaMINE may decrease the levels/effects of: Clopidogrel; Iobenguane I 123

The levels/effects of FluvoxaMINE may be decreased by: CarBAMazepine; CYP1A2 Inducers (Strong); Cyproheptadine; Peginterferon Alfa-2b

Ethanol/Nutrition/Herb Interactions

Ethanol: May increase CNS depression; monitor for increased effects with coadministration. Caution patients about effects.

Food: The bioavailability of melatonin has been reported to be increased by fluvoxamine.

Herb/Nutraceutical: Avoid valerian, St John's wort, SAMe, kava kava (may increase risk of serotonin syndrome and/or excessive sedation). Avoid alfalfa, anise, bilberry, bladderwrack, bromelain, cat's claw, celery, chamomile, coleus, cordyceps, dong quai, evening primrose, fenugreek, feverfew, garlic, ginger, ginkgo biloba, ginseng (American), ginseng (Panax), ginseng (Siberian), grape seed, green tea, guggul, horse chestnuts, horseradish, licorice, prickly ash, red clover, reishi, SAMe (S-adenosylmethionine), sweet clover, turmeric, white willow (all have additional antiplatelet activity).

Dietary Considerations May be taken with or without food.

Pharmacodynamics/Kinetics

Onset of Action Depression: The onset of action is within a week; however, individual response varies greatly and full response may not be seen until 8-12 weeks after initiation of treatment.

Half-life Elimination 15-16 hours; 17-26 hours in the elderly

Time to Peak Plasma: 3-8 hours

Pregnancy Risk Factor C

Lactation Enters breast milk/consider risk:benefit (AAP rates "of concern"; AAP 2001 update pending)

Breast-Feeding Considerations Fluvoxamine is excreted in breast milk. Based on case reports, the dose the infant receives is relatively small and adverse events have not been observed. According to the manufacturer, the decision to continue or discontinue breast-feeding during therapy should take into account the risk of exposure to the infant and the benefits of treatment to the mother.

The long-term effects on development and behavior have not been studied; therefore, fluvoxamine should be prescribed to a mother who is breast-feeding only when the benefits outweigh the potential risks.

Dosage Forms

Capsule, extended release, oral:

Luvox® CR: 100 mg, 150 mg

Tablet, oral: 25 mg, 50 mg, 100 mg

Dental Comment Problems with SSRI-induced bruxism have been reported and may preclude their use. Clinicians attempting to evaluate any patient with bruxism or involuntary muscle movement, who is simultaneously being treated with an SSRI drug, should be aware of the potential association.

References

Friedlander AH and Mahler ME, "Major Depressive Disorder. Psychopathology, Medical Management, and Dental Implications," *J Am Dent Assoc*, 2001, 132(5):629-38.

Gerber PE and Lynd LD, "Selective Serotonin Reuptake Inhibitor-induced Movement Disorders," *Ann Pharmacother*, 1998, 32(6):692-8.

Wynn RL, "New Antidepressant Medications," *Gen Dent*, 1997, 45(1):24-8.

Folic Acid (FOE lik AS id)

U.S. Brand Names Folacin-800 [OTC]

Canadian Brand Names Apo-Folic®

Generic Availability (U.S.) Yes

Pharmacologic Category Vitamin, Water Soluble

Use Treatment of megaloblastic and macrocytic anemias due to folate deficiency; dietary supplement to prevent neural tube defects

Unlabeled/Investigational Use Adjunctive cofactor therapy in methanol toxicity (alternative to leucovorin calcium)

Local Anesthetic/Vasoconstrictor Precautions No information available to require special precautions

Effects on Dental Treatment No significant effects or complications reported

Effects on Bleeding No information available to require special precautions

Adverse Effects Frequency not defined.

Allergic reaction, bronchospasm, erythema, flushing (slight), malaise (general), pruritus, rash

Dosage

Oral, I.M., I.V., SubQ: Anemia:

- Infants: 0.1 mg/day
- Children <4 years: Up to 0.3 mg/day
- Children >4 years and Adults: 0.4 mg/day
- Pregnant and lactating women: 0.8 mg/day

Oral:

RDA: Expressed as dietary folate equivalents:

Children:

- 1-3 years: 150 mcg/day
- 4-8 years: 200 mcg/day
- 9-13 years: 300 mcg/day

Children ≥14 years and Adults: 400 mcg/day

Elderly: Vitamin B_{12} deficiency must be ruled out before initiating folate therapy due to frequency of combined nutritional deficiencies: RDA requirements (1999): 400 mcg/day (0.4 mg) minimum

Prevention of neural tube defects:

Females of childbearing potential: 400-800 mcg/day (USPSTF)

Females at high risk or with family history of neural tube defects: 4 mg/day

Mechanism of Action Folic acid is necessary for formation of a number of coenzymes in many metabolic systems, particularly for purine and pyrimidine synthesis; required for nucleoprotein synthesis and maintenance in erythropoiesis; stimulates WBC and platelet production in folate deficiency anemia. Folic acid enhances the elimination of formic acid, the toxic metabolite of methanol (unlabeled use).

Contraindications Hypersensitivity to folic acid or any component of the formulation

Warnings/Precautions Not appropriate for monotherapy with pernicious, aplastic, or normocytic anemias when anemia is present with vitamin B_{12} deficiency. Doses >0.1 mg/day may obscure pernicious anemia with continuing irreversible nerve damage progression. Resistance to treatment may occur with depressed hematopoiesis, alcoholism, and deficiencies of other vitamins. Injection contains benzyl alcohol (1.5%) as preservative (use care in administration to neonates).

Drug Interactions

Avoid Concomitant Use

Avoid concomitant use of Folic Acid with any of the following: Raltitrexed

Increased Effect/Toxicity There are no known significant interactions involving an increase in effect.

Decreased Effect

Folic Acid may decrease the levels/effects of: Fosphenytoin; PHENobarbital; Phenytoin; Primidone; Raltitrexed

The levels/effects of Folic Acid may be decreased by: Green Tea

Dietary Considerations As of January 1998, the FDA has required manufacturers of enriched flour, bread, corn meal, pasta, rice, and other grain products to add folic acid to their products. The intent is to help decrease the risk of neural tube defects by increasing folic acid intake. Other foods which contain folic acid include dark green leafy vegetables, citrus fruits and juices, and lentils.

Pharmacodynamics/Kinetics

Onset of Action Peak effect: Oral: 0.5-1 hour

Pregnancy Risk Factor A

Lactation Enters breast milk/compatible

Dosage Forms

Injection, solution: 5 mg/mL (10 mL)

Tablet, oral: 0.4 mg, 0.8 mg, 1 mg

Folacin-800 [OTC]: 0.8 mg

Folic Acid, Cyanocobalamin, and Pyridoxine

(FOE lik AS id, sye an oh koe BAL a min, & peer i DOKS een)

Related Information

Cyanocobalamin *on page 444*
Folic Acid *on page 777*
Pyridoxine *on page 1436*

U.S. Brand Names FaBB; Folbee; Folbic; Folcaps™; Folgard RX®; Folgard® [OTC]; Foltabs™ 800 [OTC]; Foltx®; Homocysteine Guard [OTC]; Lev-Tov [OTC]; Tri-B® [OTC]; Tricardio B; Vita-Respa®

Pharmacologic Category Vitamin

Use Nutritional supplement in end-stage renal failure, dialysis, hyperhomocysteinemia, homocystinuria, malabsorption syndromes, dietary deficiencies

Local Anesthetic/Vasoconstrictor Precautions No information available to require special precautions

Effects on Dental Treatment No significant effects or complications reported

Effects on Bleeding No information available to require special precautions

Adverse Effects See individual agents.

General Dosage Range Oral: *Adults:* 1 tablet (folic acid 0.4-2.5 mg/cyanocobalamin 115-2000 mcg/pyridoxine 10-25 mg) daily

Follitropin Alfa (foe li TRO pin AL fa)

U.S. Brand Names Gonal-f®; Gonal-f® RFF; Gonal-f® RFF Pen

Canadian Brand Names Gonal-f®; Gonal-f® Pen

Pharmacologic Category Gonadotropin; Ovulation Stimulator

Use

Gonal-f®: Ovulation induction in patients in whom the cause of infertility is functional and not caused by primary ovarian failure; development of multiple follicles with Assisted Reproductive Technology (ART); spermatogenesis induction

Gonal-f® RFF: Ovulation induction in patients in whom the cause of infertility is functional and not caused by primary ovarian failure; development of multiple follicles with ART

Local Anesthetic/Vasoconstrictor Precautions No information available to require special precautions

Effects on Dental Treatment Key adverse event(s) related to dental treatment: Stomatitis and toothache.

Effects on Bleeding No information available to require special precautions

Adverse Effects Percentage may vary by indication, product formulation

>10%:

Central nervous system: Headache
Endocrine & metabolic: Ovarian cyst
Gastrointestinal: Abdomen enlarged, abdominal pain, nausea
Miscellaneous: Upper respiratory infection

1% to 10%:

Central nervous system: Dizziness, emotional lability, fever, malaise, migraine, pain
Dermatologic: Acne
Endocrine & metabolic: Breast pain, cervix lesion, hot flashes, intermenstrual bleeding, menstrual disorder, ovarian disorder, ovarian hyperstimulation
Gastrointestinal: Constipation, diarrhea, dyspepsia, flatulence, pelvic pain, stomatitis (ulcerative), toothache, vomiting, weight gain
Genitourinary: Cystitis, leukorrhea, micturition frequency, urinary tract infection, uterine hemorrhage, vaginal hemorrhage
Local: Injection site bruising, edema, inflammation, pain, reaction
Neuromuscular & skeletal: Back pain
Respiratory: Cough, flu-like symptoms, pharyngitis, rhinitis, sinusitis
Miscellaneous: Infection, moniliasis

General Dosage Range SubQ:

Adults (females): Initial: 75-225 int. units once daily for 5-7 days; Maintenance: Up to 300-450 int. units/day

Adults (males): Gonal-f®: Initial: 150 int. units 3 times/week; Maintenance: Up to 300 int. units 3 times/week (maximum: 18 months of therapy)

Mechanism of Action Follitropin alfa is a human FSH preparation of recombinant DNA origin. Follitropins stimulate ovarian follicular growth in women who do not have primary ovarian failure, and stimulate spermatogenesis in men with hypogonadotrophic hypogonadism. FSH is required for normal follicular growth, maturation, gonadal steroid production, and spermatogenesis.

Pharmacodynamics/Kinetics

Onset of Action Peak effect:

Spermatogenesis, median: 6.8-12.4 months (range: 2.7-15.7 months)
Follicle development: Within cycle

Half-life Elimination

I.M.: 50 hours in healthy female volunteers
SubQ: 24 hours in healthy female volunteers; 32 hours with *in vitro* fertilization/embryo transfer patients; 32-41 hours in healthy male volunteers

Time to Peak In healthy volunteers:

Females: SubQ: 8-16 hours; I.M.: 25 hours
Males: SubQ: 11-20 hours

Pregnancy Risk Factor X

Follitropin Beta (foe li TRO pin BAY ta)

U.S. Brand Names Follistim® AQ; Follistim® AQ Cartridge

Canadian Brand Names Puregon®

Pharmacologic Category Gonadotropin; Ovulation Stimulator

Use Ovulation induction in patients in whom the cause of infertility is functional and not caused by primary ovarian failure; development of multiple follicles with Assisted Reproductive Technology (ART)

Local Anesthetic/Vasoconstrictor Precautions No information available to require special precautions

Effects on Dental Treatment No significant effects or complications reported

Effects on Bleeding No information available to require special precautions

Adverse Effects Percentage may vary by indication, product formulation

>10%:

Endocrine & metabolic: Breast pain
Gastrointestinal: Abdominal pain, flatulence, nausea
Miscellaneous: Miscarriage

1% to 10%:
- Central nervous system: Headache
- Endocrine & metabolic: Ovarian hyperstimulation syndrome, ovarian pain
- Gastrointestinal: Abdomen enlarged, constipation
- Local: Injection site reaction
- Neuromuscular & skeletal: Back pain
- Respiratory: Sinusitis, upper respiratory tract infection

General Dosage Range I.M., SubQ: *Adults (females):* Initial: 75-225 int. units/day; Maintenance: Up to 175-600 int. units/day

Mechanism of Action Follitropin beta is a human FSH preparation of recombinant DNA origin. Follitropins stimulate ovarian follicular growth in women who do not have primary ovarian failure. FSH is required for normal follicular growth, maturation, gonadal steroid production, and spermatogenesis.

Pharmacodynamics/Kinetics

Onset of Action Peak effect: Follicle development: Within cycle

Half-life Elimination I.M.: 44 hours (single dose), 27-30 hours (multiple doses); SubQ: 33 hours (single dose)

Time to Peak SubQ: 13 hours

Pregnancy Risk Factor X

Fomepizole (foe ME pi zole)

U.S. Brand Names Antizol®

Pharmacologic Category Antidote

Use Treatment of methanol or ethylene glycol poisoning alone or in combination with hemodialysis

Unlabeled/Investigational Use Pediatric administration; treatment of propylene glycol toxicity

Local Anesthetic/Vasoconstrictor Precautions No information available to require special precautions

Effects on Dental Treatment Key adverse event(s) related to dental treatment: Bad/metallic taste.

Effects on Bleeding No information available to require special precautions

Adverse Effects

>10%:
- Central nervous system: Headache (14%)
- Gastrointestinal: Nausea (11%)

1% to 10% (≤3% unless otherwise noted):
- Cardiovascular: Bradycardia, facial flush, hypotension, shock, tachycardia
- Central nervous system: Dizziness (6%), drowsiness increased (6%), agitation, anxiety, fever, lightheadedness, seizure, vertigo
- Dermatologic: Rash
- Gastrointestinal: Bad/metallic taste (6%), abdominal pain, appetite decreased, diarrhea, heartburn, vomiting
- Hematologic: Anemia, disseminated intravascular coagulation (DIC), eosinophilia, lymphangitis
- Hepatic: Liver function tests increased
- Local: Application site reaction, injection site inflammation, pain during injection, phlebitis
- Neuromuscular & skeletal: Backache
- Ocular: Nystagmus, transient blurred vision, visual disturbances
- Renal: Anuria
- Respiratory: Abnormal smell, hiccups, pharyngitis
- Miscellaneous: Multiorgan failure, speech disturbances

General Dosage Range Dosage adjustment recommended in patients with renal impairment

I.V.: *Adults:* Loading dose of 15 mg/kg, followed by 10 mg/kg every 12 hours for 4 doses, then 15 mg/kg every 12 hours

Mechanism of Action Fomepizole competitively inhibits alcohol dehydrogenase, an enzyme which catalyzes the metabolism of ethanol, ethylene glycol, and methanol to their toxic metabolites. Ethylene glycol is metabolized to glycoaldehyde, then oxidized to glycolate, glyoxylate, and oxalate. Glycolate and oxalate are responsible for metabolic acidosis and renal damage. Methanol is metabolized to formaldehyde, then oxidized to formic acid. Formic acid is responsible for metabolic acidosis and visual disturbances.

Pharmacodynamics/Kinetics

Onset of Action Peak effect: Maximum: 1.5-2 hours

Half-life Elimination Has not been calculated; varies with dose

Pregnancy Risk Factor C

Fondaparinux (fon da PARE i nuks)

U.S. Brand Names Arixtra®

Canadian Brand Names Arixtra®

Pharmacologic Category Factor Xa Inhibitor

Use Prophylaxis of deep vein thrombosis (DVT) in patients undergoing surgery for hip replacement, knee replacement, hip fracture (including extended prophylaxis following hip fracture surgery), or abdominal surgery (in patients at risk for thromboembolic complications); treatment of acute pulmonary embolism (PE); treatment of acute DVT without PE

Canadian labeling: Additional uses (not approved in U.S.): Unstable angina or non-ST segment elevation myocardial infarction (UA/NSTEMI) for the prevention of death and subsequent MI; ST segment elevation MI (STEMI) for the prevention of death and myocardial reinfarction

Unlabeled/Investigational Use Prophylaxis of DVT in patients with a history of heparin-induced thrombocytopenia (HIT)

Local Anesthetic/Vasoconstrictor Precautions No information available to require special precautions

Effects on Dental Treatment Key adverse event(s) related to dental treatment: Hemorrhage may occur at any site. See Effects on Bleeding.

Effects on Bleeding As with all anticoagulants, bleeding is the major adverse effect of fondaparinux. Hemorrhage may occur at virtually any site; risk is dependent on multiple variables including the intensity of anticoagulation and patient susceptibility. Risk increased in renal dysfunction, patients >75 years and/or <50 kg; major bleeding increased as high as 5% in patients receiving initial dose <6 hours postsurgery. At the recommended doses, fondaparinux does not significantly influence platelet aggregation or affect global clotting time (ie, PT or aPTT). Medical consult is suggested.

Adverse Effects As with all anticoagulants, bleeding is the major adverse effect. Hemorrhage may occur at any site. Risk appears increased by a number of factors including renal dysfunction, age (>75 years), and weight (<50 kg).

>10%:
- Central nervous system: Fever (4% to 14%)
- Gastrointestinal: Nausea (11%)
- Hematologic: Anemia (20%)

1% to 10%:
- Cardiovascular: Edema (9%), hypotension (4%), thrombosis PCI catheter (without heparin 1%)
- Central nervous system: Insomnia (5%), dizziness (4%), headache (2% to 5%), confusion (3%), pain (2%)
- Dermatologic: Rash (8%), purpura (4%), bullous eruption (3%)
- Endocrine & metabolic: Hypokalemia (1% to 4%)
- Gastrointestinal: Constipation (5% to 9%), nausea (3%), vomiting (6%), diarrhea (3%), dyspepsia (2%)
- Genitourinary: Urinary tract infection (4%), urinary retention (3%)
- Hematologic: Moderate thrombocytopenia (50,000-100,000/mm^3: 3%), major bleeding (1% to 3%), minor bleeding (2% to 4%), hematoma (3%); risk of major bleeding increased as high as 5% in patients receiving initial dose <6 hours following surgery
- Hepatic: ALT increased (≤3%), AST increased (≤2%)
- Local: Injection site reaction (bleeding, rash, pruritus)
- Miscellaneous: Wound drainage increased (5%)

General Dosage Range SubQ:

Adults <50 kg: Treatment: 5 mg once daily

Adults 50-100 kg: Prophylaxis: 2.5 mg once daily; Treatment: 7.5 mg once daily

Adults >100 kg: Prophylaxis: 2.5 mg once daily; Treatment: 10 mg once daily

Mechanism of Action Fondaparinux is a synthetic pentasaccharide that causes an antithrombin III-mediated selective inhibition of factor Xa. Neutralization of factor Xa interrupts the blood coagulation cascade and inhibits thrombin formation and thrombus development.

Pharmacodynamics/Kinetics

Half-life Elimination 17-21 hours; prolonged with renal impairment

Time to Peak SubQ: 2-3 hours

Pregnancy Risk Factor B

Formoterol (for MOH te rol)

U.S. Brand Names Foradil® Aerolizer®; Perforomist™

Canadian Brand Names Foradil®; Oxeze® Turbuhaler®

Pharmacologic Category Beta$_2$-Adrenergic Agonist; Beta$_2$-Adrenergic Agonist, Long-Acting

Use Maintenance treatment of asthma and prevention of bronchospasm (as concomitant therapy) in patients ≥5 years of age with reversible obstructive airway disease, including patients with symptoms of nocturnal asthma; maintenance treatment of bronchoconstriction in patients with COPD; prevention of exercise-induced bronchospasm in patients ≥5 years of age (monotherapy may be indicated in patients without persistent asthma)

Canadian labeling: Oxeze®: Also approved for acute relief of symptoms ("on demand" treatment) in patients ≥6 years of age

Local Anesthetic/Vasoconstrictor Precautions No information available to require special precautions

Effects on Dental Treatment Key adverse event(s) related to dental treatment: Xerostomia (normal salivary flow resumes upon discontinuation).

Effects on Bleeding No information available to require special precautions

Adverse Effects

1% to 10%:

Cardiovascular: Chest pain (2% to 3%), palpitation

Central nervous system: Anxiety (2%), dizziness (2%), fever (2%), insomnia (2%), dysphonia (1%), headache

Dermatologic: Pruritus (2%), rash (1%)

Gastrointestinal: Diarrhea (5%), nausea (5%), xerostomia (1% to 3%), vomiting (2%), abdominal pain, dyspepsia, gastroenteritis

Neuromuscular & skeletal: Muscle cramps (2%), tremor

Respiratory: Infection (3% to 7%), asthma exacerbation (age 5-12 years: 5% to 6%; age >12 years: <4%), bronchitis (5%), pharyngitis (3% to 4%), sinusitis (3%), dyspnea (2%), tonsillitis (1%)

General Dosage Range Inhalation:

Foradil®: *Children ≥5 years and Adults:* 12 mcg capsule inhaled every 12 hours (maximum: 24 mcg/day) **or** 12 mcg capsule inhaled prior to exercise

Perforomist™: *Adults:* 20 mcg twice daily (maximum dose: 40 mcg/day)

Mechanism of Action Relaxes bronchial smooth muscle by selective action on beta$_2$ receptors with little effect on heart rate. Formoterol has a long-acting effect.

Pharmacodynamics/Kinetics

Onset of Action Powder for inhalation: Within 3 minutes

Peak effect: Powder for inhalation: 80% of peak effect within 15 minutes; Solution for nebulization: 2 hours

Duration of Action Improvement in FEV$_1$ observed for 12 hours in most patients

Half-life Elimination Powder: ~10-14 hours; Nebulized solution: ~7 hours

Time to Peak Maximum improvement in FEV$_1$ in 1-3 hours

Pregnancy Risk Factor C

Fosamprenavir (FOS am pren a veer)

Related Information

HIV Infection and AIDS *on page 1883*

U.S. Brand Names Lexiva®

Canadian Brand Names Telzir®

Pharmacologic Category Antiretroviral Agent, Protease Inhibitor

Use Treatment of HIV infections in combination with at least two other antiretroviral agents

Local Anesthetic/Vasoconstrictor Precautions No information available to require special precautions

Effects on Dental Treatment No significant effects or complications reported

Effects on Bleeding Increased bleeding has been noted with protease inhibitors in patients with hemophilia A or B. No information available to require routine special precautions relative to hemostasis in other patients.

Adverse Effects

>10%:

Dermatologic: Rash (≤19%; onset: ~11 days; duration: ~13 days)

Endocrine & metabolic: Hypertriglyceridemia (>750 mg/dL: ≤11%)

Gastrointestinal: Diarrhea (moderate-to-severe; 5% to 13%)

1% to 10%:

Central nervous system: Headache (moderate-to-severe; 2% to 4%), fatigue (moderate-to-severe; 2% to 4%)

Dermatologic: Pruritus (7% to 8%)

Endocrine & metabolic: Hyperglycemia (>251 mg/dL: ≤2%)

Gastrointestinal: Serum lipase increased (>2 times ULN: 5% to 8%), nausea (moderate-to-severe; 3% to 7%), vomiting (moderate-to-severe; 2% to 6%), abdominal pain (moderate-to-severe; ≤2%)
Hematologic: Neutropenia (<750 cells/mm^3: 3%)
Hepatic: Transaminases increased (>5 times ULN: 4% to 8%)
Frequency not defined: Diabetes mellitus, fat redistribution, and immune reconstitution syndrome have been associated with protease inhibitor therapy. Spontaneous bleeding has been reported in patients with hemophilia A or B following treatment with protease inhibitors. Acute hemolytic anemia has been reported in association with amprenavir use.

General Dosage Range Dosage adjustment recommended in patients with hepatic impairment or on concomitant therapy

Oral:

Children 2-5 years: 30 mg/kg/dose twice daily (maximum: 1400 mg twice daily)
Children ≥6 years:
Unboosted regimen: 30 mg/kg/dose twice daily (maximum: 1400 mg twice daily)
Ritonavir-boosted regimen: 18 mg/kg/dose twice daily (maximum: 700 mg twice daily)
Adults:
Unboosted regimen: 1400 mg twice daily
Ritonavir-boosted regimen: 700 mg twice daily **or** 1400 mg once daily

Mechanism of Action Fosamprenavir is rapidly and almost completely converted to amprenavir by cellular phosphatases *in vivo*. Amprenavir binds to the site of HIV-1 protease activity and inhibits cleavage of viral Gag-Pol polyprotein precursors into individual functional proteins required for infectious HIV. This results in the formation of immature, noninfectious viral particles.

Pharmacodynamics/Kinetics

Half-life Elimination ~7.7 hours (amprenavir)

Time to Peak 1.5-4 hours (median: 2.5 hours)

Pregnancy Risk Factor C

Fosaprepitant (fos a PRE pi tant)

U.S. Brand Names Emend® for Injection

Canadian Brand Names Emend® IV

Pharmacologic Category Antiemetic; Substance P/Neurokinin 1 Receptor Antagonist

Use Prevention of acute and delayed nausea and vomiting associated with moderately- and highly-emetogenic chemotherapy (in combination with other antiemetics)

Local Anesthetic/Vasoconstrictor Precautions No information available to require special precautions

Effects on Dental Treatment Key adverse event(s) related to dental treatment: Stomatitis, taste disturbances, xerostomia (normal salivary flow resumes upon discontinuation).

Effects on Bleeding No information available to require special precautions

Adverse Effects Adverse reactions reported with aprepitant and fosaprepitant (as part of a combination chemotherapy regimen) occurring at a higher frequency than standard antiemetic therapy:

1% to 10%:
Central nervous system: Fatigue (1% to 3%), headache (2%)
Gastrointestinal: Anorexia (2%), constipation 2%), dyspepsia (2%), diarrhea (1%), eructation (1%)
Hepatic: ALT increased (1% to 3%), AST increased (1%)
Local: Injection site reactions (3%; includes erythema, induration, pain, pruritus, or thrombophlebitis)
Neuromuscular & skeletal: Weakness (3%)
Miscellaneous: Hiccups (5%)

General Dosage Range I.V.: *Adults:* 115 or 150 mg as a single dose

Mechanism of Action Fosaprepitant is a prodrug of aprepitant, a substance P/neurokinin 1 (NK1) receptor antagonist. It is rapidly converted to aprepitant which prevents acute and delayed vomiting by inhibiting the substance P/neurokinin 1 (NK1) receptor; augments the antiemetic activity of the 5-HT$_3$ receptor antagonist and corticosteroid activity and inhibits chemotherapy-induced emesis.

Pharmacodynamics/Kinetics

Half-life Elimination
Half-life elimination: Fosaprepitant: ~2 minutes; Aprepitant: ~9-13 hours

Time to Peak Fosaprepitant is converted to aprepitant within 30 minutes after the end of infusion

Pregnancy Risk Factor B

Foscarnet (fos KAR net)

Related Information

Systemic Viral Diseases *on page 1904*

Canadian Brand Names Foscavir®

Generic Availability (U.S.) Yes

Pharmacologic Category Antiviral Agent

Dental Use Treatment of acyclovir-resistant mucocutaneous herpes simplex virus (HSV) infections in immunocompromised persons (eg, with advanced AIDS); treatment of CMV retinitis in persons with HIV

Use Treatment of acyclovir-resistant mucocutaneous herpes simplex virus (HSV) infections in immunocompromised persons (eg, with advanced AIDS); treatment of CMV retinitis in persons with HIV

Unlabeled/Investigational Use Other CMV infections (eg, colitis, esophagitis, neurological disease); CMV prophylaxis for cancer patients receiving alemtuzumab therapy or allogeneic stem cell transplant

Local Anesthetic/Vasoconstrictor Precautions Foscarnet is one of the drugs confirmed to prolong the QT interval and is accepted as having a risk of causing torsade de pointes. In terms of epinephrine, it is not known what effect vasoconstrictors in the local anesthetic regimen will have in patients with a known history of congenital prolonged QT interval or in patients taking any medication that prolongs the QT interval. Until more information is obtained, it is suggested that the clinician consult with the physician prior to the use of a vasoconstrictor in suspected patients, and that the vasoconstrictor (epinephrine, mepivacaine and levonordefrin [Carbocaine® 2% with Neo-Cobefrin®]) be used with caution. See Dental Comment.

Effects on Dental Treatment Key adverse event(s) related to dental treatment: Xerostomia (normal salivary flow resumes upon discontinuation), taste perversion, and ulcerative stomatitis.

Effects on Bleeding No information available to require special precautions

Adverse Effects

>10%:

- Central nervous system: Fever (65%), headache (26%)
- Endocrine & metabolic: Hypokalemia (16% to 48%), hypocalcemia (15% to 30%), hypomagnesemia (15% to 30%), hypophosphatemia (8% to 26%)
- Gastrointestinal: Nausea (47%), diarrhea (30%), vomiting (26%)
- Hematologic: Anemia (33%), granulocytopenia (17%)
- Renal: Abnormal renal function/decreased creatinine clearance (12%; without adequate hydration: 33%)

1% to 10%:

- Cardiovascular: Chest pain (1% to 5%), edema (1% to 5%), facial edema (1% to 5%), flushing (1% to 5%), hyper-/hypotension (1% to 5%), palpitation (1% to 5%), ECG changes (1% to 5%)
- Central nervous system: Seizure (includes grand mal; 8%), anxiety (≥5%), confusion (≥5%), depression (≥5%), dizziness (≥5%), fatigue (≥5%), hypoesthesia (≥5%), malaise (≥5%), pain (≥5%), aggressiveness (1% to 5%), agitation (1% to 5%), amnesia (1% to 5%), aphasia (1% to 5%), ataxia (1% to 5%), coordination abnormal (1% to 5%), dementia (1% to 5%), EEG abnormal (1% to 5%), hallucination (1% to 5%), insomnia (1% to 5%), meningitis (1% to 5%), nervousness (1% to 5%), somnolence (1% to 5%), stupor (1% to 5%)
- Dermatologic: Rash (≥5%), erythematous rash (1% to 5%), maculopapular rash (1% to 5%), pruritus (1% to 5%), seborrhea (1% to 5%), skin discoloration (1% to 5%), skin ulceration (1% to 5%)
- Endocrine & metabolic: Hyperphosphatemia (6%), acidosis (1% to 5%), hyponatremia (1% to 5%)
- Gastrointestinal: Abdominal pain (≥5%), anorexia (≥5%), constipation (1% to 5%), dyspepsia (1% to 5%), dysphasia (1% to 5%), flatulence (1% to 5%), melena (1% to 5%), pancreatitis (1% to 5%), rectal hemorrhage (1% to 5%), taste perversion (1% to 5%), ulcerative stomatitis (1% to 5%), weight loss (1% to 5%), xerostomia (1% to 5%)
- Genitourinary: Dysuria (1% to 5%), nocturia (1% to 5%), urinary retention (1% to 5%)
- Hematologic: Leukopenia (≥5%), lymphadenopathy (1% to 5%), thrombocytopenia (1% to 5%), thrombosis (1% to 5%)
- Hepatic: Alkaline phosphatase increased (1% to 5%), ALT increased (1% to 5%), AST increased (1% to 5%), hepatic function abnormal (1% to 5%), LDH increased (1% to 5%)
- Local: Injection site pain/inflammation (1% to 5%)

Neuromuscular & skeletal: Paresthesia (≥5%), involuntary muscle contractions (≥5%), rigors (≥5%), neuropathy (peripheral; ≥5%), weakness (≥5%), arthralgia (1% to 5%), back pain (1% to 5%), leg cramps (1% to 5%), myalgia (1% to 5%), tremor (1% to 5%)

Ocular: Vision abnormalities (≥5%), conjunctivitis (1% to 5%), eye pain (1% to 5%)

Renal: Acute renal failure (1% to 5%), albuminuria (1% to 5%), BUN increased (1% to 5%), polyuria (1% to 5%), urinary tract infection (1% to 5%)

Respiratory: Cough (≥5%), dyspnea (≥5%), bronchospasm (1% to 5%), hemoptysis (1% to 5%), pharyngitis (1% to 5%), pneumonia (1% to 5%), pneumothorax (1% to 5%), rhinitis (1% to 5%), sinusitis (1% to 5%), stridor (1% to 5%)

Miscellaneous: Diaphoresis (≥5%), sepsis (≥5%), infection (includes bacterial and fungal; ≥5%), flu-like syndrome (1% to 5%), malignancies (lymphoma/sarcoma 1% to 5%), thirst (1% to 5%)

Dental Usual Dosage Herpes simplex infections (acyclovir-resistant): Induction: I.V.: 40 mg/kg/dose every 8-12 hours for 14-21 days

Dosage

CMV retinitis: I.V.:

Induction treatment: 60 mg/kg/dose every 8 hours **or** 90 mg/kg every 12 hours for 14-21 days

Maintenance therapy: 90-120 mg/kg/day as a single daily infusion

Herpes simplex infections (acyclovir-resistant): Induction: I.V.: 40 mg/kg/dose every 8-12 hours for 14-21 days

Therapy of CMV infection in cancer patients (unlabeled use): I.V.:

Prophylaxis: 60 mg/kg every 8-12 hours for 7 days, followed by 90-120 mg/kg daily until day 100 after HSCT

Pre-emptive treatment: 60 mg/kg every 12 hours for 14 days; if CMV still detectable, continue with 90 mg/kg daily for 5 days/week for 2 additional weeks

Treatment: 90 mg/kg every 12 hours for 2 weeks, followed by 120 mg/kg daily for ≥2 weeks

Dosage adjustment in renal impairment: Induction and maintenance dosing schedules based on creatinine clearance (mL/minute/kg): See tables.

Induction Dosing of Foscarnet in Patients With Abnormal Renal Function

Cl_{cr} (mL/min/kg)	HSV Equivalent to 40 mg/kg q12h	HSV Equivalent to 40 mg/kg q8h	CMV Equivalent to 60 mg/kg q8h	CMV Equivalent to 90 mg/kg q12h
<0.4	Not recommended	Not recommended	Not recommended	Not recommended
≥0.4-0.5	20 mg/kg every 24 hours	35 mg/kg every 24 hours	50 mg/kg every 24 hours	50 mg/kg every 24 hours
>0.5-0.6	25 mg/kg every 24 hours	40 mg/kg every 24 hours	60 mg/kg every 24 hours	60 mg/kg every 24 hours
>0.6-0.8	35 mg/kg every 24 hours	25 mg/kg every 12 hours	40 mg/kg every 12 hours	80 mg/kg every 24 hours
>0.8-1.0	20 mg/kg every 12 hours	35 mg/kg every 12 hours	50 mg/kg every 12 hours	50 mg/kg every 12 hours
>1.0-1.4	30 mg/kg every 12 hours	30 mg/kg every 8 hours	45 mg/kg every 8 hours	70 mg/kg every 12 hours
>1.4	40 mg/kg every 12 hours	40 mg/kg every 8 hours	60 mg/kg every 8 hours	90 mg/kg every 12 hours

Maintenance Dosing of Foscarnet in Patients With Abnormal Renal Function

Cl_{cr} (mL/min/kg)	CMV Equivalent to 90 mg/kg q24h	CMV Equivalent to 120 mg/kg q24h
<0.4	Not recommended	Not recommended
≥0.4-0.5	50 mg/kg every 48 hours	65 mg/kg every 48 hours
>0.5-0.6	60 mg/kg every 48 hours	80 mg/kg every 48 hours
>0.6-0.8	80 mg/kg every 48 hours	105 mg/kg every 48 hours
>0.8-1.0	50 mg/kg every 24 hours	65 mg/kg every 24 hours
>1.0-1.4	70 mg/kg every 24 hours	90 mg/kg every 24 hours
>1.4	90 mg/kg every 24 hours	120 mg/kg every 24 hours

Hemodialysis:

Foscarnet is highly removed by hemodialysis (up to ~38% in 2.5 hours HD with high-flux membrane)

Doses of 50 mg/kg/dose posthemodialysis have been found to produce similar serum concentrations as doses of 90 mg/kg twice daily in patients with normal renal function

Doses of 60-90 mg/kg/dose loading dose (posthemodialysis) followed by 45-60 mg/kg/dose posthemodialysis (3 times/week) with the monitoring of weekly plasma concentrations to maintain peak plasma concentrations in the range of 400-800 μMolar have been recommended by some clinicians

Continuous arteriovenous or venovenous hemodiafiltration effects: Dose as for Cl_{cr} 10-50 mL/minute

Mechanism of Action Pyrophosphate analogue which acts as a noncompetitive inhibitor of many viral RNA and DNA polymerases as well as HIV reverse transcriptase. Similar to ganciclovir, foscarnet is a virostatic agent. Foscarnet does not require activation by thymidine kinase.

Contraindications Hypersensitivity to foscarnet or any component of the formulation

Warnings/Precautions [U.S. Boxed Warning]: Indicated only for immunocompromised patients with CMV retinitis and mucocutaneous acyclovir-resistant HSV infection. [U.S. Boxed Warning]: Renal impairment occurs to some degree in the majority of patients treated with foscarnet; renal impairment may occur at any time and is usually reversible within 1 week following dose adjustment or discontinuation of therapy, however, several patients have died with renal failure within 4 weeks of stopping foscarnet; therefore, renal function should be closely monitored. To reduce the risk of nephrotoxicity and the potential to administer a relative overdose, always calculate the creatine clearance even if serum creatinine is within the normal range. Adequate hydration may reduce the risk of nephrotoxicity; the manufacturer makes specific recommendations regarding this.

Imbalance of serum electrolytes or minerals occurs in at least 15% of patients (hypocalcemia, low ionized calcium, hyper/hypophosphatemia, hypomagnesemia, or hypokalemia). Correct electrolytes before initiating therapy. Use caution when administering other medications that cause electrolyte imbalances. Patients who experience signs or symptoms of an electrolyte imbalance should be assessed immediately. **[U.S. Boxed Warning]: Seizures related to plasma electrolyte/mineral imbalance may occur;** incidence has been reported in up to 10% of HIV patients. Risk factors for seizures include impaired baseline renal function, low total serum calcium, and underlying CNS conditions. May cause anemia and granulocytopenia. May cause genital/vascular tissue irritation/ulceration; adequately hydrate and administer only into vein with adequate blood flow to minimize risk. Foscarnet is deposited in teeth and bone of young, growing animals; it has adversely affected tooth enamel development in rats.

Drug Interactions

Avoid Concomitant Use

Avoid concomitant use of Foscarnet with any of the following: Artemether; Dronedarone; Lumefantrine; Nilotinib; Pimozide; QuiNINE; Tetrabenazine; Thioridazine; Toremifene; Vandetanib; Ziprasidone

Increased Effect/Toxicity

Foscarnet may increase the levels/effects of: Dronedarone; Pimozide; QTc-Prolonging Agents; QuiNINE; Tetrabenazine; Thioridazine; Toremifene; Vandetanib; Ziprasidone

The levels/effects of Foscarnet may be increased by: Alfuzosin; Artemether; Chloroquine; Ciprofloxacin; Ciprofloxacin (Systemic); Gadobutrol; Lumefantrine; Nilotinib; QuiNINE

Decreased Effect There are no known significant interactions involving a decrease in effect.

Pharmacodynamics/Kinetics

Half-life Elimination Elimination: ~3-4 hours; terminal: ~88 hours (due to bone deposition)

Pregnancy Risk Factor C

Lactation Excretion in breast milk unknown/contraindicated

Breast-Feeding Considerations The CDC recommends **not** to breast-feed if diagnosed with HIV to avoid postnatal transmission of the virus.

Dosage Forms

Injection, solution [preservative free]: 24 mg/mL (250 mL, 500 mL)

Dental Comment Foscarnet is known to prolong the QT interval. The QT interval is measured as the time and distance between the Q point of the QRS complex and the end of the T wave in the ECG tracing. After adjustment for heart rate, the QT interval is defined as prolonged if it is more than 450 msec in men and 460 msec in women. A long QT syndrome was first described in the 1950s and 60s as a congenital syndrome involving QT interval prolongation and syncope and sudden death. Some of the congenital long QT syndromes were characterized by a peculiar electrocardiographic appearance of the QRS complex involving a premature atria beat followed by a pause, then a subsequent sinus beat showing marked QT prolongation and deformity. This type of cardiac arrhythmia was originally termed "torsade de pointes" (translated from the French as "twisting of the points"). Foscarnet is considered as having a risk of causing torsade de pointes. Since it is not known what effect vasoconstrictors in the local anesthetic regimen will have in patients with a known history of congenital prolonged QT interval or in patients taking any medication that prolongs the QT interval, a medical consult is suggested.

Fosfomycin (fos foe MYE sin)

U.S. Brand Names Monurol®

Canadian Brand Names Monurol®

Pharmacologic Category Antibiotic, Miscellaneous

Use Single oral dose in the treatment of uncomplicated urinary tract infections in women due to susceptible strains of *E. coli* and *Enterococcus faecalis*

Unlabeled/Investigational Use Multiple doses have been investigated for complicated urinary tract infections in men

Local Anesthetic/Vasoconstrictor Precautions No information available to require special precautions

Effects on Dental Treatment No significant effects or complications reported

Effects on Bleeding No information available to require special precautions

Adverse Effects 1% to 10%:

Central nervous system: Headache (4% to 10%), pain (2%), dizziness (1% to 2%)
Dermatologic: Rash (1%)
Endocrine and metabolic: Dysmenorrhea (3%)
Gastrointestinal: Diarrhea (9% to 10%), nausea (4% to 5%), abdominal pain (2%), dyspepsia (1% to 2%)
Genitourinary: Vaginitis (6% to 8%)
Neuromuscular & skeletal: Back pain (3%), weakness (1% to 2%)
Respiratory: Rhinitis (5%), pharyngitis (3%)

General Dosage Range Oral: *Adults (females):* 3 g once

Mechanism of Action As a phosphoric acid derivative, fosfomycin inhibits bacterial wall synthesis (bactericidal) by inactivating the enzyme, pyruvyl transferase, which is critical in the synthesis of cell walls by bacteria

Pharmacodynamics/Kinetics

Half-life Elimination 4-8 hours; Cl_{cr} <54 mL/minute: 50 hours

Time to Peak Serum: 2 hours; within 4 hours with high-fat meal

Pregnancy Risk Factor B

Fosinopril (foe SIN oh pril)

Related Information

Cardiovascular Diseases *on page 1848*

Canadian Brand Names Apo-Fosinopril®; Monopril®; Mylan-Fosinopril; PMS-Fosinopril; RAN™-Fosinopril; Riva-Fosinopril; Teva-Fosinopril

Generic Availability (U.S.) Yes

Pharmacologic Category Angiotensin-Converting Enzyme (ACE) Inhibitor

Use Treatment of hypertension, either alone or in combination with other antihypertensive agents; treatment of heart failure (HF)

Local Anesthetic/Vasoconstrictor Precautions No information available to require special precautions

Effects on Dental Treatment Key adverse event(s) related to dental treatment: Orthostatic hypotension.

Effects on Bleeding No information available to require special precautions

Adverse Effects Note: Frequency ranges include data from hypertension and heart failure trials. Higher rates of adverse reactions have generally been noted in patients with CHF. However, the frequency of adverse effects associated with placebo is also increased in this population.

>10%: Central nervous system: Dizziness (2% to 12%)
1% to 10%:
Cardiovascular: Orthostatic hypotension (1% to 2%), palpitation (1%)
Central nervous system: Dizziness (1% to 2%; up to 12% in CHF patients), headache (3%), fatigue (1% to 2%)
Endocrine & metabolic: Hyperkalemia (2.6%)
Gastrointestinal: Diarrhea (2%), nausea/vomiting (1.2% to 2.2%)
Hepatic: Transaminases increased

Neuromuscular & skeletal: Musculoskeletal pain (<1% to 3%), noncardiac chest pain (<1% to 2%), weakness (1%)
Renal: Serum creatinine increased, renal function worsening (in patients with bilateral renal artery stenosis or hypovolemia)
Respiratory: Cough (2% to 10%)
Miscellaneous: Upper respiratory infection (2%)
>1% but ≤ frequency in patients receiving placebo: Sexual dysfunction, fever, flu-like syndrome, dyspnea, rash, headache, insomnia
Other events reported with ACE inhibitors: Neutropenia, agranulocytosis, eosinophilic pneumonitis, cardiac arrest, pancytopenia, hemolytic anemia, anemia, aplastic anemia, thrombocytopenia, acute renal failure, hepatic failure, jaundice, symptomatic hyponatremia, bullous pemphigus, exfoliative dermatitis, Stevens-Johnson syndrome. In addition, a syndrome which may include fever, myalgia, arthralgia, interstitial nephritis, vasculitis, rash, eosinophilia and positive ANA, and elevated ESR has been reported for other ACE inhibitors.

Dosage Oral:
Children ≥6 years and >50 kg: Hypertension: Initial: 5-10 mg once daily (maximum: 40 mg/day)
Adults:
Heart failure: Initial: 10 mg/day (5 mg if renal dysfunction present) and increase, as needed, to a maximum of 40 mg once daily over several weeks; usual dose: 20-40 mg/day. If hypotension, orthostasis, or azotemia occur during titration, consider decreasing concomitant diuretic dose, if any.
Hypertension: Initial: 10 mg/day; most patients are maintained on 20-40 mg/day (maximum: 80 mg/day). May need to divide the dose into two if trough effect is inadequate; discontinue the diuretic, if possible 2-3 days before initiation of therapy; resume diuretic therapy carefully, if needed.
Dosing adjustment/comments in renal impairment: None needed since hepatobiliary elimination compensates adequately diminished renal elimination.
Hemodialysis: Moderately dialyzable (20% to 50%)

Mechanism of Action Competitive inhibitor of angiotensin-converting enzyme (ACE); prevents conversion of angiotensin I to angiotensin II, a potent vasoconstrictor; results in lower levels of angiotensin II which causes an increase in plasma renin activity and a reduction in aldosterone secretion; a CNS mechanism may also be involved in hypotensive effect as angiotensin II increases adrenergic outflow from CNS; vasoactive kallikreins may be decreased in conversion to active hormones by ACE inhibitors, thus reducing blood pressure

Contraindications Hypersensitivity to fosinopril, any other ACE inhibitor, or any component of the formulation; angioedema related to previous treatment with an ACE inhibitor

Warnings/Precautions Anaphylactic reactions may occur rarely with ACE inhibitors. At any time during treatment (especially following first dose), angioedema may occur rarely with ACE inhibitors; it may involve the head and neck (potentially compromising airway) or the intestine (presenting with abdominal pain). African-Americans may be at an increased risk and patients with idiopathic or hereditary angioedema may be at an increased risk. Prolonged frequent monitoring may be required especially if tongue, glottis, or larynx are involved as they are associated with airway obstruction. Patients with a history of airway surgery may have a higher risk of airway obstruction. Aggressive early and appropriate management is critical. Use in patients with previous angioedema associated with ACE inhibitor therapy is contraindicated. Severe anaphylactoid reactions may be seen during hemodialysis (eg, CVVHD) with high-flux dialysis membranes (eg, AN69), and rarely, during low density lipoprotein apheresis with dextran sulfate cellulose. Rare cases of anaphylactoid reactions have been reported in patients undergoing sensitization treatment with hymenoptera (bee, wasp) venom while receiving ACE inhibitors.

Symptomatic hypotension with or without syncope can occur with ACE inhibitors (usually with the first several doses); effects are most often observed in volume-depleted patients; correct volume depletion prior to initiation; close monitoring of patient is required especially with initial dosing and dosing increases; blood pressure must be lowered at a rate appropriate for the patient's clinical condition. Initiation of therapy in patients with ischemic heart disease or cerebrovascular disease warrants close observation due to the potential consequences posed by falling blood pressure (eg, MI, stroke). Use with caution in hypertrophic cardiomyopathy with outflow tract obstruction, severe aortic stenosis, or before, during, or immediately after major surgery. **[U.S. Boxed Warning]: Based on human data, ACEIs can cause injury and death to the developing fetus when used in the second and third trimesters. ACEIs should be discontinued as soon as possible once pregnancy is detected.**

Hyperkalemia may occur with ACE inhibitors; risk factors include renal dysfunction, diabetes mellitus, concomitant use of potassium-sparing diuretics, potassium supplements, and/or potassium-containing salts. Use cautiously, if at all, with these agents and monitor potassium closely. Cough may occur with ACE inhibitors. Other causes of cough should be considered (eg, pulmonary congestion in patients with heart failure) and excluded prior to discontinuation.

May be associated with deterioration of renal function and/or increases in serum creatinine, particularly in patients with low renal blood flow (eg, renal artery stenosis, heart failure) whose glomerular filtration rate (GFR) is dependent on efferent arteriolar vasoconstriction by angiotensin II; deterioration may result in oliguria, acute renal failure, and progressive azotemia. Small increases in serum creatinine may occur following initiation; consider discontinuation only in patients with progressive and/or significant deterioration in renal function. Use with caution in patients with unstented unilateral/bilateral renal artery stenosis. When unstented bilateral renal artery stenosis is present, use is generally avoided due to the elevated risk of deterioration in renal function unless possible benefits outweigh risks. Concurrent use of angiotensin receptor blockers may increase the risk of clinically-significant adverse events (eg, renal dysfunction, hyperkalemia).

Rare toxicities associated with ACE inhibitors include cholestatic jaundice (which may progress to fulminant hepatic necrosis), agranulocytosis, neutropenia or leukopenia with myeloid hypoplasia. Patients with collagen vascular diseases (especially with concomitant renal impairment) or renal impairment alone may be at increased risk for hematologic toxicity; periodically monitor CBC with differential in these patients.

Drug Interactions

Avoid Concomitant Use There are no known interactions where it is recommended to avoid concomitant use.

Increased Effect/Toxicity

Fosinopril may increase the levels/effects of: Allopurinol; Amifostine; Antihypertensives; AzaTHIOprine; CycloSPORINE; CycloSPORINE (Systemic); Ferric Gluconate; Gold Sodium Thiomalate; Hypotensive Agents; Iron Dextran Complex; Lithium; Nonsteroidal Anti-Inflammatory Agents; RiTUXimab

The levels/effects of Fosinopril may be increased by: Angiotensin II Receptor Blockers; Diazoxide; DPP-IV Inhibitors; Eplerenone; Everolimus; Herbs (Hypotensive Properties); Loop Diuretics; MAO Inhibitors; Pentoxifylline; Phosphodiesterase 5 Inhibitors; Potassium Salts; Potassium-Sparing Diuretics; Prostacyclin Analogues; Sirolimus; Temsirolimus; Thiazide Diuretics; TiZANidine; Tolvaptan; Trimethoprim

Decreased Effect

The levels/effects of Fosinopril may be decreased by: Antacids; Aprotinin; Herbs (Hypertensive Properties); Methylphenidate; Nonsteroidal Anti-Inflammatory Agents; Salicylates; Yohimbine

Ethanol/Nutrition/Herb Interactions Herb/Nutraceutical: Avoid bayberry, blue cohosh, cayenne, ephedra, ginger, ginseng (American), kola, licorice (may worsen hypertension). Avoid black cohosh, california poppy, coleus, golden seal, hawthorn, mistletoe, periwinkle, quinine, shepherd's purse (may have increased antihypertensive effect).

Dietary Considerations Should not take a potassium salt supplement without the advice of healthcare provider.

Pharmacodynamics/Kinetics

Onset of Action 1 hour

Duration of Action 24 hours

Half-life Elimination Serum (fosinoprilat): 12 hours

Time to Peak Serum: ~3 hours

Pregnancy Risk Factor C (1st trimester); D (2nd and 3rd trimesters)

Lactation Enters breast milk/not recommended

Breast-Feeding Considerations Fosinoprilat is excreted in breast milk. Breast-feeding is not recommended by the manufacturer.

Dosage Forms

Tablet, oral: 10 mg, 20 mg, 40 mg

Fosinopril and Hydrochlorothiazide

(foe SIN oh pril & hye droe klor oh THYE a zide)

Related Information

Fosinopril *on page 787*

Hydrochlorothiazide *on page 854*

U.S. Brand Names Monopril-HCT® [DSC]

Canadian Brand Names Monopril-HCT®

Pharmacologic Category Angiotensin-Converting Enzyme (ACE) Inhibitor; Diuretic, Thiazide

Use Treatment of hypertension; not indicated for first-line treatment

Local Anesthetic/Vasoconstrictor Precautions No information available to require special precautions

Effects on Dental Treatment No significant effects or complications reported

Effects on Bleeding No information available to require special precautions

Adverse Effects

2% to 10%:

Central nervous system: Headache (7%, less than placebo), fatigue (4%), dizziness (3%), orthostatic hypotension (2%)

Neuromuscular & skeletal: Musculoskeletal pain (2%)

Respiratory: Cough (6%), upper respiratory infection (2%, less than placebo)

<2%: Abdominal pain, angioedema, breast mass, BUN elevation (similar to placebo), chest pain, creatinine elevation (similar to placebo), depression, diarrhea, dyspepsia, dysuria, edema, eosinophilia, esophagitis, fever, flushing, gastritis, gout, heartburn, hepatic necrosis, leukopenia, libido change, liver function test elevations (transaminases, LDH, alkaline phosphatase, serum bilirubin), muscle cramps, myalgia, nausea, neutropenia, numbness, paresthesia, pharyngitis, pruritus, rash, rhinitis, sexual dysfunction, sinus congestion, somnolence, syncope, tinnitus, urinary frequency, urinary tract infection, viral infection, vomiting, weakness

Other adverse events reported with **ACE inhibitors**: Aplastic anemia, bullous pemphigus, cardiac arrest, cholestatic jaundice, exfoliative dermatitis, hemolytic anemia, hyperkalemia, pancreatitis, pancytopenia, photosensitivity; syndrome that may include one or more of arthralgia/arthritis, vasculitis, serositis, myalgia, fever, rash or other dermopathy, positive ANA titer, leukocytosis, eosinophilia, and elevated ESR; thrombocytopenia

Other adverse events reported with **hydrochlorothiazide**: Agranulocytosis, anaphylactic reactions, anorexia, blurred vision (transient), constipation, cramping, glucosuria, hemolytic anemia, hypercalcemia, hyperglycemia, hyperuricemia, hypokalemia, jaundice (intrahepatic cholestatic), lightheadedness, muscle spasm, necrotizing angiitis, pancreatitis, photosensitivity, pneumonitis, pulmonary edema, purpura, respiratory distress, restlessness, sialadenitis, SLE, Stevens-Johnson syndrome, urticaria, vertigo, xanthopsia

General Dosage Range Oral: *Adults:* Fosinopril 10-80 mg and hydrochlorothiazide 12.5-50 mg once daily

Mechanism of Action Fosinopril is a competitive inhibitor of angiotensin-converting enzyme (ACE); prevents conversion of angiotensin I to angiotensin II, a potent vasoconstrictor; results in lower levels of angiotensin II which causes an increase in plasma renin activity and a reduction in aldosterone secretion; a CNS mechanism may also be involved in hypotensive effect as angiotensin II increases adrenergic outflow from CNS; vasoactive kallikreins may be decreased in conversion to active hormones by ACE inhibitors, thus reducing blood pressure. Hydrochlorothiazide inhibits sodium reabsorption in the distal tubules causing increased excretion of sodium and water as well as potassium and hydrogen ions.

Pregnancy Risk Factor C (1st trimester); D (2nd and 3rd trimester)

Fosphenytoin (FOS fen i toyn)

Related Information

Phenytoin *on page 1341*

U.S. Brand Names Cerebyx®

Canadian Brand Names Cerebyx®

Pharmacologic Category Anticonvulsant, Hydantoin

Use Used for the control of generalized convulsive status epilepticus and prevention and treatment of seizures occurring during neurosurgery; indicated for short-term parenteral administration when other means of phenytoin administration are unavailable, inappropriate, or deemed less advantageous (the safety and effectiveness of fosphenytoin use for more than 5 days has not been systematically evaluated)

Local Anesthetic/Vasoconstrictor Precautions No information available to require special precautions

Effects on Dental Treatment Key adverse event(s) related to dental treatment: Tongue disorder and dry mouth.

Effects on Bleeding No information available to require special precautions

Adverse Effects The more important adverse clinical events caused by the I.V. use of fosphenytoin or phenytoin are cardiovascular collapse and/or central nervous system depression. Hypotension can occur when either drug is administered rapidly by the I.V. route. Do not exceed a rate of 150 mg phenytoin equivalent/minute when administering fosphenytoin.

The adverse clinical events most commonly observed with the use of fosphenytoin in clinical trials were nystagmus, dizziness, pruritus, paresthesia, headache, somnolence, and ataxia. Paresthesia and pruritus were seen more often following fosphenytoin (versus phenytoin) administration and occurred more often with I.V. fosphenytoin than with I.M. administration. These events were dose and rate related (doses ≥15 mg/kg at a rate of 150 mg/minute). These sensations, generally described as itching, burning, or tingling are usually not at the infusion site. The location of the discomfort varied with the groin mentioned most frequently. The paresthesia and pruritus were transient events that occurred within several minutes of the start of infusion and generally resolved within 10 minutes after completion of infusion.

Transient pruritus, tinnitus, nystagmus, somnolence, and ataxia occurred 2-3 times more often at doses ≥15 mg/kg and rates ≥150 mg/minute.

I.V. administration (maximum dose/rate):

>10%:

Central nervous system: Nystagmus, dizziness, somnolence, ataxia
Dermatologic: Pruritus

1% to 10%:

Cardiovascular: Hypotension, vasodilation, tachycardia
Central nervous system: Stupor, incoordination, paresthesia, extrapyramidal syndrome, tremor, agitation, hypoesthesia, dysarthria, vertigo, brain edema, headache
Gastrointestinal: Nausea, tongue disorder, dry mouth, vomiting
Neuromuscular & skeletal: Pelvic pain, muscle weakness, back pain
Ocular: Diplopia, amblyopia
Otic: Tinnitus, deafness
Miscellaneous: Taste perversion

I.M. administration (substitute for oral phenytoin):

1% to 10%:

Central nervous system: Nystagmus, tremor, ataxia, headache, incoordination, somnolence, dizziness, paresthesia, reflexes decreased
Dermatologic: Pruritus
Gastrointestinal: Nausea, vomiting
Hematologic/lymphatic: Ecchymosis
Neuromuscular & skeletal: Muscle weakness

General Dosage Range

I.M.: *Adults:* Loading: 15-20 mg PE/kg; Maintenance: 4-6 mg PE/kg/day
I.V.: *Adults:* Loading: 10-20 mg PE/kg; Maintenance: 4-6 mg PE/kg/day

Mechanism of Action Diphosphate ester salt of phenytoin which acts as a water soluble prodrug of phenytoin; after administration, plasma esterases convert fosphenytoin to phosphate, formaldehyde, and phenytoin as the active moiety; phenytoin works by stabilizing neuronal membranes and decreasing seizure activity by increasing efflux or decreasing influx of sodium ions across cell membranes in the motor cortex during generation of nerve impulses

Pharmacodynamics/Kinetics

Half-life Elimination Fosphenytoin: 15 minutes; Phenytoin: Variable (mean: 12-29 hours); kinetics of phenytoin are saturable

Time to Peak Conversion to phenytoin: Following I.V. administration (maximum rate of administration): 15 minutes; following I.M. administration, peak phenytoin levels are reached in 3 hours

Pregnancy Risk Factor D

Fospropofol (fos PROE po fole)

U.S. Brand Names Lusedra™

Generic Availability (U.S.) No

Pharmacologic Category Sedative

Use Monitored anesthesia care (MAC) sedation in patients undergoing diagnostic or therapeutic procedures

Local Anesthetic/Vasoconstrictor Precautions No information available to require special precautions

Effects on Dental Treatment No significant effects or complications reported

Effects on Bleeding No information available to require special precautions

Adverse Effects

>10%:

Dermatologic: Pruritus (see **"Note"**; 8% to 28%)
Neuromuscular & skeletal: Paresthesia (see **"Note"**; 52% to 74%)
Respiratory: Hypoxemia (1% to 11%)

1% to 10%:
- Cardiovascular: Hypotension (2% to 7%)
- Central nervous system: Headache (1% to 2%)
- Gastrointestinal: Nausea (≤4%), vomiting (≤3%)
- Miscellaneous: Procedural pain (≤2%)

Note: Paresthesias (including perineal discomfort or burning sensation) and pruritus (including genital, perineal, and generalized pruritus) are mostly limited to the first 5 minutes of administration and usually described as mild-moderate in intensity. No pretreatments are helpful in reducing the incidence of these adverse effects.

Dosage Monitored anesthesia care (MAC) sedation: I.V.: **Note: Onset of effect is delayed as compared to propofol-emulsion due to need for conversion to active component.** If <60 kg, base dosing on 60 kg; however, lower doses may be used to achieve lower levels of sedation. If >90 kg, base dosing on 90 kg.

Healthy adults <65 years or with mild systemic disease (ASA-PS1 or -PS2): *Standard dosing regimen:* Initial: 6.5 mg/kg (maximum initial dose: 577.5 mg or 16.5 mL), followed by supplemental doses of 1.6 mg/kg (maximum supplemental dose: 140 mg or 4 mL) no more frequently than every 4 minutes as needed to achieve desired level of sedation.

Elderly patients ≥65 years or patients with severe systemic disease (ASA-PS3 or -PS4): *Modified dosing regimen:* Initial: 4.9 mg/kg (maximum initial dose: 437.5 mg or 12.5 mL), followed by supplemental doses of 1.2 mg/kg (maximum supplemental dose: 105 mg or 3 mL) no more frequently than every 4 minutes as needed to achieve desired level of sedation.

Dosage adjustment in renal impairment: No dosage adjustment recommended. Use with caution in patients with severe renal impairment (Cl_{cr} <30 mL/minute); limited safety and efficacy data available in these patients.

Dosage adjustment in hepatic impairment: No dosage adjustment recommended. Use with caution in patients with hepatic impairment; has not been adequately studied in this population.

Mechanism of Action Fospropofol disodium is a prodrug of propofol. Propofol interacts with the $GABA_A$ receptor, which is the presumed mechanism of action whereby it produces a sedative/hypnotic effect. Propofol is an alkyl-phenolic compound with intravenous general anesthetic properties.

Contraindications There are no contraindications in the manufacturer's FDA approved labeling.

Note: Applicable contraindications to propofol include: Hypersensitivity to propofol; when general anesthesia or sedation is contraindicated

Warnings/Precautions The major cardiovascular effect is hypotension; use with caution in patients who are hemodynamically unstable, hypovolemic, have abnormally low vascular tone (eg, sepsis) or compromised myocardial function (eg, heart failure). The **onset of action will be delayed** due to need for conversion to the active metabolite, propofol. If supplemental doses are administered before full effect occurs, the risk of dose-stacking may be elevated resulting in deeper sedation than intended.

Use requires careful patient monitoring; should only be administered by persons trained in the administration of general anesthesia and not involved in the conduct of the diagnostic or therapeutic procedure. Sedated patients should be continuously monitored, and facilities for maintenance of a patent airway, providing artificial ventilation, administering supplemental oxygen, and instituting cardiovascular resuscitation must be immediately available. Patients should be continuously monitored during sedation and through the recovery process for early signs of hypotension, apnea, airway obstruction, and/or oxygen desaturation. Use to induce moderate (conscious) sedation in patients warrants monitoring equivalent to that seen with general anesthesia. May cause loss of spontaneous respiration and/or hypoxemia; supplemental oxygen is recommended for all patients receiving fospropofol; monitor patient closely. The risk of these effects may be increased with the concomitant use of opioids and/or other sedatives. May cause patients to become unresponsive or minimally responsive to vigorous tactile or painful stimuli.

Use lower doses in patients ≥65 years and/or ASA-PS 3/4 patients to reduce the incidence of unwanted cardiorespiratory and neurologic depressive events. Use with caution in patients with hepatic impairment or severe renal impairment (Cl_{cr} <30 mL/minute). Use with caution in patients with respiratory disease; risk of cardiorespiratory depression may be increased. Use with caution in patients with a history of epilepsy or seizures; seizure may occur during recovery phase.

Concomitant use of opioids/sedative-hypnotics may lead to increased sedative or respiratory depressant effects of fospropofol, more pronounced decreases in systolic, diastolic, and mean arterial pressures, heart rate, and cardiac output. Fospropofol lacks analgesic properties; pain management requires specific use of analgesic agents. Fospropofol should only be used in pregnancy if clearly needed.

Not recommended for use in obstetrics, including cesarean section deliveries. Safety and efficacy have not been established in patients <18 years of age.

Drug Interactions

Metabolism/Transport Effects Substrate of CYP1A2 (minor), 2A6 (minor), 2B6 (major), 2C9 (major), 2C19 (minor), 2D6 (minor), 2E1 (minor), 3A4 (minor); **Inhibits** CYP1A2 (moderate), 2C9 (weak), 2C19 (moderate), 2D6 (weak), 2E1 (weak), 3A4 (strong)

Avoid Concomitant Use There are no known interactions where it is recommended to avoid concomitant use.

Increased Effect/Toxicity

Fospropofol may increase the levels/effects of: Ropivacaine

The levels/effects of Fospropofol may be increased by: Alfentanil; Conivaptan; CYP2B6 Inhibitors (Moderate); CYP2B6 Inhibitors (Strong); Quazepam

Decreased Effect

The levels/effects of Fospropofol may be decreased by: Tocilizumab

Pharmacodynamics/Kinetics

Onset of Action Bolus (dose dependent): Attainment of adequate sedation was achieved between 2-28 minutes (median: 8 minutes)

Duration of Action Duration of sedation: Time to fully alert: ≤1 hour (median: 5 minutes)

Half-life Elimination

Fospropofol: 0.8-0.96 hours

Propofol: 0.85-1.41 hours

Time to Peak Propofol (from fospropofol): Median: 12 minutes

Pregnancy Risk Factor B

Lactation Propofol (the active metabolite of fospropofol) enters breast milk/not recommended

Controlled Substance C-IV

Dosage Forms

Injection, solution [preservative free]:

Lusedra™: 35 mg/mL (30 mL)

References

Cohen LB, "Clinical Trial: a dose-response study of fospropofol disodium for moderate sedation during colonoscopy," *Aliment Pharmacol Ther*, 2008, 27(7):597-608.

Silvestri GA, Vincent BD, Wahidi MM, et al, "A Phase 3, Randomized, Double-blind, Study to Assess the Efficacy and Safety of Fospropofol Disodium Injection for Moderate Sedation in Patients Undergoing Flexible Bronchoscopy," *Chest*, 2009, 135(1):41-7.

Frovatriptan (froe va TRIP tan)

Related Information

Temporomandibular Dysfunction (TMD) *on page 1964*

U.S. Brand Names Frova®

Canadian Brand Names Frova®

Generic Availability (U.S.) No

Pharmacologic Category Antimigraine Agent; Serotonin 5-$HT_{1B,\ 1D}$ Receptor Agonist

Use Acute treatment of migraine with or without aura

Local Anesthetic/Vasoconstrictor Precautions No information available to require special precautions

Effects on Dental Treatment No significant effects or complications reported

Effects on Bleeding No information available to require special precautions

Adverse Effects 1% to 10%:

Cardiovascular: Flushing (4%), chest pain (2%), palpitation (1%)

Central nervous system: Dizziness (8%), fatigue (5%), headache (4%), hot or cold sensation (3%), somnolence (≥2%), anxiety (1%), dysesthesia (1%), hypoesthesia (1%), insomnia (1%), pain (1%)

Gastrointestinal: Xerostomia (3%), nausea (≥2%), dyspepsia (2%), abdominal pain (1%), diarrhea (1%), vomiting (1%)

Neuromuscular & skeletal: Paresthesia (4%), skeletal pain (3%)

Ocular: Vision abnormal (1%)

Otic: Tinnitus (1%)

Respiratory: Rhinitis (1%), sinusitis (1%)

Miscellaneous: Diaphoresis (1%)

Dosage Oral: Adults: Migraine:

U.S. labeling: 2.5 mg; if headache recurs, a second dose may be given if first dose provided relief and at least 2 hours have elapsed since the first dose (maximum daily dose: 7.5 mg)

Canadian labeling: 2.5 mg; if headache recurs, a second dose may be given if first dose provided relief and at least 4 hours have elapsed since the first dose (maximum daily dose: 5 mg)

Note: The safety of treating more than 4 migraines/month has not been established.

Dosage adjustment in renal impairment: No adjustment necessary

Dosage adjustment in hepatic impairment: No adjustment necessary in mild-to-moderate hepatic impairment; use with caution in severe impairment (has not been studied in severe impairment).

Canadian labeling (not in U.S. labeling): Use is contraindicated in severe hepatic impairment.

Mechanism of Action Selective agonist for serotonin (5-HT_{1B} and 5-HT_{1D} receptors) in cranial arteries; causes vasoconstriction and reduces sterile inflammation associated with antidromic neuronal transmission correlating with relief of migraine.

Contraindications Hypersensitivity to frovatriptan or any component of the formulation; patients with ischemic heart disease or signs or symptoms of ischemic heart disease (including Prinzmetal's angina, angina pectoris, myocardial infarction, silent myocardial ischemia); cerebrovascular syndromes (including strokes, transient ischemic attacks); peripheral vascular syndromes (including ischemic bowel disease); uncontrolled hypertension; use within 24 hours of ergotamine derivatives; use within 24 hours of another 5-HT_1 agonist; management of hemiplegic or basilar migraine

Canadian labeling: Additional contraindications (not in U.S. labeling): Cardiac arrhythmias, valvular heart disease, congenital heart disease, atherosclerotic disease; management of ophthalmoplegic migraine; severe hepatic impairment

Warnings/Precautions Not intended for migraine prophylaxis, or treatment of cluster headaches, hemiplegic or basilar migraines. Rule out underlying neurologic disease in patients with atypical headache, migraine (with no prior history of migraine) or inadequate clinical response to initial dosing. Cardiac events (coronary artery vasospasm, transient ischemia, MI, ventricular tachycardia/fibrillation, cardiac arrest, and death), cerebral/subarachnoid hemorrhage, stroke, peripheral vascular ischemia, and colonic ischemia have been reported with 5-HT_1 agonist administration. May cause vasospastic reactions resulting in colonic, peripheral, or coronary ischemia. Do not give to patients with risk factors for CAD until a cardiovascular evaluation has been performed; if evaluation is satisfactory, the healthcare provider should administer the first dose and cardiovascular status should be periodically evaluated. Significant elevation in blood pressure, including hypertensive crisis, has also been reported on rare occasions in patients using other 5-HT_{1D} agonists with and without a history of hypertension. May lower seizure threshold, use caution in epilepsy or structural brain lesions. Symptoms of agitation, confusion, hallucinations, hyper-reflexia, myoclonus, shivering, and tachycardia (serotonin syndrome) may occur with concomitant proserotonergic drugs (ie, SSRIs/SNRIs or triptans) or agents which reduce frovatriptan's metabolism. Safety and efficacy in pediatric patients have not been established.

Drug Interactions

Metabolism/Transport Effects Substrate of CYP1A2 (minor)

Avoid Concomitant Use

Avoid concomitant use of Frovatriptan with any of the following: Ergot Derivatives; Sibutramine

Increased Effect/Toxicity

Frovatriptan may increase the levels/effects of: Ergot Derivatives; Serotonin Modulators

The levels/effects of Frovatriptan may be increased by: Ergot Derivatives; Sibutramine

Decreased Effect There are no known significant interactions involving a decrease in effect.

Ethanol/Nutrition/Herb Interactions Food: Food does not affect frovatriptan bioavailability.

Pharmacodynamics/Kinetics

Half-life Elimination ~26 hours

Time to Peak 2-4 hours

Pregnancy Risk Factor C

Lactation Excretion in breast milk unknown/use caution

Dosage Forms

Tablet, oral:

Frova®: 2.5 mg

Fructose, Dextrose, and Phosphoric Acid

(FRUK tose, DEKS trose, & foss FOR ik AS id)

Related Information

Dextrose *on page 506*

U.S. Brand Names Emetrol® [OTC]; Formula EM [OTC]; Kalmz [OTC]; Nausea Relief [OTC]; Nausetrol® [OTC]

Pharmacologic Category Antiemetic

Use Relief of nausea associated with upset stomach that occurs with intestinal or stomach flu, and food indiscretions

Local Anesthetic/Vasoconstrictor Precautions No information available to require special precautions

Effects on Dental Treatment No significant effects or complications reported

Effects on Bleeding No information available to require special precautions

General Dosage Range Oral:

Children ≥2-12 years: 5-10 mL every 15 minutes as needed; do not take for more than 1 hour (5 doses)

Children ≥12 years and Adults: 15-30 mL every 15 minutes as needed; do not take for more than 1 hour (5 doses)

Fulvestrant (fool VES trant)

U.S. Brand Names Faslodex®

Canadian Brand Names Faslodex®

Pharmacologic Category Antineoplastic Agent, Estrogen Receptor Antagonist

Use Treatment of hormone receptor positive metastatic breast cancer in postmenopausal women with disease progression following antiestrogen therapy

Local Anesthetic/Vasoconstrictor Precautions No information available to require special precautions

Effects on Dental Treatment No significant effects or complications reported

Effects on Bleeding No information available to require special precautions

Adverse Effects Adverse reactions reported with 500 mg dose.

>10%:

Endocrine & metabolic: Hot flushes (7% to 13%)

Hepatic: Alkaline phosphatase increased (>15%; grades 3/4: 1 to 2%), transaminases increased (>15%; grades 3/4: 1 to 2%)

Local: Injection site pain (12% to 14%)

Neuromuscular & skeletal: Joint disorders (14% to 19%)

1% to 10%:

Cardiovascular: Ischemic disorder (1%)

Central nervous system: Fatigue (8%), headache (8%)

Gastrointestinal: Nausea (10%), anorexia (6%), vomiting (6%), constipation (5%), weight gain (≤1%)

Genitourinary: Urinary tract infection (2% to 4%)

Neuromuscular & skeletal: Bone pain (9%), arthralgia (8%), back pain (8%), extremity pain (7%), musculoskeletal pain (6%), weakness (6%)

Respiratory: Cough (5%), dyspnea (4%)

<1%, postmarketing, and/or case reports (reported with 250 mg or 500 mg dose): Angioedema, hypersensitivity reactions, leukopenia, myalgia, osteoporosis, thrombosis, urticaria, vaginal bleeding, vertigo

General Dosage Range Dosage adjustment recommended in patients with hepatic impairment

I.M.: *Adults (postmenopausal women):* Initial: 500 mg on days 1, 15, and 29; Maintenance: 500 mg once monthly

Mechanism of Action Estrogen receptor antagonist; competitively binds to estrogen receptors on tumors and other tissue targets, producing a nuclear complex that causes a dose-related down-regulation of estrogen receptors and inhibits tumor growth.

Pharmacodynamics/Kinetics

Duration of Action I.M.: Steady state concentrations reached within first month, when administered with additional dose given 2 weeks following the initial dose; plasma levels maintained for at least 1 month

Half-life Elimination 250 mg: ~40 days

Pregnancy Risk Factor D

Furosemide (fyoor OH se mide)

Related Information

Cardiovascular Diseases *on page 1848*

U.S. Brand Names Lasix®

Canadian Brand Names Apo-Furosemide®; Dom-Furosemide; Furosemide Injection, USP; Furosemide Special; Lasix®; Lasix® Special; Novo-Semide; Nu-Furosemide; PMS-Furosemide

Generic Availability (U.S.) Yes

Pharmacologic Category Diuretic, Loop

Use Management of edema associated with heart failure and hepatic or renal disease; acute pulmonary edema; treatment of hypertension (alone or in combination with other antihypertensives)

Local Anesthetic/Vasoconstrictor Precautions No information available to require special precautions

Effects on Dental Treatment No significant effects or complications reported

Effects on Bleeding No information available to require special precautions

Adverse Effects Frequency not defined.

Cardiovascular: Acute hypotension, chronic aortitis, necrotizing angiitis, orthostatic hypotension, vasculitis

Central nervous system: Dizziness, fever, headache, hepatic encephalopathy, lightheadedness, restlessness, vertigo

Dermatologic: Bullous pemphigoid, cutaneous vasculitis, erythema multiforme, exfoliative dermatitis, photosensitivity, pruritus, purpura, rash, Stevens-Johnson syndrome, toxic epidermal necrolysis, urticaria

Endocrine & metabolic: Cholesterol and triglycerides increased, glucose tolerance test altered, gout, hyperglycemia, hyperuricemia, hypocalcemia, hypochloremia, hypokalemia, hypomagnesemia, hyponatremia, metabolic alkalosis

Gastrointestinal: Anorexia, constipation, cramping, diarrhea, nausea, oral and gastric irritation, pancreatitis, vomiting

Genitourinary: Urinary bladder spasm, urinary frequency

Hematological: Agranulocytosis (rare), anemia, aplastic anemia (rare), eosinophilia, hemolytic anemia, leukopenia, thrombocytopenia

Hepatic: Intrahepatic cholestatic jaundice, ischemic hepatitis, liver enzymes increased

Local: Injection site pain (following I.M. injection), thrombophlebitis

Neuromuscular & skeletal: Muscle spasm, paresthesia, weakness

Ocular: Blurred vision, xanthopsia

Otic: Hearing impairment (reversible or permanent with rapid I.V. or I.M. administration), tinnitus

Renal: Allergic interstitial nephritis, fall in glomerular filtration rate and renal blood flow (due to overdiuresis), glycosuria, transient rise in BUN

Miscellaneous: Anaphylaxis (rare), exacerbate or activate systemic lupus erythematosus

Dosage

Infants and Children: Edema, heart failure:

Oral: Initial: 2 mg/kg/dose increased in increments of 1-2 mg/kg/dose with each succeeding dose at intervals of 6-8 hours until a satisfactory response is achieved; maximum dose: 6 mg/kg/dose

I.M., I.V.: Initial: 1 mg/kg/dose; if response not adequate, may increase dose in increments of 1 mg/kg/dose and administer not sooner than 2 hours after previous dose, until a satisfactory response is achieved; may administer maintenance dose at intervals of every 6-12 hours; maximum dose: 6 mg/kg/dose

Children 1-17 years: Hypertension, resistant (unlabeled; AAP, 2004): Oral: Initial: 0.5-2 mg/kg/dose once or twice daily; maximum dose: 6 mg/kg/dose

Adults:

Edema, heart failure:

Oral: Initial: 20-80 mg/dose; if response not adequate, may repeat the same dose or increase dose in increments of 20-40 mg/dose at intervals of 6-8 hours; usual maintenance dose interval is once or twice daily; may be titrated up to 600 mg/day with severe edematous states. **Note:** May also be given on 2-4 consecutive days every week.

I.M., I.V.: Initial: 20-40 mg/dose; if response not adequate, may repeat the same dose or increase dose in increments of 20 mg/dose and administer 1-2 hours after previous dose (maximum dose: 200 mg/dose). Individually determined dose should then be given once or twice daily although some patients may initially require dosing as frequent as every 6 hours. **Note:** ACC/AHA 2009 guidelines for heart failure recommend a maximum single dose of 160-200 mg.

Continuous I.V. infusion (Howard, 2001; Hunt, 2009): Initial: I.V. bolus dose 20-40 mg over 1-2 minutes, followed by continuous I.V. infusion doses of 10-40 mg/hour. If urine output is <1 mL/kg/hour, double as necessary to a maximum of 80-160 mg/hour. The risk associated with higher infusion rates (80-160 mg/hour) must be weighed against alternative strategies. **Note:** ACC/AHA 2009 guidelines for heart failure recommend 40 mg I.V. load, then 10-40 mg/hour infusion.

Acute pulmonary edema: I.V.: 40 mg over 1-2 minutes. If response not adequate within 1 hour, may increase dose to 80 mg. **Note:** ACC/AHA 2009 guidelines for heart failure recommend a maximum single dose of 160-200 mg.

Hypertension, resistant (Chobanian, 2003; JNC 7): Oral: 20-80 mg/day in 2 divided doses

Refractory heart failure: Oral, I.V.: Doses up to 8 g/day have been used.

Elderly: Oral, I.M., I.V.: Initial: 20 mg/day; increase slowly to desired response.

Dosing adjustment/comments in renal impairment: Acute renal failure: High doses (up to 1-3 g/day - oral/I.V.) have been used to initiate desired response; avoid use in oliguric states.

Dialysis: Not removed by hemo- or peritoneal dialysis; supplemental dose is not necessary.

Dosing adjustment/comments in hepatic disease: Diminished natriuretic effect with increased sensitivity to hypokalemia and volume depletion in cirrhosis; monitor effects, particularly with high doses.

Mechanism of Action Inhibits reabsorption of sodium and chloride in the ascending loop of Henle and distal renal tubule, interfering with the chloride-binding cotransport system, thus causing increased excretion of water, sodium, chloride, magnesium, and calcium

Contraindications Hypersensitivity to furosemide or any component of the formulation; anuria

Warnings/Precautions [U.S. Boxed Warning]: If given in excessive amounts, furosemide, similar to other loop diuretics, can lead to profound diuresis, resulting in fluid and electrolyte depletion; close medical supervision and dose evaluation are required. Watch for and correct electrolyte disturbances; adjust dose to avoid dehydration. When electrolyte depletion is present, therapy should not be initiated unless serum electrolytes, especially potassium, are normalized. In cirrhosis, avoid electrolyte and acid/base imbalances that might lead to hepatic encephalopathy; correct electrolyte and acid/base imbalances prior to initiation when hepatic coma is present. Coadministration of antihypertensives may increase the risk of hypotension.

Monitor fluid status and renal function in an attempt to prevent oliguria, azotemia, and reversible increases in BUN and creatinine; close medical supervision of aggressive diuresis is required. May increase risk of contrast-induced nephropathy. Rapid I.V. administration, renal impairment, excessive doses, hypoproteinemia, and concurrent use of other ototoxins is associated with ototoxicity. Asymptomatic hyperuricemia has been reported with use; rarely, gout may precipitate. Photosensitization may occur.

Use with caution in patients with prediabetes or diabetes mellitus; may see a change in glucose control. Use with caution in patients with systemic lupus erythematosus (SLE); may cause SLE exacerbation or activation. Use with caution in patients with prostatic hyperplasia/urinary stricture; may cause urinary retention. May lead to nephrocalcinosis or nephrolithiasis in premature infants or in children <4 years of age with chronic use. May prevent closure of patent ductus arteriosus in premature infants. Chemical similarities are present among sulfonamides, sulfonylureas, carbonic anhydrase inhibitors, thiazides, and loop diuretics (except ethacrynic acid). A risk of cross-reaction exists in patients with allergy to any of these compounds; avoid use when previous reaction has been severe. Discontinue if signs of hypersensitivity are noted.

Drug Interactions

Avoid Concomitant Use

Avoid concomitant use of Furosemide with any of the following: Ethacrynic Acid

Increased Effect/Toxicity

Furosemide may increase the levels/effects of: ACE Inhibitors; Allopurinol; Amifostine; Aminoglycosides; Antihypertensives; CISplatin; Dofetilide; Ethacrynic Acid; Hypotensive Agents; Lithium; Neuromuscular-Blocking Agents; RiTUXimab; Salicylates

The levels/effects of Furosemide may be increased by: Beta2-Agonists; Corticosteroids (Orally Inhaled); Corticosteroids (Systemic); Diazoxide; Herbs (Hypotensive Properties); Licorice; MAO Inhibitors; Pentoxifylline; Phosphodiesterase 5 Inhibitors; Probenecid; Prostacyclin Analogues

Decreased Effect

Furosemide may decrease the levels/effects of: Lithium; Neuromuscular-Blocking Agents

The levels/effects of Furosemide may be decreased by: Aliskiren; Bile Acid Sequestrants; Fosphenytoin; Herbs (Hypertensive Properties); Methylphenidate; Nonsteroidal Anti-Inflammatory Agents; Phenytoin; Probenecid; Salicylates; Yohimbine

Ethanol/Nutrition/Herb Interactions

Food: Furosemide serum levels may be decreased if taken with food.

Herb/Nutraceutical: Avoid bayberry, blue cohosh, cayenne, ephedra, ginger, ginseng (American), kola, licorice (may worsen hypertension). Avoid black cohosh, California poppy, coleus, golden seal, hawthorn, mistletoe, periwinkle, quinine, shepherd's purse (may increase antihypertensive effect). Licorice may also cause or worsen hypokalemia.

Dietary Considerations May cause potassium loss; potassium supplement or dietary changes may be required.

Pharmacodynamics/Kinetics

Onset of Action Diuresis: Oral, S.L.: 30-60 minutes; I.M.: 30 minutes; I.V.: ~5 minutes

Symptomatic improvement with acute pulmonary edema: Within 15-20 minutes; occurs prior to diuretic effect

Peak effect: Oral: 1-2 hours

Duration of Action Oral, S.L.: 6-8 hours; I.V.: 2 hours

Half-life Elimination Normal renal function: 0.5-2 hours; End-stage renal disease: 9 hours

Pregnancy Risk Factor C

Lactation Enters breast milk/use caution

Breast-Feeding Considerations Crosses into breast milk; may suppress lactation

Dosage Forms

Injection, solution [preservative free]: 10 mg/mL (2 mL, 4 mL, 10 mL)

Solution, oral: 40 mg/5 mL (5 mL, 500 mL); 10 mg/mL (4 mL, 60 mL, 120 mL)

Tablet, oral: 20 mg, 40 mg, 80 mg

Lasix®: 20 mg, 40 mg, 80 mg

Gabapentin (GA ba pen tin)

Related Information

Temporomandibular Dysfunction (TMD) *on page 1964*

U.S. Brand Names Neurontin®

Canadian Brand Names Apo-Gabapentin®; CO Gabapentin; Dom-Gabapentin; Mylan-Gabapentin; Neurontin®; PHL-Gabapentin; PMS-Gabapentin; PRO-Gabapentin; RAN™-Gabapentin; ratio-Gabapentin; Riva-Gabapentin; Teva-Gabapentin

Generic Availability (U.S.) Yes

Pharmacologic Category Anticonvulsant, Miscellaneous

Dental Use Neuropathic pain (consult with physician)

Use Adjunct for treatment of partial seizures with and without secondary generalized seizures in patients >12 years of age with epilepsy; adjunct for treatment of partial seizures in pediatric patients 3-12 years of age; management of postherpetic neuralgia (PHN) in adults

Unlabeled/Investigational Use Neuropathic pain, diabetic peripheral neuropathy, fibromyalgia, postoperative pain, bipolar disorder, restless legs syndrome (RLS), social phobia, vasomotor symptoms

Local Anesthetic/Vasoconstrictor Precautions No information available to require special precautions

Effects on Dental Treatment Key adverse event(s) related to dental treatment: Xerostomia (normal salivary flow resumes upon discontinuation), dry throat, and dental abnormalities.

Effects on Bleeding No information available to require special precautions

Adverse Effects As reported in patients >12 years of age, unless otherwise noted in children (3-12 years)

>10%:

Central nervous system: Somnolence (20%; children 8%), dizziness (17% to 28%; children 3%), ataxia (13%), fatigue (11%)

Miscellaneous: Viral infection (children 11%)

1% to 10%:

Cardiovascular: Peripheral edema (2% to 8%), vasodilatation (1%)

Central nervous system: Fever (children 10%), hostility (children 8%), emotional lability (children 4%), fatigue (children 3%), headache (3%), ataxia (3%), abnormal thinking (2% to 3%; children 2%), amnesia (2%), depression (2%), dysarthria (2%), nervousness (2%), abnormal coordination (1% to 2%), twitching (1%), hyperesthesia (1%)

Dermatologic: Pruritus (1%), rash (1%)

Endocrine & metabolic: Hyperglycemia (1%)

Gastrointestinal: Diarrhea (6%), nausea/vomiting (3% to 4%; children 8%), abdominal pain (3%), xerostomia (2% to 5%), constipation (2% to 4%), weight gain (adults and children 2% to 3%), dyspepsia (2%), flatulence (2%), dry throat (2%), dental abnormalities (2%), appetite stimulation (1%)

Genitourinary: Impotence (2%)

Hematologic: Leukopenia (1%), decreased WBC (1%)

Neuromuscular & skeletal: Tremor (7%), weakness (6%), hyperkinesia (children 3%), abnormal gait (2%), back pain (2%), myalgia (2%), fracture (1%)

Ocular: Nystagmus (8%), diplopia (1% to 6%), blurred vision (3% to 4%), conjunctivitis (1%)

Otic: Otitis media (1%)

Respiratory: Rhinitis (4%), bronchitis (children 3%), respiratory infection (children 3%), pharyngitis (1% to 3%), cough (2%)

Miscellaneous: Infection (5%)

Dental Usual Dosage

Pain (unlabeled use): Children >12 years and Adults: Oral: 300-1800 mg/day given in 3 divided doses has been the most common dosage range

Postherpetic neuralgia or neuropathic pain: Adults: Oral: Day 1: 300 mg, Day 2: 300 mg twice daily, Day 3: 300 mg 3 times/day; dose may be titrated as needed for pain relief (range: 1800-3600 mg/day, daily doses >1800 mg do not generally show greater benefit)

Dosage Oral:

Children: Anticonvulsant:

3-12 years: Initial: 10-15 mg/kg/day in 3 divided doses; titrate to effective dose over ~3 days; dosages of up to 50 mg/kg/day have been tolerated in clinical studies

3-4 years: Effective dose: 40 mg/kg/day in 3 divided doses

≥5-12 years: Effective dose: 25-35 mg/kg/day in 3 divided doses

See **"Note"** in adult dosing.

Children >12 years and Adults:

Anticonvulsant: Initial: 300 mg 3 times/day; if necessary the dose may be increased up to 1800 mg/day. Doses of up to 2400 mg/day have been tolerated in long-term clinical studies; up to 3600 mg/day has been tolerated in short-term studies.

Note: If gabapentin is discontinued or if another anticonvulsant is added to therapy, it should be done slowly over a minimum of 1 week

Pain (unlabeled use): 300-1800 mg/day given in 3 divided doses has been the most common dosage range

Adults:

Postherpetic neuralgia or neuropathic pain: Day 1: 300 mg, Day 2: 300 mg twice daily, Day 3: 300 mg 3 times/day; dose may be titrated as needed for pain relief (range: 1800-3600 mg/day, daily doses >1800 mg do not generally show greater benefit)

Diabetic neuropathy (unlabeled use): 900-3600 mg/day (Bril, 2011)

Restless legs syndrome (RLS) (unlabeled use): Initial: 300 mg once daily 2 hours before bedtime. Doses ≥600 mg/day have been given in 2 divided doses (late afternoon and 2 hours before bedtime). Dose may be titrated every 2 weeks until symptom relief achieved (range: 300-1800 mg/day). Suggested maintenance dosing schedule: One-third of total daily dose given at 12 pm, remaining two-thirds total daily dose given at 8 pm. (Garcia-Borreguero, 2002; Happe, 2003; Saletu, 2010; Vignatelli, 2006)

Vasomotor symptoms associated with menopause (unlabeled use; Butt, 2008): 300 mg 3 times/day

Elderly: Studies in elderly patients have shown a decrease in clearance as age increases. This is most likely due to age-related decreases in renal function; dose reductions may be needed.

Dosing adjustment in renal impairment: Children ≥12 years and Adults: See table.

Hemodialysis: Dialyzable

Gabapentin Dosing Adjustments in Renal Impairment

Creatinine Clearance (mL/min)	Daily Dose Range
≥60	300-1200 mg tid
>30-59	200-700 mg bid
>15-29	200-700 mg daily
15[1]	100-300 mg daily
Hemodialysis[2]	125-350 mg

[1]Cl_{cr}<15 mL/minute: Reduce daily dose in proportion to creatinine clearance.

[2]Single supplemental dose administered after each 4 hours of hemodialysis.

Mechanism of Action Gabapentin is structurally related to GABA. However, it does not bind to $GABA_A$ or $GABA_B$ receptors, and it does not appear to influence synthesis or uptake of GABA. High affinity gabapentin binding sites have been located throughout the brain; these sites correspond to the presence of voltage-gated calcium channels specifically possessing the alpha-2-delta-1 subunit. This channel appears to be located presynaptically, and may modulate the release of excitatory neurotransmitters which participate in epileptogenesis and nociception.

Contraindications Hypersensitivity to gabapentin or any component of the formulation

Warnings/Precautions Antiepileptics are associated with an increased risk of suicidal behavior/thoughts with use (regardless of indication); patients should be monitored for signs/symptoms of depression, suicidal tendencies, and other unusual behavior changes during therapy and instructed to inform their healthcare provider immediately if symptoms occur. Avoid abrupt withdrawal, may precipitate seizures; use cautiously in patients with severe renal dysfunction; male rat studies demonstrated an association with pancreatic adenocarcinoma (clinical implication unknown). May cause CNS depression, which may impair physical or mental abilities. Patients must be cautioned about performing tasks which require mental alertness (eg, operating machinery or driving). Effects with other sedative drugs or ethanol may be potentiated. Pediatric patients (3-12 years of age) have shown increased incidence of CNS-related adverse effects, including emotional lability, hostility, thought disorder, and hyperkinesia. Gabapentin products are not interchangeable with gabapentin encarbil (Horizant™) due to differences in formulation, indications, and pharmacokinetics.

Drug Interactions

Avoid Concomitant Use There are no known interactions where it is recommended to avoid concomitant use.

Increased Effect/Toxicity

Gabapentin may increase the levels/effects of: Alcohol (Ethyl); CNS Depressants; Methotrimeprazine

The levels/effects of Gabapentin may be increased by: Droperidol; Methotrimeprazine

Decreased Effect

The levels/effects of Gabapentin may be decreased by: Antacids; Ketorolac; Ketorolac (Systemic); Mefloquine

Ethanol/Nutrition/Herb Interactions

Ethanol: May increase CNS depression; monitor for increased effects with coadministration. Caution patients about effects.

Food: Does not change rate or extent of absorption.

Herb/Nutraceutical: Avoid evening primrose (seizure threshold decreased). Avoid valerian, St John's wort, kava kava, gotu kola (may increase CNS depression).

Dietary Considerations May be taken without regard to meals.

Pharmacodynamics/Kinetics

Half-life Elimination 5-7 hours; anuria 132 hours; during dialysis 3.8 hours

Pregnancy Risk Factor C

Lactation Enters breast milk/use caution

Breast-Feeding Considerations Gabapentin is excreted in human breast milk. A nursed infant could be exposed to ~1 mg/kg/day of gabapentin; the effect on the child is not known. Use in breast-feeding women only if the benefits to the mother outweigh the potential risk to the infant.

Product Availability

Gralise™: FDA approved January 2011; availability expected in late 2011

Gralise™ is a once-daily formulation of gabapentin approved for the treatment of postherpetic neuralgia.

Dosage Forms

Capsule, oral: 100 mg, 300 mg, 400 mg

Neurontin®: 100 mg, 300 mg, 400 mg

Solution, oral: 250 mg/5 mL (470 mL)

Neurontin®: 250 mg/5 mL (470 mL)

Tablet, oral: 600 mg, 800 mg

Neurontin®: 600 mg, 800 mg

References

Laird MA and Gidal BE, "Use of Gabapentin in the Treatment of Neuropathic Pain," *Ann Pharmacother*, 2000, 34(6):802-7.

Rose MA and Kam PCA, "Gabapentin: Pharmacology and Its Use in Pain Management," *Anaesthesia*, 2002, 57:451-62.

Rosenberg JM, Harrell C, Ristic H, et al, "The Effect of Gabapentin on Neuropathic Pain," *Clin J Pain*, 1997, 13(3):251-5.

Rowbotham M, Harden N, Stacey B, et al, "Gabapentin for the Treatment of Postherpetic Neuralgia: A Randomized Controlled Trial," *JAMA*, 1998, 280(21):1837-42.

Gadopentetate Dimeglumine (gad oh PEN te tate dye MEG loo meen)

U.S. Brand Names Magnevist®

Canadian Brand Names Magnevist®

Pharmacologic Category Gadolinium-Containing Contrast Agent; Radiological/Contrast Media, Ionic (High Osmolality); Radiological/Contrast Media, Paramagnetic Agent

Use Contrast medium for magnetic resonance imaging (MRI) to visualize lesions with abnormal vascularity in the brain, spine and associated tissues, head and neck, and body (excluding the heart)

Local Anesthetic/Vasoconstrictor Precautions No information available to require special precautions

Effects on Dental Treatment No significant effects or complications reported

Effects on Bleeding No information available to require special precautions

Adverse Effects 1% to 10%:

Central nervous system: Headache (5%), dizziness (1%)

Gastrointestinal: Nausea (3%)

Local: Injection site coldness/localized coldness (2%)

General Dosage Range I.V.: *Children ≥2 years and Adults:* 0.1 mmol/kg (0.2 mL/kg)

Mechanism of Action Exposure to an external magnetic field induces a large local magnetic field in gadopentetate exposed tissues. This local magnetism disrupts water protons in the vicinity, resulting in a change in proton density and spin characteristics, which can be detected by the imaging device.

Pharmacodynamics/Kinetics

Half-life Elimination 1.5-1.7 hours

Pregnancy Risk Factor C

Gadoteridol (gad oh TER i dol)

U.S. Brand Names ProHance®; ProHance® Multipack™

Pharmacologic Category Gadolinium-Containing Contrast Agent; Radiological/Contrast Media, Nonionic (Low Osmolality); Radiological/Contrast Media, Paramagnetic Agent

Use Contrast medium for magnetic resonance imaging (MRI) to visualize CNS lesions with abnormal vascularity in the brain, spine, and associated tissues and to visualize extracranial/extraspinal tissues in the head and neck

Local Anesthetic/Vasoconstrictor Precautions No information available to require special precautions

Effects on Dental Treatment No significant effects or complications reported

Effects on Bleeding No information available to require special precautions

Adverse Effects 1% to 10%: Gastrointestinal: Nausea (1%), taste perversion (1%)

General Dosage Range I.V.:

Children ≥2 years: 0.1 mmol/kg (0.2 mL/kg)

Adults: 0.1 mmol/kg (0.2 mL/kg); a second dose of 0.2 mmol/kg (0.4 mL/kg) may be repeated once if needed [CNS imaging]

Mechanism of Action Gadoteridol is a gadolinium-containing paramagnetic agent. Exposure to an external magnetic field induces a large local magnetic field in exposed tissues. This local magnetism disrupts water protons in the vicinity, resulting in a change in proton density and spin characteristics, which can be detected by the imaging device.

Pharmacodynamics/Kinetics
Half-life Elimination 1.49-1.65 hours
Pregnancy Risk Factor C

Galantamine (ga LAN ta meen)

U.S. Brand Names Razadyne®; Razadyne® ER
Canadian Brand Names Mylan-Galantamine ER; PAT-Galantamine ER; Reminyl®; Reminyl® ER
Pharmacologic Category Acetylcholinesterase Inhibitor (Central)
Use Treatment of mild-to-moderate dementia of Alzheimer's disease
Unlabeled/Investigational Use Severe dementia associated with Alzheimer's disease; mild-to-moderate dementia associated with Parkinson's disease; Lewy body dementia
Local Anesthetic/Vasoconstrictor Precautions No information available to require special precautions
Effects on Dental Treatment No significant effects or complications reported
Effects on Bleeding No information available to require special precautions
Adverse Effects
>10%: Gastrointestinal: Nausea (6% to 24%), vomiting (4% to 13%), diarrhea (6% to 12%)
1% to 10%:
Cardiovascular: Bradycardia (2% to 3%), syncope (0.4% to 2.2%: dose related), chest pain (≥1%)
Central nervous system: Dizziness (9%), headache (8%), depression (7%), fatigue (5%), insomnia (5%), somnolence (4%)
Gastrointestinal: Anorexia (7% to 9%), weight loss (5% to 7%), abdominal pain (5%), dyspepsia (5%), flatulence (≥1%)
Genitourinary: Urinary tract infection (8%), hematuria (<1% to 3%), incontinence (≥1%)
Hematologic: Anemia (3%)
Neuromuscular & skeletal: Tremor (3%)
Respiratory: Rhinitis (4%)
General Dosage Range Dosage adjustment recommended in patients with hepatic or renal impairment
Oral:
Extended-release: *Adults:* Initial: 8 mg once daily; Maintenance: 16-24 mg once daily
Immediate release: *Adults:* Initial: 4 mg twice daily; Maintenance: 16-24 mg/day in 2 divided doses
Mechanism of Action Centrally-acting cholinesterase inhibitor (competitive and reversible). It elevates acetylcholine in cerebral cortex by slowing the degradation of acetylcholine. Modulates nicotinic acetylcholine receptor to increase acetylcholine from surviving presynaptic nerve terminals. May increase glutamate and serotonin levels.
Pharmacodynamics/Kinetics
Duration of Action 3 hours; maximum inhibition of erythrocyte acetylcholinesterase ~40% at 1 hour post 8 mg oral dose; levels return to baseline at 30 hours
Half-life Elimination 7 hours
Time to Peak Immediate release: 1 hour (2.5 hours with food); extended release: 4.5-5 hours
Pregnancy Risk Factor B

Gallium Nitrate (GAL ee um NYE trate)

U.S. Brand Names Ganite™
Pharmacologic Category Calcium-Lowering Agent
Use Treatment of symptomatic cancer-related hypercalcemia
Local Anesthetic/Vasoconstrictor Precautions No information available to require special precautions
Effects on Dental Treatment No significant effects or complications reported
Effects on Bleeding Although significant myelosuppression with associated altered hemostasis has been reported for many chemotherapeutic agents, myelosuppression is not common with gallium nitrate and no specific precautions appear to necessary.
Adverse Effects Frequency not always defined.
Cardiovascular: Edema (lower extremity), hypotension, tachycardia
Central nervous system: Coma, confusion, dreams, encephalopathy, fever, hallucinations, hypothermia, lethargy

Dermatologic: Rash
Endocrine & metabolic: Hypophosphatemia (up to 79%), serum bicarbonate decreased (40% to 50%), hypocalcemia (38%), respiratory alkalosis (mild)
Hematologic: Anemia, leukopenia
Gastrointestinal: Constipation, diarrhea, nausea, vomiting
Neuromuscular & skeletal: Paresthesia, positive Cvostek's sign
Ocular: Optic neuritis
Otic: Auditory acuity decreased (<1%), tinnitus (<1%), hearing decreased
Renal: BUN increased (13%), creatinine increased (13%), acute renal failure
Respiratory: Dyspnea, pleural effusion, pulmonary infiltrates, rales, rhonchi

General Dosage Range I.V.: *Adults:* 100-200 mg/m^2/day

Mechanism of Action Inhibits bone resorption by inhibiting osteoclast function. Gallium nitrate appears to be effective in parathyroid hormone-related protein (PTHrP) and non-PTHrP-associated hypercalcemia.

Pharmacodynamics/Kinetics

Onset of Action Onset of calcium lowering: Seen within 24-48 hours of beginning therapy, with normocalcemia achieved within 4-7 days of beginning therapy

Duration of Action Normocalcemia: 7-10 days

Half-life Elimination Alpha: 1.25 hours; Beta: ~24 hours

Elimination half-life varies with method of administration (72-115 hours with prolonged intravenous infusion versus 24 hours with bolus administration); long elimination half-life may be related to slow release from tissue such as bone

Pregnancy Risk Factor C

Galsulfase (gal SUL fase)

U.S. Brand Names Naglazyme®

Pharmacologic Category Enzyme

Use Replacement therapy in mucopolysaccharidosis VI (MPS VI; Maroteaux-Lamy Syndrome) for improvement of walking and stair-climbing capacity

Local Anesthetic/Vasoconstrictor Precautions No information available to require special precautions

Effects on Dental Treatment No significant effects or complications reported

Effects on Bleeding No information available to require special precautions

Adverse Effects Note: Percentages reported are from a placebo-controlled study (39 patients, 19 on galsulfase); also included are adverse effects noted during other clinical studies.

Cardiovascular: Chest pain (16%), hypertension (11%)
Central nervous system: Pain (32%), chills (21%), malaise (11%), fever, headache
Dermatologic: Rash (21%), angioedema, pruritus, urticaria
Gastrointestinal: Abdominal pain (47%), gastroenteritis (11%), nausea, vomiting
Neuromuscular & skeletal: Arthralgia (42%), areflexia (11%)
Ocular: Conjunctivitis (21%), corneal opacification increased (11%)
Otic: Ear pain (42%), hearing impairment (11%)
Respiratory: Dyspnea (21%), pharyngitis (11%), nasal congestion (11%), laryngeal edema
Miscellaneous: Antigalsulfase antibodies (98%), infusion reactions (56%), umbilical hernia (11%)

General Dosage Range I.V.: *Children >5 years and Adults:* 1 mg/kg once weekly

Mechanism of Action Galsulfase is a recombinant form of N-acetylgalactosamine 4-sulfatase, produced in Chinese hamster cells. A deficiency of this enzyme leads to accumulation of the glycosaminoglycan dermatan sulfate in various tissues, causing progressive disease which includes decreased growth, skeletal deformities, upper airway obstruction, clouding of the cornea, heart disease, and coarse facial features. Replacement of this enzyme has been shown to improve mobility and physical function (measured by walking and stair-climbing).

Pharmacodynamics/Kinetics

Half-life Elimination

Week 1: Median 9 minutes (range: 6-21 minutes); Week 24: Median 26 minutes (range: 8-40 minutes)

Pregnancy Risk Factor B

Ganciclovir (Systemic) (gan SYE kloe veer)

Related Information

Systemic Viral Diseases *on page 1904*
ValGANciclovir *on page 1694*

U.S. Brand Names Cytovene®-IV

Canadian Brand Names Cytovene®

Generic Availability (U.S.) Yes

Pharmacologic Category Antiviral Agent

Use Treatment of CMV retinitis in immunocompromised individuals, including patients with acquired immunodeficiency syndrome; prophylaxis of CMV infection in transplant patients

Unlabeled/Investigational Use CMV retinitis: May be given in combination with foscarnet in patients who relapse after monotherapy with either drug

Local Anesthetic/Vasoconstrictor Precautions No information available to require special precautions

Effects on Dental Treatment No significant effects or complications reported

Effects on Bleeding May be associated with thrombocytopenia. No information available to require specific precautions.

Adverse Effects

>10%:

Central nervous system: Fever (48%)

Gastrointestinal: Diarrhea (44%), anorexia (14%), vomiting (13%)

Hematologic: Thrombocytopenia (57%), leukopenia (41%), anemia (16% to 26%), neutropenia with ANC <500/mm^3 (12% to 14%)

Ocular: Retinal detachment (11%; relationship to ganciclovir not established)

Renal: Serum creatinine increased (2% to 14%)

Miscellaneous: Sepsis (15%), diaphoresis (12%)

1% to 10%:

Central nervous system: Chills (10%), neuropathy (9%)

Dermatologic: Pruritus (5%)

<1%, postmarketing, and/or case reports (limited to important or life-threatening): Allergic reaction (including anaphylaxis), alopecia, arrhythmia, bronchospasm, cardiac arrest, cataracts, cholestasis, coma, dyspnea, edema, encephalopathy, exfoliative dermatitis, extrapyramidal symptoms, hepatitis, hepatic failure, pancreatitis, pancytopenia, pulmonary fibrosis, psychosis, rhabdomyolysis, seizure, alopecia, urticaria, eosinophilia, hemorrhage, Stevens-Johnson syndrome, torsade de pointes, renal failure, SIADH, visual loss

Dosage

CMV CNS infection in HIV-exposed/-infected patients (unlabeled use; CDC, 2009): Infants and Children: I.V.: 5 mg/kg/dose every 12 hours plus foscarnet until symptoms improve followed by chronic suppression

CMV retinitis:

I.V. (slow infusion): Children and Adults:

Induction therapy: 5 mg/kg/dose every 12 hours for 14-21 days followed by maintenance therapy

Maintenance therapy: 5 mg/kg/day as a single daily dose for 7 days/week or 6 mg/kg/day for 5 days/week

Prevention of CMV disease in HIV-exposed/-infected patients (unlabeled use; CDC, 2009): I.V.: Infants and Children: 5 mg/kg/dose daily

Prevention of CMV disease in transplant patients: I.V. (slow infusion): Children and Adults: Same initial and maintenance dose as CMV retinitis except duration of initial course is 7-14 days, duration of maintenance therapy is dependent on clinical condition and degree of immunosuppression

Varicella zoster: Progressive outer retinal necrosis in HIV-exposed/-infected patients (unlabeled use; CDC, 2009): Infants and Children: I.V.: 5 mg/kg/dose every 12 hours plus systemic foscarnet and intravitreal ganciclovir or intravitreal foscarnet

Elderly: Refer to adult dosing; in general, dose selection should be cautious, reflecting greater frequency of organ impairment

Dosing adjustment in renal impairment:

I.V. (Induction):

Cl_{cr} 50-69 mL/minute: Administer 2.5 mg/kg/dose every 12 hours

Cl_{cr} 25-49 mL/minute: Administer 2.5 mg/kg/dose every 24 hours

Cl_{cr} 10-24 mL/minute: Administer 1.25 mg/kg/dose every 24 hours

Cl_{cr} <10 mL/minute: Administer 1.25 mg/kg/dose 3 times/week following hemodialysis

I.V. (Maintenance):

Cl_{cr} 50-69 mL/minute: Administer 2.5 mg/kg/dose every 24 hours

Cl_{cr} 25-49 mL/minute: Administer 1.25 mg/kg/dose every 24 hours

Cl_{cr} 10-24 mL/minute: Administer 0.625 mg/kg/dose every 24 hours

Cl_{cr} <10 mL/minute: Administer 0.625 mg/kg/dose 3 times/week following hemodialysis

Hemodialysis effects: Dialyzable (50%) following hemodialysis; administer dose postdialysis. During peritoneal dialysis, dose as for Cl_{cr} <10 mL/minute. During continuous arteriovenous or venovenous hemofiltration, administer 2.5 mg/kg/dose every 24 hours.

Mechanism of Action Ganciclovir is phosphorylated to a substrate which competitively inhibits the binding of deoxyguanosine triphosphate to DNA polymerase resulting in inhibition of viral DNA synthesis

Contraindications Hypersensitivity to ganciclovir, acyclovir, or any component of the formulation

Warnings/Precautions Hazardous agent - use appropriate precautions for handling and disposal. **[U.S. Boxed Warning]: Granulocytopenia (neutropenia), anemia, and thrombocytopenia may occur.** Dosage adjustment or interruption of ganciclovir therapy may be necessary in patients with neutropenia and/or thrombocytopenia and patients with impaired renal function. **[U.S. Boxed Warning]: Animal studies have demonstrated carcinogenic and teratogenic effects, and inhibition of spermatogenesis;** contraceptive precautions for female and male patients need to be followed during and for at least 90 days after therapy with the drug; take care to administer only into veins with good blood flow. **[U.S. Boxed Warning]: Indicated only for treatment of CMV retinitis in the immunocompromised patient and CMV prevention in transplant patients at risk.**

Drug Interactions

Avoid Concomitant Use

Avoid concomitant use of Ganciclovir (Systemic) with any of the following: Imipenem

Increased Effect/Toxicity

Ganciclovir (Systemic) may increase the levels/effects of: Imipenem; Mycophenolate; Reverse Transcriptase Inhibitors (Nucleoside); Tenofovir

The levels/effects of Ganciclovir (Systemic) may be increased by: Mycophenolate; Probenecid; Tenofovir

Decreased Effect There are no known significant interactions involving a decrease in effect.

Dietary Considerations Some products may contain sodium.

Pharmacodynamics/Kinetics

Half-life Elimination 1.7-5.8 hours; prolonged with renal impairment; End-stage renal disease: 5-28 hours

Pregnancy Risk Factor C

Lactation Excretion in breast milk unknown/not recommended

Breast-Feeding Considerations Due to the carcinogenic and teratogenic effects observed in animal studies, the possibility of adverse events in a nursing infant is considered likely. Therefore, nursing should be discontinued during therapy. In addition, the CDC recommends **not** to breast-feed if diagnosed with HIV to avoid postnatal transmission of the virus.

Dosage Forms

Injection, powder for reconstitution: 500 mg

Cytovene®-IV: 500 mg

Ganirelix (ga ni REL ix)

Canadian Brand Names Orgalutran®

Pharmacologic Category Gonadotropin Releasing Hormone Antagonist

Use Inhibits premature luteinizing hormone (LH) surges in women undergoing controlled ovarian hyperstimulation

Local Anesthetic/Vasoconstrictor Precautions No information available to require special precautions

Effects on Dental Treatment No significant effects or complications reported

Effects on Bleeding No information available to require special precautions

Adverse Effects 1% to 10%:

Central nervous system: Headache (3%)

Endocrine & metabolic: Ovarian hyperstimulation syndrome (2%)

Gastrointestinal: Abdominal pain (1%), nausea (1%)

Genitourinary: Pelvic pain (5%), vaginal bleeding (2%)

Local: Injection site reaction (1%)

General Dosage Range SubQ: *Adults:* 250 mcg/day

Mechanism of Action Competitively blocks the gonadotropin-release hormone receptors on the pituitary gonadotroph and transduction pathway. This suppresses gonadotropin secretion and luteinizing hormone secretion preventing ovulation until the follicles are of adequate size.

Pharmacodynamics/Kinetics

Duration of Action <48 hours

Half-life Elimination Single dose: 12.8 hours; Multiple dosing: 16.2 hours

Time to Peak 1.1 hours

Pregnancy Risk Factor X

Gatifloxacin (gat i FLOKS a sin)

Related Information

Bacterial Infections *on page 1933*

Respiratory Diseases *on page 1876*

U.S. Brand Names Zymar® [DSC]; Zymaxid™

Canadian Brand Names Zymar®

Generic Availability (U.S.) No

Pharmacologic Category Antibiotic, Ophthalmic; Antibiotic, Quinolone

Use Treatment of bacterial conjunctivitis

Local Anesthetic/Vasoconstrictor Precautions Gatifloxacin is one of the drugs confirmed to prolong the QT interval and is accepted as having a risk of causing torsade de pointes. The risk of drug-induced torsade de pointes is extremely low when a single QT interval prolonging drug is prescribed. In terms of epinephrine, it is not known what effect vasoconstrictors in the local anesthetic regimen will have in patients with a known history of congenital prolonged QT interval or in patients taking any medication that prolongs the QT interval. Until more information is obtained, it is suggested that the clinician consult with the physician prior to the use of a vasoconstrictor in suspected patients, and that the vasoconstrictor (epinephrine, mepivacaine and levonordefrin [Carbocaine® 2% with Neo-Cobefrin®]) be used with caution.

Effects on Dental Treatment Key adverse event(s) related to dental treatment: Taste disturbance.

Effects on Bleeding No information available to require special precautions

Adverse Effects 1% to 10%:

Central nervous system: Headache

Gastrointestinal: Taste disturbance

Ocular: Chemosis, conjunctival hemorrhage, conjunctival irritation, discharge, dry eye, edema, irritation, keratitis, lacrimation increased, pain, papillary conjunctivitis, visual acuity decreased

Dosage Ophthalmic: Children ≥1 year and Adults: Bacterial conjunctivitis:

Zymar®:

Days 1 and 2: Instill 1 drop into affected eye(s) every 2 hours while awake (maximum: 8 times/day)

Days 3-7: Instill 1 drop into affected eye(s) up to 4 times/day while awake

Zymaxid™:

Day 1: Instill 1 drop into affected eye(s) every 2 hours while awake (maximum: 8 times/day)

Days 2-7: Instill 1 drop into affected eye(s) 2-4 times/day while awake

Mechanism of Action Gatifloxacin is a DNA gyrase inhibitor, and also inhibits topoisomerase IV. DNA gyrase (topoisomerase II) is an essential bacterial enzyme that maintains the superhelical structure of DNA. DNA gyrase is required for DNA replication and transcription, DNA repair, recombination, and transposition; inhibition is bactericidal.

Contraindications

Zymar®: Hypersensitivity to gatifloxacin, other quinolone antibiotics, or any component of the formulation

Zymaxid™: There are no contraindications listed in the manufacturer's labeling.

Warnings/Precautions Severe hypersensitivity reactions, including anaphylaxis, have occurred with systemic quinolone therapy. Reactions may present as typical allergic symptoms after a single dose, or may manifest as severe idiosyncratic dermatologic, vascular, pulmonary, renal, hepatic, and/or hematologic events, usually after multiple doses. Prompt discontinuation of drug should occur if skin rash or other symptoms arise. Prolonged use may result in fungal or bacterial superinfection. For topical ophthalmic use only. Do not inject ophthalmic solution subconjunctivally or introduce directly into the anterior chamber of the eye. Contact lenses should not be worn during treatment of ophthalmic infections.

Drug Interactions

Avoid Concomitant Use There are no known interactions where it is recommended to avoid concomitant use.

Increased Effect/Toxicity There are no known significant interactions involving an increase in effect.

Decreased Effect There are no known significant interactions involving a decrease in effect.

Pregnancy Risk Factor C

Lactation Excretion in breast milk unknown/use caution

Breast-Feeding Considerations Other quinolones are known to be excreted in breast milk. The manufacturer recommends using caution if gatifloxacin is administered while nursing.

Dosage Forms

Solution, ophthalmic:

Zymaxid™: 0.5% (2.5 mL)

Dental Comment Gatifloxacin is known to prolong the QT interval. The QT interval is measured as the time and distance between the Q point of the QRS complex and the end of the T wave in the ECG tracing. After adjustment for heart rate, the QT interval is defined as prolonged if it is more than 450 msec in men and 460 msec in women. A long QT syndrome was first described in the 1950s and 60s as a congenital syndrome involving QT interval prolongation and syncope and sudden death. Some of the congenital long QT syndromes were characterized by a peculiar electrocardiographic appearance of the QRS complex involving a premature atria beat followed by a pause, then a subsequent sinus beat showing marked QT prolongation and deformity. This type of cardiac arrhythmia was originally termed "torsade de pointes" (translated from the French as "twisting of the points"). Gatifloxacin is considered as having a risk of causing torsade de pointes. Since it is not known what effect vasoconstrictors in the local anesthetic regimen will have in patients with a known history of congenital prolonged QT interval or in patients taking any medication that prolongs the QT interval, a medical consult is suggested.

Gefitinib (ge FI tye nib)

U.S. Brand Names Iressa®

Canadian Brand Names IRESSA®

Pharmacologic Category Antineoplastic Agent, Tyrosine Kinase Inhibitor

Use Treatment of locally advanced or metastatic nonsmall cell lung cancer (NSCLC) after failure of platinum-based and docetaxel therapies. Treatment is limited to patients who are benefiting or have benefited from treatment with gefitinib.

Note: Due to the lack of improved survival data from clinical trials of gefitinib, and in response to positive survival data with another EGFR inhibitor, according to the U.S. labeling, physicians are advised to use treatment options other than gefitinib in patients with advanced nonsmall cell lung cancer following one or two prior chemotherapy regimens when they are refractory/intolerant to their most recent regimen.

Canada labeling: First-line treatment of locally advanced or metastatic NSCLC with activating mutations of EGFR-TK

Unlabeled/Investigational Use First-line treatment of NSCLC with known EGFR mutation

Local Anesthetic/Vasoconstrictor Precautions No information available to require special precautions

Effects on Dental Treatment Key adverse event(s) related to dental treatment: Mouth ulceration.

Effects on Bleeding Although significant myelosuppression with associated altered hemostasis has been reported for many chemotherapeutic agents, myelosuppression is not common with gefitinib and no specific precautions appear to necessary.

Adverse Effects

>10%:

- Dermatologic: Rash (43% to 54%), acne (25% to 33%), dry skin (13% to 26%), paronychia (14%)
- Gastrointestinal: Diarrhea (48% to 67%; grade 3: 1%), nausea (13% to 18%), vomiting (9% to 12%)

1% to 10%:

- Cardiovascular: Peripheral edema (2%)
- Dermatologic: Pruritus (8% to 9%)
- Gastrointestinal: Anorexia (7% to 10%), weight loss (3% to 5%), mouth ulceration (1%)
- Neuromuscular & skeletal: Weakness (4% to 6%)
- Ocular: Amblyopia (2%), conjunctivitis (1%)
- Respiratory: Dyspnea (2%), interstitial lung disease (1% to 2%; includes alveolitis, interstitial pneumonia, pneumonitis)

General Dosage Range Dosage adjustment recommended in patients on concomitant therapy or who develop toxicities.

Oral: *Adults:* 250 mg once daily

Mechanism of Action Gefitinib is a tyrosine kinase inhibitor (TKI) which inhibits numerous tyrosine kinases associated with transmembrane cell surface receptors found on both normal and cancer cells, including the tyrosine kinase associated with the epidermal growth factor receptor, EGFR. Tyrosine kinase activity appears to be vitally important to cell proliferation and survival.

Pharmacodynamics/Kinetics

Half-life Elimination Oral: 41 hours

Time to Peak Plasma: Oral: 3-7 hours

Pregnancy Risk Factor D

Prescribing and Access Restrictions As of September 15, 2005, distribution of gefitinib (IRESSA®) is limited to patients enrolled in the IRESSA® Access Program. Under this program, access to gefitinib will be limited to the following groups:

- Patients who are currently receiving and benefiting from gefitinib
- Patients who have previously received and benefited from gefitinib
- Previously-enrolled patients or new patients in non-Investigational New Drug (IND) clinical trials involving gefitinib if these protocols were approved by an IRB prior to June 17, 2005
- New patients may also receive gefitinib if the manufacturer (AstraZeneca) decides to make it available under IND, and the patients meet the criteria for enrollment under the IND

Additional information on the IRESSA® Access Program, including enrollment forms, may be obtained by calling AstraZeneca at 1-800-601-8933 or via the web at www.Iressa-access.com

Gelatin (Absorbable) (JEL a tin, ab SORB a ble)

Related Information

Antiplatelet and Anticoagulation Considerations in Dentistry *on page 1867*

U.S. Brand Names Gelfilm®; Gelfoam®

Generic Availability (U.S.) No

Pharmacologic Category Hemostatic Agent

Dental Use Adjunct to provide hemostasis in oral and dental surgery

Use Adjunct to provide hemostasis in surgery; open prostatic surgery

Local Anesthetic/Vasoconstrictor Precautions No information available to require special precautions

Effects on Dental Treatment Key adverse event(s) related to dental treatment: Local infection and abscess formation.

Effects on Bleeding Used as adjunct to enhance hemostasis.

Adverse Effects 1% to 10%: Local: Infection and abscess formation

Dosage Hemostasis: Apply packs or sponges dry or saturated with sodium chloride. When applied dry, hold in place with moderate pressure. When applied wet, squeeze to remove air bubbles. The powder is applied as a paste prepared by adding approximately 4 mL of sterile saline solution to the powder.

Contraindications Should not be used in closure of skin incisions since they may interfere with the healing of skin edges

Warnings/Precautions Do not sterilize by heat; do not use in the presence of infection

Drug Interactions

Avoid Concomitant Use There are no known interactions where it is recommended to avoid concomitant use.

Increased Effect/Toxicity There are no known significant interactions involving an increase in effect.

Decreased Effect There are no known significant interactions involving a decrease in effect.

Pregnancy Risk Factor No data reported

Dosage Forms

Film, ophthalmic:

Gelfilm®: (6s)

Film, topical:

Gelfilm®: (1s)

Powder, topical:

Gelfoam®: (1 g)

Sponge, oral, topical:

Gelfoam®: (12s)

Sponge, topical:

Gelfoam®: (4s, 6s, 12s)

Gemcitabine (jem SITE a been)

U.S. Brand Names Gemzar®

Canadian Brand Names Gemcitabine For Injection, USP; Gemzar®

Pharmacologic Category Antineoplastic Agent, Antimetabolite (Pyrimidine Analog)

Use Treatment of metastatic breast cancer; inoperable locally-advanced or metastatic nonsmall cell lung cancer (NSCLC); locally advanced or metastatic pancreatic cancer; advanced, relapsed ovarian cancer

Unlabeled/Investigational Use Treatment of biliary tract cancers (advanced), bladder cancer, cervical cancer (recurrent or persistent), Ewing's sarcoma (refractory), head and neck cancer (nasopharyngeal), Hodgkin's lymphoma (relapsed), non-Hodgkin's lymphomas (refractory), malignant pleural mesothelioma, osteosarcoma (refractory), renal cell cancer (metastatic), small cell lung cancer (refractory or relapsed), soft tissue sarcoma (advanced), testicular cancer (refractory germ cell tumors), thymic malignancies, uterine sarcoma, and unknown-primary adenocarcinoma

Local Anesthetic/Vasoconstrictor Precautions No information available to require special precautions

Effects on Dental Treatment Key adverse event(s) related to dental treatment: Stomatitis.

Effects on Bleeding Chemotherapy may result in significant myelosuppression, potentially including significant reduction in platelet counts and altered hemostasis. In patients who are under active treatment with these agents, medical consult is suggested.

Adverse Effects Frequency of adverse reactions reported for single-agent use of gemcitabine only.

>10%:

Cardiovascular: Peripheral edema (20%), edema (13%)
Central nervous system: Fever (38% to 41%), somnolence (11%)
Dermatologic: Rash (28% to 30%), alopecia (15% to 16%), pruritus (13%)
Gastrointestinal: Nausea/vomiting (69% to 71%; grade 3: 10% to 13%; grade 4: 1% to 2%), diarrhea (19% to 30%), stomatitis (10% to 11%)
Hematologic: Anemia (68% to 73%; grade 4: 1% to 2%), leukopenia (62% to 64%; grade 4: ≤1%), neutropenia (61% to 63%; grade 4: 6% to 7%), thrombocytopenia (24% to 36%; grade 4: ≤1%), hemorrhage (4% to 17%; grades 3: ≤2%; grade 4: <1%); myelosuppression is the dose-limiting toxicity
Hepatic: AST increased (67% to 78%; grade 3: 6% to 12%; grade 4: 2% to 5%), alkaline phosphatase increased (55% to 77%; grade 3: 7% to 16%; grade 4: 2% to 4%), ALT increased (68% to 72%; grade 3: 8% to 10%; grade 4: 1% to 2%), bilirubin increased (13% to 26%; grade 3: 2% to 6%; grade 4: ≤2%)
Renal: (32% to 45%; grades 3/4: <1%), hematuria (23% to 35%; grades 3/4: <1%), BUN increased (15% to 16%)
Respiratory: Dyspnea (10% to 23%)
Miscellaneous: Flu-like syndrome (19%), infection (10% to 16%; grade 3: 1% to 2%; grade 4: <1%)

1% to 10%:

Local: Injection site reactions (4%)
Neuromuscular & skeletal: Paresthesia (10%)
Renal: Creatinine increased (6% to 8%)
Respiratory: Bronchospasm (<2%)

General Dosage Range Dosage adjustment recommended in patients with hepatic impairment or who develop toxicities

I.V.: *Adults:* Dosage varies greatly depending on indication

Mechanism of Action A pyrimidine antimetabolite that inhibits DNA synthesis by inhibition of DNA polymerase and ribonucleotide reductase, specific for the S-phase of the cycle. Gemcitabine is phosphorylated intracellularly by deoxycytidine kinase to gemcitabine monophosphate, which is further phosphorylated to active metabolites gemcitabine diphosphate and gemcitabine triphosphate. Gemcitabine diphosphate inhibits DNA synthesis by inhibiting ribonucleotide reductase; gemcitabine triphosphate incorporates into DNA and inhibits DNA polymerase.

Pharmacodynamics/Kinetics

Half-life Elimination

Gemcitabine: Infusion time ≤70 minutes: 42-94 minutes; infusion time 3-4 hours: 4-10.5 hours
Metabolite (gemcitabine triphosphate), terminal phase: 1.7-19.4 hours

Time to Peak 30 minutes after completion of infusion

Pregnancy Risk Factor D

Gemfibrozil (jem FI broe zil)

Related Information

Cardiovascular Diseases *on page* 1848

U.S. Brand Names Lopid®

Canadian Brand Names Apo-Gemfibrozil®; Gen-Gemfibrozil; GMD-Gemfibrozil; Lopid®; Mylan-Gemfibrozil; Novo-Gemfibrozil; Nu-Gemfibrozil; PMS-Gemfibrozil

Generic Availability (U.S.) Yes

Pharmacologic Category Antilipemic Agent, Fibric Acid

Use Treatment of hypertriglyceridemia in Fredrickson types IV and V hyperlipidemia for patients who are at greater risk for pancreatitis and who have not responded to dietary intervention; to reduce the risk of CHD development in Fredrickson type IIb patients without a history or symptoms of existing CHD who have not responded to dietary and other interventions (including pharmacologic treatment) and who have decreased HDL, increased LDL, and increased triglycerides

Local Anesthetic/Vasoconstrictor Precautions No information available to require special precautions

Effects on Dental Treatment No significant effects or complications reported

Effects on Bleeding No information available to require special precautions

Adverse Effects

>10%: Gastrointestinal: Dyspepsia (20%)

1% to 10%:

Cardiovascular: Atrial fibrillation (1%)

Central nervous system: Fatigue (4%), vertigo (2%)

Dermatologic: Eczema (2%), rash (2%)

Gastrointestinal: Abdominal pain (10%), nausea/vomiting (3%)

Reports where causal relationship has not been established: Alopecia, anaphylaxis, cataracts, colitis, confusion, decreased fertility (male), drug-induced lupus-like syndrome, extrasystoles, hepatoma, intracranial hemorrhage, pancreatitis, peripheral vascular disease, photosensitivity, positive ANA, renal dysfunction, retinal edema, seizure, syncope, thrombocytopenia, vasculitis, weight loss

Dosage Adults: Oral: 600 mg twice daily; administer 30 minutes before breakfast and dinner

Dosage adjustment in renal impairment:

Mild-to-moderate impairment: Use caution; deterioration of renal function has been reported in patients with baseline serum creatinine >2 mg/dL

Severe impairment: Use is contraindicated

Hemodialysis: Not removed by hemodialysis; supplemental dose is not necessary

Dosage adjustment in hepatic impairment: Use is contraindicated

Mechanism of Action The exact mechanism of action of gemfibrozil is unknown, however, several theories exist regarding the VLDL effect; it can inhibit lipolysis and decrease subsequent hepatic fatty acid uptake as well as inhibit hepatic secretion of VLDL; together these actions decrease serum VLDL levels; increases HDL-cholesterol; the mechanism behind HDL elevation is currently unknown

Contraindications Hypersensitivity to gemfibrozil or any component of the formulation; hepatic or severe renal dysfunction; primary biliary cirrhosis; pre-existing gallbladder disease; concurrent use with repaglinide

Warnings/Precautions Secondary causes of hyperlipidemia should be ruled out prior to therapy. Possible increased risk of malignancy and cholelithiasis. Anemia, leukopenia, thrombocytopenia, and bone marrow hypoplasia have rarely been reported. Periodic monitoring recommended during the first year of therapy. Elevations in serum transaminases can be seen. Discontinue if lipid response not seen. Be careful in patient selection; this is not a first- or second-line choice. Other agents may be more suitable. Adjustments in warfarin therapy may be required with concurrent use. Has been associated with rare myositis or rhabdomyolysis; patients should be monitored closely. Patients should be instructed to report unexplained muscle pain, tenderness, weakness, or brown urine. Use caution when combining gemfibrozil with HMG-CoA reductase inhibitors (may lead to myopathy, rhabdomyolysis). Use with caution in patients with mild-to-moderate renal impairment; contraindicated in patients with severe impairment. Renal function deterioration has been seen when used in patients with a serum creatinine >2 mg/dL.

Drug Interactions

Metabolism/Transport Effects **Substrate** of CYP3A4 (minor); **Inhibits** CYP1A2 (moderate), 2C8 (strong), 2C9 (strong), 2C19 (strong)

Avoid Concomitant Use

Avoid concomitant use of Gemfibrozil with any of the following: Clopidogrel; Repaglinide

Increased Effect/Toxicity

Gemfibrozil may increase the levels/effects of: Antidiabetic Agents (Thiazolidinedione); Atorvastatin; Carvedilol; Colchicine; CYP1A2 Substrates; CYP2C19 Substrates; CYP2C8 Substrates (High risk); CYP2C9 Substrates (High risk); Ezetimibe; Fluvastatin; Lovastatin; Pitavastatin; Pravastatin; Repaglinide; Rosuvastatin; Simvastatin; Sulfonylureas; Treprostinil; Vitamin K Antagonists

The levels/effects of Gemfibrozil may be increased by: Conivaptan; CycloSPORINE; CycloSPORINE (Systemic)

Decreased Effect

Gemfibrozil may decrease the levels/effects of: Chenodiol; Clopidogrel; CycloSPORINE; CycloSPORINE (Systemic); Ursodiol

The levels/effects of Gemfibrozil may be decreased by: Bile Acid Sequestrants; Tocilizumab

Ethanol/Nutrition/Herb Interactions

Ethanol: Avoid ethanol to decrease triglycerides.

Food: When given after meals, the AUC of gemfibrozil is decreased.

Dietary Considerations Before initiation of therapy, patients should be placed on a standard cholesterol-lowering diet for 3-6 months and the diet should be continued during drug therapy. Should be taken 30 minutes prior to breakfast and dinner

Pharmacodynamics/Kinetics

Onset of Action May require several days

Half-life Elimination 1.5 hours

Time to Peak Serum: 1-2 hours

Pregnancy Risk Factor C

Lactation Excretion in breast milk unknown/not recommended

Dosage Forms

Tablet, oral: 600 mg

Lopid®: 600 mg

Gemifloxacin (je mi FLOKS a sin)

Related Information

Bacterial Infections *on page 1933*

U.S. Brand Names Factive®

Canadian Brand Names Factive®

Generic Availability (U.S.) No

Pharmacologic Category Antibiotic, Quinolone; Respiratory Fluoroquinolone

Use Treatment of acute exacerbation of chronic bronchitis; treatment of community-acquired pneumonia (CAP), including pneumonia caused by multidrug-resistant strains of *S. pneumoniae* (MDRSP)

Unlabeled/Investigational Use Acute sinusitis

Local Anesthetic/Vasoconstrictor Precautions No information available to require special precautions

Effects on Dental Treatment No significant effects or complications reported

Effects on Bleeding No information available to require special precautions

Adverse Effects 1% to 10%:

Central nervous system: Headache (4%), dizziness (2%)

Dermatologic: Rash (4%)

Gastrointestinal: Diarrhea (5%), nausea (4%), abdominal pain (2%), vomiting (2%)

Hepatic: Transaminases increased (1% to 4%)

Important adverse effects reported with other agents in this drug class include (not reported for gemifloxacin): Allergic reactions, CNS stimulation, hepatitis, jaundice, peripheral neuropathy, pneumonitis (eosinophilic), seizure; sensorimotor-axonal neuropathy (paresthesia, hypoesthesias, dysesthesias, weakness); severe dermatologic reactions (toxic epidermal necrolysis, Stevens-Johnson syndrome); torsade de pointes, vasculitis

Dosage

Usual dosage range:

Adults: Oral: 320 mg once daily

Indication-specific dosing:

Adults: Oral:

Acute exacerbations of chronic bronchitis: 320 mg once daily for 5 days

Community-acquired pneumonia (mild-to-moderate): 320 mg once daily for 5 or 7 days (decision to use 5- or 7-day regimen should be guided by initial sputum culture; 7 days are recommended for MDRSP, *Klebsiella*, or *M. catarrhalis* infection)

Sinusitis (unlabeled use): 320 mg once daily for 10 days

Elderly: Refer to adult dosing.

Dosage adjustment in renal impairment:

Cl_{cr} >40 mL/minute: No adjustment required

Cl_{cr} ≤40 mL/minute (or patients on hemodialysis/CAPD): 160 mg once daily (administer dose following hemodialysis)

Dosage adjustment in hepatic impairment: No adjustment required

Mechanism of Action Gemifloxacin is a DNA gyrase inhibitor and also inhibits topoisomerase IV. DNA gyrase (topoisomerase IV) is an essential bacterial enzyme that maintains the superhelical structure of DNA. DNA gyrase is required for DNA replication and transcription, DNA repair, recombination, and transposition; bactericidal

Contraindications Hypersensitivity to gemifloxacin, other fluoroquinolones, or any component of the formulation

Warnings/Precautions **[U.S. Boxed Warning]: There have been reports of tendon inflammation and/or rupture with quinolone antibiotics; risk may be increased with concurrent corticosteroids, organ transplant recipients, and in patients >60 years of age.** Rupture of the Achilles tendon sometimes requiring surgical repair has been reported most frequently; but other tendon sites (eg, rotator cuff, biceps) have also been reported. Strenuous physical activity, rheumatoid arthritis, and renal impairment may be an independent risk factor for tendonitis. Discontinue at first sign of tendon inflammation or pain. May occur even after discontinuation of therapy. Use with caution in patients with rheumatoid arthritis; may increase risk of tendon rupture. Fluoroquinolones may prolong QT_c interval; avoid use of gemifloxacin in patients with a history of QT_c prolongation, uncorrected hypokalemia, hypomagnesemia, or concurrent administration of other medications known to prolong the QT interval (including Class Ia and Class III antiarrhythmics, cisapride, erythromycin, antipsychotics, and tricyclic antidepressants). Use with caution in patients with significant bradycardia or acute myocardial ischemia. Use with caution in individuals at risk of seizures (CNS disorders or concurrent therapy with medications which may lower seizure threshold). Potential for seizures, although very rare, may be increased with concomitant NSAID therapy. Discontinue in patients who experience significant CNS adverse effects (dizziness, hallucinations, suicidal ideation or actions). Use caution in renal dysfunction; dosage adjustment required for Cl_{cr} ≤40 mL/minute.

Fluoroquinolones have been associated with the development of serious, and sometimes fatal, hypoglycemia, most often in elderly diabetics, but also in patients without diabetes. This occurred most frequently with gatifloxacin (no longer available systemically) but may occur at a lower frequency with other quinolones.

Severe hypersensitivity reactions, including anaphylaxis, have occurred with quinolone therapy. Reactions may present as typical allergic symptoms after a single dose, or may manifest as severe idiosyncratic dermatologic, vascular, pulmonary, renal, hepatic, and/or hematologic events, usually after multiple doses. May cause maculopapular rash, usually 8-10 days after treatment initiation; risk factors may include age <40 years, female gender (including postmenopausal women on HRT), and treatment duration >7 days. Prompt discontinuation of drug should occur if skin rash or other symptoms arise. **[U.S. Boxed Warning]: Quinolones may exacerbate myasthenia gravis; avoid use (rare, potentially life-threatening weakness of respiratory muscles may occur).** Avoid excessive sunlight and take precautions to limit exposure (eg, loose fitting clothing, sunscreen); may cause moderate-to-severe phototoxicity reactions. Discontinue use if photosensitivity occurs. Prolonged use may result in fungal or bacterial superinfection, including *C. difficile*-associated diarrhea (CDAD) and pseudomembranous colitis; CDAD has been observed >2 months postantibiotic treatment. Peripheral neuropathy has been linked to the use of quinolones; these cases were rare. Hemolytic reactions may (rarely) occur with quinolone use in patients with latent or actual G6PD deficiency.

Drug Interactions

Avoid Concomitant Use

Avoid concomitant use of Gemifloxacin with any of the following: BCG

Increased Effect/Toxicity

Gemifloxacin may increase the levels/effects of: Corticosteroids (Systemic); Sulfonylureas; Vitamin K Antagonists

The levels/effects of Gemifloxacin may be increased by: Insulin; Nonsteroidal Anti-Inflammatory Agents; Probenecid

Decreased Effect

Gemifloxacin may decrease the levels/effects of: BCG; Mycophenolate; Sulfonylureas; Typhoid Vaccine

The levels/effects of Gemifloxacin may be decreased by: Antacids; Calcium Salts; Didanosine; Iron Salts; Magnesium Salts; Quinapril; Sevelamer; Sucralfate; Zinc Salts

Ethanol/Nutrition/Herb Interactions Herb/Nutraceutical: Avoid dong quai, St John's wort (may also cause photosensitization).

Dietary Considerations May take tablets with or without food, milk, or calcium supplements. Gemifloxacin should be taken 3 hours before or 2 hours after supplements (including multivitamins) containing iron, zinc, or magnesium.

Pharmacodynamics/Kinetics

Half-life Elimination 7 hours (range 4-12 hours)

Time to Peak Plasma: 0.5-2 hours

Pregnancy Risk Factor C

Lactation Excretion in breast milk unknown/not recommended

Breast-Feeding Considerations It is not known if gemifloxacin is excreted in breast milk. Breast-feeding is not recommended by the manufacturer. Nondose-related effects could include modification of bowel flora.

Dosage Forms

Tablet, oral:

Factive®: 320 mg

Gemtuzumab Ozogamicin (gem TOO zoo mab oh zog a MY sin)

U.S. Brand Names Mylotarg® [DSC]

Canadian Brand Names Mylotarg®

Pharmacologic Category Antineoplastic Agent, Monoclonal Antibody

Use Treatment of relapsed CD33 positive acute myeloid leukemia (AML) in patients ≥60 years of age who are not candidates for cytotoxic chemotherapy

Note: Due to safety concerns as well as lack of clinical benefit demonstrated in a post-approval clinical trial, gemtuzumab was withdrawn from the U.S. commercial market.

Unlabeled/Investigational Use Salvage therapy for acute promyelocytic leukemia (APL), relapsed/ refractory CD33 positive acute myeloid leukemia in children and adults <60 years

Local Anesthetic/Vasoconstrictor Precautions No information available to require special precautions

Effects on Dental Treatment Key adverse event(s) related to dental treatment: Stomatitis, gingival hemorrhage, and mucositis.

Effects on Bleeding Chemotherapy may result in significant myelosuppression, potentially including significant reduction in platelet counts and altered hemostasis. In patients who are under active treatment with these agents, medical consult is suggested.

Adverse Effects Adverse reactions reported for adults of all ages. **Note:** A post-infusion symptom complex (fever, chills, less commonly hypertension, and/or dyspnea) may occur within 24 hours of administration; the incidence of infusion-related events decreases with repeat administration.

>10%:

Cardiovascular: Hypotension (20%), hypertension (16%), peripheral edema (14%)

Central nervous system: Fever (82%), chills (66%), headache (37%), pain (18%), dizziness (12%), insomnia (12%)

Dermatologic: Petechiae (19%), rash (18%)

Endocrine & metabolic: Hypokalemia (26%)

Gastrointestinal: Nausea (68%), vomiting (58%), abdominal pain (32%), diarrhea (32%), anorexia (25%), mucositis/stomatitis (25%), constipation (23%)

Hematologic: Thrombocytopenia (grades 3/4: 49% to 99%; median recovery 36-51 days), neutropenia (grades 3/4: 98%; median recovery 40-51 days), leukopenia (grades 3/4: 46% to 96%), lymphopenia (grades 3/4: 94%), anemia/hemoglobin decreased (grades 3/4: 14% to 52%), neutropenic fever (17%), hemorrhage (11% to 13%)

Hepatic: Hyperbilirubinemia (grades 3/4: 29%), veno-occlusive disease (1% to 20%; higher frequency in patients with prior history of or subsequent hematopoietic stem cell transplant), AST increased (grades 3/4: 18%), LDH increased (16%)

Local: Local reaction (22%)

Neuromuscular & skeletal: Weakness (36%), back pain (14%)

Respiratory: Epistaxis (28%; grade 3/4: 3%), dyspnea (26%), cough (17%), pneumonia (13%; grades 3/4: 8%), pharyngitis (12%)

Miscellaneous: Infection (grades 3/4: 30%), sepsis (26%; grades 3/4: 17%), cutaneous herpes simplex (21%)

1% to 10%:

Cardiovascular: Tachycardia (10%), cerebral hemorrhage (2%)

Central nervous system: Depression (9%), anxiety (8%), intracranial hemorrhage (1%)

Dermatologic: Bruising (10%), pruritus (6%)

Endocrine & metabolic: Hyperglycemia (10%), hypocalcemia (10%), hypophosphatemia (8%) hypomagnesemia (6%)

Gastrointestinal: Dyspepsia (10%), gingival hemorrhage (9%), melena (1%)

Genitourinary: Vaginal hemorrhage (4%), vaginal bleeding (3%), hematuria (grade 3/4: 1%)
Hematologic: Disseminated intravascular coagulation (DIC) (1%)
Hepatic: ALT increased (grades 3/4: 9%), prothrombin time increased (grades 3/4: 9%), alkaline phosphatase increased (8%; grades 3/4: 4%), ascites (3%), PTT increased (grades 3/4: 2%)
Neuromuscular & skeletal: Arthralgia (10%), myalgia (6%)
Renal: Creatinine increased (2%)
Respiratory: Rhinitis (8%), hypoxia (5%)

General Dosage Range I.V.: *Adults ≥60 years:* 9 mg/m^2 every 2 weeks

Mechanism of Action Antibody to CD33 antigen, which is expressed on leukemic blasts in 80% of AML patients. Binds to the CD33 antigen, resulting in internalization of the antibody-antigen complex. Following internalization, the calicheamicin derivative is released inside the myeloid cell. The calicheamicin derivative binds to DNA resulting in double strand breaks and cell death. Pluripotent stem cells and non-hematopoietic cells are not affected.

Pharmacodynamics/Kinetics

Half-life Elimination Total calicheamicin: Initial: 41-45 hours, Repeat dose: 60-64 hours; Unconjugated: 100-143 hours (no change noted in repeat dosing)

Time to Peak Immediate; higher concentrations observed after repeat dose

Pregnancy Risk Factor D

Product Availability As of June 2010, no longer commercially available in the U.S. market for new patients.

Prescribing and Access Restrictions As of June 2010, gemtuzumab has been withdrawn from the U.S. market and is no longer commercially available to new patients; thereafter, gemtuzumab will only be available in the U.S. under an Investigational New Drug (IND) protocol.

Gentamicin (Systemic) (jen ta MYE sin)

Canadian Brand Names Gentamicin Injection, USP

Pharmacologic Category Antibiotic, Aminoglycoside

Use Treatment of susceptible bacterial infections, normally gram-negative organisms, including *Pseudomonas*, *Proteus*, *Serratia*, and gram-positive *Staphylococcus*; treatment of bone infections, respiratory tract infections, skin and soft tissue infections, as well as abdominal and urinary tract infections, and septicemia; treatment of infective endocarditis

Local Anesthetic/Vasoconstrictor Precautions No information available to require special precautions

Effects on Dental Treatment No significant effects or complications reported

Effects on Bleeding No information available to require special precautions

Adverse Effects

>10%:
Central nervous system: Neurotoxicity (vertigo, ataxia)
Neuromuscular & skeletal: Gait instability
Otic: Ototoxicity (auditory), ototoxicity (vestibular)
Renal: Nephrotoxicity, decreased creatinine clearance

1% to 10%: Cardiovascular: Edema

General Dosage Range Dosage adjustment recommended for the I.M. and I.V. routes in patients with renal impairment

I.M., I.V.:
Children <5 years: 2.5 mg/kg/dose every 8 hours
Children ≥5 years: 2-2.5 mg/kg/dose every 8 hours
Adults: 1-2.5 mg/kg/dose every 8-12 hours **or** 4-7 mg/kg once daily

Intrathecal: *Adults:* 4-8 mg/day

Mechanism of Action Interferes with bacterial protein synthesis by binding to 30S and 50S ribosomal subunits resulting in a defective bacterial cell membrane

Pharmacodynamics/Kinetics

Half-life Elimination
Infants: <1 week: 3-11.5 hours; 1 week to 6 months: 3-3.5 hours
Adults: 1.5-3 hours; End-stage renal disease: 36-70 hours

Time to Peak Serum: I.M.: 30-90 minutes; I.V.: 30 minutes after 30-minute infusion

Pregnancy Risk Factor D

Gentian Violet (JEN shun VYE oh let)

Pharmacologic Category Antibiotic, Topical; Antifungal Agent, Topical

Use Treatment of cutaneous or mucocutaneous infections caused by *Candida albicans* and other superficial skin infections; external treatment of minor abrasions or cuts

Local Anesthetic/Vasoconstrictor Precautions No information available to require special precautions

Effects on Dental Treatment Key adverse event(s) related to dental treatment: Ulceration of mucous membranes.

Effects on Bleeding No information available to require special precautions

Adverse Effects Frequency not defined.

Dermatologic: Necrotic skin reactions, staining, vesicle formation

Gastrointestinal: Esophagitis, gastrointestinal irritation, ulceration of mucous membranes

Genitourinary: Hemorrhagic cystitis

Local: Burning, irritation

Ocular: Keratoconjunctivitis

Respiratory: Epistaxis, laryngitis, laryngeal obstruction, tracheitis

Miscellaneous: Allergic contact dermatitis, sensitivity reactions

General Dosage Range Topical: *Children and Adults:* Apply 0.5% to 2% to affected area once or twice daily

Mechanism of Action Topical antiseptic/germicide effective against some vegetative gram-positive bacteria, particularly *Staphylococcus* sp, and some yeast; it is much less effective against gram-negative bacteria and is ineffective against acid-fast bacteria

Pregnancy Risk Factor C

Glatiramer Acetate (gla TIR a mer AS e tate)

U.S. Brand Names Copaxone®

Canadian Brand Names Copaxone®

Pharmacologic Category Biological, Miscellaneous

Use Management of relapsing-remitting type multiple sclerosis, including patients with a first clinical episode with MRI features consistent with multiple sclerosis

Local Anesthetic/Vasoconstrictor Precautions No information available to require special precautions

Effects on Dental Treatment Key adverse event(s) related to dental treatment: Ulcerative stomatitis, salivary gland enlargement, and oral moniliasis.

Effects on Bleeding No information available to require special precautions

Adverse Effects

>10%:

Cardiovascular: Vasodilation (20%), chest pain (13%)

Central nervous system: Pain (20%), anxiety (13%)

Dermatologic: Rash (19%)

Gastrointestinal: Nausea (15%)

Local: Injection site reactions: Inflammation (49%), erythema (43%), pain (40%), pruritus (27%), mass (27%)

Neuromuscular & skeletal: Weakness (22%), back pain (12%)

Respiratory: Dyspnea (14%)

Miscellaneous: Infection (30%), flu-like syndrome (14%), diaphoresis (15%)

1% to 10%:

Cardiovascular: Edema (8%; includes peripheral and facial), palpitation (7%), tachycardia (5%), syncope (3%), hypertension (1%)

Central nervous system: Fever (6%), migraine (4%), chills (3%), nervousness (2%), speech disorder (2%), abnormal dreams (1%), emotional lability (1%), stupor (1%)

Dermatologic: Bruising (8%), pruritus (5%), erythema (4%), urticaria (3%), skin nodule (2%), eczema (1%), pustular rash (1%)

Endocrine & metabolic: Amenorrhea (1%), impotence (1%), menorrhagia (1%)

Gastrointestinal: Vomiting (7%), gastroenteritis (6%), weight gain (3%), dysphagia (2%), dental caries (1%)

Genitourinary: Urinary urgency (5%), vaginal moniliasis (4%)

Local: Injection site reactions: Hemorrhage (5%), hypersensitivity (4%), fibrosis (2%), lipoatrophy (2%), abscess (1%), edema (1%)

Neuromuscular & skeletal: Neck pain (8%), tremor (4%)

Ocular: Diplopia (3%), visual field defect (1%)

Respiratory: Rhinitis (7%), bronchitis (6%), cough (6%), laryngismus (5%), hyperventilation (1%)

Miscellaneous: Lymphadenopathy (7%), hypersensitivity (3%)

General Dosage Range SubQ: *Adults:* 20 mg daily

Mechanism of Action Glatiramer is a mixture of random polymers of four amino acids; L-alanine, L-glutamic acid, L-lysine, and L-tyrosine, the resulting mixture is antigenically similar to myelin basic protein, which is an important component of the myelin sheath of nerves; glatiramer is thought to induce and activate T-lymphocyte suppressor cells specific for a myelin antigen, it is also proposed that glatiramer interferes with the antigen-presenting function of certain immune cells opposing pathogenic T-cell function

Pregnancy Risk Factor B

Gliclazide (GLYE kla zide)

Related Information

Endocrine Disorders and Pregnancy *on page 1879*

Canadian Brand Names Apo-Gliclazide®; Apo-Gliclazide® MR; Diamicron®; Diamicron® MR; Gliclazide MR; Gliclazide-80; Mylan-Gliclazide; Novo-Gliclazide; PMS-Gliclazide

Pharmacologic Category Antidiabetic Agent, Sulfonylurea

Use Management of type 2 diabetes mellitus (noninsulin dependent, NIDDM)

Local Anesthetic/Vasoconstrictor Precautions No information available to require special precautions

Effects on Dental Treatment Gliclazide-dependent patients with diabetes (noninsulin dependent, type 2) should be appointed for dental treatment in morning in order to minimize chance of stress-induced hypoglycemia.

Effects on Bleeding No information available to require special precautions

Adverse Effects Frequency not defined.

Central nervous system: Dizziness, headache, nervousness

Dermatologic: Erythema, pruritus, rash, urticaria. Sulfonylureas have also been associated with rare photosensitivity and porphyria cutanea tarda.

Endocrine & metabolic: Hypoglycemia (dose dependent), hyponatremia (rare)

Gastrointestinal: Diarrhea, epigastric fullness, gastritis, nausea, vomiting

Hematologic: Agranulocytosis, anemia, leukopenia, thrombocytopenia

Hepatic: Jaundice, LDH increased, transaminases increased

Miscellaneous: Disulfiram reaction (very low potential)

Dosage Oral: Adults:

Immediate release tablet: Initial: 80-160 mg/day; typical dose range 80-320 mg/day; dosage of ≥160 mg should be divided into 2 equal parts for twice-daily administration; maximum dose: 320 mg/day; should be taken with meals

Sustained release tablet: 30-120 mg once daily

Note: There is no fixed dosage regimen for the management of diabetes mellitus with gliclazide or any other hypoglycemic agent. Dose must be individualized based on frequent determinations of blood glucose during dose titration and throughout maintenance.

Dosage adjustment in renal/hepatic impairment: Contraindicated in severe impairment

Mechanism of Action Stimulates insulin release from the pancreatic beta cells; reduces glucose output from the liver; lowers plasma glucose concentrations. Gliclazide has also been shown to decrease platelet aggregation at therapeutic doses.

Contraindications Hypersensitivity to gliclazide, sulfonylureas, or any component of the formulation; type 1 diabetes mellitus (insulin dependent, IDDM), diabetic ketoacidosis with or without coma; renal or hepatic impairment; pregnancy (per manufacturer); breast-feeding

Warnings/Precautions All sulfonylurea drugs are capable of producing severe hypoglycemia. Hypoglycemia is more likely to occur when caloric intake is deficient, after severe or prolonged exercise, when ethanol is ingested, or when more than one glucose-lowering drug is used. Hypoglycemia is also more likely in elderly patients, malnourished patients or in impaired renal or hepatic function.

Chemical similarities are present among sulfonamides, sulfonylureas, carbonic anhydrase inhibitors, thiazides, and loop diuretics (except ethacrynic acid). Use in patients with sulfonamide allergy is specifically contraindicated in product labeling, however, a risk of cross-reaction exists in patients with allergy to any of these compounds; avoid use when previous reaction has been severe.

Product labeling of sulfonylureas (in U.S.) states oral hypoglycemic drugs may be associated with an increased cardiovascular mortality as compared to treatment with diet alone or diet plus insulin. Data to support this association are limited, and several studies, including a large prospective trial (UKPDS), have not supported an association.

It may be necessary to discontinue therapy and administer insulin if the patient is exposed to stress (fever, trauma, infection, surgery). Safety and efficacy have not been established in children.

Drug Interactions

Metabolism/Transport Effects

Substrate of CYP2C9 (major), CYP2C19 (minor)

Avoid Concomitant Use There are no known interactions where it is recommended to avoid concomitant use.

Increased Effect/Toxicity

Gliclazide may increase the levels/effects of: Alcohol (Ethyl); Hypoglycemic Agents

The levels/effects of Gliclazide may be increased by: Beta-Blockers; Chloramphenicol; Cimetidine; Cyclic Antidepressants; CYP2C9 Inhibitors (Moderate); CYP2C9 Inhibitors (Strong); Fibric Acid Derivatives; Fluconazole; GLP-1 Agonists; Herbs (Hypoglycemic Properties); Pegvisomant; Quinolone Antibiotics; Ranitidine; Salicylates; Sulfonamide Derivatives; Voriconazole

Decreased Effect

The levels/effects of Gliclazide may be decreased by: Corticosteroids (Orally Inhaled); Corticosteroids (Systemic); CYP2C9 Inducers (Highly Effective); Luteinizing Hormone-Releasing Hormone Analogs; Peginterferon Alfa-2b; Quinolone Antibiotics; Rifampin; Somatropin; Thiazide Diuretics

Ethanol/Nutrition/Herb Interactions

Ethanol: Avoid ethanol (may cause hypoglycemia and/or rare disulfiram reactions).

Herb/Nutraceutical: Avoid chromium, garlic, gymnema (may cause hypoglycemia).

Dietary Considerations Should be taken with meals. Individualized medical nutrition therapy (MNT) based on ADA recommendations is an integral part of therapy.

Pharmacodynamics/Kinetics

Half-life Elimination 10 hours

Time to Peak 4-6 hours

Pregnancy Risk Factor Not available (similar agents rated C); manufacturer contraindicates use

Lactation Excretion in breast milk unknown/contraindicated

Breast-Feeding Considerations Potential for neonatal hypoglycemia contraindicates use.

Product Availability Not available in U.S.

Dosage Forms: Canada

Tablet:

Diamicron®: 80 mg

Tablet, sustained release:

Diamicron® MR: 30 mg, 60 mg

Glimepiride (GLYE me pye ride)

Related Information

Endocrine Disorders and Pregnancy *on page 1879*

U.S. Brand Names Amaryl®

Canadian Brand Names Amaryl®; Apo-Glimepiride®; CO Glimepiride; Novo-Glimepiride; PMS-Glimepiride; ratio-Glimepiride; Rhoxal-glimepiride; Sandoz-Glimepiride

Generic Availability (U.S.) Yes

Pharmacologic Category Antidiabetic Agent, Sulfonylurea

Use Management of type 2 diabetes mellitus (noninsulin dependent, NIDDM) as an adjunct to diet and exercise to lower blood glucose; may be used in combination with metformin or insulin in patients whose hyperglycemia cannot be controlled by diet and exercise in conjunction with a single oral hypoglycemic agent

Local Anesthetic/Vasoconstrictor Precautions No information available to require special precautions

Effects on Dental Treatment Glimepiride-dependent patients with diabetes (noninsulin dependent, type 2) should be appointed for dental treatment in morning in order to minimize chance of stress-induced hypoglycemia.

Effects on Bleeding No information available to require special precautions

Adverse Effects 1% to 10%:

Central nervous system: Dizziness (2%), headache (2%)

Endocrine & metabolic: Hypoglycemia (1% to 2%)

Gastrointestinal: Nausea (1%)

Neuromuscular & skeletal: Weakness (2%)

Dosage Oral:

Children 10-18 years (unlabeled use): Initial: 1 mg once daily; maintenance: 1-4 mg once daily

Adults: Initial: 1-2 mg once daily, administered with breakfast or the first main meal; usual maintenance dose: 1-4 mg once daily; after a dose of 2 mg once daily, increase in increments of 2 mg at 1- to 2-week intervals based upon the patient's blood glucose response to a maximum of 8 mg once daily. If inadequate response to maximal dose, combination therapy with metformin may be considered.

Combination with insulin therapy (fasting glucose level for instituting combination therapy is in the range of >150 mg/dL in plasma or serum depending on the patient): initial recommended dose: 8 mg once daily with the first main meal

After starting with low-dose insulin, upward adjustments of insulin can be done approximately weekly as guided by frequent measurements of fasting blood glucose. Once stable, combination-therapy patients should monitor their capillary blood glucose on an ongoing basis, preferably daily.

Conversion from therapy with long half-life agents: Observe patient carefully for 1-2 weeks when converting from a longer half-life agent (eg, chlorpropamide) to glimepiride due to overlapping hypoglycemic effects.

Dosing adjustment/comments in renal impairment: Cl_{cr} <22 mL/minute: Initial starting dose should be 1 mg and dosage increments should be based on fasting blood glucose levels

Dosing adjustment in hepatic impairment: No data available

Elderly: Initial: 1 mg/day; dose titration and maintenance dosing should be conservative to avoid hypoglycemia

Mechanism of Action Stimulates insulin release from the pancreatic beta cells; reduces glucose output from the liver; insulin sensitivity is increased at peripheral target sites

Contraindications Hypersensitivity to glimepiride, any component of the formulation, or sulfonamides; diabetic ketoacidosis (with or without coma)

Warnings/Precautions All sulfonylurea drugs are capable of producing severe hypoglycemia. Hypoglycemia is more likely to occur when caloric intake is deficient, after severe or prolonged exercise, when ethanol is ingested, or when more than one glucose-lowering drug is used. It is also more likely in elderly patients, malnourished patients and in patients with impaired renal or hepatic function; use with caution. Autonomic neuropathy, advanced age, and concomitant use of beta-blockers or other sympatholytic agents may impair the patient's ability to recognize the signs and symptoms of hypoglycemia; use with caution.

Chemical similarities are present among sulfonamides, sulfonylureas, carbonic anhydrase inhibitors, thiazides, and loop diuretics (except ethacrynic acid). Use in patients with sulfonamide allergy is not specifically contraindicated in product labeling, however, a risk of cross-reaction exists in patients with allergy to any of these compounds; avoid use when previous reaction has been severe.

Product labeling states oral hypoglycemic drugs may be associated with an increased cardiovascular mortality as compared to treatment with diet alone or diet plus insulin. Data to support this association are limited, and several studies, including a large prospective trial (UKPDS) have not supported an association.

It may be necessary to discontinue therapy and administer insulin if the patient is exposed to stress (fever, trauma, infection, surgery).

Drug Interactions

Metabolism/Transport Effects **Substrate** of CYP2C9 (major)

Avoid Concomitant Use There are no known interactions where it is recommended to avoid concomitant use.

Increased Effect/Toxicity

Glimepiride may increase the levels/effects of: Alcohol (Ethyl); Hypoglycemic Agents

The levels/effects of Glimepiride may be increased by: Beta-Blockers; Chloramphenicol; Cimetidine; Cyclic Antidepressants; CYP2C9 Inhibitors (Moderate); CYP2C9 Inhibitors (Strong); Fibric Acid Derivatives; Fluconazole; GLP-1 Agonists; Herbs (Hypoglycemic Properties); Pegvisomant; Quinolone Antibiotics; Ranitidine; Salicylates; Sulfonamide Derivatives; Voriconazole

Decreased Effect

The levels/effects of Glimepiride may be decreased by: Corticosteroids (Orally Inhaled); Corticosteroids (Systemic); CYP2C9 Inducers (Highly Effective); Luteinizing Hormone-Releasing Hormone Analogs; Peginterferon Alfa-2b; Quinolone Antibiotics; Rifampin; Somatropin; Thiazide Diuretics

Ethanol/Nutrition/Herb Interactions

Ethanol: Caution with ethanol (may cause hypoglycemia).

Herb/Nutraceutical: Caution with chromium, garlic, gymnema (may cause hypoglycemia).

Dietary Considerations Administer with breakfast or the first main meal of the day. Individualized medical nutrition therapy (MNT) based on ADA recommendations is an integral part of therapy.

Pharmacodynamics/Kinetics

Onset of Action Peak effect: Blood glucose reductions: 2-3 hours

Duration of Action 24 hours

Half-life Elimination 5-9 hours

Time to Peak 2-3 hours
Pregnancy Risk Factor C
Lactation Excretion in breast milk unknown/not recommended
Breast-Feeding Considerations It is not known if glimepiride is excreted in breast milk. Breast-feeding is not recommended by the manufacturer. Potentially, hypoglycemia may occur in a nursing infant exposed to a sulfonylurea via breast milk.
Dosage Forms
Tablet, oral: 1 mg, 2 mg, 4 mg
Amaryl®: 1 mg, 2 mg, 4 mg

GlipiZIDE (GLIP i zide)

Related Information
Endocrine Disorders and Pregnancy *on page 1879*
U.S. Brand Names Glucotrol XL®; Glucotrol®
Generic Availability (U.S.) Yes
Pharmacologic Category Antidiabetic Agent, Sulfonylurea
Use Management of type 2 diabetes mellitus (noninsulin dependent, NIDDM)
Local Anesthetic/Vasoconstrictor Precautions No information available to require special precautions
Effects on Dental Treatment Glipizide-dependent patients with diabetes (noninsulin dependent, type 2) should be appointed for dental treatment in morning in order to minimize chance of stress-induced hypoglycemia.
Effects on Bleeding No information available to require special precautions
Adverse Effects Frequency not defined.
Cardiovascular: Edema, syncope
Central nervous system: Anxiety, depression, dizziness, drowsiness, headache, hypoesthesia, insomnia, nervousness, pain
Dermatologic: Eczema, erythema, maculopapular eruptions, morbilliform eruptions, photosensitivity, pruritus, rash, urticaria
Endocrine & metabolic: Disulfiram-like reaction, hypoglycemia, hyponatremia, SIADH (rare)
Gastrointestinal: Anorexia, constipation, diarrhea, epigastric fullness, flatulence, gastralgia, heartburn, nausea, vomiting
Hematologic: Agranulocytopenia, aplastic anemia, blood dyscrasias, hemolytic anemia, leukopenia, pancytopenia, porphyria cutanea tarda, thrombocytopenia
Hepatic: Hepatic porphyria
Neuromuscular & skeletal: Arthralgia, leg cramps, myalgia, paresthesia, tremor
Ocular: Blurred vision
Renal: Diuretic effect (minor)
Respiratory: Rhinitis
Miscellaneous: Diaphoresis
Dosage Oral (allow several days between dose titrations): Adults: Initial: 5 mg/day; adjust dosage at 2.5-5 mg daily increments as determined by blood glucose response at intervals of several days.
Immediate release tablet: Maximum recommended once-daily dose: 15 mg; maximum recommended total daily dose: 40 mg. Doses >15 mg/day should be administered in divided doses.
Extended release tablet (Glucotrol XL®): Maximum recommended dose: 20 mg
When transferring from insulin to glipizide:
Current insulin requirement ≤20 units: Discontinue insulin and initiate glipizide at usual dose
Current insulin requirement >20 units: Decrease insulin by 50% and initiate glipizide at usual dose; gradually decrease insulin dose based on patient response. Several days should elapse between dosage changes.
Elderly: Initial: 2.5 mg/day; increase by 2.5-5 mg/day at 1- to 2-week intervals

Dosing adjustment/comments in renal impairment: Cl_{cr} <10 mL/minute: Some investigators recommend not using
Dosing adjustment in hepatic impairment: Initial dosage should be 2.5 mg/day
Mechanism of Action Stimulates insulin release from the pancreatic beta cells; reduces glucose output from the liver; insulin sensitivity is increased at peripheral target sites
Contraindications Hypersensitivity to glipizide or any component of the formulation, other sulfonamides; type 1 diabetes mellitus (insulin dependent, IDDM); diabetic ketoacidosis
Warnings/Precautions All sulfonylurea drugs are capable of producing severe hypoglycemia. Hypoglycemia is more likely to occur when caloric intake is deficient, after severe or prolonged exercise, when ethanol is ingested, or when more than one glucose-lowering drug is used. It is also more likely in elderly patients,

malnourished patients and in patients with impaired renal or hepatic function; use with caution.

Chemical similarities are present among sulfonamides, sulfonylureas, carbonic anhydrase inhibitors, thiazides, and loop diuretics (except ethacrynic acid). Use in patients with sulfonamide allergy is specifically contraindicated in product labeling, however, a risk of cross-reaction exists in patients with allergy to any of these compounds; avoid use when previous reaction has been severe.

Product labeling states oral hypoglycemic drugs may be associated with an increased cardiovascular mortality as compared to treatment with diet alone or diet plus insulin. Data to support this association are limited, and several studies, including a large prospective trial (UKPDS) have not supported an association.

Use with caution in patients with severe hepatic disease. It may be necessary to discontinue therapy and administer insulin if the patient is exposed to stress (fever, trauma, infection, surgery).

Avoid use of extended release tablets (Glucotrol XL®) in patients with known stricture/narrowing of the GI tract.

Drug Interactions

Metabolism/Transport Effects Substrate of 2C9 (major)

Avoid Concomitant Use There are no known interactions where it is recommended to avoid concomitant use.

Increased Effect/Toxicity

GlipiZIDE may increase the levels/effects of: Alcohol (Ethyl); Hypoglycemic Agents

The levels/effects of GlipiZIDE may be increased by: Beta-Blockers; Chloramphenicol; Cimetidine; Clarithromycin; Cyclic Antidepressants; CYP2C9 Inhibitors (Moderate); CYP2C9 Inhibitors (Strong); Fibric Acid Derivatives; Fluconazole; GLP-1 Agonists; Herbs (Hypoglycemic Properties); Pegvisomant; Posaconazole; Quinolone Antibiotics; Ranitidine; Salicylates; Sulfonamide Derivatives; Voriconazole

Decreased Effect

The levels/effects of GlipiZIDE may be decreased by: Corticosteroids (Orally Inhaled); Corticosteroids (Systemic); CYP2C9 Inducers (Highly Effective); Luteinizing Hormone-Releasing Hormone Analogs; Peginterferon Alfa-2b; Quinolone Antibiotics; Rifampin; Somatropin; Thiazide Diuretics

Ethanol/Nutrition/Herb Interactions

Ethanol: Caution with ethanol (may cause hypoglycemia or rare disulfiram reaction).

Food: A delayed release of insulin may occur if glipizide is taken with food. Immediate release tablets should be administered 30 minutes before meals to avoid erratic absorption.

Herb/Nutraceutical: Herbs with hypoglycemic properties may enhance the hypoglycemic effect of glipizide. This includes alfalfa, aloe, bilberry, bitter melon, burdock, celery, damiana, fenugreek, garcinia, garlic, ginger, ginseng (American), gymnema, marshmallow, stinging nettle

Dietary Considerations Take immediate release tablets 30 minutes before meals; extended release tablets should be taken with breakfast. Individualized medical nutrition therapy (MNT) based on ADA recommendations is an integral part of therapy.

Pharmacodynamics/Kinetics

Duration of Action 12-24 hours

Half-life Elimination 2-5 hours

Time to Peak 1-3 hours; extended release tablets: 6-12 hours

Pregnancy Risk Factor C

Lactation Excretion in breast milk unknown/not recommended

Breast-Feeding Considerations Data from initial studies note that glipizide was not detected in breast milk. Breast-feeding is not recommended by the manufacturer. Potentially, hypoglycemia may occur in a nursing infant exposed to a sulfonylurea via breast milk.

Dosage Forms

Tablet, oral: 5 mg, 10 mg

Glucotrol®: 5 mg, 10 mg

Tablet, extended release, oral: 2.5 mg, 5 mg, 10 mg

Glucotrol XL®: 2.5 mg, 5 mg, 10 mg

Glipizide and Metformin (GLIP i zide & met FOR min)

Related Information

Endocrine Disorders and Pregnancy *on page 1879*

GlipiZIDE *on page 819*

MetFORMIN *on page 1089*

U.S. Brand Names Metaglip™

Generic Availability (U.S.) Yes

Pharmacologic Category Antidiabetic Agent, Biguanide; Antidiabetic Agent, Sulfonylurea

Use Indicated as an adjunct to diet and exercise to improve glycemic control in adults with type 2 diabetes mellitus (noninsulin dependent, NIDDM)

Local Anesthetic/Vasoconstrictor Precautions No information available to require special precautions

Effects on Dental Treatment Key adverse event(s) related to dental treatment: Upper respiratory tract infection (8% to 10%). Dependent patients with diabetes (noninsulin dependent, type 2) should be appointed for dental treatment in the morning in order to minimize chance of stress-induced hypoglycemia.

Effects on Bleeding No information available to require special precautions

Adverse Effects Also see individual agents.

>10%:

- Central nervous system: Headache (13%)
- Endocrine & metabolic: Hypoglycemia (8% to 13%)
- Gastrointestinal: Diarrhea (2% to 18%)

1% to 10%:

- Cardiovascular: Hypertension (3% to 4%)
- Central nervous system: Dizziness (2% to 5%)
- Gastrointestinal: Nausea/vomiting (<1% to 8%), abdominal pain (6%)
- Neuromuscular & skeletal: Musculoskeletal pain (8%)
- Renal: Urinary tract infection (1%)
- Respiratory: Upper respiratory tract infection (8% to 10%)

Dosage Oral: Type 2 diabetes:

Adults:

Patients inadequately controlled on diet and exercise alone: Initial dose: Glipizide 2.5 mg/metformin 250 mg once daily with a meal. In patients with fasting plasma glucose (FPG) 280-320 mg/dL, initiate therapy with glipizide 2.5 mg/metformin 500 mg twice daily.

Note: Increase dose by 1 tablet/day every 2 weeks (maximum daily dose: Glipizide 10 mg/metformin 2000 mg in divided doses)

Patients inadequately controlled on a sulfonylurea and/or metformin: Initial dose: Glipizide 2.5 mg/metformin 500 mg or glipizide 5 mg/metformin 500 mg twice daily with morning and evening meals; starting dose should not exceed current daily dose of glipizide (or sulfonylurea equivalent) and/or metformin.

Note: Increase dose in increments of no more than glipizide 5 mg/metformin 500 mg (maximum daily dose: Glipizide 20 mg/metformin 2000 mg)

Elderly: Conservative doses are recommended in the elderly due to potentially decreased renal function; **do not titrate to maximum dose**; should not be used in patients ≥80 years unless renal function is verified as normal

Dosage adjustment in renal impairment: Contraindicated in the presence of renal disease or renal dysfunction (serum creatinine ≥1.5 mg/dL [males], ≥1.4 mg/dL [females], or abnormal creatinine clearance)

Dosage adjustment in hepatic impairment: Avoid use in patients with impaired liver function

Mechanism of Action The combination of glipizide and metformin is used to improve glycemic control in patients with type 2 diabetes mellitus (noninsulin dependent, NIDDM) by using two different, but complementary, mechanisms of action:

Glipizide: Stimulates insulin release from the pancreatic beta cells; reduces glucose output from the liver; insulin sensitivity is increased at peripheral target sites

Metformin: Decreases hepatic glucose production, decreasing intestinal absorption of glucose and improves insulin sensitivity (increases peripheral glucose uptake and utilization)

Contraindications Hypersensitivity to glipizide, metformin, or any component of the formulation; renal disease or renal dysfunction (serum creatinine ≥1.5 mg/dL in males or ≥1.4 mg/dL in females, or abnormal creatinine clearance which may also result from conditions such as cardiovascular collapse, acute myocardial infarction, and septicemia); acute or chronic metabolic acidosis with or without coma (including diabetic ketoacidosis)

Note: Temporarily discontinue in patients undergoing radiologic studies in which intravascular iodinated contrast materials are utilized.

Warnings/Precautions Age, hepatic and renal impairment are independent risk factors for hypoglycemia. Use with caution in patients with hepatic impairment, malnourished or debilitated conditions, or adrenal or pituitary insufficiency. Use caution in patients with renal impairment. Use caution in the elderly and patients taking beta-blockers; signs and symptoms of hypoglycemia may be masked. Instruct patients to avoid excessive acute or chronic ethanol use; ethanol may potentiate metformin's effect on lactate metabolism and increase risk of hypoglycemia.

[U.S. Boxed Warning]: Lactic acidosis is a rare, but potentially severe consequence of therapy with metformin. Withhold therapy in hypoxemia, dehydration, or sepsis. The risk of lactic acidosis is increased in any patient with CHF requiring pharmacologic management. This risk is particularly high during acute or unstable CHF because of the risk of hypoperfusion and hypoxemia. Metformin is substantially excreted by the kidney. The risk of accumulation and lactic acidosis increases with the degree of impairment of renal function. Patients with renal function below the limit of normal for their age should not receive metformin. In elderly patients, renal function should be monitored regularly; should not be used in any patient ≥80 years of age unless normal renal function is confirmed. Use of concomitant medications that may affect renal function (ie, affect tubular secretion) may also affect metformin disposition. Metformin should be withheld in patients with dehydration and/or prerenal azotemia. Therapy should be suspended for any surgical procedures (resume only after oral intake resumed and normal renal function is verified). Intravascular iodinated contrast media used for radiologic studies are associated with alteration of renal function and may increase risk of lactic acidosis. Discontinue Metaglip™ at the time of or prior to the procedure and withhold for 48 hours subsequent to the procedure; reinstitute only after renal function has been re-evaluated and found to be normal.

Chemical similarities are present among sulfonamides, sulfonylureas, carbonic anhydrase inhibitors, thiazides, and loop diuretics (except ethacrynic acid). Use in patients with sulfonamide allergy is not specifically contraindicated in product labeling, however, a risk of cross-reaction exists in patients with allergy to any of these compounds; avoid use when previous reaction has been severe.

Product labeling states oral hypoglycemic drugs may be associated with an increased cardiovascular mortality as compared to treatment with diet alone or diet plus insulin. Data to support this association are limited, and several studies, including a large prospective trial (UKPDS), have not supported an association.

Drug Interactions

Metabolism/Transport Effects Glipizide: **Substrate** of 2C9 (major)

Avoid Concomitant Use There are no known interactions where it is recommended to avoid concomitant use.

Increased Effect/Toxicity

Glipizide and Metformin may increase the levels/effects of: Alcohol (Ethyl); Dofetilide; Hypoglycemic Agents

The levels/effects of Glipizide and Metformin may be increased by: Beta-Blockers; Cephalexin; Chloramphenicol; Cimetidine; Clarithromycin; Cyclic Antidepressants; CYP2C9 Inhibitors (Moderate); CYP2C9 Inhibitors (Strong); Fibric Acid Derivatives; Fluconazole; GLP-1 Agonists; Glycopyrrolate; Herbs (Hypoglycemic Properties); Iodinated Contrast Agents; Pegvisomant; Posaconazole; Quinolone Antibiotics; Ranitidine; Salicylates; Sulfonamide Derivatives; Voriconazole

Decreased Effect

The levels/effects of Glipizide and Metformin may be decreased by: Corticosteroids (Orally Inhaled); Corticosteroids (Systemic); CYP2C9 Inducers (Highly Effective); Luteinizing Hormone-Releasing Hormone Analogs; Peginterferon Alfa-2b; Quinolone Antibiotics; Rifampin; Somatropin; Thiazide Diuretics

Ethanol/Nutrition/Herb Interactions See individual agents.

Dietary Considerations May cause GI upset; should be taken with food to decrease GI upset. Individualized medical nutrition therapy (MNT) based on ADA recommendations is an integral part of therapy. Monitor for signs and symptoms of vitamin B_{12} and folic acid deficiency; supplementation may be required.

Pregnancy Risk Factor C

Lactation

Glipizide: Excretion in breast milk unknown/not recommended
Metformin: Enters breast milk/not recommended

Breast-Feeding Considerations Refer to individual agents.

Dosage Forms

Tablet, oral: 2.5/250: Glipizide 2.5 mg and metformin 250 mg; 2.5/500: Glipizide 2.5 mg and metformin 500 mg; 5/500: Glipizide 5 mg and metformin 500 mg

Metaglip™: 2.5/500: Glipizide 2.5 mg and metformin 500 mg; 5/500: Glipizide 5 mg and metformin 500 mg

Glucagon (GLOO ka gon)

U.S. Brand Names GlucaGen®; GlucaGen® Diagnostic Kit; GlucaGen® HypoKit®; Glucagon Emergency Kit

Pharmacologic Category Antidote; Diagnostic Agent

Use Management of hypoglycemia; diagnostic aid in radiologic examinations to temporarily inhibit GI tract movement

Unlabeled/Investigational Use Beta-blocker- or calcium channel blocker-induced myocardial depression (with or without hypotension) unresponsive to standard measures; suspected or documented hypoglycemia secondary to insulin or sulfonylurea overdose (as adjunct to dextrose)

Local Anesthetic/Vasoconstrictor Precautions No information available to require special precautions

Effects on Dental Treatment No significant effects or complications reported

Effects on Bleeding No information available to require special precautions

Adverse Effects Frequency not defined.

Cardiovascular: Hypotension (up to 2 hours after GI procedures), hypertension, tachycardia

Gastrointestinal: Nausea, vomiting (high incidence with rapid administration of high doses)

Miscellaneous: Hypersensitivity reactions, anaphylaxis

General Dosage Range

I.M.:

Children <20 kg: 0.5 mg **or** 20-30 mcg/kg/dose, may repeat

Children ≥20 kg: 1 mg, may repeat

Adults: 1 mg, may repeat **or** 1-2 mg prior to procedure

I.V.:

Children <20 kg: 0.5 mg or 20-30 mcg/kg/dose, may repeat

Children ≥20 kg: 1 mg, may repeat

Adults: 1 mg, may repeat in 20 minutes **or** 0.25-2 mg 10 minutes prior to procedure

SubQ:

Children <20 kg: 0.5 mg **or** 20-30 mcg/kg/dose, may repeat

Children ≥20 kg and Adults: 1 mg, may repeat

Mechanism of Action Stimulates adenylate cyclase to produce increased cyclic AMP, which promotes hepatic glycogenolysis and gluconeogenesis, causing a raise in blood glucose levels

Pharmacodynamics/Kinetics

Onset of Action Peak effect: Blood glucose levels: Parenteral: I.V.: 5-20 minutes; I.M.: 30 minutes; SubQ: 30-45 minutes

Duration of Action Glucose elevation: SubQ: 60-90 minutes; I.V.: 30 minutes

Half-life Elimination Plasma: 8-18 minutes

Pregnancy Risk Factor B

Glucose Polymers (GLOO kose POL i merz)

U.S. Brand Names Moducal® [OTC]; Polycose® [OTC]

Pharmacologic Category Nutritional Supplement

Use Supplies calories for those persons not able to meet the caloric requirement with usual food intake

Local Anesthetic/Vasoconstrictor Precautions No information available to require special precautions

Effects on Dental Treatment No significant effects or complications reported

Effects on Bleeding No information available to require special precautions

General Dosage Range Oral: *Children and Adults:* Add to foods, beverages, or water as needed

Glutamic Acid (gloo TAM ik AS id)

Pharmacologic Category Gastrointestinal Agent, Miscellaneous

Use Treatment of hypochlorhydria and achlorhydria

Local Anesthetic/Vasoconstrictor Precautions No information available to require special precautions

Effects on Dental Treatment No significant effects or complications reported

Effects on Bleeding No information available to require special precautions
Adverse Effects Systemic acidosis may occur with massive overdosage
General Dosage Range Oral: *Adults:* 500-1000 mg/day in 3 divided doses
Pregnancy Risk Factor C

Glutamine (GLOO ta meen)

U.S. Brand Names Enterex® Glutapak-10® [OTC]; NutreStore™; Resource® GlutaSolve® [OTC]; Sympt-X G.I. [OTC]; Sympt-X [OTC]
Pharmacologic Category Amino Acid; Gastrointestinal Agent, Miscellaneous
Use
NutreStore™: Treatment of short bowel syndrome (SBS) when used in combination with specialized nutritional support and growth hormone therapy
OTC products: Medical food used to promote GI tract healing and nutritional supplementation with GI disorders, HIV/AIDS, cancer, and other critical illnesses
Local Anesthetic/Vasoconstrictor Precautions No information available to require special precautions
Effects on Dental Treatment No significant effects or complications reported
Effects on Bleeding No information available to require special precautions
Adverse Effects Frequency not defined.
Cardiovascular: Facial edema, peripheral edema
Central nervous system: Dizziness, fever, headache, pain
Dermatologic: Pruritus, rash
Gastrointestinal: Abdominal pain, flatulence, nausea, pancreatitis, tenesmus, vomiting
Neuromuscular & skeletal: Arthralgia, back pain, hypoesthesia
Otic: Ear or hearing symptoms
Respiratory: Rhinitis
Miscellaneous: Flu-like syndrome, infection, sepsis
General Dosage Range Oral: *Adults:* 5-30 g/day in 3 divided doses **or** 5 g 6 times/day
Mechanism of Action Glutamine regulates gastrointestinal cell growth, function, and regeneration. Considered a "conditionally essential" amino acid during metabolic stress and injury.
Pharmacodynamics/Kinetics
Half-life Elimination I.V.: 1 hour
Pregnancy Risk Factor C

GlyBURIDE (GLYE byoor ide)

Related Information
Endocrine Disorders and Pregnancy *on page 1879*
U.S. Brand Names DiaBeta®; Glynase® PresTab®
Canadian Brand Names Apo-Glyburide®; Diaβeta®; Dom-Glyburide; Euglucon®; Med-Glybe; Mylan-Glybe; Novo-Glyburide; Nu-Glyburide; PMS-Glyburide; PRO-Glyburide; ratio-Glyburide; Riva-Glyburide; Sandoz-Glyburide; Teva-Glyburide
Generic Availability (U.S.) Yes
Pharmacologic Category Antidiabetic Agent, Sulfonylurea
Use Adjunct to diet and exercise for the management of type 2 diabetes mellitus (noninsulin dependent, NIDDM)
Unlabeled/Investigational Use Alternative to insulin in women for the treatment of gestational diabetes mellitus (GDM) (11-33 weeks gestation)
Local Anesthetic/Vasoconstrictor Precautions No information available to require special precautions
Effects on Dental Treatment Glyburide-dependent patients with diabetes (noninsulin dependent, type 2) should be appointed for dental treatment in morning in order to minimize chance of stress-induced hypoglycemia.
Effects on Bleeding No information available to require special precautions
Adverse Effects Frequency not defined.
Cardiovascular: Vasculitis
Central nervous system: Dizziness, headache
Dermatologic: Angioedema, erythema, maculopapular eruptions, morbilliform eruptions, photosensitivity reaction, pruritus, purpura, rash, urticaria
Endocrine & metabolic: Disulfiram-like reaction, hypoglycemia, hyponatremia (SIADH reported with other sulfonylureas)
Gastrointestinal: Anorexia, constipation, diarrhea, epigastric fullness, heartburn, nausea
Genitourinary: Nocturia

Hematologic: Agranulocytosis, aplastic anemia, hemolytic anemia, leukopenia, pancytopenia, porphyria cutanea tarda, thrombocytopenia
Hepatic: Cholestatic jaundice, hepatitis, liver failure, transaminase increased
Neuromuscular & skeletal: Arthralgia, myalgia, paresthesia
Ocular: Blurred vision
Renal: Diuretic effect (minor)
Miscellaneous: Allergic reaction

Dosage Oral: Micronized glyburide tablets are **not** bioequivalent to conventional glyburide tablets; retitration should occur if patients are being transferred to a different glyburide formulation (eg, micronized-to-conventional or vice versa) or from other hypoglycemic agents.

DiaBeta®: Adults:
- Initial: 2.5-5 mg/day, administered with breakfast or the first main meal of the day. In patients who are more sensitive to hypoglycemic drugs, start at 1.25 mg/day.
- Increase in increments of no more than 2.5 mg/day at weekly intervals based on the patient's blood glucose response
- Maintenance: 1.25-20 mg/day given as single or divided doses. Some patients (especially those receiving >10 mg/day) may have a more satisfactory response with twice-daily dosing. Maximum: 20 mg/day
- Elderly: Initial: 1.25-2.5 mg/day, increase by 1.25-2.5 mg/day every 1-3 weeks

Micronized tablets (Glynase® PresTab®): Adults:
- Initial: 1.5-3 mg/day, administered with breakfast or the first main meal of the day in patients who are more sensitive to hypoglycemic drugs, start at 0.75 mg/day. Increase in increments of no more than 1.5 mg/day in weekly intervals based on the patient's blood glucose response.
- Maintenance: 0.75-12 mg/day given as a single dose or in divided doses. Some patients (especially those receiving >6 mg/day) may have a more satisfactory response with twice-daily dosing. Maximum: 12 mg/day

Management of noninsulin-dependent diabetes mellitus in patients previously maintained on insulin: Initial dosage dependent upon previous insulin dosage, see table.

Dose Conversion: Insulin to Glyburide

Previous Daily Insulin Dosage (units/day)	Initial Glyburide Dosage *Conventional Formulation* (mg/day)	Initial Glyburide Dosage *Micronized Formulation* (mg/day)	Insulin Dosage Change (after glyburide started)
<20	2.5-5	1.5-3	Discontinue
20-40	5	3	Discontinue
>40	5 (increase in increments of 1.25-2.5 mg every 2-10 days)	3 (increase in increments of 0.75-1.5 mg every 2-10 days)	Reduce insulin dosage by 50% (gradually taper off insulin as glyburide dosage increased)

Dosing adjustment/comments in renal impairment: Cl_{cr} <50 mL/minute: **Not recommended**

Dosing adjustment in hepatic impairment: Use conservative initial and maintenance doses and avoid use in severe disease

Mechanism of Action Stimulates insulin release from the pancreatic beta cells; reduces glucose output from the liver; insulin sensitivity is increased at peripheral target sites

Contraindications Hypersensitivity to glyburide or any component of the formulation; type 1 diabetes mellitus (insulin dependent, IDDM), diabetic ketoacidosis; concomitant use with bosentan

Warnings/Precautions All sulfonylurea drugs are capable of producing severe hypoglycemia. Hypoglycemia is more likely to occur when caloric intake is deficient, after severe or prolonged exercise, when ethanol is ingested, or when more than one glucose-lowering drug is used. It is also more likely in elderly patients, malnourished patients and in patients with impaired renal or hepatic function; use with caution.

Elderly: Rapid and prolonged hypoglycemia (>12 hours) despite hypertonic glucose injections have been reported; age and hepatic and renal impairment are independent risk factors for hypoglycemia; dosage titration should be made at weekly intervals.

Chemical similarities are present among sulfonamides, sulfonylureas, carbonic anhydrase inhibitors, thiazides, and loop diuretics (except ethacrynic acid). Use in patients with sulfonamide allergy is not specifically contraindicated in product labeling, however, a risk of cross-reaction exists in patients with allergy to any of these compounds; avoid use when previous reaction has been severe.

Product labeling states oral hypoglycemic drugs may be associated with an increased cardiovascular mortality as compared to treatment with diet alone or diet plus insulin. Data to support this association are limited, and several studies, including a large prospective trial (UKPDS) have not supported an association.

Patients with G6PD deficiency may be at an increased risk of sulfonylurea-induced hemolytic anemia; however, cases have also been described in patients without G6PD deficiency during postmarketing surveillance. Use with caution and consider a nonsulfonylurea alternative in patients with G6PD deficiency.

Micronized glyburide tablets are **not** bioequivalent to *conventional* glyburide tablets; retitration should occur if patients are being transferred to a different glyburide formulation (eg, micronized-to-conventional or vice versa) or from other hypoglycemic agents.

It may be necessary to discontinue therapy and administer insulin if the patient is exposed to stress (fever, trauma, infection, surgery).

Drug Interactions

Metabolism/Transport Effects **Substrate** of CYP2C9 (major), 3A4 (minor); **Inhibits** CYP2C8 (weak), 3A4 (weak)

Avoid Concomitant Use

Avoid concomitant use of GlyBURIDE with any of the following: Bosentan

Increased Effect/Toxicity

GlyBURIDE may increase the levels/effects of: Alcohol (Ethyl); Bosentan; CycloSPORINE; CycloSPORINE (Systemic); Hypoglycemic Agents

The levels/effects of GlyBURIDE may be increased by: Beta-Blockers; Chloramphenicol; Cimetidine; Clarithromycin; Cyclic Antidepressants; CYP2C9 Inhibitors (Moderate); CYP2C9 Inhibitors (Strong); Fibric Acid Derivatives; Fluconazole; GLP-1 Agonists; Herbs (Hypoglycemic Properties); Pegvisomant; Quinolone Antibiotics; Ranitidine; Salicylates; Sulfonamide Derivatives; Voriconazole

Decreased Effect

GlyBURIDE may decrease the levels/effects of: Bosentan

The levels/effects of GlyBURIDE may be decreased by: Bosentan; Colesevelam; Corticosteroids (Orally Inhaled); Corticosteroids (Systemic); CycloSPORINE; CycloSPORINE (Systemic); CYP2C9 Inducers (Highly Effective); Luteinizing Hormone-Releasing Hormone Analogs; Peginterferon Alfa-2b; Quinolone Antibiotics; Rifampin; Somatropin; Thiazide Diuretics

Ethanol/Nutrition/Herb Interactions

Ethanol: Caution with ethanol (may cause hypoglycemia).

Herb/Nutraceutical: Herbs with hypoglycemic properties may enhance the hypoglycemic effect of glyburide. This includes alfalfa, aloe, bilberry, bitter melon, burdock, celery, damiana, fenugreek, garcinia, garlic, ginger, ginseng (American), gymnema, marshmallow, stinging nettle

Dietary Considerations Should be taken with meals at the same time each day (twice-daily dosing may be beneficial if conventional glyburide doses are >10 mg or micronized glyburide doses are >6 mg). Individualized medical nutrition therapy (MNT) based on ADA recommendations is an integral part of therapy.

Pharmacodynamics/Kinetics

Onset of Action Serum insulin levels begin to increase 15-60 minutes after a single dose

Duration of Action ≤24 hours

Half-life Elimination Diabeta®: 10 hours; Glynase® PresTab®: ~4 hours; may be prolonged with renal or hepatic impairment

Time to Peak Serum: Adults: 2-4 hours

Pregnancy Risk Factor B/C (manufacturer dependent)

Lactation Does not enter breast milk/use caution

Breast-Feeding Considerations Data from initial studies note that glyburide was not detected in breast milk. Breast-feeding is not recommended by the manufacturer. Potentially, hypoglycemia may occur in a nursing infant exposed to a sulfonylurea via breast milk.

Dosage Forms

Tablet, oral: 1.25 mg, 1.5 mg, 2.5 mg, 3 mg, 5 mg, 6 mg

DiaBeta®: 1.25 mg, 2.5 mg, 5 mg

Glynase® PresTab®: 1.5 mg, 3 mg, 6 mg

Glyburide and Metformin (GLYE byoor ide & met FOR min)

Related Information

Endocrine Disorders and Pregnancy *on page* 1879

GlyBURIDE *on page* 824

MetFORMIN *on page* 1089

U.S. Brand Names Glucovance®

Generic Availability (U.S.) Yes

Pharmacologic Category Antidiabetic Agent, Biguanide; Antidiabetic Agent, Sulfonylurea

Use Adjunct to diet and exercise for the management of type 2 diabetes mellitus (noninsulin dependent, NIDDM)

Local Anesthetic/Vasoconstrictor Precautions No information available to require special precautions

Effects on Dental Treatment Glyburide-dependent patients with diabetes (non-insulin dependent, type 2) should be appointed for dental treatment in morning in order to minimize chance of stress-induced hypoglycemia. Metformin-dependent patients with diabetes (noninsulin dependent, type 2) should be appointed for dental treatment in morning in order to minimize chance of stress-induced hypoglycemia.

Effects on Bleeding No information available to require special precautions

Adverse Effects (Also refer to individual agents)

>10%:

Endocrine & metabolic: Hypoglycemia (11% to 38%, effects higher when increased doses were used as initial therapy)

Gastrointestinal: Diarrhea (17%)

Respiratory: Upper respiratory infection (17%)

1% to 10%:

Central nervous system: Headache (9%), dizziness (6%)

Gastrointestinal: Nausea (8%), vomiting (8%), abdominal pain (7%) (combined GI effects increased to 38% in patients taking high doses as initial therapy)

Dosage Note: Dose must be individualized. Dosages expressed as glyburide/metformin components.

Adults: Oral:

Initial therapy (no prior treatment with sulfonylurea or metformin): 1.25 mg/250 mg once daily with a meal; patients with Hb A_{1c} >9% or fasting plasma glucose (FPG) >200 mg/dL may start with 1.25 mg/250 mg twice daily with meals. **Note:** Doses of 5 mg/500 mg should not be used as initial therapy, due to risk of hypoglycemia.

Dosage may be increased in increments of 1.25 mg/250 mg, at intervals of not less than 2 weeks; maximum daily dose: 10 mg/2000 mg (limited experience with higher doses)

Previously treated with a sulfonylurea or metformin alone: Initial: 2.5 mg/500 mg or 5 mg/500 mg twice daily with meals; increase in increments no greater than 5 mg/500 mg; maximum daily dose: 20 mg/2000 mg

When switching patients previously on a sulfonylurea and metformin together, do not exceed the daily dose of glyburide (or glyburide equivalent) or metformin.

Note: May combine with a thiazolidinedione in patients with an inadequate response to glyburide/metformin therapy (risk of hypoglycemia may be increased). When adding thiazolidinedione, continue glyburide and metformin at current dose and initiate thiazolidinedione at recommended starting dose.

Elderly: Oral: Conservative doses are recommended in the elderly due to potentially decreased renal function; **do not titrate to maximum dose**; should not be used in patients ≥80 years of age unless renal function is verified as normal

Dosage adjustment in renal impairment: Risk of lactic acidosis increases with degree of renal impairment; contraindicated in renal disease or renal dysfunction (see Contraindications)

Dosage adjustment in hepatic impairment: Use conservative initial and maintenance doses and avoid use in severe hepatic disease

Mechanism of Action The combination of glyburide and metformin is used to improve glycemic control in patients with type 2 diabetes mellitus by using two different, but complementary, mechanisms of action:

Glyburide: Stimulates insulin release from the pancreatic beta cells; reduces glucose output from the liver; insulin sensitivity is increased at peripheral target sites

Metformin: Decreases hepatic glucose production, decreasing intestinal absorption of glucose and improves insulin sensitivity (increases peripheral glucose uptake and utilization)

Contraindications Hypersensitivity to glyburide, metformin, or any component of the formulation; renal disease or renal dysfunction (serum creatinine ≥1.5 mg/dL in males or ≥1.4 mg/dL in females, or abnormal creatinine clearance) which may also result from conditions such as cardiovascular collapse, acute myocardial infarction, and septicemia; acute or chronic metabolic acidosis with or without coma (including diabetic ketoacidosis)

Note: Temporarily discontinue in patients undergoing radiologic studies in which intravascular iodinated contrast materials are utilized. Temporarily discontinue for surgical procedures.

Warnings/Precautions Age, hepatic and renal impairment are independent risk factors for hypoglycemia. Use with caution in patients with hepatic impairment, malnourished or debilitated conditions, or adrenal or pituitary insufficiency. Use caution in patients with renal impairment. Use with caution in the elderly. Instruct patients to avoid excessive acute or chronic ethanol use; ethanol may potentiate metformin's effect on lactate metabolism.

[U.S. Boxed Warning]: Lactic acidosis is a rare, but potentially fatal and severe consequence of therapy with metformin. Withhold therapy in hypoxemia, dehydration, or sepsis. The risk of lactic acidosis is increased in any patient with acutely decompensated HF requiring pharmacologic management. This risk is particularly high during acute or unstable acutely decompensated HF because of the risk of hypoperfusion and hypoxemia. Metformin is substantially excreted by the kidney. The risk of accumulation and lactic acidosis increases with the degree of renal impairment. Patients with renal function below the limit of normal for their age should not receive metformin. In elderly patients, renal function should be monitored regularly; should not be used in any patient ≥80 years of age unless normal renal function is confirmed. Use of concomitant medications that may affect renal function (ie, affect tubular secretion) may also affect metformin disposition. Metformin should be withheld in patients with dehydration and/or prerenal azotemia. Therapy should be suspended for any surgical procedures requiring food or fluid restriction (resume only after normal intake resumed and normal renal function is verified). Intravascular iodinated contrast media used for radiologic studies are associated with alteration of renal function and may increase risk of lactic acidosis. Discontinue Glucovance® at the time of or prior to the procedure and withhold for 48 hours subsequent to the procedure; reinstitute only after renal function has been re-evaluated and found to be normal.

Chemical similarities are present among sulfonamides, sulfonylureas, carbonic anhydrase inhibitors, thiazides, and loop diuretics (except ethacrynic acid). Use in patients with sulfonamide allergy is not specifically contraindicated in product labeling, however a risk of cross-reaction exists in patients with allergy to any of these compounds; avoid use when previous reaction has been severe.

Product labeling states oral hypoglycemic drugs may be associated with an increased cardiovascular mortality as compared to treatment with diet alone or diet plus insulin. Data to support this association are limited, and several studies, including a large prospective trial (UKPDS), have not supported an association. Metformin does not appear to share this risk. Concurrent use with a thiazolidinedione may increase risk of hypoglycemia and/or weight gain; liver function tests should be monitored periodically with concurrent use.

Drug Interactions

Avoid Concomitant Use

Avoid concomitant use of Glyburide and Metformin with any of the following: Bosentan

Increased Effect/Toxicity

Glyburide and Metformin may increase the levels/effects of: Alcohol (Ethyl); Bosentan; CycloSPORINE; CycloSPORINE (Systemic); Dofetilide; Hypoglycemic Agents

The levels/effects of Glyburide and Metformin may be increased by: Beta-Blockers; Cephalexin; Chloramphenicol; Cimetidine; Clarithromycin; Cyclic Antidepressants; CYP2C9 Inhibitors (Moderate); CYP2C9 Inhibitors (Strong); Fibric Acid Derivatives; Fluconazole; GLP-1 Agonists; Glycopyrrolate; Herbs (Hypoglycemic Properties); Iodinated Contrast Agents; Pegvisomant; Quinolone Antibiotics; Ranitidine; Salicylates; Sulfonamide Derivatives; Voriconazole

Decreased Effect

Glyburide and Metformin may decrease the levels/effects of: Bosentan

The levels/effects of Glyburide and Metformin may be decreased by: Bosentan; Colesevelam; Corticosteroids (Orally Inhaled); Corticosteroids (Systemic); CycloSPORINE; CycloSPORINE (Systemic); CYP2C9 Inducers (Highly Effective); Luteinizing Hormone-Releasing Hormone Analogs; Peginterferon Alfa-2b; Quinolone Antibiotics; Rifampin; Somatropin; Thiazide Diuretics

Ethanol/Nutrition/Herb Interactions

Ethanol: May cause hypoglycemia; incidence of lactic acidosis may be increased; a disulfiram-like reaction characterized by flushing, headache, nausea, vomiting, sweating, or tachycardia has been reported with sulfonylureas; avoid or limit use.

Food: Metformin decreases absorption of vitamin B_{12}. Metformin decreases absorption of folic acid.

Dietary Considerations May cause GI upset; take with food to decrease GI upset. Dietary modification based on ADA recommendations is a part of therapy. Individualized medical nutrition therapy (MNT) based on ADA recommendations is an integral part of therapy. Monitor for signs and symptoms of vitamin B_{12} and folic acid deficiency; supplementation may be required.

Pharmacodynamics/Kinetics

Time to Peak Glucovance®: 2.75 hours when taken with food

Pregnancy Risk Factor B

Lactation Excretion in breast milk unknown/not recommended

Breast-Feeding Considerations Refer to individual agents.

Dosage Forms

Tablet: Glyburide 1.25 mg and metformin 250 mg; glyburide 2.5 mg and metformin 500 mg; glyburide 5 mg and metformin 500 mg

Glucovance®: 2.5 mg/500 mg: Glyburide 2.5 mg and metformin 500 mg; 5 mg/500 mg: Glyburide 5 mg and metformin 500 mg

Glycerin (GLIS er in)

U.S. Brand Names Fleet® Glycerin Maximum Strength [OTC]; Fleet® Glycerin Suppositories [OTC]; Fleet® Liquid Glycerin [OTC]; Fleet® Pedia-Lax™ Glycerin Suppositories [OTC]; Fleet® Pedia-Lax™ Liquid Glycerin Suppositories [OTC]; Orajel® Dry Mouth [OTC]; Sani-Supp® [OTC]

Pharmacologic Category Laxative, Osmotic; Ophthalmic Agent, Miscellaneous

Use Constipation; reduction of intraocular pressure; reduction of corneal edema; glycerin has been administered orally to reduce intracranial pressure

Local Anesthetic/Vasoconstrictor Precautions No information available to require special precautions

Effects on Dental Treatment No significant effects or complications reported

Effects on Bleeding No information available to require special precautions

Adverse Effects Frequency not defined.

Cardiovascular: Arrhythmias

Central nervous system: Confusion, dizziness, headache, hyperosmolar nonketotic coma

Endocrine & metabolic: Dehydration, hyperglycemia, polydipsia

Gastrointestinal: Cramping pain, diarrhea, dry mouth, nausea, rectal irritation, tenesmus, vomiting

General Dosage Range

Ophthalmic: *Children and Adults:* Instill 1-2 drops in eye(s) once or every 3-4 hours

Oral: *Children and Adults:* 1.5 g/kg/day divided every 4 hours **or** 1 g/kg/dose every 6 hours **or** 1-1.8 g/kg once

Rectal:

Children <6 years: 1 infant suppository 1-2 times/day as needed **or** 2-5 mL as an enema

Children ≥6 years and Adults: 1 adult suppository 1-2 times/day as needed **or** 5-15 mL as an enema

Mechanism of Action Osmotic dehydrating agent which increases osmotic pressure; draws fluid into colon and thus stimulates evacuation

Pharmacodynamics/Kinetics

Onset of Action

Decrease in intraocular pressure: Oral: 10-30 minutes; Peak effect: 60-90 minutes

Reduction of intracranial pressure: Oral: 10-60 minutes; Peak effect: 60-90 minutes

Constipation: Suppository: 15-30 minutes

Duration of Action

Decrease in intraocular pressure: Oral: 4-8 hours

Reduction of intracranial pressure: Oral: ~2-3 hours

Half-life Elimination Serum: 30-45 minutes

Pregnancy Risk Factor C

Glycopyrrolate (glye koe PYE roe late)

U.S. Brand Names Cuvposa™; Robinul®; Robinul® Forte

Canadian Brand Names Glycopyrrolate Injection, USP

Pharmacologic Category Anticholinergic Agent

Use Inhibit salivation and excessive secretions of the respiratory tract preoperatively; control of upper airway secretions; intraoperatively to counteract drug-induced or vagal mediated bradyarrhythmias; adjunct in treatment of peptic ulcer (indication listed in product labeling but currently has no place in management of peptic ulcer disease)

Cuvposa™: Reduce chronic, severe drooling in those with neurologic conditions (eg, cerebral palsy) associated with drooling

Unlabeled/Investigational Use Adjunct with acetylcholinesterase inhibitors (eg, neostigmine, edrophonium, pyridostigmine) to antagonize cholinergic effects

Local Anesthetic/Vasoconstrictor Precautions No information available to require special precautions

Effects on Dental Treatment Key adverse event(s) related to dental treatment: Significant xerostomia (normal salivary flow resumes upon discontinuation).

Effects on Bleeding No information available to require special precautions

Adverse Effects

>10% (as reported with Cuvposa™):

Cardiovascular: Flushing (30%)

Central nervous system: Headache (15%)

Gastrointestinal: Vomiting (40%), xerostomia (40%), constipation (35%)

Genitourinary: Urinary retention (15%)

Respiratory: Nasal congestion (30%), sinusitis (15%), upper respiratory tract infection (15%)

<10% (frequency not always defined):

Cardiovascular: Pallor (≤2%), arrhythmias, cardiac arrest, heart block, hyper-/hypotension, malignant hyperthermia, palpitation, QT_c-interval prolongation, tachycardia

Central nervous system: Aggressiveness (≤2%), agitation (≤2%), crying (abnormal; ≤2%), irritability (≤2%), mood changes (≤2%), pain (≤2%), restlessness (≤2%), confusion, dizziness, drowsiness, excitement, insomnia, nervousness, seizure

Dermatologic: Dry skin (≤2%), pruritus (≤2%), rash (≤2%), urticaria

Endocrine & metabolic: Dehydration (≤2%), lactation suppression

Gastrointestinal: Abdominal distention (≤2%), abdominal pain (≤2%), flatulence (≤2%), retching (≤2%), bloated feeling, intestinal obstruction, loss of taste, nausea, pseudo-obstruction

Genitourinary: Urinary tract infection (≤2%), impotence, urinary hesitancy

Local: Injection site reactions (edema, erythema, pain)

Neuromuscular & skeletal: Weakness

Ocular: Nystagmus (≤2%), blurred vision, cycloplegia, mydriasis, ocular tension increased, photophobia, sensitivity to light increased

Respiratory: Bronchial secretion (thickening; ≤2%), nasal dryness (≤2%), pneumonia (≤2%), respiratory depression

Miscellaneous: Anaphylactoid reactions, diaphoresis decreased, hypersensitivity reactions

General Dosage Range

I.M.:

Children <2 years: 4-9 mcg/kg once **or** 4-10 mcg/kg every 3-4 hours (maximum: 0.2 mg/dose; 0.8 mg/day)

Children ≥2 years: 4 mcg/kg once **or** 4-10 mcg/kg every 3-4 hours (maximum: 0.2 mg/dose; 0.8 mg/day)

Adults: 4 mcg/kg once **or** 0.1-0.2 mg 3-4 times/day

I.V.:

Children: 4-10 mcg/kg every 3-4 hours (maximum: 0.2 mg/dose; 0.8 mg/day) **or** 4 mcg/kg (maximum: 0.1 mg); repeat as needed

Adults: 0.1-0.2 mg 3-4 times/day **or** 0.1 mg repeated as needed

Oral: *Children 3-16 years:* 0.02-0.1 mg/kg/dose 3 times/day (maximum 3 mg/dose)

Mechanism of Action Blocks the action of acetylcholine at parasympathetic sites in smooth muscle, secretory glands, and the CNS; indirectly reduces the rate of salivation by preventing the stimulation of acetylcholine receptors

Pharmacodynamics/Kinetics

Onset of Action Oral: 50 minutes; I.M.: 15-30 minutes; I.V.: ~1 minute

Peak effect: Oral: ~1 hour; I.M.: 30-45 minutes

Duration of Action Vagal effect: 2-3 hours; Inhibition of salivation: Up to 7 hours; Anticholinergic: Oral: 8-12 hours

Half-life Elimination Infants: 22-130 minutes; Children 19-99 minutes; Adults: ~60-75 minutes; Oral solution: Adults: 3 hours

Pregnancy Risk Factor B (injection) / C (oral solution)

Gold Sodium Thiomalate (gold SOW dee um thye oh MAL ate)

U.S. Brand Names Myochrysine®
Canadian Brand Names Myochrysine®
Pharmacologic Category Gold Compound
Use Adjunctive treatment of active rheumatoid arthritis
Local Anesthetic/Vasoconstrictor Precautions No information available to require special precautions
Effects on Dental Treatment Key adverse event(s) related to dental treatment: Stomatitis, gingivitis, and glossitis.
Effects on Bleeding No information available to require special precautions
Adverse Effects Frequency not defined.
Cardiovascular: Bradycardia, syncope
Central nervous system: Confusion, fever, Guillain-Barré syndrome, hallucinations, seizure
Dermatologic: Alopecia, angioedema, dermatitis, nail shedding, pruritus, rash, urticaria
Gastrointestinal: Anorexia, abdominal cramps, diarrhea, dysphagia, enterocolitis (ulcerative), gingivitis, glossitis, nausea, stomatitis, taste disturbance (metallic), thick tongue, vomiting
Hematologic: Agranulocytosis, aplastic anemia, eosinophilia, leukopenia, purpura, thrombocytopenia
Hepatic: Cholestasis, hepatitis, hepatotoxicity, jaundice
Neuromuscular & skeletal: Arthralgia, peripheral neuropathy
Ocular: Conjunctivitis, corneal ulcers, gold deposits in ocular tissues, iritis
Respiratory: Dyspnea, gold bronchitis, interstitial pneumonitis, pulmonary fibrosis
Renal: Glomerulitis, hematuria, nephrotic syndrome, proteinuria
Miscellaneous: Anaphylactoid reaction, anaphylaxis, nitritoid reaction
General Dosage Range Dosage adjustment recommended in patients with renal impairment or who develop toxicities
I.M.:
Children: Test dose (recommended): 10 mg first week; Initial dosing: 1 mg/kg/week (maximum: 50 mg/injection); Maintenance: 1 mg/kg/dose (maximum: 50 mg/injection)
Adults: Test dose: 10 mg first week; Initial dosing: 25 mg second week, then 25-50 mg/week until 1 g cumulative dose has been given; Maintenance: 25-50 mg every other week for 2-20 weeks, then every 3-4 weeks
Mechanism of Action Unknown, may decrease prostaglandin synthesis or may alter cellular mechanisms by inhibiting sulfhydryl systems
Pharmacodynamics/Kinetics
Onset of Action Delayed; may require up to 3 months
Half-life Elimination 5 days; may be prolonged with multiple doses
Time to Peak Serum: 4-6 hours
Pregnancy Risk Factor C

Golimumab (goe LIM ue mab)

Related Information
Rheumatoid Arthritis, Osteoarthritis, and Osteoporosis *on page* 1889
U.S. Brand Names Simponi®
Canadian Brand Names Simponi®
Pharmacologic Category Antipsoriatic Agent; Antirheumatic, Disease Modifying; Monoclonal Antibody; Tumor Necrosis Factor (TNF) Blocking Agent
Use Treatment of active rheumatoid arthritis (moderate-to-severe), active psoriatic arthritis, and active ankylosing spondylitis
Local Anesthetic/Vasoconstrictor Precautions No information available to require special precautions
Effects on Dental Treatment No significant effects or complications reported
Effects on Bleeding No information available to require special precautions
Adverse Effects
>10%:
Respiratory: Upper respiratory tract infection (16%; includes laryngitis, nasopharyngitis, pharyngitis, and rhinitis)
Miscellaneous: Infection (28%)
1% to 10%:
Cardiovascular: Hypertension (3%)
Central nervous system: Dizziness (2%), fever (1%)
Gastrointestinal: Constipation (1%)
Hepatic: ALT increased (4%), AST increased (3%)

Local: Injection site reactions (6%)
Neuromuscular & skeletal: Paresthesia (2%)
Respiratory: Bronchitis (2%), sinusitis (2%)
Miscellaneous: Viral infection (5%; includes herpes and influenza), antibody formation (4%), fungal infection (superficial; 2%)

General Dosage Range SubQ: *Adults:* 50 mg once per month

Mechanism of Action Human monoclonal antibody that binds to human tumor necrosis factor alpha (TNFα), thereby interfering with endogenous TNFα activity. Biological activities of TNFα include the induction of proinflammatory cytokines (interleukin [IL]-6, IL-8, Granulocyte-colony stimulating factor, granulocyte-macrophage colony stimulating factor), expression of adhesion molecules (E-selectin, vascular cell adhesion molecule [VCAM]-1, intercellular adhesion molecule [ICAM]-1) necessary for leukocyte infiltration, activation of neutrophils and eosinophils.

Pharmacodynamics/Kinetics

Half-life Elimination ~2 weeks

Time to Peak SubQ: 2-6 days

Pregnancy Risk Factor B

Gonadorelin (goe nad oh RELL in)

Canadian Brand Names Lutrepulse™

Pharmacologic Category Gonadotropin

Use Induction of ovulation in females with hypothalamic amenorrhea

Local Anesthetic/Vasoconstrictor Precautions No information available to require special precautions

Effects on Dental Treatment No significant effects or complications reported

Effects on Bleeding No information available to require special precautions

Adverse Effects Local: Injection site irritation, superficial thrombophlebitis

General Dosage Range I.V., SubQ: *Adults:* 1-20 mcg every 90 minutes

Mechanism of Action Stimulates the release of luteinizing hormone (LH) from the anterior pituitary gland

Pharmacodynamics/Kinetics

Onset of Action Response to therapy usually observed within 2-3 weeks

Half-life Elimination Terminal: ~10-40 minutes; increased in patients with renal impairment

Product Availability Not available in U.S.

Goserelin (GOE se rel in)

U.S. Brand Names Zoladex®

Canadian Brand Names Zoladex®; Zoladex® LA

Pharmacologic Category Antineoplastic Agent, Gonadotropin-Releasing Hormone Agonist; Gonadotropin Releasing Hormone Agonist

Use Treatment of locally confined prostate cancer; palliative treatment of advanced prostate cancer; palliative treatment of advanced breast cancer in pre- and perimenopausal women; treatment of endometriosis, including pain relief and reduction of endometriotic lesions; endometrial thinning agent as part of treatment for dysfunctional uterine bleeding

Local Anesthetic/Vasoconstrictor Precautions No information available to require special precautions

Effects on Dental Treatment Key adverse event(s) related to dental treatment: Xerostomia (normal salivary flow resumes upon discontinuation) and taste disturbances.

Effects on Bleeding No information available to require special precautions

Adverse Effects Percentages reported with the 1-month implant:

>10%:

Cardiovascular: Peripheral edema (female 21%)
Central nervous system: Headache (female 32% to 75%; male 1% to 5%), emotional lability (female 60%), depression (female 54%; male 1% to 5%), pain (female 17%; male 8%), insomnia (female 11%; male 5%)
Dermatologic: Acne (female 42%), seborrhea (female 26%)
Endocrine & metabolic: Hot flashes (female 57% to 96%; male 62%), libido decreased (female 48% to 61%), sexual dysfunction (male 21%), breast atrophy (female 33%), breast enlargement (female 18%), erections decreased (18%), libido increased (female 12%)
Gastrointestinal: Nausea (female 8% to 11%; male 5%), abdominal pain (female 7% to 11%)

Genitourinary: Vaginitis (75%), pelvic symptoms (female 9% to 18%), dyspareunia (female 14%), lower urinary symptoms (male 13%)
Neuromuscular & skeletal: Bone mineral density decreased (female 23%; ~4% decrease from baseline in 6 months; postmarketing reports in males), weakness (female 11%)
Miscellaneous: Diaphoresis (female 16% to 45%; male 6%), tumor flare (female: 23%), infection (female 13%)
1% to 10%:
Cardiovascular: Arrhythmia, cerebrovascular accident, chest pain, edema, heart failure, hypertension, MI, palpitation, peripheral vascular disorder, tachycardia
Central nervous system: Abnormal thinking, anxiety, chills, dizziness, fever, lethargy, malaise, migraine, nervousness, somnolence
Dermatologic: Alopecia, bruising, dry skin, hair disorder, hirsutism, pruritus, rash, skin discoloration
Endocrine & metabolic: Breast pain, breast swelling/tenderness, dysmenorrhea, gout, hyperglycemia
Gastrointestinal: Anorexia, appetite increased, constipation, diarrhea, dyspepsia, flatulence, ulcer, vomiting, weight gain/loss, xerostomia
Genitourinary: Urinary frequency, urinary obstruction, urinary tract infection, vaginal hemorrhage, vulvovaginitis
Hematologic: Anemia, hemorrhage
Local: Application site reaction
Neuromuscular & skeletal: Arthralgia, back pain, hypertonia, joint disorder, leg cramps, myalgia, paresthesia
Ocular: Amblyopia, dry eyes
Renal: Renal insufficiency
Respiratory: Bronchitis, COPD, cough, epistaxis, pharyngitis, rhinitis, sinusitis, upper respiratory tract infection
Miscellaneous: Allergic reaction, flu-like syndrome, voice alteration

General Dosage Range SubQ: *Adults:* 3.6 mg every 28 days **or** 10.8 mg every 12 weeks

Mechanism of Action Goserelin (a gonadotropin-releasing hormone [GnRH] analog) causes an initial increase in luteinizing hormone (LH) and follicle stimulating hormone (FSH), chronic administration of goserelin results in a sustained suppression of pituitary gonadotropins. Serum testosterone falls to levels comparable to surgical castration. The exact mechanism of this effect is unknown, but may be related to changes in the control of LH or down-regulation of LH receptors.

Pharmacodynamics/Kinetics

Onset of Action

Females: Estradiol suppression reaches postmenopausal levels within 3 weeks and FSH and LH are suppressed to follicular phase levels within 4 weeks of initiation.
Males: Testosterone suppression reaches castrate levels within 2-4 weeks after initiation.

Duration of Action

Females: Estradiol, LH and FSH generally return to baseline levels within 12 weeks following the last monthly implant.
Males: Testosterone levels maintained at castrate levels throughout the duration of therapy.

Half-life Elimination SubQ: Male: ~4 hours, Female: ~2 hours; Renal impairment: Male: 12 hours

Time to Peak SubQ: Male: 12-15 days, Female: 8-22 days

Pregnancy Risk Factor X (endometriosis, endometrial thinning); D (advanced breast cancer)

Granisetron (gra NI se tron)

U.S. Brand Names Granisol™; Kytril®; Sancuso®

Canadian Brand Names Apo-Granisetron®; Kytril®

Pharmacologic Category Antiemetic; Selective 5-HT_3 Receptor Antagonist

Use Prophylaxis of nausea and vomiting associated with emetogenic chemotherapy and radiation therapy; prophylaxis and treatment of postoperative nausea and vomiting (PONV)

Unlabeled/Investigational Use Breakthrough treatment of nausea and vomiting associated with chemotherapy

Local Anesthetic/Vasoconstrictor Precautions No information available to require special precautions

Effects on Dental Treatment No significant effects or complications reported

Effects on Bleeding No information available to require special precautions

Adverse Effects

>10%:

Central nervous system: Headache (3% to 21%; transdermal patch: 1%)
Gastrointestinal: Constipation (3% to 18%)
Neuromuscular & skeletal: Weakness (5% to 18%)

1% to 10%:

Cardiovascular: QT_c prolongation (1% to 3%), hypertension (1% to 2%)
Central nervous system: Pain (10%), fever (3% to 9%), dizziness (4% to 5%), insomnia (<2% to 5%), somnolence (1% to 4%), anxiety (2%), agitation (<2%), CNS stimulation (<2%)
Dermatologic: Rash (1%)
Gastrointestinal: Diarrhea (3% to 9%), abdominal pain (4% to 6%), dyspepsia (3% to 6%), taste perversion (2%)
Hepatic: Liver enzymes increased (5% to 6%)
Renal: Oliguria (2%)
Respiratory: Cough (2%)
Miscellaneous: Infection (3%)

General Dosage Range

I.V.:

Children ≥2 years: 10 mcg/kg/dose (maximum: 1 mg/dose) as a single dose or every 12 hours
Adults: 10 mcg/kg/dose (maximum: 1 mg/dose) as a single dose or every 12 hours **or** 1 mg as a single dose

Oral: *Adults:* 2 mg/day in 1-2 divided dose

Transdermal: *Adults:* 1 patch prior to chemotherapy; Maximum duration: Patch may be worn up to 7 days

Mechanism of Action Selective $5\text{-}HT_3$-receptor antagonist, blocking serotonin, both peripherally on vagal nerve terminals and centrally in the chemoreceptor trigger zone

Pharmacodynamics/Kinetics

Duration of Action Oral, I.V.: Generally up to 24 hours

Half-life Elimination Oral: 6 hours; I.V.: 9 hours

Time to Peak Transdermal patch: Maximum systemic concentrations: ~48 hours after application (range: 24-168 hours)

Pregnancy Risk Factor B

Griseofulvin (gri see oh FUL vin)

U.S. Brand Names Grifulvin V®; Gris-PEG®

Pharmacologic Category Antifungal Agent, Oral

Use Treatment of susceptible tinea infections of the skin, hair, and nails

Local Anesthetic/Vasoconstrictor Precautions No information available to require special precautions

Effects on Dental Treatment Key adverse event(s) related to dental treatment: May cause soreness or irritation of mouth or tongue. May cause oral thrush.

Effects on Bleeding No information available to require special precautions

Adverse Effects Frequency not defined.

Central nervous system: Dizziness, fatigue, headache, insomnia, mental confusion
Dermatologic: Angioneurotic edema (rare), erythema multiforme-like drug reaction, photosensitivity, rash (most common), urticaria (most common),
Gastrointestinal: Diarrhea, epigastric distress, GI bleeding, nausea, vomiting
Genitourinary: Menstrual irregularities (rare)
Hematologic: Granulocytopenia, leukopenia
Hepatic: Hepatotoxicity
Neuromuscular & skeletal: Paresthesia (rare)
Renal: Nephrosis, proteinuria
Miscellaneous: Drug-induced lupus-like syndrome (rare), oral thrush

General Dosage Range Oral:

Microsize:

Children >2 years: 10-20 mg/kg/day in single or divided doses
Adults: 500-1000 mg/day in single or divided doses

Ultramicrosize:

Children >2 years: 5-15 mg/kg/day in single dose or 2 divided doses (maximum: 750 mg/day)
Adults: 375-750 mg/day in single or divided doses

Mechanism of Action Inhibits fungal cell mitosis at metaphase; binds to human keratin making it resistant to fungal invasion

Pharmacodynamics/Kinetics

Half-life Elimination 9-22 hours

Pregnancy Risk Factor C

GuaiFENesin (gwye FEN e sin)

U.S. Brand Names Allfen [OTC]; Bidex®-400 [OTC]; Diabetic Siltussin DAS-Na [OTC]; Diabetic Tussin® EX [OTC]; Fenesin IR [OTC]; Ganidin® NR [OTC] [DSC]; Humibid® Maximum Strength [OTC]; Mucinex® Kid's Mini-Melts™ [OTC]; Mucinex® Kid's [OTC]; Mucinex® Maximum Strength [OTC]; Mucinex® [OTC]; Mucus Relief [OTC]; Organidin® NR [OTC] [DSC]; Phanasin® Diabetic Choice® [OTC] [DSC]; Phanasin® [OTC] [DSC]; Refenesen™ 400 [OTC]; Refenesen™ [OTC]; Robafen [OTC]; Robitussin® Chest Congestion [OTC] [DSC]; Scot-Tussin® Expectorant [OTC]; Siltussin DAS [OTC] [DSC]; Siltussin SA [OTC]; Vicks® Casero™ Chest Congestion Relief [OTC]; Vicks® DayQuil® Mucus Control [OTC]; Xpect™ [OTC]

Canadian Brand Names Balminil Expectorant; Benylin® E Extra Strength; Koffex Expectorant; Robitussin®

Pharmacologic Category Expectorant

Use Help loosen phlegm and thin bronchial secretions to make coughs more productive

Local Anesthetic/Vasoconstrictor Precautions No information available to require special precautions

Effects on Dental Treatment No significant effects or complications reported

Effects on Bleeding No information available to require special precautions

Adverse Effects Frequency not defined.

Central nervous system: Dizziness, drowsiness, headache
Dermatologic: Rash
Endocrine & metabolic: Uric acid levels decreased
Gastrointestinal: Nausea, stomach pain, vomiting

General Dosage Range Oral:

Extended release: *Children ≥12 years and Adults:* 600-1200 mg every 12 hours (maximum: 2.4 g/day)

Immediate release:
- *Children 6 months to 2 years:* 25-50 mg every 4 hours (maximum: 300 mg/day)
- *Children 2-5 years:* 50-100 mg every 4 hours (maximum: 600 mg/day)
- *Children 6-11 years:* 100-200 mg every 4 hours (maximum: 1.2 g/day)
- *Children ≥12 years and Adults:* 200-400 mg every 4 hours (maximum: 2.4 g/day)

Mechanism of Action Thought to act as an expectorant by irritating the gastric mucosa and stimulating respiratory tract secretions, thereby increasing respiratory fluid volumes and decreasing mucous viscosity

Pharmacodynamics/Kinetics

Half-life Elimination ~1 hour

Pregnancy Risk Factor C

Guaifenesin and Codeine (gwye FEN e sin & KOE deen)

Related Information

Codeine *on page* 432
GuaiFENesin *on page* 835

U.S. Brand Names Allfen CD; Allfen CDX; Dex-Tuss; ExeClear-C; Gani-Tuss® NR; Mar-Cof® CG; Robafen AC; Tusso-C™

Pharmacologic Category Antitussive; Cough Preparation; Expectorant

Use Temporary control of cough due to minor throat and bronchial irritation

Local Anesthetic/Vasoconstrictor Precautions No information available to require special precautions

Effects on Dental Treatment Key adverse event(s) related to dental treatment: Xerostomia (normal salivary flow resumes upon discontinuation).

Effects on Bleeding No information available to require special precautions

Adverse Effects Frequency not defined; also see individual agents.

Cardiovascular: Bradycardia, circulatory depression, flushing, orthostatic hypotension, palpitation, syncope, tachycardia
Central nervous system: Convulsions, CNS depression, disorientation, dizziness, dysphoria, euphoria, faintness, hallucinations (transient), headache, lightheadedness, sedation
Dermatologic: Angioneurotic edema, pruritus, urticaria
Gastrointestinal: Biliary tract spasm, colonic motility increase (with chronic ulcerative colitis), constipation, nausea, stomach pain, toxic dilation (with acute ulcerative colitis), vomiting
Genitourinary: Oliguria, urinary retention
Neuromuscular & skeletal: Weakness
Ocular: Visual disturbances
Respiratory: Laryngeal edema, respiratory depression
Miscellaneous: Anaphylaxis, diaphoresis

General Dosage Range Oral: *Children ≥6 years and Adults:* Dosage varies greatly depending on product

Mechanism of Action

Guaifenesin may act as an expectorant by irritating the gastric mucosa and stimulating respiratory tract secretions, thereby increasing respiratory fluid volumes and decreasing phlegm viscosity

Codeine is an antitussive that controls cough by depressing the medullary cough center

Pregnancy Risk Factor C

Controlled Substance C-V

Guaifenesin and Dextromethorphan

(gwye FEN e sin & deks troe meth OR fan)

Related Information

Dextromethorphan *on page* 504

GuaiFENesin *on page* 835

U.S. Brand Names Allfen DM [OTC] [DSC]; Cheracol® D [OTC]; Cheracol® Plus [OTC]; Coricidin HBP® Chest Congestion and Cough [OTC]; Diabetic Siltussin-DM DAS-Na Maximum Strength [OTC]; Diabetic Siltussin-DM DAS-Na [OTC]; Diabetic Tussin® DM Maximum Strength [OTC]; Diabetic Tussin® DM [OTC]; Double Tussin DM [OTC]; Fenesin DM IR; Gani-Tuss DM NR [DSC]; Guaicon DM [OTC] [DSC]; Guaicon DMS [OTC]; Guia-D [DSC]; Guiadrine™ DX [DSC]; Kolephrin® GG/DM [OTC]; Mintab DM [DSC]; Mucinex® DM Maximum Strength [OTC]; Mucinex® DM [OTC]; Mucinex® Kid's Cough Mini-Melts™ [OTC]; Mucinex® Kid's Cough [OTC]; Phanatuss® DM [OTC] [DSC]; Refenesen™ DM [OTC]; Robafen DM Clear [OTC]; Robafen DM [OTC]; Robitussin® Cough & Chest Congestion DM Max [OTC]; Robitussin® Cough & Chest Congestion DM [OTC]; Robitussin® Cough & Chest Congestion Sugar-Free DM [OTC]; Safe Tussin® DM [OTC]; Scot-Tussin® Senior [OTC]; Silexin [OTC]; Siltussin DM DAS [OTC]; Siltussin DM [OTC]; Simuc-DM [DSC]; Su-Tuss DM [DSC]; Tussi-Bid®; Vicks® 44E [OTC]; Vicks® DayQuil® Mucus Control DM [OTC]; Vicks® Pediatric Formula 44E [OTC]

Canadian Brand Names Balminil DM E; Benylin® DM-E; Koffex DM-Expectorant; Robitussin® DM

Pharmacologic Category Antitussive; Cough Preparation; Expectorant

Use Temporary control of cough due to minor throat and bronchial irritation

Local Anesthetic/Vasoconstrictor Precautions No information available to require special precautions

Effects on Dental Treatment No significant effects or complications reported

Effects on Bleeding No information available to require special precautions

Adverse Effects See individual agents.

General Dosage Range Oral:

Children 2-6 years: Guaifenesin 50-100 mg and dextromethorphan 2.5-5 mg every 4 hours (maximum: Guaifenesin 600 mg/day; Dextromethorphan 30 mg/day)

Children 6-12 years: Guaifenesin 100-200 mg and dextromethorphan 5-10 mg every 4 hours (maximum: Guaifenesin 1200 mg/day; Dextromethorphan 60 mg/day)

Children ≥12 years and Adults: Guaifenesin 200-400 mg and dextromethorphan 10-20 mg every 4 hours (maximum: Guaifenesin 2400 mg/day; Dextromethorphan 120 mg/day)

Mechanism of Action

Guaifenesin is thought to act as an expectorant by irritating the gastric mucosa and stimulating respiratory tract secretions, thereby increasing respiratory fluid volumes and decreasing phlegm viscosity

Dextromethorphan is a chemical relative of morphine lacking narcotic properties except in overdose; controls cough by depressing the medullary cough center

Pregnancy Risk Factor C

Guaifenesin and Phenylephrine (gwye FEN e sin & fen il EF rin)

Related Information

GuaiFENesin *on page* 835

Phenylephrine (Systemic) *on page* 1339

U.S. Brand Names Ambi 10PEH/400GFN [OTC]; Crantex®; Donatussin Drops [DSC]; Fenesin PE IR; Guiatex PE™ [DSC]; Liquibid® D-R [OTC]; Liquibid® PD-R [OTC]; Maxiphen [OTC] [DSC]; Medent®-PEI [OTC]; Mucinex® Cold [OTC]; Mucus Relief Sinus [OTC]; OneTab™ Congestion & Cold [OTC]; Refenesen™ PE [OTC]; Rescon GG [OTC]; Sina-12X® [DSC]; Sudafed PE® Non-Drying Sinus [OTC]; Triaminic® Children's Chest & Nasal Congestion [OTC]

Pharmacologic Category Decongestant; Expectorant

Use Temporary relief of nasal congestion, sinusitis, rhinitis, and hay fever; temporary relief of cough associated with upper respiratory tract conditions, especially when associated with dry, nonproductive cough

Local Anesthetic/Vasoconstrictor Precautions Use with caution since phenylephrine is a sympathomimetic amine which could interact with epinephrine to cause a pressor response

Effects on Dental Treatment Key adverse event(s) related to dental treatment:

Guaifenesin: No significant effects or complications reported

Phenylephrine: Up to 10% of patients could experience tachycardia, palpitations, and xerostomia (normal salivary flow resumes upon discontinuation); use vasoconstrictor with caution

Effects on Bleeding No information available to require special precautions

Adverse Effects See individual agents.

General Dosage Range Oral: *Children >2 years and Adults:* Dosage varies greatly depending on product

Mechanism of Action See individual agents.

Pregnancy Risk Factor C

Guaifenesin and Pseudoephedrine (gwye FEN e sin & soo doe e FED rin)

Related Information

GuaiFENesin *on page 835*

Pseudoephedrine *on page 1429*

U.S. Brand Names Ambifed [OTC] [DSC]; Ambifed-G [OTC]; Congestac® [OTC]; ExeFen-IR [DSC]; Maxifed [OTC]; Maxifed-G [OTC]; Mucinex® D Maximum Strength [OTC]; Mucinex® D [OTC]; Refenesen Plus [OTC]; Respaire®-30 [DSC]; SudaTex-G [OTC]; Tenar™ PSE [DSC]

Canadian Brand Names Contac® Cold-Chest Congestion, Non Drowsy, Regular Strength; Entex® LA; Novahistex® Expectorant with Decongestant

Pharmacologic Category Alpha/Beta Agonist; Expectorant

Use Temporary relief of nasal congestion and to help loosen phlegm and thin bronchial secretions in the treatment of cough

Local Anesthetic/Vasoconstrictor Precautions Use with caution since pseudoephedrine is a sympathomimetic amine which could interact with epinephrine to cause a pressor response

Effects on Dental Treatment Key adverse event(s) related to dental treatment:

Guaifenesin: No significant effects or complications reported

Pseudoephedrine: Xerostomia (normal salivary flow resumes upon discontinuation).

Effects on Bleeding No information available to require special precautions

Adverse Effects See individual agents.

General Dosage Range Oral: *Children >2 years and Adults:* Dosage varies greatly depending on product

Pregnancy Risk Factor C

Guaifenesin, Dextromethorphan, and Phenylephrine
(gwye FEN e sin, deks troe meth OR fan, & fen il EF rin)

Related Information

Dextromethorphan *on page 504*

GuaiFENesin *on page 835*

Phenylephrine (Systemic) *on page 1339*

U.S. Brand Names Certuss-D® [DSC]; ExeCof [DSC]; ExeTuss-DM [DSC]; Giltuss Pediatric® [DSC]; Giltuss TR® [DSC]; Giltuss® [DSC]; Guaifen™ DM [DSC]; Maxiphen DM; Mucinex® Children's Multi-Symptom Cold [OTC]; Robafen CF Cough & Cold [OTC]; Robitussin® Children's Cough & Cold CF [OTC]; Robitussin® Cough & Cold CF Max [OTC]; Robitussin® Cough & Cold CF [OTC]; SINUtuss® DM [DSC]; Tusso™-DMR [DSC]

Pharmacologic Category Antitussive; Decongestant

Use Symptomatic relief of dry nonproductive coughs and upper respiratory symptoms associated with hay fever, colds, or the flu

Local Anesthetic/Vasoconstrictor Precautions Use with caution since phenylephrine is a sympathomimetic amine which could interact with epinephrine to cause a pressor response

Effects on Dental Treatment Key adverse event(s) related to dental treatment:

Dextromethorphan: No significant effects or complications reported

Guaifenesin: No significant effects or complications reported

Phenylephrine: Up to 10% of patients could experience tachycardia, palpitations, and xerostomia (normal salivary flow resumes upon discontinuation); use vasoconstrictor with caution

Effects on Bleeding No information available to require special precautions

Adverse Effects Reactions which follow have been reported with the combination product; see individual drug monographs for additional adverse reactions that may be expected from each agent.

Cardiovascular: Cardiovascular collapse, palpitation, tachycardia

Central nervous system: Anxiety, CNS depression, convulsions, dizziness, drowsiness, excitability increased, fear, hallucinations, headache, insomnia, irritability increased, lightheadedness, nervousness

Gastrointestinal: Nausea, vomiting

Neuromuscular & skeletal: Tremor, weakness

Respiratory: Respiratory difficulties

General Dosage Range Oral: *Children >4 years and Adults:* Dosage varies greatly depending on product

Mechanism of Action See individual agents.

Pregnancy Risk Factor C

Guaifenesin, Pseudoephedrine, and Codeine

(gwye FEN e sin, soo doe e FED rin, & KOE deen)

Related Information

Codeine *on page 432*

GuaiFENesin *on page 835*

Pseudoephedrine *on page 1429*

U.S. Brand Names Mytussin® DAC

Canadian Brand Names Benylin® 3.3 mg-D-E; Calmylin with Codeine

Pharmacologic Category Antitussive/Decongestant/Expectorant

Use Temporarily relieves nasal congestion and controls cough associated with upper respiratory infections and related conditions (common cold, sinusitis, bronchitis, influenza)

Local Anesthetic/Vasoconstrictor Precautions Use with caution since pseudoephedrine is a sympathomimetic amine which could interact with epinephrine to cause a pressor response

Effects on Dental Treatment Key adverse event(s) related to dental treatment:

Codeine: Xerostomia (normal salivary flow resumes upon discontinuation).

Guaifenesin: No significant effects or complications reported

Pseudoephedrine: Xerostomia (normal salivary flow resumes upon discontinuation).

Effects on Bleeding No information available to require special precautions

Adverse Effects See individual agents.

General Dosage Range Oral:

Children 6-12 years: 5 mL every 4 hours (maximum: 20 mL/24 hours)

Children >12 years and Adults: 10 mL every 4 hours (maximum: 40 mL/24 hours)

Pregnancy Risk Factor C

Controlled Substance C-V

Guaifenesin, Pseudoephedrine, and Dextromethorphan

(gwye FEN e sin, soo doe e FED rin, & deks troe meth OR fan)

Related Information

Dextromethorphan *on page 504*

GuaiFENesin *on page 835*

Pseudoephedrine *on page 1429*

U.S. Brand Names Ambifed DM [OTC]; Ambifed-G DM [OTC]; Donatussin DM; ExeFen-DMX; Maxifed DM [OTC]; Maxifed DMX [OTC]

Canadian Brand Names Balminil DM + Decongestant + Expectorant; Benylin® DM-D-E

Pharmacologic Category Antitussive/Decongestant/Expectorant

Use Temporarily relieves nasal congestion and controls cough due to minor throat and bronchial irritation; helps loosen phlegm and thin bronchial secretions to make coughs more productive

Local Anesthetic/Vasoconstrictor Precautions Use with caution since pseudoephedrine is a sympathomimetic amine which could interact with epinephrine to cause a pressor response

Effects on Dental Treatment Key adverse event(s) related to dental treatment:

Dextromethorphan: No significant effects or complications reported

Guaifenesin: No significant effects or complications reported

Pseudoephedrine: Xerostomia (normal salivary flow resumes upon discontinuation).

Effects on Bleeding No information available to require special precautions

Adverse Effects See individual agents.

General Dosage Range Oral: *Children ≥6 years and Adults:* Dosage varies greatly depending on product

Mechanism of Action See individual agents.

Pregnancy Risk Factor C

Guanabenz (GWAHN a benz)

Related Information

Cardiovascular Diseases *on page 1848*

Canadian Brand Names Wytensin®

Pharmacologic Category $Alpha_2$-Adrenergic Agonist

Use Management of hypertension

Local Anesthetic/Vasoconstrictor Precautions No information available to require special precautions

Effects on Dental Treatment Key adverse event(s) related to dental treatment: Taste disorder, nasal congestion, dyspnea, significant xerostomia (normal salivary flow resumes upon discontinuation).

Effects on Bleeding No information available to require special precautions

Adverse Effects Higher rates with larger doses

>5% (at doses of 16 mg/day):

- Cardiovascular: Orthostasis
- Central nervous system: Drowsiness or sedation (39%), dizziness (12% to 17%), headache (5%)
- Gastrointestinal: Xerostomia (28% to 38%)
- Neuromuscular & skeletal: Weakness (~10%)

≤3% (may be similar to placebo):

- Cardiovascular: Arrhythmias, chest pain, edema, palpitation
- Central nervous system: Anxiety, ataxia, depression, sleep disturbances
- Dermatologic: Pruritus, rash
- Endocrine & metabolic: Disturbances of sexual function, gynecomastia, decreased sexual function
- Gastrointestinal: Constipation, diarrhea, nausea, vomiting
- Genitourinary: Polyuria
- Neuromuscular & skeletal: Myalgia
- Ocular: Blurring of vision
- Respiratory: Dyspnea, nasal congestion
- Miscellaneous: Taste disorders

General Dosage Range Oral:

Adults: Initial: 4 mg twice daily; Maintenance: 4-32 mg twice daily

Elderly: Initial: 4 mg once daily

Mechanism of Action Stimulates $alpha_2$-adrenoreceptors in the brain stem, thus activating an inhibitory neuron, resulting in reduced sympathetic outflow, producing a decrease in vasomotor tone and heart rate

Pharmacodynamics/Kinetics

Onset of Action Antihypertensive: ~1 hour

Half-life Elimination Serum: 7-10 hours

Pregnancy Risk Factor C

GuanFACINE (GWAHN fa seen)

Related Information

Cardiovascular Diseases *on page 1848*

U.S. Brand Names Intuniv™; Tenex®

Pharmacologic Category $Alpha_2$-Adrenergic Agonist

Use

Tablet, immediate release: Management of hypertension

Tablet, extended release: Treatment of attention-deficit/hyperactivity disorder (ADHD) as monotherapy or adjunctive therapy to stimulants

Unlabeled/Investigational Use Tic disorder; aggression

Local Anesthetic/Vasoconstrictor Precautions No information available to require special precautions

Effects on Dental Treatment Key adverse event(s) related to dental treatment: Xerostomia and changes in salivation (normal salivary flow resumes upon discontinuation).

Effects on Bleeding No information available to require special precautions

Adverse Effects

>10%:

Central nervous system: Somnolence (5% to 45%; dose-related), dizziness (2% to 15%; dose-related), headache (3% to 26%), fatigue (2% to 15%)

Gastrointestinal: Xerostomia (4% to 54%; dose-related), constipation (≤16%; dose-related), abdominal pain (≤11%; dose-related)

1% to 10%:

Cardiovascular: Hypotension (≤10%; dose-related), hypertension (2% to 5%), syncope (1% to 5%), AV block (<2%), bradycardia (<2%), chest pain (<2%), orthostasis (<2%), pallor (<2%), sinus arrhythmias (<2%)

Central nervous system: Insomnia (2% to 12%), irritability (6%), lethargy (2% to 6%)

Gastrointestinal: Vomiting (9%), nausea (≤7%), weight gain (≤7%), appetite decreased (2% to 5%), diarrhea (2% to 5%), stomach discomfort (2% to 5%), dyspepsia (<2%)

Genitourinary: Impotence (≤7%), enuresis (<2%), urinary frequency (<2%)

Hepatic: ALT increased (<2%)

Neuromuscular & skeletal: Weakness (≤7%)

Respiratory: Asthma (<2%)

General Dosage Range Oral:

Immediate release: *Children ≥12 years and Adults:* 0.5-2 mg once daily

Extended release: *Children ≥6 years and Adolescents:* 1-4 mg once daily

Mechanism of Action Guanfacine is a selective $alpha_{2A}$-adrenoreceptor agonist which reduces sympathetic nerve impulses, resulting in reduced sympathetic outflow and a subsequent decrease in vasomotor tone and heart rate. In addition, guanfacine preferentially binds postsynaptic $alpha_{2A}$-adrenoreceptors in the prefrontal cortex and has been theorized to improve delay-related firing of prefrontal cortex neurons. As a result, underlying working memory and behavioral inhibition are affected; thereby improving symptoms associated with ADHD. Guanfacine is not a CNS stimulant.

Pharmacodynamics/Kinetics

Duration of Action Antihypertensive effect: 24 hours following single dose

Half-life Elimination

Immediate release: ~17 hours (range: 10-30 hours)

Extended release: 16 hours

Time to Peak Serum:

Immediate release: 2.6 hours (range: 1-4 hours)

Extended release: ~5 hours

Pregnancy Risk Factor B

Guanidine (GWAHN i deen)

Pharmacologic Category Cholinergic Agonist

Use Reduction of the symptoms of muscle weakness associated with the myasthenic syndrome of Eaton-Lambert, not for myasthenia gravis

Local Anesthetic/Vasoconstrictor Precautions No information available to require special precautions

Effects on Dental Treatment No significant effects or complications reported

Effects on Bleeding No information available to require special precautions

General Dosage Range Oral: *Adults:* Initial: 10-15 mg/kg/day in 3-4 divided doses; Maintenance: Up to 35 mg/kg/day

Haemophilus b Conjugate Vaccine

(he MOF fi lus bee KON joo gate vak SEEN)

U.S. Brand Names ActHIB®; Hiberix®; PedvaxHIB®

Canadian Brand Names ActHIB®; PedvaxHIB®

Pharmacologic Category Vaccine, Inactivated (Bacterial)

Use Routine immunization of children against invasive disease caused by *H. influenzae* type b

The Advisory Committee on Immunization Practices (ACIP) recommends routine vaccination of all children through age 59 months. Efficacy data are not available for use in older children and adults with chronic conditions associated with an increased risk of Hib disease. However, a single dose may also be considered for older children, adolescents, and adults who did not receive the childhood series and who have had splenectomies or who have sickle cell disease, leukemia, or HIV infection.

Local Anesthetic/Vasoconstrictor Precautions No information available to require special precautions

Effects on Dental Treatment No significant effects or complications reported

Effects on Bleeding No information available to require special precautions

Adverse Effects All serious adverse reactions must be reported to the U.S. Department of Health and Human Services (DHHS) Vaccine Adverse Event Reporting System (VAERS) 1-800-822-7967 or online at https://vaers.hhs.gov/esub/index. In Canada, adverse reactions may be reported to local provincial/territorial health agencies or to the Vaccine Safety Section at Public Health Agency of Canada (1-866-844-0018).

Frequency not defined:

Central nervous system: Crying (unusual, high pitched, prolonged), fever, fussiness, irritability, pain, restlessness, sleepiness

Dermatologic: Rash

Gastrointestinal: Anorexia, diarrhea, vomiting

Local: Injection site: Erythema, induration, pain, soreness, swelling

Otic: Otitis media

Respiratory: Upper respiratory tract infection

General Dosage Range I.M.: *Children:* 0.5 mL (number of doses determined by age at first dose)

Mechanism of Action Stimulates production of anticapsular antibodies and provides active immunity to *Haemophilus influenzae* type b

Pharmacodynamics/Kinetics

Onset of Action Serum antibody response: 1-2 weeks

Duration of Action Immunity: 1.5 years

Pregnancy Risk Factor C

Halcinonide (hal SIN oh nide)

U.S. Brand Names Halog®

Canadian Brand Names Halog®

Pharmacologic Category Corticosteroid, Topical

Use Inflammation of corticosteroid-responsive dermatoses [high potency topical corticosteroid]

Local Anesthetic/Vasoconstrictor Precautions No information available to require special precautions

Effects on Dental Treatment No significant effects or complications reported

Effects on Bleeding No information available to require special precautions

Adverse Effects

Frequency not defined.

Dermatologic: Acneiform eruptions, allergic contact dermatitis, dry skin, folliculitis, hypertrichosis, itching, miliaria, perioral dermatitis, skin atrophy, skin maceration, striae

Local: Burning, itching

Miscellaneous: Secondary infection

Reported with other topical corticosteroids, may occur more frequently with occlusive dressings: Cushing's syndrome, glucosuria, growth retardation (children), HPA axis suppression, hyperglycemia, intracranial hypertension (children)

General Dosage Range Topical: *Children and Adults:* Apply sparingly 1-3 times/day

Mechanism of Action Decreases inflammation by suppression of migration of polymorphonuclear leukocytes and reversal of increased capillary permeability

Pregnancy Risk Factor C

Halobetasol (hal oh BAY ta sol)

U.S. Brand Names Ultravate®

Canadian Brand Names Ultravate®

Generic Availability (U.S.) Yes

Pharmacologic Category Corticosteroid, Topical

Dental Use Relief of inflammatory and pruritic manifestations (super high potency topical corticosteroid)

Use Relief of inflammatory and pruritic manifestations of corticosteroid-response dermatoses [super high potency topical corticosteroid]

Local Anesthetic/Vasoconstrictor Precautions No information available to require special precautions

Effects on Dental Treatment No significant effects or complications reported

Effects on Bleeding No information available to require special precautions

Adverse Effects 1% to 4%: Dermatologic: Burning, itching, stinging

Dental Usual Dosage Inflammatory and pruritic manifestations: Children ≥12 years and Adults: Topical: Cream: Apply sparingly to lesion twice daily. Treatment should not exceed 2 consecutive weeks and total dosage should not exceed 50 g/week. Therapy should be discontinued when control is achieved; if no improvement is seen, reassessment of diagnosis may be necessary.

Dosage Children ≥12 years and Adults: Topical:

Inflammatory and pruritic manifestations (dental use): Cream: Apply sparingly to lesion twice daily. Treatment should not exceed 2 consecutive weeks and total dosage should not exceed 50 g/week. Therapy should be discontinued when control is achieved; if no improvement is seen, reassessment of diagnosis may be necessary.

Steroid-responsive dermatoses: Apply sparingly to skin twice daily, rub in gently and completely; treatment should not exceed 2 consecutive weeks and total dosage should not exceed 50 g/week. Therapy should be discontinued when control is achieved; if no improvement is seen, reassessment of diagnosis may be necessary.

Mechanism of Action Corticosteroids inhibit the initial manifestations of the inflammatory process (ie, capillary dilation and edema, fibrin deposition, and migration and diapedesis of leukocytes into the inflamed site) as well as later sequelae (angiogenesis, fibroblast proliferation)

Contraindications Hypersensitivity to halobetasol or any component of the formulation; viral, fungal, or tubercular skin lesions

Warnings/Precautions Systemic absorption of topical corticosteroids may cause hypothalamic-pituitary-adrenal (HPA) axis suppression (reversible) particularly in younger children. HPA axis suppression may lead to adrenal crisis. Risk is increased when used over large surface areas, for prolonged periods, or with occlusive dressings. Allergic contact dermatitis can occur, it is usually diagnosed by failure to heal rather than clinical exacerbation. Prolonged treatment with corticosteroids has been associated with the development of Kaposi's sarcoma (case reports); if noted, discontinuation of therapy should be considered. Adverse systemic effects including hyperglycemia, glycosuria, fluid and electrolyte changes, and HPA suppression may occur when used on large surface areas, for prolonged periods, or with an occlusive dressing. Not for ophthalmic use. Topical halobetasol should not be used for the treatment of rosacea or perioral dermatitis. Not recommended for application to the face, groin, or axillae. Safety and efficacy have not been established in pediatric patients; use in children <12 years of age is not recommended.

Drug Interactions

Avoid Concomitant Use

Avoid concomitant use of Halobetasol with any of the following: Aldesleukin

Increased Effect/Toxicity

Halobetasol may increase the levels/effects of: Deferasirox

Decreased Effect

Halobetasol may decrease the levels/effects of: Aldesleukin; Corticorelin

Pregnancy Risk Factor C

Lactation Excretion in breast milk unknown/use caution

Breast-Feeding Considerations Systemically administered corticosteroids appear in human milk and may cause adverse effects in a nursing infant. It is not known if the systemic absorption of topical halobetasol results in detectable quantities in human milk.

Dosage Forms

Cream, topical: 0.05% (15 g, 50 g)

Ultravate®: 0.05% (15 g, 50 g)

Ointment, topical: 0.05% (15 g, 50 g)

Ultravate®: 0.05% (15 g, 50 g)

Haloperidol (ha loe PER i dole)

Related Information

Clinical Risk Related to Drugs Prolonging QT Interval *on page* 1872

U.S. Brand Names Haldol®; Haldol® Decanoate

Canadian Brand Names Apo-Haloperidol LA®; Apo-Haloperidol®; Haloperidol Injection, USP; Haloperidol Long Acting; Haloperidol-LA; Haloperidol-LA Omega; Novo-Peridol; Peridol; PMS-Haloperidol LA

Pharmacologic Category Antipsychotic Agent, Typical

Use Management of schizophrenia; control of tics and vocal utterances of Tourette's disorder in children and adults; severe behavioral problems in children

Unlabeled/Investigational Use Treatment of non-schizophrenia psychosis; may be used for the emergency sedation of severely-agitated or delirious patients; adjunctive treatment of ethanol dependence; postoperative nausea and vomiting (alternative therapy); psychosis/agitation related to Alzheimer's dementia

Local Anesthetic/Vasoconstrictor Precautions Manufacturer's information states that haloperidol may block vasopressor activity of epinephrine. This has not been observed during use of epinephrine as a vasoconstrictor in local anesthesia. Haloperidol is one of the drugs confirmed to prolong the QT interval and is accepted as having a risk of causing torsade de pointes. The risk of drug-induced torsade de pointes is extremely low when a single QT interval prolonging drug is prescribed. In terms of epinephrine, it is not known what effect vasoconstrictors in the local anesthetic regimen will have in patients with a known history of congenital prolonged QT interval or in patients taking any medication that prolongs the QT interval. Until more information is obtained, it is suggested that the clinician consult with the physician prior to the use of a vasoconstrictor in suspected patients, and that the vasoconstrictor (epinephrine, mepivacaine and levonordefrin [Carbocaine® 2% with Neo-Cobefrin®]) be used with caution.

Effects on Dental Treatment Key adverse event(s) related to dental treatment: Xerostomia (normal salivary flow resumes upon discontinuation). Orthostatic hypotension, and nasal congestion are possible; since the drug is a dopamine antagonist, extrapyramidal symptoms of the TMJ are a possibility.

Effects on Bleeding No information available to require special precautions

Adverse Effects Frequency not defined.

Cardiovascular: Abnormal T waves with prolonged ventricular repolarization, arrhythmia, hyper-/hypotension, QT prolongation, sudden death, tachycardia, torsade de pointes

Central nervous system: Agitation, akathisia, altered central temperature regulation, anxiety, confusion, depression, drowsiness, dystonic reactions, euphoria, extrapyramidal reactions, headache, insomnia, lethargy, neuroleptic malignant syndrome (NMS), pseudoparkinsonian signs and symptoms, restlessness, seizure, tardive dyskinesia, tardive dystonia, vertigo

Dermatologic: Alopecia, contact dermatitis, hyperpigmentation, photosensitivity (rare), pruritus, rash

Endocrine & metabolic: Amenorrhea, breast engorgement, galactorrhea, gynecomastia, hyper-/hypoglycemia, hyponatremia, lactation, mastalgia, menstrual irregularities, sexual dysfunction

Gastrointestinal: Anorexia, constipation, diarrhea, dyspepsia, hypersalivation, nausea, vomiting, xerostomia

Genitourinary: Priapism, urinary retention

Hematologic: Cholestatic jaundice, obstructive jaundice

Ocular: Blurred vision

Respiratory: Bronchospasm, laryngospasm

Miscellaneous: Diaphoresis, heat stroke

General Dosage Range

I.M.:

Decanoate: *Adults:* Initial: 10-20 times daily oral dose at 4-week intervals; Maintenance: 10-15 times initial oral dose

Lactate:

Children 6-12 years: 1-3 mg/dose every 4-8 hours (maximum: 0.15 mg/kg/day)

Adults: 2-5 mg every 4-8 hours as needed

Oral:

Children 3-12 years (15-40 kg): Initial: 0.05 mg/kg/day **or** 0.25-0.5 mg/day in 2-3 divided doses; Maintenance: 0.05-0.15 mg/kg/day in 2-3 divided doses **or** 0.01-0.03 mg/kg once daily (maximum: 0.15 mg/kg/day)

Adults: Initial: 0.5-5 mg 2-3 times/day; Maintenance: Up to 30 mg/day in 2-3 divided doses

Mechanism of Action Haloperidol is a butyrophenone antipsychotic which blocks postsynaptic mesolimbic dopaminergic D_1 and D_2 receptors in the brain; depresses the release of hypothalamic and hypophyseal hormones; believed to depress the reticular activating system thus affecting basal metabolism, body temperature, wakefulness, vasomotor tone, and emesis

Pharmacodynamics/Kinetics

Onset of Action Sedation: I.M., I.V.: 30-60 minutes

Duration of Action Decanoate: ~3 weeks

Half-life Elimination 18 hours; Decanoate: 21 days

Time to Peak Oral: 2-6 hours; I.M.: 20 minutes; decanoate: 7 days

Pregnancy Risk Factor C

Dental Comment Haloperidol is known to prolong the QT interval. The QT interval is measured as the time and distance between the Q point of the QRS complex and the end of the T wave in the ECG tracing. After adjustment for heart rate, the QT interval is defined as prolonged if it is more than 450 msec in men and 460 msec in women. A long QT syndrome was first described in the 1950s and 60s as a congenital syndrome involving QT interval prolongation and syncope and sudden death. Some of the congenital long QT syndromes were characterized by a peculiar electrocardiographic appearance of the QRS complex involving a premature atria beat followed by a pause, then a subsequent sinus beat showing marked QT prolongation and deformity. This type of cardiac arrhythmia was originally termed "torsade de pointes" (translated from the French as "twisting of the points"). Haloperidol is considered as having a risk of causing torsade de pointes. Since it is not known what effect vasoconstrictors in the local anesthetic regimen will have in patients with a known history of congenital prolonged QT interval or in patients taking any medication that prolongs the QT interval, a medical consult is suggested.

Hemin (HEE min)

U.S. Brand Names Panhematin®

Pharmacologic Category Blood Modifiers; Blood Product Derivative

Use Treatment of recurrent attacks of acute intermittent porphyria (AIP)

Local Anesthetic/Vasoconstrictor Precautions No information available to require special precautions

Effects on Dental Treatment No significant effects or complications reported

Effects on Bleeding No information available to require special precautions

Adverse Effects Frequency not defined.

Central nervous system: Pyrexia

Hematologic: Leukocytosis

Local: Phlebitis

General Dosage Range I.V.: *Children ≥16 years and Adults:* 1-4 mg/kg/day divided every 12 hours (maximum: 6 mg/kg/24 hours)

Mechanism of Action Inhibits the hepatic and/or marrow synthesis of ALA synthase, the enzyme that regulates the porphyrin/heme pathway

Pregnancy Risk Factor C

Heparin (HEP a rin)

Related Information

Cardiovascular Diseases *on page 1848*

U.S. Brand Names Hep-Lock; Hep-Lock U/P; HepFlush®-10

Canadian Brand Names Hepalean®; Hepalean® Leo; Hepalean®-LOK

Pharmacologic Category Anticoagulant

Use Prophylaxis and treatment of thromboembolic disorders; as an anticoagulant for extracorporeal and dialysis procedures

Note: Heparin lock flush solution is intended only to maintain patency of I.V. devices and is **not** to be used for systemic anticoagulant therapy.

Unlabeled/Investigational Use ST-elevation myocardial infarction (STEMI) as an adjunct to thrombolysis; unstable angina/non-STEMI (UA/NSTEMI); anticoagulant used during percutaneous coronary intervention (PCI)

Local Anesthetic/Vasoconstrictor Precautions No information available to require special precautions

Effects on Dental Treatment Key adverse event(s) related to dental treatment: Bleeding from the gums. See Effects on Bleeding.

Effects on Bleeding As with all anticoagulants, bleeding is a potential adverse effect of heparin during dental surgery; risk is dependent on multiple variables, including the intensity of anticoagulation and patient susceptibility. It is unlikely that ambulatory patients presenting for dental treatment will be taking intravenous anticoagulant therapy. Medical consult is suggested.

Adverse Effects Frequency not defined.

Cardiovascular: Allergic vasospastic reaction (possibly related to thrombosis), chest pain, hemorrhagic shock, shock, thrombosis

Central nervous system: Chills, fever, headache

Dermatologic: Alopecia (delayed, transient), bruising (unexplained), cutaneous necrosis, dysesthesia pedis, erythematous plaques (case reports), eczema, urticaria, purpura

Endocrine & metabolic: Adrenal hemorrhage, hyperkalemia (suppression of aldosterone synthesis), ovarian hemorrhage, rebound hyperlipidemia on discontinuation

Gastrointestinal: Constipation, hematemesis, nausea, tarry stools, vomiting

Genitourinary: Frequent or persistent erection

Hematologic: Bleeding from gums, epistaxis, hemorrhage, ovarian hemorrhage, retroperitoneal hemorrhage, thrombocytopenia (see **"Note"**)

Hepatic: Liver enzymes increased

Local: Irritation, erythema, pain, hematoma, and ulceration have been rarely reported with deep SubQ injections; I.M. injection (not recommended) is associated with a high incidence of these effects

Neuromuscular & skeletal: Peripheral neuropathy, osteoporosis (chronic therapy effect)

Ocular: Conjunctivitis (allergic reaction), lacrimation

Renal: Hematuria

Respiratory: Asthma, bronchospasm (case reports), hemoptysis, pulmonary hemorrhage, rhinitis

Miscellaneous: Allergic reactions, anaphylactoid reactions, heparin resistance, hypersensitivity (including chills, fever, and urticaria)

Note: Thrombocytopenia has been reported to occur at an incidence between 0% and 30%. It is often of no clinical significance. However, immunologically mediated heparin-induced thrombocytopenia (HIT) has been estimated to occur in 1% to 2% of patients, and is marked by a progressive fall in platelet counts and, in some cases, thromboembolic complications (skin necrosis, pulmonary embolism, gangrene of the extremities, stroke, or MI).

General Dosage Range

I.V.:

Children: Bolus: 50-100 units/kg; Initial infusion: 15-25 units/kg/hour; Maintenance: Increase dose by 2-4 units/kg/hour every 6-8 hours as needed **or** 50-100 units/kg every 4 hours intermittently

Adults: Bolus: 60-80 units/kg; Infusion: 10-30 units/kg/hour **or** 10,000 units (initially), then 50-70 units/kg (5000-10,000 units) every 4-6 hours intermittently

SubQ: *Adults:* Thromboprophylaxis: 5000 units every 8-12 hours; Treatment: 17,500 units every 12 hours

Mechanism of Action Potentiates the action of antithrombin III and thereby inactivates thrombin (as well as activated coagulation factors IX, X, XI, XII, and plasmin) and prevents the conversion of fibrinogen to fibrin; heparin also stimulates release of lipoprotein lipase (lipoprotein lipase hydrolyzes triglycerides to glycerol and free fatty acids)

Pharmacodynamics/Kinetics

Onset of Action Anticoagulation: I.V.: Immediate; SubQ: ~20-30 minutes

Half-life Elimination

Dose-dependent: I.V. bolus: 25 units/kg: 30 minutes; 100 units/kg: 60 minutes; 400 units/kg: 150 minutes (Hirsh, 2008)

Mean: 1.5 hours; Range: 1-2 hours; affected by obesity, renal function, malignancy, presence of pulmonary embolism, and infections

Note: At therapeutic doses, elimination occurs rapidly via nonrenal mechanisms. With very high doses, renal elimination may play more of a role; however, dosage adjustment remains unnecessary for patients with renal impairment (Hirsh, 2008).

Pregnancy Risk Factor C

Hepatitis A and Hepatitis B Recombinant Vaccine

(hep a TYE tis aye & hep a TYE tis bee ree KOM be nant vak SEEN)

Related Information

Systemic Viral Diseases *on page 1904*

U.S. Brand Names Twinrix®

Canadian Brand Names Twinrix®; Twinrix® Junior

Pharmacologic Category Vaccine, Inactivated (Viral)

Use Active immunization against disease caused by hepatitis A virus and hepatitis B virus (all known subtypes) in populations desiring protection against or at high risk of exposure to these viruses.

Populations include travelers or people living in or relocating to areas of intermediate/high endemicity for **both** HAV and HBV and are at increased risk of HBV infection due to behavioral or occupational factors; patients with chronic liver disease; laboratory workers who handle live HAV and HBV; healthcare workers, police, and other personnel who render first-aid or medical assistance; workers who come in contact with sewage; employees of day care centers and correctional facilities; patients/staff of hemodialysis units; men who have sex with men; patients frequently receiving blood products; military personnel; users of injectable illicit drugs; close household contacts of patients with hepatitis A and hepatitis B infection; residents of drug and alcohol treatment centers

Local Anesthetic/Vasoconstrictor Precautions No information available to require special precautions

Effects on Dental Treatment Key adverse event(s) related to dental treatment: Flu-like syndrome and upper respiratory tract infection.

Effects on Bleeding No information available to require special precautions

Adverse Effects In the U.S., all serious adverse reactions must be reported to the U.S. Department of Health and Human Services (DHHS) Vaccine Adverse Event Reporting System (VAERS) 1-800-822-7967 or online at https://vaers.-hhs.gov/esub/index.

Incidence of adverse effects of the combination product were similar to those occurring after administration of hepatitis A vaccine and hepatitis B vaccine alone. (Incidence reported is not versus placebo.)

Adults:

>10%:

Central nervous system: Headache (13% to 22%), fatigue (11% to 14%)

Local: Injection site reaction: Soreness (35% to 41%), redness (8% to 11%)

1% to 10%:

Central nervous system: Fever (2% to 4%)

Gastrointestinal: Diarrhea (4% to 6%), nausea (2% to 4%), vomiting (≤1%)

Local: Injection site reaction: Swelling (4% to 6%), induration

Respiratory: Upper respiratory tract infection

<1%: Abdominal pain, agitation, anorexia, arthralgia, back pain, bruising at the injection site, diaphoresis, dizziness, erythema, flu-like syndrome, flushing, insomnia, irritability, migraine, myalgia, paresthesia, petechiae, pruritus at the injection site, rash, respiratory tract illness, somnolence, syncope, urticaria, vertigo, weakness

Children (as reported in Canadian labeling):

>10%: Local: Injection site pain/redness

1% to 10%:

Central nervous system: Fever (≥37.5°C), drowsiness, fatigue, headache, irritability, malaise

Gastrointestinal: Appetite decreased, diarrhea, nausea, vomiting

Local: Injection site edema

General Dosage Range I.M.: *Adults:* 3 doses (1 mL each) given on a 0-, 1-, and 6-month schedule

Mechanism of Action

Hepatitis A vaccine, an inactivated virus vaccine, offers active immunization against hepatitis A virus infection at an effective immune response rate in up to 99% of subjects.

Recombinant hepatitis B vaccine is a noninfectious subunit viral vaccine. The vaccine is derived from hepatitis B surface antigen (HB_sAg) produced through recombinant DNA techniques from yeast cells. The portion of the hepatitis B gene which codes for HB_sAg is cloned into yeast which is then cultured to produce hepatitis B vaccine.

In immunocompetent people, Twinrix® provides active immunization against hepatitis A virus infection (at an effective immune response rate >99% of subjects) and against hepatitis B virus infection (at an effective immune response rate of 93% to 97%) 30 days after completion of the 3-dose series. This is comparable to using hepatitis A vaccine and hepatitis B vaccine concomitantly.

Pharmacodynamics/Kinetics

Onset of Action Seroconversion for antibodies against HAV and HBV were detected 1 month after completion of the 3-dose series.

Duration of Action Patients remained seropositive for at least 4 years during clinical studies.

Pregnancy Risk Factor C

Hepatitis A Vaccine (hep a TYE tis aye vak SEEN)

Related Information

Systemic Viral Diseases *on page 1904*

U.S. Brand Names Havrix®; VAQTA®

Canadian Brand Names Avaxim®; Avaxim®-Pediatric; HAVRIX®; VAQTA®

Pharmacologic Category Vaccine, Inactivated (Viral)

Use

Active immunization against disease caused by hepatitis A virus (HAV)

The Advisory Committee on Immunization Practices (ACIP) recommends routine vaccination for:

- All children ≥12 months of age
- All unvaccinated adults requesting protection from HAV infection
- All unvaccinated adults at risk for HAV infection, such as:

  Behavioral risks: Men who have sex with men; injection drug users

  Occupational risks: Persons who work with HAV-infected primates or with HAV in a research laboratory setting

Medical risks: Persons with chronic liver disease; patients who receive clotting-factor concentrates

- Other risks: International travelers to regions with high or intermediate levels of endemic HAV infection (a list of countries is available at http://wwwn.cdc.gov/travel/contentdiseases.aspx)
- Unvaccinated persons who anticipate close personal contact with international adoptee from a country of intermediate to high endemicity of HAV, during their first 60 days of arrival into the United States (eg, household contacts, babysitters)

Local Anesthetic/Vasoconstrictor Precautions No information available to require special precautions

Effects on Dental Treatment No significant effects or complications reported

Effects on Bleeding No information available to require special precautions

Adverse Effects All serious adverse reactions must be reported to the U.S. Department of Health and Human Services (DHHS) Vaccine Adverse Event Reporting System (VAERS) at 1-800-822-7967 or online at https://vaers.hhs.gov/esub/index.

Frequency dependent upon age, product used, and concomitant vaccine administration. In general, headache and injection site reactions were less common in younger children.

>10%:

Central nervous system: Drowsiness, fever ≥100.4°F (1-5 days post vaccination), fever >98.6°C (1-14 days post vaccination), headache, irritability

Gastrointestinal: Appetite decreased

Local: Injection site: Erythema, pain, soreness, swelling, tenderness, warmth

1% to 10%:

Central nervous system: Chills, fatigue, fever ≥102°F (1-5 days postvaccination), insomnia, malaise

Dermatologic: Rash

Endocrine & metabolic: Menstrual disorder

Gastrointestinal: Abdominal pain, anorexia, constipation, diarrhea, gastroenteritis, nausea, vomiting

Local: Injection site bruising, induration

Neuromuscular & skeletal: Arm pain, back pain, myalgia, stiffness, weakness/fatigue

Ocular: Conjunctivitis

Otic: Otitis media

Respiratory: Asthma, cough, nasopharyngitis, nasal congestion, pharyngitis, rhinorrhea, rhinitis, upper respiratory tract infection

Miscellaneous: Crying

General Dosage Range I.M.:

Children 12 months to 18 years: 0.5 mL

Adults: 1 mL

Mechanism of Action As an inactivated virus vaccine, hepatitis A vaccine offers active immunization against hepatitis A virus infection at an effective immune response rate in up to 99% of subjects

Pharmacodynamics/Kinetics

Onset of Action Protection: 2-4 weeks after a single dose; 2 weeks after vaccine administration, 54% to 62% of patients develop neutralizing antibodies; this percentage increases to 94% to 100% at 1 month postvaccination (CDC, 2006)

Duration of Action Neutralizing antibodies have persisted for up to 8 years; based on kinetic models, antibodies may be present ≥14-20 years in children and ≥25 years in adults who receive the complete vaccination series (CDC, 2006; Van Damme, 2003).

Pregnancy Risk Factor C

Hepatitis B Immune Globulin (Human)

(hep a TYE tis bee i MYUN GLOB yoo lin YU man)

Related Information

Systemic Viral Diseases *on page 1904*

U.S. Brand Names HepaGam B®; HyperHEP B™ S/D; Nabi-HB®

Canadian Brand Names HepaGam B™; HyperHep B®

Pharmacologic Category Blood Product Derivative; Immune Globulin

Use

Passive prophylactic immunity to hepatitis B following: Acute exposure to blood containing hepatitis B surface antigen (HBsAg); perinatal exposure of infants born to HBsAg-positive mothers; sexual exposure to HBsAg-positive persons; household exposure to persons with acute HBV infection

Prevention of hepatitis B virus recurrence after liver transplantation in HBsAg-positive transplant patients

Note: Hepatitis B immune globulin is not indicated for treatment of active hepatitis B infection and is ineffective in the treatment of chronic active hepatitis B infection.

Local Anesthetic/Vasoconstrictor Precautions No information available to require special precautions

Effects on Dental Treatment No significant effects or complications reported

Effects on Bleeding No information available to require special precautions

Adverse Effects Reported with postexposure prophylaxis; frequency not defined. Adverse events reported in liver transplant patients included tremor and hypotension, were associated with a single infusion during the first week of treatment, and did not recur with additional infusions.

Central nervous system: Fainting, headache, lightheadedness, malaise
Dermatologic: Angioedema, bruising, urticaria
Gastrointestinal: Nausea, vomiting
Hematologic: WBC decreased
Hepatic: Alkaline phosphatase increased, AST increased
Local: Ache, erythema, pain, and/or tenderness at injection site
Neuromuscular & skeletal: Arthralgia, joint stiffness, myalgia
Renal: Creatinine increased
Respiratory: Cold symptoms
Miscellaneous: Anaphylaxis, flu-like syndrome

General Dosage Range

I.M.:

Newborns and Infants <12 months: 0.5 mL as a single dose

Children ≥12 months and Adults: 0.06 mL/kg as a single dose; may repeat in 28-30 days

I.V.: *Adults:* 20,000 int. units/dose daily for 8 days, then every 2 weeks, then once monthly

Mechanism of Action Hepatitis B immune globulin (HBIG) is a nonpyrogenic sterile solution containing immunoglobulin G (IgG) specific to hepatitis B surface antigen (HB_sAg). HBIG differs from immune globulin in the amount of anti-HB_s. Immune globulin is prepared from plasma that is not preselected for anti-HB_s content. HBIG is prepared from plasma preselected for high titer anti-HB_s. In the U.S., HBIG has an anti-HB_s high titer >1:100,000 by IRA.

Pharmacodynamics/Kinetics

Duration of Action Postexposure prophylaxis: 3-6 months

Half-life Elimination 17-25 days

Time to Peak Serum: I.M.: 2-10 days

Pregnancy Risk Factor C

Hepatitis B Vaccine (Recombinant)

(hep a TYE tis bee vak SEEN ree KOM be nant)

Related Information

Systemic Viral Diseases *on page 1904*

U.S. Brand Names Engerix-B®; Recombivax HB®

Canadian Brand Names Engerix-B®; Recombivax HB®

Pharmacologic Category Vaccine, Inactivated (Viral)

Use Immunization against infection caused by all known subtypes of hepatitis B virus (HBV)

The Advisory Committee on Immunization Practices (ACIP) recommends routine vaccination for the following (CDC 2006; CDC 2005):

- All infants at birth
- All infants and children (post-birth dose; refer to recommended vaccination schedule)
- All unvaccinated adults requesting protection from HBV infection
- All unvaccinated adults at risk for HBV infection such as those with:

  Behavioral risks: Sexually-active persons with >1 partner in a 6-month period; persons seeking evaluation or treatment for a sexually-transmitted disease; men who have sex with men; injection drug users

  Occupational risks: Healthcare and public safety workers with reasonably anticipated risk for exposure to blood or blood contaminated body fluids

  Medical risks: Persons with end-stage renal disease (including predialysis, hemodialysis, peritoneal dialysis, and home dialysis); persons with HIV infection; persons with chronic liver disease

Other risks: Household contacts and sex partners of persons with chronic HBV infection; residents and staff of facilities for developmentally disabled persons; international travelers to regions with high or intermediate levels of endemic HBV infection

In addition, the ACIP recommends vaccination for any persons who are wounded in bombings or similar mass casualty events who have penetrating injuries or nonintact skin exposure, or who have contact with mucous membranes (exception - superficial contact with intact skin), and who cannot confirm receipt of a hepatitis B vaccination (CDC, 2008).

Local Anesthetic/Vasoconstrictor Precautions No information available to require special precautions

Effects on Dental Treatment No significant effects or complications reported

Effects on Bleeding No information available to require special precautions

Adverse Effects All serious adverse reactions must be reported to the U.S. Department of Health and Human Services (DHHS) Vaccine Adverse Event Reporting System (VAERS) at 1-800-822-7967 or online at https://vaers.hhs.gov/esub/index.

Frequency not defined. The most common adverse effects reported with both products included injection site reactions (>10%).

Cardiovascular: Flushing, hypotension

Central nervous system: Agitation, chills, dizziness, fatigue, fever (≥37.5°C/100°F), headache, insomnia, irritability, lightheadedness, malaise, somnolence, vertigo

Dermatologic: Angioedema, petechiae, pruritus, rash, urticaria

Gastrointestinal: Abdominal pain, anorexia, appetite decreased, constipation, cramps, diarrhea, dyspepsia, nausea, vomiting

Genitourinary: Dysuria

Local: Injection site reactions: Ecchymosis, erythema, induration, pain, nodule formation, soreness, swelling, tenderness, warmth

Neuromuscular & skeletal: Achiness, arthralgia, back pain, myalgia, neck pain, neck stiffness, paresthesia, shoulder pain, tingling, weakness

Otic: Earache

Respiratory: Cough, pharyngitis, rhinitis, upper respiratory tract infection

Miscellaneous: Diaphoresis, lymphadenopathy, flu-like syndrome

General Dosage Range Dosage adjustment recommended in patients with renal impairment.

I.M.:

Birth to 19 years: 0.5 mL

Adults ≥20 years: 1 mL

Mechanism of Action Recombinant hepatitis B vaccine is a noninfectious subunit viral vaccine, which confers active immunity via formation of antihepatitis B antibodies. The vaccine is derived from hepatitis B surface antigen (HB_sAg) produced through recombinant DNA techniques from yeast cells. The portion of the hepatitis B gene which codes for HB_sAg is cloned into yeast which is then cultured to produce hepatitis B vaccine.

Pharmacodynamics/Kinetics

Duration of Action Following a 3-dose series in children, up to 50% of patients will have low or undetectable anti-HB antibody 5-15 years postvaccination. However, anamnestic increases in anti-HB have been shown up to 23 years later suggesting a lifelong immune memory response.

Pregnancy Risk Factor C

Dental Comment Immunization is recommended for dentists, oral surgeons, dental hygienists, dental nurses, and dental students

Hetastarch (HET a starch)

U.S. Brand Names Hespan®; Hextend®

Canadian Brand Names Hextend®

Pharmacologic Category Plasma Volume Expander, Colloid

Use Blood volume expander used in treatment of hypovolemia; adjunct in leukapheresis to improve harvesting and increase the yield of granulocytes by centrifugation (Hespan®)

Unlabeled/Investigational Use Priming fluid in pump oxygenators during cardiopulmonary bypass; plasma volume expansion during cardiopulmonary bypass

Local Anesthetic/Vasoconstrictor Precautions No information available to require special precautions

Effects on Dental Treatment No significant effects or complications reported

Effects on Bleeding May interefere with platelet function. Unlikely to be used in clinical situations where dental procedures are contemplated.

Adverse Effects Frequency not defined.

Cardiovascular: Bradycardia, circulatory overload, heart failure, peripheral edema, tachycardia

Central nervous system: Chills, fever, headache, intracranial bleeding

Dermatologic: Itching, pruritus (dose dependent; may be delayed), rash

Endocrine & metabolic: Metabolic acidosis, parotid gland enlargement

Gastrointestinal: Amylase levels increased, vomiting

Hematologic: Anemia, bleeding, bleeding time prolonged, clotting time prolonged, dilutional coagulopathy, disseminated intravascular coagulopathy (rare), factor VIII:C plasma levels decreased, hemolysis (rare), plasma aggregation decreased, PT prolonged, PTT prolonged, thrombocytopenia, von Willebrand factor decreased, wound hemorrhage

Hepatic: Bilirubin increased (indirect)

Neuromuscular & skeletal: Myalgia

Respiratory: Bronchospasm, pulmonary edema (noncardiac)

Miscellaneous: Anaphylactoid reactions, flu-like syndrome (mild), hypersensitivity

Postmarketing and/or case reports: Hypotension, urticaria

General Dosage Range Dosage adjustment recommended in patients with renal impairment

I.V.: *Adults:* 500-1500 mL/day **or** 20 mL/kg/day (up to 1500 mL/day)

Leukapheresis: *Adults:* 250-700 mL

Mechanism of Action Produces plasma volume expansion by virtue of its highly colloidal starch structure, similar to albumin

Pharmacodynamics/Kinetics

Onset of Action Volume expansion: I.V.: ~30 minutes

Duration of Action 6-36 hours

Pregnancy Risk Factor C

Hexachlorophene (heks a KLOR oh feen)

U.S. Brand Names pHisoHex®

Canadian Brand Names pHisoHex®

Pharmacologic Category Antibiotic, Topical

Use Surgical scrub and as a bacteriostatic skin cleanser; control an outbreak of gram-positive infection when other procedures have been unsuccessful

Local Anesthetic/Vasoconstrictor Precautions No information available to require special precautions

Effects on Dental Treatment No significant effects or complications reported

Effects on Bleeding No information available to require special precautions

General Dosage Range Topical: *Children and Adults:* Apply 5 mL cleanser and water to area to be cleansed

Mechanism of Action Bacteriostatic polychlorinated biphenyl which inhibits membrane-bound enzymes and disrupts the cell membrane

Pharmacodynamics/Kinetics

Half-life Elimination Infants: 6.1-44.2 hours

Pregnancy Risk Factor C

Hexylresorcinol (heks il re ZOR si nole)

U.S. Brand Names Sucrets® Original [OTC]

Pharmacologic Category Antiseptic, Topical; Local Anesthetic

Use Minor antiseptic and local anesthetic for sore throat; topical antiseptic for minor cuts or abrasions

Local Anesthetic/Vasoconstrictor Precautions No information available to require special precautions

Effects on Dental Treatment No significant effects or complications reported

Effects on Bleeding No information available to require special precautions

General Dosage Range Oral: *Children ≥6 years and Adults:* Up to 10 lozenges/day

Histrelin (his TREL in)

U.S. Brand Names Supprelin® LA; Vantas®

Canadian Brand Names Vantas®

Pharmacologic Category Gonadotropin Releasing Hormone Agonist

Use Palliative treatment of advanced prostate cancer; treatment of children with central precocious puberty (CPP)

Local Anesthetic/Vasoconstrictor Precautions No information available to require special precautions

Effects on Dental Treatment No significant effects or complications reported

Effects on Bleeding Although significant myelosuppression with associated altered hemostasis has been reported for many chemotherapeutic agents, myelosuppression is not common with histrelin and no specific precautions appear to necessary.

Adverse Effects

CPP:

>10%: Local: Insertion site reaction (51%; includes bruising, discomfort, itching, pain, protrusion of implant area, soreness, swelling, tingling)

>2% to 10%:

Endocrine & metabolic: Metrorrhagia (4%)

Local: Keloid scar (6%), scar (6%), suture-related complication (6%), pain at the application site (4%), post procedural pain (4%)

Prostate cancer:

>10%:

Endocrine & metabolic: Hot flashes (66%)

Local: Implant site reaction (6% to 14%; includes bruising, erythema, pain, soreness, swelling, tenderness)

2% to 10%:

Central nervous system: Fatigue (10%), headache (3%), insomnia (3%)

Endocrine & metabolic: Gynecomastia (4%), sexual dysfunction (4%), libido decreased (2%)

Gastrointestinal: Constipation (4%), weight gain (2%)

Genitourinary: Expected pharmacological consequence of testosterone suppression: Testicular atrophy (5%)

Renal: Renal impairment (5%)

General Dosage Range SubQ: *Children ≥2 years and Adults:* 50 mg implant, inserted every 12 months

Mechanism of Action Potent inhibitor of gonadotropin secretion; continuous administration results in, after an initiation phase, the suppression of luteinizing hormone (LH), follicle-stimulating hormone (FSH), and a subsequent decrease in testosterone and dihydrotestosterone (males) and estrone and estradiol (premenopausal females). Testosterone levels are reduced to castrate levels in males (treated for prostate cancer) within 2-4 weeks. Additionally, in patients with CPP, linear growth velocity is slowed (improves chance of attaining predicted adult height).

Pharmacodynamics/Kinetics

Onset of Action Prostate cancer: Chemical castration: Within 2-4 weeks; CPP: Progression of sexual development stops and growth is decreased within 1 month

Duration of Action 1 year

Half-life Elimination Adults: Terminal: ~4 hours

Time to Peak Adults: 12 hours

Pregnancy Risk Factor X

Homatropine (hoe MA troe peen)

U.S. Brand Names Isopto® Homatropine

Pharmacologic Category Anticholinergic Agent, Ophthalmic; Ophthalmic Agent, Mydriatic

Use Producing cycloplegia and mydriasis for refraction; treatment of acute inflammatory conditions of the uveal tract; optical aid in axial lens opacities

Local Anesthetic/Vasoconstrictor Precautions No information available to require special precautions

Effects on Dental Treatment Key adverse event(s) related to dental treatment: Nasal congestion.

Effects on Bleeding No information available to require special precautions

Adverse Effects

>10%: Ocular: Blurred vision, photophobia

1% to 10%:

Local: Stinging, local irritation

Ocular: Increased intraocular pressure

Respiratory: Congestion

General Dosage Range Ophthalmic:

Children: Instill 1 drop (2% solution) 2-3 times/day **or** immediately prior to procedure, repeat every 10 minutes as needed

Adults: Instill 1-2 drops (2% or 5% solution) 2-3 times/day, up to every 3-4 hours as needed **or** 1-2 drops (2% solution) or 1 drop (5% solution) prior to procedure, repeat every 5-10 minutes as needed up to 3 doses

Mechanism of Action Blocks response of iris sphincter muscle and the accommodative muscle of the ciliary body to cholinergic stimulation resulting in dilation and loss of accommodation

Pharmacodynamics/Kinetics

Onset of Action

Accommodation and pupil effect: Ophthalmic:

Maximum mydriatic effect: Within 10-30 minutes

Maximum cycloplegic effect: Within 30-90 minutes

Duration of Action

Mydriasis: 6 hours to 4 days

Cycloplegia: 10-48 hours

Pregnancy Risk Factor C

Hyaluronate and Derivatives (hye al yoor ON ate & dah RIV ah tives)

U.S. Brand Names Amvisc®; Amvisc® Plus; Bionect®; Euflexxa®; Hyalgan®; Hylira™ [DSC]; Orthovisc®; Perlane®; Provisc®; Restylane®; Supartz®; Synvisc-One®; Synvisc®

Canadian Brand Names Cystistat®; Durolane®; Eyestil; Healon GV®; Healon®; OrthoVisc®; Suplasyn®

Pharmacologic Category Antirheumatic Miscellaneous; Ophthalmic Agent, Viscoelastic; Skin and Mucous Membrane Agent, Miscellaneous

Use

Intra-articular injection: Treatment of pain in osteoarthritis in knee in patients who have failed nonpharmacologic treatment and simple analgesics

Intradermal: Correction of moderate-to-severe facial wrinkles or folds

Ophthalmic: Surgical aid in cataract extraction, intraocular implantation, corneal transplant, glaucoma filtration, and retinal attachment surgery

Topical cream, gel, spray: Management of skin ulcers and wounds

Topical lotion: Treatment of xerosis (dry, scaly skin)

Unlabeled/Investigational Use Treatment of refractory interstitial cystitis

Local Anesthetic/Vasoconstrictor Precautions No information available to require special precautions

Effects on Dental Treatment No significant effects or complications reported

Effects on Bleeding No information available to require special precautions

Adverse Effects Frequencies and/or type of local reaction may vary by formulation and site of application/injection.

>10%:

Local: Injection site (intradermal): Bruising (47% to 61%), erythema (58% to 93%), lumps/bumps (79% to 83%), pain (57% to 90%), swelling (81% to 89%); pruritus (28% to 36%), skin discoloration (31% to 34%)

Neuromuscular & skeletal: Arthralgia (intra-articular 25%)

Respiratory: Infection (12%)

1% to 10%:

Cardiovascular: Blood pressure increased (2% to 4%)

Central nervous system: Fatigue (1%)

Gastrointestinal: Nausea (≤2%)

Local: Dry skin (intradermal >1%), peeling (intradermal >1%)

Neuromuscular & skeletal: Joint effusion (intra-articular 2% to 6%), back pain (<1% to 6%), tendonitis (2%), parasthesia (1%)

Respiratory: Rhinitis (3%)

Frequency not defined:

Cardiovascular: Edema, flushing, hypotension, tachycardia

Central nervous system: Dizziness, headache

Dermatologic: Rash, hyperpigmentation, exfoliation

Local: Injection site: Nodule

Neuromuscular & skeletal: Hypokinesia (knee)

Ocular (with ophthalmic formulation): Postoperative inflammatory reactions (iritis, hypopyon), corneal edema, corneal decompensation, transient postoperative increase in IOP

Miscellaneous: Abscess formation, allergic reactions, anaphylaxis, respiratory difficulties

General Dosage Range

Intra-articular: *Adults:* 16-30 mg once weekly for 3-5 doses **or** 48 mg once per knee

Intradermal: *Adults:* Inject as required for cosmetic effect (maximum: ≤1.6 mL per injection site; 20 mL/60 kg/year [Hylaform®, Hylaform® Plus] **or** 6 mL/treatment [Perlane])

Ophthalmic: *Adults:* Depends upon procedure (slowly introduce a sufficient quantity into eye)

Topical: *Adults:* Apply to affected area 2-3 times daily

Mechanism of Action Sodium hyaluronate is a polysaccharide which is distributed widely in the extracellular matrix of connective tissue in man (vitreous and aqueous humor of the eye, synovial fluid, skin, and umbilical cord). Sodium hyaluronate and its derivatives form a viscoelastic solution in water (at physiological pH and ionic strength) which makes it suitable for aqueous and vitreous humor in ophthalmic surgery, and functions as a tissue and/or joint lubricant which plays an important role in modulating the interactions between adjacent tissues. Intradermal injection may decrease the depth of facial wrinkles.

Hyaluronidase (hye al yoor ON i dase)

U.S. Brand Names Amphadase™; Hydase™ [DSC]; Hylenex; Vitrase®

Pharmacologic Category Enzyme

Use Increase the dispersion and absorption of other injected drugs; increase rate of absorption of parenteral fluids given by subcutaneous administration (hypodermoclysis)

Unlabeled/Investigational Use Management of drug extravasations; local anesthetic adjuvant in bupivacaine-lidocaine mixture for retrobulbar/peribulbar block

Local Anesthetic/Vasoconstrictor Precautions No information available to require special precautions

Effects on Dental Treatment No significant effects or complications reported

Effects on Bleeding No information available to require special precautions

Adverse Effects Frequency not defined.

Cardiovascular: Edema

Local: Injection site reactions

General Dosage Range

Intradermal: *Children and Adults:* 0.02 mL (3 units) of a 150 units/mL solution

SubQ:

Premature Infants and Neonates: Volume of a single clysis should not exceed 25 mL/kg; rate of administration should not exceed 2 mL/minute

Children <3 years: Volume of a single clysis should not exceed 200 mL **or** 75 units over each scapula followed by injection of contrast medium at the same site

Children ≥3 years and Adults: Rate and volume of a single clysis should not exceed those used for infusion of I.V. fluids **or** 75 units over each scapula followed by injection of contrast medium at the same site

Mechanism of Action Modifies the permeability of connective tissue through hydrolysis of hyaluronic acid, one of the chief components of tissue cement which offers resistance to diffusion of liquids through tissues; hyaluronidase increases both the distribution and absorption of locally injected substances.

Pharmacodynamics/Kinetics

Onset of Action SubQ: Immediate

Duration of Action 24-48 hours

Pregnancy Risk Factor C

HydrALAZINE (hye DRAL a zeen)

Related Information

Cardiovascular Diseases *on page 1848*

Canadian Brand Names Apo-Hydralazine®; Apresoline®; Novo-Hylazin; Nu-Hydral

Pharmacologic Category Vasodilator

Use Management of moderate-to-severe hypertension

Unlabeled/Investigational Use Heart failure; hypertension secondary to pre-eclampsia/eclampsia

Local Anesthetic/Vasoconstrictor Precautions No information available to require special precautions

Effects on Dental Treatment No significant effects or complications reported

Effects on Bleeding No information available to require special precautions

Adverse Effects Frequency not defined.

Cardiovascular: Angina pectoris, flushing, orthostatic hypotension, palpitations, paradoxical hypertension, peripheral edema, tachycardia, vascular collapse

Central nervous system: Anxiety, chills, depression, disorientation, dizziness, fever, headache, increased intracranial pressure (I.V.; in patient with pre-existing increased intracranial pressure), psychotic reaction

Dermatologic: Pruritus, rash, urticaria

Gastrointestinal: Anorexia, constipation, diarrhea, nausea, paralytic ileus, vomiting

Genitourinary: Dysuria, impotence

Hematologic: Agranulocytosis, eosinophilia, erythrocyte count reduced, hemoglobin decreased, hemolytic anemia, leukopenia, thrombocytopenia (rare)

Neuromuscular & skeletal: Muscle cramps, peripheral neuritis, rheumatoid arthritis, tremor, weakness
Ocular: Conjunctivitis, lacrimation
Respiratory: Dyspnea, nasal congestion
Miscellaneous: Diaphoresis, drug-induced lupus-like syndrome (dose related; fever, arthralgia, splenomegaly, lymphadenopathy, asthenia, myalgia, malaise, pleuritic chest pain, edema, positive ANA, positive LE cells, maculopapular facial rash, positive direct Coombs' test, pericarditis, pericardial tamponade)

General Dosage Range Dosage adjustment recommended in patients with renal impairment

I.M., I.V.:

Children: 0.1-0.2 mg/kg/dose (not to exceed 20 mg) every 4-6 hours as needed (maximum: 3.5 mg/kg/day in 4-6 divided doses)

Adults: Initial: 10-20 mg/dose every 4-6 hours as needed; Maintenance: Up to 40 mg/dose every 4-6 hours **or** Eclampsia/pre-eclampsia: 5 mg/dose then 5-10 mg every 20-30 minutes as needed

Oral:

Children: Initial: 0.75-1 mg/kg/day in 2-4 divided doses; Maintenance: Up to 7.5 mg/kg/day in 2-4 divided doses (maximum: 200 mg/day)

Adults: Initial: 10-25 mg 3-4 times/day; Maintenance: 25-300 mg/day (target dose: 225-300 mg/day for CHF) in 2-4 divided doses (maximum: 300 mg/day)

Elderly: Initial: 10 mg 2-3 times/day, increase by 10-25 mg/day every 2-5 days; Target dose: 225-300 mg/day for CHF

Mechanism of Action Direct vasodilation of arterioles (with little effect on veins) with decreased systemic resistance

Pharmacodynamics/Kinetics

Onset of Action Oral: 20-30 minutes; I.V.: 5-20 minutes

Duration of Action Oral: Up to 8 hours; I.V.: 1-4 hours; **Note:** May vary depending on acetylator status of patient

Half-life Elimination Normal renal function: 2-8 hours; End-stage renal disease: 7-16 hours

Pregnancy Risk Factor C

Hydralazine and Hydrochlorothiazide

(hye DRAL a zeen & hye droe klor oh THYE a zide)

Related Information

HydrALAZINE *on page 853*
Hydrochlorothiazide *on page 854*

Pharmacologic Category Diuretic, Thiazide; Vasodilator, Direct-Acting

Use Management of moderate-to-severe hypertension and treatment of congestive heart failure

Local Anesthetic/Vasoconstrictor Precautions No information available to require special precautions

Effects on Dental Treatment No significant effects or complications reported

Effects on Bleeding No information available to require special precautions

Adverse Effects See individual agents.

General Dosage Range Oral: *Adults:* Hydralazine 25-100 mg/day and hydrochlorothiazide 25-50 mg/day in 2 divided doses (maximum: Hydrochlorothiazide: 50 mg/day)

Pregnancy Risk Factor C

Hydrochlorothiazide (hye droe klor oh THYE a zide)

Related Information

Cardiovascular Diseases *on page 1848*

U.S. Brand Names Microzide®

Canadian Brand Names Apo-Hydro®; Bio-Hydrochlorothiazide; Dom-Hydrochlorothiazide; Novo-Hydrazide; Nu-Hydro; PMS-Hydrochlorothiazide

Generic Availability (U.S.) Yes

Pharmacologic Category Diuretic, Thiazide

Use Management of mild-to-moderate hypertension; treatment of edema in heart failure and nephrotic syndrome

Unlabeled/Investigational Use Treatment of lithium-induced diabetes insipidus

Local Anesthetic/Vasoconstrictor Precautions No information available to require special precautions

Effects on Dental Treatment Key adverse event(s) related to dental treatment: Orthostatic hypotension and hypotension.

Effects on Bleeding No information available to require special precautions

Adverse Effects Frequency not defined; adverse events reported were observed at doses ≥25 mg:

Cardiovascular: Hypotension, orthostatic hypotension
Central nervous system: Dizziness, fever, headache, vertigo
Dermatologic: Alopecia, erythema multiforme, exfoliative dermatitis, photosensitivity, purpura, rash, Stevens-Johnson syndrome, toxic epidermal necrolysis, urticaria
Endocrine & metabolic: Hyperglycemia, hypokalemia, hyperuricemia
Gastrointestinal: Anorexia, constipation, cramping, diarrhea, epigastric distress, gastric irritation, nausea, pancreatitis, sialadenitis, vomiting
Genitourinary: Glycosuria, impotence
Hematologic: Agranulocytosis, aplastic anemia, hemolytic anemia, leukopenia, thrombocytopenia
Hepatic: Jaundice
Neuromuscular & skeletal: Muscle spasm, paresthesia, restlessness, weakness
Ocular: Blurred vision (transient), xanthopsia
Renal: Interstitial nephritis, renal dysfunction, renal failure
Respiratory: Respiratory distress, pneumonitis, pulmonary edema
Miscellaneous: Anaphylactic reactions, necrotizing angiitis

Dosage Oral (effect of drug may be decreased when used every day):

Children (in pediatric patients, chlorothiazide may be preferred over hydrochlorothiazide as there are more dosage formulations [eg, suspension] available): Edema, hypertension:
- <6 months: 1-3 mg/kg/day in 2 divided doses
- >6 months to 2 years: 1-3 mg/kg/day in 2 divided doses; maximum: 37.5 mg/day
- >2-17 years: Initial: 1 mg/kg/day; maximum: 3 mg/kg/day (50 mg/day)

Adults:
- Edema: 25-100 mg/day in 1-2 doses; maximum: 200 mg/day
- Hypertension: 12.5-50 mg/day; minimal increase in response and more electrolyte disturbances are seen with doses >50 mg/day

Elderly: 12.5-25 mg once daily

Dosing adjustment/comments in renal impairment: Cl_{cr} <10 mL/minute: Avoid use. Usually ineffective with GFR <30 mL/minute. Effective at lower GFR in combination with a loop diuretic.

Note: ACC/AHA 2009 Heart Failure guidelines suggest that thiazides lose their efficacy when Cl_{cr} <40 mL/minute.

Mechanism of Action Inhibits sodium reabsorption in the distal tubules causing increased excretion of sodium and water as well as potassium and hydrogen ions

Contraindications Hypersensitivity to hydrochlorothiazide or any component of the formulation, thiazides, or sulfonamide-derived drugs; anuria; renal decompensation; pregnancy

Warnings/Precautions Avoid in severe renal disease (ineffective as a diuretic). Electrolyte disturbances (hypokalemia, hypochloremic alkalosis, hyponatremia) can occur. Use with caution in severe hepatic dysfunction; hepatic encephalopathy can be caused by electrolyte disturbances. Gout may be precipitated in certain patients with a history of gout, a familial predisposition to gout, or chronic renal failure. Thiazide diuretics reduce calcium excretion; pathologic changes in the parathyroid glands with hypercalcemia and hypophosphatemia have been observed with prolonged use. Use with caution in patients with prediabetes and diabetes; may alter glucose control. May cause SLE exacerbation or activation. Use with caution in patients with moderate or high cholesterol concentrations. Photosensitization may occur. Correct hypokalemia before initiating therapy. Thiazide diuretics may decrease renal calcium excretion; consider avoiding use in patients with hypercalcemia. May cause acute transient myopia and acute angle-closure glaucoma, typically occurring within hours to weeks following initiation; discontinue therapy immediately in patients with acute decreases in visual acuity or ocular pain. Risk factors may include a history of sulfonamide or penicillin allergy.

Chemical similarities are present among sulfonamides, sulfonylureas, carbonic anhydrase inhibitors, thiazides, and loop diuretics (except ethacrynic acid). Use in patients with sulfonamide allergy is specifically contraindicated in product labeling, however, a risk of cross-reaction exists in patients with allergy to any of these compounds; avoid use when previous reaction has been severe. Discontinue if signs of hypersensitivity are noted.

Drug Interactions

Avoid Concomitant Use

Avoid concomitant use of Hydrochlorothiazide with any of the following: Dofetilide

Increased Effect/Toxicity

Hydrochlorothiazide may increase the levels/effects of: ACE Inhibitors; Allopurinol; Amifostine; Antihypertensives; Calcium Salts; CarBAMazepine; Dofetilide;

Hypotensive Agents; Lithium; OXcarbazepine; RiTUXimab; Topiramate; Toremifene; Vitamin D Analogs

The levels/effects of Hydrochlorothiazide may be increased by: Alcohol (Ethyl); Analgesics (Opioid); Barbiturates; Corticosteroids (Orally Inhaled); Corticosteroids (Systemic); Herbs (Hypotensive Properties); Licorice; MAO Inhibitors; Pentoxifylline; Phosphodiesterase 5 Inhibitors; Prostacyclin Analogues

Decreased Effect

Hydrochlorothiazide may decrease the levels/effects of: Antidiabetic Agents

The levels/effects of Hydrochlorothiazide may be decreased by: Bile Acid Sequestrants; Herbs (Hypertensive Properties); Methylphenidate; Nonsteroidal Anti-Inflammatory Agents; Yohimbine

Ethanol/Nutrition/Herb Interactions

Food: Hydrochlorothiazide peak serum levels may be decreased if taken with food. This product may deplete potassium, sodium, and magnesium.

Herb/Nutraceutical: Avoid herbs with *hypertensive* properties (bayberry, blue cohosh, cayenne, ephedra, ginger, ginseng [American], kola, licorice); may diminish the antihypertensive effect of hydrochlorothiazide. Avoid herbs with *hypotensive* properties (black cohosh, California poppy, coleus, golden seal, hawthorn, mistletoe, periwinkle, quinine, shepherd's purse); may enhance the hypotensive effect of hydrochlorothiazide.

Dietary Considerations May be taken with food or milk.

Pharmacodynamics/Kinetics

Onset of Action Diuresis: ~2 hours; Peak effect: 4-6 hours

Duration of Action 6-12 hours

Half-life Elimination 5.6-14.8 hours

Time to Peak 1-2.5 hours

Pregnancy Risk Factor B

Lactation Enters breast milk/not recommended (AAP rates "compatible"; AAP 2001 update pending)

Breast-Feeding Considerations Thiazide diuretics are found in breast milk. Following a single oral maternal dose of hydrochlorothiazide 50 mg, the mean breast milk concentration was 80 ng/mL (samples collected over 24 hours) and hydrochlorothiazide was not detected in the blood of the breast feeding infant (limit of detection 20 ng/mL). Peak plasma concentrations reported in adults following hydrochlorothiazide 12.5-100 mg are 70-490 ng/mL.

Dosage Forms

Capsule, oral: 12.5 mg

Microzide®: 12.5 mg

Tablet, oral: 12.5 mg, 25 mg, 50 mg

Hydrochlorothiazide and Spironolactone

(hye droe klor oh THYE a zide & speer on oh LAK tone)

Related Information

Hydrochlorothiazide *on page 854*

Spironolactone *on page 1550*

U.S. Brand Names Aldactazide®

Canadian Brand Names Aldactazide 25®; Aldactazide 50®; Novo-Spirozine

Pharmacologic Category Diuretic, Thiazide; Selective Aldosterone Blocker

Use Management of mild-to-moderate hypertension; treatment of edema in congestive heart failure and nephrotic syndrome, and cirrhosis of the liver accompanied by edema and/or ascites

Local Anesthetic/Vasoconstrictor Precautions No information available to require special precautions

Effects on Dental Treatment No significant effects or complications reported

Effects on Bleeding No information available to require special precautions

Adverse Effects See individual agents.

General Dosage Range Oral:

Children: 1.5-3 mg/kg/day in 2-4 divided doses (maximum: 200 mg/day)

Adults: 12.5-50 mg hydrochlorothiazide and 12.5-50 mg spironolactone/day in 1-2 divided doses

Pregnancy Risk Factor C

Hydrochlorothiazide and Triamterene

(hye droe klor oh THYE a zide & trye AM ter een)

Related Information

Hydrochlorothiazide *on page* 854

Triamterene *on page* 1674

U.S. Brand Names Dyazide®; Maxzide®; Maxzide®-25

Canadian Brand Names Apo-Triazide®; Novo-Triamzide; Nu-Triazide; Penta-Triamterene HCTZ; Riva-Zide

Generic Availability (U.S.) Yes

Pharmacologic Category Diuretic, Potassium-Sparing; Diuretic, Thiazide

Use Treatment of hypertension or edema (not recommended for initial treatment) when hypokalemia has developed on hydrochlorothiazide alone or when the development of hypokalemia must be avoided

Local Anesthetic/Vasoconstrictor Precautions No information available to require special precautions

Effects on Dental Treatment No significant effects or complications reported

Effects on Bleeding No information available to require special precautions

Adverse Effects Also see individual agents. Frequency not defined.

Cardiovascular: Angina, arrhythmia, postural hypotension, tachycardia

Central nervous system: Anxiety, dizziness, depression, fatigue, headache, insomnia, restlessness, vertigo

Dermatologic: Photosensitivity, purpura, rash, subacute cutaneous lupus erythematosus-like reactions, urticaria

Endocrine & metabolic: Acidosis, diabetes mellitus, hypercalcemia, hyperglycemia, hyper-/hypokalemia, hyperuricemia, hypochloremia, hypomagnesemia, hyponatremia

Gastrointestinal: Abdominal pain, anorexia, burning of tongue, constipation, diarrhea, loss of appetite, nausea, pancreatitis, sialadenitis, stomach cramps, taste alteration, tongue discoloration (bright orange), upset stomach, vomiting, xerostomia

Genitourinary: Impotence

Hematologic: Aplastic anemia, agranulocytosis, hemolytic anemia, leukopenia, thrombocytopenia, megaloblastic anemia

Hepatic: Jaundice, liver function tests (abnormal)

Neuromuscular & skeletal: Muscle cramping, parasthesia, weakness

Ocular: Blurred vision (transient), xanthopsia

Renal: Acute renal failure, BUN increased, glycosuria, interstitial nephritis, necrotizing vasculitis, renal stone formation, serum creatinine increased, urinary sediment abnormal, urine discoloration

Respiratory: Allergic pneumonitis, dyspnea, pulmonary edema, respiratory distress

Miscellaneous: Anaphylaxis, systemic lupus erythematosus (SLE) exacerbation

Dosage Oral: Adults:

Hydrochlorothiazide 25 mg and triamterene 37.5 mg: 1-2 tablets/capsules once daily

Hydrochlorothiazide 50 mg and triamterene 75 mg: 1/2-1 tablet daily

Mechanism of Action

Based on **triamterene** component: Interferes with potassium/sodium exchange (active transport) in the distal tubule, cortical collecting tubule and collecting duct by inhibiting sodium, potassium-ATPase; decreases calcium excretion; increases magnesium loss

Based on **hydrochlorothiazide** component: Inhibits sodium reabsorption in the distal tubules causing increased excretion of sodium and water as well as potassium and hydrogen ions

Contraindications Hypersensitivity to hydrochlorothiazide, triamterene, any component of the formulation, or sulfonamide-derived drugs; anuria; acute and chronic renal insufficiency or significant renal impairment; patients receiving other potassium-sparing diuretics, potassium-containing salt substitutes, or potassium supplements (except in severe cases of hypokalemia); preexisting hyperkalemia

Warnings/Precautions See individual agents.

Drug Interactions

Avoid Concomitant Use

Avoid concomitant use of Hydrochlorothiazide and Triamterene with any of the following: Dofetilide; Tacrolimus

Increased Effect/Toxicity

Hydrochlorothiazide and Triamterene may increase the levels/effects of: ACE Inhibitors; Allopurinol; Amifostine; Ammonium Chloride; Antihypertensives; Calcium Salts; CarBAMazepine; Cardiac Glycosides; Dofetilide; Hypotensive Agents; Lithium; OXcarbazepine; RiTUXimab; Tacrolimus; Topiramate; Toremifene; Vitamin D Analogs

The levels/effects of Hydrochlorothiazide and Triamterene may be increased by: Alcohol (Ethyl); Analgesics (Opioid); Angiotensin II Receptor Blockers; Barbiturates; Corticosteroids (Orally Inhaled); Corticosteroids (Systemic); Drospirenone; Eplerenone; Herbs (Hypotensive Properties); Indomethacin; Licorice; MAO Inhibitors; Nonsteroidal Anti-Inflammatory Agents; Pentoxifylline; Phosphodiesterase 5 Inhibitors; Potassium Salts; Prostacyclin Analogues; Tolvaptan

Decreased Effect

Hydrochlorothiazide and Triamterene may decrease the levels/effects of: Antidiabetic Agents; Cardiac Glycosides; QuiNIDine

The levels/effects of Hydrochlorothiazide and Triamterene may be decreased by: Bile Acid Sequestrants; Herbs (Hypertensive Properties); Methylphenidate; Nonsteroidal Anti-Inflammatory Agents; Yohimbine

Ethanol/Nutrition/Herb Interactions Food: Avoid food with high potassium content and potassium-containing salt substitutes.

Dietary Considerations Should be taken after meals.

Pregnancy Risk Factor C

Lactation Enters breast milk/not recommended

Breast-Feeding Considerations See individual agents.

Dosage Forms

Capsule: Hydrochlorothiazide 25 mg and triamterene 37.5 mg; hydrochlorothiazide 25 mg and triamterene 50 mg

Dyazide®: Hydrochlorothiazide 25 mg and triamterene 37.5 mg

Tablet: Hydrochlorothiazide 25 mg and triamterene 37.5 mg; hydrochlorothiazide 50 mg and triamterene 75 mg

Maxzide®: Hydrochlorothiazide 50 mg and triamterene 75 mg [scored]

Maxzide®-25: Hydrochlorothiazide 25 mg and triamterene 37.5 mg [scored]

Hydrocodone and Acetaminophen

(hye droe KOE done & a seet a MIN oh fen)

Related Information

Acetaminophen *on page 32*

Oral Pain *on page 1928*

Related Sample Prescriptions

Moderate/Moderately Severe Oral Pain *on page 1980*

U.S. Brand Names hycet®; Lorcet® 10/650; Lorcet® Plus; Lortab®; Margesic® H; Maxidone®; Norco®; Stagesic™; Vicodin®; Vicodin® ES; Vicodin® HP; Xodol® 10/300; Xodol® 5/300; Xodol® 7.5/300; Zamicet™; Zolvit™; Zydone®

Generic Availability (U.S.) Yes: Oral solution, tablet

Pharmacologic Category Analgesic Combination (Opioid)

Dental Use Treatment of postoperative pain

Use Relief of moderate-to-severe pain

Local Anesthetic/Vasoconstrictor Precautions No information available to require special precautions

Effects on Dental Treatment Key adverse event(s) related to dental treatment: Xerostomia (normal salivary flow resumes upon discontinuation). See Dental Comment.

Effects on Bleeding No information available to require special precautions

Adverse Effects Frequency not defined.

Cardiovascular: Bradycardia, cardiac arrest, circulatory collapse, coma, hypotension

Central nervous system: Anxiety, dizziness, drowsiness, dysphoria, euphoria, fear, lethargy, lightheadedness, malaise, mental clouding, mental impairment, mood changes, physiological dependence, sedation, somnolence, stupor

Dermatologic: Pruritus, rash

Endocrine & metabolic: Hypoglycemic coma

Gastrointestinal: Abdominal pain, constipation, gastric distress, heartburn, nausea, peptic ulcer, vomiting, xerostomia

Genitourinary: Ureteral spasm, urinary retention, vesical sphincter spasm

Hematologic: Agranulocytosis, bleeding time prolonged, hemolytic anemia, iron deficiency anemia, occult blood loss, thrombocytopenia

Hepatic: Hepatic necrosis, hepatitis

Neuromuscular & skeletal: Skeletal muscle rigidity

Otic: Hearing impairment or loss (chronic overdose)

Renal: Renal toxicity, renal tubular necrosis

Respiratory: Acute airway obstruction, apnea, dyspnea, respiratory depression (dose related)

Miscellaneous: Allergic reactions, clamminess, diaphoresis

Dental Usual Dosage Postoperative pain: Oral:

Children and Adults ≥50 kg: Average starting dose in opioid naive patients: Hydrocodone 5-10 mg 4 times/day; the dosage of acetaminophen should be limited to ≤4 g/day (and possibly less in patients with hepatic impairment or ethanol use).

Dosage ranges (based on specific product labeling): Hydrocodone 2.5-10 mg every 4-6 hours; maximum: 60 mg hydrocodone/day (maximum dose of hydrocodone may be limited by the acetaminophen content of specific product)

Elderly: Doses should be titrated to appropriate analgesic effect; 2.5-5 mg of the hydrocodone component every 4-6 hours. Do not exceed 4 g/day of acetaminophen.

Dosage Oral (doses should be titrated to appropriate analgesic effect): Analgesic:

Children 2-13 years or <50 kg: Hydrocodone 0.1-0.2 mg/kg/dose every 4-6 hours; do not exceed 6 doses/day or the maximum recommended dose of acetaminophen

Children and Adults ≥50 kg: Average starting dose in opioid naive patients: Hydrocodone 5-10 mg 4 times/day; the dosage of acetaminophen should be limited to ≤4 g/day (and possibly less in patients with hepatic impairment or ethanol use).

Dosage ranges (based on specific product labeling): Hydrocodone 2.5-10 mg every 4-6 hours (maximum dose of hydrocodone may be limited by the acetaminophen content of specific product)

Elderly: Doses should be titrated to appropriate analgesic effect; 2.5-5 mg of the hydrocodone component every 4-6 hours. Do not exceed 4 g/day of acetaminophen.

Dosage adjustment in hepatic impairment: Use with caution. Limited, low-dose therapy usually well tolerated in hepatic disease/cirrhosis; however, cases of hepatotoxicity at daily acetaminophen dosages <4 g/day have been reported. Avoid chronic use in hepatic impairment.

Mechanism of Action Hydrocodone, as with other narcotic (opiate) analgesics, blocks pain perception in the cerebral cortex by binding to specific receptor molecules (opiate receptors) within the neuronal membranes of synapses. This binding results in a decreased synaptic chemical transmission throughout the CNS thus inhibiting the flow of pain sensations into the higher centers. Mu and kappa are the two subtypes of the opiate receptor which hydrocodone binds to cause analgesia.

Acetaminophen inhibits the synthesis of prostaglandins in the CNS and peripherally blocks pain impulse generation; produces antipyresis from inhibition of hypothalamic heat-regulating center.

Contraindications Hypersensitivity to hydrocodone, acetaminophen, or any component of the formulation; CNS depression; severe respiratory depression

Warnings/Precautions Use with caution in patients with hypersensitivity reactions to other phenanthrene derivative opioid agonists (morphine, hydromorphone, levorphanol, oxycodone, oxymorphone); tolerance or drug dependence may result from extended use. Concurrent use of agonist/antagonist analgesics may precipitate withdrawal symptoms and/or reduced analgesic efficacy in patients following prolonged therapy with mu opioid agonists. Abrupt discontinuation following prolonged use may also lead to withdrawal symptoms.

Respiratory depressant effects may be increased with head injuries. Use caution with acute abdominal conditions; clinical course may be obscured. Use caution with adrenal insufficiency, biliary tract impairment, morbidly obese patients, toxic psychosis, thyroid dysfunction, prostatic hyperplasia, respiratory disease, hepatic or renal disease, and in the debilitated or elderly. Causes sedation; caution must be used in performing tasks which require alertness (eg, operating machinery or driving). Effects may be potentiated when used with other sedative drugs or ethanol. May cause hypotension.

Limit acetaminophen to <4 g/day. May cause severe hepatic toxicity in acute overdose; in addition, chronic daily dosing in adults has resulted in liver damage in some patients. Use with caution in patients with alcoholic liver disease; consuming ≥3 alcoholic drinks/day may increase the risk of liver damage. Use caution in patients with known G6PD deficiency.

Drug Interactions

Metabolism/Transport Effects

Hydrocodone: **Substrate** (minor) of CYP2D6, 3A

Acetaminophen: **Substrate** (minor) of CYP1A2, 2A6, 2C9, 2D6, 2E1, 3A4; **Inhibits** CYP3A4 (weak)

Avoid Concomitant Use There are no known interactions where it is recommended to avoid concomitant use.

Increased Effect/Toxicity

Hydrocodone and Acetaminophen may increase the levels/effects of: Alcohol (Ethyl); Alvimopan; CNS Depressants; Dasatinib; Desmopressin; Imatinib; Selective Serotonin Reuptake Inhibitors; SORAfenib; Thiazide Diuretics; Vitamin K Antagonists

The levels/effects of Hydrocodone and Acetaminophen may be increased by: Amphetamines; Antipsychotic Agents (Phenothiazines); Conivaptan; Dasatinib; Droperidol; Imatinib; Isoniazid; MAO Inhibitors; Metyrapone; Probenecid; SORAfenib; Succinylcholine

Decreased Effect

Hydrocodone and Acetaminophen may decrease the levels/effects of: Pegvisomant

The levels/effects of Hydrocodone and Acetaminophen may be decreased by: Ammonium Chloride; Anticonvulsants (Hydantoin); Barbiturates; CarBAMazepine; Cholestyramine Resin; Mixed Agonist / Antagonist Opioids; Peginterferon Alfa-2b; QuiNIDine; Tocilizumab

Ethanol/Nutrition/Herb Interactions

Ethanol: Consuming ≥3 alcoholic drinks/day may increase the risk of liver damage. Ethanol may also increase CNS depression; monitor for increased effects with coadministration. Caution patients about effects.

Herb/Nutraceutical: Avoid valerian, St John's wort, SAMe, kava kava (may increase risk of excessive sedation).

Pharmacodynamics/Kinetics

Onset of Action Hydrocodone: Narcotic analgesic: 10-20 minutes

Duration of Action Hydrocodone: 4-8 hours

Half-life Elimination Hydrocodone: 3.3-4.4 hours

Pregnancy Risk Factor C

Lactation Enters breast milk/not recommended

Breast-Feeding Considerations Acetaminophen and hydrocodone are excreted in breast milk. The manufacturers recommend discontinuing the medication or to discontinue nursing during therapy. Also refer to Acetaminophen monograph.

Controlled Substance C-III

Dosage Forms

Capsule, oral: Hydrocodone 5 mg and acetaminophen 500 mg

Margesic® H, Stagesic™: Hydrocodone 5 mg and acetaminophen 500 mg

Elixir, oral:

Lortab®: Hydrocodone 7.5 mg and acetaminophen 500 mg per 15 mL

Solution, oral: Hydrocodone 7.5 mg and acetaminophen 500 mg per 15 mL; hydrocodone 10 mg and acetaminophen 325 mg per 15 mL

hycet®: Hydrocodone 7.5 mg and acetaminophen 325 mg per 15 mL

Zamicet™: Hydrocodone 10 mg and acetaminophen 325 mg per 15 mL

Zolvit™: Hydrocodone 10 mg and acetaminophen 300 mg per 15 mL (480 mL)

Tablet, oral:

Generics:

Hydrocodone 2.5 mg and acetaminophen 500 mg
Hydrocodone 5 mg and acetaminophen 300 mg
Hydrocodone 5 mg and acetaminophen 325 mg
Hydrocodone 5 mg and acetaminophen 500 mg
Hydrocodone 7.5 mg and acetaminophen 300 mg
Hydrocodone 7.5 mg and acetaminophen 325 mg
Hydrocodone 7.5 mg and acetaminophen 500 mg
Hydrocodone 7.5 mg and acetaminophen 650 mg
Hydrocodone 7.5 mg and acetaminophen 750 mg
Hydrocodone 10 mg and acetaminophen 300 mg
Hydrocodone 10 mg and acetaminophen 325 mg
Hydrocodone 10 mg and acetaminophen 500 mg
Hydrocodone 10 mg and acetaminophen 650 mg
Hydrocodone 10 mg and acetaminophen 660 mg
Hydrocodone 10 mg and acetaminophen 750 mg

Brands:

Lorcet® 10/650: Hydrocodone 10 mg and acetaminophen 650 mg

Lorcet® Plus: Hydrocodone 7.5 mg and acetaminophen 650 mg

Lortab®: 5/500: Hydrocodone 5 mg and acetaminophen 500 mg; 7.5/500: Hydrocodone 7.5 mg and acetaminophen 500 mg; 10/500: Hydrocodone 10 mg and acetaminophen 500 mg

Maxidone®: Hydrocodone 10 mg and acetaminophen 750 mg

Norco®: Hydrocodone 5 mg and acetaminophen 325 mg; hydrocodone 7.5 mg and acetaminophen 325 mg; hydrocodone 10 mg and acetaminophen 325 mg

Vicodin®: Hydrocodone 5 mg and acetaminophen 500 mg

Vicodin® ES: Hydrocodone 7.5 mg and acetaminophen 750 mg

Vicodin® HP: Hydrocodone 10 mg and acetaminophen 660 mg

Xodol®: 5/300: Hydrocodone 5 mg and acetaminophen 300 mg; 7.5/300: Hydrocodone 7.5 mg and acetaminophen 300 mg; 10/300: Hydrocodone 10 mg and acetaminophen 300 mg

Zydone®: Hydrocodone 5 mg and acetaminophen 400 mg; hydrocodone 7.5 mg and acetaminophen 400 mg; hydrocodone 10 mg and acetaminophen 400 mg

Dental Comment Neither hydrocodone nor acetaminophen elicit anti-inflammatory effects. Because of addiction liability of opiate analgesics, the use of hydrocodone should be limited to 2-3 days postoperatively for treatment of dental pain. Nausea is the most common adverse effect seen after use in dental patients; sedation and constipation are second. Nausea elicited by narcotic analgesics is centrally mediated and the presence or absence of food will not affect the degree nor incidence of nausea.

Hepatotoxicity caused by acetaminophen is potentiated by chronic alcohol consumption. People who are taking acetaminophen, even at therapeutic doses, and consume alcohol are at risk of developing hepatotoxicity.

Acetaminophen may increase the levels and enhance the anticoagulant effects of vitamin K antagonists acenocoumarol and warfarin (Coumadin®). Studies have reported that acetaminophen has increased the INR in warfarin treated patients with daily acetaminophen doses as low as 2 g, particularly when taking acetaminophen for >1 week (Antlitz, 1968; Boeijinga, 1982; Gebauer, 2003; Hylek, 1998; Rubin, 1984). In addition, case reports of bleeding as a result of increased INR have been published (Bagheri, 1999; Bartle, 1991). There is no known mechanism of the interaction; furthermore, some studies have failed to demonstrate this interaction (Gadisseur, 2003; Kwan, 1995; van den Bemt, 2002). In terms of risk, the data suggest that acetaminophen and warfarin could interact in some clinically significant manner but that the benefits of concomitant use of acetaminophen for pain control in dental patients taking warfarin usually outweigh the risks. An appropriate monitoring plan should be in place to identify potential negative effects and dosage adjustments may be necessary in a minority of patients. The interaction may be more likely to occur with daily acetaminophen doses of >1.3 g for >1 week.

There are no reports of acetaminophen interacting with antiplatelet drugs such as aspirin, clopidogrel (Plavix®), or prasugrel (Effient™). Also, there are no reports of acetaminophen in combination with hydrocodone, codeine, or oxycodone interacting with warfarin (Coumadin®).

References

Antlitz AM, Mead JA Jr, and Tolentino MA, "Potentiation of Oral Anticoagulant Therapy by Acetaminophen," *Curr Ther Res Clin Exp*, 1968, 10(10):501-7.

Bagheri H, Bernhard NB, and Montastruc JL, "Potentiation of the Acenocoumarol Anticoagulant Effect by Acetaminophen," *Ann Pharmacother*, 1999, 33(4):506.

Bartle WR and Blakely JA, "Potentiation of Warfarin Anticoagulation by Acetaminophen," *JAMA*, 1991, 265(10):1260.

Bell WR, "Acetaminophen and Warfarin: Undesirable Synergy," *JAMA*, 1998, 279(9):702-3.

Boeijinga JJ, Boerstra EE, Ris P, et al, "Interaction Between Paracetamol and Coumarin Anticoagulants," *Lancet*, 1982, 1(8270):506.

Dart RC, Kuffner EK, and Rumack BH, "Treatment of Pain or Fever With Paracetamol (Acetaminophen) in the Alcoholic Patient: A Systematic Review," *Am J Ther*, 2000, 7(2):123-34.

Dionne RA, "New Approaches to Preventing and Treating Postoperative Pain," *J Am Dent Assoc*, 1992, 123(6):26-34.

Gadisseur AP, Van Der Meer FJ, and Rosendaal FR, "Sustained Intake of Paracetamol (Acetaminophen) During Oral Anticoagulant Therapy With Coumarins Does Not Cause Clinically Important INR Changes: A Randomized Double-Blind Clinical Trial," *J Thromb Haemost*, 2003, 1(4):714-7.

Gebauer MG, Nyfort-Hansen K, Henschke PJ, et al, "Warfarin and Acetaminophen Interaction," *Pharmacotherapy*, 2003, 23(1):109-12.

Gobetti JP, "Controlling Dental Pain," *J Am Dent Assoc*, 1992, 123(6):47-52.

Grant JA and Weiler JM, "A Report of a Rare Immediate Reaction After Ingestion of Acetaminophen," *Ann Allergy Asthma Immunol*, 2001, 87(3):227-9.

Hylek EM, Heiman H, Skates SJ, et al, "Acetaminophen and Other Risk factors for excessive warfarin anticoagulation," *JAMA*, 1998, 279(9):657-62.

Kwan D, Bartle WR, and Walker SE, "The Effects of Acetaminophen on Pharmacokinetics and Pharmacodynamics of Warfarin," *J Clin Pharmacol*, 1999, 39(1):68-75.

Kwan D, Bartle WR, and Walker SE, "The Effects of Acute and Chronic Acetaminophen Dosing on the Pharmacodynamics and Pharmacokinetics of (R)- and (S)-Warfarin," *Clin Pharmacol Ther*, 1995, 57:212.

McClain CJ, Price S, Barve S, et al, "Acetaminophen Hepatotoxicity: An Update," *Curr Gastroenterol Rep*, 1999, 1(1):42-9.

Rubin RN, Mentzer RL, and Budzynski AZ, "Potentiation of Anticoagulant Effect of Warfarin by Acetaminophen (Tylenol®)," *Clin Res*, 1984, 32:698a.

Shek KL, Chan LN, and Nutescu E, "Warfarin-Acetaminophen Drug Interaction Revisited," *Pharmacotherapy*, 1999, 19(10):1153-8.

Tanaka E, Yamazaki K, and Misawa S, "Update: The Clinical Importance of Acetaminophen Hepatotoxicity in Nonalcoholic and Alcoholic Subjects," *J Clin Pharm Ther*, 2000, 25(5):325-32.

van den Bemt PM, Geven LM, Kuitert NA, et al, "The Potential Interaction Between Oral Anticoagulants and Acetaminophen in Everyday Practice," *Pharm World Sci*, 2002, 24(5):201-4.

Wynn RL, "Narcotic Analgesics for Dental Pain: Available Products, Strengths, and Formulations," *Gen Dent*, 2001, 49(2):126-8, 130, 132 passim.

Hydrocodone and Chlorpheniramine
(hye droe KOE done & klor fen IR a meen)

Related Information

Chlorpheniramine *on page* 365

U.S. Brand Names TussiCaps®; Tussionex®

Pharmacologic Category Alkylamine Derivative; Alpha/Beta Agonist; Antitussive; Histamine H_1 Antagonist; Histamine H_1 Antagonist, First Generation

Use Symptomatic relief of cough and upper respiratory symptoms associated with cold and allergy

Local Anesthetic/Vasoconstrictor Precautions No information available to require special precautions

Effects on Dental Treatment Key adverse event(s) related to dental treatment: Prolonged use will cause significant xerostomia (normal salivary flow resumes upon discontinuation).

Effects on Bleeding No information available to require special precautions

Adverse Effects Also refer to Chlorpheniramine monograph. Frequency not defined.

Cardiovascular: Chest tightness

Central nervous system: Anxiety, dizziness, drowsiness, dysphoria, euphoria, fear, lethargy, mental impairment, mood changes, sedation

Dermatologic: Pruritus, rash

Gastrointestinal: Constipation, nausea, vomiting

Genitourinary: Ureteral spasm, urinary retention, vesicle sphincter spasm

Respiratory: Dryness of pharynx, respiratory depression

Miscellaneous: Psychological dependence

General Dosage Range Oral:

Children 6-12 years: TussiCaps® 5 mg/4 mg: 1 capsule every 12 hours (maximum: 2 capsules/24 hours); Tussionex®: 2.5 mL every 12 hours (maximum: 5 mL/24 hours)

Children >12 years and Adults: TussiCaps® 10 mg/8 mg: 1 capsule every 12 hours (maximum: 2 capsules/24 hours); Tussionex®: 5 mL every 12 hours (maximum: 10 mL/24 hours)

Mechanism of Action

Hydrocodone binds to opiate receptors in the CNS, altering the perception of and response to pain; suppresses cough in medullary center; produces generalized CNS depression

Chlorpheniramine competes with histamine for H_1-receptor sites on effector cells in the gastrointestinal tract, blood vessels, and respiratory tract

Pharmacodynamics/Kinetics

Duration of Action

Hydrocodone: 4-8 hours

Half-life Elimination

Hydrocodone: 3.3-4.4 hours

Pregnancy Risk Factor C

Controlled Substance C-III

Hydrocodone and Homatropine (hye droe KOE done & hoe MA troe peen)

Related Information

Homatropine *on page* 851

U.S. Brand Names Hycodan® [DSC]; Hydromet®; Tussigon®

Pharmacologic Category Antitussive

Use Symptomatic relief of cough

Local Anesthetic/Vasoconstrictor Precautions No information available to require special precautions

Effects on Dental Treatment Key adverse event(s) related to dental treatment: Xerostomia (normal salivary flow resumes upon discontinuation).

Effects on Bleeding No information available to require special precautions

Adverse Effects Frequency not defined.

Central nervous system: Anxiety, dizziness, drowsiness, dysphoria, fear, lethargy, mental clouding, mental impairment, mood changes, sedation

Dermatologic: Pruritus, rash

Gastrointestinal: Constipation, nausea, vomiting, xerostomia

Genitourinary: Urinary retention, urinary tract spasm

Respiratory: Respiratory depression

Miscellaneous: Physical and psychological dependence with prolonged use

General Dosage Range Oral:

Children 6-11 years: 1/2 tablet or 2.5 mL every 4-6 hours as needed (maximum: 3 tablets or 15 mL/24 hours)

Children ≥12 years and Adults: 1 tablet or 5 mL every 4-6 hours as needed (maximum: 6 tablets/24 hours or 30 mL/24 hours)

Mechanism of Action

Hydrocodone binds to opiate receptors in the CNS, altering the perception of and response to pain; suppresses cough in medullary center; produces generalized CNS depression.

Homatropine is an anticholinergic agent, present in a subtherapeutic amount to discourage deliberate overdose.

Pregnancy Risk Factor C

Controlled Substance C-III

Hydrocodone and Ibuprofen (hye droe KOE done & eye byoo PROE fen)

Related Information

Ibuprofen *on page 884*

Oral Pain *on page 1928*

Related Sample Prescriptions

Moderate/Moderately Severe Oral Pain *on page 1980*

U.S. Brand Names Ibudone™; Reprexain™; Vicoprofen®

Canadian Brand Names Vicoprofen®

Generic Availability (U.S.) Yes

Pharmacologic Category Analgesic, Opioid; Nonsteroidal Anti-inflammatory Drug (NSAID), Oral

Dental Use Short-term management (generally <10 days) of moderate-to-severe acute postoperative dental pain where an anti-inflammatory effect is desired

Use Short-term (generally <10 days) management of moderate-to-severe acute pain; is not indicated for treatment of such conditions as osteoarthritis or rheumatoid arthritis

Local Anesthetic/Vasoconstrictor Precautions No information available to require special precautions

Effects on Dental Treatment Key adverse event(s) related to dental treatment: Xerostomia (normal salivary flow resumes upon discontinuation). See Effects on Bleeding.

Effects on Bleeding Nonselective NSAIDs are known to reversibly decrease platelet aggregation via mechanisms different than observed with aspirin. Platelet function is restored as the drug is eliminated from the body. NSAIDs should be avoided (if possible) in general surgery patients for 3-5 half-lives of the drug (usually 1-3 days) prior to surgery to reduce the risk of excessive bleeding. However, there is no scientific evidence to warrant discontinuance of NSAIDs prior to dental surgery. In medically complicated patients or extensive oral surgery, the decision to interrupt therapy must be based on the risk to benefit in an individual patient and a medical consult is suggested. Routine interruption of NSAID therapy for most dental procedures is not warranted. If therapy is continued without interruption, the clinician should anticipate the potential for slower clotting times.

Adverse Effects

>10%:

Central nervous system: Headache (27%), somnolence (22%), dizziness (14%)

Gastrointestinal: Constipation (22%), nausea (21%), dyspepsia (12%)

1% to 10%:

Cardiovascular: Edema (3% to 9%), palpitation (<3%), vasodilation (<3%)

Central nervous system: Anxiety (3% to 9%), insomnia (3% to 9%), nervousness (3% to 9%), confusion (<3%), fever (<3%), thought abnormalities (<3%)

Dermatologic: Itching (3% to 9%)

Gastrointestinal: Abdominal pain (3% to 9%), diarrhea (3% to 9%), flatulence (3% to 9%), vomiting (3% to 9%), xerostomia (3% to 9%), gastritis (<3%), melena (<3%), mouth ulcers (<3%)

Genitourinary: Polyuria (<3%)

Neuromuscular & skeletal: Hypertonia (<3%), paresthesia (<3%)

Otic: Tinnitus (<3%)

Respiratory: Dyspnea (<3%), pharyngitis (<3%), rhinitis (<3%)

Miscellaneous: Diaphoresis (3% to 9%), infection (3% to 9%), flu-like syndrome (<3%), hiccups (<3%)

Dental Usual Dosage Moderate-to-severe acute postoperative dental pain: Adults: Oral: 1-2 tablets every 4-6 hours as needed for pain; maximum: 5 tablets/day

Dosage Oral:

Adults: 1 tablet every 4-6 hours as needed for pain; maximum: 5 tablets/day. **Note:** Short-term use is recommended (<10 days).

Elderly: Use with caution; consider reduced doses. Refer to dosing in individual monographs.

Mechanism of Action

Hydrocodone: Binds to opiate receptors in the CNS, altering the perception of and response to pain; suppresses cough in medullary center; produces generalized CNS depression

Ibuprofen: Reversibly inhibits cyclooxygenase-1 and 2 (COX-1 and 2) enzymes, which result in decreased formation of prostaglandin precursors; has antipyretic, analgesic, and anti-inflammatory properties

Contraindications Hypersensitivity to hydrocodone, ibuprofen, or any component of the formulation; patients who have experienced asthma, urticaria, or allergic-type reactions to aspirin or other NSAIDs; perioperative pain in the setting of coronary artery bypass graft (CABG) surgery

Warnings/Precautions [U.S. Boxed Warning]: NSAIDs are associated with an increased risk of adverse cardiovascular thrombotic events, including MI and stroke. Risk may be increased with duration of use or pre-existing cardiovascular risk factors or disease. May cause new-onset hypertension or worsening of existing hypertension. Use caution with fluid retention. Avoid use in heart failure. **[U.S. Boxed Warning]: Use of NSAIDs is contraindicated for treatment of perioperative pain in the setting of coronary artery bypass graft (CABG) surgery.** Risk of MI and stroke may be increased with use following CABG surgery. **[U.S. Boxed Warning]: NSAIDs may increase risk of gastrointestinal irritation, inflammation, ulceration, bleeding, and perforation.** When used concomitantly with ≤325 mg of aspirin, a substantial increase in the risk of gastrointestinal complications (eg, ulcer) occurs; concomitant gastroprotective therapy (eg, proton pump inhibitors) is recommended (Bhatt, 2008).

May increase the risk of aseptic meningitis, especially in patients with systemic lupus erythematosus (SLE) and mixed connective tissue disorders. Platelet adhesion and aggregation may be decreased; may prolong bleeding time; patients with coagulation disorders or who are receiving anticoagulants should be monitored closely. Anemia may occur; patients on long-term NSAID therapy should be monitored for anemia. Rarely, NSAID use may cause severe blood dyscrasias (eg, agranulocytosis, aplastic anemia, thrombocytopenia).

NSAIDS may cause drowsiness, dizziness, blurred vision and other neurologic effects which may impair physical or mental abilities; patients must be cautioned about performing tasks which require mental alertness (eg, operating machinery or driving). Discontinue use with blurred or diminished vision and perform ophthalmologic exam. Monitor vision with long-term therapy.

NSAID use may compromise existing renal function; dose-dependent decreases in prostaglandin synthesis may result from NSAID use, reducing renal blood flow which may cause renal decompensation. NSAID use may increase the risk for hyperkalemia. Patients with impaired renal function, dehydration, heart failure, liver dysfunction, those taking diuretics, and ACE inhibitors, and the elderly are at greater risk of renal toxicity and hyperkalemia. Rehydrate patient before starting therapy; monitor renal function closely. Not recommended for use in patients with advanced renal disease. Long-term NSAID use may result in renal papillary necrosis. NSAIDs may cause serious skin adverse events; discontinue use at first sign of skin rash or hypersensitivity. Anaphylactoid reactions may occur, even without prior exposure. Do not use in patients who experience bronchospasm, asthma, rhinitis, or urticaria with NSAID or aspirin therapy. Use caution in other forms of asthma. The elderly are at increased risk for adverse effects (especially peptic ulceration, CNS effects, renal toxicity) from NSAIDs even at low doses. Withhold for at least 4-6 half-lives prior to surgical or dental procedures.

Hydrocodone: May cause CNS depression. Effects may be potentiated when used with other sedative drugs or ethanol. May cause hypotension. Use with caution in patients with pre-existing respiratory compromise, and kyphoscoliosis or other skeletal disorder which may alter respiratory function. Use with caution in patients with hypersensitivity reactions to other phenanthrene derivative opioid agonists (codeine, hydrocodone, hydromorphone, levorphanol, oxycodone, oxymorphone). Use with extreme caution in patients with head injury, intracranial lesions, or elevated intracranial pressure. May obscure diagnosis or clinical course of patients with acute abdominal conditions. Use with caution in patients with severe hepatic dysfunction. Use with caution in patients with biliary tract dysfunction; acute pancreatitis may cause constriction of sphincter of Oddi. Use with caution in patients with adrenal insufficiency, thyroid dysfunction, seizure disorder, morbid obesity, toxic psychosis, prostatic hyperplasia and/or urinary stricture, severe hepatic dysfunction, or with a potential for or a history of drug abuse or acute alcoholism. May suppress cough reflex. Tolerance, psychological and physical dependence may occur with prolonged use. Concurrent use of agonist/antagonist analgesics may precipitate withdrawal symptoms and/or reduced analgesic efficacy in patients following prolonged therapy with mu opioid agonists. Abrupt discontinuation following prolonged use may also lead to withdrawal symptoms.

Safety and efficacy in children <16 years have not been established.

Drug Interactions

Metabolism/Transport Effects

Hydrocodone: **Substrate** (minor) of CYP2D6, 3A

Ibuprofen: **Substrate** (minor) of CYP2C9, 2C19; **Inhibits** CYP2C9 (strong)

Avoid Concomitant Use

Avoid concomitant use of Hydrocodone and Ibuprofen with any of the following: Ketorolac; Ketorolac (Systemic)

Increased Effect/Toxicity

Hydrocodone and Ibuprofen may increase the levels/effects of: Alcohol (Ethyl); Alvimopan; Aminoglycosides; Anticoagulants; Antiplatelet Agents; Bisphosphonate Derivatives; CNS Depressants; Collagenase (Systemic); CycloSPORINE; CycloSPORINE (Systemic); Deferasirox; Desmopressin; Digoxin; Drotrecogin Alfa; Eplerenone; Haloperidol; Ibritumomab; Lithium; Methotrexate; Nonsteroidal Anti-Inflammatory Agents; PEMEtrexed; Potassium-Sparing Diuretics; PRALAtrexate; Quinolone Antibiotics; Salicylates; Selective Serotonin Reuptake Inhibitors; Thiazide Diuretics; Thrombolytic Agents; Tositumomab and Iodine I 131 Tositumomab; Vancomycin; Vitamin K Antagonists

The levels/effects of Hydrocodone and Ibuprofen may be increased by: ACE Inhibitors; Amphetamines; Angiotensin II Receptor Blockers; Antidepressants (Tricyclic, Tertiary Amine); Antipsychotic Agents (Phenothiazines); Corticosteroids (Systemic); Dasatinib; Droperidol; Glucosamine; Herbs (Anticoagulant/Antiplatelet Properties); Ketorolac; Ketorolac (Systemic); MAO Inhibitors; Nonsteroidal Anti-Inflammatory Agents; Omega-3-Acid Ethyl Esters; Pentosan Polysulfate Sodium; Pentoxifylline; Probenecid; Prostacyclin Analogues; Selective Serotonin Reuptake Inhibitors; Serotonin/Norepinephrine Reuptake Inhibitors; Succinylcholine; Treprostinil; Voriconazole

Decreased Effect

Hydrocodone and Ibuprofen may decrease the levels/effects of: ACE Inhibitors; Angiotensin II Receptor Blockers; Antiplatelet Agents; Beta-Blockers; Eplerenone; HydrALAZINE; Loop Diuretics; Pegvisomant; Potassium-Sparing Diuretics; Salicylates

The levels/effects of Hydrocodone and Ibuprofen may be decreased by: Ammonium Chloride; Bile Acid Sequestrants; Mixed Agonist / Antagonist Opioids; Nonsteroidal Anti-Inflammatory Agents; QuiNIDine; Salicylates

Ethanol/Nutrition/Herb Interactions

Based on **hydrocodone** component: Ethanol: May increase CNS depression; monitor for increased effects with coadministration. Caution patients about effects.

Based on **ibuprofen** component:

Ethanol: Avoid ethanol (may enhance gastric mucosal irritation).

Food: Ibuprofen peak serum levels may be decreased if taken with food.

Herb/Nutraceutical: Avoid alfalfa, anise, bilberry, bladderwrack, bromelain, cat's claw, celery, chamomile, coleus, cordyceps, dong quai, evening primrose, fenugreek, feverfew, garlic, ginger, ginkgo biloba, ginseng (American, Panax, Siberian), grapeseed, green tea, guggul, horse chestnut seed, horseradish, licorice, prickly ash, red clover, reishi, SAMe (S-adenosylmethionine), sweet clover, turmeric, white willow (all have additional antiplatelet activity).

Pharmacodynamics/Kinetics

Onset of Action

Hydrocodone: Narcotic analgesic: 10-20 minutes

Duration of Action

Hydrocodone: 4-8 hours

Half-life Elimination

Hydrocodone: 4.5 hours

Time to Peak

Hydrocodone: 1.7 hours

Pregnancy Risk Factor C/D (3rd trimester)

Lactation Enters breast milk/not recommended

Breast-Feeding Considerations Hydrocodone and ibuprofen are excreted in breast milk. The manufacturers recommend discontinuing the medication or to discontinue nursing during therapy. Also refer to Ibuprofen monograph.

Controlled Substance C-III

Dosage Forms

Tablet: Hydrocodone 5 mg and ibuprofen 200 mg; hydrocodone 7.5 mg and ibuprofen 200 mg

Ibudone™: 5/200: Hydrocodone 5 mg and ibuprofen 200 mg; 10/200: Hydrocodone 10 mg and ibuprofen 200 mg

Reprexain™: 2.5/200: Hydrocodone 2.5 mg and ibuprofen 200 mg; 5/200: Hydrocodone 5 mg and ibuprofen 200 mg; 10/200: Hydrocodone 10 mg and ibuprofen 200 mg

Vicoprofen®: 7.5/200: Hydrocodone 7.5 mg and ibuprofen 200 mg

References

Dionne R, "To Tame the Pain?" *Compend Contin Educ Dent*, 1998, 19(4):426-8, 430-1.
Hargreaves KM, "Management of Pain in Endodontic Patients," *Tex Dent J*, 1997, 114(10):27-31.
Sunshine A, Olson NZ, O'Neill E, et al, "Analgesic Efficacy of a Hydrocodone With Ibuprofen Combination Compared With Ibuprofen Alone for the Treatment of Acute Postoperative Pain," *J Clin Pharmacol*, 1997, 37(10):908-15.
Wynn RL, "Narcotic Analgesics for Dental Pain: Available Products, Strengths, and Formulations," *Gen Dent*, 2001, 49(2):126-8, 130, 132 passim.

Hydrocortisone (Systemic) (hye droe KOR ti sone)

U.S. Brand Names A-Hydrocort®; Cortef®; Solu-CORTEF®

Canadian Brand Names Cortef®; Solu-Cortef®

Generic Availability (U.S.) Yes: Tablet

Pharmacologic Category Corticosteroid, Systemic

Dental Use Treatment of a variety of oral diseases of allergic, inflammatory, or autoimmune origin

Use Management of adrenocortical insufficiency; anti-inflammatory or immunosuppressive

Unlabeled/Investigational Use Management of septic shock when blood pressure is poorly responsive to fluid resuscitation and vasopressor therapy

Local Anesthetic/Vasoconstrictor Precautions No information available to require special precautions

Effects on Dental Treatment No significant effects or complications reported

Effects on Bleeding No information available to require special precautions

Adverse Effects Frequency not defined.

Cardiovascular: Arrhythmias, bradycardia, cardiac arrest, cardiomegaly, circulatory collapse, congestive heart failure, edema, fat embolism, hypertension, hypertrophic cardiomyopathy (premature infants), myocardial rupture (post MI), syncope, tachycardia, thromboembolism, vasculitis

Central nervous system: Delirium, depression, emotional instability, euphoria, hallucinations, headache, insomnia, intracranial pressure increased, malaise, mood swings, nervousness, neuritis, neuropathy, personality changes, pseudotumor cerebri, psychic disorders, psychoses, seizure, vertigo

Dermatologic: Acne, allergic dermatitis, alopecia, bruising, burning/tingling, dry scaly skin, edema, erythema, hirsutism, hyper-/hypopigmentation, impaired wound healing, petechiae, rash, skin atrophy, skin test reaction impaired, sterile abscess, striae, urticaria

Endocrine & metabolic: Adrenal suppression, alkalosis, amenorrhea, carbohydrate intolerance increased, Cushing's syndrome, diabetes mellitus, glucose intolerance, growth suppression, hyperglycemia, hyperlipidemia, hypokalemia, hypokalemic alkalosis, menstrual irregularities, negative nitrogen balance, pituitary-adrenal axis suppression, potassium loss, protein catabolism, sodium and water retention, sperm motility increased/decreased, spermatogenesis increased/decreased

Gastrointestinal: Abdominal distention, appetite increased, bowel dysfunction (intrathecal administration), indigestion, nausea, pancreatitis, peptic ulcer, gastrointestinal perforation, ulcerative esophagitis, vomiting, weight gain

Genitourinary: Bladder dysfunction (intrathecal administration)

Hematologic: Leukocytosis (transient)

Hepatic: Hepatomegaly, transaminases increased

Local: Atrophy (at injection site), postinjection flare (intra-articular use), thrombophlebitis

Neuromuscular & skeletal: Arthralgia, necrosis (femoral and humoral heads), Charcot-like arthropathy, fractures, muscle mass loss, muscle weakness, myopathy, osteoporosis, tendon rupture, vertebral compression fractures

Ocular: Cataracts, exophthalmoses, glaucoma, intraocular pressure increased

Miscellaneous: Abnormal fat deposits, anaphylaxis, avascular necrosis, diaphoresis, hiccups, hypersensitivity reactions, infection, secondary malignancy

Dosage Dose should be based on severity of disease and patient response

Adrenal hyperplasia (congenital): Children: Oral: Initial: 10-20 mg/m^2/day in 3 divided doses; a variety of dosing schedules have been used. **Note:** Inconsistencies have occurred with liquid formulations; tablets may provide more reliable levels. Doses must be individualized by monitoring growth, bone age, and hormonal levels. Mineralocorticoid and sodium supplementation may be required based upon electrolyte regulation and plasma renin activity.

Adrenal insufficiency (acute): I.M., I.V.:

Infants and Young Children: Succinate: 1-2 mg/kg/dose bolus, then 25-150 mg/day in divided doses every 6-8 hours

Older Children: Succinate: 1-2 mg/kg bolus then 150-250 mg/day in divided doses every 6-8 hours

Adults: Succinate: 100 mg I.V. bolus, then 300 mg/day in divided doses every 8 hours or as a continuous infusion for 48 hours; once patient is stable change to oral, 50 mg every 8 hours for 6 doses, then taper to 30-50 mg/day in divided doses

Adrenal insufficiency (chronic): Adults: Oral: 20-30 mg/day

Anti-inflammatory or immunosuppressive:

Infants and Children:

Oral: 2.5-10 mg/kg/day **or** 75-300 mg/m^2/day every 6-8 hours

I.M., I.V.: Succinate: 1-5 mg/kg/day **or** 30-150 mg/m^2/day divided every 12-24 hours

Adolescents and Adults: Oral, I.M., I.V.: Succinate: 15-240 mg every 12 hours

Physiologic replacement: Children:

Oral: 0.5-0.75 mg/kg/day **or** 20-25 mg/m^2/day every 8 hours

I.M.: Succinate: 0.25-0.35 mg/kg/day **or** 12-15 mg/m^2/day once daily

Septic shock (unlabeled use): I.V.: Succinate:

Children: Initial: 1-2 mg/kg/day (intermittent or as continuous infusion); may titrate up to 50 mg/kg/day for shock reversal (Brierley, 2009); alternative dosing suggests 50 mg/m^2/day (Dellinger, 2008). **Note:** Use recommended only in catecholamine-resistant shock and suspected or proven adrenal insufficiency.

Adults: 50 mg every 6 hours (Annane, 2002; Marik, 2008); not to exceed 300 mg/day (Dellinger, 2008). Practice guidelines also recommend alternative dosing of 100 mg bolus, followed by continuous infusion of 10 mg/hour (240 mg/day). Taper slowly (for total of 11 days) and do not stop abruptly. **Note:** Fludrocortisone is optional with use of hydrocortisone.

Status asthmaticus: Children and Adults: I.V.: Succinate: 1-2 mg/kg/dose every 6 hours for 24 hours, then maintenance of 0.5-1 mg/kg every 6 hours

Stress dosing (surgery) in patients known to be adrenally-suppressed or on chronic systemic steroids: I.V.: Adults:

Minor stress (ie, inguinal herniorrhaphy): 25 mg/day for 1 day

Moderate stress (ie, joint replacement, cholecystectomy): 50-75 mg/day (25 mg every 8-12 hours) for 1-2 days

Major stress (pancreatoduodenectomy, esophagogastrectomy, cardiac surgery): 100-150 mg/day (50 mg every 8-12 hours) for 2-3 days

Mechanism of Action Decreases inflammation by suppression of migration of polymorphonuclear leukocytes and reversal of increased capillary permeability

Contraindications Hypersensitivity to hydrocortisone or any component of the formulation; serious infections, except septic shock or tuberculous meningitis; viral, fungal, or tubercular skin lesions; I.M. administration contraindicated in idiopathic thrombocytopenia purpura; intrathecal administration of injection

Warnings/Precautions Use with caution in patients with thyroid disease, hepatic impairment, renal impairment, heart failure, hypertension, diabetes, glaucoma, cataracts, myasthenia gravis, patients at risk for osteoporosis, patients at risk for seizures, or GI diseases (diverticulitis, peptic ulcer, ulcerative colitis) due to perforation risk. Use caution following acute MI (corticosteroids have been associated with myocardial rupture). Because of the risk of adverse effects, systemic corticosteroids should be used cautiously in the elderly in the smallest possible effective dose for the shortest duration. May affect growth velocity; growth should be routinely monitored in pediatric patients. Withdraw therapy with gradual tapering of dose.

May cause hypercorticism or suppression of hypothalamic-pituitary-adrenal (HPA) axis, particularly in younger children or in patients receiving high doses for prolonged periods. HPA axis suppression may lead to adrenal crisis. Withdrawal and discontinuation of a corticosteroid should be done slowly and carefully. Particular care is required when patients are transferred from systemic corticosteroids to inhaled products due to possible adrenal insufficiency or withdrawal from steroids, including an increase in allergic symptoms. Patients receiving >20 mg per day of prednisone (or equivalent) may be most susceptible. Fatalities have occurred due to adrenal insufficiency in asthmatic patients during and after transfer from systemic corticosteroids to aerosol steroids; aerosol steroids do not provide the systemic steroid needed to treat patients having trauma, surgery, or infections.

Acute myopathy has been reported with high dose corticosteroids, usually in patients with neuromuscular transmission disorders; may involve ocular and/or respiratory muscles; monitor creatine kinase; recovery may be delayed. Corticosteroid use may cause psychiatric disturbances, including depression, euphoria, insomnia, mood swings, and personality changes. Pre-existing psychiatric conditions may be exacerbated by corticosteroid use. Prolonged use of corticosteroids may also increase the incidence of secondary infection, mask acute infection (including fungal infections), prolong or exacerbate viral infections, or limit response to vaccines. Exposure to chickenpox should be avoided; corticosteroids should not be used to treat ocular herpes simplex. Corticosteroids should not be used for cerebral malaria or viral hepatitis. Oral steroid treatment is not recommended for the treatment of acute optic neuritis. Close observation is required in patients with latent tuberculosis and/or TB reactivity; restrict use in active TB (only in conjunction with antituberculosis treatment). Prolonged treatment with corticosteroids has been associated with the development of Kaposi's sarcoma (case reports); if noted, discontinuation of therapy should be considered. High-dose corticosteroids should not be used to manage acute head injury.

Drug Interactions

Metabolism/Transport Effects **Substrate** of CYP3A4 (minor), P-glycoprotein; **Induces** CYP3A4 (weak)

Avoid Concomitant Use

Avoid concomitant use of Hydrocortisone (Systemic) with any of the following: Aldesleukin; BCG; Natalizumab; Pimecrolimus; Roflumilast; Tacrolimus (Topical)

Increased Effect/Toxicity

Hydrocortisone (Systemic) may increase the levels/effects of: Acetylcholinesterase Inhibitors; Amphotericin B; Deferasirox; Leflunomide; Loop Diuretics; Natalizumab; NSAID (COX-2 Inhibitor); NSAID (Nonselective); Thiazide Diuretics; Vaccines (Live); Warfarin

The levels/effects of Hydrocortisone (Systemic) may be increased by: Antifungal Agents (Azole Derivatives, Systemic); Aprepitant; Calcium Channel Blockers (Nondihydropyridine); Conivaptan; Denosumab; Estrogen Derivatives; Fluconazole; Fosaprepitant; Macrolide Antibiotics; Neuromuscular-Blocking Agents (Nondepolarizing); P-Glycoprotein Inhibitors; Pimecrolimus; Quinolone Antibiotics; Roflumilast; Salicylates; Tacrolimus (Topical); Trastuzumab

Decreased Effect

Hydrocortisone (Systemic) may decrease the levels/effects of: Aldesleukin; Antidiabetic Agents; BCG; Calcitriol; Corticorelin; Isoniazid; Salicylates; Sipuleucel-T; Vaccines (Inactivated)

The levels/effects of Hydrocortisone (Systemic) may be decreased by: Aminoglutethimide; Antacids; Barbiturates; Bile Acid Sequestrants; Echinacea; Mitotane; P-Glycoprotein Inducers; Primidone; Rifamycin Derivatives; Tocilizumab

Ethanol/Nutrition/Herb Interactions

Ethanol: Avoid ethanol (may enhance gastric mucosal irritation).

Food: Hydrocortisone interferes with calcium absorption.

Herb/Nutraceutical: St John's wort may decrease hydrocortisone levels. Avoid cat's claw, echinacea (have immunostimulant properties).

Dietary Considerations Systemic use of corticosteroids may require a diet with increased potassium, vitamins A, B_6, C, D, folate, calcium, zinc, phosphorus, and decreased sodium. Some products may contain sodium.

Pharmacodynamics/Kinetics

Onset of Action Hydrocortisone sodium succinate (water soluble): Rapid

Half-life Elimination Biologic: 8-12 hours

Pregnancy Risk Factor C

Lactation Enters breast milk/use caution

Breast-Feeding Considerations Corticosteroids are excreted in breast milk and endogenous hydrocortisone is also found in human milk; the effect of maternal hydrocortisone intake is not known.

Dosage Forms

Injection, powder for reconstitution:

A-Hydrocort®: 100 mg

Solu-CORTEF®: 100 mg, 250 mg, 500 mg, 1000 mg

Tablet, oral: 5 mg, 10 mg, 20 mg

Cortef®: 5 mg, 10 mg, 20 mg

Hydrocortisone (Topical) (hye droe KOR ti sone)

U.S. Brand Names Ala-Cort; Ala-Scalp; Anu-med HC; Anucort-HC™; Anusol-HC®; Aquanil HC® [OTC]; Beta-HC® [OTC]; Caldecort® [OTC]; Colocort®; Cortaid® Advanced [OTC]; Cortaid® Intensive Therapy [OTC]; Cortaid® Maximum Strength [OTC]; Cortenema®; CortiCool® [OTC]; Cortifoam®; Cortizone-10® Hydratensive Healing [OTC]; Cortizone-10® Hydratensive Soothing [OTC]; Cortizone-10® Intensive Healing Eczema [OTC]; Cortizone-10® Maximum Strength Cooling Relief [OTC]; Cortizone-10® Maximum Strength Easy Relief [OTC]; Cortizone-10®

Maximum Strength Intensive Healing Formula [OTC]; Cortizone-10® Maximum Strength [OTC]; Cortizone-10® Plus Maximum Strength [OTC]; Dermarest® Eczema Medicated [OTC]; Hemorrhoidal HC [DSC]; Hemril® -30; HYDRO-Rx [DSC]; Hydrocortisone Plus [OTC]; Hydroskin® [OTC]; HydroZone Plus [OTC] [DSC]; Ivy Soothe® [OTC] [DSC]; Locoid Lipocream®; Locoid®; Pandel®; Pedia-derm™ HC; Preparation H® Hydrocortisone [OTC]; Procto-Kit™ [DSC]; Procto-Pak™; Proctocort®; ProctoCream®-HC; Proctosol-HC®; Proctozone-HC 2.5%™; Recort [OTC]; Scalpana [OTC]; Texacort®; Tucks® Anti-Itch [OTC] [DSC]; U-Cort™; Westcort®

Canadian Brand Names Aquacort®; Cortamed®; Cortenema®; Cortifoam™; Emo-Cort®; Hycort™; Hyderm; HydroVal®; Locoid®; Prevex® HC; Sarna® HC; Westcort®

Generic Availability (U.S.) Yes: Excludes aerosol (acetate), cream (probutate), gel (base), liquid (base), lotion (base), solution (base)

Pharmacologic Category Corticosteroid, Rectal; Corticosteroid, Topical

Use Relief of inflammation of corticosteroid-responsive dermatoses (low and medium potency topical corticosteroid); adjunctive treatment of ulcerative colitis

Local Anesthetic/Vasoconstrictor Precautions No information available to require special precautions

Effects on Dental Treatment No significant effects or complications reported

Effects on Bleeding No information available to require special precautions

Adverse Effects Frequency not always defined:

Dermatologic: Acneiform eruption dermatitis, dry skin (2%), eczema (12.5%), hypertrichosis, pruritus (6%), stinging (2%)

Endocrine: HPA axis suppression; metabolic effects (hyperglycemia, hypokalemia)

Gastrointestinal: Pain (rectal), rectal bleeding (rectal)

Miscellaneous: Hypersensitivity reactions, secondary infection

Dental Usual Dosage Treatment of a variety of oral diseases of allergic, inflammatory, or autoimmune origin: Children >2 years and Adults: Topical: Apply to affected area 2-4 times/day

Dosage

Dermatosis: Children >2 years and Adults: Topical: Apply to affected area 2-4 times/day

Ulcerative colitis: Adults: Rectal: 10-100 mg 1-2 times/day for 2-3 weeks

Mechanism of Action Decreases inflammation by suppression of migration of polymorphonuclear leukocytes and reversal of increased capillary permeability

Contraindications Hypersensitivity to any component of the formulation.

Rectal suspension: Systemic fungal infections; ileocolostomy during the immediate or early postoperative period

Warnings/Precautions Topical corticosteroids may be absorbed percutaneously. Absorption may cause manifestations of Cushing's syndrome, hyperglycemia, or glycosuria. Absorption is increased by the use of occlusive dressings, application to denuded skin, or application to large surface areas. Avoid use of topical preparations with occlusive dressings or on weeping or exudative lesions. May cause hypercorticism or suppression of hypothalamic-pituitary-adrenal (HPA) axis, particularly in younger children or in patients receiving high doses for prolonged periods. HPA axis suppression may lead to adrenal crisis.

Prolonged use may result in fungal or bacterial superinfection; discontinue if dermatological infection persists despite appropriate antimicrobial therapy. Topical use has been associated with local sensitization (redness, irrritation); discontinue if sensitization is noted.

Because of the risk of adverse effects associated with systemic absorption, topical corticosteroids should be used cautiously in the elderly in the smallest possible effective dose for the shortest duration. Children may absorb proportionally larger amounts after topical application and may be more prone to systemic effects. Children may absorb proportionally larger amounts after topical application and may be more prone to systemic effects. HPA axis suppression, intracranial hypertension, and Cushing's syndrome have been reported in children receiving topical corticosteroids. Prolonged use may affect growth velocity; growth should be routinely monitored in pediatric patients.

Retention enema: Damage to the rectal wall may occur from improper or careless insertion of the enema tip. Use with caution when there is a risk of impending perforation, fresh anastomoses, obstruction, fistula, abscess, or pyogenic infection. Use with caution in patients with active or latent peptic ulcer, diverticulitis, renal insufficiency, osteoporosis, hypertension, or thyroid disease. May be associated with psychological adverse effects including euphoria and psychosis. Use caution in patients with pre-existing psychological disorders. Reduce dosage gradually when discontinuing therapy.

Drug Interactions

Metabolism/Transport Effects **Substrate** of CYP3A4 (minor), P-glycoprotein; **Induces** CYP3A4 (weak)

Avoid Concomitant Use

Avoid concomitant use of Hydrocortisone (Topical) with any of the following: Aldesleukin

Increased Effect/Toxicity

Hydrocortisone (Topical) may increase the levels/effects of: Deferasirox

The levels/effects of Hydrocortisone (Topical) may be increased by: Conivaptan

Decreased Effect

Hydrocortisone (Topical) may decrease the levels/effects of: Aldesleukin; Corticorelin

The levels/effects of Hydrocortisone (Topical) may be decreased by: Tocilizumab

Pregnancy Risk Factor C

Lactation Enters breast milk/use caution

Breast-Feeding Considerations Corticosteroids are excreted in breast milk and endogenous hydrocortisone is also found in human milk; the effect of maternal hydrocortisone intake is not known.

Dosage Forms

Aerosol, rectal:

Cortifoam®: 10% (15 g)

Cream, topical: 0.1% (15 g, 45 g); 0.2% (15 g, 45 g, 60 g); 0.5% (0.9 g, 15 g, 30 g, 60 g); 1% (0.9 g, 1 g, 1.5 g, 15 g, 20 g, 28.35 g, 28.4 g, 30 g, 114 g, 120 g, 454 g); 2% (43 g); 2.5% (20 g, 28 g, 28.35 g, 30 g, 454 g)

Ala-Cort: 1% (28.4 g, 85.2 g)
Anusol-HC®: 2.5% (30 g)
Caldecort® [OTC]: 1% (28.4 g)
Cortaid® Advanced [OTC]: 1% (42 g)
Cortaid® Intensive Therapy [OTC]: 1% (37 g, 56 g)
Cortaid® Maximum Strength [OTC]: 1% (14 g, 28 g, 37 g, 56 g)
Cortizone-10® Maximum Strength [OTC]: 1% (15 g, 28 g, 56 g)
Cortizone-10® Maximum Strength Intensive Healing Formula [OTC]: 1% (28 g, 56 g)
Cortizone-10® Plus Maximum Strength [OTC]: 1% (28 g, 56 g)
Hydrocortisone Plus [OTC]: 1% (28.4 g)
Hydroskin® [OTC]: 1% (28 g)
Locoid Lipocream®: 0.1% (15 g, 45 g, 60 g)
Locoid®: 0.1% (15 g, 45 g)
Pandel®: 0.1% (15 g, 45 g, 80 g)
Preparation H® Hydrocortisone [OTC]: 1% (26 g)
Procto-Pak™: 1% (28.4 g)
Proctocort®: 1% (28.35 g)
ProctoCream®-HC: 2.5% (30 g)
Proctosol-HC®: 2.5% (28.35 g)
Proctozone-HC 2.5%™: 2.5% (30 g)
Recort [OTC]: 1% (30 g)
U-Cort™: 1% (28 g)

Gel, topical:

CortiCool® [OTC]: 1% (0.9 g, 42.5 g)
Cortizone-10® Maximum Strength Cooling Relief [OTC]: 1% (28 g)

Liquid, topical:

Cortizone-10® Maximum Strength Easy Relief [OTC]: 1% (36 mL)
Scalpana [OTC]: 1% (85.5 mL)

Lotion, topical: 1% (114 g, 118 mL, 120 mL); 2.5% (59 mL, 60 mL, 118 mL)

Ala-Scalp: 2% (29.6 mL)
Aquanil HC® [OTC]: 1% (120 mL)
Beta-HC® [OTC]: 1% (60 mL)
Cortaid® Intensive Therapy [OTC]: 1% (98 g)
Cortizone-10® Hydratensive Healing [OTC]: 1% (113 g)
Cortizone-10® Hydratensive Soothing [OTC]: 1% (113 g)
Cortizone-10® Intensive Healing Eczema [OTC]: 1% (99 g)
Dermarest® Eczema Medicated [OTC]: 1% (118 mL)
Hydroskin® [OTC]: 1% (118 mL)
Locoid®: 0.1% (60 mL)
Pediaderm™ HC: 2% (29.6 mL)

Ointment, topical: 0.1% (15 g, 45 g); 0.2% (15 g, 45 g, 60 g); 0.5% (30 g); 1% (25 g, 28.4 g, 30 g, 110 g, 430 g, 454 g); 2.5% (20 g, 28.35 g, 30 g, 454 g)
Cortaid® Maximum Strength [OTC]: 1% (28 g, 37 g)
Cortizone-10® Maximum Strength [OTC]: 1% (28 g, 56 g)
Locoid®: 0.1% (15 g, 45 g)
Westcort®: 0.2% (15 g, 45 g, 60 g)
Powder, for prescription compounding: USP: 100% (10 g, 25 g, 50 g, 100 g, 1000 g)
Solution, topical: 0.1% (20 mL, 60 mL)
Cortaid® Intensive Therapy [OTC]: 1% (59 mL)
Locoid®: 0.1% (20 mL, 60 mL)
Texacort®: 2.5% (30 mL)
Suppository, rectal: 25 mg (12s, 24s, 1000s); 30 mg (12s)
Anu-med HC: 25 mg (12s)
Anucort-HC™: 25 mg (12s, 24s, 100s)
Anusol-HC®: 25 mg (12s, 24s)
Hemril® -30: 30 mg (12s, 24s)
Proctocort®: 30 mg (12s, 24s)
Suspension, rectal: 100 mg/60 mL (60 mL)
Colocort®: 100 mg/60 mL (60 mL)
Cortenema®: 100 mg/60 mL (60 mL)

References

Reed BR, "Dermatologic Drugs, Pregnancy, and Lactation. A Conservative guide," *Arch Dermato*, 1997, 133(7):894-8.

HYDROmorphone (hye droe MOR fone)

Related Information
Oral Pain *on page 1928*
Oxymorphone *on page 1282*

U.S. Brand Names Dilaudid-HP®; Dilaudid®; Exalgo™

Canadian Brand Names Dilaudid-HP-Plus®; Dilaudid-HP®; Dilaudid-XP®; Dilaudid®; Dilaudid® Sterile Powder; Hydromorph Contin®; Hydromorph-IR®; Hydromorphone HP; Hydromorphone HP® 10; Hydromorphone HP® 20; Hydromorphone HP® 50; Hydromorphone HP® Forte; Hydromorphone Hydrochloride Injection, USP; Jurnista™; PMS-Hydromorphone

Pharmacologic Category Analgesic, Opioid

Use Management of moderate-to-severe pain
Exalgo™: Management of moderate-to-severe pain in opioid-tolerant patients (requiring around-the-clock analgesia for an extended period of time)

Local Anesthetic/Vasoconstrictor Precautions No information available to require special precautions

Effects on Dental Treatment Key adverse event(s) related to dental treatment: Xerostomia (normal salivary flow resumes upon discontinuation).

Effects on Bleeding No information available to require special precautions

Adverse Effects Frequency not defined.
Cardiovascular: Bradycardia, extrasystoles, flushing of face, hyper-/hypotension, palpitation, peripheral edema, peripheral vasodilation, syncope, tachycardia
Central nervous system: Abnormal dreams, abnormal feelings, agitation, aggression, apprehension, attention disturbances, chills, coordination impaired, CNS depression, confusion, cognitive disorder, crying, dizziness, drowsiness, dysphoria, encephalopathy, euphoria, fatigue, hallucinations, headache, hyper-reflexia, hypo/hyperesthesia, hypothermia, increased intracranial pressure, insomnia, lightheadedness, listlessness, malaise, memory impairment, mental depression, mood alterations, nervousness, panic attacks, paranoia, psychomotor hyperactivity, restlessness, sedation, seizure, somnolence, suicide ideation, vertigo
Dermatologic: Hyperhidrosis, pruritus, rash, urticaria
Endocrine & metabolic: Amylase decreased, dehydration, erectile dysfunction, fluid retention, hyperuricemia, hypogonadism, hypokalemia, libido decreased, sexual dysfunction, testosterone decreased
Gastrointestinal: Abdominal distention, anal fissure, anorexia, appetite increased, bezoar (Exalgo™), biliary tract spasm, constipation, diarrhea, diverticulum, diverticulitis, duodenitis, dysgeusia, dysphagia, eructation, flatulence, gastric emptying impaired, gastrointestinal motility disorder (Exalgo™), gastroenteritis, hematochezia, ileus, intestinal obstruction (Exalgo™), large intestine perforation (Exalgo™), nausea, painful defecation, paralytic ileus, stomach cramps, taste perversion, vomiting, weight loss, xerostomia
Genitourinary: Dysuria, micturition disorder, ureteral spasm, urinary frequency, urinary hesitation, urinary retention, urinary tract spasm, urination decreased
Hepatic: LFTs increased
Local: Pain at injection site (I.M.), wheal/flare over vein (I.V.)

Neuromuscular & skeletal: Arthralgia, dysarthria, dyskinesia, muscle rigidity, muscle spasms, myalgia, myoclonus, paresthesia, trembling, tremor, uncoordinated muscle movements, weakness

Ocular: Blurred vision, diplopia, dry eyes, miosis, nystagmus

Otic: Tinnitus

Respiratory: Apnea, bronchospasm, dyspnea, hyperventilation, hypoxia, laryngospasm, oxygen saturation decreased, respiratory depression/distress, rhinorrhea

Miscellaneous: Antidiuretic effects, balance disorder, diaphoresis, difficulty walking, histamine release, physical and psychological dependence

General Dosage Range Dosage adjustment recommended in patients with hepatic or renal impairment

I.M., SubQ: *Children >50 kg and Adults:* 0.8-2 mg every 4-6 hours

I.V.:

Children ≥6 months and <50 kg: 0.015 mg/kg/dose every 3-6 hours as needed

Children >50 kg and Adults: 0.2-0.6 mg every 2-3 hours as needed

Adults (mechanically-ventilated): Infusion: 0.5-1 mg/hour (based on 70 kg patient) **or** 7-15 mcg/kg/hour

Epidural: *Children >50 kg and Adults:* Concentration: 0.05-0.075 mg/mL; Bolus: 1-1.5 mg; Infusion: 0.04-0.4 mg/hour; Demand dose: 0.15 mg; Lockout interval: 30 minutes

Oral:

Children ≥6 months and <50 kg: 0.03-0.08 mg/kg/dose every 3-4 hours as needed

Children >50 kg: 2-8 mg every 3-4 hours as needed

Adults: 2-8 mg every 3-4 hours as needed; Extended release: 8-64 mg every 24 hours

Elderly: 1-2 mg every 3-6 hours

PCA:

Children <50 kg: Usual concentration: 0.2 mg/mL; Demand dose: 0.003-0.005 mg/kg/dose; Lockout interval: 6-10 minutes; Usual basal rate: 0-0.004 mg/kg/hour

Children >50 kg and Adults: Usual concentration: 0.2 mg/mL; Demand dose: 0.05-0.4 mg; Lockout interval: 5-10 minutes

Rectal: *Children >50 kg and Adults:* 3 mg every 4-8 hours as needed

Mechanism of Action Binds to opiate receptors in the CNS, causing inhibition of ascending pain pathways, altering the perception of and response to pain; causes cough supression by direct central action in the medulla; produces generalized CNS depression

Pharmacodynamics/Kinetics

Onset of Action Analgesic: Immediate release formulations:

Oral: 15-30 minutes; Peak effect: 30-60 minutes

I.V.: 5 minutes; Peak effect: 10-20 minutes

Duration of Action Immediate release formulations: Oral, I.V.: 4-5 hours

Half-life Elimination

Immediate release formulations: 2-3 hours

Extended release tablets (Exalgo™): ~11 hours

Pregnancy Risk Factor C

Controlled Substance C-II

Prescribing and Access Restrictions Exalgo™: As a requirement of the REMS program, healthcare providers who prescribe Exalgo™ need to receive training on the proper use and potential risks of Exalgo™. For training, please refer to http://www.exalgorems.com. Prescribers will need retraining every 2 years or following any significant changes to the Exalgo™ REMS program.

Hydroquinone (HYE droe kwin one)

U.S. Brand Names Aclaro PD®; Aclaro®; Alphaquin HP®; Eldopaque Forte®; Eldopaque® [OTC]; Eldoquin Forte®; Eldoquin® [OTC]; EpiQuin® Micro; Esoterica® Daytime [OTC]; Esoterica® Nighttime [OTC]; Lustra-AF®; Lustra-Ultra™; Lustra®; Melanex® [DSC]; Melpaque HP®; Melquin HP®; Melquin-3®; NeoStrata® HQ Skin Lightening [OTC]; Nuquin HP®; Palmer's® Skin Success® Eventone® Fade Cream [OTC]; Palmer's® Skin Success® Eventone® Fade Milk [OTC]; Palmer's® Skin Success® Eventone® Ultra Fade Serum [OTC]

Canadian Brand Names Eldopaque®; Eldoquin®; Glyquin® XM; Lustra®; NeoStrata® HQ; Solaquin Forte®; Solaquin®; Ultraquin™

Pharmacologic Category Depigmenting Agent

Use Gradual bleaching of hyperpigmented skin conditions

Local Anesthetic/Vasoconstrictor Precautions No information available to require special precautions

Effects on Dental Treatment No significant effects or complications reported

Effects on Bleeding No information available to require special precautions

Adverse Effects Frequency not defined.

Dermatologic: Dermatitis, dryness, erythema, stinging, inflammatory reaction, sensitization

Local: Irritation

General Dosage Range Topical: *Children >12 years and Adults:* Apply thin layer and rub in twice daily

Mechanism of Action Produces reversible depigmentation of the skin by suppression of melanocyte metabolic processes, in particular the inhibition of the enzymatic oxidation of tyrosine to DOPA (3,4-dihydroxyphenylalanine); sun exposure reverses this effect and will cause repigmentation.

Pharmacodynamics/Kinetics

Onset of Action Onset of depigmentation produced by hydroquinone varies among individuals

Duration of Action Onset and duration of depigmentation produced by hydroquinone varies among individuals

Pregnancy Risk Factor C

Hydroxocobalamin (hye droks oh koe BAL a min)

U.S. Brand Names Cyanokit®

Canadian Brand Names Cyanokit®

Pharmacologic Category Antidote; Vitamin, Water Soluble

Use Treatment of pernicious anemia, vitamin B_{12} deficiency due to dietary deficiencies or malabsorption diseases, inadequate secretion of intrinsic factor, and inadequate utilization of B_{12} (eg, during neoplastic treatment); diagnostic agent for Schilling test

Cyanokit®: Treatment of cyanide poisoning (known or suspected)

Unlabeled/Investigational Use Neuropathies

Local Anesthetic/Vasoconstrictor Precautions No information available to require special precautions

Effects on Dental Treatment No significant effects or complications reported

Effects on Bleeding No information available to require special precautions

Adverse Effects

I.M. injection: Frequency not defined:

Dermatologic: Exanthema (transient), itching

Gastrointestinal: Diarrhea (mild, transient)

Local: Injection site pain

Miscellaneous: Anaphylaxis

I.V. infusion (Cyanokit®):

>10%:

Cardiovascular: Blood pressure increased (18% to 28%; systolic ≥180 mm Hg or diastolic ≥110 mm Hg)

Central nervous system: Headache (6% to 33%)

Dermatologic: Erythema (94% to 100%; may last up to 2 weeks), rash (predominantly acneiform; 20% to 44%; can appear 7-28 days after administration and usually resolves within a few weeks)

Gastrointestinal: Nausea (6% to 11%)

Genitourinary: Chromaturia (100%; may last up to 5 weeks after administration)

Hematologic: Lymphocytes decreased (8% to 17%)

Local: Infusion site reaction (6% to 39%)

Frequency not defined:

Cardiovascular: Chest discomfort, hot flashes, peripheral edema

Central nervous system: Dizziness, memory impairment, restlessness

Dermatologic: Pruritus, urticaria

Gastrointestinal: Abdominal discomfort, diarrhea, dyspepsia, dysphagia, hematochezia, vomiting

Ocular: Irritation, redness, swelling

Respiratory: Dry throat, dyspnea, throat tightness

Miscellaneous: Allergic reaction (including anaphylaxis)

General Dosage Range

I.M.:

Children: 1-5 mg given in single daily doses of 100 mcg over 2 or more weeks, followed by 30-50 mcg/month

Adults: 30 mcg/day for 5-10 days, followed by 100-200 mcg/month

I.V.: *Adults:* 5 g as single infusion; may repeat if needed (maximum: 10 g cumulative dose)

Mechanism of Action Hydroxocobalamin (vitamin B_{12a}) is a precursor to cyanocobalamin (vitamin B_{12}). Cyanocobalamin acts as a coenzyme for various metabolic functions, including fat and carbohydrate metabolism and protein synthesis, used in cell replication and hematopoiesis. In the presence of cyanide, each hydroxocobalamin molecule can bind one cyanide ion by displacing it for the hydroxo ligand linked to the trivalent cobalt ion, forming cyanocobalamin.

Pharmacodynamics/Kinetics

Half-life Elimination 26-31 hours

Pregnancy Risk Factor C

Hydroxyamphetamine and Tropicamide

(hye droks ee am FET a meen & troe PIK a mide)

Related Information

Tropicamide *on page 1685*

U.S. Brand Names Paremyd®

Pharmacologic Category Adrenergic Agonist Agent, Ophthalmic

Use Short-term pupil dilation for diagnostic procedures and exams

Local Anesthetic/Vasoconstrictor Precautions No information available to require special precautions

Effects on Dental Treatment No significant effects or complications reported

Effects on Bleeding No information available to require special precautions

Adverse Effects Frequency not defined (as reported with Paremyd® or similar medications):

Cardiovascular: Hypotension, MI, pallor, tachycardia, ventricular fibrillation
Central nervous system: Behavioral disturbances, headache, psychotic reactions
Gastrointestinal: Dry mouth, nausea, vomiting
Neuromuscular & skeletal: Muscle rigidity
Ocular: Blurred vision, intraocular pressure increased, photophobia, transient stinging
Miscellaneous: Allergic reaction, cardiorespiratory collapse, vasomotor collapse

General Dosage Range Ophthalmic: *Adults:* Instill 1-2 drops into conjunctival sac(s)

Mechanism of Action Hydroxyamphetamine hydrobromide is an indirect acting sympathomimetic agent which causes the release of norepinephrine from adrenergic nerve terminals, resulting in mydriasis. Tropicamide is a parasympatholytic agent which produces mydriasis and paralysis by blocking the sphincter muscle in the iris and the ciliary muscle.

Pharmacodynamics/Kinetics

Onset of Action 15 minutes

Duration of Action 3 hours; complete recovery usually occurs in 6-8 hours, but may take up to 24 hours

Time to Peak 60 minutes

Pregnancy Risk Factor C

Hydroxychloroquine (hye droks ee KLOR oh kwin)

Related Information

Rheumatoid Arthritis, Osteoarthritis, and Osteoporosis *on page 1889*

U.S. Brand Names Plaquenil®

Canadian Brand Names Apo-Hydroxyquine®; Gen-Hydroxychloroquine; Mylan-Hydroxychloroquine; Plaquenil®; PRO-Hydroxyquine

Pharmacologic Category Aminoquinoline (Antimalarial)

Use Suppression and treatment of acute attacks of malaria; treatment of systemic lupus erythematosus (SLE) and rheumatoid arthritis

Unlabeled/Investigational Use Porphyria cutanea tarda, polymorphous light eruptions

Local Anesthetic/Vasoconstrictor Precautions No information available to require special precautions

Effects on Dental Treatment No significant effects or complications reported

Effects on Bleeding Rare hematologic toxicity may result in thrombocytopenia. No information available to require routine special precautions.

Adverse Effects Frequency not defined.

Cardiovascular: Cardiomyopathy (rare, relationship to hydroxychloroquine unclear)
Central nervous system: Ataxia, dizziness, emotional changes, headache, irritability, lassitude, nervousness, nightmares, psychosis, seizure, vertigo
Dermatologic: Alopecia, angioedema, bleaching of hair, pigmentation changes (skin and mucosal; black-blue color), rash (acute generalized exanthematous pustulosis, erythema annulare centrifugum, exfoliative dermatitis, lichenoid, maculopapular, morbilliform, purpuric, Stevens-Johnson syndrome, urticarial), urticaria
Gastrointestinal: Abdominal cramping, anorexia, diarrhea, nausea, vomiting, weight loss

Hematologic: Agranulocytosis, aplastic anemia, hemolysis (in patients with glucose-6-phosphate deficiency), leukopenia, thrombocytopenia
Hepatic: Abnormal liver function/hepatic failure (isolated cases)
Neuromuscular & skeletal: Myopathy, palsy, or neuromyopathy leading to progressive weakness and atrophy of proximal muscle groups (may be associated with mild sensory changes, loss of deep tendon reflexes, and abnormal nerve conduction)
Ocular: Abnormal color vision, abnormal retinal pigmentation, atrophy, attenuation of retinal arterioles, corneal changes/deposits (visual disturbances, blurred vision, photophobia [reversible on discontinuation]), decreased visual acuity, disturbance in accommodation, keratopathy, macular edema, nystagmus, optic disc pallor/atrophy, pigmentary retinopathy, retinopathy (early changes reversible [may progress despite discontinuation if advanced]), scotoma
Otic: Deafness, tinnitus
Miscellaneous: Exacerbation of porphyria and nonlight sensitive psoriasis
Respiratory: Bronchospasm, respiratory failure (myopathy-related)

General Dosage Range Oral:
Children: 13 mg/kg for 1-2 doses, followed by 6.5 mg/kg for 3 doses or once weekly
Adults: Initial: 400-800 mg/day divided 1-2 times/day; Maintenance: 200-400 mg/day **or** 800 mg for 1-2 doses, followed by 400 mg for 3 doses or once weekly

Mechanism of Action Interferes with digestive vacuole function within sensitive malarial parasites by increasing the pH and interfering with lysosomal degradation of hemoglobin; inhibits locomotion of neutrophils and chemotaxis of eosinophils; impairs complement-dependent antigen-antibody reactions

Pharmacodynamics/Kinetics
Onset of Action Rheumatic disease: May require 4-6 weeks to respond
Half-life Elimination 32-50 days
Time to Peak Rheumatic disease: Several months

Hydroxyprogesterone Caproate (hye droks ee proe JES te rone CAP ro ate)

U.S. Brand Names Makena™
Pharmacologic Category Progestin
Use To reduce the risk of preterm birth in women with singleton pregnancies who have a history of spontaneous preterm birth (delivery <37 weeks gestation) with previous singleton pregnancies
Local Anesthetic/Vasoconstrictor Precautions No information available to require special precautions
Effects on Dental Treatment No significant effects or complications reported
Effects on Bleeding No information available to require special precautions
Adverse Effects
>10%:
Dermatologic: Urticaria (12%)
Local: Injection site: Pain (35%), swelling (17%)
1% to 10%:
Dermatologic: Pruritus (8%)
Gastrointestinal: Nausea (6%), diarrhea (2%)
Local: Injection site pruritus (6%), nodule (5%)
General Dosage Range I.M.: *Pregnant females:* 250 mg every 7 days
Pharmacodynamics/Kinetics
Half-life Elimination ~8 days
Time to Peak Serum: I.M.: 3-7 days
Pregnancy Risk Factor B
Prescribing and Access Restrictions The Makena Care Connection™ is a comprehensive program for patients and healthcare providers which provides administrative support (including insurance benefit investigation and prescription fulfillment); financial and co-pay assistance for eligible patients; and treatment support (including educational information, home health care service and scheduled treatment reminders). The Makena Care Connection™ is available by calling 1-800-847-3418, Monday-Friday, 8 AM to 9 PM EST.

Hydroxypropyl Cellulose (hye droks ee PROE pil SEL yoo lose)

Related Information
Hydroxypropyl Methylcellulose *on page 876*
U.S. Brand Names Lacrisert®
Canadian Brand Names Lacrisert®
Pharmacologic Category Ophthalmic Agent, Miscellaneous

Use Dry eyes (moderate-to-severe)

Local Anesthetic/Vasoconstrictor Precautions No information available to require special precautions

Effects on Dental Treatment No significant effects or complications reported

Effects on Bleeding No information available to require special precautions

Adverse Effects Frequency not defined: Ocular: Local irritation, blurred vision, edema of the eyelids

General Dosage Range Ophthalmic: *Adults:* Apply once daily

Hydroxypropyl Methylcellulose (hye droks ee PROE pil meth il SEL yoo lose)

Related Information

Hydroxypropyl Cellulose *on page 875*

U.S. Brand Names Cellugel®; GenTeal® Mild [OTC]; GenTeal® [OTC]; Gonak™; Goniosoft™ [OTC]; Isopto® Tears [OTC]; Natural Balance Tears [OTC]; Nature's Tears [OTC]; Tears Again® MC Gel Drops™ [OTC]

Canadian Brand Names Genteal®; Isopto® Tears

Pharmacologic Category Diagnostic Agent, Ophthalmic; Lubricant, Ocular

Use Relief of burning and minor irritation due to dry eyes; diagnostic agent in gonioscopic examination

Local Anesthetic/Vasoconstrictor Precautions No information available to require special precautions

Effects on Dental Treatment No significant effects or complications reported

Effects on Bleeding No information available to require special precautions

General Dosage Range Ophthalmic: *Adults:* Instill 1-2 drops in affected eye(s) as needed

Pregnancy Risk Factor C

Hydroxyurea (hye droks ee yoor EE a)

U.S. Brand Names Droxia®; Hydrea®

Canadian Brand Names Apo-Hydroxyurea®; Gen-Hydroxyurea; Hydrea®; Mylan-Hydroxyurea

Pharmacologic Category Antineoplastic Agent, Antimetabolite

Use Treatment of melanoma, refractory chronic myelocytic leukemia (CML); recurrent, metastatic, or inoperable ovarian cancer; radiosensitizing agent in the treatment of squamous cell head and neck cancer (excluding lip cancer); adjunct in the management of sickle cell patients who have had at least three painful crises in the previous 12 months (to reduce frequency of these crises and the need for blood transfusions)

Unlabeled/Investigational Use Treatment of essential thrombocythemia, polycythemia vera, hypereosinophilic syndrome; management of hyperleukocytosis due to acute myeloid leukemia; treatment of cervical cancer, treatment of meningiomas

Local Anesthetic/Vasoconstrictor Precautions No information available to require special precautions

Effects on Dental Treatment No significant effects or complications reported

Effects on Bleeding Chemotherapy may result in significant myelosuppression, potentially including significant reduction in platelet counts and altered hemostasis. In patients who are under active treatment with these agents, medical consult is suggested.

Adverse Effects Frequency not defined.

Cardiovascular: Edema

Central nervous system: Chills, disorientation, dizziness, drowsiness (dose-related), fever, hallucinations, headache, malaise, seizure

Dermatologic: Alopecia, cutaneous vasculitic toxicities, dermatomyositis-like skin changes, facial erythema, gangrene, hyperpigmentation, maculopapular rash, nail atrophy, nail discoloration, peripheral erythema, scaling, skin atrophy, skin cancer, skin ulcer, vasculitis ulcerations, violet papules

Endocrine & metabolic: Hyperuricemia

Gastrointestinal: Anorexia, constipation, diarrhea, gastrointestinal irritation and mucositis, (potentiated with radiation therapy), nausea, pancreatitis, stomatitis, vomiting

Genitourinary: Dysuria

Hematologic: Myelosuppression (anemia, leukopenia [common; reversal of WBC count occurs rapidly], thrombocytopenia); macrocytosis, megaloblastic erythropoiesis, secondary leukemias (long-term use)

Hepatic: Hepatic enzymes increased, hepatotoxicity

Neuromuscular & skeletal: Peripheral neuropathy, weakness

Renal: BUN increased, creatinine increased

Respiratory: Acute diffuse pulmonary infiltrates (rare), dyspnea, pulmonary fibrosis (rare)

General Dosage Range Dosage adjustment recommended in patients with renal impairment

Oral: *Adults:* 15-35 mg/kg/day **or** 500-3000 mg/day as single or divided dose **or** 80 mg/kg as a single dose every third day

Mechanism of Action Antimetabolite which selectively inhibits ribonucleoside diphosphate reductase, preventing the conversion of ribonucleotides to deoxyribonucleotides, halting the cell cycle at the G1/S phase and therefore has radiation sensitizing activity by maintaining cells in the G_1 phase and interfering with DNA repair. In sickle cell anemia, hydroxyurea increases red blood cell (RBC) hemoglobin F levels, RBC water content, deformability of sickled cells, and alters adhesion of RBCs to endothelium.

Pharmacodynamics/Kinetics

Onset of Action Sickle cell anemia: Fetal hemoglobin increase: 4-12 weeks

Half-life Elimination 3-4 hours

Time to Peak 1-4 hours

Pregnancy Risk Factor D

HydrOXYzine (hye DROKS i zeen)

Related Information

Management of the Patient With Anxiety or Depression *on page 1968*

Related Sample Prescriptions

Sedation (Prior to Dental Treatment) *on page 1995*

U.S. Brand Names Vistaril®

Canadian Brand Names Apo-Hydroxyzine®; Atarax®; Hydroxyzine Hydrochloride Injection, USP; Novo-Hydroxyzin; PMS-Hydroxyzine; Vistaril®

Generic Availability (U.S.) Yes

Pharmacologic Category Antiemetic; Histamine H_1 Antagonist; Histamine H_1 Antagonist, First Generation; Piperazine Derivative

Dental Use Treatment of anxiety, as a preoperative sedative in pediatric dentistry

Use Treatment of anxiety; preoperative sedative; antipruritic

Unlabeled/Investigational Use Antiemetic; ethanol withdrawal symptoms

Local Anesthetic/Vasoconstrictor Precautions No information available to require special precautions

Effects on Dental Treatment Key adverse event(s) related to dental treatment: Xerostomia (normal salivary flow resumes upon discontinuation).

Effects on Bleeding No information available to require special precautions

Adverse Effects Frequency not defined.

Central nervous system: Dizziness, drowsiness, fatigue, hallucination, headache, nervousness, seizure

Dermatologic: Pruritus, rash, urticaria

Gastrointestinal: Xerostomia

Neuromuscular & skeletal: Involuntary movements, paresthesia, tremor

Ocular: Blurred vision

Respiratory: Thickening of bronchial secretions

Miscellaneous: Allergic reaction

Dental Usual Dosage

Anxiety: Adults: Oral: 50-100 mg 4 times/day

Preoperative sedation:

- Children:
  - Oral: 0.6 mg/kg/dose
  - I.M.: 0.5-1 mg/kg/dose
- Adults:
  - Oral: 50-100 mg
  - I.M.: 25-100 mg

Dosage

- Children:
  - Preoperative sedation:
    - Oral: 0.6 mg/kg/dose
    - I.M.: 0.5-1 mg/kg/dose
  - Pruritus, anxiety: Oral:
    - <6 years: 50 mg daily in divided doses
    - ≥6 years: 50-100 mg daily in divided doses
- Adults:
  - Antiemetic (unlabeled use): I.M.: 25-100 mg/dose every 4-6 hours as needed
  - Anxiety: Oral, I.M.: 50-100 mg 4 times/day

Preoperative sedation:
Oral: 50-100 mg
I.M.: 25-100 mg
Pruritus: Oral, I.M.: 25 mg 3-4 times/day

Dosing interval in hepatic impairment: Change dosing interval to every 24 hours in patients with primary biliary cirrhosis

Mechanism of Action Competes with histamine for H_1-receptor sites on effector cells in the gastrointestinal tract, blood vessels, and respiratory tract. Possesses skeletal muscle relaxing, bronchodilator, antihistamine, antiemetic, and analgesic properties.

Contraindications Hypersensitivity to hydroxyzine or any component of the formulation; early pregnancy; SubQ, intra-arterial, or I.V. administration of injection

Warnings/Precautions Causes sedation, caution must be used in performing tasks which require alertness (eg, operating machinery or driving). Sedative effects of CNS depressants or ethanol are potentiated. SubQ, I.V., and intra-arterial administration are contraindicated since tissue damage, intravascular hemolysis, thrombosis, and digital gangrene can occur. Use with caution with narrow-angle glaucoma, prostatic hyperplasia, bladder neck obstruction, asthma, or COPD. May be inappropriate for use in the elderly due to potent anticholinergic effects; non-anticholinergic antihistamines preferred for treating allergic reactions (Beers Criteria).

Drug Interactions

Metabolism/Transport Effects Inhibits CYP2D6 (weak)

Avoid Concomitant Use There are no known interactions where it is recommended to avoid concomitant use.

Increased Effect/Toxicity

HydrOXYzine may increase the levels/effects of: Alcohol (Ethyl); Anticholinergics; CNS Depressants

The levels/effects of HydrOXYzine may be increased by: Droperidol; Pramlintide

Decreased Effect

HydrOXYzine may decrease the levels/effects of: Acetylcholinesterase Inhibitors (Central); Benzylpenicilloyl Polylysine; Betahistine

The levels/effects of HydrOXYzine may be decreased by: Acetylcholinesterase Inhibitors (Central); Amphetamines

Ethanol/Nutrition/Herb Interactions

Ethanol: May increase CNS depression; monitor for increased effects with coadministration. Caution patients about effects.

Herb/Nutraceutical: Avoid valerian, St John's wort, kava kava, gotu kola (may increase CNS depression).

Pharmacodynamics/Kinetics

Onset of Action Oral: 15-30 minutes

Duration of Action 4-6 hours

Half-life Elimination 3-7 hours

Time to Peak ~2 hours

Pregnancy Risk Factor C

Lactation Excretion in breast milk unknown/not recommended

Dosage Forms

Capsule, oral: 25 mg, 50 mg, 100 mg
Vistaril®: 25 mg, 50 mg
Injection, solution: 25 mg/mL (1 mL); 50 mg/mL (1 mL, 2 mL, 10 mL)
Solution, oral: 10 mg/5 mL (473 mL)
Syrup, oral: 10 mg/5 mL (118 mL, 473 mL, 480 mL)
Tablet, oral: 10 mg, 25 mg, 50 mg

Hyoscyamine (hye oh SYE a meen)

U.S. Brand Names Anaspaz®; HyoMax® -SR; HyoMax™-DT; HyoMax™-FT; Hyosyne; Levbid®; Levsin®; Levsin®/SL; Symax® DuoTab; Symax® FasTab; Symax® SL; Symax® SR

Canadian Brand Names Levsin®

Pharmacologic Category Anticholinergic Agent

Use

Oral: Adjunctive therapy for peptic ulcers, irritable bowel, neurogenic bladder/bowel; treatment of infant colic, GI tract disorders caused by spasm; to reduce rigidity, tremors, sialorrhea, and hyperhidrosis associated with parkinsonism; as a drying agent in acute rhinitis

Injection: Preoperative antimuscarinic to reduce secretions and block cardiac vagal inhibitory reflexes; to improve radiologic visibility of the kidneys; symptomatic relief of biliary and renal colic; reduce GI motility to facilitate diagnostic procedures (ie, endoscopy, hypotonic duodenography); reduce pain and hypersecretion in pancreatitis, certain cases of partial heart block associated with vagal activity; reversal of neuromuscular blockade

Local Anesthetic/Vasoconstrictor Precautions No information available to require special precautions

Effects on Dental Treatment Key adverse event(s) related to dental treatment: Xerostomia (normal salivary flow resumes upon discontinuation).

Effects on Bleeding No information available to require special precautions

Adverse Effects Frequency not defined.

Cardiovascular: Palpitation, tachycardia

Central nervous system: Ataxia, dizziness, drowsiness, headache, insomnia, mental confusion/excitement, nervousness, speech disorder

Dermatologic: Urticaria

Endocrine & metabolic: Lactation suppression

Gastrointestinal: Bloating, constipation, dry mouth, loss of taste, nausea, vomiting

Genitourinary: Impotence, urinary hesitancy, urinary retention

Neuromuscular & skeletal: Weakness

Ocular: Blurred vision, cycloplegia, increased ocular tension, mydriasis

Miscellaneous: Allergic reactions, sweating decreased

General Dosage Range

I.M., SubQ: *Adults:* 0.25-0.5 mg 4 times/day as needed

I.V.:

Children ≥2 years: 5 mcg/kg given 30-60 minutes prior to induction of anesthesia

Adults: 0.125-0.5 mg 4 times/day as needed **or** 0.25-0.5 mg or 5 mcg/kg as a single dose **or** 0.2 mg for every 1 mg neostigmine

Oral:

Regular release:

Children <2 years and 3.4 kg: 4 drops every 4 hours as needed (maximum: 24 drops/day)

Children <2 years and 5 kg: 5 drops every 4 hours as needed (maximum: 30 drops/day)

Children <2 years and 7 kg: 6 drops every 4 hours as needed (maximum: 36 drops/day)

Children <2 years and 10 kg: 8 drops every 4 hours as needed (maximum: 48 drops/day)

Children ≥2 years and 10 kg: 0.031-0.033 mg every 4 hours as needed (maximum: 0.75 mg/day)

Children ≥2 years and 20 kg: 0.0625 mg every 4 hours as needed (maximum: 0.75 mg/day)

Children ≥2 years and 40 kg: 0.0938 mg every 4 hours as needed (maximum: 0.75 mg/day)

Children ≥2 years and 50 kg: 0.125 mg every 4 hours as needed (maximum: 0.75 mg/day)

Adults: 0.125-0.25 mg every 4 hours or as needed (maximum: 1.5 mg/day)

Timed release: *Adults:* 0.375-0.75 mg every 12 hours (maximum: 1.5 mg/day)

S.L.:

Children ≥2 years and 10 kg: 0.031-0.033 mg every 4 hours as needed (maximum: 0.75 mg/day)

Children ≥2 years and 20 kg: 0.0625 mg every 4 hours as needed (maximum: 0.75 mg/day)

Children ≥2 years and 40 kg: 0.0938 mg every 4 hours as needed (maximum: 0.75 mg/day)

Children ≥2 years and 50 kg: 0.125 mg every 4 hours as needed (maximum: 0.75 mg/day)

Adults: 0.125-0.25 mg every 4 hours or as needed (maximum: 1.5 mg/day)

Mechanism of Action Blocks the action of acetylcholine at parasympathetic sites in smooth muscle, secretory glands and the CNS; increases cardiac output, dries secretions, antagonizes histamine and serotonin

Pharmacodynamics/Kinetics

Onset of Action 2-3 minutes

Duration of Action 4-6 hours

Half-life Elimination 3-5 hours

Pregnancy Risk Factor C

Hyoscyamine, Atropine, Scopolamine, and Phenobarbital

(hye oh SYE a meen, A troe peen, skoe POL a meen, & fee noe BAR bi tal)

Related Information

Atropine *on page* 188
Hyoscyamine *on page* 878
PHENobarbital *on page* 1333
Scopolamine (Systemic) *on page* 1513

U.S. Brand Names Donnatal Extentabs®; Donnatal®; Hyonatol

Pharmacologic Category Anticholinergic Agent; Antispasmodic Agent, Gastrointestinal

Use Adjunct in treatment of irritable bowel syndrome, acute enterocolitis, duodenal ulcer

Local Anesthetic/Vasoconstrictor Precautions No information available to require special precautions

Effects on Dental Treatment Key adverse event(s) related to dental treatment: Xerostomia (normal salivary flow resumes upon discontinuation).

Effects on Bleeding No information available to require special precautions

Adverse Effects Frequency not defined.

Cardiovascular: Palpitation, tachycardia
Central nervous system: Dizziness, drowsiness, headache, insomnia, nervousness
Dermatologic: Urticaria
Gastrointestinal: Bloating, constipation, nausea, taste loss, vomiting, xerostomia
Genitourinary: Impotence, urinary hesitancy, urinary retention
Neuromuscular & skeletal: Musculoskeletal pain, weakness
Ocular: Blurred vision, cycloplegia, mydriasis, ocular tension increased
Miscellaneous: Allergic reaction (may be severe), anaphylaxis, lactation suppressed, diaphoresis decreased

General Dosage Range Oral:

Extended release: *Adults:* 1 tablet every 8-12 hours
Regular release:
Children 4.5 kg: 0.5 mL every 4 hours **or** 0.75 mL every 6 hours
Children 10 kg: 1 mL every 4 hours **or** 1.5 mL every 6 hours
Children 14 kg: 1.5 mL every 4 hours **or** 2 mL every 6 hours
Children 23 kg: 2.5 mL every 4 hours **or** 3.8 mL every 6 hours
Children 34 kg: 3.8 mL every 4 hours **or** 5 mL every 6 hours
Children ≥45 kg: 5 mL every 4 hours **or** 7.5 mL every 6 hours
Adults: 1-2 tablets **or** 5-10 mL of elixir 3-4 times/day

Mechanism of Action A fixed combination of belladonna alkaloids and phenobarbital which provides anticholinergic/antispasmodic action and mild sedation.

Pregnancy Risk Factor C

Ibandronate (eye BAN droh nate)

Related Information

Osteonecrosis of the Jaw *on page* 1894
Rheumatoid Arthritis, Osteoarthritis, and Osteoporosis *on page* 1889

U.S. Brand Names Boniva®

Generic Availability (U.S.) No

Pharmacologic Category Bisphosphonate Derivative

Use Treatment and prevention of osteoporosis in postmenopausal females

Unlabeled/Investigational Use Hypercalcemia of malignancy; corticosteroid-induced osteoporosis; Paget's disease; reduce bone pain and skeletal complications from metastatic bone disease

Local Anesthetic/Vasoconstrictor Precautions No information available to require special precautions

Effects on Dental Treatment Key adverse event(s) related to dental treatment: Tooth disorder.

Osteonecrosis of the jaw (ONJ), generally associated with local infection and/or tooth extraction and often with delayed healing, has been reported in patients taking bisphosphonates. Symptoms included nonhealing extraction socket or an exposed jawbone. Most reported cases of bisphosphonate-associated osteonecrosis have been in cancer patients treated with intravenous bisphosphonates. However, some have occurred in patients with postmenopausal osteoporosis taking oral bisphosphonates. Dental surgery, particularly tooth extraction, may increase the risk for ONJ. Patients who develop ONJ while on bisphosphonate therapy should receive care by an oral surgeon. See Dental Comment.

Effects on Bleeding No information available to require special precautions

Adverse Effects Percentages vary based on frequency of administration (daily vs monthly). Unless specified, percentages are reported with oral use.

>10%:
- Gastrointestinal: Dyspepsia (6% to 12%)
- Neuromuscular & skeletal: Back pain (4% to 14%)

1% to 10%:
- Cardiovascular: Hypertension (6% to 7%)
- Central nervous system: Headache (3% to 7%), dizziness (1% to 4%), insomnia (1% to 2%)
- Dermatologic: Rash (1% to 2%)
- Endocrine & metabolic: Hypercholesterolemia (5%)
- Gastrointestinal: Abdominal pain (5% to 8%), diarrhea (4% to 7%), nausea (5%), tooth disorder (4%), constipation (3% to 4%), vomiting (3%)
- Genitourinary: Urinary tract infection (2% to 6%)
- Hepatic: Alkaline phosphatase decreased (frequency not defined)
- Local: Injection site reaction (<2%)
- Neuromuscular & skeletal: Pain in extremity (1% to 8%), arthralgia (4% to 6%), myalgia (1% to 6%), joint disorder (4%), weakness (4%), osteoarthritis (localized; 1% to 3%), muscle cramp (2%)
- Respiratory: Bronchitis (3% to 10%), pneumonia (6%), pharyngitis/nasopharyngitis (3% to 4%), upper respiratory infection (2%)
- Miscellaneous: Acute phase reaction (I.V. 10%; oral 3% to 9%), infection (4%), flu-like syndrome (1% to 4%), allergic reaction (3%)

Dosage

Oral:
- Treatment of postmenopausal osteoporosis: 2.5 mg once daily **or** 150 mg once a month; **Note:** Patients should receive supplemental calcium and vitamin D if dietary intake is inadequate
- Prevention of postmenopausal osteoporosis: 2.5 once daily **or** 150 mg once a month; **Note:** Patients should receive supplemental calcium and vitamin D if dietary intake is inadequate
- Metastatic bone disease (unlabeled use): 50 mg once daily

I.V.:
- Treatment of postmenopausal osteoporosis: 3 mg every 3 months; **Note:** Patients should receive supplemental calcium and vitamin D if dietary intake is inadequate
- Hypercalcemia of malignancy (unlabeled use): 2-4 mg over 2 hours
- Metastatic bone disease (unlabeled use): 6 mg over 1 hour every 3-4 weeks

Dosage adjustment in renal impairment:
- Mild or moderate impairment: Dosing adjustment not needed
- Severe impairment (Cl_{cr} <30 mL/minute): Use not recommended
- Dose adjustment in renal impairment for oncologic uses (unlabeled): Severe impairment (Cl_{cr} <30 mL/minute):
  - Oral: 50 mg once weekly
  - I.V.: 2 mg over 1 hour every 3-4 weeks

Dosage adjustment in hepatic impairment: Dosing adjustment not needed

Mechanism of Action A bisphosphonate which inhibits bone resorption via actions on osteoclasts or on osteoclast precursors; decreases the rate of bone resorption, leading to an indirect increase in bone mineral density.

Contraindications Hypersensitivity to ibandronate or any component of the formulation; hypocalcemia; oral tablets are also contraindicated in patients unable to stand or sit upright for at least 60 minutes and in patients with abnormalities of the esophagus which delay esophageal emptying, such as stricture or achalasia

Warnings/Precautions Hypocalcemia must be corrected before therapy initiation. Ensure adequate calcium and vitamin D intake. Osteonecrosis of the jaw (ONJ) has been reported in patients receiving bisphosphonates. Risk factors include invasive dental procedures (eg, tooth extraction, dental implants, boney surgery); a diagnosis of cancer, with concomitant chemotherapy or corticosteroids; poor oral hygiene, ill-fitting dentures; and comorbid disorders (anemia, coagulopathy, infection, pre-existing dental disease). Most reported cases occurred after I.V. bisphosphonate therapy; however, cases have been reported following oral therapy. A dental exam and preventative dentistry should be performed prior to placing patients with risk factors on chronic bisphosphonate therapy. The manufacturer's labeling states that discontinuing bisphosphonates in patients requiring invasive dental procedures may reduce the risk of ONJ. However, other experts suggest that there is no evidence that discontinuing therapy reduces the risk of developing ONJ (Assael, 2009). The benefit/risk must be assessed by the treating physician and/or dentist/surgeon prior to any invasive dental procedure. Patients developing ONJ while on bisphosphonates should receive care by an oral surgeon.

Atypical femur fractures have been reported in patients receiving bisphosphonates for treatment/prevention of osteoporosis. The fractures include subtrochanteric femur (bone just below the hip joint) and diaphyseal femur (long segment of the thigh bone). Some patients experience prodromal pain weeks or months before the fracture occurs. It is unclear if bisphosphonate therapy is the cause for these fractures, although the majority have been reported in patients taking bisphosphonates. Patients receiving long-term (>3-5 years) therapy may be at an increased risk. Discontinue bisphosphonate therapy in patients who develop a femoral shaft fracture.

Infrequently, severe (and occasionally debilitating) bone, joint, and/or muscle pain have been reported during bisphosphonate treatment. The onset of pain ranged from a single day to several months. Consider discontinuing therapy in patients who experience severe symptoms; symptoms usually resolve upon discontinuation. Some patients experienced recurrence when rechallenged with same drug or another bisphosphonate; avoid use in patients with a history of these symptoms in association with bisphosphonate therapy.

Oral bisphosphonates may cause dysphagia, esophagitis, esophageal or gastric ulcer; risk may increase in patients unable to comply with dosing instructions; discontinue use if new or worsening symptoms develop. Intravenous bisphosphonates may cause transient decreases in serum calcium and have also been associated with renal toxicity.

Use not recommended with severe renal impairment (Cl_{cr} <30 mL/minute).

Drug Interactions

Avoid Concomitant Use There are no known interactions where it is recommended to avoid concomitant use.

Increased Effect/Toxicity

Ibandronate may increase the levels/effects of: Deferasirox; Phosphate Supplements

The levels/effects of Ibandronate may be increased by: Aminoglycosides; Nonsteroidal Anti-Inflammatory Agents

Decreased Effect

The levels/effects of Ibandronate may be decreased by: Antacids; Calcium Salts; Iron Salts; Magnesium Salts; Proton Pump Inhibitors

Ethanol/Nutrition/Herb Interactions

Ethanol: Avoid ethanol (may increase risk of osteoporosis).

Food: May reduce absorption; mean oral bioavailability is decreased up to 90% when given with food.

Dietary Considerations Ensure adequate calcium and vitamin D intake; women and men >50 years of age should consume 1200-1500 mg/day of elemental calcium and 800-1000 int. units/day of vitamin D. Ibandronate tablet should be taken with a full glass (6-8 oz) of plain water, at least 60 minutes prior to any food, beverages, or medications. Mineral water with a high calcium content should be avoided.

Pharmacodynamics/Kinetics

Half-life Elimination

Oral: 150 mg dose: Terminal: 37-157 hours

I.V.: Terminal: ~5-25 hours

Time to Peak Oral: 0.5-2 hours

Pregnancy Risk Factor C

Lactation Excretion in breast milk unknown/use caution

Dosage Forms

Injection, solution:

Boniva®: 1 mg/mL (3 mL)

Tablet, oral:

Boniva®: 150 mg

Dental Comment According to the 2008 report by the American Dental Association (ADA), the incidence of osteonecrosis of the jawbone associated with oral bisphosphonate therapy remains low. It was also stated that the benefits of using oral bisphosphonates to prevent osteoporosis significantly outweighs the small risk of developing bisphosphonate-associated osteonecrosis (Edwards, 2008). The full 26 page report can be accessed at http://www.ada.org/sections/professionalResources/pdfs/topics_osteonecrosis_bisphosphonate_report.pdf.

The ADA review stated the incidence of oral bisphosphonate-associated osteonecrosis of the jaw was one case for every 140,000 person-years exposure to oral bisphosphonates (ADA, 2006). This figure was based on information received from Merck & Co citing 170 worldwide cases for alendronate (Fosamax®). In addition, Procter & Gamble Pharmaceuticals has cited 20 cases for risedronate (Actonel®) and Roche Laboratories, Inc has cited one case for ibandronate (Boniva®).

In addition, the ADA 2008 report reiterates that the risk of osteonecrosis of the jawbone with oral bisphosphonates is minute compared to the risks with intravenous bisphosphonates therapy in cancer patients. The ADA cites an ~20% incidence in patients receiving bisphosphonates intravenously for cancer therapy. Fewer than 10% of all cases of bisphosphonate-associated osteonecrosis of the jaw occurs in patients taking the oral drugs.

Information on alendronate (Fosamax®) use in Australia and the incidence of ONJ has been reported (Mavrokokki, 2007). A survey form was sent to all of the Australian members of the Australian and New Zealand Association of Oral and Maxillofacial Surgeons requesting cases that they had identified as ONJ in 2004 and 2005. The definition of ONJ for the survey was an area of exposed bone in the jawbone that failed to heal within 6 weeks in patients taking bisphosphonates for bone disease. The frequency of ONJ in osteoporotic patients, mainly taking weekly oral alendronate, was 1 in 8470 to 1 in 2260 (0.01% to 0.04%) patients. If extractions were carried out, the calculated frequency was 1 in 1130 to 1 in 296 (0.09% to 0.34%) patients. The minimum values in these cases were determined from the survey, whereas, the maximum values were extrapolated from survey data. The median time to onset of ONJ in alendronate patients was 24 months.

A 2010 study reported the prevalence of osteonecrosis of the jaw in patients using alendronate-type drugs was 1 out of 952 patients or ~0.1% (Lo, 2010). The study's protocol involved a survey mailed out to 13,946 members of Kaiser Permanente of Northern California healthcare delivery system; 8572 patients responded to the survey. Investigators identified respondents reporting oral problems and dental symptoms. These respondents were then interviewed by telephone for presence of dental problems including exposed bone, gingival sores, moderate periodontal disease, and persistent symptoms or complications after dental procedures. Those selected were then invited for an examination or to have their dental records reviewed. The diagnosis of ONJ was made according to the 2006 American Association of Oral and Maxillofacial Surgeons criteria which required treatment with a bisphosphonate, exposed bone in the maxillofacial region lasting >8 weeks, and no radiotherapy involving the jaw. Of the 8572 respondents, 9 cases of ONJ were identified; 5 had developed ONJ spontaneously and 4 developed ONJ after tooth extraction. Specific oral bisphosphonates were not identified. When extrapolated to patient-years of bisphosphonate exposure, this prevalence rate of 0.1% equates to a frequency of 28 cases per 100,000 person-years of oral bisphosphonate treatment.

References

American Dental Association Council on Scientific Affairs, "Dental Management of Patients Receiving Oral Bisphosphonate Therapy: Expert Panel Recommendations," *J Am Dent Assoc*, 2006, 137 (8):1144-50. Available at http://jada.ada.org/cgi/content/full/137/8/1144.

Author Unknown, "Safety Update: Bone-Building Drugs: Risks Explained," *Consumer Reports on Health*, 2006, 18(5):3.

Barrett J, Worth E, Bauss F, et al, "Ibandronate: A Clinical Pharmacological and Pharmacokinetic Update," *J Clin Pharmacol*, 2004, 44(9):951-65.

Edwards BJ, Hellstein JW, Jacobsen PL, et al, "Updated Recommendations for Managing the Care of Patients Receiving Oral Bisphosphonate Therapy: An Advisory Statement From the American Dental Association Council on Scientific Affairs," *J Am Dent Assoc*, 2008, 139(12):1674-7.

French AE, Kaplan N, Lishner M, et al, "Taking Bisphosphonates During Pregnancy," *Can Fam Physician*, 2003, 49:1281-2.

Lo JC, O'Ryan FS, Gordon NP, et al, "Prevalence of Osteonecrosis of the Jaw in Patients With Oral Bisphosphonate Exposure," *J Oral Maxillofac Surg*, 2010, 68(2):243-53.

Marx RE, Sawatari Y, Fortin M, et al, "Bisphosphonate-Induced Exposed Bone (Osteonecrosis/Osteopetrosis) of the Jaws: Risk Factors, Recognition, Prevention, and Treatment," *J Oral Maxillofac Surg*, 2005, 63(11):1567-75.

Mavrokokki T, Cheng A, Stein B, et al, "Nature and Frequency of Bisphosphonate-Associated Osteonecrosis of the Jaws in Australia," *J Oral Maxillofac Surg*, 2007, 65(3):415-23.

Ibritumomab (ib ri TYOO mo mab)

U.S. Brand Names Zevalin®

Canadian Brand Names Zevalin®

Pharmacologic Category Antineoplastic Agent, Monoclonal Antibody; Radiopharmaceutical

Use Treatment of relapsed or refractory low-grade or follicular B-cell non-Hodgkin's lymphoma (NHL); treatment of follicular NHL in patients who achieve a response (partial or complete) to first-line chemotherapy

Local Anesthetic/Vasoconstrictor Precautions No information available to require special precautions

Effects on Dental Treatment Key adverse event(s) related to dental treatment: Hypotension, cough, throat irritation, rhinitis.

Effects on Bleeding Chemotherapy may result in significant myelosuppression, potentially including significant reduction in platelet counts and altered hemostasis. In patients who are under active treatment with these agents, medical consult is suggested.

Adverse Effects Severe, potentially life-threatening allergic reactions have occurred in association with infusions. Also refer to Rituximab monograph.

>10%:

Central nervous system: Fatigue (33%), chills (24%), fever (10% to 17%), pain (13%), headache (12%)

Gastrointestinal: Nausea (18% to 31%), abdominal pain (16% to 17%), vomiting (12%), diarrhea (9% to 11%)

Hematologic: Thrombocytopenia (62% to 95%; grades 3/4: 51% to 63%; nadir: 49-53 days), neutropenia (45% to 77%; grades 3/4: 41% to 60%; nadir: 61-62 days), anemia (22% to 61%; grades 3/4: 5% to 17%; nadir: 68-69 days), leukopenia (43%; grades 3/4: 36%), lymphopenia (26%; grades 3/4: 18%), myelosuppression (nadir: 7-9 weeks; duration: 22-35 days)

Neuromuscular & skeletal: Weakness (15% to 43%)

Respiratory: Nasopharyngitis (19%), dyspnea (14%), cough (10% to 11%)

Miscellaneous: Infection (29%; serious 1% to 5%)

1% to 10%:

Cardiovascular: Peripheral edema (8%), hypertension (7%), flushing (6%), hypotension (6%)

Central nervous system: Dizziness (7% to 10%), insomnia (5%), anxiety (4%)

Dermatologic: Pruritus (7% to 9%), rash (7% to 8%), petechiae (3% to 8%), bruising (7%), angioedema (5%; grades 3/4: <1%), urticaria (4%)

Gastrointestinal: Anorexia (8%), abdominal distension (5%), constipation (5%), dyspepsia (4%), melena (2%; life threatening in 1%), gastrointestinal hemorrhage (severe: 1%)

Genitourinary: Urinary tract infection (7%)

Hematologic: Secondary malignancies (1% to 6%; includes acute myelogenous leukemia and myelodysplastic syndrome), pancytopenia (severe: 2%)

Neuromuscular & skeletal: Myalgia (7% to 9%), back pain (8%), arthralgia (7%)

Respiratory: Throat irritation (10%), bronchitis (8%), rhinitis (6% to 8%), pharyngolaryngeal pain (7%), sinusitis (7%), bronchospasm (5%), epistaxis (3% to 5%), apnea (severe: 1%)

Miscellaneous: Flu-like syndrome (8%), night sweats (8%), diaphoresis (4%), HAMA antibody formation (4%), allergic reaction (2%), infusion reaction (severe: 1%), tumor pain (severe: 1%)

General Dosage Range I.V.: *Adults:*

Day 1: In-111: 5 mCi (1.6 mg total antibody dose)

Day 7, 8, or 9: Y-90: 0.3-0.4 mCi/kg (11.1-14.8 MBq/kg actual body weight) (maximum: 32 mCi [1184 MBq])

Mechanism of Action Ibritumomab is a monoclonal antibody directed against the CD20 antigen found on B lymphocytes (normal and malignant). Ibritumomab binding induces apoptosis in B lymphocytes *in vitro*. It is combined with the chelator tiuxetan, which acts as a specific chelation site for either Indium-111 (In-111) or Yttrium-90 (Y-90). The monoclonal antibody acts as a delivery system to direct the radioactive isotope to the targeted cells, however, binding has been observed in lymphoid cells throughout the body and in lymphoid nodules in organs such as the large and small intestines. Indium-111 is a gamma-emitter used to assess biodistribution of ibritumomab, while Y-90 emits beta particles. Beta-emission induces cellular damage through the formation of free radicals (in both target cells and surrounding cells).

Pharmacodynamics/Kinetics

Duration of Action Beta cell recovery begins in ~12 weeks; generally in normal range within 9 months

Half-life Elimination Y-90 ibritumomab: 30 hours; Indium-111 decays with a physical half-life of 67 hours; Yttrium-90 decays with a physical half-life of 64 hours

Pregnancy Risk Factor D

Ibuprofen (eye byoo PROE fen)

Related Information

Antiplatelet and Anticoagulation Considerations in Dentistry *on page 1867*

Oral Pain *on page 1928*

Rheumatoid Arthritis, Osteoarthritis, and Osteoporosis *on page 1889*

Temporomandibular Dysfunction (TMD) *on page 1964*

Related Sample Prescriptions

Mild/Moderate Oral Pain *on page 1980*

Moderate/Moderately Severe Oral Pain *on page 1980*

U.S. Brand Names Addaprin [OTC]; Advil® Children's [OTC]; Advil® Infants' [OTC]; Advil® Migraine [OTC]; Advil® [OTC]; Caldolor™; I-Prin [OTC]; Ibu-200 [OTC]; Ibu®; Midol® Cramps & Body Aches [OTC]; Motrin® Children's [OTC]; Motrin® IB [OTC]; Motrin® Infants' [OTC]; Motrin® Junior [OTC]; NeoProfen®; Proprinal® [OTC]; TopCare® Junior Strength [OTC]; Ultraprin [OTC]

Canadian Brand Names Advil®; Apo-Ibuprofen®; Motrin® (Children's); Motrin® IB; Novo-Profen; Nu-Ibuprofen

Generic Availability (U.S.) Yes: Caplet, softgel capsule, suspension, tablet

Pharmacologic Category Nonsteroidal Anti-inflammatory Drug (NSAID), Oral; Nonsteroidal Anti-inflammatory Drug (NSAID), Parenteral

Dental Use Management of pain and swelling

Use

Oral: Inflammatory diseases and rheumatoid disorders including juvenile idiopathic arthritis (JIA), mild-to-moderate pain, fever, dysmenorrhea, osteoarthritis

Ibuprofen injection (Caldolor™): Management of mild-to-moderate pain; management moderate-to-severe pain when used concurrently with an opioid analgesic; reduction of fever

Ibuprofen lysine injection (NeoProfen®): To induce closure of a clinically-significant patent ductus arteriosus (PDA) in premature infants weighing between 500-1500 g and who are ≤32 weeks gestational age (GA) when usual treatments are ineffective

Unlabeled/Investigational Use Cystic fibrosis, gout, ankylosing spondylitis, acute migraine headache

Local Anesthetic/Vasoconstrictor Precautions No information available to require special precautions

Effects on Dental Treatment In a statement released on September 8, 2006, the FDA notified consumers and healthcare professionals that the administration of ibuprofen for pain relief to patients taking aspirin for cardioprotection may interfere with aspirin's cardiovascular benefits. The FDA states that ibuprofen can interfere with the antiplatelet effect of low-dose aspirin (81 mg/day). This could result in diminished effectiveness of aspirin as used for cardioprotection and stroke prevention. The FDA adds that although ibuprofen and aspirin can be taken together, it is recommended that consumers talk with their healthcare providers for additional information. For more information, including how to advise aspirin patients requiring ibuprofen for pain relief, see Effects on Bleeding and Dental Comment.

Effects on Bleeding Nonselective NSAIDs are known to reversibly decrease platelet aggregation via mechanisms different than observed with aspirin. Platelet function is restored as the drug is eliminated from the body. NSAIDs should be avoided (if possible) in general surgery patients for 3-5 half-lives of the drug (usually 1-3 days) prior to surgery to reduce the risk of excessive bleeding. However, there is no scientific evidence to warrant discontinuance of NSAIDs prior to dental surgery. In medically complicated patients or extensive oral surgery, the decision to interrupt therapy must be based on the risk to benefit in an individual patient and a medical consult is suggested. Routine interruption of NSAID therapy for most dental procedures is not warranted. If therapy is continued without interruption, the clinician should anticipate the potential for slower clotting times.

Adverse Effects

Oral:

1% to 10%:

- Cardiovascular: Edema (1% to 3%)
- Central nervous system: Dizziness (3% to 9%), headache (1% to 3%), nervousness (1% to 3%)
- Dermatologic: Rash (3% to 9%), itching (1% to 3%)
- Endocrine & metabolic: Fluid retention (1% to 3%)
- Gastrointestinal: Epigastric pain (3% to 9%), heartburn (3% to 9%), nausea (3% to 9%), abdominal pain/cramps/distress (1% to 3%), appetite decreased (1% to 3%), constipation (1% to 3%), diarrhea (1% to 3%), dyspepsia (1% to 3%), flatulence (1% to 3%), vomiting (1% to 3%)
- Otic: Tinnitus (3% to 9%)

Injection: Ibuprofen (Caldolor™): Abdominal pain, anemia, BUN increased, cough, dizziness, dyspepsia, edema, flatulence, headache, hemorrhage, hypokalemia, hypernatremia, hypertension, nausea, neutropenia, pruritus, urinary retention, vomiting

Injection: Ibuprofen lysine (NeoProfen®):

>10%:

- Cardiovascular: Intraventricular hemorrhage (29%; grade 3/4: 15%)
- Dermatologic: Skin irritation (16%)
- Endocrine & metabolic: Hypocalcemia (12%), hypoglycemia (12%)
- Gastrointestinal: GI disorders, non NEC (22%)
- Hematologic: Anemia (32%)
- Respiratory: Apnea (28%), respiratory infection (19%)
- Miscellaneous: Sepsis (43%)

1% to 10%:

- Cardiovascular: Edema (4%)
- Endocrine & metabolic: Adrenal insufficiency (7%), hypernatremia (7%)
- Genitourinary: Urinary tract infection (9%)

Renal: Urea increased (7%), renal impairment (6%), creatinine increased (3%), urine output decreased (3%; small decrease reported on days 2-6 with compensatory increase in output on day 9), renal failure (1%)
Respiratory: Respiratory failure (10%), atelectasis (4%)
Frequency not defined: Abdominal distension, cholestasis, feeding problems, gastritis, GI reflux, heart failure, hyperglycemia, hypotension, ileus, infection, inguinal hernia, injection site reaction, jaundice, neutropenia, seizure, tachycardia, thrombocytopenia

Dental Usual Dosage

Analgesic/pain/fever/dysmenorrhea: Oral:
Children: 4-10 mg/kg/dose every 6-8 hours
Adults: 200-400 mg/dose every 4-6 hours (maximum daily dose: 1.2 g, unless directed by physician; under physician supervision daily doses ≤2.4 g may be used)
OTC labeling (analgesic, antipyretic): **Note:** Treatment for >10 days is not recommended unless directed by healthcare provider. Oral:
Children 6 months to 11 years: See table; use of weight to select dose is preferred; doses may be repeated every 6-8 hours (maximum: 4 doses/day)
Children ≥12 years and Adults: 200 mg every 4-6 hours as needed (maximum: 1200 mg/24 hours)

Ibuprofen Dosing

Weight (lb)	Age	Dosage (mg)
12-17	6-11 mo	50
18-23	12-23 mo	75
24-35	2-3 y	100
36-47	4-5 y	150
48-59	6-8 y	200
60-71	9-10 y	250
72-95	11 y	300

Dosage

I.V.:
Neonates: Ibuprofen lysine (NeoProfen®): Infants between 500-1500 g and ≤32 weeks GA: Patent ductus arteriosus: Initial dose: Ibuprofen 10 mg/kg, followed by two doses of 5 mg/kg at 24 and 48 hours. Dose should be based on birth weight.
Adults (Caldolor™): **Note**: Patients should be well hydrated prior to administration
Analgesic: 400-800 mg every 6 hours as needed (maximum: 3.2 g/day)
Antipyretic: Initial: 400 mg, then every 4-6 hours or 100-200 mg every 4 hours as needed (maximum: 3.2 g/day)

Oral:
Children:
Antipyretic: 6 months to 12 years: Temperature <102.5°F (39°C): 5 mg/kg/dose; temperature >102.5°F: 10 mg/kg/dose given every 6-8 hours (maximum daily dose: 40 mg/kg/day)
Juvenile idiopathic arthritis (JIA): 30-50 mg/kg/24 hours divided every 8 hours; start at lower end of dosing range and titrate upward (maximum: 2.4 g/day)
Analgesic: 4-10 mg/kg/dose every 6-8 hours
Cystic fibrosis (unlabeled use): Chronic (>4 years) twice daily dosing adjusted to maintain serum concentration of 50-100 mcg/mL has been associated with slowing of disease progression in younger patients with mild lung disease
OTC labeling (analgesic, antipyretic): **Note:** Treatment for >10 days is not recommended unless directed by healthcare provider.
Children 6 months to 11 years: See table; use of weight to select dose is preferred; doses may be repeated every 6-8 hours (maximum: 4 doses/day)
Children ≥12 years: 200 mg every 4-6 hours as needed (maximum: 1200 mg/24 hours)
Adults:
Inflammatory disease: 400-800 mg/dose 3-4 times/day (maximum dose: 3.2 g/day)
Analgesia/pain/fever/dysmenorrhea: 200-400 mg/dose every 4-6 hours (maximum daily dose: 1.2 g, unless directed by physician; under physician supervision daily doses ≤2.4 g may be used)
OTC labeling (analgesic, antipyretic): 200 mg every 4-6 hours as needed (maximum: 1200 mg/24 hours); treatment for >10 days is not recommended unless directed by healthcare provider.
Migraine: 2 capsules at onset of symptoms (maximum: 400 mg/24 hours unless directed by healthcare provider)

Dosing adjustment/comments in renal impairment: If anuria or oliguria evident, hold dose until renal function returns to normal

Dosing adjustment/comments in severe hepatic impairment: Avoid use

Mechanism of Action Reversibly inhibits cyclooxygenase-1 and 2 (COX-1 and 2) enzymes, which results in decreased formation of prostaglandin precursors; has antipyretic, analgesic, and anti-inflammatory properties

Other proposed mechanisms not fully elucidated (and possibly contributing to the anti-inflammatory effect to varying degrees), include inhibiting chemotaxis, altering lymphocyte activity, inhibiting neutrophil aggregation/activation, and decreasing proinflammatory cytokine levels.

Contraindications Hypersensitivity to ibuprofen; history of asthma, urticaria, or allergic-type reaction to aspirin or other NSAIDs; aspirin triad (eg, bronchial asthma, aspirin intolerance, rhinitis); perioperative pain in the setting of coronary artery bypass graft (CABG) surgery

Ibuprofen lysine (NeoProfen®): Preterm infants with untreated proven or suspected infection; congenital heart disease where patency of the PDA is necessary for pulmonary or systemic blood flow; bleeding (especially with active intracranial hemorrhage or GI bleed); thrombocytopenia; coagulation defects; proven or suspected necrotizing enterocolitis (NEC); significant renal dysfunction

Warnings/Precautions [U.S. Boxed Warning]: NSAIDs are associated with an increased risk of adverse cardiovascular thrombotic events, including fatal MI and stroke. Risk may be increased with duration of use or pre-existing cardiovascular risk factors or disease. Carefully evaluate individual cardiovascular risk profiles prior to prescribing. May cause new-onset hypertension or worsening of existing hypertension. Response to ACE inhibitors, thiazides, or loop diuretics may be impaired with concurrent use of NSAIDs. Use caution with fluid retention. Avoid use in heart failure. Concurrent administration of ibuprofen, and potentially other nonselective NSAIDs, may interfere with aspirin's cardioprotective effect. **[U.S. Boxed Warning]: Use is contraindicated for treatment of perioperative pain in the setting of coronary artery bypass graft (CABG) surgery.** Risk of MI and stroke may be increased with use following CABG surgery.

May increase the risk of aseptic meningitis, especially in patients with systemic lupus erythematosus (SLE) and mixed connective tissue disorders. Platelet adhesion and aggregation may be decreased; may prolong bleeding time; patients with coagulation disorders or who are receiving anticoagulants should be monitored closely. Anemia may occur; patients on long-term NSAID therapy should be monitored for anemia. Rarely, NSAID use may cause severe blood dyscrasias (eg, agranulocytosis, aplastic anemia, thrombocytopenia).

NSAID use may compromise existing renal function; dose-dependent decreases in prostaglandin synthesis may result from NSAID use, reducing renal blood flow which may cause renal decompensation. NSAID use may increase the risk for hyperkalemia. Patients with impaired renal function, dehydration, heart failure, liver dysfunction, those taking diuretics, and ACE inhibitors, and the elderly are at greater risk of renal toxicity and hyperkalemia. Rehydrate patient before starting therapy; monitor renal function closely. Not recommended for use in patients with advanced renal disease. Long-term NSAID use may result in renal papillary necrosis.

NSAIDs may increase risk of gastrointestinal irritation, inflammation, ulceration, bleeding, and perforation. These events can be fatal and may occur at any time during therapy and without warning. Use caution with a history of GI disease (bleeding or ulcers), concurrent therapy with aspirin, anticoagulants and/or corticosteroids, smoking, use of ethanol, the elderly or debilitated patients. When used concomitantly with ≤325 mg of aspirin, a substantial increase in the risk of gastrointestinal complications (eg, ulcer) occurs; concomitant gastroprotective therapy (eg, proton pump inhibitors) is recommended (Bhatt, 2008).

Use the lowest effective dose for the shortest duration of time, consistent with individual patient goals, to reduce risk of cardiovascular or GI adverse events. Alternate therapies should be considered for patients at high risk.

NSAIDs may cause serious skin adverse events including exfoliative dermatitis, Stevens-Johnson Syndrome (SJS) and toxic epidermal necrolysis (TEN); discontinue use at first sign of skin rash or hypersensitivity. Anaphylactoid reactions may occur, even without prior exposure; patients with "aspirin triad" (bronchial asthma, aspirin intolerance, rhinitis) may be at increased risk. Do not use in patients who experience bronchospasm, asthma, rhinitis, or urticaria with NSAID or aspirin therapy. Use caution in other forms of asthma.

NSAIDS may cause drowsiness, dizziness, blurred vision and other neurologic effects which may impair physical or mental abilities; patients must be cautioned about performing tasks which require mental alertness (eg, operating machinery or driving). Monitor vision with long-term therapy. Blurred/diminished vision, scotomata, and changes in color vision have been reported. Discontinue use with altered vision and perform ophthalmologic exam.

Use with caution in patients with decreased hepatic function. Closely monitor patients with any abnormal LFT. Severe hepatic reactions (eg, fulminant hepatitis, liver failure) have occurred with NSAID use, rarely; discontinue if signs or symptoms of liver disease develop, or if systemic manifestations occur.

The elderly are at increased risk for adverse effects (especially serious gastrointestinal events, CNS effects, renal toxicity) from NSAIDs even at low doses.

Withhold for at least 4-6 half-lives prior to surgical or dental procedures. Some products may contain phenylalanine. Ibuprofen injection (Caldolor™) must be diluted prior to administration; hemolysis can occur if not diluted.

Ibuprofen lysine injection (NeoProfen®): Hold second or third doses if urinary output is <0.6 mL/kg/hour. May alter signs of infection. May inhibit platelet aggregation; monitor for signs of bleeding. May displace bilirubin; use caution when total bilirubin is elevated. Long-term evaluations of neurodevelopment, growth, or diseases associated with prematurity following treatment have not been conducted. A second course of treatment, alternative pharmacologic therapy or surgery may be needed if the ductus arteriosus fails to close or reopens following the initial course of therapy.

Self medication (OTC use): Prior to self-medication, patients should contact healthcare provider if they have had recurring stomach pain or upset, ulcers, bleeding problems, high blood pressure, heart or kidney disease, other serious medical problems, are currently taking a diuretic, aspirin, anticoagulant, or are ≥60 years of age. If patients are using for migraines, they should also contact healthcare provider if they have not had a migraine diagnosis by healthcare provider, a headache that is different from usual migraine, worst headache of life, fever and neck stiffness, headache from head injury or coughing, first headache at ≥50 years of age, daily headache, or migraine requiring bed rest. Recommended dosages should not be exceeded, due to an increased risk of GI bleeding. Stop use and consult a healthcare provider if symptoms get worse, newly appear, fever lasts for >3 days or pain lasts >3 days (children) and >10 days (adults). Do not give for >10 days unless instructed by healthcare provider. Consuming ≥3 alcoholic beverages/day or taking longer than recommended may increase the risk of GI bleeding.

Drug Interactions

Metabolism/Transport Effects Substrate (minor) of CYP2C9, 2C19; **Inhibits** CYP2C9 (strong)

Avoid Concomitant Use

Avoid concomitant use of Ibuprofen with any of the following: Ketorolac; Ketorolac (Systemic)

Increased Effect/Toxicity

Ibuprofen may increase the levels/effects of: Aminoglycosides; Anticoagulants; Antiplatelet Agents; Bisphosphonate Derivatives; Collagenase (Systemic); CycloSPORINE; CycloSPORINE (Systemic); Deferasirox; Desmopressin; Digoxin; Drotrecogin Alfa; Eplerenone; Haloperidol; Ibritumomab; Lithium; Methotrexate; Nonsteroidal Anti-Inflammatory Agents; PEMEtrexed; Potassium-Sparing Diuretics; PRALAtrexate; Quinolone Antibiotics; Salicylates; Thrombolytic Agents; Tositumomab and Iodine I 131 Tositumomab; Vancomycin; Vitamin K Antagonists

The levels/effects of Ibuprofen may be increased by: ACE Inhibitors; Angiotensin II Receptor Blockers; Antidepressants (Tricyclic, Tertiary Amine); Corticosteroids (Systemic); Dasatinib; Glucosamine; Herbs (Anticoagulant/Antiplatelet Properties); Ketorolac; Ketorolac (Systemic); Nonsteroidal Anti-Inflammatory Agents; Omega-3-Acid Ethyl Esters; Pentosan Polysulfate Sodium; Pentoxifylline; Probenecid; Prostacyclin Analogues; Selective Serotonin Reuptake Inhibitors; Serotonin/Norepinephrine Reuptake Inhibitors; Treprostinil; Voriconazole

Decreased Effect

Ibuprofen may decrease the levels/effects of: ACE Inhibitors; Angiotensin II Receptor Blockers; Antiplatelet Agents; Beta-Blockers; Eplerenone; HydrALAZINE; Loop Diuretics; Potassium-Sparing Diuretics; Salicylates; Thiazide Diuretics

The levels/effects of Ibuprofen may be decreased by: Bile Acid Sequestrants; Nonsteroidal Anti-Inflammatory Agents; Salicylates

Ethanol/Nutrition/Herb Interactions

Ethanol: Avoid ethanol (may enhance gastric mucosal irritation).

Food: Ibuprofen peak serum levels may be decreased if taken with food.

Herb/Nutraceutical: Avoid alfalfa, anise, bilberry, bladderwrack, bromelain, cat's claw, celery, chamomile, coleus, cordyceps, dong quai, evening primrose, fenugreek, feverfew, garlic, ginger, ginkgo biloba, ginseng (American, Panax, Siberian), grapeseed, green tea, guggul, horse chestnut seed, horseradish, licorice, prickly ash, red clover, reishi, SAMe (S-adenosylmethionine), sweet clover, turmeric, white willow (all have additional antiplatelet activity).

Dietary Considerations Should be taken with food. Some products may contain phenylalanine and/or potassium.

Pharmacodynamics/Kinetics

Onset of Action Oral: Analgesic: 30-60 minutes; Anti-inflammatory: ≤7 days

Duration of Action Oral: 4-6 hours

Half-life Elimination

Premature infants (highly variable between studies):
- Day 3: 35-51 hours
- Day 5: 20-33 hours

Children 3 months to 10 years: 1.6 ± 0.7 hours

Adults: 2-4 hours; End-stage renal disease: Unchanged

Time to Peak Oral: ~1-2 hours

Pregnancy Risk Factor C/D ≥30 weeks gestation

Lactation Enters breast milk/not recommended (AAP rates "compatible"; AAP 2001 update pending)

Breast-Feeding Considerations Based on limited data, only very small amounts of ibuprofen are excreted into breast milk. Adverse events have not been reported in nursing infants. Because there is a potential for adverse events to occur in nursing infants, the manufacturer does not recommend the use of ibuprofen while breast-feeding. Use with caution in nursing women with hypertensive disorders of pregnancy or pre-existing renal disease.

Dosage Forms

Caplet, oral: 200 mg
- Advil® [OTC]: 200 mg
- Motrin® IB [OTC]: 200 mg
- Motrin® Junior [OTC]: 100 mg

Capsule, liquid filled, oral:
- Advil® [OTC]: 200 mg
- Advil® Migraine [OTC]: 200 mg

Capsule, softgel, oral: 200 mg

Gelcap, oral:
- Advil® [OTC]: 200 mg

Injection, solution:
- Caldolor™: 100 mg/mL (4 mL, 8 mL)

Injection, solution [preservative free]:
- NeoProfen®: 17.1 mg/mL (2 mL)

Suspension, oral: 100 mg/5 mL (5 mL, 10 mL, 120 mL, 240 mL, 480 mL); 40 mg/mL (15 mL)
- Advil® Children's [OTC]: 100 mg/5 mL (120 mL)
- Advil® Infants' [OTC]: 40 mg/mL (15 mL)
- Motrin® Children's [OTC]: 100 mg/5 mL (60 mL, 120 mL)
- Motrin® Infants' [OTC]: 40 mg/mL (15 mL)

Tablet, oral: 200 mg, 400 mg, 600 mg, 800 mg
- Addaprin [OTC]: 200 mg
- Advil® [OTC]: 200 mg
- I-Prin [OTC]: 200 mg
- Ibu-200 [OTC]: 200 mg
- Ibu®: 400 mg, 600 mg, 800 mg
- Midol® Cramps & Body Aches [OTC]: 200 mg
- Motrin® IB [OTC]: 200 mg
- Proprinal® [OTC]: 200 mg
- Ultraprin [OTC]: 200 mg

Tablet, chewable, oral:
- Motrin® Junior [OTC]: 100 mg
- TopCare® Junior Strength [OTC]: 100 mg

Dental Comment Preoperative use of ibuprofen at a dose of 400-600 mg every 6 hours 24 hours before the appointment decreases postoperative edema and hastens healing time.

New information from the FDA states that ibuprofen can interfere with the antiplatelet effect of low-dose aspirin (81 mg/day), potentially rendering aspirin less effective when used for cardioprotection and stroke protection. In situations where these drugs could be used concomitantly, the FDA has provided the following information.

Patients who use immediate release aspirin (not enteric-coated aspirin) and take a single dose or chronic doses of ibuprofen 400 mg, should dose the ibuprofen at least **30 minutes or longer after aspirin ingestion or more than 8 hours before aspirin ingestion** to avoid attenuation of aspirin's effect.

At this time, recommendations about the timing of ibuprofen 400 mg in patients taking enteric-coated low-dose aspirin cannot be made based on available data. One study however, showed that the antiplatelet effect of enteric-coated low-dose aspirin was attenuated when ibuprofen 400 mg was dosed 2, 7, and 12 hours after aspirin (Catella-Lawson, 2001).

With occasional use of ibuprofen, there is likely to be minimal risk from any attenuation of the antiplatelet effect of low-dose aspirin, because of a long-lasting effect of aspirin on platelets.

Other over-the-counter (OTC) NSAIDs (ie, naproxen sodium and ketoprofen) should be viewed as having the potential to interfere with the antiplatelet effect of low-dose aspirin until proven otherwise. However, the FDA is unaware of any studies that have looked at the same type of interference by ketoprofen with low-dose aspirin. One study of naproxen and low-dose aspirin has suggested that naproxen may interfere with aspirin's antiplatelet activity when they are coadministered (Steinhubl, 2005). However, naproxen 500 mg administered 2 hours before or after aspirin 100 mg, did not interfere with aspirin's antiplatelet effect. The FDA stated that there is no data looking at doses of naproxen <500 mg. Naproxen OTC strength is 220 mg tablets.

Ibuprofen, prescription dose of 800 mg 3 times daily, significantly diminishes the antiplatelet effects of low-dose aspirin (baby) in healthy volunteers. Diclofenac (Systemic), 50 mg 3 times daily, did not interfere with the antiplatelet effects of low-dose aspirin (baby) in healthy volunteers. Ibuprofen, and possibly other non-selective NSAIDs, may reduce the cardioprotective effects of aspirin. It seems prudent to avoid regular, frequent use of ibuprofen in patients receiving aspirin for its cardioprotective effects. Alternative analgesics (eg, acetaminophen) or prescription diclofenac in place of prescription ibuprofen may be a safer choice.

References

Ahmad N, Grad HA, Haas DA, et al, "The Efficacy of Nonopioid Analgesics for Postoperative Dental Pain: A Meta-Analysis," *Anesth Prog*, 1997, 44(4):119-26.

Beaver WT, "Review of the Analgesic Efficacy of Ibuprofen," *Int J Clin Pract*, 2003, (Suppl 135):13-7.

Catella-Lawson F, Reilly MP, Kapoor SC, et al. "Cyclooxygenase Inhibitors and the Antiplatelet Effects of Aspirin," *N Engl J Med*, 2001, 345(25):1809-17.

Dionne R, "Additive Analgesia Without Opioid Side Effects," *Compend Contin Educ Dent*, 2000, 21 (7):572-4, 576-7.

Dionne R, "Relative Efficacy of Selective COX-2 Inhibitors Compared With Over-The-Counter Ibuprofen," *Int J Clin Pract Suppl*, 2003, (135):18-22.

Dionne RA and Berthold CW, "Therapeutic Uses of Nonsteroidal Anti-inflammatory Drugs in Dentistry," *Crit Rev Oral Biol Med*, 2001, 12(4):315-30.

Doyle G, Jayawardena S, Ashraf E, et al, "Efficacy and Tolerability of Nonprescription Ibuprofen Versus Celecoxib for Dental Pain," *J Clin Pharmacol*, 2002, 42(8):912-9.

Gobetti JP, "Controlling Dental Pain," *J Am Dent Assoc*, 1992, 123(6):47-52.

Hersh EV, Levin LM, Cooper SA, et al, "Ibuprofen Liquigel for Oral Surgery Pain," *Clin Ther*, 2000, 22 (11):1306-18.

Olson NZ, Otero AM, Marrero I, et al, "Onset of Analgesia for Liquigel Ibuprofen 400 mg, Acetaminophen 1000 mg, Ketoprofen 25 mg, and Placebo in the Treatment of Postoperative Dental Pain," *J Clin Pharmacol*, 2001, 41(11):1238-47.

Pearlman B, Boyatzis S, Daly C, et al, "The Analgesic Efficacy of Ibuprofen in Periodontal Surgery: A Multicentre Study," *Aust Dent J*, 1997, 42(5):328-34.

Nguyen AM, Graham DY, Gage T, et al, "Nonsteroidal Anti-inflammatory Drug Use in Dentistry: Gastrointestinal Implications," *Gen Dent*, 1999, 47(6):590-6.

Schuijt MP, Huntjens-Fleuren HW, de Metz M, et al, "The Interaction of Ibuprofen and Diclofenac With Aspirin in Healthy Volunteers," *Br J Pharmacol*, 2009, 157(6):931-4.

Steinhubl SR, "The Use of Anti-Inflammatory Analgesics in the Patient With Cardiovascular Disease: What a Pain," *J Am Coll Cardiol*, 2005, 45(8):1302-3.

Wynn RL, "Update on Nonprescription Pain Relievers for Dental Pain," *Gen Dent*, 2004, 52(2):94-8.

Ibutilide (i BYOO ti lide)

Related Information

Clinical Risk Related to Drugs Prolonging QT Interval *on page 1872*

U.S. Brand Names Corvert®

Pharmacologic Category Antiarrhythmic Agent, Class III

Use Acute termination of atrial fibrillation or flutter of recent onset; the effectiveness of ibutilide has not been determined in patients with arrhythmias >90 days in duration

Local Anesthetic/Vasoconstrictor Precautions Ibutilide is one of the drugs confirmed to prolong the QT interval and is accepted as having a risk of causing torsade de pointes. The risk of drug-induced torsade de pointes is extremely low when a single QT interval prolonging drug is prescribed. In terms of epinephrine, it is not known what effect vasoconstrictors in the local anesthetic regimen will have in patients with a known history of congenital prolonged QT interval or in patients taking any medication that prolongs the QT interval. Until more information is obtained, it is suggested that the clinician consult with the physician prior to the use of a vasoconstrictor in suspected patients, and that the vasoconstrictor (epinephrine, mepivacaine and levonordefrin [Carbocaine® 2% with Neo-Cobefrin®]) be used with caution.

Effects on Dental Treatment No significant effects or complications reported

Effects on Bleeding No information available to require special precautions

Adverse Effects 1% to 10%:

Cardiovascular: Ventricular extrasystoles (5.1%), nonsustained monomorphic ventricular tachycardia (4.9%), nonsustained polymorphic ventricular tachycardia (2.7%), tachycardia/supraventricular tachycardia (2.7%), hypotension (2%), bundle branch block (1.9%), sustained polymorphic ventricular tachycardia (eg, torsade de pointes) (1.7%, often requiring cardioversion), AV block (1.5%), bradycardia (1.2%), QT segment prolongation, hypertension (1.2%), palpitation (1%)

Central nervous system: Headache (3.6%)

Gastrointestinal: Nausea (>1%)

General Dosage Range I.V.:

Adults <60 kg: 0.01 mg/kg; may repeat once

Adults ≥60 kg: 1 mg; may repeat once

Mechanism of Action Exact mechanism of action is unknown; prolongs the action potential in cardiac tissue

Pharmacodynamics/Kinetics

Onset of Action ~90 minutes after start of infusion (1/2 of conversions to sinus rhythm occur during infusion)

Half-life Elimination 2-12 hours (average: 6 hours)

Pregnancy Risk Factor C

Dental Comment Ibutilide is known to prolong the QT interval. The QT interval is measured as the time and distance between the Q point of the QRS complex and the end of the T wave in the ECG tracing. After adjustment for heart rate, the QT interval is defined as prolonged if it is more than 450 msec in men and 460 msec in women. A long QT syndrome was first described in the 1950s and 60s as a congenital syndrome involving QT interval prolongation and syncope and sudden death. Some of the congenital long QT syndromes were characterized by a peculiar electrocardiographic appearance of the QRS complex involving a premature atria beat followed by a pause, then a subsequent sinus beat showing marked QT prolongation and deformity. This type of cardiac arrhythmia was originally termed "torsade de pointes" (translated from the French as "twisting of the points"). Ibutilide is considered as having a risk of causing torsade de pointes. Since it is not known what effect vasoconstrictors in the local anesthetic regimen will have in patients with a known history of congenital prolonged QT interval or in patients taking any medication that prolongs the QT interval, a medical consult is suggested.

Icodextrin (eye KOE dex trin)

U.S. Brand Names Extraneal

Pharmacologic Category Adhesiolytic; Peritoneal Dialysate, Osmotic

Use

Adept®: Reduction of postsurgical adhesions in gynecologic laparoscopic procedures

Extraneal®: Daily exchange for the long dwell (8- to 16-hour) during continuous ambulatory peritoneal dialysis (CAPD) or automated peritoneal dialysis (APD) for the management of end-stage renal disease (ESRD); improvement of long-dwell ultrafiltration and clearance of creatinine and urea nitrogen (compared to 4.25% dextrose) in patients with high/average or greater transport characteristics as measured by peritoneal equilibration test (PET)

Local Anesthetic/Vasoconstrictor Precautions No information available to require special precautions

Effects on Dental Treatment No significant effects or complications reported

Effects on Bleeding No information available to require special precautions

Adverse Effects

CAPD or APD (Extraneal®):

>10%:

Cardiovascular: Hypertension (13%)

Respiratory: Upper respiratory infection (15%)

Miscellaneous: Peritonitis (26% vs 25% in controls)

5% to 10%:

Cardiovascular: Edema (up to 6%), chest pain (5%), hypervolemia, hypotension

Central nervous system: Headache (9%), dizziness

Dermatological: Rash (10%), pruritus, skin disorder

Endocrine & metabolic: Hyperglycemia (5%), hyperphosphatemia, hypokalemia, hypoproteinemia

Gastrointestinal: Abdominal pain (8%), nausea (7%), dyspepsia (5%), diarrhea, vomiting

Hematologic: Anemia
Neuromuscular & skeletal: Arthralgia, pain, weakness
Respiratory: Cough increased (7%), dyspnea
Miscellaneous: Accidental injury (6%), flu syndrome (7%), infection

<5%:
Cardiovascular: Postural hypotension, CHF
Central nervous system: Confusion
Dermatologic: Exfoliative dermatitis, erythema multiforme, eczema, maculopapular rash, vesicobullous rash
Endocrine & metabolic: Hypercalcemia, hypochloremia, hypoglycemia, hyponatremia, alkaline phosphatase increased
Gastrointestinal: Abdominal enlargement, cramps
Hepatic: ALT increased, AST increased
Local: Infusion pain
Miscellaneous: Cloudy effluent

Laparoscopic surgery (Adept®):

>10%:
Central nervous system: Headache (35%)
Endocrine & metabolic: Dysmenorrhea (13%)
Gastrointestinal: Nausea (6% to 17%), constipation (11%)

1% to 10%:
Central nervous system: Pyrexia (6%), insomnia (5%)
Gastrointestinal: Flatulence (8%), abdominal pain (7%), abdominal distention (6%), vomiting (6%), diarrhea (1%)
Genitourinary: Dysuria (7%), urinary tract infection (7%); labial, vulvar, or vaginal swelling (6%); vaginal bleeding (6%)
Neuromuscular & skeletal: Arthralgia (9%), back pain (8%)
Respiratory: Nasopharyngitis (7%), cough (4%)

General Dosage Range Intraperitoneal: *Adults:*
CAPD or APD (Extraneal®): Given as a single daily exchange in CAPD or APD; dwell time of 8-16 hours is suggested
Laparoscopic gynecologic surgery (Adept®): Irrigate with at least 100 mL every 30 minutes during surgery; aspirate remaining fluid after surgery is completed, then instill 1 L into the cavity

Mechanism of Action When used for dialysis, icodextrin exerts osmotic pressure across small intercellular pores resulting in transcapillary ultrafiltration throughout the dwell while providing electrolytes and lactate for the maintenance of both the electrolyte and acid-base balance. When used for laparoscopic surgery, the colloidal osmotic action allows the fluid to be retained in the peritoneal cavity for 3-4 days, physically providing a temporary separation of peritoneal surfaces and minimizing adhesion formation.

Pharmacodynamics/Kinetics
Time to Peak Plasma: 13 hours

Pregnancy Risk Factor C

IDArubicin (eye da ROO bi sin)

U.S. Brand Names Idamycin PFS®
Canadian Brand Names Idamycin®
Pharmacologic Category Antineoplastic Agent, Anthracycline; Antineoplastic Agent, Antibiotic
Use Treatment of acute myeloid leukemia (AML)
Unlabeled/Investigational Use Acute lymphocytic leukemia (ALL)
Local Anesthetic/Vasoconstrictor Precautions No information available to require special precautions
Effects on Dental Treatment Key adverse event(s) related to dental treatment: Stomatitis.
Effects on Bleeding Chemotherapy may result in significant myelosuppression, potentially including significant reduction in platelet counts and altered hemostasis. In patients who are under active treatment with these agents, medical consult is suggested.

Adverse Effects

>10%:
Cardiovascular: Transient ECG abnormalities (supraventricular tachycardia, S-T wave changes, atrial or ventricular extrasystoles); generally asymptomatic and self-limiting. CHF, dose related. The relative cardiotoxicity of idarubicin compared to doxorubicin is unclear. Some investigators report no increase in cardiac toxicity at cumulative oral idarubicin doses up to 540 mg/m^2; other reports suggest a maximum cumulative intravenous dose of 150 mg/m^2.
Central nervous system: Headache

Dermatologic: Alopecia (25% to 30%), radiation recall, skin rash (11%), urticaria
Gastrointestinal: Nausea, vomiting (30% to 60%); diarrhea (9% to 22%); stomatitis (11%); GI hemorrhage (30%)
Genitourinary: Discoloration of urine (darker yellow)
Hematologic: Myelosuppression (nadir: 10-15 days; recovery: 21-28 days), primarily leukopenia; thrombocytopenia and anemia. Effects are generally less severe with oral dosing.
Hepatic: Bilirubin and transaminases increased (44%)

1% to 10%:

Central nervous system: Seizure
Neuromuscular & skeletal: Peripheral neuropathy

General Dosage Range Dosage adjustment recommended in patients with hepatic or renal impairment

I.V.: *Adults:* Induction: 12 mg/m²/day for 3 days; Consolidation: 10-12 mg/m²/day for 2 days

Mechanism of Action Similar to doxorubicin and daunorubicin; inhibition of DNA and RNA synthesis by intercalation between DNA base pairs

Pharmacodynamics/Kinetics

Half-life Elimination Oral: 14-35 hours; I.V.: 12-27 hours

Time to Peak Serum: 1-5 hours

Pregnancy Risk Factor D

Idursulfase (eye dur SUL fase)

U.S. Brand Names Elaprase®

Canadian Brand Names Elaprase®

Pharmacologic Category Enzyme

Use Replacement therapy in mucopolysaccharidosis II (MPS II, Hunter syndrome) for improvement of walking capacity

Local Anesthetic/Vasoconstrictor Precautions No information available to require special precautions

Effects on Dental Treatment No significant effects or complications reported

Effects on Bleeding No information available to require special precautions

Adverse Effects >10%:

Cardiovascular: Hypertension (25%), atrial abnormality (13%)
Central nervous system: Pyrexia (63%), headache (59%), malaise (22%), anxiety (13%), irritability (13%)
Dermatologic: Pruritus (28%), urticaria (16%), pruritic rash (13%), skin disorder (13%)
Gastrointestinal: Dyspepsia (13%)
Local: Abscess (16%), infusion-site edema (13%)
Neuromuscular & skeletal: Arthralgia (31%), limb pain (28%), chest wall musculoskeletal pain (16%), musculoskeletal dysfunction (16%)
Ocular: visual disturbance (22%)
Respiratory: Wheezing (19%)
Miscellaneous: Antibody development (51%), infusion reactions (15%), superficial injury (13%)

General Dosage Range I.V.: *Children ≥5 years and Adults:* 0.5 mg/kg once weekly

Mechanism of Action Idursulfase is a recombinant form of iduronate-2-sulfatase, an enzyme needed to hydrolyze the mucopolysaccharides dermatan sulfate and heparan sulfate in various cells. Accumulation of these polysaccharides can lead to various manifestations of disease, including physical changes, CNS involvement, cardiac, respiratory, and mobility dysfunction. Replacement of this enzyme has been shown to improve walking capacity in patients with a deficiency.

Pharmacodynamics/Kinetics

Half-life Elimination Half-life elimination: 44-48 minutes

Pregnancy Risk Factor C

Ifosfamide (eye FOSS fa mide)

U.S. Brand Names Ifex

Canadian Brand Names Ifex

Pharmacologic Category Antineoplastic Agent, Alkylating Agent; Antineoplastic Agent, Alkylating Agent (Nitrogen Mustard)

Use Treatment of testicular cancer

Unlabeled/Investigational Use Treatment of bladder cancer, cervical cancer, ovarian cancer, nonsmall cell lung cancer, small cell lung cancer, Hodgkin's and non-Hodgkin's lymphoma; acute lymphocytic leukemia; Ewing's sarcoma, osteosarcoma, and soft tissue sarcomas

Local Anesthetic/Vasoconstrictor Precautions No information available to require special precautions

Effects on Dental Treatment No significant effects or complications reported

Effects on Bleeding Chemotherapy may result in significant myelosuppression, potentially including significant reduction in platelet counts and altered hemostasis. In patients who are under active treatment with these agents, medical consult is suggested.

Adverse Effects

>10%:

Central nervous system: CNS toxicity or encephalopathy (10% to 30%; includes somnolence, agitation, confusion, delirium, hallucinations, depressive psychosis, incontinence, palsy, diplopia, aphasia, or coma)

Dermatologic: Alopecia (83%)

Endocrine & metabolic: Metabolic acidosis (31%)

Gastrointestinal: Nausea/vomiting (58%), may be more common with higher doses or bolus infusion

Hematologic: Myelosuppression (onset: 7-14 days; nadir: 21-28 days; recovery: 21-28 days), leukopenia (50% to ≤100%; grade 4: ≤50%), thrombocytopenia (20%; grades 3/4: 8%)

Renal: Hematuria (6% to 92%; grade 2 [gross hematuria]: 8% to 12%)

1% to 10%:

Central nervous system: Fever

Hepatic: Bilirubin increased (3%), liver dysfunction (3%), transaminases increased (3%)

Local: Phlebitis (2%)

Renal: Renal impairment (6%)

Miscellaneous: Infection (8%)

General Dosage Range Dosage adjustment recommended in patients with hepatic or renal impairment

I.V.: *Adults:* 4000-5000 mg/m^2/day for 1 day every 14-28 days **or** 1000-3000 mg/m^2/day for 2-5 days every 21-28 days

Mechanism of Action Causes cross-linking of strands of DNA by binding with nucleic acids and other intracellular structures; inhibits protein synthesis and DNA synthesis

Pharmacodynamics/Kinetics

Half-life Elimination

High dose (3800-5000 mg/m^2): ~15 hours

Lower dose (1600-2400 mg/m^2): ~7 hours

Pregnancy Risk Factor D

Iloperidone (eye loe PER i done)

Related Information

Clinical Risk Related to Drugs Prolonging QT Interval *on page 1872*

U.S. Brand Names Fanapt®

Generic Availability (U.S.) No

Pharmacologic Category Antipsychotic Agent, Atypical

Use Acute treatment of schizophrenia

Local Anesthetic/Vasoconstrictor Precautions Iloperidone is one of the drugs confirmed to prolong the QT interval and is accepted as having a risk of causing torsade de pointes. The risk of drug-induced torsade de pointes is extremely low when a single QT interval prolonging drug is prescribed. In terms of epinephrine, it is not known what effect vasoconstrictors in the local anesthetic regimen will have in patients with a known history of congenital prolonged QT interval or in patients taking any medication that prolongs the QT interval. Until more information is obtained, it is suggested that the clinician consult with the physician prior to the use of a vasoconstrictor in suspected patients, and that the vasoconstrictor (epinephrine, mepivacaine and levonordefrin [Carbocaine® 2% with Neo-Cobefrin®]) be used with caution.

Effects on Dental Treatment Key adverse event(s) related to dental treatment: Xerostomia and changes in salivation (normal salivary flow resumes upon discontinuation), orthostatic hypotension

Effects on Bleeding No information available to require special precautions

Adverse Effects

>10%:

Cardiovascular: Tachycardia (3% to 12%; dose related)

Central nervous system: Dizziness (10% to 20%; dose related), somnolence (9% to 15%)

1% to 10%:

Cardiovascular: Orthostatic hypotension (3% to 5%), hypotension (1% to 3%; dose related), palpitations (≥1%)

Central nervous system: Fatigue (4% to 6%), extrapyramidal symptoms (≤5%), tremor (3%), lethargy (≤3%), akathisia (2%), aggression (≥1%), delusion (≥1%), restlessness (≥1%)

Dermatologic: Rash (≤3%)

Gastrointestinal: Nausea (≤10%), xerostomia (8% to 10%), weight gain (1% to 9%; dose related), diarrhea (5% to 7%), abdominal discomfort (1% to 3%; dose related), weight loss (≥1%)

Genitourinary: Ejaculation failure (2%), urinary incontinence (≥1%), erectile dysfunction (≥1%)

Neuromuscular & skeletal: Arthralgia (3%), stiffness (1% to 3%; dose related), dyskinesia (<2%), muscle spasm (≥1%), myalgia (≥1%)

Ocular: Blurred vision (≤3%), conjunctivitis (≥1%)

Respiratory: Nasal congestion (5% to 8%), nasopharyngitis (≤4%), upper respiratory tract infection (2% to 3%), dyspnea (2%)

Dosage Oral: Adults: Schizophrenia: Initial: 1 mg twice daily; recommended dosage range: 6-12 mg twice daily (maximum: 24 mg/day)

Recommended titration schedule: Increase in 2 mg increments every 24 hours on days 2-7 (eg, Day 2: 2 mg twice daily; Day 3: 4 mg twice daily; Day 4: 6 mg twice daily; Day 5: 8 mg twice daily; Day 6: 10 mg twice daily; Day 7: 12 mg twice daily)

Note: Titrate dose to effect (to avoid orthostatic hypotensive effects); treatment >6 weeks has not been evaluated; when reinitiating treatment after discontinuation (>3 days), the initial titration schedule should be followed.

Dosage adjustment in patients receiving strong CYP2D6 inhibitors (eg, paroxetine, fluoxetine, quinidine): Decrease iloperidone dose by 50%; when the CYP2D6 inhibitor is discontinued, return to previous dose.

Dosage adjustment in patients receiving strong CYP3A4 inhibitors (eg, ketoconazole, clarithromycin): Decrease iloperidone dose by 50%; when the CYP3A4 inhibitor is discontinued, return to previous dose.

Dosage adjustment in poor metabolizers of CYP2D6: Decrease iloperidone dose by 50%.

Dosing adjustment in hepatic impairment: Not recommended in patients with hepatic impairment due to lack of data

Mechanism of Action Iloperidone is a piperidinyl-benzisoxazole atypical antipsychotic with mixed D_2/5-HT_2 antagonist activity. It exhibits high affinity for 5-HT_{2A}, D_2, and D_3 receptors, low to moderate affinity for D_1, D_4, H_1, 5-HT_{1A}, 5-HT_6, $5HT_7$, and $NE_{\alpha 1}$ receptors, and no affinity for muscarinic receptors. The addition of serotonin antagonism to dopamine antagonism (classic neuroleptic mechanism) is thought to improve negative symptoms of psychoses and reduce the incidence of extrapyramidal side effects. Iloperidone's low affinity for histamine H_1 receptors may decrease the risk for weight gain and somnolence while its affinity for $NE_{\alpha 1/\alpha 2C}$ may provide antidepressant and anxiolytic activity and improved cognitive function.

Contraindications Hypersensitivity to iloperidone or any component of the formulation

Warnings/Precautions [U.S. Boxed Warning]: Elderly patients with dementia-related psychosis treated with antipsychotics are at an increased risk of death compared to placebo. Most deaths appeared to be either cardiovascular (eg, heart failure, sudden death) or infectious (eg, pneumonia) in nature. In addition, an increased incidence of cerebrovascular effects (eg, transient ischemic attack, cerebrovascular accidents) has been reported in studies of placebo-controlled trials of antipsychotics in elderly patients with dementia-related psychosis. Iloperidone is not approved for the treatment of dementia-related psychosis.

May be sedating; use with caution in disorders where CNS depression is a feature. Caution in patients with predisposition to seizures. Use is not recommended in patients with hepatic impairment. Esophageal dysmotility and aspiration have been associated with antipsychotic use; use with caution in patients at risk of aspiration pneumonia (ie, Alzheimer's disease). Use is associated with increased prolactin levels; clinical significance of hyperprolactinemia in patients with breast cancer or other prolactin-dependent tumors is unknown. May alter temperature regulation. Leukopenia, neutropenia, and agranulocytosis (sometimes fatal) have been reported in clinical trials and postmarketing reports; presence of risk factors (eg, pre-existing low WBC or history of drug-induced leuko-/neutropenia) should prompt periodic blood count assessment and discontinuation at first signs of blood dyscrasias.

May alter cardiac conduction and prolong the QT_c interval; life-threatening arrhythmias have occurred with therapeutic doses of antipsychotics. Risks may be increased by conditions or concomitant medications which cause bradycardia, hypokalemia, and/or hypomagnesemia. Avoid use in combination with QT_c-prolonging drugs and in patients with congenital long QT syndrome, history of cardiac arrhythmia, recent MI, or uncompensated heart failure. Discontinue treatment in patients found to have persistent QT_c intervals >500 msec. Further cardiac evaluation is warranted in patients with symptoms of dizziness, palpitations, or syncope. May cause orthostatic hypotension; use with caution in patients at risk of this effect (eg, concurrent medication use which may predispose to hypotension/bradycardia or presence of hypovolemia) or in those who would not tolerate transient hypotensive episodes. Use with caution in patients with cardiovascular diseases (eg, heart failure, history of myocardial infarction or ischemia, cerebrovascular disease, conduction abnormalities).

May cause anticholinergic effects (confusion, agitation, constipation, xerostomia, blurred vision, urinary retention); therefore, use with caution in patients with decreased gastrointestinal motility, urinary retention, BPH, xerostomia, or visual problems (including narrow-angle glaucoma). May cause extrapyramidal symptoms (EPS), including pseudoparkinsonism, acute dystonic reactions, akathisia, and tardive dyskinesia. Risk of dystonia (and probably other EPS) may be greater with increased doses, use of conventional antipsychotics, males, and younger patients. Risk of neuroleptic malignant syndrome (NMS) may be increased in patients with Parkinson's disease or Lewy body dementia. May cause hyperglycemia; in some cases may be extreme and associated with ketoacidosis, hyperosmolar coma, or death. Use with caution in patients with diabetes or other disorders of glucose regulation; monitor for worsening of glucose control. Significant weight gain has been observed with antipsychotic therapy; incidence varies with product. Monitor waist circumference and BMI. Rare cases of priapism have been reported.

Dosage adjustments are recommended for iloperidone when given concomitantly with strong CYP2D6 or CYP3A4 inhibitors or in poor metabolizers of CYP2D6. The possibility of a suicide attempt is inherent in psychotic illness; use caution in high-risk patients during initiation of therapy. Prescriptions should be written for the smallest quantity consistent with good patient care. Continued use for >6 weeks has not been evaluated.

Drug Interactions

Metabolism/Transport Effects Substrate of CYP2D6 (major), 3A4 (minor)

Avoid Concomitant Use

Avoid concomitant use of Iloperidone with any of the following: Artemether; Dronedarone; Lumefantrine; Metoclopramide; Nilotinib; Pimozide; QuiNINE; Tetrabenazine; Thioridazine; Toremifene; Vandetanib; Ziprasidone

Increased Effect/Toxicity

Iloperidone may increase the levels/effects of: Alcohol (Ethyl); CNS Depressants; Dronedarone; Methylphenidate; Pimozide; QTc-Prolonging Agents; QuiNINE; Tetrabenazine; Thioridazine; Toremifene; Vandetanib; Ziprasidone

The levels/effects of Iloperidone may be increased by: Abiraterone; Acetylcholinesterase Inhibitors (Central); Alfuzosin; Artemether; Chloroquine; Ciprofloxacin; Ciprofloxacin (Systemic); Conivaptan; CYP2D6 Inhibitors (Moderate); CYP2D6 Inhibitors (Strong); Darunavir; Gadobutrol; Lithium formulations; Lumefantrine; MAO Inhibitors; Methylphenidate; Metoclopramide; Nilotinib; QuiNINE; Tetrabenazine

Decreased Effect

Iloperidone may decrease the levels/effects of: Amphetamines; Anti-Parkinson's Agents (Dopamine Agonist); Quinagolide

The levels/effects of Iloperidone may be decreased by: Lithium formulations; Peginterferon Alfa-2b; Tocilizumab

Ethanol/Nutrition/Herb Interactions

Ethanol: May increase CNS depression; monitor for increased effects with coadministration. Caution patients about effects.

Herb/Nutraceutical: Avoid St John's wort (may decrease serum levels of iloperidone). Avoid kava kava, gotu kola, valerian, St John's wort (may increase CNS depression).

Dietary Considerations May be given with or without food.

Pharmacodynamics/Kinetics

Half-life Elimination

Extensive metabolizers: Iloperidone: 18 hours; P88: 26 hours; P95: 23 hours

Poor metabolizers: Iloperidone: 33 hours; P88: 37 hours; P95: 31 hours

Time to Peak Plasma: 2-4 hours

Pregnancy Risk Factor C

Lactation Excretion in breast milk unknown/not recommended

Dosage Forms

Tablet, oral:

Fanapt®: 1 mg, 2 mg, 4 mg, 6 mg, 8 mg, 10 mg, 12 mg, 1 mg (2s), 2 mg (2s), 4 mg (2s), and 6 mg (2s)

Dental Comment Iloperidone is known to prolong the QT interval. The QT interval is measured as the time and distance between the Q point of the QRS complex and the end of the T wave in the ECG tracing. After adjustment for heart rate, the QT interval is defined as prolonged if it is more than 450 msec in men and 460 msec in women. A long QT syndrome was first described in the 1950s and 60s as a congenital syndrome involving QT interval prolongation and syncope and sudden death. Some of the congenital long QT syndromes were characterized by a peculiar electrocardiographic appearance of the QRS complex involving a premature atria beat followed by a pause, then a subsequent sinus beat showing marked QT prolongation and deformity. This type of cardiac arrhythmia was originally termed "torsade de pointes" (translated from the French as "twisting of the points"). Iloperidone is considered as having a risk of causing torsade de pointes. Since it is not known what effect vasoconstrictors in the local anesthetic regimen will have in patients with a known history of congenital prolonged QT interval or in patients taking any medication that prolongs the QT interval, a medical consult is suggested.

Iloprost (EYE loe prost)

U.S. Brand Names Ventavis®

Pharmacologic Category Prostacyclin; Prostaglandin; Vasodilator

Use Treatment of pulmonary arterial hypertension (WHO Group I) in patients with NYHA Class III or IV symptoms

Local Anesthetic/Vasoconstrictor Precautions No information available to require special precautions

Effects on Dental Treatment Key adverse event(s) related to dental treatment: Jaw pain (reported in >10% of patients).

Effects on Bleeding Iloprost is a mild inhibitor of platelet aggregation when administered by aerosol.

Adverse Effects

>10%:

- Cardiovascular: Flushing (27%), hypotension (11%)
- Central nervous system: Headache (30%)
- Gastrointestinal: Nausea (13%)
- Neuromuscular & skeletal: Trismus (12%), jaw pain (12%)
- Respiratory: Cough increased (39%)
- Miscellaneous: Flu-like syndrome (14%)

1% to 10%:

- Cardiovascular: Syncope (8%), palpitation (7%)
- Central nervous system: Insomnia (8%)
- Gastrointestinal: Vomiting (7%)
- Hepatic: Alkaline phosphatase increased (6%), GGT increased (6%)
- Neuromuscular & skeletal: Back pain (7%), muscle cramps (6%)
- Respiratory: Hemoptysis (5%), pneumonia (4%)

General Dosage Range Dosage adjustment recommended in patients with hepatic impairment.

Inhalation: *Adults:* Initial: 2.5 mcg/dose; Maintenance: 2.5-5 mcg/dose 6-9 times/day (maximum: 45 mcg/day)

Mechanism of Action Acutely, iloprost dilates systemic and pulmonary arterial vascular beds. With longer-term use, alters pulmonary vascular resistance and suppresses vascular smooth muscle proliferation. In addition, it is a mild endogenous inhibitor of platelet aggregation when aerosolized (Beghetti, 2002).

Pharmacodynamics/Kinetics

Duration of Action 30-60 minutes

Half-life Elimination 20-30 minutes (effect), 7-9 minutes (elimination)

Time to Peak Serum: Within 5 minutes after inhalation

Pregnancy Risk Factor C

Imatinib (eye MAT eh nib)

U.S. Brand Names Gleevec®

Canadian Brand Names Gleevec®

Pharmacologic Category Antineoplastic Agent, Tyrosine Kinase Inhibitor

Use Treatment of:

Gastrointestinal stromal tumors (GIST) kit-positive (CD117), including unresectable and/or metastatic malignant and adjuvant treatment following complete resection

Philadelphia chromosome-positive (Ph+) chronic myeloid leukemia (CML) in chronic phase (newly-diagnosed)
Ph+ CML in chronic phase in pediatric patients recurring following stem cell transplant or who are resistant to interferon-alpha therapy (**not** an approved use in Canada)
Ph+ CML in blast crisis, accelerated phase, or chronic phase after failure of interferon therapy
Ph+ acute lymphoblastic leukemia (ALL) (relapsed or refractory)
Aggressive systemic mastocytosis (ASM) without D816V c-Kit mutation (or c-Kit mutation status unknown)
Dermatofibrosarcoma protuberans (DFSP) (unresectable, recurrent and/or metastatic)
Hypereosinophilic syndrome (HES) and/or chronic eosinophilic leukemia (CEL)
Myelodysplastic/myeloproliferative disease (MDS/MPD) associated with platelet-derived growth factor receptor (PDGFR) gene rearrangements

Canada labeling (not an approved indication in the U.S.): Ph+ ALL induction therapy (newly diagnosed)

Unlabeled/Investigational Use Treatment of desmoid tumors (soft tissue sarcoma); post-stem cell transplant (allogeneic) follow-up treatment in CML

Local Anesthetic/Vasoconstrictor Precautions No information available to require special precautions

Effects on Dental Treatment Key adverse event(s) related to dental treatment: Mouth ulceration and taste disturbance.

Effects on Bleeding Chemotherapy may result in significant myelosuppression, potentially including significant reduction in platelet counts and altered hemostasis. In patients who are under active treatment with these agents, medical consult is suggested.

Adverse Effects Note: Adverse reactions listed as a composite of data across many trials, except where noted for a specific cancer type.

>10%:
- Cardiovascular: Edema/fluid retention (33% to 86%; grades 3/4: 3% to 13%; includes aggravated edema, anasarca, ascites, pericardial effusion, peripheral edema, pleural effusion, pulmonary edema and superficial edema); facial edema (DFSP 17%), chest pain (GIST ≤7%, CML 7% to 11%)
- Central nervous system: Fatigue (29% to 75%), fever (13% to 41%), headache (19% to 37%), dizziness (10% to 19%), insomnia (10% to 19%), depression (≤15%), anxiety (7% to 12%), chills (≤11%)
- Dermatologic: Rash (9% to 50%; grades 3/4: 1% to 9%), pruritus (8% to 19%), alopecia (GIST 10% to 15%)
- Endocrine & metabolic: Hypokalemia (6% to 13%)
- Gastrointestinal: Nausea (42% to 73%), diarrhea (25% to 59%), vomiting (23% to 58%), abdominal pain (6% to 57%), anorexia (≤36%), weight gain (5% to 32%), dyspepsia (11% to 27%), constipation (9% to 16%)
- Hematologic: Hemorrhage (12% to 53%; grades 3/4: 2% to 19%), neutropenia (grade 3: 7% to 27%; grade 4: 3% to 48%), thrombocytopenia (grade 3: 1% to 31%; grade 4: <1% to 33%), anemia (grade 3: 1% to 42%; grade 4: 1% to 11%), leukopenia (GIST 5% to 20%)
- Hepatic: ALT increased (≤17%; grade 3: 2% to 7%; grade 4: <3%), hepatotoxicity (6% to 12%; grades 3/4: 3% to 8%)
- Neuromuscular & skeletal: Muscle cramps (16% to 62%), arthralgia (≤40%), joint pain (11% to 31%), myalgia (9% to 32%), weakness (≤21%), musculoskeletal pain (children 21%; adults 12% to 49%), rigors (10% to 12%), bone pain (≤11%)
- Ocular: Periorbital edema (DFSP 33%; MPD 29%; GIST ≤47%), lacrimation increased (DFSP 25%; GIST ≤10%)
- Renal: Serum creatinine increased (≤12%; grade 3: ≤3%; DFSP: grade 4: 8%)
- Respiratory: Nasopharyngitis (10% to 31%), cough (11% to 27%), dyspnea (≤21%), upper respiratory tract infection (3% to 21%), pharyngolaryngeal pain (7% to 18%), rhinitis (DFSP 17%), pharyngitis (CML 10% to 15%), pneumonia (CML 4% to 13%), sinusitis (4% to 11%)
- Miscellaneous: Night sweats (CML 13% to 17%), infection without neutropenia (GIST ≤17%), influenza (1% to 14%), diaphoresis (GIST ≤13%)

1% to 10%:
- Cardiovascular: Flushing
- Central nervous system: CNS/cerebral hemorrhage (≤9%), hypoesthesia
- Dermatologic: Dry skin, erythema, photosensitivity reaction
- Endocrine & metabolic: Hyperglycemia (≤10%), hypocalcemia (GIST ≤6%), albumin decreased (grade 3: ≤4%)
- Gastrointestinal: Flatulence (≤10%), stomatitis/mucositis (≤10%), weight loss (≤10%), gastrointestinal hemorrhage (2% to 8%), abdominal distension, gastritis, gastroesophageal reflux, mouth ulceration, taste disturbance, xerostomia

Hematologic: Lymphopenia (GIST ≤10%), neutropenic fever, pancytopenia
Hepatic: Alkaline phosphatase increased (grade 3: ≤6%; grade 4: <1%), AST increased (grade 3: 2% to 4%; grade 4: ≤3%), bilirubin increased (grade 3: 1% to 4%; grade 4: ≤3%)
Neuromuscular & skeletal: Back pain (GIST ≤7%), limb pain (GIST ≤7%), peripheral neuropathy, joint swelling, paresthesia
Ocular: Blurred vision, conjunctival hemorrhage, conjunctivitis, dry eyes, eyelid edema
Respiratory: Epistaxis

General Dosage Range Dosage adjustment recommended in patients with hepatic or renal impairment, on concomitant therapy, and/or who develop toxicities
Oral:
Children ≥2 years: 260-340 mg/m²/day in 1-2 divided doses (maximum: 600 mg/day)
Adults: 100-800 mg/day in 1-2 divided doses

Mechanism of Action Inhibits Bcr-Abl tyrosine kinase, the constitutive abnormal gene product of the Philadelphia chromosome in chronic myeloid leukemia (CML). Inhibition of this enzyme blocks proliferation and induces apoptosis in Bcr-Abl positive cell lines as well as in fresh leukemic cells in Philadelphia chromosome positive CML. Also inhibits tyrosine kinase for platelet-derived growth factor (PDGF), stem cell factor (SCF), c-Kit, and cellular events mediated by PDGF and SCF.

Pharmacodynamics/Kinetics
Half-life Elimination Adults: Parent drug: ~18 hours; N-desmethyl metabolite: ~40 hours; Children: Parent drug: ~15 hours
Time to Peak 2-4 hours

Pregnancy Risk Factor D

Imiglucerase (i mi GLOO ser ace)

U.S. Brand Names Cerezyme®
Canadian Brand Names Cerezyme®
Pharmacologic Category Enzyme
Use Long-term enzyme replacement therapy for patients with Type 1 Gaucher's disease
Local Anesthetic/Vasoconstrictor Precautions No information available to require special precautions
Effects on Dental Treatment No significant effects or complications reported
Effects on Bleeding No information available to require special precautions
Adverse Effects
1% to 10%: Miscellaneous: Hypersensitivity reaction (7%; symptoms may include pruritus, flushing, urticaria, angioedema, bronchospasm)
Individual frequency not defined, but <1.5%:
Cardiovascular: Tachycardia
Central nervous system: Headache, dizziness, fatigue, fever
Dermatologic: Rash, pruritus
Gastrointestinal: Nausea, abdominal discomfort, vomiting, diarrhea
Local: Injection site burning, swelling, or sterile abscess (<1%)
Neuromuscular & skeletal: Backache
Miscellaneous: Anaphylactoid reactions (<1%)

General Dosage Range I.V.: *Children ≥2 years and Adults:* Initial: 30-60 units/kg every 2 weeks; Range: 2.5 units/kg 3 times/week to 60 units/kg once weekly; Average dose: 60 units/kg every 2 weeks

Mechanism of Action Imiglucerase is an analogue of glucocerebrosidase; it is produced by recombinant DNA technology using mammalian cell culture. Glucocerebrosidase is an enzyme deficient in Gaucher's disease. It is needed to catalyze the hydrolysis of glucocerebroside to glucose and ceramide.

Pharmacodynamics/Kinetics
Half-life Elimination 3.6-10.4 minutes

Pregnancy Risk Factor C

Imipenem and Cilastatin (i mi PEN em & sye la STAT in)

U.S. Brand Names Primaxin® I.M. [DSC]; Primaxin® I.V.
Canadian Brand Names Primaxin®; Primaxin® I.V.
Pharmacologic Category Antibiotic, Carbapenem

Use Treatment of lower respiratory tract, urinary tract, intra-abdominal, gynecologic, bone and joint, skin and skin structure, and polymicrobic infections as well as bacterial septicemia and endocarditis. Antibacterial activity includes resistant gram-negative bacilli (*Pseudomonas aeruginosa* and *Enterobacter* sp), gram-positive bacteria (methicillin-sensitive *Staphylococcus aureus* and *Streptococcus* sp) and anaerobes.

Unlabeled/Investigational Use Hepatic abscess; neutropenic fever; melioidosis

Local Anesthetic/Vasoconstrictor Precautions No information available to require special precautions

Effects on Dental Treatment No significant effects or complications reported

Effects on Bleeding No information available to require special precautions

Adverse Effects Adverse reactions reported with use for both I.V. and I.M. formulations in adults, except where noted.

1% to 10%:

- Cardiovascular: Tachycardia (infants 2%; adults <1%)
- Central nervous system: Seizure (infants 6%; adults <1%)
- Dermatologic: Rash (≤1%, children 2%)
- Gastrointestinal: Nausea (1% to 2%), diarrhea (children 3% to 4%; adults 1% to 2%), vomiting (≤2%)
- Genitourinary: Oliguria/anuria (infants 2%; adults <1%)
- Local: Phlebitis/thrombophlebitis (3%), pain at I.M. injection site (1.2%)

General Dosage Range Dosage adjustment recommended in patients with renal impairment

I.M.: *Adults:* 500-750 mg every 12 hours

I.V.:

Children >3 months: 15-25 mg/kg every 6 hours (maximum: 4 g/day)

Adults 30 to <70 kg: 125 mg every 12 hours up to 1000 mg every 8 hours

Adults ≥70 kg: 250-1000 mg every 6-8 hours (maximum: 50 mg/kg/day; 4 g/day)

Mechanism of Action Inhibits bacterial cell wall synthesis by binding to one or more of the penicillin-binding proteins (PBPs); which in turn inhibits the final transpeptidation step of peptidoglycan synthesis in bacterial cell walls, thus inhibiting cell wall biosynthesis. Bacteria eventually lyse due to ongoing activity of cell wall autolytic enzymes (autolysins and murein hydrolases) while cell wall assembly is arrested. Cilastatin prevents renal metabolism of imipenem by competitive inhibition of dehydropeptidase along the brush border of the renal tubules.

Pharmacodynamics/Kinetics

Half-life Elimination I.V.: Both drugs: 60 minutes; prolonged with renal impairment; I.M.: Imipenem: 2-3 hours

Time to Peak Time to peak: I.M.: 3.5 hours

Pregnancy Risk Factor C

Imipramine (im IP ra meen)

U.S. Brand Names Tofranil-PM®; Tofranil®

Canadian Brand Names Apo-Imipramine®; Novo-Pramine; Tofranil®

Pharmacologic Category Antidepressant, Tricyclic (Tertiary Amine)

Use Treatment of depression; treatment of nocturnal enuresis in children

Unlabeled/Investigational Use Analgesic for certain chronic and neuropathic pain (including diabetic neuropathy); panic disorder; attention-deficit/hyperactivity disorder (ADHD); post-traumatic stress disorder (PTSD)

Local Anesthetic/Vasoconstrictor Precautions Use with caution; epinephrine and levonordefrin have been shown to have an increased pressor response in combination with TCAs. Imipramine is one of the drugs confirmed to prolong the QT interval and is accepted as having a risk of causing torsade de pointes. The risk of drug-induced torsade de pointes is extremely low when a single QT interval prolonging drug is prescribed. In terms of epinephrine, it is not known what effect vasoconstrictors in the local anesthetic regimen will have in patients with a known history of congenital prolonged QT interval or in patients taking any medication that prolongs the QT interval. Until more information is obtained, it is suggested that the clinician consult with the physician prior to the use of a vasoconstrictor in suspected patients, and that the vasoconstrictor (epinephrine, mepivacaine and levonordefrin [Carbocaine® 2% with Neo-Cobefrin®]) be used with caution.

Effects on Dental Treatment Key adverse event(s) related to dental treatment: Xerostomia and changes in salivation (normal salivary flow resumes upon discontinuation). Long-term treatment with TCAs, such as imipramine, increases the risk of caries by reducing salivation and salivary buffer capacity. In a study by Rundergren, et al, pathological alterations were observed in the oral mucosa of 72% of 58 patients; 55% had new carious lesions after taking TCAs for a median of 5½ years. Current research is investigating the use of the salivary stimulant pilocarpine to overcome the xerostomia from imipramine.

Effects on Bleeding No information available to require special precautions

Adverse Effects Reported for tricyclic antidepressants in general. Frequency not defined.

Cardiovascular: Arrhythmia, CHF, ECG changes, heart block, hypertension, MI, orthostatic hypotension, palpitation, stroke, tachycardia

Central nervous system: Agitation, anxiety, confusion, delusions, disorientation, dizziness, drowsiness, fatigue, hallucination, headache, hypomania, insomnia, nightmares, psychosis, restlessness, seizure

Dermatologic: Alopecia, itching, petechiae, photosensitivity, purpura, rash, urticaria

Endocrine & metabolic: Breast enlargement, galactorrhea, gynecomastia, increase or decrease in blood sugar, increase or decrease in libido, SIADH

Gastrointestinal: Abdominal cramps, anorexia, black tongue, constipation, diarrhea, epigastric disorders, ileus, nausea, stomatitis, taste disturbance, vomiting, weight gain/loss, xerostomia

Genitourinary: Impotence, testicular swelling, urinary retention

Hematologic: Agranulocytosis, eosinophilia, thrombocytopenia

Hepatic: Cholestatic jaundice, transaminases increased

Neuromuscular & skeletal: Ataxia, extrapyramidal symptoms, incoordination, numbness, paresthesia, peripheral neuropathy, tingling, tremor, weakness

Ocular: Blurred vision, disturbances of accommodation, mydriasis

Otic: Tinnitus

Miscellaneous: Diaphoresis, falling, hypersensitivity (eg, drug fever, edema)

General Dosage Range Oral:

Children ≥6-12 years: Initial: 25 mg at bedtime, may increase to 50 mg at bedtime if no response (maximum: 2.5 mg/kg/day; 50 mg/day)

Children >12 years: Initial: 25 mg at bedtime, may increase to 75 mg at bedtime if not response (maximum: 75 mg/day) **or** 30-40 mg/day, increase gradually, to a maximum of 100 mg/day in single or divided doses

Adults: Initial: 75-150 mg/day, increase gradually to a maximum of 200 mg/day (outpatients) or 300 mg/day (inpatients) in divided doses or a single dose at bedtime

Elderly: Initial: 25-50 mg at bedtime (maximum: 100 mg/day)

Mechanism of Action Traditionally believed to increase the synaptic concentration of serotonin and/or norepinephrine in the central nervous system by inhibition of their reuptake by the presynaptic neuronal membrane. However, additional receptor effects have been found including desensitization of adenyl cyclase, down regulation of beta-adrenergic receptors, and down regulation of serotonin receptors.

Pharmacodynamics/Kinetics

Onset of Action Peak antidepressant effect: Usually after ≥2 weeks

Half-life Elimination 6-18 hours

Dental Comment Imipramine is known to prolong the QT interval. The QT interval is measured as the time and distance between the Q point of the QRS complex and the end of the T wave in the ECG tracing. After adjustment for heart rate, the QT interval is defined as prolonged if it is more than 450 msec in men and 460 msec in women. A long QT syndrome was first described in the 1950s and 60s as a congenital syndrome involving QT interval prolongation and syncope and sudden death. Some of the congenital long QT syndromes were characterized by a peculiar electrocardiographic appearance of the QRS complex involving a premature atria beat followed by a pause, then a subsequent sinus beat showing marked QT prolongation and deformity. This type of cardiac arrhythmia was originally termed "torsade de pointes" (translated from the French as "twisting of the points"). Imipramine is considered as having a risk of causing torsade de pointes. Since it is not known what effect vasoconstrictors in the local anesthetic regimen will have in patients with a known history of congenital prolonged QT interval or in patients taking any medication that prolongs the QT interval, a medical consult is suggested.

Imiquimod (i mi KWI mod)

Related Information

Management of Patients Undergoing Cancer Therapy *on page 1970*

Systemic Viral Diseases *on page 1904*

Viral Infections *on page 1947*

U.S. Brand Names Aldara®; Zyclara™

Canadian Brand Names Aldara®; Zyclara™

Generic Availability (U.S.) Yes

Pharmacologic Category Skin and Mucous Membrane Agent; Topical Skin Product

Use Treatment of external genital and perianal warts/condyloma acuminata; non-hyperkeratotic actinic keratosis on face or scalp; superficial basal cell carcinoma (sBCC) with a maximum tumor diameter of 2 cm located on the trunk, neck, or extremities (excluding hands or feet)

Unlabeled/Investigational Use Treatment of common warts

Local Anesthetic/Vasoconstrictor Precautions No information available to require special precautions

Effects on Dental Treatment No significant effects or complications reported

Effects on Bleeding No information available to require special precautions

Adverse Effects Note: Frequency may depend on indication/formulation.

>10%:

Local: Application site reactions are common. Frequency of reactions vary, and are related to the degree of inflammation associated with the treated disease, number of weekly applications, and individual sensitivity.

Burning, edema, erosion/ulceration, erythema, excoriation, flaking, induration, itching, scabbing/crusting, scaling/dryness, vesicles, weeping/exudate

Respiratory: Upper respiratory infection

Miscellaneous: Fungal infection

1% to 10%:

Cardiovascular: Chest pain

Central nervous system: Anxiety, dizziness, fatigue, fever, headache, pain

Dermatologic: Alopecia, eczema, seborrhoeic keratosis

Endocrine & metabolic: Blood glucose increased

Gastrointestinal: Anorexia, diarrhea, dyspepsia, nausea, vomiting

Genitourinary: Urinary tract infection

Local: Bleeding, hypopigmentation, infection, irritation, pain, papule, paresthesia, pruritus, rash, scar, sensitivity, soreness, stinging, tenderness

Neuromuscular & skeletal: Back pain, myalgia, rigors

Respiratory: Coughing, pharyngitis, rhinitis, sinusitis

Miscellaneous: Herpes simplex, influenza-like syndrome, lymphadenopathy, squamous cell carcinoma, tinea cruris

Dosage Topical: **Note:** A rest period of several days may be taken if required by the patient's discomfort or severity of the local skin reaction. Treatment may resume once the reaction subsides. Imiquimod treatment should not be prolonged beyond recommended period due to missed doses or rest periods.

Children ≥12 years and Adults (Aldara®): External genital and/or perianal warts/condyloma acuminata: Apply a thin layer 3 times/week prior to bedtime and leave on skin for 6-10 hours. Remove with mild soap and water. Examples of 3 times/week application schedules are: Monday, Wednesday, Friday; or Tuesday, Thursday, Saturday. Continue treatment until there is total clearance of the warts (maximum duration of therapy: 16 weeks).

Adults:

Aldara®:

Actinic keratosis: Apply twice weekly for 16 weeks to a treatment area on face or scalp (but not both concurrently); no more than 1 packet should be applied at each application and no more than 36 packets applied per 16 weeks; apply prior to bedtime and leave on skin for 8 hours. Remove with mild soap and water.

Common oral warts (dental use; unlabeled use): Apply once daily prior to bedtime

Common warts (unlabeled use): Apply once daily prior to bedtime for 5 days/week for up to 16 weeks (Hengge, 2000) or apply twice daily for up to 24 weeks (Grussendorf-Conen, 2002)

Superficial basal cell carcinoma: Apply once daily prior to bedtime, 5 days/week for 6 weeks. No more than 36 packets should be used during the 6-week treatment period. Treatment area should include a 1 cm margin of skin around the tumor. Leave on skin for 8 hours. Remove with mild soap and water.

Zyclara™: Actinic keratosis: Treatment consists of 2 cycles (14 days each) separated by 1 rest period (14 days) with no treatment. Apply up to 2 packets once daily at bedtime to affected area on either face or balding scalp (but not both concurrently); apply no more than 2 packets at each application and no more than 56 packets per 2 cycles of treatment. Leave on skin for 8 hours. Remove with mild soap and water. **Note:** Canadian labeling recommends avoiding application to areas larger than the face or balding scalp (~200 cm^2).

Mechanism of Action Precise mechanism of action is unknown; Toll-like receptor 7 agonist that induces cytokines, including interferon-alpha and others

Contraindications There are no contraindications listed within the approved manufacturer's labeling.

Canadian labeling (not in U.S. labeling): Hypersensitivity to imiquimod or any component of the formulation

Warnings/Precautions Imiquimod is not intended for oral, nasal, intravaginal, or ophthalmic use. Topical imiquimod administration is not recommended until tissue is healed from any previous drug or surgical treatment. Treatment should not be prolonged beyond recommended period due to missed doses or rest periods. Imiquimod has the potential to exacerbate inflammatory conditions of the skin (including chronic graft-versus-host disease). Intense inflammatory reactions may occur, and may be accompanied by systemic symptoms (fever, malaise, myalgia); interruption of therapy should be considered. May increase sunburn susceptibility; patients should protect themselves from the sun and artificial forms of sunlight. Safety and efficacy have not been established for immunosuppressed patients, or for basal cell nevus syndrome or xeroderma pigmentosum. Safety and efficacy of Zyclara™ have not been established in children <18 years of age. Safety and efficacy of Aldara® have not been established in children <12 years of age; following 2 randomized, double-blind, placebo-controlled trials, efficacy was not established for molluscum contagiosum in children 2-12 years of age. Use with caution in patients with pre-existing autoimmune disorders (onset or exacerbation of disease has been reported rarely with imiquimod).

Basal cell carcinoma: Use in basal cell carcinoma should be limited to superficial carcinomas with a maximum diameter of 2 cm. Safety and efficacy in treatment of sBCC lesions of the face, head, and anogenital area, or other subtypes of basal cell carcinoma (including nodular and morpheaform), have not been established.

Actinic keratosis: Treatment should be limited to areas ≤25 cm^2 (Aldara®) or <200 cm^2 (Zyclara™). Safety and efficacy of repeated use of Aldara® or Zyclara™ in a previously treated area have not been established. Prescribed course of therapy should be completed even if all lesions appear to be gone.

Genital warts: Safety and efficacy of Zyclara™ in the treatment of external genital warts have not been established. Imiquimod has not been evaluated for the treatment of urethral, intravaginal, cervical, rectal, or intra-anal human papilloma viral disease and is not recommended for these conditions.

Drug Interactions

Metabolism/Transport Effects Substrate (minor) of CYP1A2, 3A4

Avoid Concomitant Use

Avoid concomitant use of Imiquimod with any of the following: BCG; Natalizumab; Pimecrolimus; Roflumilast; Tacrolimus (Topical); Vaccines (Live)

Increased Effect/Toxicity

Imiquimod may increase the levels/effects of: Leflunomide; Natalizumab; Vaccines (Live)

The levels/effects of Imiquimod may be increased by: Conivaptan; Denosumab; Pimecrolimus; Roflumilast; Tacrolimus (Topical); Trastuzumab

Decreased Effect

Imiquimod may decrease the levels/effects of: BCG; Sipuleucel-T; Vaccines (Inactivated); Vaccines (Live)

The levels/effects of Imiquimod may be decreased by: Echinacea; Tocilizumab

Pharmacodynamics/Kinetics

Time to Peak 9 hours

Pregnancy Risk Factor C

Lactation Excretion in breast milk unknown/use caution

Dosage Forms

Cream, topical: 5% (24s)

Aldara®: 5% (24s)

Zyclara™: 3.75% (28s)

Dental Comment Imiquimod cream 5% has been used for actinic cheilitis or keratosis. Imiquimod 3.75% cream is FDA approved to treat actinic keratosis. Adverse events of erosion/ulcerations have been reported with topical use. Imiquimod use in the treatment of oral papilloma virus remains inadequately studied.

Immune Globulin (i MYUN GLOB yoo lin)

Related Information

Systemic Viral Diseases *on page* 1904

U.S. Brand Names Carimune® NF; Flebogamma® DIF; Flebogamma® [DSC]; GamaSTAN™ S/D; Gammagard S/D®; Gammagard® Liquid; Gammaplex®; Gamunex®; Gamunex®-C; Hizentra®; Octagam®; Privigen®; Vivaglobin® [DSC]

Canadian Brand Names BayGam®; Gamimune® N; Gammagard Liquid; Gammagard S/D; Gamunex®; IGIVnex®; Privigen®; Vivaglobin®

Generic Availability (U.S.) No

Pharmacologic Category Blood Product Derivative; Immune Globulin

Use

Treatment of primary humoral immunodeficiency syndromes (congenital agammaglobulinemia, severe combined immunodeficiency syndromes [SCIDS], common variable immunodeficiency, X-linked immunodeficiency, Wiskott-Aldrich syndrome) (Carimune® NF, Flebogamma® DIF, Gammagard® Liquid, Gammagard S/D®, Gammaplex®, Gamunex®, Gamunex®-C, Hizentra®, Octagam®, Privigen®, Vivaglobin®)

Treatment of acute and chronic immune (idiopathic) thrombocytopenic purpura (ITP) (Carimune® NF, Gammagard S/D®, Gamunex®, Gamunex®-C, Privigen® [chronic only])

Treatment of chronic inflammatory demyelinating polyneuropathy (CIDP) (Gamunex®, Gamunex®-C)

Prevention of coronary artery aneurysms associated with Kawasaki syndrome (in combination with aspirin) (Gammagard S/D®)

Prevention of bacterial infection in patients with hypogammaglobulinemia and/or recurrent bacterial infections with B-cell chronic lymphocytic leukemia (CLL) (Gammagard S/D®)

Prevention of serious infection in immunoglobulin deficiency (select agammaglobulinemias) (GamaSTAN™ S/D)

Provision of passive immunity in the following susceptible individuals (GamaSTAN™ S/D):

Hepatitis A: Pre-exposure prophylaxis; postexposure: within 14 days and/or prior to manifestation of disease

Measles: For use within 6 days of exposure in an unvaccinated person, who has not previously had measles

Rubella: Postexposure prophylaxis (within 72 hours) to reduce the risk of infection and fetal damage in exposed pregnant women who will not consider therapeutic abortion

Varicella: For immunosuppressed patients when varicella zoster immune globulin is not available

Unlabeled/Investigational Use Acquired hypogammaglobulinemia secondary to malignancy; Guillain-Barré syndrome; hematopoietic stem cell transplantation (HSCT), to prevent bacterial infections among allogeneic recipients with severe hypogammaglobulinemia (IgG <400 mg/dL) at <100 days post transplant (CDC guidelines); HIV-associated thrombocytopenia; multiple sclerosis (relapsing, remitting when other therapies cannot be used); myasthenia gravis; refractory dermatomyositis/polymyositis

Local Anesthetic/Vasoconstrictor Precautions No information available to require special precautions

Effects on Dental Treatment No significant effects or complications reported

Effects on Bleeding No information available to require special precautions

Adverse Effects Frequency not defined.

Cardiovascular: Angioedema, chest tightness, edema, flushing of the face, hyper-/hypotension, palpitation, tachycardia

Central nervous system: Anxiety, aseptic meningitis syndrome, chills, dizziness, drowsiness, fatigue, fever, headache, irritability, lethargy, lightheadedness, malaise, migraine, pain

Dermatologic: Bruising, contact dermatitis, eczema, erythema, hyperhidrosis, petechiae, pruritus, purpura, rash, urticaria

Gastrointestinal: Abdominal cramps, abdominal pain, diarrhea, discomfort, dyspepsia, gastroenteritis, nausea, sore throat, toothache, vomiting

Hematologic: Anemia, autoimmune hemolytic anemia, hematocrit decreased, hemolysis (mild), hemorrhage, thrombocytopenia

Hepatic: Bilirubin increased, LDH increased, liver function test increased

Local: Muscle stiffness at I.M. site, pain or irritation at the infusion site

Neuromuscular & skeletal: Arthralgia, back or hip pain, leg cramps, muscle cramps, myalgia, neck pain, rigors, weakness

Ocular: Conjunctivitis

Otic: Ear pain

Renal: Acute renal failure, acute tubular necrosis, anuria, BUN increased, creatinine increased, oliguria, proximal tubular nephropathy, osmotic nephrosis

Respiratory: Asthma aggravated, bronchitis, cough, dyspnea, epistaxis, nasal congestion, pharyngeal pain, pharyngitis, rhinitis, rhinorrhea, sinus headache, sinusitis, upper respiratory infection, wheezing

Miscellaneous: Anaphylaxis, diaphoresis, flu-like syndrome, hypersensitivity reactions, infusion reaction, thermal burn

Dosage According to manufacturer product labeling, intravenous formulations are for intravenous administration only. However, some clinicians may administer intravenous formulations as a subcutaneous infusion based on clinical judgment and patient tolerability. Some clinicians dose IVIG on ideal body weight or an adjusted ideal body weight in morbidly-obese patients (Siegel, 2010).

Children and Adults:

B-cell chronic lymphocytic leukemia (CLL) (Gammagard S/D®): I.V.: 400 mg/kg every 3-4 weeks

Chronic inflammatory demyelinating polyneuropathy (CIDP) (Gamunex®, Gamunex-C®): I.V.: Loading dose: 2000 mg/kg (given in divided doses over 2-4 consecutive days); Maintenance: 1000 mg/kg every 3 weeks. Alternatively, administer 500 mg/kg/day for 2 consecutive days every 3 weeks.

Hepatitis A (GamaSTAN™ S/D): I.M.:

Pre-exposure prophylaxis upon travel into endemic areas (hepatitis A vaccine preferred):

0.02 mL/kg for anticipated risk of exposure <3 months

0.06 mL/kg for anticipated risk of exposure ≥3 months; repeat every 4-6 months.

Postexposure prophylaxis: 0.02 mL/kg given within 14 days of exposure and/or prior to manifestation of disease; not needed if at least 1 dose of hepatitis A vaccine was given at ≥1 month before exposure

Immunoglobulin deficiency (GamaSTAN™ S/D): I.M.: 0.66 mL/kg (minimum dose should be 100 mg/kg) every 3-4 weeks. Administer a double dose at onset of therapy; some patients may require more frequent injections.

Immune (idiopathic) thrombocytopenic purpura (ITP):

Carimune® NF: I.V.: Initial: 400 mg/kg/day for 2-5 days; Maintenance: 400 mg/kg as needed to maintain platelet count ≥30,000/mm^3 and/or to control significant bleeding; may increase dose if needed (range: 800-1000 mg/kg)

Gammagard S/D®: I.V.: 1000 mg/kg; up to 3 additional doses may be given based on patient response and/or platelet count. **Note:** Additional doses should be given on alternate days.

Gamunex®, Gamunex-C®: I.V.: 1000 mg/kg/day for 2 consecutive days (second dose may be withheld if adequate platelet response in 24 hours) **or** 400 mg/kg once daily for 5 consecutive days

Privigen®: I.V.: 1000 mg/kg/day for 2 consecutive days

Kawasaki syndrome: I.V.:

Gammagard S/D®: 1000 mg/kg as a single dose **or** 400 mg/kg/day for 4 consecutive days. Begin within 7 days of onset of fever.

AHA guidelines (2004): 2000 mg/kg as a single dose within 10 days of disease onset

Note: Must be used in combination with aspirin: 80-100 mg/kg/day orally, divided every 6 hours for up to 14 days (until fever resolves for at least 48 hours); then decrease dose to 3-5 mg/kg/day once daily. In patients without coronary artery abnormalities, give lower dose for 6-8 weeks. In patients with coronary artery abnormalities, low-dose aspirin should be continued indefinitely.

Measles:

GamaSTAN™ S/D: I.M.:

Immunocompetent: 0.25 mL/kg given within 6 days of exposure followed by live attenuated measles vaccine in 5-6 months when indicated (Watson, 1998)

Immunocompromised children: 0.5 mL/kg (maximum dose: 15 mL) immediately following exposure

Gamunex-C®, Octagam®: I.V.:

Prophylaxis in patients with primary humoral immunodeficiency (**ONLY** if routine dose is <400 mg/kg): ≥400 mg/kg immediately before expected exposure

Treatment in patients with primary immunodeficiency: 400 mg/kg administered as soon as possible after exposure

Hizentra®: SubQ infusion: Measles exposure in patients with primary humoral immunodeficiency: Weekly dose: ≥200 mg/kg for 2 consecutive weeks for patients at risk of measles exposure (eg, during an outbreak; travel to endemic area). In patients who have been exposed to measles, administer the minimum dose as soon as possible following exposure.

Primary humoral immunodeficiency disorders:

Carimune® NF: I.V.: 400-800 mg/kg every 3-4 weeks

Flebogamma® DIF, Gammagard® Liquid, Gammagard S/D®, Gamunex®, Gamunex-C®, Octagam®: I.V.: 300-600 mg/kg every 3-4 weeks; adjusted based on dosage and interval in conjunction with monitored serum IgG concentrations and clinical response

Gammaplex®: I.V.: 300-800 mg/kg every 3-4 weeks

Gamunex-C®: SubQ infusion: Begin 1 week after last I.V. dose. Use the following equation to calculate initial dose:

Initial weekly dose (grams) = [1.37 x IGIV dose (grams)] divided by [I.V. dose interval (weeks)]

Note: For subsequent dose adjustments, refer to product labeling.

Hizentra®: SubQ infusion: Begin 1 week after last I.V. dose. Use the following equation to calculate initial dose:
Initial weekly dose (grams) = [1.53 x IGIV dose (grams)] divided by [I.V. dose interval (weeks)]
Note: For subsequent dose adjustments, refer to product labeling.
Privigen®: I.V.: 200-800 mg/kg every 3-4 weeks; adjusted based on dosage and interval in conjunction with monitored serum IgG concentrations and clinical response
Vivaglobin®: SubQ infusion: Begin 1 week after last I.V. dose; **Note:** Patient should have received an I.V. immune globulin routinely for at least 3 months before switching to SubQ. Use the following equation to calculate initial dose:
Initial weekly dose (grams) = [1.37 x IGIV dose (grams)] divided by [I.V. dose interval (weeks)]
Note: For subsequent dose adjustments, refer to product labeling.
Rubella (GamaSTAN™ S/D): I.M.: Prophylaxis during pregnancy: 0.55 mL/kg within 72 hours of exposure (Watson, 1998)
Varicella (GamaSTAN™ S/D): I.M.: Prophylaxis: 0.6-1.2 mL/kg (varicella zoster immune globulin preferred) within 72 hours of exposure

Unlabeled uses: I.V.:
Acquired hypogammaglobulinemia secondary to malignancy (unlabeled use): Adults: 400 mg/kg/dose every 3 weeks; reevaluate every 4-6 months (Anderson, 2007)
Guillain-Barré syndrome (unlabeled use): Children and Adults: Various regimens have been used, including:
400 mg/kg/day for 5 days (Hughes, 2003)
or
2000 mg/kg in divided doses administered over 2-5 days (Feasby, 2007)
Hematopoietic stem cell transplantation with hypogammaglobulinemia (CDC guidelines, 2000; unlabeled use):
Children: 400 mg/kg per month; increase dose or frequency to maintain IgG levels >400 mg/dL
Adolescents and Adults: 500 mg/kg/week
HIV-associated thrombocytopenia (unlabeled use): Adults: 1000 mg/kg/day for 2 days (Anderson, 2007)
Multiple sclerosis (relapsing-remitting, when other therapies cannot be used) (unlabeled use): Children and Adults: 1000 mg/kg per month, with or without an induction of 400 mg/kg/day for 5 days (Feasby, 2007)
Myasthenia gravis (severe exacerbation) (unlabeled use): Children and Adults: Total dose of 2000 mg/kg over 2-5 days (Feasby, 2007)
Refractory dermatomyositis/polymyositis (unlabeled uses): Children and Adults: 2000 mg/kg per treatment course administered over 2-5 days (Feasby, 2007)

Dosing adjustment/comments in renal impairment: I.V.: Cl_{cr} <10 mL/minute: Avoid use; in patients at risk of renal dysfunction, consider infusion at a rate less than maximum.

Mechanism of Action Replacement therapy for primary and secondary immunodeficiencies, and IgG antibodies against bacteria, viral, parasitic and mycoplasma antigens; interference with F_c receptors on the cells of the reticuloendothelial system for autoimmune cytopenias and ITP; provides passive immunity by increasing the antibody titer and antigen-antibody reaction potential

Contraindications Hypersensitivity to immune globulin or any component of the formulation; selective IgA deficiency; hyperprolinemia (Hizentra®, Privigen®); severe thrombocytopenia or coagulation disorders; severe thrombocytopenia or coagulation disorders where IM injections are contraindicated

Warnings/Precautions [U.S. Boxed Warning]: I.V. formulation only: Acute renal dysfunction (increased serum creatinine, oliguria, acute renal failure, osmotic nephrosis) can rarely occur; usually within 7 days of use (more likely with products stabilized with sucrose). Use with caution in the elderly, patients with renal disease, diabetes mellitus, volume depletion, sepsis, paraproteinemia, and nephrotoxic medications due to risk of renal dysfunction. In patients at risk of renal dysfunction, the rate of infusion and concentration of solution should be minimized. Discontinue if renal function deteriorates. High-dose regimens (1 g/kg for 1-2 days) are not recommended for individuals with fluid overload or where fluid volume may be of concern. Hypersensitivity and anaphylactic reactions can occur; a severe fall in blood pressure may rarely occur with anaphylactic reaction; immediate treatment (including epinephrine 1:1000) should be available. Product of human plasma; may potentially contain infectious agents which could transmit disease. Screening of donors, as well as testing and/or inactivation or removal of certain viruses, reduces the risk. Infections thought to be transmitted by this product should be reported to the manufacturer. Aseptic meningitis may occur with high doses (≥1-2 g/kg [product-dependent]) and/or rapid infusion; syndrome usually appears within several hours to 2 days following treatment; usually resolves within several days after IVIG is discontinued; patients with a migraine history may be at higher risk for AMS. Increased risk of hypersensitivity, especially in patients with anti-IgA antibodies. Increased risk of hematoma formation when administered subcutaneously for the treatment of ITP.

Intravenous immune globulin has been associated with antiglobulin hemolysis; monitor for signs of hemolytic anemia. Patients should be adequately hydrated prior to initiation of therapy. Hyperproteinemia, increased serum viscosity and hyponatremia may occur; distinguish hyponatremia from pseudohyponatremia to prevent volume depletion, a further increase in serum viscosity, and a higher risk of thrombotic events. Use caution in patients with a history of thrombotic events or a history of atherosclerosis or cardiovascular disease or patients with known/suspected hyperviscosity; there is clinical evidence of a possible association between thrombotic events and administration of intravenous immune globulin and subcutaneous immune globulin. Consider a baseline assessment of blood viscosity in patients at risk for hyperviscosity. Patients should be monitored for adverse events during and after the infusion. Stop administration with signs of infusion reaction (fever, chills, nausea, vomiting, and rarely shock). Risk may be increased with initial treatment, when switching brands of immune globulin, and with treatment interruptions of >8 weeks. Monitor for transfusion-related acute lung injury (TRALI); noncardiogenic pulmonary edema has been reported with intravenous immune globulin use. TRALI is characterized by severe respiratory distress, pulmonary edema, hypoxemia, and fever (in the presence of normal left ventricular function) and usually occurs within 1-6 hours after infusion. Response to live vaccinations may be impaired. Some clinicians may administer intravenous immune globulin products as a subcutaneous infusion based on patient tolerability and clinical judgement. SubQ infusion should begin 1 week after the last I.V. dose; dose should be individualized based on clinical response and serum IgG trough concentrations; consider premedicating with acetaminophen and diphenhydramine.

Some products may contain maltose, which may result in falsely-elevated blood glucose readings; maltose-containing products are contraindicated in patients with an allergy to corn. Some products may contain polysorbate 80, sodium, and/or sucrose. Some products may contain sorbitol; do not use in patients with fructose intolerance. Hizentra® and Privigen® contain the stabilizer L-proline and are contraindicated in patients with hyperprolinemia. Packaging of some products may contain natural latex/natural rubber; skin testing should not be performed with GamaSTAN™ S/D as local irritation can occur and be misinterpreted as a positive reaction.

Drug Interactions

Avoid Concomitant Use There are no known interactions where it is recommended to avoid concomitant use.

Increased Effect/Toxicity There are no known significant interactions involving an increase in effect.

Decreased Effect

Immune Globulin may decrease the levels/effects of: Vaccines (Live)

Dietary Considerations Some products may contain sodium.

Pharmacodynamics/Kinetics

Onset of Action I.V.: Provides immediate antibody levels

Duration of Action I.M., I.V.: Immune effects: 3-4 weeks (variable)

Half-life Elimination I.M.: ~23 days; I.V.: IgG (variable among patients): Healthy subjects: 14-24 days; Patients with congenital humoral immunodeficiencies: 26-40 days; hypermetabolism associated with fever and infection have coincided with a shortened half-life

Time to Peak

Plasma: SubQ: Hizentra®: 2.9 days; Vivaglobin®: 2.5 days

Serum: I.M.: ~48 hours

Pregnancy Risk Factor C

Lactation Excretion in breast milk unknown/use caution

Dosage Forms

Injection, powder for reconstitution [preservative free]:

Carimune® NF: 3 g, 6 g, 12 g

Gammagard S/D®: 2.5 g, 5 g, 10 g

Injection, solution [preservative free]:

Flebogamma® DIF: 5% [50 mg/mL] (10 mL, 50 mL, 100 mL, 200 mL, 400 mL); 10% [100 mg/mL] (100 mL, 200 mL)

GamaSTAN™ S/D: 15% to 18% (2 mL, 10 mL)

Gammagard® Liquid: 10% [100 mg/mL] (10 mL, 25 mL, 50 mL, 100 mL, 200 mL)

Gammaplex®: 5% [50 mg/mL] (50 mL, 100 mL, 200 mL)

Gamunex®: 10% [100 mg/mL] (10 mL, 25 mL, 50 mL, 100 mL, 200 mL)
Gamunex®-C: 10% [100 mg/mL] (10 mL, 25 mL, 50 mL, 100 mL, 200 mL)
Hizentra®: 200 mg/mL (5 mL, 10 mL, 20 mL)
Octagam®: 5% [50 mg/mL] (20 mL, 50 mL, 100 mL, 200 mL)
Privigen®: 10% [100 mg/mL] (50 mL, 100 mL, 200 mL)

Inamrinone (eye NAM ri none)

Related Information
Cardiovascular Diseases *on page 1848*

Pharmacologic Category Phosphodiesterase Enzyme Inhibitor

Use Short-term therapy in patients with intractable heart failure

Local Anesthetic/Vasoconstrictor Precautions No information available to require special precautions

Effects on Dental Treatment No significant effects or complications reported

Effects on Bleeding No information available to require special precautions

Adverse Effects 1% to 10%:
Cardiovascular: Arrhythmias (3%; especially in high-risk patients), hypotension (1% to 2%; dose related)
Gastrointestinal: Nausea (1% to 2%), vomiting (1%)
Hematologic: Thrombocytopenia (~2%; dose related)

General Dosage Range Dosage adjustment recommended in patients with renal impairment
I.V.: *Adults:* Bolus: 0.75 mg/kg; may repeat; Infusion: 5-10 mcg/kg/minute

Mechanism of Action Inhibits myocardial cyclic adenosine monophosphate (cAMP) phosphodiesterase activity and increases cellular levels of cAMP resulting in a positive inotropic effect and increased cardiac output; also possesses systemic and pulmonary vasodilator effects resulting in pre- and afterload reduction; slightly increases atrioventricular conduction

Pharmacodynamics/Kinetics
Onset of Action I.V.: 2-5 minutes; Peak effect: ~10 minutes
Duration of Action Dose dependent: Low dose: ~30 minutes; Higher doses: ~2 hours
Half-life Elimination Serum: Adults: Healthy volunteers: 3.6 hours, Congestive heart failure: 5.8 hours

Pregnancy Risk Factor C

IncobotulinumtoxinA (in kuh BOT yoo lin num TOKS in aye)

U.S. Brand Names Xeomin®

Canadian Brand Names Xeomin®

Generic Availability (U.S.) No

Pharmacologic Category Neuromuscular Blocker Agent, Toxin; Ophthalmic Agent, Toxin

Use Treatment of blepharospasm in patients previously treated with onabotulinumtoxinA (Botox®); treatment of cervical dystonia in botulinum toxin-naïve and previously treated patients

Canadian labeling: Treatment of blepharospasm, poststroke spasticity of upper limb(s), or cervical dystonia (spasmodic torticollis)

Local Anesthetic/Vasoconstrictor Precautions No information available to require special precautions

Effects on Dental Treatment Key adverse event(s) related to dental treatment: Xerostomia (normal salivary flow resumes upon discontinuation).

Effects on Bleeding No information available to require special precautions

Adverse Effects
>10%:
Gastrointestinal: Dysphagia (cervical dystonia 13% to 18%), xerostomia (blepharospasm 16%)
Neuromuscular & skeletal: Muscular weakness (cervical dystonia 7% to 11%), neck pain (cervical dystonia 7% to 15%)
Ocular: Eyelid ptosis (blepharospasm 19%), dry eye (blepharospasm 16%), vision impaired (blepharospasm 12%)
1% to 10%:
Central nervous system: Headache (blepharospasm 7%), poststroke spasticity (Canadian labeling: 1%)
Gastrointestinal: Diarrhea (blepharospasm 8%)
Local: Injection site pain (cervical dystonia 4% to 9%)
Neuromuscular & skeletal: Pain (cervical dystonia 4% to 7%)

Respiratory: Dyspnea (blepharospasm 5%), nasopharyngitis (blepharospasm 5%), respiratory tract infection (blepharospasm 5%)

Miscellaneous: Neutralizing antibody formation (1%)

<1%, postmarketing and/or case reports: Any indication: Abdominal distension, abnormal dreams, allergic dermatitis, allergic reactions, alopecia, anaphylaxis, asthma, aspiration pneumonia, blurred vision, cardiovascular insufficiency, circulatory collapse, colitis, conjunctivitis, corneal perforation, cough, diaphoresis, diplopia, dysarthria, dysphonia, edema, erythema, eye edema, eye pain, eyelid ecchymosis, eyelid edema, fatigue, herpes zoster, hypersensitivity, injection site inflammation, injection site reaction, lymphadenopathy, madarosis, muscle spasm, myalgia, nausea, paresthesia, peripheral edema, pruritus, rash, reduced blinking leading to corneal ulceration, respiratory failure, serum sickness, soft tissue edema, somnolence, tremor, trismus, urinary incontinence, urticaria, vomiting, weakness

Dosage I.M.: Adults:

Blepharospasm:

U.S. labeling: Initial: Total dose should be the same as previously administered onabotulinumtoxinA dose. If prior onabotulinumtoxinA dose is not known: 1.25-2.5 units/injection site (maximum initial dose: 35 units/eye or 70 units/both eyes). Number and location of injection sites based on disease severity and previous dose/response to onabotulinumtoxinA (in clinical trials, a mean number of 6 injections per eye were administered). Cumulative dose should not exceed 35 units/eye or 70 units/both eyes administered no more frequently than every 3 months.

Canadian labeling: Initial: 1.25-2.5 units/injection site (maximum initial dose: 25 units/eye). Dose may be increased up to twice the previous dose if the response from the initial dose lasted ≤2 months; maximum dose per site: 5 units. Cumulative dose should not exceed 35 units/eye or 70 units/both eyes administered no more frequently than every 3 months.

Cervical dystonia:

U.S. labeling: Initial total dose: 120 units (in clinical trials, similar efficacy was noted with initial total doses of 120 and 240 units and between treatment experienced and treatment naïve patients). Dose and number of injection sites should be individualized based on prior treatment, response, duration of effect, adverse events, number/location of muscle(s) to be treated and disease severity. In clinical trials most patients received a total of 2-10 injections into treated muscles. Administer no more frequently than every 3 months

Canadian labeling: Usual total dose: 200 units (maximum: 300 units; maximum dose per injection site: 50 units); administer no more frequently than every 3 months

Spasticity of upper limb (poststroke): Canadian labeling (not in U.S. labeling): Individualize dose based on patient size, extent, and location of muscle involvement, degree of spasticity, local muscle weakness, and response to prior treatment. In clinical trials, total doses up to 400 units were administered as separate injections typically divided among selected muscles; may repeat therapy at ≥3 months with appropriate dosage based upon the clinical condition of patient at time of retreatment.

Suggested guidelines for the treatment of stroke-related upper limb spasticity: **Note:** The lowest recommended starting dose should be used. Dosage and number of injection sites should be individualized. Multiple injections may minimize adverse effects. Dose listed is total dose administered to site:

Biceps: 80 units
Brachialis: 50 units
Brachioradialis: 60 units
Flexor carpi radialis: 50 units
Flexor carpi ulnaris: 40 units
Flexor digitorum profundus: 40 units
Flexor digitorum superficialis: 40 units
Adductor pollicis: 10 units
Flexor pollicis brevis: 10 units
Flexor pollicis longus: 20 units
Pronator quadratus 25 units
Pronator teres: 40 units

Elderly: Initiate therapy at lowest recommended dose and titrate upward cautiously.

Dosage adjustment in renal impairment: No specific adjustment recommended

Dosage adjustment in hepatic impairment: No specific adjustment recommended

Mechanism of Action IncobotulinumtoxinA is a neurotoxin produced from Clostridium botulinum that inhibits acetylcholine release from peripheral cholinergic nerve endings. Inhibition occurs sequentially via binding and internalization of the neurotoxin into presynaptic cholinergic nerve terminals, translocation to the nerve terminal ▶

cytosol, and enzymatic cleavage of SNAP25, a protein necessary for acetylcholine release. Inhibition of acetylcholine release at the neuromuscular junction produces a state of denervation. Muscle inactivation persists until new fibrils grow from the nerve and form junction plates on new areas of the muscle-cell walls.

Contraindications Hypersensitivity to botulinum toxin, or any component of the formulation; infection at the proposed injection site(s)

Canadian labeling: Additional contraindications (not in U.S. labeling): Generalized disorders of muscle activity (eg, myasthenia gravis, Lambert-Eaton syndrome)

Warnings/Precautions [U.S. Boxed Warning]: Distant spread of botulinum toxin beyond the site of injection has been reported; dysphagia and breathing difficulties have occurred and may be life threatening; other symptoms reported include blurred vision, diplopia, dysarthria, dysphonia, generalized muscle weakness, ptosis, and urinary incontinence which may develop within hours or weeks following injection. Risk likely greatest in children treated for the unapproved use of spasticity. Systemic effects have occurred following use in approved and unapproved uses, including low doses. Use caution in patients with underlying conditions which may predispose them to these symptoms. Immediate medical attention required if respiratory, speech, or swallowing difficulties appear. Higher doses, more frequent administration, or young age at disease onset may result in neutralizing antibody formation and loss of efficacy. Use caution in patients with bleeding disorders and/or receiving anticoagulation therapy. May impair ability to drive and/or operate machinery; if loss of strength, muscle weakness, or impaired vision occurs, patients should avoid driving or engaging in other hazardous activities.

Product contains albumin and may carry a remote risk of virus transmission. Use caution if there is excessive weakness or atrophy at the proposed injection site(s); use is contraindicated if infection is present at injection site. Have appropriate support in case of anaphylactic reaction. Use with caution in patients with neuromuscular diseases (such as myasthenia gravis or Lambert-Eaton syndrome [contraindicated in Canadian labeling]), neuropathic disorders (such as amyotrophic lateral sclerosis), patients taking aminoglycosides, neuromuscular-blocking agents, or other drugs that interfere with neuromuscular transmission and patients with pre-existing cardiovascular disease (rare reports of arrhythmia and MI). Long-term effects of chronic therapy are unknown. Botulinum products (abobotulinumtoxinA, incobotulinumtoxinA, onabotulinumtoxinA, rimabotulinumtoxinB) are not interchangeable; potency units are specific to each preparation and cannot be compared or converted to any other botulinum product.

Cervical dystonia: Dysphagia is common and may occur within hours to weeks and persist for several months after administration. If severe, alternative feeding methods may be required. Risk factors include smaller neck muscle mass or bilateral injections into the sternocleidomastoid muscle. Use extreme caution in patients with pre-existing respiratory disease; may weaken accessory muscles that are necessary for these patients to maintain adequate ventilation. Risk of aspiration resulting from severe dysphagia is increased in patients with decreased respiratory function.

Ocular disease: Blepharospasm: Reduced blinking from injection of the orbicularis muscle can lead to corneal exposure and ulceration. Careful testing of corneal sensation, avoidance of lower lid injections to prevent ectropion, and treatment of epithelial defects are necessary. Soft contact lenses, application of protective drops or ointment, or covering the affected eye may help. Gentle pressure at injection site may limit bruising of eyelid. Use caution in patients with angle-closure glaucoma.

Pharmacodynamics/Kinetics

Onset of Action Improvement: ~4-7 days

Duration of Action ~3-4 months

Pregnancy Risk Factor C

Lactation Excretion in breast milk unknown/use caution

Dosage Forms

Injection, powder for reconstitution:

Xeomin®: 50 units, 100 units

Indapamide (in DAP a mide)

Related Information

Cardiovascular Diseases *on page 1848*

Canadian Brand Names Apo-Indapamide®; Dom-Indapamide; Lozide®; Lozol®; Mylan-Indapamide; Novo-Indapamide; Nu-Indapamide; PHL-Indapamide; PMS-Indapamide; PRO-Indapamide; Riva-Indapamide

Pharmacologic Category Diuretic, Thiazide-Related

Use Management of mild-to-moderate hypertension; treatment of edema in heart failure and nephrotic syndrome

Local Anesthetic/Vasoconstrictor Precautions Indapamide is one of the drugs confirmed to prolong the QT interval and is accepted as having a risk of causing torsade de pointes. The risk of drug-induced torsade de pointes is extremely low when a single QT interval prolonging drug is prescribed. In terms of epinephrine, it is not known what effect vasoconstrictors in the local anesthetic regimen will have in patients with a known history of congenital prolonged QT interval or in patients taking any medication that prolongs the QT interval. Until more information is obtained, it is suggested that the clinician consult with the physician prior to the use of a vasoconstrictor in suspected patients, and that the vasoconstrictor (epinephrine, mepivacaine and levonordefrin [Carbocaine® 2% with Neo-Cobefrin®]) be used with caution.

Effects on Dental Treatment Key adverse event(s) related to dental treatment: Orthostatic hypotension, palpitations, flushing, xerostomia (normal salivary flow resumes upon discontinuation), and rhinorrhea.

Effects on Bleeding No information available to require special precautions

Adverse Effects 1% to 10%:

Cardiovascular: Palpitation (<5%), flushing, orthostatic hypotension

Central nervous system: Headache (≥5%), nervousness (≥5%), dizziness (<5%), drowsiness (<5%), lightheadedness (<5%), restlessness (<5%), vertigo (<5%), agitation, anxiety, depression, fatigue, lassitude, lethargy, malaise

Dermatologic: Hives (<5%), pruritus (<5%), rash (<5%)

Endocrine & metabolic: Hyperglycemia (<5%), hyperuricemia (<5%)

Gastrointestinal: Abdominal pain, anorexia, bloating, constipation, cramping, diarrhea, dry mouth, gastric irritation, nausea, vomiting, weight loss

Genitourinary: Glycosuria (<5%), impotence (<5%), libido reduced (<5%), nocturia, polyuria, urinary frequency

Neuromuscular & skeletal: Weakness (≥5%), muscle cramps, spasm

Ocular: Blurred vision (<5%)

Renal: Cutaneous vasculitis (<5%), necrotizing angiitis, vasculitis

Respiratory: Rhinorrhea (<5%)

General Dosage Range Oral: *Adults:* 1.25-5 mg once daily

Mechanism of Action Diuretic effect is localized at the proximal segment of the distal tubule of the nephron; it does not appear to have significant effect on glomerular filtration rate nor renal blood flow; like other diuretics, it enhances sodium, chloride, and water excretion by interfering with the transport of sodium ions across the renal tubular epithelium

Pharmacodynamics/Kinetics

Onset of Action 1-2 hours

Duration of Action ≤36 hours

Half-life Elimination 14-18 hours

Time to Peak 2-2.5 hours

Pregnancy Risk Factor B (manufacturer); D (expert analysis)

Dental Comment Indapamide is known to prolong the QT interval. The QT interval is measured as the time and distance between the Q point of the QRS complex and the end of the T wave in the ECG tracing. After adjustment for heart rate, the QT interval is defined as prolonged if it is more than 450 msec in men and 460 msec in women. A long QT syndrome was first described in the 1950s and 60s as a congenital syndrome involving QT interval prolongation and syncope and sudden death. Some of the congenital long QT syndromes were characterized by a peculiar electrocardiographic appearance of the QRS complex involving a premature atria beat followed by a pause, then a subsequent sinus beat showing marked QT prolongation and deformity. This type of cardiac arrhythmia was originally termed "torsade de pointes" (translated from the French as "twisting of the points"). Indapamide is considered as having a risk of causing torsade de pointes. Since it is not known what effect vasoconstrictors in the local anesthetic regimen will have in patients with a known history of congenital prolonged QT interval or in patients taking any medication that prolongs the QT interval, a medical consult is suggested.

Indinavir (in DIN a veer)

Related Information

HIV Infection and AIDS *on page 1883*

Tuberculosis *on page 1902*

U.S. Brand Names Crixivan®

Canadian Brand Names Crixivan®

Pharmacologic Category Antiretroviral Agent, Protease Inhibitor

Use Treatment of HIV infection; should always be used as part of a multidrug regimen (at least three antiretroviral agents)

Local Anesthetic/Vasoconstrictor Precautions No information available to require special precautions

Effects on Dental Treatment Key adverse event(s) related to dental treatment: Abnormal taste.

Effects on Bleeding Increased bleeding has been noted with protease inhibitors in patients with hemophilia A or B. No information available to require routine special precautions relative to hemostasis in other patients.

Adverse Effects

>10%:

- Gastrointestinal: Abdominal pain (17%), nausea (12%)
- Hepatic: Hyperbilirubinemia (14%; dose dependent)
- Renal: Nephrolithiasis/urolithiasis, including flank pain with/without hematuria (29%, pediatric patients; 12% adult patients; dose dependent)

1% to 10%:

- Central nervous system: Headache (5%), dizziness (3%), somnolence (2%), fever (2%), malaise (2%), fatigue (2%)
- Dermatologic: Pruritus (4%), rash (1%)
- Endocrine & metabolic: Hyperglycemia (1%)
- Gastrointestinal: Vomiting (8%), diarrhea (3%), taste perversion (3%), acid reflux (3%), anorexia (3%), appetite increased (2%), dyspepsia (2%), serum amylase increased (2%)
- Hematologic: Neutropenia (2%), anemia (1%), thrombocytopenia (1%)
- Hepatic: Transaminases increased (4% to 5%), jaundice (2%)
- Neuromuscular & skeletal: Back pain (8%), weakness (2%)
- Renal: Dysuria (2%)
- Respiratory: Cough (2%)

General Dosage Range Dosage adjustment recommended in patients with hepatic impairment or on concomitant therapy

Oral: *Adults:* 800 mg every 8 hours; Boosted regimen: 800 mg every 12 hours

Mechanism of Action Binds to the site of HIV-1 protease activity and inhibits cleavage of viral Gag-Pol polyprotein precursors into individual functional proteins required for infectious HIV. This results in the formation of immature, noninfectious viral particles.

Pharmacodynamics/Kinetics

Half-life Elimination 1.8 ± 0.4 hour; hepatic insufficiency: 2.8 ± 0.5 hour

Time to Peak 0.8 ± 0.3 hour

Pregnancy Risk Factor C

Indocyanine Green (in doe SYE a neen green)

U.S. Brand Names IC-Green™

Pharmacologic Category Diagnostic Agent

Use Determining hepatic function, cardiac output, and liver blood flow; ophthalmic angiography

Local Anesthetic/Vasoconstrictor Precautions No information available to require special precautions

Effects on Dental Treatment No significant effects or complications reported

Effects on Bleeding No information available to require special precautions

Adverse Effects Frequency not defined.

- Central nervous system: Headache
- Dermatologic: Pruritus, urticaria
- Gastrointestinal: Feces discoloration (green)
- Miscellaneous: Anaphylactoid reactions, diaphoresis

General Dosage Range

Cardiac catheter:

Infants: 1.25 mg (maximum total dose: 2 mg/kg)

Children: 2.5 mg (maximum total dose: 2 mg/kg)

Adults: 5 mg (maximum total dose: 2 mg/kg)

I.V.: *Adults:* Hepatic function: 0.5 mg/kg; Ophthalmic angiography: ≤40 mg bolus

Pharmacodynamics/Kinetics

Half-life Elimination 2.5-3 minutes

Pregnancy Risk Factor C

Indomethacin (in doe METH a sin)

Related Information

Rheumatoid Arthritis, Osteoarthritis, and Osteoporosis *on page 1889*

Temporomandibular Dysfunction (TMD) *on page 1964*

U.S. Brand Names Indocin®; Indocin® I.V.

Canadian Brand Names Apo-Indomethacin®; Indocid® P.D.A.; Novo-Methacin; Nu-Indo; Pro-Indo; ratio-Indomethacin; Sandoz-Indomethacin

Generic Availability (U.S.) Yes: Excludes oral suspension

Pharmacologic Category Nonsteroidal Anti-inflammatory Drug (NSAID), Oral; Nonsteroidal Anti-inflammatory Drug (NSAID), Parenteral

Use Acute gouty arthritis, acute bursitis/tendonitis, moderate-to-severe osteoarthritis, rheumatoid arthritis, ankylosing spondylitis; I.V. form used as alternative to surgery for closure of patent ductus arteriosus in neonates

Unlabeled/Investigational Use Management of preterm labor

Local Anesthetic/Vasoconstrictor Precautions No information available to require special precautions

Effects on Dental Treatment The dentist should be aware of the potential of abnormal coagulation. Caution should also be exercised in the use of NSAIDs in patients already on anticoagulant therapy with drugs such as warfarin (Coumadin®). See Effects on Bleeding.

Effects on Bleeding Nonselective NSAIDs are known to reversibly decrease platelet aggregation via mechanisms different than observed with aspirin. Platelet function is restored as the drug is eliminated from the body. NSAIDs should be avoided (if possible) in general surgery patients for 3-5 half-lives of the drug (usually 1-3 days) prior to surgery to reduce the risk of excessive bleeding. However, there is no scientific evidence to warrant discontinuance of NSAIDs prior to dental surgery. In medically complicated patients or extensive oral surgery, the decision to interrupt therapy must be based on the risk to benefit in an individual patient and a medical consult is suggested. Routine interruption of NSAID therapy for most dental procedures is not warranted. If therapy is continued without interruption, the clinician should anticipate the potential for slower clotting times.

Adverse Effects

>10%: Central nervous system: Headache (12%)

1% to 10%:

Central nervous system: Dizziness (3% to 9%), depression (<3%), fatigue (<3%), malaise (<3%), somnolence (<3%), vertigo (<3%)

Gastrointestinal: Dyspepsia (3% to 9%), epigastric pain (3% to 9%), heartburn (3% to 9%), indigestion (3% to 9%), nausea (3% to 9%), abdominal pain/cramps/ distress (<3%), constipation (<3%), diarrhea (<3%), rectal irritation (suppository), tenesmus (suppository), vomiting

Otic: Tinnitus (<3%)

Dosage

Patent ductus arteriosus:

Neonates: I.V.: Initial: 0.2 mg/kg, followed by 2 doses depending on postnatal age (PNA):

PNA **at time of first dose** <48 hours: 0.1 mg/kg at 12- to 24-hour intervals

PNA **at time of first dose** 2-7 days: 0.2 mg/kg at 12- to 24-hour intervals

PNA **at time of first dose** >7 days: 0.25 mg/kg at 12- to 24-hour intervals

In general, may use 12-hour dosing interval if urine output >1 mL/kg/hour after prior dose; use 24-hour dosing interval if urine output is <1 mL/kg/hour but >0.6 mL/kg/hour; doses should be withheld if patient has oliguria (urine output <0.6 mL/kg/hour) or anuria

Inflammatory/rheumatoid disorders: Oral: Use lowest effective dose.

Children ≥2 years: 1-2 mg/kg/day in 2-4 divided doses; maximum dose: 4 mg/kg/day; not to exceed 150-200 mg/day

Adults: 25-50 mg/dose 2-3 times/day; maximum dose: 200 mg/day; extended release capsule should be given on a 1-2 times/day schedule (maximum dose for extended release: 150 mg/day). In patients with arthritis and persistent night pain and/or morning stiffness may give the larger portion (up to 100 mg) of the total daily dose at bedtime.

Bursitis/tendonitis: Oral: Adults: Initial dose: 75-150 mg/day in 3-4 divided doses **or** 1-2 divided doses for extended release; usual treatment is 7-14 days

Acute gouty arthritis: Oral: Adults: 50 mg 3 times daily until pain is tolerable then reduce dose; usual treatment <3-5 days

Elderly: Refer to adult dosing. Use lowest recommended dose and frequency in elderly to initiate therapy for indications listed in adult dosing.

Dosage adjustment in renal impairment: Not recommended in patients with advanced renal disease

Mechanism of Action Reversibly inhibits cyclooxygenase-1 and 2 (COX-1 and 2) enzymes, which results in decreased formation of prostaglandin precursors; has antipyretic, analgesic, and anti-inflammatory properties

Other proposed mechanisms not fully elucidated (and possibly contributing to the anti-inflammatory effect to varying degrees), include inhibiting chemotaxis, altering lymphocyte activity, inhibiting neutrophil aggregation/activation, and decreasing proinflammatory cytokine levels.

Contraindications Hypersensitivity to indomethacin, aspirin, other NSAIDs, or any component of the formulation; perioperative pain in the setting of coronary artery bypass graft (CABG) surgery; patients with a history of proctitis or recent rectal bleeding (suppositories)

Neonates: Necrotizing enterocolitis; impaired renal function; active bleeding (including intracranial hemorrhage and gastrointestinal bleeding), thrombocytopenia, coagulation defects; untreated infection; congenital heart disease where patent ductus arteriosus is necessary

Warnings/Precautions [U.S. Boxed Warning]: NSAIDs are associated with an increased risk of adverse cardiovascular thrombotic events, including MI and stroke. Risk may be increased with duration of use or pre-existing cardiovascular risk factors or disease. May cause new-onset hypertension or worsening of existing hypertension. Use caution with fluid retention. Avoid use in heart failure. Concurrent administration of ibuprofen, and potentially other nonselective NSAIDs, may interfere with aspirin's cardioprotective effect. **[U.S. Boxed Warning]: Use is contraindicated for treatment of perioperative pain in the setting of coronary artery bypass graft (CABG) surgery.** Risk of MI and stroke may be increased with use following CABG surgery.

Platelet adhesion and aggregation may be decreased; may prolong bleeding time; patients with coagulation disorders or who are receiving anticoagulants should be monitored closely. Anemia may occur; patients on long-term NSAID therapy should be monitored for anemia. Rarely, NSAID use may cause severe blood dyscrasias (eg, agranulocytosis, aplastic anemia, thrombocytopenia).

NSAID use may compromise existing renal function; dose-dependent decreases in prostaglandin synthesis may result from NSAID use, reducing renal blood flow which may cause renal decompensation. NSAID use may increase the risk for hyperkalemia. Patients with impaired renal function, dehydration, heart failure, liver dysfunction, those taking diuretics, and ACE inhibitors are at greater risk of renal toxicity and hyperkalemia. Rehydrate patient before starting therapy; monitor renal function closely. Not recommended for use in patients with advanced renal disease. Long-term NSAID use may result in renal papillary necrosis.

The elderly are at increased risk for adverse effects (especially peptic ulceration, CNS effects, renal toxicity) from NSAIDs even at low doses. Risk of CNS adverse events may be higher with indomethacin compared to other NSAIDs; avoid use in this age group (Beers Criteria).

[U.S. Boxed Warning]: NSAIDs may increase risk of gastrointestinal irritation, inflammation, ulceration, bleeding, and perforation. Use caution with a history of GI disease (bleeding or ulcers), concurrent therapy with aspirin, anticoagulants and/or corticosteroids, smoking, use of alcohol, the elderly or debilitated patients. When used concomitantly with ≤325 mg of aspirin, a substantial increase in the risk of gastrointestinal complications (eg, ulcer) occurs; concomitant gastroprotective therapy (eg, proton pump inhibitors) is recommended (Bhatt, 2008).

Use the lowest effective dose for the shortest duration of time, consistent with individual patient goals, to reduce risk of cardiovascular or GI adverse events. Alternate therapies should be considered for patients at high risk.

NSAIDS may cause drowsiness, dizziness, blurred vision and other neurologic effects which may impair physical or mental abilities; patients must be cautioned about performing tasks which require mental alertness (eg, operating machinery or driving). Discontinue use with blurred or diminished vision and perform ophthalmologic exam. Monitor vision with long-term therapy.

NSAIDs may cause serious skin adverse events including exfoliative dermatitis, Stevens-Johnson syndrome (SJS) and toxic epidermal necrolysis (TEN); discontinue use at first sign of skin rash or hypersensitivity. Anaphylactoid reactions may occur, even without prior exposure; patients with "aspirin triad" (bronchial asthma, aspirin intolerance, rhinitis) may be at increased risk. Do not use in patients who experience bronchospasm, asthma, rhinitis, or urticaria with NSAID or aspirin therapy. Use caution in other forms of asthma.

Use with caution in patients with decreased hepatic function. Closely monitor patients with any abnormal LFT. Severe hepatic reactions (eg, fulminant hepatitis, liver failure) have occurred with NSAID use, rarely; discontinue if signs or symptoms of liver disease develop, or if systemic manifestations occur. The elderly are at increased risk for adverse effects (especially peptic ulceration, CNS effects, renal toxicity) from NSAIDs even at low doses. Prolonged use may cause corneal deposits and retinal disturbances; discontinue if visual changes are observed. Use caution with depression, epilepsy, or Parkinson's disease.

Withhold for at least 4-6 half-lives prior to surgical or dental procedures.

Oral: Safety and efficacy have not been established in children <14 years of age. Hepatotoxicity has been reported in younger children treated for juvenile idiopathic arthritis (JIA). Closely monitor if use is needed in children ≥2 years of age.

Drug Interactions

Metabolism/Transport Effects **Substrate** (minor) of CYP2C9, 2C19; **Inhibits** CYP2C9 (strong), 2C19 (weak)

Avoid Concomitant Use

Avoid concomitant use of Indomethacin with any of the following: Ketorolac; Ketorolac (Systemic)

Increased Effect/Toxicity

Indomethacin may increase the levels/effects of: Aminoglycosides; Anticoagulants; Antiplatelet Agents; Bisphosphonate Derivatives; Collagenase (Systemic); CycloSPORINE; CycloSPORINE (Systemic); Deferasirox; Desmopressin; Digoxin; Drotrecogin Alfa; Eplerenone; Haloperidol; Ibritumomab; Lithium; Methotrexate; Nonsteroidal Anti-Inflammatory Agents; PEMEtrexed; Potassium-Sparing Diuretics; PRALAtrexate; Quinolone Antibiotics; Salicylates; Thrombolytic Agents; Tiludronate; Tositumomab and Iodine I 131 Tositumomab; Triamterene; Vancomycin; Vitamin K Antagonists

The levels/effects of Indomethacin may be increased by: ACE Inhibitors; Angiotensin II Receptor Blockers; Antidepressants (Tricyclic, Tertiary Amine); Corticosteroids (Systemic); Dasatinib; Glucosamine; Herbs (Anticoagulant/Antiplatelet Properties); Ketorolac; Ketorolac (Systemic); Nonsteroidal Anti-Inflammatory Agents; Omega-3-Acid Ethyl Esters; Pentosan Polysulfate Sodium; Pentoxifylline; Probenecid; Prostacyclin Analogues; Selective Serotonin Reuptake Inhibitors; Serotonin/Norepinephrine Reuptake Inhibitors; Treprostinil

Decreased Effect

Indomethacin may decrease the levels/effects of: ACE Inhibitors; Angiotensin II Receptor Blockers; Antiplatelet Agents; Beta-Blockers; Eplerenone; HydrALAZINE; Loop Diuretics; Potassium-Sparing Diuretics; Salicylates; Thiazide Diuretics

The levels/effects of Indomethacin may be decreased by: Bile Acid Sequestrants; Nonsteroidal Anti-Inflammatory Agents; Salicylates

Ethanol/Nutrition/Herb Interactions

Ethanol: Avoid ethanol (may enhance gastric mucosal irritation).

Food: Food may decrease the rate but not the extent of absorption. Indomethacin peak serum levels may be delayed if taken with food.

Herb/Nutraceutical: Avoid alfalfa, anise, bilberry, bladderwrack, bromelain, cat's claw, celery, chamomile, coleus, cordyceps, dong quai, evening primrose, fenugreek, feverfew, garlic, ginger, ginkgo biloba, ginseng (American, Panax, Siberian), grapeseed, green tea, guggul, horse chestnut seed, horseradish, licorice, prickly ash, red clover, reishi, SAMe (S-adenosylmethionine), sweet clover, turmeric, white willow (all have additional antiplatelet activity).

Dietary Considerations May cause GI upset; take with food or milk to minimize

Pharmacodynamics/Kinetics

Onset of Action ~30 minutes

Duration of Action 4-6 hours

Half-life Elimination 4.5 hours; prolonged with neonates

Time to Peak Oral: Immediate release: 2 hours

Pregnancy Risk Factor C

Lactation Enters breast milk/not recommended (AAP rates "compatible"; AAP 2001 update pending)

Breast-Feeding Considerations Indomethacin is excreted into breast milk and low amounts have been measured in the plasma of nursing infants. Seizures in a nursing infant were observed in one case report, although adverse events have not been noted in other cases. Breast-feeding is not recommended by the manufacturer. (The therapeutic use of indomethacin is contraindicated in neonates with significant renal failure.) Hypertensive crisis and psychiatric side effects have been noted in case reports following use of indomethacin for analgesia in postpartum women. Use with caution in nursing women with hypertensive disorders of pregnancy or preexisting renal disease.

Dosage Forms

Capsule, oral: 25 mg, 50 mg

Capsule, extended release, oral: 75 mg

Injection, powder for reconstitution: 1 mg
Indocin® I.V.: 1 mg
Suppository, rectal: 50 mg (30s)
Suspension, oral:
Indocin®: 25 mg/5 mL (237 mL)

InFLIXimab (in FLIKS e mab)

Related Information
Rheumatoid Arthritis, Osteoarthritis, and Osteoporosis *on page 1889*

U.S. Brand Names Remicade®

Canadian Brand Names Remicade®

Pharmacologic Category Antirheumatic, Disease Modifying; Gastrointestinal Agent, Miscellaneous; Immunosuppressant Agent; Monoclonal Antibody; Tumor Necrosis Factor (TNF) Blocking Agent

Use
Treatment of moderately- to severely-active rheumatoid arthritis (with methotrexate)
Treatment of moderately- to severely-active Crohn's disease with inadequate response to conventional therapy (to reduce signs/symptoms and induce and maintain clinical remission) or to reduce the number of draining enterocutaneous and rectovaginal fistulas and maintain fistula closure
Treatment of psoriatic arthritis (to reduce signs/symptoms of active arthritis and inhibit progression of structural damage and improve physical function)
Treatment of chronic severe plaque psoriasis
Treatment of active ankylosing spondylitis (reduce signs/symptoms)
Treatment of moderately- to severely-active ulcerative colitis with inadequate response to conventional therapy (reduce signs/symptoms and induce and maintain clinical remission, mucosal healing and eliminate corticosteroid use)

Local Anesthetic/Vasoconstrictor Precautions No information available to require special precautions

Effects on Dental Treatment No significant effects or complications reported

Effects on Bleeding Has been associated with thrombocytopenia as an uncommon hematologic toxicity. No information available to require routine special precautions.

Adverse Effects **Although profile is similar, frequency of adverse effects may vary with disease state. Except where noted, percentages reported in adults with rheumatoid arthritis:**

>10%:
- Central nervous system: Headache (18%)
- Gastrointestinal: Nausea (21%), diarrhea (12%), abdominal pain (12%, Crohn's 26%)
- Hepatic: ALT increased (risk increased with concomitant methotrexate)
- Respiratory: Upper respiratory tract infection (32%), sinusitis (14%), cough (12%), pharyngitis (12%)
- Miscellaneous: Development of antinuclear antibodies (~50%), infection (36%), infusion reactions (20%; severe <1%), development of antibodies to double-stranded DNA (20%), development of new abscess (Crohn's patients with fistulizing disease: 15%), anti-infliximab antibodies (variable; ~10% to 15% [range: 6% to 61%]; Mayer, 2006)

5% to 10%:
- Cardiovascular: Hypertension (7%)
- Central nervous system: Fatigue (9%), pain (8%), fever (7%)
- Dermatologic: Rash (1% to 10%), pruritus (7%)
- Gastrointestinal: Dyspepsia (10%)
- Genitourinary: Urinary tract infection (8%)
- Neuromuscular & skeletal: Arthralgia (1% to 8%), back pain (8%)
- Respiratory: Bronchitis (10%), rhinitis (8%), dyspnea (6%)
- Miscellaneous: Moniliasis (5%)

The following adverse events were reported in children with Crohn's disease and were found more frequently in children than adults:

>10%:
- Hepatic: Liver enzymes increased (18%; ≥5 times ULN: 1%)
- Hematologic: Anemia (11%)
- Miscellaneous: Infections (56%; more common with every 8-week versus every 12-week infusions)

1% to 10%:
- Central nervous system: Flushing (9%)
- Gastrointestinal: Blood in stool (10%)
- Hematologic: Leukopenia (9%), neutropenia (7%)
- Neuromuscular & skeletal: Bone fracture (7%)

Respiratory: Respiratory tract allergic reaction (6%)

Miscellaneous: Viral infection (8%), bacterial infection (6%), antibodies to infliximab (3%)

General Dosage Range Dosage adjustment is required in heart failure patients.

I.V.:

Children ≥6 years: Initial: 5 mg/kg at 0, 2, and 6 weeks; Maintenance: 5 mg/kg every 8 weeks

Adults: Initial: 3-10 mg/kg at 0, 2, and 6 weeks; Maintenance: 3-10 mg/kg every 8 weeks **or** 5 mg/kg every 6 weeks

Mechanism of Action Infliximab is a chimeric monoclonal antibody that binds to human tumor necrosis factor alpha (TNFα), thereby interfering with endogenous TNFα activity. Elevated TNFα levels have been found in involved tissues/fluids of patients with rheumatoid arthritis, ankylosing spondylitis, psoriatic arthritis, plaque psoriasis, Crohn's disease and ulcerative colitis. Biological activities of TNFα include the induction of proinflammatory cytokines (interleukins), enhancement of leukocyte migration, activation of neutrophils and eosinophils, and the induction of acute phase reactants and tissue degrading enzymes. Animal models have shown TNFα expression causes polyarthritis, and infliximab can prevent disease as well as allow diseased joints to heal.

Pharmacodynamics/Kinetics

Onset of Action Crohn's disease: ~2 weeks

Half-life Elimination 7-12 days

Pregnancy Risk Factor B

Influenza Virus Vaccine (H5N1) (in floo EN za VYE rus vak SEEN H5N1)

Pharmacologic Category Vaccine, Inactivated (Viral)

Use Active immunization of adults at increased risk of exposure to the H5N1 viral subtype of influenza

Local Anesthetic/Vasoconstrictor Precautions No information available to require special precautions

Effects on Dental Treatment No significant effects or complications reported

Effects on Bleeding No information available to require special precautions

Adverse Effects All serious adverse reactions must be reported to the U.S. Department of Health and Human Services (DHHS) Vaccine Adverse Event Reporting System (VAERS) 1-800-822-7967 or online at https://vaers.hhs.gov/esub/index.

>10%:

Central nervous system: Headache (3% to 36%), malaise (22%)

Local: Pain (74%), tenderness (70%), erythema/redness (20%), induration/swelling (15%)

Neuromuscular & skeletal: Myalgia (16%)

1% to 10%:

Central nervous system: Fever (up to 7%)

Gastrointestinal: Nausea (10%), diarrhea (6%)

Respiratory: Nasopharyngitis (2%), upper respiratory infection (2%), nasal congestion (1%)

Additional reactions observed with other influenza vaccine formulations: Allergic reaction, anaphylaxis, angioedema, asthma, encephalopathy, facial paralysis, hives, GBS, neuropathy, optic neuritis, vasculitis

General Dosage Range I.M.: *Adults 18-64 years:* 1 mL, followed by second 1 mL dose given 28 days later

Mechanism of Action A monovalent, split virus (inactivated) preparation of the H5N1 avian strain of influenza virus (A/Vietnam/1203/2004) which promotes active immunity to avian influenza.

Pharmacodynamics/Kinetics

Onset of Action Fourfold increase in antibody titers occurred in up to 58% of patients 28 days after second dose.

Pregnancy Risk Factor C

Prescribing and Access Restrictions Commercial distribution is not planned. The vaccine will be included as part of the U.S. Strategic National Stockpile. It will be distributed by public health officials if needed.

Influenza Virus Vaccine (Inactivated)

(in floo EN za VYE rus vak SEEN, in ak ti VAY ted)

Related Information

Systemic Viral Diseases *on page 1904*

U.S. Brand Names Afluria®; Agriflu®; Fluarix®; FluLaval®; Fluvirin®; Fluzone®; Fluzone® High-Dose

Canadian Brand Names Fluviral S/F®; Vaxigrip®

Pharmacologic Category Vaccine, Inactivated (Viral)

Use Provide active immunity to influenza virus strains contained in the vaccine

The Advisory Committee on Immunization Practices (ACIP) recommends annual vaccination with the seasonal trivalent inactivated influenza vaccine (TIV) (injection) for all persons ≥6 months of age.

When vaccine supply is limited, target groups for vaccination (those at higher risk of complications from influenza infection and their close contacts) include the following:

- Persons ≥50 years of age
- Residents of nursing homes and other chronic-care facilities that house persons of any age with chronic medical conditions
- Adults and children with chronic disorders of the pulmonary or cardiovascular systems (except hypertension), including asthma
- Adults and children who have chronic metabolic diseases (including diabetes mellitus), hepatic disease, renal dysfunction, hematologic disorders, or immunosuppression (including immunosuppression caused by medications or HIV)
- Adults and children with cognitive or neurologic/neuromuscular conditions (including conditions such as spinal cord injuries or seizure disorders) which may compromise respiratory function, the handling of respiratory secretions, or that can increase the risk of aspiration
- Children and adolescents (6 months to 18 years of age) who are receiving long-term aspirin therapy, and therefore, may be at risk for developing Reye's syndrome after influenza
- Women who are or will be pregnant during the influenza season
- Children 6-59 months of age
- Healthcare personnel
- Household contacts and caregivers of children <5 years (particularly children <6 months) and adults ≥50 years
- Household contacts and caregivers of persons with medical conditions which put them at high risk of complications from influenza infection
- American Indians/Alaska Natives
- Morbidly obese (BMI ≥40)

The Advisory Committee on Immunization Practices (ACIP) states that healthy, nonpregnant persons aged 2-49 years may receive vaccination with either the seasonal live, attenuated influenza vaccine (LAIV) (nasal spray) or the seasonal trivalent inactivated influenza vaccine (TIV) (injection).

Local Anesthetic/Vasoconstrictor Precautions No information available to require special precautions

Effects on Dental Treatment No significant effects or complications reported

Effects on Bleeding No information available to require special precautions

Adverse Effects All serious adverse reactions must be reported to the U.S. Department of Health and Human Services (DHHS) Vaccine Adverse Event Reporting System (VAERS) 1-800-822-7967 or online at https://vaers.hhs.gov/esub/index. In Canada, adverse reactions may be reported to local provincial/territorial health agencies or to the Vaccine Safety Section at Public Health Agency of Canada (1-866-844-0018).

Frequency not defined. Adverse reactions in adults ≥65 years of age may be greater using the high-dose vaccine, but are typically mild and transient.

Cardiovascular: Chest tightness, facial edema

Central nervous system: Chills, drowsiness, fatigue, fever, headache, irritability, malaise, migraine, shivering

Endocrine & metabolic: Dysmenorrhea

Gastrointestinal: Appetite decreased, diarrhea, nausea, sore throat, upper abdominal pain, vomiting

Local: Injection site reactions (including bruising, erythema, induration, inflammation, pain, soreness [10% to 64%; may last up to 2 days], swelling, tenderness)

Neuromuscular & skeletal: Arthralgia, back pain, myalgia (may start within 6-12 hours and last 1-2 days; incidence equal to placebo in adults; occurs more frequently than placebo in children)

Ocular: Red eyes

Otic: Earache

Respiratory: Cough, nasal congestion, nasopharyngitis, pharyngolaryngeal pain, rhinitis, upper respiratory track infection, wheezing

Miscellaneous: Diaphoresis

General Dosage Range I.M.:

Children 6-35 months: 0.25 mL/dose (1 or 2 doses per season)

Children 3-9 years: 0.5 mL/dose (1 or 2 doses per season)

Children ≥9 years and Adults: 0.5 mL/dose (1 dose per season)

Mechanism of Action Promotes immunity to seasonal influenza virus by inducing specific antibody production. Each year the formulation is standardized according to the U.S. Public Health Service. Preparations from previous seasons must not be used.

Pharmacodynamics/Kinetics

Onset of Action Protective antibody titers achieved ~3 weeks after vaccination

Duration of Action Protective antibody titers persist approximately ≥6 months. Elderly: Protective antibody titers may fall ≤4 months after vaccination.

Pregnancy Risk Factor B/C (manufacturer specific)

Product Availability

Fluzone® Intradermal (influenza virus vaccine): FDA approved May 2011; availability expected for 2011-2012 flu season

Fluzone® Intradermal (influenza virus vaccine) is an intradermal vaccine indicated for active immunization of influenza in adults 18-64 years of age.

Influenza Virus Vaccine (Live/Attenuated)

(in floo EN za VYE rus vak SEEN)

Related Information

Systemic Viral Diseases *on page 1904*

U.S. Brand Names FluMist®

Canadian Brand Names FluMist®

Pharmacologic Category Vaccine, Live (Viral)

Use Provide active immunity to influenza virus strains contained in the vaccine

The Advisory Committee on Immunization Practices (ACIP) states that healthy, nonpregnant persons aged 2-49 years may receive vaccination with either the seasonal live, attenuated influenza vaccine (LAIV) (nasal spray) or the seasonal trivalent inactivated influenza vaccine (TIV) (injection).

Local Anesthetic/Vasoconstrictor Precautions No information available to require special precautions

Effects on Dental Treatment No significant effects or complications reported

Effects on Bleeding No information available to require special precautions

Adverse Effects All serious adverse reactions must be reported to the U.S. Department of Health and Human Services (DHHS) Vaccine Adverse Event Reporting System (VAERS) 1-800-822-7967 or online at https://vaers.hhs.gov/esub/index. In Canada, adverse reactions may be reported to local provincial/territorial health agencies or to the Vaccine Safety Section at Public Health Agency of Canada (1-866-844-0018).

Frequency of events reported within 10 days.

>10%:

Central nervous system: Headache (children 3% to 9%; adults 40%), irritability (children 12% to 21%), lethargy (children 6% to 14%)

Gastrointestinal: Appetite decreased (children 13% to 21%), abdominal pain (children 2% to 12%)

Neuromuscular & skeletal: Tiredness/weakness (adults 26%), muscle aches (children 2% to 6%; adults 17%)

Respiratory: Cough (adults 14%), nasal congestion/ runny nose (children 51% to 58%; adults 9% to 44%), sore throat (children 5% to 11%; adults 28%)

1% to 10%:

Central nervous system: Chills (children 2% to 4%, adults 9%), fever (100°F to 101°F: children 6% to 9%; >101°F: children 1% to 4%)

Otic: Otitis media (children 3%)

Respiratory: Sinusitis (adults 4%), sneezing (children 2%), wheezing (children 6-23 months 6%; children 24-59 months 2%)

General Dosage Range Intranasal:

Children 2-8 years: Previously not vaccinated: 2 doses (0.2 mL/dose) separated by at least 4 weeks; Previously vaccinated: 0.2 mL/dose (1 dose per season)

Children ≥9 years and Adults ≤49 years: 0.2 mL/dose (1 dose per season)

Mechanism of Action Promotes immunity to seasonal influenza virus by inducing specific antibody production. Each year the formulation is standardized according to the U.S. Public Health Service. Preparations from previous seasons must not be used.

Pharmacodynamics/Kinetics

Onset of Action Protective antibody titers achieved ~3 weeks after vaccination

Duration of Action Protective antibody titers persist approximately ≥6 months. Elderly: Protective antibody titers may fall ≤4 months after vaccination.

Pregnancy Risk Factor C

Insulin Aspart (IN soo lin AS part)

Related Information

Endocrine Disorders and Pregnancy *on page 1879*
Insulin Regular *on page 924*

U.S. Brand Names NovoLOG®; NovoLOG® FlexPen®; NovoLOG® Penfill®

Canadian Brand Names NovoRapid®

Pharmacologic Category Antidiabetic Agent, Insulin

Use Treatment of type 1 diabetes mellitus (insulin dependent, IDDM) and type 2 diabetes mellitus (noninsulin dependent, NIDDM) to improve glycemic control

Unlabeled/Investigational Use Gestational diabetes mellitus (GDM); mild-to-moderate diabetic ketoacidosis (DKA); mild-to-moderate hyperosmolar hyperglycemic state (HHS)

Local Anesthetic/Vasoconstrictor Precautions No information available to require special precautions

Effects on Dental Treatment Patients with type 1 diabetes (insulin dependent) should be appointed for dental treatment in the morning in order to minimize chance of stress-induced hypoglycemia.

Effects on Bleeding No information available to require special precautions

General Dosage Range Dosage adjustment recommended in patients with renal impairment

I.V.: *Adults:* Refer to Insulin Regular on page 924

SubQ: *Children ≥2 years and Adults:* Refer to Insulin Regular on page 924

Mechanism of Action Insulin aspart is a rapid-acting insulin analog.

Refer to Insulin Regular on page 924.

Pharmacodynamics/Kinetics

Onset of Action 0.2-0.3 hours; Peak effect: 1-3 hours

Duration of Action 3-5 hours

Half-life Elimination SubQ: 81 minutes

Time to Peak Plasma: 40-50 minutes

Pregnancy Risk Factor B

Insulin Aspart Protamine and Insulin Aspart

(IN soo lin AS part PROE ta meen & IN soo lin AS part)

Related Information

Insulin Regular *on page 924*

U.S. Brand Names NovoLOG® Mix 70/30; NovoLOG® Mix 70/30 FlexPen®

Canadian Brand Names NovoMix® 30

Pharmacologic Category Antidiabetic Agent, Insulin

Use Treatment of type 1 diabetes mellitus (insulin dependent, IDDM) and type 2 diabetes mellitus (noninsulin dependent, NIDDM) to improve glycemic control

Local Anesthetic/Vasoconstrictor Precautions No information available to require special precautions

Effects on Dental Treatment Patients with type 1 diabetes (insulin dependent) should be appointed for dental treatment in the morning in order to minimize chance of stress-induced hypoglycemia.

Effects on Bleeding No information available to require special precautions

Adverse Effects Refer to Insulin Regular on page 924.

General Dosage Range Dosage adjustment recommended in patients with renal impairment

SubQ: *Adults:* Refer to Insulin Regular on page 924

Mechanism of Action Insulin aspart protamine and insulin aspart is an intermediate-acting combination insulin product with a more rapid onset and similar duration of action as compared to that of insulin NPH and insulin regular combination products.

Refer to Insulin Regular on page 924.

Pharmacodynamics/Kinetics

Onset of Action 10-20 minutes; Peak effect: 1-4 hours

Duration of Action 18-24 hours

Half-life Elimination ~8-9 hours

Time to Peak 1-1.5 hours

Pregnancy Risk Factor B

Insulin Detemir (IN soo lin DE te mir)

Related Information

Endocrine Disorders and Pregnancy *on page 1879*

Insulin Regular *on page 924*

U.S. Brand Names Levemir®; Levemir® FlexPen®

Canadian Brand Names Levemir®

Pharmacologic Category Antidiabetic Agent, Insulin

Use Treatment of type 1 diabetes mellitus (insulin dependent, IDDM) and type 2 diabetes mellitus (noninsulin dependent, NIDDM) to improve glycemic control

Local Anesthetic/Vasoconstrictor Precautions No information available to require special precautions

Effects on Dental Treatment Patients with type 1 diabetes (insulin dependent) should be appointed for dental treatment in the morning in order to minimize chance of stress-induced hypoglycemia.

Effects on Bleeding No information available to require special precautions

Adverse Effects Refer to Insulin Regular on page 924.

General Dosage Range Dosage adjustment recommended in patients with renal impairment

SubQ:

Children ≥6 years: Refer to Insulin Regular on page 924

Adults: Refer to Insulin Regular on page 924; 0.1-0.2 units/kg once daily **or** 10 units once- or twice daily (manufacturer recommendations)

Mechanism of Action Insulin detemir is an intermediate- to long-acting insulin analog.

Refer to Insulin Regular on page 924.

Pharmacodynamics/Kinetics

Onset of Action 3-4 hours; Peak effect: 3-9 hours (Plank, 2005)

Duration of Action Dose dependent: 6-23 hours; **Note:** Duration is dose-dependent. At lower dosages (0.1-0.2 units/kg), mean duration is variable (5.7-12.1 hours). At 0.4 units/kg, the mean duration was 19.9 hours. At high dosages (≥0.8 units/kg) the duration is longer and less variable (mean of 22-23 hours) (Plank, 2005).

Half-life Elimination 5-7 hours (dose-dependent)

Time to Peak Plasma: 6-8 hours

Pregnancy Risk Factor C

Insulin Glargine (IN soo lin GLAR jeen)

Related Information

Endocrine Disorders and Pregnancy *on page 1879*

Insulin Regular *on page 924*

U.S. Brand Names Lantus®; Lantus® Solostar®

Canadian Brand Names Lantus®; Lantus® OptiSet®

Pharmacologic Category Antidiabetic Agent, Insulin

Use Treatment of type 1 diabetes mellitus (insulin dependent, IDDM) and type 2 diabetes mellitus (noninsulin dependent, NIDDM) to improve glycemic control

Local Anesthetic/Vasoconstrictor Precautions No information available to require special precautions

Effects on Dental Treatment Patients with type 1 diabetes (insulin dependent) should be appointed for dental treatment in the morning in order to minimize chance of stress-induced hypoglycemia.

Effects on Bleeding No information available to require special precautions

Adverse Effects Refer to Insulin Regular on page 924.

General Dosage Range Dosage adjustment recommended in patients with renal impairment

SubQ: *Children ≥6 years and Adults:* Refer to Insulin Regular on page 924

Mechanism of Action Insulin glargine is a long-acting insulin analog.

Refer to Insulin Regular on page 924.

Pharmacodynamics/Kinetics

Onset of Action 3-4 hours; Peak effect: No pronounced peak

Duration of Action Generally 24 hours or longer; reported range: 10.8 to >24 hours (up to 32 hours documented in some studies)

Time to Peak Plasma: No pronounced peak

Pregnancy Risk Factor C

Insulin Glulisine (IN soo lin gloo LIS een)

Related Information

Endocrine Disorders and Pregnancy *on page* 1879

Insulin Regular *on page* 924

U.S. Brand Names Apidra®; Apidra® SoloStar®

Canadian Brand Names Apidra®

Pharmacologic Category Antidiabetic Agent, Insulin

Use Treatment of type 1 diabetes mellitus (insulin dependent, IDDM) and type 2 diabetes mellitus (noninsulin dependent, NIDDM) to improve glycemic control

Local Anesthetic/Vasoconstrictor Precautions No information available to require special precautions

Effects on Dental Treatment Patients with type 1 diabetes (insulin dependent) should be appointed for dental treatment in the morning in order to minimize chance of stress-induced hypoglycemia.

Effects on Bleeding No information available to require special precautions

Adverse Effects Refer to Insulin Regular on page 924.

General Dosage Range Dosage adjustment recommended in patients with renal impairment

I.V.: *Adults:* Refer to Insulin Regular on page 924

SubQ: *Children ≥4 years and Adults:* Refer to Insulin Regular on page 924

Mechanism of Action Insulin glulisine is a rapid-acting insulin analog. Refer to Insulin Regular on page 924.

Pharmacodynamics/Kinetics

Onset of Action 0.2-0.5 hours; Peak effect: 1.6-2.8 hours

Duration of Action 3-4 hours

Half-life Elimination

I.V.: 13 minutes

SubQ: 42 minutes

Time to Peak Plasma: 0.6-2 hours

Pregnancy Risk Factor C

Insulin Lispro (IN soo lin LYE sproe)

Related Information

Endocrine Disorders and Pregnancy *on page* 1879

Insulin Regular *on page* 924

U.S. Brand Names HumaLOG®; HumaLOG® KwikPen™

Canadian Brand Names Humalog®

Pharmacologic Category Antidiabetic Agent, Insulin

Use Treatment of type 1 diabetes mellitus (insulin dependent, IDDM) and type 2 diabetes mellitus (noninsulin dependent, NIDDM) to improve glycemic control

Unlabeled/Investigational Use Gestational diabetes mellitus (GDM); mild-to-moderate diabetic ketoacidosis (DKA); mild-to-moderate hyperosmolar hyperglycemic state (HHS)

Local Anesthetic/Vasoconstrictor Precautions No information available to require special precautions

Effects on Dental Treatment Patients with type 1 diabetes (insulin dependent) should be appointed for dental treatment in the morning in order to minimize chance of stress-induced hypoglycemia.

Effects on Bleeding No information available to require special precautions

Adverse Effects Refer to Insulin Regular on page 924.

General Dosage Range Dosage adjustment recommended in patients with renal impairment

SubQ: *Children and Adults:* Refer to Insulin Regular on page 924

Mechanism of Action Insulin lispro is a rapid-acting insulin analog. Refer to Insulin Regular on page 924.

Pharmacodynamics/Kinetics

Onset of Action 0.25-0.5 hours; Peak effect: 0.5-2.5 hours

Duration of Action ≤5 hours

Half-life Elimination

I.V.: ~0.5-1 hour (dose-dependent)

SubQ: 1 hour

Time to Peak Plasma: 0.5-1.5 hours

Pregnancy Risk Factor B

Insulin Lispro Protamine and Insulin Lispro
(IN soo lin LYE sproe PROE ta meen & IN soo lin LYE sproe)

Related Information

Insulin Regular *on page 924*

U.S. Brand Names HumaLOG® Mix 50/50™; HumaLOG® Mix 50/50™ KwikPen™; HumaLOG® Mix 75/25™; HumaLOG® Mix 75/25™ KwikPen™

Canadian Brand Names Humalog® Mix 25

Pharmacologic Category Antidiabetic Agent, Insulin

Use Treatment of type 1 diabetes mellitus (insulin dependent, IDDM) and type 2 diabetes mellitus (noninsulin dependent, NIDDM) to improve glycemic control

Local Anesthetic/Vasoconstrictor Precautions No information available to require special precautions

Effects on Dental Treatment Patients with type 1 diabetes (insulin-dependent) should be appointed for dental treatment in the morning in order to minimize chance of stress-induced hypoglycemia.

Effects on Bleeding No information available to require special precautions

Adverse Effects Refer to Insulin Regular on page 924.

General Dosage Range Dosage adjustment recommended in patients with renal impairment

SubQ: *Adults:* Refer to Insulin Regular on page 924

Mechanism of Action Insulin lispro protamine and insulin lispro is an intermediate-acting combination product with a more rapid onset and similar duration of action as compared to that of insulin NPH and insulin regular combination products.

Refer to Insulin Regular on page 924.

Pharmacodynamics/Kinetics

Onset of Action 0.25-0.5 hours

Peak effect: Humalog® Mix 50/50™: 0.8-4.8 hours; Humalog® Mix 75/25™: 1-6.5 hours

Duration of Action 14-24 hours

Time to Peak Plasma: Humalog® Mix 50/50™: 0.75-13.5 hours; Humalog® Mix 75/25™: 0.5-4 hours

Pregnancy Risk Factor B

Insulin NPH (IN soo lin N P H)

Related Information

Endocrine Disorders and Pregnancy *on page 1879*

Insulin Regular *on page 924*

U.S. Brand Names HumuLIN® N; NovoLIN® N

Canadian Brand Names Humulin® N; Novolin® ge NPH

Pharmacologic Category Antidiabetic Agent, Insulin

Use Treatment of type 1 diabetes mellitus (insulin dependent, IDDM) and type 2 diabetes mellitus (noninsulin dependent, NIDDM) to improve glycemic control

Unlabeled/Investigational Use Gestational diabetes mellitus (GDM)

Local Anesthetic/Vasoconstrictor Precautions No information available to require special precautions

Effects on Dental Treatment Patients with type 1 diabetes (insulin dependent) should be appointed for dental treatment in the morning in order to minimize chance of stress-induced hypoglycemia.

Effects on Bleeding No information available to require special precautions

Adverse Effects Refer to Insulin Regular on page 924.

General Dosage Range Dosage adjustment recommended in patients with renal impairment

SubQ: *Children and Adults:* Refer to Insulin Regular on page 924

Mechanism of Action Insulin NPH, an isophane suspension of human insulin, is an intermediate-acting insulin.

Refer to Insulin Regular on page 924.

Pharmacodynamics/Kinetics

Onset of Action 1-2 hours; Peak effect: 4-12 hours

Duration of Action 14-24 hours

Time to Peak Plasma: 6-10 hours

Insulin NPH and Insulin Regular (IN soo lin N P H & IN soo lin REG yoo ler)

Related Information

Insulin Regular *on page 924*

U.S. Brand Names HumuLIN® 70/30; NovoLIN® 70/30

Canadian Brand Names Humulin® 20/80; Humulin® 70/30; Novolin® ge 30/70; Novolin® ge 40/60; Novolin® ge 50/50

Pharmacologic Category Antidiabetic Agent, Insulin

Use Treatment of type 1 diabetes mellitus (insulin dependent, IDDM) and type 2 diabetes mellitus (noninsulin dependent, NIDDM) to improve glycemic control

Unlabeled/Investigational Use Gestational diabetes mellitus (GDM)

Local Anesthetic/Vasoconstrictor Precautions No information available to require special precautions

Effects on Dental Treatment Patients with type 1 diabetes (insulin dependent) should be appointed for dental treatment in the morning in order to minimize chance of stress-induced hypoglycemia.

Effects on Bleeding No information available to require special precautions

Adverse Effects Refer to Insulin Regular on page 924.

General Dosage Range Dosage adjustment recommended in patients with renal impairment

SubQ: *Children and Adults:* Refer to Insulin Regular on page 924

Mechanism of Action Insulin NPH and insulin regular is an intermediate-acting combination insulin product with a more rapid onset than that of insulin NPH alone. Refer to Insulin Regular on page 924.

Pharmacodynamics/Kinetics

Onset of Action 0.5 hours; Peak effect: 2-12 hours

Duration of Action 18-24 hours

Time to Peak Based on individual components:

Insulin regular: 0.8-2 hours

Insulin NPH: 6-10 hours

Insulin Regular (IN soo lin REG yoo ler)

Related Information

Endocrine Disorders and Pregnancy *on page* 1879

Insulin Aspart *on page* 920

Insulin Aspart Protamine and Insulin Aspart *on page* 920

Insulin Detemir *on page* 921

Insulin Glargine *on page* 921

Insulin Glulisine *on page* 922

Insulin Lispro *on page* 922

Insulin Lispro Protamine and Insulin Lispro *on page* 923

Insulin NPH *on page* 923

Insulin NPH and Insulin Regular *on page* 923

U.S. Brand Names HumuLIN® R; HumuLIN® R U-500; NovoLIN® R

Canadian Brand Names Humulin® R; Novolin® ge Toronto

Pharmacologic Category Antidiabetic Agent, Insulin

Use Treatment of type 1 diabetes mellitus (insulin dependent, IDDM) and type 2 diabetes mellitus (noninsulin dependent, NIDDM) to improve glycemic control

Unlabeled/Investigational Use Hyperkalemia; gestational diabetes mellitus (GDM), diabetic ketoacidosis (DKA); hyperosmolar hyperglycemic state (HHS); adjunct of parenteral nutrition

Local Anesthetic/Vasoconstrictor Precautions No information available to require special precautions

Effects on Dental Treatment Patients with type 1 diabetes (insulin dependent) should be appointed for dental treatment in the morning in order to minimize chance of stress-induced hypoglycemia.

Effects on Bleeding No information available to require special precautions

Adverse Effects Frequency not defined.

Cardiovascular: Palpitation, pallor, peripheral edema, tachycardia

Central nervous system: Fatigue, headache, hypothermia, loss of consciousness, mental confusion

Dermatologic: Pruritus, rash, redness, urticaria

Endocrine & metabolic: Hypoglycemia, hypokalemia

Gastrointestinal: Hunger, nausea, numbness of mouth, weight gain

Local: Injection site reaction (including edema, itching, pain or warmth, stinging), lipoatrophy, lipodystrophy

Neuromuscular & skeletal: Muscle weakness, paresthesia, tremor

Ocular: Transient presbyopia or blurred vision

Miscellaneous: Anaphylaxis, antibodies to insulin (no change in efficacy), diaphoresis, local allergy, systemic allergic symptoms

General Dosage Range Dosage adjustment recommended in patients with renal impairment

I.V., SubQ: *Children and Adults:*

Diabetes mellitus, type 1: Initial: 0.5-1 unit/kg/day in divided doses; Usual maintenance: 0.5-1.2 units/kg/day in divided doses. **Note:** Generally, 50% to 75% of the total daily dose (TDD) is given as an intermediate- or long-acting form of insulin (1-2 daily injections) and the remaining portion is then divided and administered before or at mealtime (depending on the formulation) as a rapid-acting or short-acting form of insulin.

Diabetes mellitus, type 2: Initial basal insulin dose: 0.2 units/kg or 10 units/day given as an intermediate- or long-acting insulin at bedtime or long-acting insulin given in the morning

Mechanism of Action Insulin acts via specific membrane-bound receptors on target tissues to regulate metabolism of carbohydrate, protein, and fats. Target organs for insulin include the liver, skeletal muscle, and adipose tissue.

Within the liver, insulin stimulates hepatic glycogen synthesis. Insulin promotes hepatic synthesis of fatty acids, which are released into the circulation as lipoproteins. Skeletal muscle effects of insulin include increased protein synthesis and increased glycogen synthesis. Within adipose tissue, insulin stimulates the processing of circulating lipoproteins to provide free fatty acids, facilitating triglyceride synthesis and storage by adipocytes; also directly inhibits the hydrolysis of triglycerides. In addition, insulin stimulates the cellular uptake of amino acids and increases cellular permeability to several ions, including potassium, magnesium, and phosphate. By activating sodium-potassium ATPases, insulin promotes the intracellular movement of potassium.

Normally secreted by the pancreas, insulin products are manufactured for pharmacologic use through recombinant DNA technology using either *E. coli* or *Saccharomyces cerevisiae*. Insulins are categorized based on the onset, peak, and duration of effect (eg, rapid-, short-, intermediate-, and long-acting insulin).

Pharmacodynamics/Kinetics

Onset of Action SubQ: 0.5 hours; Peak effect: SubQ: 2.5-5 hours

Duration of Action SubQ:

U-100: 4-12 hours (may increase with dose)

U-500: Up to 24 hours

Half-life Elimination I.V.: ~0.5-1 hour (dose-dependent); SubQ: 1 hour

Time to Peak Plasma: SubQ: 0.8-2 hours

Interferon Alfa-2b (in ter FEER on AL fa too bee)

Related Information

Systemic Viral Diseases *on page 1904*

U.S. Brand Names Intron® A

Canadian Brand Names Intron® A

Generic Availability (U.S.) No

Pharmacologic Category Interferon

Use

Patients ≥1 year of age: Chronic hepatitis B

Patients ≥3 years of age: Chronic hepatitis C (in combination with ribavirin)

Patients ≥18 years of age: Condyloma acuminata, chronic hepatitis B, chronic hepatitis C, hairy cell leukemia, malignant melanoma, AIDS-related Kaposi's sarcoma, follicular non-Hodgkin's lymphoma

Unlabeled/Investigational Use AIDS-related thrombocytopenia, cutaneous ulcerations of Behçet's disease, neuroendocrine tumors (including carcinoid syndrome and islet cell tumor), cutaneous T-cell lymphoma, desmoid tumor, lymphomatoid granulomatosis, hepatitis D, chronic myelogenous leukemia (CML), non-Hodgkin's lymphomas (other than follicular lymphoma, see approved use), multiple myeloma, renal cell carcinoma, West Nile virus

Local Anesthetic/Vasoconstrictor Precautions No information available to require special precautions

Effects on Dental Treatment Key adverse event(s) related to dental treatment: Xerostomia (normal salivary flow resumes upon discontinuation), metallic taste, taste alteration, and gingivitis.

Effects on Bleeding Chemotherapy may result in significant myelosuppression, potentially including significant reduction in platelet counts and altered hemostasis. In patients who are under active treatment with these agents, medical consult is suggested.

Adverse Effects Note: In a majority of patients, a flu-like syndrome (fever, chills, tachycardia, malaise, myalgia, headache), occurs within 1-2 hours of administration; may last up to 24 hours and may be dose limiting.

>10%:

Cardiovascular: Chest pain (≤28%)

Central nervous system: Fatigue (8% to 96%), fever (34% to 94%), headache (21% to 62%), chills (≤54%), depression (3% to 40%; grades 3/4: 2%), somnolence (≤33%), dizziness (≤24%), irritability (≤22%), pain (≤18%), amnesia (≤14%), concentration impaired (≤14%), malaise (≤14%), confusion (≤12%), insomnia (≤12%)

Dermatologic: Alopecia (≤38%), rash (≤25%), pruritus (≤11%)

Endocrine & metabolic: Amenorrhea (≤12%)

Gastrointestinal: Anorexia (1% to 69%), nausea, (17% to 66%), diarrhea (2% to 45%), vomiting (2% to 32%), xerostomia (≤28%), taste alteration (≤24%), abdominal pain (1% to 23%), constipation (≤14%), gingivitis (≤14%), weight loss (<1% to 13%)

Hematologic: Neutropenia (≤92%; grade 4: 1% to 4%), leukopenia (≤68%), anemia (≤32%), thrombocytopenia (≤15%)

Hepatic: AST increased (≤63%; grades 3/4: 14%), ALT increased (≤15%), pain (upper right quadrant: up to 15%); alkaline phosphatase increased (≤13%)

Local: Injection site reaction (≤20%)

Neuromuscular & skeletal: Myalgia (28% to 75%), weakness (≤63%), rigors (≤42%), paresthesia (1% to 21%), skeletal pain (≤21%), arthralgia (≤19%), back pain (≤19%)

Renal: BUN increased (≤12%)

Respiratory: Dyspnea (≤34%), cough (≤31%), pharyngitis (≤31%), sinusitis (≤21%)

Miscellaneous: Flu-like syndrome (≤79%), diaphoresis (1% to 21%), moniliasis (≤17%)

5% to 10%:

Cardiovascular: Edema (≤10%), hypertension (≤9%)

Central nervous system: Hypoesthesia (≤10%), anxiety (≤9%), vertigo (≤8%), agitation (≤7%)

Dermatologic: Dry skin (≤10%), dermatitis (≤8%), purpura (≤5%)

Endocrine & metabolic: Libido decreased (≤5%)

Gastrointestinal: Loose stools (≤10%), dyspepsia (≤8%)

Genitourinary: Urinary tract infection (≤5%)

Renal: Polyuria (≤10%), serum creatinine increased (≤6%)

Respiratory: Bronchitis (≤10%), nasal congestion (≤10%), epistaxis (≤7%)

Miscellaneous: Infection (≤7%), herpes virus infections (≤5%)

Dosage Details concerning dosing in combination regimens should also be consulted. **Note:** Withhold treatment for ANC <500/mm^3 or platelets <25,000/mm^3. Consider premedication with acetaminophen prior to administration to reduce the incidence of some adverse reactions. Not all dosage forms and strengths are appropriate for all indications; refer to product labeling for details.

Children 1-17 years: **Note:** The following dosing may also be used in **infants** in the setting of HIV-exposure/-infection (CDC, 2009).

Chronic hepatitis B (including HIV coinfection): SubQ: 3 million units/m^2 3 times/week for 1 week, followed by 6 million units/m^2 3 times/week (maximum: 10 million units/dose) total duration of therapy 16-24 weeks (treat for 24 weeks in HIV-exposure/-infection)

Chronic hepatitis C with HIV coinfection: I.M., SubQ: 3-5 million units/m^2 3 times/week (maximum: 3 million units/dose) with ribavirin for 48 weeks, regardless of HCV genotype (CDC, 2009)

Adults:

Hairy cell leukemia: I.M., SubQ: 2 million units/m^2 3 times/week for up to 6 months (may continue treatment with continued treatment response)

Lymphoma (follicular): SubQ: 5 million units 3 times/week for up to 18 months

Malignant melanoma: Induction: 20 million units/m^2 I.V. for 5 consecutive days per week for 4 weeks, followed by maintenance dosing of 10 million units/m^2 SubQ 3 times/week for 48 weeks

AIDS-related Kaposi's sarcoma: I.M., SubQ: 30 million units/m^2 3 times/week

Chronic hepatitis B: I.M., SubQ: 5 million units/day or 10 million units 3 times/week for 16 weeks

Chronic hepatitis C: I.M., SubQ: 3 million units 3 times/week. In patients with normalization of ALT at 16 weeks, continue treatment (if tolerated) for 18-24 months; consider discontinuation if normalization does not occur at 16 weeks. **Note:** May be used in combination therapy with ribavirin in previously untreated patients or in patients who relapse following alpha interferon therapy.

Condyloma acuminata: Intralesionally: 1 million units/lesion (maximum: 5 lesions/treatment) 3 times/week (on alternate days) for 3 weeks; may administer a second course at 12-16 weeks

Dosage adjustment in renal impairment: Combination therapy with ribavirin (hepatitis C) should not be used in patients with reduced renal function (Cl_{cr} <50 mL/minute).

Dosage adjustment for toxicity:

Neuropsychiatric disorders (during treatment):

Clinical depression or other psychiatric problem: Monitor closely during and for 6 months after treatment

Severe depression or other psychiatric disorder: Discontinue treatment

Persistent or worsening psychiatric symptoms, suicidal ideation, aggression towards others: Discontinue treatment and follow with appropriate psychiatric intervention

Hypersensitivity reaction (acute, serious), ophthalmic disorders (new or worsening), thyroid abnormality development (which cannot be normalized with medication), signs or symptoms of liver failure: Discontinue treatment

Liver function abnormality, pulmonary infiltrate development, evidence of pulmonary function impairment, or autoimmune disorder development: Monitor closely and discontinue if appropriate

Manufacturer-recommended adjustments, listed according to indication:

Lymphoma (follicular):

Neutrophils >1000/mm^3 to <1500/mm^3: Reduce dose by 50%; may re-escalate to starting dose when neutrophils return to >1500/mm^3

Severe toxicity (neutrophils <1000/mm^3 or platelets <50,000/mm^3): Temporarily withhold

AST >5 times ULN or serum creatinine >2 mg/dL: Permanently discontinue

Hairy cell leukemia: Severe toxicity: Reduce dose by 50% or temporarily withhold and resume with 50% dose reduction; permanently discontinue if persistent or recurrent severe toxicity is noted

Chronic hepatitis B:

WBC <1500/mm^3, granulocytes <750/mm^3, or platelet count <50,000/mm^3, or other laboratory abnormality or severe adverse reaction: Reduce dose by 50%; may re-escalate to starting dose upon resolution of hematologic toxicity. Discontinue for persistent intolerance.

WBC <1000/mm^3, granulocytes <500/mm^3, or platelet count <25,000/mm^3: Permanently discontinue

Chronic hepatitis C: Severe toxicity: Reduce dose by 50% or temporarily withhold until subsides; permanently discontinue for persistent toxicities after dosage reduction

AIDS-related Kaposi sarcoma: Severe toxicity: Reduce dose by 50% or temporarily withhold; may resume at reduced dose with toxicity resolution; permanently discontinue for persistent/recurrent toxicities

Malignant melanoma:

Severe toxicity (neutrophils >250/mm^3 to <500/mm^3 or ALT/AST >5-10 times ULN): Temporarily withhold; resume with a 50% dose reduction when adverse reaction abates

Neutrophils <250/mm^3, ALT/AST >10 times ULN, or severe/persistent adverse reactions: Permanently discontinue

Mechanism of Action Following activation, multiple effects can be detected including induction of gene transcription. Inhibits cellular growth, alters the state of cellular differentiation, interferes with oncogene expression, alters cell surface antigen expression, increases phagocytic activity of macrophages, and augments cytotoxicity of lymphocytes for target cells

Contraindications Hypersensitivity to interferon alfa or any component of the formulation; decompensated liver disease; autoimmune hepatitis

Combination therapy with interferon alfa-2b and ribavirin is also contraindicated in pregnancy, males with pregnant partners; hemoglobinopathies (eg, thalassemia major, sickle-cell anemia); renal dysfunction (Cl_{cr} <50 mL/minute)

Warnings/Precautions Hazardous agent - use appropriate precautions for handling and disposal.

[U.S. Boxed Warning]: May cause or aggravate fatal or life-threatening autoimmune disorders, neuropsychiatric symptoms (including depression and/or suicidal thoughts/behaviors), ischemic, and/or infectious disorders; discontinue treatment for persistent severe or worsening symptoms.

Neuropsychiatric disorders: May cause severe psychiatric adverse events (eg, depression, psychosis, mania, suicidal behavior/ideation, homicidal ideation) in patients with and without previous psychiatric symptoms, avoid use in patients with pre-existing psychiatric condition, severe psychiatric disorder or history of severe depression; careful neuropsychiatric monitoring is required during and for 6 months after therapy. Suicidal ideation or attempts may occur more frequently in pediatric patients when compared to adults. Discontinue in patients developing severe depression or psychiatric disorders. Higher doses in elderly patients, or diseases other than hairy cell leukemia, may result in increased CNS toxicity.

Hepatic disease: May cause hepatotoxicity; monitor closely if abnormal liver function tests develop. A transient increase in ALT (≥2 times baseline) may occur in patients treated with interferon alfa-2b for chronic hepatitis B. Therapy generally may continue; monitor. Worsening and potentially fatal liver disease, including jaundice, hepatic encephalopathy, and hepatic failure have been reported in patients receiving interferon alfa for chronic hepatitis B and C with decompensated liver disease, autoimmune hepatitis, history of autoimmune disease, and immunosuppressed transplant recipients; avoid use in these patients. Chronic hepatitis B or C patients with a history of autoimmune disease or who are immunosuppressed transplant recipients should not receive interferon alfa-2b. Discontinue treatment (if appropriate) in any patient developing signs or symptoms of liver failure.

Bone marrow suppression: Causes bone marrow suppression, including potentially severe cytopenias, and very rarely, aplastic anemia. Discontinue treatment for severe neutropenia (ANC <500/mm^3) or thrombocytopenia (platelets <25,000/mm^3). Hemolytic anemia (hemoglobin <10 g/dL) was observed when combined with ribavirin; anemia occurred within 1-2 weeks of initiation of therapy. Use caution in patients with pre-existing myelosuppression and in patients with concomitant medications which cause myelosuppression.

Autoimmune disorders: Avoid use in patients with history of autoimmune disorders; development of autoimmune disorders (thrombocytopenia, vasculitis, Raynaud's disease, rheumatoid arthritis, lupus erythematosus and rhabdomyolysis) has been associated with use. Monitor closely; consider discontinuing. Worsening of psoriasis and sarcoidosis (and the development of new sarcoidosis) have been reported; use caution.

Cardiovascular disease/coagulation disorders: Use caution and monitor closely in patients with cardiovascular disease (ischemic or thromboembolic), arrhythmias, hypertension, and in patients with a history of MI or prior therapy with cardiotoxic drugs. Patients with pre-existing cardiac disease and/or advanced cancer should have baseline and periodic ECGs. May cause hypotension (during administration or delayed), arrhythmia, tachycardia, cardiomyopathy (~2% in AIDS-related Kaposi's Sarcoma patients) and/or MI. Hemorrhagic cerebrovascular events have been observed with therapy. Use caution in patients with coagulation disorders.

Endocrine disorders: Thyroid disorders (possibly reversible) have been reported; use caution in patients with pre-existing thyroid disease. Discontinue use in patients who cannot maintain normal ranges with thyroid medication. Diabetes mellitus has been reported; discontinue if cannot effectively manage with medication. Use with caution in patients with a history of diabetes mellitus, particularly if prone to DKA. Hypertriglyceridemia has been reported; discontinue if persistent and severe, and/or combined with symptoms of pancreatitis.

Pulmonary disease: Dyspnea, pulmonary infiltrates, pulmonary hypertension, interstitial pneumonitis, pneumonia, bronchiolitis obliterans, and sarcoidosis may be induced or aggravated by treatment, sometimes resulting in respiratory failure or fatality. Has been reported more in patients being treated for chronic hepatitis C, although has also occurred with use for oncology indications. Patients with fever, cough, dyspnea or other respiratory symptoms should be evaluated with a chest x-ray; monitor closely and consider discontinuing treatment with evidence of impaired pulmonary function. Use with caution in patients with a history of pulmonary disease.

Ophthalmic disorders: Decreased/loss of vision, macular edema, optic neuritis, retinal hemorrhages, cotton wool spots, papilledema, retinal detachment (serous), and retinal artery or vein thrombosis have occurred (or been aggravated) in patients receiving alpha interferons. Use caution in patients with pre-existing eye disorders; monitor closely; a complete eye exam should be done promptly in patients who develop ocular symptoms; discontinue with new or worsening ophthalmic disorders.

Commonly associated with fever and flu-like symptoms; rule out other causes/ infection with persistent fever; use with caution in patients with debilitating conditions. Acute hypersensitivity reactions have been reported. Do not treat patients with visceral AIDS-related Kaposi's sarcoma associated with rapidly-progressing or life-threatening disease. Some formulations contain albumin, which may carry a remote risk of viral transmission. Due to differences in dosage, patients should not change brands of interferons without the concurrence of their healthcare provider. Combination therapy with ribavirin is associated with birth defects and/or fetal mortality and hemolytic anemia. Do not use combination therapy with ribavirin in patients with renal dysfunction (Cl_{cr} <50 mL/minute).

Drug Interactions

Metabolism/Transport Effects Inhibits CYP1A2 (weak)

Avoid Concomitant Use

Avoid concomitant use of Interferon Alfa-2b with any of the following: Telbivudine

Increased Effect/Toxicity
Interferon Alfa-2b may increase the levels/effects of: Aldesleukin; Methadone; Ribavirin; Telbivudine; Theophylline Derivatives; Zidovudine

Decreased Effect There are no known significant interactions involving a decrease in effect.

Pharmacodynamics/Kinetics

Half-life Elimination I.V.: ~2 hours; I.M., SubQ: ~2-3 hours

Time to Peak Serum: I.M., SubQ: ~3-12 hours

Pregnancy Risk Factor C / X in combination with ribavirin

Lactation Enters breast milk/not recommended (AAP rates "compatible"; AAP 2001 update pending)

Breast-Feeding Considerations Breast milk samples obtained from a lactating mother prior to and after administration of interferon alfa-2b showed that interferon alfa is present in breast milk and administration of the medication did not significantly affect endogenous levels. Breast-feeding is not linked to the spread of hepatitis C virus; however, if nipples are cracked or bleeding, breast-feeding is not recommended. Mothers coinfected with HIV are discouraged from breast-feeding to decrease potential transmission of HIV.

Dosage Forms

Injection, powder for reconstitution [preservative free]:
Intron® A: 10 million int. units, 18 million int. units, 50 million int. units

Injection, solution:
Intron® A: 6 million int. units/mL (3 mL); 10 million int. units/mL (2.5 mL); 3 million int. units/0.2 mL (1.2 mL); 5 million int. units/0.2 mL (1.2 mL); 10 million int. units/0.2 mL (1.2 mL)

Interferon Alfa-2b and Ribavirin

(in ter FEER on AL fa too bee & rye ba VYE rin)

Related Information
Interferon Alfa-2b *on page 925*
Ribavirin *on page 1470*
Systemic Viral Diseases *on page 1904*

U.S. Brand Names Rebetron®

Pharmacologic Category Antiviral Agent; Interferon

Use Combination therapy for the treatment of chronic hepatitis C in patients with compensated liver disease previously untreated with alpha interferon or who have relapsed after alpha interferon therapy

Local Anesthetic/Vasoconstrictor Precautions No information available to require special precautions

Effects on Dental Treatment Key adverse event(s) related to dental treatment: Xerostomia (normal salivary flow resumes upon discontinuation), metallic taste, and taste perversion.

Effects on Bleeding No information available to require special precautions

Adverse Effects Note: Adverse reactions listed are specific to combination regimen in previously untreated hepatitis patients. See individual agents for additional adverse reactions reported with each agent during therapy for other diseases.

>10%:
- Central nervous system: Fatigue (children 61%; adults 68%), headache (63%), insomnia (children 14%; adults 39%), fever (children 61%; adults 37%), depression (children 13%; adults 32% to 36%), irritability (children 10%; adults 23% to 32%), dizziness (17% to 23%), emotional lability (children 16%; adults 7% to 11%), impaired concentration (5% to 14%)
- Dermatologic: Alopecia (23% to 32%), pruritus (children 12%; adults 19% to 21%), rash (17% to 28%)
- Gastrointestinal: Nausea (33% to 46%), anorexia (children 51%; adults 25% to 27%), dyspepsia (children <1%; adults 14% to 16%), vomiting (children 42%; adults 9% to 11%)
- Hematologic: Leukopenia, neutropenia (usually recovers within 4 weeks of treatment discontinuation), anemia
- Hepatic: Hyperbilirubinemia (27%; only 0.9% to 2% >3.0-6 mg/dL)
- Local: Injection site inflammation (13%)
- Neuromuscular & skeletal: Myalgia (children 32%; adults 61% to 64%), rigors (40%), arthralgia (children 15%; adults 30% to 33%), musculoskeletal pain (20% to 28%)
- Respiratory: Dyspnea (children 5%; adults 18% to 19%)
- Miscellaneous: Flu-like syndrome (children 31%; adults 14% to 18%)

1% to 10%:
- Cardiovascular: Chest pain (5% to 9%)
- Central nervous system: Nervousness (3% to 4%)

Endocrine & metabolic: Thyroid abnormalities (hyper- or hypothyroidism), serum uric acid increased, hyperglycemia
Gastrointestinal: Taste perversion (children <1%; adults 7% to 8%)
Hematologic: Hemolytic anemia (10%), thrombocytopenia, anemia
Local: Injection site reaction (7%)
Neuromuscular & skeletal: Weakness (5% to 9%)
Respiratory: Sinusitis (children <1%; adults 9% to 10%)

General Dosage Range

Oral (Rebetol®):

Children <3 years: Dosage not established
Children 3-5 years or ≤25 kg: 15 mg/kg/day in 2 divided doses
Children >5 years and 26-36 kg: 200 mg twice daily
Children >5 years and 37-49 kg: 200 mg in the morning and 400 mg in the evening
Children >5 years and 50-61 kg: 400 mg twice daily
Children >5 years and >61-75 kg: 400 mg in the morning and 600 mg in the evening
Children >5 years and >75 kg: 600 mg twice daily
Adults ≤75 kg: 400 mg in the morning and 600 mg in the evening
Adults >75 kg: 600 mg twice daily

SubQ (Intron® A):

Children <3 years: Dosage not established
Children ≥3 years and 25-61 kg: 3 million int. units/m^2 3 times/week
Children ≥3 years and >61 kg: 3 million int. units 3 times/week
Adults: 3 million int. units 3 times/week

Mechanism of Action

Interferon Alfa-2b: Alpha interferons are a family of proteins, produced by nucleated cells, that have antiviral, antiproliferative, and immune-regulating activity. There are 16 known subtypes of alpha interferons. Interferons interact with cells through high affinity cell surface receptors. Following activation, multiple effects can be detected including induction of gene transcription. Inhibits cellular growth, alters the state of cellular differentiation, interferes with oncogene expression, alters cell surface antigen expression, increases phagocytic activity of macrophages, and augments cytotoxicity of lymphocytes for target cells

Ribavirin: Inhibits replication of RNA and DNA viruses; inhibits influenza virus RNA polymerase activity and inhibits the initiation and elongation of RNA fragments resulting in inhibition of viral protein synthesis

Pregnancy Risk Factor X

Interferon Alfa-n3 (in ter FEER on AL fa en three)

Related Information

Systemic Viral Diseases *on page* 1904

U.S. Brand Names Alferon® N

Canadian Brand Names Alferon® N

Pharmacologic Category Interferon

Use Patients ≥18 years of age: Intralesional treatment of refractory or recurring genital or venereal warts (condylomata acuminata)

Local Anesthetic/Vasoconstrictor Precautions No information available to require special precautions

Effects on Dental Treatment Key adverse event(s) related to dental treatment: Xerostomia (normal salivary flow resumes upon discontinuation), metallic taste, tongue hyperesthesia, abnormal taste, thirst, rhinitis, pharyngitis, nosebleed, increased diaphoresis, taste disturbance, and gingivitis.

Effects on Bleeding No information available to require special precautions

Adverse Effects Note: Adverse reaction incidence noted below is specific to intralesional administration in patients with condylomata acuminata. Flu-like reactions, consisting of headache, fever, and/or myalgia, was reported in 30% of patients, and abated with repeated dosing.

>10%:

Central nervous system: Fever (40%), headache (31%), chills (14%), fatigue (14%)
Hematologic: Decreased WBC (11%)
Neuromuscular & skeletal: Myalgia (45%)
Miscellaneous: Flu-like syndrome (30%)

1% to 10%:

Central nervous system: Malaise (9%), dizziness (9%), depression (2%), insomnia (2%), thirst (1%)
Dermatologic: Pruritus (2%)
Gastrointestinal: Nausea (45), vomiting (3%), dyspepsia (3%), diarrhea (2%), tongue hyperesthesia (1%), taste disturbance (1%)
Genitourinary: Groin lymph node swelling (1%)

Neuromuscular & skeletal: Arthralgia (5%), back pain (4%), cramps (1%), paresthesia (1%)
Ocular: Visual disturbance (1%)
Respiratory: Rhinitis (2%), pharyngitis (1%), nosebleed (1%)
Miscellaneous: Diaphoresis increased (2%), vasovagal reaction (2%)

General Dosage Range Intralesional: *Adults:* Inject 250,000 units (0.05 mL) in each wart twice weekly (maximum: 8 weeks)

Mechanism of Action Interferons interact with cells through high affinity cell surface receptors. Following activation, multiple effects can be detected including induction of gene transcription. Inhibits cellular growth, alters the state of cellular differentiation, interferes with oncogene expression, alters cell surface antigen expression, increases phagocytic activity of macrophages, and augments cytotoxicity of lymphocytes for target cells

Pregnancy Risk Factor C

Interferon Beta-1a (in ter FEER on BAY ta won aye)

U.S. Brand Names Avonex®; Rebif®

Canadian Brand Names Avonex®; Rebif®

Pharmacologic Category Interferon

Use Treatment of relapsing forms of multiple sclerosis (MS)

Local Anesthetic/Vasoconstrictor Precautions No information available to require special precautions

Effects on Dental Treatment Key adverse event(s) related to dental treatment: Xerostomia and changes in salivation (normal salivary flow resumes upon discontinuation), and toothache.

Effects on Bleeding No information available to require special precautions

Adverse Effects Note: Adverse reactions reported as a composite of both commercially-available products. Spectrum and incidence of reactions is generally similar between products, but consult individual product labels for specific incidence.

>10%:
Central nervous system: Headache (58% to 70%), fatigue (33% to 41%), fever (20% to 28%), pain (23%), chills (19%), depression (18% to 25%), dizziness (14%)
Gastrointestinal: Nausea (23%), abdominal pain (8% to 22%)
Genitourinary: Urinary tract infection (17%)
Hematologic: Leukopenia (28% to 36%)
Hepatic: ALT increased (20% to 27%), AST increased (10% to 17%)
Local: Injection site reaction (3% to 92%)
Neuromuscular & skeletal: Myalgia (25% to 29%), back pain (23% to 25%), weakness (24%), skeletal pain (10% to 15%), rigors (6% to 13%)
Ocular: Vision abnormal (7% to 13%)
Respiratory: Sinusitis (14%), upper respiratory tract infection (14%)
Miscellaneous: Flu-like syndrome (49% to 59%), neutralizing antibodies (significance not known; Avonex® 5%; Rebif® 24%), lymphadenopathy (11% to 12%)

1% to 10%:
Cardiovascular: Chest pain (5% to 6%), vasodilation (2%)
Central nervous system: Migraine (5%), somnolence (4% to 5%), malaise (4% to 5%), seizure (1% to 5%)
Dermatologic: Erythematous rash (5% to 7%), maculopapular rash (4% to 5%), alopecia (4%), urticaria
Endocrine & metabolic: Thyroid disorder (4% to 6%)
Gastrointestinal: Xerostomia (1% to 5%), toothache (3%)
Genitourinary: Micturition frequency (2% to 7%), urinary incontinence (2% to 4%)
Hematologic: Thrombocytopenia (2% to 8%), anemia (3% to 5%)
Hepatic: Bilirubinemia (2% to 3%)
Local: Injection site pain (8%), injection site bruising (6%), injection site necrosis (1% to 3%), injection site inflammation
Neuromuscular & skeletal: Arthralgia (9%), hypertonia (6% to 7%), coordination abnormal (4% to 5%)
Ocular: Eye disorder (4%), xerophthalmia (1% to 3%)
Respiratory: Bronchitis (8%)
Miscellaneous: Infection (7%)

General Dosage Range Dosage adjustment recommended in patients who develop toxicities

I.M.: *Adults:* 30 mcg once weekly

SubQ: *Adults:* Initial: 4.4 or 8.8 mcg 3 times/week for 2 weeks; Titration: 11 or 22 mcg 3 times/week for 2 weeks; Maintenance: 22 or 44 mcg 3 times/week

Mechanism of Action Interferon beta differs from naturally occurring human protein by a single amino acid substitution and the lack of carbohydrate side chains; alters the expression and response to surface antigens and can enhance immune cell activities. Properties of interferon beta that modify biologic responses are mediated by cell surface receptor interactions; mechanism in the treatment of MS is unknown.

Pharmacodynamics/Kinetics

Onset of Action Avonex®: 12 hours (based on biological response markers)

Duration of Action Avonex®: 4 days (based on biological response markers)

Half-life Elimination Avonex®: 10 hours; Rebif®: 69 hours

Time to Peak Serum: Avonex® (I.M.): 3-15 hours; Rebif® (SubQ): 16 hours

Pregnancy Risk Factor C

Interferon Beta-1b (in ter FEER on BAY ta won bee)

U.S. Brand Names Betaseron®; Extavia®

Canadian Brand Names Betaseron®; Extavia®

Pharmacologic Category Interferon

Use Treatment of relapsing forms of multiple sclerosis (MS); treatment of first clinical episode with MRI features consistent with MS

Canadian labeling: Additional use (not in U.S. labeling): Treatment of secondary-progressive MS

Local Anesthetic/Vasoconstrictor Precautions No information available to require special precautions

Effects on Dental Treatment No significant effects or complications reported

Effects on Bleeding No information available to require special precautions

Adverse Effects Note: Flu-like syndrome (including at least two of the following - headache, fever, chills, malaise, diaphoresis, and myalgia) are reported in the majority of patients (60%) and decrease over time (average duration ~1 week).

>10%:

- Cardiovascular: Peripheral edema (15%), chest pain (11%)
- Central nervous system: Headache (57%), fever (36%), pain (51%), chills (25%), dizziness (24%), insomnia (24%)
- Dermatologic: Rash (24%), skin disorder (12%)
- Endocrine & metabolic: Metrorrhagia (11%)
- Gastrointestinal: Nausea (27%), diarrhea (19%), abdominal pain (19%), constipation (20%), dyspepsia (14%)
- Genitourinary: Urinary urgency (13%)
- Hematologic: Lymphopenia (88%), neutropenia (14%), leukopenia (14%)
- Local: Injection site reaction (85%), inflammation (53%), pain (18%)
- Neuromuscular & skeletal: Weakness (61%), myalgia (27%), hypertonia (50%), myasthenia (46%), arthralgia (31%), incoordination (21%)
- Miscellaneous: Flu-like syndrome (decreases over treatment course; 60%), neutralizing antibodies (≤45%; significance not known)

1% to 10%:

- Cardiovascular: Palpitation (4%), vasodilation (8%), hypertension (7%), tachycardia (4%), peripheral vascular disorder (6%)
- Central nervous system: Anxiety (10%), malaise (8%), nervousness (7%)
- Dermatologic: Alopecia (4%)
- Endocrine & metabolic: Menorrhagia (8%), dysmenorrhea (7%)
- Gastrointestinal: Weight gain (7%)
- Genitourinary: Impotence (9%), pelvic pain (6%), cystitis (8%), urinary frequency (7%), prostatic disorder (3%)
- Hematologic: Lymphadenopathy (8%)
- Hepatic: ALT increased >5x baseline (10%), AST increased >5x baseline (3%)
- Local: Injection site necrosis (4% to 5%), edema (3%), mass (2%)
- Neuromuscular & skeletal: Leg cramps (4%)
- Respiratory: Dyspnea (7%)
- Miscellaneous: Diaphoresis (8%), hypersensitivity (3%)

General Dosage Range SubQ: *Adults:* 0.0625-0.25 mg (2-8 million units) every other day

Mechanism of Action Interferon beta-1b differs from naturally occurring human protein by a single amino acid substitution and the lack of carbohydrate side chains; mechanism in the treatment of MS is unknown; however, immunomodulatory effects attributed to interferon beta-1b include enhancement of suppressor T cell activity, reduction of proinflammatory cytokines, down-regulation of antigen presentation, and reduced trafficking of lymphocytes into the central nervous system. Improves MRI lesions, decreases relapse rate, and disease severity in patients with secondary progressive MS.

Pharmacodynamics/Kinetics
Half-life Elimination 8 minutes to 4.3 hours
Time to Peak 1-8 hours
Pregnancy Risk Factor C

Interferon Gamma-1b (in ter FEER on GAM ah won bee)

U.S. Brand Names Actimmune®
Canadian Brand Names Actimmune®
Pharmacologic Category Interferon
Use Reduce frequency and severity of serious infections associated with chronic granulomatous disease; delay time to disease progression in patients with severe, malignant osteopetrosis
Local Anesthetic/Vasoconstrictor Precautions No information available to require special precautions
Effects on Dental Treatment No significant effects or complications reported
Effects on Bleeding No information available to require special precautions
Adverse Effects Based on 50 mcg/m² dose administered 3 times weekly for chronic granulomatous disease

>10%:
- Central nervous system: Fever (52%), headache (33%), chills (14%), fatigue (14%)
- Dermatologic: Rash (17%)
- Gastrointestinal: Diarrhea (14%), vomiting (13%)
- Local: Injection site erythema or tenderness (14%)

1% to 10%:
- Central nervous system: Depression (3%)
- Gastrointestinal: Nausea (10%), abdominal pain (8%)
- Neuromuscular & skeletal: Myalgia (6%), arthralgia (2%), back pain (2%)

Additional adverse reactions noted at doses >100 mcg/m² administered 3 times weekly: ALT increased, AST increased, autoantibodies increased, bronchospasm, chest discomfort, confusion, dermatomyositis exacerbation, disorientation, DVT, gait disturbance, GI bleeding, hallucinations, heart block, heart failure, hepatic insufficiency, hyperglycemia, hypertriglyceridemia, hyponatremia, hypotension, interstitial pneumonitis, lupus-like syndrome, MI, neutropenia, pancreatitis (may be fatal), Parkinsonian symptoms, PE, proteinuria, renal insufficiency (reversible), seizure, syncope, tachyarrhythmia, tachypnea, thrombocytopenia, TIA

General Dosage Range Dosage adjustment recommended in patients who develop toxicities
SubQ: *Children and Adults:*
- BSA ≤0.5 m²: 1.5 mcg/kg/dose 3 times/week
- BSA >0.5 m²: 50 mcg/m² (1 million int. units/m²) 3 times/week

Mechanism of Action Interferon gamma participates in immunoregulation by enhancing the oxidative metabolism of macrophages; it also enhances antibody dependent cellular cytotoxicity, activates natural killer cells and has a role in the expression of Fc receptors and histocompatibility antigens. The exact mechanism of action for the treatment of chronic granulomatous disease or osteopetrosis has not been defined.
Pharmacodynamics/Kinetics
Half-life Elimination I.V.: 38 minutes; I.M.: ~3 hours, SubQ: ~6 hours
Time to Peak Plasma: I.M.: 4 hours (1.5 ng/mL); SubQ: 7 hours (0.6 ng/mL)
Pregnancy Risk Factor C

Iodine (EYE oh dyne)

Related Information
Trace Metals *on page* 1655
U.S. Brand Names Iodex® [OTC]; Iodoflex™ [OTC]; Iodosorb® [OTC]
Pharmacologic Category Antiseptic, Topical
Use Used topically as an antiseptic in the management of minor, superficial skin wounds and has been used to disinfect the skin preoperatively
Local Anesthetic/Vasoconstrictor Precautions No information available to require special precautions
Effects on Dental Treatment No significant effects or complications reported
Effects on Bleeding No information available to require special precautions

Adverse Effects

Reactions reported following topical application: Frequency not defined:

Endocrine & metabolic: TSH increased

Local: Eczema, edema, irritation, pain, redness

Miscellaneous: Allergic reaction

Reactions reported more likely observed following large doses or chronic iodine intoxication; frequency not defined:

Central nervous system: Fever, headache

Dermatologic: Skin rash, angioedema, urticaria, acne

Endocrine & metabolic: Hypothyroidism

Gastrointestinal: Metallic taste, diarrhea

Hematologic: Eosinophilia, hemorrhage (mucosal)

Neuromuscular & skeletal: Arthralgia

Ocular: Swelling of eyelids

Respiratory: Pulmonary edema

Miscellaneous: Ioderma, lymph node enlargement

General Dosage Range Topical: *Adults:* Antiseptic: Apply to affected area 1-3 times/day; Ulcer/wound cleansing: Apply to clean wound 3 times/week (maximum: 50 g/application; 150 g/week)

Mechanism of Action Iodine is required for thyroid hormone synthesis. Iodine is also known to be a powerful broad spectrum germicidal agent effective against a wide range of bacteria, viruses, fungi, protozoa, and spores. Iodosorb® and Iodoflex™ contain iodine in hydrophilic beads of cadexomer which allows a slow release of iodine into the wound and absorption of fluid, bacteria, and other substances from the wound

Iodipamide Meglumine (eye oh DI pa mide MEG loo meen)

U.S. Brand Names Cholografin® Meglumine

Pharmacologic Category Iodinated Contrast Media; Radiological/Contrast Media, Ionic (High Osmolality)

Use Contrast medium for intravenous cholangiography and cholecystography

Local Anesthetic/Vasoconstrictor Precautions No information available to require special precautions

Effects on Dental Treatment No significant effects or complications reported

Effects on Bleeding No information available to require special precautions

Adverse Effects Frequency not defined.

Cardiovascular: Cardiac reactions (rare), cyanosis (rare), hypotension (rare)

Ocular: Edema of eyelids (rare)

Renal: Renal failure, renal function tests altered

Respiratory: Laryngospasm (rare), respiratory difficulties (rare)

Miscellaneous: Anaphylactoid reaction (rare); hypersensitivity reactions; infusion reactions (generally mild and transient; associated with rapid infusion rates; includes restlessness, sensations of warmth, sneezing, perspiration, salivation, flushing, pressure in the upper abdomen, dizziness, nausea, vomiting, chills, fever, headache, pallor, tremors)

General Dosage Range I.V.:

Infants and Children: 0.3-0.6 mL/kg (maximum: 20 mL)

Adults: 20 mL

Iodixanol (EYE oh dix an ole)

U.S. Brand Names Visipaque™

Canadian Brand Names Visipaque™

Pharmacologic Category Iodinated Contrast Media; Radiological/Contrast Media, Nonionic (Iso-Osmolality)

Use

Intra-arterial: Digital subtraction angiography, angiocardiography, peripheral arteriography, visceral arteriography, cerebral arteriography

Intravenous: Contrast enhanced computed tomography imaging, excretory urography, and peripheral venography

Local Anesthetic/Vasoconstrictor Precautions No information available to require special precautions

Effects on Dental Treatment Key adverse event(s) related to dental treatment: Taste perversion.

Effects on Bleeding No information available to require special precautions

Adverse Effects

>10%: Local: Injection site reactions (discomfort/pain/warmth 30%)

1% to 10%:

Cardiovascular: Angina/chest pain (2%)

Central nervous system: Headache/migraine (3%), vertigo (2%)

Dermatologic: Nonurticarial rash/erythema (2%), pruritus (2%)

Gastrointestinal: Taste perversion (4%), nausea (3%)

Neuromuscular & skeletal: Paresthesia (1%)

Respiratory: Parosoma (1%)

General Dosage Range

I.V.:

Children >1-12 years: Iodixanol 270 mg iodine/mL: 1-2 mL/kg (maximum: 2 mL/kg)

Children >12 years and Adults: Iodixanol 270 mg and 320 mg iodine/mL: Concentration and dose vary based on study type; refer to product labeling (maximum total dose: 80 g iodine)

Intra-arterial:

Children >1-12 years: Iodixanol 320 mg iodine/mL: 1-2 mL/kg (maximum: 4 mL/kg)

Children >12 years and Adults: Iodixanol 320 mg iodine/mL: Dose individualized based on injection site and study type; refer to product labeling (maximum total dose: 80 g iodine)

Mechanism of Action Opacifies vessels in the path of flow permitting radiographic imaging of internal structures.

Pharmacodynamics/Kinetics

Half-life Elimination Children: 2-4 hours; Adults: 2 hours

Time to Peak Immediate; peak enhancement at 15-120 seconds; optimum renal contrast at 5-15 minutes; brain contrast at up to 1 hour

Pregnancy Risk Factor B

Iodoquinol (eye oh doe KWIN ole)

U.S. Brand Names Yodoxin®

Canadian Brand Names Diodoquin®

Pharmacologic Category Amebicide

Use Treatment of acute and chronic intestinal amebiasis; asymptomatic cyst passers; *Blastocystis hominis* infections; ineffective for amebic hepatitis or hepatic abscess

Local Anesthetic/Vasoconstrictor Precautions No information available to require special precautions

Effects on Dental Treatment No significant effects or complications reported

Effects on Bleeding No information available to require special precautions

Adverse Effects Frequency not defined.

Central nervous system: Fever, chills, agitation, retrograde amnesia, headache

Dermatologic: Rash, urticaria, pruritus

Endocrine & metabolic: Thyroid gland enlargement

Gastrointestinal: Diarrhea, nausea, vomiting, stomach pain, abdominal cramps

Neuromuscular & skeletal: Peripheral neuropathy, weakness

Ocular: Optic neuritis, optic atrophy, visual impairment

Miscellaneous: Itching of rectal area

General Dosage Range Oral:

Children: 30-40 mg/kg/day in 3 divided doses (maximum: 1.95 g/day)

Adults: 650 mg 3 times/day (maximum: 2 g/day)

Mechanism of Action Contact amebicide that works in the lumen of the intestine by an unknown mechanism

Iodoquinol and Hydrocortisone

(eye oh doe KWIN ole & hye droe KOR ti sone)

Related Information

Hydrocortisone (Topical) *on page 868*

Iodoquinol *on page 935*

Related Sample Prescriptions

Angular Cheilitis *on page 1988*

U.S. Brand Names Alcortin® A; Dermazene®

Generic Availability (U.S.) Yes: Cream

Pharmacologic Category Antifungal Agent, Topical; Corticosteroid, Topical

Dental Use Reported to be useful in the treatment of angular cheilitis

IODOQUINOL AND HYDROCORTISONE

Use Treatment of eczema (including impetiginized, nuchal, and nummular); acne urticaria; anogenital pruritus, atopic dermatitis, chronic infectious dermatitis; chronic eczematoid otitis externa; folliculitis, intertrigo; lichen simplex chronicus; moniliasis; mycotic dermatoses; neurodermatitis (localized or systemic); pyoderma, stasis dermatitis

Local Anesthetic/Vasoconstrictor Precautions No information available to require special precautions

Effects on Dental Treatment No significant effects or complications reported

Effects on Bleeding No information available to require special precautions

Adverse Effects

Based on **iodoquinol** component:

- Central nervous system: Fever, chills, agitation, retrograde amnesia, headache
- Dermatologic: Rash, urticaria, pruritus
- Endocrine & metabolic: Thyroid gland enlargement
- Gastrointestinal: Diarrhea, nausea, vomiting, stomach pain, abdominal cramps
- Neuromuscular & skeletal: Peripheral neuropathy, weakness
- Ocular: Optic neuritis, optic atrophy, visual impairment
- Miscellaneous: Itching of rectal area

Based on **hydrocortisone** component:

>10%:

- Central nervous system: Insomnia, nervousness
- Gastrointestinal: Increased appetite, indigestion

1% to 10%:

- Dermatologic: Hirsutism
- Endocrine & metabolic: Diabetes mellitus
- Neuromuscular & skeletal: Arthralgia
- Ocular: Cataracts
- Respiratory: Epistaxis

Dental Usual Dosage Angular cheilitis: Adults: Topical: Apply 3-4 times/day

Dosage Topical: Children ≥12 years and Adults: Apply 3-4 times/day

Contraindications

Based on **iodoquinol** component: Hypersensitivity to iodine or iodoquinol or any component of the formulation; hepatic damage; pre-existing optic neuropathy

Based on **hydrocortisone** component: Hypersensitivity to hydrocortisone or any component of the formulation; serious infections, except septic shock or tuberculous meningitis; viral, fungal, or tubercular skin lesions

Warnings/Precautions

Based on **iodoquinol** component: Optic neuritis, optic atrophy, and peripheral neuropathy have occurred following prolonged use; avoid long-term therapy

Based on **hydrocortisone** component:

Use with caution in patients with hyperthyroidism, cirrhosis, nonspecific ulcerative colitis, hypertension, osteoporosis, thromboembolic tendencies, CHF, convulsive disorders, myasthenia gravis, thrombophlebitis, peptic ulcer, diabetes

Acute adrenal insufficiency may occur with abrupt withdrawal (depending on degree of systemic absorption) after long-term therapy or with stress; young pediatric patients may be more susceptible to adrenal axis suppression from topical therapy

Drug Interactions

Metabolism/Transport Effects Hydrocortisone: **Substrate** of CYP3A4 (minor), P-glycoprotein; **Induces** CYP3A4 (weak)

Avoid Concomitant Use

Avoid concomitant use of Iodoquinol and Hydrocortisone with any of the following: Aldesleukin; BCG; Natalizumab; Pimecrolimus; Roflumilast; Tacrolimus (Topical)

Increased Effect/Toxicity

Iodoquinol and Hydrocortisone may increase the levels/effects of: Acetylcholinesterase Inhibitors; Amphotericin B; Deferasirox; Leflunomide; Loop Diuretics; Natalizumab; NSAID (COX-2 Inhibitor); NSAID (Nonselective); Thiazide Diuretics; Vaccines (Live); Warfarin

The levels/effects of Iodoquinol and Hydrocortisone may be increased by: Antifungal Agents (Azole Derivatives, Systemic); Aprepitant; Calcium Channel Blockers (Nondihydropyridine); Conivaptan; Denosumab; Estrogen Derivatives; Fluconazole; Fosaprepitant; Macrolide Antibiotics; Neuromuscular-Blocking Agents (Nondepolarizing); P-Glycoprotein Inhibitors; Pimecrolimus; Quinolone Antibiotics; Roflumilast; Salicylates; Tacrolimus (Topical); Trastuzumab

Decreased Effect

Iodoquinol and Hydrocortisone may decrease the levels/effects of: Aldesleukin; Antidiabetic Agents; BCG; Calcitriol; Corticorelin; Isoniazid; Salicylates; Sipuleucel-T; Vaccines (Inactivated)

The levels/effects of Iodoquinol and Hydrocortisone may be decreased by: Aminoglutethimide; Antacids; Barbiturates; Bile Acid Sequestrants; Echinacea; Mitotane; P-Glycoprotein Inducers; Primidone; Rifamycin Derivatives; Tocilizumab

Pregnancy Risk Factor C

Lactation Excretion in breast milk unknown/use caution

Dosage Forms

Cream, topical: Iodoquinol 1% and hydrocortisone 1% (30 g)

Dermazene®: Iodoquinol 1% and hydrocortisone 1% (30 g)

Gel, topical:

Alcortin® A: Iodoquinol 1% and hydrocortisone 2% (2 g)

Iohexol (eye oh HEX ole)

U.S. Brand Names Omnipaque™ 140; Omnipaque™ 180; Omnipaque™ 240; Omnipaque™ 300; Omnipaque™ 350

Canadian Brand Names Omnipaque™

Pharmacologic Category Polypeptide Hormone; Radiological/Contrast Media, Nonionic (Low Osmolality)

Use

Intrathecal: Myelography; contrast enhancement for computerized tomography

Intravascular: Angiocardiography, aortography, digital subtraction angiography, peripheral arteriography, excretory urography; contrast enhancement for computed tomographic imaging

Oral/body cavity: Arthrography, GI tract examination, hysterosalpingography, pancreatography, cholangiopancreatography, herniography, cystourethrography; enhanced computed tomography of the abdomen

Local Anesthetic/Vasoconstrictor Precautions No information available to require special precautions

Effects on Dental Treatment No significant effects or complications reported

Effects on Bleeding No information available to require special precautions

Adverse Effects Frequency not defined; **Note:** Children have a lower frequency of reactions than adults.

Cardiovascular: Asystole, arrhythmia, bradycardia, cardiopulmonary collapse, edema, heart failure, hypertension (in patients with phenochromocytoma after intra-arterial injection), hypotension, syncope, transient ischemic attacks, vasovagal attacks, venous thrombosis, ventricular fibrillation, ventricular tachycardia

Central nervous system: Anxiety, confusion, dizziness, headache, loss of consciousness, seizure, vertigo

Dermatologic: Pruritus, rash, urticaria

Endocrine & metabolic: Thyrotoxicosis exacerbation

Gastrointestinal: Cramping, diarrhea, nausea, salivary gland swelling, vomiting

Local: Burning sensation, pain at injection site, thrombophlebitis

Neuromuscular & skeletal: Parasthesia, polyarthropathy, tremor

Ocular: Vision abnormalities

Renal: Contrast-associated nephropathy, creatinine increased, renal dysfunction

Respiratory: Bronchospasm, cough, dyspnea, pulmonary edema, rhinitis, sneezing

Miscellaneous: Anaphylactoid reaction, diaphoresis, hypersensitivity reactions

Mechanism of Action Opacification of vessels and anatomical structures in the path of flow of the contrast media which allows for radiographic visualization

Pharmacodynamics/Kinetics

Duration of Action

CNS: ~30 minutes following intrathecal administration, 60 minutes following intravenous administration

Serum: 15-120 seconds

Pregnancy Risk Factor B

Iopamidol (eye oh PA mi dole)

U.S. Brand Names Isovue Multipack®; Isovue-M®; Isovue®; Isovue® 200; Isovue® 300; Isovue® 370

Pharmacologic Category Iodinated Contrast Media; Radiological/Contrast Media, Nonionic (Low Osmolality)

Use

Intrathecal (Isovue-M®): Myelography contrast enhancement of computed tomographic cisternography and ventriculography; thoracolumbar myelography

Intravascular (Isovue®, Isovue Multipack®): Angiography (eg, coronary, cerebral, peripheral arteriogram), pediatric angiocardiography, excretory urography; contrast enhancement of computed tomographic imaging (in adults and children); evaluation of certain malignancies; image enhancement of non-neoplastic lesions

Local Anesthetic/Vasoconstrictor Precautions No information available to require special precautions

Effects on Dental Treatment No significant effects or complications reported

Effects on Bleeding No information available to require special precautions

Adverse Effects

>10%: Central nervous system: Headache (1% to 16%)

≥1% to 10%:

Cardiovascular: Angina pectoris (3%), flushing (2%), bradycardia (1%), hypertension (1%), hypotension (1%), arrhythmias, circulatory collapse, MI, tachycardia, ventricular fibrillation

Central nervous system: Hot flashes (3%), pain (3%), chills, faintness, fever, vasovagal reaction

Dermatologic: Hives (1%), pruritus, rash, urticaria

Gastrointestinal: Nausea (1% to 7%), vomiting (1% to 4%), anorexia, taste alterations

Genitourinary: Urinary retention

Local: Burning sensation (1%), thrombophlebitis

Neuromuscular & skeletal: Muscle pain (1% to 2%)

Ocular: Visual disturbances

Respiratory: Dyspnea, nasal congestion, pulmonary edema

Miscellaneous: Diaphoresis

Mechanism of Action Opacification of vessels and anatomical structures in the path of flow of the contrast media which allows for radiographic visualization

Pharmacodynamics/Kinetics

Half-life Elimination 2 hours; prolonged in renal impairment

Pregnancy Risk Factor B

Iopromide (eye oh PROE mide)

U.S. Brand Names Ultravist®

Pharmacologic Category Iodinated Contrast Media; Radiological/Contrast Media, Nonionic (Low Osmolality)

Use Enhance imaging in cerebral arteriography and peripheral arteriography; coronary arteriography and left ventriculography, visceral angiography and aortography; contrast-enhanced computed tomographic imaging of the head and body, excretory urography, intra-arterial digital subtraction angiography, peripheral venography

Local Anesthetic/Vasoconstrictor Precautions No information available to require special precautions

Effects on Dental Treatment Key adverse event(s) related to dental treatment: Abnormal taste.

Effects on Bleeding No information available to require special precautions

Adverse Effects 1% to 10%:

Cardiovascular: Vasodilatation (4%), chest pain (3%), hypertension (1%)

Central nervous system: Headache (6%), pain (2%), dizziness (1%)

Gastrointestinal: Nausea (4%), vomiting (2%), abnormal taste (1%),

Genitourinary: Urinary urgency (3%)

Local: Injection site hematoma (3%), injection site pain (1%)

Neuromuscular & skeletal: Back pain (3%)

Ocular: Abnormal vision (2%)

Mechanism of Action Iopromide opacifies vessels in its path of flow, permitting radiographic visualization of internal structures.

Pharmacodynamics/Kinetics

Half-life Elimination Main elimination phase: 2 hours, terminal phase: 6.2 hours

Time to Peak

Intravascular: Contrast enhancement: 15-120 seconds after bolus injection

Intravenous: Contrast enhancement: Kidneys: 5-15 minutes

Pregnancy Risk Factor B

Iothalamate Meglumine (eye oh thal A mate MEG loo meen)

U.S. Brand Names Conray®; Conray® 30; Conray® 43; Cysto-Conray® II

Pharmacologic Category Iodinated Contrast Media; Radiological/Contrast Media, Ionic (High Osmolality)

Use

Solution for injection: Arthrography, cerebral angiography, cranial computerized angiotomography, digital subtraction angiography, direct cholangiography, endoscopic retrograde cholangiopancreatography, excretory urography, peripheral arteriography, urography, venography; contrast enhancement of computed tomographic images

Solution for instillation: Retrograde cystography and cystourethrography

Local Anesthetic/Vasoconstrictor Precautions No information available to require special precautions

Effects on Dental Treatment No significant effects or complications reported

Effects on Bleeding No information available to require special precautions

Pregnancy Risk Factor B/C (product dependent)

Ioversol (EYE oh ver sole)

U.S. Brand Names Optiray® 160; Optiray® 240; Optiray® 300; Optiray® 320; Optiray® 350

Pharmacologic Category Iodinated Contrast Media; Radiological/Contrast Media, Nonionic (Low Osmolality)

Use Arteriography, angiography, angiocardiography, ventriculography, excretory urography, and venography procedures; contrast enhanced tomographic imaging; intra-arterial digital substraction angiography (Optiray® 160)

Local Anesthetic/Vasoconstrictor Precautions No information available to require special precautions

Effects on Dental Treatment No significant effects or complications reported

Effects on Bleeding No information available to require special precautions

Adverse Effects

>10%: Central nervous system: Headache (16%)

1% to 10%:

Cardiovascular: Angina pectoris (3%), flushing (2%), bradycardia (1%), hypotension (1%), arrhythmias, hypertension (in patients with phenochromocytoma after intra-arterial injection), myocardial ischemia, tachycardia, venous thrombosis, ventricular fibrillation, ventricular tachycardia

Central nervous system: Hot flashes (3%), chills, fever, transient ischemic attack

Dermatologic: Hives (1%), pruritus, rash, urticaria

Gastrointestinal: Nausea (7%), vomiting (4%), anorexia, taste alterations

Genitourinary: Urinary retention

Local: Burning sensation (1%)

Neuromuscular & skeletal: Back pain (2%), leg pain (1%), neck pain (1%), back spasm, paresthesia

Ocular: Vision abnormalities

Renal: Contrast-associated nephropathy, creatinine increased, renal dysfunction

Respiratory: Bronchospasm, cough, dyspnea, pulmonary edema, rhinitis, sneezing

Miscellaneous: Diaphoresis, hypersensitivity reactions

Mechanism of Action Opacification of vessels and anatomical structures in the path of flow of the contrast media which allows for radiographic visualization.

Pharmacodynamics/Kinetics

Half-life Elimination 2 hours

Pregnancy Risk Factor B

Ioxaglate Meglumine and Ioxaglate Sodium

(eye ox AG late MEG loo meen & eye ox AG late SOW dee um)

U.S. Brand Names Hexabrix™

Pharmacologic Category Iodinated Contrast Media; Radiological/Contrast Media, Ionic (Low Osmolality)

Use Angiocardiography, arteriography, aortography, arthrography, angiography, hysterosalpingography, venography, and urography procedures; contrast enhancement of computed tomographic imaging

Local Anesthetic/Vasoconstrictor Precautions No information available to require special precautions

Effects on Dental Treatment No significant effects or complications reported

Effects on Bleeding No information available to require special precautions

Pregnancy Risk Factor B

Ipecac Syrup (IP e kak SIR up)

Pharmacologic Category Antidote

Use Treatment of acute oral drug overdosage and in certain poisonings

Local Anesthetic/Vasoconstrictor Precautions No information available to require special precautions

Effects on Dental Treatment No significant effects or complications reported

Effects on Bleeding No information available to require special precautions

Adverse Effects Frequency not defined.

Cardiovascular: Cardiotoxicity

Central nervous system: Lethargy

Gastrointestinal: Diarrhea, protracted vomiting
Neuromuscular & skeletal: Myopathy

General Dosage Range Oral:

Children 6-12 months: 5-10 mL followed by 10-20 mL/kg of water, may repeat if vomiting does not occur within 20 minutes

Children 1-12 years: 15 mL followed by 10-20 mL/kg of water, may repeat if vomiting does not occur within 20 minutes

Adults: 15-30 mL followed by 200-300 mL of water, may repeat if vomiting does not occur within 20 minutes

Mechanism of Action Irritates the gastric mucosa and stimulates the medullary chemoreceptor trigger zone to induce vomiting

Pharmacodynamics/Kinetics

Onset of Action 15-30 minutes

Duration of Action 20-25 minutes; 60 minutes in some cases

Pregnancy Risk Factor C

Ipilimumab (ip i LIM u mab)

U.S. Brand Names Yervoy™

Pharmacologic Category Antineoplastic Agent, Monoclonal Antibody; Monoclonal Antibody

Use Treatment of unresectable or metastatic melanoma

Local Anesthetic/Vasoconstrictor Precautions No information available to require special precautions

Effects on Dental Treatment No significant effects or complications reported

Effects on Bleeding Chemotherapy may result in significant myelosuppression, potentially including significant reduction in platelet counts and altered hemostasis. In patients who are under active treatment with these agents, medical consult is suggested.

Adverse Effects

>10%:

Central nervous system: Fatigue (41% to 42%; grades 3-5: 7%), headache (14%), fever (12%)

Dermatologic: Pruritus (24% to 31%), rash (19% to 29%; grades 3-5: 2%), dermatitis (grade 2: 12%; grades 3-5: 2% to 3% [includes Stevens-Johnson syndrome, toxic epidermal necrolysis, dermal ulceration necrotic, bullous or hemorrhagic dermatitis])

Gastrointestinal: Nausea (35%), diarrhea (32% to 33%; grades 3-5: 5%), appetite decreased (27%), vomiting (24%), constipation (21%), abdominal pain (15%)

Hematologic: Anemia (12%)

Respiratory: Cough (16%), dyspnea (15%)

1% to 10%:

Dermatologic: Urticaria (2%), vitiligo (2%)

Endocrine & metabolic: Hypopituitarism (grade 2: 2%; grades 3-5: 4%), hypothyroidism (≤2%), hypophysitis (2%), adrenal insufficiency (≤2%)

Gastrointestinal: Colitis (8%; grades 3-5: 5%), enterocolitis (grade 2: 5%; grades 3-5: 7%), intestinal perforation (1%)

Hematologic: Eosinophilia (grades 3-5: 1%)

Hepatic: Hepatotoxicity (grade 2: 3%; grades 3-5: 1% to 2%), ALT increased (2%)

Renal: Nephritis (grades 3-5: 1%)

General Dosage Range Dosage adjustment recommended in patients who develop toxicities.

I.V.: *Adults:* 3 mg/kg every 3 weeks

Mechanism of Action Ipilimumab is a recombinant human IgG1 immunoglobulin monoclonal antibody which binds to the cytotoxic T-lymphocyte associated antigen 4 (CTLA-4). CTLA-4 is a down-regulator of T-cell activation pathways. Blocking CTLA-4, allows for enhanced T-cell activation and proliferation. In melanoma, ipilimumab may indirectly mediate T-cell immune responses against tumors.

Pharmacodynamics/Kinetics

Half-life Elimination Terminal: 14.7 days

Pregnancy Risk Factor C

Ipratropium (Oral Inhalation) (i pra TROE pee um)

Related Information

Respiratory Diseases *on page* 1876

U.S. Brand Names Atrovent® HFA

Canadian Brand Names Atrovent® HFA; Gen-Ipratropium; Mylan-Ipratropium Sterinebs; Novo-Ipramide; Nu-Ipratropium; PMS-Ipratropium

Pharmacologic Category Anticholinergic Agent

Use Anticholinergic bronchodilator used in bronchospasm associated with COPD, bronchitis, and emphysema

Local Anesthetic/Vasoconstrictor Precautions No information available to require special precautions

Effects on Dental Treatment Key adverse event(s) related to dental treatment: Xerostomia and changes in salivation (normal salivary flow resumes upon discontinuation), and dry mucous membranes.

Effects on Bleeding No information available to require special precautions

Adverse Effects

>10%: Respiratory: Upper respiratory tract infection (9% to 34%), bronchitis (10% to 23%), sinusitis (1% to 11%)

1% to 10%:

Cardiovascular: Chest pain (3%), palpitation

Central nervous system: Headache (6% to 7%), dizziness (2% to 3%)

Gastrointestinal: Dyspepsia (1% to 5%), nausea (4%), xerostomia (2% to 4%)

Genitourinary: Urinary tract infection (2% to 10%)

Neuromuscular & skeletal: Back pain (2% to 7%)

Respiratory: Dyspnea (7% to 10%), rhinitis (2% to 6%), cough (3% to 5%), pharyngitis (4%), bronchospasm (2%), sputum increased (1%)

Miscellaneous: Flu-like syndrome (4% to 8%)

General Dosage Range

Inhalation: *Children >12 years and Adults:* 2 inhalations 4 times/day (maximum: 12 inhalations/day)

Nebulization: *Children >12 years and Adults:* 500 mcg every 6-8 hours

Mechanism of Action Blocks the action of acetylcholine at parasympathetic sites in bronchial smooth muscle causing bronchodilation; local application to nasal mucosa inhibits serous and seromucous gland secretions.

Pharmacodynamics/Kinetics

Onset of Action Bronchodilation: Within 15 minutes; Peak effect: 1-2 hours

Duration of Action 2-5 hours

Half-life Elimination 2 hours

Pregnancy Risk Factor B

Ipratropium (Nasal) (i pra TROE pee um)

U.S. Brand Names Atrovent®

Canadian Brand Names Alti-Ipratropium; Apo-Ipravent®; Atrovent®; Mylan-Ipratropium Solution

Pharmacologic Category Anticholinergic Agent

Use Symptomatic relief of rhinorrhea associated with the common cold and allergic and nonallergic rhinitis

Local Anesthetic/Vasoconstrictor Precautions No information available to require special precautions

Effects on Dental Treatment No significant effects or complications reported

Effects on Bleeding No information available to require special precautions

Adverse Effects 1% to 10%:

Central nervous system: Headache (4% to 10%)

Gastrointestinal: Taste perversion (≤4%), xerostomia (1% to 4%), diarrhea (2%), nausea (2%)

Respiratory: Upper respiratory tract infection (5% to 10%), epistaxis (6% to 9%), pharyngitis (≤8%), nasal dryness (<1% to 5%), nasal irritation (2%), nasal congestion (1%)

General Dosage Range Intranasal:

0.03% solution: *Children ≥6 years and Adults:* 2 sprays in each nostril 2-3 times/day

0.06% solution: *Children ≥5 years and Adults:* 2 sprays in each nostril 3-4 times/day

Mechanism of Action Local application to nasal mucosa inhibits serous and seromucous gland secretions.

Pharmacodynamics/Kinetics

Half-life Elimination 1.6 hours

Pregnancy Risk Factor B

Ipratropium and Albuterol (i pra TROE pee um & al BYOO ter ole)

Related Information

Albuterol *on page 66*

Ipratropium (Oral Inhalation) *on page 940*

U.S. Brand Names Combivent®; DuoNeb®

Canadian Brand Names CO Ipra-Sal; Combivent UDV; Gen-Combo Sterinebs; ratio-Ipra Sal UDV

Generic Availability (U.S.) Yes: Solution for nebulization

Pharmacologic Category Anticholinergic Agent; $Beta_2$-Adrenergic Agonist

Use Treatment of COPD in those patients who are currently on a regular bronchodilator who continue to have bronchospasms and require a second bronchodilator

Local Anesthetic/Vasoconstrictor Precautions No information available to require special precautions

Effects on Dental Treatment Key adverse event(s) related to dental treatment: Xerostomia (normal salivary flow resumes upon discontinuation), dry mucous membrane, and unusual taste.

Effects on Bleeding No information available to require special precautions

Adverse Effects Percentages reported with either combination product (not versus placebo). Also see individual agents.

>10%: Respiratory: Bronchitis (2% to 12%), upper respiratory tract infection (11%)

1% to 10%:

Cardiovascular: Chest pain (≤3%), angina (<2%), arrhythmia (<2%), edema (<2%), hypertension (<2%), palpitation (<2%), tachycardia (<2%)

Central nervous system: Headache (6%), pain (1% to 3%), dizziness (<2%), fatigue (<2%), insomnia (<2%), nervousness (<2%), tremor (<2%)

Gastrointestinal: Diarrhea (≤2%), dyspepsia (≤2%), nausea (1% to 2%), sputum increased (<2%), taste perversion (<2%), vomiting (<2%), xerostomia (<2%)

Genitourinary: Urinary tract infection (≤2%)

Neuromuscular & skeletal: Arthralgia (<2%), paresthesia (<2%), leg cramps (1%)

Respiratory: Lung disease (6%), dyspnea (5%), cough (4%), pharyngitis (2% to 4%), respiratory disorder (3%), sinusitis (2%), pneumonia (1%), rhinitis (1%)

Miscellaneous: Dysphonia (<2%), flu-like syndrome (1%)

Dosage Adults:

Aerosol for inhalation: 2 inhalations 4 times/day (maximum: 12 inhalations/24 hours)

Solution for nebulization: Initial: 3 mL every 6 hours (maximum: 3 mL every 4 hours)

Mechanism of Action See individual agents.

Contraindications Hypersensitivity to ipratropium, albuterol, atropine (and its derivatives) or any component of the formulation

Warnings/Precautions See individual agents. The aerosol dosage form of this combination contains soya lecithin; may cause allergic reactions in patients with allergy to soya lecithin or related food products (eg, soybean and peanut)

Drug Interactions

Avoid Concomitant Use

Avoid concomitant use of Ipratropium and Albuterol with any of the following: Iobenguane I 123

Increased Effect/Toxicity

Ipratropium and Albuterol may increase the levels/effects of: AbobotulinumtoxinA; Anticholinergics; Cannabinoids; Loop Diuretics; OnabotulinumtoxinA; Potassium Chloride; RimabotulinumtoxinB; Sympathomimetics

The levels/effects of Ipratropium and Albuterol may be increased by: Atomoxetine; MAO Inhibitors; Pramlintide; Tricyclic Antidepressants

Decreased Effect

Ipratropium and Albuterol may decrease the levels/effects of: Acetylcholinesterase Inhibitors (Central); Iobenguane I 123; Secretin

The levels/effects of Ipratropium and Albuterol may be decreased by: Acetylcholinesterase Inhibitors (Central); Alpha-/Beta-Blockers; Beta-Blockers (Beta1 Selective); Beta-Blockers (Nonselective); Betahistine

Dietary Considerations The aerosol dosage form contains soya lecithin. Do not use in patients allergic to soya lecithin or related food products such as soybean and peanut.

Pregnancy Risk Factor C

Breast-Feeding Considerations See individual agents.

Dosage Forms

Aerosol for oral inhalation:

Combivent®: Ipratropium bromide 18 mcg and albuterol (base) 90 mcg per inhalation (14.7 g) [200 metered actuations]

Solution for nebulization: Ipratropium 0.5 mg and albuterol (base) 2.5 mg per 3 mL (30s, 60s)

DuoNeb®: Ipratropium 0.5 mg and albuterol (base) 2.5 mg per 3 mL (30s, 60s)

Ipratropium and Fenoterol (i pra TROE pee um & fen oh TER ole)

Related Information

Ipratropium (Oral Inhalation) *on page* 940

Canadian Brand Names Duovent® UDV

Pharmacologic Category Anticholinergic Agent; $Beta_2$-Adrenergic Agonist

Use Treatment of bronchospasm associated with acute severe exacerbation of COPD or bronchial asthma

Local Anesthetic/Vasoconstrictor Precautions No information available to require special precautions

Effects on Dental Treatment Key adverse event(s) related to dental treatment: Xerostomia (normal salivary flow resumes upon discontinuation).

Effects on Bleeding No information available to require special precautions

Adverse Effects Frequency not defined.

Cardiovascular: Arrhythmias, atrial fibrillation, cardiac arrest, hyper-/hypotension, myocardial ischemia, palpitation, QT_c prolongation, SVT, tachycardia

Central nervous system: Dizziness, headache, nervousness, psychological alterations

Gastrointestinal: Constipation, diarrhea, nausea, vomiting, xerostomia

Genitourinary: Urinary retention

Endocrine & metabolic: Hyperglycemia, hypokalemia

Neuromuscular & skeletal: Muscle cramps, myalgia, tremor, weakness

Ophthalmic: Accommodation disturbance, acute angle closure glaucoma, eye pain, intraocular pressure increased, mydriasis

Respiratory: Bronchospasm (inhalation induced), cough, pharyngitis, throat irritation

Miscellaneous: Allergic reactions (anaphylaxis, angioedema, bronchospasm, laryngospasm, oropharyngeal edema, skin rash, urticaria); diaphoresis

General Dosage Range Nebulization: *Children ≥12 years and Adults:* Usual dose: 4 mL; may repeat every 6 hours as needed

Mechanism of Action

Ipratropium: Blocks the action of acetylcholine at parasympathetic sites in bronchial smooth muscle causing bronchodilation

Fenoterol: Relaxes bronchial smooth muscle by action on $beta_2$-receptors

Pharmacodynamics/Kinetics

Onset of Action

Ipratropium: Bronchodilation: Within 15 minutes

Peak effect: 1-2 hours

Fenoterol: Bronchodilation: 5 minutes

Peak effect: 30-60 minutes

Duration of Action

Ipratropium: 6-8 hours

Fenoterol: 4-6 hours; In combination with ipratropium: 6-8 hours

Product Availability Not available in U.S.

Irbesartan (ir be SAR tan)

Related Information

Cardiovascular Diseases *on page 1848*

U.S. Brand Names Avapro®

Canadian Brand Names Avapro®

Generic Availability (U.S.) No

Pharmacologic Category Angiotensin II Receptor Blocker

Use Treatment of hypertension alone or in combination with other antihypertensives; treatment of diabetic nephropathy in patients with type 2 diabetes mellitus (non-insulin dependent, NIDDM) and hypertension

Unlabeled/Investigational Use To slow the rate of progression of aortic-root dilation in pediatric patients with Marfan's syndrome

Local Anesthetic/Vasoconstrictor Precautions No information available to require special precautions

Effects on Dental Treatment Key adverse event(s) related to dental treatment: Orthostatic hypotension.

Effects on Bleeding No information available to require special precautions

Adverse Effects Unless otherwise indicated, percentage of incidence is reported for patients with hypertension.

>10%: Endocrine & metabolic: Hyperkalemia (19%, diabetic nephropathy; rarely seen in HTN)

1% to 10%:

Cardiovascular: Orthostatic hypotension (5%, diabetic nephropathy)

Central nervous system: Fatigue (4%), dizziness (10%, diabetic nephropathy)

Gastrointestinal: Diarrhea (3%), dyspepsia (2%)

Respiratory: Upper respiratory infection (9%), cough (2.8% versus 2.7% in placebo)

>1% but frequency ≤ placebo: Abdominal pain, anxiety, chest pain, edema, headache, influenza, musculoskeletal pain, nausea, nervousness, pharyngitis, rash, rhinitis, sinus abnormality, syncope, tachycardia, urinary tract infection, vertigo, vomiting

Dosage Oral:

Hypertension:

Children:

<6 years: Safety and efficacy have not been established.

≥6-12 years: Initial: 75 mg once daily; may be titrated to a maximum of 150 mg once daily

Children ≥13 years and Adults: 150 mg once daily; patients may be titrated to 300 mg once daily

Note: Starting dose in volume-depleted patients should be 75 mg

Aortic-root dilation with Marfan's syndrome (unlabeled use): Children 14 months to 16 years: Initial: 1.4 mg/kg/day; can be increased to a maximum of 2 mg/kg/day (not to exceed adult maximum of 300 mg/day)

Nephropathy in patients with type 2 diabetes and hypertension: Adults: Target dose: 300 mg once daily

Dosage adjustment in renal impairment: No dosage adjustment necessary with mild to severe impairment unless the patient is also volume depleted.

Mechanism of Action Irbesartan is an angiotensin receptor antagonist. Angiotensin II acts as a vasoconstrictor. In addition to causing direct vasoconstriction, angiotensin II also stimulates the release of aldosterone. Once aldosterone is released, sodium as well as water are reabsorbed. The end result is an elevation in blood pressure. Irbesartan binds to the AT1 angiotensin II receptor. This binding prevents angiotensin II from binding to the receptor thereby blocking the vasoconstriction and the aldosterone secreting effects of angiotensin II.

Contraindications Hypersensitivity to irbesartan or any component of the formulation

Warnings/Precautions [U.S. Boxed Warning]: Based on human data, drugs that act on the angiotensin system can cause injury and death to the developing fetus when used in the second and third trimesters. Angiotensin receptor blockers should be discontinued as soon as possible once pregnancy is detected. May cause hyperkalemia; avoid potassium supplementation unless specifically required by healthcare provider. May be associated with deterioration of renal function and/or increases in serum creatinine, particularly in patients with low renal blood flow (eg, renal artery stenosis, heart failure) whose glomerular filtration rate (GFR) is dependent on efferent arteriolar vasoconstriction by angiotensin II. Avoid use or use a much smaller dose in patients who are intravascularly volume-depleted; use caution in patients with unstented unilateral or bilateral renal artery stenosis. When unstented bilateral renal artery stenosis is present, use is generally avoided due to the elevated risk of deterioration in renal function unless possible benefits outweigh risks. AUCs of irbesartan (not the active metabolite) are about 50% greater in patients with Cl_{cr} <30 mL/minute and are doubled in hemodialysis patients. Concurrent use of ACE inhibitors may increase the risk of clinically-significant adverse events (eg, renal dysfunction, hyperkalemia).

Drug Interactions

Metabolism/Transport Effects Substrate of CYP2C9 (minor); **Inhibits** CYP2C8 (moderate), 2C9 (moderate), 2D6 (weak), 3A4 (weak)

Avoid Concomitant Use There are no known interactions where it is recommended to avoid concomitant use.

Increased Effect/Toxicity

Irbesartan may increase the levels/effects of: ACE Inhibitors; Amifostine; Antihypertensives; Carvedilol; CYP2C8 Substrates (High risk); CYP2C9 Substrates (High risk); Hypotensive Agents; Lithium; Nonsteroidal Anti-Inflammatory Agents; Potassium-Sparing Diuretics; RiTUXimab

The levels/effects of Irbesartan may be increased by: Diazoxide; Eplerenone; Fluconazole; Herbs (Hypotensive Properties); MAO Inhibitors; Pentoxifylline; Phosphodiesterase 5 Inhibitors; Potassium Salts; Prostacyclin Analogues; Tolvaptan; Trimethoprim

Decreased Effect

The levels/effects of Irbesartan may be decreased by: Herbs (Hypertensive Properties); Methylphenidate; Nonsteroidal Anti-Inflammatory Agents; Rifamycin Derivatives; Yohimbine

Ethanol/Nutrition/Herb Interactions Herb/Nutraceutical: Avoid dong quai if using for hypertension (has estrogenic activity). Avoid ephedra, yohimbe, ginseng (may worsen hypertension). Avoid garlic (may have increased antihypertensive effect).

Dietary Considerations May be taken with or without food.

Pharmacodynamics/Kinetics

Onset of Action Peak levels in 1-2 hours

Duration of Action >24 hours
Half-life Elimination Terminal: 11-15 hours
Time to Peak Serum: 1.5-2 hours
Pregnancy Risk Factor C (1st trimester); D (2nd and 3rd trimesters)
Lactation Excretion in breast milk unknown/contraindicated
Dosage Forms
Tablet, oral:
Avapro®: 75 mg, 150 mg, 300 mg

Irbesartan and Hydrochlorothiazide
(ir be SAR tan & hye droe klor oh THYE a zide)

Related Information
Hydrochlorothiazide *on page 854*
Irbesartan *on page 943*
U.S. Brand Names Avalide®
Canadian Brand Names Avalide®
Pharmacologic Category Angiotensin II Receptor Blocker; Diuretic, Thiazide
Use Combination therapy for the management of hypertension; may be used as initial therapy in patients likely to need multiple drugs to achieve blood pressure goals
Local Anesthetic/Vasoconstrictor Precautions No information available to require special precautions
Effects on Dental Treatment No significant effects or complications reported
Effects on Bleeding No information available to require special precautions
Adverse Effects Reactions/percentages reported with combination product; also refer to individual agents.
1% to 10%:
Cardiovascular: Edema (3%), chest pain (2%), tachycardia (1%)
Central nervous system: Dizziness (8%; orthostatic: 1%), fatigue (6%)
Gastrointestinal: Nausea/vomiting (3%), abdominal pain (2%), dyspepsia (2%)
Genitourinary: Urination abnormal (2%)
Neuromuscular & skeletal: Musculoskeletal pain (6%)
Renal: BUN increased (2%), creatinine increased (1%)
Miscellaneous: Flu-like syndrome (3%)
General Dosage Range Oral: *Adults:* Irbesartan 150-300 mg and hydrochlorothiazide 12.5-25 mg once daily
Mechanism of Action
Irbesartan: Irbesartan is an angiotensin receptor antagonist. Angiotensin II acts as a vasoconstrictor. In addition to causing direct vasoconstriction, angiotensin II also stimulates the release of aldosterone. Once aldosterone is released, sodium as well as water are reabsorbed. The end result is an elevation in blood pressure. Irbesartan binds to the AT1 angiotensin II receptor. This binding prevents angiotensin II from binding to the receptor thereby blocking the vasoconstriction and the aldosterone secreting effects of angiotensin II.
Hydrochlorothiazide: Inhibits sodium reabsorption in the distal tubules causing increased excretion of sodium and water as well as potassium and hydrogen ions
Pregnancy Risk Factor D

Irinotecan (eye rye no TEE kan)

U.S. Brand Names Camptosar®
Canadian Brand Names Camptosar®; Irinotecan Hydrochloride Trihydrate
Pharmacologic Category Antineoplastic Agent, Camptothecin; Antineoplastic Agent, Natural Source (Plant) Derivative; Antineoplastic Agent, Topoisomerase I Inhibitor
Use Treatment of metastatic carcinoma of the colon or rectum
Unlabeled/Investigational Use Treatment of cervical cancer (recurrent or metastatic), central nervous system tumors (recurrent glioblastoma), esophageal cancer, Ewing's sarcoma (recurrent or progressive), gastric cancer (metastatic or locally advanced), nonsmall cell lung cancer (advanced), ovarian cancer (recurrent), pancreatic cancer (advanced), small cell lung cancer (extensive stage)
Local Anesthetic/Vasoconstrictor Precautions No information available to require special precautions
Effects on Dental Treatment Key adverse event(s) related to dental treatment: Increased salivation, mucositis, and stomatitis.
Effects on Bleeding Chemotherapy may result in significant myelosuppression, potentially including significant reduction in platelet counts and altered hemostasis. In patients who are under active treatment with these agents, medical consult is suggested.

Adverse Effects Frequency of adverse reactions reported for single-agent use of irinotecan only.

>10%:

Cardiovascular: Vasodilation (9% to 11%)

Central nervous system: Cholinergic toxicity (47% - includes rhinitis, increased salivation, miosis, lacrimation, diaphoresis, flushing and intestinal hyperperistalsis); fever (44% to 45%), pain (23% to 24%), dizziness (15% to 21%), insomnia (19%), headache (17%), chills (14%)

Dermatologic: Alopecia (46% to 72%), rash (13% to 14%)

Endocrine & metabolic: Dehydration (15%)

Gastrointestinal: Diarrhea, late (83% to 88%; grade 3/4: 14% to 31%), diarrhea, early (43% to 51%; grade 3/4: 7% to 22%), nausea (70% to 86%), abdominal pain (57% to 68%), vomiting (62% to 67%), cramps (57%), anorexia (44% to 55%), constipation (30% to 32%), mucositis (30%), weight loss (30%), flatulence (12%), stomatitis (12%)

Hematologic: Anemia (60% to 97%; grades 3/4: 5% to 7%), leukopenia (63% to 96%, grades 3/4: 14% to 28%), thrombocytopenia (96%, grades 3/4: 1% to 4%), neutropenia (30% to 96%; grades 3/4: 14% to 31%)

Hepatic: Bilirubin increased (84%), alkaline phosphatase increased (13%)

Neuromuscular & skeletal: Weakness (69% to 76%), back pain (14%)

Respiratory: Dyspnea (22%), cough (17% to 20%), rhinitis (16%)

Miscellaneous: Diaphoresis (16%), infection (14%)

1% to 10%:

Cardiovascular: Edema (10%), hypotension (6%), thromboembolic events (5%)

Central nervous system: Somnolence (9%), confusion (3%)

Gastrointestinal: Abdominal fullness (10%), dyspepsia (10%)

Hematologic: Neutropenic fever (grades 3/4: 2% to 6%), hemorrhage (grades 3/4: 1% to 5%), neutropenic infection (grades 3/4: 1% to 2%)

Hepatic: AST increased (10%), ascites and/or jaundice (grades 3/4: 9%)

Respiratory: Pneumonia (4%)

Note: In limited pediatric experience, dehydration (often associated with severe hypokalemia and hyponatremia) was among the most significant grade 3/4 adverse events, with a frequency up to 29%. In addition, grade 3/4 infection was reported in 24%.

General Dosage Range Dosage adjustment recommended in patients with hepatic impairment or who develop toxicities

I.V.: *Adults:* Dosage varies greatly depending on indication

Mechanism of Action Irinotecan and its active metabolite (SN-38) bind reversibly to topoisomerase I-DNA complex preventing religation of the cleaved DNA strand. This results in the accumulation of cleavable complexes and double-strand DNA breaks. As mammalian cells cannot efficiently repair these breaks, cell death consistent with S-phase cell cycle specificity occurs, leading to termination of cellular replication.

Pharmacodynamics/Kinetics

Half-life Elimination Irinotecan: 6-12 hours; SN-38: ~10-20 hours

Time to Peak SN-38: Following 90-minute infusion: ~1 hour

Pregnancy Risk Factor D

Iron Dextran Complex (EYE ern DEKS tran KOM pleks)

U.S. Brand Names Dexferrum®; INFeD®

Canadian Brand Names Dexiron™; Infufer®

Pharmacologic Category Iron Salt

Use Treatment of iron deficiency in patients in whom oral administration is infeasible or ineffective

Unlabeled/Investigational Use Cancer-/chemotherapy-associated anemia

Local Anesthetic/Vasoconstrictor Precautions No information available to require special precautions

Effects on Dental Treatment Key adverse event(s) related to dental treatment: Metallic taste.

Effects on Bleeding No information available to require special precautions

Adverse Effects Frequency not defined. **Note:** Adverse event risk is reported to be higher with the high-molecular-weight iron dextran formulation.

Cardiovascular: Arrhythmia, bradycardia, cardiac arrest, chest pain, chest tightness, cyanosis, flushing, hyper-/hypotension, shock, syncope, tachycardia

Central nervous system: Chills, disorientation, dizziness, fever, headache, malaise, seizure, unconsciousness, unresponsiveness

Dermatologic: Pruritus, purpura, rash, urticaria

Gastrointestinal: Abdominal pain, diarrhea, nausea, taste alteration, vomiting

Genitourinary: Discoloration of urine

Hematologic: Leukocytosis, lymphadenopathy
Local: Injection site reactions (cellulitis, inflammation, pain, phlebitis, soreness, swelling), muscle atrophy/fibrosis (with I.M. injection), skin/tissue staining (at the site of I.M. injection), sterile abscess
Neuromuscular & skeletal: Arthralgia, arthritis/arthritis exacerbation, back pain, myalgia, paresthesia, weakness
Respiratory: Bronchospasm, dyspnea, respiratory arrest, wheezing
Renal: Hematuria
Miscellaneous: Anaphylactic reactions (sudden respiratory difficulty, cardiovascular collapse), diaphoresis

General Dosage Range Note: A 0.5 mL test dose (0.25 mL in infants) should be given prior to starting iron dextran therapy.

I.M., I.V.:

Children <5 kg and >4 months: Replacement iron (mg) = blood loss (mL) x Hct; **Note:** Total dose should be divided daily at not more than 25 mg/day

Children 5-15 kg and >4 months: Total Dose (mL) = 0.0442 (desired Hgb [usually 12 g/dL] - observed Hgb) x W (in kg) + (0.26 x W [in kg]) **or** replacement iron (mg) = blood loss (mL) x hematocrit; **Note:** Total dose should be divided daily at not more than 50 mg/day (5-10 kg) or 100 mg/day (10-15 kg)

Children >15 kg: Total Dose (mL) = 0.0442 (desired Hgb [usually 14.8 g/dL] - observed Hgb) x LBW + (0.26 x LBW) **or** replacement iron (mg) = blood loss (mL) x Hct; **Note:** Total dose should be divided daily at not more than 100 mg/day

Adults: Total Dose (mL) = 0.0442 (desired Hgb [usually 14.8 g/dL] - observed Hgb) x LBW + (0.26 x LBW) **or** replacement iron (mg) = blood loss (mL) x Hct; **Note:** Total dose should be divided daily at not more than 100 mg/day

Mechanism of Action The released iron, from the plasma, eventually replenishes the depleted iron stores in the bone marrow where it is incorporated into hemoglobin

Pharmacodynamics/Kinetics

Onset of Action I.V.: Serum ferritin peak: 7-9 days after dose

Pregnancy Risk Factor C

Iron Sucrose (EYE ern SOO krose)

U.S. Brand Names Venofer®

Canadian Brand Names Venofer®

Pharmacologic Category Iron Salt

Use Treatment of iron-deficiency anemia in chronic renal failure, including non-dialysis-dependent patients (with or without erythropoietin therapy) and dialysis-dependent patients receiving erythropoietin therapy

Unlabeled/Investigational Use Cancer-/chemotherapy-associated anemia

Local Anesthetic/Vasoconstrictor Precautions No information available to require special precautions

Effects on Dental Treatment Key adverse event(s) related to dental treatment: Taste perversion.

Effects on Bleeding No information available to require special precautions

Adverse Effects

>10%:

Cardiovascular: Hypotension (1% to 7%; 39% in hemodialysis patients; may be related to total dose or rate of administration), peripheral edema (2% to 17%)
Central nervous system: Headache (3% to 13%)
Gastrointestinal: Diarrhea (1% to 17%), nausea (1% to 15%), vomiting (3% to 12%)
Neuromuscular & skeletal: Muscle cramps (1% to 3%; 29% in hemodialysis patients)

1% to 10%:

Cardiovascular: Hypertension (6% to 8%), edema (1% to 7%), chest pain (1% to 6%), murmur (<1% to 3%), heart failure (2%), myocardial infarction (1%)
Central nervous system: Dizziness (1% to 10%), fatigue (2% to 5%), fever (1% to 3%), stroke (1%)
Dermatologic: Pruritus (1% to 7%), rash (≤1%)
Endocrine & metabolic: Gout (2% to 7%), hypoglycemia (<1% to 4%), hyperglycemia (3% to 4%), fluid overload (1% to 3%)
Gastrointestinal: Taste perversion (1% to 9%), peritoneal infection (≤8%), constipation (1% to 7%), abdominal pain (1% to 4%), positive fecal occult blood (1% to 3%)
Genitourinary: Urinary tract infection (≤1%)
Local: Injection site reaction (2% to 6%), catheter site infection (≤4%)
Neuromuscular & skeletal: Arthralgia (1% to 8%), back pain (1% to 8%), muscle pain (1% to 7%), extremity pain (3% to 6%), weakness (1% to 3%)
Ocular: Conjunctivitis (<1% to 3%)
Otic: Ear pain (1% to 7%)

Respiratory: Dyspnea (1% to 10%), pharyngitis (<1% to 7%), cough (1% to 7%), sinusitis (1% to 4%), nasopharyngitis (≤3%), upper respiratory infection (1% to 3%), nasal congestion (1%), pneumonia (1%), pulmonary edema (1%), rhinitis (≤1%)

Miscellaneous: Graft complication (1% to 10%), sepsis (2%)

General Dosage Range I.V.: *Adults:* 100 mg (5 mL) 1-3 times/week during dialysis **or** 200 mg on 5 different occasions within a 14-day period **or** two 300 mg infusion 14 days apart, followed by a single 400 mg infusion 14 days later (maximum: 1000 mg cumulative total)

Mechanism of Action Iron sucrose is dissociated by the reticuloendothelial system into iron and sucrose. The released iron increases serum iron concentrations and is incorporated into hemoglobin.

Pharmacodynamics/Kinetics

Half-life Elimination Healthy adults: 6 hours

Pregnancy Risk Factor B

Isocarboxazid (eye soe kar BOKS a zid)

U.S. Brand Names Marplan®

Pharmacologic Category Antidepressant, Monoamine Oxidase Inhibitor

Use Treatment of depression

Local Anesthetic/Vasoconstrictor Precautions Attempts should be made to avoid use of vasoconstrictor due to possibility of hypertensive episodes with monoamine oxidase inhibitors

Effects on Dental Treatment Key adverse event(s) related to dental treatment: Orthostatic hypotension, xerostomia (normal salivary flow resumes upon discontinuation).

Effects on Bleeding No information available to require special precautions

Adverse Effects

>10%: Central nervous system: Dizziness (29%), headache (15%)

1% to 10%:

Cardiovascular: Orthostatic hypotension (4%), syncope (2%), palpitation (2%)

Central nervous system: Sleep disturbance (5%), drowsiness (4%), anxiety (2%), chills (2%), forgetfulness (2%), hyperactivity (2%), lethargy (2%), sedation (2%)

Gastrointestinal: Xerostomia (9%), constipation (7%), nausea (6%), diarrhea (2%)

Genitourinary: Urinary frequency (2%), impotence (2%), urinary hesitancy (1%)

Neuromuscular & skeletal: Tremor (4%), myoclonus (2%), paresthesia (2%)

Miscellaneous: Diaphoresis (2%), heavy feeling (2%)

General Dosage Range Oral: *Adults:* Initial: 10 mg 2-4 times/day; may increase to a maximum of 60 mg/day divided in 2-4 doses

Mechanism of Action Thought to act by increasing endogenous concentrations of epinephrine, norepinephrine, dopamine, and serotonin through inhibition of the enzyme (monoamine oxidase) responsible for the breakdown of these neurotransmitters

Pregnancy Risk Factor C

Isoniazid (eye soe NYE a zid)

Related Information

Tuberculosis *on page 1902*

Canadian Brand Names Isotamine®; PMS-Isoniazid

Pharmacologic Category Antitubercular Agent

Use Treatment of susceptible tuberculosis infections; treatment of latent tuberculosis infection (LTBI)

Local Anesthetic/Vasoconstrictor Precautions No information available to require special precautions

Effects on Dental Treatment Key adverse event(s) related to dental treatment: Xerostomia (normal salivary flow resumes upon discontinuation).

Effects on Bleeding Thrombocytopenia is a rare adverse effect. No information available to require routine special precautions.

Adverse Effects Frequency not defined.

Cardiovascular: Hypertension, palpitation, tachycardia, vasculitis

Central nervous system: Depression, dizziness, encephalopathy, fever, lethargy, memory impairment, psychosis, seizure, slurred speech, toxic encephalopathy

Dermatologic: Flushing, rash (morbilliform, maculopapular, pruritic, or exfoliative)

Endocrine & metabolic: Gynecomastia, hyperglycemia, metabolic acidosis, pellagra, pyridoxine deficiency

Gastrointestinal: Anorexia, epigastric distress, nausea, stomach pain, vomiting

Hematologic: Agranulocytosis, anemia (sideroblastic, hemolytic, or aplastic), eosinophilia, thrombocytopenia

Hepatic: LFTs mildly increased (10% to 20%), hyperbilirubinemia, bilirubinuria, jaundice, hepatic dysfunction, hepatitis (may involve progressive liver damage; risk increases with age; 2.3% in patients >50 years)

Neuromuscular & skeletal: Arthralgia, hyper-reflexia, paresthesia, peripheral neuropathy (dose-related incidence, 10% to 20% incidence with 10 mg/kg/day), weakness

Ocular: Blurred vision, loss of vision, optic neuritis and atrophy

Miscellaneous: Lupus-like syndrome, lymphadenopathy, rheumatic syndrome

General Dosage Range Oral, I.M.:

Children: 10-20 mg/kg/day once daily (maximum: 300 mg/day) **or** 20-40 mg/kg 2-3 times/week (maximum: 900 mg/dose)

Adults: 300 mg (5 mg/kg) once daily **or** 900 mg (15 mg/kg) 2-3 times/week

Mechanism of Action Unknown, but may include the inhibition of mycolic acid synthesis resulting in disruption of the bacterial cell wall

Pharmacodynamics/Kinetics

Half-life Elimination Fast acetylators: 30-100 minutes; Slow acetylators: 2-5 hours; may be prolonged with hepatic or severe renal impairment

Time to Peak Serum: 1-2 hours

Pregnancy Risk Factor C

Isoproterenol (eye soe proe TER e nole)

U.S. Brand Names Isuprel®

Pharmacologic Category $Beta_1$- & $Beta_2$-Adrenergic Agonist Agent

Use Manufacturer's labeled indications (see **"Note"**): Mild or transient episodes of heart block that do not require electric shock or pacemaker therapy; serious episodes of heart block and Adams-Stokes attacks (except when caused by ventricular tachycardia or fibrillation); cardiac arrest until electric shock or pacemaker therapy is available; bronchospasm during anesthesia; adjunct to fluid and electrolyte replacement therapy and other drugs and procedures in the treatment of hypovolemic or septic shock and low cardiac output states (eg, decompensated heart failure, cardiogenic shock)

Note: The use of isoproterenol in advanced cardiac life support (ACLS) has largely been supplanted by the use of other adrenergic agents (eg, epinephrine and dopamine). The use of isoproterenol for bronchospasm during anesthesia and cardiogenic, hypovolemic, or septic shock is no longer recommended. See *Unlabeled/Investigational Use* for more appropriate, yet unlabeled, uses.

Unlabeled/Investigational Use Pharmacologic overdrive pacing for refractory torsade de pointes; pharmacologic provocation during tilt table testing for syncope; temporary control of bradycardia in denervated heart transplant patients unresponsive to atropine; ventricular arrhythmias due to AV nodal block; beta-blocker overdose

Local Anesthetic/Vasoconstrictor Precautions Isoproterenol is selective for beta-adrenergic receptors and not alpha-receptors; therefore, there is no precaution in the use of vasoconstrictor such as epinephrine

Effects on Dental Treatment Key adverse event(s) related to dental treatment: Xerostomia and changes in salivation (normal salivary flow resumes upon discontinuation).

Effects on Bleeding No information available to require special precautions

Adverse Effects Frequency not defined.

Cardiovascular: Angina, flushing, hyper-/hypotension, pallor, palpitation, paradoxical bradycardia (with tilt table testing), premature ventricular beats, Stokes-Adams attacks, tachyarrhythmia, ventricular arrhythmia

Central nervous system: Dizziness, headache, nervousness, restlessness, Stokes-Adams seizure

Endocrine & metabolic: Hypokalemia, serum glucose increased

Gastrointestinal: Nausea, vomiting

Neuromuscular & skeletal: Tremor, weakness

Ocular: Blurred vision

Respiratory: Dyspnea, pulmonary edema

Miscellaneous: Diaphoresis

General Dosage Range Continuous I.V. infusion:

Children: 0.05-2 mcg/kg/minute; titrate to patient response

Adults: 2-10 mcg/minute; titrate to patient response

Mechanism of Action Stimulates $beta_1$- and $beta_2$-receptors resulting in relaxation of bronchial, GI, and uterine smooth muscle, increased heart rate and contractility, vasodilation of peripheral vasculature

Pharmacodynamics/Kinetics
Onset of Action I.V.: Immediate
Duration of Action I.V.: 10-15 minutes
Half-life Elimination 2.5-5 minutes
Pregnancy Risk Factor C

Isosorbide Dinitrate (eye soe SOR bide dye NYE trate)

Related Information
Cardiovascular Diseases *on page 1848*
Isosorbide Mononitrate *on page 952*
U.S. Brand Names Dilatrate®-SR; Isordil® Titradose™
Canadian Brand Names ISDN; Isosorbide; Novo-Sorbide; PMS-Isosorbide
Pharmacologic Category Vasodilator
Use Prevention and treatment of angina pectoris
Note: Due to slower onset of action, not the drug of choice to abort an acute anginal episode.
Unlabeled/Investigational Use Patients with heart failure (HF) who do not tolerate an ACE inhibitor or an angiotensin receptor blocker (ARB); African-American (self-identified) patients with HF remaining symptomatic despite optimal standard therapy; esophageal spastic disorders
Local Anesthetic/Vasoconstrictor Precautions No information available to require special precautions
Effects on Dental Treatment Key adverse event(s) related to dental treatment: Xerostomia and changes in salivation (normal salivary flow resumes upon discontinuation).
Effects on Bleeding No information available to require special precautions
Adverse Effects Frequency not defined.
Cardiovascular: Crescendo angina (uncommon), hypotension, postural hypotension, rebound hypertension (uncommon), syncope (uncommon)
Central nervous system: Headache (most common), lightheadedness (related to blood pressure changes)
Hematologic: Methemoglobinemia (rare, overdose)
General Dosage Range
Oral:
Immediate release: *Adults:* 5-40 mg 2-3 times/day
Sustained release: *Adults:* 40-160 mg/day in divided doses
Sublingual: *Adults:* 2.5-5 mg every 5-10 minutes for maximum of 3 doses in 15-30 minutes **or** 2.5-5 mg 15 minutes prior to activities which may provoke an anginal episode.
Mechanism of Action Stimulation of intracellular cyclic-GMP results in vascular smooth muscle relaxation of both arterial and venous vasculature with more prominent effects on the veins. Primarily reduces cardiac oxygen demand by decreasing preload (left ventricular end-diastolic pressure); may modestly reduce afterload. Additionally, coronary artery dilation improves collateral flow to ischemic regions.
Pharmacodynamics/Kinetics
Onset of Action Sublingual tablet: ~3 minutes; Oral tablet and capsule (includes extended-release formulations): ~1 hour
Duration of Action Sublingual tablet: 1-2 hours; Oral tablet and capsule (includes extended-release formulations): Up to 8 hours
Half-life Elimination Parent drug: ~1 hour; Metabolites (5-mononitrate: 5 hours; 2-mononitrate: 2 hours)
Pregnancy Risk Factor C

Isosorbide Dinitrate and Hydralazine
(eye soe SOR bide dye NYE trate & hye DRAL a zeen)

Related Information
HydrALAZINE *on page 853*
Isosorbide Dinitrate *on page 950*
U.S. Brand Names BiDil®
Generic Availability (U.S.) No
Pharmacologic Category Vasodilator
Use Treatment of heart failure, adjunct to standard therapy, in self-identified African-Americans
Local Anesthetic/Vasoconstrictor Precautions No information available to require special precautions
Effects on Dental Treatment No significant effects or complications reported

Effects on Bleeding No information available to require special precautions

Adverse Effects The following events were reported in the A-HeFT Study using the combination isosorbide dinitrate/hydralazine product. See individual drug monographs for additional information.

>10%:
- Cardiovascular: Chest pain (16%)
- Central nervous system: Headache (50%), dizziness (32%)
- Neuromuscular & skeletal: Weakness (14%)

1% to 10%:
- Cardiovascular: Hypotension (8%), palpitation (4%), ventricular tachycardia (4%), tachycardia (2%)
- Central nervous system: Malaise (1%), somnolence (1%)
- Dermatologic: Alopecia (1%), angioedema (1%)
- Endocrine & metabolic: Hyperglycemia (4%), hyperlipidemia (3%), hypercholesterolemia (1%)
- Gastrointestinal: Nausea (10%), vomiting (4%)
- Hepatic: Cholecystitis (1%)
- Neuromuscular & skeletal: Paresthesia (4%), arthralgia (1%), myalgia (1%), tendon disorder (1%)
- Ocular: Amblyopia (3%)
- Respiratory: Bronchitis (8%), sinusitis (4%), rhinitis (4%)
- Miscellaneous: Allergic reaction (1%), diaphoresis (1%)

Dosage Oral: Adults: Initial: 1 tablet 3 times/day; may titrate to a maximum dose of 2 tablets 3 times/day

Dosage adjustment for toxicity: If patient experiences intolerable side effects, dose may be reduced to as little as one-half tablet 3 times/day; dose should be titrated upward as soon as tolerated.

Mechanism of Action

Hydralazine: Direct vasodilation of arterioles (with little effect on veins) resulting in decreased systemic resistance

Isosorbide Dinitrate: Stimulation of intracellular cyclic-GMP results in vascular smooth muscle relaxation of both arterial and venous vasculature with more prominent effects on the veins. Primarily reduces cardiac oxygen demand by decreasing preload (left ventricular end-diastolic pressure); may modestly reduce afterload. Additionally, coronary artery dilation improves collateral flow to ischemic regions.

Contraindications Hypersensitivity to organic nitrates; concurrent use with phosphodiesterase-5 inhibitors (sildenafil, tadalafil, or vardenafil)

Warnings/Precautions See individual agents.

Drug Interactions

Metabolism/Transport Effects Hydralazine: **Inhibits** CYP3A4 (weak); Isosorbide dinitrate: **Substrate** of CYP3A4 (major)

Avoid Concomitant Use

Avoid concomitant use of Isosorbide Dinitrate and Hydralazine with any of the following: Phosphodiesterase 5 Inhibitors

Increased Effect/Toxicity

Isosorbide Dinitrate and Hydralazine may increase the levels/effects of: Amifostine; Antihypertensives; Hypotensive Agents; RiTUXimab; Rosiglitazone

The levels/effects of Isosorbide Dinitrate and Hydralazine may be increased by: Conivaptan; CYP3A4 Inhibitors (Moderate); CYP3A4 Inhibitors (Strong); Dasatinib; Diazoxide; Herbs (Hypotensive Properties); MAO Inhibitors; Pentoxifylline; Phosphodiesterase 5 Inhibitors; Prostacyclin Analogues

Decreased Effect

The levels/effects of Isosorbide Dinitrate and Hydralazine may be decreased by: CYP3A4 Inducers (Strong); Deferasirox; Herbs (CYP3A4 Inducers); Herbs (Hypertensive Properties); Methylphenidate; Nonsteroidal Anti-Inflammatory Agents; Tocilizumab; Yohimbine

Pharmacodynamics/Kinetics

Half-life Elimination Hydralazine: 4 hours; Isosorbide dinitrate: 2 hours

Time to Peak 1 hour (both agents)

Pregnancy Risk Factor C

Lactation See individual agents.

Breast-Feeding Considerations See individual agents.

Dosage Forms

Tablet:

BiDil®: Isosorbide dinitrate 20 mg and hydralazine 37.5 mg

Isosorbide Mononitrate (eye soe SOR bide mon oh NYE trate)

Related Information

Cardiovascular Diseases *on page 1848*
Isosorbide Dinitrate *on page 950*

U.S. Brand Names Imdur®; Ismo®; Monoket®

Canadian Brand Names Apo-ISMN®; Imdur®; PMS-ISMN; PRO-ISMN

Generic Availability (U.S.) Yes

Pharmacologic Category Vasodilator

Use Prevention of angina pectoris

Local Anesthetic/Vasoconstrictor Precautions No information available to require special precautions

Effects on Dental Treatment No significant effects or complications reported

Effects on Bleeding No information available to require special precautions

Adverse Effects

>10%: Central nervous system: Headache (13% to 35%)

1% to 10%:

- Cardiovascular: Angina (≤2%), flushing (≤2%)
- Central nervous system: Dizziness (≤4%), fatigue (≤4%), pain (≤4%), emotional lability (≤2%)
- Dermatologic: Pruritus (≤2%), rash (≤2%)
- Gastrointestinal: Nausea (≤3%), abdominal pain (≤2%), diarrhea (≤2%)
- Respiratory: Upper respiratory infection (≤4%), cough increased (≤2%)
- Miscellaneous: Allergic reaction (≤2%)

Dosage Oral:

Adults:

Regular release tablet: Initial: 5-20 mg twice daily with the 2 doses given 7 hours apart (eg, 8 AM and 3 PM) to decrease tolerance development; patients initiating therapy with 5 mg twice daily (eg, small stature) should be titrated up to 10 mg twice daily in first 2-3 days.

Extended release tablet: Initial: 30-60 mg given once daily in the morning; titrate upward as needed, giving at least 3 days between increases; maximum daily single dose: 240 mg

Elderly: Start with lowest recommended adult dose.

Dosing adjustment in renal impairment: Dose adjustment not necessary

Hemodialysis: Dose supplementation is not necessary.

Peritoneal dialysis: Dose supplementation is not necessary.

Dosing adjustment in hepatic impairment: Dose adjustment not necessary

Note: Tolerance to nitrate effects develops with chronic exposure. Dose escalation does not overcome this effect. Tolerance can only be overcome by short periods of nitrate absence from the body. Short periods of nitrate withdrawal may help minimize tolerance. Recommended twice daily dosage regimens incorporate this interval. Administer sustained release tablet once daily in the morning.

Mechanism of Action Nitroglycerin and other nitrates form free radical nitric oxide. In smooth muscle, nitric oxide activates guanylate cyclase which increases guanosine 3'5' monophosphate (cGMP) leading to dephosphorylation of myosin light chains and smooth muscle relaxation. Produces a vasodilator effect on the peripheral veins and arteries with more prominent effects on the veins. Primarily reduces cardiac oxygen demand by decreasing preload (left ventricular end-diastolic pressure); may modestly reduce afterload; dilates coronary arteries and improves collateral flow to ischemic regions.

Contraindications Hypersensitivity to isosorbide mononitrate or any component of the formulation; hypersensitivity to organic nitrates; concurrent use with phosphodiesterase-5 (PDE-5) inhibitors (sildenafil, tadalafil, or vardenafil)

Warnings/Precautions Avoid use in hypertrophic cardiomyopathy. Use with caution in volume depletion, moderate hypotension, and extreme caution with inferior wall MI and suspected right ventricular infarctions. Nitrates may precipitate or aggravate increased intracranial pressure and subsequently may worsen clinical outcomes in patients with neurologic injury (eg, intracranial hemorrhage, traumatic brain injury). Postural hypotension, transient episodes of weakness, dizziness, or syncope may occur even with small doses; ethanol accentuates these effects; tolerance and cross-tolerance to nitrate antianginal and hemodynamic effects may occur during prolonged isosorbide mononitrate therapy; (minimized by using the smallest effective dose, by alternating coronary vasodilators or offering drug-free intervals of as little as 12 hours). Excessive doses may result in severe headache, blurred vision, or xerostomia; increased anginal symptoms may be a result of dosage increases. Avoid concurrent use with PDE-5 inhibitors (eg, sildenafil, tadalafil, vardenafil). When nitrate administration becomes medically necessary, may administer nitrates only if 24 hours have elapsed after use of sildenafil or vardenafil (48 hours after tadalafil use) (O'Connor, 2010).

Drug Interactions

Metabolism/Transport Effects Substrate of CYP3A4 (major)

Avoid Concomitant Use

Avoid concomitant use of Isosorbide Mononitrate with any of the following: Phosphodiesterase 5 Inhibitors

Increased Effect/Toxicity

Isosorbide Mononitrate may increase the levels/effects of: Hypotensive Agents; Rosiglitazone

The levels/effects of Isosorbide Mononitrate may be increased by: Conivaptan; CYP3A4 Inhibitors (Moderate); CYP3A4 Inhibitors (Strong); Dasatinib; Phosphodiesterase 5 Inhibitors

Decreased Effect

The levels/effects of Isosorbide Mononitrate may be decreased by: CYP3A4 Inducers (Strong); Deferasirox; Herbs (CYP3A4 Inducers); Tocilizumab

Ethanol/Nutrition/Herb Interactions Ethanol: Caution with ethanol (may increase risk of hypotension).

Pharmacodynamics/Kinetics

Onset of Action 30-60 minutes

Duration of Action Immediate release: ≥6 hours (Thadani, 1987); Extended release: ≥12-24 hours (Anderson, 2007)

Half-life Elimination Mononitrate: ~5-6 hours

Pregnancy Risk Factor B/C (manufacturer dependent)

Lactation Excretion in breast milk unknown/use caution

Dosage Forms

Tablet, oral: 10 mg, 20 mg
Ismo®: 20 mg
Monoket®: 10 mg, 20 mg

Tablet, extended release, oral: 30 mg, 60 mg, 120 mg
Imdur®: 30 mg, 60 mg, 120 mg

ISOtretinoin (eye soe TRET i noyn)

U.S. Brand Names Amnesteem®; Claravis™; Sotret®

Canadian Brand Names Accutane®; Clarus™; Isotrex®

Pharmacologic Category Acne Products; Retinoic Acid Derivative

Use Treatment of severe recalcitrant nodular acne unresponsive to conventional therapy

Unlabeled/Investigational Use Investigational: Treatment of children with metastatic neuroblastoma or leukemia that does not respond to conventional therapy

Local Anesthetic/Vasoconstrictor Precautions No information available to require special precautions

Effects on Dental Treatment Key adverse event(s) related to dental treatment: Xerostomia and changes in salivation (normal salivary flow resumes upon discontinuation).

Effects on Bleeding No information available to require special precautions

Adverse Effects Frequency not always defined.

Cardiovascular: Chest pain, edema, flushing, palpitation, stroke, syncope, tachycardia, vascular thrombotic disease

Central nervous system: Aggressive behavior, depression, dizziness, drowsiness, emotional instability, fatigue, headache, insomnia, lethargy, malaise, nervousness, paresthesia, pseudotumor cerebri, psychosis, seizure, stroke, suicidal ideation, suicide attempts, suicide, violent behavior

Dermatologic: Abnormal wound healing acne fulminans, alopecia, bruising, cheilitis, cutaneous allergic reactions, dry nose, dry skin, eczema, eruptive xanthomas, facial erythema, fragility of skin, hair abnormalities, hirsutism, hyperpigmentation, hypopigmentation, increased sunburn susceptibility, nail dystrophy, paronychia, peeling of palms, peeling of soles, photoallergic reactions, photosensitizing reactions, pruritus, purpura, rash

Endocrine & metabolic: Triglycerides increased (25%), abnormal menses, blood glucose increased, cholesterol increased, HDL decreased, hyperuricemia

Gastrointestinal: Bleeding and inflammation of the gums, colitis, esophagitis, esophageal ulceration, inflammatory bowel disease, nausea, nonspecific gastrointestinal symptoms, pancreatitis, weight loss, xerostomia

Genitourinary: Nonspecific urogenital findings

Hematologic: Agranulocytosis (rare), anemia, neutropenia, pyogenic granuloma, thrombocytopenia

Hepatic: Alkaline phosphatase increased, ALT increased, AST increased, GGTP increased, hepatitis, LDH increased

Neuromuscular & skeletal: Back pain (29% in pediatric patients), arthralgia, arthritis, bone abnormalities, bone mineral density decreased, calcification of tendons and ligaments, CPK increased, myalgia, premature epiphyseal closure, skeletal hyperostosis, tendonitis, weakness

Ocular: Cataracts, color vision disorder, conjunctivitis, corneal opacities, dry eyes, eyelid inflammation, keratitis, night vision decreased, optic neuritis, photophobia, visual disturbances

Otic: Hearing impairment, tinnitus

Renal: Glomerulonephritis, hematuria, proteinuria, pyuria, vasculitis

Respiratory: Bronchospasms, epistaxis, respiratory infection, voice alteration, Wegener's granulomatosis

Miscellaneous: Allergic reactions, anaphylactic reactions, disseminated herpes simplex, diaphoresis, infection, lymphadenopathy

General Dosage Range Dosage adjustments recommended in patients with hepatic impairment

Oral:

Children 12-17 years: 0.05-1 mg/kg/day in 2 divided doses

Adults: 0.05-2 mg/kg/day in 2 divided doses

Mechanism of Action Reduces sebaceous gland size and reduces sebum production; regulates cell proliferation and differentiation

Pharmacodynamics/Kinetics

Half-life Elimination Terminal: Parent drug: 21 hours; Metabolite: 21-24 hours

Time to Peak Serum: 3-5 hours

Pregnancy Risk Factor X

Prescribing and Access Restrictions As a requirement of the REMS program, access to this medication is restricted. All patients (male and female), prescribers, wholesalers, and dispensing pharmacists must register and be active in the iPLEDGE™ risk management program, designed to eliminate fetal exposures to isotretinoin. This program covers all isotretinoin products (brand and generic). The iPLEDGE™ program requires that all patients meet qualification criteria and monthly program requirements (eg, pregnancy testing). Healthcare providers can only prescribe a maximum 30-day supply at each monthly visit and must counsel patients on the iPLEDGE™ program requirements and confirm counseling via the iPLEDGE™ automated system. Registration, activation, and additional information are provided at www.ipledgeprogram.com or by calling 866-495-0654.

Isoxsuprine (eye SOKS syoo preen)

Pharmacologic Category Vasodilator

Use Treatment of peripheral vascular diseases, such as arteriosclerosis obliterans and Raynaud's disease

Local Anesthetic/Vasoconstrictor Precautions No information available to require special precautions

Effects on Dental Treatment May enhance effects of other vasodilators.

Effects on Bleeding No information available to require special precautions

Adverse Effects Frequency not defined.

Cardiovascular: Chest pain, hypotension, tachycardia

Central nervous system: Dizziness

Dermatologic: Rash

Gastrointestinal: Nausea, vomiting

Neuromuscular & skeletal: Weakness

General Dosage Range Oral: *Adults:* 10-20 mg 3-4 times/day

Mechanism of Action In studies on normal human subjects, isoxsuprine increases muscle blood flow, but skin blood flow is usually unaffected. Rather than increasing muscle blood flow by beta-receptor stimulation, isoxsuprine probably has a direct action on vascular smooth muscle. The generally accepted mechanism of action of isoxsuprine on the uterus is beta-adrenergic stimulation. Isoxsuprine was shown to inhibit prostaglandin synthetase at high serum concentrations, with low concentrations there was an increase in the P-G synthesis.

Pharmacodynamics/Kinetics

Half-life Elimination Serum: Mean: 1.25 hours

Time to Peak Serum: ~1 hour

Pregnancy Risk Factor C

Isradipine (iz RA di peen)

Related Information

Calcium Channel Blockers and Gingival Hyperplasia *on page 2014*
Cardiovascular Diseases *on page 1848*

U.S. Brand Names DynaCirc CR®

Pharmacologic Category Calcium Channel Blocker; Calcium Channel Blocker, Dihydropyridine

Use Treatment of hypertension

Unlabeled/Investigational Use Pediatric hypertension

Local Anesthetic/Vasoconstrictor Precautions Isradipine is one of the drugs confirmed to prolong the QT interval and is accepted as having a risk of causing torsade de pointes. The risk of drug-induced torsade de pointes is extremely low when a single QT interval prolonging drug is prescribed. In terms of epinephrine, it is not known what effect vasoconstrictors in the local anesthetic regimen will have in patients with a known history of congenital prolonged QT interval or in patients taking any medication that prolongs the QT interval. Until more information is obtained, it is suggested that the clinician consult with the physician prior to the use of a vasoconstrictor in suspected patients, and that the vasoconstrictor (epinephrine, mepivacaine and levonordefrin [Carbocaine® 2% with Neo-Cobefrin®]) be used with caution.

Effects on Dental Treatment Unlike other calcium channel blockers, information is sparse as to whether isradipine causes gingival hyperplasia. Consultation with physician is suggested if hyperplasia is observed in patients taking isradipine.

Effects on Bleeding No information available to require special precautions

Adverse Effects Percentages reported with capsule formulation.

>10%: Central nervous system: Headache (dose related 2% to 22%)

1% to 10%:

- Cardiovascular: Edema (dose related 1% to 9%), palpitation (dose related 1% to 5%), flushing (dose related 1% to 5%), tachycardia (1% to 3%), chest pain (2% to 3%)
- Central nervous system: Dizziness (2% to 8%), fatigue (dose related 1% to 9%)
- Dermatologic: Rash (2%)
- Gastrointestinal: Nausea (1% to 5%), abdominal discomfort (≤3%), vomiting (≤1%), diarrhea (≤3%)
- Neuromuscular & skeletal: Weakness (≤1%)
- Renal: Urinary frequency (1% to 3%)
- Respiratory: Dyspnea (1% to 3%)

General Dosage Range Dosage adjustment recommended in patients with hepatic or renal impairment

Oral: *Adults:*

Capsule: Initial: 2.5 mg twice daily; Usual range: 2.5-10 mg/day

Controlled release tablet: Initial: 5 mg once daily; Maintenance: 5-20 mg once daily (maximum: 20 mg/day)

Mechanism of Action Inhibits calcium ion from entering the "slow channels" or select voltage-sensitive areas of vascular smooth muscle and myocardium during depolarization, producing a relaxation of coronary vascular smooth muscle and coronary vasodilation; increases myocardial oxygen delivery in patients with vasospastic angina

Pharmacodynamics/Kinetics

Onset of Action Immediate release: 2-3 hours

Duration of Action Immediate release: >12 hours

Half-life Elimination Terminal: 8 hours

Time to Peak Serum: 1-1.5 hours

Pregnancy Risk Factor C

Dental Comment Isradipine is known to prolong the QT interval. The QT interval is measured as the time and distance between the Q point of the QRS complex and the end of the T wave in the ECG tracing. After adjustment for heart rate, the QT interval is defined as prolonged if it is more than 450 msec in men and 460 msec in women. A long QT syndrome was first described in the 1950s and 60s as a congenital syndrome involving QT interval prolongation and syncope and sudden death. Some of the congenital long QT syndromes were characterized by a peculiar electrocardiographic appearance of the QRS complex involving a premature atria beat followed by a pause, then a subsequent sinus beat showing marked QT prolongation and deformity. This type of cardiac arrhythmia was originally termed "torsade de pointes" (translated from the French as "twisting of the points"). Isradipine is considered as having a risk of causing torsade de pointes. Since it is not known what effect vasoconstrictors in the local anesthetic regimen will have in patients with a known history of congenital prolonged QT interval or in patients taking any medication that prolongs the QT interval, a medical consult is suggested.

Itraconazole (i tra KOE na zole)

Related Information

Fungal Infections *on page 1945*

U.S. Brand Names Sporanox®

Canadian Brand Names Sporanox®

Generic Availability (U.S.) Yes: Capsule

Pharmacologic Category Antifungal Agent, Oral

Dental Use Treatment of susceptible fungal infections in immunocompromised and immunocompetent patients including blastomycosis and histoplasmosis; has activity against *Aspergillus, Candida, Coccidioides, Cryptococcus, Sporothrix,* and chromomycosis. Useful in superficial mycoses including dermatophytoses (eg, tinea capitis), pityriasis versicolor, sebopsoriasis, vaginal and chronic mucocutaneous candidiases; systemic mycoses including candidiasis, meningeal and disseminated cryptococcal infections, paracoccidioidomycosis, coccidioidomycoses; miscellaneous mycoses such as sporotrichosis, chromomycosis, leishmaniasis, fungal keratitis, alternariosis, zygomycosis.

Use

Oral capsules: Treatment of susceptible fungal infections in immunocompromised and immunocompetent patients including blastomycosis and histoplasmosis; indicated for aspergillosis (in patients intolerant/refractory to amphotericin B), and onychomycosis of the toenail and fingernail (in nonimmunocompromised patients)

Oral solution: Treatment of oral and esophageal candidiasis

Local Anesthetic/Vasoconstrictor Precautions No information available to require special precautions

Effects on Dental Treatment No significant effects or complications reported

Effects on Bleeding No information available to require special precautions

Adverse Effects

>10%: Gastrointestinal: Nausea (11%), diarrhea (3% to 11%)

1% to 10%:

- Cardiovascular: Edema (4%), hypertension (3%), chest pain (3%)
- Central nervous system: Fever (3% to 7%), headache (4%), fatigue (2% to 3%), dizziness (2%), depression (2%)
- Dermatologic: Rash (4% to 9%), pruritus (3%)
- Endocrine & metabolic: Hypokalemia (2%)
- Gastrointestinal: Vomiting (5% to 7%), abdominal pain (2% to 6%), constipation (2%)
- Hepatic: LFTs abnormal (3%)
- Respiratory: Rhinitis (5% to 9%), cough (4%), dyspnea (2%), pneumonia (2%), sinusitis (2%), sputum increased (2%)
- Miscellaneous: Diaphoresis increased (3%)

Dental Usual Dosage Oropharyngeal candidiasis: Adults: Oral solution: 200 mg once daily for 1-2 weeks; in patients unresponsive or refractory to fluconazole: 100 mg twice daily (clinical response expected in 1-2 weeks)

Dosage Oral:

Usual dosage ranges:

Children: Efficacy and safety have not been established; a small number of patients 3-16 years of age have been treated with 100 mg/day for systemic fungal infections with no serious adverse effects reported. A dose of 5 mg/kg once daily was used in a pharmacokinetic study using the oral solution in patients 6 months to 12 years; duration of study was 2 weeks.

Adults: 100-400 mg/day; doses >200 mg/day are given in 2 divided doses; length of therapy varies from 1 day to >6 months depending on the condition and mycological response

Indication-specific dosing:

Infants and Children (HIV-exposed/-positive; unlabeled use; CDC, 2009):

Candidiasis:

Oropharyngeal: Oral solution: 2.5 mg/kg/dose twice daily (maximum: 200 mg/day [400 mg/day if fluconazole-refractory]) for 7-14 days

Esophageal: Oral solution: 5 mg/kg/day once daily or divided twice daily for 4-21 days

Coccidioidomycosis:

Treatment: Oral: 5-10 mg/kg/dose twice daily for 3 days, followed by 2-5 mg/kg/dose orally twice daily (maximum: 400 mg/day)

Relapse prevention: Oral: 2-5 mg/kg/dose twice daily (maximum: 400 mg/day)

Cryptococcus: *Relapse prevention:* Oral solution: 5 mg/kg/dose once daily (maximum: 200 mg/day)

Histoplasmosis:

Treatment of mild disseminated disease: Oral solution: 2-5 mg/kg/dose 3 times daily for 3 days (9 doses), followed by twice daily for 12 months (maximum: 200 mg/dose)

Consolidation treatment for moderate-severe to severe disseminated disease, including CNS infection (following appropriate induction therapy): 2-5 mg/kg/dose 3 times daily for 3 days, followed by 2-5 mg/kg/dose (maximum: 200 mg/dose) twice daily for 12 months for non-CNS-disseminated disease or for ≥12 months for CNS infection

Relapse prevention: Oral solution: 5 mg/kg/dose twice daily (maximum: 400 mg/day)

Adults:

Aspergillosis, invasive (salvage therapy): Duration of therapy should be a minimum of 6-12 weeks or throughout period of immunosuppression: Oral: 200-400 mg/day; **Note:** 2008 IDSA guidelines recommend 600 mg/day for 3 days, followed by 400 mg/day

Appropriate use: Itraconazole should **NOT** be used for voriconazole-refractory aspergillosis since the same antifungal and/or resistance mechanism(s) may be shared by both agents. Itraconazole oral solution and capsule formulations are not bioequivalent or interchangeable. Due to variable bioavailability of oral preparations, therapeutic drug monitoring advisable.

Aspergillosis, allergic (ABPA, sinusitis): 200 mg/day; may be used in conjunction with corticosteroids

Blastomycosis: 200 mg 3 times/day for 3 days, then 200 mg twice daily for 6-12 months; in moderately-severe to severe infection, therapy should be initiated with ~2 weeks of amphotericin B (Chapman, 2008)

Brain abscess: Cerebral phaeohyphomycosis (dematiaceous): 200 mg twice daily for at least 6 months with amphotericin

Candidiasis:

Oropharyngeal: Oral solution: 200 mg once daily for 1-2 weeks; in patients unresponsive or refractory to fluconazole: 100 mg twice daily (clinical response expected in 1-2 weeks)

Esophageal: Oral solution: 100-200 mg once daily for a minimum of 3 weeks; continue dosing for 2 weeks after resolution of symptoms

Coccidioidomycosis: 200 mg twice daily

Histoplasmosis: 200 mg 3 times/day for 3 days, then 200 mg twice daily (or once daily in mild-moderate disease) for 6-12 weeks in mild-moderate disease or ≥12 months in progressive disseminated or chronic cavitary pulmonary histoplasmosis; in moderately-severe to severe infection, therapy should be initiated with ~2 weeks of a lipid formation of amphotericin B (Wheat, 2007)

Long-term suppression therapy: 200 mg/day (AIDS*info* guidelines, 2008)

Meningitis:

Coccidioides: 400-800 mg/day

Coccidioides, HIV-positive (unlabeled use): 200 mg 3 times/day for 3 days, then 200 mg twice daily; maintenance: 200 mg twice daily life-long (AIDS*info* guidelines, 2008)

Appropriate use: Fluconazole is preferred for meningeal infections.

Onychomycosis: 200 mg once daily for 12 consecutive weeks; alternative "pulse-dosing" may be considering for fingernail involvement only: 200 mg twice daily for 1 week; repeat 1-week course after 3-week off-time

Penicilliosis, HIV-positive (unlabeled use): 200 mg twice daily for 8-10 weeks (in severely-ill patients, initiate therapy with 2 weeks of amphotericin B); maintenance: 200 mg/day (*AIDSinfo* guidelines, 2008)

Pneumonia:

Coccidioides: Mild-to-moderate: 200 mg twice daily

Coccidioides, HIV-positive (focal pneumonia): 200 mg 3 times/day for 3 days, then 200 mg twice daily (AIDS*info* guidelines, 2008)

Protothecal infection: 200 mg once daily for 2 months

Sporotrichosis:

Lymphocutaneous: 100-200 mg/day for 3-6 months

Osteoarticular and pulmonary: 200 mg twice daily for 1-2 years (may use amphotericin B initially for stabilization)

Dosing adjustment in renal impairment: The FDA-approved labeling states to use with caution in patients with renal impairment. The following guidelines have been used by some clinicians:

Aronoff, 2007:

Cl_{cr} >10 mL/minute: No adjustment recommended

Cl_{cr} <10 mL/minute: Administer 50% of normal dose

Continuous renal replacement therapy (CRRT)/hemodialysis: 200 mg every 12 hours for 4 doses, then 200 mg every 24 hours (Heintz, 2009)

Hemodialysis: Not dialyzable

Dosing adjustment in hepatic impairment: Use caution in patients with hepatic impairment

Mechanism of Action Interferes with cytochrome P450 activity, decreasing ergosterol synthesis (principal sterol in fungal cell membrane) and inhibiting cell membrane formation

Contraindications Hypersensitivity to itraconazole (use caution in patients with a history of hypersensitivity to other azoles), any component of the formulation; concurrent administration with cisapride, dofetilide, ergot derivatives, levomethadyl, lovastatin, midazolam (oral), nisoldipine, pimozide, quinidine, simvastatin, or triazolam; treatment of onychomycosis (or other non-life-threatening indications) in patients with evidence of ventricular dysfunction, heart failure (HF) or a history of HF; treatment of onychomycosis in patients who are pregnant or intend on becoming pregnant

Warnings/Precautions [U.S. Boxed Warning]: Negative inotropic effects have been observed following intravenous administration. Discontinue or reassess use if signs or symptoms of HF (heart failure) occur during treatment. [U.S. Boxed Warning]: Not recommended for treatment of onychomycosis in patients with ventricular dysfunction or a history of HF. HF has been reported, particularly in patients receiving a total daily oral dose of 400 mg. Use with caution in patients with risk factors for HF (COPD, renal failure, edematous disorders, ischemic or valvular disease). Discontinue if signs or symptoms of HF or neuropathy occur during treatment. **[U.S. Boxed Warning]: Serious cardiovascular adverse events including, QT prolongation, ventricular tachycardia, torsade de pointes, cardiac arrest and/or sudden death have been observed due to increased cisapride, pimozide, quinidine or levomethadyl concentrations induced by itraconazole; concurrent use contraindicated.** Additionally, the following drugs metabolized by the CYP 3A4 isoenzyme system are also contraindicated: Ergot derivatives, lovastatin, midazolam (oral), simvastatin, and triazolam.

Calcium channel blockers (CCBs) may cause additive negative inotropic effects when used concurrently with itraconazole. Itraconazole may also inhibit the metabolism of CCBs. Use caution with concurrent use of itraconazole and CCBs due to an increased risk of HF. Concurrent use of itraconazole and nisoldipine is contraindicated.

Use with caution in patients with renal impairment. Rare cases of serious hepatotoxicity (including liver failure and death) have been reported (including some cases occurring within the first week of therapy); hepatotoxicity was reported in some patients without pre-existing liver disease or risk factors. Use with caution in patients with pre-existing hepatic impairment; monitor liver function closely and dosage adjustment may be warranted. Not recommended for use in patients with active liver disease, elevated liver enzymes, or prior hepatotoxic reactions to other drugs unless the expected benefit exceeds the risk of hepatotoxicity. Transient or permanent hearing loss has been reported. Quinidine (a contraindicated drug) was used concurrently in several of these cases. Hearing loss usually resolves after discontinuation, but may persist in some patients.

Large differences in itraconazole pharmacokinetic parameters have been observed in cystic fibrosis patients receiving the solution; if a patient with cystic fibrosis does not respond to therapy, alternate therapies should be considered. Due to differences in bioavailability, oral capsules and oral solution cannot be used interchangeably. Only the oral solution has proven efficacy for oral and esophageal candidiasis. Initiation of treatment with oral solution is not recommended in patients at immediate risk for systemic candidiasis (eg, patients with severe neutropenia).

Drug Interactions

Metabolism/Transport Effects Substrate of CYP3A4 (major); **Inhibits** CYP3A4 (strong), P-glycoprotein

Avoid Concomitant Use

Avoid concomitant use of Itraconazole with any of the following: Alfuzosin; Cisapride; Conivaptan; Dofetilide; Dronedarone; Eplerenone; Ergot Derivatives; Everolimus; Fluticasone (Oral Inhalation); Halofantrine; Lurasidone; Nilotinib; Nisoldipine; Pimozide; QuiNIDine; Ranolazine; Rivaroxaban; RomiDEPsin; Salmeterol; Silodosin; Tamsulosin; Tolvaptan; Topotecan; Toremifene

Increased Effect/Toxicity

Itraconazole may increase the levels/effects of: Alfentanil; Alfuzosin; Aliskiren; Almotriptan; Alosetron; Aprepitant; Benzodiazepines (metabolized by oxidation); Bortezomib; Bosentan; Brinzolamide; Budesonide (Nasal); Budesonide (Systemic, Oral Inhalation); BusPIRone; Busulfan; Calcium Channel Blockers; CarBAMazepine; Cardiac Glycosides; Ciclesonide; Cilostazol; Cisapride; Colchicine; Conivaptan; Corticosteroids (Orally Inhaled); Corticosteroids (Systemic); CycloSPORINE; CycloSPORINE (Systemic); CYP3A4 Substrates; Dabigatran Etexilate; Dienogest; DOCEtaxel; Dofetilide; Dronedarone; Dutasteride; Eletriptan; Eplerenone; Ergot

Derivatives; Erlotinib; Eszopiclone; Etravirine; Everolimus; FentaNYL; Fesoterodine; Fexofenadine; Fluticasone (Nasal); Fluticasone (Oral Inhalation); Fosaprepitant; Fosphenytoin; Gefitinib; GuanFACINE; Halofantrine; HMG-CoA Reductase Inhibitors; Imatinib; Irinotecan; Ixabepilone; Losartan; Lumefantrine; Lurasidone; Macrolide Antibiotics; Maraviroc; Methadone; MethylPREDNISolone; Nilotinib; Nisoldipine; Paliperidone; Paricalcitol; Pazopanib; P-Glycoprotein Substrates; Phenytoin; Phosphodiesterase 5 Inhibitors; Pimecrolimus; Pimozide; Protease Inhibitors; QuiNIDine; Ramelteon; Ranolazine; Repaglinide; Rifamycin Derivatives; Rivaroxaban; RomiDEPsin; Salmeterol; Saxagliptin; Silodosin; Sirolimus; Solifenacin; SORAfenib; SUNItinib; Tacrolimus; Tacrolimus (Systemic); Tacrolimus (Topical); Tadalafil; Tamsulosin; Temsirolimus; Tolterodine; Tolvaptan; Topotecan; Toremifene; Vilazodone; VinBLAStine; VinCRIStine; Vinorelbine; Vitamin K Antagonists; Ziprasidone; Zolpidem

The levels/effects of Itraconazole may be increased by: Etravirine; Grapefruit Juice; Macrolide Antibiotics; Protease Inhibitors

Decreased Effect

Itraconazole may decrease the levels/effects of: Amphotericin B; Prasugrel; Saccharomyces boulardii

The levels/effects of Itraconazole may be decreased by: Antacids; CYP3A4 Inducers (Strong); Deferasirox; Didanosine; Efavirenz; Etravirine; Fosphenytoin; H2-Antagonists; Herbs (CYP3A4 Inducers); Phenytoin; Proton Pump Inhibitors; Rifamycin Derivatives; Sucralfate; Tocilizumab

Ethanol/Nutrition/Herb Interactions

Food:

Capsules: Absorption enhanced by food and possibly by gastric acidity. Cola drinks have been shown to increase the absorption of the capsules in patients with achlorhydria or those taking H_2-receptor antagonists or other gastric acid suppressors. Avoid grapefruit juice.

Solution: Food decreases the bioavailability and increases the time to peak concentration.

Herb/Nutraceutical: St John's wort may decrease itraconazole levels.

Dietary Considerations

Capsule: Take with food.

Solution: Take without food, if possible.

Pharmacodynamics/Kinetics

Half-life Elimination Oral: Single dose: ~21 hours, steady state: 64 hours; Cirrhosis (single dose): 37 hours (range 20-54 hours)

Time to Peak Plasma: Capsules: 3-5 hours; Oral solution: 2-3 hours

Pregnancy Risk Factor C

Lactation Enters breast milk/not recommended

Dosage Forms

Capsule, oral: 100 mg

Sporanox®: 100 mg

Solution, oral:

Sporanox®: 10 mg/mL (150 mL)

Ivermectin (eye ver MEK tin)

U.S. Brand Names Stromectol®

Pharmacologic Category Anthelmintic

Use Treatment of the following infections: Strongyloidiasis of the intestinal tract due to the nematode parasite *Strongyloides stercoralis*. Onchocerciasis due to the immature form of the nematode parasite *Onchocerca volvulus*

Unlabeled/Investigational Use Treatment of other parasitic infections, including *Ancylostoma braziliense, Ascaris lumbricoides, Sarcoptes scabiei, Gnathostoma spinigerum, Mansonella ozzardi, Mansonella streptocerca, Pediculus humanus capitis, Pediculus humanus corporis, Phthirus pubis, Trichuris trichiura, Wucheria bancrofti*

Local Anesthetic/Vasoconstrictor Precautions No information available to require special precautions

Effects on Dental Treatment No significant effects or complications reported

Effects on Bleeding No information available to require special precautions

Adverse Effects

>10%: Miscellaneous: Mazzotti-type reaction (with onchocerciasis): Pruritus (28%), fever (23%), skin involvement (23%; including edema/urticarial rash), lymph node tenderness (1% to 14%), lymph node enlargement (3% to 13%), arthralgia/synovitis (9%)

1% to 10%:
- Cardiovascular: Tachycardia (4%), peripheral edema (3%), facial edema (1%), orthostatic hypotension (1%)
- Central nervous system: Dizziness (3%)
- Dermatologic: Pruritus (3%)
- Gastrointestinal: Diarrhea (2%), nausea (2%)
- Hematologic: Eosinophilia (3%), leukocytes decreased (3%), hemoglobin increased (1%)
- Hepatic: ALT increased (2%), AST increased (2%)

General Dosage Range Oral: *Children ≥15 kg and Adults:* 150-200 mcg/kg as a single dose

Mechanism of Action Ivermectin is a semisynthetic antihelminthic agent; it binds selectively and with strong affinity to glutamate-gated chloride ion channels which occur in invertebrate nerve and muscle cells. This leads to increased permeability of cell membranes to chloride ions then hyperpolarization of the nerve or muscle cell, and death of the parasite.

Pharmacodynamics/Kinetics

Onset of Action

Peak effect in treatment of onchocerciasis: 3-6 months

Peak effect in treatment of strongyloides: 3 months

Half-life Elimination ~18 hours

Time to Peak ~4 hours

Pregnancy Risk Factor C

Ixabepilone (ix ab EP i lone)

U.S. Brand Names Ixempra®

Pharmacologic Category Antineoplastic Agent, Antimicrotubular; Antineoplastic Agent, Epothilone B Analog

Use Treatment of metastatic or locally-advanced breast cancer (refractory or resistant)

Unlabeled/Investigational Use Treatment (second-line) of endometrial cancer

Local Anesthetic/Vasoconstrictor Precautions No information available to require special precautions

Effects on Dental Treatment Key adverse event(s) related to dental treatment: Stomatitis, mucositis, and taste perversion.

Effects on Bleeding Chemotherapy may result in significant myelosuppression, potentially including significant reduction in platelet counts and altered hemostasis. In patients who are under active treatment with these agents, medical consult is suggested.

Adverse Effects Percentages reported with monotherapy:

>10%:
- Central nervous system: Headache (11%)
- Dermatologic: Alopecia (48%)
- Gastrointestinal: Nausea (42%), vomiting (29%), mucositis/stomatitis (29%), diarrhea (22%), anorexia (19%), constipation (16%), abdominal pain (13%)
- Hematologic: Leukopenia (grade 3: 36%; grade 4: 13%), neutropenia (grade 3: 31%; grade 4: 23%)
- Neuromuscular & skeletal: Peripheral neuropathy (63%; grades 3/4: 14%; grade 3/4 median onset: cycle 4), sensory neuropathy (62%; grades 3/4: 14%), weakness (56%), myalgia/arthralgia (49%), musculoskeletal pain (20%)

1% to 10%:
- Cardiovascular: Edema (9%), chest pain (5%)
- Central nervous system: Fever (8%), pain (8%), dizziness (7%), insomnia (5%)
- Dermatologic: Nail disorder (9%), rash (9%), palmar-plantar erythrodysesthesia/hand-and-foot syndrome (8%), pruritus (6%), skin exfoliation (2%), hyperpigmentation (2%)
- Endocrine & metabolic: Hot flush (6%), dehydration (2%)
- Gastrointestinal: Gastroesophageal reflux disease (6%), taste perversion (6%), weight loss (6%)
- Hematologic: Anemia (grade 3: 6%; grade 4: 2%), neutropenic fever (3%; grade 3: 3%), thrombocytopenia (grade 3: 5%; grade 4: 2%)
- Neuromuscular & skeletal: Motor neuropathy (10%; grade 3: 1%)
- Ocular: Lacrimation increased (4%)
- Respiratory: Dyspnea (9%), upper respiratory tract infection (6%), cough (2%)
- Miscellaneous: Hypersensitivity (5%; grade 3: 1%), infection (5%)

General Dosage Range Dosage adjustment recommended in patients with hepatic impairment or who develop toxicities

I.V.: *Adults:* 40 mg/m^2 every 3 weeks (maximum dose: 88 mg)

Mechanism of Action Epothilone B analog; binds to the beta-tubulin subunit of the microtubule, stabilizing microtubular promoting tubulin polymerization and stabilizing microtubular function, thus arresting the cell cycle (at the G2/M phase) and inducing apoptosis. Activity in taxane-resistant cells has been demonstrated.

Pharmacodynamics/Kinetics

Half-life Elimination ~52 hours

Time to Peak At the end of infusion (3 hours)

Pregnancy Risk Factor D

Japanese Encephalitis Virus Vaccine (Inactivated)

(jap a NEESE en sef a LYE tis VYE rus vak SEEN, in ak ti VAY ted)

U.S. Brand Names Ixiaro®

Pharmacologic Category Vaccine, Inactivated (Viral)

Use Active immunization against Japanese encephalitis

Japanese encephalitis vaccine is not recommended for all persons traveling to or residing in Asia. The Advisory Committee on Immunization Practices (ACIP) recommends vaccination for:

- Persons spending ≥1 month in endemic areas during transmission season
- Research laboratory workers who may be exposed to the Japanese encephalitis virus

Vaccination may also be considered for the following:

- Travelers to areas with an ongoing outbreak
- Travelers spending <30 days in endemic areas during the transmission season and planning to go outside of urban areas and have an increased risk of exposure. For example, high-risk activities include extensive outdoor activity in rural areas especially at night; extensive outdoor activities such as camping, hiking, etc; staying in accommodations without air conditioning, screens or bed nets.
- Travelers to endemic areas who are unsure of specific destination, activities, or duration of travel

Local Anesthetic/Vasoconstrictor Precautions No information available to require special precautions

Effects on Dental Treatment No significant effects or complications reported

Effects on Bleeding No information available to require special precautions

Adverse Effects Report allergic or unusual adverse reactions to the Vaccine Adverse Event Reporting System (VAERS) 1-800-822-7967 or online at https://vaers.hhs.gov/esub/index. In Canada, adverse reactions may be reported to local provincial/territorial health agencies or to the Vaccine Safety Section at Public Health Agency of Canada (1-866-844-0018).

Percentage of adverse reactions reported over days 0-56. In general, incidence was similar to placebo.

>10%:

Central nervous system: Headache (28%), fatigue (11%)

Local: Injection site reaction: Tenderness (36%), pain (33%)

Neuromuscular & skeletal: Myalgia (16%)

Miscellaneous: Flu-like syndrome (12%)

1% to 10%:

Central nervous system: Pyrexia (3%)

Dermatologic: Rash (1%)

Gastrointestinal: Nausea (7%), diarrhea (2%), vomiting (1%)

Local: Injection site reaction: Erythema (10%), induration (8%), edema (4%), pruritus (4%)

Neuromuscular & skeletal: Back pain (1%)

Respiratory: Nasopharyngitis (5%), pharyngolaryngeal pain (2%), upper respiratory tract infection (2%), cough (1%), rhinitis (1%)

General Dosage Range

I.M.: *Adults ≥17 years:* 0.5 mL/dose on days 0 and 28

Pregnancy Risk Factor B

Kanamycin (kan a MYE sin)

Related Information

Tuberculosis *on page 1902*

Pharmacologic Category Antibiotic, Aminoglycoside

Use Treatment of serious infections caused by susceptible strains of *E. coli*, *Proteus* species, *Enterobacter aerogenes*, *Klebsiella pneumoniae*, *Serratia marcescens*, and *Acinetobacter* species; second-line treatment of *Mycobacterium tuberculosis*

Local Anesthetic/Vasoconstrictor Precautions No information available to require special precautions

Effects on Dental Treatment Key adverse event(s) related to dental treatment: Salivation increased.

Effects on Bleeding No information available to require special precautions

Adverse Effects Frequency not defined.

Cardiovascular: Edema
Central nervous system: Neurotoxicity, drowsiness, headache, pseudomotor cerebri
Dermatologic: Skin itching, redness, rash, photosensitivity, erythema
Gastrointestinal: Nausea, vomiting, diarrhea, malabsorption syndrome (with prolonged and high-dose therapy of hepatic coma), anorexia, weight loss, salivation increased, enterocolitis
Hematologic: Granulocytopenia, agranulocytosis, thrombocytopenia
Local: Burning, stinging
Neuromuscular & skeletal: Weakness, tremor, muscle cramps
Otic: Ototoxicity (auditory), ototoxicity (vestibular)
Renal: Nephrotoxicity
Respiratory: Dyspnea

General Dosage Range Dosage adjustment of I.M. and I.V. route recommended in patients with renal impairment

I.M., I.V.:
Children: 15 mg/kg/day divided every 8-12 hours
Adults: 5-7.5 mg/kg every 8-12 hours
Elderly: 5-7.5 mg/kg every 12-24 hours

Inhalation, aerosol: *Adults:* 250 mg 2-4 times/day
Intraperitoneal: *Adults:* 500 mg
Irrigation: *Adults:* 0.25% (maximum: 1.5 g/day)

Mechanism of Action Interferes with protein synthesis in bacterial cell by binding to ribosomal subunit

Pharmacodynamics/Kinetics

Half-life Elimination 2-4 hours; Anuria: 80 hours; End-stage renal disease: 40-96 hours

Time to Peak Serum: I.M.: 1-2 hours (decreased in burn patients)

Pregnancy Risk Factor D

Ketamine (KEET a meen)

U.S. Brand Names Ketalar®

Canadian Brand Names Ketalar®; Ketamine Hydrochloride Injection, USP

Pharmacologic Category General Anesthetic

Use Induction and maintenance of general anesthesia

Unlabeled/Investigational Use Analgesia, sedation

Local Anesthetic/Vasoconstrictor Precautions No information available to require special precautions

Effects on Dental Treatment Key adverse event(s) related to dental treatment: Increased salivation.

Effects on Bleeding No information available to require special precautions

Adverse Effects Frequency not always defined.

Cardiovascular: Arrhythmia, bradycardia/tachycardia, hyper-/hypotension
Central nervous system: CSF pressure increased
Dermatologic: Erythema (transient), morbilliform rash (transient)
Gastrointestinal: Anorexia, nausea, salivation increased, vomiting
Local: Pain at the injection site, exanthema at the injection site
Neuromuscular & skeletal: Skeletal muscle tone enhanced (tonic-clonic movements)
Ocular: Diplopia, intraocular pressure increased, nystagmus
Respiratory: Airway obstruction, apnea, bronchial secretions increased, respiratory depression, laryngospasm
Miscellaneous: Anaphylaxis, dependence with prolonged use, emergence reactions (~12%; includes confusion, delirium, dreamlike state, excitement, hallucinations, irrational behavior, vivid imagery)

General Dosage Range

I.M.: *Children ≥16 years and Adults:* 2-6 mg/kg
I.V.: *Children ≥16 years and Adults:* 0.2-2 mg/kg **or** 0.1-0.5 mg/minute as a continuous infusion

Mechanism of Action Produces a cataleptic-like state in which the patient is dissociated from the surrounding environment by direct action on the cortex and limbic system. Ketamine is a noncompetitive NMDA receptor antagonist that blocks glutamate. Low (subanesthetic) doses produce analgesia, and modulate central sensitization, hyperalgesia and opioid tolerance. Reduces polysynaptic spinal reflexes.

Pharmacodynamics/Kinetics

Onset of Action

I.V.: Anesthetic effect: 30 seconds

I.M.: Anesthetic effect: 3-4 minutes

Duration of Action Anesthetic effect: I.V.: 5-10 minutes; I.M.: 12-25 minutes

Half-life Elimination Alpha: 10-15 minutes; Beta: 2.5 hours

Controlled Substance C-III

Ketoconazole (Systemic) (kee toe KOE na zole)

Related Information

Fungal Infections *on page 1945*

Respiratory Diseases *on page 1876*

Related Sample Prescriptions

Systemic Fungal Infections *on page 1988*

Canadian Brand Names Apo-Ketoconazole®; Novo-Ketoconazole

Generic Availability (U.S.) Yes

Pharmacologic Category Antifungal Agent, Oral

Dental Use Treatment of susceptible fungal infections in the oral cavity including candidiasis, oral thrush, and chronic mucocutaneous candidiasis

Use Treatment of susceptible fungal infections, including candidiasis, oral thrush, blastomycosis, histoplasmosis, paracoccidioidomycosis, coccidioidomycosis, chromomycosis, candiduria, chronic mucocutaneous candidiasis, as well as certain recalcitrant cutaneous dermatophytoses

Unlabeled/Investigational Use Treatment of prostate cancer (androgen synthesis inhibitor)

Local Anesthetic/Vasoconstrictor Precautions No information available to require special precautions

Effects on Dental Treatment No significant effects or complications reported

Effects on Bleeding No information available to require special precautions

Adverse Effects 1% to 10%:

Dermatologic: Pruritus (2%)

Gastrointestinal: Nausea/vomiting (3% to 10%), abdominal pain (1%)

Dental Usual Dosage Oral fungal infections: Oral:

Children ≥2 years: 3.3-6.6 mg/kg/day as a single dose for 1-2 weeks for candidiasis, for at least 4 weeks in recalcitrant dermatophyte infections, and for up to 6 months for other systemic mycoses

Adults: 200-400 mg/day as a single daily dose for durations as stated above

Dosage Oral:

Fungal infections:

Children ≥2 years: 3.3-6.6 mg/kg/day as a single dose for 1-2 weeks for candidiasis, for at least 4 weeks in recalcitrant dermatophyte infections, and for up to 6 months for other systemic mycoses

Adults: 200-400 mg/day as a single daily dose for durations as stated above

Prostate cancer (unlabeled use): Adults: 400 mg 3 times/day

Dosing adjustment in renal impairment: Hemodialysis: Not dialyzable (0% to 5%)

Dosing adjustment in hepatic impairment: Dose reductions should be considered in patients with severe liver disease

Mechanism of Action Alters the permeability of the cell wall by blocking fungal cytochrome P450; inhibits biosynthesis of triglycerides and phospholipids by fungi; inhibits several fungal enzymes that results in a build-up of toxic concentrations of hydrogen peroxide; also inhibits androgen synthesis

Contraindications Hypersensitivity to ketoconazole or any component of the formulation; CNS fungal infections (due to poor CNS penetration); coadministration with ergot derivatives, cisapride, or triazolam is contraindicated due to risk of potentially fatal cardiac arrhythmias

Warnings/Precautions [U.S. Boxed Warning]: Ketoconazole has been associated with hepatotoxicity, including some fatalities; use with caution in patients with impaired hepatic function and perform periodic liver function tests. **[U.S. Boxed Warning]: Concomitant use with cisapride is contraindicated due to the occurrence of ventricular arrhythmias.** High doses of ketoconazole may depress adrenocortical function.

Drug Interactions

Metabolism/Transport Effects Substrate of CYP3A4 (major); **Inhibits** CYP1A2 (strong), CYP2A6 (moderate), CYP2B6 (weak), CYP2C8 (weak), CYP2C9 (strong), CYP2C19 (moderate), CYP2D6 (moderate), CYP3A4 (strong), P-glycoprotein

Avoid Concomitant Use

Avoid concomitant use of Ketoconazole (Systemic) with any of the following: Alfuzosin; Cisapride; Clopidogrel; Conivaptan; Dofetilide; Dronedarone; Eplerenone; Everolimus; Fluticasone (Oral Inhalation); Halofantrine; Lurasidone; Nilotinib; Nisoldipine; Pimozide; QuiNIDine; Ranolazine; Rivaroxaban; RomiDEPsin; Salmeterol; Silodosin; Tamsulosin; Thioridazine; Tolvaptan; Topotecan; Toremifene

Increased Effect/Toxicity

Ketoconazole (Systemic) may increase the levels/effects of: Alfentanil; Alfuzosin; Aliskiren; Almotriptan; Alosetron; Aprepitant; Bendamustine; Benzodiazepines (metabolized by oxidation); Bortezomib; Bosentan; Brinzolamide; Budesonide (Nasal); Budesonide (Systemic, Oral Inhalation); BusPIRone; Busulfan; Calcium Channel Blockers; CarBAMazepine; Carvedilol; Ciclesonide; Cilostazol; Cinacalcet; Cisapride; Colchicine; Conivaptan; Corticosteroids (Orally Inhaled); Corticosteroids (Systemic); CycloSPORINE; CycloSPORINE (Systemic); CYP1A2 Substrates; CYP2A6 Substrates; CYP2C19 Substrates; CYP2C9 Substrates (High risk); CYP2D6 Substrates; CYP3A4 Substrates; Dabigatran Etexilate; Dienogest; DOCEtaxel; Dofetilide; Dronedarone; Dutasteride; Eletriptan; Eplerenone; Erlotinib; Eszopiclone; Etravirine; Everolimus; FentaNYL; Fesoterodine; Fexofenadine; Fluticasone (Nasal); Fluticasone (Oral Inhalation); Fosaprepitant; Fosphenytoin; Gefitinib; GuanFACINE; Halofantrine; HMG-CoA Reductase Inhibitors; Imatinib; Irinotecan; Ixabepilone; Losartan; Lumefantrine; Lurasidone; Macrolide Antibiotics; Maraviroc; Methadone; MethylPREDNISolone; Nebivolol; Nilotinib; Nisoldipine; Paricalcitol; Pazopanib; P-Glycoprotein Substrates; Phenytoin; Phosphodiesterase 5 Inhibitors; Pimecrolimus; Pimozide; Praziquantel; Protease Inhibitors; Proton Pump Inhibitors; QuiNIDine; Ramelteon; Ranolazine; Repaglinide; Rifamycin Derivatives; Rivaroxaban; RomiDEPsin; Salmeterol; Saxagliptin; Silodosin; Sirolimus; Solifenacin; SORAfenib; SUNItinib; Tacrolimus; Tacrolimus (Systemic); Tacrolimus (Topical); Tadalafil; Tamoxifen; Tamsulosin; Temsirolimus; Thioridazine; Tolterodine; Tolvaptan; Topotecan; Toremifene; Vilazodone; Vitamin K Antagonists; Ziprasidone; Zolpidem

The levels/effects of Ketoconazole (Systemic) may be increased by: Etravirine; Grapefruit Juice; Macrolide Antibiotics; Protease Inhibitors

Decreased Effect

Ketoconazole (Systemic) may decrease the levels/effects of: Amphotericin B; Clopidogrel; Codeine; Prasugrel; Saccharomyces boulardii; TraMADol

The levels/effects of Ketoconazole (Systemic) may be decreased by: Antacids; CYP3A4 Inducers (Strong); Deferasirox; Didanosine; Etravirine; Fosphenytoin; H2-Antagonists; Herbs (CYP3A4 Inducers); Phenytoin; Proton Pump Inhibitors; Rifamycin Derivatives; Sucralfate; Tocilizumab

Ethanol/Nutrition/Herb Interactions

Food: Ketoconazole peak serum levels may be prolonged if taken with food.

Herb/Nutraceutical: St John's wort may decrease ketoconazole levels.

Dietary Considerations May be taken with food or milk to decrease GI adverse effects.

Pharmacodynamics/Kinetics

Half-life Elimination Biphasic: Initial: 2 hours; Terminal: 8 hours

Time to Peak Serum: 1-2 hours

Pregnancy Risk Factor C

Lactation Enters breast milk/not recommended

Breast-Feeding Considerations In a case report, ketoconazole in concentrations of ≤0.22 mcg/mL were detected in the breast milk of a woman 1 month post-partum. She had been taking oral ketoconazole 200 mg/day for 5 days at the time of sampling. The maximum milk concentration occurred 3.25 hours after the dose and concentrations were undetectable 24 hours after the dose. Based on the highest milk concentration, the estimated dose to the nursing infant was 1.4% of the maternal dose. Breast-feeding is not recommended by the manufacturer.

Dosage Forms

Tablet, oral: 200 mg

Ketoconazole (Topical) (kee toe KOE na zole)

Related Information

Fungal Infections *on page* 1945

Related Sample Prescriptions

Topical Fungal Infections *on page* 1988

U.S. Brand Names Extina®; Nizoral®; Nizoral® A-D [OTC]; Xolegel®

Canadian Brand Names Ketoderm®; Xolegel®

Generic Availability (U.S.) Yes: Cream, shampoo

Pharmacologic Category Antifungal Agent, Topical

Dental Use Treatment of susceptible fungal infections in the oral cavity including candidiasis, oral thrush, and chronic mucocutaneous candidiasis

Use

Cream: Treatment of tinea corporis, tinea cruris, tinea versicolor, cutaneous candidiasis, seborrheic dermatitis

Foam, gel: Treatment of seborrheic dermatitis

Shampoo: Treatment of dandruff, seborrheic dermatitis, tinea versicolor

Unlabeled/Investigational Use Cream: Treatment of susceptible fungal infections in the oral cavity including candidiasis, oral thrush, and chronic mucocutaneous candidiasis

Local Anesthetic/Vasoconstrictor Precautions No information available to require special precautions

Effects on Dental Treatment No significant effects or complications reported

Effects on Bleeding No information available to require special precautions

Adverse Effects

Topical cream/gel: Acne, allergic reaction, contact dermatitis (possibly related to sulfites or propylene glycol), discharge, dizziness, dryness, erythema, facial swelling, headache, impetigo, keratoconjunctivitis sicca, local burning (4%), nail discoloration, ocular irritation/swelling, pain, paresthesia, pruritus, pustules, pyogenic granuloma, severe irritation, stinging (~5%)

Topical foam: Application site burning (10%), application site reaction (6%), contact sensitization, dryness, erythema, pruritus, rash

Shampoo: Abnormal hair texture, alopecia, application site reaction, burning sensation, contact dermatitis, hair discoloration, hypersensitivity, itching, mild dryness of skin, oiliness/dryness of hair, pruritus, rash, scalp pustules, urticaria

Dental Usual Dosage Cream: Apply locally as directed with a thin coat to inner surface of denture and affected areas after meals

Dosage

Shampoo:

Seborrheic dermatitis (ketoconazole 1%): Children ≥12 years and Adults: Apply twice weekly for up to 8 weeks with at least 3 days between each shampoo

Tinea versicolor (ketoconazole 2%): Adults: Apply to damp skin, lather, leave on 5 minutes, and rinse (one application should be sufficient)

Topical:

Tinea infections: Adults: Cream: Rub gently into the affected area once daily. Duration of treatment: Tinea corporis, cruris: 2 weeks; tinea pedis: 6 weeks

Seborrheic dermatitis: Children ≥12 years and Adults:

Cream: Rub gently into the affected area twice daily for 4 weeks or until clinical response is noted

Foam: Apply to affected area twice daily for 4 weeks

Gel: Rub gently into the affected area once daily for 2 weeks

Susceptible fungal infections in the oral cavity (candidiasis, oral thrush, and chronic mucocutaneous candidiasis) (unlabeled use): Adults: Cream: Apply locally as directed with a thin coat to inner surface of denture and affected areas after meals

Mechanism of Action Alters the permeability of the cell wall by blocking fungal cytochrome P450; inhibits biosynthesis of triglycerides and phospholipids by fungi; inhibits several fungal enzymes that results in a build-up of toxic concentrations of hydrogen peroxide; also inhibits androgen synthesis

Contraindications Hypersensitivity to ketoconazole or any component of the formulation

Warnings/Precautions Cases of hypersensitivity reactions (including rare cases of anaphylaxis) have been reported. Formulations may contain sulfites. Avoid exposure of gel to open flames or smoking during or immediately after application. Foam formulation contains alcohol and propane/butane; do not expose to open flame or smoking during or immediately after application; do not puncture or incinerate container. Use of shampoo may remove curl from permanently wavy hair, cause hair discoloration, and changes in hair texture; avoid contact with eyes. Discontinue use if irritation occurs.

Drug Interactions

Avoid Concomitant Use There are no known interactions where it is recommended to avoid concomitant use.

Increased Effect/Toxicity There are no known significant interactions involving an increase in effect.

Decreased Effect There are no known significant interactions involving a decrease in effect.

Pregnancy Risk Factor C

Lactation Excretion in breast milk unknown/use caution

Breast-Feeding Considerations Ketoconazole has been detected in breast milk following oral dosing. Although it is not detected in the plasma following chronic use of the shampoo, and concentrations in the plasma following application of the gel are <250 times those observed with oral dosing, the manufacturers recommend that caution be used when administering to a nursing woman.

Dosage Forms

Aerosol, topical:
Extina®: 2% (50 g, 100 g)
Cream, topical: 2% (15 g, 30 g, 60 g)
Gel, topical:
Xolegel®: 2% (45 g)
Shampoo, topical: 2% (120 mL)
Nizoral®: 2% (120 mL)
Nizoral® A-D [OTC]: 1% (120 mL, 210 mL)

Ketoprofen (kee toe PROE fen)

Related Information

Oral Pain *on page 1928*
Rheumatoid Arthritis, Osteoarthritis, and Osteoporosis *on page 1889*
Temporomandibular Dysfunction (TMD) *on page 1964*

Canadian Brand Names Apo-Keto SR®; Apo-Keto-E®; Apo-Keto®; Nu-Ketoprofen; Nu-Ketoprofen-E; PMS-Ketoprofen; PMS-Ketoprofen-E

Generic Availability (U.S.) Yes

Pharmacologic Category Nonsteroidal Anti-inflammatory Drug (NSAID), Oral

Dental Use Management of pain and swelling

Use Acute and long-term treatment of rheumatoid arthritis and osteoarthritis; primary dysmenorrhea; mild-to-moderate pain

Local Anesthetic/Vasoconstrictor Precautions No information available to require special precautions

Effects on Dental Treatment Key adverse event(s) related to dental treatment: Stomatitis.

According to the FDA, the over-the-counter NSAID ketoprofen should be viewed as having the potential to interfere with the antiplatelet effect of low-dose aspirin until proven otherwise. This statement was provided in the same warning from the FDA that ibuprofen can interfere with the antiplatelet effect of low-dose aspirin (81 mg/day), potentially rendering aspirin less effective when used for cardioprotection and stroke protection. In situations where these drugs could be used concomitantly, the FDA has provided the following information: Patients who use immediate release aspirin (not enteric-coated aspirin) and take single doses of ibuprofen 400 mg, should dose the ibuprofen at least 30 minutes or longer after aspirin ingestion or more than 8 hours before aspirin ingestion to avoid attenuation of aspirin's effect. Similar recommendations may hold for concomitant ketoprofen and aspirin use. See Effects on Bleeding.

At this time, recommendations about the timing of ibuprofen 400 mg or other NSAIDs (such as ketoprofen) in patients taking enteric-coated low-dose aspirin cannot be made based on available data.

Effects on Bleeding Nonselective NSAIDs are known to reversibly decrease platelet aggregation via mechanisms different than observed with aspirin. Platelet function is restored as the drug is eliminated from the body. NSAIDs should be avoided (if possible) in general surgery patients for 3-5 half-lives of the drug (usually 1-3 days) prior to surgery to reduce the risk of excessive bleeding. However, there is no scientific evidence to warrant discontinuance of NSAIDs prior to dental surgery. In medically complicated patients or extensive oral surgery, the decision to interrupt therapy must be based on the risk to benefit in an individual patient and a medical consult is suggested. Routine interruption of NSAID therapy for most dental procedures is not warranted. If therapy is continued without interruption, the clinician should anticipate the potential for slower clotting times.

Adverse Effects

>10%:
Gastrointestinal: Dyspepsia (11%)
Hepatic: Liver function test abnormal (≤15%)

1% to 10%:
Cardiovascular: Peripheral edema (2%)
Central nervous system: Headache (3% to 9%), depression, dizziness (>1%), dreams, insomnia, malaise, nervousness, somnolence
Dermatologic: Rash (>1%)
Gastrointestinal: Abdominal pain (3% to 9%), constipation (3% to 9%), diarrhea (3% to 9%), flatulence (3% to 9%), nausea (3% to 9%), gastrointestinal bleeding (>2%), peptic ulcer (>2%), anorexia (>1%), stomatitis (>1%), vomiting (>1%)

Genitourinary: Urinary tract irritation (>1%)
Ocular: Visual disturbances (>1%)
Otic: Tinnitus (>1%)
Renal: Renal dysfunction (3% to 9%)

Dental Usual Dosage Mild-to-moderate pain: Children ≥16 years and Adults: Oral: Capsule: 25-50 mg every 6-8 hours up to a maximum of 300 mg/day

Dosage Note: The extended release formulation is not recommended for the treatment of acute pain. Oral:

Adults:

Rheumatoid arthritis, osteoarthritis (lower doses may be used in small patients or in the elderly, or debilitated):

Regular release: 50 mg 4 times/day **or** 75 mg 3 times/day; up to a maximum of 300 mg/day

Extended release: 200 mg once daily

Dysmenorrhea, mild-to-moderate pain: Regular release: 25-50 mg every 6-8 hours up to a maximum of 300 mg/day

Elderly: Initial dose should be decreased in patients >75 years; use caution when dosage changes are made

Dosage adjustment in renal impairment: In general, NSAIDs are not recommended for use in patients with advanced renal disease, but the manufacturer of ketoprofen does provide some guidelines for adjustment in renal dysfunction:

Mild impairment: Maximum dose: 150 mg/day

Severe impairment: Cl_{cr} <25 mL/minute: Maximum dose: 100 mg/day

Dosage adjustment in hepatic impairment and serum albumin <3.5 g/dL: Maximum dose: 100 mg/day

Mechanism of Action Reversibly inhibits cyclooxygenase-1 and 2 (COX-1 and 2) enzymes, which results in decreased formation of prostaglandin precursors; has antipyretic, analgesic, and anti-inflammatory properties

Other proposed mechanisms not fully elucidated (and possibly contributing to the anti-inflammatory effect to varying degrees), include inhibiting chemotaxis, altering lymphocyte activity, inhibiting neutrophil aggregation/activation, and decreasing proinflammatory cytokine levels.

Contraindications Hypersensitivity to ketoprofen, aspirin, other NSAIDs, or any component of the formulation; perioperative pain in the setting of coronary artery bypass graft (CABG) surgery

Warnings/Precautions [U.S. Boxed Warning]: NSAIDs are associated with an increased risk of adverse cardiovascular thrombotic events, including MI and stroke Risk may be increased with duration of use or pre-existing cardiovascular risk factors or disease. Carefully evaluate individual cardiovascular risk profiles prior to prescribing. May cause new-onset hypertension or worsening of existing hypertension. Use caution with fluid retention. Avoid use in heart failure. Concurrent administration of ibuprofen, and potentially other nonselective NSAIDs, may interfere with aspirin's cardioprotective effect. **[U.S. Boxed Warning]: Use is contraindicated for treatment of perioperative pain in the setting of coronary artery bypass graft (CABG) surgery.** Risk of MI and stroke may be increased with use following CABG surgery.

NSAID use may compromise existing renal function; dose-dependent decreases in prostaglandin synthesis may result from NSAID use, reducing renal blood flow which may cause renal decompensation. NSAID use may increase the risk for hyperkalemia. Patients with impaired renal function, dehydration, heart failure, liver dysfunction, those taking diuretics, and ACE inhibitors, and the elderly are at greater risk of renal toxicity and hyperkalemia. Rehydrate patient before starting therapy; monitor renal function closely. Not recommended for use in patients with advanced renal disease. Long-term NSAID use may result in renal papillary necrosis.

[U.S. Boxed Warning]: NSAIDs may increase risk of gastrointestinal irritation, inflammation, ulceration, bleeding, and perforation. These events may occur at any time during therapy and without warning. Use caution with a history of GI disease (bleeding or ulcers), concurrent therapy with aspirin, anticoagulants and/or corticosteroids, smoking, use of alcohol, the elderly or debilitated patients. When used concomitantly with ≤325 mg of aspirin, a substantial increase in the risk of gastrointestinal complications (eg, ulcer) occurs; concomitant gastroprotective therapy (eg, proton pump inhibitors) is recommended (Bhatt, 2008). Platelet adhesion and aggregation may be decreased; may prolong bleeding time; patients with coagulation disorders or who are receiving anticoagulants should be monitored closely. Anemia may occur; patients on long-term NSAID therapy should be monitored for anemia. Rarely, NSAID use may cause severe blood dyscrasias (eg, agranulocytosis, aplastic anemia, thrombocytopenia).

Use the lowest effective dose for the shortest duration of time, consistent with individual patient goals, to reduce risk of cardiovascular or GI adverse events. Alternate therapies should be considered for patients at high risk.

NSAIDS may cause drowsiness, dizziness, blurred vision and other neurologic effects which may impair physical or mental abilities; patients must be cautioned about performing tasks which require mental alertness (eg, operating machinery or driving). Discontinue use with blurred or diminished vision and perform ophthalmologic exam. Monitor vision with long-term therapy.

NSAIDs may cause serious skin adverse events including exfoliative dermatitis, Stevens-Johnson syndrome (SJS), and toxic epidermal necrolysis (TEN); discontinue use at first sign of skin rash or hypersensitivity. Anaphylactoid reactions may occur, even without prior exposure; patients with "aspirin triad" (bronchial asthma, aspirin intolerance, rhinitis) may be at increased risk. Do not use in patients who experience bronchospasm, asthma, rhinitis, or urticaria with NSAID or aspirin therapy. Use caution in other forms of asthma.

Use with caution in patients with decreased hepatic function. Closely monitor patients with any abnormal LFT. Severe hepatic reactions (eg, fulminant hepatitis, liver failure) have occurred with NSAID use, rarely; discontinue if signs or symptoms of liver disease develop, or if systemic manifestations occur. The elderly are at increased risk for adverse effects (especially peptic ulceration, CNS effects, renal toxicity) from NSAIDs, even at low doses.

Withhold for at least 4-6 half-lives prior to surgical or dental procedures. Safety and efficacy have not been established in pediatric patients.

Drug Interactions

Metabolism/Transport Effects Inhibits CYP2C9 (weak)

Avoid Concomitant Use

Avoid concomitant use of Ketoprofen with any of the following: Ketorolac; Ketorolac (Systemic)

Increased Effect/Toxicity

Ketoprofen may increase the levels/effects of: Aminoglycosides; Anticoagulants; Antiplatelet Agents; Bisphosphonate Derivatives; Collagenase (Systemic); CycloSPORINE; CycloSPORINE (Systemic); Deferasirox; Desmopressin; Digoxin; Drotrecogin Alfa; Eplerenone; Haloperidol; Ibritumomab; Lithium; Methotrexate; Nonsteroidal Anti-Inflammatory Agents; PEMEtrexed; Potassium-Sparing Diuretics; PRALAtrexate; Quinolone Antibiotics; Salicylates; Thrombolytic Agents; Tositumomab and Iodine I 131 Tositumomab; Vancomycin; Vitamin K Antagonists

The levels/effects of Ketoprofen may be increased by: ACE Inhibitors; Angiotensin II Receptor Blockers; Antidepressants (Tricyclic, Tertiary Amine); Corticosteroids (Systemic); Dasatinib; Glucosamine; Herbs (Anticoagulant/Antiplatelet Properties); Ketorolac; Ketorolac (Systemic); Nonsteroidal Anti-Inflammatory Agents; Omega-3-Acid Ethyl Esters; Pentosan Polysulfate Sodium; Pentoxifylline; Probenecid; Prostacyclin Analogues; Selective Serotonin Reuptake Inhibitors; Serotonin/Norepinephrine Reuptake Inhibitors; Treprostinil

Decreased Effect

Ketoprofen may decrease the levels/effects of: ACE Inhibitors; Angiotensin II Receptor Blockers; Antiplatelet Agents; Beta-Blockers; Eplerenone; HydrALAZINE; Loop Diuretics; Potassium-Sparing Diuretics; Salicylates; Thiazide Diuretics

The levels/effects of Ketoprofen may be decreased by: Bile Acid Sequestrants; Nonsteroidal Anti-Inflammatory Agents; Salicylates

Ethanol/Nutrition/Herb Interactions

Ethanol: Avoid ethanol (due to GI irritation).

Food: Food slows rate of absorption resulting in delayed and reduced peak serum concentrations; total bioavailability is not affected by food.

Herb/Nutraceutical: Avoid alfalfa, anise, bilberry, bladderwrack, bromelain, cat's claw, celery, chamomile, coleus, cordyceps, dong quai, evening primrose, fenugreek, feverfew, garlic, ginger, ginkgo biloba, ginseng (American, Panax, Siberian), grapeseed, green tea, guggul, horse chestnut seed, horseradish, licorice, prickly ash, red clover, reishi, SAMe (S-adenosylmethionine), sweet clover, turmeric, and white willow (all have additional antiplatelet activity).

Dietary Considerations In order to minimize gastrointestinal effects, ketoprofen can be prescribed to be taken with food or milk.

Pharmacodynamics/Kinetics

Onset of Action Regular release: <30 minutes

Duration of Action Regular release: Up to 6 hours

Half-life Elimination

Regular release: 2-4 hours; Renal impairment: Mild: 3 hours; moderate-to-severe: 5-9 hours

Extended release: ~3-7.5 hours

Time to Peak Regular release: 0.5-2 hours; Extended release: 6-7 hours

Pregnancy Risk Factor C

Lactation Enters breast milk

Breast-Feeding Considerations Small amounts of ketoprofen are found in breast milk. Breast-feeding is not recommended by the manufacturer.

Dosage Forms

Capsule, oral: 50 mg, 75 mg

Capsule, extended release, oral: 200 mg

References

Brooks PM and Day RO, "Nonsteroidal Anti-inflammatory Drugs - Differences and Similarities," *N Engl J Med*, 1991, 324(24):1716-25.

Cooper SA, "Ketoprofen in Oral Surgery Pain: A Review," *J Clin Pharmacol*, 1988, 28(12 Suppl):S40-6.

Hersh EV, "The Efficacy and Safety of Ketoprofen in Postsurgical Dental Pain," *Compendium*, 1991, 12 (4):234.

Ketorolac (Systemic) (KEE toe role ak)

Related Information

Oral Pain *on page 1928*

Rheumatoid Arthritis, Osteoarthritis, and Osteoporosis *on page 1889*

Temporomandibular Dysfunction (TMD) *on page 1964*

Canadian Brand Names Apo-Ketorolac Injectable®; Apo-Ketorolac®; Ketorolac Tromethamine Injection, USP; Novo-Ketorolac; Nu-Ketorolac; Toradol®; Toradol® IM

Generic Availability (U.S.) Yes

Pharmacologic Category Nonsteroidal Anti-inflammatory Drug (NSAID), Oral; Nonsteroidal Anti-inflammatory Drug (NSAID), Parenteral

Dental Use Short-term (≤5 days) management of moderate-to-severe acute pain requiring analgesia at the opioid level

Use Short-term (≤5 days) management of moderate-to-severe acute pain requiring analgesia at the opioid level

Local Anesthetic/Vasoconstrictor Precautions No information available to require special precautions

Effects on Dental Treatment Key adverse event(s) related to dental treatment: Xerostomia (normal salivary flow resumes upon discontinuation) and stomatitis.

NSAID formulations are known to reversibly decrease platelet aggregation via mechanisms different than observed with aspirin. The dentist should be aware of the potential of abnormal coagulation. Caution should also be exercised in the use of NSAIDs in patients already on anticoagulant therapy with drugs such as warfarin (Coumadin®). See Dental Comment.

Effects on Bleeding Nonselective NSAIDs are known to reversibly decrease platelet aggregation via mechanisms different than observed with aspirin. Platelet function is restored as the drug is eliminated from the body. NSAIDs should be avoided (if possible) in general surgery patients for 3-5 half-lives of the drug (usually 1-3 days) prior to surgery to reduce the risk of excessive bleeding. However, there is no scientific evidence to warrant discontinuance of NSAIDs prior to dental surgery. In medically complicated patients or extensive oral surgery, the decision to interrupt therapy must be based on the risk to benefit in an individual patient and a medical consult is suggested. Routine interruption of NSAID therapy for most dental procedures is not warranted. If therapy is continued without interruption, the clinician should anticipate the potential for slower clotting times.

Adverse Effects Frequencies noted for parenteral administration:

>10%:

Central nervous system: Headache (17%)

Gastrointestinal: Gastrointestinal pain (13%), dyspepsia (12%), nausea (12%)

>1% to 10%:

Cardiovascular: Edema (4%), hypertension

Central nervous system: Dizziness (7%), drowsiness (6%)

Dermatologic: Pruritus, purpura, rash

Gastrointestinal: Diarrhea (7%), constipation, flatulence, GI bleeding, GI fullness, GI perforation, GI ulcer, heartburn, stomatitis, vomiting

Hematologic: Anemia, bleeding time increased

Hepatic: Liver enzymes increased

Local: Injection site pain (2%)

Otic: Tinnitus

Renal: Renal function abnormal

Miscellaneous: Diaphoresis

Dental Usual Dosage

Short-term (≤5 days) management of moderate-to-severe acute pain requiring analgesia at the opioid level (**Note:** The maximum combined duration of treatment (for parenteral and oral) is 5 days; do not increase dose or frequency; supplement with low-dose opioids if needed for breakthrough pain). For patients <50 kg and/or ≥65 years, see Elderly dosing.

Adults:

I.M.: 60 mg as a single dose or 30 mg every 6 hours (maximum daily dose: 120 mg)

I.V.: 30 mg as a single dose or 30 mg every 6 hours (maximum daily dose: 120 mg)

Oral: 20 mg, followed by 10 mg every 4-6 hours; do not exceed 40 mg/day; oral dosing is intended to be a continuation of I.M. or I.V. therapy only

Dosage adjustments in elderly (≥65 years), renal insufficiency, or low body weight (<50 kg): Note: These groups have an increased incidence of GI bleeding, ulceration, and perforation. The maximum combined duration of treatment (for parenteral and oral) is 5 days.

I.M.: 30 mg as a single dose or 15 mg every 6 hours (maximum daily dose: 60 mg)

I.V.: 15 mg as a single dose or 15 mg every 6 hours (maximum daily dose: 60 mg)

Oral: 10 mg, followed by 10 mg every 4-6 hours; do not exceed 40 mg/day; oral dosing is intended to be a continuation of I.M. or I.V. therapy only

Dosage

Children ≥16 years and Adults (pain relief usually begins within 10 minutes with parenteral forms): **Note:** The maximum combined duration of treatment (for parenteral and oral) is 5 days; do not increase dose or frequency; supplement with low-dose opioids if needed for breakthrough pain. For patients <50 kg and/or ≥65 years, see Elderly dosing.

I.M.: 60 mg as a single dose or 30 mg every 6 hours (maximum daily dose: 120 mg)

I.V.: 30 mg as a single dose or 30 mg every 6 hours (maximum daily dose: 120 mg)

Children ≥17 years and Adults: Oral: 20 mg, followed by 10 mg every 4-6 hours; do not exceed 40 mg/day; oral dosing is intended to be a continuation of I.M. or I.V. therapy only

Note: The maximum combined duration of treatment (for parenteral and oral) is 5 days; do not increase dose or frequency; supplement with low-dose opioids if needed for breakthrough pain. Therapy should not be initiated with oral formulation. For patients <50 kg and/or ≥65 years, see Elderly dosing.

Dosage adjustments in elderly (≥65 years), renal insufficiency, or low body weight (<50 kg): Note: These groups have an increased incidence of GI bleeding, ulceration, and perforation. The maximum combined duration of treatment (for parenteral and oral) is 5 days.

I.M.: 30 mg as a single dose or 15 mg every 6 hours (maximum daily dose: 60 mg)

I.V.: 15 mg as a single dose or 15 mg every 6 hours (maximum daily dose: 60 mg)

Oral: 10 mg, followed by 10 mg every 4-6 hours; do not exceed 40 mg/day; oral dosing is intended to be a continuation of I.M. or I.V. therapy only

Dosage adjustment in renal impairment: Contraindicated in patients with advanced renal impairment. Patients with moderately-elevated serum creatinine should use half the recommended dose, not to exceed 60 mg/day I.M./I.V.

Dosage adjustment in hepatic impairment: Use with caution, may cause elevation of liver enzymes; discontinue if clinical signs and symptoms of liver disease develop

Mechanism of Action Reversibly inhibits cyclooxygenase-1 and 2 (COX-1 and 2) enzymes, which results in decreased formation of prostaglandin precursors; has antipyretic, analgesic, and anti-inflammatory properties

Other proposed mechanisms not fully elucidated (and possibly contributing to the anti-inflammatory effect to varying degrees), include inhibiting chemotaxis, altering lymphocyte activity, inhibiting neutrophil aggregation/activation, and decreasing proinflammatory cytokine levels.

Contraindications Hypersensitivity to ketorolac, aspirin, other NSAIDs, or any component of the formulation; active or history of peptic ulcer disease; recent or history of GI bleeding or perforation; patients with advanced renal disease or risk of renal failure (due to volume depletion); prophylaxis before major surgery; suspected or confirmed cerebrovascular bleeding; hemorrhagic diathesis, incomplete hemostasis, or high risk of bleeding; concurrent ASA or other NSAIDs; concomitant probenecid or pentoxifylline; epidural or intrathecal administration; perioperative pain in the setting of coronary artery bypass graft (CABG) surgery; labor and delivery; breast-feeding

Warnings/Precautions [U.S. Boxed Warning]: May inhibit platelet function; contraindicated in patients with cerebrovascular bleeding (suspected or confirmed), hemorrhagic diathesis, incomplete hemostasis and patients at high risk for bleeding. Effects on platelet adhesion and aggregation may prolong bleeding time. Anemia may occur; patients on long-term NSAID therapy should be monitored for anemia. Rarely, NSAID use has been associated with potentially severe blood dyscrasias (eg, agranulocytosis, thrombocytopenia, aplastic anemia).

[U.S. Boxed Warning]: NSAIDs are associated with an increased risk of adverse cardiovascular thrombotic events, including MI and stroke. Risk may be increased with duration of use or pre-existing cardiovascular risk factors or disease. Carefully evaluate individual cardiovascular risk profiles prior to prescribing. May cause new-onset hypertension or worsening of existing hypertension. Use caution with fluid retention. Avoid use in heart failure. Concurrent administration of ibuprofen, and potentially other nonselective NSAIDs, may interfere with aspirin's cardioprotective effect. **[U.S. Boxed Warning]: Use is contraindicated as prophylactic analgesic before any major surgery and is contraindicated for treatment of perioperative pain in the setting of coronary artery bypass graft (CABG) surgery.** Risk of MI and stroke may be increased with use following CABG surgery. Wound bleeding and postoperative hematomas have been associated with ketorolac use in the perioperative setting. Withhold for at least 4-6 half-lives prior to surgical or dental procedures.

[U.S. Boxed Warning]: Ketorolac is contraindicated in patients with advanced renal impairment and in patients at risk for renal failure due to volume depletion. NSAID use may compromise existing renal function; dose-dependent decreases in prostaglandin synthesis may result from NSAID use, reducing renal blood flow which may cause renal decompensation. NSAID use may increase the risk for hyperkalemia. Patients with impaired renal function, dehydration, heart failure, liver dysfunction, those taking diuretics and ACE inhibitors, and the elderly are at greater risk of renal toxicity. Use with caution in patients with impaired renal function or history of kidney disease; dosage adjustment is required in patients with moderate elevation in serum creatinine. Monitor renal function closely. Acute renal failure, interstitial nephritis, and nephrotic syndrome have been reported with ketorolac use; papillary necrosis and renal injury have been reported with the use of NSAIDs. Use of NSAIDs can compromise existing renal function. Rehydrate patient before starting therapy.

[U.S. Boxed Warning]: NSAIDs may increase risk of gastrointestinal irritation, inflammation, ulceration, bleeding, and perforation. These events may occur at any time during therapy and without warning. Use caution with a history of GI disease (bleeding, ulcers, inflammatory bowel disease), concurrent therapy with aspirin, anticoagulants and/or corticosteroids, smoking, use of alcohol, the elderly, or debilitated patients. When used concomitantly with ≤325 mg of aspirin, a substantial increase in the risk of gastrointestinal complications (eg, ulcer) occurs; concomitant gastroprotective therapy (eg, proton pump inhibitors) is recommended (Bhatt, 2008).

NSAIDs may cause serious skin adverse events including exfoliative dermatitis, Stevens-Johnson syndrome (SJS), and toxic epidermal necrolysis (TEN); discontinue use at first sign of skin rash or hypersensitivity. Hypersensitivity or anaphylactoid reactions may occur, even without prior exposure; patients with "aspirin triad" (bronchial asthma, aspirin intolerance, rhinitis) may be at increased risk. Do not use in patients who experience bronchospasm, asthma, rhinitis, or urticaria with NSAID or aspirin therapy. **[U.S. Boxed Warning]: Ketorolac injection is contraindicated in patients with prior hypersensitivity reaction to aspirin or NSAIDs.** Use caution in other forms of asthma.

Use with caution in patients with hepatic impairment or a history of liver disease. Closely monitor patients with any abnormal LFT. Rarely, severe hepatic reactions (eg, fulminant hepatitis, hepatic necrosis, liver failure) have occurred with NSAID use; discontinue if signs or symptoms of liver disease develop, or if systemic manifestations occur.

[U.S. Boxed Warning]: Dosage adjustment is required for patients ≥65 years of age. The elderly are at increased risk for adverse effects (especially peptic ulceration, CNS effects, renal toxicity) from NSAIDs, even at low doses. Avoid immediate and long-term use (Beers Criteria). **[U.S. Boxed Warning]: Dosage adjustment is required for patients weighing <50 kg (<110 pounds). [U.S. Boxed Warning]: May inhibit uterine contractions and affect fetal circulation; inhibits prostaglandin synthesis in neonates; use is contraindicated in labor and delivery and breast-feeding women.** Avoid use in late pregnancy. **[U.S. Boxed Warning]: Concurrent use of ketorolac with aspirin or other NSAIDs is contraindicated due to the increased risk of adverse reactions.**

[U.S. Boxed Warning]: Contraindicated for epidural or intrathecal administration. [U.S. Boxed Warning]: Systemic ketorolac is indicated for short term (≤5 days) use in adults for treatment of moderately severe acute pain requiring opioid-level analgesia. Low doses of narcotics may be needed for breakthrough pain. **[U.S. Boxed Warning]: Oral therapy is only indicated for use as continuation treatment, following parenteral ketorolac and is not indicated for minor**

or chronic painful conditions. The maximum daily oral dose is 40 mg (adults); doses above 40 mg/day do not improve efficacy but may increase the risk of serious adverse effects. The combined therapy duration (oral and parenteral) should not exceed 5 days. Use the lowest effective dose for the shortest duration of time, consistent with individual patient goals, to reduce risk of cardiovascular or GI adverse events. Alternate therapies should be considered for patients at high risk. **[U.S. Boxed Warning]: Oral ketorolac is not indicated for use in children.**

NSAIDS may cause drowsiness, dizziness, blurred vision and other neurologic effects which may impair physical or mental abilities; patients must be cautioned about performing tasks which require mental alertness (eg, operating machinery or driving). Discontinue use with blurred or diminished vision and perform ophthalmologic exam. Monitor vision with long-term therapy.

Drug Interactions

Avoid Concomitant Use

Avoid concomitant use of Ketorolac (Systemic) with any of the following: Aspirin; Ketorolac; Nonsteroidal Anti-Inflammatory Agents; Pentoxifylline; Probenecid

Increased Effect/Toxicity

Ketorolac (Systemic) may increase the levels/effects of: Aminoglycosides; Anticoagulants; Antiplatelet Agents; Aspirin; Bisphosphonate Derivatives; Collagenase (Systemic); CycloSPORINE; CycloSPORINE (Systemic); Deferasirox; Desmopressin; Digoxin; Drotrecogin Alfa; Eplerenone; Haloperidol; Ibritumomab; Lithium; Methotrexate; Neuromuscular-Blocking Agents (Nondepolarizing); Nonsteroidal Anti-Inflammatory Agents; PEMEtrexed; Pentoxifylline; Potassium-Sparing Diuretics; PRALAtrexate; Quinolone Antibiotics; Salicylates; Thrombolytic Agents; Tositumomab and Iodine I 131 Tositumomab; Vancomycin; Vitamin K Antagonists

The levels/effects of Ketorolac (Systemic) may be increased by: ACE Inhibitors; Angiotensin II Receptor Blockers; Antidepressants (Tricyclic, Tertiary Amine); Corticosteroids (Systemic); Dasatinib; Glucosamine; Herbs (Anticoagulant/Antiplatelet Properties); Ketorolac; Omega-3-Acid Ethyl Esters; Pentosan Polysulfate Sodium; Probenecid; Prostacyclin Analogues; Selective Serotonin Reuptake Inhibitors; Serotonin/Norepinephrine Reuptake Inhibitors; Treprostinil

Decreased Effect

Ketorolac (Systemic) may decrease the levels/effects of: ACE Inhibitors; Angiotensin II Receptor Blockers; Anticonvulsants; Antiplatelet Agents; Beta-Blockers; Eplerenone; HydrALAZINE; Loop Diuretics; Potassium-Sparing Diuretics; Salicylates; Thiazide Diuretics

The levels/effects of Ketorolac (Systemic) may be decreased by: Bile Acid Sequestrants; Salicylates

Ethanol/Nutrition/Herb Interactions

Ethanol: Avoid ethanol (may enhance gastric mucosal irritation).

Food: Oral: High-fat meals may delay time to peak (by ~1 hour) and decrease peak concentrations.

Herb/Nutraceutical: Avoid alfalfa, anise, bilberry, bladderwrack, bromelain, cat's claw, celery, chamomile, coleus, cordyceps, dong quai, evening primrose, fenugreek, feverfew, garlic, ginger, ginkgo biloba, ginseng (American, Panax, Siberian), grapeseed, green tea, guggul, horse chestnut seed, horseradish, licorice, prickly ash, red clover, reishi, SAMe (S-adenosylmethionine), sweet clover, turmeric, and white willow (all have additional antiplatelet activity).

Dietary Considerations Administer tablet with food or milk to decrease gastrointestinal distress.

Pharmacodynamics/Kinetics

Onset of Action Analgesic: I.M.: ~10 minutes; Peak effect: Analgesic: 2-3 hours

Duration of Action Analgesic: 6-8 hours

Half-life Elimination 2-6 hours; increased 30% to 50% in elderly; up to 19 hours in renal impairment

Time to Peak Serum: I.M.: 30-60 minutes

Pregnancy Risk Factor C

Lactation Enters breast milk/contraindicated (per manufacturer)

Breast-Feeding Considerations Low concentrations of ketorolac are found in breast milk. **[U.S. Boxed Warning]: Inhibition of prostaglandin synthesis may adversely affect neonates; use of systemic ketorolac is contraindicated in breast-feeding women.** The manufacturer of the ophthalmic product recommends that caution be used if administered to a breast-feeding woman. The maternal pharmacokinetics of ketorolac were not found to change immediately postpartum.

Dosage Forms

Injection, solution: 15 mg/mL (1 mL, 2 mL); 30 mg/mL (1 mL, 2 mL, 10 mL)

Tablet, oral: 10 mg

Dental Comment According to the manufacturer, ketorolac has been used inappropriately by physicians in the past. The drug had been prescribed to NSAID-sensitive patients, patients with GI bleeding, and for long-term use; a warning has been issued regarding increased incidence and severity of GI complications with increasing doses and duration of use. Labeling now includes the statement that ketorolac inhibits platelet function and is indicated for up to 5 days use only.

References

Ahmad N, Grad HA, Haas DA, et al, "The Efficacy of Nonopioid Analgesics for Postoperative Dental Pain: A Meta-Analysis," *Anesth Prog*, 1997, 44(4):119-26.
Balevi B, "Ketorolac Versus Ibuprofen: A Simple Cost-Efficacy Comparison for Dental Use," *J Can Dent Assoc*, 1994, 60(1):31-2.
Forbes JA, Butterworth GA, Burchfield WH, et al, "Evaluation of Ketorolac, Aspirin, and an Acetaminophen-Codeine Combination in Postoperative Oral Surgery Pain," *Pharmacotherapy*, 1990, 10(6 Pt 2):77S-93S.
Forbes JA, Kehm CJ, Grodin CD, et al, "Evaluation of Ketorolac, Ibuprofen, Acetaminophen, and an Acetaminophen-Codeine Combination in Postoperative Oral Surgery Pain," *Pharmacotherapy*, 1990, 10 (6 Pt 2):94S-105S.
Fricke JR Jr, Angelocci D, Fox K, et al, "Comparison of the Efficacy and Safety of Ketorolac and Meperidine in the Relief of Dental Pain," *J Clin Pharmacol*, 1992, 32(4):376-84.
Fricke J, Halladay SC, Bynum L, et al, "Pain Relief After Dental Impaction Surgery Using Ketorolac, Hydrocodone Plus Acetaminophen, or Placebo," *Clin Ther*, 1993, 15(3):500-9.
Pendeville PE, Van Boven MJ, Contreras V, et al, "Ketorolac Tromethamine for Postoperative Analgesia in Oral Surgery," *Acta Anaesthesiol Belg*, 1995, 46(1):25-30.
Swift JQ, Roszkowski MT, Alton T, et al, "Effect of Intra-Articular Versus Systemic Anti-inflammatory Drugs in a Rabbit Model of Temporomandibular Joint Inflammation," *J Oral Maxillofac Surg*, 1998, 56 (11):1288-95.
Walton GM, Rood JP, Snowdon AT, et al, "Ketorolac and Diclofenac for Postoperative Pain Relief Following Oral Surgery," *Br J Oral Maxillofac Surg*, 1993, 31(3):158-60.
Wynn RL, "Ketorolac (Toradol®) for Dental Pain," *Gen Dent*, 1992, 40(6):476-9.

Ketotifen (kee toe TYE fen)

U.S. Brand Names Alaway™ [OTC]; Claritin™ Eye [OTC]; Zaditor® [OTC]; ZyrTEC® Itchy Eye [OTC]

Canadian Brand Names Novo-Ketotifen; Nu-Ketotifen®; Zaditen®; Zaditor®

Pharmacologic Category Histamine H_1 Antagonist; Histamine H_1 Antagonist, Second Generation; Mast Cell Stabilizer; Piperidine Derivative

Use

Ophthalmic: Temporary relief of eye itching due to allergic conjunctivitis

Oral (Canadian use; not approved in U.S.): Adjunctive therapy in the chronic treatment of pediatric patients ≥6 months of age with mild, atopic asthma

Local Anesthetic/Vasoconstrictor Precautions No information available to require special precautions

Effects on Dental Treatment Key adverse event(s) related to dental treatment: Pharyngitis.

Effects on Bleeding No information available to require special precautions

Adverse Effects

Ophthalmic: 1% to 10%:

Ocular: Allergic reactions, burning or stinging, conjunctivitis, discharge, dry eyes, eye pain, eyelid disorder, itching, keratitis, lacrimation disorder, mydriasis, photophobia, rash

Respiratory: Pharyngitis

Miscellaneous: Flu syndrome

Oral: 1% to 10%:

Central nervous system: Sedation (8%; less than placebo), headache (1%), sleep disturbance (1%)

Dermatologic: Rash (4%), urticaria (1%)

Gastrointestinal: Weight gain (5%), abdominal pain (1%), appetite increased (1%)

Respiratory: Respiratory infection (4%), epistaxis (1%)

Miscellaneous: Flu (3%), puffy eyelid (1%)

General Dosage Range

Ophthalmic: *Children ≥3 years and Adults:* Instill 1 drop into the affected eye(s) twice daily, every 8-12 hours

Oral:

Children 6 months to 3 years: Initial: 0.025 mg/kg once daily or in 2 divided doses for 5 days; Maintenance: 0.05 mg/kg twice daily

Children >3 years: Initial: 0.5 mg once daily or in 2 divided doses for 5 days; Maintenance: 1 mg twice daily

Mechanism of Action Exhibits noncompetitive H_1-receptor antagonist and mast cell stabilizer properties. Efficacy in conjunctivitis and asthma likely results from a combination of anti-inflammatory and antihistaminergic actions including interference with chemokine-induced migration of eosinophils into inflamed conjunctiva and airways, inhibition of airway hyper-reactivity due to platelet activating factor (PAF), antagonism of leukotriene-induced bronchoconstriction.

Pharmacodynamics/Kinetics
Onset of Action Ophthalmic: Minutes
Duration of Action Ophthalmic: 8-12 hours
Half-life Elimination Oral: ~9-9.5 hours
Time to Peak Oral: 2-4 hours
Pregnancy Risk Factor C
Product Availability Oral formulation not available in U.S.

Labetalol (la BET a lole)

Related Information
Cardiovascular Diseases *on page 1848*
U.S. Brand Names Trandate®
Canadian Brand Names Apo-Labetalol®; Labetalol Hydrochloride Injection, USP; Normodyne®; Trandate®
Pharmacologic Category Beta Blocker With Alpha-Blocking Activity
Use Treatment of mild-to-severe hypertension; I.V. for severe hypertension (eg, hypertensive emergencies)
Unlabeled/Investigational Use Pediatric hypertension; management of pre-eclampsia; severe hypertension in pregnancy; hypertension during acute ischemic stroke
Local Anesthetic/Vasoconstrictor Precautions Use with caution; epinephrine has interacted with nonselective beta-blockers to result in initial hypertensive episode followed by bradycardia
Effects on Dental Treatment Key adverse event(s) related to dental treatment: Taste disorder.
Many nonsteroidal anti-inflammatory drugs, such as ibuprofen and indomethacin, can reduce the hypotensive effect of beta-blockers after 3 or more weeks of therapy with the NSAID. Short-term NSAID use (ie, 3 days) requires no special precautions in patients taking beta-blockers.
Effects on Bleeding No information available to require special precautions
Adverse Effects
>10%:
Cardiovascular: Postural hypotension (I.V. use; ≤58%)
Central nervous system: Dizziness (1% to 20%), fatigue (1% to 11%)
Gastrointestinal: Nausea (≤19%)
1% to 10%:
Cardiovascular: Hypotension (1% to 5%), edema (≤2%), flushing (1%), ventricular arrhythmia (I.V. use; 1%)
Central nervous system: Somnolence (3%), headache (2%), vertigo (1% to 2%)
Dermatologic: Scalp tingling (≤7%), pruritus (1%), rash (1%)
Gastrointestinal: Dyspepsia (≤4%), vomiting (≤3%), taste disturbance (1%)
Genitourinary: Ejaculatory failure (≤5%), impotence (1% to 4%)
Hepatic: Transaminases increased (4%)
Neuromuscular & skeletal: Paresthesia (≤5%), weakness (1%)
Ocular: Vision abnormal (1%)
Renal: BUN increased (≤8%)
Respiratory: Nasal congestion (1% to 6%), dyspnea (2%)
Miscellaneous: Diaphoresis (≤4%)
Other adverse reactions noted with beta-adrenergic blocking agents include mental depression, catatonia, disorientation, short-term memory loss, emotional lability, clouded sensorium, intensification of pre-existing AV block, laryngospasm, respiratory distress, agranulocytosis, thrombocytopenic purpura, nonthrombocytopenic purpura, mesenteric artery thrombosis, and ischemic colitis.
General Dosage Range
I.V.:
Children: 0.3-1 mg/kg/dose intermittently **or** 0.4-1 mg/kg/hour infusion (maximum: 3 mg/kg/hour)
Adults: Bolus: 20 mg, may give 40-80 mg at 10-minute intervals; Infusion: 2 mg/minute (maximum: 300 mg total cumulative dose)
Oral: *Adults:* Initial: 100 mg twice daily; Maintenance: 200-800 mg/day in 2 divided doses (maximum: 2.4 g/day)
Mechanism of Action Blocks alpha-, $beta_1$-, and $beta_2$-adrenergic receptor sites; elevated renins are reduced. The ratios of alpha- to beta-blockade differ depending on the route of administration: 1:3 (oral) and 1:7 (I.V.).
Pharmacodynamics/Kinetics
Onset of Action Oral: 20 minutes to 2 hours; I.V.: 2-5 minutes; Peak effect: Oral: 1-4 hours; I.V.: 5-15 minutes

Duration of Action Blood pressure response:
Oral: 8-12 hours (dose dependent)
I.V.: 2-18 hours (dose dependent; based on single and multiple sequential doses of 0.25-0.5 mg/kg with cumulative dosing up to 3.25 mg/kg)
Half-life Elimination Oral: 6-8 hours; I.V.: ~5.5 hours
Time to Peak Plasma: Oral: 1-2 hours
Pregnancy Risk Factor C

Lacosamide (la KOE sa mide)

U.S. Brand Names Vimpat®
Canadian Brand Names Vimpat®
Pharmacologic Category Anticonvulsant, Miscellaneous
Use Adjunctive therapy in the treatment of partial-onset seizures
Local Anesthetic/Vasoconstrictor Precautions Lacosamide may prolong PR interval resulting in cardiac conduction problems; it is not known what effect vasoconstrictors will have in patients taking medications that could prolong PR interval. It is suggested that the clinician consult with the physician prior to use of vasoconstrictor in suspected patients; use vasoconstrictor with caution.
Effects on Dental Treatment No significant effects or complications reported
Effects on Bleeding No information available to require special precautions
Adverse Effects
>10%:
Central nervous system: Dizziness (31%), headache (13%)
Gastrointestinal: Nausea (11%)
Ocular: Diplopia (11%)
1% to 10%:
Cardiovascular: Syncope (1%; dose-related: >400 mg/day)
Central nervous system: Fatigue (9%), ataxia (8%), somnolence (7%), coordination impaired (4%), vertigo (4%), depression (2%), memory impairment (2%)
Dermatologic: Pruritus (2%)
Gastrointestinal: Vomiting (9%), diarrhea (4%)
Hepatic: ALT increased (1%)
Local: Contusion (3%), skin laceration (3%), injection site pain/discomfort (2.5%), irritation (1%)
Neuromuscular & skeletal: Tremor (7%), gait instability (2%), weakness (2%)
Ocular: Blurred vision (8%), nystagmus (5%)
General Dosage Range Dosage adjustment recommended in patients with hepatic or renal impairment
Oral: *Adolescents ≥17 years and Adults:* Initial: 50 mg twice daily; Maintenance dose: 200-400 mg/day
Mechanism of Action *In vitro* studies have shown that lacosamide stabilizes hyperexcitable neuronal membranes and inhibits repetitive neuronal firing by enhancing the slow inactivation of sodium channels (with no effects on fast inactivation of sodium channels).
Pharmacodynamics/Kinetics
Half-life Elimination ~13 hours
Time to Peak Oral: 1-4 hours postdose
Pregnancy Risk Factor C
Controlled Substance C-V

Lactase (LAK tase)

U.S. Brand Names Lac-Dose® [OTC]; Lactaid® Fast Act [OTC]; Lactaid® Original [OTC]; Lactose Intolerance [OTC]; Lactrase® [OTC]
Canadian Brand Names Dairyaid®
Pharmacologic Category Enzyme
Use Help digest lactose in milk for patients with lactose intolerance
Local Anesthetic/Vasoconstrictor Precautions No information available to require special precautions
Effects on Dental Treatment No significant effects or complications reported
Effects on Bleeding No information available to require special precautions
General Dosage Range Oral: *Adults:* 1-2 capsules with meals **or** 5-15 drops or 1-2 capsules/quart of milk **or** 1-3 tablets with meals

Lactic Acid (LAK tik AS id)

Pharmacologic Category Topical Skin Product
Use Lubricate and moisturize the skin counteracting dryness and itching

Local Anesthetic/Vasoconstrictor Precautions No information available to require special precautions

Effects on Dental Treatment No significant effects or complications reported

Effects on Bleeding No information available to require special precautions

Adverse Effects Frequency not defined: Dermatologic: Burning, mild stinging, peeling

General Dosage Range Topical: *Adults:* Apply twice daily

Lactic Acid and Ammonium Hydroxide

(LAK tik AS id & a MOE nee um hye DROKS ide)

Related Information

Lactic Acid *on page 975*

U.S. Brand Names AmLactin® [OTC]; Geri-Hydrolac™ [OTC]; Geri-Hydrolac™-12 [OTC]; Lac-Hydrin®; Lac-Hydrin® Five [OTC]; LAClotion™

Pharmacologic Category Topical Skin Product

Use Treatment of moderate-to-severe xerosis and ichthyosis vulgaris

Local Anesthetic/Vasoconstrictor Precautions No information available to require special precautions

Effects on Dental Treatment No significant effects or complications reported

Effects on Bleeding No information available to require special precautions

Adverse Effects

>10%: Dermatologic: Burning/stinging (3% to 15%), rash (2% to 15%; includes erythema and irritation)

1% to 10%: Dermatologic: Itching (5%), dry skin (2%)

General Dosage Range Topical:

Cream: *Children ≥2 years and Adults:* Apply twice daily to affected area

Lotion: *Children and Adults:* Apply twice daily to affected area

Mechanism of Action Exact mechanism of action unknown; lactic acid is a normal component in blood and tissues. When applied topically to the skin, acts as a humectant.

Pregnancy Risk Factor B

Lactobacillus (lak toe ba SIL us)

Related Information

Ulcerative, Erosive, and Painful Oral Mucosal Disorders *on page 1950*

U.S. Brand Names Bacid® [OTC]; Culturelle® [OTC]; Dofus [OTC]; Flora-Q™ [OTC]; Floranex™ [OTC]; Kala® [OTC]; Lactinex™ [OTC]; Lacto-Bifidus [OTC]; Lacto-Key [OTC]; Lacto-Pectin [OTC]; Lacto-TriBlend [OTC]; Megadophilus® [OTC]; MoreDophilus® [OTC]; RisaQuad®-2 [OTC]; RisaQuad™ [OTC]; Superdophilus® [OTC]; VSL #3® [OTC]; VSL #3®-DS

Canadian Brand Names Bacid®; Fermalac

Generic Availability (U.S.) Yes

Pharmacologic Category Dietary Supplement; Probiotic

Dental Use Treatment of uncomplicated diarrhea, particularly that caused by antibiotic therapy; re-establish normal physiologic and bacterial flora of the intestinal tract

Use Promote normal bacterial flora of the intestinal tract

Local Anesthetic/Vasoconstrictor Precautions No information available to require special precautions

Effects on Dental Treatment No significant effects or complications reported

Effects on Bleeding No information available to require special precautions

Adverse Effects Gastrointestinal: Bloating (intestinal), flatulence

Dosage Dietary supplement: Oral: Dosing varies by manufacturer; consult product labeling

Children (Culturelle®): 1 capsule daily

Adults:

- Bacid®: 2 caplets/day
- Culturelle®: 1 capsule daily; may increase to twice daily
- Flora-Q™: 1 capsule/day
- Lacto-Key 100 or 600: 1-2 capsules/day
- Lactinex™: 1 packet or 4 tablets 3-4 times/day
- VSL #3®: 1-8 sachets or 2-32 capsules/day
- VSL #3®-DS: 1-4 packets/day

Mechanism of Action Helps re-establish normal intestinal flora; suppresses the growth of potentially pathogenic microorganisms by producing lactic acid which favors the establishment of an aciduric flora.

Contraindications Hypersensitivity to any component of the formulation

Warnings/Precautions *Lactobacillus* species have been studied for various gastrointestinal disorders including diarrhea, inflammatory bowel disease, gastrointestinal infection. Effectiveness may be dependent upon actual species used; studies are ongoing. Currently, there are no FDA-approved disease-prevention or therapeutic indications for these products.

Drug Interactions

Avoid Concomitant Use There are no known interactions where it is recommended to avoid concomitant use.

Increased Effect/Toxicity There are no known significant interactions involving an increase in effect.

Decreased Effect There are no known significant interactions involving a decrease in effect.

Dietary Considerations Some products may contain potassium and/or sodium.

Dosage Forms

Capsule:

Culturelle® [OTC]: *L. rhamnosus* GG 10 billion colony-forming units
Dofus [OTC]: *L. acidophilus* and *L. bifidus* 10:1 ratio
Flora-Q™ [OTC]: *L. acidophilus* and *L. paracasei* ≥8 billion colony-forming units
Lacto-Key [OTC]:
100: *L. acidophilus* 1 billion colony-forming units
600: *L. acidophilus* 6 billion colony-forming units
Lacto-Bifidus [OTC]:
100: *L. bifidus* 1 billion colony-forming units
600: *L. bifidus* 6 billion colony-forming units
Lacto-Pectin [OTC]: *L. acidophilus* and *L. casei* ≥5 billion colony-forming units
Lacto-TriBlend [OTC]:
100: *L. acidophilus, L. bifidus,* and *L. bulgaricus* 1 billion colony-forming units
600: *L. acidophilus, L. bifidus,* and *L. bulgaricus* 6 billion colony-forming units
Megadophilus® [OTC], Superdophilus® [OTC]: *L. acidophilus* 2 billion units
RisaQuad™ [OTC]: *L. acidophilus* and *L. paracasei* 8 billion colony-forming units
VSL #3® [OTC]: *L. acidophilus, L. plantarum, L. paracasei, L. bulgaricus* 112 billion live cells

Capsule, double strength:

RisaQuad®-2 [OTC]: *L. acidophilus* and *L. paracasei* 16 billion colony-forming units

Capsule, softgel: *L. acidophilus* 100 active units

Caplet:

Bacid® [OTC]: *L. acidophilus 80%* and *L. bulgaricus* 10%

Granules:

Lactinex™ [OTC]: *L. acidophilus* and *L. bulgaricus* 100 million live cells per 1 g packet (12s)

Powder:

Lacto-TriBlend [OTC]: *L. acidophilus, L. bifidus,* and *L. bulgaricus* 10 billion colony-forming units per ¼ teaspoon
Megadophilus® [OTC], Superdophilus® [OTC]: *L. acidophilus* 2 billion units per half-teaspoon
MoreDophilus® [OTC]: *L. acidophilus* 12.4 billion units per teaspoon
VSL #3® [OTC]: *L. acidophilus, L. plantarum, L. paracasei, L. bulgaricus* 450 billion live cells
VSL #3®-DS: *L. acidophilus, L. plantarum, L. paracasei, L. bulgaricus* 900 billion live cells

Tablet:

Kala® [OTC]: *L. acidophilus* 200 million units

Tablet, chewable: *L. reuteri* 100 million organisms

Floranex™ [OTC]: *L. acidophilus* and *L. bulgaricus* 1 million colony-forming units
Lactinex™ [OTC]: *L. acidophilus* and *L. bulgaricus* 1 million live cells

Wafer: *L. acidophilus* 90 mg and *L. bifidus* 25 mg (100s)

Lactulose (LAK tyoo lose)

U.S. Brand Names Constulose; Enulose; Generlac; Kristalose®

Canadian Brand Names Acilac; Apo-Lactulose®; Laxilose; PMS-Lactulose

Pharmacologic Category Ammonium Detoxicant; Laxative, Osmotic

Use Prevention and treatment of portal-systemic encephalopathy (including hepatic precoma and coma); treatment of constipation

Local Anesthetic/Vasoconstrictor Precautions No information available to require special precautions

Effects on Dental Treatment No significant effects or complications reported

Effects on Bleeding No information available to require special precautions

Adverse Effects Frequency not defined.

Endocrine & metabolic: Dehydration, hypernatremia, hypokalemia

Gastrointestinal: Abdominal discomfort, abdominal distention, belching, cramping, diarrhea (excessive dose), flatulence, nausea, vomiting

General Dosage Range

Oral:

Infants: 1.7-6.7 g/day (2.5-10 mL/day) in divided doses

Older Children and Adolescents: 26.7-60 g/day (40-90 mL/day) in divided doses

Adults: PSE: 20-30 g (30-45 mL) every hour initially, then 3-4 times/day; Constipation: 10-40 g (15-60 mL) daily

Rectal: *Adults:* Constipation: 200 g (300 mL); may repeat every 4-6 hours

Mechanism of Action The bacterial degradation of lactulose resulting in an acidic pH inhibits the diffusion of NH_3 into the blood by causing the conversion of NH_3 to NH_4+; also enhances the diffusion of NH_3 from the blood into the gut where conversion to NH_4+ occurs; produces an osmotic effect in the colon with resultant distention promoting peristalsis; reduces blood ammonia concentration to reduce the degree of portal systemic encephalopathy

Pharmacodynamics/Kinetics

Onset of Action

Constipation: Up to 24-48 hours to produce a normal bowel movement

Encephalopathy: At least 24-48 hours

Pregnancy Risk Factor B

LamiVUDine (la MI vyoo deen)

Related Information

HIV Infection and AIDS *on page* 1883

Systemic Viral Diseases *on page* 1904

U.S. Brand Names Epivir-HBV®; Epivir®

Canadian Brand Names 3TC®; Heptovir®

Pharmacologic Category Antiretroviral Agent, Reverse Transcriptase Inhibitor (Nucleoside)

Use

Epivir®: Treatment of HIV infection when antiretroviral therapy is warranted; should always be used as part of a multidrug regimen (at least three antiretroviral agents)

Epivir-HBV®: Treatment of chronic hepatitis B associated with evidence of hepatitis B viral replication and active liver inflammation. Resistance develops rapidly in hepatitis B; consider use only if other anti-HBV antiviral agents with more favorable resistance patterns cannot be used.

Unlabeled/Investigational Use Postexposure prophylaxis for HIV exposure as part of a multidrug regimen

Local Anesthetic/Vasoconstrictor Precautions No information available to require special precautions

Effects on Dental Treatment No significant effects or complications reported

Effects on Bleeding No information available to require special precautions relative to hemostasis.

Adverse Effects Reported for treatment of HIV or HBV in adults. Incidence data include patients on combination therapy with other antiretroviral agents.

>10%:

Central nervous system: Headache (21% to 35%), fatigue (24% to 27%), insomnia (11%)

Gastrointestinal: Nausea (15% to 33%), diarrhea (14% to 18%), pancreatitis (range: 0.3% to 18%; higher percentage in pediatric patients), abdominal pain (9% to 16%), vomiting (13% to 15%)

Hematologic: Neutropenia (7% to 15%)

Hepatic: Transaminases increased (2% to 11%)

Neuromuscular & skeletal: Myalgia (8% to 14%), neuropathy (12%), musculoskeletal pain (12%)

Respiratory: Nasal signs and symptoms (20%), cough (18%), sore throat (13%)

Miscellaneous: Infections (25%; includes ear, nose, and throat)

1% to 10%:

Central nervous system: Dizziness (10%), depression (9%), fever (7% to 10%), chills (7% to 10%)

Dermatologic: Rash (5% to 9%)

Gastrointestinal: Anorexia (10%), lipase increased (10%), abdominal cramps (6%), dyspepsia (5%), amylase increased (<1% to 4%), heartburn

Hematologic: Thrombocytopenia (1% to 4%), hemoglobinemia (2% to 3%)

Neuromuscular & skeletal: Creatine phosphokinase increased (9%), arthralgia (5% to 7%)

General Dosage Range Dosage adjustment recommended in patients with renal impairment

Oral:

Neonates <30 days: HIV (DHHS [pediatric], 2010): 2 mg/kg/dose twice daily

Infants 1-3 months: HIV (DHHS [pediatric], 2010): 4 mg/kg/dose twice daily

Children 3 months to 2 years: HIV: 4 mg/kg/dose twice daily (maximum: 150 mg/dose twice daily)

Children 2-16 years and >16 years and <50 kg: Hepatitis B: 3 mg/kg/dose once daily (maximum: 100 mg/day); HIV: 4 mg/kg/dose twice daily (maximum: 150 mg/dose twice daily)

Children >16 years and ≥50 kg: Hepatitis B: 3 mg/kg/dose once daily (maximum: 100 mg/day); HIV: 150 mg twice daily **or** 300 mg once daily

Adults <50 kg: Hepatitis B: 100 mg/day; HIV (DHHS [pediatric], 2010): 4 mg/kg/dose twice daily (maximum: 150 mg/dose twice daily)

Adults ≥50 kg: Hepatitis B: 100 mg/day; HIV: 150 mg twice daily **or** 300 mg once daily

Mechanism of Action Lamivudine is a cytosine analog. After lamivudine is triphosphorylated, the principle mode of action is inhibition of HIV reverse transcription via viral DNA chain termination; inhibits RNA- and DNA-dependent DNA polymerase activities of reverse transcriptase. The monophosphate form of lamivudine is incorporated into the viral DNA by hepatitis B virus polymerase, resulting in DNA chain termination.

Pharmacodynamics/Kinetics

Half-life Elimination Children: 2 hours; Adults: 5-7 hours

Time to Peak Fed: 3.2 hours; Fasted: 0.9 hours

Pregnancy Risk Factor C

Lamivudine and Zidovudine (la MI vyoo deen & zye DOE vyoo deen)

Related Information

HIV Infection and AIDS *on page* 1883

LamiVUDine *on page* 978

Zidovudine *on page* 1742

U.S. Brand Names Combivir®

Canadian Brand Names Combivir®

Pharmacologic Category Antiretroviral Agent, Reverse Transcriptase Inhibitor (Nucleoside)

Use Treatment of HIV infection when therapy is warranted based on clinical and/or immunological evidence of disease progression

Local Anesthetic/Vasoconstrictor Precautions No information available to require special precautions

Effects on Dental Treatment No significant effects or complications reported

Effects on Bleeding No information available to require special precautions relative to hemostasis.

Adverse Effects See individual agents.

General Dosage Range Oral: *Adolescents ≥30 kg and Adults:* 1 tablet (lamivudine 150 mg/zidovudine 300 mg) twice daily

Mechanism of Action The combination of zidovudine and lamivudine is believed to act synergistically to inhibit reverse transcriptase via DNA chain termination after incorporation of the nucleoside analogue as well as to delay the emergence of mutations conferring resistance

Pregnancy Risk Factor C

LamoTRIgine (la MOE tri jeen)

U.S. Brand Names LaMICtal®; LaMICtal® ODT™; LaMICtal® XR™

Canadian Brand Names Apo-Lamotrigine®; Lamictal®; Mylan-Lamotrigine; Novo-Lamotrigine; PMS-Lamotrigine; ratio-Lamotrigine; Teva-Lamotrigine

Pharmacologic Category Anticonvulsant, Miscellaneous

Use Adjunctive therapy in the treatment of generalized seizures of Lennox-Gastaut syndrome, primary generalized tonic-clonic seizures, and partial seizures; conversion to monotherapy in patients with partial seizures who are receiving treatment with valproic acid or a single enzyme-inducing antiepileptic drug (specifically carbamazepine, phenytoin, phenobarbital or primidone); maintenance treatment of bipolar I disorder

Local Anesthetic/Vasoconstrictor Precautions No information available to require special precautions

Effects on Dental Treatment Key adverse event(s) related to dental treatment: Xerostomia (normal salivary flow resumes upon discontinuation).

Effects on Bleeding Thrombocytopenia may occur as an adverse effect. No information available to require routine special precautions.

Adverse Effects Percentages reported in adults on monotherapy for epilepsy or bipolar disorder.

>10%: Gastrointestinal: Nausea (7% to 14%)

1% to 10%:

Cardiovascular: Chest pain (5%), peripheral edema (2% to 5%), edema (1% to 5%)

Central nervous system: Insomnia (5% to 10%), somnolence (9%), fatigue (8%), coordination impaired (7%), dizziness (7%), anxiety (5%), pain (5%), ataxia (2% to 5%), irritability (2% to 5%), suicidal ideation (2% to 5%), agitation (1% to 5%), amnesia (1% to 5%), depression (1% to 5%), dream abnormality (1% to 5%), emotional lability (1% to 5%), fever (1% to 5%), hypoesthesia (1% to 5%), migraine (1% to 5%), thought abnormality (1% to 5%), confusion (1%)

Dermatologic: Rash (nonserious: 7%), dermatitis (2% to 5%), dry skin (2% to 5%)

Endocrine & metabolic: Dysmenorrhea (5%), libido increased (2% to 5%)

Gastrointestinal: Vomiting (5% to 9%), dyspepsia (7%), abdominal pain (6%), xerostomia (2% to 6%), constipation (5%), weight loss (5%), anorexia (2% to 5%), peptic ulcer (2% to 5%), rectal hemorrhage (2% to 5%), flatulence (1% to 5%), weight gain (1% to 5%)

Genitourinary: Urinary frequency (1% to 5%)

Neuromuscular & skeletal: Back pain (8%), weakness (2% to 5%), arthralgia (1% to 5%), myalgia (1% to 5%), neck pain (1% to 5%), paresthesia (1%)

Ocular: Nystagmus (2% to 5%), vision abnormal (2% to 5%), amblyopia (1%)

Respiratory: Rhinitis (7%), cough (5%), pharyngitis (5%), bronchitis (2% to 5%), dyspnea (2% to 5%), epistaxis (2% to 5%), sinusitis (1% to 5%)

Miscellaneous: Infection (5%), diaphoresis (2% to 5%), reflexes increased/decreased (2% to 5%), dyspraxia (1% to 5%)

General Dosage Range Dosage adjustment recommended in patients with hepatic or renal impairment or on concomitant therapy

Oral:

Immediate release formulation:

Children 2-12 years: Dosage varies greatly depending on indication

Children ≥13 years and Adults: Dosage varies greatly depending on indication

Extended release formulation: *Children ≥13 years and Adults:* Dosage varies greatly depending on indication

Mechanism of Action A triazine derivative which inhibits release of glutamate (an excitatory amino acid) and inhibits voltage-sensitive sodium channels, which stabilizes neuronal membranes. Lamotrigine has weak inhibitory effect on the 5-HT_3 receptor; *in vitro* inhibits dihydrofolate reductase.

Pharmacodynamics/Kinetics

Half-life Elimination Immediate release: Adults: 25-33 hours, Elderly: 25-43 hours; Extended release: Similar to immediate release

Concomitant valproic acid therapy: 48-70 hours

Concomitant phenytoin, phenobarbital, primidone, or carbamazepine therapy: 13-14 hours

Chronic renal failure: 43 hours

Hemodialysis: 13 hours during dialysis; 57 hours between dialysis (~20% of a dose is eliminated in a 4-hour dialysis session)

Hepatic impairment:

Mild: 26-66 hours

Moderate: 28-116 hours

Severe without ascites: 56-78 hours

Severe with ascites: 52-148 hours

Time to Peak Plasma: Immediate release: 1-1.5 hours; Extended release: 4-11 hours (dependent on adjunct therapy)

Pregnancy Risk Factor C

Lanolin, Cetyl Alcohol, Glycerin, Petrolatum, and Mineral Oil (LAN oh lin, SEE til AL koe hol, GLIS er in, pe troe LAY tum, & MIN er al oyl)

Related Information

Glycerin *on page* 829

U.S. Brand Names Lubriderm® Fragrance Free [OTC]; Lubriderm® [OTC]

Pharmacologic Category Topical Skin Product

Use Treatment of dry skin

Local Anesthetic/Vasoconstrictor Precautions No information available to require special precautions

Effects on Dental Treatment No significant effects or complications reported

Effects on Bleeding No information available to require special precautions

Adverse Effects 1% to 10%: Local irritation

General Dosage Range Topical: *Adults:* Apply to skin as necessary

Pregnancy Risk Factor C

Lanreotide (lan REE oh tide)

U.S. Brand Names Somatuline® Depot

Canadian Brand Names Somatuline® Autogel®

Pharmacologic Category Somatostatin Analog

Use Long-term treatment of acromegaly in patients who are not candidates for or are unresponsive to surgery and/or radiotherapy

Canadian labeling: Also approved in Canada for relief of symptoms of acromegaly

Local Anesthetic/Vasoconstrictor Precautions No information available to require special precautions

Effects on Dental Treatment No significant effects or complications reported

Effects on Bleeding No information available to require special precautions

Adverse Effects

>10%:

- Cardiovascular: Bradycardia (5% to 18%)
- Gastrointestinal: Diarrhea (26% to 65%; dose related), abdominal pain (7% to 19%; dose related), flatulence (≤14%; dose related), nausea (11%), weight loss (5% to 11%)
- Hematologic: Anemia (3% to 14%)
- Hepatic: Cholelithiasis/gall bladder sludge (2% to 20%)
- Local: Injection site reaction (6% to 22%; induration 5%; pain 4%; mass 2%)

1% to 10%:

- Cardiovascular: Hypertension (5%), sinus bradycardia (3%)
- Central nervous system: Headache (7%)
- Endocrine & metabolic: Hyper-/hypoglycemia/diabetes (7%)
- Gastrointestinal: Constipation (8%), vomiting (7%), loose stools (6%)
- Neuromuscular & skeletal: Arthralgia (7%)

General Dosage Range Dosage adjustment recommended in patients with hepatic or renal impairment

SubQ: *Adults:* Initial: 90 mg once every 4 weeks for 3 months; Maintenance: 60-120 mg every 4 weeks **or** 120 mg every 6-8 weeks

Mechanism of Action Synthetic octapeptide analogue of somatostatin which is a peptide inhibitor of multiple endocrine, neuroendocrine, and exocrine mechanisms. Displays a greater affinity for somatostatin type 2 (SSTR2) and type 5 (SSTR5) receptors found in pituitary gland, pancreas, and growth hormone (GH) secreting neoplasms of pituitary gland and a lesser affinity for somatostatin receptors 1, 3, and 4. Reduces GH secretion and also reduces the levels of insulin-like growth factor 1.

Pharmacodynamics/Kinetics

Half-life Elimination 23-36 days

Time to Peak Mean: 7-12 hours

Pregnancy Risk Factor C

Lansoprazole (lan SOE pra zole)

Related Information

Gastrointestinal Disorders *on page 1874*

U.S. Brand Names Prevacid®; Prevacid® 24 HR [OTC]; Prevacid® SoluTab™

Canadian Brand Names Apo-Lansoprazole®; Mylan-Lansoprazole; Novo-Lansoprazole; Prevacid®; Prevacid® FasTab

Generic Availability (U.S.) Yes

Pharmacologic Category Proton Pump Inhibitor; Substituted Benzimidazole

Use Short-term treatment of active duodenal ulcers; maintenance treatment of healed duodenal ulcers; as part of a multidrug regimen for *H. pylori* eradication to reduce the risk of duodenal ulcer recurrence; short-term treatment of active benign gastric ulcer; treatment of NSAID-associated gastric ulcer; to reduce the risk of NSAID-associated gastric ulcer in patients with a history of gastric ulcer who require an NSAID; short-term treatment of symptomatic GERD; short-term treatment for all grades of erosive esophagitis; to maintain healing of erosive esophagitis; long-term treatment of pathological hypersecretory conditions, including Zollinger-Ellison syndrome

OTC labeling: Relief of frequent heartburn (≥2 days/week)

Local Anesthetic/Vasoconstrictor Precautions No information available to require special precautions

Effects on Dental Treatment No significant effects or complications reported

Effects on Bleeding No information available to require special precautions

Adverse Effects 1% to 10%:

Central nervous system: Headache (children 1-11 years 3%, 12-17 years 7%), dizziness (children 12-17 years 3%; adults <1%)

Gastrointestinal: Diarrhea (1% to 5%; 60 mg/day: 7%), abdominal pain (children 12-17 years 5%; adults 2%), constipation (children 1-11 years 5%; adults 1%), nausea (children 12-17 years 3%; adults 1%)

Dosage Oral:

Children 1-11 years: GERD, erosive esophagitis:

≤30 kg: 15 mg once daily for up to 12 weeks

>30 kg: 30 mg once daily for up to 12 weeks

Note: Doses were increased in some pediatric patients if still symptomatic after 2 or more weeks of treatment (maximum dose: 30 mg twice daily)

Children 12-17 years:

Nonerosive GERD: 15 mg once daily for up to 8 weeks

Erosive esophagitis: 30 mg once daily for up to 8 weeks

Adults:

Duodenal ulcer: Short-term treatment: 15 mg once daily for 4 weeks; maintenance therapy: 15 mg once daily

Gastric ulcer: Short-term treatment: 30 mg once daily for up to 8 weeks

NSAID-associated gastric ulcer (healing): 30 mg once daily for 8 weeks; controlled studies did not extend past 8 weeks of therapy

NSAID-associated gastric ulcer (to reduce risk): 15 mg once daily for up to 12 weeks; controlled studies did not extend past 12 weeks of therapy

Symptomatic GERD: Short-term treatment: 15 mg once daily for up to 8 weeks

Erosive esophagitis: Short-term treatment: 30 mg once daily for up to 8 weeks; continued treatment for an additional 8 weeks may be considered for recurrence or for patients who do not heal after the first 8 weeks of therapy; maintenance therapy: 15 mg once daily

Hypersecretory conditions: Initial: 60 mg once daily; adjust dose based upon patient response and to reduce acid secretion to <10 mEq/hour (5 mEq/hour in patients with prior gastric surgery); doses of 90 mg twice daily have been used; administer doses >120 mg/day in divided doses

Helicobacter pylori eradication:

Manufacturer labeling: 30 mg 3 times/day administered with amoxicillin 1000 mg 3 times/day for 14 days **or** 30 mg twice daily administered with amoxicillin 1000 mg *and* clarithromycin 500 mg twice daily for 10-14 days

American College of Gastroenterology guidelines (Chey, 2007):

Nonpenicillin allergy: 30 mg twice daily administered with amoxicillin 1000 mg *and* clarithromycin 500 mg twice daily for 10-14 days

Penicillin allergy: 30 mg twice daily administered with clarithromycin 500 mg *and* metronidazole 500 mg twice daily for 10-14 days **or** 30 mg once or twice daily administered with bismuth subsalicylate 525 mg *and* metronidazole 250 mg *plus* tetracycline 500 mg 4 times/day for 10-14 days

Heartburn: OTC labeling: 15 mg once daily for 14 days; may repeat 14 days of therapy every 4 months. Do not take for >14 days or more often than every 4 months, unless instructed by healthcare provider.

Dosage adjustment in renal impairment: No dosage adjustment is needed

Dosing adjustment in hepatic impairment: Severe hepatic impairment: Consider dose reduction

Mechanism of Action Decreases acid secretion in gastric parietal cells through inhibition of (H+, K+)-ATPase enzyme system, blocking the final step in gastric acid production.

Contraindications Hypersensitivity to lansoprazole or any component of the formulation

Warnings/Precautions Use of proton pump inhibitors may increase the risk of gastrointestinal infections (eg, *Salmonella, Campylobacter*). Relief of symptoms does not preclude the presence of a gastric malignancy. Atrophic gastritis (by biopsy) has been noted with long-term omeprazole therapy; this may also occur with lansoprazole. No reports of enterochromaffin-like (ECL) cell carcinoids, dysplasia, or neoplasia have occurred. Severe liver dysfunction may require dosage reductions. Decreased *H. pylori* eradication rates have been observed with short-term (≤7 days) combination therapy. The American College of Gastroenterology recommends 10-14 days of therapy (triple or quadruple) for eradication of *H. pylori* (Chey, 2007). Proton pump inhibitors may diminish the therapeutic effect of clopidogrel thought to be due to reduced formation of the active metabolite of clopidogrel; an increase in the risk of cardiovascular events may occur. The manufacturer of clopidogrel recommends avoidance of concomitant administration of another PPI (ie, omeprazole); given the potency of lansoprazole's CYP2C19 inhibitory activity, similar recommendations would appear prudent. Lansoprazole has been shown to be ineffective for the treatment of symptomatic GERD in children 1 month to <1 year.

Increased incidence of osteoporosis-related bone fractures of the hip, spine, or wrist may occur with proton pump inhibitor therapy. Patients on high-dose or long-term therapy should be monitored. Use the lowest effective dose for the shortest duration of time, use vitamin D and calcium supplementation, and follow appropriate guidelines to reduce risk of fractures in patients at risk.

When used for self-medication, patients should be instructed not to use if they have difficulty swallowing, are vomiting blood, or have bloody or black stools. Prior to use, patients should contact healthcare provider if they have liver disease, heartburn for >3 months, heartburn with dizziness, lightheadedness, or sweating, MI symptoms, frequent chest pain, frequent wheezing (especially with heartburn), unexplained weight loss, nausea/vomiting, stomach pain, or are taking antifungals, atazanavir, digoxin, tacrolimus, theophylline, or warfarin. Patients should stop use and consult a healthcare provider if heartburn continues or worsens, or if they need to take for >14 days or more often than every 4 months. Patients should be informed that it may take 1-4 days for full effect to be seen; should not be used for immediate relief.

Drug Interactions

Metabolism/Transport Effects **Substrate** of CYP2C9 (minor), 2C19 (major), 3A4 (major); **Inhibits** CYP2C9 (weak), 2C19 (moderate), 2D6 (weak), 3A4 (weak); **Induces** CYP1A2 (weak)

Avoid Concomitant Use

Avoid concomitant use of Lansoprazole with any of the following: Delavirdine; Erlotinib; Nelfinavir; Posaconazole

Increased Effect/Toxicity

Lansoprazole may increase the levels/effects of: Amphetamines; CYP2C19 Substrates; Dexmethylphenidate; Imatinib; Methotrexate; Methylphenidate; Raltegravir; Saquinavir; Tacrolimus; Tacrolimus (Systemic); Vitamin K Antagonists; Voriconazole

The levels/effects of Lansoprazole may be increased by: Conivaptan; Fluconazole; Ketoconazole; Ketoconazole (Systemic)

Decreased Effect

Lansoprazole may decrease the levels/effects of: Atazanavir; Bisphosphonate Derivatives; Cefditoren; Clopidogrel; Dabigatran Etexilate; Dasatinib; Delavirdine; Erlotinib; Gefitinib; Indinavir; Iron Salts; Itraconazole; Ketoconazole; Ketoconazole (Systemic); Mesalamine; Mycophenolate; Nelfinavir; Posaconazole

The levels/effects of Lansoprazole may be decreased by: CYP2C19 Inducers (Strong); CYP3A4 Inducers (Strong); Deferasirox; Herbs (CYP3A4 Inducers); Tipranavir; Tocilizumab

Ethanol/Nutrition/Herb Interactions

Ethanol: Avoid ethanol (may cause gastric mucosal irritation).
Food: Lansoprazole serum concentrations may be decreased if taken with food.
Herb/Nutraceutical: Avoid St John's wort (may decrease the levels/effect of lansoprazole).

Dietary Considerations Should be taken before eating; best if taken before breakfast. Some products may contain phenylalanine.

Pharmacodynamics/Kinetics

Onset of Action Gastric acid suppression: Oral: 1-3 hours
Duration of Action Gastric acid suppression: Oral: >1 day
Half-life Elimination 1.5 ± 1 hours; Elderly: 2-3 hours; Hepatic impairment: 3-7 hours
Time to Peak Plasma: 1.7 hours

Pregnancy Risk Factor B

Lactation Excretion in breast milk unknown/not recommended

Dosage Forms

Capsule, delayed release, oral: 15 mg, 30 mg
Prevacid®: 15 mg, 30 mg
Prevacid® 24 HR [OTC]: 15 mg
Tablet, delayed release, orally disintegrating, oral: 15 mg, 30 mg
Prevacid® SoluTab™: 15 mg, 30 mg

Lansoprazole, Amoxicillin, and Clarithromycin

(lan SOE pra zole, a moks i SIL in, & kla RITH roe mye sin)

Related Information

Amoxicillin *on page 124*
Clarithromycin *on page 396*
Gastrointestinal Disorders *on page 1874*
Lansoprazole *on page 981*

U.S. Brand Names Prevpac®

Canadian Brand Names Hp-PAC®

Pharmacologic Category Antibiotic, Macrolide Combination; Antibiotic, Penicillin; Gastrointestinal Agent, Miscellaneous; Proton Pump Inhibitor; Substituted Benzimidazole

Use Eradication of *H. pylori* to reduce the risk of recurrent duodenal ulcer

Local Anesthetic/Vasoconstrictor Precautions No information available to require special precautions

Effects on Dental Treatment Key adverse event(s) related to dental treatment: Taste perversion.

Effects on Bleeding No information available to require special precautions

Adverse Effects Note: Frequencies noted refer to experience with combination therapy. Also see individual agents.

3% to 10%:
- Central nervous system: Headache (6%)
- Gastrointestinal: Diarrhea (7%), taste perversion (5%)

General Dosage Range Oral: *Adults:* Lansoprazole 30 mg, amoxicillin 1 g, and clarithromycin 500 mg taken together twice daily

Pregnancy Risk Factor C (clarithromycin)

Lanthanum (LAN tha num)

U.S. Brand Names Fosrenol®

Canadian Brand Names Fosrenol®

Pharmacologic Category Phosphate Binder

Use Reduction of serum phosphate in patients with stage 5 chronic kidney disease (end-stage renal disease [ESRD]; kidney failure: GFR <15 mL/minute/1.73 m^2 or dialysis)

Local Anesthetic/Vasoconstrictor Precautions No information available to require special precautions

Effects on Dental Treatment No significant effects or complications reported

Effects on Bleeding No information available to require special precautions

Adverse Effects Reported in short-term (4-6 weeks) trials at frequency > placebo:

>10%:
- Gastrointestinal: Nausea (11%), vomiting (9%), abdominal pain (5%)
- Miscellaneous: Dialysis graft occlusion (8%)

1% to 10%: Endocrine & metabolic: Hypercalcemia was reported in longer-term trials at frequencies ≤4% (less frequently than with alternate therapy)

Note: Additional adverse effects noted in longer-term trials at rates higher than alternate therapy included constipation, diarrhea, and headache.

General Dosage Range Oral: *Adults:* Initial: 1500 mg/day in divided doses; Usual range: 1500-3000 mg/day

Mechanism of Action Disassociates in the upper gastrointestinal tract to lanthanum ions (La^{3+}) which bind to dietary phosphate resulting in insoluble lanthanum phosphate complexes and a net decrease in serum phosphate and calcium levels.

Pharmacodynamics/Kinetics

Half-life Elimination Plasma: 53 hours; Bone: 2-3.6 years

Pregnancy Risk Factor C

Lapatinib (la PA ti nib)

U.S. Brand Names Tykerb®

Canadian Brand Names Tykerb®

Pharmacologic Category Antineoplastic Agent, Tyrosine Kinase Inhibitor; Epidermal Growth Factor Receptor (EGFR) Inhibitor

Use Treatment of HER2 overexpressing advanced or metastatic breast cancer (in combination with capecitabine) in patients who have received prior therapy (with an anthracycline, a taxane, and trastuzumab) and HER2 overexpressing hormone receptor positive metastatic breast cancer in postmenopausal women (in combination with letrozole)

Unlabeled/Investigational Use Treatment (in combination with trastuzumab) of HER2 overexpressing metastatic breast cancer which had progressed on prior trastuzumab containing therapy

Local Anesthetic/Vasoconstrictor Precautions Lapatinib is one of the drugs confirmed to prolong the QT interval and is accepted as having a risk of causing torsade de pointes. The risk of drug-induced torsade de pointes is extremely low when a single QT interval prolonging drug is prescribed. In terms of epinephrine, it is not known what effect vasoconstrictors in the local anesthetic regimen will have in patients with a known history of congenital prolonged QT interval or in patients taking any medication that prolongs the QT interval. Until more information is obtained, it is suggested that the clinician consult with the physician prior to the

use of a vasoconstrictor in suspected patients, and that the vasoconstrictor (epinephrine, mepivacaine and levonordefrin [Carbocaine® 2% with Neo-Cobefrin®]) be used with caution.

Effects on Dental Treatment Key adverse event(s) related to dental treatment: Stomatitis.

Effects on Bleeding Although significant myelosuppression with associated altered hemostasis has been reported for many chemotherapeutic agents, myelosuppression is not common with lapatinib and no specific precautions appear to necessary.

Adverse Effects Percentages reported for combination therapy.

>10%:

- Central nervous system: Fatigue (10% to 20%), headache (≤14%)
- Dermatologic: Palmar-plantar erythrodysesthesia (hand-and-foot syndrome) (with capecitabine: 53%; grade 3: 12%), rash (28% to 44%), dry skin (10% to 13%), alopecia (≤13%), pruritus (≤12%), nail disorder (≤11%)
- Gastrointestinal: Diarrhea (64% to 65%; grade 3: 9% to 13%; grade 4: ≤1%), nausea (31% to 44%), vomiting (17% to 26%), abdominal pain (≤15%), mucosal inflammation (≤15%), stomatitis (≤14%), anorexia (≤11%), dyspepsia (≤11%)
- Hematologic: Anemia (with capecitabine: 56%; grade 3: <1%), neutropenia (with capecitabine: 22%; grade 3: 3%; grade 4: <1%), thrombocytopenia (with capecitabine: 18%; grade 3: <1%)
- Hepatic: AST increased (49% to 53%; grade 3: 2% to 6%; grade 4: <1%), ALT increased (37% to 46%; grade 3: 2% to 5%; grade 4<1%) total bilirubin increased (22% to 45%; grade 3: ≤4%; grade 4: <1%)
- Neuromuscular & skeletal: Limb pain (≤12%), weakness (≤12%), back pain (≤11%)
- Respiratory:Dyspnea (≤12%), epistaxis (≤11%)

1% to 10%:

- Cardiovascular: LVEF decreased (grades 1/2: 2% to 4%; grades 3/4: <1%)
- Central nervous system: Insomnia (≤10%)

General Dosage Range Dosage adjustment recommended in patients with hepatic impairment, on concomitant therapy, or who develop toxicities

Oral: *Adults:* 1250-1500 mg once daily

Mechanism of Action Tyrosine kinase (dual kinase) inhibitor; inhibits EGFR (ErbB1) and HER2 (ErbB2) by reversibly binding to tyrosine kinase, blocking phosphorylation and activation of downstream second messengers (Erk1/2 and Akt), regulating cellular proliferation and survival in ErbB- and ErbB2-expressing tumors. Combination therapy with lapatinib and endocrine therapy may overcome endocrine resistance occurring in HER2+ and hormone receptor positive disease.

Pharmacodynamics/Kinetics

Half-life Elimination ~24 hours

Time to Peak 3-6 hours

Pregnancy Risk Factor D

Prescribing and Access Restrictions Lapatinib is available **only** at specialty pharmacies through a restricted-access program, Tykerb® CARES. Information is available at www.tykerbcares.com or 1-866-489-5372.

Dental Comment Lapatinib is known to prolong the QT interval. The QT interval is measured as the time and distance between the Q point of the QRS complex and the end of the T wave in the ECG tracing. After adjustment for heart rate, the QT interval is defined as prolonged if it is more than 450 msec in men and 460 msec in women. A long QT syndrome was first described in the 1950s and 60s as a congenital syndrome involving QT interval prolongation and syncope and sudden death. Some of the congenital long QT syndromes were characterized by a peculiar electrocardiographic appearance of the QRS complex involving a premature atria beat followed by a pause, then a subsequent sinus beat showing marked QT prolongation and deformity. This type of cardiac arrhythmia was originally termed "torsade de pointes" (translated from the French as "twisting of the points"). Lapatinib is considered as having a risk of causing torsade de pointes. Since it is not known what effect vasoconstrictors in the local anesthetic regimen will have in patients with a known history of congenital prolonged QT interval or in patients taking any medication that prolongs the QT interval, a medical consult is suggested.

Laronidase (lair OH ni days)

U.S. Brand Names Aldurazyme®

Canadian Brand Names Aldurazyme®

Pharmacologic Category Enzyme

Use Treatment of Hurler and Hurler-Scheie forms of mucopolysaccharidosis I (MPS I); treatment of Scheie form of MPS I in patients with moderate-to-severe symptoms

Local Anesthetic/Vasoconstrictor Precautions No information available to require special precautions

Effects on Dental Treatment No significant effects or complications reported

Effects on Bleeding Thrombocytopenia may occur as an adverse effect. No information available to require routine special precautions.

Adverse Effects Note: Percentages reported are from a placebo-controlled study (45 patients, 22 receiving laronidase).

>10%:
- Cardiovascular: Vein disorder (14%)
- Dermatologic: Rash (36%)
- Local: Injection site reaction (18%)
- Neuromuscular & skeletal: Hyper-reflexia (14%), paresthesia (14%)
- Respiratory: Upper respiratory tract infection (32%)
- Miscellaneous: Antibody development to laronidase (91%); infusion reactions (32%; may be severe; includes flushing [23%], fever, and headache; frequency decreased over time during open-label extension period)

1% to 10%:
- Cardiovascular: Chest pain (9%), edema (9%), facial edema (9%), hypotension (9%)
- Hematologic: Thrombocytopenia (9%)
- Hepatic: Bilirubinemia (9%)
- Local: Abscess (9%), injection site pain (9%)
- Ocular: Corneal opacity (9%)
- Miscellaneous: Allergic reaction (severe/serious: 1%)

General Dosage Range I.V.: *Children ≥5 years and Adults:* 0.58 mg/kg once weekly

Mechanism of Action Laronidase is a recombinant (replacement) form of α-L-iduronidase derived from Chinese hamster cells. α-L-iduronidase is an enzyme needed to break down endogenous glycosaminoglycans (GAGs) within lysosomes. A deficiency of α-L-iduronidase leads to an accumulation of GAGs, causing cellular, tissue, and organ dysfunction as seen in MPS I. Improved pulmonary function and walking capacity have been demonstrated with the administration of laronidase to patients with Hurler, Hurler-Scheie, or Scheie (with moderate-to-severe symptoms) forms of MPS.

Pharmacodynamics/Kinetics

Half-life Elimination 1.5-3.6 hours

Pregnancy Risk Factor B

Latanoprost (la TA noe prost)

U.S. Brand Names Xalatan®

Canadian Brand Names Xalatan®

Generic Availability (U.S.) No

Pharmacologic Category Ophthalmic Agent, Antiglaucoma; Prostaglandin, Ophthalmic

Use Reduction of elevated intraocular pressure in patients with open-angle glaucoma or ocular hypertension

Local Anesthetic/Vasoconstrictor Precautions No information available to require special precautions

Effects on Dental Treatment No significant effects or complications reported

Effects on Bleeding No information available to require special precautions

Adverse Effects

>10%: Ocular: Blurred vision, burning and stinging, conjunctival hyperemia, foreign body sensation, itching, increased pigmentation of the iris, and punctate epithelial keratopathy

1% to 10%:
- Cardiovascular: Chest pain, angina pectoris
- Dermatologic: Rash, allergic skin reaction
- Neuromuscular & skeletal: Myalgia, arthralgia, back pain
- Ocular: Dry eye, excessive tearing, eye pain, lid crusting, lid edema, lid erythema, lid discomfort/pain, photophobia
- Respiratory: Upper respiratory tract infection, cold, flu

Dosage Adults: Ophthalmic: 1 drop (1.5 mcg) in the affected eye(s) once daily in the evening; do not exceed the once daily dosage because it has been shown that more frequent administration may decrease the IOP lowering effect

Note: A medication delivery device (Xal-Ease™) is available for use with Xalatan®.

Mechanism of Action Latanoprost is a prostaglandin F_2-alpha analog believed to reduce intraocular pressure by increasing the outflow of the aqueous humor

Contraindications Hypersensitivity to latanoprost or any component of the formulation

Warnings/Precautions May permanently change/increase brown pigmentation of the iris, the eyelid skin, and eyelashes. In addition, may increase the length and/or number of eyelashes (may vary between eyes); changes occur slowly and may not be noticeable for months or years. Long-term consequences and potential injury to eye are not known. Use with caution in patients with intraocular inflammation, aphakic patients, pseudophakic patients with a torn posterior lens capsule, or patients with risk factors for macular edema. Safety and efficacy have not been determined for use in patients with angle-closure-, inflammatory-, or neovascular glaucoma.

There have been reports of bacterial keratitis associated with the use of multiple-dose containers of topical ophthalmic products. Contains benzalkonium chloride which may be adsorbed by contact lenses; remove contacts prior to administration and wait 15 minutes before reinserting.

Drug Interactions

Avoid Concomitant Use There are no known interactions where it is recommended to avoid concomitant use.

Increased Effect/Toxicity

Latanoprost may increase the levels/effects of: Bimatoprost

Decreased Effect

The levels/effects of Latanoprost may be decreased by: NSAID (Ophthalmic)

Pharmacodynamics/Kinetics

Onset of Action 3-4 hours; Peak effect: Maximum: 8-12 hours

Half-life Elimination 17 minutes

Pregnancy Risk Factor C

Dosage Forms

Solution, ophthalmic:

Xalatan®: 0.005% (2.5 mL)

Latanoprost and Timolol (la TA noe prost & TIM oh lol)

Related Information

Latanoprost *on page 986*

Timolol (Ophthalmic) *on page 1633*

Canadian Brand Names Xalacom™

Pharmacologic Category Beta Blocker, Nonselective; Ophthalmic Agent, Antiglaucoma; Prostaglandin, Ophthalmic

Use Reduction of intraocular pressure (IOP) in patients with open-angle glaucoma or ocular hypertension who are insufficiently responsive to topical beta-blockers, prostaglandin analogues, or other IOP-reducing agents and in whom combination therapy is appropriate

Local Anesthetic/Vasoconstrictor Precautions No information available to require special precautions

Effects on Dental Treatment No significant effects or complications reported

Effects on Bleeding No information available to require special precautions

Adverse Effects Percentages as reported with combination product. Also see individual agents.

>10%: Ocular: Eyelash alterations (including darkening, lengthening, thickening) (≤37%), iris pigmentation increased (≤20%), eye irritation (12%)

1% to 10%:

Cardiovascular: Hypertension (≤4%), chest pain (1%)

Central nervous system: Depression (2%), headache (2%)

Dermatologic: Skin disorder (2%), rash (1%)

Endocrine & metabolic: Hypercholesterolemia (2%), diabetes mellitus (1%)

Neuromuscular & skeletal: Arthritis (2%), back pain (1%)

Ocular: Hyperemia (7%), vision abnormal (7%), visual field defect (5%), blepharitis (3%), cataract (3%), conjunctivitis (3%), corneal disorder (3%), eye pain (2%), photophobia (2%), refraction errors (2%), skin disorder (2%), conjunctival disorder (1%), keratitis (1%), meibomianitis (1%)

Respiratory: Upper respiratory infection (6%), sinusitis (2%), bronchitis (1%)

Miscellaneous: Flu-like symptoms (3%), infection (1%)

General Dosage Range Ophthalmic: *Adults:* Instill 1 drop once daily

Mechanism of Action

Latanoprost: A prostaglandin F_2-alpha analog believed to reduce intraocular pressure by increasing the outflow of the aqueous humor

Timolol: Blocks both $beta_1$- and $beta_2$-adrenergic receptors, reduces intraocular pressure by reducing aqueous humor production or possibly outflow; reduces blood pressure by blocking adrenergic receptors and decreasing sympathetic outflow, produces a negative chronotropic and inotropic activity through an unknown mechanism

Product Availability Not available in U.S.

Leflunomide (le FLOO noh mide)

Related Information

Rheumatoid Arthritis, Osteoarthritis, and Osteoporosis *on page 1889*

U.S. Brand Names Arava®

Canadian Brand Names Apo-Leflunomide®; Arava®; Mylan-Leflunomide; Novo-Leflunomide; PHL-Leflunomide; PMS-Leflunomide; Sandoz-Leflunomide

Pharmacologic Category Antirheumatic, Disease Modifying

Use Treatment of active rheumatoid arthritis; indicated to reduce signs and symptoms, and to inhibit structural damage and improve physical function

Unlabeled/Investigational Use Treatment of cytomegalovirus (CMV) disease in transplant recipients resistant to standard antivirals; prevention of acute and chronic rejection in recipients of solid organ transplants

Local Anesthetic/Vasoconstrictor Precautions No information available to require special precautions

Effects on Dental Treatment Key adverse event(s) related to dental treatment: Xerostomia (normal salivary flow resumes upon discontinuation), stomatitis, oral candidiasis, abnormal taste, tooth disorder, enlarged salivary gland, esophagitis, and gingivitis.

Effects on Bleeding Has been associated with rare thrombocytopenia. No information available to require routine special precautions.

Adverse Effects

>10%:

Gastrointestinal: Diarrhea (17%)

Respiratory: Respiratory tract infection (4% to 15%)

1% to 10%:

Cardiovascular: Hypertension (10%), chest pain (2%), edema (peripheral), palpitation, tachycardia, vasodilation, varicose vein, vasculitis

Central nervous system: Headache (7%), dizziness (4%), pain (2%), anxiety, depression, fever, insomnia, malaise, migraine, sleep disorder, vertigo

Dermatologic: Alopecia (10%), rash (10%), pruritus (4%), dry skin (2%), eczema (2%), acne, bruising, dermatitis, hair discoloration, hematoma, nail disorder, skin disorder/discoloration, skin ulcer, subcutaneous nodule

Endocrine & metabolic: Hypokalemia (1%), diabetes mellitus, hyperglycemia, hyperlipidemia, hyperthyroidism, menstrual disorder

Gastrointestinal: Nausea (9%), abdominal pain (5% to 6%), dyspepsia (5%), weight loss (4%), anorexia (3%), gastroenteritis (3%), mouth ulceration (3%), vomiting (3%), candidiasis (oral), colitis, constipation, esophagitis, flatulence, gastritis, gingivitis, melena, salivary gland enlarged, stomatitis, taste disturbance, tooth disorder, xerostomia

Genitourinary: Urinary tract infection (5%), albuminuria, cystitis, dysuria, prostate disorder, urinary frequency, vaginal candidiasis

Hematologic: Anemia

Hepatic: Abnormal LFTs (5%), cholelithiasis

Local: Abscess

Neuromuscular & skeletal: Back pain (5%), joint disorder (4%), weakness (3%), tenosynovitis (3%), synovitis (2%), paresthesia (2%), arthralgia (1%), leg cramps (1%), arthrosis, bone necrosis, bone pain, bursitis, CPK increased, myalgia, neck pain, neuralgia, neuritis, pelvic pain, tendon rupture

Ocular: Blurred vision, cataract, conjunctivitis, eye disorder

Renal: Hematuria

Respiratory: Bronchitis (7%), cough (3%), pharyngitis (3%), pneumonia (2%), rhinitis (2%), sinusitis (2%), asthma, dyspnea, epistaxis

Miscellaneous: Accidental injury (5%), allergic reactions (2%), flu-like syndrome (2%), cyst, diaphoresis, hernia, herpes infection

General Dosage Range Dosage adjustment recommended in patients who develop toxicities

Oral: *Adults:* Initial: 100 mg/day for 3 days; Maintenance range: 10-20 mg/day

Mechanism of Action Leflunomide is an immunodulatory agent that inhibits pyrimidine synthesis, resulting in antiproliferative and anti-inflammatory effects. Leflunomide is a prodrug; the active metabolite is responsible for activity. For CMV, may interfere with virion assembly.

Pharmacodynamics/Kinetics

Half-life Elimination M1: Mean: 14-15 days; enterohepatic recycling appears to contribute to the long half-life of this agent, since activated charcoal and cholestyramine substantially reduce plasma half-life

Time to Peak M1: 6-12 hours

Pregnancy Risk Factor X

Lenalidomide (le na LID oh mide)

U.S. Brand Names Revlimid®

Canadian Brand Names Revlimid®

Pharmacologic Category Angiogenesis Inhibitor; Antineoplastic Agent; Immunomodulator, Systemic

Use Treatment of low- or intermediate-risk myelodysplastic syndrome (MDS) in patients with deletion 5q (del 5q) cytogenetic abnormality with transfusion-dependent anemia (with or without other cytogenetic abnormalities); treatment of multiple myeloma (in combination with dexamethasone) in patients who have received at least one prior therapy

Unlabeled/Investigational Use Treatment of non-Hodgkin's lymphomas; systemic amyloidosis (light chain); lower-risk myelodysplastic syndrome (MDS) in transfusion-dependent patients without deletion 5q (del 5q); maintenance treatment for multiple myeloma (following autologous stem cell transplant)

Local Anesthetic/Vasoconstrictor Precautions No information available to require special precautions

Effects on Dental Treatment Key adverse event(s) related to dental treatment: Xerostomia (normal salivary flow resumes upon discontinuation), taste perversion.

Effects on Bleeding Chemotherapy may result in significant myelosuppression, potentially including significant reduction in platelet counts and altered hemostasis. In patients who are under active treatment with these agents, medical consult is suggested.

Adverse Effects

>10%:

Cardiovascular: Peripheral edema (8% to 21%)

Central nervous system: Fatigue (31% to 38%), insomnia (10% to 32%), fever (21% to 23%), dizziness (20% to 21%), headache (20% to 21%)

Dermatologic: Pruritus (42%), rash (16% to 36%; grades 3/4: 7%), dry skin (14%)

Endocrine & metabolic: Hyperglycemia (15%), hypokalemia (11%)

Gastrointestinal: Diarrhea (29% to 49%), constipation (24% to 39%), nausea (22% to 24%), weight loss (18%), dyspepsia (14%), anorexia (10% to 14%), taste perversion (6% to 13%), abdominal pain (8% to 12%)

Genitourinary: Urinary tract infection (11%)

Hematologic: Thrombocytopenia (17% to 62%; grades 3/4: 10% to 50%; onset [MDS]: 28 days [range 8-290 days]; recovery [MDS]: 22 days [range: 5-224 days]), neutropenia (28% to 59%; grades 3/4: 21% to 53%; onset [MDS]: 42 days [range 14-411 days]; recovery [MDS]: 17 days [range: 2-170 days]), anemia (12% to 24%; grades 3/4: 6% to 8%); myelosuppression is dose-dependent and reversible with treatment interruption and/or dose reduction

Neuromuscular & skeletal: Muscle cramp (18% to 30%), weakness (15% to 23%), arthralgia (10% to 22%), back pain (15% to 21%), tremor (20%), paresthesia (12%), limb pain (11%)

Ocular: Blurred vision (15%)

Respiratory: Nasopharyngitis (23%), cough (15% to 20%), dyspnea (7% to 20%), pharyngitis (16%), epistaxis (15%), upper respiratory infection (14% to 15%), pneumonia (11% to 12%)

1% to 10%:

Cardiovascular: Edema (10%), deep vein thrombosis (≤8%; grades 3/4: ≤7%), hypertension (6%), chest pain (5%), palpitation (5%), atrial fibrillation (grades 3/4: ≤3%), syncope (grade 3: 1% to 2%)

Central nervous system: Hypoesthesia (7%), pain (7%), depression (5%)

Dermatologic: Bruising (5% to 8%), cellulitis (5%), erythema (5%)

Endocrine & metabolic: Hypothyroidism (7%), hypomagnesemia (6%), hypocalcemia (grades 3/4: 4%)

Gastrointestinal: Vomiting (10%), xerostomia (7%), loose stools (6%)

Genitourinary: Dysuria (7%)

Hematologic: Leukopenia (8%; grade 3/4: ≤5%), febrile neutropenia (5%; grades 3/4: 4%), granulocytopenia (grades 3/4: 2%), lymphopenia (grade 3: 2%), pancytopenia (grades 3/4: 2%)

Hepatic: ALT increased (8%)

Neuromuscular & skeletal: Myalgia (9%), rigors (6%), peripheral neuropathy (5%)

Respiratory: Sinusitis (8%), rhinitis (7%), bronchitis (6%), pulmonary embolism (≤3%; grades 3/4: 1% to 3%), respiratory distress (grades 3/4: 2%), hypoxia (grades 3/4: 1%), pleural effusion (grades 3/4: 1%), pneumonitis (grades 3/4: 1%), pulmonary hypertension (grades 3/4: 1%)

Miscellaneous: Night sweats (8%), diaphoresis (7%), sepsis (grades 3/4: 3%)

General Dosage Range Dosage adjustment recommended in patients with renal impairment or who develop toxicities

Oral: *Adults:* 10 once daily **or** 25 mg once daily for 21 of 28 days

Mechanism of Action Immunomodulatory, antiangiogenic, and antineoplastic characteristics via multiple mechanisms. Selectively inhibits secretion of proinflammatory cytokines (potent inhibitor of tumor necrosis factor-alpha secretion); enhances cell-mediated immunity by stimulating proliferation of anti-CD3 stimulated T cells (resulting in increased IL-2 and interferon gamma secretion); inhibits trophic signals to angiogenic factors in cells. Inhibits the growth of myeloma cells by inducing cell cycle arrest and cell death.

Pharmacodynamics/Kinetics

Half-life Elimination ~3 hours; moderate-to-severe renal impairment: ~9 hours; hemodialysis patients: ~13.5 hours

Time to Peak Healthy volunteers: ~0.6-1.5 hours; Myeloma patients: 0.5-4 hours

Pregnancy Risk Factor X

Prescribing and Access Restrictions As a requirement of the REMS program, access to this medication is restricted. Lenalidomide is approved for marketing in the U.S. only under a Food and Drug Administration (FDA) approved, restricted distribution program called RevAssist® (www.REVLIMID.com or 1-888-423-5436). In Canada, distribution is restricted through RevAid® (www.RevAid.ca or 1-888-738-2431). Physicians, pharmacies, and patients must be registered; a maximum 28-day supply may be dispensed; a new prescription is required each time it is filled; pregnancy testing is required for females of childbearing potential.

Lepirudin (leh puh ROO din)

Related Information

Cardiovascular Diseases *on page 1848*

U.S. Brand Names Refludan®

Canadian Brand Names Refludan®

Pharmacologic Category Anticoagulant, Thrombin Inhibitor

Use Indicated for anticoagulation in patients with heparin-induced thrombocytopenia (HIT) and associated thromboembolic disease in order to prevent further thromboembolic complications

Unlabeled/Investigational Use Investigational: Prevention or reduction of ischemic complications associated with unstable angina

Local Anesthetic/Vasoconstrictor Precautions No information available to require special precautions

Effects on Dental Treatment Key adverse event(s) related to dental treatment: Bleeding is the major adverse effect of lepirudin. See Effects on Bleeding.

Effects on Bleeding As with all anticoagulants, bleeding is the major adverse effect of lepirudin. Hemorrhage may occur at virtually any site; risk is dependent on multiple variables including the intensity of anticoagulation and patient susceptibility. Medical consult is suggested. It is unlikely that ambulatory patients presenting for dental treatment will be receiving intravenous anticoagulant therapy.

Adverse Effects As with all anticoagulants, bleeding is the most common adverse event associated with lepirudin. Hemorrhage may occur at virtually any site. Risk is dependent on multiple variables.

HIT patients:

>10%: Hematologic: Anemia (12%), bleeding from puncture sites (11%), hematoma (11%)

1% to 10%:

- Cardiovascular: Heart failure (3%), pericardial effusion (1%), ventricular fibrillation (1%)
- Central nervous system: Fever (7%)
- Dermatologic: Maculopapular rash (4%), eczema (3%)
- Gastrointestinal: GI bleeding/rectal bleeding (5%)
- Genitourinary: Vaginal bleeding (2%)
- Hepatic: Transaminases increased (6%)
- Renal: Hematuria (4%)
- Respiratory: Epistaxis (4%)

Non-HIT populations (including those receiving thrombolytics and/or contrast media):

1% to 10%: Respiratory: Bronchospasm/stridor/dyspnea/cough

General Dosage Range Dosage adjustment recommended in patients with renal impairment

I.V.: *Adults:* Bolus: 0.2-0.4 mg/kg; Infusion: 0.1-0.15 mg/kg/hour (maximum: 0.21 mg/kg/hour)

Mechanism of Action Lepirudin is a highly specific direct inhibitor of thrombin; lepirudin is a recombinant hirudin derived from yeast cells

Pharmacodynamics/Kinetics

Half-life Elimination Initial: ~10 minutes: Terminal: Healthy volunteers: 1.3 hours; Significant renal impairment (Cl_{cr} <15 mL/minute and on hemodialysis): ≤2 days

Pregnancy Risk Factor B

Letrozole (LET roe zole)

U.S. Brand Names Femara®

Canadian Brand Names Femara®; MED-Letrozole; PMS-Letrozole; Sandoz-Letrozole

Pharmacologic Category Antineoplastic Agent, Aromatase Inhibitor

Use For use in postmenopausal women in the adjuvant treatment of hormone receptor positive early breast cancer, extended adjuvant treatment of early breast cancer after 5 years of tamoxifen, advanced breast cancer with disease progression following antiestrogen therapy, hormone receptor positive or hormone receptor unknown, locally-advanced, or first-line (or second-line) treatment of advanced or metastatic breast cancer

Unlabeled/Investigational Use Treatment of ovarian (epithelial) cancer, endometrial cancer

Local Anesthetic/Vasoconstrictor Precautions No information available to require special precautions

Effects on Dental Treatment No significant effects or complications reported

Effects on Bleeding Although significant myelosuppression with associated altered hemostasis has been reported for many chemotherapeutic agents, myelosuppression is not common with letrozole and no specific precautions appear to necessary.

Adverse Effects

>10%:

Cardiovascular: Edema (7% to 18%)

Central nervous system: Headache (4% to 20%), dizziness (3% to 14%), fatigue (8% to 13%)

Endocrine & metabolic: Hypercholesterolemia (3% to 52%), hot flashes (6% to 50%)

Gastrointestinal: Nausea (9% to 17%), weight gain (2% to 13%), constipation (2% to 11%)

Neuromuscular & skeletal: Weakness (4% to 34%), arthralgia (8% to 25%), arthritis (7% to 25%), bone pain (5% to 22%), back pain (5% to 18%), bone mineral density decreased/osteoporosis (5% to 15%), bone fracture (10% to 14%)

Respiratory: Dyspnea (6% to 18%), cough (6% to 13%)

Miscellaneous: Diaphoresis (≤24%), night sweats (15%)

1% to 10%:

Cardiovascular: Chest pain (6% to 8%), hypertension (5% to 8%), chest wall pain (6%), peripheral edema (5%), cerebrovascular accident (2% to 3%), thromboembolic event (2% to 3%), MI (1% to 2%), angina (1%)

Central nervous system: Insomnia (6% to 7%), pain (5%), anxiety (<5%), depression (<5%), vertigo (<5%),somnolence (3%)

Dermatologic: Rash (5%), alopecia (3% to 5%), pruritus (1%)

Endocrine & metabolic: Breast pain (2% to 7%), hypercalcemia (<5%)

Gastrointestinal: Diarrhea (5% to 8%), vomiting (3% to 7%), weight loss (6% to 7%), abdominal pain (6%), anorexia (1% to 5%), dyspepsia (3%)

Genitourinary: Urinary tract infection (6%), vaginal bleeding (5%), vaginal dryness (5%), vaginal hemorrhage (5%), vaginal irritation (5%)

Neuromuscular & skeletal: Limb pain (4% to 10%), myalgia (7% to 9%)

Ocular: Cataract (2%)

Renal: Renal disorder (5%)

Respiratory: Pleural effusion (<5%)

Miscellaneous: Infection (7%), influenza (6%), viral infection (6%), secondary malignancy (2% to 4%)

General Dosage Range Dosage adjustment recommended in patients with hepatic impairment

Oral: *Adults (postmenopausal females):* 2.5 mg once daily

Mechanism of Action Nonsteroidal competitive inhibitor of the aromatase enzyme system which binds to the heme group of aromatase, a cytochrome P450 enzyme which catalyzes conversion of androgens to estrogens (specifically, androstenedione to estrone and testosterone to estradiol). This leads to inhibition of the enzyme and a significant reduction in plasma estrogen (estrone, estradiol and estrone sulfate) levels. Does not affect synthesis of adrenal or thyroid hormones, aldosterone, or androgens.

Pharmacodynamics/Kinetics

Half-life Elimination Terminal: ~2 days

Time to Peak Steady state, plasma: 2-6 weeks

Pregnancy Risk Factor X

Leucovorin Calcium (loo koe VOR in KAL see um)

Canadian Brand Names Lederle Leucovorin

Pharmacologic Category Antidote; Chemotherapy Modulating Agent; Rescue Agent (Chemotherapy); Vitamin, Water Soluble

Use Antidote for folic acid antagonists (methotrexate, trimethoprim, pyrimethamine) and rescue therapy following high-dose methotrexate; in combination with fluorouracil in the treatment of colon cancer; treatment of megaloblastic anemias when folate is deficient as in infancy, sprue, pregnancy, and nutritional deficiency when oral folate therapy is not possible

Unlabeled/Investigational Use Adjunctive cofactor therapy in methanol toxicity

Local Anesthetic/Vasoconstrictor Precautions No information available to require special precautions

Effects on Dental Treatment No significant effects or complications reported

Effects on Bleeding No information available to require special precautions

Adverse Effects Frequency not defined. Toxicities (especially gastrointestinal toxicity) of fluorouracil is higher when used in combination with leucovorin.

Dermatologic: Rash, pruritus, erythema, urticaria
Hematologic: Thrombocytosis
Respiratory: Wheezing
Miscellaneous: Allergic reactions, anaphylactoid reactions

General Dosage Range

I.M.: *Children and Adults:* ≤1 mg/day [folate deficient megaloblastic anemia] **or** 15 mg (~10 mg/m^2) every 6 hours for 10 doses [methotrexate rescue dose]

I.V.:

Children: 15 mg (~10 mg/m^2) every 6 hours for 10 doses

Adults: Initial: 15 mg (~10 mg/m^2) every 6 hours for 10 doses [methotrexate rescue dose] **or** 200 mg/m^2 **or** 20 mg/m^2 as a single dose [colorectal cancer]

Oral: *Children and Adults:* 5-15 mg/day [weak folic acid antagonist overdose] **or** 15 mg (~10 mg/m^2) every 6 hours for 10 doses [methotrexate rescue dose]

Mechanism of Action A reduced form of folic acid, leucovorin supplies the necessary cofactor blocked by methotrexate. Leucovorin actively competes with methotrexate for transport sites, displaces methotrexate from intracellular binding sites, and restores active folate stores required for DNA/RNA synthesis. Stabilizes the binding of 5-dUMP and thymidylate synthetase, enhancing the activity of fluorouracil.

Methanol toxicity treatment: Formic acid (methanol's toxic metabolite) is normally metabolized to carbon dioxide and water by 10-formyltetrahydrofolate dehydrogenase after being bound to tetrahydrofolate. Administering a source of tetrahydrofolate may aid the body in eliminating formic acid.

Pharmacodynamics/Kinetics

Half-life Elimination ~4-8 hours

Time to Peak Oral: ~2 hours; I.V.: Total folates: 10 minutes; 5MTHF: ~1 hour

Pregnancy Risk Factor C

Leuprolide (loo PROE lide)

U.S. Brand Names Eligard®; Lupron Depot-Ped®; Lupron Depot®; Lupron Depot®-3 Month; Lupron Depot®-4 Month; Lupron®

Canadian Brand Names Eligard®; Lupron®; Lupron® Depot®

Pharmacologic Category Antineoplastic Agent, Gonadotropin-Releasing Hormone Agonist; Gonadotropin Releasing Hormone Agonist

Use Palliative treatment of advanced prostate cancer; management of endometriosis; treatment of anemia caused by uterine leiomyomata (fibroids); central precocious puberty

Unlabeled/Investigational Use Treatment of breast cancer; infertility; prostatic hyperplasia

Local Anesthetic/Vasoconstrictor Precautions No information available to require special precautions

Effects on Dental Treatment Key adverse event(s) related to dental treatment: Gum hemorrhage, gingivitis, dry mucous membranes, and dysphagia.

Effects on Bleeding Although significant myelosuppression with associated altered hemostasis has been reported for many chemotherapeutic agents, myelosuppression is not common with leuprolide and no specific precautions appear to necessary.

Adverse Effects

Children: 2% to 10%:

Central nervous system: Pain (2%)

Dermatologic: Acne (2%), rash (2% including erythema multiforme), seborrhea (2%)
Genitourinary: Vaginitis (2%), vaginal bleeding (2%), vaginal discharge (2%)
Local: Injection site reaction (5%)

Adults: Note: For prostate cancer treatment, an initial rise in serum testosterone concentrations may cause "tumor flare" or worsening of symptoms, including bone pain, neuropathy, hematuria, or ureteral or bladder outlet obstruction during the first 2 weeks. Similarly, an initial increase in estradiol levels, with a temporary worsening of symptoms, may occur in women treated with leuprolide.

Delayed release formulations:

10%:

Cardiovascular: Edema (≤14%)
Central nervous system: Headache (≤65%), pain (<2% to 33%), depression (≤31%), insomnia (≤31%), fatigue (≤17%), dizziness/vertigo (≤16%)
Dermatologic: Skin reaction (≤12%)
Endocrine & metabolic: Hot flashes (25% to 98%), testicular atrophy (≤20%), hyperlipidemia (≤12%), libido decreased (≤11%)
Gastrointestinal: Nausea/vomiting (≤25%), bowel function altered (≤14%), weight gain/loss (≤13%)
Genitourinary: Vaginitis (11% to 28%), urinary disorder (13% to 15%)
Local: Injection site burning/stinging (transient: ≤35%)
Neuromuscular & skeletal: Weakness (≤18%), joint disorder (≤12%)
Miscellaneous: Flu-like syndrome (≤12%)

1% to 10% (limited to important or life-threatening):

Cardiovascular: Angina (<5%), arrhythmia (<5%), atrial fibrillation (<5%), bradycardia (<5%), CHF (<5%), deep thrombophlebitis (<5%), hyper-/hypotension (<5%), palpitation (<5%), syncope (<5%), tachycardia (<5%)
Central nervous system: Nervousness (≤8%), anxiety (≤6%), confusion (<5%), delusions (<5%), dementia (<5%), fever (<5%), seizure (<5%)
Dermatologic: Acne (≤10%), alopecia (≤5%), bruising (≤5%), cellulitis (<5%), pruritus (≤3%), hirsutism (<2%), rash (<2%)
Endocrine & metabolic: Dehydration (≤8%), gynecomastia (≤7%), breast tenderness/pain (≤6%), bicarbonate decreased (≥5%), hyper-/hypocholesterolemia (≥5%), hyperglycemia (≥5%), hyperphosphatemia (≥5%), hyperuricemia (≥5%), hypoalbuminemia (≥5%), hypoproteinemia (≥5%), lactation (<5%), testicular pain (≤4%), menstrual disorder (≤2%)
Gastrointestinal: Dysphagia (<5%), gastrointestinal hemorrhage (<5%), intestinal obstruction (<5%), ulcer (<5%), gastroenteritis/colitis (≤3%), diarrhea (≤2%), constipation (≤2%)
Genitourinary: Prostatic acid phosphatase increased/decreased (≥5%), urine specific gravity increased/decreased (≥5%), impotence (≤5%), balanitis (<5%), incontinence (<5%), penile/testis disorder (<5%), urinary tract infection (<5%), nocturia (≤4%), polyuria (2% to 4%), bladder spasm (<2%), dysuria (<2%), erectile dysfunction (<2%), hematuria (<2%), urinary retention (<2%), urinary urgency (<2%)
Hematologic: Eosinophilia (≥5%), leukopenia (≥5%), platelets increased (≥5%), anemia
Hepatic: Liver function tests abnormal (≥5%), partial thromboplastin time increased (≥5%), prothrombin time increased (≥5%), hepatomegaly (<5%)
Local: Injection site pain (2% to 5%), injection site erythema (1% to 3%)
Neuromuscular & skeletal: Myalgia (≤8%), paresthesia (≤8%), neuropathy (<5%), paralysis (<5%), pathologic fracture (<5%), bone pain (<2%)
Renal: BUN increased (≥5%), creatinine increased (≥5%)
Respiratory: Emphysema (<5%), epistaxis (<5%), hemoptysis (<5%), pleural effusion (<5%), pulmonary edema (<5%), dyspnea (≤2%)
Miscellaneous: Diaphoresis (≤5%), allergic reaction (<5%), infection (5%), lymphadenopathy (<5%)

Immediate release formulation:

>10%:

Cardiovascular: ECG changes/ischemia (19%), peripheral edema (12%)
Central nervous system: Pain (13%)
Endocrine & metabolic: Hot flashes (55%)

1% to 10% (limited to important or life-threatening):

Cardiovascular: Hypertension (8%), murmur (3%), thrombosis/phlebitis (2%), CHF (1%), angina, arrhythmia, MI, syncope
Central nervous system: Headache (7%), insomnia (7%), dizziness/lightheadedness (5%), anxiety, depression, fatigue, fever, nervousness
Dermatologic: Dermatitis (5%), alopecia, bruising, itching, lesions, pigmentation
Endocrine & metabolic: Gynecomastia/breast tenderness/pain (7%), testicular size decreased (7%), diabetes, hypercalcemia, hypoglycemia, libido decreased, thyroid enlarged

Gastrointestinal: Constipation (7%), anorexia (6%), nausea/vomiting (5%), diarrhea, dysphagia, gastrointestinal bleeding, peptic ulcer, rectal polyps
Genitourinary: Urinary frequency/urgency (6%), impotence (4%), urinary tract infection (3%), bladder spasm, dysuria, incontinence, testicular pain, urinary obstruction
Hematologic: Anemia (5%)
Local: Injection site reaction
Neuromuscular & skeletal: Weakness (10%), bone pain (5%), peripheral neuropathy
Ocular: Blurred vision
Renal: Hematuria (6%), BUN increased, creatinine increased
Respiratory: Dyspnea (2%), cough, pneumonia, pulmonary embolus, pulmonary fibrosis
Miscellaneous: Infection, inflammation

General Dosage Range I.M., SubQ: *Children and Adults:* Dosage varies greatly depending on indication

Mechanism of Action Leuprolide, is an agonist of luteinizing hormone-releasing hormone (LHRH). Acting as a potent inhibitor of gonadotropin secretion; continuous administration results in suppression of ovarian and testicular steroidogenesis due to decreased levels of LH and FSH with subsequent decrease in testosterone (male) and estrogen (female) levels. In males, testosterone levels are reduced to below castrate levels. Leuprolide may also have a direct inhibitory effect on the testes, and act by a different mechanism not directly related to reduction in serum testosterone.

Pharmacodynamics/Kinetics

Onset of Action Following transient increase, testosterone suppression occurs in ~2-4 weeks of continued therapy

Pregnancy Risk Factor X

Levalbuterol (leve al BYOO ter ole)

U.S. Brand Names Xopenex HFA™; Xopenex®

Canadian Brand Names Xopenex®

Pharmacologic Category $Beta_2$-Adrenergic Agonist

Use Treatment or prevention of bronchospasm in children and adults with reversible obstructive airway disease

Local Anesthetic/Vasoconstrictor Precautions No information available to require special precautions

Effects on Dental Treatment No significant effects or complications reported

Effects on Bleeding No information available to require special precautions

Adverse Effects

>10%:

Endocrine & metabolic: Serum glucose increased, serum potassium decreased
Neuromuscular & skeletal: Tremor (≤7%)
Respiratory: Rhinitis (3% to 11%)
Miscellaneous: Viral infection (7% to 12%)

>2% to 10%:

Central nervous system: Headache (8% to 12%), nervousness (3% to 10%), dizziness (1% to 3%), anxiety (≤3%), migraine (≤3%), weakness (3%)
Cardiovascular: Tachycardia (~3%)
Dermatologic: Rash (≤8%)
Gastrointestinal: Diarrhea (2% to 6%), dyspepsia (1% to 3%)
Neuromuscular & skeletal: Leg cramps (≤3%)
Respiratory: Asthma (9%), pharyngitis (3% to 10%), cough (1% to 4%), sinusitis (1% to 4%), nasal edema (1% to 3%)
Miscellaneous: Flu-like syndrome (1% to 4%), accidental injury (≤3%)

Note: Immediate hypersensitivity reactions have occurred (including angioedema, oropharyngeal edema, urticaria, and anaphylaxis).

General Dosage Range

Inhalation (metered-dose inhaler): *Children ≥4 years and Adults:* 1-2 puffs every 4-6 hours

Nebulization (solution):

Children ≤4 years: 0.31-1.25 mg every 4-6 hours as needed
Children 5-11 years: 0.31-0.63 mg 3 times/day
Children ≥12 years and Adults: 0.63-1.25 mg every 8 hours as needed
Elderly: Initial: 0.63 mg

Mechanism of Action Relaxes bronchial smooth muscle by action on $beta_2$-receptors with little effect on heart rate

Pharmacodynamics/Kinetics

Onset of Action Measured as a 15% increase in FEV_1:

Aerosol: 5.5-10.2 minutes; Peak effect: ~77 minutes

Nebulization: 10-17 minutes; Peak effect: 1.5 hours

Duration of Action Measured as a 15% increase in FEV_1:

Aerosol: 3-4 hours (up to 6 hours in some patients)

Nebulization: 5-6 hours (up to 8 hours in some patients)

Half-life Elimination 3.3-4 hours

Time to Peak

Aerosol: Children: 0.8 hours, Adults: 0.5 hours

Nebulization: Children: 0.3-0.6 hours, Adults: 0.2 hours

Pregnancy Risk Factor C

LevETIRAcetam (lee va tye RA se tam)

U.S. Brand Names Keppra XR™; Keppra®

Canadian Brand Names Apo-Levetiracetam®; CO Levetiracetam; Dom-Levetiracetam; Keppra®; PHL-Levetiracetam; PMS-Levetiracetam; PRO-Levetiracetam

Pharmacologic Category Anticonvulsant, Miscellaneous

Use Adjunctive therapy in the treatment of partial onset, myoclonic, and/or primary generalized tonic-clonic seizures

Unlabeled/Investigational Use Bipolar disorder

Local Anesthetic/Vasoconstrictor Precautions No information available to require special precautions

Effects on Dental Treatment No significant effects or complications reported

Effects on Bleeding No information available to require special precautions

Adverse Effects

>10%:

Central nervous system: Behavioral symptoms (agitation, aggression, anger, anxiety, apathy, depersonalization, depression, emotional lability, hostility, hyperkinesias, irritability, nervousness, neurosis and personality disorder: adults 5% to 13%; children 5% to 38%), somnolence (8% to 23%), headache (14%), hostility (2% to 12%)

Gastrointestinal: Vomiting (15%), anorexia (3% to 13%)

Neuromuscular & skeletal: Weakness (9% to 15%)

Respiratory: Pharyngitis (6% to 14%), rhinitis (4% to 13%), cough (2% to 11%)

Miscellaneous: Accidental injury (17%), infection (2% to 13%)

1% to 10%:

Cardiovascular: Facial edema (2%)

Central nervous system: Fatigue (10%), nervousness (4% to 10%), dizziness (5% to 9%), personality disorder (8%), pain (6% to 7%), agitation (6%), irritability (6% to 7%), emotional lability (2% to 6%), mood swings (5%), depression (3% to 5%), vertigo (3% to 5%), ataxia (3%), amnesia (2%), anxiety (2%), confusion (2%)

Dermatologic: Bruising (4%), pruritus (2%), rash (2%), skin discoloration (2%)

Endocrine & metabolic: Dehydration (2%)

Gastrointestinal: Diarrhea (8%), nausea (5%), gastroenteritis (4%), constipation (3%)

Genitourinary: Urine abnormality (2%)

Hematologic: Leukocytes decreased (2% to 3%)

Neuromuscular & skeletal: Neck pain (2% to 8%), paresthesia (2%), reflexes increased (2%)

Ocular: Conjunctivitis (3%), diplopia (2%), amblyopia (2%)

Otic: Ear pain (2%)

Renal: Albuminuria (4%)

Respiratory: Influenza (5%), asthma (2%), sinusitis (2%)

Miscellaneous: Flu-like syndrome (3% to 8%), viral infection (2%)

General Dosage Range Dosage adjustment recommended in patients with renal impairment

Oral:

Immediate release:

Children 4-15 years: Initial: 10 mg/kg twice daily; Maintenance: 10-30 mg/kg twice daily (maximum: 60 mg/kg/day)

Children ≥12 years: Initial: 500 mg twice daily; Maintenance: 500-1500 mg twice daily (maximum: 3000 mg/day)

Adults: Initial: 500 mg twice daily; Maintenance: 500-1500 mg twice daily (maximum: 3000 mg/day)

Extended release: *Children ≥16 years and Adults:* Initial: 1000 mg once daily; Maintenance: 1000-3000 mg once daily (maximum: 3000 mg/day)

I.V.: *Children ≥16 years and Adults:* Initial: 500 mg twice daily; Maintenance: 500-1500 mg twice daily (maximum: 3000 mg/day)

Mechanism of Action The precise mechanism by which levetiracetam exerts its antiepileptic effect is unknown. However, several studies have suggested the mechanism may involve one or more of the following central pharmacologic effects: inhibition of voltage-dependent N-type calcium channels; facilitation of GABA-ergic inhibitory transmission through displacement of negative modulators; reduction of delayed rectifier potassium current; and/or binding to synaptic proteins which modulate neurotransmitter release.

Pharmacodynamics/Kinetics

Onset of Action Peak effect: Oral: 1 hour

Half-life Elimination ~6-8 hours; extended release tablet: ~7 hours; half-life increased in renal dysfunction

Time to Peak Oral: Immediate release: ~1 hour; Extended release: ~4 hours

Pregnancy Risk Factor C

Levobunolol (lee voe BYOO noe lole)

U.S. Brand Names Betagan®

Canadian Brand Names Apo-Levobunolol®; Betagan®; Novo-Levobunolol; Optho-Bunolol®; PMS-Levobunolol; Sandoz-Levobunolol

Pharmacologic Category Beta-Adrenergic Blocker, Nonselective; Ophthalmic Agent, Antiglaucoma

Use To lower intraocular pressure in chronic open-angle glaucoma or ocular hypertension

Local Anesthetic/Vasoconstrictor Precautions No information available to require special precautions

Effects on Dental Treatment Key adverse event(s) related to dental treatment: Levobunolol is a nonselective beta-blocker and may enhance the pressor response to epinephrine, resulting in hypertension and bradycardia. Many nonsteroidal anti-inflammatory drugs, such as ibuprofen and indomethacin, can reduce the hypotensive effect of beta-blockers after 3 or more weeks of therapy with the NSAID. Short-term NSAID use (ie, 3 days) requires no special precautions in patients taking beta-blockers.

Effects on Bleeding No information available to require special precautions

Adverse Effects

>10%: Ocular: Stinging/burning eyes

1% to 10%:

- Cardiovascular: Bradycardia, arrhythmia, hypotension
- Central nervous system: Dizziness, headache
- Dermatologic: Alopecia, erythema
- Local: Stinging, burning
- Ocular: Blepharoconjunctivitis, conjunctivitis
- Respiratory: Bronchospasm

General Dosage Range Ophthalmic: *Adults:* Instill 1 drop in the affected eye(s) 1-2 times/day

Mechanism of Action A nonselective beta-adrenergic blocking agent that lowers intraocular pressure by reducing aqueous humor production and possibly increases the outflow of aqueous humor

Pharmacodynamics/Kinetics

Duration of Action 1 day

Pregnancy Risk Factor C

Levocabastine (Nasal) (LEE voe kab as teen)

Canadian Brand Names Livostin®

Pharmacologic Category Histamine H_1 Antagonist; Histamine H_1 Antagonist, Second Generation; Piperidine Derivative

Use Symptomatic treatment of allergic rhinitis

Local Anesthetic/Vasoconstrictor Precautions No information available to require special precautions

Effects on Dental Treatment Key adverse event(s) related to dental treatment: Xerostomia (normal salivary flow resumes upon discontinuation)

Effects on Bleeding No information available to require special precautions

Adverse Effects Note: Most adverse reactions are transient; incidence often similar to placebo.

1% to 10%:

- Central nervous system: Somnolence (4%), headache (3%), fatigue (1%)
- Gastrointestinal: Xerostomia (3%)
- Respiratory: Nasal irritation (5%), epistaxis (1%)

General Dosage Range Intranasal: *Children ≥12 years and Adults ≤65 years:* 2 sprays in each nostril 2-4 times/day

Mechanism of Action Potent, selective histamine H_1-receptor antagonist

Pharmacodynamics/Kinetics

Onset of Action 10 minutes

Half-life Elimination 33 hours

Product Availability Not available in U.S.

Levocabastine (Ophthalmic) (LEE voe kab as teen)

Canadian Brand Names Livostin® Eye Drops

Pharmacologic Category Histamine H_1 Antagonist; Histamine H_1 Antagonist, Second Generation; Piperidine Derivative

Use Treatment of seasonal allergic conjunctivitis

Local Anesthetic/Vasoconstrictor Precautions No information available to require special precautions

Effects on Dental Treatment No significant effects or complications reported

Effects on Bleeding No information available to require special precautions

Adverse Effects

>10%: Ocular: Irritation (16%; similar to placebo)

1% to 10%:

- Central nervous system: Fatigue (2%)
- Respiratory: Epistaxis (1%)

General Dosage Range Ophthalmic: *Children ≥12 years and Adults ≤65 years:* Instill 1 drop in affected eye(s) 2-4 times/day

Mechanism of Action Potent, selective histamine H_1-receptor antagonist for topical ophthalmic use

Pharmacodynamics/Kinetics

Onset of Action 10-15 minutes

Half-life Elimination 33 hours

Product Availability Not available in U.S.

LevOCARNitine (lee voe KAR ni teen)

U.S. Brand Names Carnitine-300 [OTC]; Carnitor®; Carnitor® SF; L-Carnitine® [OTC]

Canadian Brand Names Carnitor®

Pharmacologic Category Dietary Supplement

Use

Oral: Primary systemic carnitine deficiency; acute and chronic treatment of patients with an inborn error of metabolism which results in secondary carnitine deficiency

I.V.: Acute and chronic treatment of patients with an inborn error of metabolism which results in secondary carnitine deficiency; prevention and treatment of carnitine deficiency in patients with end-stage renal disease (ESRD) who are undergoing hemodialysis.

Local Anesthetic/Vasoconstrictor Precautions No information available to require special precautions

Effects on Dental Treatment Key adverse event(s) related to dental treatment: Taste perversion.

Effects on Bleeding No information available to require special precautions

Adverse Effects Frequencies noted with I.V. therapy (hemodialysis patients).

>10%:

- Cardiovascular: Hypertension (18% to 21%), chest pain (6% to 15%)
- Central nervous system: Headache (3% to 37%), dizziness (10% to 18%), fever (5% to 12%)
- Endocrine & metabolic: Hypercalcemia (6% to 15%)
- Gastrointestinal: Diarrhea (9% to 35%), vomiting (9% to 21%), abdominal pain (5% to 21%), nausea (9% to 12%)
- Hematologic: Anemia (3% to 12%)
- Neuromuscular & skeletal: Weakness (8% to 12%), paresthesia (3% to 12%)
- Respiratory: Cough (10% to 18%), rhinitis (6% to 11%)
- Miscellaneous: Infection (10% to 24%)

1% to 10%:

- Cardiovascular: Tachycardia (5% to 9%), hemorrhage (2% to 9%), palpitation (3% to 8%), peripheral edema (3% to 6%), atrial fibrillation (2% to 6%), ECG abnormality (2% to 6%), vascular disorder (2% to 6%)
- Central nervous system: Depression (5% to 6%), vertigo (2% to 6%)
- Dermatologic: Rash (3% to 5%)
- Endocrine & metabolic: Parathyroid disorder (2% to 6%)

Gastrointestinal: Taste perversion (2% to 9%), weight loss (3% to 8%), anorexia (3% to 6%), gastrointestinal disorder (2% to 6%), melena (2% to 6%), weight gain (2% to 6%)
Ocular: Amblyopia (3% to 6%), eye disorder (3% to 6%)
Respiratory: Bronchitis (3% to 5%)
Miscellaneous: Allergic reaction (2% to 6%)

Frequency not defined: Body odor, gastritis, seizure

General Dosage Range

I.V.:

Children: 50 mg/kg/day in divided doses (maximum: 300 mg/kg/day)

Adults: 50 mg/kg/day (maximum: 300 mg/kg/day) **or** 20 mg/kg after each hemodialysis session

Oral:

Infants and Children: Initial: 50 mg/kg/day; Maintenance: 50-100 mg/kg/day in divided doses (maximum: 3 g/day)

Adults: 990 mg (tablet) 2-3 times/day **or** 1-3 g/day (solution)

Mechanism of Action Carnitine is a naturally occurring metabolic compound which functions as a carrier molecule for long-chain fatty acids within the mitochondria, facilitating energy production. Carnitine deficiency is associated with accumulation of excess acyl CoA esters and disruption of intermediary metabolism. Carnitine supplementation increases carnitine plasma concentrations. The effects on specific metabolic alterations have not been evaluated. ESRD patients on maintenance HD may have low plasma carnitine levels because of reduced intake of meat and dairy products, reduced renal synthesis, and dialytic losses. Certain clinical conditions (malaise, muscle weakness, cardiomyopathy and arrhythmias) in HD patients may be related to carnitine deficiency.

Pharmacodynamics/Kinetics

Half-life Elimination 17.4 hours

Time to Peak Oral: 3.3 hours

Pregnancy Risk Factor B

Levocetirizine (LEE vo se TI ra zeen)

U.S. Brand Names Xyzal®

Pharmacologic Category Histamine H_1 Antagonist; Histamine H_1 Antagonist, Second Generation; Piperazine Derivative

Use Relief of symptoms of perennial and seasonal allergic rhinitis; treatment of skin manifestations (uncomplicated) of chronic idiopathic urticaria

Local Anesthetic/Vasoconstrictor Precautions No information available to require special precautions

Effects on Dental Treatment Key adverse event(s) related to dental treatment: Xerostomia and changes in salivation (normal salivary flow resumes upon discontinuation).

Effects on Bleeding No information available to require special precautions

Adverse Effects

>10%: Gastrointestinal: Diarrhea (children 4% to 13%)

1% to 10%:

Central nervous system: Somnolence (2% to 6%), fever (children 4%), fatigue (1% to 4%)
Gastrointestinal: Constipation (children 7%), vomiting (children 4%), xerostomia (2% to 3%)
Neuromuscular & skeletal: Weakness (2%)
Otic: Otitis media (children 3%)
Respiratory: Nasopharyngitis (4% to 6%), cough (children 3%), epistaxis (children 2%), pharyngitis (1% to 2%)

The following potentially-severe adverse reactions have been reported with cetirizine and, therefore, may also occur with levocetirizine: Cholestasis, glomerulonephritis, hallucination, hypotension (severe), orofacial dyskinesia, suicidal ideation

General Dosage Range Dosage adjustment recommended in patients with renal impairment

Oral:

Children 6 months to 5 years: 1.25 mg once daily

Children 6-11 years: 2.5 mg once daily

Children ≥12 years and Adults: 2.5-5 mg once daily

Mechanism of Action Levocetirizine is an antihistamine which selectively competes with histamine for H_1-receptor sites on effector cells in the gastrointestinal tract, blood vessels, and respiratory tract. Levocetirizine, the active enantiomer of cetirizine, has twice the binding affinity at the H1-receptor compared to cetirizine.

Pharmacodynamics/Kinetics

Onset of Action 1 hour

Duration of Action 24 hours

Half-life Elimination Children: ~6 hours; Adults: ~8-9 hours; Renal impairment: 11-34 hours; End-stage renal disease: 46 hours

Time to Peak Children: 1.2 hours; Adults: Oral solution: 0.5 hours, Tablet: 0.9 hours

Pregnancy Risk Factor B

Levodopa, Carbidopa, and Entacapone

(lee voe DOE pa, kar bi DOE pa, & en TA ka pone)

Related Information

Carbidopa *on page 307*

Entacapone *on page 602*

U.S. Brand Names Stalevo®

Canadian Brand Names Stalevo®

Pharmacologic Category Anti-Parkinson's Agent, COMT Inhibitor; Anti-Parkinson's Agent, Decarboxylase Inhibitor; Anti-Parkinson's Agent, Dopamine Precursor

Use Treatment of idiopathic Parkinson's disease

Local Anesthetic/Vasoconstrictor Precautions No information available to require special precautions

Effects on Dental Treatment No significant effects or complications reported

Effects on Bleeding No information available to require special precautions

Adverse Effects See individual agents.

General Dosage Range Oral: *Adults:* 1 tablet (50-200 mg levodopa/12.5-50 mg carbidopa/200 mg entacapone) at each dosing interval (maximum: 1600 mg/day entacapone or 300 mg/day carbidopa)

Mechanism of Action

Levodopa: The metabolic precursor of dopamine, a chemical depleted in Parkinson's disease. Levodopa is able to circulate in the plasma and cross the blood-brain-barrier (BBB), where it is converted by striatal enzymes to dopamine.

Carbidopa: Inhibits the peripheral plasma breakdown of levodopa by inhibiting its decarboxylation; increases available levodopa at the BBB

Entacapone: A reversible and selective inhibitor of catechol-O-methyltransferase (COMT). Alters the pharmacokinetics of levodopa, resulting in more sustained levodopa serum levels and increased concentrations available for absorption across the BBB.

Pregnancy Risk Factor C

Levofloxacin (Systemic) (lee voe FLOKS a sin)

Related Information

Clinical Risk Related to Drugs Prolonging QT Interval *on page 1872*

Sexually-Transmitted Diseases *on page 1903*

Related Sample Prescriptions

Bacterial Infections and Periodontal Diseases *on page 1983*

U.S. Brand Names Levaquin®

Canadian Brand Names Levaquin®; Novo-Levofloxacin; PMS-Levofloxacin

Generic Availability (U.S.) No

Pharmacologic Category Antibiotic, Quinolone; Respiratory Fluoroquinolone

Use Treatment of community-acquired pneumonia, including multidrug resistant strains of *S. pneumoniae* (MDRSP); nosocomial pneumonia; chronic bronchitis (acute bacterial exacerbation); acute bacterial sinusitis; prostatitis, urinary tract infection (uncomplicated or complicated); acute pyelonephritis; skin or skin structure infections (uncomplicated or complicated); reduce incidence or disease progression of inhalational anthrax (postexposure)

Unlabeled/Investigational Use Diverticulitis, enterocolitis (*Shigella* spp), epididymitis (nongonococcal), gonococcal infections, complicated intra-abdominal infections (in combination with metronidazole), Legionnaires' disease, peritonitis, PID

Note: As of April 2007, the CDC no longer recommends the use of fluoroquinolones for the treatment of gonococcal disease.

Local Anesthetic/Vasoconstrictor Precautions Levofloxacin is one of the drugs confirmed to prolong the QT interval and is accepted as having a risk of causing torsade de pointes. The risk of drug-induced torsade de pointes is extremely low when a single QT interval prolonging drug is prescribed. In terms of epinephrine, it is not known what effect vasoconstrictors in the local anesthetic regimen will have in patients with a known history of congenital prolonged QT interval or in patients taking any medication that prolongs the QT interval. Until more information is obtained, it is suggested that the clinician consult with the physician prior to the use of a vasoconstrictor in suspected patients, and that the vasoconstrictor (epinephrine, mepivacaine and levonordefrin [Carbocaine® 2% with Neo-Cobefrin®]) be used with caution.

Effects on Dental Treatment No significant effects or complications reported

Effects on Bleeding No information available to require special precautions

Adverse Effects 1% to 10%:

Cardiovascular: Chest pain (1%), edema (1%)

Central nervous system: Headache (6%), insomnia (4%), dizziness (3%), fatigue (1%), pain (1%)

Dermatologic: Rash (2%), pruritus (1%)

Gastrointestinal: Nausea (7%), diarrhea (5%), constipation (3%), abdominal pain (2%), dyspepsia (2%), vomiting (2%)

Genitourinary: Vaginitis (1%)

Local: Injection site reaction (1%)

Respiratory: Pharyngitis (4%), dyspnea (1%)

Miscellaneous: Moniliasis (1%)

Dosage Note: Sequential therapy (intravenous to oral) may be instituted based on prescriber's discretion.

Usual dosage range: Adults: Oral, I.V.: 250-500 mg every 24 hours; severe or complicated infections: 750 mg every 24 hours

Indication-specific dosing:

Children ≥6 months and Adults: Oral, I.V.:

Anthrax (inhalational, postexposure):

≤50 kg: 8 mg/kg every 12 hours for 60 days (do not exceed 250 mg/dose), beginning as soon as possible after exposure

>50 kg and Adults: 500 mg every 24 hours for 60 days, beginning as soon as possible after exposure

Adults: Oral, I.V.:

Chronic bronchitis (acute bacterial exacerbation): 500 mg every 24 hours for at least 7 days

Diverticulitis, peritonitis (unlabeled use): 750 mg every 24 hours for 7-10 days; use adjunctive metronidazole therapy

Dysenteric enterocolitis, *Shigella* spp. (unlabeled use): 500 mg every 24 hours for 3-5 days

Epididymitis, nongonococcal (unlabeled use): 500 mg once daily for 10 days

Gonococcal infection (unlabeled use):

Cervicitis, urethritis: 250 mg for one dose with azithromycin or doxycycline; **Note:** As of April 2007, the CDC no longer recommends the use of fluoroquinolones for the treatment of uncomplicated gonococcal disease.

Disseminated infection: 250 mg I.V. once daily; 24 hours after symptoms improve may change to 500 mg orally every 24 hours to complete total therapy of 7 days; **Note:** As of April 2007, the CDC no longer recommends the use of fluoroquinolones for the treatment of more serious gonococcal disease, unless no other options exist and susceptibility can be confirmed via culture.

Intra-abdominal infection, complicated, community-acquired (in combination with metronidazole) (unlabeled use): I.V.: 750 mg once daily for 4-7 days (provided source controlled). **Note:** Avoid using in settings where *E. coli* susceptibility to fluoroquinolones is <90%.

Pelvic inflammatory disease (unlabeled use): 500 mg once daily for 14 days with or without adjunctive metronidazole; **Note:** The CDC recommends use only if standard cephalosporin therapy is not feasible and community prevalence of quinolone-resistant gonococcal organisms is low. Culture sensitivity must be confirmed.

Pneumonia:

Community-acquired: 500 mg every 24 hours for 7-14 days or 750 mg every 24 hours for 5 days (efficacy of 5-day regimen for MDRSP not established)

Nosocomial: 750 mg every 24 hours for 7-14 days

Prostatitis (chronic bacterial): 500 mg every 24 hours for 28 days

Sinusitis (acute bacterial): 500 mg every 24 hours for 10-14 days or 750 mg every 24 hours for 5 days

Skin and skin structure infections:

Uncomplicated: 500 mg every 24 hours for 7-10 days

Complicated: 750 mg every 24 hours for 7-14 days

Traveler's diarrhea (unlabeled use): 500 mg for one dose

Urinary tract infections:

Uncomplicated: 250 mg once daily for 3 days

Complicated, including pyelonephritis: 250 mg once daily for 10 days **or** 750 mg once daily for 5 days

Dosing adjustment in renal impairment:

Normal renal function dosing of 750 mg/day:

Cl_{cr} 20-49 mL/minute: Administer 750 mg every 48 hours

Cl_{cr} 10-19 mL/minute: Administer 750 mg initial dose, followed by 500 mg every 48 hours

Hemodialysis/CAPD: Administer 750 mg initial dose, followed by 500 mg every 48 hours

Normal renal function dosing of 500 mg/day:

Cl_{cr} 20-49 mL/minute: Administer 500 mg initial dose, followed by 250 mg every 24 hours

Cl_{cr} 10-19 mL/minute: Administer 500 mg initial dose, followed by 250 mg every 48 hours

Hemodialysis/CAPD: Administer 500 mg initial dose, followed by 250 mg every 48 hours

Normal renal function dosing of 250 mg/day:

Cl_{cr} 20-49 mL/minute: No dosage adjustment required

Cl_{cr} 10-19 mL/minute: Administer 250 mg every 48 hours (except in uncomplicated UTI, where no dosage adjustment is required)

Hemodialysis/CAPD: No information available

CRRT: **Note:** Clearance dependent on filter type, flow rates, and other variables.

CVVH/CVVHD/CVVHDF: Alternative recommendations exist:

500 mg every 48 hours **or**

250 mg every 24 hours (**Note:** This regimen has been shown to be equivalent to 500 mg/day in normal renal function. Appropriateness of this regimen for target dosing equal to 750 mg/day is not known.)

Mechanism of Action As the S(-) enantiomer of the fluoroquinolone, ofloxacin, levofloxacin, inhibits DNA-gyrase in susceptible organisms thereby inhibits relaxation of supercoiled DNA and promotes breakage of DNA strands. DNA gyrase (topoisomerase II), is an essential bacterial enzyme that maintains the superhelical structure of DNA and is required for DNA replication and transcription, DNA repair, recombination, and transposition.

Contraindications Hypersensitivity to levofloxacin, any component of the formulation, or other quinolones

Warnings/Precautions [U.S. Boxed Warning]: There have been reports of tendon inflammation and/or rupture with quinolone antibiotics; risk may be increased with concurrent corticosteroids, organ transplant recipients, and in patients >60 years of age. Rupture of the Achilles tendon sometimes requiring surgical repair has been reported most frequently; but other tendon sites (eg, rotator cuff, biceps) have also been reported. Strenuous physical activity, rheumatoid arthritis, and renal impairment may be an independent risk factor for tendonitis. Discontinue at first sign of tendon inflammation or pain. May occur even after discontinuation of therapy. Use with caution in patients with rheumatoid arthritis; may increase risk of tendon rupture. Systemic use is only recommended in children <18 years of age for the prevention of inhalational anthrax (postexposure); increased incidence of musculoskeletal disorders (eg, arthralgia, tendon rupture) has been observed in children; CNS stimulation may occur (tremor, restlessness, confusion, and very rarely hallucinations or seizures). Potential for seizures, although very rare, may be increased with concomitant NSAID therapy. Use with caution in individuals at risk of seizures, with known or suspected CNS disorders or renal dysfunction. Avoid excessive sunlight and take precautions to limit exposure (eg, loose fitting clothing, sunscreen); may cause moderate-to-severe phototoxicity reactions. Discontinue use if photosensitivity occurs.

Rare cases of torsade de pointes have been reported in patients receiving levofloxacin. Use caution in patients with known prolongation of QT interval, bradycardia, hypokalemia, hypomagnesemia, or in those receiving concurrent therapy with Class Ia or Class III antiarrhythmics.

Severe hypersensitivity reactions, including anaphylaxis, have occurred with quinolone therapy. Reactions may present as typical allergic symptoms after a single dose, or may manifest as severe idiosyncratic dermatologic, vascular, pulmonary, renal, hepatic, and/or hematologic events, usually after multiple doses. Prompt discontinuation of drug should occur if skin rash or other symptoms arise. Prolonged use may result in fungal or bacterial superinfection, including *C. difficile*-associated diarrhea (CDAD) and pseudomembranous colitis; CDAD has been observed >2 months postantibiotic treatment. Peripheral neuropathies have been linked to levofloxacin use; discontinue if numbness, tingling, or weakness develops. **[U.S. Boxed Warning]: Quinolones may exacerbate myasthenia gravis; avoid use (rare, potentially life-threatening weakness of respiratory muscles may occur).** Unrelated to hypersensitivity, severe hepatotoxicity (including acute hepatitis and fatalities) has been reported. Elderly patients may be at greater risk. Discontinue therapy immediately if signs and symptoms of hepatitis occur. Hemolytic reactions may (rarely) occur with quinolone use in patients with latent or actual G6PD deficiency.

Fluoroquinolones have been associated with the development of serious, and sometimes fatal, hypoglycemia, most often in elderly diabetics, but also in patients without diabetes. This occurred most frequently with gatifloxacin (no longer available systemically) but may occur at a lower frequency with other quinolones.

Drug Interactions

Avoid Concomitant Use

Avoid concomitant use of Levofloxacin (Systemic) with any of the following: Artemether; BCG; Dronedarone; Lumefantrine; Nilotinib; Pimozide; QuiNINE; Tetrabenazine; Thioridazine; Toremifene; Vandetanib; Ziprasidone

Increased Effect/Toxicity

Levofloxacin (Systemic) may increase the levels/effects of: Corticosteroids (Systemic); Dronedarone; Pimozide; QTc-Prolonging Agents; QuiNINE; Sulfonylureas; Tetrabenazine; Thioridazine; Toremifene; Vandetanib; Vitamin K Antagonists; Ziprasidone

The levels/effects of Levofloxacin (Systemic) may be increased by: Alfuzosin; Artemether; Chloroquine; Ciprofloxacin; Ciprofloxacin (Systemic); Gadobutrol; Insulin; Lumefantrine; Nilotinib; Nonsteroidal Anti-Inflammatory Agents; Probenecid; QuiNINE

Decreased Effect

Levofloxacin (Systemic) may decrease the levels/effects of: BCG; Mycophenolate; Sulfonylureas; Typhoid Vaccine

The levels/effects of Levofloxacin (Systemic) may be decreased by: Antacids; Calcium Salts; Didanosine; Iron Salts; Lanthanum; Magnesium Salts; Quinapril; Sevelamer; Sucralfate; Zinc Salts

Dietary Considerations Tablets may be taken without regard to meals. Oral solution should be administered on an empty stomach (1 hour before or 2 hours after a meal). Take 2 hours before or 2 hours after multiple vitamins, antacids, or other products containing magnesium, aluminum, iron, or zinc.

Pharmacodynamics/Kinetics

Half-life Elimination ~6-8 hours

Time to Peak 1-2 hours

Pregnancy Risk Factor C

Lactation Enters breast milk/not recommended

Breast-Feeding Considerations Based on data from a case report, small amounts of levofloxacin are excreted in breast milk. Breast-feeding is not recommended by the manufacturer. Levofloxacin is the L-isomer of ofloxacin. Ofloxacin has also been shown to have minimal concentrations in human milk. Nondose-related effects could include modification of bowel flora.

Dosage Forms

Infusion, premixed in D_5W [preservative free]:

Levaquin®: 250 mg (50 mL); 500 mg (100 mL); 750 mg (150 mL)

Injection, solution [preservative free]:

Levaquin®: 25 mg/mL (20 mL, 30 mL)

Solution, oral:

Levaquin®: 25 mg/mL (480 mL)

Tablet, oral:

Levaquin®: 250 mg, 500 mg, 750 mg

Dental Comment Levofloxacin is known to prolong the QT interval. The QT interval is measured as the time and distance between the Q point of the QRS complex and the end of the T wave in the ECG tracing. After adjustment for heart rate, the QT interval is defined as prolonged if it is more than 450 msec in men and 460 msec in women. A long QT syndrome was first described in the 1950s and 60s as a congenital syndrome involving QT interval prolongation and syncope and sudden death. Some of the congenital long QT syndromes were characterized by a peculiar electrocardiographic appearance of the QRS complex involving a premature atria beat followed by a pause, then a subsequent sinus beat showing marked QT prolongation and deformity. This type of cardiac arrhythmia was originally termed "torsade de pointes" (translated from the French as "twisting of the points"). Levofloxacin is considered as having a risk of causing torsade de pointes. Since it is not known what effect vasoconstrictors in the local anesthetic regimen will have in patients with a known history of congenital prolonged QT interval or in patients taking any medication that prolongs the QT interval, a medical consult is suggested.

LEVOleucovorin (lee voe loo koe VOR in)

U.S. Brand Names Fusilev™

Pharmacologic Category Antidote; Chemotherapy Modulating Agent; Rescue Agent (Chemotherapy)

Use Treatment of advanced, metastatic colorectal cancer (palliative) in combination with fluorouracil; rescue agent after high-dose methotrexate therapy in osteosarcoma; antidote for impaired methotrexate elimination and for inadvertent overdosage of folic acid antagonists

Local Anesthetic/Vasoconstrictor Precautions No information available to require special precautions

Effects on Dental Treatment Key adverse event(s) related to dental treatment: Stomatitis and taste perversion.

Effects on Bleeding No information available to require special precautions

Adverse Effects Note: Adverse reactions reported with levoleucovorin either as a part of combination chemotherapy or following chemotherapy.

>10%:

Central nervous system: Fatigue (≤29%)

Dermatologic: Dermatitis (6% to 29%), alopecia (≤26%)

Gastrointestinal: Stomatitis (38% to 72%; grades 3/4: 6% to 12%), diarrhea (6% to 70%; grades 3/4: ≤19%), nausea (19% to 62%), vomiting (38% to 40%), anorexia/appetite decreased (≤24%), abdominal pain (≤14%)

Neuromuscular & skeletal: Weakness/malaise (≤29%)

1% to 10%:

Central nervous system: Confusion (6%)

Gastrointestinal: Dyspepsia (6%), taste perversion (6%), typhlitis (6%)

Neuromuscular & skeletal: Neuropathy (6%)

Renal: Renal function abnormal (6%)

Respiratory: Dyspnea (6%)

General Dosage Range I.V.: *Children and Adults:* Dosing varies greatly depending on indication

Mechanism of Action Levoleucovorin counteracts the toxic (and therapeutic) effects of folic acid antagonists (eg, methotrexate) which act by inhibiting dihydrofolate reductase. Levoleucovorin is the levo isomeric and pharmacologic active form of leucovorin (levoleucovorin does not require reduction by dihydrofolate reductase). A reduced derivative of folic acid, leucovorin supplies the necessary cofactor blocked by methotrexate.

Leucovorin enhances the activity (and toxicity) of fluorouracil by stabilizing the binding of 5-fluoro-2'-deoxyuridine-5'-monophosphate (FdUMP; a fluorouracil metabolite) to thymidylate synthetase resulting in inhibition of this enzyme.

Pharmacodynamics/Kinetics

Half-life Elimination 15 mg: 5-7 hours; 300 mg: elimination half life: 16-30 hours

Time to Peak Serum: I.V.: 0.9 hours

Pregnancy Risk Factor C

Product Availability

Fusilev™ solution for injection: FDA approved April 2011; availability expected in the third quarter of 2011

Fusilev™ solution for injection is a ready-to-use formulation and will be available in 175 mg/17.5 mL and 250 mg/25 mL presentations.

Levonorgestrel (LEE voe nor jes trel)

Related Information

Endocrine Disorders and Pregnancy *on page 1879*

U.S. Brand Names Mirena®; Next Choice™; Plan B® One Step

Canadian Brand Names Mirena®; Plan B®

Pharmacologic Category Contraceptive; Progestin

Use

Intrauterine device (IUD): Prevention of pregnancy; treatment of heavy menstrual bleeding in women who also choose to use an IUD for contraception

Oral: Emergency contraception following unprotected intercourse or possible contraceptive failure

Plan B® One-Step is approved for OTC use by women ≥17 years of age and available by prescription only for women <17 years of age. Next Choice™ (generic of the original Plan-B® 2-dose regimen) is also approved for OTC use by women ≥17 years of age and by prescription only for women <17 years of age.

Local Anesthetic/Vasoconstrictor Precautions No information available to require special precautions

Effects on Dental Treatment No significant effects or complications reported

Effects on Bleeding No information available to require special precautions

Adverse Effects

Intrauterine device:

>5%:

Central nervous system: Headache/migraine (8%), depression (6%)

Dermatologic: Acne (7%)

Endocrine & metabolic: Amenorrhea (24%; 20% at 1 year), enlarged follicles (12%), menorrhagia (6%), breast pain/tenderness (5%), ovarian cysts

Gastrointestinal: Abdominal pain (12%)

Genitourinary: Uterine/vaginal bleeding alterations (52%), intermenstrual bleeding/spotting (23%), pelvic pain (13%), leukorrhea (5%)

Miscellaneous: Ectopic pregnancy (≤50%), IUD expulsion (5%)

Oral tablets:

>10%:

Central nervous system: Fatigue (13% to 17%), headache (10% to 17%), dizziness (10% to 11%)

Endocrine & metabolic: Heavier menstrual bleeding (14% to 31%), lighter menstrual bleeding (12%), breast tenderness (8% to 11%)

Gastrointestinal: Nausea (14% to 23%), abdominal pain (13% to 18%)

1% to 10%:

Endocrine & metabolic: Menses delayed (5%)

Gastrointestinal: Vomiting (6%), diarrhea (5%)

General Dosage Range

Intrauterine: *Adults:* Insert into uterine cavity, releases 20 mcg/day over 5 years

Oral: *Adults:* 0.75 mg every 12 hours for 2 doses **or** 1.5 mg as a single dose

Mechanism of Action Pregnancy may be prevented through several mechanisms: Thickening of cervical mucus, which inhibits sperm passage through the uterus and sperm survival; inhibition of ovulation, from a negative feedback mechanism on the hypothalamus, leading to reduced secretion of follicle stimulating hormone (FSH) and luteinizing hormone (LH); and inhibition of implantation. Levonorgestrel is not effective once the implantation process has begun.

Pharmacodynamics/Kinetics

Duration of Action Intrauterine device: Up to 5 years

Half-life Elimination Oral: ~24 hours

Time to Peak Oral: ~2 hours

Prescribing and Access Restrictions Plan B® One-Step will be limited to pharmacies or healthcare clinics with a valid license to distribute prescription products. Because there will be one package for both OTC and prescription use, pharmacies are required to keep the product behind the counter.

Levorphanol (lee VOR fa nole)

Pharmacologic Category Analgesic, Opioid

Use Relief of moderate-to-severe pain; preoperative sedation/analgesia; management of chronic pain (eg, cancer) requiring opioid therapy

Local Anesthetic/Vasoconstrictor Precautions No information available to require special precautions

Effects on Dental Treatment Key adverse event(s) related to dental treatment: Xerostomia (normal salivary flow resumes upon discontinuation).

Effects on Bleeding No information available to require special precautions

Adverse Effects Frequency not defined.

Cardiovascular: Palpitation, hypotension, bradycardia, peripheral vasodilation, cardiac arrest, shock, tachycardia

Central nervous system: CNS depression, fatigue, drowsiness, dizziness, nervousness, headache, restlessness, anorexia, malaise, confusion, coma, convulsion, insomnia, amnesia, mental depression, hallucinations, paradoxical CNS stimulation, intracranial pressure (increased)

Dermatologic: Pruritus, urticaria, rash

Endocrine & metabolic: Antidiuretic hormone release

Gastrointestinal: Nausea, vomiting, dyspepsia, stomach cramps, xerostomia, constipation, abdominal pain, dry mouth, biliary tract spasm, paralytic ileus

Genitourinary: Decreased urination, urinary tract spasm, urinary retention

Neuromuscular & skeletal: Weakness

Ocular: Miosis, diplopia

Respiratory: Respiratory depression, apnea, hypoventilation, cyanosis

Miscellaneous: Histamine release, physical and psychological dependence

General Dosage Range Dosage adjustment recommended in patients with hepatic impairment

Oral: *Adults:* 2-4 mg every 6-8 hours as needed

Mechanism of Action Levorphanol tartrate is a synthetic opioid agonist that is classified as a morphinan derivative. Opioids interact with stereospecific opioid receptors in various parts of the central nervous system and other tissues. Analgesic potency parallels the affinity for these binding sites. These drugs do not alter the threshold or responsiveness to pain, but the perception of pain.

Pharmacodynamics/Kinetics

Onset of Action Oral: 10-60 minutes

Duration of Action 4-8 hours

Half-life Elimination 11-16 hours

Pregnancy Risk Factor B/D (prolonged use or high doses at term)

Controlled Substance C-II

Levothyroxine (lee voe thye ROKS een)

Related Information

Endocrine Disorders and Pregnancy *on page 1879*

U.S. Brand Names Levothroid®; Levoxyl®; Synthroid®; Tirosint®; Unithroid®

Canadian Brand Names Eltroxin®; Euthyrox; Levothyroxine Sodium; Synthroid®

Generic Availability (U.S.) Yes

Pharmacologic Category Thyroid Product

Use Replacement or supplemental therapy in hypothyroidism; pituitary TSH suppression

Unlabeled/Investigational Use Management of hemodynamically unstable potential organ donors increasing the quantity of organs available for transplantation

Local Anesthetic/Vasoconstrictor Precautions No precautions with vasoconstrictor are necessary if patient is well controlled with levothyroxine

Effects on Dental Treatment No significant effects or complications reported

Effects on Bleeding No information available to require special precautions

Adverse Effects Frequency not defined.

Cardiovascular: Angina, arrhythmia, cardiac arrest, flushing, heart failure, hypertension, MI, palpitation, pulse increased, tachycardia

Central nervous system: Anxiety, emotional lability, fatigue, fever, headache, hyperactivity, insomnia, irritability, nervousness, pseudotumor cerebri (children), seizure (rare)

Dermatologic: Alopecia

Endocrine & metabolic: Fertility impaired, menstrual irregularities

Gastrointestinal: Abdominal cramps, appetite increased, diarrhea, vomiting, weight loss

Hepatic: Liver function tests increased

Neuromuscular & skeletal: Bone mineral density decreased, muscle weakness, tremor, slipped capital femoral epiphysis (children)

Respiratory: Dyspnea

Miscellaneous: Diaphoresis, heat intolerance, hypersensitivity (to inactive ingredients, symptoms include urticaria, pruritus, rash, flushing, angioedema, GI symptoms, fever, arthralgia, serum sickness, wheezing)

Levoxyl®: Choking, dysphagia, gagging

Dosage Doses should be adjusted based on clinical response and laboratory parameters.

Oral:

Neonates, Infants, and Children: Hypothyroidism: Daily dosage based on body weight and age as listed below:

0-3 months: 10-15 mcg/kg/day; if the infant is at risk for development of cardiac failure, use a lower starting dose of 25 mcg/day; if the initial serum T_4 is very low (<5 mcg/dL) begin treatment at a higher dosage of 50 mcg/day

3-6 months: 8-10 mcg/kg/day **or** 25-50 mcg/day

6-12 months: 6-8 mcg/kg/day **or** 50-75 mcg/day

1-5 years: 5-6 mcg/kg/day **or** 75-100 mcg/day

6-12 years: 4-5 mcg/kg/day **or** 100-125 mcg/day

>12 years: 2-3 mcg/kg/day **or** ≥150 mcg/day

Growth and puberty complete: 1.7 mcg/kg/day; refer to Adult dosing.

Dosing modifications:

Hyperactivity in older children may be minimized by starting at 1/4 of the recommended dose and increasing each week by that amount until the full dose is achieved (4 weeks).

Children with severe or chronic hypothyroidism should be started at 25 mcg/day; adjust dose by 25 mcg every 2-4 weeks.

Adults (including children in whom growth and puberty are complete, healthy adults <50 years of age, and older adults who have been recently treated for hyperthyroidism or who have been hypothyroid for only a few months):

Hypothyroidism: ~1.7 mcg/kg/day; usual doses are ≤200 mcg/day (range: 100-125 mcg/day [70 kg adult]); doses ≥300 mcg/day are rare (consider poor compliance, malabsorption, and/or drug interactions). Titrate dose every 6 weeks.

Patients >50 years or patients with cardiac disease: Refer to Elderly dosing.

Severe hypothyroidism: Initial: 12.5-25 mcg/day; adjust dose by 25 mcg/day every 2-4 weeks as appropriate

Myxedema: Oral agents are not recommended for myxedema: Refer to I.V. dosing.

Subclinical hypothyroidism (if treated): 1 mcg/kg/day

TSH suppression:

Well-differentiated thyroid cancer: Highly individualized; Doses >2 mcg/kg/day may be needed to suppress TSH to <0.1 mIU/L in intermediate- to high-risk tumors. Low-risk tumors may be maintained at or slightly below the lower limit of normal (0.1-0.5 mIU/L) (Cooper, 2009).

Benign nodules and nontoxic multinodular goiter: Routine use of T_4 for TSH suppression is not recommended in patients with benign thyroid nodules. In patients deemed appropriate candidates, treatment should never be fully suppressive (TSH <0.1 mIU/L) (Cooper, 2009; Gharib, 2010). Avoid use if TSH is already suppressed.

Elderly: Hypothyroidism (elderly patients may require <1 mcg/kg/day):

>50 years without cardiac disease **or** <50 years with cardiac disease: Initial: 25-50 mcg/day; adjust dose by 12.5-25 mcg increments at 6- to 8-week intervals as needed

>50 years with cardiac disease: Initial: 12.5-25 mcg/day; adjust dose by 12.5-25 mcg increments at 4- to 6-week intervals (many clinicians prefer to adjust at 6- to 8-week intervals)

Note: Patients with combined hypothyroidism and cardiac disease should be monitored carefully for changes in stability.

I.M., I.V.: Children, Adults, Elderly: Hypothyroidism: 50% of the oral dose

I.V.:

Adults: Myxedema coma or stupor: 200-500 mcg, then 100-300 mcg the next day if necessary; smaller doses should be considered in patients with cardiovascular disease

Elderly: Myxedema coma: Refer to adult dosing; lower doses may be needed

Mechanism of Action Levothyroxine (T_4) is a synthetic form of thyroxine, an endogenous hormone secreted by the thyroid gland. T_4 is converted to its active metabolite, L-triiodothyronine (T_3). Thyroid hormones (T_4 and T_3) then bind to thyroid receptor proteins in the cell nucleus and exert metabolic effects through control of DNA transcription and protein synthesis; involved in normal metabolism, growth, and development; promotes gluconeogenesis, increases utilization and mobilization of glycogen stores, and stimulates protein synthesis, increases basal metabolic rate

Contraindications Hypersensitivity to levothyroxine sodium or any component of the formulation; acute MI; thyrotoxicosis of any etiology; uncorrected adrenal insufficiency

Capsule: Additional contraindication: Inability to swallow capsules

Warnings/Precautions [U.S. Boxed Warning]: Thyroid supplements are ineffective and potentially toxic when used for the treatment of obesity or for weight reduction, especially in euthyroid patients. High doses may produce serious or even life-threatening toxic effects particularly when used with some anorectic drugs (eg, sympathomimetic amines). Routine use of T_4 for TSH suppression is not recommended in patients with benign thyroid nodules. In patients deemed appropriate candidates, treatment should never be fully suppressive (TSH <0.1 mIU/L). Use with caution and reduce dosage in patients with angina pectoris or other cardiovascular disease; decrease initial dose. Use cautiously in the elderly since they may be more likely to have compromised cardiovascular functions. Patients with adrenal insufficiency, myxedema, diabetes mellitus and insipidus may have symptoms exaggerated or aggravated. Chronic hypothyroidism predisposes patients to coronary artery disease. Long-term therapy can decrease bone mineral density. Levoxyl® may rapidly swell and disintegrate causing choking or gagging (should be administered with a full glass of water); use caution in patients with dysphagia or other swallowing disorders.

Drug Interactions

Avoid Concomitant Use

Avoid concomitant use of Levothyroxine with any of the following: Sodium Iodide I131

Increased Effect/Toxicity

Levothyroxine may increase the levels/effects of: Vitamin K Antagonists

Decreased Effect

Levothyroxine may decrease the levels/effects of: Sodium Iodide I131; Theophylline Derivatives

The levels/effects of Levothyroxine may be decreased by: Aluminum Hydroxide; Bile Acid Sequestrants; Calcium Polystyrene Sulfonate; Calcium Salts; CarBAMazepine; Estrogen Derivatives; Fosphenytoin; Iron Salts; Orlistat; Phenytoin; Raloxifene; Rifampin; Sevelamer; Sodium Polystyrene Sulfonate; Sucralfate

Ethanol/Nutrition/Herb Interactions Food: Taking levothyroxine with enteral nutrition may cause reduced bioavailability and may lower serum thyroxine levels leading to signs or symptoms of hypothyroidism. Soybean flour (infant formula), cottonseed meal, walnuts, and dietary fiber may decrease absorption of levothyroxine from the GI tract.

Dietary Considerations Should be taken on an empty stomach, at least 30 minutes before food.

Pharmacodynamics/Kinetics

Onset of Action Therapeutic: Oral: 3-5 days; I.V. 6-8 hours; Peak effect: I.V.: 24 hours

Half-life Elimination Euthyroid: 6-7 days; Hypothyroid: 9-10 days; Hyperthyroid: 3-4 days

Time to Peak Serum: 2-4 hours

Pregnancy Risk Factor A

Lactation Enters breast milk/compatible

Breast-Feeding Considerations Minimally excreted in human milk; adequate levels are needed to maintain normal lactation

Dosage Forms

Capsule, soft gelatin, oral:

Tirosint®: 13 mcg, 25 mcg, 50 mcg, 75 mcg, 88 mcg, 100 mcg, 112 mcg, 125 mcg, 137 mcg, 150 mcg

Injection, powder for reconstitution: 200 mcg, 500 mcg

Tablet, oral: 25 mcg, 50 mcg, 75 mcg, 88 mcg, 100 mcg, 112 mcg, 125 mcg, 137 mcg, 150 mcg, 175 mcg, 200 mcg, 300 mcg

Levothroid®: 25 mcg, 50 mcg, 75 mcg, 88 mcg, 100 mcg, 112 mcg, 125 mcg, 137 mcg, 150 mcg, 175 mcg, 200 mcg, 300 mcg

Levoxyl®: 25 mcg, 50 mcg, 75 mcg, 88 mcg, 100 mcg, 112 mcg, 125 mcg, 137 mcg, 150 mcg, 175 mcg, 200 mcg

Synthroid®: 25 mcg, 50 mcg, 75 mcg, 88 mcg, 100 mcg, 112 mcg, 125 mcg, 137 mcg, 150 mcg, 175 mcg, 200 mcg, 300 mcg

Unithroid®: 25 mcg, 50 mcg, 75 mcg, 88 mcg, 100 mcg, 112 mcg, 125 mcg, 150 mcg, 175 mcg, 200 mcg, 300 mcg

Lidocaine (Systemic) (LYE doe kane)

Related Information

Cardiovascular Diseases *on page* 1848

Oral Pain *on page* 1928

U.S. Brand Names Xylocaine®; Xylocaine® Dental; Xylocaine® MPF

Canadian Brand Names Xylocard®

Generic Availability (U.S.) Yes

Pharmacologic Category Antiarrhythmic Agent, Class Ib; Local Anesthetic

Dental Use Amide-type injectable local anesthetic

Use Local and regional anesthesia by infiltration, nerve block, epidural, or spinal techniques; acute treatment of ventricular arrhythmias from myocardial infarction or cardiac manipulation

Unlabeled/Investigational Use

ACLS guidelines: Hemodynamically stable monomorphic ventricular tachycardia (VT) (preserved ventricular function); polymorphic VT (preserved ventricular function); drug-induced monomorphic VT; when amiodarone is not available, pulseless VT or ventricular fibrillation (VF) (unresponsive to defibrillation, CPR, and vasopressor administration)

PALS guidelines: When amiodarone is not available, pulseless VT or VF (unresponsive to defibrillation, CPR, and epinephrine administration); consider in patients with cocaine overdose to prevent arrhythmias secondary to MI

I.V. infusion for chronic pain syndrome

Local Anesthetic/Vasoconstrictor Precautions No information available to require special precautions

Effects on Dental Treatment Key adverse event(s) related to dental treatment: Metallic taste.

Effects on Bleeding No information available to require special precautions

Adverse Effects Effects vary with route of administration. Many effects are dose related.

Frequency not defined.

Cardiovascular: Arrhythmia, bradycardia, arterial spasms, cardiovascular collapse, defibrillator threshold increased, edema, flushing, heart block, hypotension, sinus node supression, vascular insufficiency (periarticular injections)

Central nervous system: Agitation, anxiety, apprehension, coma, confusion, disorientation, dizziness, drowsiness, euphoria, hallucinations, headache, hyperesthesia, hypoesthesia, lethargy, lightheadedness, nervousness, psychosis, seizure, slurred speech, somnolence, unconsciousness

Gastrointestinal: Metallic taste, nausea, vomiting

Local: Thrombophlebitis

Neuromuscular & skeletal: Paresthesia, transient radicular pain (subarachnoid administration; up to 1.9%), tremor, twitching, weakness

Otic: Tinnitus

Respiratory: Bronchospasm, dyspnea, respiratory depression or arrest

Miscellaneous: Allergic reactions, anaphylactoid reaction, sensitivity to temperature extremes

Following spinal anesthesia: Positional headache (3%), shivering (2%) nausea, peripheral nerve symptoms, respiratory inadequacy and double vision (<1%), hypotension, cauda equina syndrome

Dosage

Antiarrhythmic:

Children (PALS, 2010):

I.V., intraosseous (I.O.): **Note:** For use in VF or pulseless VT if amiodarone is not available; give after defibrillation attempts, CPR, and epinephrine:

Loading dose: 1 mg/kg; follow with continuous infusion; may administer second bolus of 0.5-1 mg/kg if delay between bolus and start of infusion is >15 minutes (PALS, 2000)

Continuous infusion: 20-50 mcg/kg/minute. Per the manufacturer, use a maximum of 20 mcg/kg/minute in patients with shock, hepatic disease, cardiac arrest, or CHF

Intratracheal: 2-3 mg/kg; flush with 5 mL of NS and follow with 5 assisted manual ventilations

Adults (ACLS, 2010):

VF or pulseless VT (after defibrillation attempts, CPR, and vasopressor administration) if amiodarone is not available: I.V., intraosseous (I.O.): Initial: 1-1.5 mg/kg. If refractory VF or pulseless VT, repeat with 0.5-0.75 mg/kg bolus every 5-10 minutes (maximum cumulative dose: 3 mg/kg). Follow with continuous infusion (1-4 mg/minute) after return of perfusion. Reappearance of arrhythmia during constant infusion: 0.5 mg/kg bolus and reassessment of infusion (Zipes, 2000).

Intratracheal (loading dose only): 2-3.75 mg/kg (2-2.5 times the recommended I.V. dose); dilute in 5-10 mL NS or sterile water. **Note:** Absorption is greater with sterile water and results in less impairment of PaO_2.

Hemodynamically stable monomorphic VT: I.V.: 1-1.5 mg/kg; repeat with 0.5-0.75 mg/kg every 5-10 minutes as necessary (maximum cumulative dose: 3 mg/kg). Follow with continuous infusion of 1-4 mg/minute or 30-50 mcg/kg/minute.

Note: Dose reduction (eg, of maintenance infusion) necessary in patients with CHF, shock, or hepatic disease.

Anesthetic, local injectable: Children and Adults: Varies with procedure, degree of anesthesia needed, vascularity of tissue, duration of anesthesia required, and physical condition of patient; maximum: 4.5 mg/kg/dose not to exceed 300 mg; do not repeat within 2 hours.

Dosage adjustment in renal impairment: Not dialyzable (0% to 5%) by hemo- or peritoneal dialysis; supplemental dose is not necessary.

Dosage adjustment in hepatic impairment: Dose reduction (eg, of maintenance infusion) necessary in patients with hepatic impairment; monitor lidocaine concentrations closely.

Mechanism of Action Class Ib antiarrhythmic; suppresses automaticity of conduction tissue, by increasing electrical stimulation threshold of ventricle, His-Purkinje system, and spontaneous depolarization of the ventricles during diastole by a direct action on the tissues; blocks both the initiation and conduction of nerve impulses by decreasing the neuronal membrane's permeability to sodium ions, which results in inhibition of depolarization with resultant blockade of conduction

Contraindications Hypersensitivity to lidocaine or any component of the formulation; hypersensitivity to another local anesthetic of the amide type; Adam-Stokes syndrome; severe degrees of SA, AV, or intraventricular heart block (except in patients with a functioning artificial pacemaker); premixed injection may contain corn-derived dextrose and its use is contraindicated in patients with allergy to corn-related products

Warnings/Precautions Use caution in patients with severe hepatic dysfunction or pseudocholinesterase deficiency; may have increased risk of lidocaine toxicity.

Intravenous: Constant ECG monitoring is necessary during I.V. administration. Use cautiously in hepatic impairment, any degree of heart block, Wolff-Parkinson-White syndrome, HF, marked hypoxia, severe respiratory depression, hypovolemia, history of malignant hyperthermia, or shock. Increased ventricular rate may be seen when administered to a patient with atrial fibrillation. Correct electrolyte disturbances, especially hypokalemia or hypomagnesemia, prior to use and throughout therapy. Correct any underlying causes of ventricular arrhythmias. Monitor closely for signs and symptoms of CNS toxicity. The elderly may be prone to increased CNS and cardiovascular side effects. Reduce dose in hepatic dysfunction and CHF.

Injectable anesthetic: Follow appropriate administration techniques so as not to administer any intravascularly. Continuous intra-articular infusion of local anesthetics after arthroscopic or other surgical procedures is **not** an approved use; chondrolysis (primarily in the shoulder joint) has occurred following infusion, with some cases requiring arthroplasty or shoulder replacement. Solutions containing antimicrobial preservatives should not be used for epidural or spinal anesthesia. Some solutions contain a bisulfite; avoid in patients who are allergic to bisulfite. Resuscitative equipment, medicine and oxygen should be available in case of emergency. Use products containing epinephrine cautiously in patients with significant vascular disease, compromised blood flow, or during or following general anesthesia (increased risk of arrhythmias). Adjust the dose for the elderly, pediatric, acutely ill, and debilitated patients.

Drug Interactions

Metabolism/Transport Effects **Substrate** of CYP1A2 (minor), CYP2A6 (minor), CYP2B6 (minor), CYP2C9 (minor), CYP2D6 (major), CYP3A4 (major), P-glycoprotein; **Inhibits** CYP1A2 (strong), 2D6 (moderate), 3A4 (moderate)

Avoid Concomitant Use

Avoid concomitant use of Lidocaine (Systemic) with any of the following: Saquinavir; Thioridazine; Tolvaptan

Increased Effect/Toxicity

Lidocaine (Systemic) may increase the levels/effects of: Bendamustine; Budesonide (Systemic, Oral Inhalation); Colchicine; CYP1A2 Substrates; CYP2D6 Substrates; CYP3A4 Substrates; Eplerenone; Everolimus; Fesoterodine; Halofantrine; Lurasidone; Pimecrolimus; Ranolazine; Salmeterol; Saxagliptin; Tamoxifen; Thioridazine; Tolvaptan; Vilazodone

The levels/effects of Lidocaine (Systemic) may be increased by: Abiraterone; Amiodarone; Beta-Blockers; Conivaptan; CYP2D6 Inhibitors (Moderate); CYP2D6 Inhibitors (Strong); CYP3A4 Inhibitors (Moderate); CYP3A4 Inhibitors (Strong); Darunavir; Dasatinib; Disopyramide; P-Glycoprotein Inhibitors; Saquinavir

Decreased Effect

The levels/effects of Lidocaine (Systemic) may be decreased by: CYP3A4 Inducers (Strong); Deferasirox; Etravirine; Herbs (CYP3A4 Inducers); Peginterferon Alfa-2b; P-Glycoprotein Inducers; Tocilizumab

Ethanol/Nutrition/Herb Interactions Herb/Nutraceutical: St John's wort may decrease lidocaine levels; avoid concurrent use.

Dietary Considerations Premixed injection may contain corn-derived dextrose and its use is contraindicated in patients with allergy to corn-related products.

Pharmacodynamics/Kinetics

Onset of Action Single bolus dose: 45-90 seconds

Duration of Action 10-20 minutes

Half-life Elimination Biphasic: Prolonged with congestive heart failure, liver disease, shock, severe renal disease; Initial: 7-30 minutes; Terminal: Infants, premature: 3.2 hours, Adults: 1.5-2 hours

Pregnancy Risk Factor B

Lactation Enters breast milk/use caution (AAP rates "compatible"; AAP 2001 update pending)

Breast-Feeding Considerations Small amounts of lidocaine and the MEGX metabolite are found in breast milk. The actual amount may depend on route and duration of administration. When administered topically at recommended doses, the amount of lidocaine available to the nursing infant would not be expected to cause adverse events. Cumulative exposure from all routes of administration should be considered.

Dosage Forms

Infusion, premixed in D_5W: 0.4% [4 mg/mL] (250 mL, 500 mL); 0.8% [8 mg/mL] (250 mL, 500 mL)

Injection, solution: 0.5% [5 mg/mL] (50 mL); 1% [10 mg/mL] (2 mL, 10 mL, 20 mL, 30 mL, 50 mL); 2% [20 mg/mL] (2 mL, 5 mL, 20 mL, 50 mL)

Xylocaine®: 0.5% [5 mg/mL] (50 mL); 1% [10 mg/mL] (10 mL, 20 mL, 50 mL); 2% [20 mg/mL] (10 mL, 20 mL, 50 mL)

Xylocaine® Dental: 2% [20 mg/mL] (1.8 mL)

Injection, solution [preservative free]: 0.5% [5 mg/mL] (50 mL); 1% [10 mg/mL] (2 mL, 5 mL, 30 mL); 1.5% [15 mg/mL] (20 mL); 2% [20 mg/mL] (2 mL, 5 mL, 10 mL); 4% [40 mg/mL] (5 mL)

Xylocaine®: 2% [20 mg/mL] (5 mL)

Xylocaine® MPF: 0.5% [5 mg/mL] (50 mL); 1% [10 mg/mL] (2 mL, 5 mL, 10 mL, 30 mL); 1.5% [15 mg/mL] (10 mL, 20 mL); 2% [20 mg/mL] (2 mL, 5 mL, 10 mL); 4% [40 mg/mL] (5 mL)

Lidocaine (Topical) (LYE doe kane)

Related Information

Management of Patients Undergoing Cancer Therapy *on page 1970*
Viral Infections *on page 1947*

U.S. Brand Names AneCream™ [OTC]; Anestafoam™ [OTC]; Band-Aid® Hurt Free™ Antiseptic Wash [OTC]; Burn Jel Plus [OTC]; Burn Jel® [OTC]; L-M-X® 4 [OTC]; L-M-X® 5 [OTC]; LidaMantle®; Lidoderm®; LTA® 360; Premjact®; Regenecare®; Regenecare® HA [OTC]; Solarcaine® cool aloe Burn Relief [OTC]; Topicaine® [OTC]; Unburn® [OTC]; Xylocaine®

Canadian Brand Names Betacaine®; Lidodan™; Lidoderm®; Maxilene®; Xylocaine®

Generic Availability (U.S.) Yes: Hydrochloride cream, jelly, ointment, solution

Pharmacologic Category Analgesic, Topical; Local Anesthetic

Dental Use Topical local anesthetic

Patch: Production of mild topical anesthesia of accessible mucous membranes of the mouth prior to superficial dental procedures

Oral solution (viscous): Reduce gagging during dental impressions and x-rays

Use

Rectal: Temporary relief of pain and itching due to anorectal disorders

Topical: Local anesthetic for oral mucous membrane; use in laser/cosmetic surgeries; minor burns, cuts, and abrasions of the skin

Oral solution (viscous): Topical anesthesia of irritated oral mucous membranes and pharyngeal tissue

Patch (Lidoderm®): Relief of allodynia (painful hypersensitivity) and chronic pain in postherpetic neuralgia

Local Anesthetic/Vasoconstrictor Precautions No information available to require special precautions

Effects on Dental Treatment Key adverse event(s) related to dental treatment: Metallic taste.

Effects on Bleeding No information available to require special precautions

Adverse Effects Frequency not defined.

Cardiovascular: Cyanosis, tachycardia

Central nervous system: Anxiety, confusion, dizziness, lethargy, lightheadedness, somnolence

Dermatologic: Angioedema, bruising (topical patch), contact dermatitis, depigmentation (topical patch), edema of the skin, itching, petechia (topical patch), pruritus, rash, urticaria

Hematologic: Methemoglobinemia

Local: Irritation (topical patch)

Neuromuscular & skeletal: Pain exacerbation (topical patch), paresthesia, weakness

Respiratory: Hypoxia

Dental Usual Dosage Anesthesia, topical:

Postherpetic neuralgia: Adults: Patch: Apply patch to most painful area. Up to 3 patches may be applied in a single application. Patch may remain in place for up to 12 hours in any 24-hour period.

Dosage Anesthesia, topical:

Cream:

LidaMantle®: Skin irritation: Children and Adults: Apply a thin film to affected area 2-3 times/day as needed

L-M-X® 4: Skin irritation: Children ≥2 years and Adults: Apply up to 3-4 times daily to intact skin

L-M-X® 5: Relief of anorectal pain and itching: Children ≥12 years and Adults: Apply to affected area up to 6 times/day

Gel, ointment: Adults: Apply to affected area ≤4 times/day as needed (maximum dose: 4.5 mg/kg, not to exceed 300 mg)

Topical solution: Adults: Apply 1-5 mL (40-200 mg) to affected area

Jelly:

Children: Dose varies with age and weight (maximum dose: 4.5 mg/kg)

Adults (maximum dose: 30 mL [600 mg] in any 12-hour period):

Anesthesia of male urethra: 5-30 mL (100-600 mg)

Anesthesia of female urethra: 3-5 mL (60-100 mg)

Lubrication of endotracheal tube: Apply a moderate amount to external surface only

Oral solution (viscous):

Infants and Children <3 years: 1.25 mL applied to area with a cotton-tipped applicator no more frequently than every 3 hours (maximum: 4 doses per 12-hour period)

Children ≥3 years: Should not exceed 4.5 mg/kg/dose (or 300 mg/dose); swished in the mouth and spit out no more frequently than every 3 hours (maximum: 4 doses per 12-hour period)

Adults:

Anesthesia of the mouth: 15 mL swished in the mouth and spit out no more frequently than every 3 hours (maximum: 8 doses per 24-hour period)

Anesthesia of the pharynx: 15 mL gargled no more frequently than every 3 hours (maximum: 8 doses per 24-hour period); may be swallowed

Patch: Postherpetic neuralgia: Adults: Apply patch to most painful area. Up to 3 patches may be applied in a single application. Patch(es) may remain in place for up to 12 hours in any 24-hour period.

Mechanism of Action Blocks both the initiation and conduction of nerve impulses by decreasing the neuronal membrane's permeability to sodium ions, which results in inhibition of depolarization with resultant blockade of conduction

Contraindications Hypersensitivity to lidocaine or any component of the formulation; hypersensitivity to another local anesthetic of the amide type

Warnings/Precautions Potentially life-threatening side effects (eg, irregular heart beat, seizures, coma, respiratory depression, death) have occurred when used prior to cosmetic procedures. Excessive dosing (application to large areas, application to denuded skin, or wearing of device for longer than recommended) may lead to increased absorption and systemic toxicity. Application to broken or inflamed skin may lead to increased systemic absorption; use caution. Use caution in patients with severe hepatic disease due to diminished ability to metabolize systemically-absorbed lidocaine.

When topical anesthetics are used prior to cosmetic or medical procedures, the lowest amount of anesthetic necessary for pain relief should be applied. High systemic levels and toxic effects (eg, methemoglobinemia, irregular heart beats, respiratory depression, seizures, death) have been reported in patients who (without supervision of a trained professional) have applied topical anesthetics in large amounts (or to large areas of the skin), left these products on for prolonged periods of time, or have used wraps/dressings to cover the skin following application.

Topical cream, liquid, gel, and ointment: Do not leave on large body areas for >2 hours. Not for ophthalmic use. Some products are not recommended for use on mucous membranes; consult specific product labeling.

Topical patch: To avoid accidental ingestion by children, store and dispose of products out of the reach of children.

Drug Interactions

Metabolism/Transport Effects Substrate of CYP1A2 (minor), CYP2A6 (minor), CYP2B6 (minor), CYP2C9 (minor), CYP2D6 (major), CYP3A4 (major), P-glycoprotein; **Inhibits** CYP1A2 (strong), 2D6 (moderate), 3A4 (moderate)

Avoid Concomitant Use

Avoid concomitant use of Lidocaine (Topical) with any of the following: Thioridazine; Tolvaptan

Increased Effect/Toxicity

Lidocaine (Topical) may increase the levels/effects of: Bendamustine; Budesonide (Systemic, Oral Inhalation); Colchicine; CYP1A2 Substrates; CYP2D6 Substrates; CYP3A4 Substrates; Eplerenone; Everolimus; Fesoterodine; Halofantrine; Lurasidone; Pimecrolimus; Ranolazine; Salmeterol; Saxagliptin; Tamoxifen; Thioridazine; Tolvaptan; Vilazodone

The levels/effects of Lidocaine (Topical) may be increased by: Abiraterone; Amiodarone; Beta-Blockers; Conivaptan; CYP2D6 Inhibitors (Moderate); CYP2D6 Inhibitors (Strong); CYP3A4 Inhibitors (Moderate); CYP3A4 Inhibitors (Strong); Darunavir; Dasatinib; P-Glycoprotein Inhibitors

Decreased Effect

The levels/effects of Lidocaine (Topical) may be decreased by: CYP3A4 Inducers (Strong); Deferasirox; Herbs (CYP3A4 Inducers); Peginterferon Alfa-2b; P-Glycoprotein Inducers; Tocilizumab

Pregnancy Risk Factor B

Lactation Enters breast milk/use caution (AAP rates "compatible"; AAP 2001 update pending)

Breast-Feeding Considerations When administered topically at recommended doses, the amount of lidocaine available to the nursing infant would not be expected to cause adverse events. Cumulative exposure from all routes of administration should be considered.

Dosage Forms

Aerosol, topical:
- Anestafoam™ [OTC]: 4% (30 g)
- Solarcaine® cool aloe Burn Relief [OTC]: 0.5% (127 g)

Cream, rectal:
- L-M-X® 5 [OTC]: 5% (15 g, 30 g)

Cream, topical: 0.5% (0.9 g)
- AneCream™ [OTC]: 4% (5 g, 15 g, 30 g)
- L-M-X® 4 [OTC]: 4% (5 g, 15 g, 30 g)
- LidaMantle®: 3% (85 g)

Gel, topical:
- Burn Jel Plus [OTC]: 2.5% (118 mL)
- Burn Jel® [OTC]: 2% (59 mL, 118 mL); 2% (3.5 g)
- Regenecare®: 2% (14 g, 85 g)
- Regenecare® HA [OTC]: 2% (85 g)
- Solarcaine® cool aloe Burn Relief [OTC]: 0.5% (113 g, 226 g)
- Topicaine® [OTC]: 4% (10 g, 30 g, 113 g); 5% (10 g, 30 g, 113 g)
- Unburn® [OTC]: 2.5% (59 mL)

Jelly, topical: 2% (5 mL, 30 mL)
- Xylocaine®: 2% (5 mL, 30 mL)

Jelly, topical [preservative free]: 2% (5 mL, 10 mL, 20 mL)

Lotion, topical:
- LidaMantle®: 3% (177 mL)

Ointment, topical: 5% (30 g, 35.4 g, 50 g)

Patch, topical:
- Lidoderm®: 5% (30s)

Solution, topical: 4% [40 mg/mL] (50 mL)
- Band-Aid® Hurt Free™ Antiseptic Wash [OTC]: 2% [20 mg/mL] (177 mL)
- LTA® 360: 4% [40 mg/mL] (4 mL)
- Premjact®: 9.6% (13 mL)

Solution, topical [preservative free]: 4% [40 mg/mL] (4 mL)

Solution, viscous, oral: 2% [20 mg/mL] (20 mL, 100 mL, 500 mL)

Lidocaine and Epinephrine (LYE doe kane & ep i NEF rin)

Related Information

EPINEPHrine (Systemic, Oral Inhalation) *on page 604*
Lidocaine (Systemic) *on page 1007*
Oral Pain *on page 1928*

U.S. Brand Names Lignospan® Forte; Lignospan® Standard; Xylocaine® MPF With Epinephrine; Xylocaine® With Epinephrine

Canadian Brand Names Xylocaine® With Epinephrine

Generic Availability (U.S.) Yes

Pharmacologic Category Local Anesthetic

Dental Use Amide-type anesthetic used for local infiltration anesthesia injection near nerve trunks to produce nerve block

Use Local infiltration anesthesia; AVS for nerve block

Local Anesthetic/Vasoconstrictor Precautions No information available to require special precautions

Effects on Dental Treatment It is common to misinterpret psychogenic responses to local anesthetic injection as an allergic reaction. Intraoral injections are perceived by many patients as a stressful procedure in dentistry. Common symptoms to this stress are diaphoresis, palpitations, hyperventilation. Patients may exhibit hypersensitivity to bisulfites contained in local anesthetic solution to prevent oxidation of epinephrine. In general, patients reacting to bisulfites have a history of asthma and their airways are hyper-reactive to asthmatic syndrome.

Degree of adverse effects in the CNS and cardiovascular system is directly related to the blood levels of lidocaine: Bradycardia, hypersensitivity reactions (rare; may be manifest as dermatologic reactions and edema at injection site), asthmatic syndromes

High blood levels: Anxiety, restlessness, disorientation, confusion, dizziness, tremors, seizures, CNS depression (resulting in somnolence, unconsciousness and possible respiratory arrest), nausea, and vomiting.

Effects on Bleeding No information available to require special precautions

Adverse Effects Degree of adverse effects in the central nervous system and cardiovascular system are directly related to the blood levels of lidocaine. The effects below are more likely to occur after systemic administration rather than infiltration.

Cardiovascular: Myocardial effects include a decrease in contraction force as well as a decrease in electrical excitability and myocardial conduction rate resulting in bradycardia and reduction in cardiac output.

Central nervous system: High blood levels result in anxiety, restlessness, disorientation, confusion, dizziness, tremor, and seizure. This is followed by depression of CNS resulting in somnolence, unconsciousness and possible respiratory arrest. In some cases, symptoms of CNS stimulation may be absent and the primary CNS effects are somnolence and unconsciousness.

Gastrointestinal: Nausea and vomiting may occur

Hypersensitivity reactions: Extremely rare, but may be manifest as dermatologic reactions and edema at injection site. Asthmatic syndromes have occurred. Patients may exhibit hypersensitivity to bisulfites contained in local anesthetic solution to prevent oxidation of epinephrine. In general, patients reacting to bisulfites have a history of asthma and their airways are hyper-reactive to asthmatic syndrome.

Psychogenic reactions: It is common to misinterpret psychogenic responses to local anesthetic injection as an allergic reaction. Intraoral injections are perceived by many patients as a stressful procedure in dentistry. Common symptoms to this stress are diaphoresis, palpitation, hyperventilation, generalized pallor and a fainting feeling

Dental Usual Dosage Dosage varies with the anesthetic procedure, degree of anesthesia needed, vascularity of tissue, duration of anesthesia required, and physical condition of patient.

Dental anesthesia, infiltration, or conduction block:

Children <12 years: 20-30 mg (1-1.5 mL) of lidocaine hydrochloride as a 2% solution with epinephrine 1:100,000; maximum: 4.5 mg of lidocaine hydrochloride/kg of body weight or 100-150 mg as a single dose

Children ≥12 years and Adults: Do not exceed 7 mg/kg body weight or 300 mg of lidocaine hydrochloride and 3 mcg (0.003 mg) of epinephrine/kg of body weight or 0.2 mg epinephrine per dental appointment. The effective anesthetic dose varies with procedure, intensity of anesthesia needed, duration of anesthesia required, and physical condition of the patient. Always use the lowest effective dose along with careful aspiration.

The following numbers of dental carpules (1.7 mL or 1.8 mL) provide the indicated amounts of lidocaine hydrochloride 2% and epinephrine 1:100,000 (see table):

# of Cartridges	Lidocaine HCl (2%) (mg)		Epinephrine 1:100,000 (mg)	
(1.7 mL or 1.8 mL)	(1.7 mL cartridge)	(1.8 mL cartridge)	(1.7 mL cartridge)	(1.8 mL cartridge)
1	34	36	0.017	0.018
2	68	72	0.034	0.036
3	102	108	0.051	0.054
4	136	144	0.068	0.072
5	170	180	0.085	0.090
6	204	216	0.102	0.108
7	238	252	0.119	0.126
8	272	288	0.136	0.144
9	306	324	0.153	0.162
10	340	360	0.170	0.180

For most routine dental procedures, lidocaine hydrochloride 2% with epinephrine 1:100,000 is preferred. When a more pronounced hemostasis is required, a 1:50,000 epinephrine concentration should be used. The following numbers of dental carpules (1.7 mL or 1.8 mL) provide the indicated amounts of lidocaine hydrochloride 2% and epinephrine 1:50,000 (see table):

# of Cartridges	Lidocaine HCl (2%) (mg)		Epinephrine 1:50,000 (mg)	
(1.7 mL or 1.8 mL)	(1.7 mL cartridge)	(1.8 mL cartridge)	(1.7 mL cartridge)	(1.8 mL cartridge)
1	34	36	0.034	0.036
2	68	72	0.068	0.072
3	102	108	0.102	0.108
4	136	144	0.136	0.144
5	170	180	0.170	0.180
6	204	216	0.204	0.216

Dosage Dosage varies with the anesthetic procedure, degree of anesthesia needed, vascularity of tissue, duration of anesthesia required, and physical condition of patient.

Dental anesthesia, infiltration, or conduction block:

Children <12 years: 20-30 mg (1-1.5 mL) of lidocaine hydrochloride as a 2% solution with epinephrine 1:100,000; maximum: 4.5 mg of lidocaine hydrochloride/kg of body weight or 100-150 mg as a single dose

Children ≥12 years and Adults: Do not exceed 7 mg/kg body weight up to a maximum range of 300 mg (usual dental practice) to 500 mg (approved product labeling) of lidocaine hydrochloride and 3 mcg (0.003 mg) of epinephrine/kg of body weight or 0.2 mg epinephrine per dental appointment. The effective anesthetic dose varies with procedure, intensity of anesthesia needed, duration of anesthesia required, and physical condition of the patient. Always use the lowest effective dose along with careful aspiration.

Note: For most routine dental procedures, lidocaine hydrochloride 2% with epinephrine 1:100,000 is preferred. When a more pronounced hemostasis is required, a 1:50,000 epinephrine concentration should be used.

Mechanism of Action Lidocaine blocks both the initiation and conduction of nerve impulses via decreased permeability of sodium ions; epinephrine increases the duration of action of lidocaine by causing vasoconstriction (via alpha effects) which slows the vascular absorption of lidocaine

Contraindications Hypersensitivity to lidocaine, epinephrine, or any component of the formulation; hypersensitivity to other local anesthetics of the amide type; myasthenia gravis; shock; cardiac conduction disease; angle-closure glaucoma

Warnings/Precautions Aspirate the syringe (injection solution for infiltration formulation) after tissue penetration and before injection to minimize chance of direct vascular injection. Use caution in endocrine, hepatic, or thyroid disease. Use with caution in the elderly, debilitated, acutely ill and pediatric patients. Avoid use in presence of flammable anesthetics. Avoid in patients with uncontrolled hyperthyroidism. Use minimal amounts in patients with significant cardiovascular problems (because of epinephrine component). Careful and constant monitoring of the patient's state of consciousness should be done following each local anesthetic injection; at such times, restlessness, anxiety, tinnitus, dizziness, blurred vision, tremors, depression, or drowsiness may be early warning signs of CNS toxicity. Treatment is primarily symptomatic and supportive. Continuous intra-articular infusion of local anesthetics after arthroscopic or other surgical procedures is **not** an approved use; chondrolysis (primarily in the shoulder joint) has occurred following infusion, with some cases requiring arthroplasty or shoulder replacement. Local anesthetics have been associated with rare occurrences of sudden respiratory arrest, seizures, and cardiac arrest. May contain sodium metabisulfite; use caution in patients with a sulfite allergy. Dental practitioners and/or clinicians using local anesthetic agents should be well trained in diagnosis and management of emergencies that may arise from the use of these agents. Resuscitative equipment, oxygen, and other resuscitative drugs should be available for immediate use.

Drug Interactions

Metabolism/Transport Effects Lidocaine: **Substrate** of CYP1A2 (minor), CYP2A6 (minor), CYP2B6 (minor), CYP2C9 (minor), CYP2D6 (major), CYP3A4 (major), P-glycoprotein; **Inhibits** CYP1A2 (strong), 2D6 (moderate), 3A4 (moderate)

Avoid Concomitant Use

Avoid concomitant use of Lidocaine and Epinephrine with any of the following: Iobenguane I 123; Lurasidone

Increased Effect/Toxicity

Lidocaine and Epinephrine may increase the levels/effects of: Bromocriptine; Lurasidone; Sympathomimetics

The levels/effects of Lidocaine and Epinephrine may be increased by: Antacids; Atomoxetine; Beta-Blockers; Cannabinoids; Carbonic Anhydrase Inhibitors; COMT Inhibitors; Inhalational Anesthetics; MAO Inhibitors; Serotonin/Norepinephrine Reuptake Inhibitors; Tricyclic Antidepressants

Decreased Effect

Lidocaine and Epinephrine may decrease the levels/effects of: Benzylpenicilloyl Polylysine; Iobenguane I 123

The levels/effects of Lidocaine and Epinephrine may be decreased by: Spironolactone

Pharmacodynamics/Kinetics

Onset of Action Peak effect: ~5 minutes

Duration of Action Dose and anesthetic procedure dependent: ~2 hours

Pregnancy Risk Factor B

Lactation Lidocaine enters breast milk/use caution

Breast-Feeding Considerations Refer to Lidocaine (Systemic) monograph.

Dosage Forms

Injection, solution:

Generics:

0.5% / 1:200,000: Lidocaine hydrochloride 0.5% [5 mg/mL] and epinephrine 1:200,000 (50 mL)

1% / 1:100,000: Lidocaine hydrochloride 1% [10 mg/mL] and epinephrine 1:100,000 (20 mL, 30 mL, 50 mL)

2% / 1:100,000: Lidocaine hydrochloride 2% [20 mg/mL] and epinephrine 1:100,000 (30 mL, 50 mL)

Brands:

Xylocaine® with Epinephrine:

0.5% / 1:200,000: Lidocaine hydrochloride 0.5% [5 mg/mL] and epinephrine 1:200,000 (50 mL)

1% / 1:100,000: Lidocaine hydrochloride 1% [10 mg/mL] and epinephrine 1:100,000 (10 mL, 20 mL, 50 mL)

2% / 1:100,000: Lidocaine hydrochloride 2% [20 mg/mL] and epinephrine 1:100,000 (10 mL, 20 mL, 50 mL)

Injection, solution [preservative free]:

Generics:

1% / 1:200,000: Lidocaine hydrochloride 1% [10 mg/mL] and epinephrine 1:200,000 (30 mL)

1.5% / 1:200,000: Lidocaine hydrochloride 1.5% [15 mg/mL] and epinephrine 1:200,000 (5 mL, 30 mL)

2% / 1:200,000: Lidocaine hydrochloride 2% [20 mg/mL] and epinephrine 1:200,000 (20 mL)

Brands:

Xylocaine®-MPF with Epinephrine:

1% / 1:200,000: Lidocaine hydrochloride 1% [10 mg/mL] and epinephrine 1:200,000 (5 mL, 10 mL, 30 mL)

1.5% / 1:200,000: Lidocaine hydrochloride 1.5% [15 mg/mL] and epinephrine 1:200,000 (5 mL, 10 mL, 30 mL)

2% / 1:200,000: Lidocaine hydrochloride 2% [20 mg/mL] and epinephrine 1:200,000 (5 mL, 10 mL, 20 mL)

Injection, solution [for dental use]:

Generics:

2% / 1:50,000: Lidocaine hydrochloride 2% [20 mg/mL] and epinephrine 1:50,000 (1.7 mL, 1.8 mL)

2% / 1:100,000: Lidocaine hydrochloride 2% [20 mg/mL] and epinephrine 1:100,000 (1.7 mL, 1.8 mL)

Brands:

Lignospan® Forte: 2% / 1:50,000: Lidocaine hydrochloride 2% [20 mg/mL] and epinephrine 1:50,000 (1.7 mL)

Lignospan® Standard: 2% / 1:100,000: Lidocaine hydrochloride 2% [20 mg/mL] and epinephrine 1:100,000 (1.7 mL)

Dental Comment Oral paresthesia: The occurrence of oral paresthesia associated with 4% solutions of prilocaine or articaine, although rare, continue to be slightly more frequent than other local anesthetics. From 1999-2008, there were 182 cases of nonsurgical paresthesia (Gaffen, 2009). Of the cases, 172 involved mandibular block injection only. Another eight cases involved mandibular block combined with at least one other type of anesthetic injection. A single case involved infiltration around tooth number 35 and the final case involved infiltration and intraligamentary injection in the maxillary anterior region.

A 2010 report, reviewed adverse events submitted voluntarily over a 10-year period involving the dental local anesthetics articaine, bupivacaine, lidocaine, mepivacaine, and prilocaine in the United States. Lidocaine reported incidence: One case per 181,076,673 cartridges sold. The reported incidence of paresthesia was one case for 13,800,970 cartridges of all local anesthetics sold in the U.S. (Garisto, 2010).

References

Ayoub ST and Coleman AE, "A Review of Local Anesthetics," *Gen Dent*, 1992, 40(4):285-7, 289-90.
Budenz AW, "Local Anesthetics in Dentistry: Then and Now," *J Calif Dent Assoc*, 2003, 31(5):388-96.
Dower JS Jr, "A Review of Paresthesia in Association With Administration of Local Anesthesia," *Dent Today*, 2003, 22(2):64-9.
Finder RL and Moore PA, "Adverse Drug Reactions to Local Anesthesia," *Dent Clin North Am*, 2002, 46 (4):747-57, x.
Gaffen AS and Haas DA, "Retrospective Review of Voluntary Reports of Nonsurgical Paresthesia in Dentistry," *J Can Dent Assoc*, 2009, 75(8):579.
Garisto GA, Gaffen AS, Lawrence HP, et al, "Occurrence of Paresthesia After Dental Local Anesthetic Administration in the United States," *J Am Dent Assoc*, 2010, 141(7):836-44.
Haas DA, "An Update on Local Anesthetics in Dentistry," *J Can Dent Assoc*, 2002, 68(9):546-51.
Hawkins JM and Moore PA, "Local Anesthesia: Advances in Agents and Techniques," *Dent Clin North Am*, 2002, 46(4):719-32, ix.
"Injectable Local Anesthetics," *J Am Dent Assoc*, 2003, 134(5):628-9.
Jastak JT and Yagiela JA, "Vasoconstrictors and Local Anesthesia: A Review and Rationale for Use," *J Am Dent Assoc*, 1983, 107(4):623-30.
MacKenzie TA and Young ER, "Local Anesthetic Update," *Anesth Prog*, 1993, 40(2):29-34.
Malamed SF, "Allergy and Toxic Reactions to Local Anesthetics," *Dent Today*, 2003, 22(4):114-6, 118-21.
Nusstein J, Reader A, and Beck FM, "Anesthetic Efficacy of Different Volumes of Lidocaine With Epinephrine for Inferior Alveolar Nerve Blocks," *Gen Dent*, 2002, 50(4):372-5.
Wynn RL, "Epinephrine Interactions With Beta-Blockers," *Gen Dent*, 1994, 42(1):16, 18.
Wynn RL, "Recent Research on Mechanisms of Local Anesthetics," *Gen Dent*, 1995, 43(4):316-8.
Yagiela JA, "Local Anesthetics," *Anesth Prog*, 1991, 38(4-5):128-41.

Lidocaine and Hydrocortisone (LYE doe kane & hye droe KOR ti sone)

Related Information

Hydrocortisone (Topical) *on page 868*
Lidocaine (Topical) *on page 1010*

U.S. Brand Names AnaMantle HC® Cream; AnaMantle HC® Forte; AnaMantle HC® Gel; LidaMantle HC®; LidaMantle HC® Relief Pad™; LidoCort™; Peranex™ HC; Peranex™ HC Medi-Pad; RectaGel™ HC

Pharmacologic Category Anesthetic/Corticosteroid

Use Topical anti-inflammatory and anesthetic for skin disorders; rectal for the treatment of hemorrhoids, anal fissures, pruritus ani, or similar conditions

Local Anesthetic/Vasoconstrictor Precautions No information available to require special precautions

Effects on Dental Treatment No significant effects or complications reported

Effects on Bleeding No information available to require special precautions

General Dosage Range

Rectal: *Adults:* 1 applicatorful twice daily

Topical: *Adults:* Apply 2-3 times/day

Pregnancy Risk Factor C

Lidocaine and Prilocaine (LYE doe kane & PRIL oh kane)

Related Information

Lidocaine (Topical) *on page 1010*
Prilocaine *on page 1399*

U.S. Brand Names EMLA®; Oraqix®

Canadian Brand Names EMLA®

Generic Availability (U.S.) Yes: Cream

Pharmacologic Category Local Anesthetic

Dental Use

Periodontal gel (Oraqix®): Use in adults who require localized anesthesia in periodontal pockets during scaling and/or root planning.

Topical: Amide-type topical anesthetic for use on normal intact skin to provide local analgesia for minor procedures such as I.V. cannulation or venipuncture

Use

Topical anesthetic for use on normal intact skin to provide local analgesia for minor procedures such as I.V. cannulation or venipuncture; has also been used for painful procedures such as lumbar puncture and skin graft harvesting; for superficial minor surgery of genital mucous membranes and as an adjunct for local infiltration anesthesia in genital mucous membranes.

Periodontal gel: Topical anesthetic for use in periodontal pockets during scaling or root planning procedures

Local Anesthetic/Vasoconstrictor Precautions No information available to require special precautions

Effects on Dental Treatment Key adverse event(s) related to dental treatment: Application site reactions in the oral cavity in 52/391 patients (13%) included pain, soreness, irritation, numbness, ulcerations, vesicles, edema, abscess and/or redness in the treated area. The 13% represented adverse effects occurring in more than one patient. Each patient was counted only once per adverse event. Taste perversion also reported (2%) including complaints of bad or bitter taste for up to 4 hours after administration.

Effects on Bleeding No information available to require special precautions

Adverse Effects

Cream/patch: Frequency not defined.

Cardiovascular: Angioedema, hypotension
Central nervous system: Shock
Dermatologic: Burning, erythema, hyperpigmentation, itching, rash, urticaria
Genitourinary: Blistering of foreskin (rare)
Local: Burning, edema, stinging
Respiratory: Bronchospasm
Miscellaneous: Alteration in temperature sensation, hypersensitivity reactions

Periodontal gel:

>10%: Local: Application site reaction (1%, includes abscess, edema, irritation, numbness, pain, ulceration, vesicles)

1% to 10%:
Central nervous system: Fatigue (1%)
Gastrointestinal: Bitter taste (2%), nausea (1%)
Respiratory: Infection (1%)
Miscellaneous: Flu-like syndrome (1%), allergic reactions

Dental Usual Dosage Oraqix®: Gel: Apply on gingival margin around selected teeth using the blunt-tipped applicator included in package. Wait 30 seconds, then fill the periodontal pockets using the blunt-tipped applicator until gel becomes visible at the gingival margin. Wait another 30 seconds before starting treatment. Maximum recommended dose: One treatment session: 5 cartridges (8.5 g)

Dosage Although the incidence of systemic adverse effects is very low, caution should be exercised, particularly when applying over large areas and leaving on for >2 hours

Children (intact skin):

Cream: Should **not** be used in neonates with a gestation age <37 weeks nor in infants <12 months of age who are receiving treatment with methemoglobin-inducing agents

Dosing is based on child's age and weight:

Age 0-3 months or <5 kg: Apply a maximum of 1 g over no more than 10 cm^2 of skin; leave on for no longer than 1 hour

Age 3 months to 12 months and >5 kg: Apply no more than a maximum 2 g total over no more than 20 cm^2 of skin; leave on for no longer than 4 hours

Age 1-6 years and >10 kg: Apply no more than a maximum of 10 g total over no more than 100 cm^2 of skin; leave on for no longer than 4 hours.

Age 7-12 years and >20 kg: Apply no more than a maximum 20 g total over no more than 200 cm^2 of skin; leave on for no longer than 4 hours.

Note: If a patient >3 months of age does not meet the minimum weight requirement, the maximum total dose should be restricted to the corresponding maximum based on patient weight.

Transdermal patch: Canadian labeling (not available in U.S.): **Note:** Should not be used in neonates with a gestation age <37 weeks nor in infants <12 months of age who are receiving treatment with methemoglobin-inducing agents

Dosing is based on child's age and weight: Apply patch(es) to skin area(s) <10 cm^2:

Age 0-3 months or <5 kg: Apply 1 patch and leave on for ~1 hour (do not exceed 1-hour application time); do not apply more than 1 patch at same time; safety of repeated dosing not established

Age 3 months to 12 months and >5 kg: Apply 1-2 patches for ~1 hour (maximum application time: 4 hours); do not apply more than 2 patches at the same time

Age 1-6 years and >10 kg: Apply 1or more patches for minimum of 1 hour (maximum application time: 5 hours); maximum dose: 10 patches

Age 7-12 years and >20 kg: Apply 1 or more patches for a minimum of 1 hour (maximum application time: 5 hours); maximum dose: 20 patches

Note: If a patient >3 months of age does not meet the minimum weight requirement, the maximum total dose should be restricted to that which corresponds to the patient's weight.

Adults (intact skin): **Note:** Cream: Apply a thick layer to intact skin and cover with an occlusive dressing. Transdermal patch (CAN; not available in U.S.): Apply patch or patches to intact skin.

Minor dermal procedures (eg, I.V. cannulation or venipuncture):

Cream: Apply 2.5 g of cream (1/2 of the 5 g tube) over 20-25 cm^2 of skin surface area) for at least 1 hour

Transdermal patch: (Canadian labeling; not available in U.S.): Apply 1 or more patches to skin surface area <10 cm^2 for at least 1 hour (maximum application time: 5 hours)

Major dermal procedures (eg, more painful dermatological procedures involving a larger skin area such as split thickness skin graft harvesting): Apply 2 g of cream per 10 cm^2 of skin and allow to remain in contact with the skin for at least 2 hours.

Adult male genital skin (eg, pretreatment prior to local anesthetic infiltration): Apply a thick layer of cream (1 g/10 cm^2) to the skin surface for 15 minutes. Local anesthetic infiltration should be performed immediately after removal of cream.

Note: Dermal analgesia can be expected to increase for up to 3 hours under occlusive dressing and persist for 1-2 hours after removal of the cream

Adult female genital mucous membranes: Minor procedures (eg, removal of condylomata acuminata, pretreatment for local anesthetic infiltration): Apply 5-10 g (thick layer) of cream for 5-10 minutes

Periodontal gel (Oraqix®): Adults: Apply on gingival margin around selected teeth using the blunt-tipped applicator included in package. Wait 30 seconds, then fill the periodontal pockets using the blunt-tipped applicator until gel becomes visible at the gingival margin. Wait another 30 seconds before starting treatment. May reapply; maximum recommended dose: One treatment session: 5 cartridges (8.5 g)

Mechanism of Action Local anesthetic action occurs by stabilization of neuronal membranes and inhibiting the ionic fluxes required for the initiation and conduction of impulses

Contraindications Hypersensitivity to amide-type anesthetic agents; hypersensitivity to any component of the formulation selected; application on mucous membranes or broken or inflamed skin; infants <1 month of age if gestational age is <37 weeks; infants <12 months of age receiving therapy with methemoglobin-inducing agents; children with congenital or idiopathic methemoglobinemia, or in children who are receiving medications associated with drug-induced methemoglobinemia (eg, acetaminophen [overdosage], benzocaine, chloroquine, dapsone, nitrofurantoin, nitroglycerin, nitroprusside, phenazopyridine, phenelzine, phenobarbital, phenytoin, quinine, sulfonamides)

Warnings/Precautions Use with caution in patients with severe hepatic impairment. Use with caution in the debilitated or acutely ill patients and the elderly. Use with caution in patients receiving class I and III antiarrhythmic drugs, since systemic absorption occurs and synergistic toxicity is possible. Although the incidence of systemic adverse reactions with EMLA® is very low, caution should be exercised, particularly when applying over large areas and leaving on for longer than 2 hours. Avoid use on open wounds or near the eyes.

When topical anesthetics are used prior to cosmetic or medical procedures, the lowest amount of anesthetic necessary for pain relief should be applied. High systemic levels and toxic effects (eg, methemoglobinemia, irregular heart beats, respiratory depression, seizures, death) have been reported in patients who (without supervision of a trained professional) have applied topical anesthetics in large amounts (or to large areas of the skin), left these products on for prolonged periods of time, or have used wraps/dressings to cover the skin following application.

Drug Interactions

Metabolism/Transport Effects Lidocaine: **Substrate** of CYP1A2 (minor), CYP2A6 (minor), CYP2B6 (minor), CYP2C9 (minor), CYP2D6 (major), CYP3A4 (major), P-glycoprotein; **Inhibits** CYP1A2 (strong), 2D6 (moderate), 3A4 (moderate)

Avoid Concomitant Use There are no known interactions where it is recommended to avoid concomitant use.

Increased Effect/Toxicity There are no known significant interactions involving an increase in effect.

Decreased Effect There are no known significant interactions involving a decrease in effect.

Pharmacodynamics/Kinetics

Onset of Action EMLA®: 1 hour; Peak effect: 2-3 hours

Duration of Action EMLA®: 1-2 hours after removal; Oraqix®: ~20 minutes

Pregnancy Risk Factor B

Lactation Lidocaine enters breast milk/use caution

Breast-Feeding Considerations See individual agents.

Dosage Forms

Cream, topical: Lidocaine 2.5% and prilocaine 2.5% (5 g, 30 g)

EMLA®: Lidocaine 2.5% and prilocaine 2.5% (5 g, 30 g)

Gel, periodontal:

Oraqix®: Lidocaine 2.5% and prilocaine 2.5% (1.7 g)

Dosage Forms: Canada

Patch, transdermal:

EMLA® Patch: Lidocaine 2.5% and prilocaine 2.5% per patch (2s, 20s)

References

Broadman LM, Soliman IE, Hannallah RS, et al, "Analgesic Efficacy of Eutectic Mixture of Local Anesthetics (EMLA®) vs Intradermal Infiltration Prior to Venous Cannulation in Children," *Am J Anaesth*, 1987, 34:S56.

Friskopp J and Huledal G, "Plasma Levels of Lidocaine and Prilocaine After Application of Oraqix, a New Intrapocket Anesthetic, in Patients With Advanced Periodontitis," *J Clin Periodontol*, 2001, 28(5):425-9.

Friskopp J, Nilsson M, and Isacsson G, "The Anesthetic Onset and Duration of a New Lidocaine/Prilocaine Gel Intra-Pocket Anesthetic (Oraqix) for Periodontal Scaling/Root Planing," *J Clin Periodontol*, 2001, 28(5):453-8.

Halperin DL, Koren G, Attias D, et al, "Topical Skin Anesthesia for Venous Subcutaneous Drug Reservoir and Lumbar Puncture in Children," *Pediatrics*, 1989, 84(2):281-4.

Robieux I, Kumar R, Radhakrishnan S, et al, "Assessing Pain and Analgesia With a Lidocaine-Prilocaine Emulsion in Infants and Toddlers During Venipuncture," *J Pediatr*, 1991, 118(6):971-3.

Taddio A, Shennan AT, Stevens B, et al, "Safety of Lidocaine-Prilocaine Cream in the Treatment of Preterm Neonates," *J Pediatr*, 1995, 127(6):1002-5.

Vickers ER, Mazbani N, Gerzina TM, et al, "Pharmacokinetics of EMLA Cream 5% Application to Oral Mucosa," *Anesth Prog*, 1997, 44:32-7.

Lidocaine and Tetracaine (LYE doe kane & TET ra kane)

Related Information

Lidocaine (Topical) *on page* 1010

Tetracaine (Topical) *on page* 1610

U.S. Brand Names Pliaglis™; Synera™

Generic Availability (U.S.) No

Pharmacologic Category Analgesic, Topical; Local Anesthetic

Use Topical anesthetic for use on normal intact skin for minor procedures (eg, I.V. cannulation or venipuncture) and superficial dermatologic procedures

Local Anesthetic/Vasoconstrictor Precautions No information available to require special precautions

Effects on Dental Treatment No significant effects or complications reported

Effects on Bleeding No information available to require special precautions

Adverse Effects

>10%: Dermatologic: Erythema (47% to 71%), skin discoloration (<4% to 16%), edema (12% to 14%), blanching (12%)

1% to 10%: Dermatologic: Application site reactions (contact dermatitis, rash)

Dosage

Topical: Cream: Adults:

Superficial dermatological procedures (eg, dermal filler injection, facial laser ablation): Apply 20-30 minutes prior to procedure

Laser-assisted tattoo removal: Apply 60 minutes prior to procedure

Note: The amount of Pliaglis™ required is determined by the size of the treatment area. Use the ruler on the carton and in the packaging to measure out the proper amount (cm length of cream). Apply evenly and thinly (~1 mm or the thickness of a dime) over the area using a flat tool (eg, spatula, tongue depressor).

If surface area of treatment site:

- 10 cm^2: Apply 3 cm length Pliaglis™
- 20 cm^2: Apply 6 cm Pliaglis™
- 40 cm^2: Apply 12 cm Pliaglis™
- 80 cm^2: Apply 24 cm Pliaglis™
- 100 cm^2: Apply 30 cm Pliaglis™
- 150 cm^2: Apply 46 cm Pliaglis™
- 200 cm^2: Apply 61 cm Pliaglis™
- 250 cm^2: Apply 76 cm Pliaglis™
- 300 cm^2: Apply 91 cm Pliaglis™
- 350 cm^2: Apply 106 cm Pliaglis™
- 400 cm^2: Apply 121 cm Pliaglis™

After waiting the required application time, remove the Pliaglis™ by grasping a free edge and pulling it away from the skin.

Transdermal patch: Children ≥3 years and Adults:

Venipuncture or intravenous cannulation: Prior to procedure, apply to intact skin for 20-30 minutes; **Note:** Adults can use another patch at a new location to facilitate venous access after a failed attempt; remove previous patch.

Superficial dermatological procedures: Prior to procedure, apply to intact skin for 30 minutes

Dosage adjustment in hepatic impairment: Use caution in patients with severe hepatic dysfunction.

Mechanism of Action Local anesthetic action occurs by stabilization of neuronal membranes and inhibiting the sodium ion fluxes required for the initiation and conduction of impulses.

Synera™: A heating mechanism within the patch enhances drug delivery.

Contraindications Hypersensitivity to lidocaine, tetracaine, amide or ester-type anesthetic agents, para-aminobenzoid acid (PABA), or any other component of the formulation

Warnings/Precautions Hypersensitivity or anaphylactic reactions may occur. Use with caution in patients receiving class I antiarrhythmic drugs, since systemic absorption occurs and synergistic toxicity is possible. Use with caution in patients who may be sensitive to systemic effects (eg, acutely ill, debilitated, elderly). If being used with other products containing local anesthetic, consider potential for additive effects. Avoid contact with eye; loss of protective reflexes may predispose to corneal irritation and/or abrasion. Application to broken or inflamed skin or mucous membranes may lead to increased systemic absorption. Use caution in patients with severe hepatic disease or pseudocholinesterase deficiency. Not for use at home. Methemoglobinemia has been reported with local anesthetics including tetracaine. Use caution in patients with lung diseases (asthma, bronchitis, emphysema, in smokers), inflamed/damaged mucosa, heart disease, children <12 months of age, concurrent use with methemoglobin-inducing medications, and hemoglobin or enzyme abnormalities.

When topical anesthetics are used prior to cosmetic or medical procedures, the lowest amount of anesthetic necessary for pain relief should be applied. High systemic levels and toxic effects (eg, methhemoglobinemia, irregular heart beats, respiratory depression, seizures, death) have been reported in patients who (without supervision of a trained professional) have applied topical anesthetics in large amounts (or to large areas of the skin), left these products on for prolonged periods of time, or have used wraps/dressings to cover the skin following application.

Pliaglis™ topical cream: Safety and efficacy in children have not been established.

Synera™ transdermal patch: Use caution when applying simultaneous or sequential application of multiple patches to adults; this practice is not recommended with children. May contain conducting metal (eg, aluminum); remove patch prior to MRI. Efficacy has not been established in patients <3 years of age (safety has been documented in limited trials).

Drug Interactions

Metabolism/Transport Effects Lidocaine: **Substrate** of CYP1A2 (minor), CYP2A6 (minor), CYP2B6 (minor), CYP2C9 (minor), CYP2D6 (major), CYP3A4 (major), P-glycoprotein; **Inhibits** CYP1A2 (strong), 2D6 (moderate), 3A4 (moderate)

Avoid Concomitant Use There are no known interactions where it is recommended to avoid concomitant use.

Increased Effect/Toxicity There are no known significant interactions involving an increase in effect.

Decreased Effect There are no known significant interactions involving a decrease in effect.

Pharmacodynamics/Kinetics

Duration of Action Cream: ~11 hours

Pregnancy Risk Factor B

Lactation Lidocaine enters breast milk/use caution

Breast-Feeding Considerations Refer to Lidocaine (Topical) monograph.

Dosage Forms

Cream, topical:

Pliaglis™: Lidocaine 7% and tetracaine 7% (30 g)

Patch, transdermal:

Synera™: Lidocaine 70 mg and tetracaine 70 mg (10s)

Lincomycin (lin koe MYE sin)

U.S. Brand Names Lincocin®

Canadian Brand Names Lincocin®

Pharmacologic Category Antibiotic, Lincosamide

Use Treatment of serious susceptible bacterial infections, mainly those caused by streptococci, pneumococci, and staphylococci resistant to other agents

Local Anesthetic/Vasoconstrictor Precautions No information available to require special precautions

Effects on Dental Treatment Key adverse event(s) related to dental treatment: Glossitis and stomatitis.

Effects on Bleeding No information available to require special precautions

Adverse Effects Frequency not defined.

Cardiovascular: Cardiopulmonary arrest and hypotension (related to rapid I.V. infusion; rare)

Central nervous system: Vertigo

Dermatologic: Dermatitis (includes exfoliative and vesiculobullous; rare), erythema multiforme (rare; some resembling SJS), rash, urticaria

Gastrointestinal: Colitis, diarrhea, glossitis, nausea, pruritus ani, stomatitis, vomiting

Genitourinary: Vaginitis

Hematologic: Agranulocytosis, aplastic anemia (rare), leukopenia, neutropenia, pancytopenia (rare), thrombocytopenic purpura

Hepatic: Jaundice, liver function test abnormal

Otic: Tinnitus

Renal: Azotemia (rare), proteinuria (rare), oliguria (rare)

Miscellaneous: Hypersensitivity reactions (anaphylaxis, angioneurotic edema, serum sickness)

General Dosage Range Dosage adjustment recommended in patients with renal impairment

I.M.:

Children >1 month: 10 mg/kg every 12-24 hours

Adults: 600 mg every 12-24 hours

I.V.:

Children >1 month: 10-20 mg/kg/day divided every 8-12 hours

Adults: 600 mg to 1 g every 8-12 hours (maximum: 8 g/day)

Subconjunctival injection: *Adults:* 75 mg

Mechanism of Action Lincosamide antibiotic which was isolated from a strain of *Streptomyces lincolnensis*; lincomycin, like clindamycin, inhibits bacterial protein synthesis by specifically binding on the 50S subunit and affecting the process of peptide chain initiation. Other macrolide antibiotics (erythromycin) also bind to the 50S subunit. Since only one molecule of antibiotic can bind to a single ribosome, the concomitant use of erythromycin and lincomycin is not recommended.

Pharmacodynamics/Kinetics

Half-life Elimination Serum: ~5 hours; prolonged with renal or hepatic impairment

Time to Peak I.M.: 1 hour

Pregnancy Risk Factor C

Lindane (LIN dane)

Canadian Brand Names Hexit™; PMS-Lindane

Pharmacologic Category Antiparasitic Agent, Topical; Pediculocide; Scabicidal Agent

Use Treatment of *Sarcoptes scabiei* (scabies), *Pediculus capitis* (head lice), and *Phthirus pubis* (crab lice); FDA recommends reserving lindane as a second-line agent or with inadequate response to other therapies

Local Anesthetic/Vasoconstrictor Precautions No information available to require special precautions

Effects on Dental Treatment No significant effects or complications reported

Effects on Bleeding No information available to require special precautions

Adverse Effects Frequency not defined (includes postmarketing and/or case reports).

Cardiovascular: Cardiac arrhythmia

Central nervous system: Ataxia, dizziness, headache, restlessness, seizure, pain

Dermatologic: Alopecia, contact dermatitis, skin and adipose tissue may act as repositories, eczematous eruptions, pruritus, urticaria

Gastrointestinal: Nausea, vomiting

Hematologic: Aplastic anemia

Hepatic: Hepatitis

Local: Burning and stinging

Neuromuscular & skeletal: Paresthesia

Renal: Hematuria

Respiratory: Pulmonary edema

General Dosage Range Topical:

Lotion: *Children and Adults:* Apply a thin layer; bathe and remove drug after 8-12 hours

Shampoo: *Children and Adults:* Apply to dry hair (maximum: 60 mL)

Mechanism of Action Directly absorbed by parasites and ova through the exoskeleton; stimulates the nervous system resulting in seizures and death of parasitic arthropods

Pharmacodynamics/Kinetics

Half-life Elimination Children: 17-22 hours

Time to Peak Serum: Children: 6 hours

Pregnancy Risk Factor C

Linezolid (li NE zoh lid)

U.S. Brand Names Zyvox®

Canadian Brand Names Zyvoxam®

Pharmacologic Category Antibiotic, Oxazolidinone

Use Treatment of vancomycin-resistant *Enterococcus faecium* (VRE) infections, nosocomial pneumonia caused by *Staphylococcus aureus* (including MRSA) or *Streptococcus pneumoniae* (including multidrug-resistant strains [MDRSP]), complicated and uncomplicated skin and skin structure infections (including diabetic foot infections without concomitant osteomyelitis), and community-acquired pneumonia caused by susceptible gram-positive organisms

Local Anesthetic/Vasoconstrictor Precautions Linezolid has mild monoamine oxidase inhibitor properties. The clinician is reminded that vasoconstrictors have the potential to interact with MAO-Is to result in elevation of blood pressure. Caution is suggested.

Effects on Dental Treatment Key adverse event(s) related to dental treatment: Oral moniliasis, taste alteration, and tongue discoloration.

Effects on Bleeding No information available to require special precautions

Adverse Effects Percentages as reported in adults; frequency similar in pediatric patients

>10%:
- Central nervous system: Headache (<1% to 11%)
- Gastrointestinal: Diarrhea (3% to 11%)

1% to 10%:
- Central nervous system: Insomnia (3%), dizziness (≤2%), fever (2%)
- Dermatologic: Rash (2%)
- Gastrointestinal: Nausea (3% to 10%), lipase increased (3% to 4%), vomiting (1% to 4%), constipation (2%), taste alteration (1% to 2%), amylase increased (<1% to 2%), tongue discoloration (≤1%), oral moniliasis (≤1%), pancreatitis
- Genitourinary: Vaginal moniliasis (1% to 2%)
- Hematologic: Thrombocytopenia (<1% to 10%), hemoglobin decreased (1% to 7%), leukopenia (<1% to 2%), neutropenia (≤1%)
- Hepatic: ALT increased (2% to 10%), AST increased (2% to 5%), alkaline phosphatase increased (<1% to 4%), bilirubin increased (≤1%)
- Renal: BUN increased (≤2%)
- Miscellaneous: Fungal infection (≤1% to 2%), lactate dehydrogenase increased (<1% to 2%)

General Dosage Range

I.V.:
- *Preterm neonates (<34 weeks gestational age):* 10 mg/kg (maximum: 600 mg/dose) every 8-12 hours
- *Children ≤11 years:* 10 mg/kg (maximum dose: 600 mg) every 8 hours
- *Children ≥12 years and Adults:* 600 mg every 12 hours

Oral:
- *Preterm neonates (<34 weeks gestational age):* 10 mg/kg every 8-12 hours
- *Children <5 years:* 10 mg/kg every 8 hours (maximum: 600 mg/dose)
- *Children 5-11 years:* 10 mg/kg every 8-12 hours (maximum: 600 mg/dose)
- *Children ≥12 years and Adults:* 400-600 mg every 12 hours

Mechanism of Action Inhibits bacterial protein synthesis by binding to bacterial 23S ribosomal RNA of the 50S subunit. This prevents the formation of a functional 70S initiation complex that is essential for the bacterial translation process. Linezolid is bacteriostatic against enterococci and staphylococci and bactericidal against most strains of streptococci.

Pharmacodynamics/Kinetics

Half-life Elimination Children ≥1 week (full-term) to 11 years: 1.5-3 hours; Adults: 4-5 hours

Time to Peak Adults: Oral: 1-2 hours

Pregnancy Risk Factor C

Liothyronine (lye oh THYE roe neen)

Related Information

Endocrine Disorders and Pregnancy *on page 1879*

U.S. Brand Names Cytomel®; Triostat®

Canadian Brand Names Cytomel®

Pharmacologic Category Thyroid Product

Use

Oral: Replacement or supplemental therapy in hypothyroidism; management of nontoxic goiter; a diagnostic aid

I.V.: Treatment of myxedema coma/precoma

Unlabeled/Investigational Use Management of hemodynamically unstable potential organ donors increasing the quantity of organs available for transplantation

Local Anesthetic/Vasoconstrictor Precautions No precautions with vasoconstrictor are necessary if patient is well controlled with liothyronine

Effects on Dental Treatment No significant effects or complications reported

Effects on Bleeding No information available to require special precautions

Adverse Effects 1% to 10%: Cardiovascular: Arrhythmia (6%), tachycardia (3%), cardiopulmonary arrest (2%), hypotension (2%), MI (2%)

General Dosage Range

I.V.: *Adults:* 10-50 mcg/dose

Oral:

Infants: Initial: 5 mcg/day; Usual maintenance dose: 20 mcg/day

Children 1-3 years: Initial: 5 mcg/day; Usual maintenance dose: 50 mcg/day

Children >3 years: Initial: 5 mcg/day; Maintenance: Up to 100 mcg/day

Adults: Initial 5-25 mcg/day; Maintenance range 5-100 mcg/day

Elderly: Initial: 5 mcg/day

Mechanism of Action Exact mechanism of action is unknown; however, it is believed the thyroid hormone exerts its many metabolic effects through control of DNA transcription and protein synthesis; involved in normal metabolism, growth, and development; promotes gluconeogenesis, increases utilization and mobilization of glycogen stores, and stimulates protein synthesis, increases basal metabolic rate

Pharmacodynamics/Kinetics

Onset of Action 2-4 hours; peak response: 2-3 days

Half-life Elimination 2.5 days

Pregnancy Risk Factor A

Liotrix (LYE oh triks)

Related Information

Endocrine Disorders and Pregnancy *on page 1879*

U.S. Brand Names Thyrolar®

Canadian Brand Names Thyrolar®

Pharmacologic Category Thyroid Product

Use Replacement or supplemental therapy in hypothyroidism (uniform mixture of T_4: T_3 in 4:1 ratio by weight); little advantage to this product exists and cost is not justified

Local Anesthetic/Vasoconstrictor Precautions No precautions with vasoconstrictor are necessary if patient is well controlled with liotrix

Effects on Dental Treatment No significant effects or complications reported

Effects on Bleeding No information available to require special precautions

Adverse Effects Frequency not defined.

Cardiovascular: Cardiac arrhythmia, chest pain, palpitation, tachycardia

Central nervous system: Ataxia, fever, headache, insomnia, nervousness

Dermatologic: Alopecia

Endocrine & metabolic: Changes in menstrual cycle, increased appetite, weight loss

Gastrointestinal: Abdominal cramps, constipation, diarrhea, vomiting

Neuromuscular & skeletal: Hand tremor, myalgia, tremor

Respiratory: Dyspnea

Miscellaneous: Allergic skin reactions (rare), diaphoresis

General Dosage Range Oral:

Children 0-6 months: 8-10 mcg/kg **or** 25-50 mcg/day

Children 6-12 months: 6-8 mcg/kg **or** 50-75 mcg/day

Children 1-5 years: 5-6 mcg/kg **or** 75-100 mcg/day

Children 6-12 years: 4-5 mcg/kg **or** 100-150 mcg/day

Children >12 years: 2-3 mcg/kg **or** >150 mcg/day

Adults: Initial: 15-30 mg/day; Usual maintenance: 60-120 mg/day

Elderly: Initial: 15 mg

Mechanism of Action The primary active compound is T_3 (triiodothyronine), which may be converted from T_4 (thyroxine) and then circulates throughout the body to influence growth and maturation of various tissues. Liotrix is uniform mixture of synthetic T_4 and T_3 in 4:1 ratio; exact mechanism of action is unknown; however, it is believed the thyroid hormone exerts its many metabolic effects through control of DNA transcription and protein synthesis; involved in normal metabolism, growth, and development; promotes gluconeogenesis, increases utilization and mobilization of glycogen stores and stimulates protein synthesis, increases basal metabolic rate

Pharmacodynamics/Kinetics

Half-life Elimination 6-7 days

Time to Peak Serum: 12-48 hours

Pregnancy Risk Factor A

Liraglutide (lir a GLOO tide)

U.S. Brand Names Victoza®

Canadian Brand Names Victoza®

Pharmacologic Category Antidiabetic Agent, Glucagon-Like Peptide-1 (GLP-1) Receptor Agonist

Use Treatment of type 2 diabetes mellitus (noninsulin dependent, NIDDM) to improve glycemic control

Local Anesthetic/Vasoconstrictor Precautions No information available to require special precautions

Effects on Dental Treatment Schedule type 1 and type 2 diabetic patients for dental treatment in the morning in order to minimize chance of stress-induced hypoglycemia.

Effects on Bleeding No information available to require special precautions

Adverse Effects Percentages are as reported for monotherapy.

>10%: Gastrointestinal: Nausea (28%), diarrhea (17%), vomiting (11%)

1% to 10%:

Cardiovascular: Hypertension (3%)

Central nervous system: Headache (9%), dizziness (6%)

Gastrointestinal: Constipation (10%)

Genitourinary: Urinary tract infection (6%)

Hepatic: Hyperbilirubinemia (4%)

Local: Injection site reactions (2%; includes rash, erythema)

Neuromuscular & skeletal: Back pain (5%)

Respiratory: Upper respiratory infection (10%), sinusitis (6%), nasopharyngitis (5%)

Miscellaneous: Anti-liraglutide antibodies (low titers 9%, cross-reacting 7%), influenza (7%)

General Dosage Range SubQ: *Adults:* Initial: 0.6 mg once daily; maintenance: 1.2-1.8 mg/day

Mechanism of Action Liraglutide is a long acting analog of human glucagon-like peptide-1 (GLP-1) (an incretin hormone) which increases glucose-dependent insulin secretion, decreases inappropriate glucagon secretion, increases B-cell growth/replication, slows gastric emptying, and decreases food intake. Liraglutide administration results in decreases in hemoglobin A_{1c} by approximately 1%.

Pharmacodynamics/Kinetics

Half-life Elimination ~13 hours

Time to Peak Plasma: 8-12 hours

Pregnancy Risk Factor C

Lisdexamfetamine (lis dex am FET a meen)

U.S. Brand Names Vyvanse®

Canadian Brand Names Vyvanse™

Pharmacologic Category Stimulant

Use Treatment of attention-deficit/hyperactivity disorder (ADHD)

Local Anesthetic/Vasoconstrictor Precautions Use vasoconstrictor with caution in patients taking lisdexamfetamine. Amphetamines enhance the sympathomimetic response of epinephrine or mepivacaine and levonordefrin (Carbocaine® 2% with Neo-Cobefrin®) leading to potential hypertension and cardiotoxicity.

Effects on Dental Treatment Key adverse event(s) related to dental treatment: Xerostomia (normal salivary flow resumes upon discontinuation).

Lisdexamfetamine is a prodrug that is converted to the active component dextroamphetamine (a noncatecholamine, sympathomimetic amine); dextroamphetamine is known to increase blood pressure. Monitor blood pressure prior to using local anesthetic with vasoconstrictors.

Effects on Bleeding No information available to require special precautions

Adverse Effects

>10%:

Central nervous system: Headache (children 12%), insomnia (19% to 27%; 4% [initially])

Gastrointestinal: Appetite decreased (27% to 39%), xerostomia (children 5%; adults 26%), abdominal pain (children 12%)

1% to 10%:

Cardiovascular: Blood pressure increased (adults 3%), heart rate increased (adults 2%)

Central nervous system: Irritability (children 10%), anxiety (adults 6%), dizziness (children 5%), jitteriness (adults 4%), affect lability (children 3%), agitation (adults 3%), restlessness (adults 3%), fever (children 2%), somnolence (children 2%), tic (children 2%)

Dermatologic: Hyperhidrosis (adults 3%), rash (children 3%)

Gastrointestinal: Vomiting (children 9%), weight loss (children 9%), diarrhea (adults 7%), nausea (6% to 7%), anorexia (adult: 5%)

Genitourinary: Erectile dysfunction (adults <2%), libido decreased (adults <2%)

Neuromuscular & skeletal: Tremor (adults 2%)

Respiratory: Dyspnea (adults 2%)

Additional adverse reaction associated with amphetamines; frequency not defined:

Cardiovascular: Cardiomyopathy, hypertension, MI, sudden death, tachycardia

Central nervous system: Exacerbation of motor and phonic tics, overstimulation, stroke, Tourette's syndrome

Dermatologic: Stevens-Johnson syndrome, toxic epidermal necrolysis

Gastrointestinal: Abnormal taste, constipation

General Dosage Range Oral: *Children ≥6 years and Adults:* Initial: 30 mg once daily; Maintenance: Up to 70 mg once daily

Mechanism of Action Lisdexamfetamine dimesylate is a prodrug that is converted to the active component dextroamphetamine (a noncatecholamine, sympathomimetic amine). Amphetamines are noncatecholamine, sympathomimetic amines that cause release of catecholamines (primarily dopamine and norepinephrine) from their storage sites in the presynaptic nerve terminals. A less significant mechanism may include their ability to block the reuptake of catecholamines by competitive inhibition.

Pharmacodynamics/Kinetics

Half-life Elimination Lisdexamfetamine: <1 hour; Dextroamphetamine: 10-13 hours

Time to Peak T_{max}: Lisdexamfetamine: ~1 hour; dextroamphetamine: ~3.5 hours

Pregnancy Risk Factor C

Controlled Substance C-II

Lisinopril (lyse IN oh pril)

Related Information

Cardiovascular Diseases *on page 1848*

U.S. Brand Names Prinivil®; Zestril®

Canadian Brand Names Apo-Lisinopril®; CO Lisinopril; Dom-Lisinopril; JAMP-Lisinopril; Mint-Lisinopril; Mylan-Lisinopril; Novo-Lisinopril; PHL-Lisinopril; PMS-Lisinopril; Prinivil®; PRO-Lisinopril; RAN™-Lisinopril; ratio-Lisinopril; ratio-Lisinopril P; ratio-Lisinopril Z; Riva-Lisinopril; Sandoz-Lisinopril; Teva-Lisinopril (Type P); Teva-Lisinopril (Type Z); Zestril®; ZYM-Lisinopril

Generic Availability (U.S.) Yes

Pharmacologic Category Angiotensin-Converting Enzyme (ACE) Inhibitor

Use Treatment of hypertension, either alone or in combination with other antihypertensive agents; adjunctive therapy in treatment of heart failure (afterload reduction); treatment of acute myocardial infarction within 24 hours in hemodynamically-stable patients to improve survival; treatment of left ventricular dysfunction after myocardial infarction

Local Anesthetic/Vasoconstrictor Precautions No information available to require special precautions

Effects on Dental Treatment Key adverse event(s) related to dental treatment: Orthostatic effects.

Effects on Bleeding No information available to require special precautions

Adverse Effects Note: Frequency ranges include data from hypertension and heart failure trials. Higher rates of adverse reactions have generally been noted in patients with CHF. However, the frequency of adverse effects associated with placebo is also increased in this population.

1% to 10%:

Cardiovascular: Orthostatic effects (1%), hypotension (1% to 4%)

Central nervous system: Headache (4% to 6%), dizziness (5% to 12%), fatigue (3%)

Dermatologic: Rash (1% to 2%)

Endocrine & metabolic: Hyperkalemia (2% to 5%)

Gastrointestinal: Diarrhea (3% to 4%), nausea (2%), vomiting (1%), abdominal pain (2%)
Genitourinary: Impotence (1%)
Hematologic: Decreased hemoglobin (small)
Neuromuscular & skeletal: Chest pain (3%), weakness (1%)
Renal: BUN increased (2%); deterioration in renal function (in patients with bilateral renal artery stenosis or hypovolemia); serum creatinine increased (often transient)
Respiratory: Cough (4% to 9%), upper respiratory infection (1% to 2%)

Dosage Oral:

Heart failure: Adults: Initial: 2.5-5 mg once daily; then increase by no more than 10 mg increments at intervals no less than 2 weeks to a maximum daily dose of 40 mg. Usual maintenance: 5-40 mg/day as a single dose. Target dose: 20-40 mg once daily (ACC/AHA 2009 Heart Failure Guidelines)

Note: If patient has hyponatremia (serum sodium <130 mEq/L) or renal impairment (Cl_{cr} <30 mL/minute or creatinine >3 mg/dL), then initial dose should be 2.5 mg/day

Hypertension:

Children ≥6 years: Initial: 0.07 mg/kg once daily (up to 5 mg); increase dose at 1- to 2-week intervals; doses >0.61 mg/kg or >40 mg have not been evaluated.

Adults: Usual dosage range (JNC 7): 10-40 mg/day

Not maintained on diuretic: Initial: 10 mg/day

Maintained on diuretic: Initial: 5 mg/day

Note: Antihypertensive effect may diminish toward the end of the dosing interval especially with doses of 10 mg/day. An increased dose may aid in extending the duration of antihypertensive effect. Doses up to 80 mg/day have been used, but do not appear to give greater effect.

Elderly: Initial: 2.5-5 mg/day; increase doses 2.5-5 mg/day at 1- to 2-week intervals; maximum daily dose: 40 mg

Patients taking diuretics should have them discontinued 2-3 days prior to initiating lisinopril if possible. Restart diuretic after blood pressure is stable if needed. If diuretic cannot be discontinued prior to therapy, begin with 5 mg with close supervision until stable blood pressure. In patients with hyponatremia (<130 mEq/L), start dose at 2.5 mg/day

Acute myocardial infarction (within 24 hours in hemodynamically stable patients): Oral: 5 mg immediately, then 5 mg at 24 hours, 10 mg at 48 hours, and 10 mg every day thereafter for 6 weeks. Patients should continue to receive standard treatments such as thrombolytics, aspirin, and beta-blockers.

Dosing adjustment in renal impairment:

Heart failure: Adults: Cl_{cr} <30 mL/minute or creatinine >3 mg/dL: Initial: 2.5 mg/day

Hypertension:

Adults: Initial doses should be modified and upward titration should be cautious, based on response (maximum: 40 mg/day)

Cl_{cr} >30 mL/minute: Initial: 10 mg/day

Cl_{cr} 10-30 mL/minute: Initial: 5 mg/day

Hemodialysis: Initial: 2.5 mg/day; dialyzable (50%)

Children: Use in not recommended in pediatric patients with GFR <30 mL/minute/1.73 m^2

Mechanism of Action Competitive inhibitor of angiotensin-converting enzyme (ACE); prevents conversion of angiotensin I to angiotensin II, a potent vasoconstrictor; results in lower levels of angiotensin II which causes an increase in plasma renin activity and a reduction in aldosterone secretion; a CNS mechanism may also be involved in hypotensive effect as angiotensin II increases adrenergic outflow from CNS; vasoactive kallikreins may be decreased in conversion to active hormones by ACE inhibitors, thus reducing blood pressure

Contraindications Hypersensitivity to lisinopril or any component of the formulation; angioedema related to previous treatment with an ACE inhibitor; patients with idiopathic or hereditary angioedema

Warnings/Precautions Anaphylactic reactions may occur rarely with ACE inhibitors. At any time during treatment (especially following first dose), angioedema may occur rarely with ACE inhibitors; it may involve the head and neck (potentially compromising airway) or the intestine (presenting with abdominal pain). African-Americans may be at an increased risk. Prolonged frequent monitoring may be required especially if tongue, glottis, or larynx are involved as they are associated *with airway obstruction. Patients with a history of airway surgery may have a higher risk of airway obstruction. Aggressive early and appropriate management is critical.* Use in patients with idiopathic or hereditary angioedema or previous angioedema associated with ACE inhibitor therapy is contraindicated. Severe anaphylactoid reactions may be seen during hemodialysis (eg, CVVHD) with high-flux dialysis membranes (eg, AN69), and rarely, during low density lipoprotein apheresis with dextran sulfate cellulose. Rare cases of *anaphylactoid reactions have been reported* in patients undergoing sensitization treatment with hymenoptera (bee, wasp) venom while receiving ACE inhibitors.

Symptomatic hypotension with or without syncope can occur with ACE inhibitors (usually with the first several doses); effects are most often observed in volume depleted patients; correct volume depletion prior to initiation; close monitoring of patient is required especially with initial dosing and dosing increases; blood pressure must be lowered at a rate appropriate for the patient's clinical condition. Initiation of therapy in patients with ischemic heart disease or cerebrovascular disease warrants close observation due to the potential consequences posed by falling blood pressure (eg, MI, stroke). Use with caution in hypertrophic cardiomyopathy with outflow tract obstruction, severe aortic stenosis, or before, during, or immediately after major surgery. **[U.S. Boxed Warning]: Based on human data, ACEIs can cause injury and death to the developing fetus when used in the second and third trimesters. ACEIs should be discontinued as soon as possible once pregnancy is detected.**

Hyperkalemia may occur with ACE inhibitors; risk factors include renal dysfunction, diabetes mellitus, concomitant use of potassium-sparing diuretics, potassium supplements, and/or potassium-containing salts. Use cautiously, if at all, with these agents and monitor potassium closely. Cough may occur with ACE inhibitors. Other causes of cough should be considered (eg, pulmonary congestion in patients with heart failure) and excluded prior to discontinuation.

May be associated with deterioration of renal function and/or increases in serum creatinine, particularly in patients with low renal blood flow (eg, renal artery stenosis, heart failure) whose glomerular filtration rate (GFR) is dependent on efferent arteriolar vasoconstriction by angiotensin II; deterioration may result in oliguria, acute renal failure, and progressive azotemia. Small increases in serum creatinine may occur following initiation; consider discontinuation only in patients with progressive and/or significant deterioration in renal function. Use with caution in patients with unstented unilateral/bilateral renal artery stenosis. When unstented bilateral renal artery stenosis is present, use is generally avoided due to the elevated risk of deterioration in renal function unless possible benefits outweigh risks. Concurrent use of angiotensin receptor blockers may increase the risk of clinically-significant adverse events (eg, renal dysfunction, hyperkalemia).

Rare toxicities associated with ACE inhibitors include cholestatic jaundice (which may progress to fulminant hepatic necrosis), agranulocytosis, neutropenia, or leukopenia with myeloid hypoplasia. Patients with collagen vascular diseases (especially with concomitant renal impairment) or renal impairment alone may be at increased risk for hematologic toxicity; periodically monitor CBC with differential in these patients. Safety and efficacy have not been established in children <6 years of age or children with a Cl_{cr} ≤30 mL/minute.

Drug Interactions

Avoid Concomitant Use There are no known interactions where it is recommended to avoid concomitant use.

Increased Effect/Toxicity

Lisinopril may increase the levels/effects of: Allopurinol; Amifostine; Antihypertensives; AzaTHIOprine; CycloSPORINE; CycloSPORINE (Systemic); Ferric Gluconate; Gold Sodium Thiomalate; Hypotensive Agents; Iron Dextran Complex; Lithium; Nonsteroidal Anti-Inflammatory Agents; RiTUXimab

The levels/effects of Lisinopril may be increased by: Angiotensin II Receptor Blockers; Diazoxide; DPP-IV Inhibitors; Eplerenone; Everolimus; Herbs (Hypotensive Properties); Loop Diuretics; MAO Inhibitors; Pentoxifylline; Phosphodiesterase 5 Inhibitors; Potassium Salts; Potassium-Sparing Diuretics; Prostacyclin Analogues; Sirolimus; Temsirolimus; Thiazide Diuretics; TiZANidine; Tolvaptan; Trimethoprim

Decreased Effect

The levels/effects of Lisinopril may be decreased by: Antacids; Aprotinin; Herbs (Hypertensive Properties); Methylphenidate; Nonsteroidal Anti-Inflammatory Agents; Salicylates; Yohimbine

Ethanol/Nutrition/Herb Interactions

Food: Potassium-containing salt substitutes may increase risk of hyperkalemia.

Herb/Nutraceutical: Avoid bayberry, blue cohosh, cayenne, ephedra, ginger, ginseng (American), kola, licorice (may worsen hypertension). Avoid black cohosh, California poppy, coleus, golden seal, hawthorn, mistletoe, periwinkle, quinine, shepherd's purse (may have increased antihypertensive effect).

Dietary Considerations Use potassium-containing salt substitutes cautiously in patients with diabetes, patients with renal dysfunction, or those maintained on potassium supplements or potassium-sparing diuretics.

Pharmacodynamics/Kinetics

Onset of Action 1 hour; Peak effect: Hypotensive: Oral: ~6 hours

Duration of Action 24 hours
Half-life Elimination 11-12 hours
Time to Peak ~7 hours
Pregnancy Risk Factor C (1st trimester); D (2nd and 3rd trimesters)
Lactation Excretion in breast milk unknown/not recommended
Breast-Feeding Considerations It is not known if lisinopril is excreted in breast milk. Breast-feeding is not recommended by the manufacturer.
Dosage Forms
Tablet, oral: 2.5 mg, 5 mg, 10 mg, 20 mg, 30 mg, 40 mg
Prinivil®: 5 mg, 10 mg, 20 mg
Zestril®: 2.5 mg, 5 mg, 10 mg, 20 mg, 30 mg, 40 mg

Lisinopril and Hydrochlorothiazide

(lyse IN oh pril & hye droe klor oh THYE a zide)

Related Information
Hydrochlorothiazide *on page* 854
Lisinopril *on page* 1025
U.S. Brand Names Prinzide®; Zestoretic®
Canadian Brand Names Apo-Lisinopril®/Hctz; Mylan-Lisinopril/Hctz; Novo-Lisinopril/Hctz; Prinzide®; Sandoz-Lisinopril/Hctz; Teva-Lisinopril/Hctz (Type P); Teva-Lisinopril/Hctz (Type Z); Zestoretic®
Pharmacologic Category Angiotensin-Converting Enzyme (ACE) Inhibitor; Diuretic, Thiazide
Use Treatment of hypertension
Local Anesthetic/Vasoconstrictor Precautions No information available to require special precautions
Effects on Dental Treatment No significant effects or complications reported
Effects on Bleeding No information available to require special precautions
Adverse Effects See individual agents.
General Dosage Range Oral: *Adults:* Lisinopril 10-80 mg and hydrochlorothiazide 12.5-50 mg once daily
Pregnancy Risk Factor C/D (2nd and 3rd trimesters)

Lithium (LITH ee um)

U.S. Brand Names Lithobid®
Canadian Brand Names Apo-Lithium® Carbonate; Apo-Lithium® Carbonate SR; Carbolith™; Duralith®; Euro-Lithium; Lithane™; Lithmax; PHL-Lithium Carbonate; PMS-Lithium Carbonate; PMS-Lithium Citrate
Generic Availability (U.S.) Yes
Pharmacologic Category Antimanic Agent
Use Management of bipolar disorders; treatment of mania in individuals with bipolar disorder (maintenance treatment prevents or diminishes intensity of subsequent episodes)
Unlabeled/Investigational Use Potential augmenting agent for antidepressants; aggression, post-traumatic stress disorder, conduct disorder in children
Local Anesthetic/Vasoconstrictor Precautions No information available to require special precautions
Effects on Dental Treatment Key adverse event(s) related to dental treatment: Xerostomia and changes in salivation (normal salivary flow resumes upon discontinuation), salivary gland swelling, and metallic taste. Avoid NSAIDs if analgesics are required since lithium toxicity has been reported with concomitant administration; acetaminophen products (ie, singly or with narcotics) are recommended.
Effects on Bleeding No information available to require special precautions
Adverse Effects Frequency not defined.
Cardiovascular: Cardiac arrhythmia, hypotension, sinus node dysfunction, flattened or inverted T waves (reversible), edema, bradycardia, syncope
Central nervous system: Blackout spells, coma, confusion, dizziness, dystonia, fatigue, headache, lethargy, pseudotumor cerebri, psychomotor retardation, restlessness, sedation, seizure, slowed intellectual functioning, slurred speech, stupor, tics, vertigo
Dermatologic: Dry or thinning of hair, folliculitis, alopecia, exacerbation of psoriasis, rash
Endocrine & metabolic: Euthyroid goiter and/or hypothyroidism, hyperthyroidism, hyperglycemia, diabetes insipidus
Gastrointestinal: Polydipsia, anorexia, nausea, vomiting, diarrhea, xerostomia, metallic taste, weight gain, salivary gland swelling, excessive salivation
Genitourinary: Incontinence, polyuria, glycosuria, oliguria, albuminuria

Hematologic: Leukocytosis

Neuromuscular & skeletal: Tremor, muscle hyperirritability, ataxia, choreoathetoid movements, hyperactive deep tendon reflexes, myasthenia gravis (rare)

Ocular: Nystagmus, blurred vision, transient scotoma

Miscellaneous: Coldness and painful discoloration of fingers and toes

Postmarketing and/or case reports: Drug-induced Brugada syndrome

Dosage Oral: Monitor serum concentrations and clinical response (efficacy and toxicity) to determine proper dose

Children 6-12 years:

Bipolar disorder (unlabeled use): 15-60 mg/kg/day in 3-4 divided doses; dose not to exceed usual adult dosage

Conduct disorder (unlabeled use): 15-30 mg/kg/day in 3-4 divided doses; dose not to exceed usual adult dosage

Adults: Bipolar disorder: 900-2400 mg/day in 3-4 divided doses or 900-1800 mg/day (extended release) in 2 divided doses

Elderly: Bipolar disorder: Initial dose: 300 mg once or twice daily; increase weekly in increments of 300 mg/day, monitoring levels; rarely need >900-1200 mg/day

Dosing adjustment in renal impairment:

Cl_{cr} 10-50 mL/minute: Administer 50% to 75% of normal dose

Cl_{cr} <10 mL/minute: Administer 25% to 50% of normal dose

Hemodialysis: Dialyzable (50% to 100%); 4-7 times more efficient than peritoneal dialysis

Mechanism of Action Alters cation transport across cell membrane in nerve and muscle cells and influences reuptake of serotonin and/or norepinephrine; second messenger systems involving the phosphatidylinositol cycle are inhibited; postsynaptic D2 receptor supersensitivity is inhibited

Contraindications Hypersensitivity to lithium or any component of the formulation; avoid use in patients with severe cardiovascular or renal disease, or with severe debilitation, dehydration, or sodium depletion; pregnancy

Warnings/Precautions [U.S. Boxed Warning]: Lithium toxicity is closely related to serum levels and can occur at therapeutic doses; serum lithium determinations are required to monitor therapy. Use with caution in patients with thyroid disease, mild-moderate renal impairment, or mild-moderate cardiovascular disease. Use caution in patients receiving medications which alter sodium excretion (eg, diuretics, ACE inhibitors, NSAIDs), or in patients with significant fluid loss (protracted sweating, diarrhea, or prolonged fever); temporary reduction or cessation of therapy may be warranted. Some elderly patients may be extremely sensitive to the effects of lithium, see Dosage. Chronic therapy results in diminished renal concentrating ability (nephrogenic DI); this is usually reversible when lithium is discontinued. Changes in renal function should be monitored, and re-evaluation of treatment may be necessary. Use caution in patients at risk of suicide (suicidal thoughts or behavior).

Use with caution in patients receiving neuroleptic medications - a syndrome resembling NMS has been associated with concurrent therapy. Lithium may impair the patient's alertness, affecting the ability to operate machinery or driving a vehicle. Neuromuscular-blocking agents should be administered with caution; the response may be prolonged.

Higher serum concentrations may be required and tolerated during an acute manic phase; however, the tolerance decreases when symptoms subside. Normal fluid and salt intake must be maintained during therapy.

Drug Interactions

Avoid Concomitant Use

Avoid concomitant use of Lithium with any of the following: Sibutramine

Increased Effect/Toxicity

Lithium may increase the levels/effects of: Antipsychotics; Neuromuscular-Blocking Agents; Serotonin Modulators; Tricyclic Antidepressants

The levels/effects of Lithium may be increased by: ACE Inhibitors; Angiotensin II Receptor Blockers; Calcium Channel Blockers (Nondihydropyridine); CarBAMazepine; Desmopressin; Fosphenytoin; Loop Diuretics; MAO Inhibitors; Methyldopa; Nonsteroidal Anti-Inflammatory Agents; Phenytoin; Potassium Iodide; Selective Serotonin Reuptake Inhibitors; Sibutramine; Thiazide Diuretics; Topiramate

Decreased Effect

Lithium may decrease the levels/effects of: Amphetamines; Antipsychotics; Desmopressin

The levels/effects of Lithium may be decreased by: Calcitonin; Calcium Polystyrene Sulfonate; Carbonic Anhydrase Inhibitors; Loop Diuretics; Sodium Bicarbonate; Sodium Chloride; Sodium Polystyrene Sulfonate; Theophylline Derivatives

Ethanol/Nutrition/Herb Interactions Food: Limit caffeine.

Dietary Considerations May be taken with meals to avoid GI upset; maintain adequate fluid intake.

Pharmacodynamics/Kinetics

Half-life Elimination 18-24 hours; can increase to more than 36 hours in elderly or with renal impairment

Time to Peak Serum: Nonsustained release: ~0.5-2 hours; extended release: 4-12 hours; syrup: 15-60 minutes

Pregnancy Risk Factor D

Lactation Enters breast milk/contraindicated

Dosage Forms

Capsule, oral: 150 mg, 300 mg, 600 mg

Solution, oral: 300 mg/5 mL (5 mL, 473 mL, 500 mL)

Tablet, oral: 300 mg, 600 mg

Tablet, extended release, oral: 300 mg, 450 mg

Lithobid®: 300 mg

L-Lysine (el LYE seen)

Related Information

Viral Infections *on page* 1947

U.S. Brand Names Lysinyl [OTC]

Generic Availability (U.S.) Yes

Pharmacologic Category Nutritional Supplement

Dental Use Prevention of recurrent herpes simplex infection

Use Improves utilization of vegetable proteins; prevention of recurrent herpes simplex infection

Local Anesthetic/Vasoconstrictor Precautions No information available to require special precautions

Effects on Dental Treatment No significant effects or complications reported

Effects on Bleeding No information available to require special precautions

Dental Usual Dosage Recurrent herpes simplex infection: Adults: Oral: 500-3000 mg/day; begin treatment during early stage of recurrence.

Dosage Oral: Adults:

Supplement: 334-1500 mg/day

Prevention of recurrent herpes simplex infection: 500-3000 mg/day; begin treatment during early stage of recurrence

Dosage Forms

Capsule, oral: 500 mg

Lysinyl [OTC]: 500 mg

Powder, oral: (100 g)

Lysinyl [OTC]: (150 g)

Tablet, oral: 500 mg, 1000 mg

References

Griffith RS, Walsh DE, Myrmel KH, et al, "Success of L-Lysine Therapy in Frequently Recurrent Herpes Simplex Infection. Treatment and Prophylaxis," *Dermatologica*, 1987, 175(4):183-90.

"L-lysine," *Altern Med Rev*, 2007, 12(2):169-72.

Lodoxamide (loe DOKS a mide)

U.S. Brand Names Alomide®

Canadian Brand Names Alomide®

Pharmacologic Category Mast Cell Stabilizer

Use Treatment of vernal keratoconjunctivitis, vernal conjunctivitis, and vernal keratitis

Local Anesthetic/Vasoconstrictor Precautions No information available to require special precautions

Effects on Dental Treatment No significant effects or complications reported

Effects on Bleeding No information available to require special precautions

Adverse Effects

>10%: Local: Transient burning, stinging, discomfort

1% to 10%:

Central nervous system: Headache

Ocular: Blurred vision, corneal erosion/ulcer, eye pain, corneal abrasion, blepharitis

General Dosage Range ***Ophthalmic:*** *Children ≥2 years and Adults:* Instill 1-2 drops in eye(s) 4 times/day

Mechanism of Action Mast cell stabilizer that inhibits the *in vivo* type I immediate hypersensitivity reaction to increase cutaneous vascular permeability associated with IgE and antigen-mediated reactions

Pregnancy Risk Factor B

Lomustine (loe MUS teen)

U.S. Brand Names CeeNU®
Canadian Brand Names CeeNU®
Pharmacologic Category Antineoplastic Agent; Antineoplastic Agent, Alkylating Agent; Antineoplastic Agent, Alkylating Agent (Nitrosourea)
Use Treatment of primary and metastatic brain tumors (after surgery and/or radiation therapy); treatment of relapsed or refractory Hodgkin's disease (as part of a combination chemotherapy regimen)
Unlabeled/Investigational Use Treatment of gastric cancer, metastatic melanoma
Local Anesthetic/Vasoconstrictor Precautions No information available to require special precautions
Effects on Dental Treatment No significant effects or complications reported
Effects on Bleeding Chemotherapy may result in significant myelosuppression, potentially including significant reduction in platelet counts and altered hemostasis. In patients who are under active treatment with these agents, medical consult is suggested.
Adverse Effects
>10%:
Gastrointestinal: Nausea and vomiting, (onset: 3-6 hours after oral administration; duration: <24 hours)
Hematologic: Myelosuppression (dose-limiting, delayed, cumulative); leukopenia (65%; nadir: 5-6 weeks; recovery 6-8 weeks); thrombocytopenia (nadir: 4 weeks; recovery 5-6 weeks)
Frequency not defined: Acute leukemia, alkaline phosphatase increased, alopecia, anemia, ataxia, azotemia (progressive), bilirubin increased, blindness, bone marrow dysplasia, disorientation, dysarthria, hepatotoxicity, kidney size decreased, lethargy, optic atrophy, pulmonary fibrosis, pulmonary infiltrates, renal damage, renal failure, stomatitis, transaminases increased, visual disturbances
General Dosage Range Dosage adjustment recommended in patients with renal impairment or who develop toxicities
Oral: *Children and Adults:* 100-130 mg/m^2 as a single dose once every 6 weeks
Mechanism of Action Inhibits DNA and RNA synthesis via carbamylation of DNA polymerase, alkylation of DNA, and alteration of RNA, proteins, and enzymes
Pharmacodynamics/Kinetics
Duration of Action Marrow recovery: ~5-8 weeks
Half-life Elimination Parent drug: 16-24 hours; Active metabolite: 16-48 hours
Time to Peak Serum: Active metabolite: ~3 hours
Pregnancy Risk Factor D

Loperamide (loe PER a mide)

U.S. Brand Names Anti-Diarrheal [OTC]; Diamode [OTC]; Imodium® A-D for children [OTC]; Imodium® A-D [OTC]; Kao Paverin® [OTC] [DSC]
Canadian Brand Names Apo-Loperamide®; Diarr-Eze; Dom-Loperamide; Imodium®; Loperacap; Novo-Loperamide; PMS-Loperamine; Rhoxal-loperamide; Rho®-Loperamine; Riva-Loperamide; Sandoz-Loperamide
Pharmacologic Category Antidiarrheal
Use Treatment of chronic diarrhea associated with inflammatory bowel disease; acute nonspecific diarrhea; increased volume of ileostomy discharge
OTC labeling: Control of symptoms of diarrhea, including Traveler's diarrhea
Unlabeled/Investigational Use Cancer treatment-induced diarrhea (eg, irinotecan induced); chronic diarrhea caused by bowel resection
Local Anesthetic/Vasoconstrictor Precautions No information available to require special precautions
Effects on Dental Treatment No significant effects or complications reported
Effects on Bleeding No information available to require special precautions
Adverse Effects 1% to 10%:
Central nervous system: Dizziness (1%)
Gastrointestinal: Constipation (2% to 5%), abdominal cramping (<1% to 3%), nausea (<1% to 3%)
Postmarketing and/or case reports: Abdominal distention, abdominal pain, allergic reactions, anaphylactic shock, anaphylactoid reactions, angioedema, bullous eruption (rare), drowsiness, dry mouth, dyspepsia, erythema multiforme (rare), fatigue, flatulence, paralytic ileus, megacolon, pruritus, rash, Stevens-Johnson syndrome, toxic epidermal necrolysis, toxic megacolon, urinary retention, urticaria, vomiting

General Dosage Range Oral:

Children 2-5 years (13-20 kg): Initial: 1 mg 3 times/day for first 24 hours; Maintenance: 0.1 mg/kg after each loose stool

Children 6-8 years (20-30 kg): Initial: 2 mg twice daily for first 24 hours; Maintenance: 0.1 mg/kg after each loose stool **or** 2 mg after first loose stool, followed by 1 mg after each subsequent stool (maximum: 4 mg/day)

Children 8-12 years (>30 kg): Initial: 2 mg 3 times/day for first 24 hours; Maintenance: 0.1 mg/kg after each loose stool

Children 9-11 years: 2 mg after first loose stool, followed by 1 mg after each subsequent stool (maximum: 6 mg/day)

Children ≥12 years: Initial: 4 mg after first loose stool, followed by 2 mg after each subsequent stool (maximum: 8 mg/day)

Adults: Initial: 4 mg followed by 2 mg after each loose stool (maximum: 8-16 mg/day) **or** 4-8 mg/day in divided doses

Mechanism of Action Acts directly on circular and longitudinal intestinal muscles, through the opioid receptor, to inhibit peristalsis and prolong transit time; reduces fecal volume, increases viscosity, and diminishes fluid and electrolyte loss; demonstrates antisecretory activity. Loperamide increases tone on the anal sphincter

Pharmacodynamics/Kinetics

Half-life Elimination 7-14 hours

Time to Peak Liquid: 2.5 hours; Capsule: 5 hours

Pregnancy Risk Factor C

Loperamide and Simethicone (loe PER a mide & sye METH i kone)

Related Information

Loperamide *on page* 1031

Simethicone *on page* 1527

U.S. Brand Names Imodium® Multi-Symptom Relief [OTC]

Canadian Brand Names Imodium® Advanced Multi-Symptom

Pharmacologic Category Antidiarrheal; Antiflatulent

Use Control of symptoms of diarrhea and gas (bloating, pressure, and cramps)

Local Anesthetic/Vasoconstrictor Precautions No information available to require special precautions

Effects on Dental Treatment No significant effects or complications reported

Effects on Bleeding No information available to require special precautions

Adverse Effects See individual agents.

General Dosage Range Oral:

Children 6-8 years (48-59 lbs): 1 caplet/tablet after first loose stool, followed by 1/2 caplet/tablet with each subsequent loose stool (maximum: 2 caplets or tablets/24 hours)

Children 9-11 years (60-95 lbs): 1 caplet/tablet after first loose stool, followed by 1/2 caplet/tablet with each subsequent loose stool (maximum: 3 caplets or tablets/24 hours)

Children ≥12 years and Adults: 1 caplet/tablet after each loose stool (maximum: 4 caplets or tablets/24 hours)

Mechanism of Action

Loperamide acts by slowing intestinal motility and by affecting water and electrolyte movement through the bowel.

Simethicone acts in the stomach and intestines by altering the surface tension of gas bubbles enabling them to coalesce thereby freeing and eliminating the gas more easily by belching or passing flatus.

Lopinavir and Ritonavir (loe PIN a veer & rit ON uh veer)

Related Information

HIV Infection and AIDS *on page* 1883

Ritonavir *on page* 1488

U.S. Brand Names Kaletra®

Canadian Brand Names Kaletra®

Pharmacologic Category Antiretroviral Agent, Protease Inhibitor

Use Treatment of HIV infection in combination with other antiretroviral agents

Local Anesthetic/Vasoconstrictor Precautions No information available to require special precautions

Effects on Dental Treatment Key adverse event(s) related to dental treatment: Dysphagia.

Effects on Bleeding Increased bleeding has been noted with protease inhibitors in patients with hemophilia A or B. No information available to require routine special precautions relative to hemostasis in other patients.

Adverse Effects Data presented for short- and long-term combination antiretroviral therapy in both protease inhibitor experienced and naïve patients.

>10%:

Dermatologic: Rash (children 12%; adults ≤5%)

Endocrine & metabolic: Hypercholesterolemia (3% to 39%), triglycerides increased (3% to 36%)

Gastrointestinal: Diarrhea (7% to 28%; greater with once-daily dosing), abnormal taste/taste perversion (children 22%; adults <2%), vomiting (children 21%; adults 2% to 6%), nausea (5% to 16%), abdominal pain (1% to 11%)

Hepatic: GGT increased (10% to 29%), ALT increased (grade 3/4: 1% to 11%)

>2% to 10%:

Cardiovascular: Vasodilation (≤3%)

Central nervous system: Headache (2% to 6%), insomnia (≤3%)

Endocrine & metabolic: Hyperglycemia (≤5%), hyperuricemia (≤5%), sodium decreased or increased (children 3%),

Gastrointestinal: Amylase increased (3% to 8%), dyspepsia (≤6%), lipase increased (3% to 5%), flatulence (1% to 4%), weight loss (≤3%)

Hematologic: Platelets decreased (grade 3/4: 4% children), neutropenia (grade 3/4: 1% to 5%)

Hepatic: AST increased (grade 3/4: 2% to 10%), bilirubin increased (children 3%; adults 1%)

Neuromuscular & skeletal: Weakness (≤9%)

General Dosage Range Dosage adjustment recommended in patients on concomitant therapy

Oral:

Children 14 days to 6 months: Lopinavir 16 mg/kg or 300 mg/m^2 twice daily

Children 6 months to 18 years and <15 kg: 12 mg lopinavir/kg twice daily (maximum dose: Lopinavir 400 mg/ritonavir 100 mg)

Children 6 months to 18 years and 15-40 kg: 10 mg lopinavir/kg twice daily (maximum dose: Lopinavir 400 mg/ritonavir 100 mg)

Children 6 months to 18 years and >40 kg: Lopinavir 400 mg/ritonavir 100 mg twice daily

Adults: Lopinavir 400 mg/ritonavir 100 mg twice daily **or** lopinavir 800 mg/ritonavir 200 mg once daily

Mechanism of Action A coformulation of lopinavir and ritonavir. The lopinavir component binds to the site of HIV-1 protease activity and inhibits the cleavage of viral Gag-Pol polyprotein precursors into individual functional proteins required for infectious HIV. This results in the formation of immature, noninfectious viral particles. The ritonavir component inhibits the CYP3A metabolism of lopinavir, allowing increased plasma levels of lopinavir.

Pharmacodynamics/Kinetics

Half-life Elimination Lopinavir: 5-6 hours

Time to Peak Lopinavir: ~4 hours

Pregnancy Risk Factor C

Loratadine (lor AT a deen)

U.S. Brand Names Alavert® Allergy 24 Hour [OTC]; Alavert® Children's Allergy [OTC]; Claritin® 24 Hour Allergy [OTC]; Claritin® Children's Allergy [OTC]; Claritin® Liqui-Gels® 24 Hour Allergy [OTC]; Claritin® RediTabs® 24 Hour Allergy [OTC]; Loradamed [OTC]; Tavist® ND Allergy [OTC]

Canadian Brand Names Apo-Loratadine®; Claritin®; Claritin® Kids

Pharmacologic Category Histamine H_1 Antagonist; Histamine H_1 Antagonist, Second Generation; Piperidine Derivative

Use Relief of nasal and non-nasal symptoms of seasonal allergic rhinitis; treatment of chronic idiopathic urticaria

Local Anesthetic/Vasoconstrictor Precautions No information available to require special precautions

Effects on Dental Treatment Key adverse event(s) related to dental treatment: Xerostomia (normal salivary flow resumes upon discontinuation) and stomatitis in children (2-5 years).

Effects on Bleeding No information available to require special precautions

Adverse Effects

Adults:

Central nervous system: Headache (12%), somnolence (8%), fatigue (4%)

Gastrointestinal: Xerostomia (3%)

Children:

Central nervous system: Nervousness (4% ages 6-12 years), fatigue (3% ages 6-12 years, 2% to 3% ages 2-5 years), malaise (2% ages 6-12 years)

Dermatologic: Rash (2% to 3% ages 2-5 years)

Gastrointestinal: Abdominal pain (2% ages 6-12 years), stomatitis (2% to 3% ages 2-5 years)
Neuromuscular & skeletal: Hyperkinesia (3% ages 6-12 years)
Ocular: Conjunctivitis (2% ages 6-12 years)
Respiratory: Wheezing (4% ages 6-12 years), dysphonia (2% ages 6-12 years), upper respiratory infection (2% ages 6-12 years), epistaxis (2% to 3% ages 2-5 years), pharyngitis (2% to 3% ages 2-5 years)
Miscellaneous: Flu-like syndrome (2% to 3% ages 2-5 years), viral infection (2% to 3% ages 2-5 years)

General Dosage Range Dosage adjustment recommended in patients with hepatic or renal impairment

Oral:

Children 2-5 years: 5 mg once daily
Children ≥6 years and Adults: 10 mg once daily

Mechanism of Action Long-acting tricyclic antihistamine with selective peripheral histamine H_1-receptor antagonistic properties

Pharmacodynamics/Kinetics

Onset of Action 1-3 hours; Peak effect: 8-12 hours

Duration of Action >24 hours

Half-life Elimination 12-15 hours

Loratadine and Pseudoephedrine (lor AT a deen & soo doe e FED rin)

Related Information

Bacterial Infections *on page 1933*
Loratadine *on page 1033*
Pseudoephedrine *on page 1429*

U.S. Brand Names Alavert™ Allergy and Sinus [OTC]; Claritin-D® 12 Hour Allergy & Congestion [OTC]; Claritin-D® 24 Hour Allergy & Congestion [OTC]

Canadian Brand Names Chlor-Tripolon ND®; Claritin® Extra; Claritin® Liberator

Generic Availability (U.S.) Yes

Pharmacologic Category Alpha/Beta Agonist; Decongestant; Histamine H_1 Antagonist; Histamine H_1 Antagonist, Second Generation; Piperidine Derivative

Use Temporary relief of symptoms of seasonal allergic rhinitis, other upper respiratory allergies, or the common cold

Local Anesthetic/Vasoconstrictor Precautions Use with caution since pseudoephedrine is a sympathomimetic amine which could interact with epinephrine to cause a pressor response

Effects on Dental Treatment Key adverse event(s) related to dental treatment: Pseudoephedrine: Xerostomia (normal salivary flow resumes upon discontinuation).

Effects on Bleeding No information available to require special precautions

Adverse Effects See individual agents.

Dosage Children ≥12 years and Adults: Oral:

Claritin-D® 12-Hour: 1 tablet every 12 hours
Alavert™ Allergy and Sinus, Claritin-D® 24-Hour: 1 tablet daily

Dosage adjustment in renal impairment: Cl_{cr} ≤30 mL/minute:

Claritin-D® 12-Hour: 1 tablet daily
Claritin-D® 24-Hour: 1 tablet every other day

Dosage adjustment in hepatic impairment: Should be avoided

Contraindications Hypersensitivity to loratadine, pseudoephedrine, or any component of the formulation; use with or within 14 days of MAO inhibitors

Warnings/Precautions Use with caution in hypertension, diabetes mellitus, ischemic heart disease, increased intraocular pressure, hyperthyroidism, and prostatic hyperplasia. Use with caution in the elderly; may be more sensitive to adverse effects. Patients with swallowing difficulties (eg, upper GI narrowing or abnormal esophageal peristalsis) should not use Claritin-D® 24-Hour. Use caution with hepatic or renal impairment; dose adjustment may be required. Safety and efficacy have not been established in children <12 years of age. When used for self medication (OTC), notify healthcare provider if symptoms do not improve within 7 days or are accompanied by fever. Discontinue and contact healthcare provider if nervousness, dizziness or sleeplessness occur.

Drug Interactions

Metabolism/Transport Effects Loratadine: **Substrate** of CYP2D6 (minor), CYP3A4 (minor), P-glycoprotein; **Inhibits** CYP2C8 (weak), 2C19 (moderate), 2D6 (weak)

Avoid Concomitant Use

Avoid concomitant use of Loratadine and Pseudoephedrine with any of the following: Iobenguane I 123; MAO Inhibitors

Increased Effect/Toxicity

Loratadine and Pseudoephedrine may increase the levels/effects of: Alcohol (Ethyl); Anticholinergics; Bromocriptine; CNS Depressants; Sympathomimetics

The levels/effects of Loratadine and Pseudoephedrine may be increased by: Amiodarone; Antacids; Atomoxetine; Cannabinoids; Carbonic Anhydrase Inhibitors; Conivaptan; Droperidol; MAO Inhibitors; P-Glycoprotein Inhibitors; Pramlintide; Serotonin/Norepinephrine Reuptake Inhibitors

Decreased Effect

Loratadine and Pseudoephedrine may decrease the levels/effects of: Acetylcholinesterase Inhibitors (Central); Benzylpenicilloyl Polylysine; Betahistine; Iobenguane I 123

The levels/effects of Loratadine and Pseudoephedrine may be decreased by: Acetylcholinesterase Inhibitors (Central); Amphetamines; Peginterferon Alfa-2b; P-Glycoprotein Inducers; Spironolactone; Tocilizumab

Ethanol/Nutrition/Herb Interactions Ethanol: May increase CNS depression; monitor for increased effects with coadministration. Caution patients about effects.

Dosage Forms

Tablet, extended release: Loratadine 10 mg and pseudoephedrine 240 mg
- Alavert™ Allergy and Sinus [OTC]: Loratadine 5 mg and pseudoephedrine 120 mg
- Claritin-D® 12 Hour Allergy & Congestion [OTC]: Loratadine 5 mg and pseudoephedrine 120 mg
- Claritin-D® 24 Hour Allergy & Congestion [OTC]: Loratadine 10 mg and pseudoephedrine 240 mg

LORazepam (lor A ze pam)

Related Information

Management of the Patient With Anxiety or Depression *on page 1968*

Temporomandibular Dysfunction (TMD) *on page 1964*

Related Sample Prescriptions

Sedation (Prior to Dental Treatment) *on page 1995*

U.S. Brand Names Ativan®; Lorazepam Intensol™

Canadian Brand Names Apo-Lorazepam®; Ativan®; Dom-Lorazepam; Lorazepam Injection, USP; Novo-Lorazem; Nu-Loraz; PHL-Lorazepam; PMS-Lorazepam; PRO-Lorazepam

Generic Availability (U.S.) Yes

Pharmacologic Category Benzodiazepine

Dental Use Short-term relief of anxiety prior to dental appointment

Use

Oral: Management of anxiety disorders or short-term (≤4 months) relief of the symptoms of anxiety or anxiety associated with depressive symptoms

I.V.: Status epilepticus, amnesia, sedation

Unlabeled/Investigational Use Ethanol detoxification; insomnia; psychogenic catatonia; partial complex seizures; agitation (I.V.); antiemetic adjunct

Local Anesthetic/Vasoconstrictor Precautions No information available to require special precautions

Effects on Dental Treatment Key adverse event(s) related to dental treatment: Xerostomia (normal salivary flow resumes upon discontinuation).

Effects on Bleeding No information available to require special precautions

Adverse Effects

>10%:
- Central nervous system: Sedation
- Respiratory: Respiratory depression

1% to 10%:
- Cardiovascular: Hypotension
- Central nervous system: Akathisia, amnesia, ataxia, confusion, depression, disorientation, dizziness, headache
- Dermatologic: Dermatitis, rash
- Gastrointestinal: Changes in appetite, nausea, weight gain/loss
- Neuromuscular & skeletal: Weakness
- Ocular: Visual disturbances
- Respiratory: Apnea, hyperventilation, nasal congestion

Dental Usual Dosage

Anxiety and sedation: Adults: Oral: 1-10 mg/day in 2-3 divided doses; usual dose: 2-6 mg/day in divided doses

Preoperative: Adults:
- I.M.: 0.05 mg/kg administered 2 hours before surgery (maximum: 4 mg/dose)
- I.V.: 0.044 mg/kg 15-20 minutes before surgery (usual maximum: 2 mg/dose)

Preprocedural anxiety: Adults: Oral: 1-2 mg 1 hour before procedure

Dosage

Antiemetic (unlabeled use):
Children 2-15 years: I.V.: 0.05 mg/kg (up to 2 mg/dose) prior to chemotherapy
Adults: Oral, I.V. (**Note:** May be administered sublingually; not a labeled route): 0.5-2 mg every 4-6 hours as needed

Anxiety and sedation (unlabeled in children except for oral use in children >12 years):
Infants and Children: Oral, I.M., I.V.: Usual: 0.05 mg/kg/dose (range: 0.02-0.09 mg/kg) every 4-8 hours
I.V.: May use smaller doses (eg, 0.01-0.03 mg/kg) and repeat every 20 minutes, as needed to titrate to effect
Adults: Oral: 1-10 mg/day in 2-3 divided doses; usual dose: 2-6 mg/day in divided doses
Elderly: 0.5-4 mg/day; initial dose not to exceed 2 mg; Beers Criteria: Avoid doses >3 mg/day

Insomnia: Adults: Oral: 2-4 mg at bedtime

Preoperative: Adults:
I.M.: 0.05 mg/kg administered 2 hours before surgery (maximum: 4 mg/dose)
I.V.: 0.044 mg/kg 15-20 minutes before surgery (usual maximum: 2 mg/dose)

Preprocedural anxiety (dental use): Adults: Oral: 1-2 mg 1 hour before procedure

Operative amnesia: Adults: I.V.: Up to 0.05 mg/kg (maximum: 4 mg/dose)

Sedation (preprocedure): Infants and Children (unlabeled):
Oral, I.M., I.V.: Usual: 0.05 mg/kg (range: 0.02-0.09 mg/kg)
I.V.: May use smaller doses (eg, 0.01-0.03 mg/kg) and repeat every 20 minutes, as needed to titrate to effect

Status epilepticus: I.V.:
Infants and Children (unlabeled): 0.05-0.1 mg/kg (maximum: 4 mg/dose) slow I.V. (maximum rate: 2 mg/minute); may repeat every 10-15 minutes as needed (Hegenbarth, 2008; Sabo-Graham, 1998)
Adults: 4 mg/dose slow I.V. (maximum rate: 2 mg/minute); may repeat in 10-15 minutes; usual maximum dose: 8 mg

Rapid tranquilization of agitated patient (administer every 30-60 minutes): Adults:
Oral: 1-2 mg
I.M.: 0.5-1 mg
Average total dose for tranquilization: Oral, I.M.: 4-8 mg

Agitation in the ICU patient (unlabeled): Adults:
I.V.: 0.02-0.06 mg/kg every 2-6 hours
I.V. infusion: 0.01-0.1 mg/kg/hour
Concurrent use of probenecid or valproic acid: Reduce lorazepam dose by 50%

Dosage adjustment in renal impairment: I.V.: Risk of propylene glycol toxicity. Monitor closely if using for prolonged periods of time or at high doses.

Dosage adjustment in hepatic impairment: Use cautiously.

Mechanism of Action Binds to stereospecific benzodiazepine receptors on the postsynaptic GABA neuron at several sites within the central nervous system, including the limbic system, reticular formation. Enhancement of the inhibitory effect of GABA on neuronal excitability results by increased neuronal membrane permeability to chloride ions. This shift in chloride ions results in hyperpolarization (a less excitable state) and stabilization.

Contraindications Hypersensitivity to lorazepam or any component of the formulation (cross-sensitivity with other benzodiazepines may exist); acute narrow-angle glaucoma; sleep apnea (parenteral); intra-arterial injection of parenteral formulation; severe respiratory insufficiency (except during mechanical ventilation)

Warnings/Precautions Use with caution in elderly or debilitated patients, patients with hepatic disease (including alcoholics) or renal impairment. Due to increased sensitivity in the elderly, smaller doses of benzodiazepines may be safer and as effective; in this age group, avoid using doses >3 mg daily of lorazepam (Beers Criteria). Use with caution in patients with respiratory disease (COPD or sleep apnea) or limited pulmonary reserve, or impaired gag reflex. Initial doses in elderly or debilitated patients should be at the lower end of the dosing range. May worsen hepatic encephalopathy.

Causes CNS depression (dose-related) resulting in sedation, dizziness, confusion, or ataxia which may impair physical and mental capabilities. Patients must be cautioned about performing tasks which require mental alertness (eg, operating machinery or driving). Use with caution in patients receiving other CNS depressants or psychoactive agents. Effects with other sedative drugs or ethanol may be potentiated. Benzodiazepines have been associated with falls and traumatic injury and should be used with extreme caution in patients who are at risk of these events (especially the elderly).

Lorazepam may cause anterograde amnesia. Paradoxical reactions, including hyperactive or aggressive behavior have been reported with benzodiazepines, particularly in adolescent/pediatric or psychiatric patients. Does not have analgesic, antidepressant, or antipsychotic properties.

Use caution in patients with depression, particularly if suicidal risk may be present. Pre-existing depression may worsen or emerge during therapy. Not recommended for use in primary depressive or psychotic disorders. Use with caution in patients with a history of drug dependence, alcoholism, or significant personality disorders. Benzodiazepines have been associated with dependence and acute withdrawal symptoms on discontinuation or reduction in dose. Acute withdrawal, including seizures, may be precipitated after administration of flumazenil to patients receiving long-term benzodiazepine therapy.

As a hypnotic agent, should be used only after evaluation of potential causes of sleep disturbance. Failure of sleep disturbance to resolve after 7-10 days may indicate psychiatric or medical illness. A worsening of insomnia or the emergence of new abnormalities of thought or behavior may represent unrecognized psychiatric or medical illness and requires immediate and careful evaluation.

Parenteral formulation of lorazepam contains polyethylene glycol which has resulted in toxicity during high-dose and/or longer-term infusions. Parenteral formulation also contains propylene glycol (PG); may be associated with dose-related toxicity and can occur ≥48 hours after initiation of lorazepam. Limited data suggest increased risk of PG accumulation at doses of ≥6 mg/hour for 48 hours or more (Nelson, 2008). Consider monitoring for signs of toxicity which may include acute renal failure, lactic acidosis, and/or osmol gap. In high-risk patients requiring higher doses/extended treatment durations, use of enteral delivery of lorazepam tablets may be beneficial (Jacobi, 2002). Also contains benzyl alcohol; avoid in neonates.

Drug Interactions

Avoid Concomitant Use

Avoid concomitant use of LORazepam with any of the following: OLANZapine

Increased Effect/Toxicity

LORazepam may increase the levels/effects of: Alcohol (Ethyl); CloZAPine; CNS Depressants; Fosphenytoin; Methotrimeprazine; Phenytoin

The levels/effects of LORazepam may be increased by: Divalproex; Droperidol; Loxapine; Methotrimeprazine; OLANZapine; Probenecid; Valproic Acid

Decreased Effect

The levels/effects of LORazepam may be decreased by: Theophylline Derivatives; Yohimbine

Ethanol/Nutrition/Herb Interactions

Ethanol: May increase CNS depression; monitor for increased effects with coadministration. Caution patients about effects.

Herb/Nutraceutical: Avoid valerian, St John's wort, kava kava, gotu kola (may increase CNS depression).

Pharmacodynamics/Kinetics

Onset of Action Hypnosis: I.M.: 20-30 minutes; Sedation: I.V.: 5-20 minutes; Anticonvulsant: I.V.: 5 minutes, oral: 30-60 minutes

Duration of Action 6-8 hours

Half-life Elimination Neonates: 40.2 hours; Older children: 10.5 hours; Adults: 12.9 hours; Elderly: 15.9 hours; End-stage renal disease: 32-70 hours

Time to Peak Oral: 2 hours

Pregnancy Risk Factor D

Lactation Enters breast milk/not recommended (AAP rates "of concern"; AAP 2001 update pending)

Breast-Feeding Considerations Drowsiness, lethargy, or weight loss in nursing infants have been observed in case reports following maternal use of some benzodiazepines.

Controlled Substance C-IV

Dosage Forms

Injection, solution: 2 mg/mL (1 mL, 10 mL); 4 mg/mL (1 mL, 10 mL)

Ativan®: 2 mg/mL (1 mL, 10 mL); 4 mg/mL (1 mL, 10 mL)

Injection, solution [preservative free]: 2 mg/mL (1 mL); 4 mg/mL (1 mL)

Solution, oral: 2 mg/mL (30 mL)

Lorazepam Intensol™: 2 mg/mL (30 mL)

Tablet, oral: 0.5 mg, 1 mg, 2 mg

Ativan®: 0.5 mg, 1 mg, 2 mg

Losartan (loe SAR tan)

Related Information

Cardiovascular Diseases *on page 1848*

U.S. Brand Names Cozaar®

Canadian Brand Names Cozaar®
Generic Availability (U.S.) Yes
Pharmacologic Category Angiotensin II Receptor Blocker
Use Treatment of hypertension (HTN); treatment of diabetic nephropathy in patients with type 2 diabetes mellitus (noninsulin dependent, NIDDM) and a history of hypertension; stroke risk reduction in patients with HTN and left ventricular hypertrophy (LVH)
Unlabeled/Investigational Use To slow the rate of progression of aortic-root dilation in pediatric patients with Marfan's syndrome
Local Anesthetic/Vasoconstrictor Precautions No information available to require special precautions
Effects on Dental Treatment Key adverse event(s) related to dental treatment: Orthostatic hypotension.
Effects on Bleeding No information available to require special precautions
Adverse Effects Note: The incidence of some adverse reactions varied based on the underlying disease state. Notations are made, where applicable, for data derived from trials conducted in diabetic nephropathy and hypertensive patients, respectively.

>10%:
- Cardiovascular: Chest pain (12% diabetic nephropathy)
- Central nervous system: Fatigue (14% diabetic nephropathy)
- Endocrine: Hypoglycemia (14% diabetic nephropathy)
- Gastrointestinal: Diarrhea (2% hypertension to 15% diabetic nephropathy)
- Genitourinary: Urinary tract infection (13% diabetic nephropathy)
- Hematologic: Anemia (14% diabetic nephropathy)
- Neuromuscular & skeletal: Weakness (14% diabetic nephropathy), back pain (2% hypertension to 12% diabetic nephropathy)
- Respiratory: Cough (≤3% to 11%; similar to placebo; incidence higher in patients with previous cough related to ACE inhibitor therapy)

1% to 10%:
- Cardiovascular: Hypotension (7% diabetic nephropathy), orthostatic hypotension (4% hypertension to 4% diabetic nephropathy), first-dose hypotension (dose related: <1% with 50 mg, 2% with 100 mg)
- Central nervous system: Dizziness (4%), hypoesthesia (5% diabetic nephropathy), fever (4% diabetic nephropathy), insomnia (1%)
- Dermatology: Cellulitis (7% diabetic nephropathy)
- Endocrine: Hyperkalemia (<1% hypertension to 7% diabetic nephropathy)
- Gastrointestinal: Gastritis (5% diabetic nephropathy), weight gain (4% diabetic nephropathy), dyspepsia (1% to 4%), abdominal pain (2%), nausea (2%)
- Neuromuscular & skeletal: Muscular weakness (7% diabetic nephropathy), knee pain (5% diabetic nephropathy), leg pain (1% to 5%), muscle cramps (1%), myalgia (1%)
- Respiratory: Bronchitis (10% diabetic nephropathy), upper respiratory infection (8%), nasal congestion (2%), sinusitis (1% hypertension to 6% diabetic nephropathy)
- Miscellaneous: Infection (5% diabetic nephropathy), flu-like syndrome (10% diabetic nephropathy)

Dosage Oral:
Hypertension:
Children 6-16 years:
U.S. labeling: 0.7 mg/kg once daily (maximum: 50 mg/day); doses >1.4 mg/kg (maximum: 100 mg) have not been studied
Canadian labeling:
≥20 kg to <50 kg: 25 mg once daily (maximum: 50 mg once daily)
≥50 kg: 50 mg once daily (maximum: 100 mg once daily)
Adults: Usual starting dose: 50 mg once daily; can be administered once or twice daily with total daily doses ranging from 25-100 mg
Patients receiving diuretics or with intravascular volume depletion: Usual initial dose: 25 mg once daily
Aortic-root dilation with Marfan's syndrome (unlabeled use): Children 14 months to 16 years: Initial: 0.6 mg/kg/day; can be increased to a maximum of 1.4 mg/kg/day (not to exceed adult maximum of 100 mg/day)
Nephropathy in patients with type 2 diabetes and hypertension: Adults: Initial: 50 mg once daily; can be increased to 100 mg once daily based on blood pressure response
Stroke reduction (HTN with LVH): Adults: 50 mg once daily (maximum daily dose: 100 mg); may be used in combination with a thiazide diuretic
Dosing adjustment in renal impairment:
Children: Use is not recommended if GFR <30 mL/minute/1.73 m^2
Adults: No adjustment necessary.

Dosing adjustment in hepatic impairment:

Children 6-16 years:

U.S. labeling: No specific dosing recommendations are provided in the approved labeling, however it may be advisable to initiate therapy at a reduced dosage.

Canadian labeling: Use is not recommended.

Adults: Reduce the initial dose to 25 mg/day

Mechanism of Action As a selective and competitive, nonpeptide angiotensin II receptor antagonist, losartan blocks the vasoconstrictor and aldosterone-secreting effects of angiotensin II; losartan interacts reversibly at the AT1 and AT2 receptors of many tissues and has slow dissociation kinetics; its affinity for the AT1 receptor is 1000 times greater than the AT2 receptor. Angiotensin II receptor antagonists may induce a more complete inhibition of the renin-angiotensin system than ACE inhibitors, they do not affect the response to bradykinin, and are less likely to be associated with nonrenin-angiotensin effects (eg, cough and angioedema). Losartan increases urinary flow rate and in addition to being natriuretic and kaliuretic, increases excretion of chloride, magnesium, uric acid, calcium, and phosphate.

Contraindications Hypersensitivity to losartan or any component of the formulation

Warnings/Precautions **[U.S. Boxed Warning]: Based on human data, drugs that act on the angiotensin system can cause injury and death to the developing fetus when used in the second and third trimesters. Angiotensin receptor blockers should be discontinued as soon as possible once pregnancy is detected.** Avoid use or use a much smaller dose in patients who are volume-depleted; correct depletion first. Use with caution in patients with significant aortic/mitral stenosis. May cause hyperkalemia; avoid potassium supplementation unless specifically required by healthcare provider. May be associated with deterioration of renal function and/or increases in serum creatinine, particularly in patients with low renal blood flow (eg, renal artery stenosis, heart failure) whose glomerular filtration rate (GFR) is dependent on efferent arteriolar vasoconstriction by angiotensin II. Use caution in patients with unstented unilateral/bilateral renal artery stenosis. When unstented bilateral renal artery stenosis is present, use is generally avoided due to the elevated risk of deterioration in renal function unless possible benefits outweigh risks. Use with caution with pre-existing renal insufficiency. AUCs of losartan (not the active metabolite) are about 50% greater in patients with Cl_{cr} <30 mL/minute and are doubled in hemodialysis patients. Concurrent use of ACE inhibitors may increase the risk of clinically-significant adverse events (eg, renal dysfunction, hyperkalemia).

At any time during treatment (especially following first dose), angioedema may occur rarely; may involve the head and neck (potentially compromising airway) or the intestine (presenting with abdominal pain). Patients with idiopathic or hereditary angioedema or previous angioedema associated with ACE-inhibitor therapy may be at an increased risk. Prolonged frequent monitoring may be required, especially if tongue, glottis, or larynx are involved, as they are associated with airway obstruction. Patients with a history of airway surgery may have a higher risk of airway obstruction. Aggressive early management is critical; intramuscular (I.M.) administration of epinephrine may be necessary.

When used to reduce the risk of stroke in patients with HTN and LVH, may not be effective in African-American population. Use caution with hepatic dysfunction, dose adjustment may be needed.

Drug Interactions

Metabolism/Transport Effects **Substrate** (major) of CYP2C9, 3A4; **Inhibits** CYP1A2 (weak), 2C8 (moderate), 2C9 (moderate), 2C19 (weak), 3A4 (weak)

Avoid Concomitant Use There are no known interactions where it is recommended to avoid concomitant use.

Increased Effect/Toxicity

Losartan may increase the levels/effects of: ACE Inhibitors; Amifostine; Antihypertensives; Carvedilol; CYP2C8 Substrates (High risk); CYP2C9 Substrates (High risk); Hypoglycemic Agents; Hypotensive Agents; Lithium; Nonsteroidal Anti-Inflammatory Agents; Potassium-Sparing Diuretics; RiTUXimab

The levels/effects of Losartan may be increased by: Antifungal Agents (Azole Derivatives, Systemic); Conivaptan; CYP2C9 Inhibitors (Moderate); CYP2C9 Inhibitors (Strong); Diazoxide; Eplerenone; Fluconazole; Herbs (Hypoglycemic Properties); Herbs (Hypotensive Properties); MAO Inhibitors; Milk Thistle; Pentoxifylline; Phosphodiesterase 5 Inhibitors; Potassium Salts; Prostacyclin Analogues; Tolvaptan; Trimethoprim

Decreased Effect

The levels/effects of Losartan may be decreased by: CYP2C9 Inducers (Highly Effective); CYP3A4 Inducers (Strong); Deferasirox; Herbs (CYP3A4 Inducers); Herbs (Hypertensive Properties); Methylphenidate; Nonsteroidal Anti-Inflammatory Agents; Peginterferon Alfa-2b; Rifamycin Derivatives; Tocilizumab; Yohimbine

Ethanol/Nutrition/Herb Interactions Herb/Nutraceutical: St John's wort may decrease levels of losartan. Avoid bayberry, blue cohosh, ginseng (American), kola, licorice (may worsen hypertension). Avoid black cohosh; california poppy; coleus; golden seal; hawthorn; mistletoe; periwinkle; quinine; shepherd's purse (may increase risk for hypotension). Hypoglycemic effects of losartan may be enhanced by alfalfa; aloe; bilberry; bitter melon; burdock; celery; damiana; fenugreek; garcinia; garlic; ginger; ginseng (American); gymnema; marshmallow; stinging nettle.

Dietary Considerations May be taken without regard to meals. Some products may contain potassium.

Pharmacodynamics/Kinetics

Onset of Action 6 hours

Half-life Elimination Losartan: 1.5-2 hours; E-3174: 6-9 hours

Time to Peak Serum: Losartan: 1 hour; E-3174: 3-4 hours

Pregnancy Risk Factor C (1st trimester); D (2nd and 3rd trimesters)

Lactation Excretion in breast milk unknown/not recommended

Breast-Feeding Considerations It is not known if losartan is found in breast milk; the manufacturer recommends discontinuing the drug or discontinuing nursing based on the importance of the drug to the mother.

Dosage Forms

Tablet, oral: 25 mg, 50 mg, 100 mg

Cozaar®: 25 mg, 50 mg, 100 mg

Losartan and Hydrochlorothiazide

(loe SAR tan & hye droe klor oh THYE a zide)

Related Information

Hydrochlorothiazide *on page* 854

Losartan *on page* 1037

U.S. Brand Names Hyzaar®

Canadian Brand Names Hyzaar®; Hyzaar® DS

Generic Availability (U.S.) Yes

Pharmacologic Category Angiotensin II Receptor Blocker; Diuretic, Thiazide

Use Treatment of hypertension; stroke risk reduction in patients with HTN and left ventricular hypertrophy (LVH)

Local Anesthetic/Vasoconstrictor Precautions No information available to require special precautions

Effects on Dental Treatment No significant effects or complications reported

Effects on Bleeding No information available to require special precautions

Adverse Effects Based on clinical trials of the combination product in patients with essential hypertension. Also see individual agents.

1% to 10%:

- Cardiovascular: Edema (1%), palpitation (1%)
- Central nervous system: Dizziness (6%)
- Dermatologic: Skin rash (1%)
- Gastrointestinal: Abdominal pain (1%)
- Neuromuscular & skeletal: Back pain (2%)
- Respiratory: Upper respiratory infection (6%), cough (3%), sinusitis (1%)

Dosage Oral: Adults: Dose is individualized (combination substituted for individual components); dose may be titrated after 2-4 weeks of therapy

Hypertension/stroke reduction in hypertension (with LVH): Usual recommended starting dose of losartan: 50 mg once daily when used as monotherapy in patients who are not volume depleted

Dosage adjustment in renal impairment: Cl_{cr} ≤30 mL/minute: Use of combination formulation not recommended

Dosage adjustment in hepatic impairment: Use is not recommended

Contraindications Hypersensitivity to losartan, hydrochlorothiazide, or any component of the formulation; sulfonamide-derived drugs; anuria

Warnings/Precautions

See individual agents.

Drug Interactions

Metabolism/Transport Effects Losartan: **Substrate** (major) of CYP2C9, 3A4; **Inhibits** CYP1A2 (weak), 2C8 (moderate), 2C9 (moderate), 2C19 (weak), 3A4 (weak)

Avoid Concomitant Use

Avoid concomitant use of Losartan and Hydrochlorothiazide with any of the following: Dofetilide

Increased Effect/Toxicity

Losartan and Hydrochlorothiazide may increase the levels/effects of: ACE Inhibitors; Allopurinol; Amifostine; Antihypertensives; Calcium Salts; CarBAMazepine;

Carvedilol; CYP2C8 Substrates (High risk); CYP2C9 Substrates (High risk); Dofetilide; Hypoglycemic Agents; Hypotensive Agents; Lithium; Nonsteroidal Anti-Inflammatory Agents; OXcarbazepine; Potassium-Sparing Diuretics; RiTUXimab; Topiramate; Toremifene; Vitamin D Analogs

The levels/effects of Losartan and Hydrochlorothiazide may be increased by: Alcohol (Ethyl); Analgesics (Opioid); Antifungal Agents (Azole Derivatives, Systemic); Barbiturates; Conivaptan; Corticosteroids (Orally Inhaled); Corticosteroids (Systemic); CYP2C9 Inhibitors (Moderate); CYP2C9 Inhibitors (Strong); Eplerenone; Fluconazole; Herbs (Hypoglycemic Properties); Herbs (Hypotensive Properties); Licorice; MAO Inhibitors; Milk Thistle; Pentoxifylline; Phosphodiesterase 5 Inhibitors; Potassium Salts; Prostacyclin Analogues; Tolvaptan; Trimethoprim

Decreased Effect

Losartan and Hydrochlorothiazide may decrease the levels/effects of: Antidiabetic Agents

The levels/effects of Losartan and Hydrochlorothiazide may be decreased by: Bile Acid Sequestrants; CYP2C9 Inducers (Highly Effective); CYP3A4 Inducers (Strong); Deferasirox; Herbs (CYP3A4 Inducers); Herbs (Hypertensive Properties); Methylphenidate; Nonsteroidal Anti-Inflammatory Agents; Peginterferon Alfa-2b; Rifamycin Derivatives; Tocilizumab; Yohimbine

Dietary Considerations Some products may contain potassium.

Pregnancy Risk Factor C/D (2nd and 3rd trimesters)

Lactation Enters breast milk/contraindicated

Dosage Forms

Tablet: 50/12.5: Losartan 50 mg and hydrochlorothiazide 12.5 mg; 100/12.5: Losartan 100 mg and hydrochlorothiazide 12.5 mg; 100/25: Losartan 100 mg and hydrochlorothiazide 25 mg

Hyzaar®: 50/12.5: Losartan 50 mg and hydrochlorothiazide 12.5 mg; 100/12.5: Losartan 100 mg and hydrochlorothiazide 12.5 mg; 100/25: Losartan 100 mg and hydrochlorothiazide 25 mg

Loteprednol (loe te PRED nol)

U.S. Brand Names Alrex®; Lotemax®

Canadian Brand Names Alrex®; Lotemax®

Pharmacologic Category Corticosteroid, Ophthalmic

Use

Suspension, 0.2% (Alrex®): Temporary relief of signs and symptoms of seasonal allergic conjunctivitis

Suspension, 0.5% (Lotemax®): Inflammatory conditions (treatment of steroid-responsive inflammatory conditions of the palpebral and bulbar conjunctiva, cornea, and anterior segment of the globe such as allergic conjunctivitis, acne rosacea, superficial punctate keratitis, herpes zoster keratitis, iritis, cyclitis, selected infective conjunctivitis, when the inherent hazard of steroid use is accepted to obtain an advisable diminution in edema and inflammation) and treatment of postoperative inflammation following ocular surgery

Local Anesthetic/Vasoconstrictor Precautions No information available to require special precautions

Effects on Dental Treatment No significant effects or complications reported

Effects on Bleeding No information available to require special precautions

Adverse Effects

>10%:

Central nervous system: Headache

Respiratory: Rhinitis, pharyngitis

1% to 10%: Ocular: Abnormal vision/blurring, burning on instillation, chemosis, dry eyes, itching, injection, conjunctivitis/irritation, corneal abnormalities, eyelid erythema, papillae uveitis

General Dosage Range Ophthalmic: *Adults:* Instill 1-2 drops into affected eye(s) 4 times/day

Mechanism of Action Corticosteroids inhibit the inflammatory response including edema, capillary dilation, leukocyte migration, and scar formation. Loteprednol is highly lipid soluble and penetrates cells readily to induce the production of lipocortins. These proteins modulate the activity of prostaglandins and leukotrienes.

Pregnancy Risk Factor C

Product Availability

Lotemax® 0.5% ointment: FDA approved April 2011; expected availability undetermined

Lotemax® 0.5% ointment is a topical corticosteroid approved for the treatment of postoperative inflammation and pain following ocular surgery.

Loteprednol and Tobramycin (loe te PRED nol & toe bra MYE sin)

Related Information

Loteprednol *on page 1041*

U.S. Brand Names Zylet®

Pharmacologic Category Antibiotic/Corticosteroid, Ophthalmic

Use Treatment of steroid-responsive ocular inflammatory conditions where either a superficial bacterial ocular infection or the risk of a superficial bacterial ocular infection exists

Local Anesthetic/Vasoconstrictor Precautions No information available to require special precautions

Effects on Dental Treatment No significant effects or complications reported

Effects on Bleeding No information available to require special precautions

Adverse Effects Also see individual agents.

>10%:

Central nervous system: Headache (14%)

Ocular: Superficial punctate keratitis (15%)

4% to 10%:

Local: Burning & stinging (9%)

Ocular: Intraocular pressure increased (10%)

<4%:

Local: Discharge, itching

Ocular: Corneal deposits, eye disorders unspecified, eyelid disorder, lacrimation disorder, ocular discomfort, photophobia, secondary infection

General Dosage Range Ophthalmic: *Children and Adults:* Instill 1-2 drops into the affected eye(s) every 4-6 hours

Mechanism of Action See individual agents.

Pregnancy Risk Factor C

Lovastatin (LOE va sta tin)

Related Information

Cardiovascular Diseases *on page 1848*

U.S. Brand Names Altoprev®; Mevacor®

Canadian Brand Names Apo-Lovastatin®; CO Lovastatin; Dom-Lovastatin; Gen-Lovastatin; Mevacor®; Mylan-Lovastatin; Novo-Lovastatin; Nu-Lovastatin; PHL-Lovastatin; PMS-Lovastatin; PRO-Lovastatin; RAN™-Lovastatin; ratio-Lovastatin; Riva-Lovastatin; Sandoz-Lovastatin

Generic Availability (U.S.) Yes: Exludes extended release tablet

Pharmacologic Category Antilipemic Agent, HMG-CoA Reductase Inhibitor

Use

Adjunct to dietary therapy to decrease elevated serum total and LDL-cholesterol concentrations in primary hypercholesterolemia

Primary prevention of coronary artery disease (patients without symptomatic disease with average to moderately elevated total and LDL-cholesterol and below average HDL-cholesterol); slow progression of coronary atherosclerosis in patients with coronary heart disease

Adjunct to dietary therapy in adolescent patients (10-17 years of age, females >1 year postmenarche) with heterozygous familial hypercholesterolemia having LDL >189 mg/dL, **or** LDL >160 mg/dL with positive family history of premature cardiovascular disease (CVD), **or** LDL >160 mg/dL with the presence of at least two other CVD risk factors

Local Anesthetic/Vasoconstrictor Precautions No information available to require special precautions

Effects on Dental Treatment No significant effects or complications reported

Effects on Bleeding No information available to require special precautions

Adverse Effects Percentages as reported with immediate release tablets; similar adverse reactions seen with extended release tablets.

>10%: Neuromuscular & skeletal: CPK increased (>2x normal) (11%)

1% to 10%:

Central nervous system: Headache (2% to 3%), dizziness (≤1%)

Dermatologic: Rash (≤1%)

Gastrointestinal: Flatulence (4% to 5%), constipation (2% to 4%), abdominal pain (2% to 3%), diarrhea (2% to 3%), nausea (2% to 3%), dyspepsia (1% to 2%)

Neuromuscular & skeletal: Myalgia (2% to 3%), weakness (1% to 2%), muscle cramps (≤1%)

Ocular: Blurred vision (≤1%)

Additional class-related events or case reports (not necessarily reported with lovastatin therapy): Alkaline phosphatase increased, alteration in taste, anaphylaxis, angioedema, anorexia, anxiety, arthritis, cataracts, chills, cholestatic jaundice, cirrhosis, depression, dryness of skin/mucous membranes, dyspnea, eosinophilia, erectile dysfunction, erythema multiforme, ESR increased, facial paresis, fatty liver, fever, flushing, fulminant hepatic necrosis, GGT increased, gynecomastia, hemolytic anemia, hepatitis, hepatoma, hyperbilirubinemia, hypersensitivity reaction, impaired extraocular muscle movement, impotence, interstitial lung disease, leukopenia, libido decreased, malaise, memory loss, myopathy, nail changes, nodules, ophthalmoplegia, pancreatitis, peripheral nerve palsy, peripheral neuropathy, photosensitivity, polymyalgia rheumatica, positive ANA, psychic disturbance, purpura, renal failure (secondary to rhabdomyolysis), rhabdomyolysis, skin discoloration, Stevens-Johnson syndrome, systemic lupus erythematosus-like syndrome, thrombocytopenia, thyroid dysfunction, toxic epidermal necrolysis, transaminases increased, tremor, urticaria, vasculitis, vertigo

Dosage Oral:

Adolescents 10-17 years: Immediate release tablet:

LDL reduction <20%: Initial: 10 mg/day with evening meal

LDL reduction ≥20%: Initial: 20 mg/day with evening meal

Usual range: 10-40 mg with evening meal, then adjust dose at 4-week intervals; maximum dose per manufacturer: 40 mg/day

Adults: Initial: 20 mg with evening meal, then adjust at 4-week intervals; maximum dose: 80 mg/day immediate release tablet **or** 60 mg/day extended release tablet

Note: Doses should be individualized according to the baseline LDL-cholesterol levels, the recommended goal of therapy, and patient response.

Dosage modification/limits based on concurrent therapy:

Cyclosporine or danazol: Initial dose: 10 mg/day with a maximum recommended dose of 20 mg/day

Concurrent therapy with fibrates and/or lipid-lowering doses of niacin (≥1 g/day): Maximum recommended dose: 20 mg/day. Concurrent use with fibrates should be avoided unless risk to benefit favors use.

Concurrent therapy with amiodarone or verapamil: Maximum recommended dose: 40 mg/day of immediate release or 20 mg/day with extended release.

Dosage adjustment in renal impairment: Cl_{cr} <30 mL/minute: Use doses >20 mg/day with caution.

Mechanism of Action Lovastatin acts by competitively inhibiting 3-hydroxyl-3-methylglutaryl-coenzyme A (HMG-CoA) reductase, the enzyme that catalyzes the rate-limiting step in cholesterol biosynthesis

Contraindications Hypersensitivity to lovastatin or any component of the formulation; active liver disease; unexplained persistent elevations of serum transaminases; pregnancy; breast-feeding

Warnings/Precautions Secondary causes of hyperlipidemia should be ruled out prior to therapy. Liver function must be monitored by periodic laboratory assessment. Rhabdomyolysis with or without acute renal failure has occurred. Risk is dose-related and is increased with concurrent use of lipid-lowering agents which may cause rhabdomyolysis (gemfibrozil, fibric acid derivatives, or niacin at doses ≥1 g/day) or during concurrent use with potent CYP3A4 inhibitors. Avoid concurrent use of azole antifungals, macrolide antibiotics, and protease inhibitors. Use caution/limit dose with amiodarone, cyclosporine, danazol, gemfibrozil (or other fibrates), lipid-lowering doses of niacin, or verapamil. Monitor closely if used with other drugs associated with myopathy (eg, colchicine). Patients should be instructed to report unexplained muscle pain or weakness; lovastatin should be discontinued if myopathy is suspected/confirmed. Temporarily discontinue in any patient experiencing an acute or serious condition predisposing to renal failure secondary to rhabdomyolysis. Based upon current evidence, HMG-CoA reductase inhibitor therapy should be continued in the perioperative period unless risk outweighs cardioprotective benefit. Use with caution in patients with advanced age, these patients are predisposed to myopathy. Use with caution in patients who consume large amounts of ethanol or have a history of liver disease.

Drug Interactions

Metabolism/Transport Effects Substrate of CYP3A4 (major), P-glycoprotein; **Inhibits** CYP2C9 (weak), 2D6 (weak), 3A4 (weak)

Avoid Concomitant Use

Avoid concomitant use of Lovastatin with any of the following: Protease Inhibitors; Red Yeast Rice

Increased Effect/Toxicity

Lovastatin may increase the levels/effects of: DAPTOmycin; Diltiazem; Trabectedin; Vitamin K Antagonists

The levels/effects of Lovastatin may be increased by: Amiodarone; Antifungal Agents (Azole Derivatives, Systemic); Colchicine; Conivaptan; CycloSPORINE; CycloSPORINE (Systemic); CYP3A4 Inhibitors (Moderate); CYP3A4 Inhibitors

(Strong); Danazol; Dasatinib; Diltiazem; Dronedarone; Fenofibrate; Fenofibric Acid; Fluconazole; Gemfibrozil; Grapefruit Juice; Macrolide Antibiotics; Nefazodone; Niacin; Niacinamide; P-Glycoprotein Inhibitors; Protease Inhibitors; QuiNINE; Red Yeast Rice; Rifamycin Derivatives; Sildenafil; Verapamil

Decreased Effect

The levels/effects of Lovastatin may be decreased by: Antacids; Bosentan; CYP3A4 Inducers (Strong); Deferasirox; Efavirenz; Etravirine; Fosphenytoin; P-Glycoprotein Inducers; Phenytoin; Rifamycin Derivatives; St Johns Wort; Tocilizumab

Ethanol/Nutrition/Herb Interactions

Ethanol: Avoid excessive ethanol consumption (due to potential hepatic effects).

Food: Food **decreases** the bioavailability of lovastatin extended release tablets and **increases** the bioavailability of lovastatin immediate release tablets. Lovastatin serum concentrations may be increased if taken with grapefruit juice; avoid concurrent intake of large quantities (>1 quart/day). Red yeast rice contains an estimated 2.4 mg lovastatin per 600 mg rice.

Herb/Nutraceutical: St John's wort may decrease lovastatin levels.

Dietary Considerations Before initiation of therapy, patients should be placed on a standard cholesterol-lowering diet for 6 weeks and the diet should be continued during drug therapy. Avoid intake of large quantities of grapefruit juice (≥1 quart/day); may increase toxicity. Red yeast rice contains an estimated 2.4 mg lovastatin per 600 mg rice. Immediate release tablet should be taken with the evening meal.

Pharmacodynamics/Kinetics

Onset of Action LDL-cholesterol reductions: 3 days

Half-life Elimination 1.1-1.7 hours

Time to Peak Serum: Immediate release: 2-4 hours; extended release: 12-14 hours

Pregnancy Risk Factor X

Lactation Excretion in breast milk unknown/contraindicated

Dosage Forms

Tablet, oral: 10 mg, 20 mg, 40 mg

Mevacor®: 20 mg, 40 mg

Tablet, extended release, oral:

Altoprev®: 20 mg, 40 mg, 60 mg

Loxapine (LOKS a peen)

U.S. Brand Names Loxitane®

Canadian Brand Names Apo-Loxapine®; Loxapac® IM; Nu-Loxapine; PMS-Loxapine; Xylac

Pharmacologic Category Antipsychotic Agent, Typical

Use Management of psychotic disorders

Unlabeled/Investigational Use Psychosis/agitation related to Alzheimer's dementia

Local Anesthetic/Vasoconstrictor Precautions Most pharmacology textbooks state that in presence of phenothiazines, systemic doses of epinephrine paradoxically decrease the blood pressure. This is the so called "epinephrine reversal" phenomenon. This has never been observed when epinephrine is given by infiltration as part of the anesthesia procedure. Loxapine is one of the drugs confirmed to prolong the QT interval and is accepted as having a risk of causing torsade de pointes. The risk of drug-induced torsade de pointes is extremely low when a single QT interval prolonging drug is prescribed. In terms of epinephrine, it is not known what effect vasoconstrictors in the local anesthetic regimen will have in patients with a known history of congenital prolonged QT interval or in patients taking any medication that prolongs the QT interval. Until more information is obtained, it is suggested that the clinician consult with the physician prior to the use of a vasoconstrictor in suspected patients, and that the vasoconstrictor (epinephrine, mepivacaine and levonordefrin [Carbocaine® 2% with Neo-Cobefrin®]) be used with caution.

Effects on Dental Treatment Key adverse event(s) related to dental treatment:

Xerostomia and changes in salivation (normal salivary flow resumes upon discontinuation).

Significant hypotension may occur, especially when the drug is administered parenterally; orthostatic hypotension is due to alpha-receptor blockade, the elderly are at greater risk for orthostatic hypotension.

Tardive dyskinesia: Prevalence rate may be 40% in elderly; development of the syndrome and the irreversible nature are proportional to duration and total cumulative dose over time. Extrapyramidal reactions are more common in elderly with up to 50% developing these reactions after 60 years of age. Drug-induced

Parkinson's syndrome occurs often; akathisia is the most common extrapyramidal reaction in elderly.

Increased confusion, memory loss, psychotic behavior, and agitation frequently occur as a consequence of anticholinergic effects. Antipsychotic associated sedation in nonpsychotic patients is extremely unpleasant due to feelings of depersonalization, derealization, and dysphoria.

Effects on Bleeding No information available to require special precautions

Adverse Effects Frequency not defined.

Cardiovascular: Abnormal T waves with prolonged ventricular repolarization, arrhythmia, hyper-/hypotension, orthostatic hypotension, tachycardia, syncope

Central nervous system: Agitation, altered central temperature regulation, ataxia, confusion, dizziness, drowsiness, extrapyramidal reactions (akathisia, akinesia, dystonia, pseudoparkinsonism, tardive dyskinesia), faintness, headache, insomnia, lightheadedness, neuroleptic malignant syndrome (NMS), seizure, slurred speech, tension

Dermatologic: Alopecia, dermatitis, photosensitivity, pruritus, rash, seborrhea

Endocrine & metabolic: Amenorrhea, enlargement of breasts, galactorrhea, gynecomastia, menstrual irregularity

Gastrointestinal: Adynamic ileus, constipation, nausea, polydipsia, vomiting, weight gain/loss, xerostomia

Genitourinary: Sexual dysfunction, urinary retention

Hematologic: Agranulocytosis, leukopenia, thrombocytopenia

Neuromuscular & skeletal: Weakness

Ocular: Blurred vision

Respiratory: Nasal congestion

General Dosage Range Oral:

Adults: Initial: 10 mg twice daily; Usual range: 20-100 mg/day in 2-4 divided doses (maximum: 250 mg/day)

Elderly: 20-60 mg/day

Mechanism of Action Loxapine is a dibenzoxazepine antipsychotic which blocks postsynaptic mesolimbic D_1 and D_2 receptors in the brain, and also possesses serotonin 5-HT_2 blocking activity

Pharmacodynamics/Kinetics

Onset of Action Neuroleptic: Oral: 20-30 minutes; Peak effect: 1.5-3 hours

Duration of Action ~12 hours

Half-life Elimination Biphasic: Initial: 5 hours; Terminal: 12-19 hours

Dental Comment Loxapine is known to prolong the QT interval. The QT interval is measured as the time and distance between the Q point of the QRS complex and the end of the T wave in the ECG tracing. After adjustment for heart rate, the QT interval is defined as prolonged if it is more than 450 msec in men and 460 msec in women. A long QT syndrome was first described in the 1950s and 60s as a congenital syndrome involving QT interval prolongation and syncope and sudden death. Some of the congenital long QT syndromes were characterized by a peculiar electrocardiographic appearance of the QRS complex involving a premature atria beat followed by a pause, then a subsequent sinus beat showing marked QT prolongation and deformity. This type of cardiac arrhythmia was originally termed "torsade de pointes" (translated from the French as "twisting of the points"). Loxapine is considered as having a risk of causing torsade de pointes. Since it is not known what effect vasoconstrictors in the local anesthetic regimen will have in patients with a known history of congenital prolonged QT interval or in patients taking any medication that prolongs the QT interval, a medical consult is suggested.

Lubiprostone (loo bi PROS tone)

U.S. Brand Names Amitiza®

Pharmacologic Category Chloride Channel Activator; Gastrointestinal Agent, Miscellaneous

Use Treatment of chronic idiopathic constipation; treatment of irritable bowel syndrome with constipation in adult women

Local Anesthetic/Vasoconstrictor Precautions No information available to require special precautions

Effects on Dental Treatment Key adverse event(s) related to dental treatment: Xerostomia (normal salivary flow resumes upon discontinuation).

Effects on Bleeding No information available to require special precautions

Adverse Effects

>10%:

Central nervous system: Headache (3% to 11%)

Gastrointestinal: Nausea (7% to 29%; severe: 4%; dose related), diarrhea (7% to 12%; severe 2%)

1% to 10%:
Cardiovascular: Edema (3%), chest discomfort/pain (2%)
Central nervous system: Dizziness (3%), fatigue (2%)
Gastrointestinal: Abdominal pain (1% to 8%), abdominal distention (3% to 6%), flatulence (3% to 6%), vomiting (3%), loose stools (3%), dyspepsia (2%), xerostomia (1%)
Respiratory: Dyspnea (2% to 3%)

General Dosage Range Dosage adjustment recommended in hepatic impairment and in patients who develop toxicities

Oral:

Adults (females): 8 mcg twice daily **or** 24 mcg twice daily

Adults (males): 24 mcg twice daily

Mechanism of Action Bicyclic fatty acid that acts locally at the apical portion of the intestine as a chloride channel activator, increasing intestinal fluid secretion and intestinal motility. Does not alter serum sodium or potassium concentrations.

Pharmacodynamics/Kinetics

Half-life Elimination M3: 0.9-1.4 hours

Pregnancy Risk Factor C

Lurasidone (loo RAS i done)

U.S. Brand Names Latuda®

Pharmacologic Category Antipsychotic Agent, Atypical

Use Treatment of schizophrenia

Local Anesthetic/Vasoconstrictor Precautions No information available to require special precautions

Effects on Dental Treatment Key adverse event(s) related to dental treatment: Salivary hypersecretion has been reported (normal salivary flow resumes upon discontinuation)

Effects on Bleeding No information available to require special precautions

Adverse Effects

10%:
Central nervous system: Somnolence (dose-related: 19% to 23%), akathisia (dose-related: 11% to 15%)
Endocrine & metabolic: Fasting glucose increased (10% to 14%)
Gastrointestinal: Nausea (12%)
Neuromuscular & skeletal: Extrapyramidal symptoms (24% to 26%), parkinsonism (11%)

1% to 10%:
Cardiovascular: Tachycardia
Central nervous system: Insomnia (8%), agitation (6%), anxiety (6%), dizziness (5%), dystonia (5%), fatigue (4%), restlessness (3%)
Dermatologic: Pruritus, rash
Endocrine & metabolic: Prolactin increased (≥5 x ULN: females: 8%; males: 2%)
Gastrointestinal: Dyspepsia (8%), vomiting (8%), weight gain (≥7% increase in baseline body weight: 6%), salivary hypersecretion (2%), abdominal pain, appetite decreased, diarrhea
Neuromuscular & skeletal: Back pain (4%), CPK increased
Ocular: Blurred vision
Renal: Creatinine increased (3%)

General Dosage Range Dosage adjustment recommended in patients with hepatic or renal impairment or on concomitant therapy.

Oral: *Adults:* Initial: 40 mg once daily (maximum: 80 mg/day)

Mechanism of Action Lurasidone is a benzoisothiazol-derivative atypical antipsychotic with mixed serotonin-dopamine antagonist activity. It exhibits high affinity for D_2, 5-HT_{2A}, and 5-HT_7 receptors; moderate affinity for alpha$_{2C}$-adrenergic receptors; and is a partial agonist for 5-HT_{1A} receptors. Lurasidone has no significant affinity for muscarinic M_1 and histamine H_1 receptors. The addition of serotonin antagonism to dopamine antagonism (classic neuroleptic mechanism) is thought to improve negative symptoms of psychoses and reduce the incidence of extrapyramidal side effects as compared to typical antipsychotics.

Pharmacodynamics/Kinetics

Half-life Elimination 18 hours; Main active metabolite, ID-14283 (exo-hydroxy metabolite), exhibits a half-life of 7.5-10 hours

Time to Peak 1-3 hours; steady state concentrations achieved within 7 days

Pregnancy Risk Factor B

Lutropin Alfa (LOO troe pin AL fa)

U.S. Brand Names Luveris®

Pharmacologic Category Gonadotropin; Ovulation Stimulator

Use Stimulation of follicular development in infertile hypogonadotropic hypogonadal (HH) women with profound luteinizing hormone (LH) deficiency; to be used in combination with follitropin alfa

Local Anesthetic/Vasoconstrictor Precautions No information available to require special precautions

Effects on Dental Treatment No significant effects or complications reported

Effects on Bleeding No information available to require special precautions

Adverse Effects

1% to 10%:

Central nervous system: Headache (10%), fatigue (2% to 3%)

Endocrine & metabolic: Ovarian hyperstimulation (6%)

Gastrointestinal: Nausea (7%), constipation (2% to 3%), diarrhea (2% to 3%)

Adverse events reported with gonadotropin or menotropin therapy: Adnexal torsion, arterial thromboembolism, congenital abnormalities, ectopic pregnancy, hemoperitoneum, ovarian enlargement (mild-to-moderate), ovarian neoplasms (infrequent), postpartum fever, premature labor, pulmonary complications, spontaneous abortion, vascular complications

General Dosage Range SubQ: *Adults (females):* 75 int. units daily (maximum duration: 14 days)

Mechanism of Action Lutropin alfa is a recombinant luteinizing hormone prepared using Chinese hamster cell ovaries. Administration leads to increased follicular estradiol secretion needed for follicle stimulating hormone induced follicular development.

Pharmacodynamics/Kinetics

Half-life Elimination Terminal: ~18 hours

Time to Peak 4-16 hours

Pregnancy Risk Factor X

Mafenide (MA fe nide)

U.S. Brand Names Sulfamylon®

Pharmacologic Category Antibiotic, Topical

Use

Cream: Adjunctive antibacterial agent in the treatment of second- and third-degree burns

Solution: Adjunctive antibacterial agent for use under moist dressings over meshed autografts on excised burn wounds

Local Anesthetic/Vasoconstrictor Precautions No information available to require special precautions

Effects on Dental Treatment No significant effects or complications reported

Effects on Bleeding No information available to require special precautions

Adverse Effects Frequency not defined.

Cardiovascular: Edema, facial edema

Dermatologic: Erythema, maceration, pruritus, rash, urticaria

Endocrine & metabolic: Hyperchloremia, metabolic acidosis

Gastrointestinal: Diarrhea (following accidental ingestion)

Hematologic: Bleeding, bone marrow suppression, DIC, eosinophilia, hemolytic anemia, porphyria

Local: Blisters, burning sensation, excoriation, pain

Respiratory: Dyspnea, hyperventilation, pCO_2 decreased, tachypnea

Miscellaneous: Hypersensitivity

General Dosage Range Topical: *Children and Adults:* Apply to a thickness of approximately 1/16" once or twice daily

Mechanism of Action As a sulfonamide, mafenide interferes with bacterial folic acid synthesis through competitive inhibition of para-aminobenzoic acid. Spectrum of activity encompasses both gram positive and negative organisms, including *Pseudomonas* and some anaerobes.

Pharmacodynamics/Kinetics

Time to Peak Serum: Cream 11%: 2-4 hours; Burn tissue: Cream 11%: 2 hours, Solution 5%: 4 hours

Pregnancy Risk Factor C

Magaldrate and Simethicone (MAG al drate & sye METH i kone)

Related Information

Simethicone *on page 1527*

Pharmacologic Category Antacid; Antiflatulent

Use Relief of hyperacidity associated with peptic ulcer, gastritis, peptic esophagitis, and hiatal hernia which are accompanied by symptoms of gas

Local Anesthetic/Vasoconstrictor Precautions No information available to require special precautions

Effects on Dental Treatment Key adverse event(s) related to dental treatment: Chalky taste.

Effects on Bleeding No information available to require special precautions

Adverse Effects Frequency not defined.

Based on **magaldrate** component:

- Central nervous system: Encephalopathy
- Gastrointestinal: Constipation, chalky taste, stomach cramps, fecal impaction, diarrhea, nausea, vomiting, discoloration of feces (white speckles), rebound hyperacidity
- Endocrine & metabolic: Hypophosphatemia, hypermagnesemia, milk-alkali syndrome
- Neuromuscular & metabolic: Osteomalacia
- Miscellaneous: Aluminum intoxication

Based on **simethicone** component: No data reported

General Dosage Range Oral: *Adults:* 5-10 mL (540-1080 mg magaldrate) between meals and at bedtime

Pregnancy Risk Factor C

Magnesium Carbonate, Calcium Carbonate, and Folic Acid (mag NEE zhum KAR bun ate, KAL see um KAR bun ate, & FOE lik AS id)

Related Information

Calcium Carbonate *on page* 286

Folic Acid *on page* 777

U.S. Brand Names MagneBind® 400 Rx

Pharmacologic Category Calcium Salt; Electrolyte Supplement, Oral; Magnesium Salt; Vitamin; Vitamin, Water Soluble

Use Prevention or treatment of nutritional deficiencies

Local Anesthetic/Vasoconstrictor Precautions No information available to require special precautions

Effects on Dental Treatment No significant effects or complications reported

Effects on Bleeding No information available to require special precautions

General Dosage Range Oral: *Adults:* 1-3 tablets 3 times/day

Magnesium Chloride (mag NEE zhum KLOR ide)

U.S. Brand Names Chloromag®; Mag 64™ [OTC]; Mag Delay [OTC]; Mag-SR with Calcium [OTC] [DSC]; Slow-Mag® [OTC]

Pharmacologic Category Electrolyte Supplement, Oral; Electrolyte Supplement, Parenteral; Magnesium Salt

Use Correction or prevention of hypomagnesemia; dietary supplement

Local Anesthetic/Vasoconstrictor Precautions No information available to require special precautions

Effects on Dental Treatment Key adverse event(s) related to dental treatment: Magnesium products may prevent GI absorption of tetracyclines by forming a large ionized chelated molecule with the tetracyclines in the stomach. Tetracyclines should be given at least 1 hour before magnesium.

Effects on Bleeding No information available to require special precautions

Adverse Effects Frequency not defined: Gastrointestinal: Diarrhea (excessive oral doses)

General Dosage Range

I.V.:

- *Children <50 kg:* 0.3-0.5 mEq/kg/day
- *Children >50 kg:* 10-30 mEq/day
- *Adults:* 8-24 mEq/day added to TPN

Oral: RDA (elemental magnesium):

- *Children:* 80-240 mg/day
- *Adults:* 360-410 mg/day

Mechanism of Action Magnesium is important as a cofactor in many enzymatic reactions in the body involving protein synthesis and carbohydrate metabolism (at least 300 enzymatic reactions require magnesium). Actions on lipoprotein lipase have been found to be important in reducing serum cholesterol and on sodium/potassium ATPase in promoting polarization (eg, neuromuscular functioning).

Pregnancy Risk Factor C

Magnesium Citrate (mag NEE zhum SIT rate)

U.S. Brand Names Citroma® [OTC]

Canadian Brand Names Citro-Mag®

Pharmacologic Category Laxative, Saline; Magnesium Salt

Use Evacuation of bowel prior to certain surgical and diagnostic procedures or overdose situations

Local Anesthetic/Vasoconstrictor Precautions No information available to require special precautions

Effects on Dental Treatment Key adverse event(s) related to dental treatment: Magnesium products may prevent GI absorption of tetracyclines by forming a large ionized chelated molecule with the tetracyclines in the stomach. Tetracyclines should be given at least 1 hour before magnesium.

Effects on Bleeding No information available to require special precautions

Adverse Effects 1% to 10%:

Cardiovascular: Hypotension

Endocrine & metabolic: Hypermagnesemia

Gastrointestinal: Abdominal cramps, diarrhea, gas formation

Respiratory: Respiratory depression

General Dosage Range Oral:

Children <6 years: 2-4 mL/kg given once or in divided doses

Children 6-12 years: 100-150 mL given once or in divided doses

Children >12 years and Adults: 150-300 mL given once or in divided doses

Mechanism of Action Promotes bowel evacuation by causing osmotic retention of fluid which distends the colon with increased peristaltic activity

Pregnancy Risk Factor B

Magnesium Gluconate (mag NEE zhum GLOO koe nate)

U.S. Brand Names Magonate® [OTC]; Magtrate® [OTC]; Mag®-G [OTC]

Pharmacologic Category Electrolyte Supplement, Oral; Magnesium Salt

Use Dietary supplement

Local Anesthetic/Vasoconstrictor Precautions No information available to require special precautions

Effects on Dental Treatment Key adverse event(s) related to dental treatment: Magnesium products may prevent GI absorption of tetracyclines by forming a large ionized chelated molecule with the tetracyclines in the stomach. Tetracyclines should be given at least 1 hour before magnesium.

Effects on Bleeding No information available to require special precautions

Adverse Effects Frequency not defined: Gastrointestinal: Diarrhea (excessive oral doses)

General Dosage Range Oral: RDA (elemental magnesium):

Children 1-13 years: 80-240 mg/day

Children ≥14 years and Adults: 310-420 mg/day

Mechanism of Action Magnesium is important as a cofactor in many enzymatic reactions in the body involving protein synthesis and carbohydrate metabolism (at least 300 enzymatic reactions require magnesium). Actions on lipoprotein lipase have been found to be important in reducing serum cholesterol and on sodium/potassium ATPase in promoting polarization (eg, neuromuscular functioning).

Magnesium Hydroxide (mag NEE zhum hye DROKS ide)

U.S. Brand Names Fleet® Pedia-Lax™ Chewable Tablet [OTC]; Little Phillips'® Milk of Magnesia [OTC]; Milk of Magnesia [OTC]; Phillips'® Milk of Magnesia [OTC]

Pharmacologic Category Antacid; Laxative; Magnesium Salt

Use Short-term treatment of occasional constipation and symptoms of hyperacidity, laxative; dietary supplement

Local Anesthetic/Vasoconstrictor Precautions No information available to require special precautions

Effects on Dental Treatment Key adverse event(s) related to dental treatment: Magnesium products may prevent GI absorption of tetracyclines by forming a large ionized chelated molecule with the tetracyclines in the stomach. Tetracyclines should be given at least 1 hour before magnesium.

Effects on Bleeding No information available to require special precautions

General Dosage Range Oral:
Children 2-5 years: OTC laxative: Magnesium hydroxide 400 mg/5 mL: 5-15 mL/day
Children 6-11 years: OTC laxative: Magnesium hydroxide 400 mg/5 mL: 15-30 mL/day
Children ≥12 years and Adults: OTC laxative: Magnesium hydroxide 400 mg/5 mL: 30-60 mL/day

Mechanism of Action Promotes bowel evacuation by causing osmotic retention of fluid which distends the colon with increased peristaltic activity; reacts with hydrochloric acid in stomach to form magnesium chloride

Pharmacodynamics/Kinetics
Onset of Action Laxative: 30 minutes to 6 hours

Magnesium Hydroxide and Mineral Oil
(mag NEE zhum hye DROKS ide & MIN er al oyl)

Related Information
Magnesium Hydroxide *on page 1049*

U.S. Brand Names Phillips'® M-O [OTC]

Pharmacologic Category Laxative

Use Short-term treatment of occasional constipation

Local Anesthetic/Vasoconstrictor Precautions No information available to require special precautions

Effects on Dental Treatment Key adverse event(s) related to dental treatment: Magnesium products may prevent GI absorption of tetracyclines by forming a large ionized chelated molecule with the tetracyclines in the stomach. Tetracyclines should be given at least 1 hour before magnesium.

Effects on Bleeding No information available to require special precautions

General Dosage Range Oral:
Children 6-11 years: 20-30 mL at bedtime
Children ≥12 years and Adults: 45-60 mL at bedtime

Pharmacodynamics/Kinetics
Onset of Action Laxative: 30 minutes to 6 hours hours

Magnesium L-aspartate Hydrochloride
(mag NEE zhum el as PAR tate hye droe KLOR ide)

U.S. Brand Names Maginex™ DS [OTC]; Maginex™ [OTC]

Pharmacologic Category Electrolyte Supplement, Oral; Magnesium Salt

Use Dietary supplement

Local Anesthetic/Vasoconstrictor Precautions No information available to require special precautions

Effects on Dental Treatment Key adverse event(s) related to dental treatment: Magnesium ions prevent GI absorption of tetracycline by forming a large, ionized, chelated molecule with the magnesium ion and tetracyclines in the stomach. Magnesium supplement should not be taken within 2-4 hours of oral tetracycline or other members of the tetracycline family.

Effects on Bleeding No information available to require special precautions

Adverse Effects Frequency not defined: Gastrointestinal: Diarrhea (excessive oral doses)

General Dosage Range Oral: RDA (elemental magnesium):
Children 1-13 years: 80-240 mg/day
Children ≥14 years and Adults: 310-420 mg/day

Mechanism of Action Magnesium is important as a cofactor in many enzymatic reactions in the body involving protein synthesis and carbohydrate metabolism (at least 300 enzymatic reactions require magnesium). Actions on lipoprotein lipase have been found to be important in reducing serum cholesterol and on sodium/potassium ATPase in promoting polarization (eg, neuromuscular functioning).

Magnesium Oxide (mag NEE zhum OKS ide)

U.S. Brand Names Mag-Ox® 400 [OTC]; MagGel™ 600 [OTC]; MAGnesium-Oxide™ [OTC]; Phillips'® Laxative Dietary Supplement Cramp-Free [OTC]; Uro-Mag® [OTC]

Pharmacologic Category Electrolyte Supplement, Oral; Magnesium Salt

Use Electrolyte replacement

Local Anesthetic/Vasoconstrictor Precautions No information available to require special precautions

Effects on Dental Treatment Key adverse event(s) related to dental treatment: Magnesium products may prevent GI absorption of tetracyclines by forming a large ionized chelated molecule with the tetracyclines in the stomach. Tetracyclines should be given at least 1 hour before magnesium.

Effects on Bleeding No information available to require special precautions

Adverse Effects Frequency not defined: Gastrointestinal: Diarrhea (excessive oral doses)

General Dosage Range Oral: RDA (elemental magnesium):

Children 1-13 years: 80-240 mg/day

Children ≥14 years and Adults: 310-420 mg/day

Mechanism of Action Magnesium is important as a cofactor in many enzymatic reactions in the body involving protein synthesis and carbohydrate metabolism (at least 300 enzymatic reactions require magnesium). Actions on lipoprotein lipase have been found to be important in reducing serum cholesterol and on sodium/potassium ATPase in promoting polarization (eg, neuromuscular functioning).

Magnesium Salicylate (mag NEE zhum sa LIS i late)

Related Information

Rheumatoid Arthritis, Osteoarthritis, and Osteoporosis *on page 1889*

Temporomandibular Dysfunction (TMD) *on page 1964*

U.S. Brand Names Doan's® Extra Strength [OTC]; Keygesic [OTC]; Momentum® [OTC]; MST 600

Generic Availability (U.S.) Yes

Pharmacologic Category Salicylate

Use Mild-to-moderate pain, fever, various inflammatory conditions; relief of pain and inflammation of rheumatoid arthritis and osteoarthritis

Local Anesthetic/Vasoconstrictor Precautions No information available to require special precautions

Effects on Dental Treatment The dentist should be aware of the potential of abnormal coagulation. Caution should also be exercised in the use of NSAIDs in patients already on anticoagulant therapy with drugs such as warfarin (Coumadin®). See Effects on Bleeding.

Effects on Bleeding Nonacetylated salicylate formulations are known to reversibly decrease platelet aggregation via mechanisms different than observed with aspirin. The dentist should be aware of the potential of abnormal coagulation. Caution should also be exercised in the use of NSAIDs in patients already on anticoagulant therapy with drugs such as warfarin (Coumadin®).

Adverse Effects Refer to Aspirin monograph.

Dosage Oral:

Children ≥12 years and Adults: Relief of mild-to-moderate pain:

- Doan's® Extra Strength, Momentum®: Two caplets every 6 hours as needed (maximum: 8 caplets/24 hours)
- Keygesic: One tablet every 4 hours as needed (maximum: 4 tablets/24 hours)

Contraindications Hypersensitivity to magnesium salicylate, salicylates, other NSAIDs, or any component of the formulation; advanced chronic renal dysfunction; concomitant use with uricosuric agents

In patients ≥65 years of age: Also contraindicated with a history of chronic salicylate use, carditis, chronic liver dysfunction

Warnings/Precautions [U.S. Boxed Warnings]: Use caution with hepatic dysfunction, hypoprothrombinemia, vitamin K deficiency, and prior to surgery. Surgical patients should avoid salicylates if possible, for 1-2 weeks prior to surgery, to reduce the risk of excessive bleeding. Use with caution with bleeding disorders, renal dysfunction, dehydration, gastritis, or peptic ulcer disease. Heavy ethanol use (>3 drinks/day) can increase bleeding risks. Avoid use in renal or hepatic failure. Discontinue use if tinnitus or impaired hearing occurs. Patients with sensitivity to tartrazine dyes, nasal polyps, and asthma may have an increased risk of salicylate sensitivity. Children and teenagers who have or are recovering from chickenpox or flu-like symptoms should not use this product. Changes in behavior (along with nausea and vomiting) may be an early sign of Reye's syndrome; patients should be instructed to contact their healthcare provider if these occur. The lowest effective dose should be used in patients ≥65 years of age. Safety and efficacy have not been established in children <12 years.

Drug Interactions

Avoid Concomitant Use There are no known interactions where it is recommended to avoid concomitant use.

Increased Effect/Toxicity

Magnesium Salicylate may increase the levels/effects of: Calcium Channel Blockers; Neuromuscular-Blocking Agents

The levels/effects of Magnesium Salicylate may be increased by: Alfacalcidol; Calcitriol; Calcium Channel Blockers

Decreased Effect

Magnesium Salicylate may decrease the levels/effects of: Bisphosphonate Derivatives; Eltrombopag; Mycophenolate; Phosphate Supplements; Quinolone Antibiotics; Tetracycline Derivatives; Trientine

The levels/effects of Magnesium Salicylate may be decreased by: Trientine

Ethanol/Nutrition/Herb Interactions Refer to Aspirin monograph.

Pharmacodynamics/Kinetics

Half-life Elimination 2 hours; increased with repeated dosing

Time to Peak 1.5 hours

Pregnancy Risk Factor C

Lactation Enters breast milk/not recommended

Breast-Feeding Considerations Salicylates are excreted into human milk. Breast-feeding is not recommended by the manufacturer. Refer to Aspirin monograph for additional information.

Dosage Forms

Caplet, oral:

Doan's® Extra Strength [OTC]: 580 mg

Momentum® [OTC]: 580 mg

Tablet, oral:

Keygesic [OTC]: 650 mg

MST 600: 600 mg

Magnesium Sulfate (mag NEE zhum SUL fate)

Pharmacologic Category Anticonvulsant, Miscellaneous; Electrolyte Supplement, Parenteral; Magnesium Salt

Use Treatment and prevention of hypomagnesemia; prevention and treatment of seizures in severe pre-eclampsia or eclampsia, pediatric acute nephritis; torsade de pointes; treatment of cardiac arrhythmias (VT/VF) caused by hypomagnesemia; soaking aid

Unlabeled/Investigational Use Asthma exacerbation (life-threatening)

Local Anesthetic/Vasoconstrictor Precautions No information available to require special precautions

Effects on Dental Treatment Key adverse event(s) related to dental treatment: Magnesium products may prevent GI absorption of tetracyclines by forming a large ionized chelated molecule with the tetracyclines in the stomach. Tetracyclines should be given at least 1 hour before magnesium.

Effects on Bleeding No information available to require special precautions

Adverse Effects Adverse effects on neuromuscular function may occur at lower concentrations in patients with neuromuscular disease (eg, myasthenia gravis).

Frequency not defined:

Cardiovascular: Flushing (I.V.; dose related), hypotension (I.V.; rate related), vasodilation (I.V.; rate related)

Gastrointestinal: Diarrhea

General Dosage Range

I.V.: *Children and Adults:* Dosage varies greatly depending on indication

Oral: RDA (elemental magnesium):

Children 1-13 years: 80-240 mg/day

Children ≥14 years and Adults: 310-420 mg/day

I.M.: *Adults:* Hypomagnesemia: 1-4 g/day in divided doses

Topical: *Adults:* Soaking aid: Dissolve 2 cupfuls of powder per gallon of warm water

Mechanism of Action When taken orally, magnesium promotes bowel evacuation by causing osmotic retention of fluid which distends the colon with increased peristaltic activity; parenterally, magnesium decreases acetylcholine in motor nerve terminals and acts on myocardium by slowing rate of S-A node impulse formation and prolonging conduction time. Magnesium is necessary for the movement of calcium, sodium, and potassium in and out of cells, as well as stabilizing excitable membranes.

Intravenous magnesium may improve pulmonary function in patients with asthma; causes relaxation of bronchial smooth muscle independent of serum magnesium concentration.

Pharmacodynamics/Kinetics

Onset of Action Anticonvulsant: I.M.: 1 hour; Anticonvulsant: I.V.: Immediate

Duration of Action Anticonvulsant activity: I.M.: 3-4 hours; I.V.: 30 minutes

Pregnancy Risk Factor A/C (manufacturer dependent)

Maltodextrin (mal toe DEK strin)

U.S. Brand Names Carrington® Oral Wound Rinse [OTC]; Multidex® [OTC]
Generic Availability (U.S.) No
Pharmacologic Category Anti-inflammatory, Locally Applied
Dental Use Oral: Management and relief of pain due to oral lesions (including mucositis/stomatitis), oral ulcers, or irritation; treatment of aphthous ulcers
Use Topical: Treatment of infected or noninfected wounds
Local Anesthetic/Vasoconstrictor Precautions No information available to require special precautions
Effects on Dental Treatment No significant effects or complications reported (see Dental Comment)
Effects on Bleeding No information available to require special precautions
Dental Usual Dosage Management of pain due to oral lesions: Adults: Oral: Carrington® Oral Wound Rinse: 1 tablespoonful, swish or gargle for ~1 minute, 4 times/day or more if needed
Dosage Adults:
Oral: Management of pain due to oral lesions: Carrington® Oral Wound Rinse: 1 tablespoonful, swish or gargle for ~1 minute, 4 times/day or more if needed
Topical: Wound dressing: Multidex®: After debridement and irrigation of wound, apply and cover with a nonadherent, nonocclusive dressing. Apply 1/4" thick dressing over entire shallow wound. Completely fill in deep wounds with dressing. May be applied to moist or dry, infected or noninfected wounds. Change dressing once or twice daily.
Mechanism of Action Forms a protective barrier over wound providing an environment which promotes tissue growth.
Contraindications Third-degree burns
Warnings/Precautions Oral: Avoid eating or drinking for 1 hour; products are not harmful if accidentally swallowed; notify healthcare provider if improvement is not seen within 7 days
Dietary Considerations Some products may contain phenylalanine.
Dosage Forms
Gel, topical [preservative free]:
Multidex® [OTC]: 7.1 mL (7.1 mL); 14.2 mL (14.2 mL); 85.2 mL (85.2 mL)
Powder, topical [preservative free]:
Multidex® [OTC]: 6 g (6 g); 12 g (12 g); 25 g (25 g); 45 g (45 g)
Powder for suspension, oral:
Carrington® Oral Wound Rinse [OTC]: 23 g
Solution, topical [preservative free]:
Multidex® [OTC]: 45 mL (45 mL)
Dental Comment Carrington® Oral Wound Rinse: Fill bottle with water to first arrow; shake vigorously until suspended; continue to fill to second arrow; shake well

Maprotiline (ma PROE ti leen)

Canadian Brand Names Novo-Maprotiline
Pharmacologic Category Antidepressant, Tetracyclic
Use Treatment of depression and anxiety associated with depression
Unlabeled/Investigational Use Bulimia; duodenal ulcers; enuresis; urinary symptoms of multiple sclerosis; pain; panic attacks; tension headache; cocaine withdrawal
Local Anesthetic/Vasoconstrictor Precautions Although maprotiline is not a tricyclic antidepressant, it does block norepinephrine reuptake within CNS synapses as part of its mechanisms. It has been suggested that vasoconstrictor be administered with caution and to monitor vital signs in dental patients taking antidepressants that affect norepinephrine in this way, including maprotiline. Epinephrine and levonordefrin have been shown to have an increased pressor response in combination with TCAs. Maprotiline is one of the drugs confirmed to prolong the QT interval and is accepted as having a risk of causing torsade de pointes. The risk of drug-induced torsade de pointes is extremely low when a single QT interval prolonging drug is prescribed. In terms of epinephrine, it is not known what effect vasoconstrictors in the local anesthetic regimen will have in patients with a known history of congenital prolonged QT interval or in patients taking any medication that prolongs the QT interval. Until more information is obtained, it is suggested that the clinician consult with the physician prior to the use of a vasoconstrictor in suspected patients, and that the vasoconstrictor (epinephrine, mepivacaine and levonordefrin [Carbocaine® 2% with Neo-Cobefrin®]) be used with caution.

Effects on Dental Treatment Key adverse event(s) related to dental treatment: Xerostomia and changes in salivation (normal salivary flow resumes upon discontinuation).

Effects on Bleeding No information available to require special precautions

Adverse Effects

>10%:

Central nervous system: Drowsiness

Gastrointestinal: Xerostomia

1% to 10%:

Central nervous system: Insomnia, nervousness, anxiety, agitation, dizziness, fatigue, headache

Gastrointestinal: Constipation, nausea

Neuromuscular & skeletal: Tremor, weakness

Ocular: Blurred vision

General Dosage Range Oral:

Adults: Initial: 75 mg once daily; Maintenance: 150-225 mg/day as a single dose or in 3 divided doses

Elderly: Initial: 25 mg at bedtime; Maintenance: 50-75 mg/day

Mechanism of Action Traditionally believed to increase the synaptic concentration of norepinephrine in the central nervous system by inhibition of their reuptake by the presynaptic neuronal membrane. However, additional receptor effects have been found including desensitization of adenyl cyclase, down regulation of beta-adrenergic receptors, and down regulation of serotonin receptors.

Pharmacodynamics/Kinetics

Half-life Elimination Serum: 27-58 hours (mean: 43 hours)

Time to Peak Serum: Within 12 hours

Pregnancy Risk Factor B

Dental Comment Maprotiline is known to prolong the QT interval. The QT interval is measured as the time and distance between the Q point of the QRS complex and the end of the T wave in the ECG tracing. After adjustment for heart rate, the QT interval is defined as prolonged if it is more than 450 msec in men and 460 msec in women. A long QT syndrome was first described in the 1950s and 60s as a congenital syndrome involving QT interval prolongation and syncope and sudden death. Some of the congenital long QT syndromes were characterized by a peculiar electrocardiographic appearance of the QRS complex involving a premature atria beat followed by a pause, then a subsequent sinus beat showing marked QT prolongation and deformity. This type of cardiac arrhythmia was originally termed "torsade de pointes" (translated from the French as "twisting of the points"). Maprotiline is considered as having a risk of causing torsade de pointes. Since it is not known what effect vasoconstrictors in the local anesthetic regimen will have in patients with a known history of congenital prolonged QT interval or in patients taking any medication that prolongs the QT interval, a medical consult is suggested.

Maraviroc (mah RAV er rock)

Related Information

HIV Infection and AIDS *on page 1883*

U.S. Brand Names Selzentry™

Canadian Brand Names Celsentri™

Pharmacologic Category Antiretroviral Agent, CCR5 Antagonist

Use Treatment of CCR5-tropic HIV-1 infection, in combination with other antiretroviral agents

Local Anesthetic/Vasoconstrictor Precautions No information available to require special precautions

Effects on Dental Treatment Key adverse event(s) related to dental treatment: Stomatitis has been observed.

Effects on Bleeding No information available to require special precautions relative to hemostasis.

Adverse Effects

>10%:

Central nervous system: Fever (13%)

Dermatologic: Rash (11%)

Respiratory: Upper respiratory tract infection (23%), cough (14%)

2% to 10%:

Cardiovascular: Vascular hypertensive disorder (3%)

Central nervous system: Dizziness (9%; including postural dizziness), insomnia (8%), anxiety (4%), consciousness disturbances (4%), depression (4%), pain (4%)

Dermatologic: Folliculitis (4%), pruritus (4%), skin neoplasms (benign; 3%), erythema (2%)

Endocrine & metabolic: Lipodystrophy (3%)
Gastrointestinal: Appetite disorders (8%), constipation (6%)
Genitourinary: Urinary tract/bladder symptoms (3% to 5%), genital warts (2%)
Hematologic: Neutropenia (grades 3/4: 4%)
Hepatic: Transaminases increased (grades 3/4: 3% to 5%), bilirubin increased (grades 3/4: 6%)
Neuromuscular & skeletal: Joint disorders (7%), paresthesia (5%), peripheral neuropathy (4%), sensory abnormality (4%), muscle pain (3%)
Ocular: Conjunctivitis (2%), infection/inflammation (2%)
Otic: Otitis media (2%)
Respiratory: Bronchitis (7%), sinusitis (7%), respiratory tract/sinus disorder (3% to 6%), breathing abnormality (4%)
Miscellaneous: Herpes infection (8%), sweat gland disturbances (5%), influenza (2%)

General Dosage Range Dosage adjustment recommended in patients with renal impairment or on concomitant therapy

Oral: *Children ≥16 years and Adults:* 300 mg twice daily

Mechanism of Action Maraviroc, a CCR5 antagonist, selectively and reversibly binds to the chemokine (C-C motif receptor 5 [CCR5]) coreceptors located on human CD4 cells. CCR5 antagonism prevents interaction between the human CCR5 coreceptor and the gp120 subunit of the viral envelope glycoprotein, thereby inhibiting gp120 conformational change required for CCR5-tropic HIV-1 fusion with the CD4 cell and subsequent cell entry.

Pharmacodynamics/Kinetics

Half-life Elimination 14-18 hours

Time to Peak Plasma: 0.5-4 hours

Pregnancy Risk Factor B

m-Cresyl Acetate (em-KREE sil AS e tate)

U.S. Brand Names Cresylate™

Pharmacologic Category Otic Agent, Anti-infective

Use Provides an acid medium; for external otitis infections caused by susceptible bacteria or fungus

Local Anesthetic/Vasoconstrictor Precautions No information available to require special precautions

Effects on Dental Treatment No significant effects or complications reported

Effects on Bleeding No information available to require special precautions

General Dosage Range Otic: *Children and Adults:* Instill 2-4 drops as required

Measles, Mumps, and Rubella Virus Vaccine

(MEE zels, mumpz & roo BEL a VYE rus vak SEEN)

U.S. Brand Names M-M-R® II

Canadian Brand Names M-M-R® II; Priorix™

Pharmacologic Category Vaccine, Live (Viral)

Use Measles, mumps, and rubella prophylaxis

The Advisory Committee on Immunization Practices (ACIP) recommends routine vaccination for the following:

- All children (first dose given at 12-15 months of age)
- Adults born 1957 or later (without evidence of immunity or documentation of vaccination).
- Adults at higher risk for exposure to and transmission of measles mumps and rubella should receive special consideration for vaccination, unless an acceptable evidence of immunity exists. This includes international travelers, persons attending colleges and other post-high school education, persons working in healthcare facilities.

Local Anesthetic/Vasoconstrictor Precautions No information available to require special precautions

Effects on Dental Treatment No significant effects or complications reported

Effects on Bleeding No information available to require special precautions

Adverse Effects All serious adverse reactions must be reported to the U.S. Department of Health and Human Services (DHHS) Vaccine Adverse Event Reporting System (VAERS) 1-800-822-7967 or online at https://vaers.hhs.gov/esub/index. In Canada, adverse reactions may be reported to local provincial/territorial health agencies or to the Vaccine Safety Section at Public Health Agency of Canada (1-866-844-0018).

Frequency not defined:

Cardiovascular: Syncope, vasculitis

Central nervous system: Ataxia, dizziness, febrile seizure, fever, encephalitis, encephalopathy, Guillain-Barré syndrome, headache, irritability, malaise, measles inclusion body encephalitis, polyneuritis, polyneuropathy, seizure, subacute sclerosing panencephalitis,

Dermatologic: Angioneurotic edema, erythema multiforme, measles-like rash, pruritus, purpura, rash, Stevens-Johnson syndrome, urticaria

Endocrine & metabolic: Diabetes mellitus, parotitis

Gastrointestinal: Diarrhea, nausea, pancreatitis, sore throat, vomiting

Genitourinary: Epididymitis, orchitis

Hematologic: Leukocytosis, thrombocytopenia

Local: Injection site reactions which include burning, induration, redness, stinging, swelling, tenderness, wheal and flare, vesiculation

Neuromuscular & skeletal: Arthralgia/arthritis (variable; highest rates in women, 12% to 26% versus children, up to 3%), myalgia, paresthesia

Ocular: Conjunctivitis, ocular palsies, optic neuritis, papillitis, retinitis, retrobulbar neuritis

Otic: Nerve deafness, otitis media

Renal: Conjunctivitis, retinitis, optic neuritis, papillitis, retrobulbar neuritis

Respiratory: Bronchospasm, cough, pneumonia, pneumonitis, rhinitis

Miscellaneous: Anaphylactoid reactions, anaphylaxis, atypical measles, panniculitis, regional lymphadenopathy

General Dosage Range SubQ:

Children ≥12 months: 0.5 mL

Adults: Born ≥1957 without evidence of immunity: 0.5 mL for 1 or 2 doses

Mechanism of Action As a live, attenuated vaccine, MMR vaccine offers active immunity to disease caused by the measles, mumps, and rubella viruses.

Pregnancy Risk Factor C

Measles, Mumps, Rubella, and Varicella Virus Vaccine

(MEE zels, mumpz, roo BEL a, & var i SEL a VYE rus vak SEEN)

U.S. Brand Names ProQuad®

Canadian Brand Names Priorix-Tetra™

Pharmacologic Category Vaccine, Live (Viral)

Use To provide simultaneous active immunization against measles, mumps, rubella, and varicella

The Advisory Committee on Immunization Practices (ACIP) recommends routine vaccination against measles, mumps, rubella, and varicella in healthy children 12 months to 12 years of age. For children receiving their first dose at 12-47 months of age, either the MMRV combination vaccine or separate MMR and varicella vaccines can be used. (The ACIP prefers administration of separate MMR and varicella vaccines as the first dose in this age group unless the parent or caregiver expresses preference for the MMRV combination.) For children receiving the first dose at ≥48 months or their second dose at any age, use of MMRV is preferred.

Canadian labeling (not in U.S. labeling): MMRV combination vaccine is approved for use in healthy children 9 months to 6 years; may consider use in healthy children ≤12 years of age based upon prior experience with the separate component (live-attenuated MMR or live-attenuated varicella [OKA-strain]) vaccines.

Local Anesthetic/Vasoconstrictor Precautions No information available to require special precautions

Effects on Dental Treatment No significant effects or complications reported

Effects on Bleeding No information available to require special precautions

Adverse Effects All serious adverse reactions must be reported to the U.S. Department of Health and Human Services (DHHS) Vaccine Adverse Event Reporting System (VAERS) 1-800-822-7967 or online at https://vaers.hhs.gov/esub/index. In Canada, adverse reactions may be reported to local provincial/territorial health agencies or to the Vaccine Safety Section at Public Health Agency of Canada (1-866-844-0018). Percentages reported following one dose of ProQuad® at 12-23 months of age.

Also refer to Measles, Mumps, and Rubella Virus Vaccine (M-M-R® II) monograph for additional adverse reactions reported with those agents.

>10%:

Central nervous system: Fever ≥38.9°C (≥102°F) (22%)

Local: Injection site reaction: Pain/tenderness/soreness (22%), erythema (14%)

1% to 10%:
Central nervous system: Irritability (7%)
Dermatologic: Measles-like rash (3%), varicella-like rash (2%), rash (2%), viral exanthema (1%)
Gastrointestinal: Diarrhea (1%)
Local: Injection site reaction: Swelling (8%), bruising (2%)
Respiratory: Upper respiratory tract infection (1%)

General Dosage Range SubQ: *Children 12 months to 12 years:* 1 dose (0.5 mL)

Mechanism of Action A live, attenuated virus; offers active immunity to disease caused by the measles, mumps, rubella, and varicella-zoster virus.

Pregnancy Risk Factor C

Mebendazole (me BEN da zole)

Canadian Brand Names Vermox®

Pharmacologic Category Anthelmintic

Use Treatment of *Enterobius vermicularis* (pinworms), *Trichuris trichiura* (whipworms), *Ascaris lumbricoides* (roundworms), and *Ancylostoma duodenale* or *Necator amiericanus* (hookworms)

Unlabeled/Investigational Use
Treatment of *Ancylostoma caninum* (eosinophilic enterocolitis), *Capillaria philippinensis* (capillariasis), *Giardia duodenalis* (giardiasis), *Mansonella perstans* (filariasis), visceral larva migrans (toxocariasis)

Local Anesthetic/Vasoconstrictor Precautions No information available to require special precautions

Effects on Dental Treatment No significant effects or complications reported

Effects on Bleeding No information available to require special precautions

Adverse Effects Frequency not defined.
Central nervous system: Dizziness, drowsiness, headache, seizure
Dermatologic: Angioedema, exanthema, itching, rash, Stevens-Johnson syndrome, toxic epidermal necrolysis, urticaria
Gastrointestinal: Abdominal pain, diarrhea, nausea, vomiting
Hematologic: Agranulocytosis, eosinophilia, hemoglobin decreased, leukopenia, neutropenia
Hepatic: ALT increased, AST increased, GGT increased, hepatitis
Renal: Cylindruria, glomerulonephritis, hematuria
Miscellaneous: Hypersensitivity reactions (anaphylactic, anaphylactoid)

General Dosage Range Oral: *Children ≥2 years and Adults:* 100 mg as a single dose **or** twice daily

Mechanism of Action Inhibits the formation of helminth microtubules; selectively and irreversibly blocks glucose uptake and other nutrients in susceptible adult intestine-dwelling helminths

Pharmacodynamics/Kinetics
Half-life Elimination 1-11.5 hours
Time to Peak Serum: 2-4 hours

Pregnancy Risk Factor C

Mecasermin (mek a SER min)

U.S. Brand Names Increlex®

Pharmacologic Category Growth Hormone

Use Treatment of growth failure in children with severe primary insulin-like growth factor-1 deficiency (IGF-1 deficiency; primary IGFD), or with growth hormone (GH) gene deletions who have developed neutralizing antibodies to GH

Local Anesthetic/Vasoconstrictor Precautions No information available to require special precautions

Effects on Dental Treatment No significant effects or complications reported

Effects on Bleeding No information available to require special precautions

Adverse Effects
≥5%:
Cardiovascular: Cardiac murmur
Central nervous system: Dizziness, headache (Iplex™ 22%), seizure
Endocrine & metabolic: Hyperglycemia, hypoglycemia (Increlex® 42%; Iplex™ 31%), iron-deficiency anemia, ovarian cysts, thymus hypertrophy, thyromegaly
Gastrointestinal: Vomiting
Hepatic: Liver enzymes increased
Local: Injection site reactions: Erythema, bruising, hair growth, lipohypertrophy
Neuromuscular & skeletal: Arthralgia, bone pain, extremity pain, muscular atrophy
Ocular: Papilledema

Otic: Ear pain, hypoacusis, middle ear fluid, otitis media, serous otitis media, tympanometry abnormal
Renal: Hematuria
Respiratory: Snoring, tonsillar hypertrophy (Increlex® 15%; Iplex™ 19%)
Miscellaneous: Lymphadenopathy
<5% or frequency not defined: Anaphylaxis (case report), angioedema (case report), cardiomegaly, dyspnea (case report), hypercholesterolemia, hypersensitivity, hypertriglyceridemia, hypoglycemic seizure, intracranial hypertension, loss of consciousness secondary to hypoglycemia, obstructive sleep apnea, pruritus (case report), thickening of soft facial tissue, urticaria (case report), valvulopathy

General Dosage Range SubQ:
Children ≥2 years: Increlex®: Initial: 0.04-0.08 mg/kg twice daily; Maintenance: 0.04-0.12 mg/kg twice daily
Children ≥3 years: Iplex™: Initial: 0.5 mg/kg once daily; Maintenance: 0.5-2 mg/kg once daily

Mechanism of Action Mecasermin is an insulin-like growth factor (IGF-1) produced using recombinant DNA technology to replace endogenous IGF-1. Endogenous IGF-1 circulates predominately bound to insulin-like growth factor-binding protein-3 (IGFBP-3) and a growth hormone-dependent acid-labile subunit (ALS). Acting at receptors in the liver and other tissues, endogenous growth hormone (GH) stimulates the synthesis and secretion of IGF-1. In patients with primary severe IGF-1 deficiency, growth hormone receptors in the liver are unresponsive to GH, leading to reduced endogenous IGF-I concentrations and decreased growth (skeletal, cell, and organ). Endogenous IGF-1 also suppresses liver glucose production, stimulates peripheral glucose utilization and has an inhibitory effect on insulin secretion.
Mecasermin rinfabate is a complex of IGF-1 and IGFBP-3, both produced by recombinant DNA technology.

Pharmacodynamics/Kinetics
Half-life Elimination Severe primary IGFD: Mecasermin: 5.8 hours; Mecasermin rinfabate: >12 hours

Pregnancy Risk Factor C

Prescribing and Access Restrictions Iplex™ is not commercially available. Access is currently limited to existing patients with ALS already receiving therapy through a single-patient IND application. Additional information may be found at http://www.fda.gov/Drugs/ResourcesForYou/HealthProfessionals/ucm118117.htm.

Meclizine (MEK li zeen)

U.S. Brand Names Antivert®; Bonine® [OTC]; Dramamine® Less Drowsy Formula [OTC]; Medi-Meclizine [OTC]; Trav-L-Tabs® [OTC]

Canadian Brand Names Bonamine™; Bonine®

Pharmacologic Category Antiemetic; Histamine H_1 Antagonist; Histamine H_1 Antagonist, First Generation; Piperazine Derivative

Use Prevention and treatment of symptoms of motion sickness; management of vertigo with diseases affecting the vestibular system

Local Anesthetic/Vasoconstrictor Precautions No information available to require special precautions

Effects on Dental Treatment Key adverse event(s) related to dental treatment: Slight to moderate drowsiness, thickening of bronchial secretions, significant xerostomia (normal salivary flow resumes upon discontinuation).

Effects on Bleeding No information available to require special precautions

Adverse Effects
>10%:
Central nervous system: Slight to moderate drowsiness
Respiratory: Thickening of bronchial secretions
1% to 10%:
Central nervous system: Headache, fatigue, nervousness, dizziness
Gastrointestinal: Appetite increase, weight gain, nausea, diarrhea, abdominal pain, xerostomia
Respiratory: Pharyngitis

General Dosage Range Oral: *Children >12 years and Adults:* 12.5-50 mg 1 hour before travel, may repeat every 12-24 hours if needed **or** 25-100 mg/day in divided doses

Mechanism of Action Has central anticholinergic action by blocking chemoreceptor trigger zone; decreases excitability of the middle ear labyrinth and blocks conduction in the middle ear vestibular-cerebellar pathways

Pharmacodynamics/Kinetics

Onset of Action ~1 hour

Duration of Action 8-24 hours

Half-life Elimination 6 hours

Pregnancy Risk Factor B

Meclofenamate (me kloe fen AM ate)

Related Information

Rheumatoid Arthritis, Osteoarthritis, and Osteoporosis *on page 1889*

Temporomandibular Dysfunction (TMD) *on page 1964*

Canadian Brand Names Meclomen®

Generic Availability (U.S.) Yes

Pharmacologic Category Nonsteroidal Anti-inflammatory Drug (NSAID), Oral

Use Treatment of inflammatory disorders, arthritis, mild-to-moderate pain, dysmenorrhea

Local Anesthetic/Vasoconstrictor Precautions No information available to require special precautions

Effects on Dental Treatment The dentist should be aware of the potential of abnormal coagulation. Caution should also be exercised in the use of NSAIDs in patients already on anticoagulant therapy with drugs such as warfarin (Coumadin®). Recovery of platelet function usually occurs 1-2 days after discontinuation of NSAIDs. See Effects on Bleeding.

Effects on Bleeding Nonselective NSAIDs are known to reversibly decrease platelet aggregation via mechanisms different than observed with aspirin. Platelet function is restored as the drug is eliminated from the body. NSAIDs should be avoided (if possible) in general surgery patients for 3-5 half-lives of the drug (usually 1-3 days) prior to surgery to reduce the risk of excessive bleeding. However, there is no scientific evidence to warrant discontinuance of NSAIDs prior to dental surgery. In medically complicated patients or extensive oral surgery, the decision to interrupt therapy must be based on the risk to benefit in an individual patient and a medical consult is suggested. Routine interruption of NSAID therapy for most dental procedures is not warranted. If therapy is continued without interruption, the clinician should anticipate the potential for slower clotting times.

Adverse Effects

>10%:

Central nervous system: Dizziness

Dermatologic: Rash

Gastrointestinal: Abdominal cramps, heartburn, indigestion, nausea

1% to 10%:

Central nervous system: Headache, nervousness

Dermatologic: Itching

Endocrine & metabolic: Fluid retention

Gastrointestinal: Vomiting

Otic: Tinnitus

Dosage Children >14 years and Adults: Oral:

Mild-to-moderate pain: 50 mg every 4-6 hours; increases to 100 mg may be required; maximum dose: 400 mg

Rheumatoid arthritis and osteoarthritis: 50 mg every 4-6 hours; increase, over weeks, to 200-400 mg/day in 3-4 divided doses; do not exceed 400 mg/day; maximal benefit for any dose may not be seen for 2-3 weeks

Mechanism of Action Reversibly inhibits cyclooxygenase-1 and 2 (COX-1 and 2) enzymes, which results in decreased formation of prostaglandin precursors; has antipyretic, analgesic, and anti-inflammatory properties.

Other proposed mechanisms not fully elucidated (and possibly contributing to the anti-inflammatory effect to varying degrees) include inhibiting chemotaxis, altering lymphocyte activity, inhibiting neutrophil aggregation/activation, and decreasing proinflammatory cytokine levels.

Contraindications Hypersensitivity to meclofenamate, aspirin, other NSAIDs, or any component of the formulation; perioperative pain in the setting of coronary artery bypass graft (CABG) surgery

Warnings/Precautions NSAIDs are associated with an increased risk of adverse cardiovascular thrombotic events, including MI and stroke. Risk may be increased with duration of use or pre-existing cardiovascular risk factors or disease. Carefully evaluate individual cardiovascular risk profiles prior to prescribing. May cause new-onset hypertension or worsening of existing hypertension. Use caution with fluid retention. Avoid use in heart failure. Concurrent administration of ibuprofen, and potentially other nonselective NSAIDs, may interfere with aspirin's cardioprotective effect. Risk of MI and stroke may be increased with use following CABG surgery.

Platelet adhesion and aggregation may be decreased; may prolong bleeding time; patients with coagulation disorders or who are receiving anticoagulants should be monitored closely. Anemia may occur; patients on long-term NSAID therapy should be monitored for anemia. Rarely, NSAID use may cause severe blood dyscrasias (eg, agranulocytosis, aplastic anemia, thrombocytopenia).

NSAID use may compromise existing renal function; dose-dependent decreases in prostaglandin synthesis may result from NSAID use, reducing renal blood flow which may cause renal decompensation. NSAID use may increase the risk for hyperkalemia. Patients with impaired renal function, dehydration, heart failure, liver dysfunction, those taking diuretics, and ACE inhibitors, and the elderly are at greater risk of renal toxicity and hyperkalemia. Rehydrate patient before starting therapy; monitor renal function closely. Not recommended for use in patients with advanced renal disease. Long-term NSAID use may result in renal papillary necrosis.

NSAIDs may increase risk of gastrointestinal irritation, inflammation, ulceration, bleeding, and perforation. These events may occur at any time during therapy and without warning. Use caution with a history of GI disease (bleeding or ulcers), concurrent therapy with aspirin, anticoagulants and/or corticosteroids, smoking, use of alcohol, the elderly or debilitated patients. When used concomitantly with ≤325 mg of aspirin, a substantial increase in the risk of gastrointestinal complications (eg, ulcer) occurs; concomitant gastroprotective therapy (eg, proton pump inhibitors) is recommended (Bhatt, 2008).

Use the lowest effective dose for the shortest duration of time, consistent with individual patient goals, to reduce risk of cardiovascular or GI adverse events. Alternate therapies should be considered for patients at high risk.

NSAIDs may cause serious skin adverse events including exfoliative dermatitis, Stevens-Johnson syndrome (SJS) and toxic epidermal necrolysis (TEN); discontinue use at first sign of skin rash or hypersensitivity. Anaphylactoid reactions may occur, even without prior exposure; patients with "aspirin triad" (bronchial asthma, aspirin intolerance, rhinitis) may be at increased risk. Do not use in patients who experience bronchospasm, asthma, rhinitis, or urticaria with NSAID or aspirin therapy. Use caution in other forms of asthma.

Use with caution in patients with decreased hepatic function. Closely monitor patients with any abnormal LFT. Severe hepatic reactions (eg, fulminant hepatitis, liver failure) have occurred with NSAID use, rarely; discontinue if signs or symptoms of liver disease develop, or if systemic manifestations occur.

NSAIDS may cause drowsiness, dizziness, blurred vision and other neurologic effects which may impair physical or mental abilities; patients must be cautioned about performing tasks which require mental alertness (eg, operating machinery or driving). Discontinue use with blurred or diminished vision and perform ophthalmologic exam. Monitor vision with long-term therapy.

The elderly are at increased risk for adverse effects (especially peptic ulceration, CNS effects, renal toxicity) from NSAIDs even at low doses.

Withhold for at least 4-6 half-lives prior to surgical or dental procedures.

Drug Interactions

Avoid Concomitant Use

Avoid concomitant use of Meclofenamate with any of the following: Ketorolac; Ketorolac (Systemic)

Increased Effect/Toxicity

Meclofenamate may increase the levels/effects of: Aminoglycosides; Anticoagulants; Antiplatelet Agents; Bisphosphonate Derivatives; Collagenase (Systemic); CycloSPORINE; CycloSPORINE (Systemic); Deferasirox; Desmopressin; Digoxin; Drotrecogin Alfa; Eplerenone; Haloperidol; Ibritumomab; Lithium; Methotrexate; Nonsteroidal Anti-Inflammatory Agents; PEMEtrexed; Potassium-Sparing Diuretics; PRALAtrexate; Quinolone Antibiotics; Salicylates; Thrombolytic Agents; Tositumomab and Iodine I 131 Tositumomab; Vancomycin; Vitamin K Antagonists

The levels/effects of Meclofenamate may be increased by: ACE Inhibitors; Angiotensin II Receptor Blockers; Antidepressants (Tricyclic, Tertiary Amine); Corticosteroids (Systemic); Dasatinib; Glucosamine; Herbs (Anticoagulant/Antiplatelet Properties); Ketorolac; Ketorolac (Systemic); Nonsteroidal Anti-Inflammatory Agents; Omega-3-Acid Ethyl Esters; Pentosan Polysulfate Sodium; Pentoxifylline; Probenecid; Prostacyclin Analogues; Selective Serotonin Reuptake Inhibitors; Serotonin/Norepinephrine Reuptake Inhibitors; Treprostinil

Decreased Effect

Meclofenamate may decrease the levels/effects of: ACE Inhibitors; Angiotensin II Receptor Blockers; Antiplatelet Agents; Beta-Blockers; Eplerenone; HydrALAZINE; Loop Diuretics; Potassium-Sparing Diuretics; Salicylates; Thiazide Diuretics

The levels/effects of Meclofenamate may be decreased by: Bile Acid Sequestrants; Nonsteroidal Anti-Inflammatory Agents; Salicylates

Ethanol/Nutrition/Herb Interactions

Ethanol: Avoid ethanol (may enhance gastric mucosal irritation).

Herb/Nutraceutical: Avoid alfalfa, anise, bilberry, bladderwrack, bromelain, cat's claw, celery, chamomile, coleus, cordyceps, dong quai, evening primrose, fenugreek, feverfew, garlic, ginger, ginkgo biloba, ginseng (American, Panax, Siberian), grapeseed, green tea, guggul, horse chestnut seed, horseradish, licorice, prickly ash, red clover, reishi, SAMe (S-adenosylmethionine), sweet clover, turmeric, white willow (all have additional antiplatelet activity).

Dietary Considerations May be taken with food, milk, or antacids.

Pharmacodynamics/Kinetics

Duration of Action 2-4 hours

Half-life Elimination Meclofenamate sodium: 0.8-2.1 hours; metabolite I 15.3 hours

Time to Peak Serum: Meclofenamate sodium 0.5-1.5 hours; metabolite I 0.5-4 hours

Lactation Enters breast milk/not recommended

Breast-Feeding Considerations Meclofenamate is excreted into breast milk in trace amounts. Breast-feeding is not recommended by the manufacturer.

Dosage Forms

Capsule, oral: 50 mg, 100 mg

Medium Chain Triglycerides (mee DEE um chane trye GLIS er ides)

U.S. Brand Names MCT Oil® [OTC]

Canadian Brand Names MCT Oil®

Pharmacologic Category Nutritional Supplement

Use Dietary supplement for those who cannot digest long chain fats; malabsorption associated with disorders such as pancreatic insufficiency, bile salt deficiency, short bowel syndrome, and bacterial overgrowth of the small bowel; induce ketosis as a prevention for seizures

Local Anesthetic/Vasoconstrictor Precautions No information available to require special precautions

Effects on Dental Treatment No significant effects or complications reported

Effects on Bleeding No information available to require special precautions

Adverse Effects Frequency not defined.

Endocrine & metabolic: HDL serum levels decreased and triglycerides serum levels increased (>6 months daily use)

Gastrointestinal: Abdominal pain, bloating, cramping, diarrhea, nausea

General Dosage Range Oral:

Infants: Initial: 0.5 mL every other feeding, then advance to every feeding, then increase in increments of 0.25-0.5 mL/feeding at intervals of 2-3 days as tolerated

Children: 3 tablespoons/day in divided doses **or** ~39 mL with each meal **or** 50% to 70% (800-1120 kcal) of total calories (1600 kcal)

Adults: 3 tablespoons/day in divided doses **or** 15 mL 3-4 times/day

Mechanism of Action MCTs are saturated fatty acids in chains of 6-12 carbon atoms. They are water soluble and can pass directly through intestinal cell membranes and blood stream. Once taken up by the liver, they are used for metabolic energy before being stored.

MedroxyPROGESTERone (me DROKS ee proe JES te rone)

Related Information

Endocrine Disorders and Pregnancy *on page 1879*

U.S. Brand Names Depo-Provera®; Depo-Provera® Contraceptive; depo-subQ provera 104®; Provera®

Canadian Brand Names Alti-MPA; Apo-Medroxy®; Depo-Prevera®; Depo-Provera®; Dom-Medroxyprogesterone; Gen-Medroxy; Medroxy; Medroxyprogesterone Acetate Injectable Suspension USP; Novo-Medrone; PMS-Medroxyprogesterone; Provera-Pak; Provera®; Teva-Medroxyprogesterone

Pharmacologic Category Contraceptive; Progestin

Use Secondary amenorrhea or abnormal uterine bleeding due to hormonal imbalance; reduction of endometrial hyperplasia in nonhysterectomized postmenopausal women receiving conjugated estrogens; prevention of pregnancy; management of endometriosis-associated pain; adjunctive therapy and palliative treatment of recurrent and metastatic endometrial carcinoma

Unlabeled/Investigational Use Treatment of low-grade endometrial stromal sarcoma

Local Anesthetic/Vasoconstrictor Precautions No information available to require special precautions

Effects on Dental Treatment Progestins may predispose the patient to gingival bleeding.

Effects on Bleeding No information available to require special precautions

Adverse Effects Adverse effects as reported with any dosage form; percent ranges presented are noted with the MPA I.M. contraceptive injection:

>5%:

Central nervous system: Dizziness, headache, nervousness

Endocrine & metabolic: Libido decreased, menstrual irregularities (includes bleeding, amenorrhea, or both)

Gastrointestinal: Abdominal pain/discomfort, weight gain (>10 lbs at 24 months: 38%)

1% to 5%:

Cardiovascular: Edema

Central nervous system: Depression, fatigue, insomnia

Dermatologic: Acne, alopecia, rash

Endocrine & metabolic: Breast pain, hot flashes

Gastrointestinal: Bloating, nausea

Genitourinary: Dysmenorrhea, leukorrhea, vaginitis

Local: Injection site reaction (SubQ administration): Atrophy, induration, pain

Neuromuscular & skeletal: Arthralgia, backache, leg cramp, weakness

<1%, postmarketing, and/or case reports: Allergic reaction, anaphylaxis, anaphylactoid reactions, anemia, angioedema, anxiety, appetite changes, asthma, axillary swelling, blood dyscrasia, body odor, BMD loss, breast cancer, breast changes, cervical cancer, chest pain, chills, chloasma, cholestatic jaundice, deep vein thrombosis, diaphoresis, diarrhea, drowsiness, dry skin, dyspareunia, dyspnea, facial palsy, fainting, fever, galactorrhea, genitourinary infections, glucose tolerance decreased, hirsutism, hoarseness, jaundice, lack of return to fertility, lactation decreased, libido increased, melasma, nipple bleeding, oligomenorrhea, optic neuritis, osteoporosis, osteoporotic fractures, paralysis, paresthesia, pruritus, pulmonary embolus, rectal bleeding, retinal thrombosis, scleroderma, seizure, somnolence, syncope, tachycardia, thirst, thrombophlebitis, urticaria, uterine hyperplasia, vaginal cysts, varicose veins

In addition: Depo-Provera® aqueous suspension: Residual lump, sterile abscess, or skin discoloration at the injection

General Dosage Range Dosage adjustment recommended in patients with hepatic impairment.

I.M.:

Adolescents and Adults: Contraception: 150 mg every 3 months

Adults: Endometrial cancer: 400-1000 mg/week

Oral: *Adolescents and Adults:* 5-10 mg once daily

SubQ: *Adolescents and Adults:* 104 mg every 3 months (every 12-14 weeks)

Mechanism of Action Inhibits secretion of pituitary gonadotropins, which prevents follicular maturation and ovulation; causes endometrial thinning

Pharmacodynamics/Kinetics

Half-life Elimination Oral: 12-17 hours; I.M. (Depo-Provera® Contraceptive): ~50 days; SubQ: ~40 days

Time to Peak Oral: 2-4 hours; I.M. (Depo-Provera® Contraceptive): ~3 weeks; SubQ: ~1 week

Pregnancy Risk Factor X

Mefenamic Acid (me fe NAM ik AS id)

Related Information

Rheumatoid Arthritis, Osteoarthritis, and Osteoporosis *on page 1889*

Temporomandibular Dysfunction (TMD) *on page 1964*

U.S. Brand Names Ponstel®

Canadian Brand Names Apo-Mefenamic®; Dom-Mefenamic Acid; Mefenamic-250; Nu-Mefenamic; PMS-Mefenamic Acid; Ponstan®

Generic Availability (U.S.) Yes

Pharmacologic Category Nonsteroidal Anti-inflammatory Drug (NSAID), Oral

Use Short-term relief of mild-to-moderate pain including primary dysmenorrhea

Local Anesthetic/Vasoconstrictor Precautions No information available to require special precautions

Effects on Dental Treatment The dentist should be aware of the potential of abnormal coagulation. Caution should also be exercised in the use of NSAIDs in patients already on anticoagulant therapy with drugs such as warfarin (Coumadin®). Recovery of platelet function usually occurs 1-2 days after discontinuation of NSAIDs. See Effects on Bleeding.

Effects on Bleeding Nonselective NSAIDs are known to reversibly decrease platelet aggregation via mechanisms different than observed with aspirin. Platelet function is restored as the drug is eliminated from the body. NSAIDs should be avoided (if possible) in general surgery patients for 3-5 half-lives of the drug (usually 1-3 days) prior to surgery to reduce the risk of excessive bleeding. However, there is no scientific evidence to warrant discontinuance of NSAIDs prior to dental surgery. In medically complicated patients or extensive oral surgery, the decision to interrupt therapy must be based on the risk to benefit in an individual patient and a medical consult is suggested. Routine interruption of NSAID therapy for most dental procedures is not warranted. If therapy is continued without interruption, the clinician should anticipate the potential for slower clotting times.

Adverse Effects 1% to 10%:

Central nervous system: Headache, nervousness, dizziness (3% to 9%)

Dermatologic: Itching, rash

Endocrine & metabolic: Fluid retention

Gastrointestinal: Abdominal cramps, heartburn, indigestion, nausea (1% to 10%), vomiting (1% to 10%), diarrhea (1% to 10%), constipation (1% to 10%), abdominal distress/cramping/pain (1% to 10%), dyspepsia (1% to 10%), flatulence (1% to 10%), gastric or duodenal ulcer with bleeding or perforation (1% to 10%), gastritis (1% to 10%)

Hematologic: Bleeding (1% to 10%)

Hepatic: LFTs increased (1% to 10%)

Otic: Tinnitus (1% to 10%)

Dosage Children >14 years and Adults: Oral: 500 mg to start then 250 mg every 4 hours as needed; maximum therapy: 1 week

Dosing adjustment/comments in renal impairment: Not recommended for use

Mechanism of Action Reversibly inhibits cyclooxygenase-1 and 2 (COX-1 and 2) enzymes, which results in decreased formation of prostaglandin precursors; has antipyretic, analgesic, and anti-inflammatory properties.

Other proposed mechanisms not fully elucidated (and possibly contributing to the anti-inflammatory effect to varying degrees) include inhibiting chemotaxis, altering lymphocyte activity, inhibiting neutrophil aggregation/activation, and decreasing proinflammatory cytokine levels.

Contraindications Hypersensitivity to mefenamic acid, aspirin, other NSAIDs, or any component of the formulation; perioperative pain in the setting of coronary artery bypass graft (CABG) surgery; active ulceration or chronic inflammation of the GI tract; renal disease

Warnings/Precautions [U.S. Boxed Warning]: NSAIDs are associated with an increased risk of adverse cardiovascular thrombotic events, including MI and stroke. Risk may be increased with duration of use or pre-existing cardiovascular risk factors or disease. Carefully evaluate individual cardiovascular risk profiles prior to prescribing. May cause new-onset hypertension or worsening of existing hypertension. Use caution with fluid retention. Avoid use in heart failure. Concurrent administration of ibuprofen, and potentially other nonselective NSAIDs, may interfere with aspirin's cardioprotective effect. **[U.S. Boxed Warning]: Use is contraindicated for treatment of perioperative pain in the setting of coronary artery bypass graft (CABG) surgery.** Risk of MI and stroke may be increased with use following CABG surgery.

Platelet adhesion and aggregation may be decreased; may prolong bleeding time; patients with coagulation disorders or who are receiving anticoagulants should be monitored closely. Anemia may occur; patients on long-term NSAID therapy should be monitored for anemia. Rarely, NSAID use may cause severe blood dyscrasias (eg, agranulocytosis, aplastic anemia, thrombocytopenia).

NSAID use may compromise existing renal function; dose-dependent decreases in prostaglandin synthesis may result from NSAID use, reducing renal blood flow which may cause renal decompensation. NSAID use may increase the risk for hyperkalemia. Patients with impaired renal function, dehydration, heart failure, liver dysfunction, those taking diuretics, and ACE inhibitors, and the elderly are at greater risk of renal toxicity and hyperkalemia. Rehydrate patient before starting therapy; monitor renal function closely. Contraindicated in patients with advanced renal disease. Long-term NSAID use may result in renal papillary necrosis.

[U.S. Boxed Warning]: NSAIDs may increase risk of gastrointestinal irritation, inflammation, ulceration, bleeding, and perforation. These events may occur at any time during therapy and without warning. Use caution with a history of GI disease (bleeding or ulcers), concurrent therapy with aspirin, anticoagulants and/or corticosteroids, smoking, use of alcohol, the elderly or debilitated patients. When used concomitantly with ≤325 mg of aspirin, a substantial increase in the risk of gastrointestinal complications (eg, ulcer) occurs; concomitant gastroprotective therapy (eg, proton pump inhibitors) is recommended (Bhatt, 2008).

Use the lowest effective dose for the shortest duration of time, consistent with individual patient goals, to reduce risk of cardiovascular or GI adverse events. Alternate therapies should be considered for patients at high risk.

NSAIDs may cause serious skin adverse events including exfoliative dermatitis, Stevens-Johnson syndrome (SJS) and toxic epidermal necrolysis (TEN); discontinue use at first sign of skin rash or hypersensitivity. Anaphylactoid reactions may occur, even without prior exposure; patients with "aspirin triad" (bronchial asthma, aspirin intolerance, rhinitis) may be at increased risk. Do not use in patients who experience bronchospasm, asthma, rhinitis, or urticaria with NSAID or aspirin therapy. Use caution in other forms of asthma.

Use with caution in patients with decreased hepatic function. Closely monitor patients with any abnormal LFT. Severe hepatic reactions (eg, fulminant hepatitis, liver failure) have occurred with NSAID use, rarely; discontinue if signs or symptoms of liver disease develop, or if systemic manifestations occur.

NSAIDS may cause drowsiness, dizziness, blurred vision and other neurologic effects which may impair physical or mental abilities; patients must be cautioned about performing tasks which require mental alertness (eg, operating machinery or driving). Discontinue use with blurred or diminished vision and perform ophthalmologic exam. Monitor vision with long-term therapy.

The elderly are at increased risk for adverse effects (especially peptic ulceration, CNS effects, renal toxicity) from NSAIDs even at low doses.

Withhold for at least 4-6 half-lives prior to surgical or dental procedures.

Drug Interactions

Metabolism/Transport Effects **Substrate** of CYP2C9 (minor); **Inhibits** CYP2C9 (strong)

Avoid Concomitant Use

Avoid concomitant use of Mefenamic Acid with any of the following: Ketorolac; Ketorolac (Systemic)

Increased Effect/Toxicity

Mefenamic Acid may increase the levels/effects of: Aminoglycosides; Anticoagulants; Antiplatelet Agents; Bisphosphonate Derivatives; Collagenase (Systemic); CycloSPORINE; CycloSPORINE (Systemic); Deferasirox; Desmopressin; Digoxin; Drotrecogin Alfa; Eplerenone; Haloperidol; Ibritumomab; Lithium; Methotrexate; Nonsteroidal Anti-Inflammatory Agents; PEMEtrexed; Potassium-Sparing Diuretics; PRALAtrexate; Quinolone Antibiotics; Salicylates; Thrombolytic Agents; Tositumomab and Iodine I 131 Tositumomab; Vancomycin; Vitamin K Antagonists

The levels/effects of Mefenamic Acid may be increased by: ACE Inhibitors; Angiotensin II Receptor Blockers; Antidepressants (Tricyclic, Tertiary Amine); Corticosteroids (Systemic); Dasatinib; Glucosamine; Herbs (Anticoagulant/Antiplatelet Properties); Ketorolac; Ketorolac (Systemic); Nonsteroidal Anti-Inflammatory Agents; Omega-3-Acid Ethyl Esters; Pentosan Polysulfate Sodium; Pentoxifylline; Probenecid; Prostacyclin Analogues; Selective Serotonin Reuptake Inhibitors; Serotonin/Norepinephrine Reuptake Inhibitors; Treprostinil

Decreased Effect

Mefenamic Acid may decrease the levels/effects of: ACE Inhibitors; Angiotensin II Receptor Blockers; Antiplatelet Agents; Beta-Blockers; Eplerenone; HydrALAZINE; Loop Diuretics; Potassium-Sparing Diuretics; Salicylates; Thiazide Diuretics

The levels/effects of Mefenamic Acid may be decreased by: Bile Acid Sequestrants; Nonsteroidal Anti-Inflammatory Agents; Salicylates

Ethanol/Nutrition/Herb Interactions

Ethanol: Avoid ethanol (may enhance gastric mucosal irritation).

Herb/Nutraceutical: Avoid alfalfa, anise, bilberry, bladderwrack, bromelain, cat's claw, celery, chamomile, coleus, cordyceps, dong quai, evening primrose, fenugreek, feverfew, garlic, ginger, ginkgo biloba, ginseng (American, Panax, Siberian), grapeseed, green tea, guggul, horse chestnut seed, horseradish, licorice, prickly ash, red clover, reishi, SAMe (S-adenosylmethionine), sweet clover, turmeric, white willow (all have additional antiplatelet activity).

Dietary Considerations May be taken with food, milk, or antacids.

Pharmacodynamics/Kinetics

Onset of Action Peak effect: 2-4 hours

Duration of Action ≤6 hours

Half-life Elimination ~2 hours

Time to Peak 2-4 hours

Pregnancy Risk Factor C

Lactation Enters breast milk (trace amounts)/not recommended (AAP rates "compatible"; AAP 2001 update pending)

Breast-Feeding Considerations Trace amounts of mefenamic acid may be present in breast milk. Breast-feeding is not recommended by the manufacturer.

Dosage Forms

Capsule, oral: 250 mg

Ponstel®: 250 mg

Mefloquine (ME floe kwin)

Canadian Brand Names Apo-Mefloquine®; Lariam®

Pharmacologic Category Antimalarial Agent

Use Treatment of mild-to-moderate acute malarial infections (including treatment of chloroquine-resistant malaria) and prevention of malaria caused by *Plasmodium falciparum* or *P. vivax*

Local Anesthetic/Vasoconstrictor Precautions No information available to require special precautions

Effects on Dental Treatment No significant effects or complications reported

Effects on Bleeding No information available to require special precautions

Adverse Effects 1% to 10%:

Central nervous system: Chills, dizziness, fatigue, fever, headache

Dermatologic: Rash

Gastrointestinal: Vomiting (3%), abdominal pain, appetite decreased, diarrhea, nausea

Neuromuscular & skeletal: Myalgia

Otic: Tinnitus

General Dosage Range Oral:

Children ≥6 months: Prophylaxis: 5 mg/kg/once weekly (maximum: 250 mg/dose); Treatment: 20-25 mg/kg/day in 2 divided doses (maximum: 1250 mg)

Adults: Prophylaxis: 1 tablet (250 mg) once weekly; Treatment: 5 tablets (1250 mg) as a single dose

Mechanism of Action Mefloquine is a quinoline-methanol compound structurally similar to quinine; mefloquine's effectiveness in the treatment and prophylaxis of malaria is due to the destruction of the asexual blood forms of the malarial pathogens that affect humans, *Plasmodium falciparum, P. vivax*

Pharmacodynamics/Kinetics

Half-life Elimination ~3 weeks (range: 2-4 weeks)

Time to Peak Plasma: ~17 hours (range: 6-24 hours)

Pregnancy Risk Factor C

Megestrol (me JES trole)

U.S. Brand Names Megace®; Megace® ES

Canadian Brand Names Apo-Megestrol®; Megace®; Megace® OS; Nu-Megestrol

Pharmacologic Category Antineoplastic Agent, Hormone; Appetite Stimulant; Progestin

Use Palliative treatment of breast and endometrial carcinoma; treatment of anorexia, cachexia, or unexplained significant weight loss in patients with AIDS

Local Anesthetic/Vasoconstrictor Precautions No information available to require special precautions

Effects on Dental Treatment No significant effects or complications reported

Effects on Bleeding Although significant myelosuppression with associated altered hemostasis has been reported for many chemotherapeutic agents, myelosuppression is not common with megestrol and no specific precautions appear to necessary.

Adverse Effects Frequency not always defined.

Cardiovascular: Hypertension (≤8%), cardiomyopathy (1% to 3%), chest pain (1% to 3%), edema (1% to 3%), palpitation (1% to 3%), peripheral edema (1% to 3%), heart failure

Central nervous system: Headache (≤10%), insomnia (≤6%), fever (1% to 6%), pain (≤6%, similar to placebo), abnormal thinking (1% to 3%), confusion (1% to 3%), depression (1% to 3%), hypoesthesia (1% to 3%), seizure (1% to 3%), mood changes, malaise, lethargy

Dermatologic: Rash (2% to 12%), alopecia (1% to 3%), pruritus (1% to 3%), vesiculobullous rash (1% to 3%)

Endocrine & metabolic: Hyperglycemia (≤6%), gynecomastia (1% to 3%), adrenal insufficiency, amenorrhea, breakthrough bleeding, cervical erosion and secretions (changes), breast tenderness increased, Cushing's syndrome, diabetes, glucose intolerance, HPA axis suppression, hot flashes, hypercalcemia, menstrual flow changes, spotting, vaginal bleeding pattern changes

Gastrointestinal: Diarrhea (6% to 15%, similar to placebo), flatulence (≤10%), vomiting (≤6%), nausea (≤5%), dyspepsia (≤4%), abdominal pain (1% to 3%), constipation (1% to 3%), salivation increased (1% to 3%), xerostomia (1% to 3%), weight gain (not attributed to edema or fluid retention)

Genitourinary: Impotence (4% to 14%), decreased libido (≤5%), urinary incontinence (1% to 3%), urinary tract infection (1% to 3%), urinary frequency (≤2%)

Hematologic: Anemia (≤5%), leukopenia (1% to 3%)

Hepatic: Hepatomegaly (1% to 3%), LDH increased (1% to 3%), cholestatic jaundice, hepatotoxicity

Neuromuscular & skeletal: Weakness (2% to 6%), neuropathy (1% to 3%), paresthesia (1% to 3%), carpal tunnel syndrome

Ocular: Amblyopia (1% to 3%)

Renal: Albuminuria (1% to 3%)

Respiratory: Dyspnea (1% to 3%), cough (1% to 3%), pharyngitis (1% to 3%), pneumonia (≤2%), hyperpnea

Miscellaneous: Diaphoresis (1% to 3%), herpes infection (1% to 3%), infection (1% to 3%), moniliasis (1% to 3%), tumor flare

General Dosage Range Oral:

Adults (females): Tablet: 40-320 mg/day in divided doses

Adults (males/females): Suspension: 400-800 mg/day [Megace®] **or** 625 mg/day [Megace® ES]

Mechanism of Action A synthetic progestin with antiestrogenic properties which disrupt the estrogen receptor cycle. Megestrol interferes with the normal estrogen cycle and results in a lower LH titer. May also have a direct effect on the endometrium. Megestrol is an antineoplastic progestin thought to act through an antileutenizing effect mediated via the pituitary. May stimulate appetite by antagonizing the metabolic effects of catabolic cytokines.

Pharmacodynamics/Kinetics

Half-life Elimination 13-105 hours

Time to Peak Serum: 1-3 hours

Pregnancy Risk Factor D (tablet) / X (suspension)

Meloxicam (mel OKS i kam)

Related Information

Rheumatoid Arthritis, Osteoarthritis, and Osteoporosis *on page 1889*

U.S. Brand Names Mobic®

Canadian Brand Names Apo-Meloxicam®; CO Meloxicam; Dom-Meloxicam; Mobicox®; Mobic®; Mylan-Meloxicam; Novo-Meloxicam; PHL-Meloxicam; PMS-Meloxicam; ratio-Meloxicam; Teva-Meloxicam

Generic Availability (U.S.) Yes:

Pharmacologic Category Nonsteroidal Anti-inflammatory Drug (NSAID), Oral

Use Relief of signs and symptoms of osteoarthritis, rheumatoid arthritis, and juvenile idiopathic arthritis (JIA)

Local Anesthetic/Vasoconstrictor Precautions No information available to require special precautions

Effects on Dental Treatment Key adverse event(s) related to dental treatment: Taste perversion, ulcerative stomatitis, and xerostomia (normal salivary flow resumes upon discontinuation). The dentist should be aware of the potential of abnormal coagulation. Caution should also be exercised in the use of NSAIDs in patients already on anticoagulant therapy with drugs such as warfarin (Coumadin®). See Effects on Bleeding.

Effects on Bleeding Nonselective NSAIDs are known to reversibly decrease platelet aggregation via mechanisms different than observed with aspirin. Platelet function is restored as the drug is eliminated from the body. NSAIDs should be avoided (if possible) in general surgery patients for 3-5 half-lives of the drug (usually 1-3 days) prior to surgery to reduce the risk of excessive bleeding. However, there is no scientific evidence to warrant discontinuance of NSAIDs prior to dental surgery. In medically complicated patients or extensive oral surgery, the decision to interrupt therapy must be based on the risk to benefit in an individual patient and a medical consult is suggested. Routine interruption of NSAID therapy for most dental procedures is not warranted. If therapy is continued without interruption, the clinician should anticipate the potential for slower clotting times.

Adverse Effects Percentages reported in adult patients; abdominal pain, diarrhea, fever, headache, pyrexia, and vomiting were reported more commonly in pediatric patients

2% to 10%:

Cardiovascular: Edema (≤5%)

Central nervous system: Headache (2% to 8%), pain (1% to 5%), dizziness (≤4%), insomnia (≤4%)

Dermatologic: Pruritus (≤2%), rash (≤3%)
Gastrointestinal: Dyspepsia (4% to 10%), diarrhea (2% to 8%), nausea (2% to 7%), abdominal pain (2% to 5%), constipation (≤3%), flatulence (≤3%), vomiting (≤3%)
Genitourinary: Urinary tract infection (≤7%), micturition (≤2%)
Hematologic: Anemia (≤4%)
Neuromuscular & skeletal: Arthralgia (≤5%), back pain (≤3%)
Respiratory: Upper respiratory infection (≤8%), cough (≤2%), pharyngitis (≤3%)
Miscellaneous: Flu-like syndrome (2% to 6%), falls (≤3%)

Dosage Oral:
Children ≥2 years: Juvenile idiopathic arthritis (JIA): 0.125 mg/kg/day; maximum dose: 7.5 mg/day
Adults: Osteoarthritis, rheumatoid arthritis: Initial: 7.5 mg once daily; some patients may receive additional benefit from increasing dose to 15 mg once daily; maximum dose: 15 mg/day
Elderly: Increased concentrations may occur in elderly patients (particularly in females); however, no specific dosage adjustment is recommended

Dosage adjustment in renal impairment:
Mild-to-moderate impairment: No specific dosage recommendations
Significant impairment (Cl_{cr} ≤20 mL/minute): Patients with severe renal impairment have not been adequately studied; use not recommended.
Hemodialysis: Maximum dose: 7.5 mg/day

Dosage adjustment in hepatic impairment:
Mild (Child-Pugh class A) to moderate (Child-Pugh class B) hepatic dysfunction: No dosage adjustment is necessary
Severe hepatic impairment: Patients with severe hepatic impairment have not been adequately studied

Mechanism of Action Reversibly inhibits cyclooxygenase-1 and 2 (COX-1 and 2) enzymes, which results in decreased formation of prostaglandin precursors; has antipyretic, analgesic, and anti-inflammatory properties

Other proposed mechanisms not fully elucidated (and possibly contributing to the anti-inflammatory effect to varying degrees), include inhibiting chemotaxis, altering lymphocyte activity, inhibiting neutrophil aggregation/activation, and decreasing proinflammatory cytokine levels.

Contraindications Hypersensitivity (eg, asthma, urticaria, allergic-type reactions) to meloxicam, aspirin, other NSAIDs, or any component of the formulation; perioperative pain in the setting of coronary artery bypass graft (CABG) surgery

Warnings/Precautions [U.S. Boxed Warning]: NSAIDs are associated with an increased risk of adverse cardiovascular thrombotic events, including MI and stroke. Risk may be increased with duration of use or pre-existing cardiovascular risk factors or disease. Carefully evaluate individual cardiovascular risk profiles prior to prescribing. May cause new-onset hypertension or worsening of existing hypertension. Use caution with fluid retention. Avoid use in heart failure. Concurrent administration of ibuprofen, and potentially other nonselective NSAIDs, may interfere with aspirin's cardioprotective effect. **[U.S. Boxed Warning]: Use is contraindicated for treatment of perioperative pain in the setting of coronary artery bypass graft (CABG) surgery.** Risk of MI and stroke may be increased with use within the first 10-14 days following CABG surgery.

Platelet adhesion and aggregation may be decreased; may prolong bleeding time; patients with coagulation disorders or who are receiving anticoagulants should be monitored closely. Anemia may occur; patients on long-term NSAID therapy should be monitored for anemia. Rarely, NSAID use may cause severe blood dyscrasias (eg, agranulocytosis, aplastic anemia, thrombocytopenia).

NSAID use may compromise existing renal function; dose-dependent decreases in prostaglandin synthesis may result from NSAID use, reducing renal blood flow which may cause renal decompensation. NSAID use may increase the risk for hyperkalemia. Patients with impaired renal function, dehydration, heart failure, liver dysfunction, those taking diuretics, and ACE inhibitors, and the elderly are at greater risk of renal toxicity and hyperkalemia. Rehydrate patient before starting therapy; monitor renal function closely. Not recommended for use in patients with advanced renal disease. Long-term NSAID use may result in renal papillary necrosis.

[U.S. Boxed Warning]: NSAIDs may increase risk of gastrointestinal irritation, inflammation, ulceration, bleeding, and perforation. These events may occur at any time during therapy and without warning. Use caution with a history of GI disease (bleeding or ulcers), concurrent therapy with aspirin, anticoagulants and/or corticosteroids, smoking, use of alcohol, the elderly or debilitated patients. When used concomitantly with ≤325 mg of aspirin, a substantial increase in the risk of gastrointestinal complications (eg, ulcer) occurs; concomitant gastroprotective therapy (eg, proton pump inhibitors) is recommended (Bhatt, 2008).

Use the lowest effective dose for the shortest duration of time, consistent with individual patient goals, to reduce risk of cardiovascular or GI adverse events. Alternate therapies should be considered for patients at high risk.

NSAIDs may cause serious skin adverse events including exfoliative dermatitis, Stevens-Johnson syndrome (SJS) and toxic epidermal necrolysis (TEN); discontinue use at first sign of skin rash or hypersensitivity. Anaphylactoid reactions may occur, even without prior exposure; patients with "aspirin triad" (bronchial asthma, aspirin intolerance, rhinitis) may be at increased risk. Do not use in patients who experience bronchospasm, asthma, rhinitis, or urticaria with NSAID or aspirin therapy. Use caution in other forms of asthma.

Use with caution in patients with decreased hepatic function. Closely monitor patients with any abnormal LFT. Severe hepatic reactions (eg, fulminant hepatitis, liver failure) have occurred with NSAID use, rarely; discontinue if signs or symptoms of liver disease develop, or if systemic manifestations occur.

NSAIDS may cause drowsiness, dizziness, blurred vision and other neurologic effects which may impair physical or mental abilities; patients must be cautioned about performing tasks which require mental alertness (eg, operating machinery or driving). Discontinue use with blurred or diminished vision and perform ophthalmologic exam. Monitor vision with long-term therapy.

The elderly are at increased risk for adverse effects (especially peptic ulceration, CNS effects, renal toxicity) from NSAIDs even at low doses.

Withhold for at least 4-6 half-lives prior to surgical or dental procedures.

Drug Interactions

Metabolism/Transport Effects Substrate (minor) of CYP2C9, 3A4; **Inhibits** CYP2C9 (weak)

Avoid Concomitant Use

Avoid concomitant use of Meloxicam with any of the following: Ketorolac; Ketorolac (Systemic)

Increased Effect/Toxicity

Meloxicam may increase the levels/effects of: Aminoglycosides; Anticoagulants; Antiplatelet Agents; Bisphosphonate Derivatives; Collagenase (Systemic); CycloSPORINE; CycloSPORINE (Systemic); Deferasirox; Desmopressin; Digoxin; Drotrecogin Alfa; Eplerenone; Haloperidol; Ibritumomab; Lithium; Methotrexate; Nonsteroidal Anti-Inflammatory Agents; PEMEtrexed; Potassium-Sparing Diuretics; PRALAtrexate; Quinolone Antibiotics; Salicylates; Thrombolytic Agents; Tositumomab and Iodine I 131 Tositumomab; Vancomycin; Vitamin K Antagonists

The levels/effects of Meloxicam may be increased by: ACE Inhibitors; Angiotensin II Receptor Blockers; Antidepressants (Tricyclic, Tertiary Amine); Conivaptan; Corticosteroids (Systemic); Dasatinib; Glucosamine; Herbs (Anticoagulant/Antiplatelet Properties); Ketorolac; Ketorolac (Systemic); Nonsteroidal Anti-Inflammatory Agents; Omega-3-Acid Ethyl Esters; Pentosan Polysulfate Sodium; Pentoxifylline; Probenecid; Prostacyclin Analogues; Selective Serotonin Reuptake Inhibitors; Serotonin/Norepinephrine Reuptake Inhibitors; Treprostinil; Voriconazole

Decreased Effect

Meloxicam may decrease the levels/effects of: ACE Inhibitors; Angiotensin II Receptor Blockers; Antiplatelet Agents; Beta-Blockers; Eplerenone; HydrALAZINE; Loop Diuretics; Potassium-Sparing Diuretics; Salicylates; Thiazide Diuretics

The levels/effects of Meloxicam may be decreased by: Bile Acid Sequestrants; Nonsteroidal Anti-Inflammatory Agents; Salicylates; Tocilizumab

Ethanol/Nutrition/Herb Interactions

Ethanol: Avoid ethanol (may enhance gastric mucosal irritation).

Herb/Nutraceutical: Avoid alfalfa, anise, bilberry, bladderwrack, bromelain, cat's claw, celery, chamomile, coleus, cordyceps, dong quai, evening primrose, fenugreek, feverfew, garlic, ginger, ginkgo biloba, ginseng (American, Panax, Siberian), grapeseed, green tea, guggul, horse chestnut seed, horseradish, licorice, prickly ash, red clover, reishi, SAMe (S-adenosylmethionine), sweet clover, turmeric, white willow (all have additional antiplatelet activity).

Dietary Considerations Should be taken with food or milk to minimize gastrointestinal irritation.

Pharmacodynamics/Kinetics

Half-life Elimination Adults: 15-20 hours

Time to Peak Initial: 4-5 hours; Secondary: 12-14 hours

Pregnancy Risk Factor C /D ≥30 weeks gestation

Lactation Excretion in breast milk unknown/not recommended

Breast-Feeding Considerations It is not known whether meloxicam is excreted in human milk. Breast-feeding is not recommended by the manufacturer.

Dosage Forms

Suspension, oral: 7.5 mg/5 mL (100 mL)

Mobic®: 7.5 mg/5 mL (100 mL)

Tablet, oral: 7.5 mg, 15 mg

Mobic®: 7.5 mg, 15 mg

Melphalan (MEL fa lan)

U.S. Brand Names Alkeran®

Canadian Brand Names Alkeran®

Pharmacologic Category Antineoplastic Agent, Alkylating Agent

Use Palliative treatment of multiple myeloma and nonresectable epithelial ovarian carcinoma

Unlabeled/Investigational Use Treatment of Hodgkin's disease, amyloidosis; conditioning regimen for autologous hematopoietic stem cell transplantation in adults with hematologic disorders (eg, multiple myeloma) and autologous marrow or stem cell transplantation in pediatric neuroblastoma and Ewing's sarcoma

Local Anesthetic/Vasoconstrictor Precautions No information available to require special precautions

Effects on Dental Treatment Key adverse event(s) related to dental treatment: Stomatitis.

Effects on Bleeding Chemotherapy may result in significant myelosuppression, potentially including significant reduction in platelet counts and altered hemostasis. In patients who are under active treatment with these agents, medical consult is suggested.

Adverse Effects

>10%:

Gastrointestinal: Nausea/vomiting (oral low-dose: <10%; I.V.: 30% to 90%), oral ulceration

Hematologic: Myelosuppression, leukopenia (nadir: 14-21 days; recovery: 28-35 days), thrombocytopenia (nadir: 14-21 days; recovery: 28-35 days), anemia

Miscellaneous: Secondary malignancy (<2% to 20%; cumulative dose and duration dependent, includes acute myeloid leukemia, myeloproliferative syndrome, carcinoma)

1% to 10%: Miscellaneous: Hypersensitivity (I.V.: 2%; includes bronchospasm, dyspnea, edema, hypotension, pruritus, rash, tachycardia, urticaria)

General Dosage Range Dosage adjustment recommended in patients with renal impairment or who develop toxicities

I.V.: *Adults:* 16 mg/m^2 administered at 2-week intervals for 4 doses, then repeat at 4-week intervals

Oral: *Adults:* Dosage varies greatly depending on indication

Mechanism of Action Alkylating agent which is a derivative of mechlorethamine that inhibits DNA and RNA synthesis via formation of carbonium ions; cross-links strands of DNA; acts on both resting and rapidly dividing tumor cells.

Pharmacodynamics/Kinetics

Half-life Elimination Terminal: I.V.: 75 minutes; Oral: 1-2 hours

Time to Peak Serum: ~1-2 hours

Pregnancy Risk Factor D

Memantine (me MAN teen)

U.S. Brand Names Namenda®

Canadian Brand Names CO Memantine; Ebixa®; PMS-Memantine; ratio-Memantine; Riva-Memantine; Sandoz-Memantine

Pharmacologic Category N-Methyl-D-Aspartate Receptor Antagonist

Use Treatment of moderate-to-severe dementia of the Alzheimer's type

Unlabeled/Investigational Use Treatment of mild-to-moderate vascular dementia

Local Anesthetic/Vasoconstrictor Precautions No information available to require special precautions

Effects on Dental Treatment No significant effects or complications reported

Effects on Bleeding No information available to require special precautions

Adverse Effects 1% to 10%:

Cardiovascular: Hypertension (4%), hypotension (2%), cardiac failure, cerebrovascular accident, syncope, transient ischemic attack

Central nervous system: Dizziness (5% to 7%), confusion (6%), headache (6%), anxiety (4%), depression (3%), hallucinations (3%), pain (3%), somnolence (3%), fatigue (2%), aggressive reaction (1% to 2%), ataxia, vertigo

Dermatologic: Rash

Gastrointestinal: Constipation (3% to 5%), diarrhea (5%), weight gain (3%), vomiting (2% to 3%), abdominal pain (2%), weight loss
Genitourinary: Urinary incontinence (2%), micturition
Hematologic: Anemia
Hepatic: Alkaline phosphatase increased
Neuromuscular & skeletal: Back pain (3%), hypokinesia
Ocular: Cataract, conjunctivitis
Respiratory: Cough (4%), dyspnea (2%), pneumonia
Miscellaneous: Influenza (4%)

General Dosage Range Dosage adjustment recommended in patients with renal impairment

Oral: *Adults:* Immediate release: Initial: 5 mg once daily; Target: 20 mg/day in 2 divided doses; Extended release: Initial 7 mg once daily; Target: 28 mg/day

Mechanism of Action Glutamate, the primary excitatory amino acid in the CNS, may contribute to the pathogenesis of Alzheimer's disease (AD) by overstimulating various glutamate receptors leading to excitotoxicity and neuronal cell death. Memantine is an uncompetitive antagonist of the N-methyl-D-aspartate (NMDA) type of glutamate receptors, located ubiquitously throughout the brain. Under normal physiologic conditions, the (unstimulated) NMDA receptor ion channel is blocked by magnesium ions, which are displaced after agonist-induced depolarization. Pathologic or excessive receptor activation, as postulated to occur during AD, prevents magnesium from reentering and blocking the channel pore resulting in a chronically open state and excessive calcium influx. Memantine binds to the intra-pore magnesium site, but with longer dwell time, and thus functions as an effective receptor blocker only under conditions of excessive stimulation; memantine does not affect normal neurotransmission.

Pharmacodynamics/Kinetics

Half-life Elimination Terminal: ~60-80 hours; severe renal impairment (Cl_{cr} 5-29 mL/minute): 117-156 hours

Time to Peak Serum: Immediate release: 3-7 hours; Extended release: 9-12 hours

Pregnancy Risk Factor B

Product Availability

Namenda XR™: FDA approved in June 2010; anticipated availability is currently undetermined

Namenda XR™ is an extended release capsule (once-daily administration) approved for the treatment of moderate-to-severe dementia associated with Alzheimer's disease

Meningococcal (Groups A / C / Y and W-135) Diphtheria Conjugate Vaccine

(me NIN joe kok al groops aye, see, why & dubl yoo won thur tee fyve dif THEER ee a KON joo gate vak SEEN)

U.S. Brand Names Menactra®; Menveo®

Canadian Brand Names Menactra®; Menveo®

Pharmacologic Category Vaccine, Inactivated (Bacterial)

Use Provide active immunization of children and adults against invasive meningococcal disease caused by *N. meningitidis* serogroups A, C, Y, and W-135.

The Advisory Committee on Immunization Practices (ACIP) recommends routine vaccination of all persons at age 11 or 12 years of age, followed by a booster at age 16 years of age (CDC, 60[3], 2011).

The ACIP also recommends vaccination for persons 2 through 55 years of age at increased risk for meningococcal disease (CDC, 60[3], 2011). Meningococcal conjugate vaccine (MCV4) is preferred for persons aged 2-55 years; meningococcal polysaccharide vaccine (MPSV4) is preferred in adults ≥56 years of age (CDC, 2005).

Persons at increased risk include:

- Previously unvaccinated college freshmen living in dormitories
- Microbiologists routinely exposed to isolates of *N. meningitidis*
- Military recruits
- Persons traveling to or who reside in countries where *N. meningitidis* is hyperendemic or epidemic, particularly if contact with local population will be prolonged
- Persons with persistent complement component deficiencies (eg, C5-C9, properidin, factor H, or factor D)
- Persons with anatomic or functional asplenia
- Persons with HIV infection

Use is also recommended during meningococcal outbreaks caused by vaccine preventable serogroups.

Local Anesthetic/Vasoconstrictor Precautions No information available to require special precautions

Effects on Dental Treatment No significant effects or complications reported

Effects on Bleeding No information available to require special precautions

Adverse Effects All serious adverse reactions must be reported to the U.S. Department of Health and Human Services (DHHS) Vaccine Adverse Event Reporting System (VAERS) 1-800-822-7967 or online at https://vaers.hhs.gov/esub/index. In Canada, adverse reactions may be reported to local provincial/territorial health agencies or to the Vaccine Safety Section at Public Health Agency of Canada (1-866-844-0018).

Actual percentages may vary by product and age group:

>10%:

Central nervous system: Crying (abnormal), drowsiness, fatigue, fever, headache, irritability, malaise, sleepiness

Gastrointestinal: Anorexia, diarrhea, nausea, vomiting

Local: Injection site: Erythema, induration, pain, redness, swelling, tenderness

Neuromuscular & skeletal: Arthralgia, myalgia

1% to 10%:

Central nervous system: Chills

Dermatologic: Rash

Gastrointestinal: Eating changes

General Dosage Range I.M.:

Children 9-23 months (Menactra®):0.5 mL/dose given as a 2-dose series, 3 months apart

Children ≥2 years and Adults ≤55 years: 0.5 mL as a single dose

Mechanism of Action Induces immunity against meningococcal disease via the formation of bactericidal antibodies directed toward the polysaccharide capsular components of *Neisseria meningitidis* serogroups A, C, Y and W-135.

Pregnancy Risk Factor B/C (manufacturer dependent)

Meningococcal Polysaccharide Vaccine (Groups A, C, Y, and W-135)

(me NIN joe kok al pol i SAK a ride vak SEEN groops aye, see, why & dubl yoo won thur tee fyve)

U.S. Brand Names Menomune®-A/C/Y/W-135

Canadian Brand Names Menomune®-A/C/Y/W-135

Pharmacologic Category Vaccine, Inactivated (Bacterial)

Use Provide active immunity to meningococcal serogroups contained in the vaccine

The Advisory Committee on Immunization Practices (ACIP) recommends routine vaccination for persons at increased risk for meningococcal disease. Meningococcal conjugate vaccine (MCV4) is preferred for persons aged 2-55 years; meningococcal polysaccharide vaccine (MPSV4) is preferred in adults ≥56 years of age (CDC, 2005).

Persons at increased risk include:

- Previously unvaccinated college freshmen living in dormitories
- Microbiologists routinely exposed to isolates of *N. meningitidis*
- Military recruits
- Persons traveling to or who reside in countries where *N. meningitidis* is hyperendemic or epidemic, particularly if contact with local population will be prolonged
- Persons with persistent complement component deficiencies (eg, C5-C9, properidin, factor H, or factor D)
- Persons with anatomic or functional asplenia
- Persons with HIV infection

Use is also recommended during meningococcal outbreaks caused by vaccine preventable serogroups.

Local Anesthetic/Vasoconstrictor Precautions No information available to require special precautions

Effects on Dental Treatment No significant effects or complications reported

Effects on Bleeding No information available to require special precautions

Adverse Effects All serious adverse reactions must be reported to the U.S. Department of Health and Human Services (DHHS) Vaccine Adverse Event Reporting System (VAERS) 1-800-822-7967 or online at https://vaers.hhs.gov/esub/index. In Canada, adverse reactions may be reported to local provincial/territorial health agencies or to the Vaccine Safety Section at Public Health Agency of Canada (1-866-844-0018).

>10%:

Central nervous system: Headache (29% to 42%), fatigue (25% to 32%), malaise (17% to 22%), irritability (12%), drowsiness (11%)

Gastrointestinal: Diarrhea (10% to 14%)

Local: Injection site: Pain (26% to 48%), redness (6% to 16%), induration (4% to 11%)

Neuromuscular & skeletal: Arthralgia (5% to 16%)

1% to 10%:

Central nervous system: Chills (4% to 6%), fever (≤5%)
Dermatologic: Rash (≤3%)
Gastrointestinal: Anorexia (8% to 10%), vomiting (1% to 3%)
Local: Injection site: Swelling (3% to 8%)

General Dosage Range SubQ: *Children ≥2 years and Adults:* 0.5 mL as a single dose

Mechanism of Action Induces the formation of bactericidal antibodies to meningococcal antigens; the presence of these antibodies is strongly correlated with immunity to meningococcal disease caused by *Neisseria meningitidis* groups A, C, Y and W-135.

Pharmacodynamics/Kinetics

Onset of Action Antibody levels: 7-10 days

Duration of Action Antibodies against group A and C polysaccharides decline markedly (to prevaccination levels) over the first 3 years following a single dose of vaccine, especially in children <4 years of age

Pregnancy Risk Factor C

Menotropins (men oh TROE pins)

U.S. Brand Names Menopur®; Repronex®

Canadian Brand Names Menopur®; Repronex®

Pharmacologic Category Gonadotropin; Ovulation Stimulator

Use Female:

In conjunction with hCG to induce ovulation and pregnancy in infertile females experiencing oligoanovulation or anovulation when the cause of anovulation is functional and not caused by primary ovarian failure (Repronex®)

Stimulation of multiple follicle development in ovulatory patients as part of an assisted reproductive technology (ART) (Menopur®, Repronex®)

Unlabeled/Investigational Use Male: Stimulation of spermatogenesis in primary or secondary hypogonadotropic hypogonadism

Local Anesthetic/Vasoconstrictor Precautions No information available to require special precautions

Effects on Dental Treatment No significant effects or complications reported

Effects on Bleeding Has been associated with thrombotic events; however, no information available to require special precautions in dental procedures.

Adverse Effects Adverse effects may vary according to specific product, route, and/or dosage.

>10%:

Central nervous system: Headache (up to 34%)
Gastrointestinal: Abdominal pain (up to 18%), nausea (up to 12%)
Genitourinary: OHSS (up to 13%, dose related)
Local: Injection site reaction (4% to 12%)

1% to 10%:

Cardiovascular: Flushing
Central nervous system: Dizziness, malaise, migraine
Endocrine & metabolic: Breast tenderness, hot flashes, menstrual irregularities
Gastrointestinal: Abdominal cramping, abdominal fullness, constipation, diarrhea, enlarged abdomen, vomiting
Genitourinary: Ectopic pregnancy, ovarian disease, vaginal hemorrhage
Local: Injection site edema/pain
Neuromuscular & skeletal: Back pain
Respiratory: Cough increased, respiratory disorder
Miscellaneous: Infection, flu-like syndrome

Frequency not defined:

Cardiovascular: Stroke, tachycardia, thrombosis (venous or arterial)
Dermatologic: Angioedema, rash, urticaria
Genitourinary: Adnexal torsion, hemoperitoneum, ovarian enlargement
Neuromuscular & skeletal: Limb necrosis
Respiratory: Acute respiratory distress syndrome, atelectasis, dyspnea, embolism, laryngeal edema, pulmonary infarction, tachypnea
Miscellaneous: Allergic reaction, anaphylaxis

General Dosage Range

I.M.: *Adults:* Repronex®: Initial: 150 int. units **or** 225 int. units daily (maximum: 450 int. units/day; 12 days of therapy)

SubQ: *Adults:* Menopur®: Initial: 225 int. units daily (maximum: 450 int. units/day; 20 days of therapy); Repronex®: Initial: 150 int. units **or** 225 int. units daily (maximum: 450 int. units/day; 12 days of therapy)

Mechanism of Action Actions occur as a result of both follicle stimulating hormone (FSH) effects and luteinizing hormone (LH) effects; menotropins stimulate the development and maturation of the ovarian follicle (FSH), cause ovulation (LH), and stimulate the development of the corpus luteum (LH); in males it stimulates spermatogenesis (LH)

Pregnancy Risk Factor X

Menthol and Zinc Oxide (Topical) (MEN thole & zink OKS ide)

U.S. Brand Names Calmoseptine® [OTC]; Risamine™ [OTC]

Pharmacologic Category Protectant, Topical; Topical Skin Product

Use Provides a barrier to protect intact and/or injured skin from moisture, wound or fistula drainage, urine, or feces; diaper rash

Local Anesthetic/Vasoconstrictor Precautions No information available to require special precautions

Effects on Dental Treatment No significant effects or complications reported

Effects on Bleeding No information available to require special precautions

Adverse Effects Frequency not defined.

Dermatologic: Pruritus, rash, stinging (temporarily on application)

Miscellaneous: Hypersensitivity reactions

General Dosage Range Topical: *Children and Adults:* Apply thin layer 2-4 times/day or after each incontinent episode/diaper change

Mepenzolate (me PEN zoe late)

U.S. Brand Names Cantil®

Canadian Brand Names Cantil®

Pharmacologic Category Anticholinergic Agent; Antispasmodic Agent, Gastrointestinal

Use Adjunctive treatment of peptic ulcer disease

Local Anesthetic/Vasoconstrictor Precautions No information available to require special precautions

Effects on Dental Treatment Key adverse event(s) related to dental treatment: Xerostomia (normal salivary flow resumes upon discontinuation), dry throat, dysphagia, and loss of taste.

Effects on Bleeding No information available to require special precautions

Adverse Effects Frequency not defined.

Cardiovascular: Palpitation, tachycardia

Central nervous system: Headache, nervousness, drowsiness, dizziness, CNS stimulation may be produced with large doses, confusion, insomnia

Dermatologic: Dry skin, urticaria

Gastrointestinal: Constipation, xerostomia, dysphagia, nausea, vomiting, delayed gastric emptying, loss of taste

Genitourinary: Impotence, urinary hesitation, urinary retention

Neuromuscular & skeletal: Weakness

Ophthalmic: Cycloplegia, blurred vision, ocular tension increased, pupil dilation

Miscellaneous: Diaphoresis decreased, hypersensitivity reactions, anaphylaxis, lactation suppressed

General Dosage Range Oral: *Adults:* 25-50 mg 4 times/day

Mechanism of Action Mepenzolate is a postganglionic parasympathetic inhibitor. It decreases gastric acid and pepsin secretion and suppresses spontaneous contractions of the colon.

Pregnancy Risk Factor B

Meperidine (me PER i deen)

Related Information

Management of the Patient With Anxiety or Depression *on page 1968*

Oral Pain *on page 1928*

Related Sample Prescriptions

Severe Oral Pain *on page 1980*

U.S. Brand Names Demerol®

Canadian Brand Names Demerol®

Generic Availability (U.S.) Yes

Pharmacologic Category Analgesic, Opioid

Dental Use Adjunct in preoperative intravenous conscious sedation in patients undergoing dental surgery; alternate oral narcotic in patients allergic to codeine to treat moderate to moderate-severe pain

Use Management of moderate-to-severe pain; adjunct to anesthesia and preoperative sedation

Unlabeled/Investigational Use Reduce postoperative shivering; reduce rigors from amphotericin B (conventional)

Local Anesthetic/Vasoconstrictor Precautions No information available to require special precautions

Effects on Dental Treatment Key adverse event(s) related to dental treatment: Xerostomia (normal salivary flow resumes upon discontinuation). See Dental Comment.

Effects on Bleeding No information available to require special precautions

Adverse Effects Frequency not defined.

Cardiovascular: Hypotension

Central nervous system: Fatigue, drowsiness, dizziness, nervousness, headache, restlessness, malaise, confusion, mental depression, hallucinations, paradoxical CNS stimulation, increased intracranial pressure, seizure (associated with metabolite accumulation), serotonin syndrome

Dermatologic: Rash, urticaria

Gastrointestinal: Nausea, vomiting, constipation, anorexia, stomach cramps, xerostomia, biliary spasm, paralytic ileus, sphincter of Oddi spasm

Genitourinary: Ureteral spasms, decreased urination

Local: Pain at injection site

Neuromuscular & skeletal: Weakness

Respiratory: Dyspnea

Miscellaneous: Anaphylaxis, histamine release, hypersensitivity reactions, physical and psychological dependence

Dental Usual Dosage Pain (analgesic): Adults: Oral: Initial: Opiate-naive: 50 mg every 3-4 hours as needed; usual dosage range: 50-150 mg every 2-4 hours as needed (manufacturers recommendation; oral route is not recommended for acute pain)

Dosage Note: The American Pain Society (2008) and ISMP (2007) do not recommend meperidine's use as an analgesic.

Children: Pain: Oral, I.M., I.V., SubQ: 1-1.5 mg/kg/dose every 3-4 hours as needed; 1-2 mg/kg as a single dose preoperative medication may be used; maximum: 100 mg/dose (**Note:** Oral route is not recommended for acute pain.)

Adults: Pain:

Oral: Initial: Opiate-naive: 50 mg every 3-4 hours as needed; usual dosage range: 50-150 mg every 2-4 hours as needed (manufacturers recommendation; oral route is not recommended for acute pain)

I.M., SubQ: Initial: Opiate-naive: 50-75 mg every 3-4 hours as needed; patients with prior opiate exposure may require higher initial doses

Slow I.V.: Initial: 5-10 mg every 5 minutes as needed

Preoperatively: 50-100 mg given 30-90 minutes before the beginning of anesthesia

Postoperative shivering (unlabeled use): 25-50 mg once (Crowley, 2008; Kranke, 2002; Mercandante, 1994; Wang, 1999)

Note: If use in acute pain (in patients without renal or CNS disease) cannot be avoided, treatment should be limited to ≤48 hours and doses should not exceed 600 mg/24 hours.

Elderly:

Oral: 50 mg every 4 hours

I.M.: 25 mg every 4 hours

Dosing adjustment in renal impairment: Avoid use in renal impairment

Dosing adjustment/comments in hepatic disease: Increased narcotic effect in cirrhosis; reduction in dose more important for oral than I.V. route

Mechanism of Action Binds to opiate receptors in the CNS, causing inhibition of ascending pain pathways, altering the perception of and response to pain; produces generalized CNS depression

Contraindications Hypersensitivity to meperidine or any component of the formulation; use with or within 14 days of MAO inhibitors; pregnancy (prolonged use or high doses near term)

Warnings/Precautions Oral meperidine is not recommended for acute/chronic pain management. Meperidine should not be used for acute/cancer pain because of the risk of neurotoxicity. Normeperidine (an active metabolite and CNS stimulant) may accumulate and precipitate anxiety, tremors, or seizures; risk increases with CNS or renal dysfunction, prolonged use (>48 hours), and cumulative dose (>600 mg/24 hours). The Institute for Safe Medication Practice recommends avoiding the use of meperidine for pain control, especially in the elderly and renally-impaired (ISMP, 2007). In the elderly; meperidine is not an effective oral analgesic at commonly used doses; may cause confusion; other opioids are preferred in the elderly (Beers Criteria).

May cause CNS depression, which may impair physical or mental abilities; patients must be cautioned about performing tasks which require mental alertness (eg, operating machinery or driving). Effects may be potentiated when used with other sedative drugs or ethanol. Use only with extreme caution (if at all) in patients with head injury or increased intracranial pressure (ICP). Use caution with pulmonary, hepatic, or renal disorders, supraventricular tachycardias, acute abdominal conditions, hypothyroidism, toxic psychosis, kyphoscoliosis, morbid obesity, Addison's disease, BPH, or urethral stricture. Use with caution in patients with biliary tract dysfunction; acute pancreatitis may cause constriction of sphincter of Oddi. May cause hypotension; use with caution in patients with depleted blood volume or drugs which may exaggerate hypotensive effects (including phenothiazines or general anesthetics).

An opioid-containing analgesic regimen should be tailored to each patient's needs and based upon the type of pain being treated (acute versus chronic), the route of administration, degree of tolerance for opioids (naive versus chronic user), age, weight, and medical condition. The optimal analgesic dose varies widely among patients. Some preparations contain sulfites which may cause allergic reaction. Tolerance or drug dependence may result from extended use. Healthcare provider should be alert to problems of abuse, misuse, and diversion. Concurrent use of agonist/antagonist analgesics may precipitate withdrawal symptoms and/or reduced analgesic efficacy in patients following prolonged therapy with mu opioid agonists. Abrupt discontinuation following prolonged use may also lead to withdrawal symptoms. Avoid use in the elderly.

Drug Interactions

Metabolism/Transport Effects Substrate (minor) of CYP2B6, 2C19, 3A4

Avoid Concomitant Use

Avoid concomitant use of Meperidine with any of the following: MAO Inhibitors; Sibutramine

Increased Effect/Toxicity

Meperidine may increase the levels/effects of: Alcohol (Ethyl); Alvimopan; CNS Depressants; Desmopressin; Selective Serotonin Reuptake Inhibitors; Serotonin Modulators; Thiazide Diuretics

The levels/effects of Meperidine may be increased by: Amphetamines; Antipsychotic Agents (Phenothiazines); Barbiturates; Droperidol; MAO Inhibitors; Protease Inhibitors; Sibutramine; Succinylcholine

Decreased Effect

Meperidine may decrease the levels/effects of: Pegvisomant

The levels/effects of Meperidine may be decreased by: Ammonium Chloride; Fosphenytoin; Mixed Agonist / Antagonist Opioids; Phenytoin; Protease Inhibitors

Ethanol/Nutrition/Herb Interactions

Ethanol: May increase CNS depression; monitor for increased effects with coadministration. Caution patients about effects.

Herb/Nutraceutical: Avoid valerian, St John's wort, kava kava, gotu kola (may increase CNS depression).

Pharmacodynamics/Kinetics

Onset of Action Onset of action: Analgesic: Oral, SubQ: 10-15 minutes; I.V.: ~5 minutes. Peak effect: SubQ.: ~1 hour; Oral: 2 hours

Duration of Action Oral, SubQ.: 2-4 hours

Half-life Elimination

Parent drug: Terminal phase: Adults: 2.5-4 hours, Liver disease: 7-11 hours

Normeperidine (active metabolite): 15-30 hours; can accumulate with high doses (>600 mg/day) or renal impairment

Pregnancy Risk Factor C

Lactation Enters breast milk/not recommended (AAP rates "compatible"; AAP 2001 update pending)

Breast-Feeding Considerations Meperidine is excreted in breast milk and may cause CNS and/or respiratory depression in the nursing infant.

Controlled Substance C-II

Dosage Forms

Injection, solution: 10 mg/mL (30 mL, 50 mL, 60 mL); 25 mg/mL (1 mL); 50 mg/mL (1 mL); 100 mg/mL (1 mL)

Demerol®: 25 mg/mL (1 mL); 25 mg/0.5 mL (0.5 mL); 50 mg/mL (1 mL, 1.5 mL, 2 mL, 30 mL); 75 mg/mL (1 mL); 100 mg/mL (1 mL, 20 mL)

Solution, oral: 50 mg/5 mL (500 mL)

Tablet, oral: 50 mg, 100 mg

Demerol®: 50 mg, 100 mg

Dental Comment Meperidine is not to be used as the narcotic drug of first choice. It is recommended only to be used in codeine-allergic patients when a narcotic analgesic is indicated. Meperidine is not an anti-inflammatory agent. Meperidine, as with other narcotic analgesics, is recommended only for limited acute dosing (ie, 3 days or less); common adverse effects in the dental patient are nausea, sedation, and constipation. Meperidine has a significant addiction liability, especially when given long-term.

Mephobarbital (me foe BAR bi tal)

U.S. Brand Names Mebaral® [DSC]
Canadian Brand Names Mebaral®
Pharmacologic Category Barbiturate
Use Sedative; treatment of grand mal and petit mal epilepsy
Local Anesthetic/Vasoconstrictor Precautions No information available to require special precautions
Effects on Dental Treatment No significant effects or complications reported
Effects on Bleeding No information available to require special precautions
Adverse Effects >1%: Central nervous system: Somnolence
General Dosage Range Dosage adjustment recommended in patients with hepatic or renal impairment and on concomitant therapy.

Oral:

*Children <5 years:*16-32 mg 3-4 times/day
Children >5 years: 16-64 mg 3-4 times/day
Adults: 96-600 mg/day in 2-4 divided doses

Mechanism of Action Increases seizure threshold in the motor cortex; depresses monosynaptic and polysynaptic transmission in the CNS
Pharmacodynamics/Kinetics

Onset of Action 20-60 minutes
Duration of Action 6-8 hours
Half-life Elimination Serum: 34 hours

Pregnancy Risk Factor D
Controlled Substance C-IV

Mepivacaine (me PIV a kane)

U.S. Brand Names Carbocaine®; Polocaine®; Polocaine® Dental; Polocaine® MPF; Scandonest® 3% Plain
Canadian Brand Names Carbocaine®; Polocaine®
Generic Availability (U.S.) No
Pharmacologic Category Local Anesthetic
Dental Use Local anesthesia by nerve block, infiltration in dental procedures
Use Local or regional analgesia; anesthesia by local infiltration, peripheral and central neural techniques (epidural and caudal); **not** for use in spinal anesthesia
Local Anesthetic/Vasoconstrictor Precautions No information available to require special precautions
Effects on Dental Treatment Key adverse event(s) related to dental treatment: Degree of adverse effects in the CNS and cardiovascular system is directly related to blood levels of mepivacaine (frequency not defined; more likely to occur after systemic administration rather than infiltration): Bradycardia, cardiovascular collapse, hypotension, myocardial depression, ventricular arrhythmias, nausea, vomiting, respiratory arrest, anaphylactoid reactions, blurred vision, heart block, transient stinging or burning at injection site

High blood levels: Anxiety, restlessness, disorientation, confusion, dizziness, and seizures, followed by CNS depression resulting in somnolence, unconsciousness, and possible respiratory arrest.

In some cases, symptoms of CNS stimulation may be absent and the primary CNS effects are somnolence and unconsciousness.

Effects on Bleeding No information available to require special precautions
Adverse Effects Degree of adverse effects in the CNS and cardiovascular system is directly related to the blood levels of mepivacaine, route of administration, and physical status of the patient. The effects below are more likely to occur after systemic administration rather than infiltration.

Cardiovascular: Bradycardia, cardiac arrest, cardiac output decreased, heart block, hyper-/hypotension, myocardial depression, syncope, tachycardia, ventricular arrhythmias

Central nervous system: Anxiety, chills, convulsions, depression, dizziness, excitation, restlessness, tremors

Dermatologic: Angioneurotic edema, diaphoresis, erythema, pruritus, urticaria
Gastrointestinal: Fecal incontinence, nausea, vomiting
Genitourinary: Incontinence, urinary retention
Neuromuscular & skeletal: Chondrolysis (continuous intra-articular administration), paralysis
Ocular: Blurred vision, pupil constriction
Otic: Tinnitus
Respiratory: Apnea, hypoventilation, sneezing
Miscellaneous: Allergic reaction, anaphylactoid reaction

Dental Usual Dosage

Injectable local anesthetic: Children and Adults: Dose varies with procedure, degree of anesthesia needed, vascularity of tissue, duration of anesthesia required, and physical condition of patient. The smallest dose and concentration required to produce the desired effect should be used.

Children: Maximum dose: 5-6 mg/kg; only concentrations <2% should be used in children <3 years or <14 kg (30 lbs)

Adults: Dental anesthesia:

Single site in upper or lower jaw: 54 mg (1.8 mL) as a 3% solution

Infiltration and nerve block of entire oral cavity: 270 mg (9 mL) as a 3% solution. Manufacturer's maximum recommended dose is not more than 400 mg to normal healthy adults.

Dosage

Injectable local anesthetic: Dose varies with procedure, degree of anesthesia needed, vascularity of tissue, duration of anesthesia required, and physical condition of patient. The smallest dose and concentration required to produce the desired effect should be used.

Children: Maximum dose: 5-6 mg/kg; only concentrations <2% should be used in children <3 years or <14 kg (30 lbs)

Adults: Maximum dose: 400 mg; do not exceed 1000 mg/24 hours

Cervical, brachial, intercostal, pudendal nerve block: 5-40 mL of a 1% solution (maximum: 400 mg) **or** 5-20 mL of a 2% solution (maximum: 400 mg). For pudenal block, inject 1/2 the total dose each side.

Transvaginal block (paracervical plus pudenal): Up to 30 mL (both sides) of a 1% solution (maximum: 300 mg). Inject 1/2 the total dose each side.

Paracervical block: Up to 20 mL (both sides) of a 1% solution (maximum: 200 mg). Inject 1/2 the total dose to each side. This is the maximum recommended dose per 90-minute procedure; inject slowly with 5 minutes between sides.

Caudal and epidural block (preservative free solutions only): 15-30 mL of a 1% solution (maximum: 300 mg) **or** 10-25 mL of a 1.5% solution (maximum: 375 mg) **or** 10-20 mL of a 2% solution (maximum: 400 mg)

Infiltration: Up to 40 mL of a 1% solution (maximum: 400 mg)

Therapeutic block (pain management): 1-5 mL of a 1% solution (maximum: 50 mg) **or** 1-5 mL of a 2% solution (maximum: 100 mg)

Dental anesthesia: Adults:

Single site in upper or lower jaw: 54 mg (1.8 mL) as a 3% solution

Infiltration and nerve block of entire oral cavity: 270 mg (9 mL) as a 3% solution. Manufacturer's maximum recommended dose is not more than 400 mg to normal healthy adults.

Mechanism of Action Mepivacaine is an amide local anesthetic similar to lidocaine; like all local anesthetics, mepivacaine acts by preventing the generation and conduction of nerve impulses

Contraindications Hypersensitivity to mepivacaine, other amide-type local anesthetics, or any component of the formulation

Warnings/Precautions Careful and constant monitoring of the patient's state of consciousness should be done following each local anesthetic injection; at such times, restlessness, anxiety, tinnitus, dizziness, blurred vision, tremors, depression, or drowsiness may be early warning signs of CNS toxicity; treatment is primarily symptomatic and supportive. Continuous intra-articular infusion of local anesthetics after arthroscopic or other surgical procedures is **not** an approved use; chondrolysis (primarily in the shoulder joint) has occurred following infusion, with some cases requiring arthroplasty or shoulder replacement. Use with caution in patients with cardiac disease, hepatic or renal disease, or hyperthyroidism. Local anesthetics have been associated with rare occurrences of sudden respiratory arrest; convulsions due to systemic toxicity leading to cardiac arrest have been reported presumably due to intravascular injection. A test dose is recommended prior to epidural administration and all reinforcing doses with continuous catheter technique. Do not use solutions containing preservatives for caudal or epidural block. Use caution in debilitated, elderly, or acutely-ill patients; dose reduction may be required. Resuscitative equipment, oxygen, and other resuscitative drugs should be available for immediate use.

Drug Interactions

Avoid Concomitant Use There are no known interactions where it is recommended to avoid concomitant use.

Increased Effect/Toxicity

The levels/effects of Mepivacaine may be increased by: Beta-Blockers

Decreased Effect There are no known significant interactions involving a decrease in effect.

Pharmacodynamics/Kinetics

Onset of Action Route and dose dependent: Range: 3-20 minute

Duration of Action Route and dose dependent: 2-2.5 hours

Half-life Elimination Neonates: 8.7-9 hours; Adults: 1.9-3 hours

Pregnancy Risk Factor C

Lactation Excretion in breast milk unknown/use caution

Dosage Forms

Injection, solution: 3% [30 mg/mL] (1.8 mL)

Carbocaine®: 1% [10 mg/mL] (50 mL); 2% [20 mg/mL] (50 mL); 3% [30 mg/mL] (1.7 mL)

Polocaine®: 1% [10 mg/mL] (50 mL); 2% [20 mg/mL] (50 mL); 1% (10 mg/mL) (50 mL)

Polocaine® Dental: 3% [30 mg/mL] (1.7 mL)

Polocaine® MPF: 2% (20 mg/mL) (20 mL)

Scandonest® 3% Plain: 3% [30 mg/mL] (1.7 mL)

Injection, solution [preservative free]:

Carbocaine®: 1% [10 mg/mL] (30 mL); 1.5% [15 mg/mL] (30 mL); 2% [20 mg/mL] (20 mL)

Polocaine® MPF: 1% [10 mg/mL] (30 mL); 1.5% [15 mg/mL] (30 mL); 2% [20 mg/mL] (20 mL)

Mepivacaine (Dental Anesthetic) (me PIV a kane, DEN tl)

Related Information

Mepivacaine *on page* 1076

Oral Pain *on page* 1928

U.S. Brand Names Carbocaine®; Polocaine® Dental; Scandonest® 3% Plain

Canadian Brand Names Polocaine®

Generic Availability (U.S.) Yes

Pharmacologic Category Local Anesthetic

Dental Use Amide-type anesthetic used for local infiltration anesthesia; injection near nerve trunks to produce nerve block

Local Anesthetic/Vasoconstrictor Precautions No information available to require special precautions

Effects on Dental Treatment It is common to misinterpret psychogenic responses to local anesthetic injection as an allergic reaction. Intraoral injections are perceived by many patients as a stressful procedure in dentistry. Common symptoms to this stress are diaphoresis, palpitations, hyperventilation, generalized pallor, and a fainting feeling.

Degree of adverse effects in the CNS and cardiovascular system is directly related to the blood levels of mepivacaine.

Frequency not defined: Bradycardia and reduction in cardiac output, nausea, vomiting, tremors, asthmatic syndromes, hypersensitivity reactions (may manifest as dermatologic reactions and edema at injection site)

High blood levels: Anxiety, restlessness, disorientation, confusion, dizziness, tremors and seizures, followed by CNS depression resulting in somnolence, unconsciousness and possible respiratory arrest. In some cases, symptoms of CNS stimulation may be absent and the primary CNS effects are somnolence and unconsciousness.

Effects on Bleeding No information available to require special precautions

Adverse Effects Degree of adverse effects in the CNS and cardiovascular system are directly related to the blood levels of local anesthetic.

Cardiovascular: Myocardial effects include a decrease in contraction force as well as a decrease in electrical excitability and myocardial conduction rate resulting in bradycardia and reduction in cardiac output

Central nervous system: High blood levels result in anxiety, restlessness, disorientation, confusion, dizziness, and seizure. This is followed by depression of CNS resulting in somnolence, unconsciousness and possible respiratory arrest. In some cases, symptoms of CNS stimulation may be absent and the primary CNS effects are somnolence and unconsciousness.

Gastrointestinal: Nausea and vomiting may occur

Hypersensitivity reactions: May manifest as dermatologic reactions and edema at injection site. Asthmatic syndromes have occurred.

Neuromuscular & skeletal: Tremors

Psychogenic reactions: It is common to misinterpret psychogenic responses to local anesthetic injection as an allergic reaction. Intraoral injection is perceived by many patients as a stressful procedure in dentistry. Common symptoms to this stress are diaphoresis, palpitation, hyperventilation, generalized pallor and a fainting feeling.

Dental Usual Dosage

Children <10 years: Up to 5-6 mg/kg of body weight; maximum pediatric dosage must be carefully calculated on the basis of patient's weight but must not exceed 270 mg (9 mL) of the 3% solution

Children >10 years and Adults:

Dental anesthesia, single site in upper or lower jaw: 54 mg (1.8 mL) as a 3% solution

Infiltration and nerve block of entire oral cavity: 270 mg (9 mL) as a 3% solution; up to a maximum of 6.6 mg/kg of body weight but not to exceed 300 mg per appointment. Manufacturer's maximum recommended dose is not more than 400 mg to normal healthy adults. The effective anesthetic dose varies with procedure, intensity of anesthesia needed, duration of anesthesia required, and physical condition of the patient. Always use the lowest effective dose along with careful aspiration.

The following number of dental carpules (1.8 mL) provide the indicated amounts of mepivacaine dental anesthetic 3%. See table.

# of Cartridges (1.8 mL)	mg Mepivacaine (3%)
1	54
2	108
3	162
4	216
5	270
6	324
7	378
8	432

Note: Adult and children doses of mepivacaine dental anesthetic cited from USP Dispensing Information (USP DI), 17th ed, The United States Pharmacopeial Convention, Inc, Rockville, MD, 1997, 138-9.

Dosage

Children <10 years: Up to 5-6 mg/kg of body weight; maximum pediatric dosage must be carefully calculated on the basis of patient's weight but must not exceed 270 mg (9 mL) of the 3% solution

Children >10 years and Adults:

Dental anesthesia, single site in upper or lower jaw: 54 mg (1.8 mL) as a 3% solution

Infiltration and nerve block of entire oral cavity: 270 mg (9 mL) as a 3% solution; up to a maximum of 6.6 mg/kg of body weight but not to exceed 300 mg per appointment. Manufacturer's maximum recommended dose is not more than 400 mg to normal healthy adults. The effective anesthetic dose varies with procedure, intensity of anesthesia needed, duration of anesthesia required, and physical condition of the patient. Always use the lowest effective dose along with careful aspiration.

Note: Adult and children doses of mepivacaine dental anesthetic cited from USP Dispensing Information (USP DI), 17th ed, The United States Pharmacopeial Convention, Inc, Rockville, MD, 1997, 138-9.

Mechanism of Action Local anesthetics bind selectively to the intracellular surface of sodium channels to block influx of sodium into the axon. As a result, depolarization necessary for action potential propagation and subsequent nerve function is prevented. The block at the sodium channel is reversible. When drug diffuses away from the axon, sodium channel function is restored and nerve propagation returns.

Contraindications Hypersensitivity to local anesthetics of the amide type or any component of the formulation

Warnings/Precautions Aspirate the syringe after tissue penetration and before injection to minimize chance of direct vascular injection

Pharmacodynamics/Kinetics

Onset of Action Upper jaw: 30-120 seconds; Lower jaw: 1-4 minutes

Duration of Action Upper jaw: 20 minutes; Lower jaw: 40 minutes

Half-life Elimination Serum: 1.9 hours

Pregnancy Risk Factor C

Breast-Feeding Considerations Usual infiltration doses of mepivacaine dental anesthetic given to nursing mothers has not been shown to affect the health of the nursing infant.

Dosage Forms

Injection, solution: 3% (1.8 mL)

Carbocaine®, Polocaine® Dental, Scandonest® 3% Plain: 3% (1.7 mL)

Dental Comment Oral paresthesia: The occurrence of oral paresthesia associated with 4% solutions of prilocaine or articaine, although rare, continue to be slightly more frequent than other local anesthetics. From 1999-2008, there were 182 cases of nonsurgical paresthesia (Gaffen, 2009). Of the cases, 172 involved mandibular block injection only. Another eight cases involved mandibular block combined with at least one other type of anesthetic injection. A single case involved infiltration around tooth number 35 and the final case involved infiltration and intraligamentary injection in the maxillary anterior region.

A 2010 report, reviewed adverse events submitted voluntarily over a 10-year period involving the dental local anesthetics articaine, bupivacaine, lidocaine, mepivacaine, and prilocaine in the United States. Mepivacaine reported incidence: One case per 623,112,900 cartridges sold. The reported incidence of paresthesia was one case for 13,800,970 cartridges of all local anesthetics sold in the U.S. (Garisto, 2010).

References

Ayoub ST and Coleman AE, "A Review of Local Anesthetics," *Gen Dent*, 1992, 40(4):285-7, 289-90.
Budenz AW, "Local Anesthetics in Dentistry: Then and Now," *J Calif Dent Assoc*, 2003, 31(5):388-96.
Dower JS Jr, "A Review of Paresthesia in Association With Administration of Local Anesthesia," *Dent Today*, 2003, 22(2):64-9.
Finder RL and Moore PA, "Adverse Drug Reactions to Local Anesthesia," *Dent Clin North Am*, 2002, 46 (4):747-57, x.
Gaffen AS and Haas DA, "Retrospective Review of Voluntary Reports of Nonsurgical Paresthesia in Dentistry," *J Can Dent Assoc*, 2009, 75(8):579.
Garisto GA, Gaffen AS, Lawrence HP, et al, "Occurrence of Paresthesia After Dental Local Anesthetic Administration in the United States," *J Am Dent Assoc*, 2010, 141(7):836-44.
Haas DA, "An Update on Local Anesthetics in Dentistry," *J Can Dent Assoc*, 2002, 68(9):546-51.
Hawkins JM and Moore PA, "Local Anesthesia: Advances in Agents and Techniques," *Dent Clin North Am*, 2002, 46(4):719-32, ix.
"Injectable Local Anesthetics," *J Am Dent Assoc*, 2003, 134(5):628-9.
Malamed SF, "Allergy and Toxic Reactions to Local Anesthetics," *Dent Today*, 2003, 22(4):114-6, 118-21.
Wynn RL, "Recent Research on Mechanisms of Local Anesthetics," *Gen Dent*, 1995, 43(4):316-8.

Mepivacaine and Levonordefrin (me PIV a kane & lee voe nor DEF rin)

Related Information

Mepivacaine *on page 1076*
Oral Pain *on page 1928*

U.S. Brand Names Carbocaine® 2% with Neo-Cobefrin®; Polocaine® Dental with Levonordefrin; Scandonest® 2% L

Canadian Brand Names Polocaine® 2% and Levonordefrin 1:20,000

Generic Availability (U.S.) No

Pharmacologic Category Local Anesthetic

Dental Use Amide-type anesthetic used for local infiltration anesthesia; injection near nerve trunks to produce nerve block

Local Anesthetic/Vasoconstrictor Precautions No information available to require special precautions

Effects on Dental Treatment It is common to misinterpret psychogenic responses to local anesthetic injection as an allergic reaction. Intraoral injections are perceived by many patients as a stressful procedure in dentistry. Common symptoms to this stress are diaphoresis, palpitations, hyperventilation, generalized pallor and a fainting feeling. Patients may exhibit hypersensitivity to bisulfites contained in local anesthetic solution to prevent oxidation of levonordefrin. In general, patients reacting to bisulfites have a history of asthma and their airways are hyper-reactive to asthmatic syndrome.

Degree of adverse effects in the CNS and cardiovascular system is directly related to the blood levels of mepivacaine (frequency not defined; more likely to occur after systemic administration rather than infiltration): Bradycardia and reduction in cardiac output, nausea, vomiting, tremors, hypersensitivity reactions (extremely rare; may be manifest as dermatologic reactions and edema at injection site), asthmatic syndromes

High blood levels: Anxiety, restlessness, disorientation, confusion, dizziness, and seizures, followed by CNS depression resulting in somnolence, unconsciousness and possible respiratory arrest.

In some cases, symptoms of CNS stimulation may be absent and the primary CNS effects are somnolence and unconsciousness.

Effects on Bleeding No information available to require special precautions

Adverse Effects Degree of adverse effects in the CNS and cardiovascular system are directly related to the blood levels of mepivacaine. The effects below are more likely to occur after systemic administration rather than infiltration.

Cardiovascular: Myocardial effects include a decrease in contraction force as well as a decrease in electrical excitability and myocardial conduction rate resulting in bradycardia and reduction in cardiac output.

Central nervous system: High blood levels result in anxiety, restlessness, disorientation, confusion, dizziness, and seizure. This is followed by depression of CNS resulting in somnolence, unconsciousness and possible respiratory arrest. In some cases, symptoms of CNS stimulation may be absent and the primary CNS effects are somnolence and unconsciousness.

Gastrointestinal: Nausea and vomiting may occur

Hypersensitivity reactions: Extremely rare, but may be manifest as dermatologic reactions and edema at injection site. Asthmatic syndromes have occurred. Patients may exhibit hypersensitivity to bisulfites contained in local anesthetic solution to prevent oxidation of levonordefrin. In general, patients reacting to bisulfites have a history of asthma and their airways are hyper-reactive to asthmatic syndrome.

Neuromuscular & skeletal: Tremors

Psychogenic reactions: It is common to misinterpret psychogenic responses to local anesthetic injection as an allergic reaction. Intraoral injections are perceived by many patients as a stressful procedure in dentistry. Common symptoms to this stress are diaphoresis, palpitation, hyperventilation, generalized pallor and a fainting feeling.

Dental Usual Dosage

Children <10 years: Maximum pediatric dosage must be carefully calculated on the basis of patient's weight but should not exceed 6.6 mg/kg of body weight or 180 mg of mepivacaine hydrochloride as a 2% solution with levonordefrin 1:20,000

Children >10 years and Adults:

Dental infiltration and nerve block, single site: 36 mg (1.8 mL) of mepivacaine hydrochloride as a 2% solution with levonordefrin 1:20,000

Entire oral cavity: 180 mg (9 mL) of mepivacaine hydrochloride as a 2% solution with levonordefrin 1:20,000; up to a maximum of 6.6 mg/kg of body weight but not to exceed 400 mg of mepivacaine hydrochloride per appointment. The effective anesthetic dose varies with procedure, intensity of anesthesia needed, duration of anesthesia required, and physical condition of the patient. Always use the lowest effective dose along with careful aspiration.

The following numbers of dental carpules (1.8 mL) provide the indicated amounts of mepivacaine hydrochloride 2% and levonordefrin 1:20,000. See table.

# of Cartridges (1.8 mL)	mg Mepivacaine (2%)	mg Vasoconstrictor (Levonordefrin 1:20,000)
1	36	0.090
2	72	0.180
3	108	0.270
4	144	0.360
5	180	0.450
6	216	0.540
7	252	0.630
8	288	0.720
9	324	0.810
10	360	0.900

Note: Adult and children doses of mepivacaine hydrochloride with levonordefrin cited from USP Dispensing Information (USP DI), 17th ed, The United States Pharmacopeial Convention, Inc, Rockville, MD, 1997, 139.

Dosage

Children <10 years: Maximum pediatric dosage must be carefully calculated on the basis of patient's weight but should not exceed 6.6 mg/kg of body weight or 180 mg of mepivacaine hydrochloride as a 2% solution with levonordefrin 1:20,000

Children >10 years and Adults:

Dental infiltration and nerve block, single site: 36 mg (1.8 mL) of mepivacaine hydrochloride as a 2% solution with levonordefrin 1:20,000

Entire oral cavity: 180 mg (9 mL) of mepivacaine hydrochloride as a 2% solution with levonordefrin 1:20,000; up to a maximum of 6.6 mg/kg of body weight but not to exceed 400 mg of mepivacaine hydrochloride per appointment. The effective anesthetic dose varies with procedure, intensity of anesthesia needed, duration of anesthesia required, and physical condition of the patient. Always use the lowest effective dose along with careful aspiration.

Note: Adult and children doses of mepivacaine hydrochloride with levonordefrin cited from USP Dispensing Information (USP DI), 17th ed, The United States Pharmacopeial Convention, Inc, Rockville, MD, 1997, 139.

Mechanism of Action Local anesthetics bind selectively to the intracellular surface of sodium channels to block influx of sodium into the axon. As a result, depolarization necessary for action potential propagation and subsequent nerve function is prevented. The block at the sodium channel is reversible. When drug diffuses away from the axon, sodium channel function is restored and nerve propagation returns.

Levonordefrin prolongs the duration of the anesthetic actions of mepivacaine by causing vasoconstriction (alpha-adrenergic receptor agonist) of the vasculature surrounding the nerve axons. This prevents the diffusion of mepivacaine away from the nerves resulting in a longer retention in the axon.

Contraindications Hypersensitivity to local anesthetics of the amide-type or any component of the formulation

Warnings/Precautions Should be avoided in patients with uncontrolled hyperthyroidism. Should be used in minimal amounts in patients with significant cardiovascular problems (because of levonordefrin component). Use with caution in the elderly, debilitated, acutely ill and pediatric patients. Aspirate the syringe after tissue penetration and before injection to minimize chance of direct vascular injection. Contains sodium bisulfite which may cause allergic reactions in some individuals. Resuscitative equipment, oxygen, and other resuscitative drugs should be available for immediate use.

Drug Interactions

Avoid Concomitant Use

Avoid concomitant use of Mepivacaine and Levonordefrin with any of the following: Iobenguane I 123

Increased Effect/Toxicity

Mepivacaine and Levonordefrin may increase the levels/effects of: Bromocriptine; Sympathomimetics

The levels/effects of Mepivacaine and Levonordefrin may be increased by: Antacids; Atomoxetine; Beta-Blockers; Cannabinoids; Carbonic Anhydrase Inhibitors; MAO Inhibitors; Serotonin/Norepinephrine Reuptake Inhibitors; Tricyclic Antidepressants

Decreased Effect

Mepivacaine and Levonordefrin may decrease the levels/effects of: Benzylpenicilloyl Polylysine; Iobenguane I 123

The levels/effects of Mepivacaine and Levonordefrin may be decreased by: Spironolactone

Pharmacodynamics/Kinetics

Duration of Action Upper jaw: 1-2.5 hours; Lower jaw: 2.5-5.5 hours

Infiltration: 50 minutes

Inferior alveolar block: 60-75 minutes

Pregnancy Risk Factor C

Breast-Feeding Considerations Usual infiltration doses of mepivacaine with levonordefrin given to nursing mothers has not been shown to affect the health of the nursing infant.

Dosage Forms

Injection, solution [for dental use]:

Carbocaine® 2% with Neo-Cobefrin®: Mepivacaine 2% and levonordefrin 1:20,000 (1.7 mL)

Polocaine® Dental with Levonordefrin: Mepivacaine 2% and levonordefrin 1:20,000 (1.7 mL)

Scandonest® 2% L: Mepivacaine 2% and levonordefrin 1:20,000 (1.7 mL)

Dental Comment Oral paresthesia: The occurrence of oral paresthesia associated with 4% solutions of prilocaine or articaine, although rare, continue to be slightly more frequent than other local anesthetics. From 1999-2008, there were 182 cases of nonsurgical paresthesia (Gaffen, 2009). Of the cases, 172 involved mandibular block injection only. Another eight cases involved mandibular block combined with at least one other type of anesthetic injection. A single case involved infiltration around tooth number 35 and the final case involved infiltration and intraligamentary injection in the maxillary anterior region.

A 2010 report, reviewed adverse events submitted voluntarily over a 10-year period involving the dental local anesthetics articaine, bupivacaine, lidocaine, mepivacaine, and prilocaine in the United States. Mepivacaine reported incidence: One case per 623,112,900 cartridges sold. The reported incidence of paresthesia was one case for 13,800,970 cartridges of all local anesthetics sold in the U.S. (Garisto, 2010).

References

Ayoub ST and Coleman AE, "A Review of Local Anesthetics," *Gen Dent*, 1992, 40(4):285-7, 289-90.
Gaffen AS and Haas DA, "Retrospective Review of Voluntary Reports of Nonsurgical Paresthesia in Dentistry," *J Can Dent Assoc*, 2009, 75(8):579.
Garisto GA, Gaffen AS, Lawrence HP, et al, "Occurrence of Paresthesia After Dental Local Anesthetic Administration in the United States," *J Am Dent Assoc*, 2010, 141(7):836-44.
Jastak JT and Yagiela JA, "Vasoconstrictors and Local Anesthesia: A Review and Rationale for Use," *J Am Dent Assoc*, 1983, 107(4):623-30.
MacKenzie TA and Young ER, "Local Anesthetic Update," *Anesth Prog*, 1993, 40(2):29-34.
Wynn RL, "Epinephrine Interactions With Beta-Blockers," *Gen Dent*, 1994, 42(1):16, 18.
Wynn RL, "Recent Research on Mechanisms of Local Anesthetics," *Gen Dent*, 1995, 43(4):316-8.
Yagiela JA, "Local Anesthetics," *Anesth Prog*, 1991, 38(4-5):128-41.

Meprobamate (me proe BA mate)

Canadian Brand Names Novo-Mepro

Generic Availability (U.S.) Yes

Pharmacologic Category Antianxiety Agent, Miscellaneous

Dental Use Treatment of muscle spasm associated with acute temporomandibular joint (TMJ) pain; management of dental anxiety disorders

Use Management of anxiety disorders

Unlabeled/Investigational Use Demonstrated value for muscle contraction, headache, premenstrual tension, external sphincter spasticity, muscle rigidity, opisthotonos-associated with tetanus; treatment of muscle spasm associated with acute temporomandibular joint (TMJ) pain

Local Anesthetic/Vasoconstrictor Precautions No information available to require special precautions

Effects on Dental Treatment No significant effects or complications reported

Effects on Bleeding No information available to require special precautions

Adverse Effects Frequency not defined.

Cardiovascular: Arrhythmia EEG abnormalities, hypotensive crisis, peripheral edema, palpitation, syncope, tachycardia

Central nervous system: Ataxia, chills, dizziness, drowsiness, euphoria, fever, headache, overstimulation, paradoxical excitement, slurred speech, vertigo

Dermatologic: Angioneurotic edema, bruising, dermatitis, erythema multiforme, petechiae, purpura, rash, Stevens-Johnson syndrome

Gastrointestinal: Diarrhea, nausea, proctitis, stomatitis, vomiting

Hematologic: Agranulocytosis, aplastic anemia, eosinophilia, leukopenia, porphyria exacerbation, thrombocytopenic purpura

Neuromuscular & skeletal: Paresthesia, weakness

Ocular: Impairment of accommodation

Renal: Anuria, oliguria

Respiratory: Bronchospasm

Miscellaneous: Anaphylaxis, hypersensitivity

Dental Usual Dosage Muscle spasm (TMJ) pain or anxiety: Adults: Oral: 400 mg 3-4 times/day, up to 2400 mg/day

Dosage Oral:

Anxiety:

Children 6-12 years: 200-600 mg/day in 2-3 divided doses

Adults: 1200-1600 mg/day in 3-4 divided doses, up to 2400 mg/day

Muscle spasm (TMJ) pain (unlabeled use): Adults: 1200-1600 mg/day in 3-4 divided doses, up to 2400 mg/day

Dosing interval in renal impairment:

Cl_{cr} 10-50 mL/minute: Administer every 9-12 hours

Cl_{cr} <10 mL/minute: Administer every 12-18 hours

Hemodialysis: Moderately dialyzable (20% to 50%)

Dosing adjustment in hepatic impairment: Probably necessary in patients with liver disease

Mechanism of Action Affects the thalamus and limbic system; also appears to inhibit multineuronal spinal reflexes

Contraindications Hypersensitivity to meprobamate, related compounds (including carisoprodol), or any component of the formulation; acute intermittent porphyria

Warnings/Precautions Physical and psychological dependence and abuse may occur; abrupt cessation may precipitate withdrawal. Use with caution in patients with depression or suicidal tendencies, or in patients with a history of drug abuse. May cause CNS depression, which may impair physical or mental abilities. Patients must be cautioned about performing tasks which require mental alertness (eg, operating machinery or driving). Effects with other sedative drugs or ethanol may be potentiated. Allergic reaction may occur in patients with history of dermatological condition (usually by fourth dose). Use with caution in patients with renal or hepatic impairment, or with a history of seizures. Use with caution in the elderly; may cause confusion, cognitive impairment, excessive sedation, or addiction with prolonged use (Beers Criteria).

Drug Interactions

Avoid Concomitant Use There are no known interactions where it is recommended to avoid concomitant use.

Increased Effect/Toxicity

Meprobamate may increase the levels/effects of: Alcohol (Ethyl); CNS Depressants; Methotrimeprazine

The levels/effects of Meprobamate may be increased by: Droperidol; Methotrimeprazine

Decreased Effect

The levels/effects of Meprobamate may be decreased by: Yohimbine

Ethanol/Nutrition/Herb Interactions

Ethanol: May increase CNS depression; monitor for increased effects with coadministration. Caution patients about effects.

Herb/Nutraceutical: Avoid valerian, St John's wort, kava kava, gotu kola (may increase CNS depression).

Pharmacodynamics/Kinetics

Onset of Action Sedation: ~1 hour

Half-life Elimination 10 hours

Pregnancy Risk Factor D

Lactation Enters breast milk/not recommended

Breast-Feeding Considerations Breast milk concentrations are higher than plasma; effects are unknown.

Controlled Substance C-IV

Dosage Forms

Tablet, oral: 200 mg, 400 mg

Mequinol and Tretinoin (ME kwi nole & TRET i noyn)

U.S. Brand Names Solagé® [DSC]

Canadian Brand Names Solagé®

Pharmacologic Category Retinoic Acid Derivative; Vitamin A Derivative; Vitamin, Topical

Use Treatment of solar lentigines; the efficacy of using Solagé® daily for >24 weeks has not been established

Local Anesthetic/Vasoconstrictor Precautions No information available to require special precautions

Effects on Dental Treatment No significant effects or complications reported

Effects on Bleeding No information available to require special precautions

Adverse Effects

>10%: Dermatologic: Erythema (41%), burning, stinging or tingling (18%), desquamation (12%), pruritus (10%)

1% to 10%: Dermatologic: Skin irritation (6%), halo hypopigmentation (6%), hypopigmentation (4%), skin discomfort (4%), dry skin (3%), crusting (2%), dermatitis (2%), rash (2%), vesicular bullae rash (1%), contact allergic reaction (1%), irritant dermatitis (1%)

General Dosage Range Topical: *Adults:* Apply twice daily

Mechanism of Action Solar lentigines are localized, pigmented, macular lesions of the skin on areas of the body chronically exposed to the sun. Mequinol is a substrate for the enzyme tyrosinase and acts as a competitive inhibitor of the formation of melanin precursors. The mechanisms of depigmentation for both drugs is unknown.

Pharmacodynamics/Kinetics

Time to Peak Mequinol: 2 hours

Pregnancy Risk Factor X

Mercaptopurine (mer kap toe PYOOR een)

U.S. Brand Names Purinethol®

Canadian Brand Names Purinethol®

Pharmacologic Category Antineoplastic Agent, Antimetabolite; Antineoplastic Agent, Antimetabolite (Purine Analog); Immunosuppressant Agent

Use Treatment (maintenance and induction) of acute lymphoblastic leukemia (ALL)

Unlabeled/Investigational Use Steroid-sparing agent for corticosteroid-dependent Crohn's disease (CD) and ulcerative colitis (UC); maintenance of remission in CD; fistulizing Crohn's disease

Local Anesthetic/Vasoconstrictor Precautions No information available to require special precautions

Effects on Dental Treatment Key adverse event(s) related to dental treatment: Stomatitis and mucositis.

Effects on Bleeding Chemotherapy may result in significant myelosuppression, potentially including significant reduction in platelet counts and altered hemostasis. In patients who are under active treatment with these agents, medical consult is suggested.

Adverse Effects

>10%:

Hematologic: Myelosuppression; leukopenia, thrombocytopenia, anemia

Onset: 7-10 days

Nadir: 14-16 days

Recovery: 21-28 days

Hepatic: Intrahepatic cholestasis and focal centralobular necrosis (40%), characterized by hyperbilirubinemia, increased alkaline phosphatase and AST, jaundice, ascites, encephalopathy; more common at doses >2.5 mg/kg/day. Usually occurs within 2 months of therapy but may occur within 1 week, or be delayed up to 8 years.

1% to 10%:

Central nervous system: Drug fever

Dermatologic: Hyperpigmentation, rash

Endocrine & metabolic: Hyperuricemia

Gastrointestinal: Anorexia, diarrhea, mucositis, nausea, pancreatitis, stomach pain, stomatitis, vomiting

Renal: Renal toxicity

General Dosage Range Dosage adjustment recommended in patients on concomitant therapy

Oral:

Children: Induction: 2.5-5 mg/kg/day **or** 70-100 mg/m^2/day given once daily; Maintenance: 1.5-2.5 mg/kg/day **or** 50-75 mg/m^2/day given once daily

Adults: Induction: 2.5-5 mg/kg/day (100-200 mg); Maintenance: 1.5-2.5 mg/kg/day **or** 80-100 mg/m^2/day given once daily

Mechanism of Action Purine antagonist which inhibits DNA and RNA synthesis; acts as false metabolite and is incorporated into DNA and RNA, eventually inhibiting their synthesis; specific for the S phase of the cell cycle

Pharmacodynamics/Kinetics

Half-life Elimination Age dependent: Children: 21 minutes; Adults: 47 minutes

Time to Peak Serum: ~2 hours

Pregnancy Risk Factor D

Meropenem (mer oh PEN em)

U.S. Brand Names Merrem® I.V.

Canadian Brand Names Merrem®

Pharmacologic Category Antibiotic, Carbapenem

Use Treatment of intra-abdominal infections (complicated appendicitis and peritonitis); treatment of bacterial meningitis in pediatric patients ≥3 months of age caused by *S. pneumoniae*, *H. influenzae*, and *N. meningitidis*; treatment of complicated skin and skin structure infections caused by susceptible organisms

Unlabeled/Investigational Use *Burkholderia pseudomallei* (melioidosis), febrile neutropenia, liver abscess, meningitis (adults), otitis externa, pneumonia, urinary tract infections

Local Anesthetic/Vasoconstrictor Precautions No information available to require special precautions

Effects on Dental Treatment Key adverse event(s) related to dental treatment: Oral moniliasis (pediatric patients) and glossitis.

Effects on Bleeding No information available to require special precautions

Adverse Effects 1% to 10%:

Central nervous system: Headache (2% to 8%), pain (≤5%)

Dermatologic: Rash (2% to 3%, includes diaper-area moniliasis in pediatrics), pruritus (1%)

Endocrine & metabolic: Hypoglycemia

Gastrointestinal: Diarrhea (4% to 7%), nausea/vomiting (1% to 8%), constipation (1% to 7%), oral moniliasis (up to 2% in pediatric patients), glossitis (1%)

Hematologic: Anemia (≤6%)

Local: Inflammation at the injection site (2%), phlebitis/thrombophlebitis (1%), injection site reaction (1%)

Respiratory: Apnea (1%), pharyngitis, pneumonia

Miscellaneous: Sepsis (2%), shock (1%)

General Dosage Range Dosage adjustment recommended in patients with renal impairment

I.V.:

Children ≥3 months and <50 kg: 10-40 mg/kg every 8 hours (maximum: 2 g every 8 hours)

Children ≥50 kg and Adults: 500 mg to 2 g every 8 hours

Mechanism of Action Inhibits bacterial cell wall synthesis by binding to several of the penicillin-binding proteins, which in turn inhibit the final transpeptidation step of peptidoglycan synthesis in bacterial cell walls, thus inhibiting cell wall biosynthesis; bacteria eventually lyse due to ongoing activity of cell wall autolytic enzymes (autolysins and murein hydrolases) while cell wall assembly is arrested

Pharmacodynamics/Kinetics

Half-life Elimination

Normal renal function: 1-1.5 hours

Cl_{cr} 30-80 mL/minute: 1.9-3.3 hours

Cl_{cr} 2-30 mL/minute: 3.82-5.7 hours

Time to Peak Tissue: 1 hour following infusion

Pregnancy Risk Factor B

Mesalamine (me SAL a meen)

U.S. Brand Names Apriso™; Asacol®; Asacol® HD; Canasa®; Lialda®; Pentasa®; Rowasa®; sfRowasa™

Canadian Brand Names 5-ASA; Asacol®; Asacol® 800; Mesasal®; Mezavant®; Novo-5 ASA; Novo-5 ASA-ECT; Pentasa®; Salofalk®; Salofalk® 5-ASA

Pharmacologic Category 5-Aminosalicylic Acid Derivative

Use

Oral:

Asacol®, Pentasa®: Treatment and maintenance of remission of mildly- to moderately-active ulcerative colitis

Apriso™: Maintenance of remission of ulcerative colitis

Asacol® HD: Treatment of moderately-active ulcerative colitis

Lialda™: Treatment of mildly- to moderately-active ulcerative colitis

Rectal: Treatment of active mild-to-moderate distal ulcerative colitis, proctosigmoiditis, or proctitis

Local Anesthetic/Vasoconstrictor Precautions No information available to require special precautions

Effects on Dental Treatment Key adverse event(s) related to dental treatment: Pharyngitis.

Effects on Bleeding No information available to require special precautions

Adverse Effects Adverse effects vary depending upon dosage form. Incidence usually on lower end with enema and suppository dosage forms.

>10%:

Central nervous system: Headache (2% to 35%), pain (≤14%)

Gastrointestinal: Abdominal pain (1% to 18%), eructation (16%), nausea (3% to 13%)

Respiratory: Pharyngitis (11%)

1% to 10%:

Cardiovascular: Chest pain (3%), peripheral edema (3%), vasodilation (≥2%)

Central nervous system: Dizziness (2% to 8%), fever (1% to 6%), chills (3%), malaise (2% to 3%), fatigue (<3%), vertigo (<3%), anxiety (≥2%), migraine (≥2%), nervousness (≥2%), insomnia (2%),

Dermatologic: Rash (1% to 6%), pruritus (1% to 3%), alopecia (<3%), acne (1% to 2%)

Endocrine & metabolic: Triglyceride increased (<3%)

Gastrointestinal: Diarrhea (2% to 8%), dyspepsia (1% to 6%), flatulence (1% to 6%), constipation (5%), vomiting (1% to 5%), colitis exacerbation (1% to 3%), rectal bleeding (<3%), abdominal distention (≥2%), gastroenteritis (≥2%), gastrointestinal bleeding (≥2%), stool abnormalities (≥2%), tenesmus (≥2%), rectal pain (1% to 2%), hemorrhoids (1%)

Genitourinary: Polyuria (≥2%)

Hematologic: Hematocrit/hemoglobin decreased (<3%)

Hepatic: Cholestatic hepatitis (<3%), transaminases increased (<3%), ALT increased (1%)

Local: Pain on insertion of enema tip (1%)

Neuromuscular & skeletal: Back pain (1% to 7%), arthralgia (≤5%), hypertonia (5%), myalgia (3%), paresthesia (≥2%), weakness (≥2%), arthritis (2%), leg/joint pain (2%)

Ocular: Vision abnormalities (≥2%), conjunctivitis (2%)

Otic: Tinnitus (<3%), ear pain (≥2%)

Renal: Creatinine clearance decreased (<3%), hematuria (<3%)
Respiratory: Nasopharyngitis (1% to 4%), dyspnea (<3%), bronchitis (≥2%), sinusitis (≥2%), cough (≤2%)
Miscellaneous: Flu-like syndrome (1% to 5%), infection (≥2%), diaphoresis (3%), intolerance syndrome (3%)

General Dosage Range

Oral: *Adults:*

Capsule: Apriso™: 1.5 g once daily; Pentasa®: 1 g 4 times/day
Tablet: Asacol®: 800 mg 3 times/day or 1.6 g/day in divided doses; Asacol® HD: 1.6 g 3 times/day; Lialda™, Mezavant®: 2.4-4.8 g once daily

Rectal: *Adults:* Retention enema: 60 mL (4 g) at bedtime, retained overnight (~8 hours); Suppository: Insert 1000 mg at bedtime

Mechanism of Action Mesalamine (5-aminosalicylic acid) is the active component of sulfasalazine; the specific mechanism of action of mesalamine is unknown; however, it is thought that it modulates local chemical mediators of the inflammatory response, especially leukotrienes, and is also postulated to be a free radical scavenger or an inhibitor of tumor necrosis factor (TNF); action appears topical rather than systemic

Pharmacodynamics/Kinetics

Half-life Elimination 5-ASA: 0.5-10 hours; N-acetyl-5-ASA: 2-15 hours

Time to Peak

Capsule: Apriso™: ~4 hours; Pentasa®: 3 hours
Rectal: 4-7 hours
Tablet: Asacol®: 4-12 hours; Asacol® HD: 10-16 hours; Lialda™: 9-12 hours; Mezavant®: 8 hours

Pregnancy Risk Factor B/C (product specific)

Metaproterenol (met a proe TER e nol)

Related Information

Respiratory Diseases *on page* 1876

Canadian Brand Names Apo-Orciprenaline®; ratio-Orciprenaline®; Tanta-Orciprenaline®

Pharmacologic Category Beta$_2$-Adrenergic Agonist

Use Bronchodilator in reversible airway obstruction due to asthma or COPD

Local Anesthetic/Vasoconstrictor Precautions No information available to require special precautions

Effects on Dental Treatment Key adverse event(s) related to dental treatment: Bad taste and xerostomia (normal salivary flow resumes upon discontinuation).

Effects on Bleeding No information available to require special precautions

Adverse Effects

>10%:

Cardiovascular: Tachycardia (6% to 17%)
Central nervous system: Nervousness (5% to 20%), headache (1% to 7%)
Neuromuscular & skeletal: Tremor (2% to 17%)

1% to 10%:

Cardiovascular: Palpitation (4%)
Central nervous system: Dizziness (2%), insomnia (2%), fatigue (1%)
Gastrointestinal: Nausea (1% to 4%), diarrhea (1%)
Respiratory: Asthma exacerbation (2%)

General Dosage Range Oral:

Children <6 years: 1.3-2.6 mg/kg/day divided every 6-8 hours
Children 6-9 years (or <27 kg): 10 mg/dose 3-4 times/day
Children >9 years (or ≥27 kg) and Adults: 20 mg 3-4 times/day

Mechanism of Action Stimulates beta$_2$-receptors which increases the conversion of adenosine triphosphate (ATP) to 3'-5'-cyclic adenosine monophosphate (cAMP), resulting in bronchial smooth muscle relaxation

Pharmacodynamics/Kinetics

Onset of Action Bronchodilation: Oral: ~30 minutes; Peak effect: Oral: ~1 hour

Duration of Action ~2-6 hours

Pregnancy Risk Factor C

Metaxalone (me TAKS a lone)

U.S. Brand Names Skelaxin®

Canadian Brand Names Skelaxin®

Generic Availability (U.S.) Yes

Pharmacologic Category Skeletal Muscle Relaxant

Use Relief of discomfort associated with acute, painful musculoskeletal conditions

Local Anesthetic/Vasoconstrictor Precautions No information available to require special precautions

Effects on Dental Treatment No significant effects or complications reported

Effects on Bleeding No information available to require special precautions

Adverse Effects Frequency not defined.

Central nervous system: Dizziness, drowsiness, headache, irritability, nervousness
Dermatologic: Rash (with or without pruritus)
Gastrointestinal: Gastrointestinal upset, nausea, vomiting
Hematologic: Hemolytic anemia, leukopenia
Hepatic: Jaundice
Miscellaneous: Hypersensitivity (including rare anaphylactoid reactions)

Dosage Oral: Children >12 years and Adults: Muscle discomfort: 800 mg 3-4 times/day

Dosage adjustment in renal impairment: Use caution in patients with mild-to-moderate renal impairment; contraindicated with significant impairment. No specific recommendation are provided in approved labeling.

Dosage adjustment in hepatic impairment: Use caution in patients with mild-to-moderate hepatic impairment; contraindicated with significant impairment. No specific recommendation are provided in approved labeling.

Mechanism of Action Precise mechanism has not been established; however, efficacy appears to result from disruption of the spasm-pain-spasm cycle, probably by a general CNS depressant effect. Does not have a direct effect on skeletal muscle.

Contraindications Hypersensitivity to metaxalone or any component of the formulation; significantly impaired hepatic or renal function, history of drug-induced hemolytic anemias or other anemias

Warnings/Precautions May cause CNS depression. CNS depressant effects may be augmented when used in conjunction with other depressants (eg, barbiturates, ethanol), when taken with food, or in the elderly. May impair mental and/or physical ability to perform hazardous tasks such as operating machinery or driving a motor vehicle. Use with caution in patients with impaired renal or hepatic function (contraindicated if significant impairment); routine monitoring of transaminases is recommended. An increase in bioavailability and half-life have been observed in female patients. This class of medication is poorly tolerated by the elderly due to anticholinergic effects, sedation, and weakness. Efficacy is questionable at dosages tolerated by elderly patients (Beers Criteria). Safety and efficacy have not been established in children ≤12 years of age.

Drug Interactions

Metabolism/Transport Effects

Substrate of CYP1A2, 2C8, 2C9, 2C19, 2D6, 2E1, 3A4

Avoid Concomitant Use There are no known interactions where it is recommended to avoid concomitant use.

Increased Effect/Toxicity

Metaxalone may increase the levels/effects of: Alcohol (Ethyl); CNS Depressants; Methotrimeprazine

The levels/effects of Metaxalone may be increased by: Conivaptan; Droperidol; Methotrimeprazine

Decreased Effect

The levels/effects of Metaxalone may be decreased by: Peginterferon Alfa-2b; Tocilizumab

Ethanol/Nutrition/Herb Interactions

Ethanol: May increase CNS depression; monitor for increased effects with coadministration. Caution patients about effects.
Food: Bioavailability may be increased (may increase CNS depression).
Herb/Nutraceutical: Avoid valerian, St John's wort, kava kava, gotu kola (may increase CNS depression).

Dietary Considerations Administration with food may increase serum concentrations.

Pharmacodynamics/Kinetics

Onset of Action ~1 hour

Duration of Action ~4-6 hours

Half-life Elimination 4-14 hours

Time to Peak T_{max}: ~3 hours

Lactation Excretion in breast milk unknown/not recommended

Dosage Forms

Tablet, oral: 800 mg

Skelaxin®: 800 mg

MetFORMIN (met FOR min)

Related Information

Endocrine Disorders and Pregnancy *on page 1879*

U.S. Brand Names Fortamet®; Glucophage®; Glucophage® XR; Glumetza®; Riomet®

Canadian Brand Names Apo-Metformin®; CO Metformin; Dom-Metformin; Glucophage®; Glumetza®; Glycon; Med-Metformin; Mylan-Metformin; Novo-Metformin; Nu-Metformin; PHL-Metformin; PMS-Metformin; PRO-Metformin; RAN™-Metformin; ratio-Metformin; Riva-Metformin; Sandoz-Metformin FC

Generic Availability (U.S.) Yes: Excludes solution

Pharmacologic Category Antidiabetic Agent, Biguanide

Use Management of type 2 diabetes mellitus (noninsulin dependent, NIDDM) when hyperglycemia cannot be managed with diet and exercise alone.

Unlabeled/Investigational Use Gestational diabetes mellitus (GDM); polycystic ovary syndrome (PCOS); prevention of type 2 diabetes mellitus

Local Anesthetic/Vasoconstrictor Precautions No information available to require special precautions

Effects on Dental Treatment Key adverse event(s) related to dental treatment: Taste disorder.

Metformin-dependent patients with diabetes (noninsulin dependent, Type 2) should be appointed for dental treatment in morning in order to minimize chance of stress-induced hypoglycemia.

Effects on Bleeding No information available to require special precautions

Adverse Effects

>10%:

Gastrointestinal: Diarrhea (10% to 53%), nausea/vomiting (7% to 26%), flatulence (12%)

Neuromuscular & skeletal: Weakness (9%)

1% to 10%:

Cardiovascular: Chest discomfort, flushing, palpitation

Central nervous system: Headache (6%), chills, dizziness, lightheadedness

Dermatologic: Rash

Endocrine & metabolic: Hypoglycemia

Gastrointestinal: Indigestion (7%), abdominal discomfort (6%), abdominal distention, abnormal stools, constipation, dyspepsia/ heartburn, taste disorder

Neuromuscular & skeletal: Myalgia

Respiratory: Dyspnea, upper respiratory tract infection

Miscellaneous: Decreased vitamin B_{12} levels (7%), increased diaphoresis, flu-like syndrome, nail disorder

Dosage

Type 2 diabetes management: **Note:** Allow 1-2 weeks between dose titrations: Generally, clinically significant responses are not seen at doses <1500 mg daily; however, a lower recommended starting dose and gradual increased dosage is recommended to minimize gastrointestinal symptoms.

Immediate release tablet or solution: Oral:

Children 10-16 years: Initial: 500 mg twice daily; increases in daily dosage should be made in increments of 500 mg at weekly intervals, given in divided doses, up to a maximum of 2000 mg/day

Children ≥17 years and Adults: Initial: 500 mg twice daily **or** 850 mg once daily; titrate in increments of 500 mg weekly or 850 mg every other week; may also titrate from 500 mg twice a day to 850 mg twice a day after 2 weeks

Doses of up to 2000 mg/day may be given twice daily. If a dose >2000 mg/day is required, it may be better tolerated in three divided doses. Maximum recommended dose 2550 mg/day.

Extended release tablet: Oral: **Note:** If glycemic control is not achieved at maximum dose, may divide dose and administer twice daily.

Children ≥17 years and Adults:

Fortamet®: Initial: 500-1000 mg once daily; dosage may be increased by 500 mg weekly; maximum dose: 2500 mg once daily

Glucophage® XR: Initial: 500 mg once daily; dosage may be increased by 500 mg weekly; maximum dose: 2000 mg once daily

Adults: Glumetza®: Initial: 1000 mg once daily; dosage may be increased by 500 mg weekly; maximum dose: 2000 mg once daily

Elderly: The initial and maintenance dosing should be conservative, due to the potential for decreased renal function. Generally, elderly patients should not be titrated to the maximum dose of metformin. Do not use in patients ≥80 years of age unless normal renal function has been established.

Transfer from other antidiabetic agents: No transition period is generally necessary except when transferring from chlorpropamide. When transferring from chlorpropamide, care should be exercised during the first 2 weeks because of the prolonged retention of chlorpropamide in the body, leading to overlapping drug effects and possible hypoglycemia.

Concomitant metformin and oral sulfonylurea therapy: If patients have not responded to 4 weeks of the maximum dose of metformin monotherapy, consider a gradual addition of an oral sulfonylurea, even if prior primary or secondary failure to a sulfonylurea has occurred. Continue metformin at the maximum dose. If adequate response has not occurred following 3 months of metformin and sulfonylurea combination therapy, consider switching to insulin with or without metformin.

Failed sulfonylurea therapy: Patients with prior failure on glyburide may be treated by gradual addition of metformin. Initiate with glyburide 20 mg and metformin 500 mg daily. Metformin dosage may be increased by 500 mg/day at weekly intervals, up to a maximum metformin dose (dosage of glyburide maintained at 20 mg/day).

Concomitant metformin and insulin therapy: Initial: 500 mg metformin once daily, continue current insulin dose; increase by 500 mg metformin weekly until adequate glycemic control is achieved

Maximum daily dose: Immediate release and solution: 2550 mg metformin; Extended release: 2000-2500 mg (varies by product)

Decrease insulin dose 10% to 25% when FPG <120 mg/dL; monitor and make further adjustments as needed

Type 2 diabetes prevention (unlabeled use): **Immediate release tablet or solution:** Oral: Adults: Initial: 850 mg once daily; Target: 850 mg twice daily (Knowler, 2002)

Dosing adjustment/comments in renal impairment: The plasma and blood half-life of metformin is prolonged and the renal clearance is decreased in proportion to the decrease in creatinine clearance. Per the manufacturer, metformin is contraindicated in the presence of renal dysfunction defined as a serum creatinine ≥1.5 mg/dL in males, or ≥1.4 mg/dL in females and in patients with abnormal clearance. The Canadian labeling recommends that metformin be avoided in patients with Cl_{cr} <60 mL/minute.

Dosing adjustment in hepatic impairment: Avoid metformin; liver disease is a risk factor for the development of lactic acidosis during metformin therapy.

Mechanism of Action Decreases hepatic glucose production, decreasing intestinal absorption of glucose and improves insulin sensitivity (increases peripheral glucose uptake and utilization)

Contraindications Hypersensitivity to metformin or any component of the formulation; renal disease or renal dysfunction (serum creatinine ≥1.5 mg/dL in males or ≥1.4 mg/dL in females) or abnormal creatinine clearance from any cause, including shock, acute myocardial infarction, or septicemia; acute or chronic metabolic acidosis with or without coma (including diabetic ketoacidosis)

Note: Temporarily discontinue in patients undergoing radiologic studies in which intravascular iodinated contrast media are utilized.

Warnings/Precautions [U.S. Boxed Warning]: Lactic acidosis is a rare, but potentially severe consequence of therapy with metformin. Lactic acidosis should be suspected in any patient with diabetes receiving metformin with evidence of acidosis but without evidence of ketoacidosis. Discontinue metformin in clinical situations predisposing to hypoxemia, including conditions such as cardiovascular collapse, respiratory failure, acute myocardial infarction, acute congestive heart failure, and septicemia. Use caution in patients with congestive heart failure requiring pharmacologic management, particularly in patients with unstable or acute CHF; risk of lactic acidosis may be increased secondary to hypoperfusion.

Metformin is substantially excreted by the kidney. The risk of accumulation and lactic acidosis increases with the degree of impairment of renal function. Patients with renal function below the limit of normal for their age should not receive metformin. In elderly patients, renal function should be monitored regularly; should not be initiated in patients ≥80 years of age unless normal renal function is confirmed. Use of concomitant medications that may affect renal function (ie, affect tubular secretion) may also affect metformin disposition. Metformin should be withheld in patients with dehydration and/or prerenal azotemia. Therapy should be suspended for any surgical procedures (resume only after normal oral intake resumed and normal renal function is verified). Therapy should be temporarily discontinued prior to or at the time of intravascular administration of iodinated contrast media (potential for acute alteration in renal function). Metformin should be withheld for 48 hours after the radiologic study and restarted only after renal function has been confirmed as normal. It may be necessary to discontinue metformin and administer insulin if the patient is exposed to stress (fever, trauma, infection, surgery).

Avoid use in patients with impaired liver function. Patient must be instructed to avoid excessive acute or chronic ethanol use; ethanol may potentiate metformin's effect on lactate metabolism. Administration of oral antidiabetic drugs has been reported to be associated with increased cardiovascular mortality; metformin does not appear to share this risk. Insoluble tablet shell of Glumetza® 1000 mg extended release tablet may remain intact and be visible in the stool. Other extended released tablets (Fortamet®, Glucophage® XR, Glumetza® 500 mg) may appear in the stool as a soft mass resembling the tablet.

Drug Interactions

Avoid Concomitant Use There are no known interactions where it is recommended to avoid concomitant use.

Increased Effect/Toxicity

MetFORMIN may increase the levels/effects of: Dofetilide

The levels/effects of MetFORMIN may be increased by: Cephalexin; Cimetidine; Glycopyrrolate; Iodinated Contrast Agents; Pegvisomant

Decreased Effect

The levels/effects of MetFORMIN may be decreased by: Corticosteroids (Orally Inhaled); Corticosteroids (Systemic); Luteinizing Hormone-Releasing Hormone Analogs; Somatropin; Thiazide Diuretics

Ethanol/Nutrition/Herb Interactions

Ethanol: Avoid or limit ethanol (incidence of lactic acidosis may be increased; may cause hypoglycemia).

Food: Food decreases the extent and slightly delays the absorption. May decrease absorption of vitamin B_{12} and/or folic acid.

Herb/Nutraceutical: Caution with chromium, garlic, gymnema (may cause hypoglycemia).

Dietary Considerations Drug may cause GI upset; take with food (to decrease GI upset). Take at the same time(s) each day. Dietary modification based on ADA recommendations is a part of therapy. Monitor for signs and symptoms of vitamin B_{12} and/or folic acid deficiency; supplementation may be required.

Pharmacodynamics/Kinetics

Onset of Action Within days; maximum effects up to 2 weeks

Half-life Elimination Plasma: 4-9 hours

Time to Peak Immediate release: 2-3 hours; Extended release: 7 hours (range: 4-8 hours)

Pregnancy Risk Factor B

Lactation Enters breast milk/not recommended

Breast-Feeding Considerations Low amounts of metformin (generally ≤1% of the weight-adjusted maternal dose) are excreted into breast milk. Breast-feeding is not recommended by the manufacturer. Because breast milk concentrations of metformin stay relatively constant, avoiding nursing around peak plasma concentrations in the mother would not be helpful in reducing metformin exposure to the infant. Growth and development were not affected in infants born to mothers with PCOS and who took metformin while breast-feeding.

Dosage Forms

Solution, oral:

Riomet®: 100 mg/mL (118 mL, 473 mL)

Tablet, oral: 500 mg, 850 mg, 1000 mg

Glucophage®: 500 mg, 850 mg, 1000 mg

Tablet, extended release, oral: 500 mg, 750 mg

Fortamet®: 500 mg, 1000 mg

Glucophage® XR: 500 mg, 750 mg

Glumetza®: 500 mg, 1000 mg

Methadone (METH a done)

Related Information

Clinical Risk Related to Drugs Prolonging QT Interval *on page 1872*

U.S. Brand Names Dolophine®; Methadone Diskets®; Methadone Intensol™; Methadose®

Canadian Brand Names Metadol-D™; Metadol™

Pharmacologic Category Analgesic, Opioid

Use Management of moderate-to-severe pain; detoxification and maintenance treatment of opioid addiction as part of an FDA-approved program

Local Anesthetic/Vasoconstrictor Precautions No information available to require special precautions

Effects on Dental Treatment Key adverse event(s) related to dental treatment: Significant xerostomia (normal salivary flow resumes upon discontinuation) and glossitis.

Effects on Bleeding No information available to require special precautions

Adverse Effects Frequency not defined. During prolonged administration, adverse effects may decrease over several weeks; however, constipation and sweating may persist.

Cardiovascular: Arrhythmia, bigeminal rhythms, bradycardia, cardiac arrest, cardiomyopathy, ECG changes, edema, extrasystoles, faintness, flushing, heart failure, hypotension, palpitation,peripheral vasodilation, phlebitis, orthostatic hypotension, QT interval prolonged, shock, syncope, tachycardia, torsade de pointes, T-wave inversion, ventricular fibrillation, ventricular tachycardia,

Central nervous system: Agitation, confusion, disorientation, dizziness, drowsiness, dysphoria, euphoria, hallucination, headache, insomnia, lightheadedness, sedation, seizure

Dermatologic: Hemorrhagic urticaria, pruritus, rash, urticaria

Endocrine & metabolic: Antidiuretic effect, amenorrhea, hypokalemia, hypomagnesemia, libido decreased

Gastrointestinal: Abdominal pain, anorexia, biliary tract spasm, constipation, glossitis, nausea, stomach cramps, vomiting, weight gain, xerostomia

Genitourinary: Impotence, urinary retention or hesitancy

Hematologic: Thrombocytopenia (reversible, reported in patients with chronic hepatitis)

Neuromuscular & skeletal: Weakness

Local: I.M./SubQ injection: Erythema, pain, swelling; I.V. injection: Hemorrhagic urticaria (rare), pruritus, urticaria, rash

Ocular: Miosis, visual disturbances

Respiratory: Pulmonary edema, respiratory depression, respiratory arrest

Miscellaneous: Death, diaphoresis, physical and psychological dependence

General Dosage Range Dosage adjustment recommended in patients with renal imparment or who develop toxicities

I.M.:

Adults: Initial: 2.5-10 mg every 8-12 hours

Elderly: 2.5 mg every 8-12 hours

I.V., SubQ: *Adults:* Initial: 2.5-10 mg every 8-12 hours

Oral:

Adults: Detoxification: Initial: Up to 40 mg/day; Maintenance: 80-120 mg/day; Pain: 2.5-10 mg every 4-12 hours as needed

Elderly: 2.5 mg every 8-12 hours

Mechanism of Action Binds to opiate receptors in the CNS, causing inhibition of ascending pain pathways, altering the perception of and response to pain; produces generalized CNS depression

Pharmacodynamics/Kinetics

Onset of Action Oral: Analgesic: 0.5-1 hour; Parenteral: 10-20 minutes; Peak effect: Parenteral: 1-2 hours; Oral: Continuous dosing: 3-5 days

Duration of Action Analgesia: Oral: 4-8 hours, increases to 22-48 hours with repeated doses

Half-life Elimination 8-59 hours; may be prolonged with alkaline pH, decreased during pregnancy

Time to Peak 1-7.5 hours

Pregnancy Risk Factor C

Controlled Substance C-II

Prescribing and Access Restrictions When used for treatment of opioid addiction: May only be dispensed in accordance to guidelines established by the Substance Abuse and Mental Health Services Administration's (SAMHSA) Center for Substance Abuse Treatment (CSAT). Regulations regarding methadone use may vary by state and/or country. Obtain advice from appropriate regulatory agencies and/or consult with pain management/palliative care specialists.

Note: Regulatory Exceptions to the General Requirement to Provide Opioid Agonist Treatment (per manufacturer's labeling):

1. During inpatient care, when the patient was admitted for any condition other than concurrent opioid addiction, to facilitate the treatment of the primary admitting diagnosis.
2. During an emergency period of no longer than 3 days while definitive care for the addiction is being sought in an appropriately licensed facility.

Dental Comment This drug is known to prolong the QT interval. The QT interval is measured as the time and distance between the Q point of the QRS complex and the end of the T wave in the ECG tracing. After adjustment for heart rate, the QT interval is defined as prolonged if it is more than 450 msec in men and 460 msec in women. A long QT syndrome was first described in the 1950s and 60s as a congenital syndrome involving QT interval prolongation and syncope and sudden death. Some of the congenital long QT syndromes were characterized by a peculiar electrocardiographic appearance of the QRS complex involving a premature atria beat followed by a pause, then a subsequent sinus beat showing marked QT prolongation and deformity. This type of cardiac arrhythmia was originally termed "torsade de pointes" (translated from the French as "twisting of the points").

Prolongation of the QT interval is thought to result from delayed ventricular repolarization. The repolarization process within the myocardial cell is due to the efflux of intracellular potassium. The channels associated with this current can be blocked by many drugs and predispose the electrical propagation cycle to torsade de pointes.

Methadone is one of the drugs confirmed to prolong the QT interval and is accepted as having a risk of causing torsade de pointes. The risk of drug-induced torsade de pointes is extremely low when a single QT interval prolonging drug is prescribed. In terms of epinephrine, it is not known what effect vasoconstrictors in the local anesthetic regimen will have in patients with a known history of congenital prolonged QT interval or in patients taking any medication that prolongs the QT interval. Until more information is obtained, it is suggested that the clinician consult with the physician prior to the use of a vasoconstrictor in suspected patients, and that the vasoconstrictor (epinephrine, levonordefrin [Neo-Cobefrin®]) be used with caution.

Methamphetamine (meth am FET a meen)

U.S. Brand Names Desoxyn®

Canadian Brand Names Desoxyn®

Pharmacologic Category Anorexiant; Stimulant; Sympathomimetic

Use Treatment of attention-deficit/hyperactivity disorder (ADHD); exogenous obesity (short-term adjunct)

Pharmacotherapy for weight loss is recommended only for obese patients with a body mass index ≥30 kg/m^2, or ≥27 kg/m^2 in the presence of other risk factors such as hypertension, diabetes, and/or dyslipidemia or a high waist circumference; therapy should be used in conjunction with a comprehensive weight management program.

Unlabeled/Investigational Use Narcolepsy

Local Anesthetic/Vasoconstrictor Precautions Use vasoconstrictor with caution in patients taking methamphetamine. Amphetamines enhance the sympathomimetic response of epinephrine and norepinephrine leading to potential hypertension and cardiotoxicity.

Effects on Dental Treatment Key adverse event(s) related to dental treatment: Xerostomia (normal salivary flow resumes upon discontinuation) and unpleasant taste. Up to 10% of patients taking methamphetamine may present with hypertension. Monitor blood pressure prior to using local anesthetic with vasoconstrictors.

Effects on Bleeding No information available to require special precautions

Adverse Effects Frequency not defined.

Cardiovascular: Hypertension, palpitation, tachycardia

Central nervous system: Dizziness, dysphoria, euphoria, exacerbation of motor and phonic tics and Tourette's syndrome, headache, insomnia, overstimulation, psychosis, restlessness

Dermatologic: Rash, urticaria

Endocrine & metabolic: Change in libido

Gastrointestinal: Anorexia, constipation, diarrhea, nausea, stomach cramps, unpleasant taste, vomiting, weight loss, xerostomia

Genitourinary: Impotence

Neuromuscular & skeletal: Tremor

Miscellaneous: Suppression of growth in children, tolerance and withdrawal with prolonged use

General Dosage Range Oral:

Children ≥6-11 years: Initial: 5 mg 1-2 times/day; Maintenance: 20-25 mg/day

Children ≥12 years and Adults: ADHD: Initial: 5 mg 1-2 times/day; Maintenance: 20-25 mg/day; Obesity: 5 mg before each meal

Mechanism of Action A sympathomimetic amine related to ephedrine and amphetamine with CNS stimulant activity; causes release of catecholamines (primarily dopamine and other catecholamines) from their storage sites in the presynaptic nerve terminals. Inhibits reuptake and metabolism of catecholamines through inhibition of monoamine transporters and oxidase.

Pharmacodynamics/Kinetics

Half-life Elimination 4-5 hours

Pregnancy Risk Factor C

Controlled Substance C-II

Methazolamide (meth a ZOE la mide)

U.S. Brand Names Neptazane™

Canadian Brand Names Apo-Methazolamide®

Pharmacologic Category Carbonic Anhydrase Inhibitor; Diuretic, Carbonic Anhydrase Inhibitor; Ophthalmic Agent, Antiglaucoma

Use Treatment of chronic open-angle or secondary glaucoma; short-term therapy of acute angle-closure glaucoma prior to surgery

Local Anesthetic/Vasoconstrictor Precautions No information available to require special precautions

Effects on Dental Treatment Key adverse event(s) related to dental treatment: Xerostomia (normal salivary flow resumes upon discontinuation) and metallic taste.

Effects on Bleeding No information available to require special precautions

Adverse Effects Frequency not defined.

Central nervous system: Confusion, drowsiness, fatigue, fever, malaise, seizure
Dermatologic: Erythema multiforme, photosensitivity, rash, Stevens-Johnson syndrome, toxic epidermal necrolysis, urticaria
Endocrine & metabolic: Electrolyte imbalance, metabolic acidosis
Gastrointestinal: Appetite decreased, diarrhea, melena, nausea, taste alteration, vomiting
Genitourinary: Crystalluria, glycosuria, hematuria, polyuria, renal calculi
Hematologic: Agranulocytosis, aplastic anemia, bone marrow depression, hemolytic anemia, leukopenia, pancytopenia, thrombocytopenic purpura
Hepatic: Fulminant hepatic necrosis, hepatic insufficiency
Neuromuscular & skeletal: Flaccid paralysis, paresthesia
Ocular: Myopia
Otic: Hearing disturbance, tinnitus
Miscellaneous: Anaphylaxis, hypersensitivity

General Dosage Range Oral: *Adults:* 50-100 mg 2-3 times/day

Mechanism of Action Noncompetitive inhibition of the enzyme carbonic anhydrase; thought that carbonic anhydrase is located at the luminal border of cells of the proximal tubule. When the enzyme is inhibited, there is an increase in urine volume and a change to an alkaline pH with a subsequent decrease in the excretion of titratable acid and ammonia.

Pharmacodynamics/Kinetics

Onset of Action Slow in comparison with acetazolamide (2-4 hours); Peak effect: 6-8 hours

Duration of Action 10-18 hours

Half-life Elimination ~14 hours

Pregnancy Risk Factor C

Methenamine (meth EN a meen)

U.S. Brand Names Hiprex®

Canadian Brand Names Dehydral®; Hiprex®; Mandelamine®; Urasal®

Pharmacologic Category Antibiotic, Miscellaneous

Use Prophylaxis or suppression of recurrent urinary tract infections; urinary tract discomfort secondary to hypermotility

Local Anesthetic/Vasoconstrictor Precautions No information available to require special precautions

Effects on Dental Treatment No significant effects or complications reported

Effects on Bleeding No information available to require special precautions

Adverse Effects <4%:

Dermatologic: Pruritus, rash
Gastrointestinal: Dyspepsia, nausea, vomiting
Hepatic: ALT increased (reversible; rare), AST increased (reversible; rare)
Note: Large doses (higher than recommended) have resulted in bladder irritation, frequent/painful micturition, albuminuria, and hematuria.

General Dosage Range Oral:

Hippurate:
Children ≥6 years: 0.5-1 g twice daily
Adults: 1 g twice daily

Mandelate:
Children >2-6 years: 50-75 mg/kg/day in 3-4 divided doses **or** 0.25 g/30 lb 4 times/day
Children 6-12 years: 50-75 mg/kg/day in 3-4 divided doses **or** 0.5 g 4 times/day
Children >12 years and Adults: 1 g 4 times/day

Mechanism of Action Methenamine is hydrolyzed to formaldehyde and ammonia in acidic urine; formaldehyde has nonspecific bactericidal action. Other components, hippuric acid or mandelic acid, aid in maintaining urine acidity and may aid in suppressing bacteria.

Pharmacodynamics/Kinetics

Half-life Elimination 3-6 hours

Pregnancy Risk Factor C (methenamine mandelate)

Methenamine, Phenyl Salicylate, Methylene Blue, Benzoic Acid, and Hyoscyamine

(meth EN a meen, fen nil sa LIS i late, METH i leen bloo, ben ZOE ik AS id & hye oh SYE a meen)

Related Information

Hyoscyamine *on page 878*
Methenamine *on page 1094*

U.S. Brand Names Prosed®/DS

Pharmacologic Category Antibiotic, Miscellaneous

Use Urinary tract discomfort secondary to hypermotility resulting from infection or diagnostic procedures

Local Anesthetic/Vasoconstrictor Precautions No information available to require special precautions

Effects on Dental Treatment Key adverse event(s) related to dental treatment: Xerostomia (normal salivary flow resumes upon discontinuation).

Effects on Bleeding No information available to require special precautions

Adverse Effects Frequency not defined.

Cardiovascular: Flushing, tachycardia
Central nervous system: Dizziness
Gastrointestinal: Discoloration of stool (blue), nausea, vomiting, xerostomia
Genitourinary: Discoloration of urine (blue), micturition difficulty, urinary retention (acute)
Ocular: Blurred vision
Respiratory: Dyspnea

General Dosage Range Oral: *Adults:* 1 tablet 4 times/day

Pregnancy Risk Factor C

Methenamine, Sodium Biphosphate, Phenyl Salicylate, Methylene Blue, and Hyoscyamine

(meth EN a meen, SOW dee um bye FOS fate, fen nil sa LIS i late, METH i leen bloo, & hye oh SYE a meen)

Related Information

Hyoscyamine *on page 878*
Methenamine *on page 1094*

U.S. Brand Names Urelle®; Uribel™; Uta®; Utira™-C [DSC]; Utrona-C [DSC]

Pharmacologic Category Antibiotic, Miscellaneous

Use Treatment of symptoms of irritative voiding; relief of local symptoms associated with urinary tract infections; relief of urinary tract symptoms caused by diagnostic procedures

Local Anesthetic/Vasoconstrictor Precautions No information available to require special precautions

Effects on Dental Treatment Key adverse event(s) related to dental treatment: Xerostomia (normal salivary flow resumes upon discontinuation)

Effects on Bleeding No information available to require special precautions

Adverse Effects Frequency not defined.

Cardiovascular: Tachycardia, flushing
Central nervous system: Dizziness
Gastrointestinal: Xerostomia, nausea, vomiting
Genitourinary: Urinary retention (acute), micturition difficulty, discoloration of urine (blue)
Ocular: Blurred vision
Respiratory: Dyspnea

General Dosage Range Oral: *Adults:* 1 tablet 4 times/day

Pregnancy Risk Factor C

Methimazole (meth IM a zole)

Related Information

Endocrine Disorders and Pregnancy *on page 1879*

U.S. Brand Names Tapazole®

Canadian Brand Names Dom-Methimazole; PHL-Methimazole; Tapazole®
Pharmacologic Category Antithyroid Agent; Thioamide
Use Treatment of hyperthyroidism; improve hyperthyroidism prior to thyroidectomy or radioactive iodine therapy
Local Anesthetic/Vasoconstrictor Precautions No information available to require special precautions
Effects on Dental Treatment Key adverse event(s) related to dental treatment: Abnormal taste and salivary gland swelling.
Effects on Bleeding No information available to require special precautions
Adverse Effects Frequency not defined.
Cardiovascular: ANCA-positive vasculitis, edema, leukocytoclastic vasculitis, periarteritis
Central nervous system: Drowsiness, fever, headache, neuritis, vertigo
Dermatologic: Alopecia, exfoliative dermatitis, pruritus, skin pigmentation, skin rash, urticaria
Endocrine & metabolic: Goiter, hypoglycemic coma
Gastrointestinal: Constipation, epigastric distress, loss of taste perception, nausea, salivary gland swelling, vomiting, weight gain
Hematologic: Agranulocytosis, aplastic anemia, granulocytopenia, hypoprothrombinemia, leukopenia, thrombocytopenia
Hepatic: Hepatic necrosis, hepatitis, jaundice
Neuromuscular & skeletal: Arthralgia, myalgia, paresthesia
Renal: Nephritis
Miscellaneous: Insulin autoimmune syndrome, lymphadenopathy, SLE-like syndrome

General Dosage Range Oral:
Children: Initial: 0.4 mg/kg/day in 3 divided doses; Maintenance: 0.2 mg/kg/day in 3 divided doses
Adults: Initial: 15-60 mg/day in 3 divided doses; Maintenance: 5-15 mg/day in 1-3 divided doses

Mechanism of Action Inhibits the synthesis of thyroid hormones by blocking the oxidation of iodine in the thyroid gland. As a result, methimazole inhibits the ability of iodine to combine with tyrosine to form thyroxine and triiodothyronine (T_3); does not inactivate circulating T_4 and T_3

Pharmacodynamics/Kinetics
Onset of Action Antithyroid: Oral: 12-18 hours
Duration of Action 36-72 hours
Half-life Elimination 4-6 hours
Time to Peak Serum concentration: 1-2 hours

Pregnancy Risk Factor D

Methocarbamol (meth oh KAR ba mole)

Related Information
Temporomandibular Dysfunction (TMD) *on page 1964*
U.S. Brand Names Robaxin®; Robaxin®-750
Canadian Brand Names Robaxin®
Generic Availability (U.S.) Yes: Tablet
Pharmacologic Category Skeletal Muscle Relaxant
Dental Use Treatment of muscle spasm associated with acute temporomandibular joint pain (TMJ)
Use Adjunctive treatment of muscle spasm associated with acute painful musculoskeletal conditions (eg, tetanus)
Local Anesthetic/Vasoconstrictor Precautions No information available to require special precautions
Effects on Dental Treatment Key adverse event(s) related to dental treatment: Metallic taste.
Effects on Bleeding No information available to require special precautions
Adverse Effects Frequency not defined.
Cardiovascular: Bradycardia, flushing, hypotension, syncope
Central nervous system: Amnesia, confusion, coordination impaired (mild), dizziness, drowsiness, fever, headache, insomnia, lightheadedness, sedation, seizures, vertigo
Dermatologic: Angioneurotic edema, pruritus, rash, urticaria
Gastrointestinal: Dyspepsia, metallic taste, nausea, vomiting
Hematologic: Leukopenia
Hepatic: Jaundice
Local: Pain at injection site, thrombophlebitis
Ocular: Blurred vision, conjunctivitis, diplopia, nystagmus

Respiratory: Nasal congestion
Miscellaneous: Hypersensitivity reactions including anaphylaxis

Dental Usual Dosage Muscle spasm associated with acute TMJ pain: Children ≥16 years and Adults: Oral: 1.5 g 4 times/day for 2-3 days (up to 8 g/day may be given in severe conditions), then decrease to 4-4.5 g/day in 3-6 divided doses

Dosage

Tetanus: I.V.:

Children: Recommended **only** for use in tetanus: 15 mg/kg/dose or 500 mg/m²/dose, may repeat every 6 hours if needed; maximum dose: 1.8 g/m²/day for 3 days only

Adults: Initial dose: 1-2 g by direct I.V. injection, which may be followed by an additional 1-2 g by infusion (maximum initial dose: 3 g total); followed by 1-2 g every 6 hours until oral administration by mouth or via NG tube is possible; total oral daily doses of up to 24 g may be needed; injection should not be used for more than 3 consecutive days

Muscle spasm:

Oral: Children ≥16 years and Adults: 1.5 g 4 times/day for 2-3 days (up to 8 g/day may be given in severe conditions), then decrease to 4-4.5 g/day in 3-6 divided doses

I.M., I.V.: Adults: Initial: 1 g; may repeat every 8 hours if oral administration not possible; maximum dose: 3 g/day for no more than 3 consecutive days. If condition persists, may repeat course of therapy after a drug-free interval of 48 hours.

Dosing adjustment/comments in renal impairment: Administration of the parenteral formulation is contraindicated in patients with renal dysfunction due to the presence of polyethylene glycol.

Dosing adjustment in hepatic impairment: Specific dosing guidelines are not available.

Mechanism of Action Causes skeletal muscle relaxation by general CNS depression

Contraindications Hypersensitivity to methocarbamol or any component of the formulation; renal impairment (injection formulation)

Warnings/Precautions May cause CNS depression, which may impair physical or mental abilities; patients must be cautioned about performing tasks which require mental alertness (eg, operating machinery or driving). Effects may be potentiated when used with other sedative drugs or ethanol. Plasma protein binding and clearance are decreased and the half-life is increased in patients with hepatic impairment. This class of medication is poorly tolerated by the elderly due to anticholinergic effects, sedation, and weakness. Efficacy is questionable at dosages tolerated by elderly patients (Beers Criteria).

Injection: Contraindicated in renal impairment. Contains polyethylene glycol. Rate of injection should not exceed 3 mL/minute; solution is hypertonic; avoid extravasation. Use with caution in patients with a history of seizures. Use caution with hepatic impairment. Vial stopper contains latex. Recommended only for the treatment of tetanus in pediatric patients.

Drug Interactions

Avoid Concomitant Use There are no known interactions where it is recommended to avoid concomitant use.

Increased Effect/Toxicity

Methocarbamol may increase the levels/effects of: Alcohol (Ethyl); CNS Depressants; Methotrimeprazine

The levels/effects of Methocarbamol may be increased by: Droperidol; Methotrimeprazine

Decreased Effect

Methocarbamol may decrease the levels/effects of: Pyridostigmine

Ethanol/Nutrition/Herb Interactions

Ethanol: May increase CNS depression; monitor for increased effects with coadministration. Caution patients about effects.

Herb/Nutraceutical: Avoid valerian, St John's wort, kava kava, gotu kola (may increase CNS depression).

Pharmacodynamics/Kinetics

Onset of Action Muscle relaxation: Oral: ~30 minutes

Half-life Elimination 1-2 hours

Time to Peak Serum: Oral: 1-2 hours

Pregnancy Risk Factor C

Lactation Excretion in breast milk unknown/use caution

Dosage Forms
Injection, solution:
Robaxin®: 100 mg/mL (10 mL)
Tablet, oral: 500 mg, 750 mg
Robaxin®: 500 mg
Robaxin®-750: 750 mg

Methohexital (meth oh HEKS i tal)

U.S. Brand Names Brevital® Sodium
Canadian Brand Names Brevital®
Generic Availability (U.S.) No
Pharmacologic Category Barbiturate; General Anesthetic
Dental Use Induction and maintenance of general anesthesia for short procedures
Use For induction of anesthesia prior to the use of other general anesthetic agents; as an adjunct to subpotent inhalational anesthetic agents for short surgical procedures; for short surgical, diagnostic, or therapeutic procedures associated with minimal painful stimuli

Additional indications for adults: For use with other parenteral agents, usually narcotic analgesics, to supplement subpotent inhalational anesthetic agents for longer surgical procedures; as an agent to induce a hypnotic state

Unlabeled/Investigational Use Wada test
Local Anesthetic/Vasoconstrictor Precautions No information available to require special precautions
Effects on Dental Treatment No significant effects or complications reported
Effects on Bleeding No information available to require special precautions
Adverse Effects Frequency not defined.
Cardiovascular: Cardiorespiratory arrest, circulatory depression, hypotension, peripheral vascular collapse, tachycardia
Central nervous system: Anxiety, emergence delirium, headache, restlessness, seizure
Dermatologic: Erythema, pruritus, urticaria
Gastrointestinal: Abdominal pain, nausea, salivation, vomiting
Hepatic: Transaminases increased
Local: Injection site pain, nerve injury adjacent to injection site, thrombophlebitis
Neuromuscular & skeletal: Involuntary muscle movement, radial nerve palsy, rigidity, tremor, twitching
Respiratory: Apnea, bronchospasm, cough, dyspnea, hiccups, laryngospasm, respiratory depression, rhinitis
Miscellaneous: Anaphylaxis (rare)

Dental Usual Dosage Induction and maintenance of general anesthesia for short procedures: Doses must be titrated to effect: Adults: I.V.: Induction: 50-120 mg to start; 20-40 mg every 4-7 minutes
Dosage Doses must be titrated to effect.
Infants <1 month: Safety and efficacy not established
Infants ≥1 month and Children:
Anesthesia induction:
I.M.: 6.6-10 mg/kg of a 5% solution
Rectal: Usual: 25 mg/kg of a 1% solution
I.V. (unlabeled dose): 1-2 mg/kg/dose of a 1% solution
Procedural sedation (unlabeled dose):
I.V.: Initial: 0.5 mg/kg given immediately prior to procedure; if sedation not adequate, repeat 0.5 mg/kg to a maximum total dose of 2 mg/kg
Rectal: 25 mg/kg of a 10% (100 mg/mL) solution given 5-15 minutes prior to procedure; maximum dose 500 mg
Adults: I.V.:
Induction: 1-1.5 mg/kg; maintenance: 50-120 mcg/kg/minute (or 20-40 mg every 4-7 minutes)
Wada test (unlabeled): 2-4 mg

Dosing adjustment/comments in hepatic impairment: Lower dosage and monitor closely

Mechanism of Action Ultra short-acting I.V. barbiturate anesthetic
Contraindications Hypersensitivity to barbiturates, methohexital, or any component of the formulation; porphyria (latent or manifest); patients in whom general anesthesia is contraindicated
Warnings/Precautions Use with caution in patients with liver impairment, renal impairment, cardiovascular disease (including heart failure), severe anemia, extreme obesity, or seizure disorder, the elderly and children. May cause hypotension; use with caution in hemodynamically unstable patients (hypotension or shock) or severe hypertension. May cause respiratory depression; use with caution

in patients with pulmonary disease. Use with caution in patients with asthma and chronic obstructive pulmonary disease. Use with extreme caution in patients with ongoing status asthmaticus; hiccups, coughing, laryngospasm, and muscle twitching have occurred impairing ventilation.

Postmarketing studies have indicated that the use of hypnotic/sedative agents for sleep has been associated with hypersensitivity reactions including anaphylaxis as well as angioedema. Effects with other sedative drugs or ethanol may be potentiated. Repeated dosing or continuous infusions may cause cumulative effects. Ensure patient has intravenous access; extravasation or intra-arterial injection causes necrosis. **[U.S. Boxed Warning]: Should only be administered in hospitals or ambulatory care settings with continuous monitoring of respiratory function; resuscitative drugs, age- and size-appropriate and intubation equipment and trained personnel experienced in handling their use should be readily available. For deeply sedated patients, a healthcare provider other than the individual performing the procedure should be present to continuously monitor the patient.**

Drug Interactions

Avoid Concomitant Use There are no known interactions where it is recommended to avoid concomitant use.

Increased Effect/Toxicity

Methohexital may increase the levels/effects of: Alcohol (Ethyl); CNS Depressants; Meperidine; QuiNIDine; Thiazide Diuretics

The levels/effects of Methohexital may be increased by: Chloramphenicol; Divalproex; Droperidol; Felbamate; Primidone; Valproic Acid

Decreased Effect

Methohexital may decrease the levels/effects of: Acetaminophen; Beta-Blockers; Calcium Channel Blockers; Chloramphenicol; Contraceptives (Estrogens); Contraceptives (Progestins); Corticosteroids (Systemic); CycloSPORINE; CycloSPORINE (Systemic); Disopyramide; Divalproex; Doxycycline; Etoposide; Etoposide Phosphate; Felbamate; Fosphenytoin; LamoTRIgine; Methadone; Phenytoin; Propafenone; QuiNIDine; Teniposide; Theophylline Derivatives; Tricyclic Antidepressants; Valproic Acid; Vitamin K Antagonists

The levels/effects of Methohexital may be decreased by: Pyridoxine; Rifamycin Derivatives

Pharmacodynamics/Kinetics

Onset of Action I.V.: Immediate; I.M. (pediatrics): 2-10 minutes; Rectal (pediatrics): 5-15 minutes

Duration of Action Single dose: I.V.: 10-20 minutes; Rectal: 45 minutes

Pregnancy Risk Factor B

Lactation Enters breast milk/use caution

Breast-Feeding Considerations Methohexital is minimally excreted in breast milk and levels decline rapidly after administration. Interruption of breast-feeding is unnecessary.

Controlled Substance C-IV

Dosage Forms

Injection, powder for reconstitution:

Brevital® Sodium: 500 mg, 2.5 g

References

Buchtel HA, Passaro EA, Selwa LM, et al, "Sodium Methohexital (Brevital) as an Anesthetic in the Wada Test," *Epilepsia*, 2002, 43(9):1056-61.
Cote' CJ, "Sedation for the Pediatric Patient," *Pediatr Clin North Am*, 1994, 41(1):31-58.
Dionne RA, Yagiela JA, Moore PA, et al, "Comparing Efficacy and Safety of Four Intravenous Sedation Regimens in Dental Outpatients," *Am Dent Assoc*, 2001, 132(6):740-51.

Methotrexate (meth oh TREKS ate)

Related Information

Rheumatoid Arthritis, Osteoarthritis, and Osteoporosis *on page 1889*

U.S. Brand Names Rheumatrex®; Trexall™

Canadian Brand Names Apo-Methotrexate®; ratio-Methotrexate

Generic Availability (U.S.) Yes

Pharmacologic Category Antineoplastic Agent, Antimetabolite (Antifolate); Antirheumatic, Disease Modifying; Immunosuppressant Agent

Use

Oncology-related uses: Treatment of trophoblastic neoplasms (gestational choriocarcinoma, chorioadenoma destruens and hydatidiform mole), acute lymphocytic leukemia (ALL), meningeal leukemia, breast cancer, head and neck cancer (epidermoid), cutaneous T-Cell lymphoma (advanced mycosis fungoides), lung cancer (squamous cell and small cell), advanced non-Hodgkin's lymphomas (NHL), osteosarcoma

Nononcology uses: Treatment of psoriasis (severe, recalcitrant, disabling) and severe rheumatoid arthritis (RA), including polyarticular-course juvenile idiopathic arthritis (JIA)

Unlabeled/Investigational Use Treatment and maintenance of remission in Crohn's disease; ectopic pregnancy; dermatomyositis/polymyositis; bladder cancer, central nervous system tumors (including nonleukemic meningeal cancers), acute promyelocytic leukemia (maintenance treatment), soft tissue sarcoma (desmoid tumors); acute graft-versus-host disease (GVHD) prophylaxis; medical management of abortion; systemic lupus erythematosus; Takayasu arteritis

Local Anesthetic/Vasoconstrictor Precautions No information available to require special precautions

Effects on Dental Treatment Key adverse event(s) related to dental treatment: Ulcerative stomatitis, gingivitis, glossitis, and mucositis (dose dependent; appears 3-7 days post-therapy and resolves within 2 weeks). Dental professionals should note before prescribing NSAIDS that concurrent administration with methotrexate may cause severe bone marrow suppression, aplastic anemia, and GI toxicity (see Warnings/Precautions). Although the risk is lower at the methotrexate dosages used for rheumatoid conditions/psoriasis, the addition of an NSAID or salicylate may still lead to unexpected toxicities; caution is warranted.

Effects on Bleeding Chemotherapy may result in significant myelosuppression, potentially including significant reduction in platelet counts and altered hemostasis. Methotrexate is also used to manage rheumatoid conditions. At the dosages used in rheumatoid management, the risk of thrombocytopenia is low. In patients who are receiving this medication as a component of cancer chemotherapy, medical consult is suggested.

Adverse Effects Note: Adverse reactions vary by route and dosage. Hematologic and/or gastrointestinal toxicities may be common at dosages used in chemotherapy; these reactions are much less frequent when used at typical dosages for rheumatic diseases.

>10%:

Central nervous system (with I.T. administration or very high-dose therapy):

Arachnoiditis: Acute reaction manifested as severe headache, nuchal rigidity, vomiting, and fever; may be alleviated by reducing the dose

Subacute toxicity: 10% of patients treated with 12-15 mg/m^2 of I.T. methotrexate may develop this in the second or third week of therapy; consists of motor paralysis of extremities, cranial nerve palsy, seizure, or coma. This has also been seen in pediatric cases receiving very high-dose I.V. methotrexate.

Demyelinating encephalopathy: Seen months or years after receiving methotrexate; usually in association with cranial irradiation or other systemic chemotherapy

Dermatologic: Reddening of skin

Endocrine & metabolic: Hyperuricemia, defective oogenesis or spermatogenesis

Gastrointestinal: Ulcerative stomatitis, glossitis, gingivitis, nausea, vomiting, diarrhea, anorexia, intestinal perforation, mucositis (dose dependent; appears in 3-7 days after therapy, resolving within 2 weeks)

Hematologic: Leukopenia, myelosuppression (nadir: 7-10 days), thrombocytopenia

Renal: Renal failure, azotemia, nephropathy

Respiratory: Pharyngitis

1% to 10%:

Cardiovascular: Vasculitis

Central nervous system: Dizziness, malaise, encephalopathy, seizure, fever, chills

Dermatologic: Alopecia, rash, photosensitivity, depigmentation or hyperpigmentation of skin

Endocrine & metabolic: Diabetes

Genitourinary: Cystitis

Hematologic: Hemorrhage

Hepatic: Cirrhosis and portal fibrosis have been associated with chronic methotrexate therapy; acute elevation of liver enzymes are common after high-dose methotrexate, and usually resolve within 10 days.

Neuromuscular & skeletal: Arthralgia

Ocular: Blurred vision

Renal: Renal dysfunction: Manifested by an abrupt rise in serum creatinine and BUN and a fall in urine output; more common with high-dose methotrexate, and may be due to precipitation of the drug.

Respiratory: Pneumonitis: Associated with fever, cough, and interstitial pulmonary infiltrates; treatment is to withhold methotrexate during the acute reaction; interstitial pneumonitis has been reported to occur with an incidence of 1% in patients with RA (dose 7.5-15 mg/week)

Dosage Details concerning dosing in combination regimens should also be consulted.

Note: Doses between 100-500 mg/m^2 **may require** leucovorin calcium rescue. Doses >500 mg/m^2 **require** leucovorin calcium rescue: Oral, I.M., I.V.: Leucovorin calcium 10-15 mg/m^2 every 6 hours for 8 or 10 doses, starting 24 hours after the start of methotrexate infusion. Continue until the methotrexate level is ≤0.1 micromolar (10^{-7} M). Some clinicians continue leucovorin calcium until the methotrexate level is <0.05 micromolar (5 x 10^{-8} M) or 0.01 micromolar (10^{-8} M).

If the 48-hour methotrexate level is >1 micromolar (10^{-6} M) or the 72-hour methotrexate level is >0.2 micromolar (2 x 10^{-7} M): I.V., I.M, Oral: Leucovorin calcium 100 mg/m^2 every 6 hours until the methotrexate level is ≤0.1 micromolar (10^{-7} M). Some clinicians continue leucovorin calcium until the methotrexate level is <0.05 micromolar (5 x 10^{-8} M) or 0.01 micromolar (10^{-8} M).

Children:

Dermatomyositis (unlabeled use): Oral: 15-20 mg/m^2/week as a single dose once weekly **or** 0.3-1 mg/kg/dose once weekly

GVHD (acute) prophylaxis (unlabeled use): I.V.: Refer to adult dosing.

Juvenile idiopathic arthritis (JIA): Oral, I.M.: 10 mg/m^2 once weekly, then 5-15 mg/m^2/week as a single dose **or** as 3 divided doses given 12 hours apart

Antineoplastic dosage range:
- Oral, I.M.: 7.5-30 mg/m^2/week **or** every 2 weeks
- I.V.: 10-18,000 mg/m^2 bolus dosing **or** continuous infusion over 6-42 hours

Pediatric solid tumors (high-dose): I.V.:
- <12 years: 12-25 g/m^2
- ≥12 years: 8 g/m^2

Acute lymphocytic leukemia (intermediate-dose): I.V.: Loading: 100 mg/m^2 bolus dose, followed by 900 mg/m^2/day infusion over 23-41 hours.

Meningeal leukemia: I.T.: 6-12 mg/dose based on age. **Note:** Optimal intrathecal chemotherapy dosing should be based on age rather than on body surface area (BSA); CSF volume correlates with age and not to BSA (Bleyer, 1983; Kerr, 2001):
- <1 year: 6 mg/dose
- 1 year: 8 mg/dose
- 2 years: 10 mg/dose
- ≥3 years: 12 mg/dose

Adults:

Antineoplastic dosage range: I.V.: Range is wide from 30-40 mg/m^2/week to 100-12,000 mg/m^2 with leucovorin calcium rescue

Breast cancer: I.V.: 30-60 mg/m^2 days 1 and 8 every 3-4 weeks

Head and neck cancer: Oral, I.M., I.V.: 25-50 mg/m^2 once weekly

Lymphoma, non-Hodgkin's: I.V.:
- 30 mg/m^2 days 3 and 10 every 3 weeks **or**
- 120 mg/m^2 day 8 and 15 every 3-4 weeks **or**
- 200 mg/m^2 day 8 and 15 every 3 weeks **or**
- 400 mg/m^2 every 4 weeks for 3 cycles **or**
- 1 g/m^2 every 3 weeks **or**
- 1.5 g/m^2 every 4 weeks

Meningeal leukemia: I.T.: Usual dose: 12 mg/dose. **Note:** Optimal intrathecal chemotherapy dosing should be based on age rather than on body surface area (BSA); CSF volume correlates with age and not to BSA (Bleyer, 1983; Kerr, 2001).

Mycosis fungoides (cutaneous T-cell lymphoma): Oral, I.M.: Initial (early stages):
- 5-50 mg once weekly **or**
- 15-37.5 mg twice weekly

Osteosarcoma: I.V.: 8-12 g/m^2 weekly for 2-4 weeks

Psoriasis: **Note:** Some experts recommend concomitant folic acid 1-5 mg/day (except the day of methotrexate) to reduce hematologic, gastrointestinal, and hepatic adverse events related to methotrexate.
- Oral: 2.5-5 mg/dose every 12 hours for 3 doses given weekly **or**
- Oral, I.M., SubQ: 10-25 mg/dose given once weekly; titrate to lowest effective dose

Note: An initial test dose of 2.5-5 mg is recommended in patients with risk factors for hematologic toxicity or renal impairment (Kalb, 2009).

Rheumatoid arthritis: **Note:** Some experts recommend concomitant folic acid at a dose of least 5 mg/week (except the day of methotrexate) to reduce hematologic, gastrointestinal, and hepatic adverse events related to methotrexate.

Oral (manufacturer labeling): 7.5 mg once weekly or 2.5 mg every 12 hours for 3 doses/week (dosage exceeding 20 mg/week may cause a higher incidence and severity of adverse events); *alternatively,* 10-15 mg once weekly, increased by 5 mg every 2-4 weeks to a maximum of 20-30 mg once weekly has been recommended by some experts (Visser, 2009)

I.M., SubQ (unlabeled route): 15 mg once weekly (dosage varies, similar to oral) (Braun, 2008)

Trophoblastic neoplasms:

Oral, I.M.: 15-30 mg/day for 5 days; repeat in 7 days for 3-5 courses

I.V.: 11 mg/m² days 1 through 5 every 3 weeks

Unlabeled uses:

Active Crohn's disease (unlabeled use): Induction of remission: I.M., SubQ: 15-25 mg once weekly; remission maintenance: 15 mg once weekly

Note: Oral dosing has been reported as effective but oral absorption is highly variable. If patient relapses after a switch to oral, may consider returning to injectable.

Bladder cancer (unlabeled use): I.V.:

30 mg/m² day 1 and 8 every 3 weeks **or**

30 mg/m² day 1, 15, and 22 every 4 weeks

Dermatomyositis/polymyositis (unlabeled uses):

Oral: Initial: 7.5-15 mg/week, often adjunctively with high-dose corticosteroid therapy; may increase in weekly 2.5 mg increments to target dose of 10-25 mg/week (**Note:** Administration of folate 5-7 mg/week has been used to reduce side effects). (Briemberg, 2003; Newman, 1995; Wiendl, 2008)

I.V., I.M.: Doses of 20-60 mg/week have been employed if failure with oral therapy (doses >50 mg/week may require leucovorin calcium rescue) (Briemberg, 2003)

Ectopic pregnancy (unlabeled use): I.M.:

Single-dose regimen: Methotrexate 50 mg/m² on day 1; Measure serum hCG levels on days 4 and 7; if needed, repeat dose on day 7 (Barnhart, 2009)

Two-dose regimen: Methotrexate 50 mg/m² on day 1; Measure serum hCG levels on day 4 and administer a second dose of methotrexate 50 mg/m²; Measure serum hCG levels on day 7 and if needed, administer a third dose of 50 mg/m² (Barnhart, 2009)

Multidose regimen: Methotrexate 1 mg/kg on day 1; leucovorin calcium 0.1 mg/kg I.M. on day 2; measure serum hCG on day 2; methotrexate 1 mg/kg on day 3; leucovorin calcium 0.1 mg/kg on day 4; measure serum hCG on day 4; continue up to a total of 4 courses based on hCG concentrations (Barnhart, 2009)

GVHD (acute) prophylaxis: I.V.: 15 mg/m²/dose on day 1 and 10 mg/m²/dose on days 3 and 6 after allogeneic transplant (in combination with cyclosporine and prednisone) (Chao, 1993; Chao, 2000; Ross, 1999) **or** 15 mg/m²/dose on day 1 and 10 mg/m²/dose on days 3, 6, and 11 after allogeneic transplant (in combination with cyclosporine) (Chao, 2000)

Nonleukemic meningeal cancer (unlabeled uses): I.T.: 10-12 mg/dose twice weekly for 4 weeks, then weekly for 4 weeks, then monthly (NCCN CNS cancer guidelines v.2.2009) **or** 12 mg/dose twice weekly for 4 weeks, then weekly for 4 doses, then monthly for 4 doses (Glantz, 1998) **or** 10 mg twice weekly for 4 weeks, then weekly for 1 month, then every 2 weeks for 2 months (Glantz, 1999)

Takayasu arteritis, refractory or relapsing disease (unlabeled use): Oral: Initial dose: 0.3 mg/kg/week (maximum: 15 mg/week), titrated by 2.5 mg increments every 1-2 weeks until reaching a maximum tolerated weekly dose of 25 mg (use in combination with a corticosteroid; Hoffman, 1994)

Elderly:

Meningeal leukemia: I.T.: Consider a dose reduction (CSF volume and turnover may decrease with age)

Rheumatoid arthritis/psoriasis: Oral: Initial: 5-7.5 mg/week, not to exceed 20 mg/week

Dosing adjustment in renal impairment: The FDA-approved labeling does not contain dosage adjustment guidelines. The following guidelines have been used by some clinicians:

Cl_{cr} 61-80 mL/minute: Administer 75% of dose

Cl_{cr} 51-60 mL/minute: Administer 70% of dose

Cl_{cr} 10-50 mL/minute: Administer 30% to 50% of dose

Cl_{cr} <10 mL/minute: Avoid use

Hemodialysis: Not dialyzable (0% to 5%); supplemental dose is not necessary

Peritoneal dialysis effects: Supplemental dose is not necessary

CAVH effects: Unknown

Aronoff, 2007:
Children:
Cl_{cr} 10-50 mL/minute: Administer 50% of dose
Cl_{cr} <10 mL/minute: Administer 30% of dose
Hemodialysis: Administer 30% of dose
Continuous ambulatory peritoneal dialysis (CAPD): Administer 30% of dose
Continuous renal replacement therapy (CRRT): Administer 50% of dose
Adults:
Cl_{cr} 10-50 mL/minute: Administer 50% of dose
Cl_{cr} <10 mL/minute: Avoid use
Hemodialysis: Administer 50% of dose
Continuous renal replacement therapy (CRRT): Administer 50% of dose

Kintzel, 1995:
Cl_{cr} 46-60 mL/minute: Administer 65% of normal dose
Cl_{cr} 31-45 mL/minute: Administer 50% of normal dose
Cl_{cr} <30 mL/minute: Avoid use

Dosage adjustment in hepatic impairment: The FDA-approved labeling does not contain dosage adjustment guidelines. The following guidelines have been used by some clinicians (Floyd, 2006):
Bilirubin 3.1-5 mg/dL **or** transaminases >3 times ULN: Administer 75% of dose
Bilirubin >5 mg/dL: Avoid use

Mechanism of Action Methotrexate is a folate antimetabolite that inhibits DNA synthesis. Methotrexate irreversibly binds to dihydrofolate reductase, inhibiting the formation of reduced folates, and thymidylate synthetase, resulting in inhibition of purine and thymidylic acid synthesis. Methotrexate is cell cycle specific for the S phase of the cycle.

The MOA in the treatment of rheumatoid arthritis is unknown, but may affect immune function. In psoriasis, methotrexate is thought to target rapidly proliferating epithelial cells in the skin.

In Crohn's disease, it may have immune modulator and anti-inflammatory activity.

Contraindications Hypersensitivity to methotrexate or any component of the formulation; breast-feeding

Additional contraindications for patients with psoriasis or rheumatoid arthritis: Pregnancy, alcoholism, alcoholic liver disease or other chronic liver disease, immunodeficiency syndrome (overt or laboratory evidence); pre-existing blood dyscrasias (eg, bone marrow hypoplasia, leukopenia, thrombocytopenia, significant anemia)

Warnings/Precautions Hazardous agent - use appropriate precautions for handling and disposal.

[U.S. Boxed Warning]: Methotrexate has been associated with acute (elevated transaminases) and potentially fatal chronic (fibrosis, cirrhosis) hepatotoxicity. Risk is related to cumulative dose and prolonged exposure. Monitor closely (with liver function tests, including serum albumin) for liver toxicities. Liver enzyme elevations may be noted, but may not be predictive of hepatic disease in long term treatment for psoriasis (but generally is predictive in rheumatoid arthritis [RA] treatment). With long-term use, liver biopsy may show histologic changes, fibrosis, or cirrhosis; periodic liver biopsy is recommended with long-term use for psoriasis patients with risk factors for hepatotoxicity and for persistent abnormal liver function tests in psoriasis patients without risk factors for hepatotoxicity and in RA patients; discontinue methotrexate with moderate-to-severe change in liver biopsy. Risk factors for hepatotoxicity include history of above moderate ethanol consumption, persistent abnormal liver chemistries, history of chronic liver disease (including hepatitis B or C), family history of inheritable liver disease, diabetes, obesity, hyperlipidemia, lack of folate supplementation during methotrexate therapy, and history of significant exposure to hepatotoxic drugs. Use caution with preexisting liver impairment; may require dosage reduction. Use caution when used with other hepatotoxic agents (azathioprine, retinoids, sulfasalazine). **[U.S. Boxed Warning]: Methotrexate elimination is reduced in patients with ascites;** may require dose reduction or discontinuation. Monitor closely for toxicity.

[U.S. Boxed Warning]: May cause renal damage leading to acute renal failure, especially with high-dose methotrexate; monitor renal function and methotrexate levels closely, maintain adequate hydration and urinary alkalinization. Use caution in osteosarcoma patients treated with high-dose methotrexate in combination with nephrotoxic chemotherapy (eg, cisplatin). **[U.S. Boxed Warning]: Methotrexate elimination is reduced in patients with renal impairment;** may require dose reduction or discontinuation; monitor closely for toxicity. **[U.S. Boxed Warning]: Tumor lysis syndrome may occur in patients with high tumor burden;** use appropriate prevention and treatment.

[U.S. Boxed Warning]: May cause potentially life-threatening pneumonitis (may occur at any time during therapy and at any dosage); monitor closely for pulmonary symptoms, particularly dry, nonproductive cough. Other potential symptoms include fever, dyspnea, hypoxemia, or pulmonary infiltrate. **[U.S. Boxed Warning]: Methotrexate elimination is reduced in patients with pleural effusions;** may require dose reduction or discontinuation. Monitor closely for toxicity.

[U.S. Boxed Warning]: Bone marrow suppression may occur, resulting in anemia, aplastic anemia, pancytopenia, leukopenia, neutropenia, and/or thrombocytopenia. Use caution in patients with pre-existing bone marrow suppression. Discontinue therapy in RA or psoriasis if a significant decrease in hematologic components is noted. **[U.S. Boxed Warning]: Use of low dose methotrexate has been associated with the development of malignant lymphomas;** may regress upon discontinuation of therapy; treat lymphoma appropriately if regression is not induced by cessation of methotrexate.

[U.S. Boxed Warning]: Diarrhea and ulcerative stomatitis may require interruption of therapy; death from hemorrhagic enteritis or intestinal perforation has been reported. Use with caution in patients with peptic ulcer disease, ulcerative colitis.

May cause neurotoxicity including seizures (usually in pediatric ALL patients), leukoencephalopathy (usually with concurrent cranial irradiation) and stroke-like encephalopathy (usually with high-dose regimens). Chemical arachnoiditis (headache, back pain, nuchal rigidity, fever), myelopathy and chronic leukoencephalopathy may result from intrathecal administration.

[U.S. Boxed Warning]: Any dose level or route of administration may cause severe and potentially fatal dermatologic reactions, including toxic epidermal necrolysis, Stevens-Johnson syndrome, exfoliative dermatitis, skin necrosis, and erythema multiforme. Radiation dermatitis and sunburn may be precipitated by methotrexate administration. Psoriatic lesions may be worsened by concomitant exposure to ultraviolet radiation.

[U.S. Boxed Warning]: Concomitant administration with NSAIDs may cause severe bone marrow suppression, aplastic anemia, and GI toxicity. Do not administer NSAIDs prior to or during high dose methotrexate therapy; may increase and prolong serum methotrexate levels. Doses used for psoriasis may still lead to unexpected toxicities; use caution when administering NSAIDs or salicylates with lower doses of methotrexate for RA. Methotrexate may increase the levels and effects of mercaptopurine; may require dosage adjustments. Vitamins containing folate may decrease response to systemic methotrexate; folate deficiency may increase methotrexate toxicity. **[U.S. Boxed Warning]: Concomitant methotrexate administration with radiotherapy may increase the risk of soft tissue necrosis and osteonecrosis.**

[U.S. Boxed Warnings]: Should be administered under the supervision of a physician experienced in the use of antimetabolite therapy; serious and fatal toxicities have occurred at all dose levels. Immune suppression may lead to potentially fatal opportunistic infections. For rheumatoid arthritis and psoriasis, immunosuppressive therapy should only be used when disease is active and less toxic, traditional therapy is ineffective. Methotrexate formulations and/or diluents containing preservatives should not be used for intrathecal or high-dose therapy. May cause fetal death or congenital abnormalities; do not use for psoriasis or RA treatment in pregnant women. May cause impairment of fertility, oligospermia, and menstrual dysfunction. Toxicity from methotrexate or any immunosuppressive is increased in the elderly. Methotrexate injection may contain benzyl alcohol and should not be used in neonates.

When used for intrathecal administration, should not be prepared during the preparation of any other agents; after preparation, store intrathecal medications in an isolated location or container clearly marked with a label identifying as "intrathecal" use only; delivery of intrathecal medications to the patient should only be with other medications intended for administration into the central nervous system (Jacobson, 2009).

Drug Interactions

Metabolism/Transport Effects Substrate of P-glycoprotein, SLCO1B1

Avoid Concomitant Use

Avoid concomitant use of Methotrexate with any of the following: Acitretin; BCG; Natalizumab; Pimecrolimus; Roflumilast; Tacrolimus (Topical)

Increased Effect/Toxicity

Methotrexate may increase the levels/effects of: CycloSPORINE; CycloSPORINE (Systemic); Leflunomide; Natalizumab; Theophylline Derivatives; Vaccines (Live); Vitamin K Antagonists

The levels/effects of Methotrexate may be increased by: Acitretin; Ciprofloxacin; Ciprofloxacin (Systemic); CycloSPORINE; CycloSPORINE (Systemic); Denosumab; Eltrombopag; Nonsteroidal Anti-Inflammatory Agents; Penicillins; P-Glycoprotein Inhibitors; Pimecrolimus; Probenecid; Proton Pump Inhibitors; Roflumilast; Salicylates; Sulfonamide Derivatives; Tacrolimus (Topical); Trastuzumab; Trimethoprim

Decreased Effect

Methotrexate may decrease the levels/effects of: BCG; Cardiac Glycosides; Sapropterin; Sipuleucel-T; Vaccines (Inactivated); Vitamin K Antagonists

The levels/effects of Methotrexate may be decreased by: Bile Acid Sequestrants; Echinacea; P-Glycoprotein Inducers

Ethanol/Nutrition/Herb Interactions

Ethanol: Avoid ethanol (may be associated with increased liver injury).

Food: Methotrexate peak serum levels may be decreased if taken with food. Milk-rich foods may decrease methotrexate absorption. Folate may decrease drug response.

Herb/Nutraceutical: Avoid echinacea (has immunostimulant properties).

Dietary Considerations Some products may contain sodium.

Pharmacodynamics/Kinetics

Onset of Action Antirheumatic: 3-6 weeks; additional improvement may continue longer than 12 weeks

Half-life Elimination Low dose: 3-10 hours; High dose: 8-15 hours

Time to Peak Serum: Oral: 1-2 hours; I.M.: 30-60 minutes

Pregnancy Risk Factor X (psoriasis, rheumatoid arthritis)

Lactation Enters breast milk/contraindicated

Breast-Feeding Considerations Low amounts of methotrexate are excreted into breast milk. Due to the potential for serious adverse reactions in a breast-feeding infant, use is contraindicated in nursing mothers.

Dosage Forms

Injection, powder for reconstitution: 1 g

Injection, solution: 25 mg/mL (2 mL, 10 mL)

Injection, solution [preservative free]: 25 mg/mL (2 mL, 4 mL, 8 mL, 10 mL, 20 mL, 40 mL, 100 mL)

Tablet, oral: 2.5 mg

Rheumatrex®: 2.5 mg

Trexall™: 5 mg, 7.5 mg, 10 mg, 15 mg

Methotrimeprazine (meth oh trye MEP ra zeen)

Canadian Brand Names Apo-Methoprazine®; Novo-Meprazine; Nozinan®; PMS-Methotrimeprazine

Pharmacologic Category Analgesic, Nonopioid; Antimanic Agent; Antipsychotic Agent, Typical

Use Treatment of schizophrenia; psychosis; manic-depressive syndromes; anxiety or tension disorders; management of pain, including pain caused by neuralgia or cancer; adjunct to general anesthesia; management of nausea and vomiting; sedation

Local Anesthetic/Vasoconstrictor Precautions No information available to require special precautions (see Dental Comment)

Effects on Dental Treatment Key adverse event(s) related to dental treatment: Anticholinergic side effects can cause a reduction of saliva production or secretion, contributing to discomfort and dental disease (ie, caries, oral candidiasis, and periodontal disease). Phenothiazines can cause extrapyramidal reactions which may appear as muscle twitching or increased motor activity of the face, neck, or head.

Effects on Bleeding No information available to require special precautions

Adverse Effects Note: Frequencies not defined; some reactions listed are based on reports for other agents in this same pharmacologic class, and may not be specifically reported for methotrimeprazine.

Cardiovascular: Orthostatic hypotension, QT_c prolongation (rare), tachycardia, venous thromboembolism

Central nervous system: Dizziness, drowsiness; extrapyramidal symptoms (akathisia, dystonias, pseudoparkinsonism, tardive dyskinesia); headache, impairment of temperature regulation, neuroleptic malignant syndrome (NMS), seizure

Dermatologic: Photosensitivity (rare), rash

Endocrine & metabolic: Gynecomastia, hyperglycemia or glucose intolerance, libido changes, menstrual irregularity

Gastrointestinal: Constipation, ileus, nausea, necrotizing enterocolitis, vomiting, weight gain, xerostomia

Genitourinary: Ejaculatory disturbances or dysfunction, incontinence, polyuria, priapism, urinary retention
Hematologic: Agranulocytosis (rare), eosinophilia, hemolytic anemia, leukopenia, pancytopenia, thrombocytopenic purpura
Hepatic: Cholestatic jaundice, hepatotoxicity
Respiratory: Pulmonary embolus
Miscellaneous: Diaphoresis

General Dosage Range

I.M.:

Children: 0.063-0.125 mg/kg/day in 1-3 divided doses
Adults: 10-25 mg every 8 hours **or** 75-100 mg as a single dose

I.V.:

Children: 0.063 mg/kg in 250 mL D_5W infused at a rate of 20-40 drops/minute
Adults: 10-25 mg in 500 mL D_5W infused at a rate of 20-40 drops/minute

Oral:

Children: 0.25 mg/kg/day in 2-3 divided doses (maximum: 40 mg/day [children <12 years])
Adults: 6-75 mg/day in 2-3 divided doses (maximum: doses up to 1000 mg/day have been used) **or** 10-25 mg at bedtime

Mechanism of Action Aliphatic phenothiazine that antagonizes D1 and D2 dopamine receptor subtypes; also binds alpha-1, alpha-2, serotonin ($5\text{-}HT_1$ and $5\text{-}HT_2$), and muscarinic (M_1 and M_2) receptors

Pharmacodynamics/Kinetics

Onset of Action Injection: 1 hour
Duration of Action 2-4 hours
Half-life Elimination 15-30 hours
Time to Peak Serum: I.M.: 0.5-1.5 hours; Oral: 1-3 hours

Product Availability Not available in U.S.

Dental Comment This drug is known to prolong the QT interval. The QT interval is measured as the time and distance between the Q point of the QRS complex and the end of the T wave in the ECG tracing. After adjustment for heart rate, the QT interval is defined as prolonged if it is more than 450 msec in men and 460 msec in women. A long QT syndrome was first described in the 1950s and 60s as a congenital syndrome involving QT interval prolongation and syncope and sudden death. Some of the congenital long QT syndromes were characterized by a peculiar electrocardiographic appearance of the QRS complex involving a premature atria beat followed by a pause, then a subsequent sinus beat showing marked QT prolongation and deformity. This type of cardiac arrhythmia was originally termed "torsade de pointes" (translated from the French as "twisting of the points").

Prolongation of the QT interval is thought to result from delayed ventricular repolarization. The repolarization process within the myocardial cell is due to the efflux of intracellular potassium. The channels associated with this current can be blocked by many drugs and predispose the electrical propagation cycle to torsade de pointes.

Methotrimeprazine is one of the drugs confirmed to prolong the QT interval and is accepted as having a risk of causing torsade de pointes. The risk of drug-induced torsade de pointes is extremely low when a single QT interval prolonging drug is prescribed. In terms of epinephrine, it is not known what effect vasoconstrictors in the local anesthetic regimen will have in patients with a known history of congenital prolonged QT interval or in patients taking any medication that prolongs the QT interval. Until more information is obtained, it is suggested that the clinician consult with the physician prior to the use of a vasoconstrictor in suspected patients, and that the vasoconstrictor (epinephrine, levonordefrin [Neo-Cobefrin®]) be used with caution.

Methscopolamine (meth skoe POL a meen)

U.S. Brand Names Pamine®; Pamine® Forte
Canadian Brand Names Pamine®
Pharmacologic Category Anticholinergic Agent
Use Adjunctive therapy in the treatment of peptic ulcer
Local Anesthetic/Vasoconstrictor Precautions No information available to require special precautions
Effects on Dental Treatment Key adverse event(s) related to dental treatment: Xerostomia and changes in salivation (normal salivary flow resumes upon discontinuation), and dry throat and nose. Anticholinergic side effects can cause a reduction of saliva production or secretion, contributing to discomfort and dental disease (ie, caries, oral candidiasis and periodontal disease).
Effects on Bleeding No information available to require special precautions

Adverse Effects Frequency not defined.
Cardiovascular: Palpitation, tachycardia
Central nervous system: Headache, insomnia, flushing, nervousness, drowsiness, dizziness, confusion, fever, CNS stimulation may be produced with large doses
Dermatologic: Dry skin, urticaria
Endocrine & metabolic: Lactation suppressed
Gastrointestinal: Constipation, xerostomia, dry throat, dysphagia, nausea, vomiting, loss of taste
Genitourinary: Impotence, urinary hesitancy, urinary retention
Neuromuscular & skeletal: Weakness
Ocular: Blurred vision, cycloplegia, ocular tension increased, pupil dilation
Respiratory: Dry nose
Miscellaneous: Allergic reaction, diaphoresis decreased, hypersensitivity reactions, anaphylaxis

General Dosage Range Oral: *Adults:* 2.5-5 mg twice daily

Mechanism of Action Methscopolamine is a peripheral anticholinergic agent with limited ability to cross the blood-brain barrier and provides a peripheral blockade of muscarinic receptors. This agent reduces the volume and the total acid content of gastric secretions, inhibits salivation, and reduces gastrointestinal motility.

Pharmacodynamics/Kinetics
Onset of Action 1 hour
Duration of Action 4-6 hours

Pregnancy Risk Factor C

Methsuximide (meth SUKS i mide)

U.S. Brand Names Celontin®
Canadian Brand Names Celontin®
Pharmacologic Category Anticonvulsant, Succinimide
Use Control of absence (petit mal) seizures that are refractory to other drugs
Unlabeled/Investigational Use Partial complex (psychomotor) seizures
Local Anesthetic/Vasoconstrictor Precautions No information available to require special precautions
Effects on Dental Treatment No significant effects or complications reported
Effects on Bleeding No information available to require special precautions
Adverse Effects Frequency not defined.
Cardiovascular: Hyperemia
Central nervous system: Aggressiveness, ataxia, confusion, depression, dizziness, drowsiness, hallucinations (auditory), headache, hypochondriacal behavior, insomnia, irritability, mental instability, mental slowness, nervousness, psychosis, suicidal behavior
Dermatologic: Pruritus, rash, Stevens-Johnson syndrome, urticaria
Gastrointestinal: Abdominal pain, anorexia, constipation, diarrhea, epigastric pain, nausea, vomiting, weight loss
Genitourinary: Hematuria (microscopic), proteinuria
Hematologic: Eosinophilia, leukopenia, monocytosis, pancytopenia
Ocular: Blurred vision, periorbital edema, photophobia
Miscellaneous: Hiccups, systemic lupus erythematosus

General Dosage Range Oral: *Adults:* Initial: 300 mg/day for 1 week; Maintenance: Up to 1.2 g/day in 2-4 divided doses

Mechanism of Action Increases the seizure threshold and suppresses paroxysmal spike-and-wave pattern in absence seizures; depresses nerve transmission in the motor cortex

Pharmacodynamics/Kinetics
Half-life Elimination 2-4 hours
Time to Peak Serum: 1-3 hours

Methyclothiazide (meth i kloe THYE a zide)

Related Information
Cardiovascular Diseases *on page 1848*

Pharmacologic Category Diuretic, Thiazide
Use Management of mild-to-moderate hypertension; treatment of edema in congestive heart failure and nephrotic syndrome
Local Anesthetic/Vasoconstrictor Precautions No information available to require special precautions
Effects on Dental Treatment Key adverse event(s) related to dental treatment: Orthostatic hypotension.
Effects on Bleeding No information available to require special precautions

Adverse Effects 1% to 10%:
Cardiovascular: Orthostatic hypotension
Dermatologic: Photosensitivity
Endocrine & metabolic: Hypokalemia
Gastrointestinal: Anorexia, epigastric distress

General Dosage Range Oral: *Adults:* 2.5-10 mg once daily

Mechanism of Action Inhibits sodium reabsorption in the distal tubules causing increased excretion of sodium and water, as well as, potassium and hydrogen ions

Pharmacodynamics/Kinetics
Onset of Action Diuresis: 2 hours; Peak effect: 6 hours
Duration of Action ~1 day

Pregnancy Risk Factor B

Methyl Aminolevulinate (METH il a mee noe LEV ue lin ate)

U.S. Brand Names Metvixia™

Canadian Brand Names Metvix®

Pharmacologic Category Photosensitizing Agent, Topical; Topical Skin Product

Use Treatment of thin and moderately thick, nonhyperkeratotic, nonpigmented actinic keratoses of the face and scalp; to be used in conjunction with red light illumination

Local Anesthetic/Vasoconstrictor Precautions No information available to require special precautions

Effects on Dental Treatment No significant effects or complications reported

Effects on Bleeding No information available to require special precautions

Adverse Effects Pain and burning begin during illumination and generally resolve completely within a few minutes or hours, but may last up to a few days. Erythema and other signs generally resolve within a few days up to 3 weeks.

>10%: Dermatologic: Skin burning/pain/discomfort (86%; severe: 20%), erythema (63%; severe 6%), scabbing/crusting/blister/erosions (29%), itching (22%), skin or eyelid edema (18%), skin exfoliation (14%)

1% to 10%:
Dermatologic: Skin warm (4%), hyperpigmentation (2%), skin hemorrhage (2%), skin tightness (2%)
Local: Application site discharge (2%)

General Dosage Range Topical: *Adults:* Apply up to 1 g once; repeat in 1 week

Mechanism of Action Methyl aminolevulinate (prodrug) is metabolically converted to photoactive porphyrins (PAPs), which accumulate in the skin lesions resulting in photosensitization. When exposed to light of appropriate wavelength and energy, the accumulated PAPs produce a photodynamic reaction, releasing oxygen singlets which result in local cytotoxicity.

Pregnancy Risk Factor C

Methylcellulose (meth il SEL yoo lose)

U.S. Brand Names Citrucel® Fiber Shake [OTC] [DSC]; Citrucel® Fiber Smoothie [OTC] [DSC]; Citrucel® [OTC]; Soluble Fiber Therapy [OTC]

Pharmacologic Category Fiber Supplement; Laxative; Laxative, Bulk-Producing

Use Adjunct in treatment of constipation

Local Anesthetic/Vasoconstrictor Precautions No information available to require special precautions

Effects on Dental Treatment No significant effects or complications reported

Effects on Bleeding No information available to require special precautions

General Dosage Range Oral:
Caplet:
Children 6-11 years: 1 caplet up to 6 times/day (maximum: 6 caplets/day)
Children ≥12 years and Adults: 2 caplets up to 6 times/day (maximum: 12 caplets/day)
Powder:
Children 6-11 years: 1 g (2-2.5 level teaspoons) up to 3 times/day
Children ≥12 years and Adults: 2 g (1 rounded or heaping tablespoon) up to 3 times/day

Pregnancy Risk Factor C

Methyldopa (meth il DOE pa)

Related Information
Cardiovascular Diseases *on page 1848*

Canadian Brand Names Apo-Methyldopa®; Nu-Medopa

Pharmacologic Category Alpha-Adrenergic Inhibitor; Alpha$_2$-Adrenergic Agonist

Use Management of moderate-to-severe hypertension

Local Anesthetic/Vasoconstrictor Precautions No information available to require special precautions

Effects on Dental Treatment Key adverse event(s) related to dental treatment: Xerostomia (normal salivary flow resumes upon discontinuation). Anticholinergic side effects can cause a reduction of saliva production or secretion, contributing to discomfort and dental disease (ie, caries, oral candidiasis, and periodontal disease).

Effects on Bleeding No information available to require special precautions

Adverse Effects

>10%: Cardiovascular: Peripheral edema

1% to 10%:

Central nervous system: Drug fever, mental depression, anxiety, nightmares, drowsiness, headache

Gastrointestinal: Dry mouth

General Dosage Range Dosage adjustment recommended in patients with renal impairment

I.V.:

Children: 5-10 mg/kg/dose every 6-8 hours (maximum: 65 mg/kg/day; 3 g/day)

Adults: 250-500 mg every 6-8 hours (maximum: 1 g every 6 hours)

Oral:

Children: Initial: 10 mg/kg/day in 2-4 divided doses; Maintenance: Up to 65 mg/kg/day (maximum: 3 g/day)

Adults: Initial: 250 mg 2-3 times/day; Maintenance: 250-1000 mg/day in 2 divided doses (maximum: 3 g/day)

Elderly: Initial: 125 mg 1-2 times/day

Mechanism of Action Stimulation of central alpha-adrenergic receptors by a false transmitter that results in a decreased sympathetic outflow to the heart, kidneys, and peripheral vasculature

Pharmacodynamics/Kinetics

Onset of Action Peak effect: Hypotensive: Oral/parenteral: 3-6 hours

Duration of Action 12-24 hours

Half-life Elimination 75-80 minutes; End-stage renal disease: 6-16 hours

Pregnancy Risk Factor B

Methyldopa and Hydrochlorothiazide

(meth il DOE pa & hye droe klor oh THYE a zide)

Related Information

Hydrochlorothiazide *on page 854*

Methyldopa *on page 1108*

Canadian Brand Names Apo-Methazide®

Pharmacologic Category Alpha$_2$-Adrenergic Agonist; Diuretic, Thiazide

Use Management of moderate-to-severe hypertension

Local Anesthetic/Vasoconstrictor Precautions No information available to require special precautions

Effects on Dental Treatment Key adverse event(s) related to dental treatment: Anticholinergic side effects can cause a reduction of saliva production or secretion, contributing to discomfort and dental disease (ie, caries, oral candidiasis, and periodontal disease).

Effects on Bleeding No information available to require special precautions

Adverse Effects See individual agents.

General Dosage Range Oral: *Adults:* 1 tablet 2-3 times/day (maximum: 50 mg/day [hydrochlorothiazide]; 3 g/day [methyldopa])

Pregnancy Risk Factor C

Methylergonovine (meth il er goe NOE veen)

U.S. Brand Names Methergine®

Canadian Brand Names Methergine®

Pharmacologic Category Ergot Derivative

Use Prevention and treatment of postpartum and postabortion hemorrhage caused by uterine atony or subinvolution

Local Anesthetic/Vasoconstrictor Precautions No information available to require special precautions

Effects on Dental Treatment No significant effects or complications reported

Effects on Bleeding Rare but significant events related to hemorrhage (cerebral hemorrhage, subarachnoid hemorrhage, and stroke) have occurred following injection of some agents in this class. However, there is no information related to special precautions associated with bleeding related to dental procedures.

Adverse Effects Frequency not defined.

Cardiovascular: Acute MI, arterial spasm, bradycardia, hyper-/hypotension, palpitation, tachycardia, temporary chest pain
Central nervous system: Dizziness, hallucinations, headache, seizure
Dermatologic: Rash
Endocrine & metabolic: Water intoxication
Gastrointestinal: Diarrhea, foul taste, nausea, vomiting
Local: Thrombophlebitis
Neuromuscular & skeletal: Leg cramps
Otic: Tinnitus
Renal: Hematuria
Respiratory: Dyspnea, nasal congestion
Miscellaneous: Anaphylaxis, diaphoresis

General Dosage Range

I.M., I.V.: *Adults:* 0.2 mg after delivery; may repeat every 2-4 hours
Oral: *Adults:* 0.2 mg 3-4 times/day in the puerperium

Mechanism of Action Similar smooth muscle actions as seen with ergotamine; however, it affects primarily uterine smooth muscles producing sustained contractions and thereby shortens the third stage of labor and reduces blood loss.

Pharmacodynamics/Kinetics

Onset of Action Oxytocic: Oral: 5-10 minutes; I.M.: 2-5 minutes; I.V.: Immediately
Duration of Action Oral: ~3 hours; I.M.: ~3 hours; I.V.: 45 minutes
Half-life Elimination Biphasic: Initial: 1-5 minutes; Terminal: 0.5-2 hours
Time to Peak Serum: Oral: 0.3-2 hours; I.M.: 0.2-0.6 hours

Pregnancy Risk Factor C

Methylfolate (meth il FO late)

U.S. Brand Names Deplin™

Generic Availability (U.S.) Yes

Pharmacologic Category Dietary Supplement

Use Medicinal food for management of patients with low plasma and/or low red blood cell folate

Local Anesthetic/Vasoconstrictor Precautions No information available to require special precautions

Effects on Dental Treatment No significant effects or complications reported

Effects on Bleeding No information available to require special precautions

Dosage Oral: Adults: One tablet (7.5 mg) daily

Mechanism of Action Methylfolate, or L-methylfolate, is the active form of folate in the body, which can be transported into peripheral tissues and across the blood brain barrier. Folate is necessary for formation of numerous coenzymes in many metabolic systems, particularly for purine, pyrimidine, and nucleoprotein synthesis, and maintenance in erythropoiesis; stimulates WBC and platelet production in folate deficiency anemia.

Contraindications Hypersensitivity to any component of the formulation

Warnings/Precautions Folate administration is not appropriate for monotherapy with pernicious or other megaloblastic anemias when anemia is present with vitamin B_{12} deficiency. Doses >0.1 mg/day may obscure pernicious anemia with continuing irreversible nerve damage progression. Product is a medicinal food for use only under the supervision of a healthcare provider.

Drug Interactions

Avoid Concomitant Use

Avoid concomitant use of Methylfolate with any of the following: Raltitrexed

Increased Effect/Toxicity There are no known significant interactions involving an increase in effect.

Decreased Effect

Methylfolate may decrease the levels/effects of: CarBAMazepine; Divalproex; Fosphenytoin; PHENobarbital; Phenytoin; Primidone; Pyrimethamine; Raltitrexed; Valproic Acid

The levels/effects of Methylfolate may be decreased by: Cholestyramine Resin; Colestipol; SulfaSALAzine

Dosage Forms

Tablet, oral: 7.5 mg
Deplin™: L-methylfolate 7.5 mg

Methylfolate, Methylcobalamin, and Acetylcysteine
(meth il FO late meth il koe BAL a min & a se teel SIS teen)

Related Information
Acetylcysteine *on page 53*
Methylfolate *on page 1110*

U.S. Brand Names Cerefolin® NAC

Pharmacologic Category Dietary Supplement

Use Medicinal food for use in patients with neurovascular oxidative stress and/or hyperhomocysteinemia

Local Anesthetic/Vasoconstrictor Precautions No information available to require special precautions

Effects on Dental Treatment No significant effects or complications reported

Effects on Bleeding No information available to require special precautions

General Dosage Range Oral: *Children ≥12 years and Adults:* 1 caplet daily

Methylnaltrexone (meth il nal TREKS one)

U.S. Brand Names Relistor®

Canadian Brand Names Relistor®

Pharmacologic Category Gastrointestinal Agent, Miscellaneous; Opioid Antagonist, Peripherally-Acting

Use Treatment of opioid-induced constipation in patients with advanced illness receiving palliative care with inadequate response to conventional laxative regimens

Local Anesthetic/Vasoconstrictor Precautions No information available to require special precautions

Effects on Dental Treatment No significant effects or complications reported

Effects on Bleeding No information available to require special precautions

Adverse Effects
>10%: Gastrointestinal: Abdominal pain (29%), flatulence (13%), nausea (12%)
1% to 10%:
- Central nervous system: Dizziness (7%)
- Dermatologic: Hyperhidrosis (7%)
- Gastrointestinal: Diarrhea (6%)

General Dosage Range Dosage adjustment recommended in patients with renal impairment

SubQ:
Adults <38 kg and >114 kg: 0.15 mg/kg (round dose up to nearest 0.1 mL of volume) every other day as needed (maximum: 1 dose/24 hours)
Adults 38 to <62 kg: 8 mg every other day as needed (maximum: 1 dose/24 hours)
Adults 62-114 kg: 12 mg every other day as needed (maximum: 1 dose/24 hours)

Mechanism of Action An opioid receptor antagonist which blocks opioid binding at the mu receptor, methylnaltrexone is a quaternary derivative of naltrexone with restricted ability to cross the blood-brain barrier. It therefore functions as a peripheral acting opioid antagonist, including actions on the gastrointestinal tract to inhibit opioid-induced decreased gastrointestinal motility and delay in gastrointestinal transit time, thereby decreasing opioid-induced constipation. Does not affect opioid analgesic effects or induce opioid withdrawal symptoms.

Pharmacodynamics/Kinetics
Onset of Action Usually within 30-60 minutes (in responding patients)
Half-life Elimination Terminal: ~8 hours
Time to Peak SubQ: 30 minutes

Pregnancy Risk Factor B

Methylphenidate (meth il FEN i date)

U.S. Brand Names Concerta®; Daytrana™; Metadate CD®; Metadate® ER; Methylin®; Methylin® ER; Ritalin LA®; Ritalin-SR®; Ritalin®

Canadian Brand Names Apo-Methylphenidate®; Apo-Methylphenidate® SR; Biphentin®; Concerta®; Novo-Methylphenidate ER-C; PHL-Methylphenidate; PMS-Methylphenidate; ratio-Methylphenidate; Ritalin®; Ritalin® SR; Sandoz-Methylphenidate SR

Generic Availability (U.S.) Yes: Immediate release tablet, oral solution, sustained release tablet

Pharmacologic Category Central Nervous System Stimulant

Use Treatment of attention-deficit/hyperactivity disorder (ADHD); symptomatic management of narcolepsy

Unlabeled/Investigational Use Depression (especially elderly or medically ill)

Local Anesthetic/Vasoconstrictor Precautions No information available to require special precautions

Effects on Dental Treatment Key adverse event(s) related to dental treatment: Up to 10% of patients taking amphetamine-like drugs may present with hypertension. Monitor blood pressure prior to using local anesthetic with vasoconstrictors.

Effects on Bleeding No information available to require special precautions

Adverse Effects

Transdermal system: Frequency of adverse events as reported in trials of 7-week duration. Incidence of some events higher with extended use.

>10%:

Central nervous system: Headache (≤15%; long-term use in children: 28%), insomnia (6% to 13%; long-term use in children: 30%), irritability (7% to 11%)

Gastrointestinal: Appetite decreased (26%), nausea (10% to 12%)

Miscellaneous: Viral infection (long-term use in children: 28%)

1% to 10%:

Cardiovascular: Tachycardia (≤1%)

Central nervous system: Tic (7%), dizziness (adolescents 6%), emotional instability (6%)

Gastrointestinal: Vomiting (3% to 10%), weight loss (6% to 9%), abdominal pain (5% to 7%), anorexia (5%; long-term use in children: 46%)

Local: Application site reaction

Respiratory: Nasal congestion (6%) nasopharyngitis (5%)

Postmarketing and/or case reports (limited to important or life-threatening): Allergic contact dermatitis/sensitization, anaphylaxis, angioedema, hallucinations, seizures

All dosage forms: Frequency not defined:

Cardiovascular: Angina, cardiac arrhythmia, cerebral arteritis, cerebral hemorrhage, cerebral occlusion, cerebrovascular accidents, vasculitis, hyper-/hypotension, MI, murmur, palpitation, pulse increased/decreased, Raynaud's phenomenon, tachycardia

Central nervous system: Aggression, agitation, anger, anxiety, confusional state, depression, dizziness, drowsiness, fatigue, fever, headache, hypervigilance, insomnia, irritability, lethargy, mood alterations, nervousness, neuroleptic malignant syndrome (NMS) (rare), restlessness, stroke, tension, Tourette's syndrome (rare), toxic psychosis, tremor, vertigo

Dermatologic: Alopecia, erythema multiforme, exfoliative dermatitis, hyperhidrosis, rash, urticaria

Endocrine & metabolic: Dysmenorrhea, growth retardation, libido decreased

Gastrointestinal: Abdominal pain, anorexia, appetite decreased, bruxism, constipation, diarrhea, dyspepsia, nausea, vomiting, weight loss, xerostomia

Genitourinary: Erectile dysfunction

Hematologic: Anemia, leukopenia, pancytopenia, thrombocytopenic purpura, thrombocytopenia

Hepatic: Bilirubin increased, liver function tests abnormal, hepatic coma, transaminases increased

Neuromuscular & skeletal: Arthralgia, dyskinesia, muscle tightness, paresthesia

Ocular: Blurred vision, dry eyes, mydriasis, visual accommodation disturbance

Renal: Necrotizing vasculitis

Respiratory: Cough increased, dyspnea, pharyngitis, pharyngolaryngeal pain, rhinitis, sinusitis, upper respiratory tract infection

Miscellaneous: Accidental injury, hypersensitivity reactions

Dosage

ADHD:

Oral:

Immediate release products Children ≥6 years and Adults: Initial: 5 mg/dose (~0.3 mg/kg/dose) given twice daily before breakfast and lunch; increase by 5-10 mg/day (0.2 mg/kg/day) at weekly intervals; maximum dose: 60 mg/day (2 mg/kg/day). **Note:** Discontinue periodically to re-evaluate or if no improvement occurs within 1 month.

Extended release products:

Children ≥6 years and Adults:

Metadate® ER, Methylin® ER, Ritalin® SR: May be given in place of immediate release products, once the daily dose is titrated and the titrated 8-hour dosage corresponds to sustained or extended release tablet size; maximum: 60 mg/day

Metadate CD®, Ritalin LA®: Initial: 20 mg once daily; may be adjusted in 10-20 mg increments at weekly intervals; maximum: 60 mg/day

Children 6-12 years and Adolescents 13-17 years: *Concerta®:*

Patients not currently taking methylphenidate: Initial dose: 18 mg once daily in the morning

Patients currently taking methylphenidate: **Note:** Initial dose: Dosing based on current regimen and clinical judgment; suggested dosing listed below:
- Patients taking methylphenidate 5 mg 2-3 times/day: 18 mg once every morning
- Patients taking methylphenidate 10 mg 2-3 times/day: 36 mg once every morning
- Patients taking methylphenidate 15 mg 2-3 times/day: 54 mg once every morning

Dose adjustment: May increase dose in increments of 18 mg; dose may be adjusted at weekly intervals. A dosage strength of 27 mg is available for situations in which a dosage between 18-36 mg is desired. Maximum dose should not exceed 2 mg/kg/day **or** 54 mg/day in children 6-12 years or 72 mg/day in children 13-17 years.

Adults: *Concerta®:*

Patients not currently taking methylphenidate: Initial dose: 18-36 mg once daily in the morning

Patients currently taking methylphenidate: **Note:** Initial dose: Dosing based on current regimen and clinical judgment; suggested dosing listed below:
- Patients taking methylphenidate 5 mg 2-3 times/day: 18 mg once every morning
- Patients taking methylphenidate 10 mg 2-3 times/day: 36 mg once every morning
- Patients taking methylphenidate 15 mg 2-3 times/day: 54 mg once every morning
- Patients taking methylphenidate 20 mg 2-3 times/day: 72 mg once every morning

Dose adjustment: May increase dose in increments of 18 mg; dose may be adjusted at weekly intervals. A dosage strength of 27 mg is available for situations in which a dosage between 18-36 mg is desired. Maximum dose should not exceed 72 mg/day.

Transdermal (Daytrana™): Children 6-12 years and Adolescents 13-17 years: Initial: 10 mg patch once daily; remove up to 9 hours after application. Titrate based on response and tolerability; may increase to next transdermal dose no more frequently than every week. **Note:** Application should occur 2 hours prior to desired effect. Drug absorption may continue for a period of time after patch removal; patients converting from another formulation of methylphenidate should be initiated at 10 mg regardless of their previous dose and titrated as needed due to the differences in bioavailability of the transdermal formulation.

Narcolepsy: Oral: Adults: 10 mg 2-3 times/day, up to 60 mg/day

Depression (unlabeled use): Oral: Adults: Initial: 2.5 mg every morning before 9 AM; dosage may be increased by 2.5-5 mg every 2-3 days as tolerated to a maximum of 20 mg/day; may be divided (ie, 7 AM and 12 noon), but should not be given after noon; do not use sustained release product

Mechanism of Action Mild CNS stimulant; blocks the reuptake of norepinephrine and dopamine into presynaptic neurons; appears to stimulate the cerebral cortex and subcortical structures similar to amphetamines

Contraindications Hypersensitivity to methylphenidate, any component of the formulation, or idiosyncratic reactions to sympathomimetic amines; marked anxiety, tension, and agitation; glaucoma; use during or within 14 days following MAO inhibitor therapy; family history or diagnosis of Tourette's syndrome or tics

Metadate CD® and Metadate® ER: Additional contraindications: Severe hypertension, heart failure, arrhythmia, hyperthyroidism, recent MI or angina; concomitant use of halogenated anesthetics

Warnings/Precautions CNS stimulant use has been associated with serious cardiovascular events (eg, sudden death in children and adolescents; sudden death, stroke, and MI in adults) in patients with pre-existing structural cardiac abnormalities or other serious heart problems. These products should be avoided in patients with known serious structural cardiac abnormalities, cardiomyopathy, serious heart rhythm abnormalities, or other serious cardiac problems that could further increase their risk of sudden death. Patients should be carefully evaluated for cardiac disease prior to initiation of therapy. Use of stimulants can cause an increase in blood pressure (average 2-4 mm Hg) and increases in heart rate (average 3-6 bpm), although some patients may have larger than average increases. Use caution with hypertension, hyperthyroidism, or other cardiovascular conditions that might be exacerbated by increases in blood pressure or heart rate. Some products are contraindicated in patients with heart failure, arrhythmias, severe hypertension, hyperthyroidism, angina, or recent MI.

Has demonstrated value as part of a comprehensive treatment program for ADHD. Use with caution in patients with bipolar disorder (may induce mixed/manic episode).

May exacerbate symptoms of behavior and thought disorder in psychotic patients; new-onset psychosis or mania may occur with stimulant use; observe for symptoms of aggression and/or hostility. Use caution with seizure disorders (may reduce seizure threshold). Use caution in patients with history of ethanol or drug abuse. May exacerbate symptoms of behavior and thought disorder in psychotic patients. **[U.S. Boxed Warning]: Potential for drug dependency exists - avoid abrupt discontinuation in patients who have received for prolonged periods.** Visual disturbances have been reported (rare). Not labeled for use in children <6 years of age. Use of stimulants has been associated with suppression of growth in children; monitor growth rate during treatment.

Concerta® should not be used in patients with esophageal motility disorders or pre-existing severe gastrointestinal narrowing (small bowel disease, short gut syndrome, history of peritonitis, cystic fibrosis, chronic intestinal pseudo-obstruction, Meckel's diverticulum). Metadate CD® and Metadate® ER contain sucrose and lactose, respectively; avoid administration in hereditary galactose intolerance, Lapp lactase deficiency, or glucose-galactose malabsorption. Concomitant use with halogenated anesthetics is contraindicated; may cause sudden elevations in blood pressure; if surgery is planned, do not administer Metadate CD® or Metadate® ER on the day of surgery. Transdermal system may cause allergic contact sensitization, characterized by intense local reactions (edema, papules) that may spread beyond the patch site; sensitization may subsequently manifest systemically with other routes of methylphenidate administration; monitor closely. Avoid exposure of application site to any direct external heat sources (eg, hair dryers, heating pads, electric blankets); may increase the rate and extent of absorption and risk of overdose. Efficacy of transdermal methylphenidate therapy for >7 weeks has not been established.

Drug Interactions

Metabolism/Transport Effects Inhibits CYP2D6 (weak)

Avoid Concomitant Use

Avoid concomitant use of Methylphenidate with any of the following: Inhalational Anesthetics; Iobenguane I 123; MAO Inhibitors

Increased Effect/Toxicity

Methylphenidate may increase the levels/effects of: Anti-Parkinson's Agents (Dopamine Agonist); Antipsychotics; CloNIDine; Fosphenytoin; Inhalational Anesthetics; PHENobarbital; Phenytoin; Primidone; Sympathomimetics; Tricyclic Antidepressants; Vitamin K Antagonists

The levels/effects of Methylphenidate may be increased by: Antacids; Antipsychotics; Atomoxetine; Cannabinoids; H2-Antagonists; MAO Inhibitors; Proton Pump Inhibitors

Decreased Effect

Methylphenidate may decrease the levels/effects of: Antihypertensives; Iobenguane I 123

Ethanol/Nutrition/Herb Interactions

Ethanol: Avoid ethanol (may cause CNS depression).

Food: Food may increase oral absorption; Concerta® formulation is not affected. Food delays early peak and high-fat meals increase C_{max} and AUC of Metadate CD® formulation.

Herb/Nutraceutical: Avoid ephedra (may cause hypertension or arrhythmias) and yohimbe (also has CNS stimulatory activity).

Dietary Considerations Should be taken 30-45 minutes before meals. Concerta® is not affected by food. Some products may contain phenylalanine.

Pharmacodynamics/Kinetics

Onset of Action Peak effect:

Immediate release tablet: Cerebral stimulation: ~2 hours

Extended release capsule (Metadate CD®, Ritalin LA®): Biphasic; initial peak similar to immediate release product, followed by second rising portion (corresponding to extended release portion)

Sustained release tablet: 4-7 hours

Osmotic release tablet (Concerta®): Initial: 1-2 hours

Transdermal: ~2 hours; may be expedited by the application of external heat

Duration of Action Immediate release tablet: 3-6 hours; Sustained release tablet: 8 hours; Extended release tablet: Methylin® ER, Metadate® ER: 8 hours; Concerta®: 12 hours

Half-life Elimination *d*-methylphenidate: 3-4 hours; *l*-methylphenidate: 1-3 hours

Time to Peak Concerta®: C_{max}: 6-8 hours; Daytrana™: 7.5-10.5 hours

Pregnancy Risk Factor C

Lactation Enters breast milk/use caution

Breast-Feeding Considerations Methylphenidate excretion into breast milk has been noted in case reports. In both cases, the authors calculated the relative infant dose to be ≤0.2% of the weight adjusted maternal dose. Adverse events were not noted in either infant, however, both were older (6 months of age and 11 months of age) and exposure was limited.

Controlled Substance C-II

Dosage Forms

Capsule, extended release, oral:
Metadate CD®: 10 mg, 20 mg, 30 mg, 40 mg, 50 mg, 60 mg
Ritalin LA®: 10 mg, 20 mg, 30 mg, 40 mg

Patch, transdermal:
Daytrana™: 10 mg/9 hours (30s); 15 mg/9 hours (30s); 20 mg/9 hours (30s); 30 mg/9 hours (30s)

Solution, oral:
Methylin®: 5 mg/5 mL (500 mL); 10 mg/5 mL (500 mL)

Tablet, oral: 5 mg, 10 mg, 20 mg
Methylin®: 5 mg, 10 mg, 20 mg
Ritalin®: 5 mg, 10 mg, 20 mg

Tablet, chewable, oral:
Methylin®: 2.5 mg, 5 mg, 10 mg

Tablet, extended release, oral: 27 mg, 36 mg, 54 mg
Concerta®: 18 mg, 27 mg, 36 mg, 54 mg
Metadate® ER: 20 mg
Methylin® ER: 10 mg, 20 mg

Tablet, sustained release, oral: 20 mg
Ritalin-SR®: 20 mg

MethylPREDNISolone (meth il pred NIS oh lone)

Related Information

Respiratory Diseases *on page 1876*

Related Sample Prescriptions

Erosive Lichen Planus, Other Biopsy-Proven Desquamative Oral Diseases, and Major Aphthae *on page 1992*

U.S. Brand Names A-Methapred®; Depo-Medrol®; Medrol®; Medrol® Dosepak™; Solu-MEDROL®

Canadian Brand Names Depo-Medrol®; Medrol®; Methylprednisolone Acetate; Solu-Medrol®

Generic Availability (U.S.) Yes: Excludes preservative free injection, suspension

Pharmacologic Category Corticosteroid, Systemic

Dental Use Treatment of a variety of oral diseases of allergic, inflammatory, or autoimmune origin

Use Primarily as an anti-inflammatory or immunosuppressant agent in the treatment of a variety of diseases including those of hematologic, allergic, inflammatory, neoplastic, and autoimmune origin. Prevention and treatment of graft-versus-host disease following allogeneic bone marrow transplantation.

Unlabeled/Investigational Use Acute spinal cord injury

Local Anesthetic/Vasoconstrictor Precautions No information available to require special precautions

Effects on Dental Treatment Key adverse event(s) related to dental treatment: Ulcerative esophagitis.

Effects on Bleeding No information available to require special precautions

Adverse Effects Frequency not defined.

Cardiovascular: Arrhythmias, bradycardia, cardiac arrest, cardiomegaly, circulatory collapse, congestive heart failure, edema, fat embolism, hypertension, hypertrophic cardiomyopathy in premature infants, myocardial rupture (post MI), syncope, tachycardia, thromboembolism, vasculitis

Central nervous system: Delirium, depression, emotional instability, euphoria, hallucinations, headache, intracranial pressure increased, insomnia, malaise, mood swings, nervousness, neuritis, personality changes, psychic disorders, pseudotumor cerebri (usually following discontinuation), seizure, vertigo

Dermatologic: Acne, allergic dermatitis, alopecia, dry scaly skin, ecchymoses, edema, erythema, hirsutism, hyper-/hypopigmentation, hypertrichosis, impaired wound healing, petechiae, rash, skin atrophy, sterile abscess, skin test reaction impaired, striae, urticaria

Endocrine & metabolic: Adrenal suppression, amenorrhea, carbohydrate intolerance increased, Cushing's syndrome, diabetes mellitus, fluid retention, glucose intolerance, growth suppression (children), hyperglycemia, hyperlipidemia, hypokalemia, hypokalemic alkalosis, menstrual irregularities, negative nitrogen balance, pituitary-adrenal axis suppression, protein catabolism, sodium and water retention

Gastrointestinal: Abdominal distention, appetite increased, bowel/bladder dysfunction (after intrathecal administration), gastrointestinal hemorrhage, gastrointestinal perforation, nausea, pancreatitis, peptic ulcer, perforation of the small and large intestine, ulcerative esophagitis, vomiting, weight gain

Hematologic: Leukocytosis (transient)

Hepatic: Hepatomegaly, transaminases increased

Local: Postinjection flare (intra-articular use), thrombophlebitis

Neuromuscular & skeletal: Arthralgia, arthropathy, aseptic necrosis (femoral and humoral heads), fractures, muscle mass loss, muscle weakness, myopathy (particularly in conjunction with neuromuscular disease or neuromuscular-blocking agents), neuropathy, osteoporosis, parasthesia, tendon rupture, vertebral compression fractures, weakness

Ocular: Cataracts, exophthalmoses, glaucoma, intraocular pressure increased

Renal: Glycosuria

Respiratory: Pulmonary edema

Miscellaneous: Abnormal fat disposition, anaphylactoid reaction, anaphylaxis, angioedema, avascular necrosis, diaphoresis, hiccups, hypersensitivity reactions, infections, secondary malignancy

Dental Usual Dosage Anti-inflammatory or immunosuppressive: Adults: Oral: 2-60 mg/day in 1-4 divided doses to start, followed by gradual reduction in dosage to the lowest possible level consistent with maintaining an adequate clinical response.

Dosage Dosing should be based on the lesser of ideal body weight or actual body weight

Only sodium succinate may be given I.V.; methylprednisolone sodium succinate is highly soluble and has a rapid effect by I.M. and I.V. routes. Methylprednisolone acetate has a low solubility and has a sustained I.M. effect.

Children:

Acute spinal cord injury (unlabeled use): I.V. (sodium succinate): 30 mg/kg over 15 minutes, followed in 45 minutes by a continuous infusion of 5.4 mg/kg/hour for 23 hours. **Note:** Due to insufficient evidence of clinical efficacy (ie, preserving or improving spinal cord function), the routine use of methylprednisolone in the treatment of acute spinal cord injury is no longer recommended. If used in this setting, methylprednisolone should not be initiated >8 hours after the injury; not effective in penetrating trauma (eg, gunshot) (Consortium for Spinal Cord Medicine, 2008).

Anti-inflammatory or immunosuppressive: Oral, I.M., I.V. (sodium succinate): 0.5-1.7 mg/kg/day **or** 5-25 mg/m^2/day in divided doses every 6-12 hours; "Pulse" therapy: 15-30 mg/kg/dose over ≥30 minutes given once daily for 3 days

Asthma exacerbations, including status asthmaticus (emergency medical care or hospital doses) (NIH Asthma Guidelines, NAEPP, 2007): Children ≤12 years: Oral, I.V.: 1-2 mg/kg/day in 2 divided doses (maximum: 60 mg/day) until peak expiratory flow is 70% of predicted or personal best

Lupus nephritis: I.V. (sodium succinate): 30 mg/kg over ≥30 minutes every other day for 6 doses

Adults: **Only sodium succinate may be given I.V.;** methylprednisolone sodium succinate is highly soluble and has a rapid effect by I.M. and I.V. routes. Methylprednisolone acetate has a low solubility and has a sustained I.M. effect.

Acute spinal cord injury (unlabeled use): I.V. (sodium succinate): 30 mg/kg over 15 minutes, followed in 45 minutes by a continuous infusion of 5.4 mg/kg/hour for 23 hours. **Note:** Due to insufficient evidence of clinical efficacy (ie, preserving or improving spinal cord function), the routine use of methylprednisolone in the treatment of acute spinal cord injury is no longer recommended. If used in this setting, methylprednisolone should not be initiated >8 hours after the injury; not effective in penetrating trauma (eg, gunshot) (Consortium for Spinal Cord Medicine, 2008).

Allergic conditions: Oral: Tapered-dosage schedule:

Day 1: 24 mg on day 1 administered as 8 mg before breakfast, 4 mg after lunch, 4 mg after supper, and 8 mg at bedtime **OR** 24 mg as a single dose or divided into 2 or 3 doses upon initiation (regardless of time of day)

Day 2: 20 mg on day 2 administered as 4 mg before breakfast, 4 mg after lunch, 4 mg after supper, and 8 mg at bedtime

Day 3: 16 mg on day 3 administered as 4 mg before breakfast, 4 mg after lunch, 4 mg after supper, and 4 mg at bedtime

Day 4: 12 mg on day 4 administered as 4 mg before breakfast, 4 mg after lunch, and 4 mg at bedtime

Day 5: 8 mg on day 5 administered as 4 mg before breakfast and 4 mg at bedtime

Day 6: 4 mg on day 6 administered as 4 mg before breakfast

Anti-inflammatory or immunosuppressive:

Oral: 2-60 mg/day in 1-4 divided doses to start, followed by gradual reduction in dosage to the lowest possible level consistent with maintaining an adequate clinical response.

I.M. (sodium succinate): 10-80 mg/day once daily

I.M. (acetate): 10-80 mg every 1-2 weeks

I.V. (sodium succinate): 10-40 mg over a period of several minutes and repeated I.V. or I.M. at intervals depending on clinical response; when high dosages are needed, give 30 mg/kg over a period ≥30 minutes and may be repeated every 4-6 hours for 48 hours.

Arthritis: Intra-articular (acetate): Administer every 1-5 weeks.

Large joints (eg, knee, ankle): 20-80 mg

Medium joints (eg, elbow, wrist): 10-40 mg

Small joints: 4-10 mg

Asthma exacerbations, including status asthmaticus (emergency medical care or hospital doses): Oral, I.V.: 40-80 mg/day in 1- 2 divided doses until peak expiratory flow is 70% of predicted or personal best (NIH Asthma Guidelines, NAEPP, 2007)

Asthma, severe persistent, long-term control: Oral: 7.5-60 mg/day (or on alternate days) (NIH Asthma Guidelines, NAEPP, 2007)

Dermatitis, acute severe: I.M. (acetate): 80-120 mg as a single dose

Dermatitis, chronic: I.M. (acetate): 40-120 mg every 5-10 days

Dermatologic conditions (eg, keloids, lichen planus): Intralesional (acetate): 20-60 mg

Dermatomyositis/polymyositis: I.V. (sodium succinate): 1 g/day for 3-5 days for severe muscle weakness, followed by conversion to oral prednisone (Drake, 1996)

Lupus nephritis: High-dose "pulse" therapy: I.V. (sodium succinate): 0.5-1 g/day for 3 days (Ponticelli, 2010)

Pneumocystis pneumonia in AIDS patients: I.V.: 30 mg twice daily for 5 days, then 30 mg once daily for 5 days, then 15 mg once daily for 11 days

Mechanism of Action In a tissue-specific manner, corticosteroids regulate gene expression subsequent to binding specific intracellular receptors and translocation into the nucleus. Corticosteroids exert a wide array of physiologic effects including modulation of carbohydrate, protein, and lipid metabolism and maintenance of fluid and electrolyte homeostasis. Moreover cardiovascular, immunologic, musculoskeletal, endocrine, and neurologic physiology are influenced by corticosteroids. Decreases inflammation by suppression of migration of polymorphonuclear leukocytes and reversal of increased capillary permeability.

Contraindications Hypersensitivity to methylprednisolone or any component of the formulation; systemic fungal infection (except intra-articular injection in localized joint conditions); administration of live virus vaccines. methylprednisolone formulations containing benzyl alcohol preservative are contraindicated in premature infants; I.M. administration in idiopathic thrombocytopenia purpura; intrathecal administration

Warnings/Precautions Use with caution in patients with thyroid disease, hepatic impairment, renal impairment, cardiovascular disease, diabetes, glaucoma, cataracts, myasthenia gravis, patients at risk for osteoporosis, patients at risk for seizures, or GI diseases (diverticulitis, peptic ulcer, ulcerative colitis) due to perforation risk. Not recommended for the treatment of optic neuritis; may increase frequency of new episodes. Use caution following acute MI (corticosteroids have been associated with myocardial rupture). Cardiomegaly and congestive heart failure have been reported following concurrent use of amphotericin B and hydrocortisone for the management of fungal infections.

Because of the risk of adverse effects, systemic corticosteroids should be used cautiously in the elderly in the smallest possible effective dose for the shortest duration. May affect growth velocity; growth should be routinely monitored in pediatric patients. Withdraw therapy with gradual tapering of dose.

May cause hypercorticism or suppression of hypothalamic-pituitary-adrenal (HPA) axis, particularly in younger children or in patients receiving high doses for prolonged periods. HPA axis suppression may lead to adrenal crisis. Withdrawal and discontinuation of a corticosteroid should be done slowly and carefully. Particular care is required when patients are transferred from systemic corticosteroids to inhaled products due to possible adrenal insufficiency or withdrawal from steroids, including an increase in allergic symptoms. Patients receiving >20 mg per day of prednisone (or equivalent) may be most susceptible. Fatalities have occurred due to adrenal insufficiency in asthmatic patients during and after transfer from systemic corticosteroids to aerosol steroids; aerosol steroids do not provide the systemic steroid needed to treat patients having trauma, surgery, or infections.

Acute myopathy has been reported with high dose corticosteroids, usually in patients with neuromuscular transmission disorders; may involve ocular and/or respiratory muscles; monitor creatine kinase; recovery may be delayed. Corticosteroid use may cause psychiatric disturbances, including depression, euphoria, insomnia, mood swings, and personality changes. Pre-existing psychiatric conditions may be exacerbated by corticosteroid use. Prolonged use of corticosteroids may also increase the incidence of secondary infection, cause activation of latent infections, mask acute infection (including fungal infections), prolong or exacerbate viral or parasitic infections, or limit response to vaccines. Exposure to chickenpox or measles should be avoided; corticosteroids should not be used to treat ocular herpes simplex. Corticosteroids should not be used for cerebral malaria or viral hepatitis. Close observation is required in patients with latent tuberculosis and/or TB reactivity; restrict use in active TB (only in conjunction with antituberculosis treatment). Amebiasis should be ruled out in any patient with recent travel to tropic climates or unexplained diarrhea prior to initiation of corticosteroids. Prolonged treatment with corticosteroids has been associated with the development of Kaposi's sarcoma (case reports); discontinuation may result in clinical improvement.

High-dose corticosteroids should not be used to manage acute head injury. Rare cases of anaphylactoid reactions have been observed in patients receiving corticosteroids. Avoid injection or leakage into the dermis; dermal and/or subdermal skin depression may occur at the site of injection. Avoid deltoid muscle injection; subcutaneous atrophy may occur. Some dosage forms contain benzyl alcohol which has been associated with "gasping syndrome" in neonates.

Drug Interactions

Metabolism/Transport Effects **Substrate** of CYP3A4 (major); **Inhibits** CYP2C8 (weak), 3A4 (weak)

Avoid Concomitant Use

Avoid concomitant use of MethylPREDNISolone with any of the following: Aldesleukin; BCG; Natalizumab; Pimecrolimus; Roflumilast; Tacrolimus (Topical)

Increased Effect/Toxicity

MethylPREDNISolone may increase the levels/effects of: Acetylcholinesterase Inhibitors; Amphotericin B; CycloSPORINE; CycloSPORINE (Systemic); Deferasirox; Leflunomide; Loop Diuretics; Natalizumab; NSAID (COX-2 Inhibitor); NSAID (Nonselective); Thiazide Diuretics; Vaccines (Live); Warfarin

The levels/effects of MethylPREDNISolone may be increased by: Antifungal Agents (Azole Derivatives, Systemic); Aprepitant; Calcium Channel Blockers (Nondihydropyridine); CycloSPORINE; CycloSPORINE (Systemic); CYP3A4 Inhibitors (Strong); Denosumab; Estrogen Derivatives; Fluconazole; Fosaprepitant; Macrolide Antibiotics; Neuromuscular-Blocking Agents (Nondepolarizing); Pimecrolimus; Quinolone Antibiotics; Roflumilast; Salicylates; Tacrolimus (Topical); Trastuzumab

Decreased Effect

MethylPREDNISolone may decrease the levels/effects of: Aldesleukin; Antidiabetic Agents; BCG; Calcitriol; Corticorelin; CycloSPORINE; CycloSPORINE (Systemic); Isoniazid; Salicylates; Sipuleucel-T; Vaccines (Inactivated)

The levels/effects of MethylPREDNISolone may be decreased by: Aminoglutethimide; Antacids; Barbiturates; Bile Acid Sequestrants; Echinacea; Mitotane; Primidone; Rifamycin Derivatives; Tocilizumab

Ethanol/Nutrition/Herb Interactions

Ethanol: Avoid ethanol (may increase gastric mucosal irritation).

Food: Methylprednisolone interferes with calcium absorption. Limit caffeine.

Herb/Nutraceutical: St John's wort may decrease methylprednisolone levels. Avoid cat's claw, echinacea (have immunostimulant properties).

Dietary Considerations Take with meals to decrease GI upset.; need diet rich in pyridoxine, vitamin C, vitamin D, folate, calcium, phosphorus, and protein.

Pharmacodynamics/Kinetics

Onset of Action Peak effect (route dependent): Oral: 1-2 hours; I.M.: 4-8 days; Intra-articular: 1 week; methylprednisolone sodium succinate is highly soluble and has a rapid effect by I.M. and I.V. routes

Duration of Action Route dependent: Oral: 30-36 hours; I.M.: 1-4 weeks; Intra-articular: 1-5 weeks; methylprednisolone acetate has a low solubility and has a sustained I.M. effect

Half-life Elimination 3-3.5 hours; reduced in obese

Lactation Enters breast milk/use caution

Breast-Feeding Considerations Low levels of methylprednisolone are excreted in breast milk

Dosage Forms

Injection, powder for reconstitution: 40 mg, 125 mg, 500 mg, 1 g
A-Methapred®: 40 mg
Solu-MEDROL®: 500 mg, 1 g, 2 g

Injection, powder for reconstitution [preservative free]:
Solu-MEDROL®: 40 mg, 125 mg, 500 mg, 1 g

Injection, suspension: 40 mg/mL (1 mL, 5 mL, 10 mL); 80 mg/mL (1 mL, 5 mL)
Depo-Medrol®: 20 mg/mL (5 mL); 40 mg/mL (5 mL, 10 mL); 80 mg/mL (5 mL)

Injection, suspension [preservative free]:
Depo-Medrol®: 40 mg/mL (1 mL); 80 mg/mL (1 mL)

Tablet, oral: 4 mg, 8 mg, 16 mg, 32 mg
Medrol®: 2 mg, 4 mg, 8 mg, 16 mg, 32 mg
Medrol® Dosepak™: 4 mg

MethylTESTOSTERone (meth il tes TOS te rone)

U.S. Brand Names Android®; Methitest™; Testred®

Pharmacologic Category Androgen

Use

Male: Hypogonadism; delayed puberty; impotence and climacteric symptoms
Female: Palliative treatment of metastatic breast cancer

Unlabeled/Investigational Use Hypogonadism (male); delayed puberty (male)

Local Anesthetic/Vasoconstrictor Precautions No information available to require special precautions

Effects on Dental Treatment No significant effects or complications reported

Effects on Bleeding No information available to require special precautions

Adverse Effects Frequency not defined.

Male: Gynecomastia, impotence, oligospermia (at high doses), priapism, prostatic carcinoma, prostatic hyperplasia, testicular atrophy, virilism

Female: Atrophy, breast soreness, hirsutism, menstrual problems (amenorrhea), virilism

Cardiovascular: Edema
Central nervous system: Anxiety, depression, headache
Dermatologic: Acne, "male pattern" baldness
Endocrine & metabolic: Hypercalcemia, hypercholesterolemia, libido (changes in)
Gastrointestinal: Nausea, vomiting
Hematologic: Polycythemia, suppression of clotting factors
Hepatic: Cholestatic hepatitis, hepatic dysfunction, hepatic necrosis, hepatocellular neoplasm (rare), jaundice, liver function tests (abnormal), peliosis hepatitis
Neuromuscular & skeletal: Paresthesia
Miscellaneous: Anaphylactoid reactions (rare)

General Dosage Range

Oral:

Adults (female): 50-200 mg/day
Adults (male): 10-50 mg/day

Mechanism of Action Stimulates receptors in organs and tissues to promote growth and development of male sex organs and maintains secondary sex characteristics in androgen-deficient males

Pregnancy Risk Factor X

Controlled Substance C-III

Metipranolol (met i PRAN oh lol)

U.S. Brand Names OptiPranolol®

Canadian Brand Names OptiPranolol®

Pharmacologic Category Beta-Adrenergic Blocker, Nonselective; Ophthalmic Agent, Antiglaucoma

Use Treatment of chronic open-angle glaucoma or ocular hypertension

Local Anesthetic/Vasoconstrictor Precautions No information available to require special precautions

Effects on Dental Treatment Metipranolol is a nonselective beta-blocker and may enhance the pressor response to epinephrine, resulting in hypertension and bradycardia. Many nonsteroidal anti-inflammatory drugs, such as ibuprofen and indomethacin, can reduce the hypotensive effect of beta-blockers after 3 or more weeks of therapy with the NSAID. Short-term NSAID use (ie, 3 days) requires no special precautions in patients taking beta-blockers.

Effects on Bleeding No information available to require special precautions

Adverse Effects Frequency not defined.

Cardiovascular: Angina, atrial fibrillation, bradycardia, hypertension, MI, palpitation

Central nervous system: Anxiety, depression, dizziness, headache, nervousness, somnolence

Dermatologic: Rash

Gastrointestinal: Nausea

Neuromuscular & skeletal: Arthritis, myalgia, weakness

Ocular: Abnormal vision, blepharitis, blurred vision, browache, conjunctivitis, discomfort, edema, eyelid dermatitis, photophobia, tearing, uveitis

Respiratory: Bronchitis, cough, dyspnea, epistaxis, rhinitis

Miscellaneous: Allergic reaction

General Dosage Range Ophthalmic: *Adults:* Instill 1 drop into affected eye(s) twice daily

Mechanism of Action Beta-adrenoceptor-blocking agent; lacks intrinsic sympathomimetic activity and membrane-stabilizing effects and possesses only slight local anesthetic activity; mechanism of action of metipranolol in reducing intraocular pressure appears to be via reduced production of aqueous humor. This effect may be related to a reduction in blood flow to the iris root-ciliary body. It remains unclear if the reduction in intraocular pressure observed with beta-blockers is actually secondary to beta-adrenoceptor blockade.

Pharmacodynamics/Kinetics

Onset of Action ≤30 minutes; Peak effect: Maximum: ~2 hours

Duration of Action Intraocular pressure reduction: Up to 24 hours

Half-life Elimination ~3 hours

Pregnancy Risk Factor C

Metoclopramide (met oh KLOE pra mide)

Related Information

Endocrine Disorders and Pregnancy *on page 1879*

U.S. Brand Names Metozolv™ ODT; Reglan®

Canadian Brand Names Apo-Metoclop®; Metoclopramide Hydrochloride Injection; Metoclopramide Omega; Nu-Metoclopramide; PMS-Metoclopramide

Pharmacologic Category Antiemetic; Gastrointestinal Agent, Prokinetic

Use

Oral: Symptomatic treatment of diabetic gastroparesis; gastroesophageal reflux

I.V., I.M.: Symptomatic treatment of diabetic gastroparesis; postpyloric placement of enteral feeding tubes; prevention and/or treatment of nausea and vomiting associated with chemotherapy, or postsurgery; to stimulate gastric emptying and intestinal transit of barium during radiological examination of the stomach/small intestine

Local Anesthetic/Vasoconstrictor Precautions No information available to require special precautions

Effects on Dental Treatment Metoclopramide has relatively few adverse effects when used in low doses; however, extrapyramidal effects including akathisia (motor restlessness), acute dystonia (spasmodic contractures), pseudoparkinsonism, and tardive dyskinesia can occur. These effects are more likely in the elderly, patients taking other dopamine antagonists (including antipsychotic agents and some antiemetic agents), and patients with Parkinson's disease. Metoclopramide will increase gastric emptying which will aid in the absorption of orally administered anxiolytic or sedative agents used for minimal or moderate sedation as well as promote the emptying of the stomach following procedures during which blood may be swallowed causing GI upset.

Effects on Bleeding No information available to require special precautions

Adverse Effects Frequency not always defined.

Cardiovascular: AV block, bradycardia, HF, fluid retention, flushing (following high I.V. doses), hyper-/hypotension, supraventricular tachycardia

Central nervous system: Drowsiness (~10% to 70%; dose related), acute dystonic reactions (<1% to 25%; dose and age related), fatigue (2% to 10%), lassitude (~10%), restlessness (~10%), headache (4% to 5%), dizziness (1% to 4%), somnolence (2% to 3%), akathisia, confusion, depression, hallucinations (rare), insomnia, neuroleptic malignant syndrome (rare), Parkinsonian-like symptoms, suicidal ideation, seizure, tardive dyskinesia

Dermatologic: Angioneurotic edema (rare), rash, urticaria

Endocrine & metabolic: Amenorrhea, galactorrhea, gynecomastia, hyperprolactinemia, impotence

Gastrointestinal: Nausea (4% to 6%), vomiting (1% to 2%), diarrhea

Hematologic: Agranulocytosis, leukopenia, neutropenia, porphyria

Hepatic: Hepatotoxicity (rare)

Ocular: Visual disturbance

Respiratory: Bronchospasm, laryngeal edema (rare), laryngospasm (rare)
Miscellaneous: Allergic reactions, methemoglobinemia, sulfhemoglobinemia

General Dosage Range Dosage adjustment recommended in patients with renal impairment

I.M.: *Adults:* 10-20 mg as a single dose **or** 10 mg before each meal and at bedtime

I.V.:

Children <6 years: 0.1 mg/kg as a single dose
Children 6-14 years: 2.5-5 mg as a single dose
Children >14 years: 10 mg as a single dose
Adults: 10 mg before each meal and at bedtime **or** 1-2 mg/kg every 2-3 hours (maximum: 5 doses/day) **or** 10 mg as a single dose

Oral: *Adults:* 10-15 mg up to 4 times/day

Mechanism of Action Blocks dopamine receptors and (when given in higher doses) also blocks serotonin receptors in chemoreceptor trigger zone of the CNS; enhances the response to acetylcholine of tissue in upper GI tract causing enhanced motility and accelerated gastric emptying without stimulating gastric, biliary, or pancreatic secretions; increases lower esophageal sphincter tone

Pharmacodynamics/Kinetics

Onset of Action Oral: 30-60 minutes; I.V.: 1-3 minutes; I.M.: 10-15 minutes

Duration of Action Therapeutic: 1-2 hours, regardless of route

Half-life Elimination Normal renal function: Children: ~4 hours; Adults: 5-6 hours (may be dose dependent)

Time to Peak Serum: Oral: 1-2 hours

Pregnancy Risk Factor B

Metolazone (me TOLE a zone)

Related Information

Cardiovascular Diseases *on page 1848*

U.S. Brand Names Zaroxolyn®

Canadian Brand Names Zaroxolyn®

Pharmacologic Category Diuretic, Thiazide-Related

Use Management of mild-to-moderate hypertension; treatment of edema in heart failure and nephrotic syndrome, impaired renal function

Local Anesthetic/Vasoconstrictor Precautions No information available to require special precautions

Effects on Dental Treatment Key adverse event(s) related to dental treatment: Xerostomia (normal salivary flow resumes upon discontinuation) and orthostatic hypotension.

Effects on Bleeding No information available to require special precautions

Adverse Effects Frequency not defined.

Cardiovascular: Chest pain/discomfort, necrotizing angiitis, orthostatic hypotension, palpitation, syncope, venous thrombosis, vertigo, volume depletion
Central nervous system: Chills, depression, dizziness, drowsiness, fatigue, headache, lightheadedness, restlessness
Dermatologic: Petechiae, photosensitivity, pruritus, purpura, rash, skin necrosis, Stevens-Johnson syndrome, toxic epidermal necrolysis, urticaria
Endocrine & metabolic: Gout attacks, hypercalcemia, hyperglycemia, hyperuricemia, hypochloremia, hypochloremic alkalosis, hypokalemia, hypomagnesemia, hyponatremia, hypophosphatemia
Gastrointestinal: Abdominal bloating, abdominal pain, anorexia, constipation, diarrhea, epigastric distress, nausea, pancreatitis, vomiting, xerostomia
Genitourinary: Impotence
Hematologic: Agranulocytosis, aplastic/hypoplastic anemia, hemoconcentration, leukopenia, thrombocytopenia
Hepatic: Cholestatic jaundice, hepatitis
Neuromuscular & skeletal: Joint pain, muscle cramps/spasm, neuropathy, paresthesia, weakness
Ocular: Blurred vision (transient)
Renal: BUN increased, glucosuria

General Dosage Range Oral: *Adults:* 2.5-20 mg every 24 hours

Mechanism of Action Inhibits sodium reabsorption in the distal tubules causing increased excretion of sodium and water, as well as, potassium and hydrogen ions

Pharmacodynamics/Kinetics

Onset of Action Diuresis: ~60 minutes

Duration of Action ≥24 hours

Half-life Elimination 20 hours

Pregnancy Risk Factor B

Metoprolol (me toe PROE lole)

Related Information

Cardiovascular Diseases *on page* 1848

U.S. Brand Names Lopressor®; Toprol-XL®

Canadian Brand Names Apo-Metoprolol (Type L®); Apo-Metoprolol SR®; Apo-Metoprolol®; Betaloc®; Dom-Metoprolol; JAMP-Metoprolol-L; Lopressor®; Metoprolol Tartrate Injection, USP; Metoprolol-25; Metoprolol-L; Mylan-Metoprolol (Type L); Nu-Metop; PHL-Metoprolol; PMS-Metoprolol; Riva-Metoprolol; Sandoz-Metoprolol (Type L); Sandoz-Metoprolol SR; Teva-Metoprolol

Generic Availability (U.S.) Yes

Pharmacologic Category Beta Blocker, Beta-1 Selective

Use Treatment of angina pectoris, hypertension, or hemodynamically-stable acute myocardial infarction

Extended release: Treatment of angina pectoris or hypertension; to reduce mortality/hospitalization in patients with heart failure (stable NYHA Class II or III) already receiving ACE inhibitors, diuretics, and/or digoxin

Unlabeled/Investigational Use Treatment of ventricular arrhythmias, atrial ectopy; migraine prophylaxis, essential tremor, aggressive behavior (not recommended for dementia-associated aggression); prevention of reinfarction and sudden death after myocardial infarction; prevention and treatment of atrial fibrillation and atrial flutter; multifocal atrial tachycardia; symptomatic treatment of hypertrophic obstructive cardiomyopathy

Local Anesthetic/Vasoconstrictor Precautions No information available to require special precautions

Effects on Dental Treatment Metoprolol is a cardioselective beta-blocker. Local anesthetic with vasoconstrictor can be safely used in patients medicated with metoprolol. Nonselective beta-blockers (ie, propranolol, nadolol) enhance the pressor response to epinephrine, resulting in hypertension and bradycardia; this has not been reported for metoprolol. Many nonsteroidal anti-inflammatory drugs, such as ibuprofen and indomethacin, can reduce the hypotensive effect of beta-blockers after 3 or more weeks of therapy with the NSAID. Short-term NSAID use (ie, 3 days) requires no special precautions in patients taking beta-blockers.

Effects on Bleeding No information available to require special precautions

Adverse Effects Frequency may not be defined.

Cardiovascular: Hypotension (1% to 27%), bradycardia (2% to 16%), first-degree heart block (P-R interval ≥0.26 sec; 5%), arterial insufficiency (usually Raynaud type; 1%), chest pain (1%), CHF (1%), edema (peripheral; 1%), palpitation (1%), syncope (1%)

Central nervous system: Dizziness (2% to 10%), fatigue (1% to 10%), depression (5%), confusion, hallucinations, headache, insomnia, memory loss (short-term), nightmares, sleep disturbances, somnolence, vertigo

Dermatology: Pruritus (5%), rash (5%), photosensitivity, psoriasis exacerbated

Endocrine & metabolic: Libido decreased, Peyronie's disease (<1%), diabetes exacerbated

Gastrointestinal: Diarrhea (5%), constipation (1%), flatulence (1%), gastrointestinal pain (1%), heartburn (1%), nausea (1%), xerostomia (1%), vomiting

Hematologic: Claudication

Neuromuscular & skeletal: Musculoskeletal pain

Ocular: Blurred vision, visual disturbances

Otic: Tinnitus

Respiratory: Dyspnea (1% to 3%), bronchospasm (1%), wheezing (1%), rhinitis, shortness of breath

Miscellaneous: Cold extremities (1%)

Other events reported with beta-blockers: Catatonia, emotional lability, fever, hypersensitivity reactions, laryngospasm, nonthrombocytopenic purpura, respiratory distress, thrombocytopenic purpura

Dosage

Children: Hypertension: Oral:

1-17 years: Immediate release tablet: (National High Blood Pressure Education Program Working Group on High Blood Pressure in Children and Adolescents, 2004): Initial: 1-2 mg/kg/day; maximum 6 mg/kg/day (≤200 mg/day); administer in 2 divided doses

≥6 years: Extended release tablet: Initial: 1 mg/kg once daily (maximum initial dose: 50 mg/day). Adjust dose based on patient response (maximum: 2 mg/kg/day or 200 mg/day)

Adults:

Angina: Oral:

Immediate release: Initial: 50 mg twice daily; usual dosage range: 50-200 mg twice daily; maximum: 400 mg/day; increase dose at weekly intervals to desired effect

Extended release: Initial: 100 mg/day (maximum: 400 mg/day)

Atrial fibrillation/flutter (ventricular rate control), supraventricular tachycardia (SVT) (acute treatment; unlabeled use; Antman, 2004; Fuster, 2006; Neumar, 2010): I.V.: 2.5-5 mg every 2-5 minutes (maximum total dose: 15 mg over a 10-15 minute period). **Note:** Initiate cautiously in patients with concomitant heart failure; avoid in patients with decompensated heart failure.

Maintenance: Oral (immediate release): 25-100 mg twice daily

Heart failure: Oral (extended release): Initial: 25 mg once daily (reduce to 12.5 mg once daily in NYHA class higher than class II); may double dosage every 2 weeks as tolerated (maximum: 200 mg/day)

Hypertension: Oral:

Immediate release: Initial: 50 mg twice daily; effective dosage range: 100-450 mg/day in 2-3 divided doses; increase dose at weekly intervals to desired effect; maximum: 450 mg/day; usual dosage range (JNC 7): 50-100 mg/day

Extended release: Initial: 25-100 mg once daily; increase doses at weekly (or longer) intervals to desired effect; maximum: 400 mg/day; usual dosage range (JNC 7): 50-100 mg/day

Hypertension/ventricular rate control: I.V. (in patients having nonfunctioning GI tract): Initial: 1.25-5 mg every 6-12 hours; titrate initial dose to response. Initially, low doses may be appropriate to establish response; however, although not routine, up to 15 mg administered as frequently as every 3 hours has been employed in patients with refractory tachycardia.

Myocardial infarction:

Acute: I.V.: 5 mg every 2 minutes for 3 doses in early treatment of myocardial infarction; thereafter, give 50 mg orally every 6 hours beginning 15 minutes after last I.V. dose and continue for 48 hours; then administer a maintenance dose of 100 mg twice daily. **Note:** If initial I.V. dosing is not tolerated, may give 25-50 mg orally (depending on degree of intolerance) every 6 hours beginning 15 minutes after the last I.V. dose or as soon as clinical condition permits.

Secondary prevention (unlabeled use; Olsson, 1992): Oral: Immediate release: 25-100 mg twice daily; optimize dose based on heart rate and blood pressure; continue indefinitely.

Elderly: Initiate at the lower end of the dosage range

Note: Switching dosage forms:

When switching from immediate release metoprolol to extended release, the same total daily dose of metoprolol should be used.

When switching between oral and intravenous dosage forms, equivalent beta-blocking effect is achieved when doses in a 2.5:1 (Oral:I.V.) ratio is used. For example, if the patient is receiving an oral dose of 25 mg twice daily (50 mg/day), this would translate to 5 mg I.V. every 6 hours; consider reducing initial I.V. dose to evaluate patient response.

Dosing adjustment in renal impairment: No adjustment required.

Dosing adjustment in hepatic impairment: Reduced dose may be necessary

Mechanism of Action Selective inhibitor of $beta_1$-adrenergic receptors; competitively blocks $beta_1$-receptors, with little or no effect on $beta_2$-receptors at doses <100 mg; does not exhibit any membrane stabilizing or intrinsic sympathomimetic activity

Contraindications

Hypersensitivity to metoprolol, any component of the formulation, or other beta-blockers

Note: Additional contraindications are formulation and/or indication specific.

Immediate release tablets/injectable formulation:

Hypertension and angina: Sinus bradycardia; second- and third-degree heart block; cardiogenic shock; overt heart failure; sick sinus syndrome (except in patients with a functioning artificial pacemaker); severe peripheral arterial disease; pheochromocytoma (without alpha blockade)

Myocardial infarction: Severe sinus bradycardia (heart rate <45 beats/minute); significant first-degree heart block (P-R interval ≥0.24 seconds); second- and third-degree heart block; systolic blood pressure <100 mm Hg; moderate-to-severe cardiac failure

Extended release tablet: Severe bradycardia, second- and third degree heart block; cardiogenic shock; decompensated heart failure; sick sinus syndrome (except in patients with a functioning artificial pacemaker)

Warnings/Precautions [U.S. Boxed Warning]: Beta-blocker therapy should not be withdrawn abruptly (particularly in patients with CAD), but gradually tapered over 1-2 weeks to avoid acute tachycardia, hypertension, and/or ischemia. Consider pre-existing conditions such as sick sinus syndrome before initiating. Metoprolol commonly produces mild first-degree heart block (P-R interval >0.2-0.24 sec). May also produce severe first- (P-R interval ≥0.26 sec), second-, or third-degree heart block. Patients with acute MI (especially right ventricular MI) have a high risk of developing heart block of varying degrees. If severe heart block occurs, metoprolol should be discontinued and measures to increase heart rate should be employed. Symptomatic hypotension may occur with use. Use caution in patients with PVD (can aggravate arterial insufficiency). Use caution with concurrent use of beta-blockers and either verapamil or diltiazem; bradycardia or heart block can occur; avoid concurrent I.V. use of both agents. Use with caution in patients receiving CYP2D6 inhibitors (eg, bupropion, chlorpromazine, cimetidine, diphenhydramine, hydroxychloroquine, fluoxetine, paroxetine, propafenone, propoxyphene, quinidine, ritonavir, terbinafine, thioridazine); concurrent use may increase metoprolol plasma concentrations.

In general, beta-blockers should be avoided in patients with bronchospastic disease. Metoprolol, with B_1 selectivity, should be used cautiously in bronchospastic disease with close monitoring. Use cautiously in patients with diabetes because it can mask prominent hypoglycemic symptoms. Use caution in hyperthyroidism since beta-blockade may mask signs of thyrotoxicosis. Use caution with hepatic dysfunction. Use with caution in patients with myasthenia gravis or psychiatric disease (may cause CNS depression). Use caution with inhalation anesthetic agents which may decrease myocardial function. Although perioperative beta-blocker therapy is recommended prior to elective surgery in selected patients, use of high-dose extended release metoprolol in patients naïve to beta-blocker therapy undergoing noncardiac surgery has been associated with bradycardia, hypotension, stroke, and death. Chronic beta-blocker therapy should not be routinely withdrawn prior to major surgery. Use of beta-blockers may unmask cardiac failure in patients without a history of dysfunction. Adequate alpha-blockade is required prior to use of any beta-blocker for patients with untreated pheochromocytoma. May induce or exacerbate psoriasis. Use caution with history of severe anaphylaxis to allergens; patients taking beta-blockers may become more sensitive to repeated allergen challenges. Treatment of anaphylaxis (eg, epinephrine) in patients taking beta-blockers may be ineffective or promote undesirable effects.

Extended release: Use with caution in patients with compensated heart failure; monitor for a worsening of heart failure.

Drug Interactions

Metabolism/Transport Effects Substrate of CYP2C19 (minor), 2D6 (major); **Inhibits** CYP2D6 (weak)

Avoid Concomitant Use

Avoid concomitant use of Metoprolol with any of the following: Methacholine

Increased Effect/Toxicity

Metoprolol may increase the levels/effects of: Alpha-/Beta-Agonists (Direct-Acting); Alpha1-Blockers; Alpha2-Agonists; Amifostine; Antihypertensives; Antipsychotic Agents (Phenothiazines); Bupivacaine; Cardiac Glycosides; Fingolimod; Hypotensive Agents; Insulin; Lidocaine; Lidocaine (Systemic); Lidocaine (Topical); Mepivacaine; Methacholine; Midodrine; RiTUXimab; Sulfonylureas

The levels/effects of Metoprolol may be increased by: Abiraterone; Acetylcholinesterase Inhibitors; Aminoquinolines (Antimalarial); Amiodarone; Anilidopiperidine Opioids; Antipsychotic Agents (Phenothiazines); Calcium Channel Blockers (Nondihydropyridine); CYP2D6 Inhibitors (Moderate); CYP2D6 Inhibitors (Strong); Darunavir; Diazoxide; Dipyridamole; Disopyramide; Dronedarone; Herbs (Hypotensive Properties); MAO Inhibitors; Pentoxifylline; Phosphodiesterase 5 Inhibitors; Propafenone; Propoxyphene; Prostacyclin Analogues; QuiNIDine; Reserpine; Selective Serotonin Reuptake Inhibitors

Decreased Effect

Metoprolol may decrease the levels/effects of: Beta2-Agonists; Theophylline Derivatives

The levels/effects of Metoprolol may be decreased by: Barbiturates; Herbs (Hypertensive Properties); Methylphenidate; Nonsteroidal Anti-Inflammatory Agents; Peginterferon Alfa-2b; Rifamycin Derivatives; Yohimbine

Ethanol/Nutrition/Herb Interactions

Food: Food increases absorption. Metoprolol serum levels may be increased if taken with food.

Herb/Nutraceutical: Avoid bayberry, blue cohosh, cayenne, ephedra, ginger, ginseng (American), gotu kola, licorice, (may worsen hypertension). Avoid black cohosh, California poppy, coleus, golden seal, hawthorn, mistletoe, periwinkle, quinine, shepherd's purse (may have increased antihypertensive effect).

Dietary Considerations Regular tablets should be taken with food. Extended release tablets may be taken without regard to meals.

Pharmacodynamics/Kinetics

Onset of Action Peak effect: Oral: 1.5-4 hours; I.V.: 20 minutes (when infused over 10 minutes)

Duration of Action Oral: Immediate release: 10-20 hours, Extended release: ~24 hours; I.V.: 5-8 hours

Half-life Elimination 3-8 hours (dependent on rate of CYP2D6 metabolism)

Pregnancy Risk Factor C

Lactation Enters breast milk/use caution (AAP rates "compatible"; AAP 2001 update pending)

Breast-Feeding Considerations Small amounts of metoprolol can be detected in breast milk. The manufacturer recommends that caution be exercised when administering metoprolol to nursing women.

Dosage Forms

Injection, solution: 1 mg/mL (5 mL)

Lopressor®: 1 mg/mL (5 mL)

Injection, solution [preservative free]: 1 mg/mL (5 mL)

Tablet, oral: 25 mg, 50 mg, 100 mg

Lopressor®: 50 mg, 100 mg

Tablet, extended release, oral: 25 mg, 50 mg, 100 mg, 200 mg

Toprol-XL®: 25 mg, 50 mg, 100 mg, 200 mg

References

Foster CA and Aston SJ, "Propranolol-Epinephrine Interaction: A Potential Disaster," *Plast Reconstr Surg*, 1983, 72(1):74-8.

Wong DG, Spence JD, Lamki L, et al, "Effect of Nonsteroidal Anti-inflammatory Drugs on Control of Hypertension of Beta-Blockers and Diuretics," *Lancet*, 1986, 1(8488):997-1001.

Wynn RL, "Dental Nonsteroidal Anti-inflammatory Drugs and Prostaglandin-Based Drug Interactions, Part Two," *Gen Dent*, 1992, 40(2):104, 106, 108.

Wynn RL, "Epinephrine Interactions With Beta-Blockers," *Gen Dent*, 1994, 42(1):16, 18.

Metoprolol and Hydrochlorothiazide

(me toe PROE lole & hye droe klor oh THYE a zide)

Related Information

Hydrochlorothiazide *on page 854*

Metoprolol *on page 1122*

U.S. Brand Names Lopressor HCT®

Pharmacologic Category Beta Blocker, Beta-1 Selective; Diuretic, Thiazide

Use Treatment of hypertension (not recommended for initial treatment)

Local Anesthetic/Vasoconstrictor Precautions No information available to require special precautions

Effects on Dental Treatment

Metoprolol: Metoprolol is a cardioselective beta-blocker. Local anesthetic with vasoconstrictor can be safely used in patients medicated with metoprolol. Nonselective beta-blockers (ie, propranolol, nadolol) enhance the pressor response to epinephrine, resulting in hypertension and bradycardia; this has not been reported for metoprolol. Many nonsteroidal anti-inflammatory drugs, such as ibuprofen and indomethacin, can reduce the hypotensive effect of beta-blockers after 3 or more weeks of therapy with the NSAID. Short-term NSAID use (ie, 3 days) requires no special precautions in patients taking beta-blockers.

Hydrochlorothiazide: Key adverse event(s) related to dental treatment: Orthostatic hypotension and hypotension.

Effects on Bleeding No information available to require special precautions

Adverse Effects Reactions noted here have been reported with the combination product; see individual drug monographs for additional adverse reactions that may be expected from each agent.

1% to 10%:

- Cardiovascular: Bradycardia (6%), edema (1%)
- Central nervous system: Fatigue (10%), dizziness (10%), drowsiness (10%), headache (10%), vertigo (10%), abnormal dreams (1%)
- Dermatologic: Purpura (1%)
- Endocrine & metabolic: Hypokalemia (<10%), gout (1%)
- Gastrointestinal: Anorexia (1%), constipation (1%), diarrhea (1%), nausea (1%), vomiting (1%), xerostomia (1%)
- Genitourinary: Impotence (1%)
- Neuromuscular & skeletal: Myalgia (1%)
- Ocular: Blurred vision (1%)

Otic: Earache (1%), tinnitus (1%)
Respiratory: Dyspnea (1%)
Miscellaneous: Flu-like syndrome (10%), diaphoresis (1%), exercise tolerance decreased (1%)

General Dosage Range Oral: *Adults:* Metoprolol 50-100 mg and hydrochlorothiazide 25-50 mg administered daily as single or 2 divided doses (maximum: 50 mg/day [hydrochlorothiazide])

Mechanism of Action See individual agents.

Pregnancy Risk Factor C/D (expert analysis)

MetroNIDAZOLE (Systemic) (met roe NYE da zole)

Related Information

Bacterial Infections *on page 1933*
Gastrointestinal Disorders *on page 1874*
Periodontal Diseases *on page 1942*
Sexually-Transmitted Diseases *on page 1903*
Ulcerative, Erosive, and Painful Oral Mucosal Disorders *on page 1950*

Related Sample Prescriptions

Bacterial Infections and Periodontal Diseases *on page 1983*

U.S. Brand Names Flagyl®; Flagyl® 375; Flagyl® ER

Canadian Brand Names Apo-Metronidazole®; Flagyl®; Florazole® ER

Generic Availability (U.S.) Yes: Excludes extended release tablet

Pharmacologic Category Amebicide; Antibiotic, Miscellaneous; Antiprotozoal, Nitroimidazole

Dental Use Treatment of oral soft tissue infections due to anaerobic bacteria including all anaerobic cocci, anaerobic gram-negative bacilli (*Bacteroides*), and gram-positive spore-forming bacilli (*Clostridium*). Useful as single agent or in combination with amoxicillin, Augmentin®, or ciprofloxacin in the treatment of periodontitis associated with the presence of *Actinobacillus actinomycetemcomitans* (AA).

Use Treatment of susceptible anaerobic bacterial and protozoal infections in the following conditions: Amebiasis, symptomatic and asymptomatic trichomoniasis; skin and skin structure infections, bone and joint infections, CNS infections, endocarditis, gynecologic infections, intra-abdominal infections (as part of combination regimen), respiratory tract infections (lower), systemic anaerobic infections; treatment of antibiotic-associated pseudomembranous colitis (AAPC); as part of a multidrug regimen for *H. pylori* eradication to reduce the risk of duodenal ulcer recurrence; surgical prophylaxis (colorectal)

Unlabeled/Investigational Use Crohn's disease

Local Anesthetic/Vasoconstrictor Precautions No information available to require special precautions

Effects on Dental Treatment Key adverse event(s) related to dental treatment: Unusual/metallic taste, glossitis, stomatitis, xerostomia (normal salivary flow resumes upon discontinuation), and furry tongue.

Effects on Bleeding No information available to require special precautions

Adverse Effects Frequency not always defined.

Cardiovascular: Flattening of the T-wave, flushing, syncope
Central nervous system: Aseptic meningitis, ataxia, confusion, coordination impaired, depression, dizziness, encephalopathy, fever, headache, insomnia, irritability, seizure, vertigo
Dermatologic: Erythematous rash, pruritus, Stevens-Johnson syndrome, toxic epidermal necrolysis, urticaria
Endocrine & metabolic: Disulfiram-like reaction, dysmenorrhea
Gastrointestinal: Nausea (~12%), anorexia, abdominal cramping, constipation, diarrhea, epigastric distress, furry tongue, glossitis, pancreatitis (rare), proctitis, stomatitis, unusual/metallic taste, vomiting, xerostomia
Genitourinary: Cystitis, darkened urine (rare), dyspareunia, dysuria, incontinence, libido decreased, pelvic pressure, polyuria, vaginal dryness, vaginitis
Hematologic: Neutropenia (reversible), thrombocytopenia (reversible, rare)
Local: Thrombophlebitis
Neuromuscular & skeletal: Dysarthria, peripheral neuropathy, weakness
Ocular: Optic neuropathy
Respiratory: Nasal congestion, pharyngitis, rhinitis, sinusitis, pharyngitis
Miscellaneous: Flu-like syndrome, joint pains resembling serum sickness, moniliasis

Dental Usual Dosage

Anaerobic infections/abscess: Adults: Oral, I.V.: 500 mg every 6-8 hours, not to exceed 4 g/day

Treatment of periodontitis (monotherapy or combination) associated with the presence of *Actinobacillus actinomycetemcomitans* (AA): Adults: Oral: 500 mg every 8 hours for 8 days.

Dosage

Infants and Children:

Amebiasis: Oral: 35-50 mg/kg/day in divided doses every 8 hours for 10 days

Trichomoniasis: Oral: 15-30 mg/kg/day in divided doses every 8 hours for 7 days

Anaerobic infections:

Oral: 15-35 mg/kg/day in divided doses every 8 hours

I.V.: 30 mg/kg/day in divided doses every 6 hours

Clostridium difficile (antibiotic-associated colitis): Oral: 20 mg/kg/day divided every 6 hours

Maximum dose: 2 g/day

Adults:

Anaerobic infections (diverticulitis, intra-abdominal, peritonitis, cholangitis, or abscess): Oral, I.V.: 500 mg every 6-8 hours, not to exceed 4 g/day; **Note:** Initial: 1 g I.V. loading dose may be administered

Amebiasis: Oral: 500-750 mg every 8 hours for 5-10 days

Antibiotic-associated pseudomembranous colitis: IDSA Guidelines (Cohen, 2010):

Mild-to-moderate infection: Oral: 500 mg 3 times/day for 10-14 days

Severe complicated infection: I.V.: 500 mg 3 times/day with oral vancomycin (recommended agent) for 10-14 days

Note: Due to the emergence of a new strain of *C. difficile*, some clinicians recommend converting to oral vancomycin therapy if the patient does not show a clear clinical response after 2 days of metronidazole therapy.

Giardiasis: 500 mg twice daily for 5-7 days

Helicobacter pylori eradication: Oral: 250-500 mg with meals and at bedtime for 14 days; requires combination therapy with at least one other antibiotic and an acid-suppressing agent (proton pump inhibitor or H_2 blocker)

Intra-abdominal infection, complicated, community-acquired, mild-to-moderate (in combination with cephalosporin or fluoroquinolone): I.V.: 500 mg every 8-12 hours **or** 1.5 g every 24 hours for for 4-7 days (provided source controlled)

Bacterial vaginosis or vaginitis due to *Gardnerella, Mobiluncus*: Oral: 500 mg twice daily (regular release) or 750 mg once daily (extended release tablet) for 7 days

Pelvic inflammatory disease (unlabeled use): Oral: 500 mg twice daily for 14 days (in combination with a cephalosporin and doxycycline) (CDC, 2010)

Trichomoniasis: Oral: 250 mg every 8 hours for 7 days **or** 375 mg twice daily for 7 days **or** 2 g as a single dose **or** 1 g twice daily for 2 doses (on same day)

Urethritis (unlabeled use): Oral: 2 g as a single dose with azithromycin (CDC, 2010)

Surgical prophylaxis (colorectal): I.V. 15 mg/kg 1 hour prior to surgery; followed by 7.5 mg/kg 6 and 12 hours after initial dose

Elderly: Use lower end of dosing recommendations for adults, do not administer as a single dose

Dosing adjustment in renal impairment: Cl_{cr} <10 mL/minute, but not on dialysis: Recommendations vary: To reduce possible accumulation in patients receiving multiple doses, consider reduction to 50% of dose or every 12 hours; **Note:** Dosage reduction is unnecessary in short courses of therapy. Clinical recommendations and practice vary. Some references do not recommend reduction at any level of renal impairment (Lamp, 1999).

Hemodialysis: Extensively removed by hemodialysis and peritoneal dialysis (50% to 100%); dosage reduction not recommended; administer full dose posthemodialysis

Peritoneal dialysis: Dose as for Cl_{cr} <10 mL/minute

Continuous arteriovenous or venovenous hemofiltration: Administer usual dose

Dosing adjustment/comments in hepatic disease: Unchanged in mild liver disease; reduce dosage in severe liver disease

Mechanism of Action After diffusing into the organism, interacts with DNA to cause a loss of helical DNA structure and strand breakage resulting in inhibition of protein synthesis and cell death in susceptible organisms

Contraindications Hypersensitivity to metronidazole, nitroimidazole derivatives, or any component of the formulation; pregnancy (first trimester)

Warnings/Precautions Use with caution in patients with severe liver impairment due to potential accumulation, blood dyscrasias; history of seizures, CHF or other sodium-retaining states; reduce dosage in patients with severe liver impairment, CNS disease, and consider dosage reduction in longer-term therapy with severe renal failure (Cl_{cr} <10 mL/minute); if *H. pylori* is not eradicated in patients being treated with metronidazole in a regimen, it should be assumed that metronidazole-resistance has occurred and it should not again be used; aseptic meningitis, encephalopathy, seizures, and neuropathies have been reported especially with increased doses and chronic treatment; monitor and consider discontinuation of therapy if symptoms occur. **[U.S. Boxed Warning]: Possibly carcinogenic based**

on animal data. Prolonged use may result in fungal or bacterial superinfection, including *C. difficile*-associated diarrhea (CDAD) and pseudomembranous colitis; CDAD has been observed >2 months postantibiotic treatment. The Infectious Disease Society of America (IDSA) recommends the use of oral metronidazole for initial treatment of mild-to-moderate *C. difficile* infection and the use of oral vancomycin for initial treatment of severe *C. difficile* infection with or without I.V. metronidazole depending on the presence of complications. May treat recurrent mild-to-moderate infection once with oral metronidazole; avoid use beyond first reoccurrence due to potential cumulative neurotoxicity (Cohen, 2010). Candidiasis infection (known or unknown) maybe more prominent during metronidazole treatment, antifungal treatment required. Disulfiram-like reactions to ethanol have been reported with oral metronidazole; avoid alcoholic beverages during therapy

Drug Interactions

Metabolism/Transport Effects Inhibits CYP2C9 (weak), 3A4 (moderate)

Avoid Concomitant Use

Avoid concomitant use of MetroNIDAZOLE (Systemic) with any of the following: BCG; Tolvaptan

Increased Effect/Toxicity

MetroNIDAZOLE (Systemic) may increase the levels/effects of: Alcohol (Ethyl); Budesonide (Systemic, Oral Inhalation); Busulfan; Calcineurin Inhibitors; Colchicine; CYP3A4 Substrates; Eplerenone; Everolimus; FentaNYL; Fosphenytoin; Halofantrine; Lurasidone; Phenytoin; Pimecrolimus; Ranolazine; Salmeterol; Saxagliptin; Tipranavir; Tolvaptan; Vilazodone; Vitamin K Antagonists

The levels/effects of MetroNIDAZOLE (Systemic) may be increased by: Disulfiram; Mebendazole

Decreased Effect

MetroNIDAZOLE (Systemic) may decrease the levels/effects of: BCG; Mycophenolate; Typhoid Vaccine

The levels/effects of MetroNIDAZOLE (Systemic) may be decreased by: Fosphenytoin; PHENobarbital; Phenytoin

Ethanol/Nutrition/Herb Interactions

Ethanol: The manufacturer recommends to avoid all ethanol or any ethanol-containing drugs (may cause disulfiram-like reaction characterized by flushing, headache, nausea, vomiting, sweating, or tachycardia).

Food: Peak antibiotic serum concentration lowered and delayed, but total drug absorbed not affected.

Dietary Considerations Take on an empty stomach. Drug may cause GI upset; if GI upset occurs, take with food. Extended release tablets should be taken on an empty stomach (1 hour before or 2 hours after meals). Some products may contain sodium. The manufacturer recommends that ethanol be avoided during treatment and for 3 days after therapy is complete.

Pharmacodynamics/Kinetics

Half-life Elimination Neonates: 25-75 hours; Others: 6-8 hours, prolonged with hepatic impairment; End-stage renal disease: 21 hours

Time to Peak Serum: Oral: Immediate release: 1-2 hours

Pregnancy Risk Factor B

Lactation Enters breast milk/not recommended (AAP rates "of concern"; AAP 2001 update pending)

Breast-Feeding Considerations Metronidazole and its active metabolite are measurable in the breast milk and infant plasma. Milk concentrations are similar to those in the maternal plasma and are highly variable. Peak concentrations of metronidazole in breast milk occur ~2-4 hours after the oral dose. In studies, the calculated relative infant doses have ranged from 0.13% to 36% of the weight-adjusted maternal dose. Use of metronidazole in a lactating patient is not recommended by the manufacturer. If metronidazole is given, breast-feeding should be withheld for 12-24 hours after the dose.

Dosage Forms

Capsule, oral: 375 mg

Flagyl® 375: 375 mg

Infusion, premixed iso-osmotic sodium chloride solution: 500 mg (100 mL)

Tablet, oral: 250 mg, 500 mg

Flagyl®: 250 mg, 500 mg

Tablet, extended release, oral:

Flagyl® ER: 750 mg

References

Eisenberg L, Suchow R, Coles RS, et al, "The Effects of Metronidazole Administration on Clinical and Microbiologic Parameters of Periodontal Disease," *Clin Prev Dent*, 1991, 13(1):28-34.

Herrera D, Sanz M, Jepsen S, et al, "A Systematic Review on the Effect of Systemic Antimicrobials as an Adjunct to Scaling and Root Planing in Periodontitis Patients," *J Clin Periodontol*, 2002, 29(Suppl 3):136-59.

Jenkins WM, MacFarlane TW, Gilmour WH, et al, "Systemic Metronidazole in the Treatment of Periodontitis," *J Clin Periodontol*, 1989, 16(7):443-50.

Loesche WJ, Giordano JR, Hujoel P, et al, "Metronidazole in Periodontitis: Reduced Need for Surgery," *J Clin Periodontol*, 1992, 19(2):103-12.
Loesche WJ, Schmidt E, Smith BA, et al, "Effects of Metronidazole on Periodontal Treatment Needs," *J Periodontol*, 1991, 62(4):247-57.
Noiri Y, Okami Y, Narimatsu M, et al, "Effects of Chlorhexidine, Minocycline, and Metronidazole on Porphyromonas Gingivalis Strain 381 in Biofilms," *J Periodontol*, 2003, 74(11):1647-51.
Söder PO, Frithiof L, Wikner S, et al, "The Effect of Systemic Metronidazole After Nonsurgical Treatment in Moderate and Advanced Periodontitis in Young Adults," *J Periodontol*, 1990, 61(5):281-8.
Wynn RL, Bergman SA, Meiller TF, et al, "Antibiotics in Treating Oral-Facial Infections of Odontogenic Origin: An Update," *Gen Dent*, 2001, 49(3):238-40, 242, 244 passim.

Metronidazole and Nystatin (met roe NYE da zole & nye STAT in)

Related Information
Nystatin (Topical) *on page 1233*

Canadian Brand Names Flagystatin®

Pharmacologic Category Antifungal Agent, Vaginal; Antiprotozoal, Nitroimidazole

Use Treatment of mixed vaginal infection due to *T. vaginalis* and *C. albicans*

Local Anesthetic/Vasoconstrictor Precautions No information available to require special precautions

Effects on Dental Treatment Key adverse event(s) related to dental treatment: Taste disturbances (bitter) and coated tongue.

Effects on Bleeding No information available to require special precautions

Adverse Effects Note: Adverse effects are infrequent and generally minor.
Central nervous system: Headache
Dermatologic: Pruritus, spots on skin (around knees), welts on body
Gastrointestinal: Coated tongue, nausea, taste disturbance (bitter), vomiting
Genitourinary: Vaginal: Burning, granular sensation
Neuromuscular & skeletal: Fatigue, swelling/aching or wrists

General Dosage Range Intravaginal: *Adults:* Insert 1 applicatorful or tablet daily

Mechanism of Action See individual agents.

Product Availability Not available in U.S.

Metyrosine (me TYE roe seen)

U.S. Brand Names Demser®

Canadian Brand Names Demser®

Pharmacologic Category Tyrosine Hydroxylase Inhibitor

Use Short-term management of pheochromocytoma before surgery, long-term management when surgery is contraindicated or when chronic malignant pheochromocytoma exists

Local Anesthetic/Vasoconstrictor Precautions No information available to require special precautions

Effects on Dental Treatment Key adverse event(s) related to dental treatment: Xerostomia (normal salivary flow resumes upon discontinuation).

Effects on Bleeding No information available to require special precautions

Adverse Effects
>10%:
Central nervous system: Drowsiness, extrapyramidal symptoms
Gastrointestinal: Diarrhea
1% to 10%:
Endocrine & metabolic: Galactorrhea, edema of the breasts
Gastrointestinal: Nausea, vomiting, xerostomia
Genitourinary: Impotence
Respiratory: Nasal congestion

General Dosage Range Oral: *Children >12 years and Adults:* Initial: 250 mg 4 times/day; Maintenance: 2-3 g/day in 4 divided doses (maximum: 4 g/day)

Mechanism of Action Blocks the rate-limiting step in the biosynthetic pathway of catecholamines. It is a tyrosine hydroxylase inhibitor, blocking the conversion of tyrosine to dihydroxyphenylalanine. This inhibition results in decreased levels of endogenous catecholamines. Catecholamine biosynthesis is reduced by 35% to 80% in patients treated with metyrosine 1-4 g/day.

Pharmacodynamics/Kinetics
Half-life Elimination 3.3-3.7 hours

Pregnancy Risk Factor C

Mexiletine (meks IL e teen)

Canadian Brand Names Novo-Mexiletine

Pharmacologic Category Antiarrhythmic Agent, Class Ib

Use Management of serious ventricular arrhythmias; suppression of PVCs

Local Anesthetic/Vasoconstrictor Precautions No information available to require special precautions

Effects on Dental Treatment Key adverse event(s) related to dental treatment: Xerostomia (normal salivary flow resumes upon discontinuation).

Effects on Bleeding No information available to require special precautions

Adverse Effects

>10%:

Central nervous system: Lightheadedness (11% to 25%), dizziness (20% to 25%), nervousness (5% to 10%), incoordination (10%)

Gastrointestinal: GI distress (41%), nausea/vomiting (40%)

Neuromuscular & skeletal: Trembling, unsteady gait, tremor (13%), ataxia (10% to 20%)

1% to 10%:

Cardiovascular: Chest pain (3% to 8%), premature ventricular contractions (1% to 2%), palpitation (4% to 8%), angina (2%), proarrhythmia (10% to 15% in patients with malignant arrhythmia)

Central nervous system: Confusion, headache, insomnia (5% to 7%), depression (2%)

Dermatologic: Rash (4%)

Gastrointestinal: Constipation or diarrhea (4% to 5%), xerostomia (3%), abdominal pain (1%)

Neuromuscular & skeletal: Weakness (5%), numbness of fingers or toes (2% to 4%), paresthesia (2%), arthralgia (1%)

Ocular: Blurred vision (5% to 7%), nystagmus (6%)

Otic: Tinnitus (2% to 3%)

Respiratory: Dyspnea (3%)

General Dosage Range Dosage adjustment recommended in patients with hepatic impairment

Oral: *Adults:* Initial: 200 mg every 8 hours; Maintenance: 200-300 mg every 8 hours (maximum: 1.2 g/day)

Mechanism of Action Class IB antiarrhythmic, structurally related to lidocaine, which inhibits inward sodium current, decreases rate of rise of phase 0, increases effective refractory period/action potential duration ratio

Pharmacodynamics/Kinetics

Half-life Elimination Adults: 10-14 hours (average: 14.4 hours elderly, 12 hours younger adults); prolonged with hepatic impairment or heart failure

Time to Peak Serum: 2-3 hours

Pregnancy Risk Factor C

Micafungin (mi ka FUN gin)

Related Information

Fungal Infections *on page 1945*

U.S. Brand Names Mycamine®

Canadian Brand Names Mycamine®

Pharmacologic Category Antifungal Agent, Parenteral; Echinocandin

Use Treatment of esophageal candidiasis; *Candida* prophylaxis in patients undergoing hematopoietic stem cell transplant (HSCT); treatment of candidemia, acute disseminated candidiasis, and other *Candida* infections (peritonitis and abscesses)

Unlabeled/Investigational Use Treatment of infections due to *Aspergillus* spp; prophylaxis of HIV-related esophageal candidiasis

Local Anesthetic/Vasoconstrictor Precautions No information available to require special precautions

Effects on Dental Treatment No significant effects or complications reported

Effects on Bleeding No information available to require special precautions

Adverse Effects Percentages reflect incidence across all approved indications (prophylaxis and treatment); however, in general, a higher frequency of adverse reactions was observed in studies with HSCT patients.

>10%:

Central nervous system: Fever (20%), headache (16%)

Endocrine & metabolic: Hypokalemia (18%), hypomagnesemia (13%)

Gastrointestinal: Diarrhea (23%), nausea (22%), vomiting (22%), mucosal inflammation (14%), constipation (11%)

Hematologic: Thrombocytopenia (15%), neutropenia (14%)

1% to 10%:

Cardiovascular: Hypotension (9%), tachycardia (8%), hypertension (7%), peripheral edema (7%), phlebitis (6%), edema (5%)

Central nervous system: Insomnia (10%), anxiety (6%), fatigue (6%)

Dermatologic: Rash (9%), pruritus (6%)

Endocrine & metabolic: Hypocalcemia (7%), hyperglycemia (6%)
Gastrointestinal: Abdominal pain (10%), anorexia (6%), dyspepsia (6%)
Hematologic: Anemia (10%), febrile neutropenia (6%)
Hepatic: AST increased (6%), ALT increased (5%), serum alkaline phosphatase increased (5%)
Neuromuscular & skeletal: Rigors (9%), back pain (5%)
Respiratory: Cough (8%), dyspnea (6%), epistaxis (6%)
Miscellaneous: Bacteremia (6%), sepsis (5%)

General Dosage Range I.V.: *Adults:* Prophylaxis: 50 mg daily; Treatment: 100-150 mg daily

Mechanism of Action Concentration-dependent inhibition of 1,3-beta-D-glucan synthase resulting in reduced formation of 1,3-beta-D-glucan, an essential polysaccharide comprising 30% to 60% of *Candida* cell walls (absent in mammalian cells); decreased glucan content leads to osmotic instability and cellular lysis

Pharmacodynamics/Kinetics

Half-life Elimination 11-21 hours

Pregnancy Risk Factor C

Miconazole (Oral) (mi KON a zole)

Related Information

Fungal Infections *on page 1945*

U.S. Brand Names Oravig™

Pharmacologic Category Antifungal Agent, Oral Nonabsorbed

Use Treatment of oropharyngeal candidiasis

Adverse Effects

>10%: Local: Application site reaction (10% to 12%; including burning, discomfort, edema, glossodynia, pain, pruritus, toothache, ulceration)

1% to 10%:

Central nervous system: Headache (5% to 8%), fatigue (3%), pain (1%)
Dermatologic: Pruritus (2%)
Gastrointestinal: Diarrhea (6% to 9%), nausea (1% to 7%), vomiting (1% to 4%), abnormal taste (3% to 4%), oral discomfort (3%), xerostomia (3%), abdominal pain (1% to 3%), ageusia (2%), gastroenteritis (1%)
Hematologic: Anemia (3%), lymphopenia (2%), neutropenia (1%)
Hepatic: GGT increased (1%)
Respiratory: Cough (3%), upper respiratory infection (2%), pharyngeal pain (1%)

General Dosage Range Buccal: *Children ≥16 years and Adults:* 50 mg (1 tablet) once daily

Mechanism of Action Inhibits biosynthesis of ergosterol, damaging the fungal cell wall membrane, which increases permeability causing leaking of nutrients

Pharmacodynamics/Kinetics

Duration of Action Buccal adhesion: 15 hours

Pregnancy Risk Factor C

Miconazole (Topical) (mi KON a zole)

Related Information

Fungal Infections *on page 1945*

U.S. Brand Names 3M™ Cavilon™ Antifungal [OTC]; Aloe Vesta® Antifungal [OTC]; Baza® Antifungal [OTC]; Carrington® Antifungal [OTC]; Critic-Aid® Clear AF [OTC]; DermaFungal [OTC]; Dermagran® AF [OTC]; DiabetAid® Antifungal Foot Bath [OTC]; Fungoid® [OTC]; Lotrimin AF® [OTC]; Micaderm® [OTC]; Micatin® [OTC]; Micro-Guard® [OTC]; Miranel AF™ [OTC]; Mitrazol® [OTC]; Monistat® 1 Day or Night [OTC]; Monistat® 1 [OTC]; Monistat® 3 [OTC]; Monistat® 7 [OTC]; Neosporin® AF [OTC]; Podactin Cream [OTC]; Secura® Antifungal Extra Thick [OTC]; Secura® Antifungal Greaseless [OTC]; Ting® Spray Powder [OTC]; Zeasorb®-AF [OTC]

Canadian Brand Names Dermazole; Micatin®; Micozole; Monistat®; Monistat® 3

Pharmacologic Category Antifungal Agent, Topical; Antifungal Agent, Vaginal

Use Treatment of vulvovaginal candidiasis and a variety of skin and mucous membrane fungal infections

Local Anesthetic/Vasoconstrictor Precautions No information available to require special precautions

Effects on Dental Treatment No significant effects or complications reported

Effects on Bleeding No information available to require special precautions

Adverse Effects Frequency not defined.

Topical: Allergic contact dermatitis, burning, maceration
Vaginal: Abdominal cramps, burning, irritation, itching

General Dosage Range

Intravaginal: *Children ≥12 years and Adults:* Insert 1 applicatorful or suppository (100 mg or 200 mg) once daily at bedtime **or** insert 1 suppository (1200 mg) as a single dose.

Topical: *Children and Adults:* Apply twice daily **or** dissolve 1 effervescent tablet in ~1 gallon of water and soak feet for 15-30 minutes

Mechanism of Action Inhibits biosynthesis of ergosterol, damaging the fungal cell wall membrane, which increases permeability causing leaking of nutrients

Pregnancy Risk Factor C

Miconazole and Zinc Oxide (mi KON a zole & zink OKS ide)

Related Information

Miconazole (Topical) *on page* 1131

Zinc Oxide *on page* 1744

U.S. Brand Names Vusion®

Pharmacologic Category Antifungal Agent, Topical

Use Adjunctive treatment of diaper dermatitis complicated by *Candida albicans* infection

Local Anesthetic/Vasoconstrictor Precautions No information available to require special precautions

Effects on Dental Treatment No significant effects or complications reported

Effects on Bleeding No information available to require special precautions

General Dosage Range Topical: *Children ≥4 weeks:* Apply to affected area with each diaper change (maximum therapy: 7 days)

Mechanism of Action

Miconazole inhibits the biosynthesis of ergosterol, damaging the fungal cell wall membrane.

Zinc oxide is a mild astringent with weak antiseptic properties.

Pregnancy Risk Factor C

Midazolam (MID aye zoe lam)

Canadian Brand Names Apo-Midazolam®; Midazolam Injection

Generic Availability (U.S.) Yes

Pharmacologic Category Benzodiazepine

Dental Use Sedation component in I.V. conscious sedation in oral surgery patients; syrup formulation is used for children to help alleviate anxiety before a dental procedure

Use Preoperative sedation; moderate sedation prior to diagnostic or radiographic procedures; ICU sedation (continuous infusion); induction and maintenance of general anesthesia

Unlabeled/Investigational Use Anxiety, status epilepticus

Local Anesthetic/Vasoconstrictor Precautions No information available to require special precautions

Effects on Dental Treatment No significant effects or complications reported

Effects on Bleeding No information available to require special precautions

Adverse Effects As reported in adults unless otherwise noted:

>10%: Respiratory: Decreased tidal volume and/or respiratory rate decrease, apnea (3% children)

1% to 10%:

- Cardiovascular: Hypotension (3% children)
- Central nervous system: Drowsiness (1%), oversedation, headache (1%), seizure-like activity (1% children)
- Gastrointestinal: Nausea (3%), vomiting (3%)
- Local: Pain and local reactions at injection site (4% I.M., 5% I.V.; severity less than diazepam)
- Ocular: Nystagmus (1% children)
- Respiratory: Cough (1%)
- Miscellaneous: Physical and psychological dependence with prolonged use, hiccups (4%, 1% children), paradoxical reaction (2% children)

Dental Usual Dosage Adults:

Preoperative sedation:

I.M.: 0.07-0.08 mg/kg 30-60 minutes prior to surgery/procedure; usual dose: 5 mg; **Note:** Reduce dose in patients with COPD, high-risk patients, patients ≥60 years of age, and patients receiving other narcotics or CNS depressants

I.V.: 0.02-0.04 mg/kg; repeat every 5 minutes as needed to desired effect or up to 0.1-0.2 mg/kg

Intranasal (not an approved route): 0.2 mg/kg (up to 0.4 mg/kg in some studies); administer 30-45 minutes prior to surgery/procedure

Conscious sedation: I.V.: Initial: 0.5-2 mg slow I.V. over at least 2 minutes; slowly titrate to effect by repeating doses every 2-3 minutes if needed; usual total dose: 2.5-5 mg; use decreased doses in elderly.

Healthy Adults <60 years: Initial: Some patients respond to doses as low as 1 mg; no more than 2.5 mg should be administered over a period of 2 minutes. Additional doses of midazolam may be administered after a 2-minute waiting period and evaluation of sedation after each dose increment. A total dose >5 mg is generally not needed. If narcotics or other CNS depressants are administered concomitantly, the midazolam dose should be reduced by 30%.

Dosage The dose of midazolam needs to be individualized based on the patient's age, underlying diseases, and concurrent medications. Decrease dose (by ~30%) if narcotics or other CNS depressants are administered concomitantly. **Personnel and equipment needed for standard respiratory resuscitation should be immediately available during midazolam administration.**

Children <6 years may require higher doses and closer monitoring than older children; calculate dose on ideal body weight

Conscious sedation for procedures or preoperative sedation:

Oral: 0.25-0.5 mg/kg as a single dose preprocedure, up to a maximum of 20 mg; administer 30-45 minutes prior to procedure. Children <6 years or less cooperative patients may require as much as 1 mg/kg as a single dose; 0.25 mg/kg may suffice for children 6-16 years of age.

Intranasal (not an approved route): 0.2 mg/kg (up to 0.4 mg/kg in some studies), to a maximum of 15 mg; may be administered 30-45 minutes prior to procedure

I.M.: 0.1-0.15 mg/kg 30-60 minutes before surgery or procedure; range: 0.05-0.15 mg/kg; doses up to 0.5 mg/kg have been used in more anxious patients; maximum total dose: 10 mg

I.V.:

Infants <6 months: Limited information is available in nonintubated infants; dosing recommendations not clear; infants <6 months are at higher risk for airway obstruction and hypoventilation; titrate dose in small increments to desired effect; monitor carefully

Infants 6 months to Children 5 years: Initial: 0.05-0.1 mg/kg; titrate dose carefully; total dose of 0.6 mg/kg may be required; usual maximum total dose: 6 mg

Children 6-12 years: Initial: 0.025-0.05 mg/kg; titrate dose carefully; total doses of 0.4 mg/kg may be required; usual maximum total dose: 10 mg

Children 12-16 years: Dose as adults; usual maximum total dose: 10 mg

Conscious sedation during mechanical ventilation: Children: Loading dose: 0.05-0.2 mg/kg, followed by initial continuous infusion: 0.06-0.12 mg/kg/hour (1-2 mcg/kg/minute); titrate to the desired effect; usual range: 0.4-6 mcg/kg/minute

Status epilepticus refractory to standard therapy (unlabeled use): Infants >2 months and Children: Loading dose: 0.15 mg/kg followed by a continuous infusion of 0.06 mg/kg/hour (1 mcg/kg/minute); titrate dose upward every 5 minutes until clinical seizure activity is controlled; mean infusion rate required in 24 children was 0.14 mg/kg/hour (2.3 mcg/kg/minute) with a range of 0.06-1.1 mg/kg/hour (Rivera, 1993)

Adults:

Preoperative sedation:

I.M.: 0.07-0.08 mg/kg 30-60 minutes prior to surgery/procedure; usual dose: 5 mg; **Note:** Reduce dose in patients with COPD, high-risk patients, patients ≥60 years of age, and patients receiving other narcotics or CNS depressants

I.V.: 0.02-0.04 mg/kg; repeat every 5 minutes as needed to desired effect or up to 0.1-0.2 mg/kg

Intranasal (not an approved route): 0.2 mg/kg (up to 0.4 mg/kg in some studies); administer 30-45 minutes prior to surgery/procedure

Conscious sedation: I.V.: Initial: 0.5-2 mg slow I.V. over at least 2 minutes; slowly titrate to effect by repeating doses every 2-3 minutes if needed; usual total dose: 2.5-5 mg; use decreased doses in elderly

Healthy Adults <60 years: Some patients respond to doses as low as 1 mg; no more than 2.5 mg should be administered over a period of 2 minutes. Additional doses of midazolam may be administered after a 2-minute waiting period and evaluation of sedation after each dose increment. A total dose >5 mg is generally not needed. If narcotics or other CNS depressants are administered concomitantly, the midazolam dose should be reduced by 30%.

Anesthesia: I.V.:

Induction:

Unpremedicated patients: 0.3-0.35 mg/kg (up to 0.6 mg/kg in resistant cases)

Premedicated patients: 0.15-0.35 mg/kg

Maintenance: 0.05-0.3 mg/kg as needed, or continuous infusion 0.25-1.5 mcg/kg/minute

Sedation in mechanically-ventilated patients: I.V. continuous infusion: 100 mg in 250 mL D_5W or NS (if patient is fluid-restricted, may concentrate up to a maximum of 0.5 mg/mL); initial dose: 0.02-0.08 mg/kg (~1-5 mg in 70 kg adult) initially and repeated at 5- to 15-minute intervals until adequate sedation is achieved; may use continuous infusion to maintain sedation; usual dosage range for continuous infusion: 0.04-0.2 mg/kg/hour (Jacobi, 2002). Titrate to reach desired level of sedation.

Refractory status epilepticus (unlabeled use): I.V.: 0.15-0.3 mg/kg (usual dose: 5-15 mg); may repeat every 10-15 minutes as needed **or** continuous infusion of 0.05-0.6 mg/kg/hour

Elderly: I.V.: Conscious sedation: Initial: 0.5 mg slow I.V.; give no more than 1.5 mg in a 2-minute period; if additional titration is needed, give no more than 1 mg over 2 minutes, waiting another 2 or more minutes to evaluate sedative effect; a total dose of >3.5 mg is rarely necessary

Dosage adjustment in renal impairment:

Hemodialysis: Supplemental dose is not necessary

Peritoneal dialysis: Significant drug removal is unlikely based on physiochemical characteristics

Mechanism of Action Binds to stereospecific benzodiazepine receptors on the postsynaptic GABA neuron at several sites within the central nervous system, including the limbic system, reticular formation. Enhancement of the inhibitory effect of GABA on neuronal excitability results by increased neuronal membrane permeability to chloride ions. This shift in chloride ions results in hyperpolarization (a less excitable state) and stabilization.

Contraindications Hypersensitivity to midazolam or any component of the formulation, including benzyl alcohol (cross-sensitivity with other benzodiazepines may exist); parenteral form is not for intrathecal or epidural injection; narrow-angle glaucoma; concurrent use of potent inhibitors of CYP3A4 (amprenavir, atazanavir, or ritonavir); pregnancy

Warnings/Precautions **[U.S. Boxed Warning]: May cause severe respiratory depression, respiratory arrest, or apnea. Use with extreme caution, particularly in noncritical care settings.** Appropriate resuscitative equipment and qualified personnel must be available for administration and monitoring. Initial dosing must be cautiously titrated and individualized, particularly in elderly or debilitated patients, patients with hepatic impairment (including alcoholics), or in renal impairment, particularly if other CNS depressants (including opiates) are used concurrently. **[U.S. Boxed Warning]: Initial doses in elderly or debilitated patients should be conservative; as little as 1 mg, but not to exceed 2.5 mg.** Use with caution in patients with respiratory disease or impaired gag reflex. Use during upper airway procedures may increase risk of hypoventilation. Prolonged responses have been noted following extended administration by continuous infusion (possibly due to metabolite accumulation) or in the presence of drugs which inhibit midazolam metabolism.

Causes CNS depression (dose-related) resulting in sedation, dizziness, confusion, or ataxia which may impair physical and mental capabilities. Patients must be cautioned about performing tasks which require mental alertness (eg, operating machinery or driving). A minimum of 1 day should elapse after midazolam administration before attempting these tasks. Use with caution in patients receiving other CNS depressants or psychoactive agents. Effects with other sedative drugs or ethanol may be potentiated. Benzodiazepines have been associated with falls and traumatic injury and should be used with extreme caution in patients who are at risk of these events (especially the elderly).

May cause hypotension - hemodynamic events are more common in pediatric patients or patients with hemodynamic instability. Hypotension and/or respiratory depression may occur more frequently in patients who have received opioid analgesics. Use with caution in obese patients, chronic renal failure, and HF. Does not protect against increases in heart rate or blood pressure during intubation. Should not be used in shock, coma, or acute alcohol intoxication. **[U.S. Boxed Warning]: Parenteral form contains benzyl alcohol; avoid rapid injection in neonates or prolonged infusions.** Avoid intra-arterial administration or extravasation of parenteral formulation.

Midazolam causes anterograde amnesia. Paradoxical reactions, including hyperactive or aggressive behavior have been reported with benzodiazepines, particularly in adolescent/pediatric or psychiatric patients. Does not have analgesic, antidepressant, or antipsychotic properties.

Benzodiazepines have been associated with dependence and acute withdrawal symptoms on discontinuation or reduction in dose. Acute withdrawal, including seizures, may be precipitated after administration of flumazenil to patients receiving long-term benzodiazepine therapy.

Drug Interactions

Metabolism/Transport Effects Substrate of CYP2B6 (minor), 3A4 (major); **Inhibits** CYP2C8 (weak), 2C9 (weak), 3A4 (weak)

Avoid Concomitant Use

Avoid concomitant use of Midazolam with any of the following: Efavirenz; OLANZapine; Protease Inhibitors

Increased Effect/Toxicity

Midazolam may increase the levels/effects of: Alcohol (Ethyl); CloZAPine; CNS Depressants; Fosphenytoin; Methotrimeprazine; Phenytoin; Propofol

The levels/effects of Midazolam may be increased by: Antifungal Agents (Azole Derivatives, Systemic); Aprepitant; Atorvastatin; Calcium Channel Blockers (Nondihydropyridine); Cimetidine; Conivaptan; Contraceptives (Estrogens); Contraceptives (Progestins); CYP3A4 Inhibitors (Moderate); CYP3A4 Inhibitors (Strong); Dasatinib; Droperidol; Efavirenz; Fluconazole; Fosaprepitant; Grapefruit Juice; Isoniazid; Macrolide Antibiotics; Methotrimeprazine; Nefazodone; OLANZapine; Propofol; Protease Inhibitors; Proton Pump Inhibitors; Selective Serotonin Reuptake Inhibitors

Decreased Effect

The levels/effects of Midazolam may be decreased by: CarBAMazepine; CYP3A4 Inducers (Strong); Deferasirox; Ginkgo Biloba; Rifamycin Derivatives; St Johns Wort; Theophylline Derivatives; Tocilizumab; Yohimbine

Ethanol/Nutrition/Herb Interactions

Ethanol: May increase CNS depression; monitor for increased effects with coadministration. Caution patients about effects.

Food: Grapefruit juice may increase serum concentrations of midazolam; avoid concurrent use with oral form.

Herb/Nutraceutical: Avoid concurrent use with St John's wort (may decrease midazolam levels, may increase CNS depression). Avoid concurrent use with valerian, kava kava, gotu kola (may increase CNS depression).

Dietary Considerations Avoid grapefruit juice with oral syrup.

Pharmacodynamics/Kinetics

Onset of Action I.M.: Sedation: ~15 minutes; I.V.: 1-5 minutes; Peak effect: I.M.: 0.5-1 hour

Duration of Action I.M.: Up to 6 hours; Mean: 2 hours

Half-life Elimination 1-4 hours; prolonged with cirrhosis, congestive heart failure, obesity, elderly

Pregnancy Risk Factor D

Lactation Enters breast milk/use caution (AAP rates "of concern"; AAP 2001 update pending)

Breast-Feeding Considerations Midazolam and hydroxymidazolam can be detected in breast milk. Based on information from two women, 2-3 months postpartum, the half-life of midazolam in breast milk is ~1 hour. Milk concentrations were below the limit of detection (<5 nmol/L) 4 hours after a single maternal dose of midazolam 15 mg. Drowsiness, lethargy, or weight loss in nursing infants have been observed in case reports following maternal use of some benzodiazepines.

Controlled Substance C-IV

Dosage Forms

Injection, solution: 1 mg/mL (2 mL, 5 mL, 10 mL); 5 mg/mL (1 mL, 2 mL, 5 mL, 10 mL)

Injection, solution [preservative free]: 1 mg/mL (2 mL, 5 mL); 5 mg/mL (1 mL, 2 mL)

Syrup, oral: 2 mg/mL (118 mL)

References

Dionne RA, Yagiela JA, Moore PA, et al, "Comparing Efficacy and Safety of Four Intravenous Sedation Regimens in Dental Outpatients," *Am Dent Assoc*, 2001, 132(6):740-51.

Midodrine (MI doe dreen)

U.S. Brand Names ProAmatine® [DSC]

Canadian Brand Names Amatine®; Apo-Midodrine®

Pharmacologic Category Alpha$_1$ Agonist

Use Orphan drug: Treatment of symptomatic orthostatic hypotension

Unlabeled/Investigational Use Management of urinary incontinence; vasovagal syncope; prevention of dialysis-induced hypotension

Local Anesthetic/Vasoconstrictor Precautions No information available to require special precautions

Effects on Dental Treatment Key adverse event(s) related to dental treatment: Xerostomia (normal salivary flow resumes upon discontinuation).

Effects on Bleeding No information available to require special precautions

Adverse Effects

>10%:

Cardiovascular: Supine hypertension (7% to 13%)
Dermatologic: Piloerection (13%), pruritus (12%)
Genitourinary: Urinary urgency, retention, or polyuria, dysuria (up to 13%)
Neuromuscular & skeletal: Paresthesia (18%)

1% to 10%:

Central nervous system: Chills (5%), pain (5%)
Dermatologic: Rash (2%)
Gastrointestinal: Abdominal pain

General Dosage Range Dosage adjustment recommended in patients with renal impairment

Oral: *Adults:* 10 mg 3 times/day (maximum: 40 mg/day)

Mechanism of Action Midodrine forms an active metabolite, desglymidodrine, which is an alpha$_1$-agonist. This agent increases arteriolar and venous tone resulting in a rise in standing, sitting, and supine systolic and diastolic blood pressure in patients with orthostatic hypotension.

Pharmacodynamics/Kinetics

Onset of Action ~1 hour

Duration of Action 2-3 hours

Half-life Elimination Desglymidodrine: ~3-4 hours; Midodrine: 25 minutes

Time to Peak Desglymidodrine: 1-2 hours; Midodrine: 30 minutes

Pregnancy Risk Factor C

Mifepristone (mi FE pris tone)

Related Information

Endocrine Disorders and Pregnancy *on page* 1879

U.S. Brand Names Mifeprex®

Pharmacologic Category Abortifacient; Antineoplastic Agent, Hormone Antagonist; Antiprogestin

Use Medical termination of intrauterine pregnancy, through day 49 of pregnancy. Patients may need treatment with misoprostol and possibly surgery to complete therapy

Unlabeled/Investigational Use Treatment of unresectable meningioma; has been studied in the treatment of breast cancer, ovarian cancer, and adrenal cortical carcinoma

Local Anesthetic/Vasoconstrictor Precautions No information available to require special precautions

Effects on Dental Treatment No significant effects or complications reported

Effects on Bleeding No information available to require special precautions

Adverse Effects Vaginal bleeding and uterine cramping are expected to occur when this medication is used to terminate a pregnancy; 90% of women using this medication for this purpose also report adverse reactions. Bleeding or spotting occurs in most women for a period of 9-16 days. Up to 8% of women will experience some degree of bleeding or spotting for 30 days or more. In some cases, bleeding may be prolonged and heavy, potentially leading to hypovolemic shock.

>10%:

Central nervous system: Headache (2% to 31%), dizziness (1% to 12%)
Gastrointestinal: Abdominal pain (cramping) (96%), nausea (43% to 61%), vomiting (18% to 26%), diarrhea (12% to 20%)
Genitourinary: Uterine cramping (83%)

1% to 10%:

Cardiovascular: Syncope (1%)
Central nervous system: Fatigue (10%), fever (4%), insomnia (3%), anxiety (2%), fainting (2%)
Gastrointestinal: Dyspepsia (3%)
Genitourinary: Uterine hemorrhage (5%), vaginitis (3%), pelvic pain (2%), endometriosis/salpingitis/pelvic inflammatory disease (1%)
Hematologic: Decreased hemoglobin >2 g/dL (6%), anemia (2%), leukorrhea (2%)
Neuromuscular & skeletal: Back pain (9%), rigors (3%), leg pain (2%), weakness (2%)
Respiratory: Sinusitis (2%)
Miscellaneous: Viral infection (4%)

General Dosage Range Oral: *Adults:* Day 1: 600 mg (three 200 mg tablets) as a single dose; Day 3: 400 mcg (two 200 mcg tablets) as a single dose if needed

Mechanism of Action Mifepristone, a synthetic steroid, competitively binds to the intracellular progesterone receptor, blocking the effects of progesterone. When used for the termination of pregnancy, this leads to contraction-inducing activity in the myometrium. In the absence of progesterone, mifepristone acts as a partial progesterone agonist. Mifepristone also has weak antiglucocorticoid and antiandrogenic properties; it blocks the feedback effect of cortisol on corticotropin secretion.

Pharmacodynamics/Kinetics

Half-life Elimination Terminal: 18 hours following a slower phase where 50% eliminated between 12-72 hours

Time to Peak Oral: 90 minutes

Pregnancy Risk Factor X

Prescribing and Access Restrictions Mifepristone is deemed to have an approved REMS program. As a requirement of the REMS program, a medication guide must be given to the patient prior to receiving the medication. In addition, the manufacturer recommends distributing a patient agreement form which must be signed by the patient and prescriber confirming the patient's agreement to terminate her pregnancy. A signed copy of the patient agreement should be kept in the patient's medical record.

Mifeprex® is only available direct from Danco Laboratories' distributor. To obtain the product, please refer to, http://www.earlyoptionpill.com, or call 1-877-432-7596.

Investigators wishing to obtain the agent for use in oncology patients must apply for a patient-specific IND from the FDA.

Miglitol (MIG li tol)

Related Information

Endocrine Disorders and Pregnancy *on page 1879*

U.S. Brand Names Glyset®

Canadian Brand Names Glyset®

Pharmacologic Category Antidiabetic Agent, Alpha-Glucosidase Inhibitor

Use Type 2 diabetes mellitus (noninsulin-dependent, NIDDM):

Monotherapy as an adjunct to diet to improve glycemic control in patients with type 2 diabetes mellitus (noninsulin-dependent, NIDDM) whose hyperglycemia cannot be managed with diet alone

Combination therapy with a sulfonylurea when diet plus either miglitol or a sulfonylurea alone do not result in adequate glycemic control. The effect of miglitol to enhance glycemic control is additive to that of sulfonylureas when used in combination.

Local Anesthetic/Vasoconstrictor Precautions No information available to require special precautions

Effects on Dental Treatment Although miglitol does not cause hypoglycemia, it is frequently used in combination and may complicate the management of hypoglecemic episodes caused by other medications. As part of its therapeutic effect, miglitol slows the absorption of complex sugars or disaccharides such as sucrose. This would delay effective treatment of hypoglycemia. Simple sugars, including glucose (dextrose), are not affected. If a patient experiences hypoglycemia, use of food items such as table sugar, candy, or cookies will NOT effectively increase blood glucose. Administration of oral glucose is required in mild-moderate hypoglycemia, and parenteral glucose is required for severe hypoglycemia.

Effects on Bleeding No information available to require special precautions

Adverse Effects

>10%: Gastrointestinal: Flatulence (42%), diarrhea (29%), abdominal pain (12%)

1% to 10%: Dermatologic: Rash (4%)

General Dosage Range Oral: *Adults:* Initial: 25 mg 3 times/day; Maintenance: 25-100 mg 3 times/day (maximum: 300 mg/day)

Mechanism of Action In contrast to sulfonylureas, miglitol does not enhance insulin secretion; the antihyperglycemic action of miglitol results from a reversible inhibition of membrane-bound intestinal alpha-glucosidases which hydrolyze oligosaccharides and disaccharides to glucose and other monosaccharides in the brush border of the small intestine. In patients with diabetes, this enzyme inhibition results in delayed glucose absorption and lowering of postprandial hyperglycemia.

Pharmacodynamics/Kinetics

Half-life Elimination ~2 hours

Time to Peak 2-3 hours

Pregnancy Risk Factor B

Miglustat (MIG loo stat)

U.S. Brand Names Zavesca®

Canadian Brand Names Zavesca®

Pharmacologic Category Enzyme Inhibitor

Use Treatment of mild-to-moderate type 1 Gaucher disease when enzyme replacement therapy is not a therapeutic option

Local Anesthetic/Vasoconstrictor Precautions No information available to require special precautions

Effects on Dental Treatment No significant effects or complications reported

Effects on Bleeding No information available to require special precautions

Adverse Effects Percentages reported from open-label, uncontrolled monotherapy trials.

>10%:

Central nervous system: Headache (21% to 22%), dizziness (up to 11%)

Gastrointestinal: Diarrhea (89% to 100%), weight loss (39% to 67%), abdominal pain (18% to 67%), flatulence (29% to 50%), nausea (8% to 22%), vomiting (4% to 11%)

Neuromuscular & skeletal: Tremor (11% to 30%), weakness (17%), leg cramps (4% to 11%)

Ocular: Visual disturbances (up to 17%)

1% to 10%:

Central nervous system: Memory impairment (8%), migraine (up to 6%)

Endocrine & metabolic: Menstrual disorder (up to 6%)

Gastrointestinal: Constipation (8%), xerostomia (8%), bloating (up to 8%), anorexia (up to 7%), dyspepsia (up to 7%), epigastric pain (up to 6%)

Hematologic: Thrombocytopenia (6% to 7%)

Neuromuscular & skeletal: Paresthesia (up to 7%)

General Dosage Range Dosage adjustment recommended in patients with renal impairment

Oral: *Adults:* 100 mg 1-3 times/day

Mechanism of Action Miglustat competitively and reversibly inhibits the enzyme needed to produce glycosphingolipids and decreases the rate of glycosphingolipid glucosylceramide formation. Glucosylceramide accumulates in type 1 Gaucher disease, causing complications specific to this disease.

Pharmacodynamics/Kinetics

Half-life Elimination 6-7 hours

Time to Peak Plasma: 2-2.5 hours

Pregnancy Risk Factor X

Milnacipran (mil NAY ci pran)

U.S. Brand Names Savella®

Generic Availability (U.S.) No

Pharmacologic Category Antidepressant, Serotonin/Norepinephrine Reuptake Inhibitor

Use Management of fibromyalgia

Local Anesthetic/Vasoconstrictor Precautions Although milnacipran is not a tricyclic antidepressant, it blocks norepinephrine reuptake within the CNS synapses as part of the mechanism of action. It has been suggested that vasoconstrictors be administered with caution and vial signs monitored in dental patients taking antidepressants that affect norepinephrine in this way.

Effects on Dental Treatment Key adverse event(s) related to dental treatment: Xerostomia and changes in salivation (normal salivary flow resumes upon discontinuation) and taste perversion.

Effects on Bleeding Serotonin/norepinephrine reuptake inhibitors (SNRIs) may impair platelet aggregation resulting in increased risk of bleeding events, particularly if used concomitantly with aspirin or NSAIDs due to ulcerogenic potential

Adverse Effects

>10%:

Central nervous system: Headache (18%), insomnia (12%)

Endocrine & metabolic: Hot flashes (12%)

Gastrointestinal: Nausea (37%), constipation (16%)

1% to 10%:

Cardiovascular: Palpitation (7%), heart rate increased (6%), hypertension (5%), flushing (3%), blood pressure increased (3%), tachycardia (2%), peripheral edema (≥1%)

Central nervous system: Dizziness (10%), migraine (5%), chills (2%), tremor (2%), depression (≥1%), fatigue (≥1%), fever (≥1%), irritability (≥1%), somnolence (≥1%)

Dermatologic: Hyperhidrosis (9%), rash (3%)

Endocrine & metabolic: Hypercholesterolemia (≥1%)

Gastrointestinal: Vomiting (7%), xerostomia (5%), abdominal pain (3%), appetite decreased (2%), abdominal distension (≥1%), abnormal taste (≥1%), diarrhea (≥1%), dyspepsia (≥1%), flatulence (≥1%), gastroesophageal reflux disease (≥1%), weight changes (≥1%)

Genitourinary: Dysuria (≥2%), ejaculation disorder/failure (≥2%), erectile dysfunction (≥2%), libido decreased (≥2%), prostatitis (≥2%), scrotal pain (≥2%), testicular pain (≥2%), testicular swelling (≥2%), urethral pain (≥2%), urinary hesitation (≥2%), urinary retention (≥2%), urine flow decreased (≥2%), cystitis (≥1%), urinary tract infection (≥1%)

Neuromuscular & skeletal: Falling (≥1%)

Ocular: Blurred vision (2%)

Respiratory: Dyspnea (2%)

Miscellaneous: Night sweats (≥1%)

Dosage Oral: Adults: 50 mg twice daily (maximum dose: 200 mg/day)

Titration schedule: 12.5 mg once on day 1, then 12.5 mg twice daily on days 2-3, 25 mg twice daily on days 4-7, then 50 mg twice daily thereafter. Dose may be increased to 100 mg twice daily, based on individual response. Doses >200 mg/day have not been studied.

Discontinuation of therapy: Gradually taper dose. If intolerable symptoms occur following a dose reduction, consider resuming the previously prescribed dose and/or decrease dose at a more gradual rate.

Dosing adjustment in renal impairment:

Mild renal impairment: No dose adjustment is recommended

Moderate renal impairment: Use with caution

Severe renal impairment (Cl_{cr} ≤29 mL/minute): Reduce maintenance dose to 25 mg twice daily; dose may be increased to 50 mg twice daily, based on individual tolerance

End-stage renal disease (ESRD): Use not recommended

Dosing adjustment in hepatic impairment:

Mild-to-moderate hepatic impairment: No dose adjustment is recommended

Severe hepatic impairment: Use with caution

Mechanism of Action Potent inhibitor of norepinephrine and serotonin reuptake (3:1). Milnacipran has no significant activity for serotonergic, alpha- and beta-adrenergic, muscarinic, histaminergic, dopaminergic, opiate, benzodiazepine, and GABA receptors. It does not possess MAO-inhibitory activity.

Contraindications Concomitant use or within 2 weeks of MAO inhibitors; uncontrolled narrow-angle glaucoma

Warnings/Precautions [U.S. Boxed Warning]: Milnacipran is a serotonin/norepinephrine reuptake inhibitor (SNRI) similar to SNRIs used to treat depression and other psychiatric disorders. **Antidepressants increase the risk of suicidal thinking and behavior in children, adolescents, and young adults (18-24 years of age) with major depressive disorder (MDD) and other psychiatric disorders**; consider risk prior to prescribing. Short-term studies did not show an increased risk in patients >24 years of age and showed a decreased risk in patients ≥65 years. Closely monitor for clinical worsening, suicidality, or unusual changes in behavior; the patient's family or caregiver should be instructed to closely observe the patient and communicate condition with healthcare provider. A medication guide should be dispensed with each prescription. **Milnacipran is not FDA approved for the treatment of major depressive disorder or for use in children.**

Suicide risks should be monitored in patients treated with SNRIs regardless of the indication. The possibility of a suicide attempt is inherent in major depression and may persist until remission occurs. Monitor for worsening of depression or suicidality, especially during initiation of therapy (generally first 1-2 months) or with dose increases or decreases. Use caution in high-risk patients. Worsening depression and severe abrupt suicidality that are not part of the presenting symptoms may require discontinuation or modification of drug therapy. The patient's family or caregiver should be alerted to monitor patients for the emergence of suicidality and associated behaviors (such as agitation, irritability, hostility, impulsivity, and hypomania) and call healthcare provider.

Patients with major depressive disorder were excluded from clinical trials evaluating milnacipran for fibromyalgia; however, mania has been reported in patients with mood disorders taking similar medications. May worsen psychosis in some patients or precipitate a shift to mania or hypomania in patients with bipolar disorder. Patients presenting with depressive symptoms should be screened for bipolar disorder. Monotherapy in patients with bipolar disorder should be avoided. **Milnacipran is not FDA approved for the treatment of bipolar depression.**

Serotonin syndrome and neuroleptic malignant syndrome (NMS)-like reactions have occurred with serotonin/norepinephrine reuptake inhibitors (SNRIs) and selective serotonin reuptake inhibitors (SSRIs) when used alone, and particularly when used in combination with serotonergic agents (eg, triptans) or antidopaminergic agents (eg, antipsychotics). Concurrent use with MAO inhibitors is contraindicated. May cause sustained increase in blood pressure or heart rate. Control pre-existing hypertension and cardiovascular disease prior to initiation of milnacipran. Use caution in patients with renal impairment; dose reduction required in severe renal impairment. Use caution in patients with hepatic impairment. Avoid ethanol use. May cause hyponatremia/SIADH (elderly at increased risk); volume depletion (diuretics may increase risk). Use cautiously in patients with a history of seizures. May impair platelet aggregation, resulting in bleeding. May cause increased urinary resistance. Use caution in patients with controlled narrow-angle glaucoma; use is contraindicated with uncontrolled narrow-angle glaucoma.

Abrupt discontinuation or dosage reduction after extended therapy may lead to agitation, dysphoria, anxiety, and other symptoms. When discontinuing therapy, dosage should be tapered gradually. If intolerable symptoms occur following a decrease in dosage or upon discontinuation of therapy, then resuming the previous dose with a more gradual taper should be considered.

Drug Interactions

Avoid Concomitant Use

Avoid concomitant use of Milnacipran with any of the following: Iobenguane I 123; MAO Inhibitors; Methylene Blue; Sibutramine

Increased Effect/Toxicity

Milnacipran may increase the levels/effects of: Alcohol (Ethyl); Alpha-/Beta-Agonists; Aspirin; CNS Depressants; Digoxin; Methotrimeprazine; Methylene Blue; NSAID (Nonselective); Serotonin Modulators; Vitamin K Antagonists

The levels/effects of Milnacipran may be increased by: ClomiPRAMINE; Droperidol; MAO Inhibitors; Methotrimeprazine; Sibutramine

Decreased Effect

Milnacipran may decrease the levels/effects of: Alpha2-Agonists; Iobenguane I 123

Ethanol/Nutrition/Herb Interactions

Ethanol: May increase CNS depression; monitor for increased effects with coadministration. Caution patients about effects.

Herb/Nutraceutical: Avoid valerian, St John's wort, SAMe, kava kava, tryptophan (may increase risk of serotonin syndrome and/or excessive sedation).

Dietary Considerations May be taken with or without food; food may improve tolerability.

Pharmacodynamics/Kinetics

Half-life Elimination 6-8 hours

Time to Peak Plasma: Oral: 2-4 hours

Pregnancy Risk Factor C

Lactation Excretion in breast milk unknown/not recommended

Breast-Feeding Considerations It is unknown if milnacipran is excreted in human milk; there are no adequate and well-controlled studies in nursing mothers.

Dosage Forms

Combination package, oral:

Savella®: Tablet: 12.5 mg (5s), Tablet: 25 mg (8s), and Tablet: 50 mg (42s)

Tablet, oral:

Savella®: 12.5 mg, 25 mg, 50 mg, 100 mg

References

Gendreau RM, Thorn MD, Gendreau JF, et al, "Efficacy of Milnacipran in Patients With Fibromyalgia," *J Rheumatol*, 2005, 32(10):1975-85.

Vitton O, Gendreau M, Gendreau J, et al, "A Double-Blind Placebo-Controlled Trial of Milnacipran in the Treatment of Fibromyalgia," *Hum Psychopharmacol*, 2004, 19(Suppl 1):27-35.

Milrinone (MIL ri none)

Related Information

Cardiovascular Diseases *on page 1848*

Canadian Brand Names Milrinone Lactate Injection; Primacor®

Pharmacologic Category Phosphodiesterase Enzyme Inhibitor

Use Short-term I.V. therapy of acutely-decompensated heart failure

Unlabeled/Investigational Use Inotropic therapy for patients unresponsive to other acute heart failure therapies (eg, dobutamine); outpatient inotropic therapy for heart transplant candidates; palliation of symptoms in end-stage heart failure patients who cannot otherwise be discharged from the hospital and are not transplant candidates

Local Anesthetic/Vasoconstrictor Precautions No information available to require special precautions

Effects on Dental Treatment No significant effects or complications reported

Effects on Bleeding No information available to require special precautions

Adverse Effects

>10%: Cardiovascular: Ventricular arrhythmia (ectopy 9%, NSVT 3%, sustained ventricular tachycardia 1%, ventricular fibrillation <1%)

1% to 10%:

Cardiovascular: Supraventricular arrhythmia (4%), hypotension (3%), angina/chest pain (1%)

Central nervous system: Headache (3%)

General Dosage Range Dosage adjustment recommended in patients with renal impairment

I.V.: *Adults:* Loading dose (optional): 50 mcg/kg; Maintenance: 0.375-0.75 mcg/kg/minute

Mechanism of Action A selective phosphodiesterase inhibitor in cardiac and vascular tissue, resulting in vasodilation and inotropic effects with little chronotropic activity.

Pharmacodynamics/Kinetics

Onset of Action I.V.: 5-15 minutes

Half-life Elimination Normal renal function: ~2.5 hours; CVVH: 20.1 hours (Taniguchi, 2000)

Pregnancy Risk Factor C

Minocycline (mi noe SYE kleen)

Related Sample Prescriptions

Bacterial Infections and Periodontal Diseases *on page 1983*

U.S. Brand Names Dynacin®; Minocin®; Minocin® PAC; Solodyn®

Canadian Brand Names Apo-Minocycline®; Arestin Microspheres; Dom-Minocycline; Minocin®; Mylan-Minocycline; Novo-Minocycline; PHL-Minocycline; PMS-Minocycline; ratio-Minocycline; Riva-Minocycline; Sandoz-Minocycline

Generic Availability (U.S.) Yes: Excludes extended release tablet, injection, pellet-filled capsule

Pharmacologic Category Antibiotic, Tetracycline Derivative

Use Treatment of susceptible bacterial infections of both gram-negative and gram-positive organisms; treatment of anthrax (inhalational, cutaneous, and gastrointestinal); moderate-to-severe acne; meningococcal (asymptomatic) carrier state; Rickettsial diseases (including Rocky Mountain spotted fever, Q fever); nongonococcal urethritis, gonorrhea; acute intestinal amebiasis; respiratory tract infection; skin/soft tissue infections; chlamydial infections

Extended release (Solodyn®): Only indicated for treatment of inflammatory lesions of non-nodular moderate-to-severe acne

Unlabeled/Investigational Use Rheumatoid arthritis (patients with low disease activity of short duration); nocardiosis; alternative treatment for community-acquired MRSA infection

Local Anesthetic/Vasoconstrictor Precautions No information available to require special precautions

Effects on Dental Treatment Key adverse event(s) related to dental treatment: Discoloration of teeth (children). Opportunistic "superinfection" with *Candida albicans*; tetracyclines are not recommended for use during pregnancy or in children ≤8 years of age since they have been reported to cause enamel hypoplasia and permanent teeth discoloration. The use of tetracycline's should only be used in these patients if other agents are contraindicated or alternative antimicrobials will not eradicate the organism. Long-term use associated with oral candidiasis.

Effects on Bleeding No information available to require special precautions

Adverse Effects Frequency not defined.

Cardiovascular: Myocarditis, pericarditis, vasculitis

Central nervous system: Bulging fontanels, dizziness, fatigue, fever, headache, hypoesthesia, malaise, mood changes, paresthesia, pseudotumor cerebri, sedation, seizure, somnolence, vertigo

Dermatologic: Alopecia, angioedema, DRESS (Drug Rash with Eosinophilia and Systemic Symptoms) syndrome, erythema multiforme, erythema nodosum, erythematous rash, exfoliative dermatitis, hyperpigmentation of nails, maculopapular rash, photosensitivity, pigmentation of the skin and mucous membranes, pruritus, Stevens-Johnson syndrome, toxic epidermal necrolysis, urticaria

Endocrine & metabolic: Thyroid cancer, thyroid discoloration, thyroid dysfunction

Gastrointestinal: Anorexia, diarrhea, dyspepsia, dysphagia, enamel hypoplasia, enterocolitis, esophageal ulcerations, esophagitis, glossitis, inflammatory lesions (oral/anogenital), moniliasis, nausea, oral cavity discoloration, pancreatitis, pseudomembranous colitis, stomatitis, tooth discoloration, vomiting, xerostomia

Genitourinary: Balanitis, vulvovaginitis

Hematologic: Agranulocytosis, eosinophilia, hemolytic anemia, leukopenia, neutropenia, pancytopenia, thrombocytopenia

Hepatic: Autoimmune hepatitis, hepatic cholestasis, hepatic failure, hepatitis, hyperbilirubinemia, jaundice, liver enzyme increases
Local: Injection site reaction (I.V. administration)
Neuromuscular & skeletal: Arthralgia, arthritis, bone discoloration, joint stiffness, joint swelling, myalgia
Otic: Hearing loss, tinnitus
Renal: Acute renal failure, BUN increased, interstitial nephritis
Respiratory: Asthma, bronchospasm, cough, dyspnea, pneumonitis, pulmonary infiltrate (with eosinophilia)
Miscellaneous: Anaphylaxis, hypersensitivity, lupus erythematosus, lupus-like syndrome, serum sickness

Dosage

Usual dosage range:

I.V.:

Children >8 years: Initial: 4 mg/kg, followed by 2 mg/kg/dose every 12 hours (maximum: 400 mg/day)
Adults: Initial: 200 mg, followed by 100 mg every 12 hours (maximum: 400 mg/day)

Oral:

Capsule or immediate release tablet:
Children >8 years: Oral: Initial: 4 mg/kg, followed by 2 mg/kg/dose every 12 hours
Adults: Oral: Initial: 200 mg, followed by 100 mg every 12 hours; more frequent dosing intervals may be used (100-200 mg initially, followed by 50 mg 4 times daily)
Extended release tablet (Solodyn®): Children ≥12 years and Adults (≥45 kg): Oral: 45-135 mg once daily (weight based)

Indication-specific dosing:

Children:

Acne *(inflammatory, non-nodular, moderate-to-severe)* (Solodyn®): Oral: Children ≥12 years:
45-54 kg: 45 mg once daily
55-77 kg: 65 mg once daily
78-102 kg: 90 mg once daily
103-125 kg: 115 mg once daily
126-136 kg: 135 mg once daily
Note: Therapy should be continued for 12 weeks. Higher doses do not confer greater efficacy and may be associated with more acute vestibular side effects. Safety of use beyond 12 weeks has not been established.

Cellulitis (purulent) infection due to community-acquired MRSA (unlabeled use): Oral: Children >8 years: Initial: 4 mg/kg (maximum: 200 mg); Maintenance: 2 mg/kg/dose (maximum: 100 mg) every 12 hours for 5-10 days (Liu, 2011)

Adults:

Acne: Oral: Capsule or immediate-release tablet: 50-100 mg twice daily
Inflammatory, non-nodular, moderate-to-severe (Solodyn®):
45-54 kg: 45 mg once daily
55-77 kg: 65 mg once daily
78-102 kg: 90 mg once daily
103-125 kg: 115 mg once daily
126-136 kg: 135 mg once daily
Note: Therapy should be continued for 12 weeks. Higher doses do not confer greater efficacy and may be associated with more acute vestibular side effects. Safety of use beyond 12 weeks has not been established.

Cellulitis (purulent) due to community-acquired MRSA (unlabeled use): Oral: Initial: 200 mg; Maintenance: 100 mg twice daily for 5-10 days (Liu, 2011)

Chlamydial or *Ureaplasma urealyticum* infection, uncomplicated: Oral, I.V.: Urethral, endocervical, or rectal: 100 mg every 12 hours for at least 7 days

Gonococcal infection, uncomplicated (males): Oral, I.V.:
Without urethritis or anorectal infection: Initial: 200 mg, followed by 100 mg every 12 hours for at least 4 days (cultures 2-3 days post-therapy)
Urethritis: 100 mg every 12 hours for 5 days

Meningococcal carrier state (manufacturer's labeling): Oral: 100 mg every 12 hours for 5 days. **Note:** CDC recommendations do not mention use of minocycline for eradicating nasopharyngeal carriage of meningococcal

Mycobacterium marinum: Oral: 100 mg every 12 hours for 6-8 weeks

Nocardiosis, cutaneous (non-CNS) (unlabeled use): Oral: 100-200 mg every 12 hours

Rheumatoid arthritis (unlabeled use): Oral: 100 mg twice daily (O'Dell, 2001)

Syphilis: Oral, I.V.: Initial: 200 mg, followed by 100 mg every 12 hours for 10-15 days

Elderly: Refer to adult dosing.

Dosage adjustment in renal impairment: Use with caution; monitor BUN and creatinine clearance. Consider decreasing dose or increasing dosing interval (extended release).

Cl_{cr} <80 mL/minute: Do not exceed 200 mg/day

Mechanism of Action Inhibits bacterial protein synthesis by binding with the 30S and possibly the 50S ribosomal subunit(s) of susceptible bacteria; cell wall synthesis is not affected

Rheumatoid arthritis: The mechanism of action of minocycline in rheumatoid arthritis is not completely understood. It is thought to have antimicrobial, anti-inflammatory, immunomodulatory, and chondroprotective effects. More specifically, it is thought to be a potent inhibitor of metalloproteinases, which are active in rheumatoid arthritis joint destruction.

Contraindications Hypersensitivity to minocycline, other tetracyclines, or any component of the formulation

Warnings/Precautions May be associated with increases in BUN secondary to antianabolic effects; use caution in patients with renal impairment (Cl_{cr} <80 mL/minute). Hepatotoxicity has been reported; use caution in patients with hepatic insufficiency. Autoimmune syndromes (eg, lupus-like, hepatitis, and vasculitis) have been reported; discontinue if symptoms occur. CNS effects (lightheadedness, vertigo) may occur; patients must be cautioned about performing tasks which require mental alertness (eg, operating machinery or driving). Pseudotumor cerebri has been (rarely) reported with tetracycline use; usually resolves with discontinuation. May cause photosensitivity; discontinue if skin erythema occurs. Prolonged use may result in fungal or bacterial superinfection, including *C. difficile*-associated diarrhea (CDAD) and pseudomembranous colitis; CDAD has been observed >2 months postantibiotic treatment. May cause tissue hyperpigmentation, enamel hypoplasia, or permanent tooth discoloration; use of tetracyclines should be avoided during tooth development (children ≤8 years of age) unless other drugs are not likely to be effective or are contraindicated. However, use is recommended in treatment of anthrax exposure. Do not use during pregnancy. In addition to affecting tooth development, tetracycline use has been associated with retardation of skeletal development and reduced bone growth. Rash, along with eosinophilia, fever, and organ failure (Drug Rash with Eosinophilia and Systemic Symptoms [DRESS] syndrome) has been reported; discontinue treatment immediately if DRESS syndrome is suspected.

Drug Interactions

Avoid Concomitant Use

Avoid concomitant use of Minocycline with any of the following: BCG; Retinoic Acid Derivatives

Increased Effect/Toxicity

Minocycline may increase the levels/effects of: Neuromuscular-Blocking Agents; Retinoic Acid Derivatives; Vitamin K Antagonists

Decreased Effect

Minocycline may decrease the levels/effects of: Atazanavir; BCG; Penicillins; Typhoid Vaccine

The levels/effects of Minocycline may be decreased by: Antacids; Bile Acid Sequestrants; Bismuth; Bismuth Subsalicylate; Calcium Salts; Iron Salts; Magnesium Salts; Quinapril; Sucralfate; Zinc Salts

Ethanol/Nutrition/Herb Interactions

Food: Minocycline serum concentrations are not significantly altered if taken with food or dairy products.

Herb/Nutraceutical: Avoid dong quai, St John's wort (may also cause photosensitization).

Dietary Considerations May be taken with or without food.

Pharmacodynamics/Kinetics

Half-life Elimination I.V.: 15-23 hours; Oral: 16 hours (range: 11-22 hours)

Time to Peak Capsule, pellet filled: 1-4 hours; Extended release tablet: 3.5-4 hours

Pregnancy Risk Factor D

Lactation Enters breast milk/not recommended

Breast-Feeding Considerations Small amounts of minocycline are excreted in breast milk and therefore, breast-feeding is not recommended by the manufacturer. Minocycline absorption is not affected by dairy products. This may lead to increased absorption from maternal milk when compared to other tetracyclines which are bound by the calcium in the maternal milk. Nondose-related effects could include modification of bowel flora. There have been case reports of black discoloration of breast milk in women taking minocycline.

Dosage Forms

Capsule, oral: 50 mg, 75 mg, 100 mg

Capsule, pellet filled, oral:

Minocin®: 50 mg, 100 mg

Minocin® PAC: 50 mg, 100 mg

Injection, powder for reconstitution:

Minocin®: 100 mg

Tablet, oral: 50 mg, 75 mg, 100 mg

Dynacin®: 50 mg, 75 mg, 100 mg

Tablet, extended release, oral:

Solodyn®: 45 mg, 65 mg, 90 mg, 115 mg, 135 mg

References

Goulden V, "Guidelines for the Management of Acne Vulgaris in Adolescents," *Paediatr Drugs*, 2003, 5 (5):301-13.

Smilack JD, Wilson WR, and Cockerill FR 3d, "Tetracyclines, Chloramphenicol, Erythromycin, Clindamycin, and Metronidazole," *Mayo Clin Proc*, 1991, 66(12):1270-80.

Minocycline Hydrochloride (Periodontal)

(mi noe SYE kleen hye droe KLOR ide pair ee oh DON tol)

Related Information

Minocycline *on page 1141*

Periodontal Diseases *on page 1942*

U.S. Brand Names Arestin®

Generic Availability (U.S.) No

Pharmacologic Category Antibiotic, Tetracycline Derivative

Dental Use Adjunct to scaling and root planing procedures for reduction of pocket depth in patients with adult periodontitis. May be used as part of a periodontal maintenance program which includes good oral hygiene, scaling, and root planing.

Local Anesthetic/Vasoconstrictor Precautions No information available to require special precautions

Effects on Dental Treatment Key adverse event(s) related to dental treatment: Patients should avoid the following postadministration: Eating hard, crunchy, or sticky foods for 1 week; brushing for a 12-hour period; touching treated areas; use of interproximal cleaning devices for 10 days.

Effects on Bleeding No information available to require special precautions

Adverse Effects

>10%: Gastrointestinal: Tooth disorder (12%)

1% to 10%:

Central nervous system: Headache (9%), pain (4%)

Gastrointestinal: Dental caries (10%), dental pain (10%), gingivitis (9%), mouth ulceration (5%), dyspepsia (4%), mucous membrane disorder (3%)

Respiratory: Pharyngitis (4%)

Miscellaneous: Infection (8%), flu-like syndrome (5%)

Dental Usual Dosage Arestin® is a variable-dose product; dependent upon the size, shape, and number of pockets being treated.

Administration of Arestin® does not require local anesthesia. Professional subgingival administration is accomplished by inserting the unit-dose cartridge to the base of the periodontal pocket and then pressing the thumb ring in the handle mechanism to expel the powder while gradually withdrawing the tip from the base of the pocket. The handle mechanism should be sterilized between patients. Arestin® does not have to be removed (it is bioresorbable) nor is an adhesive dressing required.

Dosage Variable-dose product; dependent upon the size, shape, and number of pockets being treated

Mechanism of Action Minocycline, a member of the tetracycline class of antibiotics, has a broad spectrum of activity. It is bacteriostatic and exerts its antimicrobial activity by inhibiting protein synthesis.

Contraindications Known hypersensitivity to minocycline, tetracyclines, or any component of the formulation

Warnings/Precautions Hypersensitivity reactions (eg, anaphylaxis, angioneurotic edema, urticaria, rash, swelling of the face, and pruritus) have been reported. Lupus-like, hepatitis, and vasculitis autoimmune syndromes have been reported with oral minocycline use; no further treatment should be given if symptoms occur. May cause photosensitivity; discontinue if skin erythema occurs. Use skin protection and avoid prolonged exposure to sunlight; do not use tanning equipment. Prolonged use may result in fungal or bacterial superinfection, including *C. difficile*-associated diarrhea (CDAD) and pseudomembranous colitis; CDAD has been observed >2 months postantibiotic treatment. May cause tissue hyperpigmentation, enamel hypoplasia, or permanent tooth discoloration; use of tetracyclines should be avoided during tooth development (children ≤8 years of age) unless other drugs are not likely to be effective or are contraindicated. However, recommended in treatment of anthrax exposure. Do not use during pregnancy. In addition to affecting tooth development, tetracycline use has been associated with retardation of skeletal development and reduced bone growth.

Use in an acutely abscessed periodontal pocket has not been studied and is not recommended. The effects of treatment for >6 months have not been studied. Should be used with caution in patients having a history of predisposition to oral candidiasis. Safety and effectiveness have not been established for the treatment of periodontitis in patients with coexistent oral candidiasis. Not clinically tested in immunocompromised patients (such as those immunocompromised by diabetes, chemotherapy, radiation therapy, or infection with HIV). Not clinically tested for use in the regeneration of alveolar bone, either in preparation for or in conjunction with the placement of endosseous (dental) implants or in the treatment of failing implants.

Pregnancy Risk Factor D

Lactation Enters breast milk/not recommended

Dosage Forms

Powder, sustained release microspheres, subgingival:
Arestin®: 1 mg (12s)

Minoxidil (Systemic) (mi NOKS i dil)

Related Information

Cardiovascular Diseases *on page 1848*

Canadian Brand Names Loniten®

Pharmacologic Category Vasodilator, Direct-Acting

Use Management of severe hypertension (usually in combination with a diuretic and beta-blocker)

Local Anesthetic/Vasoconstrictor Precautions No information available to require special precautions

Effects on Dental Treatment No significant effects or complications reported

Effects on Bleeding No information available to require special precautions

Adverse Effects Frequency not always reported.

Cardiovascular: ECG changes (T-wave changes 60%), peripheral edema (7%), pericardial effusion with tamponade (3%), pericardial effusion without tamponade (3%), angina pectoris, heart failure, pericarditis, rebound hypertension (in children after a gradual withdrawal), sodium and water retention, tachycardia

Dermatologic: Hypertrichosis (common; 80%), bullous eruption (rare), rash, Stevens-Johnson syndrome (rare)

Endocrine & metabolic: Breast tenderness (rare; <1%)

Gastrointestinal: Nausea, vomiting, weight gain

Hematologic: Leukopenia (rare), thrombocytopenia (rare), transient decreased erythrocyte count (hemodilution), transient decreased hematocrit/hemoglobin (hemodilution)

Hepatic: Increased alkaline phosphatase

Renal: Transient increase in serum BUN and creatinine

Respiratory: Pulmonary edema

General Dosage Range Oral:

Children <12 years: Initial: 0.1-0.2 mg/kg once daily (maximum: 5 mg/day); Usual dosage range: 0.25-1 mg/kg/day in 1-2 divided doses (maximum: 50 mg/day)

Children ≥12 years and Adults: Initial: 5 mg once daily; Usual dosage range: 2.5-80 mg/day in 1-2 divided doses (maximum: 100 mg/day)

Elderly: Initial: 2.5 mg once daily

Mechanism of Action Produces vasodilation by directly relaxing arteriolar smooth muscle, with little effect on veins; effects may be mediated by cyclic AMP; stimulation of hair growth is secondary to vasodilation, increased cutaneous blood flow and stimulation of resting hair follicles

Pharmacodynamics/Kinetics

Onset of Action Hypotensive: ~30 minutes; Peak effect: 2-8 hours

Duration of Action 2-5 days

Half-life Elimination Adults: 3.5-4.2 hours

Pregnancy Risk Factor C

Mirtazapine (mir TAZ a peen)

U.S. Brand Names Remeron SolTab®; Remeron®

Canadian Brand Names Apo-Mirtazapine®; CO Mirtazapine; Dom-Mirtazapine; Mylan-Mirtazapine; Novo-Mirtazapine; PHL-Mirtazapine; PMS-Mirtazapine; PRO-Mirtazapine; ratio-Mirtazapine; Remeron®; Remeron® RD; Riva-Mirtazapine; Sandoz-Mirtazapine; Sandoz-Mirtazapine FC; ZYM-Mirtazapine

Pharmacologic Category Antidepressant, Alpha-2 Antagonist

Use Treatment of depression

Unlabeled/Investigational Use Post-traumatic stress disorder (PTSD)

Local Anesthetic/Vasoconstrictor Precautions Although mirtazapine is not a tricyclic antidepressant, it results in increased norepinephrine release as part of its mechanisms. It has been suggested that vasoconstrictor be administered with caution and to monitor vital signs in dental patients taking antidepressants that affect norepinephrine in this way, including mirtazapine.

Effects on Dental Treatment Key adverse event(s) related to dental treatment: Significant xerostomia (normal salivary flow resumes upon discontinuation).

Effects on Bleeding No information available to require special precautions

Adverse Effects

>10%:

Central nervous system: Somnolence (54%)

Endocrine & metabolic: Increased cholesterol

Gastrointestinal: Constipation (13%), xerostomia (25%), increased appetite (17%), weight gain (12%; weight gain of >7% reported in 8% of adults, ≤49% of pediatric patients)

1% to 10%:

Cardiovascular: Hypertension, vasodilatation, peripheral edema (2%), edema (1%)

Central nervous system: Dizziness (7%), abnormal dreams (4%), abnormal thoughts (3%), confusion (2%), malaise

Endocrine & metabolic: Increased triglycerides

Gastrointestinal: Vomiting, anorexia, abdominal pain

Genitourinary: Urinary frequency (2%)

Hepatic: SGPT increased (≥3 times ULN: 2%)

Neuromuscular & skeletal: Myalgia (2%), back pain (2%), arthralgia, tremor (2%), weakness (8%)

Respiratory: Dyspnea (1%)

Miscellaneous: Flu-like syndrome (5%), thirst

General Dosage Range Oral: *Adults:* Initial: 15 mg nightly; Maintenance: 15-45 mg nightly

Mechanism of Action Mirtazapine is a tetracyclic antidepressant that works by its central presynaptic alpha$_2$-adrenergic antagonist effects, which results in increased release of norepinephrine and serotonin. It is also a potent antagonist of 5-HT$_2$ and 5-HT$_3$ serotonin receptors and H1 histamine receptors and a moderate peripheral alpha$_1$-adrenergic and muscarinic antagonist; it does not inhibit the reuptake of norepinephrine or serotonin.

Pharmacodynamics/Kinetics

Half-life Elimination 20-40 hours; hampered with renal or hepatic impairment

Time to Peak Serum: 2 hours

Pregnancy Risk Factor C

Misoprostol (mye soe PROST ole)

U.S. Brand Names Cytotec®

Canadian Brand Names Apo-Misoprostol®; Novo-Misoprostol; PMS-Misoprostol

Pharmacologic Category Prostaglandin

Use Prevention of NSAID-induced gastric ulcers; medical termination of pregnancy of ≤49 days (in conjunction with mifepristone)

Unlabeled/Investigational Use Cervical ripening and labor induction (except in women with prior cesarean delivery or major uterine surgery); fat malabsorption in cystic fibrosis

Local Anesthetic/Vasoconstrictor Precautions No information available to require special precautions

Effects on Dental Treatment No significant effects or complications reported

Effects on Bleeding No information available to require special precautions

Adverse Effects

>10%: Gastrointestinal: Diarrhea, abdominal pain

1% to 10%:

Central nervous system: Headache

Gastrointestinal: Constipation, dyspepsia, flatulence, nausea, vomiting

General Dosage Range Oral:

Adults: 100-200 mcg 4 times/day

Elderly: Initial: 100 mcg/day

Mechanism of Action Misoprostol is a synthetic prostaglandin E$_1$ analog that replaces the protective prostaglandins consumed with prostaglandin-inhibiting therapies (eg, NSAIDs); has been shown to induce uterine contractions

Pharmacodynamics/Kinetics

Half-life Elimination Misoprostol acid: 20-40 minutes

Time to Peak Serum: Misoprostol acid: Fasting: 6-22 minutes

Pregnancy Risk Factor X

MitoMYcin (mye toe MYE sin)

Canadian Brand Names Mutamycin®

Pharmacologic Category Antineoplastic Agent, Antibiotic

Use Treatment of adenocarcinoma of stomach or pancreas

Unlabeled/Investigational Use Treatment of bladder cancer; prevention of excess scarring in glaucoma filtration procedures in patients at high risk of bleb failure

Local Anesthetic/Vasoconstrictor Precautions No information available to require special precautions

Effects on Dental Treatment Key adverse event(s) related to dental treatment: Stomatitis.

Effects on Bleeding Chemotherapy may result in significant myelosuppression, potentially including significant reduction in platelet counts and altered hemostasis. In patients who are under active treatment with these agents, medical consult is suggested.

Adverse Effects

>10%:

- Cardiovascular: CHF (3% to 15%) (doses >30 mg/m^2)
- Central nervous system: Fever (14%)
- Dermatologic: Alopecia, nail banding/discoloration
- Gastrointestinal: Nausea, vomiting and anorexia (14%)
- Hematologic: Anemia (19% to 24%); myelosuppression, common, dose limiting, delayed
  - Onset: 3 weeks
  - Nadir: 4-6 weeks
  - Recovery: 6-8 weeks

1% to 10%:

- Dermatologic: Rash
- Gastrointestinal: Stomatitis
- Neuromuscular: Paresthesia
- Renal: Creatinine increase (2%)
- Respiratory: Interstitial pneumonitis, infiltrates, dyspnea, cough (7%)

General Dosage Range Dosage adjustment recommended in patients with renal impairment

I.V.: *Adults:* 10-20 mg/m^2 every 6-8 weeks

Mechanism of Action Acts like an alkylating agent and produces DNA cross-linking (primarily with guanine and cytosine pairs); cell-cycle nonspecific; inhibits DNA and RNA synthesis; degrades preformed DNA, causes nuclear lysis and formation of giant cells. While not phase-specific *per se*, mitomycin has its maximum effect against cells in late G and early S phases.

Pharmacodynamics/Kinetics

Half-life Elimination 23-78 minutes; Terminal: 50 minutes

Pregnancy Risk Factor D

Mitotane (MYE toe tane)

U.S. Brand Names Lysodren®

Canadian Brand Names Lysodren®

Pharmacologic Category Antineoplastic Agent, Miscellaneous

Use Treatment of inoperable adrenocortical carcinoma

Unlabeled/Investigational Use Treatment of Cushing's syndrome

Local Anesthetic/Vasoconstrictor Precautions No information available to require special precautions

Effects on Dental Treatment No significant effects or complications reported

Effects on Bleeding Although significant myelosuppression with associated altered hemostasis has been reported for many chemotherapeutic agents, myelosuppression is not common with mitotane and no specific precautions appear to necessary.

Adverse Effects The majority of adverse events are dose-dependent.

>10%:

- Central nervous system: CNS depression (32%), lethargy/somnolence (25%), dizziness/vertigo (15%)
- Dermatologic: Skin rash (15%)
- Gastrointestinal: Anorexia (24%), nausea (39%), vomiting (37%), diarrhea (13%)
- Neuromuscular & skeletal: Weakness (12%)

1% to 10%:
- Central nervous system: Headache (5%), confusion (3%)
- Neuromuscular & skeletal: Muscle tremor (3%)

General Dosage Range Dosage adjustment recommended in patients who develop toxicities

Oral: *Adults:* Initial: 2-6 g/day in divided doses; Maintenance: 9-10 g/day in 3-4 divided doses (maximum: 18 g/day)

Mechanism of Action Adrenolytic agent which causes adrenal cortical atrophy; affects mitochondria in adrenal cortical cells and decreases production of cortisol; also alters the peripheral metabolism of steroids

Pharmacodynamics/Kinetics

Half-life Elimination 18-159 days

Time to Peak Serum: 3-5 hours

Pregnancy Risk Factor C

MitoXANtrone (mye toe ZAN trone)

U.S. Brand Names Novantrone®

Canadian Brand Names Mitoxantrone Injection®; Novantrone®

Pharmacologic Category Antineoplastic Agent, Anthracenedione

Use Treatment of acute nonlymphocytic leukemias (ANLL [includes myelogenous, promyelocytic, monocytic and erythroid leukemias]); advanced hormone-refractory prostate cancer; secondary progressive or relapsing-remitting multiple sclerosis (MS)

Unlabeled/Investigational Use Treatment of Hodgkin's lymphoma, non-Hodgkin's lymphomas (NHL), acute lymphocytic leukemia (ALL), myelodysplastic syndrome, breast cancer, pediatric acute myelogenous leukemia (AML), pediatric acute promyelocytic leukemia (APL); part of a conditioning regimen for autologous hematopoietic stem cell transplantation (HSCT)

Local Anesthetic/Vasoconstrictor Precautions No information available to require special precautions

Effects on Dental Treatment Key adverse event(s) related to dental treatment: Mucositis and stomatitis.

Effects on Bleeding Chemotherapy may result in significant myelosuppression, potentially including significant reduction in platelet counts and altered hemostasis. In patients who are under active treatment with these agents, medical consult is suggested.

Adverse Effects Includes events reported with any indication; incidence varies based on treatment, dose, and/or concomitant medications

>10%:
- Cardiovascular: Edema (10% to 30%), arrhythmia (3% to 18%), cardiac function changes (≤18%), ECG changes (≤11%)
- Central nervous system: Fever (6% to 78%), pain (8% to 41%), fatigue (≤39%), headache (6% to 13%)
- Dermatologic: Alopecia (20% to 61%), nail bed changes (≤11%), petechiae/bruising (6% to 11%)
- Endocrine & metabolic: Menstrual disorder (26% to 61%), amenorrhea (28% to 53%), hyperglycemia (10% to 31%)
- Gastrointestinal: Nausea (26% to 76%), vomiting (6% to 72%), diarrhea (14% to 47%), mucositis (10% to 29%; onset: ≤1 week), stomatitis (8% to 29%; onset: ≤1 week), anorexia (22% to 25%), weight gain/loss (13% to 17%), constipation (10% to 16%), GI bleeding (2% to 16%), abdominal pain (9% to 15%), dyspepsia (5% to 14%)
- Genitourinary: Urinary tract infection (7% to 32%), abnormal urine (5% to 11%)
- Hematologic: Neutropenia (79% to 100%; onset: ≤3 weeks; grade 4: 23% to 54%), leukopenia (9% to 100%), lymphopenia (72% to 95%), anemia/hemoglobin decreased (5% to 75%) thrombocytopenia (33% to 39%; grades 3/4: 3% to 4%), neutropenic fever (≤11%)
- Hepatic: Alkaline phosphatase increased (≤37%), transaminases increased (5% to 20%), GGT increased (3% to 15%)
- Neuromuscular & skeletal: Weakness (≤24%)
- Renal: BUN increased (≤22%), creatinine increased (≤13%), hematuria (≤11%)
- Respiratory: Upper respiratory tract infection (7% to 53%), pharyngitis (≤19%), dyspnea (6% to 18%), cough (5% to 13%)
- Miscellaneous: Infection (4% to 60%), sepsis (ANLL 31% to 34%), fungal infection (9% to 15%)

1% to 10%:
- Cardiovascular: CHF (≤5%), ischemia (≤5%), LVEF decreased (≤5%), hypertension (≤4%)

Central nervous system: Chills (≤5%), anxiety (5%), depression (5%), seizure (2% to 4%)
Dermatologic: Cutaneous mycosis (≤10%), skin infection (≤5%)
Endocrine & metabolic: Hypocalcemia (10%), hypokalemia (7% to 10%), hyponatremia (9%), menorrhagia (7%)
Gastrointestinal: Aphthosis (≤10%)
Genitourinary: Impotence (≤7%), sterility (≤5%)
Hematologic: Granulocytopenia (6%), hemorrhage (5% to 6%), secondary acute leukemias (≤3%; includes AML, APL)
Hepatic: Jaundice (3% to 7%)
Neuromuscular & skeletal: Back pain (6% to 8%), myalgia (≤5%), arthralgia (≤5%)
Ocular: Conjunctivitis (≤5%), blurred vision (≤3%)
Renal: Renal failure (≤8%), proteinuria (≤6%)
Respiratory: Rhinitis (10%), pneumonia (≤9%), sinusitis (≤6%)
Miscellaneous: Systemic infection (≤10%), diaphoresis (≤9%)

General Dosage Range **I.V.:** *Adults:* 12 mg/m^2/day once daily for 2-3 days **or** 12-14 mg/m^2 every 3 weeks **or** 12 mg/m^2 every 3 months (multiple sclerosis; maximum lifetime cumulative dose: 140 mg/m^2)

Mechanism of Action Related to the anthracyclines, mitoxantrone intercalates into DNA resulting in cross-links and strand breaks; binds to nucleic acids and inhibits DNA and RNA synthesis by template disordering and steric obstruction; replication is decreased by binding to DNA topoisomerase II and seems to inhibit the incorporation of uridine into RNA and thymidine into DNA; active throughout entire cell cycle (cell-cycle nonspecific)

Pharmacodynamics/Kinetics

Half-life Elimination Terminal: 23-215 hours (median: ~75 hours); may be prolonged with hepatic impairment

Pregnancy Risk Factor D

Modafinil (moe DAF i nil)

U.S. Brand Names Provigil®

Canadian Brand Names Alertec®; Apo-Modafinil®

Generic Availability (U.S.) No

Pharmacologic Category Stimulant

Use Improve wakefulness in patients with excessive daytime sleepiness associated with narcolepsy and shift work sleep disorder (SWSD); adjunctive therapy for obstructive sleep apnea/hypopnea syndrome (OSAHS)

Unlabeled/Investigational Use Attention-deficit/hyperactivity disorder (ADHD); treatment of fatigue in MS and other disorders

Local Anesthetic/Vasoconstrictor Precautions Use vasoconstrictor with caution. Patients may experience heart palpitations and increased heart rate when taking modafinil.

Effects on Dental Treatment Key adverse event(s) related to dental treatment: Xerostomia (normal salivary flow resumes upon discontinuation), oral ulceration, gingivitis, and taste perversion.

Effects on Bleeding No information available to require special precautions

Adverse Effects

>10%:

Central nervous system: Headache (34%, dose related)
Gastrointestinal: Nausea (11%)

1% to 10%:

Cardiovascular: Chest pain (3%), hypertension (3%), palpitation (2%), tachycardia (2%), vasodilation (2%), edema (1%)
Central nervous system: Nervousness (7%), dizziness (5%), anxiety (5%; dose related), insomnia (5%), depression (2%), somnolence (2%), chills (1%), agitation (1%), confusion (1%), emotional lability (1%), vertigo (1%)
Dermatologic: Rash (1%; includes some severe cases requiring hospitalization)
Gastrointestinal: Diarrhea (6%), dyspepsia (5%), xerostomia (4%), anorexia (4%), constipation (2%), flatulence (1%), mouth ulceration (1%), taste perversion (1%)
Genitourinary: Abnormal urine (1%), hematuria (1%), pyuria (1%)
Hematologic: Eosinophilia (1%)
Hepatic: LFTs abnormal (2%)
Neuromuscular & skeletal: Back pain (6%), paresthesia (2%), dyskinesia (1%), hyperkinesia (1%), hypertonia (1%), neck rigidity (1%), tremor (1%)
Ocular: Amblyopia (1%), eye pain (1%), vision abnormal (1%)
Respiratory: Rhinitis (7%), pharyngitis (4%), lung disorder (2%), asthma (1%), epistaxis (1%)
Miscellaneous: Flu-like syndrome (4%), thirst (1%), diaphoresis (1%), herpes simplex infection (1%)

Dosage Oral:

Adults:

ADHD (unlabeled use): 100-400 mg/day (Taylor, 2000)

Narcolepsy, obstructive sleep apnea/hypopnea syndrome (OSAHS): Initial: 200 mg as a single daily dose in the morning

Shift work sleep disorder (SWSD): Initial: 200 mg as a single dose taken ~1 hour prior to start of work shift

Note: Doses of 400 mg/day, given as a single dose, have been well tolerated, but there is no consistent evidence that this dose confers additional benefit.

Elderly: Elimination of modafinil and its metabolites may be reduced as a consequence of aging and as a result, consider initiating at lower doses in this patient population.

Dosing adjustment in renal impairment: Safety and efficacy have not been established in severe renal impairment.

Dosing adjustment in hepatic impairment: Severe hepatic impairment: Dose should be reduced to one-half of that recommended for patients with normal liver function.

Mechanism of Action The exact mechanism of action is unclear, it does not appear to alter the release of dopamine or norepinephrine, it may exert its stimulant effects by decreasing GABA-mediated neurotransmission, although this theory has not yet been fully evaluated; several studies also suggest that an intact central alpha-adrenergic system is required for modafinil's activity; the drug increases high-frequency alpha waves while decreasing both delta and theta wave activity, and these effects are consistent with generalized increases in mental alertness

Contraindications Hypersensitivity to modafinil, armodafinil, or any component of the formulation

Warnings/Precautions For use following complete evaluation of sleepiness and in conjunction with other standard treatments (eg, CPAP). The degree of sleepiness should be reassessed frequently; some patients may not return to a normal level of wakefulness. Use is not recommended with a history of angina, cardiac ischemia, recent history of myocardial infarction, left ventricular hypertrophy, or patients with mitral valve prolapse who have developed mitral valve prolapse syndrome with previous CNS stimulant use.

Serious and life-threatening rashes (including Stevens-Johnson syndrome and toxic epidermal necrolysis) have been reported with modafinil. Most cases have occurred within the first 5 weeks of therapy; however, rare cases have occurred after long-term use. No risk factors have been identified to predict occurrence or severity. Patients should be advised to discontinue at first sign of rash. The serious nature of these dermatologic adverse effects, as well reports of psychiatric events, resulted in the FDA's Pediatric Advisory Committee unanimously recommending that a specific warning against the use of modafinil in children be added to the manufacturer's labeling. Modafinil is not FDA-approved for use in pediatrics for any indication.

In addition, rare cases of multiorgan hypersensitivity reactions in association with modafinil use, and lone cases of angioedema and anaphylactoid reactions with armodafinil, have been reported. Signs and symptoms are diverse, reflecting the involvement of specific organs. Patients typically present with fever and rash associated with organ-system dysfunction. Patients should be advised to report any signs and symptoms related to these effects; discontinuation of therapy is recommended.

Caution should be exercised when modafinil is given to patients with a history of psychosis; may impair the ability to engage in potentially hazardous activities. Stimulants may unmask tics in individuals with coexisting Tourette's syndrome. Use caution with renal or hepatic impairment (dosage adjustment in severe hepatic dysfunction is recommended).

Drug Interactions

Metabolism/Transport Effects **Substrate** of CYP3A4 (major); **Inhibits** CYP1A2 (weak), 2A6 (weak), 2C9 (weak), 2C19 (strong), 2E1 (weak), 3A4 (weak); **Induces** CYP1A2 (weak), 2B6 (weak), 3A4 (weak)

Avoid Concomitant Use

Avoid concomitant use of Modafinil with any of the following: Clopidogrel; Iobenguane I 123

Increased Effect/Toxicity

Modafinil may increase the levels/effects of: CYP2C19 Substrates; Sympathomimetics

The levels/effects of Modafinil may be increased by: Atomoxetine; Cannabinoids; Conivaptan; CYP3A4 Inhibitors (Moderate); CYP3A4 Inhibitors (Strong); Dasatinib

Decreased Effect

Modafinil may decrease the levels/effects of: Clopidogrel; Contraceptives (Estrogens); CycloSPORINE; CycloSPORINE (Systemic); Iobenguane I 123; Saxagliptin

The levels/effects of Modafinil may be decreased by: CYP3A4 Inducers (Strong); Deferasirox; Herbs (CYP3A4 Inducers); Tocilizumab

Ethanol/Nutrition/Herb Interactions

Ethanol: Avoid or limit ethanol.

Food: Delays absorption, but does not affect bioavailability.

Pharmacodynamics/Kinetics

Half-life Elimination Effective half-life: 15 hours

Time to Peak Serum: 2-4 hours

Pregnancy Risk Factor C

Lactation Excretion in breast milk unknown/use caution

Controlled Substance C-IV

Dosage Forms

Tablet, oral:

Provigil®: 100 mg, 200 mg

Moexipril (mo EKS i pril)

Related Information

Cardiovascular Diseases *on page 1848*

U.S. Brand Names Univasc®

Pharmacologic Category Angiotensin-Converting Enzyme (ACE) Inhibitor

Use Treatment of hypertension, alone or in combination with thiazide diuretics

Local Anesthetic/Vasoconstrictor Precautions No information available to require special precautions

Effects on Dental Treatment No significant effects or complications reported

Effects on Bleeding No information available to require special precautions

Adverse Effects 1% to 10%:

Cardiovascular: Hypotension, peripheral edema
Central nervous system: Headache, dizziness, fatigue
Dermatologic: Flushing, rash
Endocrine & metabolic: Hyperkalemia, hyponatremia
Gastrointestinal: Diarrhea, nausea, heartburn
Genitourinary: Polyuria
Neuromuscular & skeletal: Myalgia
Renal: Reversible increases in creatinine or BUN
Respiratory: Cough, pharyngitis, upper respiratory infection, sinusitis

General Dosage Range Dosage adjustment recommended in patients with renal impairment

Oral: *Adults:* Initial: 3.75-7.5 mg once daily; Maintenance: 7.5-30 mg/day in 1 or 2 divided doses

Mechanism of Action Competitive inhibitor of angiotensin-converting enzyme (ACE); prevents conversion of angiotensin I to angiotensin II, a potent vasoconstrictor; results in lower levels of angiotensin II which causes an increase in plasma renin activity and a reduction in aldosterone secretion

Pharmacodynamics/Kinetics

Onset of Action Peak effect: 1-2 hours

Duration of Action >24 hours

Half-life Elimination Moexipril: 1 hour; Moexiprilat: 2-9 hours

Time to Peak 1.5 hours

Pregnancy Risk Factor C (1st trimester); D (2nd and 3rd trimesters)

Moexipril and Hydrochlorothiazide
(mo EKS i pril & hye droe klor oh THYE a zide)

Related Information

Hydrochlorothiazide *on page 854*
Moexipril *on page 1151*

U.S. Brand Names Uniretic®

Canadian Brand Names Uniretic®

Pharmacologic Category Angiotensin-Converting Enzyme (ACE) Inhibitor; Diuretic, Thiazide

Use Treatment of hypertension; not indicated for initial treatment of hypertension

Local Anesthetic/Vasoconstrictor Precautions No information available to require special precautions

Effects on Dental Treatment No significant effects or complications reported

Effects on Bleeding No information available to require special precautions
Adverse Effects See individual agents.
General Dosage Range Oral: *Adults:* 7.5-30 mg of moexipril/day and ≤50 mg hydrochlorothiazide/day in a single or divided dose
Mechanism of Action See individual agents.
Pregnancy Risk Factor C/D (2nd and 3rd trimesters)

Mometasone (Oral Inhalation) (moe MET a sone)

Related Information
Respiratory Diseases *on page 1876*
U.S. Brand Names Asmanex® Twisthaler®
Generic Availability (U.S.) No
Pharmacologic Category Corticosteroid, Inhalant (Oral)
Use Maintenance treatment of asthma as prophylactic therapy
Local Anesthetic/Vasoconstrictor Precautions No information available to require special precautions
Effects on Dental Treatment No significant effects or complications reported
Effects on Bleeding No information available to require special precautions
Adverse Effects
>10%:
Central nervous system: Headache (17% to 22%), fatigue (1% to 13%), depression (11%)
Neuromuscular & skeletal: Musculoskeletal pain (4% to 22%), arthralgia (13%)
Respiratory: Sinusitis (5% to 22%), rhinitis (4% to 20%), upper respiratory infection (8% to 15%), pharyngitis (8% to 13%)
Miscellaneous: Oral candidiasis (4% to 22%)
1% to 10%:
Central nervous system: Fever (children 7%), pain (1% to <3%)
Dermatologic: Bruising (children 2%)
Gastrointestinal: Abdominal pain (2% to 6%), dyspepsia (3% to 5%), nausea (1% to 3%), vomiting (1% to ≤3%), anorexia (1% to <3%), dry throat (1% to <3%), gastroenteritis (1% to <3%)
Genitourinary: Dysmenorrhea (4% to 9%), urinary tract infection (children 2%)
Neuromuscular & skeletal: Back pain (3% to 6%), myalgia (2% to 3%)
Ocular: Ocular pressure increased (3%), cataracts (1%)
Otic: Earache (1% to <3%)
Respiratory: Sinus congestion (9%), dysphonia (1% to <3%), epistaxis (1% to <3%), nasal irritation (1% to <3%)
Miscellaneous: Flu-like syndrome (1% to <3%), infection (1% to <3%)
Dosage Oral inhalation:
Children 4-11 years: 110 mcg once daily in the evening (maximum: 110 mcg/day)
Children ≥12 years and Adults: Previous therapy:
Bronchodilators or inhaled corticosteroids: Initial: 1 inhalation (220 mcg) daily (maximum: 2 inhalations or 440 mcg/day); may be given in the evening or in divided doses twice daily
Oral corticosteroids: Initial: 440 mcg twice daily (maximum: 880 mcg/day); prednisone should be reduced no faster than 2.5 mg/day on a weekly basis, beginning after at least 1 week of mometasone furoate use
NIH Asthma Guidelines (NIH, 2007): Children ≥12 years and Adults:
"Low" dose: 220 mcg/day
"Medium" dose: 440 mcg/day
"High" dose: >440 mcg/day
Note: Maximum effects may not be evident for 1-2 weeks or longer; dose should be titrated to effect, using the lowest possible dose
Mechanism of Action May depress the formation, release, and activity of endogenous chemical mediators of inflammation (kinins, histamine, liposomal enzymes, prostaglandins). Leukocytes and macrophages may have to be present for the initiation of responses mediated by the above substances. Inhibits the margination and subsequent cell migration to the area of injury, and also reverses the dilatation and increased vessel permeability in the area resulting in decreased access of cells to the sites of injury.
Contraindications Hypersensitivity to mometasone or any component of the formulation; hypersensitivity to milk proteins; primary treatment of status asthmaticus or acute bronchospasm
Warnings/Precautions May cause hypercorticism or suppression of hypothalamic-pituitary-adrenal (HPA) axis, particularly in younger children or in patients receiving high doses for prolonged periods. HPA axis suppression may lead to adrenal crisis. Withdrawal and discontinuation of a corticosteroid should be done slowly and carefully. Particular care is required when patients are transferred from systemic

corticosteroids to inhaled products due to possible adrenal insufficiency or withdrawal from steroids, including an increase in allergic symptoms. Patients receiving >20 mg per day of prednisone (or equivalent) may be most susceptible. Fatalities have occurred due to adrenal insufficiency in asthmatic patients during and after transfer from systemic corticosteroids to aerosol steroids; aerosol steroids do not provide the systemic steroid needed to treat patients having trauma, surgery, or infections. When transferring to oral inhaler, previously-suppressed allergic conditions (rhinitis, conjunctivitis, eczema) may be unmasked.

Bronchospasm may occur with wheezing after inhalation; if this occurs, stop steroid and treat with a fast-acting bronchodilator. Supplemental steroids (oral or parenteral) may be needed during stress or severe asthma attacks. Not to be used in status asthmaticus or for the relief of acute bronchospasm. Corticosteroid use may cause psychiatric disturbances, including depression, euphoria, insomnia, mood swings, and personality changes. Pre-existing psychiatric conditions may be exacerbated by corticosteroid use. Prolonged use of corticosteroids may also increase the incidence of secondary infection, mask acute infection (including fungal infections), prolong or exacerbate viral infections, or limit response to vaccines. Exposure to chickenpox should be avoided; corticosteroids should not be used to treat ocular herpes simplex. Corticosteroids should not be used for cerebral malaria or viral hepatitis. Close observation is required in patients with latent tuberculosis and/or TB reactivity; restrict use in active TB (only in conjunction with antituberculosis treatment). Prolonged treatment with corticosteroids has been associated with the development of Kaposi's sarcoma (case reports); if noted, discontinuation of therapy should be considered. Local oropharyngeal *Candida* infections have been reported; if occurs treat appropriately while continuing mometasone therapy. Patients should be instructed to rinse mouth after each use.

Reactions including, anaphylaxis, angioedema, pruritus, and rash have been reported; if these symptoms occur discontinue use. Use with caution in patients with thyroid disease, hepatic impairment, renal impairment, cardiovascular disease, diabetes, glaucoma, cataracts, myasthenia gravis, patients with or who are at risk for osteoporosis, patients at risk for seizures, or GI diseases (diverticulitis, peptic ulcer, ulcerative colitis) due to perforation risk. Use caution following acute MI (corticosteroids have been associated with myocardial rupture). Because of the risk of adverse effects, systemic corticosteroids should be used cautiously in the elderly in the smallest possible effective dose for the shortest duration.

Orally-inhaled corticosteroids may cause a reduction in growth velocity in pediatric patients (~1 centimeter per year [range: 0.3-1.8 cm per year] and related to dose and duration of exposure). To minimize the systemic effects of orally-inhaled corticosteroids, each patient should be titrated to the lowest effective dose. Growth should be routinely monitored in pediatric patients. Prior to use, the dose and duration of treatment should be based on the risk versus benefit for each individual patient. In general, use the smallest effective dose for the shortest duration of time to minimize adverse events. A gradual tapering of dose may be required prior to discontinuing therapy. There have been reports of systemic corticosteroid withdrawal symptoms (eg, joint/muscle pain, lassitude, depression) when withdrawing inhalation therapy. May contain lactose; very rare anaphylactic reactions have been reported in patients with severe milk protein allergy.

Drug Interactions

Metabolism/Transport Effects Substrate of CYP3A4 (major)

Avoid Concomitant Use

Avoid concomitant use of Mometasone (Oral Inhalation) with any of the following: Aldesleukin

Increased Effect/Toxicity

Mometasone (Oral Inhalation) may increase the levels/effects of: Amphotericin B; Deferasirox; Loop Diuretics; Thiazide Diuretics

The levels/effects of Mometasone (Oral Inhalation) may be increased by: CYP3A4 Inhibitors (Strong)

Decreased Effect

Mometasone (Oral Inhalation) may decrease the levels/effects of: Aldesleukin; Antidiabetic Agents; Corticorelin

The levels/effects of Mometasone (Oral Inhalation) may be decreased by: Tocilizumab

Dietary Considerations Asmanex® Twisthaler® contains lactose.

Pharmacodynamics/Kinetics

Half-life Elimination 5 hours

Pregnancy Risk Factor C

Lactation Excretion in breast milk unknown/use caution

Breast-Feeding Considerations Systemic corticosteroids are excreted in human milk; however, information for mometasone is not available. The use of inhaled corticosteroids is not considered a contraindication to breast-feeding.

Dosage Forms

Powder, for oral inhalation:

Asmanex® Twisthaler®: 110 mcg (30 units); 220 mcg (14 units, 30 units, 60 units, 120 units)

Mometasone (Nasal) (moe MET a sone)

U.S. Brand Names Nasonex®

Canadian Brand Names Nasonex®

Pharmacologic Category Corticosteroid, Nasal

Use Treatment of nasal symptoms of seasonal and perennial allergic rhinitis; prevention of nasal symptoms associated with seasonal allergic rhinitis; treatment of nasal polyps in adults

Local Anesthetic/Vasoconstrictor Precautions No information available to require special precautions

Effects on Dental Treatment No significant effects or complications reported

Effects on Bleeding No information available to require special precautions

Adverse Effects

>10%:

Central nervous system: Headache (17% to 26%)

Respiratory: Pharyngitis (8% to 13%), cough (nasal inhalation 7% to 13%), epistaxis (1% to 11%)

Miscellaneous: Viral infection (nasal inhalation 8% to 14%)

1% to 10%:

Gastrointestinal: Diarrhea, dyspepsia, vomiting

Genitourinary: Dysmenorrhea

Neuromuscular & skeletal: Musculoskeletal pain, myalgia

Ocular: Conjunctivitis

Otic: Otitis media

Respiratory: Asthma, nasal irritation, rhinitis, sinusitis, upper respiratory infection, wheezing

Miscellaneous: Flu-like syndrome

General Dosage Range Intranasal:

Children 2-11 years: 1 spray (50 mcg) in each nostril daily

Children ≥12 years and Adults: 2 sprays (100 mcg) in each nostril daily

Mechanism of Action May depress the formation, release, and activity of endogenous chemical mediators of inflammation (kinins, histamine, liposomal enzymes, prostaglandins). Leukocytes and macrophages may have to be present for the initiation of responses mediated by the above substances. Inhibits the margination and subsequent cell migration to the area of injury, and also reverses the dilatation and increased vessel permeability in the area resulting in decreased access of cells to the sites of injury.

Pregnancy Risk Factor C

Mometasone and Formoterol (moe MET a sone & for MOH te rol)

Related Information

Formoterol *on page 781*

Mometasone (Oral Inhalation) *on page 1152*

U.S. Brand Names Dulera®

Canadian Brand Names Zenhale™

Pharmacologic Category $Beta_2$-Adrenergic Agonist; $Beta_2$-Adrenergic Agonist, Long-Acting; Corticosteroid, Inhalant (Oral)

Use Treatment of asthma where combination therapy is indicated

Local Anesthetic/Vasoconstrictor Precautions No information available to require special precautions

Effects on Dental Treatment Key adverse event(s) related to dental treatment: Formoterol: Xerostomia (normal salivary flow resumes upon discontinuation). Localized infections with *Candida albicans* or *Aspergillus niger* have occurred frequently in the mouth and pharynx with repetitive use of oral inhaler of corticosteroids. These infections may require treatment with appropriate antifungal therapy or discontinuance of treatment with corticosteroid inhaler.

Effects on Bleeding No information available to require special precautions

Adverse Effects Also see individual agents.

1% to 10%:

Central nervous system: Headache (up to 5%)

Respiratory: Nasopharyngitis (5%), dysphonia (4% to 5%), sinusitis (2% to 3%)

General Dosage Range Inhalation: *Children ≥12 years and Adults:* 2 inhalations twice daily (maximum: 4 inhalations/day)

Mechanism of Action Formoterol relaxes bronchial smooth muscle by selective action on $beta_2$ receptors with little effect on heart rate. Formoterol has a long-acting effect. Mometasone is a corticosteroid which controls the rate of protein synthesis, depresses the migration of polymorphonuclear leukocytes/fibroblasts, and reverses capillary permeability and lysosomal stabilization at the cellular level to prevent or control inflammation.

Pregnancy Risk Factor C

Monobenzone (mon oh BEN zone)

Pharmacologic Category Topical Skin Product

Use Final depigmentation in extensive vitiligo

Local Anesthetic/Vasoconstrictor Precautions No information available to require special precautions

Effects on Dental Treatment No significant effects or complications reported

Effects on Bleeding No information available to require special precautions

Adverse Effects Frequency not defined.

Local: Burning sensation, depigmentation of skin distant to application site, dermatitis, irritation

General Dosage Range Topical: *Children ≥12 years and Adults:* Initial: Apply 2-3 times/day; once depigmentation obtained apply as needed (usually 2 times/week)

Mechanism of Action Increases excretion of melanin from melanocytes; causes melanocyte destruction and permanent depigmentation

Pharmacodynamics/Kinetics

Onset of Action 1-4 months

Pregnancy Risk Factor C

Montelukast (mon te LOO kast)

Related Information

Respiratory Diseases *on page 1876*

U.S. Brand Names Singulair®

Canadian Brand Names Singulair®

Generic Availability (U.S.) No

Pharmacologic Category Leukotriene-Receptor Antagonist

Use Prophylaxis and chronic treatment of asthma; relief of symptoms of seasonal allergic rhinitis and perennial allergic rhinitis; prevention of exercise-induced bronchospasm

Unlabeled/Investigational Use Acute asthma

Local Anesthetic/Vasoconstrictor Precautions No information available to require special precautions

Effects on Dental Treatment Key adverse event(s) related to dental treatment: Dental pain.

Effects on Bleeding No information available to require special precautions

Adverse Effects Note: Percentages and adverse events as reported in adults: 1% to 10%:

Central nervous system: Dizziness (2%), fatigue (2%), fever (2%), headache (≥1%)

Dermatologic: Rash (2%)

Gastrointestinal: Dyspepsia (2%), dental pain (2%), gastroenteritis (2%)

Hepatic: AST increased (2%), ALT increased (≥1%)

Neuromuscular & skeletal: Weakness (2%)

Respiratory: Cough (≥1%), nasal congestion (2%), epistaxis (≥1%), sinusitis (≥1%), upper respiratory infection (≥1%)

Dosage Oral:

Children:

6-23 months: Perennial allergic rhinitis: 4 mg (oral granules) once daily

12-23 months: Asthma: 4 mg (oral granules) once daily, taken in the evening

2-5 years: Asthma, seasonal or perennial allergic rhinitis: 4 mg (chewable tablet or oral granules) once daily

6-14 years: Asthma, seasonal or perennial allergic rhinitis: 5 mg (chewable tablet) once daily

Children ≥15 years and Adults:

Asthma, seasonal or perennial allergic rhinitis: 10 mg once daily

Asthma, acute (unlabeled use): 10 mg as a single dose administered with first-line therapy (Camargo, 2003; Cylly, 2003)

Bronchoconstriction, exercise-induced (prevention): 10 mg at least 2 hours prior to exercise; additional doses should not be administered within 24 hours. Daily administration to prevent exercise-induced bronchoconstriction has not been evaluated.

Dosing adjustment in renal impairment: No adjustment necessary

Dosing adjustment in hepatic impairment: Mild-to-moderate: No adjustment necessary. Patients with severe hepatic disease were **not** studied.

Mechanism of Action Selective leukotriene receptor antagonist that inhibits the cysteinyl leukotriene receptor. Cysteinyl leukotrienes and leukotriene receptor occupation have been correlated with the pathophysiology of asthma, including airway edema, smooth muscle contraction, and altered cellular activity associated with the inflammatory process, which contribute to the signs and symptoms of asthma. Cysteinyl leukotrienes are also released from the nasal mucosa following allergen exposure leading to symptoms associated with allergic rhinitis.

Contraindications Hypersensitivity to montelukast or any component of the formulation

Warnings/Precautions Montelukast is not FDA approved for use in the reversal of bronchospasm in acute asthma attacks, including status asthmaticus; some clinicians, however, support its use as adjunctive therapy (Camargo, 2003; Cylly, 2003; Ferreira, 2001; Harmancik 2006). Appropriate rescue medication should be available. Appropriate clinical monitoring and caution are recommended when systemic corticosteroid reduction is considered in patients receiving montelukast. Patients should be instructed to notify prescriber if behavioral changes occur. Inform phenylketonuric patients that the chewable tablet contains phenylalanine.

In rare cases, patients on therapy with montelukast may present with systemic eosinophilia, sometimes presenting with clinical features of vasculitis consistent with Churg-Strauss syndrome, a condition which is often treated with systemic corticosteroid therapy. Healthcare providers should be alert to eosinophilia, vasculitic rash, worsening pulmonary symptoms, cardiac complications, and/or neuropathy presenting in their patients. A causal association between montelukast and these underlying conditions has not been established. Montelukast will not interrupt bronchoconstrictor response to aspirin or other NSAIDs; aspirin sensitive asthmatics should continue to avoid these agents. Postmarketing reports of behavior changes (agitation, aggression, depression, insomnia) have been noted in children and adults.

Drug Interactions

Metabolism/Transport Effects **Substrate** (major) of CYP2C9, 3A4; **Inhibits** CYP2C8 (weak), 2C9 (weak)

Avoid Concomitant Use There are no known interactions where it is recommended to avoid concomitant use.

Increased Effect/Toxicity

The levels/effects of Montelukast may be increased by: Conivaptan; CYP2C9 Inhibitors (Moderate); CYP2C9 Inhibitors (Strong)

Decreased Effect

The levels/effects of Montelukast may be decreased by: CYP2C9 Inducers (Highly Effective); CYP3A4 Inducers (Strong); Deferasirox; Herbs (CYP3A4 Inducers); Peginterferon Alfa-2b; Tocilizumab

Ethanol/Nutrition/Herb Interactions Herb/Nutraceutical: St John's wort may decrease montelukast levels.

Dietary Considerations Some products may contain phenylalanine.

Pharmacodynamics/Kinetics

Duration of Action >24 hours

Half-life Elimination Plasma: Mean: 2.7-5.5 hours

Time to Peak Serum: Tablet: 10 mg: 3-4 hours; 5 mg: 2-2.5 hours; 4 mg: 2 hours

Pregnancy Risk Factor B

Lactation Excretion in breast milk unknown/use caution

Dosage Forms

Granules, oral:

Singulair®: 4 mg/packet (30s)

Tablet, oral:

Singulair®: 10 mg

Tablet, chewable, oral:

Singulair®: 4 mg, 5 mg

Morphine (Systemic) (MOR feen)

Related Information

Oxymorphone *on page* 1282

U.S. Brand Names Astramorph®/PF; AVINza®; Duramorph; Infumorph 200; Infumorph 500; Kadian®; MS Contin®; Oramorph® SR

Canadian Brand Names Doloral; Kadian®; M-Eslon®; M.O.S.-SR®; M.O.S.-Sulfate®; M.O.S.® 10; M.O.S.® 20; M.O.S.® 30; Morphine Extra Forte Injection; Morphine Forte Injection; Morphine HP®; Morphine LP® Epidural; Morphine SR; Morphine-EPD; MS Contin SRT; MS Contin®; MS-IR®; Novo-Morphine SR; PMS-Morphine Sulfate SR; ratio-Morphine; ratio-Morphine SR; Sandoz-Morphine SR; Statex®

Generic Availability (U.S.) Yes: Excludes capsule, sustained release tablet

Pharmacologic Category Analgesic, Opioid

Use Relief of moderate-to-severe acute and chronic pain; relief of pain of myocardial infarction; relief of dyspnea of acute left ventricular failure and pulmonary edema; preanesthetic medication

Infumorph®: Used in continuous microinfusion devices for intrathecal or epidural administration in treatment of intractable chronic pain

Controlled, extended, or sustained release products: Only intended/indicated for use when repeated doses for an extended period of time are required. The 100 mg and 200 mg tablets or capsules of Kadian®, MS Contin®, and morphine sulfate controlled-release tablets and the 60 mg, 90 mg, and 120 mg capsules of Avinza® should only be used in opioid-tolerant patients.

Local Anesthetic/Vasoconstrictor Precautions No information available to require special precautions

Effects on Dental Treatment Key adverse event(s) related to dental treatment: Xerostomia (normal salivary flow resumes upon discontinuation) and dysphagia. Anticholinergic side effects can cause a reduction of saliva production or secretion, contributing to discomfort and dental disease (ie, caries, oral candidiasis, and periodontal disease).

Effects on Bleeding No information available to require special precautions

Adverse Effects Note: Individual patient differences are unpredictable, and percentage may differ in acute pain (surgical) treatment. Reactions may be dose, formulation, and/or route dependent.

Frequency not defined:
- Cardiovascular: Circulatory depression, flushing, shock
- Central nervous system: Dysphonia, physical and psychological dependence, sedation
- Endocrine & metabolic: Antidiuretic hormone release

>10%:
- Cardiovascular: Bradycardia, hypotension
- Central nervous system: Drowsiness (9% to 48%; tolerance usually develops to drowsiness with regular dosing for 1-2 weeks), dizziness (6% to 20%), fever (<3% to >10%), confusion, headache (following epidural or intrathecal use)
- Dermatologic: Pruritus (may be dose related)
- Gastrointestinal: Xerostomia (78%), constipation (9% to 40%; tolerance develops very slowly if at all), nausea (7% to 28%; tolerance usually develops to nausea and vomiting with chronic use), vomiting
- Genitourinary: Urinary retention (16%; may be prolonged, up to 20 hours, following epidural or intrathecal use)
- Hematologic: Anemia (following intrathecal use)
- Local: Pain at injection site
- Neuromuscular & skeletal: Weakness
- Respiratory: Oxygen saturation decreased
- Miscellaneous: Histamine release

1% to 10%:
- Cardiovascular: Atrial fibrillation (<3%), chest pain (<3%), edema, hypertension, palpitation, peripheral edema, syncope, tachycardia, vasodilation
- Central nervous system: Amnesia, agitation, anxiety, apathy, apprehension, ataxia, chills, coma, delirium, depression, dream abnormalities, euphoria, false sense of well being, hallucination, hypoesthesia, insomnia, lethargy, malaise, nervousness, restlessness, seizure, slurred speech, somnolence, vertigo
- Dermatologic: Dry skin, rash, urticaria
- Endocrine & metabolic: Gynecomastia (<3%), hypokalemia, hyponatremia, libido decreased
- Gastrointestinal: Abdominal distension, abdominal pain, anorexia, biliary colic, diarrhea, dyspepsia, dysphagia, flatulence, gastroenteritis, GERD, GI irritation, paralytic ileus, rectal disorder, taste perversion, weight loss

Genitourinary: Bladder spasm, dysuria, ejaculation abnormal, impotence, urination decreased
Hematologic: Leukopenia (<3%), thrombocytopenia (<3%), hematocrit decreased
Hepatic: Liver function tests increased
Neuromuscular & skeletal: Arthralgia, back pain, bone pain, foot drop, gait abnormalities, paresthesia, rigors, skeletal muscle rigidity, tremor
Ocular: Amblyopia, conjunctivitis, eye pain, vision problems/disturbance
Renal: Oliguria
Respiratory: Asthma, atelectasis, dyspnea, hiccups, hypercapnia, hypoxia, pulmonary edema (noncardiogenic), respiratory depression, rhinitis
Miscellaneous: Diaphoresis, flu-like syndrome, infection, thirst, voice alteration, withdrawal syndrome

Dosage These are guidelines and do not represent the doses that may be required in all patients. Doses and dosage intervals should be titrated to pain relief/prevention.

Children >6 months and <50 kg: *Acute pain (moderate-to-severe):*
Oral (immediate release formulations): 0.15-0.3 mg/kg every 3-4 hours as needed. **Note:** The American Pain Society recommends an initial dose of 0.3 mg/kg for children with severe pain.
I.M., I.V.: 0.1-0.2 mg/kg every 3-4 hours as needed
I.V. infusion: Range: 10-60 mcg/kg/**hour**
Patient-controlled analgesia (PCA) (American Pain Society, 2008): **Note:** Opiate-naive: Consider lower end of dosing range:
Usual concentration: 1 mg/mL
Demand dose: Usual: 0.02 mg/kg/dose; range: 0.01-0.03 mg/kg/dose
Lockout interval: 6-8 minutes
Usual basal rate: 0-0.03 mg/kg/hour

Adults:
Acute pain (moderate-to-severe):
Oral (immediate release formulations): Opiate-naive: Initial: 10 mg every 4 hours as needed; patients with prior opiate exposure may require higher initial doses: usual dosage range: 10-30 mg every 4 hours as needed
I.M., SubQ: **Note:** Repeated SubQ administration causes local tissue irritation, pain, and induration.
Initial: Opiate-naive: 5-10 mg every 4 hours as needed; patients with prior opiate exposure may require higher initial doses; usual dosage range: 5-20 mg every 4 hours as needed
Rectal: 10-20 mg every 3-4 hours
I.V.: Initial: Opiate-naive: 2.5-5 mg every 3-4 hours; patients with prior opiate exposure may require higher initial doses. **Note:** Repeated doses (up to every 5 minutes if needed) in small increments (eg, 1-4 mg) may be preferred to larger and less frequent doses.
Acute myocardial infarction, analgesia (ACC/AHA 2004 guidelines): Initial management: 2-4 mg, give 2-8 mg every 5-15 minutes as needed.
Critically-ill patients (unlabeled dose): 0.7-10 mg (based on 70 kg patient) **or** 0.01-0.15 mg/kg every 1-2 hours as needed. **Note:** More frequent dosing may be needed (eg, mechanically-ventilated patients).
I.V., SubQ continuous infusion: 0.8-10 mg/hour; usual range: Up to 80 mg/hour
Continuous infusion: Usual dosage range: 5-35 mg/hour (based on 70 kg patient) **or** 0.07-0.5 mg/kg/hour
Patient-controlled analgesia (PCA): (Opiate-naive: Consider lower end of dosing range):
Usual concentration: 1 mg/mL
Demand dose: Usual: 1 mg; range: 0.5-2.5 mg
Lockout interval: 5-10 minutes
Intrathecal (I.T.): **Note: Must be preservative-free.** Administer with extreme caution and in reduced dosage to geriatric or debilitated patients. I.T. dose is usually 1/10 that of epidural dosage.
Opioid-naive: 0.2-1 mg/dose (may provide adequate relief for up to 24 hours); repeat doses are **not** recommended. **Note:** The American Pain Society recommends 0.1-0.3 mg/dose; adjust dose for age, injection site, and patient's medical condition and degree of opioid tolerance.
Continuous microinfusion (Infumorph®): Initial: 0.2-1 mg/day
Opioid-tolerant: 1-10 mg/day
Continuous microinfusion (Infumorph®): Initial: 1-10 mg/day, titrate to effect; usual maximum is ~20 mg/day

Epidural: Pain management: **Note: Must be preservative-free.** Administer with extreme caution and in reduced dosage to geriatric or debilitated patients. Vigilant monitoring is particularly important in these patients.

Single-dose (Astromorph/PF™, Duramorph®): Initial: 5 mg, if pain relief not achieved in 1 hour, careful administration of 1-2 mg at intervals sufficient to assess effectiveness may be given; maximum: 10 mg/24 hours (single doses may provide adequate relief for up to 24 hours)

Infusion: Bolus dose: 1-6 mg; infusion rate: 0.1-0.2 mg/hour; maximum dose: 10 mg/24 hours.

Note: The American Pain Society recommends 1-6 mg/dose as a single dose or an infusion of 0.1-1 mg/hour; adjust dose for age, injection site, and patient's medical condition and degree of opioid tolerance.

Continuous microinfusion (Infumorph®):

Opioid-naive: Initial: 0.2-1 mg/day

Opioid-tolerant: Initial: 1-10 mg/day, titrate to effect; usual maximum is ~20 mg/day

Chronic pain: **Note:** Patients taking opioids chronically may become tolerant and require doses higher than the usual dosage range to maintain the desired effect. Tolerance can be managed by appropriate dose titration. There is no optimal or maximal dose for morphine in chronic pain. The appropriate dose is one that relieves pain throughout its dosing interval without causing unmanageable side effects.

Oral: Controlled-, extended-, or sustained-release formulations: A patient's morphine requirement should be established using prompt-release formulations. Conversion to long-acting products may be considered when chronic, continuous treatment is required. Higher dosages should be reserved for use only in opioid-tolerant patients.

Capsules, extended release (Avinza®): Daily dose administered once daily (for best results, administer at same time each day)

Capsules, sustained release (Kadian®): Daily dose administered once daily or in 2 divided doses daily (every 12 hours)

Tablets, controlled release (MS Contin®), sustained release (Oramorph SR®), or extended release: Daily dose divided and administered every 8 or every 12 hours

Elderly or debilitated patients: Use with caution; may require dose reduction

Dosing adjustment in renal impairment:

Cl_{cr} 10-50 mL/minute: Children and Adults: Administer at 75% of normal dose

Cl_{cr} <10 mL/minute: Children and Adults: Administer at 50% of normal dose

Intermittent HD:

Children: Administer 50% of normal dose

Adults: No dosage adjustment necessary

Peritoneal dialysis: Children: Administer 50% of normal dose

CRRT: Children and Adults: Administer 75% of normal dose, titrate

Dosing adjustment/comments in hepatic disease: Unchanged in mild liver disease; substantial extrahepatic metabolism may occur; excessive sedation may occur in cirrhosis

Mechanism of Action Binds to opiate receptors in the CNS, causing inhibition of ascending pain pathways, altering the perception of and response to pain; produces generalized CNS depression

Contraindications Note: Some contraindications are product specific. For details, please see detailed product prescribing information.

Hypersensitivity to morphine sulfate or any component of the formulation; severe respiratory depression (without resuscitative equipment); acute or severe asthma; known or suspected paralytic ileus; sustained release products are not recommended with gastrointestinal obstruction or in acute/postoperative pain. Oral solutions contraindicated in patients with heart failure due to chronic lung disease, cardiac arrhythmias, head injuries, brain tumors, acute alcoholism, deliriums tremens, seizure disorders, Injectable solution contraindicated during labor when a premature birth is anticipated. Some products contraindicated in patients with head injuries or increased intracranial pressure. MS Contin® and Kadian® contraindicated in patients with hypercarbia. Some immediate release formulations (tablets and solution) contraindicated in post biliary tract surgery, suspected surgical abdomen, surgical anastomosis, MAO inhibitor use (concurrent or within 14 days), general CNS depression.

Warnings/Precautions An opioid-containing analgesic regimen should be tailored to each patient's needs and based upon the type of pain being treated (acute versus chronic), the route of administration, degree of tolerance for opioids (naive versus chronic user), age, weight, and medical condition. The optimal analgesic dose varies widely among patients. Doses should be titrated to pain relief/prevention. When used as an epidural injection, monitor for delayed sedation. **[U.S. Boxed Warning]: Healthcare provider should be alert to problems of abuse, misuse, and diversion.**

May cause respiratory depression; use with caution in patients (particularly elderly or debilitated) with impaired respiratory function, morbid obesity, adrenal insufficiency, prostatic hyperplasia, urinary stricture, renal impairment, or severe hepatic dysfunction and in patients with hypersensitivity reactions to other phenanthrene derivative opioid agonists (codeine, hydrocodone, hydromorphone, levorphanol, oxycodone, oxymorphone). Use with caution in patients with biliary tract dysfunction; acute pancreatitis may cause constriction of sphincter of Oddi. Some preparations contain sulfites which may cause allergic reactions; infants <3 months of age are more susceptible to respiratory depression, use with caution and generally in reduced doses in this age group.

May cause CNS depression, which may impair physical or mental abilities; patients must be cautioned about performing tasks which require mental alertness (eg, operating machinery or driving). Effects may be potentiated when used with other sedative drugs or ethanol. May cause hypotension in patients with acute myocardial infarction, volume depletion, or concurrent drug therapy which may exaggerate vasodilation. Use with extreme caution in patients with head injury, intracranial lesions, or elevated intracranial pressure; exaggerated elevation of ICP may occur. May cause seizures if high doses are used; use with caution in patients with seizure disorders. Tolerance or drug dependence may result from extended use. Concurrent use of agonist/antagonist analgesics may precipitate withdrawal symptoms and/or reduced analgesic efficacy in patients following prolonged therapy with mu opioid agonists. Abrupt discontinuation following prolonged use may also lead to withdrawal symptoms. Elderly may be particularly susceptible to adverse effects of narcotics. May obscure diagnosis or clinical course of patients with acute abdominal conditions.

Extended or sustained-release formulations:

[U.S. Boxed Warning]: Extended or sustained release dosage forms should not be crushed or chewed. Controlled-, extended-, or sustained-release products are not intended for "as needed (PRN)" use. **MS Contin® 100 or 200 mg tablets and Kadian® 100 mg or 200 mg capsules are for use only in opioid-tolerant patients.** Avinza®, Kadian®, MS Contin®: **[U.S. Boxed Warning]: Indicated for the management of moderate-to-severe pain when around the clock pain control is needed for an extended time period.**

[U.S. Boxed Warning]: Avinza®: Do not administer with alcoholic beverages or ethanol-containing products, which may disrupt extended-release characteristic of product.

Highly concentrated oral solutions: [U.S. Boxed Warning]: Check doses carefully when using highly concentrated oral solutions.

Injections: Note: Products are designed for administration by specific routes (I.V., intrathecal, epidural). Use caution when prescribing, dispensing, or administering to use formulations only by intended route(s).

[U.S. Boxed Warning]: Duramorph®: Due to the risk of severe and/or sustained cardiopulmonary depressant effects of Duramorph® must be administered in a fully equipped and staffed environment. Naloxone injection should be immediately available. Patient should remain in this environment for at least 24 hours following the initial dose.

[U.S. Boxed Warning]: Intrathecal dosage is usually 1/10 that of epidural dosage.

Infumorph® solutions are **for use in microinfusion devices only**; not for I.V., I.M., or SubQ administration, or for single-dose administration.

When used as an epidural injection, monitor for delayed sedation.

Drug Interactions

Metabolism/Transport Effects Substrate of CYP2D6 (minor)

Avoid Concomitant Use There are no known interactions where it is recommended to avoid concomitant use.

Increased Effect/Toxicity

Morphine (Systemic) may increase the levels/effects of: Alcohol (Ethyl); Alvimopan; CNS Depressants; Desmopressin; Selective Serotonin Reuptake Inhibitors; Thiazide Diuretics

The levels/effects of Morphine (Systemic) may be increased by: Amphetamines; Antipsychotic Agents (Phenothiazines); Droperidol; Succinylcholine

Decreased Effect

Morphine (Systemic) may decrease the levels/effects of: Pegvisomant

The levels/effects of Morphine (Systemic) may be decreased by: Ammonium Chloride; Mixed Agonist / Antagonist Opioids; Peginterferon Alfa-2b; Rifamycin Derivatives

Ethanol/Nutrition/Herb Interactions

Ethanol: Alcoholic beverages or ethanol-containing products may disrupt extended-release formulation resulting in rapid release of entire morphine dose. Ethanol may also increase CNS depression; monitor for increased effects with coadministration. Caution patients about effects.

Food: Administration of oral morphine solution with food may increase bioavailability (ie, a report of 34% increase in morphine AUC when morphine oral solution followed a high-fat meal). The bioavailability of Avinza®, Oramorph SR®, or Kadian® does not appear to be affected by food.

Herb/Nutraceutical: Avoid valerian, St John's wort, kava kava, gotu kola (may increase CNS depression).

Dietary Considerations Morphine may cause GI upset; take with food if GI upset occurs. Be consistent when taking morphine with or without meals.

Pharmacodynamics/Kinetics

Onset of Action Patient dependent; dosing must be individualized: Oral (immediate release): ~30 minutes; I.V.: 5-10 minutes

Duration of Action Patient dependent; dosing must be individualized: Pain relief:
Immediate release formulations: 4 hours
Extended release capsule and tablet: 8-24 hours (formulation dependent)

Half-life Elimination Adults: 2-4 hours (immediate release forms)

Time to Peak Avinza®: 30 minutes (maintained for 24 hours); Kadian®: ~10 hours; Oramorph® SR: ~4 hours

Pregnancy Risk Factor C

Lactation Enters breast milk/use caution (AAP rates "compatible"; AAP 2001 update pending)

Breast-Feeding Considerations Morphine concentrates in breast milk, with a milk to plasma AUC ratio of 2.5:1. Detectable serum levels of morphine can be found in infants following morphine administration to nursing mothers. Treatment of the mother with single doses of morphine is not expected to cause detrimental effects in nursing infants. Breast-feeding following chronic use or in neonates with hepatic or renal dysfunction may lead to higher levels of morphine in the infant and a risk of adverse effects.

Controlled Substance C-II

Dosage Forms

Capsule, extended release, oral:
AVINza®: 30 mg, 45 mg, 60 mg, 75 mg, 90 mg, 120 mg
Kadian®: 10 mg, 20 mg, 30 mg, 50 mg, 60 mg, 80 mg, 100 mg, 200 mg

Injection, solution: 1 mg/mL (10 mL, 30 mL, 50 mL); 2 mg/mL (1 mL); 4 mg/mL (1 mL); 5 mg/mL (1 mL, 30 mL, 50 mL); 8 mg/mL (1 mL); 10 mg/mL (1 mL, 10 mL); 10 mg/0.7 mL (0.7 mL); 15 mg/mL (1 mL, 20 mL); 25 mg/mL (4 mL, 10 mL, 20 mL); 50 mg/mL (20 mL, 40 mL, 50 mL)

Injection, solution [preservative free]: 0.5 mg/mL (10 mL, 30 mL); 1 mg/mL (10 mL, 30 mL); 5 mg/mL (30 mL); 25 mg/mL (4 mL, 10 mL, 20 mL)
Astramorph®/PF: 0.5 mg/mL (2 mL, 10 mL); 1 mg/mL (2 mL, 10 mL)
Duramorph: 0.5 mg/mL (10 mL); 1 mg/mL (10 mL)
Infumorph 200: 10 mg/mL (20 mL)
Infumorph 500: 25 mg/mL (20 mL)

Solution, oral: 10 mg/5 mL (5 mL, 10 mL, 100 mL, 500 mL); 20 mg/5 mL (100 mL, 500 mL); 100 mg/5 mL (1 mL, 15 mL, 30 mL, 120 mL, 240 mL)

Suppository, rectal: 5 mg (12s); 10 mg (12s); 20 mg (12s); 30 mg (12s)

Tablet, oral: 15 mg, 30 mg

Tablet, controlled release, oral:
MS Contin®: 15 mg, 30 mg, 60 mg, 100 mg, 200 mg

Tablet, extended release, oral: 15 mg, 30 mg, 60 mg, 100 mg, 200 mg

Tablet, sustained release, oral:
Oramorph® SR: 15 mg, 30 mg, 60 mg, 100 mg

Dosage Forms: Canada

Solution, oral:

Doloral: 1 mg/mL; 5 mg/mL [not available in U.S.]

Morphine and Naltrexone (MOR feen & nal TREKS one)

Related Information

Morphine (Systemic) *on page* 1157

Naltrexone *on page* 1181

U.S. Brand Names Embeda™

Generic Availability (U.S.) No

Pharmacologic Category Analgesic, Opioid; Opioid Antagonist

Use Relief of moderate-to-severe pain when continual, around-the-clock therapy is needed for an extended period of time

Local Anesthetic/Vasoconstrictor Precautions No information available to require special precautions

Effects on Dental Treatment Key adverse event(s) related to dental treatment:

Morphine sulfate: Xerostomia (normal salivary flow resumes upon discontinuation) and dysphagia. Anticholinergic side effects can cause a reduction of saliva production or secretion, contributing to discomfort and dental disease (ie, caries, oral candidiasis, and periodontal disease).

Naltrexone: Dry mouth.

Effects on Bleeding No information available to require special precautions

Adverse Effects Frequency not always defined.

>10%:

Central nervous system: Somnolence (1% to 14%)

Gastrointestinal: Constipation (7% to 31%), nausea (11% to 22%)

1% to 10%:

Cardiovascular: Flushing (≤2%), peripheral edema

Central nervous system: Dizziness (1% to 8%), headache (2% to 7%), fatigue (1% to 4%), insomnia (1% to 3%), anxiety (2%), chills, depression, irritability, lethargy, restlessness, sedation

Dermatologic: Pruritus (≤6%), hyperhidrosis (3%)

Endocrine & metabolic: Hot flashes

Gastrointestinal: Vomiting (4% to 8%), xerostomia (2% to 6%), diarrhea (≤2%), abdominal pain/discomfort, anorexia, appetite decreased, dyspepsia, flatulence

Neuromuscular & skeletal: Arthralgia, muscle spasms, tremor

Dosage Oral: Moderate-to-severe pain: **Note:** These are guidelines and do not represent the doses that may be required in all patients. Treatment should be individualized based on patient's prior analgesic treatment experience/tolerance and pain relief. Not intended for use as a PRN medication.

Adults: Opiate-naive: Initial: 20 mg/0.8 mg once or twice daily; 100 mg/4 mg strength for use in opioid-tolerant patients only

Titration: Do not increase dose more frequently than every other day. May supplement dose with a short-acting analgesic (<20% of total daily dose) for breakthrough pain. If once-daily dosing is inadequate may switch to twice daily dosing.

Conversion from other oral morphine products to Embeda™: Administer one-half of the patient's total daily oral morphine dose as Embeda™ every 12 hours or all of the patient's total daily oral morphine dose as Embeda™ once daily.

Conversion from other oral/parenteral opioids or parenteral morphine to Embeda™: Must first convert to oral morphine equivalent.

Conversion from parenteral to oral morphine: It may take 2-6 mg of oral morphine to provide pain relief equivalent to 1 mg of parenteral morphine. An oral dose 3 times the daily parenteral dose may be sufficient in chronic pain settings.

Conversion from other oral/parenteral opioids to oral morphine: Specific recommendations are not available; refer to published relative potency data realizing that such ratios are only approximations. It is generally safest to give half the estimated daily morphine requirement as the initial dose and manage inadequate relief with immediate release morphine.

Note: When converting from other opioid analgesics it is better to underestimate the patient's 24-hour oral requirement and provide breakthrough treatment than to overestimate and manage an adverse event.

Elderly or debilitated patients: Use with caution; may require dose reduction

Dosing adjustment in renal impairment: Use with caution in patients with severe impairment; no specific dosing recommendations are provided by the manufacturer.

Dosing adjustment/comments in hepatic disease: Use with caution in patients with severe impairment; no specific dosing recommendations are provided by the manufacturer.

Mechanism of Action

Morphine binds to opiate receptors in the CNS, causing inhibition of ascending pain pathways, altering the perception of and response to pain; produces generalized CNS depression.

Naltrexone (a pure opioid antagonist) is a cyclopropyl derivative of oxymorphone similar in structure to naloxone and nalorphine (a morphine derivative); it acts as a competitive antagonist at opioid receptor sites, showing the highest affinity for mu receptors. Naltrexone is not an active component unless tablet is chewed, crushed, or dissolved.

Contraindications Hypersensitivity to morphine, naltrexone, or any component of the formulation; patients with significant respiratory depression, acute/severe bronchial asthma, or hypercapnia in unmonitored settings or in the absence of resuscitative equipment; patients with or suspected of having paralytic ileus; any situation where opioids are contraindicated

Warnings/Precautions An opioid-containing analgesic regimen should be tailored to each patient's needs and based upon the type of pain being treated (acute versus chronic), the route of administration, degree of tolerance for opioids (naive versus chronic user), age, weight, and medical condition. The optimal analgesic dose varies widely among patients. Doses should be titrated to pain relief/prevention. **[U.S. Boxed Warnings]: Morphine and naltrexone is not intended for use as a prn analgesic; indicated for management of moderate-to-severe pain when a continuous, around-the-clock opioid analgesic is needed for an extended period of time. High potential for abuse; healthcare provider should be alert to problems of abuse, misuse, and diversion.**

May cause respiratory depression; use with caution in patients (particularly elderly or debilitated) with impaired respiratory function, adrenal insufficiency, prostatic hyperplasia, urinary stricture, severe renal impairment, or severe hepatic dysfunction and in patients with hypersensitivity reactions to other phenanthrene derivative opioid agonists (codeine, hydrocodone, hydromorphone, levorphanol, oxycodone, oxymorphone). Use with caution in patients with biliary tract dysfunction; acute pancreatitis may cause constriction of sphincter of Oddi.

May cause CNS depression, which may impair physical or mental abilities; patients must be cautioned about performing tasks which require mental alertness (eg, operating machinery or driving). Effects may be potentiated when used with other sedative drugs or ethanol. **[U.S. Boxed Warning]: Patients should not consume alcoholic beverages or medication containing ethanol while taking morphine and naltrexone; ethanol may increase morphine plasma levels resulting in a potentially fatal overdose.** Use caution in patients with acute alcoholism or delirium tremors. May cause hypotension in patients with acute myocardial infarction, volume depletion, or concurrent drug therapy which may exaggerate vasodilation. Use with extreme caution in patients with head injury, intracranial lesions, or elevated intracranial pressure; exaggerated elevation of ICP may occur. May cause seizures if high doses are used; use with caution in patients with seizure disorders. Tolerance or drug dependence may result from extended use. May obscure diagnosis or clinical course of patients with acute abdominal conditions. **[U.S. Boxed Warnings]: Capsules and pellets within the capsule are to be swallowed whole; do not chew, crush, or dissolve. Chewing, crushing, or dissolving capsule will result in the release of naltrexone which may precipitate withdrawal in opioid-tolerant patients.** Symptoms of withdrawal (eg, confusion, somnolence, visual hallucination, vomiting, diarrhea) usually appear within 5 minutes of naltrexone ingestion and may last for up to 48 hours. Abrupt discontinuation following prolonged use may also lead to withdrawal symptoms. Stop therapy and use parenteral short-acting opioids 24 hours prior to cordotomy. Do not use concurrently in patient taking MAO inhibitors; discontinue MAO inhibitor 14 days prior to starting morphine and naltrexone. Elderly and debilitated patients may be particularly susceptible to adverse effects of narcotics.

[U.S. Boxed Warning:] Embeda™ 100 mg/4 mg capsules are for use in opioid-tolerant patients only; may cause fatal respiratory depression in patients not already tolerant to high doses of opioids.

Drug Interactions

Avoid Concomitant Use There are no known interactions where it is recommended to avoid concomitant use.

Increased Effect/Toxicity There are no known significant interactions involving an increase in effect.

Decreased Effect There are no known significant interactions involving a decrease in effect.

Ethanol/Nutrition/Herb Interactions

Ethanol: Alcoholic beverages or ethanol-containing products may disrupt extended-release formulation resulting in rapid release of entire morphine dose. Ethanol may also increase CNS depression; monitor for increased effects with coadministration. Caution patients about effects.

Herb/Nutraceutical: Avoid valerian, St John's wort, kava kava, gotu kola (may increase CNS depression).

Dietary Considerations Morphine may cause GI upset; take with food if GI upset occurs. Be consistent when taking morphine with or without meals.

Pharmacodynamics/Kinetics

Onset of Action Patient dependent; dosing must be individualized: ~8 hours

Half-life Elimination Terminal: ~29 hours

Time to Peak 7.5 hours

Pregnancy Risk Factor C

Lactation Enters breast milk/not recommended

Breast-Feeding Considerations Morphine concentrates in breast milk, with a milk to plasma ratio of 2.5:1. Detectable serum levels of morphine can be found in infants following morphine administration to nursing mothers. Breast-feeding following chronic use or in neonates with hepatic or renal dysfunction may lead to higher levels of morphine in the infant and a risk of adverse effects.

Controlled Substance C-II

Dosage Forms

Capsule, extended release, oral:

Embeda™ 20/0.8: Morphine 20 mg and naltrexone 0.8 mg
Embeda™ 30/1.2: Morphine 30 mg and naltrexone 1.2 mg
Embeda™ 50/2: Morphine 50 mg and naltrexone 2 mg
Embeda™ 80/3.2: Morphine 80 mg and naltrexone 3.2 mg
Embeda™ 100/4: Morphine 100 mg and naltrexone 4 mg

Morrhuate Sodium (MOR yoo ate SOW dee um)

Pharmacologic Category Sclerosing Agent

Use Treatment of small, uncomplicated varicose veins of the lower extremities

Local Anesthetic/Vasoconstrictor Precautions No information available to require special precautions

Effects on Dental Treatment No significant effects or complications reported

Effects on Bleeding No information available to require special precautions

Adverse Effects Frequency not defined.

Cardiovascular: Thrombosis, valvular incompetency, vascular collapse
Central nervous system: Dizziness, drowsiness, headache
Dermatologic: Urticaria
Gastrointestinal: Nausea, vomiting
Local: Burning at the site of injection, severe extravasation effects
Neuromuscular & skeletal: Weakness
Respiratory: Asthma
Miscellaneous: Anaphylaxis, hypersensitivity reactions

General Dosage Range I.V.: *Adults:* 50-250 mg, repeated at 5- to 7-day intervals

Mechanism of Action Both varicose veins and esophageal varices are treated by the thrombotic action of morrhuate sodium. By causing inflammation of the vein's intima, a thrombus is formed. Occlusion secondary to the fibrous tissue and the thrombus results in the obliteration of the vein.

Pharmacodynamics/Kinetics

Onset of Action ~5 minutes

Pregnancy Risk Factor C

Mouthwash (Antiseptic) (MOUTH wosh)

Related Information

Bacterial Infections *on page 1933*
Dentin Hypersensitivity, Acid Erosion, High Caries Index, and Xerostomia *on page 1955*
Periodontal Diseases *on page 1942*
Ulcerative, Erosive, and Painful Oral Mucosal Disorders *on page 1950*

Related Sample Prescriptions

Antimicrobial Oral Rinses *on page 1987*

Pharmacologic Category Antimicrobial Mouth Rinse; Antiplaque Agent; Mouthwash

Dental Use Aid in prevention and reduction of plaque and gingivitis; halitosis

Local Anesthetic/Vasoconstrictor Precautions No information available to require special precautions

Effects on Dental Treatment No significant effects or complications reported (see Dental Comment)

Effects on Bleeding No information available to require special precautions

Adverse Effects No data reported

Dental Usual Dosage Plaque/gingivitis prevention: Adults: Oral: Rinse full strength for 30 seconds with 20 mL (2/3 fluid ounce or 4 teaspoonfuls) morning and night

Dosage Rinse full strength for 30 seconds with 20 mL (2/3 fluid ounce or 4 teaspoonfuls) morning and night

Contraindications Hypersensitivity to any component of the formulation

Dosage Forms

Rinse: 250 mL, 500 mL, 1000 mL

Dental Comment Active ingredients:

Listerine® Antiseptic: Thymol 0.064%, eucalyptus 0.092%, methyl salicylate 0.060%, menthol 0.042%, alcohol 26.9%, water, benzoic acid, poloxamer 407, sodium benzoate, caramel

Fresh Burst Listerine® Antiseptic: Thymol 0.064%, eucalyptus 0.092%, methyl salicylate 0.060%, menthol 0.042%, alcohol 26.9%, water, benzoic acid, poloxamer 407, sodium benzoate, flavoring, sodium, saccharin, sodium citrate, citric acid, D&C yellow #10, FD&C green #3

Cool Mint Listerine® Antiseptic: Thymol 0.064%, eucalyptus 0.092%, methyl salicylate 0.060%, menthol 0.042%, alcohol 26.9%, water, benzoic acid, poloxamer 407, sodium benzoate, flavoring, sodium, saccharin, sodium citrate, citric acid, FD&C green #3

The following information is endorsed on the label of the Listerine® products by the Council on Scientific Affairs, American Dental Association: "Listerine® Antiseptic has been shown to help prevent and reduce supragingival plaque accumulation and gingivitis when used in a conscientiously applied program of oral hygiene and regular professional care. Its effect on periodontitis has not been determined."

Moxifloxacin (Systemic) (moxs i FLOKS a sin)

Related Information

Bacterial Infections *on page 1933*

Clinical Risk Related to Drugs Prolonging QT Interval *on page 1872*

Respiratory Diseases *on page 1876*

U.S. Brand Names Avelox®; Avelox® ABC Pack; Avelox® I.V.

Canadian Brand Names Avelox®; Avelox® I.V.

Generic Availability (U.S.) No

Pharmacologic Category Antibiotic, Quinolone; Respiratory Fluoroquinolone

Use Treatment of mild-to-moderate community-acquired pneumonia, including multidrug-resistant *Streptococcus pneumoniae* (MDRSP); acute bacterial exacerbation of chronic bronchitis; acute bacterial sinusitis; complicated and uncomplicated skin and skin structure infections; complicated intra-abdominal infections

Unlabeled/Investigational Use Treatment of *Legionella* pneumonia

Local Anesthetic/Vasoconstrictor Precautions Moxifloxacin is one of the drugs confirmed to prolong the QT interval and is accepted as having a risk of causing torsade de pointes. The risk of drug-induced torsade de pointes is extremely low when a single QT interval prolonging drug is prescribed. In terms of epinephrine, it is not known what effect vasoconstrictors in the local anesthetic regimen will have in patients with a known history of congenital prolonged QT interval or in patients taking any medication that prolongs the QT interval. Until more information is obtained, it is suggested that the clinician consult with the physician prior to the use of a vasoconstrictor in suspected patients, and that the vasoconstrictor (epinephrine, mepivacaine and levonordefrin [Carbocaine® 2% with Neo-Cobefrin®]) be used with caution.

Effects on Dental Treatment Key adverse event(s) related to dental treatment: Dry mouth, glossitis, stomatitis, and taste perversion.

Effects on Bleeding No information available to require special precautions

Adverse Effects

2% to 10%:

Central nervous system: Dizziness (2%)

Endocrine & metabolic: Serum chloride increased (≥2%), serum ionized calcium increased (≥2%), serum glucose decreased (≥2%)

Gastrointestinal: Nausea (6%), diarrhea (5%), amylase decreased (≥2%)

Hematologic: Decreased serum levels of the following (≥2%): Basophils, eosinophils, hemoglobin, RBC, neutrophils; increased serum levels of the following (≥2%): MCH, neutrophils, WBC

Hepatic: Bilirubin decreased/increased (≥2%)

Renal: Serum albumin increased (≥2%)
Respiratory: PO_2 decreased (≥2%)

0.1% to <2%:

Cardiovascular: Cardiac arrhythmias, palpitation, QT_c prolongation, tachycardia, vasodilation
Central nervous system: Anxiety, headache, insomnia, malaise, nervousness, pain, somnolence, vertigo
Dermatologic: Pruritus, rash (maculopapular, purpuric, pustular), urticaria
Gastrointestinal: Abdominal pain, amylase increased, anorexia, constipation, dyspepsia, flatulence, glossitis, lactic dehydrogenase increased, stomatitis, taste perversion, vomiting, xerostomia
Genitourinary: Vaginal moniliasis, vaginitis
Hematologic: Eosinophilia, leukopenia, prothrombin time prolonged, increased INR, thrombocythemia
Hepatic: GGTP increased, liver function test abnormal
Local: Injection site reaction
Neuromuscular & skeletal: Arthralgia, myalgia, tremor, weakness
Respiratory: Pharyngitis, pneumonia, rhinitis, sinusitis
Miscellaneous: Allergic reaction, infection, diaphoresis, oral moniliasis

Dosage Adults: Oral, I.V.: Usual dosage range: 400 mg every 24 hours

Indication-specific dosing:

Acute bacterial sinusitis: 400 mg every 24 hours for 10 days

Chronic bronchitis, acute bacterial exacerbation: 400 mg every 24 hours for 5 days

Intra-abdominal infections, complicated: 400 mg every 24 hours for 5-14 days (initiate with I.V.); **Note:** 2010 IDSA guidelines recommend a treatment duration of 4-7 days (provided source controlled) for community-acquired, mild-to-moderate IAI

Pneumonia, community-acquired (including MDRSP): 400 mg every 24 hours for 7-14 days

Skin and skin structure infections:

Complicated: 400 mg every 24 hours for 7-21 days
Uncomplicated: 400 mg every 24 hours for 7 days

Elderly: No dosage adjustments are required based on age

Dosage adjustment in renal impairment: No dosage adjustment is required, including patients on hemodialysis, CRRT, or CAPD.

Dosage adjustment in hepatic impairment: No dosage adjustment is required in mild, moderate, or severe hepatic insufficiency (Child-Pugh class A, B, or C); however, use with caution in this patient population secondary to the risk of QT prolongation.

Mechanism of Action Moxifloxacin is a DNA gyrase inhibitor, and also inhibits topoisomerase IV. DNA gyrase (topoisomerase II) is an essential bacterial enzyme that maintains the superhelical structure of DNA. DNA gyrase is required for DNA replication and transcription, DNA repair, recombination, and transposition; inhibition is bactericidal.

Contraindications Hypersensitivity to moxifloxacin, other quinolone antibiotics, or any component of the formulation

Warnings/Precautions **[U.S. Boxed Warning]: There have been reports of tendon inflammation and/or rupture with quinolone antibiotics; risk may be increased with concurrent corticosteroids, organ transplant recipients, and in patients >60 years of age.** Rupture of the Achilles tendon sometimes requiring surgical repair has been reported most frequently; but other tendon sites (eg, rotator cuff, biceps) have also been reported. Strenuous physical activity, rheumatoid arthritis, and renal impairment may be an independent risk factor for tendonitis. Discontinue at first sign of tendon inflammation or pain. Tendon rupture may occur even after discontinuation of therapy. Use with caution in patients with rheumatoid arthritis or renal impairment; may increase risk of tendon rupture.

Use with caution in patients with significant bradycardia or acute myocardial ischemia. Moxifloxacin causes a concentration-dependent QT prolongation. Do not exceed recommended dose or infusion rate. Avoid use with uncorrected hypokalemia, with other drugs that prolong the QT interval or induce bradycardia, or with class Ia or III antiarrhythmic agents. Use with caution in individuals at risk of seizures (CNS disorders or concurrent therapy with medications which may lower seizure threshold). Potential for seizures, although very rare, may be increased with concomitant NSAID therapy. Discontinue in patients who experience significant CNS adverse effects (dizziness, hallucinations, suicidal ideation or actions). Use with caution in patients with mild, moderate, or severe hepatic impairment or liver cirrhosis; may increase the risk of QT prolongation. Fulminant hepatitis potentially leading to liver failure (including fatalities) has been reported with use. Use with caution in diabetes; glucose regulation may be altered.

Fluoroquinolones have been associated with the development of serious, and sometimes fatal, hypoglycemia, most often in elderly diabetics, but also in patients without diabetes. This occurred most frequently with gatifloxacin (no longer available systemically) but may occur at a lower frequency with other quinolones.

Severe hypersensitivity reactions, including anaphylaxis, have occurred with quinolone therapy. Reactions may present as typical allergic symptoms after a single dose, or may manifest as severe idiosyncratic dermatologic, vascular, pulmonary, renal, hepatic, and/or hematologic events, usually after multiple doses. Prompt discontinuation of drug should occur if skin rash or other symptoms arise. Avoid excessive sunlight and take precautions to limit exposure (eg, loose fitting clothing, sunscreen); may cause moderate-to-severe phototoxicity reactions. Discontinue use if photosensitivity occurs. Prolonged use may result in fungal or bacterial superinfection, including *C. difficile*-associated diarrhea (CDAD) and pseudomembranous colitis; CDAD has been observed >2 months postantibiotic treatment. **[U.S. Boxed Warning]: Quinolones may exacerbate myasthenia gravis; avoid use (rare, potentially life-threatening weakness of respiratory muscles may occur).** Peripheral neuropathy may rarely occur. Hemolytic reactions may (rarely) occur with quinolone use in patients with latent or actual G6PD deficiency. Adverse effects (eg, tendon rupture, QT changes) may be increased in the elderly. Some quinolones may exacerbate myasthenia gravis, use with caution (rare, potentially life-threatening weakness of respiratory muscles may occur). Safety and efficacy of systemically administered moxifloxacin (oral, intravenous) in patients <18 years of age have not been established.

Drug Interactions

Avoid Concomitant Use

Avoid concomitant use of Moxifloxacin (Systemic) with any of the following: Artemether; BCG; Dronedarone; Lumefantrine; Nilotinib; Pimozide; QuiNINE; Tetrabenazine; Thioridazine; Toremifene; Vandetanib; Ziprasidone

Increased Effect/Toxicity

Moxifloxacin (Systemic) may increase the levels/effects of: Corticosteroids (Systemic); Dronedarone; Pimozide; QTc-Prolonging Agents; QuiNINE; Sulfonylureas; Tetrabenazine; Thioridazine; Toremifene; Vandetanib; Vitamin K Antagonists; Ziprasidone

The levels/effects of Moxifloxacin (Systemic) may be increased by: Alfuzosin; Artemether; Chloroquine; Ciprofloxacin; Ciprofloxacin (Systemic); Gadobutrol; Insulin; Lumefantrine; Nilotinib; Nonsteroidal Anti-Inflammatory Agents; Probenecid; QuiNINE

Decreased Effect

Moxifloxacin (Systemic) may decrease the levels/effects of: BCG; Mycophenolate; Sulfonylureas; Typhoid Vaccine

The levels/effects of Moxifloxacin (Systemic) may be decreased by: Antacids; Didanosine; Iron Salts; Lanthanum; Magnesium Salts; Quinapril; Sevelamer; Sucralfate; Zinc Salts

Ethanol/Nutrition/Herb Interactions Food: Absorption is not affected by administration with a high-fat meal or yogurt.

Dietary Considerations May be taken without regard to meals. Take 4 hours before or 8 hours after multiple vitamins, antacids, or other products containing magnesium, aluminum, iron, or zinc.

Avelox® I.V. infusion (premixed in sodium chloride 0.8%) contains sodium 34.2 mEq (~787 mg)/250 mL.

Pharmacodynamics/Kinetics

Half-life Elimination Single dose: Oral: 12-16 hours; I.V.: 8-15 hours

Pregnancy Risk Factor C

Lactation Excretion in breast milk unknown/not recommended

Breast-Feeding Considerations It is not known if moxifloxacin is excreted into breast milk. Breast-feeding is not recommended by the manufacturer. Although there is no information on the use of moxifloxacin during breast-feeding, other quinolones are considered compatible. Nondose-related effects could include modification of bowel flora.

Dosage Forms

Infusion, premixed in sodium chloride 0.8% [preservative free]:

Avelox® I.V.: 400 mg (250 mL)

Tablet, oral:

Avelox®: 400 mg

Avelox® ABC Pack: 400 mg

Dental Comment Moxifloxacin is known to prolong the QT interval. The QT interval is measured as the time and distance between the Q point of the QRS complex and the end of the T wave in the ECG tracing. After adjustment for heart rate, the QT interval is defined as prolonged if it is more than 450 msec in men and 460 msec in women. A long QT syndrome was first described in the 1950s and 60s as a congenital syndrome involving QT interval prolongation and syncope and sudden death. Some of the congenital long QT syndromes were characterized by a peculiar electrocardiographic appearance of the QRS complex involving a premature atria beat followed by a pause, then a subsequent sinus beat showing marked QT prolongation and deformity. This type of cardiac arrhythmia was originally termed "torsade de pointes" (translated from the French as "twisting of the points"). Moxifloxacin is considered as having a risk of causing torsade de pointes. Since it is not known what effect vasoconstrictors in the local anesthetic regimen will have in patients with a known history of congenital prolonged QT interval or in patients taking any medication that prolongs the QT interval, a medical consult is suggested.

Mucosal Barrier Gel, Oral (myoo KOH sul BAR ee er GEL, OR al)

Related Information

Management of Patients Undergoing Cancer Therapy *on page 1970*

U.S. Brand Names Gelclair®

Pharmacologic Category Gastrointestinal Agent, Miscellaneous

Dental Use Management of oral mucosal pain caused by oral mucositis/stomatitis (resulting from chemotherapy or radiation therapy), irritation due to oral surgery, traumatic ulcers caused by braces/ill-fitting dentures or disease, diffuse aphthous ulcers (canker sores)

Use Management of oral mucosal pain caused by oral mucositis/stomatitis (resulting from chemotherapy or radiation therapy), irritation due to oral surgery, traumatic ulcers caused by braces/ill-fitting dentures or disease, diffuse aphthous ulcers (canker sores)

Local Anesthetic/Vasoconstrictor Precautions No information available to require special precautions

Effects on Dental Treatment No significant effects or complications reported

Effects on Bleeding No information available to require special precautions

Dental Usual Dosage Oral: Adults: Mucosal protection: Gargle and spit the mixture of 1 single-use packet (15 mL) and water 3 times daily, or as needed. Pour the contents of a single-use packet (15 mL) into a glass and mix with 1 tablespoon of water. May dilute with an additional 1-2 tablespoons of water to achieve desired thickness. Stir well and use immediately. Mixture should be rinsed around the mouth for a minimum of 1 minute (as long as possible) to coat the tongue, palate, throat, inside of cheeks, and all oral tissue thoroughly. Mixture should be gargled and spit out. Accidental ingestion is not expected to cause adverse effects. The gel may become thicker and darker over time; however, this has not been shown to affect its safety or efficacy. Any packet that is not intact should not be used. To gain maximum benefit, patients should use 30-60 minutes prior to meals.

Dosage Oral: Adults: Mucosal protection: Gargle and spit the mixture of 1 single-use packet (15 mL) and water 3 times daily, or as needed. May be used undiluted if water is unavailable.

Mechanism of Action Mechanical action for the management and relief of pain by adhering to the mucosal surface of mouth forming a protective film over the irritated areas and lesions

Contraindications Hypersensitivity to any component of the formulation

Warnings/Precautions Patients should avoid eating or drinking for a minimum of 1 hour following treatment. Consult a physician if no improvement is seen after 7 days of use.

Dosage Forms

Gel, oral:

Gelclair®: 15 mL/packet (15s)

References

Barber C, Powell R, Ellis A, et al, "Comparing Pain Control and Ability to Eat and Drink With Standard Therapy vs Gelclair: A Preliminary, Double Centre, Randomized Controlled Trial on Patients With Radiotherapy-Induced Oral Mucositis," *Support Care Cancer*, 2007, 15(4):427-40.

Hita-Iglesias P, Torres-Lagares D, and Gutiérrez-Pérez JL, "Evaluation of the Clinical Behavior of a Polyvinylpyrrolidone and Sodium Hyalonurate gel (Gelclair) in Patients Subjected to Surgical Treatment With CO2 Laser," *Int J Oral Maxillofac Surg*, 2006, 35(6):514-7.

Mupirocin (myoo PEER oh sin)

U.S. Brand Names Bactroban Cream®; Bactroban Nasal®; Bactroban®; Centany®; Centany® AT

Canadian Brand Names Bactroban®

Pharmacologic Category Antibiotic, Topical

Use

Intranasal: Eradication of nasal colonization with MRSA in adult patients and healthcare workers

Topical: Treatment of impetigo or secondary infected traumatic skin lesions due to *S. aureus* and *S. pyogenes*

Unlabeled/Investigational Use Intranasal: Surgical prophylaxis to prevent wound infections

Local Anesthetic/Vasoconstrictor Precautions No information available to require special precautions

Effects on Dental Treatment Key adverse event(s) related to dental treatment: Xerostomia (normal salivary flow resumes upon discontinuation) and taste perversion.

Effects on Bleeding No information available to require special precautions

Adverse Effects Frequency not defined.

Central nervous system: Dizziness, headache

Dermatologic: Cellulitis, dermatitis, dry skin, erythema, hives, pruritus, rash

Gastrointestinal: Abdominal pain, diarrhea, nausea, taste perversion, ulcerative stomatitis, xerostomia

Local: Burning, edema, pain, stinging, tenderness

Ocular: Blepharitis

Otic: Ear pain

Respiratory: Cough, pharyngitis, rhinitis, upper respiratory tract congestion

Miscellaneous: Secondary wound infection

General Dosage Range

Intranasal: *Children ≥12 years and Adults:* Approximately one-half of the ointment from the single-use tube should be applied into one nostril and the other half into the other nostril twice daily

Topical: *Children ≥2 months and Adults:* Apply to affected area 3 times/day

Mechanism of Action Binds to bacterial isoleucyl transfer-RNA synthetase resulting in the inhibition of protein synthesis

Pregnancy Risk Factor B

Muromonab-CD3 (myoo roe MOE nab see dee three)

U.S. Brand Names Orthoclone OKT® 3 [DSC]

Pharmacologic Category Immunosuppressant Agent; Monoclonal Antibody

Use Treatment of acute allograft rejection in renal transplant patients; treatment of steroid-resistant acute allograft rejection in cardiac or hepatic transplantation

Unlabeled/Investigational Use Treatment of acute pancreas rejection episodes resistant to conventional treatment

Local Anesthetic/Vasoconstrictor Precautions No information available to require special precautions

Effects on Dental Treatment No significant effects or complications reported

Effects on Bleeding Has been associated with thrombotic adverse events. No information available to require special precautions for dental procedures.

Adverse Effects Note: Signs and symptoms of cytokine release syndrome (characterized by pyrexia, chills, dyspnea, nausea, vomiting, chest pain, diarrhea, tremor, wheezing, headache, tachycardia, rigor, hypertension, pulmonary edema and/or other cardiorespiratory manifestations) occurs in a significant proportion of patients following the first couple of doses of muromonab-CD3. Additionally, some patients have experienced immediate hypersensitivity reactions to muromonab-CD3 (characterized by cardiovascular collapse, cardiorespiratory arrest, loss of consciousness, hypotension/shock, tachycardia, tingling, angioedema (including laryngeal, pharyngeal, or facial edema), airway obstruction, bronchospasm, dyspnea, urticaria, and/or pruritus) upon initial exposure and re-exposure.

>10%:

Cardiovascular: Tachycardia (26%), hypotension (25%), hypertension (19%), edema (12%)

Central nervous system: Pyrexia (77%), chills (43%), headache (28%)

Dermatologic: Rash (14%; erythematous 2%)

Gastrointestinal: Diarrhea (37%), nausea (32%), vomiting (25%)

Respiratory: Dyspnea (16%)

1% to 10%:

Cardiovascular: Chest pain (9%), vasodilation (7%), arrhythmia (4%), bradycardia (4%), vascular occlusion (2%)

Central nervous system: Fatigue (9%), confusion (6%), dizziness (6%), lethargy (6%), pain trunk (6%), malaise (5%), nervousness (5%), depression (3%), somnolence (2%), meningitis (1%), seizure (1%)

Dermatologic: Pruritus (7%)

Gastrointestinal: Gastrointestinal pain (7%), abdominal pain (6%), anorexia (4%)
Hematologic: Leukopenia (7%), anemia (2%), thrombocytopenia (2%), leukocytosis (1%)
Neuromuscular & skeletal: Weakness (10%), arthralgia (7%), myalgia (1%), tremor (14%)
Ocular: Photophobia (1%)
Otic: Tinnitus (1%)
Renal: Renal dysfunction (3%)
Respiratory: Abnormal chest sound (10%), hyperventilation (7%), wheezing (6%), respiratory congestion (4%), pulmonary edema (2%), hypoxia (1%), pneumonia (1%)
Miscellaneous: Diaphoresis (7%), infections (various)

General Dosage Range I.V.:
Children ≤30 kg: 2.5 mg once daily
Children >30 kg and Adults: 5 mg once daily

Mechanism of Action Reverses graft rejection by binding to T cells and interfering with their function by binding T-cell receptor-associated CD3 glycoprotein

Pharmacodynamics/Kinetics
Duration of Action 7 days after discontinuation
Time to Peak Steady-state: Trough: 3-14 days

Pregnancy Risk Factor C

Product Availability Orthoclone OKT® 3: Due to diminishing use, the manufacturer of muromonab is discontinuing production; supplies are expected to be available through the end of 2010.

Mycophenolate (mye koe FEN oh late)

U.S. Brand Names CellCept®; Myfortic®

Canadian Brand Names CellCept®; Myfortic®

Pharmacologic Category Immunosuppressant Agent

Use Prophylaxis of organ rejection concomitantly with cyclosporine and corticosteroids in patients receiving allogeneic renal (CellCept®, Myfortic®), cardiac (CellCept®), or hepatic (CellCept®) transplants

Unlabeled/Investigational Use Treatment of rejection in liver transplant patients unable to tolerate tacrolimus or cyclosporine due to neurotoxicity; mild rejection in heart transplant patients; treatment of moderate-severe psoriasis; treatment of proliferative lupus nephritis; treatment of myasthenia gravis; prevention and treatment of graft-versus-host disease (GVHD)

Local Anesthetic/Vasoconstrictor Precautions No information available to require special precautions

Effects on Dental Treatment Key adverse event(s) related to dental treatment: Mouth ulceration, gum hyperplasia, gingivitis, dry mouth, dysphagia, oral moniliasis, and stomatitis.

Effects on Bleeding May be associated with hematologic effects, potentially including significant reduction in platelet counts with altered hemostasis. In patients who are under active treatment, medical consult is suggested.

Adverse Effects Data for incidence >20% as reported in adults following oral dosing of CellCept® alone in renal, cardiac, and hepatic allograft rejection studies. Profile in 3% to <20% range reflects use in combination with cyclosporine and corticosteroids. In general, lower doses used in renal rejection patients had less adverse effects than higher doses. Rates of adverse effects were similar for each indication, except for those unique to the specific organ involved. The type of adverse effects observed in pediatric patients was similar to those seen in adults; abdominal pain, anemia, diarrhea, fever, hypertension, infection, pharyngitis, respiratory tract infection, sepsis, and vomiting were seen in higher proportion; lymphoproliferative disorder was the only type of malignancy observed. Percentages of adverse reactions were similar in studies comparing CellCept® to Myfortic® in patients following renal transplant.

>20%:
Cardiovascular: Hypertension (28% to 78%), hypotension (33%), peripheral edema (27% to 64%), edema (27% to 28%), chest pain (26%), tachycardia (20% to 22%)
Central nervous system: Pain (31% to 76%), headache (16% to 54%), insomnia (41% to 52%), fever (21% to 52%), dizziness (29%), anxiety (28%)
Dermatologic: Rash (22%)
Endocrine & metabolic: Hyperglycemia (44% to 47%), hypercholesterolemia (41%), hypomagnesemia (39%), hypokalemia (32% to 37%), hypocalcemia (30%), hyperkalemia (22%)
Gastrointestinal: Abdominal pain (25% to 63%), nausea (20% to 55%), diarrhea (31% to 51%), constipation (19% to 41%), vomiting (33% to 34%), anorexia (25%), dyspepsia (22%)

Genitourinary: Urinary tract infection (37%)
Hematologic: Leukopenia (23% to 46%), anemia (26% to 43%; hypochromic 25%), leukocytosis (22% to 41%), thrombocytopenia (24% to 38%)
Hepatic: Liver function tests abnormal (25%), ascites (24%)
Neuromuscular & skeletal: Back pain (35% to 47%), weakness (35% to 43%), tremor (24% to 34%), paresthesia (21%)
Renal: Creatinine increased (39%), BUN increased (35%), kidney function abnormal (22% to 26%)
Respiratory: Dyspnea (31% to 37%), respiratory tract infection (22% to 37%), pleural effusion (34%), cough (31%), lung disorder (22% to 30%), sinusitis (26%)
Miscellaneous: Infection (18% to 27%), sepsis (27%), lactate dehydrogenase increased (23%), *Candida* (17% to 22%), herpes simplex (10% to 21%)

3% to <20%:

Cardiovascular: Angina, arrhythmia, arterial thrombosis, atrial fibrillation, atrial flutter, bradycardia, cardiac arrest, cardiac failure, CHF, extrasystole, facial edema, hyper-/hypovolemia, pallor, palpitation, pericardial effusion, peripheral vascular disorder, postural hypotension, supraventricular extrasystoles, supraventricular tachycardia, syncope, thrombosis, vasodilation, vasospasm, venous pressure increased, ventricular extrasystole, ventricular tachycardia
Central nervous system: Agitation, chills with fever, confusion, delirium, depression, emotional lability, hallucinations, hypoesthesia, malaise, nervousness, psychosis, seizure, somnolence, thinking abnormal, vertigo
Dermatologic: Acne, alopecia, bruising, cellulitis, fungal dermatitis, hirsutism, petechia, pruritus, skin carcinoma, skin hypertrophy, skin ulcer, vesiculobullous rash
Endocrine & metabolic: Acidosis, alkalosis, Cushing's syndrome, dehydration, diabetes mellitus, gout, hypercalcemia, hyper-hypophosphatemia, hyperlipemia, hyperuricemia, hypochloremia, hypoglycemia, hyponatremia, hypoproteinemia, hypothyroidism, parathyroid disorder
Gastrointestinal: Abdomen enlarged, dysphagia, esophagitis, flatulence, gastritis, gastroenteritis, gastrointestinal hemorrhage, gastrointestinal moniliasis, gingivitis, gum hyperplasia, ileus, melena, mouth ulceration, oral moniliasis, stomach disorder, stomach ulcer, stomatitis, xerostomia, weight gain/loss
Genitourinary: Impotence, nocturia, pelvic pain, prostatic disorder, scrotal edema, urinary frequency, urinary incontinence, urinary retention, urinary tract disorder
Hematologic: Coagulation disorder, hemorrhage, neutropenia, pancytopenia, polycythemia, prothrombin time increased, thromboplastin time increased
Hepatic: Alkaline phosphatase increased, bilirubinemia, cholangitis, cholestatic jaundice, GGT increased, hepatitis, jaundice, liver damage, transaminases increased
Local: Abscess
Neuromuscular & skeletal: Arthralgia, hypertonia, joint disorder, leg cramps, myalgia, myasthenia, neck pain, neuropathy, osteoporosis
Ocular: Amblyopia, cataract, conjunctivitis, eye hemorrhage, lacrimation disorder, vision abnormal
Otic: Deafness, ear disorder, ear pain, tinnitus
Renal: Albuminuria, creatinine increased, dysuria, hematuria, hydronephrosis, oliguria, pyelonephritis, renal failure, renal tubular necrosis
Respiratory: Apnea, asthma, atelectasis, bronchitis, epistaxis, hemoptysis, hiccup, hyperventilation, hypoxia, respiratory acidosis, pharyngitis, pneumonia, pneumothorax, pulmonary edema, pulmonary hypertension, respiratory moniliasis, rhinitis, sputum increased, voice alteration
Miscellaneous: *Candida* (mucocutaneous 16% to 18%), CMV viremia/syndrome (12% to 14%), CMV tissue invasive disease (6% to 12%), herpes zoster cutaneous disease (4% to 10%), cyst, diaphoresis, flu-like syndrome, healing abnormal, hernia, ileus infection, neoplasm, peritonitis, thirst

General Dosage Range Dosage adjustment recommended in patient with renal impairment and who develop toxicities

I.V.: *Adults:* 1-1.5 g twice daily

Oral:

Cellcept®:

Children (suspension): 600 mg/m^2/dose twice daily (maximum: 1 g twice daily)
Children with BSA 1.25-1.5 m^2: 750 mg capsule twice daily
Children with BSA >1.5 m^2: 1 g capsule or tablet twice daily
Adults: 1-1.5 g twice daily

Myfortic®:

Children with BSA 1.19-1.58 m^2: 540 mg twice daily (maximum: 1080 mg/day)
Children with BSA >1.58 m^2 and Adults: 720 mg twice daily (maximum: 1440 mg/day)

Mechanism of Action MPA exhibits a cytostatic effect on T and B lymphocytes. It is an inhibitor of inosine monophosphate dehydrogenase (IMPDH) which inhibits *de novo* guanosine nucleotide synthesis. T and B lymphocytes are dependent on this pathway for proliferation.

Pharmacodynamics/Kinetics

Onset of Action Peak effect: Correlation of toxicity or efficacy is still being developed; however, one study indicated that 12-hour AUCs >40 mcg/mL/hour were correlated with efficacy and decreased episodes of rejection

Half-life Elimination

CellCept®: MPA: Oral: 18 hours; I.V.: 17 hours

Myfortic®: MPA: Oral: 8-16 hours; MPAG: 13-17 hours

Time to Peak Plasma: Oral: MPA:

CellCept®: 1-1.5 hours

Myfortic®: 1.5-2.75 hours

Pregnancy Risk Factor D

Nabumetone (na BYOO me tone)

Related Information

Rheumatoid Arthritis, Osteoarthritis, and Osteoporosis *on page 1889*

Temporomandibular Dysfunction (TMD) *on page 1964*

Canadian Brand Names Apo-Nabumetone®; Gen-Nabumetone; Mylan-Nabumetone; Novo-Nabumetone; Relafen®; Rhoxal-nabumetone; Sandoz-Nabumetone

Generic Availability (U.S.) Yes

Pharmacologic Category Nonsteroidal Anti-inflammatory Drug (NSAID), Oral

Use Management of osteoarthritis and rheumatoid arthritis

Unlabeled/Investigational Use Moderate pain

Local Anesthetic/Vasoconstrictor Precautions No information available to require special precautions

Effects on Dental Treatment Key adverse event(s) related to dental treatment: Xerostomia (normal salivary flow resumes upon discontinuation) and stomatitis. The dentist should be aware of the potential of abnormal coagulation. Caution should also be exercised in the use of NSAIDs in patients already on anticoagulant therapy with drugs such as warfarin (Coumadin®). See Effects on Bleeding.

Effects on Bleeding Nonselective NSAIDs are known to reversibly decrease platelet aggregation via mechanisms different than observed with aspirin. Platelet function is restored as the drug is eliminated from the body. NSAIDs should be avoided (if possible) in general surgery patients for 3-5 half-lives of the drug (usually 1-3 days) prior to surgery to reduce the risk of excessive bleeding. However, there is no scientific evidence to warrant discontinuance of NSAIDs prior to dental surgery. In medically complicated patients or extensive oral surgery, the decision to interrupt therapy must be based on the risk to benefit in an individual patient and a medical consult is suggested. Routine interruption of NSAID therapy for most dental procedures is not warranted. If therapy is continued without interruption, the clinician should anticipate the potential for slower clotting times.

Adverse Effects

>10%: Gastrointestinal: Diarrhea (14%), dyspepsia (13%), abdominal pain (12%)

1% to 10%:

- Cardiovascular: Edema (3% to 9%)
- Central nervous system: Dizziness (3% to 9%), headache (3% to 9%), fatigue (1% to 3%), insomnia (1% to 3%), nervousness (1% to 3%), somnolence (1% to 3%)
- Dermatologic: Pruritus (3% to 9%), rash (3% to 9%)
- Gastrointestinal: Constipation (3% to 9%), flatulence (3% to 9%), guaiac positive (3% to 9%), nausea (3% to 9%), gastritis (1% to 3%), stomatitis (1% to 3%), vomiting (1% to 3%), xerostomia (1% to 3%)
- Otic: Tinnitus
- Miscellaneous: Diaphoresis (1% to 3%)

Dosage Adults: Oral: 1000 mg/day; an additional 500-1000 mg may be needed in some patients to obtain more symptomatic relief; may be administered once or twice daily (maximum dose: 2000 mg/day)

Note: Patients <50 kg are less likely to require doses >1000 mg/day.

Dosage adjustment in renal impairment: In general, NSAIDs are not recommended for use in patients with advanced renal disease, but the manufacturer of nabumetone does provide some guidelines for adjustment in renal dysfunction:

Moderate impairment (Cl_{cr} 30-49 mL/minute): Initial dose: 750 mg/day; maximum dose: 1500 mg/day

Severe impairment (Cl_{cr} <30 mL/minute): Initial dose: 500 mg/day; maximum dose: 1000 mg/day

Mechanism of Action Reversibly inhibits cyclooxygenase-1 and 2 (COX-1 and 2) enzymes, which results in decreased formation of prostaglandin precursors; has antipyretic, analgesic, and anti-inflammatory properties

Other proposed mechanisms not fully elucidated (and possibly contributing to the anti-inflammatory effect to varying degrees), include inhibiting chemotaxis, altering lymphocyte activity, inhibiting neutrophil aggregation/activation, and decreasing proinflammatory cytokine levels.

Contraindications Hypersensitivity to nabumetone, aspirin, other NSAIDs, or any component of the formulation; perioperative pain in the setting of coronary artery bypass graft (CABG) surgery

Warnings/Precautions [U.S. Boxed Warning]: NSAIDs are associated with an increased risk of adverse cardiovascular thrombotic events, including MI and stroke. Risk may be increased with duration of use or pre-existing cardiovascular risk factors or disease. Carefully evaluate individual cardiovascular risk profiles prior to prescribing. May cause new-onset hypertension or worsening of existing hypertension. Use caution with fluid retention. Avoid use in heart failure. Concurrent administration of ibuprofen, and potentially other nonselective NSAIDs, may interfere with aspirin's cardioprotective effect. **[U.S. Boxed Warning]: Use is contraindicated for treatment of perioperative pain in the setting of coronary artery bypass graft (CABG) surgery.** Risk of MI and stroke may be increased with use following CABG surgery.

Platelet adhesion and aggregation may be decreased; may prolong bleeding time; patients with coagulation disorders or who are receiving anticoagulants should be monitored closely. Anemia may occur; patients on long-term NSAID therapy should be monitored for anemia. Rarely, NSAID use may cause severe blood dyscrasias (eg, agranulocytosis, aplastic anemia, thrombocytopenia).

NSAID use may compromise existing renal function; dose-dependent decreases in prostaglandin synthesis may result from NSAID use, reducing renal blood flow which may cause renal decompensation. NSAID use may increase the risk for hyperkalemia. Patients with impaired renal function, dehydration, heart failure, liver dysfunction, those taking diuretics, and ACE inhibitors, and the elderly are at greater risk of renal toxicity and hyperkalemia. Rehydrate patient before starting therapy; monitor renal function closely. Not recommended for use in patients with advanced renal disease. Long-term NSAID use may result in renal papillary necrosis.

[U.S. Boxed Warning]: NSAIDs may increase risk of gastrointestinal irritation, inflammation, ulceration, bleeding, and perforation. These events may occur at any time during therapy and without warning. Use caution with a history of GI disease (bleeding or ulcers), concurrent therapy with aspirin, anticoagulants and/or corticosteroids, smoking, use of alcohol, the elderly or debilitated patients. When used concomitantly with ≤325 mg of aspirin, a substantial increase in the risk of gastrointestinal complications (eg, ulcer) occurs; concomitant gastroprotective therapy (eg, proton pump inhibitors) is recommended (Bhatt, 2008).

Use the lowest effective dose for the shortest duration of time, consistent with individual patient goals, to reduce risk of cardiovascular or GI adverse events. Alternate therapies should be considered for patients at high risk.

NSAIDs may cause serious skin adverse events including exfoliative dermatitis, Stevens-Johnson syndrome (SJS) and toxic epidermal necrolysis (TEN); discontinue use at first sign of skin rash or hypersensitivity. Anaphylactoid reactions may occur, even without prior exposure; patients with "aspirin triad" (bronchial asthma, aspirin intolerance, rhinitis) may be at increased risk. Do not use in patients who experience bronchospasm, asthma, rhinitis, or urticaria with NSAID or aspirin therapy. Use caution in other forms of asthma.

Use with caution in patients with decreased hepatic function. Closely monitor patients with any abnormal LFT. Severe hepatic reactions (eg, fulminant hepatitis, liver failure) have occurred with NSAID use, rarely; discontinue if signs or symptoms of liver disease develop, or if systemic manifestations occur.

NSAIDS may cause drowsiness, dizziness, blurred vision and other neurologic effects which may impair physical or mental abilities; patients must be cautioned about performing tasks which require mental alertness (eg, operating machinery or driving). Discontinue use with blurred or diminished vision and perform ophthalmologic exam. Monitor vision with long-term therapy.

The elderly are at increased risk for adverse effects (especially peptic ulceration, CNS effects, renal toxicity) from NSAIDs even at low doses.

Withhold for at least 4-6 half-lives prior to surgical or dental procedures. May cause photosensitivity reactions.

Drug Interactions

Avoid Concomitant Use

Avoid concomitant use of Nabumetone with any of the following: Ketorolac; Ketorolac (Systemic)

Increased Effect/Toxicity

Nabumetone may increase the levels/effects of: Aminoglycosides; Anticoagulants; Antiplatelet Agents; Bisphosphonate Derivatives; Collagenase (Systemic); CycloSPORINE; CycloSPORINE (Systemic); Deferasirox; Desmopressin; Digoxin; Drotrecogin Alfa; Eplerenone; Haloperidol; Ibritumomab; Lithium; Methotrexate; Nonsteroidal Anti-Inflammatory Agents; PEMEtrexed; Potassium-Sparing Diuretics; PRALAtrexate; Quinolone Antibiotics; Salicylates; Thrombolytic Agents; Tositumomab and Iodine I 131 Tositumomab; Vancomycin; Vitamin K Antagonists

The levels/effects of Nabumetone may be increased by: ACE Inhibitors; Angiotensin II Receptor Blockers; Antidepressants (Tricyclic, Tertiary Amine); Corticosteroids (Systemic); Dasatinib; Glucosamine; Herbs (Anticoagulant/Antiplatelet Properties); Ketorolac; Ketorolac (Systemic); Nonsteroidal Anti-Inflammatory Agents; Omega-3-Acid Ethyl Esters; Pentosan Polysulfate Sodium; Pentoxifylline; Probenecid; Prostacyclin Analogues; Selective Serotonin Reuptake Inhibitors; Serotonin/Norepinephrine Reuptake Inhibitors; Treprostinil

Decreased Effect

Nabumetone may decrease the levels/effects of: ACE Inhibitors; Angiotensin II Receptor Blockers; Antiplatelet Agents; Beta-Blockers; Eplerenone; HydrALAZINE; Loop Diuretics; Potassium-Sparing Diuretics; Salicylates; Thiazide Diuretics

The levels/effects of Nabumetone may be decreased by: Bile Acid Sequestrants; Nonsteroidal Anti-Inflammatory Agents; Salicylates

Ethanol/Nutrition/Herb Interactions

Ethanol: Avoid ethanol (may enhance gastric mucosal irritation).

Food: Nabumetone peak serum concentrations may be increased if taken with food or dairy products.

Herb/Nutraceutical: Avoid alfalfa, anise, bilberry, bladderwrack, bromelain, cat's claw, celery, chamomile, coleus, cordyceps, dong quai, evening primrose, fenugreek, feverfew, garlic, ginger, ginkgo biloba, ginseng (American, Panax, Siberian), grapeseed, green tea, guggul, horse chestnut seed, horseradish, licorice, prickly ash, red clover, reishi, SAMe (S-adenosylmethionine), sweet clover, turmeric, white willow (all have additional antiplatelet activity).

Pharmacodynamics/Kinetics

Onset of Action Several days

Half-life Elimination 6MNA: ~24 hours

Time to Peak Serum: 6MNA: Oral: 2.5-4 hours; Synovial fluid: 4-12 hours

Pregnancy Risk Factor C

Lactation Excretion in breast milk unknown/not recommended

Breast-Feeding Considerations It is not known if nabumetone or 6MNA are excreted into breast milk. Breast-feeding is not recommended by the manufacturer.

Dosage Forms

Tablet, oral: 500 mg, 750 mg

Nadolol (NAY doe lol)

Related Information

Cardiovascular Diseases *on page 1848*

U.S. Brand Names Corgard®

Canadian Brand Names Alti-Nadolol; Apo-Nadol®; Corgard®; Novo-Nadolol

Pharmacologic Category Beta-Adrenergic Blocker, Nonselective

Use Treatment of hypertension and angina pectoris; prophylaxis of migraine headaches

Unlabeled/Investigational Use Primary and secondary prophylaxis of variceal hemorrhage

Local Anesthetic/Vasoconstrictor Precautions Use with caution; epinephrine has interacted with nonselective beta-blockers to result in initial hypertensive episode followed by bradycardia

Effects on Dental Treatment Nadolol is a nonselective beta-blocker and may enhance the pressor response to epinephrine, resulting in hypertension and bradycardia. Many nonsteroidal anti-inflammatory drugs, such as ibuprofen and indomethacin, can reduce the hypotensive effect of beta-blockers after 3 or more weeks of therapy with the NSAID. Short-term NSAID use (ie, 3 days) requires no special precautions in patients taking beta-blockers.

Effects on Bleeding No information available to require special precautions

Adverse Effects

>10%:

Central nervous system: Drowsiness, insomnia

Endocrine & metabolic: Decreased sexual ability

1% to 10%:

Cardiovascular: Bradycardia, palpitation, edema, CHF, reduced peripheral circulation

Central nervous system: Mental depression

Gastrointestinal: Diarrhea or constipation, nausea, vomiting, stomach discomfort

Respiratory: Bronchospasm

Miscellaneous: Cold extremities

General Dosage Range Dosage adjustment recommended in patients with renal impairment

Oral:

Adults: Initial: 40 mg once daily; Maintenance: 40-320 mg once daily

Elderly: Initial: 20 mg once daily; Maintenance: 20-240 mg once daily

Mechanism of Action Competitively blocks response to $beta_1$- and $beta_2$-adrenergic stimulation; does not exhibit any membrane stabilizing or intrinsic sympathomimetic activity. Nonselective beta-adrenergic blockers (propranolol, nadolol) reduce portal pressure by producing splanchnic vasoconstriction ($beta_2$ effect) thereby reducing portal blood flow.

Pharmacodynamics/Kinetics

Duration of Action 17-24 hours

Half-life Elimination Adults: 10-24 hours, prolonged with renal impairment; End-stage renal disease: 45 hours

Time to Peak Serum: 2-4 hours

Pregnancy Risk Factor C

Nadolol and Bendroflumethiazide

(NAY doe lol & ben droe floo meth EYE a zide)

Related Information

Nadolol *on page 1174*

U.S. Brand Names Corzide®

Pharmacologic Category Beta Blocker, Nonselective; Diuretic, Thiazide

Use Treatment of hypertension; combination product should not be used for initial therapy

Local Anesthetic/Vasoconstrictor Precautions Use with caution; epinephrine has interacted with nonselective beta-blockers to result in initial hypertensive episode followed by bradycardia

Effects on Dental Treatment Nadolol is a nonselective beta-blocker and may enhance the pressor response to epinephrine, resulting in hypertension and bradycardia. Many nonsteroidal anti-inflammatory drugs, such as ibuprofen and indomethacin, can reduce the hypotensive effect of beta-blockers after 3 or more weeks of therapy with the NSAID. Short-term NSAID use (ie, 3 days) requires no special precautions in patients taking beta-blockers.

Effects on Bleeding No information available to require special precautions

Adverse Effects See individual agents.

General Dosage Range Dosage adjustment recommended in patients with renal impairment

Oral: *Adults:* Initial: Nadolol 40 mg and bendroflumethiazide 5 mg once daily; Maintenance: Nadolol 40-80 mg and bendroflumethiazide 5 mg once daily

Mechanism of Action See individual agents.

Pregnancy Risk Factor C

Nadroparin (nad roe PA rin)

Related Information

Cardiovascular Diseases *on page 1848*

Canadian Brand Names Fraxiparine™; Fraxiparine™ Forte

Pharmacologic Category Low Molecular Weight Heparin

Use Prophylaxis of thromboembolic disorders (particularly deep venous thrombosis and pulmonary embolism) in general and orthopedic surgery; treatment of deep venous thrombosis; prevention of clotting during hemodialysis; treatment of unstable angina and non-Q-wave myocardial infarction

Local Anesthetic/Vasoconstrictor Precautions No information available to require special precautions

Effects on Dental Treatment Key adverse event(s) related to dental treatment: Bleeding is the major adverse effect of nadroparin. See Effects on Bleeding.

Effects on Bleeding As with all anticoagulants, bleeding is the major adverse effect of nadroparin. Hemorrhage may occur at virtually any site; risk is dependent on multiple variables including the intensity of anticoagulation and patient susceptibility. At the recommended doses, LMWHS do not significantly influence platelet aggregation or affect global clotting time (ie, PT or aPTT). Medical consult is suggested.

Adverse Effects Frequency not defined.

Dermatologic: Angioedema (very rare), rash

Endocrine & metabolic: Hypoaldosteronism (causing hyperkalemia and/or hyponatremia)

Genitourinary: Priapism (very rare)

Hematological: Bleeding, eosinophilia (very rare), thrombocytopenia

Hepatic: ALT increased, AST increased

Local: Calcinosis, cutaneous necrosis, injection site hematoma, pain at injection site

Neuromuscular & skeletal: Osteopenic effects

Miscellaneous: Allergic reactions, anaphylactoid reactions (very rare)

Dosage Adults:

Prevention of clotting during hemodialysis: Single dose of 65 anti-Xa int. units/kg into arterial line at start of each dialysis session; may give additional dose if session lasts longer than 4 hours; adjust dose during subsequent dialysis sessions to plasma anti-Xa levels of 0.5-1 anti-Xa int. units/mL

Patients at risk of hemorrhage: Administer 32.5 anti-Xa int. units/kg; may give additional smaller dose if session lasts longer than 4 hours; adjust dose during subsequent dialysis sessions to plasma anti-Xa levels of 0.2-0.4 anti-Xa int. units/mL.

Treatment of unstable angina and non-Q-wave myocardial infarction: Initial: I.V.: 86 anti-Xa int. units/kg bolus. Maintenance: SubQ: 86 anti-Xa int. units/kg every 12 hours (usual treatment duration: 6 days); plasma anti-Xa levels should be <1.2 anti-Xa int. units/mL 3-4 hours postinjection

Dosage adjustment in renal impairment:

Cl_{cr} ≥50 mL/minute: Dosage adjustment not required

Cl_{cr} ≥30-50 mL/minute: Reduce dose by 25% to 33%

Cl_{cr} <30 mL/minute:

Prophylaxis: Reduce dose by 25% to 33%

Treatment: Use is contraindicated

Mechanism of Action Nadroparin has high anti-Xa activity, but low anti-IIa activity. The greater ratio of anti-Xa activity has the potential to provide equivalent antithrombic efficacy with reduced hemorrhagic complications.

Contraindications Hypersensitivity to nadroparin or any component of the formulation; acute infective endocarditis; hemorrhage or increased risk of hemorrhage (hemostasis disorder); history of thrombocytopenia with heparin or positive *in vitro* test for antiplatelet antibodies in the presence of nadroparin; blood clotting disorders; organic lesions likely to bleed (active peptic ulceration); hemorrhagic cerebrovascular event (unless systemic emboli present); severe uncontrolled hypertension; diabetic or hemorrhagic retinopathy; injuries to or operations on the CNS, eyes, or ears; severe renal insufficiency (creatinine clearance <30 mL/minute when used for treatment); concomitant use of spinal/epidural anesthesia with high-dose nadroparin

Warnings/Precautions Spinal or epidural hematomas, including subsequent paralysis, may occur with recent or anticipated neuraxial anesthesia (epidural or spinal) or spinal puncture in patients anticoagulated with LMWH or heparinoids. Consider risk versus benefit prior to spinal procedures; risk is increased by concomitant agents which may alter hemostasis, the use of indwelling epidural catheters for analgesia, a history of spinal deformity or spinal surgery, as well as traumatic or repeated epidural or spinal punctures. Patient should be observed closely for bleeding if nadroparin is administered during or immediately following diagnostic lumbar puncture, epidural anesthesia, or spinal anesthesia.

Not to be used interchangeably (unit for unit) with heparin or any other low molecular weight heparins (LMWHs). Use with caution in patients with history of heparin-induced thrombocytopenia. Monitor platelet count closely. Rare thrombocytopenia may occur. Consider discontinuation of nadroparin in any patient developing significant thrombocytopenia. Rare cases of thrombocytopenia with thrombosis have occurred. Use caution in patients with congenital or drug-induced thrombocytopenia or platelet defects.

Monitor patient closely for signs or symptoms of bleeding. Certain patients are at increased risk of bleeding. Risk factors include bacterial endocarditis; congenital or acquired bleeding disorders; active ulcerative or angiodysplastic GI diseases; severe uncontrolled hypertension; hemorrhagic stroke; recent brain, spinal, or ophthalmology surgery; concomitant treatment with platelet inhibitors; recent GI bleeding; thrombocytopenia or platelet defects; severe liver disease; hypertensive or diabetic retinopathy; or in patients undergoing invasive procedures. Use with caution in patients with severe hepatic or renal disease.

Heparin can cause hyperkalemia by affecting aldosterone. Similar reactions could occur with LMWHs. Monitor for hyperkalemia. Do not use when abortion is imminent or threatened.

Drug Interactions

Avoid Concomitant Use There are no known interactions where it is recommended to avoid concomitant use.

Increased Effect/Toxicity

Nadroparin may increase the levels/effects of: Anticoagulants; Collagenase (Systemic); Deferasirox; Drotrecogin Alfa; Ibritumomab; Tositumomab and Iodine I 131 Tositumomab

The levels/effects of Nadroparin may be increased by: 5-ASA Derivatives; Antiplatelet Agents; Dasatinib; Herbs (Anticoagulant/Antiplatelet Properties); Nonsteroidal Anti-Inflammatory Agents; Pentosan Polysulfate Sodium; Pentoxifylline; Prostacyclin Analogues; Salicylates; Thrombolytic Agents

Decreased Effect There are no known significant interactions involving a decrease in effect.

Ethanol/Nutrition/Herb Interactions Herb/Nutraceutical: Avoid cat's claw, dong quai, evening primrose, garlic, ginseng (all have anticoagulant or antiplatelet activity).

Pharmacodynamics/Kinetics

Duration of Action 18 hours

Half-life Elimination Renal impairment: 3.5 hours; 6 hours

Time to Peak Serum: 3-5 hours

Pregnancy Risk Factor B

Lactation Excretion in breast milk unknown/not recommended

Product Availability Not available in U.S.

Dosage Forms: Canada

Injection, solution:

Fraxiparine™: 9500 anti-Xa int. units/mL (0.2 mL, 0.3 mL, 0.4 mL, 0.6 mL, 0.8 mL, 1 mL)

Fraxiparine™ Forte: 19,000 anti-Xa int. units/mL (0.6 mL, 0.8 mL, 1 mL)

Nafarelin (naf a REL in)

U.S. Brand Names Synarel®

Canadian Brand Names Synarel®

Pharmacologic Category Gonadotropin Releasing Hormone Agonist

Use Treatment of endometriosis, including pain and reduction of lesions; treatment of central precocious puberty (CPP; gonadotropin-dependent precocious puberty) in children of both sexes

Local Anesthetic/Vasoconstrictor Precautions No information available to require special precautions

Effects on Dental Treatment No significant effects or complications reported

Effects on Bleeding No information available to require special precautions

Adverse Effects Note: Adverse events may be more frequent in the first 6 weeks of treatment due to stimulation of the pituitary-gonadal axis. Sensitivity reactions included chest pain, pruritus, shortness of breath, rash.

CPP: 1% to 10%:

Central nervous system: Emotional lability (6%)

Dermatologic: Acne (10%), seborrhea (3%)

Endocrine & metabolic: Breast enlargement (8%; transient), vaginal bleeding (8%), hot flashes (3%; transient), vaginal discharge (3%)

Respiratory: Rhinitis (5%)

Miscellaneous: Pubic hair increased (5%; transient), body odor (4%), sensitivity reactions (3%)

Endometriosis:

>10%:

Central nervous system: Headache, emotional lability

Dermatologic: Acne

Endocrine & metabolic: Hot flashes (90%), hyperphosphatemia, hypertriglyceridemia, hypocalcemia, libido decreased

Genitourinary: Vaginal dryness

Hematologic: Leukopenia

1% to 10%:

Cardiovascular: Edema

Central nervous system: Depression, insomnia

Dermatologic: Hirsutism, seborrhea

Endocrine & metabolic: Breast size reduced, cholesterol increased, hyperlipidemia, libido increased
Gastrointestinal: Weight gain/loss
Neuromuscular & skeletal: Bone mineral density decreased, myalgia
Respiratory: Nasal irritation

General Dosage Range Nasal:
Children: 2 sprays (400 mcg) into each nostril twice daily; may increase to 3 sprays (600 mcg) into alternating nostrils 3 times/day
Adults: 1 spray (200 mcg) in 1-2 nostrils twice daily

Mechanism of Action Potent synthetic decapeptide analogue of gonadotropin-releasing hormone (GnRH; LHRH) which is approximately 200 times more potent than GnRH in terms of pituitary release of luteinizing hormone (LH) and follicle-stimulating hormone (FSH). Effects on the pituitary gland and sex hormones are dependent upon its length of administration. After acute administration, an initial stimulation of the release of LH and FSH from the pituitary is observed; an increase in androgens and estrogens subsequently follows. Continued administration of nafarelin, however, suppresses gonadotrope responsiveness to endogenous GnRH resulting in reduced secretion of LH and FSH and, secondarily, decreased ovarian and testicular steroid production.

Pharmacodynamics/Kinetics
Half-life Elimination ~3 hours; Metabolites: ~86 hours
Time to Peak Serum: 10-45 minutes

Pregnancy Risk Factor X

Nafcillin (naf SIL in)

Canadian Brand Names Nallpen®; Unipen®
Pharmacologic Category Antibiotic, Penicillin
Use Treatment of infections such as osteomyelitis, septicemia, endocarditis, and CNS infections caused by susceptible strains of staphylococci species
Local Anesthetic/Vasoconstrictor Precautions No information available to require special precautions
Effects on Dental Treatment Key adverse event(s) related to dental treatment: Prolonged use of penicillins may lead to the development of oral candidiasis.
Effects on Bleeding No information available to require special precautions
Adverse Effects Frequency not defined.
Central nervous system: Neurotoxicity (high doses)
Gastrointestinal: Pseudomembranous colitis
Hematologic: Agranulocytosis, bone marrow depression, neutropenia
Local: Inflammation, pain, phlebitis, skin sloughing, swelling, and thrombophlebitis at the injection site; oxacillin (less likely to cause phlebitis) is often preferred in pediatric patients; tissue necrosis with sloughing (SubQ extravasation)
Renal: Interstitial nephritis (rare), renal tubular damage (rare)
Miscellaneous: Anaphylaxis, hypersensitivity reactions (immediate and delayed; general incidence of 1% to 10% for penicillins), serum sickness

General Dosage Range
I.M.:
Neonates 1200-2000 g, <7 days: 50 mg/kg/day divided every 12 hours
Neonates >2000 g, <7 days: 75 mg/kg/day divided every 8 hours
Neonates 1200-2000 g, ≥7 days: 75 mg/kg/day divided every 8 hours
Neonates >2000 g, ≥7 days: 100-140 mg/kg/day divided every 6 hours
Children: 25 mg/kg twice daily
Adults: 500 mg every 4-6 hours
I.V.:
Neonates 1200-2000 g, <7 days: 50 mg/kg/day divided every 12 hours
Neonates >2000 g, <7 days: 75 mg/kg/day divided every 8 hours
Neonates 1200-2000 g, ≥7 days: 75 mg/kg/day divided every 8 hours
Neonates >2000 g, ≥7 days: 100-140 mg/kg/day divided every 6 hours
Children: 50-200 mg/kg/day in divided every 4-6 hours (maximum: 12 g/day)
Adults: 500-2000 mg every 4-6 hours

Mechanism of Action Interferes with bacterial cell wall synthesis during active multiplication, causing cell wall death and resultant bactericidal activity against susceptible bacteria

Pharmacodynamics/Kinetics
Half-life Elimination
Neonates: <3 weeks: 2.2-5.5 hours; 4-9 weeks: 1.2-2.3 hours
Children 3 months to 14 years: 0.75-1.9 hours
Adults: Normal renal/hepatic function: 30-60 minutes
Time to Peak Serum: I.M.: 30-60 minutes

Pregnancy Risk Factor B

Naftifine (NAF ti feen)

U.S. Brand Names Naftin®
Pharmacologic Category Antifungal Agent, Topical
Use Topical treatment of tinea cruris (jock itch), tinea corporis (ringworm), and tinea pedis (athlete's foot)
Local Anesthetic/Vasoconstrictor Precautions No information available to require special precautions
Effects on Dental Treatment No significant effects or complications reported
Effects on Bleeding No information available to require special precautions
Adverse Effects 1% to 10%:
Dermatologic: Burning/stinging (5% to 6%), erythema (≤2%), pruritus (1% to 2%)
Local: Dryness (3%), irritation (2%)
General Dosage Range Topical: *Adults:* Apply cream once daily and gel twice daily
Mechanism of Action Synthetic, broad-spectrum antifungal agent in the allylamine class; appears to have both fungistatic and fungicidal activity. Exhibits antifungal activity by selectively inhibiting the enzyme squalene epoxidase in a dose-dependent manner which results in a reduced synthesis of ergosterol, the primary sterol within the fungal membrane.
Pharmacodynamics/Kinetics
Half-life Elimination 2-3 days
Pregnancy Risk Factor B

Nalbuphine (NAL byoo feen)

Pharmacologic Category Analgesic, Opioid; Analgesic, Opioid Partial Agonist
Use Relief of moderate-to-severe pain; preoperative analgesia, postoperative and surgical anesthesia, and obstetrical analgesia during labor and delivery
Unlabeled/Investigational Use Opioid-induced pruritus
Local Anesthetic/Vasoconstrictor Precautions No information available to require special precautions
Effects on Dental Treatment Key adverse event(s) related to dental treatment: Xerostomia and changes in salivation (normal salivary flow resumes upon discontinuation). Anticholinergic side effects can cause a reduction of saliva production or secretion, contributing to discomfort and dental disease (ie, caries, oral candidiasis, and periodontal disease).
Effects on Bleeding No information available to require special precautions
Adverse Effects
>10%: Central nervous system: Sedation (36%)
1% to 10%:
Central nervous system: Dizziness (5%), headache (3%)
Gastrointestinal: Nausea/vomiting (6%), xerostomia (4%)
Miscellaneous: Clamminess (9%)
General Dosage Range
I.M., SubQ: *Adults:* 10 mg/70 kg every 3-6 hours (maximum: 20 mg/dose; 160 mg/day)
I.V.: *Adults:* 10 mg/70 kg every 3-6 hours (maximum: 20 mg/dose; 160 mg/day) **or** 0.3-3 mg/kg over 10-15 minutes, then 0.25-0.5 mg/kg as required for anesthesia **or** 2.5-5 mg (1-2 doses)
Mechanism of Action Agonist of kappa opiate receptors and partial antagonist of mu opiate receptors in the CNS, causing inhibition of ascending pain pathways, altering the perception of and response to pain; produces generalized CNS depression
Pharmacodynamics/Kinetics
Onset of Action Peak effect: SubQ, I.M.: <15 minutes; I.V.: 2-3 minutes
Half-life Elimination 5 hours
Pregnancy Risk Factor C
Dental Comment **Sedation:** When administered following diazepam or midazolam, the depth of sedation is rarely increased; however, recovery is somewhat less complete than that observed when diazepam or midazolam is administered alone.

Naloxone (nal OKS one)

Canadian Brand Names Naloxone Hydrochloride Injection®
Generic Availability (U.S.) Yes
Pharmacologic Category Antidote; Opioid Antagonist
Dental Use Reverse overdose effects of the two narcotic agents, fentanyl and meperidine, used in the technique of I.V. conscious sedation

Use Complete or partial reversal of opioid drug effects, including respiratory depression; management of known or suspected opioid overdose; diagnosis of suspected opioid dependence or acute opioid overdose

Unlabeled/Investigational Use Opioid-induced pruritus

Local Anesthetic/Vasoconstrictor Precautions No information available to require special precautions

Effects on Dental Treatment No significant effects or complications reported

Effects on Bleeding No information available to require special precautions

Adverse Effects Adverse reactions are related to reversing dependency and precipitating withdrawal. Withdrawal symptoms are the result of sympathetic excess. Adverse events occur secondarily to reversal (withdrawal) of narcotic analgesia and sedation.

Central nervous system: Narcotic withdrawal

Dental Usual Dosage Narcotic overdose: Adults: I.V.: 0.4-2 mg every 2-3 minutes as needed; may need to repeat doses every 20-60 minutes, if no response is observed after 10 mg, question the diagnosis. **Note:** Use 0.1-0.2 mg increments in patients who are opioid dependent and in postoperative patients to avoid large cardiovascular changes.

Dosage Note: I.M., I.V. (preferred), intranasal (adults only), and SubQ routes may be used. Intratracheal administration is the least desirable and is supported by only anecdotal evidence (case report) (ACLS, 2010):

Infants and Children: Postoperative reversal: 0.01 mg/kg; may repeat every 2-3 minutes as needed based on response (adequate ventilation without significant pain)

Children:

Opioid intoxication: Respiratory depression: I.V., intraosseous (I.O), intratracheal:

Birth (including premature infants) to 5 years or ≤20 kg (unlabeled dose): Acute: Initial: 0.1 mg/kg (maximum dose: 2 mg); repeat every 2-3 minutes if needed; consider lower initial doses of 0.01 mg/kg for non-acute situations (eg, respiratory depression during pain management) (*Drugs for Pediatric Emergencies*, 1998)

>5 years or >20 kg: Minimum dose: 2 mg/dose; if no response, repeat every 2-3 minutes (*Drugs for Pediatric Emergencies*, 1998)

Note: I.O. and intratracheal routes are alternative routes recommended by PALS 2010 guidelines. Consider using lower doses to reverse respiratory depression associated with therapeutic opioid use: 1-5 mcg/kg, titrate to effect (PALS, 2010)

Continuous infusion (unlabeled dosing): I.V.: If continuous infusion is required, calculate dosage/hour based on effective intermittent dose used and duration of adequate response seen **or** use two-thirds (2/3) of the initial effective naloxone bolus on an hourly basis; titrate dose (typically 0.04-0.16 mg/kg/hour for 2-5 days in children); one-half (1/2) of the initial bolus dose should be readministered 15 minutes after initiation of the continuous infusion to prevent a drop in naloxone levels; increase infusion rate as needed to assure adequate ventilation and prevent withdrawal symptoms

Adults:

Opioid intoxication: Respiratory depression:

I.V.: 0.4-2 mg; may need to repeat doses every 2-3 minutes; after reversal, may need to readminister dose(s) at a later interval (ie, 20-60 minutes) depending on type/duration of opioid. If no response is observed after 10 mg, consider other causes of respiratory depression. **Note:** Opioid-dependent patients may require lower doses (0.1 mg) titrated incrementally to avoid precipitating acute withdrawal.

Intranasal administration (unlabeled route): 2 mg (1 mg per nostril); may repeat in 5 minutes if respiratory depression persists. **Note:** Onset of action is slightly delayed compared to I.M. or I.V. routes (ACLS, 2010; Kelly, 2005; Robertson, 2009).

Opioid intoxication: Respiratory depression: Opioid-dependent patient: Initial: 0.04-0.4 mg; may repeat or escalate dose up to 2 mg if initial response inadequate. **Note:** Atypical opioids (eg, propoxyphene) or massive opioid overdoses may require much higher doses (ACLS, 2010).

Continuous infusion (unlabeled dosing): I.V.: Calculate dosage/hour based on effective intermittent dose used and duration of adequate response seen **or** use two-thirds (2/3) of the initial effective naloxone bolus on an hourly basis (typically 0.25-6.25 mg/hour); one-half (1/2) of the initial bolus dose should be readministered 15 minutes after initiation of the continuous infusion to prevent a drop in naloxone levels; adjust infusion rate as needed to assure adequate ventilation and prevent withdrawal symptoms

Opioid-dependent patients being treated for cancer pain (NCCN guidelines, v.1.2010): I.V.: 0.04-0.08 mg (40-80 mcg) slow I.V. push; administer every 30-60 seconds until improvement in symptoms, if no response is observed after total naloxone dose 1 mg, consider other causes of respiratory depression. **Note:** May dilute 0.4 mg/mL (1 mL) ampule into 9 mL of normal saline for a total volume of 10 mL to achieve a 0.04 mg/mL (40 mcg/mL) concentration.

Postoperative reversal: I.V.: 0.1-0.2 mg every 2-3 minutes until desired response (adequate ventilation and alertness without significant pain). **Note:** Repeat doses may be needed within 1-2 hour intervals depending on type, dose, and timing of the last dose of opioid administered.

Opioid-induced pruritus (unlabeled use): I.V. infusion: 0.25 mcg/kg/**hour**; **Note:** Monitor pain control; verify that the naloxone is not reversing analgesia (Gan, 1997)

Mechanism of Action Pure opioid antagonist that competes and displaces narcotics at opioid receptor sites

Contraindications Hypersensitivity to naloxone or any component of the formulation

Warnings/Precautions Due to an association between naloxone and acute pulmonary edema, use with caution in patients with cardiovascular disease or in patients receiving medications with potential adverse cardiovascular effects (eg, hypotension, pulmonary edema, or arrhythmias). Administration of naloxone causes the release of catecholamines; may precipitate acute withdrawal or unmask pain in those who regularly take opioids. Excessive dosages should be avoided after use of opiates in surgery. Abrupt postoperative reversal may result in nausea, vomiting, sweating, tachycardia, hypertension, seizures, and other cardiovascular events (including pulmonary edema and arrhythmias). May precipitate withdrawal symptoms in patients addicted to opiates, including pain, hypertension, sweating, agitation, irritability; in neonates: shrill cry, failure to feed; carefully titrate dose to reverse hypoventilation; do not fully awaken patient or reverse analgesic effect (postoperative patient). Use caution in patients with history of seizures; avoid use in treatment of meperidine-induced seizures. Recurrence of respiratory depression is possible if the opioid involved is long-acting; observe patients until there is no reasonable risk of recurrent respiratory depression.

Drug Interactions

Avoid Concomitant Use There are no known interactions where it is recommended to avoid concomitant use.

Increased Effect/Toxicity There are no known significant interactions involving an increase in effect.

Decreased Effect There are no known significant interactions involving a decrease in effect.

Pharmacodynamics/Kinetics

Onset of Action Endotracheal, I.M., SubQ: 2-5 minutes; Intranasal: ~8-13 minutes (Kelley, 2005; Robertson, 2009); I.V.: ~2 minutes

Duration of Action Depending on route of administration, ~30-120 minutes; I.V. has a shorter duration of action than I.M. administration; since naloxone's action is shorter than that of most opioids, repeated doses are usually needed

Half-life Elimination Neonates: 3-4 hours; Adults: 0.5-1.5 hours

Pregnancy Risk Factor C

Lactation Excretion in breast milk unknown/not recommended

Breast-Feeding Considerations No data reported. Since naloxone is used for opiate reversal the concern should be on opiate drug levels in a breast-feeding mother and transfer to the infant rather than naloxone exposure. The safest approach would be **not** to breast-feed.

Dosage Forms

Injection, solution: 0.4 mg/mL (1 mL, 10 mL)

Injection, solution [preservative free]: 1 mg/mL (2 mL)

Naltrexone (nal TREKS one)

U.S. Brand Names ReVia®; Vivitrol®

Canadian Brand Names ReVia®

Pharmacologic Category Antidote; Opioid Antagonist

Use Treatment of ethanol dependence; prevention of relapse in opioid dependent patients, following opioid detoxification

Local Anesthetic/Vasoconstrictor Precautions No information available to require special precautions

Effects on Dental Treatment Key adverse event(s) related to dental treatment: Dry mouth.

Effects on Bleeding No information available to require special precautions

Adverse Effects Combined reporting of adverse events from oral and injectable formulations:

>10%:

Cardiovascular: Syncope (13%)

Central nervous system: Headache (3% to 25%), insomnia (3% to 14%), dizziness (4% to 13%), anxiety (2% to 12%), nervousness (4% to >10%)
Gastrointestinal: Nausea (10% to 33%), vomiting (3% to 14%), appetite decreased (14%), diarrhea (13%), abdominal pain (11%), abdominal cramping
Hepatic: ALT increased (13%)
Local: Injection site reaction (≤69%; includes bruising, induration, nodules, pain, pruritus, swelling, tenderness)
Neuromuscular & skeletal: Arthralgia (12%), CPK increased (11% to 39%)
Respiratory: Pharyngitis (7% to 11%)

1% to 10%:

Cardiovascular: Hypertension (5%)
Central nervous system: Suicidal thoughts (≤10%), depression (8%), somnolence (2% to 4%), fatigue (4%), chills, energy increased, feeling down, irritability
Dermatologic: Rash (6%)
Endocrine & metabolic: Polydipsia
Gastrointestinal: Dry mouth (5%), toothache (4%)
Genitourinary: Delayed ejaculation, impotency
Hepatic: AST increased (2% to 10%), GGT increased (7%)
Neuromuscular & skeletal: Muscle cramps (8%), back pain (6%)
Miscellaneous: Influenza (5%)

General Dosage Range

I.M.: *Adults:* 380 mg once every 4 weeks

Oral: *Adults:* 25-50 mg once daily

Mechanism of Action Naltrexone (a pure opioid antagonist) is a cyclopropyl derivative of oxymorphone similar in structure to naloxone and nalorphine (a morphine derivative); it acts as a competitive antagonist at opioid receptor sites, showing the highest affinity for mu receptors.

Pharmacodynamics/Kinetics

Duration of Action Oral: 50 mg: 24 hours; 100 mg: 48 hours; 150 mg: 72 hours; I.M.: 4 weeks

Half-life Elimination Oral: 4 hours; 6-beta-naltrexol: 13 hours; I.M.: naltrexone and 6-beta-naltrexol: 5-10 days

Time to Peak Serum: Oral: ~60 minutes; I.M.: Biphasic: ~2 hours (first peak), ~2-3 days (second peak)

Pregnancy Risk Factor C

Naphazoline (Nasal) (naf AZ oh leen)

U.S. Brand Names Privine® [OTC]

Pharmacologic Category Alpha$_1$ Agonist

Use Temporary relief of nasal congestion associated with the common cold, upper respiratory allergies, or sinusitis

Local Anesthetic/Vasoconstrictor Precautions No information available to require special precautions

Effects on Dental Treatment No significant effects or complications reported

Effects on Bleeding No information available to require special precautions

Adverse Effects Frequency not defined.

Local: Transient stinging, nasal mucosa irritation, dryness, rebound congestion
Respiratory: Sneezing

General Dosage Range **Intranasal:** *Children ≥12 years and Adults:* Instill 1-2 drops or sprays every 6 hours if needed

Mechanism of Action Stimulates alpha-adrenergic receptors in the arterioles of the conjunctiva and the nasal mucosa to produce vasoconstriction

Pharmacodynamics/Kinetics

Onset of Action Decongestant: Topical: ~10 minutes

Duration of Action 2-6 hours

Naphazoline and Pheniramine (naf AZ oh leen & fen NIR a meen)

U.S. Brand Names Naphcon-A® [OTC]; Opcon-A® [OTC]; Visine-A® [OTC]

Canadian Brand Names Naphcon-A®; Visine® Advanced Allergy

Pharmacologic Category Alkylamine Derivative; Alpha$_1$ Agonist; Histamine H_1 Antagonist; Histamine H_1 Antagonist, First Generation; Imidazoline Derivative; Ophthalmic Agent, Vasoconstrictor

Use Treatment of ocular congestion, irritation, and itching

Local Anesthetic/Vasoconstrictor Precautions No information available to require special precautions

Effects on Dental Treatment No significant effects or complications reported

Effects on Bleeding No information available to require special precautions

Adverse Effects Frequency not defined.
Ocular: Pupillary dilation, increase in intraocular pressure
Systemic effects due to absorption:
Cardiovascular: Hypertension, cardiac irregularities
Endocrine & metabolic: Hyperglycemia
General Dosage Range Ophthalmic: *Children ≥6 years and Adults:* 1-2 drops up to 4 times/day
Pregnancy Risk Factor C

Naproxen (na PROKS en)

Related Information
Oral Pain *on page 1928*
Rheumatoid Arthritis, Osteoarthritis, and Osteoporosis *on page 1889*
Temporomandibular Dysfunction (TMD) *on page 1964*
Related Sample Prescriptions
Mild/Moderate Oral Pain *on page 1980*
Moderate/Moderately Severe Oral Pain *on page 1980*
U.S. Brand Names Aleve® [OTC]; Anaprox®; Anaprox® DS; EC-Naprosyn®; Mediproxen [OTC]; Midol® Extended Relief [OTC]; Naprelan®; Naprosyn®; Pamprin® Maximum Strength All Day Relief [OTC]
Canadian Brand Names Anaprox®; Anaprox® DS; Apo-Napro-Na DS®; Apo-Napro-Na®; Apo-Naproxen EC®; Apo-Naproxen SR®; Apo-Naproxen®; Mylan-Naproxen EC; Naprelan™; Naprosyn®; Naprosyn® E; Naprosyn® SR; Naproxen Sodium DS; Naproxen-NA; Naproxen-NA DF; PMS-Naproxen; PMS-Naproxen EC; PRO-Naproxen EC; Riva-Naproxen; Riva-Naproxen Sodium; Riva-Naproxen Sodium DS; Teva-Naproxen; Teva-Naproxen EC; Teva-Naproxen Sodium; Teva-Naproxen Sodium DS; Teva-Naproxen SR
Generic Availability (U.S.) Yes: Caplet, suspension, tablet
Pharmacologic Category Nonsteroidal Anti-inflammatory Drug (NSAID), Oral
Dental Use Management of pain and swelling
Use Management of ankylosing spondylitis, osteoarthritis, and rheumatoid disorders (including juvenile idiopathic arthritis [JIA]); acute gout; mild-to-moderate pain; tendonitis, bursitis; dysmenorrhea; fever
Local Anesthetic/Vasoconstrictor Precautions No information available to require special precautions
Effects on Dental Treatment Key adverse event(s) related to dental treatment: Stomatitis.

Naproxen and naproxen sodium have the potential to interfere with the antiplatelet effect of low-dose aspirin. One study of naproxen and low-dose aspirin has suggested that naproxen may interfere with aspirin's antiplatelet activity when they are coadministered (Steinhubl, 2005). However, naproxen 500 mg administered 2 hours before or after aspirin 100 mg did not interfere with aspirin's antiplatelet effect. The FDA stated that there is no data looking at doses of naproxen <500 mg. Naproxen over-the-counter strength is 220 mg tablets.

The FDA has warned that ibuprofen can interfere with the antiplatelet effect of low-dose aspirin (81 mg/day), potentially rendering aspirin less effective when used for cardioprotection and stroke protection. In situations where these drugs could be used concomitantly, the FDA has proved the following information: Patients who use immediate release aspirin (not enteric-coated aspirin) and take single doses of ibuprofen 400 mg, should dose the ibuprofen at least 30 minutes or longer after aspirin ingestion or more than 8 hours before aspirin ingestion to avoid attenuation of aspirin's effect. Similar recommendations may hold for concomitant may hold for concomitant naproxen and aspirin use. See Effects on Bleeding.

Effects on Bleeding Nonselective NSAIDs are known to reversibly decrease platelet aggregation via mechanisms different than observed with aspirin. Platelet function is restored as the drug is eliminated from the body. NSAIDs should be avoided (if possible) in general surgery patients for 3-5 half-lives of the drug (usually 1-3 days) prior to surgery to reduce the risk of excessive bleeding. However, there is no scientific evidence to warrant discontinuance of NSAIDs prior to dental surgery. In medically complicated patients or extensive oral surgery, the decision to interrupt therapy must be based on the risk to benefit in an individual patient and a medical consult is suggested. Routine interruption of NSAID therapy for most dental procedures is not warranted. If therapy is continued without interruption, the clinician should anticipate the potential for slower clotting times.

Adverse Effects 1% to 10%:
Cardiovascular: Edema (3% to 9%), palpitations (<3%)
Central nervous system: Dizziness (3% to 9%), drowsiness (3% to 9%), headache (3% to 9%), lightheadedness (<3%), vertigo (<3%)

Dermatologic: Pruritus (3% to 9%), skin eruption (3% to 9%), ecchymosis (3% to 9%), purpura (<3%), rash
Endocrine & metabolic: Fluid retention (3% to 9%)
Gastrointestinal: Abdominal pain (3% to 9%), constipation (3% to 9%), nausea (3% to 9%), heartburn (3% to 9%), diarrhea (<3%), dyspepsia (<3%), stomatitis (<3%), flatulence, gross bleeding/perforation, indigestion, ulcers, vomiting
Genitourinary: Abnormal renal function
Hematologic: Hemolysis (3% to 9%), ecchymosis (3% to 9%), anemia, bleeding time increased
Hepatic: LFTs increased
Ocular: Visual disturbances (<3%)
Otic: Tinnitus (3% to 9%), hearing disturbances (<3%)
Respiratory: Dyspnea (3% to 9%)
Miscellaneous: Diaphoresis (<3%), thirst (<3%)

Dental Usual Dosage

Mild-to-moderate pain: Adults: Initial: 500 mg, then 250 mg every 6-8 hours; maximum: 1250 mg/day naproxen base

Pain/fever (OTC labeling): Children ≥12 years and Adults: 200 mg naproxen base every 8-12 hours; if needed, may take 400 mg naproxen base for the initial dose; maximum: 400 mg naproxen base in any 8- to 12-hour period or 600 mg naproxen base/24 hours

Dosage Note: Dosage expressed as naproxen base; 200 mg naproxen base is equivalent to 220 mg naproxen sodium.

Oral:
Children >2 years: Juvenile idiopathic arthritis: 10 mg/kg/day in 2 divided doses
Adults:
Gout, acute: Initial: 750 mg, followed by 250 mg every 8 hours until attack subsides. **Note:** EC-Naprosyn® is not recommended.
Migraine, acute (unlabeled use): Initial: 500-750 mg; an additional 250-500 mg may be given if needed (maximum: 1250 mg in 24 hours). **Note:** EC-Naprosyn® is not recommended.
Pain (mild-to-moderate), dysmenorrhea, acute tendonitis, bursitis: Initial: 500 mg, then 250 mg every 6-8 hours; maximum: 1250 mg/day naproxen base
Rheumatoid arthritis, osteoarthritis, and ankylosing spondylitis: 500-1000 mg/day in 2 divided doses; may increase to 1.5 g/day of naproxen base for limited time period

OTC labeling: Pain/fever: Children ≥12 years and Adults: 200 mg naproxen base every 8-12 hours; if needed, may take 400 mg naproxen base for the initial dose; maximum: 400 mg naproxen base in any 8- to 12-hour period or 600 mg naproxen base/24 hours

Dosing adjustment in renal impairment: Cl_{cr} <30 mL/minute: Use is not recommended

Mechanism of Action Reversibly inhibits cyclooxygenase-1 and 2 (COX-1 and 2) enzymes, which results in decreased formation of prostaglandin precursors; has antipyretic, analgesic, and anti-inflammatory properties

Other proposed mechanisms not fully elucidated (and possibly contributing to the anti-inflammatory effect to varying degrees), include inhibiting chemotaxis, altering lymphocyte activity, inhibiting neutrophil aggregation/activation, and decreasing proinflammatory cytokine levels.

Contraindications Hypersensitivity to naproxen, aspirin, other NSAIDs, or any component of the formulation; perioperative pain in the setting of coronary artery bypass graft (CABG) surgery

Warnings/Precautions [U.S. Boxed Warning]: NSAIDs are associated with an increased risk of adverse cardiovascular thrombotic events, including MI and stroke. Risk may be increased with duration of use or pre-existing cardiovascular risk factors or disease. Carefully evaluate individual cardiovascular risk profiles prior to prescribing. May cause new-onset hypertension or worsening of existing hypertension. Use caution with fluid retention. Avoid use in heart failure. Use the lowest effective dose for the shortest duration of time, consistent with individual patient goals, to reduce risk of cardiovascular or GI adverse events. Alternate therapies should be considered for patients at high risk. Concurrent administration of ibuprofen, and potentially other nonselective NSAIDs, may interfere with aspirin's cardioprotective effect. **[U.S. Boxed Warning]: Use is contraindicated for treatment of perioperative pain in the setting of coronary artery bypass graft (CABG) surgery.** Risk of MI and stroke may be increased with use following CABG surgery.

[U.S. Boxed Warning]: NSAIDs may increase risk of gastrointestinal irritation, inflammation, ulceration, bleeding, and perforation. These events may occur at any time during therapy and without warning. Use caution with a history of GI disease (bleeding or ulcers), concurrent therapy with aspirin, anticoagulants and/or corticosteroids, smoking, use of alcohol, the elderly or debilitated patients. When used concomitantly with ≤325 mg of aspirin, a substantial increase in the risk of gastrointestinal complications (eg, ulcer) occurs; concomitant gastroprotective therapy (eg, proton pump inhibitors) is recommended (Bhatt, 2008).

May increase the risk of aseptic meningitis, especially in patients with systemic lupus erythematosus (SLE) and mixed connective tissue disorders. Platelet adhesion and aggregation may be decreased; may prolong bleeding time; patients with coagulation disorders or who are receiving anticoagulants should be monitored closely. Anemia may occur; patients on long-term NSAID therapy should be monitored for anemia. Rarely, NSAID use may cause severe blood dyscrasias (eg, agranulocytosis, aplastic anemia, thrombocytopenia).

NSAID use may compromise existing renal function; dose-dependent decreases in prostaglandin synthesis may result from NSAID use, reducing renal blood flow which may cause renal decompensation. NSAID use may increase the risk for hyperkalemia. Patients with impaired renal function, dehydration, heart failure, liver dysfunction, those taking diuretics, and ACE inhibitors, and the elderly are at greater risk of renal toxicity and hyperkalemia. Rehydrate patient before starting therapy; monitor renal function closely. Not recommended for use in patients with advanced renal disease. Long-term NSAID use may result in renal papillary necrosis.

NSAIDs may cause serious skin adverse events including exfoliative dermatitis, Stevens-Johnson Syndrome (SJS) and toxic epidermal necrolysis (TEN); discontinue use at first sign of skin rash or hypersensitivity. Anaphylactoid reactions may occur, even without prior exposure; patients with "aspirin triad" (bronchial asthma, aspirin intolerance, rhinitis) may be at increased risk. Do not use in patients who experience bronchospasm, asthma, rhinitis, or urticaria with NSAID or aspirin therapy. Use caution in other forms of asthma.

Use with caution in patients with decreased hepatic function. Closely monitor patients with any abnormal LFT. Severe hepatic reactions (eg, fulminant hepatitis, liver failure) have occurred with NSAID use, rarely; discontinue if signs or symptoms of liver disease develop, or if systemic manifestations occur.

NSAIDS may cause drowsiness, dizziness, blurred vision and other neurologic effects which may impair physical or mental abilities; patients must be cautioned about performing tasks which require mental alertness (eg, operating machinery or driving). Discontinue use with blurred or diminished vision and perform ophthalmologic exam. Monitor vision with long-term therapy.

In the elderly, may be inappropriate for long-term use due to potential for GI bleeding, hypertension, heart failure, and renal failure (Beers Criteria).

Withhold for at least 4-6 half-lives prior to surgical or dental procedures. Safety and efficacy have not been established in children <2 years of age.

OTC labeling: Prior to self-medication, patients should contact healthcare provider if they have had recurring stomach pain or upset, ulcers, bleeding problems, asthma, high blood pressure, heart or kidney disease, other serious medical problems, are currently taking a diuretic, anticoagulant, other NSAIDs, or are ≥60 years of age. Recommended dosages and duration should not be exceeded, due to an increased risk of GI bleeding, MI, and stroke. Patients should stop use and consult a healthcare provider if symptoms get worse, newly appear, or continue; if an allergic reaction occurs; if feeling faint, vomit blood or have bloody/black stools; if having difficulty swallowing or heartburn, or if fever lasts for >3 days or pain >10 days. Consuming ≥3 alcoholic beverages/day or taking longer than recommended may increase the risk of GI bleeding. Not for self-medication (OTC use) in children <12 years of age.

Drug Interactions

Metabolism/Transport Effects Substrate (minor) of CYP1A2, 2C9

Avoid Concomitant Use

Avoid concomitant use of Naproxen with any of the following: Ketorolac; Ketorolac (Systemic)

Increased Effect/Toxicity

Naproxen may increase the levels/effects of: Aminoglycosides; Anticoagulants; Antiplatelet Agents; Bisphosphonate Derivatives; Collagenase (Systemic); CycloSPORINE; CycloSPORINE (Systemic); Deferasirox; Desmopressin; Digoxin; Drotrecogin Alfa; Eplerenone; Haloperidol; Ibritumomab; Lithium; Methotrexate; Nonsteroidal Anti-Inflammatory Agents; PEMEtrexed; Potassium-Sparing Diuretics; PRALAtrexate; Quinolone Antibiotics; Salicylates; Thrombolytic Agents; Tositumomab and Iodine I 131 Tositumomab; Vancomycin; Vitamin K Antagonists

The levels/effects of Naproxen may be increased by: ACE Inhibitors; Angiotensin II Receptor Blockers; Antidepressants (Tricyclic, Tertiary Amine); Corticosteroids (Systemic); Dasatinib; Glucosamine; Herbs (Anticoagulant/Antiplatelet Properties); Ketorolac; Ketorolac (Systemic); Nonsteroidal Anti-Inflammatory Agents; Omega-3-Acid Ethyl Esters; Pentosan Polysulfate Sodium; Pentoxifylline; Probenecid; Prostacyclin Analogues; Selective Serotonin Reuptake Inhibitors; Serotonin/Norepinephrine Reuptake Inhibitors; Treprostinil

Decreased Effect

Naproxen may decrease the levels/effects of: ACE Inhibitors; Angiotensin II Receptor Blockers; Antiplatelet Agents; Beta-Blockers; Eplerenone; HydrALAZINE; Loop Diuretics; Potassium-Sparing Diuretics; Salicylates; Thiazide Diuretics

The levels/effects of Naproxen may be decreased by: Bile Acid Sequestrants; Nonsteroidal Anti-Inflammatory Agents; Salicylates

Ethanol/Nutrition/Herb Interactions

Ethanol: Avoid ethanol (may enhance gastric mucosal irritation).
Food: Naproxen absorption rate/levels may be decreased if taken with food.
Herb/Nutraceutical: Avoid alfalfa, anise, bilberry, bladderwrack, bromelain, cat's claw, celery, chamomile, coleus, cordyceps, dong quai, evening primrose, fenugreek, feverfew, garlic, ginger, ginkgo biloba, ginseng (American, Panax, Siberian), grapeseed, green tea, guggul, horse chestnut seed, horseradish, licorice, prickly ash, red clover, reishi, SAMe (S-adenosylmethionine), sweet clover, turmeric, white willow (all have additional antiplatelet activity).

Dietary Considerations Drug may cause GI upset, bleeding, ulceration, perforation; take with food or milk to minimize GI upset.

Pharmacodynamics/Kinetics

Onset of Action Analgesic: 1 hour; Anti-inflammatory: ~2 weeks; Peak effect: Anti-inflammatory: 2-4 weeks

Duration of Action Analgesic: ≤7 hours; Anti-inflammatory: ≤12 hours

Half-life Elimination Normal renal function: 12-17 hours; End-stage renal disease: No change

Time to Peak Serum: 1-4 hours

Pregnancy Risk Factor C

Lactation Enters breast milk/not recommended (AAP rates "compatible"; AAP 2001 update pending)

Breast-Feeding Considerations Small amounts of naproxen are excreted into breast milk. Naproxen has been detected in the urine of a breast-feeding infant. Breast-feeding is not recommended by the manufacturer. In a study which included 20 mother-infant pairs, there were two cases of drowsiness and one case of vomiting in the breast-fed infants. Maternal naproxen dose, duration, and relationship to breast-feeding were not provided.

Dosage Forms

Caplet, oral: 220 mg
Aleve® [OTC]: 220 mg
Midol® Extended Relief [OTC]: 220 mg
Pamprin® Maximum Strength All Day Relief [OTC]: 220 mg

Capsule, liquid gel, oral:
Aleve® [OTC]: 220 mg

Combination package, oral:
Naprelan®: Day 1-3: Tablet, controlled release: 825 mg [equivalent to naproxen base 750 mg] (6s) [contains sodium 75 mg] and Day 4-10: Tablet, controlled release: 550 mg [equivalent to naproxen base 500 mg] (14s) [contains sodium 50 mg]

Gelcap, oral:
Aleve® [OTC]: 220 mg

Suspension, oral: 125 mg/5 mL (500 mL)
Naprosyn®: 125 mg/5 mL (473 mL)

Tablet, oral: 220 mg, 250 mg, 275 mg, 375 mg, 500 mg, 550 mg
Aleve® [OTC]: 220 mg
Anaprox®: 275 mg
Anaprox® DS: 550 mg
Mediproxen [OTC]: 220 mg
Naprosyn®: 250 mg, 375 mg, 500 mg

Tablet, controlled release, oral:
Naprelan®: 412.5 mg, 550 mg, 825 mg

Tablet, delayed release, enteric coated, oral: 375 mg, 500 mg
EC-Naprosyn®: 375 mg, 500 mg

References

Ahmad N, Grad HA, Haas DA, et al, "The Efficacy of Nonopioid Analgesics for Postoperative Dental Pain: A Meta-Analysis," *Anesth Prog*, 1997, 44(4):119-26.
Brooks PM and Day RO, "Nonsteroidal Anti-inflammatory Drugs - Differences and Similarities," *N Engl J Med*, 1991, 324(24):1716-25.

Dionne R, "Additive Analgesia Without Opioid Side Effects," *Compend Contin Educ Dent*, 2000, 21 (7):572-4, 576-7.
Dionne RA and Berthold CW, "Therapeutic Uses of Nonsteroidal Anti-inflammatory Drugs in Dentistry," *Crit Rev Oral Biol Med*, 2001, 12(4):315-30.
Forbes JA, Keller CK, Smith JW, et al, "Analgesic Effect of Naproxen Sodium, Codeine, a Naproxen-Codeine Combination and Aspirin on the Postoperative Pain of Oral Surgery," *Pharmacotherapy*, 1986, 6(5):211-8.
Nguyen AM, Graham DY, Gage T, et al, "Nonsteroidal Anti-inflammatory Drug Use in Dentistry: Gastrointestinal Implications," *Gen Dent*, 1999, 47(6):590-6.
Steinhubl SR, "The Use of Anti-Inflammatory Analgesics in the Patient With Cardiovascular Disease: What a Pain," *J Am Coll Cardiol*, 2005, 45(8):1302-3.

Naproxen and Esomeprazole (na PROKS en & es oh ME pray zol)

Related Information

Esomeprazole *on page* 628
Naproxen *on page* 1183
Rheumatoid Arthritis, Osteoarthritis, and Osteoporosis *on page* 1889

U.S. Brand Names Vimovo™

Canadian Brand Names Vimovo™

Pharmacologic Category Nonsteroidal Anti-inflammatory Drug (NSAID), Oral; Proton Pump Inhibitor; Substituted Benzimidazole

Use Reduction of the risk of NSAID-associated gastric ulcers in patients at risk of developing gastric ulcers who require an NSAID for the treatment of rheumatoid arthritis, osteoarthritis, and ankylosing spondylitis

Local Anesthetic/Vasoconstrictor Precautions No information available to require special precautions

Effects on Dental Treatment Key adverse event(s) related to dental treatment: Esomeprazole: Xerostomia (normal salivary flow resumes upon discontinuation)

Effects on Bleeding Nonselective NSAIDs are known to reversibly decrease platelet aggregation via mechanisms different than observed with aspirin. Platelet function is restored as the drug is eliminated from the body. NSAIDs should be avoided (if possible) in general surgery patients for 3-5 half-lives of the drug (usually 1-3 days) prior to surgery to reduce the risk of excessive bleeding. However, there is no scientific evidence to warrant discontinuance of NSAIDs prior to dental surgery. In medically complicated patients or during extensive oral surgery, the decision to interrupt therapy must be based on the risk to benefit in an individual patient and a medical consult is suggested. Routine interruption of NSAID therapy for most dental procedures is not warranted. If therapy is continued without interruption, the clinician should anticipate the potential for slower clotting times.

Adverse Effects See individual agents.

General Dosage Range Oral: *Adults:* 1 tablet (naproxen 375-500 mg/esomeprazole 20 mg) twice daily; Maximum daily dose of esomeprazole: 40 mg/day

Mechanism of Action

Naproxen: Reversibly inhibits cyclooxygenase-1 and 2 (COX-1 and 2) enzymes, which result in decreased formation of prostaglandin precursors; has antipyretic, analgesic, and anti-inflammatory properties

Esomeprazole: Proton pump inhibitor which decreases acid secretion in gastric parietal cells

Pregnancy Risk Factor C; Naproxen: D/3rd trimester)

Naproxen and Pseudoephedrine (na PROKS en & soo doe e FED rin)

Related Information

Naproxen *on page* 1183
Pseudoephedrine *on page* 1429

U.S. Brand Names Aleve®-D Sinus & Cold [OTC]; Aleve®-D Sinus & Headache [OTC]; Sudafed® 12 Hour Pressure + Pain [OTC]

Pharmacologic Category Decongestant/Analgesic

Use Temporary relief of cold, sinus, and flu symptoms (including nasal congestion, sinus congestion/pressure, headache, minor body aches and pains, and fever)

Local Anesthetic/Vasoconstrictor Precautions Use with caution since pseudoephedrine is a sympathomimetic amine which could interact with epinephrine to cause a pressor response.

Effects on Dental Treatment Key adverse event(s) related to dental treatment: Pseudoephedrine: Xerostomia (normal salivary flow resumes upon discontinuation).

The dentist should be aware of the potential of abnormal coagulation. See Effects on Bleeding.

Effects on Bleeding Nonselective NSAIDs are known to reversibly decrease platelet aggregation via mechanisms different than observed with aspirin. Platelet function is restored as the drug is eliminated from the body. NSAIDs should be avoided (if possible) in general surgery patients for 3-5 half-lives of the drug (usually 1-3 days) prior to surgery to reduce the risk of excessive bleeding. However, there is no scientific evidence to warrant discontinuance of NSAIDs prior to dental surgery. In medically complicated patients or extensive oral surgery, the decision to interrupt therapy must be based on the risk to benefit in an individual patient and a medical consult is suggested. Routine interruption of NSAID therapy for most dental procedures is not warranted. If therapy is continued without interruption, the clinician should anticipate the potential for slower clotting times.

Adverse Effects See individual agents.

General Dosage Range Oral: *Children ≥12 years and Adults:* 1 caplet (naproxen sodium 220 mg/pseudoephedrine 120 mg) every 12 hours (maximum: 2 caplets/day)

Mechanism of Action

Naproxen: Reversibly inhibits cyclooxygenase-1 and 2 (COX-1 and 2) enzymes, which result in decreased formation of prostaglandin precursors; has antipyretic, analgesic, and anti-inflammatory properties

Pseudoephedrine: Directly stimulates alpha-adrenergic receptors of respiratory mucosa causing vasoconstriction; directly stimulates beta-adrenergic receptors causing bronchial relaxation

Naratriptan (NAR a trip tan)

Related Information

Temporomandibular Dysfunction (TMD) *on page* 1964

U.S. Brand Names Amerge®

Canadian Brand Names Amerge®

Pharmacologic Category Antimigraine Agent; Serotonin 5-$HT_{1B, 1D}$ Receptor Agonist

Use Treatment of acute migraine headache with or without aura

Local Anesthetic/Vasoconstrictor Precautions No information available to require special precautions

Effects on Dental Treatment No significant effects or complications reported

Effects on Bleeding No information available to require special precautions

Adverse Effects 1% to 10%:

Central nervous system: Pain/pressure (2% to 4%), malaise/fatigue (2%), dizziness (1% to 2%), drowsiness (1% to 2%), vertigo (1%)

Gastrointestinal: Nausea (4% to 5%), hyposalivation (1%), vomiting (1%)

Neuromuscular & skeletal: Paresthesia (1% to 2%)

Ocular: Photophobia (1%)

Miscellaneous: Ear/nose/throat infection (1%), pressure/tightness/heaviness sensations (1%), warm/cold temperature sensations (1%)

General Dosage Range Dosage adjustment recommended in patients with hepatic or renal impairment

Oral: *Adults:* 1-2.5 mg, may repeat after 4 hours (maximum: 5 mg/day)

Mechanism of Action Selective agonist for serotonin (5-HT_{1B} and 5-HT_{1D} receptors) in cranial arteries; causes vasoconstriction and reduces sterile inflammation associated with antidromic neuronal transmission correlating with relief of migraine

Pharmacodynamics/Kinetics

Onset of Action ~1-2 hours (Bomhof, 1999; Tfelt-Hansen, 2000)

Half-life Elimination 6 hours; increased in renal impairment (moderate impairment; mean: 11 hours; range 7-20 hours); increased in hepatic impairment (moderate impairment: 8-16 hours)

Time to Peak 2-3 hours

Pregnancy Risk Factor C

Natalizumab (na ta LIZ u mab)

U.S. Brand Names Tysabri®

Canadian Brand Names Tysabri®

Pharmacologic Category Gastrointestinal Agent, Miscellaneous; Monoclonal Antibody, Selective Adhesion-Molecule Inhibitor

Use Monotherapy for the treatment of relapsing forms of multiple sclerosis; treatment of moderately- to severely-active Crohn's disease

Canada labeling: Treatment of relapsing forms of multiple sclerosis

Local Anesthetic/Vasoconstrictor Precautions No information available to require special precautions

Effects on Dental Treatment No significant effects or complications reported

Effects on Bleeding No information available to require special precautions

Adverse Effects

>10%:

Central nervous system: Headache (32% to 38%), fatigue (10% to 27%), depression (≤19%)

Dermatologic: Rash (6% to 12%)

Gastrointestinal: Nausea (≤17%), gastroenteritis (≤11%), abdominal discomfort (≤11%)

Genitourinary: Urinary tract infection (3% to 21%)

Neuromuscular & skeletal: Arthralgia (8% to 19%), extremity pain (16%), back pain (≤12%)

Respiratory: Upper respiratory infection (≤22%), lower respiratory infection (≤17%)

Miscellaneous: Infusion-related reaction (11% to 24%), influenza (≤12%), flu-like syndrome (≤11%)

1% to 10%:

Cardiovascular: Peripheral edema (5% to 6%), chest discomfort (≤5%)

Central nervous system: Vertigo (≤6%), dysesthesia (3%), syncope (≤2%), somnolence (≤2%)

Dermatologic: Dermatitis (≤7%), pruritus (≤4%), urticaria (≤2%), dry skin (≤1%)

Endocrine & metabolic: Dysmenorrhea (2% to 6%), menstrual irregularities (≤5%), amenorrhea (≤2%), ovarian cyst (≤2%)

Gastrointestinal: Diarrhea (10%), dyspepsia (≤5%), abdominal pain (≤4%), constipation (≤4%), flatulence (≤3%), aphthous stomatitis (≤2%), weight changes (≤2%), cholelithiasis (≤1%), gingival infection (1%)

Genitourinary: Vaginitis/vaginal infections (4% to 10%), urinary frequency (≤9%), urinary incontinence (≤4%)

Hematologic: Hematoma (1%)

Hepatic: Transaminase increased (≤5%)

Local: Bleeding at injection site (≤3%)

Neuromuscular & skeletal: Muscle cramp (≤5%), tremor (1% to 3%), rigors (≤3%), joint swelling (≤2%)

Respiratory: Sinusitis (≤8%), cough (≤7%), tonsillitis (≤7%), pharyngolaryngeal pain (≤6%), epistaxis (2%)

Miscellaneous: Antibody formation (9% to 10%), tooth infection (≤9%), herpes infection (≤8%), viral infection (≤7%), hypersensitivity reactions (acute: 2% to 4%; serious acute: ≤1%; delayed: ≤5%), toothache (≤4%), serious infection (2% to 3%), night sweats (≤1%)

General Dosage Range I.V.: *Adults:* 300 mg every 4 weeks

Mechanism of Action Natalizumab is a monoclonal antibody against the alpha-4 subunit of integrin molecules. These molecules are important to adhesion and migration of cells from the vasculature into inflamed tissue. Natalizumab blocks integrin association with vascular receptors, limiting adhesion and transmigration of leukocytes. Efficacy in specific disorders may be related to reduction in specific inflammatory cell populations in target tissues. In multiple sclerosis, efficacy may be related to blockade of T-lymphocyte migration into the central nervous system; treatment results in a decreased frequency of relapse. In Crohn's disease, natalizumab decreases inflammation by binding to alpha-4 integrin, blocking adhesion and migration of leukocytes in the gut.

Pharmacodynamics/Kinetics

Half-life Elimination Crohn's disease: 3-17 days; Multiple sclerosis: 7-15 days

Pregnancy Risk Factor C

Prescribing and Access Restrictions

U.S.: Tysabri® is deemed to have an approved REMS program. As a requirement of the REMS program, access to this medication is restricted. Patients must be enrolled in the Tysabri® Outreach Unified Commitment to Health (TOUCH™) Prescribing Program (800-456-2255) to receive natalizumab (MS-TOUCH™ for multiple sclerosis or CD-TOUCH™ for Crohn's disease). Healthcare providers must also register with the program in order to prescribe, dispense or administer natalizumab. Treatment must be reauthorized every 6 months. Natalizumab is available only through infusion centers registered with the TOUCH™ program; infusion center information is available at 1-800-456-2255.

Canada: Patients receiving natalizumab therapy for multiple sclerosis are to be enrolled in the Tysabri Care Program™ (888-827-2827). This program is associated with the prescribing, administration, and monitoring of Canadian patients receiving natalizumab. Clinicians are educated on the appropriate use of natalizumab and are expected to discuss the benefits/risks of therapy. Clinicians should evaluate patients every 6 months during treatment.

Natamycin (na ta MYE sin)

U.S. Brand Names Natacyn®
Canadian Brand Names Natacyn®
Pharmacologic Category Antifungal Agent, Ophthalmic
Use Treatment of blepharitis, conjunctivitis, and keratitis caused by susceptible fungi (*Aspergillus*, *Candida*, *Cephalosporium*, *Fusarium*, and *Penicillium*)
Local Anesthetic/Vasoconstrictor Precautions No information available to require special precautions
Effects on Dental Treatment No significant effects or complications reported
Effects on Bleeding No information available to require special precautions
Adverse Effects Postmarketing and/or case reports: Allergic reaction, chest pain, corneal opacity, dyspnea, eye discomfort, edema, hyperemia, irritation and/or pain, foreign body sensation, parasthesia, tearing, vision changes
General Dosage Range Ophthalmic: *Adults:* Initial: Instill 1 drop in conjunctival sac every 1-2 hours for 3-4 days; Maintenance: 1 drop 4-8 times/day
Mechanism of Action Increases cell membrane permeability in susceptible fungi
Pregnancy Risk Factor C

Nateglinide (na te GLYE nide)

Related Information
Endocrine Disorders and Pregnancy *on page 1879*
U.S. Brand Names Starlix®
Canadian Brand Names Starlix®
Pharmacologic Category Antidiabetic Agent, Meglitinide Derivative
Use Management of type 2 diabetes mellitus (noninsulin dependent, NIDDM) as monotherapy when hyperglycemia cannot be managed by diet and exercise alone; in combination with metformin or a thiazolidinedione to lower blood glucose in patients whose hyperglycemia cannot be controlled by exercise, diet, or a single agent alone
Local Anesthetic/Vasoconstrictor Precautions No information available to require special precautions
Effects on Dental Treatment No significant effects or complications reported
Effects on Bleeding No information available to require special precautions
Adverse Effects As reported with nateglinide monotherapy: 1% to 10%:
Central nervous system: Dizziness (4%)
Endocrine & metabolic: Hypoglycemia (2%), increased uric acid
Gastrointestinal: Weight gain
Neuromuscular & skeletal: Arthropathy (3%)
Respiratory: Upper respiratory infection (10%)
Miscellaneous: Flu-like syndrome (4%)
General Dosage Range Oral: *Adults:* 60-120 mg 3 times/day
Mechanism of Action A phenylalanine derivative, nonsulfonylurea hypoglycemic agent used in the management of type 2 diabetes mellitus (noninsulin dependent, NIDDM); stimulates insulin release from the pancreatic beta cells to reduce post-prandial hyperglycemia; amount of insulin release is dependent upon existing glucose levels
Pharmacodynamics/Kinetics
Onset of Action Insulin secretion: ~20 minutes; Peak effect: 1 hour
Duration of Action 4 hours
Half-life Elimination 1.5 hours
Time to Peak ≤1 hour
Pregnancy Risk Factor C

Nebivolol (ne BIV oh lole)

Related Information
Cardiovascular Diseases *on page 1848*
U.S. Brand Names Bystolic®
Generic Availability (U.S.) No
Pharmacologic Category Beta Blocker, Beta-1 Selective
Use Treatment of hypertension, alone or in combination with other agents
Unlabeled/Investigational Use Heart failure
Local Anesthetic/Vasoconstrictor Precautions No information available to require special precautions

Effects on Dental Treatment Nebivolol is a cardioselective beta-blocker. Local anesthetic with vasoconstrictor can be safely used in patients medicated with nebivolol. Nonselective beta-blockers (ie, propranolol, nadolol) enhance the pressor response to epinephrine, resulting in hypertension and bradycardia; this has not been reported for nebivolol. Many nonsteroidal anti-inflammatory drugs, such as ibuprofen and indomethacin, can reduce the hypotensive effect of beta-blockers after 3 or more weeks of therapy with the NSAID. Short-term NSAID use (ie, 3 days) requires no special precautions in patients taking beta-blockers.

Effects on Bleeding No information available to require special precautions

Adverse Effects 1% to 10%:

Cardiovascular: Peripheral edema (1%), bradycardia (≤1%), chest pain (≤1%)

Central nervous system: Headache (6% to 9%), fatigue (dose related; 2% to 5%), dizziness (2% to 4%), insomnia (1%)

Dermatologic: Rash (≤1%)

Endocrine & metabolic: HDL levels decreased, hypercholesterolemia, triglyceride levels increased, uric acid levels increased

Gastrointestinal: Diarrhea (dose related; 2% to 3%), nausea (1% to 3%), abdominal pain

Hematologic: Platelet count decreased

Neuromuscular & skeletal: Paresthesia, weakness

Renal: BUN increased

Respiratory: Dyspnea (≤1%)

Dosage Oral:

Adults:

Hypertension: Initial: 5 mg once daily; if initial response is inadequate, may be increased at 2-week intervals to a maximum dose of 40 mg once daily

Heart failure (unlabeled use): Adults ≥70 years: Initial: 1.25 mg once daily; if tolerated, may increase by 2.5 mg at 1- to 2-week intervals to a maximum dose of 10 mg once daily (Flather, 2005). **Note:** Nebivolol has not been shown to reduce morbidity or mortality in the general HF population.

Elderly: Refer to adult dosing.

Dosing adjustment in renal impairment: Severe impairment (Cl_{cr} <30 mL/minute): Initial: 2.5 mg/day; increase cautiously

Dosage adjustment in hepatic impairment: Moderate impairment (Child-Pugh class B): Initial: 2.5 mg/day; increase cautiously

Mechanism of Action Highly-selective inhibitor of $beta_1$-adrenergic receptors; at doses ≤10 mg nebivolol preferentially blocks $beta_1$-receptors. Nebivolol, unlike other beta-blockers, also produces an endothelium-derived nitric oxide-dependent vasodilation resulting in a reduction of systemic vascular resistance.

Contraindications Hypersensitivity to nebivolol or any component of the formulation; severe bradycardia; heart block greater than first-degree (except in patients with a functioning artificial pacemaker); cardiogenic shock; decompensated cardiac failure; sick sinus syndrome (unless a permanent pacemaker is in place); severe hepatic impairment (Child-Pugh class C)

Warnings/Precautions Use caution in patients with heart failure (HF); use gradual and careful titration; monitor for symptoms of congestive heart failure. Patients should be stabilized on HF regimen prior to initiation of beta-blocker; adjustment of other medications (ACE inhibitors and/or diuretics) may be required. **Note:** Nebivolol has not been shown to reduce morbidity or mortality in the general HF population. Use with caution in patients with myasthenia gravis, psychiatric disease (may cause CNS depression), bronchospastic disease, undergoing anesthesia; and in those with impaired hepatic function. Nebivolol should not be withdrawn abruptly (particularly in patients with CAD), but gradually tapered over 1-2 weeks to avoid acute tachycardia, hypertension, and/or ischemia. Use caution in patients with PVD (can aggravate arterial insufficiency). Use caution with concurrent use of verapamil or diltiazem; bradycardia or heart block may occur. Use caution with concurrent use of CYP2D6 inhibitors.

Nebivolol, with $beta_1$-selectivity, may be used cautiously in bronchospastic disease with close monitoring. Use cautiously in patients with diabetes because it can mask prominent hypoglycemic symptoms. Use caution in hyperthyroidism since beta-blockade may mask signs of thyrotoxicosis. Dosage adjustment is required in patients with moderate hepatic or severe renal impairment. Use care with anesthetic agents which decrease myocardial function. Adequate alpha-blockade is required prior to use of any beta-blocker for patients with untreated pheochromocytoma. May induce or exacerbate psoriasis. Use caution with history of severe anaphylaxis to allergens; patients taking beta-blockers may become more sensitive to repeated challenges. Treatment of anaphylaxis (eg, epinephrine) in patients taking beta-blockers may be ineffective or promote undesirable effects.

Drug Interactions

Metabolism/Transport Effects **Substrate** of CYP2D6 (major)

Avoid Concomitant Use

Avoid concomitant use of Nebivolol with any of the following: Methacholine

Increased Effect/Toxicity

Nebivolol may increase the levels/effects of: Alpha-/Beta-Agonists (Direct-Acting); Alpha1-Blockers; Alpha2-Agonists; Amifostine; Antihypertensives; Antipsychotic Agents (Phenothiazines); Bupivacaine; Cardiac Glycosides; Fingolimod; Hypotensive Agents; Insulin; Lidocaine; Lidocaine (Systemic); Lidocaine (Topical); Mepivacaine; Methacholine; Midodrine; RiTUXimab; Sulfonylureas

The levels/effects of Nebivolol may be increased by: Acetylcholinesterase Inhibitors; Aminoquinolines (Antimalarial); Amiodarone; Anilidopiperidine Opioids; Antipsychotic Agents (Phenothiazines); Calcium Channel Blockers (Nondihydropyridine); CYP2D6 Inhibitors (Moderate); CYP2D6 Inhibitors (Strong); Diazoxide; Dipyridamole; Disopyramide; Dronedarone; Herbs (Hypotensive Properties); MAO Inhibitors; Pentoxifylline; Phosphodiesterase 5 Inhibitors; Propafenone; Propoxyphene; Prostacyclin Analogues; QuiNIDine; Reserpine; Selective Serotonin Reuptake Inhibitors

Decreased Effect

Nebivolol may decrease the levels/effects of: Beta2-Agonists; Theophylline Derivatives

The levels/effects of Nebivolol may be decreased by: Barbiturates; Herbs (Hypertensive Properties); Methylphenidate; Nonsteroidal Anti-Inflammatory Agents; Peginterferon Alfa-2b; Rifamycin Derivatives; Yohimbine

Ethanol/Nutrition/Herb Interactions Herb/Nutraceutical: Avoid bayberry, blue cohosh, cayenne, ephedra, ginger, ginseng (American), kola, licorice (may worsen hypertension). Avoid black cohosh, California poppy, coleus, golden seal, hawthorn, mistletoe, periwinkle, quinine, shepherd's purse (may increase antihypertensive effect).

Dietary Considerations May be taken without regard to meals.

Pharmacodynamics/Kinetics

Half-life Elimination Terminal: 10-12 hours (extensive metabolizers); 19-32 hours in poor metabolizers

Time to Peak 1.5-4 hours

Pregnancy Risk Factor C

Lactation Excretion in breast milk unknown/not recommended

Breast-Feeding Considerations It is not known if nebivolol is excreted into breast milk. Breast-feeding is not recommended by the manufacturer due to potential for beta-blockers to produce serious effects on nursing infants, especially bradycardia.

Dosage Forms

Tablet, oral:

Bystolic®: 2.5 mg, 5 mg, 10 mg, 20 mg

References

Brixius K, Bundkirchen A, Bolck B, et al, "Nebivolol, Bucindolol, Metoprolol and Carvedilol are Devoid of Intrinsic Sympathomimetic Activity in Human Myocardium," *Br J Pharmacol*, 2001, 133(8):1330-8.
Cazzola M, Noschese P, D'Amato M, Det al, "Comparison of the Effects of Single Oral Doses of Nebivolol and Celiprolol on Airways in Patients With Mild Asthma," *Chest*, 2000, 118(5):1322-6.
Cheymol G, Woestenborghs R, Snoeck E, et al. "Pharmacokinetic Study and Cardiovascular Monitoring of Nebivolol in Normal and Obese Subjects," *Eur J Clin Pharmacol*, 1997, 51(6):493-8.
Chobanian AV, Bakris GL, Black HR, et al, "The Seventh Report of the Joint National Committee on Prevention, Detection, Evaluation, and Treatment of High Blood Pressure: The JNC 7 Report," *JAMA*, 2003, 289(19):2560-71.
Flather MD, Shibata MC, Coats AJ, et al, "Randomized Trial to Determine the Effect of Nebivolol on Mortality and Cardiovascular Hospital Admission in Elderly Patients With Heart Failure (SENIORS)," *Eur Heart J*, 2005, 26(3):215-25.

Nedocromil (ne doe KROE mil)

Related Information

Respiratory Diseases *on page 1876*

U.S. Brand Names Alocril®

Canadian Brand Names Alocril®; Tilade®

Pharmacologic Category Mast Cell Stabilizer

Use

Aerosol: Maintenance therapy in patients with mild-to-moderate bronchial asthma

Ophthalmic: Treatment of itching associated with allergic conjunctivitis

Local Anesthetic/Vasoconstrictor Precautions No information available to require special precautions

Effects on Dental Treatment Key adverse event(s) related to dental treatment: Unpleasant taste.

Effects on Bleeding No information available to require special precautions

Adverse Effects

Inhalation aerosol:

>10%: Gastrointestinal: Unpleasant taste (12%)

1% to 10%:

Central nervous system: Headache (8%), fatigue (1%)

Gastrointestinal: Nausea (4%), vomiting (3%), dyspepsia (2%), diarrhea (1%), abdominal pain (2%)

Ocular: Conjunctivitis (1%)

Respiratory: Cough (9%), pharyngitis (8%), rhinitis (7%), upper respiratory infection

Ophthalmic solution:

>10%:

Central nervous system: Headache (40%)

Gastrointestinal: Unpleasant taste

Ocular: Burning, irritation, stinging

Respiratory: Nasal congestion

1% to 10%:

Ocular: Conjunctivitis, eye redness, photophobia

Respiratory: Asthma, rhinitis

General Dosage Range

Inhalation: *Children ≥6 years and Adults:* 2 inhalations 2-4 times/day

Ophthalmic: *Children ≥3 years and Adults:* 1-2 drops in each eye twice daily

Mechanism of Action Inhibits the activation of and mediator release from a variety of inflammatory cell types associated with asthma including eosinophils, neutrophils, macrophages, mast cells, monocytes, and platelets; it inhibits the release of histamine, leukotrienes, and slow-reacting substance of anaphylaxis; it inhibits the development of early and late bronchoconstriction responses to inhaled antigen

Pharmacodynamics/Kinetics

Onset of Action Inhalation: Full therapeutic effect may not occur until ≥1 week of therapy.

Duration of Action Therapeutic effect: 2 hours

Half-life Elimination 1.5-3.3 hours

Pregnancy Risk Factor B

Nefazodone (nef AY zoe done)

Pharmacologic Category Antidepressant, Serotonin Reuptake Inhibitor/Antagonist

Use Treatment of depression

Unlabeled/Investigational Use Post-traumatic stress disorder (PTSD)

Local Anesthetic/Vasoconstrictor Precautions Nefazodone inhibits reuptake of both serotonin and norepinephrine and also blocks some serotonin receptors. No precautions with vasoconstrictors appear to be necessary.

Effects on Dental Treatment Key adverse event(s) related to dental treatment: Significant xerostomia (normal salivary flow resumes upon discontinuation) and taste perversion.

Effects on Bleeding No information available to require special precautions

Adverse Effects

>10%:

Central nervous system: Headache, drowsiness, insomnia, agitation, dizziness

Gastrointestinal: Xerostomia, nausea, constipation

Neuromuscular & skeletal: Weakness

1% to 10%:

Cardiovascular: Bradycardia, hypotension, peripheral edema, postural hypotension, vasodilation

Central nervous system: Chills, fever, incoordination, lightheadedness, confusion, memory impairment, abnormal dreams, decreased concentration, ataxia, psychomotor retardation, tremor

Dermatologic: Pruritus, rash

Endocrine & metabolic: Breast pain, impotence, libido decreased

Gastrointestinal: Gastroenteritis, vomiting, dyspepsia, diarrhea, increased appetite, thirst, taste perversion

Genitourinary: Urinary frequency, urinary retention

Hematologic: Hematocrit decreased

Neuromuscular & skeletal: Arthralgia, hypertonia, paresthesia, neck rigidity, tremor

Ocular: Blurred vision (9%), abnormal vision (7%), eye pain, visual field defect

Otic: Tinnitus

Respiratory: Bronchitis, cough, dyspnea, pharyngitis

Miscellaneous: Flu syndrome, infection

General Dosage Range Oral:
Adults: Initial: 200 mg/day in 2 divided doses; Maintenance: 300-600 mg/day in 2 divided doses
Elderly: Initial: 50 mg twice daily; Maintenance: 200-400 mg/day in 2 divided doses

Mechanism of Action Inhibits neuronal reuptake of serotonin and norepinephrine; also blocks 5-HT_2 and $alpha_1$ receptors; has no significant affinity for $alpha_2$, beta-adrenergic, 5-HT_{1A}, cholinergic, dopaminergic, or benzodiazepine receptors

Pharmacodynamics/Kinetics
Onset of Action Therapeutic: Up to 6 weeks
Half-life Elimination Parent drug: 2-4 hours; active metabolites persist longer
Time to Peak Serum: 1 hour, prolonged in presence of food

Pregnancy Risk Factor C

Nelarabine (nel AY re been)

U.S. Brand Names Arranon®

Canadian Brand Names Atriance™

Pharmacologic Category Antineoplastic Agent, Antimetabolite

Use Treatment of relapsed or refractory T-cell acute lymphoblastic leukemia (ALL) and T-cell lymphoblastic lymphoma

Local Anesthetic/Vasoconstrictor Precautions No information available to require special precautions

Effects on Dental Treatment Key adverse event(s) related to dental treatment: Taste perversion and stomatitis.

Effects on Bleeding Chemotherapy may result in significant myelosuppression, potentially including significant reduction in platelet counts and altered hemostasis. In patients who are under active treatment with these agents, medical consult is suggested.

Adverse Effects Note: Pediatric adverse reactions fell within a range similar to adults except where noted.

>10%:
- Cardiovascular: Peripheral edema (15%), edema (11%)
- Central nervous system: Fatigue (50%), fever (23%), somnolence (7% to 23%; grades 2-4: 1% to 6%), dizziness (21%; grade 2: 8% adults), headache (15% to 17%; grades 2-4: 4% to 8%), hypoesthesia (6% to 17%; grades 2/3: children 5%, adults 12%), pain (11%)
- Dermatologic: Petechiae (12%)
- Endocrine & metabolic: Hypokalemia (11%)
- Gastrointestinal: Nausea (41%), diarrhea (22%), vomiting (10% to 22%), constipation (21%)
- Hematologic: Anemia (95% to 99%; grade 4: 10% to 14%), neutropenia (81% to 94%; grade 4: children 62%, adults 49%), thrombocytopenia (86% to 88%; grade 4: 22% to 32%), leukopenia (38%; grade 4: 7%), febrile neutropenia (12%; grade 4: 1%)
- Hepatic: Transaminases increased (12%; grade 3: 4%)
- Neuromuscular & skeletal: Peripheral neuropathy (12% to 21%; grades 2/3: 11% to 14%), weakness (6% to 17%; grade 4: 1%), paresthesia (4% to 15%; grades 2/3: 3% to 4%), myalgia (13%)
- Respiratory: Cough (25%), dyspnea (7% to 20%)

1% to 10%:
- Cardiovascular: Hypotension (8%), sinus tachycardia (8%), chest pain (5%)
- Central nervous system: Ataxia (2% to 9%; grades 2/3: children 1%, adults 8%), confusion (8%), insomnia (7%), depressed level of consciousness (6%; grades 2-4: 2%), depression (6%), seizure (grade 3: 1% adults; grade 4: 6% children), motor dysfunction (4%; grades 2/3: 2%), amnesia (3%; grade 2: 1%), balance disorder (2%; grade 2: 1%), sensory loss (1% to 2%), aphasia (grade 3: 1%), attention disturbance (1%), cerebral hemorrhage (grade 4: 1%), coma (grade 4: 1%), encephalopathy (grade 4: 1%), hemiparesis (grade 3: 1%), hydrocephalus (1%), intracranial hemorrhage (grade 4: 1%), lethargy (1%), leukoencephalopathy (grade 4: 1%), loss of consciousness (grade 3: 1%), mental impairment (1%), nerve paralysis (1%), neuropathic pain (1%), nerve palsy (1%), paralysis (1%), sciatica (1%), sensory disturbance (1%), speech disorder (1%)
- Endocrine & Metabolic: Hypocalcemia (8%), dehydration (7%), hyper-/hypoglycemia (6%), hypomagnesemia (6%)
- Gastrointestinal: Abdominal pain (9%), anorexia (9%), stomatitis (8%), abdominal distension (6%), taste perversion (3%)
- Hepatic: Albumin decreased (10%), bilirubin increased (10%; grade 3: 7%, grade 4: 2%), AST increased (6%)

Neuromuscular & skeletal: Arthralgia (9%), back pain (8%), muscle weakness (8%), rigors (8%), limb pain (7%), abnormal gait (6%), noncardiac chest pain (5%), tremor (4% to 5%; grade 2: 2% to 3%), dysarthria (1%), hyporeflexia (1%), hypertonia (1%), incoordination (1%)
Ocular: Blurred vision (4%), nystagmus (1%)
Renal: Creatinine increased (6%)
Respiratory: Pleural effusion (10%), epistaxis (8%), pneumonia (8%), sinusitis (7%), wheezing (5%), sinus headache (1%)
Miscellaneous: Infection (5% to 9%)

General Dosage Range I.V.:
Children: 650 mg/m²/dose on days 1 through 5; repeat every 21 days
Adults: 1500 mg/m²/dose on days 1, 3, and 5; repeat every 21 days

Mechanism of Action Nelarabine, a prodrug of ara-G, is demethylated by adenosine deaminase to ara-G and then converted to ara-GTP. Ara-GTP is incorporated into the DNA of the leukemic blasts, leading to inhibition of DNA synthesis and inducing apoptosis. Ara-GTP appears to accumulate at higher levels in T-cells, which correlates to clinical response.

Pharmacodynamics/Kinetics
Half-life Elimination Children: Nelarabine: 13 minutes, Ara-G: 2 hours; Adults: Nelarabine: 18 minutes, Ara-G: 3 hours
Time to Peak Adults: 3-25 hours (day 1)

Pregnancy Risk Factor D

Nelfinavir (nel FIN a veer)

Related Information
HIV Infection and AIDS *on page* *1883*
Viral Infections *on page* *1947*

U.S. Brand Names Viracept®
Canadian Brand Names Viracept®
Generic Availability (U.S.) No
Pharmacologic Category Antiretroviral Agent, Protease Inhibitor
Use In combination with other antiretroviral therapy in the treatment of HIV infection
Local Anesthetic/Vasoconstrictor Precautions No information available to require special precautions
Effects on Dental Treatment Key adverse event(s) related to dental treatment: Mouth ulcers.
Effects on Bleeding Increased bleeding has been noted with protease inhibitors in patients with hemophilia A or B. No information available to require routine special precautions relative to hemostasis in other patients.
Adverse Effects Data presented on experience in adults, unless otherwise noted.
>10%: Gastrointestinal: Diarrhea (14% to 20%; children: 39% to 47%)
2% to 10%:
Dermatologic: Rash (1% to 3%)
Gastrointestinal: Nausea (3% to 7%), flatulence (1% to 5%)
Hematologic: Lymphocytes decreased (1% to 6%), neutrophils decreased (1% to 5%)

Dosage Oral:
Children 2-13 years: 45-55 mg/kg twice daily **or** 25-35 mg/kg 3 times/day (maximum: 2500 mg/day). If tablets are unable to be taken, use oral powder in small amount of water, milk (cow's or soy), formula, or dietary supplements; do not use acidic food/juice or store for >6 hours.
Adults: 750 mg 3 times/day or 1250 mg twice daily with meals in combination with other antiretroviral therapies

Dosage adjustments for concomitant therapy: Adults:
Coadministration with bosentan:
Coadministration of bosentan in patients currently receiving nelfinavir: Begin with bosentan 62.5 mg once daily or every other day based on tolerability
Coadministration of nelfinavir in patients currently receiving bosentan: Adjust bosentan to 62.5 mg once daily or every other day based on tolerability
Coadministration with colchicine:
Familial Mediterranean fever (FMF): Maximum colchicine dose: 0.6 mg/day (0.3 mg twice daily)
Gout prophylaxis:
If original colchicine dose is 0.6 mg twice daily, adjust dose to 0.3 mg once daily
If original colchicine dose is 0.6 mg once daily, adjust dose to 0.3 mg every other day
Gout flare treatment: Initial: Colchicine 0.6 mg, followed in 1 hour by a single dose of 0.3 mg; do not repeat for at least 3 days

Coadministration with phosphodiesterase-5 enzyme (PDE-5) inhibitor:

Pulmonary arterial hypertension: Nelfinavir coadministered with tadalafil:

Patient receiving nelfinavir: Initiate tadalafil at 20 mg once daily; increase to 40 mg once daily based on individual tolerability

Patient receiving tadalafil when initiating nelfinavir: Adjust tadalafil to 20 mg once daily; increase to 40 mg once daily based on individual tolerability

Erectile dysfunction: Nelfinavir coadministered with:

Sildenafil (Viagra®): Maximum sildenafil dose: 25 mg in a 48-hour period

Tadalafil (Cialis®): Maximum tadalafil dose: 10 mg in a 72-hour period

Vardenafil: Maximum vardenafil dose: 2.5 mg in a 24-hour period

Dosing adjustment in renal impairment: No pharmacokinetic data in patients with renal impairment. However, <2% of dose excreted in urine; no dose adjustment is needed.

Dosing adjustment in hepatic impairment: No dose adjustment necessary in mild impairment (Child-Pugh class A); not recommended in patients with moderate-to-severe impairment (Child-Pugh class B or C)

Mechanism of Action Binds to the site of HIV-1 protease activity and inhibits cleavage of viral Gag-Pol polyprotein precursors into individual functional proteins required for infectious HIV. This results in the formation of immature, noninfectious viral particles.

Contraindications Hypersensitivity to nelfinavir or any component of the formulation; concurrent therapy with alfuzosin, amiodarone, ergot derivatives, midazolam, pimozide, quinidine, sildenafil (when used for pulmonary artery hypertension [eg, Revatio®]), triazolam

Warnings/Precautions Use with caution in patients taking strong CYP3A4 inhibitors, moderate or strong CYP3A4 inducers and major CYP3A4 substrates and if coadministered with QT-prolonging drugs that are metabolized by CYP3A (see Drug Interactions); consider alternative agents that avoid or lessen the potential for CYP-mediated interactions. Not recommended for use with rifampin, St John's wort, lovastatin, simvastatin, phosphodiesterase-5 (PDE-5) inhibitors, or proton pump inhibitors (based on omeprazole data). Do not coadminister colchicine in patient with renal or hepatic impairment; avoid concurrent use with salmeterol.

Use caution with hepatic impairment; use not recommended with moderate-to-severe impairment. Warn patients that redistribution of body fat can occur. New-onset diabetes mellitus, exacerbation of diabetes, and hyperglycemia have been reported in HIV-infected patients receiving protease inhibitors. Use with caution in patients with hemophilia A or B; increased bleeding during protease inhibitor therapy has been reported. Immune reconstitution syndrome has been reported; may require additional evaluation and treatment. The oral powder contains phenylalanine. Safety and efficacy have not been established in children <2 years of age.

Drug Interactions

Metabolism/Transport Effects **Substrate** of CYP2C9 (minor), CYP2C19 (major), CYP2D6 (minor), CYP3A4 (major), P-glycoprotein; **Inhibits** CYP1A2 (weak), CYP2B6 (weak), CYP2C9 (weak), CYP2C19 (weak), CYP2D6 (weak), CYP3A4 (strong), P-glycoprotein

Avoid Concomitant Use

Avoid concomitant use of Nelfinavir with any of the following: Alfuzosin; Amiodarone; Cisapride; Conivaptan; Dronedarone; Eplerenone; Ergot Derivatives; Everolimus; Fluticasone (Oral Inhalation); Halofantrine; Lovastatin; Lurasidone; Midazolam; Nilotinib; Nisoldipine; Pimozide; Proton Pump Inhibitors; QuiNIDine; Ranolazine; Rifampin; Rivaroxaban; RomiDEPsin; Salmeterol; Silodosin; Simvastatin; St Johns Wort; Tamsulosin; Tolvaptan; Topotecan; Toremifene; Triazolam

Increased Effect/Toxicity

Nelfinavir may increase the levels/effects of: Alfuzosin; Almotriptan; Alosetron; ALPRAZolam; Amiodarone; Antifungal Agents (Azole Derivatives, Systemic); Azithromycin; Azithromycin (Systemic); Bortezomib; Bosentan; Brinzolamide; Budesonide (Nasal); Budesonide (Systemic, Oral Inhalation); Calcium Channel Blockers (Dihydropyridine); Calcium Channel Blockers (Nondihydropyridine); CarBAMazepine; Ciclesonide; Cisapride; Clarithromycin; Colchicine; Conivaptan; Corticosteroids (Orally Inhaled); CycloSPORINE; CycloSPORINE (Systemic); CYP3A4 Substrates; Dabigatran Etexilate; Dienogest; Digoxin; Dronedarone; Dutasteride; Enfuvirtide; Eplerenone; Ergot Derivatives; Everolimus; FentaNYL; Fesoterodine; Fluticasone (Nasal); Fluticasone (Oral Inhalation); Fusidic Acid; GuanFACINE; Halofantrine; HMG-CoA Reductase Inhibitors; Ixabepilone; Lovastatin; Lumefantrine; Lurasidone; Maraviroc; Meperidine; MethylPREDNISolone; Midazolam; Nefazodone; Nilotinib; Nisoldipine; Paricalcitol; Pazopanib; P-Glycoprotein Substrates; Pimecrolimus; Pimozide; Protease Inhibitors; QuiNIDine; Ranolazine; Rifabutin; Rivaroxaban; RomiDEPsin; Salmeterol; Saxagliptin; Sildenafil; Silodosin; Simvastatin; Sirolimus; SORAfenib; Tacrolimus; Tacrolimus (Systemic); Tacrolimus (Topical); Tadalafil; Tamsulosin; Temsirolimus; Tenofovir;

Tolvaptan; Topotecan; Toremifene; TraZODone; Triazolam; Tricyclic Antidepressants; Vardenafil; Vilazodone; Warfarin

The levels/effects of Nelfinavir may be increased by: Antifungal Agents (Azole Derivatives, Systemic); Clarithromycin; CycloSPORINE; CycloSPORINE (Systemic); Delavirdine; Efavirenz; Enfuvirtide; Etravirine; Fusidic Acid; Lopinavir; P-Glycoprotein Inhibitors

Decreased Effect

Nelfinavir may decrease the levels/effects of: Abacavir; Clarithromycin; Contraceptives (Estrogens); Delavirdine; Divalproex; Etravirine; Lopinavir; Meperidine; Methadone; Prasugrel; Theophylline Derivatives; Valproic Acid; Warfarin; Zidovudine

The levels/effects of Nelfinavir may be decreased by: Antacids; Bosentan; CarBAMazepine; Contraceptives (Estrogens); CYP2C19 Inducers (Strong); CYP3A4 Inducers (Strong); Deferasirox; Efavirenz; Garlic; H2-Antagonists; Nevirapine; Peginterferon Alfa-2b; P-Glycoprotein Inducers; Proton Pump Inhibitors; Rifabutin; Rifampin; St Johns Wort; Tenofovir; Tocilizumab

Ethanol/Nutrition/Herb Interactions

Food: Nelfinavir taken with food increases plasma concentration time curve (AUC) by two- to threefold. Do not administer with acidic food or juice (orange juice, apple juice, or applesauce) since the combination may have a bitter taste.

Herb/Nutraceutical: St John's wort may decrease the levels/effects of protease inhibitors; concurrent use should probably be avoided.

Dietary Considerations Should be taken as scheduled with a meal. Some products may contain phenylalanine.

Pharmacodynamics/Kinetics

Half-life Elimination 3.5-5 hours

Time to Peak Serum: 2-4 hours

Pregnancy Risk Factor B

Lactation Excretion in breast milk unknown/contraindicated

Breast-Feeding Considerations In infants born to mothers who are HIV positive, HAART while breast-feeding may decrease postnatal infection. However, maternal or infant antiretroviral therapy does not completely eliminate the risk of postnatal HIV transmission. In addition, multiclass-resistant virus has been detected in breast-feeding infants despite maternal therapy.

In the United States where formula is accessible, affordable, safe, and sustainable, complete avoidance of breast-feeding by HIV-infected women is recommended to decrease potential transmission of HIV.

Dosage Forms

Powder, oral:

Viracept®: 50 mg/g (144 g)

Tablet, oral:

Viracept®: 250 mg, 625 mg

Neomycin (nee oh MYE sin)

U.S. Brand Names Neo-Fradin™; Neo-Rx [DSC]

Pharmacologic Category Ammonium Detoxicant; Antibiotic, Aminoglycoside; Antibiotic, Topical

Use Orally to prepare GI tract for surgery; treatment of diarrhea caused by *E. coli*; adjunct in the treatment of hepatic encephalopathy

Local Anesthetic/Vasoconstrictor Precautions No information available to require special precautions

Effects on Dental Treatment No significant effects or complications reported

Effects on Bleeding No information available to require special precautions

Adverse Effects

>10%: Gastrointestinal: Nausea, diarrhea, vomiting, irritation or soreness of the mouth or rectal area

General Dosage Range Oral:

Children: Encephalopathy: 50-100 mg/kg/day divided every 6-8 hours **or** 2.5-7 g/m^2/day divided every 4-6 hours (maximum: 12 g/day); Preoperative GI preparation: 75-90 mg/kg/day

Adults: Encephalopathy/hepatic insufficiency: 500 mg to 12 g/day in divided doses every 4-8 hours; Preoperative GI preparation: 1 g for 3-9 doses

Mechanism of Action Interferes with bacterial protein synthesis by binding to 30S ribosomal subunits

Pharmacodynamics/Kinetics

Half-life Elimination Age and renal function dependent: 3 hours

Time to Peak Serum: Oral: 1-4 hours

Pregnancy Risk Factor D

Neomycin and Polymyxin B (nee oh MYE sin & pol i MIKS in bee)

Related Information

Neomycin *on page 1197*

Polymyxin B *on page 1370*

U.S. Brand Names Neosporin® G.U. Irrigant

Canadian Brand Names Neosporin® Irrigating Solution

Pharmacologic Category Antibiotic, Topical; Genitourinary Irrigant

Use Short-term as a continuous irrigant or rinse in the urinary bladder to prevent bacteriuria and gram-negative rod septicemia associated with the use of indwelling catheters

Local Anesthetic/Vasoconstrictor Precautions No information available to require special precautions

Effects on Dental Treatment No significant effects or complications reported

Effects on Bleeding No information available to require special precautions

Adverse Effects Frequency not defined.

Dermatologic: Contact dermatitis, erythema, rash, urticaria

Genitourinary: Bladder irritation

Local: Burning

Neuromuscular & skeletal: Neuromuscular blockade

Otic: Ototoxicity

Renal: Nephrotoxicity

General Dosage Range Irrigation (bladder): *Children and Adults:* Add 1 mL irrigant to 1 L isotonic saline solution (maximum: Usually no more than 1 L irrigant/day)

Mechanism of Action See individual agents.

Pregnancy Risk Factor D

Neomycin, Polymyxin B, and Dexamethasone
(nee oh MYE sin, pol i MIKS in bee, & deks a METH a sone)

Related Information

Neomycin *on page 1197*

Polymyxin B *on page 1370*

U.S. Brand Names Maxitrol®; Poly-Dex™ [DSC]

Canadian Brand Names Dioptrol®; Maxitrol®

Pharmacologic Category Antibiotic/Corticosteroid, Ophthalmic

Use Steroid-responsive inflammatory ocular conditions in which a corticosteroid is indicated and where bacterial infection or a risk of bacterial infection exists

Local Anesthetic/Vasoconstrictor Precautions No information available to require special precautions

Effects on Dental Treatment No significant effects or complications reported

Effects on Bleeding No information available to require special precautions

Adverse Effects Frequency not defined: Ocular: Allergic sensitivity, cutaneous sensitization, eye pain, development of glaucoma, cataract, increased intraocular pressure, optic nerve damage, wound healing delayed

General Dosage Range Ophthalmic:

Ointment: *Children and Adults:* Place a small amount (~1/2") in the affected eye 3-4 times/day **or** at bedtime

Suspension: *Children and Adults:* Instill 1-2 drops into affected eye(s) every 3-4 hours

Mechanism of Action See individual agents.

Pregnancy Risk Factor C

Neomycin, Polymyxin B, and Gramicidin
(nee oh MYE sin, pol i MIKS in bee, & gram i SYE din)

Related Information

Neomycin *on page 1197*

Polymyxin B *on page 1370*

U.S. Brand Names Neosporin® Ophthalmic Solution

Canadian Brand Names Neosporin®; Optimyxin Plus®

Pharmacologic Category Antibiotic, Ophthalmic

Use Treatment of superficial ocular infection

Local Anesthetic/Vasoconstrictor Precautions No information available to require special precautions

Effects on Dental Treatment No significant effects or complications reported

Effects on Bleeding No information available to require special precautions

Adverse Effects Frequency not defined: Ocular: Transient irritation, burning, stinging, itching, inflammation, angioneurotic edema, urticaria, vesicular and maculopapular dermatitis

General Dosage Range Ophthalmic: *Children and Adults:* Instill 1-2 drops 4-6 times/day

Mechanism of Action Interferes with bacterial protein synthesis by binding to 30S ribosomal subunits; binds to phospholipids, alters permeability, and damages the bacterial cytoplasmic membrane permitting leakage of intracellular constituents

Pregnancy Risk Factor C

Neomycin, Polymyxin B, and Hydrocortisone

(nee oh MYE sin, pol i MIKS in bee, & hye droe KOR ti sone)

Related Information

Hydrocortisone (Topical) *on page* 868
Neomycin *on page* 1197
Polymyxin B *on page* 1370

U.S. Brand Names Cortisporin®; Cortomycin

Canadian Brand Names Cortimyxin®; Cortisporin® Otic

Pharmacologic Category Antibiotic, Ophthalmic; Antibiotic, Otic; Antibiotic, Topical; Antibiotic/Corticosteroid, Otic; Corticosteroid, Ophthalmic; Corticosteroid, Otic; Corticosteroid, Topical

Use Steroid-responsive inflammatory condition for which a corticosteroid is indicated and where bacterial infection or a risk of bacterial infection exists

Local Anesthetic/Vasoconstrictor Precautions No information available to require special precautions

Effects on Dental Treatment No significant effects or complications reported

Effects on Bleeding No information available to require special precautions

Adverse Effects Frequency not defined. For additional information, see individual agents.

Ophthalmic ointment:

Dermatologic: Delayed wound healing, rash

Ocular: Cataracts, corneal thinning, glaucoma, irritation, keratitis (bacterial), intraocular pressure increase, optic nerve damage, scleral thinning

Miscellaneous: Hypersensitivity (including anaphylaxis), secondary infection, sensitization to kanamycin, paromomycin, streptomycin, and gentamicin

Otic solution and suspension:

Dermatologic: Acneiform eruptions, allergic contact dermatitis, burning skin, dryness, folliculitis, hypertrichosis, hypopigmentation, irritation, maceration of skin, miliaria, ocular hypertension, perioral dermatitis, pruritus, skin atrophy, striae

Otic: Burning, ototoxicity, stinging

Renal: Nephrotoxicity

Miscellaneous: Hypersensitivity (including anaphylaxis), secondary infection, sensitization to karamycin, paromycin, streptomycin, and gentamicin

General Dosage Range

Ophthalmic: *Adults:* Instill 1-2 drops every 3-4 hours, or more frequently

Otic:

Children ≥2 years: Instill 3 drops into affected ear 3-4 times/day

Children ≥12 years and Adults: Instill 4 drops into affected ear 3-4 times/day

Topical: *Adults:* Apply a thin layer 1-4 times/day

Mechanism of Action See individual agents.

Pregnancy Risk Factor C

Neomycin, Polymyxin B, and Prednisolone

(nee oh MYE sin, pol i MIKS in bee, & pred NIS oh lone)

Related Information

Neomycin *on page* 1197
Polymyxin B *on page* 1370

U.S. Brand Names Poly-Pred®

Pharmacologic Category Antibiotic/Corticosteroid, Ophthalmic

Use Steroid-responsive inflammatory ocular condition in which bacterial infection or a risk of bacterial ocular infection exists

Local Anesthetic/Vasoconstrictor Precautions No information available to require special precautions

Effects on Dental Treatment No significant effects or complications reported

Effects on Bleeding No information available to require special precautions

Adverse Effects Frequency not defined.

Ocular: Allergic sensitivity, cataracts, conjunctival erythema, conjunctival hyperemia, conjunctivitis, corneal ulcers, delayed wound healing, glaucoma, globe perforation, increased intraocular pressure, itching, keratitis, optic nerve damage, secondary infection, swelling

Miscellaneous: Anaphylaxis, hypercorticoidism, hypersensitivity

General Dosage Range Ophthalmic: *Children and Adults:* Initial: 1-2 drops every 30 minutes; Maintenance: Instill 1-2 drops every 3-4 hours

Mechanism of Action See individual agents.

Pregnancy Risk Factor C

Nepafenac (ne pa FEN ak)

U.S. Brand Names Nevanac®

Canadian Brand Names Nevanac®

Pharmacologic Category Nonsteroidal Anti-inflammatory Drug (NSAID), Ophthalmic

Use Treatment of pain and inflammation associated with cataract surgery

Local Anesthetic/Vasoconstrictor Precautions No information available to require special precautions

Effects on Dental Treatment The dentist should be aware of the potential of abnormal coagulation. Caution should also be exercised in the use of NSAIDs in patients already on anticoagulant therapy with drugs such as warfarin (Coumadin®). See Effects on Bleeding.

Effects on Bleeding Nonselective NSAIDs are known to reversibly decrease platelet aggregation via mechanisms different than observed with aspirin. Platelet function is restored as the drug is eliminated from the body. NSAIDs should be avoided (if possible) in general surgery patients for 3-5 half-lives of the drug (usually 1-3 days) prior to surgery to reduce the risk of excessive bleeding. However, there is no scientific evidence to warrant discontinuance of NSAIDs prior to dental surgery. In medically complicated patients or extensive oral surgery, the decision to interrupt therapy must be based on the risk to benefit in an individual patient and a medical consult is suggested. Routine interruption of NSAID therapy for most dental procedures is not warranted. If therapy is continued without interruption, the clinician should anticipate the potential for slower clotting times.

Adverse Effects 1% to 10%:

Cardiovascular: Hypertension (1% to 4%)

Central nervous system: Headache (1% to 4%)

Gastrointestinal: Nausea (1% to 4%), vomiting (1% to 4%)

Ocular: Capsular opacity (5% to 10%), foreign body sensation (5% to 10%), intraocular pressure increased (5% to 10%), sticky sensation (5% to 10%), visual acuity decreased (5% to 10%), conjunctival edema (1% to 5%), corneal edema (1% to 5%), dry eye (1% to 5%), lid margin crusting (1% to 5%), ocular discomfort (1% to 5%), ocular hyperemia (1% to 5%), ocular pain (1% to 5%), ocular pruritus (1% to 5%), photophobia (1% to 5%), tearing (1% to 5%), vitreous detachment (1% to 5%)

Respiratory: Sinusitis (1% to 4%)

General Dosage Range Ophthalmic: *Children ≥10 years and Adults:* Instill 1 drop into affected eye(s) 3 times/day

Mechanism of Action Nepafenac is a prodrug which once converted to amfenac inhibits prostaglandin synthesis by decreasing the activity of the enzyme, cyclooxygenase, which results in decreased formation of prostaglandin precursors.

Pregnancy Risk Factor C/D (3rd trimester)

Nesiritide (ni SIR i tide)

U.S. Brand Names Natrecor®

Canadian Brand Names Natrecor®

Pharmacologic Category Natriuretic Peptide, B-Type, Human; Vasodilator

Use Treatment of acutely decompensated heart failure (HF) with dyspnea at rest or with minimal activity

Local Anesthetic/Vasoconstrictor Precautions No information available to require special precautions

Effects on Dental Treatment No significant effects or complications reported

Effects on Bleeding No information available to require special precautions

Adverse Effects Note: Frequencies cited below were recorded in VMAC trial at dosages similar to approved labeling. Higher frequencies have been observed in trials using higher dosages of nesiritide. The percentages marked with an asterisk (*) indicate frequency less than or equal to placebo or other standard therapy.

>10%:

Cardiovascular: Hypotension (total: 11%; symptomatic: 4% at recommended dose, up to 17% at higher doses)

Renal: Increased serum creatinine (28% with >0.5 mg/dL increase over baseline)

1% to 10%:

Cardiovascular: Ventricular tachycardia (3%)*, ventricular extrasystoles (3%)*, angina (2%)*, bradycardia (1%), tachycardia, atrial fibrillation, AV node conduction abnormalities

Central nervous system: Headache (8%)*, dizziness (3%), insomnia (2%)*, anxiety (3%), confusion, fever, paresthesia, somnolence, tremor

Dermatologic: Pruritus, rash

Gastrointestinal: Nausea (4%)*, abdominal pain (1%)*, vomiting (1%)*

Hematologic: Anemia

Local: Injection site reaction, catheter pain

Neuromuscular & skeletal: Back pain (4%), leg cramps

Ocular: Amblyopia

Respiratory: Apnea, cough increased, hemoptysis

Miscellaneous: Diaphoresis

Postmarketing and/or case reports: Hypersensitivity reactions (rare)

General Dosage Range I.V.: *Adults:* Bolus: 2 mcg/kg; Infusion: Initial: 0.01 mcg/kg/minute (maximum: 0.03 mcg/kg/minute)

Mechanism of Action Binds to guanylate cyclase receptor on vascular smooth muscle and endothelial cells, increasing intracellular cyclic GMP, resulting in smooth muscle cell relaxation. Has been shown to produce dose-dependent reductions in pulmonary capillary wedge pressure (PCWP) and systemic arterial pressure.

Pharmacodynamics/Kinetics

Onset of Action 15 minutes (60% of 3-hour effect achieved)

Duration of Action >60 minutes (up to several hours) for systolic blood pressure; hemodynamic effects persist longer than serum half-life would predict

Half-life Elimination Initial (distribution) 2 minutes; Terminal: 18 minutes

Time to Peak 1 hour

Pregnancy Risk Factor C

Nevirapine (ne VYE ra peen)

Related Information

HIV Infection and AIDS *on page 1883*

U.S. Brand Names Viramune®; Viramune® XR™

Canadian Brand Names Auro-Nevirapine; Viramune®

Pharmacologic Category Antiretroviral Agent, Reverse Transcriptase Inhibitor (Non-nucleoside)

Use In combination therapy with other antiretroviral agents for the treatment of HIV-1

Local Anesthetic/Vasoconstrictor Precautions No information available to require special precautions

Effects on Dental Treatment Key adverse event(s) related to dental treatment: Ulcerative stomatitis and oral lesions.

Effects on Bleeding No information available to require special precautions relative to hemostasis.

Adverse Effects Note: Potentially life-threatening nevirapine-associated adverse effects may present with the following symptoms: Abrupt onset of flu-like symptoms, abdominal pain, jaundice, or fever with or without rash; may progress to hepatic failure with encephalopathy. Skin rash is present in ~50% of cases.

Percentages of adverse effects vary by clinical trial and may vary by formulation; incidences reported below are based on immediate release formulation:

>10%:

Dermatologic: Rash (grade 1/2: 13%; grade 3/4: 2%)

Hepatic: ALT >250 units/L (5% to 14%); symptomatic hepatic events (4%, range: up to 11%)

1% to 10%:

Central nervous system: Headache (1% to 4%), fatigue (≤5%)

Gastrointestinal: Nausea (<1% to 9%), abdominal pain (≤2%), diarrhea (≤2%)

Hematologic: Neutropenia (4%)

Hepatic: AST >250 units/L (4% to 8%)

General Dosage Range Dosage adjustment recommended in patients with renal impairment

Oral, immediate release:

Neonates ≥15 days, Infants, and Children <8 years: Initial: 150-200 mg/m²/dose once daily (maximum: 200 mg/day); Maintenance: 150-200 mg/m²/dose twice daily (maximum: 400 mg/day).

Children ≥8 years: Initial: 120-150 mg/m²/dose once daily (maximum: 200 mg/day); Maintenance: 120-150 mg/m²/dose twice daily (maximum: 400 mg/day)

Adolescents and Adults: Initial: 200 mg once daily; Maintenance: 200 mg twice daily

Oral, extended release: *Adults:* Maintenance: 400 mg once daily

Mechanism of Action As a non-nucleoside reverse transcriptase inhibitor, nevirapine has activity against HIV-1 by binding to reverse transcriptase. It consequently blocks the RNA-dependent and DNA-dependent DNA polymerase activities including HIV-1 replication. It does not require intracellular phosphorylation for antiviral activity.

Pharmacodynamics/Kinetics

Half-life Elimination Decreases over 2- to 4-week time with chronic dosing due to autoinduction (ie, half-life = 45 hours initially and decreases to 25-30 hours)

Time to Peak Serum: Immediate release: 4 hours; Extended release:~24 hours

Pregnancy Risk Factor B

Niacin (NYE a sin)

Related Information

Cardiovascular Diseases *on page* 1848

U.S. Brand Names Niacin-Time® [OTC]; Niacor®; Niaspan®; Slo-Niacin® [OTC]

Canadian Brand Names Niaspan®; Niaspan® FCT; Niodan

Generic Availability (U.S.) Yes

Pharmacologic Category Antilipemic Agent, Miscellaneous; Vitamin, Water Soluble

Use Treatment of dyslipidemias (Fredrickson types IIa and IIb or primary hypercholesterolemia) as mono- or adjunctive therapy; to lower the risk of recurrent MI in patients with a history of MI and hyperlipidemia; to slow progression or promote regression of coronary artery disease; treatment of hypertriglyceridemia in patients at risk of pancreatitis

Unlabeled/Investigational Use Treatment of pellagra; dietary supplement

Local Anesthetic/Vasoconstrictor Precautions No information available to require special precautions

Effects on Dental Treatment No significant effects or complications reported

Effects on Bleeding No information available to require special precautions

Adverse Effects Frequency not defined.

Cardiovascular: Arrhythmias, atrial fibrillation, edema, flushing, hypotension, orthostasis, palpitation, syncope (rare), tachycardia

Central nervous system: Chills, dizziness, headache, insomnia, migraine, nervousness, pain

Dermatologic: Acanthosis nigricans, burning skin, dry skin, hyperpigmentation, maculopapular rash, pruritus, rash, skin discoloration, urticaria

Endocrine & metabolic: Glucose tolerance decreased, gout, phosphorous levels decreased, hyperuricemia

Gastrointestinal: Abdominal pain, amylase increased, diarrhea, dyspepsia, eructation, flatulence, nausea, peptic ulcers, vomiting

Hematologic: Platelet counts decreased

Hepatic: Hepatic necrosis (rare), hepatitis, jaundice, transaminases increased (dose-related), prothrombin time increased, total bilirubin increased

Neuromuscular & skeletal: CPK increased, leg cramps, myalgia, myasthenia, myopathy (with concurrent HMG-CoA reductase inhibitor), paresthesia, rhabdomyolysis (with concurrent HMG-CoA reductase inhibitor; rare), weakness

Ocular: Blurred vision, cystoid macular edema, toxic amblyopia

Respiratory: Cough, dyspnea

Miscellaneous: Diaphoresis, hypersensitivity reactions (rare; includes anaphylaxis, angioedema, laryngismus, vesiculobullous rash), LDH increased

Dosage Oral: **Note:** Formulations of niacin (regular release versus extended release) are not interchangeable.

Children:

Pellagra (unlabeled use): 50-100 mg/dose 3 times/day (some experts prefer niacinamide for treatment due to more favorable side effect profile)

Adequate intake (National Academy of Sciences, 1998):

0-5 months: 2 mg/day

6-11 months: 3 mg/day

Recommended daily allowances (National Academy of Sciences, 1998):
- 1-3 years: 6 mg/day
- 4-8 years: 8 mg/day
- 9-13 years: 12 mg/day
- 14-18 years: Female: 14 mg/day; Male: 16 mg/day
- ≥19 years: Refer to adult dosing

Adults:

Recommended daily allowances (National Academy of Sciences, 1998):
- ≥19 years: Female: 14 mg/day; Male: 16 mg/day
- Pregnancy (all ages): 18 mg/day
- Lactation (all ages): 17 mg/day

Dietary supplement (OTC labeling): 50 mg twice daily or 100 mg once daily. **Note:** Many over-the-counter formulations exist.

Hyperlipidemia:

Regular release formulation (Niacor®): Initial: 250 mg once daily (with evening meal); increase frequency and/or dose every 4-7 days to desired response or first-level therapeutic dose (1.5-2 g/day in 2-3 divided doses); after 2 months, may increase at 2- to 4-week intervals to 3 g/day in 3 divided doses (maximum dose: 6 g/day [NCEP recommends 4.5 g/day] in 3 divided doses). Usual daily dose after titration (NCEP, 2002): 1.5-3 g/day. **Note:** Many over-the-counter formulations exist.

Sustained release (or controlled release) formulations: **Note:** Several over-the-counter formulations exist. Usual daily dose after titration (NCEP, 2002): 1-2 g/day

Extended release formulation (Niaspan®): Initial: 500 mg at bedtime for 4 weeks, then 1 g at bedtime for 4 weeks; adjust dose to response and tolerance; may increase dose every 4 weeks by 500 mg/day to a maximum of 2 g/day. Usual daily dose after titration (NCEP, 2002): 1-2 g once daily

If additional LDL-lowering is necessary with lovastatin or simvastatin: Recommended initial lovastatin or simvastatin dose: 20 mg/day (maximum lovastatin or simvastatin dose: 40 mg/day); **Note:** Lovastatin prescribing information recommends a maximum dose of 20 mg/day with concurrent use of niacin (>1 g/day).

Pellagra (unlabeled use): 50-100 mg 3-4 times/day; maximum: 500 mg/day (some experts prefer niacinamide for treatment due to more favorable side effect profile)

Dosage adjustment in renal impairment: No dosage adjustment recommended; use with caution

Dosage adjustment in hepatic impairment: Contraindicated in patients with significant or unexplained hepatic dysfunction, active liver disease or unexplained persistent transaminase elevations.

Dosage adjustment for hepatic toxicity: Transaminases rise ≥3 times ULN, either persistent or if symptoms of nausea, fever, and/or malaise occur: Discontinue therapy.

Mechanism of Action Component of two coenzymes which is necessary for tissue respiration, lipid metabolism, and glycogenolysis; inhibits the synthesis of very low density lipoproteins (VLDL) and low density lipoproteins (LDL); may also increase the rate of chylomicron triglyceride removal from plasma.

Contraindications Hypersensitivity to niacin, niacinamide, or any component of the formulation; active hepatic disease or significant or unexplained persistent elevations in hepatic transaminases; active peptic ulcer; arterial hemorrhage

Warnings/Precautions Use with caution in patients with unstable angina or MI, diabetes (may interfere with glucose control), renal disease, active gallbladder disease (can exacerbate), gout, or with anticoagulants (may slightly increase prothrombin time). Use with caution in patients with a past history of hepatic impairment and/or who consume substantial amounts of ethanol; contraindicated with active liver disease or unexplained persistent transaminase elevation. Rare cases of rhabdomyolysis have occurred during concomitant use with HMG-CoA reductase inhibitors. With concurrent use or if symptoms suggestive of myopathy occur, monitor creatine phosphokinase (CPK) and potassium; use with caution in patients with renal impairment, inadequately treated hypothyroidism, patients with diabetes or the elderly; risk for myopathy and rhabdomyolysis may be increased.

Immediate and extended or sustained release products are not interchangeable. Cases of severe hepatotoxicity have occurred when immediate release (crystalline) niacin products have been substituted with sustained-release (modified release, timed-release) niacin products at equivalent doses. Patients should be initiated with low doses (eg, 500 mg at bedtime) with titration to achieve desired response. Flushing and pruritus, common adverse effects of niacin, may be attenuated with a gradual increase in dose, and/or by taking aspirin (adults: 325 mg) or an NSAID 30-60 minutes before dosing. Compliance is enhanced with twice-daily dosing (extended-release product excluded). Prior to initiation, secondary causes for hypercholesterolemia (eg, poorly controlled diabetes mellitus, hypothyroidism) should be excluded; management with diet and other nonpharmacologic measures (eg, exercise or weight reduction) should be attempted prior to initiation. Use has not been evaluated in Fredrickson type I or III dyslipidemias.

Drug Interactions

Avoid Concomitant Use There are no known interactions where it is recommended to avoid concomitant use.

Increased Effect/Toxicity

Niacin may increase the levels/effects of: HMG-CoA Reductase Inhibitors

Decreased Effect

The levels/effects of Niacin may be decreased by: Bile Acid Sequestrants

Ethanol/Nutrition/Herb Interactions Ethanol: Avoid heavy use; avoid use around niacin dose.

Dietary Considerations Should be taken with meal; low-fat meal if treating hyperlipidemia. Avoid hot drinks around the time of niacin dose.

Pharmacodynamics/Kinetics

Half-life Elimination 25-45 minutes

Time to Peak Serum: Immediate release formulation: 30-60 minutes; extended release formulation: 4-5 hours

Pregnancy Risk Factor A/C (dose exceeding RDA recommendation)

Lactation Enters breast milk/consider risk:benefit

Breast-Feeding Considerations Niacin is excreted in human breast milk. Because lipid-lowering doses of niacin may cause serious adverse reactions in nursing infants, a decision should be made whether to discontinue nursing or discontinue the drug, taking into account the importance of the drug to the mother.

Dosage Forms

Caplet, timed release, oral: 500 mg

Capsule, oral: 50 mg, 250 mg

Capsule, extended release, oral: 250 mg, 500 mg

Capsule, timed release, oral: 250 mg, 400 mg, 500 mg

Tablet, oral: 50 mg, 100 mg, 250 mg, 500 mg

Niacor®: 500 mg

Tablet, controlled release, oral:

Slo-Niacin® [OTC]: 250 mg, 500 mg, 750 mg

Tablet, extended release, oral:

Niaspan®: 500 mg, 750 mg, 1000 mg

Tablet, timed release, oral: 250 mg, 500 mg, 750 mg, 1000 mg

Niacin-Time® [OTC]: 500 mg

Niacinamide (nye a SIN a mide)

U.S. Brand Names Nicomide-T™ [OTC]

Pharmacologic Category Vitamin, Water Soluble

Use

Oral: Prophylaxis and treatment of pellagra

Topical: Improve the appearance of acne and decrease visible inflammation and irritation caused by acne medications

Local Anesthetic/Vasoconstrictor Precautions No information available to require special precautions

Effects on Dental Treatment No significant effects or complications reported

Effects on Bleeding No information available to require special precautions

Adverse Effects Frequency not defined.

Cardiovascular: Tachycardia

Dermatologic: Increased sebaceous gland activity, rash

Endocrine & metabolic: Hyperglycemia, hyperuricemia

Gastrointestinal: Bloating, flatulence, nausea

Neuromuscular & skeletal: Paresthesia in extremities

Ocular: Blurred vision

Respiratory: Wheezing

General Dosage Range

Oral:

Children: 10-50 mg every 6 hours

Adults: Initial: 100 mg every 6 hours; Maintenance: 50 mg every 8-12 hours

Topical: *Adults:* Apply to affected area on face twice daily

Mechanism of Action Used by the body as a source of niacin; is a component of two coenzymes which is necessary for tissue respiration, lipid metabolism, and glycogenolysis; does not have hypolipidemia or vasodilating effects. Niacinamide has anti-inflammatory properties which are believed to help decrease inflammatory acne lesions.

Pharmacodynamics/Kinetics

Half-life Elimination 45 minutes

Time to Peak Serum: 20-70 minutes

Pregnancy Risk Factor A/C (dose exceeding RDA recommendation)

Niacin and Lovastatin (NYE a sin & LOE va sta tin)

Related Information

Lovastatin *on page 1042*

Niacin *on page 1202*

U.S. Brand Names Advicor®

Canadian Brand Names Advicor®

Generic Availability (U.S.) No

Pharmacologic Category Antilipemic Agent, HMG-CoA Reductase Inhibitor; Antilipemic Agent, Miscellaneous

Use For use when treatment with both extended-release niacin and lovastatin is appropriate in combination with a standard cholesterol-lowering diet:

Extended-release niacin: Adjunctive treatment of dyslipidemias (types IIa and IIb or primary hypercholesterolemia) to lower the risk of recurrent MI and/or slow progression of coronary artery disease, including combination therapy with other antidyslipidemic agents when additional triglyceride-lowering or HDL-increasing effects are desired; treatment of hypertriglyceridemia in patients at risk of pancreatitis

Lovastatin: Treatment of primary hypercholesterolemia (Frederickson types IIa and IIb); primary and secondary prevention of cardiovascular disease

Local Anesthetic/Vasoconstrictor Precautions No information available to require special precautions

Effects on Dental Treatment No significant effects or complications reported

Effects on Bleeding No information available to require special precautions

Adverse Effects

>10%: Cardiovascular: Flushing (71%)

1% to 10%:

Central nervous system: Headache (9%), pain (8%)

Dermatologic: Pruritus (7%), rash (5%)

Endocrine & metabolic: Hyperglycemia (4%)

Gastrointestinal: Nausea (7%), diarrhea (6%), abdominal pain (4%), dyspepsia (3%), vomiting (3%)

Neuromuscular & skeletal: Back pain (5%), weakness (5%), myalgia (3%)

Miscellaneous: Flu-like syndrome (6%)

Dosage Dosage forms are a fixed combination of niacin and lovastatin.

Oral: Adults: Lowest dose: Niacin 500 mg/lovastatin 20 mg; may increase by not more than 500 mg (niacin) at 4-week intervals (maximum dose: Niacin 2000 mg/lovastatin 40 mg daily); should be taken at bedtime with a low-fat snack. **Note:** If therapy is interrupted for >7 days, reinstitution of therapy should begin with the lowest dose followed by retitration as needed.

Not for use as initial therapy of dyslipidemias. May be substituted for equivalent dose of Niaspan®, however, manufacturer does not recommend direct substitution with other niacin products.

Dosage adjustment in renal impairment:

Mild-to-moderate impairment: No dosage adjustment required

Cl_{cr} <30 mL/minute: Use doses of lovastatin >20 mg/day with caution

Dosage adjustment in hepatic impairment: Do not use in active liver disease or unexplained persistent elevations of serum transaminases.

Mechanism of Action Lovastatin acts by competitively inhibiting 3-hydroxyl-3-methylglutaryl-coenzyme A (HMG-CoA) reductase, the enzyme that catalyzes the rate-limiting step in cholesterol biosynthesis. Niacin is a component of two coenzymes which is necessary for tissue respiration, lipid metabolism, and glycogenolysis; inhibits the synthesis of very low density lipoproteins.

Contraindications Hypersensitivity to lovastatin, niacin, or any component of the formulation; active liver disease; unexplained persistent elevations of serum transaminases; active peptic ulcer disease; arterial bleeding; pregnancy; breast-feeding

Warnings/Precautions Use with caution in patients who consume large amounts of ethanol or who have a history of liver disease; use is contraindicated in patients with active liver disease or unexplained persistent elevations of serum transaminases. Obtain baseline transaminase levels prior to initiation of therapy; repeat in 6-12 weeks and with any subsequent increase in dosage, then periodically once a stable dose has been reached. Formulations of niacin (regular release versus extended release) are not interchangeable; cases of severe hepatic toxicity, including fulminant hepatic necrosis, have occurred in patients who have substituted niacin products at equivalent doses.

Myopathy and/or rhabdomyolysis with acute renal failure has occurred with HMG-CoA reductase inhibitors. Combination with niacin may increase the risk of this event, and patients should be monitored closely, particularly at higher doses (niacin >1 g/day). Risk is increased in patients with renal impairment, inadequately treated hypothyroidism, or concurrent use of potent CYP3A4 inhibitors (eg, cyclosporine, azole antifungals, macrolide antibiotics, telithromycin, protease inhibitors, nefazodone, large quantities of grapefruit juice). Monitor closely if used with other drugs associated with myopathy (eg, colchicine). Weigh the risk versus benefit when combining any of these drugs with lovastatin. Temporarily discontinue for elective major surgery, acute medical or surgical conditions, or in any patient experiencing an acute or serious condition predisposing to renal failure secondary to rhabdomyolysis. Based upon current evidence, HMG-CoA reductase inhibitor therapy should be continued in the perioperative period unless risk outweighs cardioprotective benefit. Use with caution in elderly patients as these patients are predisposed to myopathy. Patients should be instructed to report unexplained muscle pain, tenderness, weakness, or brown urine. Obtain a baseline CK level prior to initiation of therapy; repeat CK level with onset of unexplained muscle symptoms; discontinue treatment if CK levels rise to >10 times the upper limit of normal with concomitant muscle symptoms.

Use caution in unstable angina or CAD (risk of arrhythmias at high doses), diabetes (may interfere with glucose control), renal disease, active gallbladder disease (may exacerbate), or gout. Flushing and pruritus, common adverse effects of niacin, may be attenuated with a gradual increase in dose and/or by taking aspirin or another NSAID (eg, ibuprofen) 30-60 minutes before dosing.

Drug Interactions

Metabolism/Transport Effects Lovastatin: **Substrate** of CYP3A4 (major), P-glycoprotein; **Inhibits** CYP2C9 (weak), 2D6 (weak), 3A4 (weak)

Avoid Concomitant Use

Avoid concomitant use of Niacin and Lovastatin with any of the following: Protease Inhibitors; Red Yeast Rice

Increased Effect/Toxicity

Niacin and Lovastatin may increase the levels/effects of: DAPTOmycin; Diltiazem; HMG-CoA Reductase Inhibitors; Trabectedin; Vitamin K Antagonists

The levels/effects of Niacin and Lovastatin may be increased by: Amiodarone; Antifungal Agents (Azole Derivatives, Systemic); Colchicine; Conivaptan; CycloSPORINE; CycloSPORINE (Systemic); CYP3A4 Inhibitors (Moderate); CYP3A4 Inhibitors (Strong); Danazol; Dasatinib; Diltiazem; Dronedarone; Fenofibrate; Fenofibric Acid; Fluconazole; Gemfibrozil; Grapefruit Juice; Macrolide Antibiotics; Nefazodone; Niacin; Niacinamide; P-Glycoprotein Inhibitors; Protease Inhibitors; QuiNINE; Red Yeast Rice; Rifamycin Derivatives; Sildenafil; Verapamil

Decreased Effect

The levels/effects of Niacin and Lovastatin may be decreased by: Antacids; Bile Acid Sequestrants; Bosentan; CYP3A4 Inducers (Strong); Deferasirox; Efavirenz; Etravirine; Fosphenytoin; P-Glycoprotein Inducers; Phenytoin; Rifamycin Derivatives; St Johns Wort; Tocilizumab

Ethanol/Nutrition/Herb Interactions

Ethanol: Consumption of large amounts of ethanol may increase the risk of liver damage with HMG-CoA reductase inhibitors. Concurrent ingestion of ethanol may increase the risk of flushing associated with niacin.

Food: Lovastatin absorption may be decreased with food, however, the combination product is recommended to be taken with a low-fat snack at bedtime. Lovastatin serum concentrations may be increased if taken with grapefruit juice; avoid concurrent use. Concurrent ingestion of hot liquids may increase the risk of flushing associated with niacin.

Herb/Nutraceutical: St John's wort may decrease lovastatin levels. Red yeast rice contains an estimated 2.4 mg lovastatin per 600 mg rice.

Dietary Considerations Continue standard cholesterol-lowering diet during therapy. Should be taken with a low-fat snack.

Pregnancy Risk Factor X

Lactation Enters breast milk/contraindicated

Breast-Feeding Considerations Niacin is excreted in breast milk. The excretion of lovastatin is unknown, although similar agents are known to be excreted in breast milk. Use during breast-feeding is contraindicated.

Dosage Forms

Tablet, variable release:

Advicor®: 500/20: Niacin 500 mg [extended release] and lovastatin 20 mg [immediate release]; 750/20: Niacin 750 mg [extended release] and lovastatin 20 mg [immediate release]; 1000/20: Niacin 1000 mg [extended release] and lovastatin 20 mg [immediate release]; 1000/40: Niacin 1000 mg [extended release] and lovastatin 40 mg [immediate release]

Niacin and Simvastatin (NYE a sin & sim va STAT in)

Related Information

Niacin *on page* 1202

Simvastatin *on page* 1527

U.S. Brand Names Simcor®

Pharmacologic Category Antilipemic Agent, HMG-CoA Reductase Inhibitor; Antilipemic Agent, Miscellaneous

Use Reduce total cholesterol, LDL, Apo B, non-HDL, TG, and/or increase HDL in patients with primary hypercholesterolemia, mixed dyslipidemia, or hypertriglyceridemia in combination with standard cholesterol-lowering diet when simvastatin or niacin monotherapy is inadequate

Local Anesthetic/Vasoconstrictor Precautions No information available to require special precautions

Effects on Dental Treatment No significant effects or complications reported

Effects on Bleeding No information available to require special precautions

Adverse Effects Reactions/percentages reported with combination product; also refer to individual agents.

>10%: Cardiovascular: Flushing (≤59%)

1% to 10%:

- Central nervous system: Headache (5%)
- Dermatologic: Pruritus (3%)
- Gastrointestinal: Diarrhea (3%), nausea (3%)
- Neuromuscular & skeletal: Back pain (3%)

Frequency not defined: Alkaline phosphatase increased, amylase increased, bilirubin increased, creatinine kinase increased, fasting blood glucose increased, GGT increased, LDH increased, phosphorus decreased, platelets decreased, prothrombin time increased, thyroid function test abnormalities, transaminases increased, uric acid increased

General Dosage Range Oral: *Adults:* Niacin 500-2000 mg/simvastatin 20-40 mg once daily

Mechanism of Action

Niacin is a component of two coenzymes which is necessary for tissue respiration, lipid metabolism, and glycogenolysis; inhibits the synthesis of very low density lipoproteins.

Simvastatin is a derivative of lovastatin that acts by competitively inhibiting 3-hydroxy-3-methylglutaryl-coenzyme A (HMG-CoA) reductase, the enzyme that catalyzes the rate-limiting step in cholesterol biosynthesis.

Pregnancy Risk Factor X

NiCARdipine (nye KAR de peen)

Related Information

Calcium Channel Blockers and Gingival Hyperplasia *on page* 2014

Cardiovascular Diseases *on page* 1848

U.S. Brand Names Cardene® I.V.; Cardene® SR

Pharmacologic Category Calcium Channel Blocker; Calcium Channel Blocker, Dihydropyridine

Use Chronic stable angina (immediate-release product only); management of hypertension (immediate and sustained release products); parenteral only for short-term use when oral treatment is not feasible

Unlabeled/Investigational Use Congestive heart failure, control of blood pressure in acute ischemic stroke and spontaneous intracranial hemorrhage, postoperative hypertension associated with carotid endarterectomy, perioperative hypertension, prevention of migraine headaches, subarachnoid hemorrhage associated cerebral vasospasm

Local Anesthetic/Vasoconstrictor Precautions No information available to require special precautions

Effects on Dental Treatment Key adverse event(s) related to dental treatment: Xerostomia (normal salivary flow resumes upon discontinuation). Other drugs of this class can cause gingival hyperplasia (ie, nifedipine). The first case of nicardipine-induced gingival hyperplasia has been reported in a child taking 40-50 mg daily for 20 months.

Effects on Bleeding No information available to require special precautions

Adverse Effects 1% to 10%:

Cardiovascular: Cardiovascular: Flushing (6% to 10%), peripheral edema (dose related; 6% to 8%), hypotension (I.V. 6%), increased angina (dose related; 6%), palpitation (3% to 4%), tachycardia (1% to 4%), vasodilation (1% to 5%), chest pain (I.V. 1%), ECG abnormal (I.V. 1%), extrasystoles (I.V. 1%), hemopericardium (I.V. 1%), hypertension (I.V. 1%), orthostasis (1%), supraventricular tachycardia (I.V. 1%), syncope (1%), ventricular extrasystoles (I.V. 1%), ventricular tachycardia (I.V. 1%)

Central nervous system: Headache (6% to 15%), dizziness (1% to 7%), hypoesthesia (1%), intracranial hemorrhage (1%) pain (1%), somnolence (1%)

Dermatologic: Rash (1%)

Endocrine & metabolic: Hypokalemia (I.V. 1%)

Gastrointestinal: Nausea (2% to 5%), vomiting (I.V. 5%), dyspepsia (oral 2%), abdominal pain (I.V. 1%), dry mouth (1%)

Genitourinary: Polyuria (1%)

Local: Injection site pain (I.V. 1%), injection site reaction (I.V. 1%)

Neuromuscular & skeletal: Weakness (1% to 6%), myalgia (1%), paresthesia (1%)

Renal: Hematuria (1%)

Respiratory: Dyspnea (1%)

Miscellaneous: Diaphoresis (1%)

General Dosage Range Dosage adjustment recommended in patients with hepatic or renal impairment

I.V.: *Adults:* Initial: 5 mg/hour; Maintenance: 3-15 mg/hour

Oral:

Immediate release: *Adults:* Initial: 20 mg 3 times/day; Maintenance: 20-40 mg 3 times/day

Sustained release: *Adults:* Initial: 30 mg twice daily; Maintenance: Up to 60 mg twice daily

Mechanism of Action Inhibits calcium ion from entering the "slow channels" or select voltage-sensitive areas of vascular smooth muscle and myocardium during depolarization, producing a relaxation of coronary vascular smooth muscle and coronary vasodilation; increases myocardial oxygen delivery in patients with vasospastic angina

Pharmacodynamics/Kinetics

Onset of Action Oral: 0.5-2 hours; I.V.: 10 minutes; Hypotension: ~20 minutes

Duration of Action I.V.: ≤8 hours; Oral: Immediate release capsules: ≤8 hours, Sustained release capsules: 8-12 hours

Half-life Elimination 2-4 hours

Time to Peak Serum: Oral: Immediate release: 30-120 minutes; Sustained release: 60-240 minutes

Pregnancy Risk Factor C

Nicotine (nik oh TEEN)

U.S. Brand Names Commit® [OTC]; NicoDerm® CQ® [OTC]; Nicorelief [OTC]; Nicorette® [OTC]; Nicotrol® Inhaler; Nicotrol® NS; Thrive™ [OTC]

Canadian Brand Names Habitrol®; Nicoderm®; Nicorette®; Nicorette® Plus; Nicotrol®

Generic Availability (U.S.) Yes: Transdermal patch and gum

Pharmacologic Category Smoking Cessation Aid

Dental Use Treatment to aid smoking cessation for the relief of nicotine withdrawal symptoms (including nicotine craving)

Use Treatment to aid smoking cessation for the relief of nicotine withdrawal symptoms (including nicotine craving)

Unlabeled/Investigational Use Management of ulcerative colitis (transdermal)

Local Anesthetic/Vasoconstrictor Precautions No information available to require special precautions

Effects on Dental Treatment Key adverse event(s) related to dental treatment: Chewing gum: Excessive salivation, mouth/throat soreness, jaw muscle ache, hiccups, tachycardia, headache (mild), vomiting, belching, nausea, xerostomia (normal salivary flow resumes upon discontinuation), dizziness, nervousness, GI distress, hoarseness, and muscle pain.

Effects on Bleeding No information available to require special precautions

Adverse Effects

Nasal spray/inhaler:

>10%:

Central nervous system: Headache (18% to 26%)

Gastrointestinal: Inhaler: Mouth/throat irritation (66%), dyspepsia (18%)

Respiratory: Inhaler: Cough (32%), rhinitis (23%)

1% to 10%:

Dermatologic: Acne (3%)

Endocrine & metabolic: Dysmenorrhea (3%)

Gastrointestinal: Flatulence (4%), gum problems (4%), diarrhea, hiccup, nausea, taste disturbance, tooth disorder

Neuromuscular & skeletal: Back pain (6%), arthralgia (5%), jaw/neck pain

Respiratory: Nasal burning (nasal spray), sinusitis

Miscellaneous: Withdrawal symptoms

Adverse events previously reported in prescription labeling for chewing gum, lozenge and/or transdermal systems. Frequency not defined; may be product or dose specific:

Central nervous system: Concentration impaired, depression, dizziness, headache, insomnia, nervousness, pain

Gastrointestinal: Aphthous stomatitis, constipation, cough, diarrhea, dyspepsia, flatulence, gingival bleeding, glossitis, hiccups, jaw pain, nausea, salivation increased, stomatitis, taste perversion, tooth disorder, ulcerative stomatitis, xerostomia

Dermatologic: Rash

Local: Application site reaction, local edema, local erythema

Neuromuscular & skeletal: Arthralgia, myalgia, paresthesia

Respiratory: Cough, sinusitis

Miscellaneous: Allergic reaction, diaphoresis

Dental Usual Dosage

Tobacco cessation (patients should be advised to completely stop smoking upon initiation of therapy): Adults:

Gum: Chew 1 piece of gum when urge to smoke, up to 24 pieces/day. Patients who smoke <25 cigarettes/day should start with 2-mg strength; patients smoking ≥25 cigarettes/day should start with the 4-mg strength. Use according to the following 12-week dosing schedule:

Weeks 1-6: Chew 1 piece of gum every 1-2 hours; to increase chances of quitting, chew at least 9 pieces/day during the first 6 weeks

Weeks 7-9: Chew 1 piece of gum every 2-4 hours

Weeks 10-12: Chew 1 piece of gum every 4-8 hours

Inhaler: Oral: Usually 6 to 16 cartridges per day; best effect was achieved by frequent continuous puffing (20 minutes); recommended duration of treatment is 3 months, after which patients may be weaned from the inhaler by gradual reduction of the daily dose over 6-12 weeks

Lozenge: Oral: Patients who smoke their first cigarette within 30 minutes of waking should use the 4 mg strength; otherwise the 2 mg strength is recommended. Use according to the following 12-week dosing schedule:

Weeks 1-6: One lozenge every 1-2 hours

Weeks 7-9: One lozenge every 2-4 hours

Weeks 10-12: One lozenge every 4-8 hours

Note: Use at least 9 lozenges/day during first 6 weeks to improve chances of quitting; do not use more than one lozenge at a time (maximum: 5 lozenges every 6 hours, 20 lozenges/day)

Spray: Nasal: 1-2 sprays/hour; do not exceed more than 5 doses (10 sprays) per hour [maximum: 40 doses/day (80 sprays); each dose (2 sprays) contains 1 mg of nicotine]

Transdermal patch: Topical: Apply new patch every 24 hours to nonhairy, clean, dry skin on the upper body or upper outer arm; each patch should be applied to a different site. **Note:** Adjustment may be required during initial treatment (move to higher dose if experiencing withdrawal symptoms; lower dose if side effects are experienced).

NicoDerm CQ®:

Patients smoking >10 cigarettes/day: Begin with step 1 (21 mg/day) for 6 weeks, **followed by** step 2 (14 mg/day) for 2 weeks; **finish with** step 3 (7 mg/day) for 2 weeks

Patients smoking ≤10 cigarettes/day: Begin with step 2 (14 mg/day) for 6 weeks, **followed by** step 3 (7 mg/day) for 2 weeks

Note: Patients who are receiving >600 mg/day of cimetidine: Decrease to the next lower patch size

Benefits of use of nicotine transdermal patches beyond 3 months have not been demonstrated

Dosage

Smoking deterrent: Patients should be advised to completely stop smoking upon initiation of therapy.

Oral:

Gum: Chew 1 piece of gum when urge to smoke, up to 24 pieces/day. Patients who smoke <25 cigarettes/day should start with 2-mg strength; patients smoking ≥25 cigarettes/day should start with the 4-mg strength. Use according to the following 12-week dosing schedule:

Weeks 1-6: Chew 1 piece of gum every 1-2 hours; to increase chances of quitting, chew at least 9 pieces/day during the first 6 weeks

Weeks 7-9: Chew 1 piece of gum every 2-4 hours

Weeks 10-12: Chew 1 piece of gum every 4-8 hours

Inhaler: Usually 6 to 16 cartridges per day; best effect was achieved by frequent continuous puffing (20 minutes); recommended duration of treatment is 3 months, after which patients may be weaned from the inhaler by gradual reduction of the daily dose over 6-12 weeks

Lozenge: Patients who smoke their first cigarette within 30 minutes of waking should use the 4 mg strength; otherwise the 2 mg strength is recommended. Use according to the following 12-week dosing schedule:

Weeks 1-6: One lozenge every 1-2 hours

Weeks 7-9: One lozenge every 2-4 hours

Weeks 10-12: One lozenge every 4-8 hours

Note: Use at least 9 lozenges/day during first 6 weeks to improve chances of quitting; do not use more than one lozenge at a time (maximum: 5 lozenges every 6 hours, 20 lozenges/day)

Topical:

Transdermal patch: Apply new patch every 24 hours to nonhairy, clean, dry skin on the upper body or upper outer arm; each patch should be applied to a different site. **Note:** Adjustment may be required during initial treatment (move to higher dose if experiencing withdrawal symptoms; lower dose if side effects are experienced).

NicoDerm CQ®:

Patients smoking >10 cigarettes/day: Begin with **step 1** (21 mg/day) for 6 weeks, followed by **step 2** (14 mg/day) for 2 weeks; finish with **step 3** (7 mg/day) for 2 weeks

Patients smoking ≤10 cigarettes/day: Begin with **step 2** (14 mg/day) for 6 weeks, followed by **step 3** (7 mg/day) for 2 weeks

Note: Patients receiving >600 mg/day of cimetidine: Decrease to the next lower patch size

Note: Benefits of use of nicotine transdermal patches beyond 3 months have not been demonstrated.

Nasal: Spray: 1-2 sprays/hour; do not exceed more than 5 doses (10 sprays) per hour [maximum: 40 doses/day (80 sprays); each dose (2 sprays) contains 1 mg of nicotine]

Mechanism of Action Nicotine is one of two naturally-occurring alkaloids which exhibit their primary effects via autonomic ganglia stimulation. The other alkaloid is lobeline which has many actions similar to those of nicotine but is less potent. Nicotine is a potent ganglionic and central nervous system stimulant, the actions of which are mediated via nicotine-specific receptors. Biphasic actions are observed depending upon the dose administered. The main effect of nicotine in small doses is stimulation of all autonomic ganglia; with larger doses, initial stimulation is followed by blockade of transmission. Biphasic effects are also evident in the adrenal medulla; discharge of catecholamines occurs with small doses, whereas prevention of catecholamines release is seen with higher doses as a response to splanchnic nerve stimulation. Stimulation of the central nervous system (CNS) is characterized by tremors and respiratory excitation. However, convulsions may occur with higher doses, along with respiratory failure secondary to both central paralysis and peripheral blockade to respiratory muscles.

Contraindications Hypersensitivity to nicotine or any component of the formulation; patients who are smoking during the postmyocardial infarction period; patients with life-threatening arrhythmias, or severe or worsening angina pectoris; active temporomandibular joint disease (gum); pregnancy; not for use in nonsmokers

Warnings/Precautions Hazardous agent - use appropriate precautions for handling and disposal. Use caution in patients with hyperthyroidism, pheochromocytoma, or insulin-dependent diabetes. Use with caution in oropharyngeal inflammation and in patients with history of esophagitis, peptic ulcer, coronary artery disease, recent MI, serious cardiac arrhythmias, vasospastic disease, angina, hypertension, hyperthyroidism, pheochromocytoma, diabetes, severe renal dysfunction, and hepatic dysfunction. The oral inhaler and nasal spray should be used with caution in patients with bronchospastic disease (other forms of nicotine replacement may be preferred). Use of nasal product is not recommended with chronic nasal disorders (eg, allergy, rhinitis, nasal polyps, and sinusitis). Transdermal patch may contain conducting metal (eg, aluminum); remove patch prior to MRI. Cautious use of topical nicotine in patients with certain skin diseases. Hypersensitivity to the topical products can occur. Dental problems may be worsened by chewing the gum. Urge patients to stop smoking completely when initiating therapy.

Drug Interactions

Metabolism/Transport Effects Substrate (minor) of CYP1A2, 2A6, 2B6, 2C9, 2C19, 2D6, 2E1, 3A4; **Inhibits** CYP2A6 (weak), 2E1 (weak)

Avoid Concomitant Use There are no known interactions where it is recommended to avoid concomitant use.

Increased Effect/Toxicity

Nicotine may increase the levels/effects of: Adenosine

The levels/effects of Nicotine may be increased by: Cimetidine; Conivaptan

Decreased Effect

The levels/effects of Nicotine may be decreased by: Peginterferon Alfa-2b; Tocilizumab

Ethanol/Nutrition/Herb Interactions Food: Lozenge: Acidic foods/beverages decrease absorption of nicotine.

Dietary Considerations Some products may contain phenylalanine and/or sodium.

Pharmacodynamics/Kinetics

Onset of Action Intranasal: More closely approximate the time course of plasma nicotine levels observed after cigarette smoking than other dosage forms

Duration of Action Transdermal: 24 hours

Half-life Elimination 4 hours; Nasal spray: 1-2 hours

Time to Peak Serum: Transdermal: 8-9 hours; Nasal spray: 10-20 minutes

Pregnancy Risk Factor D (nasal)

Lactation Excretion in breast milk unknown/use caution

Breast-Feeding Considerations Nicotine from cigarette smoke is found in breast milk at 1.5-3 times the maternal plasma concentrations. The amount from nicotine replacement products is not known. Women who are breast-feeding are encouraged not to smoke.

Dosage Forms

Gum, chewing, oral: 2 mg (20s, 40s, 50s, 100s, 108s, 110s); 4 mg (20s, 40s, 48s, 50s, 100s, 108s, 110s)

Nicorelief [OTC]: 2 mg (50s, 110s); 4 mg (50s, 110s)

Nicorette® [OTC]: 2 mg (40s, 48s, 50s, 100s, 108s, 110s, 168s, 170s, 192s, 200s, 216s); 4 mg (40s, 48s, 50s, 100s, 108s, 110s, 168s, 170s, 192s, 200s, 216s)

Thrive™ [OTC]: 2 mg (40s); 4 mg (40s)

Lozenge, oral:

Commit® [OTC]: 2 mg (48s, 72s); 4 mg (48s, 72s)

Nicorette® [OTC]: 4 mg (50s)

Oral inhalation system, for oral inhalation:

Nicotrol® Inhaler: 10 mg (10 mL)

Patch, transdermal: 7 mg/24 hours (7s, 14s, 30s); 14 mg/24 hours (7s, 14s, 30s); 21 mg/24 hours (7s, 14s, 30s)

NicoDerm® CQ® [OTC]: 7 mg/24 hours (14s); 14 mg/24 hours (14s); 21 mg/24 hours (7s, 14s)

Solution, intranasal:

Nicotrol® NS: 10 mg/mL (10 mL)

References

Christen AG and Christen JA, "The Prescription of Transdermal Nicotine Patches for Tobacco-Using Dental Patients: Current Status in Indiana," *J Indiana Dent Assoc*, 1992, 71(6):12-8.

Davies GM, Willner P, James DL, et al, "Influence of Nicotine Gum on Acute Cravings for Cigarettes," *J Psychopharmacol*, 2004, 18(1):83-7.

Li Wan Po A, "Transdermal Nicotine in Smoking Cessation. A Meta-Analysis," *Eur J Clin Pharmacol*, 1993, 45(6):519-28.

Stafne EE, "The Nicotine Transdermal Patch: Use in the Dental Office Tobacco Cessation Program," *Northwest Dent*, 1994, 73(3):19-22.

Tonstad S and Johnston JA, "Does Bupropion Have Advantages Over Other Medical Therapies in the Cessation of Smoking?" *Expert Opin Pharmacother*, 2004, 5(4):727-34.

Transdermal Nicotine Study Group, "Transdermal Nicotine for Smoking Cessation. Six-Month Results From Two Multicenter Controlled Clinical Trials," *JAMA*, 1991, 266(22):3133-8.

Westman EC, Levin ED, and Rose JE, "The Nicotine Patch in Smoking Cessation," *Arch Intern Med*, 1993, 153(16):1917-23.

Wynn RL, "Nicotine Patches in Smoking Cessation," *AGD Impact*, 1994, 22:14.

NIFEdipine (nye FED i peen)

Related Information

Calcium Channel Blockers and Gingival Hyperplasia *on page 2014*

Cardiovascular Diseases *on page 1848*

U.S. Brand Names Adalat® CC; Afeditab® CR; Nifediac CC®; Nifedical XL®; Procardia XL®; Procardia®

Canadian Brand Names Adalat® XL®; Apo-Nifed PA®; Apo-Nifed®; Gen-Nifedipine XL; Mylan-Nifedipine Extended Release; Nifedipine PA; Nu-Nifed; Nu-Nifedipine-PA; PMS-Nifedipine

Generic Availability (U.S.) Yes

Pharmacologic Category Calcium Channel Blocker; Calcium Channel Blocker, Dihydropyridine

Use Management of chronic stable or vasospastic angina; treatment of hypertension (sustained release products only)

Unlabeled/Investigational Use Management of pulmonary hypertension, preterm labor, Raynaud's phenomenon

Local Anesthetic/Vasoconstrictor Precautions No information available to require special precautions

Effects on Dental Treatment Nifedipine has been reported to cause 10% incidence of gingival hyperplasia; effects from 30-100 mg/day have appeared after 1-9 months. Discontinuance results in complete disappearance or marked regression of symptoms; symptoms will reappear upon remedication. Marked regression occurs after 1 week and complete disappearance of symptoms has occurred within 15 days. If a gingivectomy is performed and use of the drug is continued or resumed, hyperplasia usually will recur. The success of the gingivectomy usually requires that the medication be discontinued or that a switch to a noncalcium channel blocker be made. If for some reason nifedipine cannot be discontinued, hyperplasia has not recurred after gingivectomy when extensive plaque control was performed. If nifedipine is changed to another class of cardiovascular agent, the gingival hyperplasia will probably regress and resolve. Switching to another calcium channel blocker may result in continued hyperplasia.

Effects on Bleeding No information available to require special precautions

Adverse Effects

>10%:

Cardiovascular: Flushing (10% to 25%; extended release products 3% to 4%), peripheral edema (dose related 7% to 30%)

Central nervous system: Dizziness/lightheadedness/giddiness (10% to 27%), headache (10% to 23%)

Gastrointestinal: Nausea/heartburn (10% to 11%)

≥1% to 10%:

Cardiovascular: Palpitation (≤2% to 7%), transient hypotension (dose related 5%), CHF (2%)

Central nervous system: Nervousness/mood changes (≤2% to 7%), fatigue (6%), shakiness (≤2%), jitteriness (≤2%), sleep disturbances (≤2%), difficulties in balance (≤2%), fever (≤2%), chills (≤2%)

Dermatologic: Dermatitis (≤2%), pruritus (≤2%), urticaria (≤2%)

Endocrine & metabolic: Sexual difficulties (≤2%)

Gastrointestinal: Diarrhea (≤2%), constipation (≤2%), cramps (≤2%), flatulence (≤2%), gingival hyperplasia (≤10%)

Neuromuscular & skeletal: Muscle cramps/tremor (≤2% to 8%), weakness (<3%), inflammation (≤2%), joint stiffness (≤2%)

Ocular: Blurred vision (≤2%)

Respiratory: Cough/wheezing (6%), nasal congestion/sore throat (≤2% to 6%), chest congestion (≤2%), dyspnea (≤2%)

Miscellaneous: Diaphoresis (≤2%)

Dosage Oral:

Children 1-17 years: Hypertension (unlabeled use): Extended release tablet: Initial: 0.25-0.5 mg/kg/day once daily or in 2 divided doses; maximum: 3 mg/kg/day up to 120 mg/day

Adults: **Note:** Dosage adjustments should occur at 7- to 14-day intervals, to allow for adequate assessment of new dose; when switching from immediate release to sustained release formulations, use same total daily dose.

Chronic stable or vasospastic angina:

Immediate release: Initial: 10 mg 3 times/day; usual dose: 10-20 mg 3 times/day; coronary artery spasm may require up to 20-30 mg 3-4 times/day; single doses >30 mg and total daily doses >120 mg are rarely needed; maximum: 180 mg/day; **Note:** Do not use for acute anginal episodes; may precipitate myocardial infarction

Extended release: Initial: 30 or 60 mg once daily; maximum: 120-180 mg/day

Hypertension: Extended release: Initial: 30 or 60 mg once daily; maximum: 90-120 mg/day

Pulmonary hypertension (unlabeled use; Galie, 2004): Extended release: Initial: 30 mg twice daily; may increase cautiously to 120-240 mg/day

Raynaud's phenomenon (unlabeled use; Wigley, 2002): Extended release: Dosage range: 30-120 mg once daily

Hemodialysis: Supplemental dose is not necessary

Peritoneal dialysis effects: Supplemental dose is not necessary

Dosing adjustment in hepatic impairment: Clearance of nifedipine is reduced in cirrhotic patients leading to increased systemic exposure; monitor closely for adverse effects/toxicity and consider dose adjustments.

Mechanism of Action Inhibits calcium ion from entering the "slow channels" or select voltage-sensitive areas of vascular smooth muscle and myocardium during depolarization, producing a relaxation of coronary vascular smooth muscle and coronary vasodilation; increases myocardial oxygen delivery in patients with vasospastic angina; also reduces peripheral vascular resistance, producing a reduction in arterial blood pressure.

Contraindications Hypersensitivity to nifedipine or any component of the formulation; concomitant use with strong CYP3A4 inducers (eg, rifampin); cardiogenic shock; immediate release preparation for treatment of urgent or emergent hypertension (Chobanian, 2003); acute MI (Antman, 2004)

Warnings/Precautions Symptomatic hypotension with or without syncope can rarely occur; blood pressure must be lowered at a rate appropriate for the patient's clinical condition. **The use of immediate release nifedipine (sublingually or orally) in hypertensive emergencies and urgencies is neither safe nor effective.** Serious adverse events (eg, death, cerebrovascular ischemia, syncope, stroke, acute myocardial infarction, and fetal distress) have been reported. **Immediate release nifedipine should not be used for acute blood pressure reduction.**

Blood pressure lowering should be done at a rate appropriate for the patient's condition. Rapid drops in blood pressure can lead to arterial insufficiency. Increased angina and/or MI have occurred with initiation or dosage titration of dihydropyridine calcium channel blockers; use with caution in patients with obstructive coronary disease especially in the absence of concurrent beta-blockade. Use with caution before major surgery. Cardiopulmonary bypass, intraoperative blood loss or vasodilating anesthesia may result in severe hypotension and/or increased fluid requirements. Consider withdrawing nifedipine (>36 hours) before surgery if possible.

The most common side effect is peripheral edema; occurs within 2-3 weeks of starting therapy. Reflex tachycardia may occur with use. Use with caution in HF or severe aortic stenosis (especially with concomitant beta-adrenergic blocker), severe left ventricular dysfunction, renal impairment, hypertrophic cardiomyopathy (especially obstructive), concomitant therapy with beta-blockers or digoxin, and edema. Use caution in patients with severe hepatic impairment. Clearance of nifedipine is reduced in cirrhotic patients leading to increased systemic exposure; monitor closely for adverse effects/toxicity and consider dose adjustments. Mild and transient elevations in liver function enzymes may be apparent within 8 weeks of therapy initiation. Abrupt withdrawal may cause rebound angina in patients with CAD. Short-acting nifedipine may be inappropriate for use in the elderly due to potential to cause hypotension and constipation (Beers Criteria). Immediate release formulations should not be used to manage essential hypertension, adequate studies to evaluate outcomes have not been conducted. Avoid use of extended release tablets (Procardia XL®) in patients with known stricture/narrowing of the GI tract.

Use with caution in patients taking CYP3A4 inhibitors; may result in increased nifedipine concentrations; monitor for adverse effects/toxicity and consider dose adjustments. Use with strong CYP3A4 inducers (eg, rifampin, rifabutin, phenobarbital, phenytoin, carbamazepine, St John's wort) is contraindicated due to reduced bioavailability and efficacy.

Drug Interactions

Metabolism/Transport Effects **Substrate** of CYP2D6 (minor), 3A4 (major); **Inhibits** CYP1A2 (moderate), 2C9 (weak), 2D6 (weak), 3A4 (weak)

Avoid Concomitant Use

Avoid concomitant use of NIFEdipine with any of the following: Grapefruit Juice

Increased Effect/Toxicity

NIFEdipine may increase the levels/effects of: Amifostine; Antihypertensives; Calcium Channel Blockers (Nondihydropyridine); CYP1A2 Substrates; Fosphenytoin; Hypotensive Agents; Magnesium Salts; Neuromuscular-Blocking Agents (Nondepolarizing); Nitroprusside; Phenytoin; RiTUXimab; Tacrolimus; Tacrolimus (Systemic); VinCRIStine

The levels/effects of NIFEdipine may be increased by: Alcohol (Ethyl); Alpha1-Blockers; Antifungal Agents (Azole Derivatives, Systemic); Calcium Channel Blockers (Nondihydropyridine); Cimetidine; Cisapride; Conivaptan; CycloSPORINE; CycloSPORINE (Systemic); CYP3A4 Inhibitors (Moderate); CYP3A4 Inhibitors (Strong); Dasatinib; Diazoxide; Fluconazole; Grapefruit Juice; Herbs (Hypotensive Properties); Macrolide Antibiotics; Magnesium Salts; MAO Inhibitors; Pentoxifylline; Phosphodiesterase 5 Inhibitors; Prostacyclin Analogues; Protease Inhibitors

Decreased Effect

NIFEdipine may decrease the levels/effects of: Clopidogrel; QuiNIDine

The levels/effects of NIFEdipine may be decreased by: Barbiturates; Calcium Salts; CarBAMazepine; CYP3A4 Inducers (Strong); Deferasirox; Herbs (CYP3A4 Inducers); Herbs (Hypertensive Properties); Methylphenidate; Nafcillin; Peginterferon Alfa-2b; Rifamycin Derivatives; Tocilizumab; Yohimbine

Ethanol/Nutrition/Herb Interactions

Ethanol: Avoid ethanol (may increase CNS depression and may increase the effects of nifedipine). Monitor.

Food: Nifedipine serum levels may be decreased if taken with food. Food may decrease the rate but not the extent of absorption of Procardia XL®. Increased nifedipine concentrations resulting in therapeutic and vasodilator side effects, including severe hypotension and myocardial ischemia, may occur if nifedipine is taken by patients ingesting grapefruit.

Herb/Nutraceutical: St John's wort may decrease nifedipine levels (avoid use). Avoid use of bayberry, blue cohosh, cayenne, ephedra, ginger, ginseng (American), kola, licorice (may worsen hypertension). Avoid black cohosh, California poppy, coleus, golden seal, hawthorn, mistletoe, periwinkle, quinine, shepherd's purse (may have increased antihypertensive effect).

Dietary Considerations Avoid grapefruit juice with all products.

Immediate release: Capsule is rapidly absorbed orally if it is administered without food, but may result in vasodilator side effects; if flushing is problematic, administration with low-fat meals may decrease. In general, can take with or without food.

Extended release: Adalat® CC, Afeditab® CR, Nifediac CC®: Take on an empty stomach (manufacturer recommendation). Other extended release products may not have this recommendation; consult product labeling.

Pharmacodynamics/Kinetics

Onset of Action Immediate release: ~20 minutes

Half-life Elimination Adults: Healthy: 2-5 hours; Cirrhosis: 7 hours; Elderly: 7 hours (extended release tablet)

Pregnancy Risk Factor C

Lactation Enters breast milk/not recommended (AAP considers "compatible"; AAP 2001 update pending)

Dosage Forms

Capsule, softgel, oral: 10 mg, 20 mg
Procardia®: 10 mg

Tablet, extended release, oral: 30 mg, 60 mg, 90 mg
Adalat® CC: 30 mg, 60 mg, 90 mg
Afeditab® CR: 30 mg, 60 mg
Nifediac CC®: 30 mg, 60 mg, 90 mg
Nifedical XL®: 30 mg, 60 mg
Procardia XL®: 30 mg, 60 mg, 90 mg

References

Deen-Duggins L, Fry HR, Clay JR, et al, "Nifedipine-Associated Gingival Overgrowth: A Survey of the Literature and Report of Four Cases," *Quintessence Int*, 1996, 27(3):163-70.

Desai P and Silver JG, "Drug-Induced Gingival Enlargements," *J Can Dent Assoc*, 1998, 64(4):263-8.

Harel-Raviv M, Eckler M, Lalani K, et al, "Nifedipine-Induced Gingival Hyperplasia. A Comprehensive Review and Analysis," *Oral Surg Oral Med Oral Pathol Oral Radiol Endod*, 1995, 79(6):715-22.

Lederman D, Lumerman H, Reuben S, et al, "Gingival Hyperplasia Associated With Nifedipine Therapy," *Oral Surg Oral Med Oral Pathol*, 1984, 57(6):620-2.

Lucas RM, Howell LP, and Wall BA, "Nifedipine-Induced Gingival Hyperplasia: A Histochemical and Ultrastructural Study," *J Periodontol*, 1985, 56(4):211-5.

Nery EB, Edson RG, Lee KK, et al, "Prevalence of Nifedipine-Induced Gingival Hyperplasia," *J Periodontol*, 1995, 66(7):572-8.

Nishikawa SJ, Tada H, Hamasaki A, et al, "Nifedipine-Induced Gingival Hyperplasia: A Clinical and In Vitro Study," *J Periodontol*, 1991, 62(1):30-5.

Pilloni A, Camargo PM, Carere M, et al, "Surgical Treatment of Cyclosporine A- and Nifedipine-Induced Gingival Enlargement: Gingivectomy Versus Periodontal Flap," *J Periodontol*, 1998, 69(7):791-7.

Saito K, Mori S, Iwakura M, et al, "Immunohistochemical Localization of Transforming Growth Factor Beta, Basic Fibroblast Growth Factor and Heparin Sulphate Glycosaminoglycan in Gingival Hyperplasia Induced by Nifedipine and Phenytoin," *J Periodontal Res*, 1996, 31(8):545-5.

Silverstein LH, Koch JP, Lefkove MD, et al, "Nifedipine-Induced Gingival Enlargement Around Dental Implants: A Clinical Report," *J Oral Implantol*, 1995, 21(2):116-20.

Westbrook P, Bednarczyk EM, Carlson M, et al, "Regression of Nifedipine-Induced Gingival Hyperplasia Following Switch to a Same Class Calcium Channel Blocker, Isradipine," *J Periodontol*, 1997, 68 (7):645-50.

Wynn RL, "Calcium Channel Blockers and Gingival Hyperplasia," *Gen Dent*, 1991, 39(4):240-3.

Wynn RL, "Update on Calcium Channel Blocker-Induced Gingival Hyperplasia," *Gen Dent*, 1995, 43 (3):218-22.

Nilotinib (nye LOE ti nib)

U.S. Brand Names Tasigna®

Canadian Brand Names Tasigna®

Pharmacologic Category Antineoplastic Agent, Tyrosine Kinase Inhibitor

Use Treatment of newly-diagnosed Philadelphia chromosome-positive chronic myelogenous leukemia (Ph+ CML) in chronic phase; treatment of chronic and accelerated phase Ph+ CML (refractory or intolerant to prior therapy, including imatinib)

Local Anesthetic/Vasoconstrictor Precautions Nilotinib is one of the drugs confirmed to prolong the QT interval and is accepted as having a risk of causing torsade de pointes. The risk of drug-induced torsade de pointes is extremely low when a single QT interval prolonging drug is prescribed. In terms of epinephrine, it is not known what effect vasoconstrictors in the local anesthetic regimen will have in patients with a known history of congenital prolonged QT interval or in patients taking any medication that prolongs the QT interval. Until more information is obtained, it is suggested that the clinician consult with the physician prior to the use of a vasoconstrictor in suspected patients, and that the vasoconstrictor (epinephrine, mepivacaine and levonordefrin [Carbocaine® 2% with Neo-Cobefrin®]) be used with caution.

Effects on Dental Treatment Key adverse event(s) related to dental treatment: Mouth ulcerations, stomatitis

Effects on Bleeding Chemotherapy may result in significant myelosuppression, potentially including significant reduction in platelet counts and altered hemostasis. In patients who are under active treatment with these agents, medical consult is suggested.

Adverse Effects

>10%:

Cardiovascular: Peripheral edema (8% to 11%)

Central nervous system: Headache (21% to 31%), fatigue (16% to 28%), fever (10% to 24%)

Dermatologic: Rash (28% to 36%), pruritus (19% to 29%)

Endocrine & metabolic: Hyperglycemia (grades 3/4: 4% to 11%)

Gastrointestinal: Nausea (18% to 31%), diarrhea (14% to 22%), constipation (15% to 21%), vomiting (9% to 21%), lipase increased (grades 3/4: 7% to 17%), abdominal pain (11% to 15%)

Hematologic: Neutropenia (grades 3/4: 12% to 37%; median duration: 15 days), thrombocytopenia (grade 3/4: 10% to 37%; median duration: 22 days), anemia (grades 3/4: 4% to 23%)

Neuromuscular & skeletal: Arthralgia (15% to 18%), limb pain (9% to 16%), myalgia (14%), weakness (11% to 14%), muscle spasm (10% to 14%), bone pain (11% to 13%), back pain (10% to 12%)

Respiratory: Cough (12% to 17%), nasopharyngitis (11% to 19%), upper respiratory tract infection (≤13%), dyspnea (8% to 11%)

1% to 10%:

Cardiovascular: Angina, arrhythmia (including AV block, atrial fibrillation, bradycardia, cardiac flutter, and extrasystoles), chest pain, flushing, hypertension, palpitation, pericardial effusion, QT interval prolonged

Central nervous system: Depression, dizziness, dysphonia, hypoesthesia, insomnia, pain, vertigo

Dermatologic: Acne, alopecia, bruising, dry skin, dermatitis, eczema, erythema, folliculitis, hyperhidrosis, skin papilloma, urticaria

Endocrine & metabolic: Hypophosphatemia (grades 3/4: 5% to 10%), hypokalemia (grades 3/4: ≤5%), hyperkalemia (grades 3/4: 2% to 4%), hypocalcemia (grades 3/4: ≤4%), hyponatremia (grades 3/4: ≤3%), albumin decreased (grades 3/4: ≤1%), diabetes mellitus, hypercalcemia, hypercholesterolemia, hyperlipidemia, hyperphosphatemia, hypomagnesemia

Gastrointestinal: Abdominal discomfort, amylase increased, anorexia, dyspepsia, flatulence, pancreatitis

Genitourinary: Pollakuria

Hematologic: Lymphopenia, neutropenic fever, pancytopenia

Hepatic: Hyperbilirubinemia (grades 3/4: 4% to 10%), ALT increased (grades 3/4: 2% to 4%), alkaline phosphatase increased (grades 3/4: ≤3%), AST increased (grades 3/4: 1%), GGT increased

Neuromuscular & skeletal: Musculoskeletal pain, paresthesia

Ocular: Conjunctivitis, dry eye, eye hemorrhage, eyelid edema, periorbital edema, pruritus

Respiratory: Dyspnea (exertional), epistaxis, pleural effusion (≤1%), pneumonia

Miscellaneous: Night sweats

General Dosage Range Dosage adjustment recommended in patients with hepatic impairment, on concomitant therapy, or who develop toxicities

Oral: *Adults:* 300-400 mg twice daily

Mechanism of Action Selective tyrosine kinase inhibitor that targets BCR-ABL kinase, c-KIT and platelet derived growth factor receptor (PDGFR); does not have activity against the SRC family. Inhibits BCR-ABL mediated proliferation of leukemic cell lines by binding to the ATP-binding site of BCR-ABL and inhibiting tyrosine kinase activity. Nilotinib has activity in imatinib-resistant BCR-ABL kinase mutations.

Pharmacodynamics/Kinetics

Half-life Elimination ~15-17 hour

Time to Peak 3 hours

Pregnancy Risk Factor D

Dental Comment Nilotinib is known to prolong the QT interval. The QT interval is measured as the time and distance between the Q point of the QRS complex and the end of the T wave in the ECG tracing. After adjustment for heart rate, the QT interval is defined as prolonged if it is more than 450 msec in men and 460 msec in women. A long QT syndrome was first described in the 1950s and 60s as a congenital syndrome involving QT interval prolongation and syncope and sudden death. Some of the congenital long QT syndromes were characterized by a peculiar electrocardiographic appearance of the QRS complex involving a premature atria beat followed by a pause, then a subsequent sinus beat showing marked QT prolongation and deformity. This type of cardiac arrhythmia was originally termed "torsade de pointes" (translated from the French as "twisting of the points"). Nilotinib is considered as having a risk of causing torsade de pointes. Since it is not known what effect vasoconstrictors in the local anesthetic regimen will have in patients with a known history of congenital prolonged QT interval or in patients taking any medication that prolongs the QT interval, a medical consult is suggested.

Nilutamide (ni LOO ta mide)

U.S. Brand Names Nilandron®

Canadian Brand Names Anandron®

Pharmacologic Category Antiandrogen; Antineoplastic Agent, Antiandrogen

Use Treatment of metastatic prostate cancer

Local Anesthetic/Vasoconstrictor Precautions No information available to require special precautions

Effects on Dental Treatment Key adverse event(s) related to dental treatment: Xerostomia (normal salivary flow resumes upon discontinuation).

Effects on Bleeding Although significant myelosuppression with associated altered hemostasis has been reported for many chemotherapeutic agents, myelosuppression is not common with nilutamide and no specific precautions appear to necessary.

Adverse Effects

>10%:

- Central nervous system: Headache, insomnia
- Endocrine & metabolic: Hot flashes (30% to 67%), gynecomastia (10%)
- Gastrointestinal: Nausea (mild - 10% to 32%), abdominal pain (10%), constipation, anorexia
- Genitourinary: Testicular atrophy (16%), libido decreased
- Hepatic: Transaminases increased (8% to 13%; transient)
- Ocular: Impaired dark adaptation (13% to 57%), usually reversible with dose reduction, may require discontinuation of the drug in 1% to 2% of patients
- Respiratory: Dyspnea (11%)

1% to 10%:

- Cardiovascular: Chest pain, edema, heart failure, hypertension, syncope
- Central nervous system: Dizziness, drowsiness, fever, malaise, hypoesthesia, depression
- Dermatologic: Pruritus, alopecia, dry skin, rash
- Endocrine & metabolic: Disulfiram-like reaction (hot flashes, rash) (5%)
- Gastrointestinal: Vomiting, diarrhea, dyspepsia, GI hemorrhage, melena, weight loss, xerostomia
- Genitourinary: Hematuria, nocturia
- Hematologic: Anemia
- Hepatic: Hepatitis (1%)
- Neuromuscular & skeletal: Arthritis, paresthesia
- Ocular: Chromatopsia (9%), abnormal vision (6% to 7%), cataracts, photophobia
- Respiratory: Interstitial pneumonitis (2% - typically exertional dyspnea, cough, chest pain, and fever; most often occurring within the first 3 months of treatment); rhinitis
- Miscellaneous: Diaphoresis, flu-like syndrome

General Dosage Range Oral: *Adults:* Initial: 300 mg once daily; Maintenance: 150 mg once daily

Mechanism of Action Nonsteroidal antiandrogen that inhibits androgen uptake or inhibits binding of androgen in target tissues. It specifically blocks the action of androgens by interacting with cytosolic androgen receptor F sites in target tissue

Pharmacodynamics/Kinetics

Half-life Elimination Terminal: 23-87 hours; Metabolites: 35-137 hours

Pregnancy Risk Factor C

NiMODipine (nye MOE di peen)

Related Information

Calcium Channel Blockers and Gingival Hyperplasia *on page 2014*

Canadian Brand Names Nimotop®

Pharmacologic Category Calcium Channel Blocker; Calcium Channel Blocker, Dihydropyridine

Use Vasospasm following subarachnoid hemorrhage from ruptured intracranial aneurysms

Unlabeled/Investigational Use Prevention of migraines (inconsistent data)

Local Anesthetic/Vasoconstrictor Precautions No information available to require special precautions

Effects on Dental Treatment Other drugs of this class can cause gingival hyperplasia (ie, nifedipine) but there have been no reports for nimodipine.

Effects on Bleeding No information available to require special precautions

Adverse Effects 1% to 10%:

Cardiovascular: Reductions in systemic blood pressure (1% to 8%)
Central nervous system: Headache (1% to 4%)
Dermatologic: Rash (1% to 2%)
Gastrointestinal: Diarrhea (2% to 4%), abdominal discomfort (2%)

General Dosage Range Dosage adjustment recommended in patients with hepatic impairment

Oral: *Adults:* 60 mg every 4 hours

Mechanism of Action Nimodipine shares the pharmacology of other calcium channel blockers; animal studies indicate that nimodipine has a greater effect on cerebral arterials than other arterials; this increased specificity may be due to the drug's increased lipophilicity and cerebral distribution as compared to nifedipine; inhibits calcium ion from entering the "slow channels" or select voltage sensitive areas of vascular smooth muscle and myocardium during depolarization

Pharmacodynamics/Kinetics

Half-life Elimination 1-2 hours; prolonged with renal impairment

Time to Peak Serum: ~1 hour

Pregnancy Risk Factor C

Nisoldipine (nye SOL di peen)

Related Information

Calcium Channel Blockers and Gingival Hyperplasia *on page 2014*
Cardiovascular Diseases *on page 1848*

U.S. Brand Names Sular®

Pharmacologic Category Calcium Channel Blocker; Calcium Channel Blocker, Dihydropyridine

Use Management of hypertension, alone or in combination with other antihypertensive agents

Local Anesthetic/Vasoconstrictor Precautions No information available to require special precautions

Effects on Dental Treatment Key adverse event(s) related to dental treatment: Xerostomia (normal salivary flow resumes upon discontinuation).

Unlike other calcium channel blockers, information is sparse as to whether nisoldipine causes gingival hyperplasia. Consultation with physician is suggested if hyperplasia is observed in patients taking nisoldipine.

Effects on Bleeding No information available to require special precautions

Adverse Effects

>10%:

Cardiovascular: Peripheral edema (dose related; 7% to 29%)
Central nervous system: Headache (22%)

1% to 10%:

Cardiovascular: Vasodilation (4%), palpitation (3%), angina exacerbation (2%), chest pain (2%)
Central nervous system: Dizziness (3% to 10%)

Dermatologic: Rash (2%)
Gastrointestinal: Nausea (2%)
Respiratory: Pharyngitis (5%), sinusitis (3%)

General Dosage Range Dosage adjustment recommended in patients with hepatic impairment

Oral:

Adults:

Sular® (Geomatrix® delivery system): Initial: 17 mg once daily; Maintenance: 17-34 mg once daily (maximum: 34 mg/day)

Nisoldipine extended-release (original formulation): Initial: 20 mg once daily; Maintenance: 10-40 mg once daily (maximum: 60 mg/day)

Elderly: Sular® (Geomatrix® delivery system): Initial: 8.5 mg once daily; Nisoldipine extended-release (original formulation): Initial: 10 mg once daily

Mechanism of Action As a dihydropyridine calcium channel blocker, structurally similar to nifedipine, nisoldipine impedes the movement of calcium ions into vascular smooth muscle and cardiac muscle. Dihydropyridines are potent vasodilators and are not as likely to suppress cardiac contractility and slow cardiac conduction as other calcium antagonists such as verapamil and diltiazem; nisoldipine is 5-10 times as potent a vasodilator as nifedipine.

Pharmacodynamics/Kinetics

Duration of Action >24 hours

Half-life Elimination 9-18 hours

Time to Peak 4-14 hours

Pregnancy Risk Factor C

Nitazoxanide (nye ta ZOX a nide)

U.S. Brand Names Alinia®

Pharmacologic Category Antiprotozoal

Use Treatment of diarrhea caused by *Cryptosporidium parvum* or *Giardia lamblia*

Unlabeled/Investigational Use Alternative treatment for *Clostridium difficile*-associated diarrhea (CDAD)

Local Anesthetic/Vasoconstrictor Precautions No information available to require special precautions

Effects on Dental Treatment No significant effects or complications reported

Effects on Bleeding No information available to require special precautions

Adverse Effects Rates of adverse effects were similar to those reported with placebo.

1% to 10%:

Central nervous system: Headache (1% to 3%)

Gastrointestinal: Abdominal pain (7% to 8%), diarrhea (2% to 4%), nausea (3%), vomiting (1%)

General Dosage Range Oral:

Children 1-3 years: 100 mg every 12 hours

Children 4-11 years: 200 mg every 12 hours

Children ≥12 years and Adults: 500 mg every 12 hours

Mechanism of Action Nitazoxanide is rapidly metabolized to the active metabolite tizoxanide *in vivo*. Activity may be due to interference with the pyruvate:ferredoxin oxidoreductase (PFOR) enzyme-dependent electron transfer reaction which is essential to anaerobic metabolism. *In vitro*, nitazoxanide and tizoxanide inhibit the growth of sporozoites and oocysts of *Cryptosporidium parvum* and trophozoites of *Giardia lamblia*.

Pharmacodynamics/Kinetics

Time to Peak Plasma: Tizoxanide and tizoxanide glucuronide: 1-4 hours

Pregnancy Risk Factor B

Nitisinone (ni TIS i known)

U.S. Brand Names Orfadin®

Pharmacologic Category 4-Hydroxyphenylpyruvate Dioxygenase Inhibitor

Use Treatment of hereditary tyrosinemia type 1 (HT-1) as an adjunct to dietary restriction of tyrosine and phenylalanine

Local Anesthetic/Vasoconstrictor Precautions No information available to require special precautions

Effects on Dental Treatment No significant effects or complications reported

Effects on Bleeding No information available to require special precautions

Adverse Effects 1% to 10%:

Dermatologic: Alopecia (1%), dry skin (1%), exfoliative dermatitis (1%), maculopapular rash (1%), pruritus (1%)

Hematologic: Thrombocytopenia (3%), leukopenia (3%), epistaxis (1%), granulocytopenia (1%), porphyria (1%)

Hepatic: Hepatic neoplasm (8%), hepatic failure (7%)

Ocular: Conjunctivitis (2%), corneal opacity (2%), keratitis (2%), photophobia (2%), blepharitis (1%), cataracts (1%), eye pain (1%)

General Dosage Range Oral: *Infants, Children, Adults:* 1-2 mg/kg/day in 2 divided doses

Mechanism of Action In patients with HT-1, tyrosine metabolism is interrupted due to a lack of the enzyme (fumarylacetoacetate hydrolase) needed in the last step of tyrosine degradation. Toxic metabolites of tyrosine accumulate and cause liver and kidney toxicity. Nitisinone competitively inhibits 4-hydroxyphenyl-pyruvate dioxygenase, an enzyme present early in the tyrosine degradation pathway, thereby preventing the build-up of the toxic metabolites.

Pharmacodynamics/Kinetics

Half-life Elimination Terminal: 54 hours (healthy volunteers)

Time to Peak 3 hours (healthy volunteers)

Pregnancy Risk Factor C

Prescribing and Access Restrictions Distributed by Rare Disease Therapeutics, Inc; for information regarding acquisition of product, call Accredo Health Group, Inc at 1-888-454-8860

Nitrazepam (nye TRA ze pam)

Canadian Brand Names Apo-Nitrazepam®; Mogadon; Nitrazadon®; Sandoz-Nitrazepam

Pharmacologic Category Benzodiazepine

Use Short-term management of insomnia; treatment of myoclonic seizures

Local Anesthetic/Vasoconstrictor Precautions No information available to require special precautions.

Effects on Dental Treatment Key adverse event(s) related to dental treatment: Excessive salivation has been reported. The mechanism of this effect is unknown, since many benzodiazepines cause xerostomia rather than salivation excess.

Effects on Bleeding No information available to require special precautions

Adverse Effects Frequency not defined.

Cardiovascular: Hypotension, palpitation

Central nervous system: Agitation, aggressiveness, amnesia, ataxia, confusion, delusions, disorientation, dizziness, fatigue, hallucination, hangover, headache, irritability, nightmares, psychoses, rage, restlessness, sedation

Dermatologic: Rash

Endocrine & metabolic: Changes in libido

Gastrointestinal: Constipation, diarrhea, excessive salivation, heartburn, nausea, vomiting

Hematologic: Granulocytopenia, leukopenia

Neuromuscular & skeletal: Falling, muscle weakness

Ocular: Blurred vision, double vision

Otic: Tinnitus (associated with withdrawal)

Respiratory: Aspiration, bronchial hypersecretion, dyspnea

General Dosage Range Oral:

Children ≤30 kg: 0.3-1 mg/kg/day in 3 divided doses

Adults: 5-10 mg once daily

Elderly: 2.5-5 mg once daily

Mechanism of Action Binds to stereospecific benzodiazepine receptors on the postsynaptic GABA neuron at several sites within the CNS, including the limbic system, reticular formation. Enhancement of the inhibitory effect of GABA on neuronal excitability results by increased neuronal membrane permeability to chloride ions. This shift in chloride ions results in hyperpolarization (a less excitable state) and stabilization.

Pharmacodynamics/Kinetics

Onset of Action 20-50 minutes

Half-life Elimination 30 hours, Elderly/ill patients: 40 hours

Time to Peak 2-3 hours

Product Availability Not available in U.S.

Controlled Substance CDSA IV

Nitric Oxide (NYE trik OKS ide)

U.S. Brand Names INOmax®

Canadian Brand Names INOmax®

Pharmacologic Category Vasodilator, Pulmonary

Use Treatment of term and near-term (>34 weeks) neonates with hypoxic respiratory failure associated with pulmonary hypertension; used concurrently with ventilatory support and other agents

Unlabeled/Investigational Use Treatment of adult respiratory distress syndrome (ARDS); acute vasodilator testing in pulmonary artery hypertension (PAH)

Local Anesthetic/Vasoconstrictor Precautions No information available to require special precautions

Effects on Dental Treatment No significant effects or complications reported

Effects on Bleeding No information available to require special precautions

Adverse Effects

>10%:

Cardiovascular: Hypotension (13%)

Miscellaneous: Withdrawal syndrome (12%)

1% to 10%:

Dermatologic: Cellulitis (5%)

Endocrine & metabolic: Hyperglycemia (8%)

Genitourinary: Hematuria (8%)

Respiratory: Atelectasis (9% - same as placebo), stridor (5%)

Miscellaneous: Sepsis (7%), infection (6%)

General Dosage Range Inhalation: *Neonates (up to 14 days old):* 20 ppm

Mechanism of Action In neonates with persistent pulmonary hypertension, nitric oxide improves oxygenation. Nitric oxide relaxes vascular smooth muscle by binding to the heme moiety of cytosolic guanylate cyclase, activating guanylate cyclase and increasing intracellular levels of cyclic guanosine 3',5'-monophosphate, which leads to vasodilation. When inhaled, pulmonary vasodilation occurs and an increase in the partial pressure of arterial oxygen results. Dilation of pulmonary vessels in well ventilated lung areas redistributes blood flow away from lung areas where ventilation/perfusion ratios are poor.

Pregnancy Risk Factor C

Nitrofurantoin (nye troe fyoor AN toyn)

U.S. Brand Names Furadantin®; Macrobid®; Macrodantin®

Canadian Brand Names Apo-Nitrofurantoin®; Macrobid®; Macrodantin®; Novo-Furantoin

Pharmacologic Category Antibiotic, Miscellaneous

Use Prevention and treatment of urinary tract infections caused by susceptible strains of *E. coli, S. aureus, Enterococcus, Klebsiella,* and *Enterobacter*

Local Anesthetic/Vasoconstrictor Precautions No information available to require special precautions

Effects on Dental Treatment No significant effects or complications reported

Effects on Bleeding No information available to require special precautions

Adverse Effects Frequency not defined.

Cardiovascular: Cyanosis, ECG changes (nonspecific ST/T wave changes, bundle branch block)

Central nervous system: Bulging fontanels (infants), chills, confusion, depression, dizziness, drowsiness, fever, headache, malaise, pseudotumor cerebri, psychotic reaction, vertigo

Dermatologic: Alopecia, angioedema, erythema multiforme, exfoliative dermatitis, pruritus, rash (eczematous, erythematous, maculopapular), Stevens-Johnson syndrome, urticaria

Endocrine & metabolic: Hyperphosphatemia

Gastrointestinal: Abdominal pain, anorexia, *C. difficile* colitis, constipation, diarrhea, dyspepsia, flatulence, nausea, pancreatitis, pseudomembranous colitis, sialadenitis, vomiting

Genitourinary: Urine discoloration (brown)

Hematologic: Agranulocytosis, aplastic anemia, eosinophilia, glucose-6-phosphate dehydrogenase deficiency anemia, granulocytopenia, hemoglobin decreased, hemolytic anemia, leukopenia, megaloblastic anemia, thrombocytopenia

Hepatic: Hepatitis, hepatic necrosis, transaminases increased, jaundice (cholestatic)

Neuromuscular & skeletal: Arthralgia, myalgia, numbness, paresthesia, peripheral neuropathy, weakness

Ocular: Amblyopia, nystagmus, optic neuritis

Respiratory: Cough, dyspnea, pneumonitis, pulmonary fibrosis (with long-term use), pulmonary infiltration

Miscellaneous: Acute pulmonary reaction (symptoms include chills, chest pain, cough, dyspnea, fever, and eosinophilia), anaphylaxis, hypersensitivity (including acute pulmonary hypersensitivity), lupus-like syndrome, superinfections (eg, *Pseudomonas* or *Candida*)

General Dosage Range Oral:

Children >1 month: Furadantin®, Macrodantin®: 5-7 mg/kg/day divided every 6 hours (maximum: 400 mg/day) **or** 1-2 mg/kg/day divided every 12-24 hours (maximum: 100 mg/day)

Children >12 years: Macrobid®: 100 mg twice daily

Adults: Furadantin®, Macrodantin®: 50-100 mg every 6 hours **or** once daily; Macrobid®: 100 mg twice daily

Mechanism of Action Inhibits several bacterial enzyme systems including acetyl coenzyme A interfering with metabolism and possibly cell wall synthesis

Pharmacodynamics/Kinetics

Half-life Elimination 20-60 minutes; prolonged with renal impairment

Pregnancy Risk Factor B (contraindicated at term)

Nitroglycerin (nye troe GLI ser in)

Related Information

Cardiovascular Diseases *on page 1848*

U.S. Brand Names Minitran™; Nitro-Bid®; Nitro-Dur®; Nitro-Time®; Nitrolingual®; NitroMist®; Nitrostat®

Canadian Brand Names Minitran™; Mylan-Nitro Sublingual Spray; Nitro-Dur®; Nitroglycerin Injection, USP; Nitrol®; Nitrostat®; Rho®-Nitro Pump Spray; Trans-derm-Nitro®; Trinipatch®

Generic Availability (U.S.) Yes: Capsule, injection, patch, tablet

Pharmacologic Category Vasodilator

Use Treatment or prevention of angina pectoris

Intravenous (I.V.) administration: Treatment or prevention of angina pectoris; acute decompensated heart failure (especially when associated with acute myocardial infarction); perioperative hypertension (especially during cardiovascular surgery); induction of intraoperative hypotension

Unlabeled/Investigational Use Short-term management of pulmonary hypertension (I.V.); esophageal spastic disorders

Local Anesthetic/Vasoconstrictor Precautions No information available to require special precautions

Effects on Dental Treatment Key adverse event(s) related to dental treatment: Xerostomia (normal salivary flow resumes upon discontinuation).

Effects on Bleeding No information available to require special precautions

Adverse Effects Frequency not defined.

Cardiovascular: Flushing, hypotension, peripheral edema, postural hypotension, syncope, tachycardia

Central nervous system: Headache (common), dizziness, lightheadedness

Gastrointestinal: Nausea, vomiting, xerostomia

Neuromuscular & skeletal: Paresthesia, weakness

Respiratory: Dyspnea, pharyngitis, rhinitis

Miscellaneous: Diaphoresis

Dosage Note: Hemodynamic and antianginal tolerance often develop within 24-48 hours of continuous nitrate administration. Nitrate-free interval (10-12 hours/day) is recommended to avoid tolerance development; gradually decrease dose in patients receiving NTG for prolonged period to avoid withdrawal reaction.

Adults:

Oral: Initial: 2.5-6.5 mg 3-4 times/day; may titrate up to 26 mg 4 times/day

I.V.: 5 mcg/minute, increase by 5 mcg/minute every 3-5 minutes to 20 mcg/minute; if no response at 20 mcg/minute, may increase by 10-20 mcg/minute every 3-5 minutes (generally accepted maximum dose: 400 mcg/minute)

Ointment: 1/2" upon rising and 1/2" 6 hours later; if necessary, the dose may be doubled to 1" and subsequently doubled again to 2" if response is inadequate. Doses of 1/2" to 2" were used in clinical trials. Recommended maximum: 2 doses/day; include a nitrate free-interval ~10-12 hours/day.

Patch, transdermal: Initial: 0.2-0.4 mg/hour, titrate to 0.4-0.8 mg/hour; tolerance is minimized by using a patch-on period of 12-14 hours and patch-off period of 10-12 hours

Sublingual: 0.3-0.6 mg every 5 minutes for maximum of 3 doses in 15 minutes; may also use prophylactically 5-10 minutes prior to activities which may provoke an attack

Esophageal spastic disorders (unlabeled use): 0.3-0.6 mg

Translingual: 1-2 sprays onto or under tongue every 3-5 minutes for maximum of 3 doses in 15 minutes, may also be used prophylactically 5-10 minutes prior to activities which may provoke an angina attack

Elderly: In general, dose selection should be cautious, usually starting at the low end of the dosing range

Mechanism of Action Nitroglycerin forms free radical nitric oxide. In smooth muscle, nitric oxide activates guanylate cyclase which increases guanosine 3'5' monophosphate (cGMP) leading to dephosphorylation of myosin light chains and smooth muscle relaxation. Produces a vasodilator effect on the peripheral veins and arteries with more prominent effects on the veins. Primarily reduces cardiac oxygen demand by decreasing preload (left ventricular end-diastolic pressure); may modestly reduce afterload; dilates coronary arteries and improves collateral flow to ischemic regions

Contraindications Hypersensitivity to organic nitrates or any component of the formulation (includes adhesives for transdermal product); concurrent use with phosphodiesterase-5 (PDE-5) inhibitors (sildenafil, tadalafil, or vardenafil); increased intracranial pressure; severe anemia

Additional contraindications for I.V. product: Inadequate cerebral circulation; constrictive pericarditis; pericardial tamponade; restrictive cardiomyopathy

Note: According to the 2010 American Heart Association guidelines for the treatment of acute coronary syndromes, nitrates are considered contraindicated in the following conditions: Hypotension (SBP <90 mm Hg or ≥30 mm Hg below baseline), extreme bradycardia (<50 bpm), tachycardia in the absence of heart failure (>100 bpm), and right ventricular infarction (O'Connor, 2010).

Warnings/Precautions Severe hypotension can occur. Use with caution in volume depletion, moderate hypotension, and extreme caution with inferior wall MI and suspected right ventricular involvement. Use considered contraindicated in patients with severe hypotension (SBP <90 mm Hg or ≥30 mm Hg below baseline), extreme bradycardia (<50 bpm), and right ventricular MI (O'Connor, 2010).

Paradoxical bradycardia and increased angina pectoris can accompany hypotension. Orthostatic hypotension can also occur. Ethanol can accentuate this. Tolerance does develop to nitrates and appropriate dosing is needed to minimize this (drug-free interval). Avoid use of long-acting agents in acute MI or acute HF; cannot easily reverse effects. Nitrates may aggravate angina caused by hypertrophic cardiomyopathy. Nitroglycerin may precipitate or aggravate increased intracranial pressure and subsequently may worsen clinical outcomes in patients with neurologic injury (eg, intracranial hemorrhage, traumatic brain injury). Nitroglycerin transdermal patches may contain conducting metal (eg, aluminum); remove patch prior to MRI. Avoid concurrent use with PDE-5 inhibitors. When nitrate administration becomes medically necessary, may administer nitrates only if 24 hours have elapsed after use of sildenafil or vardenafil (48 hours after tadalafil use) (Trujillo, 2007).

Drug Interactions

Avoid Concomitant Use

Avoid concomitant use of Nitroglycerin with any of the following: Ergot Derivatives; Phosphodiesterase 5 Inhibitors

Increased Effect/Toxicity

Nitroglycerin may increase the levels/effects of: Ergot Derivatives; Hypotensive Agents; Rosiglitazone

The levels/effects of Nitroglycerin may be increased by: Phosphodiesterase 5 Inhibitors

Decreased Effect

Nitroglycerin may decrease the levels/effects of: Alteplase; Heparin

The levels/effects of Nitroglycerin may be decreased by: Ergot Derivatives

Ethanol/Nutrition/Herb Interactions

Ethanol: Avoid ethanol (may increase the hypotensive effects of nitroglycerin). Monitor.

Herb/Nutraceutical: Avoid bayberry, blue cohosh, cayenne, ephedra, ginger, ginseng (American), kola, licorice (may worsen hypertension). Avoid black cohosh, California poppy, coleus, golden seal, hawthorn, mistletoe, periwinkle, quinine, shepherd's purse (may cause hypotension).

Pharmacodynamics/Kinetics

Onset of Action Sublingual tablet: 1-3 minutes; Translingual spray: Similar to sublingual tablet; Sustained release: ~60 minutes; Topical: 15-30 minutes; Transdermal: ~30 minutes; I.V.: Immediate

Peak effect: Sublingual tablet: 5 minutes; Translingual spray: 4-10 minutes; Sustained release: 2.5-4 hours; Topical: ~60 minutes; Transdermal: 120 minutes; I.V.: Immediate

Duration of Action Sublingual tablet: At least 25 minutes; Translingual spray: Similar to sublingual tablet; Sustained release: 4-8 hours; Topical: 7 hours; Transdermal: 10-12 hours; I.V.: 3-5 minutes

Half-life Elimination 1-4 minutes

Pregnancy Risk Factor C

Lactation Excretion in breast milk unknown/use caution

Dosage Forms

Aerosol, translingual:
NitroMist®: 0.4 mg/spray (8.5 g)

Capsule, extended release, oral: 2.5 mg, 6.5 mg
Nitro-Time®: 2.5 mg, 6.5 mg, 9 mg

Capsule, sustained release, oral: 2.5 mg, 6.5 mg, 9 mg

Infusion, premixed in D_5W: 25 mg (250 mL); 50 mg (250 mL, 500 mL); 100 mg (250 mL)

Injection, solution: 5 mg/mL (5 mL, 10 mL)

Ointment, topical:
Nitro-Bid®: 2% (1 g, 30 g, 60 g)

Patch, transdermal: 0.1 mg/hr (30s); 0.2 mg/hr (30s); 0.4 mg/hr (30s); 0.6 mg/hr (30s)
Minitran™: 0.1 mg/hr (30s); 0.2 mg/hr (30s); 0.4 mg/hr (30s); 0.6 mg/hr (30s)
Nitro-Dur®: 0.1 mg/hr (30s); 0.2 mg/hr (30s); 0.3 mg/hr (30s); 0.4 mg/hr (30s); 0.6 mg/hr (30s); 0.8 mg/hr (30s)

Solution, translingual:
Nitrolingual®: 0.4 mg/spray (4.9 g, 12 g)

Tablet, sublingual:
Nitrostat®: 0.3 mg, 0.4 mg, 0.6 mg

Nitroprusside (nye troe PRUS ide)

Related Information
Cardiovascular Diseases *on page 1848*

U.S. Brand Names Nitropress®

Canadian Brand Names Nipride®

Pharmacologic Category Vasodilator

Use Management of hypertensive crises; acute decompensated heart failure (HF); used for controlled hypotension to reduce bleeding during surgery

Local Anesthetic/Vasoconstrictor Precautions No information available to require special precautions

Effects on Dental Treatment No significant effects or complications reported

Effects on Bleeding No information available to require special precautions

Adverse Effects Frequency not defined.
Cardiovascular: Excessive hypotensive response, palpitation, substernal distress
Central nervous system: Disorientation, psychosis, headache, restlessness
Endocrine & metabolic: Thyroid suppression (due to thiocyanate)
Gastrointestinal: Nausea, vomiting
Neuromuscular & skeletal: Hyper-reflexia (thiocyanate toxicity), muscle spasm, weakness
Ocular: Miosis (thiocyanate toxicity)
Otic: Tinnitus (thiocyanate toxicity)
Respiratory: Hypoxia
Miscellaneous: Diaphoresis

General Dosage Range I.V.:
Children: Infusion: Initial: 1 mcg/kg/minute; Usual dose: 3 mcg/kg/minute (maximum: 5 mcg/kg/minute)
Adults: Infusion: Initial: 0.3-0.5 mcg/kg/minute; Usual dose: 3 mcg/kg/minute (maximum: 10 mcg/kg/minute)

Mechanism of Action Causes peripheral vasodilation by direct action on venous and arteriolar smooth muscle, thus reducing peripheral resistance; will increase cardiac output by decreasing afterload; reduces aortal and left ventricular impedance

Pharmacodynamics/Kinetics
Onset of Action BP reduction <2 minutes
Duration of Action 1-10 minutes
Half-life Elimination Parent drug: <10 minutes; Thiocyanate: 2.7-7 days

Pregnancy Risk Factor C

Nitrous Oxide (NYE trus OKS ide)

Related Information
Management of the Patient With Anxiety or Depression *on page 1968*

Generic Availability (U.S.) Yes

Pharmacologic Category Dental Gases; General Anesthetic

Dental Use Induction of sedation and analgesia in anxious dental patients

Use Sedation, analgesia, and amnesia; principal adjunct to inhalation and intravenous general anesthesia

Local Anesthetic/Vasoconstrictor Precautions No information available to require special precautions

Effects on Dental Treatment No significant effects or complications reported

Effects on Bleeding No information available to require special precautions

Adverse Effects An increased risk of renal and hepatic diseases and peripheral neuropathy similar to that of vitamin B_{12} deficiency have been reported in dental personnel who work in areas where nitrous oxide is frequently used without an enclosed gas scavenging system

Methionine synthase, a vitamin B_{12} dependent enzyme, is inactivated following prolonged administration of nitrous oxide, and the subsequent interference with DNA synthesis prevents production of both leukocytes and red blood cells by bone marrow. These effects do not occur within the time frame of clinical use.

Female dental personnel who were exposed to unscavenged nitrous oxide for more than 5 hours/week were significantly less fertile than women who were not exposed, or who were exposed to lower levels of scavenged or unscavenged nitrous oxide. Fertility was measured by the number of menstrual cycles, without use of contraception, required to become pregnant. Women who were exposed to nitrous oxide for more than 5 hours/week were only 41% as likely as unexposed women to conceive during each monthly cycle.

Frequency not defined:

- Cardiovascular: Hypotension
- Central nervous system: Headache, dizziness, confusion, CNS excitation
- Gastrointestinal: Possibly nausea and vomiting
- Respiratory: Apnea

Dental Usual Dosage Sedation and analgesia: Children and Adults: Concentrations of 25% to 50% nitrous oxide with oxygen

Dosage Children and Adults:

Surgical: For sedation and analgesia: Concentrations of 25% to 50% nitrous oxide with oxygen. For general anesthesia, concentrations of 40% to 70% via mask or endotracheal tube. Minimal alveolar concentration (MAC), which can be considered the ED_{50} of inhalational anesthetics, is 105%; therefore delivery in a hyperbaric chamber is necessary to use as a complete anesthetic. When administered at 70%, reduces the MAC of other anesthetics by half.

Dental: For sedation and analgesia: Concentrations of 25% to 50% nitrous oxide with oxygen

Mechanism of Action General CNS depressant action; may act similarly as inhalant general anesthetics by stabilizing axonal membranes to partially inhibit action potentials leading to sedation; may partially act on opiate receptor systems to cause mild analgesia; central sympathetic stimulating action supports blood pressure, systemic vascular resistance, and cardiac output; it does not depress carbon dioxide drive to breath. Nitrous oxide increases cerebral blood flow and intracranial pressure while decreasing hepatic and renal blood flow; has analgesic action similar to morphine.

Contraindications Hypersensitivity to nitrous oxide or any component of the formulation; nitrous oxide should not be administered without oxygen

Warnings/Precautions Nausea and vomiting occurs postoperatively in ~15% of patients. Prolonged use may produce bone marrow suppression and/or neurologic dysfunction. Oxygen should be briefly administered during emergence from prolonged anesthesia with nitrous oxide to prevent diffusion hypoxia. Patients with vitamin B_{12} deficiency (pernicious anemia) and those with other nutritional deficiencies (alcoholics) are at increased risk of developing neurologic disease and bone marrow suppression with exposure to nitrous oxide. May be associated with abuse and/or addiction.

Drug Interactions

Avoid Concomitant Use There are no known interactions where it is recommended to avoid concomitant use.

Increased Effect/Toxicity There are no known significant interactions involving an increase in effect.

Decreased Effect There are no known significant interactions involving a decrease in effect.

Pharmacodynamics/Kinetics

Onset of Action Inhalation: 2-5 minutes

Pregnancy Risk Factor No data reported

Dosage Forms

Supplied in blue cylinders

Nizatidine (ni ZA ti deen)

Related Information

Gastrointestinal Disorders *on page 1874*

U.S. Brand Names Axid®; Axid® AR [OTC] [DSC]

Canadian Brand Names Apo-Nizatidine®; Axid®; Gen-Nizatidine; Novo-Nizatidine; Nu-Nizatidine; PMS-Nizatidine

Pharmacologic Category Histamine H_2 Antagonist

Use Treatment and maintenance of duodenal ulcer; treatment of benign gastric ulcer; treatment of gastroesophageal reflux disease (GERD)

OTC labeling: Prevention of meal-induced heartburn, acid indigestion, and sour stomach

Unlabeled/Investigational Use Part of a multidrug regimen for *H. pylori* eradication to reduce the risk of duodenal ulcer recurrence

Local Anesthetic/Vasoconstrictor Precautions No information available to require special precautions

Effects on Dental Treatment Key adverse event(s) related to dental treatment: Xerostomia (normal salivary flow resumes upon discontinuation).

Effects on Bleeding No information available to require special precautions

Adverse Effects

>10%: Central nervous system: Headache (16%)

1% to 10%:

Central nervous system: Anxiety, dizziness, fever (reported in children), insomnia, irritability (reported in children), somnolence, nervousness

Dermatologic: Pruritus, rash

Gastrointestinal: Abdominal pain, anorexia, constipation, diarrhea, dry mouth, flatulence, heartburn, nausea, vomiting

Respiratory: Reported in children: Cough, nasal congestion, nasopharyngitis

General Dosage Range Dosage adjustment recommended in patients with renal impairment

Oral:

Children ≥12 years: 150 mg twice daily

Adults: 300 mg/day in 1-2 divided doses **or** 75 mg twice daily (OTC dosing)

Mechanism of Action Competitive inhibition of histamine at H_2-receptors of the gastric parietal cells resulting in reduced gastric acid secretion, gastric volume and hydrogen ion concentration reduced. In healthy volunteers, nizatidine suppresses gastric acid secretion induced by pentagastrin infusion or food.

Pharmacodynamics/Kinetics

Half-life Elimination 1-2 hours; prolonged with renal impairment

Time to Peak Plasma: 0.5-3.0 hours

Pregnancy Risk Factor B

Nonoxynol 9 (non OKS i nole nine)

U.S. Brand Names Conceptrol® [OTC]; Delfen® [OTC]; Encare® [OTC]; Gynol II® Extra Strength [OTC]; Gynol II® [OTC]; Today® [OTC]; VCF® [OTC]

Pharmacologic Category Contraceptive; Spermicide

Use Prevention of pregnancy

Local Anesthetic/Vasoconstrictor Precautions No information available to require special precautions

Effects on Dental Treatment No significant effects or complications reported

Effects on Bleeding No information available to require special precautions

Adverse Effects Frequency not defined: Genitourinary: Irritation, burning, or itching of mucous membranes (including vaginal/urethral)

General Dosage Range Intravaginal: *Adolescents and Adults:* Insert 1 applicatorful, film, suppository, or sponge 10 minutes to 3 hours prior to intercourse

Mechanism of Action Nonoxynol 9 is a surfactant which prevents pregnancy by damaging the cell membrane of sperm; some product formulations may also provide a physical barrier

Norepinephrine (nor ep i NEF rin)

U.S. Brand Names Levophed®

Canadian Brand Names Levophed®

Pharmacologic Category Alpha/Beta Agonist

Use Treatment of shock which persists after adequate fluid volume replacement; severe hypotension

Local Anesthetic/Vasoconstrictor Precautions No information available to require special precautions

Effects on Dental Treatment No significant effects or complications reported

Effects on Bleeding No information available to require special precautions

Adverse Effects Frequency not defined.

Cardiovascular: Arrhythmias, bradycardia, peripheral (digital) ischemia

Central nervous system: Anxiety, headache (transient)

Local: Skin necrosis (with extravasation)

Respiratory: Dyspnea, respiratory difficulty

General Dosage Range I.V.:

Children: Initial: 0.05-0.1 mcg/kg/minute; Maintenance: Titrate to desired effect (maximum: 2 mcg/kg/minute)

Adults: Initial: 8-12 mcg/minute; Maintenance: Titrate to desired effect (usual maintenance range: 2-4 mcg/minute)

Mechanism of Action Stimulates $beta_1$-adrenergic receptors and alpha-adrenergic receptors causing increased contractility and heart rate as well as vasoconstriction, thereby increasing systemic blood pressure and coronary blood flow; clinically, alpha effects (vasoconstriction) are greater than beta effects (inotropic and chronotropic effects)

Pharmacodynamics/Kinetics

Onset of Action I.V.: Very rapid-acting

Duration of Action Vasopressor: 1-2 minutes

Pregnancy Risk Factor C

Norethindrone (nor ETH in drone)

Related Information

Endocrine Disorders and Pregnancy *on page 1879*

U.S. Brand Names Aygestin®; Camila®; Errin®; Heather; Jolivette®; Nor-QD®; Nora-BE®; Ortho Micronor®

Canadian Brand Names Micronor®; Norlutate®

Pharmacologic Category Contraceptive; Progestin

Use Treatment of amenorrhea; abnormal uterine bleeding; endometriosis; prevention of pregnancy

Local Anesthetic/Vasoconstrictor Precautions No information available to require special precautions

Effects on Dental Treatment Until we know more about the mechanism of interaction, caution is required in prescribing antibiotics to female dental patients taking progestin-only hormonal contraceptives.

Effects on Bleeding No information available to require special precautions

Adverse Effects Frequency not defined.

Cardiovascular: Cerebral embolism, cerebral thrombosis, DVT, edema

Central nervous system: Depression, dizziness, headache, insomnia, migraine, mood swings

Dermatologic: Acne, chloasma, hirsutism, melasma, pruritus, rash, urticaria

Endocrine & metabolic: Amenorrhea, breakthrough bleeding, breast enlargement/tenderness, menstrual flow changes, spotting

Gastrointestinal: Nausea, weight gain/loss

Genitourinary: Cervical erosion changes, cervical secretion changes

Hepatic: Cholestatic jaundice, liver function test abnormalities

Ocular: Optic neuritis (with or without vision loss), retinal vascular thrombosis

Respiratory: Pulmonary embolism

Miscellaneous: Anaphylactic/anaphylactoid reactions

General Dosage Range Oral:

Norethindrone: *Children (postmenarche) and Adults:* 0.35 mg every day

Norethindrone acetate: *Adolescents and Adults:* 2.5-15 mg once daily for 5-14 days of menstrual cycle

Mechanism of Action Inhibits secretion of pituitary gonadotropin (LH) which prevents follicular maturation and ovulation

Pharmacodynamics/Kinetics

Half-life Elimination ~8 hours

Time to Peak 1-2 hours

Pregnancy Risk Factor X

Norethindrone and Mestranol (nor eth IN drone & MES tra nole)

Related Information

Endocrine Disorders and Pregnancy *on page 1879*

Norethindrone *on page 1226*

U.S. Brand Names Necon® 1/50; Norinyl® 1+50

Canadian Brand Names Ortho-Novum® 1/50

Pharmacologic Category Contraceptive; Estrogen and Progestin Combination

Use Prevention of pregnancy

Unlabeled/Investigational Use Treatment of hypermenorrhea (menorrhagia); pain associated with endometriosis; dysmenorrhea; dysfunctional uterine bleeding

Local Anesthetic/Vasoconstrictor Precautions No information available to require special precautions

Effects on Dental Treatment When prescribing antibiotics, patient must be advised to use additional methods of birth control if on hormonal contraceptives.

Effects on Bleeding No information available to require special precautions

Adverse Effects Frequency not defined.

Cardiovascular: Arterial thromboembolism, cerebral hemorrhage, cerebral thrombosis, edema, hypertension, mesenteric thrombosis, MI

Central nervous system: Depression, dizziness, headache, migraine, nervousness, premenstrual syndrome, stroke

Dermatologic: Acne, erythema multiforme, erythema nodosum, hirsutism, loss of scalp hair, melasma (may persist), rash (allergic)

Endocrine & metabolic: Amenorrhea, breakthrough bleeding, breast enlargement, breast secretion, breast tenderness, carbohydrate intolerance, lactation decreased (postpartum), glucose tolerance decreased, libido changes, menstrual flow changes, sex hormone-binding globulins (SHBG) increased, spotting, temporary infertility (following discontinuation), thyroid-binding globulin increased, triglycerides increased

Gastrointestinal: Abdominal cramps, appetite changes, bloating, cholestasis, colitis, gallbladder disease, jaundice, nausea, vomiting, weight gain/loss

Genitourinary: Cervical erosion changes, cervical secretion changes, cystitis-like syndrome, vaginal candidiasis, vaginitis

Hematologic: Antithrombin III decreased, folate levels decreased, hemolytic uremic syndrome, norepinephrine induced platelet aggregability increased, porphyria, prothrombin increased; factors VII, VIII, IX, and X increased

Hepatic: Benign liver tumors, Budd-Chiari syndrome, cholestatic jaundice, hepatic adenomas

Local: Thrombophlebitis

Ocular: Cataracts, change in corneal curvature (steepening), contact lens intolerance, optic neuritis, retinal thrombosis

Renal: Impaired renal function

Respiratory: Pulmonary thromboembolism

Miscellaneous: Hemorrhagic eruption

General Dosage Range Oral:

21-tablet package: *Children (menarche) and Adults:* 1 tablet daily for 21 days, followed by 7 days off

28-tablet package: *Children (menarche) and Adults:* 1 tablet daily

Mechanism of Action Combination oral contraceptives inhibit ovulation via a negative feedback mechanism on the hypothalamus, which alters the normal pattern of gonadotropin secretion of a follicle-stimulating hormone (FSH) and luteinizing hormone by the anterior pituitary. The follicular phase FSH and midcycle surge of gonadotropins are inhibited. In addition, combination hormonal contraceptives produce alterations in the genital tract, including changes in the cervical mucus, rendering it unfavorable for sperm penetration even if ovulation occurs. Changes in the endometrium may also occur, producing an unfavorable environment for nidation. Combination hormonal contraceptive drugs may alter the tubal transport of the ova through the fallopian tubes. Progestational agents may also alter sperm fertility.

Pregnancy Risk Factor X

Norfloxacin (nor FLOKS a sin)

U.S. Brand Names Noroxin®

Canadian Brand Names Apo-Norflox®; CO Norfloxacin; Norfloxacine®; Novo-Norfloxacin; PMS-Norfloxacin; Riva-Norfloxacin

Pharmacologic Category Antibiotic, Quinolone

Use Uncomplicated and complicated urinary tract infections caused by susceptible gram-negative and gram-positive bacteria; sexually-transmitted disease (eg, uncomplicated urethral and cervical gonorrhea) caused by *N. gonorrhoeae*; prostatitis due to *E. coli*

Note: As of April 2007, the CDC no longer recommends the use of fluoroquinolones for the treatment of gonococcal disease.

Local Anesthetic/Vasoconstrictor Precautions Norfloxacin is one of the drugs confirmed to prolong the QT interval and is accepted as having a risk of causing torsade de pointes. The risk of drug-induced torsade de pointes is extremely low when a single QT interval prolonging drug is prescribed. In terms of epinephrine, it is not known what effect vasoconstrictors in the local anesthetic regimen will have in patients with a known history of congenital prolonged QT interval or in patients taking any medication that prolongs the QT interval. Until more information is obtained, it is suggested that the clinician consult with the physician prior to the use of a vasoconstrictor in suspected patients, and that the vasoconstrictor (epinephrine, mepivacaine and levonordefrin [Carbocaine® 2% with Neo-Cobefrin®]) be used with caution.

Effects on Dental Treatment No significant effects or complications reported

Effects on Bleeding No information available to require special precautions

Adverse Effects

>1% to 10%:

Central nervous system: Headache (2% to 3%), dizziness (2% to 3%)

Gastrointestinal: Nausea (3% to 4%), abdominal cramping (2%)

Hematologic: Eosinophilia (1% to 2%)

Hepatic: Liver enzymes increased (1% to 2%)

≥0.3% to 1%:

Central nervous system: Fever, somnolence

Dermatologic: Hyperhidrosis, pruritus, rash

Gastrointestinal: Abdominal pain, anorectal pain, anorexia, constipation, diarrhea, dyspepsia, flatulence, loose stools, vomiting, xerostomia

Hematologic: Hematocrit/hemoglobin decreased (1%), leukopenia (1%), thrombocytopenia (1%)

Neuromuscular & skeletal: Back pain, paresthesia, weakness

Renal: Proteinuria (1%)

General Dosage Range Dosage adjustment recommended in patients with renal impairment

Oral: *Adults:* 400 mg every 12 hours **or** 800 mg as a single dose

Mechanism of Action Norfloxacin is a DNA gyrase inhibitor. DNA gyrase is an essential bacterial enzyme that maintains the superhelical structure of DNA. DNA gyrase is required for DNA replication and transcription, DNA repair, recombination, and transposition; bactericidal

Pharmacodynamics/Kinetics

Half-life Elimination 3-4 hours; Renal impairment (Cl_{cr} ≤30 mL/minute): 6.5 hours; Elderly: 4 hours

Time to Peak Serum: 1-2 hours

Pregnancy Risk Factor C

Dental Comment Norfloxacin is known to prolong the QT interval. The QT interval is measured as the time and distance between the Q point of the QRS complex and the end of the T wave in the ECG tracing. After adjustment for heart rate, the QT interval is defined as prolonged if it is more than 450 msec in men and 460 msec in women. A long QT syndrome was first described in the 1950s and 60s as a congenital syndrome involving QT interval prolongation and syncope and sudden death. Some of the congenital long QT syndromes were characterized by a peculiar electrocardiographic appearance of the QRS complex involving a premature atria beat followed by a pause, then a subsequent sinus beat showing marked QT prolongation and deformity. This type of cardiac arrhythmia was originally termed "torsade de pointes" (translated from the French as "twisting of the points"). Norfloxacin is considered as having a risk of causing torsade de pointes. Since it is not known what effect vasoconstrictors in the local anesthetic regimen will have in patients with a known history of congenital prolonged QT interval or in patients taking any medication that prolongs the QT interval, a medical consult is suggested.

Nortriptyline (nor TRIP ti leen)

U.S. Brand Names Pamelor®

Canadian Brand Names Alti-Nortriptyline; Apo-Nortriptyline®; Aventyl®; Gen-Nortriptyline; Norventyl; Novo-Nortriptyline; Nu-Nortriptyline; PMS-Nortriptyline

Generic Availability (U.S.) Yes: Excludes solution

Pharmacologic Category Antidepressant, Tricyclic (Secondary Amine)

Dental Use Treatment of myofascial pain, neuralgia, burning mouth syndrome

Use Treatment of symptoms of depression

Unlabeled/Investigational Use Chronic pain (including neuropathic pain), myofascial pain, burning mouth sydrome, anxiety disorders, attention-deficit/hyperactivity disorder (ADHD); enuresis; adjunctive therapy for smoking cessation

Local Anesthetic/Vasoconstrictor Precautions Nortriptyline is one of the drugs confirmed to prolong the QT interval and is accepted as having a risk of causing torsade de pointes. In terms of epinephrine, it is not known what effect vasoconstrictors in the local anesthetic regimen will have in patients with a known history of congenital prolonged QT interval or in patients taking any medication that prolongs the QT interval. Until more information is obtained, it is suggested that the clinician consult with the physician prior to the use of a vasoconstrictor in suspected patients, and that the vasoconstrictor (epinephrine, mepivacaine and levonordefrin [Carbocaine® 2% with Neo-Cobefrin®]) be used with caution. See Dental Comment.

Effects on Dental Treatment Key adverse event(s) related to dental treatment: Xerostomia (normal salivary flow resumes upon discontinuation), black tongue, and unpleasant taste. Long-term treatment with TCAs, such as nortriptyline, increases the risk of caries by reducing salivation and salivary buffer capacity.

Effects on Bleeding No information available to require special precautions

Adverse Effects Frequency not defined.

Cardiovascular: Arrhythmia, flushing, heart block, hypertension, MI, palpitation, postural hypotension, tachycardia

Central nervous system: Agitation, anxiety, ataxia, confusion, delirium, delusions, disorientation, dizziness, drowsiness, EEG changes, exacerbation of psychosis, extrapyramidal symptoms, fatigue, hallucinations, headache, hypomania, incoordination, insomnia, nightmares, panic, restlessness, seizure

Dermatologic: Alopecia, itching, petechiae, photosensitivity, rash, urticaria

Endocrine & metabolic: Blood sugar increased/decreased, breast enlargement, galactorrhea, gynecomastia, libido increased/decreased, sexual dysfunction, SIADH

Gastrointestinal: Abdominal cramps, anorexia, black tongue, constipation, diarrhea, epigastric distress, nausea, paralytic ileus, stomatitis, taste disturbance, vomiting, weight gain/loss, xerostomia

Genitourinary: Delayed micturition, impotence, nocturia, polyuria, testicular edema, urinary retention

Hematologic: Agranulocytosis (rare), eosinophilia, purpura, thrombocytopenia

Hepatic: Cholestatic jaundice, transaminases increased

Neuromuscular & skeletal: Numbness, paresthesia, peripheral neuropathy, tingling, tremor, weakness

Ocular: Blurred vision, disturbances in accommodation, eye pain, mydriasis

Otic: Tinnitus

Miscellaneous: Allergic reactions (eg, general edema or of the face/tongue), diaphoresis (excessive), withdrawal symptoms

Dental Usual Dosage Myofascial pain, neuralgia, burning mouth syndrome (unlabeled use): Adults: Initial: 10-25 mg at bedtime; dosage may be increased by 25 mg/day weekly, if tolerated; usual maintenance dose: 75 mg as a single bedtime dose or 2 divided doses

Dosage Oral:

Nocturnal enuresis: Children (unlabeled use): 10-20 mg/day; titrate to a maximum of 40 mg/day

Depression: Children (unlabeled use): 1-3 mg/kg/day

Depression:

Adults: 25 mg 3-4 times/day up to 150 mg/day; doses may be given once daily

Elderly: Initial: 30-50 mg/day, given as a single daily dose or in divided doses. **Note:** Nortriptyline is one of the best tolerated TCAs in the elderly)

Myofascial pain, neuralgia, burning mouth syndrome (unlabeled uses): Adults: Initial: 10-25 mg at bedtime; dosage may be increased by 25 mg/day weekly, if tolerated; usual maintenance dose: 75 mg as a single bedtime dose or 2 divided doses

Chronic urticaria, angioedema, nocturnal pruritus (unlabeled use): Adults: Oral: 75 mg/day

Smoking cessation (unlabeled use; Fiore, 2008): Adults: Initial: 25 mg/day; titrate dose to 75-100 mg/day 10-28 days prior to selected "quit" date; continue therapy for ≥12 weeks after "quit" day

Dosing adjustment in hepatic impairment: Lower doses and slower titration dependent on individualization of dosage is recommended

Mechanism of Action Traditionally believed to increase the synaptic concentration of serotonin and/or norepinephrine in the central nervous system by inhibition of their reuptake by the presynaptic neuronal membrane. However, additional receptor effects have been found including desensitization of adenyl cyclase, down regulation of beta-adrenergic receptors, and down regulation of serotonin receptors.

Contraindications Hypersensitivity to nortriptyline and similar chemical class, or any component of the formulation; use of MAO inhibitors within 14 days; use in a patient during the acute recovery phase of MI

Warnings/Precautions [U.S. Boxed Warning]: Antidepressants increase the risk of suicidal thinking and behavior in children, adolescents, and young adults (18-24 years of age) with major depressive disorder (MDD) and other psychiatric disorders; consider risk prior to prescribing. Short-term studies did not show an increased risk in patients >24 years of age and showed a decreased risk in patients ≥65 years. Closely monitor for clinical worsening, suicidality, or unusual changes in behavior; the patient's family or caregiver should be instructed to closely observe the patient and communicate condition with healthcare provider. A medication guide should be dispensed with each prescription. **Nortriptyline is not FDA approved for use in children.**

The possibility of a suicide attempt is inherent in major depression and may persist until remission occurs. Monitor for worsening of depression or suicidality, especially during initiation of therapy (generally first 1-2 months) or with dose increases or decreases. Use caution in high-risk patients. Worsening depression and severe abrupt suicidality that are not part of the presenting symptoms may require discontinuation or modification of drug therapy. The patient's family or caregiver should be alerted to monitor patients for the emergence of suicidality and associated behaviors (such as agitation, irritability, hostility, impulsivity, and hypomania) and call healthcare provider.

May worsen psychosis in some patients or precipitate a shift to mania or hypomania in patients with bipolar disorder. Patients presenting with depressive symptoms should be screened for bipolar disorder. Monotherapy in patients with bipolar disorder should be avoided. **Nortriptyline is not FDA approved for the treatment of bipolar depression.**

TCAs may rarely cause bone marrow suppression; monitor for any signs of infection and obtain CBC if symptoms (eg, fever, sore throat) evident. The risk of sedation and orthostatic effects are low relative to other antidepressants. However, nortriptyline may result in impaired performance of tasks requiring alertness (eg, operating machinery or driving). Sedative effects may be additive with other CNS depressants and/or ethanol. The degree of anticholinergic blockade produced by this agent is moderate relative to other cyclic antidepressants, however, caution should still be used in patients with urinary retention, benign prostatic hyperplasia, narrow-angle glaucoma, xerostomia, visual problems, constipation, or history of bowel obstruction. May cause orthostatic hypotension (risk is low relative to other antidepressants) or conduction disturbances. Use with caution in patients with a history of cardiovascular disease (including previous MI, stroke, tachycardia, or conduction abnormalities). The risk conduction abnormalities with this agent is moderate relative to other antidepressants.

Consider discontinuing, when possible, prior to elective surgery. Therapy should not be abruptly discontinued in patients receiving high doses for prolonged periods. May alter glucose regulation - use caution in patients with diabetes. Use caution in patients with a previous seizure disorder or condition predisposing to seizures such as brain damage, alcoholism, or concurrent therapy with other drugs which lower the seizure threshold. May increase the risks associated with electroconvulsive therapy. Use with caution in hyperthyroid patients or those receiving thyroid supplementation. Use with caution in patients with hepatic or renal dysfunction and in elderly patients.

Drug Interactions

Metabolism/Transport Effects Substrate of CYP1A2 (minor), 2C19 (minor), 2D6 (major), 3A4 (minor); **Inhibits** CYP2D6 (weak), 2E1 (weak)

Avoid Concomitant Use

Avoid concomitant use of Nortriptyline with any of the following: Artemether; Dronedarone; Iobenguane I 123; Lumefantrine; MAO Inhibitors; Methylene Blue; Nilotinib; Pimozide; QuiNINE; Sibutramine; Tetrabenazine; Thioridazine; Toremifene; Vandetanib; Ziprasidone

Increased Effect/Toxicity

Nortriptyline may increase the levels/effects of: Alcohol (Ethyl); Alpha-/Beta-Agonists (Direct-Acting); Alpha1-Agonists; Amphetamines; Anticholinergics; Beta2-Agonists; CNS Depressants; Desmopressin; Dronedarone; Methylene Blue; Pimozide; QTc-Prolonging Agents; QuiNIDine; QuiNINE; Serotonin Modulators; Sulfonylureas; Tetrabenazine; Thioridazine; Toremifene; TraMADol; Vandetanib; Vitamin K Antagonists; Yohimbine; Ziprasidone

The levels/effects of Nortriptyline may be increased by: Abiraterone; Alfuzosin; Altretamine; Artemether; BuPROPion; Chloroquine; Cimetidine; Cinacalcet; Ciprofloxacin; Ciprofloxacin (Systemic); Conivaptan; CYP2D6 Inhibitors (Moderate); CYP2D6 Inhibitors (Strong); Dexmethylphenidate; Divalproex; DULoxetine; Gadobutrol; Lithium; Lumefantrine; MAO Inhibitors; Methylphenidate; Metoclopramide;

Nilotinib; Pramlintide; Propoxyphene; Protease Inhibitors; QuiNIDine; QuiNINE; Selective Serotonin Reuptake Inhibitors; Sibutramine; Terbinafine; Terbinafine (Systemic); Valproic Acid

Decreased Effect

Nortriptyline may decrease the levels/effects of: Acetylcholinesterase Inhibitors (Central); Alpha2-Agonists; Iobenguane I 123

The levels/effects of Nortriptyline may be decreased by: Acetylcholinesterase Inhibitors (Central); Barbiturates; CarBAMazepine; Peginterferon Alfa-2b; St Johns Wort; Tocilizumab

Ethanol/Nutrition/Herb Interactions

Ethanol: May increase CNS depression; monitor for increased effects with coadministration. Caution patients about effects.

Herb/Nutraceutical: Avoid valerian, St John's wort, SAMe, kava kava (may increase risk of serotonin syndrome and/or excessive sedation).

Pharmacodynamics/Kinetics

Onset of Action Therapeutic: 1-3 weeks

Half-life Elimination 28-31 hours

Time to Peak Serum: 7-8.5 hours

Lactation Enters breast milk/not recommended (AAP rates "of concern"; AAP 2001 update pending)

Breast-Feeding Considerations Nortriptyline is excreted into breast milk and the M/P ratio ranged from 0.87 to 3.71 in one study. Based on available information, nortriptyline has not been detected in the serum of nursing infants, however low levels of the active metabolite E-10-hydroxynortriptyline have been detected in the serum of newborns following breast-feeding.

Dosage Forms

Capsule, oral: 10 mg, 25 mg, 50 mg, 75 mg

Pamelor®: 10 mg, 25 mg, 50 mg, 75 mg

Solution, oral: 10 mg/5 mL (473 mL, 480 mL)

Pamelor®: 10 mg/5 mL (480 mL)

Dental Comment Nortriptyline is known to prolong the QT interval. The QT interval is measured as the time and distance between the Q point of the QRS complex and the end of the T wave in the ECG tracing. After adjustment for heart rate, the QT interval is defined as prolonged if it is more than 450 msec in men and 460 msec in women. A long QT syndrome was first described in the 1950s and 60s as a congenital syndrome involving QT interval prolongation and syncope and sudden death. Some of the congenital long QT syndromes were characterized by a peculiar electrocardiographic appearance of the QRS complex involving a premature atria beat followed by a pause, then a subsequent sinus beat showing marked QT prolongation and deformity. This type of cardiac arrhythmia was originally termed "torsade de pointes" (translated from the French as "twisting of the points"). Nortriptyline is considered as having a risk of causing torsade de pointes. Since it is not known what effect vasoconstrictors in the local anesthetic regimen will have in patients with a known history of congenital prolonged QT interval or in patients taking any medication that prolongs the QT interval, a medical consult is suggested.

References

Buchanan J and Zakrzewska J, "Burning Mouth Syndrome," *Clin Evid (online)*, March 14, 2008. Available at http://www.ncbi.nlm.nih.gov/pmc/articles/PMC2907957/pdf/2008-1301.pdf.

Friedlander AH and Mahler ME, "Major Depressive Disorder. Psychopathology, Medical Management, and Dental Implications," *J Am Dent Assoc*, 2001, 132(5):629-38.

Ganzberg S, "Psychoactive Drugs," *ADA Guide to Dental Therapeutics*, 2nd ed, Chicago, IL: ADA Publishing, a Division of ADA Business Enterprises, Inc, 2000, 376-405.

Jastak JT and Yagiela JA, "Vasoconstrictors and Local Anesthesia: A Review and Rationale for Use," *J Am Dent Assoc*, 1983, 107(4):623-30.

Mínguez Serra MP, Salort Llorca C, Silvestre Donat FJ, "Pharmacological Treatment of Burning Mouth Syndrome: A Review and Update," *Med Oral Patol Oral Cir Bucal*, 2007, 12(4):E299-304.

Rundegren J, van Dijken J, Mörnstad H, et al, "Oral Conditions in Patients Receiving Long-Term Treatment With Cyclic Antidepressant Drugs," *Swed Dent J*, 1985, 9(2):55-64.

Yagiela JA, "Adverse Drug Interactions in Dental Practice: Interactions Associated With Vasoconstrictors. Part V of a Series," *J Am Dent Assoc*, 1999, 130(5):701-9.

Nylidrin (NYE li drin)

Canadian Brand Names Arlidin®

Pharmacologic Category Vasodilator, Peripheral

Use Considered "possibly effective" for increasing blood supply to treat peripheral disease (arteriosclerosis obliterans, diabetic vascular disease, nocturnal leg cramps, Raynaud's disease, frost bite, ischemic ulcer, thrombophlebitis) and circulatory disturbances of the inner ear (cochlear ischemia, macular or ampullar ischemia, etc)

Local Anesthetic/Vasoconstrictor Precautions No information available to require special precautions

Effects on Dental Treatment No significant effects or complications reported

Effects on Bleeding No information available to require special precautions

Adverse Effects
1% to 10%:
Central nervous system: Nervousness
Neuromuscular & skeletal: Trembling

General Dosage Range Oral: *Adults:* 3-12 mg 3-4 times/day

Mechanism of Action Nylidrin is a peripheral vasodilator; this results from direct relaxation of vascular smooth muscle and beta-agonist action. Nylidrin does not appear to affect cutaneous blood flow; it reportedly increases heart rate and cardiac output; cutaneous blood flow is not enhanced to any appreciable extent.

Pregnancy Risk Factor C

Nystatin (Oral) (nye STAT in)

Related Information
Fungal Infections *on page 1945*
Management of Patients Undergoing Cancer Therapy *on page 1970*

Related Sample Prescriptions
Topical Fungal Infections *on page 1988*

U.S. Brand Names Nystat-Rx [DSC]

Canadian Brand Names PMS-Nystatin

Generic Availability (U.S.) Yes

Pharmacologic Category Antifungal Agent, Oral Nonabsorbed

Dental Use Treatment of susceptible cutaneous, mucocutaneous, and oral cavity fungal infections normally caused by the *Candida* species

Use Treatment of susceptible cutaneous, mucocutaneous, and oral cavity fungal infections normally caused by the *Candida* species

Local Anesthetic/Vasoconstrictor Precautions No information available to require special precautions

Effects on Dental Treatment No significant effects or complications reported

Effects on Bleeding No information available to require special precautions

Adverse Effects 1% to 10%: Gastrointestinal: Diarrhea, nausea, stomach pain, vomiting

Dental Usual Dosage Oral candidiasis: Suspension (swish and swallow orally):
Premature infants: 100,000 units 4 times/day; paint suspension into recesses of the mouth
Infants: 200,000 units 4 times/day or 100,000 units to each side of mouth 4 times/day; paint suspension into recesses of the mouth
Children and Adults: 400,000-600,000 units 4 times/day; swish in the mouth and retain for as long as possible (several minutes) before swallowing

Dosage Oral:
Oral candidiasis:
Suspension:
Premature infants: 100,000 units 4 times/day; paint suspension into recesses of the mouth
Infants: 200,000 units 4 times/day or 100,000 units to each side of mouth 4 times/day; paint suspension into recesses of the mouth
Children and Adults: 400,000-600,000 units 4 times/day; swish in the mouth and retain for as long as possible (several minutes) before swallowing
Powder for compounding: Children and Adults: 1/8 teaspoon (500,000 units) to equal approximately 1/2 cup of water; give 4 times/day
Intestinal infections: Adults: 500,000-1,000,000 units every 8 hours

Mechanism of Action Binds to sterols in fungal cell membrane, changing the cell wall permeability allowing for leakage of cellular contents

Contraindications Hypersensitivity to nystatin or any component of the formulation

Drug Interactions

Avoid Concomitant Use There are no known interactions where it is recommended to avoid concomitant use.

Increased Effect/Toxicity There are no known significant interactions involving an increase in effect.

Decreased Effect
Nystatin (Oral) may decrease the levels/effects of: Saccharomyces boulardii

Pharmacodynamics/Kinetics

Onset of Action Symptomatic relief from candidiasis: 24-72 hours

Pregnancy Risk Factor C

Lactation Excretion in breast milk unknown/use caution

Breast-Feeding Considerations Excretion into breast milk is not known; however, absorption following oral use is poor.

Dosage Forms

Powder, for prescription compounding: 50 million units (10 g); 150 million units (30 g); 500 million units (100 g)

Suspension, oral: 100,000 units/mL (5 mL, 60 mL, 473 mL)

Tablet, oral: 500,000 units

Nystatin (Topical) (nye STAT in)

Related Information

Fungal Infections *on page* *1945*

Related Sample Prescriptions

Topical Fungal Infections *on page* *1988*

U.S. Brand Names Nyamyc®; Nystop®; Pedi-Dri®; Pediaderm™ AF

Canadian Brand Names Candistatin®; Nyaderm

Generic Availability (U.S.) Yes

Pharmacologic Category Antifungal Agent, Topical; Antifungal Agent, Vaginal

Use Treatment of susceptible cutaneous and mucocutaneous fungal infections normally caused by the *Candida* species

Local Anesthetic/Vasoconstrictor Precautions No information available to require special precautions

Effects on Dental Treatment No significant effects or complications reported

Effects on Bleeding No information available to require special precautions

Adverse Effects Frequency not defined: Dermatologic: Contact dermatitis, Stevens-Johnson syndrome

Dental Usual Dosage Mucocutaneous infections: Children and Adults: Topical: Apply 2-3 times/day to affected areas; very moist topical lesions are treated best with powder

Dosage

Mucocutaneous infections: Children and Adults: Topical: Apply 2-3 times/day to affected areas; very moist topical lesions are treated best with powder

Vaginal infections: Adults: Vaginal tablets: Insert 1 tablet/day at bedtime for 2 weeks

Mechanism of Action Binds to sterols in fungal cell membrane, changing the cell wall permeability allowing for leakage of cellular contents

Contraindications Hypersensitivity to nystatin or any component of the formulation

Drug Interactions

Avoid Concomitant Use There are no known interactions where it is recommended to avoid concomitant use.

Increased Effect/Toxicity There are no known significant interactions involving an increase in effect.

Decreased Effect There are no known significant interactions involving a decrease in effect.

Pharmacodynamics/Kinetics

Onset of Action Symptomatic relief from candidiasis: 24-72 hours

Pregnancy Risk Factor A (vaginal)/C (topical)

Lactation Excretion in breast milk unknown/not recommended

Breast-Feeding Considerations Excretion into breast milk is not known; however, absorption following oral use is poor and nystatin is not absorbed following application to mucous membranes or intact skin.

Dosage Forms

Cream, topical: 100,000 units/g (15 g, 30 g)

Pediaderm™ AF: 100,000 units/g (30 g)

Ointment, topical: 100,000 units/g (15 g, 30 g)

Powder, topical: 100,000 units/g (15 g, 30 g, 60 g)

Nyamyc®: 100,000 units/g (15 g, 30 g, 60 g)

Nystop®: 100,000 units/g (15 g, 30 g, 60 g)

Pedi-Dri®: 100,000 units/g (56.7 g)

Tablet, vaginal: 100,000 units

Nystatin and Triamcinolone (nye STAT in & trye am SIN oh lone)

Related Information

Fungal Infections *on page* *1945*

Nystatin (Topical) *on page* *1233*

Triamcinolone (Topical) *on page* *1672*

Related Sample Prescriptions

Angular Cheilitis *on page* *1988*

Generic Availability (U.S.) Yes

Pharmacologic Category Antifungal Agent, Topical; Corticosteroid, Topical

Dental Use Treatment of angular cheilitis and cutaneous candidiasis

Use Treatment of cutaneous candidiasis

Local Anesthetic/Vasoconstrictor Precautions No information available to require special precautions

Effects on Dental Treatment No significant effects or complications reported

Effects on Bleeding No information available to require special precautions

Adverse Effects 1% to 10%:

Dermatologic: Acne, allergic dermatitis, dryness, folliculitis, hypertrichosis, hypopigmentation, maceration of the skin, skin atrophy

Local: Burning, itching, irritation

Miscellaneous: Increased incidence of secondary infection

Dental Usual Dosage Angular cheilitis and cutaneous candidiasis: Children and Adults: Topical: Apply sparingly 2-4 times/day. Therapy should be discontinued when control is achieved; if no improvement is seen, reassessment of diagnosis may be necessary.

Dosage Children and Adults: Topical: Apply sparingly 2-4 times/day. Therapy should be discontinued when control is achieved; if no improvement is seen, reassessment of diagnosis may be necessary.

Mechanism of Action Nystatin is an antifungal agent that binds to sterols in fungal cell membrane, changing the cell wall permeability allowing for leakage of cellular contents. Triamcinolone is a synthetic corticosteroid; it decreases inflammation by suppression of migration of polymorphonuclear leukocytes and reversal of increased capillary permeability. It suppresses the immune system reducing activity and volume of the lymphatic system. It suppresses adrenal function at high doses.

Contraindications Hypersensitivity to nystatin, triamcinolone, or any component of the formulation

Warnings/Precautions Avoid use of occlusive dressings; limit therapy to least amount necessary for effective therapy, pediatric patients may be more susceptible to HPA axis suppression due to larger BSA to weight ratio

Drug Interactions

Avoid Concomitant Use

Avoid concomitant use of Nystatin and Triamcinolone with any of the following: Aldesleukin; BCG; Natalizumab; Pimecrolimus; Roflumilast; Tacrolimus (Topical)

Increased Effect/Toxicity

Nystatin and Triamcinolone may increase the levels/effects of: Acetylcholinesterase Inhibitors; Amphotericin B; Deferasirox; Leflunomide; Loop Diuretics; Natalizumab; NSAID (COX-2 Inhibitor); NSAID (Nonselective); Thiazide Diuretics; Vaccines (Live); Warfarin

The levels/effects of Nystatin and Triamcinolone may be increased by: Antifungal Agents (Azole Derivatives, Systemic); Aprepitant; Calcium Channel Blockers (Nondihydropyridine); Denosumab; Estrogen Derivatives; Fluconazole; Fosaprepitant; Macrolide Antibiotics; Neuromuscular-Blocking Agents (Nondepolarizing); Pimecrolimus; Quinolone Antibiotics; Roflumilast; Salicylates; Tacrolimus (Topical); Trastuzumab

Decreased Effect

Nystatin and Triamcinolone may decrease the levels/effects of: Aldesleukin; Antidiabetic Agents; BCG; Calcitriol; Corticorelin; Isoniazid; Saccharomyces boulardii; Salicylates; Sipuleucel-T; Vaccines (Inactivated)

The levels/effects of Nystatin and Triamcinolone may be decreased by: Aminoglutethimide; Barbiturates; Echinacea; Mitotane; Primidone; Rifamycin Derivatives

Pregnancy Risk Factor C

Lactation Excretion in breast milk unknown

Breast-Feeding Considerations

Nystatin: Compatible

Triamcinolone: No data reported

Dosage Forms

Cream: Nystatin 100,000 units and triamcinolone 0.1% (15 g, 30 g, 60 g)

Ointment: Nystatin 100,000 units and triamcinolone 0.1% (15 g, 30 g, 60 g)

Octreotide (ok TREE oh tide)

U.S. Brand Names SandoSTATIN LAR®; SandoSTATIN®

Canadian Brand Names Octreotide Acetate Injection; Octreotide Acetate Omega; Sandostatin LAR®; Sandostatin®

Pharmacologic Category Antidiarrheal; Antidote; Somatostatin Analog

Use Control of symptoms (diarrhea and flushing) in patients with metastatic carcinoid tumors; treatment of watery diarrhea associated with vasoactive intestinal peptide-secreting tumors (VIPomas); treatment of acromegaly

Unlabeled/Investigational Use Treatment of AIDS-associated diarrhea (including *Cryptosporidiosis*), chemotherapy-induced diarrhea, graft-versus-host disease (GVHD) associated diarrhea, postgastrectomy dumping syndrome; control of bleeding of esophageal varices; second-line treatment for thymic malignancies; Cushing's syndrome (ectopic); insulinomas; small bowel fistulas; islet cell tumors; Zollinger-Ellison syndrome; congenital hyperinsulinism; hypothalamic obesity; treatment of hypoglycemia secondary to sulfonylurea poisoning; treatment of malignant bowel obstruction

Local Anesthetic/Vasoconstrictor Precautions Octreotide is one of the drugs confirmed to prolong the QT interval and is accepted as having a risk of causing torsade de pointes. The risk of drug-induced torsade de pointes is extremely low when a single QT interval prolonging drug is prescribed. In terms of epinephrine, it is not known what effect vasoconstrictors in the local anesthetic regimen will have in patients with a known history of congenital prolonged QT interval or in patients taking any medication that prolongs the QT interval. Until more information is obtained, it is suggested that the clinician consult with the physician prior to the use of a vasoconstrictor in suspected patients, and that the vasoconstrictor (epinephrine, mepivacaine and levonordefrin [Carbocaine® 2% with Neo-Cobefrin®]) be used with caution.

Effects on Dental Treatment Key adverse event(s) related to dental treatment: Xerostomia (normal salivary flow resumes upon discontinuation), gingivitis, glossitis, stomatitis, taste perversion, and dysphagia.

Effects on Bleeding No information available to require special precautions

Adverse Effects Adverse reactions vary by route of administration and dosage form. Frequency of cardiac, endocrine, and gastrointestinal adverse reactions was generally higher in acromegalics.

>16%:

Cardiovascular: Sinus bradycardia (19% to 25%), chest pain (≤20%; non-depot formulations)

Central nervous system: Fatigue (1% to 32%), headache (6% to 30%), malaise (16% to 20%), fever (16% to 20%), dizziness (5% to 20%)

Dermatologic: Pruritus (≤18%)

Endocrine & metabolic: Hyperglycemia (2% to 27%)

Gastrointestinal: Abdominal pain (5% to 61%), loose stools (5% to 61%), nausea (5% to 61%), diarrhea (34% to 58%), flatulence (≤38%), cholelithiasis (13% to 38%; length of therapy dependent), biliary sludge (24%; length of therapy dependent), constipation (9% to 21%), vomiting (4% to 21%), biliary duct dilatation (12%)

Local: Injection site pain (2% to 50%; dose and formulation related)

Neuromuscular & skeletal: Back pain (1% to 27%), arthropathy (8% to 19%), myalgia (≤18%)

Respiratory: Upper respiratory infection (10% to 23%), dyspnea (≤20%; non-depot formulations)

Miscellaneous: Antibodies to octreotide (up to 25%; no efficacy change), flu symptoms (1% to 20%)

5% to 15%:

Cardiovascular: Hypertension (≤13%), conduction abnormalities (9% to 10%), arrhythmia (3% to 9%), palpitation, peripheral edema

Central nervous system: Pain (4% to 15%), anxiety, confusion, hypoesthesia, insomnia

Dermatologic: Rash (15%; depot formulation), alopecia (≤13%)

Endocrine & metabolic: Hypothyroidism (≤12%; non-depot formulations), goiter (≤8%; non-depot formulations)

Gastrointestinal: Anorexia, cramping, tenesmus (4% to 6%), dyspepsia (4% to 6%), steatorrhea (4% to 6%), feces discoloration (4% to 6%)

Hematologic: Anemia (≤15%; non-depot formulations: <1%)

Neuromuscular & skeletal: Arthralgia, myalgia, paresthesia, rigors, weakness

Otic: Earache

Renal: Renal calculus

Respiratory: Cough, pharyngitis, sinusitis, rhinitis

Miscellaneous: Allergy, diaphoresis

1% to 4%:

Cardiovascular: Angina, cardiac failure, edema, flushing, hematoma, phlebitis

Central nervous system: Abnormal gait, amnesia, depression, dysphonia, hallucinations, nervousness, neuralgia, somnolence, vertigo

Dermatologic: Acne, bruising, cellulitis

Endocrine & metabolic: Hypoglycemia (2% to 4%), hypokalemia, hypoproteinemia, gout, cachexia, breast pain, impotence

Gastrointestinal: Colitis, diverticulitis, dysphagia, fat malabsorption, gastritis, gastroenteritis, gingivitis, glossitis, melena, stomatitis, taste perversion, xerostomia
Genitourinary: Incontinence, pollakuria (non-depot formulations), urinary tract infection
Local: Injection site hematoma
Neuromuscular & skeletal: Hyperkinesia, hypertonia, joint pain, neuropathy, tremor
Ocular: Blurred vision, visual disturbance
Otic: Tinnitus
Renal: Albuminuria, renal abscess
Respiratory: Bronchitis, epistaxis
Miscellaneous: Bacterial infection, cold symptoms, moniliasis

General Dosage Range Dosage adjustment recommended in patients with hepatic or renal impairment

I.M.: *Adults:* Depot: 20 mg every 4 weeks (maximum: 40 mg every 2 weeks)
I.V., SubQ: *Adults:* 50-1500 mcg/day in 2-4 divided doses

Mechanism of Action Mimics natural somatostatin by inhibiting serotonin release, and the secretion of gastrin, VIP, insulin, glucagon, secretin, motilin, and pancreatic polypeptide. Decreases growth hormone and IGF-1 in acromegaly. Octreotide provides more potent inhibition of growth hormone, glucagon, and insulin as compared to endogenous somatostatin. Also suppresses LH response to GnRH, secretion of thyroid-stimulating hormone and decreases splanchnic blood flow.

Pharmacodynamics/Kinetics

Duration of Action SubQ: 6-12 hours

Half-life Elimination 1.7-1.9 hours; Increased in elderly patients; Cirrhosis: Up to 3.7 hours; Fatty liver disease: Up to 3.4 hours; Renal impairment: Up to 3.1 hours

Time to Peak Plasma: SubQ: 0.4 hours (0.7 hours acromegaly); I.M.: 1 hour

Pregnancy Risk Factor B

Dental Comment Octreotide is known to prolong the QT interval. The QT interval is measured as the time and distance between the Q point of the QRS complex and the end of the T wave in the ECG tracing. After adjustment for heart rate, the QT interval is defined as prolonged if it is more than 450 msec in men and 460 msec in women. A long QT syndrome was first described in the 1950s and 60s as a congenital syndrome involving QT interval prolongation and syncope and sudden death. Some of the congenital long QT syndromes were characterized by a peculiar electrocardiographic appearance of the QRS complex involving a premature atria beat followed by a pause, then a subsequent sinus beat showing marked QT prolongation and deformity. This type of cardiac arrhythmia was originally termed "torsade de pointes" (translated from the French as "twisting of the points"). Octreotide is considered as having a risk of causing torsade de pointes. Since it is not known what effect vasoconstrictors in the local anesthetic regimen will have in patients with a known history of congenital prolonged QT interval or in patients taking any medication that prolongs the QT interval, a medical consult is suggested.

Ofatumumab (oh fa TOOM yoo mab)

U.S. Brand Names Arzerra™

Pharmacologic Category Antineoplastic Agent, Monoclonal Antibody; Monoclonal Antibody

Use Treatment of refractory chronic lymphocytic leukemia (CLL)

Local Anesthetic/Vasoconstrictor Precautions No information available to require special precautions

Effects on Dental Treatment No significant effects or complications reported

Effects on Bleeding Chemotherapy may result in significant myelosuppression, potentially including significant reduction in platelet counts and altered hemostasis. In patients who are under active treatment with these agents, medical consult is suggested.

Adverse Effects

>10%:

Central nervous system: Fever (20%), fatigue (15%)
Dermatologic: Rash (14%)
Gastrointestinal: Diarrhea (18%), nausea (11%)
Hematologic: Neutropenia (≥grade 3: 42%; grade 4: 18%; may be prolonged >2 weeks), anemia (16%; grades 3/4: 5%)
Respiratory: Pneumonia (23%), cough (19%), dyspnea (14%), bronchitis (11%), upper respiratory tract infection (11%)
Miscellaneous: Infection (70%; includes bacterial, fungal or viral; ≥grade 3: 29%), infusion reaction (first infusion [300 mg]: 44%; second infusion [2000 mg]: 29%)

1% to 10%:

Cardiovascular: Peripheral edema (9%), hypertension (5%), hypotension (5%), tachycardia (5%)

Central nervous system: Chills (8%), insomnia (7%), headache (6%)
Dermatologic: Urticaria (8%), hyperhidrosis (5%)
Neuromuscular & skeletal: Back pain (8%), muscle spasm (5%)
Respiratory: Nasopharyngitis (8%), sinusitis (5%)
Miscellaneous: Sepsis (8%), herpes zoster (6%)

General Dosage Range Dosage adjustment recommended in patients who develop toxicities

I.V.: *Adults:* 300 mg week 1, followed 1 week later by 2000 mg once weekly for 7 doses (doses 2-8), followed 4 weeks later by 2000 mg once every 4 weeks for 4 doses (doses 9-12; for a total of 12 doses)

Mechanism of Action Ofatumumab is a monoclonal antibody which binds specifically the extracellular (large and small) loops of the CD20 molecule (which is expressed on normal B lymphocytes and in B-cell CLL) resulting in potent complement-dependent cell lysis and antibody-dependent cell-mediated toxicity in cells that overexpress CD20.

Pharmacodynamics/Kinetics

Half-life Elimination Between dose 4 and dose 12: ~14 days (range: 2-62 days)

Pregnancy Risk Factor C

Ofloxacin (Systemic) (oh FLOKS a sin)

Related Information

Sexually-Transmitted Diseases *on page 1903*

Canadian Brand Names Apo-Oflox®; Novo-Ofloxacin

Pharmacologic Category Antibiotic, Quinolone

Use Quinolone antibiotic for the treatment of acute exacerbations of chronic bronchitis, community-acquired pneumonia, skin and skin structure infections (uncomplicated), urethral and cervical gonorrhea (acute, uncomplicated), urethritis and cervicitis (nongonococcal), mixed infections of the urethra and cervix, pelvic inflammatory disease (acute), cystitis (uncomplicated), urinary tract infections (complicated), prostatitis

Note: As of April 2007, the CDC no longer recommends the use of fluoroquinolones for the treatment of gonococcal disease.

Unlabeled/Investigational Use Epididymitis (nongonococcal), leprosy, Traveler's diarrhea

Local Anesthetic/Vasoconstrictor Precautions No information available to require special precautions

Effects on Dental Treatment Key adverse event(s) related to dental treatment: Xerostomia (normal salivary flow resumes upon discontinuation) and abnormal taste.

Effects on Bleeding No information available to require special precautions

Adverse Effects 1% to 10%:

Cardiovascular: Chest pain (1% to 3%)
Central nervous system: Headache (1% to 9%), insomnia (3% to 7%), dizziness (1% to 5%), fatigue (1% to 3%), somnolence (1% to 3%), sleep disorders (1% to 3%), nervousness (1% to 3%), pyrexia (1% to 3%)
Dermatologic: Rash/pruritus (1% to 3%)
Gastrointestinal: Diarrhea (1% to 4%), vomiting (1% to 4%), GI distress (1% to 3%), abdominal cramps (1% to 3%), flatulence (1% to 3%), abnormal taste (1% to 3%), xerostomia (1% to 3%), appetite decreased (1% to 3%), nausea (3% to 10%), constipation (1% to 3%)
Genitourinary: Vaginitis (1% to 5%), external genital pruritus in women (1% to 3%)
Ocular: Visual disturbances (1% to 3%)
Respiratory: Pharyngitis (1% to 3%)
Miscellaneous: Trunk pain

General Dosage Range Dosage adjustment recommended in patients with hepatic or renal impairment

Oral: *Adults:* 200-400 mg every 12 hours

Mechanism of Action Ofloxacin is a DNA gyrase inhibitor. DNA gyrase is an essential bacterial enzyme that maintains the superhelical structure of DNA. DNA gyrase is required for DNA replication and transcription, DNA repair, recombination, and transposition; bactericidal

Pharmacodynamics/Kinetics

Half-life Elimination Biphasic: 4-5 hours and 20-25 hours (accounts for <5%); prolonged with renal impairment

Pregnancy Risk Factor C

OLANZapine (oh LAN za peen)

U.S. Brand Names ZyPREXA®; ZyPREXA® IntraMuscular; ZyPREXA® Relprevv™; ZyPREXA® Zydis®

Canadian Brand Names Apo-Olanzapine®; CO Olanzapine; CO Olanzapine ODT; Novo-Olanzapine; Olanzapine ODT; PHL-Olanzapine; PHL-Olanzapine ODT; PMS-Olanzapine; PMS-Olanzapine ODT; Sandoz-Olanzapine ODT; Teva-Olanzapine; Teva-Olanzapine OD; Zyprexa®; Zyprexa® Intramuscular; Zyprexa® Zydis®

Generic Availability (U.S.) No

Pharmacologic Category Antimanic Agent; Antipsychotic Agent, Atypical

Use

Oral: Treatment of the manifestations of schizophrenia; treatment of acute or mixed mania episodes associated with bipolar I disorder (as monotherapy or in combination with lithium or valproate); maintenance treatment of bipolar disorder; in combination with fluoxetine for treatment-resistant or bipolar I depression

I.M., extended-release (Zyprexa® Relprevv™): Treatment of schizophrenia

I.M., short-acting (Zyprexa® IntraMuscular): Treatment of acute agitation associated with schizophrenia and bipolar I mania

Unlabeled/Investigational Use Treatment of psychosis/schizophrenia in children; chronic pain; prevention of chemotherapy-associated delayed nausea or vomiting; psychosis/agitation related to Alzheimer's dementia; acute treatment of delirium

Local Anesthetic/Vasoconstrictor Precautions No information available to require special precautions

Effects on Dental Treatment No significant effects or complications reported

Effects on Bleeding No information available to require special precautions

Adverse Effects

Oral: Unless otherwise noted, adverse events are reported for placebo-controlled trials in adult patients on monotherapy:

>10%:

Central nervous system: Somnolence (dose dependent; 20% to 39%; adolescents 39% to 48%), extrapyramidal symptoms (dose dependent; ≤32%), dizziness (11% to 18%), headache (adolescents 17%), fatigue (adolescents 3% to 14%), insomnia (12%)

Endocrine & metabolic: Prolactin increased (30%; adolescents 47%)

Gastrointestinal: Weight gain (5% to 6%, has been reported as high as 40%; adolescents 29% to 31%), appetite increased (3% to 6%; adolescents 17% to 29%), xerostomia (dose dependent; 3% to 22%), constipation (9% to 11%), dyspepsia (7% to 11%)

Hepatic: ALT increased ≥3 x ULN (adolescents 12%; adults 5%)

Neuromuscular & skeletal: Weakness (dose dependent; 8% to 20%)

Miscellaneous: Accidental injury (12%)

1% to 10%:

Cardiovascular: Chest pain, hypertension, peripheral edema, postural hypotension, tachycardia

Central nervous system: Fever, personality changes, restlessness (adolescents)

Dermatologic: Bruising

Endocrine & metabolic: Breast-related events ([adolescents] discharge, enlargement, galactorrhea, gynecomastia, lactation disorder); menstrual-related events (amenorrhea, hypomenorrhea, menstruation delayed, oligomenorrhea); sexual function-related events (anorgasmia, ejaculation delayed, erectile dysfunction, changes in libido, abnormal orgasm, sexual dysfunction)

Gastrointestinal: Abdominal pain (adolescents), diarrhea (adolescents), flatulence, nausea (dose dependent), vomiting

Genitourinary: Incontinence, UTI

Hepatic: Hepatic enzymes increased

Neuromuscular & skeletal: Abnormal gait, akathisia, articulation impairment, back pain, falling, hypertonia, joint/extremity pain, muscle stiffness (adolescents), tremor (dose dependent)

Ocular: Amblyopia

Respiratory: Cough, epistaxis (adolescents), pharyngitis, respiratory tract infection (adolescents), rhinitis, sinusitis (adolescents)

Injection: Unless otherwise noted, adverse events are reported for placebo-controlled trials in adult patients on extended-release I.M. injection (Zyprexa® Relprevv™). Also refer to adverse reactions noted with oral therapy.

>10%: Central nervous system: Headache (13 to 18%), sedation (8% to 13%)

1% to 10%:

Cardiovascular: Hypertension, hypotension (short-acting), postural hypotension (short-acting), QT prolongation

Central nervous system: Abnormal dreams, abnormal thinking, auditory hallucination, dizziness, dysarthria, extrapyramidal symptoms, fatigue, fever, pain, restlessness, somnolence
Dermatologic: Acne
Gastrointestinal: Abdominal pain, appetite increased, diarrhea, flatulence, nausea, vomiting, weight gain, xerostomia
Genitourinary: Vaginal discharge
Hepatic: Liver enzymes increased
Local: Injection site pain
Neuromuscular & skeletal: Arthralgia, back pain, muscle spasms, stiffness, tremor, weakness (short-acting)
Otic: Ear pain
Respiratory: Cough, nasal congestion, nasopharyngitis, pharyngolaryngeal pain, sneezing, upper respiratory tract infection
Miscellaneous: Toothache, tooth infection, viral infection

<1%, postmarketing, and/or case reports (limited to important or life-threatening): CPK increased, post-injection delirium/sedation syndrome, syncope (short-acting)

Dosage

Adolescents ≥13 years: Schizophrenia/bipolar disorder: Oral: Initial: 2.5-5 mg once daily; adjust by 2.5-5 mg/day to target dose of 10 mg/day; dosing range: 2.5-20 mg/day

Adults:

Agitation (acute, associated with bipolar I mania or schizophrenia): Short-acting I.M. injection: Initial dose: 10 mg (a lower dose of 5-7.5 mg may be considered when clinical factors warrant); additional doses (up to 10 mg) may be considered, however, 2-4 hours should be allowed between doses to evaluate response (maximum total daily dose: 30 mg, per manufacturer's recommendation)

Bipolar I acute mixed or manic episodes: Oral:

Monotherapy: Initial: 10-15 mg once daily; increase by 5 mg/day at intervals of not less than 24 hours. Maintenance: 5-20 mg/day; recommended maximum dose: 20 mg/day.

Combination therapy (with lithium or valproate): Initial: 10 mg once daily; dosing range: 5-20 mg/day; recommended maximum dose: 20 mg/day.

Depression:

Depression associated with bipolar disorder (in combination with fluoxetine): Oral: Initial: 5 mg in the evening; adjust as tolerated to usual range of 5-12.5 mg/day. See **"Note."**

Treatment-resistant depression (in combination with fluoxetine): Oral: Initial: 5 mg in the evening; adjust as tolerated to range of 5-20 mg/day. See **"Note."**

Note: When using individual components of fluoxetine with olanzapine rather than fixed dose combination product (Symbyax®), approximate dosage correspondence is as follows:
Olanzapine 2.5 mg + fluoxetine 20 mg = Symbyax® 3/25
Olanzapine 5 mg + fluoxetine 20 mg = Symbyax® 6/25
Olanzapine 12.5 mg + fluoxetine 20 mg = Symbyax® 12/25
Olanzapine 5 mg + fluoxetine 50 mg = Symbyax® 6/50
Olanzapine 12.5 mg + fluoxetine 50 mg = Symbyax® 12/50

Schizophrenia:

Oral: Initial: 5-10 mg once daily (increase to 10 mg once daily within 5-7 days); thereafter, adjust by 5 mg/day at 1-week intervals, up to a recommended maximum of 20 mg/day. Maintenance: 10-20 mg once daily. Doses of 30-50 mg/day have been used; however, doses >10 mg/day have not demonstrated better efficacy, and safety and efficacy of doses >20 mg/day have not been evaluated.

Extended-release I.M. injection: **Note:** Establish tolerance to oral olanzapine prior to changing to extended-release I.M. injection. Maximum dose: 300 mg/2 weeks or 405 mg/4 weeks

Patients established on oral olanzapine 10 mg/day: Initial dose: 210 mg every 2 weeks for 4 doses or 405 mg every 4 weeks for 2 doses; Maintenance dose: 150 mg every 2 weeks or 300 mg every 4 weeks

Patients established on oral olanzapine 15 mg/day: Initial dose: 300 mg every 2 weeks for 4 doses; Maintenance dose: 210 mg every 2 weeks or 405 mg every 4 weeks

Patients established on oral olanzapine 20 mg/day: Initial and maintenance dose: 300 mg every 2 weeks

Delirium (unlabeled use): Oral: 5 mg daily for up to 5 days (NICE, 2010)

Prevention of chemotherapy-associated delayed nausea or vomiting (unlabeled use; in combination with a corticosteroid and serotonin [$5HT_3$] antagonist): Oral: 10 mg once daily for 3-5 days, beginning on day 1 of chemotherapy **or** 5 mg once daily for 2 days before chemotherapy, followed by 10 mg once daily (beginning on the day of chemotherapy) for 3-8 days

Elderly:

Short-acting I.M., Oral: Consider lower starting dose of 2.5-5 mg/day for elderly or debilitated patients; may increase as clinically indicated and tolerated with close monitoring of orthostatic blood pressure

Extended release I.M.: Consider lower starting dose of 150 mg every 4 weeks for elderly or debilitated patients; increase dose with caution as clinically indicated.

Delirium (unlabeled use): Patients >60 years: 2.5 mg daily for up to 5 days (NICE, 2010)

Psychosis/agitation related to Alzheimer's dementia (unlabeled use): Oral: Initial: 2.5-5 mg/day (Sultzer, 2008)

Dosage adjustment in renal impairment: No adjustment required. Not removed by dialysis.

Dosage adjustment in hepatic impairment: Dosage adjustment may be necessary; however, there are no specific recommendations. Monitor closely.

Mechanism of Action Olanzapine is a second generation thienobenzodiazepine antipsychotic which displays potent antagonism of serotonin 5-HT_{2A} and 5-HT_{2C}, dopamine D_{1-4}, histamine H_1 and alpha$_1$-adrenergic receptors. Olanzapine shows moderate antagonism of 5-HT_3 and muscarinic M_{1-5} receptors, and weak binding to GABA-A, BZD, and beta-adrenergic receptors. Although the precise mechanism of action in schizophrenia and bipolar disorder is not known, the efficacy of olanzapine is thought to be mediated through combined antagonism of dopamine and serotonin type 2 receptor sites.

Contraindications There are no contraindications listed in the manufacturer's labeling.

Canadian labeling: Hypersensitivity to olanzapine or any component of the formulation

Warnings/Precautions [U.S. Boxed Warning]: Elderly patients with dementia-related psychosis treated with antipsychotics are at an increased risk of death compared to placebo. Most deaths appeared to be either cardiovascular (eg, heart failure, sudden death) or infectious (eg, pneumonia) in nature. In addition, an increased incidence of cerebrovascular effects (eg, transient ischemic attack, stroke) has been reported in studies of placebo-controlled trials of olanzapine in elderly patients with dementia-related psychosis. Olanzapine is not approved for the treatment of dementia-related psychosis.

Moderate to highly sedating, use with caution in disorders where CNS depression is a feature; patients must be cautioned about performing tasks which require mental alertness (eg, operating machinery or driving). Use caution in patients with cardiac disease. Use with caution in Parkinson's disease, predisposition to seizures, or severe hepatic or renal disease. Life-threatening arrhythmias have occurred with therapeutic doses of some neuroleptics. May induce orthostatic hypotension; use caution with history of cardiovascular disease, hemodynamic instability, prior myocardial infarction, or ischemic heart disease. Increases in cholesterol and triglycerides have been noted. Use with caution in patients with pre-existing abnormal lipid profile. Esophageal dysmotility and aspiration have been associated with antipsychotic use; use with caution in patients at risk of aspiration pneumonia. May increase prolactin levels; clinical significance of hyperprolactinemia in patients with breast cancer or other prolactin-dependent tumors is unknown. Significant weight gain (>7% of baseline weight) may occur; monitor waist circumference and BMI. Impaired core body temperature regulation may occur; caution with strenuous exercise, heat exposure, dehydration, and concomitant medication possessing anticholinergic effects.

Leukopenia, neutropenia, and agranulocytosis (sometimes fatal) have been reported in clinical trials and postmarketing reports with antipsychotic use; presence of risk factors (eg, pre-existing low WBC or history of drug-induced leuko-/neutropenia) should prompt periodic blood count assessment. Discontinue therapy at first signs of blood dyscrasias or if absolute neutrophil count <1000/mm^3.

May cause anticholinergic effects; use with caution in patients with decreased gastrointestinal motility, urinary retention, BPH, xerostomia, or narrow-angle glaucoma. Relative to other neuroleptics, olanzapine has a moderate potency of cholinergic blockade. May cause extrapyramidal symptoms (EPS), although risk of these reactions is lower relative to other neuroleptics. Risk of dystonia (and probably other EPS) may be greater with increased doses, use of conventional antipsychotics, males, and younger patients. May be associated with neuroleptic malignant syndrome (NMS). May cause extreme and life-threatening hyperglycemia; use with caution in patients with diabetes or other disorders of glucose regulation; monitor. Olanzapine levels may be lower in patients who smoke; the manufacturer does not require dosage adjustments, although dosage adjustments may be considered. Use in adolescent patients ≥13 years of age may result in increased weight gain and sedation, as well as greater increases in LDL cholesterol, total cholesterol, triglycerides, prolactin, and liver transaminase levels when compared to adults. Adolescent patients should be maintained on the lowest dose necessary.

The possibility of a suicide attempt is inherent in psychotic illness or bipolar disorder; use caution in high-risk patients during initiation of therapy. Prescriptions should be written for the smallest quantity consistent with good patient care.

There are two Zyprexa® formulations for intramuscular injection: Zyprexa® Relprevv™ is an extended-release formulation and Zyprexa® Intramuscular is short-acting:

Extended-release I.M. injection (Zyprexa® Relprevv™): Monitor for post injection delirium/sedation syndrome; patients should be continuously watched (≥3 hours) for symptoms of olanzapine overdose. Only available through a restricted drug distribution program.

Short-acting I.M. injection (Zyprexa® IntraMuscular): Patients should remain recumbent if drowsy/dizzy until hypotension, bradycardia, and/or hypoventilation have been ruled out. Concurrent use of I.M./I.V. benzodiazepines is not recommended (fatalities have been reported, though causality not determined).

Drug Interactions

Metabolism/Transport Effects Substrate of CYP1A2 (major), 2D6 (minor); **Inhibits** CYP1A2 (weak), 2C9 (weak), 2C19 (weak), 2D6 (weak), 3A4 (weak)

Avoid Concomitant Use

Avoid concomitant use of OLANZapine with any of the following: Benzodiazepines; Metoclopramide

Increased Effect/Toxicity

OLANZapine may increase the levels/effects of: Alcohol (Ethyl); Anticholinergics; Benzodiazepines; CNS Depressants; Methotrimeprazine; Methylphenidate

The levels/effects of OLANZapine may be increased by: Abiraterone; Acetylcholinesterase Inhibitors (Central); CYP1A2 Inhibitors (Moderate); CYP1A2 Inhibitors (Strong); Deferasirox; Droperidol; FluvoxaMINE; LamoTRIgine; Lithium formulations; Methotrimeprazine; Methylphenidate; Metoclopramide; Pramlintide; Tetrabenazine

Decreased Effect

OLANZapine may decrease the levels/effects of: Amphetamines; Anti-Parkinson's Agents (Dopamine Agonist); Quinagolide

The levels/effects of OLANZapine may be decreased by: CYP1A2 Inducers (Strong); Lithium formulations; Peginterferon Alfa-2b

Ethanol/Nutrition/Herb Interactions

Ethanol: May increase CNS depression; monitor for increased effects with coadministration. Caution patients about effects.

Herb/Nutraceutical: Avoid dong quai, St John's wort (may also cause photosensitization). Avoid kava kava, gotu kola, valerian, St John's wort (may increase CNS depression).

Dietary Considerations Tablets may be taken without regard to meals. Some products may contain phenylalanine.

Pharmacodynamics/Kinetics

Half-life Elimination 21-54 hours; approximately 1.5 times greater in elderly; Extended-release injection: ~30 days

Time to Peak Maximum plasma concentrations after I.M. administration are 5 times higher than maximum plasma concentrations produced by an oral dose.

Extended-release injection: ~7 days
Short-acting injection: 15-45 minutes
Oral: ~6 hours

Pregnancy Risk Factor C

Lactation Enters breast milk/not recommended

Breast-Feeding Considerations At steady-state concentrations, it is estimated that a breast-fed infant may be exposed to ~2% of the maternal dose.

Prescribing and Access Restrictions As a requirement of the REMS program, only prescribers, healthcare facilities, and pharmacies registered with the Zyprexa® Relprevv™ Patient Care Program are able to prescribe, distribute, or dispense Zyprexa® Relprevv™ for patients who are enrolled in and meet all conditions of the program. Zyprexa® Relprevv™ must be administered at a registered healthcare facility. Prescribers will need to be recertified every 3 years. Contact the Zyprexa® Relprevv™ Patient Care Program at 1-877-772-9390.

Dosage Forms

Injection, powder for reconstitution:

ZyPREXA® IntraMuscular: 10 mg

Injection, powder for suspension, extended release:

ZyPREXA® Relprevv™: 210 mg, 300 mg, 405 mg

Tablet, oral:
ZyPREXA®: 2.5 mg, 5 mg, 7.5 mg, 10 mg, 15 mg, 20 mg
Tablet, orally disintegrating, oral:
ZyPREXA® Zydis®: 5 mg, 10 mg, 15 mg, 20 mg

Olanzapine and Fluoxetine (oh LAN za peen & floo OKS e teen)

Related Information
FLUoxetine *on page* 755
OLANZapine *on page* 1238
U.S. Brand Names Symbyax®
Pharmacologic Category Antidepressant, Selective Serotonin Reuptake Inhibitor; Antipsychotic Agent, Atypical
Use Treatment of depressive episodes associated with bipolar I disorder; treatment-resistant depression (unresponsive to 2 trials of different antidepressants in the current episode)
Local Anesthetic/Vasoconstrictor Precautions Although caution should be used in patients taking tricyclic antidepressants, no interactions have been reported with vasoconstrictors and fluoxetine, a nontricyclic antidepressant which acts to increase serotonin; no precautions appear to be needed. Fluoxetine is one of the drugs confirmed to prolong the QT interval and is accepted as having a risk of causing torsade de pointes. The risk of drug-induced torsade de pointes is extremely low when a single QT interval prolonging drug is prescribed. In terms of epinephrine, it is not known what effect vasoconstrictors in the local anesthetic regimen will have in patients with a known history of congenital prolonged QT interval or in patients taking any medication that prolongs the QT interval. Until more information is obtained, it is suggested that the clinician consult with the physician prior to the use of a vasoconstrictor in suspected patients, and that the vasoconstrictor (epinephrine, mepivacaine and levonordefrin [Carbocaine® 2% with Neo-Cobefrin®]) be used with caution.
Effects on Dental Treatment Key adverse event(s) related to dental treatment: Xerostomia or salivation increased (normal salivary flow resumes upon discontinuation), tooth disorder, and taste perversion. See Effects on Bleeding.
Effects on Bleeding May impair platelet aggregation resulting in increased risk of bleeding events, particularly if used concomitantly with aspirin, NSAIDs, warfarin, or other anticoagulants. Bleeding related to SSRI use has been reported to range from relatively minor bruising and epistaxis to life-threatening hemorrhage. Routine interruption of therapy for most dental procedures is not warranted. In medically complicated patients or extensive oral surgery, the decision to interrupt therapy must be based on the risk to benefit in an individual patient and a medical consult is suggested. If therapy is continued without interruption, the clinician should anticipate the potential for a prolonged bleeding time.
Adverse Effects As reported with combination product (also see individual agents):
>10%:
Central nervous system: Somnolence (14%), fatigue (12%)
Endocrine & metabolic: Hyperprolactinemia (28%), bicarbonate decreased (14%)
Gastrointestinal: Weight gain (25%), appetite increased (20%), xerostomia (15%)
Hepatic: Hyperbilirubinemia (15%)
1% to 10%:
Cardiovascular: Peripheral edema (9%), edema (3%), vasodilation (≥1%)
Central nervous system: Sedation (8%), attention disturbance (5%), hypersomnia (5%), restlessness (4%), lethargy (3%), pain in extremity (3%), fever (2%), nervousness (2%), pain (2%), thinking abnormal (2%), chills (≥1%), amnesia (≥1%)
Dermatologic: Photosensitivity (≥1%), ecchymosis (≥1%)
Endocrine & metabolic: Hypoalbuminemia (3%), uric acid levels increased (3%), hypophosphatemia (2%), breast pain (≥1%), menorrhagia (≥1%)
Gastrointestinal: Flatulence (3%), abdominal distension (2%), diarrhea (≥1%), taste perversion (≥1%), weight loss (≥1%)
Genitourinary: Erectile dysfunction (2%), urinary frequency (≥1%), urinary incontinence (≥1%)
Hematologic: Hemoglobin decreased (3%), lymphocytopenia (2%)
Hepatic: ALT increased (3%)
Neuromuscular & skeletal: Tremor (9%), arthralgia (4%), weakness (3%), stiffness (2%), neck rigidity (≥1%)
Ocular: Blurred vision (5%)
Renal: Glucosuria (4%)
Respiratory: Sinusitis (2%)

Frequency not defined: Alkaline phosphate increased, AST increased, cholesterol increased, GGT increased, hyperglycemia, hyponatremia, orthostatic hypotension, triglycerides increased

General Dosage Range Dosage adjustment recommended in patients with hepatic impairment

Oral:

Adults: Initial: Olanzapine 6 mg and fluoxetine 25 mg once daily; Maintenance: Olanzapine 6-12 mg and fluoxetine 25-50 mg once daily

Elderly >65 years: Initial: Olanzapine 3-6 mg and fluoxetine 25 mg once daily

Mechanism of Action Olanzapine is a second generation thienobenzodiazepine antipsychotic which displays potent antagonism of serotonin 5-HT_{2A} and 5-HT_{2C}, dopamine D_{1-4}, histamine H_1 and alpha$_1$-adrenergic receptors. Olanzapine shows moderate antagonism of 5-HT_3 and muscarinic M_{1-5} receptors, and weak binding to GABA-A, BZD, and beta-adrenergic receptors. Fluoxetine inhibits CNS neuron serotonin reuptake; minimal or no effect on reuptake of norepinephrine or dopamine; does not significantly bind to alpha-adrenergic, histamine, or cholinergic receptors. The enhanced antidepressant effect of the combination may be due to synergistic increases in serotonin, norepinephrine, and dopamine.

Pregnancy Risk Factor C

Dental Comment Fluoxetine is known to prolong the QT interval. The QT interval is measured as the time and distance between the Q point of the QRS complex and the end of the T wave in the ECG tracing. After adjustment for heart rate, the QT interval is defined as prolonged if it is more than 450 msec in men and 460 msec in women. A long QT syndrome was first described in the 1950s and 60s as a congenital syndrome involving QT interval prolongation and syncope and sudden death. Some of the congenital long QT syndromes were characterized by a peculiar electrocardiographic appearance of the QRS complex involving a premature atria beat followed by a pause, then a subsequent sinus beat showing marked QT prolongation and deformity. This type of cardiac arrhythmia was originally termed "torsade de pointes" (translated from the French as "twisting of the points"). Fluoxetine is considered as having a risk of causing torsade de pointes. Since it is not known what effect vasoconstrictors in the local anesthetic regimen will have in patients with a known history of congenital prolonged QT interval or in patients taking any medication that prolongs the QT interval, a medical consult is suggested.

Olmesartan (ole me SAR tan)

U.S. Brand Names Benicar®

Canadian Brand Names Olmetec®

Pharmacologic Category Angiotensin II Receptor Blocker

Use Treatment of hypertension with or without concurrent use of other antihypertensive agents

Local Anesthetic/Vasoconstrictor Precautions No information available to require special precautions

Effects on Dental Treatment No significant effects or complications reported

Effects on Bleeding No information available to require special precautions

Adverse Effects 1% to 10%:

Central nervous system: Dizziness (3%), headache

Endocrine & metabolic: Hyperglycemia, hypertriglyceridemia

Gastrointestinal: Diarrhea

Neuromuscular & skeletal: Back pain, CPK increased

Renal: Hematuria

Respiratory: Bronchitis, pharyngitis, rhinitis, sinusitis

Miscellaneous: Flu-like syndrome

General Dosage Range Oral:

Children 6-16 years:

20 kg to <35 kg: Initial: 10 mg once daily (maximum: 20 mg once daily)

≥35 kg: Initial: 20 mg once daily (maximum: 40 mg once daily)

Adolescents >16 years and Adults: Initial: 20 mg once daily; Maintenance: 20-40 mg once daily

Elderly: Initial: 5-20 mg once daily

Mechanism of Action As a selective and competitive, nonpeptide angiotensin II receptor antagonist, olmesartan blocks the vasoconstrictor and aldosterone-secreting effects of angiotensin II; olmesartan interacts reversibly at the AT1 and AT2 receptors of many tissues and has slow dissociation kinetics; its affinity for the AT1 receptor is 12,500 times greater than the AT2 receptor. Angiotensin II receptor antagonists may induce a more complete inhibition of the renin-angiotensin system than ACE inhibitors, they do not affect the response to bradykinin, and are less likely to be associated with nonrenin-angiotensin effects (eg, cough and angioedema). Olmesartan increases urinary flow rate and, in addition to being natriuretic and kaliuretic, increases excretion of chloride, magnesium, uric acid, calcium, and phosphate.

Pharmacodynamics/Kinetics

Half-life Elimination Terminal: 13 hours

Time to Peak 1-2 hours

Pregnancy Risk Factor C (1st trimester); D (2nd and 3rd trimesters)

Olmesartan, Amlodipine, and Hydrochlorothiazide

(ole me SAR tan, am LOE di peen, & hye droe klor oh THYE a zide)

Related Information

AmLODIPine *on page 113*

Hydrochlorothiazide *on page 854*

Olmesartan *on page 1243*

U.S. Brand Names Tribenzor™

Pharmacologic Category Angiotensin II Receptor Blocker; Calcium Channel Blocker; Calcium Channel Blocker, Dihydropyridine; Diuretic, Thiazide

Use Treatment of hypertension (not for initial therapy)

Local Anesthetic/Vasoconstrictor Precautions No information available to require special precautions

Effects on Dental Treatment Fewer reports of gingival hyperplasia with amlodipine than with other CCBs (usually resolves upon discontinuation); consultation with physician is suggested.

Effects on Bleeding No information available to require special precautions

Adverse Effects Reactions/percentages reported with combination product; also refer to individual agents.

1% to 10%:

Cardiovascular: Edema (8%), syncope (1%)

Central nervous system: Dizziness (6% to 9%), headache (6%), fatigue (4%)

Gastrointestinal: Diarrhea (3%), nausea (3%)

Neuromuscular & skeletal: Muscle spasms (3%), joint swelling (2%)

Renal: Urinary tract infection (2%)

Respiratory: Nasopharyngitis (4%), upper respiratory tract infection (3%)

General Dosage Range Oral: *Adults:* Amlodipine 5-10 mg and olmesartan 20-40 mg and hydrochlorothiazide 12.5-25 mg once daily (maximum: 10 mg/day [amlodipine]; 25 mg/day [hydrochlorothiazide]; 40 mg/day [olmesartan])

Mechanism of Action

Amlodipine inhibits calcium ion from entering the "slow channels" or select voltage-sensitive areas of vascular smooth muscle and myocardium during depolarization, producing a relaxation of coronary vascular smooth muscle and coronary vasodilation; increases myocardial oxygen delivery in patients with vasospastic angina. Amlodipine directly acts on vascular smooth muscle to produce peripheral arterial vasodilation reducing peripheral vascular resistance and blood pressure.

Olmesartan produces direct antagonism of the angiotensin II receptors, unlike the ACE inhibitors. It displaces angiotensin II from the AT1 receptor and produces its blood pressure-lowering effects by antagonizing AT1-induced vasoconstriction, aldosterone release, catecholamine release, arginine vasopressin release, water intake, and hypertrophic responses. This action results in more efficient blockade of the cardiovascular effects of angiotensin II and fewer side effects than the ACE inhibitors.

Hydrochlorothiazide inhibits sodium reabsorption in the distal tubules causing increased excretion of sodium and water as well as potassium and hydrogen ions.

Pregnancy Risk Factor C (1st trimester) / D (2nd and 3rd trimesters)

Olmesartan and Hydrochlorothiazide

(ole me SAR tan & hye droe klor oh THYE a zide)

Related Information

Hydrochlorothiazide *on page 854*

Olmesartan *on page 1243*

U.S. Brand Names Benicar HCT®

Canadian Brand Names Olmetec Plus®

Pharmacologic Category Angiotensin II Receptor Blocker; Diuretic, Thiazide

Use Treatment of hypertension (not recommended for initial treatment)

Local Anesthetic/Vasoconstrictor Precautions No information available to require special precautions

Effects on Dental Treatment No significant effects or complications reported

Effects on Bleeding No information available to require special precautions

Adverse Effects Frequencies reported with combination product. See individual monographs for additional adverse effects reported with each agent.

Cardiovascular: Chest pain, peripheral edema
Central nervous system: Dizziness (9%), vertigo
Dermatologic: Rash
Endocrine & metabolic: Hyperuricemia (4%), hyperglycemia
Gastrointestinal: Nausea (3%), abdominal pain, dyspepsia, gastroenteritis, diarrhea
Genitourinary: Hematuria
Hepatic: Transaminases increased
Neuromuscular & skeletal: Back pain, arthritis, arthralgia, myalgia
Respiratory: Upper respiratory infection (7%), cough
Miscellaneous: CPK increased

Angioedema and rhabdomyolysis have been reported with angiotensin-receptor blockers. Severe dermatologic reactions, hypokalemia, and pancreatitis have been reported with hydrochlorothiazide.

General Dosage Range Oral: *Adults:* Olmesartan 20-40 mg and hydrochlorothiazide 12.5-25 mg once daily (maximum: 25 mg/day [hydrochlorothiazide]; 40 mg/day [olmesartan])

Mechanism of Action Olmesartan blocks the vasoconstrictor and aldosterone-secreting effects of angiotensin II. Hydrochlorothiazide inhibits sodium reabsorption in the distal tubules causing increased excretion of sodium and water as well as potassium and hydrogen ions.

Pregnancy Risk Factor C/D (2nd and 3rd trimesters)

Olopatadine (Nasal) (oh la PAT a deen)

U.S. Brand Names Patanase®

Pharmacologic Category Histamine H_1 Antagonist; Histamine H_1 Antagonist, Second Generation; Piperidine Derivative

Use Treatment of the symptoms of seasonal allergic rhinitis

Local Anesthetic/Vasoconstrictor Precautions No information available to require special precautions

Effects on Dental Treatment Key adverse event(s) related to dental treatment: Taste perversion.

Effects on Bleeding No information available to require special precautions

Adverse Effects

>10%: Gastrointestinal: Bitter taste (13%)

1% to 10%:

Central nervous system: Somnolence (1%)
Gastrointestinal: Xerostomia (1%)
Genitourinary: Urinary tract infection (1%)
Neuromuscular & skeletal: CPK increased (1%)
Respiratory: Nasal ulceration (9%), epistaxis (3%), pharyngolaryngeal pain (2%), postnasal drip (2%), cough (1%), throat irritation (1%)
Miscellaneous: Influenza (1%)

General Dosage Range Intranasal: *Children ≥12 years and Adults:* 2 sprays into each nostril twice daily

Mechanism of Action Selective histamine H_1-antagonist; inhibits release of histamine from mast cells.

Pharmacodynamics/Kinetics

Onset of Action 30 minutes in seasonal allergy patients

Half-life Elimination 8-12 hours

Time to Peak Serum: 15 minutes to 2 hours

Pregnancy Risk Factor C

Olopatadine (Ophthalmic) (oh la PAT a deen)

U.S. Brand Names Pataday™; Patanol®

Canadian Brand Names Pataday™; Patanol®

Pharmacologic Category Histamine H_1 Antagonist; Histamine H_1 Antagonist, Second Generation; Piperidine Derivative

Use Treatment of the signs and symptoms of allergic conjunctivitis

Local Anesthetic/Vasoconstrictor Precautions No information available to require special precautions

Effects on Dental Treatment No significant effects or complications reported

Effects on Bleeding No information available to require special precautions

Adverse Effects

>5%:

Central nervous system: Cold syndrome (up to 10%), headache (up to 7%)
Respiratory: Pharyngitis (up to 10%)

≤5%:

Gastrointestinal: Nausea, taste perversion
Neuromuscular & skeletal: Back pain, weakness
Ocular: Blurred vision, burning, conjunctivitis, dry eyes, eye pain, eyelid edema, foreign body sensation, hyperemia, itching, keratitis, ocular pruritus, stinging
Respiratory: Cough, rhinitis, sinusitis
Miscellaneous: Flu-like syndrome, hypersensitivity, infection

General Dosage Range Ophthalmic: *Children ≥3 years and Adults:* Patanol®: Instill 1 drop into affected eye(s) twice daily; Pataday™: Instill 1 drop into affected eye(s) once daily

Mechanism of Action Selective histamine H_1-antagonist; inhibits release of histamine from mast cells. Inhibits histamine induced effects on conjunctival epithelial cells.

Pharmacodynamics/Kinetics

Half-life Elimination ~3 hours

Pregnancy Risk Factor C

Olsalazine (ole SAL a zeen)

U.S. Brand Names Dipentum®

Canadian Brand Names Dipentum®

Pharmacologic Category 5-Aminosalicylic Acid Derivative

Use Maintenance of remission of ulcerative colitis in patients intolerant to sulfasalazine

Local Anesthetic/Vasoconstrictor Precautions No information available to require special precautions

Effects on Dental Treatment No significant effects or complications reported

Effects on Bleeding No information available to require special precautions

Adverse Effects

>10%: Gastrointestinal: Diarrhea (11% to 17%; dose related)

1% to 10%:

Central nervous system: Depression (2%), dizziness/vertigo (1%)
Dermatologic: Rash (2%), pruritus (1%)
Gastrointestinal: Abdominal pain/cramps (10%), nausea (5%), bloating (2%), stomatitis (1%), vomiting (1%)
Neuromuscular & skeletal: Arthralgia (4%)
Respiratory: Upper respiratory infection (2%)

General Dosage Range Oral: *Adults:* 1 g/day in 2 divided doses

Mechanism of Action Mesalamine (5-aminosalicylic acid) is the active component of olsalazine; the specific mechanism of action of mesalamine is unknown; however, it is thought that it modulates local chemical mediators of the inflammatory response, especially leukotrienes, and is also postulated to be a free radical scavenger or an inhibitor of tumor necrosis factor (TNF); action appears topical rather than systemic.

Pharmacodynamics/Kinetics

Half-life Elimination 54 minutes

Time to Peak ~1 hour

Pregnancy Risk Factor C

Omalizumab (oh mah lye ZOO mab)

U.S. Brand Names Xolair®

Canadian Brand Names Xolair®

Pharmacologic Category Monoclonal Antibody, Anti-Asthmatic

Use Treatment of moderate-to-severe, persistent allergic asthma not adequately controlled with inhaled corticosteroids

Local Anesthetic/Vasoconstrictor Precautions No information available to require special precautions

Effects on Dental Treatment No significant effects or complications reported

Effects on Bleeding No information available to require special precautions

Adverse Effects

>10%:

Central nervous system: Headache (15%)
Local: Injection site reaction (45%; placebo 43%; severe 12%). Most reactions occurred within 1 hour, lasted <8 days, and decreased in frequency with additional dosing.

Respiratory: Upper respiratory tract infection (20%), sinusitis (16%), pharyngitis (11%)
Miscellaneous: Viral infection (23%)
1% to 10%:
Central nervous system: Pain (7%), fatigue (3%), dizziness (3%)
Dermatologic: Dermatitis (2%), pruritus (2%)
Neuromuscular & skeletal: Arthralgia (8%), leg pain (4%), arm pain (2%), fracture (2%)
Otic: Earache (2%)

General Dosage Range SubQ:
IgE ≥30-100 int. units/mL:
Children ≥12 years and Adults 30-90 kg: 150 mg every 4 weeks
Children ≥12 years and Adults >90-150 kg: 300 mg every 4 weeks
IgE >100-200 int. units/mL:
Children ≥12 years and Adults 30-90 kg: 300 mg every 4 weeks
Children ≥12 years and Adults >90-150 kg: 225 mg every 2 weeks
IgE >200-300 int. units/mL:
Children ≥12 years and Adults 30-60 kg: 300 mg every 4 weeks
Children ≥12 years and Adults >60-90 kg: 225 mg every 2 weeks
Children ≥12 years and Adults >90-150 kg: 300 mg every 2 weeks
IgE >300-400 int. units/mL:
Children ≥12 years and Adults 30-70 kg: 225 mg every 2 weeks
Children ≥12 years and Adults >70-90 kg: 300 mg every 2 weeks
IgE >400-500 int. units/mL:
Children ≥12 years and Adults 30-70 kg: 300 mg every 2 weeks
Children ≥12 years and Adults >70-90 kg: 375 mg every 2 weeks
IgE >500-600 int. units/mL:
Children ≥12 years and Adults 30-60 kg: 300 mg every 2 weeks
Children ≥12 years and Adults >60-70 kg: 375 mg every 2 weeks
IgE >600-700 int. units/mL: *Children ≥12 years and Adults 30-60 kg:* 375 mg every 2 weeks

Mechanism of Action Omalizumab is an IgG monoclonal antibody (recombinant DNA derived) which inhibits IgE binding to the high-affinity IgE receptor on mast cells and basophils. By decreasing bound IgE, the activation and release of mediators in the allergic response (early and late phase) is limited. Serum-free IgE levels and the number of high-affinity IgE receptors are decreased. Long-term treatment in patients with allergic asthma showed a decrease in asthma exacerbations and corticosteroid usage.

Pharmacodynamics/Kinetics
Half-life Elimination 26 days
Time to Peak 7-8 days

Pregnancy Risk Factor B

Omeprazole (oh MEP ra zole)

Related Information
Esomeprazole *on page 628*
Gastrointestinal Disorders *on page 1874*

U.S. Brand Names PriLOSEC OTC® [OTC]; PriLOSEC®

Canadian Brand Names Apo-Omeprazole®; Losec MUPS®; Losec®; Mylan-Omeprazole; PMS-Omeprazole; PMS-Omeprazole DR; ratio-Omeprazole; Sandoz-Omeprazole

Generic Availability (U.S.) Yes: Excludes granules for suspension

Pharmacologic Category Proton Pump Inhibitor; Substituted Benzimidazole

Use Short-term (4-8 weeks) treatment of active duodenal ulcer disease or active benign gastric ulcer; treatment of heartburn and other symptoms associated with gastroesophageal reflux disease (GERD); short-term (4-8 weeks) treatment of endoscopically-diagnosed erosive esophagitis; maintenance healing of erosive esophagitis; long-term treatment of pathological hypersecretory conditions; as part of a multidrug regimen for *H. pylori* eradication to reduce the risk of duodenal ulcer recurrence

OTC labeling: Short-term treatment of frequent, uncomplicated heartburn occurring ≥2 days/week

Unlabeled/Investigational Use Healing NSAID-induced ulcers; prevention of NSAID-induced ulcer; stress-ulcer prophylaxis in the critically-ill

Local Anesthetic/Vasoconstrictor Precautions No information available to require special precautions

Effects on Dental Treatment Key adverse event(s) related to dental treatment: Taste perversion, dry mouth, esophageal candidiasis, and mucosal atrophy (tongue).

Effects on Bleeding No information available to require special precautions

Adverse Effects 1% to 10%:

Central nervous system: Headache (7%), dizziness (2%)

Dermatologic: Rash (2%)

Gastrointestinal: Abdominal pain (5%), diarrhea (4%), nausea (4%), vomiting (3%), flatulence (3%), acid regurgitation (2%), constipation (2%)

Neuromuscular & skeletal: Back pain (1%), weakness (1%)

Respiratory: Upper respiratory infection (2%), cough (1%)

Dosage Oral:

Children 1-16 years: GERD or other acid-related disorders:

5 kg to <10 kg: 5 mg once daily

10 kg to <20 kg: 10 mg once daily

≥20 kg: 20 mg once daily

Adults:

Active duodenal ulcer: 20 mg once daily for 4-8 weeks

Gastric ulcers: 40 mg once daily for 4-8 weeks

Symptomatic GERD (without esophageal lesions): 20 mg once daily for up to 4 weeks

Erosive esophagitis: 20 mg once daily for 4-8 weeks; maintenance of healing: 20 mg once daily for up to 12 months total therapy (including treatment period of 4-8 weeks)

Helicobacter pylori eradication: Dose varies with regimen:

Manufacturer labeling: 40 mg once daily administered with clarithromycin 500 mg 3 times/day for 14 days **or** 20 mg twice daily administered with amoxicillin 1000 mg *and* clarithromycin 500 mg twice daily for 10 days. **Note:** Presence of ulcer at time of therapy initiation may necessitate an additional 14-18 days of omeprazole 20 mg/day (monotherapy) after completion of combination therapy.

American College of Gastroenterology guidelines (Chey, 2007):

Nonpenicillin allergy: 20 mg twice daily administered with amoxicillin 1000 mg *and* clarithromycin 500 mg twice daily for 10-14 days

Penicillin allergy: 20 mg twice daily administered with clarithromycin 500 mg *and* metronidazole 500 mg twice daily for 10-14 days **or** 20 mg once or twice daily administered with bismuth subsalicylate 525 mg *and* metronidazole 250 mg *plus* tetracycline 500 mg 4 times/day for 10-14 days

Pathological hypersecretory conditions: Initial: 60 mg once daily; doses up to 120 mg 3 times/day have been administered; administer daily doses >80 mg in divided doses

Stress-ulcer prophylaxis (ICU patients; unlabeled use): 40 mg once daily; periodically evaluate patient for continued need (Levy, 1997)

Frequent heartburn (OTC labeling): 20 mg once daily for 14 days; treatment may be repeated after 4 months if needed

Dosage adjustment in hepatic impairment: Bioavailability is increased with chronic liver disease. Consider dosage adjustment, especially for maintenance of erosive esophagitis. Specific guidelines are not available.

Mechanism of Action Proton pump inhibitor; suppresses gastric basal and stimulated acid secretion by inhibiting the parietal cell H+/K+ ATP pump

Contraindications Hypersensitivity to omeprazole, substituted benzimidazoles (eg, esomeprazole, lansoprazole), or any component of the formulation

Warnings/Precautions Use of proton pump inhibitors may increase the risk of gastrointestinal infections (eg, *Salmonella, Campylobacter*). Relief of symptoms does not preclude the presence of a gastric malignancy. Atrophic gastritis (by biopsy) has been noted with long-term omeprazole therapy. In long-term (2-year) studies in rats, omeprazole produced a dose-related increase in gastric carcinoid tumors. While available endoscopic evaluations and histologic examinations of biopsy specimens from human stomachs have not detected a risk from short-term exposure to omeprazole, further human data on the effect of sustained hypochlorhydria and hypergastrinemia are needed to rule out the possibility of an increased risk for the development of tumors in humans receiving long-term therapy. Proton pump inhibitors may diminish the therapeutic effect of clopidogrel thought to be due to reduced formation of the active metabolite of clopidogrel; an increase in the risk of cardiovascular events may occur. The manufacturer of clopidogrel recommends avoidance of concomitant administration of omeprazole even when scheduled 12 hours apart.

Increased incidence of osteoporosis-related bone fractures of the hip, spine, or wrist may occur with proton pump inhibitor therapy. Patients on high-dose (multiple daily doses)or long-term (≥1 year) therapy should be monitored. Use the lowest effective dose for the shortest duration of time, use vitamin D and calcium supplementation, and follow appropriate guidelines to reduce risk of fractures in patients at risk.

Decreased *H. pylori* eradication rates have been observed with short-term (≤7 days) combination therapy. The American College of Gastroenterology recommends 10-14 days of therapy (triple or quadruple) for eradication of *H. pylori* (Chey, 2007). Bioavailability may be increased in Asian populations and patients with hepatic dysfunction; consider dosage reductions, especially for maintenance healing of erosive esophagitis. Bioavailability may be increased in the elderly. When used for self-medication (OTC), do not use for >14 days.

Drug Interactions

Metabolism/Transport Effects Substrate of CYP2A6 (minor), 2C9 (minor), 2C19 (major), 2D6 (minor), 3A4 (major); **Inhibits** CYP1A2 (weak), 2C9 (moderate), 2C19 (moderate), 2D6 (weak), 3A4 (weak); **Induces** CYP1A2 (weak)

Avoid Concomitant Use

Avoid concomitant use of Omeprazole with any of the following: Clopidogrel; Delavirdine; Erlotinib; Nelfinavir; Posaconazole

Increased Effect/Toxicity

Omeprazole may increase the levels/effects of: Amphetamines; Benzodiazepines (metabolized by oxidation); Carvedilol; Cilostazol; CloZAPine; CycloSPORINE; CycloSPORINE (Systemic); CYP2C19 Substrates; CYP2C9 Substrates (High risk); Dexmethylphenidate; Fosphenytoin; Methotrexate; Methylphenidate; Phenytoin; Raltegravir; Saquinavir; Tacrolimus; Tacrolimus (Systemic); Vitamin K Antagonists; Voriconazole

The levels/effects of Omeprazole may be increased by: Conivaptan; Fluconazole; Ketoconazole; Ketoconazole (Systemic)

Decreased Effect

Omeprazole may decrease the levels/effects of: Atazanavir; Bisphosphonate Derivatives; Cefditoren; Clopidogrel; CloZAPine; Dabigatran Etexilate; Dasatinib; Delavirdine; Erlotinib; Gefitinib; Indinavir; Iron Salts; Itraconazole; Ketoconazole; Ketoconazole (Systemic); Mesalamine; Mycophenolate; Nelfinavir; Posaconazole

The levels/effects of Omeprazole may be decreased by: CYP2C19 Inducers (Strong); Peginterferon Alfa-2b; Tipranavir; Tocilizumab

Ethanol/Nutrition/Herb Interactions

Ethanol: Avoid ethanol (may cause gastric mucosal irritation).
Food: Food delays absorption.

Dietary Considerations Should be taken on an empty stomach; best if taken before breakfast.

Pharmacodynamics/Kinetics

Onset of Action Antisecretory: ~1 hour; Peak effect: Within 2 hours

Duration of Action Up to 72 hours; 50% of maximum effect at 24 hours; after stopping treatment, secretory activity gradually returns over 3-5 days

Half-life Elimination 0.5-1 hour; hepatic impairment: ~3 hours

Time to Peak Plasma: 0.5-3.5 hours

Pregnancy Risk Factor C

Lactation Enters breast milk/not recommended

Breast-Feeding Considerations Following administration of omeprazole 20 mg, peak concentrations detected in the breast milk were <7% of the maternal serum concentration.

Dosage Forms

Capsule, delayed release, oral: 10 mg, 20 mg, 40 mg
PriLOSEC®: 10 mg, 20 mg, 40 mg

Granules for suspension, delayed release, enteric coated, oral:
PriLOSEC®: 2.5 mg/packet (30s); 10 mg/packet (30s)

Tablet, delayed release, oral: 20 mg, 40 mg
PriLOSEC OTC® [OTC]: 20 mg

Omeprazole and Sodium Bicarbonate

(oh MEP ra zole & SOW dee um bye KAR bun ate)

Related Information

Omeprazole *on page 1247*
Sodium Bicarbonate *on page 1537*

U.S. Brand Names Zegerid OTC™ [OTC]; Zegerid®

Pharmacologic Category Proton Pump Inhibitor; Substituted Benzimidazole

Use Short-term (4-8 weeks) treatment of active duodenal ulcer or active benign gastric ulcer; treatment of heartburn and other symptoms associated with gastroesophageal reflux disease (GERD); short-term (4-8 weeks) treatment of endoscopically-diagnosed erosive esophagitis; maintenance healing of erosive esophagitis; reduction of risk of upper gastrointestinal bleeding in critically-ill patients

OTC labeling: Short-term (2 weeks) treatment of frequent (2 days/week), uncomplicated heartburn

Local Anesthetic/Vasoconstrictor Precautions No information available to require special precautions

Effects on Dental Treatment Key adverse event(s) related to dental treatment: Oral candidiasis.

Effects on Bleeding No information available to require special precautions

Adverse Effects Percentages of adverse events reported from a controlled clinical trial of 359 critically-ill patients receiving the oral powder for suspension

>10%:
- Central nervous system: Pyrexia (20%)
- Endocrine & metabolic: Hypokalemia (12%), hyperglycemia (11%)
- Respiratory: Nosocomial pneumonia (11%)

1% to 10%:
- Cardiovascular: Hypotension (10%), hypertension (8%), atrial fibrillation (6%), ventricular tachycardia (5%), bradycardia (4%), tachycardia (3%), supraventricular tachycardia (3%), edema (3%)
- Central nervous system: Hyperpyrexia (5%), agitation (3%)
- Dermatological: Rash (6%), decubitus ulcer (3%)
- Endocrine & metabolic: Hypomagnesemia (10%), hypocalcemia (6%), hypophosphatemia (6%), fluid overload (5%), hypoglycemia (3%), hyponatremia (4%), hypernatremia (2%), hyperkalemia (2%)
- Gastrointestinal: Constipation (5%), diarrhea (4%), hypomotility (2%)
- Genitourinary: Urinary tract infection (2%)
- Hematological: Thrombocytopenia (10%), anemia (8%), anemia increased (2%)
- Hepatic: LFTs increased (2%)
- Respiratory: ARDS (3%), respiratory failure (2%), pneumothorax (1%)
- Miscellaneous: Sepsis (5%), oral candidiasis (4%), candidal infection (2%)

General Dosage Range Oral: *Adults:* 20-40 mg/day in 1-2 divided doses

Mechanism of Action Suppresses gastric basal and stimulated acid secretion by inhibiting the parietal cell H+/K+ ATP pump

Pharmacodynamics/Kinetics

Onset of Action Antisecretory: ~1 hour; Peak antisecretory effect: 2 hours; Full therapeutic effect: 1-4 days

Duration of Action 72 hours

Half-life Elimination ~1 hour (range: 0.4-3.2 hours)

Time to Peak Serum: ~30 minutes

Pregnancy Risk Factor C

OnabotulinumtoxinA (oh nuh BOT yoo lin num TOKS in aye)

U.S. Brand Names Botox®; Botox® Cosmetic

Canadian Brand Names Botox®; Botox® Cosmetic

Generic Availability (U.S.) No

Pharmacologic Category Neuromuscular Blocker Agent, Toxin; Ophthalmic Agent, Toxin

Use Treatment of strabismus and blepharospasm associated with dystonia (including benign essential blepharospasm or VII nerve disorders) in patients ≥12 years of age; treatment of cervical dystonia (spasmodic torticollis) in patients ≥16 years of age; temporary improvement in the appearance of lines/wrinkles of the face (moderate-to-severe glabellar lines associated with corrugator and/or procerus muscle activity) in adult patients ≤65 years of age; treatment of severe primary axillary hyperhidrosis in adults not adequately controlled with topical treatments; treatment of focal spasticity (specifically upper limb spasticity) in adults; prophylaxis of chronic migraine headache (≥15 days/month with ≥4 hours/day headache duration) in adults

Canadian labeling: Additional use (not in U.S. labeling): Dynamic equinus foot deformity in pediatric cerebral palsy patients; treatment of forehead, lateral canthus, and glabellar lines in adults >65 years of age

Unlabeled/Investigational Use Treatment of oromandibular dystonia, spasmodic dysphonia (laryngeal dystonia) and other dystonias (ie, writer's cramp, focal task-specific dystonias); treatment of dynamic muscle contracture in pediatric cerebral palsy patients

Local Anesthetic/Vasoconstrictor Precautions No information available to require special precautions

Effects on Dental Treatment Key adverse event(s) related to dental treatment: Xerostomia (normal salivary flow resumes upon discontinuation), facial pain, and facial weakness. Effects occur in ~1 week and may last up to several months.

Effects on Bleeding No information available to require special precautions

Adverse Effects Adverse effects usually occur in 1 week and may last up to several months

>10%:

Cervical dystonia:

Central nervous system: Pain (32%), headache (≤11%)
Gastrointestinal: Dysphagia (19%)
Neuromuscular & skeletal: Focal weakness (17%), neck pain (11%)
Respiratory: Upper respiratory infection (12%)

Other indications (blepharospasm, primary axillary hyperhidrosis, strabismus):

Ocular: Ptosis (blepharospasm 21%; strabismus 1% to 38%), vertical deviation (strabismus 17%)

1% to 10%:

Cervical dystonia:

Central nervous system: Dizziness, drowsiness, fever, malaise, speech disorder
Gastrointestinal: Nausea, xerostomia
Local: Injection site reaction: Soreness
Neuromuscular & skeletal: Back pain, hypertonia, numbness, stiffness, weakness
Ocular: Diplopia, ptosis
Respiratory: Cough, dyspnea, rhinitis
Miscellaneous: Flu-like syndrome

Cerebral palsy spasticity:

Central nervous system: Pain (1% to 2%), fever (1%), lethargy (1%)
Neuromuscular & skeletal: Falling, weakness

Chronic migraines:

Cardiovascular: Hypertension (2%)
Central nervous system: Headache (5%), worsening migraine (4%), facial paresis (2%)
Neuromuscular & skeletal: Neck pain (9%), stiffness(4%), weakness (4%), myalgia (3%), musculoskeletal pain (3%), muscle spasm (2%)
Ocular: Eyelid ptosis (4%)
Respiratory: Bronchitis (3%)
Miscellaneous: Injection site pain (3%)

Focal spasticity:

Central nervous system: Fatigue
Gastrointestinal: Nausea
Neuromuscular & skeletal: Pain in extremity, weakness
Respiratory: Bronchitis

Other indications (blepharospasm, primary axillary hyperhidrosis, reduction of glabellar lines, strabismus):

Cardiovascular: Hypertension
Central nervous system: Anxiety, dizziness, fever, headache, pain
Dermatologic: Pruritus, rash, skin tightness
Gastrointestinal: Dyspepsia, nausea
Local: Injection site reaction: Hemorrhage, pain, soreness
Neuromuscular & skeletal: Back pain, facial pain, neck pain, weakness
Ocular: Irritation/tearing (includes dry eye, lagophthalmos, photophobia); ptosis, superficial punctate keratitis
Respiratory: Pharyngitis
Miscellaneous: Flu-like syndrome, infection, nonaxillary sweating, tooth disorder

Dosage Note: In adults treated for more than one indication, the maximum cumulative dose should be ≤360 units/3 months. Canadian labeling recommends a maximum cumulative dose of 6 units/kg (adults up to 360 units; children up to 200 units) over 3 months in patients receiving additional treatment for noncosmetic indications.

Blepharospasm:

Botox®: Children ≥12 years and Adults: I.M.: Initial dose: 1.25-2.5 units injected into the medial and lateral pretarsal orbicularis oculi of the upper lid and lateral pretarsal orbicularis oculi of lower lid

Dose may be increased up to twice the previous dose if the response from the initial dose lasted ≤2 months; maximum dose per site: 5 units. Tolerance may occur if treatments are given more often than every 3 months, but the effect is not usually permanent. Cumulative dose:

U.S. labeling: ≤200 units in 30-day period
Canadian labeling (not in U.S. labeling): Botox®: ≤200 units in 2-month period

Cervical dystonia:

Children ≥16 years and Adults: I.M.: For dosing guidance, the mean dose is 236 units (25th to 75th percentile range 198-300 units) divided among the affected muscles in patients previously treated with botulinum toxin (maximum: ≤50 units/site). Initial dose in previously untreated patients should be lower. Sequential dosing should be based on the patient's head and neck position, localization of pain, muscle hypertrophy, patient response, and previous adverse reactions. The total dose injected into the sternocleidomastoid muscles should be ≤100 units to decrease the occurrence of dysphagia.

Canadian labeling (not in U.S. labeling): Botox®: Children ≥16 years and Adults: I.M.: Effective range of 200-360 units has been used in clinical practice; administer no more frequently than every 2 months

Chronic migraine: Adults: I.M.: Administer 5 units/0.1 mL per site. Recommended total dose is 155 units once every 12 weeks. Each 155 unit dose should be equally divided and administered bilaterally, into 31 total sites as described below (refer to prescribing information for specific diagrams of recommended injection sites):

Corrugator: 5 units to each side (2 sites)
Procerus: 5 units (1 site only)
Frontalis: 10 units to each side (divided into 2 sites/side)
Temporalis: 20 units to each side (divided into 4 sites/side)
Occipitalis: 15 units to each side (divided into 3 sites/side)
Cervical paraspinal: 10 units to each side (divided into 2 sites/side)
Trapezius: 15 units to each side (divided into 3 sites/side)

Strabismus: Children ≥12 years and Adults: I.M.: **Note:** Several minutes prior to injection, administration of local anesthetic and ocular decongestant drops are recommended.

Initial dose:

Vertical muscles and for horizontal strabismus <20 prism diopters: 1.25-2.5 units in any one muscle
Horizontal strabismus of 20-50 prism diopters: 2.5-5 units in any one muscle
Persistent VI nerve palsy ≥1 month: 1.25-2.5 units in the medial rectus muscle

Re-examine patients 7-14 days after each injection to assess the effect of that dose. Subsequent doses for patients experiencing incomplete paralysis of the target may be increased up to twice the previous administered dose. The maximum recommended dose as a single injection for any one muscle is 25 units. Do not administer subsequent injections until the effects of the previous dose are gone.

Primary axillary hyperhidrosis: Adults ≥18 years: Intradermal: 50 units/axilla. Injection area should be defined by standard staining techniques. Injections should be evenly distributed into multiple sites (10-15), administered in 0.1-0.2 mL aliquots, ~1-2 cm apart. May repeat when clinical effect diminishes.

Spasticity (cerebral palsy related [dynamic equinus foot deformity]: Canadian labeling [not approved in U.S. labeling]): Children ≥2 years: I.M.: 4 units/kg (total dose) divided into two injections into medial and lateral heads of the gastrocnemius of affected leg; if clinically indicated, may repeat every 2 months (maximum dose: 200 units); in diplegia, the recommended dose is 6 units/kg (total dose) divided between affected limbs

Spasticity (focal): Adults ≥18 years: I.M.: Individualize dose based on patient size, extent, and location of muscle involvement, degree of spasticity, local muscle weakness, and response to prior treatment. In clinical trials, total doses up to 360 units (Botox®) were administered as separate injections typically divided among selected muscles; may repeat therapy at ≥3 months with appropriate dosage based upon the clinical condition of patient at time of retreatment.

Suggested guidelines for the treatment of upper limb spasticity. The lowest recommended starting dose should be used and ≤50 units/site should be administered. **Note:** Dose listed is total dose administered as individual or separate intramuscular injection(s):

Biceps brachii: 100-200 units (divided into 4 sites)
Flexor digitorum profundus: 30-50 units (1 site)
Flexor digitorum sublimes: 30-50 units (1 site)
Flexor carpi radialis: 12.5-50 units (1 site)
Flexor carpi ulnaris: 12.5-50 units (1 site)

Suggested guidelines for the treatment of stroke-related upper limb spasticity: Canadian labeling: **Note:** Dose listed is total dose administered as individual or separate intramuscular injection(s):

Biceps brachii: 100-200 units (up to 4 sites)
Flexor digitorum profundus: 15-50 units (1-2 sites)
Flexor digitorum sublimes: 15-50 units (1-2 sites)
Flexor carpi radialis: 15-60 units (1-2 sites)
Flexor carpi ulnaris: 10-50 units (1-2 sites)
Adductor pollicis: 20 units (1-2 sites)
Flexor pollicis longus: 20 units (1-2 sites)

Cosmetic uses:

Reduction of glabellar lines: Adults ≤65 years: I.M.: An effective dose is determined by gross observation of the patient's ability to activate the superficial muscles injected. The location, size and use of muscles may vary markedly among individuals. Inject 0.1 mL (4 units) dose into each of five sites, two in each corrugator muscle and one in the procerus muscle for a total dose 0.5 mL (20 units) administered no more frequently than every 3-4 months. **Note:** Treatment of adults >65 years is approved in the Canadian labeling.

Reduction of forehead lines (Canadian labeling; not in U.S. labeling): Adults: I.M.: Inject 2-6 units into each of four sites in the frontalis muscle every 1-2 cm along either side of forehead crease and 2-3 cm above eyebrows for total dose of 24 units.

Reduction of lateral canthus lines (Canadian labeling; not in U.S. labeling): Adults: I.M.: Inject 2-6 units into each of 1-3 injection sites, lateral to the lateral orbital rim.

Elderly: No specific adjustment recommended; initiate therapy at lowest recommended dose

Mechanism of Action OnabotulinumtoxinA (previously known as botulinum toxin type A) is a neurotoxin produced by *Clostridium botulinum*, spore-forming anaerobic bacillus, which appears to affect only the presynaptic membrane of the neuromuscular junction in humans, where it prevents calcium-dependent release of acetylcholine and produces a state of denervation. Muscle inactivation persists until new fibrils grow from the nerve and form junction plates on new areas of the muscle-cell walls. Intradermal injection results in temporary sweat gland denervation, reducing local sweating.

Contraindications Hypersensitivity to botulinum toxin, or any component of the formulation; infection at the proposed injection site(s)

Warnings/Precautions [U.S. Boxed Warning]: Distant spread of botulinum toxin beyond the site of injection has been reported; dysphagia and breathing difficulties have occurred and may be life threatening; other symptoms reported include blurred vision, diplopia, dysarthria, dysphonia, generalized muscle weakness, ptosis, and urinary incontinence which may develop within hours or weeks following injection. Risk likely greatest in children treated for the unapproved use of spasticity. Systemic effects have occurred following use in approved and unapproved uses, including low doses. Immediate medical attention required if respiratory, speech, or swallowing difficulties appear. Higher doses or more frequent administration may result in neutralizing antibody formation and loss of efficacy. Use caution in patients with bleeding disorders and/or receiving anticoagulation therapy. May impair ability to drive and/or operate machinery; if loss of strength, muscle weakness, or impaired vision occurs, patients should avoid driving or engaging in other hazardous activities.

Product contains albumin and may carry a remote risk of virus transmission. Use caution if there is excessive weakness or atrophy at the proposed injection site(s); use is contraindicated if infection is present at injection site. Have appropriate support in case of anaphylactic reaction. Use with caution in patients with neuromuscular diseases (such as myasthenia gravis or Lambert-Eaton syndrome), neuropathic disorders (such as amyotrophic lateral sclerosis), patients taking aminoglycosides, neuromuscular-blocking agents, or other drugs that interfere with neuromuscular transmission and patients with pre-existing cardiovascular disease (rare reports of arrhythmia and MI). Long-term effects of chronic therapy are unknown. Botulinum products (abobotulinumtoxinA, onabotulinumtoxinA, rimabotulinumtoxinB) are not interchangeable; potency units are specific to each preparation and cannot be compared or converted to any other botulinum product.

Cervical dystonia: Dysphagia is common. It may be severe requiring alternative feeding methods and may persist anywhere from 2 weeks up to 5 months after administration. Risk factors include smaller neck muscle mass, bilateral injections into the sternocleidomastoid muscle, or injections into the levator scapulae. Use extreme caution in patients with pre-existing respiratory disease; may weaken accessory muscles that are necessary for these patients to maintain adequate ventilation. Risk of aspiration resulting from severe dysphagia is increased in patients with decreased respiratory function.

Episodic migraines: Safety and efficacy have not been established in patients with 14 or fewer headaches per month.

Ocular disease: Blepharospasm: Reduced blinking from injection of the orbicularis muscle can lead to corneal exposure and ulceration. Strabismus: Retrobulbar hemorrhages may occur from needle penetration into orbit. Spatial disorientation, double vision, or past-pointing may occur if one or more extraocular muscles are paralyzed. Covering the affected eye may help. Careful testing of corneal sensation, avoidance of lower lid injections, and treatment of epithelial defects are necessary. Use with caution in angle closure glaucoma.

Primary axillary hyperhidrosis: Evaluate for secondary causes prior to treatment (eg, hyperthyroidism). Safety and efficacy for treatment of hyperhidrosis in other areas of the body have not been established.

Temporary reduction in glabellar lines: Do not use more frequently than every 3 months (Canadian labeling states not to use more frequently than every 2 months). Patients with marked facial asymmetry, ptosis, excessive dermatochalasis, deep dermal scarring, thick sebaceous skin, or the inability to substantially lessen glabellar lines by physically spreading them apart were excluded from clinical trials. Use with caution in patients with surgical alterations to the facial anatomy. Reduced blinking from injection of the orbicularis muscle can lead to corneal exposure and ulceration. Spatial disorientation, double vision, or past pointing may occur if one or more extraocular muscles are paralyzed.

Drug Interactions

Avoid Concomitant Use There are no known interactions where it is recommended to avoid concomitant use.

Increased Effect/Toxicity

OnabotulinumtoxinA may increase the levels/effects of: AbobotulinumtoxinA; RimabotulinumtoxinB

The levels/effects of OnabotulinumtoxinA may be increased by: Aminoglycosides; Anticholinergic Agents; Neuromuscular-Blocking Agents

Decreased Effect There are no known significant interactions involving a decrease in effect.

Pharmacodynamics/Kinetics

Onset of Action Blepharospasm: ~3-4 days; Cervical dystonia: ~2 weeks; Reduction of glabellar lines (Botox® Cosmetic): 1-2 days, increasing in intensity during first week; Spasticity: Focal and cerebral palsy related: <2 weeks; Strabismus: ~1-2 days

Duration of Action Blepharospasm: ~3-4 months; Cervical dystonia: ≤3-4 months; Reduction of glabellar lines (Botox® Cosmetic): ~3-4 months; Spasticity: ~3-3.5 months; Strabismus: ~2-6 weeks; Primary axillary hyperhidrosis: 201 days (mean)

Time to Peak Blepharospasm: 1-2 weeks; Cervical dystonia: ~6 weeks; Spasticity (focal): 4-6 weeks; Strabismus: Within first week

Pregnancy Risk Factor C

Lactation Excretion in breast milk unknown/use caution

Dosage Forms

Injection, powder for reconstitution [preservative free]:

Botox®: *Clostridium botulinum* type A neurotoxin complex 100 units, *Clostridium botulinum* type A neurotoxin complex 200 units

Botox® Cosmetic: *Clostridium botulinum* type A neurotoxin complex 100 units

Powder for reconstitution, for injection [preservative free]:

Botox® Cosmetic: *Clostridium botulinum* type A neurotoxin complex 50 units

Dosage Forms: Canada

Injection, powder for reconstitution [preservative free]:

Botox®: Botulinum toxin A 50 units, 100 units, 200 units

Botox Cosmetic®: Botulinum toxin A 50 unit, 100 units, 200 units

Dental Comment Cote and associates, published a paper describing all serious adverse reactions reported to the FDA (Cote, 2005). Included in the 217 serious effects reported, there were 28 deaths and 17 seizures. The deaths were attributed to heart attacks, cerebrovascular accident, pulmonary embolisms, pneumonia, or unknown causes. There were 1031 adverse effects reported after cosmetic use, 36 were of a serious nature. These included focal facial paralysis, muscle weakness, dysphagia, flu-like symptoms, and allergic reactions.

In contrast to the Cote study, the Naumann study reviewed the adverse reactions described and reported in randomized, controlled trials of onabotulinumtoxinA. They reviewed 36 studies involving 2309 subjects through the years 1966-2003. Of the 2309 subjects, 1425 received onabotulinumtoxinA treatment. No study reported severe adverse events. The only adverse event occurring significantly more often than with placebo was focal weakness.

References

Batra RS, Dover JS, and Arndt KA, "Adverse Event Reporting for Botulinum Toxin Type A," *J Am Acad Dermatol*, 2005, 53(6):1080-2.

Coté TR, Mohan AK, Polder JA, et al, "Botulinum Toxin Type A Injections: Adverse Events Reported to the U.S. Food and Drug Administration in Therapeutic and Cosmetic Cases," *J Am Acad Dermatol*, 2005, 53(3):407-15.

Naumann M and Jankovic J, "Safety of Botulinum Toxin Type A: A Systematic Review and Meta-Analysis," *Curr Med Res Opin*, 2004, 20(7):981-90.

Ondansetron (on DAN se tron)

U.S. Brand Names Zofran®; Zofran® ODT; Zuplenz®

Canadian Brand Names Apo-Ondansetron®; CO Ondansetron; Dom-Ondansetron; JAMP-Ondansetron; Mint-Ondansetron; Mylan-Ondansetron; Novo-Ondansetron; Ondansetron Injection; Ondansetron-Omega; PHL-Ondansetron; PMS-Ondansetron; RAN™-Ondansetron; ratio-Ondansetron; Sandoz-Ondansetron; Zofran®; Zofran® ODT; ZYM-Ondansetron

Pharmacologic Category Antiemetic; Selective 5-HT_3 Receptor Antagonist

Use Prevention of nausea and vomiting associated with moderately- to highly-emetogenic cancer chemotherapy; radiotherapy; prevention of postoperative nausea and vomiting (PONV); treatment of PONV if no prophylactic dose of ondansetron received

Unlabeled/Investigational Use Hyperemesis gravidarum; breakthrough treatment of nausea and vomiting associated with chemotherapy

Local Anesthetic/Vasoconstrictor Precautions No information available to require special precautions

Effects on Dental Treatment No significant effects or complications reported

Effects on Bleeding No information available to require special precautions

Adverse Effects Note: Percentages reported in adult patients.

>10%:

Central nervous system: Headache (9% to 27%), malaise/fatigue (9% to 13%)

Gastrointestinal: Constipation (6% to 11%)

1% to 10%:

Central nervous system: Drowsiness (8%), fever (2% to 8%), dizziness (4% to 7%), anxiety (6%), cold sensation (2%)

Dermatologic: Pruritus (2% to 5%), rash (1%)

Gastrointestinal: Diarrhea (2% to 7%)

Genitourinary: Gynecological disorder (7%), urinary retention (5%)

Hepatic: ALT increased (1% to 5%), AST increased (1% to 5%)

Local: Injection site reaction (4%; pain, redness, burning)

Neuromuscular & skeletal: Paresthesia (2%)

Respiratory: Hypoxia (9%)

General Dosage Range Dosage adjustment recommended in patients with hepatic impairment

I.M.: *Adults:* 4 mg as a single dose

I.V.:

Infants 1-6 months: 0.1 mg/kg as a single dose

Children 6 months to 12 years and ≤40 kg: 0.1-0.45 mg/kg as a single dose **or** 0.15 mg/kg/dose for 3 doses

Children 6 months to 12 years and >40 kg and Children >12 years to 18 years: 0.45 mg/kg **or** 4 mg as a single dose **or** 0.15 mg/kg/dose for 3 doses

Adults: Dosage varies greatly depending on indication

Oral:

Children 4-11 years: 4 mg for 3 doses, then 4 mg every 8 hours for 1-2 days

Children ≥12 years: 24 mg as a single dose **or** 8 mg every 8-12 hours

Adults: 8-24 mg as a single dose **or** 8 mg every 8-12 hours

Mechanism of Action Selective 5-HT_3-receptor antagonist, blocking serotonin, both peripherally on vagal nerve terminals and centrally in the chemoreceptor trigger zone

Pharmacodynamics/Kinetics

Onset of Action ~30 minutes

Half-life Elimination Children <15 years: 2-7 hours; Adults: 3-6 hours

Mild-to-moderate hepatic impairment (Child-Pugh classes A and B): Adults: 12 hours

Severe hepatic impairment (Child-Pugh class C): Adults: 20 hours

Time to Peak Oral: ~2 hours; Oral soluble film: ~1 hour

Pregnancy Risk Factor B

Dental Comment Ondansetron is a safer alternative than phenothiazines (ie, promethazine) for the treatment of moderate-to-severe postoperative nausea and vomiting. The cost can be a limitation.

Opium Tincture (OH pee um TING chur)

Pharmacologic Category Analgesic, Opioid; Antidiarrheal

Use Treatment of diarrhea in adults

Local Anesthetic/Vasoconstrictor Precautions No information available to require special precautions

Effects on Dental Treatment No significant effects or complications reported

Effects on Bleeding No information available to require special precautions

Adverse Effects Frequency not defined.
Cardiovascular: Palpitation, hypotension, bradycardia, peripheral vasodilation
Central nervous system: Drowsiness, dizziness, restlessness, headache, malaise, CNS depression, intracranial pressure increased, insomnia, mental depression
Gastrointestinal: Nausea, vomiting, constipation, anorexia, stomach cramps, biliary tract spasm
Genitourinary: Urination decreased, urinary tract spasm
Neuromuscular & skeletal: Weakness
Ocular: Miosis
Respiratory: Respiratory depression
Miscellaneous: Histamine release, physical and psychological dependence

General Dosage Range
Oral: Opium tincture 10% contains morphine 10 mg/mL. Use caution in ordering, dispensing, and/or administering. The following doses are expressed in **mg** (milligram) dosing units of morphine.
Adults: Usual: 6 **mg** of undiluted opium tincture (10 mg/mL) 4 times daily

Mechanism of Action Contains many narcotic alkaloids including morphine; its mechanism for gastric motility inhibition is primarily due to this morphine content; it results in a decrease in digestive secretions, an increase in GI muscle tone, and therefore a reduction in GI propulsion

Pharmacodynamics/Kinetics
Duration of Action 4-5 hours

Controlled Substance C-II

Oprelvekin (oh PREL ve kin)

U.S. Brand Names Neumega®

Pharmacologic Category Biological Response Modulator; Human Growth Factor

Use Prevention of severe thrombocytopenia; reduce the need for platelet transfusions following myelosuppressive chemotherapy for nonmyeloid malignancy

Local Anesthetic/Vasoconstrictor Precautions No information available to require special precautions

Effects on Dental Treatment Key adverse event(s) related to dental treatment: Oral moniliasis.

Effects on Bleeding No information available to require special precautions

Adverse Effects
>10%:
Cardiovascular: Tachycardia (children 84%; adults 20%), edema (59%), cardiomegaly (children 21%), vasodilation (19%), atrial arrhythmia (12% to 15%), palpitation (14%), syncope (13%)
Central nervous system: Neutropenic fever (48%), headache (41%), dizziness (38%), fever (36%), insomnia (33%)
Dermatologic: Rash (25%)
Endocrine & metabolic: Fluid retention
Gastrointestinal: Nausea/vomiting (77%), diarrhea (43%), mucositis (43%), oral moniliasis (14%), weight gain (due to fluid retention)
Hematologic: Anemia (dilutional; onset: 3-5 days; duration: ≤1 week)
Neuromuscular & skeletal: Weakness (severe 14%), periostitis (children 11%), arthralgia
Ocular: Conjunctival injection/redness/swelling (children 57%; adults 19%), papilledema (children 16%; adults 1%)
Respiratory: Dyspnea (48%), rhinitis (42%), cough (29%), pharyngitis (25%)
1% to 10%: Respiratory: Pleural effusion (10%)

General Dosage Range Dosage adjustment recommended in patients with renal impairment
SubQ: *Adults:* 50 mcg/kg once daily

Mechanism of Action Oprelvekin is a thrombopoietic growth factor which stimulates multiple stages of megakaryocytopoiesis and thrombopoiesis, resulting in proliferation of megakaryocyte progenitors and megakaryocyte maturation, thereby increasing platelet production.

Pharmacodynamics/Kinetics
Half-life Elimination Terminal: 5-9 hours
Time to Peak Serum: 1-6 hours

Pregnancy Risk Factor C

Orlistat (OR li stat)

U.S. Brand Names Alli™ [OTC]; Xenical®

Canadian Brand Names Xenical®

Pharmacologic Category Lipase Inhibitor

Use Management of obesity, including weight loss and weight management, when used in conjunction with a reduced-calorie and low-fat diet; reduce the risk of weight regain after prior weight loss; indicated for obese patients with an initial body mass index (BMI) ≥30 kg/m² or ≥27 kg/m² in the presence of other risk factors (eg, diabetes, dyslipidemia, hypertension)

Local Anesthetic/Vasoconstrictor Precautions No information available to require special precautions

Effects on Dental Treatment No significant effects or complications reported

Effects on Bleeding No information available to require special precautions

Adverse Effects Note: The frequency of most adverse reactions (especially gastrointestinal effects) decreases over time.

>10%:

Central nervous system: Headache (≤31%)

Gastrointestinal: Oily spotting (4% to 27%), abdominal pain/discomfort (≤26%), flatus with discharge (2% to 24%), fecal urgency (3% to 22%), fatty/oily stool (6% to 20%), oily evacuation (2% to 12%), defecation increased (3% to 11%)

Neuromuscular & skeletal: Back pain (≤14%)

Respiratory: Upper respiratory infection (26% to 38%)

Miscellaneous: Influenza (≤40%)

1% to 10%:

Cardiovascular: Pedal edema (≤3%)

Central nervous system: Fatigue (3% to 7%), anxiety (3% to 5%), sleep disorder (≤4%)

Dermatologic: Dry skin (≤2%)

Endocrine & metabolic: Menstrual irregularities (≤10%)

Gastrointestinal: Nausea (4% to 8%), fecal incontinence (2% to 8%), infectious diarrhea (≤5%), rectal pain/discomfort (3% to 5%), gingival disorder (2% to 4%), tooth disorder (3% to 4%)

Genitourinary: Urinary tract infection (6% to 8%), vaginitis (3% to 4%)

Neuromuscular & skeletal: Myalgia (≤4%)

Otic: Otitis (3% to 4%)

Respiratory: Lower respiratory infection (≤8%)

General Dosage Range Oral:

Children ≥12 years and Adults: Xenical®: 120 mg 3 times/day

Adults: Alli™ (OTC labeling): 60 mg 3 times/day

Mechanism of Action A reversible inhibitor of gastric and pancreatic lipases, thus inhibiting absorption of dietary fats by 30% (at doses of 120 mg 3 times/day).

Pharmacodynamics/Kinetics

Onset of Action 24-48 hours

Duration of Action 48-72 hours

Pregnancy Risk Factor B

Orphenadrine (or FEN a dreen)

Related Information

Temporomandibular Dysfunction (TMD) *on page* 1964

U.S. Brand Names Norflex™

Canadian Brand Names Norflex™; Orphenace®; Rhoxal-orphendrine

Generic Availability (U.S.) Yes

Pharmacologic Category Skeletal Muscle Relaxant

Use Treatment of muscle spasm associated with acute painful musculoskeletal conditions

Local Anesthetic/Vasoconstrictor Precautions No information available to require special precautions

Effects on Dental Treatment The peripheral anticholinergic effects of orphenadrine may decrease or inhibit salivary flow; normal salivation will return with cessation of drug therapy.

Effects on Bleeding No information available to require special precautions

Adverse Effects Frequency not defined.

Cardiovascular: Palpitation, tachycardia

Central nervous system: Agitation, dizziness, drowsiness, euphoria, hallucination, headache, mental confusion

Dermatologic: Pruritus, urticaria

Gastrointestinal: Constipation, gastric irritation, nausea, vomiting, xerostomia

Genitourinary: Urination hesitancy, urinary retention

Hematologic: Aplastic anemia (rare)

Neuromuscular & skeletal: Tremor, weakness

Ocular: Blurred vision, intraocular pressure increased, nystagmus, pupil dilation

Respiratory: Nasal congestion

Miscellaneous: Anaphylactic reaction (injection, rare), hypersensitivity

Dosage

Adults:

Oral: 100 mg twice daily

I.M., I.V.: 60 mg every 12 hours

Elderly: Use caution; generally not recommended for use in the elderly

Mechanism of Action Indirect skeletal muscle relaxant thought to work by central atropine-like effects; has some euphorigenic and analgesic properties

Contraindications Hypersensitivity to orphenadrine or any component of the formulation; glaucoma; GI obstruction, stenosing peptic ulcer; prostatic hypertrophy, bladder neck obstruction; cardiospasm; myasthenia gravis

Warnings/Precautions Use with caution in patients with HF, cardiac decompensation, coronary insufficiency, tachycardia or cardiac arrhythmias. May cause CNS depression, which may impair physical or mental abilities. May be inappropriate for use in the elderly due to excessive sedation and anticholinergic effects; alternative agents preferred (Beers Criteria). Potential for abuse; use with caution in patients with history of drug abuse. Solution for injection contains sodium bisulfite which may cause allergic reaction in some individuals. Has not been evaluated for continuous long-term use; monitor closely.

Drug Interactions

Metabolism/Transport Effects Substrate (minor) of CYP1A2, 2B6, 2D6, 3A4; **Inhibits** CYP1A2 (weak), 2A6 (weak), 2B6 (weak), 2C9 (weak), 2C19 (weak), 2D6 (weak), 2E1 (weak), 3A4 (weak)

Avoid Concomitant Use There are no known interactions where it is recommended to avoid concomitant use.

Increased Effect/Toxicity

Orphenadrine may increase the levels/effects of: AbobotulinumtoxinA; Alcohol (Ethyl); Anticholinergics; Cannabinoids; CNS Depressants; Methotrimeprazine; OnabotulinumtoxinA; Potassium Chloride; RimabotulinumtoxinB

The levels/effects of Orphenadrine may be increased by: Conivaptan; Droperidol; Methotrimeprazine; Pramlintide

Decreased Effect

Orphenadrine may decrease the levels/effects of: Acetylcholinesterase Inhibitors (Central); Secretin

The levels/effects of Orphenadrine may be decreased by: Acetylcholinesterase Inhibitors (Central); Peginterferon Alfa-2b; Tocilizumab

Ethanol/Nutrition/Herb Interactions

Ethanol: Avoid ethanol (may increase CNS depression).

Herb/Nutraceutical: Avoid valerian, St John's wort, kava kava, gotu kola (may increase CNS depression).

Pharmacodynamics/Kinetics

Onset of Action Peak effect: Oral: Within 2-4 hours

Duration of Action 4-6 hours

Half-life Elimination 14-16 hours

Pregnancy Risk Factor C

Lactation Excretion in breast milk unknown/use caution

Dosage Forms

Injection, solution: 30 mg/mL (2 mL)

Norflex™: 30 mg/mL (2 mL)

Tablet, extended release, oral: 100 mg

Orphenadrine, Aspirin, and Caffeine

(or FEN a dreen, AS pir in, & KAF een)

Related Information

Aspirin *on page 171*

Caffeine *on page 282*

Orphenadrine *on page 1257*

Pharmacologic Category Skeletal Muscle Relaxant

Use Relief of discomfort associated with skeletal muscular conditions

Local Anesthetic/Vasoconstrictor Precautions No information available to require special precautions

Effects on Dental Treatment Key adverse event(s) related to dental treatment: The peripheral anticholinergic effects of orphenadrine may decrease or inhibit salivary flow; normal salivation will return with cessation of drug therapy.

Aspirin: As with all drugs which may affect hemostasis, bleeding is associated with aspirin. Other serious reactions are idiosyncratic, related to allergy or individual sensitivity (see Effects on Bleeding).

Effects on Bleeding Aspirin inhibits platelet aggregation which prolongs bleeding times. Inhibition is irreversible; on discontinuation of ASA, normal platelet function returns only when new platelets are released from the bone marrow. Dental practitioners should note that recommendations differ between general surgery (eg, appendectomy, hip replacement) and dental surgery. Due to concerns for increased blood loss, ASA is typically avoided (if possible) in general surgery patients for 1-2 weeks prior to surgery (exception is in patients undergoing CABG or noncardiac surgery at high risk of cardiac events – per 2008 ACCP guidelines). However, in the case of dental surgery there is no scientific evidence to warrant discontinuance of aspirin.

Reports of major bleeding related to dental surgery attributed to aspirin use have not been published. Furthermore, interruption of therapy may result in a loss of therapeutic effect.

General Dosage Range Oral: *Adults:* 1-2 tablets 3-4 times/day

Pregnancy Risk Factor D

Dental Comment There is no scientific evidence to warrant discontinuance of aspirin prior to dental surgery. Patients taking one aspirin tablet daily as an antithrombotic and who require dental surgery should be given special consideration in consultation with the physician before removal of the aspirin relative to prevention of postoperative bleeding.

Oseltamivir (oh sel TAM i vir)

Related Information

Systemic Viral Diseases *on page 1904*

U.S. Brand Names Tamiflu®

Canadian Brand Names Tamiflu®

Pharmacologic Category Antiviral Agent; Neuraminidase Inhibitor

Use Treatment of uncomplicated acute illness due to influenza (A or B) infection in children ≥1 year of age and adults who have been symptomatic for no more than 2 days; prophylaxis against influenza (A or B) infection in children ≥1 year of age and adults

The Advisory Committee on Immunization Practices (ACIP) recommends that **treatment** be considered for the following:

- Persons with severe, complicated or progressive illness
- Hospitalized persons
- Persons at higher risk for influenza complications:
  - Children <2 years of age (highest risk in children <6 months of age)
  - Adults ≥65 years of age
  - Persons with chronic disorders of the pulmonary (including asthma) or cardiovascular systems (except hypertension)
  - Persons with chronic metabolic diseases (including diabetes mellitus), hepatic disease, renal dysfunction, hematologic disorders (including sickle cell disease), or immunosuppression (including immunosuppression caused by medications or HIV)
  - Persons with neurologic/neuromuscular conditions (including conditions such as spinal cord injuries, seizure disorders, cerebral palsy, stroke, mental retardation, moderate to severe developmental delay, or muscular dystrophy) which may compromise respiratory function, the handling of respiratory secretions, or that can increase the risk of aspiration
  - Pregnant or postpartum women (≤2 weeks after delivery)
  - Persons <19 years of age on long-term aspirin therapy
  - American Indians and Alaskan Natives
  - Persons who are morbidly obese (BMI ≥40)
  - Residents of nursing homes or other chronic care facilities
- Use may also be considered for previously healthy, nonhigh-risk outpatients with confirmed or suspected influenza based on clinical judgment when treatment can be started within 48 hours of illness onset.

The ACIP recommends that **prophylaxis** be considered for the following:

- Postexposure prophylaxis may be considered for family or close contacts of suspected or confirmed cases, who are at higher risk of influenza complications, and who have not been vaccinated against the circulating strain at the time of the exposure.
- Postexposure prophylaxis may be considered for unvaccinated healthcare workers who had occupational exposure without protective equipment.
- Pre-exposure prophylaxis should only be used for persons at very high risk of influenza complications who cannot be otherwise protected at times of high risk for exposure.

- Prophylaxis should also be administered to all eligible residents of institutions that house patients at high risk when needed to control outbreaks.

The ACIP recommends that treatment and prophylaxis be given to children <1 year of age when indicated.

Local Anesthetic/Vasoconstrictor Precautions No information available to require special precautions

Effects on Dental Treatment No significant effects or complications reported

Effects on Bleeding No information available to require special precautions

Adverse Effects

>10%: Gastrointestinal: Vomiting (2% to 15%)

1% to 10%:

Gastrointestinal: Nausea (4% to 10%), abdominal pain (2% to 5%), diarrhea (1% to 3%)

Ocular: Conjunctivitis (1%)

Respiratory: Epistaxis (1%)

General Dosage Range Dosage adjustment recommended in patients with renal impairment

Oral:

Children <1 year: 3 mg/kg/dose once daily

Children 1-12 years and ≤15 kg: 30 mg once or twice daily

Children 1-12 years and >15 to ≤23 kg: 45 mg once or twice daily

Children 1-12 years and >23 to ≤40 kg: 60 mg once or twice daily

Children 1-12 years and >40 kg, Children≥13 years, and Adults: 75 mg once or twice daily

Mechanism of Action Oseltamivir, a prodrug, is hydrolyzed to the active form, oseltamivir carboxylate (OC). OC inhibits influenza virus neuraminidase, an enzyme known to cleave the budding viral progeny from its cellular envelope attachment point (neuraminic acid) just prior to release.

Pharmacodynamics/Kinetics

Half-life Elimination Oseltamivir: 1-3 hours; Oseltamivir carboxylate: 6-10 hours

Pregnancy Risk Factor C

Oxacillin (oks a SIL in)

Pharmacologic Category Antibiotic, Penicillin

Use Treatment of infections such as osteomyelitis, septicemia, endocarditis, and CNS infections caused by susceptible strains of *Staphylococcus*

Local Anesthetic/Vasoconstrictor Precautions No information available to require special precautions

Effects on Dental Treatment Key adverse event(s) related to dental treatment: Prolonged use of penicillins may lead to development of oral candidiasis.

Effects on Bleeding No information available to require special precautions

Adverse Effects Frequency not defined.

Central nervous system: Fever

Dermatologic: Rash

Gastrointestinal: Nausea, diarrhea, vomiting

Hematologic: Eosinophilia, leukopenia, neutropenia, thrombocytopenia, agranulocytosis

Hepatic: Hepatotoxicity, AST increased

Renal: Acute interstitial nephritis, hematuria

Miscellaneous: Serum sickness-like reactions

General Dosage Range I.M., I.V.:

Children: 100-200 mg/kg/day in divided doses every 6 hours (maximum: 12 g/day)

Adults: 250-2000 mg every 4-6 hours

Mechanism of Action Inhibits bacterial cell wall synthesis by binding to one or more of the penicillin-binding proteins (PBPs); which in turn inhibits the final transpeptidation step of peptidoglycan synthesis in bacterial cell walls, thus inhibiting cell wall biosynthesis. Bacteria eventually lyse due to ongoing activity of cell wall autolytic enzymes (autolysins and murein hydrolases) while cell wall assembly is arrested.

Pharmacodynamics/Kinetics

Half-life Elimination Children 1 week to 2 years: 0.9-1.8 hours; Adults: 23-60 minutes; prolonged with renal impairment and in neonates

Time to Peak Serum: I.M.: 30-60 minutes

Pregnancy Risk Factor B

Oxaliplatin (ox AL i pla tin)

U.S. Brand Names Eloxatin®

Canadian Brand Names Eloxatin®

Pharmacologic Category Antineoplastic Agent, Alkylating Agent; Antineoplastic Agent, Platinum Analog

Use Treatment of stage III colon cancer (adjuvant) and advanced colorectal cancer

Unlabeled/Investigational Use Treatment of esophageal cancer, gastric cancer, hepatobiliary cancer, non-Hodgkin's lymphoma, ovarian cancer, pancreatic cancer, testicular cancer

Local Anesthetic/Vasoconstrictor Precautions No information available to require special precautions

Effects on Dental Treatment Key adverse event(s) related to dental treatment: Stomatitis, dysphagia, mucositis, and taste perversion.

Effects on Bleeding Chemotherapy may result in significant myelosuppression, potentially including significant reduction in platelet counts and altered hemostasis. In patients who are under active treatment with these agents, medical consult is suggested.

Adverse Effects Percentages reported with monotherapy.

>10%:

Central nervous system: Fatigue (61%), fever (25%), pain (14%), headache (13%), insomnia (11%)

Gastrointestinal: Nausea (64%), diarrhea (46%), vomiting (37%), abdominal pain (31%), constipation (31%), anorexia (20%), stomatitis (14%)

Hematologic: Anemia (64%; grades 3/4: 1%), thrombocytopenia (30%; grades 3/4: 3%), leukopenia (13%)

Hepatic: AST increased (54%; grades 3/4: 4%), ALT increased (36%; grades 3/4: 1%), total bilirubin increased (13%; grades 3/4: 5%)

Neuromuscular & skeletal: Peripheral neuropathy (may be dose limiting; 76%; acute 65%; grades 3/4: 5%; persistent 43%; grades 3/4: 3%), back pain (11%)

Respiratory: Dyspnea (13%), cough (11%)

1% to 10%:

Cardiovascular: Edema (10%), chest pain (5%), peripheral edema (5%), flushing (3%), thromboembolism (2%)

Central nervous system: Dizziness (7%)

Dermatologic: Rash (5%), alopecia (3%), hand-foot syndrome (1%)

Endocrine & metabolic: Dehydration (5%), hypokalemia (3%)

Gastrointestinal: Dyspepsia (7%), taste perversion (5%), flatulence (3%), mucositis (2%), gastroesophageal reflux (1%), dysphagia (acute 1% to 2%)

Genitourinary: Dysuria (1%)

Hematologic: Neutropenia (7%)

Local: Injection site reaction (9%; redness/swelling/pain)

Neuromuscular & skeletal: Rigors (9%), arthralgia (7%)

Ocular: Abnormal lacrimation (1%)

Renal: Serum creatinine increased (5% to 10%)

Respiratory: URI (7%), rhinitis (6%), epistaxis (2%), pharyngitis (2%), pharyngolaryngeal dysesthesia (grades 3/4: 1% to 2%)

Miscellaneous: Allergic reactions (3%); hypersensitivity (includes urticaria, pruritus, facial flushing, shortness of breath, bronchospasm, diaphoresis, hypotension, syncope: grades 3/4: 2% to 3%); hiccup (2%)

General Dosage Range Dosage adjustment recommended in patients who develop toxicities

I.V.: *Adults:* 85 mg/m^2 every 2 weeks

Mechanism of Action Oxaliplatin, a platinum derivative, is an alkylating agent. Following intracellular hydrolysis, the platinum compound binds to DNA forming cross-links which inhibit DNA replication and transcription, resulting in cell death. Cytotoxicity is cell-cycle nonspecific.

Pharmacodynamics/Kinetics

Half-life Elimination Terminal: 391 hours

Pregnancy Risk Factor D

Oxandrolone (oks AN droe lone)

U.S. Brand Names Oxandrin®

Pharmacologic Category Androgen

Use Adjunctive therapy to promote weight gain after weight loss following extensive surgery, chronic infections, or severe trauma, and in some patients who, without definite pathophysiologic reasons, fail to gain or to maintain normal weight; to offset protein catabolism with prolonged corticosteroid administration; relief of bone pain associated with osteoporosis

Local Anesthetic/Vasoconstrictor Precautions No information available to require special precautions

Effects on Dental Treatment No significant effects or complications reported

Effects on Bleeding No information available to require special precautions

Adverse Effects Frequency not defined.

Cardiovascular: Edema

Central nervous system: Depression, excitation, insomnia

Dermatologic: Acne (females and prepubertal males)

Also reported in females: Hirsutism, male-pattern baldness

Endocrine & metabolic: Electrolyte imbalances, glucose intolerance, gonadotropin secretion inhibited, gynecomastia, HDL decreased, LDL increased

Also reported in females: Clitoral enlargement, menstrual irregularities

Genitourinary:

Prepubertal males: Increased or persistent erections, penile enlargement

Postpubertal males: Bladder irritation, epididymitis, impotence, oligospermia, priapism (chronic), testicular atrophy, testicular function

Hepatic: Alkaline phosphatase increased, ALT increased, AST increased, bilirubin increased, cholestatic jaundice, hepatic necrosis (rare), hepatocellular neoplasms, peliosis hepatis (with long-term therapy)

Neuromuscular & skeletal: CPK increased, premature closure of epiphyses (in children)

Renal: Creatinine excretion increased

Miscellaneous: Bromsulfophthalein retention, habituation, voice alteration (deepening, in females)

General Dosage Range Oral:

Children: ≤0.1 mg/kg/day or ≤0.045 mg/lb/day

Adults: 2.5-20 mg/day in 2-4 divided doses

Elderly: 5 mg twice daily

Mechanism of Action Synthetic testosterone derivative with similar androgenic and anabolic actions

Pharmacodynamics/Kinetics

Half-life Elimination 10-13 hours

Pregnancy Risk Factor X

Controlled Substance C-III

Oxaprozin (oks a PROE zin)

Related Information

Rheumatoid Arthritis, Osteoarthritis, and Osteoporosis *on page 1889*

Temporomandibular Dysfunction (TMD) *on page 1964*

U.S. Brand Names Daypro®

Canadian Brand Names Apo-Oxaprozin®; Daypro®

Generic Availability (U.S.) Yes

Pharmacologic Category Nonsteroidal Anti-inflammatory Drug (NSAID), Oral

Use Acute and long-term use in the management of signs and symptoms of osteoarthritis and rheumatoid arthritis; juvenile idiopathic arthritis (JIA)

Local Anesthetic/Vasoconstrictor Precautions No information available to require special precautions

Effects on Dental Treatment The dentist should be aware of the potential of abnormal coagulation. Caution should also be exercised in the use of NSAIDs in patients already on anticoagulant therapy with drugs such as warfarin (Coumadin®). See Effects on Bleeding.

Effects on Bleeding Nonselective NSAIDs are known to reversibly decrease platelet aggregation via mechanisms different than observed with aspirin. Platelet function is restored as the drug is eliminated from the body. NSAIDs should be avoided (if possible) in general surgery patients for 3-5 half-lives of the drug (usually 1-3 days) prior to surgery to reduce the risk of excessive bleeding. However, there is no scientific evidence to warrant discontinuance of NSAIDs prior to dental surgery. In medically complicated patients or extensive oral surgery, the decision to interrupt therapy must be based on the risk to benefit in an individual patient and a medical consult is suggested. Routine interruption of NSAID therapy for most dental procedures is not warranted. If therapy is continued without interruption, the clinician should anticipate the potential for slower clotting times.

Adverse Effects

1% to 10%:

Cardiovascular: Edema

Central nervous system: Confusion, depression, dizziness, headache, sedation, sleep disturbance, somnolence

Dermatologic: Pruritus, rash

Gastrointestinal: Abdominal distress, abdominal pain, anorexia, constipation, diarrhea, flatulence, gastrointestinal ulcer, gross bleeding with perforation, heartburn, nausea, vomiting

Hematologic: Anemia, bleeding time increased

Hepatic: Liver enzyme elevation
Otic: Tinnitus
Renal: Dysuria, renal function abnormal, urinary frequency

Dosage Oral (individualize dosage to lowest effective dose to minimize adverse effects):

Children 6-16 years: Juvenile idiopathic arthritis (JIA):
- 22-31 kg: 600 mg once daily
- 32-54 kg: 900 mg once daily
- ≥55 kg: 1200 mg once daily

Adults:
- Osteoarthritis: 600-1200 mg once daily; patients should be titrated to lowest dose possible; patients with low body weight should start with 600 mg daily
- Rheumatoid arthritis: 1200 mg once daily; a one-time loading dose of up to 1800 mg/day or 26 mg/kg (whichever is lower) may be given
- Maximum doses:
  - Patient <50 kg: Maximum: 1200 mg/day
  - Patient >50 kg with normal renal/hepatic function and low risk of peptic ulcer: Maximum: 1800 mg or 26 mg/kg (whichever is lower) in divided doses

Dosing adjustment in renal impairment: In general, NSAIDs are not recommended for use in patients with advanced renal disease but the manufacturer of oxaprozin does provide some guidelines for adjustment in renal dysfunction.

Severe renal impairment or on dialysis: 600 mg once daily; may increase cautiously to 1200 mg/day with close monitoring

Dosing adjustment in hepatic impairment: Use caution in patients with severe dysfunction

Mechanism of Action Reversibly inhibits cyclooxygenase-1 and 2 (COX-1 and 2) enzymes, which results in decreased formation of prostaglandin precursors; has antipyretic, analgesic, and anti-inflammatory properties.

Other proposed mechanisms not fully elucidated (and possibly contributing to the anti-inflammatory effect to varying degrees) include inhibiting chemotaxis, altering lymphocyte activity, inhibiting neutrophil aggregation/activation, and decreasing proinflammatory cytokine levels.

Contraindications Hypersensitivity to oxaprozin, aspirin, other NSAIDs, or any component of the formulation; perioperative pain in the setting of coronary artery bypass graft (CABG) surgery

Warnings/Precautions **[U.S. Boxed Warning]: NSAIDs are associated with an increased risk of adverse cardiovascular thrombotic events, including MI and stroke.** Risk may be increased with duration of use or pre-existing cardiovascular risk factors or disease. Carefully evaluate individual cardiovascular risk profiles prior to prescribing. May cause new onset hypertension or worsening of existing hypertension. Use caution with fluid retention. Avoid use in heart failure. Concurrent administration of ibuprofen, and potentially other nonselective NSAIDs, may interfere with aspirin' s cardioprotective effect. **[U.S. Boxed Warning]: Use is contraindicated for treatment of perioperative pain in the setting of coronary artery bypass graft (CABG) surgery.** Risk of MI and stroke may be increased with use following CABG surgery.

Platelet adhesion and aggregation may be decreased; may prolong bleeding time; patients with coagulation disorders or who are receiving anticoagulants should be monitored closely. Anemia may occur; patients on long-term NSAID therapy should be monitored for anemia. Rarely, NSAID use may cause severe blood dyscrasias (eg, agranulocytosis, aplastic anemia, thrombocytopenia).

NSAID use may compromise existing renal function; dose-dependent decreases in prostaglandin synthesis may result from NSAID use, reducing renal blood flow which may cause renal decompensation. NSAID use may increase the risk for hyperkalemia. Patients with impaired renal function, dehydration, heart failure, liver dysfunction, those taking diuretics, and ACE inhibitors, and the elderly are at greater risk of renal toxicity and hyperkalemia. In the elderly, may be inappropriate for long-term use due to potential for GI bleeding, hypertension, heart failure, and renal failure (Beers Criteria). Rehydrate patient before starting therapy; monitor renal function closely. Not recommended for use in patients with advanced renal disease. Long-term NSAID use may result in renal papillary necrosis.

[U.S. Boxed Warning]: NSAIDs may increase risk of gastrointestinal irritation, inflammation, ulceration, bleeding, and perforation. These events may occur at any time during therapy and without warning. Use caution with a history of GI disease (bleeding or ulcers); concurrent therapy with aspirin, anticoagulants, and/or corticosteroids; smoking; use of alcohol; and the elderly or debilitated patients. When used concomitantly with ≤325 mg of aspirin, a substantial increase in the risk of gastrointestinal complications (eg, ulcer) occurs; concomitant gastroprotective therapy (eg, proton pump inhibitors) is recommended (Bhatt, 2008).

Use the lowest effective dose for the shortest duration of time, consistent with individual patient goals, to reduce risk of cardiovascular or GI adverse events. Alternate therapies should be considered for patients at high risk.

NSAIDs may cause serious skin adverse events including exfoliative dermatitis, Stevens-Johnson syndrome (SJS), and toxic epidermal necrolysis (TEN); discontinue use at first sign of skin rash or hypersensitivity. Anaphylactoid reactions may occur, even without prior exposure; patients with "aspirin triad" (bronchial asthma, aspirin intolerance, rhinitis) may be at increased risk. Do not use in patients who experience bronchospasm, asthma, rhinitis, or urticaria with NSAID or aspirin therapy. Use caution in other forms of asthma.

Use with caution in patients with decreased hepatic function. Closely monitor patients with any abnormal LFT. Severe hepatic reactions (eg, fulminant hepatitis, liver failure) have occurred with NSAID use, rarely; discontinue if signs or symptoms of liver disease develop, or if systemic manifestations occur.

NSAIDS may cause drowsiness, dizziness, blurred vision and other neurologic effects which may impair physical or mental abilities; patients must be cautioned about performing tasks which require mental alertness (eg, operating machinery or driving). Discontinue use with blurred or diminished vision and perform ophthalmologic exam. Monitor vision with long-term therapy.

The elderly are at increased risk for adverse effects (especially peptic ulceration, CNS effects, renal toxicity) from NSAIDs even at low doses.

Withhold for at least 4-6 half-lives prior to surgical or dental procedures. May cause mild photosensitivity reactions.

Drug Interactions

Avoid Concomitant Use

Avoid concomitant use of Oxaprozin with any of the following: Ketorolac; Ketorolac (Systemic)

Increased Effect/Toxicity

Oxaprozin may increase the levels/effects of: Aminoglycosides; Anticoagulants; Antiplatelet Agents; Bisphosphonate Derivatives; Collagenase (Systemic); CycloSPORINE; CycloSPORINE (Systemic); Deferasirox; Desmopressin; Digoxin; Drotrecogin Alfa; Eplerenone; Haloperidol; Ibritumomab; Lithium; Methotrexate; Nonsteroidal Anti-Inflammatory Agents; PEMEtrexed; Potassium-Sparing Diuretics; PRALAtrexate; Quinolone Antibiotics; Salicylates; Thrombolytic Agents; Tositumomab and Iodine I 131 Tositumomab; Vancomycin; Vitamin K Antagonists

The levels/effects of Oxaprozin may be increased by: ACE Inhibitors; Angiotensin II Receptor Blockers; Antidepressants (Tricyclic, Tertiary Amine); Corticosteroids (Systemic); Dasatinib; Glucosamine; Herbs (Anticoagulant/Antiplatelet Properties); Ketorolac; Ketorolac (Systemic); Nonsteroidal Anti-Inflammatory Agents; Omega-3-Acid Ethyl Esters; Pentosan Polysulfate Sodium; Pentoxifylline; Probenecid; Prostacyclin Analogues; Selective Serotonin Reuptake Inhibitors; Serotonin/Norepinephrine Reuptake Inhibitors; Treprostinil

Decreased Effect

Oxaprozin may decrease the levels/effects of: ACE Inhibitors; Angiotensin II Receptor Blockers; Antiplatelet Agents; Beta-Blockers; Eplerenone; HydrALAZINE; Loop Diuretics; Potassium-Sparing Diuretics; Salicylates; Thiazide Diuretics

The levels/effects of Oxaprozin may be decreased by: Bile Acid Sequestrants; Nonsteroidal Anti-Inflammatory Agents; Salicylates

Ethanol/Nutrition/Herb Interactions

Ethanol: Avoid ethanol (may enhance gastric mucosal irritation).

Herb/Nutraceutical: Avoid alfalfa, anise, bilberry, bladderwrack, bromelain, cat's claw, celery, chamomile, coleus, cordyceps, dong quai, evening primrose, fenugreek, feverfew, garlic, ginger, ginkgo biloba, ginseng (American, Panax, Siberian), grapeseed, green tea, guggul, horse chestnut seed, horseradish, licorice, prickly ash, red clover, reishi, SAMe (S-adenosylmethionine), sweet clover, turmeric, white willow (all have additional antiplatelet activity).

Pharmacodynamics/Kinetics

Half-life Elimination 40-50 hours

Time to Peak 2-4 hours

Pregnancy Risk Factor C

Lactation Excretion in breast milk unknown/not recommended

Breast-Feeding Considerations The amount of oxaprozin found in breast milk is not known; however, distribution into breast milk would be expected. Breast-feeding is not recommended by the manufacturer.

Dosage Forms
Caplet, oral:
Daypro®: 600 mg
Tablet, oral: 600 mg

Oxazepam (oks A ze pam)

U.S. Brand Names Serax®
Canadian Brand Names Apo-Oxazepam®; Bio-Oxazepam; Novoxapram®; Oxpam®; Oxpram®; PMS-Oxazepam; Riva-Oxazepam
Generic Availability (U.S.) Yes: Capsule
Pharmacologic Category Benzodiazepine
Use Treatment of anxiety; management of ethanol withdrawal
Unlabeled/Investigational Use Anticonvulsant in management of simple partial seizures; hypnotic
Local Anesthetic/Vasoconstrictor Precautions No information available to require special precautions
Effects on Dental Treatment Key adverse event(s) related to dental treatment: Xerostomia (normal salivary flow resumes upon discontinuation).
Effects on Bleeding No information available to require special precautions
Adverse Effects Frequency not defined.
Cardiovascular: Syncope (rare), edema
Central nervous system: Drowsiness, ataxia, dizziness, vertigo, memory impairment, headache, paradoxical reactions (excitement, stimulation of effect), lethargy, amnesia, euphoria
Dermatologic: Rash
Endocrine & metabolic: Decreased libido, menstrual irregularities
Genitourinary: Incontinence
Hematologic: Leukopenia, blood dyscrasias
Hepatic: Jaundice
Neuromuscular & skeletal: Dysarthria, tremor, reflex slowing
Ocular: Blurred vision, diplopia
Miscellaneous: Drug dependence
Dosage Oral:
Adults:
Anxiety: 10-30 mg 3-4 times/day
Ethanol withdrawal: 15-30 mg 3-4 times/day
Hypnotic: 15-30 mg
Elderly: Oral: Anxiety: 10 mg 2-3 times/day; increase gradually as needed to a total of 30-45 mg/day. Dose titration should be slow to evaluate sensitivity.
Hemodialysis: Not dialyzable (0% to 5%)
Mechanism of Action Binds to stereospecific benzodiazepine receptors on the postsynaptic GABA neuron at several sites within the central nervous system, including the limbic system, reticular formation. Enhancement of the inhibitory effect of GABA on neuronal excitability results by increased neuronal membrane permeability to chloride ions. This shift in chloride ions results in hyperpolarization (a less excitable state) and stabilization.
Contraindications Hypersensitivity to oxazepam or any component of the formulation (cross-sensitivity with other benzodiazepines may exist); narrow-angle glaucoma (not in product labeling, however, benzodiazepines are contraindicated); not indicated for use in the treatment of psychosis; pregnancy
Warnings/Precautions May cause hypotension (rare) - use with caution in patients with cardiovascular or cerebrovascular disease, or in patients who would not tolerate transient decreases in blood pressure. Serax® 15 contains tartrazine; Safety and efficacy in established in pediatric patients <6 years of age; dose has not been established between 6-12 years of age.

Use with caution in elderly or debilitated patients, patients with hepatic disease (including alcoholics), or renal impairment. Due to increased sensitivity in the elderly, smaller doses of benzodiazepines may be safer and as effective; in this age group, avoid using doses >60 mg daily of oxazepam (Beers Criteria). Use with caution in patients with respiratory disease or impaired gag reflex. Avoid use in patients with sleep apnea.

Causes CNS depression (dose-related) resulting in sedation, dizziness, confusion, or ataxia which may impair physical and mental capabilities. Patients must be cautioned about performing tasks which require mental alertness (eg, operating machinery or driving). Use with caution in patients receiving other CNS depressants or psychoactive agents. Benzodiazepines have been associated with falls and traumatic injury and should be used with extreme caution in patients who are at risk of these events (especially the elderly).

Use caution in patients with depression, particularly if suicidal risk may be present. Use with caution in patients with a history of drug dependence. Benzodiazepines have been associated with dependence and acute withdrawal symptoms on discontinuation or reduction in dose. Acute withdrawal, including seizures, may be precipitated after administration of flumazenil to patients receiving long-term benzodiazepine therapy.

Benzodiazepines have been associated with anterograde amnesia. Paradoxical reactions, including hyperactive or aggressive behavior have been reported with benzodiazepines, particularly in adolescent/pediatric or psychiatric patients. Does not have analgesic, antidepressant, or antipsychotic properties.

Drug Interactions

Avoid Concomitant Use

Avoid concomitant use of Oxazepam with any of the following: OLANZapine

Increased Effect/Toxicity

Oxazepam may increase the levels/effects of: Alcohol (Ethyl); CloZAPine; CNS Depressants; Fosphenytoin; Methotrimeprazine; Phenytoin

The levels/effects of Oxazepam may be increased by: Droperidol; Methotrimeprazine; OLANZapine

Decreased Effect

The levels/effects of Oxazepam may be decreased by: Theophylline Derivatives; Yohimbine

Ethanol/Nutrition/Herb Interactions

Ethanol: May increase CNS depression; monitor for increased effects with coadministration. Caution patients about effects.

Herb/Nutraceutical: Avoid valerian, St John's wort, kava kava, gotu kola (may increase CNS depression).

Pharmacodynamics/Kinetics

Half-life Elimination 2.8-5.7 hours

Time to Peak Serum: 2-4 hours

Breast-Feeding Considerations Drowsiness, lethargy, or weight loss in nursing infants have been observed in case reports following maternal use of some benzodiazepines.

Controlled Substance C-IV

Dosage Forms

Capsule, oral: 10 mg, 15 mg, 30 mg

Serax®: 10 mg, 15 mg, 30 mg

Tablet, oral:

Serax®: 15 mg

OXcarbazepine (ox car BAZ e peen)

U.S. Brand Names Trileptal®

Canadian Brand Names Apo-Oxcarbazepine®; Trileptal®

Pharmacologic Category Anticonvulsant, Miscellaneous

Use Monotherapy or adjunctive therapy in the treatment of partial seizures in adults and children ≥4 years of age with epilepsy; adjunctive therapy in the treatment of partial seizures in children ≥2 years of age with epilepsy

Unlabeled/Investigational Use Bipolar disorder; treatment of neuropathic pain

Local Anesthetic/Vasoconstrictor Precautions No information available to require special precautions

Effects on Dental Treatment No significant effects or complications reported

Effects on Bleeding No information available to require special precautions

Adverse Effects As reported in adults with doses of up to 2400 mg/day (includes patients on monotherapy, adjunctive therapy, and those not previously on AEDs); incidence in children was similar.

>10%:

Central nervous system: Dizziness (22% to 49%), somnolence (20% to 36%), headache (13% to 32%), ataxia (5% to 31%), fatigue (12% to 15%), vertigo (6% to 15%)

Gastrointestinal: Vomiting (7% to 36%), nausea (15% to 29%), abdominal pain (10% to 13%)

Neuromuscular & skeletal: Abnormal gait (5% to 17%), tremor (3% to 16%)

Ocular: Diplopia (14% to 40%), nystagmus (7% to 26%), abnormal vision (4% to 14%)

1% to 10%:

Cardiovascular: Hypotension (1% to 2%), leg edema (1% to 2%)

Central nervous system: Nervousness (2% to 5%), amnesia (4%), abnormal thinking (2% to 4%), insomnia (2% to 4%), speech disorder (1% to 3%), EEG abnormalities (2%), abnormal feelings (1% to 2%), agitation (1% to 2%), confusion (1% to 2%)

Dermatologic: Rash (4%), acne (1% to 2%)

Endocrine & metabolic: Hyponatremia (1% to 3%)

Gastrointestinal: Diarrhea (5% to 7%), dyspepsia (5% to 6%), constipation (2% to 6%), gastritis (1% to 2%), weight gain (1% to 2%)

Neuromuscular & skeletal: Weakness (3% to 6%), back pain (4%), falling down (4%), abnormal coordination (1% to 4%), dysmetria (1% to 3%), sprains/strains (2%), muscle weakness (1% to 2%)

Ocular: Abnormal accommodation (2%)

Respiratory: Upper respiratory tract infection (7%), rhinitis (2% to 5%), chest infection (4%), epistaxis (4%), sinusitis (4%)

General Dosage Range Dosage adjustment recommended in patients with renal impairment

Oral:

Children 2-3 years and <20 kg: Initial: 8-20 mg/kg/day (maximum: 600 mg/day) in 2 divided doses; Maintenance: maximum of 60 mg/kg/day in 2 divided doses

Children 2-3 years and ≥20 kg: Initial: 8-10 mg/kg/day (maximum: 600 mg/day) in 2 divided doses; Maintenance: maximum of 60 mg/kg/day in 2 divided doses

Children 4-16 years and <25 kg: Initial: 8-10 mg/kg/day (maximum: 600 mg/day) in 2 divided doses; Maintenance: up to 900 mg/day

Children 4-16 years and 25-30 kg: Initial: 8-10 mg/kg/day (maximum: 600 mg/day) in 2 divided doses; Maintenance: up to 1200 mg/day

Children 4-16 years and 31-39 kg: Initial: 8-10 mg/kg/day (maximum: 600 mg/day) in 2 divided doses; Maintenance: up to 1500 mg/day

Children 4-16 years and 40-55 kg: Initial: 8-10 mg/kg/day (maximum: 600 mg/day) in 2 divided doses; Maintenance: up to 1800 mg/day

Children 4-16 years and >55 kg: Initial: 8-10 mg/kg/day (maximum: 600 mg/day) in 2 divided doses; Maintenance: up to 2100 mg/day

Children >16 years and Adults: Initial: 300 mg twice daily; Maintenance: 1200-2400 mg/day in 2 divided doses (maximum: 2400 mg/day)

Mechanism of Action Pharmacological activity results from both oxcarbazepine and its monohydroxy metabolite (MHD). Precise mechanism of anticonvulsant effect has not been defined. Oxcarbazepine and MHD block voltage-sensitive sodium channels, stabilizing hyperexcited neuronal membranes, inhibiting repetitive firing, and decreasing the propagation of synaptic impulses. These actions are believed to prevent the spread of seizures. Oxcarbazepine and MHD also increase potassium conductance and modulate the activity of high-voltage activated calcium channels.

Pharmacodynamics/Kinetics

Half-life Elimination Parent drug: 2 hours; MHD: 9 hours; renal impairment (Cl_{cr} 30 mL/minute): MHD: 19 hours

Clearance of MHD is increased in younger children (~80% in children 2-4 years of age) and approaches that of adults by ~13 years of age

Time to Peak Serum (median): Tablets: 4.5 hours; oral suspension: 6 hours

Pregnancy Risk Factor C

Oxiconazole (oks i KON a zole)

U.S. Brand Names Oxistat®

Canadian Brand Names Oxistat®

Pharmacologic Category Antifungal Agent, Topical

Use Treatment of tinea pedis (athlete's foot), tinea cruris (jock itch), tinea corporis (ringworm), and tinea (pityriasis) versicolor

Local Anesthetic/Vasoconstrictor Precautions No information available to require special precautions

Effects on Dental Treatment No significant effects or complications reported

Effects on Bleeding No information available to require special precautions

Adverse Effects 1% to 10%:

Dermatologic: Pruritus (<2%)

Local: Burning (≤1%)

General Dosage Range Topical: *Children and Adults:* Apply to affected areas 1-2 times daily

Mechanism of Action The cytoplasmic membrane integrity of fungi is destroyed by oxiconazole which exerts a fungicidal activity through inhibition of ergosterol synthesis. Effective for treatment of tinea pedis, tinea cruris, tinea corporis, and tinea versicolor. Active against *Trichophyton rubrum*, *Trichophyton mentagrophytes*, *Trichophyton violaceum*, *Microsporum canis*, *Microsporum audouinii*, *Microsporum gypseum*, *Epidermophyton floccosum*, *Candida albicans*, and *Malassezia furfur*.

Pregnancy Risk Factor B

Oxybutynin (oks i BYOO ti nin)

U.S. Brand Names Ditropan XL®; Gelnique™; Oxytrol®

Canadian Brand Names Apo-Oxybutynin®; Ditropan XL®; Dom-Oxybutynin; Mylan-Oxybutynin; Novo-Oxybutynin; Nu-Oxybutyn; Oxybutyn; Oxybutynine; Oxytrol®; PHL-Oxybutynin; PMS-Oxybutynin; Riva-Oxybutynin; Uromax®

Pharmacologic Category Antispasmodic Agent, Urinary

Use Antispasmodic for neurogenic bladder (urgency, frequency, leakage, urge incontinence, dysuria); extended release formulation also indicated for treatment of symptoms associated with detrusor overactivity due to a neurological condition (eg, spina bifida)

Local Anesthetic/Vasoconstrictor Precautions No information available to require special precautions

Effects on Dental Treatment Key adverse event(s) related to dental treatment: Xerostomia and changes in salivation (normal salivary flow resumes upon discontinuation), and taste perversion.

Effects on Bleeding No information available to require special precautions

Adverse Effects

Oral:

>10%:

Central nervous system: Dizziness (4% to 17%), somnolence (2% to 14%)

Gastrointestinal: Xerostomia (29% to 71%; dose related), constipation (7% to 15%), nausea (2% to 12%)

5% to 10%:

Central nervous system: Headache (6% to 10%), pain (1% to 7%), nervousness (1% to 7%), insomnia (1% to 6%)

Gastrointestinal: Diarrhea (1% to 9%), dyspepsia (5% to 7%)

Genitourinary: Urinary hesitation (9%), urinary tract infection (5% to 7%), urinary retention (6%)

Neuromuscular & skeletal: Weakness (3% to 7%)

Ocular: Blurred vision (1% to 10%), dry eyes (3% to 6%)

Respiratory: Rhinitis (2% to 6%)

Topical gel:

1% to 10%:

Central nervous system: Dizziness (2% to 3%), fatigue (2%), headache (2%)

Dermatologic: Pruritus (1%)

Gastrointestinal: Xerostomia (7% to 8%), gastroenteritis (2%), constipation (1%)

Genitourinary: Urinary tract infection (7%)

Local: Application site reaction (5%; includes anesthesia, dermatitis, erythema, irritation, pain, papules, pruritus)

Respiratory: Nasopharyngitis (3%)

Transdermal:

>10%: Local: Application site reaction (17%), pruritus (14%)

1% to 10%:

Gastrointestinal: Xerostomia (4% to 10%), diarrhea (3%), constipation (3%)

Genitourinary: Dysuria (2%)

Local: Erythema (6% to 8%), vesicles (3%), rash (3%)

Ocular: Vision changes (3%)

General Dosage Range

Oral:

Extended release:

Children >6 years: 5 mg once daily (maximum: 20 mg/day)

Adults: Initial: 5-10 mg once daily; Maintenance: 5-30 mg once daily (maximum: 30 mg/day)

Regular release:

Children >5 years: 5 mg 2-3 times/day (maximum: 15 mg/day)

Adults: 5 mg 2-4 times/day (maximum: 20 mg/day)

Elderly: 2.5 mg 2-3 times/day

Topical gel: *Adults:* Apply contents of 1 sachet (100 mg/g) once daily

Transdermal: *Adults:* Apply one 3.9 mg/day patch twice weekly

Mechanism of Action Direct antispasmodic effect on smooth muscle, also inhibits the action of acetylcholine on smooth muscle (exhibits 1/5 the anticholinergic activity of atropine, but is 4-10 times the antispasmodic activity); does not block effects at skeletal muscle or at autonomic ganglia; increases bladder capacity, decreases uninhibited contractions, and delays desire to void, therefore, decreases urgency and frequency

Pharmacodynamics/Kinetics

Onset of Action Onset of action: Oral: 30-60 minutes; Peak effect: 3-6 hours

Duration of Action 6-10 hours (up to 24 hours for extended release oral formulation)

Half-life Elimination I.V.: ~2 hours (parent drug), 7-8 hours (metabolites); Oral: ~2-3 hours

Time to Peak Serum: Oral: Immediate release: ~60 minutes; Extended release: 4-6 hours; Transdermal: 24-48 hours

Pregnancy Risk Factor B

Oxychlorosene (oks i KLOR oh seen)

U.S. Brand Names Clorpactin® WCS-90 [OTC]

Pharmacologic Category Antibiotic, Topical

Use Treatment of localized infections

Local Anesthetic/Vasoconstrictor Precautions No information available to require special precautions

Effects on Dental Treatment No significant effects or complications reported

Effects on Bleeding No information available to require special precautions

General Dosage Range Topical: *Adults:* Apply by irrigation, instillation, spray, soaks, or wet compresses

OxyCODONE (oks i KOE done)

Related Information

Oral Pain *on page 1928*

U.S. Brand Names OxyCONTIN®; Roxicodone®

Canadian Brand Names Oxy.IR®; OxyContin®; PMS-Oxycodone; Supeudol®

Generic Availability (U.S.) Yes: Excludes liquid, controlled release tablet

Pharmacologic Category Analgesic, Opioid

Dental Use Treatment of postoperative pain

Use Management of moderate-to-severe pain, normally used in combination with nonopioid analgesics

OxyContin® is indicated for around-the-clock management of moderate-to-severe pain when an analgesic is needed for an extended period of time.

Local Anesthetic/Vasoconstrictor Precautions No information available to require special precautions

Effects on Dental Treatment Key adverse event(s) related to dental treatment: Xerostomia (normal salivary flow resumes upon discontinuation).

Effects on Bleeding No information available to require special precautions

Adverse Effects Note: Percentages as reported with OxyContin®

>10%:
- Central nervous system: Somnolence (23%), dizziness (13%)
- Dermatologic: Pruritus (13%)
- Gastrointestinal: Constipation (23%), nausea (23%), vomiting (12%)

1% to 10%:
- Cardiovascular: Postural hypotension (1% to 5%)
- Central nervous system: Headache (7%), abnormal dreams (1% to 5%), anxiety (1% to 5%), chills (1% to 5%), confusion (1% to 5%), dysphoria (1% to 5%), euphoria (1% to 5%), fever (1% to 5%), insomnia (1% to 5%), nervousness (1% to 5%), thought abnormalities (1% to 5%)
- Dermatologic: Rash (1% to 5%)
- Gastrointestinal: Xerostomia (6%), abdominal pain (1% to 5%), anorexia (1% to 5%), diarrhea (1% to 5%), dyspepsia (1% to 5%), gastritis (1% to 5%)
- Neuromuscular & skeletal: Weakness (6%), twitching (1% to 5%)
- Respiratory: Dyspnea (1% to 5%), hiccups (1% to 5%)
- Miscellaneous: Diaphoresis (5%)

Dental Usual Dosage Postoperative pain: Adults: Oral: 5 mg every 6 hours as needed

Dosage Oral: **Note:** All doses should be titrated to appropriate effect:

Children (unlabeled use): Immediate release, initial dose: 0.1-0.2 mg/kg/dose (moderate pain) or 0.2 mg/kg/dose (severe pain) (APS 6th edition). For severe chronic pain, administer on a regularly scheduled basis, every 4-6 hours, at the lowest dose that will achieve adequate analgesia.

Adults:

Immediate release: Initial: 5-15 mg every 4-6 hours as needed; dosing range: 5-20 mg/dose (APS 6th edition). For severe chronic pain, administer on a regularly scheduled basis, every 4-6 hours, at the lowest dose that will achieve adequate analgesia.

Controlled release:

Opioid naive: 10 mg every 12 hours

Concurrent CNS depressants: Reduce usual initial oxycodone dose by 1/3 to 1/2

Conversion from transdermal fentanyl: For each 25 mcg/hour transdermal dose, substitute 10 mg controlled release oxycodone every 12 hours; should be initiated 18 hours after the removal of the transdermal fentanyl patch

Currently on opioids: Use standard conversion chart to convert daily dose to oxycodone equivalent. Divide daily dose in 2 (for twice-daily dosing, usually every 12 hours) and round down to nearest dosage form.

Dose adjustment: Doses may be adjusted by changing the total daily dose (not by changing the dosing interval). Doses may be adjusted every 1-2 days and may be increased by 25% to 50%. Dose should be gradually tapered when no longer required in order to prevent withdrawal.

Note: 60 mg and 80 mg strengths, a single dose >40 mg, or a total dose of >80 mg/day are for use only in opioid-tolerant patients.

Multiplication factors for converting the daily dose of current oral opioid to the daily dose of oral oxycodone:

Current opioid mg/day dose x factor = Oxycodone mg/day dose

Codeine mg/day oral dose **x** 0.15 = Oxycodone mg/day dose
Hydrocodone mg/day oral dose **x** 0.9 = Oxycodone mg/day dose
Hydromorphone mg/day oral dose **x** 4 = Oxycodone mg/day dose
Levorphanol mg/day oral dose **x** 7.5 = Oxycodone mg/day dose
Meperidine mg/day oral dose **x** 0.1 = Oxycodone mg/day dose
Methadone mg/day oral dose **x** 1.5 = Oxycodone mg/day dose
Morphine mg/day oral dose **x** 0.5 = Oxycodone mg/day dose

Note: Divide the oxycodone mg/day dose into the appropriate dosing interval for the specific form being used.

Dosing adjustment in hepatic impairment: Reduce dosage in patients with liver disease. Decrease the dose of controlled release tablets to 1/3 to 1/2 the usual starting dose; titrate carefully.

Dosing adjustment in renal impairment: Serum concentrations are increased ~50% in patients with Cl_{cr} <60 mL/minute; adjust dose based on clinical situation.

Mechanism of Action Binds to opiate receptors in the CNS, causing inhibition of ascending pain pathways, altering the perception of and response to pain; produces generalized CNS depression

Contraindications Hypersensitivity to oxycodone or any component of the formulation; significant respiratory depression; hypercarbia; acute or severe bronchial asthma; paralytic ileus (known or suspected)

Warnings/Precautions May cause CNS depression, which may impair physical or mental abilities; patients must be cautioned about performing tasks which require mental alertness (eg, operating machinery or driving). Effects may be potentiated when used with other sedative drugs or ethanol. Use with caution in patients with hypersensitivity reactions to other phenanthrene derivative opioid agonists (morphine, hydrocodone, hydromorphone, levorphanol, oxymorphone), respiratory diseases including asthma, emphysema, or COPD. Use with caution in pancreatitis or biliary tract disease, acute alcoholism (including delirium tremens), morbid obesity, adrenocortical insufficiency, history of seizure disorders, CNS depression/coma, kyphoscoliosis (or other skeletal disorder which may alter respiratory function), hypothyroidism (including myxedema), prostatic hyperplasia, urethral stricture, and toxic psychosis. May obscure diagnosis or clinical course of patients with acute abdominal conditions.

Use with caution in the elderly, debilitated, and hepatic or renal function. Hemodynamic effects (hypotension, orthostasis) may be exaggerated in patients with hypovolemia, concurrent vasodilating drugs, or in patients with head injury. Respiratory depressant effects and capacity to elevate CSF pressure may be exaggerated in presence of head injury, other intracranial lesion, or pre-existing intracranial pressure.

[U.S. Boxed Warning]: Concomitant use with CYP3A4 inhibitors may result in increased effects and potentially fatal respiratory depression. Concurrent use of agonist/antagonist analgesics may precipitate withdrawal symptoms and/or reduced analgesic efficacy in patients following prolonged therapy with mu opioid agonists. Abrupt discontinuation following prolonged use may also lead to withdrawal symptoms. **[U.S. Boxed Warning]: Healthcare provider should be alert to problems of abuse, misuse, and diversion.** Tolerance or drug dependence may result from extended use. Patients should be assessed for risk of abuse or addition prior to therapy and all patients should be monitored for signs of misuse, abuse, and addiction.

Controlled-release formulations: [U.S. Boxed Warning]: OxyContin® is not intended for use as an "as needed" analgesic or for immediately-postoperative pain management (should be used postoperatively only if the patient has received it prior to surgery or if severe, persistent pain is anticipated). **[U.S. Boxed Warning]: Do NOT crush, break, or chew controlled-release tablets**; 60 mg and 80 mg strengths, a single dose >40 mg, or a total dose of >80 mg/day are for use only in opioid-tolerant patients.

Drug Interactions

Metabolism/Transport Effects Substrate of CYP2D6 (minor), 3A4 (major)

Avoid Concomitant Use There are no known interactions where it is recommended to avoid concomitant use.

Increased Effect/Toxicity

OxyCODONE may increase the levels/effects of: Alcohol (Ethyl); Alvimopan; CNS Depressants; Desmopressin; Selective Serotonin Reuptake Inhibitors; Thiazide Diuretics

The levels/effects of OxyCODONE may be increased by: Amphetamines; Antipsychotic Agents (Phenothiazines); Conivaptan; CYP3A4 Inhibitors (Moderate); CYP3A4 Inhibitors (Strong); Dasatinib; Droperidol; Succinylcholine; Voriconazole

Decreased Effect

OxyCODONE may decrease the levels/effects of: Pegvisomant

The levels/effects of OxyCODONE may be decreased by: Ammonium Chloride; CYP3A4 Inducers (Strong); Deferasirox; Mixed Agonist / Antagonist Opioids; Rifampin; St Johns Wort; Tocilizumab

Ethanol/Nutrition/Herb Interactions

Ethanol: May increase CNS depression; monitor for increased effects with coadministration. Caution patients about effects.

Herb/Nutraceutical: Avoid valerian, St John's wort, kava kava, gotu kola (may increase CNS depression).

Dietary Considerations Instruct patient to avoid high-fat meals when taking some products (food has no effect on the reformulated OxyContin®).

Pharmacodynamics/Kinetics

Onset of Action Pain relief: Immediate release: 10-15 minutes; Peak effect: Immediate release: 0.5-1 hour

Duration of Action Immediate release: 3-6 hours; Controlled release: ≤12 hours

Half-life Elimination Immediate release: 2-3 hours; Controlled release: ~5 hours

Time to Peak Plasma: Immediate release: 1.4-1.9 hours; Controlled release: 4-5 hours

Pregnancy Risk Factor B

Lactation Enters breast milk/not recommended

Breast-Feeding Considerations Sedation and/or respiratory depression may occur in the infant; symptoms of opioid withdrawal may occur following the cessation of breast-feeding.

Controlled Substance C-II

Prescribing and Access Restrictions As a requirement of the REMS program, healthcare providers who prescribe OxyContin® need to receive training on the proper use and potential risks of OxyContin®. For training, please refer to http://www.oxycontinrems.com. Prescribers will need retraining every 2 years or following any significant changes to the OxyContin® REMS program.

Dosage Forms

Capsule, oral: 5 mg

Solution, oral: 20 mg/mL (30 mL)

Tablet, oral: 5 mg, 10 mg, 15 mg, 20 mg, 30 mg

Roxicodone®: 5 mg, 15 mg, 30 mg

Tablet, controlled release, oral:

OxyCONTIN®: 10 mg, 15 mg, 20 mg, 30 mg, 40 mg, 60 mg, 80 mg

References

Wynn RL, "Narcotic Analgesics for Dental Pain: Available Products, Strengths, and Formulations," *Gen Dent*, 2001, 49(2)126-36.

Oxycodone and Acetaminophen (oks i KOE done & a seet a MIN oh fen)

Related Information

Acetaminophen *on page 32*
Oral Pain *on page 1928*
OxyCODONE *on page 1269*

Related Sample Prescriptions

Severe Oral Pain *on page 1980*

U.S. Brand Names Endocet®; Percocet®; Primlev™; Roxicet™; Roxicet™ 5/500; Tylox®

Canadian Brand Names Endocet®; Novo-Oxycodone Acet; Oxycocet®; Percocet®; Percocet®-Demi; PMS-Oxycodone-Acetaminophen

Generic Availability (U.S.) Yes: Excludes caplet and solution

Pharmacologic Category Analgesic, Opioid

Dental Use Treatment of postoperative pain

Use Management of moderate-to-severe pain

Local Anesthetic/Vasoconstrictor Precautions No information available to require special precautions

Effects on Dental Treatment Key adverse event(s) related to dental treatment: Nausea, sedation, constipation, and xerostomia (normal salivary flow resumes upon discontinuation). See Dental Comment.

Effects on Bleeding No information available to require special precautions

Adverse Effects Frequency not defined (also see individual agents): Allergic reaction, constipation, dizziness, dysphoria, euphoria, lightheadedness, nausea, pruritus, respiratory depression, sedation, skin rash, vomiting

Dental Usual Dosage

Note: Initial dose is based on the **oxycodone** content; however, the maximum daily dose is based on the **acetaminophen** content.

Management of pain: Doses should be given every 4-6 hours as needed and titrated to appropriate analgesic effects.

Mild-to-moderate pain:

Children: Initial dose, **based on oxycodone content:** 0.05-0.1 mg/kg/dose

Maximum acetaminophen dose: Children <45 kg: 90 mg/kg/day; children >45 kg: 4 g/day

Adults: Initial dose, **based on oxycodone content:** 2.5-5 mg

Severe pain:

Children: Initial dose, **based on oxycodone content:** 0.3 mg/kg/dose

Adults: Initial dose, **based on oxycodone content:** 10-30 mg. Do not exceed acetaminophen 4 g/day.

Elderly: Doses should be titrated to appropriate analgesic effects: Initial dose, **based on oxycodone content:** 2.5-5 mg every 6 hours. Do not exceed acetaminophen 4 g/day.

Dosage adjustment in hepatic impairment: Dose should be reduced in patients with severe liver disease.

Dosage Oral: Doses should be given every 4-6 hours as needed and titrated to appropriate analgesic effects. **Note:** Initial dose is based on the **oxycodone** content; however, the maximum daily dose is based on the **acetaminophen** content.

Children: Maximum acetaminophen dose: Children <45 kg: 90 mg/kg/day; children >45 kg: 4 g/day

Mild-to-moderate pain: Initial dose, **based on oxycodone content:** 0.05-0.1 mg/kg/dose

Severe pain: Initial dose, **based on oxycodone content:** 0.3 mg/kg/dose

Adults:

Mild-to-moderate pain: Initial dose, **based on oxycodone content:** 2.5-5 mg

Severe pain: Initial dose, **based on oxycodone content:** 10-30 mg. Do not exceed acetaminophen 4 g/day.

Elderly: Doses should be titrated to appropriate analgesic effects: Initial dose, **based on oxycodone content:** 2.5-5 mg every 6 hours. Do not exceed acetaminophen 4 g/day.

Dosage adjustment in hepatic impairment: Dose should be reduced in patients with severe liver disease.

Mechanism of Action

Oxycodone, as with other narcotic (opiate) analgesics, blocks pain perception in the cerebral cortex by binding to specific receptor molecules (opiate receptors) within the neuronal membranes of synapses. This binding results in a decreased synaptic chemical transmission throughout the CNS thus inhibiting the flow of pain sensations into the higher centers. Mu and kappa are the two subtypes of the opiate receptor to which oxycodone binds to cause analgesia.

Acetaminophen inhibits the synthesis of prostaglandins in the CNS and peripherally blocks pain impulse generation; produces antipyresis from inhibition of hypothalamic heat-regulating center.

Contraindications Hypersensitivity to oxycodone, acetaminophen, or any component of the formulation; severe respiratory depression (in absence of resuscitative equipment or ventilatory support); pregnancy (prolonged periods or high doses at term)

Warnings/Precautions Use with caution in patients with hypersensitivity reactions to other phenanthrene-derivative opioid agonists (morphine, codeine, hydrocodone, hydromorphone, levorphanol, oxymorphone); respiratory diseases including asthma, emphysema, COPD; severe liver or renal insufficiency; hypothyroidism; Addison's disease; seizure disorder; toxic psychosis; morbid obesity; CNS depression/coma; biliary tract impairment; prostatic hyperplasia; or urethral stricture. May obscure diagnosis or clinical course of patients with acute abdominal conditions. Some preparations contain sulfites which may cause allergic reactions. May be habit-forming. Causes sedation; caution must be used in performing tasks which require alertness (eg, operating machinery or driving). Effects may be potentiated when used with other sedative drugs or ethanol. May cause hypotension. Concurrent use of agonist/antagonist analgesics may precipitate withdrawal symptoms and/or reduced analgesic efficacy in patients following prolonged therapy with mu opioid agonists. Abrupt discontinuation following prolonged use may also lead to withdrawal symptoms.

Use with caution in patients with head injury and increased intracranial pressure (respiratory depressant effects increased and may also elevate CSF pressure).

Enhanced analgesia has been seen in elderly and debilitated patients on therapeutic doses of narcotics. Duration of action may be increased in the elderly. The elderly may be particularly susceptible to the CNS depressant and constipating effects of narcotics.

May cause severe hepatic toxicity on acute overdose; in addition, chronic daily dosing in adults has resulted in liver damage in some patients. Use with caution in patients with alcoholic liver disease; consuming ≥3 alcoholic drinks/day may increase the risk of liver damage. Use with caution in patients with known G6PD deficiency. Limit acetaminophen dose to <4 g/day.

Drug Interactions

Metabolism/Transport Effects

Oxycodone: **Substrate** of CYP2D6 (minor), 3A4 (major)
Acetaminophen: **Substrate** (minor) of CYP1A2, 2A6, 2C9, 2D6, 2E1, 3A4

Avoid Concomitant Use There are no known interactions where it is recommended to avoid concomitant use.

Increased Effect/Toxicity

Oxycodone and Acetaminophen may increase the levels/effects of: Alcohol (Ethyl); Alvimopan; CNS Depressants; Dasatinib; Desmopressin; Imatinib; Selective Serotonin Reuptake Inhibitors; SORAfenib; Thiazide Diuretics; Vitamin K Antagonists

The levels/effects of Oxycodone and Acetaminophen may be increased by: Amphetamines; Antipsychotic Agents (Phenothiazines); Conivaptan; CYP3A4 Inhibitors (Moderate); CYP3A4 Inhibitors (Strong); Dasatinib; Droperidol; Imatinib; Isoniazid; Metyrapone; Probenecid; SORAfenib; Succinylcholine; Voriconazole

Decreased Effect

Oxycodone and Acetaminophen may decrease the levels/effects of: Pegvisomant

The levels/effects of Oxycodone and Acetaminophen may be decreased by: Ammonium Chloride; Anticonvulsants (Hydantoin); Barbiturates; CarBAMazepine; Cholestyramine Resin; CYP3A4 Inducers (Strong); Deferasirox; Mixed Agonist / Antagonist Opioids; Peginterferon Alfa-2b; Rifampin; St Johns Wort; Tocilizumab

Ethanol/Nutrition/Herb Interactions Ethanol: Excessive intake of ethanol may increase the risk of acetaminophen-induced hepatotoxicity. Avoid ethanol or limit to <3 drinks/day. Ethanol may also increase CNS depression; monitor for increased effects with co-administration. Caution patients about effects.

Pregnancy Risk Factor C

Lactation Enters breast milk/use caution

Breast-Feeding Considerations

Oxycodone: Excreted in breast milk. If occasional doses are used during breast-feeding, monitor infant for sedation, GI effects, and changes in feeding pattern.
Acetaminophen: May be taken while breast-feeding.

Controlled Substance C-II

Dosage Forms

Caplet: Oxycodone 5 mg and acetaminophen 500 mg
Roxicet™ 5/500: Oxycodone 5 mg and acetaminophen 500 mg

Capsule: Oxycodone 5 mg and acetaminophen 500 mg
Tylox®: Oxycodone 5 mg and acetaminophen 500 mg
Solution, oral: Oxycodone 5 mg and acetaminophen 325 mg per 5 mL
Roxicet™: Oxycodone 5 mg and acetaminophen 325 mg per 5 mL
Tablet:
Generics:
Oxycodone 2.5 mg and acetaminophen 325 mg
Oxycodone 5 mg and acetaminophen 325 mg
Oxycodone 7.5 mg and acetaminophen 325 mg
Oxycodone 7.5 mg and acetaminophen 500 mg
Oxycodone 10 mg and acetaminophen 325 mg
Oxycodone 10 mg and acetaminophen 650 mg
Brands:
Endocet®:
5/325 [scored]: Oxycodone 5 mg and acetaminophen 325 mg
7.5/325: Oxycodone 7.5 mg and acetaminophen 325 mg
7.5/500: Oxycodone 7.5 mg and acetaminophen 500 mg
10/325: Oxycodone 10 mg and acetaminophen 325 mg
10/650: Oxycodone 10 mg and acetaminophen 650 mg
Percocet®:
2.5/325: Oxycodone 2.5 mg and acetaminophen 325 mg
5/325 [scored]: Oxycodone 5 mg and acetaminophen 325 mg
7.5/325: Oxycodone 7.5 mg and acetaminophen 325 mg
7.5/500: Oxycodone 7.5 mg and acetaminophen 500 mg
10/325: Oxycodone 10 mg and acetaminophen 325 mg
10/650: Oxycodone 10 mg and acetaminophen 650 mg
Primlev™:
5/300: Oxycodone 5 mg and acetaminophen 300 mg
7.5/300: Oxycodone 7.5 mg and acetaminophen 300 mg
10/300: Oxycodone 10 mg and acetaminophen 300 mg
Roxicet™ [scored]: Oxycodone 5 mg and acetaminophen 325 mg

Dental Comment Oxycodone, as with other narcotic analgesics, is recommended only for limited acute dosing (ie, 3 days or less). Oxycodone has an addictive liability, especially when given long-term. The acetaminophen component requires use with caution in patients with alcoholic liver disease.

Hepatotoxicity caused by acetaminophen is potentiated by chronic alcohol consumption. People who are taking acetaminophen, even at therapeutic doses, and consume alcohol are at risk of developing hepatotoxicity.

Acetaminophen may increase the levels and enhance the anticoagulant effects of vitamin K antagonists acenocoumarol and warfarin (Coumadin®). Studies have reported that acetaminophen has increased the INR in warfarin treated patients with daily acetaminophen doses as low as 2 g, particularly when taking acetaminophen for >1 week (Antlitz, 1968; Boeijinga, 1982; Gebauer, 2003; Hylek, 1998; Rubin, 1984). In addition, case reports of bleeding as a result of increased INR have been published (Bagheri, 1999; Bartle, 1991). There is no known mechanism of the interaction; furthermore, some studies have failed to demonstrate this interaction (Gadisseur, 2003; Kwan, 1995; van den Bemt, 2002). In terms of risk, the data suggest that acetaminophen and warfarin could interact in some clinically significant manner but that the benefits of concomitant use of acetaminophen for pain control in dental patients taking warfarin usually outweigh the risks. An appropriate monitoring plan should be in place to identify potential negative effects and dosage adjustments may be necessary in a minority of patients. The interaction may be more likely to occur with daily acetaminophen doses of >1.3 g for >1 week.

There are no reports of acetaminophen interacting with antiplatelet drugs such as aspirin, clopidogrel (Plavix®), or prasugrel (Effient™). Also, there are no reports of acetaminophen in combination with hydrocodone, codeine, or oxycodone interacting with warfarin (Coumadin®).

References

Antlitz AM, Mead JA Jr, and Tolentino MA, "Potentiation of Oral Anticoagulant Therapy by Acetaminophen," *Curr Ther Res Clin Exp*, 1968, 10(10):501-7.
Bagheri H, Bernhard NB, and Montastruc JL, "Potentiation of the Acenocoumarol Anticoagulant Effect by Acetaminophen," *Ann Pharmacother*, 1999, 33(4):506.
Bartle WR and Blakely JA, "Potentiation of Warfarin Anticoagulation by Acetaminophen," *JAMA*, 1991, 265(10):1260.
Bell WR, "Acetaminophen and Warfarin: Undesirable Synergy," *JAMA*, 1998, 279(9):702-3.
Boeijinga JJ, Boerstra EE, Ris P, et al, "Interaction Between Paracetamol and Coumarin Anticoagulants," *Lancet*, 1982, 1(8270):506.
Botting RM, "Mechanism of Action of Acetaminophen: Is There a Cyclooxygenase 3?" *Clin Infect Dis*, 2000, Suppl 5:S202-10.
Cooper SA, Precheur H, Rauch D, et al, "Evaluation of Oxycodone and Acetaminophen in Treatment of Postoperative Pain," *Oral Surg Oral Med Oral Pathol*, 1980, 50(6):496-501.
Dart RC, Kuffner EK, and Rumack BH, "Treatment of Pain or Fever With Paracetamol (Acetaminophen) in the Alcoholic Patient: A Systematic Review," *Am J Ther*, 2000, 7(2):123-34.
Dionne RA, "New Approaches to Preventing and Treating Postoperative Pain," *J Am Dent Assoc*, 1992, 123(6):26-34.

Gadisseur AP, Van Der Meer FJ, and Rosendaal FR, "Sustained Intake of Paracetamol (Acetaminophen) During Oral Anticoagulant Therapy With Coumarins Does Not Cause Clinically Important INR Changes: A Randomized Double-Blind Clinical Trial," *J Thromb Haemost*, 2003, 1(4):714-7.
Gebauer MG, Nyfort-Hansen K, Henschke PJ, et al, "Warfarin and Acetaminophen Interaction," *Pharmacotherapy*, 2003, 23(1):109-12.
Gobetti JP, "Controlling Dental Pain," *J Am Dent Assoc*, 1992, 123(6):47-52.
Grant JA and Weiler JM, "A Report of a Rare Immediate Reaction After Ingestion of Acetaminophen," *Ann Allergy Asthma Immunol*, 2001, 87(3):227-9.
Hylek EM, Heiman H, Skates SJ, et al, "Acetaminophen and Other Risk Factors for Excessive Warfarin Anticoagulation," *JAMA*, 1998, 279(9):657-62.
Kwan D, Bartle WR, and Walker SE, "The Effects of Acetaminophen on Pharmacokinetics and Pharmacodynamics of Warfarin," *J Clin Pharmacol*, 1999, 39(1):68-75.
Kwan D, Bartle WR, and Walker SE, "The Effects of Acute and Chronic Acetaminophen Dosing on the Pharmacodynamics and Pharmacokinetics of (R)- and (S)-Warfarin," *Clin Pharmacol Ther*, 1995, 57:212.
McClain CJ, Price S, Barve S, et al, "Acetaminophen Hepatotoxicity: An Update," *Curr Gastroenterol Rep*, 1999, 1(1):42-9.
Rubin RN, Mentzer RL, and Budzynski AZ, "Potentiation of Anticoagulant Effect of Warfarin by Acetaminophen (Tylenol®)," *Clin Res*, 1984, 32:698a.
Shek KL, Chan LN, and Nutescu E, "Warfarin-Acetaminophen Drug Interaction Revisited," *Pharmacotherapy*, 1999, 19(10):1153-8.
Tanaka E, Yamazaki K, and Misawa S, "Update: The Clinical Importance of Acetaminophen Hepatotoxicity in Nonalcoholic and Alcoholic Subjects," *J Clin Pharm Ther*, 2000, 25(5):325-32.
van den Bemt PM, Geven LM, Kuitert NA, et al, "The Potential Interaction Between Oral Anticoagulants and Acetaminophen in Everyday Practice," *Pharm World Sci*, 2002, 24(5):201-4.
Wynn RL, "Narcotic Analgesics for Dental Pain: Available Products, Strengths, and Formulations," *Gen Dent*, 2001, 49(2):126-8, 130, 132 passim.

Oxycodone and Aspirin (oks i KOE done & AS pir in)

Related Information

Aspirin *on page 171*
Oral Pain *on page 1928*
OxyCODONE *on page 1269*

U.S. Brand Names Endodan®; Percodan®

Canadian Brand Names Endodan®; Oxycodan®; Percodan®

Generic Availability (U.S.) Yes

Pharmacologic Category Analgesic, Opioid

Dental Use Treatment of postoperative pain

Use Management of moderate- to moderately-severe pain

Local Anesthetic/Vasoconstrictor Precautions No information available to require special precautions

Effects on Dental Treatment Key adverse event(s) related to dental treatment: Nausea, sedation, constipation, and xerostomia (normal salivary flow resumes upon discontinuation). May have anticoagulant effects which may affect bleeding time. The elderly are a high-risk population for adverse effects from NSAIDs. As many as 60% of elderly patients with GI complications from NSAIDs can develop peptic ulceration and/or hemorrhage asymptomatically. Concomitant disease and drug use contribute to the risk of GI adverse effects. Enhanced analgesia has been seen with therapeutic doses of narcotics; duration of action may be increased. Elderly may also be particularly susceptible to the CNS depressant effects of narcotics. See Effects on Bleeding and Dental Comment.

Effects on Bleeding Aspirin inhibits platelet aggregation which prolongs bleeding times. Inhibition is irreversible; on discontinuation of ASA, normal platelet function returns only when new platelets are released from the bone marrow. Dental practitioners should note that recommendations differ between general surgery (eg, appendectomy, hip replacement) and dental surgery. Due to concerns for increased blood loss, ASA is typically avoided (if possible) in general surgery patients for 1-2 weeks prior to surgery (exception is in patients undergoing CABG or noncardiac surgery at high risk of cardiac events – per 2008 ACCP guidelines). However, in the case of dental surgery there is no scientific evidence to warrant discontinuance of aspirin.

Reports of major bleeding related to dental surgery attributed to aspirin use have not been published. Furthermore, interruption of therapy may result in a loss of therapeutic effect.

Adverse Effects Note: Also refer to individual agents

Frequency not defined.

- Cardiovascular: Circulatory depression, hypotension, shock
- Central nervous system: Dizziness, drowsiness, dysphoria, euphoria, lightheadedness, sedation
- Dermatologic: Pruritus
- Gastrointestinal: Constipation, nausea, vomiting
- Respiratory: Apnea, respiratory arrest, respiratory depression

Dental Usual Dosage

Analgesic: Oral (based on oxycodone combined salts):

Children: Maximum oxycodone: 5 mg/dose; maximum aspirin dose should not exceed 4 g/day. Doses should be given every 6 hours as needed.

Mild-to-moderate pain: Initial dose, **based on oxycodone content:** 0.05-0.1 mg/kg/dose

Severe pain: Initial dose, **based on oxycodone content**: 0.3 mg/kg/dose

Adults: Percodan®: 1 tablet every 6 hours as needed for pain; maximum aspirin dose should not exceed 4 g/day.

Dosage Oral:

Children (dose based on total oxycodone content): Oxycodone 0.1-0.2 mg/kg/dose (maximum oxycodone: 5 mg/dose; maximum aspirin: 4 g/day). Doses should be given every 4-6 hours as needed (American Pain Society, 2008)

Adults: One tablet every 6 hours as needed for pain; maximum aspirin dose should not exceed 4 g/day

Dosing adjustment in renal impairment: Use with caution. Avoid use of aspirin in patients with Cl_{cr} <10 mL/minute.

Dosing adjustment in hepatic impairment: Use with caution. Avoid use of aspirin-containing products in severe impairment.

Mechanism of Action

Oxycodone, as with other narcotic (opiate) analgesics, blocks pain perception in the cerebral cortex by binding to specific receptor molecules (opiate receptors) within the neuronal membranes of synapses. This binding results in a decreased synaptic chemical transmission throughout the CNS, thus inhibiting the flow of pain sensations into the higher centers. Mu and kappa are the two subtypes of the opiate receptor to which oxycodone binds to cause analgesia.

Aspirin inhibits prostaglandin synthesis by decreasing the activity of the enzyme, cyclooxygenase, which results in decreased formation of prostaglandin precursors, acts on the hypothalamic heat-regulating center to reduce fever, blocks thromboxane synthetase action which prevents formation of the platelet-aggregating substance thromboxane A_2

Contraindications Hypersensitivity to oxycodone, salicylates, other NSAIDs, or any component of the formulation; patients with the syndrome of asthma, rhinitis, and nasal polyps; inherited or acquired bleeding disorders (including factor VII and factor IX deficiency); do not use in children and teenagers in the presence of viral infections (chickenpox or flu symptoms), with or without fever, due to a potential association with Reye's syndrome; significant respiratory depression; hypercarbia; known or suspected paralytic ileus; acute or severe bronchial asthma

Warnings/Precautions Use with caution in patients with hypersensitivity reactions to other phenanthrene-derivative opioid agonists (morphine, hydrocodone, hydromorphone, levorphanol, oxycodone, oxymorphone), respiratory diseases including asthma, emphysema, or COPD. Use with caution in pancreatitis or biliary tract disease, acute alcoholism (including delirium tremens), adrenocortical insufficiency, CNS depression/coma, kyphoscoliosis (or other skeletal disorder which may alter respiratory function), hypothyroidism (including myxedema), seizure disorder, morbid obesity, prostatic hyperplasia, urethral stricture, and toxic psychosis. May obscure diagnosis or clinical course of patients with acute abdominal conditions.

Causes sedation; caution must be used in performing tasks which require alertness (eg, operating machinery or driving). Effects may be potentiated when used with other sedative drugs or ethanol. Use with caution in elderly or debilitated patients. Use with caution in patients with renal and/or hepatic impairment; avoid use of aspirin-containing products in patients with severe hepatic or renal dysfunction. Hemodynamic effects (hypotension, orthostasis) may be exaggerated in patients with dehydration, hypovolemia, concurrent vasodilating drugs, or in patients with head injury. Respiratory depressant effects and capacity to elevate CSF pressure may be exaggerated in presence of head injury, other intracranial lesion, or pre-existing elevation of intracranial pressure. Tolerance or drug dependence may result from extended use. Healthcare provider should be alert to problems of abuse, misuse, and diversion. Taper dose gradually to avoid withdrawal symptoms in physically-dependent patients.

Use with caution in patients with platelet and bleeding disorders, erosive gastritis, or peptic ulcer disease. Heavy ethanol use (>3 drinks/day) can increase bleeding risks. Discontinue use if tinnitus or impaired hearing occurs. Patients with sensitivity to tartrazine dyes, nasal polyps, and asthma may have an increased risk of salicylate sensitivity. Surgical patients should avoid ASA if possible, for 1-2 weeks prior to surgery, to reduce the risk of excessive bleeding.

Drug Interactions

Metabolism/Transport Effects

Oxycodone: **Substrate** of CYP2D6 (minor), 3A4 (major)

Aspirin: **Substrate** of CYP2C9 (minor)

Avoid Concomitant Use

Avoid concomitant use of Oxycodone and Aspirin with any of the following: Influenza Virus Vaccine (Live/Attenuated); Ketorolac; Ketorolac (Systemic)

Increased Effect/Toxicity

Oxycodone and Aspirin may increase the levels/effects of: Alcohol (Ethyl); Alendronate; Alvimopan; Anticoagulants; Carbonic Anhydrase Inhibitors; CNS Depressants; Collagenase (Systemic); Corticosteroids (Systemic); Desmopressin; Divalproex; Drotrecogin Alfa; Heparin; Ibritumomab; Methotrexate; PRALAtrexate; Salicylates; Selective Serotonin Reuptake Inhibitors; Sulfonylureas; Thiazide Diuretics; Thrombolytic Agents; Tositumomab and Iodine I 131 Tositumomab; Valproic Acid; Varicella Virus-Containing Vaccines; Vitamin K Antagonists

The levels/effects of Oxycodone and Aspirin may be increased by: Amphetamines; Antidepressants (Tricyclic, Tertiary Amine); Antiplatelet Agents; Antipsychotic Agents (Phenothiazines); Calcium Channel Blockers (Nondihydropyridine); Conivaptan; CYP3A4 Inhibitors (Moderate); CYP3A4 Inhibitors (Strong); Dasatinib; Droperidol; Ginkgo Biloba; Glucosamine; Herbs (Anticoagulant/Antiplatelet Properties); Influenza Virus Vaccine (Live/Attenuated); Ketorolac; Ketorolac (Systemic); Loop Diuretics; Nonsteroidal Anti-Inflammatory Agents; NSAID (Nonselective); Omega-3-Acid Ethyl Esters; Pentosan Polysulfate Sodium; Pentoxifylline; Prostacyclin Analogues; Selective Serotonin Reuptake Inhibitors; Serotonin/Norepinephrine Reuptake Inhibitors; Succinylcholine; Treprostinil; Voriconazole

Decreased Effect

Oxycodone and Aspirin may decrease the levels/effects of: ACE Inhibitors; Loop Diuretics; NSAID (Nonselective); Pegvisomant; Probenecid; Tiludronate

The levels/effects of Oxycodone and Aspirin may be decreased by: Ammonium Chloride; Corticosteroids (Systemic); CYP3A4 Inducers (Strong); Deferasirox; Mixed Agonist / Antagonist Opioids; Nonsteroidal Anti-Inflammatory Agents; NSAID (Nonselective); Rifampin; St Johns Wort; Tocilizumab

Dietary Considerations Take without regard to meals.

Pregnancy Risk Factor B (oxycodone); D (aspirin)

Lactation Enters breast milk/not recommended

Breast-Feeding Considerations See individual agents.

Controlled Substance C-II

Dosage Forms

Tablet: Oxycodone hydrochloride 4.5 mg, oxycodone terephthalate 0.38 mg, and aspirin 325 mg

Endodan®, Percodan®: Oxycodone hydrochloride 4.8355 mg and aspirin 325 mg

Dental Comment Oxycodone, as with other narcotic analgesics, is recommended only for limited acute dosing (ie, 3 days or less). Oxycodone has an addictive liability, especially when given long-term. The oxycodone with aspirin could have anticoagulant effects and could possibly affect bleeding times.

There is no scientific evidence to warrant discontinuance of aspirin prior to dental surgery. Patients taking one aspirin tablet daily as an antithrombotic and who require dental surgery should be given special consideration in consultation with the physician before removal of the aspirin relative to prevention of postoperative bleeding.

References

Dionne RA, "New Approaches to Preventing and Treating Postoperative Pain," *J Am Dent Assoc*, 1992, 123(6):26-34.

Gobetti JP, "Controlling Dental Pain," *J Am Dent Assoc*, 1992, 123(6):47-52.

Wynn RL, "Narcotic Analgesics for Dental Pain: Available Products, Strengths, and Formulations," *Gen Dent*, 2001, 49(2):126-8, 130, 132 passim.

Oxycodone and Ibuprofen (oks i KOE done & eye byoo PROE fen)

Related Information

Ibuprofen *on page* 884

Oral Pain *on page* 1928

OxyCODONE *on page* 1269

Related Sample Prescriptions

Severe Oral Pain *on page* 1980

Generic Availability (U.S.) Yes

Pharmacologic Category Analgesic, Opioid; Nonsteroidal Anti-inflammatory Drug (NSAID), Oral

Dental Use Short-term (≤3-5 days) management of acute, moderate-to-severe pain

Use Short-term (≤7 days) management of acute, moderate-to-severe pain

Local Anesthetic/Vasoconstrictor Precautions No information available to require special precautions

Effects on Dental Treatment Key adverse event(s) related to dental treatment: Nausea, sedation, dizziness. See Dental Comment.

The dentist should be aware of the potential of abnormal coagulation. Caution should also be exercised in the use of NSAIDs in patients already on anticoagulant therapy with drugs such as warfarin (Coumadin®). See Effects on Bleeding.

Effects on Bleeding Nonselective NSAIDs are known to reversibly decrease platelet aggregation via mechanisms different than observed with aspirin. Platelet function is restored as the drug is eliminated from the body. NSAIDs should be avoided (if possible) in general surgery patients for 3-5 half-lives of the drug (usually 1-3 days) prior to surgery to reduce the risk of excessive bleeding. However, there is no scientific evidence to warrant discontinuance of NSAIDs prior to dental surgery. In medically complicated patients or extensive oral surgery, the decision to interrupt therapy must be based on the risk to benefit in an individual patient and a medical consult is suggested. Routine interruption of NSAID therapy for most dental procedures is not warranted. If therapy is continued without interruption, the clinician should anticipate the potential for slower clotting times.

Adverse Effects

>10%:

- Central nervous system: Dizziness (5% to 19%), somnolence (7% to 17%)
- Gastrointestinal: Nausea (9% to 25%)

2% to 10%:

- Cardiovascular: Vasodilation (<1% to 3%)
- Central nervous system: Headache (10%), fever (3%)
- Gastrointestinal: Vomiting (5%), constipation (<1% to 5%), diarrhea (2%), dyspepsia (<1% to 2%), flatulence (1%)
- Neuromuscular & skeletal: Weakness (<1% to 3%)
- Miscellaneous: Diaphoresis (2%)

Dental Usual Dosage Pain: Adults: Oral: Take 1 tablet as needed (maximum: 4 tablets/24 hours); do not take for longer than 7 days

Dosage Oral: Adults: Pain: Take 1 tablet as needed (maximum: 4 tablets/24 hours); do not take for longer than 7 days

Mechanism of Action

Oxycodone: Binds to opiate receptors in the CNS, causing inhibition of ascending pain pathways, altering the perception of and response to pain; produces generalized CNS depression

Ibuprofen: Reversibly inhibits cyclooxygenase-1 and 2 (COX-1 and 2) enzymes, which result in decreased formation of prostaglandin precursors; has antipyretic, analgesic, and anti-inflammatory properties

Contraindications Hypersensitivity to oxycodone, ibuprofen, aspirin, other NSAIDs, or any component of the formulation; paralytic ileus (known or suspected); perioperative pain in the setting of coronary artery bypass graft (CABG) surgery; significant respiratory depression, hypercarbia, acute/severe bronchial asthma

Warnings/Precautions Causes sedation; caution must be used in performing tasks which require alertness (eg, operating machinery or driving). Effects may be potentiated when used with other sedative drugs or ethanol. Use with caution in patients with hypersensitivity reactions to other phenanthrene-derivative opioid agonists and in patients with respiratory diseases. Use with caution in pancreatitis or biliary tract disease, acute alcoholism, adrenocortical insufficiency, CNS depression/coma, kyphoscoliosis (or other skeletal disorder which may alter respiratory function), hypothyroidism, seizure disorder, morbid obesity, prostatic hyperplasia, urethral stricture, and toxic psychosis. Use with caution in the elderly, debilitated, severe hepatic or renal dysfunction. Hemodynamic effects (hypotension, orthostasis) may be exaggerated in patients with hypovolemia, concurrent vasodilating drugs, or in patients with head injury. Respiratory depressant effects and capacity to elevate CSF pressure may be exaggerated in presence of head injury, other intracranial lesion, or pre-existing increased intracranial pressure. Opioids may suppress cough reflex; use with caution during postoperative period and in patients with pulmonary disease. Patients with acute abdominal condition should use this agent cautiously. Tolerance or drug dependence may result from extended use. Concurrent use of agonist/antagonist analgesics may precipitate withdrawal symptoms and/or reduced analgesic efficacy in patients following prolonged therapy with mu opioid agonists. Abrupt discontinuation following prolonged use may also lead to withdrawal symptoms.

[U.S. Boxed Warning]: NSAIDs are associated with an increased risk of adverse cardiovascular thrombotic events, including MI and stroke. New-onset or worsening of pre-existing hypertension may occur. Risk may be increased with duration of use or pre-existing cardiovascular risk factors or disease. Use caution with fluid retention. Avoid use in heart failure. Use of NSAIDs can compromise existing renal function. Rehydrate patient before starting therapy. Monitor renal function closely. Ibuprofen is not recommended for patients with advanced renal disease. **[U.S. Boxed Warning]: Use is contraindicated for treatment of perioperative pain in the setting of coronary artery bypass graft (CABG) surgery.** Risk of MI and stroke may be increased with use following CABG surgery.

[U.S. Boxed Warning]: NSAIDs may increase risk of gastrointestinal irritation, inflammation, ulceration, bleeding, and perforation. Use caution with a history of GI disease (bleeding or ulcers), concurrent therapy with aspirin, anticoagulants and/or corticosteroids, smoking, use of alcohol, the elderly or debilitated patients. When used concomitantly with ≤325 mg of aspirin, a substantial increase in the risk of gastrointestinal complications (eg, ulcer) occurs; concomitant gastroprotective therapy (eg, proton pump inhibitors) is recommended (Bhatt, 2008). May increase the risk of aseptic meningitis, especially in patients with systemic lupus erythematosus (SLE) and mixed connective tissue disorders. Platelet adhesion and aggregation may be decreased; may prolong bleeding time; patients with coagulation disorders or who are receiving anticoagulants should be monitored closely. Anemia may occur; patients on long-term NSAID therapy should be monitored for anemia. Rarely, NSAID use may cause severe blood dyscrasias (eg, agranulocytosis, aplastic anemia, thrombocytopenia).

NSAID use may compromise existing renal function; dose-dependent decreases in prostaglandin synthesis may result from NSAID use, reducing renal blood flow which may cause renal decompensation. NSAID use may increase the risk for hyperkalemia. Patients with impaired renal function, dehydration, heart failure, liver dysfunction, those taking diuretics, and ACE inhibitors, and the elderly are at greater risk of renal toxicity and hyperkalemia. Rehydrate patient before starting therapy; monitor renal function closely. Not recommended for use in patients with advanced renal disease. Long-term NSAID use may result in renal papillary necrosis.

NSAIDS may cause drowsiness, dizziness, blurred vision and other neurologic effects which may impair physical or mental abilities; patients must be cautioned about performing tasks which require mental alertness (eg, operating machinery or driving). Discontinue use with blurred or diminished vision and perform ophthalmologic exam. Monitor vision with long-term therapy.

NSAIDs may cause serious skin adverse events including exfoliative dermatitis, Stevens-Johnson Syndrome (SJS) and toxic epidermal necrolysis (TEN); discontinue use at first sign of skin rash or hypersensitivity. Anaphylactoid reactions may occur, even without prior exposure; patients with "aspirin triad" (bronchial asthma, aspirin intolerance, rhinitis) may be at increased risk. Do not use in patients who experience bronchospasm, asthma, rhinitis, or urticaria with NSAID or aspirin therapy. Use caution in other forms of asthma.

Withhold for at least 4-6 half-lives prior to surgical or dental procedures.

The elderly are at increased risk for adverse effects (especially peptic ulceration, CNS effects, renal toxicity) from NSAIDs even at low doses.

Drug Interactions

Metabolism/Transport Effects

Oxycodone: **Substrate** of CYP2D6 (minor), 3A4 (major)

Ibuprofen: **Substrate** (minor) of CYP2C9, 2C19; **Inhibits** CYP2C9 (strong)

Avoid Concomitant Use

Avoid concomitant use of Oxycodone and Ibuprofen with any of the following: Ketorolac; Ketorolac (Systemic)

Increased Effect/Toxicity

Oxycodone and Ibuprofen may increase the levels/effects of: Alcohol (Ethyl); Alvimopan; Aminoglycosides; Anticoagulants; Antiplatelet Agents; Bisphosphonate Derivatives; CNS Depressants; Collagenase (Systemic); CycloSPORINE; CycloSPORINE (Systemic); Deferasirox; Desmopressin; Digoxin; Drotrecogin Alfa; Eplerenone; Haloperidol; Ibritumomab; Lithium; Methotrexate; Nonsteroidal Anti-Inflammatory Agents; PEMEtrexed; Potassium-Sparing Diuretics; PRALAtrexate; Quinolone Antibiotics; Salicylates; Selective Serotonin Reuptake Inhibitors; Thiazide Diuretics; Thrombolytic Agents; Tositumomab and Iodine I 131 Tositumomab; Vancomycin; Vitamin K Antagonists

The levels/effects of Oxycodone and Ibuprofen may be increased by: ACE Inhibitors; Amphetamines; Angiotensin II Receptor Blockers; Antidepressants (Tricyclic, Tertiary Amine); Antipsychotic Agents (Phenothiazines); Conivaptan; Corticosteroids (Systemic); CYP3A4 Inhibitors (Moderate); CYP3A4 Inhibitors (Strong); Dasatinib; Droperidol; Glucosamine; Herbs (Anticoagulant/Antiplatelet Properties); Ketorolac; Ketorolac (Systemic); Nonsteroidal Anti-Inflammatory Agents; Omega-3-Acid Ethyl Esters; Pentosan Polysulfate Sodium; Pentoxifylline; Probenecid; Prostacyclin Analogues; Selective Serotonin Reuptake Inhibitors; Serotonin/Norepinephrine Reuptake Inhibitors; Succinylcholine; Treprostinil; Voriconazole

Decreased Effect

Oxycodone and Ibuprofen may decrease the levels/effects of: ACE Inhibitors; Angiotensin II Receptor Blockers; Antiplatelet Agents; Beta-Blockers; Eplerenone; HydrALAZINE; Loop Diuretics; Pegvisomant; Potassium-Sparing Diuretics; Salicylates

The levels/effects of Oxycodone and Ibuprofen may be decreased by: Ammonium Chloride; Bile Acid Sequestrants; CYP3A4 Inducers (Strong); Deferasirox; Mixed Agonist / Antagonist Opioids; Nonsteroidal Anti-Inflammatory Agents; Rifampin; Salicylates; St Johns Wort; Tocilizumab

Ethanol/Nutrition/Herb Interactions

Based on **oxycodone** component: Ethanol: May increase CNS depression; monitor for increased effects with coadministration. Caution patients about effects.

Based on **ibuprofen** component:

Ethanol: Avoid ethanol (may enhance gastric mucosal irritation).

Food: Food or milk are recommended to decrease gastric irritation.

Herb/Nutraceutical: Avoid alfalfa, anise, bilberry, bladderwrack, bromelain, cat's claw, celery, chamomile, coleus, cordyceps, dong quai, evening primrose, fenugreek, feverfew, garlic, ginger, ginkgo biloba, ginseng (American, Panax, Siberian), grapeseed, green tea, guggul, horse chestnut seed, horseradish, licorice, prickly ash, red clover, reishi, SAMe (S-adenosylmethionine), sweet clover, turmeric, white willow (all have additional antiplatelet activity).

Dietary Considerations Take without regard to meals.

Pharmacodynamics/Kinetics

Half-life Elimination Ibuprofen: 1.8-2.6 hours; Oxycodone: 3.1-3.7 hours

Time to Peak Serum: Ibuprofen: 1.6-3.1 hours; Oxycodone 1.3-2.1 hours

Pregnancy Risk Factor C/D ≥30 weeks gestation

Lactation Enters breast milk/not recommended

Breast-Feeding Considerations Refer to individual agents.

Controlled Substance C-II

Dosage Forms

Tablet: Oxycodone 5 mg and ibuprofen 400 mg

Dental Comment The combination of oxycodone and ibuprofen in this dose form is appropriate for the management of moderate-to-severe pain when the concomitant anti-inflammatory action of ibuprofen is desired. Oxycodone is recommended only for limited acute dosing (ie, ≤3 days). Oxycodone has an addictive liability, especially when given long term.

Oxygen (OKS i jen)

Generic Availability (U.S.) Yes

Pharmacologic Category Dental Gases

Dental Use Administered as a supplement with nitrous oxide to ensure adequate ventilation during sedation; a resuscitative agent for medical emergencies in dental office

Use Treatment of various clinical disorders, both respiratory and nonrespiratory; relief of arterial hypoxia and secondary complications; treatment of pulmonary hypertension, polycythemia secondary to hypoxemia, chronic disease states complicated by anemia, cancer, migraine headaches, coronary artery disease, seizure disorders, sickle-cell crisis, and sleep apnea

Local Anesthetic/Vasoconstrictor Precautions No information available to require special precautions

Effects on Dental Treatment No significant effects or complications reported

Effects on Bleeding No information available to require special precautions

Adverse Effects No data reported

Dental Usual Dosage Administered as a supplement with nitrous oxide to ensure adequate ventilation during sedation: Children and Adults: Average rate of 2 L/minute

Dosage Children and Adults: Average rate of 2 L/minute

Mechanism of Action Increased oxygen in tidal volume and oxygenation of tissues at molecular level

Contraindications No data reported

Warnings/Precautions Oxygen-induced hypoventilation is the greatest potential hazard of oxygen therapy. In patients with severe COPD, the respiratory drive results from hypoxic stimulation of the carotid chemoreceptors. If this hypoxic drive is diminished by excessive oxygen therapy, hypoventilation may occur and further carbon dioxide retention with possible cessation of ventilation.

Pregnancy Risk Factor No data reported

Dosage Forms

Liquid system with large reservoir holding 75-100 lb of liquid oxygen; compressed gas system consisting of high-pressure tank; tank sizes are "H" (6900 L of oxygen), "E" (622 L of oxygen) and "D" (356 L of oxygen)

Oxymetazoline (Nasal) (oks i met AZ oh leen)

Related Information

Bacterial Infections *on page 1933*

Related Sample Prescriptions

Sinus Infection Treatment *on page 1985*

U.S. Brand Names 12 Hour Nasal Relief [OTC]; 4-Way® 12 Hour [OTC]; Afrin® Extra Moisturizing [OTC]; Afrin® Original [OTC]; Afrin® Severe Congestion [OTC]; Afrin® Sinus [OTC]; Dristan® [OTC]; Duramist Plus [OTC]; Neo-Synephrine® Nighttime12-Hour [OTC]; Nostrilla® [OTC]; NRS® [OTC]; Sudafed OM® Sinus Congestion [OTC] [DSC]; Vicks® Early Defense™ [OTC] [DSC]; Vicks® Sinex® VapoSpray 12-Hour; Vicks® Sinex® VapoSpray 12-Hour UltraFine Mist [OTC]; Vicks® Sinex® VapoSpray Moisturizing 12-Hour UltraFine Mist [OTC]

Canadian Brand Names Claritin® Allergic Decongestant; Dristan® Long Lasting Nasal; Drixoral® Nasal

Generic Availability (U.S.) Yes: Intranasal solution (spray)

Pharmacologic Category Adrenergic Agonist Agent; Imidazoline Derivative

Dental Use Symptomatic relief of nasal mucosal congestion

Use Adjunctive therapy for nasal congestion, associated with acute or chronic rhinitis, the common cold, sinusitis, hay fever, or other allergies

Local Anesthetic/Vasoconstrictor Precautions No information available to require special precautions

Effects on Dental Treatment No significant effects or complications reported

Effects on Bleeding No information available to require special precautions

Adverse Effects Frequency not defined.

Respiratory: Dryness of the nasal mucosa, nasal irritation (temporary), rebound congestion (chronic use), sneezing

Dental Usual Dosage Symptomatic relief of nasal mucosal congestion: Children ≥6 years and Adults: Intranasal: Instill 2-3 sprays into each nostril twice daily for ≤3 days

Dosage Intranasal: Children ≥6 years and Adults: Instill 2-3 sprays into each nostril twice daily for ≤3 days

Mechanism of Action Stimulates alpha-adrenergic receptors in the arterioles of the nasal mucosa to produce vasoconstriction

Contraindications Hypersensitivity to oxymetazoline or any component of the formulation

Warnings/Precautions Rebound congestion may occur with extended use. Use with caution in the presence of hypertension, diabetes, hyperthyroidism, heart disease, coronary artery disease, or benign prostatic hyperplasia.

Drug Interactions

Avoid Concomitant Use

Avoid concomitant use of Oxymetazoline (Nasal) with any of the following: Iobenguane I 123; MAO Inhibitors

Increased Effect/Toxicity

Oxymetazoline (Nasal) may increase the levels/effects of: Sympathomimetics

The levels/effects of Oxymetazoline (Nasal) may be increased by: Atomoxetine; Cannabinoids; MAO Inhibitors; Tricyclic Antidepressants

Decreased Effect

Oxymetazoline (Nasal) may decrease the levels/effects of: Iobenguane I 123

Pharmacodynamics/Kinetics

Onset of Action Within seconds

Duration of Action Up to 12 hours

Dosage Forms

Solution, intranasal: 0.05% (15 mL, 30 mL)

12 Hour Nasal Relief [OTC]: 0.05% (15 mL, 30 mL)
4-Way® 12 Hour [OTC]: 0.05% (15 mL)
Afrin® Extra Moisturizing [OTC]: 0.05% (15 mL)
Afrin® Original [OTC]: 0.05% (15 mL, 30 mL)
Afrin® Severe Congestion [OTC]: 0.05% (15 mL)
Afrin® Sinus [OTC]: 0.05% (15 mL)
Dristan® [OTC]: 0.05% (15 mL)
Duramist Plus [OTC]: 0.05% (15 mL)
Neo-Synephrine® Nighttime12-Hour [OTC]: 0.05% (15 mL)
Nostrilla® [OTC]: 0.05% (15 mL)

NRS® [OTC]: 0.05% (15 mL, 30 mL)
Vicks® Sinex® VapoSpray 12-Hour: 0.05% (15 mL)
Vicks® Sinex® VapoSpray 12-Hour UltraFine Mist [OTC]: 0.05% (15 mL)
Vicks® Sinex® VapoSpray Moisturizing 12-Hour UltraFine Mist [OTC]: 0.05% (15 mL)

Oxymetholone (oks i METH oh lone)

U.S. Brand Names Anadrol®-50
Pharmacologic Category Anabolic Steroid
Use Treatment of anemias caused by deficient red cell production
Local Anesthetic/Vasoconstrictor Precautions No information available to require special precautions
Effects on Dental Treatment No significant effects or complications reported
Effects on Bleeding No information available to require special precautions
Adverse Effects Frequency not defined.
Cardiovascular: Coronary artery disease, peripheral edema
Central nervous system: Excitation, insomnia
Dermatologic: Acne (prepubertal males, women), hirsutism (women), hypercalcemia, hyperchloremia, hyperkalemia, hyperphosphatemia, hyperpigmentation, male-pattern baldness (postpubertal males, women)
Endocrine & metabolic: Amenorrhea, cholesterol increased, clitoromegaly, creatine phosphokinase increased, glucose tolerance decreased, gynecomastia, HDL-cholesterol decreased, hoarseness (women), hypernatremia, impotence (postpubertal males), LDL-cholesterol decreased, libido increased/decreased, menstrual irregularities, oligospermia, phallic enlargement (prepubertal males), priapism (postpubertal males), testicular atrophy (postpubertal males), testicular dysfunction (postpubertal males); virilism (women, high dose); voice deepening (women)
Gastrointestinal: Diarrhea, nausea, vomiting
Genitourinary: Bladder irritability (postpubertal males), epididymitis (postpubertal males), prostatic hyperplasia (elderly males), seminal volume decreased (postpubertal males)
Hematologic: Iron-deficiency anemia, polycythemia, suppression of clotting factors
Hepatic: Cholestatic hepatitis, hepatic necrosis, hepatocellular carcinoma jaundice, liver cell tumors, peliosis hepatis, transaminases increased
Neuromuscular & skeletal: Premature closure of epiphysis (children)
General Dosage Range Oral: *Children and Adults:* 1-5 mg/kg once daily
Mechanism of Action Enhances the production and urinary excretion of erythropoietin in patients with anemias due to bone marrow failure; stimulates erythropoiesis in anemias due to deficient red cell production.
Pregnancy Risk Factor X
Controlled Substance C-III

Oxymorphone (oks i MOR fone)

Related Information
Oral Pain *on page 1928*
U.S. Brand Names Opana®; Opana® ER
Pharmacologic Category Analgesic, Opioid
Use
Parenteral: Management of moderate-to-severe acute pain; relief of anxiety in patients with dyspnea associated with pulmonary edema secondary to acute left ventricular failure
Oral, regular release: Management of moderate-to-severe acute pain
Oral, extended release: Management of moderate-to-severe pain in patients requiring around-the-clock opioid treatment for an extended period of time
Local Anesthetic/Vasoconstrictor Precautions No information available to require special precautions
Effects on Dental Treatment Key adverse event(s) related to dental treatment: Xerostomia (normal salivary flow resumes upon discontinuation). Anticholinergic side effects can cause a reduction of saliva production or secretion, contributing to discomfort and dental disease (ie, caries, oral candidiasis, and periodontal disease).
Effects on Bleeding No information available to require special precautions
Adverse Effects Incidence usually on higher end with extended release tablet.
>10%:
Central nervous system: Somnolence (9% to 19%), dizziness (7% to 18%), fever (1% to 14%), headache (7% to 12%)
Dermatologic: Pruritus (8% to 15%)
Gastrointestinal: Nausea (19% to 33%), constipation (4% to 28%), vomiting (9% to 16%)

1% to 10%:

Cardiovascular: Hypotension (<10%), tachycardia (<10%), edema (<10%), flushing (<10%), hypertension (<10%)

Central nervous system: Anxiety (1% to <10%), sedation (1% to <10%), depression (<10%), disorientation (<10%), lethargy (<10%), nervousness (<10%), restlessness (<10%), fatigue (≤4%), insomnia (≤4%), confusion (3%)

Endocrine & metabolic: Dehydration (<10%)

Gastrointestinal: Abdominal distension (<10%), flatulence (1% to <10%), xerostomia (1% to <10%), dyspepsia (<10%), weight loss (<10%), diarrhea (≤4%), abdominal pain (≤3%), appetite decreased (≤3%)

Neuromuscular & skeletal: Weakness (<10%)

Ocular: Blurred vision (<10%)

Respiratory: Hypoxia (<10%), dyspnea (<10%)

Miscellaneous: Diaphoresis (1% to <10%)

General Dosage Range Dosage adjustment recommended in patients with hepatic or renal impairment

I.M., SubQ: *Adults:* Initial: 0.5 mg; Maintenance: 1-1.5 mg every 4-6 hours as needed

I.V.: *Adults:* Initial: 0.5 mg

Oral:

Extended release: *Adults (opioid-naive):* Initial: 5 mg every 12 hours; Maintenance: Titrate upward with 5-10 mg every 12 hours at 3-7 day intervals until desired response

Immediate release: *Adults (opioid-naive):* Initial: 5-20 mg every 4-6 hours; Maintenance: Titrate upward to desired response

Mechanism of Action Oxymorphone hydrochloride is a potent narcotic analgesic with uses similar to those of morphine. The drug is a semisynthetic derivative of morphine (phenanthrene derivative) and is closely related to hydromorphone chemically (Dilaudid®).

Pharmacodynamics/Kinetics

Onset of Action Parenteral: 5-10 minutes

Duration of Action Analgesic: Parenteral: 3-6 hours

Half-life Elimination Oral: Immediate release: 7-9 hours; Extended release: 9-11 hours

Pregnancy Risk Factor C

Controlled Substance C-II

Oxytocin (oks i TOE sin)

U.S. Brand Names Pitocin®

Canadian Brand Names Pitocin®; Syntocinon®

Pharmacologic Category Oxytocic Agent

Use Induction of labor at term; control of postpartum bleeding; adjunctive therapy in management of abortion

Local Anesthetic/Vasoconstrictor Precautions No information available to require special precautions

Effects on Dental Treatment No significant effects or complications reported

Effects on Bleeding No information available to require special precautions

Adverse Effects Frequency not defined.

Fetus or neonate:

Cardiovascular: Arrhythmias (including premature ventricular contractions), bradycardia

Central nervous system: Brain or CNS damage (permanent), neonatal seizure

Hepatic: Neonatal jaundice

Ocular: Neonatal retinal hemorrhage

Miscellaneous: Fetal death, low Apgar score (5 minute)

Mother:

Cardiovascular: Arrhythmias, hypertensive episodes, premature ventricular contractions

Gastrointestinal: Nausea, vomiting

Genitourinary: Pelvic hematoma, postpartum hemorrhage, uterine hypertonicity, tetanic contraction of the uterus, uterine rupture, uterine spasm

Hematologic: Afibrinogenemia (fatal)

Miscellaneous: Anaphylactic reaction, subarachnoid hemorrhage

General Dosage Range

I.M.: *Adults:* Total dose of 10 units after delivery

I.V.: *Adults:* Dosage varies greatly depending on indication

Mechanism of Action Oxytocin stimulates uterine contraction by activating G-protein-coupled receptors that trigger increases in intracellular calcium levels in uterine myofibrils. Oxytocin also increases local prostaglandin production, further stimulating uterine contraction.

Pharmacodynamics/Kinetics

Onset of Action Uterine contractions: I.M.: 3-5 minutes; I.V.: ~1 minute

Duration of Action I.M.: 2-3 hour; I.V.: 1 hour

Half-life Elimination 1-5 minutes

Pregnancy Risk Factor X

PACLitaxel (pac li TAKS el)

Canadian Brand Names Apo-Paclitaxel®; Paclitaxel For Injection; Taxol®

Pharmacologic Category Antineoplastic Agent, Antimicrotubular; Antineoplastic Agent, Natural Source (Plant) Derivative; Antineoplastic Agent, Taxane Derivative

Use Treatment of breast, nonsmall cell lung, and ovarian cancers; treatment of AIDS-related Kaposi's sarcoma (KS)

Unlabeled/Investigational Use Treatment of bladder, cervical, small cell lung, and head and neck cancers; treatment of (unknown primary) adenocarcinoma

Local Anesthetic/Vasoconstrictor Precautions No information available to require special precautions

Effects on Dental Treatment Key adverse event(s) related to dental treatment: Severe, potentially dose-limiting mucositis and stomatitis.

Effects on Bleeding Chemotherapy may result in significant myelosuppression, potentially including significant reduction in platelet counts and altered hemostasis. In patients who are under active treatment with these agents, medical consult is suggested.

Adverse Effects Percentages reported with single-agent therapy. **Note:** Myelosuppression is dose related, schedule related, and infusion-rate dependent (increased incidences with higher doses, more frequent doses, and longer infusion times) and, in general, rapidly reversible upon discontinuation.

>10%:

Cardiovascular: Flushing (28%), ECG abnormal (14% to 23%), edema (21%), hypotension (4% to 12%)

Dermatologic: Alopecia (87%), rash (12%)

Gastrointestinal: Nausea/vomiting (52%), diarrhea (38%), mucositis (17% to 35%; grades 3/4: up to 3%), stomatitis (15%; most common at doses >390 mg/m^2), abdominal pain (with intraperitoneal paclitaxel)

Hematologic: Neutropenia (78% to 98%; grade 4: 14% to 75%; onset 8-10 days, median nadir 11 days, recovery 15-21 days), leukopenia (90%; grade 4: 17%), anemia (47% to 90%; grades 3/4: 2% to 16%), thrombocytopenia (4% to 20%; grades 3/4: 1% to 7%), bleeding (14%)

Hepatic: Alkaline phosphatase increased (22%), AST increased (19%)

Local: Injection site reaction (erythema, tenderness, skin discoloration, swelling: 13%)

Neuromuscular & skeletal: Peripheral neuropathy (42% to 70%; grades 3/4: up to 7%), arthralgia/myalgia (60%), weakness (17%)

Renal: Creatinine increased (observed in KS patients only: 18% to 34%; severe: 5% to 7%)

Miscellaneous: Hypersensitivity reaction (31% to 45%; grades 3/4: up to 2%), infection (15% to 30%)

1% to 10%:

Cardiovascular: Bradycardia (3%), tachycardia (2%), hypertension (1%), rhythm abnormalities (1%), syncope (1%), venous thrombosis (1%)

Dermatologic: Nail changes (2%)

Hematologic: Febrile neutropenia (2%)

Hepatic: Bilirubin increased (7%)

Respiratory: Dyspnea (2%)

General Dosage Range Dosage adjustment recommended in patients with hepatic impairment or who develop toxicities

I.V.: *Adults:* Dosage varies greatly depending on indication

Mechanism of Action Paclitaxel promotes microtubule assembly by enhancing the action of tubulin dimers, stabilizing existing microtubules, and inhibiting their disassembly, interfering with the late G_2 mitotic phase, and inhibiting cell replication. In addition, the drug can distort mitotic spindles, resulting in the breakage of chromosomes. Paclitaxel may also suppress cell proliferation and modulate immune response.

Pharmacodynamics/Kinetics

Half-life Elimination

1- to 6-hour infusion: Mean (beta): 6.4 hours

3-hour infusion: Mean (terminal): 13.1-20.2 hours

24-hour infusion: Mean (terminal): 15.7-52.7 hours

Pregnancy Risk Factor D

PACLitaxel (Protein Bound) (pac li TAKS el PROE teen bownd)

U.S. Brand Names Abraxane®

Canadian Brand Names Abraxane®

Pharmacologic Category Antineoplastic Agent, Antimicrotubular; Antineoplastic Agent, Natural Source (Plant) Derivative; Antineoplastic Agent, Taxane Derivative

Use Treatment of refractory (metastatic) or relapsed (within 6 months of adjuvant therapy) breast cancer

Unlabeled/Investigational Use Treatment of advanced nonsmall cell lung cancer (NSCLC)

Local Anesthetic/Vasoconstrictor Precautions No information available to require special precautions

Effects on Dental Treatment Key adverse event(s) related to dental treatment: Mucositis.

Effects on Bleeding Chemotherapy may result in significant myelosuppression, potentially including significant reduction in platelet counts and altered hemostasis. In patients who are under active treatment with these agents, medical consult is suggested.

Adverse Effects

>10%:

Cardiovascular: ECG abnormal (60%; 35% in patients with a normal baseline)

Dermatologic: Alopecia (90%)

Gastrointestinal: Nausea (30%; grades 3/4: 3%), diarrhea (27%; grades 3/4: <1%), vomiting (18%; grades 3/4: 4%)

Hematologic: Neutropenia (80%; grade 4: 9%), anemia (33%; grades 3/4: 1%), myelosuppression (dose-related)

Hepatic: AST increased (39%), alkaline phosphatase increased (36%), GGT increased (grades 3/4: 14%)

Neuromuscular & skeletal: Sensory neuropathy (71%; grades 3/4: 10%; dose dependent; cumulative), weakness (47%; severe 8%), myalgia/arthralgia (44%)

Ocular: Vision disturbance (13%; severe [keratitis, blurred vision]: 1%)

Renal: Creatinine increased (11%; severe 1%)

Respiratory: Dyspnea (12%)

Miscellaneous: Infection (24%; primarily included oral candidiasis, respiratory tract infection, and pneumonia)

1% to 10%:

Cardiovascular: Edema /fluid retention (10%), hypotension (5%), cardiovascular events (grades 3/4: 3%; included chest pain, cardiac arrest, supraventricular tachycardia, thrombosis, pulmonary thromboembolism, pulmonary emboli, and hypertension)

Gastrointestinal: Mucositis (7%; grades 3/4: <1%)

Hematologic: Bleeding (2%), neutropenic fever (2%), thrombocytopenia (2%; grades 3/4: <1%)

Hepatic: Bilirubin increased (7%)

Neuromuscular & skeletal: Peripheral neuropathy (grade 3: 10%)

Respiratory: Cough (7%)

Miscellaneous: Hypersensitivity reaction (4%, includes chest pain, dyspnea, flushing, hypotension; severe: <1%)

General Dosage Range Dosage adjustment recommended in patients with hepatic impairment or who develop toxicities

I.V.: *Adults:* 260 mg/m^2 every 3 weeks

Mechanism of Action Albumin-bound paclitaxel nanoparticle formulation. Paclitaxel promotes microtubule assembly by enhancing the action of tubulin dimers, stabilizing existing microtubules, and inhibiting their disassembly, interfering with the late G_2 mitotic phase, and inhibiting cell replication. May also distort mitotic spindles, resulting in the breakage of chromosomes. Paclitaxel may also suppress cell proliferation and modulate immune response.

Pharmacodynamics/Kinetics

Half-life Elimination Terminal: 27 hours

Pregnancy Risk Factor D

Palifermin (pal ee FER min)

U.S. Brand Names Kepivance®

Canadian Brand Names Kepivance®

Generic Availability (U.S.) No

Pharmacologic Category Keratinocyte Growth Factor

Dental Use Decrease the incidence and severity of severe oral mucositis associated with hematologic malignancies in patients receiving myelotoxic therapy requiring hematopoietic stem cell support

Use Decrease the incidence and severity of severe oral mucositis associated with hematologic malignancies in patients receiving myelotoxic therapy requiring hematopoietic stem cell support

Local Anesthetic/Vasoconstrictor Precautions No information available to require special precautions

Effects on Dental Treatment Key adverse event(s) related to dental treatment: Taste alteration, mouth/tongue discoloration or thickness. See Dental Comment.

Effects on Bleeding No information available to require special precautions

Adverse Effects

>10%:

- Cardiovascular: Edema (28%), hypertension (7% to 14%)
- Central nervous system: Fever (39%); pain (16%); dysesthesia (oral hyperesthesia, hypoesthesia, and paresthesia 12%)
- Dermatologic: Rash (62%; grade 3: 3%), pruritus (35%), erythema (32%)
- Gastrointestinal: Serum amylase increased (grades 3/4: 38%), mouth/tongue discoloration or thickness (17%), taste alteration (16%), serum lipase increased (grades 3/4: 11%)
- Renal: Proteinuria (17%)
- Respiratory: Cough (32%), rhinitis (16%)

1% to 10%:

- Neuromuscular & skeletal: Arthralgia (10%)
- Miscellaneous: Antibody formation (2%)

Dental Usual Dosage Oral mucositis: Adults: I.V.: 60 mcg/kg/day for 3 consecutive days before and after myelotoxic therapy; total of 6 doses

Dosage I.V.: Adults: 60 mcg/kg/day for 3 consecutive days before and after myelotoxic therapy; total of 6 doses

Note: Administer first 3 doses prior to myelotoxic therapy, with the 3rd dose given 24-48 hours before therapy begins. The last 3 doses should be administered after myelotoxic therapy, with the first of these doses after but on the same day as hematopoietic stem cell infusion and at least 4 days after the most recent dose of palifermin.

Dosage adjustment in renal impairment: No adjustment necessary

Mechanism of Action Palifermin is a recombinant keratinocyte growth factor (KGF) produced in *E. coli*. Endogenous KGF is produced by mesenchymal cells in response to epithelial tissue injury. KGF binds to the KGF receptor resulting in proliferation, differentiation and migration of epithelial cells in multiple tissues, including (but not limited to) the tongue, buccal mucosa, esophagus, and salivary gland.

Contraindications Hypersensitivity to palifermin, *E. coli*-derived proteins, or any component of the formulation

Warnings/Precautions Hazardous agent - use appropriate precautions for handling and disposal. Edema, erythema, pruritus, rash, oral/perioral dysesthesia, taste alteration, tongue discoloration, and tongue thickening may occur; instruct patients to report mucocutaneous effects. Safety and efficacy have not been established with nonhematologic malignancies; effect on the growth of nonhematopoietic human tumors is not known. Palifermin has been shown to enhance epithelial tumor cell lines *in vitro*. Palifermin should be administered prior to and following, but not with, chemotherapy. If administered during or within 24 hours of (before or after) chemotherapy, palifermin may increase the severity and duration of mucositis due to the increased sensitivity of rapidly-dividing epithelial cells. Safety and efficacy have not been established in children.

Drug Interactions

Avoid Concomitant Use There are no known interactions where it is recommended to avoid concomitant use.

Increased Effect/Toxicity There are no known significant interactions involving an increase in effect.

Decreased Effect There are no known significant interactions involving a decrease in effect.

Pharmacodynamics/Kinetics

Onset of Action Epithelial cell proliferation (dose-dependent): 48 hours

Half-life Elimination 4.5 hours (range: 3.3-5.7 hours)

Pregnancy Risk Factor C

Lactation Excretion in breast milk unknown/use caution

Dosage Forms

Injection, powder for reconstitution [preservative free]:

Kepivance®: 6.25 mg

Dental Comment Palifermin works at the cellular level by protecting the epithelial cells lining the mouth and throat from damage caused by chemotherapy and radiation and by stimulating the growth and development of new epithelial cells to build up the mucosal barrier.

Paliperidone (pal ee PER i done)

U.S. Brand Names Invega®; Invega® Sustenna®

Canadian Brand Names Invega®; Invega® Sustenna®

Pharmacologic Category Antipsychotic Agent, Atypical

Use

Oral: Acute and maintenance treatment of schizophrenia; acute treatment of schizoaffective disorder (monotherapy or adjunctive therapy to mood stabilizers and/or antidepressants)

Injection: Acute and maintenance treatment of schizophrenia

Unlabeled/Investigational Use Psychosis/agitation related to Alzheimer's dementia

Local Anesthetic/Vasoconstrictor Precautions No information available to require special precautions

Effects on Dental Treatment Key adverse event(s) related to dental treatment: Significant xerostomia and changes in salivation (normal salivary flow resumes upon discontinuation).

Effects on Bleeding No information available to require special precautions

Adverse Effects Unless otherwise noted, frequency of adverse effects is reported for the oral/I.M. formulation in adults.

>10%:

Cardiovascular: Tachycardia (1% to 14%)

Central nervous system: EPS (≤26%; dose dependent), insomnia (10% to 15%), headache (6% to 15%), parkinsonism (3% to 14%; dose dependent), somnolence (adolescents 9% to 26%; adults 1% to 12%; dose dependent)

Neuromuscular & skeletal: Tremor (2% to 12%)

3% to 10%:

Cardiovascular: Orthostatic hypotension (1% to 4%; dose dependent), bundle branch block (≤3%)

Central nervous system: Agitation (4% to 10%), akathisia (adolescents 4% to 17%; adults 1% to 10%; dose dependent), anxiety (adolescents ≤9%; adults 3% to 8%), dizziness (1% to 6%), dystonia (1% to 5%; dose dependent), dysarthria (1% to 4%; dose dependent), fatigue (adolescents ≤4%), sleep disorder (≤3%), lethargy (adolescents ≤3%)

Endocrine & metabolic: Amenorrhea (adolescents ≤6%), galactorrhea (adolescents ≤4%), gynecomastia (adolescents ≤3%)

Gastrointestinal: Weight gain (1% to 9%; dose dependent), nausea (2% to 8%), dyspepsia (5% to 6%), vomiting (adolescents ≤11%; adults 2% to 5%), constipation (1% to 5%), salivation increased (adolescents ≤6%; adults ≤4%; dose dependent), appetite increased (2% to 3%), toothache (1% to 3%), abdominal pain (≤3%), diarrhea (≤3%), xerostomia (≤3%); tongue swelling (adolescents ≤3%), tongue paralysis (adolescents ≤3%)

Local: I.M. formulation: Injection site reaction (≤10%)

Neuromuscular & skeletal: Hyperkinesia (2% to 10% dose dependent), dyskinesia (1% to 9%), weakness (≤4%), myalgia (≤4% dose dependent), back pain (1% to 3%), extremity pain (≤3%)

Ocular: Blurred vision (adolescents ≤3%)

Respiratory: Nasopharyngitis (≤5%; dose dependent), upper respiratory tract infection (1% to 4%), cough (≤3%; dose dependent), rhinitis (1% to 3%; dose dependent)

General Dosage Range Dosage adjustment recommended in patients with renal impairment

I.M.: *Adults:* Initial: 234 mg, then 156 mg 1 week later; Maintenance: 39-234 mg/month

Oral: *Adolescents 12-17 years and Adults:* 3-12 mg once daily (maximum: 12 mg/day)

Mechanism of Action Paliperidone is considered a benzisoxazole atypical antipsychotic as it is the primary active metabolite of risperidone. As with other atypical antipsychotics, its therapeutic efficacy is believed to result from mixed central serotonergic and dopaminergic antagonism. The addition of serotonin antagonism to dopamine antagonism (classic neuroleptic mechanism) is thought to improve negative symptoms of psychoses and reduce the incidence of extrapyramidal side effects. Similar to risperidone, paliperidone demonstrates high affinity to α_1, D_2, H_1, and 5-HT_{2C} receptors, and low affinity for muscarinic and 5-HT_{1A} receptors. In contrast to risperidone, paliperidone displays nearly 10-fold lower affinity for α_2 and 5-HT_{2A} receptors, and nearly three- to fivefold less affinity for 5-HT_{1A} and 5-HT_{1D}, respectively.

Pharmacodynamics/Kinetics

Half-life Elimination

Oral: 23 hours; 24-51 hours with renal impairment (Cl_{cr} <80 mL/minute)

I.M. (following a single-dose administration): Range: 25-49 days

Time to Peak Oral: ~24 hours; I.M.: 13 days

Pregnancy Risk Factor C

Palivizumab (pah li VIZ u mab)

U.S. Brand Names Synagis®

Canadian Brand Names Synagis®

Pharmacologic Category Monoclonal Antibody

Use Prevention of serious lower respiratory tract disease caused by respiratory syncytial virus (RSV) in infants and children at high risk of RSV disease

The American Academy of Pediatrics recommends RSV prophylaxis with palivizumab during RSV season for:

- Infants <3 months of age who were born between 32 and 34 6/7 weeks gestational age and have one of the following:
  - Day care attendance
  - One or more siblings <5 years of age living in the same household
- Infants <6 months of age who were born between 29 and 31 6/7 weeks gestational age
- Infants <12 months of age who were born <28 weeks gestational age
- Infants <12 months of age with congenital airway abnormality or neuromuscular disorder that decreases the ability to manage airway secretions
- Infants and children <24 months of age with chronic lung disease (CLD) necessitating medical therapy within 6 month prior to the beginning of RSV season
- Infants and children ≤24 months of age with congenital heart disease and one of the following:
  - Receiving medication to treat congestive heart failure
  - Moderate-to-severe pulmonary hypertension
  - Cyanotic heart disease

Local Anesthetic/Vasoconstrictor Precautions No information available to require special precautions

Effects on Dental Treatment No significant effects or complications reported

Effects on Bleeding No information available to require special precautions

Adverse Effects The incidence of adverse events was similar between the palivizumab and placebo groups. >1%:

Cardiovascular: Arrhythmia, cyanosis

Central nervous system: Fever, nervousness

Dermatologic: Rash

Gastrointestinal: Diarrhea, gastroenteritis, vomiting

Hepatic: AST increased

Otic: Otitis media

Respiratory: Cough, rhinitis, upper respiratory infection, wheezing

General Dosage Range I.M.: *Children <2 years:* 15 mg/kg monthly

Mechanism of Action Exhibits neutralizing and fusion-inhibitory activity against RSV; these activities inhibit RSV replication in laboratory and clinical studies

Pharmacodynamics/Kinetics

Half-life Elimination Children <24 months: 20 days

Pregnancy Risk Factor C

Palonosetron (pal oh NOE se tron)

U.S. Brand Names Aloxi®

Pharmacologic Category Antiemetic; Selective 5-HT_3 Receptor Antagonist

Use Prevention of chemotherapy-associated nausea and vomiting; indicated for prevention of acute (highly-emetogenic therapy) as well as acute and delayed (moderately-emetogenic therapy) nausea and vomiting; prevention of postoperative nausea and vomiting (PONV)

Local Anesthetic/Vasoconstrictor Precautions No information available to require special precautions

Effects on Dental Treatment No significant effects or complications reported

Effects on Bleeding No information available to require special precautions

Adverse Effects Adverse events may vary according to indication.

1% to 10%:

Cardiovascular: QT prolongation (chemotherapy-associated <1%; PONV 1% to 5%), bradycardia (chemotherapy-associated 1%; PONV 4%), hypotension (≤1%), sinus bradycardia (≤1%), tachycardia (nonsustained) (≤1%)

Central nervous system: Headache (chemotherapy-associated 5% to 9%; PONV 3%), anxiety (1%), dizziness (≤1%)

Dermatologic: Pruritus (≤1%)

Endocrine & metabolic: Hyperkalemia (1%)

Gastrointestinal: Constipation (2% to 5%), diarrhea (≤1%), flatulence (≤1%)

Genitourinary: Urinary retention (≤1%)

Hepatic: ALT increased (≤1%; transient), AST increased (≤1%; transient)

Neuromuscular & skeletal: Weakness (1%)

General Dosage Range I.V.: *Adults:* 0.25 mg **or** 0.075 mg as a single dose

Mechanism of Action Selective 5-HT_3 receptor antagonist, blocking serotonin, both on vagal nerve terminals in the periphery and centrally in the chemoreceptor trigger zone

Pharmacodynamics/Kinetics

Half-life Elimination I.V.: Terminal: ~40 hours

Pregnancy Risk Factor B

Pamidronate (pa mi DROE nate)

Related Information

Osteonecrosis of the Jaw *on page 1894*

U.S. Brand Names Aredia®

Canadian Brand Names Aredia®; Pamidronate Disodium Omega; Pamidronate Disodium®; PMS-Pamidronate; Rhoxal-pamidronate

Pharmacologic Category Antidote; Bisphosphonate Derivative

Use Treatment of moderate or severe hypercalcemia associated with malignancy; treatment of osteolytic bone lesions associated with multiple myeloma or metastatic breast cancer; moderate-to-severe Paget's disease of bone

Unlabeled/Investigational Use Treatment of pediatric osteoporosis, treatment of osteogenesis imperfecta; treatment of symptomatic bone metastases of thyroid cancer; prevention of bone loss associated with androgen deprivation treatment in prostate cancer

Local Anesthetic/Vasoconstrictor Precautions No information available to require special precautions

Effects on Dental Treatment Osteonecrosis of the jaw (ONJ), generally associated with local infection and/or tooth extraction and often with delayed healing, has been reported in patients taking bisphosphonates. Symptoms included nonhealing extraction socket or an exposed jawbone. Most reported cases of bisphosphonate-associated osteonecrosis have been in cancer patients treated with intravenous bisphosphonates. However, some have occurred in patients with postmenopausal osteoporosis taking oral bisphosphonates. Dental surgery, particularly tooth extraction, may increase the risk for ONJ. Patients who develop ONJ while on bisphosphonate therapy should receive care by an oral surgeon. See Dental Comment.

Effects on Bleeding No information available to require special precautions

Adverse Effects Note: Actual percentages may vary by indication; treatment for multiple myeloma is associated with higher percentage.

>10%:

Central nervous system: Fatigue (≤37%), fever (18% to 39%), headache (≤26%), insomnia (≤22%)

Endocrine & metabolic: Hypophosphatemia (≤18%), hypokalemia (4% to 18%), hypomagnesemia (4% to 12%), hypocalcemia (≤12%)

Gastrointestinal: Nausea (≤54%), vomiting (≤36%), anorexia (≤26%), abdominal pain (≤23%), dyspepsia (≤23%)

Genitourinary: Urinary tract infection (≤19%)

Hematologic: Anemia (≤43%), granulocytopenia (≤20%)

Local: Infusion site reaction (≤18%; includes induration, pain, redness and swelling)

Neuromuscular & skeletal: Weakness (≤22%), myalgia (≤26%), arthralgia (≤14%), osteonecrosis of the jaw (cancer patients: 1% to 11%)
Renal: Serum creatinine increased (≤19%)
Respiratory: Dyspnea (≤30%), cough (≤26%), upper respiratory tract infection (≤24%), sinusitis (≤16%), pleural effusion (≤11%)

1% to 10%:
Cardiovascular: Atrial fibrillation (≤6%), hypertension (≤6%), syncope (≤6%), tachycardia (≤6%), atrial flutter (≤1%), cardiac failure (≤1%), edema (≤1%)
Central nervous system: Somnolence (≤6%), psychosis (≤4%)
Endocrine & metabolic: Hypothyroidism (≤6%)
Gastrointestinal: Constipation (≤6%), gastrointestinal hemorrhage (≤6%), diarrhea (≤1%), stomatitis (≤1%)
Hematologic: Leukopenia (≤4%), neutropenia (≤1%), thrombocytopenia (≤1%)
Neuromuscular & skeletal: Back pain (≤5%), bone pain (≤5%)
Renal: Uremia (≤4%)
Respiratory: Rales (≤6%), rhinitis (≤6%)
Miscellaneous: Moniliasis (≤6%)

General Dosage Range Dosage adjustment recommended in patients with renal impairment

I.V.: *Adults:* 60-90 mg as a single dose, may repeat every 3-4 weeks **or** 30 mg daily for 3 consecutive days

Mechanism of Action A bisphosphonate which inhibits bone resorption via actions on osteoclasts or on osteoclast precursors. Does not appear to produce any significant effects on renal tubular calcium handling and is poorly absorbed following oral administration (high oral doses have been reported effective); therefore, I.V. therapy is preferred.

Pharmacodynamics/Kinetics

Onset of Action 24-48 hours; Peak effect: Maximum: 5-7 days

Half-life Elimination 21-35 hours

Pregnancy Risk Factor D

Dental Comment The American Association of Oral and Maxillofacial Surgeons position paper on bisphosphonate-related osteonecrosis of the jaws, 2009 update, stated that I.V. bisphosphonate exposure in the setting of managing malignancy remains the major risk factor for the development of ONJ. After reviewing case series, case-controlled studies, and cohort studies, the estimates of the cumulative incidence of I.V. bisphosphonate-associated ONJ ranges from 0.8% to 12%.

Two reports have attempted to assess more accurately the percent of cancer patients developing ONJ after bisphosphonate treatment. Maerevoet et al, reported that among 194 patients treated with Zometa® every 3-4 weeks, nine developed ONJ. Before receiving Zometa®, six had received Aredia® 90 mg every 3-4 weeks. The median duration of treatment with Aredia® was 39 months and for Zometa® 18 months. The incidence of ONJ in these patients was calculated to be 4.6%. Durie et al, described the results of a survey by the International Myeloma Foundation in 2004 to assess the risk factors of ONJ. Out of 1203 respondents, 904 had myeloma and 299 had breast cancer. Of the myeloma patients, 62 developed ONJ and 54 had suspicious findings. Of the breast cancer patients, 13 had ONJ and 23 had suspicious findings. The total number of cases of either ONJ or suspicious findings was 152. ONJ developed in 10% of 211 patients receiving Zometa® compared to 4% of 413 receiving Aredia®. The mean time to onset of ONJ among patients taking Zometa® was 18 months; the mean time to onset after Aredia® was 6 years. It should be noted that an early report by authors from Novartis Pharmaceuticals Corporation stressed that Aredia® and Zometa® had been used in 2.5 million patients world wide and reports of ONJ during their extensive use had been rare (Tarassoff, 2003). In addition, these authors stated that review of the reported cases revealed multiple risk factors for avascular necrosis. McMahon et al, followed up with a report that, along with other factors, bisphosphonates are additional stressors of bone health that can tip the balance to osteonecrosis. They suggested that the prevention of ONJ should be stressed such as the elimination of chronic dental infections prior to chemotherapy and bisphosphonate use in cancer patients.

Pancrelipase (pan kre LYE pase)

U.S. Brand Names Creon®; Pancreaze™; Pancrelipase™; Zenpep™

Canadian Brand Names Cotazym®; Creon®; Pancrease® MT; Ultrase®; Ultrase® MT; Viokase®

Pharmacologic Category Enzyme

Use Treatment of exocrine pancreatic insufficiency (EPI) due to conditions such as cystic fibrosis (Creon®, Pancreaze™, Zenpep™); chronic pancreatitis (Creon®); or pancreatectomy (Creon®)

Local Anesthetic/Vasoconstrictor Precautions No information available to require special precautions

Effects on Dental Treatment No significant effects or complications reported

Effects on Bleeding No information available to require special precautions

Adverse Effects The following adverse reactions were reported in a short-term safety studies; actual frequency varies with different products; adverse events, particularly gastrointestinal events, were often greater with placebo:

10%:

Central nervous system: Headache (6% to 15%)

Gastrointestinal: Abdominal pain (4% to 18%)

1% to 10%:

Central nervous system: Dizziness (6%)

Endocrine & metabolic: Diabetes mellitus exacerbation (4%), hyperglycemia (4%), hypoglycemia (4%)

Gastrointestinal: Flatulence (4% to 9%), early satiety (6%), weight loss (3% to 6%), upper abdominal pain (≤5%), diarrhea (≤4%), feces abnormal (≤4%)

Respiratory: Cough (6%), nasopharyngitis (4%)

General Dosage Range Oral:

Children ≤1 year: Lipase 2000-4000 units per 120 mL of formula or breast milk

Children >1 and <4 years: Lipase 1000-2500 units/kg/meal; Maximum dose: Lipase 10,000 units/kg/day **or** lipase 4000 units/g of fat per day

Children ≥4 years and Adults: Lipase 500-2500 units/kg/meal **or** lipase 72,000 units/meal (while consuming ≥100 g of fat per day); Maximum dose: Lipase 10,000 units/kg/day **or** lipase 4000 units/g of fat per day

Mechanism of Action Pancrelipase is a natural product harvested from the porcine pancreatic glands. It contains a combination of lipase, amylase, and protease. Products are formulated to dissolve in the more basic pH of the duodenum so that they may act locally to break down fats, protein, and starch.

Pregnancy Risk Factor C

Panitumumab (pan i TOOM yoo mab)

U.S. Brand Names Vectibix®

Canadian Brand Names Vectibix®

Pharmacologic Category Antineoplastic Agent, Monoclonal Antibody; Epidermal Growth Factor Receptor (EGFR) Inhibitor

Use Monotherapy in treatment of refractory metastatic colorectal cancer

Note: Subset analyses (retrospective) in metastatic colorectal cancer trials have not shown a benefit with EGFR inhibitor treatment in patients whose tumors have codon 12 or 13 *KRAS* mutations; use is not recommended in these patients.

Local Anesthetic/Vasoconstrictor Precautions No information available to require special precautions

Effects on Dental Treatment Key adverse event(s) related to dental treatment: Stomatitis and mucositis.

Effects on Bleeding Although significant myelosuppression with associated altered hemostasis has been reported for many chemotherapeutic agents, myelosuppression is not common with panitumumab and no specific precautions appear to necessary.

Adverse Effects

>10%:

Cardiovascular: Peripheral edema (12%)

Central nervous system: Fatigue (26%)

Dermatologic: Skin toxicity (90%; grades 3/4: 14% to 16%), erythema (65%; grades 3/4: 5%), acneiform rash (57%; grades 3/4: 7%), pruritus (57%; grades 3/4: 2%), exfoliation (25%; grades 3/4: 2%), paronychia (25%), rash (22%; grades 3/4: 1%), fissures (20%; grades 3/4: 1%), acne (13%; grades 3/4: 1%)

Endocrine & metabolic: Hypomagnesemia (38%; grades 3/4: 4%)

Gastrointestinal: Abdominal pain (25%), nausea (23%), diarrhea (21%; grades 3/4: 2%), constipation (21%), vomiting (19%)

Respiratory: Cough (14%)

1% to 10%:

Dermatologic: Dry skin (10%), nail disorder (other than paronychia: 9%)

Gastrointestinal: Stomatitis (7%), mucositis (6%)

Ocular: Eyelash growth (6%), conjunctivitis (4%), ocular hyperemia (3%), lacrimation increased (2%), eye/eye lid irritation (1%)

Miscellaneous: Antibody formation (≤5%), infusion reactions (3%; grades 3/4: 1%)

General Dosage Range Dosage adjustment recommended in patients who develop toxicities

I.V.: *Adults:* 6 mg/kg every 2 weeks

Mechanism of Action Recombinant human IgG2 monoclonal antibody which binds specifically to the epidermal growth factor receptor (EGFR, HER1, c-ErbB-1) and competitively inhibits the binding of epidermal growth factor (EGF) and other ligands. Binding to the EGFR blocks phosphorylation and activation of intracellular tyrosine kinases, resulting in inhibition of cell survival, growth, proliferation and transformation. EGFR signal transduction results in *KRAS* wild-type activation; cells with *KRAS* mutations appear to be unaffected by EGFR inhibition.

Pharmacodynamics/Kinetics

Half-life Elimination ~7.5 days (range: 4-11 days)

Pregnancy Risk Factor C

Pantoprazole (pan TOE pra zole)

Related Information

Gastrointestinal Disorders *on page 1874*

U.S. Brand Names Protonix®

Canadian Brand Names Apo-Pantoprazole®; CO Pantoprazole; Mylan-Pantoprazole; Novo-Pantoprazole; Pantoloc®; Panto™ I.V.; PHL-Pantoprazole; PMS-Pantoprazole; Protonix®; RAN™-Pantoprazole; ratio-Pantoprazole; Riva-Pantoprazole; Sandoz-Pantoprazole; Tecta™; ZYM-Pantoprazole

Generic Availability (U.S.) Yes: Delayed release tablet

Pharmacologic Category Proton Pump Inhibitor; Substituted Benzimidazole

Use

Oral: Treatment and maintenance of healing of erosive esophagitis associated with GERD; reduction in relapse rates of daytime and nighttime heartburn symptoms in GERD; hypersecretory disorders associated with Zollinger-Ellison syndrome or other GI hypersecretory disorders

I.V.: Short-term treatment (7-10 days) of patients with gastroesophageal reflux disease (GERD) and a history of erosive esophagitis; hypersecretory disorders associated with Zollinger-Ellison syndrome or other neoplastic disorders

Unlabeled/Investigational Use Peptic ulcer disease, active ulcer bleeding (parenteral formulation); adjunct treatment with antibiotics for *Helicobacter pylori* eradication; stress-ulcer prophylaxis in the critically-ill

Local Anesthetic/Vasoconstrictor Precautions No information available to require special precautions

Effects on Dental Treatment No significant effects or complications reported

Effects on Bleeding No information available to require special precautions

Adverse Effects ≥1%:

Cardiovascular: Chest pain

Central nervous system: Headache (2% to 9%), insomnia (≤1%), anxiety, dizziness, migraine, pain

Dermatologic: Rash (≤2%)

Endocrine & metabolic: Hyperglycemia (≤1%), hyperlipidemia

Gastrointestinal: Diarrhea (2% to 6%), flatulence (2% to 4%), abdominal pain (1% to 4%), nausea (≤2%), vomiting (≤2%), eructation (≤1%), constipation, dyspepsia, gastroenteritis, rectal disorder

Genitourinary: Urinary frequency, UTI

Hepatic: Liver function tests abnormal (≤2%)

Local: Injection site reaction (includes thrombophlebitis and abscess)

Neuromuscular & skeletal: Arthralgia, back pain, hypertonia, neck pain, weakness

Respiratory: Bronchitis, cough, dyspnea, pharyngitis, rhinitis, sinusitis, upper respiratory tract infection

Miscellaneous: Flu syndrome, infection

Dosage

Oral:

Children ≥5 years (unlabeled use): GERD, erosive esophagitis associated with GERD: 20-40 mg once daily

Adults:

Erosive esophagitis associated with GERD:

Treatment: 40 mg once daily for up to 8 weeks; an additional 8 weeks may be used in patients who have not healed after an 8-week course

Maintenance of healing: 40 mg once daily

Note: Lower doses (20 mg once daily) have been used successfully in mild GERD treatment and maintenance of healing

Hypersecretory disorders (including Zollinger-Ellison): Initial: 40 mg twice daily; adjust dose based on patient needs; doses up to 240 mg/day have been administered

Helicobacter pylori eradication (unlabeled use): American College of Gastroenterology guidelines (Chey, 2007):

Nonpenicillin allergy: 40 mg twice daily administered with amoxicillin 1000 mg *and* clarithromycin 500 mg twice daily for 10-14 days

Penicillin allergy: 40 mg twice daily administered with clarithromycin 500 mg *and* metronidazole 500 mg twice daily for 10-14 days **or** 40 mg once or twice daily administered with bismuth subsalicylate 525 mg *and* metronidazole 250 mg *plus* tetracycline 500 mg 4 times/day for 10-14 days

I.V.:

Erosive esophagitis associated with GERD: 40 mg once daily for 7-10 days

Hypersecretory disorders: 80 mg twice daily; adjust dose based on acid output measurements; 160-240 mg/day in divided doses has been used for a limited period (up to 7 days)

Prevention of rebleeding in peptic ulcer bleed (unlabeled use): 80 mg, followed by 8 mg/hour infusion for 72 hours. **Note:** A daily infusion of 40 mg does not raise gastric pH sufficiently to enhance coagulation in active GI bleeds.

Elderly: Dosage adjustment not required

Dosage adjustment in renal impairment: Not required; pantoprazole is not removed by hemodialysis

Dosage adjustment in hepatic impairment: Not required

Mechanism of Action Suppresses gastric acid secretion by inhibiting the parietal cell H^+/K^+ ATP pump

Contraindications Hypersensitivity to pantoprazole, substituted benzamidazoles (eg, esomeprazole, lansoprazole, omeprazole, rabeprazole), or any component of the formulation

Canadian labeling: Additional contraindication (not in U.S. labeling): Concomitant use with atazanavir

Warnings/Precautions Use of proton pump inhibitors may increase the risk of gastrointestinal infections (eg, *Salmonella, Campylobacter*). Relief of symptoms does not preclude the presence of a gastric malignancy. Long-term pantoprazole therapy (especially in patients who were *H. pylori* positive) has caused biopsy-proven atrophic gastritis. No reports of enterochromaffin-like (ECL) cell carcinoids, dysplasia, or neoplasia such as those seen in rodent studies have occurred in humans. Not indicated for maintenance therapy; safety and efficacy for use beyond 16 weeks have not been established. Prolonged treatment (typically >3 years) may lead to vitamin B_{12} malabsorption and subsequent deficiency. Intravenous preparation contains edetate sodium (EDTA); use caution in patients who are at risk for zinc deficiency if other EDTA-containing solutions are coadministered. Decreased *H. pylori* eradication rates have been observed with short-term (≤7 days) combination therapy. The American College of Gastroenterology recommends 10-14 days of therapy (triple or quadruple) for eradication of *H. pylori* (Chey, 2007). Proton pump inhibitors may diminish the therapeutic effect of clopidogrel, thought to be due to reduced formation of the active metabolite of clopidogrel; an increase in the risk of cardiovascular events may occur. Of the PPIs, pantoprazole has the lowest degree of CYP2C19 inhibition and is preferred if concomitant use of a PPI is necessary.

Increased incidence of osteoporosis-related bone fractures of the hip, spine, or wrist may occur with proton pump inhibitor therapy. Patients on high-dose or long-term therapy should be monitored. Use the lowest effective dose for the shortest duration of time, use vitamin D and calcium supplementation, and follow appropriate guidelines to reduce risk of fractures in patients at risk.

Drug Interactions

Metabolism/Transport Effects Substrate of CYP2C9 (minor), 2C19 (major), 2D6 (minor), 3A4 (minor); **Inhibits** CYP2C9 (weak), 2C19 (moderate), ABCG2; **Induces** CYP1A2 (weak), 3A4 (weak)

Avoid Concomitant Use

Avoid concomitant use of Pantoprazole with any of the following: Delavirdine; Erlotinib; Nelfinavir; Posaconazole

Increased Effect/Toxicity

Pantoprazole may increase the levels/effects of: Amphetamines; CYP2C19 Substrates; Dexmethylphenidate; Methotrexate; Methylphenidate; Raltegravir; Saquinavir; Topotecan; Voriconazole

The levels/effects of Pantoprazole may be increased by: Conivaptan; Fluconazole; Ketoconazole; Ketoconazole (Systemic)

Decreased Effect

Pantoprazole may decrease the levels/effects of: Atazanavir; Bisphosphonate Derivatives; Cefditoren; Clopidogrel; Dabigatran Etexilate; Dasatinib; Delavirdine; Erlotinib; Gefitinib; Indinavir; Iron Salts; Itraconazole; Ketoconazole; Ketoconazole (Systemic); Mesalamine; Mycophenolate; Nelfinavir; Posaconazole

The levels/effects of Pantoprazole may be decreased by: CYP2C19 Inducers (Strong); Peginterferon Alfa-2b; Tipranavir; Tocilizumab

Ethanol/Nutrition/Herb Interactions

Ethanol: Avoid ethanol (may cause gastric mucosal irritation).

Herb/Nutraceutical: Prolonged treatment (typically >3 years) may lead to vitamin B_{12} malabsorption and subsequent deficiency.

Dietary Considerations

Oral: May be taken with or without food; best if taken before breakfast.

I.V.: Due to EDTA in preparation, zinc supplementation may be needed in patients prone to zinc deficiency.

Pharmacodynamics/Kinetics

Half-life Elimination 1 hour; increased to 3.5-10 hours with CYP2C19 deficiency

Time to Peak Oral: 2.5 hours

Pregnancy Risk Factor B

Lactation Enters breast milk/not recommended

Breast-Feeding Considerations Not recommended due to carcinogenicity in animal studies.

Dosage Forms

Granules for suspension, delayed release, enteric coated, oral:

Protonix®: 40 mg/packet (30s)

Injection, powder for reconstitution:

Protonix®: 40 mg

Tablet, delayed release, oral: 20 mg, 40 mg

Protonix®: 20 mg, 40 mg

Dosage Forms: Canada

Tablet, enteric coated:

Pantoloc®: 40 mg

Pantothenic Acid (pan toe THEN ik AS id)

U.S. Brand Names Panto-250 [OTC]

Pharmacologic Category Vitamin, Water Soluble

Use Pantothenic acid deficiency

Local Anesthetic/Vasoconstrictor Precautions No information available to require special precautions

Effects on Dental Treatment No significant effects or complications reported

Effects on Bleeding No information available to require special precautions

General Dosage Range Oral: *Adults:* 4-7 mg/day

Pregnancy Risk Factor A/C (dose exceeding RDA recommendation)

Papaverine (pa PAV er een)

Pharmacologic Category Vasodilator

Use Oral: Relief of peripheral and cerebral ischemia associated with arterial spasm and myocardial ischemia complicated by arrhythmias

Unlabeled/Investigational Use Investigational: Parenteral: Various vascular spasms associated with muscle spasms as in myocardial infarction, angina, peripheral and pulmonary embolism, peripheral vascular disease, angiospastic states, and visceral spasm (ureteral, biliary, and GI colic); testing for impotence

Local Anesthetic/Vasoconstrictor Precautions No information available to require special precautions

Effects on Dental Treatment No significant effects or complications reported

Effects on Bleeding No information available to require special precautions

Adverse Effects Frequency not defined.

Cardiovascular: Arrhythmias (with rapid I.V. use), flushing of the face, mild hypertension, tachycardia

Central nervous system: Drowsiness, headache, lethargy, sedation, vertigo

Gastrointestinal: Abdominal distress, anorexia, constipation, diarrhea, nausea

Hepatic: Chronic hepatitis, hepatic hypersensitivity

Respiratory: Apnea (with rapid I.V. use)

General Dosage Range

I.M., I.V.:

Children: 6 mg/kg/day in 4 divided doses

Adults: 30-65 mg, may repeat every 3 hours

Oral: *Adults:* 150-300 mg every 12 hours **or** 150 mg every 8 hours

Mechanism of Action Smooth muscle spasmolytic producing a generalized smooth muscle relaxation including: vasodilatation, gastrointestinal sphincter relaxation, bronchiolar muscle relaxation, and potentially a depressed myocardium (with large doses); muscle relaxation may occur due to inhibition or cyclic nucleotide phosphodiesterase, increasing cyclic AMP; muscle relaxation is unrelated to nerve innervation; papaverine increases cerebral blood flow in normal subjects; oxygen uptake is unaltered

Pharmacodynamics/Kinetics

Onset of Action Oral: Rapid

Half-life Elimination 0.5-1.5 hours

Pregnancy Risk Factor C

Papillomavirus (Types 6, 11, 16, 18) Vaccine (Human, Recombinant)

(pap ih LO ma VYE rus typs six e LEV en SIX teen AYE teen vak SEEN YU man ree KOM be nant)

U.S. Brand Names Gardasil®

Canadian Brand Names Gardasil®

Pharmacologic Category Vaccine, Inactivated (Viral)

Use

Females ≥9 years and ≤26 years of age: Prevention of cervical, vulvar, vaginal, and anal cancer caused by HPV types 16 and 18; genital warts caused by HPV types 6 and 11; cervical adenocarcinoma *in situ*, and vulvar, vaginal, cervical, or anal intraepithelial neoplasia caused by HPV types 6, 11, 16, 18

Males ≥9 years and ≤26 years of age: Prevention of genital warts caused by human papillomavirus (HPV) types 6 and 11; anal cancer caused by HPV types 16 and 18, and anal intraepithelial neoplasia caused by HPV types 6, 11, 16, and 18

Note: Canadian labeling: Approved for use in males ≥9 years of age and ≤17 years

The Advisory Committee on Immunization Practices (ACIP) recommends routine vaccination for females 11-12 years of age; catch-up vaccination is recommended for females 13-26 years of age; ACIP does not recommend routine use among males; however, eligible males 9-26 years of age may be vaccinated.

Unlabeled/Investigational Use Prevention of cervical, vulvar, and vaginal cancer caused by HPV types 16 and 18, genital warts caused by HPV types 6 and 11, cervical adenocarcinoma *in situ*, and vulvar, vaginal, or cervical intraepithelial neoplasia caused by HPV types 6, 11, 16, 18 in women 26-45 years of age

Local Anesthetic/Vasoconstrictor Precautions No information available to require special precautions

Effects on Dental Treatment No significant effects or complications reported

Effects on Bleeding No information available to require special precautions

Adverse Effects All serious adverse reactions must be reported to the U.S. Department of Health and Human Services (DHHS) Vaccine Adverse Event Reporting System (VAERS) 1-800-822-7967 or online at https://vaers.hhs.gov/esub/index. In Canada, adverse reactions may be reported to local provincial/territorial health agencies or to the Vaccine Safety Section at Public Health Agency of Canada (1-866-844-0018).

>10%:

Central nervous system: Headache (12% to 28%), fever (8% to 13%)

Local: Injection site: Pain (61% to 84%), erythema (17% to 25%), swelling (14% to 25%)

1% to 10%:

Central nervous system: Dizziness (1% to 4%), malaise (1%), insomnia (1%)

Gastrointestinal: Nausea (2% to 7%), diarrhea (3% to 4%), vomiting (1% to 2%), toothache (2%)

Local: Injection site: Bruising (3%), pruritus (3%), hematoma (1%)

Neuromuscular & skeletal: Arthralgia (1%), myalgia (≤1%)

Respiratory: Pharyngolaryngeal pain (3%), cough (2%), nasal congestion (1%)

General Dosage Range I.M.: *Children ≥9 years and Adults ≤26 years:* 0.5 mL initial dose, followed by 0.5 mL 2 and 6 months later

Mechanism of Action Contains inactive human papillomavirus (HPV) proteins HPV 6 L1, HPV 11 L1, HPV 16 L1, and HPV 18 L1 which produce neutralizing antibodies to prevent cervical cancer, cervical adenocarcinoma, cervical, vaginal and vulvar neoplasia, and genital warts caused by HPV.

Pharmacodynamics/Kinetics

Onset of Action Peak seroconversion was observed 1 month following the last dose of vaccine

Duration of Action Not well defined; at least 5 years

Pregnancy Risk Factor B

Papillomavirus (Types 16, 18) Vaccine (Human, Recombinant)

(pap ih LO ma VYE rus typs SIX teen AYE teen vak SEEN YU man ree KOM be nant)

U.S. Brand Names Cervarix®

Canadian Brand Names Cervarix®

Pharmacologic Category Vaccine, Inactivated (Viral)

Use Females 10 through 25 years of age: Prevention of cervical cancer, cervical adenocarcinoma *in situ*, and cervical intraepithelial neoplasia caused by human papillomavirus (HPV) types 16, 18

The Advisory Committee on Immunization Practices (ACIP) recommends routine vaccination for females 11-12 years of age; catch-up vaccination is recommended for females 13-25 years of age.

Local Anesthetic/Vasoconstrictor Precautions No information available to require special precautions

Effects on Dental Treatment No significant effects or complications reported

Effects on Bleeding No information available to require special precautions

Adverse Effects All serious adverse reactions must be reported to the U.S. Department of Health and Human Services (DHHS) Vaccine Adverse Event Reporting System (VAERS) 1-800-822-7967 or online at https://vaers.hhs.gov/esub/index. In Canada, adverse reactions may be reported to local provincial/territorial health agencies or to the Vaccine Safety Section at Public Health Agency of Canada (1-866-844-0018).

>10%:

Central nervous system: Fatigue (55%)

Local: Injection site reactions: Pain (92%), redness (48%), swelling (44%)

Neuromuscular & skeletal: Myalgia (49%), arthralgia (21%)

Headache (5% to 53%); gastrointestinal symptoms (abdominal pain, diarrhea, nausea, vomiting) (28%); fever (13%); rash (10%)

1% to 10%:

Dermatologic: Urticaria (7%)

Local: Injection site: Pruritus (1%)

Respiratory: Nasopharyngitis (4%), pharyngolaryngeal pain (3%), pharyngitis (2%), upper respiratory tract infection (2%)

Miscellaneous: Influenza (3%), chlamydia infection (2%), vaginal infection (1%)

Note: The following occurred more often with the placebo (percentages reported with Cervarix®): Headache (5% to 53%); gastrointestinal symptoms (abdominal pain, diarrhea, nausea, vomiting) (28%); fever (13%); rash (10%); dizziness (2%); injection site bruising (1%)

General Dosage Range I.M.: *Children ≥10 years and Adults ≤25 years (females):* 0.5 mL initial dose, followed by 0.5 mL 1 and 6 months later

Mechanism of Action Contains inactive human papillomavirus (HPV) proteins HPV 16 L1, and HPV 18 L1 which produce neutralizing antibodies to prevent cervical cancer, cervical adenocarcinoma, and cervical neoplasia cause by HPV.

Pharmacodynamics/Kinetics

Onset of Action Peak seroconversion was observed 1 month following the last dose of vaccine

Duration of Action Not well defined; >5 years

Pregnancy Risk Factor B

Paregoric

(par e GOR ik)

Pharmacologic Category Analgesic, Opioid

Use Treatment of diarrhea or relief of pain; neonatal opiate withdrawal

Local Anesthetic/Vasoconstrictor Precautions No information available to require special precautions

Effects on Dental Treatment No significant effects or complications reported

Effects on Bleeding No information available to require special precautions

Adverse Effects Frequency not defined.

Cardiovascular: Hypotension, peripheral vasodilation

Central nervous system: CNS depression, dizziness, drowsiness, headache, increased intracranial pressure, insomnia, malaise, mental depression, restlessness

Gastrointestinal: Anorexia, biliary tract spasm, constipation, nausea, stomach cramps, vomiting

Genitourinary: Decreased urination, ureteral spasms, urinary tract spasm

Hepatic: Increased liver function tests

Neuromuscular & skeletal: Weakness

Ocular: Miosis
Respiratory: Respiratory depression
Miscellaneous: Physical and psychological dependence, histamine release

General Dosage Range Oral:
Neonates: 3-6 drops every 3-6 hours as needed **or** 0.2-0.7 mL every 3 hours
Children: 0.25-0.5 mL/kg 1-4 times/day
Adults: 5-10 mL 1-4 times/day

Mechanism of Action Increases smooth muscle tone in GI tract, decreases motility and peristalsis, diminishes digestive secretions

Pregnancy Risk Factor B/D (prolonged use or high doses)

Controlled Substance C-III

Paricalcitol (pah ri KAL si tole)

U.S. Brand Names Zemplar®

Canadian Brand Names Zemplar®

Pharmacologic Category Vitamin D Analog

Use
I.V.: Prevention and treatment of secondary hyperparathyroidism associated with stage 5 chronic kidney disease (CKD)
Oral: Prevention and treatment of secondary hyperparathyroidism associated with stage 3 and 4 CKD and stage 5 CKD patients on hemodialysis or peritoneal dialysis

Local Anesthetic/Vasoconstrictor Precautions No information available to require special precautions

Effects on Dental Treatment Key adverse event(s) related to dental treatment: Xerostomia (normal salivary flow resumes upon discontinuation).

Effects on Bleeding No information available to require special precautions

Adverse Effects
>10%:
Gastrointestinal: Nausea (5% to 13%), diarrhea (7% to 12%)
Miscellaneous: Infection (bacterial, fungal, viral: 3% to 15%)

2% to 10%:
Cardiovascular: Edema (7%), hypertension (7%), hypervolemia (5%), hypotension (5%), palpitation (3%), chest pain (3%), peripheral edema (3%), syncope (3%)
Central nervous system: Pain (8%), dizziness (5% to 7%), chills (5%), insomnia (5%), lightheadedness (5%), vertigo (5%), fever (3% to 5%), headache (3% to 5%), anxiety (3%), depression (3%)
Dermatologic: Rash (6%), bruising (3%), skin ulcer (3%)
Endocrine & metabolic: Dehydration (3%), hypoglycemia (3%)
Gastrointestinal: Vomiting (5% to 8%), GI bleeding (5%), constipation (4% to 5%), abdominal pain (4%), dyspepsia (3%), xerostomia (3%)
Genitourinary: Urinary tract infection (3%)
Neuromuscular & skeletal: Arthritis (5%), weakness (3% to 5%), back pain (4%), leg cramps (3%)
Renal: Uremia (3%)
Respiratory: Pneumonia (5%), rhinitis (5%), oropharyngeal pain (4%), bronchitis (3%), cough (3%), sinusitis (3%)
Miscellaneous: Allergic reaction (6%), flu-like syndrome (5%), peritonitis (5%), sepsis (5%)

General Dosage Range Dosage adjustment recommended in patients with renal impairment
I.V.: *Children ≥5 years and Adults:* 0.04-0.24 mcg/kg (2.8-16.8 mcg) every other day during dialysis
Oral: *Adults:* 1-2 mcg/day **or** 2-4 mcg 3 times/week

Mechanism of Action Decreased renal conversion of vitamin D to its primary active metabolite (1,25-hydroxyvitamin D) in chronic renal failure leads to reduced activation of vitamin D receptor (VDR), which subsequently removes inhibitory suppression of parathyroid hormone (PTH) release; increased serum PTH (secondary hyperparathyroidism) reduces calcium excretion and enhances bone resorption. Paricalcitol is a synthetic vitamin D analog which binds to and activates the VDR in kidney, parathyroid gland, intestine and bone, thus reducing PTH levels and improving calcium and phosphate homeostasis.

Pharmacodynamics/Kinetics
Half-life Elimination
Healthy subjects: Oral: 4-6 hours; I.V.: 5-7 hours
Stage 3 and 4 CKD: Oral: 14-20 hours
Stage 5 CKD: Oral: 14-20 hours; I.V.: 14-15 hours

Time to Peak Plasma: 3 hours: Delayed by food

Pregnancy Risk Factor C

Paromomycin (par oh moe MYE sin)

Canadian Brand Names Humatin®

Pharmacologic Category Amebicide

Use Treatment of acute and chronic intestinal amebiasis; hepatic coma

Unlabeled/Investigational Use Treatment of cryptosporidiosis

Local Anesthetic/Vasoconstrictor Precautions No information available to require special precautions

Effects on Dental Treatment No significant effects or complications reported

Effects on Bleeding No information available to require special precautions

Adverse Effects 1% to 10%: Gastrointestinal: Diarrhea, abdominal cramps, nausea, vomiting, heartburn

General Dosage Range Oral: *Children and Adults:* Dosage varies greatly depending on indication

Mechanism of Action Acts directly on ameba; has antibacterial activity against normal and pathogenic organisms in the GI tract; interferes with bacterial protein synthesis by binding to 30S ribosomal subunits

PARoxetine (pa ROKS e teen)

Related Information

Management of the Patient With Anxiety or Depression *on page 1968*

U.S. Brand Names Paxil CR®; Paxil®; Pexeva®

Canadian Brand Names Apo-Paroxetine®; CO Paroxetine; Dom-Paroxetine; Mylan-Paroxetine; Novo-Paroxetine; Paxil CR®; Paxil®; PHL-Paroxetine; PMS-Paroxetine; ratio-Paroxetine; Riva-paroxetine; Sandoz-Paroxetine; Teva-Paroxetine

Generic Availability (U.S.) Yes: Excludes suspension, tablet (mesylate)

Pharmacologic Category Antidepressant, Selective Serotonin Reuptake Inhibitor

Use Treatment of major depressive disorder (MDD); treatment of panic disorder with or without agoraphobia; obsessive-compulsive disorder (OCD); social anxiety disorder (social phobia); generalized anxiety disorder (GAD); post-traumatic stress disorder (PTSD); premenstrual dysphoric disorder (PMDD)

Unlabeled/Investigational Use May be useful in eating disorders, impulse control disorders, self-injurious behavior; vasomotor symptoms of menopause; treatment of depression and obsessive-compulsive disorder (OCD) in children; treatment of mild dementia-associated agitation in nonpsychotic patients

Local Anesthetic/Vasoconstrictor Precautions Although caution should be used in patients taking tricyclic antidepressants, no interactions have been reported with vasoconstrictor and paroxetine, a nontricyclic antidepressant which acts to increase serotonin; no precautions appear to be needed

Effects on Dental Treatment Key adverse event(s) related to dental treatment: Xerostomia and changes in salivation (normal salivary flow resumes upon discontinuation), postural hypotension, and abnormal taste. Problems with SSRI-induced bruxism have been reported and may preclude their use; clinicians attempting to evaluate any patient with bruxism or involuntary muscle movement, who is simultaneously being treated with an SSRI drug, should be aware of the potential association. Prolonged use may decrease or inhibit salivary flow; normal salivation resumes upon discontinuation. See Effects on Bleeding.

Effects on Bleeding May impair platelet aggregation resulting in increased risk of bleeding events, particularly if used concomitantly with aspirin, NSAIDs, warfarin, or other anticoagulants. Bleeding related to SSRI use has been reported to range from relatively minor bruising and epistaxis to life-threatening hemorrhage. Routine interruption of therapy for most dental procedures is not warranted. In medically complicated patients or extensive oral surgery, the decision to interrupt therapy must be based on the risk to benefit in an individual patient and a medical consult is suggested. If therapy is continued without interruption, the clinician should anticipate the potential for a prolonged bleeding time.

Adverse Effects Frequency varies by dose and indication. Adverse reactions reported as a composite of all indications.

>10%:

- Central nervous system: Somnolence (15% to 24%), insomnia (11% to 24%), headache (17% to 18%), dizziness (6% to 14%)
- Endocrine & metabolic: Libido decreased (3% to 15%)
- Gastrointestinal: Nausea (19% to 26%), xerostomia (9% to 18%), constipation (5% to 16%), diarrhea (9% to 12%)
- Genitourinary: Ejaculatory disturbances (13% to 28%)
- Neuromuscular & skeletal: Weakness (12% to 22%), tremor (4% to 11%)
- Miscellaneous: Diaphoresis (5% to 14%)

1% to 10%:

Cardiovascular: Vasodilation (2% to 4%), chest pain (3%), palpitation (2% to 3%), hypertension (≥1%), tachycardia (≥1%)

Central nervous system: Nervousness (4% to 9%), anxiety (5%), agitation (3% to 5%), abnormal dreams (3% to 4%), concentration impaired (3% to 4%), yawning (2% to 4%), depersonalization (up to 3%), amnesia (2%), chills (2%), emotional lability (≥1%), vertigo (≥1%), confusion (1%)

Dermatologic: Rash (2% to 3%), pruritus (≥1%)

Endocrine & metabolic: Orgasmic disturbance (2% to 9%), dysmenorrhea (5%)

Gastrointestinal: Appetite decreased (5% to 9%), dyspepsia (2% to 5%), flatulence (4%), abdominal pain (4%), appetite increased (2% to 4%), vomiting (2% to 3%), taste perversion (2%), weight gain (≥1%)

Genitourinary: Genital disorder (male 10%; female 2% to 9%), impotence (2% to 9%), urinary frequency (2% to 3%), urinary tract infection (2%)

Neuromuscular & skeletal: Paresthesia (4%), myalgia (2% to 4%), back pain (3%), myoclonus (2% to 3%), myopathy (2%), myasthenia (1%), arthralgia (≥1%)

Ocular: Blurred vision (4%), abnormal vision (2% to 4%)

Otic: Tinnitus (≥1%)

Respiratory: Respiratory disorder (up to 7%), pharyngitis (4%), sinusitis (up to 4%), rhinitis (3%)

Miscellaneous: Infection (5% to 6%)

Dosage Oral:

Children:

Depression (unlabeled use; not recommended by FDA): Initial: 10 mg/day and adjusted upward on an individual basis to 20 mg/day

Obsessive-compulsive disorder (unlabeled use): Initial: 10 mg/day and titrate up as necessary to 60 mg/day

Self-injurious behavior (unlabeled use): 20 mg/day

Social anxiety disorder (unlabeled use): 2.5-15 mg/day

Adults:

Major depressive disorder:

Paxil®, Pexeva®: Initial: 20 mg once daily, preferably in the morning; increase if needed by 10 mg/day increments at intervals of at least 1 week; maximum dose: 50 mg/day

Paxil CR®: Initial: 25 mg once daily; increase if needed by 12.5 mg/day increments at intervals of at least 1 week; maximum dose: 62.5 mg/day

Generalized anxiety disorder (Paxil®, Pexeva®): Initial: 20 mg once daily, preferably in the morning (if dose is increased, adjust in increments of 10 mg/day at 1-week intervals); doses of 20-50 mg/day were used in clinical trials, however, no greater benefit was seen with doses >20 mg.

Obsessive-compulsive disorder (Paxil®, Pexeva™): Initial: 20 mg once daily, preferably in the morning; increase if needed by 10 mg/day increments at intervals of at least 1 week; recommended dose: 40 mg/day; range: 20-60 mg/day; maximum dose: 60 mg/day

Panic disorder:

Paxil®, Pexeva®: Initial: 10 mg once daily, preferably in the morning; increase if needed by 10 mg/day increments at intervals of at least 1 week; recommended dose: 40 mg/day; range: 10-60 mg/day; maximum dose: 60 mg/day

Paxil CR®: Initial: 12.5 mg once daily; increase if needed by 12.5 mg/day at intervals of at least 1 week; maximum dose: 75 mg/day

Premenstrual dysphoric disorder (Paxil CR®): Initial: 12.5 mg once daily in the morning; may be increased to 25 mg/day; dosing changes should occur at intervals of at least 1 week. May be given daily throughout the menstrual cycle or limited to the luteal phase.

Post-traumatic stress disorder (PTSD) (Paxil®): Initial: 20 mg once daily, preferably in the morning; increase if needed by 10 mg/day increments at intervals of at least 1 week; range: 20-50 mg. Limited data suggest doses of 40 mg/day were not more efficacious than 20 mg/day.

Social anxiety disorder:

Paxil®: Initial: 20 mg once daily, preferably in the morning; recommended dose: 20 mg/day; range: 20-60 mg/day; doses >20 mg may not have additional benefit

Paxil CR®: Initial: 12.5 mg once daily, preferably in the morning; may be increased by 12.5 mg/day at intervals of at least 1 week; maximum dose: 37.5 mg/day

Vasomotor symptoms of menopause (unlabeled use, Paxil CR®): 12.5-25 mg/day

Elderly:

Paxil®, Pexeva®: Initial: 10 mg/day; increase if needed by 10 mg/day increments at intervals of at least 1 week; maximum dose: 40 mg/day

Paxil CR®; Initial: 12.5 mg/day; increase if needed by 12.5 mg/day increments at intervals of at least 1 week; maximum dose: 50 mg/day

Note: Upon discontinuation of paroxetine therapy, gradually taper dose:

Paxil®, Pexeva®: 10 mg/day at weekly intervals; when 20 mg/day dose is reached, continue for 1 week before treatment is discontinued. Some patients may need to be titrated to 10 mg/day for 1 week before discontinuation.

Paxil CR®: Patients receiving 37.5 mg/day in clinical trials had their dose decreased by 12.5 mg/day to a dose of 25 mg/day and remained at a dose of 25 mg/day for 1 week before treatment was discontinued.

Dosage adjustment in renal impairment: Adults:

Cl_{cr} <30 mL/minute: Mean plasma concentration is ~4 times that seen in normal function.

Cl_{cr} 30-60 mL/minute: Plasma concentration is 2 times that seen in normal function.

Paxil®, Pexeva®: Initial: 10 mg/day; increase if needed by 10 mg/day increments at intervals of at least 1 week; maximum dose: 40 mg/day

Paxil CR®: Initial: 12.5 mg/day; increase if needed by 12.5 mg/day increments at intervals of at least 1 week; maximum dose: 50 mg/day

Dosage adjustment in severe hepatic impairment: Adults: In hepatic dysfunction, plasma concentration is 2 times that seen in normal function.

Paxil®, Pexeva®: Initial: 10 mg/day; increase if needed by 10 mg/day increments at intervals of at least 1 week; maximum dose: 40 mg/day

Paxil CR®: Initial: 12.5 mg/day; increase if needed by 12.5 mg/day increments at intervals of at least 1 week; maximum dose: 50 mg/day

Mechanism of Action Paroxetine is a selective serotonin reuptake inhibitor, chemically unrelated to tricyclic, tetracyclic, or other antidepressants; presumably, the inhibition of serotonin reuptake from brain synapse stimulated serotonin activity in the brain

Contraindications Hypersensitivity to paroxetine or any component of the formulation; use with or within 14 days of MAO inhibitors; concurrent use with thioridazine or pimozide

Warnings/Precautions Hazardous agent - use appropriate precautions for handling and disposal. **[U.S. Boxed Warning]: Antidepressants increase the risk of suicidal thinking and behavior in children, adolescents, and young adults (18-24 years of age) with major depressive disorder (MDD) and other psychiatric disorders;** consider risk prior to prescribing. Short-term studies did not show an increased risk in patients >24 years of age and showed a decreased risk in patients ≥65 years. Closely monitor patients for clinical worsening, suicidality, or unusual changes in behavior, particularly during the initial 1-2 months of therapy or during periods of dosage adjustments (increases or decreases); the patient's family or caregiver should be instructed to closely observe the patient and communicate condition with healthcare provider. A medication guide concerning the use of antidepressants should be dispensed with each prescription. **Paroxetine is not FDA approved for use in children.**

The possibility of a suicide attempt is inherent in major depression and may persist until remission occurs. Patients treated with antidepressants (for any indication) should be observed for clinical worsening and suicidality, especially during the initial few months of a course of drug therapy, or at times of dose changes, either increases or decreases. Use caution in high-risk patients. Worsening depression and severe abrupt suicidality that are not part of the presenting symptoms may require discontinuation or modification of drug therapy. The patient's family or caregiver should be alerted to monitor patients for the emergence of suicidality and associated behaviors (such as agitation, irritability, hostility, impulsivity, and hypomania) and call healthcare provider.

May worsen psychosis in some patients or precipitate a shift to mania or hypomania in patients with bipolar disorder. Patients presenting with depressive symptoms should be screened for bipolar disorder. Monotherapy in patients with bipolar disorder should be avoided. **Paroxetine is not FDA approved for the treatment of bipolar depression.**

Serotonin syndrome and neuroleptic malignant syndrome (NMS)-like reactions have occurred with serotonin/norepinephrine reuptake inhibitors (SNRIs) and selective serotonin reuptake inhibitors (SSRIs) when used alone, and particularly when used in combination with serotonergic agents (eg, triptans) or antidopaminergic agents (eg, antipsychotics). Concurrent use with MAO inhibitors is contraindicated. May increase the risks associated with electroconvulsive therapy. Has a low potential to impair cognitive or motor performance - caution operating hazardous machinery or driving. Symptoms of agitation and/or restlessness may occur during initial few weeks of therapy. Low potential for sedation or anticholinergic effects relative to cyclic antidepressants.

Use caution in patients with a previous seizure disorder or condition predisposing to seizures such as brain damage, alcoholism, or concurrent therapy with other drugs which lower the seizure threshold. Use with caution in patients with hepatic dysfunction and in elderly patients. May cause hyponatremia/SIADH (elderly at increased risk); volume depletion (diuretics may increase risk). Use caution with concomitant use of NSAIDs, ASA, or other drugs that affect coagulation; the risk of bleeding may be potentiated. Use with caution in patients with renal insufficiency or other concurrent illness (due to limited experience); dose reduction recommended with severe renal impairment. May cause or exacerbate sexual dysfunction. Use caution in patients with narrow-angle glaucoma. Avoid use in the first trimester of pregnancy.

Upon discontinuation of paroxetine therapy, gradually taper dose and monitor for discontinuation symptoms (eg, dizziness, dysphoric mood, irritability, agitation, confusion, paresthesias). If intolerable symptoms occur following a decrease in dosage or upon discontinuation of therapy, then resuming the previous dose with a more gradual taper should be considered. Safety and efficacy in children have not been established.

Drug Interactions

Metabolism/Transport Effects Substrate of CYP2D6 (major); **Inhibits** CYP1A2 (weak), 2B6 (moderate), 2C9 (weak), 2C19 (weak), 2D6 (strong), 3A4 (weak)

Avoid Concomitant Use

Avoid concomitant use of PARoxetine with any of the following: Iobenguane I 123; MAO Inhibitors; Methylene Blue; Pimozide; Sibutramine; Tamoxifen; Thioridazine; Tryptophan

Increased Effect/Toxicity

PARoxetine may increase the levels/effects of: Alcohol (Ethyl); Alpha-/Beta-Blockers; Anticoagulants; Antidepressants (Serotonin Reuptake Inhibitor/Antagonist); Antiplatelet Agents; Aspirin; Atomoxetine; Beta-Blockers; BusPIRone; CarBAMazepine; CloZAPine; CNS Depressants; Collagenase (Systemic); CYP2B6 Substrates; CYP2D6 Substrates; Desmopressin; Dextromethorphan; Drotrecogin Alfa; DULoxetine; Fesoterodine; Galantamine; Haloperidol; Ibritumomab; Lithium; Methadone; Methotrimeprazine; Methylene Blue; Mexiletine; NSAID (COX-2 Inhibitor); NSAID (Nonselective); Pimozide; Propafenone; RisperiDONE; Salicylates; Serotonin Modulators; Tamoxifen; Tetrabenazine; Thioridazine; Thrombolytic Agents; Tositumomab and Iodine I 131 Tositumomab; TraMADol; Tricyclic Antidepressants; Vitamin K Antagonists

The levels/effects of PARoxetine may be increased by: Abiraterone; Analgesics (Opioid); Asenapine; BusPIRone; Cimetidine; CYP2D6 Inhibitors (Moderate); CYP2D6 Inhibitors (Strong); Dasatinib; Droperidol; Glucosamine; Herbs (Anticoagulant/Antiplatelet Properties); MAO Inhibitors; Methotrimeprazine; Metoclopramide; Omega-3-Acid Ethyl Esters; Pentosan Polysulfate Sodium; Pentoxifylline; Prostacyclin Analogues; Sibutramine; TraMADol; Tryptophan

Decreased Effect

PARoxetine may decrease the levels/effects of: Aprepitant; Fosaprepitant; Iobenguane I 123

The levels/effects of PARoxetine may be decreased by: Aprepitant; CarBAMazepine; Cyproheptadine; Darunavir; Fosamprenavir; Fosaprepitant; Peginterferon Alfa-2b

Ethanol/Nutrition/Herb Interactions

Ethanol: May increase CNS depression; monitor for increased effects with coadministration. Caution patients about effects.

Food: Peak concentration is increased, but bioavailability is not significantly altered by food.

Herb/Nutraceutical: Avoid valerian, St John's wort, SAMe, kava kava.

Dietary Considerations May be taken without regard to meals.

Pharmacodynamics/Kinetics

Onset of Action Depression: The onset of action is within a week, however, individual response varies greatly and full response may not be seen until 8-12 weeks after initiation of treatment.

Half-life Elimination 21 hours (3-65 hours)

Time to Peak Immediate release: 5.2 hours; controlled release: 6-10 hours

Pregnancy Risk Factor D

Lactation Enters breast milk/use caution (AAP rates "of concern"; AAP 2001 update pending)

Breast-Feeding Considerations Paroxetine is excreted in breast milk and concentrations in the hindmilk are higher than in foremilk. Paroxetine has not been detected in the serum of nursing infants and adverse events have not been reported. The manufacturer recommends that caution be exercised when administering paroxetine to nursing women.

The long-term effects on development and behavior have not been studied; therefore, one should prescribe paroxetine to a mother who is breast-feeding only when the benefits outweigh the potential risks.

Dosage Forms
Suspension, oral:
Paxil®: 10 mg/5 mL (250 mL)
Tablet, oral: 10 mg, 20 mg, 30 mg, 40 mg
Paxil®: 10 mg, 20 mg, 30 mg, 40 mg
Pexeva®: 10 mg, 20 mg, 30 mg, 40 mg
Tablet, controlled release, enteric coated, oral: 12.5 mg, 25 mg, 37.5 mg
Paxil CR®: 12.5 mg, 25 mg, 37.5 mg
Tablet, extended release, enteric coated, oral: 12.5 mg, 25 mg

Pazopanib (paz OH pa nib)

Related Information
Clinical Risk Related to Drugs Prolonging QT Interval *on page 1872*
U.S. Brand Names Votrient™
Pharmacologic Category Antineoplastic Agent, Tyrosine Kinase Inhibitor; Vascular Endothelial Growth Factor (VEGF) Inhibitor
Use Treatment of advanced renal cell cancer (RCC)
Local Anesthetic/Vasoconstrictor Precautions Hypertension can occur with the use of this drug, particularly early in the treatment course. Monitor for hypertension prior to using local anesthetic with vasoconstrictor; medical consult if necessary.

Pazopanib is one of the drugs confirmed to prolong the QT interval and is accepted as having a risk of causing torsade de pointes. The risk of drug-induced torsade de pointes is extremely low when a single QT interval prolonging drug is prescribed. In terms of epinephrine, it is not known what effect vasoconstrictors in the local anesthetic regimen will have in patients with a known history of congenital prolonged QT interval or in patients taking any medication that prolongs the QT interval. Until more information is obtained, it is suggested that the clinician consult with the physician prior to the use of a vasoconstrictor in suspected patients, and that the vasoconstrictor (epinephrine, mepivacaine and levonordefrin [Carbocaine® 2% with Neo-Cobefrin®]) be used with caution.

Effects on Dental Treatment Key adverse event(s) related to dental treatment: Taste alteration.
Effects on Bleeding Chemotherapy may result in significant myelosuppression, potentially including significant reduction in platelet counts and altered hemostasis. Hemorrhagic events have been reported. In patients who are under active treatment with these agents, medical consult is suggested.

Adverse Effects
>10%:
Cardiovascular: Hypertension (40%; grade 3: 4%)
Central nervous system: Fatigue (19%)
Dermatologic: Hair color change (38%)
Endocrine & metabolic: Hyperglycemia (41%), hypophosphatemia (34%), hyponatremia (31%), hypomagnesemia (26%), hypoglycemia (17%)
Gastrointestinal: Diarrhea (52%; grade 3: 3%; grade 4: <1%), lipase increased (4% to 27%), nausea (26%), anorexia (22%), vomiting (21%), abdominal pain (11%)
Hematologic: Leukopenia (37%), neutropenia (34%; grade 3: 1%; grade 4: <1%), thrombocytopenia (32%; grades 3/4: <1%), lymphocytopenia (31%; grade 3: 4%; grade 4: <1%), hemorrhage (5% to 16%)
Hepatic: ALT increased (53%; grade 3: 10%; grade 4: 2%), AST increased (53%; grade 3: 7%; grade 4: <1%), bilirubin increased (36%; grade 3: 3%; grade 4: <1%)
Neuromuscular & skeletal: Weakness (14%)

1% to 10%:
Cardiovascular: Chest pain (5%), MI/ischemia (2%), facial edema (1%), QT prolongation (1%), transient ischemic event (1%)
Central nervous system: Headache (10%)
Dermatologic: Alopecia (8%), rash (8%), palmar-plantar erythrodysesthesia (6%), skin depigmentation (3%)
Endocrine & metabolic: Hypothyroidism (7%)
Gastrointestinal: Weight loss (9%), taste alteration (8%), dyspepsia (5%), rectal hemorrhage (1%)
Renal: Proteinuria (9%), hematuria (4%)
Respiratory: Epistaxis (2%), hemoptysis (2%)

General Dosage Range Dosage adjustment recommended in patients with hepatic impairment, on concomitant therapy, or who develop toxicities
Oral: *Adults:* 800 mg once daily
Mechanism of Action Tyrosine kinase (multikinase) inhibitor; inhibits tumor growth via angiogenesis by inhibiting cell surface vascular endothelial growth factor receptors (VEGFR-1, VEGFR-2, VEGFR-3), platelet-derived growth factor receptors

(PDGFR-alpha and -beta), fibroblast growth factor receptor (FGFR-1 and -3), cytokine receptor (cKIT), interleukin-2 receptor inducible T-cell kinase, leukocyte-specific protein tyrosine kinase (Lck), and transmembrane glycoprotein receptor tyrosine kinase (c-Fms)

Pharmacodynamics/Kinetics

Half-life Elimination ~31 hours

Time to Peak Plasma: 2-4 hours

Pregnancy Risk Factor D

Dental Comment Pazopanib is known to prolong the QT interval. The QT interval is measured as the time and distance between the Q point of the QRS complex and the end of the T wave in the ECG tracing. After adjustment for heart rate, the QT interval is defined as prolonged if it is more than 450 msec in men and 460 msec in women. A long QT syndrome was first described in the 1950s and 60s as a congenital syndrome involving QT interval prolongation and syncope and sudden death. Some of the congenital long QT syndromes were characterized by a peculiar electrocardiographic appearance of the QRS complex involving a premature atria beat followed by a pause, then a subsequent sinus beat showing marked QT prolongation and deformity. This type of cardiac arrhythmia was originally termed "torsade de pointes" (translated from the French as "twisting of the points"). Pazopanib is considered as having a risk of causing torsade de pointes. Since it is not known what effect vasoconstrictors in the local anesthetic regimen will have in patients with a known history of congenital prolonged QT interval or in patients taking any medication that prolongs the QT interval, a medical consult is suggested.

Pegademase Bovine (peg A de mase BOE vine)

U.S. Brand Names Adagen®

Canadian Brand Names Adagen®

Pharmacologic Category Enzyme

Use Enzyme replacement therapy for adenosine deaminase (ADA) deficiency in patients with severe combined immunodeficiency disease (SCID) who are not candidates for or who have failed bone marrow transplant

Local Anesthetic/Vasoconstrictor Precautions No information available to require special precautions

Effects on Dental Treatment No significant effects or complications reported

Effects on Bleeding No information available to require special precautions

Adverse Effects Postmarketing and/or case reports: Autoimmune hemolytic anemia, erythema (injection site), hemolytic anemia, thrombocythemia, urticaria

General Dosage Range I.M.: *Children:* First dose: 10 units/kg; Second dose: 15 units/kg 7 days after first dose; Third dose: 20 units/kg 7 days after second dose; Maintenance: 20 units/kg/week (maximum: 30 units/kg/week)

Mechanism of Action Adenosine deaminase is an enzyme that catalyzes the deamination of both adenosine and deoxyadenosine. Hereditary lack of adenosine deaminase activity results in severe combined immunodeficiency disease, a fatal disorder of infancy characterized by profound defects of both cellular and humoral immunity. It is estimated that 25% of patients with the autosomal recessive form of severe combined immunodeficiency lack adenosine deaminase. Pegademase bovine is a (modified) enzyme replacement for adenosine deaminase deficiency.

Pharmacodynamics/Kinetics

Half-life Elimination Plasma ADA half-life (following administration): Range: 3 to >6 days

Time to Peak Plasma adenosine deaminase activity: 2-3 days

Pregnancy Risk Factor C

Pegaptanib (peg AP ta nib)

U.S. Brand Names Macugen®

Canadian Brand Names Macugen®

Pharmacologic Category Ophthalmic Agent; Vascular Endothelial Growth Factor (VEGF) Inhibitor

Use Treatment of neovascular (wet) age-related macular degeneration (AMD)

Local Anesthetic/Vasoconstrictor Precautions No information available to require special precautions

Effects on Dental Treatment No significant effects or complications reported

Effects on Bleeding No information available to require special precautions

Adverse Effects

10% to 40%:

Cardiovascular: Hypertension

Ocular: Anterior chamber inflammation, blurred vision, cataract, conjunctival hemorrhage, corneal edema, eye discharge, eye irritation, eye pain, intraocular pressure increased, ocular discomfort, punctate keratitis, visual acuity decreased, visual disturbance, vitreous floaters, vitreous opacities

1% to 10%:

Cardiovascular: Carotid artery occlusion (1% to 5%), cerebrovascular accident (1% to 5%), chest pain (1% to 5%), transient ischemic attack (1% to 5%)

Central nervous system: Dizziness (6% to 10%), headache (6% to 10%), vertigo (1% to 5%)

Dermatologic: Contact dermatitis (1% to 5%)

Endocrine & metabolic: Diabetes mellitus (1% to 5%)

Gastrointestinal: Diarrhea (6% to 10%), nausea (6% to 10%), dyspepsia (1% to 5%), vomiting (1% to 5%)

Genitourinary: Urinary retention (1% to 5%)

Neuromuscular & skeletal: Arthritis (1% to 5%), bone spur (1% to 5%)

Ocular: Blepharitis (6% to 10%), conjunctivitis (6% to 10%), photopsia (6% to 10%), vitreous disorder (6% to 10%), allergic conjunctivitis (1% to 5%), conjunctival edema (1% to 5%), corneal abrasion (1% to 5%), corneal deposits (1% to 5%), corneal epithelium disorder (1% to 5%), endophthalmitis (1% to 5%), eye inflammation (1% to 5%), eye swelling (1% to 5%), eyelid irritation (1% to 5%), meibomianitis (1% to 5%), mydriasis (1% to 5%), periorbital hematoma (1% to 5%), retinal edema (1% to 5%), vitreous hemorrhage (1% to 5%)

Otic: Hearing loss (1% to 5%)

Renal: Urinary tract infection (6% to 10%)

Respiratory: Bronchitis (6% to 10%), pleural effusion (1% to 5%)

Miscellaneous: Contusion (1% to 5%)

General Dosage Range Intravitreous: *Adults:* 0.3 mg into affected eye every 6 weeks

Mechanism of Action Pegaptanib is an apatamer, an oligonucleotide covalently bound to polyethylene glycol, which can adopt a three-dimensional shape and bind to vascular endothelial growth factor (VEGF). Pegaptanib binds to extracellular VEGF, inhibiting VEGF from binding to its receptors and thereby suppressing neovascularization and slowing vision loss.

Pharmacodynamics/Kinetics

Half-life Elimination Plasma: 6-14 days

Pregnancy Risk Factor B

Pegaspargase (peg AS par jase)

Related Information

Asparaginase *on page 170*

U.S. Brand Names Oncaspar®

Pharmacologic Category Antineoplastic Agent, Miscellaneous

Use Treatment of acute lymphocytic leukemia (ALL); treatment of ALL with previous hypersensitivity to native L-asparaginase

Local Anesthetic/Vasoconstrictor Precautions No information available to require special precautions

Effects on Dental Treatment No significant effects or complications reported

Effects on Bleeding Although significant myelosuppression with associated altered hemostasis has been reported for many chemotherapeutic agents, myelosuppression is not common with pegaspargase and no specific precautions appear to necessary.

Adverse Effects

>5%:

Cardiovascular: Edema

Central nervous system: Fever, malaise

Dermatologic: Rash

Gastrointestinal: Nausea, vomiting

Hematologic: Coagulopathy (7%; grades 3/4: 2%)

Hepatic: Transaminases increased (11%; grades 3/4: 3%)

Miscellaneous: Allergic reactions (including bronchospasm, chills, dyspnea, edema, erythema, hypotension, rash, swelling, urticaria; no prior asparaginase hypersensitivity: 1% to 10%; grades 3/4: 2%; prior asparaginase hypersensitivity: 32%; grades 3/4: 8%)

1% to 5%:

Cardiovascular: Hypotension, peripheral edema, tachycardia, thrombosis (4%)

Central nervous system: Chills, CNS thrombosis (2% to 4%; grades 3/4: 3%), CNS hemorrhage (2%), headache, seizure

Dermatologic: Lip edema, urticaria

Endocrine & metabolic: Hyperglycemia (3% to 5%; grades 3/4: ≤5%), hyperuricemia, hypoglycemia, hypoproteinemia
Gastrointestinal: Abdominal pain, anorexia, diarrhea, pancreatitis (1% to 2%; grades 3/4: 2%)
Hematologic: Anticoagulant effect decreased, disseminated intravascular coagulation (DIC), fibrinogen decreased, hemolytic anemia, leukopenia, pancytopenia, thrombocytopenia, thromboplastin increased, myelosuppression
Hepatic: Liver function tests abnormal (grades 3/4: 5%), hyperbilirubinemia (grades 3/4: 2%), jaundice
Local: Injection site hypersensitivity, pain or reaction
Neuromuscular & skeletal: Arthralgia, limb pain, myalgia, paresthesia
Respiratory: Dyspnea
Miscellaneous: Anaphylactic reactions, night sweats

General Dosage Range I.M., I.V.: *Children and Adults:* 2500 units/m^2 every 14 days

Mechanism of Action Pegaspargase is a modified version of asparaginase. Leukemic cells, especially lymphoblasts, require exogenous asparagine; normal cells can synthesize asparagine. Asparaginase contains L-asparaginase amidohydrolase type EC-2 which inhibits protein synthesis by deaminating asparagine to aspartic acid and ammonia in the plasma and extracellular fluid and therefore deprives tumor cells of the amino acid for protein synthesis. Asparaginase is cycle-specific for the G_1 phase of the cell cycle.

Pharmacodynamics/Kinetics

Onset of Action Asparagine depletion: I.M.: Within 4 days

Duration of Action Asparagine depletion: I.M.: ~21 days; I.V. (in asparaginase naive adults): 2-4 weeks

Half-life Elimination I.M.: ~5.5-6 days; unaffected by age, renal or hepatic function; half-life decreased to 1.8-3.2 days in patients with previous hypersensitivity to native L-asparaginase; I.V.: Adults (asparaginase naive): 7 days

Time to Peak I.M.: 3-4 days

Pregnancy Risk Factor C

Pegfilgrastim (peg fil GRA stim)

U.S. Brand Names Neulasta®

Canadian Brand Names Neulasta®

Pharmacologic Category Colony Stimulating Factor

Use To decrease the incidence of infection, by stimulation of granulocyte production, in patients with nonmyeloid malignancies receiving myelosuppressive therapy associated with a significant risk of febrile neutropenia

Local Anesthetic/Vasoconstrictor Precautions No information available to require special precautions

Effects on Dental Treatment No significant effects or complications reported

Effects on Bleeding No information available to require special precautions. Medical consultation may be necessary to confirm adequate platelet counts.

Adverse Effects

>10%:
Cardiovascular: Peripheral edema (12%)
Central nervous system: Headache (16%)
Gastrointestinal: Vomiting (13%)
Neuromuscular & skeletal: Bone pain (31% to 57%), myalgia (21%), arthralgia (16%), weakness (13%)

1% to 10%:
Gastrointestinal: Constipation (10%)
Miscellaneous: Antibody formation (1% to 6%)

General Dosage Range SubQ:
Children: 100 mcg/kg (maximum dose: 6 mg) once per chemotherapy cycle
Adolescents >45 kg and Adults: 6 mg once per chemotherapy cycle

Mechanism of Action Stimulates the production, maturation, and activation of neutrophils, pegfilgrastim activates neutrophils to increase both their migration and cytotoxicity. Pegfilgrastim has a prolonged duration of effect relative to filgrastim and a reduced renal clearance.

Pharmacodynamics/Kinetics

Half-life Elimination SubQ: Adults: 15-80 hours; Children (100 mcg/kg dose): ~20-30 hours (range: up to 68 hours)

Pregnancy Risk Factor C

Peginterferon Alfa-2a (peg in ter FEER on AL fa too aye)

Related Information

Systemic Viral Diseases *on page 1904*

U.S. Brand Names Pegasys®

Canadian Brand Names Pegasys®

Pharmacologic Category Interferon

Use Treatment of chronic hepatitis C (CHC), alone or in combination with ribavirin, in patients with compensated liver disease and not previously treated with alfa interferons (includes patients with histological evidence of cirrhosis [Child-Pugh class A] and patients with clinically-stable HIV disease); treatment of patients with HBeAg positive and HBeAg negative chronic hepatitis B with compensated liver disease and evidence of viral replication and liver inflammation

Local Anesthetic/Vasoconstrictor Precautions No information available to require special precautions

Effects on Dental Treatment Key adverse event(s) related to dental treatment: Xerostomia (normal salivary flow resumes upon discontinuation).

Effects on Bleeding Chemotherapy may result in significant myelosuppression, potentially including significant reduction in platelet counts and altered hemostasis. In patients who are under active treatment with these agents, medical consult is suggested.

Adverse Effects Note: Percentages are reported for peginterferon alfa-2a in chronic hepatitis C (CHC) patients. Other percentages indicated as "with ribavirin" or "in HIV/CHC" are those which significantly exceed incidence reported for peginterferon monotherapy in CHC patients.

>10%:

Central nervous system: Headache (54%), fatigue (56%), pyrexia (37%; 41% with ribavirin; 54% in hepatitis B), insomnia (19%; 30% with ribavirin), depression (18%), dizziness (16%), irritability/anxiety/nervousness (19%; 33% with ribavirin), pain (11%)

Dermatologic: Alopecia (23%; 28% with ribavirin), pruritus (12%; 19% with ribavirin), dermatitis (16% with ribavirin)

Gastrointestinal: Nausea/vomiting (24%), anorexia (17%; 24% with ribavirin), diarrhea (16%), weight loss (16% in HIV/CHC), abdominal pain (15%)

Hematologic: Neutropenia (21%; 27% with ribavirin; 40% in HIV/CHC), lymphopenia (14% with ribavirin), anemia (11% with ribavirin; 14% in HIV/CHC)

Hepatic: ALT increases 5-10 x ULN during treatment (25% to 27% in hepatitis B); ALT increases >10 x ULN during treatment (12% to 18% in hepatitis B); ALT increases 5-10 x ULN after treatment (13% to 16% in hepatitis B); ALT increases >10 x ULN after treatment (7% to 12% in hepatitis B)

Local: Injection site reaction (22%)

Neuromuscular & skeletal: Weakness (56%; 65% with ribavirin), myalgia (37%), rigors (35%; 25% to 27% in hepatitis B), arthralgia (28%)

Respiratory: Dyspnea (13% with ribavirin)

1% to 10%:

Central nervous system: Concentration impaired (8%), memory impaired (5%), mood alteration (3%; 9% in HIV/CHC)

Dermatologic: Dermatitis (8%), rash (5%), dry skin (4%; 10% with ribavirin), eczema (1%; 5% with ribavirin)

Endocrine & metabolic: Hypothyroidism (3% to 4%), hyperthyroidism (≤1%)

Gastrointestinal: Xerostomia (6%), dyspepsia (<1%; 6% with ribavirin), weight loss (4%; 10% with ribavirin)

Hematologic: Thrombocytopenia (5%; 8% in HIV/CHC), lymphopenia (3%), anemia (2%)

Hepatic: Hepatic decompensation (2% in CHC/HIV)

Neuromuscular & skeletal: Back pain (9%)

Ocular: Blurred vision (4%)

Respiratory: Cough (4%; 10% with ribavirin), dyspnea (4%), exertional dyspnea (4% with ribavirin)

Miscellaneous: Diaphoresis (6%), bacterial infection (3%; 5% in HIV/CHC)

General Dosage Range Dosage adjustment recommended in patients with hepatic or renal impairment or who develop toxicities

SubQ: *Adults:* 180 mcg once weekly

Mechanism of Action Alpha interferons are a family of proteins, produced by nucleated cells that have antiviral, antiproliferative, and immune-regulating activity. There are 16 known subtypes of alpha interferons. Interferons interact with cells through high affinity cell surface receptors. Following activation, multiple effects can be detected including induction of gene transcription. Inhibits cellular growth, alters the state of cellular differentiation, interferes with oncogene expression, alters cell surface antigen expression, increases phagocytic activity of macrophages, and augments cytotoxicity of lymphocytes for target cells.

Pharmacodynamics/Kinetics

Half-life Elimination Terminal: 50-160 hours; increased with renal dysfunction

Time to Peak Serum: 72-96 hours

Pregnancy Risk Factor C / X in combination with ribavirin

Peginterferon Alfa-2a and Ribavirin

(peg in ter FEER on AL fa too aye & rye ba VYE rin)

Related Information

Peginterferon Alfa-2a *on page 1306*
Ribavirin *on page 1470*
Systemic Viral Diseases *on page 1904*

Canadian Brand Names Pegasys® RBV

Pharmacologic Category Antiviral Agent; Interferon

Use Combination therapy for the treatment of chronic hepatitis C (HCV) in patients without cirrhosis and patients with compensated cirrhosis; includes patients coinfected with stable HIV disease

Local Anesthetic/Vasoconstrictor Precautions No information available to require special precautions

Effects on Dental Treatment Key adverse event(s) related to dental treatment: Xerostomia (normal salivary flow resumes upon discontinuation), glossitis, stomatitis, mouth ulcerations, taste disturbances, and cheilitis.

Effects on Bleeding Chemotherapy may result in significant myelosuppression, potentially including significant reduction in platelet counts and altered hemostasis. In patients who are under active treatment with these agents, medical consult is suggested. Gingival bleeding has been reported.

Adverse Effects Adverse reactions as reported with use of the combination product. Also refer to individual agents.

>10%:

Central nervous system: Fatigue (40% to 49%), headache (35% to 48%), fever (37% to 41%), insomnia (19% to 32%), rigors (16% to 30%), irritability (15% to 28%), depression (17% to 22%), dizziness (7% to 15%)

Dermatologic: Alopecia (10% to 25%), pruritus (4% to 25%), dermatitis (1% to 16%), dry skin (4% to 13%)

Gastrointestinal: Nausea (24% to 29%), anorexia (20% to 27%), diarrhea (14% to 16%), weight loss (2% to 16%)

Hematologic: Hemolytic anemia (≤14%), neutropenia (3% to 11%)

Local: Injection site reaction (10% to 28%)

Neuromuscular & skeletal: Myalgia (32% to 42%), weakness (15% to 26%), arthralgia (16% to 22%)

Respiratory: Cough (3% to 13%), dyspnea (3% to 13%)

1% to 10%:

Cardiovascular: Chest pain (≥1% to ≤5%), flushing (≥1% to ≤5%), hypertension (≥1% to ≤5%), palpitation (≥1% to ≤5%), peripheral edema (≥1% to ≤5%), syncope (≥1% to ≤5%), tachycardia (≥1% to ≤5%)

Central nervous system: Pain (6% to 10%), impaired concentration (2% to 10%), anxiety (8%), mood altered (≤8%), malaise (3% to 6%), emotional disorder (≤5%), aggression (≥1% to ≤5%), confusion (≥1% to ≤5%), hyper-/hypoesthesia (≥1% to ≤5%), lethargy (≥1% to ≤5%), migraine (≥1% to ≤5%), nightmares (≥1% to ≤5%), somnolence (≥1% to ≤5%), suicidal ideation (≥1% to ≤5%), vertigo (≥1% to ≤5%), impaired memory (1% to 5%), nervousness (≤3%), affect lability (HIV-HCV coinfection: ≥1% to ≤3%), apathy (HIV-HCV coinfection: ≥1% to ≤3%)

Dermatologic: Rash (5% to 9%), eczema (≥1% to ≤5%), photosensitivity (≥1% to ≤5%), psoriasis (≥1% to ≤5%), urticaria (≥1% to ≤5%)

Endocrine & metabolic: Libido decreased (2% to 5%), dehydration (≥1% to ≤5%), hot flashes (≥1% to ≤5%), hyperthyroidism (≥1% to ≤5%), impotence (≥1% to ≤5%), hypothyroidism (≤4%), lactic acidosis (HIV-HCV coinfection: ≥1% to ≤3%)

Gastrointestinal: Abdominal pain (7% to 10%), vomiting (7% to 8%), xerostomia (5% to 8%), appetite decreased (≤7%), dyspepsia (2% to 6%), constipation (≥1% to ≤5%), dysphagia (≥1% to ≤5%), flatulence (≥1% to ≤5%), glossitis (≥1% to ≤5%), mouth ulceration (≥1% to ≤5%), stomatitis (≥1% to ≤5%), taste disturbance (≥1% to ≤5%), cheilitis (HIV-HCV coinfection: ≥1% to ≤3%)

Genitourinary: Chromaturia (HIV-HCV coinfection: ≥1% to ≤3%)

Hematologic: Thrombocytopenia (≥1% to 8%), bleeding (gingival) (≥1% to ≤5%)

Neuromuscular & skeletal: Back pain (3% to 5%), arthritis (≥1% to ≤5%), bone pain (≥1% to ≤5%), muscle cramps (≥1% to ≤5%), muscle weakness (≥1% to ≤5%), musculoskeletal pain (≥1% to ≤5%), neck pain (≥1% to ≤5%), paresthesia (≥1% to ≤5%), tremor (≥1% to ≤5%)

Ocular: Eye inflammation (≥1% to ≤5%), eye pain (≥1% to ≤5%), vision blurred (≥1% to ≤5%), xerophthalmia (≥1% to ≤5%)
Otic: Earache (≥1% to ≤5%), tinnitus (≥1% to ≤5%)
Respiratory: Bronchitis (≥1% to ≤5%), epistaxis (≥1% to ≤5%), nasal congestion (≥1% to ≤5%), nasopharyngitis (≥1% to ≤5%), pharyngolaryngeal pain (≥1% to ≤5%), rhinitis (≥1% to ≤5%), sinus congestion (≥1% to ≤5%), throat sore (≥1% to ≤5%), upper respiratory infection (≥1% to ≤5%), pneumonia (HIV-HCV coinfection: ≥1% to ≤3%)
Miscellaneous: Diaphoresis (2% to 5%), flu-like syndrome (≥1% to ≤5%), herpes simplex (≥1% to ≤5%), lymphadenopathy (≥1% to ≤5%), night sweats (≥1% to ≤5%), oral candidiasis (≥1% to ≤5%), thirst (≥1% to ≤5%), acquired lipodystrophy (HIV-HCV coinfection: ≥1% to ≤3%)

Use of alfa interferons has been associated with rare cases of autoimmune diseases, including idiopathic thrombocytopenic purpura, thyroiditis, rheumatoid arthritis, systemic lupus erythematosus, vasculitis, and Vogt-Koyanagi-Harada syndrome

General Dosage Range Dosage adjustment recommended in patients with hepatic or renal impairment or who develop toxicities

SubQ: Peginterferon Alfa-2a: *Adults:* 180 mcg/week

Oral: Ribavirin:
Adults <75kg: 800-1000 mg/day in 2 divided doses
Adults ≥75 kg: 800-1200 mg/day in 2 divided doses

Mechanism of Action

Peginterferon Alfa-2a: Alpha interferons are a family of proteins, produced by nucleated cells that have antiviral, antiproliferative, and immune-regulating activity. There are 16 known subtypes of alpha interferons. Interferons interact with cells through high affinity cell surface receptors. Following activation, multiple effects can be detected including induction of gene transcription. Inhibits cellular growth, alters the state of cellular differentiation, interferes with oncogene expression, alters cell surface antigen expression, increases phagocytic activity of macrophages, and augments cytotoxicity of lymphocytes for target cells.

Ribavirin: Inhibits replication of RNA and DNA viruses; inhibits influenza virus RNA polymerase activity and inhibits the initiation and elongation of RNA fragments resulting in inhibition of viral protein synthesis.

Product Availability Not available in U.S.

Peginterferon Alfa-2b (peg in ter FEER on AL fa too bee)

Related Information

Systemic Viral Diseases *on page 1904*

U.S. Brand Names PegIntron®; PegIntron™ Redipen®; Sylatron™

Canadian Brand Names PegIntron®

Pharmacologic Category Interferon

Use

PegIntron®: Treatment of chronic hepatitis C (CHC; in combination with ribavirin) in patients who have compensated liver disease; treatment of chronic hepatitis C (as monotherapy) in adult patients with compensated liver disease who have never received alfa interferons

Sylatron™: Adjuvant treatment of melanoma (with microscopic or gross nodal involvement within 84 days of definitive surgical resection, including lymphadenectomy)

Local Anesthetic/Vasoconstrictor Precautions No information available to require special precautions

Effects on Dental Treatment Key adverse event(s) related to dental treatment: Xerostomia (normal salivary flow resumes upon discontinuation).

Effects on Bleeding Chemotherapy may result in significant myelosuppression, potentially including significant reduction in platelet counts and altered hemostasis. In patients who are under active treatment with these agents, medical consult is suggested.

Adverse Effects Note: Percentages reported for adults receiving monotherapy unless noted:

>10%:

Central nervous system: Fatigue (52% to 94%), fever (22% to 75%), headache (56% to 70%), chills (≤63%), depression (29% to 59%; may be severe), dizziness (12% to 35%), anxiety/emotional liability/irritability (28%), insomnia (23%), olfactory nerve disorder (≤23%)
Dermatologic: Rash (6% to 36%), alopecia (22% to 34%), pruritus (12%), dry skin (11%)

Gastrointestinal: Anorexia (20% to 69%), nausea (26% to 64%), taste perversion (≤38%), diarrhea (18% to 37%), vomiting (7% to 26%), abdominal pain (15%), weight loss (11%)
Hematologic: Neutropenia (6% to 70%; grade 4: 1%), thrombocytopenia (7% to 20%; grades 3/4: <4%), anemia (6%; in combination with ribavirin: 12% to 47%)
Hepatic: Transaminases increased (10% to 77%), alkaline phosphatase increased (≤23%)
Local: Injection site inflammation/reaction (23% to 62%)
Neuromuscular & skeletal: Myalgia (54% to 68%), weakness (52%), arthralgia (23% to 51%), musculoskeletal pain (28%), rigors (23%), paresthesia (21%)
Miscellaneous: Viral infection (11%)

>1% to 10%:
Cardiovascular: Chest pain (6%), flushing (6%)
Central nervous system: Concentration impaired (10%), malaise (7%), nervousness (4%), agitation (2%), suicidal behavior (ideation/attempt/suicide ≤2%)
Endocrine & metabolic: Hypothyroidism (5%), menstrual disorder (4%), hyperthyroidism (3%)
Gastrointestinal: Dyspepsia (6%), xerostomia (6%), constipation (1%)
Hepatic: GGT increased (8%), hepatomegaly (6%)
Local: Injection site pain (2% to 3%)
Ocular: Conjunctivitis (4%), blurred vision (2%)
Renal: Proteinuria (≤7%)
Respiratory: Pharyngitis (10%), cough (5% to 8%), sinusitis (7%), dyspnea (4% to 6%), rhinitis (2%)
Miscellaneous: Diaphoresis (6%), neutralizing antibodies (2%)

General Dosage Range Dosage adjustment recommended in patients with renal impairment or who develop toxicities

SubQ: Melanoma:
Adults: Initial: 6 mcg/kg/week; Maintenance: 3 mcg/kg/week

SubQ: Chronic hepatitis C:
Children ≥3 years: 60 mcg/m^2/week (in combination with ribavirin)
Adults: Peginterferon monotherapy (based on average weekly dose of 1 mcg/kg):
Adults ≤45 kg: 40 mcg once weekly
Adults 46-56 kg: 50 mcg once weekly
Adults 57-72 kg: 64 mcg once weekly
Adults 73-88 kg: 80 mcg once weekly
Adults 89-106 kg: 96 mcg once weekly
Adults 107-136 kg: 120 mcg once weekly
Adults 137-160 kg: 150 mcg once weekly
Adults: Combination therapy with ribavirin (based on average weekly dose of 1.5 mcg/kg):
Adults <40 kg: 50 mcg once weekly (with ribavirin 800 mg/day)
Adults 40-50 kg: 64 mcg once weekly (with ribavirin 800 mg/day)
Adults 51-60 kg: 80 mcg once weekly (with ribavirin 800 mg/day)
Adults 61-65 kg: 96 mcg once weekly (with ribavirin 800 mg/day)
Adults 66-75 kg: 96 mcg once weekly (with ribavirin 1000 mg/day)
Adults 76-80 kg: 120 mcg once weekly (with ribavirin 1000 mg/day)
Adults 81-85 kg: 120 mcg once weekly (with ribavirin 1200 mg/day)
Adults 86-105 kg: 150 mcg once weekly (with ribavirin 1200 mg/day)
Adults >105 kg: 1.5 mcg/kg once weekly (with ribavirin 1400 mg/day)

Mechanism of Action Alpha interferons are a family of proteins, produced by nucleated cells, that have antiviral, antiproliferative, and immune-regulating activity. There are 16 known subtypes of alpha interferons. Interferons interact with cells through high affinity cell surface receptors. Following activation, multiple effects can be detected including induction of gene transcription. Inhibits cellular growth, alters the state of cellular differentiation, interferes with oncogene expression, alters cell surface antigen expression, increases phagocytic activity of macrophages, and augments cytotoxicity of lymphocytes for target cells.

Pharmacodynamics/Kinetics

Half-life Elimination CHC: ~40 hours (range: 22-60 hours); Melanoma: ~43-51 hours

Time to Peak CHC: 15-44 hours

Pregnancy Risk Factor C / X in combination with ribavirin

Pegloticase (peg LOE ti kase)

U.S. Brand Names Krystexxa™

Pharmacologic Category Enzyme; Enzyme, Urate-Oxidase (Recombinant)

Use Treatment of chronic gout refractory to conventional therapy

Local Anesthetic/Vasoconstrictor Precautions No information available to require special precautions

Effects on Dental Treatment No significant effects or complications reported

Effects on Bleeding No information available to require special precautions

Adverse Effects

>10%:

Dermatologic: Bruising (11%), urticaria (11%)

Gastrointestinal: Nausea (12%)

Miscellaneous: Antibody formation (antipegloticase antibodies: 92%; antiPEG antibodies: 42%), gout flare (74% within the first 3 months), infusion reactions (26%)

1% to 10%:

Cardiovascular: Chest pain (6% to 10%)

Dermatologic: Erythema (10%), pruritus (10%)

Gastrointestinal: Constipation (6%), vomiting (5%)

Respiratory: Dyspnea (7%), nasopharyngitis (7%)

Miscellaneous: Anaphylaxis (≤7%)

Frequency not defined: Anemia, diarrhea, headache, muscle spasms, nephrolithiasis

General Dosage Range I.V.: *Adults:* 8 mg every 2 weeks

Mechanism of Action Pegloticase is a pegylated recombinant form of urate-oxidase enzyme, also known as uricase (an enzyme normally absent in humans and high primates), which converts uric acid to allantoin (an inactive and water soluble metabolite of uric acid); it does not inhibit the formation of uric acid.

Pharmacodynamics/Kinetics

Onset of Action ~24 hours following the first dose, serum uric acid concentrations decreased

Duration of Action >300 hours (12.5 days)

Half-life Elimination Median: ~14 days

Pregnancy Risk Factor C

PEMEtrexed (pem e TREKS ed)

U.S. Brand Names Alimta®

Canadian Brand Names Alimta®

Pharmacologic Category Antineoplastic Agent, Antimetabolite; Antineoplastic Agent, Antimetabolite (Antifolate)

Use Treatment of unresectable malignant pleural mesothelioma (in combination with cisplatin); treatment of locally advanced or metastatic nonsquamous nonsmall cell lung cancer (NSCLC; as initial treatment in combination with cisplatin, as single-agent maintenance treatment after 4 cycles of initial platinum-based double therapy, and single-agent treatment after prior chemotherapy)

Unlabeled/Investigational Use Treatment of bladder cancer (metastatic), cervical cancer (recurrent or metastatic), ovarian cancer (recurrent or persistent), thymic malignancies; treatment of malignant pleural mesothelioma (either as a single agent or in combination with carboplatin)

Local Anesthetic/Vasoconstrictor Precautions No information available to require special precautions

Effects on Dental Treatment Key adverse event(s) related to dental treatment: Dysphagia, esophagitis, odynophagia, and stomatitis.

Effects on Bleeding Chemotherapy may result in significant myelosuppression, potentially including significant reduction in platelet counts and altered hemostasis. In patients who are under active treatment with these agents, medical consult is suggested.

Adverse Effects Note: Reported for single-agent therapy in patients who received folate and B_{12} supplementation.

>10%:

Central nervous system: Fatigue (25% to 34%; dose-limiting)

Dermatologic: Rash/desquamation (10% to 14%)

Gastrointestinal: Nausea (19% to 31%), anorexia (19% to 22%), vomiting (9% to 16%), stomatitis (7% to 15%), diarrhea (5% to 13%)

Hematologic: Anemia (15% to 19%; grades 3/4: 3% to 4%), leukopenia (6% to 12%; grades 3/4: 2% to 4%), neutropenia (6% to 11%; grades 3/4: 3% to 5%; nadir: 8-10 days; recovery: 12-17 days; dose-limiting)

Respiratory: Pharyngitis (15%)

1% to 10%:

Cardiovascular: Edema (1% to 5%)

Central nervous system: Fever (1% to 8%)

Dermatologic: Pruritus (1% to 7%), alopecia (1% to 6%), erythema multiforme (≤5%)

Gastrointestinal: Constipation (1% to 6%), weight loss (1%), abdominal pain (≤5%)

Hematologic: Thrombocytopenia (1% to 8%; grades 3/4: 2%; dose-limiting), febrile neutropenia (grades 3/4: 2%)

Hepatic: ALT increased (8% to 10%; grades 3/4: ≤2%), AST increased (7% to 8%; grades 3/4: ≤1%)
Neuromuscular & skeletal: Sensory neuropathy (≤9%), motor neuropathy (≤5%)
Ocular: Conjunctivitis (≤5%), lacrimation increased (≤5%)
Renal: Creatinine increased/creatinine clearance decreased (1% to 5%)
Miscellaneous: Allergic reaction/hypersensitivity (≤5%), infection (≤5%), sepsis (1%)

General Dosage Range Dosage adjustment recommended in patients with hepatic impairment, on concomitant therapy, or who develop toxicities

I.V.: *Adults:* 500 mg/m^2 on day 1 of each 21-day cycle

Mechanism of Action Antifolate; disrupts folate-dependent metabolic processes essential for cell replication. Inhibits thymidylate synthase (TS), dihydrofolate reductase (DHFR), glycinamide ribonucleotide formyltransferase (GARFT), and aminoimidazole carboxamide ribonucleotide formyltransferase (AICARFT), the enzymes involved in folate metabolism and DNA synthesis, resulting in inhibition of purine and thymidine nucleotide and protein synthesis.

Pharmacodynamics/Kinetics

Duration of Action V_{dss}: 16.1 L

Half-life Elimination Normal renal function: 3.5 hours; Cl_{cr} 40-59 mL/minute: 5.3-5.8 hours

Pregnancy Risk Factor D

Pemirolast (pe MIR oh last)

U.S. Brand Names Alamast®

Canadian Brand Names Alamast®

Pharmacologic Category Mast Cell Stabilizer; Ophthalmic Agent, Miscellaneous

Use Prevention of itching of the eye due to allergic conjunctivitis

Local Anesthetic/Vasoconstrictor Precautions No information available to require special precautions

Effects on Dental Treatment No significant effects or complications reported

Effects on Bleeding No information available to require special precautions

Adverse Effects

>10%:

Central nervous system: Headache (10% to 25%)
Respiratory: Rhinitis (10% to 25%)
Miscellaneous: Cold/flu symptoms (10% to 25%)

<5%:

Central nervous system: Fever
Endocrine & metabolic: Dysmenorrhea
Neuromuscular & skeletal: Back pain
Ocular: Burning eyes, dry eyes, foreign body sensation, ocular discomfort
Respiratory: Bronchitis, cough, sinusitis, sneezing/nasal congestion

General Dosage Range Ophthalmic: *Children >3 years and Adults:* Instill 1-2 drops in affected eye(s) 4 times/day

Mechanism of Action Mast cell stabilizer that inhibits the *in vivo* type I immediate hypersensitivity reaction; in addition, inhibits chemotaxis of eosinophils into the ocular tissue and blocks their release of mediators; also reported to prevent calcium influx into mast cells following antigen stimulation

Pharmacodynamics/Kinetics

Onset of Action A few days; Peak effect: 4 weeks

Half-life Elimination 4.5 hours

Pregnancy Risk Factor C

Penbutolol (pen BYOO toe lole)

Related Information

Cardiovascular Diseases *on page 1848*

U.S. Brand Names Levatol®

Canadian Brand Names Levatol®

Pharmacologic Category Beta Blocker With Intrinsic Sympathomimetic Activity

Use Treatment of mild-to-moderate arterial hypertension

Local Anesthetic/Vasoconstrictor Precautions No information available to require special precautions

Effects on Dental Treatment Key adverse event(s) related to dental treatment: Xerostomia (normal salivary flow resumes upon discontinuation). Penbutolol is a nonselective beta-blocker and may enhance the pressor response to epinephrine, resulting in hypertension and bradycardia. Many nonsteroidal anti-inflammatory drugs, such as ibuprofen and indomethacin, can reduce the hypotensive effect of beta-blockers after 3 or more weeks of therapy with the NSAID. Short-term NSAID use (ie, 3 days) requires no special precautions in patients taking beta-blockers.

Effects on Bleeding No information available to require special precautions

Adverse Effects 1% to 10%:

Cardiovascular: CHF, arrhythmia

Central nervous system: Mental depression, headache, dizziness, fatigue

Gastrointestinal: Nausea, diarrhea, dyspepsia

Neuromuscular & skeletal: Arthralgia

General Dosage Range Oral: *Adults:* Initial: 20 mg once daily; Maintenance: 10-40 mg once daily (maximum: 80 mg/day)

Mechanism of Action Blocks both $beta_1$- and $beta_2$-receptors and has mild intrinsic sympathomimetic activity; has negative inotropic and chronotropic effects and can significantly slow AV nodal conduction

Pharmacodynamics/Kinetics

Onset of Action Peak effect: 1.3-3 hours

Duration of Action >20 hours

Half-life Elimination Penbutolol: 5 hours; Conjugated metabolite: ~20 hours with normal renal function, 100 hours with end-stage renal disease

Time to Peak Plasma: 2-3 hours

Pregnancy Risk Factor C

Penciclovir (pen SYE kloe veer)

Related Information

Systemic Viral Diseases *on page 1904*

Viral Infections *on page 1947*

Related Sample Prescriptions

Herpes Simplex (Recurrent) *on page 1990*

U.S. Brand Names Denavir®

Generic Availability (U.S.) No

Pharmacologic Category Antiviral Agent

Dental Use Topical treatment of herpes simplex labialis (cold sores)

Use Topical treatment of herpes simplex labialis (cold sores)

Local Anesthetic/Vasoconstrictor Precautions No information available to require special precautions

Effects on Dental Treatment No significant effects or complications reported

Effects on Bleeding No information available to require special precautions

Adverse Effects

>10%: Dermatologic: Mild erythema (50%)

1% to 10%: Central nervous system: Headache (5.3%)

Dental Usual Dosage Treatment of herpes simplex labialis (cold sores): Children ≥12 years and Adults: Topical: Apply cream at the first sign or symptom of cold sore (eg, tingling, swelling); apply every 2 hours during waking hours for 4 days

Dosage Children ≥12 years and Adults: Topical: Apply cream at the first sign or symptom of cold sore (eg, tingling, swelling); apply every 2 hours during waking hours for 4 days

Mechanism of Action In cells infected with HSV-1 or HSV-2, viral thymidine kinase phosphorylates penciclovir to a monophosphate form which, in turn, is converted to penciclovir triphosphate by cellular kinases. Penciclovir triphosphate inhibits HSV polymerase competitively with deoxyguanosine triphosphate. Consequently, herpes viral DNA synthesis and, therefore, replication are selectively inhibited

Contraindications Hypersensitivity to the penciclovir or any component of the formulation; previous and significant adverse reactions to famciclovir

Warnings/Precautions Penciclovir should only be used on herpes labialis on the lips and face; because no data are available, application to mucous membranes is not recommended. Avoid application in or near eyes since it may cause irritation. The effect of penciclovir has not been established in immunocompromised patients. Safety and efficacy have not been established in children <12 years of age.

Drug Interactions

Avoid Concomitant Use There are no known interactions where it is recommended to avoid concomitant use.

Increased Effect/Toxicity There are no known significant interactions involving an increase in effect.

Decreased Effect There are no known significant interactions involving a decrease in effect.

Pregnancy Risk Factor B

Lactation Excretion in breast milk unknown

Dosage Forms

Cream, topical:

Denavir®: 1% (1.5 g)

Penicillamine (pen i SIL a meen)

U.S. Brand Names Cuprimine®; Depen®

Canadian Brand Names Cuprimine®; Depen®

Pharmacologic Category Chelating Agent

Use Treatment of Wilson's disease, cystinuria; adjunctive treatment of rheumatoid arthritis

Unlabeled/Investigational Use Chelation therapy for the treatment of lead poisoning (third-line agent)

Local Anesthetic/Vasoconstrictor Precautions No information available to require special precautions

Effects on Dental Treatment Key adverse event(s) related to dental treatment: Oral ulcerations, glossitis, gingivostomatitis, and taste alteration.

Effects on Bleeding No information available to require special precautions

Adverse Effects Frequency not defined, may vary by indication. Adverse effects requiring discontinuation of treatment have been reported in 20% to 30% of patients with Wilson's disease.

Cardiovascular: Vasculitis

Central nervous system: Anxiety, agitation, fever, hyperpyrexia, psychiatric disturbances; worsening neurologic symptoms (10% to 50% patients with Wilson's disease)

Dermatologic: Alopecia, cheilosis, dermatomyositis, exfoliative dermatitis, lichen planus, rash (early and late 5%), pemphigus, pruritus, skin friability increased, toxic epidermal necrolysis, urticaria, wrinkling (excessive), yellow nail syndrome

Endocrine & metabolic: Hypoglycemia, thyroiditis

Gastrointestinal: Anorexia, diarrhea (17%), epigastric pain, gingivostomatitis, glossitis, nausea, oral ulcerations, pancreatitis, peptic ulcer reactivation, taste alteration (12%), vomiting

Hematologic: Eosinophilia, hemolytic anemia, leukocytosis, leukopenia (2% to 5%), monocytosis, red cell aplasia, thrombocytopenia (4% to 5%), thrombotic thrombocytopenia purpura, thrombocytosis

Hepatic: Alkaline phosphatase increased, hepatic failure, intrahepatic cholestasis, toxic hepatitis

Local: Thrombophlebitis, white papules at venipuncture and surgical sites

Neuromuscular & skeletal: Arthralgia, dystonia, myasthenia gravis, muscle weakness, neuropathies, polyarthralgia (migratory, often with objective synovitis), polymyositis

Ocular: Diplopia, extraocular muscle weakness, optic neuritis, ptosis, visual disturbances

Otic: Tinnitus

Renal: Goodpasture's syndrome, hematuria, nephrotic syndrome, proteinuria (6%), renal failure, renal vasculitis

Respiratory: Asthma, interstitial pneumonitis, pulmonary fibrosis, obliterative bronchiolitis

Miscellaneous: Allergic alveolitis, anetoderma, elastosis perforans serpiginosa, lupus-like syndrome, lactic dehydrogenase increased, lymphadenopathy, mammary hyperplasia, positive ANA test

General Dosage Range Dosage adjustment recommended in patients with renal impairment

Oral:

Children: 30 mg/kg/day in 4 divided doses

Adults: Dosage varies greatly depending on indication

Mechanism of Action Chelates with lead, copper, mercury and other heavy metals to form stable, soluble complexes that are excreted in urine; depresses circulating IgM rheumatoid factor, depresses T-cell but not B-cell activity; combines with cystine to form a compound which is more soluble, thus cystine calculi are prevented

Pharmacodynamics/Kinetics

Onset of Action Rheumatoid arthritis: 2-3 months; Wilson's disease: 1-3 months

Half-life Elimination 1.7-7 hours

Time to Peak Serum: 1-3 hours

Pregnancy Risk Factor D

Penicillin G Benzathine (pen i SIL in jee BENZ a theen)

Related Information

Sexually-Transmitted Diseases *on page 1903*

U.S. Brand Names Bicillin® L-A

Canadian Brand Names Bicillin® L-A

Pharmacologic Category Antibiotic, Penicillin

Use Active against some gram-positive organisms, few gram-negative organisms such as *Neisseria gonorrhoeae*, and some anaerobes and spirochetes; used in the treatment of syphilis; used only for the treatment of mild to moderately-severe upper respiratory tract infections caused by organisms susceptible to low concentrations of penicillin G or for prophylaxis of infections caused by these organisms; primary and secondary prevention of rheumatic fever

Local Anesthetic/Vasoconstrictor Precautions No information available to require special precautions

Effects on Dental Treatment No significant effects or complications reported

Effects on Bleeding No information available to require special precautions

Adverse Effects Frequency not defined.

Cardiovascular: Cardiac arrest, cerebral vascular accident, cyanosis, gangrene, hypotension, pallor, palpitations, syncope, tachycardia, vasodilation, vasospasm, vasovagal reaction

Central nervous system: Anxiety, coma, confusion, dizziness, euphoria, fatigue, headache, nervousness, pain, seizure, somnolence

In addition, a syndrome of CNS symptoms has been reported which includes: Severe agitation with confusion, hallucinations (auditory and visual), and fear of death (Hoigne's syndrome); other symptoms include cyanosis, dizziness, palpitations, psychosis, seizures, tachycardia, taste disturbance, tinnitus

Gastrointestinal: Bloody stool, intestinal necrosis, nausea, vomiting

Genitourinary: Impotence, priapism

Hepatic: AST increased

Local: Injection site reactions: Abscess, atrophy, bruising, cellulitis, edema, hemorrhage, inflammation, lump, necrosis, pain, skin ulcer

Neuromuscular & skeletal: Arthritis exacerbation, joint disorder, neurovascular damage, numbness, periostitis, rhabdomyolysis, transverse myelitis, tremor, weakness

Ocular: Blindness, blurred vision

Renal: BUN increased, creatinine increased, hematuria, myoglobinuria, neurogenic bladder, proteinuria, renal failure

Miscellaneous: Diaphoresis, hypersensitivity reactions, Jarisch-Herxheimer reaction, lymphadenopathy, mottling, warmth

General Dosage Range I.M.:

Neonates >1200 g: 50,000 units/kg/dose

Children ≤27 kg: 600,000 units/dose

Children >27 kg: 1.2 million units/dose

Adults: 1.2-2.4 million units as a single dose

Mechanism of Action Interferes with bacterial cell wall synthesis during active multiplication, causing cell wall death and resultant bactericidal activity against susceptible bacteria

Pharmacodynamics/Kinetics

Duration of Action Dose dependent: 1-4 weeks; larger doses result in more sustained levels

Time to Peak Serum: 12-24 hours

Pregnancy Risk Factor B

Penicillin G Benzathine and Penicillin G Procaine

(pen i SIL in jee BENZ a theen & pen i SIL in jee PROE kane)

Related Information

Penicillin G Benzathine *on page 1314*

Penicillin G Procaine *on page 1315*

U.S. Brand Names Bicillin® C-R; Bicillin® C-R 900/300

Pharmacologic Category Antibiotic, Penicillin

Use May be used in specific situations in the treatment of streptococcal infections; primary prevention of rheumatic fever

Local Anesthetic/Vasoconstrictor Precautions No information available to require special precautions

Effects on Dental Treatment No significant effects or complications reported

Effects on Bleeding No information available to require special precautions

Adverse Effects See individual agents.

General Dosage Range I.M.:

Children <14 kg: 600,000 units/dose

Children 14-27 kg: 900,000 units to 1.2 million units as a single dose

Children >27 kg and Adults: 2.4 million units/dose

Mechanism of Action Inhibits bacterial cell wall synthesis by binding to one or more of the penicillin-binding proteins (PBPs); which in turn inhibits the final transpeptidation step of peptidoglycan synthesis in bacterial cell walls, thus inhibiting cell wall biosynthesis. Bacteria eventually lyse due to ongoing activity of cell wall autolytic enzymes (autolysins and murein hydrolases) while cell wall assembly is arrested.

Pharmacodynamics/Kinetics

Time to Peak Serum: I.M.: Within 3 hours

Pregnancy Risk Factor B

Penicillin G (Parenteral/Aqueous)

(pen i SIL in jee, pa REN ter al, AYE kwee us)

Related Information

Sexually-Transmitted Diseases *on page 1903*

U.S. Brand Names Pfizerpen®

Canadian Brand Names Crystapen®

Pharmacologic Category Antibiotic, Penicillin

Use Treatment of infections (including sepsis, pneumonia, pericarditis, endocarditis, meningitis, anthrax) caused by susceptible organisms; active against some gram-positive organisms, generally not *Staphylococcus aureus*; some gram-negative organisms such as *Neisseria gonorrhoeae*, and some anaerobes and spirochetes

Local Anesthetic/Vasoconstrictor Precautions No information available to require special precautions

Effects on Dental Treatment No significant effects or complications reported

Effects on Bleeding No information available to require special precautions

Adverse Effects Frequency not defined.

Central nervous system: Coma (high doses), hyper-reflexia (high doses), seizures (high doses)

Dermatologic: Contact dermatitis, rash

Endocrine & metabolic: Electrolyte imbalance (high doses)

Gastrointestinal: Pseudomembranous colitis

Hematologic: Neutropenia, positive Coombs' hemolytic anemia (rare, high doses)

Local: Injection site reaction, phlebitis, thrombophlebitis

Neuromuscular & skeletal: Myoclonus (high doses)

Renal: Acute interstitial nephritis (high doses), renal tubular damage (high doses)

Miscellaneous: Anaphylaxis, hypersensitivity reactions (immediate and delayed), Jarisch-Herxheimer reaction, serum sickness

General Dosage Range Dosage adjustment recommended in patients with renal impairment

I.M., I.V.:

Infants ≥1 month and Children: 100,000-400,000 units/kg/day in divided doses every 4-6 hours (maximum: 24 million units/day)

Adults: 2-30 million units/day in divided doses every 4-6 hours

Mechanism of Action Interferes with bacterial cell wall synthesis during active multiplication, causing cell wall death and resultant bactericidal activity against susceptible bacteria

Pharmacodynamics/Kinetics

Half-life Elimination

Neonates: <6 days old: 3.2-3.4 hours; 7-13 days old: 1.2-2.2 hours; >14 days old: 0.9-1.9 hours

Children and Adults: Normal renal function: 30-50 minutes

End-stage renal disease: 3.3-5.1 hours

Time to Peak Serum: I.M.: ~30 minutes; I.V.: ~1 hour

Pregnancy Risk Factor B

Penicillin G Procaine (pen i SIL in jee PROE kane)

Canadian Brand Names Pfizerpen-AS®; Wycillin®

Pharmacologic Category Antibiotic, Penicillin

Use Treatment of moderately-severe infections due to *Treponema pallidum* and other penicillin G-sensitive microorganisms that are susceptible to low, but prolonged serum penicillin concentrations; anthrax due to *Bacillus anthracis* (postexposure) to reduce the incidence or progression of disease following exposure to aerolized *Bacillus anthracis*

Local Anesthetic/Vasoconstrictor Precautions No information available to require special precautions

Effects on Dental Treatment No significant effects or complications reported

Effects on Bleeding No information available to require special precautions

Adverse Effects Frequency not defined.

Cardiovascular: Conduction disturbances, myocardial depression, vasodilation

Central nervous system: CNS stimulation, confusion, drowsiness, myoclonus, seizure

Hematologic: Hemolytic anemia, neutropenia, positive Coombs' reaction

Local: Pain at injection site, sterile abscess at injection site, thrombophlebitis

Renal: Interstitial nephritis

Miscellaneous: Hypersensitivity reactions, Jarisch-Herxheimer reaction, pseudoanaphylactic reactions, serum sickness

General Dosage Range Dosage adjustment recommended in patients with renal impairment

I.M.:

Children: 25,000-50,000 units/kg/day in divided doses 1-2 times/day (maximum: 4.8 million units/day)

Adults: 0.6-4.8 million units/day in divided doses every 12-24 hours

Mechanism of Action Inhibits bacterial cell wall synthesis by binding to one or more of the penicillin-binding proteins (PBPs); which in turn inhibits the final transpeptidation step of peptidoglycan synthesis in bacterial cell walls, thus inhibiting cell wall biosynthesis. Bacteria eventually lyse due to ongoing activity of cell wall autolytic enzymes (autolysins and murein hydrolases) while cell wall assembly is arrested.

Pharmacodynamics/Kinetics

Duration of Action Therapeutic: 15-24 hours

Time to Peak Serum: 1-4 hours

Pregnancy Risk Factor B

Penicillin V Potassium (pen i SIL in vee poe TASS ee um)

Related Information

Antibiotic Prophylaxis *on page 1910*

Bacterial Infections *on page 1933*

Viral Infections *on page 1947*

Related Sample Prescriptions

Bacterial Infections and Periodontal Diseases *on page 1983*

Canadian Brand Names Apo-Pen VK®; Novo-Pen-VK; Nu-Pen-VK

Generic Availability (U.S.) Yes

Pharmacologic Category Antibiotic, Penicillin

Dental Use Antibiotic of first choice in treatment of common orofacial infections caused by aerobic gram-positive cocci and anaerobes. These orofacial infections include cellulitis, periapical abscess, periodontal abscess, acute suppurative pulpitis, oronasal fistula, pericoronitis, osteitis, osteomyelitis, postsurgical and posttraumatic infection. **Note: This agent is no longer recommended for dental procedure prophylaxis.**

Use Treatment of infections caused by susceptible organisms involving the respiratory tract, otitis media, sinusitis, skin, and urinary tract; prophylaxis in rheumatic fever

Local Anesthetic/Vasoconstrictor Precautions No information available to require special precautions

Effects on Dental Treatment Key adverse event(s) related to dental treatment: Oral candidiasis (prolonged use).

Effects on Bleeding No information available to require special precautions

Adverse Effects >10%: Gastrointestinal: Mild diarrhea, vomiting, nausea, oral candidiasis

Dental Usual Dosage Note: No longer recommended for dental procedure prophylaxis

Orofacial infections: Oral:

Children <12 years: 25-50 mg/kg/day in divided doses every 6-8 hours (maximum dose: 3 g/day)

Children ≥12 years and Adults: 125-500 mg every 6-8 hours

Dosage

Usual dosage range:

Children <12 years: Oral: 25-50 mg/kg/day in divided doses every 6-8 hours (maximum dose: 3 g/day)

Children ≥12 years and Adults: Oral: 125-500 mg every 6-8 hours

Indication-specific dosing:

Children: Oral:

Pharyngitis (streptococcal): 250 mg 2-3 times/day for 10 days

Prophylaxis of pneumococcal infections:

Children <5 years: 125 mg twice daily

Children ≥5 years: 250 mg twice daily

Prophylaxis of recurrent rheumatic fever:

Children <5 years: 125 mg twice daily

Children ≥5 years: 250 mg twice daily

Adults: Oral:

Actinomycosis:

Mild: 2-4 g/day in 4 divided doses for 8 weeks

Surgical: 2-4 g/day in 4 divided doses for 6-12 months (after I.V. penicillin G therapy of 4-6 weeks)

Erysipelas: 500 mg 4 times/day

Periodontal infections: 250-500 mg every 6 hours for 5-7 days

Note: Efficacy of antimicrobial therapy in periapical abscess is questionable; the American Academy of Periodontology recommends use of antibiotic therapy only when systemic symptoms (eg, fever, lymphadenopathy) are present or in immunocompromised patients.

Pharyngitis (streptococcal): 500 mg 3-4 times/day for 10 days

Prophylaxis of pneumococcal or recurrent rheumatic fever infections: 250 mg twice daily

Dosing interval in renal impairment: Cl_{cr} <10 mL/minute: Administer 250 mg every 6 hours

Mechanism of Action Inhibits bacterial cell wall synthesis by binding to one or more of the penicillin-binding proteins (PBPs); which in turn inhibits the final transpeptidation step of peptidoglycan synthesis in bacterial cell walls, thus inhibiting cell wall biosynthesis. Bacteria eventually lyse due to ongoing activity of cell wall autolytic enzymes (autolysins and murein hydrolases) while cell wall assembly is arrested.

Contraindications Hypersensitivity to penicillin or any component of the formulation

Warnings/Precautions Use with caution in patients with severe renal impairment (modify dosage) or history of seizures. Serious and occasionally severe or fatal hypersensitivity (anaphylactoid) reactions have been reported in patients on penicillin therapy, especially with a history of beta-lactam hypersensitivity, history of sensitivity to multiple allergens, or previous IgE-mediated reactions (eg, anaphylaxis, angioedema, urticaria). Use with caution in asthmatic patients. Extended duration of therapy or use associated with high serum concentrations may be associated with an increased risk for some adverse reactions. Prolonged use may result in fungal or bacterial superinfection, including *C. difficile*-associated diarrhea (CDAD) and pseudomembranous colitis; CDAD has been observed >2 months postantibiotic treatment.

Drug Interactions

Avoid Concomitant Use

Avoid concomitant use of Penicillin V Potassium with any of the following: BCG

Increased Effect/Toxicity

Penicillin V Potassium may increase the levels/effects of: Methotrexate

The levels/effects of Penicillin V Potassium may be increased by: Probenecid

Decreased Effect

Penicillin V Potassium may decrease the levels/effects of: BCG; Mycophenolate; Typhoid Vaccine

The levels/effects of Penicillin V Potassium may be decreased by: Fusidic Acid; Tetracycline Derivatives

Ethanol/Nutrition/Herb Interactions Food: Decreases drug absorption rate; decreases drug serum concentration.

Dietary Considerations Take on an empty stomach 1 hour before or 2 hours after meals.

Pharmacodynamics/Kinetics

Half-life Elimination 30 minutes; prolonged with renal impairment

Time to Peak Serum: 0.5-1 hour

Pregnancy Risk Factor B

Lactation Enters breast milk/compatible

Breast-Feeding Considerations Penicillins are excreted in breast milk. The manufacturer recommends that caution be exercised when administering penicillin to nursing women. Nondose-related effects could include modification of bowel flora and allergic sensitization.

Dosage Forms

Powder for solution, oral: 125 mg/5 mL (100 mL, 200 mL); 250 mg/5 mL (100 mL, 200 mL)

Tablet, oral: 250 mg, 500 mg

References

Wynn RL and Bergman SA, "Antibiotics and Their Use in the Treatment of Orofacial Infections, Part I," *Gen Dent*, 1994, 42(5):398, 400, 402.
Wynn RL and Bergman SA, "Antibiotics and Their Use in the Treatment of Orofacial Infections, Part II," *Gen Dent*, 1994, 42(6):498-502.
Wynn RL, Bergman SA, Meiller TF, et al, "Antibiotics in Treating Oral-Facial Infections of Odontogenic Origin: An Update," *Gen Dent*, 2001, 49(3):238-40, 242, 244 passim.

Pentafluoropropane and Tetrafluoroethane

(pen ta flure oh PRO pane & tet ra flure oh ETH ane)

U.S. Brand Names Gebauer's Instant Ice™ [OTC]; Gebauer's Pain Ease®; Gebauer's Spray and Stretch®

Pharmacologic Category Anesthetic, Topical

Use Treatment of myofascial pain, restricted motion due to muscle tension, muscle spasm and minor sports injuries (eg, bruises, contusions, swelling, minor sprains); pain associated with injections or minor surgical procedures

Local Anesthetic/Vasoconstrictor Precautions No information available to require special precautions

Effects on Dental Treatment No significant effects or complications reported

Effects on Bleeding No information available to require special precautions

Adverse Effects Frequency not defined.

Dermatologic: Skin irritation, skin pigmentation change, frostbite

General Dosage Range Topical: *Adults:* Spray over affected area for 4-10 seconds from a distance of 3-7 inches (8-18 cm) at a rate of ~4 inches/second (10 cm/second); Reapply as needed

Mechanism of Action Vapocoolant and counterirritant

Pentamidine (pen TAM i deen)

Related Information

Clinical Risk Related to Drugs Prolonging QT Interval *on page 1872*

U.S. Brand Names Nebupent®; Pentam® 300

Pharmacologic Category Antibiotic, Miscellaneous; Antiprotozoal

Use Treatment and prevention of pneumonia caused by *Pneumocystis jiroveci* pneumonia (PCP)

Unlabeled/Investigational Use Treatment of African trypanosomiasis, cutaneous leishmaniasis, and amebic meningoencephalitis

Local Anesthetic/Vasoconstrictor Precautions Pentamidine is one of the drugs confirmed to prolong the QT interval and is accepted as having a risk of causing torsade de pointes. The risk of drug-induced torsade de pointes is extremely low when a single QT interval prolonging drug is prescribed. In terms of epinephrine, it is not known what effect vasoconstrictors in the local anesthetic regimen will have in patients with a known history of congenital prolonged QT interval or in patients taking any medication that prolongs the QT interval. Until more information is obtained, it is suggested that the clinician consult with the physician prior to the use of a vasoconstrictor in suspected patients, and that the vasoconstrictor (epinephrine, mepivacaine and levonordefrin [Carbocaine® 2% with Neo-Cobefrin®]) be used with caution.

Effects on Dental Treatment No significant effects or complications reported

Effects on Bleeding No information available to require special precautions

Adverse Effects

Aerosol:

>10%:

Central nervous system: Fatigue (66%), fever (51%), dizziness/lightheadedness (45%)
Gastrointestinal: Appetite decreased (50%)
Respiratory: Cough (1% to 63%), dyspnea (48%), wheezing (32%)
Miscellaneous: Infection (15%)

1% to 10%:

Central nervous system: Headache
Gastrointestinal: Diarrhea, nausea, oral candida, taste alteration
Hematologic: Anemia
Respiratory: Bronchitis, chest pain, pharyngitis, sinusitis, upper respiratory tract infection
Miscellaneous: Herpes infection, influenza, night sweats

Injection:

>10%:

Local: Local reactions at I.M. injection site (11%; includes sterile abscess, necrosis, pain, induration)

Renal: Renal function impaired (29%), creatinine increased (24%)

1% to 10%:

Cardiovascular: Hypotension (5%)

Central nervous system: Confusion/hallucinations (2%)

Dermatologic: Rash (3%)

Endocrine & metabolic: Hypoglycemia (6%)

Gastrointestinal: Nausea/anorexia (6%), taste alteration (2%)

Hematologic: Leukopenia (10%), thrombocytopenia (3%), anemia (1%)

Hepatic: Liver function tests increased (9%)

Renal: Azotemia (9%), BUN increased (7%)

General Dosage Range Dosage adjustment recommended in patients with renal impairment

I.M.: *Children and Adults:* 4 mg/kg once daily for 14-21 days

I.V.:

Children: 4 mg/kg once daily for 7-21 days **or** 3-4 mg/kg once daily for 21 days

Adults: 4 mg/kg once daily for 14-21 days **or** 3-4 mg/kg once daily for 21 days

Inhalation: *Children ≥5 years and Adults:* 300 mg/dose every 4 weeks

Mechanism of Action Interferes with RNA/DNA, phospholipids and protein synthesis, through inhibition of oxidative phosphorylation and/or interference with incorporation of nucleotides and nucleic acids into RNA and DNA, in protozoa

Pharmacodynamics/Kinetics

Half-life Elimination I.V.: 5-8 hours; I.M.: 7-11 hours; may be prolonged with severe renal impairment

Pregnancy Risk Factor C

Dental Comment Pentamidine is known to prolong the QT interval. The QT interval is measured as the time and distance between the Q point of the QRS complex and the end of the T wave in the ECG tracing. After adjustment for heart rate, the QT interval is defined as prolonged if it is more than 450 msec in men and 460 msec in women. A long QT syndrome was first described in the 1950s and 60s as a congenital syndrome involving QT interval prolongation and syncope and sudden death. Some of the congenital long QT syndromes were characterized by a peculiar electrocardiographic appearance of the QRS complex involving a premature atria beat followed by a pause, then a subsequent sinus beat showing marked QT prolongation and deformity. This type of cardiac arrhythmia was originally termed "torsade de pointes" (translated from the French as "twisting of the points"). Pentamidine is considered as having a risk of causing torsade de pointes. Since it is not known what effect vasoconstrictors in the local anesthetic regimen will have in patients with a known history of congenital prolonged QT interval or in patients taking any medication that prolongs the QT interval, a medical consult is suggested.

Pentastarch (PEN ta starch)

Canadian Brand Names Pentaspan®

Pharmacologic Category Plasma Volume Expander, Colloid

Use Adjunctive treatment in the management of shock

Local Anesthetic/Vasoconstrictor Precautions No information available to require special precautions

Effects on Dental Treatment No significant effects or complications reported

Effects on Bleeding No information available to require special precautions

Adverse Effects Frequency not defined.

Cardiovascular: Angina, edema, tachycardia

Central nervous system: Anxiety, chills, dizziness, fatigue, fever, headache, insomnia, malaise, shakiness

Dermatologic: Acne

Endocrine & metabolic: Amylase increased

Gastrointestinal: Diarrhea, nausea, weight gain (temporary)

Hematologic: Coagulation disorder, hemorrhage

Hepatic: Bilirubin increased

Neuromuscular & skeletal: Paresthesia, weakness

Respiratory: Nasal congestion

Miscellaneous: Anaphylactic/anaphylactoid reaction, hypersensitivity (hypotension, urticaria, wheezing)

General Dosage Range I.V.: *Adults:* 500-2000 mL/day (maximum daily dose: 28 mL/kg or 2000 mL)

Mechanism of Action Produces plasma volume expansion by virtue of its highly colloidal starch structure

Pharmacodynamics/Kinetics

Onset of Action Volume expansion: Within 1 hour

Duration of Action 18-24 hours (improves hemodynamic status for 12-18 hours)

Half-life Elimination ~2 days

Product Availability Not available in U.S.

Pentazocine (pen TAZ oh seen)

U.S. Brand Names Talwin®

Canadian Brand Names Talwin®

Pharmacologic Category Analgesic, Opioid; Analgesic, Opioid Partial Agonist

Use Relief of moderate-to-severe pain; has also been used as a sedative prior to surgery and as a supplement to surgical anesthesia

Local Anesthetic/Vasoconstrictor Precautions No information available to require special precautions

Effects on Dental Treatment Key adverse event(s) related to dental treatment: Xerostomia (normal salivary flow resumes upon discontinuation).

Effects on Bleeding No information available to require special precautions

Adverse Effects Frequency not defined.

Cardiovascular: Circulatory depression, facial edema, flushing, hyper-/hypotension, shock, syncope, systemic vascular resistance increased, tachycardia

Central nervous system: Chills, CNS depression, confusion, disorientation, dizziness, drowsiness, euphoria, excitement, hallucinations, headache, insomnia, irritability, lightheadedness, malaise, nightmares, sedation

Dermatologic: Dermatitis, erythema multiforme, pruritus, rash, Stevens-Johnson syndrome, toxic epidermal necrolysis, urticaria

Gastrointestinal: Abdominal distress, anorexia, constipation, diarrhea, nausea, taste alteration, vomiting, xerostomia

Genitourinary: Urinary retention

Hematologic: Agranulocytosis (rare), eosinophilia, WBCs decreased

Local: Injection site reaction (tissue damage and irritation)

Neuromuscular & skeletal: Paresthesia, tremor, weakness

Ocular: Blurred vision, diplopia, miosis, nystagmus

Otic: Tinnitus

Respiratory: Dyspnea, respiratory depression (rare)

Miscellaneous: Anaphylaxis, diaphoresis, physical and psychological dependence

General Dosage Range Dosage adjustment recommended in patients with renal impairment

I.M.:

Children 1-16 years: 0.5 mg/kg preoperatively

Adults: 30-60 mg every 3-4 hours (maximum: 360 mg/day; 60 mg/dose) **or** 30 mg once

I.V.: *Adults:* 30 mg every 3-4 hours (maximum: 360 mg/day; 30 mg/dose) **or** 20 mg every 2-3 hours as needed (maximum total dose: 60 mg)

SubQ: *Adults:* 30 mg every 3-4 hours (maximum: 360 mg/day; 60 mg/dose)

Mechanism of Action Binds to opiate receptors in the CNS, causing inhibition of ascending pain pathways, altering the perception of and response to pain; produces generalized CNS depression; partial agonist-antagonist

Pharmacodynamics/Kinetics

Onset of Action I.M., SubQ: 15-20 minutes; I.V.: 2-3 minutes

Duration of Action 2-3 hours

Half-life Elimination 2-3 hours; prolonged with hepatic impairment

Pregnancy Risk Factor C

Controlled Substance C-IV

Pentazocine and Acetaminophen (pen TAZ oh seen & a seet a MIN oh fen)

Related Information

Acetaminophen *on page 32*

Pentazocine *on page 1320*

Generic Availability (U.S.) Yes

Pharmacologic Category Analgesic Combination (Opioid); Analgesic, Opioid Partial Agonist

Dental Use Relief of mild-to-moderate pain

Use Relief of mild-to-moderate pain

Local Anesthetic/Vasoconstrictor Precautions No information available to require special precautions

Effects on Dental Treatment No significant effects or complications reported (see Dental Comment)

Effects on Bleeding No information available to require special precautions

Adverse Effects Adverse reactions attributed to pentazocine 50 mg. Frequency not defined. See Acetaminophen monograph for acetaminophen-related reactions.

Cardiovascular: Circulatory depression, facial edema, flushing, hyper-/hypotension, syncope, tachycardia

Central nervous system: Chills, confusion, depression, disorientation, dizziness, drowsiness, euphoria, excitement, hallucinations, headache, insomnia, intracranial pressure increased, irritability, lightheadedness, nightmares, sedation, seizure

Dermatologic: Dermatitis, erythema multiforme, pruritus, rash, Stevens-Johnson syndrome, toxic epidermal necrolysis, urticaria

Gastrointestinal: Abdominal distress, anorexia, biliary spasm, constipation, diarrhea, nausea, vomiting, xerostomia

Genitourinary: Urinary retention

Hematologic: Agranulocytosis, eosinophilia, WBCs decreased

Neuromuscular & skeletal: Paresthesia, tremor, weakness

Ocular: Blurred vision, miosis

Otic: Tinnitus

Respiratory: Respiratory depression

Miscellaneous: Anaphylaxis, diaphoresis, physical and psychological dependence, withdrawal syndrome

Dental Usual Dosage Analgesic: Adults: Oral: 1 caplet every 4 hours (maximum: 6 caplets/day)

Dosage Note: Maximum daily intake of acetaminophen from all sources should not exceed 4 g.

Oral: Children ≥12 years and Adults: Analgesic: One caplet (pentazocine 25 mg/ acetaminophen 650 mg) every 4 hours as needed (maximum: 6 caplets/day)

Dosage adjustment in renal impairment: Use with caution. Manufacturer labeling does not provide specific dosing recommendations; less frequent administration may be necessary.

Dosage adjustment in hepatic impairment: Use with caution. Manufacturer labeling does not provide specific dosing recommendations; less frequent administration may be necessary.

Mechanism of Action

Pentazocine: Binds to opiate receptors in the CNS, causing inhibition of ascending pain pathways, altering the perception of and response to pain; produces generalized CNS depression; partial agonist-antagonist

Acetaminophen: Inhibits the synthesis of prostaglandins in the central nervous system and peripherally blocks pain impulse generation

Contraindications Hypersensitivity to pentazocine, acetaminophen, or any component of the formulation; hypersensitivity to sulfites (contains metabisulfite)

Warnings/Precautions Contains sodium metabisulfite; may cause allergic-type reactions including anaphylaxis; potential for elevating CSF pressure due to respiratory effects which may be exaggerated in presence of head injury, intracranial lesions, or pre-existing increase in intracranial lesions. May cause CNS depression, which may impair physical or mental abilities; patients must be cautioned about performing tasks which require mental alertness (eg, operating machinery or driving). Effects may be potentiated when used with other sedative drugs or ethanol. Confusion, disorientation, and visual hallucinations have occurred in some patients, but usually clears within a few hours; observe patients closely. May cause severe hepatic toxicity on acute overdose; in addition, chronic daily dosing in adults has resulted in liver damage in some patients. May cause psychological and physical dependence. May obscure diagnosis or clinical course of patients with acute abdominal conditions. Use with caution in patients with respiratory depression, G6PD deficiency, biliary tract impairment, prostatic hyperplasia, urinary stricture, ethanol abuse, CNS depression, coma, myocardial infarction, porphyria, hypothyroidism, severely limited respiratory reserve, severe bronchial asthma, other obstructive respiratory conditions or cyanosis, impaired renal or hepatic function, patients prone to seizures. Use with caution in elderly or debilitated patients. Abrupt discontinuation may result in withdrawal symptoms; taper dose to decrease risk of withdrawal symptoms. Pentazocine may precipitate opiate withdrawal symptoms in patients who have been receiving opiates regularly. Pentazocine clearance may be increased in tobacco smokers.

Drug Interactions

Avoid Concomitant Use There are no known interactions where it is recommended to avoid concomitant use.

Increased Effect/Toxicity

Pentazocine and Acetaminophen may increase the levels/effects of: Alcohol (Ethyl); Alvimopan; CNS Depressants; Dasatinib; Desmopressin; Imatinib; Selective Serotonin Reuptake Inhibitors; SORAfenib; Thiazide Diuretics; Vitamin K Antagonists

The levels/effects of Pentazocine and Acetaminophen may be increased by: Amphetamines; Antipsychotic Agents (Phenothiazines); Conivaptan; Dasatinib; Droperidol; Imatinib; Isoniazid; Metyrapone; Probenecid; SORAfenib; Succinylcholine

Decreased Effect

Pentazocine and Acetaminophen may decrease the levels/effects of: Analgesics (Opioid); Pegvisomant

The levels/effects of Pentazocine and Acetaminophen may be decreased by: Ammonium Chloride; Anticonvulsants (Hydantoin); Barbiturates; CarBAMazepine; Cholestyramine Resin; Peginterferon Alfa-2b; Tocilizumab

Ethanol/Nutrition/Herb Interactions

Ethanol: Avoid ethanol (may increase CNS depression).

Herb/Nutraceutical: Avoid valerian, St John's wort, kava kava, gotu kola (may increase CNS depression).

Pregnancy Risk Factor C

Lactation Pentazocine and acetaminophen enter breast milk/use caution

Breast-Feeding Considerations See individual agents.

Controlled Substance C-IV

Dosage Forms

Tablet: Pentazocine 25 mg and acetaminophen 650 mg

Dental Comment Hepatotoxicity caused by acetaminophen is potentiated by chronic alcohol consumption. People who are taking acetaminophen, even at therapeutic doses, and consume alcohol are at risk of developing hepatotoxicity.

Acetaminophen may increase the levels and enhance the anticoagulant effects of vitamin K antagonists acenocoumarol and warfarin (Coumadin®). Studies have reported that acetaminophen has increased the INR in warfarin treated patients with daily acetaminophen doses as low as 2 g, particularly when taking acetaminophen for >1 week (Antlitz, 1968; Boeijinga, 1982; Gebauer, 2003; Hylek, 1998; Rubin, 1984). In addition, case reports of bleeding as a result of increased INR have been published (Bagheri, 1999; Bartle, 1991). There is no known mechanism of the interaction; furthermore, some studies have failed to demonstrate this interaction (Gadisseur, 2003; Kwan, 1995; van den Bemt, 2002). In terms of risk, the data suggest that acetaminophen and warfarin could interact in some clinically significant manner but that the benefits of concomitant use of acetaminophen for pain control in dental patients taking warfarin usually outweigh the risks. An appropriate monitoring plan should be in place to identify potential negative effects and dosage adjustments may be necessary in a minority of patients. The interaction may be more likely to occur with daily acetaminophen doses of >1.3 g for >1 week.

There are no reports of acetaminophen interacting with antiplatelet drugs such as aspirin, clopidogrel (Plavix®), or prasugrel (Effient™). Also, there are no reports of acetaminophen in combination with hydrocodone, codeine, or oxycodone interacting with warfarin (Coumadin®).

References

Antlitz AM, Mead JA Jr, and Tolentino MA, "Potentiation of Oral Anticoagulant Therapy by Acetaminophen," *Curr Ther Res Clin Exp*, 1968, 10(10):501-7.

Bagheri H, Bernhard NB, and Montastruc JL, "Potentiation of the Acenocoumarol Anticoagulant Effect by Acetaminophen," *Ann Pharmacother*, 1999, 33(4):506.

Bartle WR and Blakely JA, "Potentiation of Warfarin Anticoagulation by Acetaminophen," *JAMA*, 1991, 265(10):1260.

Boeijinga JJ, Boerstra EE, Ris P, et al, "Interaction Between Paracetamol and Coumarin Anticoagulants," *Lancet*, 1982, 1(8270):506.

Gadisseur AP, Van Der Meer FJ, and Rosendaal FR, "Sustained Intake of Paracetamol (Acetaminophen) During Oral Anticoagulant Therapy With Coumarins Does Not Cause Clinically Important INR Changes: A Randomized Double-Blind Clinical Trial," *J Thromb Haemost*, 2003, 1(4):714-7.

Gebauer MG, Nyfort-Hansen K, Henschke PJ, et al, "Warfarin and Acetaminophen Interaction," *Pharmacotherapy*, 2003, 23(1):109-12.

Hylek EM, Heiman H, Skates SJ, et al, "Acetaminophen and Other Risk Factors for Excessive Warfarin Anticoagulation," *JAMA*, 1998, 279(9):657-62.

Kwan D, Bartle WR, and Walker SE, "The Effects of Acute and Chronic Acetaminophen Dosing on the Pharmacodynamics and Pharmacokinetics of (R)- and (S)-Warfarin," *Clin Pharmacol Ther*, 1995, 57:212.

Rubin RN, Mentzer RL, and Budzynski AZ, "Potentiation of Anticoagulant Effect of Warfarin by Acetaminophen (Tylenol®)," *Clin Res*, 1984, 32:698a.

van den Bemt PM, Geven LM, Kuitert NA, et al, "The Potential Interaction Between Oral Anticoagulants and Acetaminophen in Everyday Practice," *Pharm World Sci*, 2002, 24(5):201-4.

PENTobarbital (pen toe BAR bi tal)

U.S. Brand Names Nembutal®

Canadian Brand Names Nembutal® Sodium

Pharmacologic Category Anticonvulsant, Barbiturate; Barbiturate

Use Sedative/hypnotic; refractory status epilepticus

Unlabeled/Investigational Use Barbiturate coma in patients with severe brain injury (eg, hemorrhagic stroke, traumatic brain injury) and increased intracranial pressure

Local Anesthetic/Vasoconstrictor Precautions No information available to require special precautions

Effects on Dental Treatment No significant effects or complications reported

Effects on Bleeding No information available to require special precautions

Adverse Effects Frequency not defined.

Cardiovascular: Bradycardia, hypotension, syncope

Central nervous system: Abnormal thinking, agitation, anxiety, ataxia, CNS excitation, confusion, depression, dizziness, drowsiness, fever, hallucinations, headache, hyperkinesia, insomnia, nervousness, nightmares, psychiatric disturbances, somnolence

Dermatologic: Angioedema, exfoliative dermatitis, rash

Gastrointestinal: Constipation, nausea, vomiting

Hematologic: Megaloblastic anemia

Hepatic: Hepatotoxicity

Local: Injection site reactions

Respiratory: Apnea (especially with rapid I.V. use), hypoventilation, laryngospasm, respiratory depression

Miscellaneous: Gangrene with inadvertent intra-arterial injection, hypersensitivity reactions

General Dosage Range

I.M.:

Children: 2-6 mg/kg (maximum: 100 mg/dose)

Adults: 150-200 mg

I.V.:

Children:

Hypnotic/sedative: 1-6 mg/kg

Refractory status epilepticus: Loading dose: 5-15 mg/kg; Maintenance infusion: 0.5-5 mg/kg/hour

Adults:

Hypnotic/sedative: 100 mg; may repeat (maximum total dose: 500 mg)

Refractory status epilepticus: Loading dose: 10-15 mg/kg; Maintenance infusion: 0.5-10 mg/kg/hour

Mechanism of Action Barbiturate with sedative, hypnotic, and anticonvulsant properties. Barbiturates depress the sensory cortex, decrease motor activity, alter cerebellar function, and produce drowsiness, sedation, and hypnosis. In high doses, barbiturates exhibit anticonvulsant activity; barbiturates produce dose-dependent respiratory depression; reduce brain metabolism and cerebral blood flow in order to decrease intracranial pressure

Pharmacodynamics/Kinetics

Onset of Action I.M.: 10-15 minutes (Krauss, 2006); I.V.: Almost immediate, within 3-5 minutes (Krauss, 2006)

Duration of Action I.V.: Variable

Half-life Elimination Terminal: Children: 26 ± 16 hours (Schaible, 1982); Adults: Healthy: 22 hours (average; Ehrnebo, 1974); (range: 15-50 hours; dose dependent)

Pregnancy Risk Factor D

Controlled Substance C-II

Pentosan Polysulfate Sodium (PEN toe san pol i SUL fate SOW dee um)

U.S. Brand Names Elmiron®

Canadian Brand Names Elmiron®

Pharmacologic Category Analgesic, Urinary

Use Relief of bladder pain or discomfort due to interstitial cystitis

Local Anesthetic/Vasoconstrictor Precautions No information available to require special precautions

Effects on Dental Treatment No significant effects or complications reported

Effects on Bleeding Pentosan polysulfate sodium is a low-molecular weight heparin-like compound with anticoagulant and fibrinolytic effects. Medical consult is suggested.

Adverse Effects 1% to 10%:

Central nervous system: Headache (3%), dizziness (1%)

Dermatologic: Alopecia (4%), rash (3%)

Gastrointestinal: Rectal hemorrhage (6%), diarrhea (4%), nausea (4%), abdominal pain (2%), dyspepsia (2%)

Hepatic: Liver function test abnormalities (1%; dose related)

General Dosage Range Oral: *Children ≥16 years and Adults:* 100 mg 3 times/day

Mechanism of Action Although pentosan polysulfate sodium is a low-molecular weight heparinoid, it is not known whether these properties play a role in its mechanism of action in treating interstitial cystitis; the drug appears to adhere to the bladder wall mucosa where it may act as a buffer to protect the tissues from irritating substances in the urine.

Pharmacodynamics/Kinetics

Half-life Elimination 20-27 hours

Time to Peak Serum: 2 hours (range: 0.6-120 hours)

Pregnancy Risk Factor B

Pentostatin (pen toe STAT in)

U.S. Brand Names Nipent®

Canadian Brand Names Nipent®

Pharmacologic Category Antineoplastic Agent, Antibiotic; Antineoplastic Agent, Antimetabolite (Purine Analog)

Use Treatment of hairy cell leukemia

Unlabeled/Investigational Use Treatment of cutaneous T-cell lymphoma, chronic lymphocytic leukemia (CLL), and acute and chronic graft-versus-host-disease (GVHD)

Local Anesthetic/Vasoconstrictor Precautions No information available to require special precautions

Effects on Dental Treatment Key adverse event(s) related to dental treatment: Stomatitis.

Effects on Bleeding Chemotherapy may result in significant myelosuppression, potentially including significant reduction in platelet counts and altered hemostasis. In patients who are under active treatment with these agents, medical consult is suggested.

Adverse Effects

>10%:

Central nervous system: Fever (42% to 46%), fatigue (29% to 42%), pain (8% to 20%), chills (11% to 19%), headache (13% to 17%), CNS toxicity (1% to 11%)

Dermatologic: Rash (26% to 43%), pruritus (10% to 21%), skin disorder (4% to 17%)

Gastrointestinal: Nausea/vomiting (22% to 63%), diarrhea (15% to 17%), anorexia (13% to 16%), abdominal pain (4% to 16%), stomatitis (5% to 12%)

Hematologic: Myelosuppression (nadir: 7 days; recovery: 10-14 days), leukopenia (22% to 60%), anemia (8% to 35%), thrombocytopenia (6% to 32%)

Hepatic: Transaminases increased (2% to 19%)

Neuromuscular & skeletal: Myalgia (11% to 19%), weakness (10% to 12%)

Respiratory: Cough (17% to 20%), upper respiratory infection (13% to 16%), rhinitis (10% to 11%), dyspnea (8% to 11%)

Miscellaneous: Infection (7% to 36%), allergic reaction (2% to 11%)

1% to 10%:

Cardiovascular: Chest pain (3% to 10%), facial edema (3% to 10%), hypotension (3% to 10%), peripheral edema (3% to 10%), angina (<3%), arrhythmia (<3%), AV block (<3%), bradycardia (<3%), cardiac arrest (<3%), deep thrombophlebitis (<3%), heart failure (<3%), hypertension (<3%), pericardial effusion (<3%), sinus arrest (<3%), syncope (<3%), tachycardia (<3%), vasculitis (<3%), ventricular extrasystoles (<3%)

Central nervous system: Anxiety (3% to 10%), confusion (3% to 10%), depression (3% to 10%), dizziness (3% to 10%), insomnia (3% to 10%), nervousness (3% to 10%), somnolence (3% to 10%), abnormal dreams/thinking (<3%), amnesia (<3%), ataxia (<3%), emotional lability (<3%), encephalitis (<3%), hallucination (<3%), hostility (<3%), meningism (<3%), neuritis (<3%), neurosis (<3%), seizure (<3%), vertigo (<3%)

Dermatologic: Cellulitis (6%), furunculosis (4%), dry skin (3% to 10%), urticaria (3% to 10%), acne (<3%), alopecia (<3%), eczema (<3%), petechial rash (<3%), photosensitivity (<3%), abscess (2%)

Endocrine & metabolic: Amenorrhea (<3%), hypercalcemia (<3%), hyponatremia (<3%), gout (<3%), libido decreased/loss (<3%)

Gastrointestinal: Dyspepsia (3% to 10%) flatulence (3% to 10%), gingivitis (3% to 10%), constipation (<3%), dysphagia (<3%), glossitis (<3%), ileus (<3%), taste perversion (<3%), oral moniliasis (2%)

Genitourinary: Urinary tract infection (3%), impotence (<3%)

Hematologic: Agranulocytosis (3% to 10%), hemorrhage (3% to 10%), acute leukemia (<3%), aplastic anemia (<3%), hemolytic anemia (<3%)

Local: Phlebitis (<3%)

Neuromuscular & skeletal: Arthralgia (3% to 10%), paresthesia (3% to 10%), arthritis (<3%), dysarthria (<3%), hyperkinesia (<3%), neuralgia (<3%), neuropathy (<3%), paralysis (<3%), twitching (<3%), osteomyelitis (1%)

Ocular: Conjunctivitis (4%), amblyopia (<3%), eyes nonreactive (<3%), lacrimation disorder (<3%), photophobia (<3%), retinopathy (<3%), vision abnormal (<3%), watery eyes (<3%), xerophthalmia (<3%)

Otic: Deafness (<3%), earache (<3%), labyrinthitis (<3%), tinnitus (<3%)

Renal: Creatinine increased (3% to 10%), nephropathy (<3%), renal failure (<3%), renal insufficiency (<3%), renal function abnormal (<3%), renal stone (<3%)

Respiratory: Pharyngitis (8% to 10%), sinusitis (6%), pneumonia (5%), asthma (3% to 10%), bronchitis (3%), bronchospasm (<3%), laryngeal edema (<3%), pulmonary embolus (<3%)

Miscellaneous: Diaphoresis (8% to 10%), herpes zoster (8%), viral infection (≤8%), bacterial infection (5%), herpes simplex (4%), sepsis (3%), flu-like syndrome (<3%)

General Dosage Range Dosage adjustment recommended in patients with renal impairment

I.V.: *Adults:* 4 mg/m^2 every 2 weeks

Mechanism of Action Pentostatin is a purine antimetabolite that inhibits adenosine deaminase, preventing the deamination of adenosine to inosine. Accumulation of deoxyadenosine (dAdo) and deoxyadenosine 5′-triphosphate (dATP) results in a reduction of purine metabolism and DNA synthesis and cell death.

Pharmacodynamics/Kinetics

Half-life Elimination

Distribution half-life: 11-85 minutes

Terminal: 3-7 hours

Renal impairment (Cl_{cr} <50 mL/minute): 4-18 hours

Pregnancy Risk Factor D

Pentoxifylline (pen toks IF i lin)

U.S. Brand Names TRENtal®

Canadian Brand Names Albert® Pentoxifylline; Apo-Pentoxifylline SR®; Nu-Pentoxifylline SR; ratio-Pentoxifylline; Trental®

Pharmacologic Category Blood Viscosity Reducer Agent

Use Treatment of intermittent claudication on the basis of chronic occlusive arterial disease of the limbs; may improve function and symptoms, but not intended to replace more definitive therapy

Unlabeled/Investigational Use Venous leg ulcers (Jull, 2007)

Local Anesthetic/Vasoconstrictor Precautions No information available to require special precautions

Effects on Dental Treatment No significant effects or complications reported

Effects on Bleeding No information available to require special precautions

Adverse Effects 1% to 10%: Gastrointestinal: Nausea (2%), vomiting (1%)

General Dosage Range Dosage adjustment recommended in patients with renal impairment

Oral: *Adults:* 400 mg 2-3 times/day

Mechanism of Action Reduces blood viscosity via increased leukocyte and erythrocyte deformability and decreased neutrophil adhesion/activation; improves peripheral tissue oxygenation presumably through enhanced blood flow.

Pharmacodynamics/Kinetics

Half-life Elimination Parent drug: 24-48 minutes; Metabolites: 60-96 minutes

Time to Peak Serum: 2-4 hours

Pregnancy Risk Factor C

Peramivir (pe RA mi veer)

Pharmacologic Category Antiviral Agent; Neuraminidase Inhibitor

Unlabeled/Investigational Use Emergency Use Authorization (EUA): Note: The EUA expired on June 23, 2010 and the use of peramivir is no longer permitted except in a clinical trial or via an FDA Emergency Investigational Drug application (E-IND).

Treatment of certain *hospitalized* patients with suspected or laboratory-confirmed 2009 H1N1 infection or infection due to nonsubtypable influenza A virus suspected to be 2009 H1N1. Eligible patients include:

- Adult or pediatric patients not responding to appropriate oral or inhaled antiviral therapy
- Adult or pediatric patients for whom drug delivery by a route other than I.V. (eg, enteral oseltamivir or inhaled zanamivir) is not feasible or not expected to be dependable

- Adult patients that the clinician judges I.V. therapy is appropriate due to other circumstances

Local Anesthetic/Vasoconstrictor Precautions No information available to require special precautions

Effects on Dental Treatment No significant effects or complications reported

Effects on Bleeding No information available to require special precautions

Adverse Effects Frequency unknown (investigational agent).

Cardiovascular: Blood pressure increased, ECG abnormalities (prolonged QT_c interval)

Central nervous system: Dizziness, headache, nervousness, neuropsychiatric events (including anxiety, confusion, delirium, depression, insomnia, nightmares, restlessness, and mood alterations), somnolence

Endocrine & metabolic: Hyperglycemia

Gastrointestinal: Anorexia, diarrhea, nausea, vomiting

Genitourinary: Cystitis, hematuria, proteinuria

Hematologic: Neutropenia

Hepatic: Hyperbilirubinemia

Mechanism of Action Peramivir, a cyclopentane analogue, selectively inhibits the neuraminidase enzyme, thus preventing the release of particles from infected cells.

Pharmacodynamics/Kinetics

Half-life Elimination Range: 8-21 hours (normal renal function)

Prescribing and Access Restrictions Investigational agent (not FDA approved) – was available in the U.S. under an Emergency Use Authorization (EUA) which expired on June 23, 2010; thereafter, clinicians wishing to prescribe peramivir to a patient will be able to do so by enrolling the patient in a clinical trial (as appropriate per inclusion/exclusion criteria) or via an FDA Emergency Investigational New Drug (E-IND) application.

Periciazine (per ee CYE ah zeen)

Canadian Brand Names Neuleptil®

Pharmacologic Category Antipsychotic Agent, Typical, Phenothiazine, Piperidine

Use Adjunctive therapy in selected psychotic patients to control prevailing hostility, impulsivity, or aggression

Local Anesthetic/Vasoconstrictor Precautions Most pharmacology textbooks state that in presence of phenothiazines, systemic doses of epinephrine paradoxically decrease the blood pressure. This is the so called "epinephrine reversal" phenomenon. This has never been observed when epinephrine is given by infiltration as part of the anesthesia procedure. See Dental Comment.

Effects on Dental Treatment Key adverse event(s) related to dental treatment:

Significant hypotension may occur, especially when the drug is administered parenterally. Orthostatic hypotension is due to alpha-receptor blockade; elderly are at greater risk.

Tardive dyskinesia: Prevalence rate may be 40% in elderly; development of the syndrome and the irreversible nature are proportional to duration and total cumulative dose over time. Extrapyramidal reactions are more common in elderly with up to 50% developing these reactions after 60 years of age. Drug-induced Parkinson's syndrome occurs often; akathisia is the most common extrapyramidal reaction in elderly.

Increased confusion, memory loss, psychotic behavior, and agitation frequently occur as a consequence of anticholinergic effects. Antipsychotic-associated sedation in nonpsychotic patients is extremely unpleasant due to feelings of depersonalization, derealization, and dysphoria.

Effects on Bleeding No information available to require special precautions

Adverse Effects Frequency not defined; listing includes adverse reactions reported with other agents from the phenothiazine class.

Cardiovascular: AV block, cardiac arrest, ECG changes, edema, hypotension, paroxysmal atrial tachycardia, QT_c prolongation, syncope, tachycardia

Central nervous system: Aggressive behavior, agitation, anxiety, bizarre dreams, cerebral edema, depression, dizziness, drowsiness, EEG changes, excitement; extrapyramidal symptoms (tremor, akathisia, dystonia, dyskinesia, oculogyric, opisthotonos, hyper-reflexia, pseudo-Parkinsonism, rigidity, sialorrhea); fatigue, fever, headache, insomnia, paradoxical psychosis, restlessness, seizures, sleep disturbance, tardive dyskinesia

Dermatologic: Angioedema, dermatitis, eczema, epithelial keratopathy, erythema, exfoliative dermatitis, photosensitivity, pruritus, rash, seborrhea, skin pigmentation (prolonged therapy), urticaria

Endocrine & metabolic: Anorexia, appetite increased, delayed ovulation, galactorrhea, gynecomastia, libido changes, menstrual irregularities, thirst, weight changes
Gastrointestinal: Adynamic ileus, constipation, fecal impaction, nausea, salivation, vomiting, xerostomia
Genitourinary: Bladder paralysis, impotence, incontinence, polyuria, urinary retention
Hematologic: Agranulocytosis, anemia, eosinophilia, leukopenia, pancytopenia, thrombocytopenia
Hepatic: Cholestasis, cholestatic jaundice, jaundice
Ocular: Blurred vision, corneal deposits (prolonged therapy), glaucoma, lenticular deposits, pigmentary retinopathy (prolonged therapy)
Respiratory: Nasal congestion, pneumonia, pneumonitis
Miscellaneous: Diaphoresis increased, lupus-like syndrome

Dosage Oral:

Children >5 years: 2.5-10 mg in the morning, followed by 5-30 mg in the evening. In general, lower dosage should be used on initiation and gradually increased based on effect and tolerance.

Adults: 5-20 mg in the morning, followed by 10-40 mg in the evening. In dividing doses, it is suggested that the larger dose should be administered in the evening. In general, lower dosage should be used on initiation and gradually increased based on effect and tolerance.

Elderly: Initial daily dose should be ~5 mg/day. May be increased gradually based on effect and tolerance. Also see adult dosing.

Dosage adjustment in renal impairment: No dosage adjustment required.

Mechanism of Action Blocks postsynaptic mesolimbic dopaminergic receptors in the brain; depresses the release of hypothalamic and hypophyseal hormones.

Contraindications Hypersensitivity to periciazine, phenothiazine derivatives, or any component of the formulation; severe CNS depression including acute intoxication with CNS depressant medications; subcortical brain damage; hepatic dysfunction; circulatory collapse; severely-depressed patients; bone marrow suppression; blood dyscrasias; coma; patients receiving spinal or regional anesthesia

Warnings/Precautions Check blood counts periodically and discontinue at first signs of blood dyscrasias; use is contraindicated in patients with bone marrow suppression. May be sedating; use with caution in disorders where CNS depression is a feature (risk may be lower than with other phenothiazines); caution patients about performing tasks which require mental alertness. Use with caution in Parkinson's disease (may be more sensitive to adverse effects), hemodynamic instability, and predisposition to seizures. Esophageal dysmotility and aspiration have been associated with antipsychotic use; use with caution in patients at risk of pneumonia (eg, Alzheimer's disease). Use with caution in breast cancer or other prolactin-dependent tumors (may elevate prolactin levels). May alter temperature regulation; use caution with strenuous exercise, heat exposure, dehydration, and concomitant medication possessing anticholinergic effects. May mask toxicity of other drugs or conditions (eg, intestinal obstruction, Reye's syndrome, brain tumor) due to antiemetic effects.

Use caution in cardiovascular disease. May alter cardiac conduction (life-threatening arrhythmias have occurred with therapeutic doses of phenothiazines); relative risk with periciazine has not been established, although rare cases of QT_c prolongation have been reported. May cause orthostatic hypotension; use with caution in patients at risk of this effect or those who would not tolerate transient hypotensive episodes (cerebrovascular disease, cardiovascular disease, or other medications which may predispose). Phenothiazines have been associated with worsening of pheochromocytoma and mitral valve prolapse; use caution.

Phenothiazines may cause anticholinergic effects (confusion, agitation, constipation, xerostomia, blurred vision, urinary retention); therefore, use with caution in patients with decreased gastrointestinal motility, urinary retention, BPH, xerostomia, or visual problems. Conditions which also may be exacerbated by cholinergic blockade include narrow-angle glaucoma (screening is recommended) and worsening of myasthenia gravis.

May cause extrapyramidal symptoms, including pseudoparkinsonism, acute dystonic reactions, akathisia, and tardive dyskinesia. May be associated with neuroleptic malignant syndrome (NMS); monitor for mental status changes, fever, muscle rigidity, and/or autonomic instability (risk may be increased in patients with Parkinson's disease or Lewy body dementia). Prolonged therapy may cause pigmentary retinopathy, corneal deposits, and/or changes in skin pigmentation. Use with caution in the elderly; risk for developing tardive dyskinesia is increased.

Drug Interactions

Metabolism/Transport Effects No published data on CYP metabolism. Based on structural analysis, may be a substrate of CYP2D6 and 3A4.

Increased Effect/Toxicity The levels/effects of periciazine may be increased by azole antifungals, chlorpromazine, ciprofloxacin, clarithromycin, delavirdine, diclofenac, doxycycline, erythromycin, fluoxetine, imatinib, isoniazid, miconazole, nefazodone, nicardipine, paroxetine, pergolide, propofol, protease inhibitors, quinidine, quinine, ritonavir, ropinirole, verapamil and other CYP2D6 or 3A4 inhibitors.

Drugs which alter the QT_c interval may be additive with periciazine, increasing the risk of malignant arrhythmias; includes type Ia antiarrhythmics, TCAs, and some quinolone antibiotics (moxifloxacin). **These agents are contraindicated with other piperidine phenothiazines (thioridazine)**. Potassium-depleting agents may increase the risk of serious arrhythmias with periciazine (includes many diuretics, aminoglycosides, and amphotericin).

Phenothiazines inhibit the ability of bromocriptine to lower serum prolactin concentrations. The sedative effects of CNS depressants or ethanol may be additive with phenothiazines. Phenothiazines and trazodone may produce additive hypotensive effects. Metoclopramide may increase risk of extrapyramidal symptoms (EPS). Concurrent use of antihypertensives may result in additive hypotensive effects (particularly orthostasis).

Phenothiazines may produce neurotoxicity with lithium; this is a rare effect. Rare cases of respiratory paralysis have been reported with concurrent use of phenothiazines and polypeptide antibiotics (eg, bacitracin). Naltrexone in combination with some phenothiazines has been reported to cause lethargy and somnolence.

Decreased Effect Aluminum salts may decrease the absorption of phenothiazines. The efficacy of amphetamines may be diminished by antipsychotics; in addition, amphetamines may increase psychotic symptoms; avoid concurrent use. Anticholinergics may inhibit the therapeutic response to phenothiazines and excess anticholinergic effects may occur (includes benztropine, trihexyphenidyl, biperiden, and drugs with significant anticholinergic activity). Low potency antipsychotics (such as periciazine) may diminish the pressor effects of epinephrine. The antihypertensive effects of guanethidine or guanadrel may be inhibited by phenothiazines. Phenothiazines may inhibit the antiparkinsonian effect of levodopa. Enzyme inducers may enhance the hepatic metabolism of phenothiazines; larger doses may be required; includes rifampin, rifabutin, barbiturates, and phenytoin.

Ethanol/Nutrition/Herb Interactions

Ethanol: Avoid ethanol (may increase CNS depression).

Herb/Nutraceutical: Avoid kava kava, valerian, St John's wort, gotu kola (may increase CNS depression). Avoid dong quai, St John's wort (may also cause photosensitization). Cigarette smoking may decrease the serum concentrations of periciazine.

Product Availability Not available in U.S.

Dosage Forms: Canada

Capsule:

Neuleptil®: 5 mg, 10 mg, 20 mg

Solution, oral drops:

Neuleptil®: 10 mg/mL

Dental Comment This drug is known to prolong the QT interval. The QT interval is measured as the time and distance between the Q point of the QRS complex and the end of the T wave in the ECG tracing. After adjustment for heart rate, the QT interval is defined as prolonged if it is more than 450 msec in men and 460 msec in women. A long QT syndrome was first described in the 1950s and 60s as a congenital syndrome involving QT interval prolongation and syncope and sudden death. Some of the congenital long QT syndromes were characterized by a peculiar electrocardiographic appearance of the QRS complex involving a premature atria beat followed by a pause, then a subsequent sinus beat showing marked QT prolongation and deformity. This type of cardiac arrhythmia was originally termed "torsade de pointes" (translated from the French as "twisting of the points").

Prolongation of the QT interval is thought to result from delayed ventricular repolarization. The repolarization process within the myocardial cell is due to the efflux of intracellular potassium. The channels associated with this current can be blocked by many drugs and predispose the electrical propagation cycle to torsade de pointes.

Periciazine is one of the drugs confirmed to prolong the QT interval and is accepted as having a risk of causing torsade de pointes. The risk of drug-induced torsade de pointes is extremely low when a single QT interval prolonging drug is prescribed. In terms of epinephrine, it is not known what effect vasoconstrictors in the local anesthetic regimen will have in patients with a known history of congenital prolonged QT interval or in patients taking any medication that prolongs the QT interval. Until more information is obtained, it is suggested that the clinician consult with the physician prior to the use of a vasoconstrictor in suspected patients, and that the vasoconstrictor (epinephrine, levonordefrin [Neo-Cobefrin®]) be used with caution.

References

Buckley NA, Whyte IM, and Dawson AH, "Cardiotoxicity More Common in Thioridazine Overdose Than With Other Neuroleptics," *J Toxicol Clin Toxicol*, 1995, 33(3):199-204.

Jaworowsky S and Zamir S, "Cardiac Arrhythmia in a Child Receiving Pericyazine," *Isr J Psychiatry Relat Sci*, 1995, 32(4):299-300.

Johnson A, Giuffre RM, and O'Malley K, "ECG Changes in Pediatric Patients on Tricyclic Antidepressants, Desipramine, and Imipramine," *Can J Psychiatry*, 1996, 41(2):102-6.

Perindopril Erbumine (per IN doe pril er BYOO meen)

Related Information

Cardiovascular Diseases *on page 1848*

U.S. Brand Names Aceon®

Canadian Brand Names Apo-Perindopril®; Coversyl®

Pharmacologic Category Angiotensin-Converting Enzyme (ACE) Inhibitor

Use Treatment of hypertension; reduction of cardiovascular mortality or nonfatal myocardial infarction in patients with stable coronary artery disease

Canadian labeling: Additional use (unlabeled use in U.S.): Treatment of mild-moderate (NYHA I-III) heart failure

Unlabeled/Investigational Use To delay the progression of nephropathy and reduce risks of cardiovascular events in hypertensive patients with type 1 or 2 diabetes mellitus

Local Anesthetic/Vasoconstrictor Precautions No information available to require special precautions

Effects on Dental Treatment No significant effects or complications reported

Effects on Bleeding No information available to require special precautions

Adverse Effects

>10%:

Central nervous system: Headache (24%)

Respiratory: Cough (incidence is higher in women, 3:1) (12%)

1% to 10%:

Cardiovascular: Edema (4%), chest pain (2%), ECG abnormal (2%), palpitation (1%)

Central nervous system: Dizziness (8%, less than placebo), sleep disorders (3%), depression (2%), fever (2%), nervousness (1%), somnolence (1%)

Dermatologic: Rash (2%)

Endocrine & metabolic: Hyperkalemia (1%, less than placebo), triglycerides increased (1%), menstrual disorder (1%)

Gastrointestinal: Diarrhea (4%), abdominal pain (3%), nausea (2%), vomiting (2%), dyspepsia (2%), flatulence (1%)

Genitourinary: Urinary tract infection (3%), sexual dysfunction (male 1%)

Hepatic: ALT increased (2%)

Neuromuscular & skeletal: Weakness (8%), back pain (6%), lower extremity pain (5%), upper extremity pain (3%), hypertonia (3%), paresthesia (2%), joint pain (1%), myalgia (1%), arthritis (1%), neck pain (1%)

Renal: Proteinuria (2%)

Respiratory: Upper respiratory tract infection (9%), sinusitis (5%), rhinitis (5%), pharyngitis (3%)

Otic: Tinnitus (2%), ear infection (1%)

Miscellaneous: Viral infection (3%), seasonal allergy (2%)

Note: Some reactions occurred at an incidence >1% but ≤ placebo.

Additional adverse effects that have been reported with **ACE inhibitors** include agranulocytosis (especially in patients with renal impairment or collagen vascular disease), neutropenia, anemia, bullous pemphigoid, cardiac arrest, eosinophilic pneumonitis, exfoliative dermatitis, falls, hepatic failure, hyponatremia, jaundice, pancreatitis (acute), pancytopenia, pemphigus, psoriasis, thrombocytopenia; decreases in creatinine clearance in some elderly hypertensive patients or those with chronic renal failure, and worsening of renal function in patients with bilateral renal artery stenosis or hypovolemic patients (diuretic therapy). In addition, a syndrome which may include fever, myalgia, arthralgia, interstitial nephritis, vasculitis, rash, eosinophilia and positive ANA, and elevated ESR has been reported with ACE inhibitors.

General Dosage Range Dosage adjustment recommended in patients with renal impairment

Oral: *Adults:* Initial: 2-4 mg once daily; Maintenance: 4-8 mg/day in 1-2 divided doses (maximum: 16 mg/day)

Mechanism of Action Perindopril is a prodrug for perindoprilat, which acts as a competitive inhibitor of angiotensin-converting enzyme (ACE); prevents conversion of angiotensin I to angiotensin II, a potent vasoconstrictor; results in lower levels of angiotensin II which, in turn, causes an increase in plasma renin activity and a reduction in aldosterone secretion

Pharmacodynamics/Kinetics

Onset of Action Peak effect: 1-2 hours

Half-life Elimination Parent drug: 1.5-3 hours; Metabolite: Effective: 3-10 hours, Terminal: 30-120 hours

Time to Peak Chronic therapy: Perindopril: 1 hour; Perindoprilat: 3-7 hours (maximum perindoprilat serum levels are 2-3 times higher and T_{max} is shorter following chronic therapy); CHF: Perindoprilat: 6 hours

Pregnancy Risk Factor D

Perindopril Erbumine and Indapamide

(per IN doe pril er BYOO meen & in DAP a mide)

Related Information

Indapamide *on page 910*
Perindopril Erbumine *on page 1329*

Canadian Brand Names Coversyl® Plus; Coversyl® Plus HD; Coversyl® Plus LD

Pharmacologic Category Angiotensin-Converting Enzyme (ACE) Inhibitor; Diuretic, Thiazide-Related

Use Treatment of hypertension

Note: Coversyl® Plus LD may be used as initial treatment; Coversyl® Plus and Coversyl® Plus HD are not indicated for initial treatment of hypertension.

Local Anesthetic/Vasoconstrictor Precautions No information available to require special precautions

Effects on Dental Treatment Key adverse event(s) related to dental treatment: Indapamide: Orthostatic hypotension, palpitations, flushing, rhinorrhea, and xerostomia and changes in salivation (normal salivary flow resumes upon discontinuation).

Effects on Bleeding No information available to require special precautions

Adverse Effects **Note:** Observed with perindopril/indapamide; also see individual agents.

1% to 10%:

- Central nervous system: Dizziness (1% to 2%)
- Endocrine & metabolic: Hypokalemia (2% to 7%), hyperkalemia (1%)
- Gastrointestinal: Nausea (2%), vomiting (2%), dyspepsia (≤1%)
- Renal: BUN increased (2% to 4%)
- Respiratory: Cough (3% to 5%), upper respiratory infection (2%)

General Dosage Range **Oral:** *Adults:* Perindopril 2-8 mg/indapamide 0.625-2.5 mg once daily

Mechanism of Action See individual agents.

Product Availability Not available in U.S.

Permethrin (per METH rin)

U.S. Brand Names A200® Lice [OTC]; Acticin® [DSC]; Elimite®; Nix® Complete Lice Treatment System [OTC]; Nix® Creme Rinse Lice Treatment [OTC]; Nix® Creme Rinse [OTC]; Nix® Lice Control Spray [OTC]; Rid® [OTC]

Canadian Brand Names Kwellada-P™; Nix®

Pharmacologic Category Antiparasitic Agent, Topical; Pediculocide; Scabicidal Agent

Use Single-application treatment of infestation with *Pediculus humanus capitis* (head louse) and its nits or *Sarcoptes scabiei* (scabies); indicated for prophylactic use during epidemics of lice

Local Anesthetic/Vasoconstrictor Precautions No information available to require special precautions

Effects on Dental Treatment No significant effects or complications reported

Effects on Bleeding No information available to require special precautions

Adverse Effects 1% to 10%:

- Dermatologic: Pruritus, erythema, rash of the scalp
- Local: Burning, stinging, tingling, numbness or scalp discomfort, edema

General Dosage Range **Topical:**

Cream:

Neonates: 5% cream was shown to be safe and effective when applied to an infant ≤1 month of age with neonatal scabies; time of application was limited to 6 hours before rinsing with soap and water

Children and Adults: Apply from head to toe, leave on 8-14 hours before washing off with water; May reapply in 1 week if live mites appear

Liquid (lotion or cream rinse): *Children >2 months and Adults:* Apply a sufficient volume to saturate the hair and scalp, leave on for 10 minutes before rinsing off with water; May reapply in 1 week if lice or nits still present

Mechanism of Action Inhibits sodium ion influx through nerve cell membrane channels in parasites resulting in delayed repolarization and thus paralysis and death of the pest

Pregnancy Risk Factor B

Perphenazine (per FEN a zeen)

Canadian Brand Names Apo-Perphenazine®

Pharmacologic Category Antiemetic; Antipsychotic Agent, Typical, Phenothiazine

Use Treatment of schizophrenia; severe nausea and vomiting

Unlabeled/Investigational Use Ethanol withdrawal; behavioral symptoms associated with dementia (elderly); Tourette's syndrome; Huntington's chorea; spasmodic torticollis; Reye's syndrome; psychosis; psychosis/agitation related to Alzheimer's dementia

Local Anesthetic/Vasoconstrictor Precautions Most pharmacology textbooks state that in presence of phenothiazines, systemic doses of epinephrine paradoxically decrease the blood pressure. This is the so called "epinephrine reversal" phenomenon. This has never been observed when epinephrine is given by infiltration as part of the anesthesia procedure.

Effects on Dental Treatment Key adverse event(s) related to dental treatment:

Significant hypotension may occur, especially when the drug is administered parenterally; orthostatic hypotension is due to alpha-receptor blockade, the elderly are at greater risk for orthostatic hypotension.

Tardive dyskinesia: Prevalence rate may be 40% in elderly; development of the syndrome and the irreversible nature are proportional to duration and total cumulative dose over time. Extrapyramidal reactions are more common in elderly with up to 50% developing these reactions after 60 years of age. Drug-induced Parkinson's syndrome occurs often; akathisia is the most common extrapyramidal reaction in elderly.

Effects on Bleeding No information available to require special precautions

Adverse Effects Frequency not defined.

Cardiovascular: Bradycardia, cardiac arrest, ECG changes, hyper-/hypotension, orthostatic hypotension, pallor, peripheral edema, sudden death, tachycardia

Central nervous system: Bizarre dreams, catatonic-like states, cerebral edema, dizziness, drowsiness, extrapyramidal symptoms (pseudoparkinsonism, akathisia, dystonias, tardive dyskinesia), faintness, headache, hyperactivity, hyperpyrexia, impairment of temperature regulation, insomnia, lethargy, neuroleptic malignant syndrome (NMS), nocturnal confusion, paradoxical excitement, paranoid reactions, restlessness, seizure

Dermatologic: Discoloration of skin (blue-gray), photosensitivity, rash

Endocrine & metabolic: Amenorrhea, breast enlargement, hyper-/hypoglycemia, galactorrhea, lactation, libido changes, gynecomastia, menstrual irregularity, parotid swelling (rare), SIADH

Gastrointestinal: Adynamic ileus, anorexia, appetite increased, constipation, diarrhea, fecal impaction, obstipation, nausea, salivation, stomach pain, vomiting, weight gain, xerostomia

Genitourinary: Bladder paralysis, ejaculatory disturbances, incontinence, polyuria, priapism, urinary retention

Hematologic: Agranulocytosis, eosinophilia, hemolytic anemia, leukopenia, pancytopenia, thrombocytopenic purpura

Hepatic: Hepatotoxicity, jaundice

Neuromuscular & skeletal: Muscle weakness, tremor

Ocular: Blurred vision, cornea and lens changes, epithelial keratopathies, glaucoma, mydriasis, myosis, pigmentary photophobia, retinopathy

Renal: Glycosuria

Respiratory: Nasal congestion

Miscellaneous: Allergic reactions, diaphoresis, systemic lupus erythematosus-like syndrome

General Dosage Range Oral: *Adults:* 4-16 mg 2-4 times/day (maximum: 64 mg/day)

Mechanism of Action Perphenazine is a piperazine phenothiazine antipsychotic which blocks postsynaptic mesolimbic dopaminergic receptors in the brain; exhibits alpha-adrenergic blocking effect and depresses the release of hypothalamic and hypophyseal hormones

Pharmacodynamics/Kinetics

Half-life Elimination Perphenazine: 9-12 hours; 7-hydroxyperphenazine: 10-19 hours

Time to Peak Serum: Perphenazine: 1-3 hours; 7-hydroxyperphenazine: 2-4 hours

Phenazopyridine (fen az oh PEER i deen)

U.S. Brand Names AZO Standard® Maximum Strength [OTC]; AZO Standard® [OTC]; Azo-Gesic™ [OTC]; Baridium [OTC]; Pyridium®; ReAzo [OTC]; UTI Relief® [OTC]

Canadian Brand Names Phenazo™

Pharmacologic Category Analgesic, Urinary

Use Symptomatic relief of urinary burning, itching, frequency, and urgency in association with urinary tract infection or following urologic procedures

Local Anesthetic/Vasoconstrictor Precautions No information available to require special precautions

Effects on Dental Treatment No significant effects or complications reported

Effects on Bleeding No information available to require special precautions

Adverse Effects 1% to 10%:

Central nervous system: Headache, dizziness

Gastrointestinal: Stomach cramps

General Dosage Range Dosage adjustment recommended in patients with renal impairment

Oral:

Children: 12 mg/kg/day in 3 divided doses

Adults: 100-200 mg 3 times/day

Mechanism of Action An azo dye which exerts local anesthetic or analgesic action on urinary tract mucosa through an unknown mechanism

Pregnancy Risk Factor B

Phendimetrazine (fen dye ME tra zeen)

U.S. Brand Names Bontril® PDM; Bontril® Slow-Release

Canadian Brand Names Bontril®; Plegine®; Statobex®

Pharmacologic Category Anorexiant; Sympathomimetic

Use Short-term (few weeks) adjunct in exogenous obesity

Pharmacotherapy for weight loss is recommended only for obese patients with a body mass index ≥30 kg/m^2, or ≥27 kg/m^2 in the presence of other risk factors such as hypertension, diabetes, and/or dyslipidemia or a high waist circumference; therapy should be used in conjunction with a comprehensive weight management program.

Local Anesthetic/Vasoconstrictor Precautions Use vasoconstrictor with caution in patients taking phendimetrazine. Phendimetrazine can enhance the sympathomimetic response to epinephrine leading to potential hypertension and cardiotoxicity.

Effects on Dental Treatment Key adverse event(s) related to dental treatment: Xerostomia (normal salivary flow resumes upon discontinuation).

Effects on Bleeding No information available to require special precautions

Adverse Effects Frequency not defined.

Cardiovascular: Flushing, hypertension, palpitation, tachycardia

Central nervous system: Agitation, dizziness, headache, insomnia, overstimulation, psychosis, restlessness

Endocrine & metabolic: Changes in libido

Gastrointestinal: Constipation, diarrhea, nausea, stomach pain, xerostomia

Genitourinary: Dysuria, urinary frequency

Neuromuscular & skeletal: Tremor

Ocular: Blurred vision, mydriasis

Miscellaneous: Diaphoresis, tachyphylaxis

General Dosage Range Oral:

Capsule: *Adults:* 105 mg once daily before breakfast

Tablet: *Adults:* 17.5-35 mg 2-3 times/day, 1 hour before meals (maximum: 70 mg 3 times/day)

Mechanism of Action Phendimetrazine is a sympathomimetic amine with pharmacologic properties similar to the amphetamines. The mechanism of action in reducing appetite appears to be secondary to CNS effects, including stimulation of the hypothalamus to release norepinephrine.

Pharmacodynamics/Kinetics

Half-life Elimination Bontril® PDM: ~2 hours; Bontril® Slow Release: ~10 hours

Pregnancy Risk Factor C

Controlled Substance C-III

Phenelzine (FEN el zeen)

U.S. Brand Names Nardil®

Canadian Brand Names Nardil®

Pharmacologic Category Antidepressant, Monoamine Oxidase Inhibitor

Use Symptomatic treatment of atypical, nonendogenous, or neurotic depression

Unlabeled/Investigational Use Selective mutism

Local Anesthetic/Vasoconstrictor Precautions Attempts should be made to avoid use of vasoconstrictor due to possibility of hypertensive episodes with monoamine oxidase inhibitors

Effects on Dental Treatment Key adverse event(s) related to dental treatment: Orthostatic hypotension, xerostomia and changes in salivation (normal salivary flow resumes upon discontinuation). Avoid use as an analgesic due to toxic reactions with MAO inhibitors.

Effects on Bleeding No information available to require special precautions

Adverse Effects Frequency not defined.

Cardiovascular: Edema, orthostatic hypotension

Central nervous system: Anxiety (acute), ataxia, coma, delirium, dizziness, drowsiness, fatigue, fever, headache, hyper-reflexia, mania, seizure, sleep disturbances, twitching

Dermatologic: Pruritus, rash

Endocrine & metabolic: Decreased sexual ability (anorgasmia, ejaculatory disturbances, impotence), hypermetabolic syndrome, hypernatremia

Gastrointestinal: Constipation, weight gain, xerostomia

Genitourinary: Urinary retention

Hematologic: Leukopenia

Hepatic: Hepatitis, jaundice, necrotizing hepatocellular necrosis (rare)

Neuromuscular & skeletal: Lupus-like syndrome, myoclonia, tremor, weakness

Ocular: Blurred vision, glaucoma

Respiratory: Edema (glottis)

Miscellaneous: Diaphoresis, transient cardiac or respiratory depression (following ECT), withdrawal syndrome (nausea, vomiting, malaise)

General Dosage Range Oral:

Adults: 45-90 mg/day in 3 divided doses

Elderly: Initial: 7.5 mg/day; Maintenance: 15-60 mg/day in 3-4 divided doses

Mechanism of Action Thought to act by increasing endogenous concentrations of norepinephrine, dopamine, and serotonin through inhibition of the enzyme (monoamine oxidase) responsible for the breakdown of these neurotransmitters

Pharmacodynamics/Kinetics

Onset of Action Therapeutic: 2-4 weeks; geriatric patients receiving an average of 55 mg/day developed a mean platelet MAO activity inhibition of about 85%.

Duration of Action May continue to have a therapeutic effect and interactions 2 weeks after discontinuing therapy

Half-life Elimination 11 hours

Pregnancy Risk Factor C

PHENobarbital (fee noe BAR bi tal)

U.S. Brand Names Luminal® Sodium [DSC]

Canadian Brand Names PMS-Phenobarbital

Generic Availability (U.S.) Yes

Pharmacologic Category Anticonvulsant, Barbiturate; Barbiturate

Use Management of generalized tonic-clonic (grand mal), status epilepticus, and partial seizures; sedative/hypnotic

Unlabeled/Investigational Use Prevention and treatment of neonatal hyperbilirubinemia and lowering of bilirubin in chronic cholestasis; neonatal seizures

Local Anesthetic/Vasoconstrictor Precautions No information available to require special precautions

Effects on Dental Treatment No significant effects or complications reported

Effects on Bleeding No information available to require special precautions

Adverse Effects Frequency not defined.

Cardiovascular: Bradycardia, hypotension, syncope

Central nervous system: Agitation, anxiety, ataxia, CNS excitation or depression, confusion, dizziness drowsiness, hallucinations, "hangover" effect, headache, hyperkinesia, impaired judgment, insomnia, lethargy, nervousness, nightmares, somnolence

Dermatologic: Exfoliative dermatitis, rash, Stevens-Johnson syndrome

Gastrointestinal: Nausea, vomiting, constipation

Hematologic: Agranulocytosis, thrombocytopenia, megaloblastic anemia

Local: Pain at injection site, thrombophlebitis with I.V. use

Renal: Oliguria

Respiratory: Laryngospasm, respiratory depression, apnea (especially with rapid I.V. use), hypoventilation

Miscellaneous: Gangrene with inadvertent intra-arterial injection

Dosage

Children:

Sedation: Oral: 2 mg/kg 3 times/day

Hypnotic: I.M., I.V.: 3-5 mg/kg at bedtime

Preoperative sedation: Oral, I.M., I.V.: 1-3 mg/kg 1-1.5 hours before procedure

Adults:

Sedation: Oral, I.M.: 30-120 mg/day in 2-3 divided doses

Hypnotic: Oral, I.M., I.V.: 100-320 mg at bedtime

Preoperative sedation: I.M.: 100-200 mg 1-1.5 hours before procedure

Anticonvulsant: Status epilepticus: **Loading dose:** I.V.:

Infants and Children: 15-20 mg/kg (maximum: 1000 mg/dose, maximum rate ≤30 mg/minute in children <60 kg); may repeat dose after 15 minutes as needed (maximum total dose: 40 mg/kg)

Adults: 10-20 mg/kg (maximum rate ≤60 mg/minute in patients ≥60 kg); may repeat dose in 20-minute intervals as needed (maximum total dose: 30 mg/kg)

Anticonvulsant maintenance dose: Oral, I.V.:

Infants: 5-8 mg/kg/day in 1-2 divided doses

Children:

1-5 years: 6-8 mg/kg/day in 1-2 divided doses

5-12 years: 4-6 mg/kg/day in 1-2 divided doses

Children >12 years and Adults: 1-3 mg/kg/day in divided doses or 50-100 mg 2-3 times/day

Sedative/hypnotic withdrawal (unlabeled use): Initial daily requirement is determined by substituting phenobarbital 30 mg for every 100 mg pentobarbital used during tolerance testing; then daily requirement is decreased by 10% of initial dose

Dosing interval in renal impairment: Cl_{cr} <10 mL/minute: Administer every 12-16 hours

Hemodialysis: Moderately dialyzable (20% to 50%)

Dosing adjustment/comments in hepatic disease: Increased side effects may occur in severe liver disease; monitor plasma levels and adjust dose accordingly

Mechanism of Action Long-acting barbiturate with sedative, hypnotic, and anticonvulsant properties. Barbiturates depress the sensory cortex, decrease motor activity, alter cerebellar function, and produce drowsiness, sedation, and hypnosis. In high doses, barbiturates exhibit anticonvulsant activity; barbiturates produce dose-dependent respiratory depression.

Contraindications Hypersensitivity to barbiturates or any component of the formulation; marked hepatic impairment; dyspnea or airway obstruction; porphyria (manifest and latent); intra-arterial administration, subcutaneous administration (not recommended); use in patients with a history of sedative/hypnotic addiction is not recommended; nephritic patients (large doses)

Warnings/Precautions Potential for drug dependency exists, abrupt cessation may precipitate withdrawal, including status epilepticus in epileptic patients. Do not administer to patients in acute pain. Use caution in elderly, debilitated, renal or hepatic dysfunction, and pediatric patients. May cause paradoxical responses, including agitation and hyperactivity, particularly in acute pain and pediatric patients. Use with caution in patients with depression or suicidal tendencies, or in patients with a history of drug abuse. Tolerance, psychological and physical dependence may occur with prolonged use. May cause CNS depression, which may impair physical or mental abilities. Effects with other sedative drugs or ethanol may be potentiated. May cause respiratory depression or hypotension, particularly when administered intravenously. Use with caution in hemodynamically unstable patients (hypovolemic shock, CHF) or patients with respiratory disease. Due to its long half-life and risk of dependence, phenobarbital is not recommended as a sedative in the elderly. Use has been associated with cognitive deficits in children. Use with caution in patients with hypoadrenalism. Intra-arterial administration may cause reactions ranging from transient pain to gangrene and is contraindicated. Subcutaneous administration may cause tissue irritation (eg, redness, tenderness, necrosis) and is not recommended.

Drug Interactions

Metabolism/Transport Effects **Substrate** of CYP2C9 (minor), 2C19 (major), 2E1 (minor); **Induces** CYP1A2 (strong), 2A6 (strong), 2B6 (strong), 2C8 (strong), 2C9 (strong), 3A4 (strong)

Avoid Concomitant Use

Avoid concomitant use of PHENobarbital with any of the following: Darunavir; Dronedarone; Etravirine; Everolimus; Lurasidone; Nilotinib; Pazopanib; Praziquantel; Ranolazine; Roflumilast; RomiDEPsin; Tolvaptan; Vandetanib; Voriconazole

Increased Effect/Toxicity

PHENobarbital may increase the levels/effects of: Alcohol (Ethyl); CNS Depressants; Meperidine; QuiNIDine; Thiazide Diuretics

The levels/effects of PHENobarbital may be increased by: Carbonic Anhydrase Inhibitors; Chloramphenicol; CYP2C19 Inhibitors (Moderate); CYP2C19 Inhibitors (Strong); Dexmethylphenidate; Divalproex; Droperidol; Felbamate; Methylphenidate; Primidone; QuiNINE; Rufinamide; Valproic Acid

Decreased Effect

PHENobarbital may decrease the levels/effects of: Acetaminophen; Bendamustine; Beta-Blockers; Calcium Channel Blockers; Chloramphenicol; Contraceptives (Estrogens); Contraceptives (Progestins); Corticosteroids (Systemic); CycloSPORINE; CycloSPORINE (Systemic); CYP1A2 Substrates; CYP2A6 Substrates; CYP2B6 Substrates; CYP2C8 Substrates (High risk); CYP2C9 Substrates (High risk); CYP3A4 Substrates; Darunavir; Deferasirox; Disopyramide; Divalproex; Doxycycline; Dronedarone; Etoposide; Etoposide Phosphate; Etravirine; Everolimus; Exemestane; Felbamate; Fosphenytoin; Gefitinib; Griseofulvin; GuanFACINE; Imatinib; Irinotecan; Ixabepilone; Lacosamide; LamoTRIgine; Lopinavir; Lurasidone; Maraviroc; Methadone; MetroNIDAZOLE; MetroNIDAZOLE (Systemic); Nilotinib; OXcarbazepine; Pazopanib; Phenytoin; Praziquantel; Propafenone; QuiNIDine; QuiNINE; Ranolazine; Roflumilast; RomiDEPsin; Rufinamide; Saxagliptin; SORAfenib; Tadalafil; Teniposide; Theophylline Derivatives; Tipranavir; Tolvaptan; Treprostinil; Tricyclic Antidepressants; Ulipristal; Valproic Acid; Vandetanib; Vitamin K Antagonists; Voriconazole; Zonisamide

The levels/effects of PHENobarbital may be decreased by: Amphetamines; Cholestyramine Resin; CYP2C19 Inducers (Strong); Folic Acid; Ketorolac; Ketorolac (Systemic); Leucovorin Calcium-Levoleucovorin; Levomefolate; Mefloquine; Methylfolate; Pyridoxine; Rifamycin Derivatives; Tipranavir

Ethanol/Nutrition/Herb Interactions

Ethanol: May increase CNS depression; monitor for increased effects with coadministration. Caution patients about effects.

Food: May cause decrease in vitamin D and calcium.

Herb/Nutraceutical: Avoid evening primrose (seizure threshold decreased). Avoid valerian, St John's wort, kava kava, gotu kola (may increase CNS depression).

Dietary Considerations Vitamin D: Loss in vitamin D due to malabsorption; increase intake of foods rich in vitamin D. Supplementation of vitamin D and/or calcium may be necessary. Injection may contain sodium.

Pharmacodynamics/Kinetics

Onset of Action Oral: Hypnosis: 20-60 minutes; I.V.: ~5 minutes; Peak effect: I.V.: ~30 minutes

Duration of Action Oral: 6-10 hours; I.V.: 4-10 hours

Half-life Elimination Neonates: 45-500 hours; Infants: 20-133 hours; Children: 37-73 hours; Adults: 53-140 hours

Time to Peak Serum: Oral: 1-6 hours

Pregnancy Risk Factor D

Lactation Enters breast milk/use caution (AAP recommends use "with caution"; AAP 2001 update pending)

Breast-Feeding Considerations Phenobarbital is excreted into breast milk. Infantile spasms and other withdrawal symptoms have been reported following the abrupt discontinuation of breast-feeding.

Controlled Substance C-IV

Dosage Forms

Elixir, oral: 20 mg/5 mL (5 mL, 7.5 mL, 15 mL)

Injection, solution: 65 mg/mL (1 mL); 130 mg/mL (1 mL)

Tablet, oral: 15 mg, 30 mg, 60 mg, 100 mg

Phenol (FEE nol)

Related Information

Management of Patients Undergoing Cancer Therapy *on page 1970*

U.S. Brand Names Castellani Paint Modified [OTC]; Cepastat® Extra Strength [OTC]; Cepastat® [OTC]; Cheracol® Spray [OTC]; Chloraseptic® Kids Sore Throat Spray [OTC]; Chloraseptic® Mouth Pain [OTC]; Chloraseptic® Sore Throat Gargle [OTC]; Chloraseptic® Sore Throat Spray [OTC]; Pain-A-Lay® [OTC]; Phenaseptic [OTC]; Phenol EZ® [OTC]; Ulcerease® [OTC]; Vicks® Formula 44® Sore Throat [OTC]

Canadian Brand Names P & S™ Liquid Phenol

Pharmacologic Category Anesthetic, Topical

Use Relief of sore throat pain, mouth, gum, and throat irritations; antiseptic; topical anesthetic

Local Anesthetic/Vasoconstrictor Precautions No information available to require special precautions

Effects on Dental Treatment No significant effects or complications reported

Effects on Bleeding No information available to require special precautions

General Dosage Range

Oral:

Children 2-12 years:

Chloraseptic®: 3 sprays onto throat or affected area; may repeat every 2 hours

Chloraseptic® for Kids: 5 sprays onto throat or affected area; may repeat every 2 hours

Children >3 years: Ulcerease®: Gargle or swish for 15 seconds, then expectorate; may repeat every 2 hours

Children 6-12 years:

Cēpastat® Extra Strength: Up to 1 lozenge every 2 hours as needed (maximum: 10 lozenges/24 hours)

Cēpastat®: Up to 1 lozenge every 2 hours as needed (maximum: 18 lozenges/24 hours)

Pain-A-Lay® Gargle: Using gauze pad, apply 10 mL to affected area, or gargle or swish for 15 seconds, then expectorate

Children ≥12 years and Adults:

Cēpastat® Extra Strength, Cēpastat®: Up to 2 lozenges every 2 hours as needed

Cheracol®, Pain-A-Lay® Spray: Spray directly in throat; rinse for 15 seconds then expectorate; may repeat every 2 hours

Chloraseptic®: 5 sprays onto throat or affected area; may repeat every 2 hours

Chloraseptic® Gargle, Cēpastat® Mouth Pain, Pain-A-Lay® Gargle, Ulcerease®: Gargle or swish for 15 seconds, then expectorate; may repeat every 2 hours

Topical: *Adults:* Apply small amount to affected area 1-3 times/day

Phenoxybenzamine (fen oks ee BEN za meen)

U.S. Brand Names Dibenzyline®

Canadian Brand Names Dibenzyline®

Pharmacologic Category $Alpha_1$ Blocker; Antidote

Use Symptomatic management of pheochromocytoma

Unlabeled/Investigational Use Micturition problems associated with neurogenic bladder, functional outlet obstruction, and partial prostate obstruction; treatment of hypertensive crisis caused by sympathomimetic amines

Local Anesthetic/Vasoconstrictor Precautions No information available to require special precautions

Effects on Dental Treatment Key adverse event(s) related to dental treatment: Xerostomia (normal salivary flow resumes upon discontinuation).

Effects on Bleeding No information available to require special precautions

Adverse Effects Frequency not defined.

Cardiovascular: Postural hypotension, tachycardia

Central nervous system: Drowsiness, fatigue

Gastrointestinal: GI irritation

Genitourinary: Inhibition of ejaculation

Ocular: Miosis

Respiratory: Nasal congestion

General Dosage Range Oral: *Adults:* Initial: 10 mg twice daily; Maintenance: 10-40 mg 1-3 times/day (maximum: 240 mg/day)

Mechanism of Action Produces long-lasting noncompetitive alpha-adrenergic blockade of postganglionic synapses in exocrine glands and smooth muscle; relaxes urethra and increases opening of the bladder

Pharmacodynamics/Kinetics

Duration of Action I.V.: ≥3 days

Half-life Elimination I.V.: 24 hours

Pregnancy Risk Factor C

Phentermine (FEN ter meen)

U.S. Brand Names Adipex-P®

Pharmacologic Category Anorexiant; Sympathomimetic

Use Short-term (few weeks) adjunct therapy in obese patients with an initial body mass index (BMI) ≥30 kg/m^2 or ≥27 kg/m^2 in the presence of other risk factors (eg, diabetes, hyperlipidemia, hypertension); therapy should be used in conjunction with a comprehensive weight management program.

Local Anesthetic/Vasoconstrictor Precautions Use vasoconstrictor with caution in patients taking phentermine. Amphetamines enhance the sympathomimetic response of epinephrine and norepinephrine leading to potential hypertension and cardiotoxicity.

Effects on Dental Treatment Key adverse event(s) related to dental treatment: Xerostomia (normal salivary flow resumes upon discontinuation) and unpleasant taste. Up to 10% of patients may present with hypertension. The use of local anesthetic without vasoconstrictor is recommended in these patients. See Dental Comment.

Effects on Bleeding No information available to require special precautions

Adverse Effects Frequency not defined.

Cardiovascular: Hypertension, palpitation, primary pulmonary hypertension and/or regurgitant cardiac valvular disease, tachycardia

Central nervous system: Dizziness, dysphoria, euphoria, headache, insomnia, overstimulation, psychosis, restlessness

Dermatologic: Urticaria

Endocrine & metabolic: Changes in libido

Gastrointestinal: Constipation, diarrhea, unpleasant taste, xerostomia

Genitourinary: Impotence

Neuromuscular & skeletal: Tremor

General Dosage Range Oral: *Children >16 years and Adults:* 15-37.5 mg/day

Mechanism of Action Phentermine is a sympathomimetic amine with pharmacologic properties similar to the amphetamines. The mechanism of action in reducing appetite appears to be secondary to CNS effects, including stimulation of the hypothalamus to release norepinephrine.

Pregnancy Risk Factor C

Controlled Substance C-IV

Dental Comment Many diet physicians have prescribed fenfluramine ("fen") and phentermine ("phen"). When taken together the combination is known as "fen-phen". The diet drug dexfenfluramine (Redux®) is chemically similar to fenfluramine (Pondimin®) and was also used in combination with phentermine called "Redux-phen". While each of the three drugs alone had approval from the FDA for sale in the treatment of obesity, neither combination had an official approval. The use of the combinations in the treatment of obesity was considered an "off-label" use. Reports in medical literature have been accumulating for some years about significant side effects associated with fenfluramine and dexfenfluramine. In 1997, the manufacturers, at the urging of the FDA, agreed to voluntarily withdraw the drugs from the market. The action was based on findings from physicians who evaluated patients taking fenfluramine and dexfenfluramine with echocardiograms. The findings indicated that approximately 30% of patients had abnormal echocardiograms, even though they had no symptoms. This was a much higher than expected percentage of abnormal test results. This conclusion was based on a sample of 291 patients examined by five different physicians. Under normal conditions, fewer than 1% of patients would be expected to show signs of heart valve disease. The findings suggested that fenfluramine and dexfenfluramine were the likely cause of heart valve problems of the type that promoted FDA's earlier warnings concerning "fen-phen". The earlier warning included the following: The mitral valve and other valves in the heart are damaged by a strange white coating and allow blood to flow back, causing heart muscle damage. In several cases, valve replacement surgery has been done. As a rule, the person must, thereafter for life, be on a blood thinner to prevent clots from the mechanical valve. This type of valve damage had only been seen before in persons who were exposed to large amounts of serotonin. The fenfluramine increases the availability of serotonin.

Phentolamine (fen TOLE a meen)

Related Information

Oral Pain *on page 1928*

Ulcerative, Erosive, and Painful Oral Mucosal Disorders *on page 1950*

U.S. Brand Names OraVerse™

Canadian Brand Names Regitine®; Rogitine®

Generic Availability (U.S.) Yes

Pharmacologic Category $Alpha_1$ Blocker

Dental Use Reversal of soft tissue anesthesia and the associated functional deficits resulting from a local dental anesthetic containing a vasoconstrictor

Use Diagnosis of pheochromocytoma and treatment of hypertension associated with pheochromocytoma or other forms of hypertension caused by excess sympathomimetic amines; treatment of dermal necrosis after extravasation of drugs with alpha-adrenergic effects (ie, dopamine, epinephrine, norepinephrine, phenylephrine)

OraVerse™: Reversal of soft tissue anesthesia and the associated functional deficits resulting from a local dental anesthetic containing a vasoconstrictor

Unlabeled/Investigational Use Treatment of pralidoxime-induced hypertension

Local Anesthetic/Vasoconstrictor Precautions Although the alpha-adrenergic blocking effects could antagonize epinephrine, there is no information available to require special precautions

Effects on Dental Treatment Key adverse event(s) related to dental treatment: The most common reaction that was greater than controls was injection site pain (~4% to 6%). A few incidences of paresthesia associated with OraVerse™ have been reported. These incidences were mild and transient, and resolved during the same time period. Orthostatic hypotension has also been reported.

Effects on Bleeding No information available to require special precautions

Adverse Effects Frequency not always defined.

Cardiovascular: Arrhythmia, flushing, hypertension (OraVerse™), hypotension, orthostatic hypotension, tachycardia (OraVerse™ ≤6%), bradycardia (OraVerse™ ≤4%)

Central nervous system: Dizziness, headache (OraVerse™ ≤6%)

Dermatologic: Pruritus (OraVerse™)

Gastrointestinal: Nausea, vomiting, diarrhea

Local: Injection site pain (OraVerse™ 4% to 6%)

Neuromuscular & skeletal: Paresthesia (OraVerse™), weakness

Respiratory: Nasal congestion

Dental Usual Dosage Reversal of soft tissue (lip, tongue) anesthesia (OraVerse™): Infiltration or block technique:submucosal oral injection:

Children: 15-30 kg: 0.2 mg maximum dose

Children >30 kg and <12 years: 0.4 mg maximum dose

Adults: **Note:** Dose is based upon the number of cartridges of local anesthetic administered. Infiltration or block injection:

0.2 mg if one-half cartridge of anesthesia was administered

0.4 mg if 1 cartridge of anesthesia was administered

0.8 mg if 2 cartridges of anesthesia were administered

Dosage

Treatment of alpha-adrenergic agonist drug extravasation: SubQ:

Children: Infiltrate area with a small amount (eg, 1 mL given in 0.2 mL aliquots) of a 0.5-1 mg/mL solution (made by diluting 5-10 mg in 10 mL of NS) within 12 hours of extravasation; in general, do not exceed 0.1-0.2 mg/kg or 5 mg total

Adults: Infiltrate area with small amount of solution made by diluting 5-10 mg in 10 mL 0.9% sodium chloride within 12 hours of extravasation; in general, do not exceed 0.1-0.2 mg/kg (5 mg total); typically doses of ≤5 mg are effective; a case using 50 mg for a large extravasation has been reported (Cooper, 1989).

If dose is effective, normal skin color should return to the blanched area within 1 hour

Diagnosis of pheochromocytoma: I.M., I.V.:

Children: 0.05-0.1 mg/kg/dose, maximum single dose: 5 mg

Adults: 5 mg

Surgery for pheochromocytoma: Hypertension: I.M., I.V.:

Children: 0.05-0.1 mg/kg/dose given 1-2 hours before procedure; repeat as needed every 2-4 hours until hypertension is controlled; maximum single dose: 5 mg

Adults: 5 mg given 1-2 hours before procedure and repeated as needed every 2-4 hours

Hypertensive crisis: Adults: 5-20 mg

Treatment of pralidoxime-induced hypertension (unlabeled use): I.V.:

Children: 1 mg

Adults and Elderly: 5 mg

Reversal of soft tissue (lip, tongue) anesthesia (OraVerse™): Infiltration or block technique: Submucosal oral injection:
Children: 15-30 kg: 0.2 mg maximum dose
Children >30 kg and <12 years: 0.4 mg maximum dose
Adults: **Note:** Dose is based upon the number of cartridges of local anesthetic administered. Infiltration or block injection:
0.2 mg if one-half cartridge of anesthesia was administered
0.4 mg if 1 cartridge of anesthesia was administered
0.8 mg if 2 cartridges of anesthesia were administered

Mechanism of Action Competitively blocks alpha-adrenergic receptors to produce brief antagonism of circulating epinephrine and norepinephrine to reduce hypertension caused by alpha effects of these catecholamines; also has a positive inotropic and chronotropic effect on the heart

OraVerse™: Causes vasodilation and increased blood flow in injection area via alpha-adrenergic blockade to accelerate reversal of soft tissue anesthetic

Contraindications Hypersensitivity to phentolamine or any component of the formulation; renal impairment; coronary or cerebral arteriosclerosis; concurrent use with phosphodiesterase-5 (PDE-5) inhibitors including sildenafil (>25 mg), tadalafil, or vardenafil

OraVerse™: There are no contraindications listed in the manufacturer's labeling.

Warnings/Precautions Myocardial infarction, cerebrovascular spasm, and cerebrovascular occlusion have occurred following administration; use with caution in patients with gastritis or peptic ulcer, tachycardia, or a history of cardiac arrhythmias. Discontinue if symptoms of angina occur or worsen. OraVerse™: Efficacy has not been established in children <6 years of age or <15 kg (33 pounds).

Drug Interactions

Avoid Concomitant Use

Avoid concomitant use of Phentolamine with any of the following: Alpha1-Blockers

Increased Effect/Toxicity

Phentolamine may increase the levels/effects of: Alpha1-Blockers; Amifostine; Antihypertensives; Calcium Channel Blockers; RiTUXimab

The levels/effects of Phentolamine may be increased by: Beta-Blockers; Diazoxide; Herbs (Hypotensive Properties); MAO Inhibitors; Pentoxifylline; Phosphodiesterase 5 Inhibitors; Prostacyclin Analogues

Decreased Effect

The levels/effects of Phentolamine may be decreased by: Herbs (Hypertensive Properties); Methylphenidate; Yohimbine

Pharmacodynamics/Kinetics

Onset of Action I.M.: 15-20 minutes; I.V.: Immediate
Peak effect: OraVerse™: 10-20 minutes

Duration of Action I.M.: 30-45 minutes; I.V.: 15-30 minutes

Half-life Elimination 19 minutes

Pregnancy Risk Factor C

Lactation Excretion in breast milk unknown

Dosage Forms

Injection, powder for reconstitution: 5 mg
Injection, solution [preservative free]:
OraVerse™: 0.4 mg/1.7 mL (1.7 mL)

Dental Comment OraVerse™ (solution for injection/dental cartridge) is administered as a submucosal injection and is not to be confused with phentolamine used as an intramuscular or intravenous injection for the treatment of hypertension associated with pheochromocytoma.

In adolescents >12 years and adults, OraVerse™ reduced the median time to recovery of normal sensation in the lower lip by 85 minutes compared to control. OraVerse™ reduced the median time to recovery of normal sensation in the upper lip by 83 minutes. Within 1 hour after administration, 41% of patients reported normal lower lip sensation as compared to 7% in the control group and 59% of patients given OraVerse™ reported normal upper lip sensation as compared to 12% in the control group.

In children 6-11 years of age, the median time to normal sensation was reduced by 75 minutes after OraVerse™ administration, a 56% acceleration of the time to normal sensation.

Phenylephrine (Systemic) (fen il EF rin)

U.S. Brand Names LuSonal™ [DSC]; Medi-First® Sinus Decongestant [OTC]; Medi-Phenyl [OTC]; PediaCare® Children's Decongestant [OTC]; Sudafed PE® Children's [OTC]; Sudafed PE® Congestion [OTC]; Sudafed PE™ Nasal

Decongestant [OTC]; Sudogest™ PE [OTC]; Triaminic Thin Strips® Children's Cold with Stuffy Nose [OTC]

Pharmacologic Category Alpha/Beta Agonist

Use Treatment of hypotension, vascular failure in shock; as a vasoconstrictor in regional analgesia; supraventricular tachycardia (**Note:** Not for routine use in treatment of supraventricular tachycardias); as a decongestant [OTC]

Local Anesthetic/Vasoconstrictor Precautions Use with caution since phenylephrine is a sympathomimetic amine which could interact with epinephrine to cause a pressor response

Effects on Dental Treatment Key adverse event(s) related to dental treatment: Tachycardia, palpitations (use vasoconstrictor with caution), and xerostomia (normal salivary flow resumes upon discontinuation).

Effects on Bleeding No information available to require special precautions

Adverse Effects Frequency not defined.

Injection:

Cardiovascular: Arrhythmia (rare), decreased cardiac output, hypertension, pallor, precordial pain or discomfort, reflex bradycardia, severe peripheral and visceral vasoconstriction

Central nervous system: Anxiety, dizziness, excitability, giddiness, headache, insomnia, nervousness, restlessness

Endocrine & metabolic: Metabolic acidosis

Gastrointestinal: Gastric irritation, nausea

Local: I.V.: Extravasation which may lead to necrosis and sloughing of surrounding tissue, blanching of skin

Neuromuscular & skeletal: Paresthesia, pilomotor response, tremor, weakness

Renal: Decreased renal perfusion, reduced urine output

Respiratory: Respiratory distress

Miscellaneous: Hypersensitivity reactions (including rash, urticaria, leukopenia, agranulocytosis, thrombocytopenia)

Oral: Central nervous system: Anxiety, dizziness, excitability, giddiness, headache, insomnia, nervousness, restlessness

General Dosage Range

I.V.:

Children: Bolus: 5-20 mcg/kg/dose every 10-15 minutes as needed; Infusion: 0.1-0.5 mcg/kg/minute

Adults: Bolus: 0.1-0.5 mg/dose every 10-15 minutes as needed (maximum: 0.5 mg); Infusion: Initial: 100-180 mcg/minute

Oral:

Children 4 to <6 years: 2.5 mg every 4 hours as needed for ≤7 days

Children 6 to <12 years: 5 mg every 4 hours as needed for ≤7 days

Children ≥12 years and Adults: 10-20 mg every 4 hours as needed for ≤7 days

Mechanism of Action Potent, direct-acting alpha-adrenergic agonist with virtually no beta-adrenergic activity; produces systemic arterial vasoconstriction. Such increases in systemic vascular resistance result in dose dependent increases in systolic and diastolic blood pressure and reductions in heart rate and cardiac output especially in patients with heart failure.

Pharmacodynamics/Kinetics

Onset of Action

Blood pressure increase/vasoconstriction: I.M., SubQ: 10-15 minutes; I.V.: Immediate

Nasal decongestant: Oral: 15-30 minutes (Kollar, 2007)

Duration of Action

Blood pressure increase/vasoconstriction: I.M.: 1-2 hours; I.V.: ~15-20 minutes; SubQ: 50 minutes

Nasal decongestant: Oral: ≤4 hours (Kollar, 2007)

Half-life Elimination Alpha phase: ~5 minutes; Terminal phase: 2-3 hours (Hengstmann, 1982; Kanfer, 1993)

Time to Peak Oral: 0.75-2 hours (Kanfer, 1993)

Pregnancy Risk Factor C

Phenylephrine (Topical) (fen il EF rin)

U.S. Brand Names Anu-Med [OTC]; Formulation R™ [OTC]; Medicone® Suppositories [OTC]; Preparation H® [OTC]; Rectacaine [OTC]; Tronolane® Suppository [OTC]

Pharmacologic Category Alpha/Beta Agonist

Use For OTC use as treatment of hemorrhoids

Local Anesthetic/Vasoconstrictor Precautions No information available to require special precautions

Effects on Dental Treatment No significant effects or complications reported

Effects on Bleeding No information available to require special precautions

Adverse Effects Rare systemic effects may occur.

General Dosage Range Rectal: *Children >12 years and Adults:* Ointment: Apply up to 4 times/day; Suppository: Insert 1 up to 4 times/day

Mechanism of Action Potent, direct-acting alpha-adrenergic agonist with virtually no beta-adrenergic activity; produces local vasoconstriction.

Phenylephrine and Zinc Sulfate (fen il EF rin & zingk SUL fate)

Related Information

Zinc Sulfate *on page 1745*

Canadian Brand Names Zincfrin®

Pharmacologic Category Adrenergic Agonist Agent

Use Soothe, moisturize, and remove redness due to minor eye irritation

Local Anesthetic/Vasoconstrictor Precautions No information available to require special precautions

Effects on Dental Treatment No significant effects or complications reported

Effects on Bleeding No information available to require special precautions

General Dosage Range Ophthalmic: *Adults:* Instill 1-2 drops in eye(s) 2-4 times/day as needed

Product Availability Not available in U.S.

Phenylephrine, Pyrilamine, and Guaifenesin
(fen il EF rin, peer IL a meen, & gwye FEN e sin)

Related Information

GuaiFENesin *on page 835*
Phenylephrine (Systemic) *on page 1339*

U.S. Brand Names Ryna-12X® [DSC]

Pharmacologic Category Alpha/Beta Agonist; Decongestant; Ethylenediamine Derivative; Expectorant; Histamine H_1 Antagonist; Histamine H_1 Antagonist, First Generation

Use Symptomatic relief of cough, nasal congestion, and discharge associated with the common cold, sinusitis, allergic rhinitis, and other respiratory tract conditions

Local Anesthetic/Vasoconstrictor Precautions Use with caution since phenylephrine is a sympathomimetic amine which could interact with epinephrine or mepivacaine and levonordefrin (Carbocaine® 2% with Neo-Cobefrin®) to cause a pressor response.

Effects on Dental Treatment Key adverse event(s) related to dental treatment:

Pyrilamine: Prolonged use will cause significant xerostomia (normal salivary flow resumes upon discontinuation).

Phenylephrine: Up to 10% of patients could experience tachycardia, palpitations, and xerostomia.

Effects on Bleeding No information available to require special precautions

Adverse Effects Frequency not defined.

Central nervous system: Dizziness (rare), drowsiness, headache, nervousness, restlessness, sedation

Dermatologic: Rash (rare), urticaria (rare)

Gastrointestinal: Dry mucous membranes, nausea, vomiting

General Dosage Range Oral:

Children 2-6 years: 2.5-5 mL of the suspension every 12 hours

Children 6-11 years: 5-10 mL of the suspension **or** 1/2 to 1 tablet every 12 hours

Children ≥12 years and Adults: 1-2 tablets every 12 hours

Mechanism of Action

Phenylephrine is a sympathomimetic agent (primarily alpha), decongestant.

Pyrilamine is an H_1-receptor antagonist.

Guaifenesin is an expectorant.

Pregnancy Risk Factor C

Phenytoin (FEN i toyn)

Related Information

Cardiovascular Diseases *on page 1848*
Fosphenytoin *on page 790*

U.S. Brand Names Dilantin-125®; Dilantin®; Phenytek®

Canadian Brand Names Dilantin®

Generic Availability (U.S.) Yes: Excludes chewable tablet

Pharmacologic Category Anticonvulsant, Hydantoin

Use Management of generalized tonic-clonic (grand mal), complex partial seizures; prevention of seizures following head trauma/neurosurgery

Local Anesthetic/Vasoconstrictor Precautions No information available to require special precautions

Effects on Dental Treatment Gingival hyperplasia is a common problem observed during the first 6 months of phenytoin therapy appearing as gingivitis or gum inflammation. To minimize severity and growth rate of gingival tissue begin a program of professional cleaning and patient plaque control within 10 days of starting anticonvulsant therapy.

Effects on Bleeding No information available to require special precautions

Adverse Effects I.V. effects: Hypotension, bradycardia, cardiac arrhythmia, cardiovascular collapse (especially with rapid I.V. use), venous irritation and pain, thrombophlebitis

Effects not related to plasma phenytoin concentrations: Hypertrichosis, gingival hypertrophy, thickening of facial features, carbohydrate intolerance, folic acid deficiency, peripheral neuropathy, vitamin D deficiency, osteomalacia, systemic lupus erythematosus

Concentration-related effects: Nystagmus, blurred vision, diplopia, ataxia, slurred speech, dizziness, drowsiness, lethargy, coma, rash, fever, nausea, vomiting, gum tenderness, confusion, mood changes, folic acid depletion, osteomalacia, hyperglycemia

Related to elevated concentrations:

>20 mcg/mL: Far lateral nystagmus

>30 mcg/mL: 45° lateral gaze nystagmus and ataxia

>40 mcg/mL: Decreased mentation

>100 mcg/mL: Death

Cardiovascular: Hypotension, bradycardia, cardiac arrhythmia, cardiovascular collapse

Central nervous system: Psychiatric changes, slurred speech, dizziness, drowsiness, headache, insomnia

Dermatologic: Rash

Gastrointestinal: Constipation, nausea, vomiting, gingival hyperplasia, enlargement of lips

Hematologic: Leukopenia, thrombocytopenia, agranulocytosis

Hepatic: Hepatitis

Local: Thrombophlebitis

Neuromuscular & skeletal: Tremor, peripheral neuropathy, paresthesia

Ocular: Diplopia, nystagmus, blurred vision

Rarely seen effects: Blood dyscrasias, coarsening of facial features, dyskinesias, hepatitis, hypertrichosis, lymphadenopathy, lymphoma, pseudolymphoma, SLE-like syndrome, Stevens-Johnson syndrome, toxic epidermal necrolysis, venous irritation and pain

Dosage Note: Phenytoin base (eg, oral suspension, chewable tablets) contains ~8% more drug than phenytoin sodium (~92 mg base is equivalent to 100 mg phenytoin sodium). Dosage adjustments and closer serum monitoring may be necessary when switching dosage forms.

Status epilepticus: I.V.:

Infants and Children: Loading dose: 15-20 mg/kg in a single or divided dose; maintenance dose: Initial: 5 mg/kg/day in 2 divided doses; usual doses:

6 months to 3 years: 8-10 mg/kg/day

4-6 years: 7.5-9 mg/kg/day

7-9 years: 7-8 mg/kg/day

10-16 years: 6-7 mg/kg/day, some patients may require every 8 hours dosing

Adults: Loading dose: Manufacturer recommends 10-15 mg/kg, however, 15-20 mg/kg is generally recommended; maximum rate: 50 mg/minute

Anticonvulsant: Children and Adults: Oral:

Loading dose: 15-20 mg/kg; based on phenytoin serum concentrations and recent dosing history; administer oral loading dose in 3 divided doses given every 2-4 hours to decrease GI adverse effects and to ensure complete oral absorption; maintenance dose: same as I.V.

Neurosurgery (prophylactic): 100-200 mg at approximately 4-hour intervals during surgery and during the immediate postoperative period

Dosage adjustment in obesity: Adults: Loading dose: Use adjusted body weight (ABW) correction based on a pharmacokinetic study of phenytoin loading doses in obese patients (Abernethy, 1985). The larger correction factor (ie, 1.33) is due to a doubling of V_d estimated in these obese patients.

ABW = [(Actual body weight – IBW) x 1.33] + IBW

Maximum loading dose: 2000 mg (Erstad, 2004)

Maintenance doses should be based on ideal body weight, conventional daily doses with adjustments based upon therapeutic drug monitoring and clinical effectiveness. (Abernethy, 1985; Erstad, 2002; Erstad, 2004)

Dosing adjustment/comments in renal impairment or hepatic disease: Safe in usual doses in mild liver disease; clearance may be substantially reduced in cirrhosis and plasma level monitoring with dose adjustment advisable. Free phenytoin levels should be monitored closely.

Mechanism of Action Stabilizes neuronal membranes and decreases seizure activity by increasing efflux or decreasing influx of sodium ions across cell membranes in the motor cortex during generation of nerve impulses; prolongs effective refractory period and suppresses ventricular pacemaker automaticity, shortens action potential in the heart

Contraindications Hypersensitivity to phenytoin, other hydantoins, or any component of the formulation; pregnancy

Warnings/Precautions Antiepileptics are associated with an increased risk of suicidal behavior/thoughts with use (regardless of indication); patients should be monitored for signs/symptoms of depression, suicidal tendencies, and other unusual behavior changes during therapy and instructed to inform their healthcare provider immediately if symptoms occur.

[U.S. Boxed Warning]: Phenytoin must be administered slowly. Intravenous administration should not exceed 50 mg/minute in adult patients. In neonates, intravenous administration rate should not exceed 1-3 mg/kg/minute (most clinicians use a lower maximum rate of infusion in neonates of 0.5-1 mg/kg/minute). Hypotension may occur with rapid administration. I.V. form may cause skin necrosis at I.V. site; avoid I.V. administration in small veins; may increase frequency of petit mal seizures; use with caution in patients with porphyria; discontinue if rash or lymphadenopathy occurs; a spectrum of hematologic effects have been reported with use (eg, neutropenia, leukopenia, thrombocytopenia, pancytopenia, and anemias); use with caution in patients with hepatic dysfunction, sinus bradycardia, S-A block, or AV block; use with caution in elderly or debilitated patients, or in any condition associated with low serum albumin levels, which will increase the free fraction of phenytoin in the serum and, therefore, the pharmacologic response. Sedation, confusional states, or cerebellar dysfunction (loss of motor coordination) may occur at higher total serum concentrations, or at lower total serum concentrations when the free fraction of phenytoin is increased. Effects with other sedative drugs or ethanol may be potentiated. Abrupt withdrawal may precipitate status epilepticus. Severe reactions, including toxic epidermal necrolysis and Stevens-Johnson syndromes, although rarely reported, have resulted in fatalities; drug should be discontinued if there are any signs of rash. Patients of Asian descent with the variant *HLA-B*1502* may be at an increased risk of developing Stevens-Johnson syndrome and/or toxic epidermal necrolysis.

Drug Interactions

Metabolism/Transport Effects **Substrate** of CYP2C9 (major), 2C19 (major), 3A4 (minor); **Induces** CYP2B6 (strong), 2C8 (strong), 2C9 (strong), 2C19 (strong), 3A4 (strong)

Avoid Concomitant Use

Avoid concomitant use of Phenytoin with any of the following: Darunavir; Dronedarone; Etravirine; Everolimus; Lurasidone; Nilotinib; Pazopanib; Praziquantel; Ranolazine; Roflumilast; RomiDEPsin; Tolvaptan; Vandetanib

Increased Effect/Toxicity

Phenytoin may increase the levels/effects of: Alcohol (Ethyl); CNS Depressants; Fosamprenavir; Lithium; Methotrimeprazine; Vecuronium; Vitamin K Antagonists

The levels/effects of Phenytoin may be increased by: Allopurinol; Amiodarone; Antifungal Agents (Azole Derivatives, Systemic); Benzodiazepines; Calcium Channel Blockers; Capecitabine; CarBAMazepine; Carbonic Anhydrase Inhibitors; CeFAZolin; Chloramphenicol; Cimetidine; Conivaptan; CYP2C19 Inhibitors (Moderate); CYP2C19 Inhibitors (Strong); CYP2C9 Inhibitors (Moderate); CYP2C9 Inhibitors (Strong); Dexmethylphenidate; Disulfiram; Droperidol; Efavirenz; Felbamate; Floxuridine; Fluconazole; Fluorouracil; Fluorouracil (Systemic); Fluorouracil (Topical); FLUoxetine; FluvoxaMINE; Isoniazid; Methotrimeprazine; Methylphenidate; MetroNIDAZOLE; MetroNIDAZOLE (Systemic); OXcarbazepine; Proton Pump Inhibitors; Rufinamide; Sertraline; Sulfonamide Derivatives; Tacrolimus; Tacrolimus (Systemic); Ticlopidine; Topiramate; Trimethoprim; Vitamin K Antagonists

Decreased Effect

Phenytoin may decrease the levels/effects of: Acetaminophen; Amiodarone; Antifungal Agents (Azole Derivatives, Systemic); CarBAMazepine; Caspofungin; Chloramphenicol; CloZAPine; Contraceptives (Estrogens); Contraceptives (Progestins); CycloSPORINE; CycloSPORINE (Systemic); CYP2B6 Substrates;

CYP2C19 Substrates; CYP2C8 Substrates (High risk); CYP2C9 Substrates (High risk); CYP3A4 Substrates; Darunavir; Deferasirox; Disopyramide; Divalproex; Doxycycline; Dronedarone; Efavirenz; Etoposide; Etoposide Phosphate; Etravirine; Everolimus; Exemestane; Felbamate; Flunarizine; Gefitinib; GuanFACINE; HMG-CoA Reductase Inhibitors; Imatinib; Irinotecan; Ixabepilone; Lacosamide; LamoTRIgine; Levodopa; Loop Diuretics; Lopinavir; Lurasidone; Maraviroc; Mebendazole; Meperidine; Methadone; MetroNIDAZOLE; MetroNIDAZOLE (Systemic); Metyrapone; Mexiletine; Nilotinib; OXcarbazepine; Pazopanib; Praziquantel; Primidone; QUEtiapine; QuiNIDine; QuiNINE; Ranolazine; Ritonavir; Roflumilast; RomiDEPsin; Rufinamide; Saxagliptin; Sertraline; Sirolimus; SORAfenib; Tacrolimus; Tacrolimus (Systemic); Tadalafil; Temsirolimus; Teniposide; Theophylline Derivatives; Thyroid Products; Tipranavir; Tolvaptan; Topiramate; Treprostinil; Ulipristal; Valproic Acid; Vandetanib; Vecuronium; Zonisamide

The levels/effects of Phenytoin may be decreased by: Amphetamines; Antacids; Barbiturates; CarBAMazepine; Ciprofloxacin; Ciprofloxacin (Systemic); CISplatin; Colesevelam; CYP2C19 Inducers (Strong); CYP2C9 Inducers (Highly Effective); Diazoxide; Divalproex; Folic Acid; Fosamprenavir; Ketorolac; Ketorolac (Systemic); Leucovorin Calcium-Levoleucovorin; Levomefolate; Lopinavir; Mefloquine; Methylfolate; Peginterferon Alfa-2b; Pyridoxine; Rifamycin Derivatives; Ritonavir; Theophylline Derivatives; Tipranavir; Tocilizumab; Valproic Acid; Vigabatrin

Ethanol/Nutrition/Herb Interactions

Ethanol:

Acute use: Avoid or limit ethanol (inhibits metabolism of phenytoin). Ethanol may also increase CNS depression; monitor for increased effects with coadministration. Caution patients about effects.

Chronic use: Avoid or limit ethanol (stimulates metabolism of phenytoin).

Food: Phenytoin serum concentrations may be altered if taken with food. If taken with enteral nutrition, phenytoin serum concentrations may be decreased. Tube feedings decrease bioavailability; hold tube feedings 1-2 hours before and 1-2 hours after phenytoin administration. May decrease calcium, folic acid, and vitamin D levels.

Herb/Nutraceutical: Avoid evening primrose (seizure threshold decreased). Avoid valerian, St John's wort, kava kava, gotu kola (may increase CNS depression).

Dietary Considerations

Folic acid: Phenytoin may decrease mucosal uptake of folic acid; to avoid folic acid deficiency and megaloblastic anemia, some clinicians recommend giving patients on anticonvulsants prophylactic doses of folic acid and cyanocobalamin. However, folate supplementation may increase seizures in some patients (dose dependent). Discuss with healthcare provider prior to using any supplements.

Calcium: Hypocalcemia has been reported in patients taking prolonged high-dose therapy with an anticonvulsant. Some clinicians have given an additional 4000 units/week of vitamin D (especially in those receiving poor nutrition and getting no sun exposure) to prevent hypocalcemia.

Vitamin D: Phenytoin interferes with vitamin D metabolism and osteomalacia may result; may need to supplement with vitamin D

Tube feedings: Tube feedings decrease phenytoin absorption. To avoid decreased serum levels with continuous NG feeds, hold feedings for 1-2 hours prior to and 1-2 hours after phenytoin administration, if possible. There is a variety of opinions on how to administer phenytoin with enteral feedings. Be **consistent** throughout therapy.

Injection may contain sodium.

Pharmacodynamics/Kinetics

Onset of Action I.V.: ~0.5-1 hour

Half-life Elimination Oral: 22 hours (range: 7-42 hours)

Time to Peak Serum (form dependent): Oral: Extended-release capsule: 4-12 hours; Immediate release preparation: 2-3 hours

Pregnancy Risk Factor D

Lactation Enters breast milk/not recommended (AAP rates "compatible"; AAP 2001 update pending)

Breast-Feeding Considerations Phenytoin is excreted in breast milk; however, the amount to which the infant is exposed is considered small. The manufacturers of phenytoin do not recommend breast-feeding during therapy. Women should be counseled of the possible risks and benefits associated with breast-feeding while on phenytoin.

Dosage Forms

Capsule, extended release, oral: 100 mg, 200 mg, 300 mg

Dilantin®: 30 mg, 100 mg

Phenytek®: 200 mg, 300 mg

Injection, solution: 50 mg/mL (2 mL, 5 mL)
Suspension, oral: 100 mg/4 mL (4 mL); 125 mg/5 mL (120 mL, 237 mL, 240 mL)
Dilantin-125®: 125 mg/5 mL (240 mL)
Tablet, chewable, oral:
Dilantin®: 50 mg

Physostigmine (fye zoe STIG meen)

Pharmacologic Category Acetylcholinesterase Inhibitor

Use Reverse toxic, life-threatening delirium caused by atropine, diphenhydramine, dimenhydrinate, *Atropa belladonna* (deadly nightshade), or jimson weed (*Datura* spp)

Local Anesthetic/Vasoconstrictor Precautions No information available to require special precautions

Effects on Dental Treatment Key adverse event(s) related to dental treatment: Salivation.

Effects on Bleeding No information available to require special precautions

Adverse Effects Frequency not defined.
Cardiovascular: Asystole, bradycardia, palpitation
Central nervous system: Hallucinations, nervousness, restlessness, seizure
Gastrointestinal: Diarrhea, nausea, salivation, stomach pain
Genitourinary: Urinary frequency
Neuromuscular & skeletal: Twitching
Ocular: Lacrimation, miosis
Respiratory: Bronchospasm, dyspnea, pulmonary edema, respiratory paralysis
Miscellaneous: Diaphoresis

General Dosage Range
I.M.: *Adults:* Initial: 0.5-2 mg, repeat every 20 minutes until response or adverse effects occur; repeat 1-4 mg every 30-60 minutes as life-threatening symptoms recur
I.V.:
Children: 0.01-0.03 mg/kg/dose, may repeat after 5-10 minutes (maximum total dose: 2 mg)
Adults: Initial: 0.5-2 mg, repeat every 20 minutes until response or adverse effects occur; repeat 1-4 mg every 30-60 minutes as life-threatening symptoms recur

Mechanism of Action Inhibits destruction of acetylcholine by acetylcholinesterase which facilitates transmission of impulses across myoneural junction and prolongs the central and peripheral effects of acetylcholine

Pharmacodynamics/Kinetics
Onset of Action ~5 minutes
Duration of Action 1-2 hours
Half-life Elimination 15-40 minutes

Pregnancy Risk Factor C

Phytonadione (fye toe na DYE one)

U.S. Brand Names Mephyton®

Canadian Brand Names AquaMEPHYTON®; Konakion; Mephyton®

Pharmacologic Category Vitamin, Fat Soluble

Use Prevention and treatment of hypoprothrombinemia caused by coumarin derivative-induced or other drug-induced vitamin K deficiency, hypoprothrombinemia caused by malabsorption or inability to synthesize vitamin K; hemorrhagic disease of the newborn

Unlabeled/Investigational Use Treatment of hypoprothrombinemia caused by anticoagulant rodenticides

Local Anesthetic/Vasoconstrictor Precautions No information available to require special precautions

Effects on Dental Treatment Key adverse event(s) related to dental treatment: Abnormal taste.

Effects on Bleeding No information available to require special precautions

Adverse Effects Parenteral administration: Frequency not defined.
Cardiovascular: Cyanosis, flushing, hypotension
Central nervous system: Dizziness
Dermatologic: Scleroderma-like lesions
Endocrine & metabolic: Hyperbilirubinemia (newborn; greater than recommended doses)
Gastrointestinal: Abnormal taste
Local: Injection site reactions
Respiratory: Dyspnea
Miscellaneous: Anaphylactoid reactions, diaphoresis, hypersensitivity reactions

General Dosage Range

I.M.:

Newborns: Prophylaxis: 0.5-1 mg within 1 hour of birth; Treatment: 1 mg/dose/day

Adults: Initial: 2.5-25 mg/dose (usual: 5-10 mg; maximum: 50 mg)

I.V.: *Adults:* Initial: 2.5-25 mg/dose (usual: 5-10 mg; maximum: 50 mg)

Oral:

Children 1-3 years: RDA: 30 mcg/day

Children 4-8 years: RDA: 55 mcg/day

Children 9-13 years: RDA: 60 mcg/day

Children 14-18 years: RDA: 75 mcg/day

Adults: Initial: 2.5-25 mg/dose (usual: 5-10 mg; maximum: 50 mg)

SubQ:

Newborns: 1 mg/dose/day

Adults: Initial: 2.5-25 mg/dose (usual: 5-10 mg; maximum: 50 mg)

Mechanism of Action Promotes liver synthesis of clotting factors (II, VII, IX, X); however, the exact mechanism as to this stimulation is unknown. Menadiol is a water soluble form of vitamin K; phytonadione has a more rapid and prolonged effect than menadione; menadiol sodium diphosphate (K_4) is half as potent as menadione (K_3).

Pharmacodynamics/Kinetics

Onset of Action

Onset of action: Increased coagulation factors: Oral: 6-10 hours; I.V.: 1-2 hours

Peak effect: INR values return to normal: Oral: 24-48 hours; I.V.: 12-14 hours

Pregnancy Risk Factor C

Pilocarpine (Systemic) (pye loe KAR peen)

Related Information

Dentin Hypersensitivity, Acid Erosion, High Caries Index, and Xerostomia *on page 1955*

Management of Patients Undergoing Cancer Therapy *on page 1970*

U.S. Brand Names Salagen®

Canadian Brand Names Salagen®

Generic Availability (U.S.) Yes

Pharmacologic Category Cholinergic Agonist

Dental Use Treatment of xerostomia caused by radiation therapy in patients with head and neck cancer and from Sjögren's syndrome

Use Symptomatic treatment of xerostomia caused by salivary gland hypofunction resulting from radiotherapy for cancer of the head and neck or Sjögren's syndrome

Local Anesthetic/Vasoconstrictor Precautions No information available to require special precautions

Effects on Dental Treatment Key adverse event(s) related to dental treatment: Increased salivation (therapeutic effect). See Dental Comment.

Effects on Bleeding No information available to require special precautions

Adverse Effects

>10%:

Cardiovascular: Flushing (8% to 13%)

Central nervous system: Chills (3% to 15%), dizziness (5% to 12%), headache (11%)

Gastrointestinal: Nausea (6% to 15%)

Genitourinary: Urinary frequency (9% to 12%)

Neuromuscular & skeletal: Weakness (2% to 12%)

Respiratory: Rhinitis (5% to 14%)

Miscellaneous: Diaphoresis (29% to 68%)

1% to 10%:

Cardiovascular: Edema (<1% to 5%), facial edema, hypertension (3%), palpitation, tachycardia

Central nervous system: Pain (4%), fever, somnolence

Dermatologic: Pruritus, rash

Gastrointestinal: Diarrhea (4% to 7%), dyspepsia (7%), vomiting (3% to 4%), constipation, flatulence, glossitis, salivation increased, stomatitis, taste perversion

Genitourinary: Vaginitis, urinary incontinence

Neuromuscular & skeletal: Myalgias, tremor

Ocular: Lacrimation (6%), amblyopia (4%), abnormal vision, blurred vision, conjunctivitis

Otic: Tinnitus

Respiratory: Cough increased, dysphagia, epistaxis, sinusitis

Miscellaneous: Allergic reaction, voice alteration

Dental Usual Dosage Treatment of xerostomia: Adults: Oral: 1-2 tablets 3-4 times/day not to exceed 30 mg/day (minimum 90-day therapy required for optimum effects)

Dosage Oral: Adults: Xerostomia:

Following head and neck cancer: 5 mg 3 times/day, titration up to 10 mg 3 times/day may be considered for patients who have not responded adequately; do not exceed 2 tablets/dose

Sjögren's syndrome: 5 mg 4 times/day

Dosage adjustment in hepatic impairment:

Moderate impairment: 5 mg 2 times/day regardless of indication; adjust dose based on response and tolerability

Severe impairment (Child-Pugh score >10): Contraindicated

Contraindications Hypersensitivity to pilocarpine or any component of the formulation; uncontrolled asthma; angle-closure glaucoma, severe hepatic impairment

Warnings/Precautions Use caution with cardiovascular disease; patients may have difficulty compensating for transient changes in hemodynamics or rhythm induced by pilocarpine. Use caution with controlled asthma, chronic bronchitis, or COPD; may increase airway resistance, bronchial smooth muscle tone, and bronchial secretions. Use caution with cholelithiasis, biliary tract disease, and nephrolithiasis; adjust dose with moderate hepatic impairment.

Drug Interactions

Metabolism/Transport Effects Inhibits CYP2A6 (weak), 2E1 (weak), 3A4 (weak)

Avoid Concomitant Use There are no known interactions where it is recommended to avoid concomitant use.

Increased Effect/Toxicity

The levels/effects of Pilocarpine (Systemic) may be increased by: Acetylcholinesterase Inhibitors

Decreased Effect There are no known significant interactions involving a decrease in effect.

Ethanol/Nutrition/Herb Interactions Food: Avoid administering with high-fat meal; fat decreases the rate of absorption, maximum concentration and increases the time it takes to reach maximum concentration.

Dietary Considerations Avoid taking with a high-fat meal.

Pharmacodynamics/Kinetics

Onset of Action 20 minutes

Duration of Action 3-5 hours

Half-life Elimination 0.76-1.35 hours; increased with hepatic impairment

Pregnancy Risk Factor C

Lactation Excretion in breast milk unknown/not recommended

Dosage Forms

Tablet, oral: 5 mg, 7.5 mg

Salagen®: 5 mg, 7.5 mg

Dental Comment Pilocarpine may have potential as a salivary stimulant in individuals suffering from xerostomia induced by antidepressants and other medications. At the present time however, the FDA has not approved pilocarpine for use in drug-induced xerostomia (clinical studies required). In an attempt to discern the efficacy of pilocarpine as a salivary stimulant in patients suffering from Sjögren's syndrome (SS), Rhodus and Schuh studied 9 patients with SS given daily doses of pilocarpine over a 6-week period. A dose of 5 mg daily produced a significant overall increase in both whole unstimulated salivary flow and parotid stimulated salivary flow. These results support the use of pilocarpine to increase salivary flow in patients with SS.

References

Davies AN and Singer J, "A Comparison of Artificial Saliva and Pilocarpine in Radiation-Induced Xerostomia," *J Laryngol Otol*, 1994, 108(8):663-5.

Fox PC, "Management of Dry Mouth," *Dent Clin North Am*, 1997, 41(4):863-75.

Fox PC, Atkinson JC, Macynski AA, et al, "Pilocarpine Treatment of Salivary Gland Hypofunction and Dry Mouth (Xerostomia)," *Arch Intern Med*, 1991, 151(6):1149-52.

Fox PC, "Salivary Enhancement Therapies," *Caries Res*, 2004, 38(3):241-6.

Garg AK and Malo M, "Manifestations and Treatment of Xerostomia and Associated Oral Effects Secondary to Head and Neck Radiation Therapy," *J Am Dent Assoc*, 1997, 128(8):1128-33.

Götrick B, Akerman S, Ericson D, et al, "Oral Pilocarpine for Treatment of Opioid-Induced Oral Dryness in Healthy Adults," *J Dent Res*, 2004, 83(5):393-7.

Hendrickson RG, Morocco AP, and Greenberg MI, "Pilocarpine Toxicity and the Treatment of Xerostomia," *J Emerg Med*, 2004, 26(4):429-32.

Johnson JT, Ferretti GA, Nethery WJ, et al, "Oral Pilocarpine for Postirradiation Xerostomia in Patients With Head and Neck Cancer," *N Engl J Med*, 1993, 329(6):390-5.

Mosqueda-Taylor A, Luna-Ortiz K, Irigoyen-Camacho ME, et al, "Effect of Pilocarpine Hydrochloride on Salivary Production in Previously Irradiated Head and Neck Cancer Patients," *Med Oral*, 2004, 9 (3):204-11.

Nagler RM and Laufer D, "Protection Against Irradiation-Induced Damage to Salivary Glands by Adrenergic Agonist Administration," *Int J Radiat Oncol Biol Phys*, 1998, 40(2):477-81.

Nelson JD, Friedlaender M, Yeatts RP, et al, "Oral Pilocarpine for Symptomatic Relief of Keratoconjunctivitis Sicca in Patients with Sjögren's Syndrome. The MGI PHARMA Sjögren's Syndrome Study Group," *Adv Exp Med Biol*, 1998, 438:979-83.

Rhodus NL and Schuh MJ, "Effects of Pilocarpine on Salivary Flow in Patients With Sjögren's Syndrome," *Oral Surg Oral Med Oral Pathol*, 1991, 72(5):545-9.

Rieke JW, Hafermann MD, Johnson JT, et al, "Oral Pilocarpine for Radiation-Induced Xerostomia: Integrated Efficacy and Safety Results From Two Prospective Randomized Clinical Trials," *Int J Radiat Oncol Biol Phys*, 1995, 31(3):661-9.
Rousseau P, "Pilocarpine in Radiation-Induced Xerostomia," *Am J Hosp Palliat Care*, 1995, 12(2):38-9.
Schuller DE, Stevens P, Clausen KP, et al, "Treatment of Radiation Side Effects With Oral Pilocarpine," *J Surg Oncol*, 1989, 42(4):272-6.
Singhal S, Mehta J, Rattenbury H, et al, "Oral Pilocarpine Hydrochloride for the Treatment of Refractory Xerostomia Associated With Chronic Graft-Versus-Host Disease," *Blood*, 1995, 85(4):1147-8.
Valdez IH, Wolff A, Atkinson JC, et al, "Use of Pilocarpine During Head and Neck Radiation Therapy to Reduce Xerostomia and Salivary Dysfunction," *Cancer*, 1993, 71(5):1848-51.
Wiseman LR and Faulds D, "Oral Pilocarpine: A Review of Its Pharmacological Properties and Clinical Potential in Xerostomia," *Drugs*, 1995, 49(1):143-55.
Wynn RL, "Oral Pilocarpine (Salagen®)-A Recently Approved Salivary Stimulant," *Gen Dent*, 1996, 44 (1):26, 29-30.
Zimmerman RP, Mark RJ, Tran LM, et al, "Concomitant Pilocarpine During Head and Neck Irradiation is Associated With Decreased Post-Treatment Xerostomia," *Int J Radiat Oncol Biol Phys*, 1997, 37 (3):571-5.

Pimecrolimus (pim e KROE li mus)

U.S. Brand Names Elidel®
Canadian Brand Names Elidel®
Generic Availability (U.S.) No
Pharmacologic Category Immunosuppressant Agent; Topical Skin Product
Use Short-term and intermittent long-term treatment of mild-to-moderate atopic dermatitis in patients not responsive to conventional therapy or when conventional therapy is not appropriate
Local Anesthetic/Vasoconstrictor Precautions No information available to require special precautions
Effects on Dental Treatment No significant effects or complications reported
Effects on Bleeding No information available to require special precautions
Adverse Effects

>10%:
- Central nervous system: Headache (7% to 25%), fever (1% to 13%)
- Local: Burning at application site (2% to 26%; tends to resolve/improve as lesions resolve)
- Respiratory: Nasopharyngitis (8% to 27%), cough (2% to 16%), upper respiratory tract infection (4% to 19%), bronchitis (≤11%)
- Miscellaneous: Influenza (3% to 13%)

1% to 10%:
- Dermatologic: Skin infection (2% to 6%), folliculitis (1% to 6%), impetigo (2% to 4%), skin papilloma (warts) (≤3%), acne (≤2%), herpes simplex dermatitis (≤2%), molluscum contagiosum (≤2%), urticaria (≤1%)
- Endocrine & metabolic: Dysmenorrhea (1% to 2%)
- Gastrointestinal: Diarrhea (1% to 8%), gastroenteritis (≤7%), abdominal pain (≤4%), constipation (≤4%)
- Local: Irritation at application site (≤6%), pruritus at application site (1% to 6%), erythema at application site (≤2%)
- Ocular: Eye infection (≤1%)
- Otic: Ear infection (1% to 6%), otitis media (1% to 3%)
- Respiratory: Pharyngitis (1% to 8%), asthma (1% to 4%), asthma aggravated (≤4%), nasal congestion (1% to 3%), sinusitis (1% to 3%), epistaxis (≤3%), dyspnea (≤2%), pneumonia (≤2%), rhinorrhea (≤2%), wheezing (≤1%)
- Miscellaneous: Viral infection (≤7%), tonsillitis (≤6%), hypersensitivity (3% to 5%), herpes simplex infection (≤4%), bacterial infection (1% to 2%)

Dosage Children ≥2 years and Adults: Topical: Apply thin layer to affected area twice daily; rub in gently and completely. **Note:** Limit application to involved areas. Continue as long as signs and symptoms persist; discontinue if resolution occurs; re-evaluate if symptoms persist >6 weeks.

Mechanism of Action Penetrates inflamed epidermis to inhibit T cell activation by blocking transcription of proinflammatory cytokine genes such as interleukin-2, interferon gamma (Th1-type), interleukin-4, and interleukin-10 (Th2-type). Pimecrolimus binds to the intracellular protein FKBP-12, inhibiting calcineurin, which blocks cytokine transcription and inhibits T-cell activation. Prevents release of inflammatory cytokines and mediators from mast cells *in vitro* after stimulation by antigen/IgE.

Contraindications Hypersensitivity to pimecrolimus or any component of the formulation

Warnings/Precautions **[U.S. Boxed Warning]: Topical calcineurin inhibitors have been associated with rare cases of lymphoma and skin malignancy.** Avoid use on malignant or premalignant skin conditions (eg, cutaneous T-cell lymphoma). Topical calcineurin agents are considered second-line therapies in the treatment of atopic dermatitis/eczema, and should be limited to use in patients who have failed treatment with other therapies. **[U.S. Boxed Warning]: They should be used for short-term and intermittent treatment using the minimum amount necessary for the control of symptoms should be used.** Application should be limited to involved areas. Diagnosis should be reconfirmed if sign/symptoms do not improve within 6 weeks of treatment. Safety of intermittent use for >1 year has not been established.

May cause local symptoms (eg, burning, soreness, stinging) during first few days of treatment; usually self-resolving. Should not be used in immunocompromised patients. Do not apply to areas of active bacterial or viral infection; infections at the treatment site should be cleared prior to therapy. Patients with atopic dermatitis are predisposed to skin infections, and pimecrolimus therapy has been associated with risk of developing eczema herpeticum, varicella zoster, and herpes simplex. Papilloma/warts have been observed with use; discontinue pimecrolimus until resolution if worsening or do not respond to conventional treatment. Pimecrolimus may be associated with development of lymphadenopathy; possible infectious causes should be investigated. Discontinue use in patients with unknown cause of lymphadenopathy or acute infectious mononucleosis. Not recommended for use in patients with skin disease which may increase the potential for systemic absorption (eg, Netherton's syndrome). Avoid artificial or natural sunlight exposure, even when Elidel® is not on the skin. Safety not established in patients with generalized erythroderma. **[U.S. Boxed Warning]: The use of Elidel® in children <2 years of age is not recommended,** particularly since the effect on immune system development is unknown.

Drug Interactions

Metabolism/Transport Effects Substrate of CYP3A4 (minor)

Avoid Concomitant Use

Avoid concomitant use of Pimecrolimus with any of the following: Immunosuppressants

Increased Effect/Toxicity

Pimecrolimus may increase the levels/effects of: Immunosuppressants

The levels/effects of Pimecrolimus may be increased by: CYP3A4 Inhibitors (Moderate); CYP3A4 Inhibitors (Strong)

Decreased Effect There are no known significant interactions involving a decrease in effect.

Ethanol/Nutrition/Herb Interactions Ethanol: Avoid ethanol (topical pimecrolimus may increase the potential for experiencing facial flushing following the consumption of alcoholic beverages).

Pregnancy Risk Factor C

Lactation Excretion in breast milk unknown/not recommended

Breast-Feeding Considerations Due to the potential for serious adverse reactions in the nursing infant, breast-feeding is not recommended.

Dosage Forms

Cream, topical:

Elidel®: 1% (30 g, 60 g, 100 g)

Pimozide (PI moe zide)

Related Information

Clinical Risk Related to Drugs Prolonging QT Interval *on page 1872*

U.S. Brand Names Orap®

Canadian Brand Names Apo-Pimozide®; Orap®; PMS-Pimozide

Pharmacologic Category Antipsychotic Agent, Typical

Use Suppression of severe motor and phonic tics in patients with Tourette's disorder who have failed to respond satisfactorily to standard treatment

Unlabeled/Investigational Use Psychosis; reported use in individuals with delusions focused on physical symptoms (ie, preoccupation with parasitic infestation); Huntington's chorea

Local Anesthetic/Vasoconstrictor Precautions Pimozide is one of the drugs confirmed to prolong the QT interval and is accepted as having a risk of causing torsade de pointes. The risk of drug-induced torsade de pointes is extremely low when a single QT interval prolonging drug is prescribed. In terms of epinephrine, it is not known what effect vasoconstrictors in the local anesthetic regimen will have in patients with a known history of congenital prolonged QT interval or in patients taking any medication that prolongs the QT interval. Until more information is obtained, it is suggested that the clinician consult with the physician prior to the use of a vasoconstrictor in suspected patients, and that the vasoconstrictor (epinephrine, mepivacaine and levonordefrin [Carbocaine® 2% with Neo-Cobefrin®]) be used with caution.

Effects on Dental Treatment Key adverse event(s) related to dental treatment: Tourette's disorder: Xerostomia and increased salivation (normal salivary flow resumes upon discontinuation), taste disturbance, and dysphagia.

Effects on Bleeding No information available to require special precautions

Adverse Effects

Frequencies as reported in adults (limited data) and/or children with Tourette's disorder:

>10%:

Central nervous system: Sedation (70%), akathisia (40%), akinesia (40%), drowsiness (35%), behavior changes (22% to 25%), somnolence (up to 25% in children)

Gastrointestinal: Xerostomia (25%), constipation (20%)

Genitourinary: Impotence (15%)

Neuromuscular & skeletal: Muscle tightness (15%), weakness (14%)

Ocular: Accommodation decreased (20%), visual disturbance (3% to 20%)

1% to 10%:

Cardiovascular: Abnormal ECG (3%)

Central nervous system: Depression (10%), insomnia (10%), speech disorder (10%), nervousness (5% to 6%), headache (3% to 5%), dreams abnormal (3%), hyperkinesias (3%)

Dermatologic: Rash (3%)

Gastrointestinal: Salivation increased (6%), appetite increased (5%), diarrhea (5%), taste disturbance (5%), thirst (5%), dysphagia (3%)

Neuromuscular & skeletal: Rigidity (10%), stooped posture (10%), handwriting change (5%), myalgia (3%), torticollis (3%), tremor (3%)

Ocular: Photophobia (5%)

Frequency not defined, postmarketing, and/or case reports (some reported for disorders other than Tourette's disorder): Anorexia, blurred vision, cataracts, chest pain, diaphoresis, dizziness, excitement; extrapyramidal symptoms (dystonia, pseudoparkinsonism, tardive dyskinesia); GI distress, gingival hyperplasia (case report), hemolytic anemia, hyper-/hypotension, hyponatremia, libido decreased, nausea, neuroleptic malignant syndrome, nocturia, palpitation, periorbital edema, polyuria, postural hypotension, QT_c prolongation, seizure, skin irritation, syncope, tachycardia, ventricular arrhythmia, vomiting, weight gain/loss

General Dosage Range Dosage adjustment recommended in patients who develop toxicities

Oral:

Children ≤12 years: Initial: 0.05 mg/kg once daily (preferably bedtime); Maintenance: 2-4 mg once daily (maximum: 10 mg/day [0.2 mg/kg/day])

Children >12 years and Adults: Initial: 1-2 mg in divided doses; Maintenance: 7-10 mg/day in divided doses (maximum: 10 mg/day [0.2 mg/kg/day])

Mechanism of Action Pimozide, a diphenylbutylperidine conventional antipsychotic, is a potent centrally-acting dopamine-receptor antagonist resulting in its characteristic neuroleptic effects

Pharmacodynamics/Kinetics

Half-life Elimination ~55 hours

Time to Peak Serum: 6-8 hours (range: 4-12 hours)

Pregnancy Risk Factor C

Dental Comment Pimozide is known to prolong the QT interval. The QT interval is measured as the time and distance between the Q point of the QRS complex and the end of the T wave in the ECG tracing. After adjustment for heart rate, the QT interval is defined as prolonged if it is more than 450 msec in men and 460 msec in women. A long QT syndrome was first described in the 1950s and 60s as a congenital syndrome involving QT interval prolongation and syncope and sudden death. Some of the congenital long QT syndromes were characterized by a peculiar electrocardiographic appearance of the QRS complex involving a premature atria beat followed by a pause, then a subsequent sinus beat showing marked QT prolongation and deformity. This type of cardiac arrhythmia was originally termed "torsade de pointes" (translated from the French as "twisting of the points"). Pimozide is considered as having a risk of causing torsade de pointes. Since it is not known what effect vasoconstrictors in the local anesthetic regimen will have in patients with a known history of congenital prolonged QT interval or in patients taking any medication that prolongs the QT interval, a medical consult is suggested.

Pindolol (PIN doe lole)

Related Information

Cardiovascular Diseases *on page 1848*

Canadian Brand Names Apo-Pindol®; Dom-Pindolol; Mylan-Pindolol; Novo-Pindol; Nu-Pindol; PMS-Pindolol; Sandoz-Pindolol; Visken®

Pharmacologic Category Beta Blocker With Intrinsic Sympathomimetic Activity

Use Treatment of hypertension, alone or in combination with other agents

Unlabeled/Investigational Use Potential augmenting agent for antidepressants; ventricular arrhythmias/tachycardia, antipsychotic-induced akathisia, situational anxiety; aggressive behavior associated with dementia

Local Anesthetic/Vasoconstrictor Precautions Use with caution; epinephrine has interacted with nonselective beta-blockers to result in initial hypertensive episode followed by bradycardia

Effects on Dental Treatment Pindolol is a nonselective beta-blocker and may enhance the pressor response to epinephrine, resulting in hypertension and bradycardia. Many nonsteroidal anti-inflammatory drugs, such as ibuprofen and indomethacin, can reduce the hypotensive effect of beta-blockers after 3 or more weeks of therapy with the NSAID. Short-term NSAID use (ie, 3 days) requires no special precautions in patients taking beta-blockers.

Effects on Bleeding No information available to require special precautions

Adverse Effects

1% to 10%:

Cardiovascular: Edema (6%), chest pain (3%), bradycardia (≤2%), heart block (≤2%), hypotension (≤2%), syncope (≤2%), tachycardia (≤2%), palpitation (≤1%)

Central nervous system: Insomnia (10%), dizziness (9%), fatigue (8%), nervousness (7%), nightmares/vivid dreams (5%), anxiety (≤2%), lethargy (≤2%)

Dermatologic: Hyperhidrosis (≤2%), pruritus (1%)

Gastrointestinal: Nausea (5%), diarrhea (≤2%), vomiting (≤2%), weight gain (≤2%)

Genitourinary: Impotence (≤2%)

Hematologic: Claudication (≤2%)

Hepatic: ALT increased (7%), AST increased (7%)

Neuromuscular & skeletal: Muscle pain (10%), arthralgia (7%), weakness (4%), paresthesia (3%), muscle cramps (3%)

Ocular: Burning eyes (≤2%), visual disturbances (≤2%), eye discomfort (≤2%)

Renal: Polyuria (≤2%)

Respiratory: Dyspnea (5%), wheezing (≤2%)

Miscellaneous: Cold extremities (≤2%)

Other adverse reactions (noted with other beta-adrenergic-blocking agents that should be considered potential adverse events with pindolol): Agranulocytosis, alopecia, catatonia, clouded sensorium, disorientation, emotional lability, fever, intensification of pre-existing AV block, ischemic colitis, laryngospasm, mental depression, mesenteric artery thrombosis, nonthrombocytopenic purpura, Peyronie's disease, rash (erythematous), respiratory distress, short-term memory loss, thrombocytopenic purpura

General Dosage Range Dosage adjustment recommended in patients with hepatic impairment

Oral:

Adults: Initial: 5 mg twice daily; Maintenance: 10-40 mg twice daily (maximum: 60 mg/day)

Elderly: Initial: 5 mg once daily

Mechanism of Action Blocks both beta$_1$- and beta$_2$-receptors and has mild intrinsic sympathomimetic activity; pindolol has negative inotropic and chronotropic effects and can significantly slow AV nodal conduction. Augmentive action of antidepressants thought to be mediated via a serotonin 1A autoreceptor antagonism.

Pharmacodynamics/Kinetics

Half-life Elimination 3-4 hours; prolonged with advanced age, and cirrhosis (range: 2.5-30 hours)

Time to Peak Serum: ~1 hour

Pregnancy Risk Factor B

Pindolol and Hydrochlorothiazide

(PIN doe lole & hye droe klor oh THYE a zide)

Related Information

Hydrochlorothiazide *on page 854*

Pindolol *on page 1350*

Canadian Brand Names Viskazide®

Pharmacologic Category Beta Blocker With Intrinsic Sympathomimetic Activity; Diuretic, Thiazide

Use Treatment of hypertension; not for initial therapy

Local Anesthetic/Vasoconstrictor Precautions Use with caution; epinephrine has interacted with nonselective beta-blockers to result in initial hypertensive episode followed by bradycardia

Effects on Dental Treatment Pindolol is a nonselective beta-blocker and may enhance the pressor response to epinephrine, resulting in hypertension and bradycardia. Many nonsteroidal anti-inflammatory drugs, such as ibuprofen and indomethacin, can reduce the hypotensive effect of beta-blockers after 3 or more weeks of therapy with the NSAID. Short-term NSAID use (ie, 3 days) requires no special precautions in patients taking beta-blockers.

Effects on Bleeding No information available to require special precautions

Adverse Effects See individual agents.

General Dosage Range Oral: *Adults:* Usual dose: Pindolol 10-20 mg and hydrochlorothiazide 25-100 mg once daily (maximum daily dose: Pindolol 20 mg/hydrochlorothiazide 100 mg)

Mechanism of Action

Pindolol: Blocks both beta$_1$- and beta$_2$-receptors and has mild intrinsic sympathomimetic activity; has negative inotropic and chronotropic effects and can significantly slow AV nodal conduction. Augmentive action of antidepressants thought to be mediated via a serotonin 1A autoreceptor antagonism.

Hydrochlorothiazide: Inhibits sodium reabsorption in the distal tubules causing increased excretion of sodium and water as well as potassium and hydrogen ions

Product Availability Not available in U.S.

Pioglitazone (pye oh GLI ta zone)

Related Information

Endocrine Disorders and Pregnancy *on page* 1879

U.S. Brand Names Actos®

Canadian Brand Names Accel-Pioglitazone; Actos®; Apo-Pioglitazone®; CO Pioglitazone; Dom-Pioglitazone; Mint-Pioglitazone; Mylan-Pioglitazone; Novo-Pioglitazone; PHL-Pioglitazone; PMS-Pioglitazone; PRO-Pioglitazone; ratio-Pioglitazone; Sandoz-Pioglitazone; Teva-Pioglitazone; ZYM-Pioglitazone

Generic Availability (U.S.) No

Pharmacologic Category Antidiabetic Agent, Thiazolidinedione

Use

Type 2 diabetes mellitus (noninsulin dependent, NIDDM), monotherapy: Adjunct to diet and exercise, to improve glycemic control

Type 2 diabetes mellitus (noninsulin dependent, NIDDM), combination therapy with sulfonylurea, metformin, or insulin: When diet, exercise, and a single agent alone does not result in adequate glycemic control

Local Anesthetic/Vasoconstrictor Precautions No information available to require special precautions

Effects on Dental Treatment Key adverse event(s) related to dental treatment: Tooth disorder. Pioglitazone-dependent diabetics should be appointed for dental treatment in morning in order to minimize chance of stress-induced hypoglycemia.

Effects on Bleeding No information available to require special precautions

Adverse Effects

>10%:

Cardiovascular: Edema (5%; in combination trials with sulfonlyureas or insulin, the incidence of edema was as high as 15%)

Respiratory: Upper respiratory tract infection (13%)

1% to 10%:

Cardiovascular: Heart failure (requiring hospitalization; up to 6% in patients with prior macrovascular disease)

Central nervous system: Headache (9%), fatigue (4%)

Gastrointestinal: Tooth disorder (5%)

Hematologic: Anemia (≤2%)

Neuromuscular & skeletal: Myalgia (5%)

Respiratory: Sinusitis (6%), pharyngitis (5%)

Frequency not defined: HDL-cholesterol increased, hematocrit/hemoglobin decreased, hypoglycemia (in combination trials with sulfonylureas or insulin), serum triglycerides decreased, weight gain/loss

Dosage Oral:

Adults:

Monotherapy: Initial: 15-30 mg once daily; if response is inadequate, the dosage may be increased in increments up to 45 mg once daily; maximum recommended dose: 45 mg once daily

Combination therapy: Maximum recommended dose: 45 mg/day

With sulfonylureas: Initial: 15-30 mg once daily; dose of sulfonylurea should be reduced if the patient reports hypoglycemia

With metformin: Initial: 15-30 mg once daily; it is unlikely that the dose of metformin will need to be reduced due to hypoglycemia

With insulin: Initial: 15-30 mg once daily; dose of insulin should be reduced by 10% to 25% if the patient reports hypoglycemia or if the plasma glucose falls to <100 mg/dL.

Dosage adjustment in patients with CHF (NYHA Class II) in mono- or combination therapy: Initial: 15 mg once daily; may be increased after several months of treatment, with close attention to heart failure symptoms

Elderly: No dosage adjustment is recommended in elderly patients.

Dosage adjustment in renal impairment: No dosage adjustment is required.

Dosage adjustment in hepatic impairment: Clearance is significantly lower in hepatic impairment (Child-Pugh Grade B/C). Therapy should not be initiated if the patient exhibits active liver disease or increased transaminases (>2.5 times ULN) at baseline. During treatment if ALT levels elevate >3 times ULN, the test should be repeated as soon as possible. If ALT levels remain >3 times ULN or if the patient is jaundiced, therapy should be discontinued.

Mechanism of Action Thiazolidinedione antidiabetic agent that lowers blood glucose by improving target cell response to insulin, without increasing pancreatic insulin secretion. It has a mechanism of action that is dependent on the presence of insulin for activity. Pioglitazone is a potent and selective agonist for peroxisome proliferator-activated receptor-gamma (PPARgamma). Activation of nuclear PPAR-gamma receptors influences the production of a number of gene products involved in glucose and lipid metabolism. PPARgamma is abundant in the cells within the renal collecting tubules; fluid retention results from stimulation by thiazolidinediones which increases sodium reabsorption.

Contraindications Hypersensitivity to pioglitazone or any component of the formulation; NYHA Class III/IV heart failure (initiation of therapy)

Canadian labeling: Additional contraindications (not is U.S. labeling): Any stage of heart failure (eg, NYHA Class I, II, III, IV); serious hepatic impairment; pregnancy

Warnings/Precautions [U.S. Boxed Warning]: Thiazolidinediones, including pioglitazone, may cause or exacerbate heart failure; closely monitor for signs and symptoms of heart failure (eg, rapid weight gain, dyspnea, edema), particularly after initiation or dose increases. Not recommended for use in any patient with symptomatic heart failure. In the U.S., initiation of therapy is contraindicated in patients with NYHA class III or IV heart failure. If used in patients with NYHA class II (systolic heart failure), initiate at lowest dosage and monitor closely. In Canada, use in any stage of heart failure (NYHA I, II, III, IV) is contraindicated. Use with caution in patients with edema; may increase plasma volume and/or cause fluid retention. Dose reduction or discontinuation is recommended if heart failure suspected. Dose-related weight gain observed with use; mechanism unknown but likely associated with fluid retention and fat accumulation.

Should not be used in diabetic ketoacidosis. Mechanism requires the presence of insulin; therefore use in type 1 diabetes is not recommended. Use with caution in premenopausal, anovulatory women - may result in a resumption of ovulation, increasing the risk of pregnancy. Use with caution in patients with anemia (may reduce hemoglobin and hematocrit). Increased incidence of bone fractures in females treated with pioglitazone; majority of fractures occurred in the lower limb and distal upper limb.

Use with caution in patients with elevated transaminases (AST or ALT); do not initiate in patients with active liver disease of ALT >2.5 times the upper limit of normal at baseline. During therapy, if ALT >3 times the upper limit of normal, re-evaluate levels promptly and discontinue if elevation persists or if jaundice occurs at any time during use. Idiosyncratic hepatotoxicity has been reported with another thiazolidinedione agent (troglitazone); avoid use in patients who previously experienced jaundice during troglitazone therapy. Monitoring should include periodic determinations of liver function. Use caution with pre-existing macular edema or diabetic retinopathy. Postmarketing reports of new-onset or worsening diabetic macular edema with decreased visual acuity has been reported. Safety and efficacy have not been established in children.

Canadian labeling (not in U.S. labeling) states use with insulin **or** as part of triple therapy (pioglitazone in combination with a sulfonylurea and metformin) is not indicated.

Drug Interactions

Metabolism/Transport Effects Substrate of CYP2C8 (major), 3A4 (minor); **Inhibits** CYP2C8 (moderate), 2C9 (weak), 2C19 (weak) **Induces** CYP3A4 (weak)

Avoid Concomitant Use There are no known interactions where it is recommended to avoid concomitant use.

Increased Effect/Toxicity

Pioglitazone may increase the levels/effects of: CYP2C8 Substrates (High risk); Hypoglycemic Agents

The levels/effects of Pioglitazone may be increased by: Conivaptan; CYP2C8 Inhibitors (Moderate); CYP2C8 Inhibitors (Strong); Deferasirox; Gemfibrozil; Herbs (Hypoglycemic Properties); Insulin; Pegvisomant; Pregabalin; Trimethoprim

Decreased Effect

Pioglitazone may decrease the levels/effects of: Saxagliptin

The levels/effects of Pioglitazone may be decreased by: Bile Acid Sequestrants; Corticosteroids (Orally Inhaled); Corticosteroids (Systemic); CYP2C8 Inducers

(Highly Effective); Luteinizing Hormone-Releasing Hormone Analogs; Rifampin; Somatropin; Thiazide Diuretics; Tocilizumab

Ethanol/Nutrition/Herb Interactions

Ethanol: Caution with ethanol (may cause hypoglycemia).

Food: Peak concentrations are delayed when administered with food, but the extent of absorption is not affected. Pioglitazone may be taken without regard to meals.

Herb/Nutraceutical: Caution with alfalfa, aloe, bilberry, bitter melon, burdock, celery, damiana, fenugreek, garcinia, garlic, ginger, ginseng (American), gymnema, marshmallow, and stinging nettle (may cause hypoglycemia).

Dietary Considerations Management of type 2 diabetes mellitus (noninsulin dependent, NIDDM) should include diet control. May be taken without regard to meals.

Pharmacodynamics/Kinetics

Onset of Action Delayed; Peak effect: Glucose control: Several weeks

Half-life Elimination Parent drug: 3-7 hours; Total: 16-24 hours

Time to Peak ~2 hours; delayed with food

Pregnancy Risk Factor C

Lactation Excretion in breast milk unknown/not recommended

Breast-Feeding Considerations It is not known if pioglitazone is excreted in breast milk. Breast-feeding is not recommended by the manufacturer.

Dosage Forms

Tablet, oral:

Actos®: 15 mg, 30 mg, 45 mg

Pioglitazone and Glimepiride (pye oh GLI ta zone & GLYE me pye ride)

Related Information

Endocrine Disorders and Pregnancy *on page* 1879
Glimepiride *on page* 817
Pioglitazone *on page* 1352

U.S. Brand Names Duetact™

Pharmacologic Category Antidiabetic Agent, Sulfonylurea; Antidiabetic Agent, Thiazolidinedione; Hypoglycemic Agent, Oral

Use Management of type 2 diabetes mellitus (noninsulin dependent, NIDDM) as an adjunct to diet and exercise

Local Anesthetic/Vasoconstrictor Precautions No information available to require special precautions

Effects on Dental Treatment Pioglitazone-dependent patients with diabetes (non-insulin dependent, type 2) or glimepiride-dependent patients with diabetes (non-insulin dependent, type 2) should be appointed for dental treatment in morning in order to minimize chance of stress-induced hypoglycemia.

Effects on Bleeding No information available to require special precautions

Adverse Effects Also see individual agents.

>10%:

Cardiovascular: Peripheral edema (6% to 12%)
Endocrine & metabolic: Hypoglycemia (13% to 16%)
Gastrointestinal: Weight gain (9% to 13%)
Respiratory: Upper respiratory tract infection (12% to 15%)

1% to 10%:

Central nervous system: Headache (4% to 7%)
Gastrointestinal: Diarrhea (4% to 6%), nausea (4% to 5%)
Genitourinary: Urinary tract infection (6% to 7%)
Hematologic: Anemia (≤2%)
Neuromuscular & skeletal: Limb pain (4% to 5%)

General Dosage Range Dosage adjustment recommended in patients with renal impairment

Oral:

Adults:

Patients inadequately controlled on **glimepiride** alone: Initial dose: Pioglitazone 30 mg and glimepiride 2-4 mg once daily (maximum: 45 mg/day [pioglitazone]; 8 mg/day [glimepiride])

Patients inadequately controlled on **pioglitazone** alone: Initial dose: Pioglitazone 30 mg and glimepiride 2 mg once daily (maximum: 45 mg/day [pioglitazone]; 8 mg/day [glimepiride])

Elderly: Initial: Glimepiride 1 mg/day prior to initiating Duetact™

Mechanism of Action

Pioglitazone: A thiazolidinedione that lowers blood glucose by improving target cell response to insulin, without increasing pancreatic insulin secretion. It has a mechanism of action that is dependent on the presence of insulin for activity.

Glimepiride: A sulfonylurea that stimulates insulin release from the pancreatic beta cells; reduces glucose output from the liver; insulin sensitivity is increased at peripheral target sites.

Pregnancy Risk Factor C

Pioglitazone and Metformin (pye oh GLI ta zone & met FOR min)

Related Information

Endocrine Disorders and Pregnancy *on page 1879*
MetFORMIN *on page 1089*
Pioglitazone *on page 1352*

U.S. Brand Names Actoplus Met®; Actoplus Met® XR

Generic Availability (U.S.) No

Pharmacologic Category Antidiabetic Agent, Biguanide; Antidiabetic Agent, Thiazolidinedione

Use Management of type 2 diabetes mellitus (noninsulin dependent, NIDDM)

Local Anesthetic/Vasoconstrictor Precautions No information available to require special precautions

Effects on Dental Treatment Pioglitazone-dependent patients with diabetes (non-insulin dependent, type 2) or metformin-dependent patients with diabetes (non-insulin dependent, type 2) should be appointed for dental treatment in morning in order to minimize chance of stress-induced hypoglycemia.

Effects on Bleeding No information available to require special precautions

Adverse Effects Also see individual agents. Percentages of adverse effects as reported with the combination product.

>10%:
- Cardiovascular: Edema (lower limb, 3% to 11%)
- Respiratory: Upper respiratory infection (12% to 16%)

1% to 10%:
- Central nervous system: Headache (2% to 6%), dizziness (5%)
- Endocrine & metabolic: Weight gain (3% to 7%)
- Gastrointestinal: Diarrhea (5% to 6%), nausea (4% to 6%)
- Genitourinary: Urinary tract infection (5% to 6%)
- Hematologic: Anemia (≤2%)
- Respiratory: Sinusitis (4% to 5%)

Dosage Oral: Type 2 diabetes mellitus:

Adults: Initial dose should be based on current dose of pioglitazone and/or metformin; metformin dose may be titrated every 1-2 weeks and pioglitazone dose may be titrated every 2-3 months as necessary to achieve goals

Immediate release tablet: **Note:** Daily doses higher than pioglitazone 15 mg plus metformin 850 mg should be divided. Initial: Pioglitazone 15 mg plus metformin 500 mg **or** pioglitazone 15 mg plus metformin 850 mg tablets once or twice daily. Maximum daily dose: Pioglitazone 45 mg/metformin 2550 mg

Variable release tablet: Pioglitazone 15 mg plus metformin 1000 mg tablet **or** pioglitazone 30 mg plus metformin 1000 mg tablet once daily with evening meal. Maximum daily dose: Pioglitazone 45 mg/metformin 2000 mg

Elderly: The initial and maintenance dosing should be conservative, due to the potential for decreased renal function (monitor). Generally, elderly patients should not be titrated to the maximum; do not use in patients ≥80 years of age unless normal renal function has been established.

Dosage adjustment in renal impairment: Do not use with renal disease or renal dysfunction (serum creatinine ≥1.5 mg/dL in males or ≥1.4 mg/dL in females or abnormal clearance).

Dosage adjustment in hepatic impairment: Do not initiate treatment with active liver disease or ALT >2.5 times ULN. During treatment, if ALT concentrations increase >3 times ULN, the test should be repeated as soon as possible. If ALT concentrations remain >3 times ULN or if the patient is jaundiced, therapy should be discontinued.

Mechanism of Action

Pioglitazone is a thiazolidinedione antidiabetic agent that lowers blood glucose by improving target cell response to insulin, without increasing pancreatic insulin secretion. It has a mechanism of action that is dependent on the presence of insulin for activity.

Metformin decreases hepatic glucose production, decreasing intestinal absorption of glucose, and improves insulin sensitivity (increases peripheral glucose uptake and utilization).

Contraindications Hypersensitivity to pioglitazone, metformin, or any component of the formulation; NYHA Class III/IV heart failure (initiation of therapy); renal disease or renal dysfunction (serum creatinine ≥1.5 mg/dL in males or ≥1.4 mg/dL in females, or abnormal creatinine clearance which may also result from conditions such as cardiovascular collapse, acute myocardial infarction, and septicemia); acute or chronic metabolic acidosis with or without coma (including diabetic ketoacidosis); concurrent iodinated radiocontrast adminstration (manufacturer recommends temporary discontinuation of metformin)

Warnings/Precautions [U.S. Boxed Warning]: Lactic acidosis is a rare, but potentially severe consequence of therapy with metformin. Lactic acidosis should be suspected in any patient with diabetes receiving metformin with evidence of acidosis but without evidence of ketoacidosis. Discontinue metformin in clinical situations predisposing to hypoxemia, including conditions such as cardiovascular collapse, respiratory failure, acute myocardial infarction, acute congestive heart failure, and septicemia.

Metformin is substantially excreted by the kidney. The risk of accumulation and lactic acidosis increases with the degree of impairment of renal function. Patients with renal function below the limit of normal for their age should not receive metformin. In elderly patients, renal function should be monitored regularly; should not be used in any patient ≥80 years of age unless normal renal function is confirmed. Use of concomitant medications that may affect renal function (ie, affect tubular secretion) may also affect metformin disposition. Metformin should be withheld in patients with dehydration and/or prerenal azotemia. Metformin therapy should be temporarily discontinued prior to or at the time of intravascular administration of iodinated contrast media (potential for acute alteration in renal function). Metformin should be withheld for 48 hours after the radiologic study and restarted only after renal function has been confirmed as normal.

[U.S. Boxed Warning]: Thiazolidinediones, including pioglitazone, may cause or exacerbate heart failure; closely monitor for signs and symptoms of heart failure (eg, rapid weight gain, dyspnea, edema), particularly after initiation or dose increases. Not recommended for use in any patient with symptomatic heart failure; initiation of therapy is contraindicated in patients with NYHA class III or IV heart failure. If used in patients with NYHA class II (systolic) heart failure, initiate at lowest dosage and monitor closely. In addition metformin should be used with caution in patients with heart failure requiring pharmacologic management, particularly in unstable or acute heart failure due to risk of lactic acidosis secondary to hypoperfusion. Use with caution in patients with edema; may increase plasma volume and/or cause fluid retention. Dose reduction or discontinuation is recommended if heart failure suspected. Dose-related weight gain observed with pioglitazone use; mechanism unknown but likely associated with fluid retention and fat accumulation.

Avoid metformin use in patients with impaired liver function due to potential for lactic acidosis. Use pioglitazone with caution in patients with elevated transaminases (AST or ALT); do not initiate in patients with active liver disease of ALT >2.5 times the upper limit of normal at baseline. During therapy, if ALT >3 times the upper limit of normal, reevaluate promptly and discontinue if elevation persists or if jaundice occurs at any time during use. Idiosyncratic hepatotoxicity has been reported with another thiazolidinedione agent (troglitazone); avoid use in patients who previously experienced jaundice during troglitazone therapy. Monitoring should include periodic determinations of liver function. Instruct patients to avoid excessive acute or chronic ethanol use; ethanol may potentiate metformin's effect on lactate metabolism.

Mechanism of pioglitazone requires the presence of insulin; therefore, use in type 1 diabetes (insulin dependent, IDDM) or diabetic ketoacidosis is not recommended. It may be necessary to discontinue metformin and administer insulin if the patient is exposed to stress (fever, trauma, infection, surgery). Increased incidence of bone fractures in females treated with pioglitazone; majority of fractures occurred in the lower limb and distal upper limb. Consider risk of fracture prior to initiation and during use. Pioglitazone may decrease hemoglobin/hematocrit; effects may be related to increased plasma volume. Metformin may impair vitamin B_{12} absorption; monitor for anemia. Use pioglitazone with caution in premenopausal, anovulatory women; may result in a resumption of ovulation, increasing the risk of pregnancy. Use pioglitazone with caution in patients with pre-existing macular edema or diabetic retinopathy; postmarketing events of new-onset or worsening diabetic macular edema with decreased visual acuity have been reported.

Drug Interactions

Metabolism/Transport Effects Pioglitazone: **Substrate** of CYP2C8 (major), 3A4 (minor); **Inhibits** CYP2C8 (moderate), 2C9 (weak), 2C19 (weak) **Induces** CYP3A4 (weak)

Avoid Concomitant Use There are no known interactions where it is recommended to avoid concomitant use.

Increased Effect/Toxicity

Pioglitazone and Metformin may increase the levels/effects of: CYP2C8 Substrates (High risk); Dofetilide; Hypoglycemic Agents

The levels/effects of Pioglitazone and Metformin may be increased by: Cephalexin; Cimetidine; Conivaptan; CYP2C8 Inhibitors (Moderate); CYP2C8 Inhibitors (Strong); Deferasirox; Gemfibrozil; Glycopyrrolate; Herbs (Hypoglycemic Properties); Insulin; Iodinated Contrast Agents; Pegvisomant; Pregabalin; Trimethoprim

Decreased Effect

Pioglitazone and Metformin may decrease the levels/effects of: Saxagliptin

The levels/effects of Pioglitazone and Metformin may be decreased by: Bile Acid Sequestrants; Corticosteroids (Orally Inhaled); Corticosteroids (Systemic); CYP2C8 Inducers (Highly Effective); Luteinizing Hormone-Releasing Hormone Analogs; Rifampin; Somatropin; Thiazide Diuretics; Tocilizumab

Ethanol/Nutrition/Herb Interactions See individual agents.

Dietary Considerations Immediate release tablets should be administered with meals. Variable release tablets should be administered with the evening meal. Avoid ethanol. Dietary modification based on ADA recommendations is a part of therapy. Monitor for signs and symptoms of vitamin B_{12} and/or folic acid deficiency; supplementation may be required.

Pregnancy Risk Factor C

Lactation

Metformin: Enters breast milk/not recommended

Pioglitazone: Excretion in breast milk unknown/not recommended

Breast-Feeding Considerations See individual agents.

Dosage Forms

Tablet, oral:

Actoplus Met®: 15/500: Pioglitazone 15 mg and metformin 500 mg; 15/850: Pioglitazone 15 mg and metformin 850 mg

Tablet, variable release, oral:

Actoplus Met® XR: 15/1000: Pioglitazone 15 mg and metformin 1000 mg; 30/1000: Pioglitazone 30 mg and metformin 1000 mg

Piperacillin (pi PER a sil in)

Canadian Brand Names Piperacillin for Injection, USP

Pharmacologic Category Antibiotic, Penicillin

Use Treatment of susceptible infections such as septicemia, acute and chronic respiratory tract infections, skin and soft tissue infections, and urinary tract infections due to susceptible strains of *Pseudomonas*, *Proteus*, and *Escherichia coli* and *Enterobacter*; active against some streptococci and some anaerobic bacteria; febrile neutropenia (as part of combination regimen)

Local Anesthetic/Vasoconstrictor Precautions No information available to require special precautions

Effects on Dental Treatment Key adverse event(s) related to dental treatment: Prolonged use of penicillins may lead to development of oral candidiasis.

Effects on Bleeding May inhibit platelet aggregation (dose related). No information available to require special precautions

Adverse Effects Frequency not defined.

Central nervous system: Confusion, convulsions, drowsiness, fever, Jarisch-Herxheimer reaction

Dermatologic: Rash, toxic epidermal necrolysis, urticaria

Endocrine & metabolic: Electrolyte imbalance, hypokalemia

Hematologic: Abnormal platelet aggregation and prolonged PT (high doses), agranulocytosis, Coombs' reaction (positive), hemolytic anemia, pancytopenia

Local: Thrombophlebitis

Neuromuscular & skeletal: Myoclonus

Renal: Acute interstitial nephritis, acute renal failure

Miscellaneous: Anaphylaxis, hypersensitivity reactions

General Dosage Range Dosage adjustment recommended in patients with renal impairment

I.M., I.V.:

Neonates: 100 mg/kg every 12 hours

Children: 200-300 mg/kg/day in divided doses every 4-6 hours

Adults: 2-4 g/dose every 4-6 hours (maximum: 24 g/day)

Mechanism of Action Inhibits bacterial cell wall synthesis by binding to one or more of the penicillin-binding proteins (PBPs); which in turn inhibits the final transpeptidation step of peptidoglycan synthesis in bacterial cell walls, thus inhibiting cell wall biosynthesis. Bacteria eventually lyse due to ongoing activity of cell wall autolytic enzymes (autolysins and murein hydrolases) while cell wall assembly is arrested.

Pharmacodynamics/Kinetics

Half-life Elimination Dose dependent; prolonged with moderately severe renal or hepatic impairment:

Neonates: 1-5 days old: 3.6 hours; >6 days old: 2.1-2.7 hours
Children: 1-6 months: 0.79 hour; 6 months to 12 years: 0.39-0.5 hour
Adults: 36-80 minutes

Time to Peak Serum: I.M.: 30-50 minutes

Pregnancy Risk Factor B

Piperacillin and Tazobactam Sodium

(pi PER a sil in & ta zoe BAK tam SOW dee um)

Related Information

Piperacillin *on page 1357*

U.S. Brand Names Zosyn®

Canadian Brand Names Tazocin®

Pharmacologic Category Antibiotic, Penicillin

Use Treatment of moderate-to-severe infections caused by susceptible organisms, including infections of the lower respiratory tract (community-acquired pneumonia, nosocomial pneumonia); urinary tract; uncomplicated and complicated skin and skin structures; gynecologic (endometritis, pelvic inflammatory disease); bone and joint infections; intra-abdominal infections (appendicitis with rupture/abscess, peritonitis); and septicemia. Tazobactam expands activity of piperacillin to include beta-lactamase producing strains of *S. aureus*, *H. influenzae*, *Bacteroides*, and other gram-negative bacteria.

Local Anesthetic/Vasoconstrictor Precautions No information available to require special precautions

Effects on Dental Treatment Key adverse event(s) related to dental treatment: Prolonged use of penicillins may lead to development of oral candidiasis.

Effects on Bleeding May inhibit platelet aggregation (dose related). No information available to require special precautions

Adverse Effects

>10%: Gastrointestinal: Diarrhea (7% to 11%)

>1% to 10%:

Cardiovascular: Hypertension (2%)
Central nervous system: Insomnia (7%), headache (8%), fever (2% to 5%), agitation (2%), pain (2%)
Dermatologic: Rash (4%), pruritus (3%)
Gastrointestinal: Constipation (1% to 8%), nausea (7%), vomiting (3% to 4%), dyspepsia (3%), stool changes (2%), abdominal pain (1% to 2%)
Hepatic: Transaminases increased
Local: Local reaction (3%), abscess (2%)
Respiratory: Pharyngitis (2%)
Miscellaneous: Moniliasis (2%), sepsis (2%), infection (2%)

General Dosage Range Dosage adjustment recommended in patients with renal impairment

I.V.:

Children 2-8 months: 80 mg/kg every 8 hours
Children ≥9 months and ≤40 kg: 100 mg/kg every 8 hours
Children >40 kg: 4.5 g every 8 hours **or** 3.375 g every 6 hours
Adults: 3.375 g every 6 hours **or** 4.5 g every 6-8 hours (maximum: 18 g/day)

Mechanism of Action Inhibits bacterial cell wall synthesis by binding to one or more of the penicillin-binding proteins (PBPs); which in turn inhibits the final transpeptidation step of peptidoglycan synthesis in bacterial cell walls, thus inhibiting cell wall biosynthesis. Bacteria eventually lyse due to ongoing activity of cell wall autolytic enzymes (autolysins and murein hydrolases) while cell wall assembly is arrested. Tazobactam inhibits many beta-lactamases, including staphylococcal penicillinase and Richmond and Sykes types II, III, IV, and V, including extended spectrum enzymes; it has only limited activity against class I beta-lactamases other than class Ic types.

Pharmacodynamics/Kinetics

Half-life Elimination Piperacillin and tazobactam: 0.7-1.2 hours

Time to Peak Immediately following infusion of 30 minutes

Pregnancy Risk Factor B

Piperazine (PI per a zeen)

Canadian Brand Names Entacyl®

Pharmacologic Category Anthelmintic

Use Treatment of pinworm and roundworm infections (used as an alternative to first-line agents, mebendazole, or pyrantel pamoate)

Local Anesthetic/Vasoconstrictor Precautions No information available to require special precautions

Effects on Dental Treatment No significant effects or complications reported

Effects on Bleeding No information available to require special precautions

General Dosage Range Oral:

Children: 65-75 mg/kg once daily (maximum: 3.5 g/day)

Adults: 65 mg/kg once daily **or** 3.5 g once daily (maximum: 3.5 g/day)

Mechanism of Action Causes muscle paralysis of the roundworm by blocking the effects of acetylcholine at the neuromuscular junction

Pharmacodynamics/Kinetics

Time to Peak Serum: 1 hour

Pregnancy Risk Factor B

Pipotiazine (pip oh TYE a zeen)

Canadian Brand Names Piportil® L_4

Pharmacologic Category Antipsychotic Agent, Typical, Phenothiazine, Piperidine

Use Maintenance treatment of schizophrenia

Local Anesthetic/Vasoconstrictor Precautions No information available to require special precautions

Effects on Dental Treatment Key adverse event(s) related to dental treatment: Xerostomia and changes in salivation (normal salivary flow resumes upon discontinuation).

Effects on Bleeding No information available to require special precautions

Adverse Effects Frequency not defined.

Cardiovascular: Cardiac arrest, ECG changes, edema, hypotension, QT_c prolongation, syncope, tachycardia, venous thromboembolism

Central nervous system: Agitation, anxiety, bizarre dreams, cerebral edema, depression, dizziness, drowsiness, EEG changes, excitement, extrapyramidal symptoms (akathisia, dyskinesia, dystonia, hyper-reflexia, oculogyric crisis, opisthotonos, pseudoparkinsonism, rigidity, sialorrhea, tremor), fatigue, fever, headache, insomnia, paradoxical psychosis, restlessness, seizure, sleep disturbance, tardive dyskinesia

Dermatologic: Angioedema, eczema, epithelial keratopathy erythema, exfoliative dermatitis, dermatitis, photosensitivity, pruritus, rash, seborrhea, skin pigmentation (prolonged therapy), urticaria

Endocrine & metabolic: Galactorrhea, glucose intolerance, gynecomastia, hyperglycemia, libido (changes in), menstrual irregularities, thirst

Gastrointestinal: Adynamic ileus, anorexia, appetite increased, constipation, fecal impaction, nausea, salivation, vomiting, weight changes, xerostomia

Genitourinary: Bladder paralysis, impotence, incontinence, polyuria, priapism, urinary retention

Hematologic: Agranulocytosis, anemia, eosinophilia, leukopenia, pancytopenia, thrombocytopenia

Hepatic: Biliary stasis, cholestatic jaundice

Ocular: Blurred vision, corneal deposits (prolonged therapy), glaucoma, lenticular deposits, pigmentary retinopathy (prolonged therapy)

Respiratory: Nasal congestion, pneumonia, pneumonitis, pulmonary embolism

Miscellaneous: Diaphoresis increased, lupus-like syndrome

General Dosage Range I.M.:

Adults: Initial: 50-100 mg; Maintenance: 25-250 mg every 3-4 weeks

Elderly >50 years: Initial: <50 mg is recommended

Mechanism of Action Blocks postsynaptic mesolimbic dopaminergic receptors in the brain; depresses the release of hypothalamic and hypophyseal hormones. Relative to other piperidine phenothiazines, pipotiazine appears to be less sedating, with less potential to potentiate other CNS depressants, and may possess a lower propensity to cause hypotension. However, it has a relatively high propensity for cause extrapyramidal reactions. Pipotiazine palmitate is an ester of pipotiazine with a prolonged duration of action.

Pharmacodynamics/Kinetics

Onset of Action I.M.: 2-3 days

Duration of Action 3-6 weeks

Product Availability Not available in U.S.

Pirbuterol (peer BYOO ter ole)

Related Information

Respiratory Diseases *on page 1876*

U.S. Brand Names Maxair® Autohaler®

Pharmacologic Category $Beta_2$-Adrenergic Agonist

Use Prevention and treatment of reversible bronchospasm including asthma

Local Anesthetic/Vasoconstrictor Precautions No information available to require special precautions

Effects on Dental Treatment Key adverse event(s) related to dental treatment: Xerostomia (normal salivary flow resumes upon discontinuation) and taste changes.

Effects on Bleeding No information available to require special precautions

Adverse Effects

>10%:

Central nervous system: Nervousness (7%)

Endocrine & metabolic: Serum glucose increased, serum potassium decreased

Neuromuscular & skeletal: Trembling (6%)

1% to 10%:

Cardiovascular: Palpitation (2%), tachycardia (1%)

Central nervous system: Headache (2%), dizziness (1%)

Gastrointestinal: Nausea (2%)

Respiratory: Cough (1%)

General Dosage Range Inhalation: *Children ≥12 years and Adults:* Prevention: 2 inhalations every 4-6 hours; Treatment: 2 inhalations at an interval of at least 1-3 minutes, followed by a third inhalation (maximum: 12 inhalations/day)

Mechanism of Action Pirbuterol is a $beta_2$-adrenergic agonist with a similar structure to albuterol, specifically a pyridine ring has been substituted for the benzene ring in albuterol. The increased $beta_2$ selectivity of pirbuterol results from the substitution of a tertiary butyl group on the nitrogen of the side chain, which additionally imparts resistance of pirbuterol to degradation by monoamine oxidase and provides a lengthened duration of action in comparison to the less selective previous beta-agonist agents.

Pharmacodynamics/Kinetics

Onset of Action Peak effect: Therapeutic: Oral: 2-3 hours with peak serum concentration of 6.2-9.8 mcg/L; Inhalation: 0.5-1 hour

Half-life Elimination 2-3 hours

Pregnancy Risk Factor C

Piroxicam (peer OKS i kam)

Related Information

Rheumatoid Arthritis, Osteoarthritis, and Osteoporosis *on page 1889*

Temporomandibular Dysfunction (TMD) *on page 1964*

U.S. Brand Names Feldene®

Canadian Brand Names Apo-Piroxicam®; Dom-Piroxicam; Gen-Piroxicam; Novo-Pirocam; Nu-Pirox; PMS-Piroxicam; PRO-Piroxicam

Generic Availability (U.S.) Yes

Pharmacologic Category Nonsteroidal Anti-inflammatory Drug (NSAID), Oral

Use Symptomatic treatment of acute and chronic rheumatoid arthritis and osteoarthritis

Unlabeled/Investigational Use Ankylosing spondylitis

Local Anesthetic/Vasoconstrictor Precautions No information available to require special precautions

Effects on Dental Treatment The dentist should be aware of the potential of abnormal coagulation. Caution should also be exercised in the use of NSAIDs in patients already on anticoagulant therapy with drugs such as warfarin (Coumadin®). See Effects on Bleeding.

Effects on Bleeding Nonselective NSAIDs are known to reversibly decrease platelet aggregation via mechanisms different than observed with aspirin. Platelet function is restored as the drug is eliminated from the body. NSAIDs should be avoided (if possible) in general surgery patients for 3-5 half-lives of the drug (usually 1-3 days) prior to surgery to reduce the risk of excessive bleeding. However, there is no scientific evidence to warrant discontinuance of NSAIDs prior to dental surgery. In medically complicated patients or extensive oral surgery, the decision to interrupt therapy must be based on the risk to benefit in an individual patient and a medical consult is suggested. Routine interruption of NSAID therapy for most dental procedures is not warranted. If therapy is continued without interruption, the clinician should anticipate the potential for slower clotting times.

Adverse Effects

>10%:

Central nervous system: Dizziness
Dermatologic: Rash
Gastrointestinal: Abdominal cramps, heartburn, indigestion, nausea

1% to 10%:

Central nervous system: Headache, nervousness
Dermatologic: Itching
Endocrine & metabolic: Fluid retention
Gastrointestinal: Vomiting
Otic: Tinnitus

Dosage Oral:

Children (unlabeled use): 0.2-0.3 mg/kg/day once daily; maximum dose: 15 mg/day

Adults: 10-20 mg/day once daily; although associated with increase in GI adverse effects, doses >20 mg/day have been used (ie, 30-40 mg/day)

Dosing adjustment in renal impairment: Not recommended in patients with advanced renal disease

Dosing adjustment in hepatic impairment: Reduction of dosage is necessary

Mechanism of Action Reversibly inhibits cyclooxygenase-1 and 2 (COX-1 and 2) enzymes, which results in decreased formation of prostaglandin precursors; has antipyretic, analgesic, and anti-inflammatory properties

Other proposed mechanisms not fully elucidated (and possibly contributing to the anti-inflammatory effect to varying degrees), include inhibiting chemotaxis, altering lymphocyte activity, inhibiting neutrophil aggregation/activation, and decreasing proinflammatory cytokine levels.

Contraindications Hypersensitivity to piroxicam, aspirin, other NSAIDs or any component of the formulation; perioperative pain in the setting of coronary artery bypass graft (CABG) surgery

Warnings/Precautions [U.S. Boxed Warning]: NSAIDs are associated with an increased risk of adverse cardiovascular thrombotic events, including MI and stroke. Risk may be increased with duration of use or pre-existing cardiovascular risk factors or disease. Carefully evaluate individual cardiovascular risk profiles prior to prescribing. May cause new-onset hypertension or worsening of existing hypertension. Use caution with fluid retention. Avoid use in heart failure. Concurrent administration of ibuprofen, and potentially other nonselective NSAIDs, may interfere with aspirin's cardioprotective effect. **[U.S. Boxed Warning]: Use is contraindicated for treatment of perioperative pain in the setting of coronary artery bypass graft (CABG) surgery.** Risk of MI and stroke may be increased with use following CABG surgery.

Platelet adhesion and aggregation may be decreased; may prolong bleeding time; patients with coagulation disorders or who are receiving anticoagulants should be monitored closely. Anemia may occur; patients on long-term NSAID therapy should be monitored for anemia. Rarely, NSAID use may cause severe blood dyscrasias (eg, agranulocytosis, aplastic anemia, thrombocytopenia).

NSAID use may compromise existing renal function; dose-dependent decreases in prostaglandin synthesis may result from NSAID use, reducing renal blood flow which may cause renal decompensation. NSAID use may increase the risk for hyperkalemia. Patients with impaired renal function, dehydration, heart failure, liver dysfunction, those taking diuretics, and ACE inhibitors, and the elderly are at greater risk of renal toxicity and hyperkalemia. Rehydrate patient before starting therapy; monitor renal function closely. Not recommended for use in patients with advanced renal disease. Long-term NSAID use may result in renal papillary necrosis.

[U.S. Boxed Warning]: NSAIDs may increase risk of gastrointestinal irritation, inflammation, ulceration, bleeding, and perforation. These events may occur at any time during therapy and without warning. Use caution with a history of GI disease (bleeding or ulcers), concurrent therapy with aspirin, anticoagulants and/or corticosteroids, smoking, use of alcohol, the elderly or debilitated patients. When used concomitantly with ≤325 mg of aspirin, a substantial increase in the risk of gastrointestinal complications (eg, ulcer) occurs; concomitant gastroprotective therapy (eg, proton pump inhibitors) is recommended (Bhatt, 2008).

Use the lowest effective dose for the shortest duration of time, consistent with individual patient goals, to reduce risk of cardiovascular or GI adverse events. Alternate therapies should be considered for patients at high risk.

NSAIDs may cause serious skin adverse events including exfoliative dermatitis, Stevens-Johnson syndrome (SJS) and toxic epidermal necrolysis (TEN); discontinue use at first sign of skin rash or hypersensitivity. Anaphylactoid reactions may occur, even without prior exposure; patients with "aspirin triad" (bronchial asthma, aspirin intolerance, rhinitis) may be at increased risk. Do not use in patients who experience bronchospasm, asthma, rhinitis, or urticaria with NSAID or aspirin therapy. Use caution with other forms of asthma. A serum sickness-like reaction can rarely occur; watch for arthralgias, pruritus, fever, fatigue, and rash.

Use with caution in patients with decreased hepatic function. Closely monitor patients with any abnormal LFT. Severe hepatic reactions (eg, fulminant hepatitis, liver failure) have occurred with NSAID use, rarely; discontinue if signs or symptoms of liver disease develop, or if systemic manifestations occur.

NSAIDS may cause drowsiness, dizziness, blurred vision and other neurologic effects which may impair physical or mental abilities; patients must be cautioned about performing tasks which require mental alertness (eg, operating machinery or driving). Discontinue use with blurred or diminished vision and perform ophthalmologic exam. Monitor vision with long-term therapy.

In the elderly, may be inappropriate for long-term use due to potential for GI bleeding, hypertension, heart failure, and renal failure (Beers Criteria).

Withhold for at least 4-6 half-lives prior to surgical or dental procedures.

Drug Interactions

Metabolism/Transport Effects Substrate of CYP2C9 (minor); **Inhibits** CYP2C9 (strong)

Avoid Concomitant Use

Avoid concomitant use of Piroxicam with any of the following: Ketorolac; Ketorolac (Systemic)

Increased Effect/Toxicity

Piroxicam may increase the levels/effects of: Aminoglycosides; Anticoagulants; Antiplatelet Agents; Bisphosphonate Derivatives; Collagenase (Systemic); CycloSPORINE; CycloSPORINE (Systemic); Deferasirox; Desmopressin; Digoxin; Drotrecogin Alfa; Eplerenone; Haloperidol; Ibritumomab; Lithium; Methotrexate; Nonsteroidal Anti-Inflammatory Agents; PEMEtrexed; Potassium-Sparing Diuretics; PRALAtrexate; Quinolone Antibiotics; Salicylates; Thrombolytic Agents; Tositumomab and Iodine I 131 Tositumomab; Vancomycin; Vitamin K Antagonists

The levels/effects of Piroxicam may be increased by: ACE Inhibitors; Angiotensin II Receptor Blockers; Antidepressants (Tricyclic, Tertiary Amine); Corticosteroids (Systemic); Dasatinib; Glucosamine; Herbs (Anticoagulant/Antiplatelet Properties); Ketorolac; Ketorolac (Systemic); Nonsteroidal Anti-Inflammatory Agents; Omega-3-Acid Ethyl Esters; Pentosan Polysulfate Sodium; Pentoxifylline; Probenecid; Prostacyclin Analogues; Selective Serotonin Reuptake Inhibitors; Serotonin/Norepinephrine Reuptake Inhibitors; Treprostinil

Decreased Effect

Piroxicam may decrease the levels/effects of: ACE Inhibitors; Angiotensin II Receptor Blockers; Antiplatelet Agents; Beta-Blockers; Eplerenone; HydrALAZINE; Loop Diuretics; Potassium-Sparing Diuretics; Salicylates; Thiazide Diuretics

The levels/effects of Piroxicam may be decreased by: Bile Acid Sequestrants; Nonsteroidal Anti-Inflammatory Agents; Salicylates

Ethanol/Nutrition/Herb Interactions

Ethanol: Avoid ethanol (may enhance gastric mucosal irritation).

Food: Onset of effect may be delayed if piroxicam is taken with food.

Herb/Nutraceutical: Avoid alfalfa, anise, bilberry, bladderwrack, bromelain, cat's claw, celery, chamomile, coleus, cordyceps, dong quai, evening primrose, fenugreek, feverfew, garlic, ginger, ginkgo biloba, ginseng (American, Panax, Siberian), grapeseed, green tea, guggul, horse chestnut seed, horseradish, licorice, prickly ash, red clover, reishi, SAMe (S-adenosylmethionine), sweet clover, turmeric, white willow (all have additional antiplatelet activity).

Dietary Considerations May be taken with food to decrease GI adverse effect.

Pharmacodynamics/Kinetics

Onset of Action Analgesic: ~1 hour

Half-life Elimination 50 hours

Time to Peak 3-5 hours

Pregnancy Risk Factor C

Lactation Enters breast milk/not recommended (AAP rates "compatible"; AAP 2001 update pending)

Breast-Feeding Considerations Piroxicam is excreted into breast milk. Breast-feeding is not recommended by the manufacturer.

Dosage Forms

Capsule, oral: 10 mg, 20 mg

Feldene®: 10 mg, 20 mg

Pitavastatin (pi TA va sta tin)

Related Information

Cardiovascular Diseases *on page 1848*

U.S. Brand Names Livalo®

Generic Availability (U.S.) No

Pharmacologic Category Antilipemic Agent, HMG-CoA Reductase Inhibitor

Use Adjunct to dietary therapy to reduce elevations in total cholesterol (TC), LDL-C, apolipoprotein B (Apo B), and triglycerides (TG), and to increase low HDL-C in patients with primary hyperlipidemia and mixed dyslipidemia

Local Anesthetic/Vasoconstrictor Precautions No information available to require special precautions

Effects on Dental Treatment No significant effects or complications reported

Effects on Bleeding No information available to require special precautions

Adverse Effects

2% to 10%:

Gastrointestinal: Constipation (2% to 4%), diarrhea (2% to 3%)

Neuromuscular & skeletal: Back pain (1% to 4%), myalgia (2% to 3%), pain in extremities (1% to 2%)

Additional class-related events or case reports (not necessarily reported with pitavastatin therapy): Cataracts, cirrhosis, dermatomyositis, eosinophilia, extraocular muscle movement impaired, fulminant hepatic necrosis, gynecomastia, hypersensitivity syndrome (symptoms may include anaphylaxis, angioedema, arthralgia, erythema multiforme, eosinophilia, hemolytic anemia, interstitial lung disease, lupus syndrome, photosensitivity, polymyalgia rheumatica, positive ANA, purpura, Stevens-Johnson syndrome, toxic epidermal necrolysis, urticaria, vasculitis), ophthalmoplegia, peripheral nerve palsy, rhabdomyolysis, renal failure (secondary to rhabdomyolysis), thyroid dysfunction, tremor, vertigo

Dosage Oral: **Note:** Doses should be individualized according to the baseline LDL-cholesterol levels, the recommended goal of therapy, and patient response; adjustments should be made at intervals of 4 weeks.

Adults: Primary hyperlipidemia and mixed dyslipidemia: Initial: 2 mg once daily; may be increased to maximum 4 mg once daily

Dosage adjustment with concomitant medications:

Erythromycin: Pitavastatin dose should not exceed 1 mg once daily

Rifampin: Pitavastatin dose should not exceed 2 mg once daily

Dosing adjustment in renal impairment:

Moderate renal impairment (Cl_{cr} 30-60 mL/minute/1.73 m^2) or end-stage renal disease receiving hemodialysis: Initial: 1 mg once daily; do not exceed 2 mg once daily

Severe renal impairment (Cl_{cr} <30 mL/minute/1.73 m^2) not receiving hemodialysis: Not recommended

Dosing adjustment in hepatic impairment: Contraindicated in active liver disease or in patients with unexplained persistent elevations of serum transaminases

Mechanism of Action Inhibitor of 3-hydroxy-3-methylglutaryl coenzyme A (HMG-CoA) reductase, the rate-limiting enzyme in cholesterol synthesis (reduces the production of mevalonic acid from HMG-CoA); this then results in a compensatory increase in the expression of LDL receptors on hepatocyte membranes and a stimulation of LDL catabolism

Contraindications Hypersensitivity to pitavastatin or any component of the formulation; active liver disease including unexplained persistent elevations of hepatic transaminases; concurrent use with cyclosporine; pregnancy; breast-feeding

Warnings/Precautions Secondary causes of hyperlipidemia should be ruled out prior to therapy. Pitavastatin has not been studied when the primary lipid abnormality is chylomicron elevation (Fredrickson types I and V) or in familial dysbetalipoproteinemia (Fredrickson type III). May cause hepatic dysfunction; in all patients, liver function must be monitored by periodic laboratory assessment. Use with caution in patients who consume large amounts of ethanol or have a history of liver disease; use is contraindicated in patients with active liver disease or unexplained persistent elevations of serum transaminases.

Myopathy and rhabdomyolysis with acute renal failure have occurred with use. Risk is dose related and is increased with concurrent use of lipid-lowering agents which may cause rhabdomyolysis (fibric acid derivatives or niacin at doses ≥1 g/day) or during concurrent use with erythromycin or protease inhibitors. Use caution in patients with renal impairment, inadequately treated hypothyroidism, and those taking other drugs associated with myopathy (eg, colchicine); these patients are predisposed to myopathy. Monitor closely if used with other drugs associated with myopathy. Weigh the risk versus benefit when combining any of these drugs with pitavastatin. Discontinue in any patient experiencing an acute or serious condition predisposing to renal failure secondary to rhabdomyolysis. Patients should be instructed to report unexplained muscle pain, tenderness, weakness, or brown urine. Concurrent use with cyclosporine is contraindicated. Ensure patient is on the lowest effective pitavastatin dose. Based upon current evidence, HMG-CoA reductase inhibitor therapy should be continued in the perioperative period unless risk outweighs cardioprotective benefit. Use with caution in elderly patients, as these patients are predisposed to myopathy.

Drug Interactions

Metabolism/Transport Effects Substrate of OATP1B1; (major) of UGT1A3 and UGT2B7; (minor) of CYP2C9, 2C8

Avoid Concomitant Use

Avoid concomitant use of Pitavastatin with any of the following: CycloSPORINE; CycloSPORINE (Systemic); Lopinavir; Red Yeast Rice; Ritonavir

Increased Effect/Toxicity

Pitavastatin may increase the levels/effects of: DAPTOmycin; Trabectedin; Vitamin K Antagonists

The levels/effects of Pitavastatin may be increased by: Atazanavir; Colchicine; CycloSPORINE; CycloSPORINE (Systemic); Danazol; Fenofibrate; Fenofibric Acid; Gemfibrozil; Grapefruit Juice; Lopinavir; Macrolide Antibiotics; Niacin; Niacinamide; Protease Inhibitors; Red Yeast Rice; Rifamycin Derivatives; Ritonavir; Sildenafil

Decreased Effect

The levels/effects of Pitavastatin may be decreased by: Antacids; Bosentan; Rifamycin Derivatives; St Johns Wort

Ethanol/Nutrition/Herb Interactions

Ethanol: Avoid excessive ethanol consumption (due to potential hepatic effects).

Food: Red yeast rice contains an estimated 2.4 mg lovastatin per 600 mg rice.

Dietary Considerations May be taken with or without food; may take without regard to time of day. Red yeast rice contains an estimated 2.4 mg lovastatin per 600 mg rice.

Pharmacodynamics/Kinetics

Half-life Elimination ~12 hours

Time to Peak ~1 hour

Pregnancy Risk Factor X

Lactation Excretion in breast milk unknown/contraindicated

Dosage Forms

Tablet, oral:

Livalo®: 1 mg, 2 mg, 4 mg

Plerixafor (pler IX a fore)

U.S. Brand Names Mozobil™

Pharmacologic Category Hematopoietic Stem Cell Mobilizer

Use Mobilization of hematopoietic stem cells (HSC) for collection and subsequent autologous transplantation (in combination with filgrastim) in patients with non-Hodgkin's lymphoma (NHL) and multiple myeloma (MM)

Local Anesthetic/Vasoconstrictor Precautions No information available to require special precautions

Effects on Dental Treatment Key adverse event(s) related to dental treatment: Xerostomia (normal salivary flow resumes upon discontinuation).

Effects on Bleeding No information available to require special precautions

Adverse Effects Adverse reactions reported with filgrastim combination therapy.

>10%:

- Central nervous system: Fatigue (27%), headache (22%), dizziness (11%)
- Gastrointestinal: Diarrhea (37%), nausea (34%)
- Local: Injection site reactions (34%, including erythema, hematoma, hemorrhage, induration, inflammation, irritation, pain, paresthesia, pruritus, rash, swelling, urticaria)
- Neuromuscular & skeletal: Arthralgia (13%)

5% to 10%:

- Central nervous system: Insomnia (7%)
- Gastrointestinal: Vomiting (10%), flatulence (7%)

General Dosage Range Dosage adjustment recommended in patients with renal impairment

SubQ: *Adults:* 0.24 mg/kg/day (maximum dose: 40 mg/day)

Mechanism of Action Reversibly inhibits binding of stromal cell-derived factor-1-alpha (SDF-1α), expressed on bone marrow stromal cells, to the CXC chemokine receptor 4 (CXCR4), resulting in mobilization of hematopoietic stem and progenitor cells from bone marrow into peripheral blood. Plerixafor used in combination with filgrastim results in synergistic increase in CD34+ cell mobilization. Mobilized CD34+ cells are capable of engrafting with extended repopulating capacity.

Pharmacodynamics/Kinetics

Onset of Action Peak CD34+ mobilization: Plerixafor monotherapy: 6-9 hours after administration; Plerixafor + filgrastim: 10-14 hours

Duration of Action WBC counts return toward baseline at ~24 after administration

Half-life Elimination Terminal: 3-6 hours

Time to Peak Plasma: SubQ: 30-60 minutes

Pregnancy Risk Factor D

Pneumococcal Conjugate Vaccine (7-Valent)

(noo moe KOK al KON ju gate vak SEEN, seven vay lent)

U.S. Brand Names Prevnar®

Canadian Brand Names Prevnar®

Pharmacologic Category Vaccine, Inactivated (Bacterial)

Use Note: In March 2010, the Advisory Committee on Immunization Practices (ACIP) released recommendations that pneumococcal 13-valent conjugate vaccine (PCV13; Prevnar 13™) replace pneumococcal 7-valent conjugate vaccine (PCV7; Prevnar®) for all doses for immunization of all children 2-59 months of age. Refer to the Pneumococcal Conjugate Vaccine (13-Valent) monograph for additional information.

Immunization of infants and toddlers against *Streptococcus pneumoniae* infection caused by serotypes included in the vaccine

Immunization of infants and toddlers against otitis media caused by serotypes included in the vaccine

The Advisory Committee on Immunization Practices (ACIP) recommends pneumococcal conjugate vaccine (PCV) for routine vaccination of all children 2-59 months and children 60-71 months with underlying medical conditions. PCV13 should be used to complete the vaccination of children who received ≥1 dose of PCV7.

Local Anesthetic/Vasoconstrictor Precautions No information available to require special precautions

Effects on Dental Treatment No significant effects or complications reported

Effects on Bleeding No information available to require special precautions

Adverse Effects All serious adverse reactions must be reported to the U.S. Department of Health and Human Services (DHHS) Vaccine Adverse Event Reporting System (VAERS) 1-800-822-7967 or online at https://vaers.hhs.gov/esub/index. In Canada, adverse reactions may be reported to local provincial/territorial health agencies or to the Vaccine Safety Section at Public Health Agency of Canada (1-866-844-0018).

>10%:

- Central nervous system: Fever, irritability, drowsiness, restlessness
- Dermatologic: Erythema
- Gastrointestinal: Decreased appetite, vomiting, diarrhea
- Local: Induration, tenderness, nodule

1% to 10%: Dermatologic: Rash

General Dosage Range I.M.: *Infants 2-6 months:* 0.5 mL at approximately 2-month intervals for 3 consecutive doses, followed by a fourth dose of 0.5 mL at 12-15 months of age

Mechanism of Action Promotes active immunization against invasive disease caused by *S. pneumoniae* capsular serotypes 4, 6B, 9V, 14, 18C, 19F, and 23F, all which are individually conjugated to CRM197 protein

Pregnancy Risk Factor C

Pneumococcal Conjugate Vaccine (13-Valent)

(noo moe KOK al KON ju gate vak SEEN, thur TEEN vay lent)

U.S. Brand Names Prevnar 13™

Canadian Brand Names Prevnar 13™

Pharmacologic Category Vaccine, Inactivated (Bacterial)

Use

Immunization of infants and children against *Streptococcus pneumoniae* infection caused by serotypes included in the vaccine

Immunization of infants and children against otitis media caused by *Streptococcus pneumoniae* serotypes 4, 6B, 9V, 14, 18C, 19F, and 23F

PNEUMOCOCCAL CONJUGATE VACCINE (13-VALENT)

The Advisory Committee on Immunization Practices (ACIP) recommends routine vaccination for the following:
All children age 2-59 months
Children 60-71 months with underlying medical conditions including: Cochlear implants, functional or anatomic asplenia (includes sickle cell disease and other hemoglobinopathies, congenital or acquired asplenia, or splenic dysfunction); immunocompromising conditions (includes HIV infection, congenital immunodeficiencies [excluding chronic granulomatous disease], chronic renal failure, nephrotic syndrome, diseases associated with immunosuppressive or radiation therapy, solid organ transplant); chronic illnesses (cardiac disease, cerebrospinal fluid leaks, diabetes mellitus, pulmonary disease [excluding asthma unless on high dose oral corticosteroids])
Children who received ≥1 dose of PCV7
Children 6-18 years of age at increased risk for invasive pneumococcal disease due to anatomic or functional asplenia (including sickle cell disease), HIV infection or other immunocompromising conditions, cochlear implant, or cerebrospinal fluid leaks (regardless of prior receipt of PCV7 or PPSV23). Routine use is not recommended for healthy children ≥5 years of age.

Local Anesthetic/Vasoconstrictor Precautions No information available to require special precautions

Effects on Dental Treatment No significant effects or complications reported

Effects on Bleeding No information available to require special precautions

Adverse Effects All serious adverse reactions must be reported to the U.S. Department of Health and Human Services (DHHS) Vaccine Adverse Event Reporting System (VAERS) 1-800-822-7967 or online at https://vaers.hhs.gov/esub/index.

>10%:
Central nervous system: Drowsiness, fever, insomnia, irritability
Gastrointestinal: Appetite decreased
Local: Erythema, swelling, tenderness

1% to 10%:
Dermatologic: Rash
Gastrointestinal: Diarrhea, vomiting

Adverse reactions observed with PCV7 which may also be seen with PCV-13: Anaphylactic reaction, angioneurotic edema, apnea, breath holding, edema, erythema multiforme, hypotonic hyporesponsive episode, injection site reaction (dermatitis, pruritus), lymphadenopathy (localized), shock

General Dosage Range I.M.:
Infants 2-6 months: 0.5 mL at approximately 2-month intervals for 3 consecutive doses, followed by a fourth dose of 0.5 mL at 12-15 months of age
Infants 7-11 months (previously unvaccinated): 0.5 mL for a total of 3 doses, 2 doses at least 4 weeks apart, followed by a third dose at 12-15 months (at least 2 months after second dose)
Children 12-23 months (previously unvaccinated) and Children 24-71 months (previously unvaccinated) with underlying conditions: 0.5 mL for a total of 2 doses, separated by at least 2 months
Healthy Children 24-59 months (previously unvaccinated) and Children 6-18 years at high risk for invasive pneumococcal disease: 0.5 mL as a single dose
Children 14 months-71 months (previously completing vaccination with PCV7): 0.5 mL supplemental dose

Mechanism of Action Promotes active immunization against invasive disease caused by *S. pneumoniae* capsular serotypes 1, 3, 4, 5, 6A, 6B, 7F, 9V, 14, 18C, 19A, 19F, and 23F, all which are individually conjugated to CRM197 protein

Pregnancy Risk Factor C

Podofilox (poe DOF il oks)

U.S. Brand Names Condylox®
Canadian Brand Names Condyline™; Wartec®
Pharmacologic Category Keratolytic Agent; Topical Skin Product
Use Treatment of external genital warts
Local Anesthetic/Vasoconstrictor Precautions No information available to require special precautions
Effects on Dental Treatment No significant effects or complications reported
Effects on Bleeding No information available to require special precautions
General Dosage Range Topical: *Adults:* Apply twice daily for 3 consecutive days, then withhold use for 4 consecutive days; May repeat cycle up to 4 times
Pregnancy Risk Factor C

Podophyllum Resin (po DOF fil um REZ in)

U.S. Brand Names Podocon-25®
Canadian Brand Names Podofilm®
Pharmacologic Category Keratolytic Agent
Use Topical treatment of soft external genital (venereal) warts (condylomata acuminate); compound benzoin tincture generally is used as the medium for topical application
Local Anesthetic/Vasoconstrictor Precautions No information available to require special precautions
Effects on Dental Treatment No significant effects or complications reported
Effects on Bleeding No information available to require special precautions
Adverse Effects
Central nervous system: Coma, fever, polyneuritis
Gastrointestinal: Paralytic ileus
Hematologic: Leukopenia, thrombocytopenia
Neuromuscular & skeletal: Paresthesia
Miscellaneous: Death
General Dosage Range Topical: *Children and Adults:* Applied by physician only
Mechanism of Action Directly affects epithelial cell metabolism by arresting mitosis through binding to a protein subunit of spindle microtubules (tubulin)
Pregnancy Risk Factor X

Polidocanol (pol i DOE kuh nol)

U.S. Brand Names Asclera™
Pharmacologic Category Sclerosing Agent
Use Treatment of small, uncomplicated varicose veins of the lower extremities
Local Anesthetic/Vasoconstrictor Precautions No information available to require special precautions
Effects on Dental Treatment No significant effects or complications reported
Effects on Bleeding No information available to require special precautions
Adverse Effects
>10%: Local: Hematoma (42%), irritation (41%), discoloration (38%), pain (24%), pruritus (19%), warmth (16%)
1% to 10%: Local: Neovascularization (8%), injection site thrombosis (6%)
General Dosage Range I.V.: *Adults:* 0.1-0.3 mL injection (0.5% or 1% solution) per session (maximum: 10 mL/session)
Mechanism of Action Acts by irritation of the vein intimal endothelium and causes thrombosis formation leading to occlusion of the injected vein
Pharmacodynamics/Kinetics
Half-life Elimination 1.5 hours
Pregnancy Risk Factor C

Poliovirus Vaccine (Inactivated)
(POE lee oh VYE rus vak SEEN, in ak ti VAY ted)

U.S. Brand Names IPOL®
Canadian Brand Names Imovax® Polio
Pharmacologic Category Vaccine, Inactivated (Viral)
Use Active immunization against poliomyelitis caused by poliovirus types 1, 2 and 3. **Note:** Combination products containing polio vaccine are also available and may be preferred in certain age groups if recipients are likely to be susceptible to the agents contained within each vaccine.

The Advisory Committee on Immunization Practices (ACIP) recommends routine vaccination for the following:
- All children (first dose given at 2 months of age)

Routine immunization of adults in the United States is generally not recommended. Adults with previous wild poliovirus disease, who have never been immunized, or those who are incompletely immunized may receive inactivated poliovirus vaccine if they fall into one of the following categories:
- Travelers to regions or countries where poliomyelitis is endemic or epidemic
- Healthcare workers in close contact with patients who may be excreting poliovirus
- Laboratory workers handling specimens that may contain poliovirus
- Members of communities or specific population groups with diseases caused by wild poliovirus

- Incompletely vaccinated or unvaccinated adults in a household or with other close contact with children receiving oral poliovirus (may be at increased risk of vaccine associated paralytic poliomyelitis)

Local Anesthetic/Vasoconstrictor Precautions No information available to require special precautions

Effects on Dental Treatment No significant effects or complications reported

Effects on Bleeding No information available to require special precautions

Adverse Effects All serious adverse reactions must be reported to the U.S. Department of Health and Human Services (DHHS) Vaccine Adverse Event Reporting System (VAERS) 1-800-822-7967 or online at https://vaers.hhs.gov/esub/index. In Canada, adverse reactions may be reported to local provincial/territorial health agencies or to the Vaccine Safety Section at Public Health Agency of Canada (1-866-844-0018).

Percentages noted with concomitant administration of DTP or DTaP vaccine and observed within 48 hours of injection.

>10%:

Central nervous system: Irritability (7% to 65%), tiredness (4% to 61%), fever ≥39°C (≤38%)

Gastrointestinal: Anorexia (1% to 17%)

Local: Injection Site: Tenderness (≤29%), swelling (≤11%)

1% to 10%:

Central nervous system: Fever >39°C (≤4%)

Gastrointestinal: Vomiting (1% to 3%)

Local: Injection site: Erythema (≤3%)

Miscellaneous: Persistent crying (up to 1% reported within 72 hours)

General Dosage Range I.M., SubQ:

Children: Primary immunization: Administer three 0.5 mL doses at 2, 4, and 6-18 months of age; do not administer more frequently than 4 weeks apart (preferably given more than 8 weeks apart). Booster dose: 0.5 mL at 4-6 years of age; Minimum interval between booster and previous dose is 6 months.

Adults (previously unvaccinated): Two 0.5 mL doses administered at 1- to 2-month intervals followed by a third dose 6-12 months later.

Pregnancy Risk Factor C

Polycarbophil (pol i KAR boe fil)

U.S. Brand Names Equalactin® [OTC]; Fiber-Lax [OTC]; Fiber-Tabs™ [OTC]; FiberCon® [OTC]; Konsyl® Fiber [OTC]

Pharmacologic Category Antidiarrheal; Fiber Supplement; Laxative, Bulk-Producing

Use Treatment of constipation or diarrhea

Local Anesthetic/Vasoconstrictor Precautions No information available to require special precautions

Effects on Dental Treatment Oral medication should be given at least 1 hour prior to taking the bulk-producing laxative in order to prevent decreased absorption of medication.

Effects on Bleeding No information available to require special precautions

Adverse Effects Frequency not defined: Gastrointestinal: Abdominal fullness

General Dosage Range Oral:

Children 6-12 years: 625 mg calcium polycarbophil 1-4 times/day

Children ≥12 years and Adults: 1250 mg calcium polycarbophil 1-4 times/day

Mechanism of Action Restoring a more normal moisture level and providing bulk in the patient's intestinal tract

Pregnancy Risk Factor C

Polyethylene Glycol 3350 (pol i ETH i leen GLY kol 3350)

U.S. Brand Names Dulcolax Balance® [OTC]; MiraLAX® [OTC]

Pharmacologic Category Laxative, Osmotic

Use Treatment of occasional constipation in adults

Unlabeled/Investigational Use Treatment of constipation in children; bowel preparation before colonoscopy

Local Anesthetic/Vasoconstrictor Precautions No information available to require special precautions

Effects on Dental Treatment No significant effects or complications reported

Effects on Bleeding No information available to require special precautions

Adverse Effects Frequency not defined.

Dermatologic: Urticaria

Gastrointestinal: Abdominal bloating, cramping, diarrhea, flatulence, nausea

General Dosage Range Oral: *Adults:* 17 g of powder (~1 heaping tablespoon) dissolved in 4-8 ounces of beverage once daily (maximum use: 1 week)

Mechanism of Action An osmotic agent, polyethylene glycol 3350 causes water retention in the stool; increases stool frequency.

Pharmacodynamics/Kinetics

Onset of Action Oral: 24-96 hours

Pregnancy Risk Factor C

Polyethylene Glycol-Electrolyte Solution

(pol i ETH i leen GLY kol ee LEK troe lite soe LOO shun)

U.S. Brand Names Colyte®; GaviLyte™-C; GaviLyte™-G; GaviLyte™-N; GoLYTELY®; MoviPrep®; NuLYTELY®; TriLyte®

Canadian Brand Names Colyte™; Klean-Prep®; PegLyte®

Pharmacologic Category Laxative, Osmotic

Use Bowel cleansing prior to GI examination

Unlabeled/Investigational Use Whole bowel irrigation (WBI) in the following toxic ingestions: Packets of illicit drugs (body packers, body stuffers), potentially toxic sustained-release or enteric-coated agents, substantial amounts of iron (AACT, 2004)

Local Anesthetic/Vasoconstrictor Precautions No information available to require special precautions

Effects on Dental Treatment No significant effects or complications reported

Effects on Bleeding No information available to require special precautions

Adverse Effects

>10%:

- Central nervous system: Malaise (18% to 27%)
- Gastrointestinal: Abdominal distension (<60%), anal irritation (<52%), nausea (14% to 47%), abdominal pain (13% to 39%), vomiting (7% to 12%)
- Neuromuscular & skeletal: Rigors (34%)
- Miscellaneous: Thirst (<47%)

1% to 10%:

- Central nervous system: Dizziness (7%), headache (2%)
- Gastrointestinal: Dyspepsia (1% to 3%)

General Dosage Range

Nasogastric tube:

Children ≥6 months: 25 mL/kg/hour until rectal effluent is clear

Adults: 20-30 mL/minute (1.2-1.8 L/hour) until rectal effluent is clear

Oral:

Children ≥6 months: (GaviLyte™-N, NuLYTELY®, TriLyte®): 25 mL/kg/hour (some studies have used up to 40 mL/kg/hour) for 4-10 hours until rectal effluent is clear (maximum total dose: 4 L)

Adults: CoLyte®, GaviLyte™-C, GaviLyte™-G, GaviLyte™-N, GoLYTELY®, NuLYTELY®, TriLyte®: 240 mL (8 oz) every 10 minutes, until 4 L are consumed or the rectal effluent is clear; MoviPrep®: 240 mL (8 oz) every 15 minutes until 1 L consumed; repeat 1 time

Mechanism of Action Induces catharsis by strong electrolyte and osmotic effects

Pharmacodynamics/Kinetics

Onset of Action Oral: ~1-2 hours

Pregnancy Risk Factor C

Poly-L-Lactic Acid (POL i el LAK tik AS id)

U.S. Brand Names Sculptra®; Sculptra® Aesthetic

Pharmacologic Category Cosmetic Agent, Implant

Use Restoration and/or correction of facial lipoatrophy in patients with HIV; correction of shallow to deep nasolabial fold contour deficiencies and other facial wrinkles in immunocompetent patients

Local Anesthetic/Vasoconstrictor Precautions No information available to require special precautions

Effects on Dental Treatment No significant effects or complications reported

Effects on Bleeding No information available to require special precautions

Adverse Effects

>10%:

- Dermatologic: Bruising (1% to 65%)
- Hematologic: Hematoma (up to 28%)
- Local: Injection site: Edema (3% to 81%), tenderness (81%), redness (78%), pain (71%), papules (3% to 52%), bleeding (34%), pruritus (20%), nodules (3%)
- Miscellaneous: Discomfort (up to 19%)

1% to 10%:

Central nervous system: Fever (<5%)

Local: erythema (up to 10%), injection site reactions (<5%)

Postmarketing/case reports: Allergic reaction, angioedema, brittle nails, colitis, ectropion, fatigue, hair breakage, hypersensitivity reaction, hypertrophy, joint aches, malaise, periorbital nodules, photosensitivity, rash, scar/skin discoloration, skin infection, skin roughness, skin sarcoidosis, telangiectasia, urticaria, visible nodules

Injection site reactions: Abscess, atrophy, discharge, fat atrophy, granuloma, induration

General Dosage Range Intradermal, SubQ:

Adults:

Sculptra® Aesthetic: 0.1-0.2 mL per individual injection to a maximum of 2.5 mL per nasolabial fold as a single treatment; may repeat treatment at ≥3-week intervals up to 4 times

Sculptra®: 0.05-0.2 mL per individual injection, ~20 injections may be needed per cheek, usually involves 3-6 treatments separated by ≥2 weeks

Mechanism of Action Poly-L-lactic acid is an immunologically inert synthetic polymer. It increases dermal thickness by causing a local reaction leading to an increase in collagen deposits. It is eventually degraded and undergoes resorption.

Pharmacodynamics/Kinetics

Onset of Action Weeks to months for full effect of treatment

Polymyxin B (pol i MIKS in bee)

U.S. Brand Names Poly-Rx

Pharmacologic Category Antibiotic, Irrigation; Antibiotic, Miscellaneous

Use Treatment of acute infections caused by susceptible strains of *Pseudomonas aeruginosa*; used occasionally for gut decontamination; parenteral use of polymyxin B has mainly been replaced by less toxic antibiotics, reserved for life-threatening infections caused by organisms resistant to the preferred drugs (eg, pseudomonal meningitis - intrathecal administration)

Local Anesthetic/Vasoconstrictor Precautions No information available to require special precautions

Effects on Dental Treatment No significant effects or complications reported

Effects on Bleeding No information available to require special precautions

Adverse Effects Frequency not defined.

Cardiovascular: Facial flushing

Central nervous system: Neurotoxicity (irritability, drowsiness, ataxia, perioral paresthesia, numbness of the extremities, and blurred vision); dizziness, drug fever, meningeal irritation with intrathecal administration

Dermatologic: Urticarial rash

Endocrine & metabolic: Hypocalcemia, hyponatremia, hypokalemia, hypochloremia

Local: Pain at injection site

Neuromuscular & skeletal: Neuromuscular blockade, weakness

Renal: Nephrotoxicity

Respiratory: Respiratory arrest

Miscellaneous: Anaphylactoid reaction

General Dosage Range Dosage adjustment recommended in patients with renal impairment

I.M.:

Children <2 years: Up to 40,000 units/kg/day divided every 6 hours

Children ≥2 years and Adults: 25,000-30,000 units/kg/day divided every 4-6 hours (maximum: 2,000,000 units/day)

I.V.:

Children <2 years: Up to 40,000 units/kg/day divided every 12 hours

Children ≥2 years and Adults: 15,000-25,000 units/kg/day divided every 12 hours (maximum: 2,000,000 units/day)

Intrathecal:

Children <2 years: 20,000 units/day for 3-4 days, then 25,000 units every other day

Children ≥2 years and Adults: 50,000 units/day for 3-4 days, then every other day

Irrigation: *Adults:*

Bladder: 20 mg (equal to 200,000 units) added to 1 L of normal saline as continuous irrigant or rinse

Topical: 500,000 units/L of normal saline (maximum: 2 million units/day)

Ophthalmic: *Children ≥2 years and Adults:* Initial: 1-3 drops/hour; Reduce to 1-2 drops 4-6 times/day based on response

Otic: *Children and Adults:* 1-2 drops 3-4 times/day

Mechanism of Action Binds to phospholipids, alters permeability, and damages the bacterial cytoplasmic membrane permitting leakage of intracellular constituents

Pharmacodynamics/Kinetics

Half-life Elimination 6 hours; 2-3 days with anuria

Time to Peak Serum: I.M.: ~2 hours

Pregnancy Risk Factor B

Polysaccharide-Iron Complex (pol i SAK a ride-EYE ern KOM pleks)

U.S. Brand Names Ferrex™ 150 Plus [OTC]; Ferrex™ 150 [OTC]; Niferex® [OTC]; Nu-Iron® 150 [OTC]; Poly-Iron 150 [OTC]; ProFe [OTC]

Pharmacologic Category Iron Salt

Use Prevention and treatment of iron-deficiency anemias

Local Anesthetic/Vasoconstrictor Precautions No information available to require special precautions

Effects on Dental Treatment No significant effects or complications reported

Effects on Bleeding No information available to require special precautions

Adverse Effects

>10%: Gastrointestinal: Stomach cramping, constipation, nausea, vomiting, dark stools, GI irritation, epigastric pain, nausea

1% to 10%:

Gastrointestinal: Heartburn, diarrhea

Genitourinary: Discolored urine

Miscellaneous: Staining of teeth

General Dosage Range Oral:

Children ≥6 years: 50-100 mg once daily or in divided doses

Adults: 100-300 mg/day in 1-2 divided doses

Polysaccharide-Iron Complex, Vitamin B12, and Folic Acid (pol i SAK a ride-EYE ern KOM pleks, VYE ta min bee twelve & FOE lik AS id)

U.S. Brand Names Ferrex™ 150 Forte; Ferrex™ 150 Forte Plus; Maxaron® Forte; Poly-Iron 150 Forte; Polysaccharide Iron 150 Forte

Pharmacologic Category Iron Salt

Use Prevention and treatment of iron-deficiency anemias and/or nutritional megaloblastic anemias

Local Anesthetic/Vasoconstrictor Precautions No information available to require special precautions

Effects on Dental Treatment No significant effects or complications reported

Effects on Bleeding No information available to require special precautions

Adverse Effects Frequency not defined.

Gastrointestinal: Abdominal pain, constipation, dark stools, diarrhea, epigastric pain, GI irritation, nausea, stomach cramping, vomiting

Genitourinary: Discolored urine

Miscellaneous: Hypersensitivity reaction

General Dosage Range Oral: *Adults:* 1-2 capsules daily

Polyvinylpyrrolidone and Sodium Hyaluronate
(pol e VI nil pi ROL i don & SOW dee um AS e tate)

Related Information

Ulcerative, Erosive, and Painful Oral Mucosal Disorders *on page 1950*

U.S. Brand Names Ameseal™

Generic Availability (U.S.) No

Pharmacologic Category Protectant, Topical

Dental Use Treatment of mouth ulcers

Local Anesthetic/Vasoconstrictor Precautions No information available to require special precautions

Effects on Dental Treatment No significant effects or complications reported

Effects on Bleeding No information available to require special precautions

Dental Usual Dosage Spray: Direct the spray applicator towards the lesions and spray 3 times or as needed to cover the affected area. Repeat throughout the day as necessary.

Mechanism of Action Polyvinylpyrrolidone (PVP) sets up a barrier at application site to protect ulcer from irritants and irritation

Dosage Forms Excipient information presented when available (limited, particularly for generics); consult specific product labeling.

Solution, topical [spray]: 15 mL

Poractant Alfa (por AKT ant AL fa)

U.S. Brand Names Curosurf®
Canadian Brand Names Curosurf®
Pharmacologic Category Lung Surfactant
Use Treatment of respiratory distress syndrome (RDS) in premature infants
Local Anesthetic/Vasoconstrictor Precautions No information available to require special precautions
Effects on Dental Treatment No significant effects or complications reported
Effects on Bleeding No information available to require special precautions
Adverse Effects Frequency not defined.
Cardiovascular: Bradycardia, hypotension
Respiratory: Endotracheal tube blockage, oxygen desaturation
General Dosage Range Intratracheal: *Premature infants:* Initial: 2.5 mL/kg of birth weight, up to 2 subsequent doses of 1.25 mL/kg birth weight can be administered at 12-hour intervals if needed; Maximum total dose: 5 mL/kg
Mechanism of Action Endogenous pulmonary surfactant reduces surface tension at the air-liquid interface of the alveoli during ventilation and stabilizes the alveoli against collapse at resting transpulmonary pressures. A deficiency of pulmonary surfactant in preterm infants results in respiratory distress syndrome characterized by poor lung expansion, inadequate gas exchange, and atelectasis. Poractant alpha compensates for the surfactant deficiency and restores surface activity to the infant's lungs. It reduces mortality and pneumothoraces associated with RDS.

Porfimer (POR fi mer)

U.S. Brand Names Photofrin®
Canadian Brand Names Photofrin®
Pharmacologic Category Antineoplastic Agent, Miscellaneous
Use Palliation in patients with obstructing (partial or complete) esophageal cancer; treatment of microinvasive endobronchial nonsmall cell lung cancer (NSCLC); reduction of obstruction and palliation in patients with obstructing (partial or complete) NSCLC; ablation of high-grade dysplasia in Barrett's esophagus
Unlabeled/Investigational Use Treatment of gastric cancer (obstruction); treatment of actinic keratoses and low-risk basal and squamous cell skin cancers
Local Anesthetic/Vasoconstrictor Precautions No information available to require special precautions
Effects on Dental Treatment Key adverse event(s) related to dental treatment: Dysphagia.
Effects on Bleeding No information available to require special precautions
Adverse Effects
>10%:
Cardiovascular: Chest pain (7% to 31%; substernal: 5%), edema (5% to 18%)
Central nervous system: Fever (8% to 31%), pain (1% to 22%), insomnia (5% to 14%)
Dermatologic: Photosensitivity reaction (19% to 22% in cancer patients; 37% to 69% in Barrett's esophagus patients; severe: 10%)
Gastrointestinal: Esophageal stricture/stenosis (6% in esophageal cancer patients; 30% to 36% in Barrett's esophagus patients), nausea (24% to 37%), vomiting (17% to 31%), constipation (5% to 24%), dysphagia (10% to 24%), mucositis (20% in superficial endobronchial cancer), abdominal pain (5% to 20%)
Hematologic: Anemia (32% in esophageal cancer patients)
Neuromuscular & skeletal: Back pain (3% to 11%)
Respiratory: Pleural effusion (32% in esophageal cancer patients; 12% in Barrett's esophagus patients; ≤5% in endobronchial cancer patients), dyspnea (7% to 30%), bronchial obstruction/mucus plug (21%), pneumonia (6% to 18%), hemoptysis (7% to 16%), cough (5% to 15%), bronchostenosis (11%), pharyngitis (11%)
5% to 10%:
Cardiovascular: Atrial fibrillation (10%), hypotension (7%), cardiac failure (7% in esophageal cancer), hypertension (6%), tachycardia (6%)
Central nervous system: Anxiety (3% to 7%), dysphonia (3% to 5%)
Endocrine & metabolic: Dehydration (7% to 10%)
Gastrointestinal: Weight loss (5% to 9%), anorexia (8%), esophageal edema (8%), hematemesis (8%), esophageal pain (7%), dyspepsia (1% to 6%), diarrhea (5%), eructation (5%), esophagitis (5%), melena (5%), odynophagia (5%)
Genitourinary: Urinary tract infection (7%)
Respiratory: Respiratory insufficiency (≤10%), bronchitis (10%), bronchial ulceration (9%), tracheoesophageal fistula (6%), fatal massive hemoptysis (≤5%)

Miscellaneous: Moniliasis (9%), tumor hemorrhage (8%), hiccups (5%), surgical complication (5% in esophageal cancer patients)

General Dosage Range **I.V.:** *Adults:* 2 mg/kg, followed by exposure to the appropriate laser light

Mechanism of Action Porfimer's cytotoxic activity is dependent on light and oxygen. Following administration, the drug is selectively retained in neoplastic tissues. Exposure of the drug to laser light at wavelengths >630 nm results in the production of oxygen free-radicals. Release of thromboxane A_2, leading to vascular occlusion and ischemic necrosis, may also occur.

Pharmacodynamics/Kinetics

Half-life Elimination Mean: 17 days (range: 13-21 days)

Time to Peak Serum: Adults: Females: ~90 minutes; Males: ~10 minutes

Pregnancy Risk Factor C

Posaconazole (poe sa KON a zole)

Related Information

Fungal Infections *on page 1945*

Related Sample Prescriptions

Systemic Fungal Infections *on page 1988*

U.S. Brand Names Noxafil®

Canadian Brand Names Posanol™

Generic Availability (U.S.) No

Pharmacologic Category Antifungal Agent, Oral

Dental Use Treatment of oropharyngeal candidiasis (including patients refractory to itraconazole and/or fluconazole)

Use Prophylaxis of invasive *Aspergillus* and *Candida* infections in severely-immunocompromised patients [eg, hematopoietic stem cell transplant (HSCT) recipients with graft-versus-host disease (GVHD) or those with prolonged neutropenia secondary to chemotherapy for hematologic malignancies]; treatment of oropharyngeal candidiasis (including patients refractory to itraconazole and/or fluconazole)

Unlabeled/Investigational Use Salvage therapy of refractory or relapsed invasive fungal infections; mucormycosis; pulmonary infection (nonimmunosuppressed)

Local Anesthetic/Vasoconstrictor Precautions No information available to require special precautions

Effects on Dental Treatment Key adverse event(s) related to dental treatment: Xerostomia (normal salivary flow resumes upon discontinuation), abnormal taste, mucositis.

Effects on Bleeding No information available to require special precautions

Adverse Effects Note: Percentages reflect data from use in comparator trials with multiple concomitant conditions and medications; some adverse reactions may be due to underlying condition(s).

>10%:

Cardiovascular: Hypertension (18%), edema (9% to 15%), hypotension (14%), tachycardia (12%)

Central nervous system: Fever (6% to 45%), headache (8% to 28%), fatigue (3% to 17%), insomnia (1% to 17%), dizziness (11%), pain (1% to 11%)

Endocrine & metabolic: Hypokalemia (≤30%), hypomagnesemia (18%), dehydration (1% to 11%), hyperglycemia (11%)

Gastrointestinal: Diarrhea (10% to 42%), nausea (9% to 38%), vomiting (7% to 29%), abdominal pain (5% to 27%), constipation (21%), anorexia (2% to 19%), mucositis (17%), weight loss (1% to 14%), oral candidiasis (1% to 12%)

Hematologic: Thrombocytopenia (29%), anemia (2% to 25%), neutropenia (4% to 23%), neutropenic fever (20%)

Hepatic: ALT increased (6% to 17%)

Neuromuscular & skeletal: Rigors (≤20%), musculoskeletal pain (16%), weakness (2% to 13%), arthralgia (11%)

Respiratory: Cough (3% to 25%), dyspnea (1% to 20%), epistaxis (14%), pharyngitis (12%)

Miscellaneous: Bacteremia (18%), herpes simplex (3% to 15%), CMV infection (14%)

1% to 10%:

Central nervous system: Anxiety (9%)

Endocrine & metabolic: Hypocalcemia (9%)

Gastrointestinal: Dyspepsia (10%)

Genitourinary: Vaginal hemorrhage (10%)

Hepatic: Hyperbilirubinemia (7% to 10%), AST increased (3% to 4%), alkaline phosphatase increased (1% to 3%)

Neuromuscular & skeletal: Back pain (10%)

Respiratory: Pneumonia (3% to 10%), upper respiratory infection (7%)
Miscellaneous: Diaphoresis (2% to 10%)

Dental Usual Dosage Children ≥13 years and Adults: Oral:
Oropharyngeal candidiasis: Initial: 100 mg twice daily for 1 day; maintenance dose: 100 mg once daily for 13 days
Refractory oropharyngeal candidiasis: 400 mg twice daily

Dosage Oral:
Children ≥13 years and Adults:
Aspergillosis, invasive:
Prophylaxis: 200 mg 3 times/day; duration of therapy is based is based on recovery from neutropenia or immunosuppression
Salvage treatment of refractory infection (unlabeled use): 200 mg 4 times/day initially; after disease stabilization may decrease frequency to 400 mg 2 times/day (Walsh, 2007). **Note:** Duration of therapy should be a minimum of 6-12 weeks or throughout period of immunosuppression (Walsh, 2008).
Candidal infections:
Prophylaxis: 200 mg 3 times/day; duration of therapy is based on recovery from neutropenia or immunosuppression
Treatment of oropharyngeal infection: Initial: 100 mg 2 times/day for 1 day; maintenance: 100 mg once daily for 13 days
Treatment of refractory oropharyngeal infection: 400 mg 2 times/day; duration of therapy is based on underlying disease and clinical response
Adults:
Mucormycosis (unlabeled use): 800 mg/day in 2 or 4 divided doses; duration of therapy is based on response and risk of relapse due to immunosuppression (Greenburg, 2006)
Cryptococcal infections:
Pulmonary, nonimmunosuppressed (unlabeled use): 400 mg 2 times/day. **Note:** Fluconazole is considered first-line treatment (Perfect, 2010).
Salvage treatment of relapsed infection (unlabeled use): 400 mg 2 times/day (or 200 mg 4 times/day) for 10-12 weeks. **Note:** Salvage treatment should only be started after an appropriate course of an induction regimen (Perfect, 2010).

Dosage adjustment in renal impairment:
Mild-to-moderate renal insufficiency (Cl_{cr} 20-80 mL/minute/1.73 m^2): No adjustment necessary
Severe renal insufficiency (Cl_{cr} <20 mL/minute/1.73 m^2): No adjustment necessary; however, monitor for breakthrough fungal infections due to variability in posaconazole exposure.
Dosage adjustment in hepatic impairment:
Mild-to-severe hepatic insufficiency (Child-Pugh classes A, B, and C): No adjustment necessary
Clinical signs and symptoms of liver disease due to posaconazole: Consider discontinuing therapy

Mechanism of Action Interferes with fungal cytochrome P450 (latosterol-14α-demethylase) activity, decreasing ergosterol synthesis (principal sterol in fungal cell membrane) and inhibiting fungal cell membrane formation.

Contraindications Hypersensitivity to posaconazole, other azole antifungals, or any component of the formulation; coadministration of cisapride, ergot alkaloids, pimozide, quinidine, simvastatin, or sirolimus

Warnings/Precautions Hepatic dysfunction has occurred, ranging from reversible mild/moderate increases of ALT, AST, alkaline phosphatase, total bilirubin, and/or clinical hepatitis to severe reactions (cholestasis, hepatic failure including death). Consider discontinuation of therapy in patients who develop clinical evidence of liver disease that may be secondary to posaconazole. Use caution in patients with an increased risk of arrhythmia (long QT syndrome, concurrent QT_c-prolonging drugs, hypokalemia). Correct electrolyte abnormalities (eg, potassium, magnesium, and calcium) before initiating therapy. Concurrent use with cyclosporine or tacrolimus may significantly increase cyclosporine/tacrolimus concentrations and may result in rare serious adverse events (eg, nephrotoxicity, leukoencephalopathy, and death); dose reduction and close monitoring are recommended with initiation of posaconazole therapy. Concurrent use with midazolam may increase midazolam concentrations and potentiate midazolam-related adverse effects.

Use caution in hypersensitivity with other azole antifungal agents; cross-reaction may occur, but has not been established. Consider alternative therapy or closely monitor for breakthrough fungal infections in patients receiving drugs that decrease absorption or increase the metabolism of posaconazole or in any patient unable to eat or tolerate an oral liquid nutritional supplement. Use caution in severe renal impairment or GI disturbances; monitor for breakthrough fungal infections.

Drug Interactions

Metabolism/Transport Effects Inhibits CYP3A4 (strong)

Avoid Concomitant Use

Avoid concomitant use of Posaconazole with any of the following: Alfuzosin; Cisapride; Conivaptan; Dofetilide; Dronedarone; Efavirenz; Eplerenone; Ergot Derivatives; Everolimus; Fluticasone (Oral Inhalation); Halofantrine; Lurasidone; Nilotinib; Nisoldipine; Pimozide; Proton Pump Inhibitors; QuiNIDine; Ranolazine; Rivaroxaban; RomiDEPsin; Salmeterol; Silodosin; Sirolimus; Tamsulosin; Tolvaptan; Toremifene

Increased Effect/Toxicity

Posaconazole may increase the levels/effects of: Alfentanil; Alfuzosin; Almotriptan; Alosetron; Antineoplastic Agents (Vinca Alkaloids); Aprepitant; Benzodiazepines (metabolized by oxidation); Bortezomib; Bosentan; Brinzolamide; Budesonide (Nasal); Budesonide (Systemic, Oral Inhalation); BusPIRone; Busulfan; Calcium Channel Blockers; CarBAMazepine; Cardiac Glycosides; Ciclesonide; Cilostazol; Cinacalcet; Cisapride; Colchicine; Conivaptan; Corticosteroids (Orally Inhaled); Corticosteroids (Systemic); CycloSPORINE; CycloSPORINE (Systemic); CYP3A4 Substrates; Dienogest; DOCEtaxel; Dofetilide; Dronedarone; Dutasteride; Eletriptan; Eplerenone; Ergot Derivatives; Erlotinib; Eszopiclone; Etravirine; Everolimus; FentaNYL; Fesoterodine; Fluticasone (Nasal); Fluticasone (Oral Inhalation); Fosamprenavir; Fosaprepitant; Fosphenytoin; Gefitinib; GlipiZIDE; GuanFACINE; Halofantrine; HMG-CoA Reductase Inhibitors; Imatinib; Irinotecan; Ixabepilone; Losartan; Lumefantrine; Lurasidone; Macrolide Antibiotics; Maraviroc; Methadone; MethylPREDNISolone; Nilotinib; Nisoldipine; Paricalcitol; Pazopanib; Phenytoin; Phosphodiesterase 5 Inhibitors; Pimecrolimus; Pimozide; Protease Inhibitors; QuiNIDine; Ramelteon; Ranolazine; Repaglinide; Rifamycin Derivatives; Rivaroxaban; RomiDEPsin; Salmeterol; Saxagliptin; Silodosin; Sirolimus; Solifenacin; SORAfenib; SUNItinib; Tacrolimus; Tacrolimus (Systemic); Tacrolimus (Topical); Tadalafil; Tamsulosin; Temsirolimus; Tolterodine; Tolvaptan; Toremifene; Vilazodone; Vitamin K Antagonists; Ziprasidone; Zolpidem

The levels/effects of Posaconazole may be increased by: Etravirine; Grapefruit Juice; Macrolide Antibiotics; Protease Inhibitors; Tacrolimus

Decreased Effect

Posaconazole may decrease the levels/effects of: Amphotericin B; Prasugrel; Saccharomyces boulardii

The levels/effects of Posaconazole may be decreased by: Didanosine; Efavirenz; Etravirine; Fosamprenavir; Fosphenytoin; H2-Antagonists; Metoclopramide; Phenytoin; Proton Pump Inhibitors; Rifamycin Derivatives; Sucralfate

Ethanol/Nutrition/Herb Interactions Food: Bioavailability increased ~3 times when posaconazole is administered with a nonfat meal or an oral liquid nutritional supplement; increased ~4 times when administered with a high-fat meal. Grapefruit juice may decrease the levels/effects of posaconazole; concurrent use should be avoided.

Dietary Considerations Give during or within 20 minutes following a full meal or liquid nutritional supplement; alternatively, posaconazole may be administered with an acidic carbonated beverage (eg, ginger ale). Consider alternative antifungal therapy in patients with inadequate oral intake or severe diarrhea/vomiting; if alternative therapy is not an option, closely monitoring for breakthrough fungal infections. Adequate posaconazole absorption from GI tract and subsequent plasma concentrations are dependent on food for efficacy. Lower average plasma concentrations have been associated with an increased risk of treatment failure.

Pharmacodynamics/Kinetics

Half-life Elimination 35 hours (range: 20-66 hours)

Time to Peak ~3-5 hours

Pregnancy Risk Factor C

Lactation Excretion in breast milk unknown/not recommended

Breast-Feeding Considerations Excretion in breast milk has not been investigated; use only if the benefit to the mother justifies potential risk to the fetus.

Dosage Forms

Suspension, oral:

Noxafil®: 40 mg/mL (123 mL)

Dental Comment This drug is known to prolong the QT interval. The QT interval is measured as the time and distance between the Q point of the QRS complex and the end of the T wave in the ECG tracing. After adjustment for heart rate, the QT interval is defined as prolonged if it is more than 450 msec in men and 460 msec in women. A long QT syndrome was first described in the 1950s and 60s as a congenital syndrome involving QT interval prolongation and syncope and sudden death. Some of the congenital long QT syndromes were characterized by a peculiar electrocardiographic appearance of the QRS complex involving a premature atria beat followed by a pause, then a subsequent sinus beat showing marked QT prolongation and deformity. This type of cardiac arrhythmia was originally termed "torsade de pointes" (translated from the French as "twisting of the points").

Prolongation of the QT interval is thought to result from delayed ventricular repolarization. The repolarization process within the myocardial cell is due to the efflux of intracellular potassium. The channels associated with this current can be blocked by many drugs and predispose the electrical propagation cycle to torsade de pointes.

Posaconazole is one of the drugs confirmed to prolong the QT interval and is accepted as having a risk of causing torsade de pointes. The risk of drug-induced torsade de pointes is extremely low when a single QT interval prolonging drug is prescribed. In terms of epinephrine, it is not known what effect vasoconstrictors in the local anesthetic regimen will have in patients with a known history of congenital prolonged QT interval or in patients taking any medication that prolongs the QT interval. Until more information is obtained, it is suggested that the clinician consult with the physician prior to the use of a vasoconstrictor in suspected patients, and that the vasoconstrictor (epinephrine, levonordefrin [Neo-Cobefrin®]) be used with caution.

Potassium Acetate (poe TASS ee um AS e tate)

Pharmacologic Category Electrolyte Supplement, Parenteral

Use Potassium deficiency; to avoid chloride when high concentration of potassium is needed, source of bicarbonate

Local Anesthetic/Vasoconstrictor Precautions No information available to require special precautions

Effects on Dental Treatment No significant effects or complications reported

Effects on Bleeding No information available to require special precautions

Adverse Effects

1% to 10%:

Cardiovascular: Bradycardia
Endocrine & metabolic: Hyperkalemia
Neuromuscular & skeletal: Weakness
Respiratory: Dyspnea
Local: Local tissue necrosis with extravasation

General Dosage Range I.V.:

Children: 2-5 mEq/kg/day; Intermittent infusion: 0.5-1 mEq/kg/dose (maximum: 30 mEq/dose) to infuse at 0.3-0.5 mEq/kg/hour (maximum: 1 mEq/kg/hour)

Adults: 40-100 mEq/day; Intermittent infusion: 5-10 mEq/dose (maximum: 40 mEq/dose) to infuse over 2-3 hours (maximum: 40 mEq over 1 hour)

Mechanism of Action Potassium is the major cation of intracellular fluid and is essential for the conduction of nerve impulses in heart, brain, and skeletal muscle; contraction of cardiac, skeletal and smooth muscles; maintenance of normal renal function, acid-base balance, carbohydrate metabolism, and gastric secretion

Pregnancy Risk Factor C

Potassium Acid Phosphate (poe TASS ee um AS id FOS fate)

U.S. Brand Names K-Phos® Original

Pharmacologic Category Urinary Acidifying Agent

Use Acidifies urine and lowers urinary calcium concentration; reduces odor and rash caused by ammoniacal urine; increases the antibacterial activity of methenamine

Local Anesthetic/Vasoconstrictor Precautions No information available to require special precautions

Effects on Dental Treatment No significant effects or complications reported

Effects on Bleeding No information available to require special precautions

Adverse Effects

>10%: Gastrointestinal: Diarrhea, nausea, stomach pain, flatulence, vomiting

1% to 10%:

Cardiovascular: Bradycardia
Endocrine & metabolic: Hyperkalemia
Local: Local tissue necrosis with extravasation
Neuromuscular & skeletal: Weakness
Respiratory: Dyspnea

General Dosage Range Oral: *Adults:* 1000 mg dissolved in 6-8 oz of water 4 times/day

Mechanism of Action The principal intracellular cation; involved in transmission of nerve impulses, muscle contractions, enzyme activity, and glucose utilization

Pregnancy Risk Factor C

Potassium Bicarbonate (poe TASS ee um bye KAR bun ate)

Pharmacologic Category Electrolyte Supplement, Oral

Use Potassium deficiency, hypokalemia

Local Anesthetic/Vasoconstrictor Precautions No information available to require special precautions

Effects on Dental Treatment No significant effects or complications reported

Effects on Bleeding No information available to require special precautions

General Dosage Range Oral:

Children: 1-4 mEq/kg/day

Adults: 25 mEq 2-4 times/day

Pregnancy Risk Factor C

Potassium Bicarbonate and Potassium Chloride

(poe TASS ee um bye KAR bun ate & poe TASS ee um KLOR ide)

Related Information

Potassium Bicarbonate *on page* 1377

Potassium Chloride *on page* 1378

Pharmacologic Category Electrolyte Supplement, Oral

Use Treatment or prevention of hypokalemia

Local Anesthetic/Vasoconstrictor Precautions No information available to require special precautions

Effects on Dental Treatment No significant effects or complications reported

Effects on Bleeding No information available to require special precautions

Adverse Effects Frequency not defined: Gastrointestinal: Abdominal discomfort, diarrhea, nausea, vomiting

General Dosage Range

Oral:

Children: 1-4 mEq/kg/day in divided doses

Adults: Prevention: 16-24 mEq/day in 2-4 divided doses; Treatment: 40-100 mEq/day in 2-4 divided doses

Pregnancy Risk Factor C

Potassium Bicarbonate and Potassium Citrate

(poe TASS ee um bye KAR bun ate & poe TASS ee um SIT rate)

Related Information

Potassium Bicarbonate *on page* 1377

Potassium Citrate *on page* 1378

U.S. Brand Names Effer-K®; Klor-Con®/EF

Pharmacologic Category Electrolyte Supplement, Oral

Use Treatment or prevention of hypokalemia

Local Anesthetic/Vasoconstrictor Precautions No information available to require special precautions

Effects on Dental Treatment No significant effects or complications reported

Effects on Bleeding No information available to require special precautions

Adverse Effects

>10%: Gastrointestinal: Diarrhea, nausea, stomach pain, flatulence, vomiting

1% to 10%:

Cardiovascular: Bradycardia

Endocrine & metabolic: Hyperkalemia

Local: Local tissue necrosis with extravasation

Neuromuscular & skeletal: Weakness

Respiratory: Dyspnea

General Dosage Range

Oral:

Children: 1-4 mEq/kg/day in divided doses

Adults: Prevention: 16-24 mEq/day in 2-4 divided doses; Treatment: 40-100 mEq/day in 2-4 divided doses

Mechanism of Action Needed for the conduction of nerve impulses in heart, brain, and skeletal muscle; contraction of cardiac, skeletal and smooth muscles; maintenance of normal renal function

Pregnancy Risk Factor C

Potassium Chloride (poe TASS ee um KLOR ide)

U.S. Brand Names Epiklor™; Epiklor™/25; K-Tab®; Kaon-CL® 10; Klor-Con®; Klor-Con® 10; Klor-Con® 8; Klor-Con® M10; Klor-Con® M15; Klor-Con® M20; Klor-Con®/25; microK®; microK® 10

Canadian Brand Names Apo-K®; K-10®; K-Dur®; Micro-K Extencaps®; Roychlor®; Slo-Pot; Slow-K®

Pharmacologic Category Electrolyte Supplement, Oral; Electrolyte Supplement, Parenteral

Use Treatment or prevention of hypokalemia

Local Anesthetic/Vasoconstrictor Precautions No information available to require special precautions

Effects on Dental Treatment No significant effects or complications reported

Effects on Bleeding No information available to require special precautions

Adverse Effects Frequency not defined.

Dermatologic: Rash

Endocrine & metabolic: Hyperkalemia

Gastrointestinal: Abdominal pain/discomfort, diarrhea, flatulence, GI bleeding (oral), GI obstruction (oral), GI perforation (oral), nausea, vomiting

General Dosage Range

I.V.:

Children: Initial: 0.5-1 mEq/kg/dose (maximum dose: 40 mEq); repeat as needed based on lab values

Adults: Intermittent infusion: ≤10 mEq/hour; repeat as needed based on lab values (maximum: 200 mEq/day)

Oral:

Children: 1-2 mEq/kg/day in 1-2 divided doses or as needed based on lab values

Adults: Initial: 6-10 mEq/dose (maximum: 40 mEq/dose); Maintenance: 40-100 mEq/day in divided doses or as needed based on lab values

Mechanism of Action Potassium is the major cation of intracellular fluid and is essential for the conduction of nerve impulses in heart, brain, and skeletal muscle; contraction of cardiac, skeletal and smooth muscles; maintenance of normal renal function, acid-base balance, carbohydrate metabolism, and gastric secretion

Pregnancy Risk Factor C

Potassium Citrate (poe TASS ee um SIT rate)

U.S. Brand Names Urocit®-K

Canadian Brand Names Urocit®-K

Pharmacologic Category Alkalinizing Agent, Oral

Use Prevention of uric acid nephrolithiasis; prevention of calcium renal stones in patients with hypocitraturia; urinary alkalinizer when sodium citrate is contraindicated

Local Anesthetic/Vasoconstrictor Precautions No information available to require special precautions

Effects on Dental Treatment No significant effects or complications reported

Effects on Bleeding No information available to require special precautions

Adverse Effects Frequency not defined.

Endocrine & metabolic: Hyperkalemia

Gastrointestinal: Abdominal discomfort, diarrhea, nausea, vomiting

General Dosage Range Oral: *Adults:* 10-20 mEq 3 times/day with meals (maximum: 100 mEq/day)

Pregnancy Risk Factor C

Potassium Citrate and Citric Acid (poe TASS ee um SIT rate & SI trik AS id)

Related Information

Potassium Citrate *on page 1378*

U.S. Brand Names Cytra-K

Pharmacologic Category Alkalinizing Agent, Oral

Use Treatment of metabolic acidosis; alkalinizing agent in conditions where long-term maintenance of an alkaline urine is desirable

Local Anesthetic/Vasoconstrictor Precautions No information available to require special precautions

Effects on Dental Treatment No significant effects or complications reported

Effects on Bleeding No information available to require special precautions

General Dosage Range Oral:
Children: 5-15 mL after meals and at bedtime
Adults: 15-30 mL **or** 1 packet dissolved in water after meals and at bedtime
Pregnancy Risk Factor A

Potassium Gluconate (poe TASS ee um GLOO coe nate)

Pharmacologic Category Electrolyte Supplement, Oral
Use Treatment or prevention of hypokalemia
Local Anesthetic/Vasoconstrictor Precautions No information available to require special precautions
Effects on Dental Treatment No significant effects or complications reported
Effects on Bleeding No information available to require special precautions
Adverse Effects
>10%: Gastrointestinal: Diarrhea, nausea, stomach pain, flatulence, vomiting (oral)
1% to 10%:
Cardiovascular: Bradycardia
Endocrine & metabolic: Hyperkalemia
Neuromuscular & skeletal: Weakness
Respiratory: Dyspnea
General Dosage Range Oral:
Children: 1-5 mEq/kg/day in 1-4 divided doses
Adults: 16-100 mEq/day in 1-4 divided doses
Mechanism of Action Potassium is the major cation of intracellular fluid and is essential for the conduction of nerve impulses in heart, brain, and skeletal muscle; contraction of cardiac, skeletal and smooth muscles; maintenance of normal renal function, acid-base balance, carbohydrate metabolism, and gastric secretion
Pregnancy Risk Factor A

Potassium Iodide (poe TASS ee um EYE oh dide)

Related Information
Endocrine Disorders and Pregnancy *on page* 1879
U.S. Brand Names iOSAT™ [OTC]; SSKI®; ThyroSafe™; Thyroshield™ [OTC]
Pharmacologic Category Antithyroid Agent; Expectorant
Use Expectorant for the symptomatic treatment of chronic pulmonary diseases complicated by mucous; block thyroidal uptake of radioactive isotopes of iodine in a radiation emergency
Unlabeled/Investigational Use Lymphocutaneous and cutaneous sporotrichosis; reduce thyroid vascularity prior to thyroidectomy; management of thyrotoxic crisis; block thyroidal uptake of radioactive isotopes of iodine after therapeutic or diagnostic exposure to radioactive iodine
Local Anesthetic/Vasoconstrictor Precautions No information available to require special precautions
Effects on Dental Treatment Key adverse event(s) related to dental treatment: Metallic taste.
Effects on Bleeding No information available to require special precautions
Adverse Effects Frequency not defined.
Cardiovascular: Irregular heart beat
Central nervous system: Confusion, tiredness, fever
Dermatologic: Skin rash
Endocrine & metabolic: Goiter, salivary gland swelling/tenderness, thyroid adenoma, swelling of neck/throat, myxedema, lymph node swelling, hyper-/hypothyroidism
Gastrointestinal: Diarrhea, gastrointestinal bleeding, metallic taste, nausea, stomach pain, stomach upset, vomiting
Neuromuscular & skeletal: Joint pain, numbness, tingling, weakness
Miscellaneous: Chronic iodine poisoning (with prolonged treatment/high doses); iodism, hypersensitivity reactions (angioedema, cutaneous and mucosal hemorrhage, serum sickness-like symptoms)
General Dosage Range Oral:
Neonates: Iosat™, ThyroSafe™, ThyroShield™: 16.25 mg once daily
Infants 1-12 months and Children 1-3 years: Iosat™, ThyroSafe™, ThyroShield™: 32.5 mg once daily
Children 3-18 years: Iosat™, ThyroSafe™, ThyroShield™: 65-130 mg once daily
Adults: Iosat™, ThyroSafe™, ThyroShield™: 130 mg once daily; SSKI®: 300-600 mg (6-12 drops) 3-4 times/day

Mechanism of Action Reduces viscosity of mucus by increasing respiratory tract secretions; inhibits secretion of thyroid hormone, fosters colloid accumulation in thyroid follicles. Following radioactive iodine exposure, potassium iodide blocks uptake of radioiodine by the thyroid, reducing the risk of thyroid cancer.

Pharmacodynamics/Kinetics

Onset of Action Hyperthyroidism: 24-48 hours; Peak effect: 10-15 days after continuous therapy

Duration of Action Radioactive iodine exposure: ~24 hours

Pregnancy Risk Factor D

Potassium Iodide and Iodine (poe TASS ee um EYE oh dide & EYE oh dine)

Related Information

Iodine *on page 933*

Potassium Iodide *on page 1379*

Pharmacologic Category Antithyroid Agent

Use Reduce thyroid vascularity prior to thyroidectomy and management of thyrotoxic crisis; block thyroidal uptake of radioactive isotopes of iodine in a radiation emergency or after therapeutic/diagnostic use of radioactive iodine; topical antiseptic

Local Anesthetic/Vasoconstrictor Precautions No information available to require special precautions

Effects on Dental Treatment Key adverse event(s) related to dental treatment: Metallic taste.

Effects on Bleeding No information available to require special precautions

Adverse Effects Frequency not defined.

Cardiovascular: Irregular heart beat

Central nervous system: Confusion, tiredness, fever

Dermatologic: Skin rash

Endocrine & metabolic: Goiter, salivary gland swelling/tenderness, thyroid adenoma, swelling of neck/throat, myxedema, lymph node swelling, hyper-/hypothyroidism

Gastrointestinal: Diarrhea, gastrointestinal bleeding, metallic taste, nausea, stomach pain, stomach upset, vomiting

Neuromuscular & skeletal: Numbness, tingling, weakness, joint pain

Miscellaneous: Chronic iodine poisoning (with prolonged treatment/high doses); iodism, hypersensitivity reactions (angioedema, cutaneous and mucosal hemorrhage, serum sickness-like symptoms)

General Dosage Range Oral:

Children: 3-8 drops 3 times/day

Adults: Dosing varies greatly depending on indication

Mechanism of Action In hyperthyroidism, iodine temporarily inhibits thyroid hormone synthesis and secretion into the circulation; use also decreases thyroid gland size and vascularity. Serum T_4 and T_3 concentrations can be reduced for several weeks with use but effect will not be maintained.

Following radioactive iodine exposure, potassium iodide blocks uptake of radioiodine by the thyroid, reducing the risk of thyroid cancer.

Pharmacodynamics/Kinetics

Onset of Action Hyperthyroidism: 24-48 hours; Peak effect: 10-15 days after continuous therapy

Pregnancy Risk Factor D (potassium iodide)

Potassium P-Aminobenzoate (poe TASS ee um pe a mee noe BEN zoe ate)

U.S. Brand Names Potaba®

Pharmacologic Category Vitamin, Water Soluble

Use Presently, all indications are classified by the FDA as "possibly effective."

Treatment of scleroderma, dermatomyositis, morphea, linear scleroderma, pemphigus, Peyronie's disease

Local Anesthetic/Vasoconstrictor Precautions No information available to require special precautions

Effects on Dental Treatment No significant effects or complications reported

Effects on Bleeding No information available to require special precautions

Adverse Effects Frequency not defined.

Central nervous system: Fever

Dermatologic: Rash

Gastrointestinal: Anorexia, nausea

Miscellaneous: Hypersensitivity reaction

General Dosage Range Oral:

Children: 1 g/10 pounds of weight/day in divided doses

Adults: 12 g/day in 4-6 divided doses

Mechanism of Action P-aminobenzoate is a member of the vitamin B complex family. It may have an antifibrotic effect due to increased oxygen uptake at the tissue level.

Potassium Phosphate (poe TASS ee um FOS fate)

U.S. Brand Names Neutra-Phos®-K [OTC] [DSC]

Pharmacologic Category Electrolyte Supplement, Parenteral

Use Treatment and prevention of hypophosphatemia; **Note:** The concomitant amount of potassium must be calculated into the total electrolyte content. For each 1 mmol of phosphate, ~1.5 mEq of potassium will be administered. Therefore, if ordering 30 mmol of potassium phosphate, the patient will receive ~45 mEq of potassium.

Local Anesthetic/Vasoconstrictor Precautions No information available to require special precautions

Effects on Dental Treatment No significant effects or complications reported

Effects on Bleeding No information available to require special precautions

Adverse Effects Frequency not defined.

Cardiovascular: Arrhythmia, bradycardia, chest pain, ECG changes, edema, heart block, hypotension

Central nervous system: Listlessness, mental confusion, tetany (with large doses of phosphate)

Endocrine & metabolic: Hyperkalemia

Gastrointestinal: Diarrhea, nausea, stomach pain, vomiting

Genitourinary: Urine output decreased

Local: Phlebitis

Neuromuscular & skeletal: Paralysis, paresthesia, weakness

Renal: Acute renal failure

Respiratory: Dyspnea

General Dosage Range

I.V.:

Children: 0.08-1 mmol phosphate/kg **or** Parenteral nutrition infusion: 0.5-2 mmol/kg/24 hours

Adults: 0.08-1 mmol phosphate/kg **or** Parenteral nutrition: Infusion: 20-40 mmol/24 hours

Pregnancy Risk Factor C

Potassium Phosphate and Sodium Phosphate

(poe TASS ee um FOS fate & SOW dee um FOS fate)

Related Information

Potassium Phosphate *on page 1381*

Sodium Phosphates *on page 1542*

U.S. Brand Names K-Phos® MF; K-Phos® Neutral; K-Phos® No. 2; Phos-NaK; Phospha 250™ Neutral; Uro-KP-Neutral®

Pharmacologic Category Electrolyte Supplement, Oral

Use Treatment of conditions associated with excessive renal phosphate loss or inadequate GI absorption of phosphate; to acidify the urine to lower calcium concentrations; to increase the antibacterial activity of methenamine; reduce odor and rash caused by ammonia in urine

Local Anesthetic/Vasoconstrictor Precautions No information available to require special precautions

Effects on Dental Treatment No significant effects or complications reported

Effects on Bleeding No information available to require special precautions

Adverse Effects Frequency not defined.

Cardiovascular: Bradycardia, arrhythmia, chest pain, edema, tachycardia

Central nervous system: Mental confusion, tetany (with large doses of phosphate), headache, dizziness, seizure

Endocrine & metabolic: Hyperkalemia, alkalosis

Gastrointestinal: Diarrhea, nausea, stomach pain, flatulence, vomiting, throat pain, weight gain

Genitourinary: Urine output decreased

Local: Phlebitis

Neuromuscular & skeletal: Weakness, arthralgia, bone pain, paralysis, paresthesia, pain/weakness of extremities, muscle cramps

Renal: Acute renal failure

Respiratory: Dyspnea

Miscellaneous: Thirst

General Dosage Range Oral: *Children ≥4 years and Adults:* Elemental phosphorus 250 mg 4 times/day after meals and at bedtime

Pregnancy Risk Factor C

Povidone-Iodine (Topical) (POE vi done EYE oh dyne)

Related Information

Management of Patients Undergoing Cancer Therapy *on page 1970*
Periodontal Diseases *on page 1942*

U.S. Brand Names Betadine® Swab Aids [OTC]; Betadine® [OTC]; Operand® Povidone-Iodine [OTC]; Povidine™ [OTC]; Summer's Eve® Medicated Douche [OTC]; Vagi-Gard® [OTC]

Canadian Brand Names Betadine®; Proviodine

Pharmacologic Category Antiseptic, Topical; Antiseptic, Vaginal; Topical Skin Product

Use External antiseptic with broad microbicidal spectrum for the prevention or treatment of topical infections associated with surgery, burns, minor cuts/scrapes; relief of minor vaginal irritation

Local Anesthetic/Vasoconstrictor Precautions No information available to require special precautions

Effects on Dental Treatment No significant effects or complications reported

Effects on Bleeding No information available to require special precautions

Adverse Effects Frequency not defined. Also refer to Iodine on page 933.

Local: Edema, irritation, pruritus, rash

General Dosage Range

Intravaginal: *Adults:* Insert 0.3% solution vaginally once daily

Topical: *Adults:* Apply to affected area as needed **or** apply to wet skin or hands, scrub for ~5 minutes, then rinse

Mechanism of Action Povidone-iodine is known to be a powerful broad spectrum germicidal agent effective against a wide range of bacteria, viruses, fungi, protozoa, and spores.

PRALAtrexate (pral a TREX ate)

U.S. Brand Names Folotyn®

Pharmacologic Category Antineoplastic Agent, Antimetabolite (Antifolate)

Use Treatment of relapsed or refractory peripheral T-cell lymphoma (PTCL)

Unlabeled/Investigational Use Treatment of relapsed or refractory cutaneous T-cell lymphoma (CTCL)

Local Anesthetic/Vasoconstrictor Precautions No information available to require special precautions

Effects on Dental Treatment Key adverse event(s) related to dental treatment: Mucositis and stomatitis

Effects on Bleeding No information available to require special precautions

Adverse Effects

>10%:

- Cardiovascular: Edema (30%)
- Central nervous system: Fatigue (36%), fever (32%)
- Dermatologic: Rash (15%; grades 3/4: 0%), pruritus (14%; grade 3: 2%; grade 4: 0%)
- Endocrine & metabolic: Hypokalemia (15%)
- Gastrointestinal: Mucositis (70%; grade 3: 17%; grade 4: 4%), nausea (40%), constipation (33%), vomiting (25%), diarrhea (21%), anorexia (15%), abdominal pain (12%)
- Hematologic: Thrombocytopenia (41%; grade 3: 14%; grade 4: 19%), anemia (34%; grade 4: 2%), neutropenia (24%; grade 3: 13%; grade 4: 7%), leukopenia (11%; grade 3: 3%; grade 4: 4%)
- Hepatic: Transaminases increased (13%; grade 3: 5%; grade 4: 0%)
- Neuromuscular & skeletal: Limb pain (12%), back pain (11%)
- Respiratory: Cough (28%), epistaxis (26%), dyspnea (19%), pharyngolaryngeal pain (14%)
- Miscellaneous: Night sweats (11%), infection

1% to 10%:

- Cardiovascular: Tachycardia (10%)
- Endocrine & metabolic: Dehydration (serious >3%)
- Hematologic: Neutropenic fever (serious >3%)
- Neuromuscular & skeletal: Weakness (10%)
- Respiratory: Upper respiratory infection (10%)
- Miscellaneous: Sepsis (serious >3%)

General Dosage Range Dosage adjustment recommended in patients who develop toxicities

I.V.: *Adults:* 30 mg/m^2 once weekly for 6 weeks of a 7-week treatment cycle

Mechanism of Action Antifolate analog; inhibits DNA, RNA, and protein synthesis by selectively entering cells expressing reduced folate carrier (RFC-1), is polyglutamylated by folylpolyglutamate synthetase (FPGS) and then competes for the DHFR-folate binding site to inhibit dihydrofolate reductase (DHFR)

Pharmacodynamics/Kinetics

Half-life Elimination 12-18 hours

Pregnancy Risk Factor D

Pramipexole (pra mi PEKS ole)

U.S. Brand Names Mirapex®; Mirapex® ER™

Canadian Brand Names Apo-Pramipexole®; CO Pramipexole; Mirapex®; Novo-Pramipexole; PHL-Pramipexole; PMS-Pramipexole; Sandoz-Pramipexole

Pharmacologic Category Anti-Parkinson's Agent, Dopamine Agonist

Use

Immediate release: Treatment of the signs and symptoms of idiopathic Parkinson's disease; treatment of moderate-to-severe primary Restless Legs Syndrome (RLS)

Extended release: Treatment of the signs and symptoms of idiopathic Parkinson's disease

Unlabeled/Investigational Use Treatment of depression; treatment of fibromyalgia

Local Anesthetic/Vasoconstrictor Precautions No information available to require special precautions

Effects on Dental Treatment Key adverse event(s) related to dental treatment: Xerostomia (normal salivary flow resumes upon discontinuation) and dysphagia.

Effects on Bleeding No information available to require special precautions

Adverse Effects

Parkinson's disease: Actual frequency may be dependent on dose and/or formulation:

>10%:

Cardiovascular: Postural hypotension (dose related; ≤53%)

Central nervous system: Somnolence (dose related; 9% to 36%), extrapyramidal syndrome (28%), insomnia (4% to 27%), dizziness (2% to 26%), hallucinations (5% to 17%), abnormal dreams (11%), headache (4% to 7%)

Gastrointestinal: Nausea (dose related; 11% to 28%), constipation (dose related; 6% to 14%)

Neuromuscular & skeletal: Dyskinesia (17% to 47%), weakness (1% to 14%)

1% to 10%:

Cardiovascular: Edema (2% to 8%), chest pain (3%)

Central nervous system: Confusion (4% to 10%), dystonia (2% to 8%), fatigue (6%), amnesia (dose related; 4% to 6%), sudden onset of sleep (3% to 6%), vertigo (2% to 4%), hypesthesia (3%), abnormal thinking (2% to 3%), akathisia (2% to 3%), malaise (2% to 3%), paranoia (2%), sleep disorder (1% to 3%), depression (≤2%), delusions (1%), fever (1%), myoclonus (1%)

Endocrine & metabolic: Libido decreased (1%)

Gastrointestinal: Xerostomia (4% to 7%), anorexia (1% to 5%), vomiting (4%), abdominal discomfort/pain (1% to 4%), dyspepsia (3%), appetite increased (2% to 3%), dysphagia (2%), weight loss (2%), salivary hypersecretion (≤2%), diarrhea (1% to 2%)

Genitourinary: Urinary frequency (6%), urinary tract infection (4%), impotence (2%), urinary incontinence (2%)

Neuromuscular & skeletal: Gait abnormalities (7%), hypertonia (7%), muscle spasm (3% to 5%), falls (4%), arthritis (3%), tremor (3%), back pain (2% to 3%), bursitis (2%), muscle twitching (2%), balance abnormalities (≤2%), CPK increased (1%), myasthenia (1%)

Ocular: Accommodation abnormalities (4%), vision abnormalities (3%), diplopia (1%)

Respiratory: Dyspnea (4%), cough (3%), rhinitis (3%), pneumonia (2%)

Restless legs syndrome: Actual frequency may be dependent on dose:

>10%:

Central nervous system: Headache (16%), insomnia (9% to 13%), abnormal dreams (1% to 8%), somnolence (6%)

Gastrointestinal: Nausea (11% to 27%), constipation (4%)

1% to 10%:

Central nervous system: Fatigue (3% to 9%)

Gastrointestinal: Diarrhea (1% to 7%), xerostomia (3%)

Neuromuscular & skeletal: Extremity pain (3% to 7%)

Respiratory: Nasal congestion (≤6%)
Miscellaneous: Influenza (1% to 7%)

General Dosage Range Dosage adjustment recommended in patients with renal impairment

Oral: Immediate release: *Adults:* Initial: 0.375 mg/day given in 3 divided doses **or** 0.125 mg once daily before bedtime; Maintenance: 1.5-4.5 mg/day in 3 divided doses **or** 0.125-0.5 mg/day

Oral: Extended release: *Adults:* Initial: 0.375-4.5 mg once daily

Mechanism of Action Pramipexole is a nonergot dopamine agonist with specificity for the D_2 subfamily dopamine receptor, and has also been shown to bind to D_3 and D_4 receptors. By binding to these receptors, it is thought that pramipexole can stimulate dopamine activity on the nerves of the striatum and substantia nigra.

Pharmacodynamics/Kinetics

Half-life Elimination 8.5 hours; Elderly: 12 hours

Time to Peak Serum: Immediate release: ~2 hours; Extended release: 6 hours

Pregnancy Risk Factor C

Pramlintide (PRAM lin tide)

U.S. Brand Names SymlinPen®; Symlin®

Pharmacologic Category Amylinomimetic; Antidiabetic Agent

Use

Adjunctive treatment with mealtime insulin in type 1 diabetes mellitus (insulin dependent, IDDM) patients who have failed to achieve desired glucose control despite optimal insulin therapy

Adjunctive treatment with mealtime insulin in type 2 diabetes mellitus (noninsulin dependent, NIDDM) patients who have failed to achieve desired glucose control despite optimal insulin therapy, with or without concurrent sulfonylurea and/or metformin

Local Anesthetic/Vasoconstrictor Precautions No information available to require special precautions

Effects on Dental Treatment No significant effects or complications reported

Effects on Bleeding No information available to require special precautions

Adverse Effects

>10%:

Central nervous system: Headache (5% to 13%)
Gastrointestinal: Nausea (28% to 48%), vomiting (7% to 11%), anorexia (≤17%)
Endocrine & metabolic: Severe hypoglycemia (type 1 diabetes ≤17%)
Miscellaneous: Inflicted injury (8% to 14%)

1% to 10%:

Central nervous system: Fatigue (3% to 7%), dizziness (2% to 6%)
Endocrine & metabolic: Severe hypoglycemia (type 2 diabetes ≤8%)
Gastrointestinal: Abdominal pain (2% to 8%)
Respiratory: Pharyngitis (3% to 5%), cough (2% to 6%)
Neuromuscular & skeletal: Arthralgia (2% to 7%)
Miscellaneous: Allergic reaction (≤6%)

General Dosage Range SubQ: *Adults:*

Type 1 diabetes mellitus (insulin dependent, IDDM): Initial: 15 mcg immediately prior to meals; Target dose: 30-60 mcg prior to meals

Type 2 diabetes mellitus (noninsulin dependent, NIDDM): Initial: 60 mcg immediately prior to meals; after 3-7 days increase to 120 mcg prior to meals

Mechanism of Action Synthetic analog of human amylin cosecreted with insulin by pancreatic beta cells; reduces postprandial glucose increases via the following mechanisms: 1) prolongation of gastric emptying time, 2) reduction of postprandial glucagon secretion, and 3) reduction of caloric intake through centrally-mediated appetite suppression

Pharmacodynamics/Kinetics

Duration of Action 3 hours

Half-life Elimination ~48 minutes

Time to Peak 20 minutes

Pregnancy Risk Factor C

Pramoxine (pra MOKS een)

U.S. Brand Names Caladryl® Clear™ [OTC]; Callergy Clear [OTC]; Curasore® [OTC]; Itch-X® [OTC]; Prax® [OTC]; Proctofoam® NS [OTC]; Sarna® Sensitive [OTC]; Sarna® Ultra [OTC]; Soothing Care™ Itch Relief [OTC]; Summer's Eve® Anti-Itch Maximum Strength [OTC]; Tronolane® Cream [OTC]; Tucks® Hemorrhoidal [OTC]

Pharmacologic Category Local Anesthetic

Use Temporary relief of pain and itching associated with anogenital pruritus or irritation; dermatosis, minor burns, or hemorrhoids

Local Anesthetic/Vasoconstrictor Precautions No information available to require special precautions

Effects on Dental Treatment No significant effects or complications reported

Effects on Bleeding No information available to require special precautions

Adverse Effects 1% to 10%:

Dermatologic: Angioedema

Local: Contact dermatitis, burning, stinging

General Dosage Range Topical: *Adults:* Apply 3-5 times/day to affected area

Mechanism of Action Pramoxine, like other anesthetics, decreases the neuronal membrane's permeability to sodium ions; both initiation and conduction of nerve impulses are blocked, thus depolarization of the neuron is inhibited

Pharmacodynamics/Kinetics

Onset of Action Therapeutic: 2-5 minutes; Peak effect: 3-5 minutes

Duration of Action Several days

Pregnancy Risk Factor C

Pramoxine and Hydrocortisone (pra MOKS een & hye droe KOR ti sone)

Related Information

Hydrocortisone (Topical) *on page 868*

Pramoxine *on page 1384*

U.S. Brand Names Analpram E™; Analpram HC®; Epifoam®; Pramosone E™; Pramosone®; ProctoFoam® HC; Zypram™

Canadian Brand Names Pramox® HC; Proctofoam™-HC

Pharmacologic Category Anesthetic/Corticosteroid

Use Relief of inflammatory and pruritic manifestations of corticosteroid-responsive dermatoses

Local Anesthetic/Vasoconstrictor Precautions No information available to require special precautions

Effects on Dental Treatment No significant effects or complications reported

Effects on Bleeding No information available to require special precautions

Adverse Effects See individual agents.

General Dosage Range Rectal, topical: *Adults:* Apply to affected areas 3-4 times/day

Pregnancy Risk Factor C

Prasugrel (PRA soo grel)

Related Information

Antiplatelet and Anticoagulation Considerations in Dentistry *on page 1867*

Cardiovascular Diseases *on page 1848*

U.S. Brand Names Effient®

Generic Availability (U.S.) No

Pharmacologic Category Antiplatelet Agent; Antiplatelet Agent, Thienopyridine

Use Reduces rate of thrombotic cardiovascular events (eg, stent thrombosis) in patients with unstable angina, non-ST-segment elevation MI, or ST-elevation MI (STEMI) managed with percutaneous coronary intervention (PCI)

Local Anesthetic/Vasoconstrictor Precautions No information available to require special precautions

Effects on Dental Treatment Key adverse event(s) related to dental treatment: May cause bleeding during invasive dental procedures nad medical consultation is suggested prior to any consideration of discontinuation. If possible, manage bleeding without discontinuing therapy; premature discontinuation of treatment may increase the risk for cardiac adverse effects.

Effects on Bleeding Prasugrel blocks platelet aggregation and may prolong bleeding time. Inhibition is irreversible; on discontinuation of prasugrel, normal platelet function returns only when new platelets are released from the bone marrow. Normal platelet function will occur within 5-9 days of discontinuation. There is no scientific evidence to warrant the discontinuance of prasugrel prior to dental surgery.

Adverse Effects As with all drugs which may affect hemostasis, bleeding is associated with prasugrel. Hemorrhage may occur at virtually any site. Risk is dependent on multiple variables, including patient susceptibility and concurrent use of multiple agents which alter hemostasis.

2% to 10%:

Cardiovascular: Hypertension (8%), hypotension (4%), atrial fibrillation (3%), bradycardia (3%), noncardiac chest pain (3%), peripheral edema (3%)

Central nervous system: Headache (6%), dizziness (4%), fatigue (4%), fever (3%), extremity pain (3%)

Dermatologic: Rash (3%)

Endocrine & metabolic: Hypercholesterolemia/hyperlipidemia (7%)

Gastrointestinal: Nausea (5%), diarrhea (2%), gastrointestinal hemorrhage (2%)

Hematologic: Leukopenia (3%), anemia (2%)

Neuromuscular & skeletal: Back pain (5%)

Respiratory: Epistaxis (6%), dyspnea (5%), cough (4%)

Dosage Oral:

Adults: Acute coronary syndrome managed with PCI: Loading dose: 60 mg administered promptly (as soon as coronary anatomy is known or before if risk for bleeding is low and need for CABG considered unlikely) and no later than 1 hour after PCI; Maintenance dose: 10 mg once daily (in combination with aspirin 81-325 mg/day). **Note:** In patients weighing <60 kg, the manufacturer suggests to consider decreasing maintenance dose to 5 mg once daily; however, prospective clinical trial data does not exist to support this recommendation and may place some patients at risk of thrombotic complications (eg, stent thrombosis); consider use of full dose while monitoring closely for bleeding complications or administration of an alternative agent (eg, clopidogrel).

Duration of prasugrel (in combination with aspirin) after stent placement: **Premature interruption of therapy may result in stent thrombosis with subsequent fatal and nonfatal MI.** With STEMI, prasugrel for at least 12 months regardless of stent type (ie, either bare metal or drug eluting stent) is recommended (Kushner, 2009). With UA/NSTEMI, at least 12 months of prasugrel regardless of stent type is recommended and for up to 15 months unless the risk of bleeding outweighs the benefits (Wright, 2011). In either setting, a duration >15 months may be considered in patients with DES placement (Kushner, 2009; Wright 2011).

Elderly: Refer to adult dosing. Patients ≥75 years: Use not recommended; may be considered in high-risk situations (eg, patients with diabetes or history of MI)

Dosing adjustment in renal impairment: No dosage adjustment necessary

Dosing adjustment in hepatic impairment: No dosage adjustment necessary for mild-to-moderate hepatic impairment; use in severe hepatic impairment has not been evaluated

Mechanism of Action Prasugrel is a prodrug that is metabolized to both active (R-138727) and inactive metabolites. The active metabolite irreversibly blocks the $P2Y_{12}$ component of ADP receptors on the platelet, which prevents activation of the GPIIb/IIIa receptor complex, thereby reducing platelet activation and aggregation. Platelet aggregation returns to baseline within 5-9 days of discontinuation.

Contraindications Active pathological bleeding such as peptic ulcer disease (PUD) or intracranial hemorrhage; history of transient ischemic attack (TIA) or stroke

Warnings/Precautions [U.S. Boxed Warning]: May cause significant or fatal bleeding. Use is contraindicated in patients with active pathological bleeding or history of TIA or stroke. Use with caution in patients who may be at risk of increased bleeding, including patients with active PUD, recent or recurrent GI bleeding, severe hepatic impairment, trauma, or surgery. Additional risk factors include body weight <60 kg, CABG or other surgical procedure, concomitant use of medications that increase risk of bleeding.

[U.S. Boxed Warning]: In patients ≥75 years of age, use is not recommended due to increased risk of fatal and intracranial bleeding and uncertain benefit; use may be considered in high-risk situations (eg, patients with diabetes or history of MI). **[U.S. Boxed Warning]: Discontinue ≥7 days before CABG;** increased risk of bleeding; do not initiate therapy in patients likely to undergo CABG.

If necessary, discontinue therapy for active bleeding, elective surgery, stroke, or TIA; reinitiate therapy as soon as possible unless patient suffers stroke or TIA where subsequent use is contraindicated. If possible, manage bleeding without discontinuing prasugrel. Use caution in concurrent treatment with oral anticoagulants (eg, warfarin), NSAIDs, or fibrinolytic agents; bleeding risk is increased. Use with caution in patients with severe liver impairment or end-stage renal disease (experience is limited). Cases of thrombotic thrombocytopenic purpura (usually occurring within the first 2 weeks of therapy), resulting in some fatalities, have been reported with other thienopyridines; urgent plasmapheresis is required. In patients <60 kg, risk of bleeding increased; consider lower maintenance dose.

Drug Interactions

Avoid Concomitant Use There are no known interactions where it is recommended to avoid concomitant use.

Increased Effect/Toxicity

Prasugrel may increase the levels/effects of: Anticoagulants; Antiplatelet Agents; Collagenase (Systemic); Drotrecogin Alfa; Ibritumomab; Salicylates; Thrombolytic Agents; Tositumomab and Iodine I 131 Tositumomab

The levels/effects of Prasugrel may be increased by: Dasatinib; Glucosamine; Herbs (Anticoagulant/Antiplatelet Properties); Nonsteroidal Anti-Inflammatory Agents; Omega-3-Acid Ethyl Esters; Pentosan Polysulfate Sodium; Pentoxifylline; Prostacyclin Analogues

Decreased Effect

The levels/effects of Prasugrel may be decreased by: CYP3A4 Inhibitors (Strong); Nonsteroidal Anti-Inflammatory Agents; Ranitidine; Rifampin; Tocilizumab

Dietary Considerations May be taken without regard to meals.

Pharmacodynamics/Kinetics

Onset of Action Inhibition of platelet aggregation (IPA): Dose dependent: 60 mg loading dose: <30 minutes; median time to reach 20% IPA: 30 minutes (Brandt, 2007)

Peak effect: Time to maximal IPA: Dose-dependent: **Note:** Degree of IPA based on adenosine diphosphate (ADP) concentration used during light aggregometry: 60 mg loading dose: Occurs 4 hours post administration; mean IPA (ADP 5 μmol/L): 78.8%: mean IPA (ADP 20 μmol/L): 84.1%

Duration of Action Duration of effect: >3 days; platelet aggregation gradually returns to baseline values over 5-9 days after discontinuation; reflective of new platelet production

Half-life Elimination Half-life elimination: Active metabolite: ~7 hours (range 2-15 hours)

Time to Peak Active metabolite: ~30 minutes (peak plasma levels begin to decrease at ~24 hours); with high-fat/high-calorie meal: 1.5 hours

Pregnancy Risk Factor B

Lactation Excretion in breast milk unknown/consider risk:benefit

Dosage Forms

Tablet, oral:

Effient®: 5 mg, 10 mg

Dental Comment There is no scientific evidence to warrant the discontinuance of prasugrel prior to dental surgery. Patients requiring dental surgery who are taking 1 tablet daily as an antithrombotic or taking 1 tablet daily in combination with aspirin should be given special consideration in consultation with their healthcare provider.

References

Brandt JT, Payne CD, Wiviott SD, et al, "A Comparison of Prasugrel and Clopidogrel Loading Doses on Platelet Function: Magnitude of Platelet Inhibition is Related to Active Metabolite Formation," *Am Heart J*, 2007, 153(1):66.e9-16.

Pravastatin (prav a STAT in)

Related Information

Cardiovascular Diseases *on page 1848*

U.S. Brand Names Pravachol®

Canadian Brand Names Apo-Pravastatin®; CO Pravastatin; Dom-Pravastatin; Mylan-Pravastatin; Novo-Pravastatin; Nu-Pravastatin; PHL-Pravastatin; PMS-Pravastatin; Pravachol®; RAN™-Pravastatin; ratio-Pravastatin; Riva-Pravastatin; Sandoz-Pravastatin; ZYM-Pravastatin

Generic Availability (U.S.) Yes

Pharmacologic Category Antilipemic Agent, HMG-CoA Reductase Inhibitor

Use Use with dietary therapy for the following:

Primary prevention of coronary events: In hypercholesterolemic patients without established coronary heart disease to reduce cardiovascular morbidity (myocardial infarction, coronary revascularization procedures) and mortality.

Secondary prevention of cardiovascular events in patients with established coronary heart disease: To slow the progression of coronary atherosclerosis; to reduce cardiovascular morbidity (myocardial infarction, coronary vascular procedures) and to reduce mortality; to reduce the risk of stroke and transient ischemic attacks

Hyperlipidemias: Reduce elevations in total cholesterol, LDL-C, apolipoprotein B, and triglycerides (elevations of 1 or more components are present in Fredrickson type IIa, IIb, III, and IV hyperlipidemias)

Heterozygous familial hypercholesterolemia (HeFH): In pediatric patients, 8-18 years of age, with HeFH having LDL-C ≥190 mg/dL **or** LDL ≥160 mg/dL with positive family history of premature cardiovascular disease (CVD) or 2 or more CVD risk factors in the pediatric patient

Local Anesthetic/Vasoconstrictor Precautions No information available to require special precautions

Effects on Dental Treatment No significant effects or complications reported

Effects on Bleeding No information available to require special precautions

Adverse Effects As reported in short-term trials; safety and tolerability with long-term use were similar to placebo

1% to 10%:

Cardiovascular: Chest pain (4%)

Central nervous system: Headache (2% to 6%), fatigue (4%), dizziness (1% to 3%)

Dermatologic: Rash (4%)

Gastrointestinal: Nausea/vomiting (7%), diarrhea (6%), heartburn (3%)

Hepatic: Transaminases increased (>3x normal on two occasions - 1%)

Neuromuscular & skeletal: Myalgia (2%)

Respiratory: Cough (3%)

Miscellaneous: Influenza (2%)

Additional class-related events or case reports (not necessarily reported with pravastatin therapy): Angioedema, cataracts, depression, dyspnea, eosinophilia, erectile dysfunction, facial paresis, hypersensitivity reaction, impaired extraocular muscle movement, impotence, interstitial lung disease, leukopenia, malaise, memory loss, ophthalmoplegia, paresthesia, peripheral neuropathy, photosensitivity, psychic disturbance, skin discoloration, thrombocytopenia, thyroid dysfunction, toxic epidermal necrolysis, transaminases increased, vomiting

Dosage Oral: **Note:** Doses should be individualized according to the baseline LDL-cholesterol levels, the recommended goal of therapy, and patient response; adjustments should be made at intervals of 4 weeks or more; doses may need adjusted based on concomitant medications

Children: HeFH:

8-13 years: 20 mg/day

14-18 years: 40 mg/day

Dosage adjustment for pravastatin based on concomitant cyclosporine: Refer to adult dosing section

Adults: Hyperlipidemias, primary prevention of coronary events, secondary prevention of cardiovascular events: Initial: 40 mg once daily; titrate dosage to response; usual range: 10-80 mg; (maximum dose: 80 mg once daily)

Dosage adjustment for pravastatin based on concomitant cyclosporine: Initial: 10 mg/day, titrate with caution (maximum dose: 20 mg/day)

Elderly: No specific dosage recommendations. Clearance is reduced in the elderly, resulting in an increase in AUC between 25% to 50%. However, substantial accumulation is not expected.

Dosing adjustment in renal impairment: Initial: 10 mg/day

Dosing adjustment in hepatic impairment: Initial: 10 mg/day

Mechanism of Action Pravastatin is a competitive inhibitor of 3-hydroxy-3-methylglutaryl coenzyme A (HMG-CoA) reductase, which is the rate-limiting enzyme involved in *de novo* cholesterol synthesis.

Contraindications Hypersensitivity to pravastatin or any component of the formulation; active liver disease; unexplained persistent elevations of serum transaminases; pregnancy; breast-feeding

Warnings/Precautions Secondary causes of hyperlipidemia should be ruled out prior to therapy. Liver function must be monitored by periodic laboratory assessment. Rhabdomyolysis with acute renal failure has occurred. Risk may be increased with concurrent use of other drugs which may cause rhabdomyolysis (including colchicine, gemfibrozil, fibric acid derivatives, or niacin at doses ≥1 g/day). Temporarily discontinue in any patient experiencing an acute or serious condition predisposing to renal failure secondary to rhabdomyolysis. Based upon current evidence, HMG-CoA reductase inhibitor therapy should be continued in the perioperative period unless risk outweighs cardioprotective benefit. Use with caution in patients with advanced age, these patients are predisposed to myopathy. Use caution in patients with previous liver disease or heavy ethanol use. Treatment in patients <8 years of age is not recommended.

Drug Interactions

Metabolism/Transport Effects **Substrate** of CYP3A4 (minor), P-glycoprotein, SLCO1B1; **Inhibits** CYP2C9 (weak), 2D6 (weak), 3A4 (weak)

Avoid Concomitant Use

Avoid concomitant use of Pravastatin with any of the following: Red Yeast Rice

Increased Effect/Toxicity

Pravastatin may increase the levels/effects of: DAPTOmycin; Trabectedin; Vitamin K Antagonists

The levels/effects of Pravastatin may be increased by: Antifungal Agents (Azole Derivatives, Systemic); Colchicine; Conivaptan; CycloSPORINE; CycloSPORINE (Systemic); Eltrombopag; Fenofibrate; Fenofibric Acid; Gemfibrozil; Niacin; Niacinamide; P-Glycoprotein Inhibitors; Protease Inhibitors; Red Yeast Rice; Rifamycin Derivatives

Decreased Effect

The levels/effects of Pravastatin may be decreased by: Antacids; Bile Acid Sequestrants; Efavirenz; Fosphenytoin; P-Glycoprotein Inducers; Phenytoin; Rifamycin Derivatives; Tocilizumab

Ethanol/Nutrition/Herb Interactions

Ethanol: Consumption of large amounts of ethanol may increase the risk of liver damage with HMG-CoA reductase inhibitors.

Food: Red yeast rice contains an estimated 2.4 mg lovastatin per 600 mg rice.

Herb/Nutraceutical: St John's wort may decrease pravastatin levels.

Dietary Considerations May be taken without regard to meals. Before initiation of therapy, patients should be placed on a standard cholesterol-lowering diet for 6 weeks and the diet should be continued during drug therapy. Red yeast rice contains an estimated 2.4 mg lovastatin per 600 mg rice.

Pharmacodynamics/Kinetics

Onset of Action Several days; Peak effect: 4 weeks

Half-life Elimination 77 hours (including all metabolites); pravastatin: ~2-3 hours (Pan, 1990); 3α-hydroxy-iso-pravastatin: ~1.5 hours (Gustavson, 2005)

Time to Peak Serum: 1-1.5 hours

Pregnancy Risk Factor X

Lactation Enters breast milk/contraindicated

Dosage Forms

Tablet, oral: 10 mg, 20 mg, 40 mg, 80 mg

Pravachol®: 10 mg, 20 mg, 40 mg, 80 mg

Praziquantel (pray zi KWON tel)

U.S. Brand Names Biltricide®

Canadian Brand Names Biltricide®

Pharmacologic Category Anthelmintic

Use Treatment of all stages of schistosomiasis caused by all *Schistosoma* species; treatment of infection (clonorchiasis and opisthorchiasis) due to liver flukes

Unlabeled/Investigational Use Cysticercosis and many intestinal tapeworms

Local Anesthetic/Vasoconstrictor Precautions No information available to require special precautions

Effects on Dental Treatment No significant effects or complications reported

Effects on Bleeding No information available to require special precautions

Adverse Effects Frequency not defined.

Central nervous system: Dizziness, fever, headache, malaise

Dermatologic: Urticaria (rare)

Gastrointestinal: Abdominal discomfort, nausea

General Dosage Range Oral: *Children ≥4 years and Adults:* 20 mg/kg/dose 2-3 times/day for 1 day at 4- to 6-hour intervals **or** 25 mg/kg 3 times/day for 1 day

Mechanism of Action Increases the cell permeability to calcium in schistosomes, causing strong contractions and paralysis of worm musculature leading to detachment of suckers from the blood vessel walls and to dislodgment

Pharmacodynamics/Kinetics

Half-life Elimination Parent drug: 0.8-1.5 hours; Metabolites: 4.5 hours

Time to Peak Serum: 1-3 hours

Pregnancy Risk Factor B

Prazosin (PRAZ oh sin)

Related Information

Cardiovascular Diseases *on page 1848*

U.S. Brand Names Minipress®

Canadian Brand Names Apo-Prazo®; Minipress®; Novo-Prazin; Nu-Prazo

Pharmacologic Category Alpha$_1$ Blocker

Use Treatment of hypertension

Unlabeled/Investigational Use Post-traumatic stress disorder (PTSD) related nightmares and sleep disruption; benign prostatic hyperplasia; Raynaud's syndrome

Local Anesthetic/Vasoconstrictor Precautions No information available to require special precautions

Effects on Dental Treatment Key adverse event(s) related to dental treatment: Significant xerostomia (normal salivary flow resumes upon discontinuation). Significant orthostatic hypotension is a possibility; monitor patient when getting out of dental chair.

Effects on Bleeding No information available to require special precautions

Adverse Effects
>4%:
Cardiovascular: Palpitation (5%)
Central nervous system: Dizziness (10%), headache (8%), drowsiness (8%)
Endocrine & metabolic: Decreased energy (7%)
Gastrointestinal: Nausea (5%)
Neuromuscular & skeletal: Weakness (7%)
1% to 4%:
Cardiovascular: Edema, orthostatic hypotension, syncope
Central nervous system: Depression, nervousness, vertigo
Dermatologic: Rash
Gastrointestinal: Constipation, diarrhea, vomiting, xerostomia
Genitourinary: Urinary frequency
Ocular: Blurred vision, reddened sclera
Respiratory: Dyspnea, epistaxis, nasal congestion

General Dosage Range Oral: *Adults:* Initial: 1 mg/dose 2-3 times/day; Maintenance: 2-20 mg/day in divided doses 2-3 times/day (maximum: 20 mg/day) (JNC 7)

Mechanism of Action Competitively inhibits postsynaptic alpha-adrenergic receptors which results in vasodilation of veins and arterioles and a decrease in total peripheral resistance and blood pressure

Pharmacodynamics/Kinetics

Onset of Action Anithypertensive: ~2 hours; Peak effect: Antihypertensive: 2-4 hours

Duration of Action 10-24 hours

Half-life Elimination 2-3 hours; prolonged with congestive heart failure

Time to Peak Plasma: ~3 hours

Pregnancy Risk Factor C

Prednicarbate (pred ni KAR bate)

U.S. Brand Names Dermatop®

Canadian Brand Names Dermatop®

Pharmacologic Category Corticosteroid, Topical

Use Relief of the inflammatory and pruritic manifestations of corticosteroid-responsive dermatoses (medium potency topical corticosteroid)

Local Anesthetic/Vasoconstrictor Precautions No information available to require special precautions

Effects on Dental Treatment No significant effects or complications reported

Effects on Bleeding No information available to require special precautions

Adverse Effects 1% to 10%: Dermatologic: Skin atrophy (children 8%; adults 1%), mild telangiectasia (children 5%), shininess (children 3%), thinness (children 3%)

General Dosage Range Topical:
Children ≥1 year and Adults: Cream: Apply a thin film to affected area twice daily
Children ≥10 year and Adults: Ointment: Apply a thin film to affected area twice daily

Mechanism of Action Topical corticosteroids have anti-inflammatory, antipruritic, vasoconstrictive, and antiproliferative actions

Pregnancy Risk Factor C

PrednisoLONE (Systemic) (pred NISS oh lone)

Related Information
PredniSONE *on page 1393*
Respiratory Diseases *on page 1876*

U.S. Brand Names Millipred™; Orapred ODT®; Orapred®; Pediapred®; Prelone®; Veripred™ 20

Canadian Brand Names Hydeltra T.B.A.®; Novo-Prednisolone; Pediapred®

Generic Availability (U.S.) Yes: Excludes orally disintegrating tablet

Pharmacologic Category Corticosteroid, Systemic

Dental Use Treatment of a variety of oral diseases of allergic, inflammatory, or autoimmune origin

Use Treatment of endocrine disorders, rheumatic disorders, collagen diseases, allergic states, respiratory diseases, hematologic disorders, neoplastic diseases, edematous states, and gastrointestinal diseases; resolution of acute exacerbations of multiple sclerosis; management of fulminating or disseminated tuberculosis and trichinosis; acute or chronic solid organ rejection

Local Anesthetic/Vasoconstrictor Precautions No information available to require special precautions

Effects on Dental Treatment Key adverse event(s) related to dental treatment: Ulcerative esophagitis.

Effects on Bleeding No information available to require special precautions

Adverse Effects Frequency not defined.

Cardiovascular: Cardiomyopathy, CHF, edema, facial edema, hypertension

Central nervous system: Headache, insomnia, malaise, nervousness, pseudotumor cerebri, psychic disorders, seizure, vertigo

Dermatologic: Bruising, facial erythema, hirsutism, petechiae, skin test reaction suppression, thin fragile skin, urticaria

Endocrine & metabolic: Carbohydrate tolerance decreased, Cushing's syndrome, diabetes mellitus, growth suppression, hyperglycemia, hypernatremia, hypokalemia, hypokalemic alkalosis, menstrual irregularities, negative nitrogen balance, pituitary adrenal axis suppression

Gastrointestinal: Abdominal distention, increased appetite, indigestion, nausea, pancreatitis, peptic ulcer, ulcerative esophagitis, weight gain

Hepatic: LFTs increased (usually reversible)

Neuromuscular & skeletal: Arthralgia, aseptic necrosis (humeral/femoral heads), fractures, muscle mass decreased, muscle weakness, osteoporosis, steroid myopathy, tendon rupture, weakness

Ocular: Cataracts, exophthalmus, eyelid edema, glaucoma, intraocular pressure increased, irritation

Respiratory: Epistaxis

Miscellaneous: Diaphoresis increased, impaired wound healing

Dental Usual Dosage Anti-inflammatory or immunosuppressive dose: Oral:

Children: 0.1-2 mg/kg/day in divided doses 1-4 times/day

Adults: Usual range: 5-60 mg/day

Dosage Dose depends upon condition being treated and response of patient; dosage for infants and children should be based on severity of the disease and response of the patient rather than on strict adherence to dosage indicated by age, weight, or body surface area. Oral dosage expressed in terms of prednisolone base. Consider alternate day therapy for long-term therapy. Discontinuation of long-term therapy requires gradual withdrawal by tapering the dose. Patients undergoing unusual stress while receiving corticosteroids should receive increased doses prior to, during, and after the stressful situation.

Children: Oral:

Acute asthma: 1-2 mg/kg/day in divided doses 1-2 times/day for 3-5 days

Anti-inflammatory or immunosuppressive dose: 0.1-2 mg/kg/day in divided doses 1-4 times/day

Nephrotic syndrome:

Initial (first 3 episodes): 2 mg/kg/day **or** 60 mg/m^2/day (maximum: 80 mg/day) in divided doses 3-4 times/day until urine is protein free for 3 consecutive days (maximum: 28 days); followed by 1-1.5 mg/kg/dose **or** 40 mg/m^2/dose given every other day for 4 weeks

Maintenance (long-term maintenance dose for frequent relapses): 0.5-1 mg/kg/dose given every other day for 3-6 months

Adults: Oral:

Usual range: 5-60 mg/day

Multiple sclerosis: 200 mg/day for 1 week followed by 80 mg every other day for 1 month

Rheumatoid arthritis: Initial: 5-7.5 mg/day; adjust dose as necessary

Elderly: Use lowest effective dose

Dosing adjustment in hyperthyroidism: Prednisolone dose may need to be increased to achieve adequate therapeutic effects

Hemodialysis: Slightly dialyzable (5% to 20%); administer dose posthemodialysis

Peritoneal dialysis: Supplemental dose is not necessary

Mechanism of Action Decreases inflammation by suppression of migration of polymorphonuclear leukocytes and reversal of increased capillary permeability; suppresses the immune system by reducing activity and volume of the lymphatic system

Contraindications Hypersensitivity to prednisolone or any component of the formulation; acute superficial herpes simplex keratitis; live or attenuated virus vaccines (with immunosuppressive doses of corticosteroids); systemic fungal infections; varicella

Warnings/Precautions May cause hypercorticism or suppression of hypothalamic-pituitary-adrenal (HPA) axis, particularly in younger children or in patients receiving high doses for prolonged periods. HPA axis suppression may lead to adrenal crisis. Withdrawal and discontinuation of a corticosteroid should be done slowly and carefully. Particular care is required when patients are transferred from systemic corticosteroids to inhaled products due to possible adrenal insufficiency or withdrawal from steroids, including an increase in allergic symptoms. Patients receiving >20 mg per day of prednisone (or equivalent) may be most susceptible. Fatalities have occurred due to adrenal insufficiency in asthmatic patients during and after transfer from systemic corticosteroids to aerosol steroids; aerosol steroids do **not** provide the systemic steroid needed to treat patients having trauma, surgery, or infections.

Acute myopathy has been reported with high dose corticosteroids, usually in patients with neuromuscular transmission disorders; may involve ocular and/or respiratory muscles; monitor creatine kinase; recovery may be delayed. Corticosteroid use may cause psychiatric disturbances, including depression, euphoria, insomnia, mood swings, and personality changes. Pre-existing psychiatric conditions may be exacerbated by corticosteroid use. Prolonged use of corticosteroids may also increase the incidence of secondary infection, mask acute infection (including fungal infections), prolong or exacerbate viral infections, or limit response to vaccines. Exposure to chickenpox should be avoided; corticosteroids should not be used to treat ocular herpes simplex. Corticosteroids should not be used for cerebral malaria or viral hepatitis. Close observation is required in patients with latent tuberculosis and/or TB reactivity; restrict use in active TB (only in conjunction with antituberculosis treatment). Prolonged use of corticosteroids may result in glaucoma; cataract formation may occur. Prolonged treatment with corticosteroids has been associated with the development of Kaposi's sarcoma (case reports); if noted, discontinuation of therapy should be considered.

Use with caution in patients with thyroid disease, hepatic impairment, renal impairment, cardiovascular disease, diabetes, glaucoma, cataracts, myasthenia gravis, patients at risk for osteoporosis, patients at risk for seizures, or GI diseases (diverticulitis, peptic ulcer, ulcerative colitis) due to perforation risk. Use caution following acute MI (corticosteroids have been associated with myocardial rupture). Because of the risk of adverse effects, systemic corticosteroids should be used cautiously in the elderly in the smallest possible effective dose for the shortest duration. Withdraw therapy with gradual tapering of dose. May affect growth velocity; growth should be routinely monitored in pediatric patients.

Drug Interactions

Metabolism/Transport Effects **Substrate** of CYP3A4 (minor); **Inhibits** CYP3A4 (weak)

Avoid Concomitant Use

Avoid concomitant use of PrednisoLONE (Systemic) with any of the following: Aldesleukin; BCG; Natalizumab; Pimecrolimus; Roflumilast; Tacrolimus (Topical)

Increased Effect/Toxicity

PrednisoLONE (Systemic) may increase the levels/effects of: Acetylcholinesterase Inhibitors; Amphotericin B; CycloSPORINE; CycloSPORINE (Systemic); Deferasirox; Leflunomide; Loop Diuretics; Natalizumab; NSAID (COX-2 Inhibitor); NSAID (Nonselective); Thiazide Diuretics; Vaccines (Live); Warfarin

The levels/effects of PrednisoLONE (Systemic) may be increased by: Antifungal Agents (Azole Derivatives, Systemic); Aprepitant; Calcium Channel Blockers (Nondihydropyridine); Conivaptan; CycloSPORINE; CycloSPORINE (Systemic); Denosumab; Estrogen Derivatives; Fluconazole; Fosaprepitant; Macrolide Antibiotics; Neuromuscular-Blocking Agents (Nondepolarizing); Pimecrolimus; Quinolone Antibiotics; Roflumilast; Salicylates; Tacrolimus (Topical); Trastuzumab

Decreased Effect

PrednisoLONE (Systemic) may decrease the levels/effects of: Aldesleukin; Antidiabetic Agents; BCG; Calcitriol; Corticorelin; CycloSPORINE; CycloSPORINE (Systemic); Isoniazid; Salicylates; Sipuleucel-T; Vaccines (Inactivated)

The levels/effects of PrednisoLONE (Systemic) may be decreased by: Aminoglutethimide; Antacids; Barbiturates; Bile Acid Sequestrants; Echinacea; Mitotane; Primidone; Rifamycin Derivatives; Tocilizumab

Ethanol/Nutrition/Herb Interactions

Ethanol: Avoid ethanol (may increase gastric mucosal irritation).

Food: Prednisolone interferes with calcium absorption. Limit caffeine.

Herb/Nutraceutical: St John's wort may decrease prednisolone levels. Avoid cat's claw, echinacea (have immunostimulant properties).

Dietary Considerations Should be taken after meals or with food or milk to decrease GI effects; increase dietary intake of pyridoxine, vitamin C, vitamin D, folate, calcium, and phosphorus.

Pharmacodynamics/Kinetics

Duration of Action 18-36 hours

Half-life Elimination 3.6 hours; End-stage renal disease: 3-5 hours

Pregnancy Risk Factor C

Lactation Enters breast milk/use caution (AAP rates "compatible"; AAP 2001 update pending)

Breast-Feeding Considerations Prednisolone is excreted into breast milk with peak concentrations occurring ~1 hour after the maternal dose. The milk/plasma ratio was found to be 0.2 with doses ≥30 mg/day and 0.1 with doses <30 mg/day.

Following a maternal dose of prednisolone 80 mg/day, a breast-feeding infant would ingest <0.1% of the dose.

Dosage Forms

Solution, oral: 5 mg/5 mL (120 mL); 15 mg/5 mL (237 mL, 240 mL, 473 mL, 480 mL)
Millipred™: 10 mg/5 mL (237 mL)
Orapred®: 15 mg/5 mL (20 mL, 237 mL)
Pediapred®: 5 mg/5 mL (120 mL)
Veripred™ 20: 20 mg/5 mL (237 mL)

Syrup, oral: 15 mg/5 mL (240 mL, 480 mL)
Prelone®: 15 mg/5 mL (240 mL, 480 mL)

Tablet, orally disintegrating, oral:
Orapred ODT®: 10 mg, 15 mg, 30 mg

Prednisolone and Gentamicin (pred NIS oh lone & jen ta MYE sin)

U.S. Brand Names Pred-G®

Pharmacologic Category Antibiotic/Corticosteroid, Ophthalmic

Use Treatment of steroid responsive inflammatory conditions and superficial ocular infections due to microorganisms susceptible to gentamicin

Local Anesthetic/Vasoconstrictor Precautions No information available to require special precautions

Effects on Dental Treatment No significant effects or complications reported

Effects on Bleeding No information available to require special precautions

Adverse Effects Frequency not defined.
Dermatologic: Delayed wound healing
Local: Burning, stinging
Ocular: Intraocular pressure increased, glaucoma, superficial punctate keratitis, optic nerve damage (infrequent), posterior subcapsular cataract formation
Miscellaneous: Secondary infection

General Dosage Range Ophthalmic: *Children and Adults:*
Ointment: Apply 1/2" ribbon in the conjunctival sac 1-3 times/day
Suspension: Initial: 1 drop every hour for 1-2 days; Maintenance: 1 drop 2-4 times/day

Pregnancy Risk Factor C

PredniSONE (PRED ni sone)

Related Information
PrednisoLONE (Systemic) *on page 1390*
Respiratory Diseases *on page 1876*
Rheumatoid Arthritis, Osteoarthritis, and Osteoporosis *on page 1889*
Ulcerative, Erosive, and Painful Oral Mucosal Disorders *on page 1950*

Related Sample Prescriptions
Erosive Lichen Planus, Other Biopsy-Proven Desquamative Oral Diseases, and Major Aphthae *on page 1992*

U.S. Brand Names PredniSONE Intensol™

Canadian Brand Names Apo-Prednisone®; Novo-Prednisone; Winpred™

Generic Availability (U.S.) Yes

Pharmacologic Category Corticosteroid, Systemic

Dental Use Treatment of a variety of oral diseases of allergic, inflammatory, or autoimmune origin

Use Treatment of a variety of diseases, including:
Allergic states (including adjunctive treatment of anaphylaxis)
Autoimmune disorders (including systemic lupus erythematosus [SLE])
Collagen diseases
Dermatologic conditions/diseases
Edematous states (including nephrotic syndrome)
Endocrine disorders
Gastrointestinal diseases
Hematologic disorders (including idiopathic thrombocytopenia purpura [ITP])
Multiple sclerosis exacerbations
Neoplastic diseases
Ophthalmic diseases
Respiratory diseases (including acute asthma exacerbation)
Rheumatic disorders (including rheumatoid arthritis)
Trichinosis with neurologic or myocardial involvement
Tuberculous meningitis

Unlabeled/Investigational Use Adjunctive therapy for *Pneumocystis jiroveci* (formerly *carinni*) pneumonia (PCP); autoimmune hepatitis; adjunctive therapy for pain management in immunocompetent patients with herpes zoster; tuberculosis (severe, paradoxical reactions); Takayasu arteritis; giant cell arteritis

Local Anesthetic/Vasoconstrictor Precautions No information available to require special precautions

Effects on Dental Treatment No significant effects or complications reported

Effects on Bleeding No information available to require special precautions

Adverse Effects Frequency not defined.

Cardiovascular: Congestive heart failure (in susceptible patients), hypertension

Central nervous system: Emotional instability, headache, intracranial pressure increased (with papilledema), psychic derangements (including euphoria, insomnia, mood swings, personality changes, severe depression), seizure, vertigo

Dermatologic: Bruising, facial erythema, petechiae, thin fragile skin, urticaria, wound healing impaired

Endocrine & metabolic: Adrenocortical and pituitary unresponsiveness (in times of stress), carbohydrate intolerance, Cushing's syndrome, diabetes mellitus, fluid retention, growth suppression (in children), hypokalemic alkalosis, hypothyroidism enhanced, menstrual irregularities, negative nitrogen balance due to protein catabolism, potassium loss, sodium retention

Gastrointestinal: Abdominal distension, pancreatitis, peptic ulcer (with possible perforation and hemorrhage), ulcerative esophagitis

Hepatic: ALT increased, AST increased, alkaline phosphatase increased

Neuromuscular & skeletal: Aseptic necrosis of femoral and humeral heads, muscle mass loss, muscle weakness, osteoporosis, pathologic fracture of long bones, steroid myopathy, tendon rupture (particularly Achilles tendon), vertebral compression fractures

Ocular: Exophthalmos, glaucoma, intraocular pressure increased, posterior subcapsular cataracts

Miscellaneous: Allergic reactions, anaphylactic reactions, diaphoresis, hypersensitivity reactions, infections, Kaposi's sarcoma

Dental Usual Dosage

Anti-inflammatory or immunosuppressive dose: Children: Oral: 0.05-2 mg/kg/day divided 1-4 times/day

Immunosuppression/chemotherapy adjunct: Adults: Oral: Range: 5-60 mg/day in divided doses 1-4 times/day

Dosage Oral:

General dosing range: Children and Adults: Initial: 5-60 mg/day: **Note:** Dose depends upon condition being treated and response of patient; dosage for infants and children should be based on severity of the disease and response of the patient rather than on strict adherence to dosage indicated by age, weight, or body surface area. Consider alternate day therapy for long-term therapy. Discontinuation of long-term therapy requires gradual withdrawal by tapering the dose.

Prednisone taper (other regimens also available):

Day 1: 30 mg divided as 10 mg before breakfast, 5 mg at lunch, 5 mg at dinner, 10 mg at bedtime

Day 2: 5 mg at breakfast, 5 mg at lunch, 5 mg at dinner, 10 mg at bedtime

Day 3: 5 mg 4 times/day (with meals and at bedtime)

Day 4: 5 mg 3 times/day (breakfast, lunch, bedtime)

Day 5: 5 mg 2 times/day (breakfast, bedtime)

Day 6: 5 mg before breakfast

Indication-specific dosing:

Children:

Acute asthma (NIH guidelines, 2007):

0-11 years 1-2 mg/kg/day for 3-10 days (maximum: 60 mg/day)

≥12 years: Refer to Adults dosing

Autoimmune hepatitis (unlabeled use; Czaja, 2002): Initial treatment: 2 mg/kg/day for 2 weeks (maximum: 60 mg/day), followed by a taper over 6-8 weeks to a dose of 0.1-0.2 mg/kg/day or 5 mg/day

Nephrotic syndrome (Pediatric Nephrology Panel recommendations [Hogg, 2000]): Initial: 2 mg/kg/day or 60 mg/m^2/day given every day in 1-3 divided doses (maximum: 80 mg/day) until urine is protein free or for 4-6 weeks; followed by maintenance dose: 2 mg/kg/dose or 40 mg/m^2/dose given every other day in the morning; gradually taper and discontinue after 4-6 weeks. **Note:** No definitive treatment guidelines exist. Dosing is dependent on institution protocols and individual response.

PCP pneumonia (AIDS*info* guidelines, 2008): 1 mg/kg twice daily for 5 days, *followed by* 0.5-1 mg/kg twice daily for 5 days, *followed by* 0.5 mg/kg once daily for 11-21 days

Adolescents and Adults:

PCP pneumonia (AIDS*info* guidelines, 2008): Note: Begin within 72 hours of PCP therapy: 40 mg twice daily for 5 days, *followed by* 40 mg once daily for 5 days, *followed by* 20 mg once daily for 11 days or until antimicrobial regimen is completed

Adults:

Acute asthma (NIH guidelines, 2007): 40-60 mg per day for 3-10 days; administer as single or 2 divided doses

Anaphylaxis, adjunctive treatment (Lieberman, 2005): 0.5 mg/kg

Antineoplastic: Usual range: 10 mg/day to 100 mg/m^2/day (depending on indication). **Note:** Details concerning dosing in combination regimens should also be consulted.

Autoimmune hepatitis (unlabeled use; Czaja, 2002): Initial treatment: 60 mg/day for 1 week, *followed by* 40 mg/day for 1 week, *then* 30 mg/day for 2 weeks, *then* 20 mg/day. Half this dose should be given when used in combination with azathioprine

Dermatomyositis/polymyositis: Oral: 1 mg/kg daily (range: 0.5-1.5 mg/kg/day), often in conjunction with steroid-sparing therapies; depending on response/tolerance, consider slow tapering after 2-8 weeks depending on response; taper regimens vary widely, but often involve 5-10 mg decrements per week and may require 6-12 months to reach a low once-daily or every-other-day dose to prevent disease flare (Briemberg, 2003; Hengstman, 2009; Iorizzo, 2008; Wiendl, 2008)

Giant cell arteritis (unlabeled use): Oral: Initial: 40-60 mg/day; typically requires 1-2 years of treatment, but may begin to taper after 2-3 months; alternative dosing of 30-40 mg/day has demonstrated similar efficacy (Hiratzka, 2010)

Herpes zoster (unlabeled use; Dworkin, 2007): 60 mg/day for 7 days, *followed by* 30 mg/day for 7 days, *then* 15 mg/day for 7 days

Idiopathic thrombocytopenia purpura (American Society of Hematology, 1997): 1-2 mg/kg/day

Rheumatoid arthritis (American College of Rheumatology, 2002): ≤10 mg/day

Systemic lupus erythematosus (American College of Rheumatology, 1999):

Mild SLE: ≤10 mg/day

Refractory or severe organ-threatening disease: 20-60 mg/day

Takayasu arteritis (unlabeled use): Oral: Initial: 40-60 mg/day; taper to lowest effective dose when ESR and CRP levels are normal; usual duration: 1-2 years (Hiratzka, 2010)

Thyrotoxicosis (type II amiodarone induced; unlabeled use): 30-40 mg/day for 7-14 days, gradually taper over 3 months

Tuberculosis, severe, paradoxical reactions (unlabeled use, AIDS*info* guidelines, 2008): 1 mg/kg/day, gradually reduce after 1-2 weeks

Elderly: Use the lowest effective dose

Dosing adjustment in hepatic impairment: Prednisone is inactive and must be metabolized by the liver to prednisolone. This conversion may be impaired in patients with liver disease, however, prednisolone levels are observed to be higher in patients with severe liver failure than in normal patients. Therefore, compensation for the inadequate conversion of prednisone to prednisolone occurs.

Dosing adjustment in hyperthyroidism: Prednisone dose may need to be increased to achieve adequate therapeutic effects

Hemodialysis: Supplemental dose is not necessary

Peritoneal dialysis: Supplemental dose is not necessary

Mechanism of Action Decreases inflammation by suppression of migration of polymorphonuclear leukocytes and reversal of increased capillary permeability; suppresses the immune system by reducing activity and volume of the lymphatic system; suppresses adrenal function at high doses. Antitumor effects may be related to inhibition of glucose transport, phosphorylation, or induction of cell death in immature lymphocytes. Antiemetic effects are thought to occur due to blockade of cerebral innervation of the emetic center via inhibition of prostaglandin synthesis.

Contraindications Hypersensitivity to any component of the formulation; systemic fungal infections; administration of live or live attenuated vaccines with immunosuppressive doses of prednisone

Warnings/Precautions May cause hypercorticism or suppression of hypothalamic-pituitary-adrenal (HPA) axis, particularly in younger children or in patients receiving high doses for prolonged periods. HPA axis suppression may lead to adrenal crisis. Withdrawal and discontinuation of a corticosteroid should be done slowly and carefully. Particular care is required when patients are transferred from systemic corticosteroids to inhaled products due to possible adrenal insufficiency or withdrawal from steroids, including an increase in allergic symptoms. Patients receiving >20 mg per day of prednisone (or equivalent) may be most susceptible. Fatalities have occurred due to adrenal insufficiency in asthmatic patients during and after transfer from systemic corticosteroids to aerosol steroids; aerosol steroids do **not** provide the systemic steroid needed to treat patients having trauma, surgery, or infections.

Acute myopathy has been reported with high dose corticosteroids, usually in patients with neuromuscular transmission disorders; may involve ocular and/or respiratory muscles; monitor creatine kinase; recovery may be delayed. Prolonged use of corticosteroids may increase the incidence of secondary infection, mask acute infection (including fungal infections), prolong or exacerbate viral infections, or limit response to vaccines. Exposure to chickenpox should be avoided. Corticosteroids should not be used to treat ocular herpes simplex or cerebral malaria. Close observation is required in patients with latent tuberculosis and/or TB reactivity; restrict use in active TB (only in conjunction with antituberculosis treatment). Prolonged treatment with corticosteroids has been associated with the development of Kaposi's sarcoma (case reports); if noted, discontinuation of therapy should be considered. Prolonged use may cause posterior subcapsular cataracts, glaucoma (with possible nerve damage) and may increase the risk for ocular infections. Corticosteroid use may cause psychiatric disturbances, including depression, euphoria, insomnia, mood swings, and personality changes. Pre-existing psychiatric conditions may be exacerbated by corticosteroid use.

Use with caution in patients with HF, diabetes, GI diseases (diverticulitis, peptic ulcer, ulcerative colitis; due to risk of perforation), hepatic impairment, myasthenia gravis, MI, patients with or who are at risk for osteoporosis, seizure disorders or thyroid disease. May affect growth velocity; growth should be routinely monitored in pediatric patients.

Prior to use, the dose and duration of treatment should be based on the risk versus benefit for each individual patient. In general, use the smallest effective dose for the shortest duration of time to minimize adverse events. A gradual tapering of dose may be required prior to discontinuing therapy.

Drug Interactions

Metabolism/Transport Effects **Substrate** of CYP3A4 (minor); **Induces** CYP2C19 (weak), 3A4 (weak)

Avoid Concomitant Use

Avoid concomitant use of PredniSONE with any of the following: Aldesleukin; BCG; Natalizumab; Pimecrolimus; Roflumilast; Tacrolimus (Topical)

Increased Effect/Toxicity

PredniSONE may increase the levels/effects of: Acetylcholinesterase Inhibitors; Amphotericin B; CycloSPORINE; CycloSPORINE (Systemic); Deferasirox; Leflunomide; Loop Diuretics; Natalizumab; NSAID (COX-2 Inhibitor); NSAID (Nonselective); Thiazide Diuretics; Vaccines (Live); Warfarin

The levels/effects of PredniSONE may be increased by: Antifungal Agents (Azole Derivatives, Systemic); Aprepitant; Calcium Channel Blockers (Nondihydropyridine); Conivaptan; CycloSPORINE; CycloSPORINE (Systemic); Denosumab; Estrogen Derivatives; Fluconazole; Fosaprepitant; Macrolide Antibiotics; Neuromuscular-Blocking Agents (Nondepolarizing); Pimecrolimus; Quinolone Antibiotics; Ritonavir; Roflumilast; Salicylates; Tacrolimus (Topical); Trastuzumab

Decreased Effect

PredniSONE may decrease the levels/effects of: Aldesleukin; Antidiabetic Agents; BCG; Calcitriol; Corticorelin; CycloSPORINE; CycloSPORINE (Systemic); Isoniazid; Salicylates; Sipuleucel-T; Vaccines (Inactivated)

The levels/effects of PredniSONE may be decreased by: Aminoglutethimide; Antacids; Barbiturates; Bile Acid Sequestrants; Echinacea; Mitotane; Primidone; Rifamycin Derivatives; Somatropin; Tesamorelin; Tocilizumab

Ethanol/Nutrition/Herb Interactions

Ethanol: Avoid ethanol (may increase gastric mucosal irritation)

Food: Prednisone interferes with calcium absorption. Limit caffeine.

Herb/Nutraceutical: St John's wort may decrease prednisone levels. Avoid cat's claw, echinacea (have immunostimulant properties).

Dietary Considerations Should be taken after meals or with food or milk; may require increased dietary intake of pyridoxine, vitamin C, vitamin D, folate, calcium, and phosphorus; may require decreased dietary intake of sodium

Pharmacodynamics/Kinetics

Half-life Elimination Normal renal function: ~3.5 hours

Lactation Enters breast milk/AAP rates "compatible" (AAP 2001 update pending)

Breast-Feeding Considerations Prednisone and its metabolite prednisolone are found in low concentrations in breast milk. Peak milk concentrations of both were found ~2 hours after the maternal dose in one case report. In a study which included 6 mother/infant pairs, adverse events were not observed in nursing infants (maternal prednisone dose not provided).

Dosage Forms

Solution, oral: 1 mg/mL (5 mL, 120 mL, 500 mL)

PredniSONE Intensol™: 5 mg/mL (30 mL)

Tablet, oral: 1 mg, 2.5 mg, 5 mg, 10 mg, 20 mg, 50 mg

Pregabalin (pre GAB a lin)

U.S. Brand Names Lyrica®

Canadian Brand Names Lyrica®

Generic Availability (U.S.) No

Pharmacologic Category Analgesic, Miscellaneous; Anticonvulsant, Miscellaneous

Use Management of pain associated with diabetic peripheral neuropathy; management of postherpetic neuralgia; adjunctive therapy for partial-onset seizure disorder in adults; management of fibromyalgia

Local Anesthetic/Vasoconstrictor Precautions No information available to require special precautions

Effects on Dental Treatment Key adverse event(s) related to dental treatment: Xerostomia and changes in salivation (normal salivary flow resumes upon discontinuation).

Effects on Bleeding May be associated with thrombocytopenia (uncommon). No information available to require routine special precautions

Adverse Effects Note: Frequency of adverse effects may be influenced by dose or concurrent therapy. In add-on trials in epilepsy, frequency of CNS and visual adverse effects were higher than those reported in pain management trials. Range noted below is inclusive of all trials.

>10%:

Cardiovascular: Peripheral edema (up to 16%)

Central nervous system: Dizziness (8% to 45%), somnolence (4% to 28%), ataxia (up to 20%), headache (up to 14%)

Gastrointestinal: Weight gain (up to 16%), xerostomia (1% to 15%)

Neuromuscular & skeletal: Tremor (up to 11%)

Ocular: Blurred vision (1% to 12%), diplopia (up to 12%)

Miscellaneous: Infection (up to 14%), accidental injury (2% to 11%)

1% to 10%:

Cardiovascular: Chest pain (up to 4%), edema (up to 6%)

Central nervous system: Neuropathy (up to 9%), thinking abnormal (up to 9%), fatigue (up to 8%), confusion (up to 7%), euphoria (up to 7%), speech disorder (up to 7%), attention disturbance (up to 6%), incoordination (up to 6%), amnesia (up to 6%), pain (up to 5%), memory impaired (up to 4%), vertigo (up to 4%), feeling abnormal (up to 3%), hypoesthesia (up to 3%), anxiety (up to 2%), depression (up to 2%), disorientation (up to 2%), lethargy (up to 2%), fever (≥1%), depersonalization (≥1%), hypertonia (≥1%), stupor (≥1%), nervousness (up to 1%)

Dermatologic: Facial edema (up to 3%), bruising (≥1%), pruritus (≥1%)

Endocrine & metabolic: Fluid retention (up to 3%), hypoglycemia (up to 3%), libido decreased (≥1%)

Gastrointestinal: Constipation (up to 10%), appetite increased (up to 7%), flatulence (up to 3%), vomiting (up to 3%), abdominal distension (up to 2%), abdominal pain (≥1%), gastroenteritis (≥1%)

Genitourinary: Incontinence (up to 2%), anorgasmia (≥1%), impotence (≥1%), urinary frequency (≥1%)

Hematologic: Thrombocytopenia (3%)

Neuromuscular & skeletal: Balance disorder (up to 9%), abnormal gait (up to 8%), weakness (up to 7%), arthralgia (up to 6%), twitching (up to 5%), back pain (up to 4%), muscle spasm (up to 4%), myoclonus (up to 4%), paresthesia (>2%), CPK increased (2%), leg cramps (≥1%), myalgia (≥1%), myasthenia (up to 1%)

Ocular: Visual abnormalities (up to 5%), visual field defect (≥2%), eye disorder (up to 2%), nystagmus (>2%), conjunctivitis (≥1%)

Otic: Otitis media (≥1%), tinnitus (≥1%)

Respiratory: Sinusitis (up to 7%), dyspnea (up to 3%), bronchitis (up to 3%), pharyngolaryngeal pain (up to 3%)

Miscellaneous: Flu-like syndrome (up to 2%), allergic reaction (≥1%)

Dosage Oral: Adults:

Fibromyalgia: Initial: 150 mg/day in divided doses (75 mg 2 times/day); may be increased to 300 mg/day (150 mg 2 times/day) within 1 week based on tolerability and effect; may be further increased to 450 mg/day (225 mg 2 times/day). Maximum dose: 450 mg/day (dosages up to 600 mg/day were evaluated with no significant additional benefit and an increase in adverse effects)

Neuropathic pain (diabetes-associated): Initial: 150 mg/day in divided doses (50 mg 3 times/day); may be increased within 1 week based on tolerability and effect; maximum dose: 300 mg/day (dosages up to 600 mg/day were evaluated with no significant additional benefit and an increase in adverse effects)

Postherpetic neuralgia: Initial: 150 mg/day in divided doses (75 mg 2 times/day or 50 mg 3 times/day); may be increased to 300 mg/day within 1 week based on tolerability and effect; further titration (to 600 mg/day) after 2-4 weeks may be considered in patients who do not experience sufficient relief of pain provided they are able to tolerate pregabalin. Maximum dose: 600 mg/day

Partial-onset seizures (adjunctive therapy): Initial: 150 mg per day in divided doses (75 mg 2 times/day or 50 mg 3 times/day); may be increased based on tolerability and effect (optimal titration schedule has not been defined). Maximum dose: 600 mg/day

Discontinuing therapy: Pregabalin should not be abruptly discontinued; taper dosage over at least 1 week

Dosage adjustment in renal impairment: In renally-impaired patients, dosage adjustment depends on renal function and daily dosage.

Pregabalin Renal Impairment Dosing

Cl_{cr} (mL/minute)	Total Pregabalin Daily Dose (mg/day)				Dosing Frequency
≥60	150	300	450	600	2-3 divided doses
30-60	75	150	225	300	2-3 divided doses
15-30	25-50	75	100-150	150	1-2 divided doses
<15	25	25-50	50-75	75	Single daily dose

Posthemodialysis supplementary dosage (as a single additional dose):
25 mg/day schedule: Single supplementary dose of 25 mg **or** 50 mg
25-50 mg/day schedule: Single supplementary dose of 50 mg **or** 75 mg
50-75 mg/day schedule: Single supplementary dose of 75 mg **or** 100 mg
75 mg/day schedule: Single supplementary dose of 100 mg **or** 150 mg

Mechanism of Action Binds to alpha$_2$-delta subunit of voltage-gated calcium channels within the CNS, inhibiting excitatory neurotransmitter release. Although structurally related to GABA, it does not bind to GABA or benzodiazepine receptors. Exerts antinociceptive and anticonvulsant activity. Decreases symptoms of painful peripheral neuropathies and, as adjunctive therapy in partial seizures, decreases the frequency of seizures.

Contraindications Hypersensitivity to pregabalin or any component of the formulation

Warnings/Precautions Antiepileptics are associated with an increased risk of suicidal behavior/thoughts with use (regardless of indication); patients should be monitored for signs/symptoms of depression, suicidal tendencies, and other unusual behavior changes during therapy and instructed to inform their healthcare provider immediately if symptoms occur.

Angioedema has been reported; may be life threatening; use with caution in patients with a history of angioedema episodes. Concurrent use with other drugs known to cause angioedema (eg, ACE inhibitors) may increase risk. Hypersensitivity reactions, including skin redness, blistering, hives, rash, dyspnea and wheezing have been reported; discontinue treatment of hypersensitivity occurs. May cause CNS depression and/or dizziness, which may impair physical or mental abilities. Patients must be cautioned about performing tasks which require mental alertness (eg, operating machinery or driving). Effects with other sedative drugs or ethanol may be potentiated. Visual disturbances (blurred vision, decreased acuity and visual field changes) have been associated with pregabalin therapy; patients should be instructed to notify their physician if these effects are noted.

Pregabalin has been associated with increases in CPK and rare cases of rhabdomyolysis. Patients should be instructed to notify their prescriber if unexplained muscle pain, tenderness, or weakness, particularly if fever and/or malaise are associated with these symptoms. Use may be associated with weight gain and peripheral edema; use caution in patients with congestive heart failure, hypertension, or diabetes. Effect on weight gain/edema may be additive to thiazolidinedione antidiabetic agent; particularly in patients with prior cardiovascular disease. May decrease platelet count or prolong PR interval.

Has been noted to be tumorigenic (increased incidence of hemangiosarcoma) in animal studies; significance of these findings in humans is unknown. Pregabalin has been associated with discontinuation symptoms following abrupt cessation, and increases in seizure frequency (when used as an antiepileptic) may occur. Should not be discontinued abruptly; dosage tapering over at least 1 week is recommended. Use caution in renal impairment; dosage adjustment required.

Drug Interactions

Avoid Concomitant Use There are no known interactions where it is recommended to avoid concomitant use.

Increased Effect/Toxicity

Pregabalin may increase the levels/effects of: Alcohol (Ethyl); Antidiabetic Agents (Thiazolidinedione); CNS Depressants; Methotrimeprazine

The levels/effects of Pregabalin may be increased by: Droperidol; Methotrimeprazine

Decreased Effect

The levels/effects of Pregabalin may be decreased by: Ketorolac; Ketorolac (Systemic); Mefloquine

Ethanol/Nutrition/Herb Interactions

Ethanol: May increase CNS depression; monitor for increased effects with coadministration. Caution patients about effects.

Herb/Nutraceutical: Avoid valerian, St John's wort, kava kava, gotu kola (may increase CNS depression).

Dietary Considerations May be taken with or without food.

Pharmacodynamics/Kinetics

Onset of Action Pain management: Effects may be noted as early as the first week of therapy

Half-life Elimination 6.3 hours

Time to Peak 1.5 hours (3 hours with food)

Pregnancy Risk Factor C

Lactation Excretion in breast milk unknown/not recommended

Product Availability Lyrica® oral solution: FDA approved December 2009; anticipated availability is currently undetermined

Controlled Substance C-V

Dosage Forms

Capsule, oral:

Lyrica®: 25 mg, 50 mg, 75 mg, 100 mg, 150 mg, 200 mg, 225 mg, 300 mg

References

Hill CM, Balkenohl M, Thomas DW, et al, "Pregabalin in Patients With Postoperative Dental Pain," *Eur J Pain*, 2001, 5(2):119-24.

Prilocaine (PRIL oh kane)

Related Information

Oral Pain *on page 1928*

U.S. Brand Names Citanest® Plain Dental

Canadian Brand Names Citanest® Plain

Generic Availability (U.S.) No

Pharmacologic Category Local Anesthetic

Dental Use Amide-type anesthetic used for local infiltration anesthesia; injection near nerve trunks to produce nerve block

Local Anesthetic/Vasoconstrictor Precautions No information available to require special precautions

Effects on Dental Treatment It is common to misinterpret psychogenic responses to local anesthetic injection as an allergic reaction. Intraoral injections are perceived by many patients as a stressful procedure in dentistry. Common symptoms to this stress are diaphoresis, palpitations, hyperventilation, generalized pallor and a fainting feeling.

Degree of adverse effects in the CNS and cardiovascular system is directly related to blood levels of prilocaine (frequency not defined; more likely to occur after systemic administration rather than infiltration): Bradycardia and reduction in cardiac output, hypersensitivity reactions (may be manifest as dermatologic reactions and edema at injection site), asthmatic syndromes

High blood levels: Anxiety, restlessness, disorientation, confusion, dizziness, tremors, and seizures, followed by CNS depression, resulting in somnolence, unconsciousness and possible respiratory arrest; nausea and vomiting

In some cases, symptoms of CNS stimulation may be absent and the primary CNS effects are somnolence and unconsciousness.

Effects on Bleeding No information available to require special precautions

Adverse Effects Degree of adverse effects in the central nervous system and cardiovascular system are directly related to the blood levels of local anesthetic. The effects below are more likely to occur after systemic administration rather than infiltration.

Cardiovascular: Myocardial effects include a decrease in contraction force as well as a decrease in electrical excitability and myocardial conduction rate resulting in bradycardia and reduction in cardiac output.

Central nervous system: High blood levels result in anxiety, restlessness, disorientation, confusion, dizziness, tremor, and seizure. This is followed by depression of CNS resulting in somnolence, unconsciousness and possible respiratory arrest. Nausea and vomiting may also occur. In some cases, symptoms of CNS stimulation may be absent and the primary CNS effects are somnolence and unconsciousness.

Hypersensitivity reactions: May be manifest as dermatologic reactions and edema at injection site. Asthmatic syndromes have occurred.

Psychogenic reactions: It is common to misinterpret psychogenic responses to local anesthetic injection as an allergic reaction. Intraoral injections are perceived by many patients as a stressful procedure in dentistry. Common symptoms to this stress are diaphoresis, palpitation, hyperventilation, generalized pallor and a fainting feeling

Dental Usual Dosage

Children <10 years: Doses >40 mg (1 mL) as a 4% solution per procedure rarely needed

Children >10 years and Adults: Dental anesthesia, infiltration, or conduction block: Initial: 40-80 mg (1-2 mL) as a 4% solution; up to a maximum of 400 mg (10 mL) as a 4% solution within a 2-hour period. Manufacturer's maximum recommended dose is not more than 600 mg to normal healthy adults. The effective anesthetic dose varies with procedure, intensity of anesthesia needed, duration of anesthesia required and physical condition of the patient. Always use the lowest effective dose along with careful aspiration.

The following numbers of dental carpules (1.8 mL) provide the indicated amounts of prilocaine hydrochloride 4%. See table.

Prilocaine

# of Cartridges (1.8 mL)	mg Prilocaine (4%)
1	72
2	144
3	216
4	288
5	360
6	432
7	504
8	576

Note: Adult and children doses of prilocaine hydrochloride cited from USP Dispensing Information (USP DI), 17th ed, The United States Pharmacopeial Convention, Inc, Rockville, MD, 1997, 139.

Dosage

Children <10 years: Doses >40 mg (1 mL) as a 4% solution per procedure rarely needed

Children >10 years and Adults: Dental anesthesia, infiltration, or conduction block: Initial: 40-80 mg (1-2 mL) as a 4% solution; up to a maximum of 400 mg (10 mL) as a 4% solution within a 2-hour period. Manufacturer's maximum recommended dose is not more than 600 mg to normal healthy adults. The effective anesthetic dose varies with procedure, intensity of anesthesia needed, duration of anesthesia required and physical condition of the patient. Always use the lowest effective dose along with careful aspiration.

Note: Adult and children doses of prilocaine hydrochloride cited from USP Dispensing Information (USP DI), 17th ed, The United States Pharmacopeial Convention, Inc, Rockville, MD, 1997, 139.

Mechanism of Action Local anesthetics bind selectively to the intracellular surface of sodium channels to block influx of sodium into the axon. As a result, depolarization necessary for action potential propagation and subsequent nerve function is prevented. The block at the sodium channel is reversible. When drug diffuses away from the axon, sodium channel function is restored and nerve propagation returns.

Contraindications Hypersensitivity to local anesthetics of the amide type or any component of the formulation

Warnings/Precautions Methemoglobinemia has been reported. Careful and constant monitoring of the patient's state of consciousness should be done following each local anesthetic injection; at such times, restlessness, anxiety, tinnitus, dizziness, blurred vision, tremors, depression, or drowsiness may be early warning signs of CNS toxicity. Treatment is primarily symptomatic and supportive. Intravascular injections should be avoided. Local anesthetics have been associated with rare occurrences of sudden respiratory arrest, seizures, and cardiac arrest. Use with caution in patients with cardiovascular disease or hepatic impairment. Use with caution in acutely ill, debilitated, pediatric or elderly patients. Aspirate the syringe after tissue penetration and before injection to minimize chance of direct vascular injection. Resuscitative equipment, oxygen, and other resuscitative drugs should be available for immediate use.

Drug Interactions

Avoid Concomitant Use There are no known interactions where it is recommended to avoid concomitant use.

Increased Effect/Toxicity There are no known significant interactions involving an increase in effect.

Decreased Effect There are no known significant interactions involving a decrease in effect.

Pharmacodynamics/Kinetics

Onset of Action Infiltration: ~2 minutes; Inferior alveolar nerve block: ~3 minutes

Duration of Action Infiltration: Complete anesthesia for procedures lasting 20 minutes; Inferior alveolar nerve block: ~2.5 hours

Half-life Elimination 10-150 minutes; prolonged with hepatic or renal impairment

Pregnancy Risk Factor B

Breast-Feeding Considerations Usual infiltration doses of prilocaine given to nursing mothers has not been shown to affect the health of the nursing infant.

Dosage Forms

Injection, solution:

Citanest® Plain Dental: 4% [40 mg/mL] (1.8 mL)

References

Budenz AW, "Local Anesthetics in Dentistry: Then and Now," *J Calif Dent Assoc*, 2003, 31(5):388-96.
Dower JS Jr, "A Review of Paresthesia in Association With Administration of Local Anesthesia," *Dent Today*, 2003, 22(2):64-9.
Finder RL and Moore PA, "Adverse Drug Reactions to Local Anesthesia," *Dent Clin North Am*, 2002, 46 (4):747-57, x.
Haas DA, "An Update on Local Anesthetics in Dentistry," *J Can Dent Assoc*, 2002, 68(9):546-51.
Hawkins JM and Moore PA, "Local Anesthesia: Advances in Agents and Techniques," *Dent Clin North Am*, 2002, 46(4):719-32, ix.
"Injectable Local Anesthetics," *J Am Dent Assoc*, 2003, 134(5):628-9.
Jastak JT and Yagiela JA, "Vasoconstrictors and Local Anesthesia: A Review and Rationale for Use," *J Am Dent Assoc*, 1983, 107(4):623-30.
MacKenzie TA and Young ER, "Local Anesthetic Update," *Anesth Prog*, 1993, 40(2):29-34.
Malamed SF, "Allergy and Toxic Reactions to Local Anesthetics," *Dent Today*, 2003, 22(4):114-6, 118-21.
Wahl MJ, Schmitt MM, Overton DA, et al, "Injection Pain of Bupivacaine With Epinephrine vs. Prilocaine Plain," *J Am Dent Assoc*, 2002, 133(12):1652-6.
Wynn RL, "Epinephrine Interactions With Beta-Blockers," *Gen Dent*, 1994, 42(1):16, 18.
Yagiela JA, "Local Anesthetics," *Anesth Prog*, 1991, 38(4-5):128-41.

Prilocaine and Epinephrine (PRIL oh kane & ep i NEF rin)

Related Information

EPINEPHrine (Systemic, Oral Inhalation) *on page 604*
Oral Pain *on page 1928*
Prilocaine *on page 1399*

U.S. Brand Names Citanest® Forte Dental

Canadian Brand Names Citanest® Forte

Generic Availability (U.S.) No

Pharmacologic Category Local Anesthetic

Dental Use Amide-type anesthetic used for local infiltration anesthesia; injection near nerve trunks to produce nerve block

Local Anesthetic/Vasoconstrictor Precautions No information available to require special precautions

Effects on Dental Treatment It is common to misinterpret psychogenic responses to local anesthetic injection as an allergic reaction. Intraoral injections are perceived by many patients as a stressful procedure in dentistry. Common symptoms to this stress are diaphoresis, palpitations, hyperventilation, generalized pallor and a fainting feeling. Patients may exhibit hypersensitivity to bisulfites contained in local anesthetic solution to prevent oxidation of epinephrine. In general, patients reacting to bisulfites have a history of asthma and their airways are hyper-reactive to asthmatic syndrome.

Degree of adverse effects in the CNS and cardiovascular system is directly related to blood levels of prilocaine (frequency not defined; more likely to occur after systemic administration rather than infiltration): Bradycardia and reduction in cardiac output, hypersensitivity reactions (extremely rare; may be manifest as dermatologic reactions and edema at injection site), asthmatic syndromes

High blood levels: Anxiety, restlessness, disorientation, confusion, dizziness, tremors, and seizures, followed by CNS depression, resulting in somnolence, unconsciousness and possible respiratory arrest; nausea and vomiting

In some cases, symptoms of CNS stimulation may be absent and the primary CNS effects are somnolence and unconsciousness.

Effects on Bleeding No information available to require special precautions

Adverse Effects Degree of adverse effects in the CNS and cardiovascular system are directly related to the blood levels of prilocaine. The effects below are more likely to occur after systemic administration rather than infiltration.

Cardiovascular: Myocardial effects include a decrease in contraction force as well as a decrease in electrical excitability and myocardial conduction rate resulting in bradycardia and reduction in cardiac output.

Central nervous system: High blood levels result in anxiety, restlessness, disorientation, confusion, dizziness, tremor and seizure. This is followed by depression of CNS resulting in somnolence, unconsciousness and possible respiratory arrest. Nausea and vomiting may also occur. In some cases, symptoms of CNS stimulation may be absent and the primary CNS effects are somnolence and unconsciousness.

Hypersensitivity reactions: Extremely rare, but may be manifest as dermatologic reactions and edema at injection site. Asthmatic syndromes have occurred. Patients may exhibit hypersensitivity to bisulfites contained in local anesthetic solution to prevent oxidation of epinephrine. In general, patients reacting to bisulfites have a history of asthma and their airways are hyper-reactive to asthmatic syndrome.

Psychogenic reactions: It is common to misinterpret psychogenic responses to local anesthetic injection as an allergic reaction. Intraoral injections are perceived by many patients as a stressful procedure in dentistry. Common symptoms to this stress are diaphoresis, palpitation, hyperventilation, generalized pallor, and a fainting feeling.

Dental Usual Dosage

Children <10 years: Doses >40 mg (1 mL) of prilocaine hydrochloride as a 4% solution with epinephrine 1:200,000 are rarely needed

Children >10 years and Adults: Dental anesthesia, infiltration, or conduction block: Initial: 40-80 mg (1-2 mL) of prilocaine hydrochloride as a 4% solution with epinephrine 1:200,000; up to a maximum of 400 mg (10 mL) of prilocaine hydrochloride within a 2-hour period. The effective anesthetic dose varies with procedure, intensity of anesthesia needed, duration of anesthesia required, and physical condition of the patient. Always use the lowest effective dose along with careful aspiration.

The following numbers of dental carpules (1.8 mL) provide the indicated amounts of prilocaine hydrochloride 4% and epinephrine 1:200,000. See table.

Prilocaine With Epinephrine

# of Cartridges (1.8 mL)	mg Prilocaine (4%)	mg Vasoconstrictor (Epinephrine 1:200,000)
1	72	0.009
2	144	0.018
3	216	0.027
4	288	0.036
5	360	0.045
6	432	0.054
7	504	0.063
8	576	0.072

Note: Adult and pediatric doses of prilocaine hydrochloride with epinephrine cited from USP Dispensing Information (USP DI), 17th ed, The United States Pharmacopeial Convention, Inc, Rockville, MD, 1997, 140.

Dosage

Children <10 years: Doses >40 mg (1 mL) of prilocaine hydrochloride as a 4% solution with epinephrine 1:200,000 are rarely needed

Children >10 years and Adults: Dental anesthesia, infiltration, or conduction block: Initial: 40-80 mg (1-2 mL) of prilocaine hydrochloride as a 4% solution with epinephrine 1:200,000; up to a maximum of 400 mg (10 mL) of prilocaine hydrochloride within a 2-hour period. The effective anesthetic dose varies with procedure, intensity of anesthesia needed, duration of anesthesia required, and physical condition of the patient. Always use the lowest effective dose along with careful aspiration.

Note: Adult and pediatric doses of prilocaine hydrochloride with epinephrine cited from USP Dispensing Information (USP DI), 17th ed, The United States Pharmacopeial Convention, Inc, Rockville, MD, 1997, 140.

Mechanism of Action Local anesthetics bind selectively to the intracellular surface of sodium channels to block influx of sodium into the axon. As a result, depolarization necessary for action potential propagation and subsequent nerve function is prevented. The block at the sodium channel is reversible. When drug diffuses away from the axon, sodium channel function is restored and nerve propagation returns.

Epinephrine prolongs the duration of the anesthetic actions of prilocaine by causing vasoconstriction (alpha-adrenergic receptor agonist) of the vasculature surrounding the nerve axons. This prevents the diffusion of prilocaine away from the nerves resulting in a longer retention in the axon.

Contraindications Hypersensitivity to local anesthetics of the amide-type or any component of the formulation

Warnings/Precautions Should be avoided in patients with uncontrolled hyperthyroidism. Should be used in minimal amounts in patients with significant cardiovascular problems (because of epinephrine component). Aspirate the syringe after tissue penetration and before injection to minimize chance of direct vascular injection

Drug Interactions

Avoid Concomitant Use

Avoid concomitant use of Prilocaine and Epinephrine with any of the following: Iobenguane I 123; Lurasidone

Increased Effect/Toxicity

Prilocaine and Epinephrine may increase the levels/effects of: Bromocriptine; Lurasidone; Sympathomimetics

The levels/effects of Prilocaine and Epinephrine may be increased by: Antacids; Atomoxetine; Beta-Blockers; Cannabinoids; Carbonic Anhydrase Inhibitors; COMT Inhibitors; Inhalational Anesthetics; MAO Inhibitors; Serotonin/Norepinephrine Reuptake Inhibitors; Tricyclic Antidepressants

Decreased Effect

Prilocaine and Epinephrine may decrease the levels/effects of: Benzylpenicilloyl Polylysine; Iobenguane I 123

The levels/effects of Prilocaine and Epinephrine may be decreased by: Spironolactone

Pharmacodynamics/Kinetics

Onset of Action Infiltration: <2 minutes; Inferior alveolar nerve block: <3 minutes

Duration of Action Infiltration: 2.25 hours; Inferior alveolar nerve block: 3 hours

Pregnancy Risk Factor C

Breast-Feeding Considerations Usual infiltration doses of prilocaine with epinephrine given to nursing mothers has not been shown to affect the health of the nursing infant.

Dosage Forms

Injection, solution [for dental use]:

Citanest® Forte Dental: Prilocaine 4% and epinephrine 1:200,000 (1.8 mL)

Dental Comment Oral paresthesia: The occurrence of oral paresthesia associated with 4% solutions of prilocaine or articaine, although rare, continue to be slightly more frequent than other local anesthetics. From 1999-2008, there were 182 cases of nonsurgical paresthesia (Gaffen, 2009). Of the cases, 172 involved mandibular block injection only. Another eight cases involved mandibular block combined with at least one other type of anesthetic injection. A single case involved infiltration around tooth number 35 and the final case involved infiltration and intraligamentary injection in the maxillary anterior region.

A 2010 report, reviewed adverse events submitted voluntarily over a 10-year period involving the dental local anesthetics articaine, bupivacaine, lidocaine, mepivacaine, and prilocaine in the United States. Prilocaine reported incidence: One case per 2,070,678 cartridges sold. The reported incidence of paresthesia was one case for 13,800,970 cartridges of all local anesthetics sold in the U.S. (Garisto, 2010).

References

Ayoub ST and Coleman AE, "A Review of Local Anesthetics," *Gen Dent*, 1992, 40(4):285-7, 289-90.
Blanton PL and Roda RS, "The Anatomy of Local Anesthesia," *J Calif Dent Assoc*, 1995, 23(4):55-65.
Budenz AW, "Local Anesthetics in Dentistry: Then and Now," *J Calif Dent Assoc*, 2003, 31(5):388-96.
Dower JS Jr, "A Review of Paresthesia in Association With Administration of Local Anesthesia," *Dent Today*, 2003, 22(2):64-9.
Finder RL and Moore PA, "Adverse Drug Reactions to Local Anesthesia," *Dent Clin North Am*, 2002, 46 (4):747-57, x.
Gaffen AS and Haas DA, "Retrospective Review of Voluntary Reports of Nonsurgical Paresthesia in Dentistry," *J Can Dent Assoc*, 2009, 75(8):579.
Garisto GA, Gaffen AS, Lawrence HP, et al, "Occurrence of Paresthesia After Dental Local Anesthetic Administration in the United States," *J Am Dent Assoc*, 2010, 141(7):836-44.
Haas DA, "An Update on Local Anesthetics in Dentistry," *J Can Dent Assoc*, 2002, 68(9):546-51.
Hawkins JM and Moore PA, "Local Anesthesia: Advances in Agents and Techniques," *Dent Clin North Am*, 2002, 46(4):719-32, ix.
"Injectable Local Anesthetics," *J Am Dent Assoc*, 2003, 134(5):628-9.
Jastak JT and Yagiela JA, "Vasoconstrictors and Local Anesthesia: A Review and Rationale for Use," *J Am Dent Assoc*, 1983, 107(4):623-30.
MacKenzie TA and Young ER, "Local Anesthetic Update," *Anesth Prog*, 1993, 40(2):29-34.
Malamed SF, "Allergy and Toxic Reactions to Local Anesthetics," *Dent Today*, 2003, 22(4):114-6, 118-21.
Wynn RL, "Epinephrine Interactions With Beta-Blockers," *Gen Dent*, 1994, 42(1):16, 18.
Yagiela JA, "Local Anesthetics," *Anesth Prog*, 1991, 38(4-5):128-41.
Yagiela JA, "Vasoconstrictor Agents for Local Anesthesia," *Anesth Prog*, 1995, 42(3-4):116-20.

Primaquine (PRIM a kween)

Pharmacologic Category Aminoquinoline (Antimalarial)

Use Prevention of relapse of *P. vivax* malaria

Unlabeled/Investigational Use Prevention of relapse of *P. ovale* malaria; treatment of *Pneumocystis jiroveci* pneumonia (PCP); prevention of chloroquine-resistant malaria

Local Anesthetic/Vasoconstrictor Precautions No information available to require special precautions

Effects on Dental Treatment No significant effects or complications reported

Effects on Bleeding No information available to require special precautions.

Adverse Effects Frequency not defined.

Cardiovascular: Arrhythmias (rare)

Central nervous system: Headache

Dermatologic: Pruritus

Gastrointestinal: Abdominal cramps, dyspepsia, nausea, vomiting

Hematologic: Agranulocytosis, anemia, hemolytic anemia (in patients with G6PD deficiency), leukopenia, leukocytosis, methemoglobinemia (in NADH-methemoglobin reductase-deficient individuals)

Ocular: Interference with visual accommodation

General Dosage Range Oral:

Children: 0.5 mg/kg once daily for 14 days (maximum dose: 30 mg/day); Alternative regimen (recommended for mild G6PD deficiency): 45 mg once weekly for 8 weeks

Adults: 30 mg once daily for 14 days; Alternative regimen (recommended for mild G6PD deficiency): 45 mg once weekly for 8 weeks

Mechanism of Action Eliminates the primary tissue exoerythrocytic forms of *P. falciparum*; disrupts mitochondria and binds to DNA

Pharmacodynamics/Kinetics

Half-life Elimination 3.7-9.6 hours

Time to Peak Serum: 1-2 hours

Primidone (PRI mi done)

U.S. Brand Names Mysoline®

Canadian Brand Names Apo-Primidone®

Pharmacologic Category Anticonvulsant, Miscellaneous; Barbiturate

Use Management of grand mal, psychomotor, and focal seizures

Unlabeled/Investigational Use Benign familial tremor (essential tremor)

Local Anesthetic/Vasoconstrictor Precautions No information available to require special precautions

Effects on Dental Treatment No significant effects or complications reported

Effects on Bleeding No information available to require special precautions

Adverse Effects Frequency not defined.

Central nervous system: Ataxia, drowsiness, emotional disturbances, fatigue, hyperirritability, suicidal ideation, vertigo

Dermatologic: Morbilliform skin eruptions

Gastrointestinal: Anorexia, nausea, vomiting

Genitourinary: Impotence

Hematologic: Agranulocytosis, granulocytopenia, megaloblastic anemia (idiosyncratic), red cell aplasia/hypoplasia

Ocular: Diplopia, nystagmus

General Dosage Range Dosage adjustment recommended in patients with renal impairment

Oral:

Children <8 years: Initial: 50 mg once daily at bedtime; Maintenance: 375-750 mg/day (10-25 mg/kg/day) in 3-4 divided doses

Children ≥8 years and Adults: Initial: 100-125 mg/day at bedtime; Maintenance: 750-1500 mg/day in 3-4 divided doses (maximum: 2 g/day)

Mechanism of Action Decreases neuron excitability, raises seizure threshold similar to phenobarbital; primidone has two active metabolites, phenobarbital and phenylethylmalonamide (PEMA); PEMA may enhance the activity of phenobarbital

Pharmacodynamics/Kinetics

Half-life Elimination Age dependent: Primidone: Mean: 5-15 hours (variable); PEMA: 16 hours (variable)

Time to Peak Serum:~3 hours (variable)

Probenecid (proe BEN e sid)

Canadian Brand Names Benuryl™

Pharmacologic Category Uricosuric Agent

Use Prevention of hyperuricemia associated with gout or gouty arthritis; prolongation and elevation of beta-lactam plasma levels

Local Anesthetic/Vasoconstrictor Precautions No information available to require special precautions

Effects on Dental Treatment Key adverse event(s) related to dental treatment: Sore gums.

Effects on Bleeding No information available to require special precautions

Adverse Effects Frequency not defined.

Cardiovascular: Flushing
Central nervous system: Dizziness, fever, headache
Dermatologic: Alopecia, dermatitis, pruritus, rash
Gastrointestinal: Anorexia, nausea, sore gums, vomiting
Genitourinary: Hematuria, polyuria
Hematologic: Anemia, aplastic anemia, hemolytic anemia, leukopenia
Hepatic: Hepatic necrosis
Neuromuscular & skeletal: Costovertebral pain, gouty arthritis (acute)
Renal: Nephrotic syndrome, renal colic
Miscellaneous: Anaphylaxis, hypersensitivity

General Dosage Range Dosage adjustment recommended in patients with renal impairment

Oral:

Children 2-14 years: Prolong penicillin serum levels: Initial: 25 mg/kg then 40 mg/kg/day given 4 times/day (maximum: 500 mg/dose)

Children >45 kg and Adults:

Gonorrhea, PID: 1 g as a single dose
Gout: Initial: 250 mg twice daily (maximum: 2-3 g/day)
Neurosyphilis: 500 mg 4 times/day for 10-14 days
Prolong PCN levels: 500 mg 4 times/day

Mechanism of Action Competitively inhibits the reabsorption of uric acid at the proximal convoluted tubule, thereby promoting its excretion and reducing serum uric acid levels; increases plasma levels of weak organic acids (penicillins, cephalosporins, or other beta-lactam antibiotics) by competitively inhibiting their renal tubular secretion

Pharmacodynamics/Kinetics

Onset of Action Effect on penicillin levels: 2 hours

Half-life Elimination Dose dependent: Normal renal function: 6-12 hours

Time to Peak Serum: 2-4 hours

Procainamide (pro KANE a mide)

Related Information

Cardiovascular Diseases *on page 1848*
Clinical Risk Related to Drugs Prolonging QT Interval *on page 1872*

Canadian Brand Names Apo-Procainamide®; Procainamide Hydrochloride Injection, USP; Procan SR®

Pharmacologic Category Antiarrhythmic Agent, Class Ia

Use

Intravenous: Treatment of life-threatening ventricular arrhythmias

Oral (Canadian labeling; not available in U.S.): Treatment of supraventricular arrhythmias. **Note:** In the treatment of atrial fibrillation, use only when preferred treatment is ineffective or cannot be used. Use in paroxysmal atrial tachycardia when reflex stimulation or other measures are ineffective.

Unlabeled/Investigational Use

Paroxysmal supraventricular tachycardia (PSVT); prevent recurrence of ventricular tachycardia; symptomatic premature ventricular contractions

ACLS guidelines: I.V.: Treatment of the following arrhythmias in patients with preserved left ventricular function: Stable monomorphic VT; pre-excited atrial fibrillation; stable wide complex regular tachycardia (likely VT)

PALS guidelines: I.V.: Tachycardia with pulses and poor perfusion (probable SVT [unresponsive to vagal maneuvers and adenosine or synchronized cardioversion]; probable VT [unresponsive to synchronized cardioversion or adenosine])

Local Anesthetic/Vasoconstrictor Precautions Procainamide is one of the drugs confirmed to prolong the QT interval and is accepted as having a risk of causing torsade de pointes. The risk of drug-induced torsade de pointes is extremely low when a single QT interval prolonging drug is prescribed. In terms of epinephrine, it is not known what effect vasoconstrictors in the local anesthetic regimen will have in patients with a known history of congenital prolonged QT interval or in patients taking any medication that prolongs the QT interval. Until more information is obtained, it is suggested that the clinician consult with the physician prior to the

use of a vasoconstrictor in suspected patients, and that the vasoconstrictor (epinephrine, mepivacaine and levonordefrin [Carbocaine® 2% with Neo-Cobefrin®]) be used with caution.

Effects on Dental Treatment Key adverse event(s) related to dental treatment: Taste disorder.

Effects on Bleeding No information available to require special precautions

Adverse Effects >1%:

Cardiovascular: Hypotension (I.V. up to 5%)

Dermatologic: Rash

Gastrointestinal: Diarrhea (oral: 3% to 4%), nausea (oral: 3% to 4%), taste disorder (oral: 3% to 4%), vomiting (oral: 3% to 4%)

Miscellaneous: Positive ANA (≤50%), SLE-like syndrome (≤30%, increased incidence with long-term therapy or slow acetylators; syndrome may include abdominal pain, arthralgia, arthritis, chills, fever, hepatomegaly, myalgia, pericarditis, pleural effusion, pulmonary infiltrates, rash)

General Dosage Range Dosage adjustment recommended in patients with hepatic or renal impairment

I.M.:

Children: 20-30 mg/kg/day divided every 4-6 hours (maximum: 4 g/day)

Adults: 50 mg/kg/day divided every 3-6 hours **or** 0.5-1 g every 4-8 hours

I.V.:

Children: Loading dose: 3-6 mg/kg/dose over 5 minutes (maximum: 100 mg/dose), may repeat every 5-10 minutes to maximum of 15 mg/kg/load; Infusion: 20-80 mcg/kg/minute (maximum: 2 g/day)

Adults: Loading dose: 15-18 mg/kg administered as slow infusion over 25-30 minutes **or** 100 mg/dose at a rate not to exceed 50 mg/minute repeated every 5 minutes as needed (maximum total dose: 1 g); Infusion: 1-4 mg/minute

Mechanism of Action Decreases myocardial excitability and conduction velocity and may depress myocardial contractility, by increasing the electrical stimulation threshold of ventricle, His-Purkinje system and through direct cardiac effects

Pharmacodynamics/Kinetics

Onset of Action I.M. 10-30 minutes

Half-life Elimination

Procainamide (hepatic acetylator, phenotype, cardiac and renal function dependent): Children: 1.7 hours; Adults: 2.5-4.7 hours; Anephric: 11 hours

NAPA (renal function dependent): Children: 6 hours; Adults: 6-8 hours; Anephric: 42 hours

Time to Peak Serum: I.M.: 15-60 minutes

Pregnancy Risk Factor C

Dental Comment Procainamide is known to prolong the QT interval. The QT interval is measured as the time and distance between the Q point of the QRS complex and the end of the T wave in the ECG tracing. After adjustment for heart rate, the QT interval is defined as prolonged if it is more than 450 msec in men and 460 msec in women. A long QT syndrome was first described in the 1950s and 60s as a congenital syndrome involving QT interval prolongation and syncope and sudden death. Some of the congenital long QT syndromes were characterized by a peculiar electrocardiographic appearance of the QRS complex involving a premature atria beat followed by a pause, then a subsequent sinus beat showing marked QT prolongation and deformity. This type of cardiac arrhythmia was originally termed "torsade de pointes" (translated from the French as "twisting of the points"). Procainamide is considered as having a risk of causing torsade de pointes. Since it is not known what effect vasoconstrictors in the local anesthetic regimen will have in patients with a known history of congenital prolonged QT interval or in patients taking any medication that prolongs the QT interval, a medical consult is suggested.

Procarbazine (proe KAR ba zeen)

U.S. Brand Names Matulane®

Canadian Brand Names Matulane®; Natulan®

Pharmacologic Category Antineoplastic Agent, Alkylating Agent

Use Treatment of Hodgkin's disease

Unlabeled/Investigational Use Treatment of non-Hodgkin's lymphoma, brain tumors

Local Anesthetic/Vasoconstrictor Precautions No information available to require special precautions

Effects on Dental Treatment Key adverse event(s) related to dental treatment: Xerostomia (normal salivary flow resumes upon discontinuation), stomatitis, and dysphagia.

Effects on Bleeding Chemotherapy may result in significant myelosuppression, potentially including significant reduction in platelet counts and altered hemostasis. In patients who are under active treatment with these agents, medical consult is suggested.

Adverse Effects Most frequencies not defined.

Cardiovascular: Edema, flushing, hypotension, syncope, tachycardia

Central nervous system: Apprehension, ataxia, chills, coma, confusion, depression, dizziness, drowsiness, fatigue, fever, hallucination, headache, insomnia, lethargy, nervousness, nightmares, pain, seizure, slurred speech

Dermatologic: Alopecia, dermatitis, hyperpigmentation, petechiae, pruritus, purpura, rash, urticaria

Endocrine & metabolic: Gynecomastia (in prepubertal and early pubertal males)

Hematologic: Eosinophilia; hemolysis (in patients with G6PD deficiency); hemolytic anemia; myelosuppression (leukopenia, anemia, thrombocytopenia); pancytopenia

Gastrointestinal: Abdominal pain, anorexia, constipation, diarrhea, dysphagia, hematemesis, melena; nausea and vomiting ([60% to 90%], increasing the dose in a stepwise fashion over several days may minimize); stomatitis, xerostomia

Genitourinary: Azoospermia (reported with combination chemotherapy), hematuria, nocturia, polyuria, reproductive dysfunction (>10%)

Hepatic: Hepatic dysfunction, jaundice

Neuromuscular & skeletal: Arthralgia, falling, foot drop, myalgia, neuropathy, paresthesia, reflex diminished, tremor, unsteadiness, weakness

Ocular: Diplopia, inability to focus, nystagmus, papilledema, photophobia, retinal hemorrhage

Otic: Hearing loss

Respiratory: Cough, epistaxis, hemoptysis, hoarseness, pleural effusion, pneumonitis, pulmonary toxicity (<1%)

Miscellaneous: Allergic reaction, diaphoresis, herpes, infection, secondary malignancies (2% to 15%; reported with combination therapy)

General Dosage Range Dosage adjustment recommended in patients with hepatic impairment

Oral:

Children: 100 mg/m^2/day for 14 days and repeated every 4 weeks

Adults: Initial: 2-4 mg/kg/day in single or divided doses for 7 days, then increase dose to 4-6 mg/kg/day; Maintenance: 1-2 mg/kg/day

Mechanism of Action Mechanism of action is not clear, methylating of nucleic acids; inhibits DNA, RNA, and protein synthesis; may damage DNA directly and suppresses mitosis; metabolic activation required by host

Pharmacodynamics/Kinetics

Half-life Elimination 1 hour

Time to Peak 1 hour

Pregnancy Risk Factor D

Prochlorperazine (proe klor PER a zeen)

Related Information

Management of the Patient With Anxiety or Depression *on page 1968*

U.S. Brand Names Compro®

Canadian Brand Names Apo-Prochlorperazine®; Nu-Prochlor; Stemetil®

Generic Availability (U.S.) Yes

Pharmacologic Category Antiemetic; Antipsychotic Agent, Typical, Phenothiazine

Use Management of nausea and vomiting; psychotic disorders, including schizophrenia and anxiety

Unlabeled/Investigational Use Behavioral syndromes in dementia; psychosis/agitation related to Alzheimer's dementia

Local Anesthetic/Vasoconstrictor Precautions May lower seizure threshold; use caution when administering prochlorperazine in combination with other agents that reduce seizure threshold (ie, local anesthetics). Due to prochlorperazine induced alpha-adrenergic blockade, administration of local anesthetics containing vasoconstrictors (epinephrine or levonordefrin), causes unopposed stimulation of beta-adrenergic receptors in heart and peripheral blood vessels that may result in tachycardia, peripheral vasodilation, or hypotension. Effects on blood pressure are greater in combination with epinephrine than levonordefrin.

Effects on Dental Treatment Key adverse event(s) related to dental treatment: Xerostomia and changes in salivation (normal salivary flow resumes upon discontinuation).

Significant hypotension may occur, especially when the drug is administered parenterally or following administration of local anesthetics containing vasoconstrictors (ie, epinephrine or levonordefrin); orthostatic hypotension is due to alpha-receptor blockade, the elderly are at greater risk for orthostatic hypotension.

Significant sedation can occur and may be increased in the elderly and in patients taking other CNS depressants (ie, opioid analgesics or benzodiazepines).

Extrapyramidal effects including akathisia (motor restlessness), acute dystonia (spasmodic contractures), pseudoparkinsonism, and tardive dyskinesia can occur with 1 dose. These effects are more likely in the elderly, patients taking other dopamine antagonists (including antipsychotic agents and some antiemetic agents), and patients with Parkinson's disease.

Due to increased risk of adverse effects and drug interactions especially with opioid analgesics, reserve use for patients with moderate-to-severe postoperative nausea and vomiting, who cannot afford ondansetron, and for whom promethazine did not provide adequate control.

Effects on Bleeding No information available to require special precautions

Adverse Effects Reported with prochlorperazine or other phenothiazines. Frequency not defined.

Cardiovascular: Cardiac arrest, hypotension, peripheral edema, Q-wave distortions, T-wave distortions

Central nervous system: Agitation, catatonia, cerebral edema, cough reflex suppressed, dizziness, drowsiness, fever (mild - I.M.), headache, hyperactivity, hyperpyrexia, impairment of temperature regulation, insomnia, neuroleptic malignant syndrome (NMS), paradoxical excitement, restlessness, seizure

Dermatologic: Angioedema, contact dermatitis, discoloration of skin (blue-gray), epithelial keratopathy, erythema, eczema, exfoliative dermatitis (injectable), itching, photosensitivity, rash, skin pigmentation, urticaria

Endocrine & metabolic: Amenorrhea, breast enlargement, galactorrhea, gynecomastia, glucosuria, hyperglycemia, hypoglycemia, lactation, libido (changes in), menstrual irregularity, SIADH

Gastrointestinal: Appetite increased, atonic colon, constipation, ileus, nausea, weight gain, xerostomia

Genitourinary: Ejaculating dysfunction, ejaculatory disturbances, impotence, incontinence, polyuria, priapism, urinary retention, urination difficulty

Hematologic: Agranulocytosis, aplastic anemia, eosinophilia, hemolytic anemia, leukopenia, pancytopenia, thrombocytopenic purpura

Hepatic: Biliary stasis, cholestatic jaundice, hepatotoxicity

Neuromuscular & skeletal: Dystonias (torticollis, opisthotonos, carpopedal spasm, trismus, oculogyric crisis, protrusion of tongue); extrapyramidal symptoms (pseudoparkinsonism, akathisia, dystonias, tardive dyskinesia); SLE-like syndrome, tremor

Ocular: blurred vision, cornea and lens changes, lenticular/corneal deposits, miosis, mydriasis, pigmentary retinopathy

Respiratory: Asthma, laryngeal edema, nasal congestion

Miscellaneous: Allergic reactions, diaphoresis

Dosage

Antiemetic: Children (therapy >1 day usually not required): **Note:** Not recommended for use in children <9 kg or <2 years:

Oral, rectal: >9 kg: 0.4 mg/kg/24 hours in 3-4 divided doses; **or**

9-13 kg: 2.5 mg every 12-24 hours as needed; maximum: 7.5 mg/day

13.1-17 kg: 2.5 mg every 8-12 hours as needed; maximum: 10 mg/day

17.1-37 kg: 2.5 mg every 8 hours or 5 mg every 12 hours as needed; maximum: 15 mg/day

I.M.: 0.13 mg/kg/dose; change to oral as soon as possible

Antiemetic: Adults:

Oral (tablet): 5-10 mg 3-4 times/day; usual maximum: 40 mg/day; larger doses may rarely be required

I.M. (deep): 5-10 mg every 3-4 hours; usual maximum: 40 mg/day

I.V.: 2.5-10 mg; maximum 10 mg/dose or 40 mg/day; may repeat dose every 3-4 hours as needed

Rectal: 25 mg twice daily

Surgical nausea/vomiting: Adults: **Note:** Should not exceed 40 mg/day

I.M.: 5-10 mg 1-2 hours before induction or to control symptoms during or after surgery; may repeat once if necessary

I.V. (administer slow IVP <5 mg/minute): 5-10 mg 15-30 minutes before induction or to control symptoms during or after surgery; may repeat once if necessary

Rectal (unlabeled use): 25 mg

Antipsychotic:

Children 2-12 years (not recommended in children <9 kg or <2 years):

Oral, rectal: 2.5 mg 2-3 times/day; do not give more than 10 mg the first day; increase dosage as needed to maximum daily dose of 20 mg for 2-5 years and 25 mg for 6-12 years

I.M.: 0.13 mg/kg/dose; change to oral as soon as possible

Adults:

Oral: 5-10 mg 3-4 times/day; titrate dose slowly every 2-3 days; doses up to 150 mg/day may be required in some patients for treatment of severe disturbances

I.M.: Initial: 10-20 mg; if necessary repeat initial dose every 1-4 hours to gain control; more than 3-4 doses are rarely needed. If parenteral administration is still required; give 10-20 mg every 4-6 hours; change to oral as soon as possible.

Nonpsychotic anxiety: Oral (tablet): Adults: Usual dose: 15-20 mg/day in divided doses; do not give doses >20 mg/day or for longer than 12 weeks

Elderly: Behavioral symptoms associated with dementia (unlabeled use): Initial: 2.5-5 mg 1-2 times/day; increase dose at 4- to 7-day intervals by 2.5-5 mg/day; increase dosing intervals (twice daily, 3 times/day, etc) as necessary to control response or side effects; maximum daily dose should probably not exceed 75 mg in elderly; gradual increases (titration) may prevent some side effects or decrease their severity

Mechanism of Action Prochlorperazine is a piperazine phenothiazine antipsychotic which blocks postsynaptic mesolimbic dopaminergic D_1 and D_2 receptors in the brain, including the chemoreceptor trigger zone; exhibits a strong alpha-adrenergic and anticholinergic blocking effect and depresses the release of hypothalamic and hypophyseal hormones; believed to depress the reticular activating system, thus affecting basal metabolism, body temperature, wakefulness, vasomotor tone and emesis

Contraindications Hypersensitivity to prochlorperazine or any component of the formulation (cross-reactivity between phenothiazines may occur); severe CNS depression; coma; pediatric surgery; Reye's syndrome; should not be used in children <2 years of age or <9 kg

Warnings/Precautions **[U.S. Boxed Warning]: Elderly patients with dementia-related psychosis treated with antipsychotics are at an increased risk of death compared to placebo.** Most deaths appeared to be either cardiovascular (eg, heart failure, sudden death) or infectious (eg, pneumonia) in nature. Prochlorperazine is not approved for the treatment of dementia-related psychosis.

Leukopenia, neutropenia, and agranulocytosis (sometimes fatal) have been reported in clinical trials and postmarketing reports with antipsychotic use; presence of risk factors (eg, pre-existing low WBC or history of drug-induced leuko-/neutropenia) should prompt periodic blood count assessment. Discontinue therapy at first signs of blood dyscrasias or if absolute neutrophil count <1000/mm^3.

May be sedating; use with caution in disorders where CNS depression is a feature. May obscure intestinal obstruction or brain tumor. May impair physical or mental abilities. Effects with other sedative drugs or ethanol may be potentiated. Use with caution in Parkinson's disease; hemodynamic instability; predisposition to seizures; subcortical brain damage; and in severe cardiac, hepatic, or renal disease. May alter temperature regulation or mask toxicity of other drugs. Use caution with exposure to heat. May alter cardiac conduction. May cause orthostatic hypotension. Hypotension may occur following administration, particularly when parenteral form is used or in high dosages. Antipsychotic use has been associated with esophageal dysmotility and aspiration; use with caution in patients at risk of pneumonia (ie, Alzheimer's disease).

May cause pigmentary retinopathy, and lenticular and corneal deposits, particularly with prolonged therapy. Use associated with increased prolactin levels; clinical significance of hyperprolactinemia in patients with breast cancer or other prolactin-dependent tumors is unknown.

Phenothiazines may cause anticholinergic effects; therefore, they should be used with caution in patients with decreased gastrointestinal motility, urinary retention, BPH, xerostomia, or visual problems. Conditions which also may be exacerbated by cholinergic blockade include narrow-angle glaucoma and worsening of myasthenia gravis. May cause extrapyramidal symptoms (EPS), including pseudoparkinsonism, acute dystonic reactions, akathisia, and tardive dyskinesia. Risk of dystonia (and possibly other EPS) may be greater with increased doses, use of conventional antipsychotics, males, and younger patients. Use caution in the elderly. Children with acute illness or dehydration are more susceptible to neuromuscular reactions; use cautiously. May be associated with neuroleptic malignant syndrome (NMS). Injection contains benzyl alcohol which has been associated with "gasping syndrome" in neonates.

Drug Interactions

Avoid Concomitant Use

Avoid concomitant use of Prochlorperazine with any of the following: Dofetilide; Metoclopramide

Increased Effect/Toxicity

Prochlorperazine may increase the levels/effects of: Alcohol (Ethyl); Analgesics (Opioid); Anticholinergics; Anti-Parkinson's Agents (Dopamine Agonist); Beta-Blockers; CNS Depressants; Dofetilide; Methotrimeprazine; Methylphenidate

The levels/effects of Prochlorperazine may be increased by: Acetylcholinesterase Inhibitors (Central); Antimalarial Agents; Beta-Blockers; Deferoxamine; Droperidol; Lithium formulations; Methotrimeprazine; Methylphenidate; Metoclopramide; Pramlintide; Tetrabenazine

Decreased Effect

Prochlorperazine may decrease the levels/effects of: Amphetamines; Quinagolide

The levels/effects of Prochlorperazine may be decreased by: Antacids; Anti-Parkinson's Agents (Dopamine Agonist); Lithium formulations

Ethanol/Nutrition/Herb Interactions

Ethanol: May increase CNS depression; monitor for increased effects with coadministration. Caution patients about effects.

Food: Limit caffeine.

Herb/Nutraceutical: Avoid dong quai, St John's wort (may also cause photosensitization). Avoid kava kava, gotu kola, valerian, St John's wort (may increase CNS depression).

Dietary Considerations Increase dietary intake of riboflavin; should be administered with food or water. Rectal suppositories may contain coconut and palm oil.

Pharmacodynamics/Kinetics

Onset of Action Oral: 30-40 minutes; I.M.: 10-20 minutes; Rectal: ~60 minutes

Peak antiemetic effect: I.V.: 30-60 minutes

Duration of Action Rectal: 12 hours; Oral: 3-4 hours; I.M., I.V.: Adults: 4-6 hours; I.M.: Children: 12 hours

Half-life Elimination Oral: 6-10 hours (single dose), 14-22 hours (repeated dosing); I.V.: 6-10 hours

Lactation Excretion in breast milk unknown/use caution

Breast-Feeding Considerations Other phenothiazines are excreted in human milk; excretion of prochlorperazine is not known.

Dosage Forms

Injection, solution: 5 mg/mL (2 mL, 10 mL)

Suppository, rectal: 25 mg (12s)

Compro®: 25 mg (12s)

Tablet, oral: 5 mg, 10 mg

Procyclidine (proe SYE kli deen)

Canadian Brand Names PHL-Procyclidine; PMS-Procyclidine

Pharmacologic Category Anti-Parkinson's Agent, Anticholinergic; Anticholinergic Agent

Use Relieves symptoms of parkinsonian syndrome and drug-induced extrapyramidal symptoms

Local Anesthetic/Vasoconstrictor Precautions No information available to require special precautions

Effects on Dental Treatment Key adverse event(s) related to dental treatment: Xerostomia (normal salivary flow resumes upon discontinuation) and dry throat and nose. Prolonged use of antidyskinetics may decrease or inhibit salivary flow, contributing to discomfort and dental disease (ie, caries, oral candidiasis, and periodontal disease).

Effects on Bleeding No information available to require special precautions

Adverse Effects Frequency not defined.

Cardiovascular: Tachycardia

Central nervous system: Acute toxic psychosis, agitation, concentration impaired, confusion, disorientation, giddiness, hallucinations, lightheadedness, memory impaired, restlessness, slurred speech

Dermatologic: Rash

Gastrointestinal: Constipation, epigastric distress, nausea, parotitis (secondary to xerostomia), vomiting, xerostomia

Genitourinary: Dysuria

Neuromuscular & skeletal: Weakness

Ocular: Blurred vision, mydriasis

Miscellaneous: Allergic reaction

General Dosage Range Oral:

Adults: Initial: 2.5 mg 3 times/day; Maintenance: Up to 30 mg/day in 3-4 divided doses

Elderly: Initial: 2.5 mg 1-2 times/day

Mechanism of Action Thought to act by blocking excess acetylcholine at cerebral synapses; many of its effects are due to its pharmacologic similarities with atropine; it exerts an antispasmodic effect on smooth muscle, is a potent mydriatic; inhibits salivation

Pharmacodynamics/Kinetics

Onset of Action 30-40 minutes

Duration of Action 4-6 hours

Half-life Elimination ~12.5 hours

Time to Peak ~1 hour

Product Availability Not available in U.S.

Progesterone (proe JES ter one)

U.S. Brand Names Crinone®; Endometrin®; First™-Progesterone VGS 100; First™-Progesterone VGS 200; First™-Progesterone VGS 25; First™-Progesterone VGS 400; First™-Progesterone VGS 50; Prochieve® [DSC]; Prometrium®

Canadian Brand Names Crinone®; Prometrium®

Pharmacologic Category Progestin

Use

Oral: Prevention of endometrial hyperplasia in nonhysterectomized, postmenopausal women who are receiving conjugated estrogen tablets; secondary amenorrhea

I.M.: Amenorrhea; abnormal uterine bleeding due to hormonal imbalance

Intravaginal gel: Part of assisted reproductive technology (ART) for infertile women with progesterone deficiency; secondary amenorrhea

Vaginal tablet: Part of ART for infertile women with progesterone deficiency

Local Anesthetic/Vasoconstrictor Precautions No information available to require special precautions

Effects on Dental Treatment Key adverse event(s) related to dental treatment: Progestins may predispose the patient to gingival bleeding.

Effects on Bleeding No information available to require special precautions

Adverse Effects

Injection (I.M.):

Cardiovascular: Cerebral edema, cerebral thrombosis, edema

Central nervous system: Depression, fever, insomnia, somnolence

Dermatologic: Acne, allergic rash (rare), alopecia, hirsutism, pruritus, rash, urticaria

Endocrine & metabolic: Amenorrhea, breakthrough bleeding, breast tenderness, galactorrhea, menstrual flow changes, spotting

Gastrointestinal: Nausea, weight gain/loss

Genitourinary: Cervical erosion changes, cervical secretion changes

Hepatic: Cholestatic jaundice

Local: Injection site: Irritation, pain, redness

Ocular: Optic neuritis, retinal thrombosis

Respiratory: Pulmonary embolism

Miscellaneous: Anaphylactoid reactions

Oral capsule (percentages reported when used in combination with or cycled with conjugated estrogens):

>10%:

Central nervous system: Headache (16% to 31%), dizziness (15% to 24%), depression (19%)

Endocrine & metabolic: Breast tenderness (27%), breast pain (6% to 16%)

Gastrointestinal: Abdominal pain (10% to 20%), abdominal bloating (8% to 12%)

Genitourinary: Urinary problems (11%)

Neuromuscular & skeletal: Joint pain (20%), musculoskeletal pain (12%)

Miscellaneous: Viral infection (12%)

5% to 10%:

Cardiovascular: Chest pain (7%)

Central nervous system: Fatigue (8%), irritability (8%), worry (8%)

Gastrointestinal: Nausea/vomiting (8%), diarrhea (7% to 8%)

Genitourinary: Vaginal discharge (10%)

Respiratory: Cough (8%)

<5%: Breast biopsy, breast cancer, cholecystectomy, constipation

Vaginal gel (percentages reported with ART); also refer to oral capsule reactions listing for additional effects noted with progesterone:

>10%:

Central nervous system: Somnolence (27%), headache (13% to 17%), nervousness (16%), depression (11%)

Endocrine & metabolic: Breast enlargement (40%), breast pain (13%), libido decreased (11%)

Gastrointestinal: Constipation (27%), nausea (7% to 22%), cramps (15%), abdominal pain (12%)
Genitourinary: Perineal pain (17%), nocturia (13%)
5% to 10%:
Central nervous system: Pain (8%), dizziness (5%)
Gastrointestinal: Diarrhea (8%), bloating (7%), vomiting (5%)
Genitourinary: Vaginal discharge (7%), dyspareunia (6%), genital moniliasis (5%), genital pruritus (5%)
Neuromuscular & skeletal: Arthralgia (8%)

Vaginal tablet (percentages reported with ART); also refer to oral capsule reactions listing for additional effects noted with progesterone:
>10%:
Gastrointestinal: Abdominal pain (12%)
Miscellaneous: Post-oocyte retrieval pain (25% to 28%)
1% to 10%:
Central nervous system: Headache (3% to 4%), fatigue (2% to 3%)
Endocrine & metabolic: Ovarian hyperstimulation syndrome (7%)
Gastrointestinal: Nausea (7% to 8%), abdominal distension (4%), constipation (2% to 3%), vomiting (2% to 3%)
Genitourinary: Uterine spasm (3% to 4%), vaginal bleeding (3%), urinary tract infection (1% to 2%)

General Dosage Range
I.M.: *Adults (females):* 5-10 mg/day for 6 doses
Intravaginal: *Adults (females):*
ART: 90 mg (8% gel) once or twice daily or 100 mg (vaginal tablet) 2-3 times/day
Secondary amenorrhea: 45 mg (4% gel) every other day, may increase to 90 mg (8% gel) every other day if needed (maximum: 6 doses)
Oral: *Adults (females):*
Amenorrhea: 400 mg once daily in the evening for 10 days
Endometrial hyperplasia prevention: 200 mg once daily in the evening for 12 days sequentially per 28-day cycle

Mechanism of Action Natural steroid hormone that induces secretory changes in the endometrium, promotes mammary gland development, relaxes uterine smooth muscle, blocks follicular maturation and ovulation, and maintains pregnancy. When used as part of an ART program in the luteal phase, progesterone supports embryo implantation.

Pharmacodynamics/Kinetics
Half-life Elimination Vaginal gel: 5-20 minutes
Time to Peak Oral: Within 3 hours; I.M.: ~8 hours; Vaginal tablet: ~17-24 hours

Pregnancy Risk Factor B (Prometrium®, per manufacturer); none established for vaginal gel, vaginal tablet, or injection

Promethazine (proe METH a zeen)

U.S. Brand Names Phenadoz®; Phenergan®; Promethegan™

Canadian Brand Names Bioniche Promethazine; Histantil; Phenergan®; PMS-Promethazine

Pharmacologic Category Antiemetic; Histamine H_1 Antagonist; Histamine H_1 Antagonist, First Generation; Phenothiazine Derivative

Use Symptomatic treatment of various allergic conditions; antiemetic; motion sickness; sedative; adjunct to postoperative analgesia and anesthesia

Local Anesthetic/Vasoconstrictor Precautions Promethazine may lower seizure threshold; use caution administering promethazine in combination with other agents that reduce seizure threshold (ie, local anesthetics). Due to promethazine induced alpha-adrenergic blockade, administration of local anesthetics containing the vasoconstrictors epinephrine or levonordefrin, causes unopposed stimulation of beta-adrenergic receptors in heart and peripheral blood vessels that may result in tachycardia and peripheral vasodilation causing hypotension. Effects on blood pressure are greater in combination with epinephrine than levonordefrin.

Effects on Dental Treatment Key adverse event(s) related to dental treatment: Xerostomia (normal salivary flow resumes upon discontinuation).

Significant hypotension may occur, especially when the drug is administered parenterally or following administration of local anesthetics containing vasoconstrictors (ie, epinephrine or levonordefrin); orthostatic hypotension is due to alpha-receptor blockade, the elderly are at greater risk for orthostatic hypotension.

Significant sedation can occur and may be increased in the elderly and in patients taking or administered other CNS depressants (ie, opioid analgesics or benzodiazepines).

Extrapyramidal effects including akathisia (motor restlessness), acute dystonia (spasmodic contractures), pseudoparkinsonism, and tardive dyskinesia can occur with a single dose. These effects are more likely in the elderly, patients taking other dopamine antagonists (including antipsychotic agents and some antiemetic agents), and patients with Parkinson's disease.

Promethazine is a less expensive alternative for moderate-to-severe postoperative nausea than ondansetron but with a greater chance of adverse effects and drug interactions especially with opioid analgesics.

Effects on Bleeding No information available to require special precautions

Adverse Effects Frequency not defined.

Cardiovascular: Bradycardia, hyper-/hypotension, nonspecific QT changes, postural hypotension, tachycardia,

Central nervous system: Agitation akathisia, catatonic states, confusion, delirium, disorientation, dizziness, drowsiness, dystonias, euphoria, excitation, extrapyramidal symptoms, faintness, fatigue, hallucinations, hysteria, insomnia, lassitude, pseudoparkinsonism, tardive dyskinesia, nervousness, neuroleptic malignant syndrome, nightmares, sedation, seizure, somnolence

Dermatologic: Angioneurotic edema, dermatitis, photosensitivity, skin pigmentation (slate gray), urticaria

Endocrine & metabolic: Amenorrhea, breast engorgement, gynecomastia, hyperglycemia, lactation

Gastrointestinal: Constipation, nausea, vomiting, xerostomia

Genitourinary: Ejaculatory disorder, impotence, urinary retention

Hematologic: Agranulocytosis, leukopenia, thrombocytopenia, thrombocytopenic purpura

Hepatic: Jaundice

Local: Abscess, distal vessel spasm, gangrene, injection site reactions (burning, edema, erythema, pain), palsies, paralysis, phlebitis, sensory loss, thrombophlebitis, tissue necrosis, venous thrombosis

Neuromuscular & skeletal: Incoordination, tremor

Ocular: Blurred vision, corneal and lenticular changes, diplopia, epithelial keratopathy, pigmentary retinopathy

Otic: Tinnitus

Respiratory: Apnea, asthma, nasal congestion, respiratory depression

General Dosage Range

I.M., I.V.:

Children ≥2 years: 0.25-1 mg/kg 4-6 times/day as needed (maximum: 25 mg/dose; sedation: 50 mg/dose)

Adults: 12.5-75 mg/dose as a single dose **or** 12.5-50 mg every 4-6 hours as needed

Oral, rectal:

Children ≥2 years:

Allergic reactions: 0.1 mg/kg every 6 hours (maximum: 12.5 mg) during the day and 0.5 mg/kg (maximum: 25 mg/dose) at bedtime as needed

Antiemetic: 0.25-1 mg/kg 4-6 times/day as needed (maximum: 25 mg/dose)

Motion sickness: 0.5 mg/kg 30 minutes to 1 hour before departure, then every 12 hours as needed (maximum: 25 mg twice daily)

Sedation: 0.5-1 mg/kg every 6 hours as needed (maximum: 50 mg/dose)

Adults: 6.25-25 mg every 4-8 hours as needed **or** 12.5-50 mg as a single dose **or** 25 mg 30-60 minutes before departure, then every 12 hours as needed

Mechanism of Action Phenothiazine derivative; blocks postsynaptic mesolimbic dopaminergic receptors in the brain; exhibits a strong alpha-adrenergic blocking effect and depresses the release of hypothalamic and hypophyseal hormones; competes with histamine for the H_1-receptor; muscarinic-blocking effect may be responsible for antiemetic activity; reduces stimuli to the brainstem reticular system

Pharmacodynamics/Kinetics

Onset of Action Oral, I.M.: ~20 minutes; I.V.: ~5 minutes

Peak effect: C_{max}: ~9 ng/mL (suppository); ~19 ng/mL (syrup)

Duration of Action Usually 4-6 hours (up to 12 hours)

Half-life Elimination 9-16 hours

Time to Peak Maximum serum concentration: ~4.5 hours (syrup); ~7-9 hours (suppositories)

Pregnancy Risk Factor C

Dental Comment **Sedation:** When used alone as a sedative agent the degree of sedation is often mild. As a sedative agent, promethazine is effective in managing pediatric patients that require mild anxiety control. It is ineffective when used alone in children with extreme apprehension or for the disruptive, unmanageable child. A more profound sedation will occur if promethazine is administered in combination with an opioid or benzodiazepine. If promethazine is combined with an opioid, the dose of the opioid should be decreased by 25% to 50%.

Promethazine and Codeine (proe METH a zeen & KOE deen)

Related Information

Codeine *on page* 432

Promethazine *on page* 1412

Pharmacologic Category Alpha/Beta Agonist; Analgesic, Opioid; Histamine H_1 Antagonist; Histamine H_1 Antagonist, First Generation; Phenothiazine Derivative

Use Temporary relief of coughs and upper respiratory symptoms associated with allergy or the common cold

Local Anesthetic/Vasoconstrictor Precautions No information available to require special precautions

Effects on Dental Treatment Although promethazine is a phenothiazine derivative, extrapyramidal reactions or tardive dyskinesias are not seen with the use of this drug.

Effects on Bleeding No information available to require special precautions

Adverse Effects See individual agents.

General Dosage Range Oral:

Children 6-11 years: 2.5-5 mL every 4-6 hours (maximum: 30 mL/day)

Children ≥12 years and Adults: 5 mL every 4-6 hours (maximum: 30 mL/day)

Pregnancy Risk Factor C

Controlled Substance C-V

Promethazine and Dextromethorphan

(proe METH a zeen & deks troe meth OR fan)

Related Information

Dextromethorphan *on page* 504

Promethazine *on page* 1412

Pharmacologic Category Antitussive; Histamine H_1 Antagonist; Histamine H_1 Antagonist, First Generation; Phenothiazine Derivative

Use Temporary relief of coughs and upper respiratory symptoms associated with allergy or the common cold

Local Anesthetic/Vasoconstrictor Precautions No information available to require special precautions

Effects on Dental Treatment Although promethazine is a phenothiazine derivative, extrapyramidal reactions or tardive dyskinesias are not seen with the use of this drug.

Effects on Bleeding No information available to require special precautions

General Dosage Range Oral:

Children 2-6 years: 1.25-2.5 mL every 4-6 hours (maximum: 10 mL/day)

Children 6-12 years: 2.5-5 mL every 4-6 hours (maximum: 20 mL/day)

Adults: 5 mL every 4-6 hours (maximum: 30 mL/day)

Pregnancy Risk Factor C

Promethazine and Phenylephrine (proe METH a zeen & fen il EF rin)

Related Information

Phenylephrine (Systemic) *on page* 1339

Promethazine *on page* 1412

Pharmacologic Category Alpha/Beta Agonist; Decongestant; Histamine H_1 Antagonist; Histamine H_1 Antagonist, First Generation; Phenothiazine Derivative

Use Temporary relief of upper respiratory symptoms associated with allergy or the common cold

Local Anesthetic/Vasoconstrictor Precautions

Phenylephrine: Use with caution since phenylephrine is a sympathomimetic amine which could interact with epinephrine to cause a pressor response

Promethazine: No information available to require special precautions

Effects on Dental Treatment Key adverse event(s) related to dental treatment: Phenylephrine: Tachycardia, palpitations, xerostomia (normal salivary flow resumes upon discontinuation); use vasoconstrictor with caution. Although promethazine is a phenothiazine derivative, extrapyramidal reactions or tardive dyskinesias are not seen with the use of this drug.

Effects on Bleeding No information available to require special precautions

General Dosage Range Oral:

Children 2-6 years: 1.25-2.5 mL every 4-6 hours (maximum: 7.5 mL/day)

Children 6-12 years: 2.5-5 mL every 4-6 hours (maximum: 30 mL/day)

Children >12 years and Adults: 5 mL every 4-6 hours (maximum: 30 mL/day)

Pregnancy Risk Factor C

Promethazine, Phenylephrine, and Codeine
(proe METH a zeen, fen il EF rin, & KOE deen)

Related Information

Codeine *on page 432*

Phenylephrine (Systemic) *on page 1339*

Promethazine *on page 1412*

Pharmacologic Category Alpha/Beta Agonist; Analgesic, Opioid; Antitussive; Decongestant; Histamine H_1 Agonist; Histamine H_1 Antagonist, First Generation; Phenothiazine Derivative

Use Temporary relief of coughs and upper respiratory symptoms including nasal congestion associated with allergy or the common cold

Local Anesthetic/Vasoconstrictor Precautions

Phenylephrine: Use with caution since phenylephrine is a sympathomimetic amine which could interact with epinephrine to cause a pressor response

Promethazine: No information available to require special precautions

Effects on Dental Treatment Key adverse event(s) related to dental treatment: Phenylephrine: Tachycardia, palpitations, xerostomia (normal salivary flow resumes upon discontinuation); use vasoconstrictor with caution. Although promethazine is a phenothiazine derivative, extrapyramidal reactions or tardive dyskinesias are not seen with the use of this drug.

Effects on Bleeding No information available to require special precautions

Adverse Effects See individual agents.

General Dosage Range Oral:

Children 6-11 years: 2.5-5 mL every 4-6 hours (maximum: 30 mL/day)

Children ≥12 years and Adults: 5 mL every 4-6 hours (maximum: 30 mL/day)

Pregnancy Risk Factor C

Controlled Substance C-V

Propafenone (pro PAF en one)

Related Information

Cardiovascular Diseases *on page 1848*

U.S. Brand Names Rythmol®; Rythmol® SR

Canadian Brand Names Apo-Propafenone®; Mylan-Propafenone; PMS-Propafenone; Rythmol® Gen-Propafenone

Pharmacologic Category Antiarrhythmic Agent, Class Ic

Use Treatment of life-threatening ventricular arrhythmias

Rythmol® SR: Maintenance of normal sinus rhythm in patients with symptomatic atrial fibrillation

Unlabeled/Investigational Use Supraventricular tachycardias, including those patients with Wolff-Parkinson-White syndrome

Local Anesthetic/Vasoconstrictor Precautions In some patients, propafenone has been reported to induce new or worsened arrhythmias (proarrhythmic effect). It is suggested that vasoconstrictors be used with caution since epinephrine has the potential to stimulate the heart rate when given in the anesthetic regimen. Propafenone is one of the drugs confirmed to prolong the QT interval and is accepted as having a risk of causing torsade de pointes. The risk of drug-induced torsade de pointes is extremely low when a single QT interval prolonging drug is prescribed. In terms of epinephrine, it is not known what effect vasoconstrictors in the local anesthetic regimen will have in patients with a known history of congenital prolonged QT interval or in patients taking any medication that prolongs the QT interval. Until more information is obtained, it is suggested that the clinician consult with the physician prior to the use of a vasoconstrictor in suspected patients, and that the vasoconstrictor (epinephrine, mepivacaine and levonordefrin [Carbocaine® 2% with Neo-Cobefrin®]) be used with caution.

Effects on Dental Treatment Key adverse event(s) related to dental treatment: Unusual taste and significant xerostomia (normal salivary flow resumes upon discontinuation).

Effects on Bleeding No information available to require special precautions

Adverse Effects 1% to 10%:

Cardiovascular: New or worsened arrhythmia (proarrhythmic effect) (2% to 10%), angina (2% to 5%), CHF (1% to 4%), ventricular tachycardia (1% to 3%), palpitation (1% to 3%), AV block (first-degree) (1% to 3%), syncope (1% to 2%), increased QRS interval (1% to 2%), chest pain (1% to 2%), PVCs (1% to 2%), bradycardia (1% to 2%), edema (0% to 1%), bundle branch block (0% to 1%), atrial fibrillation (1%), hypotension (0% to 1%), intraventricular conduction delay (0% to 1%)

Central nervous system: Dizziness (4% to 15%), fatigue (2% to 6%), headache (2% to 5%), ataxia (0% to 2%), insomnia (0% to 2%), anxiety (1% to 2%), drowsiness (1%)
Dermatologic: Rash (1% to 3%)
Gastrointestinal: Nausea/vomiting (2% to 11%), unusual taste (3% to 23%), constipation (2% to 7%), dyspepsia (1% to 3%), diarrhea (1% to 3%), xerostomia (1% to 2%), anorexia (1% to 2%), abdominal pain (1% to 2%), flatulence (0% to 1%)
Neuromuscular & skeletal: Tremor (0% to 1%), arthralgia (0% to 1%), weakness (1% to 2%)
Ocular: Blurred vision (1% to 6%)
Respiratory: Dyspnea (2% to 5%)
Miscellaneous: Diaphoresis (1%)

General Dosage Range Dosage adjustment recommended in patients with hepatic impairment

Oral:

Extended release: *Adults:* Initial: 225 mg every 12 hours; Maintenance: 225-425 mg every 12 hours

Immediate release: *Adults:* Initial: 150 mg every 8 hours; Maintenance: 150-300 mg every 8 hours

Mechanism of Action Propafenone is a class 1c antiarrhythmic agent which possesses local anesthetic properties, blocks the fast inward sodium current, and slows the rate of increase of the action potential. Prolongs conduction and refractoriness in all areas of the myocardium, with a slightly more pronounced effect on intraventricular conduction; it prolongs effective refractory period, reduces spontaneous automaticity and exhibits some beta-blockade activity.

Pharmacodynamics/Kinetics

Half-life Elimination Extensive metabolizers: 2-10 hours; Poor metabolizers: 10-32 hours

Time to Peak Serum: 3.5 hours

Pregnancy Risk Factor C

Dental Comment Propafenone is known to prolong the QT interval. The QT interval is measured as the time and distance between the Q point of the QRS complex and the end of the T wave in the ECG tracing. After adjustment for heart rate, the QT interval is defined as prolonged if it is more than 450 msec in men and 460 msec in women. A long QT syndrome was first described in the 1950s and 60s as a congenital syndrome involving QT interval prolongation and syncope and sudden death. Some of the congenital long QT syndromes were characterized by a peculiar electrocardiographic appearance of the QRS complex involving a premature atria beat followed by a pause, then a subsequent sinus beat showing marked QT prolongation and deformity. This type of cardiac arrhythmia was originally termed "torsade de pointes" (translated from the French as "twisting of the points"). Propafenone is considered as having a risk of causing torsade de pointes. Since it is not known what effect vasoconstrictors in the local anesthetic regimen will have in patients with a known history of congenital prolonged QT interval or in patients taking any medication that prolongs the QT interval, a medical consult is suggested.

Propantheline (proe PAN the leen)

Generic Availability (U.S.) Yes

Pharmacologic Category Anticholinergic Agent

Dental Use Induce dry field (xerostomia) in oral cavity

Use Adjunctive treatment of peptic ulcer

Unlabeled/Investigational Use Decreased salivation and drooling

Local Anesthetic/Vasoconstrictor Precautions No information available to require special precautions

Effects on Dental Treatment Key adverse event(s) related to dental treatment: Significant xerostomia (therapeutic effect; normal salivary flow resumes upon discontinuation), dry throat, nasal dryness, and dysphagia.

Effects on Bleeding No information available to require special precautions

Adverse Effects Frequency not defined.

Cardiovascular: Palpitation, tachycardia
Central nervous system: Confusion, dizziness, drowsiness, headache, insomnia, nervousness
Endocrine & metabolic: Suppression of lactation
Gastrointestinal: Bloated feeling, constipation, loss of taste, nausea, vomiting, xerostomia
Genitourinary: Impotence, urinary hesitancy, urinary retention
Neuromuscular & skeletal: Weakness
Ocular: Blurred vision, cycloplegia, mydriasis, ocular tension increased
Miscellaneous: Allergic reactions, anaphylaxis, diaphoresis decreased

Dental Usual Dosage Antisecretory: Oral:
Children: 1-2 mg/kg/day in 3-4 divided doses
Adults: 15 mg 3 times/day before meals or food and 30 mg at bedtime
Elderly: 7.5 mg 3 times/day before meals and at bedtime

Dosage Oral:
Antisecretory (unlabeled use):
Children: 1-2 mg/kg/day in 3-4 divided doses
Adults: 15 mg 3 times/day before meals or food and 30 mg at bedtime
Elderly: 7.5 mg 3 times/day before meals and at bedtime
Antispasmodic:
Children: 2-3 mg/kg/day in divided doses every 4-6 hours and at bedtime
Adults: 15 mg 3 times/day before meals or food and 30 mg at bedtime

Mechanism of Action Competitively blocks the action of acetylcholine at post-ganglionic parasympathetic receptor sites

Contraindications Severe ulcerative colitis, toxic megacolon, obstructive disease of the GI or urinary tract; glaucoma; myasthenia gravis; unstable cardiovascular adjustment in acute hemorrhage; intestinal atony of elderly or debilitated patients

Warnings/Precautions May cause drowsiness and/or blurred vision, which may impair physical or mental abilities; patients must be cautioned about performing tasks which require mental alertness (eg, operating machinery or driving). Use with caution in patients with hyperthyroidism, hiatal hernia with reflux esophagitis, autonomic neuropathy, hepatic, cardiac, or renal disease, hypertension, GI infections, or other endocrine diseases. In the elderly, avoid long-term use due to anticholinergic adverse effects and uncertain effectiveness (Beers Criteria). Heat prostration may occur in the presence of increased environmental temperature; use caution in hot weather and/or exercise. Diarrhea may be a sign of incomplete intestinal obstruction, treatment should be discontinued if this occurs.

Drug Interactions

Avoid Concomitant Use There are no known interactions where it is recommended to avoid concomitant use.

Increased Effect/Toxicity

Propantheline may increase the levels/effects of: AbobotulinumtoxinA; Anticholinergics; Cannabinoids; OnabotulinumtoxinA; Potassium Chloride; RimabotulinumtoxinB

The levels/effects of Propantheline may be increased by: MAO Inhibitors; Pramlintide

Decreased Effect

Propantheline may decrease the levels/effects of: Acetylcholinesterase Inhibitors (Central); Secretin

The levels/effects of Propantheline may be decreased by: Acetylcholinesterase Inhibitors (Central)

Dietary Considerations Should be taken 30 minutes before meals so that the drug's peak effect occurs at the proper time. The tablet (15 mg) contains lactose 23.2 mg.

Pharmacodynamics/Kinetics

Onset of Action 30-45 minutes

Duration of Action 4-6 hours

Half-life Elimination Serum: Average: 1.6 hours

Pregnancy Risk Factor C

Lactation Excretion in breast milk unknown/use caution

Breast-Feeding Considerations No data reported; however, atropine may be taken while breast-feeding.

Dosage Forms
Tablet, oral: 15 mg

Proparacaine (proe PAR a kane)

U.S. Brand Names Alcaine®; Parcaine™

Canadian Brand Names Alcaine®; Diocaine®

Pharmacologic Category Local Anesthetic, Ophthalmic

Use Anesthesia for tonometry, gonioscopy; suture removal from cornea; removal of corneal foreign body; cataract extraction, glaucoma surgery; short operative procedure involving the cornea and conjunctiva

Local Anesthetic/Vasoconstrictor Precautions No information available to require special precautions

Effects on Dental Treatment No significant effects or complications reported

Effects on Bleeding No information available to require special precautions

Adverse Effects 1% to 10%: Local: Burning, stinging, redness

General Dosage Range Ophthalmic: *Children and Adults:* Instill 1-2 drops of 0.5% solution in eye once **or** instill 1 drop of 0.5% solution in eye every 5-10 minutes for 5-7 doses

Mechanism of Action Prevents initiation and transmission of impulse at the nerve cell membrane by decreasing ion permeability through stabilizing

Pharmacodynamics/Kinetics

Onset of Action ~20 seconds

Duration of Action 15-20 minutes

Pregnancy Risk Factor C

Proparacaine and Fluorescein (proe PAR a kane & FLURE e seen)

Related Information

Proparacaine *on page 1417*

U.S. Brand Names Flucaine®

Pharmacologic Category Diagnostic Agent; Local Anesthetic

Use Anesthesia for tonometry, gonioscopy; suture removal from cornea; removal of corneal foreign body; cataract extraction, glaucoma surgery

Local Anesthetic/Vasoconstrictor Precautions No information available to require special precautions

Effects on Dental Treatment No significant effects or complications reported

Effects on Bleeding No information available to require special precautions

Adverse Effects 1% to 10%: Local: Burning, stinging of eye

General Dosage Range Ophthalmic: *Children and Adults:* Instill 1 drop in each eye every 5-10 minutes for 5-7 doses **or** instill 1-2 drops in each eye once

Mechanism of Action Prevents initiation and transmission of impulse at the nerve cell membrane by decreasing ion permeability through stabilizing

Pharmacodynamics/Kinetics

Onset of Action ~20 seconds

Duration of Action 15-20 minutes

Pregnancy Risk Factor C

Propofol (PROE po fole)

U.S. Brand Names Diprivan®

Canadian Brand Names Diprivan®

Pharmacologic Category General Anesthetic

Use Induction of anesthesia in patients ≥3 years of age; maintenance of anesthesia in patients >2 months of age; in adults, for monitored anesthesia care sedation during procedures; sedation in intubated, mechanically-ventilated ICU patients

Unlabeled/Investigational Use Postoperative antiemetic; refractory delirium tremens (case reports)

Local Anesthetic/Vasoconstrictor Precautions No information available to require special precautions

Effects on Dental Treatment No significant effects or complications reported

Effects on Bleeding No information available to require special precautions

Adverse Effects

>10%:

Cardiovascular: Hypotension (children 17%; adults 3% to 26%)

Central nervous system: Movement (children 17%; adults 3% to 10%)

Local: Injection site burning, stinging, or pain (children 10%; adults 18%)

Respiratory: Apnea lasting 30-60 seconds (children 10%; adults 24%), apnea lasting >60 seconds (children 5%; adults 12%)

1% to 10%:

Cardiovascular: Hypertension (children 8%), arrhythmia (1% to 3%), bradycardia (1% to 3%), cardiac output decreased (1% to 3%; concurrent opioid use increases incidence), tachycardia (1% to 3%)

Dermatologic: Pruritus (1% to 3%), rash (children 5%; adults 1% to 3%)

Endocrine & metabolic: Hypertriglyceridemia (3% to 10%)

Respiratory: Respiratory acidosis during weaning (3% to 10%)

General Dosage Range I.V.: *Children and Adults:* Dosage varies greatly depending on indication

Mechanism of Action Propofol is a short-acting, lipophilic intravenous general anesthetic. The drug is unrelated to any of the currently used barbiturate, opioid, benzodiazepine, arylcyclohexylamine, or imidazole intravenous anesthetic agents. Propofol causes global CNS depression, presumably through it's agonist actions on $GABA_A$ receptors, and perhaps also involving reduced glutamatergic activity through NMDA receptor blockade.

Pharmacodynamics/Kinetics

Onset of Action Anesthetic: Bolus infusion (dose dependent): 9-51 seconds (average: 30 seconds)

Duration of Action Dose and rate dependent: 3-10 minutes

Half-life Elimination Biphasic: Initial: 40 minutes; Terminal: 4-7 hours (after 10-day infusion, may be up to 1-3 days)

Pregnancy Risk Factor B

Propoxyphene (proe POKS i feen)

U.S. Brand Names Darvon-N® [DSC]; Darvon® [DSC]

Canadian Brand Names 642® Tablet; Darvon-N®

Pharmacologic Category Analgesic, Opioid

Use Management of mild-to-moderate pain

Local Anesthetic/Vasoconstrictor Precautions No information available to require special precautions

Effects on Dental Treatment Key adverse event(s) related to dental treatment: Xerostomia (normal salivary flow resumes upon discontinuation).

Effects on Bleeding No information available to require special precautions

Adverse Effects Frequency not defined.

Central nervous system: Dizziness, dysphoria, euphoria, hallucinations, headache, lightheadedness, sedation

Dermatologic: Rash

Gastrointestinal: Abdominal pain, constipation, nausea, vomiting

Neuromuscular & skeletal: Weakness

Ocular: Visual disturbances

General Dosage Range Oral: *Adults:* Hydrochloride: 65 mg every 4 hours as needed (maximum: 390 mg/day); Napsylate: 100 mg every 4 hours as needed (maximum: 600 mg/day)

Mechanism of Action Propoxyphene is a weak narcotic analgesic which acts through binding to opiate receptors to inhibit ascending pain pathways. Propoxyphene, as with other narcotic (opiate) analgesics, blocks pain perception in the cerebral cortex by binding to specific receptor molecules (opiate receptors) within the neuronal membranes of synapses. This binding results in a decreased synaptic chemical transmission throughout the CNS thus inhibiting the flow of pain sensations into the higher centers. Mu and kappa are the two subtypes of the opiate receptor which propoxyphene binds to cause analgesia.

Pharmacodynamics/Kinetics

Onset of Action 0.5-1 hour

Duration of Action 4-6 hours

Half-life Elimination Adults: 6-12 hours, Elderly: 13-35 hours; Norpropoxyphene: Adults: 30-36 hours, Elderly: 22-41 hours

Time to Peak Plasma: 2-2.5 hours

Pregnancy Risk Factor C

Controlled Substance C-IV

Propoxyphene and Acetaminophen
(proe POKS i feen & a seet a MIN oh fen)

Related Information

Acetaminophen *on page 32*

Propoxyphene *on page 1419*

Related Sample Prescriptions

Moderate/Moderately Severe Oral Pain *on page 1980*

U.S. Brand Names Balacet 325™ [DSC]; Darvocet A500® [DSC]; Darvocet-N® 100 [DSC]; Darvocet-N® 50 [DSC]

Canadian Brand Names Darvocet-N® 100; Darvocet-N® 50

Generic Availability (U.S.) Yes

Pharmacologic Category Analgesic Combination (Opioid)

Dental Use Management of postoperative pain

Use Management of mild-to-moderate pain

Local Anesthetic/Vasoconstrictor Precautions No information available to require special precautions

Effects on Dental Treatment Key adverse event(s) related to dental treatment: Xerostomia (normal salivary flow resumes upon discontinuation). See Dental Comment.

Effects on Bleeding No information available to require special precautions

Adverse Effects See individual agents.

Dental Usual Dosage Postoperative pain: Adults: Oral:
Darvocet A500™, Darvocet-N® 100: 1 tablet every 4 hours as needed; maximum: 600 mg propoxyphene napsylate/day
Darvocet-N® 50: 1-2 tablets every 4 hours as needed; maximum: 600 mg propoxyphene napsylate/day
Note: Dosage of acetaminophen should not exceed 4 g/day (6 tablets of Darvocet-N® 100); possibly less in patients with ethanol

Dosage Oral: Adults:
Darvocet A500®, Darvocet-N® 100: 1 tablet every 4 hours as needed; maximum: 600 mg propoxyphene napsylate/day
Darvocet-N® 50: 1-2 tablets every 4 hours as needed; maximum: 600 mg propoxyphene napsylate/day
Propoxyphene hydrochloride 65 mg and acetaminophen 650 mg: 1 tablet every 4 hours as needed; maximum: 390 mg/day propoxyphene hydrochloride, 4 g/day acetaminophen)
Note: Formulations contain significant amounts of acetaminophen; intake should be limited to <4 g acetaminophen/day (less in patients with hepatic impairment/ ethanol abuse)
Elderly: Refer to adult dosing
Concurrent use with CYP3A4 inhibitors: Monitor closely; dosage adjustment may be necessary.
Discontinuation of therapy: In patients on prolonged therapy, gradually discontinue propoxyphene and acetaminophen by reducing dose by 25% to 50% daily and carefully monitor for signs/symptoms of withdrawal.

Dosing adjustment in renal impairment: Serum concentrations of propoxyphene may be increased or elimination may be delayed. Use with caution; dosage reduction should be considered; however, no specific dosing recommendations are available.
Dosing adjustment in hepatic impairment: Serum concentrations of propoxyphene may be increased or elimination may be delayed. Use with caution; dosage reduction should be considered; however, no specific dosing recommendations are available.

Mechanism of Action
Propoxyphene, as with other narcotic (opiate) analgesics, blocks pain perception in the cerebral cortex by binding to specific receptor molecules (opiate receptors) within the neuronal membranes of synapses. This binding results in a decreased synaptic chemical transmission throughout the CNS thus inhibiting the flow of pain sensations into the higher centers. Mu and kappa are the two subtypes of the opiate receptor to which propoxyphene binds to cause analgesia.
Acetaminophen inhibits the synthesis of prostaglandins in the CNS and peripherally blocks pain impulse generation; produces antipyresis from inhibition of hypothalamic heat-regulating center

Contraindications Hypersensitivity to propoxyphene, acetaminophen, or any component of the formulation; patients with paralytic ileus, acute/severe asthma, hypercarbia, or severe respiratory depression (unless patient is mechanically ventilated)

Warnings/Precautions [U.S. Boxed Warning]: Accidental and intentional overdose has occurred (including fatalities) when propoxyphene was used alone or in combination with other CNS depressants (including ethanol). Patients with a history of emotional disturbances or suicidal ideation/attempt or who are on concurrent sedatives, tranquilizers, muscle relaxants, antidepressants, or other CNS-depressant drugs are at greatest risk of propoxyphene-related deaths. Avoid use in severely depressed or suicidal patients. Should not be prescribed in patients who are addiction prone or suicidal. **[U.S. Boxed Warning]: Use with caution in patients taking strong CYP3A4 inhibitors (see Drug Interactions); monitor patients closely. Dosage adjustments may be needed.** May cause CNS depression, which may impair physical or mental abilities; patients must be cautioned about performing tasks which require mental alertness (eg, operating machinery or driving). Use caution in patients taking CNS depressant medications or antidepressants, and in patients who use alcohol in excess.

Use caution in patients dependent on opiates, substitution may result in acute opiate withdrawal symptoms. Tolerance or drug dependence may result from extended use. Propoxyphene should be used with caution in patients with biliary tract impairment, CNS depression, coma, head trauma, prostatic hyperplasia, respiratory disease (asthma, COPD), urinary stricture, renal or hepatic dysfunction or in debilitated or elderly; consider dosing adjustment. May obscure diagnosis or clinical course of patients with acute abdominal conditions. Propoxyphene may cause hypotension; use with caution in patients with hypovolemia, cardiovascular disease (including acute MI), or drugs which may exaggerate hypotensive effects (including phenothiazines or general anesthetics).

Propoxyphene should be used with caution in patients with renal or hepatic dysfunction or in the elderly; consider dosing adjustment. May be inappropriate for use in the elderly due to adverse effects; has few advantages over acetaminophen for treating pain (Beers Criteria). Acetaminophen should be used with caution in patients with liver disease; consuming ≥3 alcoholic drinks/day may increase risk of liver damage. Use caution in patients with known G6PD deficiency.

Drug Interactions

Metabolism/Transport Effects

Propoxyphene: **Substrate** of CYP3A4 (major); **Inhibits** CYP2C9 (weak), 2D6 (weak), 3A4 (weak)

Acetaminophen: **Substrate** (minor) of CYP1A2, 2A6, 2C9, 2D6, 2E1, 3A4; **Inhibits** CYP3A4 (weak)

Avoid Concomitant Use

Avoid concomitant use of Propoxyphene and Acetaminophen with any of the following: MAO Inhibitors

Increased Effect/Toxicity

Propoxyphene and Acetaminophen may increase the levels/effects of: Alcohol (Ethyl); Alvimopan; Beta-Blockers; CarBAMazepine; CNS Depressants; Dasatinib; Desmopressin; Imatinib; MAO Inhibitors; Selective Serotonin Reuptake Inhibitors; SORAfenib; Thiazide Diuretics; Tricyclic Antidepressants; Vitamin K Antagonists

The levels/effects of Propoxyphene and Acetaminophen may be increased by: Amphetamines; Antipsychotic Agents (Phenothiazines); Conivaptan; CYP3A4 Inhibitors (Moderate); CYP3A4 Inhibitors (Strong); Dasatinib; Droperidol; Imatinib; Isoniazid; Metyrapone; Probenecid; SORAfenib; Succinylcholine

Decreased Effect

Propoxyphene and Acetaminophen may decrease the levels/effects of: Pegvisomant

The levels/effects of Propoxyphene and Acetaminophen may be decreased by: Ammonium Chloride; Anticonvulsants (Hydantoin); Barbiturates; CarBAMazepine; Cholestyramine Resin; CYP3A4 Inducers (Strong); Deferasirox; Herbs (CYP3A4 Inducers); Mixed Agonist / Antagonist Opioids; Peginterferon Alfa-2b; Tocilizumab

Ethanol/Nutrition/Herb Interactions

Based on **propoxyphene** component:

May increase CNS depression; monitor for increased effects with coadministration. Caution patients about effects.

Food: May decrease rate of absorption, but may slightly increase bioavailability. Avoid grapefruit juice (may increase levels/effects of propoxyphene).

Based on **acetaminophen** component:

Ethanol: Excessive intake of ethanol may increase the risk of acetaminophen-induced hepatotoxicity. Avoid ethanol or limit to <3 drinks/day.

Food: Rate of absorption may be decreased when given with food.

Herb/Nutraceutical: St John's wort may decrease acetaminophen levels.

Dietary Considerations Avoid grapefruit juice.

Pregnancy Risk Factor C

Lactation Enters breast milk/use caution

Breast-Feeding Considerations Refer to individual agents.

Controlled Substance C-IV

Dosage Forms

Tablet:

65/650: Propoxyphene 65 mg and acetaminophen 650 mg; 100/325: Propoxyphene 100 mg and acetaminophen 325 mg; 100/500: Propoxyphene 100 mg and acetaminophen 500 mg; 100/650: Propoxyphene 100 mg and acetaminophen 650 mg

Balacet 325™: Propoxyphene 100 mg and acetaminophen 325 mg

Darvocet A500®: Propoxyphene 100 mg and acetaminophen 500 mg

Darvocet-N® 50: Propoxyphene 50 mg and acetaminophen 325 mg

Darvocet-N® 100: Propoxyphene 100 mg and acetaminophen 650 mg

Dental Comment Propoxyphene is a narcotic analgesic and shares many properties including addiction liability. The acetaminophen component requires use with caution in patients with alcoholic liver disease.

Hepatotoxicity caused by acetaminophen is potentiated by chronic alcohol consumption. People who are taking acetaminophen, even at therapeutic doses, and consume alcohol are at risk of developing hepatotoxicity.

Acetaminophen may increase the levels and enhance the anticoagulant effects of vitamin K antagonists acenocoumarol and warfarin (Coumadin®). Studies have reported that acetaminophen has increased the INR in warfarin treated patients with daily acetaminophen doses as low as 2 g, particularly when taking acetaminophen for >1 week (Antlitz, 1968; Boeijinga, 1982; Gebauer, 2003; Hylek, 1998;

Rubin, 1984). In addition, case reports of bleeding as a result of increased INR have been published (Bagheri, 1999; Bartle, 1991). There is no known mechanism of the interaction; furthermore, some studies have failed to demonstrate this interaction (Gadisseur, 2003; Kwan, 1995; van den Bemt, 2002). In terms of risk, the data suggest that acetaminophen and warfarin could interact in some clinically significant manner but that the benefits of concomitant use of acetaminophen for pain control in dental patients taking warfarin usually outweigh the risks. An appropriate monitoring plan should be in place to identify potential negative effects and dosage adjustments may be necessary in a minority of patients. The interaction may be more likely to occur with daily acetaminophen doses of >1.3 g for >1 week.

There are no reports of acetaminophen interacting with antiplatelet drugs such as aspirin, clopidogrel (Plavix®), or prasugrel (Effient™). Also, there are no reports of acetaminophen in combination with hydrocodone, codeine, or oxycodone interacting with warfarin (Coumadin®).

References

Antlitz AM, Mead JA Jr, and Tolentino MA, "Potentiation of Oral Anticoagulant Therapy by Acetaminophen," *Curr Ther Res Clin Exp*, 1968, 10(10):501-7.

Bagheri H, Bernhard NB, and Montastruc JL, "Potentiation of the Acenocoumarol Anticoagulant Effect by Acetaminophen," *Ann Pharmacother*, 1999, 33(4):506.

Bartle WR and Blakely JA, "Potentiation of Warfarin Anticoagulation by Acetaminophen," *JAMA*, 1991, 265(10):1260.

Boeijinga JJ, Boerstra EE, Ris P, et al, "Interaction Between Paracetamol and Coumarin Anticoagulants," *Lancet*, 1982, 1(8270):506.

Botting RM, "Mechanism of Action of Acetaminophen: Is There a Cyclooxygenase 3?" *Clin Infect Dis*, 2000, Suppl 5:S202-10.

Dart RC, Kuffner EK, and Rumack BH, "Treatment of Pain or Fever with Paracetamol (Acetaminophen) in the Alcoholic Patient: A Systematic Review," *Am J Ther*, 2000, 7(2):123-34.

Gadisseur AP, Van Der Meer FJ, and Rosendaal FR, "Sustained Intake of Paracetamol (Acetaminophen) During Oral Anticoagulant Therapy With Coumarins Does Not Cause Clinically Important INR Changes: A Randomized Double-Blind Clinical Trial," *J Thromb Haemost*, 2003, 1(4):714-7.

Gebauer MG, Nyfort-Hansen K, Henschke PJ, et al, "Warfarin and Acetaminophen Interaction," *Pharmacotherapy*, 2003, 23(1):109-12.

Grant JA and Weiler JM, "A Report of a Rare Immediate Reaction After Ingestion of Acetaminophen," *Ann Allergy Asthma Immunol*, 2001, 87(3):227-9.

Hylek EM, Heiman H, Skates SJ, et al, "Acetaminophen and Other Risk Factors for Excessive Warfarin Anticoagulation," *JAMA*, 1998, 279(9):657-62.

Kwan D, Bartle WR, and Walker SE, "The Effects of Acetaminophen on Pharmacokinetics and Pharmacodynamics of Warfarin," *J Clin Pharmacol*, 1999, 39(1):68-75.

Kwan D, Bartle WR, and Walker SE, "The Effects of Acute and Chronic Acetaminophen Dosing on the Pharmacodynamics and Pharmacokinetics of (R)- and (S)-Warfarin," *Clin Pharmacol Ther*, 1995, 57:212.

McClain CJ, Price S, Barve S, et al, "Acetaminophen Hepatotoxicity: An Update," *Curr Gastroenterol Rep*, 1999, 1(1):42-9.

Rubin RN, Mentzer RL, and Budzynski AZ, "Potentiation of Anticoagulant Effect of Warfarin by Acetaminophen (Tylenol®)," *Clin Res*, 1984, 32:698a.

Shek KL, Chan LN, and Nutescu E, "Warfarin-Acetaminophen Drug Interaction Revisited," *Pharmacotherapy*, 1999, 19(10):1153-8.

Tanaka E, Yamazaki K, and Misawa S, "Update: The Clinical Importance of Acetaminophen Hepatotoxicity in Nonalcoholic and Alcoholic Subjects," *J Clin Pharm Ther*, 2000, 25(5):325-32.

van den Bemt PM, Geven LM, Kuitert NA, et al, "The Potential Interaction Between Oral Anticoagulants and Acetaminophen in Everyday Practice," *Pharm World Sci*, 2002, 24(5):201-4.

Propranolol (proe PRAN oh lole)

Related Information

Cardiovascular Diseases *on page 1848*

Endocrine Disorders and Pregnancy *on page 1879*

U.S. Brand Names Inderal® LA; InnoPran XL®

Canadian Brand Names Apo-Propranolol®; Dom-Propranolol; Inderal®; Inderal® LA; Novo-Pranol; Nu-Propranolol; PMS-Propranolol; Propranolol Hydrochloride Injection, USP

Generic Availability (U.S.) Yes

Pharmacologic Category Antiarrhythmic Agent, Class II; Beta-Adrenergic Blocker, Nonselective

Use Management of hypertension; angina pectoris; pheochromocytoma; essential tremor; supraventricular arrhythmias (such as atrial fibrillation and flutter, AV nodal re-entrant tachycardias), ventricular tachycardias (catecholamine-induced arrhythmias, digoxin toxicity); prevention of myocardial infarction; migraine headache prophylaxis; symptomatic treatment of hypertrophic subaortic stenosis (hypertrophic obstructive cardiomyopathy)

Unlabeled/Investigational Use Tremor due to Parkinson's disease; ethanol withdrawal; aggressive behavior (not recommended for dementia-associated aggression), anxiety, schizophrenia; antipsychotic-induced akathisia; primary and secondary prophylaxis of variceal hemorrhage; acute panic; thyrotoxicosis; tetralogy of Fallot (TOF) hypercyanotic spells

Local Anesthetic/Vasoconstrictor Precautions Use with caution; epinephrine has interacted with nonselective beta-blockers to result in initial hypertensive episode followed by bradycardia

Effects on Dental Treatment Propranolol is a nonselective beta-blocker and may enhance the pressor response to epinephrine, resulting in hypertension and bradycardia. Many nonsteroidal anti-inflammatory drugs, such as ibuprofen and indomethacin, can reduce the hypotensive effect of beta-blockers after 3 or more weeks of therapy with the NSAID. Short-term NSAID use (ie, 3 days) requires no special precautions in patients taking beta-blockers.

Effects on Bleeding No information available to require special precautions

Adverse Effects Frequency not defined.

Cardiovascular: Angina, arterial insufficiency, AV conduction disturbance increased, bradycardia, cardiogenic shock, CHF, hypotension, impaired myocardial contractility, mesenteric arterial thrombosis (rare), Raynaud's syndrome, syncope

Central nervous system: Amnesia, catatonia, cognitive dysfunction, confusion, depression, dizziness, emotional lability, fatigue, hallucinations, hypersomnolence, insomnia, lethargy, lightheadedness, psychosis, vertigo, vivid dreams

Dermatologic: Alopecia, contact dermatitis, cutaneous ulcers, eczematous eruptions, erythema multiforme, exfoliative dermatitis, hyperkeratosis, nail changes, oculomucocutaneous reactions, pruritus, psoriasiform eruptions, rash, Stevens-Johnson syndrome, toxic epidermal necrolysis, ulcers, ulcerative lichenoid, urticaria

Endocrine & metabolic: Hyper-/hypoglycemia, hyperkalemia, hyperlipidemia

Gastrointestinal: Anorexia, cramping, constipation, diarrhea, ischemic colitis, nausea, stomach discomfort, vomiting

Genitourinary: Impotence, interstitial nephritis (rare), oliguria (rare), Peyronie's disease, proteinuria (rare)

Hematologic: Agranulocytosis, nonthrombocytopenic purpura, thrombocytopenia, thrombocytopenic purpura

Hepatic: Alkaline phosphatase increased, transaminases increased

Neuromuscular & skeletal: Arthropathy, carpal tunnel syndrome (rare), myotonus, paresthesia, polyarthritis, weakness

Ocular: Hyperemia of the conjunctiva, mydriasis, visual acuity decreased, visual disturbances, xerophthalmia

Renal: BUN increased

Respiratory: Bronchospasm, dyspnea, laryngospasm, pharyngitis, pulmonary edema, respiratory distress, wheezing

Miscellaneous: Anaphylactic/anaphylactoid allergic reaction, cold extremities, lupus-like syndrome (rare)

Dosage

Akathisia (unlabeled use): Oral: Adults: 30-120 mg/day in 2-3 divided doses

Essential tremor: Oral: Adults: 40 mg twice daily initially; maintenance doses: Usually 120-320 mg/day

Hypertension:

Oral:

Children (unlabeled use): Initial: 0.5-1 mg/kg/day in divided doses every 6-12 hours; increase gradually every 5-7 days; maximum: 16 mg/kg/24 hours

Adults: Initial: 40 mg twice daily; increase dosage every 3-7 days; usual dose: 120-240 mg divided in 2-3 doses/day; maximum daily dose: 640 mg; usual dosage range (JNC 7): 40-160 mg/day in 2 divided doses

Extended release formulations:

Inderal® LA: Initial: 80 mg once daily; usual maintenance: 120-160 mg once daily; maximum daily dose: 640 mg; usual dosage range (JNC 7): 60-180 mg/day once daily

InnoPran XL®: Initial: 80 mg once daily at bedtime; if initial response is inadequate, may be increased at 2-3 week intervals to a maximum dose of 120 mg

Hypertrophic subaortic stenosis: Oral: Adults: 20-40 mg 3-4 times/day

Inderal® LA: 80-160 mg once daily

Migraine headache prophylaxis: Oral:

Children (unlabeled use): Initial: 2-4 mg/kg/day **or**

≤35 kg: 10-20 mg 3 times/day

>35 kg: 20-40 mg 3 times/day

Adults: Initial: 80 mg/day divided every 6-8 hours; increase by 20-40 mg/dose every 3-4 weeks to a maximum of 160-240 mg/day given in divided doses every 6-8 hours; if satisfactory response not achieved within 6 weeks of starting therapy, drug should be withdrawn gradually over several weeks

Inderal® LA: Initial: 80 mg once daily; effective dose range: 160-240 mg once daily

Post-MI mortality reduction: Oral: Adults: Initial: 40 mg 3 times/day; usual dosage range: 180-240 mg/day in 3-4 divided doses

Pheochromocytoma: Oral: Adults: 30-60 mg/day in divided doses

Stable angina: Oral: Adults: 80-320 mg/day in doses divided 2-4 times/day

Inderal® LA: Initial: 80 mg once daily; maximum dose: 320 mg once daily

Tachyarrhythmias:
Oral:
Children (unlabeled use): Initial: 0.5-1 mg/kg/day in divided doses every 6-8 hours; titrate dosage upward every 3-7 days; usual dose: 2-6 mg/kg/day; higher doses may be needed; do not exceed 16 mg/kg/day or 60 mg/day
Adults: 10-30 mg/dose every 6-8 hours
Elderly: Initial: 10 mg twice daily; increase dosage every 3-7 days; usual dosage range: 10-320 mg given in 2 divided doses
I.V.:
Children (unlabeled use): 0.01-0.1 mg/kg/dose slow IVP over 10 minutes; maximum dose: 1 mg for infants; 3 mg for children
Adults: 1-3 mg/dose slow IVP; repeat every 2-5 minutes up to a total of 5 mg; titrate initial dose to desired response
or
0.5-1 mg over 1 minute; may repeat, if necessary, up to a total maximum dose of 0.1 mg/kg (ACLS guidelines, 2010)
Note: Once response achieved or maximum dose administered, additional doses should not be given for at least 4 hours.
Elderly: Use caution; initiate at lower end of the dosing range.
Hypercyanotic spells (TOF) (unlabeled use): Children:
Oral: Palliation: Initial: 1 mg/kg/day every 6 hours; if ineffective, may increase dose after 1 week by 1 mg/kg/day to a maximum of 5 mg/kg/day; if patient becomes refractory, may increase slowly to a maximum of 10-15 mg/kg/day. Allow 24 hours between dosing changes.
I.V.: 0.01-0.2 mg/kg/dose infused over 10 minutes; maximum dose: 5 mg
Thyrotoxicosis (unlabeled use):
Oral:
Children: 2 mg/kg/day, divided every 6-8 hours, titrate to effective dose
Adolescents and Adults: Oral: 10-40 mg/dose every 6 hours
I.V.: Adults: 1-3 mg/dose slow IVP as a single dose
Variceal hemorrhage prophylaxis (unlabeled use; Garcia-Tsao, 2007): Oral: Adults:
Primary prophylaxis: Initial: 20 mg twice daily; adjust to maximal tolerated dose. **Note:** Risk factors for hemorrhage include Child-Pugh class B/C or variceal red wale markings on endoscopy.
Secondary prophylaxis: Initial: 20 mg twice daily; adjust to maximal tolerated dose

Dosing adjustment in renal impairment:
Not dialyzable (0% to 5%); supplemental dose is not necessary.
Peritoneal dialysis effects: Supplemental dose is not necessary.

Dosing adjustment in hepatic disease: Marked slowing of heart rate may occur in chronic liver disease with conventional doses; low initial dose and regular heart rate monitoring

Mechanism of Action Nonselective beta-adrenergic blocker (class II antiarrhythmic); competitively blocks response to $beta_1$- and $beta_2$-adrenergic stimulation which results in decreases in heart rate, myocardial contractility, blood pressure, and myocardial oxygen demand. Nonselective beta-adrenergic blockers (propranolol, nadolol) reduce portal pressure by producing splanchnic vasoconstriction ($beta_2$ effect) thereby reducing portal blood flow.

Contraindications Hypersensitivity to propranolol, beta-blockers, or any component of the formulation; uncompensated congestive heart failure (unless the failure is due to tachyarrhythmias being treated with propranolol), cardiogenic shock, severe sinus bradycardia or heart block greater than first-degree (except in patients with a functioning artificial pacemaker), severe hyperactive airway disease (asthma or COPD)

Warnings/Precautions Consider pre-existing conditions such as sick sinus syndrome before initiating. Administer cautiously in compensated heart failure and monitor for a worsening of the condition (efficacy of propranolol in HF has not been demonstrated). **[U.S. Boxed Warning]: Beta-blocker therapy should not be withdrawn abruptly (particularly in patients with CAD), but gradually tapered to avoid acute tachycardia, hypertension, and/or ischemia.** Use caution in patient with peripheral vascular disease (PVD). Use caution with concurrent use of beta-blockers and either verapamil or diltiazem; bradycardia or heart block can occur. Avoid concurrent I.V. use of both agents.

Use cautiously in patients with diabetes because it can mask prominent hypoglycemic symptoms. Use caution in hyperthyroidism since beta-blockade may mask signs of thyrotoxicosis. May alter thyroid-function tests. Use with caution in myasthenia gravis or psychiatric disease (may cause CNS depression). Use cautiously in renal and hepatic dysfunction; dosage adjustment required in hepatic impairment. Use care with anesthetic agents which decrease myocardial function. In general, patients with bronchospastic disease should not receive beta-blockers; if used at all, should be used cautiously with close monitoring. Adequate alpha-blockade is required prior to use of any beta-blocker for patients with untreated pheochromocytoma. May induce or exacerbate psoriasis. Use caution with history of severe anaphylaxis to allergens; patients taking beta-blockers may become more sensitive to repeated challenges. Treatment of anaphylaxis (eg, epinephrine) in patients taking beta-blockers may be ineffective or promote undesirable effects.

Drug Interactions

Metabolism/Transport Effects **Substrate** of CYP1A2 (major), 2C19 (minor), 2D6 (major), 3A4 (minor); **Inhibits** CYP1A2 (weak), CYP2D6 (weak), P-glycoprotein

Avoid Concomitant Use

Avoid concomitant use of Propranolol with any of the following: Methacholine; Topotecan

Increased Effect/Toxicity

Propranolol may increase the levels/effects of: Alpha-/Beta-Agonists (Direct-Acting); Alpha1-Blockers; Alpha2-Agonists; Amifostine; Antihypertensives; Antipsychotic Agents (Phenothiazines); Bupivacaine; Cardiac Glycosides; Colchicine; Dabigatran Etexilate; Everolimus; Fingolimod; Hypotensive Agents; Insulin; Lidocaine; Lidocaine (Systemic); Lidocaine (Topical); Mepivacaine; Methacholine; Midodrine; P-Glycoprotein Substrates; RiTUXimab; Rivaroxaban; Rizatriptan; Sulfonylureas; Topotecan; ZOLMitriptan

The levels/effects of Propranolol may be increased by: Abiraterone; Acetylcholinesterase Inhibitors; Alcohol (Ethyl); Aminoquinolines (Antimalarial); Amiodarone; Anilidopiperidine Opioids; Antipsychotic Agents (Phenothiazines); Calcium Channel Blockers (Nondihydropyridine); Conivaptan; CYP1A2 Inhibitors (Moderate); CYP1A2 Inhibitors (Strong); CYP2D6 Inhibitors (Moderate); CYP2D6 Inhibitors (Strong); Darunavir; Deferasirox; Diazoxide; Dipyridamole; Disopyramide; Dronedarone; FluvoxaMINE; Herbs (Hypotensive Properties); Lacidipine; MAO Inhibitors; Pentoxifylline; Phosphodiesterase 5 Inhibitors; Propafenone; Propoxyphene; Prostacyclin Analogues; QuiNIDine; Reserpine; Selective Serotonin Reuptake Inhibitors; Zileuton

Decreased Effect

Propranolol may decrease the levels/effects of: Beta2-Agonists; Lacidipine; Theophylline Derivatives

The levels/effects of Propranolol may be decreased by: Alcohol (Ethyl); Barbiturates; Bile Acid Sequestrants; CYP1A2 Inducers (Strong); Herbs (Hypertensive Properties); Methylphenidate; Nonsteroidal Anti-Inflammatory Agents; Peginterferon Alfa-2b; Rifamycin Derivatives; Tocilizumab; Yohimbine

Ethanol/Nutrition/Herb Interactions

Ethanol: Ethanol may increase or decrease plasma levels of propranolol. Reports are variable and have shown both enhanced as well as inhibited hepatic metabolism (of propranolol). Caution advised with consumption of alcohol and monitor for heart rate and/or blood pressure changes.

Food: Propranolol serum levels may be increased if taken with food. Protein-rich foods may increase bioavailability; a change in diet from high carbohydrate/low protein to low carbohydrate/high protein may result in increased oral clearance.

Cigarette: Smoking may decrease plasma levels of propranolol by increasing metabolism.

Herb/Nutraceutical: Avoid dong quai if using for hypertension (has estrogenic activity). Avoid bayberry, blue cohosh, cayenne, ephedra, ginger, ginseng (American), gotu kola, licorice, yohimbe (may worsen hypertension). Avoid black cohosh, california poppy, coleus, garlic, golden seal, hawthorn, mistletoe, periwinkle, quinine, shepherd's purse (have antihypertensive activity, may cause hypotension).

Dietary Considerations Tablets (immediate release) should be taken on an empty stomach; capsules (extended release) may be taken with or without food, but should always be taken consistently (with food or on an empty stomach)

Pharmacodynamics/Kinetics

Onset of Action Beta-blockade: Oral: 1-2 hours

Duration of Action Immediate release: 6-12 hours; Extended-release formulations: ~24-27 hours

Half-life Elimination Neonates and Infants: Possible increased half-life; Children: 3.9-6.4 hours; Adults: Immediate release formulation: 3-6 hours; Extended-release formulations: 8-10 hours

Time to Peak Immediate release: 1-4 hours; Extended-release formulations: ~6-14 hours

Pregnancy Risk Factor C

Lactation Enters breast milk/use caution (AAP rates "compatible"; AAP 2001 update pending)

Breast-Feeding Considerations Propranolol is excreted into breast milk with peak concentrations occurring ~2-3 hours after an oral dose. The inactive metabolites of propranolol have also been detected in breast milk. The manufacturer recommends that caution be exercised when administering propranolol to nursing women. Due to immature hepatic metabolism in newborns, breast-feeding infants should be monitored for adverse events.

Dosage Forms

Capsule, extended release, oral: 60 mg, 80 mg, 120 mg, 160 mg
InnoPran XL®: 80 mg, 120 mg

Capsule, sustained release, oral:
Inderal® LA: 60 mg, 80 mg, 120 mg, 160 mg

Injection, solution: 1 mg/mL (1 mL)

Injection, solution [preservative free]: 1 mg/mL (1 mL)

Solution, oral: 4 mg/mL (500 mL); 8 mg/mL (500 mL)

Tablet, oral: 10 mg, 20 mg, 40 mg, 60 mg, 80 mg

References

Foster CA and Aston SJ, "Propranolol-Epinephrine Interaction: A Potential Disaster," *Plast Reconstr Surg*, 1983, 72(1):74-8.

Wong DG, Spence JD, Lamki L, et al, "Effect of Nonsteroidal Anti-inflammatory Drugs on Control of Hypertension of Beta-Blockers and Diuretics," *Lancet*, 1986, 1(8488):997-1001.

Wynn RL, "Dental Nonsteroidal Anti-inflammatory Drugs and Prostaglandin-Based Drug Interactions, Part Two," *Gen Dent*, 1992, 40(2):104, 106, 108.

Wynn RL, "Epinephrine Interactions With Beta-Blockers," *Gen Dent*, 1994, 42(1):16, 18.

Propranolol and Hydrochlorothiazide

(proe PRAN oh lole & hye droe klor oh THYE a zide)

Related Information

Hydrochlorothiazide *on page 854*
Propranolol *on page 1422*

Pharmacologic Category Beta Blocker, Nonselective; Diuretic, Thiazide

Use Management of hypertension

Local Anesthetic/Vasoconstrictor Precautions Use with caution; epinephrine has interacted with nonselective beta-blockers to result in initial hypertensive episode followed by bradycardia

Effects on Dental Treatment Noncardioselective beta-blockers (ie, propranolol, nadolol) enhance the pressor response to epinephrine, resulting in hypertension and bradycardia. Many nonsteroidal anti-inflammatory drugs, such as ibuprofen and indomethacin, can reduce the hypotensive effect of beta-blockers after 3 or more weeks of therapy with the NSAID. Short-term NSAID use (ie, 3 days) requires no special precautions in patients taking beta-blockers.

Effects on Bleeding No information available to require special precautions

Adverse Effects See individual agents.

General Dosage Range Oral: *Adults:* Propranolol 80-160 mg/day and hydrochlorothiazide 12.5-50 mg/day in 2 divided doses

Pregnancy Risk Factor C

Propylhexedrine (proe pil HEKS e dreen)

U.S. Brand Names Benzedrex® [OTC]

Pharmacologic Category Adrenergic Agonist Agent

Use Topical nasal decongestant

Local Anesthetic/Vasoconstrictor Precautions No information available to require special precautions

Effects on Dental Treatment No significant effects or complications reported

Effects on Bleeding No information available to require special precautions

Adverse Effects Frequency not defined.

Local: Nasal: Burning, stinging

Respiratory: Sneezing, nasal discharge increased

General Dosage Range Oral: *Children ≥6 years and Adults:* 2 inhalations in each nostril, not more frequently than every 2 hours

Propylthiouracil (proe pil thye oh YOOR a sil)

Related Information

Endocrine Disorders and Pregnancy *on page 1879*

Canadian Brand Names Propyl-Thyracil®

Pharmacologic Category Antithyroid Agent; Thioamide

Use Adjunctive therapy in patients intolerant of methimazole to ameliorate hyperthyroidism symptoms in preparation for surgical treatment or radioactive iodine therapy; treatment of hyperthyroidism in patients intolerant of methimazole and not candidates for surgical/radiotherapy

Unlabeled/Investigational Use Management of thyrotoxic crisis

Local Anesthetic/Vasoconstrictor Precautions No information available to require special precautions

Effects on Dental Treatment Key adverse event(s) related to dental treatment: Loss of taste perception.

Effects on Bleeding No information available to require special precautions

Adverse Effects Frequency not defined.

Cardiovascular: Periarteritis, vasculitis (ANCA-positive, cutaneous, leukocytoclastic)

Central nervous system: Drowsiness, drug fever, fever, headache, neuritis, vertigo

Dermatologic: Alopecia, erythema nodosum, exfoliative dermatitis, pruritus, skin pigmentation, skin rash, skin ulcers, urticaria

Endocrine & metabolic: Goiter, weight gain

Gastrointestinal: Constipation, loss of taste, nausea, sialoadenopathy, splenomegaly, stomach pain, taste perversion, vomiting

Hematologic: Agranulocytosis, aplastic anemia, bleeding, granulopenia, hypoprothrombinemia, leukopenia, thrombocytopenia

Hepatic: Acute liver failure, cholestatic jaundice, hepatitis

Neuromuscular & skeletal: Arthralgia, myalgia, paresthesia

Renal: Acute renal failure, glomerulonephritis, nephritis

Respiratory: Alveolar hemorrhage, interstitial pneumonitis

Miscellaneous: Lymphadenopathy, SLE-like syndrome

General Dosage Range Oral:

Children 6-10 years: 50-150 mg/day

Children >10 years: 150-300 mg/day

Adults: Initial: 300-900 mg/day in 3 divided doses; Maintenance: 100-150 mg/day

Mechanism of Action Inhibits the synthesis of thyroid hormones by blocking the oxidation of iodine in the thyroid gland; blocks synthesis of thyroxine and triiodothyronine

Pharmacodynamics/Kinetics

Onset of Action Therapeutic: 24-36 hours; Peak effect: Remission: 4 months of continued therapy

Duration of Action 2-3 hours

Half-life Elimination 1.5-5 hours; End-stage renal disease: 8.5 hours

Time to Peak Serum: ~1 hour

Pregnancy Risk Factor D

Protamine Sulfate (PROE ta meen SUL fate)

Pharmacologic Category Antidote

Use Treatment of heparin overdosage; neutralize heparin during surgery or dialysis procedures

Unlabeled/Investigational Use Treatment of low molecular weight heparin (LMWH) overdose

Local Anesthetic/Vasoconstrictor Precautions No information available to require special precautions

Effects on Dental Treatment No significant effects or complications reported

Effects on Bleeding Administration reverses the effect of heparin anticoagulants to permit general surgical treatment (eg, abdominal or orthopedic surgery). Risk of bleeding is dependent on multiple variables, including the intensity of anticoagulation and patient susceptibility. The need to address the effects of anticoagulation for dental surgery is based on a complex risk to benefit assessment; medical consult is suggested.

Adverse Effects Frequency not defined.

Cardiovascular: Sudden fall in blood pressure, bradycardia, flushing, hypotension

Central nervous system: Lassitude

Gastrointestinal: Nausea, vomiting

Hematologic: Hemorrhage

Respiratory: Dyspnea, pulmonary hypertension

Miscellaneous: Hypersensitivity reactions

General Dosage Range I.V.: *Children and Adults:* 1 mg of protamine neutralizes 90 USP units of heparin (lung) and 115 USP units of heparin (intestinal) (maximum dose: 50 mg)

Mechanism of Action Combines with strongly acidic heparin to form a stable complex (salt) neutralizing the anticoagulant activity of both drugs

Pharmacodynamics/Kinetics
Onset of Action I.V.: Heparin neutralization: ~5 minutes
Pregnancy Risk Factor C

Protein C Concentrate (Human) (PROE teen cee KON suhn trate HYU man)

U.S. Brand Names Ceprotin
Pharmacologic Category Anticoagulant
Use Replacement therapy for severe congenital protein C deficiency for the prevention and/or treatment of venous thromboembolism and purpura fulminans
Local Anesthetic/Vasoconstrictor Precautions No information available to require special precautions
Effects on Dental Treatment No significant effects or complications reported
Effects on Bleeding As with all drugs which may affect hemostasis, bleeding may be associated with protein C administration. Risk is dependent on multiple variables. Medical consult is suggested.
Adverse Effects As with all drugs which may affect hemostasis, bleeding may be associated with protein C administration. Hemorrhage may occur at virtually any site. Risk is dependent on multiple variables, including the concurrent use of multiple agents that alter hemostasis and patient susceptibility. Frequency not defined.

Central nervous system: Lightheadedness
Hematologic: Bleeding
Miscellaneous: Hypersensitivity reactions (itching and rash)
Postmarketing and/or case reports: Fever, hemothorax, hypotension, hyperhidrosis, restlessness

General Dosage Range I.V.: *Children and Adults:* Initial: 100-120 int. units, followed by 60-80 int. units every 6 hours for 3 doses; maintenance: 45-60 int. units every 6 hours (short-term) or every 12 hours (short-to-long term)
Mechanism of Action Converted to activated protein C (APC). APC is a serine protease which inactivates factors Va and VIIIa, limiting thrombotic formation. *In vitro* data also suggest inhibition of plasminogen activator inhibitor-1 (PAF-1) resulting in profibrinolytic activity, inhibition of macrophage production of tumor necrosis factor, blocking of leukocyte adhesion, and limitation of thrombin-induced inflammatory responses.
Pharmacodynamics/Kinetics
Half-life Elimination Median: 9.8 hours; range 4.9-14.7 hours
Time to Peak Plasma: T_{max}: 0.5 hours
Pregnancy Risk Factor C

Protriptyline (proe TRIP ti leen)

U.S. Brand Names Vivactil®
Pharmacologic Category Antidepressant, Tricyclic (Secondary Amine)
Use Treatment of depression
Local Anesthetic/Vasoconstrictor Precautions Use with caution; epinephrine and levonordefrin have been shown to have an increased pressor response in combination with TCAs. Protriptyline is one of the drugs confirmed to prolong the QT interval and is accepted as having a risk of causing torsade de pointes. The risk of drug-induced torsade de pointes is extremely low when a single QT interval prolonging drug is prescribed. In terms of epinephrine, it is not known what effect vasoconstrictors in the local anesthetic regimen will have in patients with a known history of congenital prolonged QT interval or in patients taking any medication that prolongs the QT interval. Until more information is obtained, it is suggested that the clinician consult with the physician prior to the use of a vasoconstrictor in suspected patients, and that the vasoconstrictor (epinephrine, mepivacaine and levonordefrin [Carbocaine® 2% with Neo-Cobefrin®]) be used with caution.
Effects on Dental Treatment Key adverse event(s) related to dental treatment: Xerostomia and changes in salivation (normal salivary flow resumes upon discontinuation), unpleasant taste, and trouble with gums. Long-term treatment with TCAs, such as protriptyline, increases the risk of caries by reducing salivation and salivary buffer capacity.
Effects on Bleeding No information available to require special precautions
Adverse Effects Frequency not defined.

Cardiovascular: Arrhythmias, heart block, hyper-/hypotension, MI, palpitation, stroke, tachycardia
Central nervous system: Agitation, anxiety, ataxia, confusion, delirium, delusions, dizziness, drowsiness, EPS, exacerbation of psychosis, fatigue, hallucinations, headache, hypomania, incoordination, insomnia, nightmares, panic, restlessness, seizure

Dermatologic: Alopecia, itching, petechiae, photosensitivity, rash, urticaria
Endocrine & metabolic: Breast enlargement, galactorrhea, gynecomastia, increased or decreased libido, syndrome of inappropriate ADH secretion (SIADH)
Gastrointestinal: Anorexia, constipation, decreased lower esophageal sphincter tone may cause GE reflux, diarrhea, heartburn, increased appetite, nausea, trouble with gums, unpleasant taste, vomiting, weight gain/loss, xerostomia
Genitourinary: Difficult urination, impotence, testicular edema
Hematologic: Agranulocytosis, eosinophilia, leukopenia, purpura, thrombocytopenia
Hepatic: Cholestatic jaundice, increased liver enzymes
Neuromuscular & skeletal: Fine muscle tremor, numbness, tingling, tremor, weakness
Ocular: Blurred vision, eye pain, increased intraocular pressure
Otic: Tinnitus
Miscellaneous: Allergic reactions, excessive diaphoresis

General Dosage Range Oral:
Adolescents: 15-20 mg/day
Adults: 15-60 mg/day in 3-4 divided doses
Elderly: Initial: 5-10 mg/day; Maintenance: 15-20 mg/day

Mechanism of Action Increases the synaptic concentration of serotonin and/or norepinephrine in the central nervous system by inhibition of their reuptake by the presynaptic neuronal membrane

Pharmacodynamics/Kinetics
Half-life Elimination 54-92 hours (average: 74 hours)
Time to Peak Serum: 24-30 hours

Pregnancy Risk Factor C

Dental Comment Protriptyline is known to prolong the QT interval. The QT interval is measured as the time and distance between the Q point of the QRS complex and the end of the T wave in the ECG tracing. After adjustment for heart rate, the QT interval is defined as prolonged if it is more than 450 msec in men and 460 msec in women. A long QT syndrome was first described in the 1950s and 60s as a congenital syndrome involving QT interval prolongation and syncope and sudden death. Some of the congenital long QT syndromes were characterized by a peculiar electrocardiographic appearance of the QRS complex involving a premature atria beat followed by a pause, then a subsequent sinus beat showing marked QT prolongation and deformity. This type of cardiac arrhythmia was originally termed "torsade de pointes" (translated from the French as "twisting of the points"). Protriptyline is considered as having a risk of causing torsade de pointes. Since it is not known what effect vasoconstrictors in the local anesthetic regimen will have in patients with a known history of congenital prolonged QT interval or in patients taking any medication that prolongs the QT interval, a medical consult is suggested.

Pseudoephedrine (soo doe e FED rin)

Related Information
Bacterial Infections *on page 1933*

Related Sample Prescriptions
Sinus Infection Treatment *on page 1985*

U.S. Brand Names Children's Nasal Decongestant [OTC]; Genaphed™ [OTC]; Oranyl [OTC]; Silfedrine Children's [OTC]; Sudafed® 12 Hour [OTC]; Sudafed® 24 Hour [OTC]; Sudafed® Children's [OTC]; Sudafed® Maximum Strength Nasal Decongestant [OTC]; Sudo-Tab® [OTC]; SudoGest 12 Hour [OTC]; SudoGest Children's [OTC]; SudoGest [OTC]

Canadian Brand Names Balminil Decongestant; Benylin® D for Infants; Contac® Cold 12 Hour Relief Non Drowsy; Drixoral® ND; Eltor®; PMS-Pseudoephedrine; Pseudofrin; Robidrine®; Sudafed® Decongestant

Generic Availability (U.S.) Yes: Excludes extended release products

Pharmacologic Category Alpha/Beta Agonist

Dental Use Temporary symptomatic relief of nasal congestion due to common cold, upper respiratory allergies, and sinusitis; also promotes nasal or sinus drainage

Use Temporary symptomatic relief of nasal congestion due to common cold, upper respiratory allergies, and sinusitis; also promotes nasal or sinus drainage

Local Anesthetic/Vasoconstrictor Precautions Use with caution since pseudoephedrine is a sympathomimetic amine which could interact with epinephrine to cause a pressor response

Effects on Dental Treatment Key adverse event(s) related to dental treatment: Xerostomia (normal salivary flow resumes upon discontinuation).

Effects on Bleeding No information available to require special precautions

Adverse Effects Frequency not defined.
Cardiovascular: Arrhythmia, cardiovascular collapse with hypotension, hypertension, palpitation, tachycardia

Central nervous system: Chills, confusion, coordination impaired, dizziness, drowsiness, excitability, fatigue, hallucination, headache, insomnia, nervousness, neuritis, restlessness, seizure, transient stimulation, vertigo
Dermatologic: Photosensitivity, rash, urticaria
Gastrointestinal: Anorexia, constipation, diarrhea, dry throat, ischemic colitis, nausea, vomiting, xerostomia
Genitourinary: Difficult urination, dysuria, polyuria, urinary retention
Hematologic: Agranulocytosis, hemolytic anemia, thrombocytopenia
Neuromuscular & skeletal: Tremor, weakness
Ocular: Blurred vision, diplopia
Otic: Tinnitus
Respiratory: Chest/throat tightness, dry nose, dyspnea, nasal congestion, thickening of bronchial secretions, wheezing
Miscellaneous: Anaphylaxis, diaphoresis

Dosage Oral: General dosing guidelines:
Children:
4-5 years: 15 mg every 4-6 hours: maximum 60 mg/24 hours
6-12 years: 30 mg every 4-6 hours; maximum: 120 mg/24 hours
Children >12 years and Adults: Immediate release: 60 mg every 4-6 hours; Extended release: 120 mg every 12 hours **or** 240 mg every 24 hours; maximum: 240 mg/24 hours
Dosing adjustment in renal impairment: Consider reducing dose

Mechanism of Action Directly stimulates alpha-adrenergic receptors of respiratory mucosa causing vasoconstriction; directly stimulates beta-adrenergic receptors causing bronchial relaxation, increased heart rate and contractility

Contraindications Hypersensitivity to pseudoephedrine or any component of the formulation; with or within 14 days of MAO inhibitor therapy

Warnings/Precautions Use with caution in the elderly; may be more sensitive to adverse effects; administer with caution to patients with hypertension, hyperthyroidism, diabetes mellitus, cardiovascular disease, ischemic heart disease, increased intraocular pressure, prostatic hyperplasia, seizure disorders, or renal impairment. When used for self-medication (OTC), notify healthcare provider if symptoms do not improve within 7 days or are accompanied by fever. Discontinue and contact healthcare provider if nervousness, dizziness, or sleeplessness occur. Some products may contain sodium. Not for OTC use in children <4 years of age.

Drug Interactions

Avoid Concomitant Use

Avoid concomitant use of Pseudoephedrine with any of the following: Iobenguane I 123; MAO Inhibitors

Increased Effect/Toxicity

Pseudoephedrine may increase the levels/effects of: Bromocriptine; Sympathomimetics

The levels/effects of Pseudoephedrine may be increased by: Antacids; Atomoxetine; Cannabinoids; Carbonic Anhydrase Inhibitors; MAO Inhibitors; Serotonin/Norepinephrine Reuptake Inhibitors

Decreased Effect

Pseudoephedrine may decrease the levels/effects of: Benzylpenicilloyl Polylysine; Iobenguane I 123

The levels/effects of Pseudoephedrine may be decreased by: Spironolactone

Ethanol/Nutrition/Herb Interactions
Food: Onset of effect may be delayed if pseudoephedrine is taken with food.
Herb/Nutraceutical: Avoid ephedra, yohimbe (may cause hypertension).

Dietary Considerations Some products may contain sodium. May be taken with or without food.

Pharmacodynamics/Kinetics

Onset of Action Decongestant: Oral: 30 minutes (Chua, 1989); Peak effect: Decongestant: Oral: ~1-2 hours (Chua, 1989)

Duration of Action Immediate release tablet: 3-8 hours (Chua, 1989)

Half-life Elimination Varies by urine pH and flow rate; alkaline urine decreases renal elimination of pseudoephedrine (Kanfer, 1993)
Children: ~3 hours (urine pH ~6.5) (Simons, 1996)
Adults: 9-16 hours (pH 8); 3-6 hours (pH 5) (Chua, 1989)

Time to Peak
Children (immediate release) ~2 hours (Simons, 1996)
Adults (immediate release): 1-3 hours (dose dependent) (Kanfer, 1993)

Lactation Enters breast milk (AAP rates "compatible"; AAP 2001 update pending)

Breast-Feeding Considerations Pseudoephedrine is excreted into breast milk in concentrations that are ~4% of the weight adjusted maternal dose. The time to maximum milk concentration is ~1-2 hours after the maternal dose. Irritability has been reported in nursing infants (limited data; dose, duration, relationship to breast-feeding not provided). Milk production may be decreased in some women.

Dosage Forms

Caplet, extended release, oral:
Sudafed® 12 Hour [OTC]: 120 mg

Liquid, oral: 30 mg/5 mL (473 mL)
Children's Nasal Decongestant [OTC]: 30 mg/5 mL (118 mL)
Silfedrine Children's [OTC]: 15 mg/5 mL (118 mL, 237 mL)
Sudafed® Children's [OTC]: 15 mg/5 mL (118 mL)

Syrup, oral: 30 mg/5 mL (118 mL)
SudoGest Children's [OTC]: 15 mg/5 mL (118 mL)

Tablet, oral: 30 mg
Genaphed™ [OTC]: 30 mg
Oranyl [OTC]: 30 mg
Sudafed® Maximum Strength Nasal Decongestant [OTC]: 30 mg
Sudo-Tab® [OTC]: 30 mg
SudoGest [OTC]: 30 mg, 60 mg

Tablet, extended release, oral:
Sudafed® 24 Hour [OTC]: 240 mg
SudoGest 12 Hour [OTC]: 120 mg

Pseudoephedrine and Codeine (soo doe e FED rin & KOE deen)

Related Information

Codeine *on page 432*
Pseudoephedrine *on page 1429*

U.S. Brand Names EndaCof-DC; Notuss®-DC

Pharmacologic Category Antitussive/Decongestant

Use Temporary symptomatic relief of congestion and cough due to upper respiratory infections including common cold, bronchitis, sinusitis, and influenza

Local Anesthetic/Vasoconstrictor Precautions Use with caution since pseudoephedrine is a sympathomimetic amine which could interact with epinephrine or mepivacaine and levonordefrin (Carbocaine® 2% with Neo-Cobefrin®) to cause a pressor response.

Effects on Dental Treatment Key adverse event(s) related to dental treatment: Xerostomia (normal salivary flow resumes upon discontinuation).

Effects on Bleeding No information available to require special precautions

Adverse Effects Frequency not defined.

Cardiovascular: Arrhythmia, heart rate decreased/increased, hypertension, pallor, palpitation, tightness of chest

Central nervous system: Confusion, coordination impaired, dizziness, drowsiness, euphoria, excitation, fatigue, headache, hysteria, insomnia, irritability, lightheadedness, nervousness, neuritis, restlessness, sedation, seizure, vertigo

Dermatologic: Photosensitivity, pruritus, rash, urticaria

Endocrine & metabolic: Early menses

Gastrointestinal: Abdominal pain, anorexia, constipation, diarrhea, epigastric distress, nausea, vomiting

Genitourinary: Dysuria, polyuria, urinary retention

Neuromuscular & skeletal: Paresthesia, tremor, weakness

Ocular: Blurred vision, diplopia

Otic: Acute labyrinthitis, tinnitus

Respiratory: Dyspnea, nasal congestion, thickening of bronchial secretions, wheezing

Miscellaneous: Diaphoresis

General Dosage Range Oral:

Children 6-11 years: 2.5-5 mL every 4-6 hours as needed (maximum: 20 mL/24 hours)

Children ≥12 years and Adults: 5-10 mL every 4-6 hours as needed (maximum: 40 mL/24 hours)

Mechanism of Action

Pseudoephedrine directly stimulates alpha-adrenergic receptors of respiratory mucosa causing vasoconstriction; directly stimulates beta-adrenergic receptors causing bronchial relaxation

Codeine is an antitussive that controls cough by depressing the medullary cough center

Pregnancy Risk Factor C

Controlled Substance Liquid: C-V

Pseudoephedrine and Dextromethorphan

(soo doe e FED rin & deks troe meth OR fan)

Related Information

Dextromethorphan *on page* 504

Pseudoephedrine *on page* 1429

U.S. Brand Names Pedia Relief Cough and Cold [OTC]; Sudafed® Children's Cold & Cough [OTC]

Canadian Brand Names Balminil DM D; Benylin® DM-D; Koffex DM-D; Novahistex® DM Decongestant; Novahistine® DM Decongestant; Robitussin® Childrens Cough & Cold

Pharmacologic Category Antitussive/Decongestant

Use Temporary symptomatic relief of nasal congestion and cough due to common cold, hay fever, upper respiratory allergies

Local Anesthetic/Vasoconstrictor Precautions Use with caution since pseudoephedrine is a sympathomimetic amine which could interact with epinephrine to cause a pressor response

Effects on Dental Treatment Key adverse event(s) related to dental treatment: Pseudoephedrine: Xerostomia (normal salivary flow resumes upon discontinuation).

Effects on Bleeding No information available to require special precautions

Adverse Effects See individual agents.

General Dosage Range Oral:

Children 2-6 years: 15 mg (based on pseudoephedrine) every 4-6 hours (maximum: 60 mg/day)

Children 6-12 years: 30 mg (based on pseudoephedrine) every 4-6 hours (maximum: 120 mg/day)

Children ≥12 years and Adults: 60 mg (based on pseudoephedrine) every 4-6 hours (maximum: 240 mg/day)

Pseudoephedrine and Ibuprofen

(soo doe e FED rin & eye byoo PROE fen)

Related Information

Ibuprofen *on page* 884

Pseudoephedrine *on page* 1429

U.S. Brand Names Advil® Cold & Sinus [OTC]; Proprinal® Cold and Sinus [OTC]

Canadian Brand Names Advil® Cold & Sinus; Advil® Cold & Sinus Daytime; Children's Advil® Cold; Sudafed® Sinus Advance

Pharmacologic Category Decongestant/Analgesic

Use For temporary relief of cold, sinus, and flu symptoms (including nasal congestion, sinus pressure, headache, minor body aches and pains, and fever)

Local Anesthetic/Vasoconstrictor Precautions Use with caution since pseudoephedrine is a sympathomimetic amine which could interact with epinephrine to cause a pressor response

Effects on Dental Treatment Key adverse event(s) related to dental treatment: Pseudoephedrine: Xerostomia (normal salivary flow resumes upon discontinuation).

The dentist should be aware of the potential of abnormal coagulation. Caution should also be exercised in the use of NSAIDs in patients already on anticoagulant therapy with drugs such as warfarin (Coumadin®). See Effects on Bleeding.

Effects on Bleeding Nonselective NSAIDs are known to reversibly decrease platelet aggregation via mechanisms different than observed with aspirin. Platelet function is restored as the drug is eliminated from the body. NSAIDs should be avoided (if possible) in general surgery patients for 3-5 half-lives of the drug (usually 1-3 days) prior to surgery to reduce the risk of excessive bleeding. However, there is no scientific evidence to warrant discontinuance of NSAIDs prior to dental surgery. In medically complicated patients or extensive oral surgery, the decision to interrupt therapy must be based on the risk to benefit in an individual patient and a medical consult is suggested. Routine interruption of NSAID therapy for most dental procedures is not warranted. If therapy is continued without interruption, the clinician should anticipate the potential for slower clotting times.

Adverse Effects See individual agents.

General Dosage Range Oral: *Children ≥12 years and Adults:* 1-2 doses (ibuprofen 200 mg and pseudoephedrine 30 mg per dose) every 4-6 hours as needed (maximum: 6 doses/day)

Pregnancy Risk Factor Ibuprofen: B/D (3rd trimester)

Pseudoephedrine and Methscopolamine

(soo doe e FED rin & meth skoe POL a meen)

Related Information

Methscopolamine *on page* *1106*

Pseudoephedrine *on page* *1429*

U.S. Brand Names AlleRx™-D [DSC]

Pharmacologic Category Decongestant/Anticholingeric Combination

Use Relief of symptoms of allergic rhinitis, vasomotor rhinitis, sinusitis, and the common cold

Local Anesthetic/Vasoconstrictor Precautions Use with caution since pseudoephedrine is a sympathomimetic amine which could interact with epinephrine to cause a pressor response

Effects on Dental Treatment Key adverse event(s) related to dental treatment:

Pseudoephedrine: Xerostomia (normal salivary flow resumes upon discontinuation).

Methscopolamine: Xerostomia and changes in salivation (normal salivary flow resumes upon discontinuation), and dry throat and nose. Anticholinergic side effects can cause a reduction of saliva production or secretion, contributing to discomfort and dental disease (ie, caries, oral candidiasis and periodontal disease).

Effects on Bleeding No information available to require special precautions

Adverse Effects Frequency not defined.

Cardiovascular: Arrhythmias, bradycardia, cardiovascular collapse, flushing, hypotension, pallor, palpitation, tachycardia

Central nervous system: Anxiety, convulsions, CNS depression, dizziness, drowsiness, excitability, fear, giddiness, hallucination, headache, insomnia, irritability, lassitude, nervousness, restlessness

Gastrointestinal: Gastric irritation, nausea, xerostomia

Genitourinary: Dysuria, urinary retention

Neuromuscular & skeletal: Tremor, weakness

Ocular: Blurred vision

Respiratory: Respiratory difficulty

General Dosage Range Oral: *Children ≥12 years and Adults:* 1 tablet every 12 hours (maximum: 2 tablets/24 hours)

Mechanism of Action

Pseudoephedrine: Acts as a decongestant in respiratory tract mucous membranes.

Methscopolamine nitrate: Derivative of scopolamine; a peripheral anticholinergic agent

Pregnancy Risk Factor C

Pseudoephedrine, Dihydrocodeine, and Chlorpheniramine

(soo doe e FED rin, dye hye droe KOE deen, & klor fen IR a meen)

Related Information

Chlorpheniramine *on page* *365*

Pseudoephedrine *on page* *1429*

U.S. Brand Names Coldcough; DiHydro-CP

Pharmacologic Category Alkylamine Derivative; Alpha/Beta Agonist; Analgesic, Opioid; Antitussive; Decongestant; Histamine H_1 Antagonist; Histamine H_1 Antagonist, First Generation

Use Temporary relief of cough, congestion, and sneezing due to colds, respiratory infections, or hay fever

Local Anesthetic/Vasoconstrictor Precautions Use with caution since pseudoephedrine is a sympathomimetic amine which could interact with epinephrine to cause a pressor response

Effects on Dental Treatment Key adverse event(s) related to dental treatment:

Chlorpheniramine: Prolonged use will cause significant xerostomia (normal salivary flow resumes upon discontinuation).

Pseudoephedrine: Xerostomia (prolonged use worsens; normal salivary flow resumes upon discontinuation).

Effects on Bleeding No information available to require special precautions

Adverse Effects See individual agents.

General Dosage Range Oral:

Children 2-6 years: 1.25-2.5 mL every 4-6 hours (maximum: 4 doses/day)

Children 6-12 years: 2.5-5 mL every 4-6 hours (maximum: 4 doses/day)

Children >12 years and Adults: 5-10 mL every 4-6 hours (maximum: 4 doses/day)

Mechanism of Action
Pseudoephedrine: Directly stimulates alpha-adrenergic receptors of respiratory mucosa causing vasoconstriction; directly stimulates beta-adrenergic receptors causing bronchial relaxation
Dihydrocodeine: Binds to opiate receptors in the CNS; suppresses cough in medullary center
Chlorpheniramine: Competes with histamine for H_1-receptor sites on effector cells in the gastrointestinal tract, blood vessels, and respiratory tract
Pregnancy Risk Factor C
Controlled Substance C-III

Psyllium (SIL i yum)

U.S. Brand Names Bulk-K [OTC]; Fiberall® [OTC]; Fibro-Lax [OTC]; Fibro-XL [OTC]; Genfiber™ [OTC]; Hydrocil® Instant [OTC]; Konsyl-D™ [OTC]; Konsyl® Easy Mix™ [OTC]; Konsyl® Orange [OTC]; Konsyl® Original [OTC]; Konsyl® [OTC]; Metamucil® Plus Calcium [OTC]; Metamucil® Smooth Texture [OTC]; Metamucil® [OTC]; Natural Fiber Therapy Smooth Texture [OTC]; Natural Fiber Therapy [OTC]; Reguloid [OTC]
Canadian Brand Names Metamucil®
Pharmacologic Category Antidiarrheal; Fiber Supplement; Laxative, Bulk-Producing
Use OTC labeling: Dietary fiber supplement; treatment of occasional constipation; reduce risk of coronary heart disease (CHD)
Unlabeled/Investigational Use Treatment of diarrhea, chronic constipation, irritable bowel syndrome, inflammatory bowel disease, colon cancer, or diabetes
Local Anesthetic/Vasoconstrictor Precautions No information available to require special precautions
Effects on Dental Treatment No significant effects or complications reported
Effects on Bleeding No information available to require special precautions
Adverse Effects Frequency not defined.
Gastrointestinal: Abdominal cramps, constipation, diarrhea, esophageal or bowel obstruction
Respiratory: Bronchospasm
Miscellaneous: Anaphylaxis upon inhalation in susceptible individuals, rhinoconjunctivitis
General Dosage Range Oral:
Children 6-11 years: Psyllium 1.25-15 g/day in divided doses
Children ≥12 years and Adults: Psyllium 2.5-30 g/day in divided doses
Mechanism of Action Psyllium is a soluble fiber. It absorbs water in the intestine to form a viscous liquid which promotes peristalsis and reduces transit time.
Pharmacodynamics/Kinetics
Onset of Action Relief of constipation: 12-72 hours

Pyrantel Pamoate (pi RAN tel PAM oh ate)

U.S. Brand Names Pin-X® [OTC]; Reese's Pinworm Medicine [OTC]
Canadian Brand Names Combantrin™
Pharmacologic Category Anthelmintic
Use Treatment of pinworms (*Enterobius vermicularis*) and roundworms (*Ascaris lumbricoides*)
Unlabeled/Investigational Use Treatment of whipworms (*Trichuris trichiura*) and hookworms (*Ancylostoma duodenale*)
Local Anesthetic/Vasoconstrictor Precautions No information available to require special precautions
Effects on Dental Treatment No significant effects or complications reported
Effects on Bleeding No information available to require special precautions
Adverse Effects Frequency not defined.
Central nervous system: Dizziness, drowsiness, insomnia, headache
Dermatologic: Rash
Gastrointestinal: Abdominal cramps, anorexia, diarrhea, nausea, vomiting, tenesmus
Hepatic: Liver enzymes increased
Neuromuscular & skeletal: Weakness
General Dosage Range Oral: *Children and Adults:* 11 mg/kg as a single dose (maximum: 1 g/dose); repeat in 2 weeks for pinworm (dose is expressed as pyrantel base)
Mechanism of Action Causes the release of acetylcholine and inhibits cholinesterase; acts as a depolarizing neuromuscular blocker, paralyzing the helminths

Pharmacodynamics/Kinetics

Time to Peak Serum: 1-3 hours

Pregnancy Risk Factor C

Pyrazinamide (peer a ZIN a mide)

Related Information

Tuberculosis *on page 1902*

Canadian Brand Names Tebrazid™

Pharmacologic Category Antitubercular Agent

Use Adjunctive treatment of tuberculosis in combination with other antituberculosis agents

Local Anesthetic/Vasoconstrictor Precautions No information available to require special precautions

Effects on Dental Treatment No significant effects or complications reported

Effects on Bleeding No information available to require special precautions

Adverse Effects 1% to 10%:

Central nervous system: Malaise

Gastrointestinal: Anorexia, nausea, vomiting

Neuromuscular & skeletal: Arthralgia, myalgia

General Dosage Range Dosage adjustment recommended in patients with renal impairment

Oral:

Children: 15-30 mg/kg once daily (maximum: 2 g/day) **or** 50 mg/kg/dose twice weekly (maximum: 2 g/dose)

Adults 40-55 kg: 1000 mg once daily **or** 2000 mg twice weekly **or** 1500 mg 3 times/week

Adults 56-75 kg: 1500 mg once daily **or** 3000 mg twice weekly **or** 2500 mg 3 times/week

Adults 76-90 kg: 2000 mg once daily (maximum dose regardless of weight) **or** 4000 mg twice weekly (maximum dose regardless of weight) **or** 3000 mg 3 times/week (maximum dose regardless of weight)

Mechanism of Action Converted to pyrazinoic acid in susceptible strains of *Mycobacterium* which lowers the pH of the environment; exact mechanism of action has not been elucidated

Pharmacodynamics/Kinetics

Half-life Elimination 9-10 hours

Time to Peak Serum: Within 2 hours

Pregnancy Risk Factor C

Pyrethrins and Piperonyl Butoxide
(pye RE thrins & pi PER oh nil byo TOKS ide)

U.S. Brand Names A-200® Lice Treatment Kit [OTC]; A-200® Maximum Strength [OTC]; Licide® [OTC]; Pronto® Complete Lice Removal System [OTC]; Pronto® Plus Lice Killing Mousse Plus Vitamin E [OTC]; Pronto® Plus Lice Killing Mousse Shampoo Plus Natural Extracts and Oils [OTC]; Pronto® Plus Warm Oil Treatment and Conditioner [OTC]; RID® Maximum Strength [OTC]

Canadian Brand Names Pronto® Lice Control; R & C™ II; R & C™ Shampoo/Conditioner; RID® Mousse

Pharmacologic Category Antiparasitic Agent, Topical; Pediculocide; Shampoo, Pediculocide

Use Treatment of *Pediculus humanus* infestations (head lice, body lice, pubic lice, and their eggs)

Local Anesthetic/Vasoconstrictor Precautions No information available to require special precautions

Effects on Dental Treatment No significant effects or complications reported

Effects on Bleeding No information available to require special precautions

Adverse Effects Frequency not defined.

Dermatologic: Pruritus

Local: Burning, stinging, irritation with repeat use

General Dosage Range Topical: *Children and Adults:* Apply to infested area, keep on for 10 minutes, wash, and rinse; may repeat once in a 24-hour period and then again in 7-10 days

Mechanism of Action Pyrethrins are derived from flowers that belong to the chrysanthemum family. The mechanism of action on the neuronal membranes of lice is similar to that of DDT. Piperonyl butoxide is usually added to pyrethrin to enhance the product's activity by decreasing the metabolism of pyrethrins in arthropods.

Pharmacodynamics/Kinetics

Onset of Action ~30 minutes

Pregnancy Risk Factor C

Pyridostigmine (peer id oh STIG meen)

U.S. Brand Names Mestinon®; Mestinon® Timespan®; Regonol®

Canadian Brand Names Mestinon®; Mestinon®-SR

Pharmacologic Category Acetylcholinesterase Inhibitor

Use Symptomatic treatment of myasthenia gravis; antagonism of nondepolarizing neuromuscular blockers

Military use: Pretreatment for Soman nerve gas exposure

Local Anesthetic/Vasoconstrictor Precautions No information available to require special precautions

Effects on Dental Treatment Key adverse event(s) related to dental treatment: Dysphagia.

Effects on Bleeding No information available to require special precautions

Adverse Effects Frequency not defined.

Cardiovascular: Arrhythmias (especially bradycardia), AV block, cardiac arrest, decreased carbon monoxide, flushing, hypotension, nodal rhythm, nonspecific ECG changes, syncope, tachycardia

Central nervous system: Convulsions, dizziness, drowsiness, dysphonia, headache, loss of consciousness

Dermatologic: Skin rash, thrombophlebitis (I.V.), urticaria

Gastrointestinal: Abdominal pain, diarrhea, dysphagia, flatulence, hyperperistalsis, nausea, salivation, stomach cramps, vomiting

Genitourinary: Urinary urgency

Neuromuscular & skeletal: Arthralgia, dysarthria, fasciculations, muscle cramps, myalgia, spasms, weakness

Ocular: Amblyopia, lacrimation, small pupils

Respiratory: Bronchial secretions increased, bronchiolar constriction, bronchospasm, dyspnea, laryngospasm, respiratory arrest, respiratory depression, respiratory muscle paralysis

Miscellaneous: Allergic reactions, anaphylaxis, diaphoresis increased

General Dosage Range

I.M.:

Children: 0.05-0.15 mg/kg/dose

Adults: ~1/30th of oral dose

I.V.:

Children: 0.05-0.25 mg/kg/dose

Adults: IVP: ~1/30th of oral dose **or** 0.1-0.25 mg/kg/dose (usual: 10-20 mg); Infusion: 2 mg/hour with gradual titration in increments of 0.5-1 mg/hour (maximum: 4 mg/hour)

Oral:

Immediate release:

Children: 7 mg/kg/day divided into 5-6 doses

Adults: 60-1500 mg/day in 5-6 divided doses (usual: 600 mg/day)

Sustained release: *Adults:* 180-540 mg once or twice daily (doses separated by at least 6 hours)

Mechanism of Action Inhibits destruction of acetylcholine by acetylcholinesterase which facilitates transmission of impulses across myoneural junction

Pharmacodynamics/Kinetics

Onset of Action Oral, I.M.: 15-30 minutes; I.V. injection: 2-5 minutes

Duration of Action Oral: Up to 6-8 hours (due to slow absorption); I.V.: 2-3 hours

Half-life Elimination 1-2 hours; Renal failure: ≤6 hours

Pregnancy Risk Factor B

Pyridoxine (peer i DOKS een)

U.S. Brand Names Aminoxin® [OTC]; Pyri-500 [OTC]

Pharmacologic Category Vitamin, Water Soluble

Use Prevention and treatment of vitamin B_6 deficiency, pyridoxine-dependent seizures in infants

Unlabeled/Investigational Use Treatment and prophylaxis of neurological toxicities (ie, seizures, coma) associated with isoniazid, hydrazine, and Gyromitrin-containing mushroom (false morel) overdose/toxicity

Local Anesthetic/Vasoconstrictor Precautions No information available to require special precautions

Effects on Dental Treatment No significant effects or complications reported

Effects on Bleeding No information available to require special precautions

Adverse Effects Frequency not defined.

Central nervous system: Headache, seizure (following very large I.V. doses), somnolence

Endocrine & metabolic: Acidosis, folic acid decreased

Gastrointestinal: Nausea

Hepatic: AST increased

Neuromuscular & skeletal: Neuropathy, paresthesia

Miscellaneous: Allergic reactions

General Dosage Range

I.M., I.V., SubQ: *Infants:* Deficiency: 10-100 mg

Oral:

Infants: Deficiency: 2-100 mg/day

Children: Deficiency: 1.5-25 mg/day; Neuritis: Prophylaxis: 1-2 mg/kg/day; Treatment: 10-50 mg/day

Adults: Deficiency: 10-20 mg/day; Neuritis: Prophylaxis: 25-100 mg/day; Treatment: 100-200 mg/day

Mechanism of Action Precursor to pyridoxal, which functions in the metabolism of proteins, carbohydrates, and fats; pyridoxal also aids in the release of liver and muscle-stored glycogen and in the synthesis of GABA (within the central nervous system) and heme

Pharmacodynamics/Kinetics

Half-life Elimination Biologic: 15-20 days

Pregnancy Risk Factor A

Pyrimethamine (peer i METH a meen)

U.S. Brand Names Daraprim®

Canadian Brand Names Daraprim®

Pharmacologic Category Antimalarial Agent

Use Prophylaxis of malaria due to susceptible strains of plasmodia; used in conjunction with a sulfonamide for the treatment of uncomplicated malaria due to susceptible strains of plasmodia (alternative agent; not preferred therapy); synergistic combination with sulfonamide in treatment of toxoplasmosis

Local Anesthetic/Vasoconstrictor Precautions No information available to require special precautions

Effects on Dental Treatment Key adverse event(s) related to dental treatment: Xerostomia (normal salivary flow resumes upon discontinuation). Atrophic glossitis has been reported.

Effects on Bleeding No information available to require special precautions

Adverse Effects Frequency not defined.

Cardiovascular: Arrhythmias (large doses)

Dermatologic: Erythema multiforme, rash, Stevens-Johnson syndrome, toxic epidermal necrolysis

Gastrointestinal: Anorexia, atrophic glossitis, vomiting

Hematologic: Leukopenia, megaloblastic anemia, pancytopenia, pulmonary eosinophilia, thrombocytopenia

Genitourinary: Hematuria

Miscellaneous: Anaphylaxis

General Dosage Range Oral:

Children <4 years: Malaria prophylaxis: 6.25 mg once weekly (maximum: 25 mg/dose)

Children 4-10 years: Malaria prophylaxis: 12.5 mg once weekly (maximum: 25 mg/dose); Malaria treatment: 25 mg daily

Children >10 years: Malaria prophylaxis: 25 mg once weekly; Malaria treatment: 25 mg daily

Children: Toxoplasmosis treatment: Loading dose: 1 mg/kg/day divided into 2 equal doses for 2-4 days; Maintenance: 0.5 mg/kg/day divided into 2 doses (maximum: 25 mg/day)

Adults: Malaria prophylaxis: 25 mg once weekly; Malaria treatment: 25 mg daily; Toxoplasmosis treatment: Initial: 25-75 mg/day; Maintenance: 12.5-37.5 mg/day

Mechanism of Action Inhibits parasitic dihydrofolate reductase, resulting in inhibition of vital tetrahydrofolic acid synthesis

Pharmacodynamics/Kinetics

Onset of Action ~1 hour

Half-life Elimination 80-95 hours

Time to Peak Serum: 1.5-8 hours

Pregnancy Risk Factor C

Pyrithione Zinc (peer i THYE one zingk)

U.S. Brand Names BetaMed™ [OTC]; DermaZinc™ [OTC]; DHS™ Zinc [OTC]; Head & Shoulders® Citrus Breeze 2-in-1 [OTC]; Head & Shoulders® Citrus Breeze [OTC]; Head & Shoulders® Classic Clean 2-in-1 [OTC]; Head & Shoulders® Classic Clean [OTC]; Head & Shoulders® Dry Scalp 2-in-1 [OTC]; Head & Shoulders® Dry Scalp Care 2-in-1 [OTC]; Head & Shoulders® Dry Scalp Care [OTC]; Head & Shoulders® Dry Scalp [OTC]; Head & Shoulders® Extra Volume [OTC]; Head & Shoulders® intensive solutions 2 in 1 [OTC]; Head & Shoulders® intensive solutions for dry/damaged hair [OTC]; Head & Shoulders® intensive solutions for fine/oily hair [OTC]; Head & Shoulders® intensive solutions for normal hair [OTC]; Head & Shoulders® Ocean Lift 2-in-1 [OTC]; Head & Shoulders® Ocean Lift [OTC]; Head & Shoulders® Refresh 2-in-1 [OTC]; Head & Shoulders® Refresh [OTC]; Head & Shoulders® Restoring Shine 2 in 1 [OTC]; Head & Shoulders® Restoring Shine [OTC]; Head & Shoulders® Sensitive Care 2 in 1 [OTC]; Head & Shoulders® Sensitive Care [OTC]; Head & Shoulders® Smooth & Silky 2-in-1 [OTC]; Head & Shoulders® Smooth & Silky [OTC]; Selsun® Salon™ Classic [OTC]; Selsun® Salon™ Dandruff 2-in-1 [OTC]; Selsun® Salon™ Dandruff Moisturizing [OTC]; Selsun® Salon™ Dandruff Volumizing [OTC]; Skin Care™ [OTC]; T/Gel® Daily Control 2 in 1 Dandruff Shampoo Plus Conditioner [OTC]; T/Gel® Daily Control Dandruff Shampoo [OTC]; Zincon® [OTC]; ZNP® [OTC]

Pharmacologic Category Topical Skin Product

Use Relieves the itching, irritation, and scalp flaking associated with dandruff and/or seborrheal dermatitis

Local Anesthetic/Vasoconstrictor Precautions No information available to require special precautions

Effects on Dental Treatment No significant effects or complications reported

Effects on Bleeding No information available to require special precautions

General Dosage Range Topical: *Adults:* Apply at least twice weekly

Quazepam (KWAZ e pam)

U.S. Brand Names Doral®

Canadian Brand Names Doral®

Pharmacologic Category Benzodiazepine

Use Treatment of insomnia

Local Anesthetic/Vasoconstrictor Precautions No information available to require special precautions

Effects on Dental Treatment Key adverse event(s) related to dental treatment: Xerostomia (normal salivary flow resumes upon discontinuation) and abnormal taste perception.

Effects on Bleeding No information available to require special precautions

Adverse Effects

>10%: Central nervous system: Daytime drowsiness (12%)

<10%:

Central nervous system: Headache (5%), dizziness (2%), fatigue (2%)

Gastrointestinal: Xerostomia (2%), dyspepsia (1%)

Frequency not defined. **Note:** Asterisked (*) reactions are those reported with benzodiazepines.

Cardiovascular: Palpitation

Central nervous system: Abnormal thinking, agitation, amnesia, anxiety, apathy, ataxia, confusion, depression, dystonia*, euphoria, hallucinations*, hyper-/hypokinesia, incoordination, irritability*, malaise, nervousness, nightmare, paranoid reaction, sleep disturbances*, slurred speech*, speech disorder, stimulation*

Dermatologic: Pruritus, rash

Endocrine & metabolic: Libido decreased, menstrual irregularities*

Gastrointestinal: Abdominal pain, abnormal taste perception, anorexia, constipation, diarrhea, nausea

Genitourinary: Impotence, incontinence, urinary retention*

Hepatic: Jaundice*

Neuromuscular & skeletal: Dysarthria*, muscle spasticity*, tremor, weakness

Ocular: Abnormal vision, cataract

Miscellaneous: Drug dependence, withdrawal*

General Dosage Range Oral:

Adults: 7.5-15 mg at bedtime

Elderly: Initial: 7.5 mg at bedtime

Mechanism of Action Binds to stereospecific benzodiazepine receptors on the postsynaptic GABA neuron at several sites within the central nervous system, including the limbic system, reticular formation. Enhancement of the inhibitory effect of GABA on neuronal excitability results by increased neuronal membrane permeability to chloride ions. This shift in chloride ions results in hyperpolarization (a less excitable state) and stabilization.

Pharmacodynamics/Kinetics

Half-life Elimination Serum: Quazepam, 2-oxoquasepam: 39 hours; N-desalkyl-2-oxoquazepam: 73 hours

Time to Peak ~2 hours

Pregnancy Risk Factor X

Controlled Substance C-IV

QUEtiapine (kwe TYE a peen)

Related Information

Clinical Risk Related to Drugs Prolonging QT Interval *on page 1872*

U.S. Brand Names SEROquel XR®; SEROquel®

Canadian Brand Names Apo-Quetiapine®; CO Quetiapine; Dom-Quetiapine; JAMP-Quetiapine; Mylan-Quetiapine; Novo-Quetiapine; PHL-Quetiapine; PMS-Quetiapine; PRO-Quetiapine; ratio-Quetiapine; Riva-Quetiapine; Sandoz-Quetiapine; Seroquel XR®; Seroquel®; Teva-Quetiapine

Generic Availability (U.S.) No

Pharmacologic Category Antipsychotic Agent, Atypical

Use Treatment of schizophrenia; treatment of acute manic or mixed episodes associated with bipolar I disorder (as monotherapy or in combination with lithium or divalproex); maintenance treatment of bipolar I disorder (in combination with lithium or divalproex); treatment of acute depressive episodes associated with bipolar disorder; adjunctive treatment of major depressive disorder

Unlabeled/Investigational Use Autism; delirium in the critically-ill patient; psychosis/agitation related to Alzheimer's dementia

Local Anesthetic/Vasoconstrictor Precautions Quetiapine is one of the drugs confirmed to prolong the QT interval and is accepted as having a risk of causing torsade de pointes. The risk of drug-induced torsade de pointes is extremely low when a single QT interval prolonging drug is prescribed. In terms of epinephrine, it is not known what effect vasoconstrictors in the local anesthetic regimen will have in patients with a known history of congenital prolonged QT interval or in patients taking any medication that prolongs the QT interval. Until more information is obtained, it is suggested that the clinician consult with the physician prior to the use of a vasoconstrictor in suspected patients, and that the vasoconstrictor (epinephrine, mepivacaine and levonordefrin [Carbocaine® 2% with Neo-Cobefrin®]) be used with caution.

Effects on Dental Treatment Key adverse event(s) related to dental treatment: Xerostomia (normal salivary flow resumes upon discontinuation).

Effects on Bleeding No information available to require special precautions

Adverse Effects Actual frequency may be dependent upon dose and/or indication. Unless otherwise noted, frequency of adverse effects is reported for adult patients; spectrum and incidence of adverse effects similar in children (with significant exceptions noted).

>10%:

Cardiovascular: Diastolic blood pressure increased (children and adolescents, 41%), systolic blood pressure increased (children and adolescents, 15%)

Central nervous system: Somnolence (18% to 57%), headache (7% to 21%), agitation (5% to 20%), dizziness (1% to 18%), fatigue (3% to 14%), extrapyramidal symptoms (1% to 13%)

Endocrine & metabolic: Triglycerides increased (≥200 mg/dL, 8% to 22%), HDL cholesterol decreased (≤40 mg/dL, 6% to 19%), total cholesterol increased (≥240 mg/dL, 7% to 18%), LDL cholesterol increased (≥160 mg/dL, 4% to 17%), hyperglycemia (≥200 mg/dL post glucose challenge or fasting glucose ≥126 mg/dL, 2% to 12%)

Gastrointestinal: Xerostomia (9% to 44%), weight gain (dose related; 3% to 23%), appetite increased (2% to 12%), constipation (6% to 11%)

1% to 10%:

Cardiovascular: Orthostatic hypotension (2% to 7%; children and adolescents <1%), tachycardia (1% to 6%), syncope (<5%), palpitation (4%), peripheral edema (4%), hypotension (3%), hypertension (1% to 2%)

Central nervous system: Insomnia (9%), akathisia (≤8%), pain (1% to 7%), dystonia (≤6%), lethargy (1% to 5%), tardive dyskinesia (<5%), anxiety (2% to 4%), irritability (1% to 4%), parkinsonism (≤4%), abnormal dreams (2% to 3%), depression (1% to 3%), hypersomnia (1% to 3%), abnormal thinking (2%), ataxia (2%), attention disturbance (2%), coordination impaired (2%), disorientation (2%), hypoesthesia (2%), mental impairment (2%), migraine (2%), sluggishness (2%), vertigo (2%), confusion (1% to 2%), restlessness (1% to 2%), fever (1% to 2%), chills (1%)

Dermatologic: Rash (4%), hyperhidrosis (2%)

Endocrine & metabolic: Hyperprolactinemia (4%), libido decreased (≤2%), hypothyroidism (≤2%), female lactation (1%)

Gastrointestinal: Nausea (7% to 8%), abdominal pain (dose related; 4% to 7%), dyspepsia (dose related; 2% to 7%), vomiting (1% to 6%), drooling (<5%), gastroenteritis (2% to 4%), toothache (2% to 3%), appetite decreased (2%), dysphagia (2%), flatulence (2%), GERD (2%), anorexia (≥1%), abnormal taste (1%), abdominal distension (≤1%)

Genitourinary: Pollakiuria (2%), urinary tract infection (2%), impotence (1%)

Hematologic: Neutropenia (≤2%), leukopenia (≥1%), hemorrhage (1%)

Hepatic: Transaminases increased (1% to 6%), GGT increased (1%)

Neuromuscular & skeletal: Weakness (2% to 10%), tremor (2% to 8%), back pain (3% to 5%), dysarthria (1% to 5%), hypertonia (4%), twitching (4%), dyskinesia (≤4%), arthralgia (1% to 4%), paresthesia (3%), muscle spasm (1% to 3%), limb pain (2%), myalgia (2%), neck pain (2%), neck rigidity (1%)

Ocular: Blurred vision (1% to 4%), amblyopia (2% to 3%)

Otic: Ear pain (1% to 2%)

Respiratory: Pharyngitis (4% to 6%), nasal congestion (5%), rhinitis (3% to 4%), upper respiratory tract infection (2% to 3%), sinus congestion (2%), sinus headache (2%), sinusitis (2%), cough (3%), dyspnea (≥1%), dry throat (1%)

Miscellaneous: Diaphoresis (2%), restless legs syndrome (2%), flu-like syndrome (1% to 2%), lymphadenopathy (1%)

<1%, postmarketing, and/or case reports (limited to important or life-threatening): Acute renal failure, agranulocytosis, alkaline phosphatase increased, amnesia, anaphylactic reaction, anaphylaxis, anemia, angina, asthma, atrial arrhythmia, AV block, bradycardia, bundle branch block, cardiomyopathy, cataract formation, cerebral ischemia, cerebrovascular accident, HF, CPK increased, creatinine increased, dehydration, diabetes mellitus, dysuria, eosinophilia, epistaxis, exfoliative dermatitis, galactorrhea, hallucinations, hematemesis, hypoglycemia, hypothyroidism, hypersensitivity, hypokalemia, hyponatremia, intestinal obstruction, involuntary movements, leukocytosis, myocarditis, neuroleptic malignant syndrome, nightmares, pancreatitis, pneumonia, priapism, QRS duration increased, QT prolongation, rectal bleeding, rhabdomyolysis, seizure, SIADH, Stevens-Johnson syndrome, ST segment elevation, suicidal ideation, suicide attempt, thrombocytopenia, tinnitus, T-wave abnormal, T-wave inversion, urinary retention

Dosage Oral:

Children ≥10 years: **Note:** Total daily doses may also be divided into 3 doses per day.

Bipolar disorder:

Mania: Immediate release tablet: Initial: 25 mg twice daily on day 1; increase to 50 mg twice daily on day 2, further increasing by 100 mg/day each day until a target dose of 400 mg/day is reached on day 5. May increase up to 600 mg/day at increments ≤100 mg/day; however, no additional benefit seen with 600 mg/day. Usual dosage range: 400-600 mg/day.

Maintenance therapy: Immediate release tablet: Continue therapy at lowest dose needed to maintain remission; periodically assess maintenance treatment needs.

Autism (unlabeled use): 100-350 mg/day (1.6-5.2 mg/kg/day) (Martin, 1999)

Adolescents ≥13 years: **Note:** Total daily doses may also be divided into 3 doses per day: Schizophrenia: Immediate release tablet: Initial: 25 mg twice daily on day 1; increase to 50 mg twice daily on day 2, further increasing by 100 mg/day each day until a target dose of 400 mg/day is reached on day 5. May increase up to 800 mg/day at increments ≤100 mg/day; however, no additional benefit seen with 800 mg/day. Usual dosage range: 400-800 mg/day; periodically assess maintenance treatment needs.

Adults:

Bipolar disorder:

Depression:

Immediate release tablet: Initial: 50 mg once daily the first day; increase to 100 mg once daily on day 2, further increasing by 100 mg/day each day until a target dose of 300 mg once daily is reached by day 4. Further increases up to 600 mg once daily by day 8 have been evaluated in clinical trials, but no additional antidepressant efficacy was noted.

Extended release tablet: Initial: 50 mg/day the first day; increase to 100 mg on day 2, further increasing by 100 mg/day each day until a target dose of 300 mg/day is reached by day 4.

Mania:

Immediate release tablet: Initial: 50 mg twice daily on day 1, increase dose in increments of 100 mg/day to 200 mg twice daily on day 4; may increase to a target dose of 800 mg/day by day 6 at increments ≤200 mg/day. Usual dosage range: 400-800 mg/day.

Extended release tablet: Initial: 300 mg on day 1; increase to 600 mg on day 2 and adjust dose to 400-800 mg once daily on day 3, depending on response and tolerance.

Maintenance therapy: Immediate release tablet: 200-400 mg twice daily with lithium or divalproex; **Note:** Average time of stabilization was 15 weeks in clinical trials.

Major depressive disorder (adjunct to antidepressants): Extended release tablet: Initial: 50 mg once daily; may be increased to 150 mg on day 3. Usual dosage range: 150-300 mg/day

Schizophrenia/psychoses:

Immediate release tablet: Initial: 25 mg twice daily; followed by increases in the total daily dose on the second and third day in increments of 25-50 mg divided 2-3 times/day, if tolerated, to a target dose of 300-400 mg/day in 2-3 divided doses by day 4. Make further adjustments as needed at intervals of at least 2 days in adjustments of 25-50 mg divided twice daily. Usual maintenance range: 300-800 mg/day.

Extended release tablet: Initial: 300 mg once daily; increase in increments of up to 300 mg/day (in intervals of ≥1 day). Usual maintenance range: 400-800 mg/day.

Note: Dose reductions should be attempted periodically to establish lowest effective dose in patients with psychosis. Patients being restarted after 1 week of no drug need to be titrated as above.

ICU delirium: Initial: 50 mg twice daily; may increase as necessary on a daily basis in increments of 50 mg twice daily to a maximum dose of 400 mg/day (Devlin, 2010)

Elderly: 40% lower mean oral clearance of quetiapine in adults >65 years of age; higher plasma levels expected and, therefore, dosage adjustment may be needed; elderly patients usually require 50-200 mg/day of immediate release tablets or 50 mg/day of extended release tablets with a slower titration schedule. Increase immediate release dose by 25-50 mg/day or extended release dose by 50 mg/day to effective dose, based on clinical response and tolerability. If initiated with immediate release tablets, patient may transition to extended release formulation (at equivalent total daily dose) when effective dose has been reached. See **"Note"** in adult dosing.

Psychosis/agitation related to Alzheimer's dementia (unlabeled use): Initial: 12.5-50 mg/day; if necessary, gradually increase as tolerated not to exceed 200-300 mg/day (Rabins, 2007)

Dosing comments in renal insufficiency: 25% lower mean oral clearance of quetiapine than normal subjects; however, plasma concentrations similar to normal subjects receiving the same dose; no dosage adjustment required

Dosing comments in hepatic insufficiency: 30% lower mean oral clearance of quetiapine than normal subjects; higher plasma levels expected in hepatically impaired subjects; dosage adjustment may be needed

Immediate release tablet: Initial: 25 mg/day, increase dose by 25-50 mg/day to effective dose, based on clinical response and tolerability to patient. If initiated with immediate-release formulation, patient may transition to extended-release formulation (at equivalent total daily dose) when effective dose has been reached.

Extended release tablet: Initial: 50 mg/day; increase dose by 50 mg/day to effective dose, based on clinical response and tolerability to patient.

Mechanism of Action Quetiapine is a dibenzothiazepine atypical antipsychotic. It has been proposed that this drug's antipsychotic activity is mediated through a combination of dopamine type 2 (D_2) and serotonin type 2 (5-HT_2) antagonism. It is an antagonist at multiple neurotransmitter receptors in the brain: Serotonin 5-HT_{1A} and 5-HT_2, dopamine D_1 and D_2, histamine H_1, and adrenergic alpha$_1$- and alpha$_2$-receptors; but appears to have no appreciable affinity at cholinergic muscarinic and benzodiazepine receptors. Norquetiapine, an active metabolite, differs from its parent molecule by exhibiting high affinity for muscarinic M1 receptors.

Antagonism at receptors other than dopamine and 5-HT_2 with similar receptor affinities may explain some of the other effects of quetiapine. The drug's antagonism of histamine H_1-receptors may explain the somnolence observed. The drug's antagonism of adrenergic alpha$_1$-receptors may explain the orthostatic hypotension observed.

Contraindications There are no contraindications listed in manufacturers labeling.

Canadian labeling: Hypersensitivity to quetiapine or any component of the formulation

Warnings/Precautions [U.S. Boxed Warning]: Antidepressants increase the risk of suicidal thinking and behavior in children, adolescents, and young adults (18-24 years of age) with major depressive disorder (MDD) and other psychiatric disorders; consider risk prior to prescribing. Short-term studies did not show an increased risk in patients >24 years of age and showed a decreased risk in patients ≥65 years. Closely monitor all patients for clinical worsening, suicidality, or unusual changes in behavior; particularly during the initial 1-2 months of therapy or during periods of dosage adjustments (increased or decreases); the patient's family or caregiver should be instructed to closely observe the patient and communicate condition with healthcare provider. A medication guide concerning the use of antidepressants should be dispensed with each prescription.

[U.S. Boxed Warning]: Elderly patients with dementia-related psychosis treated with antipsychotics are at an increased risk of death compared to placebo. Most deaths appeared to be either cardiovascular (eg, heart failure, sudden death) or infectious (eg, pneumonia) in nature. Quetiapine is not approved for the treatment of dementia-related psychosis.

Leukopenia, neutropenia, and agranulocytosis (sometimes fatal) have been reported in clinical trials and postmarketing reports with antipsychotic use; presence of risk factors (eg, pre-existing low WBC or history of drug-induced leuko-/neutropenia) should prompt periodic blood count assessment. Discontinue therapy at first signs of blood dyscrasias or if absolute neutrophil count <1000/mm^3.

May be sedating, use with caution in disorders where CNS depression is a feature. Use with caution in Parkinson's disease. May induce orthostatic hypotension associated with dizziness, tachycardia, and, in some cases, syncope, especially during the initial dose titration period. Should be used with particular caution in patients with known cardiovascular disease (history of MI or ischemic heart disease, heart failure, or conduction abnormalities), cerebrovascular disease, or conditions that predispose to hypotension. Esophageal dysmotility and aspiration have been associated with antipsychotic use; use with caution in patients at risk of aspiration pneumonia (eg, Alzheimer's disease). Development of cataracts has been observed in animal studies; lens changes have been observed in humans during long-term treatment. Lens examination on initiation of therapy and every 6 months thereafter is recommended.

Due to anticholinergic effects, use with caution in patients with decreased gastrointestinal motility, urinary retention, BPH, xerostomia, visual problems, and narrow-angle glaucoma. Relative to other antipsychotics, quetiapine has a moderate potency of cholinergic blockade. May cause extrapyramidal symptoms (EPS), pseudoparkinsonism, and/or tardive dyskinesia. Risk of dystonia (and probably other EPS) may be greater with increased doses, use of conventional antipsychotics, males, and younger patients. Impaired core body temperature regulation may occur; caution with strenuous exercise, heat exposure, dehydration, and concomitant medication possessing anticholinergic effects. Neuroleptic malignant syndrome (NMS) is a potentially fatal symptom complex that has been reported in association with administration of antipsychotic drugs. Clinical manifestations of NMS are hyperpyrexia, muscle rigidity, altered mental status, and evidence of autonomic instability (irregular pulse or blood pressure, tachycardia, diaphoresis, and cardiac dysrhythmia). Management of NMS should include immediate discontinuation of antipsychotic drugs and other drugs not essential to concurrent therapy, intensive symptomatic treatment and medication monitoring, and treatment of any concomitant medical problems for which specific treatment are available.

Use caution in patients with a history of seizures. May cause decreases in total free thyroxine, elevations of liver enzymes, cholesterol levels, and/or triglyceride increases. Rare cases of priapism have been reported. May increase prolactin levels; clinical significance of hyperprolactinemia in patients with breast cancer or other prolactin-dependent tumors is unknown.

May cause hyperglycemia; in some cases may be extreme and associated with ketoacidosis, hyperosmolar coma, or death. Use with caution in patients with diabetes or other disorders of glucose regulation; monitor for worsening of glucose control. Significant weight gain has been observed with antipsychotic therapy; incidence varies with product. Monitor waist circumference and BMI. Patients using immediate release tablets may be switched to extended release tablets at the same total daily dose taken once daily. Dosage adjustments may be necessary based on response and tolerability. May cause withdrawal symptoms (rare) with abrupt cessation; gradually taper dose during discontinuation.

Drug Interactions

Metabolism/Transport Effects Substrate of CYP2D6 (minor), 3A4 (major)

Avoid Concomitant Use

Avoid concomitant use of QUEtiapine with any of the following: Artemether; Dronedarone; Lumefantrine; Metoclopramide; Nilotinib; Pimozide; QuiNINE; Tetrabenazine; Thioridazine; Toremifene; Vandetanib; Ziprasidone

Increased Effect/Toxicity

QUEtiapine may increase the levels/effects of: Alcohol (Ethyl); Anticholinergics; CNS Depressants; Dronedarone; Methylphenidate; Pimozide; QTc-Prolonging Agents; QuiNINE; Tetrabenazine; Thioridazine; Toremifene; Vandetanib; Ziprasidone

The levels/effects of QUEtiapine may be increased by: Acetylcholinesterase Inhibitors (Central); Alfuzosin; Artemether; Chloroquine; Ciprofloxacin; Ciprofloxacin (Systemic); Conivaptan; CYP3A4 Inhibitors (Moderate); CYP3A4 Inhibitors (Strong); Gadobutrol; Lithium formulations; Lumefantrine; Methylphenidate; Metoclopramide; Nilotinib; Pramlintide; QuiNINE; Tetrabenazine

Decreased Effect

QUEtiapine may decrease the levels/effects of: Amphetamines; Anti-Parkinson's Agents (Dopamine Agonist); Quinagolide

The levels/effects of QUEtiapine may be decreased by: CYP3A4 Inducers (Strong); Deferasirox; Fosphenytoin; Herbs (CYP3A4 Inducers); Lithium formulations; Peginterferon Alfa-2b; Phenytoin; Tocilizumab

Ethanol/Nutrition/Herb Interactions

Ethanol: May increase CNS depression; monitor for increased effects with coadministration. Caution patients about effects.

Food: In healthy volunteers, administration of quetiapine (immediate release) with food resulted in an increase in the peak serum concentration and AUC by 25% and 15%, respectively, compared to the fasting state. Administration of the extended release formulation with a high-fat meal (~800-1000 calories) resulted in an increase in peak serum concentration by 44% to 52% and AUC by 20% to 22% for the 50 mg and 300 mg tablets; administration with a light meal (≤300 calories) had no significant effect on the C_{max} or AUC.

Herb/Nutraceutical: St John's wort may decrease quetiapine levels. Avoid valerian, St John's wort, kava kava, gotu kola (may increase CNS depression).

Dietary Considerations Immediate-release tablet may be taken without regard to meals. Extended release tablet should be taken without food or with a light meal (≤300 calories).

Pharmacodynamics/Kinetics

Half-life Elimination

Mean: Terminal: Quetiapine: ~6 hours; Extended release: ~7 hours

Metabolite: N-desalkyl quetiapine: 9-12 hours

Time to Peak Plasma: Immediate release: 1.5 hours; Extended release: 6 hours

Pregnancy Risk Factor C

Lactation Enters breast milk/use caution

Breast-Feeding Considerations Based on information from 8 mother/infant pairs, concentrations of quetiapine in breast milk have been reported as 0-170 μg/L. The estimated exposure to the breast-feeding infant would be up to 1 mg/kg/day (relative infant dose up to 0.43% based on a weight adjusted maternal dose of 400 mg/day).

Dosage Forms

Tablet, oral:

SEROquel®: 25 mg, 50 mg, 100 mg, 200 mg, 300 mg, 400 mg

Tablet, extended release, oral:

SEROquel XR®: 50 mg, 150 mg, 200 mg, 300 mg, 400 mg

Dental Comment Quetiapine is known to prolong the QT interval. The QT interval is measured as the time and distance between the Q point of the QRS complex and the end of the T wave in the ECG tracing. After adjustment for heart rate, the QT interval is defined as prolonged if it is more than 450 msec in men and 460 msec in women. A long QT syndrome was first described in the 1950s and 60s as a congenital syndrome involving QT interval prolongation and syncope and sudden death. Some of the congenital long QT syndromes were characterized by a peculiar electrocardiographic appearance of the QRS complex involving a premature atria beat followed by a pause, then a subsequent sinus beat showing marked QT prolongation and deformity. This type of cardiac arrhythmia was originally termed "torsade de pointes" (translated from the French as "twisting of the points"). Quetiapine is considered as having a risk of causing torsade de pointes. Since it is not known what effect vasoconstrictors in the local anesthetic regimen will have in patients with a known history of congenital prolonged QT interval or in patients taking any medication that prolongs the QT interval, a medical consult is suggested.

Quinagolide (kwin AG o lide)

Canadian Brand Names Norprolac®

Pharmacologic Category Hyperprolactinemia Agent, Dopamine (D_2) Agonist

Use Treatment of hyperprolactinemia due to prolactin-secreting pituitary tumors (microadenoma or macroadenoma) or idiopathic in nature

Local Anesthetic/Vasoconstrictor Precautions No information available to require special precautions

Effects on Dental Treatment No significant effects or complications reported

Effects on Bleeding No information available to require special precautions

Adverse Effects

>10%:

- Central nervous system: Dizziness, fatigue, headache
- Gastrointestinal: Nausea, vomiting

1% to 10%:

- Cardiovascular: Edema (2%), flushing (1%), hypotension (1%), palpitation (1%), syncope (1%)
- Central nervous system: Sedation (3%), insomnia (2%), concentration decreased (1%), malaise (1%), mood lability (1%)
- Gastrointestinal: Abdominal pain/discomfort (3%), constipation (3%), anorexia (2%), dyspepsia (2%), diarrhea (1%), weight gain (1%)
- Endocrine & metabolic: Breast pain (1%)
- Neuromuscular & skeletal: Weakness (3%), extremity pain (1%)
- Respiratory: Nasal congestion (2%)

General Dosage Range Oral: *Adults:* Initial: 0.025 mg/day for 3 days followed by 0.05 mg/day for 3 days; Maintenance (begin day 7): Usual range 0.075-0.15 mg/day (maximum: 0.9 mg/day)

Mechanism of Action Selective dopamine D_2 receptor agonist that exerts a direct inhibitory effect on cells (lactotrophs) in the anterior pituitary gland which synthesize and secrete prolactin; not an ergot alkaloid

Pharmacodynamics/Kinetics

Onset of Action 2 hours; maximum effect: 4-6 hours

Duration of Action >24 hours

Half-life Elimination 11.5 hours; steady state: 17 hours

Time to Peak 30-60 minutes

Product Availability Not available in U.S.

Quinapril (KWIN a pril)

Related Information

Cardiovascular Diseases *on page 1848*

U.S. Brand Names Accupril®

Canadian Brand Names Accupril®

Generic Availability (U.S.) Yes

Pharmacologic Category Angiotensin-Converting Enzyme (ACE) Inhibitor

Use Treatment of hypertension; treatment of heart failure

Unlabeled/Investigational Use Treatment of left ventricular dysfunction after myocardial infarction; pediatric hypertension; to delay the progression of nephropathy and reduce risks of cardiovascular events in hypertensive patients with type 1 or 2 diabetes mellitus

Local Anesthetic/Vasoconstrictor Precautions No information available to require special precautions

Effects on Dental Treatment No significant effects or complications reported

Effects on Bleeding No information available to require special precautions

Adverse Effects Note: Frequency ranges include data from hypertension and heart failure trials. Higher rates of adverse reactions have generally been noted in patients with CHF. However, the frequency of adverse effects associated with placebo is also increased in this population.

1% to 10%:

- Cardiovascular: Hypotension (3%), chest pain (2%), first-dose hypotension (up to 3%)
- Central nervous system: Dizziness (4% to 8%), headache (2% to 6%), fatigue (3%)
- Dermatologic: Rash (1%)
- Endocrine & metabolic: Hyperkalemia (2%)
- Gastrointestinal: Vomiting/nausea (1% to 2%), diarrhea (2%)
- Neuromuscular & skeletal: Myalgias (2% to 5%), back pain (1%)

Renal: BUN/serum creatinine increased (2%, transient elevations may occur with a higher frequency), worsening of renal function (in patients with bilateral renal artery stenosis or hypovolemia)

Respiratory: Upper respiratory symptoms, cough (2% to 4%; up to 13% in some studies), dyspnea (2%)

Dosage Oral:

Children (unlabeled use): Hypertension: Initial 5-10 mg once daily; maximum: 80 mg/day

Adults:

Heart failure: Initial: 5 mg once or twice daily, titrated at weekly intervals to 20-40 mg daily in 2 divided doses; target dose (heart failure): 20 mg twice daily (ACC/AHA 2009 Heart Failure Guidelines)

Hypertension: Initial: 10-20 mg once daily, adjust according to blood pressure response at peak and trough blood levels; initial dose may be reduced to 5 mg in patients receiving diuretic therapy if the diuretic is continued; usual dose range (JNC 7): 10-40 mg once daily

Elderly: Initial: 2.5-5 mg/day; increase dosage at increments of 2.5-5 mg at 1- to 2-week intervals.

Dosing adjustment in renal impairment: Lower initial doses should be used; after initial dose (if tolerated), administer initial dose twice daily; may be increased at weekly intervals to optimal response:

Heart failure: Initial:

Cl_{cr} >30 mL/minute: Administer 5 mg/day

Cl_{cr} 10-30 mL/minute: Administer 2.5 mg/day

Hypertension: Initial:

Cl_{cr} >60 mL/minute: Administer 10 mg/day

Cl_{cr} 30-60 mL/minute: Administer 5 mg/day

Cl_{cr} 10-30 mL/minute: Administer 2.5 mg/day

Dosing comments in hepatic impairment: In patients with alcoholic cirrhosis, hydrolysis of quinapril to quinaprilat is impaired; however, the subsequent elimination of quinaprilat is unaltered.

Mechanism of Action Competitive inhibitor of angiotensin-converting enzyme (ACE); prevents conversion of angiotensin I to angiotensin II, a potent vasoconstrictor; results in lower levels of angiotensin II which causes an increase in plasma renin activity and a reduction in aldosterone secretion; a CNS mechanism may also be involved in hypotensive effect as angiotensin II increases adrenergic outflow from CNS; vasoactive kallikreins may be decreased in conversion to active hormones by ACE inhibitors, thus reducing blood pressure

Contraindications Hypersensitivity to quinapril or any component of the formulation; angioedema related to previous treatment with an ACE inhibitor

Warnings/Precautions Anaphylactic reactions may occur rarely with ACE inhibitors. At any time during treatment (especially following first dose) angioedema may occur rarely with ACE inhibitors; it may involve the head and neck (potentially compromising airway) or the intestine (presenting with abdominal pain). African-Americans and patients with idiopathic or hereditary angioedema may be at an increased risk. Prolonged frequent monitoring may be required especially if tongue, glottis, or larynx are involved as they are associated with airway obstruction. Patients with a history of airway surgery may have a higher risk of airway obstruction. Aggressive early and appropriate management is critical. Use in patients with previous angioedema associated with ACE inhibitor therapy is contraindicated. Severe anaphylactoid reactions may be seen during hemodialysis (eg, CVVHD) with high-flux dialysis membranes (eg, AN69), and rarely, during low density lipoprotein apheresis with dextran sulfate cellulose. Rare cases of anaphylactoid reactions have been reported in patients undergoing sensitization treatment with hymenoptera (bee, wasp) venom while receiving ACE inhibitors.

Symptomatic hypotension with or without syncope can occur with ACE inhibitors (usually with the first several doses); effects are most often observed in volume-depleted patients; close monitoring of patient is required especially with initial dosing and dosing increases; blood pressure must be lowered at a rate appropriate for the patient's clinical condition. Initiation of therapy in patients with ischemic heart disease or cerebrovascular disease warrants close observation due to the potential consequences posed by falling blood pressure (eg, MI, stroke). Use with caution in hypertrophic cardiomyopathy with outflow tract obstruction, severe aortic stenosis, or before, during, or immediately after major surgery. **[U.S. Boxed Warning]: Based on human data, ACEIs can cause injury and death to the developing fetus when used in the second and third trimesters. ACEIs should be discontinued as soon as possible once pregnancy is detected.**

Hyperkalemia may occur with ACE inhibitors; risk factors include renal dysfunction, diabetes mellitus, concomitant use of potassium-sparing diuretics, potassium supplements, and/or potassium-containing salts. Use cautiously, if at all, with these agents and monitor potassium closely. Cough may occur with ACE inhibitors. Other causes of cough should be considered (eg, pulmonary congestion in patients with heart failure) and excluded prior to discontinuation.

May be associated with deterioration of renal function and/or increases in serum creatinine, particularly in patients with low renal blood flow (eg, renal artery stenosis, heart failure) whose glomerular filtration rate (GFR) is dependent on efferent arteriolar vasoconstriction by angiotensin II; deterioration may result in oliguria, acute renal failure, and progressive azotemia. Small increases in serum creatinine may occur following initiation; consider discontinuation only in patients with progressive and/or significant deterioration in renal function. Use with caution in patients with unstented unilateral/bilateral renal artery stenosis. When unstented bilateral renal artery stenosis is present, use is generally avoided due to the elevated risk of deterioration in renal function unless possible benefits outweigh risks. Concurrent use of angiotensin receptor blockers may increase the risk of clinically-significant adverse events (eg, renal dysfunction, hyperkalemia).

Rare toxicities associated with ACE inhibitors include cholestatic jaundice (which may progress to fulminant hepatic necrosis), agranulocytosis, neutropenia, or leukopenia with myeloid hypoplasia. Patients with collagen vascular diseases (especially with concomitant renal impairment) or renal impairment alone may be at increased risk for hematologic toxicity; periodically monitor CBC with differential in these patients.

Drug Interactions

Avoid Concomitant Use There are no known interactions where it is recommended to avoid concomitant use.

Increased Effect/Toxicity

Quinapril may increase the levels/effects of: Allopurinol; Amifostine; Antihypertensives; AzaTHIOprine; CycloSPORINE; CycloSPORINE (Systemic); Ferric Gluconate; Gold Sodium Thiomalate; Hypotensive Agents; Iron Dextran Complex; Lithium; Nonsteroidal Anti-Inflammatory Agents; RiTUXimab

The levels/effects of Quinapril may be increased by: Angiotensin II Receptor Blockers; Diazoxide; DPP-IV Inhibitors; Eplerenone; Everolimus; Herbs (Hypotensive Properties); Loop Diuretics; MAO Inhibitors; Pentoxifylline; Phosphodiesterase 5 Inhibitors; Potassium Salts; Potassium-Sparing Diuretics; Prostacyclin Analogues; Sirolimus; Temsirolimus; Thiazide Diuretics; TiZANidine; Tolvaptan; Trimethoprim

Decreased Effect

Quinapril may decrease the levels/effects of: Quinolone Antibiotics; Tetracycline Derivatives

The levels/effects of Quinapril may be decreased by: Antacids; Aprotinin; Herbs (Hypertensive Properties); Methylphenidate; Nonsteroidal Anti-Inflammatory Agents; Salicylates; Yohimbine

Ethanol/Nutrition/Herb Interactions Herb/Nutraceutical: Avoid bayberry, blue cohosh, cayenne, ephedra, ginger, ginseng (American), kola, licorice (may worsen hypertension). Avoid black cohosh, California poppy, coleus, golden seal, hawthorn, mistletoe, periwinkle, quinine, shepherd's purse (may have increased antihypertensive effect).

Pharmacodynamics/Kinetics

Onset of Action 1 hour

Duration of Action 24 hours

Half-life Elimination Quinapril: 0.8 hours; Quinaprilat: 3 hours; increases as Cl_{cr} decreases

Time to Peak Serum: Quinapril: 1 hour; Quinaprilat: ~2 hours

Pregnancy Risk Factor C (1st trimester); D (2nd and 3rd trimesters)

Lactation Enters breast milk/use caution

Breast-Feeding Considerations Quinapril is excreted in breast milk. The manufacturer recommends that caution be exercised when administering quinapril to nursing women.

Dosage Forms

Tablet, oral: 5 mg, 10 mg, 20 mg, 40 mg

Accupril®: 5 mg, 10 mg, 20 mg, 40 mg

Quinapril and Hydrochlorothiazide

(KWIN a pril & hye droe klor oh THYE a zide)

Related Information

Hydrochlorothiazide *on page 854*

Quinapril *on page 1444*

U.S. Brand Names Accuretic®; Quinaretic

Canadian Brand Names Accuretic®

Pharmacologic Category Angiotensin-Converting Enzyme (ACE) Inhibitor; Diuretic, Thiazide

Use Treatment of hypertension (not for initial therapy)

Local Anesthetic/Vasoconstrictor Precautions No information available to require special precautions

Effects on Dental Treatment No significant effects or complications reported

Effects on Bleeding No information available to require special precautions

Adverse Effects 1% to 10%:

Central nervous system: Dizziness (5%), somnolence (1%)
Neuromuscular & skeletal: Weakness (1%)
Renal: Serum creatinine increased (3%), blood urea nitrogen increased (4%)
Respiratory: Cough (3%), bronchitis (1%)

General Dosage Range Oral: *Adults:* Initial: 10-20 mg quinapril and 12.5 mg hydrochlorothiazide once daily; Maintenance: 5-40 mg quinapril and 6.25-25 mg hydrochlorothiazide once daily

Pregnancy Risk Factor C (1st trimester); D (2nd and 3rd trimesters)

QuiNIDine (KWIN i deen)

Related Information

Cardiovascular Diseases *on page 1848*
Clinical Risk Related to Drugs Prolonging QT Interval *on page 1872*

Canadian Brand Names Apo-Quinidine®; BioQuin® Durules™; Novo-Quinidin; Quinate®

Pharmacologic Category Antiarrhythmic Agent, Class Ia

Use

Quinidine gluconate and sulfate salts: Conversion and prevention of relapse into atrial fibrillation and/or flutter; suppression of ventricular arrhythmias. **Note:** Due to proarrhythmic effects, use should be reserved for life-threatening arrhythmias. Moreover, the use of quinidine has largely been replaced by more effective/safer antiarrhythmic agents and/or nonpharmacologic therapies (eg, radiofrequency ablation).

Quinidine gluconate (I.V. formulation): Conversion of atrial fibrillation/flutter and ventricular tachycardia. **Note:** The use of I.V. quinidine gluconate for these indications has been replaced by more effective/safer antiarrhythmic agents (eg, amiodarone and procainamide).

Quinidine gluconate (I.V. formulation) and quinidine sulfate: Treatment of malaria (*Plasmodium falciparum*)

Unlabeled/Investigational Use Paroxysmal supraventricular tachycardia, paroxysmal AV junctional rhythm, and symptomatic atrial or ventricular premature contractions; short QT syndrome; Brugada syndrome

Local Anesthetic/Vasoconstrictor Precautions Quinidine is one of the drugs confirmed to prolong the QT interval and is accepted as having a risk of causing torsade de pointes. The risk of drug-induced torsade de pointes is extremely low when a single QT interval prolonging drug is prescribed. In terms of epinephrine, it is not known what effect vasoconstrictors in the local anesthetic regimen will have in patients with a known history of congenital prolonged QT interval or in patients taking any medication that prolongs the QT interval. Until more information is obtained, it is suggested that the clinician consult with the physician prior to the use of a vasoconstrictor in suspected patients, and that the vasoconstrictor (epinephrine, mepivacaine and levonordefrin [Carbocaine® 2% with Neo-Cobefrin®]) be used with caution.

Effects on Dental Treatment When taken over a long period of time, the anticholinergic side effects from quinidine can cause a reduction of saliva production or secretion contributing to discomfort and dental disease (ie, caries, oral candidiasis, and periodontal disease).

Effects on Bleeding No information available to require special precautions

Adverse Effects

Frequency not defined: Hypotension, syncope

>10%:

Cardiovascular: QT_c prolongation (modest prolongation is common, however, excessive prolongation is rare and indicates toxicity)
Central nervous system: Lightheadedness (15%)
Gastrointestinal: Diarrhea (35%), upper GI distress, bitter taste, diarrhea, anorexia, nausea, vomiting, stomach cramping (22%)

1% to 10%:

Cardiovascular: Angina (6%), palpitation (7%), new or worsened arrhythmia (proarrhythmic effect)

Central nervous system: Syncope (1% to 8%), headache (7%), fatigue (7%), sleep disturbance (3%), tremor (2%), nervousness (2%), incoordination (1%)
Dermatologic: Rash (5%)
Neuromuscular & skeletal: Weakness (5%)
Ocular: Blurred vision
Otic: Tinnitus
Respiratory: Wheezing

Note: Cinchonism, a syndrome which may include tinnitus, high-frequency hearing loss, deafness, vertigo, blurred vision, diplopia, photophobia, headache, confusion, and delirium has been associated with quinidine use. Usually associated with chronic toxicity, this syndrome has also been described after brief exposure to a moderate dose in sensitive patients. Vomiting and diarrhea may also occur as isolated reactions to therapeutic quinidine levels.

General Dosage Range Dosage adjustment recommended in patients with hepatic or renal impairment

I.V.: *Infants, Children, and Adults:* 10 mg/kg bolus followed by 0.02 mg/kg/minute **or** 24 mg/kg bolus followed by 12 mg/kg every 8 hours

Oral:

Gluconate: *Adults:* 324-972 mg every 8-12 hours

Sulfate:

Children: Initial: 15-60 mg/kg/day in 4-5 divided doses; Usual: 30 mg/kg/day (900 mg/m^2/day) in 5 divided doses

Adults: 100-600 mg/dose every 4-6 hours (maximum: 4 g/day)

Mechanism of Action Class Ia antiarrhythmic agent; depresses phase O of the action potential; decreases myocardial excitability and conduction velocity, and myocardial contractility by decreasing sodium influx during depolarization and potassium efflux in repolarization; also reduces calcium transport across cell membrane

Pharmacodynamics/Kinetics

Half-life Elimination Plasma: Children: 2.5-6.7 hours; Adults: 6-8 hours; prolonged with elderly, cirrhosis, and congestive heart failure

Time to Peak Serum: Sulfate: 2 hours; Gluconate: 3-5 hours

Pregnancy Risk Factor C

Dental Comment Quinidine is known to prolong the QT interval. The QT interval is measured as the time and distance between the Q point of the QRS complex and the end of the T wave in the ECG tracing. After adjustment for heart rate, the QT interval is defined as prolonged if it is more than 450 msec in men and 460 msec in women. A long QT syndrome was first described in the 1950s and 60s as a congenital syndrome involving QT interval prolongation and syncope and sudden death. Some of the congenital long QT syndromes were characterized by a peculiar electrocardiographic appearance of the QRS complex involving a premature atria beat followed by a pause, then a subsequent sinus beat showing marked QT prolongation and deformity. This type of cardiac arrhythmia was originally termed "torsade de pointes" (translated from the French as "twisting of the points"). Quinidine is considered as having a risk of causing torsade de pointes. Since it is not known what effect vasoconstrictors in the local anesthetic regimen will have in patients with a known history of congenital prolonged QT interval or in patients taking any medication that prolongs the QT interval, a medical consult is suggested.

QuiNINE (KWYE nine)

U.S. Brand Names Qualaquin®

Canadian Brand Names Apo-Quinine®; Novo-Quinine; Quinine-Odan

Pharmacologic Category Antimalarial Agent

Use In conjunction with other antimalarial agents, treatment of uncomplicated chloroquine-resistant *P. falciparum* malaria

Unlabeled/Investigational Use Treatment of *Babesia microti* infection in conjunction with clindamycin; treatment of uncomplicated chloroquine-resistant *P. vivax* malaria (in conjunction with other antimalarial agents)

Local Anesthetic/Vasoconstrictor Precautions No information available to require special precautions

Effects on Dental Treatment No significant effects or complications reported

Effects on Bleeding No information available to require special precautions

Adverse Effects Frequency not defined.

Cardiovascular: Atrial fibrillation, atrioventricular block, bradycardia, cardiac arrest, chest pain, hypotension, irregular rhythm, nodal escape beats, palpitation, postural hypotension, QT prolongation, syncope, tachycardia, torsade de pointes, unifocal premature ventricular contractions, U waves, vasodilation, ventricular fibrillation, ventricular tachycardia

Central nervous system: Aphasia, ataxia, chills, coma, confusion, disorientation, dizziness, dystonic reaction, fever, flushing, headache, mental status altered, restlessness, seizure, suicide, vertigo
Dermatologic: Acral necrosis, allergic contact dermatitis, bullous dermatitis, bruising, cutaneous rash (urticaria, papular, scarlatinal), cutaneous vasculitis, exfoliative dermatitis, erythema multiforme, petechiae, photosensitivity, pruritus, Stevens-Johnson syndrome, toxic epidermal necrolysis
Endocrine & metabolic: Hypoglycemia
Gastrointestinal: Abdominal pain, anorexia, diarrhea, esophagitis, gastric irritation, nausea, vomiting
Hematologic: Agranulocytosis, aplastic anemia, coagulopathy, disseminated intravascular coagulation, hemolytic anemia, hemolytic uremic syndrome, hemorrhage, hypoprothrombinemia, idiopathic thrombocytopenic purpura, leukopenia, neutropenia, pancytopenia, thrombocytopenia, thrombotic thrombocytopenic purpura
Hepatic: Granulomatous hepatitis, hepatitis, jaundice, liver function test abnormalities
Neuromuscular & skeletal: Myalgia, tremor, weakness
Ocular: Blindness, blurred vision (with or without scotomata), color vision disturbance, diminished visual fields, diplopia, night blindness, optic neuritis, photophobia, pupillary dilation, vision loss (sudden)
Otic: Deafness, hearing impaired, tinnitus
Renal: Acute interstitial nephritis, hemoglobinuria, renal failure, renal impairment
Respiratory: Asthma, dyspnea, pulmonary edema
Miscellaneous: Black water fever, diaphoresis, hypersensitivity reaction, lupus anticoagulant, lupus-like syndrome

General Dosage Range Dosage adjustment recommended in patients with renal impairment

Oral:

Children: 30 mg/kg/day divided every 8 hours
Adults: 648 mg every 8 hours

Mechanism of Action Depresses oxygen uptake and carbohydrate metabolism; intercalates into DNA, disrupting the parasite's replication and transcription; cardiovascular effects similar to quinidine

Pharmacodynamics/Kinetics

Half-life Elimination

Children: ~3 hours in healthy subjects; ~12 hours with malaria
Healthy adults: 10-13 hours
Healthy elderly subjects: 18 hours

Time to Peak

Children: Serum: 2 hours in healthy subjects; 4 hours with malaria
Adults: Serum: 2-4 hours in healthy subjects; 1-11 hours with malaria

Pregnancy Risk Factor C

Quinupristin and Dalfopristin (kwi NYOO pris tin & dal FOE pris tin)

U.S. Brand Names Synercid®
Canadian Brand Names Synercid®
Pharmacologic Category Antibiotic, Streptogramin
Use Treatment of complicated skin and skin structure infections caused by methicillin-susceptible *Staphylococcus aureus* or *Streptococcus pyogenes*
Local Anesthetic/Vasoconstrictor Precautions No information available to require special precautions
Effects on Dental Treatment No significant effects or complications reported
Effects on Bleeding No information available to require special precautions

Adverse Effects

>10%:

Hepatic: Hyperbilirubinemia (3% to 35%)
Local: Local pain (40% to 44%), inflammation at infusion site (38% to 42%), local edema (17% to 18%), infusion site reaction (12% to 13%)
Neuromuscular & skeletal: Arthralgia (up to 47%), myalgia (up to 47%)

1% to 10%:

Central nervous system: Pain (2% to 3%), headache (2%)
Dermatologic: Rash (3%), pruritus (2%)
Endocrine & metabolic: Hyperglycemia (1%)
Gastrointestinal: Nausea (3% to 5%), vomiting (3% to 4%), diarrhea (3%)
Hematologic: Anemia (3%)
Hepatic: GGT increased (2%), LDH increased (3%)
Local: Thrombophlebitis (2%)
Neuromuscular & skeletal: CPK increased (2%)

General Dosage Range I.V.: *Children ≥12 years and Adults:* 7.5 mg/kg every 12 hours

Mechanism of Action Quinupristin/dalfopristin inhibits bacterial protein synthesis by binding to different sites on the 50S bacterial ribosomal subunit thereby inhibiting protein synthesis

Pharmacodynamics/Kinetics

Half-life Elimination Quinupristin: 0.85 hour; Dalfopristin: 0.7 hour (mean elimination half-lives, including metabolites: 3 and 1 hours, respectively)

Pregnancy Risk Factor B

RABEprazole (ra BEP ra zole)

Related Information

Gastrointestinal Disorders *on page 1874*

U.S. Brand Names AcipHex®

Canadian Brand Names Novo-Rabeprazole EC; Pariet®; PMS-Rabeprazole EC; PRO-Rabeprazole; Rabeprazole EC; RAN™-Rabeprazole; Riva-Rabeprazole EC; Sandoz-Rabeprazole; Teva-Rabeprazole EC

Generic Availability (U.S.) No

Pharmacologic Category Proton Pump Inhibitor; Substituted Benzimidazole

Use Short-term (4-8 weeks) treatment and maintenance of erosive or ulcerative gastroesophageal reflux disease (GERD); symptomatic GERD; short-term (up to 4 weeks) treatment of duodenal ulcers; long-term treatment of pathological hypersecretory conditions, including Zollinger-Ellison syndrome; *H. pylori* eradication (in combination therapy)

Canadian labeling: Additional uses (not in U.S. labeling): Treatment of nonerosive reflux disease (NERD); treatment of gastric ulcers

Unlabeled/Investigational Use Maintenance of duodenal ulcer

Local Anesthetic/Vasoconstrictor Precautions No information available to require special precautions

Effects on Dental Treatment No significant effects or complications reported

Effects on Bleeding No information available to require special precautions

Adverse Effects 1% to 10%:

Central nervous system: Pain (3%), headache (2% to 5%)
Gastrointestinal: Diarrhea (3%), flatulence (3%), constipation (2%), nausea (2%)
Respiratory: Pharyngitis (3%)
Miscellaneous: Infection (2%)

Dosage Oral:

Children ≥12 years: *U.S. labeling:* Short-term treatment of GERD: 20 mg once daily for ≤8 weeks

Adults >18 years and Elderly:

Erosive/ulcerative GERD: Treatment: 20 mg once daily for 4-8 weeks; if inadequate response, may repeat up to an additional 8 weeks; maintenance: 20 mg once daily

Canadian labeling: 20 mg once daily for 4 weeks; if inadequate response, may repeat for an additional 4 weeks (lack of symptom control after 4 weeks warrants further evaluation); maintenance: 10 mg once daily (maximum: 20 mg once daily)

Symptomatic GERD: Treatment: 20 mg once daily for 4 weeks; if inadequate response, may repeat for an additional 4 weeks

Canadian labeling: 10 mg once daily (maximum: 20 mg once daily) for 4 weeks; lack of symptom control after 4 weeks warrants further evaluation

Duodenal ulcer: 20 mg/day before breakfast for 4 weeks; additional therapy may be required for some patients

Gastric ulcers (*Canadian labeling*): 20 mg once daily up to 6 weeks; additional therapy may be required for some patients

Helicobacter pylori eradication:

Manufacturer labeling: 20 mg twice daily administered with amoxicillin 1000 mg *and* clarithromycin 500 mg twice daily for 7 days

American College of Gastroenterology guidelines (Chey, 2007):

Nonpenicillin allergy: 20 mg twice daily administered with amoxicillin 1000 mg *and* clarithromycin 500 mg twice daily for 10-14 days

Penicillin allergy: 20 mg twice daily administered with clarithromycin 500 mg *and* metronidazole 500 mg twice daily for 10-14 days **or** 20 mg once or twice daily administered with bismuth subsalicylate 525 mg *and* metronidazole 250 mg *plus* tetracycline 500 mg 4 times/day for 10-14 days

Hypersecretory conditions: 60 mg once daily; dose may need to be adjusted as necessary. Doses as high as 100 mg once daily and 60 mg twice daily have been used, and continued as long as necessary (up to 1 year in some patients).

NERD (*Canadian labeling*): Treatment: 10 mg (maximum: 20 mg once daily) for 4 weeks; lack of symptom control after 4 weeks warrants further evaluation

Dosage adjustment in renal impairment: No dosage adjustment required

Dosage adjustment in hepatic impairment:

Mild-to-moderate: Elimination decreased; no dosage adjustment required

Severe: Use caution

Mechanism of Action Potent proton pump inhibitor; suppresses gastric acid secretion by inhibiting the parietal cell H+/K+ ATP pump

Contraindications Hypersensitivity to rabeprazole, substituted benzimidazoles (ie, esomeprazole, lansoprazole, omeprazole, pantoprazole), or any component of the formulation

Warnings/Precautions Use of proton pump inhibitors may increase the risk of gastrointestinal infections (eg, *Salmonella, Campylobacter*). Use caution in severe hepatic impairment. Relief of symptoms with rabeprazole does not preclude the presence of a gastric malignancy. Decreased *H. pylori* eradication rates have been observed with short-term (≤7 days) combination therapy. The American College of Gastroenterology recommends 10-14 days of therapy (triple or quadruple) for eradication of *H. pylori* (Chey, 2007). Proton pump inhibitors may diminish the therapeutic effect of clopidogrel, thought to be due to reduced formation of the active metabolite of clopidogrel; an increase in the risk of cardiovascular events may occur. The manufacturer of clopidogrel recommends avoidance of concomitant administration of another PPI (ie, omeprazole); given the potency of CYP2C19 inhibitory activity, similar recommendations with rabeprazole would appear prudent. Increased incidence of osteoporosis-related bone fractures of the hip, spine, or wrist may occur with proton pump inhibitor therapy. Patients on high-dose (multiple daily doses) or long-term therapy (≥1 year) should be monitored. Use the lowest effective dose for the shortest duration of time, use vitamin D and calcium supplementation, and follow appropriate guidelines to reduce risk of fractures in patients at risk.

Drug Interactions

Metabolism/Transport Effects Substrate (major) of CYP2C19, 3A4; **Inhibits** CYP2C8 (moderate), 2C19 (moderate), 2D6 (weak), 3A4 (weak)

Avoid Concomitant Use

Avoid concomitant use of RABEprazole with any of the following: Delavirdine; Erlotinib; Nelfinavir; Posaconazole

Increased Effect/Toxicity

RABEprazole may increase the levels/effects of: Amphetamines; CYP2C19 Substrates; CYP2C8 Substrates (High risk); Dexmethylphenidate; Methotrexate; Methylphenidate; Raltegravir; Saquinavir; Tacrolimus; Tacrolimus (Systemic); Voriconazole

The levels/effects of RABEprazole may be increased by: Conivaptan; Fluconazole; Ketoconazole; Ketoconazole (Systemic)

Decreased Effect

RABEprazole may decrease the levels/effects of: Atazanavir; Bisphosphonate Derivatives; Cefditoren; Clopidogrel; Dabigatran Etexilate; Dasatinib; Delavirdine; Erlotinib; Gefitinib; Indinavir; Iron Salts; Itraconazole; Ketoconazole; Ketoconazole (Systemic); Mesalamine; Mycophenolate; Nelfinavir; Posaconazole

The levels/effects of RABEprazole may be decreased by: CYP2C19 Inducers (Strong); CYP3A4 Inducers (Strong); Deferasirox; Herbs (CYP3A4 Inducers); Tipranavir; Tocilizumab

Ethanol/Nutrition/Herb Interactions

Ethanol: Avoid ethanol (may cause gastric mucosal irritation).

Food: High-fat meals may delay absorption, but C_{max} and AUC are not altered.

Herb/Nutraceutical: St John's wort may increase the metabolism and thus decrease the levels/effects of rabeprazole.

Dietary Considerations May be taken without regard to meals; best if taken before breakfast.

Pharmacodynamics/Kinetics

Onset of Action Within 1 hour

Duration of Action 24 hours

Half-life Elimination Dose dependent: 1-2 hours

Time to Peak Plasma: 2-5 hours

Pregnancy Risk Factor B

Lactation Excretion in breast milk unknown/not recommended

Dosage Forms

Tablet, delayed release, enteric coated, oral:

AcipHex®: 20 mg

Dosage Forms: Canada

Tablet, delayed release, enteric coated:

Pariet®: 10 mg, 20 mg

Rabies Immune Globulin (Human)

(RAY beez i MYUN GLOB yoo lin, HYU man)

U.S. Brand Names HyperRAB™ S/D; Imogam® Rabies-HT

Canadian Brand Names HyperRAB™ S/D; Imogam® Rabies Pasteurized

Pharmacologic Category Blood Product Derivative; Immune Globulin

Use Part of postexposure prophylaxis of persons with rabies exposure. Provides passive immunity until active immunity with rabies vaccine is established. Not for use in persons with a history of pre-exposure vaccination, history of postexposure prophylaxis, or previous vaccination with rabies vaccine and documentation of antibody response.

Local Anesthetic/Vasoconstrictor Precautions No information available to require special precautions

Effects on Dental Treatment No significant effects or complications reported

Effects on Bleeding No information available to require special precautions

Adverse Effects Frequency not defined.

Central nervous system: Fever (mild), headache, malaise
Dermatologic: Angioneurotic edema, rash
Local: Injection site: Pain, stiffness, soreness, tenderness
Renal: Nephrotic syndrome
Miscellaneous: Anaphylaxis

General Dosage Range Local wound infiltration/I.M.: *Children and Adults:* 20 units/kg in a single dose

Mechanism of Action Rabies immune globulin is a solution of globulins dried from the plasma or serum of selected adult human donors who have been immunized with rabies vaccine and have developed high titers of rabies antibody. It generally contains 10% to 18% of protein of which not less than 80% is monomeric immunoglobulin G.

Pregnancy Risk Factor C

Rabies Vaccine (RAY beez vak SEEN)

U.S. Brand Names Imovax® Rabies; RabAvert®

Canadian Brand Names Imovax® Rabies; RabAvert®

Pharmacologic Category Vaccine, Inactivated (Viral)

Use Pre-exposure and postexposure vaccination against rabies

The Advisory Committee on Immunization Practices (ACIP) recommends a primary course of prophylactic immunization (pre-exposure vaccination) for the following:

- Persons with continuous risk of infection, including rabies research laboratory and biologics production workers
- Persons with frequent risk of infection in areas where rabies is enzootic, including rabies diagnostic laboratory workers, cavers, veterinarians and their staff, and animal control and wildlife workers; persons who frequently handle bats
- Persons with infrequent risk of infection, including veterinarians and animal control staff with terrestrial animals in areas where rabies infection is rare, veterinary students, and travelers visiting areas where rabies is enzootic and immediate access to medical care and biologicals is limited

The ACIP recommends the use of postexposure vaccination for a particular person be assessed by the severity and likelihood versus the actual risk of acquiring rabies. Consideration should include the type of exposure, epidemiology of rabies in the area, species of the animal, circumstances of the incident, and the availability of the exposing animal for observation or rabies testing. Postexposure vaccination is used in both previously vaccinated and previously unvaccinated individuals.

Local Anesthetic/Vasoconstrictor Precautions No information available to require special precautions

Effects on Dental Treatment No significant effects or complications reported

Effects on Bleeding No information available to require special precautions

Adverse Effects All serious adverse reactions must be reported to the U.S. Department of Health and Human Services (DHHS) Vaccine Adverse Event Reporting System (VAERS) 1-800-822-7967 or online at https://vaers.hhs.gov/esub/index. In Canada, adverse reactions may be reported to local provincial/territorial health agencies or to the Vaccine Safety Section at Public Health Agency of Canada (1-866-844-0018).

>10%:

Central nervous system: Dizziness, headache, malaise
Gastrointestinal: Abdominal pain, nausea
Local: Erythema, itching, pain, swelling
Neuromuscular & skeletal: Myalgia

Miscellaneous: Lymphadenopathy

Uncommon, frequency not defined, postmarketing, and/or case reports:

Cardiovascular: Circulatory reactions, edema, palpitation

Central nervous system: Chills, fatigue, fever >38°C (100°F), Guillain-Barré syndrome, encephalitis, meningitis, multiple sclerosis, myelitis, neuroparalysis, vertigo

Dermatologic: Pruritus, urticaria, urticaria pigmentosa

Endocrine & metabolic: Hot flashes

Local: Limb swelling (extensive)

Neuromuscular & skeletal: Limb pain, monoarthritis, paralysis (transient), paresthesias (transient)

Ocular: Retrobulbar neuritis, visual disturbances

Respiratory: Bronchospasm

Miscellaneous: Allergic reactions, anaphylaxis, hypersensitivity reactions, swollen lymph nodes

General Dosage Range I.M.: *Children and Adults:* 1 mL

Mechanism of Action Rabies vaccine is an inactivated virus vaccine which promotes immunity by inducing an active immune response. The production of specific antibodies requires about 7-10 days to develop. Rabies immune globulin or antirabies serum, equine (ARS) is given in conjunction with rabies vaccine to provide immune protection until an antibody response can occur.

Pharmacodynamics/Kinetics

Onset of Action I.M.: Rabies antibody: ~7-10 days; Peak effect: ~30-60 days

Duration of Action ≥1 year

Pregnancy Risk Factor C

Raloxifene (ral OKS i feen)

Related Information

Endocrine Disorders and Pregnancy *on page 1879*

Rheumatoid Arthritis, Osteoarthritis, and Osteoporosis *on page 1889*

U.S. Brand Names Evista®

Canadian Brand Names Apo-Raloxifene®; Evista®; Novo-Raloxifene

Generic Availability (U.S.) No

Pharmacologic Category Selective Estrogen Receptor Modulator (SERM)

Use Prevention and treatment of osteoporosis in postmenopausal women; risk reduction for invasive breast cancer in postmenopausal women with osteoporosis and in postmenopausal women with high risk for invasive breast cancer

Local Anesthetic/Vasoconstrictor Precautions No information available to require special precautions

Effects on Dental Treatment No significant effects or complications reported

Effects on Bleeding Has been associated with thromboembolic adverse events. No information available to require routine special precautions for dental procedures.

Adverse Effects Note: Raloxifene has been associated with increased risk of thromboembolism (DVT, PE) and superficial thrombophlebitis; risk is similar to reported risk of HRT

>10%:

Cardiovascular: Peripheral edema (3% to 14%)

Endocrine & metabolic: Hot flashes (8% to 29%)

Neuromuscular & skeletal: Arthralgia (11% to 16%), leg cramps/muscle spasm (6% to 12%)

Miscellaneous: Flu syndrome (14% to 15%), infection (11%)

1% to 10%:

Cardiovascular: Chest pain (3%), venous thromboembolism (1% to 2%)

Central nervous system: Insomnia (6%)

Dermatologic: Rash (6%)

Endocrine & metabolic: Breast pain (4%)

Gastrointestinal: Weight gain (9%), abdominal pain (7%), vomiting (5%), flatulence (2% to 3%), cholelithiasis (≤3%), gastroenteritis (≤3%)

Genitourinary: Vaginal bleeding (6%), leukorrhea (3%), urinary tract disorder (3%), uterine disorder (3%), vaginal hemorrhage (3%), endometrial disorder (≤3%)

Neuromuscular & skeletal: Myalgia (8%), tendon disorder (4%)

Respiratory: Bronchitis (10%), sinusitis (10%), pharyngitis (8%), pneumonia (3%), laryngitis (≤2%)

Miscellaneous: Diaphoresis (3%)

Dosage Adults: Females: Oral:

Osteoporosis: 60 mg once daily

Invasive breast cancer risk reduction: 60 mg once daily for 5 years per ASCO guidelines (Visvanathan, 2009)

Dosage adjustment in renal impairment: Moderate-to-severe impairment: Use caution; safety and efficacy have not been established.

Dosage adjustment in hepatic impairment: Mild impairment (Child-Pugh class A): Plasma concentrations were higher and correlated with total bilirubin. Safety and efficacy in hepatic insufficiency have not been established.

Mechanism of Action A selective estrogen receptor modulator (SERM), meaning that it affects some of the same receptors that estrogen does, but not all, and in some instances, it antagonizes or blocks estrogen; it acts like estrogen to prevent bone loss and has the potential to block some estrogen effects in the breast and uterine tissues. Raloxifene decreases bone resorption, increasing bone mineral density and decreasing fracture incidence.

Contraindications History of or current venous thromboembolic disorders (including DVT, PE, and retinal vein thrombosis); pregnancy or women who could become pregnant; breast-feeding

Warnings/Precautions Hazardous agent - use appropriate precautions for handling and disposal. **[U.S. Boxed Warning]: May increase the risk for DVT or PE; use contraindicated in patients with history of or current venous thromboembolic disorders.** Use with caution in patients at high risk for venous thromboembolism; the risk for DVT and PE are higher in the first 4 months of treatment. Discontinue at least 72 hours prior to and during prolonged immobilization (postoperative recovery or prolonged bedrest). **[U.S. Boxed Warning]: The risk of death due to stroke may be increased in women with coronary heart disease or in women at risk for coronary events;** use with caution in patients with cardiovascular disease. Not be used for the prevention of cardiovascular disease. Use caution with moderate-to-severe renal dysfunction, hepatic impairment, unexplained uterine bleeding, and in women with a history of elevated triglycerides in response to treatment with oral estrogens (or estrogen/progestin). Safety with concomitant estrogen therapy has not been established. Safety and efficacy in premenopausal women or men have not been established. Not indicated for treatment of invasive breast cancer, to reduce the risk of recurrence of invasive breast cancer or to reduce the risk of noninvasive breast cancer. The efficacy (for breast cancer risk reduction) in women with inherited BRCA1 and BRCA1 mutations has not been established.

Drug Interactions

Avoid Concomitant Use There are no known interactions where it is recommended to avoid concomitant use.

Increased Effect/Toxicity There are no known significant interactions involving an increase in effect.

Decreased Effect

Raloxifene may decrease the levels/effects of: Levothyroxine

The levels/effects of Raloxifene may be decreased by: Bile Acid Sequestrants

Ethanol/Nutrition/Herb Interactions Ethanol: Avoid ethanol (may increase risk of osteoporosis).

Dietary Considerations May be taken without regard to meals. Osteoporosis prevention or treatment: Ensure adequate calcium and vitamin D intake; postmenopausal women should consume ~1500 mg/day of elemental calcium and 400-800 int. units/day of vitamin D.

Pharmacodynamics/Kinetics

Onset of Action 8 weeks

Half-life Elimination 28-33 hours

Pregnancy Risk Factor X

Lactation Excretion in breast milk unknown/contraindicated

Dosage Forms

Tablet, oral:

Evista®: 60 mg

Raltegravir (ral TEG ra vir)

Related Information

HIV Infection and AIDS *on page 1883*

U.S. Brand Names Isentress®

Canadian Brand Names Isentress®

Pharmacologic Category Antiretroviral Agent, Integrase Inhibitor

Use Treatment of HIV-1 infection in combination with other antiretroviral agents

Local Anesthetic/Vasoconstrictor Precautions No information available to require special precautions

Effects on Dental Treatment No significant effects or complications reported

Effects on Bleeding No information available to require special precautions related to hemostasis.

Adverse Effects

>10%: Endocrine & metabolic: Total cholesterol increased (grade 2: 16%; grade 3: 6%)

2% to 10%:

Cardiovascular: Hypertension (≤3%)

Central nervous system: Fatigue (<2% to 8%), dizziness (≤4%), insomnia (4%), headache (≥2%)

Dermatologic: Rash (≤5%), pruritus (≤3%), folliculitis (≤2%)

Endocrine & metabolic: LDL-cholesterol increased (grade 2: 9%; grade 3: 4%), glucose increased (126-250 mg/dL: 8%; 251-500 mg/dL: 2%), hypertriglyceridemia (grade 3: 4%)

Gastrointestinal: Abdominal pain (≤5%), lipase increased (1.6-3 x ULN: 4%), amylase increased (1.6-2 x ULN: 2%; 2.1-5 x ULN: 3%), gastroenteritis (≤3%), nausea (≥2%), constipation (≤2%)

Hepatic: AST increased (2.6-5 x ULN: 3% to 9%), hyperbilirubinemia (1.6-2.5 x ULN: 4% to 5%), ALT increased (5.1-10 x ULN: <1% to 3%), alkaline phosphatase increased (2.6-5 x ULN: <1% to 2%)

Neuromuscular & skeletal: Weakness (≥2%), creatine kinase increased (grade 4: 2%)

Renal: Creatinine increased (1.4-1.8 x ULN: 3%)

Respiratory: Nasopharyngitis (≤6%), cough (≤5%), influenza (≤3%)

Miscellaneous: Lymphadenopathy (≤3%), anogenital warts (≤2%)

Frequency <2% or not defined: Abnormal dreams, absolute neutrophil count decreased, acneiform dermatitis, allodynia, anemia, anxiety, appetite increased, arthralgia, back pain, cellulitis, central obesity, chest discomfort, chills, depression, diabetes mellitus, dry skin, dyspepsia, dyslipidemia, epistaxis, erectile dysfunction, erythema, extremity pain, facial wasting, flatulence, fever, gastritis, GERD, glossitis, gynecomastia, hepatitis, hepatomegaly, herpes simplex, herpes zoster, hyperhidrosis, hyperlactacidemia, hypersensitivity, insomnia, irritability, lipodystrophy, macrocytic anemia, maculopapular rash, MI, muscle atrophy, muscle spasms, myalgia, myopathy, myositis, nephrolithiasis, nephropathy, nephrotic syndrome, neuropathy, night sweats, nocturia, palpitation, paresthesia, platelets decreased, pollakiuria, prurigo, renal failure, renal tubular necrosis, rhabdomyolysis, somnolence, vertigo, ventricular extrasystoles, visual disturbance, vomiting, weight changes

General Dosage Range Dosage adjustment recommended in patients on concomitant therapy

Oral: *Adolescents ≥16 years and Adults:* 400 mg twice daily

Mechanism of Action Incorporation of viral DNA into the host cell's genome is required to produce a self-replicating provirus and propagation of infectious virion particles. The viral cDNA strand produced by reverse transcriptase is subsequently processed and inserted into the human genome by the enzyme HIV-1 integrase (encoded by the pol gene of HIV). Raltegravir inhibits the catalytic activity of integrase, thus preventing integration of the proviral gene into human DNA.

Pharmacodynamics/Kinetics

Half-life Elimination ~9 hours

Time to Peak ~3 hours

Pregnancy Risk Factor C

Ramelteon (ra MEL tee on)

U.S. Brand Names Rozerem™

Generic Availability (U.S.) No

Pharmacologic Category Hypnotic, Nonbenzodiazepine

Use Treatment of insomnia characterized by difficulty with sleep onset

Local Anesthetic/Vasoconstrictor Precautions No information available to require special precautions

Effects on Dental Treatment Key adverse event(s) related to dental treatment: Taste perversion.

Effects on Bleeding No information available to require special precautions

Adverse Effects 1% to 10%:

Central nervous system: Dizziness (4% to 5%), somnolence (3% to 5%), fatigue (3% to 4%), insomnia worsened (3%), depression (2%)

Endocrine & metabolic: Serum cortisol decreased (1%)

Gastrointestinal: Nausea (3%), taste perversion (2%)

Neuromuscular & skeletal: Myalgia (2%), arthralgia (2%)

Respiratory: Upper respiratory infection (3%)

Miscellaneous: Influenza (1%)

Dosage Oral: Adults: One 8 mg tablet within 30 minutes of bedtime

Dosage adjustment in renal impairment: No dosage adjustment required

Dosage adjustment in hepatic impairment: No adjustment required for mild-to-moderate impairment; use caution. Not recommended with severe impairment.

Mechanism of Action Potent, selective agonist of melatonin receptors MT_1 and MT_2 (with little affinity for MT_3) within the suprachiasmic nucleus of the hypothalamus, an area responsible for determination of circadian rhythms and synchronization of the sleep-wake cycle. Agonism of MT_1 is thought to preferentially induce sleepiness, while MT_2 receptor activation preferentially influences regulation of circadian rhythms. Ramelteon is eightfold more selective for MT_1 than MT_2 and exhibits nearly sixfold higher affinity for MT_1 than melatonin, presumably allowing for enhanced effects on sleep induction.

Contraindications History of angioedema with previous ramelteon therapy (do not rechallenge); concurrent use with fluvoxamine

Warnings/Precautions Symptomatic treatment of insomnia should be initiated only after careful evaluation of potential causes of sleep disturbance. Failure of sleep disturbance to resolve after a reasonable period of treatment may indicate psychiatric and/or medical illness. Because of the rapid onset of action, administer immediately prior to bedtime or after the patient has gone to bed and is having difficulty falling asleep. Hypnotics/sedatives have been associated with abnormal thinking and behavior changes including decreased inhibition, aggression, bizarre behavior, agitation, hallucinations, and depersonalization. These changes may occur unpredictably and may indicate previously unrecognized psychiatric disorders; evaluate appropriately. Postmarketing studies have indicated that the use of hypnotic/sedative agents (including ramelteon) for sleep has been associated with hypersensitivity reactions including anaphylaxis as well as angioedema. Do not rechallenge patients who have developed angioedema with ramelteon therapy. An increased risk for hazardous sleep-related activities such as sleep-driving; cooking and eating food, and making phone calls while asleep have also been noted. Use caution with pre-existing depression or other psychiatric conditions. Caution when using with other CNS depressants; avoid engaging in hazardous activities or activities requiring mental alertness. Not recommended for use in patients with severe sleep apnea or COPD. Use caution with moderate hepatic impairment; not recommended in patients with severe impairment. May cause disturbances of hormonal regulation. Use caution when administered concomitantly with strong CYP1A2 inhibitors.

Drug Interactions

Metabolism/Transport Effects Substrate of CYP1A2 (major), CYP3A4 (minor), CYP2C family (minor)

Avoid Concomitant Use

Avoid concomitant use of Ramelteon with any of the following: FluvoxaMINE

Increased Effect/Toxicity

Ramelteon may increase the levels/effects of: Alcohol (Ethyl); CNS Depressants; Methotrimeprazine

The levels/effects of Ramelteon may be increased by: Abiraterone; Antifungal Agents (Azole Derivatives, Systemic); Conivaptan; CYP1A2 Inhibitors (Moderate); CYP1A2 Inhibitors (Strong); Deferasirox; Droperidol; Fluconazole; FluvoxaMINE; Methotrimeprazine

Decreased Effect

The levels/effects of Ramelteon may be decreased by: Rifamycin Derivatives; Tocilizumab

Ethanol/Nutrition/Herb Interactions

Ethanol: May increase CNS depression; monitor for increased effects with coadministration. Caution patients about effects.

Food: Taking with high-fat meal delays T_{max} and increases AUC (~31%).

Herb/Nutraceutical: Avoid valerian, St John's wort, kava kava, gotu kola (may increase CNS depression).

Dietary Considerations Do not take with high-fat meal.

Pharmacodynamics/Kinetics

Onset of Action 30 minutes

Half-life Elimination Ramelteon: 1-2.6 hours; M-II: 2-5 hours

Time to Peak Median: 0.5-1.5 hours

Pregnancy Risk Factor C

Lactation Excretion in breast milk unknown/use caution

Dosage Forms

Tablet, oral:

Rozerem™: 8 mg

References

Kato K, Hirai K, Nishiyama K, et al, "Neurochemical Properties of Ramelteon (TAK-375), A Selective MT1/MT2 Receptor Agonist," *Neuropharmacology*. 2005, 48(2):301-10.

Nguyen NN, Uy SS, and Song JC, "Ramelteon: A Novel Melatonin Receptor Agonist for the Treatment of Insomnia," *Formulary*, 2005, 40:146-55.

Ramipril (RA mi pril)

Related Information

Cardiovascular Diseases *on page 1848*

U.S. Brand Names Altace®

Canadian Brand Names Altace®; Apo-Ramipril®; CO Ramipril; JAMP-Ramipril; Mylan-Ramipril; PHL-Ramipril; PMS-Ramipril; RAN™-Ramipril; ratio-Ramipril; Sandoz-Ramipril; Teva-Ramipril

Generic Availability (U.S.) Yes: Capsule

Pharmacologic Category Angiotensin-Converting Enzyme (ACE) Inhibitor

Use Treatment of hypertension, alone or in combination with thiazide diuretics; treatment of left ventricular dysfunction after MI; to reduce risk of MI, stroke, and death in patients at increased risk for these events

Unlabeled/Investigational Use Treatment of heart failure; to delay the progression of nephropathy and reduce risks of cardiovascular events in hypertensive patients with type 1 or 2 diabetes mellitus

Local Anesthetic/Vasoconstrictor Precautions No information available to require special precautions

Effects on Dental Treatment No significant effects or complications reported

Effects on Bleeding No information available to require special precautions

Adverse Effects Note: Frequency ranges include data from hypertension and heart failure trials. Higher rates of adverse reactions have generally been noted in patients with CHF. However, the frequency of adverse effects associated with placebo is also increased in this population.

>10%: Respiratory: Cough increased (7% to 12%)

1% to 10%:

Cardiovascular: Hypotension (11%), angina (up to 3%), postural hypotension (2%), syncope (up to 2%)

Central nervous system: Headache (1% to 5%), dizziness (2% to 4%), fatigue (2%), vertigo (up to 2%)

Endocrine & metabolic: Hyperkalemia (1% to 10%)

Gastrointestinal: Nausea/vomiting (1% to 2%)

Neuromuscular & skeletal: Chest pain (noncardiac) (1%)

Renal: Renal dysfunction (1%), serum creatinine increased (1% to 2%), BUN increased (<1% to 3%); transient increases of creatinine and/or BUN may occur more frequently

Respiratory: Cough (estimated 1% to 10%)

Worsening of renal function may occur in patients with bilateral renal artery stenosis or in hypovolemia. In addition, a syndrome which may include fever, myalgia, arthralgia, interstitial nephritis, vasculitis, rash, eosinophilia and positive ANA, and elevated ESR has been reported with ACE inhibitors. Risk of pancreatitis and agranulocytosis may be increased in patients with collagen vascular disease or renal impairment.

Dosage Adults: Oral:

Heart failure (unlabeled use): Initial: 1.25-2.5 mg once daily; target dose: 10 mg once daily (ACC/AHA 2009 Heart Failure Guidelines)

Hypertension: 2.5-5 mg once daily, maximum: 20 mg/day

LV dysfunction postmyocardial infarction: Initial: 2.5 mg twice daily titrated upward, if possible, to 5 mg twice daily

Reduction in risk of MI, stroke, and death from cardiovascular causes: Initial: 2.5 mg once daily for 1 week, then 5 mg once daily for the next 3 weeks, then increase as tolerated to 10 mg once daily (may be given as divided dose)

Note: The dose of any concomitant diuretic should be reduced. If the diuretic cannot be discontinued, initiate therapy with 1.25 mg. After the initial dose, the patient should be monitored carefully until blood pressure has stabilized.

Dosing adjustment in renal impairment:

Cl_{cr} <40 mL/minute: Administer 25% of normal dose.

Renal failure and heart failure: Administer 1.25 mg once daily, increasing to 1.25 mg twice daily up to 2.5 mg twice daily as tolerated.

Renal failure and hypertension: Administer 1.25 mg once daily, titrated upward as possible; maximum daily dose 5 mg

Mechanism of Action Ramipril is an ACE inhibitor which prevents the formation of angiotensin II from angiotensin I and exhibits pharmacologic effects that are similar to captopril. Ramipril must undergo enzymatic saponification by esterases in the liver to its biologically active metabolite, ramiprilat. The pharmacodynamic effects of ramipril result from the high-affinity, competitive, reversible binding of ramiprilat to angiotensin-converting enzyme, thus preventing the formation of the potent vasoconstrictor angiotensin II. This isomerized enzyme-inhibitor complex has a slow rate of dissociation, which results in high potency and a long duration of action; a CNS mechanism may also be involved in the hypotensive effect as angiotensin II increases adrenergic outflow from CNS; vasoactive kallikreins may be decreased in conversion to active hormones by ACE inhibitors, thus reducing blood pressure

Contraindications Hypersensitivity to ramipril or any component of the formulation; prior hypersensitivity (including angioedema) to ACE inhibitors

Warnings/Precautions Anaphylactic reactions may occur rarely with ACE inhibitors. At any time during treatment (especially following first dose) angioedema may occur rarely with ACE inhibitors; it may involve the head and neck (potentially compromising airway) or the intestine (presenting with abdominal pain). African-Americans and patients with idiopathic or hereditary angioedema may be at an increased risk. Prolonged frequent monitoring may be required especially if tongue, glottis, or larynx are involved as they are associated with airway obstruction. Patients with a history of airway surgery may have a higher risk of airway obstruction. Aggressive early and appropriate management is critical. Use in patients with previous angioedema associated with ACE inhibitor therapy is contraindicated. Severe anaphylactoid reactions may be seen during hemodialysis (eg, CVVHD) with high-flux dialysis membranes (eg, AN69), and rarely, during low density lipoprotein apheresis with dextran sulfate cellulose. Rare cases of anaphylactoid reactions have been reported in patients undergoing sensitization treatment with hymenoptera (bee, wasp) venom while receiving ACE inhibitors.

Symptomatic hypotension with or without syncope can occur with ACE inhibitors (usually with the first several doses); effects are most often observed in volume-depleted patients; close monitoring of patient is required especially with initial dosing and dosing increases; blood pressure must be lowered at a rate appropriate for the patient's clinical condition. Initiation of therapy in patients with ischemic heart disease or cerebrovascular disease warrants close observation due to the potential consequences posed by falling blood pressure (eg, MI, stroke). Use with caution in hypertrophic cardiomyopathy with outflow tract obstruction, severe aortic stenosis, or before, during, or immediately after major surgery. **[U.S. Boxed Warning]: Based on human data, ACEIs can cause injury and death to the developing fetus when used in the second and third trimesters. ACEIs should be discontinued as soon as possible once pregnancy is detected.**

Hyperkalemia may occur with ACE inhibitors; risk factors include renal dysfunction, diabetes mellitus, concomitant use of potassium-sparing diuretics, potassium supplements, and/or potassium containing salts. Use cautiously, if at all, with these agents and monitor potassium closely. Cough may occur with ACE inhibitors. Other causes of cough should be considered (eg, pulmonary congestion in patients with heart failure) and excluded prior to discontinuation.

May be associated with deterioration of renal function and/or increases in serum creatinine, particularly in patients with low renal blood flow (eg, renal artery stenosis, heart failure) whose glomerular filtration rate (GFR) is dependent on efferent arteriolar vasoconstriction by angiotensin II; deterioration may result in oliguria, acute renal failure, and progressive azotemia. Small increases in serum creatinine may occur following initiation; consider discontinuation only in patients with progressive and/or significant deterioration in renal function. Use with caution in patients with unstented unilateral/bilateral renal artery stenosis. When unstented bilateral renal artery stenosis is present, use is generally avoided due to the elevated risk of deterioration in renal function unless possible benefits outweigh risks. Concurrent use of angiotensin receptor blockers may increase the risk of clinically-significant adverse events (eg, renal dysfunction, hyperkalemia). Concurrent use with telmisartan is not recommended.

Rare toxicities associated with ACE inhibitors include cholestatic jaundice (which may progress to fulminant hepatic necrosis), agranulocytosis, neutropenia, or leukopenia with myeloid hypoplasia. Patients with collagen vascular diseases (especially with concomitant renal impairment) or renal impairment alone may be at increased risk for hematologic toxicity; periodically monitor CBC with differential in these patients.

Drug Interactions

Avoid Concomitant Use There are no known interactions where it is recommended to avoid concomitant use.

Increased Effect/Toxicity

Ramipril may increase the levels/effects of: Allopurinol; Amifostine; Antihypertensives; AzaTHIOprine; CycloSPORINE; CycloSPORINE (Systemic); Ferric Gluconate; Gold Sodium Thiomalate; Hypotensive Agents; Iron Dextran Complex; Lithium; Nonsteroidal Anti-Inflammatory Agents; RiTUXimab

The levels/effects of Ramipril may be increased by: Angiotensin II Receptor Blockers; Diazoxide; DPP-IV Inhibitors; Eplerenone; Everolimus; Herbs (Hypotensive Properties); Loop Diuretics; MAO Inhibitors; Pentoxifylline; Phosphodiesterase 5 Inhibitors; Potassium Salts; Potassium-Sparing Diuretics; Prostacyclin Analogues; Sirolimus; Telmisartan; Temsirolimus; Thiazide Diuretics; TiZANidine; Tolvaptan; Trimethoprim

Decreased Effect

The levels/effects of Ramipril may be decreased by: Aprotinin; Herbs (Hypertensive Properties); Methylphenidate; Nonsteroidal Anti-Inflammatory Agents; Salicylates; Yohimbine

Ethanol/Nutrition/Herb Interactions Herb/Nutraceutical: Avoid bayberry, blue cohosh, cayenne, ephedra, ginger, ginseng (American), kola, licorice (may worsen hypertension). Avoid black cohosh, California poppy, coleus, golden seal, hawthorn, mistletoe, periwinkle, quinine, shepherd's purse (may have increased antihypertensive effect).

Pharmacodynamics/Kinetics

Onset of Action 1-2 hours

Duration of Action 24 hours

Half-life Elimination Ramiprilat: Effective: 13-17 hours; Terminal: >50 hours

Time to Peak Serum: Ramipril: ~1 hour; Ramiprilat: 2-4 hours

Pregnancy Risk Factor C (1st trimester); D (2nd and 3rd trimesters)

Lactation Excretion in breast milk unknown/not recommended

Breast-Feeding Considerations Ramipril and its metabolites were not detected in breast milk following a single oral dose of 10 mg. It is not known if multiple doses will produce detectable levels. Breast-feeding is not recommended by the manufacturer.

Dosage Forms

Capsule, oral: 1.25 mg, 2.5 mg, 5 mg, 10 mg

Altace®: 1.25 mg, 2.5 mg, 5 mg, 10 mg

Ramipril and Felodipine (RA mi pril & fe LOE di peen)

Related Information

Felodipine *on page 710*

Ramipril *on page 1457*

Canadian Brand Names Altace® Plus Felodipine

Pharmacologic Category Angiotensin-Converting Enzyme (ACE) Inhibitor; Calcium Channel Blocker; Calcium Channel Blocker, Dihydropyridine

Use Treatment of hypertension when combination therapy is appropriate (not for initial therapy)

Local Anesthetic/Vasoconstrictor Precautions No information available to require special precautions

Effects on Dental Treatment No significant effects or complications reported

Effects on Bleeding No information available to require special precautions

Adverse Effects Incidence observed with combination product. Also see individual agents.

1% to 10%:

Cardiovascular: Vasodilation (3%), peripheral edema (2%), palpitation (1%)
Central nervous system: Headache (8%), dizziness (3%), vertigo (2%)
Gastrointestinal: Nausea (2%), abdominal pain (1%), diarrhea (1%)
Neuromuscular & skeletal: Back pain (2%), weakness (2%)
Respiratory: Cough (6%), bronchitis (3%), upper respiratory infection (1%)
Miscellaneous: Flu-like syndrome (2%)

General Dosage Range Dosage adjustment recommended in patients with hepatic or renal impairment

Oral:

Adults: Ramipril 2.5-10 mg and felodipine ER 2.5-10 mg once daily

Elderly: Initial: Felodipine ER: 2.5 mg daily

Mechanism of Action

Ramipril is an ACE inhibitor which first undergoes enzymatic saponification by esterases in the liver, to its active metabolite ramiprilat. The pharmacodynamic effects of ramipril result from the high-affinity, competitive, reversible binding of ramiprilat to angiotensin-converting enzyme thus preventing the formation of the potent vasoconstrictor angiotensin II from angiotensin I. This isomerized enzyme-inhibitor complex has a slow rate of dissociation, which results in high potency and a long duration of action; a CNS mechanism may also be involved in the hypotensive effect as angiotensin II increases adrenergic outflow from CNS; vasoactive kallikreins may be decreased in conversion to active hormones by ACE inhibitors, thus reducing blood pressure

Felodipine inhibits calcium ions from entering the "slow channels" or select voltage-sensitive areas of vascular smooth muscle and myocardium during depolarization, producing a relaxation of coronary vascular smooth muscle and coronary vasodilation, increases myocardial oxygen delivery in patients with vasospastic angina.

Product Availability Not available in U.S.

Ranibizumab (ra nib i ZUE mab)

U.S. Brand Names Lucentis®

Canadian Brand Names Lucentis®

Pharmacologic Category Monoclonal Antibody; Ophthalmic Agent; Vascular Endothelial Growth Factor (VEGF) Inhibitor

Use Treatment of neovascular (wet) age-related macular degeneration (AMD); treatment of macular edema following retinal vein occlusion (RVO)

Local Anesthetic/Vasoconstrictor Precautions No information available to require special precautions

Effects on Dental Treatment No significant effects or complications reported

Effects on Bleeding No information available to require special precautions in dental procedures.

Adverse Effects Note: Rates of ocular adverse reactions reported for control group when percentages overlapped with treatment group.

>10%:

Central nervous system: Headache (3% to 12%)

Neuromuscular & skeletal: Arthralgia (2% to 11%)

Ocular: Conjunctival hemorrhage (48% to 74%; control: 37% to 60%), eye pain (17% to 35%; control 12% to 30%), vitreous floaters (7% to 27%), intraocular pressure increased (7% to 24%), blurred vision/visual disturbance (5% to 18%), intraocular inflammation (1% to 18%; control 3% to 8%), blepharitis (≤12%), maculopathy (6% to 11%; control 6% to 9%), ocular hyperemia (5% to 11%; control 3% to 8%)

Note: Cataract, dry eye, eye irritation, foreign body sensation, lacrimation increased, pruritus, and vitreous detachment occurred in >10% of patients, but also occurred in similar percentages to the control; visual acuity blurred/decreased occurred more often in the control.

Respiratory: Nasopharyngitis (5% to 16%), bronchitis (≤11%)

1% to 10%:

Cardiovascular: Atrial fibrillation (1% to 5%), arterial thromboembolic events (4%; stroke ≤3%)

Gastrointestinal: Nausea (1% to 9%), viral gastroenteritis (1% to 4%)

Hematologic: Anemia (1% to 8%; control up to 7%)

Ocular: Retinal disorder (2% to 10%), retinal degeneration (1% to 8%), posterior capsule opacification (≤7%), injection site hemorrhage (≤5%)

Note: Conjunctival hyperemia and ocular discomfort occurred in 1% to 10% of patients, but also occurred in similar percentages to the control; retinal exudates occurred more often in the control.

Respiratory: Cough (2% to 9%), upper respiratory tract infection (≤9%), sinusitis (3% to 8%), chronic obstructive pulmonary disease (COPD) (≤6%), dyspnea (≤4%)

Miscellaneous: Ranibizumab antibodies (1% to 8%), influenza (3% to 7%)

General Dosage Range Intravitreal: *Adults:* 0.5 mg once every 1-3 months

Mechanism of Action Ranibizumab is a recombinant humanized monoclonal antibody fragment which binds to and inhibits human vascular endothelial growth factor A (VEGF-A). Ranibizumab inhibits VEGF from binding to its receptors and thereby suppressing neovascularization and slowing vision loss.

Pharmacodynamics/Kinetics

Half-life Elimination Vitreous: ~9 days

Pregnancy Risk Factor C

Ranitidine (ra NI ti deen)

Related Information

Gastrointestinal Disorders *on page 1874*

U.S. Brand Names Zantac 150® [OTC]; Zantac 75® [OTC]; Zantac®; Zantac® EFFERdose®

Canadian Brand Names Acid Reducer; Acid Reducer Maximum Strength Non Prescription; Apo-Ranitidine®; CO Ranitidine; Dom-Ranitidine; Med-Ranitidine; Mylan-Ranitidine; Novo-Ranidine; Nu-Ranit; PHL-Ranitidine; PMS-Ranitidine; Ranitidine Injection, USP; RAN™-Ranitidine; ratio-Ranitidine; Riva-Ranitidine; Sandoz-Ranitidine; ScheinPharm Ranitidine; Teva-Ranitidine; Zantac 75®; Zantac Maximum Strength Non-Prescription; Zantac®; ZYM-Ranitidine

Generic Availability (U.S.) Yes: Excludes effervescent tablet, premixed infusion

Pharmacologic Category Histamine H_2 Antagonist

Use

Zantac®: Short-term and maintenance therapy of duodenal ulcer, gastric ulcer, gastroesophageal reflux disease (GERD), active benign ulcer, erosive esophagitis, and pathological hypersecretory conditions; as part of a multidrug regimen for *H. pylori* eradication to reduce the risk of duodenal ulcer recurrence

Zantac 75® [OTC]: Relief of heartburn, acid indigestion, and sour stomach

Unlabeled/Investigational Use Recurrent postoperative ulcer, upper GI bleeding, prevention of acid-aspiration pneumonitis during surgery, and prevention of stress-induced ulcers

Local Anesthetic/Vasoconstrictor Precautions No information available to require special precautions

Effects on Dental Treatment No significant effects or complications reported

Effects on Bleeding No information available to require special precautions

Adverse Effects Frequency not defined.

Cardiovascular: Asystole, atrioventricular block, bradycardia (with rapid I.V. administration), premature ventricular beats, tachycardia, vasculitis

Central nervous system: Agitation, dizziness, depression, hallucinations, headache, insomnia, malaise, mental confusion, somnolence, vertigo

Dermatologic: Alopecia, erythema multiforme, rash

Endocrine & metabolic: Prolactin levels increased

Gastrointestinal: Abdominal discomfort/pain, constipation, diarrhea, nausea, pancreatitis, vomiting

Hematologic: Acquired immune hemolytic anemia, acute porphyritic attack, agranulocytosis, aplastic anemia, granulocytopenia, leukopenia, pancytopenia, thrombocytopenia

Hepatic: Cholestatic hepatitis, hepatic failure, hepatitis, jaundice

Local: Transient pain, burning or itching at the injection site

Neuromuscular & skeletal: Arthralgia, involuntary motor disturbance, myalgia

Ocular: Blurred vision

Renal: Acute interstitial nephritis, serum creatinine increased

Respiratory: Pneumonia (causal relationship not established)

Miscellaneous: Anaphylaxis, angioneurotic edema, hypersensitivity reactions (eg, bronchospasm, fever, eosinophilia)

Dosage

Children 1 month to 16 years:

Duodenal and gastric ulcer:

Oral:

Treatment: 4-8 mg/kg/day divided twice daily; maximum: 300 mg/day

Maintenance: 2-4 mg/kg/day once daily; maximum: 150 mg/day

I.V.: 2-4 mg/kg/day divided every 6-8 hours; maximum: 200 mg/day

GERD and erosive esophagitis:

Oral: 5-10 mg/kg/day divided twice daily; maximum: GERD: 300 mg/day, erosive esophagitis: 600 mg/day

I.V. (unlabeled): 2-4 mg/kg/day divided every 6-8 hours; maximum: 200 mg/day

or as an alternative

Continuous infusion: Initial: 1 mg/kg/dose for one dose followed by infusion of 0.08-0.17 mg/kg/hour or 2-4 mg/kg/day

Children ≥12 years: Prevention of heartburn: Oral: Zantac 75® [OTC]: 75 mg 30-60 minutes before eating food or drinking beverages which cause heartburn; maximum: 150 mg/24 hours; do not use for more than 14 days

Adults:

Duodenal ulcer: Oral: Treatment: 150 mg twice daily, or 300 mg once daily after the evening meal or at bedtime; maintenance: 150 mg once daily at bedtime

Helicobacter pylori eradication: 150 mg twice daily; requires combination therapy

Pathological hypersecretory conditions:

Oral: 150 mg twice daily; adjust dose or frequency as clinically indicated; doses of up to 6 g/day have been used

I.V.: Continuous infusion for Zollinger-Ellison: Initial: 1 mg/kg/hour; measure gastric acid output at 4 hours, if >10 mEq or if patient is symptomatic, increase dose in increments of 0.5 mg/kg/hour; doses of up to 2.5 mg/kg/hour (or 220 mg/hour) have been used

Gastric ulcer, benign: Oral: 150 mg twice daily; maintenance: 150 mg once daily at bedtime
GERD: Oral: 150 mg twice daily
Erosive esophagitis: Oral: Treatment: 150 mg 4 times/day; maintenance: 150 mg twice daily
Prevention of heartburn: Oral: Zantac 75® [OTC]: 75 mg 30-60 minutes before eating food or drinking beverages which cause heartburn; maximum: 150 mg in 24 hours; do not use for more than 14 days
Patients not able to take oral medication:
I.M.: 50 mg every 6-8 hours
I.V.: Intermittent bolus or infusion: 50 mg every 6-8 hours
Continuous I.V. infusion: 6.25 mg/hour

Elderly: Ulcer healing rates and incidence of adverse effects are similar in the elderly, when compared to younger patients; dosing adjustments not necessary based on age alone

Dosing adjustment in renal impairment: Adults: Cl_{cr} <50 mL/minute:
Oral: 150 mg every 24 hours; adjust dose cautiously if needed
I.V.: 50 mg every 18-24 hours; adjust dose cautiously if needed
Hemodialysis: Adjust dosing schedule so that dose coincides with the end of hemodialysis
Dosing adjustment/comments in hepatic disease: Patients with hepatic impairment may have minor changes in ranitidine half-life, distribution, clearance, and bioavailability; dosing adjustments not necessary, monitor

Mechanism of Action Competitive inhibition of histamine at H_2-receptors of the gastric parietal cells, which inhibits gastric acid secretion, gastric volume, and hydrogen ion concentration are reduced. Does not affect pepsin secretion, pentagastrin-stimulated intrinsic factor secretion, or serum gastrin.

Contraindications Hypersensitivity to ranitidine or any component of the formulation

Warnings/Precautions Ranitidine has been associated with confusional states (rare). Use with caution in patients with hepatic impairment; use with caution in renal impairment, dosage modification required. Avoid use in patients with history of acute porphyria (may precipitate attacks); long-term therapy may be associated with vitamin B_{12} deficiency. Symptoms of GI distress may be associated with a variety of conditions; symptomatic response to H_2 antagonists does not rule out the potential for significant pathology (eg, malignancy). EFFERdose® formulation contains phenylalanine.

Drug Interactions

Metabolism/Transport Effects **Substrate** of CYP1A2 (minor), CYP2C19 (minor), CYP2D6 (minor), P-glycoprotein; **Inhibits** CYP1A2 (weak), 2D6 (weak)

Avoid Concomitant Use

Avoid concomitant use of Ranitidine with any of the following: Delavirdine; Erlotinib

Increased Effect/Toxicity

Ranitidine may increase the levels/effects of: Dexmethylphenidate; Methylphenidate; Procainamide; Saquinavir; Sulfonylureas; Warfarin

The levels/effects of Ranitidine may be increased by: P-Glycoprotein Inhibitors

Decreased Effect

Ranitidine may decrease the levels/effects of: Atazanavir; Cefditoren; Cefpodoxime; Cefuroxime; Dasatinib; Delavirdine; Erlotinib; Fosamprenavir; Gefitinib; Indinavir; Iron Salts; Itraconazole; Ketoconazole; Ketoconazole (Systemic); Mesalamine; Nelfinavir; Posaconazole; Prasugrel

The levels/effects of Ranitidine may be decreased by: Peginterferon Alfa-2b; P-Glycoprotein Inducers

Ethanol/Nutrition/Herb Interactions
Ethanol: Avoid ethanol (may cause gastric mucosal irritation).
Food: Does not interfere with absorption of ranitidine.

Dietary Considerations Some products may contain phenylalanine and/or sodium. Oral dosage forms may be taken with or without food.

Pharmacodynamics/Kinetics

Half-life Elimination
Oral: Normal renal function: 2.5-3 hours; Cl_{cr} 25-35 mL/minute: 4.8 hours
I.V.: Normal renal function: 2-2.5 hours

Time to Peak Serum: Oral: 2-3 hours; I.M.: ≤15 minutes

Pregnancy Risk Factor B

Lactation Enters breast milk/use caution

Breast-Feeding Considerations Ranitidine is excreted into breast milk. The manufacturer recommends that caution be exercised when administering ranitidine to nursing women. Peak milk concentrations of ranitidine occur ~5.5 hours after the dose (case report).

Dosage Forms

Capsule, oral: 150 mg, 300 mg

Infusion, premixed in 1/2 NS [preservative free]:

Zantac®: 50 mg (50 mL)

Injection, solution: 25 mg/mL (2 mL, 6 mL, 40 mL)

Zantac®: 25 mg/mL (2 mL, 6 mL, 40 mL)

Syrup, oral: 15 mg/mL (5 mL, 10 mL, 473 mL, 480 mL)

Zantac®: 15 mg/mL (480 mL)

Tablet, oral: 75 mg, 150 mg, 300 mg

Zantac 150® [OTC]: 150 mg

Zantac 75® [OTC]: 75 mg

Zantac®: 150 mg, 300 mg

Tablet for solution, oral:

Zantac® EFFERdose®: 25 mg

Ranolazine (ra NOE la zeen)

Related Information

Clinical Risk Related to Drugs Prolonging QT Interval *on page 1872*

U.S. Brand Names Ranexa®

Pharmacologic Category Cardiovascular Agent, Miscellaneous

Use Treatment of chronic angina

Local Anesthetic/Vasoconstrictor Precautions Ranolazine is one of the drugs confirmed to prolong the QT interval and is accepted as having a risk of causing torsade de pointes. The risk of drug-induced torsade de pointes is extremely low when a single QT interval prolonging drug is prescribed. In terms of epinephrine, it is not known what effect vasoconstrictors in the local anesthetic regimen will have in patients with a known history of congenital prolonged QT interval or in patients taking any medication that prolongs the QT interval. Until more information is obtained, it is suggested that the clinician consult with the physician prior to the use of a vasoconstrictor in suspected patients, and that the vasoconstrictor (epinephrine, mepivacaine and levonordefrin [Carbocaine® 2% with Neo-Cobefrin®]) be used with caution.

Effects on Dental Treatment Key adverse event(s) related to dental treatment: Xerostomia (normal salivary flow resumes upon discontinuation).

Effects on Bleeding No information available to require special precautions

Adverse Effects

>10%:

Central nervous system: Dizziness (5% to 13%; dose related)

Gastrointestinal: Constipation (5% to 8%; 19% in the elderly)

>0.5% to 10%:

Cardiovascular: Syncope (≤3%), bradycardia (≤2%), hypotension (≤2%), orthostatic hypotension (≤2%), palpitation (≤2%), peripheral edema (≤2%), QT_c prolongation (>500 msec: ≤1%)

Central nervous system: Headache (3% to 6%), vertigo (≤2%)

Gastrointestinal: Nausea (4% to 9%), abdominal pain (≤2%), vomiting (≤2%), xerostomia (≤2%)

Hematologic: Hematocrit decreased (1%)

Otic: Tinnitus (≤2%)

Respiratory: Dyspnea (≤2%)

General Dosage Range Dosage adjustment recommended in patients on concomitant therapy

Oral: *Adults:* Initial: 500 mg twice daily; Maintenance: 500-1000 mg twice daily (maximum: 2000 mg/day)

Mechanism of Action Ranolazine exerts antianginal and anti-ischemic effects without changing hemodynamic parameters (heart rate or blood pressure). At therapeutic levels, ranolazine inhibits the late phase of the inward sodium channel (late I_{Na}) in ischemic cardiac myocytes during cardiac repolarization reducing intracellular sodium concentrations and thereby reducing calcium influx via Na^+-Ca^{2+} exchange. Decreased intracellular calcium reduces ventricular tension and myocardial oxygen consumption. It is thought that ranolazine produces myocardial relaxation and reduces anginal symptoms through this mechanism although this is uncertain. At higher concentrations, ranolazine inhibits the rapid delayed rectifier potassium current (I_{Kr}) thus prolonging the ventricular action potential duration and subsequent prolongation of the QT interval.

Pharmacodynamics/Kinetics

Half-life Elimination Terminal: 7 hours

Time to Peak 2-5 hours

Pregnancy Risk Factor C

Dental Comment Ranolazine is known to prolong the QT interval. The QT interval is measured as the time and distance between the Q point of the QRS complex and the end of the T wave in the ECG tracing. After adjustment for heart rate, the QT interval is defined as prolonged if it is more than 450 msec in men and 460 msec in women. A long QT syndrome was first described in the 1950s and 60s as a congenital syndrome involving QT interval prolongation and syncope and sudden death. Some of the congenital long QT syndromes were characterized by a peculiar electrocardiographic appearance of the QRS complex involving a premature atria beat followed by a pause, then a subsequent sinus beat showing marked QT prolongation and deformity. This type of cardiac arrhythmia was originally termed "torsade de pointes" (translated from the French as "twisting of the points"). Ranolazine is considered as having a risk of causing torsade de pointes. Since it is not known what effect vasoconstrictors in the local anesthetic regimen will have in patients with a known history of congenital prolonged QT interval or in patients taking any medication that prolongs the QT interval, a medical consult is suggested.

Rasagiline (ra SA ji leen)

U.S. Brand Names Azilect®

Pharmacologic Category Anti-Parkinson's Agent, MAO Type B Inhibitor

Use Treatment of idiopathic Parkinson's disease (initial monotherapy or as adjunct to levodopa)

Local Anesthetic/Vasoconstrictor Precautions Rasagiline in approved doses of 0.5-1 mg daily should not inhibit type-A MAO; however, the possibility exists of nonselective MAO inhibition at higher doses and/or in certain sensitive individuals. Therefore, attempts should be made to avoid use of vasoconstrictors due to possibility of hypertensive episodes.

Effects on Dental Treatment Key adverse event(s) related to dental treatment: Xerostomia and changes in salivation (normal salivary flow resumes upon discontinuation). Anticholinergic side effects can cause a reduction of saliva production or secretion, contributing to discomfort and dental disease (ie, caries, oral candidiasis, and periodontal disease). May cause orthostatic hypotension particularly during the first 2 months of therapy.

Effects on Bleeding No information available to require special precautions

Adverse Effects Unless otherwise noted, the following adverse reactions are as reported for monotherapy. Spectrum of adverse events was generally similar with adjunctive (levodopa) therapy, though the incidence tended to be higher.

>10%:

- Cardiovascular: Postural hypotension (6% to 13% adjunct therapy, dose dependent)
- Central nervous system: Dyskinesia (18% adjunct therapy), headache (14%)
- Gastrointestinal: Nausea (10% to 12% adjunct therapy)

1% to 10%:

- Cardiovascular: Angina, bundle branch block, chest pain, syncope
- Central nervous system: Depression (5%), hallucinations (4% to 5% adjunct therapy), fever (3%), malaise (2%), vertigo (2%), anxiety, dizziness
- Dermatologic: Bruising (2%), alopecia, skin carcinoma, vesiculobullous rash
- Endocrine & metabolic: Impotence, libido decreased
- Gastrointestinal: Constipation (4% to 9% adjunct therapy), weight loss (2% to 9% adjunct therapy; dose dependent), dyspepsia (7%), xerostomia (2% to 6% adjunct therapy; dose dependent), gastroenteritis (3%), anorexia, diarrhea, gastrointestinal hemorrhage, vomiting
- Genitourinary: Hematuria, urinary incontinence
- Hematologic: Leukopenia
- Hepatic: Liver function tests increased
- Neuromuscular & skeletal: Arthralgia (7%), neck pain (2%), arthritis (2%), paresthesia (2%), abnormal gait, hyperkinesias, hypertonia, neuropathy, tremor, weakness
- Ocular: Conjunctivitis (3%)
- Renal: Albuminuria
- Respiratory: Rhinitis (3%), asthma, cough increased
- Miscellaneous: Fall (5%), flu-like syndrome (5%), allergic reaction

General Dosage Range Dosage adjustment recommended in patients with hepatic impairment or on concomitant therapy

Oral: *Adults:* 0.5-1 mg once daily

Mechanism of Action Potent, irreversible and selective inhibitor of brain monoamine oxidase (MAO) type B, which plays a major role in the catabolism of dopamine. Inhibition of dopamine depletion in the striatal region of the brain reduces the symptomatic motor deficits of Parkinson's disease. There is also experimental evidence of rasagiline conferring neuroprotective effects (antioxidant, antiapoptotic), which may delay onset of symptoms and progression of neuronal deterioration.

Pharmacodynamics/Kinetics

Onset of Action Therapeutic: Within 1 hour

Duration of Action ~1 week (irreversible inhibition); may require ~14-40 days for complete restoration of (brain) MAO-B activity

Half-life Elimination ~1.3-3 hours (no correlation with biologic effect due to irreversible inhibition)

Time to Peak ~1 hour

Pregnancy Risk Factor C

Rasburicase (ras BYOOR i kayse)

U.S. Brand Names Elitek™

Canadian Brand Names Fasturtec®

Pharmacologic Category Enzyme; Enzyme, Urate-Oxidase (Recombinant)

Use Initial management of uric acid levels in patients with leukemia, lymphoma, and solid tumor malignancies receiving chemotherapy expected to result in tumor lysis and elevation of plasma uric acid

Local Anesthetic/Vasoconstrictor Precautions No information available to require special precautions

Effects on Dental Treatment Key adverse event(s) related to dental treatment: Mucositis.

Effects on Bleeding No information available to require special precautions

Adverse Effects

>10%:

Cardiovascular: Peripheral edema (≤50%), fluid overload (≤12%)

Central nervous system: Fever (46%; serious: 5%), headache (26%), anxiety (≤24%)

Dermatologic: Rash (13%; serious: 1%)

Endocrine & metabolic: Hypophosphatemia (≤17%)

Gastrointestinal: Vomiting (50%), nausea (27%), abdominal pain (20%), constipation (20%), diarrhea (20%), mucositis (15%; serious: 2%)

Hepatic: Hyperbilirubinemia (≤16%), ALT increased (≤11%)

Respiratory: Pharyngolaryngeal pain (≤14%)

Miscellaneous: Antibody formation (healthy volunteers: 61% to 64%; patients with malignancies: 11%), sepsis (≤12%; serious: 3% to 5%)

1% to 10%:

Cardiovascular: Ischemic coronary disorder, supraventricular arrhythmia

Endocrine & metabolic: Hyperphosphatemia (≤10%)

Gastrointestinal: Abdominal/gastrointestinal infection

Hematologic: Neutropenic fever (serious: 4%), neutropenia (serious: 2%)

Respiratory: Respiratory distress (serious: 3%), pulmonary hemorrhage, respiratory failure

Miscellaneous: Hypersensitivity (≤4%)

General Dosage Range I.V.: *Children and Adults:* 0.2 mg/kg once daily

Mechanism of Action Rasburicase is a recombinant urate-oxidase enzyme, which converts uric acid to allantoin (an inactive and soluble metabolite of uric acid); it does not inhibit the formation of uric acid.

Pharmacodynamics/Kinetics

Onset of Action Uric acid levels decrease within 4 hours of initial administration

Half-life Elimination ~16-23 hours

Pregnancy Risk Factor C

Remifentanil (rem i FEN ta nil)

U.S. Brand Names Ultiva®

Canadian Brand Names Ultiva®

Pharmacologic Category Analgesic, Opioid; Anilidopiperidine Opioid

Use Analgesic for use during the induction and maintenance of general anesthesia; for continued analgesia into the immediate postoperative period; analgesic component of monitored anesthesia

Unlabeled/Investigational Use Management of pain in mechanically-ventilated patients

Local Anesthetic/Vasoconstrictor Precautions No information available to require special precautions

Effects on Dental Treatment No significant effects or complications reported

Effects on Bleeding No information available to require special precautions

Adverse Effects

>10%: Gastrointestinal: Nausea, vomiting

1% to 10%:

Cardiovascular: Bradycardia (dose dependent), hypertension, hypotension (dose dependent), tachycardia

Central nervous system: Agitation, dizziness, fever, headache

Dermatologic: Pruritus

Neuromuscular & skeletal: Muscle rigidity (dose dependent)

Ocular: Visual disturbances

Respiratory: Apnea, hypoxia, respiratory depression

Miscellaneous: Postoperative pain, shivering

General Dosage Range I.V.:

Infants Birth to 2 months: Infusion: 0.4-1 mcg/kg/minute; Supplemental bolus dose: ≤1 mcg/kg

Children 1-12 years: Infusion: 0.05-1.3 mcg/kg/minute; Bolus: 1 mcg/kg every 2-5 minutes

Adults: Infusion: 0.025-4 mcg/kg/minute; Bolus: 0.5-1 mcg/kg every 2-5 minutes

Elderly: Doses should be decreased by 50% and titrated

Mechanism of Action Binds with stereospecific mu-opioid receptors at many sites within the CNS, increases pain threshold, alters pain reception, inhibits ascending pain pathways

Pharmacodynamics/Kinetics

Onset of Action I.V.: 1-3 minutes

Half-life Elimination Dose dependent: Terminal: 10-20 minutes; effective: 3-10 minutes

Pregnancy Risk Factor C

Controlled Substance C-II

Repaglinide (re PAG li nide)

Related Information

Endocrine Disorders and Pregnancy *on page 1879*

U.S. Brand Names Prandin®

Canadian Brand Names GlucoNorm®; Prandin®

Pharmacologic Category Antidiabetic Agent, Meglitinide Derivative

Use Management of type 2 diabetes mellitus (noninsulin dependent, NIDDM) as an adjunct to diet and exercise; may be used in combination with metformin or thiazolidinediones

Local Anesthetic/Vasoconstrictor Precautions No information available to require special precautions

Effects on Dental Treatment Key adverse event(s) related to dental treatment: Tooth disorder.

Effects on Bleeding No information available to require special precautions

Adverse Effects

>10%:

Central nervous system: Headache (9% to 11%)

Endocrine & metabolic: Hypoglycemia (16% to 31%)

Respiratory: Upper respiratory tract infection (10% to 16%)

1% to 10%:

Cardiovascular: Ischemia (4%), chest pain (2% to 3%)

Gastrointestinal: Diarrhea (4% to 5%), constipation (2% to 3%), tooth disorder (≤2%)

Genitourinary: Urinary tract infection (2% to 3%)

Neuromuscular & skeletal: Back pain (5% to 6%), arthralgia (3% to 6%)

Respiratory: Sinusitis (3% to 6%), bronchitis (2% to 6%)

Miscellaneous: Allergy (1% to 2%)

General Dosage Range Dosage adjustment recommended in patients with renal impairment

Oral: *Adults:* Initial: 0.5-2 mg before each meal; Maintenance: 0.5-4 mg before each meal (maximum: 16 mg/day)

Mechanism of Action Nonsulfonylurea hypoglycemic agent which blocks ATP-dependent potassium channels, depolarizing the membrane and facilitating calcium entry through calcium channels. Increased intracellular calcium stimulates insulin release from the pancreatic beta cells. Repaglinide-induced insulin release is glucose-dependent.

Pharmacodynamics/Kinetics

Onset of Action Single dose: Increased insulin levels: ~15-60 minutes

Duration of Action 4-6 hours

Half-life Elimination ~1 hour

Time to Peak Plasma: ~1 hour

Pregnancy Risk Factor C

Repaglinide and Metformin (re PAG li nide & met FOR min)

Related Information

Endocrine Disorders and Pregnancy *on page 1879*
MetFORMIN *on page 1089*
Repaglinide *on page 1466*

U.S. Brand Names PrandiMet®

Pharmacologic Category Antidiabetic Agent, Biguanide; Antidiabetic Agent, Meglitinide Derivative; Hypoglycemic Agent, Oral

Use Management of type 2 diabetes mellitus (noninsulin dependent, NIDDM), as an adjunct to diet and exercise, in patients currently receiving or not adequately controlled on metformin and/or a meglitinide

Local Anesthetic/Vasoconstrictor Precautions No information available to require special precautions

Effects on Dental Treatment Key adverse event(s) related to dental treatment: Patients with diabetes (noninsulin dependent, type 2) taking repaglinide and metformin combination should schedule dental treatment in morning in order to minimize stress-induced hypoglycemia

Effects on Bleeding No information available to require special precautions

Adverse Effects Note: The following information reflects the frequency of adverse effects experienced by patients who received the repaglinide/metformin fixed-dose combination product. Also see individual agents.

>10%:

Central nervous system: Headache (22%)
Endocrine & metabolic: Hypoglycemia (33%)
Gastrointestinal: Diarrhea (19%), nausea (15%)
Respiratory: Upper respiratory tract infection (11%)

General Dosage Range Oral: *Adults:* Repaglinide 1-2 mg and metformin 500 mg 2-3 times daily with meals (maximum single dose: 4 mg/dose [repaglinide], 1000 mg/dose [metformin]; maximum daily dose: 10 mg/day [repaglinide], 2500 mg/day [metformin])

Mechanism of Action Combination therapy; repaglinide and metformin act to improve glycemic control via two different mechanisms of action:

Repaglinide is a nonsulfonylurea hypoglycemic agent which stimulates insulin release by blocking ATP-dependent potassium channels, depolarizing the membrane and facilitating calcium entry through calcium channels; increased intracellular calcium stimulates insulin release from the pancreatic beta cells.

Metformin prevents hyperglycemia by decreasing hepatic glucose production, decreasing intestinal absorption of glucose, and improving insulin sensitivity via increased peripheral glucose uptake and utilization.

Pregnancy Risk Factor C

Reserpine (re SER peen)

Related Information

Cardiovascular Diseases *on page 1848*

Pharmacologic Category Central Monoamine-Depleting Agent; Rauwolfia Alkaloid

Use Management of mild-to-moderate hypertension; treatment of agitated psychotic states (schizophrenia)

Unlabeled/Investigational Use Management of tardive dyskinesia

Local Anesthetic/Vasoconstrictor Precautions No information available to require special precautions

Effects on Dental Treatment Key adverse event(s) related to dental treatment: Xerostomia and changes in salivation (normal salivary flow resumes upon discontinuation).

Effects on Bleeding No information available to require special precautions

Adverse Effects Frequency not defined.

Cardiovascular: Arrhythmia, bradycardia, chest pain, hypotension, peripheral edema, PVC, syncope
Central nervous system: Dizziness, drowsiness, dull sensorium, fatigue, headache, mental depression, nightmares, nervousness, parkinsonism, paradoxical anxiety
Dermatologic: Flushing of skin, pruritus, purpura, rash
Endocrine & metabolic: Gynecomastia, weight gain

Gastrointestinal: Anorexia, diarrhea, dry mouth, gastric acid secretion increased, nausea, salivation increased, vomiting
Genitourinary: Impotence, libido decreased
Hematologic: Thrombocytopenia purpura
Neuromuscular & skeletal: Muscle ache
Ocular: Blurred vision, optic atrophy
Respiratory: Dyspnea, epistaxis, nasal congstion

General Dosage Range Oral:
Adults: Initial: 0.5 mg once daily; Maintenance: 0.05-0.5 mg once daily
Elderly: Initial: 0.05 mg once daily

Mechanism of Action Reduces blood pressure via depletion of sympathetic biogenic amines (norepinephrine and dopamine); this also commonly results in sedative effects

Pharmacodynamics/Kinetics
Onset of Action Antihypertensive: 3-6 days
Duration of Action 2-6 weeks
Half-life Elimination 50-100 hours

Pregnancy Risk Factor C

Retapamulin (re te PAM ue lin)

U.S. Brand Names Altabax™

Pharmacologic Category Antibiotic, Pleuromutilin; Antibiotic, Topical

Use Treatment of impetigo caused by susceptible strains of *S. pyogenes* or methicillin-susceptible *S. aureus*

Local Anesthetic/Vasoconstrictor Precautions No information available to require special precautions

Effects on Dental Treatment No significant effects or complications reported

Effects on Bleeding No information available to require special precautions

Adverse Effects 1% to 10%:
Central nervous system: Headache (1% to 2%), pyrexia (1%)
Dermatologic: Pruritus (2%), eczema (1%)
Gastrointestinal: Diarrhea (1% to 2%), nausea (1%)
Local: Application site irritation (2%), application site pruritus (2%)
Respiratory: Nasopharyngitis (1% to 2%)

General Dosage Range Topical: *Children ≥9 months and Adults:* Apply to affected area twice daily. Total treatment area should not exceed 2% of total body surface area.

Mechanism of Action Primarily bacteriostatic. Inhibits normal bacterial protein biosynthesis by binding at a unique site (protein L3) on the ribosomal 50S subunit; prevents formation of active 50S ribosomal subunits by inhibiting peptidyl transfer and blocking P-site interactions at this site

Pregnancy Risk Factor B

Reteplase (RE ta plase)

Related Information
Cardiovascular Diseases *on page 1848*

U.S. Brand Names Retavase®

Canadian Brand Names Retavase®

Pharmacologic Category Thrombolytic Agent

Use Management of ST-elevation myocardial infarction (STEMI); improvement of ventricular function; reduction of the incidence of CHF and the reduction of mortality following AMI

Recommended criteria for treatment: STEMI: Chest pain ≥20 minutes duration, onset of chest pain within 12 hours of treatment (or within prior 12-24 hours in patients with continuing ischemic symptoms), and ST-segment elevation >0.1 mV in at least two contiguous precordial leads or two adjacent limb leads on ECG or new or presumably new left bundle branch block (LBBB)

Local Anesthetic/Vasoconstrictor Precautions No information available to require special precautions

Effects on Dental Treatment Key adverse event(s) related to dental treatment: Bleeding is the most frequent adverse effect of reteplase. See Effects on Bleeding.

Effects on Bleeding Bleeding is the most frequent adverse effect associated with reteplase. It is unlikely that ambulatory patients presenting for dental treatment will be taking intravenous anticoagulant therapy.

Adverse Effects Bleeding is the most frequent adverse effect associated with reteplase. Heparin and aspirin have been administered concurrently with reteplase in clinical trials. The incidence of adverse events is a reflection of these combined therapies, and are comparable with comparison thrombolytics.

>10%: Local: Injection site bleeding (4.6% to 48.6%)
1% to 10%:
Gastrointestinal: Bleeding (1.8% to 9.0%)
Genitourinary: Bleeding (0.9% to 9.5%)
Hematologic: Anemia (0.9% to 2.6%)
Other adverse effects noted are frequently associated with MI (and therefore may or may not be attributable to Retavase®) and include arrhythmia, hypotension, cardiogenic shock, pulmonary edema, cardiac arrest, reinfarction, pericarditis, tamponade, thrombosis, and embolism.

General Dosage Range I.V.: *Adults:* 10 units; repeat after 30 minutes

Mechanism of Action Reteplase is a nonglycosylated form of tPA produced by recombinant DNA technology using *E. coli*; it initiates local fibrinolysis by binding to fibrin in a thrombus (clot) and converts entrapped plasminogen to plasmin

Pharmacodynamics/Kinetics

Onset of Action Thrombolysis: 30-90 minutes

Half-life Elimination 13-16 minutes

Pregnancy Risk Factor C

Rh_o(D) Immune Globulin (ar aych oh (dee) i MYUN GLOB yoo lin)

U.S. Brand Names HyperRHO™ S/D Full Dose; HyperRHO™ S/D Mini-Dose; MICRhoGAM® UF Plus; RhoGAM® UF Plus; Rhophylac®; WinRho® SDF

Canadian Brand Names WinRho® SDF

Pharmacologic Category Blood Product Derivative; Immune Globulin

Use

Suppression of Rh isoimmunization: Use in the following situations when an Rh_o(D)-negative individual is exposed to Rh_o(D)-positive blood: During delivery of an Rh_o(D)-positive infant; abortion; amniocentesis; chorionic villus sampling; ruptured tubal pregnancy; abdominal trauma; hydatidiform mole; transplacental hemorrhage. Used when the mother is Rh_o(D)-negative, the father of the child is either Rh_o(D)-positive or Rh_o(D)-unknown, or the baby is either Rh_o(D)-positive or Rh_o(D)-unknown.

Transfusion: Suppression of Rh isoimmunization in Rh_o(D)-negative individuals transfused with Rh_o(D) antigen-positive RBCs or blood components containing Rh_o(D) antigen-positive RBCs

Treatment of idiopathic thrombocytopenic purpura (ITP): Used intravenously in the following nonsplenectomized Rh_o(D)-positive individuals: Children with acute or chronic ITP, adults with chronic ITP, and children and adults with ITP secondary to HIV infection

Local Anesthetic/Vasoconstrictor Precautions No information available to require special precautions

Effects on Dental Treatment No significant effects or complications reported

Effects on Bleeding No information available to require special precautions

Adverse Effects Frequency not defined.

Cardiovascular: Hyper-/hypotension, pallor, tachycardia, vasodilation
Central nervous system: Chills, dizziness, fever, headache, malaise, somnolence
Dermatologic: Pruritus, rash
Gastrointestinal: Abdominal pain, diarrhea, nausea, vomiting
Hematologic: Haptoglobin decreased, hemoglobin decreased (patients with ITP), intravascular hemolysis (patients with ITP)
Hepatic: Bilirubin increased, LDH increased
Local: Injection site reaction: Discomfort, induration, mild pain, redness, swelling
Neuromuscular & skeletal: Arthralgia, back pain, hyperkinesia, myalgia, weakness
Renal: Acute renal insufficiency
Miscellaneous: Anaphylaxis, diaphoresis, infusion-related reactions, positive anti-C antibody test (transient), shivering

General Dosage Range I.M., I.V.: *Children and Adults:* Dosage varies greatly depending on indication

Mechanism of Action

Rh suppression: Prevents isoimmunization by suppressing the immune response and antibody formation by Rh_o(D) negative individuals to Rh_o(D) positive red blood cells.

ITP: Not completely characterized; Rh_o(D) immune globulin is thought to form anti-D-coated red blood cell complexes which bind to macrophage Fc receptors within the spleen; blocking or saturating the spleens ability to clear antibody-coated cells, including platelets. In this manner, platelets are spared from destruction.

Pharmacodynamics/Kinetics

Onset of Action Onset of platelet increase: ITP: Platelets should rise within 1-2 days; Peak effect: In 7-14 days

Duration of Action Suppression of Rh isoimmunization: ~12 weeks; Treatment of ITP: 30 days (variable)

Half-life Elimination ~24-30 days

Time to Peak Plasma: I.M.: 5-10 days; I.V. (WinRho® SDF): ≤2 hours

Pregnancy Risk Factor C

Ribavirin (rye ba VYE rin)

Related Information

Systemic Viral Diseases *on page 1904*

U.S. Brand Names Copegus®; Rebetol®; Ribasphere®; Ribasphere® RibaPak®; Virazole®

Canadian Brand Names Virazole®

Pharmacologic Category Antiviral Agent

Use

Inhalation: Treatment of patients with respiratory syncytial virus (RSV) infections; specially indicated for treatment of severe lower respiratory tract RSV infections in patients with an underlying compromising condition (prematurity, bronchopulmonary dysplasia and other chronic lung conditions, congenital heart disease, immunodeficiency, immunosuppression), and recent transplant recipients

Oral capsule:

In combination with interferon alfa-2b (Intron® A) injection for the treatment of chronic hepatitis C in patients with compensated liver disease who have relapsed after alpha interferon therapy or were previously untreated with alpha interferons

In combination with peginterferon alfa-2b (PEG-Intron®) injection for the treatment of chronic hepatitis C in patients with compensated liver disease who were previously untreated with alpha interferons

Oral solution: In combination with interferon alfa 2b (Intron® A) injection for the treatment of chronic hepatitis C in patients with compensated liver disease who were previously untreated with alpha interferons or patients who have relapsed after alpha interferon therapy

Oral tablet: In combination with peginterferon alfa-2a (Pegasys®) injection for the treatment of chronic hepatitis C in patients with compensated liver disease who were previously untreated with alpha interferons (includes patients with histological evidence of cirrhosis [Child-Pugh class A] and patients with clinically-stable HIV disease)

Unlabeled/Investigational Use Used in other viral infections including influenza A and B and adenovirus

Local Anesthetic/Vasoconstrictor Precautions No information available to require special precautions

Effects on Dental Treatment Key adverse event(s) related to dental treatment: Xerostomia (normal salivary flow resumes upon discontinuation) and taste perversion.

Effects on Bleeding No information available to require special precautions

Adverse Effects

Inhalation:

1% to 10%:

Central nervous system: Fatigue, headache, insomnia

Gastrointestinal: Nausea, anorexia

Hematologic: Anemia

<1%: Hypotension, cardiac arrest, digitalis toxicity, conjunctivitis, mild bronchospasm, worsening of respiratory function, apnea

Note: Incidence of adverse effects (approximate) in healthcare workers: Headache (51%); conjunctivitis (32%); rhinitis, nausea, rash, dizziness, pharyngitis, and lacrimation (10% to 20%); bronchospasm and/or chest pain (case reports in individuals with underlying airway disease)

Oral (all adverse reactions are documented while receiving combination therapy with alfa interferons; percentages as reported in adults); asterisked (*) percentages are those similar to interferon therapy alone:

>10%:

Central nervous system: Fatigue (60% to 70%)*, headache (43% to 66%)*, fever (32% to 55%)*, insomnia (26% to 41%), depression (20% to 36%)*, irritability (23% to 33%), dizziness (14% to 26%), impaired concentration (10% to 21%)*, emotional lability (7% to 12%)*

Dermatologic: Alopecia (27% to 36%), pruritus (13% to 29%), rash (5% to 28%), dry skin (10% to 24%), dermatitis (≤16%)

Endocrine and metabolic: Hyperuricemia (33% to 38%)

Gastrointestinal: Nausea (25% to 47%), anorexia (21% to 32%), weight decrease (10% to 29%), vomiting (9% to 25%)*, diarrhea (10% to 22%), dyspepsia (6% to 16%), abdominal pain (8% to 13%), xerostomia (≤12%), RUQ pain (≤12%)
Hematologic: Leukopenia (6% to 45%), neutropenia (8% to 42%; grade 4: 2% to 11%; 40% with HIV coinfection), hemoglobin decreased (11% to 35%), anemia (11% to 17%), thrombocytopenia (<1% to 15%), lymphopenia (12% to 14%), hemolytic anemia (10% to 13%)
Hepatic: Bilirubin increase (10% to 32%)
Neuromuscular & skeletal: Myalgia (40% to 64%)*, rigors (25% to 48%), arthralgia (22% to 34%)*, musculoskeletal pain (19% to 28%)
Respiratory: Dyspnea (13% to 26%), cough (7% to 23%), pharyngitis (≤13%), sinusitis (≤12%)*
Miscellaneous: Flu-like syndrome (13% to 18%)*, viral infection (≤12%), diaphoresis (≤11%)

1% to 10%:
Cardiovascular: Chest pain (5% to 9%)*, flushing (≤4%)
Central nervous system: Pain (≤10%), mood alteration (≤6%; 9% with HIV coinfection), agitation (5% to 8%), nervousness (6%)*, memory impairment (≤6%), malaise (≤6%), suicidal ideation (adolescents: 2%; adults: 1%)
Dermatologic: Eczema (4% to 5%)
Endocrine & metabolic: Menstrual disorder (≤7%), hypothyroidism (≤5%)
Gastrointestinal: Taste perversion (4% to 9%), constipation (5%)
Hepatic: Hepatomegaly (4%), transaminases increased (1% to 3%), hepatic decompensation (2% with HIV coinfection)
Neuromuscular & skeletal: Weakness (9% to 10%), back pain (5%)
Ocular: Blurred vision (≤6%), conjunctivitis (≤5%)
Respiratory: Rhinitis (≤8%), exertional dyspnea (≤7%)
Miscellaneous: Fungal infection (≤6%), bacterial infection (3% to 5%)

Note: Incidence of anorexia, headache, fever, suicidal ideation, and vomiting are higher in children.

General Dosage Range Dosage adjustment recommended in patients who develop toxicities

Inhalation: *Children:* 20 mg/mL (6 g in 300 mL) solution; continuous: 12-18 hours/day

Oral:
Children ≥3 years and ≤25 kg: 15 mg/kg/day in 2 divided doses
Children ≥3 years and 26-36 kg: 400 mg/day in 2 divided doses
Children ≥3 years and 37-49 kg: 600 mg/day in 2 divided doses
Children ≥3 years and 50-61 kg: 800 mg/day in 2 divided doses
Children ≥3 years and >61 kg to <75 kg: 1000 mg/day in 2 divided doses
Adults ≤75 kg: 800-1000 mg/day in 2 divided doses
Adults >75 kg: 800-1200 mg/day in 2 divided doses

Mechanism of Action Inhibits replication of RNA and DNA viruses; inhibits influenza virus RNA polymerase activity and inhibits the initiation and elongation of RNA fragments resulting in inhibition of viral protein synthesis

Pharmacodynamics/Kinetics

Half-life Elimination Plasma:
Children: Inhalation: 6.5-11 hours
Adults: Oral:
Capsule, single dose (Rebetol®, Ribasphere®): 24 hours in healthy adults, 44 hours with chronic hepatitis C infection (increases to ~298 hours at steady state)
Tablet, single dose (Copegus®): ~120-170 hours

Time to Peak Serum: Inhalation: At end of inhalation period; Oral capsule: Multiple doses: 3 hours; Tablet: 2 hours

Pregnancy Risk Factor X

Riboflavin (RYE boe flay vin)

U.S. Brand Names Ribo-100 [OTC]

Generic Availability (U.S.) Yes

Pharmacologic Category Vitamin, Water Soluble

Use Prevention of riboflavin deficiency and treatment of ariboflavinosis

Local Anesthetic/Vasoconstrictor Precautions No information available to require special precautions

Effects on Dental Treatment No significant effects or complications reported

Effects on Bleeding No information available to require special precautions

Adverse Effects Frequency not defined: Genitourinary: Discoloration of urine (yellow-orange)

Dosage Oral:
Riboflavin deficiency:
Children: 2.5-10 mg/day in divided doses
Adults: 5-30 mg/day in divided doses
Recommended daily allowance:
Children: 0.4-1.8 mg
Adults: 1.2-1.7 mg

Mechanism of Action Component of flavoprotein enzymes that work together, which are necessary for normal tissue respiration; also needed for activation of pyridoxine and conversion of tryptophan to niacin

Warnings/Precautions Riboflavin deficiency often occurs in the presence of other B vitamin deficiencies.

Drug Interactions

Avoid Concomitant Use There are no known interactions where it is recommended to avoid concomitant use.

Increased Effect/Toxicity There are no known significant interactions involving an increase in effect.

Decreased Effect There are no known significant interactions involving a decrease in effect.

Pharmacodynamics/Kinetics

Half-life Elimination Biologic: 66-84 minutes

Pregnancy Risk Factor A/C (dose exceeding RDA recommendation)

Lactation Enters breast milk/compatible

Dosage Forms

Tablet, oral: 25 mg, 50 mg, 100 mg
Ribo-100 [OTC]: 100 mg

Rifabutin (rif a BYOO tin)

Related Information

Systemic Viral Diseases *on page 1904*
Tuberculosis *on page 1902*

U.S. Brand Names Mycobutin®

Canadian Brand Names Mycobutin®

Pharmacologic Category Antibiotic, Miscellaneous; Antitubercular Agent

Use Prevention of disseminated *Mycobacterium avium* complex (MAC) in patients with advanced HIV infection

Unlabeled/Investigational Use Utilized in multidrug regimens for treatment of MAC; alternative to rifampin as prophylaxis for latent tuberculosis infection (LTBI) or part of multidrug regimen for treatment active tuberculosis infection

Local Anesthetic/Vasoconstrictor Precautions No information available to require special precautions

Effects on Dental Treatment Key adverse event(s) related to dental treatment: Saliva (reddish orange).

Effects on Bleeding No information available to require special precautions

Adverse Effects

>10%:
- Dermatologic: Rash (11%)
- Genitourinary: Discoloration of urine (30%)
- Hematologic: Neutropenia (25%), leukopenia (17%)

1% to 10%:
- Central nervous system: Headache (3%), fever (2%)
- Gastrointestinal: Nausea (3% to 6%), abdominal pain (4%), dyspepsia (3%), eructation (3%), taste perversion (3%), vomiting (3%), flatulence (2%)
- Hematologic: Thrombocytopenia (5%)
- Hepatic: ALT increased (7% to 9%; incidence less than placebo), AST increased (7% to 9%; incidence less than placebo)
- Neuromuscular & skeletal: Myalgia (2%)

General Dosage Range Dosage adjustment recommended in patients with renal impairment or on concomitant therapy

Oral:
Children <6 years: 5 mg/kg once daily
Children ≥6 years and Adults: 300 mg once daily

Mechanism of Action Inhibits DNA-dependent RNA polymerase at the beta subunit which prevents chain initiation

Pharmacodynamics/Kinetics

Half-life Elimination Terminal: 45 hours (range: 16-69 hours)

Time to Peak Serum: 2-4 hours

Pregnancy Risk Factor B

Rifampin (rif AM pin)

Related Information

Rifapentine *on page 1474*

Tuberculosis *on page 1902*

U.S. Brand Names Rifadin®

Canadian Brand Names Rifadin®; Rofact™

Pharmacologic Category Antibiotic, Miscellaneous; Antitubercular Agent

Use Management of active tuberculosis in combination with other agents; elimination of meningococci from the nasopharynx in asymptomatic carriers

Unlabeled/Investigational Use Prophylaxis of *Haemophilus influenzae* type b infection; *Legionella* pneumonia; used in combination with other anti-infectives in the treatment of staphylococcal infections; treatment of *M. leprae* infections

Local Anesthetic/Vasoconstrictor Precautions No information available to require special precautions

Effects on Dental Treatment No significant effects or complications reported

Effects on Bleeding No information available to require special precautions

Adverse Effects

Frequency not defined:

- Cardiovascular: Edema, flushing
- Central nervous system: Ataxia, behavioral changes, concentration impaired, confusion, dizziness, drowsiness, fatigue, fever, headache, numbness, psychosis
- Dermatologic: Pemphigoid reaction, pruritus, urticaria
- Endocrine & metabolic: Adrenal insufficiency, menstrual disorders
- Hematologic: Agranulocytosis (rare), DIC, eosinophilia, hemoglobin decreased, hemolysis, hemolytic anemia, leukopenia, thrombocytopenia (especially with high-dose therapy)
- Hepatic: Hepatitis (rare), jaundice
- Neuromuscular & skeletal: Myalgia, osteomalacia, weakness
- Ocular: Exudative conjunctivitis, visual changes
- Renal: Acute renal failure, BUN increased, hemoglobinuria, hematuria, interstitial nephritis, uric acid increased
- Miscellaneous: Flu-like syndrome

1% to 10%:

- Dermatologic: Rash (1% to 5%)
- Gastrointestinal (1% to 2%): Anorexia, cramps, diarrhea, epigastric distress, flatulence, heartburn, nausea, pseudomembranous colitis, pancreatitis, vomiting
- Hepatic: LFTs increased (up to 14%)

General Dosage Range I.V., oral:

Children <12 years: 10-20 mg/kg/day in 1-2 divided doses **or** 10-20 mg/kg twice weekly (maximum: 600 mg/day)

Children ≥12 years and Adults: 10 mg/kg/day **or** 10 mg/kg 2-3 times/week **or** 600 mg every 12-24 hours

Mechanism of Action Inhibits bacterial RNA synthesis by binding to the beta subunit of DNA-dependent RNA polymerase, blocking RNA transcription

Pharmacodynamics/Kinetics

Duration of Action ≤24 hours

Half-life Elimination 3-4 hours, prolonged with hepatic impairment; End-stage renal disease: 1.8-11 hours

Time to Peak Serum: Oral: 2-4 hours

Pregnancy Risk Factor C

Rifampin and Isoniazid (rif AM pin & eye soe NYE a zid)

Related Information

Isoniazid *on page 948*

Rifampin *on page 1473*

U.S. Brand Names IsonaRif™; Rifamate®

Canadian Brand Names Rifamate®

Pharmacologic Category Antibiotic, Miscellaneous

Use Management of active tuberculosis; see individual agents for additional information

Local Anesthetic/Vasoconstrictor Precautions No information available to require special precautions

Effects on Dental Treatment No significant effects or complications reported

Effects on Bleeding No information available to require special precautions

General Dosage Range Oral: *Adults:* 2 capsules (rifampin 300 mg/isoniazid 150 mg/capsule) once daily

Pregnancy Risk Factor C

Rifampin, Isoniazid, and Pyrazinamide

(rif AM pin, eye soe NYE a zid, & peer a ZIN a mide)

Related Information

Isoniazid *on page 948*
Pyrazinamide *on page 1435*
Rifampin *on page 1473*

U.S. Brand Names Rifater®

Canadian Brand Names Rifater®

Pharmacologic Category Antibiotic, Miscellaneous

Use Initial phase, short-course treatment of pulmonary tuberculosis; see individual agents for additional information

Local Anesthetic/Vasoconstrictor Precautions No information available to require special precautions

Effects on Dental Treatment No significant effects or complications reported

Effects on Bleeding No information available to require special precautions

Adverse Effects See individual agents.

Note: During clinical trial evaluation, the frequency of cardiorespiratory events (eg, chest pain, hemoptysis, palpitation, chest tightness, and pneumothorax) was higher with the combination product (7%) than that reported with individual agents (2%); frequency of central and peripheral nervous system events (eg, sweating, headache, insomnia, paresthesia, and anxiety) were also higher with the combination product (4%) than that reported with individual agents (3%).

General Dosage Range Oral:

Children ≥15 years and Adults ≤44 kg: 4 tablets (rifampin 120 mg/isoniazid 50 mg/pyrazinamide 300 mg per tablet) once daily

Children ≥15 years and Adults 45-54 kg: 5 tablets (rifampin 120 mg/isoniazid 50 mg/pyrazinamide 300 mg per tablet) once daily

Children ≥15 years and Adults ≥55 kg: 6 tablets (rifampin 120 mg/isoniazid 50 mg/pyrazinamide 300 mg per tablet) once daily

Mechanism of Action

Rifampin inhibits bacterial mRNA synthesis by binding to the beta subunit of DNA-dependent RNA polymerase, blocking transcription

Isoniazid inhibits mycolic acid synthesis resulting in disruption of the bacterial cell wall

Pyrazinamide is converted to pyrazinoic acid in susceptible strains of *Mycobacterium* which lowers the pH of the environment; exact mechanism of action has not been elucidated

Pregnancy Risk Factor C

Rifapentine

(rif a PEN teen)

Related Information

Rifampin *on page 1473*
Tuberculosis *on page 1902*

U.S. Brand Names Priftin®

Canadian Brand Names Priftin®

Pharmacologic Category Antitubercular Agent

Use Treatment of pulmonary tuberculosis; rifapentine must always be used in conjunction with at least one other antituberculosis drug to which the isolate is susceptible; it may also be necessary to add a third agent (either streptomycin or ethambutol) until susceptibility is known.

Local Anesthetic/Vasoconstrictor Precautions No information available to require special precautions

Effects on Dental Treatment No significant effects or complications reported

Effects on Bleeding No information available to require special precautions

Adverse Effects

>10%: Endocrine & metabolic: Hyperuricemia (most likely due to pyrazinamide from initiation phase combination therapy)

1% to 10%:

- Cardiovascular: Hypertension
- Central nervous system: Headache, dizziness
- Dermatologic: Rash, pruritus, acne
- Gastrointestinal: Anorexia, nausea, vomiting, dyspepsia, diarrhea
- Hematologic: Neutropenia, lymphopenia, anemia, leukopenia, thrombocytosis
- Hepatic: ALT increased, AST increased
- Neuromuscular & skeletal: Arthralgia, pain
- Renal: Pyuria, proteinuria, hematuria, urinary casts

Respiratory: Hemoptysis

General Dosage Range Oral: *Adults:* 600 mg once or twice weekly

Mechanism of Action Inhibits DNA-dependent RNA polymerase in susceptible strains of *Mycobacterium tuberculosis* (but not in mammalian cells). Rifapentine is bactericidal against both intracellular and extracellular MTB organisms. MTB resistant to other rifamycins including rifampin are likely to be resistant to rifapentine. Cross-resistance does not appear between rifapentine and other nonrifamycin antimycobacterial agents.

Pharmacodynamics/Kinetics

Half-life Elimination Rifapentine: 14-17 hours; 25-desacetyl rifapentine: 13 hours

Time to Peak Serum: 5-6 hours

Pregnancy Risk Factor C

Rifaximin (rif AX i min)

U.S. Brand Names Xifaxan®

Pharmacologic Category Antibiotic, Miscellaneous

Use Treatment of travelers' diarrhea caused by noninvasive strains of *E. coli*; reduction in the risk of overt hepatic encephalopathy (HE) recurrence

Unlabeled/Investigational Use Treatment of hepatic encephalopathy; alternative treatment for *Clostridium difficile*-associated diarrhea (CDAD)

Local Anesthetic/Vasoconstrictor Precautions No information available to require special precautions

Effects on Dental Treatment No significant effects or complications reported

Effects on Bleeding No information available to require special precautions

Adverse Effects Note: Frequency of adverse events generally higher following treatment for hepatic encephalopathy (HE). Percentages are presented for HE unless otherwise stated.

>10%:

Cardiovascular: Peripheral edema (15%)

Central nervous system: Dizziness (13%), fatigue (12%)

Hepatic: Ascites (11%)

Gastrointestinal: Nausea (14%)

2% to 10%:

Cardiovascular: Chest pain (>2% to 5%), edema (>2% to 5%), hypotension (>2% to 5%)

Central nervous system: Headache (travelers' diarrhea 10%), depression (7%), fever (6%), amnesia (>2% to 5%), attention disturbance (>2% to 5%), confusion (>2% to 5%), hypoesthesia (>2% to 5%), pain (>2% to 5%), tremor (>2% to 5%), vertigo (>2% to 5%)

Dermatological: Pruritus (9%), rash (5%), cellulitis (>2% to 5%)

Endocrine and metabolism: Hyper-/hypoglycemia (>2% to 5%), hyperkalemia (>2% to 5%), hyponatremia (>2% to 5%)

Gastrointestinal: Abdominal pain (>2% to 9%), abdominal tenderness (>2% to 5%), anorexia (>2% to 5%), dehydration (>2% to 5%), esophageal varices (>2% to 5%), weight gain (>2% to 5%), xerostomia (>2% to 5%)

Hematologic: Anemia (8%)

Neuromuscular & skeletal: Muscle spasms (9%), arthralgia (6%), myalgia (>2% to 5%)

Respiratory: Nasopharyngitis (7%), dyspnea (6%), epistaxis(>2% to 5%), pneumonia (>2% to 5%), rhinitis (>2% to 5%), upper respiratory tract infection (>2% to 5%)

Miscellaneous: Influenza-like illness (>2% to 5%)

General Dosage Range Oral:

Children ≥12 years: 200 mg 3 times/day

Adults: 200 mg 3 times/day **or** 550 mg 2 times/day

Mechanism of Action Rifaximin inhibits bacterial RNA synthesis by binding to bacterial DNA-dependent RNA polymerase.

Pharmacodynamics/Kinetics

Half-life Elimination ~2-5 hours

Time to Peak Hepatic encephalopathy prevention: ~1 hour

Pregnancy Risk Factor C

Rilonacept (ri LON a sept)

U.S. Brand Names Arcalyst™

Pharmacologic Category Interleukin-1 Inhibitor

Use Orphan drug: Treatment of cryopyrin-associated periodic syndromes (CAPS) including familial cold autoinflammatory syndrome (FCAS) and Muckle-Wells syndrome (MWS)

Local Anesthetic/Vasoconstrictor Precautions No information available to require special precautions

Effects on Dental Treatment No significant effects or complications reported

Effects on Bleeding No information available to require special precautions

Adverse Effects

>10%:

Local: Injection site reactions (48%; majority mild-moderate; typically lasting 1-2 days; characterized by erythema, bruising, dermatitis, inflammation, pain, pruritus, swelling, urticaria, vesicles, warmth, and hemorrhage)

Respiratory: Upper respiratory tract infection (26%)

Miscellaneous: Infection (48% during winter months; 18% during summer months), antibody formation to rilonacept (35%)

1% to 10%:

Central nervous system: Hypoesthesia (9%)

Respiratory: Cough (9%), sinusitis (9%)

General Dosage Range SubQ:

Children ≥12 years: Loading dose 4.4 mg/kg (maximum dose: 320 mg); Maintenance dose: 2.2 mg/kg once weekly (maximum dose: 160 mg)

Adults: Loading dose: 320 mg; Maintenance dose: 160 mg once weekly

Mechanism of Action Cryopyrin-associated periodic syndromes (CAPS) refers to rare genetic syndromes caused by mutations in the nucleotide-binding domain, leucine rich family (NLR), pyrin domain containing 3 (NLRP-3) gene or the cold-induced autoinflammatory syndrome-1 (CIAS1) gene. Cryopyrin, a protein encoded by this gene, regulates interleukin-1 beta (IL-1β) activation. Deficiency of cryopyrin results in excessive inflammation. Rilonacept reduces inflammation by binding to IL-1β (some binding of IL-1α and IL-1 receptor antagonist) and preventing interaction with cell surface receptors.

Pharmacodynamics/Kinetics

Onset of Action Steady state reached by 6 weeks

Pregnancy Risk Factor C

Riluzole (RIL yoo zole)

U.S. Brand Names Rilutek®

Canadian Brand Names Rilutek®

Pharmacologic Category Glutamate Inhibitor

Use Treatment of amyotrophic lateral sclerosis (ALS); riluzole can extend survival or time to tracheostomy

Local Anesthetic/Vasoconstrictor Precautions No information available to require special precautions

Effects on Dental Treatment Key adverse event(s) related to dental treatment: Oral moniliasis and stomatitis.

Effects on Bleeding No information available to require special precautions

Adverse Effects

>10%:

Gastrointestinal: Nausea (16%)

Neuromuscular & skeletal: Weakness (19%)

1% to 10%:

Cardiovascular: Hypertension (5%), peripheral edema (3%), tachycardia (3%)

Central nervous system: Dizziness (4%), somnolence (2%), vertigo (2%), malaise (1%)

Dermatologic: Pruritus (4%), eczema (2%), exfoliative dermatitis (1%)

Gastrointestinal: Abdominal pain (5%), vomiting (4%), flatulence (3%), oral moniliasis (1%), stomatitis (1%), tooth disorder (1%)

Genitourinary: Urinary tract infection (3%), dysuria (1%)

Hepatic: Liver function tests increased (8% >3 x ULN; 2% >5 x ULN)

Neuromuscular & skeletal: Arthralgia (4%), paresthesia (circumoral; 2%), tremor (1%)

Respiratory: Lung function decreased (10%), cough increased (3%)

General Dosage Range Oral: *Adults:* 50 mg every 12 hours

Mechanism of Action Mechanism of action is not known. Pharmacologic properties include inhibitory effect on glutamate release, inactivation of voltage-dependent sodium channels; and ability to interfere with intracellular events that follow transmitter binding at excitatory amino acid receptors

Pharmacodynamics/Kinetics

Half-life Elimination 12 hours

Pregnancy Risk Factor C

RimabotulinumtoxinB (rime uh BOT yoo lin num TOKS in bee)

U.S. Brand Names Myobloc®

Pharmacologic Category Neuromuscular Blocker Agent, Toxin

Use Treatment of cervical dystonia (spasmodic torticollis)

Unlabeled/Investigational Use Treatment of cervical dystonia in patients who have developed resistance to onabotulinumtoxinA or abobotulinumtoxinA

Local Anesthetic/Vasoconstrictor Precautions No information available to require special precautions

Effects on Dental Treatment Key adverse event(s) related to dental treatment: Xerostomia (normal salivary flow resumes upon discontinuation), stomatitis, and abnormal taste.

Effects on Bleeding No information available to require special precautions

Adverse Effects

>10%:

Central nervous system: Headache (10% to 16%), pain (≤13%)

Gastrointestinal: Dysphagia (10% to 25%; severe dysphagia: 3%), xerostomia (3% to 34%; severe xerostomia: 6%)

Local: Injection site pain (12% to 16%)

Neuromuscular & skeletal: Neck pain (≤17%)

Miscellaneous: Infection (≤19%), antibody formation (~10% to 18%, at 12 and 18 months, respectively)

1% to 10%:

Cardiovascular: Chest pain, edema, peripheral edema, vasolidation

Central nervous system: Dizziness (3% to 6%), anxiety, chills, confusion, fever, hyperesthesia, malaise, migraine, somnolence, tremor, vertigo

Dermatologic: Pruritus, bruising

Endocrine & metabolic: Hypercholesterolemia

Gastrointestinal: Nausea (≤10%), dyspepsia (≤10%,) glossitis, stomatitis, taste perversion, vomiting

Genitourinary: Cystitis, urinary tract infection, vaginal moniliasis

Hematologic: Serum neutralizing activity

Neuromuscular & skeletal: Torticollis (≤8%), arthralgia (≤7%), back pain (≤7%), myasthenia (≤6%), weakness (≤6%), arthritis, hernia

Ocular: Amblyopia, vision abnormal

Otic: Otitis media, tinnitus

Respiratory: Cough (3% to 7%; placebo 3%), dyspnea, pneumonia

Miscellaneous: Flu-like syndrome (6% to 9%), abscess, allergic reaction, cyst, neoplasm, viral infection

General Dosage Range I.M.: *Adults:* Initial: 2500-5000 units divided among the affected muscles

Mechanism of Action RimabotulinumtoxinB (previously known as botulinum toxin type B) is a neurotoxin produced by *Clostridium botulinum*, spore-forming anaerobic bacillus. It cleaves synaptic Vesicle Association Membrane Protein (VAMP; synaptobrevin) which is a component of the protein complex responsible for docking and fusion of the synaptic vesicle to the presynaptic membrane. By blocking neurotransmitter release, rimabotulinumtoxinB paralyzes the muscle.

Pharmacodynamics/Kinetics

Duration of Action 12-16 weeks

Pregnancy Risk Factor C (manufacturer)

Rimantadine (ri MAN ta deen)

Related Information

Systemic Viral Diseases *on page 1904*

U.S. Brand Names Flumadine®

Canadian Brand Names Flumadine®

Pharmacologic Category Antiviral Agent; Antiviral Agent, Adamantane

Use Prophylaxis (adults and children >1 year of age) and treatment (adults) of influenza A viral infection (per manufacturer labeling; also refer to current ACIP guidelines for recommendations during current flu season)

Note: In certain circumstances, the ACIP recommends use of rimantadine in combination with oseltamivir for the treatment or prophylaxis of influenza A infection when resistance to oseltamivir is suspected.

Local Anesthetic/Vasoconstrictor Precautions No information available to require special precautions

Effects on Dental Treatment Key adverse event(s) related to dental treatment: Xerostomia (normal salivary flow resumes upon discontinuation).

Effects on Bleeding No information available to require special precautions

Adverse Effects 1% to 10%:

Central nervous system: Insomnia (2% to 3%), concentration impaired (≤2%), dizziness (1% to 2%), nervousness (1% to 2%), fatigue (1%), headache (1%)

Gastrointestinal: Nausea (3%), anorexia (2%), vomiting (2%), xerostomia (2%), abdominal pain (1%)

Neuromuscular & skeletal: Weakness (1%)

General Dosage Range Dosage adjustment recommended in patients with hepatic or renal impairment

Oral:

Children 1-9 years: 5 mg/kg/day in 1-2 divided doses (maximum: 150 mg/day)

Children ≥10 years and <40 kg: 5 mg/kg/day in 2 divided doses

Children ≥10 years and Adults: 100 mg twice daily

Elderly: 100 mg daily

Mechanism of Action Exerts its inhibitory effect on three antigenic subtypes of influenza A virus (H1N1, H2N2, H3N2) early in the viral replicative cycle, possibly inhibiting the uncoating process; it has no activity against influenza B virus and is two- to eightfold more active than amantadine

Pharmacodynamics/Kinetics

Onset of Action Antiviral activity: No data exist establishing a correlation between plasma concentration and antiviral effect

Half-life Elimination 25.4 hours; prolonged with elderly, severe liver and severe renal impairment

Time to Peak 6 hours

Pregnancy Risk Factor C

Rimexolone (ri MEKS oh lone)

U.S. Brand Names Vexol®

Canadian Brand Names Vexol®

Pharmacologic Category Corticosteroid, Ophthalmic

Use Treatment of inflammation after ocular surgery and the treatment of anterior uveitis

Local Anesthetic/Vasoconstrictor Precautions No information available to require special precautions

Effects on Dental Treatment No significant effects or complications reported

Effects on Bleeding No information available to require special precautions

Adverse Effects

1% to 5%: Ocular: Blurred vision, discharge, discomfort, pain, increased intraocular pressure, foreign body sensation, hyperemia, pruritus

<2%:

Cardiovascular: Hypotension

Central nervous system: Headache

Gastrointestinal: Taste perversion

Respiratory: Pharyngitis, rhinitis

Frequency not defined: Cataracts, damage to the optic nerve, defects in visual activity, perforation of globe, secondary ocular infection

General Dosage Range Ophthalmic: *Adults:* Instill 1-2 drops 4 times/day **or** instill 1-2 drops every 1-2 hours during waking hours

Mechanism of Action Decreases inflammation by suppression of migration of polymorphonuclear leukocytes and reversal of increased capillary permeability

Pregnancy Risk Factor C

Risedronate (ris ED roe nate)

Related Information

Osteonecrosis of the Jaw *on page 1894*

Rheumatoid Arthritis, Osteoarthritis, and Osteoporosis *on page 1889*

U.S. Brand Names Actonel®; Atelvia™

Canadian Brand Names Actonel®; Apo-Risedronate®; Dom-Risedronate; Novo-Risedronate; PMS-Risedronate; ratio-Risedronate; Riva-Risedronate; Sandoz-Risedronate

Generic Availability (U.S.) No

Pharmacologic Category Bisphosphonate Derivative

Use

Actonel®: Treatment of Paget's disease of the bone; treatment and prevention of glucocorticoid-induced osteoporosis; treatment and prevention of osteoporosis in postmenopausal women; treatment of osteoporosis in men

Atelvia™: Treatment of osteoporosis in postmenopausal women

Local Anesthetic/Vasoconstrictor Precautions No information available to require special precautions

Effects on Dental Treatment Osteonecrosis of the jaw (ONJ), generally associated with local infection and/or tooth extraction and often with delayed healing, has been reported in patients taking bisphosphonates. Symptoms included nonhealing extraction socket or an exposed jawbone. Most reported cases of bisphosphonate-associated osteonecrosis have been in cancer patients treated with intravenous bisphosphonates. However, some have occurred in patients with postmenopausal osteoporosis taking oral bisphosphonates. Dental surgery, particularly tooth extraction, may increase the risk for ONJ. Patients who develop ONJ while on bisphosphonate therapy should receive care by an oral surgeon. See Dental Comment.

Effects on Bleeding No information available to require special precautions

Adverse Effects Frequency may vary with product, dose, and indication.

>10%:

- Cardiovascular: Hypertension (11%)
- Central nervous system: Headache (3% to 18%)
- Dermatologic: Rash (8% to 12%)
- Endocrine & metabolic: Serum PTH levels increased (transient; <30%)
- Gastrointestinal: Diarrhea (5% to 20%), nausea (4% to 13%), constipation (3% to 13%), abdominal pain (2% to 12%), dyspepsia (4% to 11%)
- Genitourinary: Urinary tract infection (11%)
- Neuromuscular & skeletal: Arthralgia (7% to 33%), back pain (6% to 28%)
- Miscellaneous: Infection (≤31%)

1% to 10%:

- Cardiovascular: Peripheral edema (8%), chest pain (5% to 7%), arrhythmia (2%)
- Central nervous system: Depression (7%), dizziness (3% to 7%)
- Endocrine & metabolic: Hypocalcemia (≤5%), hypophosphatemia (<3%)
- Gastrointestinal: Vomiting (2% to 5%), gastritis (3%), duodenitis (≤1%), glossitis (≤1%)
- Genitourinary: Prostatic hyperplasia (5%; benign), nephrolithiasis (3%)
- Neuromuscular & skeletal: Joint disorder (7%), myalgia (2% to 7%), neck pain (5%), muscle spasm (1% to 2%)
- Ocular: Cataract (7%)
- Respiratory: Bronchitis (3% to 10%), pharyngitis (6%), rhinitis (6%), dyspnea (4%)
- Miscellaneous: Flu-like syndrome (10%), acute phase reaction (≤8%; includes fever, influenza-like illness)

Dosage Oral: Adults: **Note:** Patients should receive supplemental calcium and vitamin D if dietary intake is inadequate.

Immediate release tablet:

Paget's disease of bone: 30 mg once daily for 2 months

Retreatment may be considered (following post-treatment observation of at least 2 months) if relapse occurs, or if treatment fails to normalize serum alkaline phosphatase. For retreatment, the dose and duration of therapy are the same as for initial treatment. No data are available on more than one course of retreatment.

Osteoporosis (postmenopausal) prevention and treatment: 5 mg once daily **or** 35 mg once weekly **or** 150 mg once a month

Osteoporosis (male) treatment: 35 mg once weekly

Osteoporosis (glucocorticoid-induced) prevention and treatment: 5 mg once daily

Delayed release tablet: Osteoporosis (postmenopausal) treatment: 35 mg once weekly

Dosage adjustment in renal impairment:

Cl_{cr} ≥30 mL/minute: No adjustment required

Cl_{cr} <30 mL/minute: **Not** recommended for use

Dosage adjustment in hepatic impairment: No studies performed in hepatic impairment; no dosage adjustment necessary due to lack of hepatic metabolism

Mechanism of Action A bisphosphonate which inhibits bone resorption via actions on osteoclasts or on osteoclast precursors; decreases the rate of bone resorption, leading to an indirect increase in bone mineral density. In Paget's disease, characterized by disordered resorption and formation of bone, inhibition of resorption leads to an indirect decrease in bone formation; but the newly-formed bone has a more normal architecture.

Contraindications Hypersensitivity to risedronate, bisphosphonates, or any component of the formulation; hypocalcemia; inability to stand or sit upright for at least 30 minutes; abnormalities of the esophagus which delay esophageal emptying, such as stricture or achalasia

Warnings/Precautions Bisphosphonates may cause upper gastrointestinal disorders such as dysphagia, esophagitis, esophageal ulcer, and gastric ulcer; risk increases in patients unable to comply with dosing instructions. Use with caution in patients with dysphagia, esophageal disease, gastritis, duodenitis, or ulcers (may worsen underlying condition). Discontinue if new or worsening symptoms occur. Use caution in patients with renal impairment (not recommended in patients with a Cl_{cr} <30 mL/minute). Hypocalcemia must be corrected before therapy initiation with risedronate. Ensure adequate calcium and vitamin D intake, especially for patients with Paget's disease in whom the pretreatment rate of bone turnover may be greatly elevated.

Bisphosphonate therapy has been associated with osteonecrosis, primarily of the jaw. Risk factors for osteonecrosis of the jaw (ONJ) include invasive dental procedures (eg, tooth extraction, dental implants, boney surgery); a diagnosis of cancer, with concomitant chemotherapy or corticosteroids; poor oral hygiene, ill-fitting dentures; and comorbid disorders (anemia, coagulopathy, infection, pre-existing dental disease). Most reported cases occurred after I.V. bisphosphonate therapy; however, cases have been reported following oral therapy. A dental exam and preventative dentistry should be performed prior to placing patients with risk factors on chronic bisphosphonate therapy. The manufacturer's labeling states that discontinuing bisphosphonates in patients requiring invasive dental procedures may reduce the risk of ONJ. However, other experts suggest that there is no evidence that discontinuing therapy reduces the risk of developing ONJ (Assael, 2009). The benefit/risk must be assessed by the treating physician and/or dentist/surgeon prior to any invasive dental procedure. Patients developing ONJ while on bisphosphonates should receive care by an oral surgeon.

Atypical femur fractures have been reported in patients receiving bisphosphonates for treatment/prevention of osteoporosis. The fractures include subtrochanteric femur (bone just below the hip joint) and diaphyseal femur (long segment of the thigh bone). Some patients experience prodromal pain weeks or months before the fracture occurs. It is unclear if bisphosphonate therapy is the cause for these fractures, although the majority have been reported in patients taking bisphosphonates. Patients receiving long-term (>3-5 years) therapy may be at an increased risk. Discontinue bisphosphonate therapy in patients who develop a femoral shaft fracture.

Infrequently, severe (and occasionally debilitating) bone, joint, and/or muscle pain have been reported during bisphosphonate treatment. The onset of pain ranged from a single day to several months. Consider discontinuing therapy in patients who experience severe symptoms; symptoms usually resolve upon discontinuation. Some patients experienced recurrence when rechallenged with same drug or another bisphosphonate; avoid use in patients with a history of these symptoms in association with bisphosphonate therapy.

When using for glucocorticoid-induced osteoporosis, evaluate sex steroid hormonal status prior to treatment initiation; consider appropriate hormone replacement if necessary. Not approved for use in pediatric patients with osteogenesis imperfecta due to lack of efficacy in reducing the risk of fracture.

Drug Interactions

Avoid Concomitant Use There are no known interactions where it is recommended to avoid concomitant use.

Increased Effect/Toxicity

Risedronate may increase the levels/effects of: Deferasirox; Phosphate Supplements

The levels/effects of Risedronate may be increased by: Aminoglycosides; Nonsteroidal Anti-Inflammatory Agents

Decreased Effect

The levels/effects of Risedronate may be decreased by: Antacids; Calcium Salts; Iron Salts; Magnesium Salts; Proton Pump Inhibitors

Ethanol/Nutrition/Herb Interactions

Ethanol: Avoid ethanol (may increase risk of osteoporosis).

Food: Food reduces absorption (similar to other bisphosphonates); mean oral bioavailability is decreased when given with food.

Dietary Considerations Ensure adequate calcium and vitamin D intake. Take immediate release tablet with at least 6 oz of **plain water** (not mineral water) ≥30 minutes before the first food or drink of the day other than water. Take delayed release tablet with at least 4 ounces of **plain water** immediately **after** breakfast.

Pharmacodynamics/Kinetics

Onset of Action May require weeks

Half-life Elimination Initial: 1.5 hours; Terminal: 480-561 hours

Time to Peak Serum: 1-3 hours

Pregnancy Risk Factor C

Lactation Excretion in breast milk unknown/not recommended

Breast-Feeding Considerations The manufacturer recommends discontinuing nursing or discontinuing risedronate.

Dosage Forms

Tablet, oral:

Actonel®: 5 mg, 30 mg, 35 mg, 150 mg

Tablet, delayed release, oral:

Atelvia™: 35 mg

Dental Comment According to the 2008 report by the American Dental Association (ADA), the incidence of osteonecrosis of the jawbone associated with oral bisphosphonate therapy remains low. It was also stated that the benefits of using oral bisphosphonates to prevent osteoporosis significantly outweighs the small risk of developing bisphosphonate-associated osteonecrosis (Edwards, 2008). The full 26 page report can be accessed at http://www.ada.org/sections/professionalResources/pdfs/topics_osteonecrosis_bisphosphonate_report.pdf.

The ADA review stated the incidence of oral bisphosphonate-associated osteonecrosis of the jaw was one case for every 140,000 person-years exposure to oral bisphosphonates (ADA, 2006). This figure was based on information received from Merck & Co citing 170 worldwide cases for alendronate (Fosamax®). In addition, Procter & Gamble Pharmaceuticals has cited 20 cases for risedronate (Actonel®) and Roche Laboratories, Inc has cited one case for ibandronate (Boniva®).

In addition, the ADA 2008 report reiterates that the risk of osteonecrosis of the jawbone with oral bisphosphonates is minute compared to the risks with intravenous bisphosphonates therapy in cancer patients. The ADA cites an ~20% incidence in patients receiving bisphosphonates intravenously for cancer therapy. Fewer than 10% of all cases of bisphosphonate-associated osteonecrosis of the jaw occurs in patients taking the oral drugs.

Information on alendronate (Fosamax®) use in Australia and the incidence of ONJ has been reported (Mavrokokki, 2007). A survey form was sent to all of the Australian members of the Australian and New Zealand Association of Oral and Maxillofacial Surgeons requesting cases that they had identified as ONJ in 2004 and 2005. The definition of ONJ for the survey was an area of exposed bone in the jawbone that failed to heal within 6 weeks in patients taking bisphosphonates for bone disease. The frequency of ONJ in osteoporotic patients, mainly taking weekly oral alendronate, was 1 in 8470 to 1 in 2260 (0.01% to 0.04%) patients. If extractions were carried out, the calculated frequency was 1 in 1130 to 1 in 296 (0.09% to 0.34%) patients. The minimum values in these cases were determined from the survey, whereas, the maximum values were extrapolated from survey data. The median time to onset of ONJ in alendronate patients was 24 months.

A 2010 study reported the prevalence of osteonecrosis of the jaw in patients using alendronate-type drugs was 1 out of 952 patients or ~0.1% (Lo, 2010). The study's protocol involved a survey mailed out to 13,946 members of Kaiser Permanente of Northern California healthcare delivery system; 8572 patients responded to the survey. Investigators identified respondents reporting oral problems and dental symptoms. These respondents were then interviewed by telephone for presence of dental problems including exposed bone, gingival sores, moderate periodontal disease, and persistent symptoms or complications after dental procedures. Those selected were then invited for an examination or to have their dental records reviewed. The diagnosis of ONJ was made according to the 2006 American Association of Oral and Maxillofacial Surgeons criteria which required treatment with a bisphosphonate, exposed bone in the maxillofacial region lasting >8 weeks, and no radiotherapy involving the jaw. Of the 8572 respondents, 9 cases of ONJ were identified; 5 had developed ONJ spontaneously and 4 developed ONJ after tooth extraction. Specific oral bisphosphonates were not identified. When extrapolated to patient-years of bisphosphonate exposure, this prevalence rate of 0.1% equates to a frequency of 28 cases per 100,000 person-years of oral bisphosphonate treatment.

References

American Dental Association Council on Scientific Affairs, "Dental Management of Patients Receiving Oral Bisphosphonate Therapy: Expert Panel Recommendations," *J Am Dent Assoc*, 2006, 137 (8):1144-50. Available at http://jada.ada.org/cgi/content/full/137/8/1144.

Author Unknown, "Safety Update: Bone-Building Drugs: Risks Explained," *Consumer Reports on Health*, 2006, 18(5):3.

Edwards BJ, Hellstein JW, Jacobsen PL, et al, "Updated Recommendations for Managing the Care of Patients Receiving Oral Bisphosphonate Therapy: An Advisory Statement From the American Dental Association Council on Scientific Affairs," *J Am Dent Assoc*, 2008, 139(12):1674-7.

Lo JC, O'Ryan FS, Gordon NP, et al, "Prevalence of Osteonecrosis of the Jaw in Patients With Oral Bisphosphonate Exposure," *J Oral Maxillofac Surg*, 2010, 68(2):243-53.

Marx RE, Sawatari Y, Fortin M, et al, "Bisphosphonate-Induced Exposed Bone (Osteonecrosis/Osteopetrosis) of the Jaws: Risk Factors, Recognition, Prevention, and Treatment," *J Oral Maxillofac Surg*, 2005, 63(11):1567-75.

Mavrokokki T, Cheng A, Stein B, et al, "Nature and Frequency of Bisphosphonate-Associated Osteonecrosis of the Jaws in Australia," *J Oral Maxillofac Surg*, 2007, 65(3):415-23.

Ruggiero SL, Mehrotra B, Rosenberg TJ, et al, "Osteonecrosis of the Jaws Associated With the Use of Bisphosphonates: A Review of 63 Cases," *J Oral Maxillofac Surg*, 2004, 62(5):527-34.

Risedronate and Calcium (ris ED roe nate & KAL see um)

Related Information

Calcium Carbonate *on page* 286

Risedronate *on page* 1478

U.S. Brand Names Actonel® and Calcium

Canadian Brand Names Actonel Plus Calcium

Generic Availability (U.S.) No

Pharmacologic Category Bisphosphonate Derivative; Calcium Salt

Use Treatment and prevention of osteoporosis in postmenopausal women

Local Anesthetic/Vasoconstrictor Precautions No information available to require special precautions

Effects on Dental Treatment Osteonecrosis of the jaw (ONJ), generally associated with local infection and/or tooth extraction and often with delayed healing, has been reported in patients taking bisphosphonates. Symptoms included nonhealing extraction socket or an exposed jawbone. Most reported cases of bisphosphonate-associated osteonecrosis have been in cancer patients treated with intravenous bisphosphonates. However, some have occurred in patients with postmenopausal osteoporosis taking oral bisphosphonates. Dental surgery, particularly tooth extraction, may increase the risk for ONJ. Patients who develop ONJ while on bisphosphonate therapy should receive care by an oral surgeon. See Dental Comment.

Effects on Bleeding No information available to require special precautions

Adverse Effects See individual agents.

Dosage

Oral: Adults: Osteoporosis in postmenopausal females:

Risedronate: 35 mg once weekly on day 1 of 7-day treatment cycle

Calcium carbonate: 1250 mg (elemental calcium 500 mg) once daily on days 2 through 7 of 7-day treatment cycle

Dosage adjustment in renal impairment: Cl_{cr} <30 mL/minute: Not recommended for use

Mechanism of Action

Risedronate inhibits bone resorption via actions on osteoclasts or on osteoclast precursors; decreases the rate of bone resorption, leading to an indirect increase in bone mineral density.

Calcium helps to prevent or decrease the rate of bone loss.

Contraindications Hypersensitivity to risedronate, bisphosphonates, or any component of the formulation; hypocalcemia, hypercalcemia; abnormalities of the esophagus which delay esophageal emptying (eg, stricture or achalasia); inability to stand or sit upright for at least 30 minutes; severe renal impairment (Cl_{cr} <30 mL/minute)

Warnings/Precautions Bisphosphonates may cause upper gastrointestinal disorders such as dysphagia, esophageal ulcer, and gastric ulcer. Discontinue use if new or worsening symptoms develop. Use caution in patients with renal impairment (not recommended in patients with a Cl_{cr} <30 mL/minute). Hypocalcemia has been reported with the use of bisphosphonates; prior to therapy initiation, hypocalcemia must be corrected; ensure adequate calcium and vitamin D intake.

Bisphosphonate therapy has been associated with osteonecrosis, primarily of the jaw. Risk factors for osteonecrosis of the jaw (ONJ) include invasive dental procedures (eg, tooth extraction, dental implants, boney surgery); a diagnosis of cancer, with concomitant chemotherapy or corticosteroids; poor oral hygiene, ill-fitting dentures; and comorbid disorders (anemia, coagulopathy, infection, pre-existing dental disease). Most reported cases occurred after I.V. bisphosphonate therapy; however, cases have been reported following oral therapy. A dental exam and preventative dentistry should be performed prior to placing patients with risk factors on chronic bisphosphonate therapy. The manufacturer's labeling states that discontinuing bisphosphonates in patients requiring invasive dental procedures may reduce the risk of ONJ. However, other experts suggest that there is no evidence that discontinuing therapy reduces the risk of developing ONJ (Assael, 2009). The benefit/risk must be assessed by the treating physician and/or dentist/surgeon prior to any invasive dental procedure. Patients developing ONJ while on bisphosphonates should receive care by an oral surgeon.

Atypical femur fractures have been reported in patients receiving bisphosphonates for treatment/prevention of osteoporosis. The fractures include subtrochanteric femur (bone just below the hip joint) and diaphyseal femur (long segment of the thigh bone). Some patients experience prodromal pain weeks or months before the fracture occurs. It is unclear if bisphosphonate therapy is the cause for these fractures, although the majority have been reported in patients taking bisphosphonates. Patients receiving long-term (>3-5 years) therapy may be at an increased risk.

Discontinue bisphosphonate therapy in patients who develop a femoral shaft fracture.

Infrequently, severe (and occasionally debilitating) bone, joint, and/or muscle pain have been reported during bisphosphonate treatment. The onset of pain ranged from a single day to several months. Consider discontinuing therapy in patients who experience severe symptoms; symptoms usually resolve upon discontinuation. Some patients experienced recurrence when rechallenged with same drug or another bisphosphonate; avoid use in patients with a history of these symptoms in association with bisphosphonate therapy.

Calcium carbonate absorption is impaired in achlorhydria (common in elderly); administer calcium component with food. Calcium should be used with caution in patients with a history of kidney stones or hypercalciuria.

Not approved for use in pediatric patients with osteogenesis imperfecta due to lack of efficacy in reducing the risk of fracture.

Drug Interactions

Avoid Concomitant Use There are no known interactions where it is recommended to avoid concomitant use.

Increased Effect/Toxicity

Risedronate and Calcium may increase the levels/effects of: Deferasirox; Phosphate Supplements

The levels/effects of Risedronate and Calcium may be increased by: Aminoglycosides; Nonsteroidal Anti-Inflammatory Agents

Decreased Effect

The levels/effects of Risedronate and Calcium may be decreased by: Antacids; Calcium Salts; Iron Salts; Magnesium Salts; Proton Pump Inhibitors

Ethanol/Nutrition/Herb Interactions

Ethanol: Avoid ethanol (may increase risk of osteoporosis).

Food:

Risedronate: Food may reduce absorption (similar to other bisphosphonates); mean oral bioavailability is decreased when given with food.

Calcium: Food increases absorption. Calcium may decrease iron absorption. Bran, foods high in oxalates, or whole grain cereals may decrease calcium absorption

Dietary Considerations Take risedronate ≥30 minutes before the first food or drink of the day other than water. Do not take with mineral water or with other beverages. Ensure adequate calcium and vitamin D intake; women and men >50 years of age should consume 1200-1500 mg/day of elemental calcium and 800-1000 int. units/day of vitamin D.

Pregnancy Risk Factor C

Lactation Excretion of risedronate in breast milk is unknown/not recommended

Breast-Feeding Considerations See individual agents.

Dosage Forms

Combination package [each package contains]:

Actonel® and Calcium:

Tablet (Actonel®): Risedronate 35 mg (4s)

Tablet: Calcium 1250 mg (24s)

Dental Comment See Risedronate monograph.

References

Author Unknown, "Safety Update: Bone-Building Drugs: Risks Explained," *Consumer Reports on Health*, 2006, 18(5):3.

Marx RE, Sawatari Y, Fortin M, et al, "Bisphosphonate-Induced Exposed Bone (Osteonecrosis/Osteopetrosis) of the Jaws: Risk Factors, Recognition, Prevention, and Treatment," *J Oral Maxillofac Surg*, 2005, 63(11):1567-75.

Ruggiero SL, Mehrotra B, Rosenberg TJ, et al, "Osteonecrosis of the Jaws Associated With the Use of Bisphosphonates: A Review of 63 Cases," *J Oral Maxillofac Surg*, 2004, 62(5):527-34.

RisperiDONE (ris PER i done)

Related Information

Clinical Risk Related to Drugs Prolonging QT Interval *on page 1872*

U.S. Brand Names RisperDAL®; RisperDAL® Consta®; RisperDAL® M-Tab®

Canadian Brand Names Apo-Risperidone®; CO Risperidone; Dom-Risperidone; Gen-Risperidone; JAMP-Risperidone; Mint-Risperidon; Mylan-Risperidone; Novo-Risperidone; PHL-Risperidone; PMS-Risperidone; PMS-Risperidone ODT; PRO-Risperidone; RAN™-Risperidone; ratio-Risperidone; RBX-Risperidone; Risperdal®; Risperdal® Consta®; Risperdal® M-Tab®; Riva-Risperidone; Sandoz-Risperidone; ZYM-Risperidone

Generic Availability (U.S.) Yes: Excludes injection

Pharmacologic Category Antimanic Agent; Antipsychotic Agent, Atypical

Use

Oral: Treatment of schizophrenia; treatment of acute mania or mixed episodes associated with bipolar I disorder (as monotherapy in children or adults, or in combination with lithium or valproate in adults); treatment of irritability/aggression associated with autistic disorder

Injection: Treatment of schizophrenia; maintenance treatment of bipolar I disorder in adults as monotherapy or in combination with lithium or valproate

Unlabeled/Investigational Use Treatment of Tourette's syndrome; treatment of pervasive developmental disorder; psychosis/agitation related to Alzheimer's dementia; post-traumatic stress disorder (PTSD)

Local Anesthetic/Vasoconstrictor Precautions No information available to require special precautions

Effects on Dental Treatment Key adverse event(s) related to dental treatment: Significant xerostomia (normal salivary flow resumes upon discontinuation) and toothache.

Effects on Bleeding No information available to require special precautions

Adverse Effects The frequency of adverse effects is reported as absolute percentages and is not based upon net frequencies as compared to placebo. Actual frequency may be dependent upon dose and/or indication. Events are reported from placebo-controlled studies and not with combination therapy. Unless otherwise noted, frequency of adverse effects is reported for the oral formulation in adults.

>10%:

Central nervous system: Somnolence (children 12% to 67%; adults 5% to 14%; I.M. injection 5% to 6%), fatigue (children 18% to 42%; adults 1% to 3%), headache (I.M. injection 15% to 21%), fever (children 20%; adults 1% to 2%), dystonia (children 9% to 18%; adults 5% to 11%), anxiety (children ≤16%; adults 2% to 16%), dizziness (children 7% to 16%; adults 4% to 10%), Parkinsonism (children 2% to 16%; adults 12% to 20%)

Dermatologic: Rash (children ≤11%; adults 2% to 4%)

Gastrointestinal: Appetite increased (children 4% to 49%), vomiting (children 10% to 25%), salivation increased (children ≤22%; adults 1% to 3%), constipation (children 21%; adults 8% to 9%), abdominal pain (children 15% to 18%; adults 3% to 4%), nausea (children 8% to 16%; adults 4% to 9%), dyspepsia (children 5% to 16%; adults 4% to 10%), xerostomia (children 13%; adults ≤4%)

Genitourinary: Urinary incontinence (children 5% to 22%; adults <2%)

Neuromuscular & skeletal: Tremor (adults 6%; children 10% to 12%)

Respiratory: Rhinitis (children 13% to 36%; adults 7% to 11%), upper respiratory infection (children 34%; adults 2% to 3%), cough (children 34%; adults 3%)

1% to 10%:

Cardiovascular: Tachycardia (children ≤7%; adults 1% to 5%), hypertension (I.M. injection 3%), chest pain (1% to 3%), creatine phosphokinase increased (≤2%), postural hypotension (≤2%), arrhythmia (≤1%), edema (≤1%), hypotension (≤1%), syncope (≤1%)

Central nervous system: Akathisia (children ≤10%; adults 5% to 9%), automatism (children 7%), confusion (children 5%)

Dermatologic: Seborrhea (up to 2%), acne (1%)

Endocrine & metabolic: Lactation nonpuerperal (children 2% to 5%; adults 1%), ejaculation failure (≤1%)

Gastrointestinal: Diarrhea (children 7% to 8%; adults ≤3%), anorexia (children 8%; adults ≤2%;), weight gain (children 5%; adults ≤1%), toothache (I.M. injection 1% to 3%)

Genitourinary: Urinary tract infection (≤3%)

Hematologic: Neutropenia (I.M. injection <2%), anemia (I.M. injection <2%; oral ≤1%)

Hepatic: Transaminases increased (I.M. injection ≥1%; oral 1%)

Neuromuscular & skeletal: Dyskinesia (children 7%; adults 1%), arthralgia (2% to 3%), back pain (2% to 3%), myalgia (≤2%), weakness (1%)

Ocular: Abnormal vision (children 4% to 7%; adults 1% to 3%), blurred vision (I.M. injection 2% to 3%)

Otic: Earache (1%)

Respiratory: Dyspnea (children 2% to 5%; adults 2%), epistaxis (≤2%)

Dosage Note: When reinitiating treatment after discontinuation, the initial titration schedule should be followed.

Oral:

Children ≥5 years and Adolescents: Autism:

<15 kg: Use with caution; specific dosing recommendations not available

<20 kg: Initial: 0.25 mg/day; may increase dose to 0.5 mg/day after ≥4 days, maintain dose for ≥14 days. In patients not achieving sufficient clinical response, may increase dose by 0.25 mg/day in ≥2-week intervals. Therapeutic effect reached plateau at 1 mg/day in clinical trials. Following clinical response,

consider gradually lowering dose. May be administered once daily or in divided doses twice daily.

≥20 kg: Initial: 0.5 mg/day; may increase dose to 1 mg/day after ≥4 days, maintain dose for ≥14 days. In patients not achieving sufficient clinical response, may increase dose by 0.5 mg/day in ≥2-week intervals. Therapeutic effect reached plateau at 2.5 mg/day (3 mg/day in children >45 kg) in clinical trials. Following clinical response, consider gradually lowering dose. May be administered once daily or in divided doses twice daily.

Children and Adolescents:

Pervasive developmental disorder (unlabeled use):

Initial: 0.25 mg twice daily; titrate up 0.25 mg/day every 5-7 days; optimal dose range: 0.75-1.5 mg/day (Fisman, 1996)

or

Initial: 0.5 mg at bedtime; titrate up 0.5 mg/day every 7 days in a morning and bedtime dosing regimen; dose range: 1-4 mg/day (McDougal, 1997)

Schizophrenia: Adolescents 13-17 years: Initial: 0.5 mg once daily; dose may be adjusted in increments of 0.5-1 mg/day at intervals ≥24 hours to a dose of 3 mg/day. Doses ranging from 1-6 mg/day have been evaluated, however, doses >3 mg/day do not confer additional benefit and are associated with increased adverse events.

Bipolar mania: Children and Adolescents 10-17 years: Initial: 0.5 mg once daily; dose may be adjusted in increments of 0.5-1 mg/day at intervals ≥24 hours to a dose of 2.5 mg/day. Doses ranging from 0.5-6 mg/day have been evaluated, however doses >2.5 mg/day do not confer additional benefit and are associated with increased adverse events.

Maintenance: No dosing recommendation available for treatment >3 weeks duration

Adolescents and Adults: Tourette's syndrome (unlabeled use): Initial: 0.25 mg once daily for 2 days, then 0.25 mg twice daily for 3 days, then 0.5 mg twice daily for 2 days; titrate slowly thereafter in increments/decrements ≤0.5 mg twice daily and at intervals ≥3 days; maximum dose: 6 mg/day (Dion, 2002)

Adults:

Schizophrenia:

Initial: 2 mg/day in 1-2 divided doses; may be increased by 1-2 mg/day at intervals ≥24 hours to a recommended dosage range of 4-8 mg/day; may be given as a single daily dose once maintenance dose is achieved; daily dosages >6 mg do not appear to confer any additional benefit, and the incidence of extrapyramidal symptoms is higher than with lower doses. Further dose adjustments should be made in increments/decrements of 1-2 mg/day on a weekly basis. Dose range studied in clinical trials: 4-16 mg/day.

Maintenance: Recommended dosage range: 2-8 mg/day

Bipolar mania:

Initial: 2-3 mg once daily; if needed, adjust dose by 1 mg/day in intervals ≥24 hours; dosing range: 1-6 mg/day

Maintenance: No dosing recommendation available for treatment >3 weeks duration.

Post-traumatic stress disorder (PTSD) (unlabeled use): 0.5-8 mg/day (Bandelow, 2008; Benedek, 2009)

Elderly:

Initial: 0.5 mg twice daily; titration should progress slowly in increments of no more than 0.5 mg twice daily; increases to dosages >1.5 mg twice daily should occur at intervals of ≥1 week.

Note: Additional monitoring of renal function and orthostatic blood pressure may be warranted. If once-a-day dosing in the elderly or debilitated patient is considered, a twice daily regimen should be used to titrate to the target dose, and this dose should be maintained for 2-3 days prior to attempts to switch to a once-daily regimen.

Psychosis/agitation related to Alzheimer's dementia (unlabeled use): Initial: 0.25-1 mg/day; if necessary, gradually increase as tolerated not to exceed 1.5-2 mg/day; doses >1 mg/day are associated with higher rates of extrapyramidal symptoms (Rabins, 2007)

I.M.: **Note:** Oral risperidone (or other antipsychotic) should be administered with the initial injection of Risperdal® Consta® and continued for 3 weeks (then discontinued) to maintain adequate therapeutic plasma concentrations prior to main release phase of risperidone from injection site. When switching from depot administration to a short-acting formulation, administer short-acting agent in place of the next regularly-scheduled depot injection.

Adults: Schizophrenia, bipolar I maintenance (Risperdal® Consta®): Initial: 25 mg every 2 weeks; if unresponsive, some may benefit from larger doses (37.5-50 mg); maximum dose: 50 mg every 2 weeks. Dosage adjustments should not be made more frequently than every 4 weeks. A lower initial dose of 12.5 mg may be appropriate in some patients (eg, demonstrated poor tolerability to other psychotropic medications).

Elderly (Risperdal® Consta®): 25 mg every 2 weeks; a lower initial dose of 12.5 mg may be appropriate in some patients

Dosing adjustment in renal impairment:

Oral: Starting dose of 0.5 mg twice daily; titration should progress slowly in increments of no more than 0.5 mg twice daily; increases to dosages >1.5 mg twice daily should occur at intervals of ≥1 week. Clearance of the active moiety is decreased by 60% in patients with moderate-to-severe renal disease compared to healthy subjects.

I.M.: Initiate with **oral** dosing (0.5 mg twice daily for 1 week then 2 mg/day for 1 week); if tolerated, begin 25 mg **I.M.** every 2 weeks; continue oral dosing for 3 weeks after the first I.M. injection. An initial I.M. dose of 12.5 mg may also be considered.

Dosing adjustment in hepatic impairment:

Oral: Starting dose of 0.5 mg twice daily; titration should progress slowly in increments of no more than 0.5 mg twice daily; increases to dosages >1.5 mg twice daily should occur at intervals of ≥1 week. The mean free fraction of risperidone in plasma was increased by 35% in patients with hepatic impairment compared to healthy subjects.

I.M.: Initiate with **oral** dosing (0.5 mg twice daily for 1 week then 2 mg/day for 1 week); if tolerated, begin 25 mg **I.M.** every 2 weeks; continue oral dosing for 3 weeks after the first I.M. injection. An initial I.M. dose of 12.5 mg may also be considered.

Mechanism of Action Risperidone is a benzisoxazole atypical antipsychotic with mixed serotonin-dopamine antagonist activity that binds to 5-HT_2-receptors in the CNS and in the periphery with a very high affinity; binds to dopamine-D_2 receptors with less affinity. The binding affinity to the dopamine-D_2 receptor is 20 times lower than the 5-HT_2 affinity. The addition of serotonin antagonism to dopamine antagonism (classic neuroleptic mechanism) is thought to improve negative symptoms of psychoses and reduce the incidence of extrapyramidal side effects. $Alpha_1$, $alpha_2$ adrenergic, and histaminergic receptors are also antagonized with high affinity. Risperidone has low to moderate affinity for 5-HT_{1C}, 5-HT_{1D}, and 5-HT_{1A} receptors, weak affinity for D_1 and no affinity for muscarinics or $beta_1$ and $beta_2$ receptors

Contraindications Hypersensitivity to risperidone or any component of the formulation

Warnings/Precautions Hazardous agent - use appropriate precautions for handling and disposal. **[U.S. Boxed Warning]: Elderly patients with dementia-related psychosis treated with antipsychotics are at an increased risk of death compared to placebo.** Most deaths appeared to be either cardiovascular (eg, heart failure, sudden death) or infectious (eg, pneumonia) in nature. In addition, an increased incidence of cerebrovascular effects (eg, transient ischemic attack, cerebrovascular accidents) has been reported in studies of placebo-controlled trials of risperidone in elderly patients with dementia-related psychosis. Risperidone is not approved for the treatment of dementia-related psychosis.

Leukopenia, neutropenia, and agranulocytosis (sometimes fatal) have been reported in clinical trials and postmarketing reports with antipsychotic use; presence of risk factors (eg, pre-existing low WBC or history of drug-induced leuko-/neutropenia) should prompt periodic blood count assessment. Discontinue therapy at first signs of blood dyscrasias or if absolute neutrophil count <1000/mm^3.

Low to moderately sedating, use with caution in disorders where CNS depression is a feature. Use with caution in Parkinson's disease. Caution in patients with predisposition to seizures. Use with caution in renal or hepatic dysfunction; dose reduction recommended. Esophageal dysmotility and aspiration have been associated with antipsychotic use; use with caution in patients at risk of aspiration pneumonia (ie, Alzheimer's disease). Use is associated with increased prolactin levels; clinical significance of hyperprolactinemia in patients with breast cancer or other prolactin-dependent tumors is unknown. May alter temperature regulation. May mask toxicity of other drugs or conditions (eg intestinal obstruction, Reyes syndrome, brain tumor) due to antiemetic effects. Neutropenia has been reported with antipsychotic use, including fatal cases of agranulocytosis. Pre-existing myelosuppression (disease or drug-induced) increases risk and these patients should have frequent CBC monitoring; decreased blood counts in absence of other causative factors should prompt discontinuation of therapy.

Use with caution in patients with cardiovascular diseases (eg, heart failure, history of myocardial infarction or ischemia, cerebrovascular disease, conduction abnormalities). May cause orthostatic hypotension; use with caution in patients at risk of this effect (eg, concurrent medication use which may predispose to hypotension/bradycardia or presence of hypovolemia) or in those who would not tolerate transient hypotensive episodes. May alter cardiac conduction (low risk relative to other neuroleptics); life-threatening arrhythmias have occurred with therapeutic doses of neuroleptics.

May cause anticholinergic effects (confusion, agitation, constipation, xerostomia, blurred vision, urinary retention); therefore, they should be used with caution in patients with decreased gastrointestinal motility, urinary retention, BPH, xerostomia, or visual problems (including narrow-angle glaucoma). Relative to other neuroleptics, risperidone has a low potency of cholinergic blockade.

May cause extrapyramidal symptoms (EPS), including pseudoparkinsonism, acute dystonic reactions, akathisia, and tardive dyskinesia (risk of these reactions is low relative to other neuroleptics, and is dose dependent). Risk of dystonia (and probably other EPS) may be greater with increased doses, use of conventional antipsychotics, males, and younger patients. Risk of neuroleptic malignant syndrome (NMS) may be increased in patients with Parkinson's disease or Lewy body dementia; monitor for symptoms of confusion, obtundation, postural instability and extrapyramidal symptoms. May cause hyperglycemia; in some cases may be extreme and associated with ketoacidosis, hyperosmolar coma, or death. Use with caution in patients with diabetes or other disorders of glucose regulation; monitor for worsening of glucose control. Significant weight gain has been observed with antipsychotic therapy; incidence varies with product. Monitor waist circumference and BMI. Rare cases of priapism have been reported.

The possibility of a suicide attempt is inherent in psychotic illness or bipolar disorder; use caution in high-risk patients during initiation of therapy. Prescriptions should be written for the smallest quantity consistent with good patient care. Long-term effects on growth or sexual maturation have not been evaluated. Vehicle used in injectable (polylactide-co-glycolide microspheres) has rarely been associated with retinal artery occlusion in patients with abnormal arteriovenous anastomosis.

Drug Interactions

Metabolism/Transport Effects Substrate of CYP2D6 (major), 3A4 (minor); **Inhibits** CYP2D6 (weak), 3A4 (weak)

Avoid Concomitant Use

Avoid concomitant use of RisperiDONE with any of the following: Artemether; Dronedarone; Lumefantrine; Metoclopramide; Nilotinib; Pimozide; QuiNINE; Tetrabenazine; Thioridazine; Toremifene; Vandetanib; Ziprasidone

Increased Effect/Toxicity

RisperiDONE may increase the levels/effects of: Alcohol (Ethyl); Anticholinergics; CNS Depressants; Dronedarone; Methylphenidate; Paliperidone; Pimozide; QTc-Prolonging Agents; QuiNINE; Tetrabenazine; Thioridazine; Toremifene; Vandetanib; Ziprasidone

The levels/effects of RisperiDONE may be increased by: Abiraterone; Acetylcholinesterase Inhibitors (Central); Alfuzosin; Artemether; Chloroquine; Ciprofloxacin; Ciprofloxacin (Systemic); Conivaptan; CYP2D6 Inhibitors (Moderate); CYP2D6 Inhibitors (Strong); Darunavir; Divalproex; Gadobutrol; Lithium formulations; Lumefantrine; Methylphenidate; Metoclopramide; Nilotinib; Pramlintide; QuiNINE; Selective Serotonin Reuptake Inhibitors; Tetrabenazine; Valproic Acid; Verapamil

Decreased Effect

RisperiDONE may decrease the levels/effects of: Amphetamines; Anti-Parkinson's Agents (Dopamine Agonist); Quinagolide

The levels/effects of RisperiDONE may be decreased by: CarBAMazepine; Lithium formulations; Peginterferon Alfa-2b; Tocilizumab

Ethanol/Nutrition/Herb Interactions

Ethanol: May increase CNS depression; monitor for increased effects with coadministration. Caution patients about effects.

Herb/Nutraceutical: Avoid kava kava, gotu kola, valerian, St John's wort (may increase CNS depression).

Dietary Considerations May be taken without regard to meals. Some products may contain phenylalanine.

Pharmacodynamics/Kinetics

Half-life Elimination Active moiety (risperidone and its active metabolite 9-hydroxyrisperidone)

Oral: 20 hours (mean)

Extensive metabolizers: Risperidone: 3 hours; 9-hydroxyrisperidone: 21 hours
Poor metabolizers: Risperidone: 20 hours; 9-hydroxyrisperidone: 30 hours

Injection: 3-6 days; related to microsphere erosion and subsequent absorption of risperidone

Time to Peak Plasma: Oral: Risperidone: Within 1 hour; 9-hydroxyrisperidone: Extensive metabolizers: 3 hours; Poor metabolizers: 17 hours

Pregnancy Risk Factor C

Lactation Enters breast milk/not recommended

Breast-Feeding Considerations Risperidone and its metabolite are excreted in breast milk; it is recommended that women not breast-feed during therapy or for 12 weeks after the last injection if using Risperdal® Consta®.

Dosage Forms

Injection, microspheres for reconstitution, extended release:
RisperDAL® Consta®: 12.5 mg, 25 mg, 37.5 mg, 50 mg

Solution, oral: 1 mg/mL (30 mL)
RisperDAL®: 1 mg/mL (30 mL)

Tablet, oral: 0.25 mg, 0.5 mg, 1 mg, 2 mg, 3 mg, 4 mg
RisperDAL®: 0.25 mg, 0.5 mg, 1 mg, 2 mg, 3 mg, 4 mg

Tablet, orally disintegrating, oral: 0.25 mg, 0.5 mg, 1 mg, 2 mg, 3 mg, 4 mg
RisperDAL® M-Tab®: 0.5 mg, 1 mg, 2 mg, 3 mg, 4 mg

Ritonavir (ri TOE na veer)

Related Information

HIV Infection and AIDS *on page* 1883

U.S. Brand Names Norvir®

Canadian Brand Names Norvir®; Norvir® SEC

Pharmacologic Category Antiretroviral Agent, Protease Inhibitor

Use Treatment of HIV infection; should always be used as part of a multidrug regimen (at least three antiretroviral agents); may be used as a pharmacokinetic "booster" for other protease inhibitors

Local Anesthetic/Vasoconstrictor Precautions No information available to require special precautions

Effects on Dental Treatment Key adverse event(s) related to dental treatment: Xerostomia (normal salivary flow resumes upon discontinuation) and taste perversion.

Effects on Bleeding Increased bleeding has been noted with protease inhibitors in patients with hemophilia A or B. No information available to require routine special precautions relative to hemostasis in other patients.

Adverse Effects Percentages as reported for combined experiences in both treatment-naive and experienced adults:

>10%:
- Endocrine & metabolic: Hypercholesterolemia (>240 mg/dL: 37% to 45%), triglycerides increased (>800 mg/dL: 17% to 34%; >1500 mg/dL: 1% to 13%)
- Gastrointestinal: Nausea (26% to 30%), diarrhea (15% to 23%), vomiting (14% to 17%), taste perversion (7% to 11%)
- Hepatic: GGT increased (5% to 20%)
- Neuromuscular & skeletal: Weakness (10% to 15%), creatine phosphokinase increased (9% to 12%)

2% to 10%:
- Cardiovascular: Vasodilation (2%), syncope (1% to 2%)
- Central nervous system: Headache (6% to 7%), fever (1% to 5%), dizziness (3% to 4%), insomnia (2% to 3%), somnolence (2% to 3%), depression (2%), anxiety (up to 2%), malaise (1% to 2%)
- Dermatologic: Rash (up to 4%)
- Endocrine & metabolic: Uric acid increased (up to 4%)
- Gastrointestinal: Abdominal pain (6% to 8%), anorexia (2% to 8%), dyspepsia (up to 6%), local throat irritation (2% to 3%), flatulence (1% to 2%)
- Hepatic: Transaminases increased (6% to 10%)
- Neuromuscular & skeletal: Paresthesia (3% to 7%), arthralgia (up to 2%), myalgia (2%)
- Respiratory: Pharyngitis (≤1% to 3%)
- Miscellaneous: Diaphoresis (2% to 3%)

General Dosage Range Dosage adjustment recommended in patients on concurrent therapy

Oral:

Children >1 month: Initial: 250 mg/m^2 twice daily; Maintenance: 350-400 mg/m^2 twice daily (maximum dose: 1200 mg/day)

Adults: 300-600 mg twice daily (maximum: 1200 mg/day)

Mechanism of Action Binds to the site of HIV-1 protease activity and inhibits cleavage of viral Gag-Pol polyprotein precursors into individual functional proteins required for infectious HIV. This results in the formation of immature, noninfectious viral particles.

Pharmacodynamics/Kinetics

Half-life Elimination 3-5 hours

Time to Peak Oral solution: 2 hours (fasted); 4 hours (nonfasted)

Pregnancy Risk Factor B

RiTUXimab (ri TUK si mab)

U.S. Brand Names Rituxan®

Canadian Brand Names Rituxan®

Pharmacologic Category Antineoplastic Agent, Monoclonal Antibody; Monoclonal Antibody

Use

Treatment of CD20-positive non-Hodgkin's lymphomas (NHL):

- Relapsed or refractory, low-grade or follicular B-cell NHL (as a single agent)
- Follicular B-cell NHL, previously untreated (in combination with first-line chemotherapy, and as single-agent maintenance therapy if response to first-line rituximab with chemotherapy)
- Nonprogressing, low-grade B-cell NHL (as a single agent after first-line CVP treatment)
- Diffuse large B-cell NHL, previously untreated (in combination with CHOP chemotherapy [or other anthracycline-based regimen])

Treatment of CD20-positive chronic lymphocytic leukemia (CLL) (in combination with fludarabine and cyclophosphamide)

Treatment of moderately- to severely-active rheumatoid arthritis (in combination with methotrexate) in adult patients with inadequate response to one or more TNF antagonists

Treatment of Wegener's granulomatosis (WG) (in combination with glucocorticoids)

Treatment of microscopic polyangiitis (MPA) (in combination with glucocorticoids)

Unlabeled/Investigational Use Treatment of Burkitt's lymphoma, central nervous system lymphoma, Hodgkin's lymphoma (lymphocyte predominant); mucosal associated lymphoid tissue (MALT) lymphoma (gastric and nongastric), splenic marginal zone lymphoma; Waldenström's macroglobulinemia (WM); post-transplant lymphoproliferative disorder (PTLD); autoimmune hemolytic anemia (AIHA) in children; chronic immune thrombocytopenic purpura (ITP); refractory pemphigus vulgaris; treatment of steroid-refractory chronic graft-versus-host disease (GVHD)

Local Anesthetic/Vasoconstrictor Precautions No information available to require special precautions

Effects on Dental Treatment No significant effects or complications reported

Effects on Bleeding Chemotherapy may result in significant myelosuppression, potentially including significant reduction in platelet counts and altered hemostasis. In patients who are under active treatment with these agents, medical consult is suggested.

Adverse Effects Note: Patients treated with rituximab for rheumatoid arthritis (RA) may experience fewer adverse reactions.

>10%:

- Cardiovascular: Peripheral edema (8% to 16%), hypertension (6% to 12%)
- Central nervous system: Fever (5% to 53%), fatigue (13% to 39%), chills (3% to 33%), headache (17% to 19%), insomnia (≤14%), pain (12%)
- Dermatologic: Rash (10% to 17%; grades 3/4: 1%), pruritus (5% to 17%), angioedema (11%; grades 3/4: 1%)
- Gastrointestinal: Nausea (8% to 23%), diarrhea (10% to 17%), abdominal pain (2% to 14%), weight gain (11%)
- Hematologic: Cytopenias (grades 3/4: ≤48%; may be prolonged), lymphopenia (48%; grades 3/4: 40%; median duration 14 days), anemia (8% to 35%; grades 3/4: 3%), leukopenia (NHL: 14%; grades 3/4: 4%; CLL: grades 3/4: 23%; WG/MPA: 10%), neutropenia (NHL: 14%; grades 3/4: 4% to 6%; median duration 13 days; CLL: grades 3/4: 30% to 49%), neutropenic fever (CLL: grades 3/4: 9% to 15%), thrombocytopenia (12%; grades 3/4: 2% to 11%)
- Hepatic: ALT increased (≤13%)
- Neuromuscular & skeletal: Neuropathy (≤30%), weakness (2% to 26%), muscle spasm (≤17%), arthralgia (6% to 13%)
- Respiratory: Cough (13%), rhinitis (3% to 12%), epistaxis (≤11%)

Miscellaneous: Infusion-related reactions (lymphoma: first dose 77%; decreases with subsequent infusions; may include angioedema, bronchospasm, chills, dizziness, fever, headache, hyper-/hypotension, myalgia, nausea, pruritus, rash, rigors, urticaria, and vomiting; reactions reported are lower [first infusion: 32%] in RA; CLL: 59%; grades 3/4: 7% to 9%; WG/MPA: 12%); infection (19% to 62%; grades 3/4: 4%; bacterial: 19%; viral 10%; fungal: 1%), human antichimeric antibody (HACA) positive (1% to 23%), night sweats (15%)

1% to 10%:

Cardiovascular: Hypotension (10%; grades 3/4: 2%), flushing (5%)
Central nervous system: Dizziness (10%), anxiety (2% to 5%), migraine (RA: 2%)
Dermatologic: Urticaria (2% to 8%)
Endocrine & metabolic: Hyperglycemia (9%)
Gastrointestinal: Vomiting (10%), dyspepsia (RA: 3%)
Neuromuscular & skeletal: Back pain (10%), myalgia (10%), paresthesia (2%)
Respiratory: Dyspnea (≤10%), throat irritation (2% to 9%), bronchospasm (8%), dyspnea (7%), upper respiratory tract infection (RA: 7%), sinusitis (6%)
Miscellaneous: LDH increased (7%)

General Dosage Range I.V.: *Adults:* Dosage varies greatly depending on indication

Mechanism of Action Rituximab is a monoclonal antibody directed against the CD20 antigen on B-lymphocytes. CD20 regulates cell cycle initiation; and, possibly, functions as a calcium channel. Rituximab binds to the antigen on the cell surface, activating complement-dependent B-cell cytotoxicity; and to human Fc receptors, mediating cell killing through an antibody-dependent cellular toxicity. B-cells are believed to play a role in the development and progression of rheumatoid arthritis. Signs and symptoms of RA are reduced by targeting B-cells and the progression of structural damage is delayed.

Pharmacodynamics/Kinetics

Duration of Action Detectable in serum 3-6 months after completion of treatment; B-cell recovery begins ~6 months following completion of treatment; median B-cell levels return to normal by 12 months following completion of treatment

Half-life Elimination

CLL: Median terminal half-life: 32 days (range: 14-62 days)
NHL: Median terminal half-life: 22 days (range: 6-52 days)
RA: Mean terminal half-life: 18 days (range: 5-78 days)
WG/MPA: 23 days (range: 9-49 days)

Pregnancy Risk Factor C

Rivaroxaban (riv a ROX a ban)

Canadian Brand Names Xarelto®

Pharmacologic Category Factor Xa Inhibitor

Use Postoperative thromboprophylaxis in patients who have undergone elective total hip or knee replacement procedures

Local Anesthetic/Vasoconstrictor Precautions No information available to require special precautions

Effects on Dental Treatment Key adverse event(s) related to dental treatment: Surgical site bleeding may occur. See Effects on Bleeding.

Effects on Bleeding Rivaroxaban inhibits platelet activation and fibrin clot formation via direct, selective, and reversible inhibition of factor Xa. As with all anticoagulants, bleeding is the major adverse effect of rivaroxaban. Hemorrhage may occur at virtually any site; risk is dependent on multiple variables including the intensity of anticoagulation and patient susceptibility. Medical consult is suggested.

Adverse Effects 1% to 10%:

Gastrointestinal: Nausea (1%)
Hematologic: Bleeding: Major: (<1% to 2%, includes surgical site bleeding events with decreased hemoglobin or transfusion); Nonmajor: (4% to 7%), anemia (1%)
Hepatic: Transaminases increased (2%; ALT >3 X upper limit of normal [ULN] 2% to 6%), GGT increased (1%)

General Dosage Range Oral: *Adults:* 10 mg/day

Mechanism of Action Inhibits platelet activation and fibrin clot formation via direct, selective and reversible inhibition of factor Xa (FXa) in both the intrinsic and extrinsic coagulation pathways. FXa, as part of the prothrombinase complex consisting also of factor Va, calcium ions, factor II and phospholipid, catalyzes the conversion of prothrombin to thrombin. Thrombin both activates platelets and catalyzes the conversion of fibrinogen to fibrin.

Pharmacodynamics/Kinetics

Half-life Elimination Young individual: 5-9 hours; Elderly: 11-13 hours

Time to Peak Plasma: 2-4 hours

Product Availability Not available in U.S.

Rivastigmine (ri va STIG meen)

U.S. Brand Names Exelon®
Canadian Brand Names Exelon®; Mylan-Rivastigmine; Novo-Rivastigmine; PMS-Rivastigmine; ratio-Rivastigmine; Sandoz-Rivastigmine
Pharmacologic Category Acetylcholinesterase Inhibitor (Central)
Use Treatment of mild-to-moderate dementia associated with Alzheimer's disease or Parkinson's disease
Unlabeled/Investigational Use Severe dementia associated with Alzheimer's disease; Lewy body dementia
Local Anesthetic/Vasoconstrictor Precautions No information available to require special precautions
Effects on Dental Treatment No significant effects or complications reported
Effects on Bleeding No information available to require special precautions
Adverse Effects Note: Many concentration-related effects are reported at a lower frequency by transdermal route.

>10%:
Central nervous system: Dizziness (2% to 21%), headache (3% to 17%)
Gastrointestinal: Nausea (7% to 47%), vomiting (6% to 31%), diarrhea (5% to 19%), anorexia (3% to 17%), abdominal pain (1% to 13%)

1% to 10%:
Cardiovascular: Syncope (3%), hypertension (3%)
Central nervous system: Fatigue (2% to 9%), insomnia (1% to 9%), confusion (8%), depression (4% to 6%), anxiety (2% to 5%), malaise (5%), somnolence (4% to 5%), hallucinations (4%), aggressiveness (3%), parkinsonism symptoms worsening (2% to 3%), vertigo (≤2%)
Gastrointestinal: Dyspepsia (9%), constipation (5%), flatulence (4%), weight loss (3% to 8%), eructation (2%), dehydration (2%)
Genitourinary: Urinary tract infection (1% to 7%)
Neuromuscular & skeletal: Weakness (2% to 6%), tremor (1%; up to 10% in Parkinson's patients)
Respiratory: Rhinitis (4%)
Miscellaneous: Diaphoresis (4%), flu-like syndrome (3%)

General Dosage Range
Oral: *Adults:* Initial: 1.5 mg twice daily; Maintenance: 1.5-6 mg twice daily (maximum: 12 mg/day)
Transdermal patch: *Adults:* Initial: 4.6 mg/24 hours; Maintenance: 9.5 mg/24 hours (maximum dose: 9.5 mg/24 hours)

Mechanism of Action A deficiency of cortical acetylcholine is thought to account for some of the symptoms of Alzheimer's disease and the dementia of Parkinson's disease; rivastigmine increases acetylcholine in the central nervous system through reversible inhibition of its hydrolysis by cholinesterase
Pharmacodynamics/Kinetics
Duration of Action Anticholinesterase activity (CSF): ~10 hours (6 mg oral dose)
Half-life Elimination Oral: 1.5 hours; Transdermal patch: 3 hours (after removal)
Time to Peak Oral: 1 hour; Transdermal patch: 10-16 hours following first dose
Pregnancy Risk Factor B

Rizatriptan (rye za TRIP tan)

Related Information
Temporomandibular Dysfunction (TMD) *on page 1964*
U.S. Brand Names Maxalt-MLT®; Maxalt®
Canadian Brand Names Maxalt RPD™; Maxalt™
Generic Availability (U.S.) No
Pharmacologic Category Antimigraine Agent; Serotonin 5-$HT_{1B, 1D}$ Receptor Agonist
Use Acute treatment of migraine with or without aura
Local Anesthetic/Vasoconstrictor Precautions No information available to require special precautions
Effects on Dental Treatment Key adverse event(s) related to dental treatment: Xerostomia (normal salivary flow resumes upon discontinuation).
Effects on Bleeding No information available to require special precautions
Adverse Effects 1% to 10%:
Cardiovascular: Systolic/diastolic blood pressure increases (5-10 mm Hg), chest pain (5%), palpitation
Central nervous system: Dizziness, drowsiness, fatigue (13% to 30%, dose related)
Dermatologic: Skin flushing

Endocrine & metabolic: Mild increase in growth hormone, hot flashes
Gastrointestinal: Abdominal pain, dry mouth (<5%), nausea
Respiratory: Dyspnea

Dosage Note: In patients with risk factors for coronary artery disease, following adequate evaluation to establish the absence of coronary artery disease, the initial dose should be administered in a setting where response may be evaluated (physician's office or similarly staffed setting). ECG monitoring may be considered.

Oral: 5-10 mg, repeat after 2 hours if significant relief is not attained; maximum: 30 mg in a 24-hour period (use 5 mg dose in patients receiving propranolol with a maximum of 15 mg in 24 hours)

Note: For orally-disintegrating tablets (Maxalt-MLT®): Patient should be instructed to place tablet on tongue and allow to dissolve. Dissolved tablet will be swallowed with saliva.

Mechanism of Action Selective agonist for serotonin (5-HT_{1B} and 5-HT_{1D} receptors) in cranial arteries; causes vasoconstriction and reduces sterile inflammation associated with antidromic neuronal transmission correlating with relief of migraine

Contraindications Hypersensitivity to rizatriptan or any component of the formulation; documented ischemic heart disease or Prinzmetal's angina; uncontrolled hypertension; basilar or hemiplegic migraine; during or within 2 weeks of MAO inhibitors; during or within 24 hours of treatment with another 5-HT_1 agonist, or an ergot-containing or ergot-type medication (eg, methysergide, dihydroergotamine)

Warnings/Precautions Only indicated for treatment of acute migraine; if a patient does not respond to the first dose, the diagnosis of migraine should be reconsidered. Coronary artery vasospasm, transient ischemia, myocardial infarction, ventricular tachycardia/fibrillation, cardiac arrest, and death have been reported with 5-HT_1 agonist administration. Patients who experience sensations of chest pain/pressure/tightness or symptoms suggestive of angina following dosing should be evaluated for coronary artery disease or Prinzmetal's angina before receiving additional doses. Should not be given to patients who have risk factors for CAD (eg, hypertension, hypercholesterolemia, smoker, obesity, diabetes, strong family history of CAD, menopause, male >40 years of age) without adequate cardiac evaluation. Patients with suspected CAD should have cardiovascular evaluation to rule out CAD before considering use; if cardiovascular evaluation "is satisfactory," first dose should be given in the healthcare provider's office. Periodic evaluation of cardiovascular status should be done in all patients. Significant elevation in blood pressure, including hypertensive crisis, has also been reported on rare occasions in patients with and without a history of hypertension. Cerebral/subarachnoid hemorrhage, stroke, peripheral vascular ischemia, and colonic ischemia have been reported with 5-HT_1 agonist administration.

Use with caution in elderly or patients with hepatic or renal impairment (including dialysis patients). Symptoms of agitation, confusion, hallucinations, hyper-reflexia, myoclonus, shivering, and tachycardia may occur with concomitant proserotonergic drugs (eg, SSRIs/SNRIs or triptans) or agents which reduce rizatriptan's metabolism. Concurrent use of serotonin precursors (eg, tryptophan) is not recommended. Maxalt-MLT® tablets contain phenylalanine.

Drug Interactions

Avoid Concomitant Use

Avoid concomitant use of Rizatriptan with any of the following: Ergot Derivatives; MAO Inhibitors; Sibutramine

Increased Effect/Toxicity

Rizatriptan may increase the levels/effects of: Ergot Derivatives; Serotonin Modulators

The levels/effects of Rizatriptan may be increased by: Ergot Derivatives; MAO Inhibitors; Propranolol; Sibutramine

Decreased Effect There are no known significant interactions involving a decrease in effect.

Ethanol/Nutrition/Herb Interactions Food: Food delays absorption.

Dietary Considerations Some products may contain phenylalanine.

Pharmacodynamics/Kinetics

Onset of Action ~30 minutes

Duration of Action 14-16 hours

Half-life Elimination 2-3 hours

Time to Peak 1-1.5 hours

Pregnancy Risk Factor C

Lactation Excretion in breast milk unknown/use caution

Dosage Forms

Tablet, oral:

Maxalt®: 5 mg, 10 mg

Tablet, orally disintegrating, oral:

Maxalt-MLT®: 5 mg, 10 mg

Roflumilast (roe FLUE mi last)

Canadian Brand Names Daxas™

Pharmacologic Category Phosphodiesterase-4 Enzyme Inhibitor

Use Adjunct to bronchodilator therapy in the maintenance treatment of severe chronic obstructive pulmonary disease (COPD) associated with chronic bronchitis

Local Anesthetic/Vasoconstrictor Precautions No information available to require special precautions

Effects on Dental Treatment No significant effects or complications reported

Effects on Bleeding No information available to require special precautions

Adverse Effects

>10%: Gastrointestinal: Diarrhea (12%)

1% to 10%:

Cardiovascular: Supraventricular arrhythmia (1%)

Central nervous system: Headache (5%), dizziness (3%), insomnia (3%), anxiety (1%), depression (1%), fatigue (1%)

Gastrointestinal: Weight loss (7%), nausea (5%), abdominal pain (4%), appetite decreased (3%), gastritis (1%), vomiting (1%)

Neuromuscular & skeletal: Back pain (3%), muscle spasms (2%), tremor (2%)

General Dosage Range Oral: *Adults:* 500 mcg once daily

Mechanism of Action Roflumilast and its active N-oxide metabolite selectively inhibit phosphodiesterase-4 (PDE4) leading to an accumulation of cyclic AMP (cAMP) within inflammatory and structural cells important in the pathogenesis of COPD. Anti-inflammatory effects include suppression of cytokine release and inhibition of lung infiltration by neutrophils and other leukocytes. Pulmonary remodeling and mucociliary malfunction are also attenuated.

Pharmacodynamics/Kinetics

Half-life Elimination 17 hours; N-oxide metabolite: 30 hours

Time to Peak ~1 hour (delayed by food); N-oxide metabolite: ~8 hours

Product Availability

Daliresp™: FDA approved March 2011; availability expected in second quarter 2011.

Daliresp™ is an oral selective phosphodiesterase-4 inhibitor approved to reduce the risk of COPD exacerbations in patients with severe COPD secondary to chronic bronchitis with a history of exacerbations.

RomiDEPsin (roe mi DEP sin)

Related Information

Clinical Risk Related to Drugs Prolonging QT Interval *on page* 1872

U.S. Brand Names Istodax®

Pharmacologic Category Antineoplastic Agent, Histone Deacetylase Inhibitor

Use Treatment of cutaneous T-cell lymphoma (CTCL)

Local Anesthetic/Vasoconstrictor Precautions Romidepsin is one of the drugs confirmed to prolong the QT interval and is accepted as having a risk of causing torsade de pointes. The risk of drug-induced torsade de pointes is extremely low when a single QT interval prolonging drug is prescribed. In terms of epinephrine, it is not known what effect vasoconstrictors in the local anesthetic regimen will have in patients with a known history of congenital prolonged QT interval or in patients taking any medication that prolongs the QT interval. Until more information is obtained, it is suggested that the clinician consult with the physician prior to the use of a vasoconstrictor in suspected patients, and that the vasoconstrictor (epinephrine, mepivacaine and levonordefrin [Carbocaine® 2% with Neo-Cobefrin®]) be used with caution.

Effects on Dental Treatment Key adverse event(s) related to dental treatment: Taste alteration.

Effects on Bleeding Chemotherapy may result in significant myelosuppression, potentially including significant reduction in platelet counts and altered hemostasis. In patients who are under active treatment with these agents, medical consult is suggested.

Adverse Effects

>10%:

Cardiovascular: ST-T wave changes (2% to 63%, includes T-wave flattening or ST segment depression), hypotension (7% to 23%)

Central nervous system: Fatigue (53% to 77%), fever (20% to 23%)

Dermatologic: Pruritus (7% to 31%), dermatitis/exfoliative dermatitis (4% to 27%)

Endocrine & metabolic: Hypocalcemia (4% to 52%), hyperglycemia (2% to 51%), hypoalbuminemia (3% to 48%), hyperuricemia (≤33%), hypomagnesemia (22% to 28%), hypermagnesemia (≤27%), hypophosphatemia (≤27%), hypokalemia (6% to 20%), hyponatremia (≤20%)

Gastrointestinal: Nausea (56% to 86%), anorexia (23% to 54%), vomiting (34% to 52%), taste alteration (15% to 40%), constipation (12% to 39%), diarrhea (7% to 20%)

Hematologic: Anemia (19% to 72%; grades 3/4: 3% to 16%), thrombocytopenia (17% to 65%; grades 3/4: ≤14%), neutropenia (11% to 57%; grades 3/4: 4% to 27%), lymphopenia (4% to 57%; grades 3/4: ≤37%), leukopenia (4% to 46%; grades 3/4: ≤22%)

Hepatic: AST increased (3% to 28%), ALT increased (3% to 22%)

Neuromuscular & skeletal: Weakness (53% to 77%)

Miscellaneous: Infection (46% to 54%; grades 3/4: 11% to 33%)

1% to 10%:

Cardiovascular: Cardiopulmonary failure, edema, myocardial ischemia, QT prolongation, supraventricular arrhythmia, ventricular arrhythmia

Respiratory: Acute respiratory distress syndrome, dyspnea

Miscellaneous: Central line infection

General Dosage Range Dosage adjustment recommended in patients who develop toxicities

I.V.: *Adults:* 14 mg/m^2 days 1, 8, and 15 of a 28-day treatment cycle

Mechanism of Action Histone deacetylase inhibitor; catalyzes acetyl group removal from protein lysine residues (including histone and transcription factors). Inhibition of histone deacetylase results in accumulation of acetyl groups, leading to alterations in chromatin structure and transcription factor activation causing termination of cell growth (induces arrest in cell cycle at G_1 and G_2/M phases) leading to cell death.

Pharmacodynamics/Kinetics

Half-life Elimination ~3 hours

Pregnancy Risk Factor D

Dental Comment Romidepsin is known to prolong the QT interval. The QT interval is measured as the time and distance between the Q point of the QRS complex and the end of the T wave in the ECG tracing. After adjustment for heart rate, the QT interval is defined as prolonged if it is more than 450 msec in men and 460 msec in women. A long QT syndrome was first described in the 1950s and 60s as a congenital syndrome involving QT interval prolongation and syncope and sudden death. Some of the congenital long QT syndromes were characterized by a peculiar electrocardiographic appearance of the QRS complex involving a premature atria beat followed by a pause, then a subsequent sinus beat showing marked QT prolongation and deformity. This type of cardiac arrhythmia was originally termed "torsade de pointes" (translated from the French as "twisting of the points"). Romidepsin is considered as having a risk of causing torsade de pointes. Since it is not known what effect vasoconstrictors in the local anesthetic regimen will have in patients with a known history of congenital prolonged QT interval or in patients taking any medication that prolongs the QT interval, a medical consult is suggested.

RomiPLOStim (roe mi PLOE stim)

U.S. Brand Names Nplate™

Canadian Brand Names Nplate™

Pharmacologic Category Colony Stimulating Factor; Thrombopoietic Agent

Use Treatment of thrombocytopenia in patients with chronic immune (idiopathic) thrombocytopenia purpura (ITP) who have had insufficient response to corticosteroids, immune globulin, or splenectomy

Local Anesthetic/Vasoconstrictor Precautions No information available to require special precautions

Effects on Dental Treatment No significant effects or complications reported

Effects on Bleeding Romiplostim is used for treatment of thrombocytopenia; dosing is established to increase platelet counts and reduce the risk of bleeding. Bleeding is not expected with therapy; however, upon discontinuation of therapy, rebound thrombocytopenia may occur and risk of bleeding is increased; monitor closely.

Adverse Effects

>10%:

Central nervous system: Headache (35%), fatigue (33%), dizziness (17%), insomnia (16%)

Gastrointestinal: Diarrhea (17%), nausea (13%), abdominal pain (11%)

Neuromuscular & skeletal: Arthralgia (26%), myalgia (14%), back pain (13%), limb pain (13%)

Respiratory: Epistaxis (32%), upper respiratory tract infection (17%)

1% to 10%:

Gastrointestinal: Dyspepsia (7%)

Hematologic: Rebound thrombocytopenia (7%), bone marrow reticulin formation/deposition (4%)

Neuromuscular & skeletal: Shoulder pain (8%), paresthesia (6%)

Miscellaneous: Antibody formation (romiplostim 10%; TPO 5%)

General Dosage Range

SubQ:

Children: Dosage not established

Adults: Initial: 1 mcg/kg once weekly; adjust dose by 1 mcg/kg/week to achieve platelet count ≥50,000/mm^3 and reduce the risk of bleeding; Maximum: 10 mcg/kg

Mechanism of Action Thrombopoietin (TPO) peptide mimetic which increases platelet counts in ITP by binding to and activating the human TPO receptor.

Pharmacodynamics/Kinetics

Onset of Action Platelet count increase: SubQ: 4-9 days; Peak platelet count increase: Days 12-16

Duration of Action Platelet counts return to baseline by day 28

Half-life Elimination Median: 3.5 days (range: 1-34 days)

Time to Peak SubQ: Median: 14 hours (range: 7-50 hours)

Pregnancy Risk Factor C

Prescribing and Access Restrictions As a requirement of the REMS program, access to this medication is restricted. Prescribers and patients must be registered with the Nplate™ NEXUS (Network of Experts Understanding and Supporting Nplate™ and Patients) program (1-877-675-2831 or http://www.nplatenexus.com) in order to obtain the medication.

ROPINIRole (roe PIN i role)

U.S. Brand Names Requip®; Requip® XL™

Canadian Brand Names CO Ropinirole; JAMP-Ropinirole; PMS-Ropinirole; RAN™-Ropinirole; Requip®

Pharmacologic Category Anti-Parkinson's Agent, Dopamine Agonist

Use Treatment of idiopathic Parkinson's disease; in patients with early Parkinson's disease who were not receiving concomitant levodopa therapy as well as in patients with advanced disease on concomitant levodopa; treatment of moderate-to-severe primary Restless Legs Syndrome (RLS)

Local Anesthetic/Vasoconstrictor Precautions No information available to require special precautions

Effects on Dental Treatment Key adverse event(s) related to dental treatment: Xerostomia and increased salivation (normal salivary flow resumes upon discontinuation) and dysphagia.

Effects on Bleeding No information available to require special precautions

Adverse Effects

Data inclusive of trials in early Parkinson's disease (without levodopa) and Restless Legs Syndrome:

>10%:

Cardiovascular: Syncope (1% to 12%)

Central nervous system: Somnolence (11% to 40%), dizziness (6% to 40%), fatigue (8% to 11%)

Gastrointestinal: Nausea (immediate release: 40% to 60%; extended release: 19%), vomiting (11% to 12%)

Miscellaneous: Viral infection (11%)

1% to 10%:

Cardiovascular: Dependent/leg edema (2% to 7%), orthostasis (1% to 6%), hypertension (5%), chest pain (4%), flushing (3%), palpitation (3%), peripheral ischemia (2% to 3%), atrial fibrillation (2%), extrasystoles (2%), hypotension (2%), tachycardia (2%)

Central nervous system: Pain (3% to 8%), headache (extended release: 6%), confusion (5%), hallucinations (up to 5%; dose related), hypoesthesia (4%), amnesia (3%), malaise (3%), yawning (3%), concentration impaired (2%), vertigo (2%)

Dermatologic: Hyperhidrosis (3%)

Gastrointestinal: Dyspepsia (4% to 10%), abdominal pain (3% to 7%), constipation (≥5%), xerostomia (3% to 5%), diarrhea (5%), anorexia (4%), flatulence (3%)
Genitourinary: Urinary tract infection (5%), impotence (3%)
Hepatic: Alkaline phosphatase increased (3%)
Neuromuscular & skeletal: Weakness (6%), arthralgia (4%), muscle cramps (3%), paresthesia (3%), hyperkinesia (2%)
Ocular: Abnormal vision (6%), xerophthalmia (2%)
Respiratory: Pharyngitis (6% to 9%), rhinitis (4%), sinusitis (4%), bronchitis (3%), dyspnea (3%), influenza (3%), cough (3%), nasal congestion (2%)
Miscellaneous: Diaphoresis increased (3% to 6%)

Advanced Parkinson's disease (with levodopa):

>10%:

Central nervous system: Dizziness (immediate release: 26%; extended-release: 8%), somnolence (immediate release: 20%, extended release: 7%), headache (17%)
Gastrointestinal: Nausea (immediate release: 30%; extended-release: 11%)
Neuromuscular & skeletal: Dyskinesias (immediate release: 34%; extended-release: 13%; dose related)

1% to 10%:

Cardiovascular: Hypotension (2% to 5%; including orthostatic), peripheral edema (4%), syncope (3%), hypertension (3%; dose related)
Central nervous system: Hallucinations (7% to 10%; dose related), confusion (9%), anxiety (2% to 6%), amnesia (5%), nervousness (5%), pain (5%), vertigo (4%), abnormal dreaming (3%), paresis (3%), aggravated parkinsonism, insomnia
Gastrointestinal: Abdominal pain (6% to 9%), vomiting (7%), constipation (4% to 6%), diarrhea (3% to 5%), xerostomia (2% to 5%), dysphagia (2%), flatulence (2%), salivation increased (2%), weight loss (2%)
Genitourinary: Urinary tract infection (6%), pyuria (2%), urinary incontinence (2%)
Hematologic: Anemia (2%)
Neuromuscular & skeletal: Falls (2% to 10%; dose related), arthralgia (7%), tremor (6%), hypokinesia (5%), paresthesia (5%), arthritis (3%), back pain (3%)
Ocular: Diplopia (2%)
Respiratory: Upper respiratory tract infection (9%), dyspnea (3%)
Miscellaneous: Injury, diaphoresis increased (7%), viral infection, increased drug level (7%)

Other adverse effects (all phase 2/3 trials for Parkinson's disease and Restless Leg Syndrome): ≥1%: Asthma, BUN increased, depression, gastroenteritis, gastrointestinal reflux, irritability, migraine, muscle spasm, myalgia, neck pain, neuralgia, osteoarthritis, pharyngolaryngeal pain, rash, rigors, sleep disorder, tendonitis

General Dosage Range Oral: *Adults:*

Parkinson's:

Immediate release: Initial: 0.25 mg 3 times/day; Maintenance: 0.75-24 mg/day in 3 divided doses
Extended release: Initial: 2 mg once daily; Maintenance: 2-24 mg once daily (maximum: 24 mg/day)

Restless legs: Immediate release: Initial: 0.25 mg prior to bedtime; Maintenance: 0.25-4 mg prior to bedtime

Mechanism of Action Ropinirole has a high relative *in vitro* specificity and full intrinsic activity at the D_2 and D_3 dopamine receptor subtypes, binding with higher affinity to D_3 than to D_2 or D_4 receptor subtypes; relevance of D_3 receptor binding in Parkinson's disease is unknown. Ropinirole has moderate *in vitro* affinity for opioid receptors. Ropinirole and its metabolites have negligible *in vitro* affinity for dopamine D_1, 5-HT_1, 5-HT_2, benzodiazepine, GABA, muscarinic, $alpha_1$-, $alpha_2$-, and beta-adrenoreceptors. Although precise mechanism of action of ropinirole is unknown, it is believed to be due to stimulation of postsynaptic dopamine D_2-type receptors within the caudate putamen in the brain. Ropinirole caused decreases in systolic and diastolic blood pressure at doses >0.25 mg. The mechanism of ropinirole-induced postural hypotension is believed to be due to D_2-mediated blunting of the noradrenergic response to standing and subsequent decrease in peripheral vascular resistance.

Pharmacodynamics/Kinetics

Half-life Elimination ~6 hours

Time to Peak Immediate release: ~1-2 hours; Extended release: 6-10 hours; T_{max} increased by 2.5-3 hours when drug taken with food

Pregnancy Risk Factor C

Ropivacaine (roe PIV a kane)

Related Information
Oral Pain *on page* 1928
U.S. Brand Names Naropin®
Canadian Brand Names Naropin®
Pharmacologic Category Local Anesthetic
Use Local anesthetic for use in surgery, postoperative pain management, and obstetrical procedures when local or regional anesthesia is needed
Local Anesthetic/Vasoconstrictor Precautions No information available to require special precautions (see Dental Comment)
Effects on Dental Treatment No significant effects or complications reported
Effects on Bleeding No information available to require special precautions
Adverse Effects
>10%:
Cardiovascular: Hypotension (dose-related and age-related: 32% to 69%), bradycardia (6% to 20%)
Gastrointestinal: Nausea (11% to 29%), vomiting (7% to 14%)
Neuromuscular & skeletal: Back pain (7% to 16%)
1% to 10%:
Cardiovascular: Hypertension, tachycardia, chest pain (1% to 5%)
Central nervous system: Fever (3% to 9%), headache (5% to 8%), dizziness (3%), chills (2% to 3%), anxiety (1%), lightheadedness
Dermatologic: Pruritus (1% to 5%)
Endocrine & metabolic: Hypokalemia
Genitourinary: Urinary retention (1% to 5%), urinary tract infection (1% to 5%)
Hematologic: Anemia (6%)
Neuromuscular & skeletal: Paresthesia (2% to 6%), hypoesthesia, rigors, circumoral paresthesia
Renal: Oliguria
Respiratory: Dyspnea
Miscellaneous: Shivering
General Dosage Range
Epidural:
Lumbar: *Adults:* 10-30 mL of 0.2% to 1% solution **or** 15-20 mL of 0.75% solution; Infusion: 6-14 mL/hour of 0.2% solution, with incremental injections of 10-15 mL/hour of 0.2% solution
Thoracic: *Adults:* 5-15 mL of 0.5% to 0.75% solution; Infusion: 6-14 mL/hour of 0.2% solution
Field Block: *Adults:* 1-40 mL (5-200 mg) of 0.5% solution
Infiltration: *Adults:* 1-100 mL of 0.2% solution **or** 1-40 mL of 0.5% solution
Nerve Block: *Adults:* Major: 35-50 mL (175-250 mg) of 0.5 % solution **or** 10-40 mL (75-300 mg) of 0.75% solution; Minor: 1-100 mL of 0.2% solution **or** 1-40 mL of 0.5% solution
Mechanism of Action Blocks both the initiation and conduction of nerve impulses by decreasing the neuronal membrane's permeability to sodium ions, which results in inhibition of depolarization with resultant blockade of conduction
Pharmacodynamics/Kinetics
Onset of Action Anesthesia (route dependent): 3-15 minutes
Duration of Action Dose and route dependent: 3-15 hours
Half-life Elimination Epidural: 5-7 hours; I.V.: Terminal: 111 ± 62 minutes (Lee, 1989)
Pregnancy Risk Factor B
Dental Comment Not available with vasoconstrictor (epinephrine) and not available in dental (1.8 mL) carpules

Rosiglitazone (roh si GLI ta zone)

Related Information
Endocrine Disorders and Pregnancy *on page* 1879
U.S. Brand Names Avandia®
Canadian Brand Names Avandia®
Generic Availability (U.S.) No
Pharmacologic Category Antidiabetic Agent, Thiazolidinedione
Use Type 2 diabetes mellitus (noninsulin dependent, NIDDM):
Monotherapy: Improve glycemic control as an adjunct to diet and exercise
Note: Canadian labeling approves use as monotherapy only when metformin is contraindicated or not tolerated.

Combination therapy: **Note:** Use when diet, exercise, and a single agent do not result in adequate glycemic control.

U.S. labeling: In combination with a sulfonylurea, metformin, or sulfonylurea plus metformin

Canadian labeling: In combination with metformin; in combination with a sulfonylurea only when metformin use is contraindicated or not tolerated

Local Anesthetic/Vasoconstrictor Precautions No information available to require special precautions

Effects on Dental Treatment Rosiglitazone-dependent patients with diabetes should be appointed for dental treatment in morning in order to minimize chance of stress-induced hypoglycemia.

Effects on Bleeding No information available to require special precautions

Adverse Effects Note: The rate of certain adverse reactions (eg, anemia, edema, hypoglycemia) may be higher with some combination therapies.

>10%: Endocrine & metabolic: HDL-cholesterol increased, LDL-cholesterol increased, total cholesterol increased, weight gain

1% to 10%:

Cardiovascular: Edema (5%), hypertension (4%); heart failure/CHF (up to 2% to 3% in patients receiving insulin; incidence likely higher in patients with pre-existing HF; myocardial ischemia (3%; incidence likely higher in patients with preexisting CAD)

Central nervous system: Headache (6%)

Endocrine & metabolic: Hypoglycemia (1% to 3%; combination therapy with insulin: 12% to 14%)

Gastrointestinal: Diarrhea (3%)

Hematologic: Anemia (2%)

Neuromuscular & skeletal: Fractures (up to 9%; incidence greater in females; usually upper arm, hand, or foot), arthralgia (5%), back pain (4% to 5%)

Respiratory: Upper respiratory tract infection (4% to 10%), nasopharyngitis (6%)

Miscellaneous: Injury (8%)

Dosage Oral:

Adults: **Note:** All patients should be initiated at the lowest recommended dose.

Monotherapy: Initial: 4 mg daily as a single daily dose or in divided doses twice daily. If response is inadequate after 8-12 weeks of treatment, the dosage may be increased to 8 mg daily as a single daily dose or in divided doses twice daily. In clinical trials, the 4 mg twice-daily regimen resulted in the greatest reduction in fasting plasma glucose and Hb A_{1c}.

Combination therapy: When adding rosiglitazone to existing therapy, continue current dose(s) of previous agents:

U.S. labeling: With sulfonylureas or metformin (or sulfonylurea plus metformin): Initial: 4 mg daily as a single daily dose or in divided doses twice daily. If response is inadequate after 8-12 weeks of treatment, the dosage may be increased to 8 mg daily as a single daily dose or in divided doses twice daily. Reduce dose of sulfonylurea if hypoglycemia occurs. It is unlikely that the dose of metformin will need to be reduced due to hypoglycemia.

Canadian labeling:

With metformin: Initial: 4 mg daily as a single daily dose or in divided doses twice daily. If response is inadequate after 8-12 weeks of treatment, the dosage may be increased to 8 mg daily as a single daily dose or in divided doses twice daily.

With a sulfonylurea: 4 mg daily as a single daily dose or in divided doses twice daily. Dose should not exceed 4 mg daily when using in combination with a sulfonylurea. Reduce dose of sulfonylurea if hypoglycemia occurs.

Elderly: No dosage adjustment is recommended

Dosage adjustment in renal impairment: No dosage adjustment is required

Dosage comment in hepatic impairment: Clearance is significantly lower in hepatic impairment. Therapy should not be initiated if the patient exhibits active liver disease or increased transaminases (ALT >2.5 times the upper limit of normal) at baseline.

Mechanism of Action Thiazolidinedione antidiabetic agent that lowers blood glucose by improving target cell response to insulin, without increasing pancreatic insulin secretion. It has a mechanism of action that is dependent on the presence of insulin for activity. Rosiglitazone is an agonist for peroxisome proliferator-activated receptor-gamma (PPARgamma). Activation of nuclear PPARgamma receptors influences the production of a number of gene products involved in glucose and lipid metabolism. PPARgamma is abundant in the cells within the renal collecting tubules; fluid retention results from stimulation by thiazolidinediones which increases sodium reabsorption.

Contraindications NYHA Class III/IV heart failure (initiation of therapy)

Canadian labeling: Hypersensitivity to rosiglitazone or any component of the formulation; any stage of heart failure (eg, NYHA Class I, II, III, IV); serious hepatic impairment; pregnancy

Warnings/Precautions [U.S. Boxed Warning]: Thiazolidinediones, including rosiglitazone, may cause or exacerbate congestive heart failure; closely monitor for signs/symptoms of congestive heart failure (eg, rapid weight gain, dyspnea, edema), particularly after initiation or dose increases. Not recommended for use in any patient with symptomatic heart failure. In the U.S., initiation of therapy is contraindicated in patients with NYHA class III or IV heart failure; in Canada use is contraindicated in patients with any stage of heart failure (NYHA Class I, II, III, IV). Use with caution in patients with edema; may increase plasma volume and/or cause fluid retention, leading to heart failure. Dose-related weight gain observed with use; mechanism unknown but likely associated with fluid retention and fat accumulation. Use may also be associated with an increased risk of angina and MI. Use caution in patients at risk for cardiovascular events and monitor closely. Discontinue if any deterioration in cardiac status occurs.

Should not be used in diabetic ketoacidosis. Mechanism requires the presence of insulin; therefore, use in type 1 diabetes (insulin dependent, IDDM) is not recommended. Combination therapy with other hypoglycemic agents may increase risk for hypoglycemic events; dose reduction with the concomitant agent may be warranted. Concomitant use with nitrates is not recommended due to increased risk of myocardial ischemia. Avoid use with insulin due to an increased risk of edema, congestive heart failure, and myocardial ischemic events.

Use with caution in patients with elevated transaminases (AST or ALT); do not initiate in patients with active liver disease or ALT >2.5 times ULN at baseline; evaluate patients with ALT ≤2.5 times ULN at baseline or during therapy for cause of enzyme elevation; during therapy, if ALT >3 times ULN, reevaluate levels promptly and discontinue if elevation persists or if jaundice occurs at any time during use. Idiosyncratic hepatotoxicity has been reported with another thiazolidinedione agent (troglitazone); avoid use in patients who previously experienced jaundice during troglitazone therapy. Monitoring should include periodic determinations of liver function. Increased incidence of bone fractures in females treated with rosiglitazone observed during analysis of long-term trial; majority of fractures occurred in the upper arm, hand, and foot (differing from the hip or spine fractures usually associated with postmenopausal osteoporosis). May decrease hemoglobin/hematocrit and/or WBC count (slight); effects may be related to increased plasma volume and/or dose related; use with caution in patients with anemia.

Rosiglitazone has been associated with new onset and/or worsening of macular edema in patients with diabetes. Rosiglitazone should be used with caution in patients with a pre-existing macular edema or diabetic retinopathy. Discontinuation of rosiglitazone should be considered in any patient who reports visual deterioration. In addition, ophthalmological consultation should be initiated in these patients. Use with caution in premenopausal, anovulatory women; may result in resumption of ovulation, increasing the risk of pregnancy. Safety and efficacy in pediatric patients have not been established.

Additional Canadian warnings (not included in U.S. labeling): If glycemic control is inadequate, rosiglitazone may be added to metformin or a sulfonylurea (if metformin use is contraindicated or not tolerated); use of triple therapy (rosiglitazone in combination with both metformin and a sulfonylurea) is not indicated due to increased risks of heart failure and fluid retention.

Drug Interactions

Metabolism/Transport Effects Substrate of CYP2C8 (major), 2C9 (minor); **Inhibits** CYP2C8 (moderate), 2C9 (weak), 2C19 (weak)

Avoid Concomitant Use There are no known interactions where it is recommended to avoid concomitant use.

Increased Effect/Toxicity

Rosiglitazone may increase the levels/effects of: CYP2C8 Substrates (High risk); Hypoglycemic Agents

The levels/effects of Rosiglitazone may be increased by: CYP2C8 Inhibitors (Moderate); CYP2C8 Inhibitors (Strong); Deferasirox; Gemfibrozil; Herbs (Hypoglycemic Properties); Insulin; Pegvisomant; Pregabalin; Trimethoprim; Vasodilators (Organic Nitrates)

Decreased Effect

The levels/effects of Rosiglitazone may be decreased by: Bile Acid Sequestrants; Corticosteroids (Orally Inhaled); Corticosteroids (Systemic); CYP2C8 Inducers (Highly Effective); Luteinizing Hormone-Releasing Hormone Analogs; Rifampin; Somatropin; Thiazide Diuretics

Ethanol/Nutrition/Herb Interactions

Ethanol: Avoid ethanol (may cause hypoglycemia).

Food: Peak concentrations are lower by 28% and delayed when administered with food, but these effects are not believed to be clinically significant.

Herb/Nutraceutical: Avoid alfalfa, aloe, bilberry, bitter melon, burdock, celery, damiana, fenugreek, garcinia, garlic, ginger, ginseng (American), gymnema, marshmallow, stinging nettle (may cause hypoglycemia).

Dietary Considerations Management of type 2 diabetes mellitus (noninsulin dependent, NIDDM) should include diet control. May be taken without regard to meals.

Pharmacodynamics/Kinetics

Onset of Action Delayed; Maximum effect: Up to 12 weeks

Half-life Elimination 3-4 hours

Time to Peak 1 hour; delayed with food

Pregnancy Risk Factor C

Lactation Excretion in breast milk unknown/not recommended

Breast-Feeding Considerations It is not known if rosiglitazone is excreted in breast milk. Breast-feeding is not recommended by the manufacturer.

Prescribing and Access Restrictions Health Canada requires written informed consent for new and current patients receiving rosiglitazone.

Dosage Forms

Tablet, oral:

Avandia®: 2 mg, 4 mg, 8 mg

Rosiglitazone and Glimepiride (roh si GLI ta zone & GLYE me pye ride)

Related Information

Endocrine Disorders and Pregnancy *on page 1879*

Glimepiride *on page 817*

Rosiglitazone *on page 1497*

U.S. Brand Names Avandaryl®

Canadian Brand Names Avandaryl®

Pharmacologic Category Antidiabetic Agent, Sulfonylurea; Antidiabetic Agent, Thiazolidinedione

Use Management of type 2 diabetes mellitus (noninsulin dependent, NIDDM) as an adjunct to diet and exercise

Local Anesthetic/Vasoconstrictor Precautions No information available to require special precautions

Effects on Dental Treatment Dependent patients with diabetes (noninsulin dependent, type 2) should be appointed for dental treatment in the morning in order to minimize chance of stress-induced hypoglycemia.

Effects on Bleeding No information available to require special precautions

Adverse Effects Percentages below refer to combination Avandaryl®. Also see individual agents.

1% to 10%:

Cardiovascular: Edema (3%), hypertension (2% to 3%)

Central nervous system: Headache (3% to 6%)

Endocrine & metabolic: Hypoglycemia (4% to 6%)

Respiratory: Nasopharyngitis (4% to 5%)

General Dosage Range Dosage adjustment recommended in patients with hepatic or renal impairment

Oral:

Adults: Initial: Rosiglitazone 4 mg and glimepiride 1-2 mg once daily; Maintenance: Rosiglitazone 4-8 mg and glimepiride 1-4 mg once daily

Elderly: Initial: Rosiglitazone 4 mg and glimepiride 1 mg once daily

Mechanism of Action

Rosiglitazone is a thiazolidinedione antidiabetic agent that lowers blood glucose by improving target cell response to insulin, without increasing pancreatic insulin secretion. It has a mechanism of action that is dependent on the presence of insulin for activity.

Glimepiride stimulates insulin release from the pancreatic beta cells; reduces glucose output from the liver; insulin sensitivity is increased at peripheral target sites.

Pregnancy Risk Factor C

Prescribing and Access Restrictions Health Canada requires written informed consent for new and current patients receiving rosiglitazone

Rosiglitazone and Metformin (roh si GLI ta zone & met FOR min)

Related Information

Endocrine Disorders and Pregnancy *on page 1879*

MetFORMIN *on page 1089*

Rosiglitazone *on page 1497*

U.S. Brand Names Avandamet®

Canadian Brand Names Avandamet®

Pharmacologic Category Antidiabetic Agent, Biguanide; Antidiabetic Agent, Thiazolidinedione

Use Management of type 2 diabetes mellitus (noninsulin dependent, NIDDM) as an adjunct to diet and exercise in patients where dual rosiglitazone and metformin therapy is appropriate

Local Anesthetic/Vasoconstrictor Precautions No information available to require special precautions

Effects on Dental Treatment Dependent diabetics (noninsulin dependent, type 2) should be appointed for dental treatment in the morning in order to minimize chance of stress-induced hypoglycemia.

Effects on Bleeding No information available to require special precautions

Adverse Effects Also see individual agents. Percentages of adverse effects as reported with the combination product.

>10%:

Central nervous system: Headache (7% to 11%)

Gastrointestinal: Nausea/vomiting (16%), diarrhea (13% to 14%)

Respiratory: Upper respiratory tract infection (9% to 16%)

1% to 10%:

Cardiovascular: Edema (6%)

Central nervous system: Dizziness (8%), fatigue (6%)

Endocrine & metabolic: Hypoglycemia (3%)

Gastrointestinal: Dyspepsia (10%), abdominal pain (5%), loose stools (5%), constipation (5%)

Hematologic: Anemia (4% to 7%)

Neuromuscular & skeletal: Arthralgia (5%), back pain (5%)

Respiratory: Sinusitis (6%), nasopharyngitis (6%)

Miscellaneous: Injury (8%), viral infection (5%), flu-like syndrome (1%)

General Dosage Range Oral: *Adults:* Initial: Rosiglitazone 2 mg and metformin 500 mg once or twice daily; may increase by 2 mg/500 mg per day after 4 weeks (maximum: rosiglitazone 8 mg/day; metformin 2000 mg/day)

Mechanism of Action Rosiglitazone is a thiazolidinedione antidiabetic agent that lowers blood glucose by improving target cell response to insulin, without increasing pancreatic insulin secretion. It has a mechanism of action that is dependent on the presence of insulin for activity. Metformin decreases hepatic glucose production, decreases intestinal absorption of glucose, and improves insulin sensitivity (increases peripheral glucose uptake and utilization).

Pregnancy Risk Factor C

Prescribing and Access Restrictions Health Canada requires written informed consent for new and current patients receiving rosiglitazone.

Rosuvastatin (roe soo va STAT in)

Related Information

Cardiovascular Diseases *on page 1848*

U.S. Brand Names Crestor®

Canadian Brand Names Crestor®

Pharmacologic Category Antilipemic Agent, HMG-CoA Reductase Inhibitor

Use

Treatment of dyslipidemias:

Used with dietary therapy for hyperlipidemias to reduce elevations in total cholesterol (TC), LDL-C, apolipoprotein B, nonHDL-C, and triglycerides (TG) in patients with primary hypercholesterolemia (elevations of 1 or more components are present in Fredrickson type IIa, IIb, and IV hyperlipidemias); increase HDL-C; treatment of primary dysbetalipoproteinemia (Fredrickson type III hyperlipidemia); treatment of homozygous familial hypercholesterolemia (FH); to slow progression of atherosclerosis as an adjunct to diet to lower TC and LDL-C

Heterozygous familial hypercholesterolemia (HeFH): In adolescent patients (10-17 years of age, females >1 year postmenarche) with HeFH having LDL-C >190 mg/dL or LDL >160 mg/dL with positive family history of premature cardiovascular disease (CVD), or ≥2 other CVD risk factors.

Primary prevention of cardiovascular disease: To reduce the risk of stroke, myocardial infarction, or arterial revascularization procedures in patients without clinically evident coronary heart disease or lipid abnormalities but with all of the following: 1) an increased risk of cardiovascular disease based on age ≥50 years old in men and ≥60 years old in women, 2) hsCRP ≥2 mg/L, and 3) the presence of at least one additional cardiovascular disease risk factor such as hypertension, low HDL-C, smoking, or a family history of premature coronary heart disease.

Secondary prevention of cardiovascular disease: To slow progression of atherosclerosis

Local Anesthetic/Vasoconstrictor Precautions No information available to require special precautions

Effects on Dental Treatment No significant effects or complications reported

Effects on Bleeding No information available to require special precautions

Adverse Effects

>10%: Neuromuscular & skeletal: Myalgia (3% to 13%)

2% to 10%:

Central nervous system: Headache (6%), dizziness (4%)

Gastrointestinal: Nausea (3%), abdominal pain (2%), constipation (2%)

Hepatic: ALT increased (2%; >3 times ULN)

Neuromuscular & skeletal: Arthralgia (4% to 10%), CPK increased (3%; >10 x ULN: Children 3%), weakness (3%)

Adverse reactions reported with other HMG-CoA reductase inhibitors (not necessarily reported with rosuvastatin therapy) include a hypersensitivity syndrome (symptoms may include anaphylaxis, angioedema, arthralgia, erythema multiforme, eosinophilia, hemolytic anemia, interstitial lung disease, lupus syndrome, photosensitivity, polymyalgia rheumatica, positive ANA, purpura, Stevens-Johnson syndrome, toxic epidermal necrolysis, urticaria, vasculitis)

General Dosage Range Dosage adjustment recommended in patients with renal impairment, on concomitant therapy, or who develop toxicities

Oral:

Children 10-17 years (females >1 year postmenarche): Initial: 5-20 mg once daily (maximum: 20 mg/day)

Adults: Initial: 5-20 mg once daily; Maintenance: 5-40 mg once daily (maximum: 40 mg/day)

Mechanism of Action Inhibitor of 3-hydroxy-3-methylglutaryl coenzyme A (HMG-CoA) reductase, the rate-limiting enzyme in cholesterol synthesis (reduces the production of mevalonic acid from HMG-CoA); this then results in a compensatory increase in the expression of LDL receptors on hepatocyte membranes and a stimulation of LDL catabolism

Pharmacodynamics/Kinetics

Onset of Action Within 1 week; maximal at 4 weeks

Half-life Elimination 19 hours

Time to Peak Plasma: 3-5 hours

Pregnancy Risk Factor X

Rotavirus Vaccine (ROE ta vye rus vak SEEN)

U.S. Brand Names Rotarix®; RotaTeq®

Canadian Brand Names Rotarix®; RotaTeq®

Pharmacologic Category Vaccine, Live (Viral)

Use Prevention of rotavirus gastroenteritis in infants and children

The Advisory Committee on Immunization Practices (ACIP) recommends routine vaccination of all infants.

Local Anesthetic/Vasoconstrictor Precautions No information available to require special precautions

Effects on Dental Treatment No significant effects or complications reported

Effects on Bleeding No information available to require special precautions

Adverse Effects All serious adverse reactions must be reported to the U.S. Department of Health and Human Services (DHHS) Vaccine Adverse Event Reporting System (VAERS) 1-800-822-7967 or online at https://vaers.hhs.gov/esub/index.

Note: Ranges reported; actual percentage may vary between products.

>10%:

Central nervous system: Fever ≥38.1°C (17% to 43%; equal to or less than placebo), fussiness/irritability (3% to 52%)

Gastrointestinal: Diarrhea (4% to 24%), vomiting (3% to 15%)

Otic: Otitis media (15%)

1% to 10%:

Gastrointestinal: Flatulence (2%)

Respiratory: Nasopharyngitis (7%), bronchospasm (1%)

General Dosage Range Oral:

Infants 6-24 weeks: Rotarix®: A total of two 1 mL doses; the first given at 6 weeks of age and the second dose by 24 weeks of age.

Infants 6-32 weeks: RotaTeq®: A total of three 2 mL doses given at 2, 4, and 6 months of age; the first given at 6-12 weeks of age, followed by subsequent doses at 4-10 week intervals

Mechanism of Action A live vaccine; replicates in the small intestine and promotes active immunity to rotavirus gastroenteritis. Rotarix® is specifically indicated for prevention of rotavirus gastroenteritis caused by serotypes G1, G3, G4, and G9 and RotaTeq® is specifically indicated for prevention of rotavirus gastroenteritis caused by serotypes G1, G2, G3, and G4. However, vaccines may provide immunity to other serotypes.

Pharmacodynamics/Kinetics

Onset of Action Seroconversion:

Rotarix®: Antirotavirus IgA antibodies were noted 1-2 months following completion of the 2-dose series in 77% to 87% of infants.

RotaTeq®: A threefold increase in antirotavirus IgA was noted following completion of the 3-dose regimen in 93% to 100% of infants.

Duration of Action Following administration of rotavirus vaccine, efficacy of protecting against any grade of rotavirus gastroenteritis through two seasons was 70% to 79%.

Pregnancy Risk Factor C

Rufinamide (roo FIN a mide)

U.S. Brand Names Banzel®

Pharmacologic Category Anticonvulsant, Triazole Derivative

Use Adjunctive therapy in the treatment of generalized seizures of Lennox-Gastaut syndrome

Local Anesthetic/Vasoconstrictor Precautions No information available to require special precautions

Effects on Dental Treatment No significant effects or complications reported

Effects on Bleeding No information available to require special precautions

Adverse Effects

>10%:

Cardiovascular: QT shortening (46% to 65%; dose related)

Central nervous system: Headache (16% to 27%), somnolence (11% to 24%), dizziness (3% to 19%), fatigue (9% to 16%)

Gastrointestinal: Vomiting (5% to 17%), nausea (7% to 12%)

1% to 10%:

Central nervous system: Ataxia (4% to 5%), seizure (children 5%), status epilepticus (≤4%), aggression (children 3%), anxiety (adults 3%), attention disturbance (children 3%), hyperactivity (children 3%), vertigo (adults 3%)

Dermatologic: Rash (children 4%), pruritus (children 3%)

Gastrointestinal: Appetite decreased (≥1% to 5%), abdominal pain (3%), constipation (adults 3%), dyspepsia (adults 3%), appetite increased (≥1%)

Hematologic: Leukopenia (≤4%), anemia (≥1%)

Neuromuscular & skeletal: Tremor (adults 6%), back pain (adults 3%), gait disturbance (1% to 3%)

Ocular: Diplopia (4% to 9%), blurred vision (adults 6%), nystagmus (adults 6%)

Otic: Otitis media (children 3%)

Renal: Pollakiuria (≥1%)

Respiratory: Nasopharyngitis (children 5%), bronchitis (children 3%), sinusitis (children 3%)

Miscellaneous: Influenza (children 5%)

General Dosage Range Oral:

Children ≥4 years: Initial: 10 mg/kg/day in 2 equally divided doses (maximum: 45 mg/kg/day or 3200 mg/day)

Adults: Initial: 400-800 mg/day in 2 equally divided doses (maximum: 3200 mg/day)

Mechanism of Action A triazole-derivative antiepileptic whose exact mechanism is unknown. *In vitro*, it prolongs the inactive state of the sodium channels, thereby limiting repetitive firing of sodium-dependent action potentials mediating anticonvulsant effects.

Pharmacodynamics/Kinetics

Half-life Elimination ~6-10 hours

Time to Peak 4-6 hours

Pregnancy Risk Factor C

Saccharomyces boulardii (sak roe MYE sees boo LAR dee)

U.S. Brand Names Florastor® Kids [OTC]; Florastor® [OTC]
Pharmacologic Category Dietary Supplement; Probiotic
Use Promote maintenance of normal microflora in the gastrointestinal tract; used in management of bloating, gas, and diarrhea, particularly to decrease the incidence of diarrhea associated with antibiotic use
Local Anesthetic/Vasoconstrictor Precautions No information available to require special precautions
Effects on Dental Treatment No significant effects or complications reported
Effects on Bleeding No information available to require special precautions
Adverse Effects Frequency not defined.
Gastrointestinal: Constipation, flatulence
Miscellaneous: Thirst
General Dosage Range Oral: *Children and Adults:* 250 mg twice daily
Mechanism of Action *S. boulardii*, a nonpathogenic live yeast probiotic, acts as temporary flora to help re-establish the normal gastrointestinal microflora. May also modulate the immune system by inducing cytokines and suppress pathogenic bacteria growth.
Pharmacodynamics/Kinetics
Onset of Action Yeast cell release from capsules/powder: 30 minutes
Duration of Action Yeast cells cleared in 5-7 days

Sacrosidase (sak ROE si dase)

U.S. Brand Names Sucraid®
Canadian Brand Names Sucraid®
Pharmacologic Category Enzyme, Gastrointestinal
Use Orphan drug: Oral replacement therapy in sucrase deficiency, as seen in congenital sucrase-isomaltase deficiency (CSID)
Local Anesthetic/Vasoconstrictor Precautions No information available to require special precautions
Effects on Dental Treatment No significant effects or complications reported
Effects on Bleeding No information available to require special precautions
Adverse Effects 1% to 10%: Gastrointestinal: Abdominal pain, constipation, diarrhea, nausea, vomiting
General Dosage Range Oral:
Infants and Children ≥5 and <15 kg: 8500 int. units (1 mL) per meal or snack
Children >15 kg and Adults: 17,000 int. units (2 mL) per meal or snack
Mechanism of Action Sacrosidase is a naturally-occurring gastrointestinal enzyme which breaks down the disaccharide sucrose to its monosaccharide components. Hydrolysis is necessary to allow absorption of these nutrients.
Pregnancy Risk Factor C
Prescribing and Access Restrictions Sucraid® is not available in retail pharmacies or via mail-order pharmacies. To obtain the product, please refer to http://www.qolmed.com/sucraid.htm or call 1-866-740-2743.

Salicylic Acid (sal i SIL ik AS id)

U.S. Brand Names Aliclen™; Beta Sal® [OTC]; Clean & Clear® Advantage® Acne Cleanser [OTC]; Clean & Clear® Advantage® Acne Spot Treatment [OTC]; Clean & Clear® Advantage® Invisible Acne Patch [OTC]; Clean & Clear® Advantage® Oil-Free Acne [OTC]; Clean & Clear® Blackhead Clearing Daily Cleansing [OTC]; Clean & Clear® Blackhead Clearing Scrub [OTC]; Clean & Clear® Continuous Control® Acne Wash [OTC]; Clean & Clear® Deep Cleaning [OTC]; Clean & Clear® Dual Action Moisturizer [OTC]; Clean & Clear® Invisible Blemish Treatment [OTC]; Compound W® One Step Invisible Strip [OTC]; Compound W® One Step Wart Remover for Feet [OTC]; Compound W® One-Step Wart Remover for Kids [OTC]; Compound W® One-Step Wart Remover [OTC]; Compound W® [OTC]; Curad® Mediplast® [OTC]; Denorex® Extra Strength Protection 2-in-1 [OTC]; Denorex® Extra Strength Protection [OTC]; Dermarest® Psoriasis Medicated Moisturizer [OTC]; Dermarest® Psoriasis Medicated Scalp Treatment [OTC]; Dermarest® Psoriasis Medicated Shampoo/Conditioner [OTC]; Dermarest® Psoriasis Medicated Skin Treatment [OTC]; Dermarest® Psoriasis Overnight Treatment [OTC]; DHS™ Sal [OTC]; Dr. Scholl's® Callus Removers [OTC]; Dr. Scholl's® Clear Away® One Step Wart Remover [OTC]; Dr. Scholl's® Clear Away® Plantar Wart Remover For Feet [OTC]; Dr. Scholl's® Clear Away® Wart Remover Fast-Acting [OTC]; Dr. Scholl's® Clear Away® Wart Remover Invisible Strips [OTC]; Dr. Scholl's® Clear Away® Wart Remover [OTC]; Dr. Scholl's® Corn Removers [OTC]; Dr. Scholl's®

Corn/Callus Remover [OTC]; Dr. Scholl's® Extra Thick Corn Removers [OTC]; Dr. Scholl's® Extra-Thick Callus Removers [OTC]; Dr. Scholl's® For Her Corn Removers [OTC]; Dr. Scholl's® OneStep Callus Removers [OTC]; Dr. Scholl's® OneStep Corn Removers [OTC]; Dr. Scholl's® Small Corn Removers [OTC]; Dr. Scholl's® Ultra-Thin Corn Removers [OTC]; DuoFilm® [OTC]; Durasal™; Freezone® [OTC]; Fung-O® [OTC]; Gets-It® [OTC]; Gordofilm [OTC]; Hydrisalic® [OTC]; Ionil Plus® [OTC]; Ionil® [OTC]; Keralyt®; Keralyt® [OTC]; LupiCare® Dandruff [OTC]; LupiCare® Psoriasis [OTC]; MG217® Sal-Acid [OTC]; Mosco® Callus & Corn Remover [OTC]; Mosco® One Step Corn Remover [OTC]; Neutrogena® Acne Stress Control [OTC]; Neutrogena® Advanced Solutions™ [OTC]; Neutrogena® Blackhead Eliminating™ 2-in-1 Foaming Pads [OTC]; Neutrogena® Blackhead Eliminating™ Daily Scrub [OTC]; Neutrogena® Blackhead Elinimating™ [OTC]; Neutrogena® Body Clear® [OTC]; Neutrogena® Clear Pore™ Oil-Controlling Astringent [OTC]; Neutrogena® Maximum Strength T/Sal® [OTC]; Neutrogena® Oil-Free Acne Stress Control [OTC]; Neutrogena® Oil-Free Acne Wash 60 Second Mask Scrub [OTC]; Neutrogena® Oil-Free Acne Wash Cream Cleanser [OTC]; Neutrogena® Oil-Free Acne Wash Foam Cleanser [OTC]; Neutrogena® Oil-Free Acne Wash [OTC]; Neutrogena® Oil-Free Acne [OTC]; Neutrogena® Oil-Free Anti-Acne [OTC]; Neutrogena® Rapid Clear® Acne Defense [OTC]; Neutrogena® Rapid Clear® Acne Eliminating [OTC]; Neutrogena® Rapid Clear® [OTC]; OXY® Body Wash [OTC]; OXY® Chill Factor® [OTC]; OXY® Daily Cleansing [OTC]; OXY® Daily [OTC]; OXY® Face Wash [OTC]; OXY® Maximum Daily Cleansing [OTC]; OXY® Maximum [OTC]; OXY® Post-Shave [OTC]; OXY® Spot Treatment [OTC]; OXY® [OTC]; P&S® [OTC]; Palmer's® Skin Success Acne Cleanser [OTC]; Sal-Plant® [OTC]; Salactic® [OTC]; Salex®; Salitop™; Salvax; Scalpicin® Anti-Itch [OTC]; Stridex® Essential Care® [OTC]; Stridex® Facewipes To Go® [OTC]; Stridex® Maximum Strength [OTC]; Stridex® Sensitive Skin [OTC]; Thera-Sal [OTC]; Tinamed® Corn and Callus Remover [OTC]; Tinamed® Wart Remover [OTC]; Trans-Ver-Sal® [OTC]; Wart-Off® Maximum Strength [OTC]; Zapzyt® Acne Wash [OTC]; Zapzyt® Pore Treatment [OTC]

Canadian Brand Names Duofilm®; Duoforte® 27; Occlusal™-HP; Sebcur®; Soluver®; Soluver® Plus; Trans-Plantar®; Trans-Ver-Sal®

Pharmacologic Category Acne Products; Keratolytic Agent; Topical Skin Product, Acne

Use Topically for its keratolytic effect in controlling seborrheic dermatitis or psoriasis of body and scalp, dandruff, and other scaling dermatoses; also used to remove warts, corns, and calluses; acne

Local Anesthetic/Vasoconstrictor Precautions No information available to require special precautions

Effects on Dental Treatment No significant effects or complications reported

Effects on Bleeding No information available to require special precautions

Adverse Effects Frequency not defined.

Central nervous system: Dizziness, mental confusion, headache

Local: Burning and irritation at site of exposure on normal tissue, peeling, scaling

Otic: Tinnitus

Respiratory: Hyperventilation

General Dosage Range Topical: *Children and Adults:* Dosage varies greatly depending on product

Mechanism of Action Produces desquamation of hyperkeratotic epithelium via dissolution of the intercellular cement which causes the cornified tissue to swell, soften, macerate, and desquamate. Salicylic acid is keratolytic at concentrations of 3% to 6%; it becomes destructive to tissue at concentrations >6%. Concentrations of 6% to 60% are used to remove corns and warts and in the treatment of psoriasis and other hyperkeratotic disorders.

Pharmacodynamics/Kinetics

Time to Peak Serum: Within 5 hours of application with occlusion

Pregnancy Risk Factor C

Saliva Substitute (sa LYE va SUB stee tute)

Related Information

Management of Patients Undergoing Cancer Therapy *on page 1970*

Related Sample Prescriptions

Mild/Moderate Oral Pain *on page 1980*

U.S. Brand Names Aquoral™; Caphosol®; Entertainer's Secret® [OTC]; Moi-Stir® [OTC]; Mouthkote® [OTC]; Numoisyn™; Oasis®; Oral Balance® [OTC]; Salivart® [OTC] [DSC]; SalivaSure™ [OTC]

Generic Availability (U.S.) No

Pharmacologic Category Gastrointestinal Agent, Miscellaneous

Dental Use Relief of dry mouth and throat in xerostomia

Use Relief of dry mouth and throat in xerostomia or hyposalivation; adjunct to standard oral care in relief of symptoms associated with chemotherapy or radiation therapy-induced mucositis

Local Anesthetic/Vasoconstrictor Precautions No information available to require special precautions

Effects on Dental Treatment No significant effects or complications reported

Effects on Bleeding No information available to require special precautions

Dosage Adults: Use as needed or product-specific dosing:

Caphosol®:

Mucositis symptoms: Swish and spit 4-10 doses per day (begin at onset of chemo- or radiation therapy)

Xerostomia: Swish and spit 2-10 doses per day

Numoisyn™ liquid: Use 2 mL as needed

Numoisyn™ lozenges: Dissolve 1 slowly; maximum 16 lozenges/day

Oasis® mouthwash: Rinse mouth with ~30 mL twice daily or as needed; do not swallow

Oasis® spray: 1-2 sprays as needed; maximum 60 sprays/day

Oral Balance®: Use after meals, at bedtime and as needed

Mechanism of Action Protein or electrolyte mixtures which restore/replace saliva, lubricate, moisten, and provide a coating on oral mucosa

Drug Interactions

Avoid Concomitant Use There are no known interactions where it is recommended to avoid concomitant use.

Increased Effect/Toxicity There are no known significant interactions involving an increase in effect.

Decreased Effect There are no known significant interactions involving a decrease in effect.

Dietary Considerations Caphosol®: Contains sodium 75 mg/30 mL dose

Dosage Forms

Liquid:

Numoisyn™: Water, sorbitol, linseed extract, *Chondrus crispus*, methylparaben, sodium benzoate, potassium sorbate, dipotassium phosphate, propylparaben

Oral Balance® [OTC]: Water, starch, sunflower oil, propylene glycol, xylitol, glycerine, purified milk extract

Lozenge:

Numoisyn™: Sorbitol 0.3 g/lozenge, polyethylene glycol, malic acid, sodium citrate, calcium phosphate dibasic, hydrogenated cottonseed oil, citric acid, magnesium stearate, silicon dioxide

SalivaSure™ [OTC]: Xylitol, citric acid, apple acid, sodium citrate dihydrate, sodium carboxymethylcellulose, dibasic calcium phosphate, silica colloidal, magnesium stearate, stearic acid

Solution, oral:

Caphosol®: Dibasic sodium phosphate 0.032%, monobasic sodium phosphate 0.009%, calcium chloride 0.052%, sodium chloride 0.569%, purified water

Entertainer's Secret® [OTC]: Sodium carboxymethylcellulose, aloe vera gel, glycerin (60 mL)

Solution, oral [mouthwash/gargle]:

Oasis®: Water, glycerin, sorbitol, poloxamer 338, PEG-60, hydrogenated castor oil, copovidone, sodium benzoate, carboxymethycellulose

Solution, oral [spray]:

Aquoral™: Oxidized glycerol triesters and silicon dioxide

Moi-Stir® [OTC]: Water, sorbitol, sodium carboxymethylcellulose, methylparaben, propylparaben, potassium chloride, dibasic sodium phosphate, calcium chloride, magnesium chloride, sodium chloride

Mouthkote® [OTC]: Water, xylitol, sorbitol, yerba santa, citric acid, ascorbic acid, sodium saccharin, sodium benzoate

Oasis®: Glycerin, cetylpyridinium, copovidone

Salmeterol (sal ME te role)

Related Information

Respiratory Diseases *on page 1876*

U.S. Brand Names Serevent® Diskus®

Canadian Brand Names Serevent® Diskhaler® Disk; Serevent® Diskus®

Pharmacologic Category $Beta_2$-Adrenergic Agonist; $Beta_2$-Adrenergic Agonist, Long-Acting

Use Maintenance treatment of asthma and prevention of bronchospasm (as concomitant therapy) in patients with reversible obstructive airway disease, including patients with symptoms of nocturnal asthma; prevention of exercise-induced bronchospasm (monotherapy may be indicated in patients without persistent asthma); maintenance treatment of bronchospasm associated with COPD

Local Anesthetic/Vasoconstrictor Precautions No information available to require special precautions

Effects on Dental Treatment Key adverse event(s) related to dental treatment: Xerostomia (normal salivary flow resumes upon discontinuation), dental pain, and oropharyngeal candidiasis.

Effects on Bleeding No information available to require special precautions

Adverse Effects

>10%:

Central nervous system: Headache (13% to 17%)

Neuromuscular & skeletal: Pain (1% to 12%)

1% to 10%:

Cardiovascular: Hypertension (4%), edema (1% to 3%), pallor

Central nervous system: Dizziness (4%), sleep disturbance (1% to 3%), fever (1% to 3%), anxiety (1% to 3%), migraine (1% to 3%)

Dermatologic: Rash (1% to 4%), contact dermatitis (1% to 3%), eczema (1% to 3%), urticaria (3%), photodermatitis (1% to 2%)

Endocrine & metabolic: Hyperglycemia (1% to 3%)

Gastrointestinal: Throat irritation (7%), nausea (1% to 3%), dyspepsia (1% to 3%), dental pain (1% to 3%), gastrointestinal infection (1% to 3%), oropharyngeal candidiasis (1% to 3%), xerostomia (1% to 3%)

Hepatic: Liver enzymes increased

Neuromuscular & skeletal: Muscular cramps/spasm (3%), articular rheumatism (1% to 3%), arthralgia (1% to 3%), joint pain (1% to 3%), muscular stiffness (1% to 3%), paresthesia (1% to 3%), rigidity (1% to 3%)

Ocular: Keratitis/conjunctivitis (1% to 3%)

Respiratory: Nasal congestion (4% to 9%), tracheitis/bronchitis (7%), pharyngitis (≤6%), cough (5%), influenza (5%), viral respiratory tract infection (5%), sinusitis (4% to 5%), rhinitis (4% to 5%), asthma (3% to 4%)

General Dosage Range Inhalation: *Children ≥4 years and Adults:* 1 inhalation (50 mcg) twice daily

Mechanism of Action Relaxes bronchial smooth muscle by selective action on beta$_2$-receptors with little effect on heart rate; salmeterol acts locally in the lung.

Pharmacodynamics/Kinetics

Onset of Action Asthma: 30-48 minutes, COPD: 2 hours; Peak effect: Asthma: 3 hours, COPD: 2-5 hours

Duration of Action 12 hours

Half-life Elimination 5.5 hours

Time to Peak Serum: ~20 minutes

Pregnancy Risk Factor C

Salsalate (SAL sa late)

Related Information

Rheumatoid Arthritis, Osteoarthritis, and Osteoporosis *on page 1889*

Temporomandibular Dysfunction (TMD) *on page 1964*

Canadian Brand Names Amigesic®; Salflex®

Generic Availability (U.S.) Yes

Pharmacologic Category Salicylate

Use Treatment of rheumatoid arthritis, osteoarthritis, and related rheumatic disorders

Local Anesthetic/Vasoconstrictor Precautions No information available to require special precautions

Effects on Dental Treatment The dentist should be aware of the potential of abnormal coagulation. Caution should also be exercised in the use of NSAIDs in patients already on anticoagulant therapy with drugs such as warfarin (Coumadin®). See Effects on Bleeding.

Effects on Bleeding Nonacetylated salicylate formulations are known to reversibly decrease platelet aggregation via mechanisms different than observed with aspirin. Caution should also be exercised in the use of NSAIDs in patients already on anticoagulant therapy with drugs such as warfarin (Coumadin®). Unlike most salicylates/NSAIDs, salsalate does not interfere with platelet aggregation and presumably carries less risk of bleeding and/or effect on concurrent warfarin therapy.

With respect to surgery, dental practitioners should note that recommendations differ between general surgery (eg, appendectomy, hip replacement) and dental surgery. NSAIDs should be avoided (if possible) in general surgery patients for 3-5 half-lives of the drug (usually 1-3 days) prior to surgery to reduce the risk of excessive bleeding. However, there is no scientific evidence to warrant discontinuance of NSAIDs prior to dental surgery. In medically complicated patients or extensive oral surgery, the decision to interrupt therapy must be based on the risk to benefit in an individual patient and a medical consult is suggested. Routine interruption of NSAID therapy for most dental procedures is not warranted. If therapy is continued without interruption, the clinician should anticipate the potential for slower clotting times.

Adverse Effects Frequency not defined.

Cardiovascular: Hypotension

Central nervous system: Vertigo

Dermatologic: Angioedema, rash, Stevens-Johnson syndrome, toxic epidermal necrolysis, urticaria

Gastrointestinal: Abdominal pain, diarrhea, GI bleeding, GI perforation, GI ulceration, nausea

Hematologic: Anemia

Hepatic: Hepatitis, liver function abnormal

Otic: Hearing impairment, tinnitus

Renal: Creatinine clearance decreased, nephritis

Respiratory: Bronchospasm

Miscellaneous: Anaphylactic shock

Dosage Oral:

Adults: 3 g/day in 2-3 divided dose

Elderly: May require lower dosage

Mechanism of Action Weakly inhibits cyclooxygenase enzymes, which results in decreased formation of prostaglandin precursors; has antipyretic, analgesic, and anti-inflammatory properties

Other proposed mechanisms not fully elucidated (and possibly contributing to the anti-inflammatory effect to varying degrees) include inhibiting chemotaxis, altering lymphocyte activity, inhibiting neutrophil aggregation/activation, and decreasing proinflammatory cytokine levels.

Contraindications Hypersensitivity to salsalate or any component of the formulation; asthma, urticaria, or allergic reaction to aspirin or NSAIDs; perioperative pain in the setting of coronary artery bypass graft (CABG) surgery

Warnings/Precautions **[U.S. Boxed Warning]: NSAIDs are associated with an increased risk of adverse cardiovascular thrombotic events, including fatal MI and stroke.** Risk may be increased with duration of use or pre-existing cardiovascular risk factors or disease. Carefully evaluate individual cardiovascular risk profiles prior to prescribing. May cause new-onset hypertension or worsening of existing hypertension. Response to ACE inhibitors, thiazides, or loop diuretics may be impaired with concurrent use of NSAIDs. Use caution with fluid retention. Avoid use in heart failure. Concurrent administration of salsalate, and potentially other nonselective NSAIDs, may interfere with aspirin's cardioprotective effect. **[U.S. Boxed Warning]: Use is contraindicated for treatment of perioperative pain in the setting of coronary artery bypass graft (CABG) surgery.** Risk of MI and stroke may be increased with use following CABG surgery. Use the lowest effective dose for the shortest duration of time, consistent with individual patient goals, to reduce risk of cardiovascular or GI adverse events. Alternate therapies should be considered for patients at high risk.

NSAID use may compromise existing renal function; dose-dependent decreases in prostaglandin synthesis may result from NSAID use, reducing renal blood flow which may cause renal decompensation. Patients with impaired renal function, dehydration, heart failure, liver dysfunction, those taking diuretics, and ACE inhibitors, and the elderly are at greater risk of renal toxicity. Rehydrate patient before starting therapy; monitor renal function closely. Not recommended for use in patients with advanced renal disease. Long-term NSAID use may result in renal papillary necrosis.

[U.S. Boxed Warning]: NSAIDs may increase risk of gastrointestinal irritation, inflammation, ulceration, bleeding, and perforation. These events may occur at any time during therapy and without warning. Use caution with a history of GI disease (bleeding or ulcers), concurrent therapy with aspirin, anticoagulants and/or corticosteroids, smoking, use of ethanol, the elderly or debilitated patients. When used concomitantly with ≤325 mg of aspirin, a substantial increase in the risk of gastrointestinal complications (eg, ulcer) occurs; concomitant gastroprotective therapy (eg, proton pump inhibitors) is recommended (Bhatt, 2008).

Use with caution in patients with platelet and bleeding disorders.

NSAIDs may cause serious skin adverse events including exfoliative dermatitis, Stevens-Johnson Syndrome (SJS) and toxic epidermal necrolysis (TEN); discontinue use at first sign of skin rash or hypersensitivity. Patients with sensitivity to tartrazine dyes, nasal polyps, and asthma may have an increased risk of salicylate sensitivity. Anaphylactoid reactions may occur, even without prior exposure; patients with "aspirin triad" (bronchial asthma, aspirin intolerance, rhinitis) may be at increased risk. Do not use in patients who experience bronchospasm, asthma, rhinitis, or urticaria with NSAID or aspirin therapy. Use caution in other forms of asthma.

Use with caution in patients with decreased hepatic function. Closely monitor patients with any abnormal LFT. Severe hepatic reactions (eg, fulminant hepatitis, liver failure) have occurred with NSAID use, rarely; discontinue if signs or symptoms of liver disease develop, or if systemic manifestations occur.

Children and teenagers who have or are recovering from chickenpox or flu-like symptoms should not use this product. Changes in behavior (along with nausea and vomiting) may be an early sign of Reye's syndrome; patients should be instructed to contact their healthcare provider if these occur.

Drug Interactions

Avoid Concomitant Use

Avoid concomitant use of Salsalate with any of the following: Influenza Virus Vaccine (Live/Attenuated)

Increased Effect/Toxicity

Salsalate may increase the levels/effects of: Anticoagulants; Carbonic Anhydrase Inhibitors; Corticosteroids (Systemic); Divalproex; Drotrecogin Alfa; Methotrexate; PRALAtrexate; Salicylates; Sulfonylureas; Thrombolytic Agents; Valproic Acid; Varicella Virus-Containing Vaccines

The levels/effects of Salsalate may be increased by: Antiplatelet Agents; Calcium Channel Blockers (Nondihydropyridine); Ginkgo Biloba; Herbs (Anticoagulant/Antiplatelet Properties); Influenza Virus Vaccine (Live/Attenuated); Loop Diuretics; NSAID (Nonselective); Treprostinil

Decreased Effect

Salsalate may decrease the levels/effects of: ACE Inhibitors; Loop Diuretics; NSAID (Nonselective); Probenecid

The levels/effects of Salsalate may be decreased by: Corticosteroids (Systemic); NSAID (Nonselective)

Ethanol/Nutrition/Herb Interactions

Ethanol: Avoid ethanol (may enhance gastric mucosal irritation).

Food: Salsalate peak serum levels may be delayed if taken with food.

Herb/Nutraceutical: Avoid cat's claw, dong quai, evening primrose, feverfew, garlic, ginger, ginkgo, red clover, horse chestnut, green tea, ginseng (all have additional antiplatelet activity).

Dietary Considerations May be taken with food to decrease GI distress.

Pharmacodynamics/Kinetics

Onset of Action Therapeutic: 3-4 days of continuous dosing

Half-life Elimination 7-8 hours

Pregnancy Risk Factor C

Lactation Enters breast milk/use caution

Breast-Feeding Considerations Salsalate is metabolized to salicylate which is contraindicated while breast-feeding.

Dosage Forms

Tablet, oral: 500 mg, 750 mg

Sapropterin (sap roe TER in)

U.S. Brand Names Kuvan™

Pharmacologic Category Enzyme Cofactor

Use Adjunct to dietary management in the treatment of tetrahydrobiopterin (BH4) responsive phenylketonuria (PKU)

Local Anesthetic/Vasoconstrictor Precautions No information available to require special precautions

Effects on Dental Treatment No significant effects or complications reported

Effects on Bleeding No information available to require special precautions

Adverse Effects

>10%:

Central nervous system: Headache (15%)

Respiratory: Rhinorrhea (11%)

1% to 10%:

Gastrointestinal: Diarrhea (8%), vomiting (8%), nausea

Dermatologic: Bruising (5%)

Hematologic: Neutropenia (4%)

Respiratory: Pharyngolaryngeal pain (10%), cough (7%), nasal congestion (4%)

General Dosage Range Oral: *Children ≥4 years and Adults:* 10 mg/kg once daily; Maintenance range: 5-20 mg/kg/day

Mechanism of Action Sapropterin is a synthetic form of the cofactor BH4 (tetrahydrobiopterin) for the enzyme phenylalanine hydroxylase (PAH). PAH hydroxylates phenylalanine to form tyrosine. BH4 activates residual PAH enzyme, improving normal phenylalanine metabolism and decreasing phenylalanine levels in sapropterin responders.

Pharmacodynamics/Kinetics

Onset of Action Within 24 hours; maximum effect: 1-2 months

Duration of Action 24 hours

Half-life Elimination ~7 hours (range: 4-17 hours)

Pregnancy Risk Factor C

Saquinavir (sa KWIN a veer)

Related Information

HIV Infection and AIDS *on page 1883*

U.S. Brand Names Invirase®

Canadian Brand Names Invirase®

Pharmacologic Category Antiretroviral Agent, Protease Inhibitor

Use Treatment of HIV infection; used in combination with at least two other antiretroviral agents

Local Anesthetic/Vasoconstrictor Precautions No information available to require special precautions

Effects on Dental Treatment Key adverse event(s) related to dental treatment: Buccal mucosa ulceration and taste alteration.

Effects on Bleeding Increased bleeding has been noted with protease inhibitors in patients with hemophilia A or B. No information available to require routine special precautions relative to hemostasis in other patients.

Adverse Effects

Incidence data shown for saquinavir soft gel capsule formulation (no longer available) in combination with ritonavir.

10%: Gastrointestinal: Nausea (11%)

1% to 10%:

Cardiovascular: Chest pain

Central nervous system: Fatigue (6%), fever (3%), anxiety, depression, headache, insomnia, pain

Dermatologic: Pruritus (3%), rash (3%), dry lips/skin (2%), eczema (2%), verruca

Endocrine & metabolic: Lipodystrophy (5%), hyperglycemia (3%), hypoglycemia, hyperkalemia, libido disorder, serum amylase increased

Gastrointestinal: Diarrhea (8%), vomiting (7%), abdominal pain (6%), constipation (2%), abdominal discomfort, appetite decreased, buccal mucosa ulceration, dyspepsia, flatulence, taste alteration

Hepatic: AST increased, ALT increased, bilirubin increased

Neuromuscular & skeletal: Back pain (2%), CPK increased, paresthesia, weakness

Renal: Creatinine kinase increased

Respiratory: Pneumonia (5%), bronchitis (3%), sinusitis (3%)

Miscellaneous: Influenza (3%)

Incidence not currently defined (limited to significant reactions; reported for hard or soft gel capsule with/without ritonavir)

Cardiovascular: Cyanosis, heart valve disorder (including murmur), hyper-/hypotension, peripheral vasoconstriction, prolonged QT interval, prolonged PR interval, syncope, thrombophlebitis

Central nervous system: Agitation, amnesia, ataxia, confusion, hallucination, hyper-/hyporeflexia, myelopolyradiculoneuritis, neuropathies, poliomyelitis, progressive multifocal encephalopathy, psychosis, seizures, somnolence, speech disorder, suicide attempt

Dermatologic: Alopecia, bullous eruption, dermatitis, erythema, maculopapular rash, photosensitivity, Stevens-Johnson syndrome, skin ulceration, urticaria

Endocrine & metabolic: Dehydration, diabetes, electrolyte changes, TSH increased

Gastrointestinal: Ascites, colic, dysphagia, esophagitis, bloody stools, gastritis, intestinal obstruction, hemorrhage (rectal), pancreatitis, stomatitis

Genitourinary: impotence, prostate enlarged, hematuria, UTI

Hematologic; Acute myeloblastic leukemia, anemia (including hemolytic), leukopenia, neutropenia, pancytopenia, splenomegaly, thrombocytopenia

Hepatic: Alkaline phosphatase increased, GGT increased, hepatitis, hepatomegaly, hepatosplenomegaly, jaundice, liver disease exacerbation

Neuromuscular & skeletal: Arthritis, LDH increased

Ocular: Blepharitis, visual disturbance

Otic: Otitis, hearing decreased, tinnitus

Renal: Nephrolithiasis, renal calculus

Respiratory: Dyspnea, hemoptysis, pharyngitis, upper respiratory tract infection
Miscellaneous: Infections (bacterial, fungal, viral)

General Dosage Range Dosage adjustment recommended in patients on concomitant therapy

Oral: *Children >16 years and Adults:* 1000 mg twice daily

Mechanism of Action Binds to the site of HIV-1 protease activity and inhibits cleavage of viral Gag-Pol polyprotein precursors into individual functional proteins required for infectious HIV. This results in the formation of immature, noninfectious viral particles.

Pregnancy Risk Factor B

Sargramostim (sar GRAM oh stim)

U.S. Brand Names Leukine®

Canadian Brand Names Leukine®

Pharmacologic Category Colony Stimulating Factor

Use

Acute myelogenous leukemia (AML) following induction chemotherapy in older adults (≥55 years of age) to shorten time to neutrophil recovery and to reduce the incidence of severe and life-threatening infections and infections resulting in death

Bone marrow transplant (allogeneic or autologous) failure or engraftment delay

Myeloid reconstitution after allogeneic bone marrow transplantation

Myeloid reconstitution after autologous bone marrow transplantation: Non-Hodgkin's lymphoma (NHL), acute lymphoblastic leukemia (ALL), Hodgkin's lymphoma

Peripheral stem cell transplantation: Mobilization and myeloid reconstitution following autologous peripheral stem cell transplantation

Local Anesthetic/Vasoconstrictor Precautions No information available to require special precautions

Effects on Dental Treatment Key adverse event(s) related to dental treatment: Dysphagia.

Effects on Bleeding No information available to require special precautions. Medical consultation may be considered to confirm adequate platelet counts.

Adverse Effects

>10%:

Cardiovascular: Hypertension (34%), pericardial effusion (4% to 25%), edema (13% to 25%), chest pain (15%), peripheral edema (11%), tachycardia (11%)

Central nervous system: Fever (81%), malaise (57%), headache (26%), chills (25%), anxiety (11%), insomnia (11%)

Dermatologic: Rash (44%), pruritus (23%)

Endocrine & metabolic: Hyperglycemia (25%), hypercholesterolemia (17%), hypomagnesemia (15%)

Gastrointestinal: Diarrhea (≤89%), nausea (58% to 70%), vomiting (46% to 70%), abdominal pain (38%), weight loss (37%), anorexia (13%), hematemesis (13%), dysphagia (11%), gastrointestinal hemorrhage (11%)

Genitourinary: Urinary tract disorder (14%)

Hepatic: Hyperbilirubinemia (30%)

Neuromuscular & skeletal: Weakness (66%), bone pain (21%), arthralgia (11% to 21%) myalgia (18%)

Ocular: Eye hemorrhage (11%)

Renal: BUN increased (23%), serum creatinine increased (15%)

Respiratory: Pharyngitis (23%), epistaxis (17%), dyspnea (15%)

1% to 10%: Respiratory: Pleural effusion (1%)

General Dosage Range

I.V.: *Children and Adults:* Infusion: 250 mcg/m^2/day (maximum: 500 mcg/m^2/day)

SubQ: *Children and Adults:* 250 mcg/m^2 once daily

Mechanism of Action Stimulates proliferation, differentiation and functional activity of neutrophils, eosinophils, monocytes, and macrophages, as indicated.

Pharmacodynamics/Kinetics

Onset of Action Increase in WBC: 7-14 days

Duration of Action WBCs return to baseline within 1 week of discontinuing drug

Half-life Elimination I.V.: 60 minutes; SubQ: 2.7 hours

Time to Peak Serum: SubQ: 1-3 hours

Pregnancy Risk Factor C

Saxagliptin (sax a GLIP tin)

Related Information

Endocrine Disorders and Pregnancy *on page 1879*

U.S. Brand Names Onglyza™

Canadian Brand Names Onglyza™

Generic Availability (U.S.) No

Pharmacologic Category Antidiabetic Agent, Dipeptidyl Peptidase IV (DPP-IV) Inhibitor

Use Treatment of type 2 diabetes mellitus (noninsulin dependent, NIDDM) as an adjunct to diet and exercise as monotherapy or in combination therapy with other antidiabetic agents to improve glycemic control

Local Anesthetic/Vasoconstrictor Precautions No information available to require special precautions

Effects on Dental Treatment Key adverse event(s) related to dental treatment: Saxagliptin dependent patients with diabetes should be appointed for dental treatment in the morning in order to minimize chance of stress-induced hypoglycemia.

Effects on Bleeding No information available to require special precautions

Adverse Effects Note: Frequencies and adverse reactions reported with monotherapy unless otherwise noted.

1% to 10%:

- Cardiovascular: Peripheral edema (≤4%; incidence increased in conjunction with thiazolidinediones: ≤8%)
- Central nervous system: Headache (7%)
- Endocrine & metabolic: Hypoglycemia (≤6%; incidence increased in conjunction with insulin secretagogues: ≤15%)
- Gastrointestinal: Abdominal pain (2%), gastroenteritis (2%), vomiting (2%)
- Genitourinary: Urinary tract infection (7%)
- Hematologic: Lymphopenia (≤2%; dose related)
- Respiratory: Sinusitis (3%)
- Miscellaneous: Hypersensitivity reactions (2%; including urticaria and facial edema)

Dosage Oral: Adults: Type 2 diabetes: 2.5-5 mg once daily

Concomitant use with strong CYP3A4/5 inhibitors: 2.5 mg once daily

Concomitant use with insulin secretagogues: Reduced dose of the insulin secretagogue (eg, sulfonylurea) may be needed

Dosage adjustment in renal impairment:

Note: Renal function may be estimated using the Cockcroft-Gault formula or the MDRD formula for dosage adjustment purposes.

Cl_{cr} >50 mL/minute: No adjustment required

Cl_{cr} ≤50 mL/minute: 2.5 mg once daily

ESRD requiring hemodialysis: 2.5 mg once daily; administer postdialysis

Peritoneal dialysis: Not studied

Dosage adjustment in hepatic impairment: No dosage adjustment required

Mechanism of Action Saxagliptin inhibits dipeptidyl peptidase IV (DPP-IV) enzyme resulting in prolonged active incretin levels. Incretin hormones (eg, glucagon-like peptide-1 [GLP-1] and glucose-dependent insulinotropic polypeptide [GIP]) regulate glucose homeostasis by increasing insulin synthesis and release from pancreatic beta cells and decreasing glucagon secretion from pancreatic alpha cells. Decreased glucagon secretion results in decreased hepatic glucose production. Under normal physiologic circumstances, incretin hormones are released by the intestine throughout the day and levels are increased in response to a meal; incretin hormones are rapidly inactivated by the DPP-IV enzyme.

Contraindications There are no contraindications listed within the manufacturer's labeling.

Warnings/Precautions Use with caution in patients with moderate-to-severe renal dysfunction, end-stage renal disease (ESRD) requiring hemodialysis, and in patients taking strong CYP3A4/5 inhibitors (eg, atazanavir, clarithromycin, indinavir, itraconazole, nefazodone, nelfinavir, ritonavir, saquinavir, telithromycin [also see Drug Interactions]); dosing adjustment required. Use caution when used in conjunction with insulin secretagogues (eg, sulfonylureas); risk of hypoglycemia is increased. Monitor blood glucose closely; dosage adjustments of the insulin secretagogue may be necessary.

Drug Interactions

Metabolism/Transport Effects Substrate of CYP3A4 (major), P-glycoprotein

Avoid Concomitant Use There are no known interactions where it is recommended to avoid concomitant use.

Increased Effect/Toxicity

Saxagliptin may increase the levels/effects of: ACE Inhibitors; Hypoglycemic Agents

The levels/effects of Saxagliptin may be increased by: CYP3A4 Inhibitors (Moderate); CYP3A4 Inhibitors (Strong); Dasatinib; Herbs (Hypoglycemic Properties); Pegvisomant; P-Glycoprotein Inhibitors

Decreased Effect

The levels/effects of Saxagliptin may be decreased by: Corticosteroids (Orally Inhaled); Corticosteroids (Systemic); CYP3A4 Inducers; Luteinizing Hormone-Releasing Hormone Analogs; P-Glycoprotein Inducers; Somatropin; Thiazide Diuretics; Tocilizumab

Dietary Considerations May be taken without regard to meals.

Pharmacodynamics/Kinetics

Duration of Action 24 hours

Half-life Elimination Saxagliptin: 2.5 hours; 5-hydroxy saxagliptin: 3.1 hours

Time to Peak Plasma: Saxagliptin: 2 hours; 5-hydroxy saxagliptin: 4 hours

Pregnancy Risk Factor B

Lactation Excretion in breast milk unknown/use caution

Dosage Forms

Tablet, oral:

Onglyza™: 2.5 mg, 5 mg

Saxagliptin and Metformin (sax a GLIP tin & met FOR min)

Related Information

MetFORMIN *on page 1089*

Saxagliptin *on page 1512*

U.S. Brand Names Kombiglyze™ XR

Pharmacologic Category Antidiabetic Agent, Biguanide; Antidiabetic Agent, Dipeptidyl Peptidase IV (DPP-IV) Inhibitor

Use Management of type 2 diabetes mellitus (noninsulin dependent, NIDDM) as an adjunct to diet and exercise when treatment with both saxagliptin and metformin is appropriate

Local Anesthetic/Vasoconstrictor Precautions No information available to require special precautions

Effects on Dental Treatment Key adverse event(s) related to dental treatment: Saxagliptin- and metformin-dependent patients with diabetes should be appointed for dental treatment in the morning in order to minimize chance of stress-induced hypoglycemia.

Effects on Bleeding No information available to require special precautions

Adverse Effects See individual agents.

General Dosage Range Dosage adjustment recommended in patients on concomitant therapy

Oral: *Adults:* Saxagliptin 2.5-5 mg and metformin 500-2000 mg once daily (maximum: 5 mg/day [saxagliptin], 2000 mg/day [metformin])

Mechanism of Action

Saxagliptin inhibits dipeptidyl peptidase IV (DPP-IV) enzyme resulting in prolonged active incretin levels. Incretin hormones (eg, glucagon-like peptide-1 [GLP-1] and glucose-dependent insulinotropic polypeptide [GIP]) regulate glucose homeostasis by increasing insulin synthesis and release from pancreatic beta cells and decreasing glucagon secretion from pancreatic alpha cells. Decreased glucagon secretion results in decreased hepatic glucose production. Under normal physiologic circumstances, incretin hormones are released by the intestine throughout the day and levels are increased in response to a meal; incretin hormones are rapidly inactivated by the DPP-IV enzyme.

Metformin decreases hepatic glucose production, decreasing intestinal absorption of glucose and improves insulin sensitivity (increases peripheral glucose uptake and utilization).

Pregnancy Risk Factor B

Scopolamine (Systemic) (skoe POL a mee)

U.S. Brand Names Scopace™; Transderm Scōp®

Canadian Brand Names Buscopan®; Transderm-V®

Pharmacologic Category Anticholinergic Agent

Use

Scopolamine base: Transdermal: Prevention of nausea/vomiting associated with motion sickness and recovery from anesthesia and surgery

Scopolamine hydrobromide:

Injection: Preoperative medication to produce amnesia, sedation, tranquilization, antiemetic effects, and decrease salivary and respiratory secretions

Oral: Symptomatic treatment of postencephalitic parkinsonism and paralysis agitans; in spastic states; inhibits excessive motility and hypertonus of the gastrointestinal tract in such conditions as the irritable colon syndrome, mild dysentery, diverticulitis, pylorospasm, and cardiospasm

Scopolamine butylbromide [not available in the U.S.]: Oral/injection: Treatment of smooth muscle spasm of the genitourinary or gastrointestinal tract; injection may also be used to prior to radiological/diagnostic procedures to prevent spasm

Local Anesthetic/Vasoconstrictor Precautions No information available to require special precautions

Effects on Dental Treatment Key adverse event(s) related to dental treatment: Significant xerostomia (normal salivary flow resumes upon discontinuation), dry throat (transdermal), and dysphagia.

Effects on Bleeding No information available to require special precautions

Adverse Effects Frequency not defined.

Cardiovascular: Orthostatic hypotension, ventricular fibrillation, tachycardia, palpitation

Central nervous system: Confusion, drowsiness, headache, loss of memory, ataxia, fatigue

Dermatologic: Dry skin, photosensitivity increased, rash

Endocrine & metabolic: Decreased flow of breast milk

Gastrointestinal: Constipation, xerostomia, dry throat, dysphagia, bloated feeling, nausea, vomiting

Genitourinary: Dysuria

Local: Irritation at injection site

Neuromuscular & skeletal: Weakness

Ocular: Increased intraocular pain, blurred vision

Respiratory: Dry nose

Miscellaneous: Diaphoresis decreased

General Dosage Range

I.M., I.V., SubQ:

Children 6 months to 3 years: 0.1-0.15 mg

Children 3-6 years: 0.2-0.3 mg

Adults: 0.3-0.65 mg (single dose) **or** 0.6 mg 3-4 times/day

Oral: *Adults:* 0.4-0.8 mg as a single dose or every 8-12 hours as needed

Transdermal: *Adults:* Apply 1 patch every 3 days as needed

Mechanism of Action Blocks the action of acetylcholine at parasympathetic sites in smooth muscle, secretory glands and the CNS; increases cardiac output, dries secretions, antagonizes histamine and serotonin

Pharmacodynamics/Kinetics

Onset of Action Oral, I.M.: 0.5-1 hour; I.V.: 10 minutes

Peak effect: 20-60 minutes; may take 3-7 days for full recovery; transdermal: 24 hours

Duration of Action Oral, I.M.: 4-6 hours; I.V.: 2 hours

Half-life Elimination Hyoscine-N-butylbromide: 4.8 hours; Scopolamine: 9.5 hours

Pregnancy Risk Factor C

Secobarbital (see koe BAR bi tal)

U.S. Brand Names Seconal®

Pharmacologic Category Barbiturate

Use Preanesthetic agent; short-term treatment of insomnia

Local Anesthetic/Vasoconstrictor Precautions No information available to require special precautions

Effects on Dental Treatment No significant effects or complications reported

Effects on Bleeding No information available to require special precautions

Adverse Effects Frequency not defined.

Cardiovascular: Hypotension

Central nervous system: Dizziness, lightheadedness, "hangover" effect, drowsiness, CNS depression, fever, confusion, mental depression, unusual excitement, nervousness, faint feeling, headache, insomnia, nightmares, hallucinations

Dermatologic: Exfoliative dermatitis, rash, Stevens-Johnson syndrome

Gastrointestinal: Nausea, vomiting, constipation

Hematologic: Agranulocytosis, megaloblastic anemia, thrombocytopenia, thrombophlebitis, urticaria

Local: Pain at injection site

Respiratory: Apnea, laryngospasm, respiratory depression

General Dosage Range Oral:
Children: 2-6 mg/kg 1-2 hours before procedure (maximum: 100 mg/dose) **or** 6 mg/kg/day divided every 8 hours
Adults: 100-200 mg at bedtime **or** 100-300 mg 1-2 hours before procedure
Mechanism of Action Depresses CNS activity by binding to barbiturate site at GABA-receptor complex enhancing GABA activity, depressing reticular activity system; higher doses may be gabamimetic
Pharmacodynamics/Kinetics
Onset of Action Onset of hypnosis: 15-30 minutes
Duration of Action 3-4 hours with 100 mg dose
Half-life Elimination 15-40 hours, mean: 28 hours
Time to Peak Serum: Within 2-4 hours
Pregnancy Risk Factor D
Controlled Substance C-II

Secretin (SEE kr tin)

U.S. Brand Names ChiRhoStim®
Pharmacologic Category Diagnostic Agent
Use Secretin-stimulation testing to aid in diagnosis of pancreatic exocrine dysfunction; diagnosis of gastrinoma (Zollinger-Ellison syndrome); facilitation of endoscopic retrograde cholangiopancreatography (ERCP) visualization
Local Anesthetic/Vasoconstrictor Precautions No information available to require special precautions
Effects on Dental Treatment No significant effects or complications reported
Effects on Bleeding No information available to require special precautions
Adverse Effects 1% to 10%:
Cardiovascular: Flushing (1%)
Gastrointestinal: Nausea (1% to 2%), abdominal discomfort (≤1%), abdominal pain (≤1%), vomiting (≤1%)
Miscellaneous: Bleeding (sphincterectomy, 1%)
General Dosage Range I.V.: *Adults:* Test dose: 0.1 mL (0.2-0.4 mcg); Diagnostic dose: 0.2-0.4 mcg/kg
Mechanism of Action Human and porcine secretin are both synthetically derived products and are equally potent on an osmolar basis. Secretin is a hormone which is normally secreted by duodenal mucosa and upper jejunal mucosa. It increases the volume and bicarbonate content of pancreatic juice; stimulates the flow of hepatic bile with a high bicarbonate concentration; stimulates gastrin release in patients with Zollinger-Ellison syndrome.
Pharmacodynamics/Kinetics
Onset of Action Peak output of pancreatic secretions: ~30 minutes
Duration of Action Human: 1.5-2 hours; Porcine: 1-1.5 hours
Half-life Elimination Human: 45 minutes; Porcine: 27 minutes
Pregnancy Risk Factor C

Selegiline (se LE ji leen)

U.S. Brand Names Eldepryl®; Emsam®; Zelapar®
Canadian Brand Names Apo-Selegiline®; Gen-Selegiline; Mylan-Selegiline; Novo-Selegiline; Nu-Selegiline
Pharmacologic Category Anti-Parkinson's Agent, MAO Type B Inhibitor; Antidepressant, Monoamine Oxidase Inhibitor
Use Adjunct in the management of parkinsonian patients in which levodopa/carbidopa therapy is deteriorating (oral products); treatment of major depressive disorder (transdermal product)
Unlabeled/Investigational Use Early Parkinson's disease; attention-deficit/hyperactivity disorder (ADHD); negative symptoms of schizophrenia; extrapyramidal symptoms
Local Anesthetic/Vasoconstrictor Precautions Selegiline in doses of 10 mg a day or less does not inhibit type-A MAO. Therefore, there are no precautions with the use of vasoconstrictors.
Effects on Dental Treatment Key adverse event(s) related to dental treatment: Xerostomia and changes in salivation (normal salivary flow resumes upon discontinuation). Anticholinergic side effects can cause a reduction of saliva production or secretion, contributing to discomfort and dental disease (ie, caries, oral candidiasis, and periodontal disease).
Orally disintegrating tablet: Dysphagia, tooth disorder, stomatitis, and taste perversion.
Effects on Bleeding No information available to require special precautions

Adverse Effects Unless otherwise noted, the percentage of adverse events is reported for the transdermal patch (**Note:** ODT = orally disintegrating tablet, Oral = capsule/tablet)

>10%:
- Central nervous system: Headache (18%; ODT 7%; oral 2%), insomnia (12%; ODT 7%), dizziness (ODT 11%; oral 7%)
- Gastrointestinal: Nausea (ODT 11%; oral 10%)
- Local: Application site reaction (24%)

1% to 10%:
- Cardiovascular: Hypotension (including postural 3% to 10%), chest pain (≥1%; ODT 2%), hypertension (≥1%), peripheral edema (≥1%)
- Central nervous system: Pain (ODT 8%), hallucinations (ODT 4%; oral 3%), confusion (ODT 4%; oral 3%), headache (ODT 7%; oral 2%), ataxia (ODT 3%), somnolence (ODT 3%), agitation (≥1%), amnesia (≥1%), paresthesia (≥1%), thinking abnormal (≥1%), depression (<1%; ODT 2%)
- Dermatologic: Rash (4%), ecchymosis (ODT 2%), bruising (≥1%), pruritus (≥1%), acne (≥1%)
- Endocrine & metabolic: Weight loss (5%), hypokalemia (ODT 2%), sexual side effects (≤1%)
- Gastrointestinal: Diarrhea (9%; ODT 2%), xerostomia (8%; ODT 4%), stomatitis (ODT 5%), abdominal pain (oral 4%), dyspepsia (4%; ODT 5%), constipation (≥1%; ODT 4%), flatulence (≥1%; ODT 2%), anorexia (≥1%), gastroenteritis (≥1%), taste perversion (≥1%; ODT 2%), vomiting (≥1%; ODT 3%), tooth disorder (ODT 2%), dysphagia (ODT 2%)
- Genitourinary: Dysmenorrhea (≥1%), metrorrhagia (≥1%), UTI (≥1%), urinary frequency (≥1%)
- Neuromuscular & skeletal: Dyskinesia (ODT 6%), back pain (ODT 5%), ataxia (<1%; ODT 3%), leg cramps (ODT 3%), myalgia (≥1%; ODT 3%), neck pain (≥1%), tremor (<1%; ODT 3%)
- Otic: Tinnitus (≥1%)
- Respiratory: Rhinitis (ODT 7%), pharyngitis (3%; ODT 4%), sinusitis (3%), cough (≥1%), bronchitis (≥1%), dyspnea (<1%; ODT 3%)
- Miscellaneous: Diaphoresis (≥1%)

General Dosage Range

Oral:

Capsule/Tablet:
- *Adults:* 10 mg/day in 1-2 divided doses
- *Elderly:* Initial: 5 mg once daily; Maintenance: 5-10 mg once daily

Disintegrating tablet: *Adults:* Initial 1.25 mg daily for at least 6 weeks; Maintenance: 1.25-2.5 mg daily (maximum: 2.5 mg daily)

Transdermal:
- *Adults:* Initial: 6 mg once daily; Maintenance: 6-12 mg once daily (maximum: 12 mg/day)
- *Elderly:* 6 mg once daily

Mechanism of Action Potent, irreversible inhibitor of monoamine oxidase (MAO). Plasma concentrations achieved via administration of oral dosage forms in recommended doses confer selective inhibition of MAO type B, which plays a major role in the metabolism of dopamine; selegiline may also increase dopaminergic activity by interfering with dopamine reuptake at the synapse. When administered transdermally in recommended doses, selegiline achieves higher blood levels and effectively inhibits both MAO-A and MAO-B, which blocks catabolism of other centrally-active biogenic amine neurotransmitters.

Pharmacodynamics/Kinetics

Onset of Action Therapeutic: Oral: Within 1 hour

Duration of Action Oral: 24-72 hours

Half-life Elimination 18-25 hours

Pregnancy Risk Factor C

Selenium (se LEE nee um)

Related Information

Trace Metals *on page 1655*

U.S. Brand Names SE Aspartate [OTC]; Se-100 [OTC]; Selenicaps; Selenimin

Pharmacologic Category Trace Element, Parenteral

Use Trace metal supplement

Local Anesthetic/Vasoconstrictor Precautions No information available to require special precautions

Effects on Dental Treatment No significant effects or complications reported

Effects on Bleeding No information available to require special precautions

Adverse Effects Frequency not defined.
Central nervous system: Lethargy
Dermatologic: Alopecia or hair discoloration
Gastrointestinal: Abdominal pain, garlic breath, vomiting following long-term use on damaged skin
Local: Irritation
Neuromuscular & skeletal: Tremor
Miscellaneous: Diaphoresis

General Dosage Range I.V.:
Children: 3 mcg/kg/day added to TPN
Adults: Metabolically stable: 20-40 mcg/day added to TPN; Deficiency from prolonged TPN support: 100 mcg/day

Mechanism of Action Part of glutathione peroxidase which protects cell components from oxidative damage due to peroxidases produced in cellular metabolism

Pregnancy Risk Factor C

Senna (SEN na)

U.S. Brand Names Black Draught® [OTC]; Evac-U-Gen® [OTC]; ex-lax® Maximum Strength [OTC]; ex-lax® [OTC]; Fleet® Pedia-Lax™ Quick Dissolve [OTC]; Fletcher's® [OTC]; Little Tummys® Laxative [OTC]; Perdiem® Overnight Relief [OTC]; Senexon [OTC]; SennaGen [OTC]; Senokot® [OTC]

Pharmacologic Category Laxative, Stimulant

Use Short-term treatment of constipation; evacuate the colon for bowel or rectal examinations

Local Anesthetic/Vasoconstrictor Precautions No information available to require special precautions

Effects on Dental Treatment No significant effects or complications reported

Effects on Bleeding No information available to require special precautions

Adverse Effects Frequency not defined: Gastrointestinal: Abdominal cramps, diarrhea, nausea, vomiting

General Dosage Range Oral:
Children 2-6 years: Initial: 3.75 mg once daily; Maintenance: 3.75-15 mg/day in 1-2 divided doses (maximum: 15 mg/day) **or** 5-10 mL (33.3 mg/mL) up to twice daily
Children 6-12 years: Initial: 8.6 mg once daily; Maintenance: 8.6-50 mg/day in 1-2 divided doses (maximum: 50 mg/day) **or** 10-30 mL (33.3 mg/mL) up to twice daily
Children ≥12 years and Adults: Initial: 15 mg once daily; Maintenance: 15-100 mg/day in 1-2 divided doses (maximum: 100 mg/day) **or** 130 mg as a single dose

Sermorelin Acetate (ser moe REL in AS e tate)

Pharmacologic Category Diagnostic Agent; Growth Hormone

Use Geref® Diagnostic: For evaluation of the ability of the pituitary gland to secrete growth hormone (GH)

Local Anesthetic/Vasoconstrictor Precautions No information available to require special precautions

Effects on Dental Treatment Key adverse event(s) related to dental treatment: Dysphagia.

Effects on Bleeding No information available to require special precautions

Adverse Effects Frequency not defined.
Cardiovascular: Tightness in the chest
Central nervous system: Headache, dizziness, hyperactivity, somnolence
Dermatologic: Transient flushing of the face, urticaria
Gastrointestinal: Dysphagia, nausea, vomiting
Local: Pain, redness, and/or swelling at the injection site

General Dosage Range I.V.: *Children and Adults:* 1 mcg/kg as a single dose

Pharmacodynamics/Kinetics
Onset of Action Peak response: Diagnostic: Children 30 ± 27 minutes; Adults: 35 ± 29 minutes

Pregnancy Risk Factor C

Sertaconazole (ser ta KOE na zole)

U.S. Brand Names Ertaczo®

Pharmacologic Category Antifungal Agent, Topical

Use Topical treatment of tinea pedis (athlete's foot)

Local Anesthetic/Vasoconstrictor Precautions No information available to require special precautions

Effects on Dental Treatment No significant effects or complications reported
Effects on Bleeding No information available to require special precautions
Adverse Effects 1% to 10%: Dermatologic: Burning, contact dermatitis, dry skin, tenderness
General Dosage Range Topical: *Children ≥12 years and Adults:* Apply twice daily
Mechanism of Action Alters fungal cell wall membrane permeability; inhibits the CYP450-dependent synthesis of ergosterol
Pregnancy Risk Factor C

Sertraline (SER tra leen)

Related Information
Management of the Patient With Anxiety or Depression *on page 1968*
U.S. Brand Names Zoloft®
Canadian Brand Names Apo-Sertraline®; CO Sertraline; Dom-Sertraline; GD-Sertraline; Mylan-Sertraline; Nu-Sertraline; PHL-Sertraline; PMS-Sertraline; ratio-Sertraline; Riva-Sertraline; Sandoz-Sertraline; Teva-Sertraline; Zoloft®
Generic Availability (U.S.) Yes
Pharmacologic Category Antidepressant, Selective Serotonin Reuptake Inhibitor
Use Treatment of major depression; obsessive-compulsive disorder (OCD); panic disorder; post-traumatic stress disorder (PTSD); premenstrual dysphoric disorder (PMDD); social anxiety disorder
Unlabeled/Investigational Use Eating disorders; generalized anxiety disorder (GAD); impulse control disorders; treatment of mild dementia-associated agitation in nonpsychotic patients
Local Anesthetic/Vasoconstrictor Precautions Although caution should be used in patients taking tricyclic antidepressants, no interactions have been reported with vasoconstrictor and sertraline, a nontricyclic antidepressant which acts to increase serotonin; no precautions appear to be needed
Effects on Dental Treatment Key adverse event(s) related to dental treatment: Xerostomia (normal salivary flow resumes upon discontinuation) (see Effects on Bleeding and Dental Comment).
Effects on Bleeding May impair platelet aggregation resulting in increased risk of bleeding events, particularly if used concomitantly with aspirin, NSAIDs, warfarin, or other anticoagulants. Bleeding related to SSRI use has been reported to range from relatively minor bruising and epistaxis to life-threatening hemorrhage. Routine interruption of therapy for most dental procedures is not warranted. In medically complicated patients or extensive oral surgery, the decision to interrupt therapy must be based on the risk to benefit in an individual patient and a medical consult is suggested. If therapy is continued without interruption, the clinician should anticipate the potential for a prolonged bleeding time.
Adverse Effects
>10%:
Central nervous system: Dizziness, fatigue, headache, insomnia, somnolence
Endocrine & metabolic: Libido decreased
Gastrointestinal: Anorexia, diarrhea, nausea, xerostomia
Genitourinary: Ejaculatory disturbances
Neuromuscular & skeletal: Tremors
Miscellaneous: Diaphoresis
1% to 10%:
Cardiovascular: Chest pain, palpitation
Central nervous system: Agitation, anxiety, hypoesthesia, malaise, nervousness, pain
Dermatologic: Rash
Endocrine & metabolic: Impotence
Gastrointestinal: Appetite increased, constipation, dyspepsia, flatulence, vomiting, weight gain
Neuromuscular & skeletal: Back pain, hypertonia, myalgia, paresthesia, weakness
Ocular: Visual difficulty, abnormal vision
Otic: Tinnitus
Respiratory: Rhinitis
Miscellaneous: Yawning

Additional adverse reactions reported in pediatric patients (frequency >2%): Aggressiveness, epistaxis, hyperkinesia, purpura, sinusitis, urinary incontinence
Dosage Oral:
Children and Adolescents: Obsessive-compulsive disorder:
6-12 years: Initial: 25 mg once daily
13-17 years: Initial: 50 mg once daily

Note: May increase daily dose, at intervals of not less than 1 week, to a maximum of 200 mg/day. If somnolence is noted, give at bedtime.

Adults:

Depression/obsessive-compulsive disorder: Oral: Initial: 50 mg/day (see **"Note"**)

Panic disorder, post-traumatic stress disorder, social anxiety disorder: Initial: 25 mg once daily; increase to 50 mg once daily after 1 week; maximum dose: 200 mg/day

Premenstrual dysphoric disorder: 50 mg/day either daily throughout menstrual cycle **or** limited to the luteal phase of menstrual cycle, depending on physician assessment. Patients not responding to 50 mg/day may benefit from dose increases (50 mg increments per menstrual cycle) up to 150 mg/day when dosing throughout menstrual cycle **or** up to 100 mg day when dosing during luteal phase only. If a 100 mg/day dose has been established with luteal phase dosing, a 50 mg/day titration step for 3 days should be utilized at the beginning of each luteal phase dosing period.

Elderly: Depression/obsessive-compulsive disorder: Start treatment with 25 mg/day in the morning and increase by 25 mg/day increments every 2-3 days if tolerated to 50-100 mg/day; additional increases may be necessary; maximum dose: 200 mg/day. **Note:** Patients with Alzheimer's dementia-related depression may require a lower starting dosage of 12.5 mg/day, with titration intervals of 1-2 weeks, up to 150-200 mg/day maximum.

Dosage adjustment/comment in renal impairment: Multiple-dose pharmacokinetics are unaffected by renal impairment.

Hemodialysis: Not removed by hemodialysis

Dosage adjustment/comment in hepatic impairment: Sertraline is extensively metabolized by the liver; caution should be used in patients with hepatic impairment; a lower dose or less frequent dosing should be used.

Mechanism of Action Antidepressant with selective inhibitory effects on presynaptic serotonin (5-HT) reuptake and only very weak effects on norepinephrine and dopamine neuronal uptake. *In vitro* studies demonstrate no significant affinity for adrenergic, cholinergic, GABA, dopaminergic, histaminergic, serotonergic, or benzodiazepine receptors.

Contraindications Hypersensitivity to sertraline or any component of the formulation; use of MAO inhibitors within 14 days; concurrent use of pimozide; concurrent use of sertraline oral concentrate with disulfiram

Warnings/Precautions [U.S. Boxed Warning]: Antidepressants increase the risk of suicidal thinking and behavior in children, adolescents, and young adults (18-24 years of age) with major depressive disorder (MDD) and other psychiatric disorders; consider risk prior to prescribing. Short-term studies did not show an increased risk in patients >24 years of age and showed a decreased risk in patients ≥65 years. Closely monitor patients for clinical worsening, suicidality, or unusual changes in behavior, particularly during the initial 1-2 months of therapy or during periods of dosage adjustments (increases or decreases); the patient's family or caregiver should be instructed to closely observe the patient and communicate condition with healthcare provider. A medication guide concerning the use of antidepressants should be dispensed with each prescription. **Sertraline is not FDA approved for use in children with major depressive disorder (MDD). However, it is approved for the treatment of obsessive-compulsive disorder (OCD) in children ≥6 years of age.**

The possibility of a suicide attempt is inherent in major depression and may persist until remission occurs. Use caution in high-risk patients. Worsening depression and severe abrupt suicidality that are not part of the presenting symptoms may require discontinuation or modification of drug therapy. The patient's family or caregiver should be alerted to monitor patients for the emergence of suicidality and associated behaviors (such as agitation, irritability, hostility, impulsivity, and hypomania) and call healthcare provider.

May worsen psychosis in some patients or precipitate a shift to mania or hypomania in patients with bipolar disorder. Patients presenting with depressive symptoms should be screened for bipolar disorder. Monotherapy in patients with bipolar disorder should be avoided. **Sertraline is not FDA approved for the treatment of bipolar depression.**

Serotonin syndrome and neuroleptic malignant syndrome (NMS)-like reactions have occurred with serotonin/norepinephrine reuptake inhibitors (SNRIs) and selective serotonin reuptake inhibitors (SSRIs) when used alone, and particularly when used in combination with serotonergic agents (eg, triptans) or antidopaminergic agents (eg, antipsychotics). Concurrent use with MAO inhibitors is contraindicated. Has a very low potential to impair cognitive or motor performance. However, caution patients regarding activities requiring alertness until response to sertraline is known.

Does not appear to potentiate the effects of alcohol, however, ethanol use is not advised.

Use caution in patients with a previous seizure disorder or condition predisposing to seizures such as brain damage, alcoholism, or concurrent therapy with other drugs which lower the seizure threshold. May increase the risks associated with electroconvulsive therapy. Use with caution in patients with hepatic or renal dysfunction and in elderly patients. May cause hyponatremia/SIADH (elderly at increased risk); volume depletion (diuretics may increase risk). Use with caution in patients with renal insufficiency or other concurrent illness (due to limited experience). Sertraline acts as a mild uricosuric; use with caution in patients at risk of uric acid nephropathy. Use caution with concomitant use of NSAIDs, ASA, or other drugs that affect coagulation; the risk of bleeding may be potentiated. Use with caution in patients where weight loss is undesirable. May cause or exacerbate sexual dysfunction.

Use oral concentrate formulation with caution in patients with latex sensitivity; dropper dispenser contains dry natural rubber. Monitor growth in pediatric patients. Discontinuation symptoms (eg, dysphoric mood, irritability, agitation, confusion, anxiety, insomnia, hypomania) may occur upon abrupt discontinuation. Taper dose when discontinuing therapy.

Drug Interactions

Metabolism/Transport Effects Substrate of CYP2B6 (minor), 2C9 (minor), 2C19 (major), 2D6 (major), 3A4 (minor); **Inhibits** CYP1A2 (weak), 2B6 (moderate), 2C8 (weak), 2C9 (weak), 2C19 (moderate), 2D6 (moderate), 3A4 (moderate)

Avoid Concomitant Use

Avoid concomitant use of Sertraline with any of the following: Clopidogrel; Disulfiram; Iobenguane I 123; MAO Inhibitors; Methylene Blue; Pimozide; Sibutramine; Thioridazine; Tolvaptan; Tryptophan

Increased Effect/Toxicity

Sertraline may increase the levels/effects of: Alcohol (Ethyl); Alpha-/Beta-Blockers; Anticoagulants; Antidepressants (Serotonin Reuptake Inhibitor/Antagonist); Antiplatelet Agents; Aspirin; Beta-Blockers; Budesonide (Systemic, Oral Inhalation); BusPIRone; CarBAMazepine; CloZAPine; CNS Depressants; Colchicine; Collagenase (Systemic); CYP2B6 Substrates; CYP2C19 Substrates; CYP2D6 Substrates; CYP3A4 Substrates; Desmopressin; Dextromethorphan; Drotrecogin Alfa; Eplerenone; Everolimus; Fesoterodine; Fosphenytoin; Galantamine; Halofantrine; Haloperidol; Ibritumomab; Lithium; Lurasidone; Methadone; Methotrimeprazine; Methylene Blue; NSAID (COX-2 Inhibitor); NSAID (Nonselective); Phenytoin; Pimecrolimus; Pimozide; Ranolazine; RisperiDONE; Salicylates; Salmeterol; Saxagliptin; Serotonin Modulators; Tamoxifen; Thioridazine; Thrombolytic Agents; Tolvaptan; Tositumomab and Iodine I 131 Tositumomab; TraMADol; Tricyclic Antidepressants; Vitamin K Antagonists

The levels/effects of Sertraline may be increased by: Abiraterone; Analgesics (Opioid); BusPIRone; Cimetidine; Conivaptan; CYP2D6 Inhibitors (Moderate); CYP2D6 Inhibitors (Strong); Dasatinib; Disulfiram; Droperidol; Glucosamine; Herbs (Anticoagulant/Antiplatelet Properties); Macrolide Antibiotics; MAO Inhibitors; Methotrimeprazine; Metoclopramide; Omega-3-Acid Ethyl Esters; Pentosan Polysulfate Sodium; Pentoxifylline; Prostacyclin Analogues; Sibutramine; TraMADol; Tryptophan

Decreased Effect

Sertraline may decrease the levels/effects of: Clopidogrel; Iobenguane I 123

The levels/effects of Sertraline may be decreased by: CarBAMazepine; Cyproheptadine; Darunavir; Efavirenz; Fosphenytoin; Peginterferon Alfa-2b; Phenytoin; Tocilizumab

Ethanol/Nutrition/Herb Interactions

Ethanol: May increase CNS depression; monitor for increased effects with coadministration. Caution patients about effects.

Food: Sertraline average peak serum levels may be increased if taken with food.

Herb/Nutraceutical: Avoid valerian, St John's wort, kava kava, gotu kola (may increase CNS depression).

Pharmacodynamics/Kinetics

Onset of Action Depression: The onset of action is within a week, however, individual response varies greatly and full response may not be seen until 8-12 weeks after initiation of treatment.

Half-life Elimination Sertraline: 26 hours; N-desmethylsertraline: 66 hours (range: 62-104 hours)

Time to Peak Plasma: Sertraline: 4.5-8.4 hours

Pregnancy Risk Factor C

Lactation Enters breast milk/use caution (AAP rates "of concern"; AAP 2001 update pending)

Breast-Feeding Considerations Sertraline and desmethylsertraline are excreted in breast milk. Infants exposed to sertraline while breast-feeding generally receive a low relative dose and serum concentrations are not detectable in most infants. Adverse reactions have not been reported in nursing infants. Sertraline concentrations in the hindmilk are higher than in foremilk. If the benefits of the mother receiving the sertraline and breast-feeding outweigh the risks, the mother may consider pumping and discarding breast milk with the feeding 7-9 hours after the daily dose to decrease sertraline exposure to the infant. The long-term effects on development and behavior have not been studied. The manufacturer recommends that caution be exercised when administering sertraline to nursing women.

Dosage Forms

Solution, oral: 20 mg/mL (60 mL)

Zoloft®: 20 mg/mL (60 mL)

Tablet, oral: 25 mg, 50 mg, 100 mg

Zoloft®: 25 mg, 50 mg, 100 mg

Dental Comment Problems with SSRI-induced bruxism have been reported and may preclude their use; clinicians attempting to evaluate any patient with bruxism or involuntary muscle movement, who is simultaneously being treated with an SSRI drug, should be aware of the potential association.

References

Gerber PE and Lynd LD, "Selective Serotonin Reuptake Inhibitor-Induced Movement Disorders," *Ann Pharmacother*, 1998, 32(6):692-8.

Sevelamer (se VEL a mer)

U.S. Brand Names Renagel®; Renvela®

Canadian Brand Names Renagel®

Pharmacologic Category Phosphate Binder

Use Reduction or control of serum phosphorous in patients with chronic kidney disease on hemodialysis

Local Anesthetic/Vasoconstrictor Precautions No information available to require special precautions

Effects on Dental Treatment No significant effects or complications reported

Effects on Bleeding No information available to require special precautions

Adverse Effects Note: A decreased incidence of gastrointestinal adverse events was observed in a clinical trial of sevelamer carbonate compared to sevelamer hydrochloride.

>10%:

- Dermatologic: Pruritus (13%)
- Gastrointestinal: Vomiting (22%), nausea (7% to 20%), diarrhea (4% to 19%), dyspepsia (5% to 16%)
- Neuromuscular & skeletal: Limb pain (13%), arthralgia (12%)
- Respiratory: Nasopharyngitis (14%), bronchitis (11%)

1% to 10%:

- Cardiovascular: Hypertension (10%)
- Central nervous system: Headache (9%), pyrexia (5%)
- Endocrine & metabolic: Hypercalcemia (5% to 7%)
- Gastrointestinal: Abdominal pain (9%), flatulence (4% to 8%), constipation (2% to 8%)
- Neuromuscular & skeletal: Back pain (4%)
- Respiratory: Dyspnea (10%), cough (7%), upper respiratory tract infection (5%)
- Miscellaneous: Peritonitis (peritoneal dialysis: 8%)

General Dosage Range Oral: *Adults:* Initial: 800-1600 mg 3 times/day; Maintenance: Up to 2400-14,000 mg/day in 3 divided doses

Mechanism of Action Sevelamer (a polymeric compound) binds phosphate within the intestinal lumen, limiting absorption and decreasing serum phosphate concentrations without altering calcium, aluminum, or bicarbonate concentrations. Increased serum bicarbonate levels have been observed with the use of sevelamer carbonate, compared to sevelamer hydrochloride.

Pregnancy Risk Factor C

Sibutramine (si BYOO tra meen)

U.S. Brand Names Meridia® [DSC]

Canadian Brand Names Apo-Sibutramine®; Meridia®

Pharmacologic Category Anorexiant; Sympathomimetic

Use Management of obesity in patients with an initial body mass index (BMI) ≥30 kg/m^2 or ≥27 kg/m^2 in the presence of other risk factors (eg, diabetes, hyperlipidemia, hypertension)

Local Anesthetic/Vasoconstrictor Precautions No information available to require special precautions

Effects on Dental Treatment Key adverse event(s) related to dental treatment: Xerostomia (normal salivary flow resumes upon discontinuation) and taste perversion (see Dental Comment).

Effects on Bleeding No information available to require special precautions

Adverse Effects

>10%:

Central nervous system: Headache (30%), insomnia (11%)

Gastrointestinal: Xerostomia (17%), anorexia (13%), constipation (12%)

1% to 10%:

Cardiovascular: Tachycardia (3%), vasodilation (2%), hypertension (2%), palpitation (2%), chest pain (2%), peripheral edema (≥1%)

Central nervous system: Dizziness (7%), nervousness (5%), anxiety (5%), depression (4%), CNS stimulation (2%), migraine (2%), somnolence (2%), emotional lability (1%), agitation (≥1%), fever (≥1%), thinking abnormal (≥1%)

Dermatologic: Rash (4%), pruritus (≥1%)

Endocrine & metabolic: Dysmenorrhea (4%)

Gastrointestinal: Appetite increased (9%), nausea (6%), abdominal pain (5%), dyspepsia (5%), gastritis (2%), taste perversion (2%), vomiting (2%), diarrhea (≥1%), flatulence (≥1%), gastroenteritis (≥1%), tooth disorder (≥1%)

Hepatic: Abnormal LFTs (2%)

Neuromuscular & skeletal: Back pain (8%), weakness (6%), arthralgia (6%), neck pain (2%), myalgia (2%), paresthesia (2%), tenosynovitis (1%), arthritis (≥1%), hypertonia (≥1%), leg cramps (≥1%)

Ocular: Amblyopia (≥1%)

Otic: Ear disorder (2%)

Respiratory: Pharyngitis (10%), rhinitis (10%), sinusitis (5%), cough (4%), bronchitis (≥1%), dyspnea (≥1%)

Miscellaneous: Flu-like syndrome (8%), diaphoresis (3%), allergic reactions (2%), thirst (2%)

General Dosage Range Oral: *Children ≥16 years and Adults:* Initial: 10 mg once daily; Maintenance: 5-15 mg once daily

Mechanism of Action Sibutramine and its two primary metabolites block the neuronal uptake of norepinephrine, serotonin, and (to a lesser extent) dopamine. There is no monoamine-releasing (or depleting) activity.

Pharmacodynamics/Kinetics

Half-life Elimination Sibutramine: 1 hour; Metabolites: M_1: 14 hours; M_2: 16 hours

Time to Peak Sibutramine: 1.2 hours; Metabolites (M_1 and M_2): 3-4 hours

Pregnancy Risk Factor C

Controlled Substance C-IV

Dental Comment The mechanism of action is thought to be different from the "fen" drugs. Sibutramine works to suppress the appetite by inhibiting the reuptake of norepinephrine and serotonin. Unlike dexfenfluramine and fenfluramine, it is not a serotonin releaser. Sibutramine is closer chemically to the widely used antidepressants such as fluoxetine (Prozac®). The FDA approved sibutramine over the objections of its own advisory panel, who called the drug too risky. FDA reported that the drug causes blood pressure to increase, generally by a small amount, though in some patients the increases were higher. It is now recommended that patients taking sibutramine have their blood pressure evaluated regularly.

Sildenafil (sil DEN a fil)

U.S. Brand Names Revatio®; Viagra®

Canadian Brand Names ratio-Sildenafil R; Revatio®; Viagra®

Generic Availability (U.S.) No

Pharmacologic Category Phosphodiesterase-5 Enzyme Inhibitor

Use

Revatio®: Treatment of pulmonary arterial hypertension (WHO Group I) to improve exercise ability and delay clinical worsening

Viagra®: Treatment of erectile dysfunction (ED)

Unlabeled/Investigational Use Pulmonary arterial hypertension in children

Local Anesthetic/Vasoconstrictor Precautions No information available to require special precautions

Effects on Dental Treatment No significant effects or complications reported

Effects on Bleeding No information available to require special precautions

Adverse Effects Based upon normal doses for either indication or route. (Adverse effects such as flushing, diarrhea, myalgia, and visual disturbances may be increased with doses >100 mg/24 hours.)

>10%:
Central nervous system: Headache (16% to 46%)
Gastrointestinal: Dyspepsia (7% to 17%; dose related)
2% to 10%:
Cardiovascular: Flushing (10%)
Central nervous system: Insomnia (≤7%), pyrexia (6%), dizziness (2%)
Dermatologic: Erythema (6%), rash (2%)
Gastrointestinal: Diarrhea (3% to 9%), gastritis (≤3%)
Genitourinary: Urinary tract infection (3%)
Hepatic: LFTs increased
Neuromuscular & skeletal: Myalgia (≤7%), paresthesia (≤3%)
Ocular: Abnormal vision (color changes, blurred vision, or increased sensitivity to light 3% to 11%; dose related)
Respiratory: Epistaxis (9% to 13%), dyspnea exacerbated (≤7%), nasal congestion (4%), rhinitis (4%), sinusitis (3%)

Dosage

I.V.: Adults: Pulmonary arterial hypertension (Revatio®): 10 mg 3 times/day
Oral:
Children ≥1 month: Pulmonary arterial hypertension (unlabeled use): 0.25-2 mg/kg/dose every 4-6 hours. Most reports used 0.5 mg/kg/dose and titrated up to 2 mg/kg/dose
Adults:
Erectile dysfunction (Viagra®): Usual dose: 50 mg once daily 1 hour (range: 30 minutes to 4 hours) before sexual activity; dosing range: 25-100 mg once daily
Pulmonary arterial hypertension (Revatio®): 20 mg 3 times/day, taken 4-6 hours apart
Note: A delay in clinical worsening was observed in a short-term trial in which most patients achieved a target dose of 80 mg 3 times daily (unlabeled dose). The patients had an incremental dosage escalation while on a stable epoprostenol regimen (Simonneau, 2008).
Elderly >65 years: Use with caution
Revatio®: Refer to adult dosing.
Viagra®: Starting dose of 25 mg should be considered.

Dosage considerations for patients stable on alpha-blockers: Viagra®: Initial 25 mg

Dosage adjustment for concomitant use of potent CYP34A inhibitors:
Revatio®:
Erythromycin: No dosage adjustment
Itraconazole, ketoconazole: Not recommended
Viagra®:
Erythromycin, itraconazole, ketoconazole: Starting dose of 25 mg should be considered
Protease inhibitors: Maximum sildenafil dose: 25 mg every 48 hours

Dosage adjustment in renal impairment:
Revatio®: Dose adjustment not necessary
Viagra®: Cl_{cr} <30 mL/minute: Starting dose of 25 mg should be considered

Dosage adjustment in hepatic impairment:
Revatio®: Child-Pugh class A and B: Dose adjustment not necessary; not studied in severe impairment (Child-Pugh class C)
Viagra®: Child-Pugh class A and B: Starting dose of 25 mg should be considered; not studied in severe impairment (Child-Pugh class C)

Mechanism of Action

Erectile dysfunction: Does not directly cause penile erections, but affects the response to sexual stimulation. The physiologic mechanism of erection of the penis involves release of nitric oxide (NO) in the corpus cavernosum during sexual stimulation. NO then activates the enzyme guanylate cyclase, which results in increased levels of cyclic guanosine monophosphate (cGMP), producing smooth muscle relaxation and inflow of blood to the corpus cavernosum. Sildenafil enhances the effect of NO by inhibiting phosphodiesterase type 5 (PDE-5), which is responsible for degradation of cGMP in the corpus cavernosum; when sexual stimulation causes local release of NO, inhibition of PDE-5 by sildenafil causes increased levels of cGMP in the corpus cavernosum, resulting in smooth muscle relaxation and inflow of blood to the corpus cavernosum; at recommended doses, it has no effect in the absence of sexual stimulation.

Pulmonary arterial hypertension (PAH): Inhibits phosphodiesterase type 5 (PDE-5) in smooth muscle of pulmonary vasculature where PDE-5 is responsible for the degradation of cyclic guanosine monophosphate (cGMP). Increased cGMP concentration results in pulmonary vasculature relaxation; vasodilation in the pulmonary bed and the systemic circulation (to a lesser degree) may occur.

Contraindications Hypersensitivity to sildenafil or any component of the formulation; concurrent use (regularly/intermittently) of organic nitrates in any form (eg, nitroglycerin, isosorbide dinitrate); concurrent use with a protease inhibitor regimen when sildenafil used for pulmonary artery hypertension (eg, Revatio®)

Warnings/Precautions Decreases in blood pressure may occur due to vasodilator effects; use with caution in patients with left ventricular outflow obstruction (aortic stenosis or hypertrophic obstructive cardiomyopathy); may be more sensitive to hypotensive actions. Concurrent use with alpha-adrenergic antagonist therapy or substantial ethanol consumption may cause symptomatic hypotension; patients should be hemodynamically stable prior to initiating therapy at the lowest possible dose. Use with caution in patients with hypotension (<90/50 mm Hg); uncontrolled hypertension (>170/110 mm Hg); life-threatening arrhythmias, stroke or MI within the last 6 months; cardiac failure or coronary artery disease causing unstable angina; safety and efficacy have not been studied in these patients. There is a degree of cardiac risk associated with sexual activity; therefore, physicians should consider the cardiovascular status of their patients prior to initiating any treatment for erectile dysfunction. If pulmonary edema occurs when treating pulmonary arterial hypertension, consider the possibility of pulmonary veno-occlusive disease (PVOD); continued use is not recommended in patient with PVOD.

Sildenafil should be used with caution in patients with anatomical deformation of the penis (angulation, cavernosal fibrosis, or Peyronie's disease) and in patients who have conditions which may predispose them to priapism (sickle cell anemia, multiple myeloma, leukemia). All patients should be instructed to seek medical attention if erection persists >4 hours.

Vision loss may occur rarely and be a sign of nonarteritic anterior ischemic optic neuropathy (NAION). Risk may be increased with history of vision loss. Other risk factors for NAION include low cup-to-disc ratio ("crowded disc"), coronary artery disease, diabetes, hypertension, hyperlipidemia, smoking, and age >50 years. May cause dose-related impairment of color discrimination. Use caution in patients with retinitis pigmentosa; a minority have genetic disorders of retinal phosphodiesterases (no safety information available). Sudden decrease or loss of hearing has been reported rarely; hearing changes may be accompanied by tinnitus and dizziness. A direct relationship between therapy and vision or hearing loss has not been determined.

The potential underlying causes of erectile dysfunction should be evaluated prior to treatment. The safety and efficacy of sildenafil with other treatments for erectile dysfunction have not been established; use is not recommended. Efficacy with concurrent bosentan therapy has not been evaluated; use with caution. Use with caution in patients taking strong CYP3A4 inhibitors or alpha-blockers. Concomitant use with all forms of nitrates is contraindicated. If nitrate administration is medically necessary, it is not known when nitrates can be safely administered following the use of sildenafil (per manufacturer); the ACC/AHA 2007 guidelines supports administration of nitrates only if 24 hours have elapsed.

Avoid abrupt discontinuation, especially if used as monotherapy in PAH as exacerbation may occur. Use caution in patients with bleeding disorders or with active peptic ulcer disease; safety and efficacy have not been established. Efficacy has not be established for treatment of pulmonary hypertension associated with sickle cell disease. Use with caution in the elderly, or patients with renal or hepatic dysfunction; dose adjustment may be needed.

Drug Interactions

Metabolism/Transport Effects **Substrate** of CYP2C9 (minor), 3A4 (major); **Inhibits** CYP1A2 (weak), 2C9 (weak), 2C19 (weak), 2D6 (weak), 2E1 (weak), 3A4 (weak)

Avoid Concomitant Use

Avoid concomitant use of Sildenafil with any of the following: Amyl Nitrite; Phosphodiesterase 5 Inhibitors; Vasodilators (Organic Nitrates)

Increased Effect/Toxicity

Sildenafil may increase the levels/effects of: Alpha1-Blockers; Amyl Nitrite; Antihypertensives; Bosentan; HMG-CoA Reductase Inhibitors; Phosphodiesterase 5 Inhibitors; Vasodilators (Organic Nitrates)

The levels/effects of Sildenafil may be increased by: Antifungal Agents (Azole Derivatives, Systemic); Conivaptan; CYP3A4 Inhibitors (Moderate); CYP3A4 Inhibitors (Strong); Dasatinib; Macrolide Antibiotics; Protease Inhibitors; Sapropterin

Decreased Effect

The levels/effects of Sildenafil may be decreased by: Bosentan; CYP3A4 Inducers (Strong); Deferasirox; Etravirine; Herbs (CYP3A4 Inducers); Peginterferon Alfa-2b; Tocilizumab

Ethanol/Nutrition/Herb Interactions

Food: Amount and rate of absorption of sildenafil is reduced when taken with a high-fat meal. Serum concentrations/toxicity may be increased with grapefruit juice; avoid concurrent use.

Herb/Nutraceutical: St John's wort may decrease sildenafil levels.

Dietary Considerations Avoid grapefruit juice.

Pharmacodynamics/Kinetics

Onset of Action ~60 minutes

Duration of Action 2-4 hours

Half-life Elimination ~4 hours; the elderly and those with severe renal impairment have reduced clearance of sildenafil and its active N-desmethyl metabolite

Time to Peak 30-120 minutes; delayed by 60 minutes with a high-fat meal

Pregnancy Risk Factor B

Lactation Excretion in breast milk unknown/use caution

Dosage Forms

Injection, solution:

Revatio®: 0.8 mg/mL (12.5 mL)

Tablet, oral:

Revatio®: 20 mg

Viagra®: 25 mg, 50 mg, 100 mg

Silodosin (SI lo doe sin)

U.S. Brand Names Rapaflo®

Pharmacologic Category Alpha$_1$ Blocker

Use Treatment of signs and symptoms of benign prostatic hyperplasia (BPH)

Local Anesthetic/Vasoconstrictor Precautions No information available to require special precautions

Effects on Dental Treatment Key adverse event(s) related to dental treatment: Postural hypotension, particularly with initial dosing; dizziness; nasal congestion or rhinitis

Effects on Bleeding No information available to require special precautions

Adverse Effects

>10%: Miscellaneous: Retrograde ejaculation (28%)

1% to 10%:

Cardiovascular: Orthostatic hypotension (3%)

Central nervous system: Dizziness (3%), headache (2%), insomnia (1% to 2%)

Gastrointestinal: Diarrhea (3%), abdominal pain (1% to 2%)

Genitourinary: PSA increased (1% to 2%)

Neuromuscular & skeletal: Weakness (1% to 2%)

Respiratory: Nasal congestion (2%), nasopharyngitis (2%), rhinorrhea (1% to 2%), sinusitis (1% to 2%)

General Dosage Range Dosage adjustment recommended in patients with renal impairment

Oral: *Adults:* Males: 8 mg once daily

Mechanism of Action Silodosin is a selective antagonist of alpha$_{1A}$-adrenoreceptors in the prostate and bladder. Smooth muscle tone in the prostate is mediated by alpha$_{1A}$-adrenoreceptors; blocking them leads to relaxation of smooth muscle in the bladder neck and prostate causing an improvement of urine flow and decreased symptoms of BPH. Approximately 75% of the alpha1-receptors in the prostate are of the alpha$_{1A}$ subtype.

Pharmacodynamics/Kinetics

Half-life Elimination Healthy volunteers: Silodosin: 5-21 hours; KMD-3213G: ~24 hours

Time to Peak ~3 hours

Pregnancy Risk Factor B

Silver Nitrate (SIL ver NYE trate)

Generic Availability (U.S.) Yes

Pharmacologic Category Antibiotic, Topical; Cauterizing Agent, Topical; Topical Skin Product, Antibacterial

Use Cauterization of wounds and sluggish ulcers, removal of granulation tissue and warts; aseptic prophylaxis of burns

Local Anesthetic/Vasoconstrictor Precautions No information available to require special precautions

Effects on Dental Treatment No significant effects or complications reported

Effects on Bleeding No information available to require special precautions

Adverse Effects Frequency not defined.
Dermatologic: Burning and skin irritation, staining of the skin
Endocrine & metabolic: Hyponatremia
Hematologic: Methemoglobinemia

Dosage Children and Adults:
Sticks: Apply to mucous membranes and other moist skin surfaces only on area to be treated 2-3 times/week for 2-3 weeks
Topical solution: Apply a cotton applicator dipped in solution on the affected area 2-3 times/week for 2-3 weeks

Mechanism of Action Free silver ions precipitate bacterial proteins by combining with chloride in tissue forming silver chloride; coagulates cellular protein to form an eschar; silver ions or salts or colloidal silver preparations can inhibit the growth of both gram-positive and gram-negative bacteria. This germicidal action is attributed to the precipitation of bacterial proteins by liberated silver ions. Silver nitrate coagulates cellular protein to form an eschar, and this mode of action is the postulated mechanism for control of benign hematuria, rhinitis, and recurrent pneumothorax.

Contraindications Hypersensitivity to silver nitrate or any component of the formulation; not for use on broken skin, cuts, or wounds

Warnings/Precautions Do not use applicator sticks on the eyes. Prolonged use may result in skin discoloration.

Drug Interactions

Avoid Concomitant Use
Avoid concomitant use of Silver Nitrate with any of the following: BCG

Increased Effect/Toxicity There are no known significant interactions involving an increase in effect.

Decreased Effect
Silver Nitrate may decrease the levels/effects of: BCG

Pregnancy Risk Factor C

Dosage Forms
Applicator sticks, topical: Silver nitrate 75% and potassium 25% (6", 12", 18")
Solution, topical: 0.5% (960 mL); 10% (30 mL); 25% (30 mL); 50% (30 mL)

Silver Sulfadiazine (SIL ver sul fa DYE a zeen)

U.S. Brand Names Silvadene®; SSD AF®; SSD®; Thermazene®

Canadian Brand Names Flamazine®

Pharmacologic Category Antibiotic, Topical

Use Prevention and treatment of infection in second and third degree burns

Local Anesthetic/Vasoconstrictor Precautions No information available to require special precautions

Effects on Dental Treatment No significant effects or complications reported

Effects on Bleeding No information available to require special precautions

Adverse Effects Frequency not defined.
Dermatologic: Discoloration of skin, erythema multiforme, itching, photosensitivity, rash
Hematologic: Agranulocytosis, aplastic anemia, hemolytic anemia, leukopenia
Hepatic: Hepatitis
Renal: Interstitial nephritis
Miscellaneous: Allergic reactions may be related to sulfa component

General Dosage Range Topical: *Children and Adults:* Apply to a thickness of 1/16" once or twice daily

Mechanism of Action Acts upon the bacterial cell wall and cell membrane. Bactericidal for many gram-negative and gram-positive bacteria and is effective against yeast. Active against *Pseudomonas aeruginosa*, *Pseudomonas maltophilia*, *Enterobacter* species, *Klebsiella* species, *Serratia* species, *Escherichia coli*, *Proteus mirabilis*, *Morganella morganii*, *Providencia rettgeri*, *Proteus vulgaris*, *Providencia* species, *Citrobacter* species, *Acinetobacter calcoaceticus*, *Staphylococcus aureus*, *Staphylococcus epidermidis*, *Enterococcus* species, *Candida albicans*, *Corynebacterium diphtheriae*, and *Clostridium perfringens*

Pharmacodynamics/Kinetics

Half-life Elimination 10 hours; prolonged with renal impairment

Time to Peak Serum: 3-11 days of continuous therapy

Pregnancy Risk Factor B

Simethicone (sye METH i kone)

U.S. Brand Names Equalizer Gas Relief [OTC]; Gas Free Extra Strength [OTC]; Gas Relief Ultra Strength [OTC]; Gas-X® Children's Tongue Twisters™ [OTC]; Gas-X® Extra Strength [OTC]; Gas-X® Maximum Strength [OTC]; Gas-X® Thin Strips™ [OTC]; Gas-X® [OTC]; Gax-X® Infant [OTC]; Genasyme™ [OTC] [DSC]; Infantaire Gas [OTC]; Infants Gas Relief Drops [OTC]; Little Tummys® Gas Relief [OTC]; Mi-Acid Gas Relief [OTC]; Mylanta® Gas Maximum Strength [OTC]; Mylicon® Infants' [OTC]; Phazyme® Ultra Strength [OTC]

Canadian Brand Names Ovol®; Phazyme™

Pharmacologic Category Antiflatulent

Use Postoperative gas pain or for use in endoscopic examination; relief of bloating, pressure, and discomfort of gas

Local Anesthetic/Vasoconstrictor Precautions No information available to require special precautions

Effects on Dental Treatment No significant effects or complications reported

Effects on Bleeding No information available to require special precautions

Adverse Effects No data reported

General Dosage Range Oral:

Infants and Children <2 years or <11 kg: 20 mg 4 times/day, as needed

Children >2 years or >11 kg: 40 mg 4 times/day, as needed

Children >12 years and Adults: 40-360 mg after meals and at bedtime, as needed

Mechanism of Action Decreases the surface tension of gas bubbles thereby disperses and prevents gas pockets in the GI system

Simvastatin (sim va STAT in)

Related Information

Cardiovascular Diseases *on page 1848*

U.S. Brand Names Zocor®

Canadian Brand Names Apo-Simvastatin®; CO Simvastatin; Dom-Simvastatin; JAMP-Simvastatin; Mylan-Simvastatin; Nu-Simvastatin; PHL-Simvastatin; PMS-Simvastatin; RAN™-Simvastatin; ratio-Simvastatin; Riva-Simvastatin; Sandoz-Simvastatin; Taro-Simvastatin; Teva-Simvastatin; Zocor®; ZYM-Simvastatin

Generic Availability (U.S.) Yes

Pharmacologic Category Antilipemic Agent, HMG-CoA Reductase Inhibitor

Use Used with dietary therapy for the following:

Secondary prevention of cardiovascular events in hypercholesterolemic patients with established coronary heart disease (CHD) or at high risk for CHD: To reduce cardiovascular morbidity (myocardial infarction, coronary/noncoronary revascularization procedures) and mortality; to reduce the risk of stroke

Hyperlipidemias: To reduce elevations in total cholesterol (total-C), LDL-C, apolipoprotein B, triglycerides, and VLDL-C, and to increase HDL-C in patients with primary hypercholesterolemia (elevations of 1 or more components are present in Fredrickson type IIa, IIb, III, and IV hyperlipidemias); treatment of homozygous familial hypercholesterolemia

Heterozygous familial hypercholesterolemia (HeFH): In adolescent patients (10-17 years of age, females >1 year postmenarche) with HeFH having LDL-C ≥190 mg/dL **or** LDL-C ≥160 mg/dL with positive family history of premature cardiovascular disease (CVD), or 2 or more CVD risk factors in the adolescent patient

Local Anesthetic/Vasoconstrictor Precautions No information available to require special precautions

Effects on Dental Treatment No significant effects or complications reported

Effects on Bleeding No information available to require special precautions

Adverse Effects

1% to 10%:

Cardiovascular: Atrial fibrillation (6%; placebo 5%), edema (3%; placebo 2%)

Central nervous system: Headache (3% to 7%), vertigo (5%)

Dermatologic: Eczema (5%)

Gastrointestinal: Abdominal pain (7%), constipation (2% to 7%), gastritis (5%), nausea (5%)

Hepatic: Transaminases increased (>3 x ULN; 1%)

Neuromuscular & skeletal: CPK increased (>3 x normal; 5%), myalgia (4%)

Respiratory: Upper respiratory infections (9%), bronchitis (7%)

Additional class-related events or case reports (not necessarily reported with simvastatin therapy): Alteration in taste, anorexia, anxiety, bilirubin increased, cataracts, cholestatic jaundice, cirrhosis, decreased libido, depression, erectile dysfunction/impotence, facial paresis, fatty liver, fulminant hepatic necrosis, gynecomastia, hepatoma, hyperbilirubinemia, impaired extraocular muscle movement, increased CPK (>10 x normal), interstitial lung disease, ophthalmoplegia, peripheral nerve palsy, psychic disturbance, renal failure (secondary to rhabdomyolysis), thyroid dysfunction, tremor, vertigo

Dosage Oral: **Note:** Doses should be individualized according to the baseline LDL-cholesterol levels, the recommended goal of therapy, and the patient's response; adjustments should be made at intervals of 4 weeks or more; doses may need adjusted based on concomitant medications

Children 10-17 years (females >1 year postmenarche): HeFH: 10 mg once daily in the evening; range: 10-40 mg/day (maximum: 40 mg/day)

Dosage adjustment for simvastatin with concomitant amiodarone, cyclosporine, danazol, diltiazem, gemfibrozil, or verapamil: Refer to drug-specific dosing in adult dosing section

Adults:

Homozygous familial hypercholesterolemia: 40 mg once daily in the evening **or** 80 mg/day (given in 3 divided doses as 20 mg, 20 mg, and 40 mg evening dose)

Prevention of cardiovascular events, hyperlipidemias: 20-40 mg once daily in the evening; range: 5-80 mg/day

Patients requiring only moderate reduction of LDL-cholesterol may be started at 10 mg once daily in the evening

Patients requiring reduction of >45% in low-density lipoprotein (LDL) cholesterol may be started at 40 mg once daily in the evening

Patients with CHD or at high risk for CHD: Dosing should be started at 40 mg once daily in the evening; simvastatin should be started simultaneously with diet therapy.

Dosage adjustment with concomitant medications:

Cyclosporine or danazol: Initial: 5 mg simvastatin, should **not** exceed 10 mg/day

Gemfibrozil: Simvastatin dose should **not** exceed 10 mg/day

Amiodarone or verapamil: Simvastatin dose should **not** exceed 20 mg/day

Diltiazem: Simvastatin dose should **not** exceed 40 mg/day

Dosage adjustment in Chinese patients on niacin doses ≥1 g/day: Because of an increased risk of myopathy, do not administer simvastatin 80 mg concurrently.

Dosing adjustment in renal impairment: Because simvastatin does not undergo significant renal excretion, modification of dose should not be necessary in patients with mild-to-moderate renal insufficiency.

Severe renal impairment: Cl_{cr} <10 mL/minute: Initial: 5 mg/day with close monitoring.

Mechanism of Action Simvastatin is a methylated derivative of lovastatin that acts by competitively inhibiting 3-hydroxy-3-methylglutaryl-coenzyme A (HMG-CoA) reductase, the enzyme that catalyzes the rate-limiting step in cholesterol biosynthesis

Contraindications Hypersensitivity to simvastatin or any component of the formulation; active liver disease; unexplained persistent elevations of serum transaminases; pregnancy; breast-feeding

Warnings/Precautions Secondary causes of hyperlipidemia should be ruled out prior to therapy. Liver function must be monitored by laboratory assessment. Rhabdomyolysis with acute renal failure has occurred. Risk is dose-related and is increased with high doses (80 mg) or concurrent use of lipid-lowering agents which may cause rhabdomyolysis (gemfibrozil, other fibric acid derivatives, or niacin at doses ≥1 g/day), during concurrent use with danazol or moderate-to-strong CYP3A4 inhibitors (including amiodarone, cyclosporine, grapefruit juice in large quantities, or verapamil). Avoid concurrent use of strong CYP3A4 inhibitors (eg, itraconazole, ketoconazole, erythromycin, clarithromycin, telithromycin, nefazodone, and HIV protease inhibitors). Monitor closely if used with other drugs associated with myopathy (eg, colchicine). Weigh the risk versus benefit when combining any of these drugs with simvastatin. Do not initiate simvastatin-containing treatment in a patient with pre-existing therapy of cyclosporine or danazol, unless the patient has previously demonstrated tolerance to ≥5 mg/day simvastatin. Temporarily discontinue in any patient experiencing an acute or serious major medical or surgical condition which may increase the risk of rhabdomyolysis. Discontinue temporarily for elective surgical procedures. Based upon current evidence, HMG-CoA reductase inhibitor therapy should be continued in the perioperative period unless risk outweighs cardioprotective benefit. Use caution in patients with renal insufficiency. Use with caution in patients with advanced age, these patients are predisposed to myopathy. Use with caution in patients who consume large amounts of ethanol or have a history of liver disease. Use is contraindicated with active liver disease and with unexplained transaminase elevations. Concomitant use of high-dose simvastatin (80 mg) and niacin ≥1 g/day may increase risk of myopathy in Chinese patients.

Drug Interactions

Metabolism/Transport Effects Substrate of CYP3A4 (major), SLCO1B1; **Inhibits** CYP2C8 (weak), 2C9 (weak), 2D6 (weak)

Avoid Concomitant Use

Avoid concomitant use of Simvastatin with any of the following: Protease Inhibitors; Red Yeast Rice

Increased Effect/Toxicity

Simvastatin may increase the levels/effects of: DAPTOmycin; Diltiazem; Trabectedin; Vitamin K Antagonists

The levels/effects of Simvastatin may be increased by: Amiodarone; Antifungal Agents (Azole Derivatives, Systemic); Colchicine; Conivaptan; CycloSPORINE; CycloSPORINE (Systemic); CYP3A4 Inhibitors (Moderate); CYP3A4 Inhibitors (Strong); Danazol; Dasatinib; Diltiazem; Dronedarone; Eltrombopag; Fenofibrate; Fenofibric Acid; Fluconazole; Fusidic Acid; Gemfibrozil; Grapefruit Juice; Green Tea; Imatinib; Macrolide Antibiotics; Nefazodone; Niacin; Niacinamide; Protease Inhibitors; QuiNINE; Ranolazine; Red Yeast Rice; Rifamycin Derivatives; Sildenafil; Verapamil

Decreased Effect

The levels/effects of Simvastatin may be decreased by: Antacids; Bosentan; CYP3A4 Inducers (Strong); Deferasirox; Efavirenz; Etravirine; Fosphenytoin; Phenytoin; Rifamycin Derivatives; St Johns Wort; Tocilizumab

Ethanol/Nutrition/Herb Interactions

Ethanol: Avoid excessive ethanol consumption (due to potential hepatic effects).

Food: Simvastatin serum concentration may be increased when taken with grapefruit juice; avoid concurrent intake of large quantities (>1 quart/day). Red yeast rice contains an estimated 2.4 mg lovastatin per 600 mg rice.

Herb/Nutraceutical: St John's wort may decrease simvastatin levels.

Dietary Considerations May be taken without regard to meals. Red yeast rice contains an estimated 2.4 mg lovastatin per 600 mg rice.

Pharmacodynamics/Kinetics

Onset of Action >3 days; Peak effect: 2 weeks

Half-life Elimination Unknown

Time to Peak 1.3-2.4 hours

Pregnancy Risk Factor X

Lactation Excretion in breast milk unknown/contraindicated

Breast-Feeding Considerations Excretion in breast milk is unknown, but would be expected; other medications in this class are excreted in human milk. Breast-feeding is contraindicated.

Dosage Forms

Tablet, oral: 5 mg, 10 mg, 20 mg, 40 mg, 80 mg

Zocor®: 5 mg, 10 mg, 20 mg, 40 mg, 80 mg

Sincalide (SIN ka lide)

U.S. Brand Names Kinevac®

Pharmacologic Category Diagnostic Agent

Use Postevacuation cholecystography; gallbladder bile sampling; stimulate pancreatic secretion for analysis; accelerate the transit of barium through the small bowel

Local Anesthetic/Vasoconstrictor Precautions No information available to require special precautions

Effects on Dental Treatment No significant effects or complications reported

Effects on Bleeding No information available to require special precautions

Adverse Effects

>10%: Gastrointestional: Abdominal pain (20%), cramps, nausea (20%)

1% to 10%: Central nervous system: Dizziness (2%)

General Dosage Range

I.M.: *Adults:* 0.1 mcg/kg

I.V.: *Adults:* 0.02-0.04 mcg/kg as a single dose; may repeat 0.04 mcg/kg once **or** 0.12 mcg/kg as a single dose

Mechanism of Action Stimulates contraction of the gallbladder; inhibits gastric emptying by causing pyloric contraction, and increases intestinal motility; stimulates pancreatic secretion; causes smooth muscle contraction

Pharmacodynamics/Kinetics

Onset of Action Contraction of the gallbladder: ~5-15 minutes

Duration of Action ~1 hour

Pregnancy Risk Factor B

Sinecatechins (sin e KAT e kins)

U.S. Brand Names Veregen™
Pharmacologic Category Immunomodulator, Topical; Topical Skin Product
Use Treatment of external genital and perianal warts secondary to *Condylomata acuminata*
Local Anesthetic/Vasoconstrictor Precautions No information available to require special precautions
Effects on Dental Treatment No significant effects or complications reported
Effects on Bleeding No information available to require special precautions
Adverse Effects
>10%:
Dermatologic: Erythema (70%), pruritus (69%), edema (45%), vesicular rash (20%)
Local: Burning (67%), pain/discomfort (56%), erosion/ulceration (49%), induration (35%)
1% to 10%:
Dermatologic: Desquamation (5%), rash (1%), scar formation (1%)
Local: Discharge (3%), lymphadenitis (3%), bleeding (2%), reaction (2%), irritation (1%)
Miscellaneous: Phimosis (uncircumcised males; 3%), hypersensitivity (2%)
General Dosage Range Topical: *Adults:* Apply a thin layer (~0.5 cm strand) 3 times/day
Mechanism of Action The mechanism by which sinecatechins ointment aids in the clearance of genital and perianal warts is unknown. Antioxidant properties have been demonstrated *in vitro*; however, the significance of this finding is not known.
Pregnancy Risk Factor C

Sipuleucel-T (si pu LOO sel tee)

U.S. Brand Names Provenge®
Pharmacologic Category Cellular Immunotherapy, Autologous
Use Treatment of metastatic hormone-refractory prostate cancer in patients who are asymptomatic or minimally symptomatic
Local Anesthetic/Vasoconstrictor Precautions No information available to require special precautions
Effects on Dental Treatment No significant effects or complications reported
Effects on Bleeding No information available to require special precautions
Adverse Effects Note: Initial infusion-related events usually present within the first 24 hours after administration.

>10%:
Central nervous system: Chills (53%), fatigue (41%), fever (31%), headache (18%), dizziness (12%), pain (12%)
Gastrointestinal: Nausea (22%), vomiting (13%)
Hematologic: Anemia (13%)
Neuromuscular & skeletal: Back pain (30%), myalgia (12%), weakness (11%)
Miscellaneous: Acute infusion reaction (71%; grade 3: 4%), citrate toxicity (15%)
1% to 10%:
Cardiovascular: Hypertension (8%)
Central nervous system: Stroke (hemorrhagic or ischemic: 4%)
Dermatologic: Rash (5%)
Neuromuscular & skeletal: Muscle spasm (8%), neck pain (6%), tremor (5%)
Renal: Hematuria (8%)
Respiratory: Dyspnea (9%), cough (6%), upper respiratory tract infection (6%)
Miscellaneous: Flu-like syndrome (10%), diaphoresis (5%)
General Dosage Range I.V.: *Adults (males):* ≥50 million autologous CD54+ cells activated with PAP-GM-CSF; dose administered at ~2 week intervals for a total of 3 doses
Mechanism of Action Autologous cellular immunotherapy which stimulates an immune response against prostate cancer. Peripheral blood is collected (~3 days prior to infusion) from the patient via leukapheresis, from which peripheral blood mononuclear cells (PBMCs) are isolated. Antigen presenting cell (APC) precursors, consisting of CD54-positive cells that include dendritic cells are isolated from the PBMCs. The APCs are then activated (*in vitro*) with a recombinant human fusion protein, PAP-GM-CSF (also termed PA2024), composed of an antigen specific for prostate cancer, prostatic acid phosphatase (PAP) linked to granulocyte-macrophage colony-stimulating factor (GM-CSF) and cultured for ~40 hours. The final product, sipuleucel-T, is reinfused into the patient, inducing T-cell immunity to tumors that express PAP.

Prescribing and Access Restrictions Patients may currently receive Sipuleucel-T at one of the ~50 sites that participated in the clinical trials until the program is expanded to additional sites. Physicians must go through an inservice and register to prescribe the treatment; patients must also complete an enrollment form. Information on registration and enrollment is available at 1-877-336-3736.

Sirolimus (sir OH li mus)

U.S. Brand Names Rapamune®
Canadian Brand Names Rapamune®
Generic Availability (U.S.) No
Pharmacologic Category Immunosuppressant Agent; mTOR Kinase Inhibitor
Use Prophylaxis of organ rejection in patients receiving renal transplants
Unlabeled/Investigational Use Prophylaxis of organ rejection in heart transplant recipients; prevention acute graft-versus-host disease (GVHD) in allogeneic stem cell transplantation; treatment of refractory acute or chronic GVHD; treatment of soft tissue sarcoma (chordoma, angiomyolipoma, or lymphangioleiomyomatosis)
Local Anesthetic/Vasoconstrictor Precautions No information available to require special precautions
Effects on Dental Treatment Key adverse event(s) related to dental treatment: Mouth ulceration, oral moniliasis, stomatitis, gingival hyperplasia, gingivitis, and dysphagia.
Effects on Bleeding Thrombocytopenia has been associated with use; severe thrombocytopenia (rare) may be associated with delayed coagulation. Consultation to ensure adequate platelet counts may be considered in patients with signs/symptoms or a history of thrombocytopenia.
Adverse Effects Incidence of many adverse effects is dose related.

>20%:

- Cardiovascular: Peripheral edema (54% to 58%), hypertension (45% to 49%), edema (18% to 20%)
- Central nervous system: Headache (34%), pain (20% to 33%), insomnia (13% to 22%)
- Dermatologic: Acne (22%)
- Endocrine & metabolic: Hypertriglyceridemia (45% to 57%), hypercholesterolemia (43% to 46%)
- Gastrointestinal: Constipation (36% to 38%), abdominal pain (29% to 36%), diarrhea (25% to 36%), nausea (25% to 31%)
- Genitourinary: Urinary tract infection (26% to 33%)
- Hematologic: Anemia (23% to 33%), thrombocytopenia (14% to 30%)
- Neuromuscular & skeletal: Arthralgia (25% to 31%)
- Renal: Serum creatinine increased (39% to 40%)

3% to 20%:

- Cardiovascular: Atrial fibrillation, CHF, DVT, facial edema, hypervolemia, hypotension, palpitation, peripheral vascular disorder, postural hypotension, syncope, tachycardia, thrombosis, vasodilation
- Central nervous system: Anxiety, chills, confusion, depression, dizziness, emotional lability, hypoesthesia, malaise, neuropathy, somnolence
- Dermatologic: Rash (10% to 20%), skin carcinoma (up to 3%; includes basal cell carcinoma, squamous cell carcinoma, melanoma), cellulitis, dermal ulcer, dermatitis (fungal), ecchymosis, hirsutism, pruritus, skin hypertrophy, wound healing abnormal
- Endocrine & metabolic: Acidosis, Cushing's syndrome, dehydration, diabetes mellitus, glycosuria, hypercalcemia, hyperglycemia, hyperphosphatemia, hypocalcemia, hypoglycemia, hypokalemia, hypomagnesemia, hyponatremia
- Gastrointestinal: Abdomen enlarged, anorexia, dysphagia, eructation, esophagitis, flatulence, gastritis, gastroenteritis, gingival hyperplasia, gingivitis, ileus, mouth ulceration, oral moniliasis, stomatitis, weight loss
- Genitourinary: Impotence, pelvic pain, scrotal edema, testis disorder
- Hematologic: Hemolytic-uremic syndrome, hemorrhage, leukopenia, leukocytosis, polycythemia, TTP
- Hepatic: Abnormal liver function tests, alkaline phosphatase increased, LDH increased
- Local: Thrombophlebitis
- Neuromuscular & skeletal: Arthrosis, bone necrosis, CPK increased, hyper-/hypotonia, leg cramps, myalgia, osteoporosis, paresthesia, tetany
- Ocular: Abnormal vision, cataract, conjunctivitis
- Otic: Ear pain, otitis media, tinnitus
- Renal: Albuminuria, bladder pain, BUN increased, dysuria, hematuria, hydronephrosis, kidney pain, nephropathy (toxic), nocturia, oliguria, pyelonephritis, pyuria, tubular necrosis, urinary frequency, urinary incontinence, urinary retention

Respiratory: Asthma, atelectasis, bronchitis, cough, epistaxis, hypoxia, lung edema, pleural effusion, pneumonia, pulmonary embolism, rhinitis, sinusitis

Miscellaneous: Lymphoproliferative disease/lymphoma (1% to 3%), abscess, diaphoresis, flu-like syndrome, hernia, herpesvirus infection, infection (including opportunistic), lymphadenopathy, lymphocele, peritonitis, sepsis

Dosage Oral:

Low-to-moderate immunologic risk renal transplant patients: Children ≥13 years and Adults: Dosing by body weight:

<40 kg: Loading dose: 3 mg/m^2 on day 1, followed by maintenance dosing of 1 mg/m^2 once daily

≥40 kg: Loading dose: 6 mg on day 1; maintenance: 2 mg once daily

High immunologic risk renal transplant patients: Adults: Loading dose: Up to 15 mg on day 1; maintenance: 5 mg/day; obtain trough concentration between days 5-7 and adjust accordingly. Continue concurrent cyclosporine/sirolimus therapy for 1 year following transplantation. Further adjustment of the regimen must be based on clinical status.

Dosage adjustment: Sirolimus dosages should be adjusted to maintain trough concentrations within desired range based on risk and concomitant therapy. Maximum daily dose: 40 mg. Dosage should be adjusted at intervals of 7-14 days to account for the long half-life of sirolimus. In general, dose proportionality may be assumed. New sirolimus dose **equals** current dose **multiplied by** (target concentration **divided by** current concentration). **Note:** If large dose increase is required, consider loading dose calculated as:

Loading dose **equals** (new maintenance dose **minus** current maintenance dose) **multiplied by** 3

Maximum dose in 1 day: 40 mg; if required dose is >40 mg (due to loading dose), divide loading dose over 2 days. Whole blood concentrations should not be used as the sole basis for dosage adjustment (monitor clinical signs/symptoms, tissue biopsy, and laboratory parameters).

Maintenance therapy after withdrawal of cyclosporine: Cyclosporine withdrawal is not recommended in high immunological risk patients. Following 2-4 months of combined therapy, withdrawal of cyclosporine may be considered in low-to-moderate immunologic risk patients. Cyclosporine should be discontinued over 4-8 weeks, and a necessary increase in the dosage of sirolimus (up to fourfold) should be anticipated due to removal of metabolic inhibition by cyclosporine and to maintain adequate immunosuppressive effects. Dose-adjusted trough target concentrations are typically 16-24 ng/mL for the first year post-transplant and 12-20 ng/mL thereafter (measured by chromatographic methodology).

GVHD prophylaxis (unlabeled use): 12 mg loading dose on day -3, followed by 4 mg daily (target trough level: 3-12 ng/mL); taper off after 6-9 months (Armand, 2008; Cutler, 2007)

Treatment of refractory acute GVHD (unlabeled use): 4-5 mg/m^2 for 14 days (no loading dose) (Benito, 2001)

Treatment of chronic GVHD (unlabeled use): 6 mg loading dose, followed by 2 mg daily (target trough level: 7-12 ng/mL) for 6-9 months (Couriel, 2005)

Dosage adjustment in renal impairment: No dosage adjustment (in loading or maintenance dose) is necessary in renal impairment. However, adjustment of regimen (including discontinuation of therapy) should be considered when used concurrently with cyclosporine and elevated or increasing serum creatinine is noted.

Dosage adjustment in hepatic impairment:

Loading dose: No adjustment required

Maintenance dose:

Mild-to-moderate hepatic impairment: reduce maintenance dose by ~33%

Severe hepatic impairment: reduce maintenance dose by ~50%

Mechanism of Action Sirolimus inhibits T-lymphocyte activation and proliferation in response to antigenic and cytokine stimulation and inhibits antibody production. Its mechanism differs from other immunosuppressants. Sirolimus binds to FKBP-12, an intracellular protein, to form an immunosuppressive complex which inhibits the regulatory kinase, mTOR (mammalian target of rapamycin). This inhibition suppresses cytokine mediated T-cell proliferation, halting progression from the G1 to the S phase of the cell cycle. It inhibits acute rejection of allografts and prolongs graft survival.

Contraindications Hypersensitivity to sirolimus or any component of the formulation

Warnings/Precautions Hazardous agent - use appropriate precautions for handling and disposal. **[U.S. Boxed Warning]: Immunosuppressive agents, including sirolimus, increase the risk of infection and may be associated with the development of lymphoma.** Immune suppression may also increase the risk of opportunistic infections (including activation of latent viral infections including BK virus-associated nephropathy), fatal infections, and sepsis. Prophylactic treatment for *Pneumocystis jiroveci* pneumonia (PCP) should be administered for 1 year post-transplant; prophylaxis for cytomegalovirus (CMV) should be taken for 3 months post-transplant in patients at risk for CMV. Progressive multifocal leukoencephalopathy (PML), an opportunistic CNS infection caused by reactivation of the JC virus, has been reported in patients receiving immunosuppressive therapy, including sirolimus. Clinical findings of PML include apathy, ataxia, cognitive deficiency, confusion, and hemiparesis; promptly evaluate any patient presenting with neurological changes; consider decreasing the degree of immunosuppression with consideration to the risk of organ rejection in transplant patients.

[U.S. Boxed Warning]: Sirolimus is not recommended for use in liver or lung transplantation. Bronchial anastomotic dehiscence cases have been reported in lung transplant patients when sirolimus was used as part of an immunosuppressive regimen; most of these reactions were fatal. Studies indicate an association with an increase risk of hepatic artery thrombosis (HAT), graft failure, and increased mortality (with evidence of infection) in liver transplant patients when sirolimus is used in combination with cyclosporine and/or tacrolimus. Most cases of HAT occurred within 30 days of transplant.

In renal transplant patients, *de novo* use without cyclosporine has been associated with higher rates of acute rejection. Sirolimus should be used in combination with cyclosporine (and corticosteroids) initially. Cyclosporine may be withdrawn in low-to-moderate immunologic risk patients after 2-4 months, in conjunction with an increase in sirolimus dosage. In high immunologic risk patients, use in combination with cyclosporine and corticosteroids is recommended for the first year. Safety and efficacy of combination therapy with cyclosporine in high immunologic risk patients has not been studied beyond 12 months of treatment; adjustment of immunosuppressive therapy beyond 12 months should be considered based on clinical judgement. Monitor renal function closely when combined with cyclosporine; consider dosage adjustment or discontinue in patients with increasing serum creatinine.

May increase serum creatinine and decrease GFR. Use caution when used concurrently with medications which may alter renal function. May delay recovery of renal function in patients with delayed allograft function. Increased urinary protein excretion has been observed when converting renal transplant patients from calcineurin inhibitors to sirolimus during maintenance therapy. A higher level of proteinuria prior to sirolimus conversion correlates with a higher degree of proteinuria after conversion. In some patients, proteinuria may reach nephrotic levels; nephrotic syndrome (new onset) has been reported. Increased risk of BK viral-associated nephropathy which may impair renal function and cause graft loss; consider decreasing immunosuppressive burden if evidence of deteriorating renal function.

Use caution with hepatic impairment; a reduction in the maintenance dose is recommended. Has been associated with an increased risk of fluid accumulation and lymphocele; peripheral edema, lymphedema, ascites, and pleural and pericardial effusions (including significant effusions and tamponade) were reported; use with caution in patients in whom fluid accumulation may be poorly tolerated, such as in cardiovascular disease (heart failure or hypertension) and pulmonary disease. Cases of interstitial lung disease (eg, pneumonitis, bronchiolitis obliterans organizing pneumonia [BOOP], pulmonary fibrosis) have been observed; risk may be increased with higher trough levels. Avoid concurrent use of strong CYP3A4 and/or P-glycoprotein (P-gp) inhibitors (eg, clarithromycin, erythromycin, telithromycin, itraconazole, ketoconazole, voriconazole) and strong inducers of CYP3A4 and/or P-gp (eg, rifampin, rifabutin). Concurrent use with a calcineurin inhibitor (cyclosporine, tacrolimus) may increase the risk of calcineurin inhibitor-induced hemolytic uremic syndrome/thrombotic thrombocytopenic purpura/thrombotic microangiopathy (HUS/TTP/TMA).

Hypersensitivity reactions, including anaphylactic/anaphylactoid reactions, angioedema, exfoliative dermatitis, and hypersensitivity vasculitis have been reported. Concurrent use with other drugs known to cause angioedema (eg, ACE inhibitors) may increase risk. Immunosuppressant therapy is associated with an increased risk of skin cancer; limit sun and ultraviolet light exposure; use appropriate sun protection. May increase serum lipids (cholesterol and triglycerides); use with caution in patients with hyperlipidemia. May be associated with wound dehiscence and impaired healing; use caution in the perioperative period. Patients with a body mass index (BMI) >30 kg/m^2 are at increased risk for abnormal wound healing.

Sirolimus tablets and oral solution are not bioequivalent, due to differences in absorption. Clinical equivalence was seen using 2 mg tablet and 2 mg solution. It is not known if higher doses are also clinically equivalent. Monitor sirolimus levels if changes in dosage forms are made. **[U.S. Boxed Warning]: Should only be used by physicians experienced in immunosuppressive therapy and management of transplant patients. Adequate laboratory and supportive medical resources must be readily available.** Sirolimus concentrations are dependent on the assay method (eg, chromatographic and immunoassay) used; assay methods are not interchangeable. Variations in methods to determine sirolimus whole blood concentrations, as well as interlaboratory variations, may result in improper dosage adjustments, which may lead to subtherapeutic or toxic levels. Determine the assay method used to assure consistency (or accommodations if changes occur), and for monitoring purposes, be aware of alterations to assay method or reference range. The manufacturer recommends high performance liquid chromatography (HPLC) as the reference standard to determine sirolimus trough concentrations.

Drug Interactions

Metabolism/Transport Effects **Substrate** of CYP3A4 (major), P-glycoprotein; **Inhibits** CYP3A4 (weak)

Avoid Concomitant Use

Avoid concomitant use of Sirolimus with any of the following: BCG; Natalizumab; Pimecrolimus; Posaconazole; Roflumilast; Tacrolimus (Systemic); Tacrolimus (Topical); Vaccines (Live); Voriconazole

Increased Effect/Toxicity

Sirolimus may increase the levels/effects of: ACE Inhibitors; CycloSPORINE; CycloSPORINE (Systemic); Hypoglycemic Agents; Leflunomide; Natalizumab; Tacrolimus; Tacrolimus (Systemic); Tacrolimus (Topical); Vaccines (Live)

The levels/effects of Sirolimus may be increased by: Conivaptan; CycloSPORINE; CycloSPORINE (Systemic); CYP3A4 Inhibitors (Moderate); CYP3A4 Inhibitors (Strong); Dasatinib; Denosumab; Fluconazole; Herbs (Hypoglycemic Properties); Itraconazole; Ketoconazole; Ketoconazole (Systemic); Macrolide Antibiotics; P-Glycoprotein Inhibitors; Pimecrolimus; Posaconazole; Protease Inhibitors; Roflumilast; Tacrolimus; Tacrolimus (Systemic); Tacrolimus (Topical); Trastuzumab; Voriconazole

Decreased Effect

Sirolimus may decrease the levels/effects of: BCG; Sipuleucel-T; Tacrolimus; Tacrolimus (Systemic); Vaccines (Inactivated); Vaccines (Live)

The levels/effects of Sirolimus may be decreased by: CYP3A4 Inducers (Strong); Deferasirox; Echinacea; Efavirenz; Herbs (CYP3A4 Inducers); P-Glycoprotein Inducers; Phenytoin; Rifampin; Tocilizumab

Ethanol/Nutrition/Herb Interactions

Food: Avoid grapefruit juice; may decrease clearance of sirolimus. Ingestion with high-fat meals decreases peak concentrations but increases AUC by 23% to 35%. Sirolimus should be taken consistently (either with or without food) to minimize variability.

Herb/Nutraceutical: St John's wort may decrease sirolimus levels; avoid concurrent use. Avoid cat's claw, echinacea (have immunostimulant properties; consider therapy modifications). Herbs with hypoglycemic properties may increase the risk of sirolimus-induced hypoglycemia; includes alfalfa, aloe, bilberry, bitter melon, burdock, celery, damiana, fenugreek, garcinia, garlic, ginger, ginseng (American), gymnema, marshmallow, stinging nettle.

Dietary Considerations Take consistently (with or without food) to minimize variability of absorption.

Pharmacodynamics/Kinetics

Half-life Elimination Half-life elimination: Mean: 62 hours (range; 46-78 hours); extended in hepatic impairment (Child-Pugh class A or B) to 113 hours

Time to Peak Oral solution: 1-3 hours; Tablet: 1-6 hours

Pregnancy Risk Factor C

Lactation Excretion in breast milk unknown/not recommended

Breast-Feeding Considerations Due to the potential for adverse reactions in the breast-fed infant, including possible immunosuppression, breast-feeding is not recommended.

Dosage Forms

Solution, oral:

Rapamune®: 1 mg/mL (60 mL)

Tablet, oral:

Rapamune®: 0.5 mg, 1 mg, 2 mg

SitaGLIPtin (sit a GLIP tin)

Related Information

Endocrine Disorders and Pregnancy *on page 1879*

U.S. Brand Names Januvia®

Canadian Brand Names Januvia®

Generic Availability (U.S.) No

Pharmacologic Category Antidiabetic Agent, Dipeptidyl Peptidase IV (DPP-IV) Inhibitor

Use Management of type 2 diabetes mellitus (noninsulin dependent, NIDDM) as an adjunct to diet and exercise as monotherapy or in combination therapy with other antidiabetic agents

Local Anesthetic/Vasoconstrictor Precautions No information available to require special precautions

Effects on Dental Treatment Sitagliptin-dependent patients with diabetes should be appointed for dental treatment in morning in order to minimize chance of stress-induced hypoglycemia.

Effects on Bleeding No information available to require special precautions

Adverse Effects As reported with monotherapy: 1% to 10%:

Cardiovascular: Peripheral edema (2%)

Endocrine & metabolic: Hypoglycemia (1%)

Gastrointestinal: Diarrhea (4%), constipation (3%), nausea (2%)

Neuromuscular & skeletal: Osteoarthritis (1%)

Respiratory: Nasopharyngitis (5%), pharyngitis (1%), upper respiratory tract infection (viral; 1%)

Dosage Oral: Adults: Type 2 diabetes: 100 mg once daily

Concomitant use with insulin and/or insulin secretagogues (eg, sulfonylureas): Reduced dose of insulin and/or insulin secretagogues may be needed.

Dosage adjustment in renal impairment:

Cl_{cr} ≥50 mL/minute: No adjustment required

Cl_{cr} ≥30 to <50 mL/minute: 50 mg once daily

S_{cr}: Males: >1.7 to ≤3.0 mg/dL; Females: >1.5 to ≤2.5 mg/dL: 50 mg once daily

Cl_{cr}<30 mL/minute: 25 mg once daily

S_{cr}: Males: >3.0 mg/dL; Females: >2.5 mg/dL: 25 mg once daily

ESRD requiring hemodialysis or peritoneal dialysis: 25 mg once daily; administered without regard to timing of hemodialysis

Dosage adjustment in hepatic impairment:

Mild-to-moderate impairment (Child-Pugh score 7-9): No dosage adjustment required

Severe impairment (Child-Pugh score >9): Not studied

Mechanism of Action Sitagliptin inhibits dipeptidyl peptidase IV (DPP-IV) enzyme resulting in prolonged active incretin levels. Incretin hormones (eg, glucagon-like peptide-1 [GLP-1] and glucose-dependent insulinotropic polypeptide [GIP]) regulate glucose homeostasis by increasing insulin synthesis and release from pancreatic beta cells and decreasing glucagon secretion from pancreatic alpha cells. Decreased glucagon secretion results in decreased hepatic glucose production. Under normal physiologic circumstances, incretin hormones are released by the intestine throughout the day and levels are increased in response to a meal; incretin hormones are rapidly inactivated by the DPP-IV enzyme.

Contraindications Serious hypersensitivity (eg, anaphylaxis, angioedema) to sitagliptan or any component of the formulation

Warnings/Precautions Avoid use in type 1 diabetes mellitus (insulin dependent, IDDM) and diabetic ketoacidosis (DKA) due to lack of efficacy in these populations. Use caution when used in conjunction with insulin or insulin secretagogues; risk of hypoglycemia is increased. Monitor blood glucose closely; dosage adjustments of insulin or insulin secretagogues may be necessary. Use with caution in patients with moderate-to-severe renal dysfunction and end-stage renal disease (ESRD) requiring hemodialysis or peritoneal dialysis; dosing adjustment required. Safety and efficacy have not been established in severe hepatic dysfunction.

Rare hypersensitivity reactions, including anaphylaxis, angioedema, and/or severe dermatologic reactions (such as Stevens-Johnson syndrome), have been reported in postmarketing surveillance; discontinue if signs/symptoms of hypersensitivity reactions occur. Cases of acute pancreatitis (including hemorrhagic and necrotizing with some fatalities) have been reported with use; monitor for signs/symptoms of pancreatitis. Discontinue use immediately if pancreatitis is suspected and initiate appropriate management. Use with caution in patients with a history of pancreatitis (not known if this population is at greater risk).

Clinical trials included only a limited number of patients with heart failure (HF). No specific recommendations regarding this population are provided in the approved U.S. labeling (Canadian labeling recommends against use in this population). Diabetes self-management education (DSME) is essential to maximize the effectiveness of therapy.

Drug Interactions

Metabolism/Transport Effects Substrate of CYP2C8 (minor), CYP3A4 (minor), P-glycoprotein

Avoid Concomitant Use There are no known interactions where it is recommended to avoid concomitant use.

Increased Effect/Toxicity

SitaGLIPtin may increase the levels/effects of: ACE Inhibitors; Digoxin; Hypoglycemic Agents

The levels/effects of SitaGLIPtin may be increased by: Herbs (Hypoglycemic Properties); Pegvisomant; P-Glycoprotein Inhibitors

Decreased Effect

The levels/effects of SitaGLIPtin may be decreased by: Corticosteroids (Orally Inhaled); Corticosteroids (Systemic); Luteinizing Hormone-Releasing Hormone Analogs; P-Glycoprotein Inducers; Somatropin; Thiazide Diuretics

Dietary Considerations May be taken with or without food. Individualized medical nutrition therapy (MNT) based on ADA recommendations is an integral part of therapy.

Pharmacodynamics/Kinetics

Half-life Elimination 12 hours

Time to Peak 1-4 hours

Pregnancy Risk Factor B

Lactation Excretion in breast milk unknown/use caution

Breast-Feeding Considerations It is not known if sitagliptin is excreted in breast milk. The manufacturer recommends that caution be used if administered to breast-feeding women.

Dosage Forms

Tablet, oral:

Januvia®: 25 mg, 50 mg, 100 mg

Sitagliptin and Metformin (sit a GLIP tin & met FOR min)

Related Information

Endocrine Disorders and Pregnancy *on page 1879*
MetFORMIN *on page 1089*
SitaGLIPtin *on page 1534*

U.S. Brand Names Janumet®

Canadian Brand Names Janumet®

Pharmacologic Category Antidiabetic Agent, Biguanide; Antidiabetic Agent, Dipeptidyl Peptidase IV (DPP-IV) Inhibitor; Hypoglycemic Agent, Oral

Use Management of type 2 diabetes mellitus (noninsulin dependent, NIDDM) as an adjunct to diet and exercise in patients not adequately controlled on metformin or sitagliptin monotherapy

Local Anesthetic/Vasoconstrictor Precautions No information available to require special precautions

Effects on Dental Treatment Sitagliptin- and metformin-dependent patients with diabetes (noninsulin dependent, Type 2) should be appointed for dental treatment in morning in order to minimize chance of stress-induced hypoglycemia.

Effects on Bleeding No information available to require special precautions

Adverse Effects See individual agents.

General Dosage Range Oral: *Adults:* Sitagliptin 50 mg and metformin 500-1000 mg twice daily (maximum: 100 mg/day [sitagliptin], 2000 mg/day [metformin])

Mechanism of Action Sitagliptin inhibits dipeptidyl peptidase IV (DPP-IV) enzymes resulting in prolonged active incretin levels. Incretin hormones [eg, glucagon-like peptide-1 (GLP-1) and glucose-dependent insulinotropic polypeptide (GIP)] regulate glucose homeostasis by increasing insulin synthesis and release from pancreatic beta cells and decreasing glucagon secretion from pancreatic alpha cells. Decreased glucagon secretion results in decreased hepatic glucose production. Under normal physiologic circumstances, incretin hormones are released by the intestine throughout the day and levels are increased in response to a meal; incretin hormones are rapidly inactivated by DPP-IV enzymes.

Metformin decreases hepatic glucose production, decreasing intestinal absorption of glucose, and improves insulin sensitivity (increases peripheral glucose uptake and utilization).

Pregnancy Risk Factor B

Sitaxsentan (sye TACKS en tan)

Canadian Brand Names Thelin®

Pharmacologic Category Endothelin Antagonist; Vasodilator

Use Treatment of primary pulmonary arterial hypertension (PAH) or pulmonary hypertension secondary to connective tissue disease, in World Health Organization (WHO) class III patients unresponsive to conventional therapy; treatment of PAH in WHO class II patients who are unresponsive to conventional therapy and have no alternative treatment options

Local Anesthetic/Vasoconstrictor Precautions No information available to require special precautions

Effects on Dental Treatment Key adverse event(s) related to dental treatment: Bleeding gums has been reported.

Effects on Bleeding Prolongation of clotting time has been noted in some patients. Potential difficulty and/or delays in coagulation should be anticipated.

Adverse Effects

>10%: Central nervous system: Headache (15%)

1% to 10%:

Cardiovascular: Peripheral edema (9%), flushing (4%)

Central nervous system: Fatigue (3%), insomnia (2%)

Endocrine & metabolic: Menorrhagia (1%)

Gastrointestinal: Nausea (7%), constipation (3%), vomiting (3%), dyspepsia (2%), upper abdominal pain (2%), bleeding gums (1%)

Genitourinary: Vaginal hemorrhage (1%)

Hematologic: Hemoglobin decreased by >15% (dose related; 7%), INR increased (6%), PT prolonged (5%), hematoma (1%), hematocrit decreased (dose related)

Hepatic: ALT increased (2% to 3%, occurrence less then placebo), AST increased (2% to 3%, occurrence less then placebo)

Neuromuscular & skeletal: Muscle cramping (2%)

Renal: Hematuria (1%)

Respiratory: Nasal congestion (9%), epistaxis (up to 8%), hemoptysis (2%)

General Dosage Range Dosage adjustment recommended in patients who develop toxicities

Oral: *Adults:* 100 mg once daily

Mechanism of Action Sitaxsentan is a selective antagonist of the A subtype of endothelin-1 receptors (ETA) located in pulmonary smooth muscle. Stimulation of these receptors by endogenous endothelin-1 causes vasoconstriction, thus worsening symptoms of PAH. Sitaxsentan exhibits 6500-fold greater selectivity for the ET_A over the ET_B subtype, the latter of which predominates on vascular endothelial cells. Thus, preferential antagonism of ET_A reduces vasoconstriction, without compromising the vasodilatory/antiproliferative actions mediated through endothelin-1 binding to the ET_B subtype.

Pharmacodynamics/Kinetics

Half-life Elimination 10 hours

Time to Peak 1-4 hours

Product Availability Not available in U.S.

Sodium Bicarbonate (SOW dee um bye KAR bun ate)

U.S. Brand Names Brioschi® [OTC]; Neut®

Pharmacologic Category Alkalinizing Agent; Antacid; Electrolyte Supplement, Oral; Electrolyte Supplement, Parenteral

Use Management of metabolic acidosis; gastric hyperacidity; as an alkalinization agent for the urine; treatment of hyperkalemia; management of overdose of certain drugs, including tricyclic antidepressants and aspirin

Unlabeled/Investigational Use Prevention of contrast-induced nephropathy (CIN)

Local Anesthetic/Vasoconstrictor Precautions No information available to require special precautions

Effects on Dental Treatment No significant effects or complications reported

Effects on Bleeding No information available to require special precautions

Adverse Effects Frequency not defined.

Cardiovascular: Cerebral hemorrhage, CHF (aggravated), edema

Central nervous system: Tetany

Gastrointestinal: Belching, flatulence (with oral), gastric distension

Endocrine & metabolic: Hypernatremia, hyperosmolality, hypocalcemia, hypokalemia, increased affinity of hemoglobin for oxygen-reduced pH in myocardial tissue necrosis when extravasated, intracranial acidosis, metabolic alkalosis, milk-alkali syndrome (especially with renal dysfunction)

Respiratory: Pulmonary edema

General Dosage Range
I.V.: *Children and Adults:* Dosage varies greatly depending on indication
Oral:
Children: 1-10 mEq/kg/day as a single dose **or** divided every 4-6 hours
Adults <60 years: 0.5-200 mEq/kg/day in 4-5 divided doses **or** 325 mg to 2 g 1-4 times/day (maximum: 16 g [200 mEq] day)
Adults ≥60 years: 0.5-100 mEq/kg/day in 4-6 divided doses **or** 325 mg to 2 g 1-4 times/day (maximum: 8 g [100 mEq] day)

Mechanism of Action Dissociates to provide bicarbonate ion which neutralizes hydrogen ion concentration and raises blood and urinary pH

Pharmacodynamics/Kinetics
Onset of Action Oral: Rapid; I.V.: 15 minutes
Duration of Action Oral: 8-10 minutes; I.V.: 1-2 hours

Pregnancy Risk Factor C

Sodium Chloride (SOW dee um KLOR ide)

U.S. Brand Names 4-Way® Saline Moisturizing Mist [OTC]; Altachlore [OTC]; Altamist [OTC]; Ayr® Allergy Sinus [OTC]; Ayr® Baby Saline [OTC]; Ayr® Saline No-Drip [OTC]; Ayr® Saline [OTC]; Breathe Free® [OTC]; Deep Sea [OTC]; Entsol® [OTC]; HuMist® for Kids [OTC]; HuMist® [OTC]; Hyper-Sal™; Little Noses® Saline [OTC]; Little Noses® Stuffy Nose Kit [OTC]; Muro 128® [OTC]; Na-Zone® [OTC]; Nasal Moist® Saline [OTC]; Nasal Spray [OTC]; NāSal™ [OTC]; Ocean® for Kids [OTC]; Ocean® [OTC]; Pretz® [OTC]; Rhinaris® [OTC]; Saline Mist [OTC]; Simply Saline® Baby [OTC]; Simply Saline® Nasal Moist® [OTC]; Simply Saline® [OTC]; Syrex; Wound Wash Saline™ [OTC]

Pharmacologic Category Electrolyte Supplement, Parenteral; Genitourinary Irrigant; Irrigant; Lubricant, Ocular; Sodium Salt

Use
Parenteral: Restores sodium ion in patients with restricted oral intake (especially hyponatremia states or low salt syndrome).
Concentrated sodium chloride: Additive for parenteral fluid therapy
Hypertonic sodium chloride: For severe hyponatremia and hypochloremia
Hypotonic sodium chloride: Hydrating solution
Normal saline: Restores water/sodium losses
Ophthalmic: Reduces corneal edema
Inhalation: Restores moisture to pulmonary system; loosens and thins congestion caused by colds or allergies; diluent for bronchodilator solutions that require dilution before inhalation
Intranasal: Restores moisture to nasal membranes
Irrigation: Wound cleansing, irrigation, and flushing

Unlabeled/Investigational Use Parenteral: Hypertonic saline: Refractory elevated intracranial pressure (ICP) due to various etiologies (eg, subarachnoid hemorrhage, neoplasm); transtentorial herniation syndrome; traumatic brain injury with elevated ICP. **Note:** May be used in patients in whom mannitol may not be recommended (eg, renal failure).

Local Anesthetic/Vasoconstrictor Precautions No information available to require special precautions

Effects on Dental Treatment No significant effects or complications reported

Effects on Bleeding No information available to require special precautions

Adverse Effects Frequency not defined.
Cardiovascular: Congestive heart failure, transient hypotension (especially with administration of 23.4% NaCl)
Central nervous system: Central pontine myelinolysis (due to rapid correction of hyponatremia)
Endocrine & metabolic: Extravasation, hypervolemia, hypernatremia, dilution of serum electrolytes, overhydration, hypokalemia
Local: Thrombosis, phlebitis, extravasation
Respiratory: Pulmonary edema

General Dosage Range
I.V.: *Children and Adults:* Dosage varies greatly depending on indication
Inhalation: *Children ≥2 years and Adults:* 1-3 sprays (1-3 mL)
Intranasal: *Children ≥2 years and Adults:* 2-3 sprays in each nostril as needed
Irrigation: *Children ≥2 years and Adults:* 1-3 L/day **or** spray affected area
Ophthalmic: *Adults:* Ointment: Apply once or more daily; Solution: Instill 1-2 drops into affected eye(s) every 3-4 hours

Mechanism of Action Principal extracellular cation; functions in fluid and electrolyte balance, osmotic pressure control, and water distribution

Pregnancy Risk Factor C

Sodium Chondroitin Sulfate and Sodium Hyaluronate
(SOW de um kon DROY tin SUL fate & SOW de um hye al yoor ON ate)

Related Information
Chondroitin Sulfate *on page 1777*

U.S. Brand Names DisCoVisc®; Viscoat®

Pharmacologic Category Ophthalmic Agent, Viscoelastic

Use Ophthalmic surgical aid in the anterior segment during cataract extraction and intraocular lens implantation

Local Anesthetic/Vasoconstrictor Precautions No information available to require special precautions

Effects on Dental Treatment No significant effects or complications reported

Effects on Bleeding No information available to require special precautions

Adverse Effects Frequency not defined: Ocular: Intraocular pressure increased

General Dosage Range Ophthalmic: *Adults:* Carefully introduce into anterior chamber during surgery

Mechanism of Action Ophthalmic viscosurgical device which modulates the interactions between adjacent tissues by space creation, tissue stabilization, balancing pressure, and providing protection of the corneal endothelial cells during surgery.

Pregnancy Risk Factor C

Sodium Citrate and Citric Acid (SOW dee um SIT rate & SI trik AS id)

U.S. Brand Names Cytra-2; Oracit®; Shohl's Solution (Modified)

Canadian Brand Names PMS-Dicitrate

Pharmacologic Category Alkalinizing Agent, Oral

Use Treatment of metabolic acidosis; alkalinizing agent in conditions where long-term maintenance of an alkaline urine is desirable

Local Anesthetic/Vasoconstrictor Precautions No information available to require special precautions

Effects on Dental Treatment No significant effects or complications reported

Effects on Bleeding No information available to require special precautions

Adverse Effects Frequency not defined. Generally well tolerated with normal renal function.
Central nervous system: Tetany
Endocrine & metabolic: Metabolic alkalosis, hyperkalemia
Gastrointestinal: Diarrhea, nausea, vomiting

General Dosage Range Oral:
Infants and Children: 2-3 mEq/kg/day in 3-4 divided doses **or** 5-15 mL after meals and at bedtime
Adults: 10-30 mL after meals and at bedtime

Pregnancy Risk Factor Not established

Sodium Hypochlorite Solution
(SOW dee um hye poe KLOR ite soe LOO shun)

U.S. Brand Names Dakin's Solution; Di-Dak-Sol

Pharmacologic Category Disinfectant, Antibacterial (Topical)

Use Treatment of athlete's foot (0.5%); wound irrigation (0.5%); disinfection of utensils and equipment (5%)

Local Anesthetic/Vasoconstrictor Precautions No information available to require special precautions

Effects on Dental Treatment No significant effects or complications reported

Effects on Bleeding No information available to require special precautions

Adverse Effects Frequency not defined.
Dermatologic: Irritating to skin
Hematologic: Dissolves blood clots, delays clotting

General Dosage Range Topical: *Children and Adults:* Via irrigation: Lightly-to-moderately exudative wounds: Apply once daily; Highly exudative or contaminated wounds: Apply twice daily

Pregnancy Risk Factor C

Sodium Nitrite and Sodium Thiosulfate
(SOW dee um NYE trite & SOW dee um thye oh SUL fate)

U.S. Brand Names Nithiodote™

Pharmacologic Category Antidote

Use Acute, life-threatening cyanide poisoning

Local Anesthetic/Vasoconstrictor Precautions No information available to require special precautions

Effects on Dental Treatment No significant effects or complications reported

Effects on Bleeding No information available to require special precautions

Adverse Effects Frequency not defined.

Sodium nitrite:

Cardiovascular: Arrhythmias, cyanosis, flushing, hypotension, palpitation, tachycardia, syncope

Central nervous system: Anxiety, coma, confusion, dizziness, fatigue, headache, lightheadedness, seizure

Dermatologic: Urticaria

Endocrine & metabolic: Acidosis

Gastrointestinal: Abdominal pain, nausea, vomiting

Hematologic: Methemoglobinemia

Local: Injection site tingling

Neuromuscular & skeletal: Numbness, paresthesia, weakness

Ocular: Blurred vision

Respiratory: Dyspnea, tachypnea

Miscellaneous: Diaphoresis

Sodium thiosulfate:

Cardiovascular: Hypotension

Central nervous system: Disorientation, headache

Gastrointestinal: Nausea, salty taste, vomiting

Hematologic: Bleeding time prolonged

Miscellaneous: Warmth

General Dosage Range

I.V.:

Children:

Sodium nitrite: 6 mg/kg (0.2 mL/kg or 6-8 mL/m^2 of a 3% solution); maximum: 300 mg (10 mL of a 3% solution)

Sodium thiosulfate: 7 g/m^2 or 250 mg/kg (1 mL/kg or 28-40 mL/m^2 of a 25% solution); maximum: 12.5 g (50 mL of a 25% solution)

Adults:

Sodium nitrite: 300 mg (10 mL of a 3% solution)

Sodium thiosulfate: 12.5 g (50 mL of a 25% solution)

Mechanism of Action

Sodium thiosulfate serves as a sulfur donor to increase endogenous rhondanese-catalyzed thiocyanate (much less toxic than cyanide) formation.

Sodium nitrite promotes formation of methemoglobin which competes with cytochrome oxidase for the cyanide ion. Cyanide combines with methemoglobin to form cyanomethemoglobin and frees the cytochrome oxidase, allowing aerobic metabolism to continue.

Pharmacodynamics/Kinetics

Onset of Action Sodium nitrite: Peak effect: Methemoglobinemia: 30-60 minutes

Duration of Action Sodium nitrite: Methemoglobinemia: ~55 minutes

Half-life Elimination Sodium thiosulfate: ~3 hours; Renal impairment: ≤9 days

Pregnancy Risk Factor C

Product Availability Nithiodote™: FDA approved January 2011; anticipated availability is currently undetermined

Sodium Oxybate (SOW dee um ox i BATE)

U.S. Brand Names Xyrem®

Canadian Brand Names Xyrem®

Pharmacologic Category Central Nervous System Depressant

Use Treatment of cataplexy and daytime sleepiness in patients with narcolepsy

Local Anesthetic/Vasoconstrictor Precautions No information available to require special precautions

Effects on Dental Treatment Key adverse event(s) related to dental treatment: Tooth ache (see Dental Comment).

Effects on Bleeding No information available to require special precautions

Adverse Effects

>10%:

Central nervous system: Headache (9% to 37%), dizziness (8% to 37%), pain (9% to 20%), confusion (3% to 17%), sleep disorder (6% to 14%), somnolence (1% to 14%)

Gastrointestinal: Nausea (8% to 40%), vomiting (2% to 23%), abdominal pain (3% to 11%)

Genitourinary: Enuresis (3% to 17%), urinary incontinence (<1% to 14%, usually nocturnal), cystitis, metrorrhagia, urinary frequency
Miscellaneous: Diaphoresis (3% to 11%)

1% to 10%:
Cardiovascular: Hypertension (6%), chest pain, edema
Central nervous system: Disorientation (up to 9%), inebriation (up to 9%), concentration decreased (3% to 9%), dream abnormality (3% to 9%), sleepwalking (4% to 7%), depression (3% to 6%), amnesia (3% to 6%), anxiety (3% to 6%), thinking abnormality (3% to 6%), lethargy (up to 6%), insomnia (5%), agitation, ataxia, chills, fatigue, malaise, memory impairment, nervousness, pyrexia, seizure, stupor, tremor, vertigo
Dermatologic: Hyperhidrosis (3% to 6%), pruritus, rash
Endocrine & metabolic: Dysmenorrhea (3% to 6%)
Gastrointestinal: Dyspepsia (6% to 9%), diarrhea (6% to 8%), abdominal pain (6%), nausea and vomiting (6%), anorexia, constipation, tooth ache, weight gain
Hepatic: Alkaline phosphatase increased, hypercholesteremia, hypocalcemia
Neuromuscular & skeletal: Weakness (6% to 8%), hypoesthesia (6%), myasthenia (3% to 6%), pain (3% to 6%), arthritis, leg cramps, myalgia
Ocular: Amblyopia (6%), blurred vision (6%)
Otic: Tinnitus (6%), ear pain
Renal: Albuminuria, hematuria
Respiratory: Rhinitis (8%), nasopharyngitis (3% to 8%), pharyngitis (6% to 8%), infection (3% to 6%), bronchitis, cough, dyspnea
Miscellaneous: Viral infection (3% to 9%), infection (3% to 6%), allergic reaction, flu-like syndrome

General Dosage Range Dosage adjustment recommended in patients with hepatic impairment

Oral: *Children ≥16 years and Adults:* Initial: 4.5 g/day in 2 equal doses given at bedtime and 2.5-4 hours later; Maintenance: 4.5-9 g/day (maximum: 9 g/day)

Mechanism of Action Sodium oxybate is derived from gamma aminobutyric acid (GABA) and acts as an inhibitory chemical transmitter in the brain. May function through specific receptors for gamma hydroxybutyrate (GHB) and GABA (B).

Pharmacodynamics/Kinetics

Half-life Elimination 30-60 minutes

Time to Peak 30-75 minutes

Pregnancy Risk Factor B

Controlled Substance C-I (illicit use); C-III (medical use)

Prescribing and Access Restrictions Sodium oxybate is deemed to have an approved REMS program. As a requirement of the REMS program, access to this medication is restricted. Sodium oxybate oral solution will be available only to prescribers enrolled in the Xyrem® Patient Success Program® and dispensed to the patient through the designated centralized pharmacy (1-866-997-3688). Prior to dispensing the first prescription, prescribers will be sent educational materials to be reviewed with the patient and enrollment forms for the postmarketing surveillance program. Patients must be seen at least every 3 months; prescriptions can be written for a maximum of 3 months (the first prescription may only be written for a 1-month supply).

Dental Comment Sodium oxybate is a known substance of abuse. When used illegally, it has been referred to as a "date-rape drug". The dentist should be aware of patients showing signs of CNS depression, as with all other drugs in this class.

Sodium Phenylbutyrate (SOW dee um fen il BYOO ti rate)

U.S. Brand Names Buphenyl®

Pharmacologic Category Urea Cycle Disorder (UCD) Treatment Agent

Use Adjunctive therapy in the chronic management of patients with urea cycle disorder involving deficiencies of carbamoylphosphate synthetase, ornithine transcarbamylase, or argininosuccinic acid synthetase

Local Anesthetic/Vasoconstrictor Precautions No information available to require special precautions

Effects on Dental Treatment Key adverse event(s) related to dental treatment: Abnormal taste.

Effects on Bleeding No information available to require special precautions

Adverse Effects

>10%: Endocrine & metabolic: Amenorrhea/menstrual dysfunction (23%), acidosis (14%), hypoalbuminemia (11%)

1% to 10%:
Cardiovascular: Syncope (≤2%)
Central nervous system: Depression (≤2%), headache (≤2%)
Dermatologic: Rash (≤2%)

Endocrine & metabolic: Alkalosis (7%), hyperchloremia (7%), hypophosphatemia (6%), total protein decreased (3%), hyperuricemia (2%), hyperphosphatemia (2%), hypernatremia (1%), hypokalemia (1%), hyperbilirubinemia (1%)
Gastrointestinal: Anorexia (4%), abnormal taste (3%), abdominal pain (≤2%), gastritis (≤2%), nausea (≤2%), vomiting (≤2%)
Hematologic: Anemia (9%), leukocytosis (4%), leukopenia (4%), thrombocytopenia (3%), thrombocytosis (1%)
Hepatic: Alkaline phosphatase increased (6%), transaminases increased (4%)
Renal: Renal tubular acidosis (≤2%)
Miscellaneous: Offensive body odor (3%)

General Dosage Range Oral:
Children <20 kg: Powder: 450-600 mg/kg/day administered in equally divided amounts with each meal or feeding, 3-6 times daily (maximum: 20 g/day)
Children ≥20 kg and Adults: 9.9-13 g/m^2/day, administered in equally divided amounts with each meal, 3-6 times daily (maximum: 20 g/day)

Mechanism of Action Sodium phenylbutyrate is a prodrug which is rapidly converted to phenylacetate, followed by conjugation with glutamine to form phenylacetylglutamine; phenylacetylglutamine serves as a substitute for urea as it is clears nitrogenous waste from the body when excreted in the urine.

Pharmacodynamics/Kinetics
Half-life Elimination Phenylbutyrate: 0.8 hours; Phenylacetate: 1.2 hours
Time to Peak Plasma: Phenylbutyrate: ~1.4 hour; Phenylacetate: ~4 hours

Pregnancy Risk Factor C

Sodium Phosphates (SOW dee um FOS fates)

U.S. Brand Names Fleet® Enema Extra® [OTC]; Fleet® Enema [OTC]; Fleet® Pedia-Lax™ Enema [OTC]; Fleet® Phospho-soda® EZ-Prep™ [OTC] [DSC]; Fleet® Phospho-soda® [OTC] [DSC]; LaCrosse Complete [OTC]; OsmoPrep®; Visicol®

Canadian Brand Names Fleet Enema®

Pharmacologic Category Cathartic; Electrolyte Supplement, Parenteral; Laxative, Bowel Evacuant

Use
Oral, rectal: Short-term treatment of constipation and to evacuate the colon for rectal and bowel exams
I.V.: Source of phosphate in large volume I.V. fluids and parenteral nutrition; treatment and prevention of hypophosphatemia

Local Anesthetic/Vasoconstrictor Precautions No information available to require special precautions

Effects on Dental Treatment No significant effects or complications reported

Effects on Bleeding No information available to require special precautions

Adverse Effects Frequency not defined.
Cardiovascular: Edema, hypotension
Central nervous system: Dizziness, headache
Endocrine & metabolic: Hypocalcemia, hypernatremia, hyperphosphatemia, calcium phosphate precipitation
Gastrointestinal: Nausea, vomiting, diarrhea, abdominal bloating, abdominal pain, mucosal bleeding, superficial mucosal ulcerations
Renal: Acute renal failure
Postmarketing and/or case reports: Acute phosphate nephropathy, anaphylaxis, arrhythmia, atrial fibrillation (following severe vomiting [tablet formulation]), BUN increased, creatinine increased, nephrocalcinosis (oral solution), pruritus, rash, renal tubular necrosis, swelling (face, lips, tongue), urticaria, seizure

General Dosage Range
I.V.:
Children: 0.08-1 mmol phosphate/kg **or** Parenteral nutrition infusion: 0.5-2 mmol/kg/24 hours
Adults: 0.08-1 mmol phosphate/kg **or** Parenteral nutrition: Infusion: 20-40 mmol/24 hours
Oral: Solution: Fleet® Phospho-Soda®
Children 5-9 years: 7.5 mL as a single dose (maximum daily dose: 7.5 mL)
Children 10-12 years: 15 mL as a single dose (maximum daily dose: 15 mL)
Children ≥12 years and Adults: 15 mL as a single dose (maximum daily dose: 45 mL)
Rectal:
Children 2-<5 years: One-half contents of one 2.25 oz pediatric enema
Children 5-12 years: Contents of one 2.25 oz pediatric enema; may repeat
Children ≥12 years and Adults: Contents of one 4.5-ounce enema as a single dose; may repeat

Mechanism of Action As a laxative, exerts osmotic effect in the small intestine by drawing water into the lumen of the gut, producing distention and promoting peristalsis and evacuation of the bowel; phosphorous participates in bone deposition, calcium metabolism, utilization of B complex vitamins, and as a buffer in acid-base equilibrium

Pharmacodynamics/Kinetics

Onset of Action Cathartic: 3-6 hours; Rectal: 2-5 minutes

Pregnancy Risk Factor C

Sodium Tetradecyl (SOW dee um tetra DEK il)

U.S. Brand Names Sotradecol®

Canadian Brand Names Trombovar®

Pharmacologic Category Sclerosing Agent

Use Treatment of small, uncomplicated varicose veins of the lower extremities

Local Anesthetic/Vasoconstrictor Precautions No information available to require special precautions

Effects on Dental Treatment No significant effects or complications reported

Effects on Bleeding No information available to require special precautions

Adverse Effects Frequency not defined.

Central nervous system: Headache

Dermatologic: Discoloration at site of injection, sloughing and tissue necrosis following extravasation

Gastrointestinal: Nausea, vomiting

Local: Pain, itching, or ulceration at injection site

Miscellaneous: Allergic reaction (including hives, asthma, hay fever); anaphylactic shock

General Dosage Range I.V.: *Adults:* 0.5-2 mL in each vein (maximum: 10 mL per treatment session)

Mechanism of Action Acts by irritation of the vein intimal endothelium and causes thrombosis formation leading to occlusion of the injected vein

Pregnancy Risk Factor C

Sodium Thiosulfate (SOW dee um thye oh SUL fate)

U.S. Brand Names Versiclear™

Pharmacologic Category Antidote

Use

Parenteral: Used alone or with sodium nitrite or amyl nitrite in cyanide poisoning; reduce the risk of nephrotoxicity associated with cisplatin therapy; treatment of cyanide poisoning due to nitroprusside

Topical: Treatment of tinea versicolor

Unlabeled/Investigational Use Management of I.V. extravasation

Local Anesthetic/Vasoconstrictor Precautions No information available to require special precautions

Effects on Dental Treatment No significant effects or complications reported

Effects on Bleeding No information available to require special precautions

Adverse Effects Frequency not defined

Cardiovascular: Hypotension (infusion rate-dependent)

Dermatologic: Contact dermatitis, local irritation

Gastrointestinal: Nausea, vomiting

Miscellaneous: Hypersensitivity reactions

General Dosage Range

I.V.:

Children: 7 g/m^2 (maximum dose: 12.5 g) given over 10 minutes; may repeat at 1/2 the original dose if symptoms return **or** 12 g/m^2 over 6 hours or 9 g/m^2 I.V. push followed by 1.2 g/m^2 continuous infusion for 6 hours

Adults: 12.5 g; may repeat at half dose if needed **or** 0.95-1.95 mL/kg (maximum: 50 mL) **or** 12 g/m^2 over 6 hours or 9 g/m^2 I.V. push followed by 1.2 g/m^2 continuous infusion for 6 hours

Topical: *Children and Adults:* Apply a thin layer (20% to 25%) to affected areas twice daily

Mechanism of Action

Cyanide toxicity: Accelerates the clearance of cyanide via the rhodanase-catalyzed detoxification of cyanide to thiocyanate (much less toxic than cyanide). The accelerated action of rhodanase is a result of the exogenous sulfur provided by sodium thiosulfate.

Cisplatin toxicity: Complexes with cisplatin to form a compound that is nontoxic to either normal or cancerous cells

Pharmacodynamics/Kinetics
Half-life Elimination 0.65 hour
Pregnancy Risk Factor C

Solifenacin (sol i FEN a sin)

U.S. Brand Names VESIcare®
Pharmacologic Category Anticholinergic Agent
Use Treatment of overactive bladder with symptoms of urinary frequency, urgency, or urge incontinence
Local Anesthetic/Vasoconstrictor Precautions No information available to require special precautions
Effects on Dental Treatment Key adverse event(s) related to dental treatment: Xerostomia (normal salivary flow resumes upon discontinuation). Prolonged xerostomia may contribute to discomfort and dental disease (eg, caries, periodontal disease, and oral candidiasis).
Effects on Bleeding No information available to require special precautions
Adverse Effects
>10%: Gastrointestinal: Xerostomia (11% to 28%; dose-related), constipation (5% to 13%; dose-related)
1% to 10%:
Cardiovascular: Edema (≤1%), hypertension (≤1%)
Central nervous system: Headache (3% to 6%), fatigue (1% to 2%), depression (≤1%)
Gastrointestinal: Dyspepsia (1% to 4%), nausea (2% to 3%), upper abdominal pain (1% to 2%)
Genitourinary: Urinary tract infection (3% to 5%), urinary retention (≤1%)
Ocular: Blurred vision (4% to 5%), dry eyes (≤2%)
Respiratory: Cough (≤1%)
Miscellaneous: Influenza (≤2%)
General Dosage Range Dosage adjustment recommended in patients with hepatic or renal impairment and on concomitant therapy
Oral: *Adults:* 5-10 mg/day
Mechanism of Action Inhibits muscarinic receptors resulting in decreased urinary bladder contraction, increased residual urine volume, and decreased detrusor muscle pressure.
Pharmacodynamics/Kinetics
Half-life Elimination 45-68 hours following chronic dosing; prolonged in severe renal (Cl_{cr} <30 mL/minute) or moderate hepatic (Child-Pugh class B) impairment
Time to Peak Plasma: 3-8 hours
Pregnancy Risk Factor C

Somatropin (soe ma TROE pin)

U.S. Brand Names Genotropin Miniquick®; Genotropin®; Humatrope®; Norditropin FlexPro®; Norditropin®; Norditropin® NordiFlex®; Nutropin AQ Pen®; Nutropin AQ®; Nutropin AQ® NuSpin™; Nutropin®; Omnitrope®; Saizen®; Serostim®; Tev-Tropin®; Zorbtive®
Canadian Brand Names Humatrope®; Nutropin®; Nutropin® AQ; Omnitrope®; Saizen®; Serostim®
Pharmacologic Category Growth Hormone
Use
Children:
Treatment of growth failure due to inadequate endogenous growth hormone secretion (Genotropin®, Humatrope®, Norditropin®, Nutropin®, Nutropin AQ®, Omnitrope®, Saizen®, Tev-Tropin®)
Treatment of short stature associated with Turner syndrome (Genotropin®, Humatrope®, Norditropin®, Nutropin®, Nutropin AQ®)
Treatment of Prader-Willi syndrome (Genotropin®, Omnitrope®)
Treatment of growth failure associated with chronic renal insufficiency (CRI) up until the time of renal transplantation (Nutropin®, Nutropin AQ®)
Treatment of growth failure in children born small for gestational age who fail to manifest catch-up growth by 2 years of age (Genotropin®, Omnitrope®) or by 2-4 years of age (Humatrope®, Norditropin®)
Treatment of idiopathic short stature (nongrowth hormone-deficient short stature) defined by height standard deviation score (SDS) ≤-2.25 and growth rate not likely to attain normal adult height (Genotropin®, Humatrope®, Nutropin®, Nutropin AQ®, Omnitrope®)
Treatment of short stature or growth failure associated with short stature homeobox gene (SHOX) deficiency (Humatrope®)

Treatment of short stature associated with Noonan syndrome (Norditropin®)

Adults:

HIV patients with wasting or cachexia with concomitant antiviral therapy (Serostim®)

Replacement of endogenous growth hormone in patients with adult growth hormone deficiency who meet both of the following criteria (Genotropin®, Humatrope®, Norditropin®, Nutropin®, Nutropin AQ®, Omnitrope®, Saizen®):

Biochemical diagnosis of adult growth hormone deficiency by means of a subnormal response to a standard growth hormone stimulation test (peak growth hormone ≤5 mcg/L). Confirmatory testing may not be required in patients with congenital/genetic growth hormone deficiency or multiple pituitary hormone deficiencies due to organic diseases.

and

Adult-onset: Patients who have adult growth hormone deficiency whether alone or with multiple hormone deficiencies (hypopituitarism) as a result of pituitary disease, hypothalamic disease, surgery, radiation therapy, or trauma

or

Childhood-onset: Patients who were growth hormone deficient during childhood, confirmed as an adult before replacement therapy is initiated

Treatment of short-bowel syndrome (Zorbtive®)

Unlabeled/Investigational Use Investigational: Pediatric HIV patients with wasting/cachexia (Serostim®); HIV-associated adipose redistribution syndrome (HARS) (Serostim®)

Local Anesthetic/Vasoconstrictor Precautions No information available to require special precautions

Effects on Dental Treatment No significant effects or complications reported

Effects on Bleeding No information available to require special precautions

Adverse Effects

Growth hormone deficiency: Adverse reactions reported with growth hormone deficiency vary greatly by age. Generally, percentages are less in pediatric patients than adults, and many of the reactions reported in adults are dose related. Percentages reported also vary by product. Below is a listing by age group; events reported more commonly overall are noted with an asterisk (*).

Children: Antibodies development, arthralgia, benign intracranial hypertension, edema, eosinophilia, glycosuria, Hb A_{1c} increased, headache, hematoma, hematuria, hyperglycemia (mild), hypertriglyceridemia, hypoglycemia, hypothyroidism, injection site reaction, intracranial tumor, leg pain, lipoatrophy, leukemia, meningioma, muscle pain, papilledema, pseudotumor cerebri, psoriasis exacerbation, rash, scoliosis progression, seizure, slipped capital femoral epiphysis, weakness

Adults: Acne, ALT increased, AST increased, arthralgia*, back pain, bronchitis, carpal tunnel syndrome, chest pain, cough, depression, diabetes mellitus (type 2), diaphoresis, dizziness, edema*, fatigue, flu-like syndrome*, gastritis, glucose intolerance, glucosuria, headache*, hyperglycemia (mild), hypertension, hypoesthesia, hypothyroidism, infection, insomnia, insulin resistance, joint disorder, leg edema, muscle pain, myalgia*, nausea, pain in extremities, paresthesia*, peripheral edema*, pharyngitis, retinopathy, rhinitis, skeletal pain*, stiffness in extremities, surgical procedure, upper respiratory tract infection, weakness

Additional/postmarketing reactions observed with growth hormone deficiency: Gynecomastia, increased growth of pre-existing nevi, pancreatitis

HARS: Serostim®: Limited to >10%: Edema (peripheral) (19% to 45%), arthralgia (28% to 37%), pain (extremity) (5% to 19%), hypoesthesia (9% to 15%), headache (4% to 14%), blood glucose increased (4% to 14%), paresthesia (11% to 13%), myalgia (3% to 13%)

Idiopathic short stature: Percentages reported using Humatrope® versus placebo: Myalgia (24%), scoliosis (19%), otitis media (16%), arthralgia (11%), arthrosis (11%), hyperlipidemia (8%), gynecomastia (5%), hip pain (3%), hypertension (3%). Additional adverse reactions listed as reported using other products from ISS NCGS Cohort (frequencies <1%): Aggressiveness, benign intracranial hypertension, diabetes, edema, hair loss, headache, injection site reaction

Prader-Willi syndrome: Genotropin® (frequency not defined): Aggressiveness, arthralgia, edema, hair loss, headache, benign intracranial hypertension, myalgia; fatalities associated with use in this population have been reported

Turner syndrome: Percentages reported using Humatrope® compared to untreated patients. Additional adverse reactions reported from other products, frequency not specified: Surgical procedures (45%), otitis media (43%), ear disorders (18%), joint pain, respiratory illness, urinary tract infection

HIV patients with wasting or cachexia: Serostim® (limited to ≥5%): Musculoskeletal disorders (arthralgia, arthrosis, myalgia: 78%), peripheral edema (26%), headache (13%), nausea (9%), paresthesia (8%), edema (6%), gynecomastia (6%), hypoesthesia (5%)

Short-bowel syndrome: Zorbtive® (limited to >10%): Peripheral edema (69% to 81%), facial edema (44% to 50%), arthralgia (31% to 44%), nausea (13% to 31%), injection site pain (up to 31%), flatulence (25%), injection site reaction (19% to 25%), abdominal pain (13% to 25%), vomiting (19%), pain (6% to 19%), chest pain (up to 19%), dehydration (up to 19%), infection (up to 19%), rhinitis (up to 19%), hearing symptoms (13%), dizziness (6% to 13%), rash (6% to 13%), diaphoresis (up to 13%), generalized edema (up to 13%), malaise (up to 13%), moniliasis (up to 13%), myalgia (up to 13%)

SHOX deficiency: Humatrope®: Arthralgia (11%), gynecomastia (8%), excessive cutaneous nevi (7%), scoliosis (4%)

Small for gestational age: Genotropin®, Humatrope® (frequency not defined): Mild, transient hyperglycemia; benign intracranial hypertension (rare); central precocious puberty; jaw prominence (rare); aggravation of pre-existing scoliosis (rare); injection site reactions; progression of pigmented nevi; carpal tunnel syndrome (rare) diabetes mellitus (rare); otitis media; headache; slipped capital femoral epiphysis

General Dosage Range I.M., SubQ: *Children and Adults:* Dosage varies greatly depending on indication

Mechanism of Action Somatropin is a purified polypeptide hormones of recombinant DNA origin; somatropin contains the identical sequence of amino acids found in human growth hormone; human growth hormone assists growth of linear bone, skeletal muscle, and organs by stimulating chondrocyte proliferation and differentiation, lipolysis, protein synthesis, and hepatic glucose output; stimulates erythropoietin which increases red blood cell mass; exerts both insulin-like and diabetogenic effects; enhances the transmucosal transport of water, electrolytes, and nutrients across the gut

Pharmacodynamics/Kinetics

Duration of Action Maintains supraphysiologic levels for 18-20 hours

Half-life Elimination Preparation and route of administration dependent; SubQ: ~2-4 hours

Pregnancy Risk Factor B/C (depending upon manufacturer)

SORAfenib (sor AF e nib)

U.S. Brand Names NexAVAR®

Canadian Brand Names Nexavar®

Pharmacologic Category Antineoplastic Agent, Tyrosine Kinase Inhibitor; Vascular Endothelial Growth Factor (VEGF) Inhibitor

Use Treatment of advanced renal cell cancer (RCC); treatment of unresectable hepatocellular cancer (HCC)

Unlabeled/Investigational Use Treatment of advanced thyroid cancer, recurrent or metastatic angiosarcoma, resistant gastrointestinal stromal tumor (GIST)

Local Anesthetic/Vasoconstrictor Precautions Sorafenib may cause hypertension; monitor blood pressure prior to vasoconstrictor use

Effects on Dental Treatment Key adverse event(s) related to dental treatment: Mouth pain, mucositis, stomatitis, xerostomia (normal salivary flow resumes upon discontinuation), and dysphagia.

Effects on Bleeding Chemotherapy may result in significant myelosuppression, potentially including significant reduction in platelet counts and altered hemostasis. In patients who are under active treatment with these agents, medical consult is suggested.

Adverse Effects

>10%:

Cardiovascular: Hypertension (9% to 17%; grade 3: 3% to 4%; grade 4: <1%; onset: ~3 weeks)

Central nervous system: Fatigue (37% to 46%), sensory neuropathy (≤13%), pain (11%)

Dermatologic: Rash/desquamation (19% to 40%; grade 3: ≤1%), hand-foot syndrome (21% to 30%; grade 3: 6% to 8%), alopecia (14% to 27%), pruritus (14% to 19%), dry skin (10% to 11%), erythema

Endocrine & metabolic: Hypoalbuminemia (≤59%), hypophosphatemia (35% to 45%; grade 3: 11% to 13%; grade 4: <1%)

Gastrointestinal: Diarrhea (43% to 55%; grade 3: 2% to 10%; grade 4: <1%), lipase increased (40% to 41% [usually transient]), amylase increased (30% to 34% [usually transient]), abdominal pain (11% to 31%), weight loss (10% to 30%), anorexia (16% to 29%), nausea (23% to 24%), vomiting (15% to 16%), constipation (14% to 15%)

Hematologic: Lymphopenia (23% to 47%; grades 3/4: ≤13%), thrombocytopenia (12% to 46%; grades 3/4: 1% to 4%), INR increased (≤42%), neutropenia (≤18%; grades 3/4: ≤5%), hemorrhage (15% to 18%; grade 3: 2% to 3%; grade 4: ≤2%), leukopenia
Hepatic: Liver dysfunction (≤11%; grade 3: 2%; grade 4: 1%)
Neuromuscular & skeletal: Muscle pain, weakness
Respiratory: Dyspnea (≤14%), cough (≤13%)

1% to 10%:
Cardiovascular: Cardiac ischemia/infarction (≤3%), heart failure (2%; congestive), flushing
Central nervous system: Headache (≤10%), depression, fever
Dermatologic: Acne, exfoliative dermatitis
Gastrointestinal: Appetite decreased, dyspepsia, dysphagia, esophageal varices bleeding (2%), glossodynia, mucositis, stomatitis, xerostomia
Genitourinary: Erectile dysfunction
Hematologic: Anemia
Hepatic: Transaminases increased (transient)
Neuromuscular & skeletal: Joint pain (≤10%), arthralgia, myalgia
Renal: Renal failure
Respiratory: Hoarseness
Miscellaneous: Flu-like syndrome

General Dosage Range Dosage adjustments recommended in patients with hepatic or renal impairment, on concomitant therapy, or who develop toxicities
Oral: *Adults:* 400 mg twice daily

Mechanism of Action Multikinase inhibitor; inhibits tumor growth and angiogenesis by inhibiting intracellular Raf kinases (CRAF, BRAF, and mutant BRAF), and cell surface kinase receptors (VEGFR-1, VEGFR-2, VEGFR-3, PDGFR-beta, cKIT, FLT-3, and RET)

Pharmacodynamics/Kinetics
Half-life Elimination 25-48 hours
Time to Peak ~3 hours

Pregnancy Risk Factor D

Sorbitol (SOR bi tole)

Pharmacologic Category Genitourinary Irrigant; Laxative, Osmotic

Use Genitourinary irrigant in transurethral prostatic resection or other transurethral resection or other transurethral surgical procedures; diuretic; humectant; sweetening agent; hyperosmotic laxative; facilitate the passage of sodium polystyrene sulfonate through the intestinal tract

Local Anesthetic/Vasoconstrictor Precautions No information available to require special precautions

Effects on Dental Treatment Key adverse event(s) related to dental treatment: Xerostomia (normal salivary flow resumes upon discontinuation).

Effects on Bleeding No information available to require special precautions

Adverse Effects Frequency not defined.
Cardiovascular: Edema
Endocrine & metabolic: Fluid and electrolyte losses, hyperglycemia, lactic acidosis
Gastrointestinal: Abdominal discomfort, diarrhea, dry mouth, nausea, vomiting, xerostomia

General Dosage Range
Oral:
Children 2-11 years: 2 mL/kg (70% solution) as a single dose
Children ≥12 years and Adults: 30-150 mL (70% solution) as a single dose
Rectal:
Children 2-11 years: 30-60 mL (25% to 30% solution) as a single dose
Children ≥12 years and Adults: 120 mL (25% to 30% solution) as a single dose
Topical: *Adults:* 3% to 3.3% as a transurethral irrigation

Mechanism of Action A polyalcoholic sugar with osmotic cathartic actions

Pharmacodynamics/Kinetics
Onset of Action 0.25-1 hour

Pregnancy Risk Factor C

Sotalol (SOE ta lole)

Related Information
Cardiovascular Diseases *on page 1848*
Clinical Risk Related to Drugs Prolonging QT Interval *on page 1872*

U.S. Brand Names Betapace AF®; Betapace®; Sorine®

Canadian Brand Names Apo-Sotalol®; CO Sotalol; Dom-Sotalol; Med-Sotalol; Mylan-Sotalol; Novo-Sotalol; Nu-Sotalol; PHL-Sotalol; PMS-Sotalol; PRO-Sotalol; ratio-Sotalol; Rhoxal-sotalol; Riva-Sotalol; Rylosol; Sandoz-Sotalol; ZYM-Sotalol

Pharmacologic Category Antiarrhythmic Agent, Class II; Antiarrhythmic Agent, Class III; Beta-Adrenergic Blocker, Nonselective

Use Treatment of documented ventricular arrhythmias (ie, sustained ventricular tachycardia), that in the judgment of the physician are life-threatening; maintenance of normal sinus rhythm in patients with symptomatic atrial fibrillation and atrial flutter who are currently in sinus rhythm. Manufacturer states substitutions should not be made for Betapace AF® since Betapace AF® is distributed with a patient package insert specific for atrial fibrillation/flutter.

Injection: Substitution for oral sotalol in those who are unable to take sotalol orally

Unlabeled/Investigational Use Fetal tachycardia

Injection: Hemodynamically stable monomorphic ventricular tachycardia (ACLS, 2010)

Local Anesthetic/Vasoconstrictor Precautions Use with caution; epinephrine has interacted with nonselective beta-blockers to result in initial hypertensive episode followed by bradycardia. Sotalol is one of the drugs confirmed to prolong the QT interval and is accepted as having a risk of causing torsade de pointes. The risk of drug-induced torsade de pointes is extremely low when a single QT interval prolonging drug is prescribed. In terms of epinephrine, it is not known what effect vasoconstrictors in the local anesthetic regimen will have in patients with a known history of congenital prolonged QT interval or in patients taking any medication that prolongs the QT interval. Until more information is obtained, it is suggested that the clinician consult with the physician prior to the use of a vasoconstrictor in suspected patients, and that the vasoconstrictor (epinephrine, mepivacaine and levonordefrin [Carbocaine® 2% with Neo-Cobefrin®]) be used with caution.

Effects on Dental Treatment Sotalol is a nonselective beta-blocker and may enhance the pressor response to epinephrine, resulting in hypertension and bradycardia. Many nonsteroidal anti-inflammatory drugs, such as ibuprofen and indomethacin, can reduce the hypotensive effect of beta-blockers after 3 or more weeks of therapy with the NSAID. Short-term NSAID use (ie, 3 days) requires no special precautions in patients taking beta-blockers.

Adverse Effects Note: No clinical experience with I.V. sotalol; however, since exposure is similar between I.V. and oral sotalol, adverse reactions are expected to be similar.

>10%:

- Cardiovascular: Bradycardia (13% to 16%), chest pain (3% to 16%), palpitation (14%)
- Central nervous system: Fatigue (20%), dizziness (20%), lightheadedness (12%)
- Neuromuscular & skeletal: Weakness (13%)
- Respiratory: Dyspnea (21%)

1% to 10%:

- Cardiovascular: Edema (8%), abnormal ECG (7%), hypotension (6%), proarrhythmia (5%), syncope (5%), CHF (5%), torsade de pointes (dose related; 1% to 4%), peripheral vascular disorders (3%), ventricular tachycardia worsened (1%), QT_c interval prolongation (dose related)
- Central nervous system: Headache (8%), sleep problems (8%), mental confusion (6%), anxiety (4%), depression (4%)
- Dermatologic: Itching/rash (5%)
- Endocrine & metabolic: Sexual ability decreased (3%)
- Gastrointestinal: Nausea/vomiting (10%), diarrhea (7%), stomach discomfort (3% to 6%), flatulence (2%)
- Genitourinary: Impotence (2%)
- Hematologic: Bleeding (2%)
- Neuromuscular & skeletal: Extremity pain (7%), paresthesia (4%), back pain (3%)
- Ocular: Visual problems (5%)
- Respiratory: Upper respiratory problems (5% to 8%), asthma (2%)

General Dosage Range Dosage adjustment recommended in patients with renal impairment or who develop toxicities

I.V.: *Adults:* Initial: 75 mg twice daily; Maintenance: 75-150 mg twice daily (maximum: 300 mg/day)

Oral:

Children ≤2 years: Dosage should be adjusted (decreased) by plotting of the child's age on a logarithmic scale; **Note:** Refer to manufacturer's package labeling

Children >2 years: Initial: 90 mg/m²/day in 3 divided doses; Maintenance: 90-180 mg/m²/day in 3 divided doses (maximum: 180 mg/m²/day)

Adults: Initial: 80 mg twice daily; Maintenance: 240-320 mg/day in 2-3 divided doses (maximum: 320 mg/day)

Mechanism of Action

Beta-blocker which contains both beta-adrenoreceptor-blocking (Vaughan Williams Class II) and cardiac action potential duration prolongation (Vaughan Williams Class III) properties

Class II effects: Increased sinus cycle length, slowed heart rate, decreased AV nodal conduction, and increased AV nodal refractoriness

Class III effects: Prolongation of the atrial and ventricular monophasic action potentials, and effective refractory prolongation of atrial muscle, ventricular muscle, and atrioventricular accessory pathways in both the antegrade and retrograde directions

Sotalol is a racemic mixture of *d*- and *l*-sotalol; both isomers have similar Class III antiarrhythmic effects while the *l*-isomer is responsible for virtually all of the beta-blocking activity

Sotalol has both $beta_1$- and $beta_2$-receptor blocking activity. The beta-blocking effect of sotalol is a noncardioselective [half maximal at about 80 mg/day and maximal at doses of 320-640 mg/day]. Significant beta-blockade occurs at oral doses as low as 25 mg/day.

The Class III effects are seen only at oral doses ≥160 mg/day

Pharmacodynamics/Kinetics

Onset of Action Oral: Rapid, 1-2 hours; when administered I.V. for ongoing VT over 5 minutes, onset of action is ~5-10 minutes (Ho, 1994)

Duration of Action 8-16 hours

Half-life Elimination 12 hours; Children: 9.5 hours; terminal half-life decreases with age <2 years (time to steady state may be ≥1 week in neonates); increases with renal dysfunction

Time to Peak Serum: Oral: 2.5-4 hours

Pregnancy Risk Factor B

Dental Comment Sotalol is known to prolong the QT interval. The QT interval is measured as the time and distance between the Q point of the QRS complex and the end of the T wave in the ECG tracing. After adjustment for heart rate, the QT interval is defined as prolonged if it is more than 450 msec in men and 460 msec in women. A long QT syndrome was first described in the 1950s and 60s as a congenital syndrome involving QT interval prolongation and syncope and sudden death. Some of the congenital long QT syndromes were characterized by a peculiar electrocardiographic appearance of the QRS complex involving a premature atria beat followed by a pause, then a subsequent sinus beat showing marked QT prolongation and deformity. This type of cardiac arrhythmia was originally termed "torsade de pointes" (translated from the French as "twisting of the points"). Sotalol is considered as having a risk of causing torsade de pointes. Since it is not known what effect vasoconstrictors in the local anesthetic regimen will have in patients with a known history of congenital prolonged QT interval or in patients taking any medication that prolongs the QT interval, a medical consult is suggested.

Spiramycin (speer a MYE sin)

Canadian Brand Names Rovamycine®

Pharmacologic Category Antibiotic, Macrolide

Use Treatment of infections of the respiratory tract, buccal cavity, skin and soft tissues due to susceptible organisms. *N. gonorrhoeae*: as an alternate choice of treatment for gonorrhea in patients allergic to the penicillins. Before treatment of gonorrhea, the possibility of concomitant infection due to *T. pallidum* should be excluded.

Unlabeled/Investigational Use Treatment of *Toxoplasma gondii* to prevent transmission from mother to fetus

Local Anesthetic/Vasoconstrictor Precautions No information available to require special precautions

Effects on Dental Treatment No significant effects or complications reported

Effects on Bleeding No information available to require special precautions

Adverse Effects Frequency not defined.

Dermatologic: Angioedema (rare), pruritus, rash, urticaria

Gastrointestinal: Diarrhea, nausea, pseudomembranous colitis (rare), vomiting

Hepatic: Transaminases increased

Neuromuscular & skeletal: Paresthesia (rare)

Miscellaneous: Anaphylactic shock (rare)

General Dosage Range Oral:

Children: 150,000 int. units/kg/day in 2-3 divided doses

Adults: 6,000,000-15,000,000 int. units/day in 2 divided doses **or** 12,000,000-13,500,000 int. units as a single dose

Mechanism of Action Inhibits growth of susceptible organisms; mechanism not established.

Pregnancy Risk Factor Not assigned (other macrolides rated B); C per expert analysis

Product Availability Not available in U.S.

Spironolactone (speer on oh LAK tone)

Related Information

Cardiovascular Diseases *on page 1848*

U.S. Brand Names Aldactone®

Canadian Brand Names Aldactone®; Novo-Spiroton

Generic Availability (U.S.) Yes

Pharmacologic Category Diuretic, Potassium-Sparing; Selective Aldosterone Blocker

Use Management of edema associated with excessive aldosterone excretion; hypertension; primary hyperaldosteronism; hypokalemia; cirrhosis of liver accompanied by edema or ascites; nephritic syndrome; severe heart failure (NYHA class III-IV) to increase survival and reduce hospitalization when added to standard therapy

Unlabeled/Investigational Use Female acne (adjunctive therapy); hirsutism; hypertension (pediatric); diuretic (pediatric)

Local Anesthetic/Vasoconstrictor Precautions No information available to require special precautions

Effects on Dental Treatment No significant effects or complications reported

Effects on Bleeding No information available to require special precautions

Adverse Effects Frequency not always defined.

Cardiovascular: Vasculitis

Central nervous system: Ataxia, confusion, drowsiness, drug fever, fatigue, headache, lethargy

Dermatologic: Eosinophilia, maculopapular or erythematous cutaneous eruptions, urticaria

Endocrine & metabolic: Gynecomastia (men 9%), breast pain (men 2%), hyperkalemia (serious; 2%), dehydration, hyperchloremic metabolic acidosis in decompensated hepatic cirrhosis, hyponatremia, impotence, irregular menses, amenorrhea, postmenopausal bleeding

Gastrointestinal: Anorexia, cramps, diarrhea, gastritis, nausea, ulceration, vomiting, xerostomia

Hematologic: Agranulocytosis

Hepatic: Cholestatic/hepatocellular toxicity

Renal: BUN increased, renal dysfunction, renal failure

Miscellaneous: Anaphylactic reaction, breast cancer, deepening of the voice

Dosage Oral:

Children:

Diuretic, hypertension (unlabeled use): Children 1-17 years: Initial: 1 mg/kg/day divided every 12-24 hours (maximum dose: 3.3 mg/kg/day, up to 100 mg/day)

Diagnosis of primary aldosteronism (unlabeled use): 125-375 mg/m^2/day in divided doses

Adults:

Edema: 25-200 mg/day in 1-2 divided doses

Hypokalemia: 25-100 mg daily

Hypertension (JNC 7): 25-50 mg/day in 1-2 divided doses

Diagnosis of primary aldosteronism: Long test: 400 mg daily for 3-4 weeks; short test: 400 mg daily for 4 days; maintenance until surgical correction: 100-400 mg/day in 1-2 divided doses

Heart failure, severe (NYHA class III-IV; with ACE inhibitor and a loop diuretic ± digoxin): 12.5-25 mg/day; maximum daily dose: 50 mg. If 25 mg once daily not tolerated, reduce to 25 mg every other day was the lowest maintenance dose possible.

Note: If potassium >5 mEq/L or serum creatinine >4 mg/dL, discontinue or interrupt therapy.

Acne in women (unlabeled use): 25-200 mg once daily

Hirsutism in women (unlabeled use): 50-200 mg/day in 1-2 divided doses

Elderly: Indication specific: Initial: 12.5-50 mg/day in 1-2 divided doses, increasing by 25-50 mg every 5 days as needed; adjust for renal impairment

Dosing interval in renal impairment: Heart failure:

Cl_{cr} 31-50 mL/minute: Decrease initial dose to 12.5 mg once daily

Cl_{cr} <30 mL/minute: Not recommended

Mechanism of Action Competes with aldosterone for receptor sites in the distal renal tubules, increasing sodium chloride and water excretion while conserving potassium and hydrogen ions; may block the effect of aldosterone on arteriolar smooth muscle as well

Contraindications Anuria; acute renal insufficiency; significant impairment of renal excretory function; hyperkalemia

Warnings/Precautions Monitor serum potassium closely in patients being treated for heart failure. Avoid potassium supplements, potassium-containing salt substitutes, a diet rich in potassium, or other drugs that can cause hyperkalemia. Excess amounts can lead to profound diuresis with fluid and electrolyte loss; close medical supervision and dose evaluation are required. Watch for and correct electrolyte disturbances; adjust dose to avoid dehydration. In cirrhosis, avoid electrolyte and acid/base imbalances that might lead to hepatic encephalopathy. Gynecomastia is related to dose and duration of therapy. Discontinue use prior to adrenal vein catheterization. When evaluating a heart failure patient for spironolactone treatment, creatinine should be ≤2.5 mg/dL in men or ≤2 mg/dL in women and potassium <5 mEq/L. Discontinue or interrupt therapy if serum potassium >5 mEq/L or serum creatinine >4 mg/dL. **[U.S. Boxed Warning]: Shown to be a tumorigen in chronic toxicity animal studies. Avoid unnecessary use.**

Drug Interactions

Avoid Concomitant Use

Avoid concomitant use of Spironolactone with any of the following: Tacrolimus

Increased Effect/Toxicity

Spironolactone may increase the levels/effects of: ACE Inhibitors; Amifostine; Ammonium Chloride; Antihypertensives; Cardiac Glycosides; Digoxin; Hypotensive Agents; Neuromuscular-Blocking Agents (Nondepolarizing); RiTUXimab; Tacrolimus

The levels/effects of Spironolactone may be increased by: Angiotensin II Receptor Blockers; Diazoxide; Drospirenone; Eplerenone; Herbs (Hypotensive Properties); MAO Inhibitors; Nonsteroidal Anti-Inflammatory Agents; Pentoxifylline; Phosphodiesterase 5 Inhibitors; Potassium Salts; Prostacyclin Analogues; Tolvaptan

Decreased Effect

Spironolactone may decrease the levels/effects of: Alpha-/Beta-Agonists; Cardiac Glycosides; Mitotane; QuiNIDine

The levels/effects of Spironolactone may be decreased by: Herbs (Hypertensive Properties); Methylphenidate; Nonsteroidal Anti-Inflammatory Agents; Yohimbine

Ethanol/Nutrition/Herb Interactions

Ethanol: Increases risk of orthostasis.

Food: Food increases absorption.

Herb/Nutraceutical: Avoid natural licorice (due to mineralocorticoid activity)

Dietary Considerations Should be taken with food to decrease gastrointestinal irritation and to increase absorption. Excessive potassium intake (eg, salt substitutes, low-salt foods, bananas, nuts) should be avoided.

Pharmacodynamics/Kinetics

Duration of Action 2-3 days

Half-life Elimination Spironolactone: 78-84 minutes; Canrenone: 10-23 hours; 7-alpha-spirolactone: 7-20 hours

Time to Peak Serum: 3-4 hours (primarily as the active metabolite)

Pregnancy Risk Factor C

Lactation Enters breast milk/not recommended (AAP rates "compatible"; AAP 2001 update pending)

Breast-Feeding Considerations The active metabolite of spironolactone has been found in breast milk. Effects to humans are not known; however, this metabolite was found to be carcinogenic in rats. The manufacturer recommends discontinuing spironolactone or using an alternative method of feeding.

Dosage Forms

Tablet, oral: 25 mg, 50 mg, 100 mg

Aldactone®: 25 mg, 50 mg, 100 mg

Stavudine (STAV yoo deen)

Related Information

HIV Infection and AIDS *on page 1883*

U.S. Brand Names Zerit®

Canadian Brand Names Zerit®

Pharmacologic Category Antiretroviral Agent, Reverse Transcriptase Inhibitor (Nucleoside)

Use Treatment of HIV infection in combination with other antiretroviral agents

Local Anesthetic/Vasoconstrictor Precautions No information available to require special precautions

Effects on Dental Treatment No significant effects or complications reported

Effects on Bleeding No information available to require special precautions relative to hemostasis.

Adverse Effects Adverse reactions reported below represent experience with combination therapy with other nucleoside analogues and protease inhibitors.

>10%:

Central nervous system: Headache (25% to 46%)

Dermatologic: Rash (18% to 30%)

Gastrointestinal: Nausea (43% to 53%; less than comparator group), vomiting (18% to 30%; less than comparator group), diarrhea (34% to 45%)

Hepatic: Hyperbilirubinemia (65% to 68%; grade 3/4: 7% to 16%), AST increased (42% to 53%; grade 3/4: 5% to 7%), ALT increased (40% to 50%; grade 3/4: 6% to 8%), GGT increased (15% to 28%; grade 3/4: 2% to 5%)

Neuromuscular & skeletal: Peripheral neuropathy (8% to 21%)

Miscellaneous: Amylase increased (21% to 31%; grade 3/4: 4% to 8%), lipase increased (~27%; grade 3/4: 5% to 6%)

General Dosage Range Dosage adjustment recommended in patients with renal impairment.

Oral:

Newborns (Birth to 13 days): 0.5 mg/kg every 12 hours

Children ≥14 days and <30 kg: 1 mg/kg every 12 hours

Children and Adults 30-59 kg: 30 mg every 12 hours

Children and Adults ≥60 kg: 40 mg every 12 hours

Mechanism of Action Stavudine is a thymidine analog which interferes with HIV viral DNA dependent DNA polymerase resulting in inhibition of viral replication; nucleoside reverse transcriptase inhibitor

Pharmacodynamics/Kinetics

Half-life Elimination HIV-infected Children: 0.96 hours, HIV-infected Adults: 1.6 hours

Time to Peak Serum: 1 hour

Pregnancy Risk Factor C

Streptomycin (strep toe MYE sin)

Related Information

Tuberculosis *on page 1902*

Pharmacologic Category Antibiotic, Aminoglycoside; Antitubercular Agent

Use Part of combination therapy of active tuberculosis; used in combination with other agents for treatment of streptococcal or enterococcal endocarditis, mycobacterial infections, plague, tularemia, and brucellosis

Local Anesthetic/Vasoconstrictor Precautions No information available to require special precautions

Effects on Dental Treatment No significant effects or complications reported

Effects on Bleeding No information available to require special precautions

Adverse Effects Frequency not defined.

Cardiovascular: Hypotension

Central nervous system: Neurotoxicity, drowsiness, headache, drug fever, paresthesia

Dermatologic: Skin rash

Gastrointestinal: Nausea, vomiting

Hematologic: Eosinophilia, anemia

Neuromuscular & skeletal: Arthralgia, weakness, tremor

Otic: Ototoxicity (auditory), ototoxicity (vestibular)

Renal: Nephrotoxicity

Respiratory: Difficulty in breathing

General Dosage Range Dosage adjustment recommended in patients with renal impairment

I.M.:

Children: 20-40 mg/kg given daily or 2-3 times/week (maximum: 1 g/day)

Adults: Tuberculosis: 15 mg/kg/day **or** 25-30 mg/kg 2-3 times/week; Other indications: 1-4 g/day in 2 divided doses

Elderly: 10 mg/kg/day (maximum: 750 mg/day)

I.V.:

Children: 20-40 mg/kg/day **or** 20-40 mg/kg twice weekly **or** 25-30 mg/kg 3 times/week (maximum: 1 g/day)

Adults: 1-4 g/day in 2 divided doses

Mechanism of Action Inhibits bacterial protein synthesis by binding directly to the 30S ribosomal subunits causing faulty peptide sequence to form in the protein chain

Pharmacodynamics/Kinetics

Half-life Elimination Newborns: 4-10 hours; Adults: 2-4.7 hours, prolonged with renal impairment

Time to Peak I.M.: Within 1 hour

Pregnancy Risk Factor D

Streptozocin (strep toe ZOE sin)

U.S. Brand Names Zanosar®
Canadian Brand Names Zanosar®
Pharmacologic Category Antineoplastic Agent, Alkylating Agent
Use Treatment of metastatic islet cell carcinoma of the pancreas
Unlabeled/Investigational Use Treatment of adrenal tumors
Local Anesthetic/Vasoconstrictor Precautions No information available to require special precautions
Effects on Dental Treatment No significant effects or complications reported
Effects on Bleeding Chemotherapy may result in significant myelosuppression, potentially including significant reduction in platelet counts and altered hemostasis. In patients who are under active treatment with these agents, medical consult is suggested.
Adverse Effects
>10%:
Gastrointestinal: Nausea and vomiting (100%)
Hepatic: LFTs increased
Miscellaneous: Hypoalbuminemia
Renal: BUN increased, Cl_{cr} decreased, hypophosphatemia, nephrotoxicity (25% to 75%), proteinuria, renal dysfunction (65%), renal tubular acidosis
1% to 10%:
Endocrine & metabolic: Hypoglycemia (6%)
Gastrointestinal: Diarrhea (10%)
Local: Pain at injection site
General Dosage Range Dosage adjustment recommended in patients with renal impairment
I.V.: *Children and Adults:* 1-1.5 g/m^2 weekly for 6 weeks followed by a 4-week rest period **or** 0.5-1 g/m^2 for 5 consecutive days as combination therapy followed by a 4- to 6-week rest period
Mechanism of Action Interferes with the normal function of DNA by alkylation and cross-linking the strands of DNA, and by possible protein modification
Pharmacodynamics/Kinetics
Duration of Action Disappears from serum in 4 hours
Half-life Elimination 35-40 minutes
Pregnancy Risk Factor D

Succinylcholine (suks in il KOE leen)

U.S. Brand Names Anectine®; Quelicin®
Canadian Brand Names Quelicin®
Pharmacologic Category Neuromuscular Blocker Agent, Depolarizing
Use To facilitate both rapid sequence and routine endotracheal intubation and to relax skeletal muscles during surgery; to reduce the intensity of muscle contractions of pharmacologically- or electrically-induced convulsions; does not relieve pain or produce sedation
Local Anesthetic/Vasoconstrictor Precautions No information available to require special precautions
Effects on Dental Treatment No significant effects or complications reported
Effects on Bleeding No information available to require special precautions
Adverse Effects
Frequency not defined.
Cardiovascular: Arrhythmias, bradycardia (higher with second dose, more frequent in children), cardiac arrest, hyper-/hypotension, tachycardia
Dermatologic: Rash
Endocrine & metabolic: Hyperkalemia
Gastrointestinal: Salivation (excessive)
Neuromuscular & skeletal: Jaw rigidity, muscle fasciculation, postoperative muscle pain, rhabdomyolysis (with possible myoglobinuric acute renal failure)
Ocular: Intraocular pressure increased
Renal: Acute renal failure (secondary to rhabdomyolysis)
Respiratory: Apnea, respiratory depression (prolonged)
Miscellaneous: Anaphylaxis, malignant hyperthermia

Causes of prolonged neuromuscular blockade: Excessive drug administration; cumulative drug effect, decreased metabolism/excretion (hepatic and/or renal impairment); accumulation of active metabolites; electrolyte imbalance (hypokalemia, hypocalcemia, hypermagnesemia, hypernatremia); hypothermia; drug interactions; increased sensitivity to muscle relaxants (eg, neuromuscular disorders such as myasthenia gravis or polymyositis)

General Dosage Range Dosage adjustment recommended in patients with hepatic impairment

I.M.: *Children and Adults:* Up to 3-4 mg/kg (maximum: 150 mg total dose)

I.V.:

Smaller Children: Intermittent: Initial: 2 mg/kg/dose one time; Maintenance: 0.3-0.6 mg/kg/dose every 5-10 minutes as needed

Older Children and Adolescents: Intermittent: Initial: 1 mg/kg/dose one time; Maintenance: 0.3-0.6 mg/kg every 5-10 minutes as needed

Adults: Short surgical procedures: 0.6 mg/kg (range: 0.3-1.1 mg/kg); Long surgical procedures: 2.5-4.3 mg/minute continuous infusion, adjust dose based on response **or** 0.3-1.1 mg/kg followed by 0.04-0.07 mg/kg/dose as required

Mechanism of Action Acts similar to acetylcholine, produces depolarization of the motor endplate at the myoneural junction which causes sustained flaccid skeletal muscle paralysis produced by state of accommodation that develops in adjacent excitable muscle membranes

Pharmacodynamics/Kinetics

Onset of Action I.M.: 2-3 minutes; I.V.: Complete muscular relaxation: 30-60 seconds

Duration of Action I.M.: 10-30 minutes; I.V.: 4-6 minutes with single administration

Pregnancy Risk Factor C

Sucralfate (soo KRAL fate)

Related Information

Management of Patients Undergoing Cancer Therapy *on page 1970*

U.S. Brand Names Carafate®

Canadian Brand Names Novo-Sucralate; Nu-Sucralate; PMS-Sucralate; Sulcrate®; Sulcrate® Suspension Plus

Generic Availability (U.S.) Yes

Pharmacologic Category Gastrointestinal Agent, Miscellaneous

Use Short-term (≤8 weeks) management of duodenal ulcers; maintenance therapy for duodenal ulcers

Unlabeled/Investigational Use Gastric ulcers; suspension may be used topically for treatment of stomatitis due to cancer chemotherapy and other causes of esophageal and gastric erosions; GERD, esophagitis; treatment of NSAID mucosal damage; prevention of stress ulcers; postsclerotherapy for esophageal variceal bleeding

Local Anesthetic/Vasoconstrictor Precautions No information available to require special precautions

Effects on Dental Treatment No significant effects or complications reported

Effects on Bleeding No information available to require special precautions

Adverse Effects 1% to 10%: Gastrointestinal: Constipation (2%)

Dosage Oral:

Children (unlabeled use): Doses of 40-80 mg/kg/day divided every 6 hours have been used

Stomatitis (unlabeled use): 5-10 mL (1 g/10 mL suspension), swish and spit or swish and swallow 4 times/day

Adults:

Stress ulcer (unlabeled use):

Prophylaxis: 1 g 4 times/day

Treatment: 1 g every 4 hours

Duodenal ulcer:

Treatment: 1 g 4 times/day on an empty stomach and at bedtime for 4-8 weeks, or alternatively 2 g twice daily; treatment is recommended for 4-8 weeks in adults

Maintenance: Prophylaxis: 1 g twice daily

Stomatitis (unlabeled use): 10 mL (1 g/10 mL suspension), swish and spit or swish and swallow 4 times/day

Dosage comment in renal impairment: Aluminum salt is minimally absorbed (<5%), however, may accumulate in renal failure

Mechanism of Action Forms a complex by binding with positively charged proteins in exudates, forming a viscous paste-like, adhesive substance. This selectively forms a protective coating that acts locally to protect the gastric lining against peptic acid, pepsin, and bile salts.

Contraindications Hypersensitivity to sucralfate or any component of the formulation

Warnings/Precautions Because sucralfate acts locally at the ulcer site, successful therapy with sucralfate should not be expected to alter the posthealing frequency of recurrence or the severity of duodenal ulceration. Use with caution in patients with chronic renal failure; sucralfate is an aluminum complex, small amounts of aluminum are absorbed following oral administration. Excretion of aluminum may be decreased in patients with chronic renal failure. Because of the potential for sucralfate to alter the absorption of some drugs, separate administration (take other medication 2 hours before sucralfate) should be considered when alterations in bioavailability are believed to be critical.

Drug Interactions

Avoid Concomitant Use

Avoid concomitant use of Sucralfate with any of the following: Vitamin D Analogs

Increased Effect/Toxicity

The levels/effects of Sucralfate may be increased by: Vitamin D Analogs

Decreased Effect

Sucralfate may decrease the levels/effects of: Antifungal Agents (Azole Derivatives, Systemic); Digoxin; Eltrombopag; Levothyroxine; Phosphate Supplements; QuiNIDine; Quinolone Antibiotics; Tetracycline Derivatives; Vitamin K Antagonists

Ethanol/Nutrition/Herb Interactions Food: Sucralfate may interfere with absorption of vitamin A, vitamin D, vitamin E, and vitamin K.

Dietary Considerations Take with water on an empty stomach.

Pharmacodynamics/Kinetics

Onset of Action Paste formation and ulcer adhesion: 1-2 hours

Duration of Action Up to 6 hours

Pregnancy Risk Factor B

Lactation Excretion in breast milk unknown/use caution

Dosage Forms

Suspension, oral: 1 g/10 mL (10 mL)

Carafate®: 1 g/10 mL (420 mL)

Tablet, oral: 1 g

Carafate®: 1 g

SUFentanil (soo FEN ta nil)

U.S. Brand Names Sufenta®

Canadian Brand Names Sufentanil Citrate Injection, USP; Sufenta®

Pharmacologic Category Analgesic, Opioid; Anilidopiperidine Opioid; General Anesthetic

Use Analgesic supplement in maintenance of general anesthesia; epidural analgesic in conjunction with a local anesthetic

Local Anesthetic/Vasoconstrictor Precautions No information available to require special precautions

Effects on Dental Treatment Key adverse event(s) related to dental treatment: Orthostatic hypotension.

Effects on Bleeding No information available to require special precautions

Adverse Effects

>10%: Dermatologic: Pruritus (epidural: 25%)

1% to 10%:

Cardiovascular: Bradycardia (dose related; 3% to 9%), hyper-/hypotension (3% to 9%; more common with I.V. administration)

Central nervous system: Somnolence (3% to 9%), CNS depression, confusion

Gastrointestinal: Nausea (3% to 9%), vomiting (3% to 9%)

Neuromuscular & skeletal: Chest wall rigidity (dose related; 3% to 9%)

Ocular: Blurred vision

General Dosage Range

I.V.:

Children 2-12 years: 10-25 mcg/kg with 100% O_2; Maintenance: Up to 1-2 mcg/kg total dose

Adults: 1-2 mcg/kg with N_2O/O_2; Maintenance: 5-20 mcg/kg as needed

Epidural: *Adults:* 10-15 mcg (maximum: 3 doses)

Mechanism of Action Binds to opioid receptors throughout the CNS. Once receptor binding occurs, effects are exerted by opening K+ channels and inhibiting Ca++ channels. These mechanisms increase pain threshold, alter pain perception, inhibit ascending pain pathways; short-acting narcotic; dose-related inhibition of catecholamine release (up to 30 mcg/kg) controls sympathetic response to surgical stress.

Pharmacodynamics/Kinetics

Onset of Action Analgesia: I.V.: 1-3 minutes; Epidural: 10 minutes

Duration of Action Dose dependent; Epidural:10-15 mcg with bupivacaine: 1.7 hours

Half-life Elimination Neonates: 5-10 hours; Infants & Children: 55-139 minutes; Adults: 164 minutes
Pregnancy Risk Factor C
Controlled Substance C-II

Sulconazole (sul KON a zole)

U.S. Brand Names Exelderm®
Canadian Brand Names Exelderm®
Pharmacologic Category Antifungal Agent, Topical
Use Treatment of superficial fungal infections of the skin, including tinea cruris (jock itch), tinea corporis (ringworm), tinea versicolor, and tinea pedis (athlete's foot, cream only)
Local Anesthetic/Vasoconstrictor Precautions No information available to require special precautions
Effects on Dental Treatment No significant effects or complications reported
Effects on Bleeding No information available to require special precautions
Adverse Effects 1% to 10%:
Dermatologic: Itching
Local: Burning, stinging, redness
General Dosage Range Topical: *Adults:* Apply a small amount to affected area once or twice daily
Mechanism of Action Substituted imidazole derivative which inhibits metabolic reactions necessary for the synthesis of ergosterol, an essential membrane component. The end result is usually fungistatic; however, sulconazole may act as a fungicide in *Candida albicans* and *Candida parapsilosis* during certain growth phases.
Pregnancy Risk Factor C

Sulfabenzamide, Sulfacetamide, and Sulfathiazole
(sul fa BENZ a mide, sul fa SEE ta mide, & sul fa THYE a zole)

U.S. Brand Names V.V.S.®
Pharmacologic Category Antibiotic, Vaginal
Use Treatment of *Haemophilus vaginalis* vaginitis
Local Anesthetic/Vasoconstrictor Precautions No information available to require special precautions
Effects on Dental Treatment No significant effects or complications reported
Effects on Bleeding No information available to require special precautions
Adverse Effects Frequency not defined.
Dermatologic: Pruritus, urticaria, Stevens-Johnson syndrome
Local: Local irritation
Miscellaneous: Allergic reactions
General Dosage Range Intravaginal: *Adults:* Insert 1/4 to 1 applicatorful twice daily
Mechanism of Action Interferes with microbial folic acid synthesis and growth via inhibition of para-aminobenzoic acid metabolism
Pregnancy Risk Factor C (avoid if near term)

Sulfacetamide (Ophthalmic) (sul fa SEE ta mide)

U.S. Brand Names Bleph®-10; Sulfamide
Canadian Brand Names AK Sulf Liq; Bleph 10 DPS; Diosulf™; PMS-Sulfacetamide; Sodium Sulamyd
Pharmacologic Category Antibiotic, Ophthalmic
Use Treatment and prophylaxis of conjunctivitis due to susceptible organisms; corneal ulcers; adjunctive treatment with systemic sulfonamides for therapy of trachoma
Local Anesthetic/Vasoconstrictor Precautions No information available to require special precautions
Effects on Dental Treatment No significant effects or complications reported
Effects on Bleeding No information available to require special precautions
Adverse Effects Frequency not defined.
Cardiovascular: Edema
Ocular (following ophthalmic application): Burning, conjunctivitis, conjunctival hyperemia, corneal ulcers, irritation, stinging
Miscellaneous: Allergic reactions, systemic lupus erythematosus
General Dosage Range Ophthalmic: *Children >2 months and Adults:* Solution: Instill 1-2 drops up to every 2-3 hours

Mechanism of Action Interferes with bacterial growth by inhibiting bacterial folic acid synthesis through competitive antagonism of PABA

Pregnancy Risk Factor C

Sulfacetamide and Prednisolone (sul fa SEE ta mide & pred NIS oh lone)

Related Information

Sulfacetamide (Ophthalmic) *on page 1556*

U.S. Brand Names Blephamide®

Canadian Brand Names AK Cide Oph; Blephamide®; Dioptimyd®

Pharmacologic Category Antibiotic/Corticosteroid, Ophthalmic

Use Steroid-responsive inflammatory ocular conditions in which a corticosteroid is indicated and where infection is present or there is a risk of infection

Local Anesthetic/Vasoconstrictor Precautions No information available to require special precautions

Effects on Dental Treatment No significant effects or complications reported

Effects on Bleeding No information available to require special precautions

Adverse Effects Frequency not defined. Also refer to individual agents.

Dermatologic: Stevens-Johnson syndrome, toxic epidermal necrolysis, wound healing delayed

Hematologic: Agranulocytosis, aplastic anemia

Hepatic: Hepatic necrosis (fulminant)

Local: Irritation

Ocular: Accommodation loss, anterior uveitis (acute), intraocular pressure elevation, glaucoma, globe perforation, mydriasis, optic nerve damage (infrequent), posterior subcapsular cataract formation, ptosis

Miscellaneous: Allergic reactions, hypercorticoidism (systemic; rare), secondary infections (bacterial, fungal)

General Dosage Range Ophthalmic: *Children ≥6 years and Adults:*

Ointment: Apply ~1/2" ribbon 3-4 times/day and 1-2 times at night

Solution, suspension: Instill 2 drops every 4 hours

Mechanism of Action Interferes with bacterial growth by inhibiting bacterial folic acid synthesis through competitive antagonism of PABA; decreases inflammation by suppression of migration of polymorphonuclear leukocytes and reversal of increased capillary permeability; suppresses the immune system by reducing activity and volume of the lymphatic system

Pregnancy Risk Factor C

SulfADIAZINE (sul fa DYE a zeen)

Pharmacologic Category Antibiotic, Sulfonamide Derivative

Use Treatment of urinary tract infections and nocardiosis; adjunctive treatment in toxoplasmosis; uncomplicated attack of malaria

Unlabeled/Investigational Use Rheumatic fever prophylaxis

Local Anesthetic/Vasoconstrictor Precautions No information available to require special precautions

Effects on Dental Treatment No significant effects or complications reported

Effects on Bleeding No information available to require special precautions

Adverse Effects Frequency not defined.

Central nervous system: Dizziness, fever, headache

Dermatologic: Lyell's syndrome, Stevens-Johnson syndrome, itching, rash, photosensitivity

Endocrine & metabolic: Thyroid function disturbance

Gastrointestinal: Anorexia, diarrhea, nausea, vomiting

Genitourinary: Crystalluria

Hematologic: Aplastic anemia, granulocytopenia, hemolytic anemia, leukopenia, thrombocytopenia

Hepatic: Hepatitis, jaundice

Renal: Hematuria, acute nephropathy, interstitial nephritis

Miscellaneous: Serum sickness-like reactions

General Dosage Range Oral:

Newborns: 100 mg/kg/day divided every 6 hours

Children 1-2 months: 100 mg/kg/day divided every 6 hours

Children 2-12 months: Loading dose: 75 mg/kg **or** 100-200 mg/kg/day divided every 4-6 hours (maximum: 6 g/day)

Children 1-12 years: Loading dose: 75 mg/kg **or** 100-200 mg/kg/day divided every 4-6 hours (maximum: 6 g/day)

Children >12 years: Loading dose: 75 mg/kg **or** 100-200 mg/kg/day divided every 4-6 hours (maximum: 6 g/day) **or** 1 g twice daily

Adults: 2-8 g/day divided every 6 hours **or** 1 g twice daily

Mechanism of Action Interferes with bacterial growth by inhibiting bacterial folic acid synthesis through competitive antagonism of PABA

Pharmacodynamics/Kinetics

Half-life Elimination 10 hours

Time to Peak Within 3-6 hours

Pregnancy Risk Factor C

Sulfadoxine and Pyrimethamine (sul fa DOKS een & peer i METH a meen)

Related Information

Pyrimethamine *on page 1437*

U.S. Brand Names Fansidar® [DSC]

Pharmacologic Category Antimalarial Agent

Use Treatment of *Plasmodium falciparum* malaria in patients in whom chloroquine resistance is suspected; malaria prophylaxis for travelers to areas where chloroquine-resistant malaria is endemic

Local Anesthetic/Vasoconstrictor Precautions No information available to require special precautions

Effects on Dental Treatment Key adverse event(s) related to dental treatment: Atrophic glossitis.

Effects on Bleeding No information available to require special precautions

Adverse Effects Frequency not defined.

Cardiovascular: Myocarditis (allergic), pericarditis (allergic), periorbital edema

Central nervous system: Ataxia, hallucinations, headache, polyneuritis, seizure

Dermatologic: Photosensitivity, Stevens-Johnson syndrome, erythema multiforme, toxic epidermal necrolysis, rash

Endocrine & metabolic: Thyroid function dysfunction

Gastrointestinal: Anorexia, atrophic glossitis, gastritis, pancreatitis, vomiting

Genitourinary: Crystalluria

Hematologic: Megaloblastic anemia, leukopenia, thrombocytopenia, pancytopenia

Hepatic: Hepatic necrosis, hepatitis

Neuromuscular & skeletal: Tremors

Renal: BUN increased, interstitial nephritis, renal failure, serum creatinine increased

Respiratory: Respiratory failure, alveolitis (resembling eosinophilic or allergic)

Miscellaneous: Anaphylactoid reaction, drug fever, hypersensitivity, Lupus-like syndrome, periarteritis nodosum

General Dosage Range Oral:

Children 2-11 months: 1/4 tablet as a single dose

Children 1-3 years: 1/2 tablet as a single dose

Children 4-8 years: 1 tablet as a single dose

Children 9-14 years: 2 tablets as a single dose

Children >14 years and Adults: 3 tablets as a single dose

Mechanism of Action Sulfadoxine interferes with bacterial folic acid synthesis and growth via competitive inhibition of para-aminiobenzoic acid; pyrimethamine inhibits microbial dihydrofolate reductase, resulting in inhibition of tetrahydrofolic acid synthesis

Pharmacodynamics/Kinetics

Half-life Elimination Pyrimethamine: 80-95 hours; Sulfadoxine: 5-8 days

Time to Peak Serum: 2-8 hours

Pregnancy Risk Factor C/D (at term)

Sulfamethoxazole and Trimethoprim
(sul fa meth OKS a zole & trye METH oh prim)

Related Information

Trimethoprim *on page 1681*

U.S. Brand Names Bactrim™; Bactrim™ DS; Septra® DS; Septra® [DSC]; Sulfatrim®

Canadian Brand Names Apo-Sulfatrim®; Apo-Sulfatrim® DS; Apo-Sulfatrim® Pediatric; Novo-Trimel; Novo-Trimel D.S.; Nu-Cotrimox; Septra® Injection

Generic Availability (U.S.) Yes

Pharmacologic Category Antibiotic, Miscellaneous; Antibiotic, Sulfonamide Derivative

Use

Oral treatment of urinary tract infections due to *E. coli*, *Klebsiella* and *Enterobacter* sp, *M. morganii*, *P. mirabilis* and *P. vulgaris*; acute otitis media in children; acute exacerbations of chronic bronchitis in adults due to susceptible strains of *H. influenzae* or *S. pneumoniae*; treatment and prophylaxis of *Pneumocystis jiroveci* pneumonitis (PCP); traveler's diarrhea due to enterotoxigenic *E. coli*; treatment of enteritis caused by *Shigella flexneri* or *Shigella sonnei*

I.V. treatment of severe or complicated infections when oral therapy is not feasible, for documented PCP, empiric treatment of PCP in immune compromised patients; treatment of documented or suspected shigellosis, typhoid fever, *Nocardia asteroides* infection, or other infections caused by susceptible bacteria

Unlabeled/Investigational Use Cholera and *Salmonella*-type infections and nocardiosis; chronic prostatitis; as prophylaxis in neutropenic patients with *P. jiroveci* infections, in leukemia patients, and in patients following renal transplantation, to decrease incidence of PCP; treatment of *Cyclospora* infection, typhoid fever, *Nocardia asteroides* infection; prophylaxis against urinary tract infection; alternative treatment for MRSA infections

Local Anesthetic/Vasoconstrictor Precautions No information available to require special precautions

Effects on Dental Treatment Key adverse event(s) related to dental treatment: Stomatitis.

Effects on Bleeding No information available to require special precautions

Adverse Effects The most common adverse reactions include gastrointestinal upset (nausea, vomiting, anorexia) and dermatologic reactions (rash or urticaria). Rare, life-threatening reactions have been associated with co-trimoxazole, including severe dermatologic reactions, blood dyscrasias, and hepatotoxic reactions. Most other reactions listed are rare, however, frequency cannot be accurately estimated.

Cardiovascular: Allergic myocarditis

Central nervous system: Apathy, aseptic meningitis, ataxia, chills, depression, fatigue, fever, hallucinations, headache, insomnia, kernicterus (in neonates), nervousness, peripheral neuritis, seizure, vertigo

Dermatologic: Photosensitivity, pruritus, rash, skin eruptions, urticaria; rare reactions include erythema multiforme, exfoliative dermatitis, Henoch-Schönlein purpura, Stevens-Johnson syndrome, and toxic epidermal necrolysis

Endocrine & metabolic: Hyperkalemia (generally at high dosages), hypoglycemia (rare), hyponatremia

Gastrointestinal: Abdominal pain, anorexia, diarrhea, glottitis, nausea, pancreatitis, pseudomembranous colitis, stomatitis, vomiting

Hematologic: Agranulocytosis, aplastic anemia, eosinophilia, hemolysis (with G6PD deficiency), hemolytic anemia, hypoprothrombinemia, leukopenia, megaloblastic anemia, methemoglobinemia, neutropenia, thrombocytopenia

Hepatic: Hepatotoxicity (including hepatitis, cholestasis, and hepatic necrosis), hyperbilirubinemia, transaminases increased

Neuromuscular & skeletal: Arthralgia, myalgia, rhabdomyolysis, weakness

Otic: Tinnitus

Renal: BUN increased, crystalluria, diuresis (rare), interstitial nephritis, nephrotoxicity (in association with cyclosporine), renal failure, serum creatinine increased, toxic nephrosis (with anuria and oliguria)

Respiratory: Cough, dyspnea, pulmonary infiltrates

Miscellaneous: Allergic reaction, anaphylaxis, angioedema, periarteritis nodosa (rare), serum sickness, systemic lupus erythematosus (rare)

Dosage Dosage recommendations are based on the trimethoprim component. Double-strength tablets are equivalent to sulfamethoxazole 800 mg and trimethoprim 160 mg.

Usual dosage ranges:

Children >2 months:

Mild-to-moderate infections: Oral: 8-12 mg TMP/kg/day in divided doses every 12 hours

Serious infection:

Oral: 20 mg TMP/kg/day in divided doses every 6 hours

I.V.: 8-12 mg TMP/kg/day in divided doses every 6 hours

Adults:

Oral: 1-2 double-strength tablets (sulfamethoxazole 800 mg; trimethoprim 160 mg) every 12-24 hours

I.V.: 8-20 mg TMP/kg/day divided every 6-12 hours

Indication-specific dosing:

Children >2 months:

Acute otitis media: Oral: 8 mg TMP/kg/day in divided doses every 12 hours for 10 days. **Note:** Recommended by the American Academy of Pediatrics as an alternative agent in penicillin-allergic patients at a dose of 6-10 mg TMP/kg/day (AOM guidelines, 2004).

Cyclosporiasis (unlabeled use): Oral, I.V.: 5 mg TMP/kg twice daily for 7-10 days

Pneumocystis jiroveci:

Treatment: Oral, I.V.: 15-20 mg TMP/kg/day in divided doses every 6-8 hours for 21 days

Prophylaxis: Oral, 150 mg TMP/m^2/day in divided doses every 12 hours and administered for 3 days/week on consecutive or alternate days; an alternative dosing regimen allows for same dose to be administered in 2 divided doses daily (maximum: trimethoprim 320 mg and sulfamethoxazole 1600 mg daily) (CDC, 2009)

Shigellosis:

Oral: 8 mg TMP/kg/day in divided doses every 12 hours for 5 days

I.V.: 8-10 mg TMP/kg/day in divided doses every 6, 8, or 12 hours for up to 5 days

Skin/soft tissue infection due to community-acquired MRSA (unlabeled use): Oral: 4-6 mg TMP/kg/dose every 12 hours for 5-10 days (Liu, 2011); **Note:** If beta-hemolytic *Streptococcus* spp are also suspected, a beta-lactam antibiotic should be added to the regimen (Liu, 2011)

Toxoplasmosis primary prophylaxis (HIV-exposed/infected): Oral: 150 mg TMP/m^2/day in 2 divided doses (CDC, 2009)

Urinary tract infection:

Treatment:

Oral: 6-12 mg TMP/kg/day in divided doses every 12 hours

I.V.: 8-10 mg TMP/kg/day in divided doses every 6, 8, or 12 hours for up to 14 days with serious infections

Prophylaxis: Oral: 2 mg TMP/kg/dose daily or 5 mg TMP/kg/dose twice weekly

Adults:

Chronic bronchitis (acute): Oral: One double-strength tablet every 12 hours for 10-14 days

Cyclosporiasis (unlabeled use): Oral, I.V.: 160 mg TMP twice daily for 7-10 days. **Note:** AIDS patients: Oral: One double-strength tablet 2-4 times/day for 10 days, then 1 double-strength tablet 3 times/week for 10 weeks (Pape, 1994; Verdier, 2000)

Granuloma inguinale (donovanosis) (unlabeled use): Oral: One double-strength tablet every 12 hours for at least 3 weeks and until lesions have healed (CDC, 2010)

Meningitis (bacterial): I.V.: 10-20 mg TMP/kg/day in divided doses every 6-12 hours

Nocardia (unlabeled use): Oral, I.V.:

Cutaneous infections: 5-10 mg TMP/kg/day in 2-4 divided doses

Severe infections (pulmonary/cerebral): 15 mg TMP/kg/day in 2-4 divided doses for 3-4 weeks, then 10 mg TMP/kg/day in 2-4 divided doses. Treatment duration is controversial; an average of 7 months has been reported.

Note: Therapy for severe infection may be initiated I.V. and converted to oral therapy (frequently converted to approximate dosages of oral solid dosage forms: 2 DS tablets every 8-12 hours). Although not widely available, sulfonamide levels should be considered in patients with questionable absorption, at risk for dose-related toxicity, or those with poor therapeutic response.

Osteomyelitis due to MRSA (unlabeled use): Oral, I.V.: 3.5-4 mg TMP/kg/dose every 8-12 hours for a minimum of 8 weeks with rifampin 600 mg once daily (Liu, 2011)

***Pneumocystis jiroveci*:**

Prophylaxis: Oral: One double-strength tablet daily or 3 times/week

Treatment: Oral, I.V.: 15-20 mg TMP/kg/day in 3-4 divided doses

Sepsis: I.V.: 20 TMP/kg/day divided every 6 hours

Septic arthritis due to MRSA (unlabeled use): Oral, I.V.: 3.5-4 mg TMP/kg/dose every 8-12 hours for 3-4 weeks (some experts combine with rifampin) (Liu, 2011)

Shigellosis:

Oral: One double-strength tablet every 12 hours for 5 days

I.V.: 8-10 mg TMP/kg/day in divided doses every 6, 8, or 12 hours for up to 5 days

Skin/soft tissue infection due to community-acquired MRSA (unlabeled use): Oral: 1-2 double-strength tablets every 12 hours for 5-10 days (Liu, 2011); **Note:** If beta-hemolytic *Streptococcus* spp are also suspected, a beta-lactam antibiotic should be added to the regimen (Liu, 2011)

***Stenotrophomonas maltophilia* (ventilator-associated pneumonia):** I.V.: Most clinicians have utilized 12-15 mg TMP/kg/day for the treatment of VAP caused by *Stenotrophomonas maltophilia*. Higher doses (up to 20 mg TMP/kg/day) have been mentioned for treatment of severe infection in patients with normal renal function (Vartivarian, 1989; Looney, 2009; Wood, 2010)

Travelers' diarrhea: Oral: One double-strength tablet every 12 hours for 5 days

Urinary tract infection:

Oral: One double-strength tablet every 12 hours

Duration of therapy: Uncomplicated: 3-5 days; Complicated: 7-10 days

Pyelonephritis: 14 days

Prostatitis: Acute: 2 weeks; Chronic: 2-3 months

I.V.: 8-10 mg TMP/kg/day in divided doses every 6, 8, or 12 hours for up to 14 days with severe infections

Dosing adjustment in renal impairment: Oral, I.V.:

Manufacturer's recommendation: Children and Adults:

Cl_{cr} 15-30 mL/minute: Administer 50% of recommended dose

Cl_{cr} <15 mL/minute: Use is not recommended

Alternate recommendations:

Cl_{cr} 15-30 mL/minute:

Treatment: Administer full daily dose (divided every 12 hours) for 24-48 hours, then decrease daily dose by 50% and administer every 24 hours (**Note:** For serious infections including *Pneumocystis jiroveci* pneumonia (PCP), full daily dose is given in divided doses every 6-8 hours for 2 days, followed by reduction to 50% daily dose divided every 12 hours) (Nahata, 1995).

PCP prophylaxis: One-half single-strength tablet (40 mg trimethoprim) daily **or** 1 single-strength tablet (80 mg trimethoprim) daily or 3 times weekly (Masur, 2002).

Cl_{cr} <15 mL/minute:

Treatment: Administer full daily dose every 48 hours (Nahata, 1995)

PCP prophylaxis: One-half single-strength tablet (40 mg trimethoprim) daily **or** 1 single-strength tablet (80 mg trimethoprim) 3 times weekly (Masur, 2002). While the guidelines do acknowledge the alternative of giving 1 single-strength tablet daily, this may be inadvisable in the uremic/ESRD patient.

Hemodialysis:

Treatment: Full daily dose before dialysis and 50% dose after dialysis (Nahata, 1995)

Children: GFR <10 mL/minute/1.73 m^2: Not recommended, but if required 5-10 mg TMP/kg every 24 hours (Arnoff, 2007)

PCP prophylaxis: One single-strength tablet (80 mg trimethoprim) after each dialysis session (Masur, 2002)

CAPD:

Use Cl_{cr} <15 mL/minute dosing recommendations. Not significantly removed by CAPD; supplemental dosing is not required (Aronoff, 2007):

Exit-site and tunnel infections: Oral: One single-strength tablet daily (Li, 2010)

Peritonitis: Oral: One double-strength tablet twice daily (Li, 2010)

Children: GFR <10 mL/minute/1.73 m^2: Not recommended, but if required 5-10 mg TMP/kg every 24 hours. Intraperitoneal: Loading dose: TMP-SMX 320/1600 mg/L; Maintenance: TMP-SMX 80/400 mg/L (Arnoff, 2007; Warady, 2000)

CRRT: 2.5-10 mg TMP/kg/dose every 12 hours (Heintz, 2009)

Mechanism of Action Sulfamethoxazole interferes with bacterial folic acid synthesis and growth via inhibition of dihydrofolic acid formation from para-aminobenzoic acid; trimethoprim inhibits dihydrofolic acid reduction to tetrahydrofolate resulting in sequential inhibition of enzymes of the folic acid pathway

Contraindications Hypersensitivity to any sulfa drug, trimethoprim, or any component of the formulation; megaloblastic anemia due to folate deficiency; infants <2 months of age; marked hepatic damage or severe renal disease (if patient not monitored); pregnancy (at term); breast-feeding

Warnings/Precautions Use with caution in patients with G6PD deficiency, impaired renal or hepatic function or potential folate deficiency (malnourished, chronic anticonvulsant therapy, or elderly); maintain adequate hydration to prevent crystalluria; adjust dosage in patients with renal impairment. Injection vehicle contains benzyl alcohol and sodium metabisulfite.

Chemical similarities are present among sulfonamides, sulfonylureas, carbonic anhydrase inhibitors, thiazides, and loop diuretics (except ethacrynic acid). Use in patients with sulfonamide allergy is specifically contraindicated in product labeling, however, a risk of cross-reaction exists in patients with allergy to any of these compounds; avoid use when previous reaction has been severe.

Fatalities associated with severe reactions including Stevens-Johnson syndrome, toxic epidermal necrolysis, hepatic necrosis, agranulocytosis, aplastic anemia, and other blood dyscrasias; discontinue use at first sign of rash or serious adverse reactions. Elderly patients appear at greater risk for more severe adverse reactions. May cause hypoglycemia, particularly in malnourished, or patients with renal or hepatic impairment. Use with caution in patients with porphyria or thyroid dysfunction. Slow acetylators may be more prone to adverse reactions. Caution in patients with allergies or asthma. May cause hyperkalemia (associated with high doses of trimethoprim). Incidence of adverse effects appears to be increased in patients with AIDS. Prolonged use may result in fungal or bacterial superinfection, including *C. difficile*-associated diarrhea (CDAD) and pseudomembranous colitis; CDAD has been observed >2 months postantibiotic treatment.

Drug Interactions

Metabolism/Transport Effects

Sulfamethoxazole: **Substrate** of CYP2C9 (major), 3A4 (minor); **Inhibits** CYP2C9 (moderate)

Trimethoprim: **Substrate** (major) of CYP2C9, 3A4; **Inhibits** CYP2C8 (moderate), 2C9 (moderate)

Avoid Concomitant Use

Avoid concomitant use of Sulfamethoxazole and Trimethoprim with any of the following: BCG; Dofetilide; Methenamine; Potassium P-Aminobenzoate; Procaine

Increased Effect/Toxicity

Sulfamethoxazole and Trimethoprim may increase the levels/effects of: ACE Inhibitors; Amantadine; Angiotensin II Receptor Blockers; Antidiabetic Agents (Thiazolidinedione); AzaTHIOprine; Carvedilol; CycloSPORINE; CycloSPORINE (Systemic); CYP2C8 Substrates (High risk); CYP2C9 Substrates (High risk); Dapsone; Dapsone (Systemic); Dapsone (Topical); Dofetilide; Fosphenytoin; LamiVUDine; Memantine; Methotrexate; Phenytoin; PRALAtrexate; Procainamide; Repaglinide; Sulfonylureas; Vitamin K Antagonists

The levels/effects of Sulfamethoxazole and Trimethoprim may be increased by: Amantadine; Conivaptan; CYP2C9 Inhibitors (Moderate); CYP2C9 Inhibitors (Strong); Dapsone; Dapsone (Systemic); Memantine; Methenamine

Decreased Effect

Sulfamethoxazole and Trimethoprim may decrease the levels/effects of: BCG; CycloSPORINE; CycloSPORINE (Systemic); Typhoid Vaccine

The levels/effects of Sulfamethoxazole and Trimethoprim may be decreased by: CYP2C9 Inducers (Highly Effective); CYP3A4 Inducers (Strong); Deferasirox; Herbs (CYP3A4 Inducers); Leucovorin Calcium-Levoleucovorin; Peginterferon Alfa-2b; Potassium P-Aminobenzoate; Procaine; Tocilizumab

Ethanol/Nutrition/Herb Interactions Herb/Nutraceutical: Avoid dong quai; St John's wort (may diminish effects and also cause photosensitization).

Dietary Considerations Should be taken with 8 oz of water. May be taken without regard to meals.

Pharmacodynamics/Kinetics

Half-life Elimination SMX: 9 hours, TMP: 6-17 hours; both are prolonged in renal failure

Time to Peak Serum: Within 1-4 hours

Pregnancy Risk Factor C

Lactation Enters breast milk/contraindicated (AAP rates "compatible"; AAP 2001 update pending)

Breast-Feeding Considerations Small amounts of TMP and SMX are transferred to breast milk. Per the manufacturer, TMP-SMX is contraindicated in nursing mothers since sulfonamides cross into the milk and may cause kernicterus in the newborn. Because TMP-SMX has therapeutic indications for infants ≥2 months of age, kernicterus after exposure via breast-feeding would not be expected in healthy infants of this age group; however, sulfonamides should not be used while nursing an infant with G6PD deficiency or hyperbilirubinemia. Nondose related effects could include modification of bowel flora.

Dosage Forms The 5:1 ratio (SMX:TMP) remains constant in all dosage forms.

Injection, solution: Sulfamethoxazole 80 mg and trimethoprim 16 mg per mL (5 mL, 10 mL, 30 mL)

Suspension, oral: Sulfamethoxazole 200 mg and trimethoprim 40 mg per 5 mL

Sulfatrim®: Sulfamethoxazole 200 mg and trimethoprim 40 mg per 5 mL

Tablet: Sulfamethoxazole 400 mg and trimethoprim 80 mg

Bactrim™: Sulfamethoxazole 400 mg and trimethoprim 80 mg

Tablet, double-strength: Sulfamethoxazole 800 mg and trimethoprim 160 mg

Bactrim™ DS, Septra® DS: Sulfamethoxazole 800 mg and trimethoprim 160 mg

Sulfanilamide (sul fa NIL a mide)

U.S. Brand Names AVC™

Pharmacologic Category Antifungal Agent, Vaginal

Use Treatment of vulvovaginitis caused by *Candida albicans*

Local Anesthetic/Vasoconstrictor Precautions No information available to require special precautions

Effects on Dental Treatment No significant effects or complications reported

Effects on Bleeding No information available to require special precautions

General Dosage Range Intravaginal: *Adults:* 1 applicatorful once or twice daily

Mechanism of Action Interferes with microbial folic acid synthesis and growth via inhibition of para-aminiobenzoic acid metabolism; exerts a bacteriostatic action

Pregnancy Risk Factor C

SulfaSALAzine (sul fa SAL a zeen)

U.S. Brand Names Azulfidine EN-tabs®; Azulfidine®

Canadian Brand Names Alti-Sulfasalazine; Salazopyrin En-Tabs®; Salazopyrin®

Pharmacologic Category 5-Aminosalicylic Acid Derivative

Use Treatment of mild-to-moderate ulcerative colitis or as adjunctive therapy in severe ulcerative colitis; enteric coated tablets are also used for rheumatoid arthritis (including juvenile idiopathic arthritis [JIA]) in patients who inadequately respond to analgesics and NSAIDs

Unlabeled/Investigational Use Ankylosing spondylitis, Crohn's disease, psoriasis, psoriatic arthritis

Local Anesthetic/Vasoconstrictor Precautions No information available to require special precautions

Effects on Dental Treatment No significant effects or complications reported

Effects on Bleeding No information available to require special precautions

Adverse Effects

>10%:

Central nervous system: Headache
Dermatologic: Rash
Gastrointestinal: Anorexia, dyspepsia, gastric distress, nausea, vomiting
Genitourinary: Oligospermia (reversible)

1% to 10%:

Cardiovascular: Cyanosis
Central nervous system: Dizziness, fever
Dermatologic: Pruritus, urticaria
Gastrointestinal: Abdominal pain, stomatitis
Hematologic: Heinz body anemia, hemolytic anemia, leukopenia, thrombocytopenia
Hepatic: Liver function tests abnormal

General Dosage Range Oral:

Delayed release:

Children ≥6 years: Initial: 1/4 to 1/3 of expected maintenance dose; Maintenance: 30-50 mg/kg/day in 2 divided doses (maximum: 2 g/day)

Adults: Initial: 0.5-1 g/day; Maintenance: 2 g/day in 2 divided doses (maximum: 3 g/day)

Immediate release:

Children ≥6 years: Initial: 40-60 mg/kg/day in 3-6 divided doses; Maintenance: 30 mg/kg/day in 4 divided doses

Adults: Initial: 3-4 g/day in evenly divided doses at ≤8-hour intervals; Maintenance: 2 g/day in divided doses at ≤8-hour intervals

Mechanism of Action Acts locally in the colon to decrease the inflammatory response and systemically interferes with secretion by inhibiting prostaglandin synthesis

Pharmacodynamics/Kinetics

Half-life Elimination 5.7-10 hours (prolonged in elderly); sulfapyridine half-life prolonged in slow acetylators (14.8 hours)

Time to Peak Sulfasalazine: 3-12 hours (mean: 6 hours); metabolites: ~10 hours

Pregnancy Risk Factor B

Sulfonated Phenolics in Aqueous Solution

(SUL fo NATE ed fe NOL iks in AYE kwee us so LU shun)

Related Information

Ulcerative, Erosive, and Painful Oral Mucosal Disorders *on page 1950*

U.S. Brand Names Debacterol®

Generic Availability (U.S.) No

Pharmacologic Category Aphthous Ulcer Treatment Agent

Dental Use Therapeutic cauterization in the treatment of oral mucosal lesions (aphthous stomatitis, gingivitis, moderate-to-severe periodontitis)

Local Anesthetic/Vasoconstrictor Precautions No information available to require special precautions

Effects on Dental Treatment No significant effects or complications reported

Effects on Bleeding No information available to require special precautions

Dental Usual Dosage Apply applicator tip to the lesion as directed (see Dental Comment)

Mechanism of Action Semiviscous, chemical cautery agent which provides controlled, focal debridement and sterilization of necrotic tissues; relieving pain, sealing damaged tissue, and providing local antiseptic action

Contraindications Hypersensitivity to sulfur; for external use only

Warnings/Precautions For topical use only. Debacterol® is not intended for the treatment of cold sores and fever blisters. Prolonged use of Debacterol® on normal tissue should be avoided. If ingested, do not induce vomiting; immediately dilute with milk or water and get medical help or contact a Poison Control Center. If eye exposure occurs, immediately remove contact lenses, irrigate eyes for at least 15 minutes with lukewarm water, and contact a physician. Safety and efficacy in children <12 years of age have not been established.

Drug Interactions

Avoid Concomitant Use There are no known interactions where it is recommended to avoid concomitant use.

Increased Effect/Toxicity There are no known significant interactions involving an increase in effect.

Decreased Effect There are no known significant interactions involving a decrease in effect.

Pregnancy Risk Factor C

Breast-Feeding Considerations Unknown if excreted in breast milk; use with caution

Dosage Forms

Solution, topical:

Debacterol®: Sulfonated phenolics 50% and sulfuric acid 30% (1.5 mL) [for professional use only]

Swab, topical [for oral mucosa]:

Debacterol®: Sulfonated phenolics 50% and sulfuric acid 30% (0.2 mL) [for professional use only]

Dental Comment Prior to application/treatment, the ulcerated mucosal area should be thoroughly dried using the drying swab. After drying lesion, hold applicator "swab" with the colored ring end up. Bend the colored ring tip gently to the side until it snaps to release liquid inside. Liquid flows down into the white tip applicator. Apply the Debacterol® coated applicator tip to the dried ulcer area for at least 5 seconds, but no more than 10 seconds. Use rolling motion to completely cover the entire ulcer bed and ulcer rim. A "stinging" sensation is experienced immediately upon application. Debacterol® will not harm normal mucosa when used as directed. Thoroughly rinse out the mouth with water and spit out the rinse water. If the ulcer pain returns shortly after rinsing with water, it is an indication that some part of the ulcer was not covered. Repeat application one more time following directions above. One application per ulcer is usually sufficient. If excess irritation occurs during use, a rinse with sodium bicarbonate (baking soda) solution will neutralize the reaction (use 0.5 teaspoon in 120 mL water). It is not recommended that more than one Debacterol® treatment session be performed on an individual ulcer.

References

Rhodus NL and Bereuter J, "An Evaluation of a Chemical Cautery Agent and an Anti-inflammatory Ointment for the Treatment of Recurrent Aphthous Stomatitis: A Pilot Study," *Quintessence Int*, 1998, 29 (12):769-73.

Sulindac (SUL in dak)

Related Information

Rheumatoid Arthritis, Osteoarthritis, and Osteoporosis *on page 1889*

Temporomandibular Dysfunction (TMD) *on page 1964*

U.S. Brand Names Clinoril®

Canadian Brand Names Apo-Sulin®; Novo-Sundac; Nu-Sundac

Generic Availability (U.S.) Yes

Pharmacologic Category Nonsteroidal Anti-inflammatory Drug (NSAID), Oral

Use Management of inflammatory diseases including osteoarthritis, rheumatoid arthritis, acute gouty arthritis, ankylosing spondylitis, acute painful shoulder (bursitis/tendonitis)

Unlabeled/Investigational Use Management of preterm labor

Local Anesthetic/Vasoconstrictor Precautions No information available to require special precautions

Effects on Dental Treatment The dentist should be aware of the potential of abnormal coagulation. Caution should also be exercised in the use of NSAIDs in patients already on anticoagulant therapy with drugs such as warfarin (Coumadin®). See Effects on Bleeding.

Effects on Bleeding Nonselective NSAIDs are known to reversibly decrease platelet aggregation via mechanisms different than observed with aspirin. Platelet function is restored as the drug is eliminated from the body. NSAIDs should be avoided (if possible) in general surgery patients for 3-5 half-lives of the drug (usually 1-3 days) prior to surgery to reduce the risk of excessive bleeding. However, there is no scientific evidence to warrant discontinuance of NSAIDs prior to dental surgery. In medically complicated patients or extensive oral surgery, the decision to interrupt therapy must be based on the risk to benefit in an individual patient and a medical consult is suggested. Routine interruption of NSAID therapy for most dental procedures is not warranted. If therapy is continued without interruption, the clinician should anticipate the potential for slower clotting times.

Adverse Effects 1% to 10%:

Cardiovascular: Edema (1% to 3%)

Central nervous system: Dizziness (3% to 9%), headache (3% to 9%), nervousness (1% to 3%)

Dermatologic: Rash (3% to 9%), pruritus (1% to 3%)

Gastrointestinal: GI pain (10%), constipation (3% to 9%), diarrhea (3% to 9%), dyspepsia (3% to 9%), nausea (3% to 9%), abdominal cramps (1% to 3%), anorexia (1% to 3%), flatulence (1% to 3%), vomiting (1% to 3%)

Otic: Tinnitus (1% to 3%)

Dosage Oral:

Children: Dose not established

Adults: **Note:** Maximum daily dose: 400 mg

Osteoarthritis, rheumatoid arthritis, ankylosing spondylitis: 150 mg twice daily

Acute painful shoulder (bursitis/tendonitis): 200 mg twice daily; usual treatment: 7-14 days

Acute gouty arthritis: 200 mg twice daily; usual treatment: 7 days

Dosing adjustment in renal impairment: Not recommended with advanced renal impairment; if required, decrease dose and monitor closely

Dosing adjustment in hepatic impairment: Dose reduction is necessary; discontinue if abnormal liver function tests occur

Mechanism of Action Reversibly inhibits cyclooxygenase-1 and 2 (COX-1 and 2) enzymes, which results in decreased formation of prostaglandin precursors; has antipyretic, analgesic, and anti-inflammatory properties

Other proposed mechanisms not fully elucidated (and possibly contributing to the anti-inflammatory effect to varying degrees), include inhibiting chemotaxis, altering lymphocyte activity, inhibiting neutrophil aggregation/activation, and decreasing proinflammatory cytokine levels.

Contraindications Hypersensitivity or allergic-type reactions to sulindac, aspirin, other NSAIDs, or any component of the formulation; perioperative pain in the setting of coronary artery bypass graft (CABG) surgery

Warnings/Precautions **[U.S. Boxed Warning]: NSAIDs are associated with an increased risk of adverse cardiovascular thrombotic events, including MI and stroke.** Use caution with fluid retention. Avoid use in heart failure. Concurrent administration of ibuprofen, and potentially other nonselective NSAIDs, may interfere with aspirin's cardioprotective effect. May cause new-onset hypertension or worsening of existing hypertension. NSAID use may compromise existing renal function; dose-dependent decreases in prostaglandin synthesis may result from NSAID use, reducing renal blood flow which may cause renal decompensation. NSAID use may increase the risk for hyperkalemia. Patients with impaired renal function, dehydration, heart failure, liver dysfunction, those taking diuretics, and ACE inhibitors, and the elderly are at greater risk of renal toxicity and hyperkalemia. Rehydrate patient before starting therapy; monitor renal function closely. Not recommended for use in patients with advanced renal disease. Long-term NSAID use may result in renal papillary necrosis. Use caution in patients with renal lithiasis; sulindac metabolites have been reported as components of renal stones. Maintain adequate hydration in patients with a history of renal stones. Use with caution in patients with decreased hepatic function. May require dosage adjustment in hepatic dysfunction; sulfide and sulfone metabolites may accumulate. The elderly are at increased risk for adverse effects. **[U.S. Boxed Warning]: Use is contraindicated for treatment of perioperative pain in the setting of coronary artery bypass graft (CABG) surgery.** Risk of MI and stroke may be increased with use following CABG surgery.

[U.S. Boxed Warning]: NSAIDs may increase risk of gastrointestinal irritation, inflammation, ulceration, bleeding, and perforation. Use the lowest effective dose for the shortest duration of time, consistent with individual patient goals, to reduce risk of cardiovascular or GI adverse events. When used concomitantly with ≤325 mg of aspirin, a substantial increase in the risk of gastrointestinal complications (eg, ulcer) occurs; concomitant gastroprotective therapy (eg, proton pump inhibitors) is recommended (Bhatt, 2008). Pancreatitis has been reported; discontinue with suspected pancreatitis.

NSAIDS may cause drowsiness, dizziness, blurred vision and other neurologic effects which may impair physical or mental abilities; patients must be cautioned about performing tasks which require mental alertness (eg, operating machinery or driving). Discontinue use with blurred or diminished vision and perform ophthalmologic exam. Monitor vision with long-term therapy.

Platelet adhesion and aggregation may be decreased, may prolong bleeding time; patients with coagulation disorders or who are receiving anticoagulants should be monitored closely. Anemia may occur; patients on long-term NSAID therapy should be monitored for anemia. Rarely, NSAID use may cause severe blood dyscrasias (eg, agranulocytosis, aplastic anemia, thrombocytopenia). NSAIDs may cause serious skin adverse events including exfoliative dermatitis, Stevens-Johnson syndrome (SJS) and toxic epidermal necrolysis (TEN); discontinue use at first sign of skin rash or hypersensitivity. Anaphylactoid reactions may occur. Do not use in patients who experience bronchospasm, asthma, rhinitis, or urticaria with NSAID or aspirin therapy. Use caution in other forms of asthma. May increase the risk of aseptic meningitis, especially in patients with systemic lupus erythematosus (SLE) and mixed connective tissue disorders.

Withhold for at least 4-6 half-lives prior to surgical or dental procedures.

Drug Interactions

Avoid Concomitant Use

Avoid concomitant use of Sulindac with any of the following: Ketorolac; Ketorolac (Systemic)

Increased Effect/Toxicity

Sulindac may increase the levels/effects of: Aminoglycosides; Anticoagulants; Antiplatelet Agents; Bisphosphonate Derivatives; Collagenase (Systemic); CycloSPORINE; CycloSPORINE (Systemic); Deferasirox; Desmopressin; Digoxin; Drotrecogin Alfa; Eplerenone; Haloperidol; Ibritumomab; Methotrexate; Nonsteroidal Anti-Inflammatory Agents; PEMEtrexed; Potassium-Sparing Diuretics; PRALAtrexate; Quinolone Antibiotics; Salicylates; Thrombolytic Agents; Tositumomab and Iodine I 131 Tositumomab; Vancomycin; Vitamin K Antagonists

The levels/effects of Sulindac may be increased by: ACE Inhibitors; Angiotensin II Receptor Blockers; Antidepressants (Tricyclic, Tertiary Amine); Corticosteroids (Systemic); Dasatinib; Dimethyl Sulfoxide; Glucosamine; Herbs (Anticoagulant/Antiplatelet Properties); Ketorolac; Ketorolac (Systemic); Nonsteroidal Anti-Inflammatory Agents; Omega-3-Acid Ethyl Esters; Pentosan Polysulfate Sodium; Pentoxifylline; Probenecid; Prostacyclin Analogues; Selective Serotonin Reuptake Inhibitors; Serotonin/Norepinephrine Reuptake Inhibitors; Treprostinil

Decreased Effect

Sulindac may decrease the levels/effects of: ACE Inhibitors; Angiotensin II Receptor Blockers; Antiplatelet Agents; Beta-Blockers; Eplerenone; HydrALAZINE; Loop Diuretics; Potassium-Sparing Diuretics; Salicylates; Thiazide Diuretics

The levels/effects of Sulindac may be decreased by: Bile Acid Sequestrants; Nonsteroidal Anti-Inflammatory Agents; Salicylates

Ethanol/Nutrition/Herb Interactions

Ethanol: Avoid ethanol (may enhance gastric mucosal irritation).

Herb/Nutraceutical: Avoid alfalfa, anise, bilberry, bladderwrack, bromelain, cat's claw, celery, chamomile, coleus, cordyceps, dong quai, evening primrose, fenugreek, feverfew, garlic, ginger, ginkgo biloba, ginseng (American, Panax, Siberian), grapeseed, green tea, guggul, horse chestnut seed, horseradish, licorice, prickly ash, red clover, reishi, SAMe (S-adenosylmethionine), sweet clover, turmeric, white willow (all have additional antiplatelet activity).

Dietary Considerations Drug may cause GI upset, bleeding, ulceration, perforation; take with food or milk to minimize GI upset.

Pharmacodynamics/Kinetics

Half-life Elimination Sulindac: ~8 hours; Sulfide metabolite: ~16 hours

Time to Peak Sulindac: 3-4 hours; Sulfide and sulfone metabolites: 5-6 hours

Pregnancy Risk Factor C

Lactation Excretion in breast milk unknown/not recommended

Breast-Feeding Considerations It is not known if sulindac is excreted into breast milk. Breast-feeding is not recommended by the manufacturer.

Dosage Forms

Tablet, oral: 150 mg, 200 mg

Clinoril®: 200 mg

SUMAtriptan (soo ma TRIP tan)

Related Information

Temporomandibular Dysfunction (TMD) *on page 1964*

U.S. Brand Names Alsuma™; Imitrex®; Sumavel™ DosePro™

Canadian Brand Names Apo-Sumatriptan®; CO Sumatriptan; Dom-Sumatriptan; Gen-Sumatriptan; Imitrex®; Imitrex® DF; Imitrex® Nasal Spray; Mylan-Sumatriptan; Novo-Sumatriptan; PHL-Sumatriptan; PMS-Sumatriptan; ratio-Sumatriptan; Rhoxal-sumatriptan; Riva-Sumatriptan; Sandoz-Sumatriptan; Sumatryx

Generic Availability (U.S.) Yes

Pharmacologic Category Antimigraine Agent; Serotonin 5-$HT_{1B, 1D}$ Receptor Agonist

Use

Intranasal, Oral, SubQ: Acute treatment of migraine with or without aura

SubQ: Acute treatment of cluster headache episodes

Local Anesthetic/Vasoconstrictor Precautions No information available to require special precautions

Effects on Dental Treatment Key adverse event(s) related to dental treatment: Bad taste, dysphagia, hyposalivation (tablet), mouth/tongue discomfort (injection).

Effects on Bleeding No information available to require special precautions

Adverse Effects

Injection:

>10%:

Central nervous system: Dizziness (12%), warm/hot sensation (11%)

Local: Injection site reaction (≤86%; includes bleeding, bruising, edema, and erythema)

Neuromuscular & skeletal: Paresthesia (5% to 14%)

1% to 10%:

Cardiovascular: Chest discomfort/tightness/pressure (2% to 5%)

Central nervous system: Burning sensation (7%), feeling of heaviness (7%), flushing (7%), pressure sensation (7%), feeling of tightness (5%), drowsiness (3%), feeling strange (2%), headache (2%), tight feeling in head (2%), anxiety (1%), cold sensation (1%), malaise/fatigue (1%)

Gastrointestinal: Nausea/vomiting (4%), abdominal discomfort (1%), dysphagia (1%)

Neuromuscular & skeletal: Neck pain/stiffness (5%), numbness (5%), weakness (5%), jaw discomfort (2%), myalgia (2%), muscle cramps (1%)

Ocular: Vision alterations (1%)

Respiratory: Throat discomfort (3%), nasal disorder/discomfort (2%), bronchospasm (1%)

Miscellaneous: Diaphoresis (2%)

Nasal spray:

>10%: Gastrointestinal: Bad taste (13% to 24%), nausea (11% to 13%), vomiting (11% to 13%)

1% to 10%:

Central nervous system: Dizziness (1% to 2%)

Respiratory: Nasal disorder/discomfort (2% to 4%), throat discomfort (1% to 2%)

Tablet:

1% to 10%:

Cardiovascular: Chest pain/tightness/heaviness/pressure (1% to 2%), palpitation (1%), syncope (1%)

Central nervous system: Burning (1%), dizziness (>1%), drowsiness (>1%), malaise/fatigue (2% to 3%), headache (>1%), nonspecified pain (1% to 2%, placebo 1%), vertigo (<1% to 2%), migraine (>1%), sleepiness (>1%)

Gastrointestinal: Diarrhea (1%), nausea (>1%), vomiting (>1%), hyposalivation (>1%)

Genitourinary: Hematuria (1%)

Hematologic: Hemolytic anemia (1%)

Neuromuscular & skeletal: Neck, throat, and jaw pain/tightness/pressure (2% to 3%), paresthesia (3% to 5%), myalgia (1%), numbness (1%)

Otic: Ear hemorrhage (1%), hearing loss (1%), sensitivity to noise (1%), tinnitus (1%)

Respiratory: Allergic rhinitis (1%), dyspnea (1%), nasal inflammation (1%), nose/throat hemorrhage (1%), sinusitis (1%), upper respiratory inflammation (1%)

Miscellaneous: Hypersensitivity reactions (1%), nonspecified pressure/tightness/heaviness (1% to 3%, placebo 2%); warm/cold sensation (2% to 3%, placebo 2%)

Dosage

Adults:

Oral: A single dose of 25 mg, 50 mg, or 100 mg (taken with fluids). If a satisfactory response has not been obtained at 2 hours, a second dose may be administered. Results from clinical trials show that initial doses of 50 mg and 100 mg are more effective than doses of 25 mg, and that 100 mg doses do not provide a greater effect than 50 mg and may have increased incidence of side effects. Although doses of up to 300 mg/day have been studied, the total daily dose should not exceed 200 mg. The safety of treating an average of >4 headaches in a 30-day period have not been established.

Intranasal: A single dose of 5 mg, 10 mg, or 20 mg administered in one nostril. A 10 mg dose may be achieved by administering a single 5 mg dose in each nostril. If headache returns, the dose may be repeated once after 2 hours, not to exceed a total daily dose of 40 mg. In clinical trials, a greater number of patients responded to initial doses of 20 mg versus 5 or 10 mg. The safety of treating an average of >4 headaches in a 30-day period has not been established.

SubQ: Initial: Up to 6 mg; may repeat if needed ≥1 hour after initial dose (maximum: Two 6 mg injections per 24-hour period). However, controlled clinical trials have failed to document a benefit with administration of a second 6 mg dose in nonresponders.

Elderly: Not recommended due to increased potential for adverse effects.

Dosage adjustment in renal impairment: Dosage adjustment not necessary

Dosage adjustment in hepatic impairment:

Mild-to-moderate hepatic impairment:

Oral: Bioavailability of oral sumatriptan is increased with liver disease. If treatment is needed, do not exceed single doses of 50 mg.

Nasal spray: Has not been studied in patients with hepatic impairment, however, because the spray does not undergo first-pass metabolism, levels would not be expected to be altered.

Subcutaneous: Has been studied and pharmacokinetics were not altered in patients with hepatic impairment compared to healthy patients.

Severe hepatic impairment: Oral, nasal, and subcutaneous (limited to Imitrex® injection, per prescribing information) formulations are contraindicated with severe hepatic impairment.

Mechanism of Action Selective agonist for serotonin (5-HT_{1B} and 5-HT_{1D}receptors) in cranial arteries; causes vasoconstriction and reduces neurogenic inflammation associated with antidromic neuronal transmission correlating with relief of migraine

Contraindications Hypersensitivity to sumatriptan or any component of the formulation; patients with ischemic heart disease or signs or symptoms of ischemic heart disease (including Prinzmetal's angina, angina pectoris, myocardial infarction, silent myocardial ischemia); cerebrovascular syndromes (including strokes, transient ischemic attacks); peripheral vascular disease (including ischemic bowel disease); uncontrolled hypertension; use within 24 hours of ergotamine derivatives; use within 24 hours of another 5-HT_1 agonist; concurrent administration or within 2 weeks of discontinuing an MAO type A inhibitors (oral and nasal sumatriptan only; see Warnings/Precautions); management of hemiplegic or basilar migraine; severe hepatic impairment (oral and nasal sumatriptan, and injectable Imitrex® only); not for I.V. administration

Warnings/Precautions Sumatriptan is only indicated for the acute treatment of migraine or cluster headache; not indicated for migraine prophylaxis, or for the treatment of hemiplegic or basilar migraine. If a patient does not respond to the first dose, the diagnosis of migraine or cluster headache should be reconsidered; rule out underlying neurologic disease in patients with atypical headache and in patients with no prior history of migraine or cluster headache. Cardiac events (coronary artery vasospasm, transient ischemia, myocardial infarction, ventricular tachycardia/fibrillation, cardiac arrest and death), cerebral/subarachnoid hemorrhage, and stroke have been reported with 5-HT_1 agonist administration. Do not give to patients with risk factors for CAD until a cardiovascular evaluation has been performed; if evaluation is satisfactory, the healthcare provider should administer the first dose and cardiovascular status should be periodically evaluated.

Significant elevation in blood pressure, including hypertensive crisis, has also been reported on rare occasions in patients with and without a history of hypertension; use is contraindicated in patients with uncontrolled hypertension. Vasospasm-related reactions have been reported other than coronary artery vasospasm. Peripheral vascular ischemia and colonic ischemia with abdominal pain and bloody diarrhea have occurred. Transient and permanent blindness and significant partial vision loss have been very rarely reported. Use with caution in patients with a history of seizure disorder or in patients with a lowered seizure threshold. Use the oral formulation with caution in patients with hepatic impairment. Presystemic clearance of orally administered sumatriptan is reduced in hepatic impairment, leading to increased plasma concentrations; dosage reduction of the oral product is recommended. Non-oral routes of administration (nasal, subcutaneous formulations) do not undergo similar hepatic first-pass metabolism and are not expected to result in significantly altered pharmacokinetics in patients with hepatic impairment. Use of the oral, nasal, or Imitrex® injectable is contraindicated in severe hepatic impairment.

Symptoms of agitation, confusion, hallucinations, hyper-reflexia, myoclonus, shivering, and tachycardia (serotonin syndrome) may occur with concomitant proserotonergic drugs (ie, SSRIs/SNRIs or triptans) or agents which reduce sumatriptan's metabolism. Concurrent use of serotonin precursors (eg, tryptophan) is not recommended. Concurrent use with an MAO inhibitor may result in increased sumatriptan concentrations and increased risk for dose-related adverse effects (eg, serotonin syndrome); use with oral or nasal sumatriptan is contraindicated. Although generally not recommended, if concomitant use with injectable sumatriptan is deemed necessary, careful monitoring and appropriate dosage adjustments are required. I.V. administration is contraindicated due to the potential to cause coronary vasospasm. Not recommended for use in elderly patients; older adults are at a higher risk for coronary artery disease and may be more likely to have reduced hepatic function.

Drug Interactions

Avoid Concomitant Use

Avoid concomitant use of SUMAtriptan with any of the following: Ergot Derivatives; MAO Inhibitors; Sibutramine

Increased Effect/Toxicity

SUMAtriptan may increase the levels/effects of: Ergot Derivatives; Serotonin Modulators

The levels/effects of SUMAtriptan may be increased by: Ergot Derivatives; MAO Inhibitors; Sibutramine

Decreased Effect There are no known significant interactions involving a decrease in effect.

Pharmacodynamics/Kinetics

Onset of Action Oral: ~30 minutes; Nasal: ~15-30 minutes; SubQ: ~10 minutes

Half-life Elimination ~2-2.5 hours

Time to Peak Oral: 2-2.5 hours; SubQ: 12 minutes (range: 4-20 minutes)

Pregnancy Risk Factor C

Lactation Enters breast milk/use caution (AAP rates "compatible"; AAP 2001 update pending)

Breast-Feeding Considerations The amount of sumatriptan an infant would be exposed to following breast-feeding is considered to be small (although the mean milk-to-plasma ratio is ~4.9, weight adjusted doses estimates suggest breast-fed infants receive 3.5% of a maternal dose). Expressing and discarding the milk for 8-12 hours after a single dose is suggested to reduce the amount present even further. The half-life of sumatriptan in breast milk is 2.22 hours.

Dosage Forms

Injection, solution: 4 mg/0.5 mL (0.5 mL); 6 mg/0.5 mL (0.5 mL)
Alsuma™: 6 mg/0.5 mL (0.5 mL)
Imitrex®: 4 mg/0.5 mL (0.5 mL); 6 mg/0.5 mL (0.5 mL)
Sumavel™ DosePro™: 6 mg/0.5 mL (0.5 mL)

Solution, intranasal: 5 mg/0.1 mL (6s); 20 mg/0.1 mL (6s)
Imitrex®: 5 mg/0.1 mL (6s); 20 mg/0.1 mL (6s)

Tablet, oral: 25 mg, 50 mg, 100 mg
Imitrex®: 25 mg, 50 mg, 100 mg

Sumatriptan and Naproxen (soo ma TRIP tan & na PROKS en)

Related Information

Naproxen *on page 1183*
SUMAtriptan *on page 1566*

U.S. Brand Names Treximet™

Pharmacologic Category Antimigraine Agent; Nonsteroidal Anti-inflammatory Drug (NSAID), Oral; Serotonin 5-HT$_{1B,\ 1D}$ Receptor Agonist

Use Acute treatment of migraine with or without aura

Local Anesthetic/Vasoconstrictor Precautions No information available to require special precautions

Effects on Dental Treatment The dentist should be aware of the potential of abnormal coagulation. Caution should also be exercised in the use of NSAIDs in patients already on anticoagulant therapy with drugs such as warfarin (Coumadin®). See Effects on Bleeding.

Effects on Bleeding Nonselective NSAIDs are known to reversibly decrease platelet aggregation via mechanisms different than observed with aspirin. Platelet function is restored as the drug is eliminated from the body. NSAIDs should be avoided (if possible) in general surgery patients for 3-5 half-lives of the drug (usually 1-3 days) prior to surgery to reduce the risk of excessive bleeding. However, there is no scientific evidence to warrant discontinuance of NSAIDs prior to dental surgery. In medically complicated patients or extensive oral surgery, the decision to interrupt therapy must be based on the risk to benefit in an individual patient and a medical consult is suggested. Routine interruption of NSAID therapy for most dental procedures is not warranted. If therapy is continued without interruption, the clinician should anticipate the potential for slower clotting times.

Adverse Effects >1% to 10%:

Cardiovascular: Chest pain/discomfort (3%), palpitation (>1%)
Central nervous system: Dizziness (4%), somnolence (3%), fatigue (≥1%)
Gastrointestinal: Nausea (3%), dyspepsia (2%), xerostomia (2%), abdominal pain (≥1%)

Neuromuscular & skeletal: Neck, throat, and jaw pain/tightness/pressure (3%), paresthesia (2%), weakness (≥1%), muscle tightness (>1%)
Miscellaneous: Feeling hot (>1%)

General Dosage Range Oral: *Adults:* 1 tablet (sumatriptan 85 mg and naproxen 500 mg); may repeat in 2 hours if needed (maximum: 2 tablets/24 hours)

Mechanism of Action

Sumatriptan: Selective agonist for serotonin (5-HT_{1B} and 5-HT_{1D} receptors) in cranial arteries; causes vasoconstriction and reduces sterile inflammation associated with antidromic neuronal transmission correlating with relief of migraine

Naproxen: Reversibly inhibits cyclooxygenase-1 and 2 (COX-1 and 2) enzymes, which result in decreased formation of prostaglandin precursors; has antipyretic, analgesic, and anti-inflammatory properties

Pregnancy Risk Factor C

SUNItinib (su NIT e nib)

Related Information

Clinical Risk Related to Drugs Prolonging QT Interval *on page 1872*

U.S. Brand Names Sutent®

Canadian Brand Names Sutent®

Pharmacologic Category Antineoplastic Agent, Tyrosine Kinase Inhibitor; Vascular Endothelial Growth Factor (VEGF) Inhibitor

Use Treatment of gastrointestinal stromal tumor (GIST) intolerant to or with disease progression on imatinib; treatment of advanced renal cell cancer (RCC)

Unlabeled/Investigational Use Treatment of advanced thyroid cancer, treatment of pancreatic neuroendocrine tumors, treatment of non-GIST soft tissue sarcomas

Local Anesthetic/Vasoconstrictor Precautions Hypertension can occur with the use of this drug, particularly early in the treatment course. Monitor for hypertension prior to using local anesthetic with vasoconstrictor; medical consult if necessary.

Sunitinib is one of the drugs confirmed to prolong the QT interval and is accepted as having a risk of causing torsade de pointes. The risk of drug-induced torsade de pointes is extremely low when a single QT interval prolonging drug is prescribed. In terms of epinephrine, it is not known what effect vasoconstrictors in the local anesthetic regimen will have in patients with a known history of congenital prolonged QT interval or in patients taking any medication that prolongs the QT interval. Until more information is obtained, it is suggested that the clinician consult with the physician prior to the use of a vasoconstrictor in suspected patients, and that the vasoconstrictor (epinephrine, mepivacaine and levonordefrin [Carbocaine® 2% with Neo-Cobefrin®]) be used with caution.

Effects on Dental Treatment Key adverse event(s) related to dental treatment: Xerostomia (normal salivary flow resumes upon discontinuation), mucositis/stomatitis, taste perversion, and oral pain.

Effects on Bleeding Chemotherapy may result in significant myelosuppression, potentially including significant reduction in platelet counts and altered hemostasis. In patients who are under active treatment with these agents, medical consult is suggested.

Adverse Effects

>10%:

Cardiovascular: Hypertension (15% to 34%; grade 3: 4% to 13%), peripheral edema (24%), LVEF decreased (11% to 16%; grades 3/4: 1% to 3%), heart failure (≤15%), chest pain (13%)

Central nervous system: Fatigue (34% to 62%), headache (≤23%), fever (≤22%), insomnia (15%), chills (14%), depression (11%), dizziness (11%)

Dermatologic: Skin discoloration (25% to 30%), rash (14% to 29%), hand-foot syndrome (14% to 29%; grades 3/4: 4% to 8%), dry skin (≤23%), hair color changes (7% to 20%), alopecia (5% to 14%), erythema (12%), pruritus (12%)

Endocrine & metabolic: Hyperuricemia (≤46%), hypocalcemia (42%), hypophosphatemia (≤31%), hypoalbuminemia (28%), hyperglycemia (23%), hyponatremia (≤20%), hypoglycemia (17%), hyperkalemia (≤16%), hypothyroidism (4% to 16%; grades 3/4: ≤2%), hypercalcemia (13%), hypokalemia (12% to 13%), hypernatremia (10% to 13%)

Gastrointestinal: Diarrhea (40% to 66%), nausea (24% to 58%), lipase increased (25% to 56%), anorexia (33% to 48%), mucositis/stomatitis (29% to 47%), taste perversion (21% to 47%), vomiting (16% to 39%), amylase increased (17% to 35%), dyspepsia (34%), abdominal pain (≤30%), constipation (20% to 23%), weight loss (16%), flatulence (14%), oral pain (6% to 14%), xerostomia (13%), GERD/reflux (12%), glossodynia (11%)

Hematologic: Anemia (26% to 79%; grades 3/4: 3% to 8%), leukopenia (78%; grades 3/4: 8%), neutropenia (53% to 77%; grades 3/4: 10% to 17%), lymphopenia (38% to 68%; grades 3/4: ≤18%), thrombocytopenia (38% to 68%; grades 3/4: 5% to 9%), hemorrhage/bleeding (18% to 37%)
Hepatic: AST increased (39% to 56%; grades 3/4: 2%), ALT increased (39% to 51%; grades 3/4: 2% to 3%), alkaline phosphatase increased (24% to 46%; grades 3/4: 2% to 4%), hyperbilirubinemia (10% to 20%; grades 3/4 ≤1%)
Neuromuscular & skeletal: Creatine kinase increased (49%), limb pain (14% to 40%), arthralgia (≤30%), back pain (≤28%), weakness (22% to 26%), myalgia (14%)
Renal: Creatinine increased (12% to 70%)
Respiratory: Cough (27%), dyspnea (26%), nasopharyngitis (14%), upper respiratory tract infection (11%)

1% to 10%:
Cardiovascular: Venous thrombotic events (3%), DVT (2% to 3%)
Gastrointestinal: Hemorrhoids (10%), pancreatitis (1%)
Respiratory: Pulmonary embolism (2%)
Miscellaneous: Flu-like syndrome (5%)

General Dosage Range Dosage adjustment recommended in patients with renal impairment, on concomitant therapy, or who develop toxicities
Oral: *Adults:* 50 mg once daily for 4 weeks of a 6-week treatment cycle

Mechanism of Action Exhibits antitumor and antiangiogenic properties by inhibiting multiple receptor tyrosine kinases, including platelet-derived growth factors (PDGFRα and PDGFRβ), vascular endothelial growth factors (VEGFR1, VEGFR2, and VEGFR3), FMS-like tyrosine kinase-3 (FLT3), colony-stimulating factor type 1 (CSF-1R), and glial cell-line-derived neurotrophic factor receptor (RET).

Pharmacodynamics/Kinetics
Half-life Elimination Terminal: Sunitinib: 40-60 hours; SU12662: 80-110 hours
Time to Peak 6-12 hours

Pregnancy Risk Factor D

Dental Comment Sunitinib is known to prolong the QT interval. The QT interval is measured as the time and distance between the Q point of the QRS complex and the end of the T wave in the ECG tracing. After adjustment for heart rate, the QT interval is defined as prolonged if it is more than 450 msec in men and 460 msec in women. A long QT syndrome was first described in the 1950s and 60s as a congenital syndrome involving QT interval prolongation and syncope and sudden death. Some of the congenital long QT syndromes were characterized by a peculiar electrocardiographic appearance of the QRS complex involving a premature atria beat followed by a pause, then a subsequent sinus beat showing marked QT prolongation and deformity. This type of cardiac arrhythmia was originally termed "torsade de pointes" (translated from the French as "twisting of the points"). Sunitinib is considered as having a risk of causing torsade de pointes. Since it is not known what effect vasoconstrictors in the local anesthetic regimen will have in patients with a known history of congenital prolonged QT interval or in patients taking any medication that prolongs the QT interval, a medical consult is suggested.

Tacrolimus (Systemic) (ta KROE li mus)

U.S. Brand Names Prograf®
Canadian Brand Names Advagraf™; Prograf®
Generic Availability (U.S.) Yes: Capsule
Pharmacologic Category Calcineurin Inhibitor; Immunosuppressant Agent
Use Prevention of organ rejection in heart, kidney, or liver transplant recipients
Unlabeled/Investigational Use Prevention of organ rejection in lung, small bowel transplant recipients; prevention and treatment of graft-versus-host disease (GVHD) in allogenic hematopoietic stem cell transplantation
Local Anesthetic/Vasoconstrictor Precautions No information available to require special precautions
Effects on Dental Treatment Key adverse event(s) related to dental treatment: Stomatitis, oral moniliasis, dysphagia, and esophagitis (including ulcerative).
Effects on Bleeding Thrombocytopenia has been associated with use; severe thrombocytopenia (rare) may be associated with delayed coagulation. Consultation to ensure adequate platelet counts may be considered in patients with signs/symptoms or a history of thrombocytopenia.
Adverse Effects As reported for kidney, liver, and heart transplantation:
≥15%:
Cardiovascular: Hypertension (13% to 62%), edema (peripheral 11% to 36%), chest pain (19%), edema (18%), pericardial effusion (heart transplant 15%)

Central nervous system: Headache (25% to 64%), insomnia (30% to 64%), pain (24% to 63%), fever (19% to 48%), postprocedural pain (kidney transplant 29%), dizziness (19%)
Dermatologic: Pruritus (15% to 36%), rash (10% to 24%)
Endocrine & metabolic: Hypophosphatemia (28% to 49%), hypomagnesemia (16% to 48%), hyperglycemia (21% to 47%), hyperkalemia (8% to 45%), hyperlipemia (10% to 31%), hypokalemia (13% to 29%), diabetes mellitus (24% to 26%)
Gastrointestinal: Diarrhea (24% to 72%), abdominal pain (29% to 59%), nausea (32% to 46%), constipation (23% to 36%), anorexia (7% to 34%), vomiting (14% to 29%), dyspepsia (18% to 28%)
Genitourinary: Urinary tract infection (16% to 34%)
Hematologic: Anemia (5% to 50%), leukopenia (13% to 48%), leukocytosis (8% to 32%), thrombocytopenia (14% to 24%)
Hepatic: Liver function tests abnormal (6% to 36%), ascites (7% to 27%)
Local: Incision site complication (kidney transplant 28%)
Neuromuscular & skeletal: Tremor (34% to 56%; heart transplant 15%), weakness (11% to 52%), paresthesia (17% to 40%), back pain (17% to 30%), arthralgia (25%)
Renal: Abnormal kidney function (36% to 56%), creatinine increased (23% to 45%), BUN increased (12% to 30%), oliguria (18% to 19%)
Respiratory: Atelectasis (5% to 28%), pleural effusion (30% to 36%), dyspnea (5% to 29%), cough increased (18%), bronchitis (17%)
Miscellaneous: Infection (24% to 45%), CMV infection (32%), graft dysfunction (kidney transplant 24%)

<15%:

Cardiovascular: Abnormal ECG (QRS or ST segment abnormal), arrhythmia, atrial fibrillation, atrial flutter, bradycardia, cardiopulmonary failure, deep thrombophlebitis, heart failure, heart rate decreased, hemorrhage, hemorrhagic stroke, hypervolemia, hypotension, peripheral vascular disorder, phlebitis, postural hypotension, syncope, tachycardia, thrombosis, vasodilation, ventricular fibrillation
Central nervous system: Abnormal dreams, abnormal thinking, agitation, amnesia, anxiety, chills, confusion, depression, emotional lability, encephalopathy, flaccid paralysis, hallucinations, mood elevated, nervousness, psychosis, quadriparesis, seizure, somnolence
Dermatologic: Acne, alopecia, bruising, cellulitis, exfoliative dermatitis, fungal dermatitis, hirsutism, photosensitivity reaction, skin discoloration, skin disorder, skin neoplasm, skin ulcer, wound healing impaired
Endocrine & metabolic: Acidosis, alkalosis, bicarbonate decreased, Cushing's syndrome, dehydration, gout, hypercholesterolemia, hyper-/hypocalcemia, hyperphosphatemia, hyperuricemia, hypoproteinemia, serum iron decreased
Gastrointestinal: Appetite increased, cramps, duodenitis, dysphagia, enlarged abdomen, esophagitis (including ulcerative), flatulence, gastritis, gastroesophagitis, GI perforation/hemorrhage, ileus, oral moniliasis, pancreatic pseudocyst, rectal disorder, stomatitis, weight gain
Genitourinary: Bladder spasm, cystitis, dysuria, nocturia, urge incontinence, urinary frequency, urinary incontinence, urinary retention, vaginitis
Hematologic: Coagulation disorder, decreased prothrombin, hypochromic anemia, polycythemia
Hepatic: Alkaline phosphatase increased, bilirubinemia, cholangitis, cholestatic jaundice, GGT increased, hepatitis (including granulomatous), jaundice, LDH increased, liver damage
Local: Phlebitis
Neuromuscular & skeletal: Hypertonia, incoordination, joint disorder, leg cramps, myalgia, myasthenia, myoclonus, nerve compression, neuropathy, osteoporosis
Ocular: Abnormal vision, amblyopia
Otic: Ear pain, otitis media, tinnitus
Renal: Acute renal failure, albuminuria, BK nephropathy, hematuria, hydronephrosis, renal tubular necrosis, toxic nephropathy
Respiratory: Asthma, lung disorder, pharyngitis, pneumonia, pneumothorax, pulmonary edema, respiratory disorder, rhinitis, sinusitis, voice alteration
Miscellaneous: Abscess, abnormal healing, allergic reaction, crying, diaphoresis, flu-like syndrome, generalized spasm, hernia, herpes simplex, peritonitis, sepsis, writing impaired

Dosage

Oral:

Prevention of organ rejection in transplant recipients: The initial dose of tacrolimus should begin no sooner than 6 hours post-transplant; adjunctive therapy with corticosteroids is recommended early post-transplant. I.V. route should only be used in patients not able to take oral medications and continued only until oral medication can be tolerated; anaphylaxis has been reported with I.V. administration. If switching from I.V. to oral, the oral dose should be started 8-12 hours after stopping the infusion.

Children: Patients without pre-existing renal or hepatic dysfunction have required (and tolerated) higher doses than adults to achieve similar blood concentrations. It is recommended that therapy be initiated at ***high end*** of the recommended adult I.V. and oral dosing ranges; dosage adjustments may be required.

Liver transplant: Initial dose: 0.15-0.20 mg/kg/day in 2 divided doses, given every 12 hours

Adults:

Heart transplant: Initial dose: 0.075 mg/kg/day in 2 divided doses, given every 12 hours. Use in combination with azathioprine or mycophenolate mofetil is recommended.

Kidney transplant: Initial dose: 0.2 mg/kg/day in combination with azathioprine **or** 0.1 mg/kg/day in combination with mycophenolate mofetil. Administer in 2 divided doses, given every 12 hours; initial dose may be given within 24 hours of transplant, but should be delayed until renal function has recovered; African-American patients may require larger doses to maintain trough concentration.

Liver transplant: Initial dose: 0.1-0.15 mg/kg/day in 2 divided doses, given every 12 hours

Prevention of graft-versus-host disease (unlabeled use): Children and Adults: Convert from I.V. to oral dose (1:4 ratio): Multiply total daily I.V. dose times 4 and administer in 2 divided oral doses per day, every 12 hours (Uberti, 1999; Yanik, 2000).

Treatment of graft-versus-host disease (unlabeled use): Adults: 0.06 mg/kg twice daily (Furlong, 2000; Przepiorka, 1999)

I.V.:

Prevention of organ rejection in transplant recipients: The initial dose of tacrolimus should begin no sooner than 6 hours post-transplant; adjunctive therapy with corticosteroids is recommended early post-transplant. I.V. route should only be used in patients not able to take oral medications and continued only until oral medication can be tolerated; anaphylaxis has been reported with I.V. administration. If switching from I.V. to oral, the oral dose should be started 8-12 hours after stopping the infusion.

Children: It is recommended that therapy be initiated at the ***high end*** of the dosing range.

Liver transplant: Initial dose: 0.03-0.05 mg/kg/day as a continuous infusion

Adults: It is recommended that therapy be initiated at the ***lower end*** of the dosing range.

Heart transplant: Initial dose: 0.01 mg/kg/day as a continuous infusion. Use in combination with azathioprine or mycophenolate mofetil is recommended.

Kidney transplant: Initial dose: 0.03-0.05 mg/kg/day as a continuous infusion. Use in combination with azathioprine or mycophenolate mofetil is recommended.

Liver transplant: Initial dose: 0.03-0.05 mg/kg/day as a continuous infusion.

Prevention of graft-versus-host disease (unlabeled use): Children and Adults: Initial: 0.03 mg/kg/day (based on lean body weight) as continuous infusion. Treatment should begin at least 24 hours prior to stem cell infusion and continued only until oral medication can be tolerated (Przepiorka, 1999; Yanik, 2000).

Treatment of graft-versus-host disease (unlabeled use): Adults: Initial: 0.03 mg/kg/day (based on lean body weight) as continuous infusion (Furlong, 2000; Przepiorka, 1999)

Dosing adjustment in renal impairment: Systemic therapy: Evidence suggests that lower doses should be used; patients should receive doses at the lowest value of the recommended I.V. and oral dosing ranges; further reductions in dose below these ranges may be required.

Tacrolimus therapy should usually be delayed up to 48 hours or longer in patients with postoperative oliguria.

Hemodialysis: Not removed by hemodialysis; supplemental dose is not necessary.

Peritoneal dialysis: Significant drug removal is unlikely based on physiochemical characteristics.

Dosing adjustment in hepatic impairment: Systemic therapy: Use of tacrolimus in liver transplant recipients experiencing post-transplant hepatic impairment may be associated with increased risk of developing renal insufficiency related to high whole blood levels of tacrolimus. The presence of moderate-to-severe hepatic dysfunction (serum bilirubin >2 mg/dL; Child-Pugh score ≥10) appears to affect the metabolism of tacrolimus. The half-life of the drug was prolonged and the clearance reduced after I.V. administration. The bioavailability of tacrolimus was also increased after oral administration. The higher plasma concentrations as determined by ELISA, in patients with severe hepatic dysfunction are probably due to the accumulation of metabolites of lower activity. These patients should be monitored closely and dosage adjustments should be considered. Some evidence indicates that lower doses could be used in these patients.

Mechanism of Action Suppresses cellular immunity (inhibits T-lymphocyte activation), by binding to an intracellular protein, FKBP-12 and complexes with calcineurin dependent proteins to inhibit calcineurin phosphatase activity

Contraindications Hypersensitivity to tacrolimus or any component of the formulation

Warnings/Precautions Hazardous agent - use appropriate precautions for handling and disposal. **[U.S. Boxed Warning]: Increased susceptibility to infection and the possible development of lymphoma may result from immunosuppression with tacrolimus.** The risk of developing other malignancies may also be increased. Insulin-dependent post-transplant diabetes mellitus (PTDM) has been reported including in patients without pretransplant history of diabetes mellitus; risk increases in African-American and Hispanic kidney transplant patients. Posterior reversible encephalopathy syndrome (PRES) may occur with therapy; symptoms are reversible with dose reduction or discontinuation of immunosuppressant therapy; stabilize blood pressure and reduce dose with suspected or confirmed diagnosis. Nephrotoxicity has has been reported, especially with higher doses; to avoid excess nephrotoxicity do not administer simultaneously with other nephrotoxic drugs (eg sirolimus, cyclosporine). Neurotoxicity may occur especially when used in high doses; tremor headache, coma and delirium have been reported and are associated with serum concentrations. Seizures may also occur. Monitoring of serum concentrations (trough for oral therapy) is essential to prevent organ rejection and reduce drug-related toxicity. Variable absorption is seen in bone marrow transplantation relative to total body radiation and/or methotrexate use. A period of ≥24 hours should elapse between discontinuation of cyclosporine and the initiation of tacrolimus. Delay initiation further with persistently elevated tacrolimus/cyclosporine levels. Use caution in renal or hepatic dysfunction, dosing adjustments may be required. Delay initiation if postoperative oliguria occurs. Use may be associated with the development of hypertension (common); hyperkalemia has been reported; avoid use of potassium-sparing diuretics. Myocardial hypertrophy has been reported (rare). Each mL of injection contains polyoxyl 60 hydrogenated castor oil (HCO-60) (200 mg) and dehydrated alcohol USP 80% v/v. Anaphylaxis has been reported with the injection, use should be reserved for those patients not able to take oral medications. **[U.S. Boxed Warning]: Should be administered under the supervision of a physician experienced in immunosuppressive therapy and organ transplantation in a facility appropriate for monitoring and managing therapy.**

Drug Interactions

Metabolism/Transport Effects **Substrate** of CYP3A4 (major), P-glycoprotein; **Inhibits** CYP3A4 (weak), P-glycoprotein

Avoid Concomitant Use

Avoid concomitant use of Tacrolimus (Systemic) with any of the following: Artemether; BCG; CycloSPORINE (Systemic); Dronedarone; Grapefruit Juice; Lumefantrine; Natalizumab; Nilotinib; Pimecrolimus; Pimozide; QuiNINE; Roflumilast; Silodosin; Sirolimus; Tacrolimus (Topical); Temsirolimus; Tetrabenazine; Thioridazine; Topotecan; Toremifene; Vaccines (Live); Vandetanib; Ziprasidone

Increased Effect/Toxicity

Tacrolimus (Systemic) may increase the levels/effects of: Colchicine; CycloSPORINE (Systemic); Dabigatran Etexilate; Dronedarone; Everolimus; Fosphenytoin; Leflunomide; Natalizumab; P-Glycoprotein Substrates; Phenytoin; Pimozide; QTc-Prolonging Agents; QuiNINE; Rivaroxaban; Silodosin; Sirolimus; Temsirolimus; Tetrabenazine; Thioridazine; Topotecan; Toremifene; Vaccines (Live); Vandetanib; Ziprasidone

The levels/effects of Tacrolimus (Systemic) may be increased by: Alfuzosin; Antidepressants (Serotonin Reuptake Inhibitor/Antagonist); Artemether; Calcium Channel Blockers (Dihydropyridine); Calcium Channel Blockers (Nondihydropyridine); Chloroquine; Ciprofloxacin; Ciprofloxacin (Systemic); Clotrimazole; Clotrimazole (Oral); Conivaptan; CycloSPORINE (Systemic); CYP3A4 Inhibitors (Moderate); CYP3A4 Inhibitors (Strong); Denosumab; Fluconazole; Gadobutrol; Grapefruit Juice; Itraconazole; Ketoconazole; Ketoconazole (Systemic); Lumefantrine; Macrolide Antibiotics; MetroNIDAZOLE; MetroNIDAZOLE (Systemic); Nilotinib; P-Glycoprotein Inhibitors; Pimecrolimus; Posaconazole; Protease Inhibitors; Proton Pump Inhibitors; QuiNINE; Ranolazine; Roflumilast; Sirolimus; Tacrolimus (Topical); Temsirolimus; Trastuzumab; Voriconazole

Decreased Effect

Tacrolimus (Systemic) may decrease the levels/effects of: BCG; Sipuleucel-T; Vaccines (Inactivated); Vaccines (Live)

The levels/effects of Tacrolimus (Systemic) may be decreased by: Caspofungin; Cinacalcet; CYP3A4 Inducers (Strong); Deferasirox; Echinacea; Efavirenz; Fosphenytoin; P-Glycoprotein Inducers; Phenytoin; Rifamycin Derivatives; Sirolimus; St Johns Wort; Temsirolimus; Tocilizumab

Ethanol/Nutrition/Herb Interactions

Food: Decreases rate and extent of absorption. High-fat meals have most pronounced effect (37% decrease in AUC, 77% decrease in C_{max}). Grapefruit juice, CYP3A4 inhibitor, may increase serum level and/or toxicity of tacrolimus; avoid concurrent use.

Herb/Nutraceutical: St John's wort: May reduce tacrolimus serum concentrations (avoid concurrent use).

Dietary Considerations Capsule: Take on an empty stomach; be consistent with timing and composition of meals if GI intolerance occurs and administration with food becomes necessary (per manufacturer). Avoid grapefruit juice.

Pharmacodynamics/Kinetics

Half-life Elimination Variable, 23-46 hours in healthy volunteers; 2.1-36 hours in transplant patients

Time to Peak 0.5-6 hours

Pregnancy Risk Factor C

Lactation Enters breast milk/not recommended

Breast-Feeding Considerations Concentrations of tacrolimus in breast milk are lower than that of the maternal serum. The low bioavailability of tacrolimus following oral absorption may also decrease the amount of exposure to a nursing infant.

Dosage Forms

Capsule, oral: 0.5 mg, 1 mg, 5 mg

Prograf®: 0.5 mg, 1 mg, 5 mg

Injection, solution:

Prograf®: 5 mg/mL (1 mL)

Tacrolimus (Topical) (ta KROE li mus)

U.S. Brand Names Protopic®

Canadian Brand Names Protopic®

Generic Availability (U.S.) No

Pharmacologic Category Calcineurin Inhibitor; Topical Skin Product

Dental Use Treatment of severe ulcerative or vesicobullous lesions (usually in consult with patient's physician)

Use Moderate-to-severe atopic dermatitis in immunocompetent patients not responsive to conventional therapy or when conventional therapy is not appropriate

Canadian labeling: Additional use (not in U.S. labeling): Maintenance therapy to prevent flares and extend flare-free intervals in patients with moderate-to-severe atopic dermatitis who are responsive to initial therapy and experiencing ≥5 flares per year

Local Anesthetic/Vasoconstrictor Precautions No information available to require special precautions

Effects on Dental Treatment No significant effects or complications reported

Effects on Bleeding No information available to require special precautions

Adverse Effects As reported in children and adults, unless otherwise noted:

>10%:

Central nervous system: Headache (5% to 20%), fever (1% to 21%)

Dermatologic: Skin burning (43% to 58%; tends to improve as lesions resolve), pruritus (41% to 46%), erythema (12% to 28%)

Respiratory: Increased cough (children 18%)

Miscellaneous: Flu-like syndrome (23% to 31%), allergic reaction (4% to 12%)

1% to 10%:

Cardiovascular: Peripheral edema (adults 3% to 4%)

Central nervous system: Hyperesthesia (adults 3% to 7%), pain (1% to 2%)

Dermatologic: Skin tingling (2% to 8%), acne (adults 4% to 7%), localized flushing (following ethanol consumption; adults 3% to 7%), folliculitis (2% to 6%), urticaria (1% to 6%), rash (2% to 5%), pustular rash (2% to 4%), vesiculobullous rash (children 4%), contact dermatitis (3% to 4%), cyst (adults 1% to 3%), eczema herpeticum (1% to 2%), fungal dermatitis (adults 1% to 2%), sunburn (adults 1% to 2%), alopecia (adults 1%), dry skin (children 1%)

Endocrine & metabolic: Dysmenorrhea (adult females 4%)

Gastrointestinal: Diarrhea (3% to 5%), dyspepsia (adults 1% to 4%), abdominal pain (children 3%), vomiting (adults 1%), gastroenteritis (adults 2%), nausea (children 1%), tooth disorder (adults 1%)
Neuromuscular & skeletal: Paresthesia (adults 3%), myalgia (adults 2% to 3%), weakness (adults 2% to 3%), arthralgia (adults 1% to 3%), back pain (adults 2%)
Ocular: Conjunctivitis (2% adults)
Otic: Otitis media (12% children)
Respiratory: Rhinitis (6% children), sinusitis (2% to 4% adults), bronchitis (2% adults), pneumonia (1% adults)
Miscellaneous: Varicella/herpes zoster (1% to 5%), lymphadenopathy (3% children)

Dosage Topical: Atopic dermatitis (moderate-to-severe):
Treatment:
Children ≥2-15 years: Apply thin layer of 0.03% ointment to affected area twice daily; rub in gently and completely. Discontinue use when symptoms have cleared. If no improvement within 6 weeks, patients should be re-examined to confirm diagnosis.
Children >15 years and Adults: Apply thin layer of 0.03% or 0.1% ointment to affected area twice daily; rub in gently and completely. Discontinue use when symptoms have cleared. If no improvement within 6 weeks, patients should be re-examined to confirm diagnosis.
Maintenance therapy (Canadian labeling; not in U.S. labeling):
Children ≥2-15 years: Apply one application (thin layer of 0.03% ointment) to areas usually affected twice a week, allowing 2-3 days between applications (eg, one application on Monday and Thursday). Reevaluate after 12 months. Safety of maintenance therapy >12 months has not been established.
Children >15 years and Adults: Apply one application (thin layer of 0.03% or 0.1% ointment) to areas usually affected twice a week, allowing 2-3 days between applications (eg, one application on Monday and Thursday). Reevaluate after 12 months. Safety of maintenance therapy >12 months has not been established.
Note: Patients experiencing flares should resume twice daily treatment.

Mechanism of Action Suppresses cellular immunity (inhibits T-lymphocyte activation), by binding to an intracellular protein, FKBP-12 and complexes with calcineurin dependent proteins to inhibit calcineurin phosphatase activity

Contraindications Hypersensitivity to tacrolimus or any component of the formulation

Warnings/Precautions [U.S. Boxed Warning]: Topical calcineurin inhibitors have been associated with rare cases of malignancy (including skin and lymphoma); therefore, it should be limited to short-term and intermittent treatment using the minimum amount necessary for the control of symptoms and only on involved areas. Use in children <2 years of age is not recommended, children ages 2-15 should only use the 0.03% ointment. Avoid use on malignant or premalignant skin conditions (eg cutaneous T-cell lymphoma). Should not be used in immunocompromised patients. Do not apply to areas of active bacterial or viral infection; infections at the treatment site should be cleared prior to therapy. Topical calcineurin agents are considered second-line therapies in the treatment of atopic dermatitis/eczema, and should be limited to use in patients who have failed treatment with other therapies. Patients with atopic dermatitis are predisposed to skin infections, and tacrolimus therapy has been associated with risk of developing eczema herpeticum, varicella zoster, and herpes simplex. If atopic dermatitis is not improved in <6 weeks, re-evaluate to confirm diagnosis. May be associated with development of lymphadenopathy; possible infectious causes should be investigated. Discontinue use in patients with unknown cause of lymphadenopathy or acute infectious mononucleosis. Acute renal failure has been observed (rarely) with topical use. Not recommended for use in patients with skin disease which may increase systemic absorption (eg, Netherton's syndrome). Minimize sunlight exposure during treatment. Safety not established in patients with generalized erythroderma. Safety of intermittent use for >1 year has not been established, particularly since the effect on immune system development is unknown. Should not be used in immunocompromised patients; safety and efficacy have not been evaluated.

Drug Interactions

Metabolism/Transport Effects Substrate of CYP3A4 (major), P-glycoprotein; **Inhibits** CYP3A4 (weak), P-glycoprotein

Avoid Concomitant Use

Avoid concomitant use of Tacrolimus (Topical) with any of the following: Immunosuppressants

Increased Effect/Toxicity

Tacrolimus (Topical) may increase the levels/effects of: Alcohol (Ethyl); CycloSPORINE; CycloSPORINE (Systemic); Immunosuppressants; Sirolimus; Temsirolimus

The levels/effects of Tacrolimus (Topical) may be increased by: Antidepressants (Serotonin Reuptake Inhibitor/Antagonist); Antifungal Agents (Azole Derivatives, Systemic); Calcium Channel Blockers (Nondihydropyridine); Conivaptan; CycloSPORINE; CycloSPORINE (Systemic); Fluconazole; Grapefruit Juice; Macrolide Antibiotics; Protease Inhibitors; Sirolimus; Temsirolimus

Decreased Effect There are no known significant interactions involving a decrease in effect.

Ethanol/Nutrition/Herb Interactions Ethanol: Localized flushing (redness, warm sensation) may occur at application site of topical tacrolimus following ethanol consumption.

Pregnancy Risk Factor C

Lactation Enters breast milk/not recommended

Breast-Feeding Considerations Tacrolimus is excreted into breast milk following systemic administration. Refer to the Tacrolimus (Systemic) monograph for additional information.

Dosage Forms

Ointment, topical:

Protopic®: 0.03% (30 g, 60 g, 100 g); 0.1% (30 g, 60 g, 100 g)

Tadalafil (tah DA la fil)

U.S. Brand Names Adcirca®; Cialis®

Canadian Brand Names Adcirca®; Cialis®

Generic Availability (U.S.) No

Pharmacologic Category Phosphodiesterase-5 Enzyme Inhibitor

Use

Adcirca®: Treatment of pulmonary arterial hypertension (PAH) (WHO Group I) to improve exercise ability

Cialis®: Treatment of erectile dysfunction (ED)

Local Anesthetic/Vasoconstrictor Precautions No information available to require special precautions

Effects on Dental Treatment No significant effects or complications reported

Effects on Bleeding No information available to require special precautions

Adverse Effects Based upon usual doses for either indication. For erectile dysfunction, similar adverse events are reported with once-daily versus intermittent dosing, but are generally lower than with doses used intermittently.

>10%:

- Cardiovascular: Flushing (1% to 13%; dose related)
- Central nervous system: Headache (3% to 42%; dose related)
- Gastrointestinal: Dyspepsia (1% to 13%), nausea (10% to 11%)
- Neuromuscular & skeletal: Myalgia (1% to 14%; dose related), back pain (2% to 12%), extremity pain (1% to 11%)
- Respiratory: Respiratory tract infection (3% to 13%), nasopharyngitis (2% to 13%)

2% to 10%:

- Cardiovascular: Hypertension (1% to 3%)
- Gastrointestinal: Gastroenteritis (viral; 3% to 5%), GERD (1% to 3%), abdominal pain (1% to 2%), diarrhea (1% to 2%)
- Genitourinary: Urinary tract infection (≤2%)
- Respiratory: Nasal congestion (≤9%), cough (2% to 4%), bronchitis (≤2%)
- Miscellaneous: Flu-like syndrome (2% to 5%)

Dosage Oral: Adults:

Erectile dysfunction (Cialis®):

As-needed dosing: 10 mg at least 30 minutes prior to anticipated sexual activity (dosing range: 5-20 mg); to be given as one single dose and not given more than once daily. **Note:** Erectile function may be improved for up to 36 hours following a single dose; adjust dose.

Once-daily dosing: 2.5 mg once daily (dosing range: 2.5-5 mg/day) to be given at approximately the same time daily without regard to timing of sexual activity

Dosing adjustment with concomitant medications:

$Alpha_1$-blockers: If stabilized on either alpha-blockers or tadalafil therapy, initiate new therapy with the other agent at the lowest possible dose.

Protease inhibitors: Maximum tadalafil dose: 10 mg in a 72-hour period

Other CYP3A4 inhibitors: Dose reduction of tadalafil is recommended with strong CYP3A4 inhibitors. When used on an as-needed basis, the dose of tadalafil should not exceed 10 mg, and tadalafil should not be taken more frequently than once every 72 hours. When used on a once-daily basis, the dose of tadalafil should not exceed 2.5 mg. Examples of such inhibitors include clarithromycin, conivaptan, delavirdine, diclofenac, imatinib, isoniazid, itraconazole, ketoconazole, miconazole, nefazodone, nicardipine, propofol, quinidine, and telithromycin.

Pulmonary arterial hypertension (Adcirca®): 40 mg once daily
Dosing adjustment with concomitant medications:
Coadministration with protease inhibitor regimen:
Concurrent use with atazanavir/ritonavir, darunavir/ritonavir, fosamprenavir, ritonavir, saquinavir/ritonavir, tipranavir/ritonavir:
Coadministration of tadalafil in patients currently receiving one of these protease inhibitor regimens for at least 1 week: Initiate tadalafil at 20 mg once daily; increase to 40 mg once daily based on individual tolerability.
Coadministration of one of these protease inhibitor regimens in patients currently receiving tadalafil: Discontinue tadalafil at least 24 hours prior to the initiation of the protease inhibitor regimen. After at least 1 week of the protease inhibitor regimen, resume tadalafil at 20 mg once daily; increase to 40 mg once daily based on individual tolerability.
Concurrent use with indinavir or nelfinavir:
Patient receiving indinavir/nelfinavir when initiating tadalafil: Initiate tadalafil at 20 mg once daily; increase to 40 mg once daily based on individual tolerability
Patient receiving tadalafil when initiating indinavir/nelfinavir: Adjust tadalafil to 20 mg once daily; increase to 40 mg once daily based on individual tolerability
Other potent CYP3A4 inhibitors: Avoid concurrent use when tadalafil used for PAH. Examples of such inhibitors include clarithromycin, conivaptan, delavirdine, diclofenac, imatinib, isoniazid, itraconazole, ketoconazole, miconazole, nefazodone, nicardipine, propofol, quinidine, and telithromycin.
Potent CYP3A4 inducers (eg, rifampin): Avoid concurrent use when tadalafil used for PAH.

Elderly: No dose adjustment for patients >65 years of age in the absence of renal or hepatic impairment

Dosage adjustment in renal impairment:
Erectile dysfunction (Cialis®):
As-needed use:
Cl_{cr} ≥51 mL/minute: Dosage adjustment not required
Cl_{cr} 31-50 mL/minute: Initial: 5 mg once daily; maximum: 10 mg (not to be given more frequently than every 48 hours)
Cl_{cr} <30 mL/minute and on hemodialysis: Maximum: 5 mg (not to be given more frequently than every 72 hours)
Once-daily use:
Cl_{cr} ≥31 mL/minute: Dose adjustment not required
Cl_{cr} <30 mL/minute and on hemodialysis: Use not recommended
Pulmonary arterial hypertension (Adcirca®):
Cl_{cr} 31-80 mL/minute: Initial: 20 mg once daily; increase to 40 mg once daily based on individual tolerability
Cl_{cr} <30 mL/minute and on hemodialysis: Avoid use due to increased tadalafil exposure, limited clinical experience, and lack of ability to influence clearance by dialysis.
Dosage adjustment in hepatic impairment:
Erectile dysfunction (Cialis®):
As-needed use:
Mild-to-moderate hepatic impairment (Child-Pugh class A or B): Use with caution; dose should not exceed 10 mg once daily
Severe hepatic impairment (Child-Pugh class C): Use is not recommended
Once-daily use:
Mild-to-moderate hepatic impairment (Child-Pugh class A or B): Use with caution
Severe hepatic impairment (Child-Pugh class C): Use is not recommended
Pulmonary arterial hypertension (Adcirca®):
Mild-to-moderate hepatic impairment (Child-Pugh class A or B): Use with caution; consider initial dose of 20 mg once daily
Severe hepatic impairment (Child-Pugh class C): Avoid use; has not been studied in patients with severe hepatic cirrhosis.

Mechanism of Action

Erectile dysfunction: Does not directly cause penile erections, but affects the response to sexual stimulation. The physiologic mechanism of erection of the penis involves release of nitric oxide (NO) in the corpus cavernosum during sexual stimulation. NO then activates the enzyme guanylate cyclase, which results in increased levels of cyclic guanosine monophosphate (cGMP), producing smooth muscle relaxation and inflow of blood to the corpus cavernosum. Tadalafil enhances the effect of NO by inhibiting phosphodiesterase type 5 (PDE-5), which is responsible for degradation of cGMP in the corpus cavernosum; when sexual stimulation causes local release of NO, inhibition of PDE-5 by tadalafil causes increased levels of cGMP in the corpus cavernosum, resulting in smooth muscle relaxation and inflow of blood to the corpus cavernosum. At recommended doses, it has no effect in the absence of sexual stimulation.

PAH: Inhibits phosphodiesterase type 5 (PDE-5) in smooth muscle of pulmonary vasculature where PDE-5 is responsible for the degradation of cyclic guanosine monophosphate (cGMP). Increased cGMP concentration results in pulmonary vasculature relaxation; vasodilation in the pulmonary bed and the systemic circulation (to a lesser degree) may occur.

Contraindications Known serious hypersensitivity to tadalafil; concurrent use (regularly/intermittently) of organic nitrates in any form (eg, nitroglycerin, isosorbide dinitrate)

Warnings/Precautions There is a degree of cardiac risk associated with sexual activity; therefore, physicians should consider the cardiovascular status of their patients prior to initiation. Use for erectile dysfunction is not recommended in patients with hypotension (<90/50 mm Hg), uncontrolled hypertension (>170/100 mm Hg), NYHA class II-IV heart failure within the last 6 months, uncontrolled arrhythmias, stroke within the last 6 months, MI within the last 3 months, unstable angina or angina during sexual intercourse; safety and efficacy have not been evaluated in these patients. Safety and efficacy in PAH have not been evaluated in patients with clinically significant aortic and/or mitral valve disease, life-threatening arrhythmias, hypotension (<90/50 mm Hg), uncontrolled hypertension, significant left ventricular dysfunction, pericardial constriction, restrictive or congestive cardiomyopathy, symptomatic coronary artery disease. Use caution in patients with left ventricular outflow obstruction (eg, aortic stenosis, hypertrophic obstructive cardiomyopathy); may be more sensitive to vasodilator effects.

Patients experiencing anginal chest pain after tadalafil administration should seek immediate medical attention. Concomitant use (regularly/intermittently) with all forms of nitrates is contraindicated. When used for either erectile dysfunction or PAH and nitrate administration is medically necessary following use, at least 48 hours should elapse after the tadalafil dose and nitrate administration. When used for PAH, per the manufacturer, nitrate may be administered within 48 hours of tadalafil. For both situations, administration of nitrates should only be done under close medical supervision with hemodynamic monitoring.

Concurrent use with alpha-adrenergic antagonist therapy or substantial alcohol consumption may cause symptomatic hypotension; patients should be hemodynamically stable prior to initiating tadalafil therapy at the lowest possible dose. When used for erectile dysfunction, use caution in patients receiving strong CYP3A4 inhibitors. When used for PAH, avoid use in patients taking strong CYP3A4 inducers/inhibitors. Use in patients receiving or about to receive ritonavir requires dosage adjustment or interruption of therapy, respectively. Pulmonary vasodilators may exacerbate the cardiovascular status in patients with pulmonary veno-occlusive disease (PVOD); use is not recommended. In patients with unrecognized PVOD, signs of pulmonary edema should prompt investigation into this diagnosis. Use with caution in patients with mild-to-moderate hepatic impairment; dosage adjustment/limitation is needed. Use is not recommended in patients with severe hepatic impairment or cirrhosis. Use with caution in patients with renal impairment; dosage adjustment/limitation is needed. Safety and efficacy with other tadalafil brands or other PDE-5 inhibitors (ie, sildenafil and vardenafil) have not been established. Patients should be informed not to take with other tadalafil brands or other PDE-5 inhibitors. Use caution in patients with bleeding disorders or peptic ulcer disease due to effect on platelets (bleeding).

When used to treat erectile dysfunction, potential underlying causes of erectile dysfunction should be evaluated prior to treatment. Use with caution in patients with anatomical deformation of the penis (angulation, cavernosal fibrosis, or Peyronie's disease), or who have conditions which may predispose them to priapism (sickle cell anemia, multiple myeloma, leukemia). Instruct patients to seek immediate medical attention if erection persists >4 hours. Safety and efficacy with other tadalafil brands or other PDE-5 inhibitors (ie, sildenafil and vardenafil) have not been established. Patients should be informed not to take with other tadalafil brands or other PDE-5 inhibitors. The safety and efficacy of tadalafil with other treatments for erectile dysfunction have not been studied and are, therefore, not recommended as combination therapy.

Rare cases of nonarteritic anterior ischemic optic neuropathy (NAION) have been reported; risk may be increased with history of vision loss or NAION in one eye. Other risk factors for NAION include heart disease, diabetes, hypertension, smoking, age >50 years, or history of certain eye problems. Sudden decrease or loss of hearing has been reported rarely; hearing changes may be accompanied by tinnitus and dizziness. A direct relationship between therapy and vision or hearing loss has not been determined. Instruct patients to seek medical assistance for sudden loss of vision in one or both eyes, sudden decrease in hearing, or sudden loss of hearing.

Patients with genetic retinal disorders (eg, retinitis pigmentosa) were not evaluated in clinical trials; use is not recommended. Use with caution in the elderly.

Drug Interactions

Metabolism/Transport Effects **Substrate** of CYP3A4 (major)

Avoid Concomitant Use

Avoid concomitant use of Tadalafil with any of the following: Amyl Nitrite; Phosphodiesterase 5 Inhibitors; Vasodilators (Organic Nitrates)

Increased Effect/Toxicity

Tadalafil may increase the levels/effects of: Alpha1-Blockers; Amyl Nitrite; Antihypertensives; Bosentan; Phosphodiesterase 5 Inhibitors; Vasodilators (Organic Nitrates)

The levels/effects of Tadalafil may be increased by: Antifungal Agents (Azole Derivatives, Systemic); CYP3A4 Inhibitors (Moderate); CYP3A4 Inhibitors (Strong); Dasatinib; Macrolide Antibiotics; Ritonavir; Sapropterin

Decreased Effect

The levels/effects of Tadalafil may be decreased by: Bosentan; CYP3A4 Inducers (Strong); Etravirine; Tocilizumab

Ethanol/Nutrition/Herb Interactions

Ethanol: Substantial consumption of ethanol may increase the risk of hypotension and orthostasis. Lower ethanol consumption has not been associated with significant changes in blood pressure or increase in orthostatic symptoms.

Food: Rate and extent of absorption are not affected by food. Grapefruit juice may increase serum levels/toxicity of tadalafil. Use tadalafil with caution in patients who regularly consume grapefruit juice. In general, use of grapefruit juice should be limited or avoided; the manufacturer does not give specific recommendations.

Herb/Nutraceutical: St John's wort: Use caution with concomitant use.

Dietary Considerations May be taken with or without food.

Pharmacodynamics/Kinetics

Onset of Action Within 1 hour

Peak effect: Pulmonary artery vasodilation: 75-90 minutes (Ghofrani, 2004)

Duration of Action Erectile dysfunction: Up to 36 hours

Half-life Elimination 15-17.5 hours; Pulmonary hypertension (not receiving bosentan): 35 hours

Time to Peak Plasma: ~2-4 hours (range: 30 minutes to 8 hours)

Pregnancy Risk Factor B

Lactation Excretion in breast milk unknown/use caution

Dosage Forms

Tablet, oral:

Adcirca®: 20 mg

Cialis®: 2.5 mg, 5 mg, 10 mg, 20 mg

Tamoxifen (ta MOKS i fen)

Canadian Brand Names Apo-Tamox®; Mylan-Tamoxifen; Nolvadex®-D; Novo-Tamoxifen; PMS-Tamoxifen; Tamofen®

Generic Availability (U.S.) Yes

Pharmacologic Category Antineoplastic Agent, Estrogen Receptor Antagonist; Selective Estrogen Receptor Modulator (SERM)

Use Treatment of metastatic (female and male) breast cancer; adjuvant treatment of breast cancer after primary treatment with surgery and radiation; reduce risk of invasive breast cancer in women with ductal carcinoma *in situ* (DCIS) after surgery and radiation; reduce the incidence of breast cancer in women at high risk

Unlabeled/Investigational Use Treatment of mastalgia, gynecomastia, ovarian cancer, endometrial cancer, uterine sarcoma, and desmoid tumors; risk reduction in women with Paget's disease of the breast (with DCIS or without associated cancer); induction of ovulation; treatment of precocious puberty in females, secondary to McCune-Albright syndrome

Local Anesthetic/Vasoconstrictor Precautions No information available to require special precautions

Effects on Dental Treatment No significant effects or complications reported

Effects on Bleeding Although significant myelosuppression with associated altered hemostasis has been reported for many chemotherapeutic agents, myelosuppression is not common with tamoxifen and no specific precautions appear to necessary.

Adverse Effects

>10%:

Cardiovascular: Vasodilation (41%), flushing (33%), hypertension (11%), peripheral edema (11%)

Central nervous system: Mood changes (12% to 18%), pain (3% to 16%), depression (2% to 12%)

Dermatologic: Skin changes (6% to 19%), rash (13%)

Endocrine & metabolic: Hot flashes (3% to 80%), fluid retention (32%), altered menses (13% to 25%), amenorrhea (16%)
Gastrointestinal: Nausea (5% to 26%), weight loss (23%), vomiting (12%)
Genitourinary: Vaginal discharge (13% to 55%), vaginal bleeding (2% to 23%)
Neuromuscular & skeletal: Weakness (18%), arthritis (14%), arthralgia (11%)
Respiratory: Pharyngitis (14%)
Miscellaneous: Lymphedema (11%)

1% to 10%:
Cardiovascular: Chest pain (5%), venous thrombotic events (5%), edema (4%), cardiovascular ischemia (3%), angina (2%), deep venous thrombus (≤2%), MI (1%)
Central nervous system: Insomnia (9%), dizziness (8%), headache (8%), anxiety (6%), fatigue (4%)
Dermatologic: Alopecia (≤5%)
Endocrine & metabolic: Oligomenorrhea (9%), breast pain (6%), menstrual disorder (6%), breast neoplasm (5%), hypercholesterolemia (4%)
Gastrointestinal: Abdominal pain (9%), weight gain (9%), constipation (4% to 8%), diarrhea (7%), dyspepsia (6%), throat irritation (oral solution 5%), abdominal cramps (1%), anorexia (1%)
Genitourinary: Urinary tract infection (10%), leukorrhea (9%), vaginal hemorrhage (6%), vaginitis (5%), vulvovaginitis (5%), ovarian cyst (3%)
Hematologic: Thrombocytopenia (≤10%), anemia (5%)
Hepatic: AST increased (5%), serum bilirubin increased (2%)
Neuromuscular & skeletal: Back pain (10%), bone pain (6% to 10%), osteoporosis (7%), fracture (7%), arthrosis (5%), joint disorder (5%), myalgia (5%), paresthesia (5%), musculoskeletal pain (3%)
Ocular: Cataract (7%)
Renal: Serum creatinine increased (≤2%)
Respiratory: Cough (4% to 9%), dyspnea (8%), bronchitis (5%), sinusitis (5%)
Miscellaneous: Infection/sepsis (≤9%), diaphoresis (6%), flu-like syndrome (6%), cyst (5%), neoplasm (5%), allergic reaction (3%)

Dosage Oral: **Note:** For the treatment of breast cancer, patients receiving both tamoxifen and chemotherapy, should receive treatment sequentially, with tamoxifen following completion of chemotherapy.

Children: Females: Precocious puberty and McCune-Albright syndrome (unlabeled use): A dose of 20 mg/day has been reported in patients 2-10 years of age; safety and efficacy have not been established for treatment of longer than 1 year duration (Eugster, 2003)

Adults:
Breast cancer treatment:
Adjuvant therapy (females): 20 mg once daily for 5 years
Metastatic (males and females): 20-40 mg/day (doses >20 mg should be given in 2 divided doses). **Note:** Although the FDA-approved labeling recommends dosing up to 40 mg/day, clinical benefit has not been demonstrated with doses above 20 mg/day (Bratherton, 1984).
Premenopausal women: Duration of treatment is 5 years (NCCN Breast Cancer guidelines v.1.2011)
Postmenopausal women: Duration of tamoxifen treatment is 2-3 years followed by an aromatase inhibitor (AI) to complete 5 years; if contraindications or intolerant to AI, may take tamoxifen for the full 5 years **or** extended therapy: 4.5-6 years of tamoxifen followed by 5 years of an AI (NCCN Breast Cancer guidelines v.1.2011)
DCIS (females), to reduce the risk for invasive breast cancer: 20 mg once daily for 5 years
Breast cancer risk reduction (pre- and postmenopausal high-risk females): 20 mg once daily for 5 years
Induction of ovulation (unlabeled use): 20 mg once daily (range: 20-80 mg once daily) for 5 days (Steiner, 2005)
Paget's disease of the breast (risk reduction; with DCIS or without associated cancer): 20 mg once daily for 5 years (NCCN Breast Cancer Guidelines, v.1.2011)
Dosage adjustment for DVT, pulmonary embolism, cerebrovascular accident, or prolonged immobilization: Discontinue tamoxifen (NCCN Breast Cancer Risk Reduction Guidelines, v.2.2010)

Mechanism of Action Competitively binds to estrogen receptors on tumors and other tissue targets, producing a nuclear complex that decreases DNA synthesis and inhibits estrogen effects; nonsteroidal agent with potent antiestrogenic properties which compete with estrogen for binding sites in breast and other tissues; cells accumulate in the G_0 and G_1 phases; therefore, tamoxifen is cytostatic rather than cytocidal.

Contraindications Hypersensitivity to tamoxifen or any component of the formulation; concurrent warfarin therapy or history of deep vein thrombosis or pulmonary embolism (when tamoxifen is used for cancer risk reduction in women at high-risk for breast cancer and in women with DCIS)

Warnings/Precautions Hazardous agent - use appropriate precautions for handling and disposal. **[U.S. Boxed Warning]: Serious and life-threatening events (including stroke, pulmonary emboli, and uterine malignancy) have occurred at an incidence greater than placebo during use for breast cancer risk reduction in women at high-risk for breast cancer and in women with DCIS;** these events are rare, but require consideration in risk:benefit evaluation. An increased incidence of thromboembolic events, including DVT and pulmonary embolism, has been associated with use for breast cancer; risk is increased with concomitant chemotherapy; use with caution in individuals with a history of thromboembolic events. Thrombocytopenia and/or leukopenia may occur; neutropenia and pancytopenia have been reported rarely. Although the relationship to tamoxifen therapy is uncertain, rare hemorrhagic episodes have occurred in patients with significant thrombocytopenia. Use with caution in patients with hyperlipidemias; infrequent postmarketing cases of hyperlipidemias have been reported. Decreased visual acuity, retinal vein thrombosis, retinopathy, corneal changes, color perception changes, and increased incidence of cataracts (and the need for cataract surgery), have been reported. Hypercalcemia has occurred in patients with bone metastasis, usually within a few weeks of therapy initiation; institute appropriate hypercalcemia management; discontinue if severe. Local disease flare and increased bone and tumor pain may occur in patients with metastatic breast cancer; may be associated with (good) tumor response.

Tamoxifen is associated with a high potential for drug interactions, including CYP- and Pgp-mediated interactions. Decreased efficacy and an increased risk of breast cancer recurrence has been reported with concurrent moderate or strong CYP2D6 inhibitors (Aubert, 2009; Dezentje, 2009). Concomitant use with select SSRIs may result in decreased tamoxifen efficacy. Strong CYP2D6 inhibitors (eg, fluoxetine, paroxetine) and moderate CYP2D6 inhibitors (eg, sertraline) are reported to interfere with transformation to the active metabolite endoxifen. Weak CYP2D6 inhibitors (eg, venlafaxine, citalopram) have minimal effect on the conversion to endoxifen (Jin, 2005; NCCN Breast Cancer Risk Reduction Guidelines v.2.2010); escitalopram is also a weak CYP2D6 inhibitor. Lower plasma concentrations of endoxifen (active metabolite) have been observed in patients associated with reduced CYP2D6 activity (Jin, 2005) and may be associated with reduced efficacy. In a retrospective analysis of breast cancer patients taking tamoxifen and SSRIs, concomitant use of paroxetine and tamoxifen was associated with an increased risk of death due to breast cancer (Kelly, 2010).

Tamoxifen use may be associated with changes in bone mineral density (BMD) and the effects may be dependent upon menstrual status. In postmenopausal women, tamoxifen use is associated with a protective effect on bone mineral density (BMD), preventing loss of BMD which lasts over the 5-year treatment period. In premenopausal women, a decline (from baseline) in BMD mineral density has been observed in women who continued to menstruate; may be associated with an increased risk of fractures. Liver abnormalities such as cholestasis, fatty liver, hepatitis, and hepatic necrosis have occurred. Hepatocellular carcinomas have been reported in some studies; relationship to treatment is unclear. Tamoxifen is associated with an increased incidence of uterine or endometrial cancers. Endometrial hyperplasia, polyps, endometriosis, uterine fibroids, and ovarian cysts have occurred. Monitor and promptly evaluate any report of abnormal vaginal bleeding. Amenorrhea and menstrual irregularities have been reported with tamoxifen use.

Drug Interactions

Metabolism/Transport Effects Substrate of CYP2A6 (minor), 2B6 (minor), 2C9 (major), 2D6 (major), 2E1 (minor), 3A4 (major); **Inhibits** CYP2B6 (weak), 2C8 (moderate), 2C9 (weak), 3A4 (weak), p-glycoprotein

Avoid Concomitant Use

Avoid concomitant use of Tamoxifen with any of the following: CYP2D6 Inhibitors (Strong); Silodosin; Topotecan; Vitamin K Antagonists

Increased Effect/Toxicity

Tamoxifen may increase the levels/effects of: Colchicine; CYP2C8 Substrates (High risk); Dabigatran Etexilate; Everolimus; P-Glycoprotein Substrates; Rivaroxaban; Silodosin; Topotecan; Vitamin K Antagonists

The levels/effects of Tamoxifen may be increased by: Abiraterone; Conivaptan; CYP2C9 Inhibitors (Moderate); CYP2C9 Inhibitors (Strong); CYP2D6 Inhibitors (Moderate); CYP2D6 Inhibitors (Strong); CYP3A4 Inhibitors (Moderate); CYP3A4 Inhibitors (Strong); Darunavir; Dasatinib

Decreased Effect

Tamoxifen may decrease the levels/effects of: Anastrozole; Letrozole

The levels/effects of Tamoxifen may be decreased by: Aminoglutethimide; CYP2C9 Inducers (Highly Effective); CYP3A4 Inducers (Strong); Deferasirox; Herbs (CYP3A4 Inducers); Peginterferon Alfa-2b; Rifamycin Derivatives; Tocilizumab

Ethanol/Nutrition/Herb Interactions

Food: Avoid grapefruit juice (may decrease the metabolism of tamoxifen).

Herb/Nutraceutical: Avoid black cohosh, dong quai in estrogen-dependent tumors. Avoid St John's wort (may decrease levels/effects of tamoxifen).

Dietary Considerations May be taken with or without food. Avoid grapefruit and grapefruit juice.

Pharmacodynamics/Kinetics

Half-life Elimination Tamoxifen: ~5-7 days; N-desmethyl tamoxifen: ~14 days

Time to Peak Serum: ~5 hours

Pregnancy Risk Factor D

Lactation Excretion in breast milk unknown/not recommended

Breast-Feeding Considerations It is not known if tamoxifen is excreted in breast milk, however, it has been shown to inhibit lactation. Due to the potential for adverse reactions, women taking tamoxifen should not breast-feed.

Dosage Forms

Tablet, oral: 10 mg, 20 mg

Tamsulosin (tam SOO loe sin)

U.S. Brand Names Flomax®

Canadian Brand Names Flomax® CR; JAMP-Tamsulosin; Mylan-Tamsulosin; Novo-Tamsulosin; RAN™-Tamsulosin; ratio-Tamsulosin; Sandoz-Tamsulosin; Sandoz-Tamsulosin CR

Generic Availability (U.S.) Yes

Pharmacologic Category $Alpha_1$ Blocker

Use Treatment of signs and symptoms of benign prostatic hyperplasia (BPH)

Unlabeled/Investigational Use Symptomatic treatment of bladder outlet obstruction or dysfunction

Local Anesthetic/Vasoconstrictor Precautions No information available to require special precautions

Effects on Dental Treatment Key adverse event(s) related to dental treatment: Orthostatic hypotension and tooth disorder.

Effects on Bleeding No information available to require special precautions

Adverse Effects

>10%:

Cardiovascular: Orthostatic hypotension (6 % to 19%)

Central nervous system: Headache (19% to 21%), dizziness (15% to 17%)

Genitourinary: Abnormal ejaculation (8% to 18%)

Respiratory: Rhinitis (13% to 18%)

Miscellaneous: Infection (9% to 11%)

1% to 10%:

Cardiovascular: Chest pain (4%)

Central nervous system: Somnolence (3% to 4%), insomnia (1% to 2%), vertigo (≤1%)

Endocrine & metabolic: Libido decreased (1% to 2%)

Gastrointestinal: Diarrhea (4% to 6%), nausea (3% to 4%), gum pain, toothache

Neuromuscular & skeletal: Weakness (8% to 9%), back pain (7% to 8%)

Ocular: Blurred vision (≤2%)

Respiratory: Pharyngitis (5% to 6%), cough (3% to 5%), sinusitis (2% to 4%)

Dosage Oral: Adults:

BPH: 0.4 mg once daily ~30 minutes after the same meal each day; dose may be increased after 2-4 weeks to 0.8 mg once daily in patients who fail to respond. If therapy is interrupted for several days, restart with 0.4 mg once daily.

Bladder outlet obstruction (unlabeled use): 0.4 mg once daily ~30 minutes after the same meal each day

Dosage adjustment in renal impairment:

Cl_{cr} ≥10 mL/minute: No adjustment needed

Cl_{cr} <10 mL/minute: Not studied

Dosage adjustment in hepatic impairment:

Mild-to-moderate impairment: No adjustment needed

Severe impairment: Not studied

Mechanism of Action Tamsulosin is an antagonist of $alpha_{1A}$-adrenoreceptors in the prostate. Smooth muscle tone in the prostate is mediated by $alpha_{1A}$-adrenoreceptors; blocking them leads to relaxation of smooth muscle in the bladder neck and prostate causing an improvement of urine flow and decreased symptoms of BPH. Approximately 75% of the $alpha_1$-receptors in the prostate are of the $alpha_{1A}$ subtype.

Contraindications Hypersensitivity to tamsulosin or any component of the formulation

Warnings/Precautions Not intended for use as an antihypertensive drug. May cause significant orthostatic hypotension and syncope, especially with first dose; anticipate a similar effect if therapy is interrupted for a few days, if dosage is rapidly increased, or if another antihypertensive drug (particularly vasodilators) or a PDE-5 inhibitor (eg, sildenafil, tadalafil, vardenafil) is introduced. "First-dose" orthostatic hypotension may occur 4-8 hours after dosing; may be dose related. Patients should be cautioned about performing hazardous tasks when starting new therapy or adjusting dosage upward. Discontinue if symptoms of angina occur or worsen. Rule out prostatic carcinoma before beginning therapy with tamsulosin. Intraoperative floppy iris syndrome has been observed in cataract surgery patients who were on or were previously treated with $alpha_1$-blockers; causality has not been established and there appears to be no benefit in discontinuing alpha-blocker therapy prior to surgery; instruct patients to inform ophthalmologist of tamsulosin use when considering eye surgery. Priapism has been associated with use (rarely). Rarely, patients with a sulfa allergy have also developed an allergic reaction to tamsulosin; avoid use when previous reaction has been severe. Not indicated for use in women.

Drug Interactions

Metabolism/Transport Effects Substrate (major) of CYP2D6, 3A4

Avoid Concomitant Use

Avoid concomitant use of Tamsulosin with any of the following: Alpha1-Blockers; CYP3A4 Inhibitors (Strong)

Increased Effect/Toxicity

Tamsulosin may increase the levels/effects of: Alpha1-Blockers; Calcium Channel Blockers

The levels/effects of Tamsulosin may be increased by: Abiraterone; Beta-Blockers; CYP2D6 Inhibitors (Moderate); CYP2D6 Inhibitors (Strong); CYP3A4 Inhibitors (Moderate); CYP3A4 Inhibitors (Strong); Dasatinib; MAO Inhibitors; Phosphodiesterase 5 Inhibitors

Decreased Effect

The levels/effects of Tamsulosin may be decreased by: CYP3A4 Inducers (Strong); Deferasirox; Herbs (CYP3A4 Inducers); Peginterferon Alfa-2b; Tocilizumab

Ethanol/Nutrition/Herb Interactions

Food: Fasting increases bioavailability by 30% and peak concentration 40% to 70%.

Herb/Nutraceutical: St John's wort: May decrease the levels/effects of tamsulosin. Avoid herbs with hypotensive properties (black cohosh, California poppy, coleus, golden seal, hawthorn, mistletoe, periwinkle, quinine, Shepherd's purse); may enhance the hypotensive effect of tamsulosin. Avoid saw palmetto (due to limited experience with this combination).

Dietary Considerations Take once daily, 30 minutes after the same meal each day.

Pharmacodynamics/Kinetics

Half-life Elimination Healthy volunteers: 9-13 hours; Target population: 14-15 hours

Time to Peak Fasting: 4-5 hours; With food: 6-7 hours

Steady-state: By the fifth day of once daily dosing

Pregnancy Risk Factor B

Dosage Forms

Capsule, oral: 0.4 mg

Flomax®: 0.4 mg

Tablet, oral: 0.4 mg

Tapentadol (ta PEN ta dol)

Related Information

Oral Pain *on page 1928*

U.S. Brand Names Nucynta®

Canadian Brand Names Nucynta™ CR

Generic Availability (U.S.) No

Pharmacologic Category Analgesic, Opioid

Dental Use Management of moderate-to-severe acute pain

Use Relief of moderate-to-severe acute pain

Local Anesthetic/Vasoconstrictor Precautions Although part of the mechanism of tapentadol inhibits the reuptake of norepinephrine, there is no information available to require any special precautions.

Effects on Dental Treatment Key adverse effect(s) related to dental treatment: Xerostomia (normal salivary flow resumes upon discontinuation)

Effects on Bleeding No information available to require special precautions

Adverse Effects

>10%:

Central nervous system: Dizziness (24%), somnolence (15%)

Gastrointestinal: Nausea (30%), vomiting (18%)

1% to 10%:

Central nervous system: Fatigue (3%), insomnia (2%), anxiety (1%), confusion (1%), dreams abnormal (1%), lethargy (1%)

Dermatologic: Pruritus (3% to 5%), hyperhidrosis (3%), rash (1%)

Endocrine & metabolic: Hot flushes (1%)

Gastrointestinal: Constipation (8%), xerostomia (4%), appetite decreased (2%), dyspepsia (2%)

Genitourinary: Urinary tract infection (1%)

Neuromuscular & skeletal: Arthralgia (1%), tremor (1%)

Respiratory: Nasopharyngitis (1%), upper respiratory tract infection (1%)

Dental Usual Dosage Adults: 50-100 mg every 4-6 hours as need for acute pain

Dosage Oral: **Note:** Dose and dosage intervals should be individualized according to pain severity with respect to patient's previous experience with similar opioid analgesics. Dosage form availability differs between the U.S. (immediate release formulation) and Canada (controlled release formulation).

Adults: Acute moderate-severe pain:

U.S. labeling (immediate release formulation): Day 1: 50-100 mg every 4-6 hours as needed; may administer a second dose ≥1 hour after the initial dose (maximum dose on first day: 700 mg/day); Day 2 and subsequent dosing: 50-100 mg every 4-6 hours as needed (maximum: 600 mg/day)

Canadian labeling (controlled release formulation):

Opioid naive: Initial: 50 mg twice daily (recommended interval: ~12 hours); titrate to effective dose (therapeutic range: 100-250 mg twice daily)

Opioid experienced (**Note:** Decrease initial dose by 50% when switching from other opioid analgesics): Titrate in increments of 50 mg twice daily every 3 days to recommended dosing range of 100-250 mg twice daily (maximum dose should not exceed 500 mg/day)

Elderly: Initial: Consider initiating at lower range of dosing. Refer to adult dosing.

Dosage adjustment in renal impairment:

Mild-moderate renal impairment: No adjustment necessary

Severe renal impairment: Not recommended (not studied); use is contraindicated in the Canadian labeling

Dosage adjustment in hepatic impairment:

Mild hepatic impairment: No adjustment necessary

Moderate hepatic impairment:

U.S. labeling (immediate release formulation): Initial: 50 mg every 8 hours or longer (maximum: 3 doses/24 hours). Further treatment for maintenance of analgesia may be achieved by either shortening or lengthening the dosing interval.

Canadian labeling (controlled release formulation): Initial: 50 mg once daily; titrate dose cautiously; manufacturer labeling does not provide specific recommendations.

Severe hepatic impairment: Not recommended (not studied); use is contraindicated in the Canadian labeling

Mechanism of Action Binds to μ-opiate receptors in the CNS causing inhibition of ascending pain pathways, altering the perception of and response to pain; also inhibits the reuptake of norepinephrine, which also modifies the ascending pain pathway

Contraindications Impaired pulmonary function (severe respiratory depression, acute or severe asthma or hypercapnia) in unmonitored settings or in absence of resuscitative equipment or ventilatory support; paralytic ileus; use of MAO inhibitors within 14 days

Canadian labeling: Additional contraindications (not in U.S. labeling): Hypersensitivity to tapentadol, opioids, or any component of the formulation or container; any disease/condition that affects bowel transit (eg, ileus of any type, strictures); severe renal impairment (Cl_{cr} <30 mL/minute); severe hepatic impairment (Child-Pugh class C); mild, intermittent, or short-duration pain that can be managed with alternative pain medication; management of perioperative pain; acute alcoholism, delirium tremens, and seizure disorders; severe CNS depression, increased cerebrospinal or intracranial pressure or head injury; pregnancy; breast-feeding; use during labor/delivery

Warnings/Precautions Use with caution in patients with respiratory disease or respiratory compromise (eg, asthma, chronic obstructive pulmonary disease [COPD], cor pulmonale, sleep apnea, severe obesity, kyphoscoliosis, hypoxia, hypercapnia); critical respiratory depression may occur, even at therapeutic dosages. May cause CNS depression, which may impair physical or mental abilities; patients must be cautioned about performing tasks which require mental alertness (eg, operating machinery or driving). Use with caution in patients with CNS depression or coma. Effects may be potentiated when used with other sedative drugs or ethanol.

Serotonin syndrome (SS) may occur with serotonin/norepinephrine reuptake inhibitors (SNRIs), including tapentadol. Signs of SS may include agitation, tachycardia, hyperthermia, nausea, and vomiting. Avoid use with serotonergic agents such as TCAs, triptans, venlafaxine, trazodone, lithium, sibutramine, meperidine, dextromethorphan, St John's wort, SNRIs, and SSRIs; concomitant use has been associated with the development of serotonin syndrome. Contraindicated with MAO inhibitor use within 14 days.

Use caution in patients with biliary tract dysfunction or acute pancreatitis; opioids may cause spasm of the sphincter of Oddi. Opioid use may obscure diagnosis or clinical course of patients with acute abdominal conditions. Use with extreme caution in patients with head injury, intracranial lesions, or elevated intracranial pressure (ICP); exaggerated elevation of ICP may occur. Serum concentrations are increased in hepatic impairment; use with caution in patients with moderate hepatic impairment (dosage adjustment required). Not recommended for use in severe hepatic impairment (not studied). Use with caution in patients with mild-to-moderate renal impairment (no dosage adjustment recommended). Not recommended for use in severe renal impairment (not studied). Use caution in patients with a history of seizures or conditions predisposing patients to seizures; patients with a history of seizures were excluded in clinical trials of tapentadol. Tramadol, an analgesic with similar pharmacologic properties to tapentadol, has been associated with seizures, particularly in patients with predisposing factors.

Approved for acute pain (not approved for chronic use); prolonged use increases risk of abuse, addiction, and withdrawal symptoms. An opioid-containing regimen should be tailored to each patient's needs with respect to degree of tolerance for opioids (naïve versus chronic user), age, weight, and medical condition. Healthcare provider should be alert to problems of abuse, misuse, and diversion. Abrupt discontinuation may lead to withdrawal symptoms. Symptoms may be decreased by tapering prior to discontinuation. Use opioids with caution in elderly; consider decreasing initial dose. Use caution in debilitated patients; there is a greater potential for critical respiratory depression, even at therapeutic dosages.

During dosage adjustments, the Canadian labeling recommends that immediate release tramadol may be used as rescue medication (maximum dose: 400 mg/day) and that fentanyl should not be used as rescue medication. Controlled-release tablets (Canadian availability; not available in U.S.) must be swallowed whole and should **not** be crushed, broken, chewed, or dissolved.

Drug Interactions

Avoid Concomitant Use

Avoid concomitant use of Tapentadol with any of the following: MAO Inhibitors; Sibutramine

Increased Effect/Toxicity

Tapentadol may increase the levels/effects of: Alcohol (Ethyl); Alvimopan; CNS Depressants; Desmopressin; MAO Inhibitors; Selective Serotonin Reuptake Inhibitors; Serotonin Modulators; Thiazide Diuretics

The levels/effects of Tapentadol may be increased by: Amphetamines; Antipsychotic Agents (Phenothiazines); Droperidol; Sibutramine; Succinylcholine

Decreased Effect

Tapentadol may decrease the levels/effects of: Pegvisomant

The levels/effects of Tapentadol may be decreased by: Ammonium Chloride; Mixed Agonist / Antagonist Opioids; Peginterferon Alfa-2b

Ethanol/Nutrition/Herb Interactions

Ethanol: May increase CNS depression; monitor for increased effects with coadministration. Caution patients about effects.

Food: When administered after a high fat/calorie meal, the AUC and C_{max} increased by 25% and 16%, respectively; may administer without regard to meals.

Herb/Nutraceutical: Avoid St John's wort (may increase CNS depression and risk of serotonin syndrome).

Dietary Considerations May be taken without regard to meals.

Pharmacodynamics/Kinetics

Half-life Elimination Immediate release: ~4 hours; Controlled release: ~4-8 hours

Time to Peak Plasma: Immediate release: 1.25 hours; Controlled release: 3-6 hours

Pregnancy Risk Factor C

Lactation Excretion in breast milk unknown/not recommended

Breast-Feeding Considerations Limited information available on the excretion of tapentadol in human milk; however, data suggests it may be excreted in human milk. The possibility of sedation or respiratory depression in the nursing infant should be considered.

Controlled Substance C-II

Dosage Forms

Tablet, oral:

Nucynta®: 50 mg, 75 mg, 100 mg

Dosage Forms: Canada

Tablet, controlled release, oral:

Nucynta™ CR: 50 mg, 100 mg, 150 mg, 200 mg, 250 mg

Dental Comment Tapentadol is classified as a narcotic analgesic having a unique ability to bind to μ-opiate receptors and to also inhibit the reuptake of norepinephrine. It shares many properties of the traditional narcotic drugs including addiction liability. A report by Kleinert et al, showed that single doses of tapentadol ≥75 mg effectively reduced moderate-to-severe postoperative dental pain in a dose related fashion and were well tolerated compared to 60 mg morphine. The study showed that tapentadol was a highly effective, centrally acting analgesic with a favorable side effect profile with rapid onset of action.

References

Kleinert R, Lange C, Steup A, et al, "Single Dose Analgesic Efficacy of Tapentadol in Postsurgical Dental Pain: The Results of a Randomized, Double-Blind, Placebo-Controlled Study," *Anesth Analg*, 2008, 107 (6):2048-55.

Tazarotene (taz AR oh teen)

U.S. Brand Names Avage®; Tazorac®

Canadian Brand Names Tazorac®

Pharmacologic Category Acne Products; Keratolytic Agent; Topical Skin Product, Acne

Use Topical treatment of facial acne vulgaris; topical treatment of stable plaque psoriasis; mitigation (palliation) of facial skin wrinkling, facial mottled hyper-/hypo-pigmentation, and benign facial lentigines

Local Anesthetic/Vasoconstrictor Precautions No information available to require special precautions

Effects on Dental Treatment No significant effects or complications reported

Effects on Bleeding No information available to require special precautions

Adverse Effects Percentage of incidence varies with formulation and/or strength:

>10%: Dermatologic: Burning/stinging, desquamation, dry skin, erythema, irritation, pruritus, skin pain, worsening of psoriasis

1% to 10%:

Cardiovascular: Peripheral edema

Dermatologic: Cheilitis, contact dermatitis, discoloration, eczema, fissuring, inflammation, localized bleeding, rash

Endocrine & metabolic: Hypertriglyceridemia

Frequency not defined: Dermatologic: Photosensitization

General Dosage Range Topical: *Children ≥12 years and Adults:* Apply a pea-sized amount or thin film **or** 2 mg/cm^2 once daily

Mechanism of Action Synthetic, acetylenic retinoid which modulates differentiation and proliferation of epithelial tissue and exerts some degree of anti-inflammatory and immunological activity

Pharmacodynamics/Kinetics

Duration of Action Therapeutic: Psoriasis: Effects have been observed for up to 3 months after a 3-month course of topical treatment

Half-life Elimination 18 hours

Pregnancy Risk Factor X

Tegaserod (teg a SER od)

U.S. Brand Names Zelnorm®

Canadian Brand Names Zelnorm® [DSC]

Pharmacologic Category Serotonin 5-HT$_4$ Receptor Agonist

Use Emergency treatment of irritable bowel syndrome with constipation (IBS-C) and chronic idiopathic constipation (CIC) in women (<55 years of age) in which no alternative therapy exists

Local Anesthetic/Vasoconstrictor Precautions No information available to require special precautions

Effects on Dental Treatment No significant effects or complications reported

Effects on Bleeding No information available to require special precautions

Adverse Effects

>10%:

Central nervous system: Headache (15%)

Gastrointestinal: Abdominal pain (12%)

1% to 10%:

Central nervous system: Dizziness (4%), migraine (2%)

Gastrointestinal: Diarrhea (9%; severe <1%), nausea (8%), flatulence (6%)

Neuromuscular & skeletal: Back pain (5%), arthropathy (2%), leg pain (1%)

General Dosage Range Oral: *Adults (females <55 years of age):* 6 mg twice daily

Mechanism of Action Tegaserod is a partial neuronal 5-HT_4 receptor agonist. Its action at the receptor site leads to stimulation of the peristaltic reflex and intestinal secretion, and moderation of visceral sensitivity.

Pharmacodynamics/Kinetics

Half-life Elimination I.V.: 11 ± 5 hours

Time to Peak 1 hour

Pregnancy Risk Factor B

Prescribing and Access Restrictions Available in U.S. under an emergency investigational new drug (IND) process. Emergency situations are defined as immediately life-threatening or requiring hospitalization. Physicians with patients who may qualify can contact the FDA's Division of Drug Information via email (druginfo@fda.hhs.gov). The FDA may either deny the request or authorize shipment of Zelnorm® by Novartis. Additional information can be found at http://www.-fda.gov/Drugs/DrugSafety/PostmarketDrugSafetyInformationforPatientsandProviders/ucm103223.htm.

Telavancin (tel a VAN sin)

Related Information

Clinical Risk Related to Drugs Prolonging QT Interval *on page 1872*

U.S. Brand Names Vibativ™

Pharmacologic Category Glycopeptide

Use Treatment of complicated skin and skin structure infections caused by susceptible gram-positive organisms including methicillin-susceptible or -resistant *Staphylococcus aureus*, vancomycin-susceptible *Enterococcus faecalis*, and *Streptococcus pyogenes*, *Streptococcus agalactiae*, or *Streptococcus anginosus* group

Local Anesthetic/Vasoconstrictor Precautions Telavancin is one of the drugs confirmed to prolong the QT interval and is accepted as having a risk of causing torsade de pointes. The risk of drug-induced torsade de pointes is extremely low when a single QT interval prolonging drug is prescribed. In terms of epinephrine, it is not known what effect vasoconstrictors in the local anesthetic regimen will have in patients with a known history of congenital prolonged QT interval or in patients taking any medication that prolongs the QT interval. Until more information is obtained, it is suggested that the clinician consult with the physician prior to the use of a vasoconstrictor in suspected patients, and that the vasoconstrictor (epinephrine, mepivacaine and levonordefrin [Carbocaine® 2% with Neo-Cobefrin®]) be used with caution.

Effects on Dental Treatment Key adverse event(s) related to dental treatment: Metallic or abnormal taste

Effects on Bleeding Although there are no reports of enhanced bleeding, telavancin may interfere with test used to monitor coagulation (eg, prothrombin time, INR, activated partial thromboplastin time, activated clotting time, and coagulation based factor Xa tests).

Adverse Effects

>10%:

Central nervous system: Insomnia (13%), psychiatric disorder (12%), headache (11%)

Gastrointestinal: Metallic/soapy taste (33%), nausea (27%), vomiting (14%)

Genitourinary: Foamy urine (13%)

1% to 10%:

Central nervous system: Dizziness (6%)

Dermatologic: Pruritus (3% to 6%), rash (4%)

Endocrine & metabolic: Hypokalemia (7%)

Gastrointestinal: Diarrhea (7%), appetite decreased (3%), abdominal pain (2%)
Hematologic: Thrombocytopenia (7%)
Local: Infusion site pain (4%), infusion site erythema (3%)
Neuromuscular & skeletal: Paresthesia (5%), rigors (4%)
Renal: Serum creatinine increased (8%), microalbuminuria (7%)
Respiratory: Dyspnea (8%)

General Dosage Range Dosage adjustment recommended in patients with renal impairment

I.V.: *Adults:* 10 mg/kg every 24 hours

Mechanism of Action Exerts concentration-dependent bactericidal activity; inhibits bacterial cell wall synthesis by blocking polymerization and cross-linking of peptidoglycan by binding to D-Ala-D-Ala portion of cell wall. Unlike vancomycin, additional mechanism involves disruption of membrane potential and changes cell permeability due to presence of lipophilic side chain moiety.

Pharmacodynamics/Kinetics

Half-life Elimination 6.6-9.6 hours

Pregnancy Risk Factor C

Dental Comment Telavancin is known to prolong the QT interval. The QT interval is measured as the time and distance between the Q point of the QRS complex and the end of the T wave in the ECG tracing. After adjustment for heart rate, the QT interval is defined as prolonged if it is more than 450 msec in men and 460 msec in women. A long QT syndrome was first described in the 1950s and 60s as a congenital syndrome involving QT interval prolongation and syncope and sudden death. Some of the congenital long QT syndromes were characterized by a peculiar electrocardiographic appearance of the QRS complex involving a premature atria beat followed by a pause, then a subsequent sinus beat showing marked QT prolongation and deformity. This type of cardiac arrhythmia was originally termed "torsade de pointes" (translated from the French as "twisting of the points"). Telavancin is considered as having a risk of causing torsade de pointes. Since it is not known what effect vasoconstrictors in the local anesthetic regimen will have in patients with a known history of congenital prolonged QT interval or in patients taking any medication that prolongs the QT interval, a medical consult is suggested.

Telbivudine (tel BI vyoo deen)

Related Information

HIV Infection and AIDS *on page 1883*
Systemic Viral Diseases *on page 1904*

U.S. Brand Names Tyzeka®

Canadian Brand Names Sebivo®

Pharmacologic Category Antiretroviral Agent, Reverse Transcriptase Inhibitor (Nucleoside)

Use Treatment of chronic hepatitis B with evidence of viral replication and either persistent transaminase elevations or histologically-active disease

Local Anesthetic/Vasoconstrictor Precautions No information available to require special precautions

Effects on Dental Treatment No significant effects or complications reported

Effects on Bleeding No information available to require special precautions regarding hemostasis.

Adverse Effects

>10%:
Central nervous system: Fatigue (13%), headache (10%)
Neuromuscular & skeletal: CPK increased (79%; grades 3/4: 13%)

1% to 10%:
Central nervous system: Dizziness (4%), fever (4%), insomnia (3%)
Dermatologic: Rash (4%), pruritus (2%)
Endocrine & metabolic: Lipase increased (grades 3/4: 2%)
Gastrointestinal: Abdominal pain (3% to 6%), diarrhea (6%), nausea (5%), abdominal distension (3%), dyspepsia (3%)
Hematologic: Neutropenia (grades 3/4: 2%)
Hepatic: ALT increased (grades 3/4: 5% to 7%), AST increased (grades 3/4: 6%)
Neuromuscular & skeletal: Arthralgia (4%), back pain (4%), myalgia (3%)
Respiratory: Cough (6%), pharyngolaryngeal pain (5%)

General Dosage Range Dosage adjustment recommended in patients with renal impairment

Oral: *Children ≥16 years and Adults:* 600 mg once daily

Mechanism of Action Telbivudine, a synthetic thymidine nucleoside analogue (L-enantiomer of thymidine), is intracellularly phosphorylated to the active triphosphate form, which competes with the natural substrate, thymidine 5'-triphosphate, to inhibit hepatitis B viral DNA polymerase; enzyme inhibition blocks reverse transcriptase activity thereby reducing viral DNA replication.

Pharmacodynamics/Kinetics

Half-life Elimination Terminal: 40-49 hours

Time to Peak 1-4 hours

Pregnancy Risk Factor B

Product Availability Tyzeka® oral solution: FDA approved April 2009; anticipated availability is currently undetermined

Telithromycin (tel ith roe MYE sin)

Related Information

Clinical Risk Related to Drugs Prolonging QT Interval *on page* 1872

U.S. Brand Names Ketek®

Canadian Brand Names Ketek®

Generic Availability (U.S.) No

Pharmacologic Category Antibiotic, Ketolide

Use Treatment of community-acquired pneumonia (mild-to-moderate) caused by susceptible strains of *Streptococcus pneumoniae* (including multidrug-resistant isolates), *Haemophilus influenzae*, *Chlamydophila pneumoniae*, *Moraxella catarrhalis*, and *Mycoplasma pneumoniae*

Local Anesthetic/Vasoconstrictor Precautions Telithromycin is one of the drugs confirmed to prolong the QT interval and is accepted as having a risk of causing torsade de pointes. The risk of drug-induced torsade de pointes is extremely low when a single QT interval prolonging drug is prescribed. In terms of epinephrine, it is not known what effect vasoconstrictors in the local anesthetic regimen will have in patients with a known history of congenital prolonged QT interval or in patients taking any medication that prolongs the QT interval. Until more information is obtained, it is suggested that the clinician consult with the physician prior to the use of a vasoconstrictor in suspected patients, and that the vasoconstrictor (epinephrine, mepivacaine and levonordefrin [Carbocaine® 2% with Neo-Cobefrin®]) be used with caution.

Effects on Dental Treatment Key adverse event(s) related to dental treatment: Xerostomia (normal salivary flow resumes upon discontinuation), glossitis, stomatitis, and tooth discoloration.

Effects on Bleeding No information available to require special precautions

Adverse Effects

>10%: Gastrointestinal: Diarrhea (10% to 11%)

2% to 10%:

- Central nervous system: Headache (2% to 6%), dizziness (3% to 4%)
- Gastrointestinal: Nausea (7% to 8%), vomiting (2% to 3%), loose stools (2%), dysgeusia (2%)

≥0.2% to <2%:

- Central nervous system: Fatigue, insomnia, somnolence, vertigo
- Dermatologic: Rash
- Gastrointestinal: Abdominal distension, abdominal pain, anorexia, constipation, dyspepsia, flatulence, gastritis, gastroenteritis, GI upset, glossitis, stomatitis, watery stools, xerostomia
- Genitourinary: Vaginal candidiasis
- Hematologic: Platelets increased
- Hepatic: Transaminases increased
- Ocular: Blurred vision, accommodation delayed, diplopia
- Miscellaneous: Candidiasis, diaphoresis increased

Dosage Oral:

Children ≥13 years and Adults: Tonsillitis/pharyngitis (unlabeled use; Canadian indication): 800 mg once daily for 5 days

Adults: Community-acquired pneumonia: 800 mg once daily for 7-10 days

Dosage adjustment in renal impairment:

U.S. product labeling: Cl_{cr} <30 mL/minute, including dialysis: 600 mg once daily; when renal impairment is accompanied by hepatic impairment, reduce dosage to 400 mg once daily

Canadian product labeling: Cl_{cr} <30 mL/minute: Reduce dose to 400 mg once daily

Hemodialysis: Administer following dialysis

Dosage adjustment in hepatic impairment: No adjustment recommended, unless concurrent severe renal impairment is present

Mechanism of Action Inhibits bacterial protein synthesis by binding to two sites on the 50S ribosomal subunit. Telithromycin has also been demonstrated to alter secretion of IL-1alpha and TNF-alpha; the clinical significance of this immunomodulatory effect has not been evaluated.

Contraindications Hypersensitivity to telithromycin, macrolide antibiotics, or any component of the formulation; myasthenia gravis; history of hepatitis and/or jaundice associated with telithromycin or other macrolide antibiotic use; concurrent use of cisapride or pimozide

Warnings/Precautions Acute hepatic failure and severe liver injury, including hepatitis and hepatic necrosis (leading to some fatalities) have been reported, in some cases after only a few doses; if signs/symptoms of hepatitis or liver damage occur, discontinue therapy and initiate liver function tests. **[U.S. Boxed Warning]: Life-threatening (including fatal) respiratory failure has occurred in patients with myasthenia gravis;** use in these patients is contraindicated. May prolong QT_c interval, leading to a risk of ventricular arrhythmias; closely-related antibiotics have been associated with malignant ventricular arrhythmias and torsade de pointes. Avoid in patients with prolongation of QTc interval due to congenital causes, history of long QT syndrome, uncorrected electrolyte disturbances (hypokalemia or hypomagnesemia), significant bradycardia (<50 bpm), or concurrent therapy with QT_c-prolonging drugs (eg, class Ia and class III antiarrhythmics). Avoid use in patients with a prior history of confirmed cardiogenic syncope or ventricular arrhythmias while receiving macrolide antibiotics or other QT_c-prolonging drugs. May cause severe visual disturbances (eg, changes in accommodation ability, diplopia, blurred vision). May cause loss of consciousness (possibly vagal-related); caution patients that these events may interfere with ability to operate machinery or drive, and to use caution until effects are known. Use caution in renal impairment; severe impairment (Cl_{cr} <30 mL/minute) requires dosage adjustment. Pseudomembranous colitis has been reported. Safety and efficacy not established in pediatric patients <13 years of age per Canadian approved labeling and <18 years of age per U.S. approved labeling.

Drug Interactions

Metabolism/Transport Effects **Substrate** of CYP1A2 (minor), 3A4 (major); **Inhibits** CYP2D6 (weak), 3A4 (strong)

Avoid Concomitant Use

Avoid concomitant use of Telithromycin with any of the following: Alfuzosin; Artemether; BCG; Cisapride; Conivaptan; Disopyramide; Dronedarone; Eplerenone; Everolimus; Fluticasone (Oral Inhalation); Halofantrine; Lumefantrine; Lurasidone; Nilotinib; Nisoldipine; Pimozide; QuiNINE; Ranolazine; Rivaroxaban; RomiDEPsin; Salmeterol; Silodosin; Tamsulosin; Tetrabenazine; Thioridazine; Tolvaptan; Toremifene; Vandetanib; Ziprasidone

Increased Effect/Toxicity

Telithromycin may increase the levels/effects of: Alfentanil; Alfuzosin; Almotriptan; Alosetron; Antifungal Agents (Azole Derivatives, Systemic); Antineoplastic Agents (Vinca Alkaloids); Benzodiazepines (metabolized by oxidation); Bortezomib; Brinzolamide; Budesonide (Nasal); Budesonide (Systemic, Oral Inhalation); BusPIRone; Calcium Channel Blockers; CarBAMazepine; Cardiac Glycosides; Ciclesonide; Cilostazol; Cisapride; CloZAPine; Colchicine; Conivaptan; Corticosteroids (Orally Inhaled); Corticosteroids (Systemic); CycloSPORINE; CycloSPORINE (Systemic); CYP3A4 Substrates; Dienogest; Disopyramide; Dronedarone; Dutasteride; Eletriptan; Eplerenone; Ergot Derivatives; Everolimus; FentaNYL; Fesoterodine; Fluticasone (Nasal); Fluticasone (Oral Inhalation); GuanFACINE; Halofantrine; HMG-CoA Reductase Inhibitors; Ixabepilone; Lumefantrine; Lurasidone; Maraviroc; MethylPREDNISolone; Nilotinib; Nisoldipine; Paricalcitol; Pazopanib; Phosphodiesterase 5 Inhibitors; Pimecrolimus; Pimozide; QTc-Prolonging Agents; QuiNIDine; QuiNINE; Ranolazine; Repaglinide; Rifamycin Derivatives; Rivaroxaban; RomiDEPsin; Salmeterol; Saxagliptin; Selective Serotonin Reuptake Inhibitors; Silodosin; Sirolimus; SORAfenib; Tacrolimus; Tacrolimus (Systemic); Tacrolimus (Topical); Tadalafil; Tamsulosin; Temsirolimus; Tetrabenazine; Thioridazine; Tolvaptan; Toremifene; Vandetanib; Verapamil; Vilazodone; Vitamin K Antagonists; Ziprasidone; Zopiclone

The levels/effects of Telithromycin may be increased by: Alfuzosin; Antifungal Agents (Azole Derivatives, Systemic); Artemether; Chloroquine; Ciprofloxacin; Ciprofloxacin (Systemic); CYP3A4 Inhibitors (Moderate); CYP3A4 Inhibitors (Strong); Gadobutrol; Lumefantrine; Nilotinib; QuiNINE

Decreased Effect

Telithromycin may decrease the levels/effects of: BCG; Clopidogrel; Prasugrel; Typhoid Vaccine

The levels/effects of Telithromycin may be decreased by: CYP3A4 Inducers (Strong); Deferasirox; Etravirine; Herbs (CYP3A4 Inducers); Tocilizumab

Ethanol/Nutrition/Herb Interactions Herb/nutraceutical: St John's wort: May decrease the levels/effects of telithromycin.

Dietary Considerations May be taken with or without food.

Pharmacodynamics/Kinetics

Half-life Elimination 10 hours

Time to Peak Plasma: 1 hour

Pregnancy Risk Factor C

Lactation Excretion in breast milk unknown/use caution

Breast-Feeding Considerations It is not known if telithromycin is excreted in breast milk. The manufacturer recommends caution if using telithromycin in a breast-feeding woman.

Dosage Forms

Tablet, oral:

Ketek®: 300 mg, 400 mg

Dosage Forms: Canada

Tablet:

Ketek®: 400 mg

Dental Comment Telithromycin is known to prolong the QT interval. The QT interval is measured as the time and distance between the Q point of the QRS complex and the end of the T wave in the ECG tracing. After adjustment for heart rate, the QT interval is defined as prolonged if it is more than 450 msec in men and 460 msec in women. A long QT syndrome was first described in the 1950s and 60s as a congenital syndrome involving QT interval prolongation and syncope and sudden death. Some of the congenital long QT syndromes were characterized by a peculiar electrocardiographic appearance of the QRS complex involving a premature atria beat followed by a pause, then a subsequent sinus beat showing marked QT prolongation and deformity. This type of cardiac arrhythmia was originally termed "torsade de pointes" (translated from the French as "twisting of the points"). Telithromycin is considered as having a risk of causing torsade de pointes. Since it is not known what effect vasoconstrictors in the local anesthetic regimen will have in patients with a known history of congenital prolonged QT interval or in patients taking any medication that prolongs the QT interval, a medical consult is suggested.

References

Carbon C, "A Pooled Analysis of Telithromycin in the Treatment of Community-Acquired Respiratory Tract Infections in Adults," *Infection*, 2003, 31(5):308-17.

Demolis JL, Vacheron F, Cardus S, et al, "Effect of Single and Repeated Oral Doses of Telithromycin on Cardiac QT Interval in Healthy Subjects," *Clin Pharmacol Ther*, 2003, 73(3):242-52.

Quinn J, Ruoff GE, and Ziter PS, "Efficacy and tolerability of 5-day, once-daily telithromycin compared with 10-day, twice-daily clarithromycin for the treatment of group A beta-hemolytic streptococcal tonsillitis/pharyngitis: a multicenter, randomized, double-blind, parallel-group study," *Clin Ther*, 2003, 25(2):422-43.

Ubukata K, Iwata S, and Sunakawa K, "*In vitro* Activities of New Ketolide, Telithromycin, and Eight Other Macrolide Antibiotics Against *Streptococcus pneumoniae* Having mefA and ermB Genes That Mediate Macrolide Resistance," *J Infect Chemother*, 2003, 9(3):221-6.

Telmisartan (tel mi SAR tan)

Related Information

Cardiovascular Diseases *on page 1848*

U.S. Brand Names Micardis®

Canadian Brand Names Micardis®

Generic Availability (U.S.) No

Pharmacologic Category Angiotensin II Receptor Blocker

Use Treatment of hypertension (may be used alone or in combination with other antihypertensive agents); cardiovascular risk reduction in patients ≥55 years of age unable to take ACE inhibitors and who are at high risk of major cardiovascular events (eg, MI, stroke, death)

Local Anesthetic/Vasoconstrictor Precautions No information available to require special precautions

Effects on Dental Treatment No significant effects or complications reported

Effects on Bleeding No information available to require special precautions

Adverse Effects May be associated with worsening of renal function in patients dependent on renin-angiotensin-aldosterone system.

1% to 10%:

Cardiovascular: Intermittent claudication (7%; placebo 6%), chest pain (≥1%), hypertension (≥1%), peripheral edema (≥1%)

Central nervous system: Dizziness (≥1%), fatigue (≥1%), headache (≥1%), pain (≥1%)

Dermatologic: Skin ulcer (3%; placebo 2%)

Gastrointestinal: Diarrhea (3%), abdominal pain (≥1%), dyspepsia (≥1%), nausea (≥1%)

Genitourinary: Urinary tract infection (≥1%)

Neuromuscular & skeletal: Back pain (3%), myalgia (≥1%)

Respiratory: Upper respiratory infection (7%), sinusitis (3%), cough (≥1%), pharyngitis (1%)

Dosage Oral:

Adults:

Hypertension: Initial: 40 mg once daily; usual maintenance dose range: 20-80 mg/day. Patients with volume depletion should be initiated on the lower dosage with close supervision.

Cardiovascular risk reduction: Initial: 80 mg once daily. **Note:** It is unknown whether doses <80 mg/day are associated with a reduction in risk of cardiovascular morbidity or mortality.

Elderly:

Hypertension: Initial: 20 mg/day; usual maintenance dose range: 20-80 mg/day

Cardiovascular risk reduction: Initial 80 mg once daily

Dosage adjustment in renal impairment: No adjustment required; hemodialysis patients are more susceptible to orthostatic hypotension

Dosage adjustment in hepatic impairment: Initiate therapy with low dose; titrate slowly and monitor closely.

Canadian labeling: Recommended initial dose: 40 mg/day

Mechanism of Action Angiotensin II acts as a vasoconstrictor. In addition to causing direct vasoconstriction, angiotensin II also stimulates the release of aldosterone. Once aldosterone is released, sodium as well as water are reabsorbed. The end result is an elevation in blood pressure. Telmisartan is a nonpeptide AT1 angiotensin II receptor antagonist. This binding prevents angiotensin II from binding to the receptor thereby blocking the vasoconstriction and the aldosterone secreting effects of angiotensin II.

Contraindications There are no contraindications listed in manufacturer's labeling.

Canadian labeling: Hypersensitivity to telmisartan or any component of the formulation; second and third trimesters of pregnancy; breast-feeding; fructose intolerance

Warnings/Precautions [U.S. Boxed Warning]: Based on human data, drugs that act on the angiotensin system can cause injury and death to the developing fetus when used in the second and third trimesters. Angiotensin receptor blockers should be discontinued as soon as possible once pregnancy is detected. May cause hyperkalemia; avoid potassium supplementation unless specifically required by healthcare provider. Avoid use or use a smaller dose in patients who are volume depleted; correct depletion first. May be associated with deterioration of renal function and/or increases in serum creatinine, particularly in patients with low renal blood flow (eg, renal artery stenosis, heart failure) whose glomerular filtration rate (GFR) is dependent on efferent arteriolar vasoconstriction by angiotensin II. Use with caution in unstented unilateral/bilateral renal artery stenosis. When unstented bilateral renal artery stenosis is present, use is generally avoided due to the elevated risk of deterioration in renal function unless possible benefits outweigh risks. Use with caution with pre-existing renal insufficiency; significant aortic/mitral stenosis. Concurrent use of ACE inhibitors may increase the risk of clinically-significant adverse events (eg, renal dysfunction, hyperkalemia). Concurrent use with ramipril is not recommended. Use with caution in patients who have biliary obstructive disorders or hepatic dysfunction. Product contains sorbitol. The Canadian labeling (not in U.S. labeling) contraindicates use in fructose intolerant patients.

Drug Interactions

Metabolism/Transport Effects Inhibits CYP2C19 (weak)

Avoid Concomitant Use There are no known interactions where it is recommended to avoid concomitant use.

Increased Effect/Toxicity

Telmisartan may increase the levels/effects of: ACE Inhibitors; Amifostine; Antihypertensives; Cardiac Glycosides; Hypotensive Agents; Lithium; Nonsteroidal Anti-Inflammatory Agents; Potassium-Sparing Diuretics; Ramipril; RiTUXimab

The levels/effects of Telmisartan may be increased by: Diazoxide; Eplerenone; Herbs (Hypotensive Properties); MAO Inhibitors; Pentoxifylline; Phosphodiesterase 5 Inhibitors; Potassium Salts; Prostacyclin Analogues; Tolvaptan; Trimethoprim

Decreased Effect

The levels/effects of Telmisartan may be decreased by: Herbs (Hypertensive Properties); Methylphenidate; Nonsteroidal Anti-Inflammatory Agents; Yohimbine

Ethanol/Nutrition/Herb Interactions Herb/Nutraceutical: Avoid herbs with hypertensive properties (bayberry, blue cohosh, cayenne, ephedra, ginger, ginseng [American], kola, licorice); may diminish the antihypertensive effect of telmisartan. Avoid herbs with hypotensive properties (black cohosh, California poppy, coleus, golden seal, hawthorn, mistletoe, periwinkle, quinine, shepherd's purse); may enhance the hypotensive effect of telmisartan.

Dietary Considerations May be taken without regard to meals. Product contains sorbitol.

Pharmacodynamics/Kinetics

Onset of Action 1-2 hours; Peak effect: 0.5-1 hours

Duration of Action Up to 24 hours

Half-life Elimination Terminal: 24 hours

Time to Peak Plasma: 0.5-1 hours

Pregnancy Risk Factor C (1st trimester); D (2nd and 3rd trimesters)

Lactation Excretion in breast milk unknown/not recommended

Dosage Forms

Tablet, oral:

Micardis®: 20 mg, 40 mg, 80 mg

Telmisartan and Amlodipine (tel mi SAR tan & am LOE di peen)

Related Information

AmLODIPine *on page* 113

Telmisartan *on page* 1592

U.S. Brand Names Twynsta®

Pharmacologic Category Angiotensin II Receptor Blocker; Calcium Channel Blocker; Calcium Channel Blocker, Dihydropyridine

Use Treatment of hypertension, including initial treatment in patients who will require multiple antihypertensives for adequate control

Local Anesthetic/Vasoconstrictor Precautions No information available to require special precautions

Effects on Dental Treatment Key adverse event(s) related to dental treatment: Fewer reports of gingival hyperplasia reported with amlodipine use than with other calcium channel blockers (usually resolves upon discontinuation); consult with healthcare provider. Orthostatic hypotension has been reported; monitor patient for dizziness while rising from dental chair.

Effects on Bleeding No information available to require special precautions

Adverse Effects Reactions/percentages reported with combination product; also see individual agents.

>10%: Cardiovascular: Peripheral edema (dose related: 1% to 11%)

1% to 10%:

Cardiovascular: Orthostatic hypotension (6%), edema (<2%), hypotension (<2%), syncope (<2%)

Central nervous system: Dizziness (3%)

Neuromuscular & skeletal: Back pain (2%)

General Dosage Range Oral: *Adults:* Amlodipine 5-10 mg and telmisartan 40-80 mg once daily (maximum: 10 mg/day [amlodipine]; 80 mg/day [telmisartan])

Mechanism of Action

Telmisartan is a nonpeptide AT1 (angiotensin II type 1) receptor antagonist. Angiotensin II acts as a vasoconstrictor. In addition to causing direct vasoconstriction, angiotensin II also stimulates the release of aldosterone. Once aldosterone is released, sodium and water are reabsorbed. The end result is an elevation in blood pressure. Telmisartan binding to AT1 prevents angiotensin II from binding to the receptor thereby blocking the vasoconstriction and the aldosterone secreting effects of angiotensin II.

Amlodipine inhibits calcium ion from entering the "slow channels" or select voltage-sensitive areas of vascular smooth muscle and myocardium during depolarization, producing a relaxation of coronary vascular smooth muscle and coronary vasodilation; increases myocardial oxygen delivery in patients with vasospastic angina. Amlodipine directly acts on vascular smooth muscle to produce peripheral arterial vasodilation reducing peripheral vascular resistance and blood pressure.

Pregnancy Risk Factor C (1st trimester); D (2nd and 3rd trimesters)

Telmisartan and Hydrochlorothiazide
(tel mi SAR tan & hye droe klor oh THYE a zide)

Related Information

Hydrochlorothiazide *on page* 854

Telmisartan *on page* 1592

U.S. Brand Names Micardis® HCT

Canadian Brand Names Micardis® Plus

Pharmacologic Category Angiotensin II Receptor Blocker; Diuretic, Thiazide

Use Treatment of hypertension; combination product should not be used for initial therapy

Local Anesthetic/Vasoconstrictor Precautions No information available to require special precautions

Effects on Dental Treatment No significant effects or complications reported

Effects on Bleeding No information available to require special precautions

Adverse Effects The following reactions have been reported with the combination product; see individual agents for additional adverse reactions that may be expected from each agent.

2% to 10%:

- Central nervous system: Dizziness (5%), fatigue (3%)
- Gastrointestinal: Diarrhea (3%), nausea (2%)
- Renal: BUN increased (3%)
- Respiratory: Upper respiratory tract infection (8%), sinusitis (4%)
- Miscellaneous: Flu-like syndrome (2%)

<2%: Abdominal pain, back pain, bilirubin increased, bronchitis, dyspepsia, hematocrit decreased, hemoglobin decreased, hypokalemia, liver enzymes increased, pharyngitis, postural hypotension, rash, serum creatinine increased, tachycardia, vomiting; rhabdomyolysis has been reported (rarely) with angiotensin-receptor antagonists

General Dosage Range Oral: *Adults:* Initial: Telmisartan 80 mg and hydrochlorothiazide 12.5-25 mg once daily; Maintenance: Telmisartan 80-160 mg and hydrochlorothiazide 12.5-25 mg once daily

Mechanism of Action

Telmisartan: Telmisartan is an angiotensin receptor antagonist. Angiotensin II acts as a vasoconstrictor. In addition to causing direct vasoconstriction, angiotensin II also stimulates the release of aldosterone. Once aldosterone is released, sodium as well as water are reabsorbed. The end result is an elevation in blood pressure. Telmisartan binds to the AT1 angiotensin II receptor. This binding prevents angiotensin II from binding to the receptor thereby blocking the vasoconstriction and the aldosterone secreting effects of angiotensin II.

Hydrochlorothiazide: Inhibits sodium reabsorption in the distal tubules causing increased excretion of sodium and water as well as potassium and hydrogen ions

Pregnancy Risk Factor C (1st trimester); D (2nd and 3rd trimesters)

Temazepam (te MAZ e pam)

U.S. Brand Names Restoril™

Canadian Brand Names Apo-Temazepam®; CO Temazepam; Dom-Temazepam; Gen-Temazepam; Novo-Temazepam; Nu-Temazepam; PHL-Temazepam; PMS-Temazepam; ratio-Temazepam; Restoril™

Generic Availability (U.S.) Yes

Pharmacologic Category Hypnotic, Benzodiazepine

Use Short-term treatment of insomnia

Unlabeled/Investigational Use Treatment of anxiety

Local Anesthetic/Vasoconstrictor Precautions No information available to require special precautions

Effects on Dental Treatment Key adverse event(s) related to dental treatment: Significant xerostomia (normal salivary flow resumes upon discontinuation).

Effects on Bleeding No information available to require special precautions

Adverse Effects 1% to 10%:

- Central nervous system: Anxiety, confusion, dizziness, drowsiness, euphoria, fatigue, hangover, headache, lethargy, vertigo
- Dermatologic: Rash
- Endocrine & metabolic: Libido decreased
- Gastrointestinal: Diarrhea
- Neuromuscular & skeletal: Dysarthria, weakness
- Ocular: Blurred vision
- Miscellaneous: Diaphoresis

Dosage Oral:

Adults: Usual dose: 15-30 mg at bedtime; some patients may respond to 7.5 mg in transient insomnia

Elderly or debilitated patients: Initial: 7.5 mg at bedtime

Mechanism of Action Binds to stereospecific benzodiazepine receptors on the postsynaptic GABA neuron at several sites within the central nervous system, including the limbic system, reticular formation. Enhancement of the inhibitory effect of GABA on neuronal excitability results by increased neuronal membrane permeability to chloride ions. This shift in chloride ions results in hyperpolarization (a less excitable state) and stabilization.

Contraindications Hypersensitivity to temazepam or any component of the formulation (cross-sensitivity with other benzodiazepines may exist); narrow-angle glaucoma (not in product labeling, however, benzodiazepines are contraindicated); pregnancy

Warnings/Precautions As a hypnotic, should be used only after evaluation of potential causes of sleep disturbance. Failure of sleep disturbance to resolve after 7-10 days may indicate psychiatric or medical illness. A worsening of insomnia or the emergence of new abnormalities of thought or behavior may represent unrecognized psychiatric or medical illness and requires immediate and careful evaluation.

Use with caution in elderly or debilitated patients, patients with hepatic disease (including alcoholics), or renal impairment. Due to increased sensitivity in the elderly, smaller doses of benzodiazepines may be safer and as effective. Avoid using doses >15 mg daily of temazepam (Beers Criteria). Use with caution in patients with respiratory disease, or impaired gag reflex. Avoid use inpatients with sleep apnea.

Causes CNS depression (dose-related) resulting in sedation, dizziness, confusion, or ataxia which may impair physical and mental capabilities. Patients must be cautioned about performing tasks which require mental alertness (eg, operating machinery or driving). Use with caution in patients receiving other CNS depressants or psychoactive agents. Postmarketing studies have indicated that the use of hypnotic/sedative agents for sleep has been associated with hypersensitivity reactions including anaphylaxis as well as angioedema. An increased risk for hazardous sleep-related activities such as sleep-driving; cooking and eating food, and making phone calls while asleep have also been noted. Effects with other sedative drugs or ethanol may be potentiated. Benzodiazepines have been associated with falls and traumatic injury and should be used with extreme caution in patients who are at risk of these events (especially the elderly).

Use caution in patients with suicidal risk. Use with caution in patients with a history of drug dependence. Benzodiazepines have been associated with dependence and acute withdrawal symptoms on discontinuation or reduction in dose (may occur after as little as 10 days). Acute withdrawal, including seizures, may be precipitated after administration of flumazenil to patients receiving long-term benzodiazepine therapy.

Benzodiazepines have been associated with anterograde amnesia. Paradoxical reactions, including hyperactive or aggressive behavior, have been reported with benzodiazepines, particularly in adolescent/pediatric or psychiatric patients. Does not have analgesic, antidepressant, or antipsychotic properties.

Drug Interactions

Metabolism/Transport Effects **Substrate** (minor) of CYP2B6, 2C9, 2C19, 3A4

Avoid Concomitant Use

Avoid concomitant use of Temazepam with any of the following: OLANZapine

Increased Effect/Toxicity

Temazepam may increase the levels/effects of: Alcohol (Ethyl); CloZAPine; CNS Depressants; Fosphenytoin; Methotrimeprazine; Phenytoin

The levels/effects of Temazepam may be increased by: Conivaptan; Droperidol; Methotrimeprazine; OLANZapine

Decreased Effect

The levels/effects of Temazepam may be decreased by: Theophylline Derivatives; Tocilizumab; Yohimbine

Ethanol/Nutrition/Herb Interactions

Ethanol: May increase CNS depression; monitor for increased effects with coadministration. Caution patients about effects.

Food: Serum levels may be increased by grapefruit juice.

Herb/Nutraceutical: St John's wort may decrease temazepam levels. Avoid valerian, St John's wort, kava kava, gotu kola (may increase CNS depression).

Pharmacodynamics/Kinetics

Half-life Elimination 9.5-12.4 hours

Time to Peak Serum: 2-3 hours

Pregnancy Risk Factor X

Lactation Enters breast milk/use caution (AAP rates "of concern"; AAP 2001 update pending)

Breast-Feeding Considerations Information is available from a study conducted in 10 nursing women, <2 weeks postpartum. All women were given temazepam 10-20 mg at bedtime for ≥2 nights. Samples were obtained 10-21 hours after a dose. Temazepam was not found in the milk of nine mothers (maternal serum concentrations 8-59 mcg/L). Temazepam was detected in the milk of one patient whose serum concentration was 234 mcg/mL at ~14 hours after the dose; milk concentrations were 28 mcg/L (pre-feed) and 26 mcg/L (post-feed). Oxazepam concentrations were 9 mcg/mL in the maternal serum and below the limit of detection in breast milk. Adverse events were not noted in any nursing infants. Drowsiness, lethargy, or weight loss in nursing infants have been observed in case reports following maternal use of some benzodiazepines.

Controlled Substance C-IV

Dosage Forms

Capsule, oral: 7.5 mg, 15 mg, 22.5 mg, 30 mg
Restoril™: 7.5 mg, 15 mg, 22.5 mg, 30 mg

Temozolomide (te moe ZOE loe mide)

U.S. Brand Names Temodar®

Canadian Brand Names Temodal®

Pharmacologic Category Antineoplastic Agent, Alkylating Agent (Triazene)

Use Treatment of newly-diagnosed glioblastoma multiforme (initially in combination with radiotherapy, then as maintenance treatment); treatment of refractory anaplastic astrocytoma

Canadian labeling (not an approved indication in the U.S.): Treatment of recurrent or progressive glioblastoma multiforme

Unlabeled/Investigational Use Treatment of recurrent glioblastoma multiforme, low-grade astrocytoma, low-grade oligodendroglioma, anaplastic oligodendroglioma, metastatic CNS lesions, refractory primary CNS lymphoma, advanced or metastatic melanoma, cutaneous T-cell lymphomas (mycosis fungoides [MF] and Sézary syndrome [SS]), advanced neuroendocrine tumors (carcinoid or islet cell), Ewing's sarcoma (recurrent or progressive), soft tissue sarcomas (extremity/retroperitoneal/intra-abdominal or hemangiopericytoma/solitary fibrous tumor), treatment of pediatric neuroblastoma

Local Anesthetic/Vasoconstrictor Precautions No information available to require special precautions

Effects on Dental Treatment Key adverse event(s) related to dental treatment: Stomatitis, dysphagia, and taste perversion.

Effects on Bleeding Chemotherapy may result in significant myelosuppression, potentially including significant reduction in platelet counts and altered hemostasis. In patients who are under active treatment with these agents, medical consult is suggested.

Adverse Effects Note: With CNS malignancies, it may be difficult to distinguish between CNS adverse events caused by temozolomide versus the effects of progressive disease.

>10%:

Cardiovascular: Peripheral edema (11%)
Central nervous system: Fatigue (34% to 61%), headache (23% to 41%), seizure (6% to 23%), hemiparesis (18%), fever (13%), dizziness (5% to 12%), coordination abnormality (11%)
Dermatologic: Alopecia (55%), rash (8% to 13%)
Gastrointestinal: Nausea (49% to 53%; grades 3/4: 1% to 10%), vomiting (29% to 42%; grades 3/4: 2% to 6%), constipation (22% to 33%), anorexia (9% to 27%), diarrhea (10% to 16%)
Hematologic: Lymphopenia (grades 3/4: 55%), thrombocytopenia (grades 3/4: adults: 4% to 19%; children: 25%), neutropenia (grades 3/4: adults: 8% to 14%; children: 20%), leukopenia (grades 3/4: 11%)
Neuromuscular & skeletal: Weakness (7% to 13%)
Miscellaneous: Viral infection (11%)

1% to 10%:

Central nervous system: Amnesia (10%), insomnia (4% to 10%), somnolence (9%), ataxia (8%), paresis (8%), anxiety (7%), memory impairment (7%), depression (6%), confusion (5%)
Dermatologic: Pruritus (5% to 8%), dry skin (5%), radiation injury (2% maintenance phase after radiotherapy), erythema (1%)
Endocrine & metabolic: Hypercorticism (8%), breast pain (females 6%)
Gastrointestinal: Stomatitis (9%), abdominal pain (5% to 9%), dysphagia (7%), taste perversion (5%), weight gain (5%)
Genitourinary: Incontinence (8%), urinary tract infection (8%), urinary frequency (6%)
Hematologic: Anemia (grades 3/4: 4%)
Neuromuscular & skeletal: Paresthesia (9%), back pain (8%), abnormal gait (6%), arthralgia (6%), myalgia (5%)
Ocular: Blurred vision (5% to 8%), diplopia (5%), vision abnormality (visual deficit/vision changes 5%)
Respiratory: Pharyngitis (8%), upper respiratory tract infection (8%), cough (5% to 8%), sinusitis (6%), dyspnea (5%)
Miscellaneous: Allergic reaction (≤3%)

General Dosage Range Dosage adjustment recommended in patients who develop toxicities.

I.V., Oral: *Adults:* Dosage varies greatly depending on indication

Mechanism of Action Like dacarbazine, temozolomide (a prodrug) is rapidly and nonenzymatically converted to the active alkylating metabolite MTIC [(methyl-triazene-1-yl)-imidazole-4-carboxamide]. Unlike dacarbazine, however, this conversion is spontaneous, nonenzymatic, and occurs under physiologic conditions in all tissues to which it distributes. The cytotoxic effects of MTIC are manifested through alkylation of DNA at the O^6, N^7 guanine positions.

Pharmacodynamics/Kinetics

Half-life Elimination Mean: Parent drug: 1.8 hours

Time to Peak Oral: Empty stomach: 1 hour; with food (high-fat meal): 2.25 hours

Pregnancy Risk Factor D

Temsirolimus (tem sir OH li mus)

U.S. Brand Names Torisel®

Canadian Brand Names Torisel®

Pharmacologic Category Antineoplastic Agent, mTOR Kinase Inhibitor

Use Treatment of advanced renal cell cancer (RCC)

Local Anesthetic/Vasoconstrictor Precautions No information available to require special precautions

Effects on Dental Treatment Key adverse event(s) related to dental treatment: Effects on oral cavity including mucositis, stomatitis, and taste disturbances.

Effects on Bleeding Thrombocytopenia has been associated with use; severe thrombocytopenia (rare) may be associated with delayed coagulation. Consultation to ensure adequate platelet counts may be considered in patients with signs/symptoms or a history of thrombocytopenia.

Adverse Effects

>10%:

- Cardiovascular: Edema (35%), peripheral edema (27%), chest pain (16%)
- Central nervous system: Pain (28%), fever (24%), headache (15%), insomnia (12%)
- Dermatologic: Rash (47%), pruritus (19%), nail disorder/thinning (14%), dry skin (11%)
- Endocrine & metabolic: Hyperglycemia (26% to 89%; grades 3/4: 16%), hypercholesterolemia (24% to 87%; grades 3/4: 2%), hypertriglyceridemia (83%; grades 3/4: 44%), hypophosphatemia (49%; grades 3/4: 18%), hyperlipidemia (27%), hypokalemia (21%; grades 3/4: 5%)
- Gastrointestinal: Mucositis (41%), nausea (37%), anorexia (32%), diarrhea (27%), abdominal pain (21%), constipation (20%), stomatitis (20%), taste disturbance (20%), vomiting (19%), weight loss (19%)
- Genitourinary: Urinary tract infection (15%)
- Hematologic: Anemia (45% to 94%; grades 3/4: 20%), lymphopenia (53%; grades 3/4: 16%), thrombocytopenia (14% to 40%; grades 3/4: 1%; dose-limiting toxicity), leukopenia (6% to 32%; grades 3/4: 1%), neutropenia (7% to 19%; grades 3/4: 3% to 5%)
- Hepatic: Alkaline phosphatase increased (68%; grades 3/4: 3%), AST increased (8% to 38%; grades 3/4: 1% to 2%)
- Neuromuscular & skeletal: Weakness (51%), back pain (20%), arthralgia (18%)
- Renal: Creatinine increased (14% to 57%; grades 3/4: 3%)
- Respiratory: Dyspnea (28%), cough (26%), epistaxis (12%), pharyngitis (12%)
- Miscellaneous: Infection (20% to 27%; includes abscess, bronchitis, cellulitis, herpes simplex, herpes zoster)

1% to 10%:

- Cardiovascular: Hypertension (7%), venous thromboembolism (2%, includes DVT and PE), thrombophlebitis (1%)
- Central nervous system: Chills (8%), depression (4%)
- Dermatologic: Acne (10%), wound healing impaired (1%)
- Gastrointestinal: Bowel perforation (fatal: 1%)
- Hepatic: Hyperbilirubinemia (8%; grades 3/4: 1%)
- Neuromuscular & skeletal: Myalgia (8%)
- Ocular: Conjunctivitis (7%)
- Respiratory: Rhinitis (10%), pneumonia (8%), upper respiratory tract infection (7%), interstitial lung disease (2%)
- Miscellaneous: Allergic/hypersensitivity/infusion reaction (9%; includes anaphylaxis, apnea, chest pain, dyspnea, flushing, hypotension, loss of consciousness)

General Dosage Range Dosage adjustment recommended in patients with hepatic impairment, on concomitant therapy, or who develop toxicities

I.V.: *Adults:* 25 mg once weekly

Mechanism of Action Temsirolimus and its active metabolite, sirolimus, are targeted inhibitors of mTOR (mammalian target of rapamycin) kinase activity. Temsirolimus (and sirolimus) bind to FKBP-12, an intracellular protein, to form a complex which inhibits mTOR signaling, halting the cell cycle at the G1 phase in tumor cells. In renal cell carcinoma, mTOR inhibition also exhibits anti-angiogenesis activity by reducing levels of HIF-1 and HIF-2 alpha (hypoxia inducible factors) and vascular endothelial growth factor (VEGF).

Pharmacodynamics/Kinetics

Half-life Elimination Temsirolimus: ~17 hours; Sirolimus: ~55 hours

Time to Peak Temsirolimus: At end of infusion; Sirolimus: 0.5-2 hours after temsirolimus infusion

Pregnancy Risk Factor D

Tenecteplase (ten EK te plase)

Related Information

Cardiovascular Diseases *on page* 1848

U.S. Brand Names TNKase®

Canadian Brand Names TNKase®

Pharmacologic Category Thrombolytic Agent

Use Thrombolytic agent used in the management of ST-elevation myocardial infarction (STEMI) for the lysis of thrombi in the coronary vasculature to restore perfusion and reduce mortality.

Recommended criteria for treatment: STEMI: Chest pain ≥20 minutes duration, onset of chest pain within 12 hours of treatment (or within prior 12-24 hours in patients with continuing ischemic symptoms), and S-T segment elevation >0.1 mV in at least two contiguous precordial leads or two adjacent limb leads on ECG or new or presumably new left bundle branch block (LBBB)

Unlabeled/Investigational Use Acute MI - combination regimen of tenecteplase (unlabeled dose), abciximab, and heparin (unlabeled dose)

Local Anesthetic/Vasoconstrictor Precautions No information available to require special precautions

Effects on Dental Treatment Key adverse event(s) related to dental treatment: Bleeding is the most frequent adverse effect of tenecteplase. See Effects on Bleeding.

Effects on Bleeding Bleeding is the most frequent adverse effect associated with tenecteplase. It is unlikely that ambulatory patients presenting for dental treatment will be taking intravenous anticoagulant therapy.

Adverse Effects As with all drugs which may affect hemostasis, bleeding is the major adverse effect associated with tenecteplase. Hemorrhage may occur at virtually any site. Risk is dependent on multiple variables, including the dosage administered, concurrent use of multiple agents which alter hemostasis, and patient predisposition. Rapid lysis of coronary artery thrombi by thrombolytic agents may be associated with reperfusion-related arterial and/or ventricular arrhythmia. The incidence of stroke and bleeding increase in patients >65 years.

>10%:
- Hematologic: Bleeding (22% minor: ASSENT-2 trial)
- Local: Hematoma (12% minor)

1% to 10%:
- Central nervous system: Stroke (2%)
- Gastrointestinal: GI hemorrhage (1% major, 2% minor), epistaxis (2% minor)
- Genitourinary: GU bleeding (4% minor)
- Hematologic: Bleeding (5% major: ASSENT-2 trial)
- Local: Bleeding at catheter puncture site (4% minor), hematoma (2% major)
- Respiratory: Pharyngeal bleeding (3% minor)

Additional cardiovascular events associated with use in MI: Cardiogenic shock, arrhythmia, AV block, pulmonary edema, heart failure, cardiac arrest, recurrent myocardial ischemia, myocardial reinfarction, myocardial rupture, cardiac tamponade, pericarditis, pericardial effusion, mitral regurgitation, thrombosis, embolism, electromechanical dissociation, hypotension, fever, nausea, vomiting

General Dosage Range I.V.:

Adults <60 kg: 30 mg as a single dose
Adults ≥60 to <70 kg: 35 mg as a single dose
Adults ≥70 to <80 kg: 40 mg as a single dose
Adults ≥80 to <90 kg: 45 mg as a single dose
Adults ≥90 kg: 50 mg as a single dose

Mechanism of Action Initiates fibrinolysis by binding to fibrin and converting plasminogen to plasmin.

Pharmacodynamics/Kinetics
Half-life Elimination 90-130 minutes
Pregnancy Risk Factor C

Teniposide (ten i POE side)

U.S. Brand Names Vumon®
Canadian Brand Names Vumon®
Pharmacologic Category Antineoplastic Agent, Podophyllotoxin Derivative
Use Treatment of refractory childhood acute lymphoblastic leukemia (ALL) in combination with other chemotherapy
Unlabeled/Investigational Use Treatment of refractory acute lymphoblastic leukemia (ALL) in adults
Local Anesthetic/Vasoconstrictor Precautions No information available to require special precautions
Effects on Dental Treatment Key adverse event(s) related to dental treatment: Mucositis.
Effects on Bleeding Chemotherapy may result in significant myelosuppression, potentially including significant reduction in platelet counts and altered hemostasis. In patients who are under active treatment with these agents, medical consult is suggested.
Adverse Effects
>10%:
Gastrointestinal: Mucositis (76%), diarrhea (33%), nausea/vomiting (29%; mild to moderate)
Hematologic: Neutropenia (95%), leukopenia (89%), anemia (88%), thrombocytopenia (85%), myelosuppression (75%)
Miscellaneous: Infection (12%)
1% to 10%:
Cardiovascular: Hypotension (2%; associated with rapid [<30 minutes] infusions)
Central nervous system: Fever (3%)
Dermatologic: Alopecia (9%; usually reversible), rash (3%)
Hematologic: Bleeding (5%)
Miscellaneous: Hypersensitivity reactions (5%; includes bronchospasm, chills, dyspnea, fever, flushing, hyper-/hypotension, tachycardia, or urticaria)
General Dosage Range I.V.: *Children:* 165 mg/m^2 twice weekly for 8-9 doses **or** 250 mg/m^2 weekly for 4-8 weeks
Mechanism of Action Teniposide does not inhibit microtubular assembly; it has been shown to delay transit of cells through the S phase and arrest cells in late S or early G_2 phase, preventing cells from entering mitosis. Teniposide is a topoisomerase II inhibitor, and appears to cause DNA strand breaks by inhibition of strand-passing and DNA ligase action.
Pharmacodynamics/Kinetics
Half-life Elimination Children: 5 hours
Pregnancy Risk Factor D

Tenofovir (te NOE fo veer)

Related Information
HIV Infection and AIDS *on page 1883*
Systemic Viral Diseases *on page 1904*
U.S. Brand Names Viread®
Canadian Brand Names Viread®
Pharmacologic Category Antiretroviral Agent, Reverse Transcriptase Inhibitor (Nucleotide)
Use Management of HIV infections in combination with at least two other antiretroviral agents; treatment of chronic hepatitis B virus (HBV) in patients with compensated or decompensated liver disease
Local Anesthetic/Vasoconstrictor Precautions No information available to require special precautions
Effects on Dental Treatment No significant effects or complications reported
Effects on Bleeding No information available to require special precautions regarding hemostasis.
Adverse Effects Frequencies listed are treatment-emergent adverse effects noted at higher frequency than in the placebo group or comparator group. Only adverse events from treatment-naive studies which varied significantly were noted (eg, rash event). Patients treated for chronic hepatitis B had similar reactions and frequencies.

>10%:

Central nervous system: Insomnia (3% to 4%; decompensated liver disease 18%), pain (7% to 13%), dizziness (3%; treatment naive 8%; decompensated liver disease 13%), depression (4% to 8%; treatment naive 9% to 11%), fever (2% to 4%; treatment naive 8%; decompensated liver disease 11%)

Dermatologic: Rash event (includes maculopapular, pustular, or vesiculobullous rash, pruritus or urticaria 5% to 7%; treatment naive 18%)

Endocrine & metabolic: Triglycerides increased (grades 3/4: 11%; treatment naive 4%)

Gastrointestinal: Abdominal pain (4% to 7%; decompensated liver disease 22%), nausea (8% to 11%; decompensated liver disease 20%), diarrhea (11% to 16%), vomiting (4% to 7%; decompensated liver disease 13%)

Neuromuscular & skeletal: Creatine kinase increased (9% to 12%), weakness (7% to 11%)

1% to 10%:

Cardiovascular: Chest pain (3%)

Central nervous system: Fatigue (9%), headache (5% to 8%), anxiety (6%)

Endocrine & metabolic: Hyperglycemia (grades 3/4: 3%)

Gastrointestinal: Serum amylase increased (grades 3/4: 4% to 7%; treatment naive 8% to 9%), anorexia (3% to 4%), dyspepsia (3% to 4%), flatulence (3% to 4%), weight loss (2% to 4%)

Genitourinary: Hematuria (grades 3/4: 3% to 7%)

Hematologic: Neutropenia (1% to 3%)

Hepatic: Transaminases increased (2% to 5%), alkaline phosphatase increased (1%)

Neuromuscular & skeletal: Back pain (3% to 4%; treatment naive 9%), peripheral neuropathy (3% to 5%), myalgia (3% to 4%)

Renal: Serum creatinine increased (decompensated liver disease 9%), renal failure (decompensated liver disease 7%), glycosuria (grades 3/4: 3%)

Respiratory: Upper respiratory tract infection (8%), sinusitis (8%), nasopharyngitis (5%), pneumonia (2% to 3%; treatment naive 5%)

Miscellaneous: Diaphoresis (3%)

General Dosage Range Dosage adjustment recommended in patients with renal impairment

Oral: *Children ≥12 years and ≥35 kg and Adults:* 300 mg once daily

Mechanism of Action Tenofovir disoproxil fumarate (TDF) is an analog of adenosine 5'-monophosphate; it interferes with the HIV viral RNA dependent DNA polymerase resulting in inhibition of viral replication. TDF is first converted intracellularly by hydrolysis to tenofovir and subsequently phosphorylated to the active tenofovir diphosphate; nucleotide reverse transcriptase inhibitor. Tenofovir inhibits replication of HBV by inhibiting HBV polymerase.

Pharmacodynamics/Kinetics

Half-life Elimination ~17 hours

Time to Peak Serum: Fasting: 36-84 minutes; With food: 96-144 minutes

Pregnancy Risk Factor B

Terazosin (ter AY zoe sin)

Related Information

Cardiovascular Diseases *on page 1848*

Canadian Brand Names Apo-Terazosin®; Dom-Terazosin; Hytrin®; Nu-Terazosin; PHL-Terazosin; PMS-Terazosin; ratio-Terazosin; Teva-Terazosin

Generic Availability (U.S.) Yes

Pharmacologic Category Alpha$_1$ Blocker

Use Management of mild-to-moderate hypertension; alone or in combination with other agents such as diuretics or beta-blockers; benign prostate hyperplasia (BPH)

Unlabeled/Investigational Use Pediatric hypertension

Local Anesthetic/Vasoconstrictor Precautions No information available to require special precautions

Effects on Dental Treatment Key adverse event(s) related to dental treatment: Xerostomia (normal salivary flow resumes upon discontinuation) and orthostatic hypotension.

Effects on Bleeding No information available to require special precautions

Adverse Effects

>10%:

Central nervous system: Dizziness (9% to 19%)

Neuromuscular & skeletal: Muscle weakness (7% to 11%)

1% to 10%:

Cardiovascular: Peripheral edema (1% to 6%), orthostatic hypotension (1% to 4%), palpitation (≤4%), tachycardia (≤2%), syncope (≤1%)

Central nervous system: Somnolence (4% to 5%), vertigo (1%)
Gastrointestinal: Nausea (2% to 4%)
Genitourinary: Impotence (≤2%), libido decreased (≤1%)
Neuromuscular & skeletal: Extremity pain (≤4%), paresthesia (≤3%), back pain (≤2%)
Ocular: Blurred vision (≤2%)
Respiratory: Nasal congestion (2% to 6%), dyspnea (2% to 3%), sinusitis (≤3%)

Dosage Oral:

Hypertension:

Children (unlabeled use): Initial: 1 mg once daily; gradually increase dose as necessary, up to maximum of 20 mg/day

Adults: Initial: 1 mg at bedtime; slowly increase dose to achieve desired blood pressure, up to 20 mg/day; usual dose range (JNC 7): 1-20 mg once daily

Benign prostatic hyperplasia: Adults: Initial: 1 mg at bedtime; thereafter, titrate upwards, if needed, over several weeks, balancing therapeutic benefit with terazosin-induced postural hypotension; most patients require 10 mg day; if no response after 4-6 weeks of 10 mg/day, may increase to 20 mg/day

Concurrent use with a diuretic or other antihypertensive agent (especially verapamil): Dosage reduction may be needed when adding

Concurrent use with PDE-5 inhibitors: Initiate PDE-5 inhibitor therapy at the lowest dose due to additive orthostatic and blood pressure lowering effects

Note: If drug is discontinued for greater than several days, consider beginning with initial dose and retitrate as needed; dosage may be given on a twice daily regimen if response is diminished at 24 hours and hypotension is observed at 2-4 hours following a dose.

Mechanism of Action $Alpha_1$-specific blocking agent with minimal $alpha_2$ effects; this allows peripheral postsynaptic blockade, with the resultant decrease in arterial tone, while preserving the negative feedback loop which is mediated by the peripheral presynaptic $alpha_2$-receptors; terazosin relaxes the smooth muscle of the bladder neck, thus reducing bladder outlet obstruction

Contraindications Hypersensitivity to terazosin or any component of the formulation

Warnings/Precautions Can cause significant orthostatic hypotension and syncope, especially with first dose; anticipate a similar effect if therapy is interrupted for a few days, if dosage is rapidly increased, or if another antihypertensive drug (particularly vasodilators) or a PDE-5 inhibitor is introduced. Discontinue if symptoms of angina occur or worsen. Patients should be cautioned about performing hazardous tasks when starting new therapy or adjusting dosage upward. Prostate cancer should be ruled out before starting for BPH. Intraoperative floppy iris syndrome has been observed in cataract surgery patients who were on or were previously treated with $alpha_1$-blockers. Causality has not been established and there appears to be no benefit in discontinuing alpha-blocker therapy prior to surgery. Priapism has been associated with use (rarely).

Drug Interactions

Avoid Concomitant Use

Avoid concomitant use of Terazosin with any of the following: Alpha1-Blockers

Increased Effect/Toxicity

Terazosin may increase the levels/effects of: Alpha1-Blockers; Amifostine; Antihypertensives; Calcium Channel Blockers; Hypotensive Agents; RiTUXimab

The levels/effects of Terazosin may be increased by: Beta-Blockers; Diazoxide; Herbs (Hypotensive Properties); MAO Inhibitors; Pentoxifylline; Phosphodiesterase 5 Inhibitors; Prostacyclin Analogues

Decreased Effect

The levels/effects of Terazosin may be decreased by: Herbs (Hypertensive Properties); Methylphenidate; Yohimbine

Ethanol/Nutrition/Herb Interactions Herb/Nutraceutical: Avoid dong quai if using for hypertension (has estrogenic activity). Avoid ephedra, yohimbe, ginseng (may worsen hypertension). Avoid saw palmetto. Avoid garlic (may have increased antihypertensive effect).

Dietary Considerations May be taken without regard to meals at the same time each day.

Pharmacodynamics/Kinetics

Onset of Action 1-2 hours

Half-life Elimination ~12 hours

Time to Peak Serum: ~1 hour

Pregnancy Risk Factor C

Lactation Excretion in breast milk unknown/use caution

Dosage Forms

Capsule, oral: 1 mg, 2 mg, 5 mg, 10 mg

Terbinafine (Systemic) (TER bin a feen)

U.S. Brand Names LamISIL®

Canadian Brand Names Apo-Terbinafine®; CO Terbinafine; JAMP-Terbinafine; Lamisil®; Novo-Terbinafine; Nu-Terbinafine; PHL-Terbinafine; PMS-Terbinafine; Riva-Terbinafine; Sandoz-Terbinafine

Pharmacologic Category Antifungal Agent, Oral

Use Active against most strains of *Trichophyton mentagrophytes*, *Trichophyton rubrum*; may be effective for infections of *Microsporum gypseum* and *M. nanum*, *Trichophyton verrucosum*, *Epidermophyton floccosum*, *Candida albicans*, and *Scopulariopsis brevicaulis*

Onychomycosis of the toenail or fingernail due to susceptible dermatophytes; treatment of tinea capitis

Local Anesthetic/Vasoconstrictor Precautions No information available to require special precautions

Effects on Dental Treatment Key adverse event(s) related to dental treatment: Taste disturbance.

Effects on Bleeding No information available to require special precautions

Adverse Effects Adverse events listed for tablets unless otherwise specified. Granules were studied in patients 4-12 years of age.

>10%: Central nervous system: Headache (13%; granules 7%)

1% to 10%:

Central nervous system: Fever (granules 7%)

Dermatologic: Rash (6%; granules 2%), pruritus (3%; granules 1%), urticaria (1%)

Gastrointestinal: Diarrhea (6%; granules 3%), vomiting (granules 5%), dyspepsia (4%), nausea (3%; granules 2%), taste disturbance (3%), abdominal pain (2%; granules 2% to 4%), toothache (granules 1%)

Hepatic: Liver enzyme abnormalities (3%)

Respiratory: Nasopharyngitis (granules 10%), cough (granules 6%), nasal congestion (granules 2%), pharyngeal pain (granules 2%), rhinorrhea (granules 2%)

General Dosage Range

Oral granules: *Children ≥4 years:*

<25 kg: 125 mg once daily for 6 weeks

25-35 kg: 187.5 mg once daily for 6 weeks

>35 kg: 250 mg once daily for 6 weeks

Oral tablet: *Adults:* 250-500 mg daily in 1-2 divided doses

Mechanism of Action Synthetic allylamine derivative which inhibits squalene epoxidase, a key enzyme in sterol biosynthesis in fungi. This results in a deficiency in ergosterol within the fungal cell wall and results in fungal cell death.

Pharmacodynamics/Kinetics

Half-life Elimination Terminal half-life: 200-400 hours; very slow release of drug from skin and adipose tissues occurs; effective half-life: ~36 hours; Children 27-31 hours

Time to Peak Plasma: Children and Adults: 1-2 hours

Pregnancy Risk Factor B

Terbutaline (ter BYOO ta leen)

Related Information

Respiratory Diseases *on page 1876*

Canadian Brand Names Bricanyl®

Pharmacologic Category Beta$_2$-Adrenergic Agonist

Use Bronchodilator in reversible airway obstruction and bronchial asthma

Unlabeled/Investigational Use Injection: Tocolytic agent (short-term [≤72 hours] prevention or management of preterm labor

Local Anesthetic/Vasoconstrictor Precautions No information available to require special precautions

Effects on Dental Treatment Key adverse event(s) related to dental treatment: Xerostomia (normal salivary flow resumes upon discontinuation) and bad taste in mouth.

Effects on Bleeding No information available to require special precautions

Adverse Effects

>10%:

Central nervous system: Nervousness, restlessness

Endocrine & metabolic: Serum glucose increased, serum potassium decreased

Neuromuscular & skeletal: Trembling

1% to 10%:

Cardiovascular: Tachycardia, hypertension

Central nervous system: Dizziness, drowsiness, headache, insomnia
Gastrointestinal: Xerostomia, nausea, vomiting, bad taste in mouth
Neuromuscular & skeletal: Muscle cramps, weakness
Miscellaneous: Diaphoresis

General Dosage Range Dosage adjustment recommended in patients with renal impairment

Oral:

Children 12-15 years: 2.5 mg every 6 hours 3 times/day (maximum: 7.5 mg/day)
Children >15 years and Adults: 2.5-5 mg every 6 hours 3 times/day (maximum: 15 mg/day)

SubQ:

Children <12 years: 0.005-0.01 mg/kg/dose to a maximum of 0.4 mg/dose; may repeat in 15-20 minutes
Children ≥12 years and Adults: 0.25 mg/dose; may repeat in 15-30 minutes (maximum: 0.5 mg/4-hour period)

Mechanism of Action Relaxes bronchial smooth muscle by action on $beta_2$-receptors with less effect on heart rate

Pharmacodynamics/Kinetics

Onset of Action Oral: 30-45 minutes; SubQ: 6-15 minutes

Half-life Elimination 11-16 hours

Pregnancy Risk Factor B

Terconazole (ter KONE a zole)

U.S. Brand Names Terazol® 3; Terazol® 7; Zazole™ [DSC]

Canadian Brand Names Terazol®

Pharmacologic Category Antifungal Agent, Vaginal

Use Local treatment of vulvovaginal candidiasis

Local Anesthetic/Vasoconstrictor Precautions No information available to require special precautions

Effects on Dental Treatment No significant effects or complications reported

Effects on Bleeding No information available to require special precautions

Adverse Effects 1% to 10%:

Central nervous system; Fever, chills
Gastrointestinal: Abdominal pain
Genitourinary: Vulvar/vaginal burning, dysmenorrhea

General Dosage Range Intravaginal: *Adults:* Insert 1 applicatorful or suppository at bedtime

Mechanism of Action Triazole ketal antifungal agent; involves inhibition of fungal cytochrome P450. Specifically, terconazole inhibits cytochrome P450-dependent 14-alpha-demethylase which results in accumulation of membrane disturbing 14-alpha-demethylsterols and ergosterol depletion.

Pregnancy Risk Factor C

Teriparatide (ter i PAR a tide)

Related Information

Rheumatoid Arthritis, Osteoarthritis, and Osteoporosis *on page* 1889

U.S. Brand Names Forteo®

Canadian Brand Names Forteo®

Pharmacologic Category Parathyroid Hormone Analog

Use Treatment of osteoporosis in postmenopausal women at high risk of fracture; treatment of primary or hypogonadal osteoporosis in men at high risk of fracture; treatment of glucocorticoid-induced osteoporosis in men and women at high risk for fracture

Local Anesthetic/Vasoconstrictor Precautions No information available to require special precautions

Effects on Dental Treatment Key adverse event(s) related to dental treatment: Tooth disorder.

Effects on Bleeding No information available to require special precautions

Adverse Effects

>10%: Endocrine & metabolic: Hypercalcemia (transient increases noted 4-6 hours postdose [women 11%; men 6%])

1% to 10%:

Cardiovascular: Orthostatic hypotension (5%; transient), chest pain (3%), syncope (3%)
Central nervous system: Dizziness (8%), insomnia (4% to 5%), anxiety (≤4%), depression (4%), vertigo (4%)
Dermatologic: Rash (5%)

Endocrine & metabolic: Hyperuricemia (3%)
Gastrointestinal: Nausea (9% to 14%), gastritis (≤7%), dyspepsia (5%), vomiting (3%), tooth disorder (2%)
Neuromuscular & skeletal: Arthralgia (10%), weakness (9%), leg cramps (3%)
Respiratory: Rhinitis (10%), pharyngitis (6%), dyspnea (4% to 6%), pneumonia (4% to 6%)
Miscellaneous: Antibodies to teriparatide (3% of women in long-term treatment; hypersensitivity reactions or decreased efficacy were not associated in preclinical trials), herpes zoster (≤3%)

General Dosage Range
SubQ: *Adults:* 20 mcg once daily

Mechanism of Action Teriparatide is a recombinant formulation of endogenous parathyroid hormone (PTH), containing a 34-amino-acid sequence which is identical to the N-terminal portion of this hormone. The pharmacologic activity of teriparatide, which is similar to the physiologic activity of PTH, includes stimulating osteoblast function, increasing gastrointestinal calcium absorption, and increasing renal tubular reabsorption of calcium. Treatment with teriparatide results in increased bone mineral density, bone mass, and strength. In postmenopausal women, teriparatide has been shown to decrease osteoporosis-related fractures.

Pharmacodynamics/Kinetics
Half-life Elimination I.V.: 5 minutes; SubQ: ~1 hour
Time to Peak Serum: ~30 minutes

Pregnancy Risk Factor C

Tesamorelin (tes a moe REL in)

U.S. Brand Names Egrifta™

Pharmacologic Category Growth Hormone Releasing Factor

Use Reduction of excess abdominal fat in HIV-infected patients with lipodystrophy

Local Anesthetic/Vasoconstrictor Precautions No information available to require special precautions

Effects on Dental Treatment No significant effects or complications reported

Effects on Bleeding No information available to require special precautions

Adverse Effects Note: The incidence of adverse reactions generally decreases with treatment continued beyond 26 weeks.

10%:
Local: Injection site reactions (6% to 25%; includes erythema [1% to 9%], pruritus [2% to 8%], pain [4%], irritation [3%], hemorrhage [2%], swelling [2%], urticaria [2%], rash [1%])
Neuromuscular & skeletal: Arthralgia (13%)

1% to 10%:
Cardiovascular: Peripheral edema (2% to 6%), hypertension (1% to 2%), chest pain (1%), palpitation (1%)
Central nervous system: Hypoesthesia (2% to 4%), depression (2%), pain (2%), insomnia (1%)
Dermatologic: Rash (4%), pruritus (1% to 2%), urticaria (1%)
Endocrine & metabolic: Hb A_{1c} increased (5%), hot flush (1%), hyperglycemia
Gastrointestinal: Nausea (4%), vomiting (2% to 3%), dyspepsia (2%), abdominal pain (1%)
Neuromuscular & skeletal: Pain in extremity (3% to 6%), myalgia (1% to 6%), paresthesia (2% to 5%), carpal tunnel syndrome (2%), creatine phosphokinase increased (2%), muscle stiffness (2%), musculoskeletal pain (2%), joint stiffness (2%), peripheral neuropathy (2%), joint swelling (1%), muscle spasm (1%), muscle strain (1%)
Miscellaneous: Hypersensitivity reactions (1% to 4%), night sweats (1%)

General Dosage Range SubQ: *Adults:* 2 mg once daily

Mechanism of Action Tesamorelin binds to pituitary growth hormone-releasing factor (GRF) receptors and stimulates the secretion of endogenous growth hormone which has anabolic and lipolytic properties. Growth hormone exerts its effects by interacting with receptors on target cells such as osteoblasts, myocytes, hepatocytes, and adipocytes to promote the reduction of total fat mass. These effects are primarily mediated by IGF-1 produced in the liver and in peripheral tissues.

Pharmacodynamics/Kinetics
Half-life Elimination Healthy adults: 26 minutes; HIV-infected patients: 38 minutes
Time to Peak 9 minutes

Pregnancy Risk Factor X

Prescribing and Access Restrictions In order to prescribe Egrifta™, healthcare providers must call the Axis Center at 1-877-714-2947. Egrifta™ is only available through specialty pharmacy distribution.

Testosterone (tes TOS ter one)

U.S. Brand Names Androderm®; AndroGel®; Axiron®; Delatestryl®; Depo®-Testosterone; First®-Testosterone; First®-Testosterone MC; Fortesta™; Striant®; Testim®; Testopel®

Canadian Brand Names Andriol®; Androderm®; AndroGel®; Andropository; Delatestryl®; Depotest® 100; Everone® 200; PMS-Testosterone; Testim®

Pharmacologic Category Androgen

Use

Injection: Androgen replacement therapy in the treatment of delayed male puberty; male hypogonadism (primary or hypogonadotropic); inoperable metastatic female breast cancer (enanthate only)

Pellet: Androgen replacement therapy in the treatment of delayed male puberty; male hypogonadism (primary or hypogonadotropic)

Buccal system, topical gel, topical solution, transdermal system: Male hypogonadism (primary or hypogonadotropic)

Capsule (not available in U.S.): Conditions associated with a deficiency or absence of endogenous testosterone

Unlabeled/Investigational Use Androgen deficiency in men with AIDS wasting; postmenopausal women (short-term use in select cases)

Local Anesthetic/Vasoconstrictor Precautions No information available to require special precautions

Effects on Dental Treatment Key adverse event(s) related to dental treatment: Buccal administration: Bitter taste, gum edema, gum or mouth irritation, gum tenderness, and taste perversion.

Effects on Bleeding No information available to require special precautions

Adverse Effects Frequency not always defined.

Cardiovascular: Deep venous thrombosis, edema, hypertension, vasodilation

Central nervous system: Abnormal dreams, aggressive behavior, anger, amnesia, anxiety, blood pressure decreased, depression, dizziness, emotional lability, excitation, headache, hostility, insomnia, malaise, memory loss, mood swings, nervousness, seizure, sleep apnea, sleeplessness

Dermatologic: Acne, alopecia, dry skin, folliculitis, hair discoloration, hirsutism (increase in pubic hair growth), pruritus, rash, seborrhea

Endocrine & metabolic: Breast pain/soreness, gonadotropin secretion decreased, growth acceleration, gynecomastia, hot flashes, hypercalcemia, hyperchloremia, hypercholesterolemia, hyper-/hypoglycemia, hyper-/hypokalemia, hyperlipidemia, hypernatremia, inorganic phosphate retention, libido changes, menstrual problems (including amenorrhea), virilism, water retention

Gastrointestinal: Appetite increased, diarrhea, GI bleeding, GI irritation, nausea, taste disorder, vomiting, weight gain

Following buccal administration (most common): Bitter taste, gum edema, gum or mouth irritation, gum pain, gum tenderness, taste perversion

Genitourinary: Bladder irritability, impotence, oligospermia, penile erections (spontaneous), priapism, prostatic carcinoma, prostatic hyperplasia, PSA increased, testicular atrophy, urination impaired

Hepatic: Bilirubin increased, cholestatic hepatitis, cholestatic jaundice, hepatic dysfunction, hepatic necrosis, hepatocellular neoplasms, liver function test changes, peliosis hepatis

Hematologic: Anemia, bleeding, hematocrit/hemoglobin increased, leukopenia, polycythemia, suppression of clotting factors

Local: Application site reaction (gel, solution), injection site inflammation/pain

Transdermal system: Pruritus at application site (37%), burn-like blisters under system (12%), erythema at application site (7%), vesicles at application site (6%), allergic contact dermatitis to system (4%), burning at application site (3%), induration at application site (3%)

Neuromuscular & skeletal: Hyperkinesias, paresthesia, weakness

Ocular: Lacrimation increased

Renal: Creatinine increased

Respiratory: Dyspnea, nasopharyngitis

Miscellaneous: Anaphylactoid reactions, diaphoresis, hypersensitivity reactions, smell disorder

General Dosage Range

Buccal: *Adults (males):* 30 mg every 12 hours

I.M.: *Adolescents and Adults (males):* 50-400 mg every 2-4 weeks

SubQ: *Adolescents and Adults (males):* 150-450 mg every 3-6 months

Transdermal: *Adults (males):* Androderm®: Apply 2.5-7.5 mg/day; AndroGel®, Testim®: 5-10 g (50-100 mg testosterone) applied once daily (maximum: 10 g/day); Axiron®: Apply 30-120 mg/day; Fortesta™: Apply 10-70 mg/day

Mechanism of Action Principal endogenous androgen responsible for promoting the growth and development of the male sex organs and maintaining secondary sex characteristics in androgen-deficient males

Pharmacodynamics/Kinetics

Duration of Action Route and ester dependent; I.M.: Cypionate and enanthate esters have longest duration, ≤2-4 weeks; gel: 24-48 hours

Half-life Elimination Variable: 10-100 minutes

Pregnancy Risk Factor X

Product Availability AndroGel® 1.62%: FDA approved April 2011, availability expected in the second quarter 2011

Controlled Substance C-III

Tetanus Immune Globulin (Human)

(TET a nus i MYUN GLOB yoo lin HYU man)

U.S. Brand Names HyperTET™ S/D

Canadian Brand Names HyperTET™ S/D

Pharmacologic Category Immune Globulin

Use Prophylaxis against tetanus following injury in patients where immunization status is not known or uncertain

The Advisory Committee on Immunization Practices (ACIP) recommends passive immunization with TIG for the following:

- Persons with a wound that is not clean or minor and in whom contraindications to a tetanus-toxoid containing vaccine exist and they have not completed a primary series of tetanus toxoid immunization.
- Persons who are wounded in bombings or similar mass casualty events who have penetrating injuries or nonintact skin exposure and who cannot confirm receipt of a tetanus booster within the previous 5 years. In case of shortage, use should be reserved for persons ≥60 years of age.

Local Anesthetic/Vasoconstrictor Precautions No information available to require special precautions

Effects on Dental Treatment No significant effects or complications reported

Effects on Bleeding No information available to require special precautions

Adverse Effects Frequency not defined.

Central nervous system: Temperature increased

Dermatologic: Angioneurotic edema (rare)

Local: Injection site: pain, soreness, tenderness

Renal: Nephritic syndrome (rare)

Miscellaneous: Anaphylactic shock (rare)

General Dosage Range I.M.:

Children <7 years: Prophylaxis: 4 units/kg

Children ≥7 years: Prophylaxis: 250 units

Children: Treatment: 500-6000 units

Adults: Prophylaxis: 250 units; Treatment: 500-6000 units

Mechanism of Action Passive immunity toward tetanus

Pregnancy Risk Factor C

Tetanus Toxoid (Adsorbed) (TET a nus TOKS oyd, ad SORBED)

Pharmacologic Category Vaccine, Inactivated (Bacterial)

Use Active immunization against tetanus when combination antigen preparations are not indicated; tetanus prophylaxis in wound management. **Note:** Tetanus and diphtheria toxoids for adult use (Td) is the preferred immunizing agent for most adults and for children after their seventh birthday. Young children should receive trivalent DTaP (diphtheria/tetanus/acellular pertussis) as part of their childhood immunization program, unless pertussis is contraindicated, then DT is warranted.

Local Anesthetic/Vasoconstrictor Precautions No information available to require special precautions

Effects on Dental Treatment No significant effects or complications reported

Effects on Bleeding No information available to require special precautions

Adverse Effects All serious adverse reactions must be reported to the U.S. Department of Health and Human Services (DHHS) Vaccine Adverse Event Reporting System (VAERS) 1-800-822-7967 or online at https://vaers.hhs.gov/esub/index.

Frequency not defined.

Cardiovascular: Hypotension

Central nervous system: Brachial neuritis, fever, malaise, pain

Gastrointestinal: Nausea

Local: Edema, induration (with or without tenderness), rash, redness, urticaria, warmth

Neuromuscular: Arthralgia, Guillain-Barré syndrome

Miscellaneous: Anaphylactic reaction, Arthus-type hypersensitivity reaction

General Dosage Range I.M.: *Children ≥7 years and Adults:* Initial: 0.5 mL; repeat at 4-8 weeks after first dose and 6-12 months after second dose

Mechanism of Action Tetanus toxoid preparations contain the toxin produced by virulent tetanus bacilli (detoxified growth products of *Clostridium tetani*). The toxin has been modified by treatment with formaldehyde so that it has lost toxicity but still retains ability to act as antigen and produce active immunity; the aluminum salt, a mineral adjuvant, delays the rate of absorption and prolongs and enhances its properties; duration ~10 years.

Pharmacodynamics/Kinetics

Duration of Action Primary immunization: ~10 years

Pregnancy Risk Factor C

Tetrabenazine (tet ra BEN a zeen)

U.S. Brand Names Xenazine®

Canadian Brand Names Nitoman™

Pharmacologic Category Central Monoamine-Depleting Agent

Use Treatment of chorea associated with Huntington's disease

Canadian labeling: Treatment of hyperkinetic movement disorders, including Huntington's chorea, hemiballismus, senile chorea, Tourette syndrome, and tardive dyskinesia

Local Anesthetic/Vasoconstrictor Precautions No information available to require special precautions

Effects on Dental Treatment Key adverse event(s) related to dental treatment: Orthostatic hypotension has been reported; monitor patient during erect posture from dental chair and dysphagia.

Effects on Bleeding No information available to require special precautions

Adverse Effects Note: Many adverse effects are dose-related and may resolve at lower dosages. Adverse effects reported for adults with chorea associated with Huntington's disease.

>10%:

Central nervous system: Extrapyramidal symptoms (15% to 33%), sedation (31%), somnolence (31%), fatigue (22%), insomnia (22%), akathisia (19%), depression (19%), anxiety (15%)

Gastrointestinal: Nausea (13%)

Neuromuscular & skeletal: Falls (15%)

Respiratory: Upper respiratory tract infection (11%)

1% to 10%:

Central nervous system: Parkinsonism (3% to 10%), irritability (9%), dizziness (4%), headache (4%), obsessive reaction (4%)

Dermatologic: Bruising (6%)

Gastrointestinal: Dysphagia (4% to 10%), vomiting (6%), appetite decreased (4%), diarrhea (2%)

Genitourinary: Dysuria (4%)

Neuromuscular & skeletal: Balance difficulty (9%), bradykinesia (9%), dysarthria (4%), gait disturbance (4%)

Respiratory: Bronchitis (4%), dyspnea (4%)

General Dosage Range Dosage adjustment recommended in patients on concomitant therapy or who develop toxicities

Oral: *Adults:* 12.5 mg once daily; Maintenance: 25-100 mg/day in 2-3 divided doses

Mechanism of Action Within basal ganglia, interferes with and depletes monoamine neurotransmitters (including dopamine, serotonin, and norepinephrine) in presynaptic vesicles (likely through actions on vesicle monoamine transporter). Tetrabenazine inhibits presynaptic dopamine release and also blocks CNS dopamine receptors. The effects resemble reserpine but with less peripheral activity and a shorter duration of action. Treatment results in symptomatic improvement of hyperkinetic movement disorders, including Huntington's chorea, hemiballismus, senile chorea, Tic and Hille's de la Tourette syndrome, and tardive dyskinesia.

Pharmacodynamics/Kinetics

Duration of Action 16-24 hours (at steady-state); chorea may recur within 12-18 hours after discontinuation

Half-life Elimination Alpha-HTBZ: 4-8 hours; Beta-HTBZ: 2-4 hours (increased with hepatic impairment)

Time to Peak Within 1-1.5 hours

Pregnancy Risk Factor C

Prescribing and Access Restrictions Xenazine® is available only through specialty pharmacies. For more information regarding the procurement of Xenazine®, healthcare providers, patients, and caregivers may contact the Xenazine® Information Center (XIC) at 1-888-882-6013 or at:

Healthcare providers: http://www.xenazineusa.com/HCP/PrescribingXenazine/Default.aspx

Patients and caregivers: http://www.xenazineusa.com/AboutXenazine/Getting-Your-Prescription.aspx

Tetracaine (Systemic) (TET ra kane)

U.S. Brand Names Pontocaine® Niphanoid® [DSC]; Pontocaine® [DSC]

Canadian Brand Names Pontocaine®

Generic Availability (U.S.) Yes

Pharmacologic Category Local Anesthetic

Dental Use Ester-type local anesthetic

Use Spinal anesthesia

Local Anesthetic/Vasoconstrictor Precautions No information available to require special precautions

Effects on Dental Treatment No significant effects or complications reported

Effects on Bleeding No information available to require special precautions

Adverse Effects Frequency not defined. **Note:** Adverse effects listed are those characteristics of local anesthetics. Systemic adverse effects are generally associated with excessive doses or rapid absorption.

Cardiovascular: Cardiac arrest, hypotension

Central nervous system: Chills, convulsions, dizziness, drowsiness, nervousness, unconsciousness

Dermatologic: Urticaria

Gastrointestinal: Nausea, vomiting

Hematologic: Methemoglobinemia

Neuromuscular & skeletal: Tremors

Ocular: Blurred vision, pupil constriction

Otic: Tinnitus

Respiratory: Respiratory arrest

Miscellaneous: Allergic reaction, anaphylaxis

Dosage Injection: Adults: Spinal anesthesia: **Note:** Dosage varies with the anesthetic procedure, the degree of anesthesia required, and the individual patient response; it is administered by subarachnoid injection for spinal anesthesia.

Perineal anesthesia: 5 mg

Perineal and lower extremities: 10 mg

Anesthesia extending up to costal margin: 15 mg; doses up to 20 mg may be given, but are reserved for exceptional cases

Low spinal anesthesia (saddle block): 2-5 mg

Mechanism of Action Ester local anesthetic blocks both the initiation and conduction of nerve impulses by decreasing the neuronal membrane's permeability to sodium ions, which results in inhibition of depolarization with resultant blockade of conduction

Contraindications Hypersensitivity to tetracaine, ester-type anesthetics, aminobenzoic acid, or any component of the formulation; injection should not be used when spinal anesthesia is contraindicated

Warnings/Precautions Use with caution in patients with cardiac disease (especially rhythm disturbances, heart block, or shock), hyperthyroidism, and abnormal or decreased levels of plasma esterases. Use of the lowest effective dose is recommended. Acutely ill, elderly, debilitated, obstetric patients, or patients with increased intra-abdominal pressure may require decreased doses. Products may contain sodium bisulfite which may cause allergic reactions in some individuals. Dental practitioners and/or clinicians using local anesthetic agents should be well-trained in diagnosis and management of emergencies that may arise from the use of these agents. Resuscitative equipment, oxygen, and other resuscitative drugs should be available for immediate use.

Drug Interactions

Avoid Concomitant Use There are no known interactions where it is recommended to avoid concomitant use.

Increased Effect/Toxicity There are no known significant interactions involving an increase in effect.

Decreased Effect There are no known significant interactions involving a decrease in effect.

Pregnancy Risk Factor C
Lactation Excretion in breast milk unknown/use caution
Dosage Forms
Injection, solution [preservative free]: 1% [10 mg/mL] (2 mL)

Tetracaine (Topical) (TET ra kane)

Related Information
Oral Pain *on page 1928*
Ulcerative, Erosive, and Painful Oral Mucosal Disorders *on page 1950*
U.S. Brand Names Pontocaine® [DSC]
Canadian Brand Names Ametop™; Pontocaine®
Generic Availability (U.S.) No
Pharmacologic Category Local Anesthetic
Dental Use Ester-type local anesthetic; applied to throat for various diagnostic procedures and on cold sores and fever blisters for pain
Use Applied to nose and throat for diagnostic procedures
Local Anesthetic/Vasoconstrictor Precautions No information available to require special precautions
Effects on Dental Treatment No significant effects or complications reported
Effects on Bleeding No information available to require special precautions
Adverse Effects Frequency not defined. **Note:** Adverse effects listed are those characteristics of local anesthetics. Systemic adverse effects are generally associated with excessive doses or rapid absorption.

Cardiovascular: Cardiac arrest, hypotension
Central nervous system: Chills, convulsions, dizziness, drowsiness, nervousness, unconsciousness
Dermatologic: Urticaria
Gastrointestinal: Nausea, vomiting
Hematologic: Methemoglobinemia
Neuromuscular & skeletal: Tremors
Ocular: Blurred vision, pupil constriction
Otic: Tinnitus
Respiratory: Respiratory arrest
Miscellaneous: Allergic reaction, anaphylaxis

Dental Usual Dosage Topical mucous membranes (rhinolaryngology): Adults: Used as a 0.25% or 0.5% solution by direct application or nebulization; total dose should not exceed 20 mg
Dosage Adults: Topical mucous membranes (rhinolaryngology): Used as a 0.25% or 0.5% solution by direct application or nebulization; total dose should not exceed 20 mg
Mechanism of Action Ester local anesthetic blocks both the initiation and conduction of nerve impulses by decreasing the neuronal membrane's permeability to sodium ions, which results in inhibition of depolarization with resultant blockade of conduction
Contraindications Hypersensitivity to tetracaine, ester-type anesthetics, aminobenzoic acid, or any component of the formulation
Warnings/Precautions For topical use only. Use with caution in patients with cardiac disease, hyperthyroidism, and abnormal or decreased levels of plasma esterases. Use of the lowest effective dose is recommended. Use caution in acutely ill, elderly, debilitated, or obstetric patients. Dental practitioners and/or clinicians using local anesthetic agents should be well trained in diagnosis and management of emergencies that may arise from the use of these agents. Resuscitative equipment, oxygen, and other resuscitative drugs should be available for immediate use.
Drug Interactions
Avoid Concomitant Use There are no known interactions where it is recommended to avoid concomitant use.
Increased Effect/Toxicity There are no known significant interactions involving an increase in effect.
Decreased Effect There are no known significant interactions involving a decrease in effect.
Pharmacodynamics/Kinetics
Onset of Action Anesthetic: Rhinolaryngology: 5-10 minutes
Duration of Action Rhinolaryngology: ~30 minutes
Pregnancy Risk Factor C
Lactation Excretion in breast milk unknown/use caution
Dosage Forms
Solution, topical:
Pontocaine®: 2% [20 mg/mL] (30 mL, 118 mL)

Tetracycline (tet ra SYE kleen)

Related Information

Bacterial Infections *on page* 1933
Gastrointestinal Disorders *on page* 1874
Periodontal Diseases *on page* 1942
Ulcerative, Erosive, and Painful Oral Mucosal Disorders *on page* 1950

Canadian Brand Names Apo-Tetra®; Nu-Tetra

Generic Availability (U.S.) Yes: Capsule

Pharmacologic Category Antibiotic, Tetracycline Derivative

Dental Use Treatment of periodontitis associated with presence of *Actinobacillus actinomycetemcomitans* (AA); as adjunctive therapy in recurrent aphthous ulcers

Use Treatment of susceptible bacterial infections of both gram-positive and gram-negative organisms; also infections due to *Mycoplasma*, *Chlamydia*, and *Rickettsia*; indicated for acne, exacerbations of chronic bronchitis, and treatment of gonorrhea and syphilis in patients who are allergic to penicillin; as part of a multidrug regimen for *H. pylori* eradication to reduce the risk of duodenal ulcer recurrence

Unlabeled/Investigational Use Treatment of periodontitis associated with presence of *Actinobacillus actinomycetemcomitans* (AA)

Local Anesthetic/Vasoconstrictor Precautions No information available to require special precautions

Effects on Dental Treatment Key adverse event(s) related to dental treatment: Esophagitis, superinfections, and candidal superinfection. Opportunistic "superinfection" with *Candida albicans*; tetracyclines are not recommended for use during pregnancy or in children ≤8 years of age since they have been reported to cause enamel hypoplasia and permanent teeth discoloration. The use of tetracyclines should only be used in these patients if other agents are contraindicated or alternative antimicrobials will not eradicate the organism. Long-term use associated with oral candidiasis.

Effects on Bleeding No information available to require special precautions

Adverse Effects Frequency not defined.

Cardiovascular: Pericarditis

Central nervous system: Intracranial pressure increased, bulging fontanels in infants, pseudotumor cerebri, paresthesia

Dermatologic: Photosensitivity, pruritus, pigmentation of nails, exfoliative dermatitis

Endocrine & metabolic: Diabetes insipidus syndrome

Gastrointestinal: Discoloration of teeth and enamel hypoplasia (young children), nausea, diarrhea, vomiting, esophagitis, anorexia, abdominal cramps, antibiotic-associated pseudomembranous colitis, staphylococcal enterocolitis, pancreatitis

Hematologic: Thrombophlebitis

Hepatic: Hepatotoxicity

Renal: Acute renal failure, azotemia, renal damage

Miscellaneous: Superinfection, anaphylaxis, hypersensitivity reactions, candidal superinfection

Dental Usual Dosage Periodontitis: Adults: Oral: 250 mg every 6 hours until improvement (usually 10 days)

Dosage

Usual dosage range:

Children >8 years: Oral: 25-50 mg/kg/day in divided doses every 6 hours

Adults: Oral: 250-500 mg/dose every 6 hours

Indication-specific dosing:

Adults: Oral:

Acne: 250-500 twice daily

Chronic bronchitis, acute exacerbation: 500 mg 4 times/day

Erlichiosis: 500 mg 4 times/day for 7-14 days

Peptic ulcer disease: Eradication of *Helicobacter pylori*: 500 mg 2-4 times/day depending on regimen; requires combination therapy with at least one other antibiotic and an acid-suppressing agent (proton pump inhibitor or H_2 blocker)

Periodontitis (unlabeled use): 250 mg every 6 hours until improvement (usually 10 days)

Vibrio cholerae: 500 mg 4 times/day for 3 days

Dosing interval in renal impairment:

Cl_{cr} 50-80 mL/minute: Administer every 8-12 hours

Cl_{cr} 10-50 mL/minute: Administer every 12-24 hours

Cl_{cr} <10 mL/minute: Administer every 24 hours

Dialysis: Slightly dialyzable (5% to 20%) via hemo- and peritoneal dialysis or via continuous arteriovenous or venovenous hemofiltration; no supplemental dosage necessary

Dosing adjustment in hepatic impairment: Use caution; no dosing adjustment required

Mechanism of Action Inhibits bacterial protein synthesis by binding with the 30S and possibly the 50S ribosomal subunit(s) of susceptible bacteria; may also cause alterations in the cytoplasmic membrane

Contraindications Hypersensitivity to tetracycline or any component of the formulation; do not administer to children ≤8 years of age; pregnancy

Warnings/Precautions Use with caution in patients with renal or hepatic impairment (eg, elderly); dosage modification required in patients with renal impairment since it may increase BUN as an antianabolic agent. Hepatotoxicity has been reported rarely; risk may be increased in patients with pre-existing hepatic or renal impairment. Pseudotumor cerebri has been reported with tetracycline use (usually resolves with discontinuation); outdated drug can cause nephropathy; use protective measure to avoid photosensitivity. Prolonged use may result in fungal or bacterial superinfection, including *C. difficile*-associated diarrhea (CDAD) and pseudomembranous colitis; CDAD has been observed >2 months postantibiotic treatment. May cause tissue hyperpigmentation, enamel hypoplasia, or permanent tooth discoloration; use of tetracyclines should be avoided during tooth development (children ≤8 years of age) unless other drugs are not likely to be effective or are contraindicated. However, recommended in treatment of anthrax exposure. Do not use during pregnancy. In addition to affecting tooth development, tetracycline use has been associated with retardation of skeletal development and reduced bone growth.

Drug Interactions

Metabolism/Transport Effects Substrate of CYP3A4 (major); **Inhibits** CYP3A4 (moderate)

Avoid Concomitant Use

Avoid concomitant use of Tetracycline with any of the following: BCG; Retinoic Acid Derivatives; Tolvaptan

Increased Effect/Toxicity

Tetracycline may increase the levels/effects of: Budesonide (Systemic, Oral Inhalation); Colchicine; CYP3A4 Substrates; Eplerenone; Everolimus; FentaNYL; Halofantrine; Lurasidone; Neuromuscular-Blocking Agents; Pimecrolimus; Ranolazine; Retinoic Acid Derivatives; Salmeterol; Saxagliptin; Tolvaptan; Vilazodone; Vitamin K Antagonists

The levels/effects of Tetracycline may be increased by: Conivaptan

Decreased Effect

Tetracycline may decrease the levels/effects of: Atovaquone; BCG; Penicillins; Typhoid Vaccine

The levels/effects of Tetracycline may be decreased by: Antacids; Bile Acid Sequestrants; Bismuth; Bismuth Subsalicylate; Calcium Salts; CYP3A4 Inducers (Strong); Deferasirox; Herbs (CYP3A4 Inducers); Iron Salts; Magnesium Salts; Quinapril; Sucralfate; Tocilizumab; Zinc Salts

Ethanol/Nutrition/Herb Interactions

Food: Serum concentrations may be decreased if taken with dairy products.

Herb/Nutraceutical: Avoid dong quai, St John's wort (may also cause photosensitization)

Dietary Considerations Take on an empty stomach (ie, 1 hour prior to, or 2 hours after meals). Take at least 1-2 hours prior to, or 4 hours after antacid.

Pharmacodynamics/Kinetics

Half-life Elimination Normal renal function: 8-11 hours; End-stage renal disease: 57-108 hours

Time to Peak Serum: Oral: 2-4 hours

Pregnancy Risk Factor D

Lactation Enters breast milk/not recommended (AAP rates "compatible"; AAP 2001 update pending)

Breast-Feeding Considerations Tetracyclines are excreted in breast milk. Tetracycline binds to calcium. The calcium in the maternal milk will decrease the amount of tetracycline absorbed by the breast-feeding infant. Nondose-related effects could include modification of bowel flora.

Dosage Forms

Capsule, oral: 250 mg, 500 mg

References

Gordon JM and Walker CB, "Current Status of Systemic Antibiotic Usage in Destructive Periodontal Disease," *J Periodontol*, 1993, 64(8 Suppl): 760-71.

Rams TE and Slots J, "Antibiotics in Periodontal Therapy: An Update," *Compendium*, 1992, 13(12):1130, 1132, 1134.

Seymour RA and Heasman PA, "Tetracyclines in the Management of Periodontal Diseases. A Review," *J Clin Periodontol*, 1995, 22(1):22-35.

Seymour RA and Heasman PA, "Pharmacological Control of Periodontal Disease. II. Antimicrobial Agents," *J Dent*, 1995, 23(1):5-14

Tetracycline Periodontal Fibers

(tet ra SYE kleen per ee oh DON tal FYE bers)

U.S. Brand Names Actisite®

Generic Availability (U.S.) No

Pharmacologic Category Antibacterial, Dental

Dental Use Treatment of adult periodontitis; as an adjunct to scaling and root planing for the reduction of pocket depth and bleeding on probing in selected patients with adult periodontitis

Use Used exclusively in dental applications

Local Anesthetic/Vasoconstrictor Precautions No information available to require special precautions

Effects on Dental Treatment Key adverse event(s) related to dental treatment: Gingival inflammation, mouth pain, glossitis, candidiasis, staining of tongue, local erythema following removal, and discomfort from fiber placement.

Effects on Bleeding No information available to require special precautions

Adverse Effects 1% to 10%:

Dermatologic: Local erythema following removal

Miscellaneous: Discomfort from fiber placement

Dosage

Children: Has not been established

Adults: Insert fiber to fill the periodontal pocket; each fiber contains 12.7 mg of tetracycline in 23 cm (9 inches) and provides continuous release of drug for 10 days; fibers are to be secured in pocket with cyanoacrylate adhesive and left in place for 10 days

Mechanism of Action Tetracycline is an antibiotic which inhibits growth of susceptible microorganisms. Tetracycline binds primarily to the 30S subunits of bacterial ribosomes, and appears to prevent access of aminoacyl tRNA to the acceptor site on the mRNA-ribosome complex. The fiber releases tetracycline into the periodontal site at a rate of 2 mcg/cm/hour.

Contraindications Hypersensitivity to tetracyclines or any component of the formulation

Drug Interactions

Avoid Concomitant Use There are no known interactions where it is recommended to avoid concomitant use.

Increased Effect/Toxicity There are no known significant interactions involving an increase in effect.

Decreased Effect There are no known significant interactions involving a decrease in effect.

Pregnancy Risk Factor C

Lactation Excretion in breast milk unknown

Dosage Forms

Fibers:

Actisite®: 23 cm (9") in length

References

Baer PN, "Actisite (Tetracycline Hydrochloride Periodontal Fiber): A Critique," *Periodontal Clin Investig*, 1994, 16(2):5-7.

Greenstein G, "Treating Periodontal Diseases With Tetracycline-Impregnated Fibers: Data and Controversies," *Compend Contin Educ Dent*, 1995, 16(5)448-55.

Kerry G, "Tetracycline-Loaded Fibers as Adjunctive Treatment in Periodontal Disease," *J Am Dent Assoc*, 1994, 125(9):1199-203.

Michalowicz BS, Pihlstrom BL, Drisko CL, et al, "Evaluation of Periodontal Treatments Using Controlled-Release Tetracycline Fibers: Maintenance Response," *J Periodontol*, 1995, 66(8):708-15.

Mombelli A, Lehmann B, Tonetti M, et al, "Clinical Response to Local Delivery of Tetracycline in Relation to Overall and Local Periodontal Conditions," *J Clin Periodontol*, 1997, 24(7):470-77.

Vandekerckhove BN, Quirynen M, and van Steenberghe D, "The Use of Tetracycline-Containing Controlled-Release Fibers in the Treatment of Refractory Periodontitis," *J Periodontol*, 1997, 68 (4):353-61.

Tetrahydrocannabinol and Cannabidiol

(TET ra hye droe can NAB e nol & can nab e DYE ol)

Canadian Brand Names Sativex®

Pharmacologic Category Analgesic, Miscellaneous

Use Adjunctive treatment of neuropathic pain or spasticity in multiple sclerosis; adjunctive treatment of moderate-to-severe pain in advanced cancer

Local Anesthetic/Vasoconstrictor Precautions No information available to require special precautions

Effects on Dental Treatment Key adverse event(s) related to dental treatment: Xerostomia and changes in salivation (normal salivary flow resumes upon discontinuation), abnormal taste, oral pain, orthostatic hypotension; administered as buccal spray, associated with irritation to the buccal (oral) mucosa.

Effects on Bleeding No information available to require special precautions

Adverse Effects

>10%:

Central nervous system: Dizziness (12% to 25%), somnolence (8% to 15%), fatigue (13%)

Gastrointestinal: Nausea (10% to 12%)

1% to 10%:

Cardiovascular: Hypotension (5%), palpitation (1%), syncope (1%), tachycardia (1%)

Central nervous system: Confusion (7%), vertigo (5% to 7%), disorientation (4%), attention disturbance (3% to 4%), depression (3%), headache (3%), impaired balance (3%), insomnia (3%), panic attack (3%), euphoria (2% to 3%), hallucination (≤3%), dissociation (2%), feeling abnormal (2%), lethargy (2%), amnesia (1%), malaise (1%), memory impairment (1%), paranoia (1%), suicidal ideation (1%)

Gastrointestinal: Vomiting (4% to 8%), diarrhea (6% to 7%), xerostomia (6%), glossodynia (3%), oral candidiasis (3%), taste abnormal (3%), anorexia (2%), constipation (2%), mouth ulceration (2%), oral mucosal disorder (2%), tooth discoloration (2%), abdominal pain (1%), appetite increased (1%)

Genitourinary: Urinary retention (5%)

Hepatic: Hepatic function tests abnormal (5%)

Neuromuscular & skeletal: Weakness (5% to 6%), dysarthria (2%), fall (2%)

Ocular: Vision blurred (2%)

Renal: Hematuria (3%)

Respiratory: Throat irritation (1%)

Miscellaneous: Drunken feeling (3%)

General Dosage Range Dosage adjustment recommended in patients who develop toxicities

Buccal: *Adults:* Initial: 1 spray twice daily; Maintenance: Usual maximum: 12 sprays/day

Mechanism of Action Stimulates cannabinoid receptors CB1 and CB2 in the CNS and dorsal root ganglia as well as other sites in the body. Cannabinoid receptors in the pain pathways of the brain and spinal cord mediate cannabinoid-induced analgesia. Peripheral CB2 receptors modulate immune function through cytokine release.

Pharmacodynamics/Kinetics

Half-life Elimination Biphasic: Initial: 1-2 hours; Terminal: 24-36 hours (or longer) secondary to redistribution from fatty tissue

Time to Peak 2-4 hours

Product Availability Not available in U.S.

Controlled Substance CDSA-II

Tetrahydrozoline (Nasal) (tet ra hye DROZ a leen)

U.S. Brand Names Tyzine®; Tyzine® Pediatric

Pharmacologic Category Adrenergic Agonist Agent; Imidazoline Derivative

Use Symptomatic relief of nasal congestion

Local Anesthetic/Vasoconstrictor Precautions No information available to require special precautions

Effects on Dental Treatment No significant effects or complications reported

Effects on Bleeding No information available to require special precautions

Adverse Effects

>10%:

Local: Transient stinging

Respiratory: Sneezing

1% to 10%:

Cardiovascular: Hypertension, palpitation, tachycardia

Central nervous system: Headache

Neuromuscular & skeletal: Tremor

Ocular: Blurred vision

General Dosage Range Intranasal:

Children 2-6 years: Instill 2-3 drops (0.05%) into each nostril every 4-6 hours as needed (maximum: Every 3 hours)

Children >6 years and Adults: Instill 2-4 drops (0.1%) **or** 3-4 sprays (0.1%) into each nostril every 3-4 hours as needed (maximum: Every 3 hours)

Mechanism of Action Stimulates alpha-adrenergic receptors in the arterioles of the nasal mucosa to produce vasoconstriction

Pharmacodynamics/Kinetics

Onset of Action Decongestant: 4-8 hours

Pregnancy Risk Factor C

Tetrastarch (TET ra starch)

U.S. Brand Names Voluven®

Canadian Brand Names Voluven®

Pharmacologic Category Plasma Volume Expander, Colloid

Use Blood volume expander used in treatment and prevention of hypovolemia

Local Anesthetic/Vasoconstrictor Precautions No information available to require special precautions

Effects on Dental Treatment No significant effects or complications reported

Effects on Bleeding Tetrastarch has caused prolongation of activated partial thromboplastin time (aPPT); coagulation factors prolonged. Monitor patient for increased bleeding; medical consult is suggested. It is unlikely that ambulatory patients presenting for dental treatment will be receiving intravenous blood volume expander.

Adverse Effects 1% to 10%

Dermatologic: Pruritus (dose dependent; may be delayed), rash

Gastrointestinal: Amylase levels increased

Hematologic: Anemia, aPTT increased, coagulation factors prolonged, hemorrhage from wound site, PT prolonged

General Dosage Range I.V. infusion:

Children <2 years: Average dose: 7-25 mL/kg

Children >12 years and Adults: Maximum dose: 50 mL/kg/day

Mechanism of Action Expands plasma volume via the hydroxyethyl starch colloidal solution

Pharmacodynamics/Kinetics

Duration of Action ≥6 hours

Half-life Elimination 12 hours

Pregnancy Risk Factor C

Thalidomide (tha LI doe mide)

Related Information

HIV Infection and AIDS *on page 1883*

Ulcerative, Erosive, and Painful Oral Mucosal Disorders *on page 1950*

U.S. Brand Names Thalomid®

Canadian Brand Names Thalomid®

Generic Availability (U.S.) No

Pharmacologic Category Angiogenesis Inhibitor; Immunomodulator, Systemic; Tumor Necrosis Factor (TNF) Blocking Agent

Use Treatment of newly-diagnosed multiple myeloma; treatment and maintenance of cutaneous manifestations of erythema nodosum leprosum (ENL)

Unlabeled/Investigational Use Treatment of refractory Crohn's disease; treatment of chronic graft-versus-host disease (GVHD) in hematopoietic stem cell transplantation; AIDS-related aphthous stomatitis; Waldenström's macroglobulinemia; maintenance therapy of multiple myeloma (following autologous stem cell transplant)

Local Anesthetic/Vasoconstrictor Precautions No information available to require special precautions

Effects on Dental Treatment Key adverse event(s) related to dental treatment: Oral moniliasis (HIV-seropositive patients), toothache, xerostomia (normal salivary flow resumes upon discontinuation), and aphthous stomatitis.

Effects on Bleeding No information available to require special precautions

Adverse Effects

>10%:

Cardiovascular: Edema (57%), thrombosis/embolism (23%; grade 3: 13%, grade 4: 9%), hypotension (16%)

Central nervous system: Fatigue (79%; grade 3: 14%, grade 4: 3%), somnolence (36% to 38%), dizziness (4% to 20%), sensory neuropathy (54%), confusion (28%), anxiety/agitation (9% to 26%), fever (19% to 23%), motor neuropathy (22%), headache (13% to 19%)

Dermatologic: Rash/desquamation (21% to 30%; grade 3: 4%), dry skin (21%), maculopapular rash (4% to 19%), acne (3% to 11%)

Endocrine & metabolic: Hypocalcemia (72%)

Gastrointestinal: Constipation (3% to 55%), nausea (4% to 28%), anorexia (3% to 28%), weight loss (23%), weight gain (22%), diarrhea (4% to 19%), oral moniliasis (4% to 11%)

Hematologic: Leukopenia (17% to 35%), neutropenia (31%), anemia (6% to 13%), lymphadenopathy (6% to 13%)

Hepatic: AST increased (3% to 25%), bilirubin increased (14%)

Neuromuscular & skeletal: Muscle weakness (40%), tremor (4% to 26%), weakness (6% to 22%), myalgia (17%), paresthesia (6% to 16%), arthralgia (13%)
Renal: Hematuria (11%)
Respiratory: Dyspnea (42%)
Miscellaneous: Diaphoresis (13%)

1% to 10%:
Cardiovascular: Peripheral edema (3% to 8%), facial edema (4%)
Central nervous system: Insomnia (9%), nervousness (3% to 9%), malaise (8%), vertigo (8%), pain (3% to 8%)
Dermatologic: Dermatitis (fungal 4% to 9%), pruritus (3% to 8%), nail disorder (3% to 4%)
Endocrine & metabolic: Hyperlipemia (6% to 9%)
Gastrointestinal: Xerostomia (8% to 9%), flatulence (8%), tooth pain (4%)
Genitourinary: Impotence (3% to 8%)
Hepatic: LFTs abnormal (9%)
Neuromuscular & skeletal: Neuropathy (8%), back pain (4% to 6%), neck pain (4%), neck rigidity (4%)
Renal: Albuminuria (3% to 8%)
Respiratory: Pharyngitis (4% to 8%), rhinitis (4%), sinusitis (3% to 8%)
Miscellaneous: Infection (6% to 8%)

Dosage Oral:
Children ≥3 years: Chronic graft-versus-host disease (refractory), treatment (unlabeled second-line use; limited data): 3 mg/kg 4 times/day (dose adjusted to goal thalidomide concentration of ≥5 mcg/mL 2 hours postdose) (Vogelsang, 1992) **or** Initial: 3-6 mg/kg/day in 2-4 divided doses; target dose 12 mg/kg/day; Maximum daily dose: 800 mg (Rovelli, 1998)
Children ≥12 years and Adults: Cutaneous ENL: Initial: 100-300 mg once daily
Adjustments to initial dose:
Patients weighing <50 kg: Initiate at lower end of the dosing range
Severe cutaneous reaction or patients previously requiring high dose may be initiated at 400 mg/day; doses may be divided, but taken 1 hour after meals
Duration and tapering/maintenance:
Maintenance: Dosing should continue until active reaction subsides (usually at least 2 weeks), then tapered in 50 mg decrements every 2-4 weeks
Patients who flare during tapering or with a history of requiring prolonged maintenance should be maintained on the minimum dosage necessary to control the reaction. Efforts to taper should be repeated every 3-6 months, in decrements of 50 mg every 2-4 weeks.
Adults:
Multiple myeloma: **Note:** Details concerning dosing for multiple myeloma with combination regimens should also be consulted.
200 mg once daily at bedtime (in combination with dexamethasone 40 mg daily on days 1-4, 9-12, and 17-20 of a 28-day treatment cycle)
In combination with melphalan and prednisone (unlabeled combination in U.S.): 200-400 mg once daily (Facon, 2007) **or** 100 mg once daily (Palumbo, 2008)
Canadian labeling: Adults ≥65 years: 200 mg once daily (in combination with melphalan and prednisone)
AIDS-related aphthous stomatitis (unlabeled use): 200 mg once daily at bedtime for up to 8 weeks, if no response, then 200 mg twice daily for 4 weeks (Jacobson, 1997)
Chronic graft-versus-host disease (refractory), treatment (unlabeled second-line use; optimum dose not determined): Initial: 100 mg at bedtime, with dose escalation up to 400 mg/day in 3-4 divided doses (Wolff, 2010) **or** Initial: 50-100 mg 3 times/day; maximum dose: 600-1200 mg/day (Kulkarni, 2003) **or** 200 mg 4 times/day (dose adjusted to goal thalidomide concentration of ≥5 mcg/mL 2 hours postdose) (Vogelsang, 1992) **or** 100-300 mg 4 times/day (Parker, 1995)
Crohn's disease, refractory (unlabeled use): 50-100 mg/day at bedtime (Vasiliauskas, 1999) **or** 200-300 mg/day at bedtime (Ehrenpreis, 1999)
Multiple myeloma, maintenance (following autologous stem cell transplant; unlabeled use): 200 mg/day starting 3-6 months after transplant; continue until disease progression or unacceptable toxicity (Brinker, 2006) **or** 100 mg/day starting 42-60 days following transplant; increase to 200 mg/day after 2 weeks if tolerated; continue for up to 12 months (in combination with prednisolone) (Spencer, 2009)
Waldenström's macroglobulinemia (unlabeled use): 200 mg/day for up to 52 weeks (in combination with rituximab) (Treon, 2008)

Dosing adjustment for toxicity:
ANC ≤750/mm^3: Withhold treatment if clinically appropriate

Multiple myeloma:

U.S. labeling: Constipation, oversedation, peripheral neuropathy: Temporarily withhold or continue with a reduced dose

Canadian labeling:

ANC $<1500/mm^3$: Withhold melphalan and prednisone for 1 week; resume melphalan and prednisone after 1 week if ANC $>1500/mm^3$ **or** if ANC $1000\text{-}1500/mm^3$ reduce melphalan dose by 50% **or** if ANC $<1000/mm^3$ adjust chemotherapy dose based on clinical status of patient.

Constipation, oversedation: Temporarily withhold thalidomide treatment or continue with a reduced dose

Peripheral neuropathy, Grade 1 (paresthesia, weakness and/or loss of reflexes) without loss of function): Evaluate patient and consider dose reduction with worsening of symptoms; symptom improvement may not follow dose reduction, however.

Peripheral neuropathy, Grade 2 (interferes with function but not with daily activities), Grade 3 (interferes with daily activities), or Grade 4 (disabling neuropathy): Discontinue thalidomide treatment

Thromboembolic events: Withhold therapy and initiate standard anticoagulant treatment; may resume thalidomide therapy at original dose following stabilization of patient and resolution of thromboembolic event; maintain anticoagulant treatment for duration of thalidomide therapy

Mechanism of Action Has immunomodulatory and antiangiogenic characteristics. Immunologic effects may vary based on conditions; may suppress excessive tumor necrosis factor-alpha production in patients with ENL, yet may increase plasma tumor necrosis factor-alpha levels in HIV-positive patients. In multiple myeloma, thalidomide is associated with an increase in natural killer cells and increased levels of interleukin-2 and interferon gamma. Other proposed mechanisms of action include suppression of angiogenesis, prevention of free-radical-mediated DNA damage, increased cell mediated cytotoxic effects, and altered expression of cellular adhesion molecules.

Contraindications Hypersensitivity to thalidomide or any component of the formulation; patient unable to comply with STEPS® program (including males); women of childbearing potential unless alternative therapies are inappropriate and adequate precautions are taken to avoid pregnancy; pregnancy

Canadian labeling: Additional contraindications (not in U.S. labeling): Hypersensitivity to lenalidomide; breast-feeding

Warnings/Precautions Hazardous agent - use appropriate precautions for handling and disposal. **[U.S. Boxed Warning]: Thalidomide should only be prescribed to patients (male and female) who can understand and comply with the conditions of the S.T.E.P.S.® program. Distribution is restricted; physicians, pharmacists, and patients must be registered with the S.T.E.P.S.® program. [U.S. Boxed Warning]: Thalidomide is a known teratogen; effective contraception must be used for at least 4 weeks before initiating therapy, during therapy, and for 4 weeks following discontinuation of thalidomide for women of childbearing potential.** Use caution with drugs which may decrease the efficacy of hormonal contraceptives.

[U.S. Boxed Warning]: Thrombotic events have been reported, generally in patients with other risk factors for thrombosis (neoplastic disease, inflammatory disease, or concurrent therapy with combination chemotherapy. Use in combination with dexamethasone is associated with increased risk for deep vein thrombosis (DVT) and pulmonary embolism (PE), monitor for signs and symptoms of thromboembolism; patients at risk may benefit from prophylactic anticoagulation or aspirin. The NCCN multiple myeloma guidelines (v.1.2011) recommend anticoagulant prophylaxis with thalidomide-based therapy. Anticoagulant prophylaxis should be individualized and selected based on the venous thromboembolism risk of the combination treatment regimen, using the safest and easiest to administer (Palumbo, 2008). The Canadian labeling recommends anticoagulant prophylaxis for at least the first 5 months of thalidomide-based therapy.

May cause sedation; patients must be warned to use caution when performing tasks which require alertness. Use caution in patients with renal or hepatic impairment, neurological disorders, or constipation. Thalidomide has been associated with the development of peripheral neuropathy, which may be irreversible; generally occurs following chronic use (over months), but may occur with short-term use; use caution with other medications which may cause peripheral neuropathy. Consider immediate discontinuation (if clinically appropriate) in patients who develop neuropathy. May cause seizures; use caution in patients with a history of seizures, concurrent therapy with drugs which alter seizure threshold, or conditions which predispose to seizures. May cause neutropenia; discontinue therapy if absolute neutrophil count decreases to $<750/mm^3$. Use caution in patients with HIV infection; has been associated with increased viral loads. May cause orthostasis and/or bradycardia; use with caution in patients with cardiovascular disease or in patients who would not tolerate transient hypotensive episodes. Hypersensitivity, Stevens-Johnson syndrome (SJS) and toxic epidermal necrolysis (TEN) have been reported; withhold therapy and evaluate with skin rashes; permanently discontinue if rash is exfoliative, purpuric, bullous or if SJS or TEN is suspected.

Drug Interactions

Avoid Concomitant Use

Avoid concomitant use of Thalidomide with any of the following: Abatacept; Anakinra; BCG; Canakinumab; Certolizumab Pegol; Natalizumab; Pimecrolimus; Rilonacept; Roflumilast; Tacrolimus (Topical); Vaccines (Live)

Increased Effect/Toxicity

Thalidomide may increase the levels/effects of: Abatacept; Alcohol (Ethyl); Anakinra; Canakinumab; Certolizumab Pegol; CNS Depressants; Leflunomide; Methotrimeprazine; Natalizumab; Pamidronate; Rilonacept; Vaccines (Live); Zoledronic Acid

The levels/effects of Thalidomide may be increased by: Denosumab; Dexamethasone; Dexamethasone (Systemic); Droperidol; Methotrimeprazine; Pimecrolimus; Roflumilast; Tacrolimus (Topical); Trastuzumab

Decreased Effect

Thalidomide may decrease the levels/effects of: BCG; Sipuleucel-T; Vaccines (Inactivated); Vaccines (Live)

The levels/effects of Thalidomide may be decreased by: Echinacea

Ethanol/Nutrition/Herb Interactions

Ethanol: May increase CNS depression; monitor for increased effects with coadministration. Caution patients about effects.

Herb/Nutraceutical: Avoid cat's claw and echinacea (have immunostimulant properties; consider therapy modifications).

Dietary Considerations Should be taken at least 1 hour after the evening meal.

Pharmacodynamics/Kinetics

Half-life Elimination 5-7 hours

Time to Peak Plasma: 3-6 hours

Pregnancy Risk Factor X

Lactation Excretion in breast milk unknown/not recommended

Breast-Feeding Considerations Due to the potential for serious adverse reactions in the infant, a decision should be made to discontinue nursing or discontinue treatment with thalidomide. Use in breast-feeding women is contraindicated in the Canadian labeling.

Prescribing and Access Restrictions U.S.: As a requirement of the REMS program, access to this medication is restricted. Thalidomide is approved for marketing only under a special distribution program. This program, called the "System for Thalidomide Education and Prescribing Safety" (STEPS® 1-888-423-5436), has been approved by the FDA. Prescribers and pharmacist must be registered with the program. No more than a 4-week supply should be dispensed. Blister packs should be dispensed intact (do not repackage capsules). Prescriptions must be filled within 7 days. Subsequent prescriptions may be filled only if fewer than 7 days of therapy remain on the previous prescription. A new prescription is required for further dispensing (a telephone prescription may not be accepted.) Pregnancy testing is required for females of childbearing potential.

Canada: Access to thalidomide is restricted through a controlled distribution program called RevAid®. Only physicians and pharmacists enrolled in this program are authorized to prescribe or dispense thalidomide. Patients must be enrolled in the program by their physicians. Further information is available by calling 1-888-738-2431.

Dosage Forms

Capsule, oral:

Thalomid®: 50 mg, 100 mg, 150 mg, 200 mg

References

Beckman DA and Brent RL, "Mechanism of Known Environmental Teratogens: Drugs and Chemicals," *Clin Perinatol*, 1986, 13(3):649-87.

Gunzler V, "Thalidomide in Human Immunodeficiency Virus (HIV) Patients. A Review of Safety Considerations," *Drug Saf*, 1992, 7(2):116-34.

Hamuryudan V, Mat C, Saip S, et al, "Thalidomide in the Treatment of the Mucocutaneous Lesions of the Behçet Syndrome. A Randomized, Double-Blind, Placebo-Controlled Trial," *Ann Intern Med*, 1998, 128 (6):443-50.

Jacobson JM, Greenspan JS, Spritzler J, et al, "Thalidomide for the Treatment of Oral Aphthous Ulcers in Patients With Human Immunodeficiency Virus Infection. National Institute of Allergy and Infectious Diseases AIDS Clinical Trials Group," *N Engl J Med*, 1997, 336(21):1487-93.

Levien T, Baker DE, and Ballasiotes AA, "Reviews of Dexrazoxane and Thalidomide," *Hosp Pharm*, 1996, 31(5):487-8, 493-4, 499-500, 504, 508, 510.

Schuler U and Ehninger G, "Thalidomide: Rationale for Renewed Use in Immunological Disorders," *Drug Saf*, 1995, 12(6):364-9.

"Thalidomide," *Med Lett Drugs Ther*, 1998, 40(1038):103-4.

Theophylline (thee OFF i lin)

Related Information

Aminophylline *on page* 100
Respiratory Diseases *on page* 1876

U.S. Brand Names Elixophyllin® Elixir; Theo-24®; Theochron™

Canadian Brand Names Apo-Theo LA®; Novo-Theophyl SR; PMS-Theophylline; Pulmophylline; ratio-Theo-Bronc; Theochron® SR; Uniphyl® SRT

Pharmacologic Category Theophylline Derivative

Use Treatment of symptoms and reversible airway obstruction due to chronic asthma, or other chronic lung diseases; apnea of prematurity

Note: The Global Initiative for Asthma Guidelines (2009) and the National Heart, Lung and Blood Institute Guidelines (2007) do not recommend oral theophylline as a long-term control medication for asthma in children ≤5 years of age; use has been shown to be effective as an add-on (but not preferred) agent in older children and adults with severe asthma treated with inhaled or oral glucocorticoids. The guidelines do not recommend theophylline for the treatment of exacerbations of asthma.

The Global Initiative for Chronic Obstructive Lung Disease Guidelines (2009) suggest that while higher doses of slow release formulations of theophylline have been proven to be effective for use in COPD, it is not a preferred agent due to its potential for toxicity.

Local Anesthetic/Vasoconstrictor Precautions No information available to require special precautions

Effects on Dental Treatment Prescribe erythromycin products with caution to patients taking theophylline products. Erythromycin will delay the normal metabolic inactivation of theophyllines leading to increased blood levels; this has resulted in nausea, vomiting, and CNS restlessness. Azithromycin does not cause these effects in combination with theophylline products.

Effects on Bleeding No information available to require special precautions

Adverse Effects Frequency not defined. Adverse events observed at therapeutic serum levels:

Cardiovascular: Flutter, tachycardia
Central nervous system: Headache, hyperactivity (children), insomnia, restlessness, seizures
Endocrine & metabolic: Hypercalcemia (with concomitant hyperthyroid disease)
Gastrointestinal: Nausea, reflux or ulcer aggravation, vomiting
Genitourinary: Difficulty urinating (elderly males with prostatism)
Neuromuscular & skeletal: Tremor
Renal: Diuresis (transient)

General Dosage Range

I.V.:

Neonates ≤24 days: 1 mg/kg every 12 hours
Neonates >24 days: 1.5 mg/kg every 12 hours
Infants 6-52 weeks: mg/kg/hour = (0.008) (age in weeks) + 0.21
Children 1-9 years: 0.8 mg/kg/hour
Children 9-12 years and Adolescents 12-16 years (cigarette or marijuana smokers): 0.7 mg/kg/hour
Adolescents 12-16 years (nonsmokers): 0.5 mg/kg/hour; maximum 900 mg/day unless serum levels indicate need for larger dose
Adults 16-60 years (otherwise healthy, nonsmokers): 0.4 mg/kg/hour; maximum 900 mg/day unless serum levels indicate need for larger dose
Adults >60 years: 0.3 mg/kg/hour; maximum 400 mg/day unless serum levels indicate need for larger dose

Oral solution:

Premature Neonates <24 days postnatal age: 1 mg/kg/dose every 12 hours
Premature Neonates ≥24 days postnatal age: 1.5 mg/kg/dose every 12 hours
Full-term Infants and Infants <26 weeks: Total daily dose (mg) = [(0.2 x age in weeks) +5] x (weight in kg); divide dose into 3 equal amounts and administer at 8-hour intervals
Full-term Infants and Infants ≥26 weeks and <52 weeks: Total daily dose (mg) = [(0.2 x age in weeks) +5] x (weight in kg); divide dose into 4 equal amounts and administer at 6-hour intervals
Children ≥1 year and <45 kg: Initial: 10-14 mg/kg/day in divided doses (maximum dose: 300 mg/day); titrate to maintenance dose: 20 mg/kg/day in divided doses every 4-6 hours (maximum dose: 600 mg/day)
Children >45 kg and Adults: Initial: 300 mg/day in divided doses; titrate to maintenance dose: 600 mg/day in divided doses every 6-8 hours

Oral extended release formulations:

Children ≥1 year and <45 kg: Initial: 10-14 mg/kg once daily (maximum dose: 300 mg/day); titrate to maintenance dose: 20 mg/kg once daily (maximum dose: 600 mg/day)

Children >45 kg and Adults: 300-600 mg once daily

Mechanism of Action Causes bronchodilatation, diuresis, CNS and cardiac stimulation, and gastric acid secretion by blocking phosphodiesterase which increases tissue concentrations of cyclic adenine monophosphate (cAMP) which in turn promotes catecholamine stimulation of lipolysis, glycogenolysis, and gluconeogenesis and induces release of epinephrine from adrenal medulla cells

Pharmacodynamics/Kinetics

Onset of Action I.V.: <30 minutes

Half-life Elimination Highly variable and age, liver and cardiac function, lung disease, and smoking history dependent

Premature infants, postnatal age 3-15 days: 30 hours (range: 17-43 hours)

Premature infants, postnatal age 25-57 days: 20 hours (range: 9.4-30.6 hours)

Children 6-17 years: 3.7 hours (range: 1.5-5.9 hours)

Adults 16-60 years with asthma, nonsmoking, otherwise healthy: 8.7 hours (range: 6.1-12.8 hours)

Time to Peak Serum: Oral: Liquid: 1 hour

Pregnancy Risk Factor C

Thiamine (THYE a min)

Canadian Brand Names Betaxin®

Pharmacologic Category Vitamin, Water Soluble

Use Treatment of thiamine deficiency including beriberi, Wernicke's encephalopathy, Korsakoff's syndrome, neuritis associated with pregnancy, or in alcoholic patients; dietary supplement

Local Anesthetic/Vasoconstrictor Precautions No information available to require special precautions

Effects on Dental Treatment Key adverse event(s) related to dental treatment: Tightness of the throat.

Effects on Bleeding No information available to require special precautions

Adverse Effects Adverse reactions reported with injection. Frequency not defined.

Cardiovascular: Cyanosis

Central nervous system: Restlessness

Dermatologic: Angioneurotic edema, pruritus, urticaria

Gastrointestinal: Hemorrharge into GI tract, nausea, tightness of the throat

Local: Induration and/or tenderness at the injection site (following I.M. administration)

Neuromuscular & skeletal: Weakness

Respiratory: Pulmonary edema

Miscellaneous: Anaphylactic/hypersensitivity reactions (following I.V. administration), diaphoresis, warmth

General Dosage Range

I.M., I.V.:

Children: 10-25 mg/dose daily (thiamine deficiency)

Adults: 5-30 mg/dose 3 times/day (thiamine deficiency) **or** 50-250 mg/day (Wernicke's encephalopathy)

Oral:

Infants: 0.2-0.3 mg/day (adequate intake)

Children: 0.5-1.4 mg/day (recommended daily intake) **or** 5-50 mg/day (thiamine deficiency)

Adults: 1.1-1.4 mg/day (recommended daily intake) **or** 5-30 mg/day in 1-3 divided doses (thiamine deficiency)

Mechanism of Action An essential coenzyme in carbohydrate metabolism by combining with adenosine triphosphate to form thiamine pyrophosphate

Pregnancy Risk Factor A

Thioguanine (thye oh GWAH neen)

U.S. Brand Names Tabloid®

Canadian Brand Names Lanvis®

Pharmacologic Category Antineoplastic Agent, Antimetabolite (Purine Analog)

Use Treatment of acute myelogenous (nonlymphocytic) leukemia (AML)

Unlabeled/Investigational Use Treatment of pediatric acute lymphoblastic leukemia (ALL)

Local Anesthetic/Vasoconstrictor Precautions No information available to require special precautions

Effects on Dental Treatment Key adverse event(s) related to dental treatment: Stomatitis.

Effects on Bleeding Chemotherapy may result in significant myelosuppression, potentially including significant reduction in platelet counts and altered hemostasis. In patients who are under active treatment with these agents, medical consult is suggested.

Adverse Effects Frequency not defined.

Endocrine & metabolic: Fluid retention, hyperuricemia (common)

Gastrointestinal: Anorexia, intestinal necrosis, intestinal perforation, nausea, splenomegaly, stomatitis, vomiting, weight gain

Hematologic: Anemia (may be delayed), bleeding, granulocytopenia, leukopenia (common; may be delayed), marrow hypoplasia, pancytopenia, thrombocytopenia (common; may be delayed)

Hepatic: Ascites, esophageal varices, hepatic necrosis (centrilobular), hepatic veno-occlusive disease (VOD), hepatitis, hepatomegaly [tender], hepatoportal sclerosis, hepatotoxicity, hyperbilirubinemia, jaundice, LFTs increased, nodular regenerative hyperplasia, peliosis hepatitis, periportal fibrosis, portal hypertension

Miscellaneous: Infection

Mechanism of Action Purine analog that is incorporated into DNA and RNA resulting in the blockage of synthesis and metabolism of purine nucleotides

Pharmacodynamics/Kinetics

Half-life Elimination Terminal: 5-9 hours

Time to Peak Serum: Within 8 hours; predominantly metabolite(s)

Pregnancy Risk Factor D

Thiopental (thye oh PEN tal)

U.S. Brand Names Pentothal® [DSC]

Canadian Brand Names Pentothal®

Pharmacologic Category Anticonvulsant, Barbiturate; Barbiturate; General Anesthetic

Use Induction of anesthesia; control of convulsive states; treatment of elevated intracranial pressure

Local Anesthetic/Vasoconstrictor Precautions No information available to require special precautions

Effects on Dental Treatment No significant effects or complications reported

Effects on Bleeding No information available to require special precautions

Adverse Effects Frequency not defined.

Cardiovascular: Bradycardia, hypotension, syncope

Central nervous system: Drowsiness, lethargy, CNS excitation or depression, impaired judgment, "hangover" effect, confusion, somnolence, agitation, hyperkinesia, ataxia, nervousness, headache, insomnia, nightmares, hallucinations, anxiety, dizziness, shivering

Dermatologic: Rash, exfoliative dermatitis, Stevens-Johnson syndrome

Gastrointestinal: Nausea, vomiting, constipation

Hematologic: Agranulocytosis, thrombocytopenia, megaloblastic anemia, immune hemolytic anemia (rare)

Local: Pain at injection site, thrombophlebitis with I.V. use

Renal: Oliguria

Respiratory: Laryngospasm, respiratory depression, apnea (especially with rapid I.V. use), hypoventilation, apnea, sneezing, cough, bronchospasm

Miscellaneous: Gangrene with inadvertent intra-arterial injection, anaphylaxis, anaphylactic reactions

General Dosage Range Dosage adjustment recommended in patients with renal impairment

I.V.:

Infants <1 year: Anesthesia induction: 5-8 mg/kg

Children 1-12 years: Anesthesia induction: 5-6 mg/kg; Maintenance: 1 mg/kg as needed **or** 1.5-5 mg/kg/dose, repeat as needed

Children >12 years: Maintenance: 1 mg/kg as needed **or** 1.5-5 mg/kg/dose, repeat as needed

Adults: Anesthesia induction: 3-5 mg/kg; Maintenance: 25-100 mg as needed **or** 1.5-5 mg/kg/dose, repeat as needed **or** 75-250 mg/dose, repeat as needed

Mechanism of Action Short-acting barbiturate with sedative, hypnotic, and anticonvulsant properties. Barbiturates depress the sensory cortex, decrease motor activity, alter cerebellar function, and produce drowsiness, sedation, and hypnosis. In high doses, barbiturates exhibit anticonvulsant activity; barbiturates produce dose-dependent respiratory depression.

Pharmacodynamics/Kinetics

Onset of Action Anesthetic: I.V.: 30-60 seconds

Duration of Action 5-30 minutes

Half-life Elimination 3-11.5 hours; decreased in children

Pregnancy Risk Factor C

Controlled Substance C-III

Thioridazine (thye oh RID a zeen)

Related Information

Clinical Risk Related to Drugs Prolonging QT Interval *on page 1872*

Pharmacologic Category Antipsychotic Agent, Typical, Phenothiazine

Use Management of schizophrenic patients who fail to respond adequately to treatment with other antipsychotic drugs, either because of insufficient effectiveness or the inability to achieve an effective dose due to intolerable adverse effects from those medications

Unlabeled/Investigational Use Behavior problems (children); severe psychoses (children); schizophrenia/psychoses (children); depressive disorders/dementia (children and adults); behavioral symptoms associated with dementia (elderly); psychosis/agitation related to Alzheimer's dementia

Local Anesthetic/Vasoconstrictor Precautions Most pharmacology textbooks state that in presence of phenothiazines, systemic doses of epinephrine paradoxically decrease the blood pressure. This is the so called "epinephrine reversal" phenomenon. This has never been observed when epinephrine is given by infiltration as part of the anesthesia procedure. Thioridazine is one of the drugs confirmed to prolong the QT interval and is accepted as having a risk of causing torsade de pointes. The risk of drug-induced torsade de pointes is extremely low when a single QT interval prolonging drug is prescribed. In terms of epinephrine, it is not known what effect vasoconstrictors in the local anesthetic regimen will have in patients with a known history of congenital prolonged QT interval or in patients taking any medication that prolongs the QT interval. Until more information is obtained, it is suggested that the clinician consult with the physician prior to the use of a vasoconstrictor in suspected patients, and that the vasoconstrictor (epinephrine, mepivacaine and levonordefrin [Carbocaine® 2% with Neo-Cobefrin®]) be used with caution.

Effects on Dental Treatment Key adverse event(s) related to dental treatment: Xerostomia and changes in salivation (normal salivary flow resumes upon discontinuation). Significant hypotension may occur, especially when the drug is administered parenterally; orthostatic hypotension is due to alpha-receptor blockade, the elderly are at greater risk for orthostatic hypotension.

Tardive dyskinesia; Prevalence rate may be 40% in elderly; development of the syndrome and the irreversible nature are proportional to duration and total cumulative dose over time. Extrapyramidal reactions are more common in elderly with up to 50% developing these reactions after 60 years of age. Drug-induced Parkinson's syndrome occurs often; akathisia is the most common extrapyramidal reaction in elderly.

Effects on Bleeding No information available to require special precautions

Adverse Effects Frequency not defined.

Cardiovascular: Hypotension, orthostatic hypotension, peripheral edema, ECG changes

Central nervous system: EPS (pseudoparkinsonism, akathisia, dystonias, tardive dyskinesia), dizziness, drowsiness, neuroleptic malignant syndrome (NMS), impairment of temperature regulation, lowering of seizure threshold, seizure

Dermatologic: Increased sensitivity to sun, rash, discoloration of skin (blue-gray)

Endocrine & metabolic: Changes in menstrual cycle, libido (changes in), breast pain, galactorrhea, amenorrhea

Gastrointestinal: Constipation, weight gain, nausea, vomiting, stomach pain, xerostomia, nausea, vomiting, diarrhea

Genitourinary: Difficulty in urination, ejaculatory disturbances, urinary retention, priapism

Hematologic: Agranulocytosis, leukopenia

Hepatic: Cholestatic jaundice, hepatotoxicity

Neuromuscular & skeletal: Tremor

Ocular: Pigmentary retinopathy, blurred vision, cornea and lens changes

Respiratory: Nasal congestion

General Dosage Range Oral:

Children >2-12 years: 0.5-3 mg/kg/day in 2-3 divided doses **or** 10-25 mg 2-3 times/day (maximum: 3 mg/kg/day)

Children >12 years and Adults: Initial: 50-100 mg 3 times/day; Maintenance: 150-800 mg/day in 2-4 divided doses (maximum: 800 mg/day) **or** Initial: 25 mg 3 times/day; Maintenance: 20-200 mg/day

Elderly: Initial: 10-25 mg 1-2 times/day; Maintenance: 10-400 mg/day in 1-2 divided doses (maximum: 400 mg/day)

Mechanism of Action Thioridazine is a piperidine phenothiazine which blocks postsynaptic mesolimbic dopaminergic receptors in the brain; exhibits a strong alpha-adrenergic blocking effect and depresses the release of hypothalamic and hypophyseal hormones

Pharmacodynamics/Kinetics

Duration of Action 4-5 days

Half-life Elimination 21-25 hours

Time to Peak Serum: ~1 hour

Pregnancy Risk Factor C

Dental Comment Thioridazine is known to prolong the QT interval. The QT interval is measured as the time and distance between the Q point of the QRS complex and the end of the T wave in the ECG tracing. After adjustment for heart rate, the QT interval is defined as prolonged if it is more than 450 msec in men and 460 msec in women. A long QT syndrome was first described in the 1950s and 60s as a congenital syndrome involving QT interval prolongation and syncope and sudden death. Some of the congenital long QT syndromes were characterized by a peculiar electrocardiographic appearance of the QRS complex involving a premature atria beat followed by a pause, then a subsequent sinus beat showing marked QT prolongation and deformity. This type of cardiac arrhythmia was originally termed "torsade de pointes" (translated from the French as "twisting of the points"). Thioridazine is considered as having a risk of causing torsade de pointes. Since it is not known what effect vasoconstrictors in the local anesthetic regimen will have in patients with a known history of congenital prolonged QT interval or in patients taking any medication that prolongs the QT interval, a medical consult is suggested.

Thiotepa (thye oh TEP a)

Pharmacologic Category Antineoplastic Agent, Alkylating Agent

Use Treatment of superficial papillary bladder cancer; palliative treatment of adenocarcinoma of breast or ovary; controlling intracavitary effusions caused by metastatic tumors

Unlabeled/Investigational Use Intrathecal treatment of leptomeningeal metastases

Local Anesthetic/Vasoconstrictor Precautions No information available to require special precautions

Effects on Dental Treatment No significant effects or complications reported

Effects on Bleeding Chemotherapy may result in significant myelosuppression, potentially including significant reduction in platelet counts and altered hemostasis. In patients who are under active treatment with these agents, medical consult is suggested.

Adverse Effects Frequency not defined.

Central nervous system: Chills, dizziness, fatigue, fever, headache

Dermatologic: Alopecia, contact dermatitis, depigmentation (with topical treatment), dermatitis, rash, urticaria

Endocrine & metabolic: Amenorrhea, spermatogenesis inhibition

Gastrointestinal: Abdominal pain, anorexia, nausea, vomiting

Genitourinary: Dysuria, urinary retention

Hematologic: Anemia, bleeding, leukopenia, thrombocytopenia

Local: Injection site pain

Neuromuscular & skeletal: Weakness

Ocular: Blurred vision, conjunctivitis

Renal: Hematuria

Respiratory: Asthma, epistaxis, laryngeal edema, wheezing

Miscellaneous: Allergic reaction, anaphylactic shock, infection

General Dosage Range Dosage adjustment recommended in patients who develop toxicities

I.V.: *Adults:* 0.3-0.4 mg/kg every 1-4 weeks

Intracavitary: *Adults:* 0.6-0.8 mg/kg

Intravesical: *Adults:* 60 mg retained for 2 hours once weekly for 4 weeks

Mechanism of Action Alkylating agent that reacts with DNA phosphate groups to produce cross-linking of DNA strands leading to inhibition of DNA, RNA, and protein synthesis; mechanism of action has not been explored as thoroughly as the other alkylating agents, it is presumed that the aziridine rings open and react as nitrogen mustard; reactivity is enhanced at a lower pH

Pharmacodynamics/Kinetics
Half-life Elimination Terminal: Dose-dependent clearance: ~2 hours
Pregnancy Risk Factor D

Thiothixene (thye oh THIKS een)

U.S. Brand Names Navane®
Canadian Brand Names Navane®
Pharmacologic Category Antipsychotic Agent, Typical
Use Management of schizophrenia
Unlabeled/Investigational Use Psychotic disorders (children); rapid tranquilization of the agitated patient (children); nonpsychotic patient, dementia behavior (elderly); psychosis/agitation related to Alzheimer's dementia
Local Anesthetic/Vasoconstrictor Precautions Most pharmacology textbooks state that in presence of phenothiazines, systemic doses of epinephrine paradoxically decrease the blood pressure. This is the so called "epinephrine reversal" phenomenon. This has never been observed when epinephrine is given by infiltration as part of the anesthesia procedure. Thiothixene is one of the drugs confirmed to prolong the QT interval and is accepted as having a risk of causing torsade de pointes. The risk of drug-induced torsade de pointes is extremely low when a single QT interval prolonging drug is prescribed. In terms of epinephrine, it is not known what effect vasoconstrictors in the local anesthetic regimen will have in patients with a known history of congenital prolonged QT interval or in patients taking any medication that prolongs the QT interval. Until more information is obtained, it is suggested that the clinician consult with the physician prior to the use of a vasoconstrictor in suspected patients, and that the vasoconstrictor (epinephrine, mepivacaine and levonordefrin [Carbocaine® 2% with Neo-Cobefrin®]) be used with caution.
Effects on Dental Treatment Key adverse event(s) related to dental treatment: Xerostomia and changes in salivation (normal salivary flow resumes upon discontinuation), significant hypotension may occur, especially when the drug is administered parenterally; orthostatic hypotension is due to alpha-receptor blockade, the elderly are at greater risk for orthostatic hypotension.

Tardive dyskinesia: Prevalence rate may be 40% in elderly; development of the syndrome and the irreversible nature are proportional to duration and total cumulative dose over time. Extrapyramidal reactions are more common in elderly with up to 50% developing these reactions after 60 years of age. Drug-induced Parkinson's syndrome occurs often; akathisia is the most common extrapyramidal reaction in elderly.
Effects on Bleeding No information available to require special precautions
Adverse Effects Frequency not defined.
Cardiovascular: Hypotension, nonspecific ECG changes, syncope, tachycardia
Central nervous system: Agitation, dizziness, drowsiness, extrapyramidal symptoms (akathisia, dystonias, lightheadedness, pseudoparkinsonism, tardive dyskinesia), insomnia restlessness
Dermatologic: Discoloration of skin (blue-gray), photosensitivity, pruritus, rash, urticaria
Endocrine & metabolic: Amenorrhea, breast pain, libido (changes in), changes in menstrual cycle, galactorrhea, gynecomastia, hyper-/hypoglycemia, hyperprolactinemia, lactation
Gastrointestinal: Constipation, nausea, salivation increased, stomach pain, vomiting, weight gain, xerostomia
Genitourinary: Difficulty in urination, ejaculatory disturbances, impotence
Hematologic: Leukocytes, leukopenia
Neuromuscular & skeletal: Tremors
Ocular: Blurred vision, pigmentary retinopathy
Respiratory: Nasal congestion
Miscellaneous: Diaphoresis
General Dosage Range Oral: *Adults:* Initial: 6-10 mg/day in 2-3 divided doses; Maintenance: 20-60 mg/day in 2-3 divided doses (maximum: 60 mg/day)
Mechanism of Action Thiothixene is a thioxanthene antipsychotic which elicits antipsychotic activity by postsynaptic blockade of CNS dopamine receptors resulting in inhibition of dopamine-mediated effects; also has alpha-adrenergic blocking activity
Pharmacodynamics/Kinetics
Half-life Elimination >24 hours with chronic use

Dental Comment Thiothixene is known to prolong the QT interval. The QT interval is measured as the time and distance between the Q point of the QRS complex and the end of the T wave in the ECG tracing. After adjustment for heart rate, the QT interval is defined as prolonged if it is more than 450 msec in men and 460 msec in women. A long QT syndrome was first described in the 1950s and 60s as a congenital syndrome involving QT interval prolongation and syncope and sudden death. Some of the congenital long QT syndromes were characterized by a peculiar electrocardiographic appearance of the QRS complex involving a premature atria beat followed by a pause, then a subsequent sinus beat showing marked QT prolongation and deformity. This type of cardiac arrhythmia was originally termed "torsade de pointes" (translated from the French as "twisting of the points"). Thiothixene is considered as having a risk of causing torsade de pointes. Since it is not known what effect vasoconstrictors in the local anesthetic regimen will have in patients with a known history of congenital prolonged QT interval or in patients taking any medication that prolongs the QT interval, a medical consult is suggested.

Thrombin (Topical) (THROM bin, TOP i kal)

Related Information

Antiplatelet and Anticoagulation Considerations in Dentistry *on page 1867*

U.S. Brand Names Evithrom™; Recothrom™; Thrombi-Gel®; Thrombi-Pad®; Thrombin-JMI®; Thrombin-JMI® Epistaxis Kit; Thrombin-JMI® Spray Kit; Thrombin-JMI® Syringe Spray Kit

Generic Availability (U.S.) No

Pharmacologic Category Blood Product Derivative; Hemostatic Agent

Dental Use Hemostasis whenever minor bleeding from capillaries and small venules is accessible

Use Hemostasis whenever minor bleeding from capillaries and small venules is accessible

Thrombi-Gel®; Thrombi-Pad®: Temporary control as trauma dressing for moderate-to-severe bleeding wounds; control of surface bleeding from vascular access sites and percutaneous catheter/tubes

Local Anesthetic/Vasoconstrictor Precautions No information available to require special precautions

Effects on Dental Treatment No significant effects or complications reported

Effects on Bleeding General dental procedures and simple restorative procedures are not associated with bleeding; therefore, there is no contraindication to general dental treatment for most patients with bleeding disorders. However, after dental extractions and other dental surgeries including deep scaling, block anesthesia, and large fillings, in patients with hemophilia, drugs such as topical thrombin may be useful in controlling bleeding. A carefully coordinated strategy between the dental and medical team may be required to ensure adequate procedures for hemostasis.

Adverse Effects Frequency not defined.

Dermatologic: Pruritus

Gastrointestinal: Nausea, vomiting

Hematologic: Bleeding, aPTT increased, INR increased, lymphocyte count decreased, neutrophil count increased, PT prolonged

Local: Incision site complication

Miscellaneous: Antibody development, hypersensitivity reactions

Dental Usual Dosage Topical: Hemostasis: **Note:** For topical use only; do not administer intravenously or intra-arterially:

Evithrom™: Children and Adults: Dose depends on area to be treated; up to 10 mL was used with absorbable gelatin sponge in clinical studies

Recothrom™: Adults: Dose depends on area to be treated

Thrombi-Gel® 10, 40, 100: Adults: Wet product with up to 3 mL, 10 mL, or 20 mL, respectively, of 0.9% sodium chloride or SWFI; apply directly over source of the bleeding with manual pressure

Thrombi-Pad®: Adults: Apply pad directly over source of bleeding; may apply dry or wetted with up to 10 mL of 0.9% sodium chloride. If desired, product may be left in place for up to 24 hours; do not leave in the body.

Thrombin-JMI®: Adults:

Solution: Use 1000-2000 int. units/mL of solution where bleeding is profuse; use 100 int. units/mL for bleeding from skin or mucosal surfaces

Powder: May apply powder directly to the site of bleeding or on oozing surfaces

Dosage Topical: Hemostasis: **Note:** For topical use only; do not administer intravenously or intra-arterially:

Evithrom™: Children and Adults: Dose depends on area to be treated; up to 10 mL was used with absorbable gelatin sponge in clinical studies

Recothrom™: Adults: Dose depends on area to be treated

Thrombi-Gel® 10, 40, 100: Adults: Wet product with up to 3 mL, 10 mL, or 20 mL, respectively, of 0.9% sodium chloride or SWFI; apply directly over source of the bleeding with manual pressure

Thrombi-Pad®: Adults: Apply pad directly over source of bleeding; may apply dry or wetted with up to 10 mL of 0.9% sodium chloride. If desired, product may be left in place for up to 24 hours; do not leave in the body.

Thrombin-JMI®: Adults:

Solution: Use 1000-2000 int. units/mL of solution where bleeding is profuse; use 100 int. units/mL for bleeding from skin or mucosal surfaces

Powder: May apply powder directly to the site of bleeding or on oozing surfaces

Mechanism of Action Activates platelets and catalyzes the conversion of fibrinogen to fibrin to promote hemostasis.

Contraindications Hypersensitivity to thrombin or any component of the formulation; not for direct injection into the circulatory system (for topical use only); additionally,

Evithrom™ is also contraindicated in patients with known anaphylactic or severe systemic reactions to blood products; also contraindicated for the treatment of severe or brisk arterial bleeding

Recothrom™ is also contraindicated in patients with hypersensitivity to hamster proteins; also contraindicated for the treatment of severe or brisk arterial bleeding

Thrombi-Gel®: Should not be used in closure of skin incisions, due to possible interference with healing of skin edges.

Thrombin-JMI® and Thrombi-Pad® are also contraindicated in patients with hypersensitivity to material of bovine origin.

Warnings/Precautions For topical use only. Do not inject intravenously or intra-arterially. Intravascular clotting, possibly leading to death, may occur following injection. Powder and solution formulations may be used in combination with absorbable gelatin sponges

[U.S. Boxed Warning]: Bovine-source topical thrombin may be associated with abnormal hemostasis, ranging from asymptomatic laboratory alterations to severe bleeding and/or thrombosis. Abnormalities appear to be immunologically mediated; repeated applications increase risk. Consult expert in coagulation disorders if laboratory evidence and/or signs and symptoms of bleeding are noted. Re-exposure of patients who develop antibodies to bovine thrombin preparations should be avoided. Evithrom™ is a product of human plasma; may potentially contain infectious agents which could transmit disease. Screening of donors, as well as testing and/or inactivation or removal of certain viruses, reduces the risk. Infections thought to be transmitted by this product should be reported to the manufacturer. Recothrom™ should be used with caution in patients with known hypersensitivity to snake proteins; the potential for allergic reaction exists. Do not use Thrombi-Gel® or Thrombi-Pad® in the presence of infection; use caution in areas of contamination. Thrombi-Pad® is nonabsorbable; do not leave in the body.

Drug Interactions

Avoid Concomitant Use There are no known interactions where it is recommended to avoid concomitant use.

Increased Effect/Toxicity There are no known significant interactions involving an increase in effect.

Decreased Effect There are no known significant interactions involving a decrease in effect.

Pregnancy Risk Factor C

Dosage Forms

Pad, topical [preservative free]:

Thrombi-Pad® 3x3: ≥200 units

Powder for reconstitution, topical:

Thrombin-JMI®: 5000 int. units, 20,000 int. units

Thrombin-JMI® Epistaxis kit: 5000 int. units

Thrombin-JMI® Spray Kit, Thrombin-JMI® Syringe Spray Kit: 20,000 int. units

Powder for reconstitution, topical [preservative free]:

Recothrom™: 5000 int. units; 20,000 int. units

Solution, topical:

Evithrom™: 800-1200 int. units/mL (2 mL, 5 mL, 20 mL)

Sponge, topical [preservative free]:

Thrombi-Gel® 10: ≥1000 units (10s)

Thrombi-Gel® 40: ≥1000 units (5s)

Thrombi-Gel® 100: ≥2000 units (5s)

Thyroid, Desiccated (THYE roid DES i kay tid)

Related Information

Endocrine Disorders and Pregnancy *on page* 1879

U.S. Brand Names Armour® Thyroid; Nature-Throid™; Westhroid™

Pharmacologic Category Thyroid Product

Use Replacement or supplemental therapy in hypothyroidism; pituitary TSH suppressants (thyroid nodules, thyroiditis, multinodular goiter, thyroid cancer), thyrotoxicosis, diagnostic suppression tests

Local Anesthetic/Vasoconstrictor Precautions No precautions with vasoconstrictor are necessary if patient is well controlled with thyroid preparations

Effects on Dental Treatment No significant effects or complications reported

Effects on Bleeding No information available to require special precautions

General Dosage Range Oral:

Children 0-6 months: 15-30 mg/day **or** 4.8-6 mg/kg/day

Children 6-12 months: 30-45 mg/day **or** 3.6-4.8 mg/kg/day

Children 1-5 years: 45-60 mg/day **or** 3-3.6 mg/kg/day

Children 6-12 years: 60-90 mg/day **or** 2.4-3 mg/kg/day

Children >12 years: >90 mg/day **or** 1.2-1.8 mg/kg/day

Adults: Initial: 15-30 mg/day; Maintenance: 60-120 mg/day

Mechanism of Action The primary active compound is T_3 (triiodothyronine), which may be converted from T_4 (thyroxine) and then circulates throughout the body to influence growth and maturation of various tissues; exact mechanism of action is unknown; however, it is believed the thyroid hormone exerts its many metabolic effects through control of DNA transcription and protein synthesis; involved in normal metabolism, growth, and development; promotes gluconeogenesis, increases utilization and mobilization of glycogen stores and stimulates protein synthesis, increases basal metabolic rate

Pharmacodynamics/Kinetics

Half-life Elimination Serum: Liothyronine: 1-2 days; Thyroxine: 6-7 days

Pregnancy Risk Factor A

Thyrotropin Alpha (thye roe TROH pin AL fa)

U.S. Brand Names Thyrogen®

Canadian Brand Names Thyrogen®

Pharmacologic Category Diagnostic Agent

Use As an adjunctive diagnostic tool for serum thyroglobulin (Tg) testing; adjunctive treatment for radioiodine ablation of thyroid tissue remnants after total or near-total thyroidectomy in patients with well-differentiated thyroid cancer without evidence of metastatic disease

Potential clinical uses include: Patients with an undetectable Tg on thyroid hormone suppressive therapy to exclude the diagnosis of residual or recurrent thyroid cancer, patients requiring serum Tg testing and radioiodine imaging who are unwilling to undergo thyroid hormone withdrawal testing and whose treating physician believes that use of a less sensitive test is justified, patients who are either unable to mount an adequate endogenous TSH response to thyroid hormone withdrawal or in whom withdrawal is medically contraindicated, and patients without evidence of metastatic disease to ablate thyroid remnants (in combination with radioiodine [I^{131}]) following near-total thyroidectomy.

Local Anesthetic/Vasoconstrictor Precautions No information available to require special precautions

Effects on Dental Treatment No significant effects or complications reported

Effects on Bleeding No information available to require special precautions

Adverse Effects

>10%: Gastrointestinal: Nausea (3% to 12%)

1% to 10%:

Central nervous system: Headache (1% to 7%), dizziness (≤3%), fatigue (1% to 3%), insomnia (≤2%)

Endocrine & metabolic: Hypercholesterolemia (≤3%), cholesterol abnormal (≤1%)

Gastrointestinal: Vomiting (1% to 3%), diarrhea (≤1%)

Neuromuscular & skeletal: Paresthesia (≤2%), weakness (≤2%)

Respiratory: Nasopharyngitis (≤1%)

Adverse reactions which may be related to local edema or hemorrhage at metastatic sites: Acute visual loss, enlargement of locally-recurring papillary carcinoma (accompanied by dyspnea, stridor, or dysphonia), hemiplegia, hemiparesis, laryngeal edema with respiratory distress, pain

General Dosage Range I.M.: *Children >16 years and Adults:* 0.9 mg, followed 24 hours later by a second 0.9 mg dose

Mechanism of Action Thyrotropin alfa, derived from a recombinant DNA source, has the identical amino acid sequence as endogenous human thyroid stimulating hormone (TSH). As a diagnostic tool in conjunction with serum thyroglobulin (Tg) testing, thyrotropin alfa stimulates the secretion of Tg from any remaining thyroid tissues (remnants). Under conditions of successful thyroidectomy and complete ablation, very little serum Tg should be detected under TSH stimulatory conditions; conversely, elevated Tg levels suggest the presence of remnant thyroid tissues. Since the source of TSH is exogenous, stimulation of Tg synthesis can be achieved in euthyroid patients, avoiding the need for thyroid hormone withdrawal.

As an adjunctive agent for radioiodine ablation treatment of thyroid cancer tissue remnants, thyrotropin alfa binds to TSH receptors on these tissues, stimulating the uptake and organification of iodine, including radiolabeled iodine (I^{131}). Cancerous tissue is destroyed via gamma emission from the radioiodine concentrated in these tissues.

Pharmacodynamics/Kinetics

Half-life Elimination 25 ± 10 hours

Time to Peak Median: 10 hours (range: 3-24 hours)

Pregnancy Risk Factor C

TiaGABine (tye AG a been)

U.S. Brand Names Gabitril®

Canadian Brand Names Gabitril®

Pharmacologic Category Anticonvulsant, Miscellaneous

Use Adjunctive therapy in adults and children ≥12 years of age in the treatment of partial seizures

Local Anesthetic/Vasoconstrictor Precautions No information available to require special precautions

Effects on Dental Treatment Key adverse event(s) related to dental treatment: Stomatitis, gingivitis, and mouth ulceration.

Effects on Bleeding No information available to require special precautions

Adverse Effects

>10%:

- Central nervous system: Concentration decreased, dizziness, nervousness, somnolence
- Gastrointestinal: Nausea
- Neuromuscular & skeletal: Weakness, tremor

1% to 10%:

- Cardiovascular: Chest pain, edema, hypertension, palpitation, peripheral edema, syncope, tachycardia, vasodilation
- Central nervous system: Agitation, ataxia, chills, confusion, difficulty with memory, confusion, depersonalization, depression, euphoria, hallucination, hostility, insomnia, malaise, migraine, paranoid reaction, personality disorder, speech disorder
- Dermatologic: Alopecia, bruising, dry skin, pruritus, rash
- Gastrointestinal: Abdominal pain, diarrhea, gingivitis, increased appetite, mouth ulceration, stomatitis, vomiting, weight gain/loss
- Neuromuscular & skeletal: Abnormal gait, arthralgia, dysarthria, hyper-/hypokinesia, hyper-/hypotonia, myasthenia, myalgia, myoclonus, neck pain, paresthesia, reflexes decreased, stupor, twitching, vertigo
- Ocular: Abnormal vision, amblyopia, nystagmus
- Otic: Ear pain, hearing impairment, otitis media, tinnitus
- Respiratory: Bronchitis, cough, dyspnea, epistaxis, pneumonia
- Miscellaneous: Allergic reaction, cyst, diaphoresis, flu-like syndrome, lymphadenopathy

General Dosage Range Dosage adjustment recommended in patients on concomitant therapy

Oral:

Children 12-18 years: Initial: 4 mg once daily; Maintenance: 8-32 mg/day in 2-4 divided doses

Adults: Initial: 4 mg once daily; Maintenance: 8-56 mg/day in 2-4 divided doses

Mechanism of Action The exact mechanism by which tiagabine exerts antiseizure activity is not definitively known; however, *in vitro* experiments demonstrate that it enhances the activity of gamma aminobutyric acid (GABA), the major neuroinhibitory transmitter in the nervous system; it is thought that binding to the GABA uptake carrier inhibits the uptake of GABA into presynaptic neurons, allowing an increased amount of GABA to be available to postsynaptic neurons; based on *in vitro* studies, tiagabine does not inhibit the uptake of dopamine, norepinephrine, serotonin, glutamate, or choline

Pharmacodynamics/Kinetics

Half-life Elimination 2-5 hours when administered with enzyme inducers; 7-9 hours when administered without enzyme inducers

Time to Peak Plasma: 45 minutes

Pregnancy Risk Factor C

Ticarcillin and Clavulanate Potassium

(tye kar SIL in & klav yoo LAN ate poe TASS ee um)

U.S. Brand Names Timentin®

Canadian Brand Names Timentin®

Pharmacologic Category Antibiotic, Penicillin

Use Treatment of lower respiratory tract, urinary tract, skin and skin structures, bone and joint, gynecologic (endometritis) and intra-abdominal (peritonitis) infections, and septicemia caused by susceptible organisms. Clavulanate expands activity of ticarcillin to include beta-lactamase producing strains of *S. aureus*, *H. influenzae*, *Bacteroides* species, and some other gram-negative bacilli

Local Anesthetic/Vasoconstrictor Precautions No information available to require special precautions

Effects on Dental Treatment Key adverse event(s) related to dental treatment: Prolonged use of penicillins may lead to development of oral candidiasis.

Effects on Bleeding May inhibit platelet aggregation (dose related). No information available to require special precautions

Adverse Effects Frequency not defined.

Central nervous system: Confusion, drowsiness, fever, headache, Jarisch-Herxheimer reaction, seizure

Dermatologic: Erythema multiforme, pruritus, rash, Stevens-Johnson syndrome, toxic epidermal necrolysis, urticaria

Endocrine & metabolic: Electrolyte imbalance

Gastrointestinal: *Clostridium difficile* colitis, diarrhea, nausea, vomiting

Hematologic: Bleeding, eosinophilia, hemolytic anemia, leukopenia, neutropenia, positive Coombs' reaction, prothrombin time prolonged, thrombocytopenia

Hepatic: Hepatotoxicity, jaundice

Local: Injection site reaction (pain, burning, induration); thrombophlebitis

Neuromuscular & skeletal: Myoclonus

Renal: BUN increased, interstitial nephritis (acute), serum creatinine increased

Miscellaneous: Anaphylaxis, hypersensitivity reactions

General Dosage Range Dosage adjustment recommended in patients with hepatic or renal impairment

I.V.:

Children and Adults <60 kg: 200-300 mg of ticarcillin component/kg/day in divided doses every 4-6 hours

Children ≥60 kg and Adults: 3.1 g (ticarcillin 3 g plus clavulanic acid 0.1 g) every 4-6 hours (maximum: 24 g of ticarcillin component/day)

Mechanism of Action Inhibits bacterial cell wall synthesis by binding to one or more of the penicillin-binding proteins (PBPs); which in turn inhibits the final transpeptidation step of peptidoglycan synthesis in bacterial cell walls, thus inhibiting cell wall biosynthesis. Bacteria eventually lyse due to ongoing activity of cell wall autolytic enzymes (autolysins and murein hydrolases) while cell wall assembly is arrested.

Pharmacodynamics/Kinetics

Half-life Elimination Ticarcillin: 1.1 hours; Clavulanic acid: 1.1 hours

Pregnancy Risk Factor B

Ticlopidine (tye KLOE pi deen)

Canadian Brand Names Alti-Ticlopidine; Apo-Ticlopidine®; Gen-Ticlopidine; Mylan-Ticlopidine; Novo-Ticlopidine; Nu-Ticlopidine; Rhoxal-ticlopidine; Sandoz-Ticlopidine; Ticlid®

Pharmacologic Category Antiplatelet Agent; Antiplatelet Agent, Thienopyridine

Use Platelet aggregation inhibitor that reduces the risk of thrombotic stroke in patients who have had a stroke or stroke precursors. **Note:** Due to its association with life-threatening hematologic disorders, ticlopidine should be reserved for patients who are intolerant to aspirin, or who have failed aspirin therapy. Adjunctive therapy (with aspirin) following successful coronary stent implantation to reduce the incidence of subacute stent thrombosis.

Unlabeled/Investigational Use Protection of aortocoronary bypass grafts, diabetic microangiopathy, ischemic heart disease, prevention of postoperative DVT, reduction of graft loss following renal transplant

Local Anesthetic/Vasoconstrictor Precautions No information available to require special precautions

Effects on Dental Treatment No significant effects or complications reported; if a patient is to undergo elective surgery and an antiplatelet effect is not desired, ticlopidine should be discontinued at least 7 days prior to surgery.

Effects on Bleeding Ticlopidine blocks platelet aggregation and may prolong bleeding time. Inhibition is irreversible; on discontinuation, normal platelet function returns only when new platelets are released from the bone marrow. Dental practitioners should note that recommendations differ between general surgery (eg, appendectomy, hip replacement) and dental surgery. Prior to elective general surgery, it may be temporarily discontinued (usually for 5-10 days) to restore platelet function. However, routine interruption of therapy for noninvasive dental procedures is NOT warranted and there is no scientific evidence to warrant the discontinuance of ticlopidine prior to dental surgery. In particular, ticlopidine should NOT be discontinued in patients with cardiac stents that have not completed their full course of dual antiplatelet therapy (aspirin, clopidogrel/ticlopidine); patient specific situations need to be discussed with cardiologist. When feasible, postponement of dental surgery until the completion of dual antiplatelet therapy should be considered.

Adverse Effects As with all drugs which may affect hemostasis, bleeding is associated with ticlopidine. Hemorrhage may occur at virtually any site. Risk is dependent on multiple variables, including the use of multiple agents which alter hemostasis and patient susceptibility.

>10%:
- Endocrine & metabolic: Total cholesterol increased (increases of ~8% to 10% within 1 month of therapy), triglycerides increased
- Gastrointestinal: Diarrhea (13%)

1% to 10%:
- Central nervous system: Dizziness (1%)
- Dermatologic: Rash (5%), purpura (2%), pruritus (1%)
- Gastrointestinal: Nausea (7%), dyspepsia (7%), gastrointestinal pain (4%), vomiting (2%), flatulence (2%), anorexia (1%)
- Hematologic: Neutropenia (2%)
- Hepatic: Alkaline phosphatase increased (>2 x upper limit of normal; 8%), abnormal liver function test (1%)

General Dosage Range Oral: *Adults:* 250 mg twice daily

Mechanism of Action Ticlopidine requires *in vivo* biotransformation to an unidentified active metabolite. This active metabolite irreversibly blocks the P2Y12 component of ADP receptors, which prevents activation of the GPIIb/IIIa receptor complex, thereby reducing platelet aggregation. Platelets blocked by ticlopidine are affected for the remainder of their lifespan.

Pharmacodynamics/Kinetics

Onset of Action ~6 hours; Peak effect: 3-5 days; serum levels do not correlate with clinical antiplatelet activity

Half-life Elimination 13 hours

Time to Peak ~2 hours

Pregnancy Risk Factor B

Tigecycline (tye ge SYE kleen)

U.S. Brand Names Tygacil®

Canadian Brand Names Tygacil®

Pharmacologic Category Antibiotic, Glycylcycline

Use Treatment of complicated skin and skin structure infections caused by susceptible organisms, including methicillin-resistant *Staphylococcus aureus* and vancomycin-sensitive *Enterococcus faecalis*; complicated intra-abdominal infections (cIAI); community-acquired pneumonia

Local Anesthetic/Vasoconstrictor Precautions No information available to require special precautions

Effects on Dental Treatment Key adverse events(s) related to dental treatment: Tigecycline is structurally similar to tetracycline. Therefore, tigecycline is not recommended for use in pregnancy or in children ≤8 years of age. Permanent discoloration of the teeth may occur if used during tooth development.

Effects on Bleeding No information available to require special precautions

Adverse Effects Note: Frequencies relative to placebo are not available; some frequencies are lower than those experienced with comparator drugs.

>10%: Gastrointestinal: Nausea (26%; severe: 1%), vomiting (18%; severe: 1%), diarrhea (12%)

2% to 10%:

Central nervous system: Headache (6%), dizziness (3%)
Dermatologic: Rash (3%)
Endocrine & metabolic: Hypoproteinemia (5%)
Gastrointestinal: Abdominal pain (6%), dyspepsia (2%)
Hematologic: Anemia (4%)
Hepatic: ALT increased (5%), AST increased (4%), alkaline phosphatase increased (4%), amylase increased (3%), bilirubin increased (2%)
Local: Phlebitis (3%)
Neuromuscular & skeletal: Weakness (3%)
Renal: BUN increased (3%)
Miscellaneous: Infection (8%), abnormal healing (4%), abscess (3%)

General Dosage Range Dosage adjustment recommended in patients with hepatic impairment

I.V.: *Adults:* Initial: 100 mg as a single dose; Maintenance: 50 mg every 12 hours

Mechanism of Action A glycylcycline antibiotic that binds to the 30S ribosomal subunit of susceptible bacteria, thereby, inhibiting protein synthesis. Generally considered bacteriostatic; however, bactericidal activity has been demonstrated against isolates of *S. pneumoniae* and *L. pneumophila.* Tigecycline is a derivative of minocycline (9-t-butylglycylamido minocycline), and while not classified as a tetracycline, it may share some class-associated adverse effects. Tigecycline has demonstrated activity against a variety of gram-positive and -negative bacterial pathogens including methicillin-resistant staphylococci.

Pharmacodynamics/Kinetics

Half-life Elimination Single dose: 27 hours; following multiple doses: 42 hours

Pregnancy Risk Factor D

Tiludronate (tye LOO droe nate)

Related Information

Osteonecrosis of the Jaw *on page* 1894

U.S. Brand Names Skelid®

Pharmacologic Category Bisphosphonate Derivative

Use Treatment of Paget's disease of the bone (osteitis deformans) in patients who have a level of serum alkaline phosphatase (SAP) at least twice the upper limit of normal, or who are symptomatic, or who are at risk for future complications of their disease

Local Anesthetic/Vasoconstrictor Precautions No information available to require special precautions

Effects on Dental Treatment Osteonecrosis of the jaw (ONJ), generally associated with local infection and/or tooth extraction and often with delayed healing, has been reported in patients taking bisphosphonates. Symptoms included nonhealing extraction socket or an exposed jawbone. Most reported cases of bisphosphonate-associated osteonecrosis have been in cancer patients treated with intravenous bisphosphonates. However, some have occurred in patients with postmenopausal osteoporosis taking oral bisphosphonates. Dental surgery, particularly tooth extraction, may increase the risk for ONJ. Patients who develop ONJ while on bisphosphonate therapy should receive care by an oral surgeon. See Dental Comment.

Effects on Bleeding No information available to require special precautions

Adverse Effects 1% to 10%:

Cardiovascular: Chest pain (3%), edema (3%), peripheral edema (3%), flushing, hypertension, syncope
Central nervous system: Anxiety, fatigue, insomnia, nervousness, somnolence, vertigo
Dermatologic: Rash (3%), skin disorder (3%), pruritus
Endocrine & metabolic: Hyperparathyroidism (3%)
Gastrointestinal: Nausea (9%), diarrhea (9%), dyspepsia (5%), vomiting (4%), flatulence (3%), tooth disorder (3%), abdominal pain, anorexia, constipation, gastritis, xerostomia
Genitourinary: Urinary tract infection
Neuromuscular & skeletal: Paresthesia (4%), arthrosis (3%), fractures, muscle spasm, weakness
Ocular: Cataract (3%), conjunctivitis (3%), glaucoma (3%)
Respiratory: Rhinitis (5%), sinusitis (5%), pharyngitis (3%), bronchitis
Miscellaneous: Accidental injury (4%), infection (3%), diaphoresis

General Dosage Range Oral: *Adults:* 400 mg once daily

Mechanism of Action Inhibition of normal and abnormal bone resorption. Inhibits osteoclasts through at least two mechanisms: disruption of the cytoskeletal ring structure, possibly by inhibition of protein-tyrosine-phosphatase, thus leading to the detachment of osteoclasts from the bone surface area and the inhibition of the osteoclast proton pump.

Pharmacodynamics/Kinetics

Onset of Action Delayed, may require several weeks

Half-life Elimination Healthy volunteers: Single dose: 50 hours; Cl_{cr} 11-18 mL/minute: 205 hours; Pagetic patients: Repeated dosing: 150 hours

Time to Peak Plasma: Within 2 hours

Pregnancy Risk Factor C

Dental Comment According to the 2008 report by the American Dental Association (ADA), the incidence of osteonecrosis of the jawbone associated with oral bisphosphonate therapy remains low. It was also stated that the benefits of using oral bisphosphonates to prevent osteoporosis significantly outweighs the small risk of developing bisphosphonate-associated osteonecrosis (Edwards, 2008). The full 26 page report can be accessed at http://www.ada.org/sections/professionalResources/pdfs/topics_osteonecrosis_bisphosphonate_report.pdf.

The ADA review stated the incidence of oral bisphosphonate-associated osteonecrosis of the jaw was one case for every 140,000 person-years exposure to oral bisphosphonates (ADA, 2006). This figure was based on information received from Merck & Co citing 170 worldwide cases for alendronate (Fosamax®). In addition, Procter & Gamble Pharmaceuticals has cited 20 cases for risedronate (Actonel®) and Roche Laboratories, Inc has cited one case for ibandronate (Boniva®).

In addition, the ADA 2008 report reiterates that the risk of osteonecrosis of the jawbone with oral bisphosphonates is minute compared to the risks with intravenous bisphosphonates therapy in cancer patients. The ADA cites an ~20% incidence in patients receiving bisphosphonates intravenously for cancer therapy. Fewer than 10% of all cases of bisphosphonate-associated osteonecrosis of the jaw occurs in patients taking the oral drugs.

Information on alendronate (Fosamax®) use in Australia and the incidence of ONJ has been reported (Mavrokokki, 2007). A survey form was sent to all of the Australian members of the Australian and New Zealand Association of Oral and Maxillofacial Surgeons requesting cases that they had identified as ONJ in 2004 and 2005. The definition of ONJ for the survey was an area of exposed bone in the jawbone that failed to heal within 6 weeks in patients taking bisphosphonates for bone disease. The frequency of ONJ in osteoporotic patients, mainly taking weekly oral alendronate, was 1 in 8470 to 1 in 2260 (0.01% to 0.04%) patients. If extractions were carried out, the calculated frequency was 1 in 1130 to 1 in 296 (0.09% to 0.34%) patients. The minimum values in these cases were determined from the survey, whereas, the maximum values were extrapolated from survey data. The median time to onset of ONJ in alendronate patients was 24 months.

A 2010 study reported the prevalence of osteonecrosis of the jaw in patients using alendronate-type drugs was 1 out of 952 patients or ~0.1% (Lo, 2010). The study's protocol involved a survey mailed out to 13,946 members of Kaiser Permanente of Northern California healthcare delivery system; 8572 patients responded to the survey. Investigators identified respondents reporting oral problems and dental symptoms. These respondents were then interviewed by telephone for presence of dental problems including exposed bone, gingival sores, moderate periodontal disease, and persistent symptoms or complications after dental procedures. Those selected were then invited for an examination or to have their dental records reviewed. The diagnosis of ONJ was made according to the 2006 American Association of Oral and Maxillofacial Surgeons criteria which required treatment with a bisphosphonate, exposed bone in the maxillofacial region lasting >8 weeks, and no radiotherapy involving the jaw. Of the 8572 respondents, 9 cases of ONJ were identified; 5 had developed ONJ spontaneously and 4 developed ONJ after tooth extraction. Specific oral bisphosphonates were not identified. When extrapolated to patient-years of bisphosphonate exposure, this prevalence rate of 0.1% equates to a frequency of 28 cases per 100,000 person-years of oral bisphosphonate treatment.

Timolol (Systemic) (TIM oh lol)

Related Information

Cardiovascular Diseases *on page* 1848

Canadian Brand Names Apo-Timol®; Nu-Timolol

Pharmacologic Category Beta-Adrenergic Blocker, Nonselective

Use Treatment of hypertension and angina; to reduce mortality following myocardial infarction; prophylaxis of migraine

Local Anesthetic/Vasoconstrictor Precautions Epinephrine has interacted with nonselective beta-blockers, such as propranolol, to result in initial hypertensive episode followed by bradycardia. Timolol is also a nonselective beta-blocker. The significance of a potential systemic interaction is well known and cautionary use of epinephrine is advised.

Effects on Dental Treatment Key adverse event(s) related to dental treatment: Xerostomia (normal salivary flow resumes upon discontinuation).

Timolol is a nonselective beta-blocker and may enhance the pressor response to epinephrine, resulting in hypertension and bradycardia. Many nonsteroidal anti-inflammatory drugs, such as ibuprofen and indomethacin, can reduce the hypotensive effect of beta-blockers after 3 or more weeks of therapy with the NSAID. Short-term NSAID use (ie, 3 days) requires no special precautions in patients taking beta-blockers.

Effects on Bleeding No information available to require special precautions

Adverse Effects 1% to 10%:

Cardiovascular: Bradycardia

Central nervous system: Fatigue, dizziness

Respiratory: Dyspnea

Frequency not defined:

Cardiovascular: Angina pectoris, arrhythmia, cardiac failure, cardiac arrest, cerebral vascular accident, cerebral ischemia, edema, hypotension, heart block, palpitation, Raynaud's phenomenon

Central nervous system: Anxiety, confusion, depression, disorientation, hallucinations, insomnia, memory loss, nervousness, nightmares, somnolence

Dermatologic: Alopecia, angioedema, pseudopemphigoid, psoriasiform rash, psoriasis exacerbation, rash, urticaria

Endocrine & metabolic: Hypoglycemia masked, libido decreased

Gastrointestinal: Anorexia, diarrhea, dyspepsia, nausea, xerostomia

Genitourinary: Impotence, retoperitoneal fibrosis

Hematologic: Claudication

Neuromuscular & skeletal: Myasthenia gravis exacerbation, paresthesia

Ocular: Blepharitis, conjunctivitis, corneal sensitivity decreased, cystoid macular edema, diplopia, dry eyes, foreign body sensation, keratitis, ocular discharge, ocular pain, ptosis, refractive changes, tearing, visual disturbances

Otic: Tinnitus

Respiratory: Bronchospasm, cough, nasal congestion, pulmonary edema, respiratory failure

Miscellaneous: Allergic reactions, cold hands/feet, Peyronie's disease, systemic lupus erythematosus

General Dosage Range Oral: *Adults:* Initial: 10 mg twice daily; Maintenance: 20-60 mg/day in 2 divided doses (maximum: 60 mg/day)

Mechanism of Action Blocks both $beta_1$- and $beta_2$-adrenergic receptors; reduces blood pressure by blocking adrenergic receptors and decreasing sympathetic outflow, produces a negative chronotropic and inotropic activity through an unknown mechanism

Pharmacodynamics/Kinetics

Onset of Action Hypotensive: 15-45 minutes; Peak effect: 0.5-2.5 hours

Duration of Action ~4 hours

Half-life Elimination 2-2.7 hours; prolonged with renal impairment

Time to Peak Plasma: 1-2 hours

Pregnancy Risk Factor C

Timolol (Ophthalmic) (TIM oh lol)

U.S. Brand Names Betimol®; Istalol®; Timolol GFS; Timoptic-XE®; Timoptic®; Timoptic® in OcuDose®

Canadian Brand Names Apo-Timop®; Dom-Timolol; Med-Timolol; Mylan-Timolol; PMS-Timolol; Rhoxal-Timolol; Sandoz-Timolol; Tim-AK; Timoptic-XE®; Timoptic®

Pharmacologic Category Beta-Adrenergic Blocker, Nonselective; Ophthalmic Agent, Antiglaucoma

Use Treatment of elevated intraocular pressure such as glaucoma or ocular hypertension

Local Anesthetic/Vasoconstrictor Precautions Epinephrine has interacted with nonselective beta-blockers, such as propranolol, to result in initial hypertensive episode followed by bradycardia. Timolol is also a nonselective beta-blocker. The significance of a potential systemic interaction with epinephrine is unknown. However, it is suggested that cautionary procedures be used, particularly if vasoconstrictor is used immediately following a dose of timolol taken by the patient.

Effects on Dental Treatment Key adverse event(s) related to dental treatment: Xerostomia (normal salivary flow resumes upon discontinuation).

Timolol is a nonselective beta-blocker and may enhance the pressor response to epinephrine, resulting in hypertension and bradycardia.

Effects on Bleeding No information available to require special precautions

Adverse Effects

>10%: Ocular: Burning, stinging

Frequency not defined:

Cardiovascular: Angina pectoris, arrhythmia, bradycardia, cardiac arrest, cardiac failure, cerebral ischemia, cerebral vascular accident, edema, heart block, hypertension, hypotension, palpitation, Raynaud's phenomenon

Central nervous system: Anxiety, confusion, depression, disorientation, dizziness, hallucinations, headache, insomnia, memory loss, nervousness, nightmares, somnolence

Dermatologic: Alopecia, angioedema, pseudopemphigoid, psoriasiform rash, psoriasis exacerbation, rash, urticaria

Endocrine & metabolic: Hypoglycemia masked, libido decreased

Gastrointestinal: Anorexia, diarrhea, dyspepsia, nausea, xerostomia

Genitourinary: Impotence, retoperitoneal fibrosis

Hematologic: Claudication

Neuromuscular & skeletal: Myasthenia gravis exacerbation, paresthesia

Ocular: Blepharitis, blurred vision, cataract, choroidal detachment (following filtration surgery), conjunctival injection, conjunctivitis, corneal sensitivity decreased, cystoid macular edema, diplopia, dry eyes, foreign body sensation, hyperemia, itching, keratitis, ocular discharge, ocular pain, ptosis, tearing, visual acuity decreased refractive changes, visual disturbances

Otic: Tinnitus

Respiratory: Bronchospasm, cough, dyspnea, nasal congestion, pulmonary edema, respiratory failure

Miscellaneous: Allergic reactions, cold hands/feet, Peyronie's disease, systemic lupus erythematosus

General Dosage Range Ophthalmic:

Gel-forming solution: *Children and Adults:* Instill 1 drop (0.25% or 0.5%) once daily

Solution: *Children and Adults:* Initial: Instill 1 drop (0.25%) twice daily; Maintenance: Instill 1 drop (0.25% or 0.5%) 1-2 times daily (maximum: 2 drops/day [0.5%])

Mechanism of Action Blocks both $beta_1$- and $beta_2$-adrenergic receptors, reduces intraocular pressure by reducing aqueous humor production or possibly outflow; reduces blood pressure by blocking adrenergic receptors and decreasing sympathetic outflow, produces a negative chronotropic and inotropic activity through an unknown mechanism

Pharmacodynamics/Kinetics

Onset of Action Intraocular pressure reduction: 30 minutes; Peak effect: 1-2 hours

Duration of Action ~4 hours; Intraocular: 24 hours

Pregnancy Risk Factor C

Tinidazole (tye NI da zole)

U.S. Brand Names Tindamax®

Pharmacologic Category Amebicide; Antibiotic, Miscellaneous; Antiprotozoal, Nitroimidazole

Use Treatment of trichomoniasis caused by *T. vaginalis*; treatment of giardiasis caused by *G. duodenalis* (*G. lamblia*); treatment of intestinal amebiasis and amebic liver abscess caused by *E. histolytica*; treatment of bacterial vaginosis caused by *Bacteroides* spp, *Gardnerella vaginalis*, and *Prevotella* spp in nonpregnant females

Local Anesthetic/Vasoconstrictor Precautions No information available to require special precautions

Effects on Dental Treatment Key adverse event(s) related to dental treatment: Xerostomia and changes in salivation (normal salivary flow resumes upon discontinuation), metallic/bitter taste, oral candidiasis, tongue discoloration, stomatitis, furry tongue. See Dental Comment.

Effects on Bleeding No information available to require special precautions

Adverse Effects

1% to 10%:

Central nervous system: Fatigue/malaise (1% to 2%), dizziness (≤1%), headache (≤1%)

Endocrine & metabolic: Menorrhagia (>2%)

Gastrointestinal: Metallic/bitter taste (4% to 6%), nausea (3% to 5%), anorexia (2% to 3%), appetite decreased (>2%), flatulence (>2%), dyspepsia/cramps/epigastric discomfort (1% to 2%), vomiting (1% to 2%), constipation (≤1%)

Genitourinary: *Candida* vaginitis (5%), painful urination (>2%), pelvic pain (>2%), urine abnormality (>2%), vaginal odor (>2%), vulvovaginal discomfort (>2%)
Neuromuscular & skeletal: Weakness (1% to 2%)
Renal: Urinary tract infection (>2%)
Respiratory: Upper respiratory tract infection (>2%)

Frequency not defined:
Cardiovascular: Flushing, palpitation
Central nervous system: Ataxia, coma (rare), confusion (rare), depression (rare), drowsiness, fever, giddiness, insomnia, seizure, vertigo
Dermatologic: Angioedema, pruritus, rash, urticaria
Gastrointestinal: Abdominal pain, diarrhea, furry tongue (rare), oral candidiasis, salivation, stomatitis, thirst, tongue discoloration, xerostomia
Genitourinary: Urine darkened, vaginal discharge increased
Hematologic: Leukopenia (transient), neutropenia (transient), thrombocytopenia (reversible; rare)
Hepatic: Transaminases increased
Neuromuscular & skeletal: Arthralgia, arthritis, myalgia, peripheral neuropathy (transient, includes numbness and paresthesia)
Respiratory: Bronchospasm (rare), dyspnea (rare), pharyngitis (rare)
Miscellaneous: Burning sensation, *Candida* overgrowth, diaphoresis

General Dosage Range Oral:
Children >3 years: 50 mg/kg/day (maximum: 2 g/day)
Adults: 1-2 g/day

Mechanism of Action After diffusing into the organism, it is proposed that tinidazole causes cytotoxicity by damaging DNA and preventing further DNA synthesis.

Pharmacodynamics/Kinetics
Half-life Elimination 13 hours
Time to Peak 1.6 hours

Pregnancy Risk Factor C

Dental Comment Although this drug is a member of the metronidazole family, there is no specific dental indication for its use. Just as with metronidazole, alcohol in any form is contraindicated while the patient is on this medication because of the danger of a disulfiram-type reaction.

Tinzaparin (tin ZA pa rin)

Related Information
Cardiovascular Diseases *on page 1848*

U.S. Brand Names Innohep®

Canadian Brand Names Innohep®

Pharmacologic Category Low Molecular Weight Heparin

Use Treatment of acute symptomatic deep vein thrombosis, with or without pulmonary embolism, in conjunction with warfarin sodium

Unlabeled/Investigational Use Prophylaxis of deep vein thrombosis following hip or knee replacement surgery, and general surgery

Local Anesthetic/Vasoconstrictor Precautions No information available to require special precautions

Effects on Dental Treatment Key adverse event(s) related to dental treatment: Bleeding is the major adverse effect of tinzaparin. See Effects on Bleeding.

Effects on Bleeding As with all anticoagulants, bleeding is the major adverse effect of tinzaparin. Hemorrhage may occur at virtually any site; risk is dependent on multiple variables including the intensity of anticoagulation and patient susceptibility. At the recommended doses, LMWHS do not significantly influence platelet aggregation or affect global clotting time (ie, PT or aPTT). Medical consult is suggested.

Adverse Effects As with all anticoagulants, bleeding is the major adverse effect of tinzaparin. Hemorrhage may occur at virtually any site. Risk is dependent on multiple variables.

>10%:
Hepatic: ALT increased (13%)
Local: Injection site hematoma (16%)

1% to 10%:
Cardiovascular: Angina pectoris, chest pain (2%), hyper-/hypotension, tachycardia
Central nervous system: Confusion, dizziness, fever (2%), headache (2%), insomnia, pain (2%)
Dermatologic: Bullous eruption, pruritus, rash (1%), skin disorder
Gastrointestinal: Constipation (1%), dyspepsia, flatulence, nausea (2%), nonspecified gastrointestinal disorder, vomiting (1%)
Genitourinary: Dysuria, urinary retention, urinary tract infection (4%)

Hematologic: Anemia, hematoma, hemorrhage (2%), thrombocytopenia (1%)
Hepatic: AST increased (9%)
Local: Thrombophlebitis (deep)
Neuromuscular & skeletal: Back pain (2%)
Renal: Hematuria (1%)
Respiratory: Dyspnea (1%), epistaxis (2%), pneumonia, pulmonary embolism (2%), respiratory disorder
Miscellaneous: Impaired healing, infection, unclassified reactions

General Dosage Range SubQ: *Adults:* 175 anti-Xa int. units/kg of body weight once daily

Mechanism of Action Standard heparin consists of components with molecular weights ranging from 4000-30,000 daltons with a mean of 16,000 daltons. Heparin acts as an anticoagulant by enhancing the inhibition rate of clotting proteases by antithrombin III, impairing normal hemostasis and inhibition of factor Xa. Low molecular weight heparins have a small effect on the activated partial thromboplastin time and strongly inhibit factor Xa. The primary inhibitory activity of tinzaparin is through antithrombin. Tinzaparin is derived from porcine heparin that undergoes controlled enzymatic depolymerization. The average molecular weight of tinzaparin ranges between 5500 and 7500 daltons which is distributed as <2000 daltons (<10%), 2000-8000 daltons (60% to 72%), and >8000 daltons (22% to 36%). The anti-Xa activity is approximately 100 int. units/mg.

Pharmacodynamics/Kinetics

Onset of Action 2-3 hours

Half-life Elimination 3-4 hours

Time to Peak 4-5 hours

Pregnancy Risk Factor B

Tioconazole (tye oh KONE a zole)

U.S. Brand Names 1-Day™ [OTC]; Vagistat®-1 [OTC]

Pharmacologic Category Antifungal Agent, Vaginal

Use Local treatment of vulvovaginal candidiasis

Local Anesthetic/Vasoconstrictor Precautions No information available to require special precautions

Effects on Dental Treatment No significant effects or complications reported

Effects on Bleeding No information available to require special precautions

Adverse Effects Frequency not defined.

Central nervous system: Headache
Gastrointestinal: Abdominal pain
Dermatologic: Burning, desquamation
Genitourinary: Discharge, dyspareunia, dysuria, irritation, itching, nocturia, vaginal pain, vaginitis, vulvar swelling

General Dosage Range Intravaginal: *Adults:* Insert 1 applicatorful prior to bedtime, as a single dose

Mechanism of Action A 1-substituted imidazole derivative with a broad antifungal spectrum against a wide variety of dermatophytes and yeasts, including *Trichophyton mentagrophytes*, *T. rubrum*, *T. erinacei*, *T. tonsurans*, *Microsporum canis*, *Microsporum gypseum*, and *Candida albicans*. Both agents appear to be similarly effective against *Epidermophyton floccosum*.

Pharmacodynamics/Kinetics

Onset of Action Some improvement: Within 24 hours; Complete relief: Within 7 days

Pregnancy Risk Factor C

Tiopronin (tye oh PROE nin)

U.S. Brand Names Thiola®

Pharmacologic Category Urinary Tract Product

Use Prevention of kidney stone (cystine) formation in patients with severe homozygous cystinuria who have urinary cystine >500 mg/day who are resistant to treatment with high fluid intake, alkali and diet modification, or who have had adverse reactions to penicillamine

Local Anesthetic/Vasoconstrictor Precautions No information available to require special precautions

Effects on Dental Treatment No significant effects or complications reported

Effects on Bleeding No information available to require special precautions

Adverse Effects Frequency not defined.

Central nervous system: Chills, fatigue, fever

Dermatologic: Bruising, pemphigus, pruritus, rash, skin friability/wrinkling, urticaria, warts

Gastrointestinal: Abdominal pain, anorexia, bloating, diarrhea, flatulence, loss of taste perception, nausea, oral ulceration, vomiting

Hematologic: Anemia, bleeding, eosinophilia, leukopenia, thrombocytopenia

Hepatic: Jaundice, liver function tests abnormal

Neuromuscular & skeletal: Arthralgia, myalgia, myasthenia gravis, weakness

Renal: Goodpasture's syndrome, hematuria, nephrotic syndrome, proteinuria

Respiratory: Bronchiolitis, dyspnea, hemoptysis, laryngeal edema, pharyngitis, pulmonary infiltrates, respiratory distress

Miscellaneous: Elastosis perforans serpiginosa, hypersensitivity, loss of smell, lupus-like syndrome, lymphadenopathy, positive ANA test

General Dosage Range Oral:

Children ≥9 years: Initial: 15 mg/kg/day in 3 divided doses

Adults: Initial: 800 mg/day in 3 divided doses; average dose: 1000 mg/day

Mechanism of Action As an active reducing agent, tiopronin undergoes thiol-disulfide exchange with cystine to form tiopronin-cystine disulfide, which is more water soluble than cystine. As a result, the amount of sparingly soluble cystine in the urine is decreased and the formation of cystine calculi is reduced.

Pregnancy Risk Factor C

Tiotropium (ty oh TRO pee um)

Related Information

Respiratory Diseases *on page 1876*

U.S. Brand Names Spiriva® HandiHaler®

Canadian Brand Names Spiriva®

Pharmacologic Category Anticholinergic Agent

Use Maintenance treatment of bronchospasm associated with COPD (including bronchitis and emphysema); reduction of COPD exacerbations

Local Anesthetic/Vasoconstrictor Precautions No information available to require special precautions

Effects on Dental Treatment Key adverse event(s) related to dental treatment: Xerostomia (normal salivary flow resumes upon discontinuation) and ulcerative stomatitis.

Effects on Bleeding No information available to require special precautions

Adverse Effects

>10%:

Gastrointestinal: Xerostomia (5% to 16%)

Respiratory: Upper respiratory tract infection (41%), pharyngitis (9% to 13%), sinusitis (7% to 11%)

1% to 10%:

Cardiovascular: Chest pain (1% to 7%), edema (dependent, 5%)

Central nervous system: Headache (6%), insomnia (4%), depression (1% to 4%), dysphonia (1% to 3%)

Dermatologic: Rash (4%)

Endocrine & metabolic: Hypercholesterolemia (1% to 3%), hyperglycemia (1% to 3%)

Gastrointestinal: Dyspepsia (6%), abdominal pain (5%), constipation (4% to 5%), vomiting (4%), gastroesophageal reflux (1% to 3%), stomatitis (including ulcerative; 1% to 3%)

Genitourinary: Urinary tract infection (7%)

Neuromuscular & skeletal: Arthralgia (4%), myalgia (4%), arthritis (≥3%), leg pain (1% to 3%), paresthesia (1% to 3%), skeletal pain (1% to 3%)

Ocular: Cataract (1% to 3%)

Respiratory: Rhinitis (6%), epistaxis (4%), cough (≥3%), laryngitis (1% to 3%)

Miscellaneous: Infection (4%), moniliasis (4%), flu-like syndrome (≥3%), allergic reaction (1% to 3%), herpes zoster (1% to 3%)

General Dosage Range Inhalation: *Adults:* Contents of 1 capsule (18 mcg) once daily

Mechanism of Action Competitively and reversibly inhibits the action of acetylcholine at type 3 muscarinic (M_3) receptors in bronchial smooth muscle causing bronchodilation

Pharmacodynamics/Kinetics

Half-life Elimination 5-6 days

Time to Peak Plasma: 5 minutes (following inhalation)

Pregnancy Risk Factor C

Tipranavir (tip RA na veer)

Related Information

HIV Infection and AIDS *on page 1883*

U.S. Brand Names Aptivus®

Canadian Brand Names Aptivus®

Pharmacologic Category Antiretroviral Agent, Protease Inhibitor

Use Treatment of HIV-1 infections in combination with ritonavir and other antiretroviral agents; limited to highly treatment-experienced or multiprotease inhibitor-resistant patients.

Local Anesthetic/Vasoconstrictor Precautions No information available to require special precautions

Effects on Dental Treatment No significant effects or complications reported

Effects on Bleeding Increased bleeding has been noted with protease inhibitors in patients with hemophilia A or B. No information available to require routine special precautions relative to hemostasis in other patients.

Adverse Effects

>10%:

- Dermatologic: Rash (children 21%; adults 3% to 10%)
- Endocrine & metabolic: Hypertriglyceridemia (>400 mg/dL: 61%), hypercholesterolemia (>300 mg/dL: 22%)
- Gastrointestinal: Diarrhea (15%)
- Hepatic: Transaminases increased (>2.5 x ULN: 26% to 32%; grade 3/4: 10% to 20%)
- Neuromuscular & skeletal: CPK increased (grade 3/4: children 11%)

2% to 10%:

- Central nervous system: Fever (6% to 8%), fatigue (6%), headache (5%)
- Endocrine & metabolic: Dehydration (2%)
- Gastrointestinal: Nausea (5% to 9%), amylase increased (grade 3: 6% to 8%), vomiting (6%), abdominal pain (4%), diarrhea (children 4%), weight loss (3%)
- Hematologic: Bleeding (children 8%), WBC decreased (grades 3: 5%), anemia (3%), neutropenia (2%)
- Hepatic: ALT increased (2%, grades 3/4: 10%), AST increased (grades 3/4: 6%), GGT increased (2%)
- Neuromuscular & skeletal: Myalgia (2%)
- Respiratory: Cough (children 6%), dyspnea (2%), epistaxis (children 4%)

General Dosage Range Dosage adjustment recommended in patients on concomitant therapy

Oral:

Children ≥2 years: 12-14 mg/kg or 290-375 mg/m^2 (maximum: 500 mg/dose) twice daily

Adults: 500 mg twice daily

Mechanism of Action Binds to the site of HIV-1 protease activity and inhibits cleavage of viral Gag-Pol polyprotein precursors into individual functional proteins required for infectious HIV. This results in the formation of immature, noninfectious viral particles.

Pharmacodynamics/Kinetics

Half-life Elimination Children 2-<6 years of age: ~8 hours, 6-<12 years of age: ~7 hours, 12-18 years: ~5 hours; Adults: 6 hours

Time to Peak 3 hours

Pregnancy Risk Factor C

Tirofiban (tye roe FYE ban)

Related Information

Cardiovascular Diseases *on page 1848*

U.S. Brand Names Aggrastat®

Canadian Brand Names Aggrastat®

Pharmacologic Category Antiplatelet Agent, Glycoprotein IIb/IIIa Inhibitor

Use Treatment of acute coronary syndrome (ie, unstable angina/non-ST-elevation myocardial infarction [UA/NSTEMI]) in combination with heparin

Unlabeled/Investigational Use To support PCI during ST-elevation myocardial infarction (STEMI) (administered at the time of primary PCI)

Local Anesthetic/Vasoconstrictor Precautions No information available to require special precautions

Effects on Dental Treatment Key adverse event(s) related to dental treatment: Bleeding is a potential adverse effect of tirofiban. See Effects on Bleeding.

Effects on Bleeding As with all anticoagulants, bleeding is a potential adverse effect of tirofiban during dental surgery; risk is dependent on multiple variables, including the intensity of anticoagulation and patient susceptibility. Medical consult is suggested. It is unlikely that ambulatory patients presenting for dental treatment will be taking intravenous anticoagulant therapy.

Adverse Effects Bleeding is the major drug-related adverse effect. Patients received background treatment with aspirin and heparin. Major bleeding was reported in 1.4% to 2.2%; minor bleeding in 10.5% to 12%; transfusion was required in 4% to 4.3%.

>1% (nonbleeding adverse events):
- Cardiovascular: Coronary artery dissection (5%), bradycardia (4%), edema (2%)
- Central nervous system: Dizziness (3%), vasovagal reaction (2%), fever (>1%), headache (>1%)
- Gastrointestinal: Nausea (>1%)
- Genitourinary: Pelvic pain (6%)
- Hematologic: Thrombocytopenia: <90,000/mm^3 (1.5%), <50,000/mm^3 (0.3%)
- Neuromuscular & skeletal: Leg pain (3%)
- Miscellaneous: Diaphoresis (2%)

General Dosage Range Dosage adjustment recommended in patients with renal impairment

I.V.: *Adults:* Initial: 0.4 mcg/kg/minute for 30 minutes; Maintenance infusion: 0.1 mcg/kg/minute

Mechanism of Action A reversible antagonist of fibrinogen binding to the GP IIb/IIIa receptor, the major platelet surface receptor involved in platelet aggregation. When administered intravenously, it inhibits *ex vivo* platelet aggregation in a dose- and concentration-dependent manner. When given according to the recommended regimen, >90% inhibition is attained by the end of the 30-minute infusion. Platelet aggregation inhibition is reversible following cessation of the infusion.

Pharmacodynamics/Kinetics

Half-life Elimination 2 hours

Pregnancy Risk Factor B

TiZANidine (tye ZAN i deen)

U.S. Brand Names Zanaflex Capsules®; Zanaflex®

Canadian Brand Names Apo-Tizanidine®; Gen-Tizanidine; Mylan-Tizanidine; Zanaflex®

Generic Availability (U.S.) Yes: Tablet

Pharmacologic Category Alpha$_2$-Adrenergic Agonist

Use Skeletal muscle relaxant used for treatment of muscle spasticity

Unlabeled/Investigational Use Tension headaches, low back pain, and trigeminal neuralgia

Local Anesthetic/Vasoconstrictor Precautions No information available to require special precautions

Effects on Dental Treatment Key adverse event(s) related to dental treatment: Significant xerostomia (normal salivary flow resumes upon discontinuation).

Effects on Bleeding No information available to require special precautions

Adverse Effects Frequency percentages below reported during multiple-dose studies, unless specified otherwise.

>10%:
- Cardiovascular: Hypotension (single-dose study with doses ≥8 mg: 16% to 33%)
- Central nervous system: Somnolence (48%), dizziness (16%)
- Gastrointestinal: Xerostomia (49%)
- Neuromuscular & skeletal: Weakness (41%)

1% to 10%:
- Cardiovascular: Bradycardia (single-dose study with doses ≥8 mg: 2% to 10%)
- Central nervous system: Nervousness (3%), speech disorder (3%), visual hallucinations/delusions (3%; generally occurring in first 6 weeks of therapy), anxiety (1%), depression (1%), fever (1%)
- Dermatologic: Rash (1%), skin ulcer (1%)
- Gastrointestinal: Constipation (4%), vomiting (3%), abdominal pain (1%), diarrhea (1%), dyspepsia (1%)
- Genitourinary: UTI (10%), urinary frequency (3%)
- Hepatic: Liver enzymes increased (3% to 5%)
- Neuromuscular & skeletal: Dyskinesia (3%), back pain (1%), myasthenia (1%), paresthesia (1%)
- Ocular: Blurred vision (3%)
- Respiratory: Pharyngitis (3%), rhinitis (3%)
- Miscellaneous: Infection (6%), flu-like syndrome (3%), diaphoresis (1%)

Dosage

Adults: 2-4 mg 3 times/day

Usual initial dose: 4 mg, may increase by 2-4 mg as needed for satisfactory reduction of muscle tone every 6-8 hours to a maximum of 3 doses in any 24-hour period

Maximum: 36 mg/day

Elderly: No specific dosing guidelines exist; clearance is decreased; dose cautiously

Dosing adjustment in renal impairment: Cl_{cr} <25 mL/minute: Use with caution; clearance reduced >50%. During initial dose titration, use reduced doses. If higher doses necessary, increase dose instead of increasing dosing frequency.

Dosing adjustment in hepatic impairment: Avoid use in hepatic impairment; if used, lowest possible dose should be used initially with close monitoring for adverse effects (eg, hypotension).

Mechanism of Action An alpha$_2$-adrenergic agonist agent which decreases excitatory input to alpha motor neurons; an imidazole derivative chemically-related to clonidine, which acts as a centrally acting muscle relaxant with alpha$_2$-adrenergic agonist properties; acts on the level of the spinal cord

Contraindications Hypersensitivity to tizanidine or any component of the formulation; concomitant therapy with ciprofloxacin or fluvoxamine (potent CYP1A2 inhibitors)

Warnings/Precautions Significant hypotension (possibly with bradycardia or orthostatic hypotension) and sedation may occur; use caution in patients with cardiac disease or those at risk for severe hypotensive or sedative effects. Avoid concomitant administration with CYP1A2 inhibitors; increased tizanidine levels/effects (severe hypotension and sedation) may occur. These effects may also be increased with concomitant administration with other CNS depressants and/or antihypertensives; use caution. Elderly patients are at risk due to decreased clearance, particulary in elderly patients with renal insufficiency (Cl_{cr} <25 mL/minute) compared to healthy elderly subjects; this may lead to an increased risk of adverse effects and/or a longer duration of effects. Use caution in any patient with renal impairment; reduced initial doses recommended in patient with Cl_{cr} <25 mL/minute. Use with extreme caution or avoid in hepatic impairment due to extensive hepatic metabolism and potential hepatotoxicity; AST/ALT elevations (≥2 times baseline) and rarely hepatic failure have occurred; monitoring recommended.

Use has been associated with visual hallucinations or delusions, generally in first 6 weeks of therapy; use caution in patients with psychiatric disorders. Withdrawal resulting in rebound hypertension, tachycardia, and hypertonia may occur upon discontinuation; doses should be decreased slowly, particularly in patients receiving high doses for prolonged periods. Pharmacokinetics and bioequivalence between capsules and tablets altered by nonfasting vs fasting conditions. Limited data exists for chronic use of single doses >8 mg and multiple doses >24 mg/day.

Drug Interactions

Metabolism/Transport Effects Substrate of CYP1A2 (major)

Avoid Concomitant Use

Avoid concomitant use of TiZANidine with any of the following: Ciprofloxacin; Ciprofloxacin (Systemic); FluvoxaMINE; Iobenguane I 123

Increased Effect/Toxicity

TiZANidine may increase the levels/effects of: ACE Inhibitors; Alcohol (Ethyl); CNS Depressants; Hypotensive Agents; Lisinopril; Methotrimeprazine

The levels/effects of TiZANidine may be increased by: Abiraterone; Beta-Blockers; Ciprofloxacin; Ciprofloxacin (Systemic); Contraceptives (Estrogens); CYP1A2 Inhibitors (Moderate); CYP1A2 Inhibitors (Strong); Deferasirox; Droperidol; FluvoxaMINE; MAO Inhibitors; Methotrimeprazine

Decreased Effect

TiZANidine may decrease the levels/effects of: Iobenguane I 123

The levels/effects of TiZANidine may be decreased by: Antidepressants (Alpha2-Antagonist); Serotonin/Norepinephrine Reuptake Inhibitors; Tricyclic Antidepressants

Ethanol/Nutrition/Herb Interactions

Ethanol: May increase CNS depression; monitor for increased effects with coadministration. Caution patients about effects.

Food: The tablet and capsule dosage forms are not bioequivalent when administered with food. Food increases both the time to peak concentration and the extent of absorption for both the tablet and capsule. However, maximal concentrations of tizanidine achieved when administered with food were increased by 30% for the tablet, but decreased by 20% for the capsule. Under fed conditions, the capsule is approximately 80% bioavailable relative to the tablet.

Herb/Nutraceutical: Avoid valerian, St John's wort, kava kava, gotu kola (may increase CNS depression). Avoid black cohosh, California poppy, coleus, golden seal, hawthorn, mistletoe, periwinkle, quinine, shepherd's purse (may increase hypotensive effects).

Dietary Considerations Administration with food compared to administration in the fasting state results in clinically-significant differences in absorption and other pharmacokinetic parameters. Patients should be consistent and should not switch administration of the tablets or the capsules between the fasting and nonfasting state. In addition, switching between the capsules and the tablets in the fed state will also result in significant differences. Opening capsule contents to sprinkle on applesauce compared to swallowing intact capsules whole will also result in significant absorption differences. Patients should be consistent with regards to administration.

Pharmacodynamics/Kinetics

Duration of Action 3-6 hours

Half-life Elimination 2.5 hours

Time to Peak

Fasting state: Capsule, tablet: 1 hour

Fed state: Capsule: 3-4 hours, Tablet: 1.5 hours

Pregnancy Risk Factor C

Lactation Excretion in breast milk unknown/not recommended

Dosage Forms

Capsule, oral:

Zanaflex Capsules®: 2 mg, 4 mg, 6 mg

Tablet, oral: 2 mg, 4 mg

Zanaflex®: 4 mg

Tobramycin (Systemic, Oral Inhalation) (toe bra MYE sin)

U.S. Brand Names TOBI®

Canadian Brand Names TOBI®; Tobramycin Injection, USP

Pharmacologic Category Antibiotic, Aminoglycoside

Use Treatment of documented or suspected infections caused by susceptible gram-negative bacilli, including *Pseudomonas aeruginosa*. Tobramycin solution for inhalation is indicated for the management of cystic fibrosis patients (>6 years of age) with *Pseudomonas aeruginosa*.

Local Anesthetic/Vasoconstrictor Precautions No information available to require special precautions

Effects on Dental Treatment No significant effects or complications reported

Effects on Bleeding No information available to require special precautions

Adverse Effects

Injection: Frequency not defined:

Central nervous system: Confusion, disorientation, dizziness, fever, headache, lethargy, vertigo

Dermatologic: Exfoliative dermatitis, itching, rash, urticaria

Endocrine & metabolic: Serum calcium, magnesium, potassium, and/or sodium decreased

Gastrointestinal: Diarrhea, nausea, vomiting

Hematologic: Anemia, eosinophilia, granulocytopenia, leukocytosis, leukopenia, thrombocytopenia

Hepatic: ALT increased, AST increased, bilirubin increased, LDH increased

Local: Pain at the injection site

Otic: Hearing loss, tinnitus, ototoxicity (auditory), ototoxicity (vestibular), roaring in the ears

Renal: BUN increased, cylindruria, serum creatinine increased, oliguria, proteinuria

Inhalation:

>10%:

Gastrointestinal: Sputum discoloration (21%)

Respiratory: Voice alteration (13%)

1% to 10%:

Central nervous system: Malaise (6%)

Otic: Tinnitus (3%)

General Dosage Range Dosage adjustment recommended for the I.M. and I.V. routes in patients with renal impairment

I.M.:

Infants and Children <5 years: 2.5 mg/kg every 8 hours

Children ≥5 years: 2-3.3 mg/kg every 6-8 hours

Adults: 1-2.5 mg/kg every 8-12 hours (1 mg/kg used for synergy) **or** 4-7 mg/kg/day as a single daily dose

Elderly: 1.5-5 mg/kg/day in 1-2 divided doses

I.V.:

Infants and Children <5 years: 2.5 mg/kg every 8 hours
Children ≥5 years: 2-3.3 mg/kg every 6-8 hours
Adults: 1-2.5 mg/kg every 8-12 hours (1 mg/kg/dose used for synergy) **or** 4-7 mg/kg/day as a single daily dose
Elderly: 1.5-5 mg/kg/day in 1-2 divided doses **or** 5-7 mg/kg given every 24, 36, or 48 hours based on Cl_{cr}

Inhalation: *Children ≥6 years and Adults:* 300 mg every 12 hours [TOBI®]

Mechanism of Action Interferes with bacterial protein synthesis by binding to 30S and 50S ribosomal subunits, resulting in a defective bacterial cell membrane

Pharmacodynamics/Kinetics

Half-life Elimination

Neonates: ≤1200 g: 11 hours; >1200 g: 2-9 hours
Adults: 2-3 hours; directly dependent upon glomerular filtration rate
Adults with impaired renal function: 5-70 hours

Time to Peak Serum: I.M.: 30-60 minutes; I.V.: ~30 minutes

Pregnancy Risk Factor D

Tobramycin and Dexamethasone (toe bra MYE sin & deks a METH a sone)

U.S. Brand Names TobraDex®

Canadian Brand Names Tobradex®

Pharmacologic Category Antibiotic/Corticosteroid, Ophthalmic

Use Treatment of external ocular infection caused by susceptible gram-negative bacteria and steroid responsive inflammatory conditions of the palpebral and bulbar conjunctiva, cornea, and anterior segment of the globe

Local Anesthetic/Vasoconstrictor Precautions No information available to require special precautions

Effects on Dental Treatment No significant effects or complications reported

Effects on Bleeding No information available to require special precautions

Adverse Effects Unless otherwise noted, frequency not defined.

Dermatologic: Allergic contact dermatitis, delayed wound healing
Ocular: Cataract formation, conjunctival erythema (<4%), glaucoma, intraocular pressure increased, keratitis, lacrimation, lid itching (<4%), lid swelling (<4%), optic nerve damage, secondary infection

General Dosage Range Ophthalmic: *Children ≥2 years and Adults:* Ointment: Apply ~1/2" ribbon up to 3-4 times/day; Suspension: Instill 1-2 drops every every 4-6 hours, may increase to 1-2 drops every 2 hours for 24-48 hours

Mechanism of Action See individual agents.

Pregnancy Risk Factor C

Tocilizumab (toe si LIZ oo mab)

Related Information

Rheumatoid Arthritis, Osteoarthritis, and Osteoporosis *on page* 1889

U.S. Brand Names Actemra®

Canadian Brand Names Actemra®

Pharmacologic Category Antirheumatic, Disease Modifying; Interleukin-6 Receptor Antagonist

Use Treatment of moderately- to severely-active rheumatoid arthritis in adult patients who have had an inadequate response to one or more TNF antagonists (as monotherapy or in combination with nonbiological disease modifying antirheumatic drugs [DMARDs]); treatment of active systemic juvenile idiopathic arthritis (SJIA) (as monotherapy or in combination with methotrexate)

Local Anesthetic/Vasoconstrictor Precautions No information available to require special precautions

Effects on Dental Treatment Key adverse event(s) related to dental treatment: Mouth ulcerations and stomatitis

Effects on Bleeding No information available to require special precautions

Adverse Effects Incidence as reported for monotherapy, except where noted. Combination therapy refers to use in rheumatoid arthritis with nonbiological DMARDs or use in SJIA in trials where most patients (~70%) were taking methotrexate at baseline.

>10%: Hepatic: ALT increased (≤36%; grades 3/4: <1%), AST increased (≤22%; grades 3/4: <1%)

1% to 10%:

Cardiovascular: Hypertension (1% to 6%), peripheral edema (<2%)
Central nervous system: Headache (1% to 7%), dizziness (3%)

Dermatologic: Rash (2%), skin reaction (combination therapy; 1% [includes pruritus, urticaria])
Endocrine & metabolic: LDL cholesterol increased (>1.5-2 x ULN; combination therapy; children 2%), total cholesterol increased (>1.5-2 x ULN; combination therapy; children 2%), hypothyroidism (<2%)
Gastrointestinal: Diarrhea (children ≤5%), abdominal pain (2%), mouth ulceration (2%), gastric ulcer (<2%), stomatitis (<2%), weight gain (<2%), gastritis (1%)
Hematologic: Neutropenia (combination therapy; grade 3: 2% to 7%; grade 4: <1%), thrombocytopenia (combination therapy; 1% to 2%), leukopenia (<2%)
Hepatic: Bilirubin increased (<2%)
Local: Infusion-related reactions (combination therapy; 4% to 16%)
Ocular: Conjunctivitis (<2%)
Renal: Nephrolithiasis (<2%)
Respiratory: Upper respiratory tract infection (7%), nasopharyngitis (7%), bronchitis (3%), cough (<2%), dyspnea (<2%)
Miscellaneous: Anti-tocilizumab antibody formation (2%), herpes simplex (<2%)

General Dosage Range Dosage adjustment recommended in patients who develop toxicities

I.V.:

Children ≥2 years and <30 kg: 12 mg/kg every 2 weeks
Children ≥2 years and ≥30 kg: 8 mg/kg every 2 weeks
Adults: 4-8 mg/kg every 4 weeks (maximum: 800 mg per infusion)

Mechanism of Action Antagonist of the interleukin-6 (IL-6) receptor. Endogenous IL-6 is induced by inflammatory stimuli and mediates a variety of immunological responses. Inhibition of IL-6 receptors by tocilizumab leads to a reduction in cytokine and acute phase reactant production.

Pharmacodynamics/Kinetics

Half-life Elimination Terminal, single dose: 6.3 days (concentration-dependent; may be increased up to 23 days [children] or 13 days [adults] at steady state)

Pregnancy Risk Factor C

TOLAZamide (tole AZ a mide)

Related Information

Endocrine Disorders and Pregnancy *on page 1879*

Canadian Brand Names Tolinase®

Pharmacologic Category Antidiabetic Agent, Sulfonylurea

Use Adjunct to diet for the management of mild-to-moderately severe, stable, type 2 diabetes mellitus (noninsulin dependent, NIDDM)

Local Anesthetic/Vasoconstrictor Precautions No information available to require special precautions

Effects on Dental Treatment Use salicylates with caution in patients taking tolazamide due to potential increased hypoglycemia; NSAIDs such as ibuprofen and naproxen may be safely used. Tolazamide-dependent patients with diabetes (noninsulin dependent, type 2) should be appointed for dental treatment in morning in order to minimize chance of stress-induced hypoglycemia.

Effects on Bleeding No information available to require special precautions

Adverse Effects Frequency not defined.

Central nervous system: Dizziness, fatigue, headache, malaise, vertigo
Dermatologic: Maculopapular eruptions, morbilliform eruptions, photosensitivity, pruritus, rash, urticaria
Endocrine & metabolic: Disulfiram-like reaction, hypoglycemia, hyponatremia, SIADH
Gastrointestinal: Anorexia, constipation, diarrhea, epigastric fullness, heartburn, nausea, vomiting
Hematologic: Agranulocytosis, aplastic anemia, hemolytic anemia, leukopenia, pancytopenia, porphyria cutanea tarda, thrombocytopenia
Hepatic: Cholestatic jaundice, hepatic porphyria
Neuromuscular & skeletal: Weakness
Renal: Diuretic effect

General Dosage Range Oral: *Adults:* Initial: 100-250 mg/day with first main meal of day; Maintenance: 100-1000 mg/day in 1-2 (doses >500 mg) divided doses (maximum: 1 g/day)

Mechanism of Action Stimulates insulin release from the pancreatic beta cells; reduces glucose output from the liver; insulin sensitivity is increased at peripheral target sites

Pharmacodynamics/Kinetics

Onset of Action Hypoglycemic effect: 20 minutes; Peak hypoglycemic effect: 4-6 hours

Duration of Action 10-24 hours

Half-life Elimination 7 hours

Time to Peak Serum: 3-4 hours

Pregnancy Risk Factor C

TOLBUTamide (tole BYOO ta mide)

Related Information

Endocrine Disorders and Pregnancy *on page* 1879

Canadian Brand Names Apo-Tolbutamide®

Pharmacologic Category Antidiabetic Agent, Sulfonylurea

Use Adjunct to diet for the management of type 2 diabetes mellitus (noninsulin dependent, NIDDM)

Local Anesthetic/Vasoconstrictor Precautions No information available to require special precautions

Effects on Dental Treatment Key adverse event(s) related to dental treatment: Taste alteration.

Use salicylates with caution in patients taking tolazamide due to potential increased hypoglycemia; NSAIDs such as ibuprofen and naproxen may be safely used. Tolbutamide-dependent patients with diabetes (noninsulin dependent, type 2) should be appointed for dental treatment in morning in order to minimize chance of stress-induced hypoglycemia.

Effects on Bleeding No information available to require special precautions

Adverse Effects Frequency not defined.

Central nervous system: Headache

Dermatologic: Erythema, maculopapular rash, morbilliform rash, pruritus, urticaria, photosensitivity

Endocrine & metabolic: Disulfiram-like reactions, hypoglycemia, hyponatremia, SIADH

Gastrointestinal: Epigastric fullness, heartburn, nausea, taste alteration

Hematologic: Agranulocytosis, aplastic anemia, hemolytic anemia, leukopenia, pancytopenia, thrombocytopenia

Hepatic: Cholestatic jaundice, hepatic porphyria, porphyria cutanea tarda

Miscellaneous: Hypersensitivity reaction

General Dosage Range Oral:

Adults: Initial: 1-2 g/day as a single dose or divided doses; Maintenance: 0.25-3 g/day as a single dose or divided doses

Elderly: Initial: 0.25 g 1-3 times/day; Maintenance: 0.5-2 g/day in 1-3 divided doses (maximum: 3 g/day)

Mechanism of Action Stimulates insulin release from the pancreatic beta cells; reduces glucose output from the liver; insulin sensitivity is increased at peripheral target sites, suppression of glucagon may also contribute

Pharmacodynamics/Kinetics

Onset of Action 1 hour

Duration of Action Oral: 6-24 hours

Half-life Elimination 4.5-6.5 hours (range: 4-25 hours)

Time to Peak Serum: 3-4 hours

Pregnancy Risk Factor C

Tolcapone (TOLE ka pone)

U.S. Brand Names Tasmar®

Pharmacologic Category Anti-Parkinson's Agent, COMT Inhibitor

Use Adjunct to levodopa and carbidopa for the treatment of signs and symptoms of idiopathic Parkinson's disease in patients with motor fluctuations not responsive to other therapies

Local Anesthetic/Vasoconstrictor Precautions No information available to require special precautions

Effects on Dental Treatment Key adverse event(s) related to dental treatment: Significant xerostomia (normal salivary flow resumes upon discontinuation) and tooth disorder.

Dopaminergic therapy in Parkinson's disease (ie, treatment with levodopa) is associated with orthostatic hypotension. Tolcapone enhances levodopa bioavailability and may increase the occurrence of hypotension/syncope in the dental patient. The patient should be carefully assisted from the chair and observed for signs of orthostatic hypotension.

Effects on Bleeding No information available to require special precautions

Adverse Effects

>10%:

Cardiovascular: Orthostatic hypotension (17%)

Central nervous system: Somnolence (14% to 32%), sleep disorder (24% to 25%), hallucinations (8% to 24%), excessive dreaming (16% to 21%), dizziness (6% to 13%), headache (10% to 11%), confusion (10% to 11%)

Gastrointestinal: Nausea (28% to 50%), diarrhea (16% to 34%; approximately 3% to 4% severe), anorexia (19% to 23%)

Neuromuscular & skeletal: Dyskinesia (42% to 51%), dystonia (19% to 22%), muscle cramps (17% to 18%)

1% to 10%:

Cardiovascular: Syncope (4% to 5%), chest pain (1% to 3%), hypotension (2%), palpitation

Central nervous system: Fatigue (3% to 7%), loss of balance (2% to 3%), agitation (1%), euphoria (1%), hyperactivity (1%), malaise (1%), panic reaction (1%), irritability (1%), mental deficiency (1%), fever (1%), depression, hypoesthesia, tremor, speech disorder, vertigo, emotional lability, hyperkinesia

Dermatologic: Alopecia (1%), bleeding (1%), tumor (1%), rash

Gastrointestinal: Vomiting (8% to 10%), constipation (6% to 8%), xerostomia (5% to 6%), abdominal pain (5% to 6%), dyspepsia (3% to 4%), flatulence (2% to 4%), tooth disorder

Genitourinary: UTI (5%), hematuria (4% to 5%), urine discoloration (2% to 3%), urination disorder (1% to 2%), uterine tumor (1%), incontinence, impotence

Hepatic: Transaminases increased (1% to 3%; 3 times ULN, usually with first 6 months of therapy)

Neuromuscular & skeletal: Paresthesia (1% to 3%), hyper-/hypokinesia (1% to 3%), arthritis (1% to 2%), neck pain (2%), stiffness (2%), myalgia, rhabdomyolysis

Ocular: Cataract (1%), eye inflammation (1%)

Otic: Tinnitus

Respiratory: Upper respiratory infection (5% to 7%), dyspnea (3%), sinus congestion (1% to 2%), bronchitis, pharyngitis

Miscellaneous: Diaphoresis (4% to 7%), influenza (3% to 4%), burning (1% to 2%), flank pain, injury, infection

General Dosage Range Oral: *Adults:* Initial: 100 mg 3 times/day; Maintenance: 100-200 mg 3 times/day

Mechanism of Action Tolcapone is a selective and reversible inhibitor of catechol-o-methyltransferase (COMT). In the presence of a decarboxylase inhibitor (eg, carbidopa), COMT is the major degradation pathway for levodopa. Inhibition of COMT leads to more sustained plasma levels of levodopa and enhanced central dopaminergic activity.

Pharmacodynamics/Kinetics

Half-life Elimination 2-3 hours

Time to Peak ~2 hours

Pregnancy Risk Factor C

Prescribing and Access Restrictions A patient signed consent form acknowledging the risks of hepatic injury should be obtained by the treating physician.

Tolmetin (TOLE met in)

Related Information

Rheumatoid Arthritis, Osteoarthritis, and Osteoporosis *on page 1889*
Temporomandibular Dysfunction (TMD) *on page 1964*

Generic Availability (U.S.) Yes

Pharmacologic Category Nonsteroidal Anti-inflammatory Drug (NSAID), Oral

Use Treatment of rheumatoid arthritis and osteoarthritis, juvenile idiopathic arthritis (JIA)

Local Anesthetic/Vasoconstrictor Precautions No information available to require special precautions

Effects on Dental Treatment The dentist should be aware of the potential of abnormal coagulation. Caution should also be exercised in the use of NSAIDs in patients already on anticoagulant therapy with drugs such as warfarin (Coumadin®). See Effects on Bleeding.

Effects on Bleeding Nonselective NSAIDs are known to reversibly decrease platelet aggregation via mechanisms different than observed with aspirin. Platelet function is restored as the drug is eliminated from the body. NSAIDs should be avoided (if possible) in general surgery patients for 3-5 half-lives of the drug (usually 1-3 days) prior to surgery to reduce the risk of excessive bleeding. However, there is no scientific evidence to warrant discontinuance of NSAIDs prior to dental surgery. In medically complicated patients or extensive oral surgery, the decision to interrupt therapy must be based on the risk to benefit in an individual patient and a medical consult is suggested. Routine interruption of NSAID therapy for most dental procedures is not warranted. If therapy is continued without interruption, the clinician should anticipate the potential for slower clotting times.

Adverse Effects

>10%: Gastrointestinal: Nausea (11%)

1% to 10%:

Cardiovascular: Edema (3% to 9%), hypertension (3% to 9%), chest pain (1% to 3%)

Central nervous system: Dizziness (3% to 9%), headache (3% to 9%), depression (1% to 3%), drowsiness (1% to 3%)

Dermatologic: Skin irritation (1% to 3%)

Endocrine & metabolic: Weight gain/loss (3% to 9%)

Gastrointestinal: Abdominal pain (3% to 9%), diarrhea (3% to 9%), dyspepsia (3% to 9%), flatulence (3% to 9%), gastrointestinal distress (3% to 9%), vomiting (3% to 9%), constipation (1% to 3%), gastritis (1% to 3%), peptic ulcer (1% to 3%)

Genitourinary: Urinary tract infection (1% to 3%)

Hematologic: Hemoglobin/hematocrit decreased (transient; 1% to 3%)

Neuromuscular & skeletal: Weakness (3% to 9%)

Ocular: Visual disturbances (1% to 3%)

Otic: Tinnitus (1% to 3%)

Renal: BUN increased (1% to 3%)

Dosage Oral:

Children ≥2 years:

Juvenile idiopathic arthritis (JIA): Initial: 20 mg/kg/day in 3-4 divided doses, then 15-30 mg/kg/day in 3-4 divided doses (maximum dose: 30 mg/kg/day)

Analgesic (unlabeled use): 5-7 mg/kg/dose every 6-8 hours

Adults: RA, osteoarthritis: 400 mg 3 times/day; usual dose: 600 mg to 1.8 g/day; maximum: 1.8 g/day

Mechanism of Action Reversibly inhibits cyclooxygenase-1 and 2 (COX-1 and 2) enzymes, which results in decreased formation of prostaglandin precursors; has antipyretic, analgesic, and anti-inflammatory properties.

Other proposed mechanisms not fully elucidated (and possibly contributing to the anti-inflammatory effect to varying degrees) include inhibiting chemotaxis, altering lymphocyte activity, inhibiting neutrophil aggregation/activation, and decreasing proinflammatory cytokine levels.

Contraindications Hypersensitivity to tolmetin, aspirin, other NSAIDs, or any component of the formulation; perioperative pain in the setting of coronary artery bypass graft (CABG) surgery

Warnings/Precautions [U.S. Boxed Warning]: NSAIDs are associated with an increased risk of adverse cardiovascular thrombotic events, including MI and stroke. Risk may be increased with duration of use or pre-existing cardiovascular risk factors or disease. Carefully evaluate individual cardiovascular risk profiles prior to prescribing. May cause new-onset hypertension or worsening of existing hypertension. Use caution with fluid retention. Avoid use in heart failure. Concurrent administration of ibuprofen, and potentially other nonselective NSAIDs, may interfere with aspirin's cardioprotective effect. **[U.S. Boxed Warning]: Use is contraindicated for treatment of perioperative pain in the setting of coronary artery bypass graft (CABG) surgery.** Risk of MI and stroke may be increased with use following CABG surgery.

Platelet adhesion and aggregation may be decreased; may prolong bleeding time; patients with coagulation disorders or who are receiving anticoagulants should be monitored closely. Anemia may occur; patients on long-term NSAID therapy should be monitored for anemia. Rarely, NSAID use may cause severe blood dyscrasias (eg, agranulocytosis, aplastic anemia, thrombocytopenia).

NSAID use may compromise existing renal function; dose-dependent decreases in prostaglandin synthesis may result from NSAID use, reducing renal blood flow which may cause renal decompensation. NSAID use may increase the risk for hyperkalemia. Patients with impaired renal function, dehydration, heart failure, liver dysfunction, those taking diuretics, and ACE inhibitors, and the elderly are at greater risk of renal toxicity and hyperkalemia. Rehydrate patient before starting therapy; monitor renal function closely. Not recommended for use in patients with advanced renal disease. Long-term NSAID use may result in renal papillary necrosis. Acute interstitial nephritis and nephritic syndrome have been reported with tolmetin.

[U.S. Boxed Warning]: NSAIDs may increase risk of gastrointestinal irritation, inflammation, ulceration, bleeding, and perforation. These events may occur at any time during therapy and without warning. Use caution with a history of GI disease (bleeding or ulcers), concurrent therapy with aspirin, anticoagulants and/or corticosteroids, smoking, use of alcohol, the elderly or debilitated patients. When used concomitantly with ≤325 mg of aspirin, a substantial increase in the risk of gastrointestinal complications (eg, ulcer) occurs; concomitant gastroprotective therapy (eg, proton pump inhibitors) is recommended (Bhatt, 2008).

Use the lowest effective dose for the shortest duration of time, consistent with individual patient goals, to reduce risk of cardiovascular or GI adverse events. Alternate therapies should be considered for patients at high risk.

NSAIDs may cause serious skin adverse events including exfoliative dermatitis, Stevens-Johnson syndrome (SJS) and toxic epidermal necrolysis (TEN); discontinue use at first sign of skin rash or hypersensitivity. Anaphylactoid reactions may occur, even without prior exposure; patients with "aspirin triad" (bronchial asthma, aspirin intolerance, rhinitis) may be at increased risk. Do not use in patients who experience bronchospasm, asthma, rhinitis, or urticaria with NSAID or aspirin therapy.

Use with caution in patients with decreased hepatic function. Closely monitor patients with any abnormal LFT. Severe hepatic reactions (eg, fulminant hepatitis, liver failure) have occurred with NSAID use, rarely; discontinue if signs or symptoms of liver disease develop, or if systemic manifestations occur.

NSAIDS may cause drowsiness, dizziness, blurred vision and other neurologic effects which may impair physical or mental abilities; patients must be cautioned about performing tasks which require mental alertness (eg, operating machinery or driving). Discontinue use with blurred or diminished vision and perform ophthalmologic exam. Monitor vision with long-term therapy.

The elderly are at increased risk for adverse effects (especially peptic ulceration, CNS effects, renal toxicity) from NSAIDs even at low doses.

Withhold for at least 4-6 half-lives prior to surgical or dental procedures.

Drug Interactions

Avoid Concomitant Use

Avoid concomitant use of Tolmetin with any of the following: Ketorolac; Ketorolac (Systemic)

Increased Effect/Toxicity

Tolmetin may increase the levels/effects of: Aminoglycosides; Anticoagulants; Antiplatelet Agents; Bisphosphonate Derivatives; Collagenase (Systemic); CycloSPORINE; CycloSPORINE (Systemic); Deferasirox; Desmopressin; Digoxin; Drotrecogin Alfa; Eplerenone; Haloperidol; Ibritumomab; Lithium; Methotrexate; Nonsteroidal Anti-Inflammatory Agents; PEMEtrexed; Potassium-Sparing Diuretics; PRALAtrexate; Quinolone Antibiotics; Salicylates; Thrombolytic Agents; Tositumomab and Iodine I 131 Tositumomab; Vancomycin; Vitamin K Antagonists

The levels/effects of Tolmetin may be increased by: ACE Inhibitors; Angiotensin II Receptor Blockers; Antidepressants (Tricyclic, Tertiary Amine); Corticosteroids (Systemic); Dasatinib; Glucosamine; Herbs (Anticoagulant/Antiplatelet Properties); Ketorolac; Ketorolac (Systemic); Nonsteroidal Anti-Inflammatory Agents; Omega-3-Acid Ethyl Esters; Pentosan Polysulfate Sodium; Pentoxifylline; Probenecid; Prostacyclin Analogues; Selective Serotonin Reuptake Inhibitors; Serotonin/Norepinephrine Reuptake Inhibitors; Treprostinil

Decreased Effect

Tolmetin may decrease the levels/effects of: ACE Inhibitors; Angiotensin II Receptor Blockers; Antiplatelet Agents; Beta-Blockers; Eplerenone; HydrALAZINE; Loop Diuretics; Potassium-Sparing Diuretics; Salicylates; Thiazide Diuretics

The levels/effects of Tolmetin may be decreased by: Bile Acid Sequestrants; Nonsteroidal Anti-Inflammatory Agents; Salicylates

Ethanol/Nutrition/Herb Interactions

Ethanol: Avoid ethanol (may enhance gastric mucosal irritation).

Food: Tolmetin peak serum concentrations may be decreased if taken with food or milk.

Herb/Nutraceutical: Avoid alfalfa, anise, bilberry, bladderwrack, bromelain, cat's claw, celery, chamomile, coleus, cordyceps, dong quai, evening primrose, fenugreek, feverfew, fenugreek, garlic, ginger, ginkgo biloba, ginseng (American, Panax, Siberian), grapeseed, green tea, guggul, horse chestnut seed, horseradish, licorice, prickly ash, red clover, reishi, SAMe (S-adenosylmethionine), sweet clover, turmeric, white willow (all have additional antiplatelet activity).

Dietary Considerations May be taken with antacids to minimize stomach upset. Administration with food or milk decreases bioavailability by 16%. Some products may contain sodium.

Pharmacodynamics/Kinetics

Onset of Action Analgesic: 1-2 hours; Anti-inflammatory: Days to weeks

Half-life Elimination Biphasic: Rapid: 1-2 hours; Slow: 5 hours

Time to Peak Serum: 30-60 minutes

Pregnancy Risk Factor C

Lactation Enters breast milk/not recommended (AAP rates "compatible"; AAP 2001 update pending)

Breast-Feeding Considerations Tolmetin is found in breast milk and breast-feeding is not recommended by the manufacturer.

Dosage Forms

Capsule, oral: 400 mg

Tablet, oral: 200 mg, 600 mg

Tolnaftate (tole NAF tate)

U.S. Brand Names Blis-To-Sol® [OTC]; Mycocide® NS [OTC]; Podactin Powder [OTC]; Tinactin® Antifungal Deodorant [OTC]; Tinactin® Antifungal Jock Itch [OTC]; Tinactin® Antifungal [OTC]; Tinaderm [OTC]; Ting® Cream [OTC]; Ting® Spray Liquid [OTC]

Canadian Brand Names Pitrex

Pharmacologic Category Antifungal Agent, Topical

Use Treatment of tinea pedis, tinea cruris, tinea corporis

Local Anesthetic/Vasoconstrictor Precautions No information available to require special precautions

Effects on Dental Treatment No significant effects or complications reported

Effects on Bleeding No information available to require special precautions

Adverse Effects Frequency not defined.

Dermatologic: Pruritus, contact dermatitis

Local: Irritation, stinging

General Dosage Range Topical: *Children ≥2 years and Adults:* Apply to affected areas 2 times/day

Mechanism of Action Distorts the hyphae and stunts mycelial growth in susceptible fungi

Pharmacodynamics/Kinetics

Onset of Action 24-72 hours

Pregnancy Risk Factor C

Tolterodine (tole TER oh deen)

U.S. Brand Names Detrol®; Detrol® LA

Canadian Brand Names Detrol®; Detrol® LA; Unidet®

Generic Availability (U.S.) No

Pharmacologic Category Anticholinergic Agent

Use Treatment of patients with an overactive bladder with symptoms of urinary frequency, urgency, or urge incontinence

Local Anesthetic/Vasoconstrictor Precautions No information available to require special precautions

Effects on Dental Treatment The anticholinergic effects of tolterodine are selective for the urinary bladder rather than salivary glands; xerostomia and changes in salivation (normal salivary flow resumes upon discontinuation).

Effects on Bleeding No information available to require special precautions

Adverse Effects As reported with immediate release tablet, unless otherwise specified

>10%: Gastrointestinal: Dry mouth (35%; extended release capsules 23%)

1% to 10%:

Cardiovascular: Chest pain (2%)

Central nervous system: Headache (7%; extended release capsules 6%), somnolence (3%; extended release capsules 3%), fatigue (4%; extended release capsules 2%), dizziness (5%; extended release capsules 2%), anxiety (extended release capsules 1%)

Dermatologic: Dry skin (1%)

Gastrointestinal: Abdominal pain (5%; extended release capsules 4%), constipation (7%; extended release capsules 6%), dyspepsia (4%; extended release capsules 3%), diarrhea (4%), weight gain (1%)

Genitourinary: Dysuria (2%; extended release capsules 1%)

Neuromuscular & skeletal: Arthralgia (2%)

Ocular: Abnormal vision (2%; extended release capsules 1%), dry eyes (3%; extended release capsules 3%)

Respiratory: Bronchitis (2%), sinusitis (extended release capsules 2%)

Miscellaneous: Flu-like syndrome (3%), infection (1%)

Dosage

Oral: Adults: Treatment of overactive bladder:

Immediate release tablet: 2 mg twice daily; the dose may be lowered to 1 mg twice daily based on individual response and tolerability

Dosing adjustment in patients concurrently taking CYP3A4 inhibitors: 1 mg twice daily

Extended release capsule: 4 mg once a day; dose may be lowered to 2 mg daily based on individual response and tolerability

Dosing adjustment in patients concurrently taking CYP3A4 inhibitors: 2 mg daily

Elderly: Safety and efficacy in patients >64 years was found to be similar to that in younger patients; no dosage adjustment is needed based on age

Dosing adjustment in renal impairment: Use with caution (studies conducted in patients with Cl_{cr} 10-30 mL/minute):

Immediate release tablet: 1 mg twice daily

Extended release capsule: 2 mg daily

Dosing adjustment in hepatic impairment:

Immediate release tablet: 1 mg twice daily

Extended release capsule: 2 mg daily

Mechanism of Action Tolterodine is a competitive antagonist of muscarinic receptors. In animal models, tolterodine demonstrates selectivity for urinary bladder receptors over salivary receptors. Urinary bladder contraction is mediated by muscarinic receptors. Tolterodine increases residual urine volume and decreases detrusor muscle pressure.

Contraindications Hypersensitivity to tolterodine or any component of the formulation; urinary retention; gastric retention; uncontrolled narrow-angle glaucoma

Warnings/Precautions May cause drowsiness and/or blurred vision, which may impair physical or mental abilities; patients must be cautioned about performing tasks which require mental alertness (eg, operating machinery or driving). Use with caution in patients with bladder flow obstruction, may increase the risk of urinary retention. Use with caution in patients with gastrointestinal obstructive disorders (ie, pyloric stenosis), may increase the risk of gastric retention. Use with caution in patients with myasthenia gravis and controlled (treated) narrow-angle glaucoma; metabolized in the liver and excreted in the urine and feces, dosage adjustment is required for patients with renal or hepatic impairment. Tolterodine has been associated with QT_c prolongation at high (supratherapeutic) doses. The manufacturer recommends caution in patients with congenital prolonged QT or in patients receiving concurrent therapy with QT_c-prolonging drugs (class Ia or III antiarrhythmics). However, the mean change in QT_c even at supratherapeutic dosages was less than 15 msec. Individuals who are CYP2D6 poor metabolizers or in the presence of inhibitors of CYP2D6 and CYP3A4 may be more likely to exhibit prolongation. Dosage adjustment is recommended in patients receiving CYP3A4 inhibitors (a lower dose of tolterodine is recommended).

Drug Interactions

Metabolism/Transport Effects **Substrate** of CYP2C9 (minor), 2C19 (minor), 2D6 (major), 3A4 (major)

Avoid Concomitant Use There are no known interactions where it is recommended to avoid concomitant use.

Increased Effect/Toxicity

Tolterodine may increase the levels/effects of: AbobotulinumtoxinA; Anticholinergics; Cannabinoids; OnabotulinumtoxinA; Potassium Chloride; RimabotulinumtoxinB; Warfarin

The levels/effects of Tolterodine may be increased by: Abiraterone; Antifungal Agents (Azole Derivatives, Systemic); Conivaptan; CYP2D6 Inhibitors (Moderate); CYP2D6 Inhibitors (Strong); CYP3A4 Inhibitors (Moderate); CYP3A4 Inhibitors (Strong); Darunavir; Dasatinib; Fluconazole; Pramlintide; VinBLAStine

Decreased Effect

Tolterodine may decrease the levels/effects of: Acetylcholinesterase Inhibitors (Central); Secretin

The levels/effects of Tolterodine may be decreased by: Acetylcholinesterase Inhibitors (Central); CYP3A4 Inducers (Strong); Deferasirox; Herbs (CYP3A4 Inducers); Peginterferon Alfa-2b; Tocilizumab

Ethanol/Nutrition/Herb Interactions

Food: Increases bioavailability (~53% increase) of tolterodine tablets (dose adjustment not necessary); does not affect the pharmacokinetics of tolterodine extended release capsules. As a CYP3A4 inhibitor, grapefruit juice may increase the serum level and/or toxicity of tolterodine, but unlikely secondary to high oral bioavailability.

Herb/Nutraceutical: St John's wort (*Hypericum*) appears to induce CYP3A enzymes.

Pharmacodynamics/Kinetics

Half-life Elimination

Immediate release tablet: Extensive metabolizers: ~2 hours; Poor metabolizers: ~10 hours

Extended release capsule: Extensive metabolizers: ~7 hours; Poor metabolizers: ~18 hours

Time to Peak Immediate release tablet: 1-2 hours; Extended release tablet: 2-6 hours

Pregnancy Risk Factor C

Lactation Excretion in breast milk unknown/not recommended

Dosage Forms

Capsule, extended release, oral:
Detrol® LA: 2 mg, 4 mg

Tablet, oral:
Detrol®: 1 mg, 2 mg

Tolvaptan (tol VAP tan)

U.S. Brand Names Samsca™

Pharmacologic Category Vasopressin Antagonist

Use Treatment of clinically significant hypervolemic or euvolemic hyponatremia (associated with heart failure, cirrhosis or SIADH) with either a serum sodium <125 mEq/L or less marked hyponatremia that is symptomatic and resistant to fluid restriction

Local Anesthetic/Vasoconstrictor Precautions No information available to require special precautions

Effects on Dental Treatment No significant effects or complications reported

Effects on Bleeding No information available to require special precautions

Adverse Effects

>10%:
- Gastrointestinal: Nausea (21%), xerostomia (7% to 13%)
- Renal: Pollakiuria (4% to 11%), polyuria (4% to 11%)
- Miscellaneous: Thirst (12% to 16%)

2% to 10%:
- Central nervous system: Pyrexia (4%)
- Endocrine & metabolic: Hyperglycemia (6%)
- Gastrointestinal: Constipation (7%), anorexia (4%)
- Neuromuscular & skeletal: Weakness (9%)

General Dosage Range Oral: *Adults:* 15-60 mg once daily

Mechanism of Action An arginine vasopressin (AVP) receptor antagonist with affinity for AVP receptor subtypes V_2 and V_{1a} in a ratio of 29:1. Antagonism of the V_2 receptor by tolvaptan promotes the excretion of free water (without loss of serum electrolytes) resulting in net fluid loss, increased urine output, decreased urine osmolality, and subsequent restoration of normal serum sodium levels.

Pharmacodynamics/Kinetics

Onset of Action 2-4 hour; Peak effect: 4-8 hours

Duration of Action 60% peak serum sodium elevation is retained at 24 hours; urinary excretion of free water is no longer elevated

Half-life Elimination 5-12 hours; dominant half-life <12 hours

Time to Peak Plasma: 2-4 hours

Pregnancy Risk Factor C

Topiramate (toe PYRE a mate)

U.S. Brand Names Topamax®

Canadian Brand Names Apo-Topiramate®; CO Topiramate; Dom-Topiramate; Mint-Topiramate; Mylan-Topiramate; Novo-Topiramate; PHL-Topiramate; PMS-Topiramate; PRO-Topiramate; ratio-Topiramate; Sandoz-Topiramate; Topamax®; ZYM-Topiramate

Generic Availability (U.S.) Yes

Pharmacologic Category Anticonvulsant, Miscellaneous

Use Monotherapy or adjunctive therapy for partial onset seizures and primary generalized tonic-clonic seizures; adjunctive treatment of seizures associated with Lennox-Gastaut syndrome; prophylaxis of migraine headache

Unlabeled/Investigational Use Diabetic neuropathy, infantile spasms, neuropathic pain; prophylaxis of cluster headache

Local Anesthetic/Vasoconstrictor Precautions No information available to require special precautions

Effects on Dental Treatment Key adverse event(s) related to dental treatment: Gingivitis, dysphagia, glossitis, gum hyperplasia, and xerostomia (normal salivary flow resumes upon discontinuation).

Effects on Bleeding No information available to require special precautions

Adverse Effects Adverse events are reported for placebo-controlled trials of adjunctive therapy in adult and pediatric patients. Unless otherwise noted, the percentages refer to incidence in epilepsy trials. **Note:** A wide range of dosages were studied; incidence of adverse events was frequently lower in the pediatric population studied.

>10%:

Central nervous system: Somnolence (15% to 29%), dizziness (4% to 25%; dose dependent), fatigue (9% to 16%; dose-dependent), nervousness (9% to 18%), ataxia (6% to 16%), psychomotor slowing (3% to 13%; dose dependent), speech problems (2% to 13%), memory difficulties (2% to 12%), behavior problems (children 11%), confusion (4% to 11%)

Endocrine & metabolic: Serum bicarbonate decreased (dose related: 7% to 67%; marked reductions [to <17 mEq/L] 1% to 11%)

Gastrointestinal: Anorexia (4% to 24%; dose dependent), nausea (6% to 10%; migraine trial: 9% to 14%)

Neuromuscular & skeletal: Paresthesia (1% to 11%; migraine trial: 35% to 51%)

Ocular: Abnormal vision (2% to 13%)

Respiratory: Upper respiratory infection (migraine trial: 12% to 14%)

Miscellaneous: Injury (14%)

1% to 10%:

Cardiovascular: Chest pain (2% to 4%), edema (2%), hypertension (1% to 2%), bradycardia (1%), pallor (1%), syncope (1%)

Central nervous system: Difficulty concentrating (5% to 10%), aggressive reactions (2% to 9%), depression (5% to 9%; dose dependent, insomnia (4% to 8%), mood problems (≤6%), abnormal coordination (4%), agitation (3%), cognitive problems (3%), emotional lability (3%), anxiety (2% to 3%; dose dependent), hypoesthesia (2%; migraine trial: 6% to 8%), stupor (2%), vertigo (2%), fever (migraine trial: 1% to 2%), apathy (1%), hallucination (1%), neurosis (1%), psychosis (1%), seizure (1%), suicide attempt (1%)

Dermatologic: Pruritus (migraine trial: 2% to 4%), skin disorder (2% to 3%), alopecia (2%), dermatitis (2%), hypertrichosis (2%), rash erythematous (1% to 2%), eczema (1%), seborrhea (1%), skin discoloration (1%)

Endocrine & metabolic: Breast pain (4%), hot flashes (1% to 2%), libido decreased (<1% to 2%), menstrual irregularities (1% to 2%), hypoglycemia (1%), metabolic acidosis (hyperchloremia, nonanion gap)

Gastrointestinal: Weight loss (4% to 9%), dyspepsia (2% to 7%), abdominal pain (5% to 6%), salivation increased (6%), constipation (4% to 5%), gastroenteritis (2% to 3%), vomiting (migraine trial: 1% to 3%), diarrhea (2%; migraine trial: 9% to 11%), dysgeusia (2%; migraine trial: 8% to 15%), xerostomia (2%), loss of taste (migraine trial: ≤2%), appetite increased (1%), dysphagia (1%), fecal incontinence (1%), flatulence (1%), GERD (1%), gingivitis (1%), glossitis (1%), gum hyperplasia (1%), weight gain (1%)

Genitourinary: Incontinence (2% to 4%), UTI (2%), premature ejaculation (migraine trial: ≤3%), cystitis (2%), leukorrhea (2%), impotence (1%), nocturia (1%)

Hematologic: Purpura (8%), leukopenia (2%), anemia (1%), hematoma (1%), prothrombin time increased (1%), thrombocytopenia (1%)

Neuromuscular & skeletal: Tremor (3% to 9%), gait abnormal (3% to 8%), arthralgia (migraine trial: 1% to 7%), weakness (6%), hyperkinesia (5%), back pain (1% to 5%), involuntary muscle contractions (2%; migraine trial: 2% to 4%), leg cramps (2%), leg pain (2%), myalgia (2%), hyporeflexia (2%), rigors (1%), skeletal pain (1%)

Ocular: Diplopia (1% to 10%), nystagmus (10%), conjunctivitis (1%), lacrimation abnormal (1%), myopia (1%)

Otic: Hearing decreased (2%), tinnitus (2%), otitis media (migraine trial: 1% to 2%)

Renal: Hematuria (2%), renal calculus (migraine trial ≤2%)

Respiratory: Rhinitis (4% to 7%), pharyngitis (6%), sinusitis (5%; migraine trial: 6% to 10%), pneumonia (5%), epistaxis (2% to 4%), cough (migraine trial: 2% to 4%), bronchitis (migraine trial: 3%), dyspnea (migraine trial: 1% to 3%)

Miscellaneous: Viral infection (2% to 7%: migraine trial: 3% to 4%), flu-like syndrome (3%), allergy (2%), infection (2%), thirst (2%), body odor (1%), diaphoresis (1%), moniliasis (1%)

Dosage Oral: **Note:** Do not abruptly discontinue therapy; taper dosage gradually to prevent rebound effects. (In clinical trials, adult doses were withdrawn by decreasing in weekly intervals of 50-100 mg/day gradually over 2-8 weeks for seizure treatment, and by decreasing in weekly intervals by 25-50 mg/day for migraine prophylaxis.)

Epilepsy, monotherapy: Children ≥10 years and Adults: Partial onset seizure and primary generalized tonic-clonic seizure: Initial: 25 mg twice daily; may increase weekly by 50 mg/day up to 100 mg twice daily (week 4 dose); thereafter, may further increase weekly by 100 mg/day up to the recommended maximum of 200 mg twice daily.

Canadian labeling: Children ≥6 years and Adults: Initial: 25 mg once daily (in evening); may increase to 25 mg twice daily in weeks 2 or 3, and up to 50 mg twice daily by weeks 3 or 4; may further increase weekly in increments of 50 mg/day up to recommended maximum of 200 mg twice daily.

Epilepsy, adjunctive therapy:

Children 2-16 years:

Partial onset seizure or seizure associated with Lennox-Gastaut syndrome: Initial: 25 mg (1-3 mg/kg/day) once daily (in evening); may increase every 1-2 weeks in increments of 1-3 mg/kg/day up to the recommended maximum of 5-9 mg/kg/day in 2 divided doses

Primary generalized tonic-clonic seizure: Use initial dose listed above for partial onset seizures, but use slower initial titration rate; titrate to the recommended maintenance dose of 6 mg/kg/day by the end of 8 weeks

Canadian labeling: Initial: 25 mg (1-3 mg/kg/day) once daily (in evening); may increase every 1-2 weeks in increments of 1-3 mg/kg/day up to the recommended maximum of 5-9 mg/kg/day in two divided doses

Adolescents ≥17 years and Adults:

Partial onset seizures: Initial: 25 mg once or twice daily for 1 week; may increase weekly by 25-50 mg/day until response; usual maintenance dose: 100-200 mg twice daily. Doses >1600 mg/day have not been studied.

Primary generalized tonic-clonic seizures: Use initial dose as listed above for partial onset seizures, but use slower initial titration rate; titrate upwards to recommended dose by the end of 8 weeks; usual maintenance dose: 200 mg twice daily. Doses >1600 mg/day have not been studied.

Canadian labeling: Initial: 25 mg once or twice daily; may increase weekly by 50 mg/day up to the recommended dose of 100-200 mg twice daily (maximum recommended dose: 800 mg/day; doses >400 mg/day have shown no additional benefit)

Migraine prophylaxis: Adults: Initial: 25 mg once daily (in evening); may increase weekly by 25 mg/day, up to the recommended dose of 100 mg/day given in 2 divided doses. Doses >100 mg/day have shown no additional benefit.

Cluster headache prophylaxis (unlabeled use): Adults: Initial: 25 mg/day, titrated at weekly intervals in 25 mg increments, up to 200 mg/day (Pascual, 2007)

Diabetic neuropathy (unlabeled use): Adults: Initial: 25 mg/day, titrated at weekly intervals in 25-50 mg increments to target dose of 400 mg daily in 2 divided doses (Raskin, 2004; Thienel, 2004)

Dosing adjustment in renal impairment: Cl_{cr} <70 mL/minute/1.73 m^2: Administer 50% dose and titrate more slowly

Hemodialysis: Supplemental dose may be needed during hemodialysis

Dosing adjustment in hepatic impairment: Clearance may be reduced; however the manufacturer's labeling provides no specific dosing recommendations

Mechanism of Action Anticonvulsant activity may be due to a combination of potential mechanisms: Blocks neuronal voltage-dependent sodium channels, enhances GABA(A) activity, antagonizes AMPA/kainate glutamate receptors, and weakly inhibits carbonic anhydrase.

Contraindications There are no contraindications listed in the manufacturers' labeling.

Canadian labeling (not in U.S. labeling): Hypersensitivity to topiramate or any component of the formulation or container; pregnancy and women in childbearing years not using effective contraception (migraine prophylaxis only)

Warnings/Precautions Antiepileptics are associated with an increased risk of suicidal behavior/thoughts with use (regardless of indication); patients should be monitored for signs/symptoms of depression, suicidal tendencies, and other unusual behavior changes during therapy and instructed to inform their healthcare provider immediately if symptoms occur. Use with caution in patients with hepatic, respiratory, or renal impairment. Topiramate may decrease serum bicarbonate concentrations (up to 67% of patients); treatment-emergent metabolic acidosis is less common. Risk may be increased in patients with a predisposing condition (organ dysfunction, ketogenic diet, or concurrent treatment with other drugs which may cause acidosis). Metabolic acidosis may occur at dosages as low as 50 mg/day. Monitor serum bicarbonate as well as potential complications of chronic acidosis (nephrolithiasis, osteomalacia, and reduced growth rates in children). Kidney stones have been reported in both children and adults; the risk of kidney stones is about 2-4 times that of the untreated population; the risk of this event may be reduced by increasing fluid intake.

Cognitive dysfunction, psychiatric disturbances (mood disorders), and sedation (somnolence or fatigue) may occur with topiramate use; incidence may be related to rapid titration and higher doses. Patients must be cautioned about performing tasks which require mental alertness (eg, operating machinery or driving). Topiramate may also cause paresthesia, dizziness, and ataxia. Topiramate has been associated with acute myopia and secondary angle-closure glaucoma in adults and children, typically within 1 month of initiation; discontinue in patients with acute onset of decreased visual acuity or ocular pain. Hyperammonemia with or without encephalopathy may occur with or without concomitant valproate administration;

valproic acid dose-dependency was observed in limited pediatric studies; use with caution in patients with inborn errors of metabolism or decreased hepatic mitochondrial activity. Topiramate may be associated (rarely) with severe oligohydrosis and hyperthermia, most frequently in children; use caution and monitor closely during strenuous exercise, during exposure to high environmental temperature, or in patients receiving receiving other carbonic anhydrase inhibitors and drugs with anticholinergic activity. Concurrent use of topiramate and hydrochlorothiazide may increase the risk for hypokalemia; monitor potassium closely.

Avoid abrupt withdrawal of topiramate therapy, it should be withdrawn/tapered slowly to minimize the potential of increased seizure frequency. Doses were also gradually withdrawn in migraine prophylaxis studies. Effects with other sedative drugs or ethanol may be potentiated. Safety and efficacy have not been established in children <2 years of age for adjunctive treatment of seizures and <10 years of age for monotherapy treatment of seizures. In pediatric patients, weight loss may occur most often early in therapy; in clinical trials of at least 1 year, the majority of patients with weight loss had a resumption of weight gain within the study period. Safety and efficacy have not been established in children for migraine prophylaxis.

Drug Interactions

Metabolism/Transport Effects **Inhibits** CYP2C19 (weak); **Induces** CYP3A4 (weak)

Avoid Concomitant Use There are no known interactions where it is recommended to avoid concomitant use.

Increased Effect/Toxicity

Topiramate may increase the levels/effects of: Alcohol (Ethyl); CNS Depressants; Divalproex; Fosphenytoin; Lithium; Methotrimeprazine; Phenytoin; Valproic Acid

The levels/effects of Topiramate may be increased by: Droperidol; Methotrimeprazine; Thiazide Diuretics

Decreased Effect

Topiramate may decrease the levels/effects of: Contraceptives (Estrogens); Contraceptives (Progestins); Saxagliptin

The levels/effects of Topiramate may be decreased by: CarBAMazepine; Fosphenytoin; Ketorolac; Ketorolac (Systemic); Mefloquine; Phenytoin

Ethanol/Nutrition/Herb Interactions

Ethanol: May increase CNS depression; monitor for increased effects with coadministration. Caution patients about effects.

Food: Ketogenic diet may increase the possibility of acidosis and/or kidney stones.

Herb/Nutraceutical: Avoid evening primrose (seizure threshold decreased).

Pharmacodynamics/Kinetics

Half-life Elimination Mean: Adults: Normal renal function: 21 hours; shorter in pediatric patients; clearance is 50% higher in pediatric patients; Elderly: ~24 hours

Time to Peak Serum: ~1-4 hours

Pregnancy Risk Factor D

Lactation Enters breast milk/use caution

Breast-Feeding Considerations Based on limited data, topiramate was found in breast milk. Infant plasma concentrations of topiramate have been reported as 10% to 20% of the maternal plasma concentration.

Dosage Forms

Capsule, sprinkle, oral: 15 mg, 25 mg

Topamax®: 15 mg, 25 mg

Tablet, oral: 25 mg, 50 mg, 100 mg, 200 mg

Topamax®: 25 mg, 50 mg, 100 mg, 200 mg

Topotecan (toe poe TEE kan)

U.S. Brand Names Hycamtin®

Canadian Brand Names Hycamtin®; Topotecan For Injection

Pharmacologic Category Antineoplastic Agent, Camptothecin; Antineoplastic Agent, Natural Source (Plant) Derivative; Antineoplastic Agent, Topoisomerase I Inhibitor

Use Treatment of metastatic ovarian cancer, relapsed or refractory small cell lung cancer, recurrent or resistant cervical cancer (in combination with cisplatin)

Unlabeled/Investigational Use Treatment of nonsmall cell lung cancer, sarcoma (pediatrics), neuroblastoma (pediatrics), refractory solid tumors (pediatrics)

Local Anesthetic/Vasoconstrictor Precautions No information available to require special precautions

Effects on Dental Treatment Key adverse event(s) related to dental treatment: Stomatitis.

Effects on Bleeding Chemotherapy may result in significant myelosuppression, potentially including significant reduction in platelet counts and altered hemostasis. In patients who are under active treatment with these agents, medical consult is suggested.

Adverse Effects

>10%:

Central nervous system: Fatigue (11% to 29%), fever (5% to 28%), pain (23%), headache (18%)

Dermatologic: Alopecia (10% to 49%), rash (16%)

Gastrointestinal: Nausea (27% to 64%), vomiting (19% to 45%), diarrhea (14% to 32%; Oral: grade 3: 4%; grade 4: ≤1%; onset: 9 days), constipation (29%), abdominal pain (22%), anorexia (7% to 19%), stomatitis (18%)

Hematologic: Neutropenia (83% to 97%; grade 4: 32% to 80%; nadir 8-11 days; duration: 7 days; recovery <21 days), leukopenia (86% to 97%; grade 4: 15% to 32%), anemia (89% to 98%; grade 4: 7% to 10%), thrombocytopenia (69% to 81%; grade 4: 6% to 29%; duration: 3 days), neutropenic fever/sepsis (2% to 28%)

Neuromuscular & skeletal: Weakness (3% to 25%)

Respiratory: Dyspnea (22%), cough (15%)

1% to 10%:

Hepatic: Liver enzymes increased (transient; 8%)

Neuromuscular & skeletal: Paresthesia (7%)

Miscellaneous: Sepsis (grades 3/4: 5%)

General Dosage Range Dosage adjustment recommended in patients with renal impairment or who develop toxicities

Oral: *Adults:* 2.3 mg/m^2/day for 5 days; repeated every 21 days

I.V.: *Adults:* IVPB: 1.5 mg/m^2/day for 5 days; repeated every 21 days **or** 0.75 mg/m^2/day for 3 days every 21 days

Mechanism of Action Binds to topoisomerase I and stabilizes the cleavable complex so that religation of the cleaved DNA strand cannot occur. This results in the accumulation of cleavable complexes and single-strand DNA breaks. Topotecan acts in S phase of the cell cycle.

Pharmacodynamics/Kinetics

Half-life Elimination I.V.: 2-3 hours; renal impairment: 5 hours; Oral: 3-6 hours

Time to Peak Oral 1-2 hours; delayed with high-fat meal (1.5-4 hours)

Pregnancy Risk Factor D

Toremifene (tore EM i feen)

U.S. Brand Names Fareston®

Canadian Brand Names Fareston®

Pharmacologic Category Antineoplastic Agent, Estrogen Receptor Antagonist; Selective Estrogen Receptor Modulator (SERM)

Use Treatment of metastatic breast cancer in postmenopausal women with estrogen receptor positive or estrogen receptor status unknown

Unlabeled/Investigational Use Treatment of soft tissue sarcoma (desmoid tumors)

Local Anesthetic/Vasoconstrictor Precautions No information available to require special precautions

Effects on Dental Treatment No significant effects or complications reported

Effects on Bleeding Although significant myelosuppression with associated altered hemostasis has been reported for many chemotherapeutic agents, myelosuppression is not common with toremifene and no specific precautions appear to necessary.

Adverse Effects

>10%:

Endocrine & metabolic: Hot flashes (35%)

Gastrointestinal: Nausea (14%)

Genitourinary: Vaginal discharge (13%)

Hepatic: Alkaline phosphatase increased (8% to 19%), AST increased (5% to 19%)

Miscellaneous: Diaphoresis (20%)

1% to 10%:

Cardiovascular: Edema (5%), arrhythmia (≤2%), CVA/TIA (≤2%), thrombosis (≤2%), cardiac failure (≤1%), MI (≤1%)

Central nervous system: Dizziness (9%)

Endocrine & metabolic: Hypercalcemia (≤3%)

Gastrointestinal: Vomiting (4%)

Genitourinary: Vaginal bleeding (2%)

Hepatic: Bilirubin increased (1% to 2%)

Local: Thrombophlebitis (≤2%)

Ocular: Cataracts (≤10%), xerophthalmia (≤9%), visual field abnormal (≤4%), corneal keratopathy (≤2%), glaucoma (≤2%), vision abnormal/diplopia (≤2%)
Respiratory: Pulmonary embolism (≤2%)

General Dosage Range Oral: *Adults:* 60 mg once daily

Mechanism of Action Nonsteroidal, triphenylethylene derivative with potent anti-estrogenic properties (also has estrogenic effects). Competitively binds to estrogen receptors on tumors and other tissue targets, producing a nuclear complex that decreases DNA synthesis and inhibits estrogen effects. Competes with estrogen for binding sites in breast and other tissues; cells accumulate in the G_0 and G_1 phases; therefore, toremifene is cytostatic rather than cytocidal.

Pharmacodynamics/Kinetics

Half-life Elimination Toremifene: ~5 days; N-demethyltoremifene: 6 days

Time to Peak Serum: ≤3 hours

Pregnancy Risk Factor D

Torsemide (TORE se mide)

Related Information

Cardiovascular Diseases *on page* 1848

U.S. Brand Names Demadex®

Pharmacologic Category Diuretic, Loop

Use Management of edema associated with heart failure and hepatic or renal disease (including chronic renal failure); treatment of hypertension

Local Anesthetic/Vasoconstrictor Precautions No information available to require special precautions

Effects on Dental Treatment No significant effects or complications reported

Effects on Bleeding No information available to require special precautions

Adverse Effects

1% to 10%:
Cardiovascular: ECG abnormality (2%), chest pain (1%)
Central nervous system: Nervousness (1%)
Gastrointestinal: Constipation (2%), diarrhea (2%), dyspepsia (2%), nausea (2%), sore throat (2%)
Genitourinary: Excessive urination (7%)
Neuromuscular & skeletal: Arthralgia (2%), myalgia (2%), weakness (2%)
Respiratory: Rhinitis (3%), cough (2%)

General Dosage Range

I.V.: *Adults:* 10-200 mg once daily

Oral: *Adults:* 5-200 mg once daily (maximum: 200 mg/day)

Mechanism of Action Inhibits reabsorption of sodium and chloride in the ascending loop of Henle and distal renal tubule, interfering with the chloride-binding cotransport system, thus causing increased excretion of water, sodium, chloride, magnesium, and calcium; does not alter GFR, renal plasma flow, or acid-base balance

Pharmacodynamics/Kinetics

Onset of Action Diuresis: Oral: Within 1 hour; Peak effect: Diuresis: Oral: 1-2 hours; Antihypertensive: Oral: 4-6 weeks (up to 12 weeks)

Duration of Action Diuresis: Oral: ~6-8 hours

Half-life Elimination ~3.5 hours; Cirrhosis: 7-8 hours

Time to Peak Plasma: Oral: 1 hour; delayed ~30 minutes when administered with food

Pregnancy Risk Factor B

Trace Metals (trase MET als)

Related Information

Chromium *on page* 1778
Iodine *on page* 933
Selenium *on page* 1516

U.S. Brand Names 4 Trace Elements; Multitrace®-4; Multitrace®-4 Concentrate; Multitrace®-4 Neonatal; Multitrace®-4 Pediatric; Multitrace®-5; Multitrace®-5 Concentrate; Trace Elements 4 Pediatric

Pharmacologic Category Trace Element, Parenteral

Use Prevention and correction of trace metal deficiencies

Local Anesthetic/Vasoconstrictor Precautions No information available to require special precautions

Effects on Dental Treatment No significant effects or complications reported

Effects on Bleeding No information available to require special precautions

General Dosage Range I.V.: *Infants, Children, and Adults:* Dosage varies greatly depending on indication

Pregnancy Risk Factor C

TraMADol (TRA ma dole)

Related Sample Prescriptions
Moderate/Moderately Severe Oral Pain *on page 1980*

U.S. Brand Names Rybix™ ODT; Ryzolt™; Ultram®; Ultram® ER

Canadian Brand Names Ralivia™ ER; Tridural™; Zytram® XL

Generic Availability (U.S.) Yes: Excludes orally disintegrating tablet

Pharmacologic Category Analgesic, Opioid

Dental Use Relief of moderate to moderately-severe dental pain

Use Relief of moderate to moderately-severe pain

Extended release formulations are indicated for patients requiring around-the-clock management of moderate to moderately-severe pain for an extended period of time

Local Anesthetic/Vasoconstrictor Precautions No information available to require special precautions

Effects on Dental Treatment Key adverse event(s) related to dental treatment: Xerostomia and changes in salivation (normal salivary flow resumes upon discontinuation). See Dental Comment.

Effects on Bleeding No information available to require special precautions

Adverse Effects

>10%:

Cardiovascular: Flushing (8% to 16%)

Central nervous system: Dizziness (10% to 33%), headache (4% to 32%), somnolence (7% to 25%), insomnia (2% to 11%)

Dermatologic: Pruritus (5% to 12%)

Gastrointestinal: Constipation (10% to 46%), nausea (15% to 40%), vomiting (5% to 17%), dyspepsia (1% to 13%)

Neuromuscular & skeletal: Weakness (4% to 12%)

1% to 10%:

Cardiovascular: Postural hypotension (2% to 5%), chest pain (1% to <5%), vasodilation (1% to <5%)

Central nervous system: Anxiety (1% to <5%), confusion (1% to <5%), coordination impaired (1% to <5%), depression (1% to <5%), euphoria (1% to <5%), hypoesthesia (1% to <5%), lethargy (1% to <5%), nervousness (1% to <5%), pain (1% to <5%), pyrexia (1% to <5%), restlessness (1% to <5%), malaise (<1% to <5%), fatigue (2%), vertigo (2%)

Dermatologic: Dermatitis (1% to <5%), rash (1% to <5%)

Endocrine & metabolic: Hot flashes (2% to 9%), menopausal symptoms (1% to <5%)

Gastrointestinal: Diarrhea (5% to 10%), xerostomia (3% to 10%), anorexia (1% to <6%), abdominal pain (1% to <5%), appetite decreased (1% to <5%), weight loss (1% to <5%), flatulence (<1% to <5%)

Genitourinary: Urinary tract infection (1% to <5%), urinary frequency (<1% to <5%), urinary retention (<1% to <5%)

Neuromuscular & skeletal: Arthralgia (1% to <5%), back pain (1% to <5%), hypertonia (1% to <5%), rigors (1% to <5%), paresthesia (1% to <5%), tremor (1% to <5%), creatine phosphokinase increased (1% to <5%)

Ocular: Blurred vision (1% to <5%), miosis (1% to <5%)

Respiratory: Bronchitis (1% to <5%), congestion (nasal/sinus) (1% to <5%), cough (1% to <5%), dyspnea (1% to <5%), nasopharyngitis (1% to <5%), rhinorrhea (1% to <5%), sinusitis (1% to <5%), sneezing (1% to <5%), sore throat (1% to <5%), upper respiratory infection (1% to <5%)

Miscellaneous: Diaphoresis (2% to 9%), flu-like syndrome (1% to < 5%), shivering (<1% to <5%)

A withdrawal syndrome may occur with abrupt discontinuation; includes anxiety, diarrhea, hallucinations (rare), nausea, pain, piloerection, rigors, sweating, and tremor. Uncommon discontinuation symptoms may include severe anxiety, panic attacks, or paresthesia.

Dental Usual Dosage Moderate-to-severe chronic pain: Oral:

Adults:

Immediate release formulation: 50-100 mg every 4-6 hours (not to exceed 400 mg/day)

For patients not requiring rapid onset of effect, tolerability may be improved by starting dose at 25 mg/day and titrating dose by 25 mg every 3 days, until reaching 25 mg 4 times/day. The total daily dose may then be increased by 50 mg every 3 days as tolerated, to reach dose of 50 mg 4 times/day. After titration, 50-100 mg may be given every 4-6 hours as needed up to a maximum 400 mg/day.

Extended release formulations:

Ultram® ER:

Patients not currently on immediate-release: 100 mg once daily; titrate every 5 days (maximum: 300 mg/day)

Patients currently on immediate-release: Calculate 24-hour immediate release total and initiate total daily dose (round dose to the next lowest 100 mg increment); titrate (maximum: 300 mg/day)

Ralivia™ ER (Canadian labeling, not available in U.S.): 100 mg once daily; titrate every 5 days as needed based on clinical response and severity of pain (maximum: 300 mg/day)

Ryzolt™:

Patients not currently on immediate-release: 100 mg once daily; titrate every 2-3 days by 100 mg/day increments; usual daily dose: 200-300 mg/day (maximum: 300 mg/day)

Patients currently on immediate-release: Calculate 24 hour immediate release total dose and initiate total extended release daily dose (round dose to the next lowest 100 mg increment); titrate (maximum: 300 mg/day)

Tridural™ (Canadian labeling, not available in U.S.): 100 mg once daily; titrate by 100 mg/day every 2 days as needed based on clinical response and severity of pain (maximum: 300 mg/day)

Zytram® XL (Canadian labeling, not available in U.S.): 150 mg once daily; if pain relief is not achieved may titrate by increasing dosage incrementally, with sufficient time to evaluate effect of increased dosage; generally not more often than every 7 days (maximum: 400 mg/day)

Elderly >75 years:

Immediate release: 50 mg every 6 hours (not to exceed 300 mg/day); see dosing adjustments for renal and hepatic impairment.

Extended release formulation: Use with great caution. See adult dosing.

Dosage Oral: Moderate-to-severe pain:

Children 7-16 years (unlabeled use): 1-2 mg/kg/dose every 4-6 hours; maximum: 400 mg/day

Children ≥17 years and Adults: Immediate release formulation: 50-100 mg every 4-6 hours (not to exceed 400 mg/day)

For patients not requiring rapid onset of effect, tolerability may be improved by starting dose at 25 mg/day and titrating dose by 25 mg every 3 days, until reaching 25 mg 4 times/day. The total daily dose may then be increased by 50 mg every 3 days as tolerated, to reach dose of 50 mg 4 times/day. After titration, 50-100 mg may be given every 4-6 hours as needed up to a maximum 400 mg/day.

Adults: Extended release formulations:

Ultram® ER:

Patients not currently on immediate-release: 100 mg once daily; titrate every 5 days (maximum: 300 mg/day)

Patients currently on immediate-release: Calculate 24-hour immediate release total dose and initiate total extended release daily dose (round dose to the next lowest 100 mg increment); titrate (maximum: 300 mg/day)

Ralivia™ ER (Canadian labeling, not available in U.S.): 100 mg once daily; titrate every 5 days as needed based on clinical response and severity of pain (maximum: 300 mg/day)

Ryzolt™:

Patients not currently on immediate-release: 100 mg once daily; titrate every 2-3 days by 100 mg/day increments; usual daily dose: 200-300 mg/day (maximum: 300 mg/day)

Patients currently on immediate-release: Calculate 24 hour immediate release total dose and initiate total extended release daily dose (round dose to the next lowest 100 mg increment); titrate (maximum: 300 mg/day)

Tridural™ (Canadian labeling, not available in U.S.): 100 mg once daily; titrate by 100 mg/day every 2 days as needed based on clinical response and severity of pain (maximum: 300 mg/day)

Zytram® XL (Canadian labeling, not available in U.S.): 150 mg once daily; if pain relief is not achieved may titrate by increasing dosage incrementally, with sufficient time to evaluate effect of increased dosage; generally not more often than every 7 days (maximum: 400 mg/day)

Elderly >65 years: Use caution and initiate at the lower end of the dosing range

Immediate release: Elderly >75 years: Do not exceed 300 mg/day; see dosing adjustments for renal and hepatic impairment.

Extended release formulation: Elderly >75 years: Use with great caution. See adult, renal, and hepatic dosing.

Dosing adjustment in renal impairment:

Immediate release: Cl_{cr} <30 mL/minute: Administer 50-100 mg dose every 12 hours (maximum: 200 mg/day)

Extended release: Should not be used in patients with Cl_{cr} <30 mL/minute

Dosing adjustment in hepatic impairment:

Immediate release: Cirrhosis: Recommended dose: 50 mg every 12 hours

Extended release: Should not be used in patients with severe (Child-Pugh class C) hepatic dysfunction; Ryzolt™ should not be used in any degree of hepatic impairment

Mechanism of Action Tramadol and its active metabolite (M1) binds to μ-opiate receptors in the CNS causing inhibition of ascending pain pathways, altering the perception of and response to pain; also inhibits the reuptake of norepinephrine and serotonin, which also modifies the ascending pain pathway

Contraindications Hypersensitivity to tramadol, opioids, or any component of the formulation; opioid-dependent patients; acute intoxication with alcohol, hypnotics, centrally-acting analgesics, opioids, or psychotropic drugs

Additional contraindications for Ryzolt™: Severe/acute bronchial asthma, hypercapnia, or significant respiratory depression in the absence of appropriately monitored setting and/or resuscitative equipment

Canadian product labeling:

Tramadol is contraindicated during or within 14 days following MAO inhibitor therapy

Extended release formulations (Ralivia™ ER [CAN], Tridural™[CAN], and Zytram® XL [CAN]): Additional contraindications: Severe (Cl_{cr} <30 mL/minute) renal dysfunction, severe (Child-Pugh class C) hepatic dysfunction

Warnings/Precautions Rare but serious anaphylactoid reactions (including fatalities) often following initial dosing have been reported. Pruritus, hives, bronchospasm, angioedema, toxic epidermal necrolysis (TEN) and Stevens-Johnson syndrome also have been reported with use. Previous anaphylactoid reactions to opioids may increase risks for similar reactions to tramadol. Caution patients to swallow extended release tablets whole. Rapid release and absorption of tramadol from extended release tablets that are broken, crushed, or chewed may lead to a potentially lethal overdose. May cause CNS depression, which may impair physical or mental abilities; patients must be cautioned about performing tasks which require mental alertness (eg, operating machinery or driving). May cause CNS depression and/or respiratory depression, particularly when combined with other CNS depressants. Use with caution and reduce dosage when administered to patients receiving other CNS depressants. An increased risk of seizures may occur in patients receiving serotonin reuptake inhibitors (SSRIs or anorectics), tricyclic antidepressants or other cyclic compounds (including cyclobenzaprine, promethazine), neuroleptics, drugs which may lower seizure threshold, or drugs which impair metabolism of tramadol (ie, CYP2D6 and 3A4 inhibitors). Patients with a history of seizures, or with a risk of seizures (head trauma, metabolic disorders, CNS infection, or malignancy, or during ethanol/drug withdrawal) are also at increased risk. Avoid use, if possible, with serotonergic agents such as TCAs, MAO inhibitors (use with extreme caution; contraindicated in Canadian product labeling), triptans, venlafaxine, trazodone, lithium, sibutramine, meperidine, dextromethorphan, St John's wort, SNRIs, and SSRIs; use caution with drugs which impair metabolism of tramadol (ie, CYP2D6 and 3A4 inhibitors); concomitant may increase the risk of serotonin syndrome.

Elderly (particularly >75 years of age), debilitated patients and patients with chronic respiratory disorders may be at greater risk of adverse events. Use with caution in patients with increased intracranial pressure or head injury. Avoid use in patients who are suicidal or addiction prone; use with caution in patients taking tranquilizers and/or antidepressants, or those with an emotional disturbance including depression. Healthcare provider should be alert to problems of abuse, misuse, and diversion. Use caution in heavy alcohol users. Use caution in treatment of acute abdominal conditions; may mask pain. Use tramadol with caution and reduce dosage in patients with liver disease or renal dysfunction. Avoid using extended release tablets in severe hepatic impairment. Do not use Ryzolt™ in any degree of hepatic impairment. Tolerance or drug dependence may result from extended use (withdrawal symptoms have been reported); abrupt discontinuation should be avoided. Tapering of dose at the time of discontinuation limits the risk of withdrawal symptoms. Some products may contain phenylalanine.

Drug Interactions

Metabolism/Transport Effects Substrate of CYP2D6 (major), 3A4 (major)

Avoid Concomitant Use

Avoid concomitant use of TraMADol with any of the following: Sibutramine

Increased Effect/Toxicity

TraMADol may increase the levels/effects of: Alcohol (Ethyl); Alvimopan; CNS Depressants; Desmopressin; MAO Inhibitors; Selective Serotonin Reuptake Inhibitors; Serotonin Modulators; Thiazide Diuretics; Vitamin K Antagonists

The levels/effects of TraMADol may be increased by: Amphetamines; Antipsychotic Agents (Phenothiazines); Conivaptan; CYP3A4 Inhibitors (Moderate); CYP3A4 Inhibitors (Strong); Dasatinib; Droperidol; Selective Serotonin Reuptake Inhibitors; Sibutramine; Succinylcholine; Tricyclic Antidepressants

Decreased Effect

TraMADol may decrease the levels/effects of: Pegvisomant

The levels/effects of TraMADol may be decreased by: Ammonium Chloride; CYP2D6 Inhibitors (Moderate); CYP2D6 Inhibitors (Strong); CYP3A4 Inducers (Strong); Deferasirox; Mixed Agonist / Antagonist Opioids; Tocilizumab

Ethanol/Nutrition/Herb Interactions

Ethanol: May increase CNS depression; monitor for increased effects with coadministration. Caution patients about effects.

Food:

Immediate release: Does not affect the rate or extent of absorption.

Extended release: Reduced C_{max} and AUC and T_{max} occurred 3 hours earlier when taken with a high-fat meal.

Ryzolt™: Increased C_{max}; no effect on AUC.

Herb/Nutraceutical: Avoid valerian, St John's wort, kava kava, gotu kola (may increase CNS depression).

Dietary Considerations May be taken without regard to meals. Ultram® ER: Be consistent; always give with food or always give on an empty stomach. Some products may contain phenylalanine.

Pharmacodynamics/Kinetics

Onset of Action Immediate release: ~1 hour

Duration of Action 9 hours

Half-life Elimination Tramadol: ~6-8 hours; Active metabolite: 7-9 hours, prolonged in elderly, hepatic, or renal impairment; Zytram® XL: ~16 hours; Ralivia™ ER, Ryzolt™, Tridural™: ~5-9 hours

Time to Peak Immediate release: ~2 hours; Extended release: Ultram® ER: ~12 hours, Ryzolt™, Tridural™: ~4 hours

Pregnancy Risk Factor C

Lactation Enters breast milk/not recommended

Breast-Feeding Considerations Sixteen hours following a single 100 mg I.V. dose, the amount of tramadol found in breast milk was 0.1% of the maternal dose. Use is not recommended by the manufacturer for postdelivery analgesia in nursing mothers.

Dosage Forms

Tablet, oral: 50 mg

Ultram®: 50 mg

Tablet, extended release, oral: 100 mg, 200 mg

Ryzolt™: 100 mg, 200 mg, 300 mg

Ultram® ER: 100 mg, 200 mg, 300 mg

Tablet, orally disintegrating, oral:

Rybix™ ODT: 50 mg

Dosage Forms: Canada

Tablet, extended release:

Ralivia™ ER, Tridural™: 100 mg, 200 mg, 300 mg

Zytram® XL: 75 mg, 100 mg, 150 mg, 200 mg, 300 mg, 400 mg

Dental Comment Literature reports suggest that the efficacy of tramadol in oral surgery pain is equivalent to the combination of aspirin and codeine. One study (Olson, 1990) showed acetaminophen and dextropropoxyphene combination to be superior to tramadol and another study showed tramadol to be superior to acetaminophen and dextropropoxyphene combination. Tramadol appears to be at least equal to if not better than codeine alone. Seizures have been reported with the use of tramadol.

References

Collins M, Young I, Sweeney P, et al, "The Effect of Tramadol on Dento-Alveolar Surgical Pain," *Br J Oral Maxillofac Surg*, 1997, 35(1):54-8.

Doroschak AM, Bowles WR, and Hargreaves KM, "Evaluation of the Combination of Flurbiprofen and Tramadol for Management of Endodontic Pain," *J Endod*, 1999, 25(10):660-3.

Kahn LH, Alderfer RJ, and Graham DJ, "Seizures Reported With Tramadol," *JAMA*, 1997, 278(20):1661.

Lewis KS and Han NH, "Tramadol: A New Centrally Acting Analgesic," *Am J Health Syst Pharm*, 1997, 54 (6):643-52.

Moore PA, "Pain Management in Dental Practice: Tramadol vs. Codeine Combinations," *J Am Dent Assoc*, 1999, 130(7):1075-9.

Moore PA, Crout RJ, Jackson DL, et al, "Tramadol Hydrochloride: Analgesic Efficacy Compared With Codeine, Aspirin With Codeine, and Placebo After Dental Extraction," *J Clin Pharmacol*, 1998, 38 (6):554-60.

Olson NZ, Sunshine A, O'Neill, et al, *Tramadol Hydrochloride: Oral Efficacy in Postoperative Pain*, American Pain Society 9th Annual Scientific Meeting, St Louis, MO, October, 1990.

Roelofse JA and Payne KA, "Oral Tramadol: Analgesic Efficacy in Children Following Multiple Dental Extractions," *Eur J Anaesthesiol*, 1999, 16(7):441-7.
Sunshine A, "New Clinical Experience With Tramadol," *Drugs*, 1994, 47(Suppl 1):8-18.
Sunshine A, Olson NZ, Zighelboim I, et al, "Analgesic Oral Efficacy of Tramadol Hydrochloride in Postoperative Pain," *Clin Pharmacol Ther*, 1992, 51(6):740-6.
Wynn RL, "Tramadol (Ultram) - A New Kind of Analgesic," *Gen Dent*, 1996, 44(3):216-8,220.

Trandolapril (tran DOE la pril)

Related Information
Cardiovascular Diseases *on page 1848*

U.S. Brand Names Mavik®

Canadian Brand Names Mavik®

Pharmacologic Category Angiotensin-Converting Enzyme (ACE) Inhibitor

Use Treatment of hypertension alone or in combination with other antihypertensive agents; treatment of heart failure (HF) or left ventricular (LV) dysfunction after myocardial infarction (MI)

Unlabeled/Investigational Use To delay the progression of nephropathy and reduce risks of cardiovascular events in hypertensive patients with type 1 or 2 diabetes mellitus

Local Anesthetic/Vasoconstrictor Precautions No information available to require special precautions

Effects on Dental Treatment No significant effects or complications reported

Effects on Bleeding No information available to require special precautions

Adverse Effects Note: Frequency ranges include data from hypertension and heart failure trials. Higher rates of adverse reactions have generally been noted in patients with CHF. However, the frequency of adverse effects associated with placebo is also increased in this population.

>1%:
- Cardiovascular: Hypotension (<1% to 11%), syncope (6%), bradycardia (<1% to 5%), intermittent claudication (4%)
- Central nervous system: Dizziness (1% to 23%)
- Endocrine & metabolic: Uric acid increased (15%), hyperkalemia (5%), hypocalcemia (5%)
- Gastrointestinal: Diarrhea (1%)
- Neuromuscular & skeletal: Myalgia (5%)
- Renal: BUN increased (9%), serum creatinine increased (1% to 5%)
- Respiratory: Cough (2% to 35%)

Worsening of renal function may occur in patients with bilateral renal artery stenosis or hypovolemia. In addition, a syndrome which may include fever, myalgia, arthralgia, interstitial nephritis, vasculitis, rash, eosinophilia and positive ANA, and elevated ESR has been reported with ACE inhibitors. Eosinophilic pneumonitis has also been reported with other ACE inhibitors.

General Dosage Range Dosage adjustment recommended in patients with hepatic or renal impairment

Oral: *Adults:* Initial: 1-2 mg once daily; Maintenance: 1-4 mg once daily

Mechanism of Action Trandolapril is an ACE inhibitor which prevents the formation of angiotensin II from angiotensin I. Trandolapril must undergo enzymatic hydrolysis, mainly in liver, to its biologically active metabolite, trandolaprilat. A CNS mechanism may also be involved in the hypotensive effect as angiotensin II increases adrenergic outflow from the CNS. Vasoactive kallikrein's may be decreased in conversion to active hormones by ACE inhibitors, thus reducing blood pressure.

Pharmacodynamics/Kinetics

Onset of Action 1-2 hours; Peak effect: Reduction in blood pressure: 6 hours

Duration of Action Prolonged; 72 hours after single dose

Half-life Elimination
Trandolapril: 6 hours; Trandolaprilat: Effective: 22.5 hours

Time to Peak Parent: 1 hour; Active metabolite trandolaprilat: 4-10 hours

Pregnancy Risk Factor C (1st trimester); D (2nd and 3rd trimesters)

Trandolapril and Verapamil (tran DOE la pril & ver AP a mil)

Related Information
Trandolapril *on page 1660*
Verapamil *on page 1716*

U.S. Brand Names Tarka®

Canadian Brand Names Tarka®

Pharmacologic Category Angiotensin-Converting Enzyme (ACE) Inhibitor; Calcium Channel Blocker

Use Treatment of hypertension; however, not indicated for initial treatment of hypertension

Local Anesthetic/Vasoconstrictor Precautions No information available to require special precautions

Effects on Dental Treatment No significant effects or complications reported

Effects on Bleeding No information available to require special precautions

Adverse Effects See individual agents.

General Dosage Range Dosage adjustment recommended in patients with hepatic or renal impairment

Oral: *Adults:* Trandolapril 1-4 mg and verapamil 180-240 mg once daily

Pregnancy Risk Factor C/D (2nd and 3rd trimesters)

Tranexamic Acid (tran eks AM ik AS id)

Related Information

Antiplatelet and Anticoagulation Considerations in Dentistry *on page 1867*

U.S. Brand Names Cyklokapron®; Lysteda™

Canadian Brand Names Cyklokapron®; Tranexamic Acid Injection BP

Pharmacologic Category Antifibrinolytic Agent; Antihemophilic Agent; Hemostatic Agent; Lysine Analog

Use

Solution for injection: Short-term use (2-8 days) in hemophilia patients to reduce or prevent hemorrhage and reduce need for replacement therapy during and following tooth extraction

Tablet: Treatment of cyclic heavy menstrual bleeding

Unlabeled/Investigational Use Trauma-associated hemorrhage

Local Anesthetic/Vasoconstrictor Precautions No information available to require special precautions

Effects on Dental Treatment No significant effects or complications reported. See Effects on Bleeding and Dental Comment.

Effects on Bleeding General dental procedures and simple restorative procedures are not associated with bleeding; therefore, there is no contraindication to general dental treatment for most patients with bleeding disorders. However, after dental extractions and other dental surgeries including deep scaling, block anesthesia, and large fillings, in patients with hemophilia, antifibrinolytic drugs such as tranexamic acid are useful in controlling bleeding. A carefully coordinated strategy between the dental and medical team may be required to ensure adequate procedures for hemostasis. As preparation for selected dental procedures tranexamic acid may be required.

Immediately before dental extraction in hemophilic patients, administer 10 mg/kg tranexamic acid I.V. together with replacement therapy. Presently there is no oral dosage form commercially available for tranexamic acid.

Adverse Effects

Injection: Frequency not defined:

Cardiovascular: Hypotension (with rapid I.V. injection)
Central nervous system: Giddiness
Dermatologic: Allergic dermatitis
Endocrine & metabolic: Unusual menstrual discomfort
Gastrointestinal: Diarrhea, nausea, vomiting
Ocular: Blurred vision

Oral:

>10%:

Central nervous system: Headache (50%)
Gastrointestinal: Abdominal pain (20%)
Neuromuscular & skeletal: Back pain (21%), muscle pain (11%)
Respiratory: Nasal/sinus symptoms (25%)

1% to 10%:

Central nervous system: Fatigue (5%)
Hematologic: Anemia (6%)
Neuromuscular & skeletal: Arthralgia (7%), muscle cramps/spasms (7%)

General Dosage Range Dosage adjustment recommended in patients with renal impairment

I.V.: *Children and Adults:* Initial: 10 mg/kg as a single dose; Maintenance: 10 mg/kg/dose 3-4 times/day

Oral: *Adults:* 1300 mg 3 times daily (3900 mg/day)

Mechanism of Action Forms a reversible complex that displaces plasminogen from fibrin resulting in inhibition of fibrinolysis; it also inhibits the proteolytic activity of plasmin

Pharmacodynamics/Kinetics

Half-life Elimination ~2-11 hours

Time to Peak Oral: ~3 hours

Pregnancy Risk Factor B

Dental Comment Antifibrinolytic drugs are useful for the control of bleeding after dental extractions in patients with hemophilia because the oral mucosa and saliva are rich in plasminogen activators.

Tranylcypromine (tran il SIP roe meen)

U.S. Brand Names Parnate®

Canadian Brand Names Parnate®

Pharmacologic Category Antidepressant, Monoamine Oxidase Inhibitor

Use Treatment of major depressive episode without melancholia

Local Anesthetic/Vasoconstrictor Precautions Attempts should be made to avoid use of vasoconstrictor due to possibility of hypertensive episodes with monoamine oxidase inhibitors

Effects on Dental Treatment Key adverse event(s) related to dental treatment: Orthostatic hypotension. Avoid use as an analgesic due to toxic reactions with MAO inhibitors. Xerostomia (normal salivary flow resumes upon discontinuation).

Effects on Bleeding No information available to require special precautions

Adverse Effects Frequency not defined.

Cardiovascular: Edema, orthostatic hypotension, palpitation, tachycardia

Central nervous system: Agitation, anxiety, chills, dizziness, drowsiness, headache, insomnia, mania, restlessness

Dermatologic: Alopecia (rare), rash (rare), urticaria

Endocrine & metabolic: Sexual dysfunction (anorgasmia, ejaculatory disturbances, impotence); SIADH

Gastrointestinal: Abdominal pain, anorexia, constipation, diarrhea, nausea, xerostomia

Genitourinary: Urinary retention

Hematologic: Agranulocytosis, anemia, leukopenia, thrombocytopenia

Hepatic: Hepatitis (rare)

Neuromuscular & skeletal: Muscle spasm, myoclonus, numbness, paresthesia, tremor, weakness

Ocular: Blurred vision

Otic: Tinnitus

Miscellaneous: Diaphoresis

General Dosage Range Oral: *Adults:* 10-30 mg twice daily (maximum: 60 mg/day)

Mechanism of Action Tranylcypromine is a nonhydrazine monoamine oxidase inhibitor. It increases endogenous concentrations of epinephrine, norepinephrine, dopamine, and serotonin through inhibition of the enzyme (monoamine oxidase) responsible for the breakdown of these neurotransmitters.

Pharmacodynamics/Kinetics

Onset of Action Therapeutic: 2 days to 3 weeks continued dosing

Duration of Action MAO inhibition may persist for up to 10 days following discontinuation.

Half-life Elimination 90-190 minutes

Time to Peak Serum: ~2 hours

Trastuzumab (tras TU zoo mab)

U.S. Brand Names Herceptin®

Canadian Brand Names Herceptin®

Pharmacologic Category Antineoplastic Agent, Monoclonal Antibody; Monoclonal Antibody

Use Treatment (adjuvant) of HER-2 overexpressing breast cancer; treatment of HER-2 overexpressing metastatic breast cancer; treatment of HER-2 overexpressing metastatic gastric or gastroesophageal junction adenocarcinoma (in patients who have not received prior treatment)

Local Anesthetic/Vasoconstrictor Precautions No information available to require special precautions

Effects on Dental Treatment No significant effects or complications reported

Effects on Bleeding Although significant myelosuppression with associated altered hemostasis has been reported for many chemotherapeutic agents, myelosuppression is not common with trastuzumab and no specific precautions appear to necessary.

Adverse Effects Note: Percentages reported with single-agent therapy.

>10%:

Cardiovascular: LVEF decreased (4% to 22%)

Central nervous system: Pain (47%), fever (6% to 36%), chills (5% to 32%), headache (10% to 26%), insomnia (14%), dizziness (4% to 13%)

Dermatologic: Rash (4% to 18%)

Gastrointestinal: Nausea (6% to 33%), diarrhea (7% to 25%), vomiting (4% to 23%), abdominal pain (2% to 22%), anorexia (14%)

Neuromuscular & skeletal: Weakness (4% to 42%), back pain (5% to 22%)

Respiratory: Cough (5% to 26%), dyspnea (3% to 22%), rhinitis (2% to 14%), pharyngitis (12%)

Miscellaneous: Infusion reaction (21% to 40%, chills and fever most common; severe: 1%), infection (20%)

1% to 10%:

Cardiovascular: Peripheral edema (5% to 10%), edema (8%), HF (2% to 7%; severe: <1%), tachycardia (5%), hypertension (4%), arrhythmia (3%), palpitation (3%)

Central nervous system: Depression (6%)

Dermatologic: Acne (2%), nail disorder (2%), pruritus (2%)

Gastrointestinal: Constipation (2%), dyspepsia (2%)

Genitourinary: Urinary tract infection (3% to 5%)

Hematologic: Anemia (4%), leukopenia (3%)

Neuromuscular & skeletal: Paresthesia (2% to 9%), bone pain (3% to 7%), arthralgia (6% to 8%), myalgia (4%), muscle spasm (3%), peripheral neuritis (2%), neuropathy (1%)

Respiratory: Sinusitis (2% to 9%), nasopharyngitis (8%), upper respiratory infection (3%), epistaxis (2%), pharyngolaryngeal pain (2%)

Miscellaneous: Flu-like syndrome (2% to 10%), accidental injury (6%), influenza (4%), allergic reaction (3%), herpes simplex (2%)

General Dosage Range Dosage adjustment recommended in patients who develop toxicities

I.V.: *Adults:* Loading dose: 4 mg/kg; Maintenance: 2 mg/kg once weekly **or** Loading dose: 8 mg/kg; Maintenance: 6 mg/kg every 3 weeks

Mechanism of Action Trastuzumab is a monoclonal antibody which binds to the extracellular domain of the human epidermal growth factor receptor 2 protein (HER-2); it mediates antibody-dependent cellular cytotoxicity by inhibiting proliferation of cells which overexpress HER-2 protein.

Pharmacodynamics/Kinetics

Half-life Elimination Weekly dosing: Mean: 6 days (range: 1-32 days); every 3 week regimen: Mean: 16 days (range: 11-23 days)

Pregnancy Risk Factor D

Travoprost (TRA voe prost)

U.S. Brand Names Travatan Z®; Travatan® [DSC]

Canadian Brand Names Travatan Z®; Travatan®

Pharmacologic Category Ophthalmic Agent, Antiglaucoma; Prostaglandin, Ophthalmic

Use Reduction of elevated intraocular pressure in patients with open-angle glaucoma or ocular hypertension who are intolerant of the other IOP-lowering medications or insufficiently responsive (failed to achieve target IOP determined after multiple measurements over time) to another IOP-lowering medication

Local Anesthetic/Vasoconstrictor Precautions No significant effects or complications reported

Effects on Dental Treatment No information available to require special precautions

Effects on Bleeding No information available to require special precautions

Adverse Effects

>10%: Ocular: Hyperemia (35% to 50%)

5% to 10%: Ocular: Decreased visual acuity, eye discomfort, foreign body sensation, pain, pruritus

1% to 5%:

Cardiovascular: Angina pectoris, bradycardia, hyper-/hypotension

Central nervous system: Depression, pain, anxiety, headache

Endocrine & metabolic: Hypercholesterolemia

Gastrointestinal: Dyspepsia

Genitourinary: Prostate disorder, urinary incontinence

Neuromuscular & skeletal: Arthritis, back pain, chest pain

Ocular (1% to 4%): Abnormal vision, blepharitis, blurred vision, conjunctivitis, dry eye, iris discoloration, keratitis, lid margin crusting, photophobia, subconjunctival hemorrhage, cataract, tearing, periorbital skin discoloration (darkening), eyelash darkening, eyelash growth increased

Respiratory: Bronchitis, sinusitis

General Dosage Range Ophthalmic: *Adults:* Instill 1 drop into affected eye(s) once daily

Mechanism of Action A selective FP prostanoid receptor agonist which lowers intraocular pressure by increasing trabecular meshwork and outflow

Pharmacodynamics/Kinetics

Onset of Action ~2 hours; Peak effect: 12 hours

Duration of Action Plasma levels decrease to <10 pg/mL within 1 hour

Pregnancy Risk Factor C

TraZODone (TRAZ oh done)

Related Information

Management of the Patient With Anxiety or Depression *on page 1968*

U.S. Brand Names Oleptro™

Canadian Brand Names Apo-Trazodone D®; Apo-Trazodone®; Dom-Trazodone; Mylan-Trazodone; Novo-Trazodone; Nu-Trazodone; Nu-Trazodone D; Oleptro™; PHL-Trazodone; PMS-Trazodone; ratio-Trazodone; Trazorel®; ZYM-Trazodone

Generic Availability (U.S.) Yes: Excludes extended release tablet

Pharmacologic Category Antidepressant, Serotonin Reuptake Inhibitor/Antagonist

Use Treatment of major depressive disorder

Unlabeled/Investigational Use Potential augmenting agent for antidepressants, hypnotic

Local Anesthetic/Vasoconstrictor Precautions Trazodone inhibits reuptake of both serotonin and norepinephrine and also blocks some serotonin receptors. No precautions with vasoconstrictors appear to be necessary.

Effects on Dental Treatment Key adverse event(s) related to dental treatment: Significant xerostomia (normal salivary flow resumes upon discontinuation).

Effects on Bleeding No information available to require special precautions

Adverse Effects

>10%:

Central nervous system: Sedation (≤46%), headache (10% to 33%), dizziness (20% to 28%), fatigue (6% to 15%)

Gastrointestinal: Xerostomia (15% to 34%), nausea (10% to 21%)

Ocular: Blurred vision (5% to 15%)

1% to 10%:

Cardiovascular: Edema (3% to 7%), hypotension (≤7%), syncope (≤5%), hypertension (1% to 2%)

Central nervous system: Confusion (5% to 6%), incoordination (2% to 5%), concentration decreased (1% to 3%), disorientation (≤2%), memory impairment (≤1%), agitation, migraine

Endocrine & metabolic: Libido decreased (1% to 2%)

Gastrointestinal: Diarrhea (5% to 9%), constipation (7% to 8%), abdominal pain, abnormal taste, flatulence, vomiting, weight gain/loss

Genitourinary: Ejaculation disorder (2%), urinary urgency

Neuromuscular & skeletal: Back pain (≤5%), tremor (1% to 5%), paresthesia (≤1%), myalgia

Ocular: Visual disturbance

Respiratory: Nasal congestion (3% to 6%), dyspnea

Miscellaneous: Night sweats

Dosage Oral: Therapeutic effects may take up to 6 weeks to occur; therapy is normally maintained for 6-12 months after optimum response is reached to prevent recurrence of depression

Children 6-12 years: Depression (unlabeled use): Initial: 1.5-2 mg/kg/day in divided doses; increase gradually every 3-4 days as needed; maximum: 6 mg/kg/day in 3 divided doses

Adolescents: Depression (unlabeled use): Initial: 25-50 mg/day; increase to 100-150 mg/day in divided doses

Adults:

Depression: Initial: 150 mg/day in 3 divided doses (may increase by 50 mg/day every 3-7 days); maximum dose: 600 mg/day

Extended release formulation: Initial: 150 mg once daily at bedtime (may increase by 75 mg/day every 3 days); maximum dose: 375 mg/day; once adequate response obtained, gradually reduce with adjustment based on therapeutic response

Note: Therapeutic effects may take up to 6 weeks. Therapy is normally maintained for 6-12 months after optimum response is reached to prevent recurrence of depression.

Sedation/hypnotic (unlabeled use): 25-50 mg at bedtime (often in combination with daytime SSRIs); may increase up to 200 mg at bedtime

Elderly: 25-50 mg at bedtime with 25-50 mg/day dose increase every 3 days for inpatients and weekly for outpatients, if tolerated; usual dose: 75-150 mg/day

Mechanism of Action Inhibits reuptake of serotonin, causes adrenoreceptor subsensitivity, and induces significant changes in 5-HT presynaptic receptor adrenoreceptors. Trazodone also significantly blocks histamine (H_1) and alpha$_1$-adrenergic receptors.

Contraindications Hypersensitivity to trazodone or any component of the formulation

Warnings/Precautions [U.S. Boxed Warning]: Antidepressants increase the risk of suicidal thinking and behavior in children, adolescents, and young adults (18-24 years of age) with major depressive disorder (MDD) and other psychiatric disorders; consider risk prior to prescribing. Short-term studies did not show an increased risk in patients >24 years of age and showed a decreased risk in patients ≥65 years of age. Closely monitor for clinical worsening, suicidality, or unusual changes in behavior; the patient's family or caregiver should be instructed to closely observe the patient and communicate condition with healthcare provider. A medication guide should be dispensed with each prescription. **Trazodone is not FDA approved for use in children.**

The possibility of a suicide attempt is inherent in major depression and may persist until remission occurs. Monitor for worsening of depression or suicidality, especially during initiation of therapy (generally first 1-2 months) or with dose increases or decreases. Use caution in high-risk patients. Worsening depression and severe abrupt suicidality that are not part of the presenting symptoms may require discontinuation or modification of drug therapy. The patient's family or caregiver should be alerted to monitor patients for the emergence of suicidality and associated behaviors (such as agitation, irritability, hostility, impulsivity, and hypomania) and call healthcare provider.

May worsen psychosis in some patients or precipitate a shift to mania or hypomania in patients with bipolar disorder. Patients presenting with depressive symptoms should be screened for bipolar disorder. Monotherapy in patients with bipolar disorder should be avoided. **Trazodone is not FDA approved for the treatment of bipolar depression.**

Priapism, including cases resulting in permanent dysfunction, has occurred with the use of trazodone. Instruct patient to seek medical assistance for erection lasting >4 hours; use with caution in patients who have conditions which may predispose them to priapism (eg, sickle cell anemia, multiple myeloma, leukemia). Not recommended for use in a patient during the acute recovery phase of MI. The risks of sedation, postural hypotension, and/or syncope are high relative to other antidepressants. Trazodone frequently causes sedation, which may result in impaired performance of tasks requiring alertness (eg, operating machinery or driving). Sedative effects may be additive with other CNS depressants and ethanol.

Use with caution in patients with a history of cardiovascular disease (including previous MI, stroke, tachycardia, or conduction abnormalities). Although the risk of conduction abnormalities with this agent is low relative to other antidepressants, QT prolongation (with or without torsade de pointes), ventricular tachycardia, and other arrhythmias have been observed with the use of trazodone (reports limited to immediate-release formulation); use with caution in patients with pre-existing cardiac disease. Concurrent use of CYP3A4 inhibitors may increase the risk of QT prolongation and/or proarrhythmia. Concurrent use with other drugs known to prolong QT_c interval is not recommended. May impair platelet aggregation resulting in increased risk of bleeding events (eg, epistaxis, life threatening bleeding), particularly if used concomitantly with aspirin, NSAIDs, warfarin or other anticoagulants. Trazodone should be initiated with caution in patients who are receiving concurrent or recent therapy with a MAO inhibitor. Oleptro™: Avoid use in combination with or within 14 days of an MAO inhibitor.

Serotonin syndrome (SS)/neuroleptic malignant syndrome (NMS)-like reactions may occur with trazodone when used alone, particularly if used with other serotonergic agents (eg, serotonin/norepinephrine reuptake inhibitors [SNRIs], selective serotonin reuptake inhibitors [SSRIs], or triptans), drugs that impair serotonin metabolism (eg, MAO inhibitors), or antidopaminergic agents (eg, antipsychotics). If concurrent use is clinically warranted, carefully observe patient during treatment initiation and dose increases. Do not use concurrently with serotonin precursors (eg, tryptophan).

May cause SIADH and hyponatremia, predominantly in the elderly; volume depletion and/or concurrent use of diuretics likely increases risk. Use with caution in patients taking antihypertensives; may increase the risk of hypotension or syncope. Use with caution in patients taking strong CYP3A4 inhibitors and moderate or strong CYP3A4 inducers; monitor or consider alternative agents that avoid or lessen the potential for CYP-mediated interactions.

Therapy should not be abruptly discontinued in patients receiving high doses for prolonged periods; gradually reduce dosage prior to complete discontinuation to avoid withdrawal symptoms (eg, anxiety, agitation, sleep disturbance). Use caution in patients with a previous seizure disorder or condition predisposing to seizures such as brain damage, alcoholism, or concurrent therapy with other drugs which lower the seizure threshold. Use with caution in patients with hepatic or renal dysfunction and in elderly patients.

Drug Interactions

Metabolism/Transport Effects Substrate of CYP2D6 (minor), 3A4 (major); **Inhibits** CYP3A4 (weak); **Induces** P-glycoprotein

Avoid Concomitant Use

Avoid concomitant use of TraZODone with any of the following: Dabigatran Etexilate; Methylene Blue; Saquinavir; Sibutramine

Increased Effect/Toxicity

TraZODone may increase the levels/effects of: Alcohol (Ethyl); CNS Depressants; Methylene Blue; Serotonin Modulators

The levels/effects of TraZODone may be increased by: BusPIRone; Conivaptan; CYP3A4 Inhibitors (Moderate); CYP3A4 Inhibitors (Strong); Dasatinib; Droperidol; MAO Inhibitors; Protease Inhibitors; Saquinavir; Selective Serotonin Reuptake Inhibitors; Sibutramine; Venlafaxine

Decreased Effect

TraZODone may decrease the levels/effects of: Dabigatran Etexilate; P-Glycoprotein Substrates

The levels/effects of TraZODone may be decreased by: CYP3A4 Inducers (Strong); Deferasirox; Peginterferon Alfa-2b; Tocilizumab

Ethanol/Nutrition/Herb Interactions

Ethanol: May increase CNS depression; monitor for increased effects with coadministration. Caution patients about effects.

Food: Time to peak serum levels may be increased if immediate release trazodone is taken with food.

Herb/Nutraceutical: Avoid valerian, St John's wort, SAMe, kava kava (may increase risk of serotonin syndrome and/or excessive sedation).

Pharmacodynamics/Kinetics

Onset of Action Therapeutic (antidepressant): Up to 6 weeks; sleep aid: 1-3 hours

Half-life Elimination 7-10 hours

Time to Peak

Immediate release: 30-100 minutes; delayed with food (up to 2.5 hours)

Extended release: 9 hours; not significantly affected by food

Pregnancy Risk Factor C

Lactation Enters breast milk/use caution (AAP rates "of concern"; AAP 2001 update pending)

Breast-Feeding Considerations Trazodone is excreted into breast milk; breast milk concentrations peak ~2 hours following administration. It is not known if the trazodone metabolite is found in breast milk. The long-term effects on neurobehavior have not been studied. The manufacturer recommends that caution be exercised when administering trazodone to nursing women.

Dosage Forms

Tablet, oral: 50 mg, 100 mg, 150 mg, 300 mg

Tablet, extended release, oral:

Oleptro™: 150 mg, 300 mg

Treprostinil (tre PROST in il)

U.S. Brand Names Remodulin®; Tyvaso™

Canadian Brand Names Remodulin®

Pharmacologic Category Prostacyclin; Prostaglandin; Vasodilator

Use

Injection: Treatment of pulmonary arterial hypertension (PAH) in patients with NYHA Class II-IV symptoms to decrease exercise-associated symptoms; to diminish clinical deterioration when transitioning from epoprostenol (I.V.)

Inhalation: Treatment of pulmonary arterial hypertension (PAH) in patients with NYHA Class III symptoms to increase walk distance. **Note:** Nearly all controlled clinical trial experience has been with concomitant bosentan or sildenafil.

Local Anesthetic/Vasoconstrictor Precautions No information available to require special precautions

Effects on Dental Treatment No significant effects or complications reported. Treprostinil may enhance the risk of bleeding associated with other antiplatelet agents (aspirin or NSAIDs).

Effects on Bleeding Treprostinil is an inhibitor of platelet aggregation and may prolong bleeding times.

Adverse Effects

>10%:

Cardiovascular: Flushing (inhalation: 15%), vasodilation (11%)

Central nervous system: Headache (27% to 41%)

Dermatologic: Rash (14%)

Gastrointestinal: Diarrhea (25%), nausea (19% to 22%)

Local: Infusion site pain (SubQ: 85%; may improve after several months of therapy); infusion site reaction (SubQ: 83%)

Neuromuscular & skeletal: Jaw pain (13%)

Respiratory: Cough (inhalation: 54%), throat irritation/pharyngolaryngeal pain (inhalation: 25%)

1% to 10%:

Cardiovascular: Edema (9%), syncope (inhalation: 6%), hypotension (4%), epistaxis (inhalation), wheezing (inhalation)

Central nervous system: Dizziness (9%)

Dermatologic: Pruritus (8%)

Respiratory: Pneumonia (inhalation: 4%), hemoptysis (inhalation: 2%)

General Dosage Range Dosage adjustment recommended for the I.V. infusion and SubQ routes in patients with hepatic impairment

Inhalation: *Adults:* Initial: 18 mcg (or 3 inhalations) every 4 hours 4 times/day; Maintenance: Maximum dose: 54 mcg (or 9 inhalations) 4 times/day

I.V. Infusion, SubQ: *Adults:* Initial: 0.625-1.25 ng/kg/minute; Maintenance: 1.25-40 ng/kg/minute

Mechanism of Action Treprostinil is a direct vasodilator of both pulmonary and systemic arterial vascular beds; also inhibits platelet aggregation.

Pharmacodynamics/Kinetics

Half-life Elimination Terminal: ~4 hours

Pregnancy Risk Factor B

Tretinoin (Systemic) (TRET i noyn, sis TEM ik)

Canadian Brand Names Vesanoid®

Pharmacologic Category Antineoplastic Agent, Miscellaneous; Retinoic Acid Derivative

Use Induction of remission in patients with acute promyelocytic leukemia (APL), French American British (FAB) classification M3 (including the M3 variant) characterized by t(15;17) translocation and/or PML/RARα gene presence

Unlabeled/Investigational Use Post consolidation and maintenance therapy in APL; combination therapy (with arsenic trioxide) for remission induction in APL

Local Anesthetic/Vasoconstrictor Precautions No information available to require special precautions

Effects on Dental Treatment Key adverse event(s) related to dental treatment: Xerostomia (normal salivary flow resumes upon discontinuation).

Effects on Bleeding Although significant myelosuppression with associated altered hemostasis has been reported for many chemotherapeutic agents, myelosuppression is not common with tretinoin and no specific precautions appear to necessary.

Adverse Effects Most patients will experience drug-related toxicity, especially headache, fever, weakness and fatigue. These are seldom permanent or irreversible and do not typically require therapy interruption.

>10%:

Cardiovascular: Peripheral edema (52%), chest discomfort (32%), edema (29%), arrhythmias (23%), flushing (23%), hypotension (14%), hypertension (11%)

Central nervous system: Headache (86%), fever (83%), malaise (66%), pain (37%), dizziness (20%), anxiety (17%), depression (14%), insomnia (14%), confusion (11%)

Dermatologic: Skin/mucous membrane dryness (77%), rash (54%), pruritus (20%), alopecia (14%), skin changes (14%)

Endocrine & metabolic: Hypercholesterolemia and/or hypertriglyceridemia (≤60%)

Gastrointestinal: Nausea/vomiting (57%), GI hemorrhage (34%), abdominal pain (31%), mucositis (26%), diarrhea (23%), weight gain (23%), anorexia (17%), constipation (17%), weight loss (17%), dyspepsia (14%), abdominal distention (11%)
Hematologic: Hemorrhage (60%), leukocytosis (40%), disseminated intravascular coagulation (DIC) (26%)
Hepatic: Liver function tests increased (50% to 60%)
Local: Phlebitis (11%)
Neuromuscular & skeletal: Bone pain (77%), paresthesia (17%), myalgia (14%)
Ocular: Ocular disorder (17%), visual disturbances (17%)
Otic: Earache/ear fullness (23%)
Renal: Renal insufficiency (11%)
Respiratory: Upper respiratory tract disorders (63%), dyspnea (60%), respiratory insufficiency (26%), pleural effusion (20%), expiratory wheezing (14%), pneumonia (14%), rales (14%)
Miscellaneous: Shivering (63%), infections (58%), retinoic acid-acute promyelocytic leukemia syndrome differentiation syndrome (≤25%), diaphoresis (20%)

1% to 10%:
Cardiovascular: Cerebral hemorrhage (9%), cardiac failure (6%), facial edema (6%), pallor (6%), cardiac arrest (3%), cardiomyopathy (3%), heart enlarged (3%), heart murmur (3%), ischemia (3%), MI (3%), myocarditis (3%), pericarditis (3%), stroke (3%)
Central nervous system: Agitation (9%), intracranial hypertension (9%), hallucination (6%), aphasia (3%), cerebellar edema (3%), CNS depression (3%), coma (3%), dementia (3%), encephalopathy (3%), facial paralysis (3%), forgetfulness (3%), hypotaxia (3%), hypothermia (3%), light reflex absent (3%), seizure (3%), slow speech (3%), somnolence (3%), spinal cord disorder (3%), unconsciousness (3%)
Dermatologic: Cellulitis (8%)
Endocrine & metabolic: Fluid imbalance (6%), acidosis (3%)
Gastrointestinal: Hepatosplenomegaly (9%), ulcer (3%)
Genitourinary: Dysuria (9%), micturition frequency (3%), prostate enlarged (3%)
Hepatic: Ascites (3%), hepatitis (3%)
Neuromuscular & skeletal: Flank pain (9%), abnormal gait (3%), asterixis (3%), bone inflammation (3%), dysarthria (3%), hemiplegia (3%), hyporeflexia (3%), leg weakness (3%), tremor (3%)
Ocular: Visual acuity change (6%), agnosia (3%), visual field deficit (3%)
Otic: Hearing loss (6%)
Renal: Acute renal failure (3%), renal tubular necrosis (3%)
Respiratory: Lower respiratory tract disorders (9%), pulmonary infiltration (6%), bronchial asthma (3%), larynx edema (3%), pulmonary hypertension (3%)
Miscellaneous: Lymph disorder (6%)

General Dosage Range Dosage adjustment recommended in patients who develop toxicities

Oral: *Children and Adults:* Induction: 45 mg/m^2/day in 2 divided doses (maximum duration of treatment: 90 days)

Mechanism of Action Tretinoin appears to bind one or more nuclear receptors and decreases proliferation and induces differentiation of APL cells; initially produces maturation of primitive promyelocytes and repopulates the marrow and peripheral blood with normal hematopoietic cells to achieve complete remission

Pharmacodynamics/Kinetics

Half-life Elimination Terminal: Parent drug: 0.5-2 hours

Time to Peak Serum: 1-2 hours

Pregnancy Risk Factor D

Tretinoin (Topical) (TRET i noyn, TOP i kal)

U.S. Brand Names Atralin™; Avita®; Refissa™; Renova®; Retin-A Micro®; Retin-A®; Tretin-X™

Canadian Brand Names Rejuva-A®; Renova®; Retin-A Micro®; Retin-A®; Retinova®; Stieva-A

Pharmacologic Category Acne Products; Retinoic Acid Derivative; Topical Skin Product, Acne

Use Treatment of acne vulgaris; photodamaged skin; palliation of fine wrinkles, mottled hyperpigmentation, and tactile roughness of facial skin as part of a comprehensive skin care and sun avoidance program

Unlabeled/Investigational Use Some skin cancers

Local Anesthetic/Vasoconstrictor Precautions No information available to require special precautions

Effects on Dental Treatment No significant effects or complications reported

Effects on Bleeding No information available to require special precautions

Adverse Effects

>10%: Dermatologic: Excessive dryness, erythema, scaling of the skin, pruritus

1% to 10%:

Dermatologic: Hyperpigmentation or hypopigmentation, photosensitivity, initial acne flare-up

Local: Edema, blistering, stinging

General Dosage Range Topical: *Children >12 years and Adults:* Apply once daily **or** every other day

Mechanism of Action Keratinocytes in the sebaceous follicle become less adherent which allows for easy removal; inhibits microcomedone formation and eliminates lesions already present

Pregnancy Risk Factor C

Triacetin (trye a SEE tin)

U.S. Brand Names Myco-Nail [OTC]

Pharmacologic Category Antifungal Agent, Topical

Use Fungistat for athlete's foot and other superficial fungal infections

Local Anesthetic/Vasoconstrictor Precautions No information available to require special precautions

Effects on Dental Treatment No significant effects or complications reported

Effects on Bleeding No information available to require special precautions

General Dosage Range Topical: *Adults*: Apply twice daily to affected areas

Triamcinolone (Systemic) (trye am SIN oh lone)

Related Information

Respiratory Diseases *on page 1876*

U.S. Brand Names Aristospan®; Kenalog®-10; Kenalog®-40

Canadian Brand Names Aristospan®

Generic Availability (U.S.) No

Pharmacologic Category Corticosteroid, Systemic

Dental Use Adjunctive treatment and temporary relief of symptoms associated with oral inflammatory lesions and ulcerative lesions resulting from trauma

Use

Intra-articular (soft tissue): Acute gouty arthritis, acute/subacute bursitis, acute tenosynovitis, epicondylitis, rheumatoid arthritis, synovitis of osteoarthritis

Intralesional: Alopecia areata, discoid lupus erythematosus, keloids, granuloma annulare lesions (localized hypertrophic, infiltrated, or inflammatory), lichen planus plaques, lichen simplex chronicus plaques, psoriatic plaques, necrobiosis lipoidica diabeticorum, cystic tumors of aponeurosis or tendon (ganglia)

Systemic: Adrenocortical insufficiency, dermatologic diseases, endocrine disorders, gastrointestinal diseases, hematologic and neoplastic disorders, nervous system disorders, nephrotic syndrome, rheumatic disorders, allergic states, respiratory diseases, systemic lupus erythematosus (SLE), and other diseases requiring anti-inflammatory or immunosuppressive effects

Local Anesthetic/Vasoconstrictor Precautions No information available to require special precautions

Effects on Dental Treatment Key adverse event(s) related to dental treatment: Ulcerative esophagitis, perioral dermatitis, atrophy of oral mucosa, burning, irritation, and oral monilia (oral inhaler).

Effects on Bleeding No information available to require special precautions

Adverse Effects Frequency not defined; reactions reported with corticosteroid therapy in general:

Cardiovascular: Arrhythmia, bradycardia, cardiac arrest, cardiac enlargement, CHF, circulatory collapse, edema, hypertension, hypertrophic cardiomyopathy (premature infants), myocardial rupture (following recent MI), syncope, tachycardia, thromboembolism, vasculitis

Central nervous system: Arachnoiditis (I.T.), depression, emotional instability, euphoria, headache, insomnia, intracranial pressure increased, malaise, meningitis (I.T.), mood changes, neuritis, neuropathy, personality change, pseudotumor cerebri (with discontinuation), seizure, vertigo

Dermatologic: Abscess (sterile), acne, allergic dermatitis, angioedema, atrophy (cutaneous/subcutaneous), bruising, dry skin, erythema, hair thinning, hirsutism, hyper-/hypopigmentation, hypertrichosis, impaired wound healing, lupus erythematosus-like lesions, petechiae, purpura, rash, skin test suppression, striae, thin skin

Endocrine & metabolic: Carbohydrate intolerance, Cushingoid state, diabetes mellitus, fluid retention, glucose intolerance, growth suppression (children), hypokalemia, hypokalemic alkalosis, menstrual irregularities, negative nitrogen balance, sodium retention, sperm motility altered

Gastrointestinal: Abdominal distention, appetite increased, GI hemorrhage, GI perforation, nausea, pancreatitis, peptic ulcer, ulcerative esophagitis, weight gain

Hepatic: Hepatomegaly, liver function tests increased

Local: Thrombophlebitis

Neuromuscular & skeletal: Aseptic necrosis of femoral and humeral heads, calcinosis, Charcot-like arthropathy, fractures, joint tissue damage, muscle mass loss, myopathy, osteoporosis, parasthesia, tendon rupture, vertebral compression fractures, weakness

Ocular: Cataracts, exophthalmos, glaucoma, ocular pressure increased, papilledema

Renal: Glycosuria

Respiratory: Pulmonary edema

Miscellaneous: Abnormal fat deposits, anaphylactoid reaction, anaphylaxis, diaphoresis, hiccups, infection, moon face

Dosage The lowest possible dose should be used to control the condition; when dose reduction is possible, the dose should be reduced gradually.

Injection:

Acetonide:

Intra-articular, intrabursal, tendon sheaths: Adults: Initial: Smaller joints: 2.5-5 mg, larger joints: 5-15 mg; may require up to 10 mg for small joints and up to 40 mg for large joints; maximum dose/treatment (several joints at one time): 20-80 mg

Intradermal: Adults: Initial: 1 mg

I.M.: Range: 2.5-100 mg/day

Children: Initial: 0.11-1.6 mg/kg/day in 3-4 divided doses

Children 6-12 years: Initial: 40 mg

Children >12 years and Adults: Initial: 60 mg

Hay fever/pollen asthma: 40-100 mg as a single injection/season

Multiple sclerosis (acute exacerbation): 160 mg daily for 1 week, followed by 64 mg every other day for 1 month

Hexacetonide: Adults:

Intralesional, sublesional: Up to 0.5 mg/square inch of affected skin; range: 2-48 mg/day

Intra-articular: Average dose: 2-20 mg; smaller joints: 2-6 mg; larger joints: 10-20 mg. Frequency of injection into a single joint is every 3-4 weeks as necessary; to avoid possible joint destruction use as infrequently as possible.

Triamcinolone Dosing

	Acetonide	Hexacetonide
Intrasynovial	5-40 mg	
Intralesional	1-30 mg (usually 1 mg per injection site); 10 mg/mL suspension usually used	Up to 0.5 mg/sq inch affected area
Sublesional	1-30 mg	
Systemic I.M.	2.5-60 mg/dose (usual adult dose: 60 mg; may repeat with 20-100 mg dose when symptoms recur)	
Intra-articular	2.5-40 mg	2-20 mg average
large joints	5-15 mg	10-20 mg
small joints	2.5-5 mg	2-6 mg
Tendon sheaths	2.5-10 mg	
Intradermal	1 mg/site	

Mechanism of Action Decreases inflammation by suppression of migration of polymorphonuclear leukocytes and reversal of increased capillary permeability; suppresses the immune system by reducing activity and volume of the lymphatic system; suppresses adrenal function at high doses

Contraindications Hypersensitivity to triamcinolone or any component of the formulation; systemic fungal infections; cerebral malaria; idiopathic thrombocytopenic purpura (I.M. injection)

Warnings/Precautions May cause hypercorticism or suppression of hypothalamic-pituitary-adrenal (HPA) axis, particularly in younger children or in patients receiving high doses for prolonged periods. HPA axis suppression may lead to adrenal crisis. Withdrawal and discontinuation of a corticosteroid should be done slowly and carefully.

Acute myopathy has been reported with high-dose corticosteroids, usually in patients with neuromuscular transmission disorders; may involve ocular and/or respiratory muscles; monitor creatine kinase; recovery may be delayed. Corticosteroid use may cause psychiatric disturbances, including depression, euphoria, insomnia, mood swings, and personality changes. Pre-existing psychiatric conditions may be exacerbated by corticosteroid use. Prolonged use of corticosteroids may also increase the incidence of secondary infection, mask acute infection (including fungal infections), prolong or exacerbate viral infections, or limit response to vaccines. Exposure to chickenpox should be avoided; corticosteroids should not be used to treat ocular herpes simplex. Corticosteroids should not be used for cerebral malaria or viral hepatitis. Close observation is required in patients with latent tuberculosis and/or TB reactivity; restrict use in active TB (only in conjunction with antituberculosis treatment). Use with caution in patients with threadworm infection; may cause serious hyperinfection. Prolonged treatment with corticosteroids has been associated with the development of Kaposi's sarcoma (case reports); if noted, discontinuation of therapy should be considered. Avoid use in head injury patients.

Use with caution in patients with thyroid disease, hepatic impairment, renal impairment, cardiovascular disease, diabetes, myasthenia gravis, patients at risk for osteoporosis, patients at risk for seizures, or GI diseases (diverticulitis, peptic ulcer, ulcerative colitis) due to perforation risk. Avoid use in head injury patients. Use caution following acute MI (corticosteroids have been associated with myocardial rupture). Because of the risk of adverse effects, systemic corticosteroids should be used cautiously in the elderly in the smallest possible effective dose for the shortest duration. Patients should not be immunized with live, viral vaccines while receiving immunosuppressive doses of corticosteroids. The ability to respond to dead viral vaccines is unknown.

Withdraw therapy with gradual tapering of dose. There have been reports of systemic corticosteroid withdrawal symptoms (eg, joint/muscle pain, lassitude, depression) when withdrawing oral inhalation therapy. Injection suspension contains benzyl alcohol; benzyl alcohol has been associated with the "gasping syndrome" in neonates and low-birth-weight infants.

Drug Interactions

Avoid Concomitant Use

Avoid concomitant use of Triamcinolone (Systemic) with any of the following: Aldesleukin; BCG; Natalizumab; Pimecrolimus; Roflumilast; Tacrolimus (Topical)

Increased Effect/Toxicity

Triamcinolone (Systemic) may increase the levels/effects of: Acetylcholinesterase Inhibitors; Amphotericin B; Deferasirox; Leflunomide; Loop Diuretics; Natalizumab; NSAID (COX-2 Inhibitor); NSAID (Nonselective); Thiazide Diuretics; Vaccines (Live); Warfarin

The levels/effects of Triamcinolone (Systemic) may be increased by: Antifungal Agents (Azole Derivatives, Systemic); Aprepitant; Calcium Channel Blockers (Nondihydropyridine); Denosumab; Estrogen Derivatives; Fluconazole; Fosaprepitant; Macrolide Antibiotics; Neuromuscular-Blocking Agents (Nondepolarizing); Pimecrolimus; Quinolone Antibiotics; Roflumilast; Salicylates; Tacrolimus (Topical); Trastuzumab

Decreased Effect

Triamcinolone (Systemic) may decrease the levels/effects of: Aldesleukin; Antidiabetic Agents; BCG; Calcitriol; Corticorelin; Isoniazid; Salicylates; Sipuleucel-T; Vaccines (Inactivated)

The levels/effects of Triamcinolone (Systemic) may be decreased by: Aminoglutethimide; Barbiturates; Echinacea; Mitotane; Primidone; Rifamycin Derivatives

Dietary Considerations Ensure adequate intake of calcium and vitamins (or consider supplementation) in patients on medium-to-high doses of systemic corticosteroids.

Pharmacodynamics/Kinetics

Half-life Elimination Biologic: 18-36 hours

Time to Peak I.M.: 8-10 hours

Pregnancy Risk Factor C

Lactation Excretion in breast milk unknown/use caution

Breast-Feeding Considerations Corticosteroids are excreted in human milk; information specific to triamcinolone has not been located.

Dosage Forms

Injection, suspension:

Aristospan®: 5 mg/mL (5 mL); 20 mg/mL (1 mL, 5 mL)

Kenalog®-10: 10 mg/mL (5 mL)

Kenalog®-40: 40 mg/mL (1 mL, 5 mL, 10 mL)

Triamcinolone (Nasal) (trye am SIN oh lone)

U.S. Brand Names Nasacort® AQ

Canadian Brand Names Nasacort® AQ; Trinasal®

Pharmacologic Category Corticosteroid, Nasal

Use Management of seasonal and perennial allergic rhinitis

Local Anesthetic/Vasoconstrictor Precautions No information available to require special precautions

Effects on Dental Treatment No significant effects or complications reported

Effects on Bleeding No information available to require special precautions

Adverse Effects

>10%:

Central nervous system: Headache (2% to 51%)

Respiratory: Pharyngitis (5% to 25%)

1% to 10%:

Cardiovascular: Facial edema (1% to 3%)

Central nervous system: Pain (1% to 3%)

Dermatologic: Photosensitivity (1% to 3%), rash (1% to 3%)

Endocrine & metabolic: Dysmenorrhea (≥2%)

Gastrointestinal: Taste perversion (5% to 8%), dyspepsia (3% to 5%), abdominal pain (1% to 5%), nausea (2% to 3%), diarrhea (1% to 3%), oral moniliasis (1% to 3%), toothache (1% to 3%), vomiting (1% to 3%), weight gain (1% to 3%), xerostomia (1% to 3%)

Genitourinary: Cystitis (1% to 3%), urinary tract infection (1% to 3%), vaginal moniliasis (1% to 3%)

Local: Nasal burning (≥2%; transient), nasal stinging (≥2%; transient)

Neuromuscular & skeletal: Back pain (2% to 8%), bursitis (1% to 3%), myalgia (1% to 3%), tenosynovitis (1% to 3%)

Ocular: Conjunctivitis (1% to 4%)

Otic: Otitis media (≥2%)

Respiratory: Sinusitis (2% to 9%), cough (≤8%), epistaxis (≤5%), bronchitis (children 3%), chest congestion (1% to 3%), asthma (≥2%), rhinitis (≥2%)

Miscellaneous: Flu-like syndrome (2% to 59%), voice alteration (1% to 3%), allergic reaction (≥2%), infection (≥2%)

General Dosage Range Inhalation:

Nasal inhaler:

Children 6-11 years: 220 mcg/day as 2 sprays in each nostril once daily

Children ≥12 years and Adults: 220-440 mcg/day as 2-4 sprays in each nostril 1-4 times/day

Nasal spray:

Children 2-5 years: 110 mcg/day as 1 spray in each nostril once daily (maximum: 110 mcg/day)

Children 6-11 years: Initial: 110 mcg/day as 1 spray in each nostril once daily; Maintenance: 110-220 mcg/day as 1-2 sprays in each nostril

Children ≥12 years and Adults: 110-220 mcg/day as 1-2 sprays in each nostril once daily

Mechanism of Action Suppresses the immune system by reducing activity and volume of the lymphatic system

Pharmacodynamics/Kinetics

Half-life Elimination Biologic: 18-36 hours

Pregnancy Risk Factor C

Triamcinolone (Topical) (trye am SIN oh lone)

Related Information

Ulcerative, Erosive, and Painful Oral Mucosal Disorders *on page* 1950

Related Sample Prescriptions

Mild Lichen Planus *on page* 1992

Recurrent Aphthous Stomatitis *on page* 1992

U.S. Brand Names Kenalog®; Oralone®; Pediaderm™ TA; Triderm®; Zytopic™

Canadian Brand Names Kenalog®; Oracort; Triaderm

Generic Availability (U.S.) Yes: Excludes aerosol

Pharmacologic Category Corticosteroid, Topical

Dental Use Oral topical: Adjunctive treatment and temporary relief of symptoms associated with oral inflammatory lesions and ulcerative lesions resulting from trauma

Use

Oral topical: Adjunctive treatment and temporary relief of symptoms associated with oral inflammatory lesions and ulcerative lesions resulting from trauma

Topical: Inflammatory dermatoses responsive to steroids

Local Anesthetic/Vasoconstrictor Precautions No information available to require special precautions

Effects on Dental Treatment Key adverse event(s) related to dental treatment: Ulcerative esophagitis, perioral dermatitis, atrophy of oral mucosa, burning, and irritation.

Effects on Bleeding No information available to require special precautions

Adverse Effects Frequency not defined.

Dermatologic: Acneiform eruptions, allergic contact dermatitis, dryness, folliculitis,, hypertrichosis, hypopigmentation, itching, miliaria, perioral dermatitis, skin atrophy, skin infection (secondary), skin maceration, striae

Endocrine: HPA axis suppression; metabolic effects (hyperglycemia, hypokalemia)

Local: Burning, irritation

Dental Usual Dosage Oral inflammatory lesions/ulcers: Adults: Oral topical: Press a small dab (about 1/4 inch) to the lesion until a thin film develops; a larger quantity may be required for coverage of some lesions. For optimal results, use only enough to coat the lesion with a thin film; do not rub in.

Dosage

Oral topical: Oral inflammatory lesions/ulcers: Press a small dab (about 1/4 inch) to the lesion until a thin film develops. A larger quantity may be required for coverage of some lesions. For optimal results use only enough to coat the lesion with a thin film; do not rub in.

Topical:

Cream, Ointment:

0.025%: Apply thin film to affected areas 2-4 times/day

0.1% or 0.5%: Apply thin film to affected areas 2-3 times/day

Spray: Apply to affected area 3-4 times/day

Mechanism of Action Decreases inflammation by suppression of migration of polymorphonuclear leukocytes and reversal of increased capillary permeability; suppresses the immune system by reducing activity and volume of the lymphatic system

Contraindications Hypersensitivity to triamcinolone or any component of the formulation; fungal, viral, or bacterial infections of the mouth or throat (oral topical formulation)

Warnings/Precautions Topical corticosteroids may be absorbed percutaneously. Absorption may cause manifestations of Cushing's syndrome, hyperglycemia, or glycosuria. Absorption is increased by the use of occlusive dressings, application to denuded skin, or application to large surface areas. Do not use occlusive dressings on weeping or exudative lesions and general caution with occlusive dressings should be observed; discontinue if skin irritation or contact dermatitis should occur; do not use in patients with decreased skin circulation. May cause hypercorticism or suppression of hypothalamic-pituitary-adrenal (HPA) axis, particularly in younger children or in patients receiving high doses for prolonged periods. HPA axis suppression may lead to adrenal crisis.

Prolonged use may result in fungal or bacterial superinfection; discontinue if dermatological infection persists despite appropriate antimicrobial therapy. Topical use has been associated with local sensitization (redness, irritation); discontinue if sensitization is noted. When used as a topical agent in the oral cavity, if significant regeneration or repair of oral tissues has not occurred in seven days, re-evaluation of the etiology of the oral lesion is advised.

Because of the risk of adverse effects associated with systemic absorption, topical corticosteroids should be used cautiously in the elderly in the smallest possible effective dose for the shortest duration. Children may absorb proportionally larger amounts after topical application and may be more prone to systemic effects. HPA axis suppression, intracranial hypertension, and Cushing's syndrome have been reported in children receiving topical corticosteroids. Prolonged use may affect growth velocity; growth should be routinely monitored in pediatric patients.

Drug Interactions

Avoid Concomitant Use

Avoid concomitant use of Triamcinolone (Topical) with any of the following: Aldesleukin

Increased Effect/Toxicity

Triamcinolone (Topical) may increase the levels/effects of: Deferasirox

Decreased Effect
Triamcinolone (Topical) may decrease the levels/effects of: Aldesleukin; Corticorelin

Pharmacodynamics/Kinetics
Half-life Elimination Biologic: 18-36 hours

Pregnancy Risk Factor C

Lactation Excretion in breast milk unknown/use caution

Breast-Feeding Considerations Corticosteroids are excreted in human milk; information specific to triamcinolone has not been located. The amount of triamcinolone absorbed systemically following topical administration is variable. Hypertension in the nursing infant has been reported following corticosteroid ointment applied to the nipples. Use with caution.

Dosage Forms
Aerosol, topical:
Kenalog®: 0.2 mg/2-second spray (63 g)
Cream, topical: 0.025% (15 g, 80 g, 454 g); 0.1% (15 g, 30 g, 80 g, 454 g, 2240 g, 2270 g); 0.5% (15 g)
Pediaderm™ TA: 0.1% (30 g)
Triderm®: 0.1% (30 g, 85 g)
Zytopic™: 0.1% (85 g)
Lotion, topical: 0.025% (60 mL); 0.1% (60 mL)
Ointment, topical: 0.025% (15 g, 80 g, 454 g); 0.05% (430 g); 0.1% (15 g, 80 g, 454 g); 0.5% (15 g)
Paste, oral, topical: 0.1% (5 g)
Oralone®: 0.1% (5 g)

Triamterene (trye AM ter een)

Related Information
Cardiovascular Diseases *on page 1848*

U.S. Brand Names Dyrenium®

Pharmacologic Category Diuretic, Potassium-Sparing

Use Alone or in combination with other diuretics in treatment of edema and hypertension; decreases potassium excretion caused by kaliuretic diuretics

Local Anesthetic/Vasoconstrictor Precautions No information available to require special precautions

Effects on Dental Treatment No significant effects or complications reported

Effects on Bleeding No information available to require special precautions

Adverse Effects 1% to 10%:
Cardiovascular: Hypotension, edema, CHF, bradycardia
Central nervous system: Dizziness, headache, fatigue
Gastrointestinal: Constipation, nausea
Respiratory: Dyspnea

General Dosage Range Oral: *Adults:* 50-300 mg/day in 1-2 divided doses (maximum: 300 mg/day)

Mechanism of Action Interferes with potassium/sodium exchange (active transport) in the distal tubule, cortical collecting tubule and collecting duct by inhibiting sodium, potassium-ATPase; decreases calcium excretion; increases magnesium loss

Pharmacodynamics/Kinetics
Onset of Action Diuresis: 2-4 hours
Duration of Action 7-9 hours

Pregnancy Risk Factor C

Triazolam (trye AY zoe lam)

Related Information
Management of the Patient With Anxiety or Depression *on page 1968*

Related Sample Prescriptions
Sedation (Prior to Dental Treatment) *on page 1995*

U.S. Brand Names Halcion®

Canadian Brand Names Apo-Triazo®; Gen-Triazolam; Halcion®; Mylan-Triazolam

Generic Availability (U.S.) Yes

Pharmacologic Category Hypnotic, Benzodiazepine

Dental Use Oral premedication before dental procedures

Use Short-term treatment of insomnia

Unlabeled/Investigational Use Treatment of anxiety before dental procedures

Local Anesthetic/Vasoconstrictor Precautions No information available to require special precautions

Effects on Dental Treatment No significant effects or complications reported (see Dental Comment)

Effects on Bleeding No information available to require special precautions

Adverse Effects

>10%: Central nervous system: Drowsiness (14%)

1% to 10%:

Central nervous system: Headache (10%), dizziness (8%), nervousness (5%), lightheadedness (5%), ataxia (5%)

Gastrointestinal: Nausea (5%), vomiting (5%)

Dental Usual Dosage Note: Onset of action is rapid, patient should be in bed when taking medication

Preprocedure sedation: Adults: Oral: 0.25 mg taken the evening before oral surgery; or 0.25 mg 1 hour before procedure

Dosage Oral (onset of action is rapid, patient should be in bed when taking medication):

Children <18 years: Dosage not established

Adults:

Insomnia (short-term): 0.125-0.25 mg at bedtime (maximum dose: 0.5 mg/day)

Preprocedure sedation (unlabeled use): 0.25 mg taken the evening before oral surgery; or 0.25 mg 1 hour before procedure

Elderly: Insomnia (short-term use): Initial: 0.125 mg at bedtime; maximum dose: 0.25 mg/day

Dosing adjustment/comments in hepatic impairment: Reduce dose or avoid use in cirrhosis

Mechanism of Action Binds to stereospecific benzodiazepine receptors on the postsynaptic GABA neuron at several sites within the central nervous system, including the limbic system, reticular formation. Enhancement of the inhibitory effect of GABA on neuronal excitability results by increased neuronal membrane permeability to chloride ions. This shift in chloride ions results in hyperpolarization (a less excitable state) and stabilization.

Contraindications Hypersensitivity to triazolam or any component of the formulation (cross-sensitivity with other benzodiazepines may exist); concurrent therapy with itraconazole, ketoconazole, nefazodone, and other moderate/strong CYP3A4 inhibitors; pregnancy

Warnings/Precautions As a hypnotic, should be used only after evaluation of potential causes of sleep disturbance. Failure of sleep disturbance to resolve after 7-10 days may indicate psychiatric or medical illness. A worsening of insomnia or the emergence of new abnormalities of thought or behavior may represent unrecognized psychiatric or medical illness and requires immediate and careful evaluation. Prescription should be written for a maximum of 7-10 days and should not be prescribed in quantities exceeding a 1-month supply. Abrupt discontinuation after sustained use (generally >10 days) may cause withdrawal symptoms.

An increase in daytime anxiety may occur after as few as 10 days of continuous use, which may be related to withdrawal reaction in some patients. Anterograde amnesia may occur at a higher rate with triazolam than with other benzodiazepines. Use with caution in elderly or debilitated patients, patients with hepatic disease (including alcoholics), or renal impairment. Due to increased sensitivity in the elderly, smaller doses of benzodiazepines may be safer and as effective. Avoid using doses >0.25 mg daily of triazolam (Beers Criteria). Use with caution in patients with respiratory disease or impaired gag reflex. Avoid use in patients with sleep apnea.

Causes CNS depression (dose-related) resulting in sedation, dizziness, confusion, or ataxia which may impair physical and mental capabilities. Patients must be cautioned about performing tasks which require mental alertness (eg, operating machinery or driving). Use with caution in patients receiving other CNS depressants or psychoactive agents. Postmarketing studies have indicated that the use of hypnotic/sedative agents for sleep has been associated with hypersensitivity reactions including anaphylaxis as well as angioedema. An increased risk for hazardous sleep-related activities such as sleep-driving; cooking and eating food, and making phone calls while asleep have also been noted. Effects with other sedative drugs or ethanol may be potentiated. Benzodiazepines have been associated with falls and traumatic injury and should be used with extreme caution in patients who are at risk of these events (especially the elderly).

Use caution with potent CYP3A4 inhibitors, as they may significantly decreased the clearance of triazolam. Use caution in patients with suicidal risk. Use with caution in patients with a history of drug dependence. Benzodiazepines have been associated with dependence and acute withdrawal symptoms on discontinuation or reduction in dose. Acute withdrawal, including seizures, may be precipitated after administration of flumazenil to patients receiving long-term benzodiazepine therapy.

Paradoxical reactions, including hyperactive or aggressive behavior have been reported with benzodiazepines, particularly in adolescent/pediatric or psychiatric patients. Does not have analgesic, antidepressant, or antipsychotic properties.

Drug Interactions

Metabolism/Transport Effects Substrate of CYP3A4 (major); **Inhibits** CYP2C8 (weak), 2C9 (weak)

Avoid Concomitant Use

Avoid concomitant use of Triazolam with any of the following: Efavirenz; OLANZapine; Protease Inhibitors

Increased Effect/Toxicity

Triazolam may increase the levels/effects of: Alcohol (Ethyl); CloZAPine; CNS Depressants; Fosphenytoin; Methotrimeprazine; Phenytoin

The levels/effects of Triazolam may be increased by: Antifungal Agents (Azole Derivatives, Systemic); Aprepitant; Calcium Channel Blockers (Nondihydropyridine); Cimetidine; Conivaptan; Contraceptives (Estrogens); Contraceptives (Progestins); CYP3A4 Inhibitors (Moderate); CYP3A4 Inhibitors (Strong); Dasatinib; Droperidol; Efavirenz; Fluconazole; Fosaprepitant; Grapefruit Juice; Isoniazid; Macrolide Antibiotics; Methotrimeprazine; Nefazodone; OLANZapine; Protease Inhibitors; Proton Pump Inhibitors; Selective Serotonin Reuptake Inhibitors

Decreased Effect

The levels/effects of Triazolam may be decreased by: CarBAMazepine; CYP3A4 Inducers (Strong); Deferasirox; Rifamycin Derivatives; St Johns Wort; Theophylline Derivatives; Tocilizumab; Yohimbine

Ethanol/Nutrition/Herb Interactions

Ethanol: May increase CNS depression; monitor for increased effects with coadministration. Caution patients about effects.

Food: Food may decrease the rate of absorption. Benzodiazepine serum concentrations may be increased by grapefruit juice; monitor.

Herb/Nutraceutical: St John's wort may decrease levels/effects of benzodiazepines. Avoid valerian, St John's wort, kava kava, gotu kola (may increase CNS depression).

Pharmacodynamics/Kinetics

Onset of Action Hypnotic: 15-30 minutes

Duration of Action 6-7 hours

Half-life Elimination 1.5-5.5 hours

Pregnancy Risk Factor X

Lactation Excretion in breast milk unknown/not recommended

Breast-Feeding Considerations Drowsiness, lethargy, or weight loss in nursing infants have been observed in case reports following maternal use of some benzodiazepines.

Controlled Substance C-IV

Dosage Forms

Tablet, oral: 0.125 mg, 0.25 mg

Halcion®: 0.25 mg

Dental Comment Triazolam (0.25 mg) 1 hour prior to dental procedure has been used as an oral preop sedative.

Triazolam is a benzodiazepine and is being used in dentistry as a preprocedural oral sedative. There has been recent interest in its use as an orally titratable sedative to render anxious patients at ease during difficult dental procedures. This technique has been referred to as enteral conscious sedation (ECS) and oral conscious sedation (OCS).

Triazolam has the shortest half-life of all the orally administered benzodiazepines. Although midazolam is shorter, it is used parenterally, not orally. The relatively fast onset of action (15-30 minutes) of triazolam offers an advantage in its use as an oral sedative. The clinician is reminded that no kinetic data has been reported with multiple titration doses of triazolam, a technique often used in the ECS/OCS regimen.

References

Berthold CW, Dionne RA, and Corey SE, "Comparison of Sublingually and Orally Administered Triazolam for Premedication Before Oral Surgery," *Oral Surg Oral Med Oral Pathol Oral Radiol Endod*, 1997, 84 (2):119-24.

Berthold CW, Schneider A, and Dionne RA, "Using Triazolam to Reduce Dental Anxiety," *J Am Dent Assoc*, 1993, 124(11):58-64.

Dionne R, "Oral Sedation," *Compend Contin Educ Dent*, 1998, 19(9):868-70.

Flanagan D, "Oral Triazolam Sedation in Implant Dentistry," *J Oral Implantol*, 2004, 30(2):93-7.

Goodchild JH, Feck AS, and Silverman MD, "Anxiolysis in General Dental Practice," *Dent Today*, 2003, 22(3):106-11.

Kaufman E, Hargreaves KM, and Dionne RA, "Comparison of Oral Triazolam and Nitrous Oxide With Placebo and Intravenous Diazepam for Outpatient Premedication," *Oral Surg Oral Med Oral Pathol*, 1993, 75(2):156-64.

Kurzrock M, "Triazolam and Dental Anxiety," *J Am Dent Assoc*, 1994, 125(4):358, 360.

Lieblich SE and Horswell B, "Attenuation of Anxiety in Ambulatory Oral Surgery Patients With Oral Triazolam," *J Oral Maxillofac Surg*, 1991, 49(8):792-7.

Matear DW and Clarke D, "Considerations for the Use of Oral Sedation in the Institutionalized Geriatric Patient During Dental Interventions: A Review of the Literature," *Spec Care Dentist*, 1999, 19(2):56-63.
Milgrom P, Quarnstrom FC, Longley A, et al, "The Efficacy and Memory Effects of Oral Triazolam Premedication in Highly Anxious Dental Patients," *Anesth Prog*, 1994, 41(3):70-6.
Quarnstrom F, "Should Dentists Do Oral Sedation?" *Dent Today*, 2004, 23(3):16-8.

Trichloroacetic Acid (trye klor oh a SEE tik AS id)

U.S. Brand Names Tri-Chlor®
Pharmacologic Category Keratolytic Agent
Use Chemical used in compounding agents for the treatment of warts, skin resurfacing (chemical peels)
Local Anesthetic/Vasoconstrictor Precautions No information available to require special precautions
Effects on Dental Treatment No significant effects or complications reported
Effects on Bleeding No information available to require special precautions

Triclosan and Fluoride (trye KLOE san & FLOR ide)

Related Information

Fluoride *on page 752*
Periodontal Diseases *on page 1942*

U.S. Brand Names Colgate Total®
Generic Availability (U.S.) No
Pharmacologic Category Antibacterial, Dental; Mineral, Oral (Topical)
Dental Use Anticavity, antigingivitis, antiplaque toothpaste
Use Used exclusively in dental applications
Local Anesthetic/Vasoconstrictor Precautions No information available to require special precautions
Effects on Dental Treatment No significant effects or complications reported (see Dental Comment)
Effects on Bleeding No information available to require special precautions
Adverse Effects No data reported
Dental Usual Dosage Prevention of dental caries and gingivitis: Adults: Oral: Brush teeth thoroughly after each meal or at least twice daily
Dosage Brush teeth thoroughly after each meal or at least twice daily
Mechanism of Action Triclosan is an antibacterial agent which helps to prevent gingivitis with regular use. Fluoride promotes remineralization of decalcified enamel, inhibits the cariogenic microbial process in dental plaque, and increases tooth resistance to acid dissolution
Warnings/Precautions Antigingivitis and antiplaque effects have not been determined in children <6 years of age. If an amount greater than used for brushing is swallowed, seek professional assistance of contact a poison control center immediately
Drug Interactions
Avoid Concomitant Use There are no known interactions where it is recommended to avoid concomitant use.
Increased Effect/Toxicity There are no known significant interactions involving an increase in effect.
Decreased Effect There are no known significant interactions involving a decrease in effect.
Pregnancy Risk Factor No data reported
Dosage Forms
Gel, oral [toothpaste]:
Colgate Total®: Triclosan 0.30% and fluoride 0.24% (119 g, 170 g, 221 g)
Paste, oral [toothpaste]:
Colgate Total®: Triclosan 0.30% and fluoride 0.24% (119 g, 170 g, 221 g)
Dental Comment It has been shown that stannous fluoride and triclosan when formulated into a toothpaste vehicle provide plaque inhibitory effects. To provide a longer retention time of the triclosan in plaque, a polymer has been added to the toothpaste vehicle. The polymer is known as PVM/MA which stands for polyvinylmethyl ether/maleic acid copolymer, and is listed as an inactive ingredient (PVM/MA Copolymer) on the manufacturer's label. Studies have reported that the retention of triclosan in plaque (exceeding the minimal inhibitory concentration) after polymer application was 14 hours after brushing. Ongoing studies are evaluating the effects of triclosan/copolymer on alveolar bone loss. Rosling et al. have reported that the daily use of Colgate Total® reduced (1) the frequency of deep periodontal pockets and (2) the number of sites that exhibited additional probing attachment and bone loss.

References

Binney A, Addy M, Owens J, et al, "A Comparison of Triclosan and Stannous Fluoride Toothpastes for Inhibition of Plaque Regrowth. A Crossover Study Designed to Access Carry Over," *J Clin Periodontol*, 1997, 24(3):166-70.

Ellwood RP, Worthington HV, Blinkhorn AS, et al, "Effect of a Triclosan/Copolymer Dentifrice on the Incidence of Periodontal Attachment Loss in Adolescents," *J Clin Periodontol*, 1998, 25(5):363-7.

Mandel ID, "The New Toothpastes," *J Calif Dent Assoc*, 1998, 26(3):186-90.

Rosling B, Wannfors B, Volpe AR, et al, "The Use of a Triclosan/Copolymer Dentifrice May Retard the Progression of Periodontitis," *J Clin Periodontol*, 1997, 24(12):873-80.

Trifluoperazine (trye floo oh PER a zeen)

Canadian Brand Names Apo-Trifluoperazine®; Novo-Trifluzine; PMS-Trifluoperazine; Terfluzine

Pharmacologic Category Antipsychotic Agent, Typical, Phenothiazine

Use Treatment of schizophrenia; short-term treatment of generalized nonpsychotic anxiety

Unlabeled/Investigational Use Management of psychotic disorders; behavioral symptoms associated with dementia behavior (elderly); psychosis/agitation related to Alzheimer's dementia

Local Anesthetic/Vasoconstrictor Precautions Most pharmacology textbooks state that in presence of phenothiazines, systemic doses of epinephrine paradoxically decrease the blood pressure. This is the so called "epinephrine reversal" phenomenon. This has never been observed when epinephrine is given by infiltration as part of the anesthesia procedure.

Effects on Dental Treatment Key adverse event(s) related to dental treatment: Significant hypotension may occur, especially when the drug is administered parenterally; orthostatic hypotension is due to alpha-receptor blockade, the elderly are at greater risk for orthostatic hypotension. Xerostomia (normal salivary flow resumes upon discontinuation).

Tardive dyskinesia: Prevalence rate may be 40% in elderly; development of the syndrome and the irreversible nature are proportional to duration and total cumulative dose over time. Extrapyramidal reactions are more common in elderly with up to 50% developing these reactions after 60 years of age. Drug-induced Parkinson's syndrome occurs often; akathisia is the most common extrapyramidal reaction in elderly.

Effects on Bleeding No information available to require special precautions

Adverse Effects Frequency not defined.

Cardiovascular: Hypotension, orthostatic hypotension, cardiac arrest

Central nervous system: Extrapyramidal signs (pseudoparkinsonism, akathisia, dystonias, tardive dyskinesia), dizziness, headache, neuroleptic malignant syndrome (NMS), impairment of temperature regulation, lowering of seizure threshold

Dermatologic: Increased sensitivity to sun, rash, discoloration of skin (blue-gray), photosensitivity

Endocrine & metabolic: Changes in menstrual cycle, libido (changes in), breast pain, hyperglycemia, hypoglycemia, gynecomastia, lactation, galactorrhea

Gastrointestinal: Constipation, weight gain, nausea, vomiting, stomach pain, xerostomia

Genitourinary: Difficulty in urination, ejaculatory disturbances, urinary retention, priapism

Hematologic: Agranulocytosis, leukopenia, pancytopenia, thrombocytopenic purpura, eosinophilia, hemolytic anemia, aplastic anemia

Hepatic: Cholestatic jaundice, hepatotoxicity

Neuromuscular & skeletal: Tremor

Ocular: Pigmentary retinopathy, cornea and lens changes

Respiratory: Nasal congestion

General Dosage Range Oral:

Children 6-12 years: Initial: 1 mg 1-2 times/day; Maintenance: 1-15 mg/day in 1-2 divided doses (maximum: 15 mg/day)

Adults: Inpatient: Initial: 2-5 mg twice daily; Maintenance: 15-40 mg/day in 2 divided doses (maximum: 40 mg/day); Outpatient: Initial: 1-3 mg twice daily (maximum: 40 mg/day)

Mechanism of Action Trifluoperazine is a piperazine phenothiazine antipsychotic which blocks postsynaptic mesolimbic dopaminergic receptors in the brain; exhibits alpha-adrenergic blocking effect and depresses the release of hypothalamic and hypophyseal hormones

Pharmacodynamics/Kinetics

Half-life Elimination >24 hours with chronic use

Trifluridine (trye FLURE i deen)

Related Information

Systemic Viral Diseases *on page 1904*

U.S. Brand Names Viroptic®

Canadian Brand Names Sandoz-Trifluridine; Viroptic®

Pharmacologic Category Antiviral Agent, Ophthalmic

Use Treatment of primary keratoconjunctivitis and recurrent epithelial keratitis caused by herpes simplex virus types I and II

Local Anesthetic/Vasoconstrictor Precautions No information available to require special precautions

Effects on Dental Treatment No significant effects or complications reported

Effects on Bleeding No information available to require special precautions

Adverse Effects 1% to 10%: Local: Burning, stinging

General Dosage Range Ophthalmic: *Adults:* Initial: Instill 1 drop into affected eye(s) every 2 hours while awake (maximum: 9 drops/day); After re-epithelialization of corneal ulcer: 1 drop every 4 hours (maximum: 21 days of treatment)

Mechanism of Action Interferes with viral replication by incorporating into viral DNA in place of thymidine, inhibiting thymidylate synthetase resulting in the formation of defective proteins

Pregnancy Risk Factor C

Trihexyphenidyl (trye heks ee FEN i dil)

Canadian Brand Names PMS-Trihexyphenidyl; Trihexyphen; Trihexyphenidyl

Generic Availability (U.S.) Yes

Pharmacologic Category Anti-Parkinson's Agent, Anticholinergic; Anticholinergic Agent

Use Adjunctive treatment of Parkinson's disease; treatment of drug-induced extrapyramidal symptoms

Local Anesthetic/Vasoconstrictor Precautions No information available to require special precautions

Effects on Dental Treatment Key adverse event(s) related to dental treatment: Xerostomia, dry throat (normal salivary flow resumes upon discontinuation). Prolonged xerostomia may contribute to discomfort and dental disease (ie, caries, periodontal disease, and oral candidiasis).

Effects on Bleeding No information available to require special precautions

Adverse Effects Frequency not defined.

Cardiovascular: Tachycardia

Central nervous system: Agitation, confusion, delusions, dizziness, drowsiness, euphoria, hallucinations, headache, nervousness, paranoia, psychiatric disturbances

Dermatologic: Rash

Gastrointestinal: Constipation, dilatation of colon, ileus, nausea, parotitis, vomiting, xerostomia

Genitourinary: Urinary retention

Neuromuscular & skeletal: Weakness

Ocular: Blurred vision, glaucoma, intraocular pressure increased, mydriasis

Dosage Oral:

Adults:

Parkinson's disease: Initial: 1 mg/day, increase by 2 mg increments at intervals of 3-5 days; usual dose: 6-10 mg/day in 3-4 divided doses; doses of 12-15 mg/day may be required

Drug-induced EPS: Initial: 1 mg/day; increase as necessary to usual range: 5-15 mg/day in 3-4 divided doses

Use in combination with levodopa: Usual range: 3-6 mg/day in divided doses

Elderly: Parkinson's disease: Refer to adult dosing. **Note:** Conservative initial doses and gradual titration is especially important in patients >60 years of age.

Mechanism of Action Exerts a direct inhibitory effect on the parasympathetic nervous system. It also has a relaxing effect on smooth musculature; exerted both directly on the muscle itself and indirectly through parasympathetic nervous system (inhibitory effect)

Contraindications There are no contraindications listed within the manufacturer's labeling.

Warnings/Precautions Use with caution in hot weather or during exercise, especially when administered concomitantly with other atropine-like drugs to chronically-ill patients, alcoholics, patients with CNS disease, or persons doing manual labor in a hot environment. Use with caution in patients with cardiovascular disease (including hypertension), glaucoma, prostatic hyperplasia or any tendency toward urinary retention, liver or kidney disorders, and obstructive disease of the GI tract. May exacerbate mental symptoms when used to treat extrapyramidal symptoms. When given in large doses or to susceptible patients, may cause weakness. May impair physical or mental abilities; patients must be cautioned about performing tasks which require mental alertness (eg, operating machinery or driving). Does not improve symptoms of tardive dyskinesias. Elderly patients require strict dosage regulation.

Drug Interactions

Avoid Concomitant Use There are no known interactions where it is recommended to avoid concomitant use.

Increased Effect/Toxicity

Trihexyphenidyl may increase the levels/effects of: AbobotulinumtoxinA; Anticholinergics; Cannabinoids; OnabotulinumtoxinA; Potassium Chloride; RimabotulinumtoxinB

The levels/effects of Trihexyphenidyl may be increased by: Pramlintide

Decreased Effect

Trihexyphenidyl may decrease the levels/effects of: Acetylcholinesterase Inhibitors (Central); Secretin

The levels/effects of Trihexyphenidyl may be decreased by: Acetylcholinesterase Inhibitors (Central)

Ethanol/Nutrition/Herb Interactions Ethanol: Avoid ethanol (may increase CNS depression).

Dietary Considerations May be taken before or after meals; tolerated best if given with food.

Pharmacodynamics/Kinetics

Half-life Elimination 33 hours

Time to Peak Serum: 1.3 hours

Lactation Excretion in breast milk unknown/use caution

Breast-Feeding Considerations Anticholinergic agents may suppress lactation.

Dosage Forms

Elixir, oral: 2 mg/5 mL (473 mL)

Tablet, oral: 2 mg, 5 mg

Trimethobenzamide (trye meth oh BEN za mide)

U.S. Brand Names Tigan®

Canadian Brand Names Tigan®

Pharmacologic Category Antiemetic

Use Treatment of postoperative nausea and vomiting; treatment of nausea associated with gastroenteritis

Local Anesthetic/Vasoconstrictor Precautions No information available to require special precautions

Effects on Dental Treatment No significant effects or complications reported

Effects on Bleeding No information available to require special precautions

Adverse Effects Frequency not defined.

Cardiovascular: Hypotension (I.V. administration)

Central nervous system: Coma, depression, disorientation, dizziness, drowsiness, EPS, headache, Parkinson-like symptoms, seizure

Dermatologic: Allergic-type skin reactions

Gastrointestinal: Diarrhea

Hematologic: Blood dyscrasias

Hepatic: Jaundice

Local: Injection site burning, pain, redness, stinging, or swelling

Neuromuscular & skeletal: Muscle cramps, opisthotonos

Ocular: Blurred vision

Miscellaneous: Hypersensitivity reactions

General Dosage Range

I.M.: *Adults:* 200 mg 3-4 times/day **or** 200 mg as a single dose, repeat 1 hour later

Oral: *Children >40 kg and Adults:* 300 mg 3-4 times/day

Mechanism of Action Acts centrally to inhibit the medullary chemoreceptor trigger zone by blocking emetic impulses to the vomiting center

Pharmacodynamics/Kinetics

Onset of Action Antiemetic: Oral: 10-40 minutes; I.M.: 15-35 minutes

Duration of Action 3-4 hours

Half-life Elimination 7-9 hours

Time to Peak Oral: ~45 minutes; I.M.: ~30 minutes

Dental Comment Consider trimethobenzamide as a safer alternative to phenothiazines (ie, promethazine) to prevent nausea and vomiting or treat mild nausea and vomiting.

Trimethoprim (trye METH oh prim)

U.S. Brand Names Primsol®

Canadian Brand Names Apo-Trimethoprim®

Pharmacologic Category Antibiotic, Miscellaneous

Use Treatment of urinary tract infections due to susceptible strains of *E. coli*, *P. mirabilis*, *K. pneumoniae*, *Enterobacter* spp and coagulase-negative *Staphylococcus* including *S. saprophyticus*; acute otitis media due to susceptible strains of *S. pneumoniae* and *H. influenzae* in children

Unlabeled/Investigational Use Alternative agent for *Pneumocystis jirovecii* pneumonia (in combination with dapsone)

Local Anesthetic/Vasoconstrictor Precautions No information available to require special precautions

Effects on Dental Treatment Key adverse event(s) related to dental treatment: Glossitis.

Effects on Bleeding No information available to require special precautions

Adverse Effects Frequency not defined.

Central nervous system: Aseptic meningitis (rare), fever

Dermatologic: Maculopapular rash (3% to 7% at 200 mg/day; incidence higher with larger daily doses), erythema multiforme (rare), exfoliative dermatitis (rare), pruritus (common), phototoxic skin eruptions, Stevens-Johnson syndrome (rare), toxic epidermal necrolysis (rare)

Endocrine & metabolic: Hyperkalemia, hyponatremia

Gastrointestinal: Epigastric distress, glossitis, nausea, vomiting

Hematologic: Leukopenia, megaloblastic anemia, methemoglobinemia, neutropenia, thrombocytopenia

Hepatic: Cholestatic jaundice (rare), liver enzymes increased

Renal: BUN and creatinine increased

Miscellaneous: Anaphylaxis, hypersensitivity reactions

General Dosage Range Dosage adjustment recommended in patients with renal impairment

Oral:

Children ≥2 months: 4-12 mg/kg/day in divided doses every 12 hours

Adults: 100 mg once daily **or** 100 mg every 12 hours **or** 200 mg every 24 hours; up to 15mg/kg/day

Mechanism of Action Inhibits folic acid reduction to tetrahydrofolate, and thereby inhibits microbial growth

Pharmacodynamics/Kinetics

Half-life Elimination 8-14 hours; prolonged with renal impairment

Time to Peak Serum: 1-4 hours

Pregnancy Risk Factor C

Trimethoprim and Polymyxin B (trye METH oh prim & pol i MIKS in bee)

Related Information

Polymyxin B *on page* 1370

Trimethoprim *on page* 1681

U.S. Brand Names Polytrim®

Canadian Brand Names PMS-Polytrimethoprim; Polytrim™

Pharmacologic Category Antibiotic, Ophthalmic

Use Treatment of surface ocular bacterial conjunctivitis and blepharoconjunctivitis

Local Anesthetic/Vasoconstrictor Precautions No information available to require special precautions

Effects on Dental Treatment No significant effects or complications reported

Effects on Bleeding No information available to require special precautions

Adverse Effects Frequency not defined: Ocular: Burning, itching, edema, rash, redness increased, stinging, tearing

General Dosage Range Ophthalmic: *Children ≥2 months and Adults:* Instill 1 drop in affected eye(s) every 3 hours (maximum: 6 doses per day) for 7-10 days

Pregnancy Risk Factor C

Trimipramine (trye MI pra meen)

U.S. Brand Names Surmontil®

Canadian Brand Names Apo-Trimip®; Nu-Trimipramine; Rhotrimine®; Surmontil®

Pharmacologic Category Antidepressant, Tricyclic (Tertiary Amine)

Use Treatment of depression

Local Anesthetic/Vasoconstrictor Precautions Use with caution; epinephrine and levonordefrin have been shown to have an increased pressor response in combination with TCAs. Trimipramine is one of the drugs confirmed to prolong the QT interval and is accepted as having a risk of causing torsade de pointes. The risk of drug-induced torsade de pointes is extremely low when a single QT interval prolonging drug is prescribed. In terms of epinephrine, it is not known what effect vasoconstrictors in the local anesthetic regimen will have in patients with a known history of congenital prolonged QT interval or in patients taking any medication that prolongs the QT interval. Until more information is obtained, it is suggested that the clinician consult with the physician prior to the use of a vasoconstrictor in suspected patients, and that the vasoconstrictor (epinephrine, mepivacaine and levonordefrin [Carbocaine® 2% with Neo-Cobefrin®]) be used with caution.

Effects on Dental Treatment Key adverse event(s) related to dental treatment: Xerostomia (normal salivary flow resumes upon discontinuation) and unpleasant taste. Long-term treatment with TCAs, such as trimipramine, increases the risk of caries by reducing salivation and salivary buffer capacity.

Effects on Bleeding No information available to require special precautions

Adverse Effects Frequency not defined.

Cardiovascular: Arrhythmias, facial edema, flushing, heart block, hyper-/hypotension, MI, palpitation, stroke, tachycardia

Central nervous system: Agitation, anxiety, confusion, delusions, disorientation, dizziness, drowsiness, EEG abnormalities, exacerbation of psychosis, fatigue, hallucinations, headache, hypomania, insomnia, nightmares, restlessness, seizure

Dermatologic: Alopecia, itching, petechiae, photosensitivity, rash, urticaria

Endocrine & metabolic: Breast enlargement, galactorrhea, gynecomastia, hyper-/hypoglycemia, libido (changes in), parotid swelling, syndrome of inappropriate ADH secretion (SIADH)

Gastrointestinal: Abdominal cramps, anorexia, black tongue, constipation, diarrhea, epigastric distress, nausea, paralytic ileus, stomatitis, tongue edema, unpleasant taste, tongue edema, vomiting, weight gain/loss, xerostomia

Genitourinary: Delayed/difficult urination, impotence, polyuria, testicular edema, urinary retention

Hematologic: Agranulocytosis, eosinophilia, purpura, thrombocytopenia

Hepatic: Cholestatic jaundice, liver enzymes increased

Neuromuscular & skeletal: Ataxia, extrapyramidal symptoms, incoordination, numbness, paresthesia, peripheral neuropathy, tingling, tremor, weakness

Ocular: Blurred vision, disturbances in accommodation, mydriasis

Otic: Tinnitus

Miscellaneous: Diaphoresis, withdrawal syndrome

General Dosage Range

Oral:

Adolescents: Initial: 50 mg/day (maximum: 100 mg/day)

Adults: 50-200 mg at bedtime (maximum: 200 mg/day [outpatient] or 300 mg/day [inpatient])

Elderly: 50-100 mg at bedtime (maximum: 100 mg/day)

Mechanism of Action Increases the synaptic concentration of serotonin and/or norepinephrine in the central nervous system by inhibition of their reuptake by the presynaptic neuronal membrane

Pharmacodynamics/Kinetics

Half-life Elimination 16-40 hours

Pregnancy Risk Factor C

Dental Comment Trimipramine is known to prolong the QT interval. The QT interval is measured as the time and distance between the Q point of the QRS complex and the end of the T wave in the ECG tracing. After adjustment for heart rate, the QT interval is defined as prolonged if it is more than 450 msec in men and 460 msec in women. A long QT syndrome was first described in the 1950s and 60s as a congenital syndrome involving QT interval prolongation and syncope and sudden death. Some of the congenital long QT syndromes were characterized by a peculiar electrocardiographic appearance of the QRS complex involving a premature atria beat followed by a pause, then a subsequent sinus beat showing marked QT prolongation and deformity. This type of cardiac arrhythmia was originally termed "torsade de pointes" (translated from the French as "twisting of the points"). Trimipramine is considered as having a risk of causing torsade de pointes. Since it is not known what effect vasoconstrictors in the local anesthetic regimen will have in patients with a known history of congenital prolonged QT interval or in patients taking any medication that prolongs the QT interval, a medical consult is suggested.

Triprolidine and Pseudoephedrine (trye PROE li deen & soo doe e FED rin)

Related Information

Pseudoephedrine *on page* 1429

U.S. Brand Names Allerfrim [OTC]; Aprodine [OTC]; Genac™ [OTC]; Pediatex® TD; Silafed [OTC]; Tripohist™ D

Canadian Brand Names Actifed®

Pharmacologic Category Alkylamine Derivative; Alpha/Beta Agonist; Decongestant; Histamine H_1 Antagonist; Histamine H_1 Antagonist, First Generation

Use Temporary relief of nasal congestion, decongest sinus openings, running nose, sneezing, itching of nose or throat and itchy, watery eyes due to common cold, hay fever, or other upper respiratory allergies

Local Anesthetic/Vasoconstrictor Precautions Use with caution since pseudoephedrine is a sympathomimetic amine which could interact with epinephrine to cause a pressor response

Effects on Dental Treatment Key adverse event(s) related to dental treatment: Pseudoephedrine: Xerostomia (normal salivary flow resumes upon discontinuation). Chronic use of antihistamines will inhibit salivary flow, particularly in elderly patients; this may contribute to periodontal disease and oral discomfort.

Effects on Bleeding No information available to require special precautions

Adverse Effects Frequency not defined.

Cardiovascular: Tachycardia

Central nervous system: Dizziness, drowsiness, fatigue, headache, insomnia, nervousness, transient stimulation

Gastrointestinal: Abdominal pain, appetite increase, diarrhea, nausea, weight gain, xerostomia

Genitourinary: Dysuria

Neuromuscular & skeletal: Arthralgia, weakness

Respiratory: Pharyngitis, thickening of bronchial secretions

Miscellaneous: Diaphoresis

General Dosage Range Oral: *Children ≥6 years and Adults:* Dosage varies greatly depending on product

Mechanism of Action Refer to Pseudoephedrine monograph

Triprolidine is a member of the propylamine (alkylamine) chemical class of H_1-antagonist antihistamines. As such, it is considered to be relatively less sedating than traditional antihistamines of the ethanolamine, phenothiazine, and ethylenediamine classes of antihistamines. Triprolidine has a shorter half-life and duration of action than most of the other alkylamine antihistamines. Like all H_1-antagonist antihistamines, the mechanism of action of triprolidine is believed to involve competitive blockade of H_1-receptor sites resulting in the inability of histamine to combine with its receptor sites and exert its usual effects on target cells. Antihistamines do not interrupt any effects of histamine which have already occurred. Therefore, these agents are used more successfully in the prevention rather than the treatment of histamine-induced reactions.

Pregnancy Risk Factor C

Triprolidine, Pseudoephedrine, and Codeine
(trye PROE li deen, soo doe e FED rin, & KOE deen)

Related Information

Codeine *on page* 432

Pseudoephedrine *on page* 1429

Canadian Brand Names CoActifed®; Covan®; ratio-Cotridin

Pharmacologic Category Alkylamine Derivative; Alpha/Beta Agonist; Analgesic, Opioid; Antitussive; Decongestant; Histamine H_1 Antagonist; Histamine H_1 Antagonist, First Generation

Use Symptomatic relief of upper respiratory symptoms and cough

Local Anesthetic/Vasoconstrictor Precautions Use with caution since pseudoephedrine is a sympathomimetic amine which could interact with epinephrine to cause a pressor response

Effects on Dental Treatment Key adverse event(s) related to dental treatment: Pseudoephedrine: Xerostomia (normal salivary flow resumes upon discontinuation) and taste disturbance.

Effects on Bleeding No information available to require special precautions

Adverse Effects Frequency not defined.

Cardiovascular: Hypotension

Central nervous system: Agitation, dizziness, drowsiness, dysphoria, euphoria, hallucination, headache, ICP increased, lightheadedness, sedation, seizure

Dermatologic: Pruritus, rash

Gastrointestinal: Constipation, nausea, vomiting, anorexia, xerostomia, taste disturbance, biliary tract spasm
Genitourinary: Urinary retention, urinary tract spasm
Neuromuscular & skeletal: Muscle tremor, paresthesia, muscular rigidity (rare)
Ocular: Blurred vision, nystagmus
Respiratory: Respiratory depression
Miscellaneous: Diaphoresis, physical or psychological dependence with continued use, withdrawal syndrome

General Dosage Range Oral:
Children 2-6 years: 2.5 mL 4 times/day
Children 7-12 years: 5 mL 4 times/day **or** 1/2 tablet 4 times/day
Children >12 years and Adults: 10 mL 4 times/day **or** 1 tablet 4 times/day

Pregnancy Risk Factor C

Product Availability Not available in U.S.

Controlled Substance CDSA-I

Triptorelin (trip toe REL in)

U.S. Brand Names Trelstar®

Canadian Brand Names Trelstar®

Pharmacologic Category Gonadotropin Releasing Hormone Agonist

Use Palliative treatment of advanced prostate cancer

Unlabeled/Investigational Use Treatment of endometriosis, *in vitro* fertilization, precocious puberty, uterine sarcoma

Local Anesthetic/Vasoconstrictor Precautions No information available to require special precautions

Effects on Dental Treatment No significant effects or complications reported

Effects on Bleeding Although significant myelosuppression with associated altered hemostasis has been reported for many chemotherapeutic agents, myelosuppression is not common with triptorelin and no specific precautions appear to necessary.

Adverse Effects As reported with all strengths; frequency of effect may vary by strength:

>10%:
Endocrine & metabolic: Hot flashes (59% to 73%), glucose increased, testosterone levels increased (peak: days 2-4; decline to low levels by weeks 3-4)
Hematologic: Hemoglobin decreased, RBC count decreased
Hepatic: Alkaline phosphatase increased (2% to >10%), ALT increased, AST increased
Neuromuscular & skeletal: Skeletal pain (12% to 13%)
Renal: BUN increased

1% to 10%:
Cardiovascular: Leg edema (6%), hypertension (1% to 4%), chest pain (2%), edema (2%), peripheral edema (≤1%)
Central nervous system: Headache (2% to 7%), pain (2% to 3%), dizziness (1% to 3%), fatigue (2%), insomnia (1% to 2%), emotional lability (1%)
Dermatologic: Rash (2%), pruritus (1%)
Endocrine & metabolic: Breast pain (2%), gynecomastia (2%), libido decreased (2%)
Gastrointestinal: Nausea (3%), anorexia (2%), constipation (2%), dyspepsia (2%), vomiting (2%), abdominal pain (1%), diarrhea (1%)
Genitourinary: Erectile dysfunction (10%), testicular atrophy (8%), impotence (2% to 7%), dysuria (5%), urinary retention (≤1%), urinary tract infection (≤1%)
Hematologic: Anemia (1%)
Local: Injection site pain (4%)
Neuromuscular & skeletal: Leg pain (2% to 5%), back pain (1% to 3%), leg cramps (2%), arthralgia (1% to 2%), extremity pain (1%), myalgia (1%), weakness (1%)
Ocular: Conjunctivitis (1%), eye pain (1%)
Respiratory: Cough (2%), dyspnea (1%), pharyngitis (1%)

General Dosage Range I.M.: *Adults:* 3.75 mg once every 4 weeks **or** 11.25 mg once every 12 weeks **or** 22.5 mg once every 24 weeks

Mechanism of Action Causes suppression of ovarian and testicular steroidogenesis due to decreased levels of LH and FSH with subsequent decrease in testosterone (male) and estrogen (female) levels. After chronic and continuous administration, usually 2-4 weeks after initiation, a sustained decrease in LH and FSH secretion occurs.

Pharmacodynamics/Kinetics
Half-life Elimination 2.8 ± 1.2 hours
Moderate-to-severe renal impairment: 6.5-7.7 hours
Hepatic impairment: 7.6 hours
Time to Peak 1-3 hours
Pregnancy Risk Factor X

Trolamine (TROLE a meen)

U.S. Brand Names Aspercreme® [OTC]; Flex-Power [OTC]; Mobisyl® [OTC]; Myoflex® [OTC]; Sportscreme® [OTC]
Canadian Brand Names Antiphlogistine Rub A-535 No Odour; Myoflex®
Pharmacologic Category Analgesic, Topical; Salicylate; Topical Skin Product
Use Relief of pain of muscular aches, rheumatism, neuralgia, sprains, arthritis on intact skin
Local Anesthetic/Vasoconstrictor Precautions No information available to require special precautions
Effects on Dental Treatment No significant effects or complications reported
Effects on Bleeding No information available to require special precautions
Adverse Effects 1% to 10%:
Central nervous system: Confusion, drowsiness
Gastrointestinal: Nausea, vomiting, diarrhea
Respiratory: Hyperventilation
General Dosage Range Topical: *Children ≥12 years and Adults:* Apply to affected area as needed up to 3-4 times/day

Tromethamine (troe METH a meen)

U.S. Brand Names THAM®
Pharmacologic Category Alkalinizing Agent, Parenteral
Use Correction of metabolic acidosis associated with cardiac bypass surgery or cardiac arrest; to correct excess acidity of stored blood that is preserved with acid citrate dextrose (ACD); indicated in infants needing alkalinization after receiving maximum sodium bicarbonate (8-10 mEq/kg/24 hours)
Local Anesthetic/Vasoconstrictor Precautions No information available to require special precautions
Effects on Dental Treatment No significant effects or complications reported
Effects on Bleeding No information available to require special precautions
Adverse Effects Frequency not defined.
Cardiovascular: Hypervolemia, venospasm
Endocrine & metabolic: Hyperkalemia, hypoglycemia (usually doses >500 mg/kg administered over <1 hour)
Hepatic: Hepatic necrosis (resulted during delivery via umbilical venous catheter)
Local: Necrosis with extravasation, phlebitis, tissue irritation
Respiratory: Apnea, pulmonary edema, respiratory depression
General Dosage Range
I.V.:
Neonates and Infants: Initial: Approximately 1 mL/kg for each pH unit below 7.4; additional doses determined by changes in PaO_2, pH, and pCO_2
Adults: 3.6-10.8 g (111-333 mL) **or** 9 mL/kg (maximum: 500 mg/kg) **or** 15-77 mL added to each 500 mL of blood
Intraventricular: *Adults:* 3.6-10.8 g (111-333 mL) **or** 9 mL/kg (maximum: 500 mg/kg) **or** 15-77 mL added to each 500 mL of blood
Mechanism of Action Acts as a proton acceptor, which combines with hydrogen ions, liberating bicarbonate buffer, to correct acidosis. It buffers both metabolic and respiratory acids, limiting carbon dioxide generation. Also an osmotic diuretic.
Pharmacodynamics/Kinetics
Half-life Elimination 5.6 hours
Pregnancy Risk Factor C

Tropicamide (troe PIK a mide)

U.S. Brand Names Mydral™ [DSC]; Mydriacyl®; Tropicacyl®
Canadian Brand Names Diotrope®; Mydriacyl®
Pharmacologic Category Ophthalmic Agent, Mydriatic
Use Short-acting mydriatic used in diagnostic procedures; as well as preoperatively and postoperatively; treatment of some cases of acute iritis, iridocyclitis, and keratitis
Local Anesthetic/Vasoconstrictor Precautions No information available to require special precautions

Effects on Dental Treatment Key adverse event(s) related to dental treatment: Dryness of mouth.

Effects on Bleeding No information available to require special precautions

Adverse Effects Frequency not defined.

Cardiovascular: Edema, tachycardia, vascular congestion
Central nervous system: Headache, parasympathetic stimulations, somnolence
Dermatologic: Eczematoid dermatitis
Gastrointestinal: Dryness of mouth
Local: Transient stinging
Ocular: Blurred vision, follicular conjunctivitis, increased intraocular pressure, photophobia with or without corneal staining

General Dosage Range Ophthalmic: *Children and Adults:* 0.5%: Instill 1-2 drops 15-20 minutes before exam, may repeat; 1%: Instill 1-2 drops, may repeat in 5 minutes

Mechanism of Action Prevents the sphincter muscle of the iris and the muscle of the ciliary body from responding to cholinergic stimulation

Pharmacodynamics/Kinetics

Onset of Action Mydriasis: ~20-40 minutes; Cycloplegia: ~30 minutes

Duration of Action Mydriasis: ~6-7 hours; Cycloplegia: <6 hours

Pregnancy Risk Factor C

Trospium (TROSE pee um)

U.S. Brand Names Sanctura®; Sanctura® XR

Canadian Brand Names Sanctura® XR; Trosec

Pharmacologic Category Anticholinergic Agent

Use Treatment of overactive bladder with symptoms of urgency, incontinence, and urinary frequency

Local Anesthetic/Vasoconstrictor Precautions No information available to require special precautions

Effects on Dental Treatment Key adverse event(s) related to dental treatment: Significant xerostomia and changes in salivation (normal salivary flow resumes upon discontinuation).

Effects on Bleeding No information available to require special precautions

Adverse Effects

>10%: Gastrointestinal: Xerostomia (9% to 22%)

1% to 10%:

Cardiovascular: Tachycardia
Central nervous system: Headache (4% to 7%), fatigue (2%)
Dermatologic: Dry skin
Gastrointestinal: Constipation (9% to 10%), abdominal pain (1% to 3%), dyspepsia (1% to 2%), flatulence (1% to 2%), nausea (1%), abdominal distention (<2%), taste abnormal, vomiting
Genitourinary: Urinary tract infection (1% to 7%), urinary retention (≤1%)
Ocular: Dry eyes (1% to 2%), blurred vision (1%)
Respiratory: Nasopharyngitis (3%), nasal dryness (1%)
Miscellaneous: Influenza (2%)

General Dosage Range Dosage adjustment recommended in patients with renal impairment

Oral:

Adults: Immediate release formulation: 20 mg twice daily; Extended release formulation: 60 mg once daily

Elderly ≥75 years: Immediate release formulation: Initial: 20 mg at bedtime

Mechanism of Action Trospium antagonizes the effects of acetylcholine on muscarinic receptors in cholinergically innervated organs. It reduces the smooth muscle tone of the bladder.

Pharmacodynamics/Kinetics

Half-life Elimination Immediate release formulation: 20 hours

Severe renal insufficiency (Cl_{cr} <30 mL/minute): ~33 hours; extended release formulation: ~35 hours

Time to Peak 5-6 hours

Pregnancy Risk Factor C

Trypsin, Balsam Peru, and Castor Oil
(TRIP sin, BAL sam pe RUE, & KAS tor oyl)

Related Information

Castor Oil *on page* 322

U.S. Brand Names Allanderm-T™ [DSC]; Granulex®; Optase™; Xenaderm™

Pharmacologic Category Protectant, Topical

Use Treatment of decubitus ulcers, varicose ulcers, debridement of eschar, dehiscent wounds and sunburn; promote wound healing; reduce odor from necrotic wounds

Local Anesthetic/Vasoconstrictor Precautions No information available to require special precautions

Effects on Dental Treatment No significant effects or complications reported

Effects on Bleeding No information available to require special precautions

Adverse Effects Frequency not defined: Local: Temporary stinging at application site

General Dosage Range Topical: *Adults:* Apply a minimum of twice daily or as often as necessary

Mechanism of Action Trypsin is used to debride necrotic tissue; balsam peru stimulates circulation at the wound site and may be mildly bactericidal; castor oil improves epithelialization, acts as a protectant covering and helps reduce pain

Tuberculin Tests (too BER kyoo lin tests)

U.S. Brand Names Aplisol®; Tubersol®

Pharmacologic Category Diagnostic Agent

Use Skin test in diagnosis of tuberculosis

Local Anesthetic/Vasoconstrictor Precautions No information available to require special precautions

Effects on Dental Treatment No significant effects or complications reported

Effects on Bleeding No information available to require special precautions

Adverse Effects Suspected adverse reactions should be reported to the Food and Drug Administration (FDA) MedWatch Program at 1-800-332-1088

Frequency not defined:

Dermatologic: Rash

Local: Injection site reactions: Bleeding, bruising, discomfort, erythematous reaction, hematoma, necrosis, pain, pruritus, redness, scarring, ulceration, vesiculation

Miscellaneous: Anaphylaxis

General Dosage Range Intradermal: *Children and Adults:* 0.1 mL

Mechanism of Action Tuberculosis results in individuals becoming sensitized to certain antigenic components of the *M. tuberculosis* organism. Culture extracts called tuberculins are contained in tuberculin skin test preparations. Upon intracutaneous injection of these culture extracts, a classic delayed (cellular) hypersensitivity reaction occurs. This reaction is characteristic of a delayed course (peak occurs >24 hours after injection, induration of the skin secondary to cell infiltration, and occasional vesiculation and necrosis). Delayed hypersensitivity reactions to tuberculin may indicate infection with a variety of nontuberculosis mycobacteria, or vaccination with the live attenuated mycobacterial strain of *M. bovis* vaccine, BCG, in addition to previous natural infection with *M. tuberculosis*.

Pharmacodynamics/Kinetics

Onset of Action Delayed hypersensitivity reactions: 5-6 hours; Peak effect: 48-72 hours

Duration of Action Reactions subside over a few days

Pregnancy Risk Factor C

Typhoid Vaccine (TYE foid vak SEEN)

U.S. Brand Names Typhim Vi®; Vivotif®

Canadian Brand Names Typherix®; Typhim Vi®; Vivotif®

Pharmacologic Category Vaccine, Inactivated (Bacterial); Vaccine, Live (Bacterial)

Use Active immunization against typhoid fever caused by *Salmonella typhi*

Not for routine vaccination. In the United States and Canada, use should be limited to:

- Travelers to areas with a prolonged risk of exposure to *S. typhi*
- Persons with intimate exposure to a *S. typhi* carrier
- Laboratory technicians with exposure to *S. typhi*
- Travelers with achlorhydria or hypochlorhydria (Canadian recommendation)

Local Anesthetic/Vasoconstrictor Precautions No information available to require special precautions

Effects on Dental Treatment No significant effects or complications reported

Effects on Bleeding No information available to require special precautions

Adverse Effects In the U.S., all serious adverse reactions must be reported to the Department of Health and Human Services (DHHS) Vaccine Adverse Event Reporting System (VAERS) 1-800-822-7967 or online at https://vaers.hhs.gov/esub/index. In Canada, adverse reactions may be reported to local provincial/territorial health agencies or to the Vaccine Safety Section at Public Health Agency of Canada (1-866-844-0018).

Oral:

1% to 10%:

Central nervous system: Headache (5%), fever (3%)

Dermatologic: Rash (1%)

Gastrointestinal: Abdominal pain (6%), nausea (6%), diarrhea (3%), vomiting (2%)

Postmarketing and/or case reports: Anaphylactic reaction, demyelinating disease, myalgia, pain, RA, urticaria, sepsis, weakness

Injection (incidence may vary based on age and/or product used):

>10%:

Central nervous system: Fever (undefined; 2% to 32%), malaise (4% to 24%), headache (16% to 20%)

Local: Injection site: Tenderness (97% to 98%), pain (27% to 41%), soreness (up to 16%), induration (5% to 15%)

Neuromuscular & skeletal: General aches (1% to 13%)

1% to 10%:

Central nervous system: Fever ≥100°F (2%), >102°F (2%)

Dermatologic: Pruritus (up to 8%)

Gastrointestinal: Nausea (up to 8%), vomiting (2%)

Local: Injection site: Erythema (up to 5%), swelling (up to 4%)

Neuromuscular & skeletal: Myalgia (3% to 7%)

General Dosage Range

I.M.: *Children ≥2 years and Adults:* 0.5 mL given at least 2 weeks prior to expected exposure; may repeat every 2 years

Oral: *Children ≥6 years and Adults:* 1 capsule on alternate days for a total of 4 doses; may repeat full course every 5 years

Mechanism of Action Virulent strains of *Salmonella typhi* cause disease by penetrating the intestinal mucosa and entering the systemic circulation via the lymphatic vasculature. One possible mechanism of conferring immunity may be the provocation of a local immune response in the intestinal tract induced by oral ingesting of a live strain with subsequent aborted infection. The ability of *Salmonella typhi* to produce clinical disease (and to elicit an immune response) is dependent on the bacteria having a complete lipopolysaccharide. The live attenuate Ty21a strain lacks the enzyme UDP-4-galactose epimerase so that lipopolysaccharide is only synthesized under conditions that induce bacterial autolysis. Thus, the strain remains avirulent despite the production of sufficient lipopolysaccharide to evoke a protective immune response. Despite low levels of lipopolysaccharide synthesis, cells lyse before gaining a virulent phenotype due to the intracellular accumulation of metabolic intermediates.

Pharmacodynamics/Kinetics

Onset of Action Immunity to *Salmonella typhi*: Oral: ~1 week

Duration of Action Immunity: Oral: ~4-7 years; Parenteral: Typhim Vi®: >17-21 months, Typherix®: ~3 years

Pregnancy Risk Factor C

Ulipristal (ue li PRIS tal)

U.S. Brand Names ella®

Pharmacologic Category Contraceptive; Progestin Receptor Modulator

Use Emergency contraception following unprotected intercourse or possible contraceptive failure

Local Anesthetic/Vasoconstrictor Precautions No information available to require special precautions

Effects on Dental Treatment No significant effects or complications reported

Effects on Bleeding No information available to require special precautions

Adverse Effects

>10%:

Central nervous system: Headache (18% to 19%)

Endocrine & metabolic: Menstruation occurring ≥7 days later than expected (19%), dysmenorrhea (7% to 13%)

Gastrointestinal: Abdominal pain (8% to 15%), nausea (12% to 13%)

1% to 10%:

Central nervous system: Fatigue (6%), dizziness (5%)

Endocrine & metabolic: Intermenstrual bleeding (9%), menstruation occurring ≥7 days earlier than expected (7%)

General Dosage Range Oral: *Adults:* 1 tablet (30 mg) as a single dose

Mechanism of Action Prevents progestin from binding to the progesterone receptor. Ulipristal postpones follicular rupture when administered prior to ovulation, thereby inhibiting or delaying ovulation. May also alter the normal endometrium, impairing implantation.

Pharmacodynamics/Kinetics

Half-life Elimination Ulipristal: ~32 hours; Monodemethylated metabolite: ~27 hours

Time to Peak Serum: 1 hour (ulipristal and monodemethylated metabolite)

Pregnancy Risk Factor X

Undecylenic Acid and Derivatives (un de sil EN ik AS id & dah RIV ah tivs)

U.S. Brand Names Fungi-Nail® [OTC]

Pharmacologic Category Antifungal Agent, Topical

Use Treatment of athlete's foot (tinea pedis); ringworm (except nails and scalp)

Local Anesthetic/Vasoconstrictor Precautions No information available to require special precautions

Effects on Dental Treatment No significant effects or complications reported

Effects on Bleeding No information available to require special precautions

General Dosage Range Topical: *Children ≥2 years and Adults:* Apply twice daily to affected area

Urea (yoor EE a)

U.S. Brand Names Aqua Care® [OTC]; Aquaphilic® with Carbamide [OTC]; BP 50%; Carmol® 10 [OTC]; Carmol® 20 [OTC]; Carmol® 40; Carmol® Deep Cleansing [OTC]; DPM™ [OTC]; Gordon's® Urea [OTC]; Gormel® Ten [OTC]; Gormel® [OTC]; Hydro 35™; Hydro 40™; Kerafoam®; Kerafoam® 42; Keralac™; Keralac™ Nailstik; Keratol 40™ [DSC]; Kerol™; Kerol™ AD; Kerol™ Redi-Cloths; Kerol™ ZX; Lanaphilic® with Urea [OTC]; Nutraplus® [OTC]; Quinnostik; Rea Lo® 30 [OTC]; Rea Lo® 40; Remeven™; RevitaDERM® 40; U-Kera E™ [DSC]; Ultra Mide 25® [OTC]; Umecta PD™; Umecta®; Umecta® Nail Film; Uramaxin®; Uramaxin® GT; Ureacin-10® [OTC]; Ureacin-20® [OTC]; X-Viate™

Canadian Brand Names UltraMide 25™; Uremol®; Urisec®

Pharmacologic Category Diuretic, Osmotic; Keratolytic Agent; Topical Skin Product

Use Keratolytic agent to soften nails or skin; OTC: Moisturizer for dry, rough skin

Local Anesthetic/Vasoconstrictor Precautions No information available to require special precautions

Effects on Dental Treatment No significant effects or complications reported

Effects on Bleeding No information available to require special precautions

Adverse Effects Frequency not defined: Local: Transient stinging, local irritation

General Dosage Range Topical: *Adults:* Apply 1-3 times/day

Mechanism of Action Urea softens hyperkeratotic areas by dissolving the intracellular matrix, resulting in loosening the horny layer of the skin, or softening and debridement of the nail plate

Pregnancy Risk Factor C

Urea and Hydrocortisone (yoor EE a & hye droe KOR ti sone)

Related Information

Hydrocortisone (Topical) *on page 868*
Urea *on page 1689*

U.S. Brand Names Carmol-HC®

Canadian Brand Names Ti-U-Lac® H; Uremol® HC

Pharmacologic Category Corticosteroid, Topical

Use Inflammation of corticosteroid-responsive dermatoses

Local Anesthetic/Vasoconstrictor Precautions No information available to require special precautions

Effects on Dental Treatment No significant effects or complications reported

Effects on Bleeding No information available to require special precautions

General Dosage Range Topical: *Children and Adults:* Apply thin film and rub in well 2-4 times/day

Pregnancy Risk Factor C

Urofollitropin (yoor oh fol li TROE pin)

U.S. Brand Names Bravelle®

Canadian Brand Names Bravelle®; Fertinorm® H.P.

Pharmacologic Category Gonadotropin; Ovulation Stimulator

Use Ovulation induction in patients who previously received pituitary suppression; development of multiple follicles with Assisted Reproductive Technologies (ART)

Local Anesthetic/Vasoconstrictor Precautions No information available to require special precautions

Effects on Dental Treatment No significant effects or complications reported

Effects on Bleeding Medical consult is suggested.

Adverse Effects Percentage may vary by indication, route of administration.

>10%:

- Central nervous system: Headache
- Endocrine & metabolic: Ovarian enlargement, ovarian hyperstimulation syndrome
- Gastrointestinal: Abdominal cramps

1% to 10%:

- Cardiovascular: Hypertension
- Central nervous system: Depression, emotional lability, fever, pain
- Dermatologic: Acne, exfoliative dermatitis, rash
- Endocrine & metabolic: Breast tenderness, hot flashes, ovarian disorder (pain, cyst)
- Gastrointestinal: Abdomen enlarged, abdominal pain, constipation, diarrhea, dehydration, nausea, vomiting, weight gain
- Genitourinary: Cervical disorder, urinary tract infection, pelvic pain/cramps, uterine spasms, vaginal discharge, vaginal hemorrhage, vaginal spotting
- Local: Injection site reaction
- Neuromuscular & skeletal: Neck pain
- Respiratory: Respiratory disorder, sinusitis
- Miscellaneous: Infection, post retrieval pain

General Dosage Range

I.M.: *Adults (females):* Initial: 150 int. units once daily for 5 days; Maintenance: Up to 450 int. units/day (maximum: 12 days therapy)

SubQ: *Adults (females):* Initial: 150-225 int. units once daily for 5 days; Maintenance: Up to 450 int. units/day (maximum: 12 days therapy)

Mechanism of Action Urofollitropin is a preparation of highly purified follicle-stimulating hormone (FSH) extracted from the urine of postmenopausal women. Follitropins stimulate ovarian follicular growth in women who do not have primary ovarian failure. FSH is required for normal follicular growth, maturation, gonadal steroid production, and spermatogenesis.

Pharmacodynamics/Kinetics

Half-life Elimination

- I.M.: 37 hours, 15 hours following multiple doses
- SubQ: 32 hours, 21 hours following multiple doses

Time to Peak

- I.M.: 17 hours, 11 hours following multiple doses
- SubQ: 21 hours, 10 hours following multiple doses

Pregnancy Risk Factor X

Ursodiol (ur soe DYE ol)

U.S. Brand Names Actigall®; Urso 250®; Urso Forte®

Canadian Brand Names Dom-Ursodiol C; PHL-Ursodiol C; PMS-Ursodiol C; Urso®; Urso® DS

Pharmacologic Category Gallstone Dissolution Agent

Use

- Actigall®: Gallbladder stone dissolution; prevention of gallstones in obese patients experiencing rapid weight loss
- Urso®, Urso Forte®: Primary biliary cirrhosis

Local Anesthetic/Vasoconstrictor Precautions No information available to require special precautions

Effects on Dental Treatment No significant effects or complications reported

Effects on Bleeding Medical consult is suggested.

Adverse Effects

>10%:

- Central nervous system: Headache (up to 25%), dizziness (17%)
- Gastrointestinal: Diarrhea (up to 27%), constipation (up to 26%), dyspepsia (17%), nausea (up to 17%), vomiting (up to 14%)
- Neuromuscular & skeletal: Back pain (up to 12%)

Respiratory: Upper respiratory tract infection (up to 16%)

1% to 10%:

Dermatologic: Alopecia (5%), rash (3%)

Endocrine & metabolic: Hyperglycemia (1%)

Gastrointestinal: Flatulence (up to 8%), peptic ulcer (1%)

Genitourinary: Urinary tract infection (7%)

Hematologic: Leukopenia (3%), thrombocytopenia (1%)

Hepatic: Cholecystitis (5%)

Neuromuscular & skeletal: Arthritis (6%), myalgia (6%)

Renal: Serum creatinine increased (1%)

Respiratory: Pharyngitis (up to 8%), bronchitis (7%), cough (7%)

Miscellaneous: Viral infection (9%), flu-like syndrome (7%), allergy (5%)

General Dosage Range Oral: *Adults:* 8-15 mg/kg/day in 2-4 divided doses **or** 300 mg twice daily

Mechanism of Action Decreases the cholesterol content of bile and bile stones by reducing the secretion of cholesterol from the liver and the fractional reabsorption of cholesterol by the intestines. Mechanism of action in primary biliary cirrhosis is not clearly defined.

Pregnancy Risk Factor B

Ustekinumab (yoo stek in YOO mab)

U.S. Brand Names Stelara™

Canadian Brand Names Stelara™

Pharmacologic Category Antipsoriatic Agent; Interleukin-12 Inhibitor; Interleukin-23 Inhibitor; Monoclonal Antibody

Use Treatment of moderate-to-severe plaque psoriasis

Local Anesthetic/Vasoconstrictor Precautions No information available to require special precautions

Effects on Dental Treatment No significant effects or complications reported

Effects on Bleeding No information available to require special precautions

Adverse Effects

>10%: Miscellaneous: Infection (27% to 61%)

1% to 10%:

Central nervous system: Headache (5%), fatigue (3%), dizziness (1% to 2%), depression (1%)

Dermatologic: Pruritus (1% to 2%), rash (<2%), urticaria (<2%)

Local: Injection site erythema (1% to 2%)

Neuromuscular & skeletal: Back pain (1% to 2%)

Respiratory: Pharyngolaryngeal pain (1% to 2%)

Miscellaneous: Antibody formation (3% to 5%)

General Dosage Range Oral: *Adults:* ≤100 kg: 45 mg at 0- and 4 weeks, and then every 12 weeks; >100 kg: 45 mg or 90 mg at 0- and 4 weeks, and then every 12 weeks

Mechanism of Action Ustekinumab is a human monoclonal antibody that binds to and interferes with the proinflammatory cytokines, interleukin (IL)-12 and IL-23. Biological effects of IL-12 and IL-23 include natural killer (NK) cell activation, CD4+ T-cell differentiation and activation. Ustekinumab also interferes with the expression of monocyte chemotactic protein-1 (MCP-1), tumor necrosis factor-alpha (TNF-α), interferon-inducible protein-10 (IP-10), and interleukin-8 (IL-8). Significant clinical improvement in psoriasis patients is seen in association with reduction of these proinflammatory signalers.

Pharmacodynamics/Kinetics

Half-life Elimination 10-126 days

Time to Peak Plasma: 7-13.5 days

Pregnancy Risk Factor B

Vaccinia Immune Globulin (Intravenous)

(vax IN ee a i MYUN GLOB yoo lin IN tra VEE nus)

U.S. Brand Names CNJ-016®

Pharmacologic Category Blood Product Derivative; Immune Globulin

Use Treatment of infectious complications of smallpox (vaccinia virus) vaccination, such as eczema vaccinatum, progressive vaccinia, and severe generalized vaccinia; treatment of vaccinia infections in individuals with concurrent skin conditions or accidental virus exposure to eyes (except vaccinia keratitis), mouth, or other areas where viral infection would pose significant risk

CDC guidelines for use:
Use is recommended for:
- Inadvertent inoculation (considering severity, toxicity of affected person, and pain)
- Eczema vaccinatum
- Generalized vaccinia (severe form or if underlying illness is present)
- Progressive vaccinia

Use may be considered for:
- Severe ocular complications except isolated keratitis

Use is not recommended for:
- Inadvertent inoculation that is not severe
- Mild or limited generalized vaccinia
- Nonspecific rashes, erythema multiforme, or Stevens-Johnson syndrome
- Postvaccinial encephalitis or encephalomyelitis

Local Anesthetic/Vasoconstrictor Precautions No information available to require special precautions

Effects on Dental Treatment No significant effects or complications reported

Effects on Bleeding No information available to require special precautions

Adverse Effects Note: Actual frequency varies by dose and rate of infusion
Cardiovascular: Peripheral edema
Central nervous system: Cold or hot feeling, dizziness, fatigue, headache, pain, pallor, pyrexia
Dermatologic: Erythema
Gastrointestinal: Appetite decreased, nausea, vomiting
Local: Injection site reaction
Neuromuscular & skeletal: Back pain, paraesthesia, muscle spasm, rigors, tremor, weakness
Miscellaneous: Diaphoresis

General Dosage Range I.V.: *Adults:* Initial: 6000 units/kg; may repeat 6000-9000 units/kg if needed (maximum: 24,000 units/kg)

Mechanism of Action Antibodies obtained from pooled human plasma of individuals immunized with the smallpox vaccine provide passive immunity

Pharmacodynamics/Kinetics
Half-life Elimination 30 days (range 13-67 days)
Time to Peak Plasma: ≤2 hours

Pregnancy Risk Factor C

Prescribing and Access Restrictions Vaccinia immune globulin is not available for general public use. All supplies are currently owned by the federal government for inclusion in the Strategic National Stockpile. The CDC Smallpox Adverse Events Clinical Consultation team will coordinate shipment. The State Health Department should be contacted first concerning severe or unexpected adverse events from smallpox vaccination.

ValACYclovir (val ay SYE kloe veer)

Related Information
Acyclovir (Systemic) *on page* 55
Systemic Viral Diseases *on page* 1904
Viral Infections *on page* 1947

Related Sample Prescriptions
Herpes Simplex (Recurrent) *on page* 1990

U.S. Brand Names Valtrex®

Canadian Brand Names Apo-Valacyclovir®; Mylan-Valacyclovir; PHL-Valacyclovir; PMS-Valacyclovir; PRO-Valacyclovir; Riva-Valacyclovir; Valtrex®

Generic Availability (U.S.) Yes

Pharmacologic Category Antiviral Agent; Antiviral Agent, Oral

Dental Use Treatment of herpes labialis (cold sores)

Use Treatment of herpes zoster (shingles) in immunocompetent patients; treatment of first-episode and recurrent genital herpes; suppression of recurrent genital herpes and reduction of heterosexual transmission of genital herpes in immunocompetent patients; suppression of genital herpes in HIV-infected individuals; treatment of herpes labialis (cold sores); chickenpox in immunocompetent children

Unlabeled/Investigational Use Prophylaxis of cancer-related HSV, VZV, and CMV infections; treatment of cancer-related HSV, VZV infection

Local Anesthetic/Vasoconstrictor Precautions No information available to require special precautions

Effects on Dental Treatment No significant effects or complications reported

Effects on Bleeding Medical consult is suggested.

Adverse Effects

>10%:

Central nervous system: Headache (13% to 38%)

Gastrointestinal: Nausea (5% to 15%), abdominal pain (1% to 11%)

Hematologic: Neutropenia (≤18%)

Hepatic: ALT increased (≤14%), AST increased (2% to 16%)

Respiratory: Nasopharyngitis (≤16%)

1% to 10%:

Central nervous system: Fatigue (≤8%), depression (≤7%), fever (children 4%), dizziness (2% to 4%)

Dermatologic: Rash (≤8%)

Endocrine: Dysmenorrhea (≤1% to 8%), dehydration (children 2%)

Gastrointestinal: Vomiting (<1% to 6%), diarrhea (children 5%; adults <1%)

Hematologic: Thrombocytopenia (≤3%)

Hepatic: Alkaline phosphatase increased (≤4%)

Neuromuscular & skeletal: Arthralgia (<1 to 6%)

Respiratory: Rhinorrhea (children 2%)

Miscellaneous: Herpes simplex (children 2%)

Dental Usual Dosage Herpes labialis (cold sores): Adolescents and Adults: Oral: 2 g twice daily for 1 day (separate doses by ~12 hours)

Dosage Oral:

Children 2 to <18 years: Chickenpox: 20 mg/kg/dose 3 times/day for 5 days (maximum: 1 g 3 times/day)

Children ≥12 and Adults: Herpes labialis (cold sores): 2 g twice daily for 1 day (separate doses by ~12 hours)

Adults:

CMV prophylaxis in allogeneic HSCT recipients (unlabeled use): 2 g 4 times/day

Herpes zoster (shingles): 1 g 3 times/day for 7 days

HSV, VZV in cancer patients (unlabeled use): Prophylaxis: 500 mg 2-3 times/day; Treatment: 1 g 3 times/day

Genital herpes:

Initial episode: 1 g twice daily for 10 days

Recurrent episode: 500 mg twice daily for 3 days

Reduction of transmission: 500 mg once daily (source partner)

Suppressive therapy:

Immunocompetent patients: 1000 mg once daily (500 mg once daily in patients with <9 recurrences per year)

HIV-infected patients (CD4 ≥100 cells/mm^3): 500 mg twice daily

Dosing adjustment in renal impairment:

Herpes zoster: Adults:

Cl_{cr} 30-49 mL/minute: 1 g every 12 hours

Cl_{cr} 10-29 mL/minute: 1 g every 24 hours

Cl_{cr} <10 mL/minute: 500 mg every 24 hours

Genital herpes: Adults:

Initial episode:

Cl_{cr} 10-29 mL/minute: 1 g every 24 hours

Cl_{cr} <10 mL/minute: 500 mg every 24 hours

Recurrent episode: Cl_{cr} <29 mL/minute: 500 mg every 24 hours

Suppressive therapy: Cl_{cr} <29 mL/minute:

For usual dose of 1 g every 24 hours, decrease dose to 500 mg every 24 hours

For usual dose of 500 mg every 24 hours, decrease dose to 500 mg every 48 hours

HIV-infected patients: 500 mg every 24 hours

Herpes labialis: Adolescents and Adults:

Cl_{cr} 30-49 mL/minute: 1 g every 12 hours for 2 doses

Cl_{cr} 10-29 mL/minute: 500 mg every 12 hours for 2 doses

Cl_{cr} <10 mL/minute: 500 mg as a single dose

Hemodialysis: Dialyzable (~33% removed during 4-hour session); administer dose postdialysis

Chronic ambulatory peritoneal dialysis/continuous arteriovenous hemofiltration dialysis: Pharmacokinetic parameters are similar to those in patients with ESRD; supplemental dose not needed following dialysis

Dosing adjustment in hepatic impairment: No adjustment required.

Mechanism of Action Valacyclovir is rapidly and nearly completely converted to acyclovir by intestinal and hepatic metabolism. Acyclovir is converted to acyclovir monophosphate by virus-specific thymidine kinase then further converted to acyclovir triphosphate by other cellular enzymes. Acyclovir triphosphate inhibits DNA synthesis and viral replication by competing with deoxyguanosine triphosphate for viral DNA polymerase and being incorporated into viral DNA.

Contraindications Hypersensitivity to valacyclovir, acyclovir, or any component of the formulation

Warnings/Precautions Thrombotic thrombocytopenic purpura/hemolytic uremic syndrome has occurred in immunocompromised patients (at doses of 8 g/day). Safety and efficacy have not been established for treatment/suppression of recurrent genital herpes or disseminated herpes in patients with profound immunosuppression (eg, advanced HIV with CD4 <100 cells/mm^3). CNS adverse effects (including agitation, hallucinations, confusion, delirium, seizures, and encephalopathy) have been reported. Use caution in patients with renal impairment, the elderly, and/or those receiving nephrotoxic agents. Acute renal failure has been observed in patients with renal dysfunction; dose adjustment may be required. Decreased precipitation in renal tubules may occur leading to urinary precipitation; adequately hydrate patient. For cold sores, treatment should begin at with earliest symptom (tingling, itching, burning). For genital herpes, treatment should begin as soon as possible after the first signs and symptoms (within 72 hours of onset of first diagnosis or within 24 hours of onset of recurrent episodes). For herpes zoster, treatment should begin within 72 hours of onset of rash. For chickenpox, treatment should begin with earliest sign or symptom. Use with caution in the elderly; CNS effects have been reported. Safety and efficacy have not been established in patients <2 years of age.

Drug Interactions

Avoid Concomitant Use

Avoid concomitant use of ValACYclovir with any of the following: Zoster Vaccine

Increased Effect/Toxicity

ValACYclovir may increase the levels/effects of: Mycophenolate; Tenofovir; Zidovudine

The levels/effects of ValACYclovir may be increased by: Mycophenolate

Decreased Effect

ValACYclovir may decrease the levels/effects of: Zoster Vaccine

Dietary Considerations May be taken with or without food.

Pharmacodynamics/Kinetics

Half-life Elimination Normal renal function: Adults: 2.5-3.3 hours (acyclovir), ~30 minutes (valacyclovir); End-stage renal disease: 14-20 hours (acyclovir); During hemodialysis: 4 hours

Pregnancy Risk Factor B

Lactation Enters breast milk/use caution

Breast-Feeding Considerations Peak concentrations in breast milk range from 0.5-2.3 times the corresponding maternal acyclovir serum concentration. This is expected to provide a nursing infant with a dose of acyclovir equivalent to ~0.6 mg/kg/day following ingestion of valacyclovir 500 mg twice daily by the mother. Use with caution while breast-feeding.

Dosage Forms

Caplet, oral: 500 mg, 1 g

Valtrex®: 500 mg, 1 g

Tablet, oral: 500 mg, 1 g

ValGANciclovir (val gan SYE kloh veer)

Related Information

Ganciclovir (Systemic) *on page 803*

Systemic Viral Diseases *on page 1904*

U.S. Brand Names Valcyte®

Canadian Brand Names Valcyte®

Pharmacologic Category Antiviral Agent

Use Treatment of cytomegalovirus (CMV) retinitis in patients with acquired immunodeficiency syndrome (AIDS); prevention of CMV disease in high-risk patients (donor CMV positive/recipient CMV negative) undergoing kidney, heart, or kidney/pancreas transplantation

Local Anesthetic/Vasoconstrictor Precautions No information available to require special precautions

Effects on Dental Treatment No significant effects or complications reported

Effects on Bleeding Medical consult is suggested.

Adverse Effects

>10%:

Cardiovascular: Hypertension (12% to 18%)

Central nervous system: Fever (9% to 31%), headache (6% to 22%), insomnia (6% to 20%)

Gastrointestinal: Diarrhea (16% to 41%), nausea (8% to 30%), vomiting (3% to 21%), abdominal pain (15%), constipation

Hematologic: Anemia (≤31%), thrombocytopenia (≤22%), neutropenia (3% to 19%)

Neuromuscular & skeletal: Tremor (12% to 28%)

Ocular: Retinal detachment (15%)
Renal: Serum creatinine increased (S_{cr} >1.5-2.5 mg/dL: 12% to 50%; S_{cr} >2.5: 3% to 17%)
Respiratory: Cough, upper respiratory tract infection
5% to 10%: Central nervous system: Peripheral neuropathy (9%), paresthesia (8%)
<5%:
Cardiovascular: Edema, hypotension, peripheral edema
Central nervous system: Agitation, confusion, depression, dizziness, fatigue, hallucination, pain, psychosis, seizure
Dermatologic: Acne, dermatitis, pruritus
Endocrine & metabolic: Dehydration, hyperglycemia, hyper-/hypokalemia, hypocalcemia, hypomagnesemia, hypophosphatemia
Gastrointestinal: Abdominal distention/pain, appetite (decreased), dyspepsia
Genitourinary: Urinary tract infection
Hematologic: Aplastic anemia, bleeding (potentially life-threatening due to thrombocytopenia), bone marrow depression, pancytopenia
Hepatic: Ascites
Neuromuscular & skeletal: Arthralgia, back pain, limb pain, muscle cramps, weakness
Renal: Creatinine clearance (decreased), dysuria, renal impairment
Respiratory: Dyspnea, nasopharyngitis, pharyngitis, pleural effusion, rhinorrhea
Miscellaneous: Allergic reaction, local and systemic infection (including sepsis)

General Dosage Range Dosage adjustment recommended in patients with renal impairment

Oral:

Children 4 months to 16 years: Dose (mg) = 7 x body surface area x creatinine clearance once daily

Children >16 years and Adults: 900 mg 1-2 times/day

Mechanism of Action Valganciclovir is rapidly converted to ganciclovir in the body. The bioavailability of ganciclovir from valganciclovir is increased 10-fold compared to oral ganciclovir. A dose of 900 mg achieved systemic exposure of ganciclovir comparable to that achieved with the recommended doses of intravenous ganciclovir of 5 mg/kg. Ganciclovir is phosphorylated to a substrate which competitively inhibits the binding of deoxyguanosine triphosphate to DNA polymerase resulting in inhibition of viral DNA synthesis.

Pharmacodynamics/Kinetics

Half-life Elimination Ganciclovir: 4.08 hours, prolonged with renal impairment; Severe renal impairment: Up to 68 hours

Time to Peak Ganciclovir: 1-3 hours

Pregnancy Risk Factor C

Valproic Acid (val PROE ik AS id)

U.S. Brand Names Depacon®; Depakene®; Stavzor™

Canadian Brand Names Apo-Valproic®; Depakene®; Epival® I.V.; Mylan-Valproic; PHL-Valproic Acid; PHL-Valproic Acid E.C.; PMS-Valproic Acid; PMS-Valproic Acid E.C.; ratio-Valproic; ratio-Valproic ECC; Rhoxal-valproic; Sandoz-Valproic

Generic Availability (U.S.) Yes: Excludes delayed release capsule

Pharmacologic Category Anticonvulsant, Miscellaneous; Antimanic Agent; Histone Deacetylase Inhibitor

Use Monotherapy and adjunctive therapy in the treatment of patients with complex partial seizures; monotherapy and adjunctive therapy of simple and complex absence seizures; adjunctive therapy in patients with multiple seizure types that include absence seizures

Stavzor™: Mania associated with bipolar disorder; migraine prophylaxis

Unlabeled/Investigational Use Status epilepticus, diabetic neuropathy

Local Anesthetic/Vasoconstrictor Precautions No information available to require special precautions

Effects on Dental Treatment Key adverse event(s) related to dental treatment: Periodontal abscess and taste perversion.

Effects on Bleeding Has been associated with dose-related thrombocytopenia. Normal coagulation may generally be expected unless thrombocytopenia is present and severe.

Adverse Effects

>10%:
Central nervous system: Headache (≤31%), somnolence (≤30%), dizziness (12% to 25%), insomnia (>1% to 15%), nervousness (>1% to 11%), pain (1% to 11%)
Dermatologic: Alopecia (>1% to 24%)

Gastrointestinal: Nausea (15% to 48%), vomiting (7% to 27%), diarrhea (7% to 23%), abdominal pain (7% to 23%), dyspepsia (7% to 23%), anorexia (>1% to 12%)
Hematologic: Thrombocytopenia (1% to 24%; dose related)
Neuromuscular & skeletal: Tremor (≤57%), weakness (6% to 27%)
Ocular: Diplopia (>1% to 16%), amblyopia/blurred vision (≤12%)
Miscellaneous: Infection (≤20%), flu-like syndrome (12%)

1% to 10%:
Cardiovascular: Peripheral edema (>1% to 8%), chest pain (>1% to <5%), edema (>1% to <5%), facial edema (>1% to <5%), hypertension (>1% to <5%), hypotension (>1% to <5%), palpitation (>1% to <5%), postural hypotension (>1% to <5%), tachycardia (>1% to <5%), vasodilation (>1% to <5%), arrhythmia
Central nervous system: Ataxia (>1% to 8%), amnesia (>1% to 7%), emotional lability (>1% to 6%), fever (>1% to 6%), abnormal thinking (≤6%), depression (>1% to 5%), abnormal dreams (>1% to <5%), agitation (>1% to <5%), anxiety (>1% to <5%), catatonia (>1% to <5%), chills (>1% to <5%), confusion (>1% to <5%), coordination abnormal (>1% to <5%), hallucination (>1% to <5%), malaise (>1% to <5%), personality disorder (>1% to <5%), speech disorder (>1% to <5%), tardive dyskinesia (>1% to <5%), vertigo (>1% to <5%), euphoria (1%), hypoesthesia (1%)
Dermatologic: Rash (>1% to 6%), bruising (>1% to 5%), discoid lupus erythematosus (>1% to <5%), dry skin (>1% to <5%), furunculosis (>1% to <5%), petechia (>1% to <5%), pruritus (>1% to <5), seborrhea (>1% to <5%)
Endocrine & metabolic: Amenorrhea (>1% to <5%), dysmenorrhea (>1% to <5%), metrorrhagia (>1% to <5%), hypoproteinemia
Gastrointestinal: Weight gain (4% to 9%), weight loss (6%), appetite increased (≤6%), constipation (>1% to 5%), xerostomia (>1% to 5%), eructation (>1% to <5%), fecal incontinence (>1% to <5%), flatulence (>1% to <5%), gastroenteritis (>1% to <5%), glossitis (>1% to <5%), hematemesis (>1% to <5%), pancreatitis (>1% to <5%), periodontal abscess (>1% to <5%), stomatitis (>1% to <5%), taste perversion (>1% to <5%), dysphagia, gum hemorrhage, mouth ulceration
Genitourinary: Cystitis (>1% to 5%), dysuria (>1% to 5%), urinary frequency (>1% to <5%), urinary incontinence (>1% to <5%), vaginal hemorrhage (>1% to 5%), vaginitis (>1% to <5%)
Hepatic: ALT increased (>1% to <5%), AST increased (>1% to <5%)
Local: Injection site pain (3%), injection site reaction (2%), injection site inflammation (1%)
Neuromuscular & skeletal: Back pain (≤8%), abnormal gait (>1% to <5%), arthralgia (>1% to <5%), arthrosis (>1% to <5%), dysarthria (>1% to <5%), hypertonia (>1% to <5%), hypokinesia (>1% to <5%), leg cramps (>1% to <5%), myalgia (>1% to <5%), myasthenia (>1% to <5%), neck pain (>1% to <5%), neck rigidity (>1% to <5%), paresthesia (>1% to <5%), reflex increased (>1% to <5%), twitching (>1% to <5%)
Ocular: Nystagmus (1% to 8%), dry eyes (>1% to 5%), eye pain (>1% to 5%), abnormal vision (>1% to <5%), conjunctivitis (>1% to <5%)
Otic: Tinnitus (1% to 7%), ear pain (>1% to 5%), deafness (>1% to <5%), otitis media (>1% to <5%)
Respiratory: Pharyngitis (2% to 8%), bronchitis (5%), rhinitis (>1% to 5%), dyspnea (1% to 5%), cough (>1% to <5%), epistaxis (>1% to <5%), pneumonia (>1% to <5%), sinusitis (>1% to <5%)
Miscellaneous: Diaphoresis (1%), hiccups

Dosage

Seizure disorders: **Note:** Administer doses >250 mg/day in divided doses.

Oral:

Simple and complex absence seizures: Children and Adults: Initial: 15 mg/kg/day; increase by 5-10 mg/kg/day at weekly intervals until therapeutic levels are achieved; maximum: 60 mg/kg/day. Larger maintenance doses may be required in younger children.

Complex partial seizures: Children ≥10 years and Adults: Initial: 10-15 mg/kg/day; increase by 5-10 mg/kg/day at weekly intervals until therapeutic levels are achieved; maximum: 60 mg/kg/day. Larger maintenance doses may be required in younger children.

Note: Regular release and delayed release formulations are usually given in 2-4 divided doses/day.

I.V.: Administer as a 60-minute infusion (≤20 mg/minute) with the same frequency as oral products; switch patient to oral products as soon as possible. Rapid infusions ≤45 mg/kg over 5-10 minutes (1.5-6 mg/kg/minute) were generally well tolerated in a clinical trial.

Rectal (unlabeled): Dilute syrup 1:1 with water for use as a retention enema; loading dose: 17-20 mg/kg one time; maintenance: 10-15 mg/kg/dose every 8 hours

Status epilepticus (unlabeled use): Adults:

Loading dose: I.V.: 15-45 mg/kg administered at ≤6 mg/kg/minute.

Maintenance dose: I.V. infusion: 1-4 mg/kg/hour; titrate dose as needed based upon patient response and evaluation of drug-drug interactions

Mania (Stavzor™): Adults: Oral: Initial: 750 mg/day in divided doses; dose should be adjusted as rapidly as possible to desired clinical effect; maximum recommended dosage: 60 mg/kg/day

Migraine prophylaxis (Stavzor™): Children ≥12 years: Oral: 250 mg twice daily; adjust dose based on patient response, up to 1000 mg/day

Diabetic neuropathy (unlabeled use): Adults: Oral: 500-1200 mg/day (Bril, 2011)

Elderly: Elimination is decreased in the elderly. Studies of elderly patients with dementia show a high incidence of somnolence. In some patients, this was associated with weight loss. Starting doses should be lower and increases should be slow, with careful monitoring of nutritional intake and dehydration. Safety and efficacy for use in patients >65 years have not been studied for migraine prophylaxis.

Dosing adjustment in renal impairment: A 27% reduction in clearance of unbound valproate is seen in patients with Cl_{cr} <10 mL/minute. Hemodialysis reduces valproate concentrations by 20%, therefore no dose adjustment is needed in patients with renal failure. Protein binding is reduced, monitoring only total valproate concentrations may be misleading.

Dosing adjustment/comments in hepatic impairment: Reduce dose. Clearance is decreased with liver impairment. Hepatic disease is also associated with decreased albumin concentrations and 2- to 2.6-fold increase in the unbound fraction. Free concentrations of valproate may be elevated while total concentrations appear normal. Use is contraindicated in severe impairment.

Mechanism of Action Causes increased availability of gamma-aminobutyric acid (GABA), an inhibitory neurotransmitter, to brain neurons or may enhance the action of GABA or mimic its action at postsynaptic receptor sites

Contraindications Hypersensitivity to valproic acid, derivatives, or any component of the formulation; hepatic disease or significant impairment; urea cycle disorders

Warnings/Precautions [U.S. Boxed Warning]: Hepatic failure resulting in fatalities has occurred in patients; children <2 years of age are at considerable risk. Other risk factors include organic brain disease, mental retardation with severe seizure disorders, congenital metabolic disorders, and patients on multiple anticonvulsants. Hepatotoxicity has usually been reported within 6 months of therapy initiation. Monitor patients closely for appearance of malaise, weakness, facial edema, anorexia, jaundice, and vomiting; discontinue immediately with signs/symptom of significant or suspected impairment. Liver function tests should be performed at baseline and at regular intervals after initiation of therapy, especially within the first 6 months. Hepatic dysfunction may progress despite discontinuing treatment. Should only be used as monotherapy in children <2 years of age and patients at high risk for hepatotoxicity. Contraindicated with severe impairment.

[U.S. Boxed Warning]: Cases of life-threatening pancreatitis, occurring at the start of therapy or following years of use, have been reported in adults and children. Some cases have been hemorrhagic with rapid progression of initial symptoms to death. Promptly evaluate symptoms of abdominal pain, nausea, vomiting, and/or anorexia; should generally be discontinued if pancreatitis is diagnosed.

[U.S. Boxed Warning]: May cause teratogenic effects such as neural tube defects (eg, spina bifida). Use in women of childbearing potential requires that benefits of use in mother be weighed against the potential risk to fetus, especially when used for conditions not associated with permanent injury or risk of death (eg, migraine).

May cause severe thrombocytopenia, inhibition of platelet aggregation, and bleeding. Tremors may indicate overdosage; use with caution in patients receiving other anticonvulsants. Hypersensitivity reactions affecting multiple organs have been reported in association with valproic acid use; may include dermatologic and/or hematologic changes (eosinophilia, neutropenia, thrombocytopenia) or symptoms of organ dysfunction.

Hyperammonemia and/or encephalopathy, sometimes fatal, have been reported following the initiation of valproic acid therapy and may be present with normal transaminase levels. Ammonia levels should be measured in patients who develop unexplained lethargy and vomiting, changes in mental status, or in patients who present with hypothermia (unintentional drop in core body temperature to <35°C/95°F). Discontinue therapy if ammonia levels are increased and evaluate for possible urea cycle disorder (UCD); contraindicated in patients with UCD.

Evaluation of UCD should be considered for the following patients prior to the start of therapy: History of unexplained encephalopathy or coma; encephalopathy associated with protein load; pregnancy or postpartum encephalopathy; unexplained mental retardation; history of elevated plasma ammonia or glutamine; history of cyclical vomiting and lethargy; episodic extreme irritability, ataxia; low BUN or protein avoidance; family history of UCD or unexplained infant deaths (particularly male); or signs or symptoms of UCD (hyperammonemia, encephalopathy, respiratory alkalosis). Hypothermia has been reported with valproic acid therapy; may or may not be associated with hyperammonemia; may also occur with concomitant topiramate therapy.

In vitro studies have suggested valproic acid stimulates the replication of HIV and CMV viruses under experimental conditions. The clinical consequence of this is unknown, but should be considered when monitoring affected patients.

Antiepileptics are associated with an increased risk of suicidal behavior/thoughts with use (regardless of indication); patients should be monitored for signs/symptoms of depression, suicidal tendencies, and other unusual behavior changes during therapy and instructed to inform their healthcare provider immediately if symptoms occur.

Use of Depacon® injection is not recommended for post-traumatic seizure prophylaxis following acute head trauma. Anticonvulsants should not be discontinued abruptly because of the possibility of increasing seizure frequency; valproic acid should be withdrawn gradually to minimize the potential of increased seizure frequency, unless safety concerns require a more rapid withdrawal. Concomitant use with carbapenem antibiotics may reduce valproic acid levels to subtherapeutic levels; monitor levels frequently and consider alternate therapy if levels drop significantly or lack of seizure control occurs. Concomitant use with clonazepam may induce absence status. Patients treated for bipolar disorder should be monitored closely for clinical worsening or suicidality; prescriptions should be written for the smallest quantity consistent with good patient care.

CNS depression may occur with valproic acid use. Patients must be cautioned about performing tasks which require mental alertness (operating machinery or driving). Effects with other sedative drugs or ethanol may be potentiated. Use with caution in the elderly.

Drug Interactions

Metabolism/Transport Effects For valproic acid: **Substrate** (minor) of CYP2A6, 2B6, 2C9, 2C19, 2E1; **Inhibits** CYP2C9 (weak), 2C19 (weak), 2D6 (weak), 3A4 (weak); **Induces** CYP2A6 (weak)

Avoid Concomitant Use There are no known interactions where it is recommended to avoid concomitant use.

Increased Effect/Toxicity

Valproic Acid may increase the levels/effects of: Barbiturates; Ethosuximide; LamoTRIgine; LORazepam; Paliperidone; Primidone; RisperiDONE; Rufinamide; Temozolomide; Tricyclic Antidepressants; Vorinostat; Zidovudine

The levels/effects of Valproic Acid may be increased by: ChlorproMAZINE; Felbamate; GuanFACINE; Salicylates; Topiramate

Decreased Effect

Valproic Acid may decrease the levels/effects of: CarBAMazepine; Fosphenytoin; OXcarbazepine; Phenytoin

The levels/effects of Valproic Acid may be decreased by: Barbiturates; CarBAMazepine; Carbapenems; Ethosuximide; Fosphenytoin; Methylfolate; Phenytoin; Primidone; Protease Inhibitors; Rifampin

Ethanol/Nutrition/Herb Interactions

Ethanol: Avoid ethanol (may increase CNS depression).

Food: Food may delay but does not affect the extent of absorption. Valproic acid serum concentrations may be decreased if taken with food. Milk has no effect on absorption.

Herb/Nutraceutical: Avoid evening primrose (seizure threshold decreased).

Dietary Considerations Valproic acid may cause GI upset; take with large amount of water or food to decrease GI upset. May need to split doses to avoid GI upset. Valproate sodium oral solution will generate valproic acid in carbonated beverages and may cause mouth and throat irritation; do not mix valproate sodium oral solution with carbonated beverages.

Pharmacodynamics/Kinetics

Half-life Elimination Increased in neonates and with liver disease; Children >2 months: 7-13 hours; Adults: 9-16 hours

Time to Peak Serum: Stavzor™: 2 hours

Pregnancy Risk Factor D

Lactation Enters breast milk/not recommended (AAP considers "compatible"; AAP 2001 update pending)

Breast-Feeding Considerations Breast milk concentrations of valproic acid have been reported as 1% to 10% of maternal concentration. The weight-adjusted dose to the infant has been calculated to be ~4%.

Dosage Forms

Capsule, softgel, oral: 250 mg
Depakene®: 250 mg

Capsule, softgel, delayed release, oral:
Stavzor™: 125 mg, 250 mg, 500 mg

Injection, solution [preservative free]: 100 mg/mL (5 mL)
Depacon®: 100 mg/mL (5 mL)

Solution, oral: 250 mg/5 mL (473 mL, 480 mL)

Syrup, oral: 250 mg/5 mL (5 mL, 10 mL, 473 mL, 480 mL)
Depakene®: 250 mg/5 mL (473 mL)

Valrubicin (val ROO bi sin)

U.S. Brand Names Valstar®

Canadian Brand Names Valtaxin®

Pharmacologic Category Antineoplastic Agent, Anthracycline

Use Intravesical therapy of BCG-refractory bladder carcinoma *in situ*

Local Anesthetic/Vasoconstrictor Precautions No information available to require special precautions

Effects on Dental Treatment No significant effects or complications reported

Effects on Bleeding Chemotherapy may result in significant myelosuppression, potentially including significant reduction in platelet counts and altered hemostasis. In patients who are under active treatment with these agents, medical consult is suggested.

Adverse Effects Note: In general, local adverse reactions occur during or shortly after instillation and resolve within 1-7 days.

>10%: Genitourinary: Bladder irritation (88%), urinary frequency (61%), urinary urgency (57%), dysuria (56%), bladder spasm (31%), hematuria (29%; gross: 1%), bladder pain (28%), urinary incontinence (22%), cystitis (15%), urinary tract infection (15%), urine red-tinged

1% to 10%:

Cardiovascular: Chest pain (3%), vasodilation (2%), peripheral edema (1%)
Central nervous system: Headache (4%), malaise (4%), dizziness (3%), fever (2%)
Dermatologic: Rash (3%)
Endocrine & metabolic: Hyperglycemia (1%)
Gastrointestinal: Abdominal pain (5%), nausea (5%), diarrhea (3%), vomiting (2%), flatulence (1%)
Genitourinary: Nocturia (7%), burning symptoms (5%), urinary retention (4%), urethral pain (3%), pelvic pain (1%), hematuria (microscopic) (3%)
Hematologic: Anemia (2%)
Neuromuscular & skeletal: Weakness (4%), back pain (3%), myalgia (1%)
Respiratory: Pneumonia (1%)

General Dosage Range Dosage adjustment recommended in patients who develop toxicities

Intravesical: *Adults:* 800 mg once weekly for 6 weeks

Mechanism of Action Blocks function of DNA topoisomerase II; inhibits DNA synthesis, causes extensive chromosomal damage, and arrests cell development; unlike other anthracyclines, does not appear to intercalate DNA; readily penetrates cells.

Pregnancy Risk Factor C

Valsartan (val SAR tan)

Related Information

Cardiovascular Diseases *on page* 1848

U.S. Brand Names Diovan®

Canadian Brand Names Diovan®; Ran-Valsartan; Sandoz-Valsartan; Teva-Valsartan

Generic Availability (U.S.) No

Pharmacologic Category Angiotensin II Receptor Blocker

Use Alone or in combination with other antihypertensive agents in the treatment of essential hypertension; reduction of cardiovascular mortality in patients with left ventricular dysfunction postmyocardial infarction; treatment of heart failure (NYHA Class II-IV)

Local Anesthetic/Vasoconstrictor Precautions No information available to require special precautions

Effects on Dental Treatment No significant effects or complications reported

Effects on Bleeding No information available to require special precautions

Adverse Effects

>10%:

Central nervous system: Dizziness (heart failure trials 17%)

Renal: BUN increased >50% (heart failure trials 17%)

1% to 10%:

Cardiovascular: Hypotension (heart failure trials 7%; MI trial 1%), postural hypotension (heart failure trials 2%), syncope (up to >1%)

Central nervous system: Dizziness (hypertension trial 2% to 8%), fatigue (heart failure trials 3%; hypertension trial 2%), postural dizziness (heart failure trials 2%), headache (heart failure trials >1%), vertigo (up to >1%)

Endocrine & metabolic: Serum potassium increased by >20% (4% to 10%), hyperkalemia (heart failure trials 2%)

Gastrointestinal: Diarrhea (heart failure trials 5%), abdominal pain (2%), nausea (heart failure trials >1%), upper abdominal pain (heart failure trials >1%)

Hematologic: Neutropenia (2%)

Neuromuscular & skeletal: Arthralgia (heart failure trials 3%), back pain (up to 3%)

Ocular: Blurred vision (heart failure trials >1%)

Renal: Creatinine doubled (MI trial 4%), creatinine increased >50% (heart failure trials 4%), renal dysfunction (up to >1%)

Respiratory: Cough (1% to 3%)

Miscellaneous: Viral infection (3%)

Dosage Oral:

Hypertension:

Children 6-16 years: Initial: 1.3 mg/kg once daily (maximum: 40 mg/day); dose may be increased to achieve desired effect; doses >2.7 mg/kg (maximum: 160 mg) have not been studied

Adults: Initial: 80 mg or 160 mg once daily (in patients who are not volume depleted); dose may be increased to achieve desired effect; maximum recommended dose: 320 mg/day

Heart failure: Adults: Initial: 40 mg twice daily; titrate dose to 80-160 mg twice daily, as tolerated; maximum daily dose: 320 mg

Left ventricular dysfunction after MI: Adults: Initial: 20 mg twice daily; titrate dose to target of 160 mg twice daily as tolerated; may initiate ≥12 hours following MI

Dosing adjustment in renal impairment:

Children: Use is not recommended if Cl_{cr} <30 mL/minute.

Adults: No dosage adjustment necessary if Cl_{cr} >10 mL/minute.

Dialysis: Not significantly removed

Dosing adjustment in hepatic impairment In mild-to-moderate liver disease no adjustment is needed. Use caution in patients with liver disease. Patients with mild-to-moderate chronic disease have twice the exposure as healthy volunteers.

Mechanism of Action Valsartan produces direct antagonism of the angiotensin II (AT2) receptors, unlike the ACE inhibitors. It displaces angiotensin II from the AT1 receptor and produces its blood pressure-lowering effects by antagonizing AT1-induced vasoconstriction, aldosterone release, catecholamine release, arginine vasopressin release, water intake, and hypertrophic responses. This action results in more efficient blockade of the cardiovascular effects of angiotensin II and fewer side effects than the ACE inhibitors.

Contraindications There are no contraindications listed in manufacturer's labeling.

Canadian labeling: Hypersensitivity to valsartan or any component of the formulation

Warnings/Precautions **[U.S. Boxed Warning]: Based on human data, drugs that act on the angiotensin system can cause injury and death to the developing fetus when used in the second and third trimesters. Angiotensin receptor blockers should be discontinued as soon as possible once pregnancy is detected.** May cause hyperkalemia; avoid potassium supplementation unless specifically required by healthcare provider. During the initiation of therapy, hypotension may occur, particularly in patients with heart failure or post-MI patients. Use extreme caution with concurrent administration of potassium-sparing diuretics or potassium supplements, in patients with mild-to-moderate hepatic dysfunction (adjust dose), in those who may be sodium/water depleted (eg, on high-dose diuretics), and in the elderly; correct depletion first.

Use caution with unstented unilateral/bilateral renal artery stenosis. When unstented bilateral renal artery stenosis is present, use is generally avoided due to the elevated risk of deterioration in renal function unless possible benefits outweigh risks. Use with caution with preexisting renal insufficiency; significant aortic/mitral stenosis. May be associated with deterioration of renal function and/or increases in serum creatinine, particularly in patients with low renal blood flow (eg, renal artery stenosis, heart failure) whose glomerular filtration rate (GFR) is dependent on efferent arteriolar vasoconstriction by angiotensin II. Use caution in patients with severe renal impairment or significant hepatic dysfunction. Monitor renal function closely in patients with severe heart failure; changes in renal function should be anticipated and dosage adjustments of valsartan or concomitant medications may be needed. Concurrent use of ACE inhibitors may increase the risk of clinically-significant adverse events (eg, renal dysfunction, hyperkalemia). In Canada, use is not approved in patients <18 years of age.

Drug Interactions

Metabolism/Transport Effects **Substrate** of SLCO1B1; **Inhibits** CYP2C9 (weak)

Avoid Concomitant Use There are no known interactions where it is recommended to avoid concomitant use.

Increased Effect/Toxicity

Valsartan may increase the levels/effects of: ACE Inhibitors; Amifostine; Antihypertensives; Hypotensive Agents; Lithium; Nonsteroidal Anti-Inflammatory Agents; Potassium-Sparing Diuretics; RiTUXimab

The levels/effects of Valsartan may be increased by: Diazoxide; Eltrombopag; Eplerenone; Herbs (Hypotensive Properties); MAO Inhibitors; Pentoxifylline; Phosphodiesterase 5 Inhibitors; Potassium Salts; Prostacyclin Analogues; Tolvaptan; Trimethoprim

Decreased Effect

The levels/effects of Valsartan may be decreased by: Herbs (Hypertensive Properties); Methylphenidate; Nonsteroidal Anti-Inflammatory Agents; Yohimbine

Ethanol/Nutrition/Herb Interactions

Food: Decreases the peak plasma concentration and extent of absorption by 50% and 40%, respectively.

Herb/Nutraceutical: Avoid bayberry, blue cohosh, cayenne, ephedra, ginger, ginseng (American), kola, licorice (may worsen hypertension). Avoid black cohosh, California poppy, coleus, golden seal, hawthorn, mistletoe, periwinkle, quinine, shepherd's purse (may have increased antihypertensive effect).

Dietary Considerations Avoid salt substitutes which contain potassium. May be taken with or without food.

Pharmacodynamics/Kinetics

Onset of Action ~2 hours

Duration of Action 24 hours

Half-life Elimination ~6 hours

Time to Peak Serum: 2-4 hours

Pregnancy Risk Factor D

Lactation Excretion in breast milk unknown/not recommended

Breast-Feeding Considerations It is not known if valsartan is found in breast milk; the manufacturer recommends discontinuing the drug or discontinuing nursing based on the importance of the drug to the mother.

Dosage Forms

Tablet, oral:

Diovan®: 40 mg, 80 mg, 160 mg, 320 mg

Valsartan and Hydrochlorothiazide

(val SAR tan & hye droe klor oh THYE a zide)

Related Information

Hydrochlorothiazide *on page 854*

Valsartan *on page 1699*

U.S. Brand Names Diovan HCT®

Canadian Brand Names Diovan HCT®; Sandoz Valsartan HCT

Pharmacologic Category Angiotensin II Receptor Blocker; Diuretic, Thiazide

Use Treatment of hypertension

Local Anesthetic/Vasoconstrictor Precautions No information available to require special precautions

Effects on Dental Treatment No significant effects or complications reported

Effects on Bleeding No information available to require special precautions

Adverse Effects Percentages reported with combination product; other reactions have been reported (see individual agents for additional information)

>10%: Renal: BUN increased (15%)

1% to 10%:

Cardiovascular: Hypotension (1%)

Central nervous system: Dizziness (6%; dose related)

Endocrine & metabolic: Hypokalemia (3%)

Renal: Creatinine increased (2%)
Respiratory: Nasopharyngitis (2%)

General Dosage Range Oral: *Adults:* Valsartan 80-160 mg and hydrochlorothiazide 12.5-25 mg once daily (maximum: 25 mg/day [hydrochlorothiazide]; 320 mg/day [valsartan])

Mechanism of Action

Valsartan produces direct antagonism of the angiotensin II (AT2) receptors, unlike the ACE inhibitors. It displaces angiotensin II from the AT1 receptor and produces its blood pressure-lowering effects by antagonizing AT1-induced vasoconstriction, aldosterone release, catecholamine release, arginine vasopressin release, water intake, and hypertrophic responses. This action results in more efficient blockade of the cardiovascular effects of angiotensin II and fewer side effects than the ACE inhibitors.

Hydrochlorothiazide inhibits sodium reabsorption in the distal tubules causing increased excretion of sodium and water as well as potassium and hydrogen ions

Pregnancy Risk Factor D

Vancomycin (van koe MYE sin)

U.S. Brand Names Vancocin®

Canadian Brand Names Vancocin®

Generic Availability (U.S.) Yes: Excludes capsule

Pharmacologic Category Glycopeptide

Use Treatment of patients with infections caused by staphylococcal species and streptococcal species; used orally for staphylococcal enterocolitis or for antibiotic-associated pseudomembranous colitis produced by *C. difficile*

Unlabeled/Investigational Use Bacterial endophthalmitis; treatment of infections caused by gram-positive organisms in patients who have serious allergies to beta-lactam agents; treatment of beta-lactam resistant gram-positive infections

Local Anesthetic/Vasoconstrictor Precautions No information available to require special precautions

Effects on Dental Treatment Key adverse event(s) related to dental treatment: Bitter taste. "Red man syndrome", characterized by skin rash and hypotension, is not an allergic reaction but rather is associated with too rapid infusion of the drug. To alleviate or prevent the reaction, infuse vancomycin at a rate of ≥30 minutes for each 500 mg of drug being administered (eg, 1 g over ≥60 minutes); 1.5 g over ≥90 minutes.

Effects on Bleeding No information available to require special precautions

Adverse Effects

Oral:
- >10%: Gastrointestinal: Bitter taste, nausea, vomiting
- 1% to 10%:
  - Central nervous system: Chills, drug fever
  - Hematologic: Eosinophilia

Parenteral:
- >10%:
  - Cardiovascular: Hypotension accompanied by flushing
  - Dermatologic: Erythematous rash on face and upper body (red neck or red man syndrome - infusion rate related)
- 1% to 10%:
  - Central nervous system: Chills, drug fever
  - Dermatologic: Rash
  - Hematologic: Eosinophilia, reversible neutropenia
  - Local: Phlebitis

Dental Usual Dosage Prophylaxis against infective endocarditis: I.V.:

Infants >1 month and Children:

Dental, oral, or upper respiratory tract surgery: 20 mg/kg 1 hour prior to the procedure. **Note:** American Heart Association (AHA) guidelines now recommend prophylaxis only in patients undergoing invasive procedures and in whom underlying cardiac conditions may predispose to a higher risk of adverse outcomes should infection occur.

GI/GU procedure: 20 mg/kg plus gentamicin 2 mg/kg 1 hour prior to surgery. **Note:** As of April 2007, routine prophylaxis no longer recommended by the AHA.

Adults:

Dental, oral, or upper respiratory tract surgery: 1 g 1 hour before surgery. **Note:** AHA guidelines now recommend prophylaxis only in patients undergoing invasive procedures and in whom underlying cardiac conditions may predispose to a higher risk of adverse outcomes should infection occur

GI/GU procedure: 1 g plus 1.5 mg/kg gentamicin 1 hour prior to surgery. **Note:** As of April 2007, routine prophylaxis no longer recommended by the AHA.

Dosage

Usual dosage range:

Infants >1 month and Children: I.V.: 10-15 mg/kg every 6 hours

Adults: Initial intravenous dosing should be based on actual body weight; subsequent dosing adjusted based on serum trough vancomycin concentrations.

I.V.: 2-3 g/day (or 30-60 mg/kg/day) in divided doses every 8-12 hours (Rybak, 2009); **Note:** Dose requires adjustment in renal impairment

Oral: 500-2000 mg/day in divided doses every 6 hours

Indication-specific dosing:

Catheter-related infections: Adults: Antibiotic lock technique (Mermel, 2009): 2 mg/mL ± 10 units heparin/mL **or** 2.5 mg/mL ± 2500 **or** 5000 units heparin/mL **or** 5 mg/mL ± 5000 units heparin/mL (preferred regimen); instill into catheter port with a volume sufficient to fill the catheter (2-5 mL). **Note:** May use SWFI/NS or D_5W as diluents. Do not mix with any other solutions. Dwell times generally should not exceed 48 hours before renewal of lock solution. Remove lock solution prior to catheter use, then replace.

C. difficile **-associated diarrhea (CDAD):**

Infants >1 month and Children: Oral: 40 mg/kg/day in 3-4 divided doses added to fluids for 7-10 days (maximum: 2000 mg/day)

Adults: Oral:

Manufacturer recommendations: 500-2000 mg/day in 3-4 divided doses for 7-10 days (usual dose: 125-500 mg every 6 hours)

IDSA guideline recommendations: Severe infection: 125 mg 4 times/day for 10-14 days; Severe, complicated infection: 500 mg 4 times/day with or without concurrent I.V. metronidazole. May consider vancomycin retention enema (in patients with complete ileus) (Cohen, 2010).

Complicated infections in seriously-ill patients: Adults: I.V.: Loading dose: 25-30 mg/kg (based on actual body weight) may be used to rapidly achieve target concentration; then 15-20 mg/kg/dose every 8-12 hours (Rybak, 2009)

Enterocolitis *(S. aureus):*

Infants >1 months and Children: Oral: 40 mg/kg/day in 3-4 divided doses added to fluids for 7-10 days (maximum: 2000 mg/day)

Adults: Oral: 500-2000 mg/day in 3-4 divided doses for 7-10 days (usual dose: 125-500 mg every 6 hours)

Endophthalmitis (unlabeled use): Adults: Intravitreal: Usual dose: 1 mg/0.1 mL NS instilled into vitreum; may repeat administration if necessary in 3-4 days, usually in combination with ceftazidime or an aminoglycoside. **Note:** Some clinicians have recommended using a lower dose of 0.2 mg/0.1 mL, based on concerns for retinotoxicity.

Hospital-acquired pneumonia (HAP): Adults: I.V.: 15-20 mg/kg/dose every 8-12 hours (American Thoracic Society [ATS], 2005 guidelines; Rybak 2009)

Meningitis:

Infants >1 month and Children:

I.V.: 15 mg/kg every 6 hours (Tunkel, 2004)

Intrathecal, intraventricular (unlabeled route): 5-20 mg/day (Tunkel, 2004)

Adults:

I.V.: 30-60 mg/kg/day in divided doses every 8-12 hours (Rybak, 2009) **or** 500-750 mg every 6 hours. **Note:** For PCN-resistant *Streptococcus pneumoniae* (MIC ≥2 mcg/mL), combine with a third-generation cephalosporin.

Intrathecal, intraventricular (unlabeled route): 5-20 mg/day

MRSA infections:

Bacteremia (Liu, 2011): I.V.:

Children: 15 mg/kg/dose every 6 hours for 2-6 weeks depending on severity

Adults: 15-20 mg/kg/dose every 8-12 hours for 2-6 weeks depending on severity

Brain abscess, subdural empyema, spinal epidural abscess (Liu, 2011): I.V.:

Children.: 15 mg/kg/dose every 6 hours for 4-6 weeks (some experts combine with rifampin)

Adults: 15-20 mg/kg/dose every 8-12 hours for 4-6 weeks (some experts combine with rifampin)

Complicated skin and skin structure infections (Liu, 2011): I.V.:

Children: 15 mg/kg/dose every 6 hours for 7-14 days

Adults: 15-20 mg/kg/dose every 8-12 hours for 7-14 days

Endocarditis, native valve (Liu, 2011): I.V.:

Children: 15 mg/kg/dose every 6 hours for 6 weeks

Adults: 15-20 mg/kg/dose every 8-12 hours for 6 weeks

Endocarditis, prosthetic valve (Liu, 2011): I.V.:

Children: 15 mg/kg/dose every 6 hours for at least 6 weeks

Adults: 15-20 mg/kg/dose every 8-12 hours for at least 6 weeks (combine with rifampin for the entire duration of therapy and gentamicin for the first 2 weeks)

Meningitis (Liu, 2011): I.V.:
Children: 15 mg/kg/dose every 6 hours for 2 weeks (some experts combine with rifampin)
Adults: 15-20 mg/kg/dose every 8-12 hours for 2 weeks (some experts combine with rifampin)
Osteomyelitis (Liu, 2011): I.V.:
Children: 15 mg/kg/dose every 6 hours for 4-6 weeks
Adults: 15-20 mg/kg/dose every 8-12 hours for a minimum of 8 weeks (some experts combine with rifampin)
Pneumonia (Liu, 2011): I.V.:
Children: 15 mg/kg/dose every 6 hours for 7-21 days depending on severity
Adults: 15-20 mg/kg/dose every 8-12 hours for 7-21 days depending on severity
Septic arthritis (Liu, 2011): I.V.:
Children: 15 mg/kg/dose every 6 hours for minimum of 3-4 weeks
Adults: 15-20 mg/kg/dose every 8-12 hours for 3-4 weeks
Septic thrombosis of cavernous or dural venous sinus (Liu, 2011): I.V.:
Children: 15 mg/kg/dose every 6 hours for 4-6 weeks (some experts combine with rifampin)
Adults: 15-20 mg/kg/dose every 8-12 hours for 4-6 weeks (some experts combine with rifampin)

Prophylaxis against infective endocarditis: I.V.:
Children:
Dental, oral, or upper respiratory tract surgery: 20 mg/kg/dose administered 1 hour prior to the procedure. **Note:** American Heart Association (AHA) guidelines recommend prophylaxis only in patients undergoing invasive procedures and in whom underlying cardiac conditions may predispose to a higher risk of adverse outcomes should infection occur.
GI/GU procedure: 20 mg/kg (plus gentamicin 1.5 mg/kg) administered 1 hour prior to surgery. **Note:** Routine prophylaxis no longer recommended by the AHA.
Adults:
Dental, oral, or upper respiratory tract surgery: 1 g 1 hour before surgery. **Note:** AHA guidelines now recommend prophylaxis only in patients undergoing invasive procedures and in whom underlying cardiac conditions may predispose to a higher risk of adverse outcomes should infection occur
GI/GU procedure: 1 g plus 1.5 mg/kg gentamicin 1 hour prior to surgery. **Note:** As of April 2007, routine prophylaxis no longer recommended by the AHA.

Susceptible (MIC ≤1 mcg/mL; Rybak, 2009) gram-positive infections: I.V.:
Infants >1 month and Children: 10 mg/kg every 6 hours (manufacturer recommendations) **or** 15 mg/kg every 6 hours (Liu, 2011)
Adults: 15-20 mg/kg/dose (usual: 750-1500 mg) every 8-12 hours
Note: If MIC ≥2 mcg/mL, alternative therapies are recommended.

Dosing interval in renal impairment (vancomycin levels should be monitored in patients with any renal impairment):
Cl_{cr} >50 mL/minute: Start with 15-20 mg/kg/dose (usual: 750-1500 mg) every 8-12 hours
Cl_{cr} 20-49 mL/minute: Start with 15-20 mg/kg/dose (usual: 750-1500 mg) every 24 hours
Cl_{cr} <20 mL/minute: Will need longer intervals; determine by serum concentration monitoring
Note: In the critically-ill patient with renal insufficiency, the initial loading dose (25-30 mg/kg) should not be reduced. However, subsequent dosage adjustments should be made based on renal function and trough serum concentrations.

Dialysis: Variable, depending on method; poorly dialyzable by conventional hemodialysis (0% to 5%). Use of high-flux membranes and continuous renal replacement therapy (CRRT) increases vancomycin clearance, and generally requires replacement dosing.
Hemodialysis (HD): Following loading dose of 15-20 mg/kg, give 500 mg to 1 g after each dialysis session, depending on factors such as HD membrane type and flow rate; monitor levels closely.
Continuous ambulatory peritoneal dialysis (CAPD):
Administration via CAPD fluid: 15-30 mg/L (15-30 mcg/mL) of CAPD fluid
Systemic: 1 g loading dose, followed by 500 mg to 1 g every 48-72 hours with close monitoring of levels
Continuous renal replacement therapy (CRRT): Removal of vancomycin is highly dependent on the method of replacement, filter type, and flow rate. Appropriate dosing requires close monitoring of levels in relation to target trough. The following are general recommendations only (Heintz, 2009; Trotman, 2005), and require consideration of the aforementioned parameters.

CVVH: Following loading dose of 15-25 mg/kg, give 1 g every 48 hours **or** 10-15 mg/kg every 24-48 hours

CVVHD or CVVHDF: Following loading dose of 15-25 mg/kg, give 1 g every 24 hours **or** 10-15 mg/kg every 24 hours (for CVVHD) **or** 7.5-10 mg/kg every 12 hours (CVVHDF)

Mechanism of Action Inhibits bacterial cell wall synthesis by blocking glycopeptide polymerization through binding tightly to D-alanyl-D-alanine portion of cell wall precursor

Contraindications Hypersensitivity to vancomycin or any component of the formulation; avoid in patients with previous severe hearing loss

Warnings/Precautions May cause nephrotoxicity although limited data suggest direct causal relationship; usual risk factors include pre-existing renal impairment, concomitant nephrotoxic medications, advanced age, and dehydration. If multiple sequential (≥2) serum creatinine concentrations demonstrate an increase of 0.5 mg/dL or ≥50% increase from baseline (whichever is greater) in the absence of an alternative explanation, the patient should be identified as having vancomycin-induced nephrotoxicity (Rybak, 2009). Discontinue treatment if signs of nephrotoxicity occur; renal damage is usually reversible. May cause neurotoxicity; usual risk factors include pre-existing renal impairment, concomitant neuro-/nephrotoxic medications, advanced age, and dehydration. Ototoxicity, although rarely associated with monotherapy, is proportional to the amount of drug given and the duration of treatment. Tinnitus or vertigo may be indications of vestibular injury and impending bilateral irreversible damage. Discontinue treatment if signs of ototoxicity occur. Prolonged therapy (>1 week) or total doses exceeding 25 g may increase the risk of neutropenia; prompt reversal of neutropenia is expected after discontinuation of therapy. Prolonged use may result in fungal or bacterial superinfection, including *C. difficile*-associated diarrhea (CDAD) and pseudomembranous colitis; CDAD has been observed >2 months postantibiotic treatment. Use with caution in patients with renal impairment or those receiving other nephrotoxic or ototoxic drugs; dosage modification required in patients with impaired renal function (especially elderly). Rapid I.V. administration may result in hypotension, flushing, erythema, urticaria, and/or pruritus. Oral vancomycin is only indicated for the treatment of pseudomembranous colitis due to *C. difficile* and enterocolitis due to *S. aureus* and is not effective for systemic infections; parenteral vancomycin is not effective for the treatment of colitis due to *C. difficile* and enterocolitis due to *S. aureus*. **Note:** The Infectious Disease Society of America (IDSA) recommends the use of oral metronidazole for initial treatment of mild-to-moderate *C. difficile* infection and the use of oral vancomycin for initial treatment of severe *C. difficile* infection (Cohen, 2010).

Drug Interactions

Avoid Concomitant Use

Avoid concomitant use of Vancomycin with any of the following: BCG; Gallium Nitrate

Increased Effect/Toxicity

Vancomycin may increase the levels/effects of: Aminoglycosides; Colistimethate; Gallium Nitrate; Neuromuscular-Blocking Agents

The levels/effects of Vancomycin may be increased by: Nonsteroidal Anti-Inflammatory Agents

Decreased Effect

Vancomycin may decrease the levels/effects of: BCG; Typhoid Vaccine

Dietary Considerations May be taken with food.

Pharmacodynamics/Kinetics

Half-life Elimination Biphasic: Terminal:

Newborns: 6-10 hours
Infants and Children 3 months to 4 years: 4 hours
Children >3 years: 2.2-3 hours
Adults: 5-11 hours; significantly prolonged with renal impairment
End-stage renal disease: 200-250 hours

Time to Peak Serum: I.V.: Immediately after completion of infusion

Pregnancy Risk Factor B (oral); C (injection)

Lactation Enters breast milk/not recommended

Breast-Feeding Considerations Small amounts of vancomycin are excreted in human milk and use during breast-feeding is not recommended by the manufacturer. If given orally to the mother, the minimal systemic absorption of the dose would limit the amount available to pass into the milk. If given intravenously, the small amount that distributes to the milk would not be expected to cause systemic toxicity due to the lack of GI absorption. Nondose-related effects could include modification of bowel flora.

Dosage Forms

Capsule, oral:

Vancocin®: 125 mg, 250 mg

Infusion, premixed iso-osmotic dextrose solution: 500 mg (100 mL); 750 mg (150 mL); 1 g (200 mL)

Injection, powder for reconstitution: 500 mg, 750 mg, 1 g, 5 g, 10 g

References

Wilson W, Taubert KA, Gewitz M, et al, "Prevention of Infective Endocarditis: Guidelines From the American Heart Association: A Guideline From the American Heart Association Rheumatic Fever, Endocarditis, and Kawasaki Disease Committee, Council on Cardiovascular Disease in the Young, and the Council on Clinical Cardiology, Council on Cardiovascular Surgery and Anesthesia, and the Quality of Care and Outcomes Research Interdisciplinary Working Group," *Circulation*, 2007, 116(15):1736-54. Available at http://circ.ahajournals.org/cgi/reprint/CIRCULATIONAHA.106.183095v1; last accessed July 26, 2007.

Vandetanib (van DET a nib)

Related Information

Clinical Risk Related to Drugs Prolonging QT Interval *on page 1872*

Pharmacologic Category Antineoplastic Agent, Tyrosine Kinase Inhibitor; Epidermal Growth Factor Receptor (EGFR) Inhibitor; Vascular Endothelial Growth Factor (VEGF) Inhibitor

Use Treatment of metastatic or unresectable locally advanced medullary thyroid cancer (symptomatic or progressive)

Local Anesthetic/Vasoconstrictor Precautions Hypertension can occur with the use of this drug, particularly early in the treatment course. Monitor for hypertension prior to using local anesthetic with vasoconstrictor; medical consult if necessary.

Vandetanib is one of the drugs confirmed to prolong the QT interval and is accepted as having a risk of causing torsade de pointes. The risk of drug-induced torsade de pointes is extremely low when a single QT interval prolonging drug is prescribed. In terms of epinephrine, it is not known what effect vasoconstrictors in the local anesthetic regimen will have in patients with a known history of congenital prolonged QT interval or in patients taking any medication that prolongs the QT interval. Until more information is obtained, it is suggested that the clinician consult with the physician prior to the use of a vasoconstrictor in suspected patients, and that the vasoconstrictor (epinephrine, mepivacaine and levonordefrin [Carbocaine® 2% with Neo-Cobefrin®]) be used with caution.

Effects on Dental Treatment Key adverse event(s) related to dental treatment: Xerostomia (normal salivary flow resumes upon discontinuation), mucositis/stomatitis, taste perversion, and oral pain.

Effects on Bleeding Chemotherapy may result in significant myelosuppression, potentially including significant reduction in platelet counts and altered hemostasis. In patients who are under active treatment with these agents, medical consult is suggested.

Adverse Effects

>10%:

Cardiovascular: Hypertension (33%; grades 3/4: 9%), QT prolongation (14%; grades 3/4: 8%)

Central nervous system: Headache (26%), fatigue (24%), insomnia (13%)

Dermatologic: Rash (53%; grades 3/4: 5%), dermatitis acneiform/acne (35%; grades 3/4: 1%), dry skin (15%), photosensitivity (13%), pruritus (11%)

Endocrine & metabolic: Hypocalcemia (11% to 57%), hypoglycemia (24%)

Gastrointestinal: Diarrhea/colitis (57%; grades 3/4: 11%), nausea (33%), abdominal pain (21%), appetite decreased (21%), vomiting (15%), dyspepsia (11%)

Hematologic: Leukopenia (19%), anemia (13%; grades 3/4: <1%), hemorrhage (13% to 14%)

Hepatic: ALT increased (51%), bilirubin increased (13%)

Neuromuscular & skeletal: Weakness (15%)

Renal: Creatinine increased (16%)

Respiratory: Cough (11%), nasopharyngitis (11%)

1% to 10%:

Cardiovascular: Cardiac failure (2%)

Central nervous system: Depression (10%)

Endocrine & metabolic: Hypercalcemia (7%), hypomagnesemia (7%), hyperkalemia (6%), hypokalemia (6%), hyperglycemia (5%), hypermagnesemia (3%)

Gastrointestinal: Weight loss (10%)

Hematologic: Neutropenia (10%; grades 3/4: <1%), thrombocytopenia (9%)

Ocular: Blurred vision (9%)

Renal: Proteinuria (10%)

Respiratory: Aspiration pneumonia (2%), respiratory arrest (2%), respiratory failure (2%)

Miscellaneous: Sepsis (2%)

Mechanism of Action Multikinase inhibitor; inhibits tyrosine kinases including epidermal growth factor reception (EGFR), vascular endothelial growth factor (VEGF), rearranged during transfection (RET), protein tyrosine kinase 6 (BRK), TIE2, EPH kinase receptors and SRC kinase receptors, selectively blocking intracellular signaling, angiogenesis and cellular proliferation

Pharmacodynamics/Kinetics

Half-life Elimination 19 days

Time to Peak 6 hours (range: 4-10 hours)

Pregnancy Risk Factor D

Prescribing and Access Restrictions As a requirement of the REMS program, access to vandetanib is restricted. Vandetanib is approved for marketing under a Food and Drug Administration (FDA) approved, risk management program, and through a restricted distribution program, the Vandetanib REMS Program (1-800-236-9933). Prescribers and pharmacies must be certified with the program to prescribe or dispense vandetanib.

Dental Comment Vandetanib is known to prolong the QT interval. The QT interval is measured as the time and distance between the Q point of the QRS complex and the end of the T wave in the ECG tracing. After adjustment for heart rate, the QT interval is defined as prolonged if it is more than 450 msec in men and 460 msec in women. A long QT syndrome was first described in the 1950s and 60s as a congenital syndrome involving QT interval prolongation and syncope and sudden death. Some of the congenital long QT syndromes were characterized by a peculiar electrocardiographic appearance of the QRS complex involving a premature atria beat followed by a pause, then a subsequent sinus beat showing marked QT prolongation and deformity. This type of cardiac arrhythmia was originally termed "torsade de pointes" (translated from the French as "twisting of the points"). Vandetanib is considered as having a risk of causing torsade de pointes. Since it is not known what effect vasoconstrictors in the local anesthetic regimen will have in patients with a known history of congenital prolonged QT interval or in patients taking any medication that prolongs the QT interval, a medical consult is suggested.

Vardenafil (var DEN a fil)

U.S. Brand Names Levitra®; Staxyn™

Canadian Brand Names Levitra®

Generic Availability (U.S.) No

Pharmacologic Category Phosphodiesterase-5 Enzyme Inhibitor

Use Treatment of erectile dysfunction (ED)

Local Anesthetic/Vasoconstrictor Precautions No information available to require special precautions

Effects on Dental Treatment No significant effects or complications reported

Effects on Bleeding No information available to require special precautions

Adverse Effects

>10%:

Cardiovascular: Flushing (8% to 11%)

Central nervous system: Headache (14% to 15%)

2% to 10%:

Central nervous system: Dizziness (2%)

Gastrointestinal: Dyspepsia (3% to 4%), nausea (2%)

Neuromuscular & skeletal: Back pain (2%), CPK increased (2%)

Respiratory: Rhinitis (9%), nasal congestion (3%), sinusitis (3%)

Miscellaneous: Flu-like syndrome (3%)

Dosage Note: Oral disintegrating tablets should not be used interchangeably with film-coated tablets; patients requiring a dose other than 10 mg should use the film-coated tablets.

Oral: Erectile dysfunction:

Adults:

Film-coated tablet (Levitra®): 10 mg 60 minutes prior to sexual activity; dosing range: 5-20 mg; to be given as one single dose and not given more than once daily

Oral disintegrating tablet (Staxyn™): 10 mg 60 minutes prior to sexual activity; maximum: 10 mg/day

Elderly ≥65 years: Initial: 5 mg 60 minutes prior to sexual activity; to be given as one single dose and not given more than once daily

Dosing adjustment with concomitant medications:

Alpha-blocker (dose should be stable at time of vardenafil initiation):

Film-coated tablet (Levitra®): Initial vardenafil dose: 5 mg/24 hours; if an alpha-blocker is added to vardenafil therapy, it should be initiated at the smallest possible dose and titrated carefully.

Oral disintegrating tablet (Staxyn™): Do not use to initiate therapy. Initial therapy should be with film-coated tablets at lower doses. Patients who have previously used film-coated tablets may be switched to oral disintegrating tablets as recommended by healthcare provider.

Film-coated tablet (Levitra®):

Atazanavir: Maximum vardenafil dose: 2.5 mg/24 hours

Clarithromycin: Maximum vardenafil dose: 2.5 mg/24 hours

Darunavir: Maximum vardenafil dose: 2.5 mg/72 hours

Erythromycin: Maximum vardenafil dose: 5 mg/24 hours

Fosamprenavir: Maximum vardenafil dose: 2.5 mg/24 hours

Fosamprenavir/ritonavir: Maximum vardenafil dose: 2.5 mg/72 hours

Indinavir: Maximum vardenafil dose: 2.5 mg/24 hours

Itraconazole:

200 mg/day: Maximum vardenafil dose: 5 mg/24 hours

400 mg/day: Maximum vardenafil dose: 2.5 mg/24 hours

Ketoconazole:

200 mg/day: Maximum vardenafil dose: 5 mg/24 hours

400 mg/day: Maximum vardenafil dose: 2.5 mg/24 hours

Lopinavir/ritonavir: Maximum vardenafil dose: 2.5 mg/72 hours

Nelfinavir: Maximum vardenafil dose: 2.5 mg/24 hours

Ritonavir: Maximum vardenafil dose: 2.5 mg/72 hours

Saquinavir: Maximum vardenafil dose: 2.5 mg/24 hours

Tipranavir: Maximum vardenafil dose: 2.5 mg/72 hours

Oral disintegrating tablet (Staxyn™): Concurrent use not recommended with potent or moderate CYP3A4 inhibitors (atazanavir, clarithromycin, erythromycin, indinavir, itraconazole, ketoconazole, ritonavir, saquinavir)

Dosage adjustment in renal impairment: Dose adjustment not needed for mild, moderate, or severe impairment; use not recommended in patients on hemodialysis

Dosage adjustment in hepatic impairment:

Child-Pugh class A: No adjustment required

Child-Pugh class B:

Film-coated tablet (Levitra®): Initial: 5 mg 60 minutes prior to sexual activity (maximum dose: 10 mg); to be given as one single dose and not given more than once daily

Oral disintegrating tablet (Staxyn™): Use not recommended

Child-Pugh class C: Has not been studied; use is not recommended by the manufacturer

Mechanism of Action Does not directly cause penile erections, but affects the response to sexual stimulation. The physiologic mechanism of erection of the penis involves release of nitric oxide (NO) in the corpus cavernosum during sexual stimulation. NO then activates the enzyme guanylate cyclase, which results in increased levels of cyclic guanosine monophosphate (cGMP), producing smooth muscle relaxation and inflow of blood to the corpus cavernosum. Vardenafil enhances the effect of NO by inhibiting phosphodiesterase type 5 (PDE-5), which is responsible for degradation of cGMP in the corpus cavernosum; when sexual stimulation causes local release of NO, inhibition of PDE-5 by vardenafil causes increased levels of cGMP in the corpus cavernosum, resulting in smooth muscle relaxation and inflow of blood to the corpus cavernosum; at recommended doses, it has no effect in the absence of sexual stimulation.

Contraindications Hypersensitivity to vardenafil or any component of the formulation; concurrent (regular or intermittent) use of organic nitrates in any form (eg, nitroglycerin, isosorbide dinitrate)

Warnings/Precautions There is a degree of cardiac risk associated with sexual activity; therefore, physicians may wish to consider the patient's cardiovascular status prior to initiating any treatment for erectile dysfunction. Use caution in patients with anatomical deformation of the penis (angulation, cavernosal fibrosis, or Peyronie's disease) and in patients who have conditions which may predispose them to priapism (sickle cell anemia, multiple myeloma, leukemia). Instruct patients to seek immediate medical attention if erection persists >4 hours.

Use is not recommended in patients with hypotension (<90/50 mm Hg); uncontrolled hypertension (>170/100 mm Hg); unstable angina or angina during intercourse; life-threatening arrhythmias, stroke, or MI within the last 6 months; cardiac failure or coronary artery disease causing unstable angina. Safety and efficacy have not been studied in these patients. Use caution in patients with left ventricular outflow obstruction (eg, aortic stenosis). Use caution with alpha-blockers, effective CYP3A4 inhibitors, the elderly, or those with hepatic impairment (Child-Pugh class B); dosage adjustment is needed.

Rare cases of nonarteritic ischemic optic neuropathy (NAION) have been reported; risk may be increased with history of vision loss. Other risk factors for NAION include heart disease, diabetes, hypertension, smoking, age >50 years, or history of certain eye problems. Sudden decrease or loss of hearing has been reported rarely; hearing changes may be accompanied by tinnitus and dizziness.

Safety and efficacy have not been studied in patients with the following conditions, therefore, use in these patients is not recommended at this time: Congenital QT prolongation, patients taking medications known to prolong the QT interval (avoid use in patients taking Class Ia or III antiarrhythmics); severe hepatic impairment (Child-Pugh class C); end-stage renal disease requiring dialysis; retinitis pigmentosa or other degenerative retinal disorders. The safety and efficacy of vardenafil with other treatments for erectile dysfunction have not been studied and are not recommended as combination therapy. Concomitant use with all forms of nitrates is contraindicated. If nitrate administration is medically necessary, it is not known when nitrates can be safely administered following the use of vardenafil; the ACC/AHA 2007 guidelines support administration of nitrates only if 24 hours have elapsed. Potential underlying causes of erectile dysfunction should be evaluated prior to treatment. Some products may contain phylalanine. Some products may contain sorbitol; do not use in patients with fructose intolerance.

Drug Interactions

Metabolism/Transport Effects **Substrate** of CYP2C (minor), 3A4 (major)

Avoid Concomitant Use

Avoid concomitant use of Vardenafil with any of the following: Amyl Nitrite; Phosphodiesterase 5 Inhibitors; Vasodilators (Organic Nitrates)

Increased Effect/Toxicity

Vardenafil may increase the levels/effects of: Alpha1-Blockers; Amyl Nitrite; Antihypertensives; Bosentan; Phosphodiesterase 5 Inhibitors; Vasodilators (Organic Nitrates)

The levels/effects of Vardenafil may be increased by: Antifungal Agents (Azole Derivatives, Systemic); Conivaptan; CYP3A4 Inhibitors (Moderate); CYP3A4 Inhibitors (Strong); Dasatinib; Macrolide Antibiotics; Protease Inhibitors; Sapropterin

Decreased Effect

The levels/effects of Vardenafil may be decreased by: Bosentan; Etravirine; Tocilizumab

Ethanol/Nutrition/Herb Interactions Food: High-fat meals decrease maximum serum concentration 18% to 50%. Serum concentrations/toxicity may be increased with grapefruit juice; avoid concurrent use.

Dietary Considerations May take with or without food. Avoid grapefruit juice. Some products may contain phenylalanine. Some products may contain sorbitol; do not use in patients with fructose intolerance.

Pharmacodynamics/Kinetics

Onset of Action ~60 minutes

Half-life Elimination Terminal: Vardenafil and metabolite: 3-6 hours

Time to Peak Plasma: 0.5-2 hours

Pregnancy Risk Factor B

Lactation Excretion in breast milk unknown/not indicated for use in women.

Dosage Forms

Tablet, oral:

Levitra®: 2.5 mg, 5 mg, 10 mg, 20 mg

Tablet, orally disintegrating, oral:

Staxyn™: 10 mg

Varenicline (var e NI kleen)

U.S. Brand Names Chantix®

Canadian Brand Names Champix®

Generic Availability (U.S.) No

Pharmacologic Category Partial Nicotine Agonist; Smoking Cessation Aid

Use Treatment to aid in smoking cessation

Local Anesthetic/Vasoconstrictor Precautions No information available to require special precautions

Effects on Dental Treatment Key adverse event(s) related to dental treatment: Xerostomia (normal salivary flow resumes upon discontinuation).

Effects on Bleeding No information available to require special precautions

Adverse Effects

>10%:

Central nervous system: Insomnia (18% to 19%), headache (15% to 19%), abnormal dreams (9% to 13%)

Gastrointestinal: Nausea (16% to 40%; dose related)

1% to 10%:

Central nervous system: Malaise (≤7%), sleep disorder (≤5%), somnolence (3%), nightmares (1% to 2%), lethargy (1% to 2%)

Dermatologic: Rash (≤3%)

Gastrointestinal: Flatulence (6% to 9%), constipation (5% to 8%), abnormal taste (5% to 8%), abdominal pain (≤7%), xerostomia (≤6%), dyspepsia (5%), vomiting (≤5%), appetite increased (3% to 4%), anorexia (≤2%), gastroesophageal reflux (1%)

Respiratory: Upper respiratory tract disorder (5% to 7%), dyspnea (≤2%), rhinorrhea (≤1%)

Dosage Oral: Adults:

Initial:

Days 1-3: 0.5 mg once daily

Days 4-7: 0.5 mg twice daily

Maintenance (≥ Day 8): 1 mg twice daily

Note: Start 1 week before target quit date. Patients who cannot tolerate adverse events may require temporary (or permanent) reduction in dose. If patient successfully quits smoking at the end of the 12 weeks, may continue for another 12 weeks to help maintain success. If not successful in first 12 weeks, then stop medication and reassess factors contributing to failure.

Dosage adjustment for toxicity: Lower dose for a period of time, then may increase dose again or remain on lower dose

Dosage adjustment in renal impairment:

Cl_{cr} ≥30 mL/minute: No adjustment required

Cl_{cr} <30 mL/minute: Initial: 0.5 mg once daily; maximum dose: 0.5 mg twice daily

Hemodialysis: Maximum dose: 0.5 mg once daily

Dosage adjustment in hepatic impairment: No adjustment required

Mechanism of Action Partial neuronal α_4 β_2 nicotinic receptor agonist; prevents nicotine stimulation of mesolimbic dopamine system associated with nicotine addiction. Also binds to 5 HT_3 receptor (significance not determined) with moderate affinity. Varenicline stimulates dopamine activity but to a much smaller degree than nicotine does, resulting in decreased craving and withdrawal symptoms.

Contraindications Known history of serious hypersensitivity or skin reactions to varenicline

Warnings/Precautions [U.S. Boxed Warning]: Serious neuropsychiatric events (including depression, suicidal thoughts, and suicide) have been reported with use; some cases may have been complicated by symptoms of nicotine withdrawal following smoking cessation. Smoking cessation (with or without treatment) is associated with nicotine withdrawal symptoms and the exacerbation of underlying psychiatric illness; however, some of the behavioral disturbances were reported in treated patients who continued to smoke. Neuropsychiatric symptoms (eg, mood disturbances, psychosis, hostility) have occurred in patients with and without pre-existing psychiatric disease; many cases resolved following therapy discontinuation although in some cases, symptoms persisted. Monitor all patients for behavioral changes and psychiatric symptoms (eg, agitation, depression, suicidal behavior, suicidal ideation); inform patients to discontinue treatment and contact their healthcare provider immediately if they experience any behavioral and/or mood changes. **[U.S. Boxed Warning]: Before prescribing, the risks of serious neuropsychiatric events must be weighed against the immediate and long term benefits of smoking abstinence for each patient.**

Hypersensitivity reactions (including angioedema) and rare cases of serious skin reactions (including Stevens-Johnson syndrome and erythema multiforme) have been reported. Patients should be instructed to discontinue use and contact healthcare provider if signs/symptoms occur. Dose-dependent nausea may occur; both transient and persistent nausea has been reported. Dosage reduction may be considered for intolerable nausea. May cause sedation, which may impair physical or mental abilities; patients must be cautioned about performing tasks which require mental alertness (eg, operating machinery or driving).

Use caution in renal dysfunction; dosage adjustment required. Safety and efficacy of varenicline with other smoking cessation therapies have not been established; increased adverse events when used concurrently with nicotine replacement therapy.

Drug Interactions

Avoid Concomitant Use There are no known interactions where it is recommended to avoid concomitant use.

Increased Effect/Toxicity There are no known significant interactions involving an increase in effect.

Decreased Effect There are no known significant interactions involving a decrease in effect.

Dietary Considerations Should be given with food and a full glass of water to decrease gastric upset.

Pharmacodynamics/Kinetics

Half-life Elimination ~24 hours

Time to Peak Plasma: ~3-4 hours

Pregnancy Risk Factor C

Lactation Excretion in breast milk unknown/not recommended

Dosage Forms

Combination package, oral:

Chantix®: Tablet: 0.5 mg (11s) [white tablets] and Tablet: 1 mg (42s) [light blue tablets]

Tablet, oral:

Chantix®: 0.5 mg, 1 mg

Varicella-Zoster Immune Globulin (Human)

(var i SEL a- ZOS ter i MYUN GLOB yoo lin HYU man)

Canadian Brand Names VariZIG™

Pharmacologic Category Blood Product Derivative; Immune Globulin

Use In pregnant women, for the prevention or reduction in severity of maternal infection within 4 days of exposure to the varicella zoster virus.

Unlabeled/Investigational Use In the United States, the Centers for Disease Control and Prevention (CDC) recommends varicella-zoster immune globulin (VZIG) for the passive immunization of patients who are at a greater risk of complications following significant exposure to varicella and do not have evidence of immunity. Guidelines restrict administration to those patients meeting the following criteria:

- Immunocompromised patients without evidence of immunity, including those with neoplastic disease (eg, leukemia or lymphoma); primary or acquired immunodeficiency; immunosuppressive therapy (including steroid therapy equivalent to prednisone ≥2 mg/kg or 20 mg/day)
- Newborn of mother who had onset of varicella (chickenpox) within 5 days before delivery or within 48 hours after delivery
- Premature infants (≥28 weeks gestation) whose mother has no evidence of immunity
- Premature infants (<28 weeks gestation or ≤1000 g) regardless of maternal history
- Pregnant women without evidence of immunity

Significant exposure includes:

Continuous household contact

Face-to-face indoor contact (>5 minutes or >1 hour depending on reference)

Hospital contact (in same 2-4 bedroom or adjacent beds in a large ward or prolonged face-to-face contact with an infectious staff member or patient)

Local Anesthetic/Vasoconstrictor Precautions No information available to require special precautions

Effects on Dental Treatment No significant effects or complications reported

Effects on Bleeding No information available to require special precautions

Adverse Effects

>10%:

Central nervous system: Headache (7% to 11%)

Local: Injection site pain (17% to 47%)

1% to 10%:

Central nervous system: Dizziness (up to 5%), fever (up to 5%), pain (up to 5%), chills (up to 2%), fatigue (up to 2%), flushing (up to 2%), insomnia (up to 2%)

Dermatologic: Rash (up to 4%), dermatitis (up to 2%), erythematous rash (up to 2%)

Gastrointestinal: Nausea (2% to 5%), dysgeusia (up to 2%)

Local: Injection site bruising, itching, or tenderness (up to 2%)

Neuromuscular & skeletal: Neck pain (up to 5%), myalgia (up to 2%)

General Dosage Range I.M., I.V.: *Adults:* 125 int. units/10 kg (minimum dose: 125 int. units; maximum dose: 625 int. units)

Mechanism of Action Antibodies obtained from pooled human plasma of individuals with high titers of varicella-zoster provide passive immunity.

Pharmacodynamics/Kinetics

Duration of Action ≥6 weeks

Half-life Elimination I.V.: 18-24 days; I.M.: 24-30 days

Time to Peak I.V.: <3 hours; I.M.: 2-7 days

Prescribing and Access Restrictions Varicella-zoster immune globulin (VZIG) was discontinued in the United States in 2005. It is currently available as VariZIG™ under an Investigational New Drug Application Expanded Access protocol. Inventory for anticipated patients may be obtained by contacting FFF Enterprises at 800-843-7477. Additional information is available at http://www.fffenterprises.com/Products/VariZIGINDProtocolPre.aspx

Vasopressin (vay soe PRES in)

U.S. Brand Names Pitressin®

Canadian Brand Names Pressyn®; Pressyn® AR

Pharmacologic Category Antidiuretic Hormone Analog; Hormone, Posterior Pituitary

Use Treatment of central diabetes insipidus; differential diagnosis of diabetes insipidus

Unlabeled/Investigational Use ACLS guidelines: Pulseless arrest (ventricular tachycardia [VT]/ventricular fibrillation [VF], asystole/pulseless electrical activity [PEA]); cardiac arrest secondary to anaphylaxis (unresponsive to epinephrine)

Adjunct in the treatment of GI hemorrhage and esophageal varices; adjunct in the treatment of vasodilatory shock (septic shock); donor management in brain-dead patients (hormone replacement therapy)

Local Anesthetic/Vasoconstrictor Precautions No information available to require special precautions

Effects on Dental Treatment No significant effects or complications reported

Effects on Bleeding No information available to require special precautions

Adverse Effects Frequency not defined.

Cardiovascular: Arrhythmia, asystole (>0.04 units/minute), blood pressure increased, cardiac output decreased (>0.04 units/minute), chest pain, MI, vasoconstriction (with higher doses), venous thrombosis

Central nervous system: Pounding in the head, fever, vertigo

Dermatologic: Ischemic skin lesions, circumoral pallor, urticaria

Gastrointestinal: Abdominal cramps, flatulence, mesenteric ischemia, nausea, vomiting

Genitourinary: Uterine contraction

Neuromuscular & skeletal: Tremor

Respiratory: Bronchial constriction

Miscellaneous: Diaphoresis

General Dosage Range I.M., SubQ:

Children: 2.5-10 units 2-4 times/day as needed

Adults: 5-10 units 2-4 times/day as needed

Mechanism of Action Increases cyclic adenosine monophosphate (cAMP) which increases water permeability at the renal tubule resulting in decreased urine volume and increased osmolality; causes peristalsis by directly stimulating the smooth muscle in the GI tract; direct vasoconstrictor without inotropic or chronotropic effects

Pharmacodynamics/Kinetics

Onset of Action Nasal: 1 hour

Duration of Action Nasal: 3-8 hours; I.M., SubQ: 2-8 hours

Half-life Elimination Nasal: 15 minutes; Parenteral: 10-20 minutes

Pregnancy Risk Factor C

Velaglucerase Alfa (vel a GLOO ser ase AL fa)

U.S. Brand Names VPRIV™

Canadian Brand Names VPRIV™

Pharmacologic Category Enzyme

Use Long-term enzyme replacement therapy for patients with type 1 Gaucher's disease

Local Anesthetic/Vasoconstrictor Precautions No information available to require special precautions

Effects on Dental Treatment No significant effects or complications reported

Effects on Bleeding No information available to require special precautions

Adverse Effects

>10%:

Central nervous system: Headache (30% to 35%), fatigue (13%), fever (13% to 22%; more common in children), dizziness (8% to 22%)

Gastrointestinal: Abdominal pain (15% to 19%)

Hematologic: aPPT prolonged (5% to 11%; more common in children)

Respiratory: Upper respiratory tract infections (30% to 32%; more common in children)

Miscellaneous: Infusion-related reactions (23% to 52%)

1% to 10%:

Cardiovascular: Flushing (>2%), hyper-/hypotension (>2%), tachycardia (>2%)

Dermatologic: Rash (>2%; more common in children), urticaria (>2%)

Gastrointestinal: Nausea (6% to 10%)

Miscellaneous: Hypersensitivity reactions

General Dosage Range I.V.: *Children ≥4 years and Adults:* 15-60 units/kg every other week

Mechanism of Action Velaglucerase alfa, an analogue of endogenous glucocerebrosidase, contains the native human enzyme sequence. In patients with type 1 Gaucher's disease, glucocerebrosidase deficiency results in accumulation of glucocerebroside in macrophages, thereby causing the associated signs and symptoms. Velaglucerase alfa is used to diminish hepatosplenomegaly and improve anemia, thrombocytopenia, and bone disease.

Pharmacodynamics/Kinetics

Half-life Elimination 11-12 minutes

Pregnancy Risk Factor B

Venlafaxine (ven la FAX een)

U.S. Brand Names Effexor XR®; Effexor®

Canadian Brand Names CO Venlafaxine XR; Effexor XR®; Mylan-Venlafaxine XR; PMS-Venlafaxine XR; ratio-Venlafaxine XR; Riva-Venlafaxine XR; Sandoz-Venlafaxine XR; Teva-Venlafaxine XR; Venlafaxine XR

Generic Availability (U.S.) Yes

Pharmacologic Category Antidepressant, Serotonin/Norepinephrine Reuptake Inhibitor

Use Treatment of major depressive disorder, generalized anxiety disorder (GAD), social anxiety disorder (social phobia), panic disorder

Unlabeled/Investigational Use Obsessive-compulsive disorder (OCD); hot flashes; neuropathic pain (including diabetic neuropathy); attention attention-deficit/hyperactivity disorder (ADHD); post-traumatic stress disorder (PTSD)

Local Anesthetic/Vasoconstrictor Precautions Although venlafaxine is not a tricyclic antidepressant, it does block norepinephrine reuptake within CNS synapses as part of its mechanisms. It has been suggested that vasoconstrictor be administered with caution and to monitor vital signs in dental patients taking antidepressants that affect norepinephrine in this way. This is particularly important in patients taking venlafaxine, which has been noted to produce a sustained increase in diastolic blood pressure and heart rate as a side effect.

Effects on Dental Treatment Key adverse event(s) related to dental treatment: Significant xerostomia (normal salivary flow resumes upon discontinuation); may contribute to oral discomfort, especially in the elderly; taste perversion. See Effects on Bleeding.

Effects on Bleeding May impair platelet aggregation resulting in increased risk of bleeding events, particularly if used concomitantly with aspirin, NSAIDs, warfarin, or other anticoagulants. Bleeding related to SSRI use has been reported to range from relatively minor bruising and epistaxis to life-threatening hemorrhage. Routine interruption of therapy for most dental procedures is not warranted. In medically complicated patients or extensive oral surgery, the decision to interrupt therapy must be based on the risk to benefit in an individual patient and a medical consult is suggested. If therapy is continued without interruption, the clinician should anticipate the potential for a prolonged bleeding time.

Adverse Effects Note: Actual frequency may be dependent upon formulation and/or indication

>10%:

Central nervous system: Headache (25% to 38%), somnolence (12% to 26%), dizziness (11% to 24%), insomnia (15% to 24%), nervousness (6% to 21%), anxiety (2% to 11%),

Gastrointestinal: Nausea (21% to 58%), xerostomia (12% to 22%), anorexia (8% to 17%), constipation (8% to 15%)

Genitourinary: Abnormal ejaculation/orgasm (2% to 19%)

Neuromuscular & skeletal: Weakness (8% to 19%)

Miscellaneous: Diaphoresis (7% to 19%)

1% to 10%:

Cardiovascular: Vasodilation (2% to 6%), hypertension (dose related; 3% in patients receiving <100 mg/day, up to 13% in patients receiving >300 mg/day), palpitation (3%), tachycardia (2%), chest pain (2%), postural hypotension (1%), edema

Central nervous system: Yawning (3% to 8%), abnormal dreams (3% to 7%), chills (2% to 7%), agitation (2% to 5%), confusion (2%), abnormal thinking (2%), depersonalization (1%), depression (1% to 3%), fever, migraine, amnesia, hypoesthesia, vertigo
Dermatologic: Rash (3%), pruritus (1%), bruising
Endocrine & metabolic: Libido decreased (2% to 8%), hypercholesterolemia (5%), triglycerides increased
Gastrointestinal: Abdominal pain (8%), diarrhea (8%), vomiting (3% to 8%), dyspepsia (5% to 7%), weight loss (1% to 6%), flatulence (3% to 4%), taste perversion (2%), appetite increased, belching, weight gain
Genitourinary: Impotence (4% to 6%), urinary frequency (3%), urination impaired (2%), urinary retention (1%), metrorrhagia, prostatic disorder, vaginitis
Neuromuscular & skeletal: Tremor (1% to 10%), hypertonia (3%), paresthesia (2% to 3%), twitching (1% to 3%), arthralgia, neck pain, trismus
Ocular: Accommodation abnormal (6% to 9%), abnormal or blurred vision (4% to 6%), mydriasis (2%)
Otic: Tinnitus (2%)
Renal: Albuminuria
Respiratory: Pharyngitis (7%), sinusitis (2%), bronchitis, cough increased, dyspnea
Miscellaneous: Infection (6%), flu-like syndrome (2%), trauma (2%)

Dosage Oral:

Children and Adolescents:

Attention-deficit/hyperactivity disorder (unlabeled use; Olvera, 1996): Initial: 12.5 mg/day

Children <40 kg: Increase by 12.5 mg/week to maximum of 50 mg/day in 2 divided doses

Children ≥40 kg: Increase by 25 mg/week to maximum of 75 mg/day in 3 divided doses.

Mean dose: 60 mg or 1.4 mg/kg administered in 2-3 divided doses

Adults:

Depression:

Immediate-release tablets: Initial: 75 mg/day, administered in 2 or 3 divided doses; may increase in ≤75 mg/day increments at intervals of ≥4 days as tolerated (maximum daily dose: 225-375 mg)

Extended-release capsules or tablets: Initial: 37.5-75 mg once daily; in patients who are initiated at 37.5 mg once daily, may increase to 75 mg once daily after 4-7 days; dose may then be increased by ≤75 mg/day increments at intervals of ≥4 days as tolerated (maximum daily dose: 225 mg)

Generalized anxiety disorder: Extended-release capsules: Initial: 37.5-75 mg once daily; in patients who are initiated at 37.5 mg once daily, may increase to 75 mg once daily after 4-7 days; may then be increased by ≤75 mg/day increments at intervals of ≥4 days as tolerated (maximum daily dose: 225 mg)

Panic disorder: Extended-release capsules: Initial: 37.5 mg once daily for 1 week; may increase to 75 mg once daily after 7 days, may then be increased by ≤75 mg/day increments at intervals of ≥7 days (maximum daily dose: 225 mg).

Social anxiety disorder: Extended-release capsules or tablets: 75 mg once daily (maximum daily dose: 75 mg); no evidence that doses >75 mg/day offer any additional benefit

Obsessive-compulsive disorder (unlabeled use): Titrate to usual dosage range of 150-300 mg/day; however, doses up to 375 mg/day have been used; response may be seen in 4 weeks (Phelps, 2005)

Neuropathic pain (unlabeled use): Dosages evaluated varied considerably based on etiology of chronic pain, but efficacy has been shown for many conditions in the range of 75-225 mg/day; onset of relief may occur in 1-2 weeks, or take up to 6 weeks for full benefit (Grothe, 2004).

Diabetic neuropathy (unlabeled use): 75-225 mg/day (Bril, 2011)

Hot flashes (unlabeled use): Doses of 37.5-75 mg/day have demonstrated significant improvement of vasomotor symptoms after 4-8 weeks of treatment; in one study, doses >75 mg/day offered no additional benefit (Evans, 2005; Loprinzi, 2000); however, higher doses (225 mg/day) may be beneficial in patients with perimenopausal depression

Attention-deficit disorder (unlabeled use): Initial: Doses vary between 18.75 to 75 mg/day; may increase after 4 weeks to 150 mg/day; if tolerated, doses up to 225 mg/day have been used (Maidment, 2003)

Post-traumatic stress disorder (PTSD) (unlabeled use): Extended release formulation: 37.5-300 mg/day (Bandelow, 2008; Benedek, 2009)

Note: When discontinuing this medication after more than 1 week of treatment, it is generally recommended that the dose be tapered. If venlafaxine is used for 6 weeks or longer, the dose should be tapered over 2 weeks when discontinuing its use.

Elderly: Alzheimer's dementia-related depression (unlabeled use; Rabins, 2007):
Immediate-release tablets: Initial: 25 mg/day; may increase at weekly intervals to maximum of 375 mg/day in divided doses
Extended-release capsules: Initial: 37.5 mg/day; may increase at weekly intervals to maximum of 225 mg/day

Dosing adjustment in renal impairment:
GFR: 10-70 mL/minute: Reduce total daily dose by 25% to 50%
Hemodialysis: Reduce total daily dose by 50%

Dosing adjustment in hepatic impairment: Mild-to-moderate hepatic impairment: Reduce total daily dose by 50%; further reductions may be necessary in some patients

Mechanism of Action Venlafaxine and its active metabolite, O-desmethylvenlafaxine (ODV), are potent inhibitors of neuronal serotonin and norepinephrine reuptake and weak inhibitors of dopamine reuptake. Venlafaxine and ODV have no significant activity for muscarinic cholinergic, H_1-histaminergic, or alpha$_2$-adrenergic receptors. Venlafaxine and ODV do not possess MAO-inhibitory activity.

Contraindications Hypersensitivity to venlafaxine or any component of the formulation; use of MAO inhibitors within 14 days; should not initiate MAO inhibitor within 7 days of discontinuing venlafaxine

Warnings/Precautions [U.S. Boxed Warning]: Antidepressants increase the risk of suicidal thinking and behavior in children, adolescents, and young adults (18-24 years of age) with major depressive disorder (MDD) and other psychiatric disorders; consider risk prior to prescribing. Short-term studies did not show an increased risk in patients >24 years of age and showed a decreased risk in patients ≥65 years. Closely monitor for clinical worsening, suicidality, or unusual changes in behavior; the patient's family or caregiver should be instructed to closely observe the patient and communicate condition with healthcare provider. Reduced growth rate has been observed with venlafaxine therapy in children. A medication guide should be dispensed with each prescription. **Venlafaxine is not FDA approved for use in children.**

The possibility of a suicide attempt is inherent in major depression and may persist until remission occurs. Monitor for worsening of depression or suicidality, especially during initiation of therapy (generally first 1-2 months) or with dose increases or decreases. Use caution in high-risk patients. Worsening depression and severe abrupt suicidality that are not part of the presenting symptoms may require discontinuation or modification of drug therapy. The patient's family or caregiver should be alerted to monitor patients for the emergence of suicidality and associated behaviors (such as agitation, irritability, hostility, impulsivity, and hypomania) and call healthcare provider.

May worsen psychosis in some patients or precipitate a shift to mania or hypomania in patients with bipolar disorder. Patients presenting with depressive symptoms should be screened for bipolar disorder. Monotherapy in patients with bipolar disorder should be avoided. **Venlafaxine is not FDA approved for the treatment of bipolar depression.**

Serotonin syndrome and neuroleptic malignant syndrome (NMS)-like reactions have occurred with serotonin/norepinephrine reuptake inhibitors (SNRIs) and selective serotonin reuptake inhibitors (SSRIs) when used alone, and particularly when used in combination with serotonergic agents (eg, triptans) or antidopaminergic agents (eg, antipsychotics). Concurrent use with MAO inhibitors is contraindicated. May cause sustained increase in blood pressure or tachycardia; dose related and increases are generally modest (12-15 mm Hg diastolic). Control pre-existing hypertension prior to initiation of venlafaxine. Use caution in patients with recent history of MI, unstable heart disease, or hyperthyroidism; may cause increase in anxiety, nervousness, insomnia; may cause weight loss (use with caution in patients where weight loss is undesirable); may cause increases in serum cholesterol. Use caution with hepatic or renal impairment; dosage adjustments recommended. May cause hyponatremia/SIADH (elderly at increased risk); volume depletion (diuretics may increase risk).

May impair platelet aggregation resulting in increased risk of bleeding events, particularly if used concomitantly with aspirin or NSAIDs. Bleeding related to SSRI or SNRI use has been reported to range from relatively minor bruising and epistaxis to life-threatening hemorrhage. Interstitial lung disease and eosinophilic pneumonia have been rarely reported; may present as progressive dyspnea, cough, and/or chest pain. Prompt evaluation and possible discontinuation of therapy may be necessary. Venlafaxine may increase the risks associated with electroconvulsive therapy. Use cautiously in patients with a history of seizures. The risks of cognitive or motor impairment, as well as the potential for anticholinergic effects are very low. May cause or exacerbate sexual dysfunction.

Abrupt discontinuation or dosage reduction after extended (≥6 weeks) therapy may lead to agitation, dysphoria, nervousness, anxiety, and other symptoms. When discontinuing therapy, dosage should be tapered gradually over at least a 2-week period. If intolerable symptoms occur following a decrease in dosage or upon discontinuation of therapy, then resuming the previous dose with a more gradual taper should be considered. Use caution in patients with increased intraocular pressure or at risk of acute narrow-angle glaucoma.

Drug Interactions

Metabolism/Transport Effects Substrate of CYP2C9 (minor), 2C19 (minor), 2D6 (major), 3A4 (major); **Inhibits** CYP2B6 (weak), 2D6 (weak), 3A4 (weak)

Avoid Concomitant Use

Avoid concomitant use of Venlafaxine with any of the following: Iobenguane I 123; MAO Inhibitors; Methylene Blue; Sibutramine

Increased Effect/Toxicity

Venlafaxine may increase the levels/effects of: Alcohol (Ethyl); Alpha-/Beta-Agonists; Aspirin; CNS Depressants; Methotrimeprazine; Methylene Blue; NSAID (Nonselective); Serotonin Modulators; TraZODone; Vitamin K Antagonists

The levels/effects of Venlafaxine may be increased by: Abiraterone; Conivaptan; CYP2D6 Inhibitors (Moderate); CYP2D6 Inhibitors (Strong); CYP3A4 Inhibitors (Moderate); CYP3A4 Inhibitors (Strong); Darunavir; Dasatinib; Droperidol; MAO Inhibitors; Methotrimeprazine; Metoclopramide; Propafenone; Sibutramine; Voriconazole

Decreased Effect

Venlafaxine may decrease the levels/effects of: Alpha2-Agonists; Indinavir; Iobenguane I 123

The levels/effects of Venlafaxine may be decreased by: CYP3A4 Inducers (Strong); Deferasirox; Peginterferon Alfa-2b; Tocilizumab

Ethanol/Nutrition/Herb Interactions

Ethanol: May increase CNS depression; monitor for increased effects with coadministration. Caution patients about effects.

Herb/Nutraceutical: Avoid valerian, St John's wort, SAMe, kava kava, tryptophan (may increase risk of serotonin syndrome and/or excessive sedation).

Dietary Considerations Should be taken with food.

Pharmacodynamics/Kinetics

Half-life Elimination Venlafaxine: 5 ± 2 hours; ODV: 11 ± 2 hours; prolonged with cirrhosis (venlafaxine: ~30%, ODV: ~60%), renal impairment (venlafaxine: ~50%, ODV: ~40%), and during dialysis (venlafaxine: ~180%, ODV: ~142%)

Time to Peak

Immediate release: Venlafaxine: 2 hours, ODV: 3 hours

Extended release: Venlafaxine: 5.5 hours, ODV: 9 hours

Pregnancy Risk Factor C

Lactation Enters breast milk/not recommended

Breast-Feeding Considerations Venlafaxine and ODV are found in human milk. Low concentrations of ODV have been found in the serum of nursing infants whose mothers are taking venlafaxine; venlafaxine has also been detected in some infants. Adverse events have not been observed; however, it is recommended to monitor the infant for adverse events if the decision to breast-feed has been made. The long-term effects on neurobehavior have not been studied, thus one should prescribe venlafaxine to a mother who is breast-feeding only when the benefits outweigh the potential risks. The manufacturer does not recommend breast-feeding during therapy.

Dosage Forms

Capsule, extended release, oral: 37.5 mg, 75 mg, 150 mg

Effexor XR®: 37.5 mg, 75 mg, 150 mg

Tablet, oral: 25 mg, 37.5 mg, 50 mg, 75 mg, 100 mg

Effexor®: 50 mg

Tablet, extended release, oral: 37.5 mg, 75 mg, 150 mg, 225 mg

References

Ganzber S, "Psychoactive Drugs," *ADA Guide to Dental Therapeutics*, 2nd edition, Chapter 21, Chicago, IL: ADA Publishing, 2000, 381.

Verapamil (ver AP a mil)

Related Information

Calcium Channel Blockers and Gingival Hyperplasia *on page 2014*

Cardiovascular Diseases *on page 1848*

U.S. Brand Names Calan®; Calan® SR; Covera-HS®; Isoptin® SR; Verelan®; Verelan® PM

Canadian Brand Names Apo-Verap®; Apo-Verap® SR; Calan®; Chronovera®; Covera-HS®; Covera®; Dom-Verapamil SR; Gen-Verapamil; Gen-Verapamil SR; Isoptin® SR; Med-Verapamil; Mylan-Verapamil; Mylan-Verapamil SR; Novo-Veramil; Novo-Veramil SR; Nu-Verap; Nu-Verap SR; PHL-Verapamil SR; PMS-Verapamil SR; PRO-Verapamil SR; Riva-Verapamil SR; Verapamil Hydrochloride Injection, USP; Verapamil SR; Verelan SRC

Generic Availability (U.S.) Yes: Excludes caplet (sustained release) and tablet (extended release, controlled onset)

Pharmacologic Category Antiarrhythmic Agent, Class IV; Calcium Channel Blocker; Calcium Channel Blocker, Nondihydropyridine

Use

Oral: Treatment of hypertension; angina pectoris (vasospastic, chronic stable, unstable) (Calan®, Covera-HS®); supraventricular tachyarrhythmia (PSVT, atrial fibrillation/flutter [rate control])

I.V.: Supraventricular tachyarrhythmia (PSVT, atrial fibrillation/flutter [rate control])

Unlabeled/Investigational Use Migraine; hypertrophic cardiomyopathy; bipolar disorder (manic manifestations)

Local Anesthetic/Vasoconstrictor Precautions No information available to require special precautions

Effects on Dental Treatment Key adverse event(s) related to dental treatment: Gingival hyperplasia. Calcium channel blockers (CCB) have been reported to cause gingival hyperplasia (GH). Verapamil-induced GH has appeared 11 months or more after subjects took daily doses of 240-360 mg. The severity of hyperplastic syndrome does not seem to be dose dependent. Gingivectomy is only successful if CCB therapy is discontinued. GH regresses markedly 1 week after CCB discontinuance with all symptoms resolving in 2 months. If a patient must continue CCB therapy, begin a program of professional cleaning and patient plaque control to minimize severity and growth rate of gingival tissue.

Effects on Bleeding No information available to require special precautions

Adverse Effects

>10%:

Central nervous system: Headache (1% to 12%)

Gastrointestinal: Gingival hyperplasia (≤19%), constipation (7% to 12%)

1% to 10%:

Cardiovascular: Peripheral edema (1% to 4%), hypotension (3%), CHF/pulmonary edema (2%), AV block (1% to 2%), bradycardia (HR <50 bpm: 1%), flushing (1%)

Central nervous system: Fatigue (2% to 5%), dizziness (1% to 5%), lethargy (3%), pain (2%), sleep disturbance (1%)

Dermatologic: Rash (1% to 2%)

Gastrointestinal: Dyspepsia (3%), nausea (1% to 3%), diarrhea (2%)

Hepatic: Liver enzymes increased (1%)

Neuromuscular & skeletal: Myalgia (1%), paresthesia (1%)

Respiratory: Dyspnea (1%)

Miscellaneous: Flu-like syndrome (4%)

Dosage

Children: **Note:** Verapamil is no longer included in the Pediatric Advanced Life Support (PALS) tachyarrhythmia algorithm.

Children: 1-15 years: SVT: I.V.: 0.1-0.3 mg/kg/dose over 2 minutes; maximum: 5 mg/dose, may repeat dose in 30 minutes if inadequate response; maximum for second dose: 10 mg

Adults:

SVT (ACLS, 2010): I.V.: 2.5-5 mg over 2 minutes; second dose of 5-10 mg (~0.15 mg/kg) may be given 15-30 minutes after the initial dose if patient tolerates, but does not respond to initial dose; maximum total dose: 20-30 mg

Angina: Oral: **Note:** When switching from immediate-release to extended/sustained release formulations, the total daily dose remains the same unless formulation strength does not allow for equal conversion.

Immediate release: Initial: 80-120 mg 3 times/day (elderly or small stature: 40 mg 3 times/day); Usual dose range (Gibbons, 2002): 80-160 mg 3 times/day

Extended release (Covera-HS®): Initial: 180 mg once daily at bedtime; if inadequate response, may increase dose at weekly intervals to 240 mg once daily, then 360 mg once daily, then 480 mg once daily; maximum dose: 480 mg/day

Chronic atrial fibrillation (rate-control), PSVT prophylaxis: Oral: Immediate release: 240-480 mg/day in 3-4 divided doses; Usual dose range (Fuster, 2006): 120-360 mg/day in divided doses

Hypertension: Oral: **Note:** When switching from immediate-release to extended/sustained release formulations, the total daily dose remains the same unless formulation strength does not allow for equal conversion.

Immediate release: 80 mg 3 times/day; usual dose range (JNC 7): 80-320 mg/day in 2 divided doses

Sustained release: Usual dose range (JNC 7): 120-480 mg/day in 1-2 divided doses; **Note:** There is no evidence of additional benefit with doses >360 mg/day.

Calan® SR, Isoptin® SR: Initial: 180 mg once daily in the morning (elderly or small stature: 120 mg/day); if inadequate response, may increase dose at weekly intervals to 240 mg once daily, then 180 mg twice daily (or 240 mg in the morning followed by 120 mg in the evening); maximum dose: 240 mg twice daily.

Verelan®: Initial: 180 mg once daily in the morning (elderly or small stature: 120 mg/day); if inadequate response, may increase dose at weekly intervals to 240 mg once daily, then 360 mg once daily, then 480 mg once daily; maximum dose: 480 mg/day

Extended release: Usual dose range (JNC 7): 120-360 mg once daily (once-daily dosing is recommended at bedtime)

Covera-HS®: Initial: 180 mg once daily at bedtime; if inadequate response, may increase dose at weekly intervals to 240 mg once daily, then 360 mg once daily, then 480 mg once daily; maximum dose: 480 mg/day

Verelan® PM: Initial: 200 mg once daily at bedtime (elderly or small stature: 100 mg/day); if inadequate response, may increase dose at weekly intervals to 300 mg once daily, then 400 mg once daily; maximum dose: 400 mg/day

Dosing adjustment in renal impairment: Manufacturer recommends caution and additional ECG monitoring in patients with renal insufficiency. The manufacturer of Verelan PM® recommends an initial dose of 100 mg/day at bedtime. **Note:** A multiple dose study in adults suggests reduced renal clearance of verapamil and its metabolite (norverapamil) with advanced renal failure (Storstein, 1984). Additionally, several clinical papers report adverse effects of verapamil in patients with chronic renal failure receiving recommended doses of verapamil (Pritza, 1991; Váquez, 1996). In contrast, a number of single dose studies show no difference in verapamil (or norverapamil metabolite) disposition between chronic renal failure and control patients (Beyerlein, 1990; Hanyok, 1988; Mooy, 1985; Zachariah, 1991).

Dialysis: Not removed by hemodialysis (Mooy, 1985); supplemental dose is not necessary.

Dosing adjustment/comments in hepatic disease: In cirrhosis, reduce dose to 20% and 50% of normal for oral and intravenous administration, respectively, and monitor ECG (Somogyi, 1981). The manufacturer of Verelan PM® recommends an initial adult dose of 100 mg/day at bedtime. The manufacturers of Calan®, Calan® SR, Covera-HS®, Isoptin® SR, and Verelan® recommend giving 30% of the normal dose to patients with severe hepatic impairment.

Mechanism of Action Inhibits calcium ion from entering the "slow channels" or select voltage-sensitive areas of vascular smooth muscle and myocardium during depolarization; produces relaxation of coronary vascular smooth muscle and coronary vasodilation; increases myocardial oxygen delivery in patients with vasospastic angina; slows automaticity and conduction of AV node.

Contraindications Hypersensitivity to verapamil or any component of the formulation; severe left ventricular dysfunction; hypotension (systolic pressure <90 mm Hg) or cardiogenic shock; sick sinus syndrome (except in patients with a functioning artificial ventricular pacemaker); second- or third-degree AV block (except in patients with a functioning artificial ventricular pacemaker); atrial flutter or fibrillation and an accessory bypass tract (Wolff-Parkinson-White [WPW] syndrome, Lown-Ganong-Levine syndrome)

I.V.: Additional contraindications include concurrent use of I.V. beta-blocking agents; ventricular tachycardia

Warnings/Precautions Avoid use in heart failure; can exacerbate condition; use is contraindicated in severe left ventricular dysfunction. Symptomatic hypotension with or without syncope can rarely occur; blood pressure must be lowered at a rate appropriate for the patient's clinical condition. Rare increases in hepatic enzymes can be observed. Can cause first-degree AV block or sinus bradycardia; use is contraindicated in patients with sick sinus syndrome, second- or third-degree AV block (except in patients with a functioning artificial pacemaker), or an accessory bypass tract (eg, WPW syndrome). Other conduction abnormalities are rare. Considered contraindicated in patients with wide complex tachycardias unless known to be supraventricular in origin; severe hypotension likely to occur upon administration (ACLS, 2010). Use caution when using verapamil together with a beta-blocker. Administration of I.V. verapamil and an I.V. beta-blocker within a few hours of each other may result in asystole and should be avoided; simultaneous administration is contraindicated. Use with other agents known to reduce SA node function and/or AV nodal conduction (eg, digoxin) or reduce sympathetic outflow (eg, clonidine) may increase the risk of serious bradycardia. Verapamil significantly increases digoxin serum concentrations; adjust digoxin dose. Use with caution in patients with hypertrophic cardiomyopathy with outflow tract obstruction (especially those with resting outflow obstruction and severe limiting symptoms); may be used in patients who cannot tolerate beta-blockade.

Decreased neuromuscular transmission has been reported with verapamil; use with caution in patients with attenuated neuromuscular transmission (Duchenne's muscular dystrophy, myasthenia gravis); dosage reduction may be required. Use with caution in renal impairment; monitor hemodynamics and possibly ECG if severe impairment, particularly if concomitant hepatic impairment. Use with caution in patients with hepatic impairment; dosage reduction may be required; monitor hemodynamics and possibly ECG if severe impairment. May prolong recovery from nondepolarizing neuromuscular-blocking agents. Use Covera-HS® (extended-release delivery system) with caution in patients with severe GI narrowing. In patients with extremely short GI transit times (eg, <7 hours), dosage adjustment may be required; inadequate pharmacokinetic data. I.V. use for SVT for is not recommended in infants; use with caution in children as myocardial depression/hypotension may occur.

Drug Interactions

Metabolism/Transport Effects **Substrate** of CYP1A2 (minor), CYP2B6 (minor), CYP2C9 (minor), CYP2C18 (minor), CYP2E1 (minor), CYP3A4 (major), P-glycoprotein; **Inhibits** CYP1A2 (weak), CYP2C9 (weak), CYP2D6 (weak), CYP3A4 (moderate), P-glycoprotein

Avoid Concomitant Use

Avoid concomitant use of Verapamil with any of the following: Disopyramide; Dofetilide; Tolvaptan; Topotecan

Increased Effect/Toxicity

Verapamil may increase the levels/effects of: Alcohol (Ethyl); Aliskiren; Amifostine; Amiodarone; Antihypertensives; Atorvastatin; Benzodiazepines (metabolized by oxidation); Beta-Blockers; Budesonide (Systemic, Oral Inhalation); BusPIRone; Calcium Channel Blockers (Dihydropyridine); CarBAMazepine; Cardiac Glycosides; Colchicine; Corticosteroids (Systemic); CycloSPORINE; CycloSPORINE (Systemic); CYP3A4 Substrates; Dabigatran Etexilate; Disopyramide; Dofetilide; Dronedarone; Eletriptan; Eplerenone; Everolimus; Fexofenadine; Fingolimod; Flecainide; Fosphenytoin; Halofantrine; Hypotensive Agents; Lithium; Lovastatin; Lurasidone; Magnesium Salts; Midodrine; Neuromuscular-Blocking Agents (Nondepolarizing); Nitroprusside; P-Glycoprotein Substrates; Phenytoin; Pimecrolimus; QuiNIDine; Ranolazine; Red Yeast Rice; RisperiDONE; RiTUXimab; Rivaroxaban; Salicylates; Salmeterol; Saxagliptin; Simvastatin; Tacrolimus; Tacrolimus (Systemic); Tacrolimus (Topical); Tolvaptan; Topotecan; Vilazodone

The levels/effects of Verapamil may be increased by: Alpha1-Blockers; Anilidopiperidine Opioids; Antifungal Agents (Azole Derivatives, Systemic); Atorvastatin; Calcium Channel Blockers (Dihydropyridine); Cimetidine; Conivaptan; CycloSPORINE; CycloSPORINE (Systemic); CYP3A4 Inhibitors (Moderate); CYP3A4 Inhibitors (Strong); Dasatinib; Diazoxide; Dronedarone; Fluconazole; Grapefruit Juice; Herbs (Hypotensive Properties); Macrolide Antibiotics; Magnesium Salts; MAO Inhibitors; Pentoxifylline; P-Glycoprotein Inhibitors; Phosphodiesterase 5 Inhibitors; Prostacyclin Analogues; Protease Inhibitors; QuiNIDine; Telithromycin

Decreased Effect

Verapamil may decrease the levels/effects of: Clopidogrel

The levels/effects of Verapamil may be decreased by: Barbiturates; Calcium Salts; CarBAMazepine; CYP3A4 Inducers (Strong); Deferasirox; Herbs (CYP3A4 Inducers); Herbs (Hypertensive Properties); Methylphenidate; Nafcillin; P-Glycoprotein Inducers; Rifamycin Derivatives; Tocilizumab; Yohimbine

Ethanol/Nutrition/Herb Interactions

Ethanol: Avoid or limit ethanol (may increase ethanol levels).

Food: Grapefruit juice may increase the serum concentration of verapamil; use with caution and monitor for increased verapamil effects.

Herb/Nutraceutical: St John's wort may decrease levels. Avoid herbs with hypertensive properties (bayberry, blue cohosh, cayenne, ephedra, ginger, ginseng [American], kola, licorice); may diminish the antihypertensive effect of verapamil. Avoid herbs with hypotensive properties (black cohosh, California poppy, coleus, golden seal, hawthorn, mistletoe, periwinkle, quinine, shepherd's purse); may enhance the hypotensive effect of verapamil.

Dietary Considerations Calan® SR and Isoptin® SR products may be taken with food or milk, other formulations may be administered without regard to meals; sprinkling contents of Verelan® or Verelan® PM capsule onto applesauce does not affect oral absorption.

Pharmacodynamics/Kinetics

Onset of Action Oral (immediate release tablets): Peak effect: 1-2 hours; I.V.: Peak effect: 1-5 minutes

Duration of Action Oral: Immediate release tablets: 6-8 hours; I.V.: 10-20 minutes

Half-life Elimination Infants: 4.4-6.9 hours; Adults: Single dose: 3-7 hours, Multiple doses: 4.5-12 hours; severe hepatic impairment: 14-16 hours

Time to Peak Serum: Oral:

Immediate release: 1-2 hours

Extended release (Covera-HS®, Verelan PM®): ~11 hours, drug release delayed ~4-5 hours

Sustained release: 5.21 hours (Calan® SR, Isoptin® SR); 7-9 hours (Verelan®)

Pregnancy Risk Factor C

Lactation Enters breast milk/not recommended (AAP considers "compatible"; AAP 2001 update pending)

Breast-Feeding Considerations Crosses into breast milk; manufacturer recommends to discontinue breast-feeding while taking verapamil.

Dosage Forms

Caplet, sustained release, oral:

Calan® SR: 120 mg, 180 mg, 240 mg

Capsule, extended release, oral: 120 mg, 180 mg, 240 mg

Capsule, extended release, controlled onset, oral: 100 mg, 200 mg, 300 mg

Verelan® PM: 100 mg, 200 mg, 300 mg

Capsule, sustained release, oral: 120 mg, 180 mg, 240 mg, 360 mg

Verelan®: 120 mg, 180 mg, 240 mg, 360 mg

Injection, solution: 2.5 mg/mL (2 mL, 4 mL)

Tablet, oral: 40 mg, 80 mg, 120 mg

Calan®: 80 mg, 120 mg

Tablet, extended release, oral: 120 mg, 180 mg, 240 mg

Tablet, extended release, controlled onset, oral:

Covera-HS®: 180 mg, 240 mg

Tablet, sustained release, oral: 240 mg

Isoptin® SR: 120 mg, 180 mg, 240 mg

References

Wynn RL, "Update on Calcium Channel Blocker Induced Gingival Hyperplasia," *Gen Dent*, 1995, 43 (3):218-22.

Verteporfin (ver te POR fin)

U.S. Brand Names Visudyne®

Canadian Brand Names Visudyne®

Pharmacologic Category Ophthalmic Agent

Use Treatment of predominantly classic subfoveal choroidal neovascularization due to macular degeneration, presumed ocular histoplasmosis, or pathologic myopia

Unlabeled/Investigational Use Predominantly **occult** subfoveal choroidal neovascularization

Local Anesthetic/Vasoconstrictor Precautions No information available to require special precautions

Effects on Dental Treatment No significant effects or complications reported

Effects on Bleeding No information available to require special precautions

Adverse Effects

>10%:

Central nervous system: Headache

Local: Injection site reactions (including injection site extravasation, injection site rash)

Ocular: Blurred vision, visual acuity decreased, visual field defects, visual disturbances

1% to 10%:

Cardiovascular: Atrial fibrillation, hypertension, peripheral vascular disorder, varicose veins

Central nervous system: Fever, hypoesthesia, sleep disturbance, vertigo

Dermatologic: Eczema, photosensitivity

Gastrointestinal: Constipation, gastrointestinal cancers, nausea

Genitourinary: Prostatic disorder

Hematologic: Anemia, leukocytosis, leukopenia

Hepatic: Liver function tests increased

Neuromuscular & skeletal: Arthralgia, arthrosis, back pain (primarily during infusion), myasthenia, weakness

Ocular: Diplopia, lacrimation disorder

Treatment site: Blepharitis, cataracts, conjunctivitis/conjunctival injection, dry eyes, ocular itching, severe vision loss (1% to 4%, decrease in 4 lines or more within 7 days of treatment, partial recovery seen in many patients), subconjunctival, subretinal or vitreous hemorrhage.

Otic: Hearing loss

Renal: Albuminuria, creatinine increased

Respiratory: Cough, pharyngitis, pneumonia

Miscellaneous: Flu-like syndrome

General Dosage Range I.V.: *Adults:* 6 mg/m^2 body surface area

Mechanism of Action Following intravenous administration, verteporfin is transported by lipoproteins to the neovascular endothelium in the affected eye(s), including choroidal neovasculature and the retina. Verteporfin then needs to be activated by nonthermal red light, which results in local damage to the endothelium, leading to temporary choroidal vessel occlusion.

Pharmacodynamics/Kinetics

Half-life Elimination Terminal: 5-6 hours, biexponential

Pregnancy Risk Factor C

Vigabatrin (vye GA ba trin)

U.S. Brand Names Sabril®

Canadian Brand Names Sabril®

Pharmacologic Category Anticonvulsant, Miscellaneous

Use Treatment of infantile spasms; refractory complex partial seizures not controlled by usual treatments

Canadian labeling: Additional uses (not in U.S. labeling): Active management of partial or secondary generalized seizures not controlled by usual treatments

Unlabeled/Investigational Use Spasticity, tardive dyskinesias

Local Anesthetic/Vasoconstrictor Precautions No information available to require special precautions

Effects on Dental Treatment No significant effects or complications reported

Effects on Bleeding No information available to require special precautions

Adverse Effects Note: Adult and pediatric information presented combined unless significantly different.

>10%:

Central nervous system: Somnolence (adults 17% to 24%; infants 17% to 45%), headache (18% to 33%), fatigue (16% to 28%), fever (adults 4% to 6%; infants 19% to 29%), dizziness (15% to 24%), irritability (adults 7%; infants 16% to 23%), sedation (adults 4%; infants 17% to 19%), nystagmus (7% to 15%), tremor (7% to 15%), insomnia (10% to 12%), seizure (4% to 11%)

Dermatologic: Rash (4% to 11%)

Gastrointestinal: Vomiting (adults 6% to 7%; infants 14% to 20%), weight gain (6% to 17%), constipation (6% to 14%), diarrhea (7% to 13%)

Neuromuscular & skeletal: Tremor (7% to 15%)

Ocular: Blurred vision (6% to 13%)

Otic: Otitis media (infants 7% to 44%)

Respiratory: Upper respiratory tract infection (adults 7% to 10%; infants 46% to 51%), bronchitis (infants 30%), pharyngitis (10% to 14%), pneumonia (infants 11% to 13%), nasal congestion (infants 4% to 13%)

Miscellaneous: Viral infection (infants 19% to 20%)

1% to 10%:

Cardiovascular: Peripheral edema (2% to 5%), chest pain (1%)

Central nervous system: Irritability (adults 7% to 10%; infants 16% to 23%), memory impairment (7% to 10%), coordination impaired (7% to 9%), disturbance in attention (5% to 9%), depression (4% to 8%), lethargy (4% to 7%), confusional state (4% to 6%), hypotonia (4% to 6%), status epilepticus (2% to 6%), weakness (5%), hyporeflexia (4% to 5%), sensory disturbance (4% to 5%), anxiety (4%), hypoesthesia (3% to 4%), abnormal behavior (3%), abnormal thinking (3%), aggression (2%), nervousness (2%), postictal state (2%), vertigo (2%), abnormal dreams (1%), dystonia (1%), expressive language disorder (1%), hypertonia (1%)

Dermatologic: Contusion (3% to 4%)

Endocrine & metabolic: Dysmenorrhea (7% to 9%), fluid retention (2%)

Gastrointestinal: Nausea (7% to 10%), decreased appetite (7% to 9%), viral gastroenteritis (infants 5% to 6%), abdominal pain (3% to 5%), dyspepsia (4%), abdominal distention (2%), hemorrhoidal symptoms (2%), toothache (2%), increased appetite (1% to 2%)

Genitourinary: Urinary tract infection (4% to 6%)

Neuromuscular & skeletal: Arthralgia (8% to 10%), gait disturbance (6%), paresthesia (5% to 7%), pain in extremity (5% to 6%), back pain (4% to 6%), hyperreflexia (4%), myalgia (3%), muscle spasms (2% to 3%), dysarthria (2%), joint swelling (2%), shoulder pain (2%), joint sprain (1%), muscle strain (1%), muscle twitching (1%)

Ocular: Visual field defect (9%), diplopia (3% to 7%), strabismus (5%), conjunctivitis (2% to 5%), eye strain (2%)

Otic: Tinnitus (2%)

Respiratory: Pharyngolaryngeal pain (7% to 9%), sinusitis (5% to 9%), cough (2% to 8%), sinus headache (4% to 6%), dyspnea (2%)
Miscellaneous: Candidiasis (3% to 8%), influenza (3% to 6%), croup (1% to 5%), thirst (2%)

General Dosage Range Dosage adjustment recommended in patients with renal impairment

Oral:
Infants: 50-150 mg/kg/day in 2 divided doses
Adults: 1-3 g/day in 2 divided doses

Mechanism of Action Irreversibly inhibits gamma-aminobutyric acid transaminase (GABA-T), increasing the levels of the inhibitory compound gamma amino butyric acid (GABA) within the brain. Duration of effect is dependent upon rate of GABA-T resynthesis.

Pharmacodynamics/Kinetics

Duration of Action Resynthesis of GABA-T dependent: Variable (not strictly correlated to serum concentrations)

Half-life Elimination Infants: 5.7 hours; Adults: 7.5 hours; Elderly: 12-13 hours

Time to Peak Infants: 2.5 hours; Children: 1 hour; Adults: 1 hour

Pregnancy Risk Factor C

Prescribing and Access Restrictions As a requirement of the REMS program, access to this medication is restricted. Vigabatrin is only available in the U.S. under a special restricted distribution program (SHARE). Under the SHARE program, only prescribers and pharmacies registered with the program are able to prescribe and distribute vigabatrin. Vigabatrin may only be dispensed to patients who are enrolled in and meet all conditions of SHARE. Contact the SHARE program at 1-888-45-SHARE.

Vilazodone (vil AZ oh done)

U.S. Brand Names Viibryd™

Pharmacologic Category Antidepressant, Selective Serotonin Reuptake Inhibitor/ 5-HT_{1A} Receptor Partial Agonist

Use Treatment of major depressive disorder

Local Anesthetic/Vasoconstrictor Precautions Although caution should be used in patients taking tricyclic antidepressants, no interactions have been reported with vasoconstrictors and vilazodone, a nontricyclic antidepressant which acts to increase serotonin; no precautions appear to be needed

Effects on Dental Treatment Key adverse event(s) related to dental treatment: Xerostomia (normal salivary flow resumes upon discontinuation) and abnormal taste. See Effects on Bleeding.

Effects on Bleeding May impair platelet aggregation resulting in increased risk of bleeding events, particularly if used concomitantly with aspirin, NSAIDs, warfarin, or other anticoagulants. Bleeding related to SSRI use has been reported to range from relatively minor bruising and epistaxis to life-threatening hemorrhage. Routine interruption of therapy for most dental procedures is not warranted. In medically complicated patients or extensive oral surgery, the decision to interrupt therapy must be based on the risk to benefit in an individual patient and a medical consult is suggested. If therapy is continued without interruption, the clinician should anticipate the potential for a prolonged bleeding time.

Adverse Effects

>10%:
Gastrointestinal: Diarrhea (28%), nausea (23%)

1% to 10%:
Cardiovascular: Palpitation (2%)
Central nervous system: Dizziness (9%), insomnia (6%), dreams abnormal (4%), fatigue (4%), restlessness (3%), somnolence (3%), migraine (≥1%), sedation (≥1%)
Dermatologic: Hyperhidrosis (≥1%)
Endocrine & metabolic: Libido decreased (3% to 5%), orgasm abnormal (2% to 4%), sexual dysfunction (≤2%)
Gastrointestinal: Xerostomia (8%), vomiting (5%), dyspepsia (3%), flatulence (3%), gastroenteritis (3%), appetite increased (2%), appetite decreased (≥1%)
Genitourinary: Ejaculation delayed (2%), erectile dysfunction (2%)
Neuromuscular & skeletal: Arthralgia (3%), paresthesia (3%), jittery (2%), tremor (2%)
Ocular: Blurred vision (≥1%), dry eyes (≥1%)
Miscellaneous: Night sweats (≥1%)

General Dosage Range Dosage adjustment recommended in patients on concomitant therapy

Oral: *Adults:* 10-40 mg once daily

Mechanism of Action Vilazodone inhibits CNS neuron serotonin uptake; minimal or no effect on reuptake of norepinephrine or dopamine. It also binds selectively with high affinity to 5-HT_{1A} receptors and is a 5-HT_{1A} receptor partial agonist. 5-HT_{1A} receptor activity may be altered in depression and anxiety.

Pharmacodynamics/Kinetics

Half-life Elimination Terminal: ~25 hours

Time to Peak Serum: 4-5 hours

Pregnancy Risk Factor C

Product Availability Viibryd™: FDA approved January 2011; availability expected during the second quarter of 2011; consult prescribing information for additional information

VinBLAStine (vin BLAS teen)

Pharmacologic Category Antineoplastic Agent, Natural Source (Plant) Derivative; Antineoplastic Agent, Vinca Alkaloid

Use Treatment of Hodgkin's and non-Hodgkin's lymphoma; testicular cancer; breast cancer; mycosis fungoides; Kaposi's sarcoma; histiocytosis (Letterer-Siwe disease); choriocarcinoma

Unlabeled/Investigational Use Treatment of bladder cancer, melanoma, non-small cell lung cancer (NSCLC), ovarian cancer, soft tissue sarcoma (desmoid tumors)

Local Anesthetic/Vasoconstrictor Precautions No information available to require special precautions

Effects on Dental Treatment Key adverse event(s) related to dental treatment: Stomatitis, metallic taste, and jaw pain.

Effects on Bleeding Chemotherapy may result in significant myelosuppression, potentially including significant reduction in platelet counts and altered hemostasis. In patients who are under active treatment with these agents, medical consult is suggested.

Adverse Effects Frequency not defined.

Common:

Cardiovascular: Hypertension

Central nervous system: Malaise

Dermatologic: Alopecia

Gastrointestinal: Constipation

Hematologic: Myelosuppression, leukopenia/granulocytopenia (nadir: 5-10 days; recovery: 7-14 days; dose-limiting toxicity)

Neuromuscular & skeletal: Bone pain, jaw pain, tumor pain

Less common:

Cardiovascular: Angina, cerebrovascular accident, coronary ischemia, ECG abnormalities, limb ischemia, MI, myocardial ischemia, Raynaud's phenomenon

Central nervous system: Depression, dizziness, headache, neurotoxicity (duration: >24 hours), seizure, vertigo

Dermatologic: Dermatitis, photosensitivity (rare), rash, skin blistering

Endocrine & metabolic: Aspermia, hyperuricemia, SIADH

Gastrointestinal: Abdominal pain, anorexia, diarrhea, gastrointestinal bleeding, hemorrhagic enterocolitis, ileus, metallic taste, nausea (mild), paralytic ileus, rectal bleeding, stomatitis, toxic megacolon, vomiting (mild)

Genitourinary: Urinary retention

Hematologic: Anemia, thrombocytopenia (recovery within a few days), thrombotic thrombocytopenic purpura

Local: Cellulitis (with extravasation), irritation, phlebitis (with extravasation), radiation recall

Neuromuscular & skeletal: Deep tendon reflex loss, myalgia, paresthesia, peripheral neuritis, weakness

Ocular: Nystagmus

Otic: Auditory damage, deafness, vestibular damage

Renal: Hemolytic uremic syndrome

Respiratory: Bronchospasm, dyspnea, pharyngitis

General Dosage Range Dosage adjustment recommended in patients with hepatic impairment

I.V.:

Children: Initial dose: 3-6.5 mg/m² every 7 days as needed

Adults: Initial: 3.7 mg/m²; adjust dose every 7 days; Second dose: 5.5 mg/m²; Third dose: 7.4 mg/m²; Fourth dose: 9.25 mg/m²; Fifth dose: 11.1 mg/m²; Usual range: 5.5-7.4 mg/m² every 7 days; Maximum dose: 18.5 mg/m²

Mechanism of Action Vinblastine binds to tubulin and inhibits microtubule formation, therefore, arresting the cell at metaphase by disrupting the formation of the mitotic spindle; it is specific for the M and S phases. Vinblastine may also interfere with nucleic acid and protein synthesis by blocking glutamic acid utilization.

Pharmacodynamics/Kinetics

Half-life Elimination Biphasic: Initial: 4 minutes; Terminal: 25 hours

Pregnancy Risk Factor D

VinCRIStine (vin KRIS teen)

U.S. Brand Names Vincasar PFS®

Canadian Brand Names Vincristine Sulfate Injection

Pharmacologic Category Antineoplastic Agent, Natural Source (Plant) Derivative; Antineoplastic Agent, Vinca Alkaloid

Use Treatment of acute lymphocytic leukemia (ALL), Hodgkin's lymphoma, non-Hodgkin's lymphomas, Wilms' tumor, neuroblastoma, rhabdomyosarcoma

Unlabeled/Investigational Use Treatment of multiple myeloma, chronic lymphocytic leukemia (CLL), brain tumors, small cell lung cancer, ovarian germ cell tumors

Local Anesthetic/Vasoconstrictor Precautions No information available to require special precautions

Effects on Dental Treatment Key adverse event(s) related to dental treatment: Oral ulceration, metallic taste, orthostatic hypotension or hypertension.

Effects on Bleeding Although significant myelosuppression with associated altered hemostasis has been reported for many chemotherapeutic agents, myelosuppression is not common with vincristine and no specific precautions appear to necessary.

Adverse Effects Frequency not defined.

Cardiovascular: Edema, hyper-/hypotension, MI, myocardial ischemia

Central nervous system: Ataxia, coma, cranial nerve dysfunction (auditory damage, extraocular muscle impairment, laryngeal muscle impairment, paralysis, paresis, vestibular damage, vocal cord paralysis), dizziness, fever, headache, neurotoxicity, neuropathic pain (common), seizure, vertigo

Dermatologic toxicity: Alopecia (common), rash

Endocrine & metabolic: Hyperuricemia, parotid pain, SIADH (rare)

Gastrointestinal: Abdominal cramps, abdominal pain, anorexia, constipation (common), diarrhea, intestinal necrosis, intestinal perforation, nausea, oral ulcers, paralytic ileus, vomiting, weight loss

Genitourinary: Bladder atony, dysuria, polyuria, urinary retention

Hematologic: Anemia (mild), leukopenia (mild), thrombocytopenia (mild), thrombotic thrombocytopenic purpura

Hepatic: Veno-occlusive liver disease (VOD)

Local: Phlebitis, tissue irritation/necrosis (if infiltrated)

Neuromuscular & skeletal: Back pain, bone pain, deep tendon reflex loss, difficulty walking, foot drop, gait changes, jaw pain, limb pain, motor difficulties, muscle wasting, myalgia, paralysis, paresthesia, peripheral neuropathy (common), sensorimotor dysfunction, sensory loss

Ocular: Cortical blindness (transient), nystagmus, optic atrophy with blindness

Otic: Deafness

Renal: Acute uric acid nephropathy, hemolytic uremic syndrome

Respiratory: Bronchospasm, dyspnea, pharyngeal pain

Miscellaneous: Allergic reactions (rare), anaphylaxis (rare), hypersensitivity (rare)

General Dosage Range Dosage adjustment recommended in patients with hepatic impairment

I.V.:

Children ≤10 kg: 0.05 mg/kg once weekly (maximum: 2 mg/dose)

Children >10 kg: 1.5-2 mg/m²/dose (maximum: 2 mg/dose)

Adults: 1.4 mg/m²/dose (maximum: 2 mg/dose)

Mechanism of Action Binds to tubulin and inhibits microtubule formation, therefore, arresting the cell at metaphase by disrupting the formation of the mitotic spindle; it is specific for the M and S phases. Vincristine may also interfere with nucleic acid and protein synthesis by blocking glutamic acid utilization.

Pharmacodynamics/Kinetics

Half-life Elimination Terminal: 85 hours (range: 19-155 hours)

Pregnancy Risk Factor D

Vinorelbine (vi NOR el been)

U.S. Brand Names Navelbine®

Canadian Brand Names Navelbine®; Vinorelbine Injection, USP; Vinorelbine Tartrate for Injection

Pharmacologic Category Antineoplastic Agent, Natural Source (Plant) Derivative; Antineoplastic Agent, Vinca Alkaloid

Use Treatment of nonsmall cell lung cancer (NSCLC)

Unlabeled/Investigational Use Treatment of breast cancer (metastatic), cervical cancer, ovarian cancer, malignant pleural mesothelioma, and soft tissue sarcoma

Local Anesthetic/Vasoconstrictor Precautions No information available to require special precautions

Effects on Dental Treatment No significant effects or complications reported

Effects on Bleeding Chemotherapy may result in significant myelosuppression, potentially including significant reduction in platelet counts and altered hemostasis. In patients who are under active treatment with these agents, medical consult is suggested.

Adverse Effects Note: Reported with single-agent therapy.

>10%:

- Central nervous system: Fatigue (27%)
- Dermatologic: Alopecia (12% to 30%)
- Gastrointestinal: Nausea (31% to 44%; grade 3: 1% to 2%), constipation (35%; grade 3: 3%), vomiting (20% to 31%; grade 3: 1% to 2%), diarrhea (12% to 17%)
- Hematologic: Leukopenia (83% to 92%; grade 4: 6% to 15%), granulocytopenia (90%; grade 4: 36%; nadir: 7-10 days; recovery 14-21 days; dose-limiting), neutropenia (85%; grade 4: 28%), anemia (83%; grades 3/4: 9%)
- Hepatic: AST increased (67%; grade 3: 5%; grade 4: 1%), total bilirubin increased (5% to 13%; grade 3: 4%; grade 4: 3%)
- Local: Injection site reaction (22% to 28%; includes erythema, vein discoloration), injection site pain (16%)
- Neuromuscular & skeletal: Weakness (36%), peripheral neuropathy (25%; grade 3: 1%; grade 4: <1%)
- Renal: Creatinine increased (13%)

1% to 10%:

- Cardiovascular: Chest pain (5%)
- Dermatologic: Rash (<5%)
- Gastrointestinal: Paralytic ileus (1%)
- Hematologic: Neutropenic fever/sepsis (8%; grade 4: 4%), thrombocytopenia (3% to 5%; grades 3/4: 1%)
- Local: Phlebitis (7% to 10%)
- Neuromuscular & skeletal: Loss of deep tendon reflexes (<5%), myalgia (<5%), arthralgia (<5%), jaw pain (<5%)
- Otic: Ototoxicity (≤1%)
- Respiratory: Dyspnea (7%)

General Dosage Range Dosage adjustment recommended in patients with hepatic impairment or who develop toxicities

I.V.: *Adults:* 25-30 mg/m^2/dose every 7 days

Mechanism of Action Semisynthetic vinca alkaloid which binds to tubulin and inhibits microtubule formation, therefore, arresting the cell at metaphase by disrupting the formation of the mitotic spindle; it is specific for the M and S phases. Vinorelbine may also interfere with nucleic acid and protein synthesis by blocking glutamic acid utilization.

Pharmacodynamics/Kinetics

Half-life Elimination Triphasic: Terminal: 28-44 hours

Pregnancy Risk Factor D

Vitamin A (VYE ta min aye)

U.S. Brand Names A-25 [OTC]; A-Natural [OTC]; A-Natural-25 [OTC]; Aquasol A®

Pharmacologic Category Vitamin, Fat Soluble

Use Treatment and prevention of vitamin A deficiency; parenteral (I.M.) route is indicated when oral administration is not feasible or when absorption is insufficient (malabsorption syndrome)

Local Anesthetic/Vasoconstrictor Precautions No information available to require special precautions

Effects on Dental Treatment No significant effects or complications reported

Effects on Bleeding No information available to require special precautions

Adverse Effects 1% to 10%:

- Central nervous system: Fever, headache, irritability, lethargy, malaise, vertigo
- Dermatologic: Drying or cracking of skin
- Endocrine & metabolic: Hypercalcemia
- Gastrointestinal: Weight loss
- Ocular: Visual changes
- Miscellaneous: Hypervitaminosis A

General Dosage Range I.M., oral: *Children and Adults:* Dosage varies greatly depending on indication

Mechanism of Action Needed for bone development, growth, visual adaptation to darkness, testicular and ovarian function, and as a cofactor in many biochemical processes

Pregnancy Risk Factor A/X (dose exceeding RDA recommendation)

Vitamin A and Vitamin D (VYE ta min aye & VYE ta min dee)

Related Information

Vitamin A *on page 1725*

U.S. Brand Names A and D® Original [OTC]; Baza® Clear [OTC]; Sween Cream® [OTC]

Pharmacologic Category Topical Skin Product

Use Temporary relief of discomfort due to chapped skin, diaper rash, minor burns, abrasions, as well as irritations associated with ostomy skin care

Local Anesthetic/Vasoconstrictor Precautions No information available to require special precautions

Effects on Dental Treatment No significant effects or complications reported

Effects on Bleeding No information available to require special precautions

Adverse Effects Frequency not defined: Local: Irritation

General Dosage Range Topical: *Children and Adults:* Apply locally as needed

Pregnancy Risk Factor B

Vitamin B Complex Combinations
(VYE ta min bee KOM pleks kom bi NAY shuns)

Pharmacologic Category Vitamin

Use Supplement for use in the wasting syndrome in chronic renal failure, uremia, impaired metabolic functions of the kidney, dialysis; labeled for OTC use as a dietary supplement

Local Anesthetic/Vasoconstrictor Precautions No information available to require special precautions

Effects on Dental Treatment No significant effects or complications reported

Effects on Bleeding No information available to require special precautions

Adverse Effects Frequency not defined.

Central nervous system: Somnolence
Dermatologic: Itching
Gastrointestinal: Bloating, constipation, diarrhea, flatulence, nausea, vomiting
Hematologic: Peripheral vascular thrombosis, polycythemia vera
Neuromuscular & skeletal: Paresthesia
Miscellaneous: Allergic reaction

General Dosage Range

Oral: *Adults:* Dosage varies greatly depending on product

Pregnancy Risk Factor A (RDA recommended doses)

Vitamin E (VYE ta min ee)

U.S. Brand Names Alph-E [OTC]; Alph-E-Mixed [OTC]; Aqua Gem-E™ [OTC]; Aquasol E® [OTC]; Aquavit-E [OTC] [DSC]; d-Alpha Gems™ [OTC]; E-Gems® Elite [OTC]; E-Gems® Plus [OTC]; E-Gems® [OTC]; E-Gem® Lip Care [OTC]; E-Gem® [OTC]; Ester-E™ [OTC]; Gamma E-Gems® [OTC]; Gamma-E PLUS [OTC]; High Gamma Vitamin E Complete™ [OTC]; Key-E® Kaps [OTC]; Key-E® Powder [OTC]; Key-E® [OTC]

Pharmacologic Category Vitamin, Fat Soluble

Use Dietary supplement

Unlabeled/Investigational Use To reduce the risk of bronchopulmonary dysplasia or retrolental fibroplasia in infants exposed to high concentrations of oxygen; prevention and treatment of tardive dyskinesia; prevention and treatment of hemolytic anemia secondary to vitamin E deficiency

Local Anesthetic/Vasoconstrictor Precautions No information available to require special precautions

Effects on Dental Treatment No significant effects or complications reported

Effects on Bleeding No information available to require special precautions

Adverse Effects Frequency not defined.

Central nervous system: Fatigue, headache
Dermatologic: Contact dermatitis with topical preparation
Endocrine & metabolic: Gonadal dysfunction
Gastrointestinal: Diarrhea, intestinal cramps, nausea

Neuromuscular & skeletal: Weakness
Ocular: Blurred vision

General Dosage Range

Oral:

Children: 1 unit/kg/day **or** 100-750 units/day
Adults: 30-1600 units/day **or** 1000 units twice daily

Topical: *Adults:* Apply a thin layer over affected area

Mechanism of Action Prevents oxidation of vitamin A and C; protects polyunsaturated fatty acids in membranes from attack by free radicals and protects red blood cells against hemolysis

Pregnancy Risk Factor A/C (dose exceeding RDA recommendation)

Vitamins (Fluoride) (VYE ta mins, FLOOR ide)

U.S. Brand Names Poly-Vi-Flor®; Poly-Vi-Flor® With Iron; Soluvite-F; Tri-Vi-Flor®; Tri-Vi-Flor® with Iron; Vi-Daylin®/F + Iron [DSC]; Vi-Daylin®/F ADC [DSC]; Vi-Daylin®/F ADC + Iron [DSC]; Vi-Daylin®/F [DSC]

Pharmacologic Category Vitamin

Use Prevention/treatment of vitamin deficiency; products containing fluoride are used to prevent dental caries; labeled for OTC use as a dietary supplement

Local Anesthetic/Vasoconstrictor Precautions No information available to require special precautions

Effects on Dental Treatment No significant effects or complications reported

Dosage Daily dose varies by product; refer to package insert for specific product labeling

Contraindications Hypersensitivity to any component of the formulation; pre-existing hypervitaminosis

Warnings/Precautions Not all products can be used in children of all age groups; consult specific product labeling prior to use. Do not exceed recommended doses. Use caution with severe renal or hepatic dysfunction or failure. **[U.S. Boxed Warning]: Products may contain iron. Severe iron toxicity may occur in overdose, particularly when ingested by children; iron is a leading cause of fatal poisoning in children; store out of children's reach and in child-resistant containers.**

Dietary Considerations May take with food to decrease stomach upset.

Dosage Forms Content varies depending on product used. For more detailed information on ingredients in these and other multivitamins, please refer to package labeling.

Dental Comment Chronic overdose of fluoride may result in mottling of tooth enamel and osseous changes.

Vitamins (Multiple/Oral) (VYE ta mins, MUL ti pul/OR al)

U.S. Brand Names Androvite® [OTC]; CalciFolic-D™; Centamin [OTC]; Centrum Cardio® [OTC]; Centrum Performance® [OTC]; Centrum® Silver® Ultra Men's [OTC]; Centrum® Silver® Ultra Women's [OTC]; Centrum® Silver® [OTC]; Centrum® Ultra Men's [OTC]; Centrum® Ultra Women's [OTC]; Centrum® [OTC]; Diatx®Zn; Drinkables® Fruits and Vegetables [OTC]; Drinkables® MultiVitamins [OTC]; Encora®; Foltrin®; Freedavite [OTC]; Geri-Freeda [OTC]; Geriation [OTC]; Geritol Complete® [OTC]; Geritol Extend® [OTC]; Geritol® Tonic [OTC]; Glutofac®-MX; Glutofac®-ZX; Gynovite® Plus [OTC]; Hemocyte Plus®; Hi-Kovite [OTC]; Iberet®-500 [OTC] [DSC]; Monocaps [OTC]; Myadec® [OTC]; Nutrimin-Plus [OTC]; Ocuvite® Adult 50+ [OTC]; Ocuvite® Extra® [OTC]; Ocuvite® Lutein [OTC]; Ocuvite® [OTC]; One A Day® Cholesterol Plus [OTC]; One A Day® Energy [OTC]; One A Day® Essential [OTC]; One A Day® Maximum [OTC]; One A Day® Men's 50+ Advantage [OTC]; One A Day® Men's Health Formula [OTC]; One A Day® Teen Advantage for Her [OTC]; One A Day® Teen Advantage for Him [OTC]; One A Day® Weight Smart® Advanced [OTC]; One A Day® Women's 50+ Advantage [OTC]; One A Day® Women's Active Mind & Body [OTC]; One A Day® Women's [OTC]; Optivite® P.M.T. [OTC]; PreserVision® AREDS [OTC]; PreserVision® Lutein [OTC]; Quintabs [OTC]; Quintabs-M Iron-Free [OTC]; Quintabs-M [OTC]; Renax®; Renax® 5.5; Replace Without Iron [OTC]; Replace [OTC]; Repliva 21/7®; SourceCF®; Strovite®; Strovite® Advance; Strovite® Forte; Strovite® Plus; T-Vites [OTC]; Ultra Freeda A-Free [OTC]; Ultra Freeda Iron-Free [OTC]; Ultra Freeda With Iron [OTC]; Viactiv® Calcium Flavor Glides™ [OTC]; Viactiv® Flavor Glides [OTC]; Viactiv® for Teens [OTC]; Viactiv® With Calcium [OTC]; Viactiv® [OTC]; Vitafol®; Xtramins [OTC]; Yelets [OTC]

Pharmacologic Category Vitamin

Use Prevention/treatment of vitamin and mineral deficiencies; labeled for OTC use as a dietary supplement

Local Anesthetic/Vasoconstrictor Precautions No information available to require special precautions

Effects on Dental Treatment No significant effects or complications reported

Effects on Bleeding No information available to require special precautions

Adverse Effects Refer to individual vitamin monographs.

General Dosage Range Oral: *Adults:* 1 tablet/capsule **or** 5-15 mL once daily

Pregnancy Risk Factor A (at RDA recommended dose)

Voriconazole (vor i KOE na zole)

Related Information

Clinical Risk Related to Drugs Prolonging QT Interval *on page* 1872

Fungal Infections *on page* 1945

U.S. Brand Names VFEND®

Canadian Brand Names VFEND®

Generic Availability (U.S.) Yes: Tablet

Pharmacologic Category Antifungal Agent, Oral; Antifungal Agent, Parenteral

Use Treatment of invasive aspergillosis; treatment of esophageal candidiasis; treatment of candidemia (in non-neutropenic patients); treatment of disseminated *Candida* infections of the skin and viscera; treatment of serious fungal infections caused by *Scedosporium apiospermum* and *Fusarium* spp (including *Fusarium solani*) in patients intolerant of, or refractory to, other therapy

Unlabeled/Investigational Use Fungal infection prophylaxis in intermediate or high risk neutropenic cancer patients with myelodysplastic syndrome (MDS) or acute myelogenous leukemia (AML), neutropenic allogeneic hematopoietic stem cell recipients, and patients with significant graft-versus-host disease; empiric antifungal therapy (second-line) for persistent neutropenic fever

Local Anesthetic/Vasoconstrictor Precautions Voriconazole is one of the drugs confirmed to prolong the QT interval and is accepted as having a risk of causing torsade de pointes. The risk of drug-induced torsade de pointes is extremely low when a single QT interval prolonging drug is prescribed. In terms of epinephrine, it is not known what effect vasoconstrictors in the local anesthetic regimen will have in patients with a known history of congenital prolonged QT interval or in patients taking any medication that prolongs the QT interval. Until more information is obtained, it is suggested that the clinician consult with the physician prior to the use of a vasoconstrictor in suspected patients, and that the vasoconstrictor (epinephrine, mepivacaine and levonordefrin [Carbocaine® 2% with Neo-Cobefrin®]) be used with caution.

Effects on Dental Treatment Key adverse event(s) related to dental treatment: Xerostomia (normal salivary flow resumes upon discontinuation).

Effects on Bleeding No information available to require special precautions

Adverse Effects

>10%:

- Central nervous system: Hallucinations (4% to 12%; auditory and/or visual and likely serum concentration-dependent)
- Ocular: Visual changes (dose related; photophobia, color changes, increased or decreased visual acuity, or blurred vision occur in ~21%)
- Renal: Creatinine increased (1% to 21%)

2% to 10%:

- Cardiovascular: Tachycardia (≤2%)
- Central nervous system: Fever (≤6%), chills (≤4%), headache (≤3%)
- Dermatologic: Rash (≤7%)
- Endocrine & metabolic: Hypokalemia (≤2%)
- Gastrointestinal: Nausea (1% to 5%), vomiting (1% to 4%)
- Hepatic: Alkaline phosphatase increased (4% to 5%), AST increased (2% to 4%), ALT increased (2% to 3%), cholestatic jaundice (1% to 2%)
- Ocular: Photophobia (2% to 3%)

Dosage

Usual dosage ranges:

Children <12 years: Dosage not established

Children ≥12 years and Adults:

- Oral: 100-300 mg every 12 hours
- I.V.: 6 mg/kg every 12 hours for 2 doses; followed by maintenance dose of 4 mg/kg every 12 hours

Indication-specific dosing:

Infants and Children:

Aspergillosis, invasive including disseminated and extrapulmonary infection in HIV-exposed/-positive patients: (unlabeled; CDC, 2009):

Oral: Loading dose: 8 mg/kg/dose (maximum: 400 mg/dose) every 12 hours for 2 doses on day 1, followed by maintenance dose of 7 mg/kg/dose (maximum: 200 mg/dose) every 12 hours for ≥12 weeks

I.V.: Loading dose: 6-8 mg/kg/dose (maximum: 400 mg/dose) every 12 hours for 2 doses on day 1, followed by maintenance dose of 7 mg/kg/dose (maximum: 200 mg/dose) every 12 hours for ≥12 weeks

Children ≥12 years and Adults:

Aspergillosis, invasive, including disseminated and extrapulmonary infection: Duration of therapy should be a minimum of 6-12 weeks or throughout period of immunosuppression (Walsh, 2008):

I.V.: Initial: Loading dose: 6 mg/kg every 12 hours for 2 doses; followed by maintenance dose of 4 mg/kg every 12 hours

Oral: Maintenance dose:

Manufacturer's recommendations:

Patients <40 kg: 100 mg every 12 hours; maximum 300 mg/day

Patients ≥40 kg: 200 mg every 12 hours; maximum: 600 mg/day

IDSA recommendations (Walsh, 2008): May consider oral therapy in place of I.V. with dosing of 4 mg/kg (rounded up to convenient tablet dosage form) every 12 hours; however, I.V. administration is preferred in serious infections since comparative efficacy with the oral formulation has not been established.

Scedosporiosis, fusariosis:

I.V.: Initial: Loading dose: 6 mg/kg every 12 hours for 2 doses; followed by maintenance dose of 4 mg/kg every 12 hours

Oral: Maintenance dose:

Patients <40 kg: 100 mg every 12 hours; maximum: 300 mg/day

Patients ≥40 kg: 200 mg every 12 hours; maximum: 600 mg/day

Candidemia and other deep tissue *Candida* infections: Treatment should continue for a minimum of 14 days following resolution of symptoms or following last positive culture, whichever is longer.

I.V.: Initial: Loading dose 6 mg/kg every 12 hours for 2 doses; followed by maintenance dose of 3-4 mg/kg every 12 hours

Oral:

Manufacturer's recommendations: Maintenance dose:

Patients <40 kg: 100 mg every 12 hours; maximum: 300 mg/day

Patients ≥40 kg: 200 mg every 12 hours; maximum: 600 mg/day

IDSA recommendations (Pappas, 2009): Initial: Loading dose: 400 mg every 12 hours for 2 doses; followed by 200 mg every 12 hours

Endophthalmitis, fungal (unlabeled use, Pappas, 2009): I.V.: 6 mg/kg every 12 hours for 2 doses, then 3-4 mg/kg every 12 hours

Esophageal candidiasis: Oral: Treatment should continue for a minimum of 14 days, and for at least 7 days following resolution of symptoms:

Patients <40 kg: 100 mg every 12 hours; maximum: 300 mg/day

Patients ≥40 kg: 200 mg every 12 hours; maximum: 600 mg/day

Dosage adjustment in patients unable to tolerate treatment:

I.V.: Dose may be reduced to 3 mg/kg every 12 hours

Oral: Dose may be reduced in 50 mg decrements to a minimum dosage of 200 mg every 12 hours in patients weighing ≥40 kg (100 mg every 12 hours in patients <40 kg)

Dosage adjustment in patients receiving concomitant CYP450 enzyme inducers or substrates:

Cyclosporine: Reduce cyclosporine dose by one-half and monitor closely; upon discontinuation of voriconazole, monitor cyclosporine concentrations and escalate the cyclosporine dose as needed

Efavirenz: Oral: Increase maintenance dose of voriconazole to 400 mg every 12 hours and reduce efavirenz dose to 300 mg once daily; upon discontinuation of voriconazole, return to the initial dose of efavirenz

Omeprazole: Reduce omeprazole dose by one-half in patients maintained on ≥40 mg/day of omeprazole

Phenytoin:

I.V.: Increase voriconazole maintenance dosage to 5 mg/kg every 12 hours

Oral: Increase voriconazole dose to 400 mg every 12 hours in patients ≥40 kg (200 mg every 12 hours in patients <40 kg)

Tacrolimus: Reduce tacrolimus dose by one-third and monitor closely; upon discontinuation of voriconazole, monitor tacrolimus concentrations and escalate the tacrolimus dose as needed.

Dosage adjustment in renal impairment: In patients with Cl_{cr} <50 mL/minute, accumulation of the intravenous vehicle (cyclodextrin) occurs. After initial I.V. loading dose, oral voriconazole should be administered to these patients, unless an assessment of the benefit:risk to the patient justifies the use of I.V. voriconazole. Monitor serum creatinine and change to oral voriconazole therapy when possible.

Hemodialysis: Oral dosage adjustment not required; I.V. dosing not recommended since cyclodextrin vehicle is cleared at half the rate of voriconazole and may accumulate

Dosage adjustment in hepatic impairment:

Mild-to-moderate hepatic dysfunction (Child-Pugh class A and B): Following standard loading dose, reduce maintenance dosage by 50%

Severe hepatic impairment: Should only be used if benefit outweighs risk; monitor closely for toxicity

Mechanism of Action Interferes with fungal cytochrome P450 activity (selectively inhibits 14-alpha-lanosterol demethylation), decreasing ergosterol synthesis (principal sterol in fungal cell membrane) and inhibiting fungal cell membrane formation.

Contraindications Hypersensitivity to voriconazole or any component of the formulation (cross-reaction with other azole antifungal agents may occur but has not been established, use caution); coadministration of CYP3A4 substrates which may lead to QT_c prolongation (cisapride, pimozide, or quinidine); coadministration with barbiturates (long acting), carbamazepine, efavirenz (with standard [eg, not adjusted] voriconazole and efavirenz doses), ergot derivatives, rifampin, rifabutin, ritonavir (≥800 mg/day), sirolimus, St John's wort

Warnings/Precautions Visual changes, including blurred vision, changes in visual acuity, color perception, and photophobia, are commonly associated with treatment; postmarketing cases of optic neuritis and papilledema (lasting >1 month) have also been reported. Patients should be warned to avoid tasks which depend on vision, including operating machinery or driving. Changes are reversible on discontinuation following brief exposure/treatment regimens (≤28 days).

Serious hepatic reactions (including hepatitis, cholestasis, and fulminant hepatic failure) have occurred during treatment, primarily in patients with serious concomitant medical conditions. However, hepatotoxicity has occurred in patients with no identifiable risk factors. Use caution in patients with pre-existing hepatic impairment (dose adjustment or discontinuation may be required).

Voriconazole tablets contain lactose; avoid administration in hereditary galactose intolerance, Lapp lactase deficiency, or glucose-galactose malabsorption. Suspension contains sucrose; use caution with fructose intolerance, sucrose-isomaltase deficiency, or glucose-galactose malabsorption. Avoid/limit use of intravenous formulation in patients with renal impairment; intravenous formulation contains excipient cyclodextrin (sulfobutyl ether beta-cyclodextrin), which may accumulate in renal insufficiency. Acute renal failure has been observed in severely ill patients; use with caution in patients receiving concomitant nephrotoxic medications. Anaphylactoid-type infusion-related reactions may occur with intravenous dosing. Consider discontinuation of infusion if reaction is severe.

Use caution in patients taking strong cytochrome P450 inducers, CYP2C9 inhibitors, and major 3A4 substrates (see Drug Interactions); consider alternative agents that avoid or lessen the potential for CYP-mediated interactions. QT interval prolongation has been associated with voriconazole use; rare cases of arrhythmia (including torsade de pointes), cardiac arrest, and sudden death have been reported, usually in seriously ill patients with comorbidities and/or risk factors (eg, prior cardiotoxic chemotherapy, cardiomyopathy, electrolyte imbalance, or concomitant QT_c-prolonging drugs). Use with caution in these patient populations; correct electrolyte abnormalities (eg, hypokalemia, hypomagnesemia, hypocalcemia) prior to initiating therapy. Do not infuse concomitantly with blood products or short-term concentrated electrolyte solutions, even if the two infusions are running in separate intravenous lines (or cannulas).

Rare cases of malignancy (melanoma, squamous cell carcinoma) have been reported in patients (mostly immunocompromised) with prior onset of severe photosensitivity reactions and exposure to long-term voriconazole therapy. Other serious exfoliative cutaneous reactions, including Stevens-Johnson syndrome, have also been reported. Patient should avoid strong, direct exposure to sunlight; may cause photosensitivity, especially with long-term use. Discontinue use in patients who develop an exfoliative cutaneous reaction or a skin lesion consistent with squamous cell carcinoma or melanoma. Periodic total body skin examinations should be performed, particularly with prolonged use.

Monitor pancreatic function in patients (children and adults) at risk for acute pancreatitis (eg, recent chemotherapy or hematopoietic stem cell transplantation); there have been postmarketing reports of pancreatitis in children.

Drug Interactions

Metabolism/Transport Effects **Substrate** of CYP2C9 (major), 2C19 (major), 3A4 (minor); **Inhibits** CYP2C9 (moderate), 2C19 (weak), 3A4 (moderate)

Avoid Concomitant Use

Avoid concomitant use of Voriconazole with any of the following: Alfuzosin; Artemether; Barbiturates; CarBAMazepine; Cisapride; Conivaptan; Darunavir; Dofetilide; Dronedarone; Eplerenone; Ergot Derivatives; Everolimus; Fluconazole; Fluticasone (Oral Inhalation); Halofantrine; Lopinavir; Lumefantrine; Lurasidone; Nilotinib; Nisoldipine; Pimozide; QuiNIDine; QuiNINE; Ranolazine; Rifamycin Derivatives; Ritonavir; Rivaroxaban; RomiDEPsin; Salmeterol; Silodosin; Sirolimus; St Johns Wort; Tamsulosin; Tetrabenazine; Thioridazine; Tolvaptan; Toremifene; Vandetanib; Ziprasidone

Increased Effect/Toxicity

Voriconazole may increase the levels/effects of: Alfentanil; Alfuzosin; Almotriptan; Alosetron; Antineoplastic Agents (Vinca Alkaloids); Aprepitant; Benzodiazepines (metabolized by oxidation); Bortezomib; Bosentan; Brinzolamide; Budesonide (Nasal); Budesonide (Systemic, Oral Inhalation); BusPIRone; Busulfan; Calcium Channel Blockers; CarBAMazepine; Carvedilol; Ciclesonide; Cilostazol; Cinacalcet; Cisapride; Colchicine; Conivaptan; Contraceptives (Estrogens); Contraceptives (Progestins); Corticosteroids (Orally Inhaled); Corticosteroids (Systemic); CycloSPORINE; CycloSPORINE (Systemic); CYP2C9 Substrates (High risk); CYP3A4 Substrates; Diclofenac; Diclofenac (Systemic); Diclofenac (Topical); Dienogest; DOCEtaxel; Dofetilide; Dronedarone; Dutasteride; Eletriptan; Eplerenone; Ergot Derivatives; Erlotinib; Eszopiclone; Etravirine; Everolimus; FentaNYL; Fesoterodine; Fluticasone (Nasal); Fluticasone (Oral Inhalation); Fosaprepitant; Fosphenytoin; Gefitinib; GuanFACINE; Halofantrine; HMG-CoA Reductase Inhibitors; Ibuprofen; Imatinib; Irinotecan; Ixabepilone; Losartan; Lumefantrine; Lurasidone; Macrolide Antibiotics; Maraviroc; Meloxicam; Methadone; MethylPREDNISolone; Nilotinib; Nisoldipine; OxyCODONE; Paricalcitol; Pazopanib; Phenytoin; Phosphodiesterase 5 Inhibitors; Pimecrolimus; Pimozide; Protease Inhibitors; QTc-Prolonging Agents; QuiNIDine; QuiNINE; Ramelteon; Ranolazine; Repaglinide; Reverse Transcriptase Inhibitors (Non-Nucleoside); Rifamycin Derivatives; Rivaroxaban; RomiDEPsin; Salmeterol; Saxagliptin; Silodosin; Sirolimus; Solifenacin; SORAfenib; Sulfonylureas; SUNItinib; Tacrolimus; Tacrolimus (Systemic); Tacrolimus (Topical); Tadalafil; Tamsulosin; Tetrabenazine; Thioridazine; Tolterodine; Tolvaptan; Toremifene; Vandetanib; Venlafaxine; Vilazodone; Vitamin K Antagonists; Ziprasidone; Zolpidem

The levels/effects of Voriconazole may be increased by: Alfuzosin; Artemether; Chloramphenicol; Chloroquine; Ciprofloxacin; Ciprofloxacin (Systemic); Contraceptives (Estrogens); Contraceptives (Progestins); CYP2C19 Inhibitors (Moderate); CYP2C19 Inhibitors (Strong); CYP2C9 Inhibitors (Moderate); CYP2C9 Inhibitors (Strong); Etravirine; Fluconazole; Gadobutrol; Grapefruit Juice; Lumefantrine; Macrolide Antibiotics; Nilotinib; Protease Inhibitors; Proton Pump Inhibitors; QuiNINE

Decreased Effect

Voriconazole may decrease the levels/effects of: Amphotericin B; Prasugrel; Saccharomyces boulardii

The levels/effects of Voriconazole may be decreased by: Barbiturates; CarBAMazepine; CYP2C19 Inducers (Strong); CYP2C9 Inducers (Highly Effective); Darunavir; Didanosine; Etravirine; Fosphenytoin; Lopinavir; Peginterferon Alfa-2b; Phenytoin; Reverse Transcriptase Inhibitors (Non-Nucleoside); Rifamycin Derivatives; Ritonavir; St Johns Wort; Sucralfate; Tocilizumab

Ethanol/Nutrition/Herb Interactions

Food: May decrease voriconazole absorption. Oral voriconazole should be taken 1 hour before or 1 hour after a meal. Avoid grapefruit juice (may decrease voriconazole levels).

Herb/Nutraceutical: St John's wort may decrease voriconazole levels; concurrent use with voriconazole is contraindicated.

Dietary Considerations Oral: Should be taken 1 hour before or 1 hour after a meal. Voriconazole tablets contain lactose; avoid administration in hereditary galactose intolerance, Lapp lactase deficiency, or glucose-galactose malabsorption. Suspension contains sucrose; use caution with fructose intolerance, sucrose-isomaltase deficiency, or glucose-galactose malabsorption.

Pharmacodynamics/Kinetics

Half-life Elimination Variable, dose dependent

Time to Peak Oral: 1-2 hours; 0.5 hours (crushed tablet)

Pregnancy Risk Factor D

Lactation Excretion in breast milk unknown/not recommended

Breast-Feeding Considerations Excretion in breast milk has not been investigated; avoid breast-feeding until additional data are available.

Dosage Forms

Injection, powder for reconstitution:
VFEND®: 200 mg

Powder for suspension, oral:
VFEND®: 40 mg/mL (70 mL)

Tablet, oral: 50 mg, 200 mg
VFEND®: 50 mg, 200 mg

Dental Comment Voriconazole is known to prolong the QT interval. The QT interval is measured as the time and distance between the Q point of the QRS complex and the end of the T wave in the ECG tracing. After adjustment for heart rate, the QT interval is defined as prolonged if it is more than 450 msec in men and 460 msec in women. A long QT syndrome was first described in the 1950s and 60s as a congenital syndrome involving QT interval prolongation and syncope and sudden death. Some of the congenital long QT syndromes were characterized by a peculiar electrocardiographic appearance of the QRS complex involving a premature atria beat followed by a pause, then a subsequent sinus beat showing marked QT prolongation and deformity. This type of cardiac arrhythmia was originally termed "torsade de pointes" (translated from the French as "twisting of the points"). Voriconazole is considered as having a risk of causing torsade de pointes. Since it is not known what effect vasoconstrictors in the local anesthetic regimen will have in patients with a known history of congenital prolonged QT interval or in patients taking any medication that prolongs the QT interval, a medical consult is suggested.

Vorinostat (vor IN oh stat)

U.S. Brand Names Zolinza™

Canadian Brand Names Zolinza®

Pharmacologic Category Antineoplastic Agent, Histone Deacetylase Inhibitor

Use Treatment of progressive, persistent, or recurrent cutaneous T-cell lymphoma (CTCL)

Local Anesthetic/Vasoconstrictor Precautions No information available to require special precautions

Effects on Dental Treatment Key adverse event(s) related to dental treatment: High incidence of xerostomia (normal salivary flow resumes upon discontinuation) and taste perversion.

Effects on Bleeding Chemotherapy may result in significant myelosuppression, potentially including significant reduction in platelet counts and altered hemostasis. In patients who are under active treatment with these agents, medical consult is suggested.

Adverse Effects

>10%:

Cardiovascular: Peripheral edema (13%)

Central nervous system: Fatigue (52%), chills (16%), dizziness (15%), headache (12%), fever (11%)

Dermatologic: Alopecia (19%), pruritus (12%)

Endocrine & metabolic: Hyperglycemia (8% to 69%; grade 3: 5%), dehydration (1% to 16%)

Gastrointestinal: Diarrhea (52%), nausea (41%), taste alteration (28%), anorexia (24%), weight loss (21%), xerostomia (16%), constipation (15%), vomiting (15%), appetite decreased (14%)

Hematologic: Thrombocytopenia (26%; grades 3/4: 6%), anemia (14%; grades 3/4: 2%)

Neuromuscular & skeletal: Muscle spasm (20%)

Renal: Proteinuria (51%), creatinine increased (16% to 47%)

Respiratory: Cough (11%), upper respiratory infection (11%)

1% to 10%:

Cardiovascular: QT_c prolongation (3% to 4%)

Dermatologic: Squamous cell carcinoma (4%)

Respiratory: Pulmonary embolism (5%)

General Dosage Range Dosage adjustment recommended in patients who develop toxicities

Oral: *Adults:* 400 mg once daily

Mechanism of Action Inhibition of histone deacetylase enzymes, HDAC1, HDAC2, HDAC3, and HDAC6, which catalyze acetyl group removal from protein lysine residues (including histones and transcription factors). Inhibition of histone deacetylase results in accumulation of acetyl groups, leading to alterations in chromatin structure and transcription factor activation causing termination of cell growth leading to cell death.

Pharmacodynamics/Kinetics

Half-life Elimination ~2 hours

Time to Peak Plasma: With high-fat meal: ~4 hours (range: 2-10 hours)

Pregnancy Risk Factor D

Dental Comment This drug is known to prolong the QT interval. The QT interval is measured as the time and distance between the Q point of the QRS complex and the end of the T wave in the ECG tracing. After adjustment for heart rate, the QT interval is defined as prolonged if it is more than 450 msec in men and 460 msec in women. A long QT syndrome was first described in the 1950s and 60s as a congenital syndrome involving QT interval prolongation and syncope and sudden death. Some of the congenital long QT syndromes were characterized by a peculiar electrocardiographic appearance of the QRS complex involving a premature atria beat followed by a pause, then a subsequent sinus beat showing marked QT prolongation and deformity. This type of cardiac arrhythmia was originally termed "torsade de pointes" (translated from the French as "twisting of the points").

Prolongation of the QT interval is thought to result from delayed ventricular repolarization. The repolarization process within the myocardial cell is due to the efflux of intracellular potassium. The channels associated with this current can be blocked by many drugs and predispose the electrical propagation cycle to torsade de pointes.

Vorinostat is one of the drugs confirmed to prolong the QT interval and is accepted as having a risk of causing torsade de pointes. The risk of drug-induced torsade de pointes is extremely low when a single QT interval prolonging drug is prescribed. In terms of epinephrine, it is not known what effect vasoconstrictors in the local anesthetic regimen will have in patients with a known history of congenital prolonged QT interval or in patients taking any medication that prolongs the QT interval. Until more information is obtained, it is suggested that the clinician consult with the physician prior to the use of a vasoconstrictor in suspected patients, and that the vasoconstrictor (epinephrine, levonordefrin [Neo-Cobefrin®]) be used with caution.

Warfarin (WAR far in)

Related Information

Antiplatelet and Anticoagulation Considerations in Dentistry *on page 1867*
Cardiovascular Diseases *on page 1848*

U.S. Brand Names Coumadin®; Jantoven®

Canadian Brand Names Apo-Warfarin®; Coumadin®; Mylan-Warfarin; Novo-Warfarin; Taro-Warfarin

Generic Availability (U.S.) Yes: Tablet

Pharmacologic Category Anticoagulant, Coumarin Derivative; Vitamin K Antagonist

Use Prophylaxis and treatment of thromboembolic disorders (eg, venous, pulmonary) and embolic complications arising from atrial fibrillation or cardiac valve replacement; adjunct to reduce risk of systemic embolism (eg, recurrent MI, stroke) after myocardial infarction

Unlabeled/Investigational Use Prevention of recurrent transient ischemic attacks

Local Anesthetic/Vasoconstrictor Precautions No information available to require special precautions

Effects on Dental Treatment Key adverse event(s) related to dental treatment: Mouth ulcers and taste disturbance.

Signs of warfarin overdose may first appear as bleeding from gingival tissue. See Effects on Bleeding.

Effects on Bleeding As with all anticoagulants, bleeding is a potential adverse effect of warfarin during dental surgery; risk is dependent on multiple variables, including the intensity of anticoagulation and patient susceptibility. Consultation with prescribing physician is advisable prior to surgery to determine temporary dose reduction or withdrawal of medication.

Adverse Effects Bleeding is the major adverse effect of warfarin. Hemorrhage may occur at virtually any site. Risk is dependent on multiple variables, including the intensity of anticoagulation and patient susceptibility.

Cardiovascular: Angina, chest pain, edema, hemorrhagic shock, hypotension, pallor, syncope, vasculitis

Central nervous system: Coma, dizziness, fatigue, fever, headache, lethargy, malaise, pain, stroke

Dermatologic: Alopecia, bullous eruptions, dermatitis, rash, pruritus, urticaria

Gastrointestinal: Abdominal cramps, abdominal pain, anorexia, diarrhea, flatulence, gastrointestinal bleeding, mouth ulcers, nausea, taste disturbance, vomiting

Genitourinary: Hematuria, priapism

Hematologic: Agranulocytosis, anemia, leukopenia, retroperitoneal hematoma, unrecognized bleeding sites (eg, colon cancer) may be uncovered by anticoagulation
Hepatic: Cholestatic jaundice, hepatic injury, hepatitis, transaminases increased
Neuromuscular & skeletal: Joint pain, muscle pain, osteoporosis (potential association with long-term use), paralysis, paresthesia, weakness
Respiratory: Dyspnea, tracheobronchial calcification
Miscellaneous: Anaphylactic reaction, cold intolerance, hypersensitivity/allergic reactions, skin necrosis, gangrene, "purple toes" syndrome

Dosage Note: Labeling identifies genetic factors which may increase patient sensitivity to warfarin. Specifically, genetic variations in the proteins CYP2C9 and VKORC1, responsible for warfarin's primary metabolism and pharmacodynamic activity, respectively, have been identified as predisposing factors associated with decreased dose requirement and increased bleeding risk. Genotyping tests are available, and may provide important guidance on initiation of anticoagulant therapy.

Oral:

Infants and Children (unlabeled use): Initial loading dose (if baseline INR is 1-1.3): 0.2 mg/kg (maximum: 10 mg/dose); adjust dose based on INR (reported ranges to maintain INR of 2-3: 0.09-0.33 mg/kg/day). Infants <12 months of age may require doses at or near the high end of this range; consistent anticoagulation may be difficult to maintain in children <5 years of age.

Adults: Initial dosing must be individualized. Consider the patient (hepatic function, cardiac function, age, nutritional status, concurrent therapy, risk of bleeding) in addition to prior dose response (if available) and the clinical situation. Start 2-5 mg daily for 2 days **or** 5-10 mg daily for 1-2 days (Ansell, 2008). Adjust dose according to INR results; usual maintenance dose ranges from 2-10 mg daily (individual patients may require loading and maintenance doses outside these general guidelines).

Note: Lower starting doses may be required for patients with hepatic impairment, poor nutrition, CHF, elderly, high risk of bleeding, or patients who are debilitated, or those with reduced function genomic variants of the catabolic enzymes CYP2C9 (*2 or *3 alleles) or VKORC1 (-1639 polymorphism); see table. Higher initial doses may be reasonable in selected patients (ie, receiving enzyme-inducing agents and with low risk of bleeding).

Range[1] of Expected Therapeutic Maintenance Dose Based on CYP2C9[2] and VKORC1[3] Genotypes

VKORC1	CYP2C9					
	*1/*1	*1/*2	*1/*3	*2/*2	*2/*3	*3/*3
GG	5-7 mg	5-7 mg	3-4 mg	3-4 mg	3-4 mg	0.5-2 mg
AG	5-7 mg	3-4 mg	3-4 mg	3-4 mg	0.5-2 mg	0.5-2 mg
AA	3-4 mg	3-4 mg	0.5-2 mg	0.5-2 mg	0.5-2 mg	0.5-2 mg

Note: Must also take into account other patient related factors when determining initial dose (eg, age, body weight, concomitant medications, comorbidities).

[1]Ranges derived from multiple published clinical studies.

[2]Patients with CYP2C9 *1/*3, *2/*2, *2/*3, and *3/*3 alleles may take up to 4 weeks to achieve maximum INR with a given dose regimen.

[3]VKORC1 -1639G>A (rs 9923231) variant is used in this table; other VKORC1 variants may also be important determinants of dose.

I.V.: Adults: 2-5 mg/day administered as a slow bolus injection

Dosing adjustment in renal disease: No adjustment required, however, patients with renal failure have an increased risk of bleeding complications. Monitor closely.

Dosing adjustment in hepatic disease: Monitor effect at usual doses; the response to oral anticoagulants may be markedly enhanced in obstructive jaundice (due to reduced vitamin K absorption) and also in hepatitis and cirrhosis (due to decreased production of vitamin K-dependent clotting factors); INR should be closely monitored

Mechanism of Action Hepatic synthesis of coagulation factors II, VII, IX, and X, as well as proteins C and S, requires the presence of vitamin K. These clotting factors are biologically activated by the addition of carboxyl groups to key glutamic acid residues within the proteins' structure. In the process, "active" vitamin K is oxidatively converted to an "inactive" form, which is then subsequently reactivated by vitamin K epoxide reductase complex 1 (VKORC1). Warfarin competitively inhibits the subunit 1 of the multi-unit VKOR complex, thus depleting functional vitamin K reserves and hence reduces synthesis of active clotting factors.

Contraindications Hypersensitivity to warfarin or any component of the formulation; hemorrhagic tendencies (eg, patients bleeding from the GI, respiratory, or GU tract; aneurysm; cerebrovascular hemorrhage; following spinal puncture and other diagnostic or therapeutic procedures with potential for significant bleeding; history of bleeding diathesis); recent or potential surgery of the eye or CNS; major regional lumbar block anesthesia or surgery resulting in large, open surfaces; blood dyscrasias; severe uncontrolled or malignant hypertension; pericarditis or pericardial effusion; subacute bacterial endocarditis; history of warfarin-induced necrosis; an unreliable, noncompliant patient; alcoholism; patient who has a history of falls or is a significant fall risk; unsupervised senile or psychotic patient; eclampsia/pre-eclampsia, threatened abortion, pregnancy

Warnings/Precautions Hazardous agent - use appropriate precautions for handling and disposal. Use care in the selection of patients appropriate for this treatment. Ensure patient cooperation especially from the alcoholic, illicit drug user, demented, or psychotic patient; ability to comply with routine laboratory monitoring is essential. Use with caution in trauma, acute infection, moderate-severe renal insufficiency, prolonged dietary insufficiencies, moderate-severe hypertension, polycythemia vera, vasculitis, open wound, active TB, any disruption in normal GI flora, history of PUD, anaphylactic disorders, indwelling catheters, severe diabetes, thyroid disease, and menstruating and postpartum women. Use with caution in protein C deficiency. Use with caution in patients with heparin-induced thrombocytopenia and DVT. Warfarin monotherapy is contraindicated in the initial treatment of active HIT. Reduced liver function, regardless of etiology, may impair synthesis of coagulation factors leading to increased warfarin sensitivity.

[U.S. Boxed Warning]: May cause major or fatal bleeding. Risk factors for bleeding include high intensity anticoagulation (INR >4), age (>65 years), variable INRs, history of GI bleeding, hypertension, cerebrovascular disease, serious heart disease, anemia, malignancy, trauma, renal insufficiency, drug-drug interactions, long duration of therapy, or known genetic deficiency in CYP2C9 activity. Patient must be instructed to report bleeding, accidents, or falls. Unrecognized bleeding sites (eg, colon cancer) may be uncovered by anticoagulation. Patient must also report any new or discontinued medications, herbal or alternative products used, or significant changes in smoking or dietary habits. Necrosis or gangrene of the skin and other tissue can occur, usually in conjunction with protein C or S deficiency. "Purple toes syndrome," due to cholesterol microembolization, may rarely occur. Women may be at risk of developing ovarian hemorrhage at the time of ovulation. The elderly may be more sensitive to anticoagulant therapy. Safety and efficacy have not been established in children; monitor closely.

Presence of the CYP2C9*2 or *3 allele and/or polymorphism of the vitamin K oxidoreductase (VKORC1) gene may increase the risk of bleeding. Lower doses may be required in these patients; genetic testing may help determine appropriate dosing.

Drug Interactions

Metabolism/Transport Effects **Substrate** of CYP1A2 (minor), 2C9 (major), 2C19 (minor), 3A4 (minor); **Inhibits** CYP2C9 (moderate), 2C19 (weak)

Avoid Concomitant Use

Avoid concomitant use of Warfarin with any of the following: Tamoxifen

Increased Effect/Toxicity

Warfarin may increase the levels/effects of: Anticoagulants; Collagenase (Systemic); Deferasirox; Drotrecogin Alfa; Ethotoin; Fosphenytoin; Phenytoin

The levels/effects of Warfarin may be increased by: Acetaminophen; Allopurinol; Amiodarone; Androgens; Antineoplastic Agents; Antiplatelet Agents; Atazanavir; Bicalutamide; Capecitabine; Cephalosporins; Chloral Hydrate; Chloramphenicol; Cimetidine; Clopidogrel; Corticosteroids (Systemic); Cranberry; CYP2C9 Inhibitors (Moderate); CYP2C9 Inhibitors (Strong); Desvenlafaxine; Dexmethylphenidate; Disulfiram; Dronedarone; Efavirenz; Erythromycin (Ophthalmic); Esomeprazole; Ethacrynic Acid; Ethotoin; Etoposide; Exenatide; Fenofibrate; Fenofibric Acid; Fenugreek; Fibric Acid Derivatives; Fluconazole; Fluorouracil; Fluorouracil (Systemic); Fluorouracil (Topical); Fosamprenavir; Fosphenytoin; Gefitinib; Ginkgo Biloba; Glucagon; Green Tea; Herbs (Anticoagulant/Antiplatelet Properties); HMG-CoA Reductase Inhibitors; Ifosfamide; Imatinib; Itraconazole; Ivermectin; Ketoconazole; Ketoconazole (Systemic); Lansoprazole; Leflunomide; Macrolide Antibiotics; Methylphenidate; MetroNIDAZOLE; MetroNIDAZOLE (Systemic); Miconazole (Oral); Miconazole (Topical); Milnacipran; Mirtazapine; Nelfinavir; Neomycin; NSAID (COX-2 Inhibitor); NSAID (Nonselective); Omega-3-Acid Ethyl Esters; Omeprazole; Orlistat; Pentosan Polysulfate Sodium; Pentoxifylline; Phenytoin; Posaconazole; Propafenone; Propoxyphene; Prostacyclin Analogues; QuiNIDine; QuiNINE; Quinolone Antibiotics; Ranitidine; Salicylates; Saquinavir; Selective Serotonin Reuptake Inhibitors; Sitaxentan; SORAfenib; Sulfinpyrazone [Off Market]; Sulfonamide Derivatives; Tamoxifen; Tetracycline Derivatives; Thrombolytic Agents; Thyroid Products; Tigecycline; Tolterodine; Toremifene; Torsemide; TraMADol; Tricyclic Antidepressants; Venlafaxine; Vitamin E; Voriconazole; Vorinostat; Zafirlukast; Zileuton

Decreased Effect
The levels/effects of Warfarin may be decreased by: Aminoglutethimide; Antineoplastic Agents; Antithyroid Agents; Aprepitant; AzaTHIOprine; Barbiturates; Bile Acid Sequestrants; Bosentan; CarBAMazepine; Coenzyme Q-10; Contraceptives (Estrogens); Contraceptives (Progestins); CYP2C9 Inducers (Highly Effective); Darunavir; Dicloxacillin; Efavirenz; Fosaprepitant; Ginseng (American); Glutethimide; Green Tea; Griseofulvin; Lopinavir; Mercaptopurine; Nafcillin; Nelfinavir; Peginterferon Alfa-2b; Phytonadione; Rifamycin Derivatives; Ritonavir; St Johns Wort; Sucralfate; Tocilizumab

Ethanol/Nutrition/Herb Interactions
Ethanol: Avoid ethanol. Acute ethanol ingestion (binge drinking) decreases the metabolism of warfarin and increases PT/INR. Chronic daily ethanol use increases the metabolism of warfarin and decreases PT/INR.

Food: The anticoagulant effects of warfarin may be decreased if taken with foods rich in vitamin K. Vitamin E may increase warfarin effect. Cranberry juice may increase warfarin effect.

Herb/Nutraceutical: Cranberry, fenugreek, ginkgo biloba, glucosamine, may enhance bleeding or increase warfarin's effect. Ginseng (American), coenzyme Q_{10}, and St John's wort may decrease warfarin levels and effects. Avoid alfalfa, anise, bilberry, bladderwrack, bromelain, cat's claw, celery, chamomile, coleus, cordyceps, dong quai, evening primrose oil, fenugreek, feverfew, garlic, ginger, ginkgo biloba, ginseng (American), ginseng (Panax), ginseng (Siberian), grapeseed, green tea, guggul, horse chestnut seed, horseradish, licorice, omega-3-acids, prickly ash, red clover, reishi, SAMe (s-adenosylmethionine), sweet clover, turmeric, and white willow (all have additional antiplatelet activity).

Dietary Considerations Foods high in vitamin K (eg, beef liver, pork liver, green tea, and leafy green vegetables) inhibit anticoagulant effect. Do not change dietary habits once stabilized on warfarin therapy. A balanced diet with a consistent intake of vitamin K is essential. Avoid large amounts of alfalfa, asparagus, broccoli, Brussels sprouts, cabbage, cauliflower, green teas, kale, lettuce, spinach, turnip greens, and watercress; decreased efficacy of warfarin. It is recommended that the diet contain a CONSISTENT vitamin K content of 70-140 mcg/day. Check with healthcare provider before changing diet.

Pharmacodynamics/Kinetics
Onset of Action Anticoagulation: Oral: 24-72 hours; Peak effect: Full therapeutic effect: 5-7 days; INR may increase in 36-72 hours

Duration of Action 2-5 days

Half-life Elimination 20-60 hours; Mean: 40 hours; highly variable among individuals

Time to Peak Oral: ~4 hours

Pregnancy Risk Factor X

Lactation Does not enter breast milk (AAP rates "compatible"; AAP 2001 update pending)

Breast-Feeding Considerations Breast-feeding women may be treated with warfarin. Based on limited data, warfarin does not pass into breast milk; however, prolonged PT may occur in some infants (product labeling). Women who are breast-feeding should be carefully monitored to avoid excessive anticoagulation. ACCP guidelines recommend continuation of warfarin in lactating women who wish to breast-feed their infants (Bates, 2008). Warfarin was not detected in breast milk in 2 reports of warfarin exposure during breast-feeding in 9 infants. Evaluation of coagulation tests and vitamin K status of breast-feeding infant is considered prudent (product labeling).

Dosage Forms
Injection, powder for reconstitution:
Coumadin®: 5 mg

Tablet, oral: 1 mg, 2 mg, 2.5 mg, 3 mg, 4 mg, 5 mg, 6 mg, 7.5 mg, 10 mg
Coumadin®: 1 mg, 2 mg, 2.5 mg, 3 mg, 4 mg, 5 mg, 6 mg, 7.5 mg, 10 mg
Jantoven®: 1 mg, 2 mg, 2.5 mg, 3 mg, 4 mg, 5 mg, 6 mg, 7.5 mg, 10 mg

References
Jeske AH, Suchko GD, ADA Council on Scientific Affairs and Division of Science, et al, "Lack of a Scientific Basis for Routine Discontinuation of Oral Anticoagulation Therapy Before Dental Treatment," *J Am Dent Assoc*, 2003, 134(11):1492-7.
Little JW, Miller CS, Henry RG, et al, "Antithrombotic Agents: Implications in Dentistry," *Oral Surg Oral Med Oral Pathol Oral Radiol Endod*, 2002, 93(5):544-51.
Scully C and Wolff A, "Oral Surgery in Patients on Anticoagulant Therapy," *Oral Surg Oral Med Oral Pathol Oral Radiol Endod*, 2002, 94(1):57-64.

Wheat Dextrin (weet DEKS trin)

U.S. Brand Names Benefiber® Plus Calcium [OTC]; Benefiber® [OTC]
Pharmacologic Category Fiber Supplement; Laxative, Bulk-Producing
Use OTC labeling: Dietary fiber supplement

Unlabeled/Investigational Use Treatment of constipation; aid to enhance LDL lowering to reduce the risk of coronary heart disease

Local Anesthetic/Vasoconstrictor Precautions No information available to require special precautions

Effects on Dental Treatment No significant effects or complications reported

Effects on Bleeding No information available to require special precautions

Adverse Effects Frequency not defined: Gastrointestinal: Bloating, flatulence, GI discomfort

General Dosage Range Oral: *Children and Adults:* Dosage varies greatly depending on product

Mechanism of Action Wheat dextrin is a soluble fiber. It absorbs water in the intestine to form a viscous liquid which promotes peristalsis and reduces transit time.

Zafirlukast (za FIR loo kast)

Related Information

Respiratory Diseases *on page 1876*

U.S. Brand Names Accolate®

Canadian Brand Names Accolate®

Generic Availability (U.S.) Yes

Pharmacologic Category Leukotriene-Receptor Antagonist

Use Prophylaxis and chronic treatment of asthma in adults and children ≥5 years of age

Local Anesthetic/Vasoconstrictor Precautions No information available to require special precautions

Effects on Dental Treatment No significant effects or complications reported

Effects on Bleeding No information available to require special precautions

Adverse Effects

>10%: Central nervous system: Headache (13%)

1% to 10%:

Central nervous system: Dizziness (2%), pain (2%), fever (2%)

Gastrointestinal: Nausea (3%), diarrhea (3%), abdominal pain (2%), vomiting (2%), dyspepsia (1%)

Hepatic: ALT increased (2%)

Neuromuscular & skeletal: Back pain (2%), myalgia (2%), weakness (2%)

Miscellaneous: Infection (4%)

Dosage Oral:

Children <5 years: Safety and effectiveness have not been established

Children 5-11 years: 10 mg twice daily

Children ≥12 years and Adults: 20 mg twice daily

Elderly: The mean dose (mg/kg) normalized AUC and C_{max} increase and plasma clearance decreases with increasing age. In patients >65 years of age, there is a two- to threefold greater C_{max} and AUC compared to younger adults.

Dosing adjustment in renal impairment: Dosage adjustment not required.

Dosing adjustment in hepatic impairment: In patients with hepatic impairment (ie, biopsy-proven cirrhosis), there is a 50% to 60% greater C_{max} and AUC compared to normal subjects.

Mechanism of Action Zafirlukast is a selectively and competitive leukotriene-receptor antagonist (LTRA) of leukotriene D4 and E4 (LTD4 and LTE4), components of slow-reacting substance of anaphylaxis (SRSA). Cysteinyl leukotriene production and receptor occupation have been correlated with the pathophysiology of asthma, including airway edema, smooth muscle constriction, and altered cellular activity associated with the inflammatory process, which contribute to the signs and symptoms of asthma.

Contraindications Hypersensitivity to zafirlukast or any component of the formulation

Warnings/Precautions Zafirlukast is not FDA approved for use in the reversal of bronchospasm in acute asthma attacks, including status asthmaticus. Therapy with zafirlukast can be continued during acute exacerbations of asthma.

Hepatic adverse events (including hepatitis, hyperbilirubinemia, and hepatic failure) have been reported; female patients may be at greater risk. Discontinue immediately if liver dysfunction is suspected. Periodic testing of liver function may be considered (early detection is generally believed to improve the likelihood of recovery). If hepatic dysfunction is suspected (due to clinical signs/symptoms), liver function tests should be measured immediately. Do not resume or restart if hepatic function studies are consistent with dysfunction. Use caution in patients with alcoholic cirrhosis; clearance is reduced. Postmarketing reports of behavioral changes (ie, depression, insomnia) have been noted. Monitor INR closely with concomitant warfarin use. Rare cases of eosinophilic vasculitis (Churg-Strauss) have been reported in patients receiving zafirlukast (usually, but not always, associated with reduction in concurrent steroid dosage). No causal relationship established. Monitor for eosinophilic vasculitis, rash, pulmonary symptoms, cardiac symptoms, or neuropathy.

An increased proportion of zafirlukast patients >55 years of age reported infections as compared to placebo-treated patients. These infections were mostly mild or moderate in intensity and predominantly affected the respiratory tract. Infections occurred equally in both sexes, were dose-proportional to total milligrams of zafirlukast exposure, and were associated with coadministration of inhaled corticosteroids.

Drug Interactions

Metabolism/Transport Effects Substrate of CYP2C9 (major); **Inhibits** CYP1A2 (weak), 2C8 (weak), 2C9 (moderate), 2C19 (weak), 2D6 (weak), 3A4 (weak)

Avoid Concomitant Use There are no known interactions where it is recommended to avoid concomitant use.

Increased Effect/Toxicity

Zafirlukast may increase the levels/effects of: Carvedilol; CYP2C9 Substrates (High risk); Theophylline Derivatives; Vitamin K Antagonists

The levels/effects of Zafirlukast may be increased by: CYP2C9 Inhibitors (Moderate); CYP2C9 Inhibitors (Strong)

Decreased Effect

The levels/effects of Zafirlukast may be decreased by: CYP2C9 Inducers (Highly Effective); Erythromycin; Erythromycin (Systemic); Peginterferon Alfa-2b; Theophylline Derivatives

Ethanol/Nutrition/Herb Interactions Food: Decreases bioavailability of zafirlukast by 40%.

Dietary Considerations Should be taken on an empty stomach (1 hour before or 2 hours after meals).

Pharmacodynamics/Kinetics

Half-life Elimination 10 hours

Time to Peak Serum: 3 hours

Pregnancy Risk Factor B

Lactation Enters breast milk/contraindicated

Breast-Feeding Considerations The manufacturer does not recommend breast-feeding due to tumorigenicity observed in animal studies.

Dosage Forms

Tablet, oral: 10 mg, 20 mg

Accolate®: 10 mg, 20 mg

Zaleplon (ZAL e plon)

U.S. Brand Names Sonata®

Generic Availability (U.S.) Yes

Pharmacologic Category Hypnotic, Nonbenzodiazepine

Use Short-term (7-10 days) treatment of insomnia (has been demonstrated to be effective for up to 5 weeks in controlled trial)

Local Anesthetic/Vasoconstrictor Precautions No information available to require special precautions

Effects on Dental Treatment Key adverse event(s) related to dental treatment: Xerostomia (normal salivary flow resumes upon discontinuation).

Effects on Bleeding No information available to require special precautions

Adverse Effects

>10%: Central nervous system: Headache (30% to 42%)

1% to 10%:

Cardiovascular: Chest pain (≥1%), peripheral edema (≤1%)

Central nervous system: Dizziness (7% to 9%), somnolence (5% to 6%), amnesia (2% to 4%), depersonalization (<1% to 2%), hypoesthesia (<1% to 2%), malaise (<1% to 2%), abnormal thinking (≥1%), anxiety (≥1%), depression (≥1%), fever (≥1%), migraine (≥1%), nervousness (≥1%), confusion (≤1%), hallucination (≤1%), vertigo (≤1%)

Dermatologic: Pruritus (≥1%), rash (≥1%), photosensitivity reaction (≤1%)

Endocrine & metabolic: Dysmenorrhea (3% to 4%)

Gastrointestinal: Nausea (6% to 8%), abdominal pain (6%), anorexia (<1% to 2%), constipation (≥1%), dyspepsia (≥1%), taste perversion (≥1%), xerostomia (≥1%), colitis (up to 1%)

Neuromuscular & skeletal: Weakness (5% to 7%), paresthesia (3%), tremor (2%), arthralgia (≥1%), arthritis (≥1%), back pain (≥1%), myalgia (≥1%), hypertonia (1%)

Ocular: Eye pain (3% to 4%), abnormal vision (<1% to 2%), conjunctivitis (≥1%)

Otic: Hyperacusis (1% to 2%), ear pain (≤1%)

Respiratory: Bronchitis (≥1%), epistaxis (≤1%)

Miscellaneous: Parosmia (<1% to 2%)

Dosage Oral:

Adults: 10 mg at bedtime (range: 5-20 mg); has been used for up to 5 weeks of treatment in controlled trial setting

Elderly: 5 mg at bedtime; recommended maximum: 10 mg/day

Dosage adjustment in renal impairment: No adjustment for mild-to-moderate renal impairment; use in severe renal impairment has not been adequately studied

Dosage adjustment in hepatic impairment: Mild-to-moderate impairment: 5 mg; not recommended for use in patients with severe hepatic impairment

Mechanism of Action Zaleplon is unrelated to benzodiazepines, barbiturates, or other hypnotics. However, it interacts with the benzodiazepine GABA receptor complex. Nonclinical studies have shown that it binds selectively to the brain omega-1 receptor situated on the alpha subunit of the GABA-A receptor complex.

Contraindications Hypersensitivity to zaleplon or any component of the formulation

Warnings/Precautions Symptomatic treatment of insomnia should be initiated only after careful evaluation of potential causes of sleep disturbance. Failure of sleep disturbance to resolve after 7-10 days may indicate psychiatric and/or medical illness.

Use with caution in patients with depression, particularly if suicidal risk may be present. Use with caution in patients with a history of drug dependence. Abrupt discontinuance may lead to withdrawal symptoms. Hypnotics/sedatives have been associated with abnormal thinking and behavior changes including decreased inhibition, aggression, bizarre behavior, agitation, hallucinations, and depersonalization. These changes may occur unpredictably and may indicate previously unrecognized psychiatric disorders; evaluate appropriately. May impair physical and mental capabilities. Patients must be cautioned about performing tasks which require mental alertness (operating machinery or driving). Amnesia can occur. Use with caution in patients receiving other CNS depressants or psychoactive medications. Effects with other sedative drugs or ethanol may be potentiated. Postmarketing studies have indicated that the use of hypnotic/sedative agents for sleep has been associated with hypersensitivity reactions including anaphylaxis as well as angioedema. An increased risk for hazardous sleep-related activities such as sleep-driving, cooking and eating food, and making phone calls while asleep have been noted.

Use with caution in the elderly, those with compromised respiratory function, or hepatic impairment (dosage adjustment recommended in mild-to-moderate hepatic impairment; avoid use in severe impairment). Because of the rapid onset of action, zaleplon should be administered immediately prior to bedtime or after the patient has gone to bed and is having difficulty falling asleep. Capsules contain tartrazine (FDC yellow #5); avoid in patients with sensitivity (caution in patients with asthma).

Drug Interactions

Metabolism/Transport Effects **Substrate** of CYP3A4 (minor)

Avoid Concomitant Use There are no known interactions where it is recommended to avoid concomitant use.

Increased Effect/Toxicity

Zaleplon may increase the levels/effects of: Alcohol (Ethyl); CNS Depressants; Methotrimeprazine

The levels/effects of Zaleplon may be increased by: Cimetidine; Conivaptan; Droperidol; Methotrimeprazine

Decreased Effect

The levels/effects of Zaleplon may be decreased by: Flumazenil; Rifamycin Derivatives; Tocilizumab

Ethanol/Nutrition/Herb Interactions

Ethanol: May increase CNS depression; monitor for increased effects with coadministration. Caution patients about effects.

Food: High fat meal prolonged absorption; delayed T_{max} by 2 hours, and reduced C_{max} by 35%.

Herb/Nutraceutical: St John's wort may decrease zaleplon levels. Avoid valerian, St John's wort, kava kava, gotu kola (may increase CNS depression).

Dietary Considerations Avoid taking with or after a heavy, high-fat meal; reduces absorption.

Pharmacodynamics/Kinetics

Onset of Action Rapid

Duration of Action 6-8 hours

Half-life Elimination 1 hour

Time to Peak Serum: 1 hour

Pregnancy Risk Factor C

Lactation Enters breast milk/not recommended

Controlled Substance C-IV

Dosage Forms
Capsule, oral: 5 mg, 10 mg
Sonata®: 5 mg, 10 mg

Zanamivir (za NA mi veer)

Related Information
Systemic Viral Diseases *on page* 1904

U.S. Brand Names Relenza®

Canadian Brand Names Relenza®

Pharmacologic Category Antiviral Agent; Neuraminidase Inhibitor

Use Treatment of uncomplicated acute illness due to influenza virus A and B in patients who have been symptomatic for no more than 2 days; prophylaxis against influenza virus A and B

The Advisory Committee on Immunization Practices (ACIP) recommends that **treatment** be considered for the following:
- Persons with severe, complicated or progressive illness
- Hospitalized persons
- Persons at higher risk for influenza complications:
  - Children <2 years of age (highest risk in children <6 months of age)
  - Adults ≥65 years of age
  - Persons with chronic disorders of the pulmonary (including asthma) or cardiovascular systems (except hypertension)
  - Persons with chronic metabolic diseases (including diabetes mellitus), hepatic disease, renal dysfunction, hematologic disorders (including sickle cell disease), or immunosuppression (including immunosuppression caused by medications or HIV)
  - Persons with neurologic/neuromuscular conditions (including conditions such as spinal cord injuries, seizure disorders, cerebral palsy, stroke, mental retardation, moderate to severe developmental delay, or muscular dystrophy) which may compromise respiratory function, the handling of respiratory secretions, or that can increase the risk of aspiration
  - Pregnant or postpartum women (≤2 weeks after delivery)
  - Persons <19 years of age on long-term aspirin therapy
  - American Indians and Alaskan Natives
  - Persons who are morbidly obese (BMI ≥40)
  - Residents of nursing homes or other chronic care facilities
- Use may also be considered for previously healthy, nonhigh-risk outpatients with confirmed or suspected influenza based on clinical judgment when treatment can be started within 48 hours of illness onset.

The ACIP recommends that **prophylaxis** be considered for the following:
- Postexposure prophylaxis may be considered for family or close contacts of suspected or confirmed cases, who are at higher risk of influenza complications, and who have not been vaccinated against the circulating strain at the time of the exposure.
- Postexposure prophylaxis may be considered for unvaccinated healthcare workers who had occupational exposure without protective equipment.
- Pre-exposure prophylaxis should only be used for persons at very high risk of influenza complications who cannot be otherwise protected at times of high risk for exposure.
- Prophylaxis should also be administered to all eligible residents of institutions that house patients at high risk when needed to control outbreaks.

Local Anesthetic/Vasoconstrictor Precautions No information available to require special precautions

Effects on Dental Treatment No significant effects or complications reported

Effects on Bleeding No information available to require special precautions

Adverse Effects Most adverse reactions occurred at a frequency which was less than or equal to the control (lactose vehicle).

>10%:
Central nervous system: Headache (prophylaxis 13% to 24%; treatment 2%)
Gastrointestinal: Throat/tonsil discomfort/pain (prophylaxis 8% to 19%)
Respiratory: Nasal signs and symptoms (prophylaxis 12% to 20%; treatment 2%), cough (prophylaxis 7% to 17%; treatment ≤2%)
Miscellaneous: Viral infection (prophylaxis 3% to 13%)

1% to 10%:
Central nervous system: Fever/chills (prophylaxis 5% to 9%; treatment <1.5%), fatigue (prophylaxis 5% to 8%; treatment <1.5%), malaise (prophylaxis 5% to 8%; treatment <1.5%), dizziness (treatment 1% to 2%)
Dermatologic: Urticaria (treatment <1.5%)

Gastrointestinal: Anorexia/appetite decreased (prophylaxis 2% to 4%), appetite increased (prophylaxis 2% to 4%), nausea (prophylaxis 1% to 2%; treatment ≤3%), diarrhea (prophylaxis 2%; treatment 2% to 3%), vomiting (prophylaxis 1% to 2%; treatment 1% to 2%), abdominal pain (treatment <1.5%)

Neuromuscular & skeletal: Muscle pain (prophylaxis 3% to 8%), musculoskeletal pain (prophylaxis 6%), arthralgia/articular rheumatism (prophylaxis 2%), arthralgia (treatment <1.5%), myalgia (treatment <1.5%)

Respiratory: Infection (ear/nose/throat; prophylaxis 2%; treatment 1% to 5%), sinusitis (treatment 3%), bronchitis (treatment 2%), nasal inflammation (prophylaxis 1%)

General Dosage Range Oral inhalation:

Children ≥5 years: Prophylaxis: 10 mg once daily

Children ≥7 years: Treatment: 10 mg twice daily

Adolescents and Adults: Prophylaxis: 10 mg once to twice daily; Treatment: 10 mg twice daily

Mechanism of Action Zanamivir inhibits influenza virus neuraminidase enzymes, potentially altering virus particle aggregation and release.

Pharmacodynamics/Kinetics

Half-life Elimination Serum: 2.5-5.1 hours; Mild-to-moderate renal impairment: 4.7 hours; Severe renal impairment: 18.5 hours

Time to Peak 1-2 hours

Pregnancy Risk Factor C

Prescribing and Access Restrictions Zanamivir *aqueous solution* intended for nebulization or intravenous (I.V.) administration is **not** currently approved for use. Data on safety and efficacy via these routes of administration are limited. However, limited supplies of zanamivir aqueous solution may be made available through the Zanamivir Compassionate Use Program for qualifying patients for the treatment of serious influenza illness. For information, contact the GlaxoSmithKline Clinical Support Help Desk at 1-866-341-9160 or gskclinicalsupportHD@gsk.com.

Ziconotide (zi KOE no tide)

U.S. Brand Names Prialt®

Pharmacologic Category Analgesic, Nonopioid; Calcium Channel Blocker, N-Type

Use Management of severe chronic pain in patients requiring intrathecal (I.T.) therapy and who are intolerant or refractory to other therapies

Local Anesthetic/Vasoconstrictor Precautions No information available to require special precautions

Effects on Dental Treatment Key adverse event(s) related to dental treatment: Xerostomia (normal salivary flow resumes upon discontinuation) and taste perversion.

Effects on Bleeding No information available to require special precautions

Adverse Effects

>10%:

Central nervous system: Dizziness (46%), confusion (15% to 33%), memory impairment (7% to 22%), somnolence (17%), ataxia (14%), speech disorder (14%), headache (13%), aphasia (12%), hallucination (12%; including auditory and visual)

Gastrointestinal: Nausea (40%), diarrhea (18%), vomiting (16%)

Neuromuscular & skeletal: Creatine kinase increased (40%; ≥3 times ULN: 11%), weakness (18%), gait disturbances (14%)

Ocular: Blurred vision (12%)

2% to 10%:

Cardiovascular: Hypotension, peripheral edema, postural hypotension

Central nervous system: Abnormal thinking (8%), amnesia (8%), anxiety (8%), vertigo (7%), insomnia (6%), fever (5%), paranoid reaction (3%), delirium (2%), hostility (2%), stupor (2%), agitation, attention disturbance, balance impaired, burning sensation, coordination abnormal, depression, disorientation, fatigue, fever, hypoesthesia, irritability, lethargy, mental impairment, mood disorder, nervousness, pain, sedation

Dermatologic: Pruritus (7%)

Gastrointestinal: Anorexia (6%), taste perversion (5%), abdominal pain, appetite decreased, constipation, xerostomia

Genitourinary: Urinary retention (9%), dysuria, urinary hesitance

Neuromuscular & skeletal: Dysarthria (7%), paresthesia (7%), rigors (7%), tremor (7%), muscle spasm (6%), limb pain (5%), areflexia, muscle cramp, muscle weakness, myalgia

Ocular: Nystagmus (8%), diplopia, visual disturbance

Respiratory: Sinusitis (5%)

Miscellaneous: Diaphoresis (5%)

General Dosage Range Dosage adjustment recommended in patients who develop toxicities

I.T.: *Adults:* Initial dose: ≤2.4 mcg/day (0.1 mcg/hour); Maintenance range: 2.4-19.2 mcg/day (0.1-0.8 mcg/hour) (maximum: 19.2 mcg/day [0.8 mcg/hour])

Mechanism of Action Ziconotide selectively binds to N-type voltage-sensitive calcium channels located on the nociceptive afferent nerves of the dorsal horn in the spinal cord. This binding is thought to block N-type calcium channels, leading to a blockade of excitatory neurotransmitter release and reducing sensitivity to painful stimuli.

Pharmacodynamics/Kinetics

Half-life Elimination I.V.: 1-1.6 hours (plasma); I.T.: 2.9-6.5 hours (CSF)

Pregnancy Risk Factor C

Zidovudine (zye DOE vyoo deen)

Related Information

HIV Infection and AIDS *on page 1883*
Systemic Viral Diseases *on page 1904*

U.S. Brand Names Retrovir®

Canadian Brand Names Apo-Zidovudine®; AZT™; Novo-AZT; Retrovir®; Retrovir® (AZT™)

Pharmacologic Category Antiretroviral Agent, Reverse Transcriptase Inhibitor (Nucleoside)

Use Treatment of HIV infection in combination with at least two other antiretroviral agents; prevention of maternal/fetal HIV transmission as monotherapy

Unlabeled/Investigational Use Postexposure prophylaxis for HIV exposure as part of a multidrug regimen

Local Anesthetic/Vasoconstrictor Precautions No information available to require special precautions

Effects on Dental Treatment Key adverse event(s) related to dental treatment: Taste perversion, oral mucosa pigmentation, dysphagia, and mouth ulcer.

Effects on Bleeding No information available to require special precautions relative to hemostasis.

Adverse Effects As reported in adult patients with asymptomatic HIV infection. Frequency and severity may increase with advanced disease.

>10%:

Central nervous system: Headache (63%), malaise (53%)

Gastrointestinal: Nausea (51%), anorexia (20%), vomiting (17%)

1% to 10%:

Gastrointestinal: Constipation (6%)

Hematologic: Granulocytopenia (2%; onset 6-8 weeks), anemia (1%; onset 2-4 weeks)

Hepatic: Transaminases increased (1% to 3%)

Neuromuscular & skeletal: Weakness (9%)

Frequency not defined:

Cardiovascular: Cardiomyopathy, chest pain, syncope, vasculitis

Central nervous system: Anxiety, chills, confusion, depression, dizziness, fatigue, insomnia, loss of mental acuity, mania, seizure, somnolence, vertigo

Dermatologic: Pruritus, rash, skin/nail pigmentation changes, Stevens-Johnson syndrome, toxic epidermal necrolysis, urticaria

Endocrine & metabolic: Body fat redistribution, diabetes, dyslipidemias, gynecomastia, insulin resistance

Gastrointestinal: Abdominal cramps, abdominal pain, dyspepsia, dysphagia, flatulence, mouth ulcer, oral mucosa pigmentation, pancreatitis, taste perversion

Genitourinary: Urinary frequency, urinary hesitancy

Hematologic: Aplastic anemia, hemolytic anemia, leukopenia, lymphadenopathy, pancytopenia with marrow hypoplasia, pure red cell aplasia

Hepatic: Hepatitis, hepatomegaly with steatosis, hyperbilirubinemia, jaundice, lactic acidosis

Neuromuscular & skeletal: Arthralgia, back pain, CPK increased, LDH increased, musculoskeletal pain, myalgia, neuropathy, muscle spasm, myopathy, myositis, paresthesia, rhabdomyolysis, tremor

Ocular: Amblyopia, macular edema, photophobia

Otic: Hearing loss

Respiratory: Cough, dyspnea, rhinitis, sinusitis

Miscellaneous: Allergic reactions, anaphylaxis, angioedema, diaphoresis, flu-like syndrome, immune reconstitution syndrome

General Dosage Range Dosage adjustment recommended in patients with renal impairment or who develop toxicities

I.V.:

Infants <30 weeks gestation at birth: 1.5 mg/kg/dose every 12 hours; at 4 weeks of age advance to 1.5 mg/kg/dose every 8 hours

Infants ≥30 weeks and <35 weeks gestation at birth: 2 mg/kg/dose every 12 hours; at 2 weeks of age, advance to 1.5 mg/kg/dose every 8 hours

Infants (full term): 1.5 mg/kg/dose every 6 hours

Children 6 weeks to <12 years: 120 mg/m^2/dose every 6 hours **or** 20 mg/m^2/hour as a continuous infusion

Children ≥12 years and Adults: 1 mg/kg/dose every 4 hours around-the-clock **or** 2 mg/kg bolus followed by 1 mg/kg/hour continuous infusion

Oral:

Infants <30 weeks gestation at birth: 2 mg/kg/dose every 12 hours; at 4 weeks of age advance to 2 mg/kg/dose every 8 hours

Infants ≥30 weeks and <35 weeks gestation at birth: 2 mg/kg/dose every 12 hours; at 2 weeks of age, advance to 2 mg/kg/dose every 8 hours

Infants (full term): 2 mg/kg/dose every 6 hours

Children 4 weeks to <18 years: 240 mg/m^2 every 12 hours (maximum 300 mg every 12 hours) **or** 160 mg/m^2/dose every 8 hours (maximum: 200 mg every 8 hours)

4 to <9 kg: 12 mg/kg/dose twice daily **or** 8 mg/kg/dose 3 times/day

≥9 to <30 kg: 9 mg/kg/dose twice daily **or** 6 mg/kg/dose 3 times/day

≥30 kg and Adults: 300 mg twice daily **or** 200 mg 3 times/day

Mechanism of Action Zidovudine is a thymidine analog which interferes with the HIV viral RNA-dependent DNA polymerase resulting in inhibition of viral replication; nucleoside reverse transcriptase inhibitor

Pharmacodynamics/Kinetics

Half-life Elimination Terminal: 0.5-3 hours

Time to Peak Serum: 30-90 minutes

Pregnancy Risk Factor C

Zileuton (zye LOO ton)

Related Information

Respiratory Diseases *on page 1876*

U.S. Brand Names Zyflo CR®; Zyflo®

Pharmacologic Category 5-Lipoxygenase Inhibitor

Use Prophylaxis and chronic treatment of asthma

Local Anesthetic/Vasoconstrictor Precautions No information available to require special precautions

Effects on Dental Treatment No significant effects or complications reported

Effects on Bleeding No information available to require special precautions

Adverse Effects

>10%: Central nervous system: Headache (23% to 25%)

1% to 10%:

Cardiovascular: Chest pain

Central nervous system: Pain (8%), dizziness, fever, insomnia, malaise, nervousness, somnolence

Dermatologic: Pruritus, rash

Gastrointestinal: Dyspepsia (8%), diarrhea (5%), nausea (5% to 6%), abdominal pain (5%), constipation, flatulence, vomiting

Genitourinary: Urinary tract infection, vaginitis

Hematologic: Leukopenia (1% to 3%)

Hepatic: ALT increased (≥3 x ULN: 2% to 5%), hepatotoxicity

Neuromuscular & skeletal: Myalgia (7%), weakness (4%), arthralgia, hypertonia, neck pain/rigidity

Ocular: Conjunctivitis

Respiratory: Upper respiratory tract infection (9%), sinusitis (7%), pharyngolaryngeal pain (5%)

Miscellaneous: Hypersensitivity reactions, lymphadenopathy

General Dosage Range Oral:

Extended release: *Children ≥12 years and Adults:* 1200 mg twice daily

Immediate release: *Children ≥12 years and Adults:* 600 mg 4 times/day

Mechanism of Action Specific 5-lipoxygenase inhibitor which inhibits leukotriene formation. Leukotrienes augment neutrophil and eosinophil migration, neutrophil and monocyte aggregation, leukocyte adhesion, increased capillary permeability, and smooth muscle contraction (which contribute to inflammation, edema, mucous secretion, and bronchoconstriction in the airway of the asthmatic.)

Pharmacodynamics/Kinetics
Half-life Elimination ~3 hours
Time to Peak Immediate release: 1.7 hours
Pregnancy Risk Factor C

Zinc Acetate (zink AS e tate)

U.S. Brand Names Galzin®
Pharmacologic Category Trace Element
Use Maintenance treatment of Wilson's disease following initial chelation therapy
Local Anesthetic/Vasoconstrictor Precautions No information available to require special precautions
Effects on Dental Treatment No significant effects or complications reported
Effects on Bleeding No information available to require special precautions
Adverse Effects Frequency not defined.
Central nervous system: Neurologic deterioration (uncommon)
Endocrine & metabolic: Amylase increased, lipase increased
Gastrointestinal: Gastric irritation
Hepatic: Alkaline phosphatase increased, hepatic function decreased (rare)
General Dosage Range Oral:
Children ≥10 years and Adults (pregnant females): 75-150 mg/day in 3 divided doses
Adults (males and nonpregnant females): 150 mg/day in 3 divided doses
Mechanism of Action Zinc induces production of the copper binding protein metallothionein in enterocytes. Copper binding within enterocytes results in an impairment of the intestinal absorption of dietary copper and reabsorption of endogenously secreted copper in saliva, bile, gastric acid. Following enterocyte desquamation, bound copper is eliminated in the feces.
Pharmacodynamics/Kinetics
Onset of Action Slow
Half-life Elimination Inhibition of copper uptake: ~11 days following cessation of therapy
Pregnancy Risk Factor A

Zinc Chloride (zink KLOR ide)

Pharmacologic Category Trace Element
Use Cofactor for replacement therapy to different enzymes; helps maintain normal growth rates, normal skin hydration, and senses of taste and smell
Local Anesthetic/Vasoconstrictor Precautions No information available to require special precautions
Effects on Dental Treatment No significant effects or complications reported
Effects on Bleeding No information available to require special precautions
General Dosage Range I.V.:
Premature infants <1500 g up to 3 kg: 300 mcg/kg/day
Infants (full term) and Children ≤5 years: 100 mcg/kg/day to I.V. fluid
Adults: 2-6 mg/day, up to 12.2 mg/L TPN **or** 17.1 mg/kg of stool or ileostomy output
Pregnancy Risk Factor C

Zinc Gelatin (zink JEL ah tin)

U.S. Brand Names Gelucast®
Pharmacologic Category Topical Skin Product
Use As a protectant and to support varicosities and similar lesions of the lower limbs
Local Anesthetic/Vasoconstrictor Precautions No information available to require special precautions
Effects on Dental Treatment No significant effects or complications reported
Effects on Bleeding No information available to require special precautions
Adverse Effects 1% to 10%: Local: Irritation
General Dosage Range Topical: *Adults:* Apply externally as an occlusive boot

Zinc Oxide (zink OKS ide)

U.S. Brand Names Ammens® Original Medicated [OTC]; Ammens® Shower Fresh [OTC]; Balmex® [OTC]; Boudreaux's® Butt Paste [OTC]; Critic-Aid Skin Care® [OTC]; Desitin® Creamy [OTC]; Desitin® [OTC]
Canadian Brand Names Zincofax®
Pharmacologic Category Topical Skin Product

Use Protective coating for mild skin irritations and abrasions; soothing and protective ointment to promote healing of chapped skin, diaper rash

Local Anesthetic/Vasoconstrictor Precautions No information available to require special precautions

Effects on Dental Treatment No significant effects or complications reported

Effects on Bleeding No information available to require special precautions

Adverse Effects 1% to 10%: Local: Skin sensitivity, irritation

General Dosage Range Topical: *Children and Adults:* Apply as required to affected areas several times daily

Mechanism of Action Mild astringent with weak antiseptic properties

Zinc Sulfate (zink SUL fate)

U.S. Brand Names Orazinc® 110 [OTC]; Orazinc® 220 [OTC]; Zinc 15 [OTC]; Zincate®

Canadian Brand Names Anuzinc; Rivasol

Pharmacologic Category Trace Element

Use Zinc supplement (oral and parenteral); may improve wound healing in those who are deficient

Local Anesthetic/Vasoconstrictor Precautions No information available to require special precautions

Effects on Dental Treatment No significant effects or complications reported

Effects on Bleeding No information available to require special precautions

Adverse Effects Frequency not defined.

Central nervous system: Dizziness, restlessness

Gastrointestinal: Diarrhea, gastric ulcers, nausea, vomiting

General Dosage Range

I.V.:

Premature infants (<1500 g up to 3 kg): 300 mcg/kg/day

Infants (full term) and Children ≤5 years: 100 mcg/kg/day

Adults: 2.5-6 mg/day **or** 12.2 mg/L of TPN **or** 17.1 mg/kg of stool or ileostomy output

Oral:

Children: 0.5-1 mg elemental zinc/kg/day divided in 1-3 doses

Adults: 110-220 mg (25-50 mg elemental zinc) 3 times/day

Pregnancy Risk Factor C

Ziprasidone (zi PRAS i done)

Related Information

Clinical Risk Related to Drugs Prolonging QT Interval *on page* 1872

U.S. Brand Names Geodon®

Canadian Brand Names Zeldox®

Pharmacologic Category Antipsychotic Agent, Atypical

Use Treatment of schizophrenia; treatment of acute manic or mixed episodes associated with bipolar disorder with or without psychosis; maintenance treatment of bipolar disorder as an adjunct to lithium or valproate; acute agitation in patients with schizophrenia

Unlabeled/Investigational Use Tourette's syndrome; psychosis/agitation related to Alzheimer's dementia

Local Anesthetic/Vasoconstrictor Precautions Ziprasidone is one of the drugs confirmed to prolong the QT interval and is accepted as having a risk of causing torsade de pointes. The risk of drug-induced torsade de pointes is extremely low when a single QT interval prolonging drug is prescribed. In terms of epinephrine, it is not known what effect vasoconstrictors in the local anesthetic regimen will have in patients with a known history of congenital prolonged QT interval or in patients taking any medication that prolongs the QT interval. Until more information is obtained, it is suggested that the clinician consult with the physician prior to the use of a vasoconstrictor in suspected patients, and that the vasoconstrictor (epinephrine, mepivacaine and levonordefrin [Carbocaine® 2% with Neo-Cobefrin®]) be used with caution.

Effects on Dental Treatment Key adverse event(s) related to dental treatment: Xerostomia and changes in salivation (normal salivary flow resumes upon discontinuation), orthostatic hypotension, tongue edema, dysphagia, and tooth disorder.

Effects on Bleeding No information available to require special precautions

Adverse Effects Note: Although minor QT_c prolongation (mean: 10 msec at 160 mg/day) may occur more frequently (incidence not specified), clinically-relevant prolongation (>500 msec) was rare (0.06%) and less than placebo (0.23%).

>10%:

Central nervous system: Extrapyramidal symptoms (2% to 31%), somnolence (8% to 31%), headache (3% to 18%), dizziness (3% to 16%)

Gastrointestinal: Nausea (4% to 12%)

1% to 10%:

Cardiovascular: Postural hypotension (5%), chest pain (3%), hypertension (2% to 3%), tachycardia (2%), bradycardia (≤2%), facial edema (1%), vasodilation (≤1%), orthostatic hypotension

Central nervous system: Akathisia (2% to 10%), anxiety (2% to 5%), insomnia (3%), agitation (2%), speech disorder (2%), personality disorder (2%), akinesia (≥1%), amnesia (≥1%), ataxia (≥1%), confusion (≥1%), coordination abnormal (≥1%), delirium (≥1%), dystonia (≥1%), hostility (≥1%), oculogyric crisis (≥1%), vertigo (≥1%), chills (1%), fever (1%), hypothermia (1%), psychosis (1%)

Dermatologic: Rash (4% to 5%), fungal dermatitis (2%)

Endocrine & metabolic: Dysmenorrhea (2%)

Gastrointestinal: Weight gain (6% to 10%), constipation (2% to 9%), dyspepsia (1% to 8%), diarrhea (3% to 5%), vomiting (3% to 5%), xerostomia (1% to 5%), salivation increased (4%), tongue edema (≤3%), anorexia (2%), abdominal pain (≤2%), dysphagia (≤2%), rectal hemorrhage (≤2%), buccoglossal syndrome (≥1%), tooth disorder (1%)

Genitourinary: Priapism (1%)

Local: Injection site pain (7% to 9%)

Neuromuscular & skeletal: Weakness (2% to 6%), hypoesthesia (2%), myalgia (2%), paresthesia (2%), abnormal gait (≥1%), choreoathetosis (≥1%), dysarthria (≥1%), dyskinesia (≥1%), hyper-/hypokinesia (≥1%), hypotonia (≥1%), neuropathy (≥1%), tremor (≥1%), twitching (≥1%), back pain (1%), cogwheel rigidity (1%), hypertonia (1%)

Ocular: Vision abnormal (3% to 6%), diplopia (≥1%)

Respiratory: Infection (8%), rhinitis (1% to 4%), cough (3%), pharyngitis (3%), dyspnea (2%)

Miscellaneous: Diaphoresis (2%), furunculosis (2%), withdrawal syndrome (≥1%), flank pain (1%), flu-like syndrome (1%), photosensitivity reaction (1%),

General Dosage Range

I.M.: *Adults:* 10 mg every 2 hours **or** 20 mg every 4 hours (maximum: 40 mg/day)

Oral: *Adults:* Initial: 20-40 mg twice daily; Maintenance: 20-80 mg twice daily (maximum: 200 mg/day)

Mechanism of Action Ziprasidone is a benzylisothiazolylpiperazine antipsychotic. The exact mechanism of action is unknown. However, *in vitro* radioligand studies show that ziprasidone has high affinity for D_2, D_3, 5-HT_{2A}, 5-HT_{1A}, 5-HT_{2C}, 5-HT_{1D}, and alpha$_1$-adrenergic; moderate affinity for histamine H_1 receptors; and no appreciable affinity for alpha$_2$-adrenergic receptors, beta-adrenergic, 5-HT_3, 5-HT_4, cholinergic, mu, sigma, or benzodiazepine receptors. Ziprasidone functions as an antagonist at the D_2, 5-HT_{2A}, and 5-HT_{1D} receptors and as an agonist at the 5-HT_{1A} receptor. Ziprasidone moderately inhibits the reuptake of serotonin and norepinephrine.

Pharmacodynamics/Kinetics

Half-life Elimination 2-7 hours

Time to Peak Oral: 6-8 hours; I.M.: ≤60 minutes

Pregnancy Risk Factor C

Dental Comment Ziprasidone is known to prolong the QT interval. The QT interval is measured as the time and distance between the Q point of the QRS complex and the end of the T wave in the ECG tracing. After adjustment for heart rate, the QT interval is defined as prolonged if it is more than 450 msec in men and 460 msec in women. A long QT syndrome was first described in the 1950s and 60s as a congenital syndrome involving QT interval prolongation and syncope and sudden death. Some of the congenital long QT syndromes were characterized by a peculiar electrocardiographic appearance of the QRS complex involving a premature atria beat followed by a pause, then a subsequent sinus beat showing marked QT prolongation and deformity. This type of cardiac arrhythmia was originally termed "torsade de pointes" (translated from the French as "twisting of the points"). Ziprasidone is considered as having a risk of causing torsade de pointes. Since it is not known what effect vasoconstrictors in the local anesthetic regimen will have in patients with a known history of congenital prolonged QT interval or in patients taking any medication that prolongs the QT interval, a medical consult is suggested.

Zoledronic Acid (zoe le DRON ik AS id)

Related Information

Osteonecrosis of the Jaw *on page* 1894

Rheumatoid Arthritis, Osteoarthritis, and Osteoporosis *on page* 1889

U.S. Brand Names Reclast®; Zometa®

Canadian Brand Names Aclasta®; Zometa®

Generic Availability (U.S.) No

Pharmacologic Category Antidote; Bisphosphonate Derivative

Use

Oncology-related uses: Treatment of hypercalcemia of malignancy (albumin-corrected serum calcium >12 mg/dL); treatment of multiple myeloma; treatment of bone metastases of solid tumors

Nononcology uses: Treatment of Paget's disease of bone; treatment of osteoporosis in postmenopausal women (to reduce the incidence of fractures or to reduce the incidence of new clinical fractures in patients with low-trauma hip fracture); prevention of osteoporosis in postmenopausal women, treatment of osteoporosis in men (to increase bone mass); treatment and prevention of glucocorticoid-induced osteoporosis (in patients initiating or continuing prednisone ≥7.5 mg/day [or equivalent] and expected to remain on glucocorticoids for at least 12 months)

Unlabeled/Investigational Use Prevention of bone loss associated with aromatase inhibitor therapy in postmenopausal women with breast cancer; prevention of bone loss associated with androgen deprivation therapy in prostate cancer

Local Anesthetic/Vasoconstrictor Precautions No information available to require special precautions

Effects on Dental Treatment Key adverse event(s) related to dental treatment: Mucositis, dysphagia, stomatitis, and sore throat.

Osteonecrosis of the jaw (ONJ), generally associated with local infection and/or tooth extraction and often with delayed healing, has been reported in patients taking bisphosphonates. Symptoms included nonhealing extraction socket or an exposed jawbone. Most reported cases of bisphosphonate-associated osteonecrosis have been in cancer patients treated with intravenous bisphosphonates. However, some have occurred in patients with postmenopausal osteoporosis taking oral bisphosphonates. Dental surgery, particularly tooth extraction, may increase the risk for ONJ. Patients who develop ONJ while on bisphosphonate therapy should receive care by an oral surgeon. See Dental Comment.

Effects on Bleeding No information available to require special precautions

Adverse Effects Note: An acute reaction (eg, arthralgia, fever, flu-like symptoms, myalgia) may occur within the first 3 days following infusion in up to 44% of patients; usually resolves within 3-4 days of onset, although may take up to 14 days to resolve. The incidence may be decreased with acetaminophen (prior to infusion and for 72 hours postinfusion).

Zometa®:

>10%:

Cardiovascular: Leg edema (5% to 21%), hypotension (11%)

Central nervous system: Fatigue (39%), fever (32% to 44%), headache (5% to 19%), dizziness (18%), insomnia (15% to 16%), anxiety (11% to 14%), depression (14%), agitation (13%), confusion (7% to 13%), hypoesthesia (12%)

Dermatologic: Alopecia (12%), dermatitis (11%)

Endocrine & metabolic: Dehydration (5% to 14%), hypophosphatemia (12% to 13%), hypokalemia (12%), hypomagnesemia (11%)

Gastrointestinal: Nausea (29% to 46%), vomiting (14% to 32%), constipation (27% to 31%), diarrhea (17% to 24%), anorexia (9% to 22%), abdominal pain (14% to 16%), weight loss (16%), appetite decreased (13%)

Genitourinary: Urinary tract infection (12% to 14%)

Hematologic: Anemia (22% to 33%), neutropenia (12%)

Neuromuscular & skeletal: Bone pain (55%), weakness (5% to 24%), myalgia (23%), arthralgia (5% to 21%), back pain (15%), paresthesia (15%), limb pain (14%), skeletal pain (12%), rigors (11%)

Renal: Renal deterioration (8% to 17%; up to 40% in patients with abnormal baseline creatinine)

Respiratory: Dyspnea (22% to 27%), cough (12% to 22%)

Miscellaneous: Cancer progression (16%), moniliasis (12%)

1% to 10%:

Cardiovascular: Chest pain (5% to 10%)

Central nervous system: Somnolence (5% to 10%)

Endocrine & metabolic: Hypocalcemia (5% to 10%; grades 3/4: ≤1%), hypermagnesemia (2%)

Gastrointestinal: Dysphagia (5% to 10%), dyspepsia (10%), mucositis (5% to 10%), stomatitis (8%), sore throat (8%)

Hematologic: Granulocytopenia (5% to 10%), pancytopenia (5% to 10%), thrombocytopenia (5% to 10%)

Renal: Serum creatinine increased (grades 3/4: ≤2%)

Respiratory: Pleural effusion, upper respiratory tract infection (10%)

Miscellaneous: Infection (nonspecific; 5% to 10%), metastases (5% to 10%)

Reclast®:

>10%:

Cardiovascular: Hypertension (5% to 13%)

Central nervous system: Pain (2% to 24%), fever (9% to 22%), headache (4% to 20%), chills (2% to 18%), fatigue (2% to 18%)

Endocrine & metabolic: Hypocalcemia (≤3%; Paget's disease 21%)

Gastrointestinal: Nausea (5% to 18%)

Neuromuscular & skeletal: Arthralgia (9% to 27%), myalgia (5% to 23%), back pain (4% to 18%), limb pain (3% to 16%), musculoskeletal pain (≤12%)

Miscellaneous: Acute phase reaction (4% to 25%), flu-like syndrome (1% to 11%)

1% to 10%:

Cardiovascular: Chest pain (1% to 8%), peripheral edema (3% to 6%), atrial fibrillation (1% to 3%), palpitation (≤3%)

Central nervous system: Dizziness (2% to 9%), malaise (1% to 7%), hypoesthesia (≤6%), lethargy (3% to 5%), vertigo (1% to 4%), hyperthermia (≤2%)

Dermatologic: Rash (2% to 3%), hyperhidrosis (≤3%)

Gastrointestinal: Abdominal pain (1% to 9%), diarrhea (5% to 8%), vomiting (2% to 8%), constipation (6% to 7%), dyspepsia (2% to 7%), abdominal discomfort/distension (1% to 2%), anorexia (1% to 2%)

Neuromuscular & skeletal: Bone pain (3% to 9%), arthritis (2% to 9%), rigors (8%), shoulder pain (≤7%), neck pain (1% to 7%), weakness (2% to 6%), muscle spasm (2% to 6%), stiffness (1% to 5%), jaw pain (2% to 4%), joint swelling (≤3%), paresthesia (2%)

Ocular: Eye pain (≤2%)

Renal: Serum creatinine increased (2%)

Respiratory: Dyspnea (5% to 7%)

Miscellaneous: C-reactive protein increased (≤5%)

Dosage I.V.: Adults: **Note:** Acetaminophen administration after the infusion may reduce symptoms of acute-phase reactions. Patients treated for multiple myeloma, osteoporosis, and Paget's disease should receive a daily calcium supplement and multivitamin containing vitamin D (if dietary intake is inadequate).

Hypercalcemia of malignancy (albumin-corrected serum calcium ≥12 mg/dL) (Zometa®): 4 mg (maximum) given as a single dose. Wait at least 7 days before considering retreatment. Dosage adjustment may be needed in patients with decreased renal function following treatment.

Multiple myeloma or metastatic bone lesions from solid tumors (Zometa®): 4 mg every 3-4 weeks

Osteoporosis, glucocorticoid-induced, treatment and prevention (Reclast®, Aclasta® [CAN]): 5 mg infused over at least 15 minutes once a year

Osteoporosis, prevention (Reclast®): 5 mg infused over at least 15 minutes every 2 years

Osteoporosis, treatment (Reclast®, Aclasta® [CAN]): 5 mg infused over at least 15 minutes once a year

Paget's disease: 5 mg infused over at least 15 minutes. **Note:** Data concerning retreatment is not available; retreatment may be considered for relapse if appropriate, for inadequate response, or in patients who are symptomatic.

Prevention of aromatase inhibitor-induced bone loss in breast cancer (unlabeled use): 4 mg every 6 months (Brufsky, 2007)

Prevention of androgen deprivation-induced bone loss in nonmetastatic prostate cancer (unlabeled use): 4 mg every 3 months for 1 year (Smith, 2003) or 4 mg every 12 months (Michaelson, 2007)

Dosage adjustment in renal impairment (at treatment initiation):

Reclast®:

Cl_{cr} ≥35 mL/minute: No adjustment required

Cl_{cr} <35 mL/minute: Use is not recommended

Zometa®: Multiple myeloma and bone metastases:

Cl_{cr} >60 mL/minute: 4 mg

Cl_{cr} 50-60 mL/minute: 3.5 mg

Cl_{cr} 40-49 mL/minute: 3.3 mg

Cl_{cr} 30-39 mL/minute: 3 mg

Cl_{cr} <30 mL/minute: Not recommended

Zometa®: Hypercalcemia of malignancy:

Mild-to-moderate impairment: No adjustment necessary

Severe impairment (serum creatinine >4.5 mg/dL): Evaluate risk versus benefit

Aclasta® [CAN]:

Cl_{cr} ≥30 mL/minute: No adjustment required

Cl_{cr} <30 mL/minute: Use is not recommended

Dosage adjustment for renal toxicity (during treatment):

Hypercalcemia of malignancy: Evidence of renal deterioration: Evaluate risk versus benefit.

Multiple myeloma and bone metastases: Evidence of renal deterioration: Withhold dose until renal function returns to within 10% of baseline: renal deterioration defined as follows:

Normal baseline creatinine: Increase of 0.5 mg/dL

Abnormal baseline creatinine: Increase of 1 mg/dL

Reinitiate dose at the same dose administered prior to treatment interruption.

Multiple myeloma: Albuminuria >500 mg/24 hours (unexplained): Withhold dose until return to baseline, then re-evaluate every 3-4 weeks; consider reinitiating with a longer infusion time of at least 30 minutes (Kyle, 2007).

Dosage adjustment in hepatic impairment: Specific guidelines are not available.

Mechanism of Action A bisphosphonate which inhibits bone resorption via actions on osteoclasts or on osteoclast precursors; inhibits osteoclastic activity and skeletal calcium release induced by tumors. Decreases serum calcium and phosphorus, and increases their elimination. In osteoporosis, zoledronic acid inhibits osteoclast-mediated resorption, therefore reducing bone turnover.

Contraindications Hypersensitivity to zoledronic acid, other bisphosphonates, or any component of the formulation; hypocalcemia (Reclast®)

Canadian labeling: Aclasta® is also contraindicated with uncorrected hypocalcemia at the time of infusion and in pregnancy and breast-feeding.

Warnings/Precautions Osteonecrosis of the jaw (ONJ) has been reported in patients receiving bisphosphonates. Risk factors include invasive dental procedures (eg, tooth extraction, dental implants, boney surgery); a diagnosis of cancer, with concomitant chemotherapy or corticosteroids; poor oral hygiene, ill-fitting dentures; and comorbid disorders (anemia, coagulopathy, infection, pre-existing dental disease). Most reported cases occurred after I.V. bisphosphonate therapy; however, cases have been reported following oral therapy. A dental exam and preventative dentistry should be performed prior to placing patients with risk factors on chronic bisphosphonate therapy. The manufacturer's labeling states that discontinuing bisphosphonates in patients requiring invasive dental procedures may reduce the risk of ONJ. However, other experts suggest that there is no evidence that discontinuing therapy reduces the risk of developing ONJ (Assael, 2009). The benefit/risk must be assessed by the treating physician and/or dentist/surgeon prior to any invasive dental procedure. Patients developing ONJ while on bisphosphonates should receive care by an oral surgeon.

Atypical femur fractures have been reported in patients receiving bisphosphonates for treatment/prevention of osteoporosis. The fractures include subtrochanteric femur (bone just below the hip joint) and diaphyseal femur (long segment of the thigh bone). Some patients experience prodromal pain weeks or months before the fracture occurs. It is unclear if bisphosphonate therapy is the cause for these fractures, although the majority have been reported in patients taking bisphosphonates. Patients receiving long-term (>3-5 years) therapy may be at an increased risk. Discontinue bisphosphonate therapy in patients who develop a femoral shaft fracture.

Infrequently, severe (and occasionally debilitating) musculoskeletal (bone, joint, and/or muscle) pain have been reported during bisphosphonate treatment. The onset of pain ranged from a single day to several months. Consider discontinuing therapy in patients who experience severe symptoms; symptoms usually resolve upon discontinuation. Some patients experienced recurrence when rechallenged with same drug or another bisphosphonate; avoid use in patients with a history of these symptoms in association with bisphosphonate therapy.

May cause hypocalcemia in patients with Paget's disease, in whom the pretreatment rate of bone turnover may be greatly elevated. Hypocalcemia must be corrected before initiation of therapy in patients with Paget's disease and osteoporosis. Ensure adequate calcium and vitamin D intake during therapy. Use caution in patients with disturbances of calcium and mineral metabolism (eg, hypoparathyroidism, thyroid surgery, malabsorption syndromes).

Reclast®: Use is not recommended in patients with Cl_{cr} <35 mL/minute.

Zometa®: Use caution in mild-to-moderate renal dysfunction; dosage adjustment required. In cancer patients, renal toxicity has been reported with doses >4 mg or infusions administered over 15 minutes. Risk factors for renal deterioration include pre-existing renal insufficiency and repeated doses of zoledronic acid and other bisphosphonates. Dehydration and the use of other nephrotoxic drugs which may contribute to renal deterioration should be identified and managed. Use is not recommended in patients with severe renal impairment (serum creatinine >3 mg/dL or Cl_{cr} <30 mL/minute) and bone metastases (limited data); use in patients with hypercalcemia of malignancy and severe renal impairment (serum creatinine >4.5 mg/dL for hypercalcemia of malignancy) should only be done if the benefits outweigh the risks. Renal function should be assessed prior to treatment; if decreased after treatment, additional treatments should be withheld until renal function returns to within 10% of baseline. Diuretics should not be used before correcting hypovolemia. Renal deterioration, resulting in renal failure and dialysis has occurred in patients treated with zoledronic acid after single and multiple infusions at recommended doses of 4 mg over 15 minutes.

Aclasta® [CAN; not available in U.S.]: Use is not recommended in patients with Cl_{cr} <30 mL/minute.

According to the American Society of Clinical Oncology (ASCO) guidelines for bisphosphonates in multiple myeloma, treatment with zoledronic acid is not recommended for asymptomatic (smoldering) or indolent myeloma or with solitary plasmacytoma (Kyle, 2007). The National Comprehensive Cancer Network® (NCCN) multiple myeloma guidelines (v.2.2009) also do not recommend zoledronic acid use in stage 1 or smoldering disease, unless part of a clinical trial.

Adequate hydration is required during treatment (urine output ~2 L/day); avoid overhydration, especially in patients with heart failure. Pre-existing renal compromise, severe dehydration, and concurrent use with diuretics or other nephrotoxic drugs may increase the risk for renal impairment. Single and multiple infusions in patients with both normal and impaired renal function have been associated with renal deterioration, resulting in renal failure and dialysis (rare). Use caution in patients with aspirin-sensitive asthma (may cause bronchoconstriction) and the elderly. Women of childbearing age should be advised against becoming pregnant. Not approved for use in children.

Drug Interactions

Avoid Concomitant Use There are no known interactions where it is recommended to avoid concomitant use.

Increased Effect/Toxicity

Zoledronic Acid may increase the levels/effects of: Deferasirox; Phosphate Supplements

The levels/effects of Zoledronic Acid may be increased by: Aminoglycosides; Nonsteroidal Anti-Inflammatory Agents; Thalidomide

Decreased Effect

The levels/effects of Zoledronic Acid may be decreased by: Proton Pump Inhibitors

Dietary Considerations

Multiple myeloma or metastatic bone lesions from solid tumors: Take daily calcium supplement (500 mg) and daily multivitamin (with 400 int. units vitamin D).

Osteoporosis: Ensure adequate calcium and vitamin D supplementation; general requirements are calcium 1200 mg/day and vitamin D 800-1000 int. units/day.

Paget's disease: Take calcium 1500 mg/day and vitamin D 800 units/day, particularly during the first 2 weeks after administration.

Pharmacodynamics/Kinetics

Half-life Elimination Triphasic; Terminal: 146 hours

Pregnancy Risk Factor D

Lactation Excretion in breast milk unknown/not recommended

Breast-Feeding Considerations Because it binds to bone long term, zoledronic acid use is not recommended in nursing women.

Dosage Forms

Infusion, solution, premixed:

Reclast®: 5 mg (100 mL)

Injection, solution:

Zometa®: 4 mg/5 mL (5 mL)

Dosage Forms: Canada

Infusion, solution [premixed]:

Aclasta®: 5 mg (100 mL)

Dental Comment Zoledronic acid (Reclast®) is administered once annually for the treatment of osteoporosis. A single, large prospective, placebo-controlled study established its efficacy for this indication through 3 years of treatment (Black, 2007). Two cases of ONJ were reported, one each in the treatment and control groups, suggesting a low risk of ONJ with this treatment protocol through 3 years.

The American Association of Oral and Maxillofacial Surgeons position paper on bisphosphonate-related osteonecrosis of the jaws, 2009 update, stated that I.V. bisphosphonate exposure in the setting of managing malignancy remains the major risk factor for the development of ONJ. After reviewing case series, case-controlled studies, and cohort studies, the estimates of the cumulative incidence of I.V. bisphosphonate-associated ONJ ranges from 0.8% to 12%.

Two reports have attempted to assess more accurately the percent of cancer patients developing ONJ after bisphosphonate treatment. Maerevoet et al, reported that among 194 patients treated with Zometa® every 3-4 weeks, nine developed ONJ. Before receiving Zometa®, six had received Aredia® 90 mg every 3-4 weeks.

The median duration of treatment with Aredia® was 39 months and for Zometa® 18 months. The incidence of ONJ in these patients was calculated to be 4.6%. Durie et al, described the results of a survey by the International Myeloma Foundation in 2004 to assess the risk factors of ONJ. Out of 1203 respondents, 904 had myeloma and 299 had breast cancer. Of the myeloma patients, 62 developed ONJ and 54 had suspicious findings. Of the breast cancer patients, 13 had ONJ and 23 had suspicious findings. The total number of cases of either ONJ or suspicious findings was 152. ONJ developed in 10% of 211 patients receiving Zometa® compared to 4% of 413 receiving Aredia®. The mean time to onset of ONJ among patients taking Zometa® was 18 months; the mean time to onset after Aredia® was 6 years. It should be noted that an early report by authors from Novartis Pharmaceuticals Corporation stressed that Aredia® and Zometa® had been used in 2.5 million patients world wide and reports of ONJ during their extensive use had been rare (Tarassoff, 2003). In addition, these authors stated that review of the reported cases revealed multiple risk factors for avascular necrosis. McMahon et al, followed up with a report that, along with other factors, bisphosphonates are additional stressors of bone health that can tip the balance to osteonecrosis. They suggested that the prevention of ONJ should be stressed such as the elimination of chronic dental infections prior to chemotherapy and bisphosphonate use in cancer patients.

References

American Dental Association Council on Scientific Affairs, "Dental Management of Patients Receiving Oral Bisphosphonate Therapy," *JADA*, 2006, 137(8):1144-50. Available at: http://www.ada.org/prof/resources/pubs/jada/reports/report bisphosphonate.pdf.

Black DM, Delmas PD, Eastell R, et al, "Once-Yearly Zoledronic Acid for Treatment of Postmenopausal Osteoporosis," *New Engl J Med*, 2007, 356(18):1809-22.

Durie BG, Katz M, and Crowley J, "Osteonecrosis of the Jaw and Bisphosphonates," *N Engl J Med*, 2005, 353(1):99-102.

Maerevoet M, Martin C, and Duck L, "Osteonecrosis of the Jaw and Bisphosphonates," *N Engl J Med*, 2005, 353(1):99-102.

McMahon RE, Bouquot JE, Glueck CJ, et al, "Osteonecrosis: A Multifactorial Etiology," *J Oral Maxillofac Surg*, 2004, 62(7):904-5.

Ruggiero SL, Dodson TB, Assael LA, et al, "American Association of Oral and Maxillofacial Surgeons Position Paper on Bisphosphonate-Related Osteonecrosis of the Jaws-2009 Update," *J Oral Maxillofac Surg*, 2009, 67(5 Suppl):2-12.

Ruggiero S, Gralow J, Marx RE, et al, "Practical Guidelines for the Prevention, Diagnosis, and Treatment of Osteonecrosis of the Jaw in Patients With Cancer," *J Clin Oncol*, 2006, 2(1):7-14.

Tarassoff P and Csermak K, "Avascular Necrosis of the Jaws: Risk Factors in Metastatic Cancer Patients," *J Oral Maxillofac Surg*, 2003, 61(10):1238-9.

ZOLMitriptan (zohl mi TRIP tan)

Related Information

Temporomandibular Dysfunction (TMD) *on page 1964*

U.S. Brand Names Zomig-ZMT®; Zomig®

Canadian Brand Names Zomig®; Zomig® Nasal Spray; Zomig® Rapimelt

Pharmacologic Category Antimigraine Agent; Serotonin 5-HT$_{1B,\ 1D}$ Receptor Agonist

Use Acute treatment of migraine with or without aura

Local Anesthetic/Vasoconstrictor Precautions No information available to require special precautions

Effects on Dental Treatment Key adverse event(s) related to dental treatment: Xerostomia (normal salivary flow resumes upon discontinuation) and dysphagia.

Effects on Bleeding No information available to require special precautions

Adverse Effects Percentages noted from oral preparations.

1% to 10%:

Cardiovascular: Chest pain (2% to 4%), palpitation (up to 2%)

Central nervous system: Dizziness (6% to 10%), somnolence (5% to 8%), pain (2% to 3%), vertigo (≤2%)

Gastrointestinal: Nausea (4% to 9%), xerostomia (3% to 5%), dyspepsia (1% to 3%), dysphagia (≤2%)

Neuromuscular & skeletal: Paresthesia (5% to 9%), weakness (3% to 9%), warm/cold sensation (5% to 7%), hypoesthesia (1% to 2%), myalgia (1% to 2%), myasthenia (up to 2%)

Miscellaneous: Neck/throat/jaw pain (4% to 10%), diaphoresis (up to 3%), allergic reaction (up to 1%)

General Dosage Range Dosage adjustment recommended in patients with hepatic impairment

Nasal inhalation: *Adults:* 1 spray (5 mg) at the onset of migraine headache; may repeat in 2 hours if no relief (maximum: 10 mg/24 hours)

Oral: *Adults:* 1.25-2.5 mg at the onset of migraine headache; may repeat in 2 hours if no relief (maximum: 10 mg/24 hours)

Mechanism of Action Selective agonist for serotonin (5-HT$_{1B}$ and 5-HT$_{1D}$ receptors) in cranial arteries; causes vasoconstriction and reduces sterile inflammation associated with antidromic neuronal transmission correlating with relief of migraine

Pharmacodynamics/Kinetics

Onset of Action 0.5-1 hour

Half-life Elimination 2.8-3.7 hours

Time to Peak Serum: Tablet: 1.5 hours; Orally-disintegrating tablet and nasal spray: 3 hours

Pregnancy Risk Factor C

Zolpidem (zole PI dem)

U.S. Brand Names Ambien CR®; Ambien®; Edluar™; Zolpimist®

Generic Availability (U.S.) Yes: Excludes oral spray, sublingual tablet

Pharmacologic Category Hypnotic, Nonbenzodiazepine

Use

Ambien®, Edluar™, Zolpimist®: Short-term treatment of insomnia (with difficulty of sleep onset)

Ambien CR®: Treatment of insomnia (with difficulty of sleep onset and/or sleep maintenance)

Local Anesthetic/Vasoconstrictor Precautions No information available to require special precautions

Effects on Dental Treatment Key adverse event(s) related to dental treatment: Xerostomia (normal salivary flow resumes upon discontinuation).

Effects on Bleeding No information available to require special precautions

Adverse Effects Actual frequency may be dosage form, dose, and/or age dependent

>10%: Central nervous system: Headache (7% to 19%), somnolence (6% to 15%), dizziness (1% to 12%)

1% to 10%:

Cardiovascular: Blood pressure increased, chest discomfort/pain, palpitation

Central nervous system: Abnormal dreams, anxiety, apathy, amnesia, ataxia, attention disturbance, body temperature increased, burning sensation, confusion, depersonalization, depression, disinhibition, disorientation, drowsiness, drugged feeling, euphoria, fatigue, fever, hallucinations, hypoesthesia, insomnia, lethargy, lightheadedness, memory disorder, mood swings, sleep disorder, stress

Dermatologic: Rash, urticaria, wrinkling

Endocrine & metabolic: Menorrhagia

Gastrointestinal: Abdominal discomfort, abdominal pain, abdominal tenderness, appetite disorder, constipation, diarrhea, dyspepsia, flatulence, gastroenteritis, gastroesophageal reflux, hiccup, nausea, vomiting, xerostomia

Genitourinary: Urinary tract infection, vulvovaginal dryness

Neuromuscular & skeletal: Arthralgia, back pain, balance disorder, involuntary muscle contractions, myalgia, neck pain, paresthesia, psychomotor retardation, tremor, weakness

Ocular: Asthenopia, blurred vision, depth perception altered, diplopia, red eye, visual disturbance

Otic: Labyrinthitis, tinnitus, vertigo

Renal: Dysuria

Respiratory: Pharyngitis, sinusitis, throat irritation, upper respiratory tract infection

Miscellaneous: Allergy, binge eating, flu-like syndrome

Dosage Oral:

Adults:

Immediate release tablet, spray, sublingual tablet: 10 mg immediately before bedtime; maximum dose: 10 mg

Extended release tablet: 12.5 mg immediately before bedtime

Elderly:

Immediate release tablet, spray, sublingual tablet: 5 mg immediately before bedtime

Extended release tablet: 6.25 mg immediately before bedtime

Dosing adjustment in renal impairment: Dose adjustment not required; monitor closely

Hemodialysis: Not dialyzable

Dosing adjustment in hepatic impairment:

Immediate release tablet, spray, sublingual tablet: 5 mg

Extended release tablet: 6.25 mg

Mechanism of Action Zolpidem, an imidazopyridine hypnotic that is structurally dissimilar to benzodiazepines, enhances the activity of the inhibitory neurotransmitter, γ-aminobutyric acid (GABA), via selective agonism at the benzodiazepine-1 (BZ_1) receptor; the result is increased chloride conductance, neuronal hyperpolarization, inhibition of the action potential, and a decrease in neuronal excitability leading to sedative and hypnotic effects. Because of its selectivity for the BZ_1 receptor site over the BZ_2 receptor site, zolpidem exhibits minimal anxiolytic, myorelaxant, and anticonvulsant properties (effects largely attributed to agonism at the BZ_2 receptor site).

Contraindications Hypersensitivity to zolpidem or any component of the formulation

Warnings/Precautions Should be used only after evaluation of potential causes of sleep disturbance. Failure of sleep disturbance to resolve after 7-10 days may indicate psychiatric or medical illness. Hypnotics/sedatives have been associated with abnormal thinking and behavior changes including decreased inhibition, aggression, bizarre behavior, agitation, hallucinations, and depersonalization. These changes may occur unpredictably and may indicate previously unrecognized psychiatric disorders; evaluate appropriately. Sedative/hypnotics may produce withdrawal symptoms following abrupt discontinuation. Use with caution in patients with depression; worsening of depression, including suicide or suicidal ideation has been reported with the use of hypnotics. Intentional overdose may be an issue in this population. The minimum dose that will effectively treat the individual patient should be used. Prescriptions should be written for the smallest quantity consistent with good patient care. Causes CNS depression, which may impair physical and mental capabilities. Zolpidem should only be administered when the patient is able to stay in bed a full night (7-8 hours) before being active again. Effects with other sedative drugs or ethanol may be potentiated.

Use caution in patients with myasthenia gravis. Avoid use in patients with sleep apnea or a history of sedative-hypnotic abuse. Postmarketing studies have indicated that the use of hypnotic/sedative agents for sleep has been associated with hypersensitivity reactions including anaphylaxis as well as angioedema. An increased risk for hazardous sleep-related activities such as sleep-driving; cooking and eating food, and making phone calls while asleep have also been noted; amnesia may also occur. Discontinue treatment in patients who report any sleep-related episodes.

Use caution with respiratory disease. Use caution with hepatic impairment; dose adjustment required. Because of the rapid onset of action, administer immediately prior to bedtime or after the patient has gone to bed and is having difficulty falling asleep.

Use caution in the elderly; dose adjustment recommended. Closely monitor elderly or debilitated patients for impaired cognitive or motor performance. When studied for the unapproved use of insomnia associated with ADHD in children, a higher incidence (~7%) of hallucinations was reported. In addition, sleep latency did not decrease compared to placebo. Zolpidem is **not** FDA-approved for use in pediatric patients.

Drug Interactions

Metabolism/Transport Effects Substrate of CYP1A2 (minor), 2C9 (minor), 2C19 (minor), 2D6 (minor), 3A4 (major)

Avoid Concomitant Use There are no known interactions where it is recommended to avoid concomitant use.

Increased Effect/Toxicity

Zolpidem may increase the levels/effects of: Alcohol (Ethyl); CarBAMazepine; CNS Depressants; Methotrimeprazine

The levels/effects of Zolpidem may be increased by: Antifungal Agents (Azole Derivatives, Systemic); Conivaptan; CYP3A4 Inhibitors (Moderate); CYP3A4 Inhibitors (Strong); Dasatinib; Droperidol; Methotrimeprazine

Decreased Effect

The levels/effects of Zolpidem may be decreased by: CarBAMazepine; CYP3A4 Inducers (Strong); Deferasirox; Flumazenil; Herbs (CYP3A4 Inducers); Peginterferon Alfa-2b; Rifamycin Derivatives; Tocilizumab

Ethanol/Nutrition/Herb Interactions

Ethanol: May enhance the adverse/toxic effects of zolpidem; avoid use.

Food: Maximum plasma concentration and bioavailability are decreased with food; time to peak plasma concentration is increased; half-life remains unchanged. Grapefruit juice may decrease the metabolism of zolpidem.

Herb/Nutraceutical: St John's wort may decrease the levels/effects of zolpidem; avoid concomitant use. In addition, concomitant use of valerian, kava kava, and gotu kola should be avoided due to the risk of increased CNS depression.

Dietary Considerations For faster sleep onset, do not administer with (or immediately after) a meal.

Pharmacodynamics/Kinetics

Onset of Action Immediate release: 30 minutes

Duration of Action Immediate release: 6-8 hours

Half-life Elimination

Immediate release, Extended release: ~2.5 hours (range 1.4-4.5 hours); Cirrhosis: Up to 9.9 hours; Elderly: Prolonged up to 32%

Spray: ~3 hours (range: 1.7-8.4)

Sublingual: ~3 hours (range: 1.6-6.7 hours)

Time to Peak

Immediate release: 1.6 hours; 2.2 hours with food

Extended release: 1.5 hours; 4 hours with food

Spray: ~0.9 hours

Sublingual: ~1.4 hours; ~1.8 hours with food

Pregnancy Risk Factor C

Lactation Enters breast milk/use caution (AAP rates "compatible"; AAP 2001 update pending)

Controlled Substance C-IV

Dosage Forms

Solution, oral:

Zolpimist®: 5 mg/actuation (8.2 g)

Tablet, oral: 5 mg, 10 mg

Ambien®: 5 mg, 10 mg

Tablet, sublingual:

Edluar™: 5 mg, 10 mg

Tablet, extended release, oral: 6.25 mg

Ambien CR®: 6.25 mg, 12.5 mg

References

Garnier R, Guerault E, Muzard D, et al, "Acute Zolpidem Poisoning - Analysis of 344 Cases," *J Toxicol Clin Toxicol*, 1994, 32(4):391-404.

Holm KJ and Goa KL, "Zolpidem: An Update of Its Pharmacology, Therapeutic Efficacy and Tolerability in the Treatment of Insomnia," *Drugs*, 2000, 59(4):865-89.

Lange CL, "Medication-Associated Somnambulism," *J Am Acad Child Adolesc Psychiatry*, 2005, 44 (3):211-2.

Langtry HD and Benfield P, "Zolpidem: A Review of Its Pharmacodynamic and Pharmacokinetic Properties and Therapeutic Potential," *Drugs*, 1990, 40(2):291-313.

Lheureux P, Debailleul G, De Witte O, et al, "Zolpidem Intoxication Mimicking Narcotic Overdose: Response to Flumazenil," *Hum Exp Toxicol*, 1990, 9(2):105-7.

Meram D and Descotes J, "Acute Poisoning By Zolpidem," *Rev Med Interne*, 1989, 10(5):466.

Mercurio M, De Roos F, and Hoffman RS, "Zolpidem (Ambien®): Exposure Assessment of a New Nonbenzodiazepine GABA Agonist," *Vet Hum Toxicol*, 1994, 36:371.

Pacifici GM, Viani A, Rizzo G, et al, "Plasma Protein Binding of Zolpidem in Liver and Renal Insufficiency," *Int J Clin Pharmacol Ther Toxicol*, 1988, 26(9):439-43.

Queneau PE, Koch S, Hrusovsky S, et al, "Cytolytic Hepatitis Related to Zolpidem," 1st International Symposium on Hepatology and Clinical Pharmacology Liver and Drugs, Abstract, 1994, 39.

Salva P and Costa J, "Clinical Pharmacokinetics and Pharmacodynamics of Zolpidem. Therapeutic Implications," *Clin Pharmacokinet*, 1995, 29(3):142-53.

Sanger DJ, "The Pharmacology and Mechanisms of Action of New Generation, Non-Benzodiazepine Hypnotic Agents," *CNS Drugs*, 2004, 18 (Suppl 1):9-15.

Simcox DA, "Zolpidem-Associated Falls," *Consult Pharm*, 1995, 10:1378-80.

Zonisamide (zoe NIS a mide)

U.S. Brand Names Zonegran®

Pharmacologic Category Anticonvulsant, Miscellaneous

Use Adjunct treatment of partial seizures in children >16 years of age and adults with epilepsy

Unlabeled/Investigational Use Bipolar disorder

Local Anesthetic/Vasoconstrictor Precautions No information available to require special precautions

Effects on Dental Treatment Key adverse event(s) related to dental treatment: Xerostomia (normal salivary flow resumes upon discontinuation) and abnormal taste.

Effects on Bleeding No information available to require special precautions

Adverse Effects Adjunctive therapy: Frequencies noted in patients receiving other anticonvulsants:

>10%:

Central nervous system: Somnolence (17%), dizziness (13%)

Gastrointestinal: Anorexia (13%)

1% to 10%:

Central nervous system: Headache (10%), agitation/irritability (9%), fatigue (8%), tiredness (7%), ataxia (6%), confusion (6%), concentration decreased (6%), memory impairment (6%), depression (6%), insomnia (6%), speech disorders (5%), mental slowing (4%), anxiety (3%), nervousness (2%), schizophrenic/schizophreniform behavior (2%), difficulty in verbal expression (2%), status epilepticus (1%), convulsion (1%), hyperesthesia (1%), incoordination (1%)

Dermatologic: Rash (3%), bruising (2%), pruritus (1%)

Gastrointestinal: Nausea (9%), abdominal pain (6%), diarrhea (5%), dyspepsia (3%), weight loss (3%), constipation (2%), taste perversion (2%), xerostomia (2%), vomiting (1%)

Neuromuscular & skeletal: Paresthesia (4%), abnormal gait (1%), tremor (1%), weakness (1%)

Ocular: Diplopia (6%), nystagmus (4%), amblyopia (1%)

Otic: Tinnitus (1%)
Respiratory: Rhinitis (2%), pharyngitis (1%), increased cough (1%)
Miscellaneous: Flu-like syndrome (4%) accidental injury (1%)

General Dosage Range Oral: *Children >16 years and Adults:* Initial: 100 mg/day; Maintenance: 100-600 mg/day (maximum: 600 mg/day)

Mechanism of Action The exact mechanism of action is not known. May stabilize neuronal membranes and suppress neuronal hypersynchronization through action at sodium and calcium channels. Does not affect GABA activity.

Pharmacodynamics/Kinetics

Half-life Elimination Plasma: ~63 hours

Time to Peak 2-6 hours

Pregnancy Risk Factor C

Zopiclone (ZOE pi clone)

Canadian Brand Names Apo-Zopiclone®; CO Zopiclone; Dom-Zopiclone; Imovane®; Mylan-Zopiclone; Novo-Zopiclone; Nu-Zopiclone; PHL-Zopiclone; PMS-Zopiclone; PRO-Zopiclone; RAN™-Zopiclone; ratio-Zopiclone; Rhovane®; Riva-Zopiclone; Sandoz-Zopiclone

Pharmacologic Category Hypnotic, Nonbenzodiazepine

Use Symptomatic relief of transient and short-term insomnia

Local Anesthetic/Vasoconstrictor Precautions No information available to require special precautions

Effects on Dental Treatment Key adverse event(s) related to dental treatment: Coated tongue, dry mouth, halitosis, taste alteration (bitter taste, common).

Effects on Bleeding No information available to require special precautions

Adverse Effects Frequency not defined.

Cardiovascular: Palpitations
Central nervous system: Agitation, anterograde amnesia, anxiety, asthenia, chills, confusion, depression, dizziness, drowsiness, euphoria, headache, hostility, memory impairment, nervousness, nightmares, somnolence, speech abnormalities
Dermatological: Rash, spots on skin
Endocrine & metabolic: Anorexia; libido decreased; alkaline phosphatase, ALT, and AST increased; appetite increased
Gastrointestinal: Constipation, coated tongue, diarrhea, dry mouth, dyspepsia, halitosis, nausea, taste alteration (bitter taste, common), vomiting
Neuromuscular & skeletal: Coordination impaired, hypotonia, limb heaviness, muscle spasms, paresthesia, tremor
Ocular: Amblyopia
Respiratory: Dyspnea
Miscellaneous: Diaphoresis

General Dosage Range Dosage adjustment recommended in patients with hepatic impairment

Oral:

Adults: 3.75-7.5 mg at bedtime
Elderly: Initial: 3.75 mg at bedtime

Mechanism of Action Zopiclone is a cyclopyrrolone derivative and has a pharmacological profile similar to benzodiazepines. Zopiclone reduces sleep latency, increases duration of sleep, and decreases the number of nocturnal awakenings.

Pharmacodynamics/Kinetics

Half-life Elimination 5 hours; Elderly: 7 hours; Hepatic impairment: 11.9 hours

Time to Peak Serum: <2 hours; Hepatic impairment: 3.5 hours

Pregnancy Risk Factor Not assigned; similar agents rated D

Product Availability Not available in U.S.

Zoster Vaccine (ZOS ter vak SEEN)

U.S. Brand Names Zostavax®

Pharmacologic Category Vaccine, Live (Viral)

Use Prevention of herpes zoster (shingles) in patients ≥50 years of age

The Advisory Committee on Immunization Practices (ACIP) recommends routine vaccination of all patients ≥60 years of age, including:

- Patients who report a previous episode of zoster.
- Patients with chronic medical conditions (eg, chronic renal failure, diabetes mellitus, rheumatoid arthritis, chronic pulmonary disease) unless those conditions are contraindications.
- Residents of nursing homes and other long-term care facilities ≥60 years of age, without contraindications.

Local Anesthetic/Vasoconstrictor Precautions No information available to require special precautions

Effects on Dental Treatment No significant effects or complications reported

Effects on Bleeding No information available to require special precautions

Adverse Effects All serious adverse reactions must be reported to the U.S. Department of Health and Human Services (DHHS) Vaccine Adverse Event Reporting System (VAERS) 1-800-822-7967 or online at https://vaers.hhs.gov/esub/index.

>10%: Local: Injection site reaction (48% to 64%; includes erythema, tenderness, pain, swelling, hematoma, pruritus, and/or warmth)

1% to 10% (**Note:** Rates similar to placebo):

Central nervous system: Fever (2%), headache (1% to 9%)

Dermatologic: Skin disorder (1%)

Gastrointestinal: Diarrhea (2%)

Neuromuscular & skeletal: Weakness (1%)

Respiratory: Respiratory tract infection (2%), rhinitis (1%)

Miscellaneous: Flu-like syndrome (2%)

General Dosage Range SubQ: *Adults ≥50 years:* 0.65 mL as a single dose

Mechanism of Action As a live, attenuated vaccine (Oka/Merck strain of varicella-zoster virus), zoster virus vaccine stimulates active immunity to disease caused by the varicella-zoster virus. Administration has been demonstrated to protect against the development of herpes zoster, with the highest efficacy in patients 60-69 years of age. It may also reduce the severity of complications, including postherpetic neuralgia, in patients who develop zoster following vaccination.

Pharmacodynamics/Kinetics

Onset of Action Seroconversion: ~6 weeks

Duration of Action Not established; protection has been demonstrated for at least 4 years

NATURAL PRODUCTS: HERBAL AND DIETARY SUPPLEMENTS

Medical problem: "I have a toothache."
2000 BC response: "Here, eat this root."
1000 AD: "That root is heathen; here, say this prayer."
1850 AD: "That prayer is superstitious; here, drink this potion."
1940 AD: "That potion is snake oil; here, swallow this pill."
1985 AD: "That pill is ineffective; here, take this new antibiotic."
2000 AD: "That antibiotic is artificial; here, eat this root."
Adapted from an anonymous Internet communication.

INTRODUCTION

For centuries, Eastern and Western civilizations have attributed a large number of medical uses to plants and herbs. Over time, modern scientific methodologies have emerged from some of these remedies. Conversely, some of these agents have fallen into less popularity as more medical knowledge has evolved. In spite of this dichotomy, herbal and natural therapies for treatment of common medical ailments have become exceedingly popular. In America, people consistently seek out natural products that may be able to offset some perceived ailment or assist in the prevention of an ailment. One area of particular interest to those individuals using herbal or natural remedies has commonly been weight loss. There are numerous systemic considerations when some of the natural products that have been attributed weight loss powers are utilized. Many of these products are sold under the blanket of dietary supplements and, therefore, have avoided some of the more stringent Food and Drug Administration legislation. However, in 1994, that legislation was modified to include herbs, vitamins, minerals, and amino acids that may be taken as dietary supplements and the federal guidelines were further modified in 1999. This information must be made available to patients taking these types of products.

The real concern lies in the fact that health claims need not be approved by the FDA, but advertisements must include a disclaimer saying that the product has not yet been fully evaluated. Claims of medicinal use/value are often drawn from popular use, not necessarily from scientific studies. Safety is a concern when these agents are taken in combination with other prescription drugs due to the medical risk which might result. Many of these natural products may have real medicinal value but caution on the part of the dental clinician is prudent. It is impossible to cover all of the natural products, therefore, this chapter has been limited to some of the most popular dietary and herbal supplements and natural remedies used by patients you might treat and what we know about the effects of some of these agents on the body's various systems.

EFFECTS ON VARIOUS SYSTEMS

CARDIOVASCULAR SYSTEM

CONGESTIVE HEART FAILURE

(Diuretics, Xanthine derivatives, Licorice, Ginseng, Aconite)

Alisma plantago, bearberry *(Arctostaphylos uva-ursi)*, buchu *(Barosma betulina)*, couch grass, dandelion, horsetail rush, juniper, licorice, and xanthine derivatives exert varying degrees of diuretic action. Many patients with congestive heart failure (CHF) are already taking a diuretic medication. By taking products containing one or more of these components, patients already on diuretic medications may increase their risk for dehydration.

Ginseng and licorice can potentially worsen congestive heart failure and edema by causing fluid retention. Aconite has varying effects on the heart that itself could lead to heart failure. Patients with CHF should be advised to consult with their healthcare provider before using products containing any of these components.

HYPERTENSION/HYPOTENSION

(Diuretics, Ginkgo biloba, Ginseng, Hawthorn, Ma-huang, Xanthine derivatives)

The stimulant properties of ginseng and ma-huang could worsen pre-existing hypertension. Elevated blood pressure has been reported as a side effect of ginseng. Although ma-huang contains ephedrine, a known vasoconstrictor, ma-huang's effect on blood pressure varies between individuals. Ma-huang can cause hypotension or hypertension. Due to its unpredictable effects, patients with pre-existing hypertension should use caution when using natural products containing ma-huang. Providers should caution patients with labile hypertension against the use of ginseng.

The diuretic effect of xanthine derivatives and other diuretic components could increase the effects of antihypertensive medications, increasing the risk for hypotension. Hawthorn and ginkgo biloba can cause vasodilation increasing the hypotensive effects of antihypertensive medication. Patients susceptible to hypotension or patients taking antihypertensive medication should use caution when taking products containing xanthine derivatives or diuretics. Patients with pre-existing hypertension or hypotension who wish to use products containing these components should be closely monitored by a healthcare professional for changes in blood pressure control.

ARRHYTHMIAS

(Ginseng)

It has been reported that ginseng may increase the risk of arrhythmias, although it is unclear whether this effect is due to the actual ingredient (ginseng) or other possible impurities. Patients at risk for arrhythmias should be cautioned against the use of products containing ginseng without first consulting with their healthcare provider.

CENTRAL NERVOUS SYSTEM

(Aconite, Ginseng, Xanthine derivatives)

Aconite and hawthorn have potentially sedating effects, and aconite also contains various alkaloids and traces of ephedrine. Some documented central nervous system (CNS) effects of aconite include sedation, vertigo, and incoordination. Hawthorn has been reported to exert a depressive effect on the CNS leading to sedation.

Ginseng, ma-huang, and xanthine derivatives can exert a stimulant effect on the central nervous system. Some of the CNS effects of ginseng include nervousness, insomnia, and euphoria. The action of ma-huang is due to the presence of ephedrine and pseudoephedrine. Ma-huang exerts a stimulant action on the CNS similar to decongestant/weight loss products (Dexatrim®, etc) thus causing nervousness, insomnia, and anxiety. Kola nut, green tea, guarana, and yerba mate contain varying amounts of caffeine, a xanthine derivative. Stimulant properties exerted by these herbs are expected to be comparable to those of caffeine, including insomnia, nervousness, and anxiety.

Products containing aconite and hawthorn should be used with caution in patients with known history of depression, vertigo, or syncope. Ginseng or xanthine derivatives should be avoided in patients with history of insomnia or anxiety. Use of natural products with these components may contribute to a worsening of a patient's pre-existing medical condition. Patients taking CNS-active medications should avoid or use extreme caution when using preparations containing any of the above components. These components may interact directly or indirectly with CNS-active medications causing an increase or decrease in overall effect.

ENDOCRINE SYSTEM

DIABETES MELLITUS

(Chromium, Glucomannan, Ginseng, Hawthorn, Ma-huang, Periploca, Spirulina)

Ma-huang and spirulina both may increase glucose levels. This could cause a decrease in glucose control, thereby, increasing a patient's risk for hyperglycemia. Patients with diabetes or glucose intolerance should avoid using ma-huang and spirulina containing products.

Chromium, ginseng, glucomannan, periploca *(gymneme sylvestre)*, and hawthorn should be used with caution in patients being treated for diabetes. These ingredients may reduce glucose levels increasing the risk for hypoglycemia in patients who are already taking a hypoglycemic agent. Patients with diabetes who wish to use products containing these ingredients should be closely monitored for fluctuations in blood glucose levels.

GASTROINTESTINAL SYSTEM

PEPTIC ULCER DISEASE

(Betaine Hydrochloride, White Willow)

Betaine hydrochloride is a source of hydrochloric acid. The acid released from betaine hydrochloride could aggravate an existing ulcer. White willow, like aspirin, contains salicylates.

Aspirin has been known to induce gastric damage by direct irritation on the gastric mucosa and by an indirect systemic effect. As a result, patients with a history of peptic ulcer disease or gastritis are informed to avoid use of aspirin and other salicylate derivatives. These precautions should also apply to white willow. Patients with a history of peptic ulcer disease or gastritis should not use products containing white willow or betaine hydrochloride as either could exacerbate ulcers.

INFLAMMATORY BOWEL DISEASE

(Cascara Sagrada, Senna, Dandelion)

Cascara sagrada and senna are stimulant laxatives. Their laxative effect is exerted by stimulation of peristalsis in the colon and by inhibition of water and electrolyte secretion. The laxative effect produced by these herbs could induce an exacerbation of inflammatory bowel disease. Patients with a history of inflammatory bowel disease should avoid using products containing cascara sagrada or senna, and use caution when taking products containing dandelion which may also have a laxative effect.

OBSTRUCTION/ILEUS

(Glucomannan, Kelp, Psyllium)

Glucomannan, kelp, and psyllium act as bulk laxatives. In the presence of water, bulk laxatives swell or form a viscous solution adding extra bulk in the gastrointestinal tract. The resulting mass is thought to stimulate peristalsis. In the presence of an ileus, these laxatives could cause an obstruction.

If sufficient water is not consumed when taking a bulk laxative, a semisolid mass can form resulting in an obstruction. Any patient who wishes to take a natural product containing kelp, psyllium, or glucomannan should drink sufficient water to decrease the risk of obstruction. This may be of concern in particular disease states such as CHF or other cases where excess fluid intake may influence the existing disease presentation. Patients with a suspected obstruction or ileus should avoid using products containing kelp, psyllium, or glucomannan without consent of their primary healthcare provider.

HEMATOLOGIC SYSTEM

ANTICOAGULATION THERAPY & COAGULATION DISORDERS

(Horsetail Rush, Ginseng, Ginkgo Biloba, Guarana, White Willow)

Horsetail rush, ginseng, ginkgo biloba, guarana, and white willow can potentially affect platelet aggregation and bleeding time. Ginkgo biloba, ginseng, guarana, and white willow inhibit platelet aggregation resulting in an increase in bleeding time. Horsetail rush, on the other hand, may decrease bleeding time. Patients with coagulation disorders or patients on anticoagulation therapy may be sensitive to the effects on coagulation by these components and should, therefore, avoid use of products containing any of these components.

OTHER

PHENYLKETONURIA

(Aspartame, Spirulina)

Patients with phenylketonuria should not use products containing aspartame or spirulina. Aspartame, a common artificial sweetener, is metabolized to phenylalanine, while spirulina contains phenylalanine.

GOUT

(Diuretics, White Willow)

Patients with a history of gout should avoid using natural products containing components with diuretic action or white willow. By increasing urine output, ingredients with diuretic action may concentrate uric acid in the blood increasing the risk of gout in these patients. White willow, like aspirin, may inhibit excretion of urate resulting in an increase in uric acid concentration. The increase in urate levels could cause precipitation of uric acid resulting in an exacerbation of gout.

ALPHABETICAL LISTING OF NATURAL PRODUCTS

Aloe

Pharmacologic Category Herb; Topical Skin Product

Reported Use

Aphthous stomatitis (Garnick, 1998)
Arthritis (review) (Cowan, 2010)
Cancer (prevention) (Sakai, 1989)
Constipation (Odes, 1991)
Diabetes (Bunyapraphatsara, 1996; Ngo, 2010; Yongchaiyudha, 1996)
Dry skin (Dal'Belo, 2006)
Dyslipidemia (Ngo, 2010)
Genital herpes (Syed, 1996; Syed, 1997)
Gingivitis (pharmacologic activity)
Healing agent for wounds, minor burns, and other minor skin irritations (Davis, 1989; Heggers, 1996)
Human Immunodeficiency Virus (HIV) (McDaniel, 1987; McDaniel, 1990; Montaner, 1996)
Irritable bowel syndrome (Davis, 2006)
Lichen planus (Choonhakarn, 2008)
Mucositis (Worthington, 2007; Worthington, 2010; Su, 2004)
Pressure ulcers (Thomas, 1998)
Psoriasis vulgaris (Syed, 1996)
Radiation dermatitis (Heggie, 2002; Merchant, 2007; Olsen, 2001; Williams, 1996)
Seborrheic dermatitis (Vardy, 1999)
Skin burns (Visuthikosol, 1995)
Ulcerative colitis (Langmead, 2004)

Local Anesthetic/Vasoconstrictor Precautions No information available to require special precautions.

Effects on Bleeding None reported

Warnings/Precautions Based on animal/*in vitro* studies, some wound healing may be delayed when using topical *Aloe vera* gel (Schmidt, 1991). Use with caution in individuals receiving laxatives, digoxin and other medications used for heart rhythm disturbances, diuretics, or steroids due to increased risk of dehydration, potassium depletion, and electrolyte imbalance when taking oral aloe. Preliminary reports suggest that levels of zidovudine may be increased by intake of aloe.

References

Bunyapraphatsara N, Yongchaiyudha S, Rungpitarangsi V, et al, "Antidiabetic Activity of *Aloe vera* L. Juice. II. Clinical Trial in Diabetes Mellitus Patients in Combination With Glibenclamide," *Phytomed*, 1996, 3(3):245-8.

Choonhakarn C, Busaracome P, Sripanidkulchai B, et al, "The Efficacy of *Aloe vera* Gel in the Treatment of Oral Lichen Planus: A Randomized Controlled Trial," *Br J Dermatol*, 2008, 158(3):573-7.

Cowan D, "Oral Aloe Vera as a Treatment for Osteoarthritis: A Summary," *Br J Community Nurs*, 2010, 15 (6):280-2.

Dal'Belo SE, Gaspar LR, and Maia Campos PM, "Moisturizing Effect of Cosmetic Formulations Containing *Aloe vera* Extract in Different Concentrations Assessed by Skin Bioengineering Techniques," *Skin Res Technol*, 2006, 12(4):241-6.

Davis K, Philpott S, Kumar D, et al, "Randomised Double-Blind Placebo-Controlled Trial of *Aloe vera* for Irritable Bowel Syndrome," *Int J Clin Pract*, 2006, 60(9):1080-6.

Davis RH, Leitner MG, Russo JM, et al, "Wound Healing. Oral and Topical Activity of *Aloe vera*," *J Am Podiatr Med Assoc*, 1989, 79(11):559-62.

Garnick JJ, Singh B, and Winkley G, "Effectiveness of a Medicament Containing Silicon Dioxide, Aloe, and Allantoin on Aphthous Stomatitis," *Oral Surg Oral Med Oral Pathol Oral Radiol Endod*, 1998, 86 (5):550-6.

Heggers JP, Kucukcelebi A, Listengarten D, et al, "Beneficial Effect of Aloe on Wound Healing in an Excisional Wound Model," *J Altern Complement Med*, 1996, 2(2):271-7.

Langmead L, Feakins RM, Goldthorpe S, et al, "Randomized, Double-Blind, Placebo-Controlled Trial of Oral *Aloe vera* Gel for Active Ulcerative Colitis," Aliment Pharmacol Ther, 2004, 19(7):739-47.

McDaniel HR and McAnalley BH, "Evaluation of Polymannoacetate (Carrisyn) in the Treatment of AIDS," *Clin Research*, 1987, 35(3):483a.

McDaniel HR, Combs C, McDaniel HR, et al, "An Increase in Circulating Monocyte/Macrophages (M/M) Is Induced by Oral Acemannan (ACE-M) in HIV-1 Patients," *Amer J Clin Pathol*, 1990, 94(4):516-517.

Merchant TE, Bosley C, Smith J, et al, "A Phase III Trial Comparing an Anionic Phospholipid-Based Cream and Aloe Vera-Based Gel in the Prevention of Radiation Dermatitis in Pediatric Patients," *Radiat Oncol*, 2007, 2:45.

Montaner JS, Gill J, Singer J, et al, "Double-Blind Placebo-Controlled Pilot Trial of Acemannan in Advanced Human Immunodeficiency Virus Disease," J Acquir Immune Defic Syndr Hum Retrovirol, 1996, 12(2):153-7.

Natural Standard Research Collaboration, Chief Editors: Ulbricht C, Basch E, *Natural Standard Herb and Supplement Reference - Evidence-Based Clinical Reviews*, USA: Elsevier/Mosby, 2005.

Ngo MQ, Nguyen NN, and Shah SA, "Oral Aloe Vera for Treatment of Diabetes Mellitus and Dyslipidemia," *Am J Health Syst Pharm*, 2010, 67(21):1804-08.

Odes HS and Madar Z, "A Double-Blind Trial of a Celandin, *Aloe vera* and Psyllium Laxative Preparation in Adult Patients With Constipation," *Digestion*, 1991, 49(2):65-71.

Olsen DL, Raub W Jr, Bradley C, et al, "The Effect of Aloe Vera Gel/Mild Soap Versus Mild Soap Alone in Preventing Skin Reactions in Patients Undergoing Radiation Therapy," *Oncol Nurs Forum*, 2001, 28 (3):543-7.

Richardson J, Smith JE, McIntyre M, et al, "Aloe Vera for Preventing Radiation-Induced Skin Reactions: A Systematic Literature Review," *Clin Oncol (R Coll Radiol)*, 2005, 17(6):478-84.

Sakai R, "Epidemiologic Survey on Lung Cancer With Respect to Cigarette Smoking and Plant Diet," *Jpn J Cancer Res*, 1989, 80(6):513-20.

Schmidt JM and Greenspoon JS, "*Aloe vera* Dermal Wound Gel is Associated With a Delay in Wound Healing," *Obstet Gynecol*, 1991, 78(1):115-7.

Su CK, Mehta V, Ravikumar L, et al, "Phase II Double-Blind Randomized Study Comparing Oral Aloe Vera Versus Placebo to Prevent Radiation-Related Mucositis in Patients With Head-and-Neck Neoplasms," *Int J Radiat Oncol Biol Phys*, 2004, 60(1):171-7.

Syed TA, Afzal M, and Ashfaq AS, "Management of Genital Herpes in Men With 0.5% *Aloe vera* Extract in a Hydrophilic Cream. A Placebo-Controlled Double-Blind Study," *J Derm Treatment*, 1997, 8(2):99-102.
Syed TA, Ahmad SA, Holt AH, et al, "Management of Psoriasis With *Aloe vera* Extract in a Hydrophilic Cream: A Placebo-Controlled, Double-Blind Study," *Trop Med Int Health*, 1996, 1(4):505-9.
Syed TA, Cheema KM, Ahmad SA, et al, "*Aloe vera* Extract 0.5% in Hydrophilic Cream Versus *Aloe vera* Gel for the Measurement of Genital Herpes in Males. A Placebo-Controlled, Double-Blind, Comparative Study," *Journal of the European Academy of Dermatology & Venerology*, 1996, 7(3):294-5.
Thomas DR, Goode PS, LaMaster K, et al, "Acemannan Hydrogel Dressing Versus Saline Dressing for Pressure Ulcers. A Randomized, Controlled Trial," *Adv Wound Care*, 1998, 11(6):273-6.
Vardy AD, Cohen AD, and Tchetov T, "A Double-Blind, Placebo-Controlled Trial of *Aloe vera* (A. barbadensis) Emulsion in the Ttreatment of Seborrheic Dermatitis," *J Derm Treatment*, 1999, 10 (1):7-11.
Visuthikosol V, Chowchuen B, Sukwanarat Y, et al, "Effect of *Aloe vera* Gel to Healing of Burn Wound: A Clinical and Histologic Study," *J Med Assoc Thai*, 1995, 78(8):403-9.
Williams MS, Burk M, Loprinzi CL, et al, "Phase III Double-Blind Evaluation of an Aloe Vera Gel as a Prophylactic Agent for Radiation-Induced Skin Toxicity," *Int J Radiat Oncol Biol Phys*, 1996, 36 (2):345-9.
Worthington HV, Clarkson JE, and Eden OB, "Interventions for Preventing Oral Mucositis for Patients With Cancer Receiving Treatment," *Cochrane Database Syst Rev*, 2007, (4):CD000978.
Worthington HV, Clarkson JE, Bryan G, et al, "Interventions for Preventing Oral Mucositis for Patients With Cancer Receiving Treatment," *Cochrane Database Syst Rev*, 2010, (12):CD000978.
Yongchaiyudha S, Rungpitarangsi V, Bunyapraphatsara A, et al, "Antidiabetic Activity of *Aloe vera* L. Juice. I Clinical Trial in New Cases of Diabetes Mellitus," *Phytomedicine*, 1996, 3(3):241-3.

Alpha-Lipoic Acid

Related Information

Ulcerative, Erosive, and Painful Oral Mucosal Disorders *on page 1950*

Pharmacologic Category Nutritional Supplement

Reported Use

Alcohol-induced liver damage (Loginov, 1989)
Alzheimer's disease (Hager, 2007)
Antioxidant (Huang, 2008; Zembron-Lacny, 2007)
Burning mouth syndrome (Femiano, 2004)
Cancer (Berkson, 2006; Berkson, 2009)
Cardiovascular outcomes (in end-state renal disease) (Chang, 2007)
Carpal tunnel syndrome (DiGeronimo, 2009)
Cataract prevention (Packer, 1995)
Chemotherapy and radiation (adjunct) (pharmacologic activity)
Circulation (pharmacologic activity)
Cognitive function (Anonymous, 1998)
Coronary artery disease (McMackin, 2007)
Diabetes, diabetic peripheral neuropathy; insulin resistance (Bashan, 1999; Borcea, 1999; Haak, 2000; Jacob, 1999; Kamenova, 2006; Kishi, 1999; Konrad, 1999; Nagamatsu, 1995; Nardino, 2000; Reljanovic, 1999; Tang, 2007; Ziegler, 1997; Ziegler, 1997; Ziegler, 2006)
Drug-induced cardiotoxicity (Al-Majed, 2002)
Glaucoma (Filina, 1995)
Hypertension (pharmacologic activity)
Liver protective effects (Dünschede, 2006)
Migraine (prophylaxis) (Magis, 2007)
Multiple sclerosis (pharmacologic activity)
Neuralgias (Sladki, 1962; Sladki, 1967)
Neurologic disorders, including stroke (preventive) (Packer, 1997)
Peripheral artery disease (Vincent, 2007)
Radiation injuries (Korkina, 1993)
Skin aging (Thom, 2005)
Weight loss (Kim, 2008; Koh, 2011)
Wound healing (Alleva, 2005)

Local Anesthetic/Vasoconstrictor Precautions No information available to require special precautions

Effects on Bleeding None reported

Warnings/Precautions Use with caution in individuals who may be predisposed to hypoglycemia (including individuals receiving antidiabetic agents). Dermatologic reactions (rashes) have been reported with alpha-lipoic acid. Caution should be used among patients with type 2 diabetes, due to the possibility of changes in insulin sensitivity.

May alter glucose regulation. Use with caution in individuals with diabetes or in those who may be predisposed to hypoglycemia. Effects of drugs with hypoglycemic activity may be potentiated (including insulin and oral hypoglycemics). Blood sugar should be closely monitored, and the dosage of hypoglycemic medications may require adjustment. This should be carefully coordinated among the individuals' healthcare providers. Use with caution in individuals receiving adriamycin, doxorubicin, and drugs broken down in the liver. Use with caution in individuals receiving thiamine (B_1) or vitamin C.

References

Alleva R, Nasole E, Di Donato F, et al, "Alpha-Lipoic Acid Supplementation Inhibits Oxidative Damage, Accelerating Chronic Wound Healing in Patients Undergoing Hyperbaric Oxygen Therapy," *Biochem Biophys Res Commun*, 2005, 333(2):404-10.
Al-Majed A, Gdo A, Al-Shabanah O, et al, "Alpha-lipoic Acid Ameliorates Myocardial Toxicity Induced by Doxorubicin," *Pharmacol Res*, 2002, 46(6):499-503.
Anonymous, "A Randomized, Double-Blind, Placebo-Controlled Trial of Deprenyl and Thioctic Acid in Human Immunodeficiency Virus-Associated Cognitive Impairment. Dana Consortium on the Therapy of HIV Dementia and Related Cognitive Disorders," *Neurology*, 1998, 50(3):645-51.
Bashan N, et al, "Lipoic Acid Protects Against Oxidation-Induced Insulin Resistance in 3T3 L1 Adipocytes," *Diabetes*, 1999, 48(Suppl):A261.
Berkson BM, Rubin DM, and Berkson AJ, "Revisiting the ALA/N (Alpha-Lipoic Acid/Low-Dose Naltrexone) Protocol for People With Metastatic and Nonmetastatic Pancreatic Cancer: A Report of 3 New Cases," *Integr Cancer Ther*, 2009, 8(4):416-22.
Berkson BM, Rubin DM, and Berkson AJ, The Long-Term Survival of a Patient With Pancreatic Cancer With Metastases to the Liver After Treatment With the Intravenous Alpha-Lipoic Acid/Low-Dose Naltrexone Protocol," *Integr Cancer Ther*, 2006, 5(1):83-9.
Borcea V, Nourooz-Zadeh J, Wolff SP, et al, "Alpha-Lipoic Acid Decreases Oxidative Stress Even in Diabetic Patients With Poor Glycemic Control and Albuminuria," *Free Radic Biol Med*, 1999, 26 (11-12):1495-500.
Chang JW, Lee EK, Kim TH, et al, "Effects of Alpha-Lipoic Acid on the Plasma Levels of Asymmetric Dimethylarginine in Diabetic End-Stage Renal Disease Patients on Hemodialysis: A Pilot Study," *Am J Nephrol*, 2007, 27(1):70-4.
Di Geronimo G, Caccese AF, Caruso L, et al, "Treatment of Carpal Tunnel Syndrome With Alpha-Lipoic Acid," *Eur Rev Med Pharmacol Sci*, 2009, 13(2):133-9.
Dünschede F, Erbes K, Kircher A, et al, "Reduction of Ischemia Reperfusion Injury After Liver Resection and Hepatic Inflow Occlusion by Alpha-Lipoic Acid in Humans," *World J Gastroenterol*, 2006, 12 (42):6812-7.
Femiano F, Gombos F, and Scully C, "Burning Mouth Syndrome: The Efficacy of Lipoic Acid on Subgroups," *J Eur Acad Dermatol Venereol*, 2004, 18(6):676-8.
Filina AA, Davydova NG, Endrikhovskii SN, et al, "Lipoic Acid as a Means of Metabolic Therapy of Open-Angle Glaucoma," *Vestn Oftalmol*, 1995, 111(4):6-8.
Haak E, Usadel KH, Kusterer K, et al, "Effects of Alpha-Lipoic Acid on Microcirculation in Patients With Peripheral Diabetic Neuropathy," *Exp Clin Endocrinol Diabetes*, 2000, 108(3):168-74.
Hager K, Kenklies M, McAfoose J, et al, "Alpha-Lipoic Acid as a New Treatment Option for Alzheimer's Disease - A 48 Months Follow-Up Analysis," *J Neural Transm Suppl*, 2007, (72):189-93.
Huang EA and Gitelman SE, "The Effect of Oral Alpha-Lipoic Acid on Oxidative Stress in Adolescents With Type 1 Diabetes Mellitus," *Pediatr Diabetes*, 2008, 9(3 Pt 2):69-73.
Jacob S, Ruus P, Hermann R, et al, "Oral Administration of RAC-Alpha-Lipoic Acid Modulates Insulin Sensitivity in Patients With Type-2 Diabetes Mellitus: A Placebo-Controlled Pilot Trial," *Free Radic Biol Med*, 1999, 27(3-4):309-14.
Kamenova P, "Improvement of Insulin Sensitivity in Patients With Type 2 Diabetes Mellitus After Oral Administration of Alpha-Lipoic Acid," *Hormones (Athens)*, 2006, 5(4):251-8.
Kim E, Park DW, Choi SH, et al, "A Preliminary Investigation of Alpha-Lipoic Acid Treatment of Antipsychotic Drug-Induced Weight Gain in Patients With Schizophrenia," *J Clin Psychopharmacol*, 2008, 28(2):138-46.
Kishi Y, Schmelzer JD, Yao JK, et al, "Alpha-Lipoic Acid: Effect on Glucose Uptake, Sorbitol Pathway, and Energy Metabolism in Experimental Diabetic Neuropathy," *Diabetes*, 1999, 48(10):2045-51.
Koh EH, Lee WJ, Lee SA, et al, "Effects of Alpha-Lipoic Acid on Body Weight in Obese Subjects," *Am J Med*, 2011, 124(1):85.e1-8.
Konrad T, Vicini P, Kusterer K, et al, "Alpha-Lipoic Acid Treatment Decreases Serum Lactate and Pyruvate Concentrations and Improves Glucose Effectiveness in Lean and Obese Patients With Type 2 Diabetes," *Diabetes Care*, 1999, 22(2):280-7.
Korkina LG, Afanas'ef IB, and Diplock AT, "Antioxidant Therapy in Children Affected by Irradiation From the Chernobyl Nuclear Accident," *Biochem Soc Trans*, 1993, 21 (Pt 3)(3):314S.
Loginov AS, Nilova TV, Bendikov EA, et al, "Pharmacokinetics of Preparations of Lipoic Acid and Their Effect on ATP Synthesis, Processes of Microsomal and Cytosol Oxidation in Hepatocytes in Liver Damage in Man," *Farmakol Toksikol*, 1989, 52(4):78-82.
Magis D, Ambrosini A, Sándor P, et al, "A Randomized Double-Blind Placebo-Controlled Trial of Thioctic Acid in Migraine Prophylaxis," *Headache*, 2007, 47(1):52-7.
McMackin CJ, Widlansky ME, Hamburg NM, et al, "Effect of Combined Treatment With Alpha-Lipoic Acid and Acetyl-L-Carnitine on Vascular Function and Blood Pressure in Patients With Coronary Artery Disease," *J Clin Hypertens (Greenwich)*, 2007, 9(4):249-55.
Nagamatsu M, Nickander KK, Schmelzer JD, et al, "Lipoic Acid Improves Nerve Blood Flow, Reduces Oxidative Stress, and Improves Distal Nerve Conduction in Experimental Diabetic Neuropathy," *Diabetes Care*, 1995, 18(8):1160-7.
Nardino RJ, et al, "Alpha-Lipoic Acid for the Prevention and Treatment of Diabetic Neuropathy," *Alter Med Alert*, 2000, 3(7):73-7.
Natural Standard Research Collaboration, Chief Editors: Ulbricht C, Basch E, *Natural Standard Herb and Supplement Reference - Evidence-Based Clinical Reviews*, USA: Elsevier/Mosby, 2005.
Packer L, Tritschler HJ, Wessel K, et al, "Neuroprotection by the Metabolic Antioxidant Alpha-Lipoic Acid," *Free Radic Biol Med*, 1997, 22(1-2):359-78.
Packer L, Witt EH, Tritschler HJ, et al, "Alpha-Lipoic Acid as a Biological Antioxidant," *Free Radic Biol Med*, 1995, 19(2):227-50.
Reljanovic M, Reichel G, Rett K, et al, "Treatment of Diabetic Polyneuropathy With the Antioxidant Thioctic Acid (Alpha-Lipoic Acid): A Two-Year Multicenter Randomized Double-Blind Placebo-Controlled Trial (ALADIN II). Alpha Lipoic Acid in Diabetic Neuropathy," *Free Radic Res*, 1999, 31(3):171-9.
Sladki E, Sladka H, and Prusinski A, "Studies on the Value of Local Injections of Thioctic Acid in the Treatment of Trigeminal Neuralgia and Upon Etiopathogenesis of This Disease in the Light of the Author's Own Observations," *Czas Stomatol*, 1967, 20(9):981-6.
Sladki E, "Trials of the Treatment of Trigeminal Neuralgia With Local Administration of Thioctic Acid," *Med Welt*, 1962, 52:2783-4.
Tang J, Wingerchuk DM, Crum BA, et al, "Alpha-Lipoic Acid May Improve Symptomatic Diabetic Polyneuropathy," *Neurologist*, 2007, 13(3):164-7.
Thom E, "A Randomized, Double-Blind, Placebo-Controlled Study on the Clinical Efficacy of Oral Treatment With DermaVite on Ageing Symptoms of the Skin," *J Int Med Res*, 2005, 33(3):267-72.
Vincent HK, Bourguignon CM, Vincent KR, et al, "Effects of Alpha-Lipoic Acid Supplementation in Peripheral Arterial Disease: A Pilot Study," *J Altern Complement Med*, 2007, 13(5):577-84.
Zembron-Lacny A, Szyszka K, and Szygula Z, "Effect of Cysteine Derivatives Administration in Healthy Men Exposed to Intense Resistance Exercise by Evaluation of Pro-Antioxidant Ratio," *J Physiol Sci*, 2007, 57(6):343-8.
Ziegler D, Ametov A, Barinov A, et al, "Oral Treatment With Alpha-Lipoic Acid Improves Symptomatic Diabetic Polyneuropathy: The SYDNEY 2 Trial," *Diabetes Care*, 2006, 29(11):2365-70.
Ziegler D and Gries FA, "Alpha-Lipoic Acid in the Treatment of Diabetic Peripheral and Cardiac Autonomic Neuropathy," *Diabetes*, 1997, 46(Suppl 2):S62-6.
Ziegler D, Schatz H, Conrad F, et al, "Effects of Treatment With the Anti-Oxidant Alpha-Lipoic Acid on Cardiac Autonomic Neuropathy in NIDDM Patients. A 4-Month Randomized Controlled Multicenter Trial (DEKAN Study)," *Diabetes Care*, 1997, 20(3):369-73.

Arnica

Pharmacologic Category Herb

Reported Use

Bruising (Seeley, 2006)
Coagulation (Baillargeon, 1993)
Diabetic retinopathy (Zicari, 1995; Zicari, 1997)
Muscle soreness (Tveiten, 1998)
Osteoarthritis (Knuesel, 2002)
Pain (Lüdtke, 2005); Robertson, 2007)
Swelling (postoperative) (Brinkhaus, 2006)
Trauma (Jeffrey, 2002)

Local Anesthetic/Vasoconstrictor Precautions May cause serious interactions with anesthetic drugs

Effects on Bleeding May see increased bleeding due to inhibition of platelet aggregation

Warnings/Precautions Avoid full strength arnica tinctures on hypersensitive or broken skin. Use with caution in individuals with a history of bleeding, hemostatic disorders, or drug-related hemostatic problems. Use with caution in individuals taking anticoagulant medications, including warfarin, aspirin, aspirin-containing products, NSAIDs, or antiplatelet agents (eg, ticlopidine, clopidogrel, dipyridamole). Discontinue use prior to dental or surgical procedures (generally at least 14 days before). Use with caution in individuals taking anesthetic drugs. Use with caution with antihypertensive agents.

References

Baillargeon L, Drouin J, Desjardins L, et al, "The Effects of *Arnica montana* on Blood Coagulation. Randomized Controlled Trial," *Can Fam Physician*, 1993, 39:2362-7.
Brinkhaus B, Wilkens JM, Lüdtke R, et al, "Homeopathic Arnica Therapy in Patients Receiving Knee Surgery: Results of Three Randomised Double-Blind Trials," *Complement Ther Med*, 2006, 14 (4):237-46.
Hall IH, Starnes CO Jr, Lee KH, et al, "Mode of Action of Sesquiterpene Lactones as Anti-Inflammatory Agents," *J Pharm Sci*, 1980, 69(5):537-43.
Jeffrey SL and Belcher HJ, "Use of Arnica to Relieve Pain After Carpal-Tunnel Release Surgery," *Altern Ther Health Med*, 2002, 8(2):66-8.
Knuesel O, Weber M, and Suter A, "*Arnica montana* Gel in Osteoarthritis of the Knee: An Open, Multicenter Clinical Trial," *Adv Ther*, 2002, 19(5):209-18.
Lüdtke R and Hacke D, "On the Effectiveness of the Homeopathic Remedy Arnica Montana," *Wien Med Wochenschr*, 2005, 155(21-22):482-90.
Merfort I, "Arnica: New Insights on the Molecular Mode of Action of a Traditional Medicinal Plant," *Forsch Komplementarmed Klass Naturheilkd*, 2003, 1(10 Suppl):45-8.
Natural Standard Research Collaboration, Chief Editors: Ulbricht C, Basch E, *Natural Standard Herb and Supplement Reference - Evidence-Based Clinical Reviews*, USA: Elsevier/Mosby, 2005.
Robertson A, Suryanarayanan R, and Banerjee A, "Homeopathic *Arnica montana* for Post-Tonsillectomy Analgesia: A Randomised Placebo Control Trial," *Homeopathy*, 2007, 96(1):17-21.
Seeley BM, Denton AB, Ahn MS, et al, "Effect of Homeopathic *Arnica montana* on Bruising in Face-Lifts: Results of a Randomized, Double-Blind, Placebo-Controlled Clinical Trial," *Arch Facial Plast Surg*, 2006, 8(1):54-9.
Tveiten D, Bruseth S, Borchgrevink CF, et al, "Effects of the Homoeopathic Remedy Arnica D30 on Marathon Runners: A Randomized, Double-Blind Study During the 1995 Oslo Marathon," *Comp Ther Med*, 1998, 6:71-4.
Zicari D, Agneni F, Ricciotti F, et al, "Angioprotective Action of Arnica 5 CH: Preliminary Data," *Invest Ophthalmol Visual Science*, 1995, 36:S479.
Zicari D, Cumps P, Del Beato P, et al, "Arnica 5 CH Activity on Retinal Function," *Invest Opthalmol Visual Science*, 1997, 38:767.

Astragalus

Pharmacologic Category Herb

Reported Use

Adaptogen/tonic (promote wellness) (Chang, 1986)
Antiviral activity (Batey, 1998; Gu, 1996; Liu, 2004; Mao, 2004; Qian, 1990; Sun, 2004; Yan, 1991; Zhang, 1993)
Athletic performance (enhancement) (Chen, 2002; Su, 2001)
Burns (Shi, 2001)
Chemotherapy and radiation (adjunct) (McCulloch, 2006; Zhao, 1990)
Coronary artery disease (Chen, 1995; Lei, 1994; Liao, 1989; Lu, 1994; Zhang, 2002)
Diabetes (Chen 2003; Xia, 1999; Yin, 2001; Zhang, 1986)
Heart failure (Li, 1995; Li, 2003; Liu, 2003; Luo, 1995; Zhang, 2002; Zhang, 2005; Zhou 2000; Zhou, 2001)
Immune support (Geng, 1986; Wang, 2007; Wu, 2006)
Liver protection (Chen, 2000; Tan, 2001)
Mental performance (Zhang, 1990)
Multiple sclerosis (pharmacologic activity)
Otitis media (pharmacologic activity)
Renal failure (Sheng, 1994; Su, 1993)
Smoking cessation (Lee, 2005)
Tissue oxygenation (Griga, 1977)
Tuberculosis (Niu, 2001)

Local Anesthetic/Vasoconstrictor Precautions No information available to require special precautions

Effects on Bleeding Astragalus may increase the risk of bleeding.

Warnings/Precautions Use with caution in individuals receiving immunosuppressants or antivirals and individuals with diabetes or receiving antidiabetic agents. Use with caution in patients receiving antihypertensives, anticoagulants, or cholesteral-lowering agents. Use with caution in individuals with renal disorders.

References

Batey RG, Bensoussan A, Fan YY, et al, "Preliminary Report of a Randomized, Double-Blind Placebo-Controlled Trial of a Chinese Herbal Medicine Preparation CH-100 in the Treatment of Chronic Hepatitis C," *Journal of Gastroenterol Hepatology*, 1998, 13(3):244-7.

Chang H, *Pharmacology and Application of Chinese Materia Medica*, Philadelphia, PA: World Scientific, 1986, 4.

Chen H and Weng L, "Comparison on Efficacy in Treating Liver Fibrosis of Chronic Hepatitis B Between Astragalus Polygonum Anti-Fibrosis Decoction and Jinshuibao Capsule," *Zhongguo Zhong Xi Yi Jie He Za Zhi*, 2000, 20(4):255-7.

Chen KT, Su CH, Hsin LH, et al, "Reducing Fatigue of Athletes Following Oral Administration of Huangqi Jianzhong Tang," *Acta Pharmacol Sin*, 2002, 23(8):757-61.

Chen LX, Liao JZ, and Guo WQ, "Effects of *Astragalus membranaceus* on Left Ventricular Function and Oxygen Free Radical in Acute Myocardial Infarction Patients and Mechanism of Its Cardiotonic Action," *Zhongguo Zhong Xi Yi Jie He Za Zhi*, 1995, 15(3):141-3.

Chen ML, Liu WJ, Wang CY, et al, "Effects of Yishenjiangyafang on Blood Pressure and Protecting Renal Function in RPH Rats," *Zhongguo Zhong Yao Za Zhi*, 2003, 28(8):746-51.

Chu DT, Sun Y, and Lin JR, "Immune Restoration of Local Xenogeneic Graft-Versus-Host Reaction in Cancer Patients *In Vitro* and Reversal of Cyclophosphamide-Induced Immune Suppression in the Rat *In Vivo* by Fractionated *Astragalus membranaceus*," *Chung Hsi I Chieh Ho Tsa Chih*, 1989, 9(6):326, 351-4.

Geng CS, "Advances in Immuno-Pharmacological Studies on *Astragalus membranaceus*," *Chung Hsi I Chieh Ho Tsa Chih*, 1986, 6(1):62-4.

Griga IV, "Effect of a Summary Preparation of *Astragalus cicer* on the Blood Pressure of Rats With Renal Hypertension and on the Oxygen Consumption by the Tissues," *Farm Zh*, 1977, 6:64-6.

Gu W, Yang YZ, and He MX, "A Study on Combination Therapy of Western and Traditional Chinese Medicine of Acute Viral Myocarditis," *Zhongguo Zhong Xi Yi Jie He Za Zhi*, 1996, 16(12):713-6.

Khoo KS and Ang PT, "Extract of *Astragalus membranaceus* and *Ligustrum lucidum* Does Not Prevent Cyclophosamide-Induced Myelosuppression," *Singapore Med J*, 1995, 36(4):387-90.

Lee HJ and Lee JH, "Effects of Medicinal Herb Tea on the Smoking Cessation and Reducing Smoking Withdrawal Symptoms," *Am J Chin Med*, 2005, 33(1):127-38.

Lei ZY, Qin H, and Liao JZ, "Action of *Astragalus membranaceus* on Left Ventricular Function of Angina Pectoris," *Zhongguo Zhong Xi Yi Jie He Za Zhi*, 1994, 14(4):199-202.

Li C, Luo J, Li L, et al, "The Collagenolytic Effects of the Traditional Chinese Medicine Preparation, Han-Dan-Gan-Le, Contribute to Reversal of Chemical-Induced Liver Fibrosis in Rats," *Life Sci*, 2003, 72 (14):1563-71.

Li SQ, Yuan RX, and Gao H, "Clinical Observation on the Treatment of Ischemic Heart Disease With *Astragalus membranaceus*," *Zhongguo Zhong Xi Yi Jie He Za Zhi*, 1995, 15(2):77-80.

Liao JZ, Chen JJ, Wu ZM, et al, "Clinical and Experimental Studies of Coronary Heart Disease Treated With Yi-Qi Huo-Xue Injection," *J Tradit Chin Med*, 1989, 9(3):193-8.

Liu JP, Yang M, and Du XM, "Herbal Medicines for Viral Myocarditis," *Cochrane Database Syst Rev*, 2004, (3):CD003711.

Liu ZG, Xiong ZM, and Yu XY, "Effect of Astragalus Injection on Immune Function in Patients With Congestive Heart Failure," *Zhongguo Zhong Xi Yi Jie He Za Zhi*, 2003, 23(5):351-3.

Lu DC, Su ZJ, and Rui T, "Effect of Jian Yan Ling on Serum Lipids, Apoprotein and Lipoprotein-a," *Zhonguo Zhong Xi Yi Jie He Za Zi*, 1994, 14(3):142-4, 131-2.

Luo HM, Dai RH, and Li Y, "Nuclear Cardiology Study on Effective Ingredients of *Astragalus membranaceus* in Treating Heart Failure," *Zhongguo Zhong Xi Yi Jie He Za Zhi*, 1995, 15(12):707-9.

Mao SP, Cheng KL, and Zhou YF, "Modulatory Effect of *Astragalus membranaceus* on Th1/Th2 Cytokine in Patients With Herpes Simplex Keratitis," *Zhongguo Zhong Xi Yi Jie He Za Zhi*, 2004, 24(2):121-3.

McCulloch M, See C, Shu XJ, et al, "Astragalus-Based Chinese Herbs and Platinum-Based Chemotherapy for Advanced Non-Small-Cell Lung Cancer: Meta-Analysis of Randomized Trials," *J Clin Oncol*, 2006, 24(3):419-30.

Natural Standard Research Collaboration, Chief Editors: Ulbricht C, Basch E, *Natural Standard Herb and Supplement Reference - Evidence-Based Clinical Reviews*, USA: Elsevier/Mosby, 2005.

Niu HR, Lai ZH, and Yuan L, "Observation on Effect of Supplementary Treatment by Astragalus Injection in Treating Senile Pulmonary Tuberculosis Patients," *Zhongguo Zhong Xi Yi Jie He Za Zhi*, 2001, 21 (5):349-50.

Qian ZW, Mao SJ, Cai XC, et al, "Viral Etiology of Chronic Cervicitis and Its Therapeutic Response to a Recombinant Interferon," *Chin Med J (Engl)*, 1990, 103(8):647-51.

Sheng ZL, Li NY, and Ge XP, "Clinical Study of Baoyuan Dahuang Decoction in the Treatment of Chronic Renal Failure," *Zhongguo Zhong Xi Yi Jie He Za Zhi*, 1994, 14(5):268-70, 259.

Shi FS, Yang ZG, and Di GP, "Effect of *Astragalus saponin* on Vascular Endothelial Cell and Its Function in Burn Patients," *Zhongguo Zhong Xi Yi Jie He Za Zhi*, 2001, 21(10):750-1.

Su YC, Lin CJ, Chen KT, et al, "Effects of Huangqi Jianzhong Tang on Hematological and Biochemical Parameters in Judo Athletes," *Acta Pharmacol Sin*, 2001, 22(12):1154-8.

Su ZZ, He YY, and Chen G, "Clinical and Experimental Study on Effects of Man-shen-ling Oral Liquid in the Treatment of 100 Cases of Chronic Nephritis," *Zhongguo Zhong Xi Yi Jie He Za Zhi*, 1993, 13 (5):269-72.

Sun Y and Yang J, "Experimental Study of the Effect of *Astragalus membranaceus* Against Herpes Simplex Virus Type 1," *Di Yi Jun Yi Da Xue Xue Bao*, 2004, 24(1):57-8.

Tan YW, Yin YM, and Yu XJ, "Influence of *Salvia miltiorrhizae* and *Astragalus membranaceus* on Hemodynamics and Liver Fibrosis Indexes in Liver Cirrhotic Patients With Portal Hypertension," *Zhongguo Zhong Xi Yi Jie He Za Zhi*, 2001, 21(5):351-3.

Wang MS, Li J, Di HX, et al, "Clinical Study on Effect of Astragalus Injection and Its Immuno-Regulation Action in Treating Chronic Aplastic Anemia," *Chin J Integr Med*, 2007, 13(2):98-102.

Wu J, Wang YX, Su WL, et al, "Effect of Astragalus Injection on Serious Abdominal Traumatic Patients' Cellular Immunity," *Chin J Integr Med*, 2006, 12(1):29-31.

Xia D, Zeng Y, amd Liao Z, "Clinical and Experimental Study of Yushen Jiangtang Tablet in Treating Non-Insulin Dependent Diabetes Mellitus," *Zhongguo Zhong Xi Yi Jie He Za Zhi*, 1999, 19(2):90-2.

Yan HJ, "Clinical and Experimental Study of the Effect of Kang Er Xin-I on Viral Myocarditis," *Zhong Xi Yi Jie He Za Zhi*, 1991, 11(8):468-70, 452.

Yin X, Zhang S, Kong Y, et al, "Observation on Efficiency of Jiangtang Capsule in Treating Diabetes Mellitus Type 2 With Hyperlipidemia," *Chinese Journal of Interated Traditional and Western Medicine*, 2001, 7(3):214-6.

Zhang BZ, Ding F, and Tan LW, "Clinical and Experimental Study on Yi-gan-ning Granule in Treating Chronic Hepatitis B," *Zhongguo Zhong Xi Yi Jie He Za Zhi*, 1993, 13(10):597-9, 580.

Zhang HE, et al, "Treatment of Adult Diabetes With Jiangtangjia Tablet," *Journal of Traditional Chinese Medicine*, 1986, 27(4):37-9.

Zhang JG, Gao DS, and Wei GH, "Clinical Study on Effect of Astragalus Injection on Left Ventricular Remodeling and Left Ventricular Function in Patients With Acute Myocardial Infarction," *Zhongguo Zhong Xi Yi Jie He Za Zhi*, 2002, 22(5):346-8.

Zhang JG, Yang N, and He H, "Effect of Astraglus Injection on Serum Apoptosis Relevant Factors in Patients With Chronic Heart Failure," *Zhongguo Zhong Xi Yi Jie He Za Zhi*, 2005, 25(5):400-3.
Zhang ZL, Wen QZ, and Liu CX, "Hepatoprotective Effects of Astraglus Root," *J Ethnopharmacology*, 1990, 30(2):145-9.
Zhao KS, Mancini C, and Doria G, "Enhancement of the Immune Response in Mice by *Astragalus membranaceus* Extracts," *Immunopharmacology*, 1990, 20(3):225-33.
Zhou JY, Fan Y, Kong JL, et al, "Effects of Components Isolated From *Astragalus membranaceus* Bunge on Cardiac Function Injured by Myocardial Ischemia Reperfusion in Rats," *Zhongguo Zhong Yao Za Zhi*, 2000, 25(5):300-2.
Zhou Y, Huang Z, Huang T, et al, "Clinical Study of Shengxue Mixture in Treating Aplastic Anemia," *Chinese Journal of Integrated Traditional and Western Medicine*, 2001, 7(3):186-9.

Barberry

Pharmacologic Category Herb

Reported Use

Bladder infection (pharmacologic activity)
Bronchitis (pharmacologic activity)
Diabetes (Ni, 1988)
Diarrhea (pharmacologic activity) (Desai, 1971)
Giardiasis (Choudry, 1972; Gupte, 1975)
Heart failure (Marin-Neto, 1988)
Hypertension (pharmacologic activity) (Chun, 1979)
Inflammation (pharmacologic activity) (Ivanovska, 1996)
Sore throat (pharmacologic activity)
Trachoma (Babbar, 1982; Mohan, 1982)
Yeast infection (pharmacologic activity)

Local Anesthetic/Vasoconstrictor Precautions No information available to require special precautions

Effects on Bleeding May see increased bleeding due to inhibition of platelet aggregation

Warnings/Precautions Avoid in women who are pregnant or lactating. Barberry has exhibited uterine stimulant properties, and berberine has been shown to have antifertility activity. Use with caution in individuals with cardiovascular disease; has been shown to cause hypotension and bradycardia. Use with caution in individuals with gastrointestinal disease; may irritate the gastrointestinal tract. Use with caution in individuals with kidney disease; may cause kidney irritation and nephritis.

Use with caution in individuals with a history of bleeding, hemostatic disorders, or drug-related hemostatic problems. Use with caution in individuals taking anticoagulant medications, including warfarin, aspirin, aspirin-containing products, NSAIDs, or antiplatelet agents (eg, ticlopidine, clopidogrel, dipyridamole). Discontinue use prior to dental or surgical procedures (generally at least 14 days before).

References

Babbar OP, Chhatwal VK, Ray IB, et al, "Effect of Berberine Chloride Eye Drops on Clinically Positive Trachoma Patients," *Indian J Med Res*, 1982, 76 Suppl:83-8.
Choudhry VP, Sabir M, and Bhide VN, "Berberine in Giardiasis," *Indian Pediatr*, 1972, 9(3):143-6.
Chun YT, Yip TT, Lau KL, et al, "A Biochemical Study on the Hypotensive Effect of Berberine in Rats," *Gen Pharmacol*, 1979,10(3):177-82.
Desai AB, Shah KM, and Shah DM, "Berberine in Treatment of Diarrhoea," *Indian Pediatr*, 1971, 8 (9):462-5.
Freile ML, Giannini F, Pucci G, et al, "Antimicrobial Activity of Aqueous Extracts and of Berberine Isolated From *Berberis heterophylla*," *Fitoterapia*, 2003, 74(7-8):702-5.
Gupte S, "Use of Berberine in Treatment of Giardiasis," *Am J Dis Child*, 1975, 129(7):866.
Ivanovska N and Philipov S, "Study on the Anti-Inflammatory Action of *Berberis vulgaris* Root Extract, Alkaloid Fractions and Pure Alkaloids," *Int J Immunopharmacol*, 1996, 18(10):553-61.
Marin-Neto JA, Maciel BC, Secches AL, et al, "Cardiovascular Effects of Berberine in Patients With Severe Congestive Heart Failure," *Clin Cardiol*, 1988, 11(4):253-60.
Mohan M, Pant CR, Angra SK, et al, "Berberine in Trachoma. (A Clinical Trial)," *Indian J Ophthalmol*, 1982, 30(2):69-75.
Natural Standard Research Collaboration, Chief Editors: Ulbricht C, Basch E, *Natural Standard Herb and Supplement Reference - Evidence-Based Clinical Reviews*, USA: Elsevier/Mosby, 2005.
Ni YX, "Therapeutic Effect of Berberine on 60 Patients With Type II Diabetes Mellitus and Experimental Research," *Zhong Xi Yi Jie He Za Zhi*, 1988, 8(12):711-3, 707.

Bilberry

Pharmacologic Category Herb

Reported Use

Circulation, peripheral: Vascular disorders: Varicose veins, capillary permeability/stability, phlebitis (Bottecchia, 1977; Gatta, 1988)
Diabetes (Cignarella, 1996)
Diarrhea (pharmacologic activity)
Dysmenorrhea (Bettini, 1984; Bettini, 1984; Colantuoni, 1991; Colombo, 1985)
Fibrocystic breast disease (FBD) (Leonardi, 1993)
Hemorrhoids (pharmacologic activity)
Ophthalmologic disorders (antioxidant): Myopia, diminished acuity, glaucoma, dark adaptation, macular degeneration, night blindness, diabetic retinopathy, cataracts (Morazonni, 1996; Perossini, 1987); contradictory study (Muth, 2000)

Peptic ulcer disease (Lietti, 1976; Lietti, 1976; Magistretti, 1988; Mertz-Nielsen, 1990)
Scleroderma (pharmacologic activity)

Local Anesthetic/Vasoconstrictor Precautions No information available to require special precautions

Effects on Bleeding May see increased bleeding due to inhibition of platelet aggregation

Warnings/Precautions If pregnant or nursing, use caution; based on *in vitro* or animal studies (Morazzoni, 1991). Use bilberry leaf with caution in individuals with diabetes (*in vitro* or animal studies indicate potential to alter glucose regulation).

Based on pharmacologic activity, this herb may be contraindicated in individuals with active bleeding (eg, peptic ulcer, intracranial bleeding). Use with caution in individuals with a history of bleeding, hemostatic disorders, or drug-related hemostatic problems. Use with caution in individuals taking anticoagulant medications, including warfarin, aspirin, aspirin-containing products, NSAIDs, or antiplatelet agents (eg, ticlopidine, clopidogrel, dipyridamole). Discontinue use prior to dental or surgical procedures (generally at least 14 days before). Use with caution in individuals taking insulin or oral hypoglycemic drugs.

References

Bettini V, "Effects of *Vaccinium myrtillus* Anthocyanosides on Vascular Smooth Muscle," *Fitoterapia*, 1984, 55(5):265-72.
Bettini V, Mayellaro F, Ton P, et al, "Interactions Between *Vaccinium myrtillus* Anthocyanosides and Serotonin on Splenic Artery Smooth Muscle," *Fitoterapia*, 1984, 55(4):201-8.
Bottecchia D, et al, "*Vaccinium myrtillus*," *Fitoterapia*, 1977, 48:3-8.
Cignarella A, Nastasi M, Cavalli E, et al, "Novel Lipid-Lowering Properties of *Vaccinium myrtillus* L. Leaves, a Traditional Antidiabetic Treatment, in Several Models of Rat Dyslipidaemia: A Comparison With Ciprofibrate," *Thromb Res*, 1996, 84(5):311-22.
Colantuoni A, Bertuglia S, Magistretti MJ, et al, "Effects of *Vaccinium myrtillus* Anthocyanosides on Arterial Vasomotion," *Arzneimittelforschung*, 1991, 41(9):905-9.
Colombo D and Vescovini R, "Controlled Clinical Trial of Anthocyanosides From *Vaccinium myrtillus* in Primary Dysmenorrhea," *G Ital Obstet Ginecol*, 1985, 7:1033-8.
Gatta L, "Experimental Single-Blind Study: 60 Pts with Venous Insufficiency Received Bilberry Extract Equivalent to 173 mg Anthocyanins Daily or Placebo for 30 Days," *Fitoterapia*, 1988, 59(Suppl 1):19.
Leonardi M, "Treatment of Fibrocystic Disease of the Breast With Myrtillus Anthocyanins. Our Experience," *Minerva Ginecol*, 1993, 45(12):617-21.
Lietti A and Forni G, "Studies on *Vaccinium myrtillus* Anthocyanosides. II. Aspects of Anthocyanins Pharmacokinetics in the Rat," *Arzneimittelforschung*, 1976, 26(5):832-5.
Lietti A, Cristoni A, and Picci M, "Studies on *Vaccinium myrtillus* Anthocyanosides. I. Vasoprotective and Antiinflammatory Activity," *Arzneimittelforschung*, 1976, 26(5):829-32.
Magistretti MJ, Conti M, and Cristoni A, "Antiulcer Activity of an Anthocyanidin From *Vaccinium myrtillus*," *Arzneimittelforschung*, 1988, 38(5):686-90.
Mertz-Nielsen A, Munck LK, Bukhave K, et al, "A Natural Flavonoid, IdB 1027, Increases Gastric Luminal Release of Prostaglandin E_2 in Healthy Subjects," *Ital J Gastroenterol*, 1990, 22(5):288-90.
Morazzoni P, "*Vaccinium myrtillus* Anthocyanosides Pharmacokinetics in Rats," *Arzneimittelforschung*, 1991, 41(2):128-31.
Morazzoni P and Bombardelli E, "*Vaccinium myrtillus*," *Fitoterapia*, 1996, 67(1):3-29.
Muth ER, Laurent JM, Jasper P, "The Effect of Bilberry Nutritional Supplementation on Night Visual Acuity and Contrast Sensitivity," *Altern Med Rev*, 2000, 5(2):164-73.
Natural Standard Research Collaboration, Chief Editors: Ulbricht C, Basch E, *Natural Standard Herb and Supplement Reference - Evidence-Based Clinical Reviews*, USA: Elsevier/Mosby, 2005.
Perossini M, et al, "Diabetic and Hypertensive Retinopathy Therapy With *Vacciniuum myrtillus* Anthocyanosides (Tegens): Double Blind Placebo Controlled Clinical Trial," *Ann Ottalmol Clin Ocul*, 1987, 113:1173.

Black Cohosh

Pharmacologic Category Herb

Reported Use

Hot flashes, related to breast cancer treatment (Jacobson, 2001)
Menopause symptoms (including vasomotor); premenstrual syndrome (PMS); depression (mild); arthritis (Chung, 2007; Jarry, 1985; Lieberman, 1998; McKenna, 2001; Newall, 1996; Oktem, 2007; Pockaj, 2006; Radowicki, 2006; Shibata, 1980; Wuttke, 2006)
Migraine (Burke, 2002)

Local Anesthetic/Vasoconstrictor Precautions No information available to require special precautions

Effects on Bleeding None reported

Warnings/Precautions Contraindicated in individuals with a history of estrogen-dependent tumors or endometrial cancer. Black cohosh may cause nausea, vomiting, headache, and hypotension at higher dosages. Use with caution in individuals allergic to salicylates; it is not known whether the amount of salicylic acid is likely to affect platelet aggregation or have other effects associated with salicylates. Use with caution in individuals with hypotension or those taking antihypertensive medications. Use with caution in individuals receiving anticoagulant medications. Monitoring of serum hormone levels is recommended after 6 months of use with black cohosh. Use with caution in individuals with liver disease due to cases of liver damage (Cohen, 2004; Lontos, 2003; Lynch, 2006). Use with caution in patients with seizure disorder (Shuster, 1996). Contraindicated in pregnancy (based on *in vitro* or animal studies, may stimulate uterine contractions) and lactation (Duker, 1991).

To date, phytoestrogen-containing herbs have not been associated with the negative health effects seen with synthetic estrogen. However, use with caution in individuals on hormone replacement therapy or oral contraceptives, or a history of thromboembolic disease or stroke.

References

Burke BE, Olson RD, and Cusack BJ, "Randomized, Controlled Trial of Phytoestrogen in the Prophylactic Treatment of Menstrual Migraine," *Biomed Pharmacother*, 2002, 56(6):283-8.
Chung DJ, Kim HY, Park KH, et al, "Black Cohosh and St. John's Wort (GYNO-Plus) for Flimacteric Symptoms," *Yonsei Med J*, 2007, 48(2):289-94.
Cohen SM, O'Connor AM, Hart J, et al, "Autoimmune Hepatitis Associated With the Use of Black Cohosh: A Case Study," *Menopause*, 2004, 11(5):575-7.
Combest WL, "Black Cohosh," *U.S. Pharmacist*, 1999, 24(9):46-55.
Duker EM, Kopanski L, Jarry H, et al, "Effects of Extracts From *Cimicifuga racemosa* on Gonadotropin Release in Menopausal Women and Ovariectomized Rats," *Planta Med*, 1991, 57(5):420-4.
Jacobson JS, Troxel AB, Evans J, et al, "Randomized Trial of Black Cohosh for the Treatment of Hot Flashes Among Women With a History of Breast Cancer," *J Clin Oncol*, 2001, 19(10):2739-45.
Jarry H, Harnischfeger G, and Duker E, "The Endocrine Effects of Constituents of *Cimicifuga racemosa* 2. *In vitro* Binding of Constituents to Estrogen Receptors," *Planta Med*, 1985, (4):316-9.
Kennelly EJ, Baggett S, Nuntanakorn P, et al, "Analysis of Thirteen Populations of Black Cohosh for Formononetin," *Phytomedicine*, 2002, 9(5):461-7.
Lieberman S, "A Review of the Effectiveness of *Cimicifuga racemosa* (Black Cohosh) for the Symptoms of Menopause," *J Womens Health*, 1998, 7(5):525-9.
Lontos S, Jones RM, Angus PW, et al, "Acute Liver Failure Associated With the Use of Herbal Preparations Containing Black Cohosh," *Med J Aust*, 2003, 179(7):390-1.
Lynch CR, Folkers ME, and Hutson WR, "Fulminant Hepatic Failure Associated With the Use of Black Cohosh: A Case Report," *Liver Transpl*, 2006, 12(6):989-92.
McKenna DJ, Jones K, Humphrey S, et al, "Black Cohosh: Efficacy, Safety, and Use in Clinical and Preclinical Applications," *Altern Ther Health Med*, 2001, 7(3):93-100.
Natural Standard Research Collaboration, Chief Editors: Ulbricht C, Basch E, *Natural Standard Herb and Supplement Reference - Evidence-Based Clinical Reviews*, USA: Elsevier/Mosby, 2005.
Newall CA, Anderson LA, and Phillipson JD, *Herbal Medicines: A Guide for Health Care Professionals*, London, England: The Pharmaceutical Press, 1996, 250-2.
Oktem M, Eroglu D, Karahan HB, et al, "Black Cohosh and Fluoxetine in the Treatment of Postmenopausal Symptoms: A Prospective, Randomized Trial," *Adv Ther*, 2007, 24(2):448-61.
Pockaj BA, Gallagher JG, Loprinzi CL, et al, "Phase III Double-Blind, Randomized, Placebo-Controlled Crossover Trial of Black Cohosh in the Management of Hot Flashes: NCCTG Trial N01CC1," *J Clin Oncol*, 2006, 24(18):2836-41.
Radowicki S, Skórzewska K, Rudnicka E, et al, "Effectiveness and Safety of the Treatment of Menopausal Syndrome With Cimicifuga Racemosa Dry Extract," *Ginekol Pol*, 2006, 77(9):678-83.
Shibata M, Ikoma M, Onoda M, et al, "Pharmacological Studies on the Chinese Crude Drug 'Shoma.' III. Central Depressant and Antispasmodic Actions of *Cimicifuga rhizoma, Cimicifuga simplex* Wormsk," *Yakugaku Zasshi*, 1980, 100(11):1143-50.
Shuster J, "Heparin and Thrombocytopenia. Black Cohosh Root? Chasteberry Tree? Seizures!" *Hosp Pharm*, 1996, 1553-4.
Umland EM, Cauffield JS, Kirk JK, et al, "Phytoestrogens As Therapeutic Alternatives to Traditional Hormone Replacement in Postmenopausal Women," *Pharmacotherapy*, 2000, 20(8):981-90.
Wuttke W, Gorkow C, and Seidlová-Wuttke D, "Effects of Black Cohosh (Cimicifuga Racemosa) on Bone Turnover, Vaginal Mucosa, and Various Blood Parameters in Postmenopausal Women: A Double-Blind, Placebo-Controlled, and Conjugated Estrogens-Controlled Study," *Menopause*, 2006, 13(2):185-96.

Bladderwrack

Pharmacologic Category Herb

Reported Use

Anticoagulant (Maruyama, 1987; Soeda, 1992; Springer, 1957)
Antioxidant (Le Tutour, 1998)
Bacterial and fungal infections (Criado, 1983; Criado, 1984)
Cancer (Ellouali, 1993; Riou, 1996; Yamamoto, 1977)
Diabetes (Lamela, 1989)
Fibrocystic breast disease (FBD) (Bradley, 1992)
Hypothyroidism (Bradley, 1992)
Nutrient (rich source of iodine, potassium, magnesium, calcium, and iron) (Bradley, 1992)
Weight loss (theoretical)

Local Anesthetic/Vasoconstrictor Precautions No information available to require special precautions

Effects on Bleeding May see increased bleeding due to anticoagulant properties.

Warnings/Precautions Use with caution with anticoagulants; may increase bleeding risk. Use with caution in individuals taking thyroid agents; do not use in hyperthyroidism. Use with caution in individuals with kidney failure (may alter potassium levels). Use with caution in individuals taking insulin or oral hypoglycemic drugs, laxatives, diuretics, lithium, or stimulants. Avoid use in individuals with iodine sensitivity.

References

Bradley PR, ed, *British Herbal Compendium*, Vol 1, Bournemouth, England: British Herbal Medicine Association, 1992, 37-9.
Criado MT and Ferreiros CM, "Selective Interaction of a *Fucus vesiculosus* Lectin-Like Mucopolysaccharide With Several *Candida* Species," *Ann Microbiol (Paris)*, 1983, 134A(2):149-54.
Criado MT and Ferreiros CM, "Toxicity of an Algal Mucopolysaccharide for *Escherichia coli* and *Neisseria meningitidis* Strains," *Rev Esp Fisiol*, 1984, 40(2):227-30.
Ellouali M, Boisson-Vidal C, Durand P, et al, "Antitumor Activity of Low Molecular Weight Fucans Extracted From Brown Seaweed *Ascophyllum nodosum*," *Anticancer Res*, 1993, 13(6A):2011-9.
Lamela M, Anca J, Villar R, et al, "Hypoglycemic Activity of Several Seaweed Extracts," *J Ethnopharmacol*, 1989, 27(1-2):35-43.
Le Tutour B, Benslimane F, Gouleau MP, et al, "Antioxidant and Pro-Oxidant Activities of the Brown Algae, *Laminaria digitata*, *Himanthalia elongata*, *Fucus vesiculosus*, *Fucus serratus*, and *Ascophyllum nodosum*," *J Applied Phycology*, 1998, 10(2):121-9.

Maruyama H, Nakajima J, and Yamamoto I, "A Study on the Anticoagulant and Fibrinolytic Activities of a Crude Fucoidan From the Edible Brown Seaweed *Laminaria religiosa*, With Special Reference to Its Inhibitory Effect on the Growth of Sarcoma-180 Ascites Cells Subcutaneously Implanted Into Mice," *Kitasato Arch Exp Med*, 1987, 60(3):105-21.
Natural Standard Research Collaboration, Chief Editors: Ulbricht C, Basch E, *Natural Standard Herb and Supplement Reference - Evidence-Based Clinical Reviews*, USA: Elsevier/Mosby, 2005.
Riou D, Colliec-Jouault S, Pinczon du Sel D, et al, "Antitumor and Antiproliferative Effects of a Fucan Extracted From *Ascophyllum Nodosum* Against a Non-Small-Cell Bronchopulmonary Carcinoma Line," *Anticancer Res*, 1996, 16(3A):1213-8.
Soeda S, Sakaguchi S, Shimeno H, et al, "Fibrinolytic and Anticoagulant Activities of Highly Sulfated Fucoidan," *Biochem Pharmacol*, 1992, 43(8):1853-8.
Springer GF, Wurzel HA, McNeal GM, et al, "Isolation of Anticoagulant Fractions From Crude Fucoidin," *Proc Soc Exp Biol Med*, 1957, 94(2):404-9.
Yamamoto I, Nagumo T, Fujihara M, et al. "Antitumor Effect of Seaweeds. II. Fractionation and Partial Characterization of the Polysaccharide With Antitumor Activity From *Sargassum fulvellum*," *Jpn J Exp Med*, 1977, 47(3):133-40.

Bromelain

Pharmacologic Category Herb

Reported Use

Arthritis (anti-inflammatory; proteolytic) (Taussig, 1980)
Burn debridement (Rosenberg, 2004)
Cancer (Gerard, 1972)
Cervical dysplasia (pharmacologic activity)
Chronic obstructive pulmonary disease (COPD) (Weiss, 1972)
Digestive enzyme (Barbarino, 1982)
Inflammation/pain (Hotz, 1989; Zatuchni, 1967)
Muscle soreness (Stone, 2002)
Osteoarthritis of the knee (Akhtar, 2004; Brien, 2006)
Rash (Massimiliano, 2007)
Rheumatoid arthritis (Cohen, 1964)
Sinusitis (Leung, 1996; Seltzer, 1967; Taub, 1966; Taub, 1967)
Steatorrhea (Balakrishnan, 1981)
Urinary tract infection (UTI) (Mori, 1972)

Local Anesthetic/Vasoconstrictor Precautions No information available to require special precautions

Effects on Bleeding May cause increased bleeding due to inhibition of platelet aggregation

Warnings/Precautions Use with caution in GI ulceration (based on case reports) and in individuals with hypertension or other cardiovascular disorders (based on case reports and *in vitro* or animal data) (Gutfreund, 1978).

Based on *in vitro* or animal studies, bromelain may have effects on platelet aggregation (Heinicke, 1972). Based on pharmacologic activity, this herb may be contraindicated in individuals with active bleeding (eg, peptic ulcer, intracranial bleeding). Use with caution in individuals with a history of bleeding, hemostatic disorders, or drug-related hemostatic problems. Use with caution in individuals taking anticoagulant medications, including warfarin, aspirin, aspirin-containing products, NSAIDs, or antiplatelet agents (eg, ticlopidine, clopidogrel, dipyridamole). Discontinue use prior to dental or surgical procedures (generally at least 14 days before). Bromelain may increase heart rate at higher doses and should be used with caution in people with heart disease.

References

Akhtar NM, Naseer R, Farooqi AZ, et al, "Oral Enzyme Combination Versus Diclofenac in the Treatment of Osteoarthritis of the Knee - A Double-Blind Prospective Randomized Study," *Clin Rheumatol*, 2004, 23(5):410-5.
Balakrishnan V, Hareendran A, and Nair CS, "Double-Blind Cross-Over Trial of an Enzyme Preparation in Pancreatic Steatorrhoea," *J Assoc Physicians India*, 1981, 29(3):207-9.
Barbarino F, Szabo P, and Neumann E, "The Influence of Bromelin on Digestion and Absorption in Control Animals and in Methotrexate-Induced 'Cytostatic' Enteropathy," *J Nucl Med Allied Sci*, 1982, 26 (2):97-103.
Brien S, Lewith G, Walker AF, et al, "Bromelain as an Adjunctive Treatment for Moderate-to-Severe Osteoarthritis of the Knee: A Randomized Placebo-Controlled Pilot Study," *QJM*, 2006, 99(12):841-50.
Cohen A and Goldman J, "Bromelains Therapy in Rheumatoid Arthritis," *Pa Med J*, 1964, 67:27-30.
Gerard G, "Anticancer Treatment and Bromelains," *Agressologie*, 1972, 13(4):261-74.
Gutfreund AE, Taussig SJ, and Morris AK, "Effect of Oral Bromelain on Blood Pressure and Heart Rate of Hypertensive Patients," *Hawaii Med J*, 1978, 37(5):143-6.
Heinicke RM, van der Wal L, and Yokoyama M, "Effect of Bromelain (Anase) on Human Platelet Aggregation," *Experientia*, 1972, 28(7):844-5.
Hotz G, Frank T, Zöller J, et al, "Antiphlogistic Effect of Bromelaine Following Third Molar Removal," *Dtsch Zahnarztl Z*, 1989, 44(11):830-2.
Leung AY and Foster S, *Encyclopedia of Common Natural Ingredients Used in Foods, Drugs, and Cosmetics*, New York, NY: Wiley, 1996, 100-3.
Massimiliano R, Pietro R, Paolo S, et al, "Role of Bromelain in the Treatment of Patients With Pityriasis Lichenoides Chronica," *J Dermatolog Treat*, 2007, 18(4):219-22.
Mori S, Ojima Y, Hirose T, et al, "The Clinical Effect of Proteolytic Enzyme Containing Bromelain and Trypsin on Urinary Tract Infection Evaluated by Double Blind Method," *Acta Obstet Gynaecol Jpn*, 1972, 19(3):147-53.
Natural Standard Research Collaboration, Chief Editors: Ulbricht C, Basch E, *Natural Standard Herb and Supplement Reference - Evidence-Based Clinical Reviews*, USA: Elsevier/Mosby, 2005.
Rosenberg L, Lapid O, Bogdanov-Berezovsky A, et al, "Safety and Efficacy of a Proteolytic Enzyme for Enzymatic Burn Debridement: A Preliminary Report," *Burns*, 2004, 30(8):843-50.
Seltzer AP, "Adjunctive Use of Bromelains in Sinusitis: A Controlled Study," *Eye Ear Nose Throat Mon*, 1967, 46(10):1281-8.

Stone MB, Merrick MA, Ingersoll CD, et al, "Preliminary Comparison of Bromelain and Ibuprofen for Delayed Onset Muscle Soreness Management," *Clin J Sport Med*, 2002, 12(6):373-8.
Taub SJ, "The Use of Bromelains in Sinusitis: A Double-Blind Clinical Evaluation," *Eye Ear Nose Throat Mon*, 1967, 46(3):361-2.
Taub SJ, "The Use of Ananase in Sinusitis. A Study of 60 Patients," *Eye Ear Nose Throat Mon*, 1966, 45 (6):96.
Taussig SJ, "The Mechanism of the Physiological Action of Bromelain," *Med Hypotheses*, 1980, 6 (1):99-104.
Weiss S and Scherrer M, "Crossed Double-Blind Trial of Potassium Iodide and Bromelain (Traumanase) in Chronic Bronchitis," *Schweiz Rundsch Med Prax*, 1972, 61(43):1331-3.
Zatuchni GI and Colombi DJ, "Bromelains Therapy for the Prevention of Episiotomy Pain," *Obstet Gynecol*, 1967, 29(2):275-8.

Calendula

Pharmacologic Category Herb

Reported Use

Antibacterial, antifungal, antiviral, antiprotozoal (Klouchek-Popova, 1982; Leung, 1996)
Otitis media (Sarrell, 2001; Sarrell, 2003)
Radiation dermatitis (Pommier, 2004)
Skin inflammation (Della, 1994)
Venous leg ulcers (Duran, 2005)
Wound healing (Kartikeyan, 1990; Leung, 1996)

Local Anesthetic/Vasoconstrictor Precautions No information available to require special precautions

Effects on Bleeding None reported

Warnings/Precautions High doses of calendula may be sedative, hypotensive, and cholesterol-lowering. Use with caution in individuals taking sedative, antihypertensive, or antilipemic agents.

References

Al-Achi A and Greenwood R, "Calendula Herb," *U.S. Pharmacist*, 2001, 26(1):66-8.
Della LR, Tubaro A, Sosa S, et al, "The Role of Triterpenoids in the Topical Anti-Inflammatory Activity of *Calendula officinalis* Flowers," *Planta Med*, 1994, 60(6):516-20.
Duran V, Matic M, Jovanovć M, et al, "Results of the Clinical Examination of an Ointment With Marigold (*Calendula officinalis*) Extract in the Treatment of Venous Leg Ulcers," *Int J Tissue React*, 2005, 27 (3):101-6.
Kartikeyan S, Chaturvedi RM, and Narkar SV, "Effect of Calendula on Trophic Ulcers," *Lepr Rev*, 1990, 61 (4):399.
Klouchek-Popova E, Popov A, Pavlova N, et al, "Influence of the Physiological Regeneration and Epithelialization Using Fractions Isolated From *Calendula officinalis*," *Acta Physiol Pharmacol Bulg*, 1982, 8(4):63-7.
Leung AY and Foster S, *Encyclopedia of Common Natural Ingredients Used in Foods, Drugs, and Cosmetics*, New York, NY: Wiley, 1996, 113-5.
Natural Standard Research Collaboration, Chief Editors: Ulbricht C, Basch E, *Natural Standard Herb and Supplement Reference - Evidence-Based Clinical Reviews*, USA: Elsevier/Mosby, 2005.
Pommier P, Gomez F, Sunyach MP, et al, "Phase III Randomized Trial of *Calendula officinalis* Compared With Trolamine for the Prevention of Acute Dermatitis During Irradiation for Breast Cancer," *J Clin Oncol*, 2004, 22(8):1447-53.
Sarrell EM, Cohen HA, and Kahan E, "Naturopathic Treatment for Ear Pain in Children," *Pediatrics*, 2003, 111(5 Pt 1):e574-9.
Sarrell EM, Mandelberg A, and Cohen HA, "Efficacy of Naturopathic Extracts in the Management of Ear Pain Associated With Acute Otitis Media," *Arch Pediatr Adolesc Med*, 2001, 155(7):796-9.

Carnitine

Pharmacologic Category Amino Acid

Reported Use

Acute myocardial infarction (mortality) (Tarantini, 2006)
Angina (Cacciatore, 1991; Cherchi, 1985; Iyer, 2000)
Arrhythmia (Mondillo, 1995; Palazzuoli, 1993)
Athletic performance (enhancement) (Giamberardino, 1996)
Attention-deficit hyperactivity disorder (ADHD) (Van Oudheusden, 2002)
Chronic obstructive pulmonary disease (COPD) (Borghi-Silva, 2006)
Congestive heart failure (CHF) (Ghidini, 1988)
Diabetes (Mingrone, 1999; Rahbar, 2005)
Dialysis (Rogerson, 1998; Thomas, 1999)
Diphtheria (Ramos, 1984; Ramos, 1992)
Erectile dysfunction (Cavallini, 2004; Gentile, 2004)
Exercise performance (Colombani, 1996; Dal Negro, 1986)
Fatigue (Lebrun, 2006)
Hepatic encephalopathy (Malaguarnera, 2003; Malaguarnera, 2005)
HIV/AIDS (De Simone, 1993; Moretti, 1998)
Huntington's disease (Goety, 1990)
Hypercholesterolemia (Abdel-Azid, 1984)
Hyperlipoproteinemia (Sirtori, 2000)
Hyperthyroidism (Benvenga, 2001)
Male infertility (Costa, 1994)
Myocardial infarction (Iliceto, 1995; Singh, 1996)
Neonatal growth and breathing (Crill, 2006)
Obesity (Villani, 2000)

Peripheral vascular disease (Brevetti, 1988; Brevetti, 1989)
Postexercise metabolic stress and muscle damage (Spiering, 2007)
Quality of life (maintenance hemodialysis patients) (Rathod, 2006)
Renal failure/dialysis (Ahmad, 1990; Gunal, 1999)
Respiratory distress (Dal Negro, 1988)
Sperm motility (Li, 2005; Sigman, 2006)
Surgical uses (Bohles, 1986)
Weight loss (pharmacologic activity)
Contradictory study (Elmslie, 2006)

Local Anesthetic/Vasoconstrictor Precautions No information available to require special precautions

Effects on Bleeding None reported

Warnings/Precautions No significant toxicity has been reported. Occasionally, gastrointestinal complaints are noted. L-Carnitine is often used as a supplement with breast milk or infant formula for low birth weight infants (either preterm or full-term). Avoid D-carnitine, which may be employed in some preparations of carnitine, since this may cause a deficiency of L-carnitine. In addition, DL-carnitine has been associated with myasthenia-like adverse effects when administered intravenously to dialysis patients. Use with caution in individuals with chronic liver disease. Use with caution in patients with peripheral vascular disease. Use with caution in patients with hypertension.

References

Abdel-Azid MT, et al, "Effect of Carnitine on Blood Lipid Pattern in Diabetic Patients," *Nutr Rep Internat*, 1984, 29:1071-9.

Ahmad S, Robertson HT, Golper TA, et al, "Multicenter Trial of L-Carnitine in Maintenance Hemodialysis Patients. II. Clinical and Biochemical Effects," *Kidney Int*, 1990, 38(5):912-8.

Benvenga S, Ruggeri RM, Russo A, et al, "Usefulness of L-Carnitine, a Naturally Occurring Peripheral Antagonist of Thyroid Hormone Action, in Latrogenic Hyperthyroidism: A Randomized, Double-Blind, Placebo-Controlled Clinical Trial," *J Clin Endocrinol Metab*, 2001, 86(8):3579-94.

Bohles H, Noppeney T, Akcetin Z, et al, "The Effect of Preoperative L-Carnitine Supplementation on Myocardial Metabolism During Aorto-Coronary-Bypass Surgery," *Current Therapeutic Research*, 1986, 39(3):429-35.

Borghi-Silva A, Baldissera V, Sampaio LM, et al, "L-Carnitine as an Ergogenic Aid for Patients With Chronic Obstructive Pulmonary Disease Submitted to Whole-Body and Respiratory Muscle Training Programs," *Braz J Med Biol Res*, 2006, 39(4):465-74.

Brevetti G, Attisano T, Perna S, et al, "Effect of L-Carnitine on the Reactive Hyperemia in Patients Affected by Peripheral Vascular Disease: A Double-Blind, Crossover Study," *Angiology*, 1989, 40 (10):857-62.

Brevetti G, Chiariello M, Ferulano G, et al, "Increases in Walking Distance in Patients With Peripheral Vascular Disease Treated With L-Carnitine: A Double-Blind, Cross-Over Study," *Circulation*, 1988, 77 (4):767-73.

Cacciatore L, Cerio R, Ciarimboli M, et al, "The Therapeutic Effect of L-Carnitine in Patients With Exercise-Induced Stable Angina: A Controlled Study," *Drugs Exp Clin Res*, 1991, 17(4):225-35.

Cavallini G, Ferraretti AP, Gianaroli L, et al, "Cinnoxicam and L-Carnitine/Acetyl-L-Carnitine Treatment for Idiopathic and Varicocele-Associated Oligoasthenospermia," *J Androl*, 2004, 25(5):761-70.

Cherchi A, Lai C, Angelino F, et al, "Effects of L-Carnitine on Exercise Tolerance in Chronic Stable Angina: A Multicenter, Double-Blind, Randomized, Placebo Controlled Crossover Study," *Int J Clin Pharmacol Ther Toxicol*, 1985, 23(10):569-72.

Colombani P, Wenk C, Kunz I, et al, "Effects of L-Carnitine Supplementation on Physical Performance and Energy Metabolism of Endurance-Trained Athletes: A Double-Blind Crossover Field Study," *Eur J Appl Physiol Occup Physiol*, 1996, 73(5):434-9.

Costa M, Canale D, Filicori M, et al, "L-Carnitine in Idiopathic Asthenozoospermia: A Multicenter Study. Italian Study Group on Carnitine and Male Infertility," *Andrologia*, 1994, 26(3):155-9.

Crill CM, Storm MC, Christensen ML, et al, "Carnitine Supplementation in Premature Neonates: Effect on Plasma and Red Blood Cell Total Carnitine Concentrations, Nutrition Parameters and Morbidity," *Clin Nutr*, 2006, 25(6):886-96.

Dal Negro R, Pomari G, Zoccatelli O, et al, "Changes in Physical Performance of Untrained Volunteers; Effects of L-Carnitine," *Clinical Trials Journal*, 1986, 23(4):242-8.

Dal Negro R, Turco P, Pomari C, et al, "Effects of L-Carnitine on Physical Performance in Chronic Respiratory Insufficiency," *Int J Clin Pharmacol Ther Toxicol*, 1988, 26(5):269-72.

De Simone C, Tzantzoglou S, Famularo G, et al, "High Dose L-Carnitine Improves Immunologic and Metabolic Parameters in AIDS Patients," *Immunopharmacol Immunotoxicol*, 1993, 15(1):1-12.

Elmslie JL, Porter RJ, Joyce PR, et al, "Carnitine Does Not Improve Weight Loss Outcomes in Valproate-Treated Bipolar Patients Consuming an Energy-Restricted, Low-Fat Diet," *Bipolar Disord*, 2006, 8(5 Pt 1):503-7.

Gentile V, Vicini P, Prigiotti G, et al, "Preliminary Observations on the Use of Propionyl-L-Carnitine in Combination With Sildenafil in Patients With Erectile Dysfunction and Diabetes," *Curr Med Res Opin*, 2004, 20(9):1377-84.

Ghidini O, Azzurro M, Vita G, et al, "Evaluation of the Therapeutic Efficacy of L-Carnitine in Congestive Heart Failure," *Int J Clin Pharmacol Ther Toxicol*, 1988, 26(4):217-20.

Giamberardino MA, Dragani L, Valente R, et al, "Effects of Prolonged L-Carnitine Administration on Delayed Muscle Pain and CK Release After Eccentric Effort," *Int J Sports Med*, 1996, 17(5):320-4.

Goety CG, Tanner CM, Cohen JA, et al, "L-Acetyl-Carnitine in Huntington's Disease: Double-Blind Placebo Controlled Crossover Study of Drug Effects on Movement Disorder and Dementia," *Mov Disord*, 1990, 5(3):263-5.

Gunal AI, Celiker H, Donder E, et al, "The Effect of L-Carnitine on Insulin Resistance in Hemodialysed Patients With Chronic Renal Failure," *J Nephrol*, 1999, 12(1):38-40.

Iliceto S, Scrutinio D, Bruzzi P, et al, "Effects of L-Carnitine Administration on Left Ventricular Remodeling After Acute Anterior Myocardial Infarction: The L-Carnitine Ecocardiografia Digitalizzata Infarto Miocardico (CEDIM) Trial," *J Am Coll Cardiol*, 1995, 26(2):380-7.

Iyer RN, Khan AA, Gupta A, et al, "L-Carnitine Moderately Improves the Exercise Tolerance in Chronic Stable Angina," *J Assoc Physicians India*, 2000, 48(11):1050-2.

Lebrun C, Alchaar H, Candito M, et al, "Levocarnitine Administration in Multiple Sclerosis Patients With Immunosuppressive Therapy-Induced Fatigue," *Mult Scler*, 2006, 12(3):321-4.

Li Z, Chen GW, Shang XJ, et al, "A Controlled Randomized Trial of the Use of Combined L-Carnitine and Acetyl-L-Carnitine Treatment in Men With Oligoasthenozoospermia," *Zhonghua Nan Ke Xue*, 2005, 11 (10):761-4.

Malaguarnera M, Pistone G, Astuto M, et al, "L-Carnitine in the Treatment of Mild or Moderate Hepatic Encephalopathy," *Dig Dis*, 2003, 21(3):271-5.

Malaguarnera M, Pistone G, Elvira R, et al, "Effects of L-Carnitine in Patients With Hepatic Encephalopathy," *World J Gastroenterol*, 2005, 11(45):7197-202.

Mingrone G, Greco AV, Capristo E, et al, "L-Carnitine Improves Glucose Disposal in Type 2 Diabetic Patients," *J Am Coll Nutr*, 1999, 18(1):77-82.
Mondillo S, Faglia S, D'Aprile N, et al, "Therapy of Arrhythmia Induced by Myocardial Ischemia. Association of L-Carnitine, Propafenone and Mexiletine," *Clin Ter*, 1995, 146(12):769-74.
Moretti S, Alesse E, Di Marzio L, et al, "Effect of L-Carnitine on Human Immunodeficiency Virus-1 Infection-Associated Apoptosis: A Pilot Study," *Blood*, 1998, 91(10):3817-24.
Natural Standard Research Collaboration, Chief Editors: Ulbricht C, Basch E, *Natural Standard Herb and Supplement Reference - Evidence-Based Clinical Reviews*, USA: Elsevier/Mosby, 2005.
Palazzuoli V, Mondillo S, Faglia S, et al, "The Evaluation of the Antiarrhythmic Activity of L-Carnitine and Propafenone in Ischemic Cardiopathy," *Clin Ter*, 1993, 142(2):155-9.
Rahbar AR, Shakerhosseini R, Saadat N, et al, "Effect of L-Carnitine on Plasma Glycemic and Lipidemic Profile in Patients With Type II Diabetes Mellitus," *Eur J Clin Nutr*, 2005, 59(4):592-6.
Ramos AC, Barrucand L, Elias PR, et al, "Carnitine Supplementation in Diphtheria," *Indian Pediatr*, 1992, 29(12):1501-5.
Ramos AC, Elias PR, Barrucand L, et al, "The Protective Effect of Carnitine in Human Diphtheric Myocarditis," *Pediatr Res*, 1984, 18(9):815-9.
Rathod R, Baig MS, Khandelwal PN, et al, "Results of a Single Blind, Randomized, Placebo-Controlled Clinical Trial to Study the Effect of Intravenous L-Carnitine Supplementation on Health-Related Quality of Life in Indian Patients on Maintenance Hemodialysis," *Indian J Med Sci*, 2006, 60(4):143-53.
Rogerson ME, Rylance PB, Wilson R, et al, "Carnitine and Weakness in Haemodialysis Patients," *Nephrol Dial Transplant*, 1989, 4(5):366-71.
Sigman M, Glass S, Campagnone J, et al, "Carnitine for the Treatment of Idiopathic Asthenospermia: A Randomized, Double-Blind, Placebo-Controlled Trial," *Fertil Steril*, 2006, 85(5):1409-14.
Singh RB, Niaz MA, Agarwal P, et al, "A Randomised, Double-Blind, Placebo-Controlled Trial of L-Carnitine in Suspected Acute Myocardial Infarction," *Postgrad Med J*, 1996, 72(843):45-50.
Sirtori CR, Calabresi L, Ferrara S, et al, "L-Carnitine Reduces Plasma Lipoprotein(a) Levels in Patients With Hyper Lp(a)," *Nutr Metab Cardiovasc Dis*, 2000, 10(5):247-51.
Spiering BA, Kraemer WJ, Vingren JL, et al, "Responses of Criterion Variables to Different Supplemental Doses of L-Carnitine L-Tartrate," *J Strength Cond Res*, 2007, 21(1):259-64.
Tarantini G, Scrutinio D, Bruzzi P, et al, "Metabolic Treatment With L-Carnitine in Acute Anterior ST Segment Elevation Myocardial Infarction. A Randomized Controlled Trial," *Cardiology*, 2006, 106 (4):215-23.
Thomas S, Fischer FP, Mettang T, et al, "Effects of L-Carnitine on Leukocyte Function and Viability in Hemodialysis Patients: A Double-Blind Randomized Trial," *Am J Kidney Dis*, 1999, 34(4):678-87.
Van Oudheusden LJ and Scholte HR, "Efficacy of Carnitine in the Treatment of Children With Attention-Deficit Hyperactivity Disorder," *Prostaglandins Leukot Essent Fatty Acids*, 2002, 67(1):33-8.
Villani RG, Gannon J, Self M, et al, "L-Carnitine Supplementation Combined With Aerobic Training Does Not Promote Weight Loss in Moderately Obese Women," *Int J Sport Nutr Exerc Metab*, 2000, 10 (2):199-207.

Cascara

Pharmacologic Category Laxative

Reported Use

Laxative (Petticrew, 1997)

Local Anesthetic/Vasoconstrictor Precautions No information available to require special precautions

Effects on Bleeding None reported

Warnings/Precautions Avoid use in children <12 years of age. Contraindicated in bowel obstruction, diarrhea, or dehydration. Use with caution in bowel disorders, inflammatory bowel disease (ulcerative colitis, Crohn's disease), and appendicitis. The pharmacologic activity of this agent suggests it may decrease absorption of certain oral medications by decreasing bowel transit time; excessive use may lead to potassium loss and other electrolyte disturbances. Use with caution in cardiovascular disease; overuse may cause electrolyte disorders. Use caution with digitalis glycosides, corticosteroids, or diuretics due to increased risk of hypokalemia. Cascara may potentiate anticoagulant therapy by reducing absorption or vitamin K from the gut. Use with caution in patients taking vitamin K. Cascara induces increased speed of intestinal emptying, which may result in decreased absorption of vitamin K. May potentiate the effects of various pharmaceutical drugs with narrow therapeutic windows (Bradley, 1992).

References

Bradley PR, ed, *British Herbal Compendium*, Vol 1, Bournemouth, England: British Herbal Medicine Association, 1992, 52-4.
Natural Standard Research Collaboration, Chief Editors: Ulbricht C, Basch E, *Natural Standard Herb and Supplement Reference - Evidence-Based Clinical Reviews*, USA: Elsevier/Mosby, 2005.
Petticrew M, Watt I, and Sheldon T, "Systematic Review of the Effectiveness of Laxatives in the Elderly," *Health Technol Assess*, 1997, 1(13):i-iv,1-52.

Cat's Claw

Pharmacologic Category Herb

Reported Use

Allergies (Immodal Pharmaka GmbH, 1996)
Anti-inflammatory (Aquino, 1991)
Antimicrobial (antibacterial, antifungal, antiviral) (Aquino, 1989; Senatore, 1989)
Antioxidant (Aquino, 1990)
Arthritis (Mur, 2002; Piscoya, 2001)
Cancer (Leon, 1996)
Cervical dysplasia (pharmacologic activity)
Crohn's disease (pharmacologic activity)
Diverticulitis (pharmacologic activity)
Endometriosis (pharmacologic activity)
Fibromyalgia (pharmacologic activity)

Immune support (Wagner, 1985)
Multiple sclerosis (pharmacologic activity)
Rosacea (pharmacologic activity)
Systemic lupus erythematosus (SLE) (pharmacologic activity)

Local Anesthetic/Vasoconstrictor Precautions No information available to require special precautions

Effects on Bleeding May cause increased bleeding due to inhibition of platelet aggregation

Warnings/Precautions Do not use during pregnancy. Use with caution in transplant recipients or others taking therapeutic immunosuppression or I.V. immunoglobulin therapy (Aquino, 1990).

Pharmacologic activity includes potential antiplatelet effects (Haginiwa, 1973). Based on pharmacologic activity, this herb may be contraindicated in individuals with active bleeding (eg, peptic ulcer, intracranial bleeding). Use with caution in individuals with a history of bleeding, hemostatic disorders, or drug-related hemostatic problems. Use with caution in individuals taking anticoagulant medications, including warfarin, aspirin, aspirin-containing products, NSAIDs, or antiplatelet agents (eg, ticlopidine, clopidogrel, dipyridamole). Discontinue use prior to dental or surgical procedures (generally at least 14 days before). Use with caution in individuals taking antiarrhythmic agents. Use with caution in individuals taking antihypertensives, diuretics, immunomodulators, corticosteroids, antilipemics, or cytochrome P450 metabolized agents.

References

Aquino R, De Feo V, De Simone F, et al, "Plant Metabolites. New Compounds and Anti-Inflammatory Activity of *Uncaria tomentosa*," *J Nat Prod*, 1991, 54(2):453-9.

Aquino R, De Simone F, Pizza C, et al, "Plant Metabolites. Structure and *In Vitro* Antiviral Activity of Quinovic Acid Glycosides From *Uncaria tomentosa* and *Guettarda platypoda*," *J Nat Prod*, 1989, 52 (4):679-85.

Aquino R, De Simone F, Vincieri FF, et al, "New Polyhydroxylated Triterpenes From *Uncaria tomentosa*," *J Nat Prod*, 1990, 53(3):559-64.

Haginiwa J, Sakai S, Aimi N, et al, "Studies of Plants Containing Indole Alkaloids. 2. On the Alkaloids of *Uncaria rhynchophylla* Miq," *Yakugaku Zasshi*, 1973, 93(4):448-52.

Immodal Pharmaka GmbH, Krallendorn®, *Uncaria tomentosa* (Willd.) DC mod. pent, "Root Exract: Report on Experiences With Probands," *Volders/Tirol*, 1996, Austria:20.

Leon FR, Ortiz N, Antunez de Mayolo A, et al, "Antimutagenic Activity of a Freeze-Dried Aquous Extract of *Unceria tomentosa* in Smokers and Non-Smokers," 3rd European Colloquium on Ethnopharmacology/1st International Conference of Anthropology and History and Disease Societe Europeenne d'Ethnopharmacologie Strasbourg (France)/Dipartimento di Scienze Antropologiche Universita di Genova (Italia), 1996, 255.

Mur E, Hartig F, Eibl G, et al, "Randomized Double Blind Trial of an Extract From the Pentacyclic Alkaloid-chemotype of *Uncaria tomentosa* for the Treatment of Rheumatoid Arthritis," *J Rheumatol*, 2002, 29 (4):678-81.

Natural Standard Research Collaboration, Chief Editors: Ulbricht C, Basch E, *Natural Standard Herb and Supplement Reference - Evidence-Based Clinical Reviews*, USA: Elsevier/Mosby, 2005.

Piscoya J, Rodriguez Z, Bustamante SA, et al, "Efficacy and Safety of Freeze-Dried Cat's Claw in Osteoarthritis of the Knee: Mechanisms of Action of the Species *Uncaria guianensis*," *Inflamm Res*, 2001, 50(9):442-8.

Senatore A, Cataldo A, Iaccarino FP, et al, "Phytochemical and Biological Study of *Uncaria tomentosa*," *Boll Soc Ital Biol Sper*, 1989, 65(6):517-20.

Wagner H, Kreutzkamp B, and Jurcic K, "The Alkaloids of *Uncaria tomentosa* and Their Phagocytosis-Stimulating Action," *Planta Med*, 1985, (5):419-23.

Cayenne

Related Information

Capsaicin *on page 296*

Pharmacologic Category Herb

Reported Use

Anti-inflammatory and analgesic (topical) (Magnusson, 1996; Nagy, 1982; Rains, 1995; Tandan, 1992)
Cardiovascular circulatory support (Newall, 1996)
Cluster headache (Fusco, 1994; Marks 1993)
Concentration/stimulant (Meyer-Bahlburg, 1972)
Digestive stimulant (Newall, 1996)
Duodenal ulcer (Kumar, 1984)
Dyspepsia (Bortolotti, 2002)
Fibromyalgia (McCarty, 1994)
H. pylori (Graham, 1999)
Low back pain (Frerick, 2003; Gagnier, 2006; Gagnier 2007; Keitel, 2001; Stam, 2001)
Nausea/vomiting (postoperative) (Kim, 2001; Misra, 2005)
Pain (postoperative) (Kim, 2006; Kim, 2006; Kim, 2009)
Postherpetic neuralgia (Bernstein, 1989)
Pruritus (Cho, 1997; Tarng, 1996)
Rhinitis (Blom, 1997; Gerth Van Wijk, 2000)

Local Anesthetic/Vasoconstrictor Precautions No information available to require special precautions

Effects on Bleeding None reported

Warnings/Precautions Use with caution in individuals with GI ulceration (based on case reports). Due to pharmacologic activity, may interfere with MAO inhibitors and antihypertensive therapies due to increased catecholamine secretion (Newall, 1996).

References

Bernstein JE, Korman NJ, Bickers DR, et al, "Topical Capsaicin Treatment of Chronic Postherpetic Neuralgia," *J Am Acad Dermatol*, 1989, 21(2 Pt 1):265-70.
Blom HM, Van Rijswijk JB, Garrelds IM, et al, "Intranasal Capsaicin Is Efficacious in Non-Allergic, Non-Infectious Perennial Rhinitis. A Placebo-Controlled Study," *Clin Exp Allergy*, 1997, 27(7):796-801.
Bortolotti M, Coccia G, Grossi G, et al, "The Treatment of Functional Dyspepsia With Red Pepper," *Aliment Pharmacol Ther*, 2002, 16(6):1075-82.
Cho YL, Liu HN, Huang TP, et al, "Uremic Pruritus: Roles of Parathyroid Hormone and Substance P," *J Am Acad Dermatol*, 1997, 36(4):538-43
Frerick H, Keitel W, Kuhn U, et al, "Topical Treatment of Chronic Low Back Pain With a Capsicum Plaster," *Pain*, 2003, 106(1-2):59-64.
Fusco BM, Marabini S, Maggi CA, et al, "Preventative Effect of Repeated Nasal Applications of Capsaicin in Cluster Headache," *Pain*, 1994, 59(3):321-5.
Gagnier JJ, van Tulder MW, Berman B, et al, "Herbal Medicine for Low Back Pain: A Cochrane Review," *Spine* (Phila Pa 1976), 2007, 32(1):82-92.
Gagnier JJ, van Tulder M, Berman B, et al, "Herbal Medicine for Low Back Pain," *Cochrane Database Syst Rev*, 2006, (2):CD004504.
Gerth Van Wijk R, Terreehorst IT, Mulder PG, et al, "Intranasal Capsaicin Is Lacking Therapeutic Effect in Perennial Allergic Rhinitis to House Dust Mite. A Placebo-Controlled Study," *Clin Exp Allergy*, 2000, 30 (12):1792-8.
Graham DY, Anderson SY, and Lang T, "Garlic or Jalapeno Peppers for Treatment of *Helicobacter Pylori* Infection," *Am J Gastroenterol*, 1999, 94(5):1200-2.
Keitel W, Frerick H, Kuhn U, et al, "Capsicum Pain Plaster in Chronic Non-Specific Low Back Pain," *Arzneimittelforschung*, 2001, 51(11):896-903.
Kim KS, Kim KN, Hwang KG, et al, "Capsicum Plaster at the Hegu Point Reduces Postoperative Analgesic Requirement After Orthognathic Surgery," *Anesth Analg*, 2009, 108(3):992-6.
Kim KS, Kim DW, and Yu YK, "The Effect of Capsicum Plaster in Pain After Inguinal Hernia Repair in Children," *Paediatr Anaesth*, 2006, 16(10):1036-41.
Kim KS and Nam YM, "The Analgesic Effects of Capsicum Plaster at the Zusanli Point After Abdominal Hysterectomy," *Anesth Analg*, 2006, 103(3):709-13.
Kim KS, Koo MS, Jeon JW, et al, "Capsicum Plaster at the Korean Hand Acupuncture Point Reduces Postoperative Nausea and Vomiting After Abdominal Hysterectomy," *Anesth Analg*, 2002, 95(4):1103-7, table of contents.
Kumar N, Vij JC, Sarin SK, et al, "Do Chillies Influence Healing of Duodenal Ulcer?" *Br Med J (Clin Res Ed)*, 1984, 288(6433):1803-4.
Magnusson BM and Kaskinen LD, "Effects of Topical Application of Capsaicin to Human Skin: A Comparison of Effects Evaluated by Visual Assessment, Sensation Registration, Skin Blood Flow and Cutaneous Impedance Measurements," *Acta Derm Venereol*, 1996, 76(2):129-32.
Marks DR, Rapoport A, Padla D, et al, "A Double-Blind Placebo-Controlled Trial of Intranasal Capsaicin for Cluster Headache," *Cephalalgia*, 1993, 13(2):114-6.
McCarty DJ, Csuka M, McCarthy G, et al, "Treatment of Pain Due to Fibromyalgia With Topical Capsaicin: A Pilot Study," *Semin Arthr Rheum*, 1994, 23:41-7.
Meyer-Bahlburg HF, "Pilot Studies on Stimulant Effects of Capsicum Spices," *Nutr Metab*, 1972, 14 (4):245-54.
Misra MN, Pullani AJ, and Mohamed ZU, "Prevention of PONV by Acustimulation With Capsicum Plaster Is Comparable to Ondansetron After Middle Ear Surgery," *Can J Anaesth*, 2005, 52(5):485-9.
Nagy, JI, et al, "Fluoride-Resistant Acid Phosphatase-Containing Neurones in Dorsal Root Ganglia are Separate from Those Containing Substance P or Somatostatin," *Neuroscience*, 1982, 7(1):89-97.
Natural Standard Research Collaboration, Chief Editors: Ulbricht C, Basch E, *Natural Standard Herb and Supplement Reference - Evidence-Based Clinical Reviews*, USA: Elsevier/Mosby, 2005.
Newall CA, Anderson LA, and Phillipson JD, *Herbal Medicines: A Guide for Health Care Professionals*, London, England: The Pharmaceutical Press, 1996, 60-61.
Rains C and Bryson HM, "Topical Capsaicin. A Review of Its Pharmacological Properties and Therapeutic Potential in Post-Herpetic Neuralgia, Diabetic Neuropathy and Osteoarthritis," *Drugs Aging*, 1995, 7 (4):317-28.
Stam C, Bonnet MS, and van Haselen RA, "The Efficacy and Safety of a Homeopathic Gel in the Treatment of Acute Low Back Pain: A Multi-Centre, Randomised, Double-Blind Comparative Clinical Trial," *Br Homeopath J*, 2001, 90(1):21-8.
Tandan R, Lewis GA, Krusinski PB, et al, "Topical Capsaicin in Painful Diabetic Neuropathy. Controlled Study With Long-Term Follow-up," *Diabetes Care*, 1992, 15(1):8-14.
Tarng DC, Cho YL, Liu HN, et al, "Hemodialysis-Related Pruritus: A Double-Blind, Placebo-Controlled, Crossover Study of Capsaicin 0.025% Cream," *Nephron*, 1996, 72(4):617-22.

Chamomile

Pharmacologic Category Herb

Reported Use

Acute radiation skin reaction (Maiche,1991)
Cardiovascular conditions (Gould, 1973)
Carminative, antispasmotic; insomnia (mild sedative); anxiolytic (Newall, 1996)
Colic (pharmacologic activity)
Common cold (Saller, 1990)
Diaper rash (pharmacologic activity)
Diarrhea (children); diarrhea (children, combination product) (Becker, 2006)
Eczema (Patzelt-Wenczler, 2000)
Hemorrhagic cystitis (Barsom, 1993)
Hemorrhoids (Förster, 1996)
Indigestion (pharmacologic activity)
Minor injury (topical anti-inflammatory) (Bradley, 1992)
Mucositis (from chemotherapy) (Carl, 1991)
Nausea/vomiting (pharmacologic activity)
Oral health (as mouth rinse/gargle) (Bradley, 1992)

Stress/anxiety (pharmacologic activity)
Teething (pharmacologic activity)
Uterine tonic (Shipochiliev, 1981)
Vaginitis (Benetti, 1985)

Local Anesthetic/Vasoconstrictor Precautions No information available to require special precautions

Effects on Bleeding None reported

Warnings/Precautions Avoid use in individuals with allergies to members of the *Asteraceae/Compositae* family (chrysanthemum, daisy) or ragweed pollens (Subiza, 1989). Do not use in pregnancy and lactation (Bradley, 1992). Based on pharmacologic activity, may cause drowsiness in some individuals. Caution individuals to avoid hazardous tasks (eg, driving or operating machinery). Caution individuals taking sedative medications (eg, anxiolytics, benzodiazepines). Based on pharmacologic activity, this herb should be avoided in individuals with active bleeding (eg, peptic ulcer, intracranial bleeding). Use with caution in individuals with a history of bleeding, hemostatic disorders, or drug-related hemostatic problems. Use caution in individuals taking anticoagulant medications, including warfarin, aspirin or aspirin-containing products, NSAIDs, or antiplatelet agents (eg, ticlopidine, clopidogrel, dipyridamole). Discontinue use prior to dental or surgical procedures (generally at least 14 days before). Use with caution in individuals using cytochrome P450 metabolized agents.

References

Barsom VS, Moosmayr A, and Sakka M, "Behandlung der Hamorrhagischen Systitis (Harnblasens-chleimhautblutungen) Mit Kamillenextrakt," *Erfahrungsheilkunde*, 1993, 3:138-9.
Becker B, Kuhn U, and Hardewig-Budny B, "Double-Blind, Randomized Evaluation of Clinical Efficacy and Tolerability of an Apple Pectin-Chamomile Extract in Children With Unspecific Diarrhea," *Arzneimittelforschung*, 2006, 56(6):387-93.
Benetti C and Manganelli F, "Clinical Experiences in the Pharmacological Treatment of Vaginitis With a Camomile-Extract Vaginal Douche," *Minerva Ginecol*, 1985, 37(12):799-801.
Bradley PR, ed, *British Herbal Compendium*, Vol 1, Bournemouth, England: British Herbal Medicine Association, 1992, 154-7.
Carl W and Emrich LS, "Management of Oral Mucositis During Local Radiation and Systemic Chemotherapy: A Study of 98 Patients," *J Prosthet Dent*, 1991, 66(3):361-9.
Förster CF, Süssmann HE, and Patzelt-Wenczler R, "Optimization of the Barron Ligature Treatment of 2nd and 3rd-Degree Hemorrhoids Using a Therapeutic Troika," *Praxis*, 1996, 85(46):1476-81.
Gould L, Reddy CV, and Gomprecht RF, "Cardiac Effects of Chamomile Tea," *J Clin Pharmacol*, 1973, 13 (11):475-9.
Maiche AG, Gröhn P, and Mäki-Hokkonen H, "Effect of Chamomile Cream and Almond Ointment on Acute Radiation Skin Reaction," *Acta Oncol*, 1991, 30(3):395-6.
Natural Standard Research Collaboration, Chief Editors: Ulbricht C, Basch E, *Natural Standard Herb and Supplement Reference - Evidence-Based Clinical Reviews*, USA: Elsevier/Mosby, 2005.
Newall CA, Anderson LA, and Phillipson JD, *Herbal Medicines: A Guide for Health Care Professionals*, London, England: The Pharmaceutical Press, 1996, 69-71.
Patzelt-Wenczler R and Ponce-Pöschl E, "Proof of Efficacy of Kamillosan® Cream in Atopic Eczema," *Eur J Med Res*, 2000, 5(4):171-5.
Saller R, Beschomer M, Hellenbrecht D, et al, "Dose Dependency of Symptomatic Relief of Complaints by Chamomile Steam Inhalation in Patients With Common Cold," *Eur J Pharmacol*, 1990, 183:728-9.
Shipochiliev T, "Extracts From a Group of Medicinal Plants Enhancing Uterine Tonus," *Vet Med Nauk*, 1981, 18:94-8.
Subiza J, Subiza JL, Hinojosa M, et al, "Anaphylactic Reaction After Ingestion of Chamomile Tea: A Study of Cross-Reactivity With Other Composite Pollens," *Clin Immunol*, 1989, 84(3):353-8.

Chasteberry

Pharmacologic Category Herb

Reported Use

Acne vulgaris (Amann, 1975)
Cervical dysplasia (pharmacologic activity)
Corpus luteum insufficiency; hyperprolactinemia and insufficient lactation (Milewicz, 1993; Sliutz, 1993)
Cyclic mastalgia (Halaska, 1998; Kubista, 1987; Wuttke, 1997)
Menopause (Newall, 1996)
Menorrhagia (pharmacologic activity)
Menstrual disorders (including amenorrhea, endometriosis, premenstrual syndrome [PMS]) (Amann, 1979; Lauritzen, 1997; Schellenberg, 2001; Turner, 1993)
Rosacea (pharmacologic activity)

Local Anesthetic/Vasoconstrictor Precautions No information available to require special precautions

Effects on Bleeding None reported

Warnings/Precautions Contraindicated in pregnancy and lactation, based on case reports of uterine stimulation and emmenagogue effects (Newall, 1996). Based on pharmacologic activity, may interact with medications that increase dopaminergic activity (bromocriptine, levodopa) or alter the effects of dopamine antagonists (metoclopramide, antipsychotic agents). Use with caution in individuals receiving hormonal therapy. Use with caution in individuals taking oral contraceptives or hormone replacement therapy.

References

Amann W, "Acne Vulgaris and *Agnus castus*," *Z Allgemeinmed*, 1975, 51(35):1645-8.
Amann W, "Premenstrual Water Retention. Favorable Effect of *Agnus castus* (Agnolyt) on Premenstrual Water Retention," *ZFA (Stuttgart)*, 1979, 55(1):48-51.

Halaska M, Raus K, Beles P, et al, "Treatment of Cyclical Mastodynia Using an Extract of *Vitex agnus castus*: Results of a Double-Blind Comparison With a Placebo," *Ceska Gynekol*, 1998, 63(5):388-92.
Kubista E, Muller G, and Spona J, "Treatment of Mastopathies With Cyclic Mastodynia. Clinical Results and Hormonal Profiles," *Rev Fr Gynecol Obstet*, 1987, 82(4):221-7.
Lauritzen CH, Reuter HD, Repges, et al, "Treatment of Premenstrual Tension Syndrome With *Vitex agnus castus*," *Phytomedicine*, 1997, 4:183-9.
Milewicz A, Gejdel E, Sworen H, et al, "*Vitex agnus castus* Extract in the Treatment of Luteal Phase Defects Due to Latent Hyperprolactinemia. Results of a Randomized Placebo-Controlled Double-Blind Study," *Arzneimittelforschung*, 1993, 43(7):752-6.
Natural Standard Research Collaboration, Chief Editors: Ulbricht C, Basch E, *Natural Standard Herb and Supplement Reference - Evidence-Based Clinical Reviews*, USA: Elsevier/Mosby, 2005.
Newall CA, Anderson LA, and Phillipson JD, *Herbal Medicines: A Guide for Health Care Professionals*, London, England: The Pharmaceutical Press, 1996, 19-20.
Schellenberg R, "Treatment for the Premenstrual Syndrome With *Agnus castus* Fruit Extract: Prospective, Randomised, Placebo Controlled Study," *BMJ*, 2001, 322(7279):134-7.
Sliutz G, Speiser P, Schultz AM, et al, "*Agnus castus* Extracts Inhibit Prolactin Secretion of Rat Pituitary Cells," *Horm Metab Res*, 1993, 25(5):253-5.
Snow JM, "*Vitex agnus-castus* L (Verbenaceae)," *Protocol J Botanical Med*, 1996, 1(4):20-3.
Turner S and Mills S, "A Double Blind Clinical Trial on a Herbal Remedy for Premenstrual Syndrome: A Case Study," *Complement Ther Med*, 1993, 1:73-7.
Umland EM, Cauffield JS, Kirk JK, et al, "Phytoestrogens as Therapeutic Alternatives to Traditional Hormone Replacement in Postmenopausal Women," *Pharmacotherapy*, 2000, 20(8):981-90.
Wuttke W, Splitt G, Gorkow C, et al, "Behandlung Zyklusabhangiger Brustschmerzen Mit Einem Agnus Castus-Haltigen Arzneimittel," *Geburtsh u Frauenheilk*, 1997, 57:569-74.

Chondroitin Sulfate

Pharmacologic Category Nutraceutical

Reported Use

Coronary artery disease (Morrison, 1973; Nakazawa, 1969; Nakazawa, 1970; Nakazawa, 1979)
Interstitial cystitis (Erickson, 1997; Steinhoff, 2002)
Iron absorption enhancement (Balbi, 1979)
Muscle soreness, delayed onset (contradictory study) (Braun, 2005)
Ophthalmologic uses (Burke, 1990; Embriano, 1989; Lane, 1991)
Osteoarthritis (Clegg, 2006; Das, 2000; Leeb, 2000; Mazières, 2007; McAlindon, 2000; Reginster, 2003; Reichenbach, 2007; Richy, 2003; Towheed, 2000; Uebelhart, 1998)
Overactive bladder (Gauruder-Burmester, 2006)
Psoriasis (Verges, 2004; Verges, 2005)

Local Anesthetic/Vasoconstrictor Precautions No information available to require special precautions

Effects on Bleeding None reported

Warnings/Precautions Use with caution in individuals with a history of bleeding, hemostatic disorders, or drug-related hemostatic problems. Use with caution in individuals taking anticoagulant medications, including warfarin, aspirin, aspirin-containing products, NSAIDs, or antiplatelet agents (eg, ticlopidine, clopidogrel, dipyridamole). Discontinue use prior to dental or surgical procedures (generally at least 14 days before).

References

Balbi C, D'Ajello M, and Nappa L, "Clinical Study of a Drug Containing the Chondroitin-Sulfonic Ferric Acid Complex in Iron-Deficiency Anemias in the Puerperium," *Minerva Ginecol*, 1979, 31(11):821-4.
Braun WA, Flynn MG, Armstrong WJ, et al, "The Effects of Chondroitin Sulfate Supplementation on Indices of Muscle Damage Induced by Eccentric Arm Exercise," *J Sports Med Phys Fitness*, 2005, 45 (4):553-60.
Burke S, Sugar J, and Farber MD, "Comparison of the Effects of Two Viscoelastic Agents, Healon and Viscoat, on Postoperative Intraocular Pressure After Penetrating Keratoplasty," *Ophthalmic Surg*, 1990, 21(12):821-6.
Clegg DO, Reda DJ, Harris CL, et al, "Glucosamine, Chondroitin Sulfate, and the Two in Combination for Painful Knee Osteoarthritis," *N Engl J Med*, 2006, 354(8):795-808.
Das A Jr and Hammad TA, "Efficacy of a Combination of FCHG49 Glucosamine Hydrochloride, TRH122 Low Molecular Weight Sodium Chondroitin Sulfate and Manganese Ascorbate in the Management of Knee Osteoarthritis," *Osteoarthritis Cartilage*, 2000, 8(5):343-50.
Embriano PJ, "Postoperative Pressures After Phacoemulsification: Sodium Hyaluronate vs Sodium Chondroitin Sulfate-Sodium Hyaluronate," *Ann Ophthalmol*, 1989, 21(3):85-8, 90.
Erickson DR, Ordille S, Martin A, et al, "Urinary Chondroitin Sulfates, Heparan Sulfate and Total Sulfated Glycosaminoglycans in Interstitial Cystitis," *J Urol*, 1997, 157(1):61-4.
Gauruder-Burmester A, Wildt B, and Tunn R, "Treatment of Overactive Bladder With Sodium Chondroitin Sulphate," *Zentralbl Gynakol*, 2006, 128(6):336-40.
Lane SS, Naylor DW, Kullerstrand LJ, et al, "Prospective Comparison of the Effects of Occucoat, Viscoat, and Healon on Intraocular Pressure and Endothelial Cell Loss," *J Cataract Refract Surg*, 1991, 17 (1):21-6.
Leeb BF, Schweitzer H, Montag K, et al, "A Metaanalysis of Chondroitin Sulfate in the Treatment of Osteoarthritis," *J Rheumatol*, 2000, 27(1):205-11.
Mazières B, Hucher M, Zaïm M, et al, "Effect of Chondroitin Sulphate in Symptomatic Knee Osteoarthritis: A Multicentre, Randomised, Double-Blind, Placebo-Controlled Study," *Ann Rheum Dis*, 2007, 66 (5):639-45.
McAlindon TE, LaValley MP, Gulin JP, et al, "Glucosamine and Chondroitin for Treatment of Osteoarthritis: A Systematic Quality Assessment and Meta-Analysis," *JAMA*, 2000, 283(11):1469-75.
Morrison LM and Enrick N, "Coronary Heart Disease: Reduction of Death Rate by Chondroitin Sulfate A," *Angiology*, 1973, 24(5):269-87.
Nakazawa K, "Effect of Chondroitin Sulfates on Atherosclerosis. I. Long Term Oral Administration of Chondroitin Sulfates to Atherosclerotic Subjects," *Nippon Naika Gakkai Zasshi*, 1970, 59(10):1084-92.
Nakazawa K and Murata K, "Comparative Study of the Effects of Chondroitin Sulfate Isomers on Atherosclerotic Subjects," *ZFA*, 1979, 34(2):153-9.
Nakazawa K, Murata K, Izuka K, et al, "The Short-Term Effects of Chondroitin Sulfates A and C on Coronary Atherosclerotic Subjects: With Reference to Its Anti-Thrombogenic Activities," *Jpn Heart J*, 1969, 10(4):289-96.
Natural Standard Research Collaboration, Chief Editors: Ulbricht C, Basch E, *Natural Standard Herb and Supplement Reference - Evidence-Based Clinical Reviews*, USA: Elsevier/Mosby, 2005.

Reginster JY, Bruyere O, Lecart MP, et al, "Naturocetic (Glucosamine and Chondroitin Sulfate) Compounds as Structure-Modifying Drugs in the Treatment of Osteoarthritis," *Curr Opin Rheumatol*, 2003, 15(5):651-5.
Reichenbach S, Sterchi R, Scherer M, et al, "Meta-Analysis: Chondroitin for Osteoarthritis of the Knee or Hip," *Ann Intern Med*, 2007, 146(8):580-90.
Richy F, Bruyere O, Ethgen O, et al, "Structural and Symptomatic Efficacy of Glucosamine and Chondroitin in Knee Osteoarthritis: A Comprehensive Meta-Analysis," *Arch Intern Med*, 2003, 163 (13):1514-22.
Steinhoff G, Ittah B, and Rowan S, "The Efficacy of Chondroitin Sulfate 0.2% in Treating Interstitial Cystitis," *Can J Urol*, 2002, 9(1):1454-8.
Towheed TE and Anastassiades TP, "Glucosamine and Chondroitin for Treating Symptoms of Osteoarthritis: Evidence Is Widely Touted but Incomplete," *JAMA*, 2000, 283(11):1483-4.
Uebelhart D, Thonar EJ, Delmas PD, et al, "Effects of Oral Chondroitin Sulfate on the Progression of Knee Osteoarthritis: A Pilot Study," *Osteoarthritis Cartilage*, 1998, 6(Suppl A):39-46.
Verges J, Montell E, Herrero M, et al, "Clinical and Histopathological Improvement of Psoriasis in Patients With Osteoarthritis Treated With Chondroitin Sulfate: Report of 3 Cases," *Med Clin (Barc)*, 2004, 123 (19):739-42.
Verges J, Montell E, Herrero M, et al, "Clinical and Histopathological Improvement of Psoriasis With Oral Chondroitin Sulfate: A Serendipitous Finding," *Dermatol Online J*, 2005, 11(1):31.

Chromium

Related Information

Trace Metals *on page* 1655

Pharmacologic Category Nutraceutical

Reported Use

Atherosclerosis (Newman, 1978)
Bipolar disorder (Amann, 2007)
Bone loss (postmenopausal women) (Evans, 1993)
Cardiovascular disease (risk reduction; in combination) (Albarracin, 2007)
Depression (Docherty, 2005)
Diabetes (Albarracin, 2007; Althuis, 2002, no effect; Anderson 1997; Morris, 2000; Singer, 2006)
Diabetes, type 1 (Fox, 1998)
Diabetes, type 2 (Anderson, 1987)
Glaucoma (Lane, 1991)
Hypercholesterolemia (Balk, 2007; Press, 1990; Roeback, 1991)
Hypertriglyceridemia (Anderson, 1986)
Hypothyroidism (pharmacologic activity)
Immunosuppression (Chang, 1996)
Insulin sensitivity (obese women with polycystic ovarian syndrome) (Lucidi, 2005; Lydic, 2006)
Premenstrual syndrome (PMS) (pharmacologic activity)
Weight loss (Anderson, 1998)

Local Anesthetic/Vasoconstrictor Precautions No information available to require special precautions

Effects on Bleeding None reported

Warnings/Precautions Use with caution in individuals receiving oral hypoglycemics or insulin. Blood glucose should be closely monitored, and the dosage of diabetic agents may need to be reduced. This should be carefully coordinated among the individual's healthcare providers. Excess intake can result in tissue accumulation and can inhibit rather than enhance insulin activity. Extreme excesses may be carcinogenic. Use with caution in patients with iron deficiency. Use with caution in patients with hepatic or renal impairment.

References

Albarracin C, Fuqua B, Geohas J, et al, "Combination of Chromium and Biotin Improves Coronary Risk Factors in Hypercholesterolemic Type 2 Diabetes Mellitus: A Placebo-Controlled, Double-Blind Randomized Clinical Trial," *J Cardiometab Syndr*, 2007, 2(2):91-7.
Althuis MD, Jordan NE, Ludington EA, et al, "Glucose and Insulin Responses to Dietary Chromium Supplements: A Meta-Analyis," *Am J Clin Nutr*, 2002, 76(1):148-55.
Amann BL, Mergl R, Vieta E, et al, "A 2-Year, Open-Label Pilot Study of Adjunctive Chromium in Patients With Treatment-Resistant Rapid-Cycling Bipolar Disorder, *J Clin Psychopharmacol*, 2007, 27(1):104-6.
Anderson RA, "Effects of Chromium on Body Composition and Weight Loss," *Nutr Rev*, 1998, 56 (9):266-70.
Anderson RA, "Trace Elements and Cardiovascular Diseases," *Acta Pharmacol Toxicol (Copenh)*, 1986, 59(Supp 7):317-24.
Anderson RA, Cheng N, Bryden NA, et al, "Elevated Intakes of Supplemental Chromium Improve Glucose and Insulin Variables in Individuals With Type 2 Diabetes," *Diabetes*, 1997, 46(11):1786-91.
Anderson RA, Polansky MM, Bryden NA, et al, "Effects of Supplemental Chromium on Patients With Symptoms of Reactive Hypoglycemia," *Metabolism*, 1987, 36(4):351-5.
Balk EM, Tatsioni A, Lichtenstein AH, et al, "Effect of Chromium Supplementation on Glucose Metabolism and Lipids: A Systematic Review of Randomized Controlled Trials," *Diabetes Care*, 2007, 30 (8):2154-63.
Chang GX, Mallard BA, Mowat DN, et al, "Effect of Supplemental Chromium on Antibody Responses of Newly Arrived Feeder Calves to Vaccines and Ovalbumin," *Can J Vet Res*, 1996, 60(2):140-4.
Docherty JP, Sack DA, Roffman M, et al, "A Double-Blind, Placebo-Controlled, Exploratory Trial of Chromium Picolinate in Atypical Depression: Effect on Carbohydrate Craving," *J Psychiatr Pract*, 2005, 11(5):302-14.
Evans GW and Pouchnik DJ, "Composition and Biological Activity of Chromium-Pyridine Carboxylate Complexes," *J Inorg Biochem*, 1993, 49(3):177-87.
Fox GN and Sabovic Z, "Chromium Picolinate Supplementation for Diabetes Mellitus," *J Fam Pract*, 1998, 46(1):83-6.
Lane BC, "Diet and the Glaucomas," *J Am Coll Nutr*, 1991, 10(5):536.
Lucidi RS, Thyer AC, Easton CA, et al, "Effect of Chromium Supplementation on Insulin Resistance and Ovarian and Menstrual Cyclicity in Women With Polycystic Ovary Syndrome," *Fertil Steril*, 2005, 84 (6):1755-7.

Lydic ML, McNurlan M, Bembo S, et al, "Chromium Picolinate Improves Insulin Sensitivity in Obese Subjects With Polycystic Ovary Syndrome," *Fertil Steril*, 2006, 86(1):243-6.
Morris BW, Kouta S, Robinson R, et al, "Chromium Supplementation Improves Insulin Resistance in Patients With Type 2 Diabetes Mellitus," *Diabet Med*, 2000, 17(9):684-5.
Natural Standard Research Collaboration, Chief Editors: Ulbricht C, Basch E, *Natural Standard Herb and Supplement Reference - Evidence-Based Clinical Reviews*, USA: Elsevier/Mosby, 2005.
Newman HA, Leighton RF, Lanese RR, et al, "Serum Chromium and Angiographically Determined Coronary Artery Disease," *Clin Chem*, 1978, 24(4):541-4.
Press RI, Geller J, and Evans GW, "The Effect of Chromium Picolinate on Serum Cholesterol and Apolipoprotein Fractions in Human Subjects," *West J Med*, 1990, 152(1):41-5.
Roeback JR Jr, Hla KM, Chambless LE, et al, "Effects of Chromium Supplementation on Serum High-Density Lipoprotein Cholesterol Levels in Men Taking Beta-Blockers. A Randomized, Controlled Trial," *Ann Intern Med*, 1991, 115(12):917-24.
Singer GM and Geohas J, "The Effect of Chromium Picolinate and Biotin Supplementation on Glycemic Control in Poorly Controlled Patients With Type 2 Diabetes Mellitus: A Placebo-Controlled, Double-Blinded, Randomized Trial," *Diabetes Technol Ther*, 2006, 8(6):636-43.

Coenzyme Q_{10}

Pharmacologic Category Nutraceutical

Reported Use

Acute myocardial infarction (Singh, 1998; Singh 2003)
AIDS (Folkers, 1988; Folkers 1991)
Alzheimer's disease (Gutzmann, 1998; Mazzola, 1987)
Amyotrophic lateral sclerosis (ALS) (Levy, 2006)
Angina (Kamikawa, 1985)
Antioxidant (Niklowitz, 2007)
Asthenozoospermia (idiopathic) (Balercia, 2000)
Cancer (preventive) (Portakal, 2000)
Cardiomyopathy (Langsjoen, 1985; Langsjoen, 1990; Langsjoen, 1994; Pogessi, 1991)
Cardioprotection during surgery (Chello, 1994; Chello, 1996; Taggart, 1996)
Chemotherapy (adjunct) (Kokawa, 1983)
Chronic fatigue syndrome (Langsjoen, 1993)
Congestive heart failure (CHF) (Belardinelli, 2006; Pogessi, 1991; Rosenfeldt, 2003; Sinatra, 1997; Tran, 2001)
Down syndrome (Miles, 2006)
Exercise performance (Fujimoto, 1993; Ylikoski, 1997)
Fibromyalgia (pharmacologic activity)
Friedreich's ataxia (Hart, 2005; Lodi, 2001; Musumeci, 2001)
Gingivitis (pharmacologic activity)
Hypercholesterolemia (pharmacologic activity)
Hypertension (Langsjoen, 1994; Okamoto, 1991; Rosenfeldt, 2003; Rosenfeldt, 2007; Singh, 1999)
Migraine (Sandor, 2005); pediatric migraine (Hershey, 2007)
Mitochondrial disease and Kearns-Sayre syndrome (Chen, 1997)
Multiple sclerosis (pharmacologic activity)
Muscle pain (associated with HMG-CoA reductase inhibitors) (Caso, 2007)
Muscular dystrophy (Folkers, 1995)
Myelodysplastic syndromes (Galili, 2007)
Parkinson's disease (The NINDS NET-PD Investigators, 2007; Shults, 2002; Storch, 2007)
Periodontal disease (Hansen, 1976)
Renal failure (Singh, 2000)
Tinnitus (Khan, 2007)
Weight loss (van Gaal, 1984)

Local Anesthetic/Vasoconstrictor Precautions No information available to require special precautions

Effects on Bleeding May increase the risk of bleeding

Warnings/Precautions May increase bleeding risk. May decrease response to warfarin (Combs, 1976; Landbo, 1998; Spigset, 1994). Use with caution with antidiabetic, psychiatric, and cardiovascular drugs, herbs, and supplements. Potential adverse effects include abdominal discomfort, headache, nausea, and vomiting (Singh, 1999). Concurrent use with doxorubicin (Adriamycin®) is contraindicated (Shinozawa, 1991).

References

Balercia G, Arnaldi G, Lucarelli G, et al, "Effects of Exogenous CoQ_{10} Administration in Patients With Idiopathic Asthenozoospermia," *International Journal of Andrology*, 2000, Suppl 23-43.
Belardinelli R, Muçaj A, Lacalaprice F, et al, "Coenzyme Q_{10} and Exercise Training in Chronic Heart Failure," *Eur Heart J*, 2006, 27(22):2675-81.
Berthold HK, Naini A, Di Mauro S, et al, "Effect of Ezetimibe and/or Simvastatin on Coenzyme Q_{10} Levels in Plasma: A Randomised Trial," *Drug Saf*, 2006, 29(8):703-12.
Caso G, Kelly P, McNurlan MA, et al, "Effect of Coenzyme Q_{10} on Myopathic Symptoms in Patients Treated With Statins," *Am J Cardiol*, 2007, 99(10):1409-12.
Chello M, Mastroroberto P, Romano R, et al, "Protection by Coenzyme Q_{10} From Myocardial Reperfusion Injury During Coronary Artery Bypass Grafting," *Ann Thorac Surg*, 1994, 58(5):1427-32.
Chello M, Mastroroberto P, Romano R, et al, "Protection by Coenzyme Q_{10} of Tissue Reperfusion Injury During Abdominal Aortic Cross-clamping," *J Cardiovasc Surg (Torino)*, 1996, 37(3):229-35.
Chen RS, Huang CC, and Chu NS, "Coenzyme Q_{10} Treatment in Mitochondrial Encephalomyopathies. Short-Term Double-Blind, Crossover Study," *Eur Neurol*, 1997, 37(4):212-8.

Combs AB, Porter TH, and Folkers K, "Anticoagulant Activity of Naphthoquinone Analog of Vitamin K and an Inhibitor of Coenzyme Q_{10}-Enzyme Systems," *Res Commun Chem Pathol Pharmacol*, 1976, 13 (1):109-14.

De Pinieux G, Chariot P, Ammi-Said M, et al, "Lipid-Lowering Drugs and Mitochondrial Function: Effects of HMG-CoA Reductase Inhibitors on Serum Ubiquinone and Blood Lactate/Pyruvate Ratio," *Br J Clin Pharmacol*, 1996, 42(3):333-7.

Folkers K and Simonsen R, "Two Successful Double-Blind Trials With Coenzyme Q_{10} (Vitamin Q_{10}) on Muscular Dystrophies and Neurogenic Atrophies," *Biochim Biophys Acta*, 1995, 1271(1):281-6.

Folkers K, Hanioka T, Xia LJ, et al, "Coenzyme Q_{10} Increases T4/T8 Ratios of Lymphocytes in Ordinary Subjects and Relevance to Patients Having the AIDS Related Complex," *Biochem Biophys Res Commun*, 1991, 176(2):786-91.

Folkers K, Langsjoen P, Nara Y, et al, "Biochemical Deficiencies of Coenzyme Q_{10} in HIV-Infection and Exploratory Treatment," *Biochem Biophys Res Commun*, 1988, 153(2):888-96.

Folkers K, Langsjoen P, Willis R, et al, "Lovastatin Decreases Coenzyme Q Levels in Humans," *Proc Natl Acad Sci USA*, 1990, 87(22):8931-4.

Fujimoto S, Kurihara N, Hirata K, et al, "Effects of Coenzyme Q_{10} Administration on Pulmonary Function and Exercise Performance in Patients With Chronic Lung Diseases," *Clin Investig*, 1993, 71(8 Suppl): S162-6.

Fuke C, Krikorian SA, and Couris RR, "Coenzyme Q_{10}: A Review of Essential Functions and Clinical Trials," *U.S. Pharmacist*, 2000, 25(10):28-41.

Galili N, Sechman EV, Cerny J, et al, "Clinical Response of Myelodysplastic Syndromes Patients to Treatment With Coenzyme Q_{10}," *Leuk Res*, 2007, 31(1):19-26.

Ghirlanda G, Oradei A, Manto A, et al, "Evidence of Plasma CoQ_{10}-Lowering Effect by HMG-CoA Reductase Inhibitors: A Double-Blind, Placebo-Controlled Study," *J Clin Pharmacol*, 1993, 33(3):226-9.

Gutzmann H and Hadler D, "Sustained Efficacy and Safety of Idebenone in the Treatment of Alzheimer's Disease: Update on a 2-Year Double-Blind Multicentre Study," *J Neural Transm Suppl*, 1998, 54:301-10.

Hansen IL, Iwamoto Y, Kishi T, et al, "Bioenergetics in Clinical Medicine. IX. Gingival and Leucocytic Deficiencies of Coenzyme Q_{10} in Patients With Periodontal Disease," *Res Commun Chem Pathol Pharmacol*, 1976, 14(4):729-38.

Hart PE, Lodi R, Rajagopalan B, et al, "Antioxidant Treatment of Patients With Friedreich Ataxia: Four-Year Follow-Up," *Arch Neurol*, 2005, 62(4):621-6.

Hershey AD, Powers SW, Vockell AL, et al, "Coenzyme Q_{10} Deficiency and Response to Supplementation in Pediatric and Adolescent Migraine," *Headache*, 2007, 47(1):73-80.

Kamikawa T, Kobayashi A, Yamashita T, et al, "Effects of Coenzyme Q_{10} on Exercise Tolerance in Chronic Stable Angina Pectoris," *Am J Cardiol*, 1985, 56(4):247-51.

Khan M, Gross J, Haupt H, et al, "A Pilot Clinical Trial of the Effects of Coenzyme Q_{10} on Chronic Tinnitus Aurium," *Otolaryngol Head Neck Surg*, 2007, 136(1):72-7.

Kishi T, Watanabe T, and Folkers K, "Bioenergetics in Clinical Medicine XV. Inhibition of Coenzyme Q_{10} - Enzymes by Clinically Used Adrenergic Blockers of Beta-Receptors," 1977, 17(1):157-64.

Kokawa T, Shiota K, Oda K, et al, "Coenzyme Q_{10} in Cancer Chemotherapy - Experimental Studies on Augmentation of the Effects of Masked Compounds, Especially in the Combined Chemotherapy With Immunopotentiators," *Gan To Kagaku Ryoho*, 1983, 10(3):768-74.

Landbo C and Almdal TP, "Interaction Between Warfarin and Coenzyme Q_{10}," *Ugeskr Laeger*, 1998, 160 (22):3226-7.

Langsjoen H, Langsjoen P, Langsjoen P, et al, "Usefulness of Coenzyme Q_{10} in Clinical Cardiology: A Long-Term Study," *Mol Aspects Med*, 1994, 15(Suppl):S165-75.

Langsjoen P, Langsjoen P, Willis R, et al, "Treatment of Essential Hypertension With Coenzyme Q_{10}," *Mol Aspects Med*, 1994, 15(Suppl): S265-72.

Langsjoen PH, Folkers K, Lyson K, et al, "Pronounced Increase of Survival of Patients With Cardiomyopathy When Treated With Coenzyme Q_{10} and Conventional Therapy," *Int J Tissue React*, 1990, 12 (3):163-8.

Langsjoen PH, Langsjoen PH, and Folkers K, "Isolated Diastolic Dysfunction of the Myocardium and Its Response to CoQ_{10} Treatment," *Clin Investig*, 1993, 71(8 Suppl):S140-4.

Langsjoen PH, Vadhanavikit S, and Folkers K, "Response of Patients in Classes III and IV of Cardiomyopathy to Therapy in a Blind and Crossover Trial With Coenzyme Q_{10}," *Proc Natl Acad Sci USA*, 1985, 82(12):4240-4.

Levy G, Kaufmann P, Buchsbaum R, et al, "A Two-Stage Design for a Phase II Clinical Trial of Coenzyme Q_{10} in ALS," *Neurology*, 2006, 66(5):660-3.

Lodi R, Hart PE, Rajagopalan B, et al, "Antioxidant Treatment Improves *in vivo* Cardiac and Skeletal Muscle Bioenergetics in Patients With Friedreich's Ataxia," *Ann Neurol*, 2001, 49(5):590-6.

Mazzola C, Guffanti EE, Vaccarella A, et al, "Noninvasive Assessment of Coenzyme Q_{10} Patients With Chronic Stable Effort Angina and Moderate Heart Failure," *Current Therapeutic Research*, 1987, 41 (6):923-32.

Migliore L, Molinu S, Naccarati A, et al, "Evaluation of Cytogenetic and DNA Damage in Mitochondrial Disease Patients: Effects of Coenzyme Q_{10} Therapy," *Mutagenesis*, 2004, 19(1):43-9.

Miles MV, Patterson BJ, Schapiro MB, et al, "Coenzyme Q_{10} Absorption and Tolerance in Children With Down Syndrome: A Dose-Ranging Trial," *Pediatr Neurol*, 2006, 35(1):30-7.

Mortensen SA, Leth A, Agner E, et al, "Dose-Related Decrease of Serum Coenzyme Q_{10} During Treatment With HMG-CoA Reductase Inhibitors," *Mol Aspects Med*, 1997, 18 Suppl:S137-44.

Musumeci O, Naini A, Slonim AE, et al, "Familial Cerebellar Ataxia With Muscle Coenzyme Q_{10} Deficiency," *Neurology*, 2001, 56(7):849-55.

Natural Standard Research Collaboration, Chief Editors: Ulbricht C, Basch E, *Natural Standard Herb and Supplement Reference - Evidence-Based Clinical Reviews*, USA: Elsevier/Mosby, 2005.

Niklowitz P, Sonnenschein A, Janetzky B, et al, "Enrichment of Coenzyme Q_{10} in Plasma and Blood Cells: Defense Against Oxidative Damage," *Int J Biol Sci*, 2007, 3(4):257-62.

The NINDS NET-PD Investigators, "A Randomized Clinical Trial of Coenzyme Q_{10} and GPI-1485 in Early Parkinson Disease," *Neurology*, 2007, 68(1):20-8.

Oda T, "Effect of Coenzyme Q_{10} on Stress-Induced Cardiac Dysfunction in Paediatric Patients With Mitral Valve Prolapse: A Study by Stress Echocardiography," *Drugs Exp Clin Res*, 1985, 11(8):557-76.

Okamoto H, Kawaguchi H, Togashi H, et al, "Effect of Coenzyme Q_{10} on Structural Alterations in the Renal Membrane of Stroke-Prone Spontaneously Hypertensive Rats," *Biochem Med Metab Biol*, 1991, 45(2):216-26.

Pogessi L, Galanti G, Comeglio M, et al, "Effect of Coenzyme Q_{10} on Left Ventricular Function in Patients With Dilative Cardiomyopathy: A Medium-Term Randomized Double-Blind Study Versus Placebo," *Curr Ther Res*, 1991, 49:878-86.

Portakal O, Ozkaya O, Erden Inal M, et al, "Coenzyme Q_{10} Concentrations and Antioxidant Status in Tissues of Breast Cancer Patients," *Clin Biochem*, 2000, 33(4):279-84.

Rosenfeldt FL, Haas SJ, Krum H, et al, "Coenzyme Q_{10} in the Treatment of Hypertension: A Meta-Analysis of the Clinical Trials," *J Hum Hypertens*, 2007, 21(4):297-306.

Rosenfeldt F, Hilton D, Pepe S, et al, "Systematic Review of Effect of Coenzyme Q_{10} in Physical Exercise, Hypertension and Heart Failure," *Biofactors*, 2003, 18(1-4):91-100.

Sandor PS, Di Clemente L, Coppola G, et al, "Efficacy of Coenzyme Q_{10} in Migraine Prophylaxis: A Randomized Controlled Trial," *Neurology*, 2005, 64(4):713-5.

Shinozawa S, Gomita Y, and Araki Y, "Tissue Concentration of Doxorubicin (Adriamycin®) in Mouse Pretreated With Alpha-Tocopherol or Coenzyme Q_{10}," *Acta Med Okayama*, 1991, 45(3):195-9.

Shults CW, Oakes D, Kieburtz K, et al, "Effects of Coenzyme Q_{10} in Early Parkinson Disease: Evidence of Slowing of the Functional Decline," *Arch Neurol*, 2002, 59(10):1541-50.

Sinatra ST, "Coenzyme Q_{10}: A Vital Therapeutic Nutrient for the Heart With Special Application in Congestive Heart Failure," *Conn Med*, 1997, 61(11):707-11.

Singh RB, Khanna HK, and Niaz MA, "Randomized, Double-Blind Placebo-Controlled Trial of Coenzyme Q_{10} in Chronic Renal Failure: Discovery of a New Role," *J Nutr Environ Med*, 2000, 10:281-8.

Singh RB, Neki NS, Kartikey K, et al, "Effect of Coenzyme Q_{10} on Risk of Atherosclerosis in Patients With Recent Myocardial Infarction," *Mol Cell Biochem*, 2003, 246(1-2):75-82.
Singh RB, Niaz MA, Rastogi SS, et al, "Effect of Hydrosoluble Coenzyme Q_{10} on Blood Pressures and Insulin Resistance in Hypertensive Patients With Coronary Artery Disease," *J Hum Hypertens*, 1999, 13 (3):203-8.
Singh RB, Wander GS, Rastogi A, et al, "Randomized, Double-Blind Placebo-Controlled Trial of Coenzyme Q_{10} in Patients With Acute Myocardial Infarction," *Cardiovasc Drugs Ther*, 1998, 12 (4):347-53.
Spigset O, "Reduced Effect of Warfarin Caused by Ubidecarenone," *Lancet*, 1994, 344(8933):1372-3.
Storch A, Jost WH, Vieregge P, et al, "Randomized, Double-Blind, Placebo-Controlled Trial on Symptomatic Effects of Coenzyme Q_{10} in Parkinson Disease," *Arch Neurol*, 2007, 64(7):938-44.
Taggart DP, Jenkins M, Hooper J, et al, "Effects of Short-Term Supplementation With Coenzyme Q_{10} on Myocardial Protection During Cardiac Operations," *Ann Thorac Surg*, 1996, 61(3):829-33.
Tran MT, Mitchell TM, Kennedy DT, et al, "Role of Coenzyme Q_{10} in Chronic Heart Failure, Angina, and Hypertension," *Pharmacotherapy*, 2001, 21(7):797-806.
van Gaal L, Folkers K, and Yamamura Y, eds, *Explatory Study of Coenzyme Q_{10} in Obesity, Biomedical and Clinical Aspects of Coenzyme Q, Vol 4, Amsterdam: Elsevier Science Publications*, 1984, 369-73.
Watson PS, Scalia GM, Galbraith A, et al, "Lack of Effect of Coenzyme Q on Left Ventricular Function in Patients With Congestive Heart Failure," *J Am Coll Cardiol*, 1999, 33(6):1549-52.
Watts GF, Castelluccio C, Rice-Evans C, et al, "Plasma Coenzyme Q (Ubiquinone) Concentrations in Patients Treated With Simvastatin," *J Clin Pathol*, 1993, 46(11):1055-7.
Ylikoski T, Piirainen J, Hanninen O, et al, "The Effect of Coenzyme Q_{10} on the Exercise Performance of Cross-Country Skiers," *Mol Aspects Med*, 1997, 18 Suppl:S283-90.

Cranberry

Pharmacologic Category Herb

Reported Use

Achlorhydria and B_{12} absorption (Saltzman, 1994)
Antioxidant (Pedersen, 2000; Wilson, 1998; Yan, 2002)
Bacterial and fungal infections (Konowalchuk, 1978; Swartz, 1968)
Cancer (prevention) (Bomser, 1996)
H. pylori infection (Burger, 2000; Shmuely, 2007)
Plaque (Terris, 2001)
Reduction of urinary odors (DuGan, 1966)
Urinary tract infection, including prevention (Bailey, 2007; Di Martino, 2006; Kontiokari, 2001; Kontiokari, 2005; Zafriri, 1989)

Local Anesthetic/Vasoconstrictor Precautions No information available to require special precautions

Effects on Bleeding None reported

Warnings/Precautions Use with caution in individuals with diabetes or glucose intolerance, due to risk of hyperglycemia. Some commercially available cranberry juice products contain large amounts of sugar. Sugar-free cranberry juice products are also available. Use with caution in individuals with a history of nephrolithiasis (kidney stones) due to its high oxalate content (Terris, 2001). Cranberry may contain salicylic acid and should be used cautiously in individuals with allergy to aspirin (Duthie, 2005).

References

Bailey DT, Dalton C, Joseph Daugherty F, et al, "Can a Concentrated Cranberry Extract Prevent Recurrent Urinary Tract Infections in Women? A Pilot Study," *Phytomedicine*, 2007, 14(4):237-41.
Bomser J, Madhavi DL, Singletary K, et al, "*In vitro* Anticancer Activity of Fruit Extracts From *Vaccinium* Species," *Planta Med*, 1996, 62(3):212-6.
Burger O, Ofek I, Tabak M, et al, "A High Molecular Mass Constituent of Cranberry Juice Inhibits *Helicobacter pylori* Adhesion to Human Gastric Mucus," *FEMS Immunol Med Microbiol*, 2000, 29 (4):295-301.
Di Martino P, Agniel R, David K, et al, "Reduction of Escherichia Coli Adherence to Uroepithelial Bladder Cells After Consumption of Cranberry Juice: A Double-Blind Randomized Placebo-Controlled Cross-Over Trial," *World J Urol*, 2006, 24(1):21-7.
Duthie GG, Kyle JA, Jenkinson AM, et al, "Increased Salicylate Concentrations in Urine of Human Volunteers After Consumption of Cranberry Juice," *J Agric Food Chem*, 2005, 53(8):2897-900.
Grant P, "Warfarin and Cranberry Juice: An Interaction?" *J Heart Valve Dis*, 2004, 13(1):25-6.
Hodek P, Trefil P, Stiborova M, "Flavonoids-Potent and Versatile Biologically Active Compounds Interacting With Cytochromes P450," *Chem Biol Interact*, 2002, 139(1):1-21.
Konowalchuk J and Speirs JI, "Antiviral Effect of Commercial Juices and Beverages," *Appl Environ Microbiol*, 1978, 35(6):1219-20.
Kontiokari T, Salo J, Eerola E, et al, "Cranberry Juice and Bacterial Colonization in Children - A Placebo-Controlled Randomized Trial," *Clin Nutr*, 2005, 24(6):1065-72.
Kontiokari T, Sundqvist K, Nuutinen M, et al, "Randomised Trial of Cranberry-Lingonberry Juice and *Lactobacillus* GG Drink for the Prevention of Urinary Tract Infections in Women," *BMJ*, 2001, 322 (7302):1571.
Leung AY and Foster S, *Encyclopedia of Common Natural Ingredients Used in Foods, Drugs, and Cosmetics*, New York, NY: Wiley, 1996, 198-9.
Natural Standard Research Collaboration, Chief Editors: Ulbricht C, Basch E, *Natural Standard Herb and Supplement Reference - Evidence-Based Clinical Reviews*, USA: Elsevier/Mosby, 2005.
Pedersen CB, Kyle J, Jenkinson AM, et al, "Effects of Blueberry and Cranberry Juice Consumption on the Plasma Antioxidant Capacity of Healthy Female Volunteers," *Eur J Clin Nutr*, 2000, 54(5):405-8.
Rettie AE, Korzekwa KR, Kunze KL, et al, "Hydroxylation of Warfarin by Human cDNA-Expressed Cytochrome P450: A Role for P4502C9 in the Etiology of (S)-Warfarin-Drug Interactions," *Chem Res Toxicol*, 1992, 5(1):54-9.
Saltzman JR, Kemp JA, Golner BB, et al, "Effect of Hypochlorhydria Due to Omeprazole Treatment or Atrophic Gastritis on Protein-Bound Vitamin B_{12} Absorption," *J Am Coll Nutr*, 1994, 13(6):584-91.
Shmuely H, Yahav J, Samra Z, et al, "Effect of Cranberry Juice on Eradication of *Helicobacter pylori* in Patients Treated With Antibiotics and a Proton Pump Inhibitor," *Mol Nutr Food Res*, 2007, 51(6):746-51.
Suvarna R, Pirmohamed M, Henderson L, "Possible Interaction Between Warfarin and Cranberry Juice," *BMJ*, 2003, 327(7429):1454.
Swartz JH and Medrek TF, "Antifungal Properties of Cranberry Juice," *Appl Microbiol*, 1968, 16 (10):1524-7.
Terris MK, Issa MM, and Tacker JR, "Dietary Supplementation With Cranberry Concentrate Tablets May Increase the Risk of Nephrolithiasis," *Urology*, 2001, 57(1):26-9.
Wilson T, Porcari JP, and Harbin D, "Cranberry Extract Inhibits Low Density Lipoprotein Oxidation," *Life Sci*, 1998, 62(24):L381-6.

Yan X, Murphy BT, Hammond GB, et al, "Antioxidant Activities and Antitumor Screening of Extracts From Cranberry Fruit (*Vaccinium macrocarpon*)," *J Agric Food Chem*, 2002, 50(21):5844-9.
Zafriri D, Ofek I, Adar R, et al, "Inhibitory Activity of Cranberry Juice on Adherence of Type 1 and Type P Fimbriated *Escherichia coli* to Eucaryotic Cells," *Antimicrob Agents Chemother*, 1989, 33(1):92-8.

Creatine

Pharmacologic Category Nutraceutical

Reported Use

Athletic performance (enhancement): Energy production and protein synthesis for muscle building (Barnes, 2001; Bemben, 2001; Chilibeck, 2004; Greenhaff, 1995; Silva, 2007); in older adults (Brose, 2003; Chrusch, 2001)
  Contradictory studies (Cornish, 2006; Glaister, 2006; Pluim, 2006); resistance training (Ferguson, 2006)
Bone density (Chilibeck, 2005)
Chronic obstructive pulmonary disease (Fuld, 2005)
  Contradictory study (Faager, 2006)
Congestive heart failure (CHF) (Andrews, 1998; Ferraro,1996)
Dermatomyositis/polymyositis (Alexanderson, 2009; Chung, 2007)
GAMT deficiency (Schulze, 2003)
Hemodialysis-associated muscle cramps (Chang, 2002)
Huntington's disease (Tabrizi, 2005; Verbessem, 2003)
Hyperlipidemia (Earnest, 1996)
Ischemic heart disease (Pedone, 1984)
McArdle's disease (Vorgerd, 2000; Vorgerd, 2002)
Mitochondrial diseases (Tarnopolsky, 1997)
Muscle function and strength (Chung, 2007; Kuethe, 2006)
  Contradictory study (Norman, 2006)
Mood (McMorris, 2006)
Muscular dystrophy (Escolar, 2005)
Parkinson's disease (Bender, 2006; NINDS NET-PD Investigators); resistance training in patients with Parkinson's disease (Hass, 2007)
Schizophrenia (contradictory study) (Kaptsan, 2007)
Spinal cord injury (Jacobs, 2002; Kendall, 2005)
Surgery (adjunct) (Chambers, 1996; Cisowski, 1996; Semenovsky, 1987)
Traumatic brain injury, prevention of complications (children) (Sakellaris, 2006)

Local Anesthetic/Vasoconstrictor Precautions No information available to require special precautions

Effects on Bleeding None reported

Warnings/Precautions Weight gain, muscle cramps, gastrointestinal upset, diarrhea, dizziness, heat intolerance, fever, dehydration, reduced blood volume, or electrolyte imbalances may occur. May cause elevation of serum creatinine (not a reflection of renal dysfunction). Use with caution in individuals with renal or hepatic disease. No known toxicity or serious side effects.

References

Alexanderson H, "Exercise Effects in Patients With Adult Idiopathic Inflammatory Myopathies," *Curr Opin Rheumatol*, 2009, 21(2):158-63.
Andrews R, Greenhaff P, Curtis S, et al, "The Effect of Dietary Creatine Supplementation on Skeletal Muscle Metabolism in Congestive Heart Failure," *Eur Heart J*, 1998, 19(4):617-22.
Barnes CL and Kushner JM, "Use of Creatine and Androstenedione to Enhance Athletic Performance," *US Pharmacist*, 2001, 26(08):47-9.
Bemben MG, Bemben DA, Loftiss DD, et al, "Creatine Supplementation During Resistance Training in College Football Athletes," *Med Sci Sports Exerc*, 2001, 33(10):1667-73.
Bender A, Koch W, Elstner M, et al, "Creatine Supplementation in Parkinson Disease: A Placebo-Controlled Randomized Pilot Trial," *Neurology*, 2006, 67(7):1262-4.
Brose A, Parise G, and Tarnopolsky MA, "Creatine Supplementation Enhances Isometric Strength and Body Composition Improvements Following Strength Exercise Training in Older Adults," *J Gerontol A Biol Sci Med Sci*, 2003, 58(1):11-9.
Chambers DJ, Haire K, Morley N, et al, "St. Thomas' Hospital Cardioplegia: Enhanced Protection With Exogenous Creatine Phosphate," *Ann Thorac Surg*, 1996, 61(1):67-75.
Chang CT, Wu CH, Yang CW, et al, "Creatine Monohydrate Treatment Alleviates Muscle Cramps Associated With Haemodialysis," *Nephrol Dial Transplant*, 2002, 17(11):1978-81.
Chilibeck PD, Chrusch MJ, Chad KE, et al, "Creatine Monohydrate and Resistance Training Increase Bone Mineral Content and Density in Older Men," *J Nutr Health Aging*, 2005, 9(5):352-3.
Chilibeck PD, Stride D, Farthing JP, et al, "Effect of Creatine Ingestion After Exercise on Muscle Thickness in Males and Females," *Med Sci Sports Exerc*, 2004, 36(10):1781-8.
Chrusch MJ, Chilibeck PD, Chad KE, et al, "Creatine Supplementation Combined With Resistance Training in Older Men," *Med Sci Sports Exerc*, 2001, 33(12):2111-7.
Chung YL, Alexanderson H, Pipitone N, et al, "Creatine Supplements in Patients With Idiopathic Inflammatory Myopathies Who Are Clinically Weak After Conventional Pharmacologic Treatment: Six-Month, Double-Blind, Randomized, Placebo-Controlled Trial," *Arthritis Rheum*, 2007, 57 (4):694-702.
Cisowski M, Bochenek A, Kucewicz E, et al, "The Use of Exogenous Creatine Phosphate for Myocardial Protection in Patients Undergoing Coronary Artery Bypass Surgery," *J Cardiovasc Surg*, 1996, 37(6 Suppl 1):75-80.
Cornish SM, Chilibeck PD, and Burke DG, "The Effect of Creatine Monohydrate Supplementation on Sprint Skating in Ice-Hockey Players," *J Sports Med Phys Fitness*, 2006, 46(1):90-8.
Earnest CP, Almada AL, and Mitchell TL, "High-Performance Capillary Electrophoresis-Pure Creatine Monohydrate Reduces Blood Lipids in Men and Women," *Clin Sci*, 1996, 91(1):113-8.
Escolar DM, Buyse G, Henricson E, et al, "CINRG Randomized Controlled Trial of Creatine and Glutamine in Duchenne Muscular Dystrophy," *Ann Neurol*, 2005, 58(1):151-5.
Faager G, Söderlund K, Sköld CM, et al, "Creatine Supplementation and Physical Training in Patients With COPD: A Double Blind, Placebo-Controlled Study," *Int J Chron Obstruct Pulmon Dis*, 2006, 1 (4):445-53.

Ferguson TB and Syrotuik DG, "Effects of Creatine Monohydrate Supplementation on Body Composition and Strength Indices in Experienced Resistance Trained Women," *J Strength Cond Res*, 2006, 20 (4):939-46.
Ferraro S, Codella C, Palumbo F, et al, "Hemodynamic Effects of Creatine Phosphate in Patients With Congestive Heart Failure: A Double-Blind Comparison Trial Versus Placebo," *Clin Cardiol*, 1996, 19 (9):699-703.
Fuld JP, Kilduff LP, Neder JA, et al, "Creatine Supplementation During Pulmonary Rehabilitation in Chronic Obstructive Pulmonary Disease," *Thorax*, 2005, 60(7):531-7.
Glaister M, Lockey RA, Abraham CS, et al, "Creatine Supplementation and Multiple Sprint Running Performance," *J Strength Cond Res*, 2006, 20(2):273-7.
Greenhaff PL, "Creatine and Its Application as an Erogenic Aid," *Int J Sport Nutr*, 1995, 5(Suppl):S100-10.
Hass CJ, Collins MA, and Juncos JL, "Resistance Training With Creatine Monohydrate Improves Upper-Body Strength in Patients With Parkinson Disease: A Randomized Trial," *Neurorehabil Neural Repair*, 2007, 21(2):107-15.
Jacobs PL, Mahoney ET, Cohn KA, et al, "Oral Creatine Supplementation Enhances Upper Extremity Work Capacity in Persons With Cervical-Level Spinal Cord Injury," *Arch Phys Med Rehabil*, 2002, 83 (1):19-23.
Kaptsan A, Odessky A, Osher Y, et al, "Lack of Efficacy of 5 Grams Daily of Creatine in Schizophrenia: A Randomized, Double-Blind, Placebo-Controlled Trial," *J Clin Psychiatry*, 2007, 68(6):881-4.
Kendall RW, Jacquemin G, Frost R, et al, "Creatine Supplementation for Weak Muscles in Persons With Chronic Tetraplegia: A Randomized Double-Blind Placebo-Controlled Crossover Trial," *J Spinal Cord Med*, 2005, 28(3):208-13.
Kuethe F, Krack A, Richartz BM, et al, "Creatine Supplementation Improves Muscle Strength in Patients With Congestive Heart Failure," *Pharmazie*, 2006, 61(3):218-22.
McMorris T, Harris RC, Swain J, et al, "Effect of Creatine Supplementation and Sleep Deprivation, With Mild Exercise, on Cognitive and Psychomotor Performance, Mood State, and Plasma Concentrations of Catecholamines and Cortisol," *Psychopharmacology (Berl)*, 2006, 185(1):93-103.
Natural Standard Research Collaboration, Chief Editors: Ulbricht C, Basch E, *Natural Standard Herb and Supplement Reference - Evidence-Based Clinical Reviews*, USA: Elsevier/Mosby, 2005.
NINDS NET-PD Investigators, "A Randomized, Double-Blind, Futility Clinical Trial of Creatine and Minocycline in Early Parkinson Disease," *Neurology*, 2006, 66(5):664-71.
Norman K, Stübler D, Baier P, et al, "Effects of Creatine Supplementation on Nutritional Status, Muscle Function and Quality of Life in Patients With Colorectal Cancer - A Double Blind Randomised Controlled Trial," *Clin Nutr*, 2006, 25(4):596-605.
Pedone V, Corbelli C, Frondini C, et al, "Myocardial T1-201 Scintigraphy in the Study of the Development of Acute Myocardial Infarction. Evaluation of the Effects of a Drug With Metabolic Action: Creatine Phosphate," *Clin Ter*, 1984, 111(6):531-8.
Pluim BM, Ferrauti A, Broekhof F, et al, "The Effects of Creatine Supplementation on Selected Factors of Tennis Specific Training," *Br J Sports Med*, 2006, 40(6):507-11.
Sakellaris G, Kotsiou M, Tamiolaki M, et al, "Prevention of Complications Related to Traumatic Brain Injury in Children and Adolescents With Creatine Administration: An Open Label Randomized Pilot Study," *J Trauma*, 2006, 61(2):322-9.
Schulze A, Bachert P, Schlemmer H, et al, "Lack of Creatine in Muscle and Brain in an Adult With GAMT Deficiency," *Ann Neurol*, 2003, 53(2):248-51.
Semenovsky ML, Shumakov VI, Sharov VG, et al, "Protection of Ischemic Myocardium by Exogenous Phosphocreatine. II. Clinical, Ultrastructural, and Biochemical Evaluations," *J Thorac Cardiovasc Surg*, 1987, 94(5):762-9.
Silva AJ, Machado Reis V, Guidetti L, et al, "Effect of Creatine on Swimming Velocity, Body Composition and Hydrodynamic Variables," *J Sports Med Phys Fitness*, 2007, 47(1):58-64.
Tabrizi SJ, Blamire AM, Manners DN, et al, "High-Dose Creatine Therapy for Huntington Disease: A 2-Year Clinical and MRS Study," *Neurology*, 2005, 64(9):1655-6.
Tarnopolsky MA, Roy BD, and MacDonald JR, "A Randomized, Controlled Trial of Creatine Monohydrate in Patients With Mitochondrial Cytopathies," *Muscle Nerve*, 1997, 20(12):1502-9.
Verbessem P, Lemiere J, Eijnde BO, et al, "Creatine Supplementation in Huntington's Disease: A Placebo-Controlled Pilot Trial," *Neurology*, 2003, 61(7):925-30.
Vorgerd M, Grehl T, Jager M, et al, "Creatine Therapy in Myophosphorylase Deficiency (McArdle Disease): A Placebo-Controlled Crossover Trial," *Arch Neurol*, 2000, 57(7):956-63.
Vorgerd M, Zange J, Kley R, et al, "Effect of High-Dose Creatine Therapy on Symptoms of Exercise Intolerance in McArdle Disease: Double-Blind, Placebo-Controlled Crossover Study," *Arch Neurol*, 2002, 59(1):97-101.

Damiana

Pharmacologic Category Herb

Reported Use

Female sexual dysfunction (Ito, 2001)
Weight loss/obesity (Andersen, 2001)

Local Anesthetic/Vasoconstrictor Precautions No information available to require special precautions

Effects on Bleeding None reported

Warnings/Precautions Avoid in individuals with Alzheimer's disease or Parkinson's disease; ethanol extracts of the leaves and stem have exhibited CNS depressant activity. Use with caution in individuals with a history of breast cancer (may interact with progesterone receptors on cells), individuals with psychiatric disorders (may cause hallucinations and mood changes), and individuals with diabetes or in those taking medications to control blood sugar levels (may affect blood sugar levels).

References

Alarcon-Aguilara FJ, Roman-Ramos R, Perez-Gutierrez S, et al, "Study of the Anti-Hyperglycemic Effect of Plants Used as Antidiabetics," *J Ethnopharmacol*, 1998, 61(2):101-10.
Andersen T and Fogh J, "Weight Loss and Delayed Gastric Emptying Following a South American Herbal Preparation in Overweight Patients," *J Hum Nutr Diet*, 2001, 14(3):243-50.
Arletti R, Benelli A, Cavazzuti E, et al, "Stimulating Property of *Turnera diffusa* and *Pfaffia paniculata* Extracts on the Sexual-Behavior of Male Rats," *Psychopharmacology (Berl)*, 1999, 143(1):15-9.
Ito TY, Trant AS, and Polan ML, "A Double-Blind Placebo-Controlled Study of ArginMax, a Nutritional Supplement for Enhancement of Female Sexual Function," *J Sex Marital Ther*, 2001, 27(5):541-9.
Natural Standard Research Collaboration, Chief Editors: Ulbricht C, Basch E, *Natural Standard Herb and Supplement Reference - Evidence-Based Clinical Reviews*, USA: Elsevier/Mosby, 2005.
Zava DT, Dollbaum CM, and Blen M, "Estrogen and Progestin Bioactivity of Foods, Herbs, and Spices," *Proc Soc Exp Biol Med*, 1998, 217(3):369-78.

Dehydroepiandrosterone

Pharmacologic Category Nutraceutical

Reported Use

Adrenal insufficiency (Arlt, 1999; Bilger, 2005; Hunt, 2000; Johannsson, 2002; Munarriz, 2001; Munarriz, 2002)
AIDS/HIV (Abrams, 2007; Dyner, 1990)
Anti-aging (Yen, 1995)
Cardiovascular disease (Fassati, 1970; Fassati, 1971; Kawano, 2003; Koo, 1983)
Cervical cancer (Suh-Burgmann, 2003)
Chronic fatigue syndrome (Himmel, 1999)
Cocaine withdrawal (Shoptaw, 2004)
Cognitive function (Parsons, 2006)
Crohn's disease (Andus, 2003)
Dementia (Azuma, 1999; Huppert, 2001; Wolkowitz, 2003)
  Contradictory studies (Van Niekerk, 2001; Wolf, 1998; Wolf, 1998)
Depression (Rabkin, 2006; Wolkowitz, 1997)
Diabetes, type 2 (Casson, 1995)
Erectile dysfunction (Reiter, 1999)
Extrapyramidal symptoms (Strous, 2007)
Fatigue (Scott, 1999)
Fibromyalgia (Finckh, 2005)
Induction of labor (Ishikawa, 1989; Mochizuki, 1978; Mochizuki, 1985; Sasaki, 1982)
Infertility (Casson, 1998; Casson, 2000)
Libido (premenopausal women) (Barnhart, 1999)
Lupus (Van Vollenhoven, 1996)
Muscle mass and strength (Villareal, 2006)
  Contradictory studies (Percheron, 2003; Wallace, 1999)
Obesity (Colker, 1999; Kalman, 2000; Morales, 1998; Shun, 1999; Villareal, 2004)
Perimenopausal symptoms (Barnhart, 1999)
Psoriasis (Holzmann, 1973)
Rheumatoid arthritis (Giltay, 1999)
Schizophrenia (Strous, 2003)
Sjögren's syndrome (Pillemer, 2004)

Local Anesthetic/Vasoconstrictor Precautions No information available to require special precautions

Effects on Bleeding None reported

Warnings/Precautions Acne is a common adverse effect associated with DHEA use but is generally mild and treatable. DHEA and DHEAS may cause elevated blood pressure and decreases in high-density lipoprotein (HDL) levels. Use with caution in individuals with psychiatric disorders; agitation, confusion, anxiety, paranoia, and suicidal thoughts have been reported. Use of hormones like DHEA may cause erythrocytosis.

References

Abrams DI, Shade SB, Couey P, et al, "Dehydroepiandrosterone (DHEA) Effects on HIV Replication and Host Immunity: A Randomized Placebo-Controlled Study," *AIDS Res Hum Retroviruses*, 2007, 23 (1):77-85.
Andus T, Klebl F, Rogler G, et al, "Patients With Refractory Crohn's Disease or Ulcerative Colitis Respond to Dehydroepiandrosterone: A Pilot Study," *Aliment Pharmacol Ther*, 2003, 17(3):409-14.
Arlt W, Callies F, van Vlijmen JC, et al, "Dehydroepiandrosterone Replacement in Women With Adrenal insufficiency," *N Engl J Med*, 1999, 341(14):1013-20.
Azuma T, Nagai Y, Saito T, et al, "The Effect of Dehydroepiandrosterone Sulfate Administration to Patients With Multi-Infarct Dementia," *J Neurol Sci*, 1999, 162(1):69-73.
Barnhart KT, Freeman E, Grisso JA, et al, "The Effect of Dehydroepiandrosterone Supplementation to Symptomatic Perimenopausal Women on Serum Endocrine Profiles, Lipid Parameters, and Health-Related Quality of Life," *J Clin Endocrinol Metab*, 1999, 84(11):3896-902.
Bilger M, Speraw S, LaFranchi SH, et al, "Androgen Replacement in Adolescents and Young Women With Hypopituitarism," *J Pediatr Endocrinol Metab*, 2005, 18(4):355-62.
Casson PR, Faguin LC, Stentz FB, et al, "Replacement of Dehydroepiandrosterone Enhances T-Lymphocyte Insulin Binding in Postmenopausal Women," *Fertil Steril*, 1995, 63(5):1027-31.
Casson PR, Lindsay MS, Pisarska MD, et al, "Dehydroepiandrosterone Supplementation Augments Ovarian Stimulation in Poor Responders: A Case Series," *Hum Reprod*, 2000, 15(10):2129-32.
Casson PR, Santoro N, Elkind-Hirsch K, et al, "Postmenopausal Dehydroepiandrosterone Administration Increases Free Insulin-Like Growth Factor-I and Decreases High-Density Lipoprotein: A Six-Month Trial," *Fertil Steril*, 1998, 70(1):107-10.
Colker C, Torina G, Swain M, et al, "Double-Blind, Placebo-Controlled, Randomized Clinical Trial Evaluating the Effects of Exercise Plus 3-Acetyl-7-Oxo-Dehydroepiandrosterone on Body Composition and the Endocrine System in Overweight Adults," *Journal of Exercise Physiology*, 1999, 2(4).
Dean CE, "Prasterone (DHEA) and Mania," *Ann Pharmacother*, 2000, 34(12):1419-22.
Dyner T, Lang W, Geaga JV, et al, ""Phase I Study of Dehydroepiandrosterone (EL-10) Therapy in Symptomatic HIV Disease," *6th Intl Conf on AIDS*, 1990, 3:208.
Fassati P, Fassati M, Sonka J, et al, "Dehydroepiandrosterone Sulphate - A New Approach to Some Cases of Angina Pectoris Therapy," *Agressologie*, 1970, 11(5):445-8.
Fassati P, Fassati M, Sonka J, et al, "New Approach to the Treatment of Angina Pectoris by Dehydroepiandrosterone-Sulfate," *Cas Lek Cesk*, 1971, 110(26):606-9.
Finckh A, Berner IC, Aubry-Rozier B, et al, "A Randomized Controlled Trial of Dehydroepiandrosterone in Postmenopausal Women With Fibromyalgia," *J Rheumatol*, 2005, 32(7):1336-40.
Giltay EJ, van Schaardenburg D, Gooren LJ, et al, "Dehydroepiandrosterone Sulfate in Patients With Rheumatoid Arthritis," *Ann NY Acad Sci*, 1999, 22;876:152-4.
Himmel P and Seligman TM, "A Pilot Study Employing Dehydroepiandrosterone (DHEA) in the Treatment of Chronic Fatigue Syndrome," *J Clin Rheumatol*, 1999, 5(2):56-9.

Holzmann H, Morsches B, Krapp R, et al, "Therapy of Psoriasis With Dehydroepiandrosterone-Enanthate. II. Intramuscular Depot Application of 300 mg Weekly," *Arch Dermatol Forsch*, 1973, 247 (1):23-8.

Hunt PJ, Gurnell EM, Huppert FA, et al, "Improvement in Mood and Fatigue After Dehydroepiandrosterone Replacement in Addison's Disease in a Randomized, Double Blind Trial," *J Clin Endocrinol Metab*, 2000, 85(12):4650-6.

Huppert FA and Van Niekerk JK, "Dehydroepiandrosterone (DHEA) Supplementation for Cognitive Function," *Cochrane Database Syst Rev*, 2001, (2):CD000304.

Ishikawa M and Shimizu T, "Dehydroepiandrosterone Sulfate and Induction of Labor," *Am J Perinatol*, 1989, 6(2):173-5.

Johannsson G, Burman P, Wiren L, et al, "Low Dose Dehydroepiandrosterone Affects Behavior in Hypopituitary Androgen-Deficient Women: A Placebo-Controlled Trial," *J Clin Endocrinol Metab*, 2002, 87(5):2046-52.

Kalman DS, Colker CM, Swain MA, et al, "A Randomized, Double-Blind, Placebo-Controlled Study of 3-Acetyl-7-Oxo-Dehydroepiandrosterone in Healthy Overweight Adults," *Current Therapeutic Research*, 2000, 61(7):435-42.

Kawano H, Yasue H, Kitagawa A, et al, "Dehydroepiandrosterone Supplementation Improves Endothelial Function and Insulin Sensitivity in Men," *J Clin Endocrinol Metab*, 2003, 88(7):3190-5.

Koo E, Feher KG, Feher T, et al, "Effect of Dehydroepiandrosterone on Hereditary Angioedema," *Klin Wochenschr*, 1983, 61(14):715-7.

The Mayo Clinic, "Dermatomyositis," 2009. Available at: http://www.mayoclinic.com/health/dermatomyositis.

Mochizuki M and Maruo T, "Effect of Dehydroepiandrosterone Sulfate on Uterine Cervical Ripening in Late Pregnancy," *Acta Physiol Hung*, 1985, 65(3):267-74.

Mochizuki M, Honda T, Deguchi M,et al, "A Study on the Effect of Dehydroepiandrosterone Sulfate on So-Called Cervical Ripening," *Acta Obstet Gynecol Scand*, 1978, 57(5):397-401.

Morales AJ, Haubrich RH, Hwang JY, et al, "The Effect of Six Months Treatment With a 100 mg Daily Dose of Dehydroepiandrosterone (DHEA) on Circulating Sex Steroids, Body Composition and Muscle Strength in Age-Advanced Men and Women," *Clin Endocrinol (Oxf)*, 1998, 49(4):421-32.

Munarriz R, Talakoub L, Flaherty E, et al, "Androgen Replacement Therapy With Dehydroepiandrosterone for Androgen Insufficiency and Female Sexual Dysfunction: Androgen and Questionnaire Results," *J Sex Marital Ther*, 2002, 28(Suppl 1):165-73.

Munarriz R, Talakoub L, Flaherty E, et al, "Hormone, Sexual Function and Personal Sexual Distress Outcomes Following Dehydroepiandosterone (DHEA) Treatment for Multi-Dimensional Female Sexual Dysfunction and Androgen Deficiency Syndrome," American Urological Association Annual Meeting, June 2-7, 2001.

Natural Standard Research Collaboration, Chief Editors: Ulbricht C, Basch E, *Natural Standard Herb and Supplement Reference - Evidence-Based Clinical Reviews*, USA: Elsevier/Mosby, 2005.

Parsons TD, Kratz KM, Thompson E, et al, "Dhea Supplementation and Cognition in Postmenopausal Women," *Int J Neurosci*, 2006, 116(2):141-55.

Percheron G, Hogrel JY, Denot-Ledunois S, et al, "Effect of 1-Year Oral Administration of Dehydroepiandrosterone to 60- to 80-Year-Old Individuals on Muscle Function and Cross-Sectional Area: A Double-Blind Placebo-Controlled Trial," *Arch Intern Med*, 2003, 163(6):720-7.

Pillemer SR, Brennan MT, Sankar V, et al, "Pilot Clinical Trial of Dehydroepiandrosterone (DHEA) Versus Placebo for Sjogren's Syndrome," *Arthritis Rheum*, 2004, 51(4):601-4.

Rabkin JG, McElhiney MC, Rabkin R, et al, "Placebo-Controlled Trial of Dehydroepiandrosterone (DHEA) for Treatment of Nonmajor Depression in Patients With HIV/AIDS," *Am J Psychiatry*, 2006, 163 (1):59-66.

Reiter WJ, Pycha A, Schatzl G, et al, "Dehydroepiandrosterone in the Treatment of Erectile Dysfunction: A Prospective, Double-Blind, Randomized, Placebo-Controlled Study," *Urology*, 1999, 53(3):590-5.

Sasaki K, Nakano R, Kadoya Y, et al, "Cervical Ripening With Dehydroepiandrosterone Sulphate," *Br J Obstet Gynaecol*, 1982, 89(3):195-8.

Scott, LV, Salahuddin F, Cooney J, et al, "Differences in Adrenal Steroid Profile in Chronic Fatigue Syndrome, In Depression and in Health," *J Affect Disord*, 1999, 54(1-2):129-37.

Shoptaw S, Majewska MD, Wilkins J, et al, "Participants Receiving Dehydroepiandrosterone During Treatment for Cocaine Dependence Show High Rates of Cocaine Use in a Placebo-Controlled Pilot Study," *Exp Clin Psychopharmacol*, 2004, 12(2):126-35.

Shun YP, Shun LH, Feng YY, et al, "The Effect of DHEA on Body Fat Distribution and Serum Lipids in Elderly Overweight Males," *Practical Geriatrics*, 1999, 13(1):31-3.

Strous RD, Maayan R, Lapidus R, et al, "Dehydroepiandrosterone Augmentation in the Management of Negative, Depressive, and Anxiety Symptoms in Schizophrenia," *Arch Gen Psychiatry*, 2003, 60 (2):133-41.

Strous RD, Stryjer R, Maayan R, et al, "Analysis of Clinical Symptomatology, Extrapyramidal Symptoms and Neurocognitive Dysfunction Following Dehydroepiandrosterone (DHEA) Administration in Olanzapine Treated Schizophrenia Patients: A Randomized, Double-Blind Placebo Controlled Trial," *Psychoneuroendocrinology*, 2007, 32(2):96-105.

Suh-Burgmann E, Sivret J, Duska LR, et al, "Long-Term Administration of Intravaginal Dehydroepiandrosterone on Regression of Low-Grade Cervical Dysplasia - A Pilot Study," *Gynecol Obstet Invest*, 2003, 55(1):25-31.

van Niekerk JK, Huppert FA, and Herbert J, "Salivary Cortisol and DHEA: Association With Measures of Cognition and Well-Being in Normal Older Men, and Effects of Three Months of DHEA Supplementation," *Psychoneuroendocrinology*, 2001, 26(6):591-612.

van Vollenhoven RF and McGuire JL, "Studies of Dehydroepiandrosterone (DHEA) as a Therapeutic Agent in Systemic Lupus Erythematosus," *Ann Med Interne (Paris)*, 1996, 147(4):290-6.

van Vollenhoven RF, Park JL, Genovese MC, et al, "A Double-Blind, Placebo-Controlled, Clinical Trial of Dehydroepiandrosterone in Severe Systemic Lupus Erythematosus," *Lupus*, 1999, 8(3):181-7.

Villareal DT and Holloszy JO, "DHEA Enhances Effects of Weight Training on Muscle Mass and Strength in Elderly Women and Men," *Am J Physiol Endocrinol Metab*, 2006, 291(5):E1003-8.

Villareal DT and Holloszy JO, "Effect of DHEA on Abdominal Fat and Insulin Action in Elderly Women and Men: A Randomized Controlled Trial," *JAMA*, 2004, 292(18):2243-8.

Wallace MB, Lim J, Cutler A, et al, "Effects of Dehydroepiandrosterone vs Androstenedione Supplementation in Men," *Med Sci Sports Exerc*, 1999, 31(12):1788-92.

Wolf OT, Kudielka BM, Hellhammer DH, et al, "Opposing Effects of DHEA Replacement in Elderly Subjects on Declarative Memory and Attention After Exposure to a Laboratory Stressor," *Psychoneuroendocrinology*, 1998, 23(6):617-29.

Wolf OT, Naumann E, Hellhammer DH, et al, "Effects of Dehydroepiandrosterone Replacement in Elderly Men on Event-Related Potentials, Memory, and Well-Being," *J Gerontol A Biol Sci Med Sci*, 1998, 53(5): M385-90.

Wolkowitz OM, Kramer JH, Reus VI, et al, "DHEA Treatment of Alzheimer's Disease: A Randomized, Double-Blind, Placebo-Controlled Study," *Neurology*, 2003, 60(7):1071-6.

Wolkowitz OM, Reus VI, Roberts E, et al, "Dehydroepiandrosterone (DHEA) Treatment of Depression," *Biol Psychiatry*, 1997, 41(3):311-8.

Yen SS, Morales AJ, and Khorram O, "Replacement of DHEA in Aging Men and Women. Potential Remedial Effects," *Ann N Y Acad Sci*, 1995, 774:128-42.

Devil's Claw

Pharmacologic Category Herb

Reported Use

Anti-inflammatory (Erdos, 1978; Lanhers, 1992)
Contradictory study (Whitehouse, 1983)
Back pain (Chrubasik, 1999)
Osteoarthritis, gout, and other inflammatory conditions (Grahame 1981; Lanhers, 1992)

Local Anesthetic/Vasoconstrictor Precautions No information available to require special precautions

Effects on Bleeding May see increased bleeding due to inhibition of platelet aggregation

Warnings/Precautions Avoid in patients with peptic ulcer disease. Use of devil's claw is contraindicated in pregnancy and lactation; case reports indicate potential to stimulate uterine contractions (Newall, 1996). Based on pharmacologic activity, use caution in individuals receiving antiarrhythmic medications or cardiac glycosides (Shaw, 1997). Use with caution in individuals with GI disorders (De Smet, 1993). Use caution in individuals with diabetes as devil's claw may lower blood glucose levels.

Based on pharmacologic activity, may alter hemostasis (Shaw, 1997) and may be contraindicated in individuals with active bleeding (eg, peptic ulcer, intracranial bleeding). Use with caution in individuals with a history of bleeding, hemostatic disorders, or drug-related hemostatic problems; or in individuals taking anticoagulant medications, including warfarin, aspirin, aspirin-containing products, NSAIDs, or antiplatelet agents (eg, ticlopidine, clopidogrel, dipyridamole). Discontinue use prior to dental or surgical procedures (generally at least 14 days before).

References

Chrubasik S, Junck H, Breitschwerdt H, et al, "Effectiveness of Harpagophytum Extract WS 1531 in the Treatment of Exacerbation of Low Back Pain: A Randomized, Placebo-Controlled, Double-Blind Study," *Eur J Anaesthesiol*, 1999, 16(2):118-29.
De Smet PA, Hansel R, Keller K, et al, *Adverse Effects of Herbal Drugs*, Vol 2, New York, NY: Springer-Verlag, 1993.
Erdos A, Fontaine R, Friehe H, et al, "Contribution to the Pharmacology and Toxicology of Different Extracts as Well as the Harpagoside From *Harpagophytum procumbens* DC," *Planta Med*, 1978, 34 (1):97-108.
Grahame R and Robinson BV, "Devil's Claw (*Harpagophytum procumbens*): Pharmacological and Clinical Studies," *Ann Rheum Dis*, 1981, 40(6):632.
Lanhers MC, Fleurentin J, Mortier F, et al, "Anti-Inflammatory and Analgesic Effects of an Aqueous Extract of *Harpagophytum procumbens*," *Planta Med*, 1992, 58(2):117-23.
Natural Standard Research Collaboration, Chief Editors: Ulbricht C, Basch E, *Natural Standard Herb and Supplement Reference - Evidence-Based Clinical Reviews*, USA: Elsevier/Mosby, 2005.
Newall CA, Anderson LA, and Phillipson JD, *Herbal Medicines: A Guide for Health Care Professionals*, London, England: The Pharmaceutical Press, 1996, 98-100.
Shaw D, Leon C, Kolev S, et al, "Traditional Remedies and Food Supplements. A 5-Year Toxicological Study (1991-1995)," *Drug Saf*, 1997, 17(5):342-56.
Whitehouse LW, Znamirowska M, and Paul CJ, "Devil's Claw (*Harapogophytum procumbens*): No Evidence for Anti-Inflammatory Activity in the Treatment of Arthritic Disease," *Can Med Assoc J*, 1983, 129(3):249-51.

Docosahexaenoic Acid

Pharmacologic Category Nutraceutical

Reported Use

Alzheimer's disease (Kyle, 1999)
Angina pectoris (Aucamp, 1993; Kristensen, 1987)
Appetite (López-Alarcón, 2006)
Arrhythmias (Christensen, 1995; Christensen, 1996; Sellmayer, 1995)
Asthma (Anon, 2004; Dry, 1991; Masuev, 1997; Mihrshahi, 2004; Nagakura, 2000; Oddy, 2004; Okamoto, 2000)
Attention-deficit disorder and attention-deficit hyperactivity disorder (ADD/ADHD) (Aman, 1987; Stevens, 1995)
Bipolar disorder (Calabrese, 1999; Stoll, 1999; Tanskanen, 2001)
Cancer (prevention): colon cancer (Augustsson, 2003; Caygill, 1995; de Deckere, 1999; Klein, 2000; Mehrotra, 2002; Norrish, 1999; Rose, 1999; Terry 2001)
Cardiovascular disease (Din, 2004; Pepe, 2002; Woodman, 2002)
Coronary heart disease (risk reduction) (O'Keefe, 2000)
Crohn's disease (Belluzzi, 1996)
Cystic fibrosis (Beckles, 2001; Beckles, 2002; De Vizia, 2003; Katz, 1996; Kurlandsky, 1994; Lawrence, 1993)
Depression (Chiu, 2003; Frasure-Smith, 2004; Jacka, 2004; Logan, 2004; Mischoulon, 2000; Mischoulon, 2008; Nemets, 2002; Nemets, 2004; Su, 2003); postpartum depression (Otto, 2003)
Diabetes (McManus, 1996)
Diabetes, type 2 (Woodman, 2002)
Dysmenorrhea (Deutch, 1996; Deutch, 2000; Harel, 1996)
Eczema (Bjorneboe, 1989; Koch, 2008; Takwale, 2003)
Hypercholesterolemia (Kalmijn, 2004)
Hypertension (Morris, 1993; Theobald, 2007)
Hypertriglyceridemia (Aldámiz-Echevarria, 2006; Pritchard, 1995)

IgA nephropathy (Alexopoulos, 2004; Dillon, 1997; Donadio, 2000; Donadio, 2001; Donadio, 2004; Parinyasiri, 2004; Sulikowska, 2004)
Immune support (Dunstan, 2003)
Infant eye/brain development (Birch, 1992; Carlson, 1987; Carlson, 1993; Carlson, 1996; Carlson, 1996; Fewtrell, 2004; Hoffman, 1993; Judge, 2007; Judge, 2007; Smithers, 2008)
Infection (López-Alarcón, 2006)
Lupus (Clark, 1993; Clark, 1994; Duffy, 2004; Walton, 1991)
Nephrotic syndrome (Bakker, 1989; Stacpoole, 1989)
Pre-eclampsia (Bulstra-Ramakers, 1994; D'Almeida, 1992; Olsen, 1992; Olsen, 2000; Olsen, 2002; Onwude, 1995; Salvig, 1996)
Prevention of graft failure after heart bypass surgery (Eritsland, 1996; Roy, 1991)
Protection from cyclosporine toxicity in organ transplant patients (Andreassen, 1997; Badalamenti, 1995; Berthoux, 1992; Brouwer, 1991; Homan, 1989; Homan, 1990; Homan, 1992; Maachi, 1995; Stoof, 1989; Sweny, 1989; van der Heide, 1993; Ventura, 1993)
Psoriasis (Bittiner, 1988)
Rheumatoid arthritis (Kremer, 1991)
Schizophrenia (Fenton, 2001; Joy, 2000; Mellor, 1996; Peet, 1998)
Stroke (risk reduction) (Iso, 2001)
Ulcerative colitis (Aslan, 1992; Belluzzi, 1997; Dichi, 2000; Greenfield, 1993; Hawthorne, 1990, Hawthorne, 1992; Loeschke, 1996; Lorenz, 1989; Lorenz, 1994; Ross, 1993; Stenson, 1990; Stenson, 1992)

Local Anesthetic/Vasoconstrictor Precautions No information available to require special precautions

Effects on Bleeding None reported

References

Aldámiz-Echevarría L, Sanjurjo P, Elorz J, et al, "Effect of Docosahexaenoic Acid Administration on Plasma Lipid Profile and Metabolic Parameters of Children With Methylmalonic Acidaemia," *J Inherit Metab Dis*, 2006, 29(1):58-63.

Alexopoulos E, Stangou M, Pantzaki A, et al, "Treatment of Severe IgA Nephropathy With Omega-3 Fatty Acids: The Effect of a 'Very Low Dose' Regimen,"*Ren Fail* , 2004, 26(4):453-9.

Aman MG, Mitchell EA, and Turbott SH, "The Effects of Essential Fatty Acid Supplementation by Efamol in Hyperactive Children," *J Abnorm Child Psychol*, 1987, 15(1):75-90.

Andreassen AK, Hartmann A, Offstad J, et al, "Hypertension Prophylaxis With Omega-3 Fatty Acids in Heart Transplant Recipients," *J Am Coll Cardiol*, 1997, 29(6):1324-31.

Anon, "Health Effects of Omega-3 Fatty Acids on Asthma," *Evid Rep Technol Assess*, 2004, (91):1-7.

Aslan A and Triadafilopoulos G, "Fish Oil Fatty Acid Supplementation in Active Ulcerative Colitis: A Double-Blind, Placebo-Controlled, Crossover Study," *Am J Gastroenterol*, 1992, 87(4):432-7.

Aucamp AK, Schoeman HS, and Coetzee JH, "Pilot Trial to Determine the Efficacy of a Low Dose of Fish Oil in the Treatment of Angina Pectoris in the Geriatric Patient," *Prostaglandins Leukot Essent Fatty Acids*, 1993, 49(3):687-9.

Augustsson K, Michaud DS, Rimm EB, et al, "A Prospective Study of Intake of Fish and Marine Fatty Acids and Prostate Cancer," *Cancer Epidemiol Biomarkers Prev*, 2003, 12(1):64-7.

Badalamenti S, Salerno F, Lorenzano E, et al, "Renal Effects of Dietary Supplementation With Fish Oil in Cyclosporine-Treated Liver Transplant Recipients," *Hepatology*, 1995, 22(6):1695-71.

Bakker DJ, Haberstroh BN, Philbrick DJ, et al, "Triglyceride Lowering in Nephrotic Syndrome Patients Consuming a Fish Oil Concentrate," *Nutrit Res*, 1989, 9:27-34.

Beckles WN, Elliott TM, and Everard ML, "Omega-3 Fatty Acids for Cystic Fibrosis (Protocol for a Cochrane Review)," *The Cochrane Library*, 2001, (3).

Beckles WI, Elliott TM, and Everard ML, "Omega-3 Fatty Acids (From Fish Oils) for Cystic Fibrosis," *Cochrane Database Syst Rev*, 2002, (3):CD002201.

Belluzzi A, Brignola C, Boschi S, et al, "A Novel Enteric Coated Preparation of Omega-3 Fatty Acids in a Group of Steroid-Dependent Ulcerative Colitis: An Open Study," *Gastroenterology*, 1997, 112(Suppl): A930.

Belluzzi A, Brignola C, Campieri M, et al, "Effect of an Enteric-Coated Fish Oil Preparation on Relapses in Crohn's Disease," *N Engl J Med*, 1996, 334(24):1557-60.

Bender NK, Kraynak MA, Chiquette E, et al, "Effects of Marine Fish Oils on the Anticoagulation Status of Patients Receiving Chronic Warfarin Therapy," *J Thromb Thrombolysis*, 1998, 5(3):257-61.

Berthoux FC, Guerin C, Burgard G, et al, "One-Year Randomized Controlled Trial With Omega-3 Fatty Acid-Fish Oil in Clinical Renal Transplantation," *Transplant Proc*, 1992, 24(6):2578-82.

Birch DG, Birch EE, Hoffman DR, et al, "Retinal Development in Very-Low-Birth-Weight Infants Fed Diets Differing in Omega-3 Fatty Acids," *Invest Ophthalmol Vis Sci*, 1992, 33(8):2365-76.

Bittiner SB, Tucker WF, Cartwright I, et al, "A Double-Blind, Randomised, Placebo-Controlled Trial of Fish Oil in Psoriasis," *Lancet*, 1988, 1(8582):378-80.

Bjorneboe A, Soyland R, Bjorneboe GE, et al, "Effect of N-3 Fatty Acid Supplement to Patients With Atopic Dermatitis," *J Intern Med Suppl*, 1989, 225(731):233-6.

Brouwer RM, Wenting GJ, Pos B, et al, "Fish Oil Ameliorates Established Cyclosporin A Nephrotoxicity After Heart Transplantation," *Kidney Int*, 1991, 40:347-8.

Buckley MS, Goff AD, and Knapp WE, "Fish Oil Interaction With Warfarin," *Ann Pharmacother*, 2004, 38 (1):50-2.

Bulstra-Ramakers MT, Huisjes HJ, and Visser GH, "The Effects of 3g Eicosapentaenoic Acid Daily on Recurrence of Intrauterine Growth Retardation and Pregnancy Induced Hypertension," *Br J Obstet Gynaecol*, 1994, 102:123-6.

Calabrese JR, Rapport DJ, and Shelton MD, "Fish Oils and Bipolar Disorder: A Promising But Untested Treatment," *Arch Gen Psychiatry*, 1999, 56(5):413-4.

Carlson SE and Werkman SH, "A Randomized Trial of Visual Attention of Preterm Infants Fed Docosahexaenoic Acid Until Two Months," *Lipids*, 1996, 31(1):85-90.

Carlson SE, Rhodes PG, Rao VS, et al, "Effect of Fish Oil Supplementation on the N-3 Fatty Acid Content of Red Blood Cell Membranes in Preterm Infants," *Pediatr Res*, 1987, 21(5):507-10.

Carlson SE, Werkman SH, and Tolley EA, "Effect of Long-Chain N-3 Fatty Acid Supplementation on Visual Acuity and Growth of Preterm Infants With and Without Bronchopulmonary Dysplasia," *Am J Clin Nutr*, 1996, 63(5):687-97.

Carlson SE, Werkman SH, Rhodes PG, et al, "Visual-Acuity Development in Healthy Preterm Infants: Effect of Marine-Oil Supplementation," *Am J Clin Nutr*, 1993, 58(1):35-42.

Caygill CP and Hill MJ, "Fish, N-3 Fatty Acids and Human Colorectal and Breast Cancer Mortality," *Eur J Cancer Prev*, 1995, 4(4):329-32.

Chiu CC, Huang SY, Shen WW, et al, "Omega-3 Fatty Acids for Depression in Pregnancy," *Am J Psychiatry*, 2003, 160(2):385.

Christensen JH, Gustenhoff P, Ejlersen E, et al, "N-3 Fatty Acids and Ventricular Extrasystoles in Patients With Ventricular Tachyarrhythmias," *Nutr Res*, 1995, 15(1):1-8.
Christensen JH, Gustenhoff P, Korup E, et al, "Effect of Fish Oil on Heart Rate Variability in Survivors of Myocardial Infarction: A Double Blind Randomised Controlled Trial," *BMJ*, 1996, 312(7032):677-8.
Clark WF and Parbtani A, "Omega-3 Fatty Acid Supplementation in Clinical and Experimental Lupus Nephritis," *Am J Kidney Dis*, 1994, 23(5):644-7.
Clark WF, Parbtani A, Naylor CD, et al, "Fish Oil in Lupus Nephritis: Clinical Findings and Methodological Implications," *Kidney Int*, 1993, 44(1):75-86.
D'Almeida A, Carter JP, Anatol A, et al, "Effects of a Combination of Evening Primrose Oil (Gamma Linolenic Acid) and Fish Oil (Eicosapentaenoic + Docahexaenoic Acid) Versus Magnesium, and Versus Placebo in Preventing Pre-Eclampsia," *Women Health*, 1992, 19(2-3):117-31.
de Deckere EA, "Possible Beneficial Effect of Fish and Fish N-3 Polyunsaturated Fatty Acids in Breast and Colorectal Cancer," *Eur J Cancer Prev*, 1999, 8(3):213-21.
De Vizia B, Raia V, Spano C, et al, "Effect of an 8-Month Treatment With Omega-3 Fatty Acids (Eicosapentaenoic and Docosahexaenoic) in Patients With Cystic Fibrosis," *JPEN J Parenter Enteral Nutr*, 2003, 27(1):52-7.
Deutch B, "Painful Menstruation and Low Intake of N-3 Fatty Acids," *Ugeskr Laeger*, 1996, 158 (29):4195-8.
Deutch B, Jorgensen EB, and Hansen JC, "Menstrual Discomfort in Danish Women Reduced by Dietary Supplements of Omega-3 PUFA and B12 (Fish Oil or Seal Oil Capsules)," *Nutr Res*, 2000, 20 (5):621-31.
Dichi I, Frenhane P, Dichi JB, et al, "Comparison of Omega-3 Fatty Acids and Sulfasalazine in Ulcerative Colitis," *Nutrition*, 2000, 16(2):87-90.
"Dietary Supplementation With N-3 Polyunsaturated Fatty Acids and Vitamin E After Myocardial Infarction: Results of the GISSI-Prevenzione Trial. Gruppo Italiano per lo Studio della Sopravvivenza Nell'Infarto Miocardico," *Lancet*, 1999, 354(9177):447-55.
Dillon JJ, "Fish Oil Therapy for IgA Nephropathy: Efficacy and Interstudy Variability," *J Am Soc Nephrol*, 1997, 8(11):1739-44.
Din JN, "Omega 3 Fatty Acids and Cardiovascular Disease - Fishing for a Natural Treatment," *BMJ*, 2004, 328(7430):30-5.
Donadio JV, "The Emerging Role of Omega-3 Polyunsaturated Fatty Acids in the Management of Patients With IgA Nephropathy," *J Ren Nutr*, 2001, 11(3):122-8.
Donadio JV Jr, "Use of Fish Oil to Treat Patients With Immunoglobulin a Nephropathy," *Am J Clin Nutr*, 2000, 71(1 Suppl):373S-5S.
Donadio JV and Grande JP, "The Role of Fish Oil/Omega-3 Fatty Acids in the Treatment of IgA Nephropathy," *Semin Nephrol*, 2004, 24(3):225-43.
Dry J and Vincent D, "Effect of a Fish Oil Diet on Asthma: Results of a 1-Year Double-Blind Study," *Int Arch Allergy Appl Immunol*, 1991, 95(2-3):156-7.
Duffy EM, Meenagh GK, McMillan SA, et al, "The Clinical Effect of Dietary Supplementation With Omega-3 Fish Oils and/or Copper in Systemic Lupus Erythematosus," *J Rheumatol*, 2004, 31(8):1551-6.
Dunstan JA, Mori TA, Barden A, et al, " Fish Oil Supplementation in Pregnancy Modifies Neonatal Allergen-Specific Immune Responses and Clinical Outcomes in Infants at High Risk of Atopy: A Randomized, Controlled Trial," *J Allergy Clin Immunol*, 2003, 112(6):1178-84.
Eritsland J, Arnesen H, Gronseth K, et al, "Effect of Dietary Supplementation With N-3 Fatty Acids on Coronary Artery Bypass Graft Patency," *Am J Cardiol*, 1996, 77(1):31-6.
Fenton WS, Dickerson F, Boronow J, et al, "A Placebo-Controlled Trial of Omega-3 Fatty Acid (Ethyl Eicosapentaenoic Acid) Supplementation for Residual Symptoms and Cognitive Impairment in Schizophrenia," *Am J Psychiatry*, 2001, 158(12):2071-4.
Fewtrell MS, Abbott RA, Kennedy K, et al, "Randomized, Double-Blind Trial of Long-Chain Polyunsaturated Fatty Acid Supplementation With Fish Oil and Borage Oil in Preterm Infants," *J Pediatr*, 2004, 144 (4):471-9.
Frasure-Smith N, Lesperance F, and Julien P, "Major Depression Is Associated With Lower Omega-3 Fatty Acid Levels in Patients With Recent Acute Coronary Syndromes," *Biol Psychiatry*, 2004, 55 (9):891-6.
Greenfield SM, Green AT, Teare JP, et al, "A Randomized Controlled Study of Evening Primrose Oil and Fish Oil in Ulcerative Colitis," *Aliment Pharmacol Ther*, 1993, 7(2):159-66.
Harel Z, Biro FM, Kottenhahn RK, et al, "Supplementation With Omega-3 Polyunsaturated Fatty Acids in the Management of Dysmenorrhea in Adolescents," *Am J Obstet Gynecol*, 1996, 174(4):1335-8.
Hawthorne AB, Daneshmend TK, Hawkey CJ, et al, "Fish Oil in Ulcerative Colitis: Final Results of a Controlled Clinical Trial," *Gastroenterology*, 1990, 98(5 pt 2):A174.
Hawthorne AB, Daneshmend TK, Hawkey CJ, et al, "Treatment of Ulcerative Colitis With Fish Oil Supplementation: A Prospective 12 Month Randomised Controlled Trial," *Gut*, 1992, 33(7):922-8.
Henderson WR Jr, Astley SJ, McCready MM, et al, "Oral Absorption of Omega-3 Fatty Acids in Patients With Cystic Fibrosis Who Have Pancreatic Insufficiency and in Healthy Control Subjects," *J Pediatr*, 1994, 124(3):400-8.
Hoffman DR, Birch EE, Birch DG, et al, "Effects of Supplementation With Omega 3 Long-Chain Polyunsaturated Fatty Acids on Retinal and Cortical Development in Premature Infants," *Am J Clin Nutr*, 1993, 57(5 Suppl):807S-812S.
Holub BJ, "Clinical Nutrition: 4. Omega-3 Fatty Acids in Cardiovascular Care," *CMAJ*, 2002, 166 (5):608-15.
Homan van der Heide JJ, Bilo HJ, Donker AJ, et al, "Dietary Supplementation With Fish Oil Modifies Renal Reserve Filtration Capacity in Postoperative, Cyclosporin A-Treated Renal Transplant Recipients," *Transpl Int*, 1990, 3(3):171-5.
Homan van der Heide JJ, Bilo HJ, Donker AJ, et al, "The Effects of Dietary Supplementation With Fish Oil on Renal Function and the Course of Early Postoperative Rejection Episodes in Cyclosorine-Treated Renal Transplant Recipients," *Transplantation*, 1992, 54(2):257-63.
Homan van der Heide JJ, Bilo HJ, Tegzess AM, et al, "Omega-3 Polyunsaturated Fatty Acids Improve Renal Function in Renal Transplant Recipients Treated With Cyclosporin-A," *Kidney Int*, 1989, 35:516A.
Iso H, Rexrode KM, Stampfer MJ, et al, "Intake of Fish and Omega-3 Fatty Acids and Risk of Stroke in Women," *JAMA*, 2001, 285(3):304-12.
Jacka FN, Pasco JA, Henry MJ, et al, "Dietary Omega-3 Fatty Acids and Depression in a Community Sample," *Nutr Neurosci*, 2004, 7(2):101-6.
Joy CB, Mumby-Croft R, and Joy LA, "Polyunsaturated Fatty Acid (Fish or Evening Primrose Oil) for Schizophrenia," *Cochrane Database Syst Rev*, 2000, (2):CD001257.
Judge MP, Harel O, and Lammi-Keefe CJ, "A Docosahexaenoic Acid-Functional Food During Pregnancy Benefits Infant Visual Acuity at Four But Not Six Months of Age," *Lipids*, 2007, 42(2):117-22.
Judge MP, Harel O, and Lammi-Keefe CJ, "Maternal Consumption of a Docosahexaenoic Acid-Containing Functional Food During Pregnancy: Benefit for Infant Performance on Problem-Solving But Not on Recognition Memory Tasks at Age 9 Mo.," *Am J Clin Nutr*, 2007, 85(6):1572-7.
Kalmijn S, van Boxtel MP, Ocke M, et al, "Dietary Intake of Fatty Acids and Fish in Relation to Cognitive Performance at Middle Age," *Neurology*, 2004, 62(2):275-80.
Katz DP, Manner T, Furst P, et al, "The Use of an Intravenous Fish Oil Emulsion Enriched With Omega-3 Fatty Acids in Patients With Cystic Fibrosis," *Nutrition*, 1996, 12(5):334-9.
Klein V, Chajes V, Germain E, et al, "Low Alpha-Linolenic Acid Content of Adipose Breast Tissue Is Associated With an Increased Risk of Breast Cancer," *Eur J Cancer*, 2000, 36(3):335-40.
Koch C, Dölle S, Metzger M, et al, "Docosahexaenoic Acid (DHA) Supplementation in Atopic Eczema: A Randomized, Double-Blind, Controlled Trial," *Br J Dermatol*, 2008, 158(4):786-92.
Kremer JM, "Clinical Studies of Omega-3 Fatty Acid Supplementation in Patients Who Have Rheumatoid Arthritis," *Rheum Dis Clin North Am*, 1991, 17(2):391-402.
Kristensen SD, Schmidt EB, Andersen HR, et al, "Fish Oil in Angina Pectoris," *Atherosclerosis*, 1987, 64 (1):13-9.

Kurlandsky LE, Bennink MR, Webb PM, et al, "The Absorption and Effect of Dietary Supplementation With Omega-3 Fatty Acids on Serum Leukotriene B_4 in Patients With Cystic Fibrosis," *Pediatr Pulmonol*, 1994, 18(4):211-7.
Kyle DJ, Schaefer E, Patton G, et al, "Low Serum Docosahexaenoic Acid Is a Significant Risk Factor for Alzheimer's Dementia," *Lipids*, 1999, 34(Suppl):S245.
Lawrence R and Sorrell T, "Eicosapentaenoic Acid in Cystic Fibrosis: Evidence of a Pathogenetic Role for Leukotriene B_4," *Lancet*, 1993, 342(8869):465-9.
Loeschke K, Ueberschaer B, Pietsch A, et al, "N-3 Fatty Acids Only Delay Early Relapse of Ulcerative Colitis in Remission," *Dig Dis Sci*, 1996, 41(10):2087-94.
Logan AC, "Omega-3 Fatty Acids and Major Depression: A Primer for the Mental Health Professional," *Lipids Health Dis*, 2004, 3:25.
López-Alarcón M, Furuya-Meguro MM, García-Zúñiga PA, et al, "The Effect of Docosahexaenoic Acid on the Loss of Appetite in Pediatric Patients With Pneumonia," *Rev Med Inst Mex Seguro Soc*, 2006, 44 (1):5-11.
Lorenz R and Loeschke K, "Placebo-Controlled Trials of Omega 3 Fatty Acids in Chronic Inflammatory Bowel Disease," *World Rev Nutr Diet*, 1994, 76:143-5.
Lorenz R, Weber PC, Szimnau P, et al, "Supplementation With N-3 Fatty Acids From Fish Oil in Chronic Inflammatory Bowel Disease - A Randomized, Placebo-Controlled, Double-Blind Cross-Over Trial," *J Intern Med Suppl*, 1989, 731:225-32.
Maachi K, Berthoux P, Burgard G, et al, "Results of a 1-Year Randomized Controlled Trial With Omega-3 Fatty Acid Fish Oil in Renal Transplantation Under Triple Immunosuppressive Therapy," *Transplant Proc*, 1995, 27(1):846-9.
Masuev KA, "The Effect of Polyunsaturated Fatty Acids of the Omega-3 Class on the Late Phase of the Allergic Reaction in Bronchial Asthma Patients," *Ter Arkh*, 1997, 69(3):31-3.
McManus RM, Jumpson J, Finegood DT, et al, "A Comparison of the Effects of N-3 Fatty Acids From Linseed Oil and Fish Oil in Well-Controlled Type II Diabetes," *Diabetes Care*, 1996, 19(5):463-7.
Mehrotra B and Ronquillo J, "Dietary Supplementation in Hem/Onc Outpatients at a Tertiary Care Hospital," American Society of Clinical Oncology 38th Annual Meeting, Orlando, Florida, May 18-21, 2002.
Mellor J, Laugharne JD, and Peet M, "Omega-3 Fatty Acid Supplementation in Schizophrenic Patients," *Human Psychopharmacol*, 1996, 11:39-46.
Mihrshahi S, Peat JK, Webb K, et al, "Effect of Omega-3 Fatty Acid Concentrations in Plasma on Symptoms of Asthma at 18 Months of Age," *Pediatr Allergy Immunol*, 2004, 15(6):517-22.
Mischoulon D and Fava M, "Docosahexanoic Acid and Omega-3 Fatty Acids in Depression," *Psychiatr Clin North Am*, 2000, 23(4):785-94.
Mischoulon D, Best-Popescu C, Laposata M, et al, "A Double-Blind Dose-Finding Pilot Study of Docosahexaenoic Acid (DHA) for Major Depressive Disorder," *Eur Neuropsychopharmacol*, 2008, 18 (9):639-45.
Morris MC, Sacks F, and Rosner B, et al, "Does Fish Oil Lower Blood Pressure? A Meta-Analysis of Controlled Trials," *Circulation*, 1993, 88(2):523-33.
Nagakura T, Matsuda S, Shichijyo K, et al, "Dietary Supplementation With Fish Oil Rich in Omega-3 Polyunsaturated Fatty Acids in Children With Bronchial Asthma," *Eur Respir J*, 2000, 16(5):861-5.
Natural Standard Research Collaboration, Chief Editors: Ulbricht C, Basch E, *Natural Standard Herb and Supplement Reference - Evidence-Based Clinical Reviews*, USA: Elsevier/Mosby, 2005.
Nemets B, Osher Y, and Belmaker RH, "Omega-3 Fatty Acids and Augmentation Strategies in Treating Resistant Depression," *Essent Psychopharmacol*, 2004, 6(1):59-64.
Nemets B, Stahl Z, and Belmaker RH, "Addition of Omega-3 Fatty Acid to Maintenance Medication Treatment for Recurrent Unipolar Depressive Disorder," *Am J Psychiatry*, 2002, 159(3):477-9.
Norrish AE, Skeaff CM, Arribas GL, et al, "Prostate Cancer Risk and Consumption of Fish Oils: A Dietary Biomarker-Based Case-Control Study," *Br J Cancer*, 1999, 81(7):1238-42.
O'Keefe JH Jr and Harris WS, "From Inuit to Implementation: Omega-3 Fatty Acids Come of Age," *Mayo Clin Proc*, 2000, 75(6):607-14.
Oddy WH, de Klerk NH, Kendall GE, el al, "Ratio of Omega-6 to Omega-3 Fatty Acids and Childhood Asthma," *J Asthma*, 2004, 41(3):319-26.
Okamoto M, Mitsunobu F, Ashida K, et al, "Effects of Dietary Supplementation With N-3 Fatty Acids Compared With N-6 Fatty Acids on Bronchial Asthma," *Intern Med*, 2000, 39(2):107-11.
Olsen SF and Secher NJ, "Low Consumption of Seafood in Early Pregnancy as a Risk Factor for Preterm Delivery: Prospective Cohort Study," *BMJ*, 2002, 324(7335):447.
Olsen SF, Secher NJ, Tabor A, et al, "Randomised Clinical Trials of Fish Oil Supplementation in High Risk Pregnancies. Fish Oil Trials in Pregnancy (FOTIP) Team," *BJOG*, 2000, 107(3):382-95.
Olsen SF, Sorensen JD, Secher NJ, et al, "Randomised Controlled Trial of Effect of Fish-Oil Supplementation on Pregnancy Duration," *Lancet*, 1992, 339(8800):1003-7.
Onwude JL, Lilford RJ, Hjartardottir H, et al, "A Randomised Double Blind Placebo Controlled Trial of Fish Oil in High Risk Pregnancy," *Br J Obstet Gynaecol*, 1995, 102(2):95-100.
Otto SJ, de Groot RH, and Hornstra G, "Increased Risk of Postpartum Depressive Symptoms Is Associated With Slower Normalization After Pregnancy of the Functional Docosahexaenoic Acid Status," *Prostaglandins Leukot Essent Fatty Acids*, 2003, 69(4):237-43.
Parinyasiri U, Ong-Ajyooth L, Parichatikanond P, et al, "Effect of Fish Oil on Oxidative Stress, Lipid Profile and Renal Function in IgA Nephropathy," *J Med Assoc Thai*, 2004, 87(2):143-9.
Peet M and Mellor J, "Double-Blind Placebo Controlled Trial of N-3 Polyunsaturated Fatty Acids as an Adjunct to Neuroleptics," *Schizophrenia Res*, 1998, 29(1-2):160-1.
Pepe S and McLennan PL, "Cardiac Membrane Fatty Acid Composition Modulates Myocardial Oxygen Consumption and Postischemic Recovery of Contractile Function," *Circulation*, 2002, 105(19):2303-8.
Pritchard BN, Smith CC, Ling KL, et al, "Fish Oils and Cardiovascular Disease," *BMJ*, 1995, 310 (6983):819-20.
Rose DP and Connolly JM, "Omega-3 Fatty Acids as Cancer Chemopreventive Agents," *Pharmacol Ther*, 1999, 83(3):217-44.
Ross E, "The Role of Marine Fish Oils in the Treatment of Ulcerative Colitis," *Nutr Rev*, 1993, 51(2):47-9.
Roy I, Meyer F, Gingras L, et al, "A Double Blind Randomized Controlled Study Comparing the Efficacy of Fish Oil and Low dose ASA to Prevent Coronary Saphenous Vein Graft Obstruction After CABG," *Circulation*, 1991, 84:II-285.
Salvig JD, Olsen SF, and Secher NJ, "Effects of Fish Oil Supplementation in Late Pregnancy on Blood Pressure: A Randomised Controlled Trial," *Br J Obstet Gynaecol*, 1996, 103(6):529-33.
Sellmayer A, Witzgall H, Lorenz RL, et al, "Effects of Dietary Fish Oil on Ventricular Premature Complexes," *Am J Cardiol*, 1995, 76(12):974-7.
Smithers LG, Gibson RA, McPhee A, et al, "Higher Dose of Docosahexaenoic Acid in the Neonatal Period Improves Visual Acuity of Preterm Infants: Results of a Randomized Controlled Trial," *Am J Clin Nutr*, 2008, 88(4):1049-56.
Song MK, Rosenthal MJ, Naliboff BD, et al, "Effects of Bovine Prostate Powder on Zinc, Glucose, and Insulin Metabolism in Old Patients With Non-Insulin-Dependent Diabetes Mellitus," *Metabolism*, 1998, 47(1):39-43.
Stacpoole PW, Alig J, Ammon L, et al, "Dose-Response Effects of Dietary Marine Oil on Carbohydrate and Lipid Metabolism in Normal Subjects and Patients With Hypertriglyceridemia," *Metabolism*, 1989, 38(10):946-56.
Stenson WF, Cort D, Beeken W, et al, "A Trial of Fish Oil Supplemented Diet in Ulcerative Colitis," *Gastroenterology*, 1990, 98(Suppl):A475.
Stenson WF, Cort D, Rodgers J, et al, "Dietary Supplementation With Fish Oil in Ulcerative Colitis," *Ann Intern Med*, 1992, 116(8):609-14.
Stevens LJ, Zentall SS, Deck JL, et al, "Essential Fatty Acid Metabolism in Boys with Attention-Deficit Hyperactivity Disorder," *Am J Clin Nutr*, 1995, 62(4):761-8.
Stoll AL, Severus WE, Freeman MP, et al, "Omega 3 Fatty Acids in Bipolar Disorder: A Preliminary Double-Blind, Placebo-Controlled Trial," *Arch Gen Psychiatry*, 1999, 56(5):407-12.

Stoof TJ, Korstanje MJ, Bilo HJ, et al, "Does Fish Oil Protect Renal Function in Cyclosporin-Treated Psoriasis Patients?" *J Intern Med*, 1989, 226(6):437-41.
Su KP, Huang SY, Chiu CC, et al, "Omega-3 Fatty Acids in Major Depressive Disorder. A Preliminary Double-Blind, Placebo-Controlled Trial," *Eur Neuropsychopharmacol*, 2003, 13(4):267-71.
Sulikowska B, Nieweglowski T, Manitius J, et al, "Effect of 12-Month Therapy With Omega-3 Polyunsaturated Acids on Glomerular Filtration Response to Dopamine in IgA Nephropathy," *Am J Nephrol*, 2004, 24(5):474-82.
Sweny P, Wheeler DC, Lui SF, et al, "Dietary Fish Oil Supplements Preserve Renal Function in Renal Transplant Recipients With Chronic Vascular Rejection," *Nephrol Dial Transplant*, 1989, 4(12):1070-5.
Takwale A, Tan E, Agarwal S, et al, "Efficacy and Tolerability of Borage Oil in Adults and Children With Atopic Eczema: Randomised, Double Blind, Placebo Controlled, Parallel Group Trial," *Br Med J*, 2003, 327(7428):1385.
Tanskanen A, Hibbeln JR, Hintikka J, et al "Fish Consumption, Depression, and Suicidality in a General Population," *Arch Gen Psychiatry*, 2001, 58(5):512-3.
Terry P, Lichtenstein P, Feychting M, et al, "Fatty Fish Consumption and Risk of Prostate Cancer," *Lancet*, 2001, 357(9270):1764-6.
Theobald HE, Goodall AH, Sattar N, et al, "Low-Dose Docosahexaenoic Acid Lowers Diastolic Blood Pressure in Middle-Aged Men and Women," *J Nutr*, 2007, 137(4):973-8.
van der Heide JJ, Bilo HJ, Donker JM, et al, "Effect of Dietary Fish Oil on Renal Function and Rejection in Cyclosporine-Treated Recipients of Renal Transplants," *N Engl J Med*, 1993, 329(11):769-73.
Ventura HO, Milani RV, Lavie CJ, et al, "Cyclosporine-Induced Hypertension. Efficacy of Omega-3 Fatty Acids in Patients After Cardiac Transplantation," *Circulation*, 1993, 88(5 Pt 2):II281-5.
Walton AJ, Snaith ML, Locniskar M, et al, "Dietary Fish Oil and the Severity of Symptoms in Patients With Systemic Lupus Erythematosus," *Ann Rheum Dis*, 1991, 50(7):463-6.
Woodman RJ, Mori TA, Burke V, et al, "Effects of Purified Eicosapentaenoic and Docosahexaenoic Acids on Glycemic Control, Blood Pressure, and Serum Lipids in Type 2 Diabetic Patients With Treated Hypertension," *Am J Clin Nutri*, 2002, 76(5):1007-15.

Dong Quai

Pharmacologic Category Herb

Reported Use

Anemia (Zhu, 1987)
Energy enhancement (particularly in females) (Zhu, 1987)
Hypertension (Zhu, 1987)
Menopause, dysmenorrhea, premenstrual syndrome (PMS), and amenorrhea (Hirata, 1997; Xu, 1981)
  Contradictory study (Hirata,1997)
Menorrhagia (pharmacologic activity)
Phytoestrogen (Lin, 1979)
Pulmonary hypertension (Xu, 1992; Xu, 2000; Zhao, 1990)

Local Anesthetic/Vasoconstrictor Precautions No information available to require special precautions

Effects on Bleeding Has potential for decreasing platelet aggregation and may increase bleeding

Warnings/Precautions Based on potential interference with platelet aggregation (observed with related species), dong quai may alter hemostasis. Based on pharmacologic activity, this herb may be contraindicated in individuals with active bleeding (eg, peptic ulcer, intracranial bleeding). Use with caution in individuals with a history of bleeding, hemostatic disorders, or drug-related hemostatic problems. Use with caution in individuals taking anticoagulant medications, including warfarin, aspirin, aspirin-containing products, NSAIDs, or antiplatelet agents (eg, ticlopidine, clopidogrel, dipyridamole). Discontinue use prior to dental or surgical procedures (generally at least 14 days before).

Use with caution in pregnancy and lactation. May cause photosensitization (Leung, 1996); avoid prolonged exposure to sunlight or other sources of ultraviolet radiation (ie, tanning booths). Based on pharmacologic activity (Zhu, 1987), use with caution in individuals at risk of hypotension or in those who would tolerate hypotension poorly (cerebrovascular or cardiovascular disease). Use with caution in individuals taking antihypertensive medications.

To date, phytoestrogen-containing herbs have not been associated with the negative health effects seen with synthetic estrogen. However, use with caution in individuals on hormone replacement therapy, oral contraceptives, or those with a history of estrogen-dependent tumors, endometrial cancer, thromboembolic disease, or stroke.

References

Chou CT and Kuo SC, "The Anti-Inflammatory and Anti-Hyperuricemic Effects of Chinese Herbal Formula Danggui-Nian-Tong-Tang on Acute Gouty Arthritis: A Comparative Study With Indomethacin and Allopurinol," *Am J Chin Med*, 1995, 23(3-4):261-71.
Hirata JD, Swiersz LM, Zell B, et al, "Does Dong Quai Have Estrogenic Effects in Postmenopausal Women? A Double-Blind, Placebo-Controlled Trial," *Fertil Steril*, 1997, 68(6):981-6.
Leung AY and Foster S, *Encyclopedia of Common Natural Ingredients Used in Foods, Drugs, and Cosmetics*, New York, NY: Wiley, 1996, 32-3.
Lin M, Zhu GD, Sun QM, et al, "Chemical Studies of *Angelica sinensis*," *Yao Hsueh Hsueh Pao*, 1979, 14 (9):529-34.
Lo AC, Chan K, Yeung JH, et al, "Danggui (*Angelica sinensis*) Affects the Pharmacodynamics But Not the Pharmacokinetics of Warfarin in Rabbits," *Eur J Drug Metab Pharmacokinet*, 1995, 20(1):55-60.
Natural Standard Research Collaboration, Chief Editors: Ulbricht C, Basch E, *Natural Standard Herb and Supplement Reference - Evidence-Based Clinical Reviews*, USA: Elsevier/Mosby, 2005.
Page RL 2nd and Lawrence JD, "Potentiation of Warfarin by Dong Quai," *Pharmacotherapy*, 1999, 19 (7):870-6.
Umland EM, Cauffield JS, Kirk JK, et al, "Phytoestrogens As Therapeutic Alternatives to Traditional Hormone Replacement in Postmenopausal Women," *Pharmacotherapy*, 2000, 20(8):981-90.

Xu J and Li G, "Observation on Short-Term Effects of Angelica Injection on Chronic Obstructive Pulmonary Disease Patients With Pulmonary Hypertension," *Zhongguo Zhong Xi Yi Jie He Za Zhi*, 2000, 20(3):187-9.
Xu JY, Li BX, and Cheng SY, "Short-Term Effects of Angelica Sinensis and Nifedipine on Chronic Obstructive Pulmonary Disease in Patients With Pulmonary Hypertension," *Zhongguo Zhong Xi Yi Jie He Za Zhi* , 1992, 12(12):716-8, 707.
Xu LN, Ouyang R, Yin ZZ, et al, "The Effect of Dang-gui (*Angelica sinensis*) and Its Constituent Ferulic Acid on Phagocytosis in Mice," *Yao Hsueh Hsueh Pao*, 1981, 16(6):411-4.
Zhao L, "Prevention of Hypoxic Pulmonary Hypertension With 'Qi-Xue' Injection," *Zhongguo Yi Xue Ke Xue Yuan Xue Bao*, 1990, 12(1):51-5.
Zhu DP, "Dong Quai," *Am J Chin Med*, 1987, 15(3-4):117-25.

Echinacea

Pharmacologic Category Herb

Reported Use

Antibacterial (topical: Boils, abscesses, tonsillitis, poison ivy) (Leung, 1996)
Antiviral (Orinda, 1973)
Arthritis (*E. augustifolia*) (Tubaro, 1987)
Genital herpes (Vonau, 2001)
Immune support (cold and other upper respiratory infections) (Bauer, 1996; Brinkeborn, 1999; Luettig, 1989)
Otitis media (pharmacologic activity)
Radiation-associated leucopenia (Bendel, 1989; Pohl, 1970; Sartor, 1972)
Upper respiratory infection (Schoop, 2006; Shah, 2007; Taylor, 2003)
Uveitis (Neri, 2006)

Local Anesthetic/Vasoconstrictor Precautions No information available to require special precautions

Effects on Bleeding None reported

Warnings/Precautions Based on this agent's pharmacologic activity, use for more than 10 days in acute infections or in immunosuppressed individuals is not recommended (Bradley, 1992). When used as prophylaxis, ingestion should be cycled for 3 weeks on and 1 week off (Brown, 1999). Use with caution in individuals with renal disease or impairment; may cause electrolyte imbalance (Murray, 1995). Use with caution in individuals allergic to members of the *Asteraceae/Compositae* family (ragweed, daisy, aster, chrysanthemum) and other pollens; rare but severe reactions have been reported (Mullins, 1998). Use tinctures cautiously with alcoholic patients and in patients taking disulfiram or metronidazole; many tinctures contain significant concentrations of alcohol (range: 15% to 90%).

References

Barrett B, Brown R, Rakel D, et al, "Echinacea for Treating the Common Cold: A Randomized Trial," *Ann Intern Med*, 2010, 153(12):769-77.
Bauer R, "Echinacea Drugs - Effects and Active Ingredients," *Z Arztl Fortbild (Jena)*, 1996, 90(2):111-5.
Bendel R, Bendel V, Renner K, et al, "Additional Treatment With Esberitox N in Patients With Chemo-Radiotherapy Treatment of Advanced Breast Cancer," *Onkologie*, 1989, 12 Suppl 3:32-8.
Bradley PR, ed, *British Herbal Compendium*, Vol 1, Bournemouth, England: British Herbal Medicine Association, 1992, 81-3.
Brinkeborn RM, Shah DV, and Degenring FH, "Echinaforce and other Echinacea Fresh Plant Preparations in the Treatment of the Common Cold: A Randomized, Placebo Controlled, Double-Blind Clinical Trial," *Phytomedicine*, 1999, 6:1-5.
Brown D, "Echinacea Root Fails to Prevent Upper Respiratory Tract Infections," *HealthNotes Rev Complement Alternative Med*, 1999, 6(1):6-7.
Grimm W and Müller HH, "A Randomized Controlled Trial of the Effect of Fluid Extract of *Echinacea purpurea* on the Incidence and Severity of Colds and Respiratory Infections," *Am J Med*, 1999, 106 (2):138-43.
Hoheisel O, Sandbers M, Bertram S, et al, "Echinacea Root Extracts for the Prevention of Upper Respiratory Tract Infections: A Double-Blind, Placebo Controlled Trial," *Eur J Clin Res*, 1997, 2:261-8.
Leung AY and Foster S, *Encyclopedia of Common Natural Ingredients Used in Foods, Drugs, and Cosmetics*, New York, NY: Wiley, 1996, 216-20.
Luettig B, Steinmuller C, Gifford GE, et al, "Macrophage Activation by the Polysaccharide Arabinogalactan Isolated From Plant Cell Cultures of *Echinacea purpurea*," *Natl Cancer Inst*, 1989, 81(9):669-75.
Mullins RJ, "Echinacea-Associated Anaphylaxis," *Med J Aust*, 1998, 168(4):170-1.
Murray MT, "Echinacea: Pharmacology and Clinical Applications," *Am J Natural Med*, 1995, 2:18-24.
Natural Standard Research Collaboration, Chief Editors: Ulbricht C, Basch E, *Natural Standard Herb and Supplement Reference - Evidence-Based Clinical Reviews*, USA: Elsevier/Mosby, 2005.
Neri PG, Stagni E, Filippello M, et al, "Oral *Echinacea purpurea* Extract in Low-Grade, Steroid-Dependent, Autoimmune Idiopathic Uveitis: A Pilot Study," *J Ocul Pharmacol Ther*, 2006, 22(6):431-6.
Orinda D, Diederich J, and Wacker A, "Antiviral Activity of Components of *Echinacea purpurea*," *Arzneimittelforschung*, 1973, 23(8):1119-20.
Pohl P, "Treatment of Radiation-Induced Leukopenia With Esberitox," *Ther Ggw*, 1970, 109(6):902.
Sartor KJ, "Efficacy of Esberitox in the Treatment of Radiation-Induced Leukopenia," *Ther Ggw*, 1972, 111 (8):1147-50.
Schoop R, Klein P, Suter A, et al, "Echinacea in the Prevention of Induced Rhinovirus Colds: A Meta-Analysis," *Clin Ther*, 2006, 28(2):174-83.
Shah SA, Sander S, White CM, et al, "Evaluation of Echinacea for the Prevention and Treatment of the Common Cold: A Meta-Analysis," *Lancet Infect Dis*, 2007, 7(7):473-80.
Taylor JA, Weber W, Standish L, et al, "Efficacy and Safety of Echinacea in Treating Upper Respiratory Tract Infections in Children: A Randomized Controlled Trial," *JAMA*, 2003, 290(21):2824-30.
Tubaro A, Tragni E, Del Negro P, et al, "Anti-inflammatory Activity of a Polysaccharidic Fraction of *Echinacea angustifolia*," *J Pharm Pharmacol*, 1987, 39(7):567-9.
Vonau B, Chard S, Mandalia S, et al, "Does the Extract of the Plant *Echinacea purpurea* Influence the Clinical Course of Recurrent Genital Herpes?" *Int J STD AIDS*, 2001, 12(3):154-8.

Evening Primrose

Pharmacologic Category Herb

Reported Use
Amenorrhea (pharmacologic activity)
Atopic dermatitis (Berth-Jones, 1993; Humphreys, 1994; Morse, 1989)
Attention-deficit disorder, contradictory studies (Aman, 1987; Arnold, 1989; Colquhoun, 1981)
Bronchitis (combined with thyme) (Gruenwald, 2005; Kemmerich, 2007)
Depression (pharmacologic activity)
Diabetes (van Doormaal, 1988)
Diabetic peripheral neuropathy (Dines, 1995; Keen, 1993)
Eczema, dermatitis, and psoriasis (Horrobin, 1992; Li Wan Po, 1991)
Endometriosis (Horrobin, 1990)
Fatigue (pharmacologic activity)
Fibrocystic breast disease (FBD) (pharmacologic activity)
Hypercholesterolemia (pharmacologic activity)
Ichthyosis vulgaris (Chalmers, 1983)
Irritable bowel syndrome (IBS) (Cotterell, 1990)
Mastalgia (Blommers, 2002; Gateley, 1990; Gateley, 1992; Pashby, 1981)
Menorrhagia (pharmacologic activity)
Multiple sclerosis (Dworkin, 1984)
Obesity (Haslett, 1983)
Omega-6 fatty acid supplementation (pharmacologic activity)
Pre-eclampsia (D'Almeida, 1992; Moodley, 1989)
Premenstrual syndrome (PMS) and menopause (Khoo, 1990)
Raynaud's phenomenon (Belch, 1985; Belch, 1986)
Rheumatoid arthritis (Horrobin, 1992; Li Wan Po, 1991)
Rosacea (pharmacologic activity)
Scleroderma (pharmacologic activity)

Local Anesthetic/Vasoconstrictor Precautions No information available to require special precautions

Effects on Bleeding May see increased bleeding due to inhibition of platelet aggregation

Warnings/Precautions Evening primrose oil may lower seizure threshold (based on animal studies); use is contraindicated in individuals with seizure disorders, schizophrenia, or in individuals receiving anticonvulsant or antipsychotic medications (based on evidence from human studies) (Dines, 1995; Miller, 1998; Vaddadi, 1981).

May inhibit platelet aggregation (De La Cruz, 1997). Based on pharmacologic activity, this herb may be contraindicated in individuals with active bleeding (eg, peptic ulcer, intracranial bleeding). Use with caution in individuals with a history of bleeding, hemostatic disorders, or drug-related hemostatic problems. Use with caution in individuals taking anticoagulant medications, including warfarin, aspirin, aspirin-containing products, NSAIDs, or antiplatelet agents (eg, ticlopidine, clopidogrel, dipyridamole). Discontinue use prior to dental or surgical procedures (generally at least 14 days before).

Based on pharmacologic activity, it may alter glucose regulation. Use with caution in individuals with diabetes or in those who may be predisposed to hypoglycemia. Effects of drugs with hypoglycemic activity may be potentiated (including insulin and oral hypoglycemics). Blood sugar should be closely monitored, and the dosage of hypoglycemic medications may require adjustment. This should be carefully coordinated among the individual's healthcare providers.

Based on pharmacologic activity, use caution in individuals at risk of hypotension (including those taking antihypertensive medication or agents that predispose to orthostasis), elderly individuals, or those who would not tolerate transient hypotensive episodes (ie, cerebrovascular or cardiovascular disease). May potentiate antihypertensive effects.

References

Aman MG, Mitchell EA, and Turbott SH, "The Effects of Essential Fatty Acid Supplementation by Efamol in Hyperactive Children," *J Abnorm Child Psychol*, 1987, 15(1):75-90.
Arnold LE, Kleykamp D, Votolato NA, et al, "Gamma-Linolenic Acid for Attention-Deficit Hyperactivity Disorder: Placebo-Controlled Comparison to D-Amphetamine," *Biol Psychiatry*, 1989, 25(2):222-8.
Belch JJ, Shaw B, O'Dowd A, et al, "Evening Primrose Oil (Efamol) as a Treatment for Cold-Induced Vasospasm (Raynaud's Phenomenon)," *Pre Lipid Res*, 1986, 25:335-40.
Belch JJ, Shaw B, O'Dowd A, et al, "Evening Primrose Oil (Efamol) in the Treatment of Raynaud's Phenomenon: A Double Blind Study," *Thromb Haemost*, 1985, 54(2):490-4.
Berth-Jones J and Graham-Brown RA, "Placebo-Controlled Trial of Essential Fatty Acid Supplementation in Atopic Dermatitis," *Lancet*, 1993, 341(8860):1557-60.
Blommers J, de Lange-De Klerk ES, and Kuik DJ, "Evening Primrose Oil and Fish Oil for Severe Chronic Mastalgia: A Randomized, Double-Blind, Controlled Trial," *Am J Obstet Gynecol*, 2002, 187(5):1389-94.
Chalmers RJ and Shuster S, "Evening Primrose Seed Oil in Ichthyosis Vulgaris," *Lancet*, 1983, 1 (8318):236-7.
Colquhoun I and Bunday S, "A Lack of Essential Fatty Acids as a Possible Cause of Hyperactivity in Children," *Med Hypotheses*, 1981, 7(5):673-9.
Cotterell JC, Lee AJ, and Hunter JO, "Double-Blind Cross-Over Trial of Evening Primrose Oil in Women With Menstrually-Related Irritable Bowel Syndrome," *Omega-6 Essential Fatty Acids: Pathophysiology and Roles in Clinical Medicine*, Horrobin DF, ed, New York, NY: Wiley-Liss, 1990, 421-6.

D'Almeida A, Carter JP, Anatol A, et al, "Effects of a Combination of Evening Primrose Oil (Gamma Linolenic Acid) and Fish Oil (Eicosapentaenoic + Docahexaenoic Acid) Versus Magnesium, and Versus Placebo in Preventing Pre-Eclampsia," *Women Health*, 1992, 19(2-3):117-31.
De La Cruz JP, Martin-Romero M, Carmona JA, et al, "Effect of Evening Primrose Oil on Platelet Aggregation in Rabbits Fed an Atherogenic Diet," *Thromb Res*, 1997, 87(1):141-9.
Dines CD, Cotter MA, and Cameron NE, "Nerve Function in Galactosaemic Rats: Effects of Evening Primrose Oil and Doxazosin," *Eur J Pharmacol*, 1995, 281(3):303-9.
Dworkin RH, Bates D, Millar JH, et al, "Linoleic Acid and Multiple Sclerosis: A Reanalysis of Three Double-Blind Trials," *Neurology*, 1984, 34(11):1441-5.
Gateley CA, Maddox PR, Mansel RE, et al, "Mastalgia Refractory to Drug Treatment," *Br J Surg*, 1990, 77 (10):1110-2.
Gateley CA, Maddox PR, Pritchard GA, et al, "Plasma Fatty Acid Profiles in Benign Breast Disorders," *Br J Surg*, 1992, 79(5):407-9.
Gruenwald J, Graubaum HJ, and Busch R, "Efficacy and Tolerability of a Fixed Combination of Thyme and Primrose Root in Patients With Acute Bronchitis. A Double-Blind, Randomized, Placebo-Controlled Clinical Trial," *Arzneimittelforschung*, 2005, 55(11):669-76.
Haslett C, Douglas JG, Chalmers SR, et al, "A Double-Blind Evaluation of Evening Primrose Oil as an Antiobesity Agent," *Int J Obes*, 1983, 7(6):549-53.
Horrobin DF, "Gamma-Linolenic Acid; An Intermediate in Essential Fatty Acid Metabolism With Potential as an Ethical Pharmaceutical and as a Food," *Rev Contemp Pharmacother*, 1990:1-45.
Horrobin DF, "Nutritional and Medical Importance of Gamma-Linoleic Acid," *Prog Lipid Res*, 1992, 31 (2):163-94.
Humphreys F, Symons J, Brown H, et al, "The Effects of Gamolenic Acid on Adult Atopic Eczema and Premenstrual Exacerbation of Eczema," *Eur J Dermatol*, 1994, 4(598):603.
Keen H, Payan J, Allawi J, et al, "Treatment of Diabetic Neuropathy With Gamma-Linolenic Acid. The Gamma-Linolenic Acid Multicenter Trial Group," *Diabetes Care*, 1993, 16(1):8-15.
Kemmerich B, "Evaluation of Efficacy and Tolerability of a Fixed Combination of Dry Extracts of Thyme Herb and Primrose Root in Adults Suffering From Acute Bronchitis With Productive Cough. A Prospective, Double-Blind, Placebo-Controlled Multicentre Clinical Trial," *Arzneimittelforschung*, 2007, 57(9):607-15.
Khoo SK, Munro C, and Battistutta D, "Evening Primrose Oil and Treatment of Premenstrual Syndrome," *Med J Aust*, 1990, 153(4):189-92.
Li Wan Po A, "Evening Primrose Oil," *Pharm J*, 1991, 246:670-6.
Miller LG, "Herbal Medicinals: Selected Clinical Considerations Focusing on Known or Potential Drug-Herb Interactions," *Arch Intern Med*, 1998, 158(20):2200-11.
Moodley J and Norman RJ, "Attempts at Dietary Alteration of Prostaglandin Pathways in the Management of Pre-Eclampsia," *Prostaglandins Leukot Essent Fatty Acids*, 1989, 37(3):145-7.
Morse PF, Horrobin DF, Manku MS, et al, "Meta-Analysis of Placebo-Controlled Studies of the Efficacy of Epogam in the Treatment of Atopic Eczema. Relationship Between Plasma Essential Fatty Acid Changes and Clinical Response," *Br J Dermatol*, 1989, 121(1):75-90.
Natural Standard Research Collaboration, Chief Editors: Ulbricht C, Basch E, *Natural Standard Herb and Supplement Reference - Evidence-Based Clinical Reviews*, USA: Elsevier/Mosby, 2005.
Pashby N, Mansel R, Hughes L, et al, "A Clinical Trial of Evening Primrose in Mastalgia," *Br J Surg*, 1981, 68:801.
Vaddadi KS, "The Use of Gamma-Linolenic Acid and Linoleic Acid to Differentiate Between Temporal Lobe Epilepsy and Schizophrenia," *Prostaglandins Med*, 1981, 6(4):375-9.
van Doormaal JJ, Idema IG, Muskiet FA, et al, "Effects of Short-Term High Dose Intake of Evening Primrose Oil on Plasma and Cellular Fatty Acid Compositions, Alpha-Tocopherol Levels, and Erythropoiesis in Normal and Type 1 (Insulin-Dependent) Diabetic Men," *Diabetologia*, 1988, 31(8):576-84.

Fennel

Pharmacologic Category Herb

Reported Use

ACE inhibitor-associated cough (Arya, 1999)
Colic, infantile (Alexandrovich, 2003; Weizman, 1993)
Dysmenorrhea (Modaress Nejad, 2006; Namavar, 2003)
Ultraviolet skin protection (Dres, 1999)

Local Anesthetic/Vasoconstrictor Precautions No information available to require special precautions

Effects on Bleeding May see increased bleeding

Warnings/Precautions Use with caution in individuals with diabetes or in those taking antidiabetic agents. Fennel preparations, other than fennel seed infusions and fennel honey, should be avoided in infants and toddlers. Use with caution in individuals with a history of bleeding, hemostatic disorders, or drug-related hemostatic problems. Use with caution in individuals taking anticoagulant medications, including warfarin, aspirin, aspirin-containing products, NSAIDs, or antiplatelet agents (eg, ticlopidine, clopidogrel, dipyridamole). Discontinue use prior to dental or surgical procedures (generally at least 14 days before). Use cautiously in patients with celery, carrot, or mugwort allergy (risk of cross sensitivity).

References

Alexandrovich I, Rakovitskaya O, Kolmo E, et al, "The Effect of Fennel (*Foeniculum vulgare*) Seed Oil Emulsion in Infantile Colic: A Randomized, Placebo-Controlled Study," *Altern Ther Health Med*, 2003, 9 (4):58-61.
Arya S, "Controlling Angiotensin-Converting-Enzyme-Inhibitor Induced Cough by Fennel Fruit," *Indian J Pharmacol*, 1999, 31(2):159.
Dres C, Johnson C, and Loda L, "Enzymes and Erythema Reduction," *SPC*, 1999, 71(313):33.
Modaress Nejad V and Asadipour M, "Comparison of the Effectiveness of Fennel and Mefenamic Acid on Pain Intensity in Dysmenorrhoea," *East Mediterr Health J*, 2006, 12(3-4):423-7.
Namavar JB, Tartifizadeh A, and Khabnadideh S, "Comparison of Fennel and Mefenamic Acid for the Treatment of Primary Dysmenorrhea," *Int J Gynaecol Obstet*, 2003, 80(2):153-7.
Natural Standard Research Collaboration, Chief Editors: Ulbricht C, Basch E, *Natural Standard Herb and Supplement Reference - Evidence-Based Clinical Reviews*, USA: Elsevier/Mosby, 2005.
Weizman Z, Alkrinawi S, Goldfarb D, et al, "Efficacy of Herbal Tea Preparation in Infantile Colic," *J Pediatr*, 1993, 122(4):650-2.

Feverfew

Pharmacologic Category Herb

Reported Use

Anti-inflammatory, rheumatoid arthritis (Pattrick, 1989)
Migraine headache (preventive) (Diener, 2005; Johnson, 1985)
Muscle soreness (pharmacologic activity)

Local Anesthetic/Vasoconstrictor Precautions No information available to require special precautions

Effects on Bleeding May see increased bleeding due to inhibition of platelet aggregation

Warnings/Precautions Use of feverfew is contraindicated in pregnancy (animal data suggests emmenagogue activity) (Bradley, 1992) or in individuals with allergies to members of the *Asteraceae/Compositae* family (chrysanthemum, daisy). The onset of feverfew's effects may be delayed for several weeks. Abrupt discontinuation may increase migraine frequency, rebound headaches, and anxiety. A "post-feverfew syndrome" has been described, including nervousness, insomnia, joint stiffness, and pain which may occur following discontinuation in some individuals.

Pharmacologic activity may include inhibition of platelet aggregation (Makheja, 1982). Based on pharmacologic activity, this herb may be contraindicated in individuals with active bleeding (eg, peptic ulcer, intracranial bleeding). Use with caution in individuals with a history of bleeding, hemostatic disorders, or drug-related hemostatic problems. Use with caution in individuals taking anticoagulant medications, including warfarin, aspirin, aspirin-containing products, NSAIDs, or antiplatelet agents (eg, ticlopidine, clopidogrel, dipyridamole). Discontinue use prior to dental or surgical procedures (generally at least 14 days before).

This herb may also cause gastrointestinal upset and irritation of oral mucosa/tongue.

Feverfew may increase the risk of photosensitivity. Use caution in individuals taking photosensitizing agents.

References

Bradley PR, ed, *British Herbal Compendium*, Vol 1, Bournemouth, England: British Herbal Medicine Association, 1992, 96-8.
Diener HC, Pfaffenrath V, Schnitker J, et al, "Efficacy and Safety of 6.25 mg t.i.d. Feverfew CO2-Extract (MIG-99) in Migraine Prevention - A Randomized, Double-Blind, Multicentre, Placebo-Controlled Study," *Cephalalgia*, 2005, 25(11):1031-41.
Johnson ES, Kadam NP, Hylands DM, et al, "Efficacy of Feverfew as Prophylactic Treatment of Migraine," *Br Med J (Clin Res Ed)*, 1985, 291(6495):569-73.
Makheja AN and Bailey JM, "A Platelet Phospholipase Inhibitor From the Medicinal Herb Feverfew (*Tanacetum parthenium*)," *Prostaglandins Leukot Med*, 1982, 8(6):653-60.
Natural Standard Research Collaboration, Chief Editors: Ulbricht C, Basch E, *Natural Standard Herb and Supplement Reference - Evidence-Based Clinical Reviews*, USA: Elsevier/Mosby, 2005.
Newall CA, Anderson LA, and Phillipson JD, *Herbal Medicines: A Guide for Health Care Professionals*, London, England: The Pharmaceutical Press, 1996, 119-21.
Pattrick M, Heptinstall S, and Doherty M, "Feverfew in Rheumatoid Arthritis: A Double-Blind Placebo Controlled Study," *Ann Rheum Dis*, 1989, 48(7):547-49.

Flaxseed Oil

Pharmacologic Category Nutraceutical

Reported Use

Acne vulgaris (pharmacologic activity)
Arthritis (rheumatoid) (pharmacologic activity)
Asthma (pharmacologic activity)
Attention deficit hyperactivity disorder (ADHD) (Joshi, 2006)
Constipation (pharmacologic activity)
Coronary heart disease (risk reduction) (O'Keefe, 2000)
Diabetes (Glauber, 1988; Nestel, 1997)
Dry eyes (Sjogren's syndrome) (Pinheiro, 2007)
Hemorrhoids (pharmacologic activity)
Hyperlipidemia (Singer, 1990)
Hypertension (pharmacologic activity)
Menopausal symptoms (Lemay, 2002)
Multiple sclerosis (pharmacologic activity)
Omega-3 essential fatty acid source (cell wall and cellular membrane structure; cholesterol transport and oxidation) (pharmacologic activity)
Premenstrual syndrome (PMS) (pharmacologic activity)
Prostaglandins production (Sinclair, 1984)
Psoriasis (pharmacologic activity)
Stroke (risk reduction) (Iso, 2001)
Systemic lupus erythematosus (SLE) (pharmacologic activity)

Local Anesthetic/Vasoconstrictor Precautions No information available to require special precautions

Effects on Bleeding None reported

Warnings/Precautions Use with caution in individuals with a history of bleeding, hemostatic disorders, or drug-related hemostatic problems. Use with caution in individuals taking anticoagulant medications, including warfarin, aspirin, aspirin-containing products, NSAIDs, or antiplatelet agents (eg, ticlopidine, clopidogrel, dipyridamole) based on trial evidence; however, no clinical cases are reported in the available literature. Discontinue use prior to dental or surgical procedures (generally at least 14 days before).

Use with caution in individuals with diabetes or in those who may be predisposed to hypoglycemia; may alter glucose regulation. Effects of drugs with hypoglycemic activity may be potentiated (including insulin and oral hypoglycemics). Blood sugar should be closely monitored, and the dosage of hypoglycemic medications may require adjustment. This should be carefully coordinated among the individuals' healthcare providers.

Use with caution in individuals using antihypertensive agents. Flaxseed oil may lower blood pressure and have additive effects. Use with caution in individuals using laxatives; flaxseed oil may enhance the laxative effects. Use with caution in individuals using lithium because flaxseed may increase episodes of mania and in individuals using oral contraceptives or hormone replacement therapy; may interact with these agents.

References

Arjmandi BH, Khan DA, Juma S, et al, "Whole Flaxseed Consumption Lowers Serum LDL-Cholesterol and Lipoprotein (a) Concentrations in Postmenopausal Women," *Nutrit Res*, 1998, 18(7):1203-14.
Bougnoux P, Koscielny S, Chajes V, et al, "Alpha-Linolenic Acid Content of Adipose Breast Tissue: A Host Determinant of the Risk of Early Metastasis in Breast Cancer," *Br J Cancer*, 1994, 70(2):330-4.
Clark WF and Parbtani A, "Omega-3 Fatty Acid Supplementation in Clinical and Experimental Lupus Nephritis," *Am J Kidney Dis*, 1994, 23(5):644-7.
Clark WF, Kortas C, Heidenheim AP, et al, "Flaxseed in Lupus Nephritis: A Two-Year Nonplacebo-Controlled Crossover Study," *J Am Coll Nutr*, 2001, 20(2 Suppl):143-8.
Clark WF, Parbtani A, Huff MW, et al, "Flaxseed: A Potential Treatment for Lupus Nephritis," *Kidney Int*, 1995, 48(2):475-80.
Cunnane SC, Ganguli S, Menard C, et al, "High Alpha-Linolenic Acid Flaxseed (*Linum usitatissimum*): Some Nutritional Properties in Humans," *Br J Nutr*, 1993, 69(2):443-53.
Cunnane SC, Hamadeh MJ, Liede AC, et al, "Nutritional Attributes of Traditional Flaxseed in Healthy Young Adults," *Am J Clin Nutr*, 1995, 61(1):62-8.
Glauber H, Wallace P, Griver K, et al, "Adverse Metabolic Effect of Omega-3 Fatty Acids in Non-Insulin-Dependent Diabetes Mellitus," *Ann Intern Med*, 1988, 108(5):663-8.
Goss PE, Li T, Theriault M, et al, "Effects of Dietary Flaxseed in Women With Cyclical Mastalgia," *Breast Cancer Res Treat*, 2000, 64:49.
Haggans CJ, Travelli EJ, Thomas W, et al, "The Effect of Flaxseed and Wheat Bran Consumption on Urinary Estrogen Metabolites in Premenopausal Women," *Cancer Epidemiol Biomarkers Prev*, 2000, 9 (7):719-25.
Hutchins AM, Martini MC, Olson BA, et al, "Flaxseed Consumption Influences Endogenous Hormone Concentrations in Postmenopausal Women," *Nutr Cancer*, 2001, 39(1):58-65.
Iso H, Rexrode KM, Stampfer MJ, et al, "Intake of Fish and Omega-3 Fatty Acids and Risk of Stroke in Women," *JAMA*, 2001, 285(3):304-12.
Jenkins DJ, Kendall CW, Vidgen E, et al, "Health Aspects of Partially Defatted Flaxseed, Including Effects on Serum Lipids, Oxidative Measures, and *ex vivo* Androgen and Progestin Activity: A Controlled Crossover Trial," *Am J Clin Nutr*, 1999, 69(3):395-402.
Lemay A, Dodin S, Kadri N, et al, "Flaxseed Dietary Supplement Versus Hormone Replacement Therapy in Hypercholesterolemic Menopausal Women," *Obstet Gynecol*, 2002, 100(3):495-504.
Lin X, Gingrich JR, Bao W, et al, "Effect of Flaxseed Supplementation on Prostatic Carcinoma in Transgenic Mice," *Urology*, 2002, 60(5):919-24.
Lucas EA, Wild RD, Hammond LJ, et al, "Flaxseed Improves Lipid Profile Without Altering Biomarkers of Bone Metabolism in Postmenopausal Women," *J Clin Endocrinol Metab*, 2002, 87(4):1527-32.
Natural Standard Research Collaboration, Chief Editors: Ulbricht C, Basch E, *Natural Standard Herb and Supplement Reference - Evidence-Based Clinical Reviews*, USA: Elsevier/Mosby, 2005.
Nestel PJ, Pomeroy SE, Sasahara T, et al, "Arterial Compliance in Obese Subjects Is Improved With Dietary Plant N-3 Fatty Acid From Flaxseed Oil Despite Increased LDL Oxidizability," *Arterioscler Thromb Vasc Biol*, 1997, 17(6):1163-70.
O'Keefe JH Jr and Harris WS, "From Inuit to Implementation: Omega-3 Fatty Acids Come of Age," *Mayo Clin Proc*, 2000, 75(6):607-14.
Phipps WR, Martini MC, Lampe JW, et al, "Effect of Flax Seed Ingestion on the Menstrual Cycle," *J Clin Endocrinol Metab*, 1993, 77(5):1215-9.
Plu-Bureau G, Thalabard JC, Sitruk-Ware R, et al, "Cyclical Mastalgia as a Marker of Breast Cancer Susceptibility: Results of a Case-Control Study Among French Women," *Br J Cancer*, 1992, 65 (6):945-9.
Sinclair HM, "Essential Fatty Acids in Perspective," *Hum Nutr Clin Nutr*, 1984, 38(4):245-60.
Singer P, Jaeger W, Berger I, et al, "Effects of Dietary Oleic, Linoleic and Alpha-Linolenic Acids on Blood Pressure, Serum Lipids, Lipoproteins and the Formation of Eicosanoid Precursors in Patients With Mild Essential Hypertension," *J Hum Hypertens*, 1990, 4(3):227-33.
Tarpila S, Aro A, Salminen I, et al, "The Effect of Flaxseed Supplementation in Processed Foods on Serum Fatty Acids and Enterolactone," *Eur J Clin Nutr*, 2002, 56(2):157-65.

Gamma Linolenic Acid

Pharmacologic Category Nutraceutical

Reported Use

Acute respiratory distress syndrome (Gadek, 1999; Pacht, 2003)
Atopic dermatitis (Takwale, 2003; van Gool, 2003)
Attention-deficit hyperactivity disorder (ADHD) (Stevens, 2003)
Blood pressure control (Deferne, 1992; Deferne, 1996; Leng, 1998)
Cancer treatment (adjunct) (McIllmurray, 1987)
Diabetic neuropathy (Jamal, 1986; Keen 1993)
Immune enhancement (Miles, 2004; Wu, 1999)
Mastalgia (Goyal, 2005)

Menopausal hot flashes (Chenoy, 1994)
Migraine (Wagner, 1997)
Osteoporosis (Kruger, 1998)
Pre-eclampsia (D'Almeida, 1992)
Premenstrual syndrome (PMS) (Puolakka, 1985)
Pruritus (Yoshimoto-Furuie, 1999)
Rheumatoid arthritis (Belch, 1988; Leventhal, 1993; Zurier, 1996)
Sjogren's syndrome (Manthorpe, 1984)
Ulcerative colitis (Middleton, 2002)

Local Anesthetic/Vasoconstrictor Precautions No information available to require special precautions

Effects on Bleeding None reported

Warnings/Precautions High doses may cause gastrointestinal upset, loose stools, and nausea.

Contraindicated in individuals with active bleeding (eg, peptic ulcer, intracranial bleeding). Use with caution in individuals with a history of bleeding, hemostatic disorders, or drug-related hemostatic problems. Use with caution in individuals taking anticoagulant medications, including warfarin, aspirin, aspirin-containing products, NSAIDs, or antiplatelet agents (eg, ticlopidine, clopidogrel, dipyridamole). Discontinue use prior to dental or surgical procedures (generally at least 14 days before).

References

Belch JJ, Ansell D, Madhok R, et al, "Effects of Altering Dietary Essential Fatty Acids on Requirements for Non-Steroidal Anti-Inflammatory Drugs in Patients With Rheumatoid Arthritis: A Double Blind Placebo Controlled Study," *Ann Rheum Dis*, 1988, 47(2):96-104.

Chenoy R, Hussain S, Tayob Y, et al, "Effect of Oral Gamolenic Acid From Evening Primrose Oil on Menopausal Flushing," *BMJ*, 1994, 308(6927):501-3.

D'Almeida A, Carter JP, Anatol A, et al, "Effects of a Combination of Evening Primrose Oil (Gamma Linolenic Acid) and Fish Oil (Eicosapentaenoic + Docahexaenoic Acid) Versus Magnesium, and Versus Placebo in Preventing Pre-Eclampsia," *Women Health*, 1992, 19(2-3):117-31.

Deferne JL and Leeds AR, "Resting Blood Pressure and Cardiovascular Reactivity to Mental Arithmetic in Mild Hypertensive Males Supplemented With Blackcurrant Seed Oil," *J Hum Hypertens*, 1996, 10 (8):531-7.

Deferne JL and Leeds AR, "The Antihypertensive Effect of Dietary Supplementation With a 6-Desaturated Essential Fatty Acid Concentrate as Compared With Sunflower Seed Oil," *J Hum Hypertens*, 1992, 6 (2):113-9.

Gadek JE, DeMichele SJ, Karlstad MD, et al, "Effect of Enteral Feeding With Eicosapentaenoic Acid, Gamma-Linolenic Acid, and Antioxidants in Patients With Acute Respiratory Distress Syndrome. Enteral Nutrition in ARDS Study Group," *Crit Care Med*, 1999, 27(8):1409-20.

Goyal A, Mansel RE, and Efamast Study Group, "A Randomized Multicenter Study of Gamolenic Acid (Efamast) With and Without Antioxidant Vitamins and Minerals in the Management of Mastalgia," *Breast J*, 2005, 11(1):41-7.

Jamal GA, Carmichael H and Weir AI, "Gamma-Linolenic Acid in Diabetic Neuropathy," *Lancet* , 1986, 1 (8489):1098.

Keen H, Payan J, Allawi J, et al, "Treatment of Diabetic Neuropathy With Gamma-Linolenic Acid. The Gamma-Linolenic Acid Multicenter Trial Group," *Diabetes Care*, 1993, 16(1):8-15.

Kruger MC, Coetzer H, de Winter R, et al, "Calcium, Gamma-Linolenic Acid and Eicosapentaenoic Acid Supplementation in Senile Osteoporosis," *Aging (Milano)*, 1998, 10(5):385-94.

Leng GC, Lee AJ, Fowkes FG, et al, "Randomized Controlled Trial of Gamma-Linolenic Acid and Eicosapentaenoic Acid in Peripheral Arterial Disease," *Clin Nutr*, 1998, 17(6):265-71.

Leventhal LJ, Boyce EG, and Zurier RB, "Treatment of Rheumatoid Arthritis With Gammalinolenic Acid," *Ann Intern Med*, 1993, 119(9):867-73.

Manthorpe R, Hagen Petersen S, and Prause JU, "Primary Sjogren's Syndrome Treated With Efamol/Efavit. A Double-Blind Cross-Over Investigation," *Rheumatol Int*, 1984, 4(4):165-7.

The Mayo Clinic, "Dermatomyositis," 2009. Available at: http://www.mayoclinic.com/health/dermatomyositis.

McIllmurray MB and Turkie W, "Controlled Trial of Gamma Linolenic Acid in Duke's C Colorectal Cancer," *Br Med J (Clin Res Ed)*, 1987, 16;294(6582):1260.

Middleton SJ, Naylor S, Woolner J, et al, "A Double-Blind, Randomized, Placebo-Controlled Trial of Essential Fatty Acid Supplementation in the Maintenance of Remission of Ulcerative Colitis," *Aliment Pharmacol Ther*, 2002, 16(6):1131-5.

Miles EA, Banerjee T, Dooper MM, et al, "The Influence of Different Combinations of Gamma-Linolenic Acid, Stearidonic Acid and EPA on Immune Function in Healthy Young Male Subjects," *Br J Nutr*, 2004, 91(6):893-903.

Natural Standard Research Collaboration, Chief Editors: Ulbricht C, Basch E, *Natural Standard Herb and Supplement Reference - Evidence-Based Clinical Reviews*, USA: Elsevier/Mosby, 2005.

Pacht ER, DeMichele SJ, Nelson JL, et al, "Enteral Nutrition With Eicosapentaenoic Acid, Gamma-Linolenic Acid, and Antioxidants Reduces Alveolar Inflammatory Mediators and Protein Influx in Patients With Acute Respiratory Distress Syndrome," *Crit Care Med*, 2003, 31(2):491-500.

Puolakka J, Makarainen L, Viinikka L, et al, "Biochemical and Clinical Effects of Treating the Premenstrual Syndrome With Prostaglandin Synthesis Precursors," *J Reprod Med*, 1985, 30(3):149-53.

Stevens L, Zhang W, Peck L, et al, "EFA Supplementation in Children With Inattention, Hyperactivity, and Other Disruptive Behaviors," *Lipids*, 2003, 38(10):1007-21

Takwale A, Tan E, Agarwal S, et al, "Efficacy and Tolerability of Borage Oil in Adults and Children With Atopic Eczema: Randomised, Double Blind, Placebo Controlled, Parallel Group Trial," *BMJ*, 2003, 327 (7428):1385.

van Gool CJ, Thijs C, Henquet CJ, et al, "Gamma-Linolenic Acid Supplementation for Prophylaxis of Atopic Dermatitis - A Randomized Controlled Trial in Infants at High Familial Risk," *Am J Clin Nutr* , 2003, 77(4):943-51.

Wagner W and Nootbaar-Wagner U, "Prophylactic Treatment of Migraine With Gamma-Linolenic and Alpha-Linolenic Acids," *Cephalalgia*, 1997, 17(2):127-30.

Wu D, Meydani M, Leka LS, et al, "Effect of Dietary Supplementation With Black Currant Seed Oil on the Immune Response of Healthy Elderly Subjects," *Am J Clin Nutr*, 1999, 70(4):536-43.

Yoshimoto-Furuie K, Yoshimoto K, Tanaka T, et al, "Effects of Oral Supplementation With Evening Primrose Oil for Six Weeks on Plasma Essential Fatty Acids and Uremic Skin Symptoms in Hemodialysis Patients," *Nephron*, 1999, 81(2):151-9.

Zurier RB, Rossetti RG, Jacobson EW, et al, "Gamma-Linolenic Acid Treatment of Rheumatoid Arthritis. A Randomized, Placebo-Controlled Trial," *Arthritis Rheum*, 1996, 39(11):1808-17.

Garlic

Pharmacologic Category Herb

Reported Use

Alopecia (Hajheydari, 2007)

Antimicrobial (bacterial and fungal) (Adetumbi, 1983; Pai, 1995); *Helicobacter pylori* infection (contradictory studies) (Graham, 1999; McNulty, 2001); Tinea pedis (Ledezma, 1999)

Antioxidant (practitioners should be aware that aged garlic extracts have been reported to improve this benefit) (Munday, 1999; Steiner, 1996)

Atherosclerosis (Orekhov, 1996; Siegel, 2000; Siegel 2001)

Cancer (prevention) (Buiatti, 1989; Cook-Mozaffari, 1979; Dorant, 1995; Dorant, 1996; Gail, 1998; Gao, 1999; Ishikawa, 2006; Levi, 1993; Shu, 1993; Steinmatz, 1994; Swanson, 1992; Takezaki, 1999; Tanaka, 2006; Wang, 1990; Witte, 1996; You, 1998)

Coagulation (mild inhibitor of platelet-activating factor) (Bordia, 1998)

Cryptococcal meningitis (Anonymous, 1980)

Cutaneous microcirculation (Jung, 1991)

Diabetes (contradictory study) (Sitprija, 1987)

Hyperlipidemia (Ackermann, 2001; Agarwal, 1996; Bordia, 1981; Kojuri, 2007; Mulrow, 2000; Neil, 1996; Simons, 1995; Steiner, 1996)

Contradictory studies: See Summary (Bertold, 1998; Byrne, 1999; Gardner, 2007; Isaacsohn, 1998)

Hypertension (Ernst, 1987; Neil, 1996; Silagy, 1994)

Immune support (Salman, 1999)

Peripheral vascular disease (Czerny, 1996; Jepson, 2001; Jung, 1991; Jung, 1991; Kiesewetter, 1993)

Tick repellant (Stjernberg, 2000)

Upper respiratory tract infection (Andrianova, 2003; Josling, 2001)

Local Anesthetic/Vasoconstrictor Precautions No information available to require special precautions

Effects on Bleeding May see increased bleeding due to potent platelet inhibition

Warnings/Precautions Garlic may cause GI distress or irritation in some individuals during the initiation of therapy.

Garlic has *in vitro* effects on platelet aggregation (Kiesewetter, 1993) and has been associated with reports of bleeding. Based on pharmacologic activity, this herb may be contraindicated in individuals with active bleeding (eg, peptic ulcer, intracranial bleeding). Use with caution in individuals with a history of bleeding, hemostatic disorders, or drug-related hemostatic problems and in individuals taking anticoagulant medications, including warfarin, aspirin, aspirin-containing products, NSAIDs, or antiplatelet agents (eg, ticlopidine, clopidogrel, dipyridamole). Discontinue use prior to dental or surgical procedures (generally at least 14 days before).

Based on pharmacologic activity, use caution in individuals at risk of hypotension (including those taking antihypertensive medication or agents that predispose to orthostasis), elderly individuals, or those who would not tolerate transient hypotensive episodes (ie, cerebrovascular or cardiovascular disease); may potentiate effects of antihypertensives.

Use with caution in individuals with diabetes or in those who may be predisposed to hypoglycemia; pharmacologic activity may alter glucose regulation. Effects of drugs with hypoglycemic activity may be potentiated (including insulin and oral hypoglycemics). Blood sugar should be closely monitored and the dosage of hypoglycemic medications may require adjustment. This should be carefully coordinated among the individual's healthcare providers.

Effects of drugs with hypolipidemic activity may be potentiated. Blood lipid levels should be closely monitored and the dosage of hypolipidemic medications may require adjustment. This should be carefully coordinated among the individual's healthcare providers. Use caution in individuals taking hypolipidemic agents (based on pharmacologic activity, the effects may be additive).

References

Ackermann RT, Mulrow CD, Ramirez G, et al, "Garlic Shows Promise for Improving Some Cardiovascular Risk Factors," *Arch Intern Med*, 2001, 161(6):813-24.

Adetumbi MA and Lau BH, "*Allium sativum* (Garlic)-A Natural Antibiotic," *Med Hypotheses* 1983, 12 (3):227-37.

Agarwal KC, "Therapeutic Actions of Garlic Constituents," *Med Res Rev*, 1996, 16(1):111-24.

Andrianova IV, Sobenin IA, Sereda EV, et al, "Effect of Long-Acting Garlic Tablets 'Allicor' on the Incidence of Acute Respiratory Viral Infections in Children," *Ter Arkh*, 2003, 75(3):53-6.

Anonymous, "Garlic in Cryptococcal Meningitis: A Preliminary Report of 21 Cases," *Chin Med J (Engl)*, 1980, 93(2):123-6.

Berthold HK, Sudhop T, and von Bergmann K, "Effect of a Garlic Oil Preparation on Serum Lipoproteins and Cholesterol Metabolism: A Randomized Controlled Trial," *JAMA*, 1998, 279(23):1900-2.

Bordia A, "Effect of Garlic on Blood Lipids in Patients With Coronary Heart Disease," *Am J Clin Nutr*, 1981, 34(10):2100-3.

Bordia A, Verma SK, and Srivastava KC, "Effect of Garlic (*Allium sativum*) on Blood Lipids, Blood Sugar, Fibrinogen and Fibrinolytic Activity in Patients With Coronary Artery Disease," *Prostaglandins Leukot Essent Fatty Acids*, 1998, 58(4):257-63.
Buiatti E, Palli D, Decarli A, et al, "A Case-Control Study of Gastric Cancer and Diet in Italy," *Int J Cancer*, 1989, 44(4):611-6.
Byrne DJ, Neil HA, Vallance DT, et al, "A Pilot Study of Garlic Consumption Shows No Significant Effect on Markers of Oxidation or Sub-Fraction Composition of Low-Density Lipoprotein Including Lipoprotein (a) After Allowance for Non-Compliance and the Placebo Effect," *Clin Chim Acta*, 1999, 285(1-2):21-33.
Chi MS, "Effects of Garlic Products on Lipid Metabolism in Cholesterol-Fed Rats (41494)," *Proc Soc Exp Biol Med*, 1982, 171(2):174-8.
Cook-Mozaffari PJ, Azordegan F, Day NE, et al, "Esophageal Cancer Studies in the Caspian Littoral of Iran: Results of a Case-Control Study," *Br J Cancer*, 1979, 39(3):293-309.
Czerny B and Samochowiec J, "Klinische Untersuchungen Mit Einem Knoblauch-Lezithin-Praparat," *Arztezeitschr Naturheilverf*, 1996, 37:126-9.
Davis LE, Shen J, and Royer RE, "*In vitro* Synergism of Concentrated *Allium sativum* Extract and Amphotericin B Against *Cryptococcus neoformans*," *Planta Med*, 1994, 60(6):546-9.
Dorant E, van den Brandt PA, and Goldbohm RA, "A Prospective Cohort Study on the Relationship Between Onion and Leek Consumption, Garlic Supplement Use and the Risk of Colorectal Carcinoma in the Netherlands," *Carcinogenesis*, 1996, 17(3):477-84.
Dorant E, van den Brandt PA, and Goldbohm RA, "Allium Vegetable Consumption, Garlic Supplement Intake, and Female Breast Carcinoma Incidence," *Breast Cancer Res Treat*, 1995, 33(2):163-70.
Ernst E, "Cardiovascular Effects of Garlic (*Allium sativum*): A Review," *Pharmatherapeutica*, 1987, 5 (2):83-9.
Gail MH, You WC, Chang YS, et al, "Factorial Trial of Three Interventions to Reduce the Progression of Precancerous Gastric Lesions in Shandong, China: Design Issues and Initial Data," *Control Clin Trials*, 1998, 19(4):352-69.
Gao CM, Takezaki T, Ding JH, et al, "Protective Effect of Allium Vegetables Against Both Esophageal and Stomach Cancer: A Simultaneous Case-Referent Study of a High-Epidemic Area in Jiangsu Province, China," *Jpn J Cancer Res*, 1999, 90(6):614-21.
Gardner CD, Lawson LD, Block E, et al, "Effect of Raw Garlic vs Commercial Garlic Supplements on Plasma Lipid Concentrations in Adults With Moderate Hypercholesterolemia: A Randomized Clinical Trial," *Arch Intern Med*, 2007, 167(4):346-53.
Gebhardt R, Beck H, and Wagner KG, "Inhibition of Cholesterol Biosynthesis by Allicin and Ajoene in Rat Hepatocytes and HepG2 Cells," *Biochim Biophys Acta*, 1994, 1213(1):57-62.
Graham DY, Anderson SY, and Lang T, "Garlic or Jalapeño Peppers for Treatment of *Helicobacter pylori* Infection," *Am J Gastroenterol*, 1999, 94(5):1200-2.
Hajheydari Z, Jamshidi M, Akbari J, et al, "Combination of Topical Garlic Gel and Betamethasone Valerate Cream in the Treatment of Localized Alopecia Areata: A Double-Blind Randomized Controlled Study," *Indian J Dermatol Venereol Leprol*, 2007, 73(1):29-32.
Isaacsohn JL, Moser M, Stein EA, et al, "Garlic Powder and Plasma Lipids and Lipoproteins: A Multicenter, Randomized, Placebo-Controlled Trial," *Arch Intern Med*, 1998, 158(11):1189-94.
Ishikawa H, Saeki T, Otani T, et al, "Aged Garlic Extract Prevents a Decline of NK Cell Number and Activity in Patients With Advanced Cancer," *J Nutr*, 2006, 136(3 Suppl):816S-820S.
Jepson RG, Kleijnen J, and Leng GC, "Garlic for Peripheral Arterial Occlusive Disease (Cochrane Review)," *The Cochrane Library*, 2001, 2.
Josling P, "Preventing the Common Cold With a Garlic Supplement: A Double-Blind, Placebo-Controlled Survey," *Adv Ther*, 2001, 18(4):189-93.
Jung EM, Jung F, Mrowietz C, et al, "Influence of Garlic Powder on Cutaneous Microcirculation. A Randomized Placebo-Controlled Double-Blind Cross-Over Study in Apparently Healthy Subjects," *Arzneimittelforschung*, 1991, 41(6):626-30.
Jung F, Jung EM, Mrowietz C, et al, "The Effects of Garlic Powder on Cutaneous Microcirculation. A Cross-Over Test With Healthy Test Persons," *Med Welt*, 1991, 42:28-30.
Kiesewetter H, Jung F, Jung EM, et al, "Effects of Garlic Coated Tablets in Peripheral Arterial Occlusive Disease," *Clin Investig*, 1993, 71(5):383-6.
Kojuri J, Vosoughi AR, and Akrami M, "Effects of *Anethum graveolens* and Garlic on Lipid Profile in Hyperlipidemic Patients," *Lipids Health Dis*, 2007, 6:5.
Ledezma E, López JC, Marin P, et al, "Ajoene in the Topical Short-Term Treatment of *Tinea cruris* and *Tinea corporis* in Humans. Randomized Comparative Study With Terbinafine," *Arzneimittelforschung*, 1999, 49(6):544-7.
Levi F, Franceschi S, Negri E, et al, "Dietary Factors and the Risk of Endometrial Cancer," *Cancer*, 1993, 71(11):3575-81.
McNulty CA, Wilson MP, Havinga W, et al, "A Pilot Study to Determine the Effectiveness of Garlic Oil Capsules in the Treatment of Dyspeptic Patients With *Helicobacter pylori*," *Helicobacter*, 2001, 6 (3):249-53.
Mulrow C, Lawrence V, Ackermann R, et al, "Garlic: Effects on Cardiovascular Risks and Disease, Protective Effects Against Cancer, and Clinical Adverse Effects," *Evid Rep Technol Assess (Summ)*, 2000, (20):1-4.
Munday JS, James KA, Fray LM, et al, "Daily Supplementation With Aged Garlic Extract, but Not Raw Garlic, Protects Low Density Lipoprotein Against *In vitro*, Oxidation," *Atherosclerosis*, 1999, 143 (2):399-404.
Natural Standard Research Collaboration, Chief Editors: Ulbricht C, Basch E, *Natural Standard Herb and Supplement Reference - Evidence-Based Clinical Reviews*, USA: Elsevier/Mosby, 2005.
Neil HA, Silagy CA, Lancaster T, et al, "Garlic Powder in the Treatment of Moderate Hyperlipidaemia: A Controlled Trial and Meta-Analysis," *J R Coll Physicians Lond*, 1996, 30(4):329-34.
Orekhov AN, Pivovarova EM, and Tertov VV, "Garlic Powder Tablets Reduce Atherogenicity of Low Density Lipoprotein. A Placebo-Controlled Double-Blind Study," *Nutr Metab Cardiovascular Dis*, 1996, 6:21-31.
Pai ST and Platt MW, "Antifungal Effects of *Allium sativum* (Garlic) Extract Against the *Aspergillus* Species Involved in Otomycosis," *Lett Appl Microbiol*, 1995, 20(1):14-8.
Piscitelli SC, Burstein AH, Welden N, et al, "The Effect of Garlic Supplements on the Pharmacokinetics of Saquinavir," *Clin Infect Dis*, 2002, 34(2):234-8.
Qureshi AA, Abuirmeileh N, Din ZZ, et al, "Inhibition of Cholesterol and Fatty Acid Biosynthesis in Liver Enzymes and Chicken Hepatocytes by Polar Fractions of Garlic," *Lipids*, 1983, 18(5):343-8.
Salman H, Beyman M, Bessler H, et al, "Effect of Garlic Derivative (Alliin) on Peripheral Blood Cell Immune Responses," *Int J Immunopharmacol*, 1999, 21(9):589-97.
Shu XO, Zheng W, Potischman N, et al, "A Population-Based Case-Control Study of Dietary Factors and Endometrial Cancer in Shanghai, People's Republic of China," *Am J Epidemiol*, 1993, 137(2):155-65.
Siegel G, "Long-Term Effect of Garlic in Preventing Arteriosclerosis - Results of Two Controlled Clinical Trials," *Eur Phytojournal*, 2001, Symposium posters (1):1.
Siegel G and Klussendorf D, "The Anti-Atheroslerotic Effect of *Allium sativum*: Statistics Re-evaluated," *Atherosclerosis*, 2000, 150(2):437-8.
Silagy C and Neil A, "Garlic as a Lipid Lowering Agent - A Meta-Analysis," *J R Coll Physicians Lond*, 1994, 28(1):39-45.
Simons LA, Balasubramaniam S, von Konigsmark M, et al, "On the Effect of Garlic on Plasma Lipids and Lipoproteins in Mild Cholesterolaemia," *Atherosclerosis*, 1995, 113(2):219-25.
Sitprija S, Plengvidhya C, Kangkaya V, et al, "Garlic and Diabetes Mellitus Phase II Clinical Trial," *J Med Assoc Thai*, 1987, 70(Suppl 2):223-7.
Steiner M, Khan AH, Holbert D, et al, "A Double-Blind Crossover Study in Moderately Hypercholesterolemic Men That Compared the Effect of Aged Garlic Extract and Placebo Administration on Blood Lipids," *Am J Clin Nutr*, 1996, 64(6):866-70.
Steinmetz KA, Kushi LH, Bostick RM, et al, "Vegetables, Fruit, and Colon Cancer in the Iowa Women's Health Study," *Am J Epidemiol*, 1994, 139(1):1-15.

Stjernberg L and Berglund J, "Garlic as an Insect Repellent," *JAMA*, 2000, 284(7):831.
Swanson CA, Mao BL, Li JY, et al, "Dietary Determinants of Lung-Cancer Risk: Results From a Case-Control Study in Yunnan Province, China," *Int J Cancer*, 1992, 50(6):876-80.
Takezaki T, Gao CM, Ding JH, et al, "Comparative Study of Lifestyles of Residents in High and Low Risk Areas for Gastric Cancer in Jiangsu Province, China; With Special Reference to Allium Vegetables," *J Epidemiol*, 1999, 9(5):297-305.
Tanaka S, Haruma K, Yoshihara M, et al, "Aged Garlic Extract Has Potential Suppressive Effect on Colorectal Adenomas in Humans," *J Nutr*, 2006, 136(3 Suppl):821S-826S.
Wang ZY, Boice JD Jr, Wei LX, et al, "Thyroid Nodularity and Chromosome Aberrations Among Women in Areas of High Background Radiation in China," *J Natl Cancer Inst*, 1990, 82(6):478-85.
Witte JS, Longnecker MP, Bird CL, et al, "Relation of Vegetable, Fruit, and Grain Consumption to Colorectal Adenomatous Polyps," *Am J Epidemiol*, 1996, 144(11):1015-25.
You WC, Zhang L, Gail MH, et al, "*Helicobacter pylori* Infection, Garlic Intake and Precancerous Lesions in a Chinese Population at Low Risk of Gastric Cancer," *Int J Epidemiol*, 1998, 27(6):941-4.

Ginger

Pharmacologic Category Herb

Reported Use

Antiemetic; for nausea and vomiting in pregnancy; motion sickness; chemotherapy (Betz, 2005; Bone, 1990; Borrelli, 2005; Grontved, 1988; Keating, 2002; Pace, 1987; Vutyavanich, 2001; Willetts, 2003)
Anti-inflammatory (musculoskeletal) (Srivastava, 1992)
Diverticulitis (pharmacologic activity)
Indigestion/heartburn (Newall, 1996)
Osteoarthritis, gonarthritis, rheumatoid arthritis (Altman, 2001; Srivastava, 1989; Wigler, 2003)
Shortening duration of labor (Calvert, 2005)

Local Anesthetic/Vasoconstrictor Precautions No information available to require special precautions

Effects on Bleeding Very high doses may inhibit platelet aggregation.

Warnings/Precautions Pharmacologic activity may include alteration of platelet aggregation (Guh, 1995). Based on pharmacologic activity, ginger may be contraindicated in individuals with active bleeding (eg, peptic ulcer, intracranial bleeding). Use with caution in individuals with a history of bleeding, hemostatic disorders, or drug-related hemostatic problems; in individuals taking anticoagulant medications, including warfarin, aspirin, aspirin-containing products, NSAIDs, or antiplatelet agents (eg, ticlopidine, clopidogrel, dipyridamole); and in individuals with inflammatory bowel disease, history of intestinal obstruction, or gastric or duodenal ulcers. Discontinue use prior to dental or surgical procedures (generally at least 14 days before).

References

Altman RD and Marcussen KC, "Effects of a Ginger Extract on Knee Pain in Patients With Osteoarthritis," *Arthritis Rheum*, 2001, 44(11):2531-8.
Betz O, Kranke P, Geldner G, et al, "Is Ginger a Clinically Relevant Antiemetic? A Systematic Review of Randomized Controlled Trials," *Forsch Komplementarmed Klass Naturheilkd*, 2005, 12(1):14-23.
Bone ME, Wilkinson DJ, Young JR, et al, "Ginger Root - A New Antiemetic. The Effect of Ginger Root on Postoperative Nausea and Vomiting After Major Gynaecological Surgery," *Anaesthesia*, 1990, 45 (8):669-71.
Borrelli F, Capasso R, Aviello G, et al, "Effectiveness and Safety of Ginger in the Treatment of Pregnancy-Induced Nausea and Vomiting," *Obstet Gynecol*, 2005, 105(4):849-56.
Calvert I, "Ginger: An Essential Oil for Shortening Labour?" *Pract Midwife*, 2005, 8(1):30-4.
Grontved A, Brask T, Kambskard J, et al, "Ginger Root Against Seasickness. A Controlled Trial on the Open Sea," *Acta Otolaryngol (Stockh)*, 1988, 105(1-2):45-9.
Guh JH, Kof N, Jong TT, et al, "Antiplatelet Effect of Gingerol Isolated From *Zingiber officinale*," *J Pharm Pharmacol*, 1995, 47(4):329-32.
Keating A and Chez RA, "Ginger Syrup as an Antiemetic in Early Pregnancy," *Altern Ther Health Med*, 2002, 8(5):89-91.
Meyer K, Schwartz J, Crater D, et al, "*Zingiber officinale* (Ginger) Used to Prevent 8-Mop Associated Nausea," *Dermatol Nurs*, 1995, 7(4):242-4.
Natural Standard Research Collaboration, Chief Editors: Ulbricht C, Basch E, *Natural Standard Herb and Supplement Reference - Evidence-Based Clinical Reviews*, USA: Elsevier/Mosby, 2005.
Newall CA, Anderson LA, and Phillipson JD, *Herbal Medicines: A Guide for Health Care Professionals*, London, England: The Pharmaceutical Press, 1996, 135-7.
Pace J and Conlin DS, "Oral Ingestion of Encapsulated Ginger and Reported Self-Care Actions for the Relief of Chemotherapy-Associated Nausea and Vomiting," *Dissertation Abstracts International*, 1987, 47(8):3297-B.
Sharma SS and Gupta YK, "Reversal of Cisplatin-Induced Delay in Gastric Emptying in Rats by Ginger (*Zingiber officinale*)," *J Ethnopharmacol*, 1998, 62(1):49-55.
Srivastava KC and Mustafa T, "Ginger (*Zingiber officinale*) in Rheumatism and Musculoskeletal Disorders," *Med Hypotheses*, 1992, 39(4):342-8.
Srivastava K and Mustafa T, "Ginger (*Zingiber officinale*) and Rheumatic Disorders," *Med Hypotheses*, 1989, 29(1):25-8.
Vutyavanich T, Kraisarin T, and Ruangsri R, "Ginger for Nausea and Vomiting in Pregnancy: Randomized, Double-Masked, Placebo-Controlled Trial," *Obstet Gynecol*, 2001, 97(4):577-82.
Wigler I, Grotto I, Caspi D, et al, "The Effects of Zintona EC (a Ginger Extract) on Symptomatic Gonarthritis," *Osteoarthritis Cartilage*, 2003, 11(11):783-9.
Willetts KE, Ekangaki A, and Eden JA, "Effect of a Ginger Extract on Pregnancy-Induced Nausea: A Randomised Controlled Trial," *Aust N Z J Obstet Gynaecol*, 2003, 43(2):139-44.

Ginkgo Biloba

Pharmacologic Category Herb

Reported Use

Acute ischemic stroke (Garg, 1995; Zeng, 2005)

Alzheimer's disease, dementia, age-related memory impairment (Birks, 2002; Brautigam, 1998; Ernst, 1999; Itil, 1998; Le Bars, 1997; Napryeyenko, 2007; Oken, 1998)
Contradictory study (Schneider, 2005; van Dongen, 2000)
Anxiety (Woelk, 2007)
Asthma (Braquet, 1987)
Cerebral insufficiency (Hopfenmüller, 1994; Kleijnen, 1992)
Chemotherapy (adjunct) (Hauns, 1999)
Chronic cochleovestibular disorders (Hahn, 2000)
Cocaine dependence, contradictory study (Kampman, 2003)
Cognitive function (Carlson, 2007)
Depression (Schubert, 1993); seasonal affective disorder (SAD), contradictory study (Lingaerde, 1999)
Diabetic neuropathy (Lu, 2005)
Dyslexia (Donfrancesco, 2007)
Epilepsy (pharmacologic activity)
Functional measures (in patients with multiple sclerosis) (Johnson, 2006)
Gastric cancer (Xu, 2003)
Glaucoma (Quaranta, 2003)
Headache (pharmacologic activity)
Intermittent claudication (Ernst, 1996; Peters, 1998; Pittler, 2000)
Macular degeneration (Lebuisson, 1986)
Memory enhancement (Allain, 1993; Kleijnen, 1992)
Mountain sickness (Roncin, 1996)
Multiple sclerosis (Brochet, 1992; Brochet, 1995; Lovera, 2007)
Ocular blood flow (contradictory study) (Wimpissinger, 2007)
Parkinson's disease (pharmacologic activity)
Peripheral blood flow: Cerebral vascular disease, peripheral vascular insufficiency, impotence, tinnitus, and depression (Kleijnen, 1992)
Premenstrual syndrome (PMS) (Tamborini, 1993)
Quality of life (Cockle, 2000; Trick, 2004)
Raynaud's phenomenon (Muir, 2002)
Retinopathy (Huang, 2004)
Schizophrenia (Atmaca, 2005)
Seizures (pharmacologic activity)
Sexual dysfunction (antidepressant-induced) (Cohen, 1998)
Tinnitus (Drew, 2001; Holgers, 1994; Meyer, 1986; Morgenstern, 2002; Rejali, 2004)
Vertigo (Haguenauer, 1986)
Vitiligo (Parsad, 2003)

Local Anesthetic/Vasoconstrictor Precautions No information available to require special precautions

Effects on Bleeding May see increased bleeding due to inhibition of platelet aggregation; antagonizes platelet activating factor (PAF)

Warnings/Precautions May cause abdominal problems, nausea, and dyspepsia (Pittler, 2000). Avoid in patients with seizure disorders as ginkgo may lower the seizure threshold. Avoid in patients at risk of bleeding, taking anticoagulants, or with clotting disorders, based on reports of bleeding.

Ginkgo demonstrates *in vitro* inhibition of platelet aggregation and has been associated with case reports of bleeding (Matthews, 1998; Odawara, 1997; Rosenblatt, 1997; Skogh, 1998; Vale, 1998). Based on pharmacologic activity, this herb may be contraindicated in individuals with active bleeding (eg, peptic ulcer, intracranial bleeding). Avoid in individuals with a history of bleeding, hemostatic disorders, or drug-related hemostatic problems, and in individuals taking anticoagulant medications, including warfarin, aspirin, aspirin-containing products, NSAIDs, or antiplatelet agents (eg, ticlopidine, clopidogrel, dipyridamole). Discontinue use prior to dental or surgical procedures (generally at least 14 days before).

Based on pharmacologic activity, may increase effect or toxicity of monoamine oxidase inhibitors (MAOIs) (White, 1966; Wu 1999).

References

Allain H, Raoul P, Lieury A, et al, "Effect of Two Doses of *Ginkgo biloba* Extract (EGb 761) on the Dual-Coding Test in Elderly Subjects," *Clin Ther*, 1993, 15(3):549-58.
Atmaca M, Tezcan E, Kuloglu M, et al, "The Effect of Extract of *Ginkgo biloba* Addition to Olanzapine on Therapeutic Effect and Antioxidant Enzyme Levels in Patients With Schizophrenia," *Psychiatry Clin Neurosci*, 2005, 59(6):652-6.
Balon R, "*Ginkgo biloba* for Antidepressant-Induced Sexual Dysfunction," *J Sex Marital Ther*, 1999, 25 (1):1-2.
Birks J, Grimley EV, and Van Dongen M, "*Ginkgo biloba* for Cognitive Impairment and Dementia," *Cochrane Database Syst Rev*, 2002, (4):CD003120.
Braquet P, "The Ginkgolides: Potent Platelet-Activating Factor Antagonists Isolated from *Ginkgo biloba* L.: Chemistry, Pharmacology, and Clinical Applications," *Drugs of the Future*, 1987, 12:643-99.
Brautigm MR, Blommaert FA, Verleye G, et al, "Treatment of Age-Related Memory Complaints With *Ginkgo biloba* Extract: A Randomized Double Blind Placebo-Controlled Study," *Phytomed*, 1998, 5 (6):425-34.

Brochet B, Guinot P, Orgogozo JM, et al, "Double Blind Placebo Controlled Multicentre Study of Ginkgolide B in Treatment of Acute Exacerbations of Multiple Sclerosis. The Ginkgolide Study Group in Multiple Sclerosis," *J Neurol Neurosurg Psychiatry*, 1995, 58(3):360-2.
Brochet B, Orgogozo JM, Guinot P, et al, "Pilot Study of Ginkgolide B, a PAF-acether Specific Inhibitor in the Treatment of Acute Outbreaks of Multiple Sclerosis," *Rev Neurol (Paris)*, 1992, 148(4):299-301.
Carlson JJ, Farquhar JW, DiNucci E, et al, "Safety and Efficacy of a *Ginkgo biloba*-Containing Dietary Supplement on Cognitive Function, Quality of Life, and Platelet Function in Healthy, Cognitively Intact Older Adults," *J Am Diet Assoc*, 2007, 107(3):422-32.
Cockle SM, Kimber S, and Hindmarch I, "The Effects of *Ginkgo biloba* Extract (LI 1370) Supplementation on Activities of Daily Living in Free Living Older Volunteers: A Questionnaire Survey," *Hum Psychopharmacol*, 2000, 15(4):227-35.
Cohen AJ and Bartlik B, "*Ginkgo biloba* for Antidepressant-Induced Sexual Dysfunction," *J Sex Marital Ther*, 1998, 24(2):139-43.
Donfrancesco R and Ferrante L, "*Ginkgo biloba* in Dyslexia: A Pilot Study," *Phytomedicine*, 2007, 14 (6):367-70.
Drew S and Davies E, "Effectiveness of *Ginkgo biloba* in Treating Tinnitus: Double Blind, Placebo Controlled Trial," *BMJ*, 2001, 322(7278):73.
Ernst E, "*Ginkgo biloba* in Treatment of Intermittent Claudication. A Systematic Research Based on Controlled Studies in the Literature," *Fortschr Med*, 1996, 114(8):85-7.
Ernst E and Pittler MH, "*Ginkgo biloba* for Dementia: A Systematic Review of Double-Blind, Placebo-Controlled Trials," *Clin Drug Invest*, 1999, 17(4):301-8.
Galluzzi S, Zanetti O, Binetti G, et al, "Coma in a Patient With Alzheimer's Disease Taking Low Dose Trazodone and Gingko Biloba," *J Neurol Neurosurg Psychiatry*, 2000, 68(5):679-80.
Garg RK, Nag D, and Agrawal A, "A Double Blind Placebo Controlled Trial of *Ginkgo biloba* Extract in Acute Cerebral Ischaemia," *J Assoc Physicians India*, 1995, 43(11):760-3.
Haguenauer JP, Cantenot F, Koskas H, et al, "Treatment of Equilibrium Disorders With *Ginkgo biloba* Extract. A Multicenter Double-Blind Drug Vs. Placebo Study," *Presse Med*, 1986, 15(31):1569-72.
Hahn A and Stolbova K, "*Ginkgo biloba*: Local Experiences," *Int Tinnitus J*, 2000, 6(1):54-5.
Hauns B, Haring B, Kohler S, et al, "Phase II Study With 5-Fluorouracil and *Ginkgo biloba* Extract (GBE 761 ONC) in Patients With Pancreatic Cancer," *Arzneimittelforschung*, 1999, 49(12):1030-4.
Holgers KM, Axelsson A, and Pringle I, "*Ginkgo biloba* Extract for the Treatment of Tinnitus," *Audiology*, 1994, 33(2):85-92.
Hopfenmüller W, "Evidence for a Therapeutic Effect of *Ginkgo biloba* Special Extract. Meta-Analysis of 11 Clinical Studies in Patients With Cerebrovascular Insufficiency in Old Age," *Arzneimittelforschung*, 1994, 44(9):1005-13.
Huang SY, Jeng C, Kao SC, et al, "Improved Haemorrheological Properties by *Ginkgo biloba* Extract (Egb 761) in Type 2 Diabetes Mellitus Complicated With Retinopathy," *Clin Nutr*, 2004, 23(4):615-21.
Itil TM, Erlap E, Ahmed I, et al, "The Pharmacological Effects of *Ginkgo biloba*, a Plant Extract, on the Brain of Dementia Patients in Comparison With Tacrine," *Psychopharmacol Bull*, 1998, 34(3):391-7.
Johnson SK, Diamond BJ, Rausch S, et al, "The Effect of *Ginkgo biloba* on Functional Measures in Multiple Sclerosis: A Pilot Randomized Controlled Trial," *Explore (NY)*, 2006, 2(1):19-24.
Kampman K, Majewska MD, Tourian K, et al, "A Pilot Trial of Piracetam and *Ginkgo biloba* For the Treatment of Cocaine Dependence," *Addict Behav*, 2003, 28(3):437-48.
Kleijnen J and Knipschild P, "*Ginkgo biloba* For Cerebral Insufficiency," *Br J Clin Pharmacol*, 1992, 34 (4):352-8.
Kleijnen J and Knipschild P, "*Ginkgo biloba*," *Lancet*, 1992, 340(8828):1136-9.
Le Bars PL, Katz MM, Berman N, et al, "A Placebo-Controlled, Double-Blind, Randomized Trial of an Extract of *Ginkgo biloba* for Dementia. North American EGb Study Group," *JAMA*, 1997, 278 (16):1327-32.
Lebuissen DA, Leroy L, and Rigal G, "Treatment of Senile Macular Degeneration With *Ginkgo biloba* Extract. A Preliminary Double-Blind Drug vs Placebo Study," *Presse Med*, 1986, 15(31):1556-8.
Lingaerde O, Foreland AR, and Magnusson A, "Can Winter Depression Be Prevented by *Ginkgo biloba* Extract? A Placebo-Controlled Trial," *Acta Psychiatr Scand*, 1999, 100(1):62-6.
Lovera J, Bagert B, Smoot K, et al, "*Ginkgo biloba* for the Improvement of Cognitive Performance in Multiple Sclerosis: A Randomized, Placebo-Controlled Trial," *Mult Scler*, 2007, 13(3):376-85.
Lu J and He H, "Clinical Observation of *Ginkgo biloba* Extract Injection in Treating Early Diabetic Nephropathy," *Chin J Integr Med*, 2005, 11(3):226-8.
Matthews MK Jr, "Association of *Ginkgo biloba* With Intracerebral Hemorrhage," *Neurology*, 1998, 50 (6):1933-4.
Meyer B, "Multicenter Randomized Double-Blind Drug vs Placebo Study of the Treatment of Tinnitus With *Ginkgo biloba* Extract," *Presse Med*, 1986, 15(31):1562-4.
Morgenstern C and Biermann E, "The Efficacy of Ginkgo Special Extract EGb 761 in Patients With Tinnitus," *Int J Clin Pharmacol Ther*, 2002, 40(5):188-97.
Muir AH, Robb R, McLaren M, et al, "The Use of *Ginkgo biloba* in Raynaud's Disease: A Double-Blind Placebo-Controlled Trial," *Vasc Med*, 2002, 7(4):265-7.
Napryeyenko O, Borzenko I, and GINDEM-NP Study Group, "*Ginkgo biloba* Special Extract in Dementia With Neuropsychiatric Features. A Randomised, Placebo-Controlled, Double-Blind Clinical Trial," *Arzneimittelforschung*, 2007, 57(1):4-11.
Natural Standard Research Collaboration, Chief Editors: Ulbricht C, Basch E, *Natural Standard Herb and Supplement Reference - Evidence-Based Clinical Reviews*, USA: Elsevier/Mosby, 2005.
Odawara M, Tamaoka A, and Yamashita K, "*Ginkgo biloba*," *Neurology*, 1997, 48(3):789-90.
Oken BS, Storzbach DM, and Kaye JA, "The Efficacy of *Ginkgo biloba* on Cognitive Function in Alzheimer Disease," *Arch Neurol*, 1998, 55(11):1409-15.
Parsad D, Pandhi R, and Juneja A, "Effectiveness of Oral *Ginkgo biloba* in Treating Limited, Slowly Spreading Vitiligo," *Clin Exp Dermatol*, 2003, 28(3):285-7.
Peters H, Kieser M, and Holscher U, "Demonstration of the Efficacy of *Ginkgo biloba* Special Extract EGb 761 on Intermittent Claudication - A Placebo-Controlled, Double-Blind Multicenter Trial," *Vasa*, 1998, 27 (2):106-10.
Pittler MH and Ernst E, "*Ginkgo biloba* Extract for the Treatment of Intermittent Claudication: A Meta-analysis of Randomized Trials," *Am J Med*, 2000, 108(4):276-81.
Quaranta L, Bettelli S, Uva MG, et al, "Effect of Ginkgo Biloba Extract on Preexisting Visual Field Damage in Normal Tension Glaucoma," *Ophthalmology*, 2003, 110(2):359-62.
Rejali D, Sivakumar A, and Balaji N, "*Ginkgo biloba* Does Not Benefit Patients With Tinnitus: A Randomized Placebo-Controlled Double-Blind Trial and Meta-Analysis of Randomized Trials," *Clin Otolaryngol Allied Sci*, 2004, 29(3):226-31.
Roncin JP, Schwartz F, and D'Arbigny P, "EGb 761 in Control of Acute Mountain Sickness and Vascular Reactivity to Cold Exposure," *Aviat Space Environ Med*, 1996, 67(5):445-52.
Rosenblatt M and Mindel J, "Spontaneous Hyphema Associated With Ingestion of *Ginko biloba* Extract," *N Engl J Med*, 1997, 336(15):1108.
Sasaki K, Hatta S, Haga M, et al, "Effects of Bilobalide on Gamma-Aminobutyric Acid Levels and Glutamic Acid Decarboxylase in Mouse Brain," *Eur J Pharmacol*, 1999, 367(2-3):165-73.
Schneider LS, DeKosky ST, Farlow MR, et al, "A Randomized, Double-Blind, Placebo-Controlled Trial of Two Doses of *Ginkgo biloba* Extract in Dementia of the Alzheimer's Type," *Curr Alzheimer Res*, 2005, 2 (5):541-51.
Schubert H and Halama P, "Depressive Episode Primarily Unresponsive to Therapy in Elderly Patients. Efficacy of *Ginkgo biloba* in Combination With Antidepressants," *Geriatre Forschung*, 1993, 3(1):45-53.
Skogh M, "Extracts of *Ginkgo biloba*, and Bleeding or Haemorrhage," *Lancet*, 1998, 352(9134):1145-6.
Tamborini A and Taurelle R, "Value of Standardized *Ginkgo biloba* Extract (EGb 761) in the Management of Congestive Symptoms of Premenstrual Syndrome," *Rev Fr Gynecol Obstet*, 1993, 88(7-9):447-57.
Trick L, Boyle J, and Hindmarch I, "The Effects of *Ginkgo biloba* Extract (LI 1370) Supplementation and Discontinuation on Activities of Daily Living and Mood in Free Living Older Volunteers," *Phytother Res*, 2004, 18(7):531-7.

Vale S, "Subarachnoid Haemorrhage Associated With *Ginkgo biloba*," *Lancet*, 1998, 352(9121):36.
van Dongen MC, van Rossum E, Kessels AG, et al, "The Efficacy of Ginkgo for Elderly People With Dementia and Age-Associated Memory Impairment: New Results of a Randomized Clinical Trial," *J Am Geriatr Soc*, 2000, 48(10):1183-94.
White HL, Scates PW, and Cooper BR, "Extracts of *Ginkgo biloba* Leaves Inhibit Monoamine Oxidase," *Life Sci*, 1966, 58(16):1315-21.
Wimpissinger B, Berisha F, Garhoefer G, et al, "Influence of *Ginkgo biloba* on Ocular Blood Flow," *Acta Ophthalmol Scand*, 2007, 85(4):445-9.
Woelk H, Arnoldt KH, Kieser M, et al, "*Ginkgo biloba* Special Extract EGB 761 in Generalized Anxiety Disorder and Adjustment Disorder With Anxious Mood: A Randomized, Double-Blind, Placebo-Controlled Trial," *J Psychiatr Res*, 2007, 41(6):472-80.
Wu WR and Zhu XZ, "Involvement of Monoamine Oxidase Inhibition in Neuroprotective and Neurorestorative Effects of *Ginkgo biloba* Extract Against MPTP-Induced Nigrostriatal Dopaminergic Toxicity in C57 Mice," *Life Sci*, 1999, 65(2):157-64.
Xu AH, Chen HS, Sun BC, et al, "Therapeutic Mechanism of *Ginkgo biloba* Exocarp Polysaccharides on Gastric Cancer," *World J Gastroenterol*, 2003, 9(11):2424-7.
Zeng X, Liu M, Yang Y, et al, "*Ginkgo biloba* for Acute Ischaemic Stroke," *Cochrane Database Syst Rev*, 2005, (4):CD003691.

Ginseng, Panax

Pharmacologic Category Herb

Reported Use

Adrenal tonic (Hiai, 1979)
Brain injury (Ai, 2003)
Bronchitis (Scaglione, 2001)
Cancer (Suh, 2002)
Congestive heart failure (Ding, 1995)
COPD (Gross, 2002)
Dementia (Zhao, 1990)
Diabetes (Ng, 1985; Reay, 2006; Vuksan, 2000)
Diabetic nephropathy (Jiangming, 2000)
Erectile dysfunction (Choi, 1995; de Andrade, 2007)
Hepatoprotection (Cui, 1994; Zuin, 1987)
Hyperlipidemia (Kim, 2003)
Hypertension (Han, 1998; Sung, 2000)
Immune support (Kim, 1990; Scaglione, 1990; Scaglione, 1996)
Mental health (Reay, 2005)
Physical and mental performance; energy enhancement (Cherdrungsi, 1995; Chong, 1988; Forgo, 1983; Pieralisi, 1991; Van Schepdael, 1993)
Radiation therapy side effects (Chang, 1980; Fang-yun, 2001)

Local Anesthetic/Vasoconstrictor Precautions Has potential to interact with epinephrine and levonordefrin to result in increased BP; use vasoconstrictor with caution

Effects on Bleeding May have antiplatelet effects

Warnings/Precautions Use of *Panax ginseng* is contraindicated in renal failure and acute infection. Avoid in pregnancy and lactation (Bradley, 1992). Use with caution in individuals receiving MAO inhibitors (based on pharmacologic activity and case reports). Use caution with stimulant medications, including decongestants, caffeine, and caffeine-containing beverages (based on pharmacologic activity). May be associated with a syndrome of diarrhea, hypertension, nervousness, dermatologic eruptions, and insomnia (Ginseng Abuse Syndrome) after prolonged use or high dosages (Chen, 1981). May also cause mastalgia in prolonged, high-dose use (case reports, Dukes, 1978). May cause vaginal breakthrough bleeding (case reports, Hopkins, 1988). Due to pharmacologic activity, may interfere with hormonal therapy.

May cause palpitations and tachycardia in sensitive individuals or in high doses. Based on pharmacologic activity, use with caution in individuals with hypertension or in those receiving antihypertensives (Siegel, 1980). Also use caution in individuals at risk of hypotension (including those taking antihypertensive medication or agents that predispose to orthostasis), elderly individuals, or those who would not tolerate transient hyper- or hypotensive episodes (ie, cerebrovascular or cardiovascular disease). May increase the QT_c interval (Caron, 2002).

May alter glucose regulation. Use with caution in individuals with diabetes or in those who may be predisposed to hypoglycemia. Effects of drugs with hypoglycemic activity may be potentiated (including insulin and oral hypoglycemics). Blood sugar should be closely monitored, and the dosage of hypoglycemic medications may require adjustment. This should be carefully coordinated among the individual's healthcare providers.

Based on pharmacologic activity and case reports, may alter hemostasis (Janetsky, 1997; Teng, 1989) and may be contraindicated in individuals with active bleeding (eg, peptic ulcer, intracranial bleeding). Use with caution in individuals with a history of bleeding, hemostatic disorders, or drug-related hemostatic problems; and in individuals taking anticoagulant medications, including warfarin, aspirin, aspirin-containing products, NSAIDs, antiplatelet agents (eg, ticlopidine, clopidogrel, dipyridamole). Discontinue use prior to dental or surgical procedures (generally at least 14 days before).

References

Ai WB, Chen YH, and Yang QJ, "Clinical Observation on Effect of Xuesaitong Injection as Auxiliary Treatment of Severe Craniocerebral Injury," *Zhongguo Zhong Xi Yi Jie He Za Zhi*, 2004, 24(3):213-5.
Caron MF, Hotsko AL, Robertson S, et al, "Electrocardiographic and Hemodynamic Effects of *Panax Ginseng*," *Ann Pharmacother*, 2002, 36(5):758-63.
Chan LY, Chiu PY, and Lau TK, "An *In vitro* Study of Ginsenoside Rb1-Induced Teratogenicity Using a Whole Rat Embryo Culture Model," *Hum Reprod*, 2003, 18(10):2166-8.
Chang YS and Park CI, "The Effect of *Panax ginseng* on the Postoperative Radiation Complication in Cervical Cancer Patients," *Seoul J Med*, 1980, 21:187-93.
Chen KJ, "The Effect and Abuse Syndrome of Ginseng," *J Tradit Chin Med*, 1981, 1(1):69-72.
Cherdrungsi P and Rungroeng K, "Effects of Standardized Ginseng Extract and Exercise Training on Aerobic and Anaerobic Exercise Capacities in Humans," *Korean J Ginseng Sci*, 1995, 19(2):93-100.
Choi HK, Seong DH, and Rha KH, "Clinical Efficacy of Korean Red Ginseng for Erectile Dysfunction," *Int J Impot Res*, 1995, 7(3):181-6.
Chong SK and Oberholzer VG, "Ginseng - Is There a Use in Clinical Medicine?" *Postgrad Med J*, 1988, 64(757):841-6.
Cui XD and Wang BP, "Panax Pseudo-Ginseng Powder for the Treatment of 30 Patients With Chronica Active Hepatitis," *Chinese Journal of Integrated Traditional and Western Medicine on Liver Diseases*, 1994, 4(2):37-38.
de Andrade E, de Mesquita AA, Claro Jde A, et al, "Study of the Efficacy of Korean Red Ginseng in the Treatment of Erectile Dysfunction," *Asian J Androl*, 2007, 9(2):241-4.
Ding DZ, Shen TK, and Cui YZ, "Effects of Red Ginseng on the Congestive Heart Failure and Its Mechanism," *Zhongguo Zhong Xi Yi Jie He Za Zhi*, 1995, 15(6):325-7.
Dukes MN, "Ginseng and Mastalgia," *Br Med J*, 1978, 1(6127):1621.
Fang-yun X, Zhi-fan Z, Hui-ying H, et al, "Clinical Observation on Nasopharyngeal Carcinoma Treated With Combined Therapy of Radiotherapy and Ginseng Polysaccharide Injection," *Chinese Journal of Integrated Traditional and Western Medicine*, 2001, 7(4):273-6.
Forgo I, "Effect of Drugs on Physical Exertion and the Hormonal System of Athletes," *MMW Munch Med Wochenschr*, 1983, 125(38):822-4.
Gross D, Shenkman Z, Bleiberg B, et al, "Ginseng Improves Pulmonary Functions and Exercise Capacity in Patients With COPD," *Monaldi Arch Chest Dis*, 2002, 57(5-6):242-6.
Han KH, Choe SC, Kim HS, et al, "Effect of Red Ginseng on Blood Pressure in Patients With Essential Hypertension and White Coat Hypertension," *Am J Chin Med*, 1998, 26(2):199-209.
Hiai S, et al, "Stimulation of Pituitary-Adrenocortical System by Ginseng Saponin," *J Endocrinol Jpn*, 1979, 26(6):661-5.
Hopkins MP, Androff L, and Benninghoff AS, "Ginseng Face Cream and Unexplained Vaginal Bleeding," *Am J Obstet Gynecol*, 1988, 159(5):1121-2
Janetzky K and Morreale AP, "Probable Interaction Between Warfarin and Ginseng," *Am J Health Syst Pharm*, 1997, 54(6):692-3.
Jiangming L, Haiwei C, Aisheng W, et al, "Comparative Study Effect of *Panax notoginseng* and Ticlid in Treating Early Diabetes Nephropathy," *Diabetes*, 2000, 49:A376.
Jones BD and Runikis AM, "Interaction of Ginseng With Phenelzine," *J Clin Psychopharmacol*, 1987, 7 (3):201-2.
Kim JY, Germolec DR, and Luster MI, "*Panax ginseng* as a Potential Immunomodulator: Studies in Mice," *Immunopharmacol Immunotoxicol*, 1990, 12(2):257-76.
Kim SH and Park KS, "Effects of Panax Ginseng Extract on Lipid Metabolism in Humans," *Pharmacol Res*, 2003, 48(5):511-3.
Natural Standard Research Collaboration, Chief Editors: Ulbricht C, Basch E, *Natural Standard Herb and Supplement Reference - Evidence-Based Clinical Reviews*, USA: Elsevier/Mosby, 2005.
Ng TB and Yeung HW, "Hypoglycemic Constituents of *Panax ginseng*," *Gen Pharmacol*, 1985, 16 (6):549-52.
Palop-Larrea V, Gonzálvez-Perales JL, Catálan-Oliver C, et al, "Metrorrhagia and Ginseng," *Ann Pharmacother*, 2000, 34(11):1347-8.
Pieralisi G, Ripari P, and Vecchiet L, "Effects of a Standardized Ginseng Extract Combined With Dimethylaminoethanol Bitartrate, Vitamins, Minerals, and Trace Elements on Physical Performance During Exercise," *Clin Ther*, 1991, 13(3):373-82.
Reay JL, Kennedy DO, and Scholey AB, "The Glycaemic Effects of Single Doses of *Panax ginseng* in Young Healthy Volunteers," *Br J Nutr*, 2006, 96(4):639-42.
Reay JL, Kennedy DO, and Scholey AB, "Single Doses of Panax Ginseng (G115) Reduce Blood Glucose Levels and Improve Cognitive Performance During Sustained Mental Activity," *J Psychopharmacol*, 2005, 19(4):357-65.
Scaglione F, Weiser K, and Alessandria M, "Effects of the Standardised Ginseng Extract G115(R) in Patients With Chronic Bronchitis: A Nonblinded, Randomised, Comparative Pilot Study," *Clinical Drug Investigations*, 2001, 21(1):41-5.
Scaglione F, Cattaneo G, Alessandria M, et al, "Efficacy and Safety of the Standardised Ginseng Extract G115 for Potentiating Vaccination Against the Influenza Syndrome and Protection Against the Common Cold," *Drugs Exp Clin Res*, 1996, 22(2):65-72.
Scaglione F, Ferrara F, Dugnani S, et al, "Immunomodulatory Effects of Two Extracts of *Panax ginseng* C.A. Meyer," *Drugs Exp Clin Res*, 1990, 16(10):537-42.
Siegel RK, "Ginseng and High Blood Pressure," *JAMA*, 1980, 243(1):32.
Suh SO, Kroh M, Kim NR, et al, "Effects of Red Ginseng Upon Postoperative Immunity and Survival in Patients With Stage III Gastric Cancer," *Am J Chin Med*, 2002, 30(4):483-94.
Sung J, Han KH, Zo JH, et al, "Effects of Red Ginseng Upon Vascular Endothelial Function in Patients With Essential Hypertension," *Am J Chin Med*, 2000, 28(2):205-16.
Teng CM, Kuo SC, Kof N, et al, "Antiplatelet Actions of Panaxynol and Ginsenosides Isolated From Ginseng," *Biochim Biophys Acta*, 1989, 990(3):315-20.
Van Schepdael P, "Les Effets du Ginseng G115 sur la Capacite Physique de Sportifs d'Endurance," *Acta Therapeutica*, 1993, 19:337-347.
Vuksan V, Sievenpiper JL, Koo VY, et al, "American Ginseng (*Panax quinquefolius* L) Reduces Postprandial Glycemia in Nondiabetic Subjects and Subjects With Type 2 Diabetes Mellitus," *Arch Intern Med*, 2000, 160(7):1009-13.
Vuksan V, Stavro MP, Sievenpiper JL, et al, "Similar Postprandial Glycemic Reductions With Escalation of Dose and Administration Time of American Ginseng in Type 2 Diabetes," *Diabetes Care*, 2000, 23 (9):1221-6.
Zhao XZ, "Antisenility Effect of Ginseng-Rhizome Saponin," *Zhong Xi Yi Jie He Za Zhi*, 1990, 10 (10):579,586-9.
Zuin M, Battezzati PM, Camisasca M, et al, "Effects of a Preparation Containing a Standardized Ginseng Extract Combined With Trace Elements and Multivitamins Against Hepatotoxin-Induced Chronic Liver Disease in the Elderly," *J Int Med Res*, 1987, 15(5):276-81.

Ginseng, Siberian

Pharmacologic Category Herb

Reported Use

Adaptogen/tonic (promote wellness) (Brekhman, 1965; Brekhman, 1969)

Athletic performance (enhancement); stress (decrease fatigue); immune support (Hikino, 1986; Huang, 2005; Szołomicki, 2000)
Herpes simplex, type 2 (Williams, 1995)
Neurocirculatory hypotension (Kaloeva, 1986)

Local Anesthetic/Vasoconstrictor Precautions Has potential to interact with epinephrine and levonordefrin to result in increased BP; use vasoconstrictor with caution

Effects on Bleeding May have antiplatelet effects

Warnings/Precautions Based on pharmacologic activity, use with caution with stimulant products, including decongestants, caffeine, and caffeine-containing beverages.

Based on pharmacologic activity, use with caution in individuals with hypertension or in individuals receiving antihypertensive medications; and in individuals at risk of hypotension (including those taking antihypertensive medication or agents that predispose to orthostasis), elderly individuals, or those who would not tolerate transient hyper- or hypotensive episodes (ie, cerebrovascular or cardiovascular disease). May potentiate effects of antihypertensives.

Use with caution in individuals taking barbiturates (based on *in vitro* or animal studies) (McRae, 1996; Medon, 1984).

Use with caution in individuals with diabetes or in those who may be predisposed to hypoglycemia; may alter glucose regulation. Effects of drugs with hypoglycemic activity may be potentiated (including insulin and oral hypoglycemics). Blood sugar should be closely monitored and the dosage of hypoglycemic medications may require adjustment. This should be carefully coordinated among the individual's healthcare providers.

Based on pharmacologic activity and case reports, hemostasis may be affected. Based on pharmacologic activity, this herb may be contraindicated in individuals with active bleeding (eg, peptic ulcer, intracranial bleeding). Use with caution in individuals with a history of bleeding, hemostatic disorders, or drug-related hemostatic problems; and in individuals taking anticoagulant medications, including warfarin, aspirin, aspirin-containing products, NSAIDs, or antiplatelet agents (eg, ticlopidine, clopidogrel, dipyridamole). Discontinue use prior to dental or surgical procedures (generally at least 14 days before).

Extensive or prolonged use may heighten estrogenic activity (based on pharmacologic activity).

References

Brekhman II and Kirillov OI, "Effect of *Eleutherococcus* on Alarm-Phase of Stress," *Life Sci*, 1969, 8 (3):113-21.
Brekhman II and Maianskii GM, "*Eleutherococcus* - a Means of Increasing the Nonspecific Resistance of the Organism," *Izv Akad Nauk SSSR Biol*, 1965, 5:762-5.
Chan LY, Chiu PY, and Lau TK, "An *In-Vitro* Study of Ginsenoside Rb1-Induced Teratogenicity Using a Whole Rat Embryo Culture Model," *Hum Reprod*, 2003, 18(10):2166-8.
Hikino H, Takahashi M, Otakek, et al, "Isolation and Hypoglycemic Activity of Eleutherans A, B, C, D, E, F and G: Glycans of *Eleutherococcus senticosus* Roots," *J Nat Prod*, 1986, 49(2):293-7.
Huang DB, Ran RZ, and Yu ZF, "Effect of Acanthopanax Senticosus Injection on the Activities of Human Tumor Necrosis Factor and Natural Killer Cell in Blood in the Patients With Lung Cancer," *Zhongguo Zhong Yao Za Zhi*, 2005, 30(8):621-4.
Kaloeva ZD, "Effect of the Glycosides of Eleutherococcus Senticosus on the Hemodynamic Indices of Children With Hypotensive States," *Farmakol Toksikol*, 1986, 49(5):73.
McRae S, "Elevated Serum Digoxin Levels in a Patient Taking Digoxin and Siberian Ginseng," *CMAJ*, 1996, 155(3):293-5.
Medon PJ, Ferguson PW, and Watson CF, "Effects of *Eleutherococcus senticosus* Extracts on Hexobarbital Metabolism *In Vivo* and *In Vitro*," *J Ethnopharmacol*, 1984, 10(2):235-41.
Natural Standard Research Collaboration, Chief Editors: Ulbricht C, Basch E, *Natural Standard Herb and Supplement Reference - Evidence-Based Clinical Reviews*, USA: Elsevier/Mosby, 2005.
Szołomicki J, Samochowiec L, Wójcicki J, et al, "The Influence of Active Components of Eleutherococcus Senticosus on Cellular Defence and Physical Fitness in Man," *Phytother Res*, 2000, 14(1):30-5.
Williams M, "Immunoprotection Against Herpes Simplex Type II Infection by Eleutherococcus Root Extract," *J Alt Comp Med*, 1995, 13:9-12.

Glucosamine

Pharmacologic Category Nutraceutical

Reported Use

Chronic venous insufficiency (Gossetti, 1986)
Inflammatory bowel disease (Salvatore, 2000)
Knee injury recovery (Ostojic, 2007)
Osteoarthritis and joint structure support (Das, 2000; Herrero-Beaumont, 2007; McAlindon, 2000; Muller, 1994; Noack, 1994; Phillipi, 1999; Pujalte, 1980; Qiu, 1998; Reginster, 2001; Reginster, 2003; Richy, 2003; Shankland, 1998; Towheed, 2000)
Rheumatoid arthritis and other inflammatory conditions (McCarty, 1998)
Temporomandibular joint (TMJ) disorders (Shankland, 1998)

Local Anesthetic/Vasoconstrictor Precautions No information available to require special precautions

Effects on Bleeding None reported

Warnings/Precautions Use with caution in individuals with allergy to shellfish.

No known toxicity or serious side effects reported. Occasional reports of mild gastrointestinal discomfort or stomach upset. Based on animal studies, may alter glucose regulation/insulin sensitivity; use with caution in individuals with diabetes.

Contraindicated in individuals with active bleeding (eg, peptic ulcer, intracranial bleeding). Use with caution in individuals with a history of bleeding, hemostatic disorders, or drug-related hemostatic problems. Use with caution in individuals taking anticoagulant medications, including warfarin, aspirin, aspirin-containing products, NSAIDs, or antiplatelet agents (eg, ticlopidine, clopidogrel, dipyridamole). Discontinue use prior to dental or surgical procedures (generally at least 14 days before).

May cause drowsiness, somnolence, or insomnia. Use with caution when driving or operating heavy machinery.

Use with caution in individuals with renal impairment.

References

Das A Jr and Hammad TA, "Efficacy of a Combination of FCHG49 Glucosamine Hydrochloride, TRH122 Low Molecular Weight Sodium Chondroitin Sulfate and Manganese Ascorbate in the Management of Knee Osteoarthritis," *Osteoarthritis Cartilage*, 2000, 8(5):343-50.

Gossetti B, Gattuso R, Irace L, et al, "Venous Insufficiency of the Legs. Pharmacologic Treatment With Glycosamine-Glycan (Perclar)," *Minerva Med*, 1986, 77(41):1915-8.

Herrero-Beaumont G, Ivorra JA, Del Carmen Trabado M, et al, "Glucosamine Sulfate in the Treatment of Knee Osteoarthritis Symptoms: A Randomized, Double-Blind, Placebo-Controlled Study Using Acetaminophen as a Side Comparator," *Arthritis Rheum*, 2007, 56(2):555-67.

McAlindon TE, LaValley MP, Gulin JP, et al, "Glucosamine and Chondroitin for Treatment of Osteoarthritis: A Systematic Quality Assessment and Meta-Analysis," *JAMA*, 2000, 283(11):1469-75.

McCarty MF, "Vascular Heparan Sulfates May Limit the Ability of Leukocytes to Penetrate the Endothelial Barrier - Implications for Use of Glucosamine in Inflammatory Disorders," *Med Hypotheses*, 1998, 51 (1):11-15.

Muller H, Bach GL, Haase W, et al, "Glucosamine Sulfate Compared to Ibuprofen in Osteoarthritis of the Knee," *Osto and Cart*, 1994, 2:61-9.

Natural Standard Research Collaboration, Chief Editors: Ulbricht C, Basch E, *Natural Standard Herb and Supplement Reference - Evidence-Based Clinical Reviews*, USA: Elsevier/Mosby, 2005.

Nelson BA, Robinson KA, and Buse MG, "High Glucose and Glucosamine Induce Insulin Resistance Via Different Mechanisms in 3T3-L1 Adipocytes," *Diabetes*, 2000, 49(6):981-91.

Noack W, Fischer M, Forster KK, et al, "Glucosamine Sulfate in Osteoarthritis of the Knee," *Osto and Cart*, 1994, 2:51-9.

Ostojic SM, Arsic M, Prodanovic S, et al, "Glucosamine Administration in Athletes: Effects on Recovery of Acute Knee Injury," *Res Sports Med*, 2007, 15(2):113-24.

Phillipi AF, Leffler CT, Leffler SG, et al, "Glucosamine, Chondroitin, and Manganese Ascorbate for Degenerative Joint Disease of the Knee or Low Back: A Randomized, Double-Blind, Placebo-Controlled Pilot Study," *Military Medicine*, 1999, 164:85-91.

Pujalte JM, Llavore EP, and Ylescupidez FR, "Double-Blind Clinical Evaluation of Oral Glucosamine Sulfate in the Basic Treatment of Osteoarthrosis," *Curr Med Res Opin*, 1980, 7(2):110-14.

Qui GX, Gao SN, Giacovelli G, et al, "Efficacy and Safety of Glucosamine Sulfate Versus Ibuprofen in Patients With Knee Osteoarthritis," *Arzneimittelforschung*, 1998, 48(5):469-74.

Reginster JY, Bruyere O, Lecart MP, et al, "Naturocetic (Glucosamine and Chrondroitin Sulfate) Compounds as Structure-Modifying Drugs in the Treatment of Osteoarthritis," *Curr Opin Rheumatol*, 2003, 15(5):651-5.

Reginster JY, Deroisy R, Rovati LC, et al, "Long-Term Effects of Glucosamine Sulphate on Osteoarthritis Progression: A Randomised, Placebo-Controlled Clinical Trial," *Lancet*, 2001, 357(9252):251-6.

Richy F, Bruyere O, Ethgen O, et al, "Structural and Symptomatic Efficacy of Glucosamine and Chondroitin in Knee Osteoarthritis: A Comprehensive Meta-Analysis," *Arch Intern Med*, 2003, 163 (13):1514-22.

Russell AS, Aghazadeh-Habashi A, and Jamali F, "Active Ingredient Consistency of Commercially Available Glucosamine Sulfate Products," *J Rheumatol*, 2002, 29(11):2407-9.

Salvatore S, Heuschkel R, Tomlin S, et al, "A Pilot Study of N-acetyl Glucosamine, a Nutritional Substrate for Glycosaminoglycan Synthesis, in Paediatric Chronic Inflammatory Bowel Disease," *Aliment Pharmacol Ther*, 2000, 14(12):1567-79.

Shankland WE 2nd, "The Effects of Glucosamine and Chondroitin Sulfate on Osteoarthritis of the TMJ: A Preliminary Report of 50 Patients," *Cranio*, 1998, 16(4):230-5.

Steensma, DP, "The Kiss of Death: A Severe Allergic Reaction to a Shellfish Induced by a Good-Night Kiss," *Mayo Clin Proc*, 2003, 78(2):221-2.

Towheed TE and Anastassiades TP, "Glucosamine and Chondroitin for Treating Symptoms of Osteoarthritis: Evidence Is Widely Touted but Incomplete," *JAMA*, 2000, 283(11):1483-4.

Yue QY, Strandell J, and Myrberg O, "Concomitant Use of Glucosamine May Potentiate the Effect of Warfarin." Available at http://www.who-umc.org/graphics/9722.pdf.

Glutathione

Pharmacologic Category Nutraceutical

Reported Use

Antioxidant (Kim, 2002)

Chemoprotection (Cascinu, 1995; Cascinu, 1997; Cascinu, 1998; Cascinu, 2002; Colombo, 1995; Smyth, 1997)

Hepatoprotection (alcohol-induced liver damage) (Altomare, 1988)

Immune support (Spallholz, 1990)

Male infertility (Lenzi, 1993)

Peptic ulcer disease (Hirokawa, 1995)

Peripheral artery disease (Arosio, 2002)

Local Anesthetic/Vasoconstrictor Precautions No information available to require special precautions

Effects on Bleeding None reported

Warnings/Precautions Acetaminophen and alcohol may decrease the effects of glutathione.

References

Altomare E, Vendemiale G, and Albano O, "Hepatic Glutathione Content in Patients With Alcoholic and Non-Alcoholic Liver Diseases," *Life Sci*, 1988, 43(12):991-8.

Arosio E, De Marchi S, Zannoni M, et al, "Effect of Glutathione Infusion on Leg Arterial Circulation, Cutaneous Microcirculation, and Pain-Free Walking Distance in Patients With Peripheral Obstructive Arterial Disease: A Randomized, Double-Blind, Placebo-Controlled Trial," *Mayo Clin Proc*, 2002, 77 (8):754-9.

Cascinu S, Catalano V, Cordella L, et al, "Neuroprotective Effect of Reduced Glutathione on Oxaliplatin-Based Chemotherapy in Advanced Colorectal Cancer: A Randomized, Double-Blind, Placebo-Controlled Trial," *J Clin Oncol*, 2002, 20(16):3478-83.

Cascinu S, Cordella L, Del Ferro E, et al, "Neuroprotective Effect of Reduced Glutathione on Cisplatin-Based Chemotherapy in Advanced Gastric Cancer: A Randomized Double-Blind Placebo-Controlled Trial," *J Clin Oncol*, 1995, 13(1):26-32.

Cascinu S, Labianca R, Alessandroni P, et al, "Intensive Weekly Chemotherapy for Advanced Gastric Cancer Using Fluorouracil, Cisplatin, Epi-Doxorubicin, 6S-Leucovorin, Glutathione, and Filgrastim: A Report From the Italian Group for the Study of Digestive Tract Cancer," *J Clin Oncol*, 1997, 15 (11):3313-9.

Cascinu S, Labianca R, Graziano F, et al, "Intensive Weekly Chemotherapy for Locally Advanced Gastric Cancer Using 5-Fluorouracil, Cisplatin, Epidoxorubicin, 6S-Leucovorin, Glutathione and Filgrastim: A Report From the Italian Group for the Study of Digestive Tract Cancer (GISCAD)," *Br J Cancer*, 1998, 78 (3):390-3.

Colombo N, Bini S, Miceli D, et al, "Weekly Cisplatin +/- Glutathione in Relapsed Ovarian Carcinoma," *Int J Gynecol Cancer*, 1995, 5(2):81-86.

Hirokawa K and Kawasaki H, "Changes in Glutathione in Gastric Mucosa of Gastric Ulcer Patients," *Res Commun Mol Pathol Pharmacol*, 1995, 88(2):163-76.

Kim HJ, Liu X, Wang H, et al, "Glutathione Prevents Inhibition of Fibroblast-Mediated Collagen Gel Contraction by Cigarette Smoke," *Amer J of Physiol Lung Cell Mol Physiol*, 2002, 283(2):L409-L417.

Lenzi A, Culasso F, Gandini L, et al, "Placebo-Controlled, Double-Blind, Cross-Over Trial of Glutathione Therapy in Male Infertility," *Hum Reprod*, 1993, 8(10):1657-62.

Natural Standard Research Collaboration, Chief Editors: Ulbricht C, Basch E, *Natural Standard Herb and Supplement Reference - Evidence-Based Clinical Reviews*, USA: Elsevier/Mosby, 2005.

Smyth JF, Bowman A, Perren T, et al, "Glutathione Reduces the Toxicity and Improves Quality of Life of Women Diagnosed With Ovarian Cancer Treated With Cisplatin: Results of a Double-Blind, Randomised Trial," *Ann Oncol*, 1997, 8(6):569-73.

Spallholz JE, "Selenium and Glutathione Peroxidase: Essential Nutrient and Antioxidant Component of the Immune System," *Adv Exp Med Biol*, 1990, 262:145-58.

Golden Seal

Pharmacologic Category Herb

Reported Use

- Fever (pharmacologic activity)
- Gallbladder (pharmacologic activity)
- Heart failure (Marin-Neto, 1988; Zeng, 2003)
- Hypercholesterolemia (Kong, 2004)
- Immune stimulation (Liu, 1991)
- Infectious diarrhea (Rabbani, 1987)
- Malaria (chloroquine-resistant) (Sheng, 1997)
- Mucous membrane tonifying (used in inflammation of mucosal membranes); gastritis; antimicrobial (antibacterial/antifungal); bronchitis, cystitis, and infectious diarrhea (Bradley, 1992)
- Narcotic concealment (urine analysis) (Cone, 1998)
- Sinusitis (pharmacologic activity)
- Sore throat (pharmacologic activity)
- Trachoma (Babbar, 1982; Khosla, 1992; Mohan, 1982; Sabir, 1976)
- Urinary tract infection (UTI) (pharmacologic activity)

Local Anesthetic/Vasoconstrictor Precautions No information available to require special precautions

Effects on Bleeding None reported

Warnings/Precautions Use of golden seal is contraindicated in pregnancy (based on animal studies) (De Smet, 1992). The berberine constituent of golden seal may cause kernicterus in newborns. Use with caution in individuals with cardiovascular disease. High doses may cause hypotension or bradycardia (based on animal studies) (Sabir, 1971). Doses in the range of 2-3 g may cause gastrointestinal distress or bradycardia. Extremely high-dose ingestion (18 g) has been reported to induce CNS depression. High-dose hydrastine has been associated with hypertension, hyper-reflexia, and seizures (Genest, 1969). Extended use of high doses has been associated in some reports with neuroexcitation, hallucinations, delirium, and gastrointestinal disorders. Overdose has been associated with myocardial damage and respiratory failure (Genest, 1969).

References

Babbar OP, Chatwal VK, Ray IB, et al, "Effect of Berberine Chloride Eye Drops on Clinically Positive Trachoma Patients," *Indian J Med Res*, 1982, 76(Suppl):83-8.

Bradley PR, ed, *British Herbal Compendium*, Vol 1, Bournemouth, England: British Herbal Medicine Association, 1992, 119-20.

Cone EJ, Lange R, Darwin WD, "*In vivo* Adulteration: Excess Fluid Ingestion Causes False-Negative Marijuana and Cocaine Urine Test Results," *J Anal Toxicol*, 1998, 22(6):460-73.

Genest, K et al, "Natural Products in Canadian Pharmaceuticals, *Hydrastis canadensis*," *Can J Pharm Sci*, 1969, 4:41-45.

Khosla PK, Neeraj VI, Gupta SK, et al, "Berberine, a Potential Drug for Trachoma," *Rev Int Trach Pathol Ocul Trop Subtrop Sante Publique*, 1992, 69:147-65.

Kong W, Wei J, Abidi P, et al, "Berberine Is a Novel Cholesterol-Lowering Drug Working Through a Unique Mechanism Distinct From Statins," *Nat Med*, 2004, 10(12):1344-51.

Liu CX, Xiao PG, and Liu GS, "Studies on Plant Resources, Pharmacology and Clinical Treatment With Berbamine," *Phytotheraphy Research*, 1991, 5:228-30.
Marin-Neto JA, Maciel BC, Secches AL, et al, "Cardiovascular Effects of Berberine in Patients With Severe Congestive Heart Failure," *Clin Cardiol*, 1988, 11(4):253-60.
Mohan M, Pant CR, Angra SK, et al, "Berberine in Trachoma. (A Clinical Trial)," *Indian J Ophthalmol*, 1982, 30(2):69-75.
Natural Standard Research Collaboration, Chief Editors: Ulbricht C, Basch E, *Natural Standard Herb and Supplement Reference - Evidence-Based Clinical Reviews*, USA: Elsevier/Mosby, 2005.
Newall CA, Anderson LA, and Phillipson JD, *Herbal Medicines: A Guide for Health Care Professionals*, London, England: The Pharmaceutical Press, 1996, 151-2.
Rabbani GH, Butler T, Knight J, et al, "Randomized Controlled Trial of Berberine Sulfate Therapy for Diarrhea Due to Enterotoxigenic *Escherichia coli* and *Vibrio cholerae*," *J Infect Dis*, 1987, 155 (5):979-84.
Sabir M and Bhide NK, "Study of Some Pharmacological Actions of Berberine," *Indian J Physiol Pharmacol*, 1971, 15(3):111-32.
Sabir M, Mahajan VM, Mohapatra LN, et al, "Experimental Study of the Antitrachoma Action of Berberine," *Indian J Med Res*, 1976, 64(8):1160-7.
Sheng WD, Jiddawi MS, Hong XQ, et al, "Treatment of Chloroquine-Resistant Malaria Using Pyrimethamine in Combination With Berberine, Tetracycline or Cotrimoxazole," *East Afr Med J*, 1997, 74 (5):283-4.
Zeng XH, Zeng XJ, and Li YY, "Efficacy and Safety of Berberine for Congestive Heart Failure Secondary to Ischemic or Idiopathic Dilated Cardiomyopathy," *Am J Cardiol*, 2003, 92(2):173-6.

Gotu Kola

Pharmacologic Category Herb

Reported Use

Anxiety (Bradwejn, 1998; Bradwejn, 1999; Bradwejn, 2000)
Cirrhosis (Kaziulin, 2006)
Connective tissue (support) (Newall, 1996)
Diabetic microangiopathy (Belcaro, 1989; Cesarone, 2001; Incandela, 2001)
Hemorrhoids (topical) (Suguna, 1996; Tenni, 1988)
Macular degeneration (pharmacologic activity)
Memory enhancement (Newall, 1996)
Psoriasis (Natarajan, 1973)
Venous insufficiency (Cesarone, 1994; Pointel, 1987)
Wound healing (topical) (Suguna, 1996; Tenni, 1988)

Local Anesthetic/Vasoconstrictor Precautions No information available to require special precautions

Effects on Bleeding None reported

Warnings/Precautions Use of gotu kola is contraindicated during pregnancy (emmenagogue and abortifacient in animal studies) (Ramswamy, 1970). Large doses may be sedating (Ramswamy, 1970). Caution individuals to avoid hazardous tasks (eg, driving or operating machinery). Use with caution in individuals taking sedative medications (eg, anxiolytics, benzodiazepines). Effects may be additive with other CNS depressants. Topical administration may cause contact dermatitis in sensitive individuals (Danese, 1994). High doses of gotu kola may elevate cholesterol levels (Ramswamy, 1970). Use with caution in individuals with diabetes or in those taking antidiabetic agents because gotu kola may cause hyperglycemia (Ramswamy, 1970). Use with caution in individuals taking antilipemic agents because gotu kola may elevate cholesterol (Ramswamy, 1970). Hepatotoxicity has been reported with gotu kola use (Jorge, 2005).

References

Belcaro G, Laurora G, Cesarone MR, et al, "Efficacy of Centellase® in the Treatment of Venous Hypertension Evaluated by a Combined Microcirculatory Model," *Curr Ther Res*, 1989, 46(6);1015-26.
Bradwejn J, Kosycki D, Shlik J, et al, "*Centella asiatica* Decreases the Acoustic Startle Response," 152nd Annual Meeting of the American Psychiatric Association, Washington, DC, USA (May 15-20), 1999.
Bradwejn J, Zhou Y, Koszycki, et al, "Effect of Acute Administration of Gotu-Kola (*Centella asiatica*) on Acoustic Startle Response in Healthy Volunteers," XXIst Collegium Internationale Neuro-Psychopharmacologicum, Glascow, Scotland (July 12-16), 1998.
Bradwejn J, Zhou Y, and Koszycki D, "A Double-Blind, Placebo-Controlled Study on the Effects of Gotu Kola (*Centella asiatica*) on Acoustic Startle Response in Healthy Subjects," *J Clin Psychopharmacol*, 2000, 20(6):680-4.
Cesarone MR, Incandela L, De Sanctis MT, et al, "Evaluation of Treatment of Diabetic Microangiopathy With Total Triterpenic Fraction of *Centella asiatica*: A Clinical Prospective Randomized Trial With a Microcirculatory Model," *Angiology*, 2001, 52(2 Suppl):S49-54.
Cesarone MR, Laurora G, De Santis MT, et al, "The Microcirculatory Activity of *Centella asiatica* in Venous Insufficiency. A Double-Blind Study," *Minerva Cardioangiol*, 1994, 42(6):299-304.
Danese P, Carnevali C, and Bertazzoni MG, "Allergic Contact Dermatitis Due to *Centella asiatica* Extract," *Contact Dermatitis*, 1994, 31(3):201.
Incandela L, Belcaro G, Cesarone MR, et al, "Treatment of Diabetic Microangiopathy and Edema With Total Triterpenic Fraction of *Centella asiatica*: A Prospective, Placebo-Controlled Randomized Study," *Angiology*, 2001, 52(2 Suppl):S27-31.
Jorge OA and Jorge AD, "Hepatotoxicity Associated With the Ingestion of *Centella asiatica*," *Rev Esp Enferm Dig*, 2005, 97(2):115-24.
Kaziulin AN, Petukhov AB, and Kucheriavyĭ IuA, "Efficiency of Includes of Bioactive Substances in Diet of Patient With Hepatic Encephalopathy," *Vopr Pitan*, 2006, 75(2):40-4.
Natarajan S and Paily PP, "Effect of Topical *Hydrocotyle asiatica* in Psoriasis," *Indian J Dermatol*, 1973, 18(4):82-5.
Natural Standard Research Collaboration, Chief Editors: Ulbricht C, Basch E, *Natural Standard Herb and Supplement Reference - Evidence-Based Clinical Reviews*, USA: Elsevier/Mosby, 2005.
Newall CA, Anderson LA, and Phillipson JD, *Herbal Medicines: A Guide for Health Care Professionals*, London, England: The Pharmaceutical Press, 1996, 170-2.
Pointel JP, Boccalon H, Cloarec M, et al, "Titrated Extract of *Centella asiatica* (TECA) in the Treatment of Venous Insufficiency of the Lower Limbs," *Angiology*, 1987, 38(1 Pt 1):46-50.
Ramswamy AS, et al, "Pharmacological Studies of *Centella asiatica*," *Indian J Med Res*, 1970, 4:160-75.
Suguna L, Sivakumar P, and Chandrakasan G, "Effects of *Centella asiatica* Extract on Dermal Wound Healing in Rats," *Indian J Exp Biol*, 1996, 34(12):1208-11.

Tenni R, Zanaboni G, De Agostini MP, et al, "Effect of the Triterpenoid Fraction of *Centella asiatica* on Macromolecules of the Connective Matrix in Human Skin Fibroblast Cultures," *Ital J Biochem*, 1988, 37 (2):69-77.

Grapefruit Seed

Pharmacologic Category Herb

Reported Use

Antifungal, antibacterial, antiparasitic agent (Ionescu, 1990)
Diarrhea (pharmacologic activity)
Diverticulitis (pharmacologic activity)
Eczema (pharmacologic activity)
Endometriosis (pharmacologic activity)
Heart disease (Cerda, 1988)
Irritable bowl syndrome (IBS) (pharmacologic activity)
Kidney stones (Trinchieri, 2002)
Metabolic syndrome (Fujioka, 2006)
Rosacea (pharmacologic activity)
Sinusitis (pharmacologic activity)
Sore throat (pharmacologic activity)
Ulcerative colitis (pharmacologic activity)
Urinary tract infection (UTI) (pharmacologic activity)

Local Anesthetic/Vasoconstrictor Precautions No information available to require special precautions

Effects on Bleeding None reported

Warnings/Precautions Grapefruit seed extract is not the equivalent of grapefruit juice. Grapefruit juice/pulp has been associated with the inhibition of drug metabolism via cytochrome P450 isoenzyme 3A4 (CYP3A4), resulting in a number of drug interactions. It may also inhibit CYP 1A2, 2C9, and 2C19, as well as the drug transporters. P-glycoprotein (P-gp) and organic anion transporting peptide (OATP). It is not known whether extracts of grapefruit seed share in this potential to alter drug metabolism. Until further information is available, it is reasonable to avoid the concurrent use of grapefruit seed extract in individuals receiving calcium channel blockers, benzodiazepines, immunosuppressants, HMG-CoA reductase inhibitors, and other medications metabolized by this pathway. Caution is warranted.

References

Cerda JJ, Robbins FL, Burgin CW, et al, "The Effects of Grapefruit Pectin on Patients at Risk for Coronary Heart Disease Without Altering Diet or Lifestyle," *Clin Cardiol*, 1988, 11(9):589-94.
Fujioka K, Greenway F, Sheard J, et al, "The Effects of Grapefruit on Weight and Insulin Resistance: Relationship to the Metabolic Syndrome," *J Med Food*, 2006, 9(1):49-54.
Ionescu G, Kiehl R, Wichmann-Kunz F, et al, "Oral Citrus Seed Extract in Atopic Eczema: *In vitro* and *In vivo* Studies on Intestinal Microflora," *Journal of Orthomolecular Medicine*, 1990, 5:72-3.
Natural Standard Research Collaboration, Chief Editors: Ulbricht C, Basch E, *Natural Standard Herb and Supplement Reference - Evidence-Based Clinical Reviews*, USA: Elsevier/Mosby, 2005.
Trinchieri A, Lizzano R, Bernardini P, et al, "Effect of Acute Load of Grapefruit Juice on Urinary Excretion of Citrate and Urinary Risk Factors for Renal Stone Formation," *Dig Liver Dis*, 2002, 34(Suppl 2): S160-3.

Grapeseed

Pharmacologic Category Herb

Reported Use

Agitation (aromatherapy) (Snow, 2004)
Allergies, anti-inflammatory, asthma (Frankel, 1993)
Antioxidant (Maffei Facino, 1997)
Cardiovascular health (Vinson, 2002)
Chloasma (Yamakoshi, 2004)
Circulation, platelet aggregation inhibitor, capillary fragility, arterial/venous insufficiency (intermittent claudification, varicose veins) (Delacroix, 1981; Jonadet, 1983; Thebaut, 1985)
Diabetic retinopathy (Arne, 1982)
Edema (Baruch, 1984; Parienti, 1983; Sarrat, 1981)
Gingivitis (pharmacologic activity)
Glaucoma (pharmacologic activity)
Hyperlipidemia (Sano, 2007)
Macular degeneration (pharmacologic activity)
Multiple sclerosis (pharmacologic activity)
Pancreatitis (Banerjee, 2001)
Premenstrual syndrome (Amsellem, 1987)
Parkinson's disease (pharmacologic activity)
Scleroderma (pharmacologic activity)
Sun protection (Mittal, 2003)
Vision problems (Boissin, 1988; Corbé, 1988)

Local Anesthetic/Vasoconstrictor Precautions No information available to require special precautions

Effects on Bleeding May see increase in bleeding due to inhibition of platelet aggregation

Warnings/Precautions Based on pharmacologic activity, grapeseed may inhibit platelet aggregation (Chang, 1989) and may be contraindicated in individuals with active bleeding (eg, peptic ulcer, intracranial bleeding). Use with caution in individuals with a history of bleeding, hemostatic disorders, or drug-related hemostatic problems. Use with caution in individuals taking anticoagulant medications, including warfarin, aspirin, aspirin-containing products, NSAIDs, or antiplatelet agents (eg, ticlopidine, clopidogrel, dipyridamole). Discontinue use prior to dental or surgical procedures (generally at least 14 days before).

In vitro studies indicate grapeseed may inhibit xanthine oxidase (Bombardelli, 1995). It may increase toxicity of methotrexate.

References

Amsellem M, Masson JM, Negui B, et al, "Endotelon in the Treatment of Venolymphatic Problems in Premenstrual Syndrome. Multicenter Study on 165 Patients," *Tempo Med*, 1987, 282:46-51.

Arne JL, "Contribution to the Study of Procyanidolic Oligomers: Endotelon in Diabetic Retinopathy (Based on 30 Cases)," *Gaz Med France*, 1982, 89(30):3610-4.

Banerjee B and Bagchi D, "Beneficial Effects of a Novel IH636 Grape Seed Proanthocyanidin Extract in the Treatment of Chronic Pancreatitis," *Digestion*, 2001, 63(3):203-6.

Baruch J, "Effect of Endotelon in Postoperative Edema. Results of a Double-Blind Study Versus Placebo in 32 Female Patients," *Ann Chir Plast Esthet*, 1984, 29(4):393-5.

Boissin JP, Corbe C, and Siou A, "Chorioretinal Circulation and Dazzling Use of Procyanidol Oligomers (Endotelon)" *Bull Soc Ophtalmol Fr*, 1988, 88(2):173-4, 177-9.

Bombardelli E, "*Vitus vinifera* L," *Fitoterapia*, 1995, 66(4):291-7.

Chang WC and Hsu FL, "Inhibition of Platelet Aggregation and Arachidonate Metabolism in Platelets by Procyanidins," *Prostaglandins Leukot Essent Fatty Acids*, 1989, 38(3):181-8.

Corbé C, Boissin JP, and Siou A, "Light Vision and Chorioretinal Circulation. Study of the Effect of Procyanidolic Oligomers (Endotelon)," *J Fr Ophtalmol*, 1988, 11(5):453-60.

Delacroix P, "Double-Blind Study of Endotelon in Chronic Venous Insufficiency," *La Revue de Medecine*, 1981, 31(27-8):1793-1802.

Frankel EN, Kanner J, German JB, et al, "Inhibition of Oxidation of Human Low-Density Lipoprotein by Phenolic Substances in Red Wine," *Lancet*, 1993, 341(8843):454-7.

Jonadet M, Meunier MT, Bastide J, et al, "Anthocyanosides Extracted From *Vitis vinifera, Vaccinium myrtillus* and *Pinus maritimus*. I. Elastase-Inhibiting Activities *In vitro*. II. Compared Angioprotective Activities *In vivo*," *J Pharm Belg*, 1983, 38(1):41-6.

Maffei Facino R, Carini M, Aldini G, et al, "Regeneration of Endogenous Antioxidants, Ascorbic Acid, Alpha Tocopherol, by the Oligomeric Procyanide Fraction of *Vitus vinifera L*: ESR Study," *Boll Chim Farm*, 1997, 136(4):340-4.

Mittal A, Elmets CA, and Katiyar SK, "Dietary Feeding of Proanthocyanidins From Grape Seeds Prevents Photocarcinogenesis in SKH-1 Hairless Mice: Relationship to Decreased Fat and Lipid Peroxidation," *Carcinogenesis*, 2003, 24(8):1379-88.

Natural Standard Research Collaboration, Chief Editors: Ulbricht C, Basch E, *Natural Standard Herb and Supplement Reference - Evidence-Based Clinical Reviews*, USA: Elsevier/Mosby, 2005.

Parienti J and Pareinti-Amsellem J, "Post-Traumatic Edemas in Sports: A Controlled Test of Endotelon," *Gaz Med France*, 1983, 90(3):231-5.

Sano A, Uchida R, Saito M, et al, "Beneficial Effects of Grape Seed Extract on Malondialdehyde-Modified LDL," *J Nutr Sci Vitaminol (Tokyo)*, 2007, 53(2):174-82.

Sarrat L, "Therapeutic Relief of Functional Problems of the Lower Legs by Endotelon, a Microangioprotector," *Bordeaux Med*, 1981, 14:685-8.

Snow LA, Hovanec L, and Brandt J, "A Controlled Trial of Aromatherapy for Agitation in Nursing Home Patients With Dementia," *J Altrn Complement Med*, 2004, 10(3):431-7.

Thebaut JF, Thebaut P, and Vin F, "Study of Endotelon in the Functional Manifestations of Peripheral Venous Insufficiency. Results of a Double-Blind Study of 92 Patients," *Gazette Medicale*, 1985, 92 (1):96-100.

Vinson JA, Mandarano MA, Shuta DL, et al, "Beneficial Effects of a Novel IH636 Grape Seed Proanthocyanidin Extract and a Niacin-Bound Chromium in a Hamster Atherosclerosis Model," *Mol Cell Biochem*, 2002, 240(1-2):99-103.

Yamakoshi J, Sano A, Tokutake S, et al, "Oral Intake of Proanthocyanidin-Rich Extract From Grape Seeds Improves Chloasma," *Phytother Res*, 2004, 18(11):895-9.

Green Tea

Pharmacologic Category Herb

Reported Use

Antioxidant; cancer and cardiovascular disease (preventive) (Stoner, 1995; Yokozawa, 1997)
Cancer (prevention) (Bettuzzi, 2006; Hirohata, 1997; Mukhtar, 2000; Okabayashi, 2000; Snow, 1995; Theuer, 2000; Tsubono, 2001; Vermeer, 1999)
Cardiovascular disease (reduction of risks) (Nagao, 2007)
Chemotherapy and radiation (adjunct) (Mitscher, 1997)
Common cold (prevention) (Rowe, 2007)
Diabetes (Fukino, 2005)
Diarrhea (pharmacologic activity)
Genital warts (Gross, 2007; Stockfleth, 2008)
Gingivitis (prevention) (Krahwinkel, 2000)
Human T-cell lymphocytic virus (Sonoda, 2004)
Hypercholesterolemia (Yang, 1997)
Hypertension (Hodgson, 1999)
Hypertriglyceridemia (Unno, 2005)
Macular degeneration (pharmacologic activity)
Photoprotection (Chiu, 2005)
Platelet aggregation inhibition (Sagesake-Mitane, 1990)
Weight loss (Chantre, 2002; Diepvens, 2006; Kovacs, 2004)

Local Anesthetic/Vasoconstrictor Precautions No information available to require special precautions

Effects on Bleeding May see increased bleeding due to inhibition of platelet aggregation

Warnings/Precautions If product is not decaffeinated, caffeine may cause gastric irritation, decreased appetite, insomnia, tachycardia, palpitations, and nervousness in sensitive individuals. Caffeinated products should be used with caution in individuals with peptic ulcer disease or cardiovascular disease. At high doses, caffeine-containing products may interact with many medications.

Based on *in vitro* effects on platelet aggregation (Sagesaka-Mitane, 1990), green tea is contraindicated in individuals with active bleeding (eg, peptic ulcer, intracerebral bleeding). Use with caution in individuals with a history of bleeding, hemostatic disorders, or drug-related hemostatic problems and in individuals taking anticoagulant medications, aspirin, aspirin-containing products, NSAIDs, or antiplatelet agents (eg, ticlopidine, clopidogrel, dipyridamole). Discontinue use prior to dental or surgical procedures (generally at least 14 days before). Green tea has also been reported to antagonize the effects of warfarin (Taylor, 1999).

Use with caution when taking other stimulants such as caffeine and decongestants, unless a caffeine-free product is used. It is important to note that the addition of milk to any tea may significantly lower the antioxidant potential of this agent.

Reports exist of hepatoxicity with use of a green tea extract supplement and may worsen liver damage in patients with liver disease (Bonkovsky, 2006; Gloro, 2005).

Green tea polyphenols may negate the therapeutic efficacy of bortezomib and other boronic acid-based proteasome inhibitors (Golden, 2009).

References

Bettuzzi S, Brausi M, Rizzi F, et al, "Chemoprevention of Human Prostate Cancer by Oral Administration of Green Tea Catechins in Volunteers With High-Grade Prostate Intraepithelial Neoplasia: A Preliminary Report From a One-Year Proof-of-Principle Study," *Cancer Res*, 2006, 66(2):1234-40.

Bonkovsky HL, "Hepatotoxicity Associated With Supplements Containing Chinese Green Tea (*Camellia sinensis*)," *Ann Intern Med*, 2006, 144(1):68-71.

Chantre P and Lairon D, "Recent Findings of Green Tea Extract AR25 (Exolise) and Its Activity for the Treatment of Obesity," *Phytomedicine*, 2002, 9(1):3-8.

Chiu AE, Chan JL, Kern DG, et al, "Double-Blinded, Placebo-Controlled Trial of Green Tea Extracts in the Clinical and Histologic Appearance of Photoaging Skin," *Dermatol Surg*, 2005, 31:855-60.

Diepvens K, Kovacs EM, Vogels N, et al, "Metabolic Effects of Green Tea and of Phases of Weight Loss," *Physiol Behav*, 2006, 87(1):185-91.

Fukino Y, Shimbo M, Aoki N, et al, "Randomized Controlled Trial for an Effect of Green Tea Consumption on Insulin Resistance and Inflammation Markers," *J Nutr Sci Vitaminol (Tokyo)*, 2005, 51(5):335-42.

Gloro R, Hourmand-Ollivier I, Mosquet B, et al, "Fulminant Hepatitis During Self-Medication With Hydroalcoholic Extract of Green Tea," *Eur J Gastroenterol Hepatol*, 2005, 17(10):1135-7.

Golden EB, Lam PY, Kardosh A, et al, "Green Tea Polyphenols Block the Anticancer Effects of Bortezomib and Other Boronic Acid-Based Proteasome Inhibitors," *Blood*, 2009.

Gross G, Meyer KG, Pres H, et al, "A Randomized, Double-Blind, Four-Arm Parallel-Group, Placebo-Controlled Phase II/III Study to Investigate the Clinical Efficacy of Two Galenic Formulations of Polyphenon E in the Treatment of External Genital Warts," *J Eur Acad Dermatol Venereol*, 2007, 21 (10):1404-12.

Hirohata T and Kono S, "Diet/Nutrition and Stomach Cancer in Japan," *Int J Cancer*, 1997, Suppl 10:34-6.

Hodgson JM, Puddey IB, Burke V, et al, "Effects on Blood Pressure of Drinking Green and Black Tea," *J Hypertens*, 1999, 17(4):457-63.

Kovacs EM, Lejeune MP, Nijs I, et al, "Effects of Green Tea on Weight Maintenance After Body-Weight Loss," *Br J Nutr*, 2004, 91(3):431-7.

Krahwinkel T and Willershausen B, "The Effect of Sugar-Free Green Tea Chew Candies on the Degree of Inflammation of the Gingiva," *Eur J Med Res*, 2000, 5(11):463-7.

Mitscher LA, Jung M, Shankel D, et al, "Chemoprotection: A Review of the Potential Therapeutic Antioxidant Properties of Green Tea (*Camellia sinensis*) and Certain of Its Constituents," *Med Res Rev*, 1997, 17(4):327-65.

Mukhtar H and Ahmad N, "Tea Polyphenols: Prevention of Cancer and Optimizing Health," *Am J Clin Nutr*, 2000, 71(6 Suppl):1698S-702S.

Nagao T, Hase T, and Tokimitsu I, "A Green Tea Extract High in Catechins Reduces Body Fat and Cardiovascular Risks in Humans," *Obesity (Silver Spring)*, 2007, 15(6):1473-83.

Natural Standard Research Collaboration, Chief Editors: Ulbricht C, Basch E, *Natural Standard Herb and Supplement Reference - Evidence-Based Clinical Reviews*, USA: Elsevier/Mosby, 2005.

Okabayashi T, Gotoda T, Kondo H, et al, "Early Carcinoma of the Gastric Cardia in Japan: Is It Different From That in the West?" *Cancer*, 2000, 89(12):2555-9.

Rowe CA, Nantz MP, Bukowski JF, et al, "Specific Formulation of *Camellia sinensis* Prevents Cold and Flu Symptoms and Enhances Gamma, Delta T Cell Function: A Randomized, Double-Blind, Placebo-Controlled Study," *J Am Coll Nutr*, 2007, 26(5):445-52.

Sadzuka Y, Sugiyama T, Miyagishima A, et al, "The Effects of Theanine, as a Novel Biochemical Modulator, on the Antitumor Activity of Adriamycin," *Cancer Lett*, 1996, 105(2):203-9.

Sagesaka-Mitane Y, Miwa M, and Okada S, "Platelet Aggregation Inhibitors in Hot Water Extract of Green Tea," *Chem Pharm Bull (Tokyo)*, 1990, 38(3):790-3.

Snow J, "*Camellia sinensis* (L) Kuntze (Theaceae)," *Protocol J Botanical Med*, 1995, 47-51.

Sonoda J, Koriyama C, Yamamoto S, et al, "HTLV-1 Provirus Load in Peripheral Blood Lymphocytes of HTLV-1 Carriers Is Diminished by Green Tea Drinking," *Cancer Sci*, 2004, 95(7):596-601.

Stammler G and Volm M, "Green Tea Catechins (EGCG and EGC) Have Modulating Effects on the Activity of Doxorubicin in Drug-Resistant Cell Lines," *Anticancer Drugs*, 1997, 8(3):265-8.

Stockfleth E, Beti H, Orasan R, et al, "Topical Polyphenon E in the Treatment of External Genital and Perianal Warts: A Randomized Controlled Trial," *Br J Dermatol*, 2008, 158(6):1329-38.

Stoner GD and Mukhtar H, "Polyphenols as Cancer Chemopreventive Agents," *J Cell Biochem Suppl*, 1995, 22:169-80.

Taylor JR, Wilt VM, "Probable Antagonism of Warfarin by Green Tea," *Ann Pharmacother*, 1999, 33 (4):426-8.

Theuer CP, Kurosaki T, Ziogas A, et al, "Asian Patients With Gastric Carcinoma in the United States Exhibit Unique Clinical Features and Superior Overall and Cancer Specific Survival Rates," *Cancer*, 2000, 89(9):1883-92.

Tsubono Y, Nishino Y, Komatsu S, et al, "Green Tea and the Risk of Gastric Cancer in Japan," *N Engl J Med*, 2001, 344(9):632-6.

Unno T, Tago M, Suzuki Y, et al, "Effect of Tea Catechins on Postprandial Plasma Lipid Responses in Human Subjects," *Br J Nutr*, 2005, 93(4):543-7.
Vermeer IT, Moonen EJ, Dallinga JW, et al, "Effect of Ascorbic Acid and Green Tea on Endogenous Formation of N-Nitrosodimethylamine and N-Nitrosopiperidine in Humans," *Mutat Res*, 1999, 428 (1-2):353-61.
Yang TT and Koo MW, "Hypocholesterolemic Effects of Chinese Tea," *Pharmacol Res*, 1997, 35 (6):505-12.
Yokozawa T and Dong E, "Influence of Green Tea and Its Three Major Components Upon Low-Density Lipoprotein Oxidation," *Exp Toxicol Pathol*, 1997, 49(5):329-35.

Hawthorn

Pharmacologic Category Herb

Reported Use

Angina, hypotension, hypertension, peripheral vascular disease, tachycardia; cardiotonic; congestive heart failure (Schussler, 1995; Walker, 2006; Weihmayr, 1996)

Heart failure (Bodigheimer, 1994; Forster, 1994; Holubarsch, 2008; Iwamoto, 1981; O'Conolly, 1986; O'Conolly, 1987; Pittler, 2003; Schmidt, 1994)

Contradictory study (Zick, 2008)

Local Anesthetic/Vasoconstrictor Precautions No information available to require special precautions

Effects on Bleeding None reported

Warnings/Precautions Contraindicated in pregnancy (based on animal studies and human case reports) (Ammon, 1981). Due to pharmacologic activity, use with caution in individuals receiving antihypertensive medications, including vasodilators and angiotensin converting enzyme inhibitors (Ammon, 1981), and in individuals receiving cardiac glycosides. It has been used in Europe to decrease the need for digoxin. May cause dizziness, headache, or hypotension. Use caution in individuals at risk of hypotension including those taking antihypertensive medication or agents that predispose to orthostasis, elderly individuals, or those who would not tolerate transient hypotensive episodes (ie, cerebrovascular or cardiovascular disease).

Theoretically, based on its proposed pharmacologic activity, hawthorn has the potential to share some effects associated with ACE inhibitors. Cough is frequently associated with ACE inhibition and serious, rare reactions (including angioedema and renal impairment) have been attributed to these agents; however, these have not been reported with hawthorn despite broad experience.

References

Ammon HP and Handel M, "Crataegus, Toxicology and Pharmacology, Part I: Toxicity," *Plant Med*, 1981, 43(2):105-20.
Bodigheimer K and Chase D, "Effectiveness of Hawthorn Extract at a Dosage of 3x100 mg Per Day," *Munch Med Wschr*, 1994, 136(suppl 1):s7-11.
Forster A, Forster K, Buhring M, et al, "Crataegus for Moderately Reduced Left Ventricular Ejection Fraction. Ergospirometric Monitoring Study With 72 Patients in a Double-Blind Comparison With Placebo," *Munch Med Wschr*, 1994, 136(Suppl 1):s21-6.
Holubarsch CJ, Colucci WS, Meinertz T, et al, "The Efficacy and Safety of Crataegus Extract WS 1442 in Patients With Heart Failure: The SPICE Trial," *Eur J Heart Fail*, 2008, 10(12):1255-63.
Iwamoto M, Sato T, and Ishizaki T, "The Clinical Effect of Crataegutt in Heart Disease of Ischemic or Hypertensive Origin. A Multicenter Double-Blind Study," *Planta Med*, 1981, 42(1):1-16.
McGuffin M, et al, eds, *American Herbal Products Association's Botanical Safety Handbook*, Boca Raton, FL: CRC Press, 1997, 37.
Natural Standard Research Collaboration, Chief Editors: Ulbricht C, Basch E, *Natural Standard Herb and Supplement Reference - Evidence-Based Clinical Reviews*, USA: Elsevier/Mosby, 2005.
O'Conolly M, Bernhoft G, and Bartsch G, "Treatment of Stenocardia (Angina pectoris) Pain in Advanced Age Patients With Multi-Morbidity," *Therapiewoche*, 1987, 37:3587-3600.
O'Conolly M, Jansen W, Bernhöft G, et al, "Treatment of Decreasing Cardiac Performance. Therapy Using Standardized Crataegus Extract in Advanced Age," *Fortschr Med*, 1986, 104(42):805-8.
Pittler MH, Schmidt K, and Ernst E, "Hawthorn Extract for Treating Chronic Heart Failure: Meta-Analysis of Randomized Trials," *Am J Med*, 2003, 114(8):665-74.
Schmidt U, Kuhn U, Ploch M, et al, "Efficacy of Hawthorn (Crataegus) Preparation LI 132 in 78 Patients With Chronic Congestive Heart Failure Defined as NYHA Functional Class II," *Phytomedicine*, 1994, 1:17-24.
Schussler M, Holzl J, and Fricke U, "Myocardial Effects of Flavonoids From *Crataegus* Species," *Arzneimittelforschung*, 1995, 45(8):842-5.
Walker AF, Marakis G, Simpson F, et al, "Hypotensive Effects of Hawthorn for Patients With Diabetes Taking Prescription Drugs: A Randomised Controlled Trial," *BR J Gen Pract*, 2006, 56(527):437-43.
Weihmayr T and Ernst E, "Therapeutic Effectiveness of *Crataegus*," *Fortschr Med*, 1996, 114(1-2):27-9.
Zick SM, Gillespie B, and Aaronson KD, "The Effect of *Crataegus oxycantha* Special Extract WS 1442 on Clinical Progression in Patients With Mild to Moderate Symptoms of Heart Failure," *Eur J Heart Fail*, 2008, 10(6):587-93.

Horse Chestnut

Pharmacologic Category Herb

Reported Use

Scleroderma (pharmacologic activity)

Venous insufficiency [varicose veins, hemorrhoids, deep venous thrombosis, lower extremity edema (oral and topical)] (Bisler, 1986; Pittler, 1998; Rudofsky, 1986; Siebert, 2002; Simini, 1996)

Local Anesthetic/Vasoconstrictor Precautions No information available to require special precautions

Effects on Bleeding Inhibits platelet aggregation; may see increased bleeding

Warnings/Precautions Based on pharmacologic activity (inhibition of platelet aggregation) (Urbaniuk, 1967), may be contraindicated in individuals with active bleeding (eg, peptic ulcer, intracranial bleeding). Use with caution in individuals with a history of bleeding, hemostatic disorders, or drug-related hemostatic problems. Use with caution in individuals taking anticoagulant medications, including warfarin, aspirin, aspirin-containing products, NSAIDs, or antiplatelet agents (eg, ticlopidine, clopidogrel, dipyridamole). Discontinue use prior to dental or surgical procedures (generally at least 14 days before).

Use with caution in individuals with hepatic or renal impairment; may cause gastrointestinal upset. Based on pharmacologic activity, may alter glucose regulation (Yoshikawa, 1998). Use with caution in individuals with diabetes or those predisposed to hypoglycemia. Effects of drugs with hypoglycemic activity may be potentiated (including insulin and oral hypoglycemics). Blood sugar should be closely monitored and the dosage of hypoglycemic medications may require adjustment. This should be carefully coordinated among the individual's healthcare providers.

References

Bisler H, Pfeifer R, Klüken N, et al, "Effects of Horse-Chestnut Seed Extract on Transcapillary Filtration in Chronic Venous Insufficiency," *Dtsch Med Wochenschr*, 1986, 111(35):1321-9.
Natural Standard Research Collaboration, Chief Editors: Ulbricht C, Basch E, *Natural Standard Herb and Supplement Reference - Evidence-Based Clinical Reviews*, USA: Elsevier/Mosby, 2005.
Pittler MH and Ernst E, "Horse-Chestnut Seed Extract for Chronic Venous Insufficiency. A Criteria-Based Systematic Review," *Arch Dermatol* 1998, 134(11):1356-60.
Rudofsky G, et al, "Odemprotektive Wirkung und Klinische Wirksamkeit von ro Kastaniensamenextrakt im Doppeltblindversuch," *Phleb Prokto*, 1986, 15:47-54.
Siebert U, Brach M, Sroczynski G, et al, "Efficacy, Routine Effectiveness, and Safety of Horsechestnut Seed Extract in the Treatment of Chronic Venous Insufficiency. A Meta-Analysis of Randomized Controlled Trials and Large Observational Studies," *Int Angiol*, 2002, 21(4):305-15.
Simini B, "Horse-Chestnut Seed Extract for Chronic Venous Insufficiency," *Lancet*, 1996, 347 (9009):1182-3.
Urbaniuk KG and Gorelov KP, "The Anticoagulant Action of Horse Chestnut and Eskuzan," *Klin Med (Mosk)*, 1967, 45(2):129-33.
Yoshikawa M, Murakami T, Yamahara J, et al, "Bioactive Saponins and Glycosides. XII. Horse Chestnut. (2): Structures of Escins IIIb, IV, V, and VI and Isoescins Ia, Ib, and V, Acylated Polyhydroxyoleanene Triterpene Oligoglycosides, From the Seeds of Horse Chestnut Tree (*Aesculus hippocastanum* L., Hippocastanaceae)," *Chem Pharm Bull* (Tokyo), 1998, 46(11):1764-9.

HuperzineA

Pharmacologic Category Herb

Reported Use

Myasthenia gravis (Cheng, 1986)
Senile dementia and Alzheimer's disease (Wang, 1998)

Local Anesthetic/Vasoconstrictor Precautions No information available to require special precautions

Effects on Bleeding None reported

Warnings/Precautions Based on pharmacologic activity, use with caution in individuals taking other acetylcholinesterase inhibitors

References

Cheng YS, Lu CZ, Ying ZL, et al, "128 Cases of Myasthenia Gravis Treated With Huperzine A," *New Drugs Clin Rem*, 1986, 5:260-2.
Natural Standard Research Collaboration, Chief Editors: Ulbricht C, Basch E, *Natural Standard Herb and Supplement Reference - Evidence-Based Clinical Reviews*, USA: Elsevier/Mosby, 2005.
Wang H and Tang XC, "Anticholinesterase Effects of HuperzineA, E2020, and Tacrine in Rats," *Chung Kuo Yao Li Hsueh Pao*, 1998, 19(1):27-30.

Hyssop

Pharmacologic Category Herb

Reported Use

Kidney inflammation (Deng, 2004)

Local Anesthetic/Vasoconstrictor Precautions No information available to require special precautions

Effects on Bleeding None reported

Warnings/Precautions Avoid in individuals with epilepsy, fever, hypertension, or pregnancy. Children should avoid hyssop; may cause seizures. Use with caution in individuals taking antidiabetic agents or in those who have diabetes; may lower blood sugar levels. Due to the possible immunomodulatory activity, hyssop may interact with immunosuppressant medications.

References

Deng YY, Chen YP, Wang L, et al, "Clinical Study on Treatment of Mid-Advanced Crescentic Nephritis by Qingre Huoxue Recipe," *Zhongguo Zhong Xi Yi Jie He Za Zhi*, 2004, 24(12):1084-6.
Natural Standard Research Collaboration, Chief Editors: Ulbricht C, Basch E, *Natural Standard Herb and Supplement Reference - Evidence-Based Clinical Reviews*, USA: Elsevier/Mosby, 2005.

Kava Kava

Pharmacologic Category Herb

Reported Use

Fibromyalgia (pharmacologic activity)

Insomnia; anxiety/stress, skeletal muscle relaxation, postischemic episodes (Connor, 2006; Davies, 1992; Ernst, 2006; Geller, 2007; Kinzler, 1991; Lehmann, 1996; Malsch, 2001; Pittler, 2000; Singh, 1992; Warnecke, 1991)

Muscle soreness (pharmacologic activity)

Local Anesthetic/Vasoconstrictor Precautions No information available to require special precautions

Effects on Bleeding None reported

Warnings/Precautions The U.S. Food and Drug Administration (FDA) is attempting to determine whether dietary supplements containing the herbal extract kava (*Piper methysticum*) are directly responsible for causing certain types of hepatotoxicity. Recently, more than 20 cases of hepatitis, cirrhosis, and liver failure have been reported in Europe, with at least one individual requiring a liver transplant. Healthcare providers are urged to query their patients about the use of kava and to evaluate closely these individuals for potential liver complications. In addition, physicians are urged to review all their cases of liver toxicity to determine if kava-containing products may be involved. Kava is marketed for a variety of uses, including stress relief, tension, anxiety, insomnia, and postmenstrual syndrome (PMS).

Use of kava kava is contraindicated in pregnancy and lactation (based on case reports) (Meyer). Due to the potential for dopamine antagonism, use is also contraindicated in Parkinson's disease (Schelosky, 1995). Use with caution in individuals receiving antianxiety agents (ie, alprazolam), antidepressants, antipsychotics, or other agents which cause CNS depression such as sedative/hypnotics (based on pharmacologic activity and case reports) (Almeida, 1996). May potentiate the effects of concurrent ethanol (Jamieson, 1990). Some conflicting evidence concerning effects with ethanol have been published (Herberg, 1993). May cause drowsiness or sedation in higher doses; use caution when performing tasks which require alertness (driving or operating heavy machinery). Long-term use of high doses may cause rash.

References

Almeida JC and Grimsley EW, "Coma From the Health Food Store: Interaction Between Kava and Alprazolam," *Ann Intern Med*, 1996, 125(11):940-1.

Davies LP, Drew CA, Duffield P, et al, "Kava Pyrones and Resin: Studies on GABAA, GABAB and Benzodiazepine Binding Sites in Rodent Brain," *Pharmacol Toxicol*, 1992, 71(2):120-6.

Herberg KW, "Effect of Kava-Special Extract WS 1490 Combined With Ethyl Alcohol on Safety-Relevant Performance Parameters," *Blutalkohol*, 1993, 30(2):96-105.

Jamieson DD and Duffield PH, "Positive Interaction of Ethanol and Kava Resin in Mice," *Clin Exp Pharmacol Physiol*, 1990, 17(7):509-14.

Kinzler E, Krömer J, and Lehmann E, "Effect of a Special Kava Extract in Patients With Anxiety-, Tension-, and Excitation States of Non-Psychotic Genesis. Double Blind Study With Placebos Over 4 Weeks," *Arzneimittelforschung*, 1991, 41(6):584-8.

Lehmann E, Kinzler E, and Friedemann J, "Efficacy of a Special Kava Extract (*Piper methysticum*) in Patients With States of Anxiety, Tension and Excitedness of Non-Mental Origin - A Double-Blind Placebo-Controlled Study of Four Weeks Treatment," *Phytomedicine*, 1996, 3(2):113-9.

Malsch U and Kieser M, "Efficacy of Kava-Kava in the Treatment of Non-Psychotic Anxiety, Following Pretreatment With Benzodiazepines," *Psychopharmacology (Berl)*, 2001, 157(3):277-83.

Meyer JJ, "Pharmacology of Kava," Ethnopharmacologic Search for Psychoactive Drugs, U.S. Dept Health, Education, and Welfare, Pub No 1645, Washington, DC: Government Printing Office, 133-40.

Natural Standard Research Collaboration, Chief Editors: Ulbricht C, Basch E, *Natural Standard Herb and Supplement Reference - Evidence-Based Clinical Reviews*, USA: Elsevier/Mosby, 2005.

Pittler MH and Ernst E, "Efficacy of Kava Extract for Treating Anxiety: Systematic Review and Meta-Analysis," *J Clin Psychopharmacol*, 2000, 20(1):84-9.

Schelosky L, Raffauf C, Jendroska K, et al, "Kava and Dopamine Antagonism," *J Neurol Neurosurg Psychiatry*, 1995, 58(5):639-40.

Singh YN, "Kava: An Overview," *J Ethnopharmacol*, 1992, 37(1):13-45.

Warnecke G, "Psychosomatic Dysfunctions in the Female Climacteric. Clinical Effectiveness and Tolerance of Kava Extract WS 1490," *Fortschr Med*, 1991, 109(4):119-22.

Kudzu

Pharmacologic Category Herb

Reported Use

Alcoholism (Shebek, 2000)

Cardiovascular disease/angina (Xie, 2003; Zhao, 1998)

Deafness (Liu, 2002)

Diabetes (Shi, 2002)

Diabetic retinopathy (Ren, 2000)

Glaucoma (Kang, 1993)

Ischemic stroke (Tan, 2008)

Menopausal symptoms (Lamlertkittikul, 2004)

Local Anesthetic/Vasoconstrictor Precautions No information available to require special precautions

Effects on Bleeding May see increased bleeding due to inhibition of platelet aggregation

Warnings/Precautions Use with caution in individuals taking antiarrhythmic agents; the kudzu constituent, daidzein, may have antiarrhythmic properties. Use with caution in individuals with a history of bleeding, hemostatic disorders, or drug-related hemostatic problems. Use with caution in individuals taking anticoagulant medications, including warfarin, aspirin, aspirin-containing products, NSAIDs, or antiplatelet agents (eg, ticlopidine, clopidogrel, dipyridamole). Use with caution in individuals with diabetes or who are taking antidiabetic drugs; kudzu may lower blood glucose levels and have additive effects. Use with caution in individuals using agents with estrogenic activity; kudzu may competitively inhibit the effects of estrogen therapy.

References

Kang RX, "The Intraocular Pressure Depressive Effect of Puerarin," *Zhonghua Yan Ke Za Zhi*, 1993, 29 (6):336-9.
Keung WM and Vallee BL, "Kudzu Root: An Ancient Chinese Source of Modern Antidipsotropic Agents," *Phytochemistry*, 1998, 47(4):499-506.
Lamlertkittikul S and Chandeying V, "Efficacy and Safety of Pueraria Mirifica (Kwao Kruea Khao) for the Treatment of Vasomotor Symptoms in Perimenopausal Women: Phase II Study," *J Med Assoc Thai*, 2004, 87(1):33-40.
Liu JM, Ma L, and He WP, "Therapeutic Effect of Puerarin Therapy on Sudden Deafness," *Di Yi Jun Yi Da Xue Xue Bao*, 2002, 22(11):1044-5.
Natural Standard Research Collaboration, Chief Editors: Ulbricht C, Basch E, *Natural Standard Herb and Supplement Reference - Evidence-Based Clinical Reviews*, USA: Elsevier/Mosby, 2005.
Ren P, Hu H, and Zhang R, "Observation on Efficacy of Puerarin in Treating Diabetic Retinopathy," *Zhongguo Zhong Xi Yi Jie He Za Zhi*, 2000, 20(8):574-6.
Shebek J and Rindone JP, "A Pilot Study Exploring the Effect of Kudzu Root on the Drinking Habits of Patients With Chronic Alcoholism," *J Altern Complement Med*, 2000, 6(1):45-8.
Shi WG, Qu L, and Wang JW, "Study on Interventing Effect of Puerarin on Insulin Resistance in Patients With Coronary Heart Disease," *Zhongguo Zhong Xi Yi Jie He Za Zhi*, 2002, 22(1):21-4.
Tan Y, Liu M, and Wu B, "Puerarin for Acute Ischaemic Stroke," *Cochrane Database Syst Rev*, 2008, (1): CD004955.
Xie RQ, Du J, and Hao YM, "Myocardial Protection and Mechanism of Puerarin Injection on Patients of Coronary Heart Disease With Ischemia/Reperfusion," *Zhongguo Zhong Xi Yi Jie He Za Zhi*, 2003, 23 (12):895-7.
Zhao Z, Yang X, and Zhang Y, "Clinical Study of Puerarin in Treatment of Patients With Unstable Angina," *Zhongguo Zhong Xi Yi Jie He Za Zhi*, 1998, 18(5):282-4.

Lemon Balm/Melissa

Pharmacologic Category Herb

Reported Use

Agitation in dementia (Ballard, 2002)
Antiviral (oral herpes virus) (Dimitrova, 1993; Grauds, 2001; Vogt, 1991; Wölbling, 1994)
Anxiety (Buchner, 1974; Lagoni, 1998; Schmidt, 1992)
Attention-deficit hyperactivity disorder (ADHD) (Klein, 1998)
Cognitive performance (Akhondzadeh, 2003; Kennedy, 2001; Kennedy, 2003)
Colitis (Chakurski, 1981)
Dyspepsia (Borho, 1991; Madisch, 2001; Madisch, 2004)
Sedation (pediatrics) (Leung, 1996)
Sleep quality (Cerny, 1999; Dressing, 1992; Dressing, 1996; Lindahl, 1989; Orth-Wagner, 1995; Widy-Tyszkiewicz, 1997)
Teething (topical) (pharmacologic activity)

Local Anesthetic/Vasoconstrictor Precautions No information available to require special precautions

Effects on Bleeding None reported

Warnings/Precautions Use with caution in individuals receiving sedative medications. May cause drowsiness or sedation in higher doses; use caution when performing tasks which require alertness (driving or operating heavy machinery). Use with caution in individuals with thyroid problems such as Graves' disease due to potential for thyroid hormone inhibition (Auf'mkolk, 1985).

References

Akhondzadeh S, Noroozian M, Mohammadi M, et al, "*Melissa officinalis* Extract in the Treatment of Patients With Mild-to-Moderate Alzheimer's Disease: A Double Blind, Randomised, Placebo Controlled Trial," *J Neurol Neurosurg Psychiatry*, 2003, 74(7):863-6.
Auf'mkolk M, Ingbar JC, Kubota K, et al, "Extracts and Auto-Oxidized Constituents of Certain Plants Inhibit the Receptor-Binding and the Biological Activity of Graves' Immunoglobulins," *Endocrinology*, 1985, 116(5):1687-93.
Ballard CG, O'Brien JT, Reichelt K, et al, "Aromatherapy as a Safe and Effective Treatment for the Management of Agitation in Severe Dementia: The Results of a Double-Blind, Placebo-Controlled Trial With *Melissa*," *J Clin Psychiatry*, 2002, 63(7):553-8.
Borho B, "Biologische Therapie Von Funktionellen Magenerkrankungen," 1991, 6:501-9.
Buchner KH, Hellings H, Huber M, et al, "Double Blind Study as Evidence of the Therapeutic Effect of Melissengeist on Psycho-Vegetative Syndromes," *Medizinische Klinik*, 1974, 69(23):1032-6.
Cerny AS and Schmid K, "Tolerability and Efficacy of Valerian/Lemon Balm in Healthy Volunteers: A Double-Blind Placebo-Controlled, Multicentre Study," *Fitoterapia*, 1999, 70(3):221-8.
Chakurski I, Matev M, Koichev A, et al, "Treatment of Chronic Colitis With an Herbal Combination of *Taraxacum officinale*, *Hipericum perforatum*, *Melissa officinaliss*, *Calendula officinalis*, and *Foeniculum vulgare*," *Vutr Boles*, 1981, 20(6):51-4.
Dimitrova Z, Dimov B, Manolova N, et al, "Antiherpes Effect of *Melissa officinalis* L. Extracts," *Acta Microbiol Bulg*, 1993, 29:65-72.
Dressing H, "Valerian Combination Therapy vs Benzodiazepine: Same Efficacy in the Treatment of Sleeping Disorders?" *Therapiewoche*, 1992, 42(12):726-36.
Dressing H, Kohler S, and Muller WF, "Improvement in Sleep Quality With a High Dose Valerian-Mellissa Preparation," *Psychopharmakotherapie*, 1996, 3:123-30.
Grauds C, "Lemon Balm for the Treatment of Oral Herpes," *Pharm Times*, 2001, May:40.

Kennedy D, Scholey A, Tildeslev N, et al, "Dose-Dependent Changes in Mood and Cognitive Performance Following Single Doses of *Melissa officinalis* (Lemon Balm) to Healthy Young Adults," Proceedings of the British Psychological Society, 2001, 9(2):209.
Kennedy DO, Wake G, Savelev S, et al, "Modulation of Mood and Cognitive Performance Following Acute Administration of Single Doses of *Melissa officinalis* (Lemon Balm) With Human CNS Nicotinic and Muscarinic Receptor-Binding Properties," *Neuropsychopharmacology*, 2003, 28(10):1871-81.
Klein R, "Herbal Immune Support for Children," *Health Nutr Breakthroughs*, 1998, 3:37-8.
Lagoni N, "Wirksamkeitsprüfung Eines Pflanzlichen Tagessedativums in Einer Multizentrischen Studie," 1998, 39(3):166-9.
Leung AY and Foster S, *Encyclopedia of Common Natural Ingredients Used in Foods, Drugs, and Cosmetics*, New York, NY: Wiley, 1996, 57-58.
Lindahl O and Lindwall L, "Double Blind Study of a Valerian Preparation," *Pharmacol Biochem Behav*, 1989, 32(4):1065-6.
Madisch A, Holtmann G, Mayr G, et al, "Treatment of Functional Dyspepsia With a Herbal Preparation. A Double-Blind, Randomized, Placebo-Controlled, Multicenter Trial," *Digestion*, 2004, 69(1):45-52.
Madisch A, Melderis H, Mayr G, et al, "A Plant Extract and Its Modified Preparation in Functional Dyspepsia. Results of a Double-Blind Placebo Controlled Comparative Study," *Z Gastroenterol*, 2001, 39(7):511-7.
Natural Standard Research Collaboration, Chief Editors: Ulbricht C, Basch E, *Natural Standard Herb and Supplement Reference - Evidence-Based Clinical Reviews*, USA: Elsevier/Mosby, 2005.
Orth-Wagner S, Ressin W, and Friedrich I, "Phytosedativum Gegen Schlafstörungen / Klinische Wirksamkeit und Verträglichkeit Eines Phytosedativums Mit Auszügen Aus Baldrianwurzel," *Hopfenzapfen und Melissenblättern*, 1995, 16(147):156.
Schmidt U, Krieger W, Freerick H, et al, "Psychosomatische und Psychische Störungen / Baldrian und Melisse Statt Synthetischer," *Psychopharmaka*, 1992, 14:15-9.
Vogt M, Tausch I, Wölbling RH, et al, "Melissa Extract in Herpes Simplex: A Double-Blind Placebo-Controlled Study," *Der Allgemeinarzt*, 1991, 13:832-41.
Widy-Tyszkiewicz E and Schminda R, "A Randomized Double Blind Study of Sedative Effects of Phytotherapeutic Containing Valerian, Hops, Balm, and Motherwort Versus Placebo," *Herb Polon*, 1997, 2:154-9.
Wölbling RH and Leonhardt K, "Local Therapy of Herpes Simplex With Dried Extract From *Melissa officinalis*," *Phytomedicine*, 1994, 1:25-31.

Licorice

Pharmacologic Category Herb

Reported Use

Adrenal insufficiency (licorice) (Davis, 1991)
Aphthous ulcers/canker sores (Worner, 1974)
Atopic dermatitis (Saeedi, 2003)
Body fat mass reduction (Armanini, 2003)
Crohn's disease (pharmacologic activity)
Croup (pharmacologic activity)
Expectorant and antitussive (licorice) (Bradley, 1992)
Familial Mediterranean Fever (FMF) (Amaryan, 2003)
Gastrointestinal ulceration (DGL chewable products), peptic ulcer disease (Dehpour, 1994), gastric mucosal damage by aspirin (Rees, 1979)
Contradictory studies (anonymous, 1971; Balakrishnan, 1978; Engqvist, 1973; Nussbaumer, 1977)
Herpes simplex (Sekizawa, 2001)
HIV/AIDS (Hattori, 1989)
Hyperkalemia (Murakami, 1993)
Sore throat (postoperative) (Agarwal, 2009)
Viral hepatitis (Arase, 1997; Fujioka, 2003; Liu, 2003; van Rossum, 1999; van Rossum, 2001)

Local Anesthetic/Vasoconstrictor Precautions No information available to require special precautions

Effects on Bleeding None reported

Warnings/Precautions May cause retinal or occipital vasospasms (Dobbins, 2000).

May alter platelet aggregation (Tawata, 1990). Based on pharmacologic activity, this herb may be contraindicated in individuals with active bleeding (eg, peptic ulcer, intracranial bleeding). Use with caution in individuals with a history of bleeding, hemostatic disorders, or drug-related hemostatic problems. Use with caution in individuals taking anticoagulant medications, including warfarin, aspirin, aspirin-containing products, NSAIDs, or antiplatelet agents (eg, ticlopidine, clopidogrel, dipyridamole). Discontinue use prior to dental or surgical procedures (generally at least 14 days before).

Licorice: Contraindicated in pregnancy and lactation. Based on pharmacologic activity, use is contraindicated in individuals with hepatic or renal impairment. Avoid use in hypertension, arrhythmias, congestive heart failure, or edematous states; may cause sodium and water retention (based on human studies and case reports) (de Klerk, 1997; Stormer, 1993). Do not use in individuals receiving antihypertensives, diuretics, digoxin, or potassium supplements; due to mineralocorticoid effects, licorice may deplete potassium. Avoid use in hypokalemic states. High doses may cause pseudoaldosteronism.

Phytoestrogen-containing herbs have not been associated with the negative health effects seen with synthetic estrogen; however, use with caution in individuals on hormone replacement therapy or oral contraceptives or with a history of estrogen-dependent tumors, endometrial cancer, thromboembolic disease, or stroke.

DGL Licorice: Use DGL licorice with caution in individuals receiving nitrofurantoin (increases excretion).

References

Amaryan G, Astvatsatryan V, Gabrielyan E, et al, "Double-Blind, Placebo-Controlled, Randomized, Pilot Clinical Trial of ImmunoGuard™ - A Standardized Fixed Combination of *Andrographis paniculata* Nees, With *Eleutherococcus senticosus* Maxim, *Schizandra chinensis* Bail, and *Glycyrrhiza glabra* L. Extracts in Patients With Familial Mediterranean Fever," *Phytomedicine*, 2003, 10(4):271-85.

Anonymous, "Treatment of Duodenal Ulcer With Glycyrrhizinic-Acid-Reduced Liquorice. A Multicentre Trial," *Br Med J*, 1971, 3(5773):501-3.

Arase Y, Ikeda K, Murashima N, et al, "The Long Term Efficacy of Glycyrrhizin in Chronic Hepatitis C Patients," *Cancer*, 1997, 79(8):1494-500.

Armanini D, De Palo CB, Mattarello MJ, et al, "Effect of Licorice on the Reduction of Body Fat Mass in Healthy Subjects," *J Endocrinol Invest*, 2003, 26(7):646-50.

Balakrishnan V, Pillai MV, Raveendran PM, et al, "Deglycyrrhizinated Liquorice in the Treatment of Chronic Duodenal Ulcer," *J Assoc Physicians India*, 1978, 26(9):811-4.

Bradley PR, ed, *British Herbal Compendium*, Vol 1, Bournemouth, England: British Herbal Medicine Association, 1992, 145-8.

Davis EA and Morris DJ, "Medicinal Uses of Licorice Through the Millennia: The Good and Plenty of It," *Mol Cell Endocrinol*, 1991, 78(1-2):1-6.

de Klerk GJ, Nieuwenhuis MG, and Beutler JJ, "Hypokalaemia and Hypertension Associated With Use of Liquorice Flavoured Chewing Gum," *BMJ*, 1997, 314(7082):731-2.

Dehpour AR, Zolfaghari ME, Samadian T, et al, "The Protective Effect of Liquorice Components and Their Derivatives Against Gastric Ulcer Induced by Aspirin in Rats," *J Pharm Pharmacol*, 1994, 46(2):148-9.

Dobbins KR and Saul RF, "Transient Visual Loss After Licorice Ingestion," *J Neuroophthalmol*, 2000, 20 (1):38-41.

Engqvist A, von Feilitzen F, Pyk E, et al, "Double-Blind Trial of Deglycyrrhizinated Liquorice in Gastric Ulcer," *Gut*, 1973, 14(9):711-5.

Fujioka T, Kondou T, Fukuhara A, et al, "Efficacy of a Glycyrrhizin Suppository for the Treatment of Chronic Hepatitis C: A Pilot Study," *Hepatol Res*, 2003, 26(1):10-14.

Liu J, Manheimer E, Tsutani K, et al, "Medicinal Herbs for Hepatitis C Virus Infection: A Cochrane Hepatobiliary Systematic Review of Randomized Trials," *Am J Gastroenterol*, 2003, 98(3):538-44.

Murakami T and Uchikawa T, "Effect of Glycyrrhizine on Hyperkalemia Due to Hyporeninemic Hypoaldosteronism in Diabetes Mellitus," *Life Sci*, 1993, 53(5):PL63-8.

Natural Standard Research Collaboration, Chief Editors: Ulbricht C, Basch E, *Natural Standard Herb and Supplement Reference - Evidence-Based Clinical Reviews*, USA: Elsevier/Mosby, 2005.

Newall CA, Anderson La, and Phillipson JD, *Herbal Medicines: A Guide for Health Care Professionals*, London, England: The Pharmaceutical Press, 1996, 183-6.

Nussbaumer U, Landolt M, Röthlisberger G, et al, "Postoperative Stress Hemorrhage: Ineffective Prevention With Pepsin Inhibitor and Deglycyrrhizinized Licorice Extract. Prospective Study," *Schweiz Med Wochenschr*, 1977, 107(8):276-9.

Saeedi M, Morteza-Semnani K, and Ghoreishi MR, "The Treatment of Atopic Dermatitis With Licorice Gel," *J Dermatolog Treat*, 2003, 14(3):153-7.

Sekizawa T, Yanagi K, and Itoyama Y, "Glycyrrhizin Increases Survival of Mice With Herpes Simplex Encephalitis," *Acta Virol*, 2001, 45(1):51-4.

Stormer FC, Reistad R, and Alexander J, "Glycyrrhizic Acid in Liquorice-Evaluation of Health Hazard," *Food Chem Toxicol*, 1993, 31(4): 303-12.

Tawata M, Yoda Y, Aida K, et al, "Anti-Platelet Action of GU-7, a 3-Arylcoumarin Derivative, Purified from *Glycyrrhizae radix*." *Planta Med*, 1990, 56(3):259-63.

van Rossum TG, Vulto AG, Hop WC, et al, "Glycyrrhizin-Induced Reduction of ALT in European Patients With Chronic Hepatitis C," *Am J Gastroenterol*, 2001, 96(8):2432-7.

van Rossum TG, Vulto AG, Hop WC, et al, "Intravenous Glycyrrhizin for the Treatment of Chronic Hepatitis C: A Double-Blind, Randomized, Placebo-Controlled Phase I/II Trial," *J Gastroenterol Hepatol*, 1999, 14(11):1093-9.

Worner H, Rolffs J, and Schmelzle R, "Aphthous and Ulcerating Changes of the Mouth Mucosa. Treatment With Carbenoxolone-Sodium," *Fortschr Med*, 1974, 92(2):81-3.

Lutein

Pharmacologic Category Nutraceutical

Reported Use

Antioxidant (Zhao, 2006)
Breast cancer (Kim, 2001)
Cardiovascular disease, contradictory study (Knekt, 2004)
Cataracts (Lyle, 1999)
Colon cancer (Slattery, 2000)
Diabetes, contradictory study (Montonen, 2004)
Macular degeneration (Hammond, 1997)
Pre-eclampsia (Williams, 2003)
Visual acuity and function (Bahrami, 2006; Ma, 2009); retinal degeneration (Dagnelie, 2000)

Local Anesthetic/Vasoconstrictor Precautions No information available to require special precautions

Effects on Bleeding None reported

Warnings/Precautions No known toxicity or serious side effects reported.

References

Bahrami H, Melia M, and Dagnelie G, "Lutein Supplementation in Retinitis Pigmentosa: PC-Based Vision Assessment in a Randomized Double-Masked Placebo-Controlled Clinical Trial," *BMC Ophthalmol*, 2006, 6:23.

Hammond BR Jr, Johnson EJ, Russell RM, et al, "Dietary Modification of Human Macular Pigment Density," *Invest Ophthalmol Vis Sci*, 1997, 38(9):1795-801.

Lyle BJ, Mares-Perlman JA, Klein BE, et al, "Antioxidant Intake and Risk of Incident Age-Related Nuclear Cataracts in the Beaver Dam Eye Study," *Am J Epidemiol*, 1999, 149(9):801-9.

Natural Standard Research Collaboration, Chief Editors: Ulbricht C, Basch E, *Natural Standard Herb and Supplement Reference - Evidence-Based Clinical Reviews*, USA: Elsevier/Mosby, 2005.

Slattery ML, Benson J, Curtin K, et al, "Carotenoids and Colon Cancer," *Am J Clin Nutr*, 2000, 71 (2):575-82.
Williams MA, Woelk GB, King IB, et al, "Plasma Carotenoids, Retinol, Tocopherols, and Lipoproteins in Preeclamptic and Normotensive Pregnant Zimbabwean Women," *Am J Hypertens*, 2003, 16(8):665-72.
Zhao X, Aldini G, Johnson EJ, et al, "Modification of Lymphocyte DNA Damage by Carotenoid Supplementation in Postmenopausal Women," *Am J Clin Nutr*, 2006, 83(1):163-9.

Lycopene

Pharmacologic Category Nutraceutical

Reported Use

Asthma (exercise-induced) (Neuman, 2000)
Atherosclerosis (Agarwal, 1998)
Benign prostate hypertrophy (BPH) (Schwarz, 2008)
Cancer (preventive; especially colon, lung, prostate, and kidney) (Bosetti, 2007; Bunker, 2007; Giovannucci, 1999; Michaud, 2000; Walfisch, 2007)
Diabetes, contradictory study (Wang, 2006)
Gingivitis (Chandra, 2007)
Hypertension (Engelard, 2006)
Immune enhancement (contradictory study) (Corridan, 2001)
Infertility (Gupta, 2002)
Macular degeneration (Mares-Perlman, 1995)
Oral submucous fibrosis (Kumar, 2007)
Pre-eclampsia (Sharma, 2003)
Contradictory study (Banerjee, 2009)

Local Anesthetic/Vasoconstrictor Precautions No information available to require special precautions

Effects on Bleeding None reported

Warnings/Precautions Lycopene supplements should be avoided in individuals with known allergy/hypersensitivity to lycopene or tomatoes.

References

Agarwal S and Rao AV, "Tomato Lycopene and Low Density Lipoprotein Oxidation: A Human Dietary Intervention Study," *Lipids*, 1998, 33(10):981-4.
Bunker CH, McDonald AC, Evans RW, et al, "A Randomized Trial of Lycopene Supplementation in Tobago Men With High Prostate Cancer Risk," *Nutr Cancer*, 2007, 57(2):130-7.
Corridan BM, O'Donoghue M, Hughes DA, et al, "Low-Dose Supplementation With Lycopene or Beta-Carotene Does Not Enhance Cell-Mediated Immunity in Healthy Free-Living Elderly Humans," *Eur J Clin Nutr*, 2001, 55(8):627-35.
Giovannucci E, "Tomatoes, Tomato-Based Products, Lycopene, and Cancer: Review of the Epidemiologic Literature," *J Natl Cancer Inst*, 1999, 91(4):317-31.
Kumar A, Bagewadi A, Keluskar V, et al, "Efficacy of Lycopene in the Management of Oral Submucous Fibrosis," *Oral Surg Oral Med Oral Pathol Oral Radiol Endod*, 2007, 103(2):207-13.
Mares-Perlman JA, Brady WE, Klein R, et al, "Serum Antioxidants and Age-Related Macular Degeneration in a Population-Based Case-Control Study," *Arch Ophthalmol*, 1995, 113(12):1518-23.
Michaud DS, Feskanich D, Rimm EB, et al, "Intake of Specific Carotenoids and Risk of Lung Cancer in 2 Prospective U.S. Cohorts," *Am J Clin Nutr*, 2000, 72(4):990-7.
Natural Standard Research Collaboration, Chief Editors: Ulbricht C, Basch E, *Natural Standard Herb and Supplement Reference - Evidence-Based Clinical Reviews*, USA: Elsevier/Mosby, 2005.
Neuman I, Nahum H, and Ben-Amotz A, "Reduction of Exercise-Induced Asthma Oxidative Stress by Lycopene, a Natural Antioxidant," *Allergy*, 2000, 55(12):1184-9.
Walfisch S, Walfisch Y, Kirilov E, et al, "Tomato Lycopene Extract Supplementation Decreases Insulin-Like Growth Factor-I Levels in Colon Cancer Patients," *Eur J Cancer Prev*, 2007, 16(4):298-303.

Maitake

Pharmacologic Category Herb

Reported Use

Cancer (Kodama, 2002)
Diabetes (animal)
Immune stimulation (animal)

Local Anesthetic/Vasoconstrictor Precautions No information available to require special precautions

Effects on Bleeding None reported

Warnings/Precautions Use with caution in individuals taking hypotensive/hypertensive agents; may decrease blood pressure. Use with caution in individuals taking hypoglycemic agents; research suggests maitake has hypoglycemic properties.

References

Kodama N, Komuta K, and Nanba H, "Can Maitake MD-Fraction Aid Cancer Patients?" *Altern Med Rev*, 2002, 7(3):236-9.
Natural Standard Research Collaboration, Chief Editors: Ulbricht C, Basch E, *Natural Standard Herb and Supplement Reference - Evidence-Based Clinical Reviews*, USA: Elsevier/Mosby, 2005.

Mastic

Pharmacologic Category Herb

Reported Use

Dental plaque (Takahashi, 2003)
H. pylori inhibitor; peptic ulcer disease (Al Habbal, 1984; Huwez, 1998)

Local Anesthetic/Vasoconstrictor Precautions No information available to require special precautions

Effects on Bleeding None reported

Warnings/Precautions Use with caution in individuals taking hypotensive/hypertensive agents; may decrease blood pressure.

References

Huwez FU, Thirlwell D, Cockayne A, et al, "Mastic Gum Kills *Helicobacter pylori*," *N Engl J Med*, 1998, 339(26):1946.
Natural Standard Research Collaboration, Chief Editors: Ulbricht C, Basch E, *Natural Standard Herb and Supplement Reference - Evidence-Based Clinical Reviews*, USA: Elsevier/Mosby, 2005.
Takahashi K, Fukazawa M, Motohira H, et al, "A Pilot Study on Antiplaque Effects of Mastic Chewing Gum in the Oral Cavity," *J Periodontol*, 2003, 74(4):501-5.

Melatonin

Pharmacologic Category Nutraceutical

Reported Use

Age-related macular degeneration (Yi, 2005)
Alzheimer's disease (sleep disorders) (Brusco, 1998; Cardinali, 2002; Singer, 1997)
Anxiety (preoperative) (Capuzzo, 2006; Caumo, 2007)
Athletic performance (Mero, 2006)
Autism (sleep disorders) (Garstang, 2006)
Benzodiazepine tapering (Cardinali, 2002; Dagan, 1997; Garfinkel, 1999; Rasmussen, 1997)
Bipolar disorder (Leibenluft, 1997; Robertson, 1997)
Cancer (Barni, 1995; Ernst, 2006; Lissoni, 1995; Lissoni, 2001; Neri, 1998; Todisco, 2001)
Cardioprotection (Dominguez-Rodriguez, 2007)
Chemotherapy adverse effects (Barni, 1996; Lissoni, 1996; Lissoni, 1997; Lissoni, 1997; Viviani, 1990)
Chronic fatigue syndrome (van Heukelom, 2006)
Cognitive impairment (Jansen, 2006; Peck, 2004)
Delayed sleep phase syndrome (Buscemi, 2005; Dagan, 1998; Kayumov, 2001; Mundey, 2005; Wasdell, 2008)
Depression (sleep disturbances) (Dalton, 2000; deVries, 1997; Dolberg, 1998; Kripke, 2003)
Duodenal ulcer (Malinovskaia, 2006)
Dyspepsia (Klupińska, 2007)
Glaucoma (Samples, 1988; Viggiano, 1994)
Glycemic control (Hussain, 2006)
Headache prevention (Claustrat, 1997; Gagnier, 2001; Leone, 1996; Nagtegaal, 1998)
HIV/AIDS (Lissoni, 1995)
Hypertension (Birau, 1981; Cagnacci, 1997; Zaslavskaia, 1999; Zaslavskaia, 2000; Zaslavaskaia, 2000); nocturnal hypertension (Cagnacci, 2005; Grossman, 2006)
Insomnia (Brezezinski, 2005; Zisapel, 1999); elderly (Dawson, 1998; Garfinkel, 1995; Wade, 2007; Zhdanova, 2001) children (Smits, 2001; Smits, 2003); individuals with intellectual disabilities (Braam, 2008)
Irritable bowel syndrome (Lu, 2005; Saha, 2007)
Jet lag (Arendt, 1986; Herxheimer, 2001; Herxheimer, 2002; Petrie, 1993; Suhner, 1998)
Menopause (Bellipanni, 2001)
Nocturia (Sugaya, 2007)
Oxidative stress in dialysis patients (preventive) (Herrera, 2001)
Parkinson's disease (Antolin, 2002; Bordet, 2003; Shaw, 1973)
Periodic limb movement disorder (Kunz, 2001)
Preoperative sedation/anxiolysis (Naguib, 1999; Naguib, 2000; Naguib, 2003; Naguib, 2003)
Rett syndrome (McArthur, 1998; Miyamoto, 1999)
Sarcoidosis, chronic (Pignone, 2006)
Schizophrenia (sleep disorders) (Shamir, 2000; Shamir, 2000; Suresh Kumar, 2007)
Seasonal affective disorder (SAD) (Avery, 1998; Leppanmaki, 2003; Lewy, 1998; Sherer, 1985; Wirz-Justice, 1990)
Sedation (children) (Schmidt, 2007)
Seizure disorders (Brueske, 1981; Fauteck, 1999; Jan, 1999; Molina-Carballo, 1997; Rufo-Campos, 2002; Siddiqui, 2001)
Skin damage (Bangha, 1996, Bangha, 1997; Dreher, 1998; Fischer, 1999)
Sleep disturbances, in blind people (Hack, 2003; Sack, 2000); in children with developmental disabilities (Phillips, 2004; Van der Heijden, 2007; Weiss, 2006)
Stroke (Adams, 2002; Chaudhary, 2003; Gupta, 2002; Pei, 2002; Pei, 2002; Pei, 2003; Pei, 2003; Reiter, 2003)
Tardive dyskinesia (Bhattacharya, 2002; Naidu, 2003; Naidu, 2003; Nelson, 2003; Shamir, 2000; Shamir, 2001)

Thermoregulation (Gubin, 2006)
Thrombocytopenia (Barni, 1996; Lissoni, 1995; Lissoni, 1995; Lissoni, 1997; Lissoni, 1999; Lissoni, 2001)
Tinnitus (sleep disorders) (Megwalu, 2006)
Tuberous sclerosis (Hancock, 2005)
Work-shift sleep disorder (Folkard, 1993; Jorgensen, 1998)

Local Anesthetic/Vasoconstrictor Precautions No information available to require special precautions

Effects on Bleeding None reported

Warnings/Precautions No known toxicity or serious side effects reported; however, long-term human studies have not been conducted. Excessive dosages may cause morning sedation or drowsiness.

Use with caution in individuals with a history of bleeding, hemostatic disorders, or drug-related hemostatic problems; in individuals taking anticoagulant medications, including warfarin, aspirin, aspirin-containing products, NSAIDs, or antiplatelet agents (eg, ticlopidine, clopidogrel, dipyridamole); and in individuals taking antidiabetic agents. Melatonin may reduce glucose tolerance and insulin sensitivity.

References

Adams JD Jr, Yang J, Mishra LC, et al, "Effects of Ashwagandha in a Rat Model of Stroke," *Altern Ther Health Med*, 2002, 8(5):18-9.
Antolin I, Mayo JC, Sainz RM, et al, "Protective Effect of Melatonin in a Chronic Experimental Model of Parkinson's Disease," *Brain Res*, 2002, 943(2):163-73.
Arendt J, Aldhous M, and Marks V, "Alleviation of Jet Lag by Melatonin: Preliminary Results of Controlled Double Blind Trial," *Br Med J (Clin Res Ed)*, 1986, 292(6529):1170.
Avery D, Lenz M, and Landis C, "Guidelines for Prescribing Melatonin," *Ann Med*, 1998, 30(1):122-30.
Bangha E, Elsner P, and Kistler GS, "Suppression of UV-Induced Erythema by Topical Treatment With Melatonin (N-Acetyl-5-Methoxytryptamine). A Dose Response Study," *Arch Dermatol Res*, 1996, 288 (9):522-6.
Bangha E, Elsner P, and Kistler GS, "Suppression of UV-Induced Erythema by Topical Treatment With Melatonin (N-Acetyl-5-Methoxytryptamine). Influence of the Application Time Point," *Dermatology*, 1997, 195(3):248-52.
Barni S, Lissoni P, Cazzaniga M, et al, "A Randomized Study of Low-Dose Subcutaneous Interleukin-2 Plus Melatonin Versus Supportive Care Alone in Metastatic Colorectal Cancer Patients Progressing Under 5-Fluorouracil and Folates," *Oncology*, 1995, 52(3):243-5.
Barni S, Lissoni P, Paolorossi F, et al, "Prevention of Chemotherapy-Induced Thrombocytopenia by the Pineal Hormore Melatonin (MLT)," *Proc Annu Meet Am Soc Clin Oncol*, 1996, 15:528.
Bellipanni G, Bianchi P, Pierpaoli W, et al, "Effects of Melatonin in Perimenopausal and Menopausal Women: A Randomized and Placebo Controlled Study," *Exp Gerontol*, 2001, 36(2):297-310.
Bhattacharya SK, Bhattacharya D, Sairam K, et al, "Effect of *Withania somnifera* Glycowithanolides on a Rat Model of Tardive Dyskinesia," *Phytomedicine*, 2002, 9(2):167-70.
Birau N, Petersen U, Meyer C, et al, "Hypotensive Effect of Melatonin in Essential Hypertension," *IRCS Med Sci*, 1981, 9:905-6.
Bordet R, Devos D, Brique S, et al, "Study of Circadian Melatonin Secretion Pattern at Different Stages of Parkinson's Disease," *Clin Neuropharmacol*, 2003, 26(2):65-72.
Braam W, Didden R, Smits M, et al, "Melatonin Treatment in Individuals With Intellectual Disability and Chronic Insomnia: A Randomized Placebo-Controlled Study," *J Intellect Disabil Res*, 2008, 52(Pt 3):256-64.
Brueske V, Allen J, Kepic T, et al, "Melatonin Inhibition of Seizure Activity in Man," *Electroencephalog Clin Neurophysiol*, 1981, 51:20.
Brusco LI, Marquez M, and Cardinali DP, "Monozygotic Twins With Alzheimer's Disease Treated With Melatonin: Case Report," *J Pineal Res*, 1998, 25(4):260-3.
Brzezinski A, Vangel MG, Wurtman RJ, et al, "Effects of Exogenous Melatonin on Sleep: A Meta-Analysis," *Sleep Med Rev*, 2005, 9(1):41-50.
Buscemi N, Vandermeer B, Hooton N, et al, "The Efficacy and Safety of Exogenous Melatonin for Primary Sleep Disorders. A Meta-Analysis," *J Gen Intern Med*, 2005, 20(12):1151-8.
Cagnacci A, Arangino S, Angiolucci M, et al, "Potentially Beneficial Cardiovascular Effects of Melatonin Administration in Women," *J Pineal Res*, 1997, 22(1):16-9.
Cagnacci A, Cannoletta M, Renzi A, et al, "Prolonged Melatonin Administration Decreases Nocturnal Blood Pressure in Women," *Am J Hypertens*, 2005, 18(12 Pt 1):1614-8.
Capuzzo M, Zanardi B, Schiffino E, et al, "Melatonin Does Not Reduce Anxiety More Than Placebo in the Elderly Undergoing Surgery," *Anesth Analg*, 2006, 103(1):121-3.
Cardinali DP, Brusco LI, Liberczuk C, et al, "The Use of Melatonin in Alzheimer's Disease," *Neuro Endocrinol Lett*, 2002, 23 Suppl 1:20-3.
Cardinali DP, Gvozdenovich E, Kaplan MR, et al, "A Double Blind-Placebo Controlled Study on Melatonin Efficacy to Reduce Anxiolytic Benzodiazepine Use in the Elderly," *Neuro Endocrinol Lett*, 2002, 23 (1):55-60.
Caumo W, Torres F, Moreira NL Jr, et al, "The Clinical Impact of Preoperative Melatonin on Postoperative Outcomes in Patients Undergoing Abdominal Hysterectomy," *Anesth Analg*, 2007, 105(5):1263-71.
Chaudhary G, Sharma U, Jagannathan NR, et al, "Evaluation of *Withania somnifera* in a Middle Cerebral Artery Occlusion Model of Stroke in Rats," *Clin Exp Pharmacol Physiol*, 2003, 30(5-6):399-404.
Claustrat B, Brun J, Geoffriau M, et al, "Nocturnal Plasma Melatonin Profile and Melatonin Kinetics During Infusion in Status Migrainosus," *Cephalalgia*, 1997, 17(4):511-7.
Dagan Y, Yovel I, Hallis D, et al, "Evaluating the Role of Melatonin in the Long-Term Treatment of Delayed Sleep Phase Syndrome (DSPS)," *Chronobiol Int*, 1998, 15(2):181-90.
Dagan Y, Zisapel N, Nof D, et al, "Rapid Reversal of Tolerance to Benzodiazepine Hypnotics by Treatment With Oral Melatonin: A Case Report," *Eur Neuropsychopharmacol*, 1997, 7(2):157-60.
Dalton EJ, Rotondi D, Levitan RD, et al, "Use of Slow-Release Melatonin in Treatment-Resistant Depression," *J Psychiatry Neurosci*, 2000, 25(1):48-52.
Dawson D, Rogers NL, van den Heuvel CJ, et al, "Effect of Sustained Nocturnal Transbuccal Melatonin Administration on Sleep and Temperature in Elderly Insomniacs," *J Biol Rhythms*, 1998, 13(6):532-8.
deVries MW and Peeters FP, "Melatonin as a Therapeutic Agent in the Treatment of Sleep Disturbance in Depression," *J Nerv Ment Dis*, 1997, 185(3):201-2.
Dolberg OT, Hirschmann S, and Grunhaus L, "Melatonin for the Treatment of Sleep Disturbances in Major Depressive Disorder," *Am J Psychiatry*, 1998, 155(8):1119-21.
Dominguez-Rodriguez A, Abreu-Gonzalez P, Garcia-Gonzalez MJ, et al, "A Unicenter, Randomized, Double-Blind, Parallel-Group, Placebo-Controlled Study of Melatonin as an Adjunct in Patients With Acute Myocardial Infarction Undergoing Primary Angioplasty the Melatonin Adjunct in the Acute Myocardial Infarction Treated With Angioplasty (MARIA) Trial: Study Design and Rationale," *Contemp Clin Trials*, 2007, 28(4):532-9.
Dreher F, Gabard B, Schwindt DA, et al, "Topical Melatonin in Combination With Vitamins E and C Protects Skin From Ultraviolet-Induced Erythema: A Human Study *in vivo*," *Br J Dermatol*, 1998, 139 (2):332-9.

Fauteck J, Schmidt H, Lerchl A, et al, "Melatonin in Epilepsy: First Results of Replacement Therapy and First Clinical Results," *Biol Signals Recept*, 1999, 8(1-2):105-10.
Fischer T, Bangha E, Elsner P, et al, "Suppression of UV-Induced Erythema by Topical Treatment With Melatonin. Influence of the Application Time Point," *Biol Signals Recept*, 1999, 8(1-2):132-5.
Folkard S, Arendt J, and Clark M, "Can Melatonin Improve Shift Workers' Tolerance of the Night Shift? Some Preliminary Findings," *Chronobiol Int*, 1993, 10(5):315-20.
Gagnier JJ, "The Therapeutic Potential of Melatonin in Migraines and Other Headache Types," *Altern Med Rev*, 2001, 6(4):383-9.
Garfinkel D, Zisapel N, Wainstein J, et al, "Facilitation of Benzodiazepine Discontinuation by Melatonin: A New Clinical Approach," *Arch Intern Med*, 1999, 159(20):2456-60.
Garstang J and Wallis M, "Randomized Controlled Trial of Melatonin for Children With Autistic Spectrum Disorders and Sleep Problems," *Child Care Health Dev*, 2006, 32(5):585-9.
Grossman E, Laudon M, Yalcin R, et al, "Melatonin Reduces Night Blood Pressure in Patients With Nocturnal Hypertension," *Am J Med*, 2006, 119(10):898-902.
Gupta YK, Chaudhary G, and Sinha K, "Enhanced Protection by Melatonin and Meloxicam Combination in a Middle Cerebral Artery Occlusion Model of Acute Ischemic Stroke in Rat," *Can J Physiol Pharmacol*, 2002, 80(3):210-7.
Hack LM, Lockley SW, Arendt J, et al, "The Effects of Low-Dose 0.5-mg Melatonin on the Free-Running Circadian Rhythms of Blind Subjects," *J Biol Rhythms*, 2003, 18(5):420-9.
Hancock E, O'Callaghan F, and Osborne JP, "Effect of Melatonin Dosage on Sleep Disorder in Tuberous Sclerosis Complex," *J Child Neurol*, 2005, 20(1):78-80.
Herrera J, Nava M, Romero F, et al, "Melatonin Prevents Oxidative Stress Resulting From Iron and Erythropoietin Administration," *Am J Kidney Dis*, 2001, 37(4):750-7.
Hussain SA, Khadim HM, Khalaf BH, et al, "Effects of Melatonin and Zinc on Glycemic Control in Type 2 Diabetic Patients Poorly Controlled With Metformin," *Saudi Med J*, 2006, 27(10):1483-8.
Jan JE, Connolly MB, Hamilton D, et al, "Melatonin Treatment of Non-Epileptic Myoclonus in Children," *Dev Med Child Neurol*, 1999, 41(4):255-9.
Jorgensen KM and Witting MD, "Does Exogenous Melatonin Improve Day Sleep or Night Alertness in Emergency Physicians Working Night Shifts?," *Ann Emerg Med*, 1998, 31(6):699-704.
Kayumov L, Brown G, Jindal R, et al," A Randomized, Double-Blind, Placebo-Controlled Crossover Study of the Effect of Exogenous Melatonin on Delayed Sleep Phase Syndrome," *Psychosom Med*, 2001, 63 (1):40-8.
Klupińska G, Poplawski T, Drzewoski J, et al, "Therapeutic Effect of Melatonin in Patients With Functional Dyspepsia," *J Clin Gastroenterol*, 2007, 41(3):270-4.
Kripke DF, Youngstedt SD, Rex KM, et al, "Melatonin Excretion With Affect Disorders Over Age 60," *Psychiatry Res*, 2003, 118(1):47-54.
Kunz D and Bes F, "Exogenous Melatonin in Periodic Limb Movement Disorder: An Open Clinical Trial and a Hypothesis," *Sleep*, 2001, 24(2):183-7.
Leibenluft E, Feldman-Naim S, Turner EH, et al, "Effects of Exogenous Melatonin Administration and Withdrawal in Five Patients With Rapid-Cycling Bipolar Disorder," *J Clin Psychiatry*, 1997, 58(9):383-8.
Leone M, D'Amico D, Moschiano F, et al, "Melatonin Versus Placebo in the Prophylaxis of Cluster Headache: A Double-Blind Pilot Study With Parallel Groups," *Cephalalgia*, 1996, 16(7):494-6.
Leppamaki S, Partonen T, Vakkuri O, et al, "Effect of Controlled-Release Melatonin on Sleep Quality, Mood, and Quality of Life in Subjects With Seasonal or Weather-Associated Changes in Mood and Behaviour," *Eur Neuropsychopharmacol*, 2003, 13(3):137-45.
Lewy AJ, Bauer VK, Cutler NL, et al, "Melatonin Treatment of Winter Depression: A Pilot Study," *Psychiatry Res*, 1998, 77(1):57-61.
Lissoni P, Ardizzoia A, Barni S, et al, "Randomized Study of Tamoxifen Alone Versus Tamoxifen Plus Melatonin in Estrogen Receptor-Negative Heavily Pretreated Metastatic Breast Cancer Patients," *Oncology Reports*, 1995, 2:871-3.
Lissoni P, Barni S, Brivio F, et al, "A Biological Study on the Efficacy of Low-Dose Subcutaneous Interleukin-2 Plus Melatonin in the Treatment of Cancer-Related Thrombocytopenia," *Oncology*, 1995, 52(5):360-2.
Lissoni P, Barni S, Brivio F, et al, "Treatment of Cancer-Related Thrombocytopenia by Low-Dose Subcutaneous Interleukin-2 Plus the Pineal Hormone Melatonin: A Biological Phase II Study," *J Biol Regul Homeost Agents*, 1995, 9(2):52-4.
Lissoni P, Bucovec R, Bonfanti A, et al, "Thrombopoietic Properties of 5-Methoxytryptamine Plus Melatonin Versus Melatonin Alone in the Treatment of Cancer-Related Thrombocytopenia," *J Pineal Res*, 2001, 30(2):123-6.
Lissoni P, Cazzaniga M, Tancini G, et al, "Reversal of Clinical Resistance to LHRH Analogue in Metastatic Prostate Cancer by the Pineal Hormone Melatonin: Efficacy of LHRH Analogue Plus Melatonin in Patients Progressing on LHRH Analogue Alone," *Eur Urol*, 1997, 31(2):178-81.
Lissoni P, Paolorossi F, Tancini G, et al, "Is There a Role for Melatonin in the Treatment of Neoplastic Cachexia?," *Eur J Cancer*, 1996, 32A(8):1340-3.
Lissoni P, Rovelli F, Malugani F, et al, "Anti-Angiogenic Activity of Melatonin in Advanced Cancer Patients," *Neuro Endocrinol Lett*, 2001, 22(1):45-7.
Lissoni P, Tancini G, Barni S, et al, "Treatment of Cancer Chemotherapy-Induced Toxicity With the Pineal Hormone Melatonin," *Support Care Cancer*, 1997, 5(2):126-9.
Lissoni P, Tancini G, Paolorossi F, et al, "Chemoneuroendocrine Therapy of Metastatic Breast Cancer With Persistent Thrombocytopenia With Weekly Low-Dose Epirubicin Plus Melatonin: A Phase II Study," *J Pineal Res*, 1999, 26(3):169-73.
Lissoni P, Vigore L, Rescaldani R, et al, "Neuroimmunotherapy With Low-Dose Subcutaneous Interleukin-2 Plus Melatonin in AIDS Patients With CD4 Cell Number Below 200/mm^3: A Biological Phase-II Study," *J Biol Regul Homeost Agents*, 1995, 9(4):155-8.
Lu WZ, Gwee KA, Moochhalla S, et al, "Melatonin Improves Bowel Symptoms in Female Patients With Irritable Bowel Syndrome: A Double-Blind Placebo-Controlled Study," *Aliment Pharmacol Ther*, 2005, 22(10):927-34.
Lusardi P, Piazza E, and Fogari R, "Cardiovascular Effects of Melatonin in Hypertensive Patients Well Controlled by Nifedipine: A 24-Hour Study," *Br J Clin Pharmacol*, 2000, 49(5):423-7.
Malinovskaia NK, Komarova FI, Rapoport SI, et al, "Melatonin in Treatment of Duodenal Ulcer," *Klin Med (Mosk)*, 2006, 84(1):5-11.
McArthur AJ and Budden SS, "Sleep Dysfunction in Rett Syndrome: A Trial of Exogenous Melatonin Treatment," *Dev Med Child Neurol*, 1998, 40(3):186-92.
Megwalu UC, Finnell JE, and Piccirillo JF, "The Effects of Melatonin on Tinnitus and Sleep," *Otolaryngol Head Neck Surg*, 2006, 134(2):210-3.
Miyamoto A, Oki J, Takahashi S, et al, "Serum Melatonin Kinetics and Long-Term Melatonin Treatment for Sleep Disorders in Rett Syndrome," *Brain Dev*, 1999, 21(1):59-62.
Molina-Carballo A, Munoz-Hoyos A, Reiter RJ, et al, "Utility of High Doses of Melatonin as Adjunctive Anticonvulsant Therapy in a Child With Severe Myoclonic Epilepsy: Two Years' Experience," *J Pineal Res*, 1997, 23(2):97-105.
Nagtegaal JE, Smits MG, Swart AC, et al, "Melatonin-Responsive Headache in Delayed Sleep Phase Syndrome: Preliminary Observations," *Headache*, 1998, 38(4):303-7.
Naguib M and Samarkandi AH, "Premedication With Melatonin: A Double-Blind, Placebo-Controlled Comparison With Midazolam," *Br J Anaesth*, 1999, 82(6):875-80.
Naguib M and Samarkandi AH, "The Comparative Dose-Response Effects of Melatonin and Midazolam for Premedication of Adult Patients: A Double-Blinded, Placebo-Controlled Study," *Anesth Analg*, 2000, 91(2):473-9.
Naguib M, Hammond DL, Schmid PG 3rd, et al, "Pharmacological Effects of Intravenous Melatonin: Comparative Studies With Thiopental and Propofol," *Br J Anaesth*, 2003, 90(4):504-7.
Naguib M, Schmid PG 3rd, and Baker MT, "The Electroencephalographic Effects of I.V. Anesthetic Doses of Melatonin: Comparative Studies With Thiopental and Propofol," *Anesth Analg*, 2003, 97(1):238-43.

Naidu PS, Singh A, and Kulkarni SK, "Effect of *Withania somnifera* Root Extract on Haloperidol-Induced Orofacial Dyskinesia: Possible Mechanisms of Action," *J Med Food*, 2003, 6(2):107-14.
Naidu PS, Singh A, Kaur P, et al, "Possible Mechanism of Action in Melatonin Attenuation of Haloperidol-Induced Orofacial Dyskinesia," *Pharmacol Biochem Behav*, 2003, 74(3):641-8.
Natural Standard Research Collaboration, Chief Editors: Ulbricht C, Basch E, *Natural Standard Herb and Supplement Reference - Evidence-Based Clinical Reviews*, USA: Elsevier/Mosby, 2005.
Nelson LA, McGuire JM, and Hausafus SN, "Melatonin for the Treatment of Tardive Dyskinesia," *Ann Pharmacother*, 2003, 37(7-8):1128-31.
Neri B, de Leonardis V, Gemelli MT, et al, "Melatonin as Biological Response Modifier in Cancer Patients," *Anticancer Res*, 1998, 18(2B):1329-32.
Peck JS, LeGoff DB, Ahmed I, et al, "Cognitive Effects of Exogenous Melatonin Administration in Elderly Persons: A Pilot Study," *Am J Geriatr Psychiatry*, 2004, 12(4):432-6.
Pei Z, Fung PC, and Cheung RT, "Melatonin Reduces Nitric Oxide Level During Ischemia But Not Blood-Brain Barrier Breakdown During Reperfusion in a Rat Middle Cerebral Artery Occlusion Stroke Model," *J Pineal Res*, 2003, 34(2):110-8.
Pei Z, Ho HT, and Cheung RT, "Pretreatment With Melatonin Reduces Volume of Cerebral Infarction in a Permanent Middle Cerebral Artery Occlusion Stroke Model in the Rat," *Neurosci Lett*, 2002, 318 (3):141-4.
Pei Z, Pang SF, and Cheung RT, "Administration of Melatonin After Onset of Ischemia Reduces the Volume of Cerebral Infarction in a Rat Middle Cerebral Artery Occlusion Stroke Model," *Stroke*, 2003, 34 (3):770-5.
Pei Z, Pang SF, and Cheung RT, "Pretreatment With Melatonin Reduces Volume of Cerebral Infarction in a Rat Middle Cerebral Artery Occlusion Stroke Model," *J Pineal Res*, 2002, 32(3):168-72.
Petrie K, Dawson AG, Thompson L, et al, "A Double-Blind Trial of Melatonin as a Treatment for Jet Lag in International Cabin Crew," *Biol Psychiatry*, 1993, 33(7):526-30.
Pignone AM, Rosso AD, Fiori G, et al, "Melatonin Is a Safe and Effective Treatment for Chronic Pulmonary and Extrapulmonary Sarcoidosis," *J Pineal Res*, 2006, 41(2):95-100.
Rasmussen P, "A Role of Phytotherapy Treatment of Benzodiazepine and Opiate Drug Withdrawal," *The European Journal of Herbal Medicine*, 1997, 3(1):11-21.
Reiter RJ, Sainz RM, Lopez-Burillo S, et al, "Melatonin Ameliorates Neurologic Damage and Neurophysiologic Deficits in Experimental Models of Stroke," *Ann N Y Acad Sci*, 2003, 993:35-47.
Robertson JM and Tanguay PE, "Case Study: The Use of Melatonin in a Boy With Refractory Bipolar Disorder," *J Am Acad Child Adolesc Psychiatry*, 1997, 36(6):822-5.
Rufo-Campos M, "Melatonin and Epilepsy," *Rev Neurol*, 2002, 35(1 Suppl):S51-8.
Sack RL, Brandes RW, Kendall AR, et al, "Entrainment of Free-Running Circadian Rhythms by Melatonin in Blind People," *N Engl J Med*, 2000, 343(15):1070-7.
Saha L, Malhotra S, Rana S, et al, "A Preliminary Study of Melatonin in Irritable Bowel Syndrome," *J Clin Gastroenterol*, 2007, 41(1):29-32.
Samples JR, Krause G, and Lewy AJ, "Effect of Melatonin on Intraocular Pressure," *Curr Eye Res*, 1988, 7(7):649-53.
Schmidt CM, Knief A, Deuster D, et al, "Melatonin Is a Useful Alternative to Sedation in Children Undergoing Brainstem Audiometry With an Age Dependent Success Rate - A Field Report of 250 Investigations," *Neuropediatrics*, 2007, 38(1):2-4.
Shamir E, Barak Y, Plopsky I, et al, "Is Melatonin Treatment Effective for Tardive Dyskinesia?" *J Clin Psychiatry*, 2000, 61(8):556-8.
Shamir E, Barak Y, Shalman I, et al, "Melatonin Treatment for Tardive Dyskinesia: A Double-Blind, Placebo-Controlled, Crossover Study," *Arch Gen Psychiatry*, 2001, 58(11):1049-52.
Shamir E, Laudon M, Barak Y, et al, "Melatonin Improves Sleep Quality of Patients With Chronic Schizophrenia," *J Clin Psychiatry*, 2000, 61(5):373-7.
Shamir E, Rotenberg VS, Laudon M, et al, "First-Night Effect of Melatonin Treatment in Patients With Chronic Schizophrenia," *J Clin Psychopharmacol*, 2000, 20(6):691-4.
Shaw KM, Stern GM, and Sandler M, "Melatonin and Parkinsonism," *Lancet*, 1973, 1(7797):271.
Sherer MA, Weingartner H, James SP, et al, "Effects of Melatonin on Performance Testing in Patients With Seasonal Affective Disorder," *Neurosci Lett*, 1985, 58(3):277-82.
Siddiqui MA, Nazmi AS, Karim S, et al, "Effect of Melatonin and Valproate in Epilepsy and Depression," *Indian J Pharmacol*, 2001, 33:378-81.
Singer CM, Moffit MT, Colling ED, et al, "Low Dose Melatonin Administration and Nocturnal Activity Levels in Patients With Alzheimer's Disease," *Sleep Res*, 1997, 26:752.
Smits MG, Nagtegaal EE, van der Heijden J, et al, "Melatonin for Chronic Sleep Onset Insomnia in Children: A Randomized Placebo-Controlled Trial," *J Child Neurol*, 2001, 16(2):86-92.
Smits MG, van Stel HF, van der Heijden K, et al, "Melatonin Improves Health Status and Sleep in Children With Idiopathic Chronic Sleep-Onset Insomnia: A Randomized Placebo-Controlled Trial," *J Am Acad Child Adolesc Psychiatry*, 2003, 42(11):1286-93.
Sugaya K, Nishijima S, Miyazato M, et al, "Effects of Melatonin and Rilmazafone on Nocturia in the Elderly," *J Int Med Res*, 2007, 35(5):685-91.
Suhner A, Schlagenhauf P, Johnson R, et al, "Comparative Study to Determine the Optimal Melatonin Dosage Form for the Alleviation of Jet Lag," *Chronobiol Int*, 1998, 15(6):655-66.
Suresh Kumar PN, Andrade C, Bhakta SG, et al, "Melatonin in Schizophrenic Outpatients With Insomnia: A Double-Blind, Placebo-Controlled Study," *J Clin Psychiatry*, 2007, 68(2):237-41.
Todisco M, Casaccia P, and Rossi N, "Cyclophosphamide Plus Somatostatin, Bromocriptin, Retinoids, Melatonin and ACTH in the Treatment of Low-Grade Non-Hodgkin's Lymphomas at Advanced Stage: Results of a Phase II Trial," *Cancer Biother Radiopharm*, 2001, 16(2):171-7.
Van der Heijden KB, Smits MG, Van Someren EJ, et al, "Effect of Melatonin on Sleep, Behavior, and Cognition in ADHD and Chronic Sleep-Onset Insomnia," *J Am Acad Child Adolesc Psychiatry*, 2007, 46 (2):233-41.
van Heukelom RO, Prins JB, Smits MG, et al, "Influence of Melatonin on Fatigue Severity in Patients With Chronic Fatigue Syndrome and Late Melatonin Secretion," *Eur J Neurol*, 2006, 13(1):55-60.
Viggiano SR, Koskela TK, Klee GG, et al, "The Effect of Melatonin on Aqueous Humor Flow in Humans During the Day," *Ophthalmology*, 1994, 101(2):326-31.
Viviani S, Negretti E, Orazi A, et al, "Preliminary Studies on Melatonin in the Treatment of Myelodysplastic Syndromes Following Cancer Chemotherapy," *J Pineal Res*, 1990, 8(4):347-54.
Von Bahr C, Ursing C, Yasui N, et al, "Fluvoxamine But Not Citalopram Increases Serum Melatonin in Healthy Subjects - An Indication That Cytochrome P450 CYP1A2 and CYP2C19 Hydroxylate Melatonin," *Eur J Clin Pharmacol*, 2000, 56(2):123-7.
Wade AG, Ford I, Crawford G, et al, "Efficacy of Prolonged Release Melatonin in Insomnia Patients Aged 55-80 Years: Quality of Sleep and Next-Day Alertness Outcomes," *Curr Med Res Opin*, 2007, 23 (10):2597-605.
Wasdell MB, Jan JE, Bomben MM, et al, "A Randomized, Placebo-Controlled Trial of Controlled Release Melatonin Treatment of Delayed Sleep Phase Syndrome and Impaired Sleep Maintenance in Children With Neurodevelopmental Disabilities," *J Pineal Res*, 2008, 44(1):57-64.
Weiss MD, Wasdell MB, Bomben MM, et al, "Sleep Hygiene and Melatonin Treatment for Children and Adolescents With ADHD and Initial Insomnia," *J Am Acad Child Adolesc Psychiatry*, 2006, 45(5):512-9.
Wirz-Justice A, Graw P, Krauchi K, et al, "Morning or Night-Time Melatonin Is Ineffective in Seasonal Affective Disorder," *J Psychiatr Res*, 1990, 24(2):129-37.
Yi C, Pan X, Yan H, et al, "Effects of Melatonin in Age-Related Macular Degeneration," *Ann N Y Acad Sci*, 2005, 1057:384-92.
Zaslavskaia RM, Biiasilov NS, Akhmetov KZh, et al, "Capozide-50 Alone and in Combination With Melatonin in Therapy of Hypertension," *Klin Med (Mosk)*, 2000, 78(11):39-41.
Zaslavskaia RM, Komarov FI, Shakirova AN, et al, "Effect of Moxonidine Monotherapy and in Combination With Melatonin on Hemodynamic Parameters in Patients With Arterial Hypertension," *Klin Med (Mosk)*, 2000, 78(4):41-4.

Zaslavskaia RM, Shakirova AN, Komarov FI, et al, "Effects of Melatonin Alone and in Combination With Aceten on Chronostructure of Diurnal Hemodynamic Rhythms in Patients With Hypertension Stage II," *Ter Arkh*, 1999, 71(12):21-4.
Zhdanova IV, Wurtman RJ, Regan MM, et al "Melatonin Treatment for Age-Related Insomnia," *J Clin Endocrinol Metab*, 2001, 86(10):4727-30.
Zisapel N, "The Use of Melatonin for the Treatment of Insomnia," *Biol Signals Recept*, 1999, 8(1-2):84-9.

Methyl Sulfonyl Methane

Pharmacologic Category Nutraceutical

Reported Use

Allergies (pharmacologic activity)
Analgesia (Jacob, 1999)
Arthritis (osteo and rheumatoid) (Rizzo, 1995; Usha, 2004)
Interstitial cystitis (Childs, 1994)
Lupus (Morton, 1986)
Seasonal allergic rhinitis (Barrager, 2002)

Local Anesthetic/Vasoconstrictor Precautions No information available to require special precautions

Effects on Bleeding None reported

Warnings/Precautions No known toxicity or serious side effects reported.

References

Barrager E, Veltmann JR Jr, Schauss AG, et al, "A Multicentered, Open-Label Trial on the Safety and Efficacy of Methylsulfonylmethane in the Treatment of Seasonal Allergic Rhinitis," *J Altern Complement Med*, 2002, 8(2):167-73.
Childs SJ, "Dimethyl Sulfone (DMSO2) in the Treatment of Interstitial Cystitis," *Urol Clin North Am*, 1994, 21(1):85-8.
Jacob SW, *The Miracle of MSM: The Natural Solution for Pain*, New York, NY: Putnam, 1999, 57-8.
Morton JI and Moore RD, "Lupus Nephritis and Deaths Are Diminished in B/W Mice Drinking 3% Water Solutions of Dimethyl Sulfoxide (DMSO) and Dimethyl Sulfone ($DMSO_2$)," *J Leukocyte Biol*, 1986, 40 (3):322.
Natural Standard Research Collaboration, Chief Editors: Ulbricht C, Basch E, *Natural Standard Herb and Supplement Reference - Evidence-Based Clinical Reviews*, USA: Elsevier/Mosby, 2005.
Rizzo R, "Calcium, Sulfur and Zinc Distribution in Normal and Arthritic Articular Equine Cartilage: A Synchrotron Radiation Induced X-Ray Emission Study (SRIXE)," *J Exp Zool*,1995, 273(1):82-6.
Usha PR and Naidu MU, "Randomised, Double-Blind, Parallel, Placebo-Controlled Study of Oral Glucosamine, Methylsulfonylmethane and Their Combination in Osteoarthritis," *Clin Drug Investig*, 2004, 24 (6):353-63.

Milk Thistle

Pharmacologic Category Herb

Reported Use

Amanita phalloides mushroom toxicity (Carducci, 1996; Floersheim, 1982; Hruby, 1984)
Antidote: Death Cup mushroom (Vogel, 1984)
Antioxidant (specifically hepatic cells): Acute/chronic hepatitis, jaundice, and stimulation of bile secretion/cholagogue (Carrescia, 1980; Flora, 1998; Kropacova, 1998)
Chemotherapy and radiation (adjunct) (pharmacologic activity)
Cirrhosis (Benda, 1980; Ferenci, 1989; Jacobs, 2002; Lang, 1988; Lang, 1990; Lawrence, 2000; Lucena, 2002; Pares, 1998); liver disease (chronic, alcoholic, viral) (Buzzelli, 1993; Kiesewetter, 1977; Magliulo, 1978; Marcelli, 1992)
Contradictory studies (Rambaldi, 2005; Rambaldi, 2007); drug-/toxin-induced (Boari, 1981; Magula, 1996)
Constipation (pharmacologic activity)
Diabetes (Velussi, 1993; Velussi, 1997; Zhang, 1993)
Eczema (pharmacologic activity)
Gallbladder (pharmacologic activity)
Halitosis (pharmacologic activity)
Hepatoprotection (including drug toxicities): Phenothiazines, butyrophenones, ethanol, and acetaminophen (Morazzoni, 1995)
Hyperlipidemia (Nassuato, 1991; Somogyi, 1989)
Hyperthyroidism (pharmacologic activity)
Psoriasis (pharmacologic activity)
Rosacea (pharmacologic activity)

Local Anesthetic/Vasoconstrictor Precautions No information available to require special precautions

Effects on Bleeding None reported

Warnings/Precautions Use with caution in individuals taking medications metabolized by cytochrome P450 due to possible inhibition of enzymes CYP3A4 and CYP2C9. Use with caution in individuals taking antidiabetic medications due to possible additive effects. Avoid in patients with known allergy to members of the *Compositeal/Asteraceae* family.

Avoid use of above-ground parts of the plant in women with hormone-sensitive conditions because milk thistle plant extract might have estrogenic effects. Some of these conditions include breast, uterine, and ovarian cancer; endometriosis; and uterine fibroids. The more commonly used milk thistle seed extracts are not known to have estrogenic effects.

References

Benda L, Dittrich H, Ferenzi P, et al, "The Influence of Therapy With Silymarin on the Survival Rate of Patients With Liver Cirrhosis," *Wien Klin Wochenschr*, 1980, 92(19):678-83.
Carducci R, Armellino MF, Volpe C, et al, "Silibinin and Acute Poisoning With Amanita Phalloides," *Minerva Anestesiol*, 1996, 62(5):187-93.
Carrescia O, Benelli L, Saraceni F, et al, "Silymarin in the Prevention of Hepatic Damage by Psychopharmacologic Drugs. Experimental Premises and Clinical Evaluations," *Clin Ter*, 1980, 95 (2):157-64.
Ferenci P, Dragosics B, Dittrich H, et al, "Randomized Controlled Trial of Silymarin Treatment in Patients With Cirrhosis of the Liver," *J Hepatol*, 1989, 9(1):105-13.
Floersheim GL, Weber O, Tschumi P, et al, "Clinical Death-Cap (*Amanita phalloides*) Poisoning: Prognostic Factors and Therapeutic Measures. Analysis of 205 cases," *Schweiz Med Wochenschr*, 1982, 112(34):1164-77.
Flora K, Hahn M, Rosen H, et al, "Milk Thistle (*Silybum marianum*) for the Therapy of Liver Disease," *Am J Gastroenterol*, 1998, 93(2):139-43.
Hruby K, Caomos G, and Thaler H, "Silbinin in the Treatment of Deathcap Fungus Poisoning," Forum, 1984, 6:23-6.
Kropacova K, Misurova E, and Hakova H, "Protective and Therapeutic Effect of Silymarin on the Development of Latent Liver Damage," *Radiats Biol Radioecol*, 1998, 38(3):411-5.
Lang I, Deak G, Nekam K, et al, "Hepatoprotective and Immunomodulatory Effects of Antioxidant Therapy," *Acta Med Hung*, 1988, 45(3-4):287-95.
Lang I, Nekam K, Gonzalez-Cabello R, et al, "Hepatoprotective and Immunological Effects of Antioxidant Drugs," *Tokai J Exp Clin Med*, 1990, 15(2-3):123-7.
Lucena MI, Andrade RJ, de la Cruz JP, et al, "Effects of Silymarin MZ-80 on Oxidative Stress in Patients With Alcoholic Cirrhosis. Results of a Randomized, Double-Blind, Placebo-Controlled Clinical Study," *Int J Clin Pharmacol Ther*, 2002, 40(1):2-8.
Morazzoni P, et al, "*Silybum marianum*," *Fitoterapia*, 1995, 66:3-42.
Nassuato G, Iemmolo RM, Strazzabosco M, et al, "Effect of Silibinin on Biliary Lipid Composition. Experimental and Clinical Study," *J Hepatol*, 1991, 12(3):290-5.
Natural Standard Research Collaboration, Chief Editors: Ulbricht C, Basch E, *Natural Standard Herb and Supplement Reference - Evidence-Based Clinical Reviews*, USA: Elsevier/Mosby, 2005.
Pares A, Planas R, Torres M, et al, "Effects of Silymarin in Alcoholic Patients With Cirrhosis of the Liver: Results of a Controlled, Double-Blind, Randomized and Multicenter Trial," *J Hepatol*, 1998, 28 (4):615-21.
Somogyi A, Ecsedi GG, Blazovics A, et al, "Short Term Treatment of Type II Hyperlipoproteinaemia With Silymarin," *Acta Med Hung*, 1989, 46(4):289-95.
Velussi M, Cernigoi AM, De Monte A, et al, "Long-Term (12 Months) Treatment With an Anti-Oxidant Drug (Silymarin) Is Effective on Hyperinsulinemia, Exogenous Insulin Need and Malondialdehyde Levels in Cirrhotic Diabetic Patients," *J Hepatol*, 1997, 26(4):871-9.
Velussi M, Cernigoi AM, Viezzoli L, et al, "Silymarin Reduces Hyperinsulinemia, Malondialdehyde Levels, and Daily Insulin Need in Cirrhotic Diabetic Patients," *Curr Ther Res*, 1993, 53(5):533-45.
Vogel G, Tuchweber B, Trost W, et al, "Protection by Silibinin Against *Amanita phalloides* Intoxication in Beagles," *Toxicol Appl Pharmacol*, 1984, 73(3):355-62.
Zhang JQ, Mao XM, and Zhou YP," Effects of Silybin on Red Blood Cell Sorbitol and Nerve Conduction Velocity in Diabetic Patients," *Zhongguo Zhong Xi Yi Jie He Za Zhi*, 1993, 13(12):725-6, 708.

Nicotinamide Adenine Dinucleotide

Pharmacologic Category Nutraceutical

Reported Use

Chronic fatigue syndrome (Forsyth, 1999)
Dementia (Birkmayer, 1996)
Diabetes, type 1 (Gale, 2004)
Hepatitis (Colombi, 1969)
Parkinson's disease (Swerdlow, 1998)
Stamina and energy (Forsyth, 1999)

Local Anesthetic/Vasoconstrictor Precautions No information available to require special precautions

Effects on Bleeding None reported

Warnings/Precautions No known toxicity or serious side effects reported.

References

Birkmayer JG, "Coenzyme Nicotinamide Adenine Dinucleotide: New Therapeutic Approach for Improving Dementia of the Alzheimer Type," *Ann Clin Lab Sci*, 1996, 26(1):1-9.
Colombi A, Tholen H, and Huber F, "Influence of Coenzyme A, Nicotinamide Adenine Dinucleotide (NAD), Alpha-Lipoic Acid and Cocarboxylase on Acute Hepatitis (Double Blind Experiment)," *Int Z Klin Pharmakol Ther Toxikol*, 1969, 2(2):133-8.
Forsyth LM, Preuss HG, MacDowell AL, et al, "Therapeutic Effects of Oral NADH on the Symptoms of Patients With Chronic Fatigue Syndrome," *Ann Allergy Asthma Immunol*, 1999, 82(2):185-91.
Gale EA, Bingley PJ, Emmett CL, et al, "European Nicotinamide Diabetes Intervention Trial (ENDIT): A Randomized Controlled Trial of Intervention Before the Onset of Type 1 Diabetes," *Lancet*, 2004, 363 (9413):925-31.
Natural Standard Research Collaboration, Chief Editors: Ulbricht C, Basch E, *Natural Standard Herb and Supplement Reference - Evidence-Based Clinical Reviews*, USA: Elsevier/Mosby, 2005.
Swerdlow RH, "Is NADH Effective in the Treatment of Parkinson's Disease?" *Drugs Aging*, 1998, 13 (4):263-8.

Omega-3-Acid Ethyl Esters

Pharmacologic Category Nutraceutical

Reported Use

Acne vulgaris (pharmacologic activity)
Angina pectoris (Aucamp, 1993; Kristensen, 1987)
Arrhythmias (Christensen, 1995; Christensen, 1996; Sellmayer, 1995)

- Asthma (Anon, 2004; Dry, 1991; Masuev, 1997; Mihrshahi, 2004; Nagakura, 2000; Oddy, 2004; Okamoto, 2000)
- Bipolar disorder (Calabrese, 1999; Stoll, 1999; Tanskanen, 2001)
- Body weight improvement (Mehra, 2006)
- Cancer (prevention)
- Cardiac death (sudden; preventive) (Albert, 2002)
- Cardiac support (general; proposed benefits) (Rosenberg, 2002)
- Cardiovascular disease (Din, 2004; Pepe, 2002; Woodman, 2002)
- Circulation (pharmacologic activity)
- Cognitive performance (Kalmijn, 2004)
- Colon cancer (Augustsson, 2003; Caygill, 1995; de Deckere, 1999; Klein, 2000; Mehrotra, 2002; Norrish, 1999; Rose, 1999; Terry, 2001)
- Coronary heart disease (preventive) (Bucher, 2002; Burr, 1989; Burr, 1994; GISSI - Prevenzione trial, 1999; Kris-Etherton, 2003; Kromhout, 1985; Kromhout, 1995; O'Keefe, 2000; Marchioli, 2002; Mizushima, 1997; Shekelle, 1985; Singh, 1997; Stone, 1996)
  - Contradictory study (Sacks, 1995)
- Crohn's disease (Belluzzi, 1996)
- Cystic fibrosis (Beckles, 2001; Beckles, 2002; De Vizia, 2003; Katz, 1996; Kurlandsky, 1994; Lawrence, 1993)
- Depression (Chiu, 2003; Frasure-Smith, 2004; Jacka, 2004; Logan, 2004; Mischoulon, 2000; Nemets, 2002; Nemets, 2004; Su, 2003)
- Diabetes, type 2 (McManus, 1996; Patti, 1999; Woodman, 2002)
- Dysmenorrhea (Deutch, 1996; Deutch, 2000; Harel, 1996)
- Eczema, psoriasis (Takwale, 2003; Bjorneboe, 1989)
- Fatigue (pharmacologic activity)
- Headache (pharmacologic activity)
- Heart disease and heart attack (risk reduction) (Daviglus, 1997), including women (Hu, 1999; Hu, 2002); anti-inflammatory effects in heart failure patients (Mehra, 2006)
- Herpes simplex 2 (pharmacologic activity)
- Hypercholesterolemia (Kalmijn, 2004; Nordoy, 2000; Nordoy, 2001)
- Hypertension (Appel, 1993; Bønaa, 1990; Howe, 1997; Knapp, 1989; Morris, 1993)
- Hypertriglyceridemia (Grimsgaard, 1997; Harris, 1988; Harris, 1997; Montori, 2000; Prichard, 1995; Roche, 1996; Sanders, 1997)
- IgA nephropathy (Alexopoulos, 2004; Dillon, 1997; Donadio, 2000; Donadio, 2001; Donadio, 2004; Parinyasiri, 2004; Sulikowska, 2004)
- Immune support (Dunstan, 2003)
- Infant eye-brain development (Birch, 1992; Carlson, 1987; Carlson, 1993; Carlson, 1996; Carlson, 1996; Fewtrell, 2004; Hoffman, 1993)
- Lupus (Clark, 1993; Clark, 1994; Duffy, 2004; Walton, 1991)
- Memory enhancement (Gamoh, 1999)
- Multiple sclerosis (pharmacologic activity)
- Nephrotic syndrome (Bakker, 1989; Stacpoole, 1989)
- Pre-eclampsia (Bulstra-Ramakers, 1994; D'Almeida, 1992; Olsen, 1992; Olsen, 2000; Olsen, 2002; Onwude, 1995; Salvig, 1996)
- Premenstrual syndrome (PMS) (pharmacologic activity)
- Prevention of graft failure after heart bypass surgery (Eritsland, 1996; Roy, 1991)
- Protection from cyclosporine toxicity in organ transplant patients (Andreassen, 1997; Badalamenti, 1995; Berthoux, 1992; Brouwer, 1991; Homan, 1989; Homan, 1990; Homan, 1992; Maachi, 1995; Stoof, 1989; Sweny, 1989; van der Heide, 1993; Ventura, 1993)
- Psoriasis (Bittiner, 1988; Danno, 1998; Mayser, 1998)
- Raynaud's phenomenon (DiGiacomo, 1989)
- Rheumatoid arthritis (Cleland, 1988; Fortin, 1995; Geusens, 1994; Kjeldsen-Kragh, 1992; Kremer, 1985; Kremer, 1987; Kremer, 1990; Kremer, 1991; Kremer, 1995; Lau, 1993; Nielsen, 1992; Skoldstam, 1992; Sperling, 1987; Tulleken, 1990; van der Tempel, 1990; Volker, 2000)
- Rosacea (pharmacologic activity)
- Schizophrenia (Fenton, 2001; Joy, 2000; Mellor, 1996; Peet, 1998)
- Scleroderma (pharmacologic activity)
- Stroke (risk reduction) (Iso, 2001)
- Ulcerative colitis (Aslan, 1992; Belluzzi, 1997; Dichi, 2000; Greenfield, 1993; Hawthorne, 1990; Hawthorne, 1992; Loeschke, 1996; Lorenz, 1989; Lorenz, 1994; Ross, 1993; Stenson, 1990; Stenson, 1992)

Local Anesthetic/Vasoconstrictor Precautions No information available to require special precautions

Effects on Bleeding None reported

Warnings/Precautions High doses may cause gastrointestinal upset, loose stools, and nausea.

Use with caution in individuals with diabetes or in those who may be predisposed to hypoglycemia; may alter glucose regulation. Effects of drugs with hypoglycemic activity may be potentiated (including insulin and oral hypoglycemics). Blood sugar should be closely monitored, and the dosage of hypoglycemic medications may require adjustment. This should be carefully coordinated among the individuals' healthcare providers.

Contraindicated in individuals with active bleeding (eg, peptic ulcer, intracranial bleeding). Use with caution in individuals with a history of bleeding, hemostatic disorders, or drug-related hemostatic problems; and in individuals taking anticoagulant medications, including warfarin, aspirin, aspirin-containing products, NSAIDs, or antiplatelet agents (eg, ticlopidine, clopidogrel, dipyridamole). Discontinue use prior to dental or surgical procedures (generally at least 14 days before).

Use with caution in individuals using antihypertensive agents. Fish oils may lower blood pressure and have additive effects.

References

Albert CM, Campos H, Stampfer MJ, et al, "Blood Levels of Long-Chain N-3 Fatty Acids and the Risk of Sudden Death," *N Engl J Med*, 2002, 346(15):1113-8.

Alexopoulos E, Stangou M, Pantzaki A, et al, "Treatment of Severe IgA Nephropathy With Omega-3 Fatty Acids: The Effect of a "Very Low Dose" Regimen," *Ren Fail*, 2004, 26(4):453-9.

Andreassen AK, Hartmann A, Offstad J, et al, "Hypertension Prophylaxis With Omega-3 Fatty Acids in Heart Transplant Recipients," *J Am Coll Cardiol*, 1997, 29(6):1324-31.

Anon, "Health Effects of Omega-3 Fatty Acids on Asthma," *Evid Rep Technol Assess (Summ)*, 2004, (91):1-7.

Appel LJ, Miller ER 3rd, Seidler AJ, et al, "Does Supplementation of Diet With 'Fish Oil' Reduce Blood Pressure? A Meta-Analysis of Controlled Clinical Trials," *Arch Intern Med*, 1993, 153(12):1429-38.

Aslan A and Triadafilopoulos G, "Fish Oil Fatty Acid Supplementation in Active Ulcerative Colitis: A Double-Blind, Placebo-Controlled, Crossover Study," *Am J Gastroenterol*, 1992, 87(4):432-7.

Aucamp AK, Schoeman HS, and Coetzee JH, "Pilot Trial to Determine the Efficacy of a Low Dose of Fish Oil in the Treatment of Angina Pectoris in the Geriatric Patient," *Prostaglandins Leukot Essent Fatty Acids*, 1993, 49(3):687-9.

Augustsson K, Michaud DS, Rimm EB, et al, "A Prospective Study of Intake of Fish and Marine Fatty Acids and Prostate Cancer," *Cancer Epidemiol Biomarkers Prev*, 2003, 12(1):64-7.

Badalamenti S, Salerno F, Lorenzano E, et al, "Renal Effects of Dietary Supplementation With Fish Oil in Cyclosporine-Treated Liver Transplant Recipients," *Hepatology*, 1995, 22(6):1695-71.

Bakker DJ, Haberstroh BN, Philbrick DJ, et al, "Triglyceride Lowering in Nephrotic Syndrome Patients Consuming a Fish Oil Concentrate," *Nutrit Res*, 1989, 9:27-34.

Beckles WN, Elliott TM, and Everard ML, "Omega-3 Fatty Acids for Cystic Fibrosis (Protocol for a Cochrane Review)," *The Cochrane Library*, 2001, (3).

Beckles WI, Elliott TM, and Everard ML, "Omega-3 Fatty Acids (From Fish Oils) for Cystic Fibrosis," *Cochrane Database Syst Rev*, 2002, (3):CD002201.

Belluzzi A, Brignola C, Boschi S, et al, "A Novel Enteric Coated Preparation of Omega-3 Fatty Acids in a Group of Steroid-Dependent Ulcerative Colitis: An Open Study [Abstract]," *Gastroenterology*, 1997, 112 (Suppl):A930.

Belluzzi A, Brignola C, Campieri M, et al, "Effect of an Enteric-Coated Fish Oil Preparation on Relapses in Crohn's Disease," *N Engl J Med*, 1996, 334(24):1557-60.

Bender NK, Kraynak MA, Chiquette E, et al, "Effects of Marine Fish Oils on the Anticoagulation Status of Patients Receiving Chronic Warfarin Therapy," *J Thromb Thrombolysis*, 1998, 5(3):257-61.

Berthoux FC, Guerin C, Burgard G, et al, "One-Year Randomized Controlled Trial With Omega-3 Fatty Acid-Fish Oil in Clinical Renal Transplantation," *Transplant Proc*, 1992, 24(6):2578-82.

Birch DG, Birch EE, Hoffman DR, et al, "Retinal Development in Very-Low-Birth-Weight Infants Fed Diets Differing in Omega-3 Fatty Acids," *Invest Ophthalmol Vis Sci*, 1992, 33(8):2365-76.

Bittiner SB, Tucker WF, Cartwright I, et al, "A Double-Blind, Randomised, Placebo-Controlled Trial of Fish Oil in Psoriasis," *Lancet*, 1988, 1(8582):378-80.

Bjorneboe A, Soyland R, Bjorneboe GE, et al, "Effect of N-3 Fatty Acid Supplement to Patients With Atopic Dermatitis," *J Intern Med Suppl*, 1989, 225(731):233-6.

Bønaa KH, Bjerve KS, Straume B, et al, "Effect of Eicosapentaenoic and Docosahexaenoic Acids on Blood Pressure in Hypertension. A Population-Based Intervention Trial From the Tromsø Study," *N Engl J Med*, 1990, 322(12):795-801.

Brouwer RM, Wenting GJ, Pos B, et al, "Fish Oil Ameliorates Established Cyclosporin A Nephrotoxicity After Heart Transplantation," *Kidney Int*, 1991, 40:347-8.

Bucher HC, Hengstler P, Schindler C, et al, "N-3 Polyunsaturated Fatty Acids in Coronary Heart Disease: A Meta-Analysis of Randomized Controlled Trials," *Am J Med*, 2002, 112(4):298-304.

Buckley MS, Goff AD, Knapp WE, "Fish Oil Interaction With Warfarin," *Ann Pharmacother*, 2004, 38 (1):50-2.

Bulstra-Ramakers MT, Huisjes HJ, and Visser GH, "The Effects of 3g Eicosapentaenoic Acid Daily on Recurrence of Intrauterine Growth Retardation and Pregnancy Induced Hypertension," *Br J Obstet Gynaecol*, 1994, 102:123-6.

Burr ML, Fehily AM, Gilbert JF, et al, "Effects of Changes in Fat, Fish, and Fibre Intakes on Death and Myocardial Reinfarction: Diet and Reinfarction Trial (DART)," *Lancet*, 1989, 2(8666):757-61.

Burr ML, Sweetham PM, and Fehily AM, "Diet and Reinfarction," *Eur Heart J*, 1994, 15(8):1152-3.

Calabrese JR, Rapport DJ, and Shelton MD, "Fish Oils and Bipolar Disorder: A Promising But Untested Treatment," *Arch Gen Psychiatry*, 1999, 56(5):413-4.

Carlson SE, Rhodes PG, Rao VS, et al, "Effect of Fish Oil Supplementation on the N-3 Fatty Acid Content of Red Blood Cell Membranes in Preterm Infants," *Pediatr Res*, 1987, 21(5):507-10.

Carlson SE and Werkman SH, "A Randomized Trial of Visual Attention of Preterm Infants Fed Docosahexaenoic Acid Until Two Months," *Lipids*, 1996, 31(1):85-90.

Carlson SE, Werkman SH, Rhodes PG, et al, "Visual-Acuity Development in Healthy Preterm Infants: Effect of Marine-Oil Supplementation," *Am J Clin Nutr*, 1993, 58(1):35-42.

Carlson SE, Werkman SH, and Tolley EA, "Effect of Long-Chain N-3 Fatty Acid Supplementation on Visual Acuity and Growth of Preterm Infants With and Without Bronchopulmonary Dysplasia," *Am J Clin Nutr*, 1996, 63(5):687-97.

Caygill CP and Hill MJ, "Fish, N-3 Fatty Acids and Human Colorectal and Breast Cancer Mortality," *Eur J Cancer Prev*, 1995, 4(4):329-32.

Chiu CC, Huang SY, Shen WW, et al, "Omega-3 Fatty Acids for Depression in Pregnancy," *Am J Psychiatry*, 2003, 160(2):385.

Christensen JH, Gustenhoff P, Ejlersen E, et al, "N-3 Fatty Acids and Ventricular Extrasystoles in Patients With Ventricular Tachyarrhythmias," *Nutr Res*, 1995, 15(1):1-8.

Christensen JH, Gustenhoff P, Korup E, et al, "Effect of Fish Oil on Heart Rate Variability in Survivors of Myocardial Infarction: A Double Blind Randomised Controlled Trial," *BMJ*, 1996, 312(7032):677-8.

Clark WF and Parbtani A, "Omega-3 Fatty Acid Supplementation in Clinical and Experimental Lupus Nephritis," *Am J Kidney Dis*, 1994, 23(5):644-7.

Clark WF, Parbtani A, Naylor CD, et al, "Fish Oil in Lupus Nephritis: Clinical Findings and Methodological Implications," *Kidney Int*, 1993, 44(1):75-86.

Cleland LG, French JK, Betts WH, et al, "Clinical and Biochemical Effects of Dietary Fish Oil Supplements in Rheumatoid Arthritis," *J Rheumatol*, 1988, 15(10):1471-5.
D'Almeida A, Carter JP, Anatol A, et al, "Effects of a Combination of Evening Primrose Oil (Gamma Linolenic Acid) and Fish Oil (Eicosapentaenoic + Docahexaenoic Acid) Versus Magnesium, and Versus Placebo in Preventing Pre-Eclampsia," *Women Health*, 1992, 19(2-3):117-31.
Danno K and Sugie N, "Combination Therapy With Low-Dose Etretinate and Eicosapentaenoic Acid for Psoriasis Vulgaris," *J Dermatol*, 1998, 25(11):703-5.
Daviglus ML, Stamler J, Orencia AJ, et al, "Fish Consumption and the 30-Year Risk of Fatal Myocardial Infarction," *N Engl J Med*, 1997, 336(15):1046-53.
de Deckere EA, "Possible Beneficial Effect of Fish and Fish N-3 Polyunsaturated Fatty Acids in Breast and Colorectal Cancer," *Eur J Cancer Prev*, 1999, 8(3):213-21.
Deutch B, "Painful Menstruation and Low Intake of N-3 Fatty Acids," *Ugeskr Laeger*, 1996, 158 (29):4195-8.
Deutch B, Jorgensen EB, and Hansen JC, "Menstrual Discomfort in Danish Women Reduced by Dietary Supplements of Omega-3 PUFA and B12 (Fish Oil or Seal Oil Capsules)," *Nutr Res*, 2000, 20 (5):621-31.
De Vizia B, Raia V, Spano C, et al, "Effect of an 8-Month Treatment With Omega-3 Fatty Acids (Eicosapentaenoic and Docosahexaenoic) in Patients With Cystic Fibrosis," *JPEN J Parenter Enteral Nutr*, 2003, 27(1):52-7.
Dichi I, Frenhane P, Dichi JB, et al, "Comparison of Omega-3 Fatty Acids and Sulfasalazine in Ulcerative Colitis," *Nutrition*, 2000, 16(2):87-90.
"Dietary Supplementation With N-3 Polyunsaturated Fatty Acids and Vitamin E After Myocardial Infarction: Results of the GISSI-Prevenzione Trial. Gruppo Italiano per lo Studio della Sopravvivenza Nell'Infarto Miocardico," *Lancet*, 1999, 354(9177):447-55.
DiGiacomo RA, Kremer JM, and Shah DM, "Fish-Oil Dietary Supplementation in Patients With Raynaud's Phenomenon: A Double-Blind, Controlled, Prospective Study," *Am J Med*, 1989, 86(2):158-64.
Dillon JJ, "Fish Oil Therapy for IgA Nephropathy: Efficacy and Interstudy Variability," *J Am Soc Nephrol*, 1997, 8(11):1739-44.
Din JN, "Omega 3 Fatty Acids and Cardiovascular Disease - Fishing for a Natural Treatment," *Br Med J*, 2004, 328(7430):30-5.
Donadio JV, "The Emerging Role of Omega-3 Polyunsaturated Fatty Acids in the Management of Patients With IgA Nephropathy," *J Ren Nutr*, 2001, 11(3):122-8.
Donadio JV Jr, "Use of Fish Oil to Treat Patients With Immunoglobulin a Nephropathy," *Am J Clin Nutr*, 2000, 71(1 Suppl):373S-5S.
Donadio JV and Grande JP, "The Role of Fish Oil/Omega-3 Fatty Acids in the Treatment of IgA Nephropathy," *Semin Nephrol*, 2004, 24(3):225-43.
Dry J and Vincent D, "Effect of a Fish Oil Diet on Asthma: Results of a 1-Year Double-Blind Study," *Int Arch Allergy Appl Immunol*, 1991, 95(2-3):156-7.
Duffy EM, Meenagh GK, McMillan SA, et al, "The Clinical Effect of Dietary Supplementation With Omega-3 Fish Oils and/or Copper in Systemic Lupus Erythematosus," *J Rheumatol*, 2004, 31(8):1551-6.
Dunstan JA, Mori TA, Barden A, et al, "Fish Oil Supplementation in Pregnancy Modifies Neonatal Allergen-Specific Immune Responses and Clinical Outcomes in Infants at High Risk of Atopy: a Randomized, Controlled Trial," *J Allergy Clin Immunol*, 2003, 112(6):1178-84.
Eritsland J, Arnesen H, Gronseth K, et al, "Effect of Dietary Supplementation With N-3 Fatty Acids on Coronary Artery Bypass Graft Patency," *Am J Cardiol*, 1996, 77(1):31-6.
Fenton WS, Dickerson F, Boronow J, et al, "A Placebo-Controlled Trial of Omega-3 Fatty Acid (Ethyl Eicosapentaenoic Acid) Supplementation for Residual Symptoms and Cognitive Impairment in Schizophrenia," *Am J Psychiatry*, 2001, 158(12):2071-4.
Fewtrell MS, Abbott RA, Kennedy K, et al, "Randomized, Double-Blind Trial of Long-Chain Polyunsaturated Fatty Acid Supplementation With Fish Oil and Borage Oil in Preterm Infants," *J Pediatr*, 2004, 144 (4):471-9.
"Fish Consumption and Mortality From Coronary Heart Disease," *N Engl J Med*, 1985, 313(13):820-4.
Fortin PR, Lew RA, Liang MH, et al, "Validation of a Meta-Analysis: The Effects of Fish Oil in Rheumatoid Arthritis," *J Clin Epidemiol*, 1995, 48(11):1379-90.
Frasure-Smith N, Lesperance F, and Julien P, "Major Depression Is Associated With Lower Omega-3 Fatty Acid Levels in Patients With Recent Acute Coronary Syndromes," *Biol Psychiatry*, 2004, 55 (9):891-6.
Gamoh S, Hashimoto M, Sugioka K, et al, "Chronic Administration of Docosahexaenoic Acid Improves Reference Memory-Related Learning Ability in Young Rats," *Neuroscience*, 1999, 93(1):237-41.
Geusens P, Wouters C, Nijs J, et al, "Long-Term Effect of Omega-3 Fatty Acid Supplementation in Active Rheumatoid Arthritis. A 12-Month, Double-Blind, Controlled Study," *Arthritis Rheum*, 1994, 37(6):824-9.
Goldstein MR, "Sudden Death Due to Cardiac Arrhythmias," *N Engl J Med*, 2002, 346(12):946-7.
Greenfield SM, Green AT, Teare JP, et al, "A Randomized Controlled Study of Evening Primrose Oil and Fish Oil in Ulcerative Colitis," *Aliment Pharmacol Ther*, 1993, 7(2):159-66.
Grimsgaard S, Bonaa KH, Hansen JB, et al, "Highly Purified Eicosapentaenoic Acid and Docosahexaenoic Acid in Humans Have Similar Triacylglycerol-Lowering Effects But Divergent Effects on Serum Fatty Acids," *Am J Clin Nutr*, 1997, 66(3):649-59.
Harel Z, Biro FM, Kottenhahn RK, et al, "Supplementation With Omega-3 Polyunsaturated Fatty Acids in the Management of Dysmenorrhea in Adolescents," *Am J Obstet Gynecol*, 1996, 174(4):1335-8.
Harris WS, "N-3 Fatty Acids and Serum Lipoproteins: Human Studies," *Am J Clin Nutr*, 1997, 65(5 Suppl):1645S-1654S.
Harris WS, Dujovne CA, Zucker M, et al, "Effects of a Low Saturated Fat, Low Cholesterol Fish Oil Supplement in Hypertriglyceridemic Patients. A Placebo-Controlled Trial," *Ann Intern Med*, 1988, 109 (6):465-70.
Hawthorne AB, Daneshmend TK, Hawkey CJ, et al, "Fish Oil in Ulcerative Colitis: Final Results of a Controlled Clinical Trial [Abstract]," *Gastroenterology*, 1990, 98(5 pt 2):A174.
Hawthorne AB, Daneshmend TK, Hawkey CJ, et al, "Treatment of Ulcerative Colitis With Fish Oil Supplementation: A Prospective 12 Month Randomised Controlled Trial," *Gut*, 1992, 33(7):922-8.
Henderson WR Jr, Astley SJ, McCready MM, et al, "Oral Absorption of Omega-3 Fatty Acids in Patients With Cystic Fibrosis Who Have Pancreatic Insufficiency and in Healthy Control Subjects.
Hoffman DR, Birch EE, Birch DG, et al, "Effects of Supplementation With Omega 3 Long-Chain Polyunsaturated Fatty Acids on Retinal and Cortical Development in Premature Infants," *Am J Clin Nutr*, 1993, 57(5 Suppl):807S-812S.
Holub BJ, "Clinical Nutrition: 4. Omega-3 Fatty Acids in Cardiovascular Care," *CMAJ*, 2002, 166 (5):608-15.
Homan van der Heide JJ, Bilo HJ, Donker AJ, et al, "Dietary Supplementation With Fish Oil Modifies Renal Reserve Filtration Capacity in Postoperative, Cyclosporin A-Treated Renal Transplant Recipients," *Transpl Int*, 1990, 3(3):171-5.
Homan van der Heide JJ, Bilo HJ, Donker AJ, et al, "The Effects of Dietary Supplementation With Fish Oil on Renal Function and the Course of Early Postoperative Rejection Episodes in Cyclosorine-Treated Renal Transplant Recipients," *Transplantation*, 1992, 54(2):257-63.
Homan van der Heide JJ, Bilo HJ, Tegzess AM, et al, "Omega-3 Polyunsaturated Fatty Acids Improve Renal Function in Renal Transplant Recipients Treated With Cyclosporin-A," *Kidney Int*, 1989, 35:516A.
Howe PR, "Dietary Fats and Hypertension. Focus on Fish Oil," *Ann N Y Acad Sci*, 1997, 827:339-52.
Hu FB, Bronner L, Willett WC, et al, "Fish and Omega-3 Fatty Acid Intake and Risk of Coronary Heart Disease in Women," *JAMA*, 2002, 287(14):1815-21.
Hu FB, Stampfer MJ, Manson JE, et al, "Dietary Intake of Alpha-Linolenic Acid and Risk of Fatal Ischemic Heart Disease Among Women," *Am J Clin Nutr*, 1999, 69(5):890-7.
Iso H, Rexrode KM, Stampfer MJ, et al, "Intake of Fish and Omega-3 Fatty Acids and Risk of Stroke in Women," *JAMA*, 2001, 285(3):304-12.
Jacka FN, Pasco JA, Henry MJ, et al, "Dietary Omega-3 Fatty Acids and Depression in a Community Sample," *Nutr Neurosci*, 2004, 7(2):101-6.

Joy CB, Mumby-Croft R, and Joy LA, "Polyunsaturated Fatty Acid (Fish or Evening Primrose Oil) for Schizophrenia," *Cochrane Database Syst Rev*, 2000, (2):CD001257.
Kalmijn S, van Boxtel MP, Ocke M, et al, "Dietary Intake of Fatty Acids and Fish in Relation to Cognitive Performance at Middle Age," *Neurology*, 2004, 62(2):275-80.
Katz DP, Manner T, Furst P, et al, "The Use of an Intravenous Fish Oil Emulsion Enriched With Omega-3 Fatty Acids in Patients With Cystic Fibrosis," *Nutrition*, 1996, 12(5):334-9.
Kjeldsen-Kragh J, Lund JA, Riise T, "Dietary Omega-3 Fatty Acid Supplementation and Naproxen Treatment in Patients With Rheumatoid Arthritis," *J Rheumatol*, 1992, 19(10):1531-6.
Klein V, Chajes V, Germain E, et al, "Low Alpha-Linolenic Acid Content of Adipose Breast Tissue Is Associated With an Increased Risk of Breast Cancer," *Eur J Cancer*, 2000, 36(3):335-40.
Knapp HR and FitzGerald GA, "The Antihypertensive Effects of Fish Oil. A Controlled Study of Polyunsaturated Fatty Acid Supplements in Essential Hypertension," *N Engl J Med*, 1989, 320 (16):1037-43.
Kremer JM, "Clinical Studies of Omega-3 Fatty Acid Supplementation in Patients Who Have Rheumatoid Arthritis," *Rheum Dis Clin North Am*, 1991, 17(2):391-402.
Kremer JM, Bigauoette J, Michalek AV, et al, "Effects of Manipulation of Dietary Fatty Acids on Clinical Manifestations of Rheumatoid Arthritis," *Lancet*, 1985, 1(8422):184-7.
Kremer JM, Jubiz W, Michalek A, et al, "Fish-Oil Fatty Acid Supplementation in Active Rheumatoid Arthritis. A Double-Blinded, Controlled, Crossover Study," *Ann Intern Med*, 1987, 106(4):497-503.
Kremer JM, Lawrence DA, Jubiz W, et al, "Dietary Fish Oil and Olive Oil Supplementation in Patients With Rheumatoid Arthritis. Clinical and Immunologic Effects," *Arthritis Rheum*, 1990, 33(6):810-20.
Kremer JM, Lawrence DA, Petrillo GF, et al, "Effects of High-Dose Fish Oil on Rheumatoid Arthritis After Stopping Nonsteroidal Antiinflammatory Drugs. Clinical and Immune Correlates," *Arthritis Rheum*, 1995, 38(8):1107-14.
Kris-Etherton PM, Harris WS, Appel LJ, et al, "Fish Consumption, Fish Oil, Omega-3 Fatty Acids, and Cardiovascular Disease," *Arterioscler Thromb Vasc Biol*, 2003, 23(2):e20-30.
Kristensen SD, Schmidt EB, Andersen HR, et al, "Fish Oil in Angina Pectoris," *Atherosclerosis*, 1987, 64 (1):13-9.
Kromhout D, Bosschieter EB, and de Lezenne Coulander C, "The Inverse Relation Between Fish Consumption and 20-Year Mortality From Coronary Heart Disease," *N Engl J Med*, 1985, 312 (19):1205-9.
Kromhout D, Menotti A, Bloemberg B, et al, "Dietary Saturated and Trans Fatty Acids and Cholesterol and 25-Year Mortality From Coronary Heart Disease: The Seven Countries Study," *Prev Med*, 1995, 24 (3):308-15.
Kurlandsky LE, Bennink MR, Webb PM, et al, "The Absorption and Effect of Dietary Supplementation With Omega-3 Fatty Acids on Serum Leukotriene B4 in Patients With Cystic Fibrosis," *Pediatr Pulmonol*, 1994, 18(4):211-7.
Lau CS, Morley KD, and Belch JJ, "Effects of Fish Oil Supplementation on Non-steroidal Anti-inflammatory Drug Requirement in Patients With Mild Rheumatoid Arthritis - A Double-Blind Placebo Controlled Study," *Br J Rheumatol*, 1993, 32(11):982-9.
Lawrence R and Sorrell T, "Eicosapentaenoic Acid in Cystic Fibrosis: Evidence of a Pathogenetic Role for Leukotriene B4," *Lancet*, 1993, 342(8869):465-9.
Loeschke K, Ueberschaer B, Pietsch A, et al, "N-3 Fatty Acids Only Delay Early Relapse of Ulcerative Colitis in Remission," *Dig Dis Sci*, 1996, 41(10):2087-94.
Logan AC, "Omega-3 Fatty Acids and Major Depression: A Primer for the Mental Health Professional," *Lipids Health Dis*, 2004, 3:25.
Lorenz R and Loeschke K, "Placebo-Controlled Trials of Omega 3 Fatty Acids in Chronic Inflammatory Bowel Disease," *World Rev Nutr Diet*, 1994, 76:143-5.
Lorenz R, Weber PC, Szimnau P, et al, "Supplementation With N-3 Fatty Acids From Fish Oil in Chronic Inflammatory Bowel Disease - A Randomized, Placebo-Controlled, Double-Blind Cross-Over Trial," *J Intern Med Suppl*, 1989, 731:225-32.
Maachi K, Berthoux P, Burgard G, et al, "Results of a 1-Year Randomized Controlled Trial With Omega-3 Fatty Acid Fish Oil in Renal Transplantation Under Triple Immunosuppressive Therapy," *Transplant Proc*, 1995, 27(1):846-9.
Marchioli R, Barzi F, Bomba E, et al, "Early Protection Against Sudden Death by n-3 Polyunsaturated Fatty Acids After Myocardial Infarction: Time-Course Analysis of the Results of the Gruppo Italiano per lo Studio della Sopravvivenza nell'Infarto Miocardico (GISSI)-Prevenzione," *Circulation*, 2002, 105 (16):1897-903.
Masuev KA, "The Effect of Polyunsaturated Fatty Acids of the Omega-3 Class on the Late Phase of the Allergic Reaction in Bronchial Asthma Patients," *Ter Arkh*, 1997, 69(3):31-3.
The Mayo Clinic, "Dermatomyositis," 2009. Available at: http://www.mayoclinic.com/health/dermatomyositis.
Mayser P, Mrowietz U, Arenberger P, et al, "Omega-3 Fatty Acid-Based Lipid Infusion in Patients With Chronic Plaque Psoriasis: Results of a Double-Blind, Randomized, Placebo-Controlled, Multicenter Trial," *J Am Acad Dermatol*, 1998, 38(4):539-47.
McManus RM, Jumpson J, Finegood DT, et al, "A Comparison of the Effects of n-3 Fatty Acids From Linseed Oil and Fish Oil in Well-Controlled Type II Diabetes," *Diabetes Care*, 1996, 19(5):463-7.
Mehra MR, Lavie CJ, Ventura HO, et al, "Fish Oils Produce Anti-Inflammatory Effects and Improve Body Weight in Severe Heart Failure," *J Heart Lung Transplant*, 2006, 25(7):834-8.
Mehrotra B and Ronquillo J, "Dietary Supplementation in Hem/Onc Outpatients at a Tertiary Care Hospital," American Society of clinicla Oncology 38th Annual Meeting, Orlando, Florida, May 18-21, 2002.
Mellor J, Laugharne JD, and Peet M, "Omega-3 Fatty Acid Supplementation in Schizophrenic Patients," *Human Psychopharmacol*, 1996, 11:39-46.
Mihrshahi S, Peat JK, Webb K, et al, "Effect of Omega-3 Fatty Acid Concentrations in Plasma on Symptoms of Asthma at 18 Months of Age," *Pediatr Allergy Immunol*, 2004, 15(6):517-22.
Mischoulon D and Fava M, "Docosahexanoic Acid and Omega-3 Fatty Acids in Depression," *Psychiatr Clin North Am*, 2000, 23(4):785-94.
Mizushima S, Moriguchi EH, Ishikawa P, et al, "Fish Intake and Cardiovascular Risk Among Middle-Aged Japanese in Japan and Brazil," *J Cardiovasc Risk*, 1997, 4(3):191-9.
Montori VM, Farmer A, Wollan PC, et al, "Fish Oil Supplementation in Type 2 Diabetes: A Quantitative Systematic Review," *Diabetes Care*, 2000, 23(9):1407-15.
Morris MC, Sacks F, and Rosner B, et al, "Does Fish Oil Lower Blood Pressure? A Meta-analysis of Controlled Trials," *Circulation*, 1993, 88(2):523-33.
Nagakura T, Matsuda S, Shichijyo K, et al, "Dietary Supplementation With Fish Oil Rich in Omega-3 Polyunsaturated Fatty Acids in Children With Bronchial Asthma," *Eur Respir J*, 2000, 16(5):861-5.
Natural Standard Research Collaboration, Chief Editors: Ulbricht C, Basch E, *Natural Standard Herb and Supplement Reference - Evidence-Based Clinical Reviews*, USA: Elsevier/Mosby, 2005.
Nemets B, Osher Y, and Belmaker RH, "Omega-3 Fatty Acids and Augmentation Strategies in Treating Resistant Depression," *Essent Psychopharmacol*, 2004, 6(1):59-64.
Nemets B, Stahl Z, and Belmaker RH, "Addition of Omega-3 Fatty Acid to Maintenance Medication Treatment for Recurrent Unipolar Depressive Disorder," *Am J Psychiatry*, 2002, 159(3):477-9.
Nielsen GL, Faarvang KL, Thomsen BS, et al, "The Effects of Dietary Supplementation With n-3 Polyunsaturated Fatty Acids in Patients With Rheumatoid Arthritis: A Randomized, Double Blind Trial," *Eur J Clin Invest*, 1992, 22(10):687-91.
Nordoy A, Bonaa KH, Sandset PM, et al, "Effect of Omega-3 Fatty Acids and Simvastatin on Hemostatic Risk Factors and Postprandial Hyperlipemia in Patients With Combined Hyperlipemia," *Arterioscler Thromb Vasc Biol*, 2000, 20(1):259-65.
Nordoy A, Hansen JB, Brox J, et al, "Effects of Atorvastatin and Omega-3 Fatty Acids on LDL Subfractions and Postprandial Hyperlipemia in Patients With Combined Hyperlipemia," *Nutr Metab Cardiovasc Dis*, 2001, 11(1):7-16.

Norrish AE, Skeaff CM, Arribas GL, et al, "Prostate Cancer Risk and Consumption of Fish Oils: A Dietary Biomarker-Based Case-Control Study," *Br J Cancer*, 1999, 81(7):1238-42.
Oddy WH, de Klerk NH, Kendall GE, el al, "Ratio of Omega-6 to Omega-3 Fatty Acids and Childhood Asthma," *J Asthma*, 2004, 41(3):319-26.
Okamoto M, Mitsunobu F, Ashida K, et al, "Effects of Dietary Supplementation With N-3 Fatty Acids Compared With N-6 Fatty Acids on Bronchial Asthma," *Intern Med*, 2000, 39(2):107-11.
O'Keefe JH Jr and Harris WS, "From Inuit to Implementation: Omega-3 Fatty Acids Come of Age," *Mayo Clin Proc*, 2000, 75(6):607-14.
Olsen SF and Secher NJ, "Low Consumption of Seafood in Early Pregnancy as a Risk Factor for Preterm Delivery: Prospective Cohort Study," *BMJ*, 2002, 324(7335):447.
Olsen SF, Secher NJ, Tabor A, et al, "Randomised Clinical Trials of Fish Oil Supplementation in High Risk Pregnancies. Fish Oil Trials in Pregnancy (FOTIP) Team," *BJOG*, 2000, 107(3):382-95.
Olsen SF, Sorensen JD, Secher NJ, et al, "Randomised Controlled Trial of Effect of Fish-Oil Supplementation on Pregnancy Duration," *Lancet*, 1992, 339(8800):1003-7.
Onwude JL, Lilford RJ, Hjartardottir H, et al, "A Randomised Double Blind Placebo Controlled Trial of Fish Oil in High Risk Pregnancy," *Br J Obstet Gynaecol*, 1995, 102(2):95-100.
Parinyasiri U, Ong-Ajyooth L, Parichatikanond P, et al, "Effect of Fish Oil on Oxidative Stress, Lipid Profile and Renal Function in IgA Nephropathy," *J Med Assoc Thai*, 2004, 87(2):143-9.
Patti L, Maffettone A, Iovine C, et al, "Long-Term Effects of Fish Oil on Lipoprotein Subfractions and Low-Density Lipoprotein Size in Non-Insulin-Dependent Diabetic Patients With Hypertriglyceridemia," *Atherosclerosis*, 1999, 146(2):361-7.
Peet M and Mellor J, "Double-Blind Placebo Controlled Trial of N-3 Polyunsaturated Fatty Acids as an Adjunct to Neuroleptics [Abstract]," *Schizophrenia Res*, 1998, 29(1-2):160-1.
Pepe S and McLennan PL, "Cardiac Membrane Fatty Acid Composition Modulates Myocardial Oxygen Consumption and Postischemic Recovery of Contractile Function," *Circulation*, 2002, 105(19):2303-8.
Prichard BN, Smith CC, Ling KL, et al, "Fish Oils and Cardiovascular Disease," *BMJ*, 1995, 310 (6983):819-20.
Roche HM and Gibney MJ, "Postprandial Triacylglycerolaemia: The Effect of Low-Fat Dietary Treatment With and Without Fish Oil Supplementation," *Eur J Clin Nutr*, 1996, 50(9):617-24.
Rose DP and Connolly JM, "Omega-3 Fatty Acids as Cancer Chemopreventive Agents," *Pharmacol Ther*, 1999, 83(3):217-44.
Rosenberg IH, "Fish - Food to Calm the Heart," *N Engl J Med*, 2002, 346(15):1102-3.
Ross E, "The Role of Marine Fish Oils in the Treatment of Ulcerative Colitis," *Nutr Rev*, 1993, 51(2):47-9.
Roy I, Meyer F, Gingras L, et al, "A Double Blind Randomized Controlled Study Comparing the Efficacy of Fish Oil and Low dose ASA to Prevent Coronary Saphenous Vein Graft obstruction After CABG [Abstract]," *Circulation*, 1991, 84:II-285.
Sacks FM, Stone PH, Gibson CM, et al, "Controlled Trial of Fish Oil for Regression of Human Coronary Atherosclerosis. HARP Research Group," *J Am Coll Cardiol*, 1995, 25(7):1492-8.
Salvig JD, Olsen SF, and Secher NJ, "Effects of Fish Oil Supplementation in Late Pregnancy on Blood Pressure: A Randomised Controlled Trial," *Br J Obstet Gynaecol*, 1996, 103(6):529-33.
Sanders TA, Oakley FR, Miller GJ, et al, "Influence of n-6 Versus n-3 Polyunsaturated Fatty Acids in Diets Low in Saturated Fatty Acids on Plasma Lipoproteins and Hemostatic Factors," *Arterioscler Thromb Vasc Biol*, 1997, 17(12):3449-60.
Sellmayer A, Witzgall H, Lorenz RL, et al, "Effects of Dietary Fish Oil on Ventricular Premature Complexes," *Am J Cardiol*, 1995, 76(12):974-7.
Singh RB, Niaz MA, Sharma JP, et al, "Randomized, Double-Blind, Placebo-Controlled Trial of Fish Oil and Mustard Oil in Patients With Suspected Acute Myocardial Infarction: The Indian Experiment of Infarct Survival - 4," *Cardiovasc Drugs Ther*, 1997, 11(3):485-91.
Sköldstam L, Börjesson O, Kjällman A, et al, "Effect of Six Months of Fish Oil Supplementation in Stable Rheumatoid Arthritis. A Double-Blind, Controlled Study," *Scand J Rheumatol*, 1992, 21(4):178-85.
Sperling RI, Weinblatt M, Robin JL, et al, "Effects of Dietary Supplementation With Marine Fish Oil on Leukocyte Lipid Mediator Generation and Function in Rheumatoid Arthritis," *Arthritis Rheum*, 1987, 30 (9):988-97.
Stacpoole PW, Alig J, Ammon L, et al, "Dose-Response Effects of Dietary Marine Oil on Carbohydrate and Lipid Metabolism in Normal Subjects and Patients With Hypertriglyceridemia," *Metabolism*, 1989, 38(10):946-56.
Stenson WF, Cort D, Beeken W, et al, "A Trial of Fish Oil Supplemented Diet in Ulcerative Colitis [Abstract]," *Gastroenterology*, 1990, 98(Suppl):A475.
Stenson WF, Cort D, Rodgers J, et al, "Dietary Supplementation With Fish Oil in Ulcerative Colitis," *Ann Intern Med*, 1992, 116(8):609-14.
Stoll AL, Severus WE, Freeman MP, et al, "Omega 3 Fatty Acids in Bipolar Disorder: A Preliminary Double-Blind, Placebo-Controlled Trial," *Arch Gen Psychiatry*, 1999, 56(5):407-12.
Stone NJ, "Fish Consumption, Fish Oil, Lipids, and Coronary Heart Disease," *Circulation*, 1996, 94 (9):2337-40.
Stoof TJ, Korstanje MJ, Bilo HJ, et al, "Does Fish Oil Protect Renal Function in Cyclosporin-Treated Psoriasis Patients?" *J Intern Med*, 1989, 226(6):437-41.
Su KP, Huang SY, Chiu CC, et al, "Omega-3 Fatty Acids in Major Depressive Disorder. A Preliminary Double-Blind, Placebo-Controlled Trial," *Eur Neuropsychopharmacol*, 2003, 13(4):267-71.
Sulikowska B, Nieweglowski T, Manitius J, et al, "Effect of 12-Month Therapy With Omega-3 Polyunsaturated Acids on Glomerular Filtration Response to Dopamine in IgA Nephropathy," *Am J Nephrol*, 2004, 24(5):474-82.
Sweny P, Wheeler DC, Lui SF, et al, "Dietary Fish Oil Supplements Preserve Renal Function in Renal Transplant Recipients With Chronic Vascular Rejection," *Nephrol Dial Transplant*, 1989, 4(12):1070-5.
Takwale A, Tan E, Agarwal S, et al, "Efficacy and Tolerability of Borage Oil in Adults and Children With Atopic Eczema: Randomised, Double Blind, Placebo Controlled, Parallel Group Trial," *Br Med J*, 2003, 327(7428):1385.
Tanskanen A, Hibbeln JR, Hintikka J, et al, "Fish Consumption, Depression, and Suicidality in a General Population," *Arch Gen Psychiatry* , 2001, 58(5):512-3.
Terry P, Lichtenstein P, Feychting M, et al, "Fatty Fish Consumption and Risk of Prostate Cancer," *Lancet*, 2001, 357(9270):1764-6.
Tulleken JE, Limburg PC, Muskiet FA, et al, "Vitamin E Status During Dietary Fish Oil Supplementation in Rheumatoid Arthritis," *Arthritis Rheum*, 1990, 33(9):1416-9.
van der Heide JJ, Bilo HJ, Donker JM, et al, "Effect of Dietary Fish Oil on Renal Function and Rejection in Cyclosporine-Treated Recipients of Renal Transplants," *N Engl J Med*, 1993, 329(11):769-73.
van der Tempel H, Tulleken JE, Limburg PC, et al, "Effects of Fish Oil Supplementation in Rheumatoid Arthritis," *Ann Rheum Dis*, 1990, 49(2):76-80.
Ventura HO, Milani RV, Lavie CJ, et al, "Cyclosporine-Induced Hypertension. Efficacy of Omega-3 Fatty Acids in Patients After Cardiac Transplantation," *Circulation*, 1993, 88(5 Pt 2):II281-5.
Volker D, Fitzgerald P, Major G, et al, "Efficacy of Fish Oil Concentrate in the Treatment of Rheumatoid Arthritis," *J Rheumatol*, 2000, 27(10):2343-6.
Walton AJ, Snaith ML, Locniskar M, et al, "Dietary Fish Oil and the Severity of Symptoms in Patients With Systemic Lupus Erythematosus," *Ann Rheum Dis*, 1991, 50(7):463-6.
Woodman RJ, Mori TA, Burke V, et al, "Effects of Purified Eicosapentaenoic and Docosahexaenoic Acids on Glycemic Control, Blood Pressure, and Serum Lipids in Type 2 Diabetic Patients With Treated Hypertension," *Am J Clin Nutri*, 2002, 76(5):1007-15.

Parsley

Pharmacologic Category Herb

Reported Use

Halitosis; antibacterial, antifungal (Newall, 1996)

Local Anesthetic/Vasoconstrictor Precautions No information available to require special precautions

Effects on Bleeding None reported

Warnings/Precautions Encapsulated parsley products: Extremely large doses of constituents (apiole and myristicin) have been associated with hematologic, renal, and hepatic toxicity (based on *in vitro* or animal studies) (Buchanan, 1978). Use with caution in individuals receiving MAO inhibitors, anticoagulant/antiplatelet drugs, or diuretics.

References

Buchanan RL, "Toxicity of Species Containing Methylenedioxygenzene Derivatives," *J Food Safety*, 1978, 1:275-293.

Natural Standard Research Collaboration, Chief Editors: Ulbricht C, Basch E, *Natural Standard Herb and Supplement Reference - Evidence-Based Clinical Reviews*, USA: Elsevier/Mosby, 2005.

Newall CA, Anderson LA, and Phillipson JD, *Herbal Medicines: A Guide for Health Care Professionals*, London, England: The Pharmaceutical Press, 1996, 203-4.

Passion Flower

Pharmacologic Category Herb

Reported Use

Anxiety (Akhondzadeh, 2001)
Congestive heart failure (CHF) (Von Eiff, 1994)
Hyperthyroidism (pharmacologic activity)
Insomnia (sedative) (Speroni, 1988; Wolfman, 1994)
Opiate withdrawal (Akhondzadeh, 2001)

Local Anesthetic/Vasoconstrictor Precautions No information available to require special precautions

Effects on Bleeding None reported

Warnings/Precautions Based on pharmacologic effects, may cause drowsiness; use caution when driving an automobile or operating heavy machinery. Use with caution in individuals taking antianxiety agents, antidepressants, hypnotics, or sedatives. Reported in animal studies to increase sleeping time induced by hexobarbital (Aoyagi, 1974).

Use with caution in individuals with a history of bleeding, hemostatic disorders, or drug-related hemostatic problems. Use with caution in individuals taking anticoagulant medications, including warfarin, aspirin, aspirin-containing products, NSAIDs, or antiplatelet agents (eg, ticlopidine, clopidogrel, dipyridamole).

References

Akhondzadeh S, Kashani L, Mobaseri M, et al, "Passionflower in the Treatment of Opiates Withdrawal: A Double-Blind Randomized Controlled Trial," *J Clin Pharm Ther*, 2001, 26(5):369-73.

Aoyagi N, Kimura R, and Murata T, "Studies on *Passiflora incarnata* Dry Extract, Isolation of Maltol and Pharmacological Action of Maltol and Ethyl Maltol," *Chem Pharm Bull (Tokyo)*, 1974, 22(5):1008-13.

Natural Standard Research Collaboration, Chief Editors: Ulbricht C, Basch E, *Natural Standard Herb and Supplement Reference - Evidence-Based Clinical Reviews*, USA: Elsevier/Mosby, 2005.

Speroni E and Minghetti A, "Neuropharmacological Activity of Extracts From *Passiflora incarnata*," *Planta Med*, 1988, 54(6):488-91.

Von Eiff M, Brunner H, Haegeli A, et al, "Hawthorn/Passion Flower Extract and Improvement in Physical Exercise Capacity of Patients With Dyspnoea Class II of the NYHA Functional Classifications," *Acta Therapeutica*, 1994, 20:47-66.

Wolfman C, Viola H, Paladini A, et al, "Possible Anxiolytic Effects of Chrysin, a Central Benzodiazepine Receptor Ligand Isolated From *Passiflora coerulea*," *Pharmacol Biochem Behav*, 1994, 47(1):1-4.

Policosanol

Pharmacologic Category Nutraceutical

Reported Use

Coronary heart disease (Stusser, 1998)
Hypercholesterolemia (Alcocer, 1999; Arruzazabala, 2002; Batista, 1996; Canetti, 1995; Castano, 1999; Castano, 2000; Castano, 2001; Castano 2001; Castano, 2002; Castano, 2002; Castano, 2002; Castano, 2003; Castano, 2004; Castano, 2004; Chen, 2005; Crespo, 1999; Francini-Pesenti, 2008; Mas, 1999; Mas, 2004; Mas, 2004; Mirkin, 2001; Pons, 1994; Torres, 1995); contradictory studies (Berthold, 2006; Cubeddu, 2006; Dulin, 2006; Greyling, 2006)
Intermittent claudication (Castano, 1999; Castano, 2001; Illnait, 2008)
Platelet aggregation inhibition (Arruzazabala, 1996; Arruzazabala, 1997; Arruzazabala, 1998; Carbajal, 1998; Valdes, 1996)
Contradictory study (Reiner, 2007)
Reactivity/brain activity (Fontani, 2000)

Local Anesthetic/Vasoconstrictor Precautions No information available to require special precautions

Effects on Bleeding May see increased bleeding due to inhibition of platelet aggregation

Warnings/Precautions Use with caution in individuals with a history of bleeding, hemostatic disorders, or drug-related hemostatic problems; and in individuals taking anticoagulant medications, including antiplatelet agents (eg, clopidogrel, dipyridamole, ticlopidine), aspirin, aspirin-containing products, NSAIDs, or warfarin. Discontinue use prior to dental or surgical procedures (generally at least 14 days before).

Use with caution in individuals taking antidiabetic agents; policosanol may alter glucose levels. Use with caution in individuals using antihypertensive agents.

References

Alcocer L, Fernandez L, Campos E, et al, "A Comparative Study of Policosanol Versus Acipimox in Patients With Type II Hypercholesterolemia," *Int J Tissue React*, 1999, 21(3):85-92.

Arruzazabala ML, Mas R, Molina V, et al, "Effect of Policosanol on Platelet Aggregation in Type II Hypercholesterolemic Patients," *Int J Tissue React*, 1998, 20(4):119-24.

Arruzazabala ML, Molina V, Mas R, et al, "Antiplatelet Effects of Policosanol (20 and 40 mg/day) in Healthy Volunteers and Dyslipidaemic Patients," *Clin Exp Pharmacol Physiol*, 2002, 29(10):891-7.

Arruzazabala ML, Valdes S, Mas R, et al, "Comparative Study of Policosanol, Aspirin and the Combination Therapy Policosanol-Aspirin on Platelet Aggregation in Healthy Volunteers," *Pharmacol Res*, 1997, 36(4):293-7.

Arruzazabala ML, Valdes S, Mas R, et al, "Effect of Policosanol Successive Dose Increases on Platelet Aggregation in Healthy Volunteers," *Pharmacol Res*, 1996, 34(5-6):181-5.

Batista J, Stusser R, Saez F, et al, "Effect of Policosanol on Hyperlipidemia and Coronary Heart Disease in Middle-Aged Patients. A 14-Month Pilot Study," *Int J Clin Pharmacol Ther*, 1996, 34(3):134-7.

Berthold HK, Unverdorben S, Degenhardt R, et al, "Effect of Policosanol on Lipid Levels Among Patients With Hypercholesterolemia or Combined Hyperlipidemia: A Randomized Controlled Trial," *JAMA*, 2006, 295(19):2262-9.

Canetti M, Moreira M, Mas R, et al, "A Two-Year Study on the Efficacy and Tolerability of Policosanol in Patients With Type II Hyperlipoproteinaemia," *Int J Clin Pharmacol Res*, 1995, 15(4):159-65.

Carbajal D, Arruzazabala ML, Valdes S, et al, "Effect of Policosanol on Platelet Aggregation and Serum Levels of Arachidonic Acid Metabolites in Healthy Volunteers," *Prostaglandins Leukot Essent Fatty Acids*, 1998, 58(1):61-4.

Castano G, Fernandez L, Mas R, et al, "Comparison of the Efficacy, Safety and Tolerability of Original Policosanol Versus Other Mixtures of Higher Aliphatic Primary Alcohols in Patients With Type II Hypercholesterolemia," *Int J Clin Pharmacol Res*, 2002, 22(2):55-66.

Castano G, Mas Ferreiro R, Fernandez L, et al, "A Long-Term Study of Policosanol in the Treatment of Intermittent Claudication," *Angiology*, 2001, 52(2):115-25.

Castano G, Mas R, Arruzazabala ML, et al, "Effects of Policosanol and Pravastatin on Lipid Profile, Platelet Aggregation and Endothelemia in Older Hypercholesterolemic Patients," *Int J Clin Pharmacol Res*, 1999, 19(4):105-16.

Castano G, Mas R, Fernandez JC, et al, "Effects of Policosanol in Older Patients With Type II Hypercholesterolemia and High Coronary Risk," *J Gerontol A Biol Sci Med Sci*, 2001, 56(3):M186-92.

Castano G, Mas R, Fernandez JC, et al, "Effects of Policosanol on Older Patients With Hypertension and Type II Hypercholesterolaemia," *Drugs R D*, 2002, 3(3):159-72.

Castano G, Mas R, Fernandez L, et al, "Comparison of the Efficacy and Tolerability of Policosanol With Atorvastatin in Elderly Patients With Type II Hypercholesterolaemia," *Drugs Aging*, 2003, 20(2):153-63.

Castano G, Mas R, Fernandez L, et al, "Effects of Policosanol 20 Versus 40 mg/day in the Treatment of Patients With Type II Hypercholesterolemia: A 6-Month Double-Blind Study," *Int J Clin Pharmacol Res*, 2001, 21(1):43-57.

Castano G, Mas R, Fernandez L, et al, "Effects of Policosanol on Postmenopausal Women With Type II Hypercholesterolemia," *Gynecol Endocrinol*, 2000, 14(3):187-95.

Castano G, Mas R, Fernandez L, et al, "Effects of Policosanol 20 Versus 40 mg/day in the Treatment of Patients With Type II Hypercholesterolemia: A 6-Month Double-Blind Study," *Int J Clin Pharmacol Res* , 2001, 21(1):43-57.

Castano G, Mas R, Gamez R, et al, "Concomitant Use of Policosanol and Beta-Blockers in Older Patients," *Int J Clin Pharmacol Res*, 2004, 24(2-3):65-77.

Castano G, Mas R, Gamez R, et al, "Effects of Policosanol and Ticlopidine in Patients With Intermittent Claudication: A Double-Blinded Pilot Comparative Study," *Angiology*, 2004, 55(4):361-71.

Castano G, Mas R, Roca J, et al, "A Double-Blind, Placebo-Controlled Study of the Effects of Policosanol in Patients With Intermittent Claudication," *Angiology*, 1999, 50(2):123-30.

Castano G, Menendez R, Mas R, et al, "Effects of Policosanol and Lovastatin on Lipid Profile and Lipid Peroxidation in Patients With Dyslipidemia Associated With Type 2 Diabetes Mellitus," *Int J Clin Pharmacol Res*, 2002, 22(3-4):89-99.

Chen JT, Wesley R, Shamburek RD, et al, "Meta-Analysis of Natural Therapies for Hyperlipidemia: Plant Sterols and Stanols Versus Policosanol," *Pharmacotherapy*, 2005, 25(2):171-83.

Crespo N, Illnait J, Mas R, et al, "Comparative Study of the Efficacy and Tolerability of Policosanol and Lovastatin in Patients With Hypercholesterolemia and Noninsulin Dependent Diabetes Mellitus," *Int J Clin Pharmacol Res*, 1999, 19(4):117-27.

Cubeddu LX, Cubeddu RJ, Heimowitz T, et al, "Comparative Lipid-Lowering Effects of Policosanol and Atorvastatin: A Randomized, Parallel, Double-Blind, Placebo-Controlled Trial," *Am Heart J*, 2006, 152 (5):982.e1-5.

Dulin MF, Hatcher LF, Sasser HC, et al, "Policosanol Is Ineffective in the Treatment of Hypercholesterolemia: A Randomized Controlled Trial," *Am J Clin Nutr*, 2006, 84(6):1543-8.

Fontani G, Maffei D, and Lodi L, "Policosanol, Reaction Time and Event-Related Potentials," *Neuropsychobiology*, 2000, 41(3):158-65.

Francini-Pesenti F, Brocadello F, Beltramolli D, et al, "Sugar Cane Policosanol Failed to Lower Plasma Cholesterol in Primitive, Diet-Resistant Hypercholesterolaemia: A Double Blind, Controlled Study," *Complement Ther Med*, 2008, 16(2):61-5.

Greyling A, De Witt C, Oosthuizen W, et al, "Effects of a Policosanol Supplement on Serum Lipid Concentrations in Hypercholesterolaemic and Heterozygous Familial Hypercholesterolaemic Subjects," *Br J Nutr*, 2006, 95(5):968-75.

Illnait J, Castaño G, Alvarez E, et al, "Effects of Policosanol (10 mg/d) Versus Aspirin (100 mg/d) in Patients With Intermittent Claudication: A 10-Week, Randomized, Comparative Study," *Angiology*, 2008, 59(3):269-77.

Mas R, Castano G, Fernandez J, et al, "Long-Term Effects of Policosanol on Obese Patients With Type II Hypercholesterolemia," *Asia Pac J Clin Nutr*, 2004, 13(Suppl):S102.

Mas R, Castano G, Fernandez J, et al, "Long-Term Effects of Policosanol on Older Patients With Type 2 Diabetes," *Asia Pac J Clin Nutr*, 2004, 13(Suppl):S101.

Mas R, Castano G, Illnait J, et al, "Effects of Policosanol in Patients With Type II Hypercholesterolemia and Additional Coronary Risk Factors," *Clin Pharmacol Ther*, 1999, 65(4):439-47.

Mirkin A, Mas R, Martinto M, et al, "Efficacy and Tolerability of Policosanol in Hypercholesterolemic Postmenopausal Women," *Int J Clin Pharmacol Res*, 2001, 21(1):31-41.

Natural Standard Research Collaboration, Chief Editors: Ulbricht C, Basch E, *Natural Standard Herb and Supplement Reference - Evidence-Based Clinical Reviews*, USA: Elsevier/Mosby, 2005.

Pons P, Rodriguez M, Robaina C, et al, "Effects of Successive Dose Increases of Policosanol on the Lipid Profile of Patients With Type II Hypercholesterolaemia and Tolerability to Treatment," *Int J Clin Pharmacol Res*, 1994, 14(1):27-33.

Reiner Z and Tedeschi-Reiner E, "Rice Policosanol Does Not Have Any Effects on Blood Coagulation Factors in Hypercholesterolemic Patients," *Coll Antropol*, 2007, 31(4):1061-4.

Stusser R, Batista J, Padron R, et al, "Long-Term Therapy With Policosanol Improves Treadmill Exercise-ECG Testing Performance of Coronary Heart Disease Patients," *Int J Clin Pharmacol Ther*, 1998, 36 (9):469-73.
Torres O, Agramonte AJ, Illnait J, et al, "Treatment of Hypercholesterolemia in NIDDM With Policosanol," *Diabetes Care*, 1995, 18(3):393-7.
Valdes S, Arruzazabala ML, Fernandez L, et al, "Effect of Policosanol on Platelet Aggregation in Healthy Volunteers," *Int J Clin Pharmacol Res*, 1996, 16(2-3):67-72.

Pycnogenol

Pharmacologic Category Nutraceutical

Reported Use

Aging (Ryan, 2008)
Asthma (Hosseini, 2001; Lau, 2004)
Attention-deficit hyperactivity disorder (ADHD) (Trebaticka, 2006)
Chronic venous insufficiency (Arcangeli, 2000; Cesarone, 2006; Petrassi, 2000)
Climacteric syndrome (Yang, 2007)
Diabetes, type 2 (Liu, 2004)
Diabetic microangiopathy (Cesarone, 2006)
Erectile dysfunction (Durackova, 2003)
Gingival bleeding/plaque (Kimbrough, 2002)
Hypertension (Hosseini, 2001; Liu, 2004)
Osteoarthritis (Belcaro, 2008; Cisár, 2008)
Platelet aggregation (smokers) (Araghi-Niknam, 2000)
Prevention of blood clots during long airplane flights (Belcaro, 2004; Cesarone, 2005)
Retinopathy (Spadea, 2001)
Systemic lupus erythematosus (SLE) (Stefanescu, 2001)
Venous leg ulcers (Belcaro, 2005; Belcaro, 2006)

Local Anesthetic/Vasoconstrictor Precautions No information available to require special precautions

Effects on Bleeding May see increased bleeding due to inhibition of platelet aggregation

Warnings/Precautions Use with caution in individuals with diabetes or hypoglycemia; poor theoretical potential for blood glucose lowering. Use with caution in individuals using hypolipidemics; may significantly decrease serum cholesterol and LDL. Use with caution in individuals with a history of bleeding, hemostatic disorders, or drug-related hemostatic problems. Use with caution in individuals taking anticoagulant medications, including warfarin, aspirin, aspirin-containing products, NSAIDs, or antiplatelet agents (eg, ticlopidine, clopidogrel, dipyridamole). Discontinue use prior to dental or surgical procedures (generally at least 14 days before). Use with caution in individuals taking hypertensive medications; potential for additive hypotensive effects. Use with caution in individuals using immune-stimulating or -inhibiting drugs; potential for immune modulating effects.

References

Araghi-Niknam M, Hosseini S, Larson D, et al, "Pine Bark Extract Reduces Platelet Aggregation," *Integr Med*, 2000, 2(2):73-77.
Arcangeli P, "Pycnogenol in Chronic Venous Insufficiency," *Fitoterapia*, 2000, 71(3):236-44.
Belcaro G, Cesarone MR, Errichi BM, et al, "Diabetic Ulcers: Microcirculatory Improvement and Faster Healing With Pycnogenol," *Clin Appl Thromb Hemost*, 2006, 12(3):318-23.
Belcaro G, Cesarone MR, Errichi BM, et al, "Venous Ulcers: Microcirculatory Improvement and Faster Healing With Local Use of Pycnogenol," *Angiology*, 2005, 56(6):699-705.
Belcaro G, Cesarone MR, Errichi S, et al, "Treatment of Osteoarthritis With Pycnogenol. The SVOS (San Valentino Osteo-Arthrosis Study). Evaluation of Signs, Symptoms, Physical Performance and Vascular Aspects," *Phytother Res*, 2008, 22(4):518-23.
Belcaro G, Cesarone MR, Rohdewald P, et al, "Prevention of Venous Thrombosis and Thrombophlebitis in Long-Haul Flights With Pycnogenol," *Clin Appl Thromb Hemost*, 2004, 10(4):373-7.
Cesarone MR, Belcaro G, Rohdewald P, et al, "Improvement of Diabetic Microangiopathy With Pycnogenol: A Prospective, Controlled Study," *Angiology*, 2006, 57(4):431-6.
Cesarone MR, Belcaro G, Rohdewald P, et al, "Prevention of Edema in Long Flights With Pycnogenol," *Clin Appl Thromb Hemost*, 2005, 11(3):289-94.
Cesarone MR, Belcaro G, Rohdewald P, et al, "Rapid Relief of Signs/Symptoms in Chronic Venous Microangiopathy With Pycnogenol: A Prospective, Controlled Study," *Angiology*, 2006, 57(5):569-76.
Cisár P, Jány R, Waczulíková I, et al, "Effect of Pine Bark Extract (Pycnogenol) on Symptoms of Knee Osteoarthritis," *Phytother Res*, 2008, 22(8):1087-92.
Durackova Z, Trebaticky B, Novotny V, et al, "Lipid Metabolism and Erectile Dysfunction Improvement by Pycnogenol® Extract From the Bark of *Pinus pinaster* in Patients Suffering From Erectile Dysfunction - A Pilot Study," *Nutr Res*, 2003, 23:1189-98.
Hosseini S, Lee J, Sepulveda RT, et al, "A Randomized, Double Blind, Placebo Controlled Prospective 16 Week Crossover Study to Determine the Role of Pycnogenol® in Modifying Blood Pressure in Mildly Hypertensive Patients," *Nutr Res*, 2001, 21(9):67-76.
Hosseini S, Pishnamazi S, Sadrzadeh SM, et al, "Pycnogenol (R) in the Management of Asthma," *J Med Food*, 2001, 4(4):201-9.
Kimbrough C, Chun M, dela Roca G, et al, "PYCNOGENOL Chewing Gum Minimizes Gingival Bleeding and Plaque Formation," *Phytomedicine*, 2002, 9(5):410-3.
Lau BH, Riesen SK, Truong KP, et al, "Pycnogenol as an Adjunct in the Management of Childhood Asthma," *J Asthma*, 2004, 41(8):825-32.
Liu X, Wei J, Tan F, et al, "Antidiabetic Effect of Pycnogenol French Maritime Pine Bark Extract in Patients With Diabetes Type II," *Life Sci*, 2004, 75(21):2505-13.
Liu X, Wei J, Tan F, et al, "Pycnogenol, French Maritime Pine Bark Extract, Improves Endothelial Function of Hypertensive Patients," *Life Sci*, 2004, 74(7):855-62.
Natural Standard Research Collaboration, Chief Editors: Ulbricht C, Basch E, *Natural Standard Herb and Supplement Reference - Evidence-Based Clinical Reviews*, USA: Elsevier/Mosby, 2005.
Petrassi C, Mastromarino A, and Spartera C, "PYCNOGENOL in Chronic Cenous Insufficiency," *Phytomedicine*, 2000, 7(5):383-8.

Ryan J, Croft K, Mori T, et al, "An Examination of the Effects of the Antioxidant Pycnogenol on Cognitive Performance, Serum Lipid Profile, Endocrinological and Oxidative Stress Biomarkers in an Elderly Population," *J Psychopharmacol*, 2008, 22(5):553-62.
Spadea L and Balestrazzi E, "Treatment of Vascular Retinopathies With Pycnogenol," *Phytother Res*, 2001, 15(3):219-23.
Stefanescu M, Matache C, Onu A, et al, "Pycnogenol Efficacy in the Treatment of Systemic Lupus Erythematosus Patients," *Phytother Res*, 2001, 15(8):698-704.
Trebaticka J, Kopasova S, Hradecna Z, et al, "Treatment of ADHD With French Maritime Pine Bark Extract, Pycnogenol," *Eur Child Adolesc Psychiatry*, 2006, 15(6):329-35.
Yang HM, Liao MF, Zhu SY, et al, "A Randomised, Double-Blind, Placebo-Controlled Trial on the Effect of Pycnogenol on the Climacteric Syndrome in Peri-Menopausal Women," *Acta Obstet Gynecol Scand*, 2007, 86(8):978-85.

Quercetin

Pharmacologic Category Nutraceutical

Reported Use

Allergies (Bronner, 1985)
Asthma (pharmacologic activity)
Atherosclerosis (Negre-Salvayre, 1992)
Cancer, prevention (lung, ovarian, pancreatic) (Bobe, 2008; Gates, 2007; Nöthlings, 2007)
Cardiovascular disease (Conquer, 1998)
Cataracts (Beyer-Mears, 1979)
Hypertension (Edwards, 2007)
Immune function (Nieman, 2007; Nieman, 2007)
Kidney transplant (Shoskes, 2005)
Peptic ulcer disease (Alarcon de la Lastra, 1994)
Prostatitis (Shoskes, 1999)
Sinusitis (pharmacologic activity)

Local Anesthetic/Vasoconstrictor Precautions No information available to require special precautions

Effects on Bleeding None reported

Warnings/Precautions Use with caution in individuals with a history of bleeding, hemostatic disorders, or drug-related hemostatic problems. Use with caution in individuals taking anticoagulant medications, including warfarin, aspirin, aspirin-containing products, NSAIDs, or antiplatelet agents (eg, ticlopidine, clopidogrel, dipyridamole). Discontinue use prior to dental or surgical procedures (generally at least 14 days before).

References

Alarcon de la Lastra C, Martin MJ, and Motilva V, "Antiulcer and Gastroprotective Effects of Quercetin: A Gross and Histologic Study," *Pharmacology*, 1994, 48(1):56-62.
Beyer-Mears A and Farnsworth PN, "Diminished Sugar Cataractogenesis by Quercetin," *Exp Eye Res*, 1979, 28(6):709-16.
Bronner C and Landry Y, "Kinetics of the Inhibitory Effect of Flavonoids on Histamine Secretion From Mast Cells," *Agents Actions*, 1985, 16(3-4):147-51.
Castillo MH, Perkins E, Campbell JH, et al, "The Effects of the Bioflavonoid Quercetin on Squamous Cell Carcinoma of Head and Neck Origin," *Am J Surg*, 1989, 158(4):351-5.
Conquer JA, Maiani G, Azzini E, et al, "Supplementation With Quercetin Markedly Increases Plasma Quercetin Concentration Without Effect on Selected Risk Factors for Heart Disease in Healthy Subjects," *J Nutr*, 1998, 128(3):593-7.
ElAttar TM and Virji AS, "Modulating Effect of Resveratrol and Quercetin on Oral Cancer Cell Growth and Proliferation," *Anticancer Drugs*, 1999, 10(2):187-93.
Ferry DR, Smith A, Malkhandi J, et al, "Phase I Clinical Trial of the Flavonoid Quercetin: Pharmacokinetics and Evidence for *in vivo* Tyrosine Kinase Inhibition," *Clin Cancer Res*, 1996, 2(4):659-68.
Hayashi A, Gillen AC, and Lott JR, "Effects of Daily Oral Administration of Quercetin Chalcone and Modified Citrus Pectin on Implanted Colon-25 Tumor Growth in Balb-c Mice," *Altern Med Rev*, 2000, 5 (6):546-52.
Hoffman R, Graham L, and Newlands ES, "Enhanced Anti-Proliferative Action of Busulphan by Quercetin on the Human Leukaemia Cell Line K562," *Br J Cancer*, 1989, 59(3):347-8.
Makita H, Tanaka T, Fujitsuka H, et al, "Chemoprevention of 4-Nitroquinoline 1-Oxide-Induced Rat Oral Carcinogenesis by the Dietary Flavonoids Chalcone, 2-Hydroxychalcone, and Quercetin," *Cancer Res*, 1996, 56(21):4904-9.
Morrow DM, Fitzsimmons PE, Chopra M, et al, "Dietary Supplementation With the Anti-Tumour Promoter Quercetin: Its Effects on Matrix Metalloproteinase Gene Regulation," *Mutat Res*, 2001, 480-481:269-76.
Natural Standard Research Collaboration, Chief Editors: Ulbricht C, Basch E, *Natural Standard Herb and Supplement Reference - Evidence-Based Clinical Reviews*, USA: Elsevier/Mosby, 2005.
Negre-Salvayre A and Salvayre R, "Quercetin Prevents the Cytotoxicity of Oxidized LDL on Lymphoid Cell Lines," *Free Radic Biol Med*, 1992, 12(2):101-6.
Nieman DC, Henson DA, Davis JM, et al, "Quercetin's Influence on Exercise-Induced Changes in Plasma Cytokines and Muscle and Leukocyte Cytokine mRNA," *J Appl Physiol*, 2007, 103(5):1728-35.
Nieman DC, Henson DA, Gross SJ, et al, "Quercetin Reduces Illness But Not Immune Perturbations After Intensive Exercise," *Med Sci Sports Exerc*, 2007, 39(9):1561-9.
Nöthlings U, Murphy SP, Wilkens LR, et al, "Flavonols and Pancreatic Cancer Risk: The Multiethnic Cohort Study," *Am J Epidemiol*, 2007, 166(8):924-31.
Shoskes DA, Zeitlin SI, Shahed A, et al, "Quercetin in Men With Category III Chronic Prostatitis: A Preliminary Prospective, Double-Blind, Placebo-Controlled Trial," *Urology*, 1999, 54(6):960-3.
Yoshida M, Sakai T, Hosokawa N, et al, "The Effect of Quercetin on Cell Cycle Progression and Growth of Human Gastric Cancer Cells," *FEBS Lett*, 1990, 260(1):10-3.

Red Yeast Rice

Pharmacologic Category Herb

Reported Use

Coronary heart disease (Wang, 2004; Zhao, 2004; Zhao, 2007)
Diabetes (Fang, 2000)

Hypercholesterolemia (Endo, 1986; Heber, 1999; Keithley, 2002; Lin, 2005; Thompson Coon, 2003)

Local Anesthetic/Vasoconstrictor Precautions No information available to require special precautions

Effects on Bleeding None reported

Warnings/Precautions Based on pharmacologic activity, use is contraindicated in pregnancy or lactation (or if trying to become pregnant). In addition, the use of red yeast rice is contraindicated in individuals with known hypersensitivity to rice or yeast. Use with caution in individuals currently receiving other cholesterol-lowering medications. Keep out of reach of children; do not use if <20 years of age. Adverse effects include gastrointestinal upset.

HMG-CoA reductase inhibitors have been associated with rare (less than 1% to 2% incidence) but serious adverse effects, including hepatic and skeletal muscle disorders (myopathy, rhabdomyolysis). The risk of these disorders may be increased by concomitant therapy with specific medications. These effects have not been specifically reported for red yeast rice. Do not use in individuals with hepatic disease, a history of liver disease, or in those who may be at risk of liver disease; in individuals with serious infection, recent major surgery, other serious disease, or organ transplant individuals; and in any individual who consumes more than 1-2 alcohol-containing drinks per day. Discontinue use at the first sign of hepatic dysfunction or muscle problems.

References

Endo A, Komagata D, and Shimada H, "Monacolin M, a New Inhibitor of Cholesterol Biosynthesis," *J Antibiot (Tokyo)*, 1986, 39(12):1670-3.

Fang Y and Li W, "Effect of Xuezhikang on Lipid Metabolism and Islet 3 Cell Function in Type II Diabetic Patients," *Journal of Capital Medicine*, 2000, 7(2):44-5.

Gordon RY, Cooperman T, Obermeyer W, et al, "Marked Variability of Monacolin Levels in Commercial Red Yeast Rice Products: Buyer Beware!" *Arch Intern Med*, 2010, 170(19):1722-7.

Heber D, Yip I, Ashley JM, et al, "Cholesterol-Lowering Effects of a Proprietary Chinese Red-Yeast-Rice Dietary Supplement," *Am J Clin Nutr*, 1999, 69(2):231-6.

Keithley JK, Swanson B, Sha BE, et al, "A Pilot Study of the Safety and Efficacy of Cholestin in Treating HIV-Related Dyslipidemia," *Nutrition*, 2002, 18(2):201-4.

Lin CC, Li TC, and Lai MM, "Efficacy and Safety of *Monascus purpureus* Went Rice in Subjects With Hyperlipidemia," *Eur J Endocrinol*, 2005, 153(5):679-86.

Natural Standard Research Collaboration, Chief Editors: Ulbricht C, Basch E, *Natural Standard Herb and Supplement Reference - Evidence-Based Clinical Reviews*, USA: Elsevier/Mosby, 2005.

Thompson Coon JS and Ernst E, "Herbs for Serum Cholesterol Reduction: A Systematic View," *J Fam Pract*, 2003, 52(6):468-78.

Wang WH, Zhang H, Yu YL, et al, "Intervention of Xuezhikang on Patients of Acute Coronary Syndrome With Different Levels of Blood Lipids," *Zhongguo Zhong Xi Yi Jie He Za Zhi*, 2004, 24(12):1073-6.

Zhao SP, Liu L, Cheng YC, et al, "Xuezhikang, An Extract of Cholestin, Protects Endothelial Function Through Antiinflammatory and Lipid-Lowering Mechanisms in Patients With Coronary Heart Disease," *Circulation*, 2004, 24;110(8):915-20.

Zhao SP, Lu ZL, Du BM, et al, "Xuezhikang, an Extract of Cholestin, Reduces Cardiovascular Events in Type 2 Diabetes Patients With Coronary Heart Disease: Subgroup Analysis of Patients With Type 2 Diabetes From China Coronary Secondary Prevention Study (CCSPS)," *J Cardiovasc Pharmacol*, 2007, 49(2):81-4.

SAMe

Pharmacologic Category Nutritional Supplement

Reported Use

AIDS-related myelopathy (Castagna, 1995; Tan, 1998)

Attention-deficit/hyperactivity disorder (ADHD) (Shekim, 1990)

Cardiovascular disease (Loehrer, 1996)

Cholestasis (Anonymous, 2002; Manzillo, 1992; Qin, 2000); pregnancy (Anonymous, 2002; Frezza, 1984; Frezza, 1987; Frezza, 1990; Lafuenti, 1988; Nicastri, 1998; Ribalta, 1991)

Depression (Anonymous, 2002; Bressa, 1994; Fava, 1995; Kagan, 1990; Rosenbaum, 1990)

Fibromyalgia (Jacobsen, 1991; Volkmann, 1997)

Headache (pharmacologic activity)

Insomnia (Sitaram, 1995)

Liver disease (Anonymous, 2002; Mato, 1999; Miglio, 1975)

Osteoarthritis (Anonymous, 2002; di Padova, 1987; Soeken, 2002)

Rheumatoid arthritis (Polli, 1975)

Local Anesthetic/Vasoconstrictor Precautions No information available to require special precautions

Effects on Bleeding None reported

Warnings/Precautions Minor side effects, including dry mouth, nausea, and restlessness, are occasionally reported. Use caution when combining SAMe with other antidepressants, tryptophan, or 5-HTP. SAMe is not effective for the depressive symptoms associated with bipolar disorder.

SAMe has been reported to block platelet aggregation *in vitro* (De la Cruz, 1997; De la Cruz, 1997); contraindicated in individuals with active bleeding (eg, peptic ulcer, intracranial bleeding). Use with caution in individuals with a history of bleeding, hemostatic disorders, or drug-related hemostatic problems and in individuals taking anticoagulant medications, including warfarin, aspirin, aspirin-containing products, NSAIDs, or antiplatelet agents (eg, ticlopidine, clopidogrel, dipyridamole). Discontinue use prior to dental or surgical procedures (generally at least 14 days before).

References

American Psychiatric Association, "Practice Guideline for the Treatment of Patients with Major Depressive Disorder," May 2010. Available at: http://www.psychiatryonline.com/pracGuide/pracGuideTopic_7.aspx.

Anonymous, "S-Adenosyl-L-Methionine for Treatment of Depression, Osteoarthritis, and Liver Disease," Evidence Report/Technology Assessment, Number 64, 2002.

Binder T, Salaj P, Zima T, et al, "Randomized Prospective Comparative Study of Ursodeoxycholic Acid and S-Adenosyl-L-Methionine in the Treatment of Intrahepatic Cholestasis of Pregnancy," *J Perinat Med*, 2006, 34(5):383-91.

Bressa GM, "S-Adenosyl-L-Methionine (SAMe) as Antidepressant: Meta-Analysis of Clinical Studies," *Acta Neurol Scand*, Suppl 1994, 154:7-14.

Castagna A, Le Grazie C, Accordini A, et al, "Cerebrospinal Fluid S-Adenosylmethionine (SAMe) and Glutathione Concentrations in HIV Infection: Effect of Parenteral Treatment With SAMe," *Neurology*, 1995, 45(9):1678-83.

De la Cruz JP, Gonzalez-Correa JA, Martin-Aurioles E, et al, "Effects of S-Adenosyl-L-Methionine on Platelet Thromboxane and Vascular Prostacyclin," *Biochem Pharmacol*, 1997, 53(11):1761-3.

De la Cruz JP, Merida M, Gonzalez-Correa JA, et al, "Effects of S-Adenosyl-L-Methionine on Blood Platelet Activation," *Gen Pharmacol*, 1997, 29(4):651-5.

di Padova C, "S-Adenosylmethionine in the Treatment of Osteoarthritis. Review of the Clinical Studies," *Am J Med*, 1987, 83(5A):60-5.

Fava M, Giannelli A, Rapisarda V, et al, "Rapidity of Onset of the Antidepressant Effect of Parenteral S-Adenosyl-L-Methionine," *Psychiatry Res*, 1995, 56(3):295-7.

Frezza M, Centini G, Cammareri G, et al, "S-Adenosylmethionine for the Treatment of Intrahepatic Cholestasis of Pregnancy. Results of a Controlled Clinical Trial," *Hepatogastroenterology*, 1990, 37(2 Suppl):122-5.

Frezza M, Di Padova C, and Italian Study Group for SAMe, "Multicenter Placebo Controlled Clinical Trial of Intravenous and Oral S-Adenosyl-L-Methionine (SAMe) in Cholestatic Patients With Liver Disease," *Hepatology*, 1987, 7(5):1105.

Frezza M, Pozzato G, Chiesa L, el al, "Reversal of Intrahepatic Cholestasis of Pregnancy in Women After High Dose S-Adenosyl-L-Methionine Administration," *Hepatology*, 1984, 4(2):274-8.

Jacobsen S, Danneskiold-Samsoe B, and Anderson BB, "Oral S-Adenosylmethionine in Primary Fibromyalgia. Double-Blind Clinical Evaluation," *Scand J Rheumatol*, 1991, 20(4):294-302.

Kagan BL, Sultzer DL, Rosenlicht, et al, "Oral S-Adenosylmethionine in Depression: A Randomized, Double-Blind, Placebo-Controlled Trial," *Am J Psychiatry*, 1990, 147(5):591-5.

Lafuenti G, Plotti G, Nicolanti G, et al, "Evaluation of the Obstetrical Risk in Pregnant Women With Intrahepatic Cholestasis Treated With S-Adenosyl-L-Methionine," *Recenti Prog Med*, 1988, 79 (10):420-3.

Loehrer FM, Angst CP, Haefeli WE, et al, "Low Whole-Blood S-Adenosylmethionine and Correlation Between 5-Methyltetrahydrofolate and Homocysteine in Coronary Artery Disease," *Arterioscler Thromb Vasc Biol*, 1996, 16(6):727-33.

Manzillo G, Piccinino F, Surrenti C, et al, "Multicentre Double-Blind Placebo-Controlled Study of Intravenous and Oral S-Adenosyl-L-Methionine (SAMe) in Cholestatic Patients With Liver Disease," *Drug Invest*, 1992, 4(Suppl 4)90-100.

Mato JM, Cámara J, Fernández de Paz J, et al, "S-Adenosylmethionine in Alcoholic Liver Cirrhosis: A Randomized, Placebo-Controlled, Double-Blind, Multicenter Clinical Trial," *J Hepatol*, 1999, 30 (6):1081-9.

Miglio F, Stefanini GF, Corazza GR, et al, "Double-Blind Studies of the Therapeutic Action of S-Adenosylmethionine (SAMe) in Oral Administration, in Liver Cirrhosis and Other Chronic Hepatitides," *Minerva Med*, 1975, 66(33):1595-9.

Natural Standard Research Collaboration, Chief Editors: Ulbricht C, Basch E, *Natural Standard Herb and Supplement Reference - Evidence-Based Clinical Reviews*, USA: Elsevier/Mosby, 2005.

Nicastri PL, Diaferia A, Tartagni M, et al, "A Randomised Placebo-Controlled Trial of Ursodeoxycholic Acid and S-Adenosylmethionine in the Treatment of Intrahepatic Cholestasis of Pregnancy," *Br J Obstet Gynaecol*, 1998, 105(11):1205-7.

Polli E, Cortellareo M, Parrini L, et al, "Pharmacological and Clinical Aspects of S-Adenosylmethionine (SAMe) in Primary Degenerative Arthropathy," *Minerva Med*, 1975, 66(83):4443-59.

Qin B, Guo S, Zhao Y, et al, "A Trial of Ademetionine in the Treatment of Intrahepatic Biliary Stasis Viral Hepatitis," *Zhonghua Gan Zang Bing Za Zhi*, 2000, 8(3):158-60.

Ribalta J, Reyes H, Gonzalez MC, et al, "S-Adenosyl-L-Methionine in the Treatment of Patients With Intrahepatic Cholestasis of Pregnancy: A Randomized, Double-Blind, Placebo-Controlled Study With Negative Results," *Hepatology*, 1991, 13(6):1084-9.

Rosenbaum JF, Fava M, Falk WE, et al, "The Antidepressant Potential of Oral S-Adenosyl-L-Methionine," *Acta Psychiatr Scand*, 1990, 81(5):432-6.

Shekim WO, Antun F, Hanna GL, et al, "S-Adenosyl-L-Methionine (SAM) in Adults With ADHD, RS: Preliminary Results From an Open Trial," *Psychopharmacol Bull*, 1990, 26(2):249-53.

Sitaram BR, Sitaram M, Traut M, et al, "Nyctohemeral Rhythm in the Levels of S-Adenosylmethionine in the Rat Pineal Gland and Its Relationship to Melatonin Biosynthesis," *J Neurochem*, 1995, 65 (4):1887-94.

Soeken KL, Lee WL, Bausell RB, et al, "Safety and Efficacy of S-Adenosylmethionine (SAMe) for Osteoarthritis," *J Fam Pract*, 2002, 51(5):425-30.

Tan SV and Guiloff RJ, "Hypothesis on the Pathogenesis of Vacuolar Myelopathy, Dementia, and Peripheral Neuropathy in AIDS," *J Neurol Neurosurg Psychiatry*, 1998, 65(1):23-8.

Volkmann H, Nørregaard J, Jacobsen S, et al, "Double-Blind, Placebo-Controlled Cross-Over Study of Intravenous S-Adenosyl-L-Methionine in Patients With Fibromyalgia," *Scand J Rheumatol*, 1997, 26 (3):206-11.

Saw Palmetto

Pharmacologic Category Herb

Reported Use

Androgenetic alopecia (topical) (Morganti, 1998)

Benign prostatic hyperplasia (BPH) (Boyle, 2000; Braeckman, 1994; Plosker, 1996; Reece Smith, 1986; Strauch, 1994; Wilt, 1998; Wilt, 2000)

Contradictory study (Bent, 2006)

Prostatitis (Aliaev, 2006)

Contradictory study (Kaplan, 2004)

Local Anesthetic/Vasoconstrictor Precautions No information available to require special precautions

Effects on Bleeding None reported

Warnings/Precautions Adverse effects reported with the use of saw palmetto include mild gastrointestinal complaints such as diarrhea, vomiting, nausea, and constipation; headache; mild sexual dysfunction; and pruritus.

Use with caution in individuals with hormone-sensitive conditions or in those taking hormonal agents. Based on its pharmacologic activity, use with caution in individuals receiving treatments for BPH (alpha-adrenergic blocking agents, finasteride) (Goepel, 1999). Individuals should have a prostatic exam and laboratory studies (PSA) to rule out cancer and other conditions prior to use for symptoms of BPH. Based on the proposed anti-androgenic mechanism of action of saw palmetto, therapy may decrease the effectiveness of therapeutic androgens.

Use with caution in individuals with a history of bleeding, hemostatic disorders, or drug-related hemostatic problems. Use with caution in individuals taking anticoagulant medications, including warfarin, aspirin, aspirin-containing products, NSAIDs, or antiplatelet agents (eg, ticlopidine, clopidogrel, dipyridamole). Discontinue use prior to dental or surgical procedures (generally at least 14 days before). Use with caution in individuals taking antihypertensive medications.

References

Bent S, Kane C, Shinohara K, et al, "Saw Palmetto for Benign Prostatic Hyperplasia," *N Engl J Med*, 2006, 354(6):557-66.

Boyle P, Robertson C, Lowe F, et al, "Meta-Analysis of Clinical Trials of Permixon in the Treatment of Symptomatic Benign Prostatic Hyperplasia," *Urology*, 2000, 55(4):533-9.

Braeckman J, "The Extract of *Serenoa repens* in the Treatment of Benign Prostatic Hyperplasia: A Multicenter Open Study," *Curr Ther Res*, 1994, 55(7):76-84.

Gerber GS, Zagaja GP, Bales GT, et al, "Saw Palmetto (*Serenoa repens*) in Men in Lower Urinary Tract Symptoms: Effects on Urodynamics Parameters and Voiding Symptoms," *Urology*, 1998, 51(6):1003-7.

Goepel M, Hecker U, Krege S, et al, "Saw Palmetto Extracts Potently and Non-Competitively Inhibit Human Alpha 1-Adrenoceptors *In Vitro*," *Prostate*, 1999, 38(3):208-15.

Kaplan SA, Volpe MA, and Te AE, "A Prospective, 1-Year Trial Using Saw Palmetto Versus Finasteride in the Treatment of Category III Prostatitis/Chronic Pelvic Pain Syndrome," *J Urol*, 2004, 171(1):284-8.

Morganti P, Fabrizi G, James B, et al, "Effect of Gelatin-Cystine and *Serenoa repens* Extract on Free Radicals Level and Hair Growth," *J Appl Cosmetol*, 1998, 16:57-64.

Natural Standard Research Collaboration, Chief Editors: Ulbricht C, Basch E, *Natural Standard Herb and Supplement Reference - Evidence-Based Clinical Reviews*, USA: Elsevier/Mosby, 2005.

Plosker GL and Brogden RN, "*Serenoa repens* (Permixon). A Review of Its Pharmacology and Therapeutic Efficacy in Benign Prostatic Hyperplasia," *Drugs Aging*, 1996, 9(5):379-95.

Reece Smith H, Memon A, Smart CJ, et al, "The Value of Permixon in Benign Prostatic Hypertrophy," *Br J Urol*, 1986, 58(1):36-40.

Strauch G, Perles P, Vergult G, et al, "Comparison of Finasteride (Proscar) and *Serenoa repens* (Permixon) in the Inhibition of 5-Alpha Reductase in Healthy Male Volunteers," *Eur Urol*, 1994, 26 (3):247-52.

Wilt TJ, Ishani A, Stark G, et al, "Saw Palmetto Extracts for Treatment of Benign Prostatic Hyperplasia: A Systematic Review," *JAMA*, 1998, 280(18):1604-9.

Wilt T, Ishani A, Stark G, et al, "Serenoa Repens for Benign Prostatic Hyperplasia," *Cochrane Database Syst Rev*, 2000, (2):CD001423.

Schisandra

Pharmacologic Category Herb

Reported Use

Adaptogen/tonic (to promote wellness); hepatic protection and detoxification (Liu, 1989; Yamada, 1993)

Chemotherapy and radiation (adjunct) (Lin, 1991)

Endurance, stamina, and work performance (enhancement); decreases fatigue (Suekawa, 1987; Volicer, 1965)

Local Anesthetic/Vasoconstrictor Precautions No information available to require special precautions

Effects on Bleeding None reported

Warnings/Precautions Contraindicated in pregnancy due to uterine stimulation in animal studies (Liu, 1989). Theoretically, enzyme enhancement may alter metabolism of many drugs; caution with drugs which may have a narrow therapeutic window. Use with caution in individuals on calcium channel blockers (Suekawa, 1987).

References

Lin TJ, "Antioxidation Mechanism of Schizandrin and Tanshinonatic Acid A and Their Effects on the Protection of Cardiotoxic Action of Adriamycin," *Sheng Li Ko Hsueh Chin Chan*, 1991, 22(4):342-5.

Liu GT, "Pharmacological Actions and Clinical Use of *Fructus schizandrae*," *Chin Med J (Engl)*, 1989, 102 (10):740-9.

Natural Standard Research Collaboration, Chief Editors: Ulbricht C, Basch E, *Natural Standard Herb and Supplement Reference - Evidence-Based Clinical Reviews*, USA: Elsevier/Mosby, 2005.

Suekawa M, Shiga T, Sone H, "Effects of Gomisin J and Analogous Lignan Compounds in Schisandra Fruits on Isolated Smooth Muscles," *Yakugaku Zasshi*, 1987, 107(9):720-6.

Volicer L, Janku I, Motl O, "The Mode of Action of *Schisandra chinesis*," in Pharmacology of Oriental Plants (New York: Pergamon Press Books, Macmillan Company, 1965).

Yamada S, Murawaki Y, and Kawasaki H, "Preventive Effect of Gomisin A, a Lignan Component of Shizandra Fruits, on Acetaminophen-Induced Hepatotoxicity in Rats," *Biochem Pharmacol*, 1993, 46 (6):1081-5.

Shark Cartilage

Pharmacologic Category Nutraceutical

Reported Use

Analgesia (Fontenele, 1996; Fontenele, 1997)
Cancer therapy (Escudier, 2007; Lane, 1992; Prudden, 1985)
Kaposi sarcoma (Hillman, 2001)
Macular degeneration (Turcotte, 1999)
Osteoarthritis, rheumatoid arthritis (Lane, 1992)
Psoriasis (Dupont, 1998)

Local Anesthetic/Vasoconstrictor Precautions No information available to require special precautions

Effects on Bleeding None reported

Warnings/Precautions May cause gastrointestinal upset (nausea). Use with caution in individuals with diabetes or who are using antidiabetic agents due to possible additive hypoglycemic effects. Based on theoretical inhibition of collateral neovascularization due to the antiangiogenesis properties of shark cartilage, use with caution in individuals with coronary artery disease and peripheral vascular disease. Shark cartilage preparations contain up to 25% calcium. Concomitant use of shark cartilage with calcium may increase the risk of hypercalcemia.

References

Dupont E, Savard PE, Jourdain C, et al, "Antiangiogenic Properties of a Novel Shark Cartilage Extract: Potential Role in the Treatment of Psoriasis," *J Cutan Med Surg*, 1998, 2(3):146-52.
Escudier B, Choueiri TK, Oudard S, et al, "Prognostic Factors of Metastatic Renal Cell Carcinoma After Failure of Immunotherapy: New Paradigm From a Large Phase III Trial With Shark Cartilage Extract AE 941," *J Urol*, 2007, 178(5):1901-5.
Fontenele JB, Araujo GB, de Alencar JW, et al, "The Analgesic and Anti-Inflammatory Effects of Shark Cartilage Are Due to a Peptide Molecule and Are Nitric Oxide (NO) System Dependent," *Biol Pharm Bull*, 1997, 20(11):1151-4.
Fontenele JB, Viana GS, Xavier-Filho J, et al, "Anti-Inflammatory and Analgesic Activity of a Water-Soluble Fraction From Shark Cartilage," *Braz J Med Biol Res*, 1996, 29(5):643-6.
Lane IW, *Sharks Don't Get Cancer*, Garden City Park, New York: Avery Publishing Group, 1992, 107-18.
Natural Standard Research Collaboration, Chief Editors: Ulbricht C, Basch E, *Natural Standard Herb and Supplement Reference - Evidence-Based Clinical Reviews*, USA: Elsevier/Mosby, 2005.
Prudden JF, "The Treatment of Human Cancer With Agents Prepared From Bovine Cartilage," *J Biol Response Mod*, 1985, 4(6):551-84.
Turcotte P, "Phase I Dose Escalation Study of AE-941, an Antiangiogenic Agent, in Age-Related Macular Degeneration Patient," Retina Society Conference (Hawaii, December 2, 1999).

Slippery Elm

Pharmacologic Category Herb

Reported Use

Cancer (pharmacologic activity)
Diarrhea (pharmacologic activity)
Gastrointestinal disorders (pharmacologic activity)
Sore throat (pharmacologic activity)

Local Anesthetic/Vasoconstrictor Precautions No information available to require special precautions

Effects on Bleeding None reported

Warnings/Precautions Avoid during pregnancy due to risk of contamination with slippery elm whole bark; may have abortifacient properties.

References

Gallagher R, "Use of Herbal Preparations for Intractable Cough," *J Pain Symptom Manage*, 1997, 14 (1):1-2.
Kaegi E, "Unconventional Therapies for Cancer: 1. Essiac. The Task Force on Alternative Therapies of the Canadian Breast Cancer Research Initiative," *CMAJ* 1998 Apr 7;158(7):897-902.
Kato A, Ando K, Tamura G, et al, "Effects of Some Fatty Acid Esters on the Viability and Transplantability of Ehrlich Ascites Tumor Cells," *Cancer Res*, 1971, 31(5):501-4.
Natural Standard Research Collaboration, Chief Editors: Ulbricht C, Basch E, *Natural Standard Herb and Supplement Reference - Evidence-Based Clinical Reviews*, USA: Elsevier/Mosby, 2005.

Soy Isoflavones

Pharmacologic Category Nutraceutical

Reported Use

Antioxidant (Azadbakht, 2007; Bertipaglio de Santana, 2008; Siefker, 2006)
Athletic performance (Candow, 2006; Dragan, 1992)
Benign prostatic hyperplasia (BPH) (Weber, 2001)
Bone mineral density (increase) (Greendale, 2002)
Cancer (prevention) (Horn-Ross, 2003; Kennedy, 1998; Messina, 1994; Murray, 2003; Trock, 2006; van Erp-Baart, 2003)
Cardiovascular effects (Hooper, 2008; Sacks, 2006; Teede, 2001)
  Contradictory study (van der Schouw, 2005)
Cervical dysplasia (pharmacologic activity)
Chemotherapy (adjunct) (Lei, 1999)
Cognitive function (Kreijkamp-Kaspers, 2004)
  Contradictory study (Fournier, 2007)
Crohn's disease (Capristo, 2000)
Cyclical breast pain (McFadyen, 2000)
Diabetes (Fujita, 2001; Hiroyuki, 2001; Jayagopal, 2002)

Diarrhea (Allen, 1994; Burks, 2001; Santosham, 1991)
Endometriosis (pharmacologic activity)
Food allergies (Osborn, 2006)
Hypercholesterolemia (Allen, 2007; Chester, 2001; Crouse, 1999; Devi, 1972; Hooper, 2008; Meng, 1999; Weggemans, 2003; Zhan, 2005; Zhuo, 2004)
Hypertension (Rivas, 2002)
Immune function (Ryan-Borchers, 2006)
Kidney disease (Azadbakht, 2003; Soroka, 1998)
Menopausal symptoms (Albert, 2002; Albertazzi, 1998; Alekel, 2000; Crisafulli, 2004; Duncan, 1999; Hidalgo, 2005; Howes, 2006; Kaari, 2006; Mei, 2001; Nagata, 2001; Petri Nahas, 2004; Scambia, 2000; Secreto, 2004; Upmalis, 2000; Washburn, 1999)
Menstrual migraine (Burke, 2002)
Osteoarthritis (Soeken, 2002)
Osteoporosis (Alekel, 2000; Schreiber, 1999); prevention of bone loss (Wu, 2006)
Platelet function (Garrido, 2006)
Premenstrual syndrome (PMS) (pharmacologic activity)
Skin aging (Izumi, 2007)
Weight loss (Allison, 2003)

Local Anesthetic/Vasoconstrictor Precautions No information available to require special precautions

Effects on Bleeding None reported

Warnings/Precautions Women who are taking estrogen-containing medications or who have current or history of estrogen-dependent tumors (including breast cancer) should consult their physician prior to use. Use cautiously in adults and infants with decreased thyroid function. Use cautiously in individuals with gastrointestinal problems.

References

Albertazzi P, Pansini F, Bonaccorsi G, et al, "The Effect of Dietary Soy Supplementation on Hot Flushes," *Obstet Gynecol*, 1998, 91(1):6-11.

Alekel DL, St. Germain A, Peterson CT, et al, "Isoflavone-Rich Soy Protein Isolate Attenuates Bone Loss in the Lumbar Spine of Perimonopausal Women," *Am J Clin Nutr*, 2000, 72(3):844-53.

Allen JK, Becker DM, Kwiterovich PO, et al, "Effect of Soy Protein-Containing Isoflavones on Lipoproteins in Postmenopausal Women," *Menopause*, 2007, 14(1):106-14.

Allison DB, Gadbury G, Schwartz LG, et al, "A Novel Soy-Based Meal Replacement Formula for Weight Lloss Among Obese Individuals: A Randomized Controlled Clinical Trial," *Eur J Clin Nutr*, 2003, 57 (4):514-22.

Burke BE, Olson RD, and Cusack BJ, "Randomized, Controlled Trial of Phytoestrogen in the Prophylactic Treatment of Menstrual Migraine," *Biomed Pharmacother*, 2002, 56(6):283-8.

Burks AW, Vanderhoof JA, Mehra S, et al, "Randomized Clinical Trial of Soy Formula With and Without Added Fiber in Antibiotic-Induced Diarrhea," *J Pediatr*, 2001, 139(4):578-82.

Chester EA, "Soy for Cardiovascular Indications," *Am J Health Syst Pharm*, 2001, 58(8):663, 666.

Crouse JR, Morgan T, Terry JG, et al, "A Randomized Trial Comparing the Effect of Casein with that of Soy Protein Containing Varying Amounts of Isoflavones on Plasma Concentrations of Lipids and Lipoproteins," *Arch Intern Med*, 1999; 159(17):2070-6.

de Lemos ML, "Effects of Soy Phytoestrogens Genistein and Daidzein on Breast Cancer Growth," *Ann Pharmacother*, 2001, 35(9):1118-21.

Devi KS and Kurup PA, "Hypolipaemic Activity of *Phaseolus Mungo* (Blackgram) in Rats Fed a High-Fat, High-Cholesterol Diet. Isolation of a Protein and Polysaccharide Fraction," *Atherosclerosis*, 1972, 15 (2):223-30.

Duncan AM, Underhill KE, Xu X, et al, "Modest Hormonal Effects of Soy Isoflavones in Postmenopausal Women," *J Clin Endocrinol Metab*, 1999, 84(10):3479-84.

Garrido A, De la Maza MP, Hirsch S, et al, "Soy Isoflavones Affect Platelet Thromboxane A2 Receptor Density But Not Plasma Lipids in Menopausal Women," *Maturitas*, 2006, 54(3):270-6.

Greendale GA, FitzGerald G, Huang MH, et al, "Dietary Soy Isoflavones and Bone Mineral Density: Results From the Study of Women's Health Across the Nation," *Am J Epidemiol*, 2002, 155(8):746-54.

Hidalgo LA, Chedraui PA, Morocho N, et al, "The Effect of Red Clover Isoflavones on Menopausal Symptoms, Lipids and Vaginal Cytology in Menopausal Women: A Randomized, Double-Blind, Placebo-Controlled Study," *Gynecol Endocrinol*, 2005, 21(5):257-64.

Kaari C, Haidar MA, Júnior JM, et al, "Randomized Clinical Trial Comparing Conjugated Equine Estrogens and Isoflavones in Postmenopausal Women: A Pilot Study," *Maturitas*, 2006, 53(1):49-58.

Kennedy AR, "The Bowman-Birk Inhibitor From Soybeans as an Anticarcinogenic Agent," *Am J Clin Nutr*, 1998, 68(6 Suppl):1406S-1412S.

Kreijkamp-Kaspers S, Kok L, Grobbee DE, et al, "Effect of Soy Protein Containing Isoflavones on Cognitive Function, Bone Mineral Density, and Plasma Lipids in Post-Menopausal Women: A Randomized Controlled Trial," *JAMA*, 2004, 292(1):65-74.

Lei W, Mayotte JE, Levitt ML, et al "Enhancement of Chemosensitivity and Programmed Cell Death by Tyrosine Kinase Inhibitors Correlates With EGFR Expression in Non-Small Cell Lung Cancer Cells," *Anticancer Res*, 1999, 19:221-8.

Mei J, Yeung SS, and Kung AW, "High Dietary Phytoestrogen Intake is Associated With Higher Bone Mineral Density in Postmenopausal but not Premenopausal Women," *J Clin Endocrinol Metab*, 2001, 86 (11):5217-21.

Meng QH, Lewis P, Wahala K, et al, "Incorporation of Esterified Soybean Isoflavones With Antioxidant Activity Into Low Density Lipoprotein," *Biochim Biophys Acta*, 1999, 1438(3):369-76.

Messina M, Messina V, and Setchell K, *The Simple Soybean and Your Health*, Garden City Park, NY: Avery Publishing Group, 1994, 75-6.

Natural Standard Research Collaboration, Chief Editors: Ulbricht C, Basch E, *Natural Standard Herb and Supplement Reference - Evidence-Based Clinical Reviews*, USA: Elsevier/Mosby, 2005.

Ryan-Borchers TA, Park JS, Chew BP, et al, "Soy Isoflavones Modulate Immune Function in Healthy Postmenopausal Women," *Am J Clin Nutr*, 2006, 83(5):1118-25.

Schreiber MD and Rebar RW, "Isoflavones and Postmenopausal Bone Health: A Viable Alternative to Estrogen Therapy?" *Menopause*, 1999, 6(3):233-41.

Soeken KL, Lee WL, Bausell RB, et al, "Safety and Efficacy of S-Adenosylmethionine (SAMe) for Osteoarthritis," *J Fam Pract*, 2002, 51(5):425-30.

Takahashi J, Kawakatsu K, Wakayama T, et al, "Elevation of Serum Theophylline Levels by Ipriflavone in a Patient With Chronic Obstructive Pulmonary Disease," *Eur J Clin Pharmacol*, 1992, 43(2):207-8.

Teede HJ, Dalais FS, Kotsopoulos D, et al, "Dietary Soy Has Both Beneficial and Potentially Adverse Cardiovascular Effects: A Placebo-Controlled Study in Men and Post-Menopausal Women," *J Clin Endocrinol Metab*, 2001, 86(7):3053-60.

Weber KS, Setchell KD, Stocco DM, et al, "Dietary Soy-Phytoestrogens Decrease Testosterone Levels and Prostate Weight Without Altering LH, Prostate 5Alpha-Reductase or Testicular Steroidogenic Acute Regulatory Peptide Levels in Adult Male Sprague-Dawley Rats," *J Endocrinol*, 2001, 170(3):591-9.
Wu J, Oka J, Higuchi M, et al, "Cooperative Effects of Isoflavones and Exercise on Bone and Lipid Metabolism in Postmenopausal Japanese Women: A Randomized Placebo-Controlled Trial," *Metabolism*, 2006, 55(4):423-33.

Spirulina

Pharmacologic Category Nutraceutical

Reported Use

Allergic rhinitis (Karkos, 2007)
Arsenic poisoning (Misbahuddin, 2006)
Blepharospasm (Vitale, 2004)
Chronic viral hepatitis (contradictory study) (Băicuş, 2002)
Diabetes, type 2 (Mani, 2000)
Fatigue (contradictory study) (Baicus, 2007)
Hypercholesterolemia (Nakaya, 1988; Samuels, 2002)
Malnutrition (Branger, 2003)
Oral leukoplakia/cancer (Mathew, 1995)
Skeletal muscle damage (Lu, 2006)
Weight loss (Becker, 1986)

Local Anesthetic/Vasoconstrictor Precautions No information available to require special precautions

Effects on Bleeding None reported

Warnings/Precautions Use with caution in individuals with phenylketonuria; content in blue-green algae theoretically may exacerbate this condition. Use with caution in individuals with compromised immune systems. Hepatotoxicity has been reported.

Use with caution in individuals with a history of bleeding, hemostatic disorders, or drug-related hemostatic problems. Use with caution in individuals taking anticoagulant medications, including warfarin, aspirin, aspirin-containing products, NSAIDs, or antiplatelet agents (eg, ticlopidine, clopidogrel, dipyridamole). Discontinue use prior to dental or surgical procedures (generally at least 14 days before). Use with caution in individuals taking antihypertensive medications.

References

Baicus C and Baicus A, "Spirulina Did Not Ameliorate Idiopathic Chronic Fatigue in Four N-of-1 Randomized Controlled Trials," *Phytother Res*, 2007, 21(6):570-3.
Băicuş C and Tănăsescu C, "Chronic Viral Hepatitis, the Treatment With Spiruline for One Month Has No Effect on the Aminotransferases," *Rom J Intern Med*, 2002, 40(1-4):89-94.
Becker EW, Jakober B, Luft D, et al, "Clinical and Biochemical Evaluations of the Alga Spirulina With Regard to Its Application in the Treatment of Obesity. A Double-Blind Cross-Over Study," *Nutr Report Internat*, 1986, 33(4):565-74.
Branger B, Cadudal JL, Delobel M, et al, "Spiruline as a Food Supplement in Case of Infant Malnutrition in Burkina-Faso," *Arch Pediatr*, 2003, 10(5):424-31.
Karkos PD, Leong SC, Arya AK, et al, "'Complementary ENT': A Systematic Review of Commonly Used Supplements," *J Laryngol Otol*, 2007, 121(8):779-82.
Lu HK, Hsieh CC, Hsu JJ, et al, "Preventive Effects of *Spirulina platensis* on Skeletal Muscle Damage Under Exercise-Induced Oxidative Stress," *Eur J Appl Physiol*, 2006, 98(2):220-6.
Mani UV, Desai S, and Iyer U, "Studies on the Long-Term Effect of Spirulina Supplementation and Serum Lipid Profile and Glycated Proteins in NIDDM Patients," *J Nutraceut*, 2000, 2(3):25-32.
Mathew B, Sankaranarayanan R, Nair PP, et al, "Evaluation of Chemoprevention of Oral Cancer With *Spirulina fusiformis*," *Nutr Cancer*, 1995, 24(2):197-202.
Misbahuddin M, Islam AZ, Khandker S, et al, "Efficacy of Spirulina Extract Plus Zinc in Patients of Chronic Arsenic Poisoning: A Randomized Placebo-Controlled Study," *Clin Toxicol (Phila)*, 2006, 44(2):135-41.
Nakaya N, Homma Y, and Goto Y, "Cholesterol Lowering Effect of Spirulina," *Nutr Report Internat*, 1988, 37(6):1329-37.
Natural Standard Research Collaboration, Chief Editors: Ulbricht C, Basch E, *Natural Standard Herb and Supplement Reference - Evidence-Based Clinical Reviews*, USA: Elsevier/Mosby, 2005.
Samuels R, Mani UV, Iyer UM, et al, "Hypocholesterolemic Effect of Spirulina in Patients With Hyperlipidemic Nephrotic Syndrome," *J Med Food*, 2002, 5(2):91-6.
Vitale S, Miller NR, Mejico LJ, et al, "A Randomized, Placebo-Controlled, Crossover Clinical Trial of Super Blue-Green Algae in Patients With Essential Blepharospasm or Meige Syndrome," *Am J Ophthalmol*, 2004, 138(1):18-32.

St John's Wort

Pharmacologic Category Herb

Reported Use

ADHD, contradictory study (Weber, 2008)
Antibacterial, anti-inflammatory (topical: minor wounds, infections, bruises, muscle soreness, and sprains) (Newall, 1996)
Antiviral (Miller, 1998)
Anxiety (Panijel, 1985)
Atopic dermatitis (Schempp, 2003; Schempp, 2003)
Autism (Niederhofer, 2009)
Burning mouth syndrome (Sardella, 2008)
Climacteric symptoms (combination therapy) (Chung, 2007; Uebelhack, 2006)

Depression (mild to moderate only) (Linde, 2005; Randløv, 2006; Röder, 2004; Werneke, 2004); depression (children) (Findling, 2003; Hubner, 2001; Kobak, 2003); seasonal affective disorder (SAD) (Kasper, 1997; Stevinson, 2000); melancholia, stress, and anxiety (Cott, 1998; Gaster, 2000; Harrer, 1999; Hippius, 1998; Lenoir, 1999; Linde, 1996; Volz, 1997; Vorbach, 1997; Woelk, 2000); major depression (Kasper, 2006)

No reported benefit (Hypericum Depression Trial Study Group, 2002; Shelton, 2001)

HIV (contradictory study) (Gulick, 1999)

Irritable bowel syndrome (IBS), contradictory study (Saito, 2010)

Obsessive-compulsive disorder (OCD) (Kobak, 2005; Simeon, 2005)

Perimenopausal symptoms (Abdali, 2010; Al-Akoum, 2009; Grube, 1999; Steger, 1985; Taylor, 2000)

Premenstrual syndrome (PMS) (Hicks, 2004)

Smoking cessation (Lawvere, 2006)

Contradictory study (Barnes, 2006)

Social phobia (Kobak, 2005; Wheatley, 1999)

Somatoform disorders (Maisenbacher, 1992; Muller, 2004; Volz, 2002)

Local Anesthetic/Vasoconstrictor Precautions No information available to require special precautions

Effects on Bleeding None reported

Warnings/Precautions St John's wort is contraindicated in pregnancy (based on animal studies) (Grush 1998). Use with caution in individuals taking digoxin (may alter levels of this medication) (Johne 1999). It is not for use in severe depression. Use with caution in individuals taking other antidepressants (Gordon, 1998). Based on its pharmacologic activity, St John's wort may alter the actions of monoamine oxidase (MAO) inhibitors, tricyclic antidepressants, and selective serotonin reuptake inhibitors (SSRIs) (Bennett, 1998; Chatterjee, 1998). May elevate hepatic transaminases (noted animal studies at high doses) (Brockmoller, 1990). May cause photosensitivity (Brockmoller, 1997; Schempp, 2003). Use with caution in individuals on reserpine (effects may be antagonized by St John's wort) (Okpanyi, 1987). Use with caution in individuals on narcotic medications (based on animal studies, may enhance sedation from these drugs) (Okpanyi, 1987).

May cause drowsiness (mild). Based on pharmacologic activity, use with caution while driving or operating machinery. Use caution in individuals taking sedative medications (eg, anxiolytics, benzodiazepines). Effects may be additive with other CNS depressants or natural products with sedative properties.

Antidepressant therapy may precipitate a shift to mania or hypomania in individuals with bipolar affective disorder (Schneck, 1998).

Three patients experienced mania after short-term St John's wort use. All returned to normal after discontinuing the product.

St John's wort may induce the cytochrome P450 enzyme system, although there is conflicting information about this claim. Specifically, data indicates probable interactions between St John's wort and the HIV-1 protease inhibitor indinavir (Piscitelli, 2000), the antirejection medication cyclosporine (Ruschitzka, 2000), midazolam (Wang, 2001), and nifedipine (Smith, 2001). Additionally, enzyme induction may result in decreased estrogen levels in individuals taking oral contraceptives (Yue, 2000). While the FDA has issued a public health advisory regarding this issue, the authors recommend considerable caution be exercised before adding St John's wort to any medication regimen containing a cytochrome P-450 3A substrate.

St John's wort may also induce cytochrome P450, 1A2, and 2C9 but to a lesser extent than cytochrome P450 and 3A4 (Henderson, 2002). There are reports of St John's wort reducing the effects of warfarin and lowering the INR (Cott, 2001; Jiang, 2004; Yue, 2000).

St John's wort may cause an increase in thyroid-stimulating hormone (Ferko, 2001; Hauben, 2002).

Concurrent use of St John's wort with 5-HT1 agonists or "triptans" (eg, sumatriptan) can increase the risk of serotonergic adverse effects, including serotonin syndrome.

References

Abdali K, Khajehei M, and Tabatabaee HR, "Effect of St John's Wort on Severity, Frequency, and Duration of Hot Flashes in Premenopausal, Perimenopausal and Postmenopausal Women: A Randomized, Double-Blind, Placebo-Controlled Study," *Menopause*, 2010, 17(2):326-31.

Al-Akoum M, Maunsell E, Verreault R, et al, "Effects of *Hypericum perforatum* (St. John's Wort) on Hot Flashes and Quality of Life in Perimenopausal Women: A Randomized Pilot Trial," *Menopause*, 2009, 16(2):307-14.

American Psychiatric Association, "Practice Guideline for the Treatment of Patients with Major Depressive Disorder," May 2010. Available at: http://www.psychiatryonline.com/pracGuide/pracGuideTopic_7.aspx.

Barnes J, Barber N, Wheatley D, et al, "A Pilot Randomised, Open, Uncontrolled, Clinical Study of Two Dosages of St John's Wort (*Hypericum perforatum*) Herb Extract (LI-160) as an Aid to Motivational/Behavioural Support in Smoking Cessation," *Planta Med*, 2006, 72(4):378-82.

Bennett DA Jr, Phun L, Polk JF, et al, "Neuropharmacology of St John's Wort (*Hypericum*)," *Ann Pharmacother*, 1998, 32(11):1201-8.
Brockmoller J, Reum T, Bauer S, et al, "Hypericin and Pseudohypericin: Pharmacokinetics and Effects of Photosensitivity in Humans," *Pharmacopsychiatry*, 1997, 30(Supp 2):94-101.
Brown TM, "Acute St. John's Wort Toxicity," *Am J Emerg Med*, 2000, 18(2):231-2.
Chatterjee SS, Bhattacharya SK, Wonnemann M, et al, "Hyperforin as a Possible Antidepressant Component of *Hypericum* Extracts," *Life Sci*, 1998, 63(6):499-510.
Chung DJ, Kim HY, Park KH, et al, "Black Cohosh and St John's Wort (GYNO-Plus) for Climacteric Symptoms," *Yonsei Med J*, 2007, 48(2):289-94.
Cott JM, "Herb-Drug Interactions: Focus on Pharmacokinetics," *CNS Spectr*, 2001, 6(10):827-32.
Cott JM and Fugh-Berman A, "Is St John's Wort (*Hypericum perforatum*) an Effective Antidepressant?" *J Nerv Ment Dis*, 1998, 186(8):500-1.
Dresser GK, Schwarz UI, Wilkinson GR, et al, "Coordinate Induction of Both Cytochrome P4503A and MDR1 by St John's Wort in Healthy Subjects," *Clin Pharmacol Ther*, 2003, 73(1):41-50.
Eggertsen R, Andreasson A, and Andrén L, "Effects of Treatment With a Commercially Available St John's Wort Product (Movina) on Cholesterol Levels in Patients With Hypercholesterolemia Treated With Simvastatin," *Scand J Prim Health Care*, 2007, 25(3):154-9.
Eich-Hochli D, Oppliger R, Golay KP, et al, "Methadone Maintenance Treatment and St. John's Wort - A Case Report," *Pharmacopsychiatry*, 2003, 36(1):35-7.
Ferko N and Levine MA, "Evaluation of the Association Between St John's Wort and Elevated Thyroid-Stimulating Hormone," *Pharmacotherapy*, 2001, 21(12):1574-8.
Findling RL, McNamara NK, O'Riordan MA, et al, "An Open-Label Pilot Study of St. John's Wort in Juvenile Depression," *J Am Acad Child Adolesc Psychiatry*, 2003, 42(8):908-14.
Frye RF, Fitzgerald SM, Lagattuta TF, et al, "Effect of St John's Wort on Imatinib Mesylate Pharmacokinetics," P96 American Society for Clinical Pharmacology and Therapeutics, PDII-B-4, February 2004.
Gaster B and Holroyd J, "St John's Wort for Depression: A Systematic Review," *Arch Intern Med*, 2000, 160(2):152-6.
Goldman P, "Herbal Medicines Today and the Roots of Modern Pharmacology," *Ann Intern Med*, 2001, 135(8 Pt 1):594-600.
Gordon JB, "SSRIs and St John's Wort: Possible Toxicity?" *Am Fam Physician*, 1998, 57(5):950, 953.
Grube B, Walper A, and Wheatley D, "St. John's Wort Extract: Efficacy for Menopausal Symptoms of Psychological Origin," *Adv Ther*, 1999, 16(4):177-86.
Grush LR, Nierenberg A, Keefe B, et al, "St John's Wort During Pregnancy," *JAMA*, 1998, 280(18):1566.
Gulick RM, McAuliffe V, Holden-Wiltse J, et al, "Phase I Studies of Hypericin, the Active Compound in St. John's Wort, as an Antiretroviral Agent in HIV-Infected Adults. AIDS Clinical Trials Group Protocols 150 and 258," *Ann Intern Med*, 1999, 130(6):510-4.
Harrer G, Schmidt U, Kuhn U, et al, "Comparison of Equivalence Between the St John's Wort Extract LoHyp-57 and Fluoxetine," *Arzneimittelforschung*, 1999, 49(4):289-96.
Hauben M, "The Association of St John's Wort With Elevated Thyroid-Stimulating Hormone," *Pharmacotherapy*, 2002, 22(5):673-5.
Henderson L, Yue QY, Bergquist C, et al, "St John's Wort (*Hypericum perforatum*): Drug Interactions and Clinical Outcomes," *Br J Clin Pharmacol*, 2002, 54(4):349-56.
Hennessy M, Kelleher D, Spiers JP, et al, "St Johns Wort Increases Expression of P-Glycoprotein: Implications for Drug Interactions," *Br J Clin Pharmacol*, 2002, 53(1):75-82.
Hicks SM, Walker AF, Gallagher J, et al, "The Significance of 'Nonsignificance' in Randomized Controlled Studies: A Discussion Inspired by a Double-Blinded Study on St. John's Wort (*Hypericum perforatum* L.) for Premenstrual Symptoms," *J Altern Complement Med*, 2004, 10(6):925-32.
Hippius H, "St John's Wort (*Hypericum perforatum*) - A Herbal Antidepressant," *Curr Med Res Opin*, 1998, 14(3):171-84.
Hubner WD and Kirste T, "Experience With St John's Wort (*Hypericum perforatum*) in Children Under 12 Years With Symptoms of Depression and Psychovegetative Disturbances," *Phytother Res*, 2001, 15 (4):367-70.
Hypericum Depression Trial Study Group, "Effect of *Hypericum perforatum* (St John's Wort) in Major Depressive Disorder: A Randomized Controlled Trial," *JAMA*, 2002, 287(14):1807-14.
Jiang X, Williams KM, Liauw WS, et al, "Effect of St John's Wort and Ginseng on the Pharmacokinetics and Pharmacodynamics of Warfarin in Healthy Subjects," *Br J Clin Pharmacol*, 2004, 57(5):592-9.
Johne A, Brockmoller J, Bauer S, et al, "Pharmacokinetic Interaction of Digoxin With an Herbal Extract from St John's Wort," *Clin Pharmacol Ther*, 1999, 66(4):338-45.
Johne A, Schmider J, Brockmöller J, et al, "Decreased Plasma Levels of Amitriptyline and Its Metabolites on Comedication With an Extract From St. John's Wort (*Hypericum perforatum*)," *J Clin Psychopharmacol*, 2002, 22(1):46-54.
Kasper S, Anghelescu IG, Szegedi A, et al, "Superior Efficacy of St John's Wort Extract WS 5570 Compared to Placebo in Patients With Major Depression: A Randomized, Double-Blind, Placebo-Controlled, Multi-Center Trial [ISRCTN77277298]," *BMC Med*, 2006, 4:14.
Kasper S, "Treatment of Seasonal Affective Disorder (SAD) With *Hypericum* Extract," *Pharmacopsychiatry*, 1997, 2(30 Suppl):89-93.
Kawaguchi A, Ohmori M, Tsuruoka S, et al, "Drug Interaction Between St John's Wort and Quazepam," *Br J Clin Pharmacol*, 2004, 58(4):403-10.
Kobak KA, Taylor L, Futterer R, et al, "St. John's Wort in Generalized Anxiety Disorder: Three More Case Reports," *J Clin Psychopharmacol*, 2003, 23(5):531-2.
Kobak KA, Taylor LV, Bystritsky A, et al, "St John's Wort Versus Placebo in Obsessive-Compulsive Disorder: Results From a Double-Blind Study," *Int Clin Psychopharmacol*, 2005, 20(6):299-304.
Kobak KA, Taylor LV, Warner G, et al, "St. John's Wort Versus Placebo in Social Phobia: Results From a Placebo-Controlled Pilot Study," *J Clin Psychopharmacol*, 2005, 25(1):51-8.
Lawvere S, Mahoney MC, Cummings KM, et al, "A Phase II Study of St John's Wort for Smoking Cessation," *Complement Ther Med*, 2006, 14(3):175-84.
Lenoir S, Degenring FH, and Saller R, "A Double-Blind Randomised Trial to Investigate Three Different Concentrations of a Standardised Fresh Plant Extract Obtained From the Shoot Tips of *Hypericum perforatum* L," *Phytomedicine*, 1999, 6(3):141-6.
Linde K, Berner MM, and Kriston L, "St John's Wort for Major Depression," *Cochrane Database Syst Rev*, 2008, (4):CD000448.
Linde K, Mulrow CD, Berner M, et al, "St John's Wort for Depression," *Cochrane Database Syst Rev*, 2005, (2):CD000448.
Linde K, Ramirez G, Mulrow CD, et al, "St John's Wort for Depression - An Overview and Meta-Analysis of Randomised Clinical Trials," *BMJ*, 1996 313(7052):253-8.
Mai I, Stormer E, Bauer S, et al, "Impact of St John's Wort Treatment on the Pharmacokinetics of Tacrolimus and Mycophenolic Acid in Renal Transplant Patients," *Nephrol Dial Transplant*, 2003, 18 (4):819-22.
Maisenbacher HJ and Kuhn U, "The Therapy of Depressions in Practice: Results of a Post-Marketing Surveillance Study With Herba Hyperici," *Natura Medica*, 1992, 7(5):394-9.
Miller AL, "St John's Wort (*Hypericum perforatum*): Clinical Effects on Depression and Other Conditions," *Altern Med Rev*, 1998, 3(1):18-26.
Moses EL and Mallinger AG, "St John's Wort: Three Cases of Possible Mania Induction," *J Clin Psychopharmacol*, 2000, 20(1):115-7.
Muller T, Mannel M, Murck H, et al, "Treatment of Somatoform Disorders With St. John's Wort: A Randomized, Double-Blind and Placebo-Controlled Trial," *Psychosom Med*, 2004, 66(4):538-47.
Natural Standard Research Collaboration, Chief Editors: Ulbricht C, Basch E, *Natural Standard Herb and Supplement Reference - Evidence-Based Clinical Reviews*, USA: Elsevier/Mosby, 2005.
Newall CA, Anderson LA, and Phillipson JD, *Herbal Medicines: A Guide for Health Care Professionals*, London, England: The Pharmaceutical Press, 1996, 250-2.
Niederhofer H, "St John's Wort Treating Patients With Autistic Disorder," *Phytother Res*, 2009, 23 (11):1521-3.

Okpanyi SN and Weischer ML, "Animal Experiments on the Psychotropic Action of a *Hypericum* Extract," *Arzneimittelforschung*, 1987, 37(1):10-3.
Panijel M, "Treatment of Moderately Severe Anxiety States," *Therapiewoche*, 1985, 35(41):4659-68.
Parker V, Wong AH, Boon HS, et al, "Adverse Reactions to St John's Wort," *Can J Psychiatry*, 2001, 46 (1):77-9.
Patel S, Robinson R and Burk M, "Hypertensive Crisis Associated With St John's Wort," *Am J Med*, 2002, 112(6):507-8.
Piscitelli SC, Burstein AH, Chaitt D, et al, "Indinavir Concentration and St John's Wort," *Lancet*, 2000, 355:547-8.
Randløv C, Mehlsen J, Thomsen CF, et al, "The Efficacy of St John's Wort in Patients With Minor Depressive Symptoms or Dysthymia - a Double-Blind Placebo-Controlled Study," *Phytomedicine*, 2006, 13(4):215-21.
Rengelshausen J, Banfield M, Riedel KD, et al, "Opposite Effects of Short-Term and Long-Term St John's Wort Intake on Voriconazole Pharmacokinetics," *Clin Pharmacol Ther*, 2005, 78(1):25-33.
Röder C, Schaefer M, and Leucht S, "Meta-Analysis of Effectiveness and Tolerability of Treatment of Mild to Moderate Depression With St. John's Wort," *Fortschr Neurol Psychiatr*, 2004, 72(6):330-43.
Roots I, Johne A, Schmider, J, et al, "Interaction of a Herbal Extract From St. John's Wort With Amitriptyline and Its Metabolites," *Clin Pharm Ther*, 2000, 67(2):159.
Ruschitzka F, Meier PJ, Turina M, et al, "Acute Heart Transplant Rejection Due to St John's Wort," *Lancet*, 2000, 355:548-9.
Saito YA, Rey E, Almazar-Elder AE, et al, "A Randomized, Double-Blind, Placebo-Controlled Trial of St John's Wort for Treating Irritable Bowel Syndrome," *Am J Gastroenterol*, 2010, 105(1):170-7.
Sardella A, Lodi G, Demarosi F, et al, "*Hypericum perforatum* Extract in Burning Mouth Syndrome: A Randomized Placebo-Controlled Study," *J Oral Pathol Med*, 2008, 37(7):395-401.
Schempp CM, Hezel S, and Simon JC, "Topical Treatment of Atopic Dermatitis With *Hypericum* Cream. A Randomised, Placebo-Controlled, Double-Blind Half-Side Comparison Study," *Hautarzt*, 2003, 54 (3):248-53.
Schempp CM, Winghofer B, Muller K, et al, "Effect of Oral Administration of *Hypericum perforatum* Extract (St. John's Wort) on Skin Erythema and Pigmentation Induced by UVB, UVA, Visible Light and Solar Simulated Radiation," *Phytother Res*, 2003, 17(2):141-6.
Schneck C, "St John's Wort and Hypomania," *J Clin Psychiatry*, 1998 59(12):689.
Shelton RC, Keller MB, Gelenberg A, et al, "Effectiveness of St John's Wort in Major Depression: A Randomized Controlled Trial," *JAMA*, 2001, 285(15):1978-86.
Simeon J, Nixon MK, Milin R, et al, "Open-Label Pilot Study of St. John's Wort in Adolescent Depression," *J Child Adolesc Psychopharmacol*, 2005, 15(2):293-301.
Smith M, Lin KM, and Zheng YP, "PIII-89 an Open Trial of Nifedipine-Herb Interactions: Nifedipine With St. John's Wort, Ginseng or *Ginkgo biloba*," Clin Pharm Ther, 2001, 69:P86.
Steger W, "Depressive Verstimmungen," *Z Allg Med*, 1985, 61:914-8.
Stevinson C and Ernst E, "A Pilot Study of *Hypericum perforatum* for the Treatment of Premenstrual Syndrome," *BJOG*, 2000, 107(7):870-6.
Tannergren C, Engman H, Knutson L, et al, "St John's Wort Decreases the Bioavailability of R- and S-Verapamil Through Induction of the First-Pass Metabolism," *Clin Pharmacol Ther*, 2004, 75(4):298-309.
Taylor LH and Kobak KA, "An Open-Label Trial of St. John's Wort (*Hypericum perforatum*) in Obsessive-Compulsive Disorder," *J Clin Psychiatry*, 2000, 61(8):575-8.
Uebelhack R, Blohmer JU, Graubaum HJ, et al, "Black Cohosh and St John's Wort for Climacteric Complaints: A Randomized Trial," *Obstet Gynecol*, 2006, 107:247-55.
Volz HP, "Controlled Clinical Trials of *Hypericum* Extracts in Depressed Patients - An Overview," *Pharmacopsychiatry*, 1997, 30(Suppl 2):72-6.
Volz HP, Murck H, Kasper S, et al, "St John's Wort Extract (LI 160) in Somatoform Disorders: Results of a Placebo-Controlled Trial," *Psychopharmacology (Berl)*, 2002, 164(3):294-300.
Vorbach EU, Arnoldt KH, and Hubner WD, "Efficacy and Tolerability of St John's Wort Extract LI 160 Versus Imipramine in Patients With Severe Depressive Episodes According to ICD-10," *Pharmacopsychiatry*, 1997, Suppl 2:81-5.
Wang Z, Gorski JC, Hamman MA, et al, "The Effects of St John's Wort (*Hypericum perforatum*) on Human Cytochrome P450 Activity," *Clin Pharmacol Ther*, 2001, 70(4):317-26.
Wang Z, Hamman MA, Huang SM, et al, "Effect of St John's Wort on the Pharmacokinetics of Fexofenadine," *Clin Pharmacol Ther*, 2002, 71(6):414-20.
Weber W, Vander Stoep A, McCarty RL, et al, "*Hypericum perforatum* (St John's Wort) for Attention-Deficit/Hyperactivity Disorder in Children and Adolescents: A Randomized Controlled Trial," *JAMA*, 2008, 299(22):2633-41.
Werneke U, Horn O, and Taylor DM, "How Effective Is St John's Wort? The Evidence Revisited," *J Clin Psychiatry*, 2004, 65(5):611-7.
Wheatley D, "Hypericum in Seasonal Affective Disorder (SAD)," *Curr Med Res Opin*, 1999, 15(1):33-7.
Woelk H, "Comparison of St John's Wort and Imipramine for Treating Depression: Randomised Controlled Trial," *BMJ*, 2000, 321(7260):536-9.
Wurglics M, Westerhoff K, Kaunzinger A, et al, "Comparison of German St John's Wort Products According to Hyperforin and Total Hypericin Content," *J Am Pharm Assoc (Wash)*, 2001, 41(4):560-6.
Yue QY, Bergquist C, and Gerden B, "Safety of St John's Wort," *Lancet*, 2000, 355(9203):576-7.

Tea Tree

Pharmacologic Category Herb

Reported Use Not for ingestion:

Acne vulgaris (Bassett, 1990)

Contradictory study (Enshaieh, 2007)

Antifungal, antibacterial; dental and oral health (mouthwash); burns, cuts, scrapes, insect bites, dandruff, lice, MRSA, onychomycosis, thrush (Bagg, 2006; Buck, 1994; Canyon, 2007; Carson, 1998; Concha, 1998; Jandourek, 1998; Soukoulis, 2004; Tong, 1992)

Contradictory studies (Caelli, 1998; Caelli, 2000; Dryden, 2004; Satchell, 2002)

Local Anesthetic/Vasoconstrictor Precautions No information available to require special precautions

Effects on Bleeding None reported

Warnings/Precautions Not for ingestion. May cause allergic dermatitis in sensitive individuals (Rubel, 1998). Use with caution in patients with known allergy/hypersensitivity to tea tree oil (*Melaleuca alternifolia*), any of its constituents, Balsam of Peru, benzoin, colophony (rosin) tinctures, eucalyptol, or other members of the Myrtle (*Myrtaceae*) family. Use with caution in individuals using topical drying agents or astringents due to additive drying effects.

References

Bagg J, Jackson MS, Petrina Sweeney M, et al, "Susceptibility to *Melaleuca alternifolia* (Tea Tree) Oil of Yeasts Isolated From the Mouths of Patients With Advanced Cancer," *Oral Oncol*, 2006, 42(5):487-92.

Bassett IB, Pannowitz DL, and Barnetson RS, "A Comparative Study of Tea-Tree Oil Versus Benzoylperoxide in the Treatment of Acne," *Med J Aust*, 1990, 153(8):455-8.
Buck DS, Nidorf DM, and Addino JG, "Comparison of Two Topical Preparations for the Treatment of Onychomycosis: *Melaleuca alternifolia* (Tea Tree) Oil and Clotrimazole," *J Fam Pract*, 1994, 38 (6):601-5.
Caelli M and Riley T, "Tea Tree Oil – An Alternative Topical Decolonisation Agent for Adult Inpatients With Methicillin-Resistant Staphylococcus Aureus (MRSA) – A Pilot Study," *J Hosp Infect*, 1998, 40(Suppl A):9.
Caelli M, Porteous J, Carson CF, et al, "Tea Tree Oil as an Alternative Topical Decolonization Agent for Methicillin-Resistant Staphylococcus Aureus," *J Hosp Infect*, 2000, 46(3):236-7.
Canyon DV and Speare R, "A Comparison of Botanical and Synthetic Substances Commonly Used to Prevent Head Lice (*Pediculus humanus* var. *capitis*) Infestation," *Int J Dermatol*, 2007, 46(4):422-6.
Carson CF, Riley TV, and Cookson BD, "Efficacy and Safety of Tea Tree Oil as a Topical Antimicrobial Agent," *J Hosp Infect*, 1998, 40(3):175-8.
Concha JM, Moore LS, and Holloway WJ, "1998 William J. Stickel Bronze Award. Antifungal Activity of *Melaleuca alternifolia* (Tea-Tree) Oil Against Various Pathogenic Organisms," *J Am Podiatr Med Assoc*, 1998, 88(10):489-92.
Dryden MS, Dailly S, and Crouch M, "A Randomized, Controlled Trial of Tea Tree Topical Preparations Versus a Standard Topical Regimen for the Clearance of MRSA Colonization," *J Hosp Infect*, 2004, 56 (4):283-6.
Enshaieh S, Jooya A, Siadat AH, et al, "The Efficacy of 5% Topical Tea Tree Oil Gel in Mild to Moderate Acne Vulgaris: A Randomized, Double-Blind Placebo-Controlled Study," *Indian J Dermatol Venereol Leprol*, 2007, 73(1):22-5.
Jandourek A, Vaishampayan JK, and Vazquez JA, "Efficacy of Melaleuca Oral Solution for the Treatment of Fluconazole Refractory Oral Candidiasis in AIDS Patients," *AIDS*, 1998, 12(9):1033-7.
Natural Standard Research Collaboration, Chief Editors: Ulbricht C, Basch E, *Natural Standard Herb and Supplement Reference - Evidence-Based Clinical Reviews*, USA: Elsevier/Mosby, 2005.
Rubel DM, Freeman S, and Southwell IA, "Tea Tree Oil Allergy: What Is the Offending Agent? Report of Three Cases of Tea Tree Oil Allergy and Review of the Literature," *Australas J Dermatol*, 1998, 39 (4):244-7.
Satchell AC, Saurajen A, Bell C, et al, "Treatment of Dandruff With 5% Tea Tree Oil Shampoo," *J Am Acad Dermatol*, 2002, 47(6):852-5.
Soukoulis S and Hirsch R, "The Effects of a Tea Tree Oil-Containing Gel on Plaque and Chronic Gingivitis," *Aust Dent J*, 2004, 49(2):78-83.
Syed TA, Qureshi ZA, Ali SM, et al, "Treatment of Toenail Onychomycosis With 2% Butenafine and 5% *Melaleuca alternifolia* (Tea Tree) Oil in Cream," *Trop Med Int Health*, 1999, 4(4):284-7.
Tong MM, Altman PM, and Barnetson RS, "Tea Tree Oil in the Treatment of Tinea Pedis," *Australas J Dermatol*, 1992, 33(3):145-9.

Turmeric

Pharmacologic Category Herb

Reported Use

Antioxidant; anti-inflammatory (Ammon, 1993; Usharani, 2008)
Antirheumatic; hypercholesterolemia (Ammon, 1991)
Cancer (Kuttan, 1987; Polasa, 1992)
Cholelithiasis prevention, gallbladder disease (Niederau, 1999; Rasyid, 1999)
Dysmenorrhea (pharmacologic activity)
Dyspepsia (Thamlikitkul, 1989)
HIV (Copeland, 1994; Hellinger, 1996)
Muscle soreness (pharmacologic activity)
Osteoarthritis (Kulkarni, 1991)
Peptic ulcer disease (Kositchaiwat, 1993; Van Dau, 1998)
Rheumatoid arthritis (Deodhar, 1980)
Scabies (Charles, 1992)
Uveitis (Lal, 1999)

Local Anesthetic/Vasoconstrictor Precautions No information available to require special precautions

Effects on Bleeding May see increased bleeding due to inhibition of platelet aggregation

Warnings/Precautions Based on its pharmacologic activity, turmeric is contraindicated in biliary obstruction (Ammon, 1991). Use with caution in individuals with gastrointestinal disease (peptic ulcer disease, ulcerative colitis, Crohn's). May potentiate lipid-lowering therapies.

Avoid in patients with known allergy/hypersensitivity to turmeric, any of its constituents (including curcumin), yellow food colorings, or other members of the *Zingiberaceae* (ginger) family.

May alter platelet aggregation (Srivastava, 1995). Based on pharmacologic activity, this herb may be contraindicated in individuals with active bleeding (eg, peptic ulcer, intracranial bleeding). Use with caution in individuals with a history of bleeding, hemostatic disorders, or drug-related hemostatic problems. Use with caution in individuals taking anticoagulant medications, including warfarin, aspirin, aspirin-containing products, NSAIDs, or antiplatelet agents (eg, ticlopidine, clopidogrel, dipyridamole). Discontinue use prior to dental or surgical procedures (generally at least 14 days before).

References

Ammon HP and Wahl MA, "Pharmacology of *Curcuma longa*," *Planta Med*, 1991, 57(1):1-7.
Ammon HP, Safayhi H, Mack T, et al, "Mechanism of Anti-Inflammatory Actions of Curcumin and Boswellic Acids," *J Ethnopharmacol*, 1993, 38(2-3):113-9.
Charles V and Charles SX, "The Use and Efficacy of *Azadirachta indica* ADR ('Neem') and *Curcuma longa* ('Turmeric') in Scabies. A Pilot Study," *Trop Geogr Med*, 1992, 44(1-2):178-81.
Copeland R, "Curcumin Therapy in HIV-Infected Patients Initially Increased CD-4 and CD-8 Cell Counts," *X Int Conf AIDS*, 1994, 10:216.

Deodhar SD, Sethi R, and Srimal RC, "Preliminary Study on Antirheumatic Activity of Curcumin (Diferuloyl Methane)," *Indian J Med Res*, 1980, 71:632-4.
Hellinger JA, Cohen CJ, Dugan ME, et al, "Phase I/II Randomized, Open-Label Study of Oral Curcumin Safety, and Antiviral Effects on HIV-RT PCR in HIV+ Individuals," 3rd Conference on Retroviruses and Opportunistic Infections (January 28 - February 1, 1996, Washington DC).
Kositchaiwat C, Kositchaiwat S, and Havanondha J, "*Curcuma longa* Linn. in the Treatment of Gastric Ulcer Comparison to Liquid Antacid: A Controlled Clinical Trial," *J Med Assoc Thai*, 1993, 76(11):601-5.
Kulkarni RR, Patki PS, Jog VP, et al, "Treatment of Osteoarthritis With a Herbomineral Formulation: A Double-Blind, Placebo-Controlled, Cross-Over Study," *J Ethnopharmacol*, 1991, 33(1-2):91-5.
Kuttan R, Sudheeran PC, and Josph CD, "Turmeric and Curcumin as Topical Agents in Cancer Therapy," *Tumori*, 1987, 73(1):29-31.
Lal B, Kapoor AK, Asthana OP, et al, "Efficacy of Curcumin in the Management of Chronic Anterior Uveitis," *Phytother Res*, 1999, 13(4):318-22.
Natural Standard Research Collaboration, Chief Editors: Ulbricht C, Basch E, *Natural Standard Herb and Supplement Reference - Evidence-Based Clinical Reviews*, USA: Elsevier/Mosby, 2005.
Niederau C and Gopfert E, "The Effect of Chelidonium- and Turmeric Root Extract on Upper Abdominal Pain Due to Functional Disorders of the Biliary System. Results From a Placebo-Controlled Double-Blind Study," *Med Klin (Munich)*, 1999, 94(8):425-30.
Polasa K, Raghuram TC, Krishna TP, et al, "Effect of Turmeric on Urinary Mutagens in Smokers," *Mutagenesis*, 1992, 7(2):107-9.
Rasyid A and Lelo A, "The Effect of Curcumin and Placebo on Human Gall-Bladder Function: An Ultrasound Study," *Aliment Pharmacol Ther*, 1999, 13(2):245-9.
Snow JM, "*Curcuma Longa* L (Zingiberaceae)," *Protocol J Botanical Med*, 1995, 1(2):43-6.
Srivastava KC, Bordia A, and Verma SK, "A Major Component of Food Spice Turmeric (*Curcuma longa*) Inhibits Aggregation and Alters Eicosanoid Metabolism In Human Blood Platelets," *Prostaglandins Leukot Essent Fatty Acids*, 1995, 52(4):223-7.
Thamlikitkul V, Bunyapraphatsara N, Dechatiwongse T, et al, "Randomized Double Blind Study of *Curcuma domestica* Val. for Dyspepsia," *J Med Assoc Thai*, 1989, 72(11):613-20.
Van Dau N, Ngoc Ham N, Huy Khac D, et al, "The Effects of a Traditional Drug, Tumeric (*Curcuma longa*), and Placebo on the Healing of Duodenal Ulcer," *Phytomed*, 1998, 5(1):29-34.

Uva Ursi

Pharmacologic Category Herb

Reported Use

Hyperpigmentation (Arndt, 1965; Sugai, 1992)

Urinary tract infections and kidney stone (preventive) (Bradley, 1992)

Local Anesthetic/Vasoconstrictor Precautions No information available to require special precautions

Effects on Bleeding None reported

Warnings/Precautions Contraindicated in pregnancy and lactation (based on animal studies) (Bradley, 1992). Contraindicated in renal failure (based on pharmacologic activity). Anecdotal reports state that drinking 1 teaspoonful of baking soda in water prior to use may promote conversion of hydroquinones to their active form. May cause green-brown discoloration of urine. Do not use for more than 7-10 days.

References

Arndt KA and Fitzpatrick TB, "Topical Use of Hydroquinone as a Depigmenting Agent," *JAMA*, 1965, 194 (9):965-7.
Bradley PR, ed, *British Herbal Compendium*, Vol 1, Bournemouth, England: British Herbal Medicine Association, 1992, 211-13.
Natural Standard Research Collaboration, Chief Editors: Ulbricht C, Basch E, *Natural Standard Herb and Supplement Reference - Evidence-Based Clinical Reviews*, USA: Elsevier/Mosby, 2005.
Sugai T, "Clinical Effects of Arbutin in Patients With Chloasma," *Skin Research*, 1992, 34:522-9.

Valerian

Pharmacologic Category Herb

Reported Use

Anxiety (Andreatini, 2002; Delsignore, 1980; Kohnen, 1988; Müller, 2003; Sousa, 1992)

Depression (Müller, 2003)

Hyperthyroidism (pharmacologic activity)

Insomnia (sedative/hypnotic) (Balderer, 1985; Bent, 2006; Cerny, 1999; Dominguez, 2000; Koetter, 2007; Leathwood, 1982; Morin, 2005; Müller, 2006; Vorbach, 1996) Contradictory studies (Coxeter, 2003; Diaper, 2004; Oxman, 2007)

Premenstrual syndrome (PMS), menopause; restless motor syndromes and muscle spasms (Houghton, 1988)

Local Anesthetic/Vasoconstrictor Precautions No information available to require special precautions

Effects on Bleeding None reported

Warnings/Precautions Based on pharmacologic activities, may cause drowsiness or sedation. Use with caution when driving or operating heavy machinery (German Commission E, 1985). Use caution in individuals taking medications that cause CNS depression, including sedative-hypnotics, antihistamines, antidepressants, and anxiolytics. May increase sleeping time from hypnotic agents (reported with pentobarbital in animal studies) (Hendriks, 1985).

Note: Do not use valerian supplements in children <3 years of age. Use only valepotriate and baldrinal-free in children <12 years of age due to potential mutagenic properties.

References

Andreatini R, Sartori VA, Seabra ML, et al, "Effect of Valepotriates (Valerian Extract) in Generalized Anxiety Disorder: A Randomized Placebo-Controlled Pilot Study," *Phytother Res*, 2002, 16(7):650-4.
Balderer G and Borbely AA, "Effect of Valerian on Human Sleep," *Psychopharmacology (Berl)*, 1985, 87(4):406-9.
Bent S, Padula A, Moore D, et al, "Valerian for Sleep: A Systematic Review and Meta-Analysis," *Am J Med*, 2006, 119(12):1005-12.
Cerny AS and Schmid K, "Tolerability and Efficacy of Valerian/Lemon Balm in Healthy Volunteers: A Double Blind Placebo Controlled, Multicentre Study," *Fitoterapia*, 1999, 70(3):221-8.
Coxeter PD, Schluter PJ, Eastwood HL, et al, "Valerian Does Not Appear to Reduce Symptoms for Patients With Chronic Insomnia in General Practice Using a Series of Randomised N-of-1 Trials," *Complement Ther Med*, 2003, 11(4):215-22.
Delsignore R, Orlando S, Costi D, et al, "Placebo Controlled Clinical Trial With Valerian," *Settimana Medica*, 1980, 68(9):437-47.
Diaper A and Hindmarch I, "A Double-Blind, Placebo-Controlled Investigation of the Effects of Two Doses of a Valerian Preparation on the Sleep, Cognitive and Psychomotor Function of Sleep-Disturbed Older Adults," *Phytother Res*, 2004, 18(10):831-6.
Dominguez RA, Bravo-Valverde RL, Kaplowitz BR, et al, "Valerian As a Hypnotic for Hispanic Patients," *Cultur Divers Ethni Minor Psychol*, 2000, 6(1):84-92.
Hendriks H, Bos R, Woerdenbag, HJ, et al, "Central Nervous Depressant Activity of Valerenic Acid in the Mouse," *Planta Med*, 1985, (1):28-31.
Houghton PJ, "The Biological Activity of Valerian and Related Plants," *J Ethnopharmacol*, 1988, 22(2):121-42.
Koetter U, Schrader E, Käufeler R, et al, "A Randomized, Double Blind, Placebo-Controlled, Prospective Clinical Study to Demonstrate Clinical Efficacy of a Fixed Valerian Hops Extract Combination (Ze 91019) in Patients Suffering From Non-Organic Sleep Disorder," *Phytother Res*, 2007, 21(9):847-51.
Kohnen R and Oswald WD, "The Effects of Valerian, Propranolol, and Their Combination on Activation, Performance, and Mood of Healthy Volunteers Under Social Stress Conditions," *Pharmacopsychiatry*, 1988, 21(6):447-8.
Leathwood PD, Chauffard F, Heck E, et al, "Aqueous Extract of Valerian Root (*Valeriana officinalis L.*) Improves Sleep Quality in Man," *Pharmacol Biochem Behav*, 1982, 17(1):65-71.
Morin CM, Koetter U, Bastien C, et al, "Valerian-Hops Combination and Diphenhydramine for Treating Insomnia: A Randomized Placebo-Controlled Clinical Trial," *Sleep*, 2005, 28(11):1465-71.
Müller SF and Klement S, "A Combination of Valerian and Lemon Balm Is Effective in the Treatment of Restlessness and Dyssomnia in Children," *Phytomedicine*, 2006, 13(6):383-7.
Müller D, Pfeil T, and von den Driesch V, "Treating Depression Comorbid With Anxiety – Results of an Open, Practice-Oriented Study With St John's Wort WS 5572 and Valerian Extract in High Doses," *Phytomedicine*, 2003, 10(Suppl 4):25-30.
Natural Standard Research Collaboration, Chief Editors: Ulbricht C, Basch E, *Natural Standard Herb and Supplement Reference - Evidence-Based Clinical Reviews*, USA: Elsevier/Mosby, 2005.
Oxman AD, Flottorp S, Håvelsrud K, et al, "A Televised, Web-Based Randomised Trial of an Herbal Remedy (Valerian) for Insomnia," *PLoS ONE*, 2007, 2(10):e1040.
Sousa MPd, Pacheco P, and Roldao V, "Double-Blind Comparative Study of the Efficacy and Safety of Valdispert vs Clobazepam," *KlaiChemi Med Research Info*, 1992.
"*Valerianae radix*," German Commission E Monograph, Bundesanzeiger, 1985, No 90.
Vorbach EU, Darmstadt R, Gortelmeyer, et al, "Therapie von Insomnien," *Psychopharmakotherapie*, 1996, 3:109-15.

Vanadium

Pharmacologic Category Mineral

Reported Use

Allergic rhinitis (Tsiklauri, 2009)
Diabetes, type 1 (Badmaev, 1999)
Diabetes, type 2 (Boden, 1996)
Hypercholesterolemia (Dimond, 1963; Harland, 1994)
Hypoglycemia (pharmacologic activity)
Pneumonia (Tarkhan-Mouravi, 2006)

Local Anesthetic/Vasoconstrictor Precautions No information available to require special precautions

Effects on Bleeding None reported

Warnings/Precautions No dietary toxicity or serious side effects reported; however, industrial exposure has resulted in toxicity. May alter glucose regulation. Use with caution in individuals with diabetes or in those who may be predisposed to hypoglycemia. Effects of drugs with hypoglycemic activity may be potentiated (including insulin and oral hypoglycemics). Blood sugar should be closely monitored and the dosage of hypoglycemic medications may require adjustment. This should be carefully coordinated among the individuals' healthcare providers. Use with caution in individuals taking anticoagulant or antiplatelet medications. Theoretically, vanadium may enhance anticoagulant effects.

References

Badmaev V, Prakash S, and Majeed M, "Vanadium: A Review of Its Potential Role in the Fight Against Diabetes," *J Altern Complement Med*, 1999, 5(3):273-91.
Boden G, Chen X, Ruiz J, et al, "Effects of Vanadyl Sulfate on Carbohydrate and Lipid Metabolism in Patients With Non-Insulin-Dependent Diabetes Mellitus," *Metabolism*, 1996, 45(9):1130-5.
Dimond EG, Caravaca J, and Benchimola, "Vanadium, Excretion, Toxicity, Lipid Effect in Man," *Am J Clin Nutr*, 1963, 12:49-53
Harland BF and Harden-Williams BA, "Is Vanadium of Human Nutritional Importance Yet?" *J Am Diet Assoc*, 1994, 94(8):891-4.
Natural Standard Research Collaboration, Chief Editors: Ulbricht C, Basch E, *Natural Standard Herb and Supplement Reference - Evidence-Based Clinical Reviews*, USA: Elsevier/Mosby, 2005.
Tarkhan-Mouravi ID and Abkhazi MN, "Influence of Treatment of Vanadium Electrophoresis on Certain-bio-Chemical and Immunological Indicators in Patients With Prolonged Cases of Pneumonia," *Georgian Med News*, 2006, (137):42-7.

Wild Yam

Pharmacologic Category Herb

Reported Use
Female vitality (conversion to progesterone in the body is poor) (Weiss, 1988)
Hyperlipidemia (Zakharov, 1977)
Menopause (Hudson, 1997; Komesaroff, 2001)

Local Anesthetic/Vasoconstrictor Precautions No information available to require special precautions

Effects on Bleeding None reported

Warnings/Precautions Use with caution in individuals taking steroidal medications. Phytoestrogen-containing herbs have not been associated with the negative health effects seen with synthetic estrogen. However, use with caution in individuals on hormone replacement therapy or oral contraceptives, or in those with a history of thromboembolic disease or stroke. Contraindicated in individuals with a history of estrogen-dependent tumors or endometrial cancer.

References

Hudson T, Standish L, Breed C, et al, "Clinical and Endocrinological Effects of a Menopausal Botanical Formula," *Journal of Naturopathic Medicine*, 1997, 7:73-7.
Komesaroff PA, Black CV, Cable V, et al, "Effects of Wild Yam Extract on Menopausal Symptoms, Lipids and Sex Hormones in Healthy Menopausal Women," *Climacteric*, 2001, 4(2):144-50.
Natural Standard Research Collaboration, Chief Editors: Ulbricht C, Basch E, *Natural Standard Herb and Supplement Reference - Evidence-Based Clinical Reviews*, USA: Elsevier/Mosby, 2005.
Umland EM, Cauffield JS, Kirk JK, et al, "Phytoestrogens as Therapeutic Alternatives to Traditional Hormone Replacement in Postmenopausal Women," *Pharmacotherapy*, 2000, 20(8):981-90.
Weiss RF, *Herbal Medicine*, Beaconsfield, England: Beaconsfield Publishers LTD, 1988, 330.
Zakharov VN, "Hypolipemic Effect of Diosponine in Ischemic Heart Disease Depending on the Type of Hyperlipoproteinemia," *Kardiologiia*, 1977, 17(6):136-7.

Yohimbe

Pharmacologic Category Herb

Reported Use
Athletic performance (Ostojic, 2006)
Autonomic failure (Jordan, 1998; Montastruc, 1981)
Platelet aggregation inhibition (Boon, 1983)
Sexual side effects of SSRIs (Hollander, 1992; Jacobsen, 1992; Montorsi, 1994; Reid, 1987)
Sexual vitality (men and women); male erectile dysfunction (Carey, 1996; Ernst, 1998; Mann, 1996; Riley, 1994; Rowland, 1997; Yan, 2000)
Xerostomia (psychotropic drug-induced) (Bagheri, 1997)

Local Anesthetic/Vasoconstrictor Precautions Has potential to interact with epinephrine and levonordefrin to result in increased BP; use vasoconstrictor with caution

Effects on Bleeding None reported

Warnings/Precautions Contraindicated in pregnancy. Do not use in individuals taking MAO inhibitors or antihypertensives; do not use in hypertensive individuals (De Smet, 1994) or cardiovascular disease. Toxic doses may trigger psychosis, hypotension, and cardiac failure. Based on pharmacologic activity, use with caution in individuals receiving $alpha_2$ blockers; may cause CNS stimulation (anxiety, insomnia), hypertension, and tachycardia. Avoid using in individuals with benign prostatic hypertrophy (BPH) because yohimbine, the active constituent of yohimbe, may exacerbate symptoms of BPH due to its presynaptic $alpha_2$ blocking ability.

References

Bagheri H, Schmitt L, Berlan M, et al, "A Comparative Study of the Effects of Yohimbine and Anetholtrithione on Salivary Secretion in Depressed Patients Treated With Psychotropic Drugs," *Eur J Clin Pharmacol*, 1997, 52(5):339-42.
Boon NA, Elliott JM, Grahame-Smith DG, et al, "A Comparison of Alpha 2-Adrenoreceptor Binding Characteristics of Intact Human Platelets Identified by [3H]-Yohimbine and [3H]-Dihydroergocryptine," *J Auton Pharmacol*, 1983, 3(2):89-95.
Carey MP and Johnson BT, "Effectiveness of Yohimbine in the Treatment of Erectile Disorder: Four Meta-Analytic Integrations," *Arch Sex Behav*, 1996, 25(4):341-60.
De Smet PA and Smeets OS, "Potential Risks of Health Food Products Containing Yohimbe Extracts," *BMJ*, 1994, 309(6959):958.
Ernst E and Pittler MH, "Yohimbine for Erectile Dysfunction: A Systematic Review and Meta-Analysis of Randomized Clinical Trials," *J Urol*, 1998, 159(2):433-6.
Hollander E and McCarley A, "Yohimbine Treatment of Sexual Side Effects Induced by Serotonin Reuptake Blockers," *J Clin Psychiatry*, 1992, 53(6):207-9.
Jacobsen FM, "Fluoxetine-Induced Sexual Dysfunction and an Open Trial of Yohimbine," *J Clin Psychiatry*, 1992, 53(4):119-22.
Jordan J, Shannon JR, Biaggioni I, et al, "Contrasting Actions of Pressor Agents in Severe Autonomic Failure," *Am J Med*, 1998, 105(2):116-24.
Mann K, Klingler T, Noe S, et al, "Effects of Yohimbine on Sexual Experiences and Nocturnal Penile Tumescence and Rigidity in Erectile Dysfunction," *Arch Sex Behav*, 1996, 25(1):1-16.
Montastruc JL, Puech AJ, Clanet M, et al, "Yohimbine in Treatment of Parkinson's Disease. Preliminary Results," *Nouv Presse Med*, 1981, 10(16):1331-2.
Montorsi F, Strambi LF, Guazzoni G, et al, "Effect of Yohimbine-Trazodone on Psychogenic Impotence: A Randomized, Double-Blind, Placebo-Controlled Study," *Urology*, 1994, 44(5):732-6.
Natural Standard Research Collaboration, Chief Editors: Ulbricht C, Basch E, *Natural Standard Herb and Supplement Reference - Evidence-Based Clinical Reviews*, USA: Elsevier/Mosby, 2005.
Reid K, Surridge DH, Morales A, et al, "Double-Blind Trial of Yohimbine in Treatment of Psychogenic Impotence," *Lancet*, 1987, 2(8556):421-3.
Riley AJ, "Yohimbine in the Treatment of Erectile Disorder," *Br J Clin Pract*, 1994, 48(3):133-6.
Rowland DL, Kallan K, and Slob AK, "Yohimbine, Erectile Capacity, and Sexual Response in Men," *Arch Sex Behav*, 1997, 26(1):49-62.

ORAL MEDICINE TOPICS

PART I:

DENTAL MANAGEMENT AND THERAPEUTIC CONSIDERATIONS IN MEDICALLY-COMPROMISED PATIENTS

This first part of the chapter focuses on common medical conditions and their associated drug therapies with which the dentist must be familiar. Patient profiles with commonly associated drug regimens are described.

TABLE OF CONTENTS

CARDIOVASCULAR DISEASES

Cardiovascular disease is the most prevalent human disease affecting over 60 million Americans, accounting for >50% of all deaths in the United States. Surgical and pharmacological therapies have resulted in many cardiovascular patients living healthy and profitable lives. Consequently, patients presenting to the dental office may require treatment planning modifications related to the medical management of their cardiovascular disease. For the purposes of this text, we will cover coronary artery disease (CAD) including angina pectoris, myocardial infarction, cardiac arrhythmias, heart failure, and hypertension.

CARDIOVASCULAR DRUGS AND DENTAL CONSIDERATIONS

Some of the drug listings are redundant because the drugs are used to treat more than one cardiovascular disorder. As a convenience to the reader, each table has been constructed as a stand alone listing of drugs for the given disorder. The dental implications of these cardiovascular drugs are listed in Tables 7 and 8. Each of these two tables is a consolidation of the drugs from Tables 1-6. The more frequent cardiovascular, respiratory, and central nervous system adverse reactions which you may see in the dental patient are described in Table 7. Table 8 describes the effects on dental treatment reported for these drugs. It is suggested that the reader use Tables 7 and 8 to check for potential effects which could occur in the medicated cardiovascular dental patients.

CORONARY ARTERY DISEASE

Any long-term decrease in the delivery of oxygen to the heart muscle can lead to the condition ischemic heart disease. Often arteriosclerosis and atherosclerosis result in a narrowing of the coronary vessels' luminae and are the most common causes of vascular ischemic heart disease. Other causes such as previous infarct, mitral valve regurgitation, and ruptured septa may also lead to ischemia in the heart muscle. The two most common major conditions that result from ischemic heart disease are angina pectoris and myocardial infarction. Sudden death can likewise result from ischemia.

To the physician, the most common presenting sign or symptom of ischemic heart disease is chest pain. This chest pain can be of a transient nature as in angina pectoris or the result of a myocardial infarction. It is now believed that sudden death represents a separate occurrence that essentially involves the development of a lethal cardiac arrhythmia or coronary artery spasm leading to an acute shutdown of the heart muscle blood supply. Risk factors in patients for coronary atherosclerosis include age (males ≥45, females ≥55 years), family history of premature development, hypertension, hypercholesterolemia, low HDL, cigarette smoking, and diabetes mellitus.

CAD is the cause of about half of all deaths in the United States. CAD has been shown to be correlated with the levels of plasma cholesterol and/or triacylglycerol-containing lipoprotein particles. Primary prevention focuses on averting the development of CAD. In contrast, secondary prevention of CAD focuses on therapies to reduce morbidity and mortality in patients with clinically documented CAD.

Lipid-lowering and cardioprotective drugs provide significant risk-reducing benefits in the secondary prevention of CAD. By reducing the levels of total and low density cholesterol through the inhibition of hydroxymethylglutaryl-coenzyme A (HMG-CoA) reductase, statin drugs significantly improve survival. Cardioprotective drug therapy includes antiplatelet/anticoagulant agents to inhibit platelet adhesion; aggregation and blood coagulation; beta-blockers to lower heart rate, contractility and blood pressure; and the angiotensin-converting enzyme (ACE) inhibitors to lower peripheral resistance and workload. For a listing of lipid lowering drugs, see Table 1.

Table 1. DRUGS USED IN THE TREATMENT OF HYPERLIPIDEMIA

Reduction of Total and Low-Density Cholesterol Levels

Bile Acid Sequestrant

Colesevelam on page 435

HMG-CoA Reductase Inhibitors

Fluvastatin on page 773

Lovastatin on page 1042

Pitavastatin on page 1363

Pravastatin on page 1387

Rosuvastatin on page 1501

Simvastatin on page 1527

Atorvastatin on page 184

Fibrate Group

Fenofibrate on page 711

Gemfibrozil on page 809

Bile Acid Resins

Cholestyramine Resin on page 375

Colesevelam on page 435

Colestipol on page 437

Nicotinic Acid

Niacin on page 1202

Antilipemic Agent, 2-Azetidinone

Ezetimibe on page 700

Antilipemic Agent, Miscellaneous

Omega-3-Acid Ethyl Esters (Fish Oils) on page 1823

ANGINA PECTORIS
(EMPHASIS ON UNSTABLE ANGINA)

Numerous physiologic triggers can initiate the rupture of plaque in coronary blood vessels. Rupture leads to the activation, adhesion and aggregation of platelets, and the activation of the clotting cascade, resulting in the formation of occlusive thrombus. If this process leads to the complete occlusion of the artery, acute myocardial infarction with ST-segment elevation occurs. Alternatively, if the process leads to severe stenosis and the artery remains patent, unstable angina occurs. Triggers which induce unstable angina include physical exertion, mechanical stress due to an increase in cardiac contractility, pulse rate, blood pressure, and vasoconstriction.

Unstable angina accounts for more than 1 million hospital admissions annually. In 1989, Braunwald devised a system to classify the severity of the clinical manifestations of angina. These manifestations are defined as acute angina while at rest (within the 48 hours before presentation), subacute angina while at rest (within the previous month but not within the 48 hours before presentation), or new onset of accelerated (progressively more severe) angina. The system also classifies angina according to the clinical circumstances in which unstable angina develops, defined as either angina in the presence or absence of other conditions (ie, fever, hypoxia, tachycardia, thyrotoxicosis) and whether or not ECG abnormalities are present. Recently, the term "acute coronary syndrome" has been used to describe the range of conditions that includes unstable angina, ST-elevation myocardial infarction, and non-ST-elevation myocardial infarction.

Pharmacologic therapy to treat unstable angina includes antiplatelet drugs, antithrombin therapy, and conventional antianginal therapy with beta-blockers, nitrates, and calcium channel blockers. These drug groups and selected agents are listed in Table 2 and see Antiplatelet and Anticoagulation Considerations in Dentistry on page 1867.

Conventional Antianginal Therapy: Beta-Blockers, Nitrates, Calcium Channel Blockers

The pharmacotherapeutic strategy in treating angina is directed at improving myocardial oxygen supply and/or decreasing myocardial oxygen demand. Myocardial oxygen supply can be increased through enhancing coronary blood flow. Myocardial oxygen demand can be reduced by decreasing heart rate, contractility, and myocardial wall tension. Preload, afterload, and myocardial wall thickness are determinants of myocardial wall tension.

Organic Nitrates

Organic nitrates benefit angina by enhancing coronary blood flow via vasodilation of both large epicardial vessels and neighboring collateral vessels and decreasing myocardial oxygen demand by dilating veins and reducing preload. In order to be effective for the chronic prevention of angina, organic nitrates need to be dosed in a manner that does not induce nitrate tolerance.

Beta-Blockers

Beta-blockers are beneficial in treating angina since they decrease heart rate and contractility. Beta-blockers without intrinsic sympathomimetic activity (ISA) are preferred and those with ISA generally should be avoided when treating angina (such beta-blockers may actually increase myocardial workload). Beta-blockers are useful in the treatment of stable and unstable angina; but, since they can induce coronary vasospasm, they should be avoided in patients with variant angina.

Caution should be used when using beta-blockers in patients with difficult-to-control diabetes mellitus, bronchospastic disease, or peripheral vascular disease. The medications may be dosed as high as possible without inducing symptomatic bradycardia, hypotension, and/or heart blocks. Some patients on beta-blockers will experience fatigue and other adverse effects related to the central nervous system. Abrupt withdrawal of beta-blockers in patients with angina has been known to cause a rebound effect.

Calcium Channel Blockers

Three "types" of agents comprise calcium channel blockers: Diltiazem, verapamil, and the dihydropyridine family. These agents are useful in treating stable and unstable angina and are the drugs of choice in treating variant angina. All three agents increase coronary blood flow. Verapamil and diltiazem reduce contractility, heart rate, and, to some extent, afterload (thus reducing wall tension). Dihydropyridines are potent afterload reducers and several older agents may reduce contractility. Dihydropyridines have no impact on reducing heart rate. In fact, some older dihydropyridines may actually increase heart rate in patients not on a beta-blocker.

Stable and Unstable Angina

Beta-blockers are the preferred initial choice, often used in conjunction with an organic nitrate to more positively address the hemodynamic imbalances causing the angina. If the patient cannot tolerate the beta-blocker or if the beta-blocker therapy is contraindicated, a calcium channel blocker with or without an organic nitrate can be considered. If the beta-blocker is ineffective in preventing angina, an organic nitrate (if it has yet to be used) may be added. If dual combination therapy is ineffective, a calcium channel blocker may be added. Since the combination of a beta-blocker and either verapamil or diltiazem frequently induces undesirable bradycardia, a dihydropyridine is often selected in combination with a beta-blocker.

Since stable and unstable angina are nearly always related to coronary artery disease, patients should be placed on aspirin and an angiotensin-converting enzyme inhibitor (especially if the patient has heart failure or diabetes mellitus) in addition to antianginal therapy. Clopidogrel may be considered if the patient is allergic to aspirin. If applicable, weight reduction, smoking cessation, and following an appropriate low-cholesterol, low-fat diet should be encouraged as well as an effort to reduce other CAD risk factors. The lipid profile of these patients should be determined and, if needed, treated aggressively - LDL-C <100 mg/dL or, in high-risk patients, <70 mg/dL.

Dental Management

The dental management of the patient with angina pectoris may include sedation techniques for complicated procedures (see the Sedation section in Management of the Patient With Anxiety or Depression on page 1968), to limit the extent of procedures, and to limit the use of local anesthesia containing 1:100,000 epinephrine to two carpules. Anesthesia without a vasoconstrictor might also be selected. The appropriate use of a vasoconstrictor in anesthesia, however, should be weighed against the necessity to maximize anesthesia. Complete history, appropriate referral, and consultation with the patient's physician should be done for patients who are known to be at risk for angina pectoris.

MYOCARDIAL INFARCTION

Myocardial infarction is the leading cause of death in the United States. It is an acute irreversible ischemic event that produces an area of myocardial necrosis in the heart tissue. If a patient has a previous history of myocardial infarction, he/she may be taking a variety of drugs (ie, antihypertensives, lipid lowering drugs, ACE inhibitors, and antianginal medications) to not only prevent a second infarct, but to treat the long-term effects associated ischemic heart disease. Postmyocardial infarction patients are often taking anticoagulants, such as warfarin, and antiplatelet agents, such as aspirin, clopidogrel, or prasugrel. Consultation with the prescribing physician by the dentist is necessary prior to invasive procedures. Temporary dose reduction may allow the dentist to proceed with very invasive procedures. Most procedures, however, can be accomplished without changing the anticoagulant therapy at all, using local hemostasis techniques and thereby keeping the thromboembolic risk to a minimum.

Aspirin on page 171
Warfarin on page 1733

Thrombolytic drugs, which might dissolve hemostatic plugs, may also be given on a short-term basis immediately following an infarct and include:

Alteplase on page 89
Reteplase on page 1468
Tenecteplase on page 1599

Alteplase (tissue plasminogen activator [TPA]) is also currently in use for acute myocardial infarction. Following myocardial infarction and rehabilitation, outpatients may be placed on anticoagulants (such as Coumadin®), diuretics, beta-adrenergic blockers, ACE inhibitors or angiotensin receptor blockers, lipid-lowering therapies, and possibly aldosterone inhibitors if significant heart failure is associated with the MI. Depending on the presence or absence of continued angina pectoris, patients may also be taking nitrates, beta-blockers, or calcium channel blockers as indicated for treatment of angina.

BETA-ADRENERGIC BLOCKING AGENTS CATEGORIZED ACCORDING TO SPECIFIC PROPERTIES

Alpha-Adrenergic Blocking Activity

Labetalol on page 974

Intrinsic Sympathomimetic Activity

Acebutolol on page 29
Pindolol on page 1350

Long Duration of Action and Fewer CNS Effects

Acebutolol on page 29
Atenolol on page 179
Betaxolol (Systemic) on page 233
Nadolol on page 1174

Beta$_1$-Receptor Selectivity

Acebutolol on page 29
Atenolol on page 179
Metoprolol on page 1122

Nonselective (blocks both beta$_1$- and beta$_2$-receptors)

Betaxolol (Systemic) on page 233
Labetalol on page 974
Nadolol on page 1174
Pindolol on page 1350
Propranolol on page 1422
Timolol (Systemic) on page 1632

ARRHYTHMIAS

Abnormal cardiac rhythm can develop spontaneously and survivors of a myocardial infarction are often left with an arrhythmia. An arrhythmia is any alteration or disturbance in the normal rate, rhythm, or conduction through the cardiac tissue. Abnormalities in rhythm can occur in either the atria or the ventricles. Various valvular deformities, drug effects, and chemical derangements can initiate arrhythmias. These arrhythmias can be a slowing of the heart rate (<60 beats/minute) as defined in bradycardia or tachycardia resulting in a rapid heart beat (usually >150 beats/minute). The dentist will encounter a variety of treatments for management of arrhythmias. Usually, underlying causes such as reduced cardiac output, hypertension, and irregular ventricular beats will require treatment. Pacemaker therapy is also sometimes used. Indwelling pacemakers may require supplementation with antibiotics, and consultation with the physician is certainly appropriate.

Beta-blockers are often used to slow cardiac rate and diazepam may be helpful when anxiety is a contributing factor in arrhythmia. When atrial flutter and atrial fibrillation are diagnosed, drug therapy is usually required.

Digoxin on page 527

Atrial fibrillation (AF) is an arrhythmia characterized by multiple electrical activations in the atria resulting in scattered and disorganized depolarization and repolarization of the myocardium. Atrial contraction can lead to an irregular and rapid rate of ventricular contraction. The prevalence of AF within the US population ranges between 1% and 4%, with the incidence increasing with age. It is often associated with rheumatic valvular disease and nonvalvular conditions including coronary artery disease and hypertension. Coronary artery disease is present in about one-half of the patients with AF. Atrial fibrillation is a major risk factor for systemic and cerebral embolism. It is thought that thrombi develop as a result of stasis in the dilated left atrium and is dislodged by sudden changes in cardiac rhythm. About 10% of all strokes in patients >60 years of age are caused by AF.

The cornerstones of drug therapy for atrial fibrillation are the restoration and maintenance of a normal sinus rhythm through the use of antiarrhythmic drugs, ventricular rate control through the use of beta-blockers, digitalis drugs or calcium channel blockers, and stroke prevention through the use of anticoagulants.

Antiarrhythmic Drugs

Cardiac rhythm is conducted through the sinoatrial (SA) and atrioventricular (AV) nodes, bundle branches, and Purkinje fibers. Electrical impulses are transmitted within this system by the opening and closing of sodium and potassium channels. Antiarrhythmic drugs are classified by which channel they act upon, a classification known as Vaughan Williams. The Class I agents act primarily on sodium channels, and the Class III agents act on potassium channels. In addition, there are subclassifications within the Class I agents according to effects of the drug on conduction and refractoriness within the Purkinje and ventricular tissues. Class IA agents show moderate depression of conduction and prolongation of repolarization.

Atrial Fibrillation: Restoring and Maintaining Normal Sinus Rhythm

Pharmacologic cardioversion may be attempted in hemodynamically stable patients whose ventricular rate is controlled. If a patient has been in atrial fibrillation for >48 hours, anticoagulation should be considered prior to cardioversion. Drugs more commonly used for pharmacologic cardioversion include amiodarone or sotalol, depending upon patient's specific characteristics (eg, heart failure).

Ventricular Rate Control

It is accepted practice to treat patients with medication when the resting ventricular rate is >110 beats/minute. Digoxin, calcium channel blockers, and beta-adrenergic blockers are used in the regulation of ventricular rate. Digoxin increases the vagal tone to the AV node, calcium channel blockers slow the AV nodal conduction, and the beta-adrenergic blocking drugs decrease the sympathetic activation of the AV nodal conduction.

Table 2. DRUGS USED TO MANAGE UNSTABLE ANGINA

Antiplatelet Drugs

- Aspirin on page 171
- Clopidogrel on page 421
- Prasugrel on page 1385
- Ticlopidine on page 1629
- **Glycoprotein IIb / IIIa Receptor Antagonists**
  - Abciximab on page 26
  - Eptifibatide on page 615
  - Tirofiban on page 1638

Antithrombin Drugs

- **Indirect Thrombin Inhibitors**
  - Heparin (unfractionated) on page 844
- **Low molecular weight heparins**
  - Dalteparin on page 464
  - Enoxaparin on page 601
  - Nadroparin on page 1175
  - Tinzaparin on page 1635
- **Direct Thrombin Inhibitors**
  - Argatroban on page 156
  - Lepirudin on page 990
  - Bivalirudin on page 241
  - Dabigatran Etexilate on page 461
  - Desirudin on page 486
- **Vitamin K Antagonist**
  - Warfarin on page 1733

REFERENCES

American Diabetes Association, "Standards of Medical Care in Diabetes-2010," *Diabetes Care*, 2010, 33 (Suppl 1):S11-61.

Anderson JL, Adams CD, Antman EM, et al, "ACC/AHA 2007 Guidelines for the Management of Patients With Unstable Angina/Non-ST-Elevation Myocardial Infarction: A Report of the American College of Cardiology/American Heart Association Task Force on Practice Guidelines (Writing Committee to Revise the 2002 Guidelines for the Management of Patients With Unstable Angina/Non-ST-Elevation Myocardial Infarction) Developed in Collaboration With the American College of Emergency Physicians, the Society for Cardiovascular Angiography and Interventions, and the Society of Thoracic Surgeons Endorsed by the American Association of Cardiovascular and Pulmonary Rehabilitation and the Society for Academic Emergency Medicine," *J Am Coll Cardiol*, 2007, 50(7):e1-e157.

Brunzell JD, Davidson M, Furberg CD, et al, "Lipoprotein Management in Patients With Cardiometabolic Risk: Consensus Statement From the American Diabetes Association and the American College of Cardiology Foundation," *Diabetes Care*, 2008, 31(4):811-22.

Expert Panel on Detection, Evaluation, and Treatment of High Blood Cholesterol in Adults, "Executive Summary of The Third Report of The National Cholesterol Education Program (NCEP) Expert Panel on Detection, Evaluation, and Treatment of High Blood Cholesterol in Adults (Adult Treatment Panel III)," *JAMA*, 2001, 285(19):2486-97.

Fuster V, Rydén LE, Cannom DS, et al, "ACC/AHA/ESC 2006 Guidelines for the Management of Patients With Atrial Fibrillation: Full Text: A Report of the American College of Cardiology/American Heart Association Task Force on Practice Guidelines and the European Society of Cardiology Committee for Practice Guidelines (Writing Committee to Revise the 2001 Guidelines for the Management of Patients With Atrial Fibrillation) Developed in Collaboration With the European Heart Rhythm Association and the Heart Rhythm Society," *Europace*, 2006, 8(9):651-745.

Gibbons RJ, Chatterjee K, Daley J, et al, "ACC/AHA/ACP-ASIM Guidelines for the Management of Patients With Chronic Stable Angina: A Report of the American College of Cardiology/American Heart Association Task Force on Practice Guidelines (Committee on Management of Patients With Chronic Stable Angina)," *J Am Coll Cardiol*, 1999, 33(7):2092-197.

Grundy SM, Cleeman JI, Merz CN, et al, "Implications of Recent Clinical Trials for the National Cholesterol Education Program Adult Treatment Panel III Guidelines," *J Am Coll Cardiol*, 2004, 44 (3):720-32.

Kushner FG, Hand M, Smith SC Jr, et al, "2009 Focused Updates: ACC/AHA Guidelines for the Management of Patients With ST-Elevation Myocardial Infarction (Updating the 2004 Guideline and 2007 Focused Update) and ACC/AHA/SCAI Guidelines on Percutaneous Coronary Intervention (Updating the 2005 Guideline and 2007 Focused Update) a Report of the American College of Cardiology Foundation/American Heart Association Task Force on Practice Guidelines," *J Am Coll Cardiol*, 2009, 54(23):2205-41.

HEART FAILURE

Heart failure is a condition in which the heart is unable to pump sufficient blood to meet the needs of the body. It is caused by an impaired ability of the cardiac muscle to contract or by an increased workload imposed on the heart. Most frequently, the underlying cause of heart failure is coronary artery disease. Other contributory causes include hypertension, diabetes, idiopathic dilated cardiomyopathy, and valvular heart disease. It is estimated that heart failure affects approximately 5 million Americans. The New York Heart Association functional classification is regarded as the standard measure to describe the severity of a patient's symptom. Class I is characterized by having no limitation of physical activity. There is no dyspnea, fatigue, palpitations, or angina with ordinary physical activity. There is no objective evidence of cardiovascular dysfunction. Class II includes those patients having slight limitation of physical activity. These patients experience fatigue, palpitations, dyspnea, or angina with ordinary physical activity, but are comfortable at rest. There is evidence of minimal cardiovascular dysfunction. Class III is characterized by marked limitation of activity. Less-than-ordinary physical activity causes fatigue, palpitations, dyspnea, or angina, but patients are comfortable at rest. There is objective evidence of moderately severe cardiovascular dysfunction. Class IV is characterized by the inability to carry out any physical activity without discomfort. Symptoms of heart failure or anginal syndrome may be present even at rest, and any physical activity undertaken increases discomfort. There is objective evidence of severe cardiovascular dysfunction. Drug classes and the specific agents used to treat heart failure are listed in Table 3.

Table 3. DRUGS USED IN THE TREATMENT OF HEART FAILURE

Angiotensin-Converting Enzyme (ACE) Inhibitors[1]

- Benazepril on page 213
- Captopril on page 297
- Enalapril on page 596
- Fosinopril on page 787
- Lisinopril on page 1025
- Perindopril Erbumine on page 1329
- Quinapril on page 1444
- Ramipril on page 1457
- Trandolapril on page 1660

Angiotensin II Receptor Blockers

- Candesartan on page 292
- Losartan on page 1037
- Valsartan on page 1699

Diuretics

Thiazides

- Hydrochlorothiazide on page 854

Loop Diuretics

- Furosemide on page 796

Aldosterone Blocker (Selective)

- Eplerenone on page 610
- Spironolactone on page 1550

Digitalis Glycosides

- Digoxin on page 527

Beta-Adrenergic Receptor Blockers

- Bisoprolol on page 240
- Carvedilol on page 318
- Metoprolol on page 1122

Catecholamines

- DOBUTamine on page 554
- DOPamine

Supplemental Agents

Direct-Acting Vasodilators

- HydrALAZINE on page 853
- Isosorbide Dinitrate on page 950
- Isosorbide Mononitrate on page 952
- Nitroglycerin on page 1221
- Nitroprusside on page 1223

Table 3. DRUGS USED IN THE TREATMENT OF HEART FAILURE *(continued)*

Phosphodiesterase Inhibitors
Inamrinone on page 908
Milrinone on page 1140

[1]Regarded as the cornerstone of heart failure treatment and should be used routinely and early in all patients.

Drug Classes and Specific Agents Used to Treat Heart Failure

Angiotensin-converting enzyme (ACE) inhibitors reduce left ventricular volume and filling pressure while decreasing total peripheral resistance. They induce cardiac output (modestly) and natriuresis. ACE inhibitors are usually used in all patients with heart failure if no contraindication or intolerance exists. This group of drugs is considered the cornerstone of treatment and is used routinely and early if pharmacologic treatment is indicated. Angiotensin receptor blockers may be used if a patient cannot tolerate and ACE inhibitor.

Diuretics increase sodium chloride and water excretion resulting in reduction of preload, thus relieving the symptoms of pulmonary congestion associated with heart failure. They may also reduce myocardial oxygen demand. The thiazides, loop diuretics, and potassium-sparing agents are all useful in reducing preload by way of their diuretic actions.

Digitalis glycosides have been used in the treatment of heart failure for more than 200 years. Digitalis drugs increase cardiac output by a direct positive inotropic action on the myocardium. This increased cardiac output results in decreased venous pressure, reduced heart size, and diminished compensatory tachycardia.

Beta-adrenergic receptor blocking drugs (beta-blockers) are used in the treatment of heart failure because of their beneficial effect in reducing mortality. A meta-analysis of randomized clinical trials showed that the beta-blockers significantly reduced all causes of cardiac-related deaths, with carvedilol (Coreg®) showing the greatest efficacy. The overall risk of death was reduced by >30%.

Other drugs used in the treatment of heart failure include aldosterone blockers, catecholamines, and direct-acting vasodilators and phosphodiesterase inhibitors. Direct-acting vasodilators (hydralazine, isosorbide) may be used in place of an ACE inhibitor. The direct-acting vasodilators reduce excessive vasoconstriction and reduce workload of the failing heart. Aldosterone blockers may be used in severe forms of heart failure to enhance survival; close attention to introduction and monitoring is essential to prevent hyperkalemia. The catecholamines and phosphodiesterase inhibitors are alternative agents with positive inotropic effects, are effective for short-term therapy, and have not been demonstrated to prolong life during long-term therapy.

HYPERTENSION

In the United States, almost 50 million adults, 25-74 years of age, have hypertension. Hypertension is defined as systolic blood pressure ≥140 mm Hg, and/or diastolic pressure >90 mm Hg. People with blood pressure above normal are considered at increased risk of developing damage to the heart, kidney, brain, and eyes, resulting in premature morbidity and mortality.

The Joint National Committee on Prevention, Detection, Evaluation, and Treatment of High Blood Pressure, released its 7th Report in the summer of 2003. The highlights of the report are that several of the categories have been renamed to connote changes in philosophy towards earlier treatment and intervention for patients with elevated blood pressure.

Also, there is an increased importance in the elevation of systolic blood pressure for people >50 years of age. The category of high normal blood pressure has now been replaced with the term prehypertension for those patients with systolic blood pressure of 120-139 mm Hg and for those with diastolic blood pressure of 80-89 mm Hg. The remaining stages of hypertension have been broken into simply two categories: Stage 1 and Stage 2. Stage 1 diastolic pressure is 90-99 mm Hg and systolic pressure is 140-159 mm Hg, whereas in Stage 2, diastolic pressure >100 mm Hg or systolic pressure >160 mm Hg are the respective cut-off for treatment decisions. This greatly simplifies the classification of blood pressure.

In addition, the 7th Joint National Committee Report highlights the importance of lifestyle modifications in controlling blood pressure along with pharmacologic intervention. Thiazide diuretics have been considered one of the most important treatments in uncomplicated hypertension and their benefits of lowering blood pressure have been greatly emphasized. The role of dentistry in detection, as well as assisting in compliance for patients, has been clearly emphasized in this report.

The suggested initial goals of drug therapy are the maintenance of an arterial pressure of ≤140/90 mm Hg with concurrent control of other modifiable cardiovascular risk factors. Further reduction to 130/85 mm Hg should be pursued if cardiovascular and cerebrovascular function is not compromised. The Hypertension Optimal Treatment (HOT) randomized trial using patients 50-80 years of age found that the lowest incidence of major cardiovascular events and the lowest risk of cardiovascular mortality occurred at a mean diastolic blood pressure of 82.6 and 86.5 mm Hg, respectively.

Table 4. CLASSIFICATION OF BLOOD PRESSURE FOR ADULTS ≥18 YEARS OF AGE

BP Classification	Systolic BP (mm Hg)	Diastolic BP (mm Hg)
Normotensive	<120	<80
Prehypertension[1]	120-139	80-89
Stage 1 hypertension[2]	140-159	90-99
Stage 2 hypertension[3]	≥160	≥100

[1]Not taking antihypertensive drugs and not acutely ill. When systolic and diastolic blood pressures fall into different categories, the higher category should be selected to classify the individual's blood pressure status. In addition to classifying stages of hypertension on the basis of average blood pressure levels, clinicians should specify presence or absence of target organ disease and additional risk factors. The specificity is important for risk classification and treatment.

[2]Optimal blood pressure with respect to cardiovascular risk is below 120/80 mm Hg. However, unusually low readings should be evaluated for clinical significance.

[3]Based on the average of two or more readings taken at each of two or more visits after an initial screening.

Adapted from Chobanian AV, Bakris GL, Black HR, et al, "Joint National Committee on Prevention, Detection, Evaluation, and Treatment of High Blood Pressure. National Heart, Lung, and Blood Institute; National High Blood Pressure Education Program Coordinating Committee. Seventh Report of the Joint National Committee on Prevention, Detection, Evaluation, and Treatment of High Blood Pressure," *Hypertension*, 2003, 42(6):1206-52.

Table 5. LIFESTYLE MODIFICATIONS TO MANAGE HYPERTENSION[1-3]

Modification	Recommendation	Approximate Systolic Reduction (Range)
Weight reduction	Maintain normal body weight (body mass index 18.5-24.9 kg/m^2)	5-20 mm of mercury/ 10 kg weight loss[4]
Adopt DASH[5] eating plan	Consume a diet rich in fruits, vegetables, and low fat dairy products with a reduced content of saturated and total fat	8-14 mm Hg[6]
Dietary sodium reduction	Reduce dietary sodium intake to ≤100 mmol/day (2.4 g sodium or 6 g sodium chloride)	2-8 mm Hg[7]
Physical activity	Engage in regular aerobic physical activity such as brisk walking (≥30 minutes/day, most days of the week)	4-9 mm Hg[8]
Moderation of alcohol consumption	Limit consumption to ≤2 drinks (1 oz or 30 mL ethanol); (eg, 24 oz beer, 10 oz wine, or 3 oz 80-proof whiskey) per day in most men and to ≤1 drink/day in women and lighter weight people	2-4 mm Hg[9]

[1]Adapted from U.S. Department of Health and Human Services; National Institutes of Health; National Heart, Lung, and Blood Institute; National High Blood Pressure Education Program

[2]Overall cardiovascular risk education can be achieved by cessation of smoking.

[3]The effects of implementing these modifications are dose- and time-dependent and could be greater for some people.

[4]The trials of Hypertension Prevention Collaborative Research Group; He and colleagues

[5]DASH: Dietary Approaches to Stop Hypertension

[6]Sacks and colleagues; Vollmer and colleagues

[7]Sacks and colleagues; Vollmer and colleagues; Chobanian and Hill

[8]Kelley and Kelley; Whelton and colleagues

[9]Xin and colleagues

CLASSES OF DRUGS USED IN THE TREATMENT OF HYPERTENSION

- Diuretics
- Beta-adrenergic receptor blocking agents (beta-blockers)
- Alpha$_1$-adrenergic receptor blocking agents (alpha$_1$-blockers)
- Agents which have both alpha- and beta-adrenergic blocking properties (alpha-/beta-blockers)
- Angiotensin-converting enzyme (ACE) inhibitors
- Angiotensin II receptor blockers
- Calcium channel blocking agents
- Supplemental agents such as central-acting alpha$_2$-adrenergic receptor agonists and direct-acting peripheral vasodilators.

Table 6 lists the drug categories and representative agents used to treat hypertension. Combination drugs are now available to supply several classes of these drugs.

Table 6. DRUG CATEGORIES AND REPRESENTATIVE AGENTS USED IN THE TREATMENT OF HYPERTENSION[1]

Diuretics

Thiazide Types

Chlorothiazide on page 365

Chlorthalidone on page 373

Hydrochlorothiazide on page 854

Indapamide on page 910

Methyclothiazide on page 1107

Metolazone on page 1121

Loops

Bumetanide on page 255

Ethacrynic Acid on page 648

Furosemide on page 796

Torsemide on page 1655

Potassium-Sparing

AMILoride on page 97

Spironolactone on page 1550

Triamterene on page 1674

Beta-Blockers

Cardioselective

Acebutolol on page 29

Atenolol on page 179

Betaxolol (Systemic) on page 233

Bisoprolol on page 240

Metoprolol on page 1122

Nebivolol on page 1190

Sotalol on page 1547

Noncardioselective

Carvedilol on page 318

Nadolol on page 1174

Penbutolol on page 1311

Pindolol on page 1350

Propranolol on page 1422

Timolol (Systemic) on page 1632

Alpha$_1$-Blocker

Doxazosin on page 564

Prazosin on page 1389

Reserpine on page 1467

Terazosin on page 1601

Alpha- / Beta-Blocker

Carvedilol on page 318

Labetalol on page 974

Table 6. DRUG CATEGORIES AND REPRESENTATIVE AGENTS USED IN THE TREATMENT OF HYPERTENSION[1] *(continued)*

Angiotensin-Converting Enzyme (ACE) Inhibitors

Benazepril on page 213

Captopril on page 297

Enalapril on page 596

Fosinopril on page 787

Lisinopril on page 1025

Moexipril on page 1151

Quinapril on page 1444

Ramipril on page 1457

Trandolapril on page 1660

Angiotensin II Receptor Blockers

Candesartan on page 292

Eprosartan on page 613

Irbesartan on page 943

Losartan on page 1037

Telmisartan on page 1592

Valsartan on page 1699

Renin Inhibitor

Aliskiren on page 78

Calcium Channel Blockers

AmLODIPine on page 113

Diltiazem on page 535

Felodipine on page 710

Isradipine on page 955

NiCARdipine on page 1207

NIFEdipine on page 1212

Nisoldipine on page 1217

Verapamil on page 1716

Supplemental Agents

Central-Acting Alpha$_2$-Agonist

CloNIDine on page 416

Guanabenz on page 839

GuanFACINE on page 839

Methyldopa on page 1108

Direct-Acting Peripheral Vasodilator

HydrALAZINE on page 853

Minoxidil (Systemic) on page 1145

Current Thinking Regarding Antihypertensive Drug Selection

Medications in the first eight categories in Table 6 were held to be equally effective in two large-scale studies reported in the *New England Journal of Medicine* and the *Journal of the American Medical Association*, and that any of the medications could be used initially for monotherapy. According to the Seventh Report of the Joint National Committee on Prevention, Detection, Evaluation, and Treatment of High Blood Pressure (JNC VI), diuretics or beta-blockers are recommended as initial therapy for uncomplicated hypertension. If a diuretic is selected as initial therapy, a thiazide diuretic is preferred in patients with normal renal function. If necessary, potassium replacement or concurrent treatment with a potassium-sparing agent may prevent hypokalemia. Loop diuretics are used in patients with impaired renal function or who cannot tolerate thiazides. Diuretics are well-tolerated and inexpensive. They are considered the drugs of choice for treating isolated systolic hypertension in the elderly.

Beta-blockers are the agents of choice in patients with coronary artery disease or supraventricular arrhythmia, and in young patients with hyperdynamic circulation. Beta-blockers are alternatives for initial therapy and are more effective in Caucasian patients than in African-American patients. Beta-blockers are not considered first choice drugs in elderly patients with uncomplicated hypertension. The beta-blocking drug carvedilol also selectively blocks $alpha_1$ receptors and has been shown to reduce mortality in hypertensive patients.

$Alpha_1$-adrenergic blocking agents can be used as initial therapy. The $alpha_1$-blocking agent prazosin and related drugs have an added advantage in treating hypertensive patients with coexisting hyperlipidemia since these medications seem to have beneficial effects on lipid levels. Selective blockade of the postsynaptic $alpha_1$-receptors by prazosin and related agents reduces peripheral vascular resistance and systemic blood pressure. In addition, all $alpha_1$-adrenergic blocking agents relieve symptoms of benign prostatic hyperplasia.

ACE inhibitors are the preferred drugs for patients with coexisting heart failure. They are useful as initial therapy in hypertensive patients with kidney damage or diabetes mellitus with proteinuria, and in Caucasian patients. No clinically relevant differences have been found among the available ACE inhibitors. The ACE inhibitors are well-tolerated by young, physically active patients and the elderly. The most common adverse effect of the ACE inhibitors is dry cough. Angiotensin II receptor blockers produce hemodynamic effects similar to ACE inhibitors while avoiding dry cough. These agents are similar to the ACE inhibitors in potency and are useful for initial therapy.

Calcium channel blocking agents are effective as initial therapy in both African-American and Caucasian patients, and are well-tolerated by the elderly. These agents inhibit entry of calcium ion into cardiac cells and smooth muscle cells of the coronary and systemic vasculature. Nifedipine (Procardia®) and amlodipine (Norvasc®) are more potent as peripheral vasodilators than diltiazem (Cardizem®). Long-acting formulations of the calcium channel blockers have been shown to be very safe despite some earlier reports that short-acting calcium channel blockers were associated with a 60% increase in heart attacks among hypertensive patients given a short-acting calcium antagonist.

Supplemental antihypertensive agents include the central-acting $alpha_2$ agonists and direct-acting vasodilators. These agents are less commonly prescribed for initial therapy because of the impressive effectiveness of the other drug groups. Clonidine (Catapres®) lowers blood pressure by activating inhibitory $alpha_2$ receptors in the CNS, thus reducing sympathetic outflow. It lowers both supine and standing blood pressure by reducing total peripheral resistance. Hydralazine reduces blood pressure by directly relaxing arteriolar smooth muscle. Hydralazine is given orally for the management of chronic hypertension, usually with a diuretic and a beta-blocker.

The most common oral side effects of the management of the hypertensive patient are related to the antihypertensive drug therapy. A dry, sore mouth can be caused by diuretics and central-acting adrenergic inhibitors. Occasionally, lichenoid reactions can occur in patients taking quinidine and methyldopa. The thiazides are occasionally also implicated. Lupus-like face rashes can be seen in patients taking calcium channel blockers as well.

Table 7. CARDIOVASCULAR / RESPIRATORY / NERVOUS SYSTEM EFFECTS CAUSED BY DRUGS USED FOR CARDIOVASCULAR DISORDERS[1]

Agent	Incidence	Adverse Effect
$Alpha_1$-Blocker		
Prazosin (Minipress®)	*More frequent*	Orthostatic hypotension, dizziness
	Less frequent	Heart Palpitations
	Rare	Angina
Alpha- / Beta-Blocker		
Carvedilol (Coreg®)	*More frequent*	Bradycardia, postural hypotension, dizziness
	Rare	A-V block, hypertension, hypotension, palpitations, vertigo, nervousness, asthma
Angiotensin-Converting Enzyme (ACE) Inhibitors		
Benazepril (Lotensin®)	*Less frequent*	Dizziness, insomnia, headache
	Rare	Hypotension, bronchitis
Captopril (Capoten®)	*Less frequent*	Tachycardia, insomnia, transient cough, dizziness, headache
	Rare	Hypotension

(continued)

Agent	Incidence	Adverse Effect
Enalapril (Vasotec®)	*Less frequent*	Chest pain, palpitations, tachycardia, syncope, dizziness, dyspnea
	Rare	Angina pectoris, asthma
Fosinopril (Monopril®)	*Less frequent*	Orthostatic hypotension, dizziness, cough, headache
	Rare	Syncope, insomnia
Lisinopril (Prinivil®)	*Less frequent*	Hypotension, dizziness
	Rare	Angina pectoris, orthostatic hypotension, rhythm disturbances, tachycardia
Moexipril (Univasc®)	*Less frequent*	Hypotension, peripheral edema, headache, dizziness, fatigue, cough, pharyngitis, upper respiratory infection, sinusitis
	Rare	Chest pain, myocardial infarction, palpitations, arrhythmias, syncope, CVA, orthostatic hypotension, dyspnea, bronchospasm
Perindopril Erbumine (Aceon®)	*Less frequent*	Headache, dizziness, cough[2]
	Rare	Hypotension
Quinapril (Accupril®)	*Less frequent*	Hypotension, dizziness, headache, cough
	Rare	Orthostatic hypotension, angina, insomnia
Ramipril (Altace®)	*Less frequent*	Tachycardia, dizziness, headache, cough
	Rare	Hypotension
Trandolapril (Mavik®)	*Less frequent*	Tachycardia, headache, dizziness, cough[3]
	Rare	Hypotension
Angiotensin-Converting Enzyme (ACE) Inhibitor / Diuretic Combination		
Captopril/HCTZ (Capozide®)	*Less frequent*	Tachycardia, palpitations, chest pain, dizziness
	Rare	Hypotension
Angiotensin II Receptor Blockers		
Candesartan (Atacand®)	*Less frequent*	Chest pain, flushing
	Rare	Myocardial infarction, tachycardia, angina, palpitations, dyspnea
Losartan (Cozaar®)	*Less frequent*	Hypotension without reflex tachycardia, dizziness
	Rare	Orthostatic hypotension, angina, A-V block (second degree), CVA, palpitations, tachycardia, sinus bradycardia, flushing, dyspnea
Angiotensin II Receptor Blocker / Diuretic Combination		
Candesartan (Atacand HCT™) + HCTZ	*Less frequent*	Chest pain, flushing
	Rare	Myocardial infarction, tachycardia, angina, palpitations, dyspnea
Irbesartan/HCTZ (Avalide®)		Effects unavailable
Valsartan/HCTZ (Diovan HCT®)		Effects unavailable
Antiplatelet / Anticoagulant Agents		
Abciximab (ReoPro®)	*More frequent*	Hypotension, pain
	Less frequent	Bradycardia
Aspirin	*Less frequent or Rare*	Anaphylactoid reaction, bronchospastic allergic reaction
Clopidogrel (Plavix®)	*Less frequent*	Chest pain, edema, hypertension, headache, dizziness, depression, fatigue, dyspnea, rhinitis, bronchitis, coughing, upper respiratory infection, syncope, palpitations, cardiac failure, paresthesia, vertigo, atrial fibrillation, neuralgia
Eptifibatide (Integrilin®)	*More frequent*	Hypotension, bleeding
Ticlopidine (Ticlid®)	*Less frequent*	Dizziness
	Rare	Peripheral neuropathy, angioedema, vasculitis, allergic pneumonitis
Tirofiban (Aggrastat®)	*More frequent*	Bleeding
	Less frequent	Bradycardia, dizziness, headache

(continued)

Agent	Incidence	Adverse Effect
Warfarin (Coumadin®)	*Less frequent*	Hemoptysis
	Rare	Fever, purple toes syndrome
Beta-Blockers		
Acebutolol (Sectral®)	*Less frequent*	Chest pain, bradycardia, hypotension, dizziness, dyspepsia, dyspnea
	Rare	Ventricular arrhythmias
Atenolol (Tenormin®)	*Less frequent*	Bradycardia, hypotension, chest pain, dizziness, dyspepsia, dyspnea
	Rare	Ventricular arrhythmias
Betaxolol (Kerlone®)	*Less frequent*	Bradycardia, palpitations, dizziness
	Rare	Chest pain
Bisoprolol (Zebeta®)	*More frequent*	Lethargy
	Less frequent	Hypotension, chest pain, bradycardia, headache, dizziness, insomnia, cough
Labetalol (Trandate®)	*Less frequent*	Orthostatic hypotension, dizziness, nasal congestion
	Rare	Bradycardia, chest pain
Metoprolol (Lopressor®)	*More frequent*	Dizziness
	Less frequent	Bradycardia, heartburn, wheezing
	Rare	Chest pain, confusion
Nadolol (Corgard®)	*More frequent*	Bradycardia
	Less frequent	Dizziness, dyspepsia, wheezing
	Rare	Congestive heart failure, orthostatic hypotension, confusion, paresthesia
Penbutolol (Levatol®)	*Less frequent*	Congestive heart failure, dizziness
	Rare	Bradycardia, chest pain, hypotension, confusion
Pindolol	*More frequent*	Dizziness
	Less frequent	Congestive heart failure, dyspnea
Propranolol (Inderal®)	*More frequent*	Bradycardia
	Less frequent	Congestive heart failure, dizziness, wheezing
	Rare	Chest pain, hypotension, bronchospasm
Timolol (Blocadren®)	*Less frequent*	Bradycardia, dizziness, dyspnea
	Rare	Chest pain, congestive heart failure
Calcium Channel Blockers		
AmLODIPine (Norvasc®)	*Less frequent*	Palpitations, dizziness, dyspnea
	Rare	Hypotension, bradycardia, arrhythmias
Diltiazem (Cardizem®)	*Less frequent*	Bradycardia, dizziness
	Rare	Dyspepsia, paresthesia, tremor
NIFEdipine (Procardia®)	*More frequent*	Flushing, dizziness
	Less frequent	Palpitations, hypotension, dyspnea
	Rare	Tachycardia, syncope
Verapamil (Calan®)	*Less frequent*	Bradycardia, congestive heart failure, hypotension
	Rare	Chest pain, hypotension (excessive)
Class I Antiarrhythmics		
Disopyramide (Norpace®)	*More frequent*	Exacerbation of angina pectoris, dizziness
	Less frequent	Hypotension, hypertension, tachycardia, dyspnea
	Rare	Syncope, flushing, hyperventilation
Flecainide (Tambocor™)	*More frequent*	Dizziness, dyspnea
	Less frequent	Palpitations, chest pain, tachycardia, tremor
	Rare	Bradycardia, nervousness, paresthesia
Procainamide (Procanbid®)	*Less frequent*	Tachycardia, dizziness, lightheadedness
	Rare	Hypotension, confusion, disorientation

(continued)

Agent	Incidence	Adverse Effect
Propafenone (Rythmol®)	*More frequent*	Dizziness
	Less frequent	Palpitations, angina, bradycardia, loss of balance, dyspepsia, dyspnea
	Rare	Paresthesia
QuiNIDine	*Less frequent*	Hypotension, syncope, lightheadedness, wheezing
	Rare	Confusion, vertigo, angina, edema
Class III Antiarrhythmics		
Amiodarone (Cordarone®)	*More frequent*	Dizziness, tremor, paresthesia, dyspnea
	Less frequent	Congestive heart failure, bradycardia, tachycardia
	Rare	Hypotension
Sotalol (Betapace®)	*More frequent*	Bradycardia, chest pain, palpitations, fatigue, dizziness, lightheadedness, dyspnea
	Less frequent	Congestive heart failure, hypotension, proarrhythmia, syncope, reduced peripheral circulation, edema, asthma, upper respiratory problems
	Rare	Diaphoresis, clouded sensorium, fever, lack of coordination
Digitalis Glycosides		
Digoxin (Lanoxicaps®, Lanoxin®)	*Rare*	Atrial tachycardia, sinus bradycardia, ventricular fibrillation, vertigo
Diuretics		
Thiazide type	*Rare*	Hypotension
Loops	*More frequent*	Orthostatic hypotension, dizziness
Potassium-sparing	*Less frequent*	Hypotension, bradycardia, dizziness
	Rare	Flushing
Potassium-sparing combination	*Rare*	Dizziness
HMG-CoA Reductase Inhibitors		
Atorvastatin Fluvastatin Lovastatin Pravastatin Simvastatin	*Less frequent*	Headache, dizziness
Nitrates		
Nitroglycerins	*More frequent*	Postural hypotension, flushing, headache, dizziness
	Rare	Reflex tachycardia, bradycardia, arrhythmia
Supplemental Drugs for Heart Failure		
Inamrinone	*Less frequent*	Arrhythmia, chest pain
DOBUTamine	*Less frequent*	Tachycardia, chest pain
	Rare	Headache, dyspnea
HydrALAZINE	*More frequent*	Tachycardia, headache
	Less frequent	Hypotension, nasal congestion
	Rare	Edema, dizziness
Milrinone (Primacor®)	*More frequent*	Arrhythmias
	Less frequent	Chest pain
Nitroprusside sodium (Nitropress®)	*Less frequent*	Palpitations, headache
Supplemental Drugs for Hypertension		
Central-Acting Alpha$_2$-Agonists		
CloNIDine (Catapres®)	*More frequent*	Dizziness
	Less frequent	Orthostatic hypotension, nervousness/agitation
	Rare	Palpitations, tachycardia, bradycardia, congestive heart failure

(continued)

Agent	Incidence	Adverse Effect
Direct-Acting		
HydrALAZINE	*More frequent*	Tachycardia, headache
	Less frequent	Hypotension, nasal congestion
	Rare	Edema, dizziness

Legend: % of incidence: More frequent = >10%, less frequent = 1% to 10%, rare = <1%.

[1]Source: Professional package insert for individual agents or United States Pharmacopeial Dispensing Information. *Drug Information for the Health Care Professional*, Vol I, 19th ed, Rockville, MD: The United States Pharmacopeial Convention, Inc, 1999.

[2]Incidence greater in women 3:1.

[3]More frequent in women.

Table 8. CARDIOVASCULAR DRUGS DENTAL DRUG INTERACTIONS AND EFFECTS ON DENTAL TREATMENT

Alpha$_1$-Blocker	
Prazosin (Minipress®)	Significant orthostatic hypotension a possibility; monitor patient when getting out of dental chair; significant dry mouth in up to 10% of patients.
Alpha- / Beta-Blocker	
Carvedilol (Coreg®)	See Nonselective Beta-Blockers
ACE Inhibitors	The NSAID indomethacin reduces the hypotensive effects of ACE inhibitors. Effects of other NSAIDs, such as ibuprofen, are not considered significant.
Angiotensin-Converting Enzyme (ACE) Inhibitor / Diuretic Combination	
Captopril/HCTZ (Capozide®)	No effect or complications on dental treatment reported.
Angiotensin II Receptor Blockers	
Candesartan (Atacand®)	No effect or complications on dental treatment reported.
Losartan (Cozaar®)	
Antiplatelet / Anticoagulant Agents	
Aspirin	May cause a reduction in the serum levels of NSAIDs if they are used to manage postoperative pain.
Clopidogrel (Plavix®)	If a patient is to undergo elective surgery and an antiplatelet effect is not desired, clopidogrel should be discontinued 7-14 days prior to surgery, but thromboembolic risk must be considered and any alteration should be done only with medical agreement.
Prasugrel (Effient™)	
Eptifibatide (Integrilin®)	Bleeding may occur while patient is medicated with eptifibatide; platelet function is restored in about 4 hours following discontinuation.
Warfarin (Coumadin®)	Signs of warfarin overdose may first appear as bleeding from gingival tissue; consultation with prescribing physician is advisable prior to surgery to determine temporary dose reduction or withdrawal of medication.
Beta-Blockers	
Cardioselective	Cardioselective beta-blockers (ie, atenolol) have no effect or complications on dental treatment reported.
Noncardioselective	Any of the noncardioselective beta-blockers (ie, nadolol, penbutolol, pindolol, propranolol, timolol) may enhance the pressor response to vasoconstrictor epinephrine resulting in hypertension and reflex bradycardia. Although not reported, it is assumed that similar effects could be caused with levonordefrin (Neo-Cobefrin®). Use either vasoconstrictor with caution in hypertensive patients medicated with noncardioselective beta-adrenergic blockers.
Calcium Channel Blockers (CB)	Cause gingival hyperplasia in approximately 1% of the general population taking these drugs. There have been fewer reports with diltiazem and amlodipine than with other CBs such as nifedipine. The hyperplasia will usually disappear with cessation of drug therapy. Consultation with the physician is suggested.

(continued)

Class I Antiarrhythmics	
Disopyramide (Norpace®)	Increased serum levels and toxicity with erythromycin. High incidence of anticholinergic effect manifested as dry mouth and throat.
Flecainide (Tambocor™)	No effect or complications on dental treatment reported.
Procainamide (Procanbid®)	Systemic lupus-like syndrome has been reported resulting in joint pain and swelling, pains with breathing, skin rash.
Propafenone (Rythmol®)	Greater than 10% experience significantly reduced salivary flow; taste disturbance, bitter or metallic taste
QuiNIDine	Secondary anticholinergic effects may decrease salivary flow, especially in middle-aged and elderly patients; known to contribute to caries, periodontal disease, and oral candidiasis.
Class III Antiarrhythmics	
Amiodarone	Bitter or metallic taste has been reported.
Digitalis Glycosides	Use vasoconstrictor with caution due to risk of cardiac arrhythmias. Sensitive gag reflex induced by digitalis drugs may cause difficulty in taking dental impressions.
Diuretics	
Thiazide type	No effect or complications on dental treatment reported.
Loops	NSAIDs may increase chloride and tubular water reuptake to counteract loop type diuretics.
Potassium-sparing	No effect or complications on dental treatment reported.
Potassium-sparing combination	No effect or complications on dental treatment reported.
HMG-CoA Reductase Inhibitors	Concurrent use of erythromycin, clarithromycin, and some of the statin drugs may result in rhabdomyolysis.
Nitrates	No effect or complications on dental treatment reported.
Supplemental Drugs for Heart Failure	
Inamrinone Milrinone (Primacor®)	No effect or complications on dental treatment reported
Supplemental Drugs for Hypertension	
Central-Acting Alpha$_2$-Agonists	
CloNIDine (Catapres®)	Greater than 10% of patients experience significant dry mouth.
Direct-Acting	
HydrALAZINE	No effect or complications on dental treatment reported.

REFERENCES

Bader JD, Bonito AJ, and Shugars DA, "A Systematic Review of Cardiovascular Effects of Epinephrine on Hypertensive Dental Patients," *Oral Surg Oral Med Oral Pathol Oral Radiol Endod*, 2002, 93(6):647-53.

Beck JD and Offenbacher S, "Systemic Effects of Periodontitis: Epidemiology of Periodontal Disease and Cardiovascular Disease," *J Periodontol*, 2005, 76(11 Suppl):2089-100.

Chobanian AV and Hill M, "National Heart, Lung, and Blood Institute Workshop on Sodium and Blood Pressure: A Critical Review of Current Scientific Evidence," *Hypertension*, 2000, 35(4):858-63.

Chobanian AV, Bakris GL, Black HR, et al, "The Seventh Report of the Joint National Committee on Prevention, Detection, Evaluation, and Treatment of High Blood Pressure: The JNC 7 Report," *JAMA*, 2003, 289(19):2560-72.

Colucci WS and Braunwald E, "Pathophysiology of Heart Failure," *Braunwald's Heart Disease: A Textbook Of Cardiovascular Medicine*, 7th ed, Zipes D, Libby P, and Bonow RO, eds, Philadelphia, PA: WB Saunders Co, 2005.

"Effects of Weight Loss and Sodium Reduction Intervention on Blood Pressure and Hypertension Incidence in Overweight People With High-Normal Blood Pressure. The Trials of Hypertension Prevention, Phase II. The Trials of Hypertension Prevention Collaborative Research Group," *Arch Intern Med*, 1997, 157(6):657-67.

Hajjar I, Kotchen JM, and Kotchen TA, "Hypertension: Trends in Prevalence, Incidence, and Control," *Annu Rev Public Health*, 2006, 27:465-90.

He J, Whelton PK, Appel LJ, et al, "Long-Term Effects of Weight Loss and Dietary Sodium Reduction on Incidence of Hypertension," *Hypertension*, 2000, 35(2):544-9.

Hunt SA, Abraham WT, Chin MH, et al, "2009 Focused Update Incorporated into the ACC/AHA 2005 Guidelines for the Diagnosis and Management of Heart Failure in Adults A Report of the American College of Cardiology Foundation/American Heart Association Task Force on Practice Guidelines Developed in Collaboration With the International Society for Heart and Lung Transplantation," *J Am Coll Cardiol*, 2009, 53(15):e1-e90.

Kelley GA and Kelley KS, "Progressive Resistance Exercise and Resting Blood Pressure: A Meta-Analysis of Randomized Controlled Trials," *Hypertension*, 2000, 35(3):838-43.

Pickering TG, Hall JE, Appel LJ, et al, "Recommendations for Blood Pressure Measurement in Humans and Experimental Animals: Part 1: Blood Pressure Measurement in Humans: A Statement for Professionals From the Subcommittee of Professional and Public Education of the American Heart Association Council on High Blood Pressure Research," *Circulation*, 2005, 111(5):697-716.

Sacks FM, Svetkey LP, Vollmer WM, et al, "Effects on Blood Pressure of Reduced Dietary Sodium and the Dietary Approaches to Stop Hypertension (DASH) Diet. DASH-Sodium Collaborative Research Group," *N Engl J Med*, 2001, 344(1):3-10.

Vollmer WM, Sacks FM, Ard J, et al, "Effects of Diet and Sodium Intake on Blood Pressure: Subgroup Analysis of the DASH-Sodium Trial," *Ann Intern Med*, 2001, 135(12):1019-28.
Whelton SP, Chin A, Xin X, et al, "Effect of Aerobic Exercise on Blood Pressure: A Meta-Analysis of Randomized, Controlled Trials," *Ann Intern Med*, 2002, 136(7):493-503.
Xin X, He J, Frontini MG, et al, "Effects of Alcohol Reduction on Blood Pressure: A Meta-Analysis of Randomized Controlled Trials," *Hypertension*, 2001, 38(5):1112-7.

CARDIOVASCULAR DISEASE IN WOMEN

AMERICAN HEART ASSOCIATION GUIDELINES FOR REDUCING CARDIOVASCULAR RISK IN WOMEN

Most cardiovascular disease (CVD) in women is preventable, according to the American Heart Association (AHA). In 1999, the AHA published a set of guidelines based on a 1997 review of the literature that described risk factor management and occurrence of CVD in women. The AHA has updated the 1999 guidelines, making specific recommendations, which provide a general approach to the female patient according to risk.

Cardiovascular disease is the largest single cause of death among women worldwide and accounts for one-third of all deaths. New reports have shown that in the United States, more women than men die every year of CVD. In the United States, $403 billion was estimated to be spent in 2006 on health care or in lost productivity as a result of CVD, compared to $190 billion for cancer and $29 billion for human immunodeficiency virus (HIV).

In general the women who are at risk of CVD are those that have more than one major risk factor for CVD including:

- Cigarette smoking
- Poor diet
- Inactive physically
- Obesity
- Family history of CVD at <55 years of age in male relative and <65 years of age in female relative
- Hypertension
- Dyslipidemia
- Evidence of subclinical vascular disease (eg, coronary calcification)
- Metabolic syndrome
- Poor exercise capacity on treadmill test
- Abnormal heart rate recovery after stopping exercise

Specific Recommendations:

Aspirin:

Aspirin use in high risk women

As a preventive drug intervention in women, aspirin therapy at a dose of 75-325 mg/day should be used in high risk women unless contraindicated. High risk women were defined as those with established coronary artery disease, cerebrovascular disease, or peripheral artery disease.

It was noted that the upper dosage of aspirin for high risk women increases to 325 mg/day rather than 162 mg.

Aspirin use for other at risk or healthy women

In women ≥65 years of age, consider aspirin therapy 81 mg/day or 100 mg every other day if blood pressure is controlled and benefit for ischemic stroke and myocardial infarction (MI) prevention is likely to outweigh the risk of gastrointestinal bleeding and hemorrhagic stroke. The same aspirin regimen can be used in women <65 years of age when benefit for ischemic stroke prevention is likely to outweigh adverse effects of therapy. However, the new guidelines suggested that the routine use of aspirin in healthy women <65 years of age is not recommended to prevent MI. It was noted in these new guidelines that previous guidelines by the AHA did not recommend aspirin at all in lower risk or healthy women.

Smoking Cessation: The new guidelines suggest smokers try behavioral modification programs, counseling, nicotine replacement therapy, or prescription smoking cessation medications such as varenicline (Chantix™) or bupropion (Zyban®). Also, women should avoid environmental tobacco smoke.

Exercise: Women should accumulate a minimum of 30 minutes of moderate-intensity physical activity on most, and preferably all, days of the week.

Obesity and Exercise: Women who need to lose weight or sustain weight loss should accumulate a minimum of 60-90 minutes of moderate-intensity physical activity, such as brisk walking, on most days of the week.

Dietary Intake: Consume a diet rich in fruits and vegetables. Choose whole grain, high fiber foods. Consume fish, especially oily fish, such as mackerel or salmon at least twice a week. Limit intake of dietary saturated fat to <10% of caloric intake. Limit cholesterol intake to <300 mg/day. Limit sodium intake to no more than 1 teaspoonful daily. Limit consumption of trans-fatty acids to <1% of caloric intake.

Alcohol Consumption: Limit to no more than one drink per day. A drink is equivalent to a 12 ounce bottle of beer, a 5 ounce glass of wine, or a 1.5 ounce shot of 80 proof spirit. It does not matter what form of alcohol is consumed. In contrast to the recommendations by the AHA for moderate alcohol intake as part of the updated guidelines for heart disease prevention in women, a recent report showed that alcohol consumption increases the risk of breast cancer. One to two drinks per day increased the risk of breast cancer by 10% and excessive drinking defined as three or more drinks per day increased the risk by 30%. The researchers examined data from 70,033 women who gave health information during medical examinations during 1978-1985. In 2004, follow ups indicated that 2829 of the women in the study were diagnosed with breast cancer. The study examined alcohol preferences, frequency of drinking one type of alcohol, and overall alcohol consumption. High consumption of any alcohol was linked with a significant increased risk of being diagnosed with breast cancer.

Omega-3 Fatty Acids: As an adjunct to diet, omega-3 fatty acids in capsule form (approximately 850-1000 mg of EPA [eicosapentaenoic acid] and DHA [docosahexaenoic acid] should be considered in those with coronary heart disease and higher doses [2-4 g]) may be used for treatment of women with high triglyceride levels.

In addition, the new guidelines suggested that the following interventions were not useful and may be harmful for CVD or MI in women.

Menopausal Therapy: Hormone replacement therapy, such as Premarin® and Prempro™, and selective estrogen-receptor modulators (SERMs), such as raloxifene (Evista®), should not be used for the primary prevention or secondary prevention of CVD.

Antioxidant Supplements: Antioxidant vitamin supplements such as vitamin E, C, or beta-carotene should not be used for the primary or secondary prevention of CVD.

Folic Acid: Folic acid, with or without vitamin B_6 and B_{12} supplementation, should not be used for the primary or secondary prevention of CVD.

REFERENCES

Mosca L, Grundy SM, Judelson D, et al, "Guide to Preventive Cardiology for Women. AHA/ACC Scientific Statement Consensus Panel Statement," *Circulation*, 1999, 99(18):2480-4.

Mosca L, Linfante AH, Benjamin EJ, et al, "National Study of Physician Awareness and Adherence to Cardiovascular Disease Prevention Guidelines," *Circulation*, 2005, 111(4):499-510.

ANTIPLATELET AND ANTICOAGULATION CONSIDERATIONS IN DENTISTRY

Over the last 30 years, there has been an increasing use of drugs that relate to the clotting mechanisms in patients. These drugs have included the widespread use of aspirin, as well as an increasing use of anticoagulants found in warfarin and synthetic drugs that also have anticoagulation effects. Many patients with ischemic heart disease, atherosclerosis, atrial fibrillation, and in patients at high risk for stroke, we find the increased use of these anticoagulants. Large numbers of these patients are receiving oral anticoagulation therapy as outpatients. The dental clinician is often faced with the decision as to how to manage these patients prior to dental procedures. Key factors regarding the patient receiving any form of anticoagulation therapy include:

- Is the surgery urgent or elective?
- Can the procedure be done safely without discontinuing the drug?
- Does the patient understand the nature of the dental procedure and the risks associated with continuing or discontinuing the drug?
- What degree of risk are the patient and the provider willing to accept?
- Is the patient on a single antiplatelet drug or on combination therapy with another drug?
- What is the thromboembolic risk for this patient?
- What is the bleeding risk of the dental procedure planned?
- If an invasive procedure is planned in the face of a high thromboembolic risk, what is the managing physician's opinion on altering the dosage of anticoagulation therapy?

Often, in order to determine these factors, consultation with a patient's physician is necessary. However, recent reviews have argued that inappropriate adjustments in anticoagulation therapy create far greater risk for the patient than the risk of hemorrhage during most dental procedures (Jeske, 2003 and others in the reference list). Therefore, the scientific evidence does not support changing regimens of anticoagulation therapy in most instances. This decision can only be determined by weighing the factors described above and discussing the situation with the patient's physician.

Antiplatelet Drugs Used in Cardiovascular Diseases

Aspirin reduces platelet aggregation by blocking platelet cyclo-oxygenase through irreversible acetylation. This action prevents the formation of thromboxane A_2. A number of studies have confirmed that aspirin reduces the risk of death from cardiac causes and fatal and nonfatal myocardial infarction by ~50% to 70% in patients presenting with unstable angina (see Aspirin Alert Update for Dentistry at the end of this chapter).

Clopidogrel inhibits platelet aggregation by affecting the ADP-dependent activation of the glycoprotein IIb/IIIa complex. Clopidogrel is chemically related to ticlopidine but has fewer side effects.

Prasugrel is a prodrug and has no biological activity but is metabolized in the body to an active molecule exhibiting antiplatelet action. The active compound irreversibly blocks P2Y12 component of adenosine diphosphate (ADP) receptors on the platelet for their lifespan, inhibiting activation and decreasing subsequent platelet aggregation. Normal platelet aggregation returns only when new platelets are produced (5-9 days after discontinuation of prasugrel).

Platelet Glycoprotein IIb / IIIa Receptor Antagonists

Antagonists of glycoprotein IIb/IIIa, a receptor on the platelet for adhesive proteins, inhibit the final common pathway involved in adhesion, activation, and aggregation. Presently, there exist three classes of inhibitors. One class is murine-human chimeric antibodies of which abciximab is the prototype. The other two classes are the synthetic peptide forms (eg, eptifibatide) and the synthetic nonpeptide forms (eg, tirofiban). These agents, in combination with heparin and aspirin, have been used to treat unstable angina, significantly reducing the incidence of death or myocardial infarction.

Antithrombin Drugs

Unfractionated heparin, in combination with aspirin, is used to treat unstable angina. Unfractionated heparin consists of polysaccharide chains which bind to antithrombin III, causing a conformational change that accelerates the inhibition of thrombin and factor Xa. Unfractionated heparin is therefore an indirect thrombin inhibitor. Unfractionated heparin can only be administered intravenously. Low-molecular-weight heparins (LMWH) have a more predictable pharmacokinetic profile than unfractionated heparin and can be administered subcutaneously. These heparins have a mechanism of action and use similar to unfractionated heparin.

The direct antithrombins decrease thrombin activity in a manner independent of any actions on antithrombin III. Two such direct antithrombins are lepirudin (also known as recombinant hirudin) and argatroban. These agents are highly specific. They bind directly to thrombin (circulating and clot bound) and inhibit thrombogenic activity. Direct antithrombins are used for the prevention or reduction of ischemic complications associated with unstable angina.

Warfarin (Coumadin®) elicits its anticoagulant effect by interfering with the hepatic synthesis of vitamin K-dependent coagulation factors II, VII, IX, and X. Although warfarin appears to be somewhat effective after myocardial infarction in preventing death or recurrent myocardial infarction, its effectiveness in the treatment of acute coronary syndrome is questionable. Combination therapy with aspirin and heparin, followed by warfarin, has resulted in reduced incidence of recurrent angina, myocardial infarction, death, or all three at 14 days as compared with aspirin alone. In contrast, another study failed to show any additional benefit in the treatment of acute coronary syndrome using a combination of aspirin and warfarin compared to aspirin alone.

Recently, the FDA approved Dabigatran (Pradaxa®) for the prevention of stroke and systemic embolism in patients with atrial fibrillation. Dabigatran is the first FDA-approved replacement available for warfarin.

Dabigatran is an anticoagulant that acts by inhibiting thrombin, an enzyme in the blood that is involved in blood clotting. Thrombin (serine protease) enables the conversion of fibrinogen to fibrin during the coagulation cascade preventing the development of thrombus. The recommended oral dose is 150 mg twice daily for patients with a creatinine clearance >30 mL/minute. For patients with a creatinine clearance 15-30 mL/minute, the recommended oral dose is 75 mg twice daily.

Dental clinicians should consider consultation with patient's healthcare provider prior to invasive therapies. However, recent reviews have argued that inappropriate adjustments in anticoagulation therapy places the patient at far greater risk of stroke than hemorrhage during most dental procedures (Jeske, 2003). Therefore, scientific evidence does not support changing regimens of anticoagulation therapy in most instances.

Evaluating Antiplatelet Response

Partial thromboplastin time and bleeding time (IVY) are appropriate measures for platelet dysfunction. Aspirin, Clopidogrel (Plavix®), Prasugrel (Effient™), and other drugs, such as ticlopidine (Ticlid®) are considered antiplatelet drugs, whereas oral Coumadin® is considered an oral anticoagulant. Aspirin works by inhibiting cyclooxygenase which is an enzyme involved in the platelet system associated with clot formation. As little as one aspirin (300 mg dose) can result in an alteration in this enzyme pathway. Although aspirin is cleared from the circulation very quickly (within 15-30 minutes), the effect on the life of the platelet may last up to 7-10 days. Most routine dental procedures can be accomplished with no change in these medications using aggressive local hemostasis efforts and prudent treatment planning.

Evaluating Coumadin® Response

The effects of Coumadin® on the coagulation within patients occur by way of the vitamin K-dependent clotting mechanism and are generally monitored by measuring the prothrombin time known as the PT. Often, to prevent venous thrombosis, a patient will be maintained at approximately 2.5 times their normal prothrombin time. Other anticoagulant goals, such as prevention of arterial thromboembolism as in patients with artificial heart valves, may require 2.5-3.5 times the normal prothrombin time. It is important for the clinician to obtain not only the accurate PT but also the International Normalized Ratio (INR) for the patient. This ratio is calculated by dividing the patient's PT by the mean normal PT for the laboratory, which is determined by using the International Sensitivity Index (ISI) to adjust for the lab's reagents.

The response to oral anticoagulants varies greatly in patients and should be monitored regularly. The dental clinician planning an invasive procedure should consider not only what the patient can tell them from a historical point-of-view, but also when the last monitoring test was performed. In general, all dental procedures can be performed in patients that are 3 times normal or less. Most researchers further suggest that even less than 4 times normal pose little risk in most dental patients and procedures, but these values may be misleading unless the INR is also determined at a time close to the actual planned dental procedure. When in doubt, the prudent dental clinician will consult with the patient's physician and obtain current prothrombin time and INR in order to evaluate fully and plan for his patients.

At recommended therapeutic doses, dabigatran (Pradaxa™) prolongs the activated partial thromboplastin time (aPTT). For an oral dose of 150 mg twice daily, the median peak aPTT is approximately twice that of control values. Twelve hours after the last dose, the median aPTT is 1.5 times the control values. The INR test is relatively insensitive to the activity of dabigatran and may not be elevated in patients on this medication.

Regarding dental management patients that are already taking warfarin, the use of analgesics is implicated as a potential source of drug interaction. In an article by Hayek in *JAMA*, it was found that patients taking warfarin for anticoagulation identified the use of dangerously elevated INRs and the fact was discovered that they concomitantly had been taking acetaminophen (not necessarily with their physician's recommendation). The study of the international normalized ratio (INR) in these patients has indicated that additional factors independently influence the INR, as well as the potential interaction with acetaminophen. Potential effects on the INR are greatest in patients taking acetaminophen at high doses over a protracted time period. Short-term pain management with acetaminophen poses little risk. These factors included advanced malignancy, patients who did not take their warfarin properly (therefore, took more than was necessary), changes in oral intake of liquids or solids, acute diarrhea leading to dehydration, alcohol consumption, and vitamin K intake.

The mechanisms of these augmenting factors for enhancement of the INR are that the cytochrome P450 system is also affected by changes in metabolism associated with these factors. For instance, the metabolism of alcohol in the liver alters its ability to manage the CYP450 enzyme system necessary for warfarin; therefore, enhancing its presence and potentially increasing the half-life of warfarin. As oral intake of nutrients declines in patients with either diarrhea or reduced intake of liquids and/or solids, absorption of vitamin K is reduced and the vitamin K-dependent system of metabolism of warfarin changes, therefore increases warfarin blood levels. These factors, along with the liver metabolism of acetaminophen, have resulted in the increased concern that patients, who may be taking acetaminophen as an analgesic or for other reasons, may be at risk for enhancing or elevating, inadvertently, their anticoagulation effect of warfarin. The dentist should be aware of these potential interactions in prescribing any drug containing acetaminophen or in recommending that a patient use an analgesic for relief of even mild pain on a prolonged basis.

Acetaminophen on page 32

It should also be noted that as we learn more about herbal and nutritional supplements, we will find that some of these products have affects on coagulation. Patients sometimes do not include this information in their normal history and it is important for the practitioner to delve into all types of over-the-counter, as well as prescription drugs, that the patient may be taking.

Although not used specifically for this purpose, numerous herbal medicines and natural dietary supplements have been associated with inhibition of platelet aggregation or other anticoagulation effects, and therefore may lead to increased bleeding during invasive dental procedures. Current reports include bilberry, bromelain, cat's claw, devil's claw, dong quai, evening primrose, feverfew, garlic (irreversible inhibition), ginger (only at very high doses), ginkgo biloba, ginseng, grape seed, green tea, horse chestnut, and turmeric.

ASPIRIN ALERT UPDATE FOR DENTISTRY

There are three special alerts provided by the FDA of clinical importance relative to the aspirin patient:

Special Alert 1: Sudden aspirin discontinuation may elevate the risk of myocardial infarction

It was reported in 2004 by Collett et al, that patients with acute coronary syndrome (ACS) who discontinued aspirin use had worse short-term outcomes than individuals not previously on aspirin therapy. Fischer et al, have also reported similar findings and have suggested that discontinuation of aspirin by daily aspirin users may increase the risk of myocardial infarction. A Harvard Health Letter in 2005 also stated that quitting aspirin "cold turkey" could be dangerous and studies have linked aspirin withdrawal to heart attacks.

A more recent review updated the risks associated with discontinuing aspirin antiplatelet therapy and the bleeding risks associated with continuing aspirin during surgical procedures (Lordkipanidze, 2009). The article review confirmed the possibility of a pharmacological rebound phenomenon which could lead to adverse ischemic events and supports the warning against premature discontinuation of aspirin issued previously. An analysis of data obtained from 50,279 patients, reported that the increased risk of major adverse cardiac events attributed to aspirin withdrawal/nonadherence was approximately threefold (Biondi-Zoccai, 2006).

Special Alert 2: Ibuprofen may interfere with aspirin's cardioprotection

In a statement released on September 8, 2006, the Food and Drug Administration (FDA) notified consumers and healthcare professionals that the administration of ibuprofen for pain relief to patients taking aspirin for cardioprotection may interfere with aspirin's cardiovascular benefits. The report stated that ibuprofen can interfere with the antiplatelet effect of low-dose aspirin (81 mg daily). This could result in diminished effectiveness of aspirin as used for cardioprotection and stroke prevention. The FDA added that although ibuprofen and aspirin can be taken together, it is recommended that consumers talk with their healthcare providers for additional information.

Special Alert 3: Strong advisory warning against the discontinuation of dual aspirin and clopidogrel (Plavix®) antiplatelet therapy in patients with coronary artery stents

Aspirin and clopidogrel (Plavix®) in combination is the primary prevention strategy against stent thrombosis after placement of drug-eluting metal stents in coronary patients (Grines, 2007). Premature discontinuation of this drug combination strongly increases the risk of a catastrophic event of stent thrombosis leading to myocardial infarction and/or death (Grines, 2007). The AHA stresses a 12-month therapy of aspirin and Plavix® combination after placement of a drug-eluting stent in order to prevent thrombosis at the stent site. The AHA also stresses educating both the patient and the healthcare provider about the hazards of premature antiplatelet drug discontinuation. Any elective surgery should be postponed for 1 year after stent implantation, and if surgery must be performed, consideration should be given to continuing the antiplatelet therapy during the perioperative period in high risk patients with drug-eluting stents.

The recommendations from the AHA advisory panel were summarized for the dental professional according to the following:

> Dental professionals and other healthcare providers who perform invasive or surgical procedures and are concerned about periprocedural and postoperative bleeding must be made aware of the potential catastrophic risks of premature discontinuation of dual antiplatelet (aspirin and Plavix®) therapy. The dental professional should contact the patient's cardiologist if issues regarding the patient's antiplatelet therapy are unclear, in order to discuss optimal patient management strategy.
>
> Elective procedures for which there is significant risk of perioperative or postoperative bleeding should be deferred until patients have completed an appropriate course of dual antiplatelet therapy. The course of this therapy is suggested as 12 months after drug-eluting stent implantation if patient is not at high risk of bleeding.

Agents Useful to Aid in Hemostasis During or Prior to Perioperative Bleeding

Aluminum Chloride on page 90
Aminocaproic Acid on page 98
Cellulose (Oxidized/Regenerated) on page 346
Collagen (Absorbable) on page 438
Collagen Hemostat on page 439
Fibrin Sealant on page 733
Gelatin (Absorbable) on page 808
Thrombin (Topical) on page 1625
Tranexamic Acid on page 1661

Hemostatic agents inhibit the activation of plasminogen to plasmin, producing antifibrinolytic activity. These agents have been used systemically and locally for treatment and prevention of various bleeding disorders. The oral mucosa tissues are rich in plasminogen activators, making hemostatic agents potentially effective for controlling oral bleeding. Although many hemostatic agents are available, only tranexamic acid and epsilon aminocaproic acid can be prepared and used as mouthwashes. Tranexamic acid is available as an intravenous injection (100 mg/mL). Aminocaproic acid is available as a 500 mg tablet, an injectable solution (250 mg/mL), and a raspberry-flavored oral syrup (250 mg/mL). A potentially critical difference between these drugs is that tranexamic acid is 6-10 times more potent that aminocaproic acid, as show in both *in vitro* and *in vivo* assays. Neither agent is commercially available as a mouthwash.

The EACA oral syrup is most readily usable as a mouthwash; however, due to cost the tablet is usually compounded to form a mouthwash. In addition, the solution for injection may be diluted with sterile water and used as a mouthwash. To ensure stability and sterility, this is commonly prepared the day of surgery. The adverse effects of these agents are dose dependent and generally manifest as nausea, vomiting, abdominal pain, and diarrhea. Theoretically, adverse effects are more likely to occur with systemic use than with local use.

REFERENCES

"Aspirin: Quitting Cold Turkey Could Be Dangerous. Studies Have Linked Aspirin Withdrawal to Heart Attacks," *Harv Health Lett*, 2005, 30(12):6.

Biondi-Zoccai GG, Lotrionte M, Agostoni P, et al, "A Systematic Review and Meta-Analysis on the Hazards of Discontinuing or Not Adhering to Aspirin Among 50,279 Patients at Risk for Coronary Artery Disease," *Eur Heart J*, 2006, 27(22):2667-74.

Brennan MT, Wynn RL, and Miller CS, "Aspirin and Bleeding in Dentistry: An Update and Recommendations," *Oral Surg Oral Med Oral Pathol Oral Radiol Endod*, 2007, 104(3):316-23.

Carter G, Goss AN, Lloyd J, et al, "Current Concepts of the Management of Dental Extractions for Patients Taking Warfarin," *Aust Dent J*, 2003, 48(2):89-96.

Chhatriwalla AK and Bhatt DL, "Should Dual Antiplatelet Therapy After Drug-Eluting Stents Be Continued for More Than 1 Year?: Dual Antiplatelet Therapy After Drug-Eluting Stents Should Be Continued for More Than One Year and Preferably Indefinitely," *Circ Cardiovasc Interv*, 2008, 1(3):217-25.

Collet JP, Montalescot G, Blanchet B, et al, "Impact of Prior Use or Recent Withdrawal of Oral Antiplatelet Agents on Acute Coronary Syndromes," *Circulation*, 2004, 110(16):2361-7.

Connolly SJ, Ezekowitz MD, Yusuf S, et al, "Dabigatran Versus Warfarin in Patients With Atrial Fibrillation," *N Engl J Med*, 2009, 361(12):1139-51.

Culić V, Eterović D, Mirić D, et al, "Triggering of Ventricular Tachycardia by Meteorologic and Emotional Stress: Protective Effect of Beta-Blockers and Anxiolytics in Men and Elderly," *Am J Epidemiol*, 2004, 160(11):1047-58.

DiMarco JP, Flaker G, Waldo AL, et al, "Factors Affecting Bleeding Risk During Anticoagulant Therapy in Patients With Atrial Fibrillation: Observations From the Atrial Fibrillation Follow-Up Investigation of Rhythm Management (AFFIRM) Study," *Am Heart J*, 2005, 149(4):650-6.

Eisenberg MJ, Richard PR, Libersan D, et al, "Safety of Short-Term Discontinuation of Antiplatelet Therapy in Patients With Drug-Eluting Stents," *Circulation*, 2009, 119(12):1634-42.

FDA, "Ibuprofen and Aspirin Taken Together," available at http://www.fda.gov/Safety/MedWatch/SafetyInformation/SafetyAlertsforHumanMedicalProducts/ucm150611.htm.

Fischer LM, Schlienger RG, Matter CM, et al, "Discontinuation of Nonsteroidal Anti-Inflammatory Drug Therapy and Risk of Acute Myocardial Infarction," *Arch Intern Med*, 2004, 164(22):2472-6.

Gengo FM, Rubin L, Robson M, et al, "Effects of Ibuprofen on the Magnitude and Duration of Aspirin's Inhibition of Platelet Aggregation: Clinical Consequences in Stroke Prophylaxis," *J Clin Pharmacol*, 2008, 48(1):117-22.

Gladding PA, Webster MW, Farrell HB, et al, "The Antiplatelet Effect of Six Nonsteroidal Anti-Inflammatory Drugs and Their Pharmacodynamic Interaction With Aspirin in Healthy Volunteers," *Am J Cardiol*, 2008, 101(7):1060-3.

Grines CL, Bonow RO, Casey DE Jr, et al, "Prevention of Premature Discontinuation of Dual Antiplatelet Therapy in Patients With Coronary Artery Stents: A Science Advisory From the American Heart Association, American College of Cardiology, Society for Cardiovascular Angiography and Interventions, American College of Surgeons, and American Dental Association, With Representation From the American College of Physicians," *Circulation*, 2007, 115(6):813-8.

Grosset ABM and Rodgers GM, "Acquired Coagulation Disorders," *Wintrobe's Clinical Hematology*, 10th ed, Lee GR, Foerster J, Lukens J, et al, eds, Baltimore, MD: Williams and Wilkins, 1999, 1733-81.

Harder S, Klinkhardt U, and Alvarez JM, "Avoidance of Bleeding During Surgery in Patients Receiving Anticoagulant and/or Antiplatelet Therapy: Pharmacokinetic and Pharmacodynamic Considerations," *Clin Pharmacokinet*, 2004, 43(14):963-81.

Homoncik M, Jilma B, Hergovich N, et al, "Monitoring of Aspirin (ASA) Pharmacodynamics With the Platelet Function Analyzer PFA-100," *Thromb Haemost*, 2000, 83(2):316-21.

Jafri SM, "Periprocedural Thromboprophylaxis in Patients Receiving Chronic Anticoagulation Therapy," *Am Heart J*, 2004, 147(1):3-15.

Jeske AH, Suchko GD, ADA Council on Scientific Affairs and Division of Science, et al, "Lack of a Scientific Basis for Routine Discontinuation of Oral Anticoagulation Therapy Before Dental Treatment," *J Am Dent Assoc*, 2003, 134(11):1492-7.

Kessler CM, "Hemorrhagic Disorders: Coagulation Factor Deficiencies," *Cecil Textbook of Medicine*, 22nd ed, Goldman L and Ausiello D, eds, Philadelphia, PA: Saunders, 2004, 1069-78.

Lermann BB, "Ventricular Arrhythmias and Sudden Death," *Cecil Textbook of Medicine*, 22nd ed, Goldman L and Ausiello D, eds, Philadelphia, PA: WB Saunders Co, 2004.

Levine SP, "Qualitative Disorders of Platelet Function," *Wintrobe's Clinical Hematology*, 10th ed, Lee GR, Foerster J, Lukens J, et al, eds, Baltimore, MD: Williams and Wilkins, 1999, 1661-82.

Libby P and Theroux P, "Pathophysiology of Coronary Artery Disease," *Circulation*, 2005, 111(25):3481-8.

Lippert S and Gutschik E, "Views of Cardiac-Valve Prosthesis Patients and Their Dentists on Anticoagulation Therapy," *Scand J Dent Res*, 1994, 102(3):168-71.

Little JW, Miller CS, Henry RG, et al, "Antithrombotic Agents: Implications in Dentistry," *Oral Surg Oral Med Oral Pathol Oral Radiol Endod*, 2002, 93(5):544-51.

Lockhart PB, Gibson J, Pond SH, et al, "Dental Management Considerations for the Patient With an Acquired Coagulopathy. Part 2: Coagulopathies From Drugs," *Br Dent J*, 2003, 195(9):495-501.

Lordkipanidzé M, Diodati JG, and Pharand C, "Possibility of a Rebound Phenomenon Following Antiplatelet Therapy Withdrawal: A Look at the Clinical and Pharmacological Evidence," *Pharmacol Ther*, 2009, 123(2):178-86.

Madan GA, Madan SG, Madan G, et al, "Minor Oral Surgery Without Stopping Daily Low-Dose Aspirin Therapy: A Study of 51 Patients," *J Oral Maxillofac Surg*, 2005, 63(9):1262-5.

Shuman M, "Hemorrhagic Disorders: Abnormalities of Platelet and Vascular Function," *Cecil Textbook of Medicine*, 22nd ed, Goldman L and Ausiello D, eds, Philadelphia, PA: Saunders, 2004, 1060-9.

Thom T, Haase N, Rosamond W, et al, "Heart Disease and Stroke Statistics-2006 Update: A Report From the American Heart Association Statistics Committee and Stroke Statistics Subcommittee," *Circulation*, 2006, 113(6):e85-151.

Thompson AR, "Congenital Bleeding Disorders From Other Coagulation Protein Deficiencies," *Clinical Hematology*, Young NS, Gerson SL, and High KA, eds, Philadelphia, PA: Mosby Elsevier, 2006, 855-67.

CLINICAL RISK RELATED TO DRUGS PROLONGING QT INTERVAL

The QT interval is measured as the time and distance between the Q point of the QRS complex and the end of the T wave in the ECG tracing. After adjustment for heart rate, the QT interval is defined as prolonged if it is more than 450 msec in men and 460 msec in women. A long QT syndrome was first described in the 1950s and 60s as a congenital syndrome involving QT interval prolongation, syncope, and sudden death. Some of the congenital long QT syndromes were characterized by a peculiar electrocardiographic appearance of the QRS complex involving a premature atria beat, followed by a pause, then a subsequent sinus beat showing marked QT prolongation and deformity. This type of cardiac arrhythmia was originally termed "torsade de pointes" (translated from the French as "twisting of the points").

Prolongation of the QT interval is thought to result from delayed ventricular repolarization. The repolarization process within the myocardial cell is due to the efflux of intracellular potassium. The channels associated with this current can be blocked by many drugs and predispose the electrical propagation cycle to torsade de pointes.

Erythromycin, a drug often associated with dental antibiotics, is considered as having a risk of causing torsade de pointes. The risk of drug-induced torsade de pointes is extremely low when a single QT interval prolonging drug is prescribed. It is not known what effect vasoconstrictors in the local anesthetic regimen will have in patients with a known history of congenital prolonged QT interval or in patients taking any medication that prolongs the QT interval. Until more information is obtained, it is suggested that the clinician consult with the physician prior to the use of a vasoconstrictor in suspected patients, and that the vasoconstrictor (epinephrine, levonordefrin [Neo-Cobefrin®]) be used with caution.

Thioridazine is another drug confirmed to prolong the QT interval and is accepted as having a risk of causing torsade de pointes. The risk of drug-induced torsade de pointes is extremely low when a single QT interval prolonging drug is prescribed. In terms of epinephrine, it is not known what effect vasoconstrictors in the local anesthetic regimen will have in patients with a known history of congenital prolonged QT interval or in patients taking any medication that prolongs the QT interval. Until more information is obtained, it is suggested that the clinician consult with the physician prior to the use of a vasoconstrictor in suspected patients, and that the vasoconstrictor (epinephrine, levonordefrin [Neo-Cobefrin®]) be used with caution.

Table 10. DRUGS GENERALLY ACCEPTED AS HAVING A RISK OF CAUSING TORSADE DE POINTES

Generic Name	Brand Name	Use
Amiodarone	Cordarone®	Antiarrhythmic
Arsenic Trioxide	Trisenox®	Antileukemic agent
Artemether and Lumefantrine	Coartem®	Antimalarial Agent
Asenapine	Saphris®	Antipsychotic
Azithromycin (Systemic)	**Zithromax®**	**Antibiotic**
Chloroquine	Aralen®	Antimalarial
ChlorproMAZINE	-	Antipsychotic
Clarithromycin	**Biaxin®**	**Antibiotic**
Dasatinib	Sprycel®	Antineoplastic
Disopyramide	Norpace®	Antiarrhythmic
Dofetilide	Tikosyn®	Antiarrhythmic
Droperidol	-	Antiemetic
Escitalopram	Lexapro®	Antidepressant
Erythromycin (Systemic)	**Various brand names available**	**Antibiotic**
Fluconazole	**Diflucan®**	**Antifungal**
FLUoxetine	PROzac®	Antidepressant
Haloperidol	Haldol®	Antipsychotic
Ibutilide	Corvert®	Antiarrhythmic

Table 10. DRUGS GENERALLY ACCEPTED AS HAVING A RISK OF CAUSING TORSADE DE POINTES *(continued)*

Generic Name	Brand Name	Use
Iloperidone	Fanapt™	Antipsychotic
Levofloxacin (Systemic)	**Levaquin®**	**Antibiotic**
Methadone	Various brand names available	Analgesic, Opioid
Moxifloxacin (Systemic)	**Avelox®**	**Antibiotic**
Pazopanib	Votrient™	Antineoplastic Agent, Tyrosine Kinase Inhibitor
Pentamidine	NebuPent®	Antibiotic
Pimozide	Orap®	Antipsychotic
Procainamide	Procanbid®	Antiarrhythmic
QUEtiapine	SEROquel®	Antipsychotic
QuiNIDine	-	Antiarrhythmic
Ranolazine	Ranexa®	Antianginal
RisperiDONE	RisperDAL®	Antipsychotic
RomiDEPsin	Istodax®	Antineoplastic Agent, Histone Deacetylase Inhibitor
Sotalol	Betapace®	Antiarrhythmic
SUNItinib	Sutent®	Antineoplastic
Telavancin	Vibativ™	Glycopeptide
Telithromycin	**Ketek®**	**Antibiotic**
Thioridazine	-	Antipsychotic
Vandetanib	-	Medullary thyroid cancer (symptomatic or progressive)
Voriconazole	**VFEND®**	**Antifungal**
Ziprasidone	Geodon®	Antipsychotic
Zuclopenthixol	Clopixol®	Antipsychotic

Note: Dental drugs are identified by bold print. This is not a comprehensive list; additional resources should be consulted.

GASTROINTESTINAL DISORDERS

The oral cavity and related structures comprise the first part of the gastrointestinal tract. Diseases affecting the oral cavity are often reflected in GI disturbances. In addition, the oral cavity may indeed reflect diseases of the GI tract, including ulcers, polyps, and liver and gallbladder diseases. The first oral condition that may reflect or be reflected in GI disturbances is taste. Typically, complaints of taste abnormalities are presented to the dentist. The sweet, saline, sour, and bitter taste sensations all vary in quality and intensity and are affected by the olfactory system. Often, anemic conditions are reflected in changes in the tongue, resulting in taste aberrations.

Gastric and duodenal ulcers represent the primary diseases that can be reflected in the oral cavity. Gastric reflux and problems with food metabolism often present as acid erosions to the teeth and occasionally, changes in the mucosal surface as well. Patients may be identified, upon diagnosis, as harboring the organism *Helicobacter pylori*. Treatment with antibiotics can oftentimes aid in correcting the ulcerative disease.

PROTON PUMP AND GASTRIC ACID SECRETION INHIBITORS

Dexlansoprazole on page 497
Esomeprazole on page 628
Lansoprazole on page 981
Lansoprazole, Amoxicillin, and Clarithromycin on page 983
Omeprazole on page 1247
Pantoprazole on page 1292
RABEprazole on page 1450

HISTAMINE H_2 ANTAGONIST

Cimetidine on page 384
Famotidine on page 706
Nizatidine on page 1225
Ranitidine on page 1460

The oral aspects of gastrointestinal disease are often nonspecific and are related to the patient's gastric reflux problems. Intestinal polyps occasionally present as part of the "Peutz-Jeghers Syndrome," resulting in pigmented areas of the perioral region that resemble freckles. The astute dentist will need to differentiate these from melanin pigmentation, while at the same time encouraging the patient to seek evaluation for an intestinal disorder.

Diseases of the liver and gallbladder system are complex. Most of the disorders of interest to the dentist are covered in the section on Systemic Viral Diseases on page 1904. All of the new drugs, including interferons, are mentioned in this section.

Multiple Drug Regimens for the Treatment of *H. pylori* Infection

Drug	Dosages	Duration of Therapy
H_2-receptor antagonist[1]	Any one given at appropriate dose	4 weeks
plus		
Bismuth on page 239	525 mg 4 times/day	2 weeks
plus		
MetroNIDAZOLE (Systemic) on page 1126	250 mg 4 times/day	2 weeks
plus		
Tetracycline on page 1611	500 mg 4 times/day	2 weeks
Proton pump inhibitor[1]	Esomeprazole 40 mg once daily	10 days
plus		
Clarithromycin on page 396	500 mg twice daily	10 days
plus		
Amoxicillin on page 124	1000 mg twice daily	10 days
Proton pump inhibitor[1]	Lansoprazole 30 mg twice daily or Omeprazole 20 mg twice daily	10-14 days
plus		
Clarithromycin on page 396	500 mg twice daily	10-14 days
plus		
Amoxicillin on page 124	1000 mg twice daily	10-14 days
Proton pump inhibitor[1]	RABEprazole 20 mg twice daily	7 days
plus		
Clarithromycin on page 396	500 mg twice daily	7 days
plus		
Amoxicillin on page 124	1000 mg twice daily	7 days
Proton pump inhibitor	Lansoprazole 30 mg twice daily or Omeprazole 20 mg twice daily	2 weeks
plus		
Clarithromycin on page 396	500 mg twice daily	2 weeks
plus		
MetroNIDAZOLE (Systemic) on page 1126	500 mg twice daily	2 weeks
Proton pump inhibitor	Lansoprazole 30 mg once daily or Omeprazole 20 mg once daily	2 weeks
plus		
Bismuth on page 239	525 mg 4 times/day	2 weeks
plus		
MetroNIDAZOLE (Systemic) on page 1126	500 mg 3 times/day	2 weeks
plus		
Tetracycline on page 1611	500 mg 4 times/day	2 weeks

[1]FDA-approved regimen

Modified from Howden CS and Hunt RH, "Guidelines for the Management of *Helicobacter pylori* Infection," *AJG*, 1998, 93:2336.

REFERENCES

Cobrin GM and Abreu MT, "Defects in Mucosal Immunity Leading to Crohn's Disease," *Immunol Rev*, 2005, 206:277-95.

Permin H and Andersen LP, "Inflammation, Immunity, and Vaccines for *Helicobacter* Infection," *Helicobacter*, 2005, 10(Suppl 1):21-5.

Schreiber S, Rosenstiel P, Albrecht M, et al, "Genetics of Crohn Disease, an Archetypal Inflammatory Barrier Disease," *Nat Rev Genet*, 2005, 6(5):376-88.

Tummala S, Keates S, and Kelly CP, "Update on the Immunologic Basis of *Helicobacter pylori* Gastritis," *Curr Opin Gastroenterol*, 2004, 20(6):592-7.

Yuan Y, Padol IT, and Hunt RH, "Peptic Ulcer Disease Today," *Nat Clin Pract Gastroenterol Hepatol*, 2006, 3(2):80-9.

RESPIRATORY DISEASES

Diseases of the respiratory system put dental patients at increased risk in the dental office because of their decreased pulmonary reserve, the medications they may be taking, drug interactions between these medications, medications the dentist may prescribe, and in some patients with infectious respiratory diseases, a risk of disease transmission.

The respiratory system consists of the nasal cavity, the nasopharynx, the trachea, and the components of the lung including, the bronchi, the bronchioles, and the alveoli. The diseases that affect the lungs and the respiratory system can be separated by location of affected tissue. Diseases that affect the lower respiratory tract are often chronic, although infections can also occur. Three major diseases that affect the lower respiratory tract are often encountered in the medical history for dental patients. These include chronic bronchitis, emphysema, and asthma. Diseases that affect the upper respiratory tract are usually of the infectious nature and include sinusitis and the common cold. The upper respiratory tract infections may also include a wide variety of nonspecific infections, most of which are also caused by viruses. Influenza produces upper respiratory type symptoms and is often caused by orthomyxoviruses. Herpangina is caused by the Coxsackie type viruses and results in upper respiratory infections in addition to pharyngitis or sore throat. One serious condition, known as croup, has been associated with *Haemophilus influenzae* infections. Other more serious infections might include respiratory syncytial virus, adenoviruses, and parainfluenza viruses.

The respiratory symptoms that are often encountered in both upper respiratory and lower respiratory disorders include cough, dyspnea (difficulty in breathing), the production of sputum, hemoptysis (coughing up blood), a wheeze, and occasionally chest pain. One additional symptom, orthopnea (difficulty in breathing when lying down), is often used by the dentist to assist in evaluating the patient with the condition pulmonary edema. This condition results from either respiratory disease or congestive heart failure.

No effective drug treatments are available for the management of many of the upper respiratory tract viral infections. However, amantadine (Symmetrel®) is a synthetic drug given orally (200 mg/day) and has been found to be effective against some strains of influenza. Treatment other than for influenza includes supportive care products, available over-the-counter. These might include antihistamines for symptomatic relief of the upper respiratory congestion, antibiotics to combat secondary bacterial infections, and in severe cases, fluids, when patients have become dehydrated during the illness (see Pharmacologic Category Index for selection). The treatment of herpangina may include management of the painful ulcerations of the oropharynx. The dentist may become involved in managing these lesions in a similar way to those seen in other acute viral infections (see Systemic Viral Diseases on page 1904).

SINUSITIS

Sinusitis represents an upper respiratory condition that often comes under the purview of the practicing dentist. Acute sinusitis is characterized by nasal obstruction, fever, chills, and midface head pain. Oftentimes there is only evidence of inflammation rather than true infection. This condition may be discovered as part of a differential workup for other facial or dental pain since the symptoms are often referred to teeth adjacent to the affected sinus. Chronic sinusitis may likewise produce similar dental symptoms. Dental drugs of choice may include ephedrine or nasal drops, antihistamines, and analgesics. When infection accompanies the inflammation of sinusitis, antibiotics may be required. Most commonly, broad spectrum antibiotics such as ampicillin are prescribed. These are often combined with antral lavage to re-establish drainage from the sinus area. Surgical intervention, such as a Caldwell-Luc procedure opening into the sinus, is rarely necessary and many of the second generation antibiotics, such as cephalosporins, are used successfully in treating the acute and chronic sinusitis patient (see Antibiotic Prophylaxis on page 1910).

Gatifloxacin on page 806
Moxifloxacin (Systemic) on page 1165

LOWER RESPIRATORY DISEASES

Lower respiratory tract diseases, including asthma, chronic bronchitis, and emphysema are often identified in dental patients. Asthma is an intermittent respiratory disorder that produces recurrent bronchial smooth muscle spasm, inflammation of the bronchial mucosa, and hypersecretion of mucus. The incidence of childhood asthma appears to be increasing and may be related to the presence of pollutants such as sulfur dioxide and indoor cigarette smoke. The end result is widespread narrowing of the airways and decreased ventilation with increased airway resistance, especially to expiration.

Asthmatic patients often suffer asthmatic attacks when stimulated by respiratory tract infections, exercise, and cold air. Medications such as aspirin and some NSAIDs, as well as cholinergic and beta-adrenergic blocking drugs, can also trigger asthmatic attacks in addition to chemicals, smoke, and emotional anxiety.

The classical chronic obstructive pulmonary diseases (COPD) of chronic bronchitis and emphysema are both characterized by chronic airflow obstructions during normal ventilatory efforts. They often occur in combination in the same patient and their treatment is similar. One common finding is that the patient is often a smoker. The dentist can play a role in reinforcement of smoking cessation in patients with chronic respiratory diseases.

Treatments include a variety of drugs depending on the severity of the symptoms and the respiratory compromise upon full respiratory evaluation. Patients who are having acute and chronic obstructive pulmonary attacks may be susceptible to infection and antibiotics such as penicillin, ampicillin, tetracycline, or sulfamethoxazole-trimethoprim are often used to eradicate susceptible infective organisms. Corticosteroids, as well as a wide variety of respiratory stimulants, are available in inhalant and/or oral forms. In patients using inhalant medication, oral candidiasis is occasionally encountered.

Analgesics
Antibiotics
Antihistamines
Decongestants

SPECIFIC DRUGS USED IN THE TREATMENT OF CHRONIC RESPIRATORY CONDITIONS

Beta$_2$-Selective Agonists

Albuterol on page 66
Metaproterenol on page 1087
Pirbuterol on page 1360
Salmeterol on page 1506
Terbutaline on page 1603

Methylxanthines

Aminophylline on page 100
Theophylline on page 1619

Mast Cell Stabilizer

Cromolyn (Systemic, Oral Inhalation) on page 443
Nedocromil on page 1192

Corticosteroids

Beclomethasone (Oral Inhalation) on page 209
Dexamethasone (Systemic) on page 492
Flunisolide (Oral Inhalation) on page 748
Fluticasone (Oral Inhalation) on page 766
Mometasone (Oral Inhalation) on page 1152
PredniSONE on page 1393
Triamcinolone (Systemic) on page 1669

Anticholinergics

Ipratropium (Oral Inhalation) on page 940
Tiotropium on page 1637

Leukotriene Receptor Antagonists

Montelukast on page 1155
Zafirlukast on page 1737

5-Lipoxygenase Inhibitors

Zileuton on page 1743

Other respiratory diseases include tuberculosis and sarcoidosis which are considered to be restrictive granulomatous respiratory diseases (see Tuberculosis on page 1902). Sarcoidosis is a condition that at one time was thought to be similar to tuberculosis; however, it is a multisystem disorder of unknown origin which has as a characteristic lymphocytic and mononuclear phagocytic accumulation in epithelioid granulomas within the lung. It occurs worldwide but shows a slight increased prevalence in temperate climates. The treatment of sarcoidosis is usually one that corresponds to its usually benign course; however, many patients are placed on corticosteroids at the level of 40-60 mg of prednisone daily. This treatment is continued for a protracted period of time. As in any disease requiring steroid therapy, consideration of adrenal suppression is necessary. Alteration of steroid dosage prior to stressful dental procedures may be necessary, usually increasing the steroid dosage prior to and during the stressful procedures and then gradually returning the patient to the original dosage over several days. Many dentists prefer to use the Medrol® Dosepak®; however, consultation with the patient's physician regarding dose selection is always advised. Even in the absence of evidence of adrenal suppression, consultation with the prescribing physician for appropriate dosing and timing of procedures is advisable.

PredniSONE on page 1393

RELATIVE POTENCY OF ENDOGENOUS AND SYNTHETIC CORTICOSTEROIDS

Agent	Equivalent Dose (mg)
Short-Acting (8-12 h)	
Cortisol	20
Cortisone acetate	25
Intermediate-Acting (18-36 h)	
PrednisoLONE	5
PredniSONE	5
MethylPREDNISolone	4
Triamcinolone	4
Long-Acting (36-54 h)	
Betamethasone	0.75
Dexamethasone	0.75

Potential drug interactions for the respiratory disease patient exist. An acute sensitivity to aspirin-containing drugs and some of the nonsteroidal anti-inflammatory drugs is a threat for the asthmatic patient. Barbiturates and narcotics may occasionally precipitate asthmatic attacks as well. Erythromycin, clarithromycin, and ketoconazole are contraindicated in patients who are taking theophylline due to potential enhancement of theophylline toxicity. Patients that are taking steroid preparations as part of their respiratory therapy may require alteration in dosing prior to stressful dental procedures. The physician should be consulted.

Barbiturates
Clarithromycin on page 396
Erythromycin (Systemic) on page 620
Ketoconazole (Systemic) on page 963

REFERENCES AND SELECTED READINGS

de Almeida FR, Lowe AA, Tsuiki S, et al, "Long-Term Compliance and Side Effects of Oral Appliances Used for the Treatment of Snoring and Obstructive Sleep Apnea Syndrome," *J Clin Sleep Med*, 2005, 1 (2):143-52.

Dincer HE and O'Neill W, "Deleterious Effects of Sleep-Disordered Breathing on the Heart and Vascular System," *Respiration*, 2006, 73(1):124-30.

Doll R, Peto R, Boreham J, et al, "Mortality in Relation to Smoking: 50 Years' Observations on Male British Doctors," *BMJ*, 2004, 328(7455):1519.

Expert Panel Report 3, "Guidelines for the Diagnosis and Management of Asthma." Available at http://www.nhlbi.nih.gov/guidelines/asthma/asthgdln.pdf.

Ferguson KA, Cartwright R, Rogers R, et al, "Oral Appliances for Snoring and Obstructive Sleep Apnea: A Review," *Sleep*, 2006, 29(2):244-62.

Gay P, Weaver T, Loube D, et al, "Evaluation of Positive Airway Pressure Treatment for Sleep Related Breathing Disorders in Adults," *Sleep*, 2006, 29(3):381-401.

Hu S, Pallonen U, McAlister AL, et al, "Knowing How to Help Tobacco Users. Dentists' Familiarity and Compliance With the Clinical Practice Guideline," *J Am Dent Assoc*, 2006, 137(2):170-9.

Javaheri S, "Sleep and Cardiovascular Disease: Present and Future," *Principles and Practice of Sleep Medicine*, 4th ed, Kryger MH, Roth T, and Dement WC, Philadelphia, PA: Elsevier, 2005, 1157-60.

Ryan CF, "Sleep X 9: An Approach to Treatment of Obstructive Sleep Apnoea/Hypopnoea Syndrome Including Upper Airway Surgery," *Thorax*, 2005, 60(7):595-604.

Schroeder SA, "Tobacco Control in the Wake of the 1998 Master Settlement Agreement," *N Engl J Med*, 2004, 350(3):293-301.

Schwab R, Kuna S, and Remmers JE, "Anatomy and Physiology of Upper Airway Obstruction," *Principles and Practice of Sleep Medicine*, 4th ed, Kryger MH, Roth T, and Dement WC, Philadelphia, PA: Elsevier, 2005, 983-1000.

The International Classification of Sleep Disorders: Diagnostic and Coding Manual, 2nd ed, Westchester, IL: American Academy of Sleep Medicine, 2005.

ENDOCRINE DISORDERS AND PREGNANCY

The human endocrine system manages metabolism and homeostasis. Numerous glandular tissues produce hormones that act in broad reactions with tissues throughout the body. Cells in various organ systems may be sensitive to the hormone, or they release, in reaction to the hormone, a second hormone that acts directly on another organ. Diseases of the endocrine system may have importance in dentistry. For the purposes of this section, we will limit our discussion to diseases of the thyroid tissues, diabetes mellitus, conditions requiring the administration of synthetic hormones, and pregnancy.

THYROID

Thyroid diseases can be classified into conditions that cause the thyroid to be overactive (hyperthyroidism) and those that cause the thyroid to be underactive (hypothyroidism). Clinical signs and symptoms associated with hyperthyroidism may include goiter, heat intolerance, tremor, weight loss, diarrhea, and hyperactivity. Thyroid hormone production can be tested by TSH levels and additional screens may include radioactive iodine uptake or a pre-T_4 (tetraiodothyronine, thyroxine) assay or iodine index or total serum T_3 (triiodothyronine). The results of thyroid function tests may be altered by ingestion of antithyroid drugs such as propylthiouracil, estrogen-containing drugs, and organic and inorganic iodides. When a diagnosis of hyperthyroidism has been made, treatment usually begins with antithyroid drugs which may include propranolol coupled with radioactive iodides, as well as surgical procedures, to reduce thyroid tissue. Generally, the beta-blockers are used to control cardiovascular effects of excessive T_4. Propylthiouracil or methimazole are the most common antithyroid drugs used. The dentist should be aware that epinephrine is definitely contraindicated in patients with uncontrolled hyperthyroidism.

Diseases and conditions associated with hypothyroidism may include bradycardia, drowsiness, cold intolerance, thick dry skin, and constipation. Generally, hypothyroidism is treated with replacement thyroid hormone until a euthyroid state is achieved. Various preparations are available, the most common is levothyroxine and is generally the drug of choice for thyroid replacement therapy.

Drugs to Treat Hypothyroidism

Levothyroxine on page 1005
Liothyronine on page 1022
Liotrix on page 1023
Thyroid, Desiccated on page 1627

Drugs to Treat Hyperthyroidism

Methimazole on page 1095
Potassium Iodide on page 1379
Propranolol on page 1422
Propylthiouracil on page 1426

DIABETES

Diabetes mellitus refers to a condition of prolonged hyperglycemia associated with either abnormal production or lack of production of insulin. Commonly known as Type 1 diabetes, insulin-dependent diabetes (IDDM) is a condition where there are absent or deficient levels of circulating insulin therefore triggering tissue reactions associated with prolonged hyperglycemia. The kidney's attempt to excrete the excess glucose and the organs that do not receive adequate glucose essentially are damaged. Small vessels and arterial vessels in the eye, kidney, and brain are usually at the greatest risk. Generally, blood sugar levels between 70-120 mg/dL are considered to be normal. Inadequate insulin levels allow glucose to rise to greater than the renal threshold which is 180 mg/dL, and such elevations prolonged lead to organ damage.

The goals of treatment of the diabetic are to maintain metabolic control of the blood glucose levels and to reduce the morbid effects of periodic hyperglycemia. Insulin therapy is the primary mechanism to attain management of consistent insulin levels. Insulin preparations are categorized according to their duration of action. Generally, intermediate-acting insulin and long-acting insulin can be used in combination with short-acting or rapid-acting insulins to maintain levels consistent throughout the day.

In Type 2 or noninsulin-dependent diabetes (NIDDM), the receptor for insulin in the tissues is generally down regulated; therefore, the glucose is not utilized at an appropriate rate. There is perhaps a stronger genetic basis for noninsulin-dependent diabetes than for Type 1. Treatment of the diabetes Type 2 patient is generally directed toward early nonpharmacologic intervention, mainly weight reduction, moderate exercise, and lower plasma-glucose concentrations. Oral hypoglycemic agents as seen in the following list are often used to maintain blood sugar levels. Thirty percent of Type 2 diabetics require insulin, as well as oral hypoglycemics, in order to manage their diabetes. Generally, the two classes of oral hypoglycemics are the sulfonylureas and the biguanides. The sulfonylureas are prescribed more frequently. They stimulate beta cell production of insulin, increase glucose utilization, and tend to normalize glucose metabolism in the liver. The uncontrolled diabetic may represent a challenge to the dental practitioner.

Glycosylated hemoglobin or glycol-hemoglobin assays have emerged as a "gold standard" by which glycemic control is measured in diabetic patients. The test does not rely on the patient's ability to monitor their daily blood glucose levels and is not influenced by acute changes in blood glucose or by the interval since the last meal. Glycohemoglobin is formed when glucose reacts with hemoglobin A in the blood and is composed of several fractions. Numerous assay methods have been developed, however, they vary in their precision. Dental clinicians are advised to be aware of the laboratory's particular standardization procedures when requesting glycosylated hemoglobin values. One major advantage of the glycosylated hemoglobin assay is that it provides an overview of the level of glucose in the life span of the red blood cell population in the patient, and therefore is a measure of overall glycemic control for the previous six to twelve weeks. Thus, clinicians use glycosylated hemoglobin values to determine whether their patient is under good control, on average. These assays have less value in medication dosing decisions. Blood glucose monitoring methods are actually better in that respect. The values of glycosylated hemoglobin are expressed as a percentage of the total hemoglobin in the red blood cell population and a normal value is considered to be <6%. The goal is generally for diabetic patients to remain at <7% and values >8% would constitute a worrisome signal. Medical conditions such as anemias or any red blood cell disease, numerous levels of myelosuppression, or pregnancy can artificially lower glycosylated hemoglobin values.

Rapid-Acting Insulins

Insulin Lispro (HumaLOG®) on page 922
Insulin Aspart (NovoLOG®) on page 920
Insulin Glulisine (Apidra®) on page 922

Short-Acting Insulin

Insulin Regular on page 924

Intermediate-Acting Insulin

Insulin NPH on page 923

Intermediate- to Long-Acting Insulin

Insulin Detemir on page 921

Long-Acting Insulin

Insulin Glargine on page 921

Oral Hypoglycemic Agents

Acarbose on page 29
ChlorproPAMIDE on page 373
Gliclazide on page 816
Glimepiride on page 817
GlipiZIDE on page 819
Glipizide and Metformin on page 821
GlyBURIDE on page 824
Glyburide and Metformin on page 827
MetFORMIN on page 1089
Miglitol on page 1137
Nateglinide on page 1190
Pioglitazone on page 1352
Pioglitazone and Glimepiride on page 1354
Pioglitazone and Metformin on page 1355
Repaglinide on page 1466
Repaglinide and Metformin on page 1467
Rosiglitazone on page 1497
Rosiglitazone and Glimepiride on page 1500
Rosiglitazone and Metformin on page 1501
Saxagliptin on page 1512

SitaGLIPtin on page 1534
Sitagliptin and Metformin on page 1536
TOLAZamide on page 1643
TOLBUTamide on page 1644

Adjunct Therapy

Metoclopramide on page 1120

Oral manifestations of uncontrolled diabetes might include abnormal neutrophil function resulting in a poor response to periodontal pathogens. Increased risk of gingivitis and periodontitis in these patients is common. Candidiasis is also a frequent occurrence. Denture-sore mouth may be more prominent. Poor wound-healing following extractions may be one of the complications encountered.

HORMONAL THERAPY

Two uses of hormonal supplementation include oral contraceptives and estrogen replacement therapy. Drugs used for contraception interfere with fertility by inhibiting release of follicle stimulating hormone, luteinizing hormone, and by preventing ovulation. There are few oral side effects; however, moderate gingivitis, similar to that seen during pregnancy, has been reported. The dentist should be aware that decreased effect of oral contraceptives has been reported with most antibiotics (see individual monographs for specific details). It is therefore recommended that dental professionals, when prescribing antibiotics to oral contraceptive users, advise them of this interaction and suggest consulting their physician for additional barrier contraception during antibiotic therapy.

Drugs commonly encountered include:

Estradiol (Systemic) on page 631
Ethinyl Estradiol and Drospirenone on page 653
Ethinyl Estradiol and Etonogestrel on page 659
Ethinyl Estradiol and Norethindrone on page 670
Ethinyl Estradiol and Norgestimate on page 677
MedroxyPROGESTERone on page 1061
Norethindrone on page 1226
Norethindrone and Mestranol on page 1227

Estrogens or derivatives are usually prescribed as replacement therapy following menopause or cyclic irregularities and to inhibit osteoporosis. The following list of drugs may interact with antidepressants and barbiturates. New tissue-specific estrogens like Evista® may help with the problem of osteoporosis.

Estrogens (Conjugated/Equine, Systemic) on page 638
Estrogens (Conjugated A/Synthetic) on page 636
Estrogens (Esterified) on page 642
Estrogens (Conjugated/Equine) and Medroxyprogesterone on page 641
Estrogens (Esterified) and Methyltestosterone on page 643
Estropipate on page 644
Raloxifene on page 1453

PREGNANCY

Normal endocrine and physiologic functions are altered during pregnancy. Endogenous estrogens and progesterone increase and placental hormones are secreted. Thyroid stimulating hormone and growth hormone also increase. Cardiovascular changes can result and increased blood volume can lead to blood pressure elevations and transient heart murmurs. Generally, in a normal pregnancy, oral gingival changes will be limited to gingivitis. Alteration of treatment plans might include limiting administration of all drugs to emergency procedures only during the first and third trimesters and medical consultation regarding the patients' status for all elective procedures. Limiting dental care throughout pregnancy to preventive procedures is reasonable. The effects on dental treatment of the "morning after pill" (Plan B® and PREVEN®) and the abortifacient, mifepristone on page 1136, have not been documented at this time. Please also review the Dental Drug Use in Pregnancy and Breast-Feeding table on page 2018 in the appendix for potential interactions. This reference is only a summary and consultation of other sources of information is recommended. Consultation with the patient's internist and obstetrician for evaluation of medication safety in pregnancy is advised.

REFERENCES AND SELECTED READINGS

Bloomgarden ZT, "Developments in Diabetes and Insulin Resistance," *Diabetes Care*, 2006, 29(1):161-7.

Booth GL, Kapral MK, Fung K, et al, "Recent Trends in Cardiovascular Complications Among Men and Women With and Without Diabetes," *Diabetes Care*, 2006, 29(1):32-7.

Courtney CH and Olefsky JM, "Type 2 Diabetes Mellitus: Etiology, Pathogenesis and Natural History," *Endocrinology*, 5th ed, De Groot LJ and Jameson JL, eds, Philadelphia, PA: Elsevier Saunders, 2006.

Geiss LS, Pan L, Cadwell B, et al, "Changes in Incidence of Diabetes in U.S. Adults, 1997-2003," *Am J Prev Med*, 2006, 30(5):371-7.

Germain DLS, "Thyroid Hormone Metabolism," *Endocrinology*, 5th ed, De Groot LJ and Jameson JL, eds, Philadelphia, PA: Elsevier Saunders, 2006, 1861-73.

Hoogwerf BJ, "Exenatide and Pramlintide: New Glucose-Lowering Agents for Treating Diabetes Mellitus," *Cleve Clin J Med*, 2006, 73(5):477-84.

Jameson JL and Weetman AP, "Disease of the Thyroid Gland," *Harrison's Online Principles of Medicine*, 16th ed, Kasper DL, ed, New York, NY: McGraw-Hill, 2005, 2104-27.

Kaaja RJ and Greer IA, "Manifestations of Chronic Disease During Pregnancy," *JAMA*, 2005, 294 (21):2751-7.

Lalla E, Park DB, Papapanou PN, et al, "Oral Disease Burden in Northern Manhattan Patients With Diabetes Mellitus," *Am J Public Health*, 2004, 94(5):755-8.

Little JW, "Thyroid Disorders. Part I: Hyperthyroidism," *Oral Surg Oral Med Oral Pathol Oral Radiol Endod*, 2006, 101(3):276-84.

Mario M, Chiovato L, and Pinchera A, "Graves' Disease," *Endocrinology*, 5th ed, De Groot LJ and Jameson JL, eds, Philadelphia, PA: Elsevier Saunders, 2006, 1995-2029.

Nathan DM, Cleary PA, Backlund JY, et al, "Intensive Diabetes Treatment and Cardiovascular Disease in Patients With Type 1 Diabetes," *N Engl J Med*, 2005, 353(25):2643-53.

Norris AW and Svoren BM, "Complications and Comorbidities of Type 2 Diabetes," *Pediatr Ann*, 2005, 34 (9):710-8.

Novak KF, Taylor GW, Dawson DR, et al, "Periodontitis and Gestational Diabetes Mellitus: Exploring the Link in NHANES III," *J Public Health Dent*, 2006, 66(3):163-8.

Offenbacher S, Boggess KA, Murtha AP, et al, "Progressive Periodontal Disease and Risk of Very Preterm Delivery," *Obstet Gynecol*, 2006, 107(1):29-36.

Perkins BA and Bril V, "Early Vascular Risk Factor Modification in Type 1 Diabetes," *N Engl J Med*, 2005, 352(4):408-9.

Rhodus NL, Vibeto BM, and Hamamoto DT, "Glycemic Control in Patients With Diabetes Mellitus Upon Admission to a Dental Clinic: Considerations for Dental Management," *Quintessence Int*, 2005, 36 (6):474-82.

Schwartz SL, Wu JF, and Berner B, "Metformin Extended Release for the Treatment of Type 2 Diabetes Mellitus," *Expert Opin Pharmacother*, 2006, 7(6):803-9.

Zammitt NN and Frier BM, "Hypoglycemia in Type 2 Diabetes: Pathophysiology, Frequency, and Effects of Different Treatment Modalities," *Diabetes Care*, 2005, 28(12):2948-61.

HIV INFECTION AND AIDS

Human immunodeficiency virus (HIV) represents agents HIV-1 and HIV-2 that produce a devastating systemic disease. The virus causes disease by leading to elevated risk of infections in patients and, from our experience over the last 18 years, there clearly are oral manifestations associated with these patients. Also, there has been a revolution in infection control in our dental offices over the last two decades due to our expanding knowledge of this infectious agent. Infection control practices have been elevated to include all of the infectious agents with which dentists often come into contact. These might include, in addition to HIV, hepatitis viruses (of which the serotypes include A, B, C, D, E, F, and G), the herpes viruses (see Systemic Viral Diseases on page 1904); STDs such as syphilis, gonorrhea, and papillomavirus (see Sexually-Transmitted Diseases on page 1903).

Acquired immunodeficiency syndrome (AIDS) has been recognized since early 1981 as a unique clinical syndrome manifest by opportunistic infections or by neoplasms complicating the underlying defect in the cellular immune system. These defects are now known to be brought on by infection and pathogenesis with human immunodeficiency virus 1 or 2 (HIV-1 is the predominant serotype identified). The major cellular defect brought on by infection with HIV is a depletion of T-cells, primarily the subtype, T-helper cells, known as CD4+ cells. When the CD4 cell count falls below 200 cells/µL, patients are at high risk for life-threatening AIDS-defining opportunistic infections (eg, *Pneumocystis jiroveci* pneumonia, *Toxoplasma gondii* encephalitis, disseminated *Mycobacterium avium* complex disease, tuberculosis, bacterial pneumonia). Over these years, our knowledge regarding HIV infection and the oral manifestations often associated with patients with HIV or AIDS, has increased dramatically. Populations of individuals known to be at high risk of HIV transmission include homosexuals, intravenous drug abuse patients, transfusion recipients, patients with other sexually transmitted diseases, and patients practicing promiscuous sex.

The definitions of AIDS have also evolved over this period of time. The natural history of HIV infection along with some of the oral manifestations can be reviewed in Table 1. The risk of developing these opportunistic infections increases as the patient progresses to AIDS.

Table 1. NATURAL HISTORY OF HIV INFECTION/ORAL MANIFESTATIONS

Time From Transmission (Average)	Observation	CD4 Cell Count
0	Viral transmissions	Normal: 1000 (±500/mm^3)
2-4 weeks	Self-limited infectious mononucleosis-like illness with fever, rash, leukopenia, mucocutaneous ulcerations (mouth, genitals, etc), thrush	Transient decrease
6-12 weeks	Seroconversion (rarely requires ≥3 months for seroconversion)	Normal
0-8 years	Healthy/asymptomatic HIV infection; peripheral/ persistent generalized lymphadenopathy; HPV, thrush, OHL; RAU, periodontal diseases, salivary gland diseases; dermatitis	≥500/mm^3 gradual reduction with average decrease of 50-80/mm^3/ year
4-8 years	Early symptomatic HIV infection previously called (AIDS-related complex): Thrush, vaginal candidiasis (persistent, frequent and/or severe), cervical dysplasia/CA Hodgkin's lymphoma, B-cell lymphoma, oral hairy leukoplakia, salivary gland diseases, ITP, xerostomia, dermatitis, shingles; RAU, herpes simplex, HPV, bacterial infections, periodontal diseases, molluscum contagiosum, other physical symptoms: fever, weight loss, fatigue	≥300-500/mm^3
6-10 years	AIDS: Wasting syndrome, *Candida* esophagitis, Kaposi's sarcoma, HIV-associated dementia, disseminated *M. avium*, Hodgkin's or B-cell lymphoma, herpes simplex >30 days; PCP; cryptococcal meningitis, other systemic fungal infections; CMV	<200/mm^3

Natural history indicates course of HIV infection in absence of antiretroviral treatment. Adapted from Bartlett JG, "A Guide to HIV Care from the AIDS Care Program of the Johns Hopkins Medical Institutions," 2nd ed.

PCP - *Pneumocystis carinii* pneumonia; ITP - idiopathic thrombocytopenia purpura; HPV - human papilloma virus; OHL - oral hairy leukoplakia; RAU - recurrent aphthous ulcer

Patients with HIV infection and/or AIDS are seen in dental offices throughout the country. In general, it is the dentist's obligation to treat HIV individuals including patients of record and other patients who may seek treatment when the office is accepting new patients. These patients are protected under the Americans with Disabilities Act and the dentist has an obligation as described. Two excellent publications, one by the American Dental Association and the other by the American Academy of Oral Medicine, outline the dentist's responsibility as well as a very detailed explanation of dental management protocols for HIV patients. These protocols, however, are evolving just as our knowledge of HIV has evolved. New drugs and their interactions present the dentist with continuous need for updates regarding the appropriate management of HIV patients. Diagnostic tests, including determining viral load in combination with the CD4 status, now are used to modify a patient's treatment in ways that allow them to remain relatively illness-free for longer periods of time. This places more of a responsibility on the dental practice team to be aware of drug changes, of new drugs, and of the appropriate oral management in such patients.

Our knowledge of AIDS allows us to properly treat these patients while protecting ourselves, our staff, and other patients in the office. All types of infectious disease require consistent practices in our dental offices known as Standard/Universal Precautions. These agents include sexually transmitted disease agents, the highly virulent hepatitis viruses, and the less virulent but always worrisome HIV. In general, an office that is practicing standard/universal precautions is one that is considered safe for patients and staff. Throughout this spectrum, HIV is placed somewhere in the middle, in terms of infection risk in the dental office. Other sexually transmitted diseases and infectious diseases such as tuberculosis represent a greater threat to the dentist than HIV itself. However, due to the grave danger of HIV infection, many of our precautions have been instituted to assist the dentist in protecting himself, his staff, and other patients in situations where the office may be involved in treating a patient that is HIV positive.

As in the management of all medically-compromised patients, the appropriate care of HIV patients begins with a complete and thorough history. This history must allow the dentist to identify risk factors in the development of HIV as well as identify those patients known to be HIV positive. Knowledge of all medications prescribed to patients at risk is also important.

The current antiretroviral therapy used to treat patients with HIV infection and/or AIDS includes three primary classifications of drugs. These are the nucleoside analogs, protease inhibitors, and the non-nucleoside/nucleotide analogs (analogs refers to chemicals that can substitute competitively for naturally produced cell components such as found in DNA, RNA, or proteins). The newest drugs include several nucleoside analogs, abacavir (Ziagen®), subprotease inhibitors, amprenavir, and several non-nucleoside analogs, efavirenz (Sustiva®), and adefovir. Finding the perfect "cocktail" of anti-HIV medications still eludes clinicians. This is partly due to the fact that therapies are still too novel and the patient's years too few to study. Numerous studies have indicated that combinations of drugs are far better than individual drug therapy. Several of these studies have looked at two drug combinations, particularly between nucleoside analogs in combination with protease inhibitors. The newer drugs (non-nucleoside analogs) have added the possibility of a triple "cocktail". Recently several studies indicated that this three-drug combination may be the best in managing HIV infection.

When HIV was first discovered, the efforts for monitoring HIV infection focused on the CD4 blood levels and the ratios between the helper cells, suppressor cells within the patient's immune system. These markers were used to indicate success or failure of drug therapies as patients moved through HIV pathogenesis toward AIDS. More recently, however, the advent of protease inhibitors has allowed clinicians to monitor the actual presence of viral RNA within the patient and the term viral load has become the focus of therapy monitoring. The availability of better therapies and our rapidly expanding knowledge of molecular biology of the HIV virus have created new opportunities to control the AIDS epidemic. Cases can be monitored closely looking at the number of copy units or virions within the patient's bloodstream as an indication in combination with other infections and/or declining or increasing CD4 numbers to establish prognostic values for the patient's success. Long-term survival of patients infected with HIV has been accomplished by monitoring and adjusting therapy to these numbers.

Comprehensive coordinated approaches, that have been advocated by researchers, have sought to establish national standards for HIV reporting, greater access to effective newly approved medications, improved access to individual physicians treating HIV patients, and continued protection of patient's privacy. These goals allow the reporting of studies that suggest that combination therapies, some of which have been tried in less controlled individual patient treatments, may prove useful in larger populations of HIV-infected individuals. As these studies are reported, the dental clinician should be aware that patients' drug therapies change rapidly, various combinations may be tried, and the side effects and interactions as described in the chapter on drug interactions and the CYP system will also emerge. The dentist must be aware of these potential interactions with seemingly innocuous drugs such as clarithromycin, erythromycin, and some of the sedative drugs that a dentist may utilize in their practice as well as some of the analgesics. These drug interactions may be the most important part of monitoring that the dentist provides in helping to manage a situation. Some of the antiviral drugs more commonly used for HIV, AIDS, Asymptomatic, CD4 <500, and the newer drugs (ie, protease inhibitors, nucleoside analogs, and non-nucleoside nucleotide analogs) are listed in Table 2.

Table 2. EXAMPLES OF DRUGS

Nucleoside Analogs	Protease Inhibitors	Non-nucleoside Analogs	Nucleotide Analogs	Fusion Protein Inhibitor
Zidovudine (Retrovir®, AZT, SDV)	Saquinavir (Invirase®)	Nevirapine (Viramune®)	Adefovir (Hepsera™)	Enfuvirtide (Fuzeon®)
Didanosine (Videx®, ddi)	Ritonavir (Norvir®)	Delavirdine (Rescriptor®)	Tenofovir (Viread®)	Maraviroc (Selzentry®)
Zalcitabine (Hivid® [DSC], ddc)	Indinavir (Crixivan®)	Efavirenz (Sustiva®)		
Stavudine (Zerit®, d4T)	Nelfinavir (Viracept®)			
LamiVUDine (Epivir®)	Fosamprenavir (Lexiva™)			
Abacavir (Ziagen®)	Atazanavir (Reyataz®)			
Emtricitabine (Emtriva®)	Darunavir (Prezista®)			
Entecavir (Baraclude®)	Tipranavir (Aptivus®)			
Telbivudine (Tyzeka®)				

The presence of other infections is an important part of the health history. Appropriate medical consultation may be mandated after a health history in order to accomplish a complete evaluation of the patients at risk. Uniformity in the taking of a history from a patient is the dentist's best plan for all patients so that no selectivity or discrimination can be implicated.

An appropriate review of symptoms may also identify oral and systemic conditions that may be present in aggressive HIV disease. Medical physical examination may reveal pre-existing or developing intra- or extra-oral signs/symptoms of progressive disease. Aggressive herpes simplex, herpes zoster, papillomavirus, Kaposi's sarcoma or lymphoma are among the disorders that might be identified. In addition to these, intra-oral examination may raise suspicion regarding fungal infections, angular cheilitis, squamous cell carcinoma, and recurrent aphthous ulcers. The dentist should be vigilant in all patients regardless of HIV risk.

It will always be up to the dental practitioner to determine whether testing for HIV should be recommended following the history and physical examination of a new patient. Because of the severe psychological implications of learning of HIV positivity for a patient, the dentist should be aware that there are appropriate referral sites where psychological counseling and appropriate discrete testing for the patient is available. The dentist's office should have these sites available for referral should the patient be interested. Candid discussions, however, with the patient regarding risk factors and/or other signs or symptoms in their history and physical condition that may indicate a higher HIV risk than the normal population, should be an area the dentist feels comfortable in broaching with any new patient. Oftentimes, it is appropriate to recommend testing for other infectious diseases should risk factors be present. For example, testing for hepatitis B may be appropriate for the patient and along with this the dentist could recommend that the patient consider HIV testing. Because of the legal issues involved, anonymity for HIV testing may be appropriate and it is always up to the patient to follow the doctor's recommendations.

When a patient has either given a positive history of knowing that they are HIV positive or it has been determined after referral for consultation, the dentist should be aware of the AIDS-defining illnesses. Of course, current medical status and drug therapy that the patient may be undergoing is of equal importance. The dentist, through medical consultation and regular follow-up with the patient's physician, should be made aware of the CD4 count (Table 3), the viral load, and the drugs that the patient is taking. The presence of other AIDS-defining illnesses as well as complications, such as higher risk of endocarditis and the risk of other systemic infections such as tuberculosis, are extremely important for the dentist. These may make an impact on the dental treatment plan in terms of the selection of preprocedural antibiotics or the use of oral medications to treat opportunistic infections in or around the oral cavity.

Table 3. CD4+ LYMPHOCYTE COUNT AND PERCENTAGE AS RELATED TO THE RISK OF OPPORTUNISTIC INFECTION

CD4+ Cells/mm^3	CD4+ Percentage[1]	Risk of Opportunistic Infection
>600	32-60	No increased risk
400-500	<29	Initial immune suppression
200-400	14-28	Appearance of opportunistic infections, some may be major
<200	<14	Severe immune suppression. AIDS diagnosis. Major opportunistic infections. Although variable, prognosis for surviving greater than 3 years is poor
<50	—	Although variable, prognosis for surviving greater than 1 year is poor

[1]Several studies have suggested that the CD4+ percentage demonstrates less variability between measurements, as compared to the absolute CD4+ cell count. CD4+ percentages may therefore give a clearer impression of the course of disease.

Adapted from Glick M and Silverman S, "Dental Management of HIV-Infected Patients," *J Am Dent Assoc* (Supplement to Reviewers), 1995.

AIDS-defining illnesses such as candidiasis, recurrent pneumonia, or lymphoma are clearly important to the dentist. Chemotherapy that might be being given to the patient for treatment for any or all of these disorders can have implications in terms of the patient's response to simple dental procedures.

Drug therapies have become complex in the treatment of HIV/AIDS. Because of the moderate successes with protease inhibitors and the drug combination therapies, more patients are living longer and receiving more dental care throughout their lives. Drug therapies are often tailored to the current CD4 count in combination with the viral load. In general, patients with high CD4 counts are usually at lower risk for complications in the dental office than patients with low CD4 counts. However, the presence of a high viral load with or without a stable CD4 count may be indicative or a more rapid progression of the HIV/AIDS disease process than had previously been thought. Patients with a high viral load and a declining CD4 count are considered to have the greatest risk and the poorest prognosis of all the groups.

In HIV infections, a new drug known as raltegravir is an integrase inhibitor which works by interrupting HIV integration into the host cell DNA. In addition, in 2007, a new class of anti-HIV drugs was introduced, these are the chemokine receptor 5 antagonists or the CCR5 receptor blockers. The drug of interest for this class is maraviroc. This antiviral drug has shown great promise as an adjuvant therapy along with other anti-HIV drugs.

Other organ damage, such as liver compromise potentially leading to bleeding disorders, can be found as the disease progresses to AIDS. Liver dysfunction may be related to pre-existing hepatic diseases due to previous infection with a hepatitis virus such as hepatitis B or other drug toxicities associated with the treatment of AIDS. The dentist must have available current prothrombin and partial thromboplastin times (PT and PTT) in order to accurately evaluate any risk of bleeding abnormality. Platelet count and liver function studies are also important. Potential drug interactions include some antibiotics, as well as any anticoagulating drugs, which may be contraindicated in such patients. It may be necessary to avoid NSAIDs, as well as aspirin. (See Drug Interactions: Metabolism/Transport Effects on page 2008).

The use of preprocedural antibiotics is another issue in the HIV patient. As the absolute neutrophil count declines during the progression of AIDS, the use of antibiotics as a preprocedural step prior to dental care may be necessary. If protracted treatment plans are necessary, the dentist should receive updated information as the patient receives such from their physician. It is always important that the dentist have current CD4 counts, viral load assay, as well as liver function studies, AST and ALT, and bleeding indicators including platelet count, PT, and PTT. If any other existing conditions such as cardiac involvement or joint prostheses are involved, antibiotic coverage may also be necessary. However, these determinations are no different than in the non-HIV population and this subject is covered in Antibiotic Prophylaxis - Preprocedural Guidelines for Dental Patients on page 1910. Use the table of Normal Blood Values on page 2011 as a general guideline for provision of dental care.

The consideration of current blood values is important in long-term care of any medically compromised patient and in particular the HIV-positive patient. Preventive dental care is likewise valuable in these patients, however, the dentist's approach should be no different than as with all patients. See Table 4 for oral lesions commonly associated with HIV disease and a brief description of their usual treatment (see Part II of this Oral Medicine chapter for more detailed descriptions of these common oral lesions).

The clinician should be aware that several of the protease inhibitors have now been associated with drug interactions. Some of these drug interactions include therapies that the dentist may be utilizing. The basis for these drug interactions with protease inhibitors is the inhibition of cytochrome P450 isoforms, which are important in normal liver function and metabolism of drugs. A detailed description of the mechanisms of inhibition can be found in Drug Interactions: Metabolism/Transport Effects on page 2008, as well as a table illustrating some known drug interactions with antiviral therapy and drugs commonly prescribed in the dental office. The metabolism of these drugs could be affected by the patient's antiviral therapy.

Every dental office should have in place protocols for standard/universal precautions during patient care and for emergency procedures in case of occupational exposure to blood-borne pathogens.

Table 4. ORAL LESIONS COMMONLY SEEN IN HIV/AIDS

Condition	Management
Oral candidiasis	See Fungal Infections on page 1945
Angular cheilitis	
Oral hairy leukoplakia	See Systemic Viral Diseases on page 1904
Periodontal diseases Linear gingivitis Ulcerative periodontitis	See Bacterial Infections on page 1933
Herpes simplex	Acyclovir - see Systemic Viral Diseases on page 1904
Herpes zoster	
Chronic aphthous ulceration	Palliation / Thalidomide (Thalomid®)
Salivary gland disease	Referral
Human papillomavirus	Laser / Surgical excision
Kaposi's sarcoma	See Antibiotic Prophylaxis on page 1910; Biopsy / Laser
Non-Hodgkin's lymphoma	Biopsy / Referral
Tuberculosis	Referral

Abacavir on page 24
Adefovir on page 62
Dapsone (Systemic) on page 467
Delavirdine on page 480
Didanosine on page 521
Efavirenz on page 591
Efavirenz, Emtricitabine, and Tenofovir on page 592
Emtricitabine on page 595
Emtricitabine and Tenofovir on page 596
Enfuvirtide on page 600
Etravirine on page 696
Indinavir on page 911
LamiVUDine on page 978
Lopinavir and Ritonavir on page 1032
Maraviroc on page 1054
Nelfinavir on page 1195
Ritonavir on page 1488
Stavudine on page 1551
Telbivudine on page 1589
Tenofovir on page 1600
Thalidomide on page 1615
Zidovudine on page 1742
Lamivudine and Zidovudine on page 979

Several new classes of drugs have been developed as antiretroviral drug classifications in the management of HIV infection. These are fusion inhibitors, CCR5 receptor blockers, and integrase inhibitors. The prototype fusion inhibitor is enfuvirtide (Fuzeon®). There are no significant drug interactions; however, there are numerous side effects and toxicities including Guillain-Barré syndrome, as well as taste aberrations with this drug. The prototype CCR5 receptor blocker is maraviroc (Selzentry®) and the integrase inhibitor is raltegravir (Isentress™) both with no specific oral side effects.

FREQUENTLY ASKED QUESTIONS

How does one get AIDS, aside from having unprotected sex?

Our current knowledge about the immunodeficiency virus is that it is carried via semen, contaminated needles, blood products, transfusion products not tested, and potentially in other fluids of the body. Patients at highest risk include I.V. drug-abusers, those receiving multiple transfusions with blood that has not been screened for HIV, or patients practicing unprotected sex with multiple partners, where the history of the partner may not be as clear as the patient would like.

Are patients safe from AIDS or HIV infection when they present to the dentist office?

Our current knowledge indicates that the answer is an unequivocal "yes". The patient is protected because dental offices are practicing standard/universal precautions, using antimicrobial handwashing agents, gloves, face masks, eye protection, special clothing, aerosol control, and instrument soaking and autoclaving. All of these procedures stop potential transmission to a new patient, as well as, allow for easy disposal of contaminated office supplies for elimination of microbes by an antimicrobial technique, should they be contaminated through treatment of another patient. These precautions are mandated by OSHA requirements.

What is the most common opportunistic infection that HIV-positive patients suffer that may be important in dentistry?

The most common opportunistic infection important to dentistry is oral candidiasis. This disease can present as white plaques, red areas, or angular cheilitis occurring at the corners of the mouth. Management of such lesions is appropriate by the dentist and is described in this handbook (see Fungal Infections on page 1945). Other oral complications include HIV-associated periodontal disease, as well as the other conditions outlined in Table 4. Of great concern to the dentist is the risk of tuberculosis. In many HIV-positive patients, tuberculosis has become a serious, life-threatening opportunistic infection. The dentist should be aware that appropriate referral for anyone showing such respiratory signs and symptoms would be prudent.

Can one patient infect another through unprotected sex if the other patient has tested negative for HIV?

Yes, there is always the possibility that a sexual partner may be in the early window of time when plasma viremia is not at a detectable level. The antibody response to plasma viremia may be slightly delayed and diagnostic testing may not indicate HIV positivity. This window of time represents a period when the patient may be infectious but not show up yet on normal diagnostic testing.

Can HIV be passed by oral fluids?

As our knowledge about HIV has evolved, we have thought that HIV is inactivated in saliva by an agent possibly associated with secretory leukocyte protease inhibitors known as SLPI. There is, however, a current resurgence in our interest in oral transmission because some research indicates that in moderate to advanced periodontal lesions or other oral lesions where there is tissue damage, the presence of a serous exudate may increase the risk of transmission. The dentist should be aware of this ongoing research and attempt to renew knowledge regularly so that any future breakthroughs will be noted.

REFERENCES AND SELECTED READINGS

Barouch DH, Baden LR, and Dolin R, "Human Immunodeficiency Virus Vaccines," *Principles and Practice of Infectious Disease*, 6th ed, Mandell GL, Bennett JE, and Dolin R, eds, Philadelphia, PA: Churchhill Livingstone, 2005, 1707-17.

Merson MH, "The HIV-AIDS Pandemic at 25-The Global Response," *N Engl J Med*, 2006, 354 (23):2414-7.

Panel on Antiretroviral Guidelines for Adults and Adolescents, "Guidelines for the Use of Antiretroviral Agents in HIV-Infected Adults and Adolescents, Department of Health and Human Services," 2011, 1-166. Available at http://www.aidsinfo.nih.gov

Sax PE and Walker BD, "Immunology Related to AIDS," *Cecil Textbook of Medicine*, 22nd ed, Goldman L and Ausiello D, eds, Philadelphia, PA: Saunders, 2004, 2137-8.

Workowski KA, Berman S, and Centers for Disease Control and Prevention (CDC), "Sexually Transmitted Diseases Treatment Guidelines, 2010," *MMWR Recomm Rep*, 2010, 59(RR-12):1-110. Available at http://www.cdc.gov/std/treatment/2010/STD-Treatment-2010-RR5912.pdf

RHEUMATOID ARTHRITIS, OSTEOARTHRITIS, AND OSTEOPOROSIS

RA AND OSTEOARTHRITIS MANAGEMENT

Arthritis and its variations represent the most common chronic musculoskeletal disorders of man. The conditions can essentially be divided into rheumatoid, osteoarthritic, and polyarthritic presentations. Differences in age of onset and joint involvement exist and it is now currently believed that the diagnosis of each may be less clear than previously thought. These autoinflammatory diseases have now been shown to affect young and old alike. Criteria for a diagnosis of rheumatoid arthritis include a positive serologic test for rheumatoid factor, subcutaneous nodules, affected joints on opposite sides of the body, and clear radiographic changes. The hematologic picture includes moderate normocytic hypochromic anemia, mild leukocytosis, and mild thrombocytopenia. During acute inflammatory periods, C-reactive protein is elevated and IgG and IgM (rheumatoid factors) can be detected. Osteoarthritis lacks these diagnostic features.

Other systemic conditions, such as systemic lupus erythematosus and Sjögren's syndrome, are often found simultaneously with some of the arthritic conditions. The treatment of arthritis includes the use of slow-acting and rapid-acting anti-inflammatory agents ranging from the gold salts to aspirin (see following listings). Long-term usage of these drugs can lead to numerous adverse effects including bone marrow suppression, platelet suppression, and oral ulcerations. The dentist should be aware that steroids (usually prednisone) are often prescribed along with the listed drugs and are often used in dosages sufficient to induce adrenal suppression. Adjustment of dosing prior to invasive dental procedures may be indicated along with consultation with the managing physician. Alteration of steroid dosage prior to stressful dental procedures may be necessary, usually increasing the steroid dosage prior to and during the stressful procedures and then gradually returning the patient to the original dosage over several days. Even in the absence of evidence of adrenal suppression, consultation with the prescribing physician for appropriate dosing and timing of procedures is advisable.

Antirheumatic, Disease Modifying

Abatacept on page 26
Adalimumab on page 59
Anakinra on page 143
Certolizumab Pegol on page 350
Etanercept on page 646
Golimumab on page 831
InFLIXimab on page 916
Tocilizumab on page 1642

Gold Salts

Auranofin on page 191

Metabolic Inhibitor

Leflunomide on page 988
Methotrexate on page 1099

Nonsteroidal Anti-inflammatory Agents

Diclofenac (Systemic) on page 513
Diflunisal on page 524
Etodolac on page 690
Fenoprofen on page 715
Flurbiprofen (Systemic) on page 763
Ibuprofen on page 884
Indomethacin on page 912
Ketoprofen on page 966
Ketorolac (Systemic) on page 969
Meclofenamate on page 1059
Mefenamic Acid on page 1062
Meloxicam on page 1066

Nabumetone on page 1172
Naproxen on page 1183
Oxaprozin on page 1262
Piroxicam on page 1360
Sulindac on page 1564
Tiaprofenic Acid
Tolmetin on page 1645

COX-2 Inhibitor NSAID

Celecoxib on page 342

Combination NSAID Product to Prevent GI Distress

Diclofenac and Misoprostol on page 519
Naproxen and Esomeprazole on page 1187

Salicylates

Aminosalicylic Acid on page 101
Aspirin on page 171
Choline Magnesium Trisalicylate on page 376
Magnesium Salicylate on page 1051
Salsalate on page 1507

Other

Hydroxychloroquine on page 874
PredniSONE on page 1393

OSTEOPOROSIS MANAGEMENT

Prevalence

Osteoporosis effects 25 million Americans of which 80% are women; 27% of American women >80 years of age have osteopenia and 70% of American women >80 years of age have osteoporosis.

Consequences

1.3 million bone fractures annually (low impact/nontraumatic) and pain, pulmonary insufficiency, decreased quality of life, and economic costs; >250,000 hip fractures per year with a 20% mortality rate.

Risk Factors

Advanced age, female, chronic renal disease, hyperparathyroidism, Cushing's disease, hypogonadism/anorexia, hyperprolactinemia, cancer, large and prolonged dose heparin or glucocorticoids, anticonvulsants, hyperthyroidism (current or history, or excessive thyroid supplements), sedentary, excessive exercise, early menopause, oophorectomy without hormone replacement, excessive aluminum-containing antacid, smoking, methotrexate.

Diagnosis / Monitoring

DXA bone density, history of fracture (low impact or nontraumatic), compressed vertebrae, decreased height, hump-back appearance. Osteomark® urine assay measures bone breakdown fragments and may help assess therapy response earlier than DXA but diagnostic value is uncertain as Osteomark® does not reveal extent of bone loss. Bone markers may be tested to evaluate effectiveness of antiresorptive urine therapy. The clinician is referred to Osteonecrosis of the Jaw on page 1894 since the bisphosphonates are associated with this adverse event.

Prevention

1. Adequate dietary calcium (eg, dairy products)
2. Vitamin D (eg, fortified dairy products, cod, fatty fish)
3. Weight-bearing exercise (eg, walking) as tolerated
4. Fall prevention (eg, visual/hearing checks, minimizing pharmacologic agents that contribute to fall risk, checking environment for safety hazards)
5. Avoidance of tobacco use and excessive alcohol intake

6. Calcium: Adequate intake of at least 1200 mg **elemental** calcium daily in the form of dietary calcium or calcium supplementation, particularly women ≥50 years of age. Intakes exceeding 1200-1500 mg offer limited additional benefit and may increase the risk for cardiovascular disease or kidney stones. To minimize constipation add fiber and start with 500 mg/day for several months, then increase to 500 mg twice daily taken at different times than fiber. Chewable and liquid products are available. Calcium carbonate is given with food to enhance bioavailability. Calcium citrate may be given without regards to meals.
   - Contraindications: Hypercalcemia, ventricular fibrillation
   - Side effects: Constipation, anorexia
   - Drug interactions: Fiber, tetracycline, iron supplement, minerals
7. Vitamin D Supplement: Adequate intake of at least 800-1000 int. units of vitamin D for adults ≥50 years of age. Measuring serum vitamin D concentrations may be warranted, particularly in those at greatest risk for deficiency, to allow for the administration of vitamin D replacement. **Note:** Certain patients at risk for vitamin D deficiency (eg, elderly, diseases associated with malabsorption, chronic renal insufficiency) may require higher intakes. Some elderly, especially with significant renal or liver disease cannot metabolize (activate) vitamin D and require calcitriol 0.25 mcg orally twice daily or adjusted per serum calcium level, the active form of vitamin D.
   - Contraindications: Hypercalcemia (weakness, headache, drowsiness, nausea, diarrhea), hypercalciuria and renal stones
   - Side effects (uncommon): Hypercalcemia (see above)
   - Monitor 24-hour urine and serum calcium if using >1000 units/day
8. Bisphosphonates: Osteoporosis prevention: Postmenopausal Females:
   - Alendronate: Oral: 5 mg once daily **or** 35 mg once weekly
   - Ibandronate: Oral: 2.5 mg once daily **or** 150 mg once per month
   - Risedronate: Oral: 5 mg once daily **or** 35 mg once weekly **or** one 75 mg tablet once daily on two consecutive days per month (total: 2 tablets/month) or 150 mg once per month
   - Zoledronic acid (Reclast®): I.V.: 5 mg infused over at least 15 minutes every 2 years
9. Glucocorticoid-induced osteoporosis prevention: Males and Females:
   - Risedronate: Oral: 5 mg once daily
   - Zoledronic acid (Reclast®): I.V.: 5 mg infused over at least 15 minutes every 12 months (in patients initiating or continuing prednisone ≥7.5 mg/day [or equivalent] and expected to remain on glucocorticoids for at least 12 months)
10. Estrogen agonist/antagonist (previously known as selective estrogen receptor modulators):
    - Postmenopausal Females: Raloxifene: Oral: 60 mg once daily; may be taken any time of the day without regard to meals but should be stopped 72 hours prior to or during immobilization due to risk of thromboembolic events.
11. Parathyroid hormone: Initial administration of teriparatide should occur under circumstances in which the patient may sit or lie down, in the event of orthostasis
    - Glucocorticoid-induced osteoporosis prevention: Males and Females: Teriparatide: SubQ: 20 mcg once daily
12. Estrogens/hormone therapy: Should not be considered first agents for preventing osteoporosis due to increased risk of breast cancer, heart disease, stroke, and deep-vein thrombosis (DVT) found in the Women's Health Initiative study. Estrogens, as well as various combination therapies, including ethinyl estradiol and norethindrone (femhrt®) and estradiol and norgestimate (Prefest™), have been approved for the prevention of osteoporosis. The FDA recommends that approved nonestrogen treatments should be considered before the use of estrogen/hormone therapy for the sole purpose of prevention of osteoporosis. **Note:** In women with an intact uterus, administer estrogen with oral progesterone; unopposed estrogen can cause endometrial cancer.

Treatment

1. Calcium, vitamin D, exercise, and estrogen: As above
2. Bisphosphonates: Oral bisphosphonates should be administered ≥30 minutes before first food or drink (except water) with 6-8 ounces tap water (**not** mineral water) and patients should remain upright (or raise head of bed to at least a 30° angle) to avoid ulcerative esophagitis. Consult individual monographs for details regarding use, precautions, dosing, and administration of any of the specific drugs mentioned below.
   - Alendronate: Males and Postmenopausal Females: Oral: 10 mg once daily or 70 mg once weekly
   - Ibandronate: Postmenopausal Females:
     - Oral: 2.5 mg once daily or 150 mg once per month
     - I.V.: 3 mg every 3 months
   - Risedronate:
     - Postmenopausal Females: Oral: 5 mg once daily or 35 mg once weekly or one 75 mg tablet once daily on two consecutive days per month (total: 2 tablets/month) or 150 mg once monthly
     - Males: Oral: 35 mg once weekly
   - Zoledronic acid (Reclast®): Males and Postmenopausal Females: I.V.: 5 mg infused over at least 15 minutes every 12 months
   - Glucocorticoid-induced osteoporosis treatment:
     - Alendronate: Oral: 5 mg once daily; Postmenopausal females not receiving estrogen: 10 mg once daily
     - Risedronate: Oral: 5 mg once daily
     - Zoledronic acid (Reclast®): I.V.: 5 mg infused over at least 15 minutes every 12 months (in patients initiating or continuing prednisone ≥7.5 mg/day [or equivalent] and expected to remain on glucocorticoids for at least 12 months)
3. Estrogen agonist/antagonist (previously known as selective estrogen receptor modulators):
   - Postmenopausal Females: Raloxifene: Oral: 60 mg once daily; may be taken any time of the day without regard to meals but should be stopped 72 hours prior to or during immobilization due to risk of thromboembolic events.
4. Calcitonin: Adequate dietary or supplemental calcium and vitamin D are essential.
   - Osteoporosis treatment: Postmenopausal Females (>5 years postmenopause):
     - Calcitonin (Miacalcin®): I.M., SubQ: 100 units every other day (I.M. route is preferred if volume exceeds 2 mL)
     - Calcitonin (Fortical®, Miacalcin®): Intranasal: 200 units (1 spray) in one nostril daily, alternate right and left nostril
5. Parathyroid hormone: Initial administration of teriparatide should occur under circumstances in which the patient may sit or lie down, in the event of orthostasis.
   - Osteoporosis treatment: Postmenopausal females at high risk of fracture or treatment of primary or hypogonadal osteoporosis in men at high risk of fracture:
     - Teriparatide: SubQ: 20 mcg once daily
   - Glucocorticoid-induced osteoporosis treatment: Males and Females: Teriparatide: SubQ: 20 mcg once daily
6. Fall prevention: Minimize psychoactive and cardiovascular drugs (monitor BP for orthostasis), give diuretics early in the day, environmental safety check.

	% Elemental Calcium	Elemental Calcium
Calcium gluconate (various)	9	500 mg = 45 mg
Calcium glubionate (Calcionate)	6.5	1.8 g = 115 g/5 mL
Calcium lactate (various)	13	325 mg = 42.25 mg
Calcium citrate (Citrical®)	21	950 mg = 200 mg
Effervescent tabs (Citrical Liquitab®)		2376 mg = 500 mg
Calcium acetate		
Phos-Ex 250®	25	1000 mg = 250 mg
Phos-Lo®		667 mg = 169 mg
Calcium phosphate, tribasic (Posture®)	39	1565.2 mg = 600 mg
Calcium carbonate		
Tums®	40	1.2 g = 500 mg
Oscal-500® oral suspension		1.2 g/5 mL = 500 mg
Caltrate 600®		1.5 g = 600 mg

REFERENCES AND SELECTED READINGS

Saag KG, Teng GG, Patkar NM, et al, "American College of Rheumatology 2008 Recommendations for the Use of Nonbiologic and Biologic Disease-Modifying Antirheumatic Drugs in Rheumatoid Arthritis," *Arthritis Rheum*, 2008, 59(6):762-84.

National Osteoporosis Foundation, "Clinician's Guide to Prevention and Treatment of Osteoporosis," Washington, DC, 2010. Available at http://www.nof.org

OSTEONECROSIS OF THE JAW

Osteonecrosis of the jaw (ONJ), which is relevant to the discussion of osteoporosis as well as Management of Patients Undergoing Cancer Therapy on page 1970 is an uncommon condition that results in exposure of bone in the oral cavity. Other signs and symptoms may be associated with changes in bone metabolism and/or poor wound healing, but also can develop spontaneously, such as along the mylohyoid ridge, away from teeth, or any site where obvious trauma could have occurred. Cases of ONJ began to emerge in approximately 2003 and were linked primarily with patients with cancer and those receiving the drugs zoledronic acid (Zometa®) and/or pamidronate (Aredia®) which are bisphosphonates administered by an intravenous route. A third intravenous bisphosphonate, clodronate (Bonefos®), is encountered much less commonly. Other bisphosphonates have been used for many years in the treatment of osteoporosis, Paget's disease, and other bone mineralization diseases, including a group of bisphosphonates administered orally.

Bone disease occurs in many patients with cancer, particularly those with multiple myeloma and metastatic lesions associated with breast cancer, prostate cancer, and other cancers. These changes are often associated with pain and pathologic fractures. This bone destruction often results from changes in the osteoclast and osteoblast activities related to bone remodeling and healing following trauma. Bisphosphonates act at sites of active bone remodeling, changing the activity of the cells necessary for osteoclastic activity. There are no data that indicate that bisphosphonates directly change mineralization of the bone; however, these drugs do result in changes in the vascularity of the bone and cell activity.

Since the emergence of numerous cases of ONJ and their documentation, the American Dental Association through its Council on Scientific Affairs has released various news reports and position statements related to the state of the current knowledge and recommendations for the practicing dental professionals to manage patients who may be at risk for ONJ. Most of the data that exist are related to the use of intravenous bisphosphonates in cancer patients. Recently, data has begun to emerge related to oral bisphosphonates and the risk of ONJ in patients who are receiving a significantly lower dosage of bisphosphonate via the oral route. Also refer to Management of Patients Undergoing Cancer Therapy on page 1970

A panel of experts convened by the American Dental Association believes that dental patients who are taking oral bisphosphonates should discuss with their dentist the risks that they face when undergoing procedures that involve the jaw bone, such as tooth extraction or placement of implants. The ADA recommends that a comprehensive oral evaluation be carried out on all patients and if they are about to begin oral bisphosphonates, patients should be made aware of the potential long-term risks. However, the ADA notes that dentists generally will not need to modify dental treatments based solely on bisphosphonate therapy. Furthermore, patients must understand that the risk for developing ONJ is considered very small and the vast majority of patients taking oral bisphosphonates will never develop any particular oral complication.

Orally Administered Bisphosphonates

Alendronate (Fosamax®) on page 72
Clodronate (Clasteon®) (Canada only) on page 410
Etidronate (Didronel®) on page 689
Ibandronate (Boniva®) on page 880
Risedronate (Actonel®) on page 1478
Tiludronate (Skelid®) on page 1631

The current dental management recommendations for patients on oral bisphosphonates comprised by the American Dental Association's Council on Scientific Affairs was released, in 2006. The risk of developing ONJ is very low, however, millions of patients take these drugs; therefore, the recommendations must be disseminated to the dental community. The Panel's recommendations focus on conservative dental procedures, proper sterile technique, appropriate use of oral disinfectants, and principles of effective antibiotic therapy. There are currently no data from clinical trials evaluating dental management of patients on oral bisphosphonates and therefore these recommendations are based on expert opinion only.

The dentist must always carry out a comprehensive oral evaluation and should stay active in reviewing the literature as new data emerge. The reference list below refers primarily to intravenous bisphosphonate therapy since this is where most of the data have been accumulated. The various drug manufacturers have placed precautionary statements in their product inserts and the dentist should be familiar with these precaution statements since the wording is very carefully based on the data that are available.

The latest reference on the management treatment of patients with ONJ has been published in the *Journal of Oncology Practice*. All of the information contained in these recommendations is available through the drug companies' precautionary statements as well as doctor letters which have been disseminated to every practicing dentist in the world. In addition, new information is emerging as data develop.

FREQUENTLY ASKED QUESTIONS

According to the latest literature, what is the incidence of ONJ in oral bisphosphonates users?

Presently, the current estimates of the frequency of occurrence of ONJ in oral bisphosphonate users are the following: Merck drug company, the manufacturer of Fosamax® calculated the incidence of ONJ to be 0.7 cases per 100,000 person-years of exposure to oral bisphosphonates. The Medical Consultants of Consumer Reports On-Health Bulletin reported an incidence of one case for every 20,000 users of oral bisphosphonates (0.005%). A recent report from Australia estimated that the frequency of ONJ in osteoporotic patients mainly on weekly oral alendronate (Fosamax®) ranged from a minimum of 1 in 8470 to a maximum of 1 in 2260 (0.01% to 0.04%) patients. If extractions were performed, the frequency increased to 0.09% to 0.34%.

What numbers can practitioners use to tell the dental patient their risk of developing ONJ with oral bisphosphonates?

The recommendations from the Expert Panel of the American Dental Association suggest that the patient be informed that there is a very low risk of developing ONJ. The true risk posed by oral bisphosphonates remains uncertain, but appears to be very small. All the data seem to point to a risk of ~0.1% of total users and that the risk increases with dental extractions to ~0.3%. Also, be aware that the risks of developing ONJ can be minimized but never totally eliminated. Good oral hygiene along with regular dental care is the best way to lower the risk of developing ONJ. The current data on incidence of ONJ in patients taking oral bisphosphonates is retrospective information derived primarily from surveys and the number of reported cases in patients taking the drugs. More meaningful assessment of incidence of ONJ in the population at risk must come from retrospective or prospective cohort investigations. To date, no such studies have been reported.

Is the risk of acquiring osteonecrosis of the jaw bone diminished with the use of other oral bisphosphonates compared to Fosamax®?

In addition to alendronate (Fosamax®), cases of ONJ, albeit rare, have been reported in patients taking either risedronate (Actonel®) or ibandronate (Boniva®). Among the class of oral bisphosphonates, more cases have been associated with Fosamax® than with Actonel® or Boniva®. Also, there is no evidence to suggest that the risk of ONJ is less when taking monthly doses of Boniva®. Zoledronic acid under the band name of Reclast® has recently been approved as a once annual 15 minute intravenous infusion of a dose of 5 mg to prevent osteoporosis. This dosing was associated with a significant improvement in bone mineral density and bone metabolism markers. It is unknown whether this dosing schedule places the patient at risk for ONJ; however, data do show a higher risk of serious atrial fibrillation in patients receiving Reclast® compared to patients receiving placebo.

Will Fosamax® or the other oral bisphosphonates continue to be the standard treatment for osteoporosis?

Yes. The oral bisphosphonates continue to be the most effective class of drugs in reducing the risk of osteoporotic fractures and are the first line therapy in the treatment of osteoporosis. Fosamax® has been shown to prevent bone loss at the spine and hip in postmenopausal women and to reduce fractures by ~50%. Risedronate (Actonel®) produced a 30% reduction in hip fractures. Fosamax® continues to be in the top 50 of the most widely prescribed drugs in this country. By 2006, over 190 million prescriptions were dispensed worldwide.

Do we know the pathogenesis of ONJ?

This question has not been answered and information is only speculative at this time. Osteoporosis can occur due to age-related changes in the number of osteoclasts and bone resorption sites. This overwhelms the production of new bone by osteoblasts and a decrease in bone mass occurs. By inhibiting osteoclastic activity, the oral bisphosphonates seemingly arrest the osteoporotic syndrome. In the process, however, the maxilla and mandible, upon continued exposure to the bisphosphonates, are unable to repair themselves from injury from mechanical forces or invasive surgery such as tooth extraction. This coupled with a reduction in bone blood supply by the bisphosphonates (antiangiogenic effect) leads to jaw bone necrosis. Ruggiero and Drew have suggested that a preferential deposition of the bisphosphonates in the mandible and maxilla may contribute to the necrosis appearing within the jaw rather than within bones outside the craniofacial skeleton.

What are the factors that increase the risk of ONJ in oral bisphosphonate users?

Patients with a history of periodontal disease and dental abscesses are at increased risk of developing ONJ if taking oral bisphosphonates. Also, dentoalveolar trauma will increase the risk. The use of chronic steroids such as prednisone has been identified as a risk factor. Other factors are the duration of exposure and age, with longer treatment regimens and age >65 years associated with a greater risk of developing the disease. Patients identified with jaw bone necrosis typically were exposed to oral bisphosphonates for 3 years or longer.

What are the symptoms that an oral bisphosphonates patient would experience which could indicate necrotic jaw bone?

Tooth mobility, mucosal swelling, and/or ulceration. Clinical symptoms would include a nonhealing extraction site, exposed bone surrounded by inflamed soft tissue, and purulent discharge at site of exposed bone. Exposed bone is usually more prevalent in areas such as the tori and the mylohyoid ridge.

What kind of dental procedures can be performed in oral bisphosphonate users with no increase in risk for ONJ?

According to the American Dental Association, all routine procedures can be carried out. Routine dental treatment should not be modified on the basis of oral bisphosphonates on board the patient. However, presence of risk factors such as steroid use, >65 years of age, or prolonged exposure to the oral bisphosphonates may require consultation with an expert in metabolic bone disease prior to routine dental treatment.

Is dentoalveolar surgery contraindicated in Fosamax® users?

According to both Ruggiero et al, and Marx et al, no alteration or delay in planned surgery is typically necessary in patients taking an oral bisphosphonate for <3 years and having no other risk factors for ONJ. In asymptomatic patients receiving oral bisphosphonate therapy, dentoalveolar surgery is not contraindicated. Also surgery common to periodontists and other dental providers need not be delayed.

In addition, Marx suggested that if dental implants are placed, informed consent should be obtained related to the potential for implant failure and possible ONJ if the patient continues to take an oral bisphosphonate.

Is a so-called "drug holiday" an effective way to reduce the risks of ONJ?

Although a "drug holiday" has been suggested by some groups, there is no statistically significant evidence indicating in the cancer patient population that this is beneficial in reducing ONJ risk and in fact may be detrimental if the chance of a skeletal related event increases. The data in oral bisphosphonates use are even less compelling since the incidence is so low to begin with that subjective drug holidays can not be documented with any degree of confidence. As mentioned earlier, for individuals who have taken a bisphosphonate for <3 years and have no other risk factors for ONJ, no alteration or delay in the planned surgery is necessary.

In patients about to begin oral bisphosphonate therapy, should the bisphosphonate be delayed until dental health is optimized?

No. It does not appear necessary for patients to initiate prophylactic dental treatment prior to initiating oral bisphosphonate therapy for osteoporosis. It would be prudent, however, to encourage these patients to maintain an optimal level of dental health.

Is diagnostic imaging useful in assessing oral bisphosphonate individuals at risk for ONJ?

Imaging modalities have proved helpful in determining the extent of existing necrotic process, but have not been able to demonstrate any efficacy in assessing patients at risk for ONJ. It has been reported that panoramic and periapical radiographs probably will not reveal significant changes in early stages of osteonecrosis and they are poor screening tools for prediction. Computerized tomography (CT) scan also has not proved helpful with early identification of osteonecrosis in asymptomatic patients.

Do the Fosamax®-type drugs increase the risk of ONJ in patients receiving dental implants?

A conclusive cause and effect relationship between bisphosphonate therapy and ONJ still has not been established. Evidence does suggest, however, that such an association may exist, particularly with intravenous bisphosphonate use in cancer patients. Oral bisphosphonates are widely used for the treatment of osteoporosis. It is estimated that 22-30 million prescriptions were written for alendronate (Fosamax®), the most widely used oral bisphosphonate in the United States, between May 2003 and April 2004. For many years, dental implants have been placed in many patients taking oral bisphosphonates. Prior to the reports on the risk of bisphosphonate-associated ONJ, these patients were treated without any modification of the surgically placed implant procedure. Recently, however, guidelines from the American Dental Association (ADA) and the American Association of Oral and Maxillofacial Surgeons (AAOMS) have suggested a cautious approach to implant surgery and extractions for patients receiving bisphosphonate therapy.

Regarding dental implants, the ADA report cautions practitioners that patients may be at increased risk of developing osteonecrosis of the jaw bone when extensive implant placement or guided bone regeneration is necessary.

If dental implants are to be placed, the AAOMS Task Force suggested contacting the physician who prescribed the oral bisphosphonate prior to surgery to suggest an alternate dosing schedule, a drug holiday (discontinuance of the drug for a short time period), or an alternative to bisphosphonate therapy. It is important to remember that any beneficial or detrimental effects of these drug holidays have not been prospectively studied.

In addition, Marx has suggested the following precautions. Dental implant, if elected, can be placed in the patient about to begin oral bisphosphonate therapy. However, informed consent concerning the potential for implant loss and/or exposed bone related to the bisphosphonates should be obtained as the patient continues bisphosphonate therapy and exceeds 3 years of continuous use. For individuals who have taken an oral bisphosphonate for <3 years and have no clinical or radiographic risk factors, no alteration or delay is necessary for planned dental surgeries. If dental implants are placed, inform consent should be obtained related to the potential for implant failure and possible ONJ if the patient continues to take the bisphosphonate.

For patients who have taken an oral bisphosphonates for >3 years, it is advised that the prescribing physician be contacted and a recommendation made to discontinue the oral bisphosphonate for 3 months prior to the procedure and refrain from reinstating use until 3 months after the procedure.

One report from the UK suggested an even more conservative approach. Scully et al, suggested that where possible, extractions should be avoided in patients receiving oral bisphosphonates and it is best to avoid all elective surgery in these patients including endosseous implant placement or treatment should be performed well in advance prior to bisphosphonate therapy. If surgery is performed on patients taking bisphosphonates, they must be counseled about the risk.

A new report showed that implant surgery on patients receiving Fosamax®-type drugs did not result in bisphosphonate-associated ONJ. This study, out of the Dentistry/Oral Surgery Group at Montefiore Medical Center, Albert Einstein College of Medicine, reported that of 115 patients taking oral bisphosphonates, none showed evidence or had symptoms of osteonecrosis after implant placement. This report had findings similar to a previous report by Dr Jeffcoat, who showed success in implant placement and no signs of necrosis in patients taking oral bisphosphonates.

The Montefiore study, by Grant et al, used a survey to collect information from patients who had received dental implants and were taking oral bisphosphonates. The study, reported in the *Journal of Oral and Maxillofacial Surgery*, identified 1319 female patients >40 years of age who had implant surgery between January 1998 and December 2006. A survey was mailed to each of these individuals asking about current and past use of oral bisphosphonates. Of the 1319 surveys mailed out, 458 (35%) were returned. From those returned, 115 individuals reported taking oral bisphosphonates before or after implant surgery. None reported receiving intravenous bisphosphonates. In this population, it was then determined that a total of 468 implants had been placed in the 115 individuals. This population that responded to the survey was then compared to a random sample of individuals who did not respond with regard to age and number of implants. It was found that only five among 100 nonresponders to the survey had a history of bisphosphonate use compared to the 115 of the 458 responders. The remaining 343 patients indicated that they had not received bisphosphonate therapy. From the pool of 458 responders, there were 1450 implants placed in these patients and 1436 had integrated successfully. Implant success was defined using criteria which included the absence of symptoms such as pain, infection, paresthesia, or neuropathies and that the dental implant should provide functional service for 5 years in 75% of the cases.

The results were the following:

1. None of the 458 responders to the survey reported symptoms of bisphosphonate-associated ONJ.
2. Since 115 of the 458 responders indicated they were treated with bisphosphonates, it was assumed that none of the 115 responders treated with bisphosphonates had ONJ.
3. Out of the pool of 115 patients, there was a total of 468 implants placed. It was found that 466 of those implants were in function and were considered successful. Only two implants failed. In one case of failure, the patient had taken oral bisphosphonates for 3 years prior to implant placement but no longer was taking any drug at the time of implant placement or thereafter. The investigators removed and replaced the implant and it was still in function for more than 4 years. In the second case, the patient had been taking bisphosphonates for more than 8 years and the failure occurred in one implant out of a total of 13 in place. The failed implant was removed, not replaced, and the area healed uneventfully.
4. There were no reports of ONJ from any of the 861 patients who did not return the survey.

This report from Montefiore is consistent with that of the findings of Jeffcoat. She also reported success in implant placement and no signs of necrosis in patients taking oral bisphosphonates. Her method was a single blind controlled study using 50 postmenopausal female dental implant patients. Twenty-five had taken oral bisphosphonates for 1-4 years and the other 25 patients did not take oral bisphosphonates prior to or during the study. In the bisphosphonate group, there was a total of 102 implants that were placed and in the nondrug group, there were 108 implants that were placed. After 3 years, there was 100% success rate with no evidence of infection, pain, or necrosis in patients receiving bisphosphonates. There was 99.2% success rate in the group not taking oral bisphosphonates.

A further review of the literature found only two cases of dental implant failure associated with oral bisphosphonate use. One was a case report from 1995 that suggested that failure of five implants was caused by bisphosphonate therapy. In that case, five implants were placed and successfully integrated in the mandible. The patient then began bisphosphonate therapy 28 months after implant placement and after 4 months, a panoramic radiograph revealed osteolysis around all implants and all five were removed one month later.

In the report by Wang et al, a patient developed a significant bone defect with necrosis after proper implant placement. The patient was a 65-year old female who had taken Fosamax® for 10 years. She received five implants in the mandible. Ten days after surgery, healing appeared to be progression uneventfully. Four weeks later upon evaluation, bone defects were observed and noted around two of the implants. The defects were repaired with mineralized human cancellous bone mixed with tetracycline and covered with collagen membrane. Eventually after some further antibiotics and chlorhexidine daily rinsing, complete uneventful healing occurred.

Is the CTX bone marker useful to assess the risk of ONJ in oral bisphosphonate users?

CTX is an acronym for C-terminal telopeptide. During bone resorption, the dominant type 1 collagen is degraded and, during this collagen breakdown, the telopeptide (CTX) is released. Thus, serum levels of CTX can be used as an indicator of bone breakdown/resorption. The CTX blood test, as a risk marker for ONJ, first proposed by Marx in 2007, was used in an Australian study to determine its effectiveness in the prevention and management of ONJ in patient taking bisphosphonates. Essentially, this test was found to be able to identify groups of those individuals in the "risk zone" for developing ONJ, which was defined as a blood level of 150 picograms/mL (pg/mL) to 200 picograms/mL (pg/mL). It was, however, not found to be predictive of the development of ONJ in any individual patient. The CTX test requires a 1 mL sample of whole blood drawn in the morning in fasted individuals. Marx used Quest Diagnostics Nichols East Lab in San Juan Capistrano California to perform the analysis on the samples. Values lower than 100 pg/mL were correlated with a high risk of ONJ; values between 100 pg/mL and 150 pg/mL correlated to a moderate risk and values >150 pg/mL associated with minimal or no risk. According to Ruggiero and Drew, low bone turnover in the jaw due to osteoclastic inhibition by bisphosphonates results in the inability of the bone to repair local microdamage from normal mechanical loading or injury. This ultimately results in bone necrosis. Thus, individuals with low CTX values while taking bisphosphonates are assumed to have jaw bones which may not be able to normally repair themselves and these individuals would have a relatively higher risk of developing ONJ compared to individuals having higher CTX serum values.

Rigorous prospective studies on greater numbers of individuals are required before the use of the CTX serum test could be suggested with any confidence.

Do the new anti-RANK-L drugs such as denosumab (Prolia™, Xgeva™) increase the risk of ONJ?

ONJ has been rarely reported in clinical studies in patients receiving denosumab at FDA-approved doses for osteoporosis. In clinical studies, patients with advanced cancer treated with 120 mg denosumab administered monthly, have reported a 2% incidence of ONJ. Known risk factors for ONJ include a diagnosis of cancer with bone lesions, concomitant therapies (eg, chemotherapy, antiangiogenic biologics, corticosteroids, radiotherapy to the head and neck), poor oral hygiene, dental extractions, comorbid disorders (eg, pre-existing dental disease, anaemia, coagulopathy, infection) and previous treatment with bisphosphonates.

A dental examination with appropriate preventive dentistry should be considered prior to initiating denosumab treatment in patients with concomitant risk factors. These patients should avoid invasive dental procedures if possible during treatment with denosumab. Patients should maintain good oral hygiene during treatment. For patients who develop ONJ while on denosumab therapy, dental surgery may exacerbate the condition. Use clinical judgement and guide the management plan of each patient based on individual risk:benefit evaluation.

Denosumab on page 483

CLINICAL DENTAL MANAGEMENT CONSIDERATIONS

Suggested Preventive Dentistry Before Initiating Chemotherapy, Immunotherapy, or Bisphosphonate Therapy

- Remove abscessed and nonrestorable teeth and teeth with severe periodontal disease involvement
- Remove teeth with poor long-term prognosis
- Functionally rehabilitate salvageable dentition, including endodontic therapy
- Perform dental prophylaxis, caries control, and stabilizing restorative dental care
- Examine dentures to ensure proper fit (dentures should be removed at night)
- Educate patients on oral self-care hygiene

Patients at Risk of ONJ Due to Bisphosphonate Therapy (Without Any Signs of ONJ):

Invasive dental procedures should be avoided in patients receiving intravenous bisphosphonate therapy. These procedures should also be performed ideally prior to a patient starting bisphosphonate I.V. therapy. The treating physician should guide the management plan of each patient based on individual benefit:risk assessment and communication with the dentist. For patients requiring dental procedures, there are no prospective data available to suggest whether discontinuation of bisphosphonate treatment reduces the risk of ONJ.

There are five primary actions in this management plan:

1. Patients should be educated on maintaining excellent oral hygiene to reduce the risk of need for invasive procedures in the future.
2. Patients should check and adjust removable appliances such as prostheses to avoid soft tissue injury.
3. Routine cleaning should be performed with care, attempting to reduce any soft tissue injury; however, since hygiene is important, the normal recall planning and treatment should continue.
4. Dental infection should be managed aggressively and nonsurgically when possible. Alternatives such as endodontic therapy or over extraction may be advisable.
5. Endodontic therapy is preferable to extractions; treatment with endodontics followed by coronal amputation and root canal therapy on the retained roots may be necessary.

If a Patient Develops Osteonecrosis of the Jaw: Consultations between oral surgeons/dental oncologists and the treating physician are strongly recommended:

- A nonsurgical approach is recommended to prevent further osseous injury.
- Only minimal bony debridement to reduce sharp and rough surfaces to prevent further trauma to adjacent or opposing tissues is recommended.
- A removable appliance or protective stent may be used to protect exposed bone or adjacent tissues.
- Before discontinuing bisphosphonate therapy, patient should be evaluated for potential risk of further osteonecrosis versus the risk of skeletal complications.
- Hyperbaric oxygen therapy is not recommended.
- Biopsy is not recommended unless metastasis to the jaw is suspected.
- Cultures should be taken for directed antimicrobial therapy.
- Prophylactic antibiotic therapy may be considered for pain and disease control.

SAMPLE PRESCRIPTIONS FOR PROPHYLACTIC ANTIBIOTIC THERAPY

Rx:
Amoxicillin 875 mg tablets
Disp: 60 tablets
Sig: Take 1 tablet twice daily

Note: Alternatively, 500 mg tablet 3 times daily can be prescribed and may be continued for >1 month. Patients should be cautioned regarding gastrointestinal side effects with long-term use of any antibiotic. Probiotics may help but evidence is conflicted on true efficacy.

Rx:
Clindamycin (Systemic) 300 mg capsules
Disp: 40 capsules
Sig: Take 1 capsule 3 or 4 times/day for 7-10 days

Note: Prescription usually selected for patients allergic to penicillin; may be prescribed for 3 or 4 times/day. This prescription can be continued for >1 month; however, risk of *Clostridium difficile* colitis increases. Patients should be cautioned to take clindamycin with food and monitor for gastrointestinal side effects with long-term use. Probiotics may help but evidence is conflicted on true efficacy.

Rx:
Chlorhexidine Oral Rinse
Disp: 1 bottle
Sig: Rinse with 20 cc twice daily for 30 seconds and expectorate

ONJ Diagnosis and Definition

- Intraoral pain is variable
- Complaint of roughness along the teeth or ridge
- History of dental procedures eg, extractions, but may occur on tissues
- Complaint of ill-fitting denture(s)
- Diagnosis made clinically with presence of exposed bone in maxillofacial region (>8 weeks duration [with no history of radiation therapy])
- If the presence of exposed bone in maxillofacial region is noted but is <8 weeks duration (with no history of radiation therapy), the clinician must consider a differential diagnosis of:
  - Spontaneous lingual mandibular sequestration with ulceration
  - Trauma
  - Advanced periodontal disease with dehiscence
  - Local malignancy
  - Metastatic cancer

REFERENCES AND SELECTED READINGS

Advisory Task Force on Bisphosphonate-Related Osteonecrosis of the Jaws, American Association of Oral and Maxillofacial Surgeons, "American Association of Oral and Maxillofacial Surgeons Position Paper on Bisphosphonate-Related Osteonecrosis of the Jaws," *J Oral Maxillofac Surg*, 2007, 65 (3):369-76.

Aghaloo TL, Felsenfeld AL, and Tetradis S, "Osteonecrosis of the Jaw in a Patient on Denosumab," *J Oral Maxillofac Surg*, 2010, 68(5):959-63.

Almubarak H, Jones A, Chaisuparat R, et al, "Zoledronic Acid Directly Suppresses Cell Proliferation and Induces Apoptosis in Highly Tumorigenic Prostate and Breast Cancers," *J Carcinog*, 2011, 10:2.

American Dental Association Council on Scientific Affairs, "Dental Management of Patients Receiving Oral Bisphosphonate Therapy: Expert Panel Recommendations," *J Am Dent Assoc*, 2006, 137 (8):1144-50.

Arthritis and Allied Conditions: A Textbook of Rheumatology, Vol 1, 15th ed, Koopman WJ and Moreland LW, eds, Philadelphia, PA: Lippincott, Williams and Wilkins, 2005, 1448.

Badros A, Weikel D, Salama A, et al, "Osteonecrosis of the Jaw in Multiple Myeloma Patients: Clinical Features and Risk Factors," *J Clin Oncol*, 2006, 24(6):945-52.

Black DM, Delmas PD, Eastell R, et al, "Once-Yearly Zoledronic Acid for Treatment of Postmenopausal Osteoporosis," *N Engl J Med*, 2007, 356(18):1809-22.

Bone HG, Hosking D, Devogelaer JP, et al, "Ten Years' Experience With Alendronate for Osteoporosis in Postmenopausal Women," *N Engl J Med*, 2004, 350(12):1189-99.

Durie BG, Katz M, and Crowley J, "Osteonecrosis of the Jaw and Bisphosphonates," *N Engl J Med*, 2005, 353(1):99-102.

Grant BT, Amenedo C, Freeman K, et al, "Outcomes of Placing Dental Implants in Patients Taking Oral Bisphosphonates: A Review of 115 Cases," *J Oral Maxillofac Surg*, 2008, 66(2):223-30.

Hoff AO, Toth BB, Altundag K, et al, "Osteonecrosis of the Jaw in Patients Receiving Intravenous Bisphosphonate Therapy," *J Clin Oncol*, 2006, 24:8528; available at http://meeting.jco.org/content/abstract/24/18_suppl/8528.

Jeffcoat MK, "Safety of Oral Bisphosphonates: Controlled Studies on Alveolar Bone," *Int J Oral Maxillofac Implants*, 2006, 21(3):349-53.

Johnston CC Jr, Bjarnason NH, Cohen FJ, et al, "Long-Term Effects of Raloxifene on Bone Mineral Density, Bone Turnover, and Serum Lipid Levels in Early Postmenopausal Women: Three-Year Data From 2 Double-Blind, Randomized, Placebo-Controlled Trials," *Arch Intern Med*, 2000, 160 (22):3444-50.

Kyrgidis A and Toulis KA, "Denosumab-Related Osteonecrosis of the Jaws," *Osteoporos Int*, 2011, 22 (1):369-70.

Marx RE, Cillo JE Jr, and Ulloa JJ, "Oral Bisphosphonate-Induced Osteonecrosis: Risk Factors, Prediction of Risk Using Serum CTX Testing, Prevention, and Treatment," *J Oral Maxillofac Surg*, 2007, 65(12):2397-410.

Marx RE, *Oral and Intravenous Bisphosphonate-Induced Osteonecrosis of the Jaws: History, Etiology, Prevention and Treatment*, Chicago, IL: Quintessence Publishing Company, 2007, 87-91.

Marx RE, Sawatari Y, Fortin M, et al, "Bisphosphonate-Induced Exposed Bone (Osteonecrosis/Osteopetrosis) of the Jaws: Risk Factors, Recognition, Prevention, and Treatment," *J Oral Maxillofac Surg*, 2005, 63(11):1567-75.

Mavrokokki T, Cheng A, Stein B, et al, "Nature and Frequency of Bisphosphonate-Associated Osteonecrosis of the Jaws in Australia," *J Oral Maxillofac Surg*, 2007, 65(3):415-23.

Migliorati CA, Casiglia J, Epstein J, et al, "Managing the Care of Patients With Bisphosphonate-Associated Osteonecrosis: An American Academy of Oral Medicine Position Paper," *J Am Dent Assoc*, 2005, 136(12):1658-68.

Ott SM, "Long-Term Safety of Bisphosphonates," *J Clin Endocrinol Metab*, 2005, 90(3):1897-9.

Reginster J, Minne HW, Sorensen OH, et al, "Randomized Trial of the Effects of Risedronate on Vertebral Fractures in Women With Established Postmenopausal Osteoporosis. Vertebral Efficacy With Risedronate Therapy (VERT) Study Group," *Osteoporos Int*, 2000, 11(1):83-91.

Rosen HN, Moses AC, Garber J, et al, "Serum CTX: A New Marker of Bone Resorption That Shows Treatment Effect More Often Than Other Markers Because of Low Coefficient of Variability and Large Changes With Bisphosphonate Therapy," *Calcif Tissue Int*, 2000, 66(2):100-3.

Ruggiero S, Gralow J, Marx RE, "Practical Guidelines for the Prevention, Diagnosis, and Treatment of Osteonecrosis of the Jaw in Patients With Cancer," *J Oncol Pract*, 2006, 2(1):7-14.

Ruggiero SL and Drew SJ, "Osteonecrosis of the Jaws and Bisphosphonate Therapy," *J Dent Res*, 2007, 86(11):1013-21.

Ruggiero SL, Dodson TB, Assael LA, et al, "American Association of Oral and Maxillofacial Surgeons Position Paper on Bisphosphonate-Related Osteonecrosis of the Jaw - 2009 Update," *Aust Endod J*, 2009, 35(3):119-30.

Ruggiero SL, Fantasia J, and Carlson E, "Bisphosphonate-Related Osteonecrosis of the Jaw: Background and Guidelines for Diagnosis, Staging and Management," *Oral Surg Oral Med Oral Pathol Oral Radiol Endod*, 2006, 102(4):433-41.

Ruggiero SL, Mehrotra B, Rosenberg TJ, et al, "Osteonecrosis of the Jaws Associated With the Use of Bisphosphonates: A Review of 63 Cases," *J Oral Maxillofac Surg*, 2004, 62(5):527-34.

Scheper MA, Badros A, Chaisuparat R, et al, "Effect of Zoledronic Acid on Oral Fibroblasts and Epithelial Cells: A Potential Mechanism of Bisphosphonate-Associated Osteonecrosis," *Br J Haematol*, 2009, 144 (5):667-76.

Scheper MA, Badros A, Salama AR, et al, "A Novel Bioassay Model to Determine Clinically Significant Bisphosphonate Levels," *Support Care Cancer*, 2009, 17(12):1553-7.

Scheper M, Chaisuparat R, Cullen K, et al, "A Novel Soft-Tissue *in vitro* Model for Bisphosphonate-Associated Osteonecrosis," *Fibrogenesis Tissue Repair*, 2010, 3:6.

Scully C, Madrid C, and Bagan J, "Dental Endosseous Implants in Patients on Bisphosphonate Therapy," *Implant Dent*, 2006, 15(3):212-8.

Starck WJ and Epker BN, "Failure of Osseointegrated Dental Implants After Diphosphonate Therapy for Osteoporosis: A Case Report," *Int J Oral Maxillofac Implants*, 1995, 10(1):74-8.

Tarassoff P and Hei YJ, "Osteonecrosis of the Jaw and Bisphosphonates," *N Engl J Med*, 2005, 353:101-2.

Taylor KH, Middlefell LS, and Mizen KD, "Osteonecrosis of the Jaws Induced by Anti-RANK Ligand Therapy," *Br J Oral Maxillofac Surg*, 2010, 48(3):221-3.

Verispan, VONA, "The Top 200 Brand-Name Drugs by Units in 2006," *Drug Topics*, 2007.

Wang HL, Weber D, and McCauley LK, "Effect of Long-Term Oral Bisphosphonates on Implant Wound Healing: Literature Review and a Case Report," *J Periodontol*, 2007, 78(3):584-94.

TUBERCULOSIS

Tuberculosis is caused by the organism *Mycobacterium tuberculosis* as well as a variety of other mycobacteria including *M. bovis*, *M. avium-intracellulare*, and *M. kansasii*. Diagnosis of tuberculosis can be made from a skin test and a positive chest x-ray as well as acid-fast smears of cultures from respiratory secretions. Nucleic acid probes and polymerase chain reaction (PCR) to identify nucleic acid of *M. tuberculosis* have recently become useful.

The treatment of tuberculosis is based on the general principle that multiple drugs should reduce infectivity within 2 weeks and that failures in therapy may be due to noncompliance with the long-term regimens necessary. General treatment regimens last 6-12 months.

Isoniazid-resistant and multidrug-resistant mycobacterial infections have become an increasingly significant problem in recent years. TB as an opportunistic disease in HIV-positive patients has also risen. Combination drug therapy has always been popular in TB management and the advent of new antibiotics has not diminished this need.

ANTITUBERCULOSIS DRUGS

Bactericidal Agents

Capreomycin on page 295
*Isoniazid on page 948
Kanamycin on page 961
*Pyrazinamide on page 1435
Rifabutin on page 1472
Rifapentine on page 1474
*Rifampin on page 1473
*Streptomycin on page 1552

Bacteriostatic Agents

CycloSERINE on page 451
*Ethambutol on page 649
Ethionamide on page 687
Aminosalicylic Acid on page 101

*Drugs of choice.

REFERENCES AND SELECTED READINGS

Cohn DL, "Treatment of Latent Tuberculosis Infection," *Semin Respir Infect*, 2003, 18(4):249-62.

Kaplan JE, Benson C, Holmes KH, et al, "Guidelines for Prevention and Treatment of Opportunistic Infections in HIV-Infected Adults and Adolescents: Recommendations From CDC, the National Institutes of Health, and the HIV Medicine Association of the Infectious Diseases Society of America," *MMWR Recomm Rep*, 2009, 58(RR-4):1-207.

Van den Brande P, "Revised Guidelines for the Diagnosis and Control of Tuberculosis: Impact on Management in the Elderly," *Drugs Aging*, 2005, 22(8):663-86.

SEXUALLY-TRANSMITTED DISEASES

Sexually transmitted diseases (STDs) represent a group of infectious diseases that include bacterial, fungal, and viral etiologies. Several related infections are covered elsewhere. Several viral STDs can be effectively prevented through vaccination with widely available vaccines, including hepatitis A, hepatitis B, and human papilloma virus vaccines. Vaccines for other STDs (eg, HIV and herpes simplex virus) are under development or undergoing clinical trials. Vaccines are not available for bacterial or fungal STDs.

The management of a patient with an STD begins with identification. Paramount to the correct management of patients with a history of gonorrhea or syphilis is when the condition was diagnosed, how and with what agent it was treated, did the condition recur, and are there any residual signs and symptoms potentially indicating active or recurrent disease. With standard/universal precautions, the patient with *Neisseria gonorrhoea* or *Treponema pallidum* infection poses little threat to the dentist; however, diagnosis of oral lesions may be problematic. Gonococcal pharyngitis, primary syphilitic lesions (chancre), secondary syphilitic lesions (mucous patch), and tertiary lesions (gumma) may be identified by the dentist. All patients who have gonorrhea should also be tested for other STDs, including chlamydia, syphilis, and HIV. Most gonococcal infections of the pharynx are asymptomatic and can be relatively common in some populations. Gonococcal infections of the pharynx are more difficult to eradicate than urogenital and anorectal infections. Few antimicrobial regimens, including those involving oral cephalosporins, can reliably cure >90% of gonococcal pharyngeal infections. Chlamydial coinfection of the pharynx is unusual; however, because coinfection at genital sites sometimes occurs, treatment for both gonorrhea and chlamydia is recommended.

Gonorrhea is the second most commonly reported bacterial STD. The majority of urethral infections caused by *N. gonorrhoeae* among men produce symptoms that cause them to seek curative treatment soon enough to prevent serious sequelae, but treatment may not be soon enough to prevent transmission to others. Among women, gonococcal infections may not produce recognizable symptoms until complications (eg, pelvic inflammatory disease [PID]) have occurred. PID can result in tubal scarring that can lead to infertility or ectopic pregnancy. Treatment of uncomplicated gonococcal infections of the cervix, urethra, and rectum include ceftriaxone, cefixime, azithromycin, and doxycycline.

Chlamydial genital infection is the most frequently reported infectious disease in the United States and is found more commonly in patients ≤25 years of age. Several important sequelae can result from *C. trachomatous* infection in women including PID, infertility, and ectopic pregnancy. Chlamydia treatment should be provided promptly for all patients testing positive for infection. Coinfection with *C. trachomatous* frequently occurs among patients who have gonococcal infection; therefore, concurrent treatment for both infections is recommended. Chlamydial infections can be treated with azithromycin or doxycycline. Alternative treatments include erythromycin, levofloxacin, or ofloxacin (systemic). If treating gonorrhea concurrently, would not consider use of a fluoroquinolone as resistance is high.

DRUGS USED IN TREATMENT OF CHLAMYDIA, GONORRHEA/ SYPHILIS INCLUDE:

Azithromycin (Systemic) on page 197
Cefixime on page 331
CefTRIAXone on page 339
Doxycycline on page 573
Ofloxacin (Systemic) on page 1237
Penicillin G Benzathine on page 1314
Penicillin G (Parenteral/Aqueous) on page 1315

The drugs listed above are often used alone or in stepped regimens, particularly when there is concomitant *Chlamydia* infection or when there is evidence of disseminated disease. The proper treatment for syphilis depends on the state of the disease.

REFERENCES AND SELECTED READINGS

Little JW, "Gonorrhea: Update," *Oral Surg Oral Med Oral Pathol Oral Radiol Endod*, 2006, 101(2):137-43.
Little JW, "Syphilis: An Update," *Oral Surg Oral Med Oral Pathol Oral Radiol Endod*, 2005, 100(1):3-9.
Miller WC and Zenilman JM, "Epidemiology of Chlamydial Infection, Gonorrhea, and Trichomoniasis in the United States-2005," *Infect Dis Clin North Am*, 2005, 19(2):281-96.
Workowski KA, Berman S, and Centers for Disease Control and Prevention (CDC), "Sexually Transmitted Diseases Treatment Guidelines, 2010," *MMWR Recomm Rep*, 2010, 59(RR-12):1-110. Available at http://www.cdc.gov/std/treatment/2010/STD-Treatment-2010-RR5912.pdf

SYSTEMIC VIRAL DISEASES

HEPATITIS

The hepatitis viruses are a group of DNA and RNA viruses that produce symptoms associated with inflammation of the liver. Currently, hepatitis A through G have been identified by immunological testing; however, hepatitis A through E have received most attention in terms of disease identification. Recently, there has been increased interest in hepatitis viruses F and G, particularly as related to healthcare professionals. Our knowledge is expanding rapidly in this area and the clinician should be alert to changes in the literature that might update their knowledge. Hepatitis F, for instance, remains a diagnosis of exclusion, effectively being non-A, B, C, D, E, or G. Hepatitis G has serologic testing available; however, it is not commercially at this time. Research evaluations of various antibody and RT-PCR tests for hepatitis G are under development at this time.

Signs and symptoms of viral hepatitis in general are quite variable. Patients infected may range from asymptomatic to experiencing flu-like symptoms only. In addition, fever, nausea, joint muscle pain, jaundice, and hepatomegaly along with abdominal pain can result from infection with one of the hepatitis viruses. The virus also can create an acute or chronic infection. Usually following these early symptoms or the asymptomatic period, the patient may recover or may go on to develop chronic liver dysfunction. Liver dysfunction may be represented primarily by changes in liver function tests known as LFTs and these primarily include aspartate aminotransferase known as AST and alanine aminotransferase known as ALT. In addition, for A, B, C, D, and E, there are serologic tests for either antigen, antibody, or both. Of hepatitis A through G, five forms have both acute and chronic forms whereas A and E appear to only create acute disease. There are differences in the way clinicians may approach a known post-exposure to one of the hepatitis viruses. In many instances, gamma globulin may be used; however, the indications for gamma globulin as a drug limit their use to several of the viruses only. The dental clinician should be aware that the gastroenterologist may choose to give gamma globulin off-label.

Hepatitis A

Hepatitis A virus is an enteric virus that is a member of the Picornavirus family along with Coxsackie viruses and poliovirus. Previously known as infectious hepatitis, hepatitis A has been detected in humans for centuries. It causes acute hepatitis, often transmitted by oral-fecal contamination and having an incubation period of approximately 30 days. Typically, constitutional symptoms are present and jaundice may occur. Drug therapy that the dentist may encounter in a patient being treated for hepatitis A would primarily include immunoglobulin. Hepatitis A vaccine (inactivated) is an FDA-approved vaccine indicated in the prevention of contracting hepatitis A in exposed or high-risk individuals. Candidates at high-risk for HAV infection include persons traveling internationally to highly endemic areas, individuals with chronic liver disease, individuals engaging in high-risk sexual behavior, illicit drug users, persons with high-risk occupational exposure, hemophiliacs or other persons receiving blood products, and pediatric populations. Hepatitis A, caused by infection with HAV, has an incubation period of ~28 days (range: 15-50 days). HAV replicates in the liver and is shed in high concentrations in feces from 2 weeks before to 1 week after the onset of clinical illness. HAV infection produces a self-limited disease that does not result in chronic infection or chronic liver disease; however, 10% to 15% of patients experience relapse symptoms during the 6 months after acute illness. Patients with acute hepatitis A usually require only supportive care with no restrictions in diet or activity. Hospitalization may be necessary for patients who become dehydrated due to nausea and vomiting, but is critical for patients with signs or symptoms of acute liver failure. Medications that may cause liver damage or are metabolized by the liver should be used with caution among patients with hepatitis A.

Two products are available for the prevention of HAV infection: Hepatitis A vaccine and immune globulin (IG) for I.M. administration. Patients recently exposed (within 14 days and prior to development of illness) to HAV and have not received a hepatitis A vaccine should be administered a single dose of single-antigen vaccine or IG ([GamaSTAN™ S/D] 0.02 mL/kg) as soon as possible.

Hepatitis B

Hepatitis B virus is previously known as serum hepatitis and has particular trophism for liver cells. Hepatitis B virus causes both acute and chronic disease in susceptible patients. The incubation period is often long and the diagnosis might be made by serologic markers even in the absence of symptoms.

Hepatitis B is caused by infection with the hepatitis B virus (HBV). The incubation period from the time of exposure to onset of symptoms is 6 weeks to 6 months. The highest concentrations of HBV are found in blood with lower concentrations found in other body fluids.

HBV infection can be self-limited or chronic. In adults, only ~1/2 of newly acquired HBV infections are symptomatic and ~1% of reported cases result in acute liver failure. HBV is efficiently transmitted by percutaneous or mucous membrane exposure to blood or body fluids that contain blood. Preventing disease after exposure in a person without previous hepatitis B vaccine protection is important. Passive-active postexposure prophylaxis (PEP) occurs with administration of hepatitis B immune globulin and hepatitis B vaccine.

Hepatitis C

Hepatitis C virus was described in 1988 and has been formerly classified as non-A/non-B. It is clear that hepatitis C represents a high percentage of the transfusion-associated hepatitis that is seen. Treatment of acute hepatitis C infection is generally supportive. Interferon Alfa-2a therapy has been used with some success recently and interferon-alfa may be beneficial with hepatitis C-related chronic hepatitis.

Hepatitis C virus (HCV) infection is the most common chronic blood-borne infection in the United States. HCV is transmitted through parenteral exposures to contaminated blood usually through use of injection drugs (sharing of needles or works) and to a lesser extent through exposures in healthcare settings. No vaccine is available for hepatitis C and prophylaxis with immune globulin is not effective in preventing HCV infection after exposure. Testing to determine whether HCV infection has developed is recommended for healthcare workers after percutaneous or perimucosal exposure to HCV-positive blood.

Hepatitis D

Hepatitis D, previously known as the delta agent, is a virus that is incomplete in that it requires previous infection with hepatitis B in order to be manifested. Antiviral therapy is not indicated for an acute infection.

Hepatitis E

Hepatitis E virus is an RNA virus that represents a proportion of the previously classified non-A/non-B diagnoses. There is currently no antiviral therapy against hepatitis E.

Hepatitis F

Hepatitis F remains a diagnosis of exclusion. There are no known immunological tests available for identification of hepatitis F at present and currently the Centers for Disease Control have not come out with specific guidelines or recommendations. It is thought that hepatitis F is a blood-borne virus and it has been used as a diagnosis in several cases of post-transfusion hepatitis.

Hepatitis G

Hepatitis G virus (HGV) is the newest hepatitis and is also assumed to be a blood-borne virus. Similar in family to hepatitis C, it is thought to occur concomitantly with hepatitis C and appears to be even more prevalent in some blood donors than hepatitis C. Occupational transmission of HGV is currently under study (see the references for updated information) and currently there are no specific CDC recommendations for postexposure to an HGV individual as the testing for identification remains experimental.

For further information, refer to the following:

Hepatitis A Vaccine on page 846
Hepatitis A and Hepatitis B Recombinant Vaccine on page 845
Hepatitis B Immune Globulin (Human) on page 847
Hepatitis B Vaccine (Recombinant) on page 848
Immune Globulin on page 903
Interferon Alfa-2b on page 925
Peginterferon Alfa-2a on page 1306
Peginterferon Alfa-2a and Ribavirin on page 1307
Peginterferon Alfa-2b on page 1308
Peginterferon Alfa-2b and Ribavirin

TYPES OF HEPATITIS VIRUS

Features	A	B	C	D	E	F	G
Incubation Period	2-6 wks	8-24 wks	2-52 wks	3-13 wks	3-6 wks	Unknown	Unknown
Onset	Abrupt	Insidious	Insidious	Abrupt	Abrupt	Insidious	Insidious
Symptoms							
Jaundice	Adults: 70% to 80%; Children: 10%	25%	25%	Varies	Unknown	Unknown	Unknown
Asymptomatic patients	Adults: 50%; Children: Most	~75%	~75%	Rare	Rare	Common	Common
Routes of Transmission							
Fecal/Oral	Yes	No	No	No	Yes	Unknown	Unknown
Parenteral	Rare	Yes	Yes	Yes	No		
Sexual	No	Yes	Possible	Yes	No		
Perinatal	No	Yes	Possible	Possible	No		
Water/Food	Yes	No	No	No	Yes		
Sequelae (% of patients)							
Chronic state	No	Adults: 6% to 10%; Children: 25% to 50%; Infants: 70% to 90%	>75%	10% to 15%	No	Unknown	Likely
Case-Fatality Rate	0.6%	1.4%	1% to 2%	30%	1% to 2% Pregnant women: 20%	Unknown	Unknown

PRE-EXPOSURE RISK FACTORS FOR HEPATITIS B

Healthcare factors:

- Healthcare workers[1]
- Special patient groups (eg, adolescents, infants born to HB_sAg–positive mothers, military personnel, etc)
  - Hemodialysis patients[2]
  - Recipients of certain blood products[3]

Lifestyle factors:

- Homosexual and bisexual men
- Intravenous drug-abusers
- Heterosexually active persons with multiple sexual partners or recently acquired sexually transmitted diseases

Environmental factors:

- Household and sexual contacts of HBV carriers
- Prison inmates
- Clients and staff of institutions for the mentally handicapped
- Residents, immigrants, and refugees from areas with endemic HBV infection
- International travelers at increased risk of acquiring HBV infection

[1]The risk of hepatitis B virus (HBV) infection for healthcare workers varies both between hospitals and within hospitals. Hepatitis B vaccination is recommended for all healthcare workers with blood exposure.

[2]Hemodialysis patients often respond poorly to hepatitis B vaccination; higher vaccine doses or increased number of doses are required. A special formulation of one vaccine is now available for such persons (Recombivax HB®, 40 mcg/mL). The anti-HB_s (antibody to hepatitis B surface antigen) response of such persons should be tested after they are vaccinated, and those who have not responded should be revaccinated with 1-3 additional doses.

Patients with chronic renal disease should be vaccinated as early as possible, ideally before they require hemodialysis. In addition, their anti-HB_s levels should be monitored at 6- to 12-month intervals to assess the need for revaccination.

[3]Patients with hemophilia should be immunized subcutaneously, not intramuscularly.

POSTEXPOSURE PROPHYLAXIS FOR HEPATITIS B[1]

Exposure	Hepatitis B Immune Globulin	Hepatitis B Vaccine
Perinatal	0.5 mL I.M. within 12 hours of birth	0.5 mL[2] I.M. within 12 hours of birth (no later than 7 days), and at 1 and 6 months[3]; test for HB_sAg and anti-HB_s at 12-15 months
Sexual	0.06 mL/kg I.M. within 14 days of sexual contact; a second dose should be given if the index patient remains HB_sAg-positive after 3 months and hepatitis B vaccine was not given initially	1 mL I.M. at 0, 1, and 6 months for homosexual and bisexual men and regular sexual contacts of persons with acute and chronic hepatitis B
Percutaneous; exposed person unvaccinated		
Source known HB_sAg-positive	0.06 mL/kg I.M. within 24 hours	1 mL I.M. within 7 days, and at 1 and 6 months[4]
Source known, HB_sAg status unknown	Test source for HB_sAg; if source is positive, give exposed person 0.06 mL/kg I.M. once within 7 days	1 mL I.M. within 7 days, and at 1 and 6 months[4]
Source not tested or unknown	Nothing required	1 mL I.M. within 7 days, and at 1 and 6 months
Percutaneous; exposed person vaccinated		
Source known HB_sAg-positive	Test exposed person for anti-HB_s[5]. If titer is protective, nothing is required; if titer is not protective, give 0.06 mL/kg within 24 hours	Review vaccination status[6]
Source known, HB_sAg status unknown	Test source for HB_sAg and exposed person for anti-HB_s. If source is HB_sAg-negative, or if source is HB_sAg-positive but anti-HB_s titer is protective, nothing is required. If source is HB_sAg-positive and anti-HB_s titer is not protective or if exposed person is a known nonresponder, give 0.06 mL/kg I.M. within 24 hours. A second dose of hepatitis B immune globulin can be given 1 month later if a booster dose of hepatitis B vaccine is not given.	Review vaccination status[6]
Source not tested or unknown	Test exposed person for anti-HB_s. If anti-HB_s titer is protective, nothing is required. If anti-HB_s titer is not protective, 0.06 mL/kg may be given along with a booster dose of hepatitis B vaccine.	Review vaccination status[6]

[1]HB_sAg = hepatitis B surface antigen; anti-HB_s = antibody to hepatitis B surface antigen; I.M. = intramuscularly; SRU = standard ratio units.

[2]Each 0.5 mL dose of plasma-derived hepatitis B vaccine contains 10 mcg of HB_sAg; each 0.5 mL dose of recombinant hepatitis B vaccine contains 5 mcg or 10 mcg of HB_sAg.

[3]If hepatitis B immune globulin and hepatitis B vaccine are given simultaneously, they should be given at separate sites.

[4]If hepatitis B vaccine is not given, a second dose of hepatitis B immune globulin should be given 1 month later.

[5]Anti-HB_s titers <10 SRU by radioimmunoassay or negative by enzyme immunoassay indicate lack of protection. Testing the exposed person for anti-HB_s is not necessary if a protective level of antibody has been shown within the previous 24 months.

[6]If the exposed person has not completed a three-dose series of hepatitis B vaccine, the series should be completed. Test the exposed person for anti-HB_s. If the antibody level is protective, nothing is required. If an adequate antibody response in the past is shown on retesting to have declined to an inadequate level, a booster dose (1 mL) of hepatitis B vaccine should be given. If the exposed person has inadequate antibody or is a known nonresponder to vaccination, a booster dose can be given along with one dose of hepatitis B immune globulin.

Pre-exposure Vaccination

Pre-exposure vaccination is one of the most effective methods for preventing transmission of some STDs. Two human papillomavirus (HPV) vaccines are available for females 9-26 years of age to prevent cervical precancer and cancer, quadrivalent HPV vaccine (Gardasil®) and the bivalent HPV vaccine (Cervarix®). Routine vaccination for females 11-12 years of age is recommended with either vaccine. A catch-up vaccination for females 13-26 years of age is also recommended. Gardasil® can be administered to males 9-26 years of age to prevent genital warts. Details regarding HPV vaccination are available at www.cdc.gov/std/hpv.

Hepatitis B vaccination is recommended for all unvaccinated and uninfected patients being evaluated for an STD. In addition, hepatitis A and B vaccines are recommended for men who have sex with men and injection drug users; each of these vaccines should also be administered to HIV-infected patients not yet infected with one or both types of hepatitis virus. Details regarding hepatitis A and B vaccination are available at http://www.cdc.gov/hepatitis.

HERPES

The herpes viruses not only represent a topic of specific interest to the dentist due to oral manifestations, but are widespread as systemic infections. Herpes simplex virus is also of interest because of its central nervous system infections and its relationship as one of the viral infections commonly found in AIDS patients. Oral herpes infections will be covered elsewhere. Current recommended drug therapy includes acyclovir, valacyclovir, or famciclovir; alternative includes cidofovir, foscarnet, ganciclovir, or valganciclovir. Epstein-Barr virus is a member of the herpesvirus family and produces syndromes important in dentistry, including infectious mononucleosis with the commonly found oral pharyngitis and petechial hemorrhages, as well as being the causative agent of Burkitt's lymphoma. The relationship between Epstein-Barr virus to oral hairy leukoplakia in AIDS patients has not been shown to be one of cause and effect; however, the presence of Epstein-Barr in these lesions is consistent. Currently, there is no accepted treatment for Epstein-Barr virus, although acyclovir has been shown in *in vitro* studies to have some efficacy. Varicella-zoster virus is another member of the herpesvirus family and is the causative agent of two clinical entities, chickenpox and shingles, or herpes zoster. Oral manifestations of both chickenpox and herpes zoster include vesicular eruptions often leading to confluent mucosal ulcerations. Acyclovir is the drug of choice for treatment of herpes zoster infections. Other drugs include valacyclovir and famciclovir.

There are other herpes viruses that produce disease in man and animals. These viruses have no specific treatment; therefore, incidence is thought to be less common than those mentioned and the specific treatment is not determined at present. The role of some of these viruses in concomitant infection with the HIV and other coinfection viruses is still under study.

ANTIVIRALS

AGENTS OF ESTABLISHED EFFECTIVENESS

Viral Infection	Drug
Cytomegalovirus	
Retinitis	Ganciclovir (Systemic), Foscarnet, Cidofovir, ValGANciclovir
Pneumonia	Ganciclovir (Systemic), Foscarnet, Cidofovir
Hepatitis viruses	
Chronic hepatitis A & B	Hepatitis A and Hepatitis B Recombinant Vaccine, Immune Globulin
Chronic hepatitis C (Kaplan, 2009; Mofenson, 2009)	Peginterferon Alfa-2a and Ribavirin, Peginterferon Alfa-2b and Ribavirin
Chronic hepatitis B (Kaplan, 2009; Mofenson, 2009)	Interferon Alfa-2b, Peginterferon Alfa-2a, LamiVUDine, Adefovir, Entecavir, Tenofovir, Telbivudine
Herpes simplex virus	
Orofacial herpes	
First episode	Acyclovir[1], Famciclovir, ValACYclovir
Recurrence	Acyclovir[1], Penciclovir, ValACYclovir
Genital herpes	
First episode, recurrence, suppression	Acyclovir, Famciclovir, ValACYclovir
Encephalitis	Acyclovir
Mucocutaneous disease in immunocompromised	Acyclovir
Neonatal	Acyclovir
Keratoconjunctivitis	Trifluridine
Influenza A virus	Amantadine, Influenza Virus Vaccine (Inactivated), Influenza Virus Vaccine (Live/Attenuated), Oseltamivir, Rimantadine, Zanamivir
Papillomavirus	
Condyloma acuminatum	Interferon Alfa-2b, Imiquimod (Aldara™): (use for oral lesions is under study)
Respiratory syncytial virus	Ribavirin (inhalation)
Varicella-zoster virus	
Varicella in normal children	Acyclovir
Varicella in immunocompromised	Acyclovir, ValACYclovir, Famciclovir
Herpes zoster in immunocompromised	Acyclovir, ValACYclovir, Famciclovir
Herpes zoster in normal hosts	Acyclovir, Famciclovir, ValACYclovir

[1]Although acyclovir is often used for these infections, penciclovir and valacyclovir are specifically approved for herpes labialis. The clinician is referred to the monographs.

Acyclovir (Systemic) on page 55
Acyclovir (Topical) on page 58
Amantadine on page 94
Atovaquone on page 186
Cidofovir on page 381
Famciclovir on page 704
Foscarnet on page 784
Ganciclovir (Systemic) on page 803
Hepatitis B Immune Globulin (Human) on page 847
Imiquimod on page 901

Immune Globulin on page 903
Interferon Alfa-2b on page 925
Interferon Alfa-2b and Ribavirin
Interferon Alfa-n3 on page 930
Oseltamivir on page 1259
Peginterferon Alfa-2a on page 1306
Peginterferon Alfa-2b on page 1308
Penciclovir on page 1312
Ribavirin on page 1470
Rifabutin on page 1472
Rimantadine on page 1477
Trifluridine on page 1679
ValACYclovir on page 1692
Zanamivir on page 1740

REFERENCES

Advisory Committee on Immunization Practices (ACIP), "Prevention of Hepatitis A Through Active or Passive Immunization: Recommendations of the Advisory Committee on Immunization Practices (ACIP)," *MMWR Recomm Rep*, 2006, 55(RR-7):1-23.

Centers for Disease Control and Prevention (CDC), "Recommendations of the Advisory Committee on Immunization Practices (ACIP): General Recommendations on Immunization," *MMWR Recomm Rep*, 2011, 60(2):1-64.

Corey L, Wald A, Patel R, et al, "Once-Daily Valacyclovir to Reduce the Risk of Transmission of Genital Herpes," *N Engl J Med*, 2004, 350(1):11-20.

Ghany MG, Strader DB, Thomas DL, et al, "Diagnosis, Management, and Treatment of Hepatitis C: An Update," *Hepatology*, 2009, 49(4):1335-74.

Kaplan JE, Benson C, Holmes KH, et al, "Guidelines for Prevention and Treatment of Opportunistic Infections in HIV-Infected Adults and Adolescents: Recommendations From CDC, the National Institutes of Health, and the HIV Medicine Association of the Infectious Diseases Society of America," *MMWR Recomm Rep*, 2009, 58(RR-4):1-207.

Mast EE, Margolis HS, Fiore AE, et al, "A Comprehensive Immunization Strategy to Eliminate Transmission of Hepatitis B Virus Infection in the United States: Recommendations of the Advisory Committee on Immunization Practices (ACIP) Part 1: Immunization of Infants, Children, and Adolescents," *MMWR Recomm Rep*, 2005, 54(RR-16):1-31.

Miller CS, Avdiushko SA, Kryscio RJ, et al, "Effect of Prophylactic Valacyclovir on the Presence of Human Herpesvirus DNA in Saliva of Healthy Individuals After Dental Treatment," *J Clin Microbiol* , 2005, 43 (5):2173-80.

Mofenson LM, Brady MT, Danner SP, et al, "Guidelines for the Prevention and Treatment of Opportunistic Infections Among HIV-Exposed and HIV-Infected Children: Recommendations From CDC, the National Institutes of Health, the HIV Medicine Association of The Infectious Diseases Society of America, the Pediatric Infectious Diseases Society, and the American Academy of Pediatrics," *MMWR Recomm Rep*, 2009, 58(RR-11):1-166.

Workowski KA, Berman S, and Centers for Disease Control and Prevention (CDC), "Sexually Transmitted Diseases Treatment Guidelines, 2010," *MMWR Recomm Rep*, 2010, 59(RR-12):1-110. Available at http://www.cdc.gov/std/treatment/2010/STD-Treatment-2010-RR5912.pdf

ANTIBIOTIC PROPHYLAXIS

PREPROCEDURAL GUIDELINES FOR DENTAL PATIENTS

INTRODUCTION

In dental practice, the clinician is often confronted with a decision to prescribe antibiotics. The focus of this section is on the use of antibiotics as a preprocedural treatment in the prevention of adverse infectious sequelae in two commonly encountered situations: Prevention of infective endocarditis and prevention of late infections of prosthetic implants.

The criteria for preprocedural decisions begins with patient evaluation. An accurate and complete medical history is always the initial basis for any prescriptive treatments on the part of the dentist. These prescriptive treatments can include ordering appropriate laboratory tests, referral to the patient's physician for consultation, or an immediate decision to prescribe preprocedural antibiotics. The dentist should also be aware that antibiotic coverage of the patient might be appropriate due to diseases covered elsewhere in this text, such as human immunodeficiency virus, cavernous thrombosis, undiagnosed or uncontrolled diabetes, lupus, renal failure, and periods of neutropenia as are often associated with cancer chemotherapy. In these instances, medical consultation is almost always necessary in making antibiotic decisions in order to tailor the treatment and dosing to the individual patient's needs. When in doubt regarding a patient's medical status, communicating with the physician is always an appropriate and prudent step.

Note: The ADA Council on Scientific Affairs recently restated the dentist's responsibility when prescribing antibiotics to oral contraceptive users (*JADA*, 2002, 133:880). It is recommended that dental professionals advise these patients to consult their physician for additional barrier contraception due to potential reduction in the efficacy of oral contraceptives from antibiotic interaction.

PREVENTION OF INFECTIVE ENDOCARDITIS

In one of the most significant examples of Evidence Based Science, the American Heart Association (AHA), in conjunction with the American Dental Association (ADA) and other experts in both medicine and dentistry, reviewed the evidence regarding the use of antibiotic prophylaxis to prevent infective endocarditis (IE) prior to dental appointments. The reviewers concluded that IE is more frequently caused by a patient's susceptibility to bacteremias associated with normal activities rather than bacteremia caused by dental procedures. Therefore, maintaining oral health to reduce bacteremia is more effective in reducing the risk of IE than the use of prophylactic antibiotics before dental procedures. Since the mid-1950s, patients at risk for IE from a variety of conditions have been routinely premedicated with antibiotics prior to dental and other procedures. After a review of the evidence, it has been concluded that the majority of patients did not benefit from this prophylaxis. The incidence of IE was not changed when compared to patients who received IE prophylaxis and those who did not and the risk for adverse effects from antibiotic use exceeded the benefit of therapy. Therefore, based on the evidence, a change in the Guidelines has been recommended by AHA, the ADA, as well as the Infectious Disease Society. The AHA/ADA recommends that most patients no longer need short-term antibiotics as a preventive measure before their dental treatment. Only those patients with the highest risk should receive prophylaxis.

Antibiotic prophylaxis with dental procedures is recommended for patients at high risk of IE due to specific cardiac conditions:

- prosthetic cardiac valve
- a prior incidence of IE
- prophylaxis is also required for heart transplant patients who develop cardiac valvulopathy
- patients with congenital heart disease (CHD) are only required prophylaxis with the following conditions:
    1. unrepaired cyanotic CHD, including palliative shunts and conduits
    2. CHD repaired by prosthetic material or device (for first 6 months after procedure)
    3. **or** if there are residual defects after repair (inhibiting endothelialization)

These patients with high-risk cardiac conditions are recommended for prophylaxis for all dental procedures involving manipulation of gingival tissue or the periapical region of teeth or perforation of the oral mucosa.

Dental procedures that do not require prophylaxis include:

- routine anesthetic injection into noninfected tissue
- taking dental radiographs
- placement of removable prosthodontic or orthodontic appliances
- adjustment of orthodontic appliances, placement of orthodontic brackets
- shedding of deciduous teeth
- bleeding from trauma to the lips or oral mucosa

ANTIBIOTIC SELECTION

For examples of sample prescriptions, see Infective Endocarditis (Prevention). The dentist should be vigilant in reviewing literature for updates.

Amoxicillin is an amino-type penicillin with an extended spectrum of antibacterial action compared to penicillin VK. The pharmacology of amoxicillin as a dental antibiotic has been reviewed previously in *General Dentistry*. The suggested regimen for standard general prophylaxis is a dose of 2 g 30-60 minutes before the procedure. A follow-up dose is no longer necessary. The pediatric dose is 50 mg/kg orally 30-60 minutes before the procedure and not to exceed the adult dose. Amoxicillin is available in capsules (250 mg and 500 mg), chewable tablets (125 mg, 200 mg, 250 mg, 400 mg), tablets (500 mg, 875 mg), and liquid suspension (125 mg/5 mL, 200 mg/5 mL, 250 mg/ 5 mL, 400 mg/5 mL).

For individuals unable to take oral medications, intramuscular or intravenous ampicillin is recommended for both adults and children. It is to be given at the same doses used for the oral amoxicillin medication. Ampicillin is also an amino-type penicillin having an antibacterial spectrum similar to amoxicillin. Ampicillin is not absorbed from the GI tract as effectively as amoxicillin and, therefore, is not recommended for oral use. Cefazolin or ceftriaxone are alternatives.

Table 1. PROPHYLACTIC REGIMENS FOR INFECTIVE ENDOCARDITIS FOR DENTAL PROCEDURES

Situation	Drug	Single Dosage 30-60 minutes prior to procedure
Oral	Amoxicillin on page 124	Children: 50 mg/kg Adults: 2 g
Unable to take oral medications	Ampicillin on page 136 **or**	Children: 50 mg/kg I.M. or I.V. Adults: 2 g I.M. or I.V.
	CeFAZolin on page 325 **or** CefTRIAXone on page 339	Children: 50 mg/kg I.M. or I.V. Adults: 1 g I.M. or I.V.
Allergic to penicillins or ampicillin (oral)	Cephalexin on page 347[1,2] **or**	Children: 50 mg/kg Adults: 2 g
	Clindamycin (Systemic) on page 402 **or**	Children: 20 mg/kg Adults: 600 mg
	Azithromycin (Systemic) on page 197 **or** Clarithromycin on page 396	Children: 15 mg/kg Adults: 500 mg
Allergic to penicillins or ampicillin and unable to take oral medications	CeFAZolin on page 325 **or** CefTRIAXone on page 339[2]	Children: 50 mg/kg I.M. or I.V. Adults: 1 g I.M. or I.V.
	Clindamycin (Systemic) on page 402	Children: 20 mg/kg I.M. or I.V. Adults: 600 mg I.M. or I.V.

Note: Intramuscular injections should be avoided in patients receiving anticoagulant therapy.

[1]Can use first- or second-generation oral cephalosporins in equivalent doses.

[2]Cephalosporins should not be used in individuals with immediate-type hypersensitivity reaction (urticaria, angioedema, or anaphylaxis) to penicillins.

Individuals who are allergic to the penicillins, such as amoxicillin or ampicillin, should be treated with an alternate antibiotic. The new guidelines have suggested a number of alternate agents including clindamycin, cephalosporins, azithromycin, and clarithromycin. Clindamycin (Cleocin®) occupies an important niche in dentistry as a useful and effective antibiotic and it was a recommended alternative agent for the prevention of bacterial endocarditis in the previous guidelines. In the new guidelines, the oral adult dose is 600 mg 30-60 minutes before the procedure. A follow-up dose is not necessary. Clindamycin is available as 300 mg capsules; thus two capsules will provide the recommended dose. The children's oral dose for clindamycin is 20 mg/kg 30-60 minutes before the procedure. Clindamycin is also available as flavored granules for oral solution. When reconstituted with water, each bottle yields a solution containing 75 mg/5 mL. Intravenous clindamycin is recommended in adults and children who are allergic to penicillin and unable to take oral medications.

Clindamycin was developed in the 1960s as a semisynthetic derivative of lincomycin which was found in the soil organism, *Streptomyces lincolnensis*, near Lincoln, Nebraska. It is commercially available as the hydrochloride salt to improve solubility in the GI tract. Clindamycin is antibacterial against most aerobic gram-positive cocci, including staphylococci and streptococci, and against many types of anaerobic gram-negative and gram-positive organisms. It has been used over the years in dentistry as an alternative to penicillin and erythromycins for the treatment of oral-facial infections.

The mechanism of antibacterial action of clindamycin is the same as erythromycin. It inhibits protein synthesis in susceptible bacteria resulting in the inhibition of bacterial growth and replication. Following oral administration of a single dose of clindamycin (150 mg, 300 mg, or 600 mg) on an empty stomach, 90% of the dose is rapidly absorbed into the bloodstream and peak serum concentrations are attained within 45-80 minutes. Administration with food does not markedly impair absorption into the bloodstream. Clindamycin serum levels exceed the minimum inhibitory concentration (MIC) for bacterial growth for at least 6 hours after the recommended dose of 600 mg. The serum half-life is 2-3 hours.

Adverse effects of clindamycin after a single dose are virtually nonexistent. Although it is estimated that 1% of patients taking clindamycin will develop symptoms of pseudomembranous colitis, these symptoms usually develop after 9-14 days of clindamycin therapy. These symptoms are rare and only one case has been reported in a patient taking an acute dose for the prevention of endocarditis.

In lieu of clindamycin, penicillin-allergic individuals may receive cephalexin (Keflex®) provided that they have not had an immediate-type sensitivity reaction such as anaphylaxis, urticaria, or angioedema to penicillins. These antibiotics are first-generation cephalosporins having an antibacterial spectrum of action similar to amoxicillin and ampicillin. They elicit a bactericidal action by inhibiting cell wall synthesis in susceptible bacteria. The recommended adult prophylaxis dose for either of these drugs is 2 g 30-60 minutes before the procedure. Again, no follow-up dose is needed. The children's oral dose for cephalexin is 50 mg/kg 30-60 minutes before the procedure. Cephalexin is supplied as capsules (250 mg, 500 mg, 750 mg) and is available in the form of powder for oral suspension at concentrations of 125 mg/5 mL and 250 mg/5 mL.

For those individuals (adults and children) allergic to penicillin and unable to take oral medicines, parenteral cefazolin (Ancef®) may be used, provided they do not have the sensitivities described previously. Cefazolin is also a first-generation cephalosporin. Please note that parenteral cefazolin can be given I.M. or I.V. (refer to Table 1, for the adult and children's doses of parenteral cefazolin).

Azithromycin (Zithromax®) and clarithromycin (Biaxin®) are members of the class of antibiotics known as macrolides. The pharmacology of these drugs has been reviewed previously in *General Dentistry*. Erythromycins have been available for use in dentistry and medicine since the mid 1950s. Azithromycin and clarithromycin represent the first additions to this class in more than 40 years. The adult prophylactic dose for either drug is 500 mg 30-60 minutes before the procedure with no follow-up dose. The pediatric prophylactic dose of azithromycin and clarithromycin is 15 mg/kg orally 30-60 minutes before the procedure. Although the erythromycin family of drugs is known to inhibit the hepatic metabolism of theophylline and carbamazepine to enhance their effects, azithromycin has not been shown to affect the liver metabolism of these drugs.

Azithromycin is well absorbed from the gastrointestinal tract and is extensively taken up from circulation into tissues with a slow release from those tissues. It reaches peak serum levels in 2-4 hours and serum half-life is 68 hours. Zithromax® is supplied as 250 mg, 500 mg, and 600 mg tablets. It is also available for oral suspension at concentrations of 100 mg/5 mL, 200 mg/5 mL, and single-dose packets containing 1 g.

Clarithromycin (Biaxin®) achieves peak plasma concentrations in 3 hours and maintains effective serum concentrations over a 12-hour period. Reports indicate that it probably interacts with theophylline and carbamazepine by elevating the plasma concentrations of the two drugs. Biaxin® is supplied as 250 mg and 500 mg tablets and 500 mg extended release tablets. It is also available as granules for oral suspension at concentrations of 125 mg/5 mL and 250 mg/5 mL.

Amoxicillin on page 124
Ampicillin on page 136
Azithromycin (Systemic) on page 197
CeFAZolin on page 325
CefTRIAXone on page 339
Cephalexin on page 347
Clarithromycin on page 396
Clindamycin (Systemic) on page 402

Clinical Considerations for Dentistry

See Figure 1.

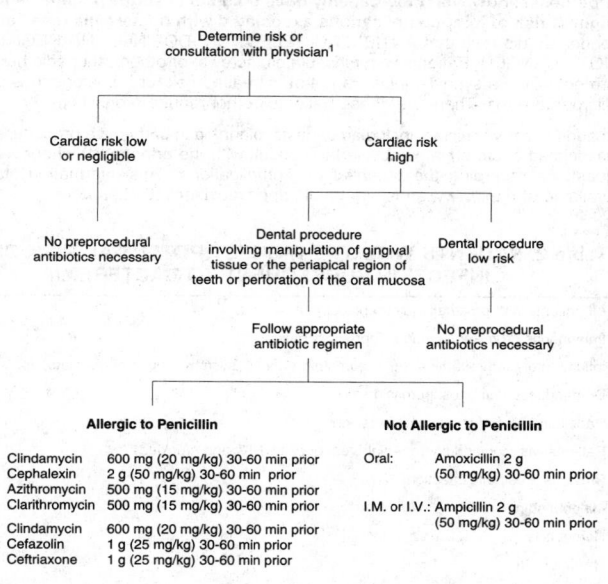

Figure 1
Preprocedural Dental Action Plan for Patients With a History Indicative of Elevated Endocarditis Risk

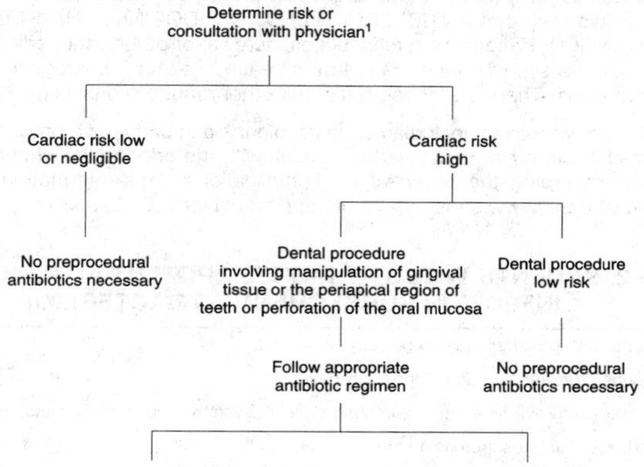

Allergic to Penicillin

Oral:	Clindamycin	600 mg (20 mg/kg) 30-60 min prior
	Cephalexin	2 g (50 mg/kg) 30-60 min prior
	Azithromycin	500 mg (15 mg/kg) 30-60 min prior
	Clarithromycin	500 mg (15 mg/kg) 30-60 min prior
I.V.:	Clindamycin	600 mg (20 mg/kg) 30-60 min prior
I.M. or I.V.:	Cefazolin	1 g (25 mg/kg) 30-60 min prior
	Ceftriaxone	1 g (25 mg/kg) 30-60 min prior

Not Allergic to Penicillin

Oral:	Amoxicillin 2 g (50 mg/kg) 30-60 min prior
I.M. or I.V.:	Ampicillin 2 g (50 mg/kg) 30-60 min prior

Dosages for children are in parentheses and should never exceed adult dose. Cephalosporins should be avoided in patients with previous Type I hypersensitivity reactions to penicillin due to some evidence of cross-allergenicity.

[1]For Emergency Dental Care, the clinician should attempt phone consultation. If unable to contact patient's physician or determine risk, the patient should be treated as though there is a high risk of cardiac complication and follow the algorithm.

Patients with a suspicious history of one of the high-risk cardiac conditions, who are in need of an immediate dental procedure, should be prophylaxed with an appropriate antibiotic prior to the procedure(s) until medical evaluation has been completed and the risk level determined. If unanticipated dental risk develops during a procedure in a cardiac at-risk patient, appropriate antibiotics should be given immediately.

If a series of dental procedures is planned, the clinician must judge whether an interval between procedures, requiring prophylaxis, should be scheduled. The literature supports 9- to 14-day intervals as ideal to minimize the risk of emergence of resistant organisms. Since serum levels of the standard amoxicillin dose may be adequate for 6-14 hours depending on the specific organism challenge, the clinician may have to consider the efficacy of a second dose if multiple procedures are planned over the course of a single day.

PREPROCEDURAL ANTIBIOTICS FOR PROSTHETIC IMPLANTS

A significant number of dental patients have had total joint replacements or other implanted prosthetic devices. Prior to performing dental procedures that might induce bacteremia, the dentist must consider the use of antibiotic prophylaxis in these patients. In February 2009, the American Academy of Orthopedic Surgeons released an updated information statement regarding antibiotic prophylaxis for bacteremia in patients with joint replacements. The guidelines are modestly, but significantly, altered from the guidelines released by the Joint Commission of the Academy of Orthopedic Surgeons and the American Dental Association in 1997 and revised in 2003. The American Dental Association is still considering this new 2009 Information Statement; therefore, the reader is advised to be vigilant for updates.

The most important modification, the 2-year rule for need for prophylaxis, has been eliminated. Prophylaxis is now recommended for all patients with joint prostheses; however, the Academy does go on to describe patients who have the highest risk of joint complications associated with bacteremia (see Table 2). The reader should note that ANTIBIOTIC SELECTION, DOSING, AND REGIMINS HAVE NOT CHANGED. Patients with pins, plates, screws, or other orthopedic hardware that are not within a synovial joint are not at increased risk for hematogenous seeding by microorganisms. Therefore, these patients do not require prophylaxis.

In addition, any clinician, including dentists, planning to carry out a procedure with likely associated bacteremia, is advised to consult with the orthopedist whenever there are questions regarding the potential for complications. This information statement is available at http://www.aaos.org/about/papers/advistmt/1033.asp.

Table 2. PATIENTS WITH THE HIGHEST POTENTIAL RISK OF JOINT INFECTION SUBSEQUENT TO BACTEREMIA

All patients with prosthetic joint replacement
Immunocompromised/immunosuppressed patients
Inflammatory arthropathies (eg, rheumatoid arthritis, systemic lupus erythematosus)
Drug-induced immunosuppression
Radiation-induced immunosuppression
Patients with comorbidity (eg, diabetes, obesity, HIV, and smoking)
Previous prosthetic infections
Malnourishment
Hemophilia
HIV infection
Type 1 diabetes mellitus (insulin dependent, IDDM)
Malignancy
Megaprosthesis

Source: February 2009 AAOS Information Statement. Available at http://www.aaos.org/about/papers/advistmt/1033.asp. Original source: American Dental Association; American Academy of Orthopedic Surgeons, "Antibiotic Prophylaxis for Dental Patients With Total Joint Replacements," *J Am Dent Assoc*, 2003, 134(7):895-9.

The use of antibiotics in patients with prosthetic devices, including total joint replacements, has remained controversial because of several issues. Late infections of implanted prosthetic devices have rarely been associated with microbial organisms of oral origin. Secondly, since late infections in such patients are often not reported, data is lacking to substantiate or refute this potential. There is however, general acceptance that patients with acute infections at distant sites such as the oral cavity may be at greater risk of infection of an implanted prosthetic device. Periodontal disease has been implicated as a distant site infection. Since antibiotics are associated with allergies and other adverse reactions, and because the frequent use of antibiotics may lead to emergence of resistant organisms, any perceived benefit of antibiotic prophylaxis must always be weighed against known risks of toxicity, allergy, or potential microbial resistance.

ANTIBIOTIC REGIMENS

The antibiotic prophylaxis regimens as suggested by the advisory panel are listed in Table 3. These regimens are not exactly the same as those listed in Table 1 (for prevention of endocarditis) and must be reviewed carefully to avoid confusion. Cephalexin or amoxicillin may be used in patients not allergic to penicillin. The selected antibiotic is given as a single 2 g dose 1 hour before the procedure. A follow-up dose is not recommended. Cephalexin (Keflex®) and amoxicillin were described earlier in this section.

Parenteral cefazolin (Ancef®) or ampicillin is the recommended antibiotic for patients unable to take oral medications (see Table 3 for doses). Cefazolin is a first-generation cephalosporin, effective against anaerobes and aerobic gram-positive bacteria. Ampicillin is an aminopenicillin (described earlier). For patients allergic to penicillin, clindamycin is the recommended antibiotic of choice. Clindamycin is active against aerobic and anaerobic streptococci, most staphylococci, the *Bacteroides*, and the *Actinomyces* families of bacteria. The recommended oral and parenteral doses of clindamycin in the joint prosthetic patient are listed in Table 3 below.

Table 3. ANTIBIOTIC REGIMENS FOR PATIENTS WITH PROSTHETIC IMPLANTS

Patients not allergic to penicillin:	Cephalexin or amoxicillin:	2 g orally 1 hour prior to the procedure
Patients not allergic to penicillin and unable to take oral medications:	CeFAZolin:	1 g I.M. or I.V. 1 hour prior to the procedure
	or Ampicillin:	2 g I.M. or I.V. 1 hour prior to the procedure
Patients allergic to penicillin:	Clindamycin (Systemic):	600 mg orally 1 hour prior to dental procedure
Patients allergic to penicillin and unable to take oral medications:	Clindamycin (Systemic):	600 mg I.V. 1 hour prior to the procedure

For examples of sample prescriptions see Prosthetic Joint Late Infections (Prevention) on page 1979

Amoxicillin on page 124
Ampicillin on page 136
CeFAZolin on page 325
Cephalexin on page 347
Clindamycin (Systemic) on page 402

Clinical Considerations for Dentistry

See Figure 2.

Figure 2
Preprocedural Dental Action Plan for Patients With Prosthetic Implants

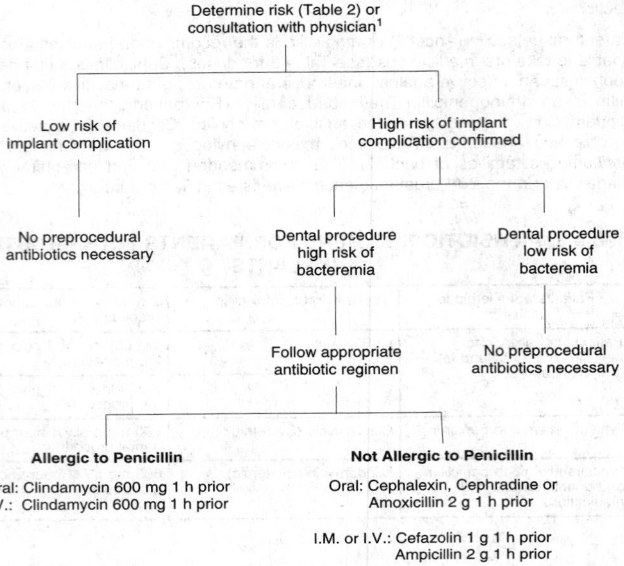

Cephalosporins should be avoided in patients with previous Type I hypersensitivity reactions to penicillin due to some evidence of cross allergenicity.

[1]For Emergency Dental Care the clinician should attempt phone consultation. If unable to contact patient's physician or determine risk, the patient should be treated as though there is high risk of implant complication and follow the algorithm.

The frequency of postinsertion infections in patients who have undergone total joint replacement or prosthetic device placement is variable. The most common cause of infection with all devices is found to be from contamination at the time of surgical insertions. The presence of an acute distant infection at a site other than the joint, however, appears to be a risk factor for late infection of these devices. As more evidence and data are collected, these recommendations may be revised; however, it is thought to be prudent for the dental clinician to fully evaluate all patients with respect to history and/or physical findings prior to determining the risk.

If a dental procedure considered to be low risk for bacteremia is performed in a patient at risk for joint complications, and inadvertent bleeding occurs, then an appropriate antibiotic should be given immediately. Although this is not ideal, animal studies suggest that it may be useful. Likewise, in patients where concern exists over joint complications and a medical consultation cannot be immediately obtained, the patient should be treated as though antibiotic coverage is necessary until such time that an appropriate consultation can be completed. The presence of an acute oral infection, in addition to any pre-existing dental conditions, may increase the risk of late infection at the prosthetic joint. Even though most late joint infections are caused by *Staphylococcus* sp, the risk of bacteremia involving another organism, predominant in an acute infection, may increase the risk of joint infection.

The dentist may also need to consider the question of multiple procedures over a period of time, rescheduling procedures at intervals of 9-14 days is best. The risk of emergence of resistant organisms in patients receiving multiple short-term doses of antibiotics has been shown to be greater than with those receiving antibiotics over longer intervals of time.

FREQUENTLY ASKED QUESTIONS FOR INFECTIVE ENDOCARDITIS (IE) AND PROSTHETIC IMPLANTS

When should we start following the new prevention of IE guidelines?

Immediately, since the latest guidelines as described herein were released in April, 2007.

What should we do for patients who have been premedicated in the past?

Most patients will no longer require premedication. If the patient does not fall into one of the highest risk groups, premedication should be discontinued. If it cannot be clearly determined if the patient is in the highest risk group, a medical consultation should be sent to determine if prophylaxis should be continued.

Are there different drugs and regimens?

The drugs have undergone minor revisions (see Table 1) and the dosing regimens for all drugs has been changed from 1 hour prior to 30-60 minutes prior to procedure.

Should I just premedicate to be safe?

No, the new guidelines are based on evidence which documents that the risk of adverse side effects from the antibiotics (allergy, GI upset, development of microbial resistance, etc) outweigh the benefits in most patients who previously received SBE/IE prophylaxis. The new Guidelines clearly recommend the use of prophylactic antibiotics only for those with the highest risk.

Has there been any change in the Guidelines for prophylaxis for patients with prosthetic joint replacements?

No, continue to use the published Guidelines.

What if a patient did not meet the new high-risk criteria outlined in the new Guidelines and the patient's physician still recommends IE prophylaxis?

Please contact the physician to see if there are compelling medical reasons for continuing IE prophylaxis.

What if a patient who has received IE prophylaxis in the past for a condition that is now deemed as NOT being high risk for IE prophylaxis still insists on being premedicate?

Recommend that the patient contacts the physician to see if there are compelling medical reasons for continuing IE prophylaxis.

If the patient is presently taking antibiotics for some other ailment, is prophylaxis still necessary?

If a patient is already taking antibiotics for another condition, prophylaxis (when deemed necessary under the new guidelines) should be accomplished with a drug from another class. For example, in the patient who is not allergic to penicillin who is taking a macrolide antibiotic for a medical condition, such as *Mycoplasma* infection, amoxicillin would be the drug of choice for prophylaxis. Also, in the penicillin-allergic patient taking clindamycin, prophylaxis would best be accomplished with azithromycin or clarithromycin.

Can clindamycin be used safely in patients with gastrointestinal disorders?

If a patient has a history of inflammatory bowel disease and is allergic to penicillin, azithromycin or clarithromycin should be selected over clindamycin. In patients with a negative history of inflammatory bowel disease, clindamycin has not been shown to induce colitis following a single-dose administration.

Why do the suggested drug regimens for patients with joint prostheses resemble so closely the regimens for the prevention of endocarditis?

Bacteremia is the predisposing risk factor for the development of endocarditis in those patients at high risk due to a cardiac condition. Likewise, the potential of bacteremia during dental procedures is considered to be the risk factor in some late-joint prostheses infections, even though this risk is presumed to be much lower.

How do we determine those patients who have had joint replacement complications?

Patients who have had complications during the initial placement of a total joint would be those who had infection following placement, those with recurrent pain, or those who have had previous joint replacement failures. If the patient reports even minor complications, a medical consultation with the orthopedist would be the most appropriate action for the dentist.

Is prophylaxis required in patients with pins, screws, or plates often used in orthopedic repairs?

There is currently no evidence supporting use of antibiotics following the placement of pins, plates, or screws. Breast implants, dental implants, and implanted lenses in the eye following cataract surgery are also all thought to be at minimal risk for infection following dental procedures. Therefore, no antibiotic prophylaxis is recommended in these situations. There is, however, some evidence indicating elevated risk of infection following some types of penile implants and some vascular access devices, used during chemotherapy. It is recommended that the dentist discuss such patients with the physician prior to determining the need for antibiotics.

What should I do if medical consultation results in a recommendation that differs from the published guidelines endorsed by the American Dental Association?

The dentist is ultimately responsible for treatment recommendations. Ideally, by communicating with the physician, a consensus can be achieved that is either in agreement with the guidelines or is based on other established medical reasoning.

What is the best antibiotic modality for treating dental infections?

Penicillin is still the drug of choice for treatment of infections in and around the oral cavity. Phenoxymethyl penicillin (Pen VK®) has long been the most commonly selected antibiotic. In penicillin-allergic individuals, erythromycin may be an appropriate consideration. If another drug is sought, clindamycin prescribed 300 mg as a loading dose followed by 150 mg 4 times/day would be an appropriate regimen for a dental infection. In general, if there is no response to Pen VK®, then Augmentin® may be a good alternative in the nonpenicillin-allergic patient because of its slightly altered spectrum. Recommendations would include that the patient take the drug with food.

Is there cross-allergenicity between the cephalosporins and penicillin?

The incidence of cross-allergenicity is 5% to 8% in the overall population. If a patient has demonstrated a Type I hypersensitivity reaction to penicillin, namely urticaria or anaphylaxis, then this incidence would increase to 20%.

Is there definitely an interaction between contraception agents and antibiotics?

There are well-founded interactions between contraceptives and antibiotics. The best instructions that a patient could be given by his/her dentist are that should an antibiotic be necessary, and the dentist is aware that the patient is on contraceptives, and if the patient is using chemical contraceptives, the patient should seriously consider additional means of contraception during the antibiotic management.

Are antibiotics necessary in diabetic patients?

In the management of diabetes, control of the diabetic status is the key factor relative to all morbidity issues. If a patient is well controlled, then antibiotics will likely not be necessary; however, in patients where the control is questionable or where they have recently been given a different drug regimen for their diabetes or if they are being titrated to an appropriate level of either insulin or oral hypoglycemic agents during these periods of time, the dentist might consider preprocedural antibiotics to be efficacious.

Do nonsteroidal anti-inflammatory drugs (NSAIDs) interfere with blood pressure medication?

At the current time there is no clear evidence that NSAIDs interfere with any of the blood pressure medications that are currently in use.

Some materials in this chapter were adapted from the guidelines of Wilson W, Taubert KA, Gewitz M, et al, "Prevention of Infective Endocarditis: Guidelines From the American Heart Association: A Guideline From the American Heart Association Rheumatic Fever, Endocarditis, and Kawasaki Disease Committee, Council on Cardiovascular Disease in the Young, and the Council on Clinical Cardiology, Council on Cardiovascular Surgery and Anesthesia, and the Quality of Care and Outcomes Research Interdisciplinary Working Group," *Circulation*, 2007, 116(15):1736-54.

PROBIOTICS TO REDUCE GASTRIC SYMPTOMS DURING LONG-TERM ANTIBIOTIC THERAPY

Cultures of direct-fed microorganisms or probiotics are able to multiply in the intestinal tract to create a balance of microflora. Some lactobacillus species used in probiotic applications include *L. acidophilus*, *L. casei*, *L. reuteri*, *L. rhamnosus*, and *Bifidobacterium bifidum*. These and other organisms form a symbiotic or mutual relationship with their host. Each species develops a resistance to the disease-causing potential of such organisms and form mutual beneficial relationships with these organisms. The familiar *L. acidophilus* produces lactic acid, reduces gut pH, and acts as a colonizer. Some forms of antibiotics, such as cephalosporins, clindamycin, or fluoroquinolones, induce colitis, an inflammation of the large intestine, in some individuals. This type of colitis is caused by a toxin produced by the bacteria *Clostridium difficile*, which is resistant to many antibiotics and proliferates in the intestines when other normal bacterial flora in the intestine are altered by the antibiotics.

It is usually recommended to take probiotics at least 3 hours apart from antibiotics. Taking both at the same time defeats the purpose as the friendly bacteria will be totally destroyed by the drug. During antibiotic therapy, a good dose of viable probiotic cells is 6-25 billion colony-forming units per day. Probiotics are also being studied as adjunctive therapy to periodontal treatment and treatment of other bacterial infections.

REFERENCES

Baddour LM, Bettmann MA, Bolger AF, et al, "Nonvalvular Cardiovascular Device-Related Infections," *Circulation*, 2003, 108(16):2015-31.

Bashore TM, Cabell C, and Fowler V Jr, "Update on Infective Endocarditis," *Curr Probl Cardiol*, 2006, 31 (4):274-352.

Brennan MT, Kent ML, Fox PC, et al, "The Impact of Oral Disease and Nonsurgical Treatment on Bacteremia in Children," *J Am Dent Assoc*, 2007, 138(1):80-5.

Burton JP, Chilcott CN, Moore CJ, et al, "A Preliminary Study of the Effect of Probiotic *Streptococcus salivarius* K12 on Oral Malodour Parameters," *J Appl Microbiol*, 2006, 100(4):754-64.

Duval X, Alla F, Hoen B, et al, "Estimated Risk of Endocarditis in Adults With Predisposing Cardiac Conditions Undergoing Dental Procedures With or Without Antibiotic Prophylaxis," *Clin Infect Dis*, 2006, 42(12):e102-7.

Gould FK, Elliott TS, Foweraker J, et al, "Guidelines for the Prevention of Endocarditis: Report of the Working Party of the British Society for Antimicrobial Chemotherapy," *J Antimicrob Chemother*, 2006, 57 (6):1035-42.

Karchmer AW, "Infective Endocarditis," *Braunwald's Heart Disease: A Textbook Of Cardiovascular Medicine*, 7th ed, Zipes D, Libby P, and Bonow RO, eds, Philadelphia, PA: WB Saunders Co, 2005, 1633-58.

Krasse P, Carlsson B, Dahl C, et al, "Decreased Gum Bleeding and Reduced Gingivitis by the Probiotic *Lactobacillus reuteri*," *Swed Dent J*, 2006, 30(2):55-60.

Lockhart PB, "The Risk for Endocarditis in Dental Practice," *Periodontol 2000*, 2000, 23:127-35.

Meurman JH and Stamatova I, "Probiotics: Contributions to Oral Health," *Oral Dis*, 2007, 13(5):443-5.

Teughels W, Van Essche M, Sliepen I, et al, "Probiotics and Oral Healthcare," *Periodontol 2000*, 2008, 48:111-47.

Twetman S and Stecksén-Blicks C, "Probiotics and Oral Health Effects in Children," *Int J Paediatr Dent*, 2008, 18(1):3-10.

Wilson W, Taubert KA, Gewitz M, et al, "Prevention of Infective Endocarditis: Guidelines From the American Heart Association: A Guideline From the American Heart Association Rheumatic Fever, Endocarditis, and Kawasaki Disease Committee, Council on Cardiovascular Disease in the Young, and the Council on Clinical Cardiology, Council on Cardiovascular Surgery and Anesthesia, and the Quality of Care and Outcomes Research Interdisciplinary Working Group," *Circulation*, 2007, 116(15):1736-54.

MANAGEMENT OF THE CHEMICALLY DEPENDENT PATIENT

INTRODUCTION

As long as history has been recorded, man has used drugs to alter mood, thought, and feeling. The financial and emotional cost to society due to the abuse and addiction of these substances is staggering. Some reports place the cost to society of alcoholism and alcohol abuse as high as $185 billion dollars annually. Increased on-the-job accidents, absenteeism, welfare costs, and alcohol-related auto fatalities contribute to this cost.

In 1986, the American Dental Association (ADA) passed a policy statement recognizing chemical dependency as a disease. In recognizing this disease, the Association mandated that dentists have a responsibility to include questions relating to a history of chemical dependency, or more broadly, substance abuse in their health history questionnaire. This policy statement included patients who are actively abusing drugs as well as patients who are in recovery. An affirmative response was an alert to the dentist and dental team to use caution with certain medications and that the treatment plan may have to be altered. This policy statement was revised in 1989 and 1991 with minor changes. In October 2005 at the annual ADA session, the House of Delegates passed several resolutions encompassing the use of opioids in management of dental pain, alcohol, and other substance use by pregnant and postpartum patients, and guidelines related to alcohol, nicotine, and/or drug use by child or adolescent patients. The House of Delegates in 2005 reaffirmed the disease concept of alcoholism and other substance use disorders and provided a more current statement on provision of dental treatment for patients with substance use disorders. For an in-depth review of these resolutions, refer to www.ada.org. At the minimum, the patient's past medical history questionnaire should include a question asking if there is a history of chemical dependency and if so, how long they have been in recovery. The dental office should have a list available of local resources for drug counseling in the event the patient admits drug use and seeks some help.

This chapter reviews substances of abuse, where they come from, signs and symptoms of the substance abuser, and some of the dental implications of treating patients actively using or in recovery from these substances. There are many books and articles devoted to this topic that provide greater detail. The intent of this chapter is to provide an overview of some of the most prevalent drugs, how abuse of these substances by patients may influence dental treatment, and how to recognize some signs and symptoms of substance abuse and withdrawal.

Substances of abuse originate from many sources. They may be naturally occurring, semisynthetic, synthetic, over-the-counter, or prescription drugs. There is a paucity of information in the dental literature correlating substance abuse with dental manifestations for a simple reason. Most substance abusers do not seek routine dental care because obtaining their drug of choice is their top priority. Most often they will be episodic patients. In fact, that is one of the cardinal signs of addiction, a preoccupation with obtaining the drug or sex or gambling or whatever the addiction. Again, it is not the intent of this chapter to explore addiction or abuse in detail. The reader is referred to several comprehensive texts on this disease.

As a general rule, the stimulant (uppers) abusing dental patient will not be going to the dentist while under the influence of the drug because the upper will increase their already existing anxiety. It is more likely that a patient will use or abuse a depressant (downer) substance to self-medicate anxiety. This is important to the dentist because uppers such as cocaine, methamphetamine, and ecstacy are sympathomimetics and in combination with vasoconstrictor could result in a hypertensive crisis (stroke). **Plain local anesthetic without vasoconstrictor is not contraindicated in that patient.** Patients who self-medicate with depressant drugs such as alcohol, opiates, barbiturates, or marijuana are generally more compliant while in the dental chair, and the drug combination does not pose a serious threat.

ALCOHOL

Ethyl alcohol (referred to as alcohol) is the most abused drug in the United States today and the number one most abused drug by dentists. As mentioned above, the cost to society for the treatment of alcoholism and alcohol abuse is billions of dollars annually. Alcohol is a depressant drug (downer) and not a stimulant as many people (particularly the adolescent population) believe. Its effect on the central nervous system is dose-dependent and correlated with the rising blood alcohol concentration rather than the falling concentration. Cognitive ability, reaction time, memory, psychomotor, and perceptual ability are impaired to varying degrees.

The majority of consumed alcohol is absorbed from the small intestine and is, therefore, affected by the gastric emptying time and the consumption of food. Alcohol is metabolized by the liver and excess consumption of alcohol can result in hepatic damage that may affect the patient's ability to metabolize medications. Doses of medications that are metabolized by the liver, such as acetaminophen, may have to be reduced when treating a patient with confirmed hepatic damage from alcohol or other substance abuse. Alcohol readily crosses the placental barrier and has the potential of producing fetal alcohol syndrome (FAS) resulting in mental retardation, supernumerary teeth, and facial deformities to name a few. There are many resources that provide greater detail about this preventable syndrome and the reader is referred to those sources.

Excessive alcohol use has been associated with an increased incidence of periodontal disease, poor wound healing, chronic orofacial infections, iatrogenic injury, and an increased incidence of oral cancer. Since alcohol is a depressant drug, any medication that causes respiratory depression should be prescribed or administered with caution or not at all. Patients who present to the dental office and are obviously intoxicated should not be provided dental treatment. The major concern with the intoxicated patient is a failure to follow directions while in the chair, and the inability to follow postoperative instructions. An additional concern is the aggressive, combative behavior exhibited by some that are intoxicated.

Signs and Symptoms of Alcohol Use or Abuse	
Lethargic, slow to respond	Odor on breath and/or clothes
Slurred speech	Inability to respond to commands
Telangiectasia	Psychomotor impairment

MARIJUANA

The most abused illegal drug by high school students today is marijuana. Marijuana is a plant that grows throughout the world, but is particularly suited for a warm, humid environment. There are three species of plants but the two most frequently cited are *Cannabis sativa* and *Cannabis indica*. All species possess a female and male plant. Although approximately 450 chemicals have been isolated from the plant, the major psychoactive ingredient is delta-9-tetrahydrocannabinol (THC). Of these 450 chemicals, there are approximately 23 psychoactive chemicals, THC being the most abundant. The highest concentration of THC is found in the bud of the female plant (hashish). The concentration of THC varies according to growing conditions and the part of the plant but has increased from approximately 2% to 3% in marijuana sold in the 1950s to approximately 40% sold on the streets today. Marijuana can be smoked in cigarettes (joints), pipes, water pipes (bongs), or baked in brownies, cakes, etc, and then ingested. However, smoking marijuana is more efficient and the "high" has a quicker onset. Marijuana is a Schedule I drug but has been promoted as medicinal for the treatment of glaucoma, for increasing appetite in patients who have HIV disease, to prevent the nausea associated with cancer chemotherapy, and as an analgesic for chronic pain. In response to this request, the FDA approved dronabinol (Marinol®), a synthetic THC, and placed this drug in Schedule III to be prescribed by physicians for the indicated medical conditions. The synthetic THC does not produce a "high" and in fact is not well absorbed from the gastrointestinal tract.

An individual under the influence of marijuana may exhibit no signs or symptoms of intoxication. The pharmacologic effects are dose-dependent and depend to a large extent on the set and setting of the intoxicated individual. As the dose of THC increases, the person experiences euphoria or a state of well-being, often referred to as "mellowing out". Everything becomes comical, problems disappear, and their appetite for snack foods increases. This is called the "munchies". Additionally, marijuana produces time and spatial distortion, which contribute, as the dose increases, to a dysphoria characterized by paranoia and fear. Although there has never been a death reported from marijuana overdose, certainly the higher doses may produce such bizarre circumstances as to increase the chances of accidental death. THC is fat soluble. Daily consumption of marijuana will result in THC being stored in body fat which will result in detectable amounts of THC being found in the urine for as long as 60 days in some cases.

Because of anxiety associated with dental visits, marijuana would be the most likely drug, after alcohol, to be used when coming to the dental office. But, unlike alcohol, marijuana may not produce any detectable odor on the breath nor signs of intoxication. Fortunately, local anesthetics, analgesics, and antibiotics used by the general dentist do not interact with marijuana. The major concern with the marijuana-intoxicated patient, similar to the alcohol-intoxicated patient, is a failure to follow directions while in the chair, and the inability to follow postoperative instructions.

Signs and Symptoms of Marijuana Use	
Blood shot eyes	Odor on breath and clothes
Lethargic, slow to respond	Inability to respond to commands
Slurred speech	Memory impairment

OPIATES

The opiates are most often called narcotics. The word "narcosis" means sleep. These drugs are referred to on the street as "downers", the most common being heroin. Heroin is the diacetyl derivative of morphine which is extracted from opium. Although commercial production of morphine involves extraction from the dried opium plant which grows in many parts of the world, some areas still harvest opium by making slits in the unripened seed pod. The pod secretes a white, viscous material which upon contact with the air turns a blackish-brown color. It is this off-white material that is called opium. The opium is then dried and smoked or processed to yield morphine and codeine. Actually, the raw opium contains several chemicals that are used medicinally or commercially. Much (approximately 50%) of morphine is converted chemically into heroin which finds its way into the United States and then on the street. Heroin is a Schedule I drug and has no acceptable use in the United States today. In fact, possession is a violation of the Controlled Substances Act of 1970. The majority of the heroin found on the streets in the United States is from Colombia, South America (65%) and can be as pure as 50% to 60%.

The heroin user goes through many phases once the drug has been administered. When administered intravenously, the user initially feels a "rush" often described as an "orgasmic rush". This initial feeling is most likely due to the release of histamine resulting in cutaneous vasodilation, itching, and a flushed appearance. Shortly after this "rush" the user becomes euphoric. This euphoric stage often called "stoned" or being "high" lasts approximately 3-4 hours. During this stage, the user is lethargic, slow to react to stimuli, speech is slurred, pain reaction threshold is elevated, exhibits xerostomia, experiences slowed heart rate, and his/hers pupils may be constricted. Following the "high", the abuser is "straight" for about 2 hours, with no tell-tale signs of abuse. Approximately 6-8 hours following the last injection of heroin, the user begins to experience a runny nose, lacrimation, and abdominal muscle cramps as the withdrawal from the drug begins. During this stage and the one that follows, the person may become agitated as he/she develops anxiety about where the next "hit" will come from. The withdrawal signs and symptoms become more intense. For the next 3 days, the abuser begins to sweat profusely in combination with cutaneous vasoconstriction. The skin becomes cold and clammy, hence the term "cold turkey". Tachycardia, pupillary dilation, diarrhea, and salivation occur for 3 days following the last injection. Withdrawal signs and symptoms may last longer than the average of 3 days or they may be more abrupt.

Many patients who have been abusing opiates will exhibit multiple carious lesions, particularly class V lesions. This increased caries rate is probably a result of the heroin-induced xerostomia, high intake of sweets, and lack of daily oral hygiene. Patients who are recovering from heroin or any opiate addiction should not be given any kind of opiate analgesic, whether it is for sedation or as a postoperative analgesic because of the increased chance of relapse. Nonsteroidal anti-inflammatory drugs (NSAIDs) should be used to control any postoperative discomfort. Patients who admit to a past history of intravenous heroin use, or any intravenous drug for that matter, are at higher risk for subacute bacterial endocarditis (SBE), HIV disease, and hepatitis, with the exception of postoperative analgesia should present no special problem for dental care.

Signs and Symptoms of Narcotic Use	
Pin point pupils	Glazed eyes
Lethargic, slow to respond	Inability to respond to commands
Slurred speech	Xerostomia

METHAMPHETAMINE

Methamphetamine has been available clinically for 45 years as a medication to curb appetite. Today it is one of the most widely abused drugs on the street. Methamphetamine can be smoked in the form of "ice", snorted, injected, or consumed orally. The onset of action varies with the route of administration, smoking providing the most rapid onset of action. Clandestine methamphetamine is usually synthesized from pseudoephedrine or ephedrine. The methamphetamine molecule can exist in either the "D" isomer or the "L" isomer. The latter isomer has its greatest effect on the cardiovascular system and, in fact, is available commercially over-the-counter as a nasal decongestant. The "D" isomer has its principle effects on the central nervous system as a stimulant (upper) and can not be converted from the "L" form. It is a sympathomimetic and as such raises blood pressure. This effect on the autonomic nervous system results in increased basal metabolic rate (BMR) and increased body temperature resulting in the "sweats". Methamphetamine users crave sweets possibly as a source of energy to fuel the increased BMR. As a consequence of the increased sweating the individual becomes dehydrated and thirsty. The sympathetic stimulation produces a thick, ropey saliva. This lack of saliva, increased consumption of sweets in the form of soda pop, and lack of routine dental care no doubt is the primary cause of "meth mouth". Initially the meth user experiences a feeling of exhilaration, alertness, and incredible energy. With successive uses, tolerance occurs and the user abuses increasing amounts of methamphetamine looking for the same high they experienced on the first time. They never quite attain it. This has been referred to on the street as "chasing the monkey". As a substitute, the user continues their high for several hours or days in some cases. This is called bingeing. A binge may last for 5 or 6 days. The user becomes very paranoid, develops psychotic episodes, and has the potential of becoming violent. stereotypical behavior develops such as rocking back and forth in a chair, picking their fingernails, or other behavior. During this stage the user begins "tweaking", using small amounts to stay high, and begins to hallucinate. Characteristically, they will describe the feeling that bugs are crawling under their skin and they scratch their arms, face, and any other exposed part of their body. The street term for this hallucination is called "coke bugs". Usually, the user will collapse from the physical exhaustion. Withdrawal can take weeks after the last use. As mentioned above, vasoconstrictor is contraindicated if there has been methamphetamine use within the last 24 hours.

Methamphetamine Signs and Symptoms in the Dental Office	
Dilated pupils	Jittery, irritable behavior
Rapid speech	Unable to sit still, twitching
Tremendous anxiety	Difficult to anesthetize

BENZODIAZEPINES AND OTHER NONALCOHOL SEDATIVES

These drugs are used mainly for treatment of anxiety disorders and, in some instances, insomnia. These drugs are commonly abused, either by themselves or as adjunct to the opiates. They have the ability to produce a strong physical dependency on the use of the medication. As tolerance builds up to the drug, the physical dependency increases dramatically. Unlike street drugs, where addiction is a primary consideration, the overuse of benzodiazepine lies in their ability to induce physical dependency. When these drugs are taken for several weeks, there is relatively little tolerance induced. However, after several months, the proportion of patients who become tolerant increases and reducing the dose or stopping the medication produces severe withdrawal symptoms often resulting in death.

It is extremely difficult for the physician to distinguish between the withdrawal symptoms and the reappearance of the myriad anxiety symptoms that cause the drug to be prescribed initially. Many patients increase their dose over time because tolerance develops to at least the sedative effects of the drug. The antianxiety benefits of the benzodiazepines continue to occur long after tolerance to the sedating effects. Patients often take these drugs for many years with relatively few ill effects other than the risk of withdrawal. The dentist should be keenly aware of the signs and symptoms and the historical pattern in patients taking benzodiazepines.

NICOTINE

Cigarette (nicotine) addiction is influenced by multiple variables. Nicotine itself produces reinforcement; users compare nicotine to stimulants such as cocaine or amphetamine, although its effects are of lower magnitude.

Nicotine is absorbed readily through the skin, mucous membranes, and of course, through the lungs. The pulmonary route produces discernible central nervous system effects in as little as 7 seconds. Thus, each puff produces some discrete reinforcement. With 10 puffs per cigarette, the 1 pack per day smoker reinforces the habit 200 times daily. The timing, setting, situation, and preparation all become associated repetitively with the effects of nicotine.

Nicotine has both stimulant and depressant actions. The smoker feels alert, yet there is some muscle relaxation. Nicotine activates the nucleus accumbens reward system in the brain. Increased extracellular dopamine has been found in this region after nicotine injections in rats. Nicotine affects other systems as well, including the release of endogenous opioids and glucocorticoids.

Nicotine Withdrawal Syndrome Signs and Symptoms	
Irritability, impatience, hostility	Restlessness
Anxiety	Decreased heart rate
Dysphoric or depressed mood	Increased appetite or weight gain
Difficulty concentrating	

SMOKING CESSATION PRODUCTS

Several years ago, the journal, *Science*, stated that approximately 80% of smokers say they want to quit, but each year <1 in 10 actually succeed. Nicotine transdermal delivery preparations (or nicotine patches) were approved by the U.S. Food and Drug Administration in 1992 as aids to smoking cessation for the relief of nicotine withdrawal symptoms. Four preparations were approved simultaneously: Habitrol®, Nicoderm®, Nicotrol®, and ProStep®. These products differ in how much nicotine is released and whether they provide a 24- or 16-hour release time.

Studies are still being reported on the effectiveness of nicotine patches on tobacco cessation. Most previous studies had good entry criteria including definition of the Fagerstrom score. Dr Fred Cowan of Oregon Health Sciences University described these Fagerstrom criteria in a previous report on nicotine substitutes in AGD *Impact*. Abstinence of smoking cessation has usually been assessed by self-report, measurement of carbon monoxide in breath, and plasma or urine nicotine products.

In numerous protocols, percentages of study subjects who abstained from smoking after 3-10 weeks of patch treatment with nicotine compared to placebo, have never exceeded 40%. After the initial assessment, six studies continued to follow the study subjects through 24-52 weeks of patch treatment. The results were even poorer with <25% sustained success. A review of these and additional studies, reveals some general conclusions regarding the effectiveness of nicotine patches in tobacco cessation. In every study, many smokers abstained after treatment with placebo patches; nicotine treatment was initially more effective than placebo; and improved abstinence rates were more marked in the short term (10 weeks) than in the long term (52 weeks). Subjects undergoing tobacco cessation trials tended to gain weight irrespective of whether placebo or nicotine patches were worn. Patients often favor the nicotine polacrilex gum (Nicorette®) which releases nicotine into the blood stream via the oral mucosa.

Data are now available from tobacco cessation studies carried out in general medical practices. The effectiveness of nicotine patch substitution under these conditions is similar to the results described previous. Most patch systems and gum are now available as over-the-counter products; only Habitrol® remains prescription. bupropion (Zyban®) is another approach to the treatment of tobacco cessation. This drug is a norepinephrine/serotonin/dopamine reuptake inhibitor and its action directly affects the craving for tobacco. Another new product just introduced is varenicline (Chantix®). This product targets certain nicotine receptors to prevent nicotine access and diminishes the mesolimbic dopamine reward associated with nicotine use. The reader is referred to more comprehensive information about these products and the treatment of tobacco cessation. In addition, the reader should familiarize themselves with the supportive ADA posture on the role of the dental team in tobacco cessation treatment.

COCAINE

Cocaine, referred to on the street as "snow", "nose candy", "girl", and many other euphemisms, has created an epidemic. This drug is like no other local anesthetic. Known for about the last 2000 years, cocaine has been used and abused by politicians, scientists, farmers, warriors, and of course, on the street. Cocaine is derived from the leaves of a plant called *Erythroxylon* coca which grows in South America. Ninety percent of the world's supply of cocaine originates in Peru, Bolivia, and Colombia. At last estimate, the United States consumes 75% of the world's supply. The plant grows to a height of approximately 4 feet and produces a red berry. Farmers go through the fields stripping the leaves from the plant three times a year. During the working day, the farmers chew the coca leaves to suppress appetite and fight the fatigue of working the fields. The leaves are transported to a laboratory site where the cocaine is extracted by a process called maceration. It takes approximately 7-8 pounds of leaves to produce 1 ounce of cocaine.

On the streets of the United States, cocaine can be found in two forms - one is the hydrochloride salt which can be "snorted" or dissolved in water and injected intravenously, the other is the free base form which can be smoked and is sometimes referred to as "crack", "rock", or "free base". It is called crack because it cracks or pops when large pieces are smoked. It is called rock because it is hard and difficult to break into smaller pieces. The most popular method of administration of cocaine is "snorting" in which small amounts of cocaine hydrochloride are divided into segments or "lines" and any straw-like device can be used to inhale one or more lines of the cocaine into the nose. Although cocaine does not reach the lungs, enough cocaine is absorbed through nasal mucosa to provide a "high" within 3-5 minutes. Rock or crack, on the other hand, is heated and inhaled from any device available. This form of cocaine does reach the lungs and provides a much faster onset of action as well as a more intense stimulation. There are dangers to the user with any form of cocaine. Undoubtedly, the most dangerous form is the intravenous route.

Signs and Symptoms of Cocaine Use	
Dilated pupils	Tremors
Jitteriness	Talkative
Irritability	Increased blood pressure

The cocaine user, regardless of how the cocaine was administered, presents a potential life-threatening situation in the dental operatory. The patient under the influence of cocaine could be compared to a car going 100 miles per hour. Blood pressure is elevated and heart rate is likely increased. Use of a local anesthetic with epinephrine in such a patient may result in a medical emergency. Such patients can be identified by jitteriness, irritability, talkativeness, tremors, and short abrupt speech patterns. These same signs and symptoms may also be seen in a normal dental patient with preoperative dental anxiety; therefore, the dentist must be particularly alert to identify the potential cocaine abuser. If a patient is suspected, they should never be given a local anesthetic with vasoconstrictor for fear of exacerbating cocaine-induced sympathetic response. Life-threatening episodes of cardiac arrhythmias and hypertensive crises have been reported when local anesthetic with vasoconstrictor was administered to a patient under the influence of cocaine. No local anesthetic used by any dentist can interfere with, nor test positive for cocaine in any urine testing screen. Therefore, the dentist need not be concerned with any false drug use accusations associated with dental anesthesia.

CLUB DRUGS

Perceptual distortions that include hallucinations, illusions, and disorders of thinking such as paranoia can be produced by toxic doses of many drugs. These phenomena also may be seen during toxic withdrawal from sedatives such as alcohol. There are, however, certain drugs that have as their primary effect the production of perception, thought, or mood disturbances at low doses with minimal effects on memory and orientation. These are commonly called *hallucinogenic drugs*, but their use does not always result in frank hallucinations.

Ecstasy (MDMA) and Phenylethylamines (MDA): MDA and MDMA have stimulant, as well as, psychedelic effects and produce degeneration of serotonergic nerve cells and axons. While nerve degeneration has not been well-demonstrated in human beings, the potential remains. Thus, there is possible neurotoxicity with overuse of these drugs. Ecstasy became popular during the 1980s on college campuses and it is still recommended by some psychotherapists as an aid to the process of therapy, although very little controlled data is available. Acute effects are dose-dependent and include dry mouth, jaw clinching, muscle aches, and tachycardia. At higher doses, effects include agitation, hyperthermia, panic attacks, and visual hallucinations. Frequent, repeated use of psychedelic drugs is unusual and, therefore, tolerance is not commonly seen. However, tolerance does develop to the behavioral effects of various psychedelic drugs, and after numerous doses, the tendency towards behavioral tolerance can be observed.

Lysergic Acid Diethylamide (LSD): LSD is the most potent hallucinogenic drug and produces significant psychedelic effects with a total dose of as little as 25-50 mcg. This drug is over 3000 times more potent than mescaline. It is sold on the illicit market in a variety of forms, as a tablet, capsule, sugar cube, or on blotting paper, a popular contemporary system involving postage stamp-sized papers impregnated with varying doses of LSD (50-300 mcg). A majority of street samples sold as LSD actually do contain LSD, while mushrooms and other botanicals sold as sources of psilocybin and other psychedelics have a low probability of containing the advertised hallucinogenics. Adverse effects which may affect treatment include visual and auditory hallucinations, tachycardia, psychosis, fear, tremors, delirium, hyperglycemia, fever, sweating, flushing, euphoria, hypertonia, nausea, vomiting, coma, seizures, tachypnea, and respiratory arrest.

INHALANTS

Anesthetic gases such as nitrous oxide or halothane are sometimes used as intoxicants by medical personnel. Nitrous oxide also is abused by food service employees because it is supplied for use as a propellant in disposable aluminum minitanks for whipping cream canisters. Nitrous oxide produces euphoria and analgesia and then loss of consciousness. Compulsive use and chronic toxicity rarely are reported, but there are obvious risks of overdose associated with the abuse of this anesthetic. Chronic use has been reported to cause peripheral neuropathy. Glue, correction fluid, gasoline, aerosol key board cleaners, model paint, in fact, any volatile substance has the potential to cause a "high" and like all of the above can become very addictive and deadly.

The dental team should be alert to the signs and symptoms of drug abuse and withdrawal. Further reading is recommended.

ORAL MEDICINE TOPICS

PART II:

DENTAL MANAGEMENT AND THERAPEUTIC CONSIDERATIONS IN PATIENTS WITH SPECIFIC ORAL CONDITIONS AND OTHER MEDICINE TOPICS

The second part of the chapter focuses on therapies the dentist may choose to prescribe for patients suffering from oral disease or who are in need of special care. Some overlap between these sections has resulted from systemic conditions that have oral manifestations and vice-versa. Cross-references to the descriptions and the monographs for individual drugs described elsewhere in this handbook allow for easy retrieval of information. Example prescriptions of selected drug therapies for each condition are presented so that the clinician can evaluate alternate approaches to treatment, since there is seldom a single drug of choice.

Drug prescriptions shown represent prototype drugs and popular prescriptions and are examples only. The pharmacologic category index is available for cross-referencing if alternatives and additional drugs are sought.

TABLE OF CONTENTS

ORAL PAIN

PAIN PREVENTION

For the dental patient, the prevention of pain aids in relieving anxiety and reduces the probability of stress during dental care. For the practitioner, dental procedures can be accomplished more efficiently in a "painless" situation. Appropriate selection and use of local anesthetics is one of the foundations for success in this arena. Local anesthetics listed below include drugs for the most commonly confronted dental procedures. Ester anesthetics are no longer available in dose form for dental injections, and historically had a higher incidence of allergic manifestations due to the formation of the metabolic byproduct, para-aminobenzoic acid. Articaine, which has an ester side chain, is rapidly metabolized to a non-PABA acid and functions as an amide and has a low allergic potential. The amides, in general, have a nearly negligible incidence of true allergic reactions, and only one well-documented case of amide allergy has been reported by Seng, et al. Although injectable diphenhydramine (Benadryl®) has been used in an attempt to provide anesthesia in patients allergic to all the local anesthetics, it is no longer recommended in this context. The vehicle for injectable diphenhydramine can cause tissue necrosis.

LOCAL ANESTHETICS

Articaine and Epinephrine on page 162
Bupivacaine on page 256
Bupivacaine and Epinephrine on page 257
Chloroprocaine on page 363
Lidocaine and Epinephrine on page 1012
Lidocaine (Systemic) on page 1007
Mepivacaine Dental Anesthetic on page 1078
Mepivacaine and Levonordefrin on page 1080
Prilocaine on page 1399
Prilocaine and Epinephrine on page 1401
Ropivacaine on page 1497
Tetracaine (Topical) on page 1610

The selection of a vasoconstrictor with the local anesthetic must be based on the length of the procedure to be performed, the patient's medical status (epinephrine is contraindicated in patients with uncontrolled hyperthyroidism), and the need for hemorrhage control. The following table lists some of the common drugs with their duration of action. The long-acting amide injectable, Ropivacaine (Naropin®) may be useful for postoperative pain management.

DENTAL ANESTHETICS (Average Duration by Route)

Product	Infiltration	Inferior Alveolar Block
Articaine HCl 4% and epinephrine 1:100,000	60 minutes	~60 minutes
Articaine HCl 4% and epinephrine 1:200,000	40 minutes	50 minutes
Carbocaine® HCl 2% with Neo-Cobefrin® 1:20,000 (mepivacaine HCl and levonordefrin)	50 minutes	60-75 minutes
Carbocaine® Plain 3%	20 minutes	40 minutes
Citanest® Plain 4% (prilocaine)	20 minutes	2.5 hours
Citanest Forte® with epinephrine 1:200,000 (prilocaine with epinephrine)	2.25 hours	3 hours
Lidocaine HCl 2% and epinephrine 1:100,000	60 minutes	90 minutes
Marcaine® HCl 0.5% with epinephrine 1:200,000 (bupivacaine and epinephrine)	60 minutes	5-7 hours
Vivacaine™ 0.5% with epinephrine 1:200,000 (bupivacaine and epinephrine)	60 minutes	5-7 hours

The use of articaine 4% with epinephrine 1:100,000 solution for mandibular blocks has been associated occasionally with paresthesia (*J Am Dent Assoc*, 2001, 132 (2):177-85).

The use of preinjection topical anesthetics can assist in pain prevention (see also Viral Infections on page 1947 and Ulcerative, Erosive, and Painful Oral Mucosal Disorders on page 1950). It should be noted that the FDA recently warned healthcare professionals regarding potential risks associated with unsupervised patient cutaneous use of topical anesthetic products. Life-threatening adverse events such as arrhythmias, seizures, coma, and respiratory complications have been reported. Thus, healthcare professionals are advised to prescribe FDA-approved topical anesthetics in the lowest concentration consistent with pain relief goals. It is not known if oral mucosa misuse may pose the same risk factors.

Clinicians are also using a eutectic mixture of 2.5% lidocaine with 2.5% prilocaine in a periodontal gel form in adults who require localized anesthesia in periodontal pockets during scaling and/or root planing. However, the same mixture available as a skin patch (EMLA®) from Astra is not currently approved for oral use.

Recently, Phase 2 and 3 clinical trials have been completed and FDA approval of the local anesthetic reversal agent OraVerse™ has now occurred. OraVerse™ (phentolamine mesylate) injection is a local anesthetic reversal agent that accelerates the return to normal sensation and function following restorative and periodontal maintenance procedures. OraVerse™ is indicated for the reversal of soft tissue anesthesia (ie, anesthesia of the lip, tongue, and the associated functional deficits resulting from an intraoral submucosal injection of a local anesthetic containing a vasoconstrictor. OraVerse™ is not recommended for use in children <6 years of age or weighing <15 kg (33 lbs).

Phentolamine (OraVerse™), as used in its original context as a medical hypotensive agent, could be expected to cause significant hypotension and reflex tachycardia when used as the anesthetic reversal agent in children. Studies have shown, however, that neither of these reactions occurred in the children receiving the drug. According to the authors of the study, there was an impressive benefit:risk ratio suggesting a safe approach in accelerating recovery from soft tissue anesthesia in children (Tavares, et al, *JADA*, 2008, 139(8):1095-1104). There were no serious adverse events observed. The adverse reactions were observed from study populations of 484 adults and 152 children. It should be anticipated that more adverse effects could occur as OraVerse™ is used in a larger number of patients. The clinical studies used a maximum of 2 cartridges of OraVerse™ (0.8 mg phentolamine). There is no information published on effects that occur with higher doses of OraVerse™. Phentolamine is a very powerful alpha-adrenergic receptor blocker which can cause cardiovascular effects if inadvertently injected in high doses. The manufacturer advises to adhere to the recommended dosing for the OraVerse™ formulation. The dosing for OraVerse™ is based on the number of cartridges of local anesthetic with vasoconstrictor administered, with 1 cartridge of OraVerse™ containing 0.4 mg of phentolamine and 2 cartridges containing 0.8 mg phentolamine. Dosing is as a 1:1 cartridge ratio to local anesthetic using the same injection site and administration technique as that used for the local anesthetic. The manufacturer advises to report any adverse reactions observed and deemed significant to the manufacturer at Novalar Pharmaceuticals, Inc. 12555 High Bluff Drive, Suite 300, San Diego, CA 92130 (888-888-1441).

Benzocaine on page 218
Lidocaine (Systemic) on page 1007
Phentolamine on page 1338
Tetracaine (Topical) on page 1610

PAIN MANAGEMENT

The patient with existing acute or chronic oral pain requires appropriate treatment and sensitivity on the part of the dentist, all for the purpose of achieving relief from the oral source of pain. Pain can be divided into mild, moderate, and severe levels and requires a subjective assessment by the dentist based on knowledge of the dental procedures to be performed, the presenting signs and symptoms of the patient, and the realization that most dental procedures are invasive often leading to pain once the patient has left the dental office. The practitioner must be aware that the treatment of the source of the pain is usually the best management. If infection is present, treatment of the infection will directly alleviate the patient's discomfort. However, a patient who is not in pain tends to heal better and it is wise to adequately cover the patient for any residual or recurrent discomfort suffered. Likewise, many of the procedures that the dentist performs have pain associated with them. Much of this pain occurs after leaving the dentist office due to an inflammatory process or a healing process that has been initiated. It is difficult to assign specific pain levels (mild, moderate, or severe) for specific procedures; however, the dentist should use his or her prescribing capacity judiciously so that overmedication is avoided.

The potential interaction between acetaminophen and warfarin has been recently raised in the literature. The cytochrome P450 system of drug metabolism for these vitamin K-dependent metabolic pathways has raised the possibility that prolonged use of acetaminophen may inadvertently enhance, to dangerous levels, the anticoagulation effect of warfarin. As monitored by the INR, the effects of these drugs may be one and one-half to two times greater than as expected from the warfarin dosage alone. This potential interaction could be of importance in selecting an analgesic/antipyretic drug for the dental patient.

The following categories of drugs and appropriate example prescriptions for each can be found in the example prescriptions quick reference section, following the chapters. These include management of mild pain with aspirin products, acetaminophen, and some of the nonsteroidal noninflammatory agents (eg, ibuprofen). Management of moderate pain includes codeine, Toradol®, Vicodin®, Vicodin ES®, Lorcet® 10/650, Opana®; and Motrin® in the 800 mg dosage. Etodolac is approved as an NSAID for mild-to-moderate acute and chronic pain, as well as, for pain of osteo and rheumatoid arthritis. Severe pain may require treatment with Percodan® or Percocet®. A new drug, tapentadol is similar to tramadol in its actions and was approved in November 2008 for moderate-to-severe acute pain. Tapentadol is classified as a narcotic analgesic having a unique ability to bind to μ-opiate receptors and inhibit the reuptake of norepinephrine. It shares many properties of traditional narcotic drugs including addiction liability. A report by Kleinert et al, showed that a single dose of tapentadol ≥75 mg effectively reduced moderate-to-severe postoperative dental pain in a dose related fashion and was well tolerated compared to 60 mg morphine. Their study showed that tapentadol was a highly effective, central-acting analgesic with a favorable side effect profile with rapid onset of action (Kleinert, 2008). All prescription pain preparations should be closely monitored for efficacy and discontinued if the pain persists or requires a higher level formulation. Combination drugs such as the recently released Combunox™ containing 5 mg of oxycodone and 400 mg of ibuprofen have proven usefulness in acute moderately severe to severe pain management.

The chronic pain patient represents a particular challenge for the practitioner. Some additional drugs that may be useful in managing the patient with chronic pain of neuropathic origin are covered in the temporomandibular dysfunction section. It is always incumbent on the practitioner to reevaluate the diagnosis, source of pain, and treatment, whenever prolonged use of analgesics (narcotic or non-narcotic) is contemplated. Drugs such as Dilaudid® are not recommended for management of dental pain in most states.

Recently, the FDA has formally requested manufacturers to limit the amount of acetaminophen in prescription combination products to no more than 325 mg in each tablet or capsule. The FDA is also requiring manufacturers to update labeling of all prescription combination acetaminophen products to warn of the potential risk for severe liver injury. The over-the-counter acetaminophen products are not affected by this ruling.

Overdose from prescription combination products containing acetaminophen account for nearly half of all cases of acetaminophen-related liver failure in the United States. Many cases result in liver transplant or death. There is no immediate danger to patients taking these combination pain medications. Patients should continue to take them as directed by healthcare provider. The risk of liver injury primarily occurs when patients take multiple products containing acetaminophen at one time and exceed the current maximum adult dose of 4000 mg within a 24-hour period. The elimination of higher-dose prescription combination acetaminophen products will be phased in over 3 years and should not create shortages. For more information and a complete list of affected products see www.fda.gov/acetaminophen.

Narcotic analgesics can be used on a short-term basis or intermittently in combination with non-narcotic therapy in the chronic pain patient. Judicious prescribing, monitoring, and maintenance by the practitioner are imperative, particularly whenever considering the use of a narcotic analgesic due to the abuse and addiction liabilities.

MILD PAIN

Acetaminophen on page 32
Aspirin (various products) on page 171
Diflunisal on page 524
Etodolac on page 690
Ibuprofen on page 884
Ketoprofen on page 966
Naproxen on page 1183

MODERATE / MODERATELY SEVERE PAIN

Dihydrocodeine, Aspirin, and Caffeine on page 531
Hydrocodone and Acetaminophen on page 858
Hydrocodone and Ibuprofen on page 863
Acetaminophen and Tramadol on page 43
Ibuprofen (various products) on page 884
Ketorolac (Systemic) on page 969
Oxymorphone on page 1282
Tapentadol on page 1584

An additional class of NSAIDs has been approved and indicated in the treatment of arthritis, COX-2 inhibitors. Celecoxib (Celebrex®) has been approved for use in oral pain management.

The following is a guideline to use when prescribing codeine with either aspirin or acetaminophen (Tylenol®):

Codeine No. 2 = codeine 15 mg
Codeine No. 3 = codeine 30 mg
Codeine No. 4 = codeine 60 mg

Example: ASA No. 3 = aspirin 325 mg + codeine 30 mg

HYDROCODONE PRODUCTS

Available hydrocodone oral products are listed in the following table and are scheduled as C-III controlled substances, indicating that prescriptions may either be oral or written. Thus, the prescriber may call in a prescription to the pharmacy for any of these hydrocodone products. All the formulations are combined with acetaminophen except for Vicoprofen®, which contains ibuprofen, and Lortab® ASA and Damason-P®, which all contain aspirin. Most of these brand name drugs are available generically and the pharmacist will dispense the generic equivalent if available, unless the prescriber indicates otherwise.

HYDROCODONE ANALGESIC COMBINATION ORAL PRODUCTS (All Products DEA Schedule C-III)

Hydrocodone is available under numerous brand names with varying dosages and in combination with aspirin or ibuprofen.					
Hydrocodone Bitartrate	**Acetaminophen (APAP[1])**	**Other**	**Brand Name**	**Generic Available**	**Form**
2.5 mg	500 mg	–	–	Yes	Tablet
5 mg	400 mg	–	Zydone®	No	Tablet
5 mg	500 mg	–	Vicodin®; Lortab®5/500	Yes	Tablet
5 mg	500 mg	–	Margesic® H; Stagesic™	No	Capsule
7.5 mg	400 mg	–	Zydone®	No	Tablet
7.5 mg	500 mg	–	Lortab® 7.5/500	Yes	Tablet
7.5 mg	650 mg	–	Lorcet Plus®	Yes	Tablet
7.5 mg	750 mg	–	Vicodin ES®	Yes	Tablet
10 mg	400 mg	–	Zydone®	No	Tablet
10 mg	325 mg	–	Norco®	Yes	Tablet
10 mg	500 mg	–	Lortab® 10/500	Yes	Tablet
10 mg	650 mg	–	Lorcet® 10/650	Yes	Tablet
10 mg	660 mg	–	Vicodin HP®	Yes	Tablet
10 mg	750 mg	–	Maxidone™	Yes	Tablet
7.5 mg/15 mL	500 mg/15 mL	–	Lortab® Elixir	Yes	Elixir
7.5 mg	–	Ibuprofen 200 mg	Vicoprofen®	Yes	Tablet
5 mg	–	Ibuprofen 200 mg	Ibudone™; Reprexain™	Yes	Tablet

Note: Although all of these products are currently available, the FDA is requesting the elimination of prescription combination drugs containing more than 325 mg of acetaminophen over the next 3 years. A complete list of affected products is available at www.fda.gov/acetaminophen

[1]APAP is the common acronym for acetaminophen and is the abbreviation of the chemical name N-acetylparaminophenol.

The following are the usual adult doses of the hydrocodone oral products as listed by the most recent edition of the Drug Information for the Health Care Professional (USPDI).

1 or 2 tablets containing 2.5 mg of hydrocodone and 500 mg of acetaminophen every 4-6 hours; or

1 tablet containing 5 mg of hydrocodone and 500 mg acetaminophen every 4-6 hours as needed, with dosage being increased to 2 tablets every 6 hours, if necessary; or

1 capsule containing 5 mg of hydrocodone and 500 mg of acetaminophen every 4-6 hours as needed, with dosage being increased to 2 capsules every 6 hours if necessary; or

1 tablet containing 7.5 mg hydrocodone and 650 mg of acetaminophen every 4-6 hours as needed, with dosage being increased to 2 tablets every 6 hours if necessary; or

1 tablet containing 7.5 mg hydrocodone and 750 mg of acetaminophen every 4-6 hours as needed; or

1 tablet containing 10 mg of hydrocodone and 650 mg acetaminophen every 4-6 hours as needed.

For the elixir (Lortab®), the recommended dose is 1 tablespoonful every 4-6 hours when necessary for pain.

For the aspirin products (Lortab® ASA and Damason-P®), the recommended dose is 1 or 2 tablets every 4-6 hours as needed.

For the ibuprofen product (Vicoprofen®), the recommended dose is 1 or 2 tablets every 4-6 hours as needed. The manufacturer recommends that the maximum dose of Vicoprofen® should not exceed 5 tablets in 24 hours.

The usual adult prescribing limits for the combination hydrocodone-acetaminophen products is up to 40 mg of hydrocodone and up to 4000 mg (4 g) of acetaminophen in a 24-hour period.

SEVERE PAIN

HYDROmorphone on page 871
Meperidine on page 1073
OxyCODONE on page 1269
Oxycodone and Acetaminophen on page 1272
Oxycodone and Aspirin on page 1275
Oxycodone and Ibuprofen on page 1277

Oxycodone is available in a variety of dosages and combinations under numerous brand names.

SAMPLE PRESCRIPTIONS

Rx:
Ibuprofen 800 mg tablets
Disp: 16 tablets
Sig: Take 1 tablet 3 times/day as needed for pain

Note: For severe pain, can be given up to 4 times/day. Also available as 600 mg tablets

Rx:
Norco® 10 mg
Disp: 16 tablets
Sig: Take 1 or 2 tablets every 4 hours as needed for pain; not to exceed 8 tablets in 24 hours

Note: Restrictions: C-III; no refills
Ingredients: Hydrocodone 10 mg and acetaminophen 325 mg; available as generic equivalent

For additional sample prescriptions see Oral Pain on page 1980

REFERENCE

Kleinert R, Lange C, Steup A, et al, "Single Dose Analgesic Efficacy of Tapentadol in Postsurgical Dental Pain: The Results of a Randomized, Double-Blind, Placebo-Controlled Study," *Anesth Analg*, 2008, 107 (6):2048-55.

BACTERIAL INFECTIONS

Dental infection can occur for any number of reasons, primarily involving pulpal and periodontal infections. Secondary infections of the soft tissues as well as sinus infections pose special treatment challenges. The drugs of choice in treating most oral infections have been selected because of their efficacy in providing adequate blood levels for delivery to the oral tissues and their proven usefulness in managing dental infections. Penicillin remains the primary drug for treatment of dental infections of pulpal origin. The management of soft tissue infections may require the use of additional drugs.

OROFACIAL INFECTIONS

The basis of all infections is the successful multiplication of a microbial pathogen on or within a host. The pathogen is usually defined as any microorganism that has the capacity to cause disease. If the pathogen is bacterial in nature, antibiotic therapy is often indicated.

DIFFERENTIAL DIAGNOSIS OF ODONTOGENIC INFECTIONS

In choosing the appropriate antibiotic for therapy of a given infection, a number of important factors must be considered. First, the identity of the organism must be known. In odontogenic infections involving dental or periodontal structures, this is seldom the case. Secondly, accurate information regarding antibiotic susceptibility is required. Again, unless the organism has been identified, this is not possible. And thirdly, host factors must be taken into account, in terms of ability to absorb an antibiotic, to achieve appropriate host response. When clinical evidence of cellulitis or odontogenic infection has been found and the cardinal signs of swelling, inflammation, pain, and perhaps fever are present, the selection by the clinician of the appropriate antibiotic agent may lead to eradication.

CAUSES OF ODONTOGENIC INFECTIONS

Most acute orofacial infections are of odontogenic origin. Dental caries, resulting in infection of dental pulp, is the leading cause of odontogenic infection.

The major causative organisms involved in dental caries have been identified as members of the viridans (alpha-hemolytic) streptococci and include *Streptococcus mutans, Streptococcus sobrinus,* and *Streptococcus milleri*. Once the bacteria have breached the enamel they invade the dentin and eventually the dental pulp. An inflammatory reaction occurs in the pulp tissue resulting in necrosis and a lower tissue oxidation-reduction potential. At this point, the bacterial flora changes from predominantly aerobic to a more obligate anaerobic flora. The anaerobic gram-positive cocci *(Peptostreptococcus* species), and the anaerobic gram-negative rods, including *Bacteroides, Prevotella, Porphyromonas,* and *Fusobacterium* are most frequently present. An abscess usually forms at the apex of the involved tooth resulting in destruction of bone. Depending on the effectiveness of the host resistance and the virulence of the bacteria, the infection may spread through the marrow spaces, perforate the cortical plate, and enter the surrounding soft tissues.

The other major source of odontogenic infection arises from the anaerobic bacterial flora that inhabits the periodontal and supporting structures of the teeth. The most important potential pathogenic anaerobes within these structures are *Actinobacillus actinomycetemcomitans, Prevotella intermedius, Porphyromonas gingivalis, Fusobacterium nucleatum,* and *Eikenella corrodens*.

Most odontogenic infections (70%) have mixed aerobic and anaerobic flora. Pure aerobic infections are much less common and comprise ~5% incidence. Pure anaerobic infections make up the remaining 25% of odontogenic infections. Clinical correlates suggest that early odontogenic infections are characterized by rapid spreading and cellulitis with the absence of abscess formation. The bacteria are predominantly aerobic with gram-positive, alpha-hemolytic streptococci *(S. viridans)* the predominant pathogen. As the infection matures and becomes more severe, the microbial flora becomes a mix of aerobes and anaerobes. The anaerobes present are determined by the characteristic flora associated with the site of origin, whether it is pulpal or periodontal. Finally, as the infectious process becomes controlled by host defenses, the flora becomes primarily anaerobic. For example, Lewis and MacFarlane found a predominance of facultative oral streptococci in the early infections (<3 days of symptoms) with the later predominance of obligate anaerobes.

In a review of severe odontogenic infections, it was reported that Brook, et al, observed that 50% of odontogenic deep facial space infections yielded anaerobic bacteria only.

Also, 44% of these infections yielded a mix of aerobic and anaerobic flora. The results of a study published in 1998 by Sakamoto, et al, were also described in the review. The study confirmed that odontogenic infections usually result from a synergistic interaction among several bacterial species and usually consist of an oral streptococcus and an oral anaerobic gram-negative rod. Sakamoto and his group reported a high level of the *Streptococcus milleri* group of aerobic gram-positive cocci, and high levels of oral anaerobes, including the *Peptostreptococcus* species and the *Prevotella, Porphyromonas,* and *Fusobacterium* species.

Oral streptococci, especially of the *Streptococcus milleri* group, can invade soft tissues initially, thus preparing an environment conducive to growth of anaerobic bacteria. Obligate oral anaerobes are dependent on nutrients synthesized by the aerobes. Thus the anaerobes appear approximately 3 days after onset of symptoms. Early infections are thus caused primarily by the aerobic streptococci (exquisitely sensitive to penicillin) and late infections are caused by the anaerobes (frequently resistant to penicillin).

It appears logical, as Flynn has noted, to separate infections presenting early in their course from those presenting later when selecting empiric antibiotics of choice for odontogenic infections.

If the patient is not allergic to penicillin, penicillin VK still remains the empiric antibiotic of first choice to treat mild or early odontogenic infections (see Table 1). In patients allergic to penicillin, clindamycin clearly remains the alternative antibiotic for treatment of mild or early infections. Secondary alternative antibiotics still recognized as useful in these conditions are cephalexin (Keflex®), or other first generation cephalosporins available in oral dose forms. The first generation cephalosporins can be used in both penicillin-allergic and nonallergic patients, providing that the penicillin allergy is not the anaphylactoid type.

PENICILLIN VK

The spectrum of antibacterial action of penicillin VK is consistent with most of the organisms identified in odontogenic infections (see Table 2). Penicillin VK is a beta-lactam antibiotic, as are all the penicillins and cephalosporins, and is bactericidal against gram-positive cocci and the major pathogens of mixed anaerobic infections. It elicits virtually no adverse effects in the absence of allergy and is relatively low in cost. Adverse drug reactions occurring in >10% of patients include mild diarrhea, nausea, and oral candidiasis. To treat odontogenic infections and other orofacial infections, the usual dose for adults and children >12 years of age is 500 mg every 6 hours for at least 7 days (see Table 4). The daily dose for children ≤12 years of age is 25-50 mg/kg of body weight in divided doses every 6-8 hours (see Table 4). The patient must be instructed to take the penicillin continuously for the duration of therapy.

After oral dosing, penicillin VK achieves peak serum levels within 1 hour. Penicillin VK may be given with meals; however, blood concentrations may be slightly higher when penicillin is given on an empty stomach. The preferred dosing is 1 hour before meals or 2 hours after meals to ensure maximum serum levels. Penicillin VK diffuses into most body tissues, including oral tissues, soon after dosing. Hepatic metabolism accounts for <30% of the elimination of penicillins. Elimination is primarily renal. The non-metabolized penicillin is excreted largely unchanged in the urine by glomerular filtration and active tubular secretion. Penicillins cross the placenta and are distributed in breast milk. Penicillin VK, like all beta-lactam antibiotics, causes death of bacteria by inhibiting synthesis of the bacterial cell wall during cell division. This action is dependent on the ability of penicillins to reach and bind to penicillin-binding proteins (PBPs) located on the inner membrane of the bacterial cell wall. PBPs (which include transpeptidases, carboxypeptidases, and endopeptidases) are enzymes that are involved in the terminal stages of assembling and reshaping the bacterial cell wall during growth. Penicillins and beta-lactams bind to and inactivate PBPs resulting in lysis of the cell due to weakening of the cell wall.

Penicillin VK is considered a "narrow spectrum" antibiotic. This class of antibiotics produces less alteration of normal microflora thereby reducing the incidence of super-infection. Also, its bactericidal action will reduce the numbers of microorganisms resulting in less reliance on host-phagocyte mechanisms for eradication of the pathogen.

Among patients, 0.7% to 10% are allergic to penicillins. There is no evidence that any single penicillin derivative differs from others in terms of incidence or severity when administered orally. About 85% of allergic reactions associated with penicillin VK are delayed and take >2 days to develop. This allergic response manifests as skin rashes characterized as erythema and bullous eruptions. This type of allergic reaction is mild, reversible, and usually responds to concurrent antihistamine therapy, such as diphenhydramine (Benadryl®). Severe reactions of angioedema have occurred, characterized by marked swelling of the lips, tongue, face, and periorbital tissues. Patients with a history of penicillin allergy must never be given penicillin VK for treatment of infections.

The alternative antibiotic is clindamycin. If the allergy is the delayed type and not the anaphylactoid type, a first generation cephalosporin may be used as an alternate antibiotic.

CLINDAMYCIN

In the event of penicillin allergy, clindamycin is clearly an alternative of choice in treating mild or early odontogenic infections (see Table 1). It is highly effective against almost all oral pathogens. Clindamycin is active against most aerobic gram-positive cocci, including staphylococci, *S. pneumoniae*, other streptococci, and anaerobic gram-negative and gram-positive organisms, including bacteroides (see Table 3). Clindamycin is not effective against mycoplasma or gram-negative aerobes. It inhibits protein synthesis in bacteria through binding to the 50 S subunit of bacterial ribosomes. Clindamycin has bacteriostatic actions at low concentrations, but is known to elicit bactericidal effects against susceptible bacteria at higher concentrations of drug at the site of infection.

The usual adult oral dose of clindamycin to treat orofacial infections of odontogenic origin is 150-450 mg every 6 hours for 7-10 days. The usual daily oral dose for children is 8-25 mg/kg in 3-4 equally divided doses (see Table 4).

Following oral administration of a 150 mg or a 300 mg dose on an empty stomach, 90% of the dose is rapidly absorbed into the bloodstream and peak serum concentrations are attained in 45-60 minutes. Administration with food does not markedly impair absorption into the bloodstream. Clindamycin serum levels exceed the minimum inhibitory concentration for bacterial growth for at least 6 hours after the recommended doses. The serum half-life is 2-3 hours. Clindamycin is distributed effectively to most body tissues, including saliva and bone. Its small molecular weight enables it to more readily enter bacterial cytoplasm and to penetrate bone. It is partially metabolized in the liver to active and inactive metabolites and is excreted in the urine, bile, and feces.

Adverse effects caused by clindamycin can include abdominal pain, nausea, vomiting, and diarrhea. Hypersensitivity reactions are rare, but have resulted in skin rash. Approximately 1% of clindamycin users develop pseudomembranous colitis characterized by severe diarrhea, abdominal cramps, and excretion of blood or mucus in the stools. The mechanism is disruption of normal bacterial flora of the colon, which leads to colonization of the bacterium *Clostridium difficile*. This bacterium releases endotoxins that cause mucosal damage and inflammation. Symptoms usually develop 2-9 days after initiation of therapy, but may not occur until several weeks after taking the drug. If significant diarrhea develops, clindamycin therapy should be discontinued immediately. Theoretically, any antibiotic can cause antibiotic-associated colitis and clindamycin probably has an undeserved reputation associated with this condition.

Sandor, et al, also notes that odontogenic infections are typically polymicrobial and that anaerobes outnumber aerobes by at least four-fold. The penicillins have historically been used as the first-line therapy in these cases, but increasing rates of resistance have lowered their usefulness. Bacterial resistance to penicillins is predominantly achieved through production of beta-lactamases. Clindamycin, because of its relatively broad spectrum of activity and resistance to beta-lactamase degradation, is an attractive first-line therapy in treatment of odontogenic infections. Recently, researchers have established a causal link between exposure to antibiotics and antibiotic resistance and they also have established evidence that the development of resistance to one class of antibiotic may confer persistent increased resistance to other antibiotic classes.

FIRST GENERATION CEPHALOSPORINS

Antibiotics of this class, which are available in oral dosage forms, include cefadroxil (Duricef®) and cephalexin (Keflex®). The first generation cephalosporins are alternates to penicillin VK in the treatment of odontogenic infections based on bactericidal effectiveness against the oral streptococci. These drugs are most active against gram-positive cocci, but are not very active against many anaerobes. First generation cephalosporins are indicated as alternatives in early infections because they are effective in killing the aerobes. First generation cephalosporins are active against gram-positive staphylococci and streptococci, but not enterococci. They are active against many gram-negative aerobic bacilli, including *E. coli, Klebsiella,* and *Proteus mirabilis*. They are inactive against methicillin-resistant *S. aureus* and penicillin-resistant *S. pneumoniae*. The gram-negative aerobic cocci, *Moraxella catarrhalis*, portrays variable sensitivity to first generation cephalosporins.

Cephalexin (Keflex®) is the first generation cephalosporin often used to treat odontogenic infections. The usual adult dose is 250-1000 mg every 6 hours with a maximum of 4 g/day. Children's dose is 25-50 mg/kg/day in divided doses every 6 hours; for severe infections: 50-100 mg/kg/day in divided doses every 6 hours with a maximum dose of 3 g/day (see Table 4).

Cephalexin (Keflex®) causes diarrhea in about 1% to 10% of patients. About 90% of the cephalexin is excreted unchanged in urine.

SECOND GENERATION CEPHALOSPORINS

The second generation cephalosporins such as cefaclor (Ceclor®) have better activity against some of the anaerobes including some *Bacteroides, Peptococcus,* and *Peptostreptococcus* species. Cefaclor (Ceclor®) and cefuroxime (Ceftin®) have been used to treat early stage infections. These antibiotics have the advantage of twice-a-day dosing. The usual oral adult dose of cefaclor is 250-500 mg every 8 hours (or daily dose can be given in 2 divided doses) for at least 7 days. Children's dose is 20-40 mg/kg/day divided every 8-12 hours with a maximum dose of 2 g/day. The usual adult oral dose of cefuroxime is 250-500 mg twice daily. Children's dose is 20 mg/kg/day (maximum: 500 mg/day) in 2 divided doses.

The cephalosporins inhibit bacterial cell wall synthesis by binding to one or more of the penicillin-binding proteins (PBPs), which in turn inhibit the final transpeptidation step of peptidoglycan synthesis in bacterial cell walls, thus inhibiting cell wall biosynthesis. Bacteria eventually lyse due to ongoing activity of cell wall autolytic enzymes while cell wall assembly is arrested.

BACTERIAL RESISTANCE TO ANTIBIOTICS

If a patient with an early stage odontogenic infection does not respond to penicillin VK within 24-36 hours, it is evidence of the presence of resistant bacteria. Bacterial resistance to the penicillins is predominantly achieved through the production of beta-lactamase. A switch to beta-lactamase-stable antibiotics should be made. For example, Kuriyama, et al, reported that past beta-lactam administration increases the emergence of beta-lactamase-producing bacteria and that beta-lactamase-stable antibiotics should be prescribed to patients with unresolved infections who have received beta-lactams. These include either clindamycin or amoxicillin/clavulanic acid (Augmentin®). Doses are listed in Table 4.

In the past, all *S. viridans* species were uniformly susceptible to beta-lactam antibiotics. However, over the years, there has been a significant increase in resistant strains. Resistance may also be due to alteration of penicillin-binding proteins. Consequently, drugs which combine a beta-lactam antibiotic with a beta-lactamase inhibitor, such as amoxicillin/clavulanic acid (Augmentin®), may no longer be more effective than the penicillin VK alone. In these situations, clindamycin is the recommended alternate antibiotic.

Evidence suggests that empirical use of penicillin VK as the first-line drug in treating early odontogenic infections is still the best way to ensure the minimal production of resistant bacteria to other classes of antibiotics, since any overuse of clindamycin or amoxicillin/clavulanic acid (Augmentin®) is minimized in these situations. There is concern that overuse of clindamycin could contribute to development of clindamycin-resistant pathogens.

In late odontogenic infections, it is suggested that clindamycin be considered the first-line antibiotic to treat these infections. The dose of clindamycin would be the same as that used to treat early infections (see Table 4). In these infections, anaerobic bacteria usually predominate. Since penicillin spectrum includes anaerobes, penicillin VK is also useful as an empiric drug of first choice in these infections. It has been reported, however, that the penicillin resistance rate among patients with serious and late infections is in the 35% to 50% range. Therefore, if penicillin is the drug of first choice and the patient does not respond within 24-36 hours, a resistant pathogen should be suspected and a switch to clindamycin be made. Clindamycin, because of its relatively broad spectrum of activity and resistance to beta-lactamase degradation, is an attractive first-line therapy in the treatment of these infections. Another alternative is to add a second drug to the penicillin (eg, metronidazole [Flagyl®]). Consequently, for those infections not responding to treatment with penicillin, the addition of a second drug (eg, metronidazole), not a beta-lactam or macrolide, is likely to be more effective. Bacterial resistance to metronidazole is very rare. The metronidazole dose is listed in Table 4.

Nonionized metronidazole is readily taken up by anaerobic organisms. Its selectivity for anaerobic bacteria is a result of the ability of these organisms to reduce metronidazole to its active form within the bacterial cell. The electron transport proteins necessary for this reaction are found only in anaerobic bacteria. Reduced metronidazole then disrupts DNA's helical structure, thereby inhibiting bacterial nucleic acid synthesis leading to death of the organism. Consequently, metronidazole is not effective against gram-positive aerobic cocci and most *Actinomyces, Lactobacillus,* and *Proprionibacterium* species. Since most odontogenic infections are mixed aerobic and anaerobic, metronidazole should rarely be used as a single agent but it can be useful when combined with penicillins. Alternatively, one can switch to a beta-lactamase resistant drug (eg, amoxicillin/clavulanic acid [Augmentin®]). The beta-lactamase resistant penicillins including methicillin, oxacillin, cloxacillin, dicloxacillin, and nafcillin, are only effective against gram-positive cocci and have no activity against anaerobes, hence, should not be used to treat the late stage odontogenic infections.

RESISTANCE IN ODONTOGENIC INFECTIONS

Recently, there has been an alarming increase in the incidence of resistant bacterial isolates in odontogenic infections. Many anaerobic bacteria have developed resistance to beta-lactam antibiotics via production of beta-lactamase enzymes. These include several species of *Prevotella, Porphyromonas, Fusobacterium nucleatum,* and *Campylobacter gracilus. Fusobacterium*, especially in combination with *S. viridans* species, has been associated with severe odontogenic infections. Often, they are resistant to macrolides. Clindamycin is the empiric drug of first choice in these patients.

SEVERE INFECTIONS

In patients hospitalized for severe odontogenic infections, I.V. antibiotics are indicated and clindamycin is the clear empiric antibiotic of choice. Alternative antibiotics include an I.V. combination of penicillin and metronidazole or I.V. ampicillin-sulbactam (Unasyn®). Clindamycin, I.V. cephalosporins (if penicillin allergy is not the anaphylactoid type), and ciprofloxacin have been used in patients allergic to penicillins. Flynn notes that *Eikenella corrodens*, an occasional oral pathogen, is resistant to clindamycin. Ciprofloxacin is an excellent antibiotic for this organism.

ERYTHROMYCIN, CLARITHROMYCIN, AND AZITHROMYCIN

In the past, erythromycins were considered highly effective antibiotics for treating odontogenic infections, especially in penicillin allergy. At the present time, however, the current high resistance rates of both oral streptococci and oral anaerobes have rendered the entire macrolide family of antibiotics obsolete for odontogenic infections. Montgomery has noted that resistance develops rapidly to macrolides and there may be cross-resistance between erythromycin and newer macrolides, particularly among streptococci and staphylococci. Hardee has stated that erythromycin is no longer very useful because of resistant pathogens. The antibacterial spectrum of the erythromycin family is similar to penicillin VK. Erythromycins are effective against streptococcus, staphylococcus, and gram-negative aerobes, such as *H. influenzae, M. catarrhalis, N. gonorrhoeae, Bordetella pertussis,* and *Legionella pneumophilia*. Erythromycins are considered narrow spectrum antibiotics.

Both azithromycin and clarithromycin have been used to treat acute odontogenic infections. This is because of the following spectrum of actions: Clarithromycin shows good activity against many gram-positive and gram-negative aerobic and anaerobic organisms. It is active against methicillin-sensitive *S. aureus* and most streptococcus species. *S. aureus* strains resistant to erythromycin are resistant to clarithromycin. Clarithromycin is active against *H. influenzae*. It is similar to erythromycin in effectiveness against anaerobic gram-positive cocci and *Bacteroides sp*. Clarithromycin has been suggested as an alternative antibiotic if the prescriber wants to give an antibiotic from the macrolide family (see Table 3). The recommended oral adult dose is 500 mg twice daily for 7 days.

Azithromycin is active against staphylococci, including *S. aureus* and *S. epidermitis*, as well as streptococci, such as *S. pyogenes* and *S. pneumoniae*. Erythromycin-resistant strains of staphylococcus, enterococcus, and streptococcus, including methicillin-resistant *S. aureus*, are also resistant to azithromycin. It has excellent activity against *H. influenzae*. Inhibition of anaerobes, such as *Clostridium perfringens*, is better with azithromycin than with erythromycin. Inhibition of *Bacteroides fragilis* and other bacteroides species by azithromycin is comparable to erythromycin. Both azithromycin and clarithromycin are presently recommended as alternatives in the prophylactic regimen for prevention of bacterial endocarditis.

AMOXICILLIN

Some clinicians select amoxicillin over penicillin VK as the penicillin of choice to empirically treat odontogenic infections. Except for coverage of *Haemophilus influenzae* in acute sinus and otitis media infections, amoxicillin does not offer any advantage over penicillin VK for treatment of odontogenic infections. It is less effective than penicillin VK for aerobic gram-positive cocci, and similar to penicillin for coverage of anaerobes. Although it does provide coverage against gram-negative enteric bacteria, this is not needed to treat odontogenic infections, except in immunosuppressed patients where these organisms may be present. If one adheres to the principle of using the most effective narrow spectrum antibiotic, amoxicillin should not be favored over penicillin VK.

Note: The ADA Council on Scientific Affairs has published a review on the subject of antibiotic interaction with oral contraceptives in which a clear statement of the dental professional's responsibility was made. In essence, it was concluded that in any situation where a dentist is planning to prescribe a course of antibiotics, alternative/additional means of contraception should be recommended to the oral contraceptive users. Specifically, patients should be told about the potential for antibiotics to lower the usefulness of oral contraceptives and advised to consult their physician about non-hormonal contraceptive techniques while continuing their oral contraceptive regimen. Even though there is minimal scientific data supporting this position, the risk of possible unwanted pregnancies warrants this simple approach for professionals licensed to prescribe antibiotics (*JADA*, 2002, 133:880).

The following tables have been adapted from Wynn RL, Bergman SA, Meiller TF, et al. "Antibiotics in Treating Orofacial Infections of Odontogenic Origin," *Gen Dent*, 2001, 47 (3):238-52.

Amoxicillin and Clavulanate Potassium on page 127
Amoxicillin on page 124
Cephalexin on page 347
Cefditoren on page 328
Ceftibuten on page 338
Chlorpheniramine on page 365
Chlorhexidine Gluconate on page 360
Clarithromycin on page 396
Clindamycin (Systemic) on page 402
Dicloxacillin on page 519
Erythromycin (Systemic) on page 620
Gatifloxacin on page 806
Gemifloxacin on page 811
Loratadine and Pseudoephedrine on page 1034
MetroNIDAZOLE (Systemic) on page 1126
Mouthwash, Antiseptic on page 1164
Moxifloxacin (Systemic) on page 1165
Oxymetazoline (Nasal) on page 1281
Penicillin V Potassium on page 1316
Pseudoephedrine on page 1429
Tetracycline on page 1611

Table 1. EMPIRIC ANTIBIOTICS OF CHOICE FOR ODONTOGENIC INFECTIONS

Type of Infection	Antibiotic of Choice
Early (first 3 days of symptoms)	Penicillin VK, amoxicillin Clindamycin Cephalexin (or other first generation cephalosporin)[1]
No improvement in 24-36 hours	Beta-lactamase-stable antibiotic: Clindamycin or amoxicillin / clavulanic acid
Penicillin allergy	Clindamycin Cephalexin (if penicillin allergy is not anaphylactoid type) Clarithromycin (Biaxin®)[2]
Late (>3 days)	Clindamycin Penicillin VK-metroNIDZOLE, amoxicillin-metroNIDAZOLE
Penicillin allergy	Clindamycin

[1]For better patient compliance, second generation cephalosporins (cefaclor; cefuroxime) at twice daily dosing have been used; see text.

[2]A macrolide useful in patients allergic to penicillin, given as twice daily dosing for better patient compliance; see text.

Table 2. PENICILLIN VK: ANTIBACTERIAL SPECTRUM

Gram-Positive Cocci	**Oral Anaerobes**
Streptococci	*Bacteroides*
Nonresistant staphylococci[1]	*Porphyromonas*
Pneumococci	*Prevotella*
	Peptococci
Gram-Negative Cocci	Peptostreptococci
Neisseria meningitides	*Actinomyces*
Neisseria gonorrhoeae	*Veillonella*
	Eubacterium
Gram-Positive Rods	*Eikenella*
Bacillus	*Capnocytophaga*
Corynebacterium	*Campylobacter*
Clostridium	*Fusobacterium*
	Others

[1]Nonresistant staphylococcus represents a small portion of community-acquired strains of *S. aureus* (5% to 15%). Most strains of *S. aureus* and *S. epidermitis* produce beta-lactamases, which destroy penicillins.

Table 3. CLINDAMYCIN: ANTIBACTERIAL SPECTRUM[1]

Gram-Positive Cocci	Anaerobes[2]
Streptococci[3]	**Gram-Negative Bacilli**
S. aureus[4]	*Bacteroides* species including *B. fragilis*
Penicillinase and nonpenicillinase-producing staphylococcus	*B. melaninogenicus* *Fusobacterium species*
S. epidermitis	**Gram-Positive Nonsporeforming Bacilli**
Pneumococci	*Propionibacterium*
	Eubacterium
	Actinomyces species
	Gram-Positive Cocci
	Peptococcus
	Peptostreptococcus
	Microaerophilic streptococci

[1]*In vitro* activity against isolates; information from manufacturer's package insert

[2]*Clostridia* are more resistant than most anaerobes to clindamycin. Most *Clostridium perfringens* are susceptible but *C. sporogens* and *C. tertium* are frequently resistant.

[3]Except *S. faecalis*

[4]Some staph strains originally resistant to erythromycin rapidly develop resistance to clindamycin.

Table 4. ORAL DOSE RANGES OF ANTIBIOTICS USEFUL IN TREATING ODONTOGENIC INFECTIONS[1]

Clinicians must select specific dose and regimen from ranges available to be prescribed based on clinical judgment		
Antibiotic	Dosage	
	Children	Adults
Penicillin VK	≤12 years: 25-50 mg/kg body weight in equally divided doses q6-8h for at least 7 days; maximum dose: 3 g/day	>12 years: 500 mg q6h for at least 7 days
Clindamycin	8-25 mg/kg in 3-4 equally divided doses	150-450 mg q6h for at least 7 days; maximum dose: 1.8 g/day
Cephalexin (Keflex®)	25-50 mg/kg/d in divided doses q6h severe infection: 50-100 mg/kg/d in divided doses q6h; maximum dose: 3 g/24 h	250-1000 mg q6h; maximum dose: 4 g/day
Amoxicillin	<40 kg: 20-40 mg (amoxicillin)/kg/d in divided doses q8h >40 kg: 250-500 mg q8h or 875 mg q12h for at least 7 days; maximum dose 2 g/day	>40 kg: 250-500 mg q8h or 875 mg q12h for at least 7 days; maximum dose: 2 g/day

Table 4. ORAL DOSE RANGES OF ANTIBIOTICS USEFUL IN TREATING ODONTOGENIC INFECTIONS[1] *(continued)*

Clinicians must select specific dose and regimen from ranges available to be prescribed based on clinical judgment		
Antibiotic	**Dosage**	
	Children	**Adults**
Amoxicillin/ clavulanic acid (Augmentin®)	<40 kg: 20-40 mg (amoxicillin)/kg/d in divided doses q8h >40 kg: 250-500 mg q8h or 875 mg q12h for at least 7 days; maximum dose 2 g/day	>40 kg: 250-500 mg q8h or 875 mg q12h for at least 7 days; maximum dose: 2 g/day
MetroNIDAZOLE (Flagyl®)		500 mg q6-8h for 7-10 days; maximum dose: 4 g/day

[1]For doses of other antibiotics, see monographs

SAMPLE PRESCRIPTIONS

Rx:

Penicillin V potassium 500 mg

Disp: 40 tablets

Sig: Take 1 tablet 4 times/day for 7-10 days (consider a loading dose of 1 g for acute infection)

Rx:

Clindamycin 300 mg

Disp: 40 capsules

Sig: Take 1 capsule 4 times/day for 7-10 days

Note: Prescription usually selected for patients allergic to penicillin; may be prescribed for 3 or 4 times/day. This prescription can be continued for treatment of some infections >1 month; however, risk of *Clostridium difficile* infection increases with long-term clindamycin use. Patient should be cautioned to take clindamycin with food and contact healthcare provider if diarrhea develops even after antibiotic course is completed. Probiotics may help but evidence is conflicted on true efficacy.

Rx:

Amoxicillin 500 mg

Disp: 30 capsules or tablets

Sig: Take 1 capsule or tablet 3 times/day for 7-10 days

For additional sample prescriptions see Bacterial Infections and Periodontal Diseases on page 1983

SINUS INFECTION TREATMENT

Sinus infections represent a common condition which may present with confounding dental complaints. Treatment is sometimes instituted by the dentist, but due to the often chronic and recurrent nature of sinus infections, early involvement of an otolaryngologist is advised. These infections may require antibiotics of varying spectrum as well as requiring the management of sinus congestion. Although amoxicillin is usually adequate, many otolaryngologists initially prescribe Augmentin®. Second-generation cephalosporins and clarithromycin are sometimes used depending on the chronicity of the problem.

For examples of sample prescriptions see Sinus Infection Treatment on page 1985

FREQUENTLY ASKED QUESTIONS

What is the best antibiotic modality for treating dental infections?

Penicillin is still the drug of choice for treatment of infections in and around the oral cavity. Phenoxymethyl penicillin (Pen VK) long has been the most commonly selected antibiotic. In penicillin-allergic individuals, clindamycin may be an appropriate consideration, prescribing 300 mg as a loading dose followed by 150 mg 4 times/day would be an appropriate regimen for a dental infection. In general, if there is no response to Pen VK, then Augmentin® may be a good alternative in the nonpenicillin-allergic patient because of its slightly altered spectrum. Recommendations would include that the patient should take the drug with food.

Is there cross-allergenicity between the cephalosporins and penicillin?

The incidence of cross-allergenicity is 5% to 8% in the overall population. If a patient has demonstrated a Type I hypersensitivity reaction to penicillin, namely urticaria or anaphylaxis, then this incidence would increase to 20%.

Is there definitely an interaction between contraception agents and antibiotics?

There are well founded interactions between contraceptives and antibiotics. The best instructions that a patient could be given by their dentist are that should an antibiotic be necessary and the dentist is aware that the patient is on contraceptives, and if the patient is using chemical contraceptives, the patient should seriously consider additional means of contraception during the antibiotic management.

Are antibiotics necessary in diabetic mellitus patients?

In the management of diabetes, control of the diabetic status is the key factor relative to all morbidity issues. If a patient is well controlled, then antibiotics will likely not be necessary. However, in patients where the control is questionable or where they have recently been given a different drug regimen for their diabetes or if they are being titrated to an appropriate level of either insulin or oral hypoglycemic agents during these periods of time, the dentist might consider preprocedural antibiotics to be efficacious.

Do nonsteroidal anti-inflammatory drugs interfere with blood pressure medication?

At the current time there is no clear evidence that NSAIDs interfere with any of the blood pressure medications that are currently in usage.

REFERENCES AND SELECTED READINGS

Flynn TR, "The Swollen Face. Severe Odontogenic Infections," *Emerg Med Clin North Am*, 2000, 18 (3):481-519.

Hardee WM, "Tried-and-True Medication," *Practical Endodontics*, 1997, 7(5):38.

Kuriyama T, Nakagawa K, Karasawa T, et al, "Past Administration of Beta-lactam Antibiotics and Increase in the Emergence of Beta-lactamase-producing Bacteria in Patients With Orofacial Odontogenic Infections," *Oral Surg Oral Med Oral Path Oral Radiol Endod*, 2000, 89(2):186-92.

Lewis MA, Parkhurst CL, Douglas CW, et al, "Prevalence of Penicillin Resistant Bacteria in Acute Suppurative Oral Infection," *J Antimicrob Chemother*, 1995, 35(6):785-91.

Montgomery EH, "Antimicrobial Agents in the Prevention and Treatment of Infection," *Pharmacology and Therapeutics for Dentistry*, 4th ed, Yagiela JA, Neidle EA, Dowd FJ, eds, St. Louis, MO: Mosby-Year Book, Inc, 1998, 637.

Petri WA, "Penicillins, Cephalosporins, and Other β-Lactam Antibiotics," *Goodman and Gilman's the Pharmacological Basis of Therapeutics*, 11th ed, Brunton LL, Lazo JS, and Parker KL, eds, New York, NY: McGraw Hill, 2006, 1127-54.

PERIODONTAL DISEASES

Periodontal diseases are common to mankind affecting, according to some epidemiologic studies, greater than 80% of the worldwide population. The conditions refer primarily to diseases that are caused by accumulations of dental plaque and the subsequent immune response of the host to the bacteria and toxins present in this plaque. Although most of the organisms that have been implicated in advanced periodontal diseases are anaerobic in nature, some aerobes contribute by either coaggregation with the anaerobic species or direct involvement with specific disease types.

Periodontal condition, as a group of diseases, affects the soft tissues supporting the teeth (ie, gingiva) leading to the term gingivitis or inflammation of gingival structures and those conditions that affect the bone and ligament supporting the teeth (ie, periodontitis) resulting from the infection and/or inflammation of these structures. Diseases of the periodontia can be further subdivided into various types including chronic periodontitis (localized and generalized, mainly in adults), aggressive periodontitis (localized and generalized, including previously classified), early onset periodontitis, prepubertal periodontitis, and rapidly progressing periodontitis. In addition, periodontitis as a manifestation of systemic diseases (hematologic, genetic disorders, not otherwise specified) as well as a necrotizing type due to specific conditions associated with predisposing immunodeficiency disease, such as those found in HIV-infected patients, create further subclassifications of the periodontal diseases, some of which are covered in those chapters associated with those conditions.

It is well accepted that control of most periodontal diseases requires, at the very minimum, appropriate mechanical cleansing of the dentition and the supporting structures by the patient. These efforts include brushing, some type of interdental cleaning, preferably with either floss or other aids, as well as appropriate sulcular cleaning usually with a brush.

Following appropriate dental treatment by the general dental practitioner and/or the periodontist, aids to these efforts by the patient might include the use of chemical agents to assist in the control of the periodontal diseases, or to prevent periodontal diseases. There are many available chemical agents on the market, only some of which are approved by the American Dental Association (ADA). Several have been tested utilizing guidelines published in 1986 by the ADA for assessment of agents that claim efficacy in the management of periodontal diseases. These chemical agents including chlorhexidine (Peridex®, PerioGard®), a quaternary compound, are bisbiguanides. Chlorhexidine, in various concentrations, has shown efficacy in reducing plaque and gingivitis in patients with short-term utilization. Some side effects include staining of the dentition which is reversible by dental prophylaxis. Chlorhexidine demonstrates the concept of substantivity, indicating that after its use, it has a continued effect in reducing the ability of plaque to form. It has been shown to be useful in a variety of periodontal conditions including acute necrotizing ulcerative gingivitis and healing studies. Some disturbances in taste and accumulation of calculus have been reported; however, chlorhexidine is the most applicable chemical agent of the bisbiguanides that has been studied to date.

Other chemical agents available as mouthwashes include the phenol compound Listerine Antiseptic®. These compounds are primarily restricted to prototype agents; the first to be approved by the ADA being Listerine Antiseptic®. Listerine Antiseptic® has been shown to be effective against plaque and gingivitis in long-term studies and comparable to chlorhexidine in these long-term investigations. However, chlorhexidine performs better than Listerine Antiseptic® in short-term investigations. Triclosan, the chemical agent found in the toothpaste Total®, has been recently approved by the FDA and is an aid in the prevention of gingivitis. Antiplaque activity of triclosan is enhanced with the addition of zinc citrate and there are no serious side effects to the use of triclosan. Sanguinarine is a principle herbal extract used for antiplaque activity. It is an alkaloid from the plant *Sanguinaria canadensis* and has some antimicrobial properties perhaps due to its enzyme activity although a relationship was found between epithelial mucosa premalignant changes and sanguinarine use in mouth rinse. Zinc citrate and zinc chloride have often been added to toothpastes as well as enzymes such as mucinase, mutanase, and dextrinase which have demonstrated varying results in studies. Some commercial anionic surfactants are available on the market which include aminoalcohols and the agent Plax® which essentially is comprised of sodium thiosulfate as a surfactant. Recent studies have shown Plax® to have some efficacy when it is added to triclosan.

Long-term use of prescription medications, including antibiotics, is seldom recommended and is not in any way a substitute for general dental/periodontal therapies. As adjunctive therapy, however, benefit has been shown and the new formulations of doxycycline (Periostat® and Atridox™), are recommended for long-term or repetitive treatments. It should be noted that the manufacturer's claims indicate that Periostat® functions as a collagenase inhibitor not as an antibiotic at recommended low doses for long-term therapy. Atridox™ functions as an antibiotic and is not recommended for constant long-term therapy, but rather in repetitive applications as necessary. Prescription medications used in efforts to treat periodontal diseases have historically included the use of antibiotics such as tetracycline although complications with use with young patients (ie, teeth intrinsic staining) have often precluded their prescription. Doxycycline is often preferred to tetracycline in low doses. This broad-spectrum bacteriostatic agent has shown efficacy against a wide variety of bacterial organisms found in periodontal disease. Minocycline slow-release (Arestin™) has recently been approved.

The drug metronidazole is a nitroimidazole, an agent that was originally used in treatment of protozoan infections and some anaerobic bacteria. It is bactericidal and has a good absorption and distribution throughout the body. The studies using metronidazole have suggested that it has a variety of uses in periodontal treatment and can be used as adjunct in both acute necrotizing ulcerative gingivitis and has specific efficacy against spirochetes, bacteria, and some *Porphyromonas* species. Metronidazole has also been useful alone or with clavulanic acid when combined with amoxicillin for management of acute periodontal infections and in cases of gingival hyperplasia. Recently, it has been used in combination with amoxicillin alone or with clavulanic acid in the management of osteomyelitis associated with bisphosphonate use.

Clindamycin is a derivative of vancomycin and has been useful in treatment of suppurative periodontal lesions. Long-term use is precluded by its complicating toxicities associated with colitis and gastrointestinal problems; however, recent studies have shown that a variety of antibiotics can result in colitis, thus, clindamycin should not be singled out as the sole or main culprit of this reported complication.

When severe gingival inflammation appears to be refractory to routine periodontal therapies the clinician should consider a biopsy since autoimmune conditions that comprise desquamative gingivitis diseases must be considered.

Research has also shown that various combination therapies of metronidazole and tetracycline for localized aggressive periodontitis and metronidazole with amoxicillin for rapidly progressive disease can be useful. The use of other prescription drugs including nonsteroidal anti-inflammatory, as well as other antibacterial agents, have been under study. Effects on prostaglandins of NSAIDs may indirectly slow periodontal disease progression. New research is currently underway in this regard. Perhaps, in combination therapy with some of the antibiotics, these drugs may assist in reducing the patient's immune response or inflammatory response to the presence of disease-causing bacteria.

Of greatest interest has been the improvement in technology for delivery of chemical agents to the periodontally-diseased site. These systems include biodegradable gelatins and biodegradable chips that can be placed under the gingiva and deliver antibacterial agents directly to the site as an adjunct to periodontal treatment. The initial therapy of mechanical debridement by the periodontal therapist is essential prior to using any chemical agent, and the dentist should be aware that the development of newer agents does not substitute for appropriate periodontal therapy and maintenance. The trade names of the gelatin chips and subgingival delivery systems include Periochip®, Atridox®, and Periostat®.

In addition to the periodontal therapy, consideration of the patient's pre-existing or developing medical conditions are important in the management of the periodontal patient. Several diseases illustrate these points most acutely. The reader is referred to the chapters on Diabetes, Cardiovascular Disease, Pregnancy, Respiratory Disease, HIV, and Cancer Chemotherapy. It has long been accepted that uncontrolled diabetes mellitus may predispose to periodontal lesions. Now, under current investigation is the hypothesis that pre-existing periodontal diseases may make it more difficult for a diabetic patient to come under control. In addition, the inflammatory response and immune challenge that is ongoing in periodontal disease appears to be implicated in the development of coronary artery disease as well as an increased risk of myocardial infarction and/or stroke. The accumulation of intra-arterial plaques appears enhanced by the presence of the inflammatory response often seen systemically in patients suffering with periodontal disease. In addition, the clinician is referred to the section on preprocedural antibiotics in the text for a consideration of antibiotic usage in patients that may be at risk for infective endocarditis. Other conditions including pregnancy and respiratory diseases such as COPD, HIV, and cancer therapy must be considered in the overall view of periodontal diseases. The reader is referred to the sections within the text.

NECROTIZING ULCERATING PERIODONTITIS (HIV Periodontal Disease)

Initial Treatment *(In-Office)*

Gentle debridement

Note: Ensure patient has no iodine allergies

Betadine® rinse on page 1382

At-Home Treatment

Listerine® antiseptic rinse (20 mL for 30 seconds twice daily)

Peridex® rinse on page 360

MetroNIDAZOLE (Systemic) (Flagyl®) 7-10 days on page 1126

Follow-Up Therapy

Proper dental cleaning, including scaling and root planing (repeat as needed)

Continue Peridex® and Listerine® rinse (indefinitely)

Amoxicillin on page 124
Chlorhexidine Gluconate on page 360
Ciprofloxacin (Systemic) on page 385
Clindamycin (Systemic) on page 402
Doxycycline Hyclate Periodontal Extended-Release Liquid on page 578
Listerine Antiseptic® on page 1164
MetroNIDAZOLE (Systemic) on page 1126
Minocycline Hydrochloride (Periodontal) on page 1144
NSAIDs see Oral Pain section on page 1928
Tetracycline on page 1611
Triclosan and Fluoride on page 1677

For examples of sample prescriptions see Bacterial Infections and Periodontal Diseases on page 1983

PHARMACOLOGIC MANAGEMENT OF PERIODONTAL DISEASES

Antibiotic	Adult Dosage
Azithromycin	500 mg once daily for 4-7 days
Ciprofloxacin (Systemic)	500 mg bid for 8 days
Clindamycin (Systemic)	300 mg tid for 8 days
Doxycycline or minocycline	100-200 mg once daily for 21 days
MetroNIDAZOLE (Systemic)	500 mg tid for 8 days
Metronidazole + amoxicillin	250 mg tid for 8 days of each drug
Metronidazole + ciprofloxacin (systemic)	500 mg bid for 8 days of each drug

Adapted from: Recommendations from the American Academy of Periodontology. Available at: www.perio.org.

FUNGAL INFECTIONS

Oral fungal infections can result from alteration in oral flora, immunosuppression, and underlying systemic diseases that may allow the overgrowth of these opportunistic organisms. These systemic conditions might include diabetes mellitus, long-term xerostomia, adrenal suppression, anemia, and chemotherapy-induced myelosuppression for the management of cancer. Long-term administration of antibiotics such as doripenem used to treat advanced systemic infections, has been implicated in elevating the risk of fungal infections. Also, the use of oral inhalers that include steroids, such as Advair™ Diskus®, have been implicated in the enhancing of the risk of fungal overgrowth. Clinical presentation might include pseudomembranous, erythematous, and hyperkeratotic forms. Fungus has also been implicated in denture stomatitis, angular cheilitis, and symptomatic geographic tongue (erythema migrans). Patients being treated for fungal skin infections or common oral conditions (eg, angular cheilitis) may also be using topical antifungal preparations coupled with a steroid such as triamcinolone.

Nystatin (Mycostatin®) is effective topically in the treatment of candidal infections of the skin and mucous membrane. The drug is extremely well tolerated and appears to be nonsensitizing although gastrointestinal upset and nausea are fairly common side effects. Clotrimazole troches are also useful as a topical therapy. Due to the significant sugar content in nystatin, patients with salivary gland hypofunction should be prescribed an alternative medication, such as clotrimazole, in order to lessen the caries risk. Clotrimazole is also available as an over-the-counter product in vaginal suppository formulations. In persons with denture stomatitis in which *Candida albicans* plays at least a contributory role, it is important to soak the prosthesis (laden with organisms) overnight in a nystatin liquid suspension besides treatment of the affected oral mucosa. Nystatin ointment can be placed in the denture during the daytime much like a denture adhesive. Antifungal medication should be continued for at least 14 days in order to prevent relapse and the patient must be re-evaluated. Predisposing systemic factors must be reconsidered if the oral fungal infection persists. Topical applications rely on contact of the drug with the organism within the lesions; therefore, 4-5 times daily with a dissolving troche or pastille is appropriate.

Oravig™ (miconazole) is now approved by the FDA. This unique bioadhesive tablet uses slow-dissolving delivery of miconazole to manage oropharyngeal fungal infections. Several other drugs of different classes can also be used in treating systemic and localized fungal infections including, amphotericin B, anidulafungin, caspofungin, ciclopirox olamine, clotrimazole, fluconazole, itraconazole, ketoconazole, micafungin, miconazole, naftifine hydrochloride, nystatin, oxiconazole, posaconazole, and voriconazole.

MANAGEMENT OF FUNGAL INFECTIONS REQUIRING SYSTEMIC MEDICATION

If the patient is refractory to topical treatment, consideration of a systemic route usually includes fluconazole (Diflucan®) or ketoconazole. Also, when the patient cannot tolerate topical therapy, these choices are effective, well-tolerated, systematic drugs for mucocutaneous candidiasis. Concern over liver function and possible drug interactions must be considered.

In patients that appear to be refractory to itraconazole or fluconazole related to the treatment of oropharyngeal candidiasis, posaconazole has been approved for usage. Anidulafungin (Eraxis™), caspofungin (Cancidas®), micafungin (Mycamine®), or voriconazole (VFEND®) are also indicated for treatment of serious fungal infections in patients intolerant of, or refractory to, other therapy.

Amphotericin B (Conventional) on page 131
Anidulafungin on page 145
Caspofungin on page 321
Clotrimazole (Oral) on page 425
Fluconazole on page 739
Ketoconazole (Systemic) on page 963
Ketoconazole (Topical) on page 964
Micafungin on page 1130
Nystatin (Oral) on page 1232
Nystatin (Topical) on page 1233
Nystatin and Triamcinolone on page 1233
Posaconazole on page 1373
Voriconazole on page 1728

Note: Consider Peridex® oral rinse or Listerine® antiseptic oral rinse for long-term control in immunosuppressed patients.

SAMPLE PRESCRIPTIONS FOR SYSTEMIC TREATMENT

Rx:

Diflucan® 100 mg tablets
Disp: 16 tablets
Sig: Take 2 tablets day 1, then 1 tablet/day until gone

Note: Sometimes a shorter course is adequate; however, oral infections commonly are more difficult to eradicate often a 21-day (3-week) course, or and even a second course, may be necessary.

Ingredient: Fluconazole

Rx:

Ketoconazole (Systemic) 200 mg
Disp: 14 tablets
Sig: Take 1 tablet daily, with a meal, for 2 weeks

Note: May cause irreversible liver damage; liver function should be monitored with long-term use (ie, >3 weeks)

Ingredient: Ketoconazole

SAMPLE PRESCRIPTIONS FOR TOPICAL TREATMENT

Rx:

Nystatin 100,000 units/mL oral suspension
Disp: 300 mL
Sig: Rinse with 1 teaspoon (5 mL) for 2 minutes 4-5 times/day and expectorate

Rx:

Mycelex® 10 mg troches
Disp: 70 troches
Sig: Dissolve 1 troche in mouth 5 times/day until gone; leave any prostheses out during treatment and soak prosthesis in nystatin liquid suspension overnight

Ingredient: Clotrimazole (Oral)

For additional sample prescriptions see Fungal Infections on page 1988

MANAGEMENT OF ANGULAR CHEILITIS

Angular cheilitis may represent the clinical manifestation of a multitude of etiologic factors. Cheilitis-like lesions may result from local habits, from a decrease in the intermaxillary space, or from nutritional deficiency. More commonly, angular cheilitis represents a mixed infection coupled with an inflammatory response involving *Candida albicans* and other organisms (most frequently *Staphylococcus aureus*). The drug of choice is now formulated to contain nystatin and triamcinolone and the effect is excellent. In addition, an off-label use of iodoquinol and hydrocortisone has also been reported to be effective in the treatment of angular cheilitis.

VIRAL INFECTIONS

Oropharyngeal viral infections are most commonly caused by herpes simplex viruses and Coxsackie viruses. Infections of the oropharynx and upper respiratory infections are commonly caused by the Coxsackie group A viruses. Oral cavity proper soft tissue viral infections, on the other hand, are most often caused by the herpes simplex viruses. Herpes zoster or varicella-zoster virus, which is one of the herpes family of viruses, can likewise cause similar viral eruptions involving the oral mucosa. Oral manifestations of mononucleosis caused by Epstein-Barr virus (another Herpes family virus) usually do not require direct therapy but resolve as the systemic condition improves.

The diagnosis of an acute viral infection begins by ruling out bacterial etiology and having an awareness of the presenting signs and symptoms associated with viral infection. Acute onset and vesicular eruption on the soft tissues generally favors a diagnosis of viral infection. Unfortunately, vesicles do not remain for a great length of time in the oral cavity; therefore, the short-lived vesicles rupture leaving ulcerated bases as the only indication of their presence. These ulcers are generally small in size and only when left unmanaged, coalesce to form larger, irregular ulcerations. Distinction must be made between the commonly recurring intraoral atraumatic ulcers (aphthous ulcerations) which do not have a viral etiology and the lesions associated with intraoral recurrent herpes since their effective treatment is distinctly different.

The management of an oral viral infection may be palliative for the most part; however, with the advent of improved antiviral prescription medications there now exists a family of drugs that can assist in managing primary and secondary infection. Human *Papillomavirus* is causative in a number of oral lesions, the most common of which are *Condyloma acuminatum* and Verruca vulgaris. Within the past few years certain subtypes of human Papillomavirus already proven to cause uterine cervical carcinoma are suspected of also being responsible for some posterior oral squamous cell carcinomas. Aldara® has been approved for treatment of genital warts (superficial basal cell carcinomas and actinic keratosis); oral mucosa use is still under study.

It should be noted that herpes can present as a primary infection (gingivostomatitis or pharyngo stomatitis), recurrent lip lesions (herpes labialis of the skin and adjacent vermilion border), and intraoral ulcers (recurrent intraoral herpes), involving the oral and perioral tissues. Primary infection is a systemic infection that leads to acute gingivostomatitis that may involve all moveable and nonmovable sites of the oral cavity (buccal mucosa, lips, tongue, floor of the mouth, palate, and the gingiva). Treatment of primary infections utilizes prescription antivirals such as acyclovir in combination with supportive care. Topical anesthetics, such as lidocaine 1% or dyclonine HCl 1%, used in combination with Benadryl® 0.5% in a saline vehicle was found to be an effective oral rinse in the symptomatic treatment of primary herpetic gingivostomatitis. Other agents for symptomatic and supportive treatment include commercially available elixir of Benadryl®, Xylocaine® viscous, Orajel® (OTC), and antibiotics to prevent secondary infections. Systemic supportive therapy should include forced fluids, high concentration protein, vitamin and mineral food supplements, and rest.

Antivirals

Abreva™ (OTC) on page 556
Acyclovir (Systemic) on page 55
Acyclovir (Topical) on page 58
Famciclovir on page 704
Imiquimod on page 901
L-Lysine on page 1030
Nelfinavir on page 1195
Penciclovir on page 1312
ValACYclovir on page 1692
Viroxyn® on page 217

Supportive Therapy

DiphenhydrAMINE (Systemic) on page 540
Lidocaine (Topical) on page 1010

Prevention of Secondary Bacterial Infection

Penicillin V Potassium on page 1316

SUPPORTIVE CARE FOR PAIN AND PREVENTION OF SECONDARY INFECTION

Primary infections often become secondarily infected with bacteria, requiring antibiotics. Dietary supplement may be necessary. Options are presented due to variability in patient compliance and response.

RECURRENT HERPETIC INFECTIONS

Following the primary herpetic infection, the herpesvirus remains latent until such time as it has the opportunity to recur. The etiology of this latent period and the degree of viral shedding present during latency is currently under study; however, it is thought that some trigger in the mucosa or the skin causes the virus to begin to replicate. This process may involve Langerhans cells which are immunocompetent antigen-presenting cells resident in all epidermal and epithelial surfaces. The virus replication then leads to physical movement of the virus along the sensory axon leading to eruptions in innervated tissues surrounding the mouth or within. The most common form of recurrence is the lip lesion or herpes labialis; however, intraoral recurrent herpes also occurs with some frequency (attached gingival and hard palate preferentially). Prevention of recurrences has been attempted with lysine (OTC) 500-1000 mg/day and acyclovir but response has been variable. Herpes zoster outbreaks can also involve the oral and facial tissues although this is less common. Valacyclovir or famciclovir are the drugs of choice. Of the two medications, famciclovir is reported to be more effective against postherpetic neuralgia. Valacyclovir HCl in 500 mg and 1 g tablets has recently been approved by the FDA for first time generic formulations.

Water-soluble bioflavonoid-ascorbic acid complex, now available as Peridin-C®, may be helpful in reducing the signs and symptoms associated with recurrent herpes simplex virus infections. As with all agents used, the therapy is more effective when instituted in the early prodromal stage of the disease process.

PREVENTATIVE SAMPLE PRESCRIPTIONS

Rx:
L-Lysine (OTC) 500 mg
Sig: Take 2 tablets/day as preventive; increase to 4 tablets/day if prodrome or recurrence begins

Rx:
Citrus bioflavonoids and ascorbic acid tablets 400 mg (Peridin-C®)
Disp: 10 tablets
Sig: Take 2 tablets at once, then 1 tablet 3 times/day for 3 days

Where a recurrence is usually precipitated by exposure to sunlight, the lesion may be prevented by the application to the area of a sunscreen, with a high skin protection factor (SPF) in the range of ≥25.

SUPPORTIVE CARE FOR PAIN AND MAINTENANCE OF NUTRITION DURING ORAL VIRAL INFECTIONS

Rx:
Benadryl® liquid 12.5 mg/5 mL
Disp: 4 oz bottle
Sig: Rinse with 1-2 teaspoonfuls every 2 hours and expectorate

Note: Benadryl® is available as a generic diphenhydramine liquid.

Rx:
Benadryl® liquid 12.5 mg/5 mL (mix 50/50) with Kaopectate®
Disp: 8 oz total
Sig: Rinse with 1-2 teaspoonfuls every 2 hours and expectorate.

Note: Maalox® can be used in place of Kaopectate® if constipation is a problem. Benadryl® is available as a generic diphenhydramine liquid.

Rx:
Xylocaine® viscous 2%
Disp: 450 mL bottle
Sig: Swish with 1 tablespoon 4 times/day and spit out
Ingredient: Lidocaine (Topical)

Rx:

Meritene®
Disp: 1 lb can (plain, chocolate, eggnog flavors)
Sig: Take 3 servings daily; prepare as indicated on can

Ingredient: Protein-vitamin-mineral food supplement

PRESCRIPTIVE TREATMENT

Acyclovir (Zovirax®) possesses antiviral activity against herpes simplex types 1 and 2. Historically, ophthalmic ointments were used topically to treat recurrent mucosal and skin lesions. These do not penetrate well on the skin lesions, thereby providing questionable relief of symptoms. If recommended, use should be closely monitored. Penciclovir, an active metabolite of famciclovir, has been specifically approved in a cream for treatment of recurrent herpes lesions. Valacyclovir and famciclovir have also been approved for treatment of herpes labialis (see monograph for dosing). The FDA has also approved acyclovir cream 5 % for treatment of herpes labialis in adults and adolescents. Recently, in addition to docosanol (Abreva®), another over-the-counter preparation for treatment of recurrent herpes labialis has been approved. Benzalkonium chloride and isopropyl alcohol (Viroxyn®) is an alcohol/benzalkonium chloride medication in a single dose applicator kit (3 pack) that is marketed to reduce the duration and symptoms of cold sores. Other over-the-counter preparations include 2% tetracaine gel and L-lysine 500 mg tablets.

SAMPLE PRESCRIPTIONS

Rx:

Zovirax® 200 mg capsules
Disp: 50 or 60 capsules
Sig: Take 1 capsule 5 times/day for 10 days or 2 capsules 3 times/day for 10 days

Ingredient: Acyclovir (Systemic)

Rx:

Valtrex® 500 mg caplets
Disp: 42 caplets
Sig: Take 2 caplets 3 times/day for 7 days without regard to meals

Ingredient: ValACYclovir

Rx:

Famvir® 500 mg tablets
Disp: 3 tablets
Sig: Take 1500 mg as a single dose

Ingredient: Famciclovir; available as generic equivalent

Rx:

Denavir® topical cream 1%
Disp: 1.5 g tube
Sig: Apply locally as directed to lesion every 2 hours during waking hours (begin when symptoms first occur)

Ingredient: Penciclovir

For additional sample prescriptions see Viral Infections on page 1990

ULCERATIVE, EROSIVE, AND PAINFUL ORAL MUCOSAL DISORDERS

RECURRENT APHTHOUS STOMATITIS - MINOR, MAJOR, AND HERPETIFORM TYPES

Recurrent aphthous stomatitis is an extremely common mucosal disease. Although it is not considered a classic autoimmune disorder, the conditions that have been termed minor, major, and herpetiform types have in common a cellular-mediated event with underlying T-cells activation. This cytotoxicity leads to a destruction of the mucosal surface and is mediated by inflammatory cytokines throughout the oral tissues. The term herpetiform ulcerations is a misnomer and implies a herpes-type appearance to the ulcers when they are present. This is as far as the connection goes since there has never been a viral or bacterial etiology cited for any of the aphthous forms of ulcerations. The different subsets of patients have different triggering factors (eg, stress, hormonal, fluctuations and minor chemical irritations) and thus no one product or technique is universally effective in all patients. For minor or major aphthous ulcers that severely affect daily living and quality of life, corticosteroids seem to be the mainstay drug. It is believed that the immunomodulating effect of a short-term regimen of corticosteroids in an immunocompetent sufferer is effective without creating the well-known side effects of long-term or high-dose corticosteroid therapy. Sufferers of the herpetiform type of aphthae, in which as many as a hundred small ulcers appear per outbreak, may also obtain relief from an oral suspension corticosteroid, although management may be more protracted.

Triamcinolone (Oralone®) paste is indicated for the temporary relief of minor symptoms associated with infrequent recurrences of minor aphthous lesions and ulcerative lesions resulting from trauma. Some clinicians prescribe a soothing rinse containing corticosteroid (eg, dexamethasone), an antifungal agent (eg, nystatin), a topical anesthetic (eg, viscous lidocaine), an antihistamine (eg, diphenhydramine), an antimicrobial/antibiotic (chlorhexidine), and/or coating agent such as attapulgite creating a so-called "magic elixir." The most popular combination contains 1.5 g tetracycline; 60 mg hydrocortisone; nystatin 6 million international units and an equal volume elixir of Benadryl® and has been called Mary's Magic potion. Numerous other mixtures have been formulated by clinicians but there are insufficient data to provide evidence for selection of any of these combinations over others. All of the combinations do, however, have reasonable anecdotal evidence of palliative effects. More severe forms of recurrent aphthous stomatitis may be treated with topical corticosteroids of higher strength (eg, fluocinonide, clobetasol) alone or mixed with Orabase®. An oral suspension of tetracycline may be prescribed for avoidance of secondary infection. Tetracycline use is contraindicated during pregnancy, infancy, and childhood to the age of 8 years due to intrinsic staining of teeth. *Lactobacillus acidophilus* preparations (Bacid®, Lactinex™) are occasionally effective for reducing the frequency and severity of the minor lesions. With professional oversight, a cauterizing agent, such as Debacterol® may markedly decrease the pain associated with the aphthous ulcer. Clinician and patient must be extremely careful in using cauterizing agents within the oral cavity. Patients with long-standing history of recurrent aphthous stomatitis should be evaluated for iron, folic acid, and vitamin B_{12} deficiencies as well as hematological assessments for anemia. One subset of recurrent aphthous stomatitis sufferers markedly improve when tooth dentifrices lacking sodium lauryl sulfate are used.

A noncorticosteroid prescription medication, 5% Aphthasol® paste, has been approved for recurrent aphthous stomatitis and published studies indicate it hastens the healing of these lesions by more than a day. In patients with medical contraindications for corticosteroid use and when Aphthasol® has not been effective, alternatives (eg, colchicine, dapsone, immune globulin [intravenous], methotrexate, misoprostol, mycophenolate mofetil, pentoxifylline, tacrolimus, and tretinoin) have had anecdotal reports of effectiveness. These alternative drugs should only be considered in consultation with the patient's physician. Regular use of Listerine® antiseptic has been shown in clinical trials to reduce the severity, duration, and frequency of aphthous stomatitis. An antimicrobial such as chlorhexidine oral rinses (20 mL for 30 seconds 2-3 times/day) has also demonstrated efficacy in reducing the duration of aphthae. With both of these products, however, patient intolerance of the burning from the alcohol content is of concern. The newer alcohol-free antimicrobial rinses have not been evaluated. Immunocompromised patients, such as those with AIDS, may have severe ulcer recurrences and thalidomide has been approved for these patients on an FDA orphan drug approved basis. See Periodontal Diseases on page 1942 for HIV related periodontal considerations.

Two other conditions should be mentioned here since their diagnosis and management requires consideration of all of the ulcerative, erosive, and painful oral mucosal disorders. Necrotizing ulcerative gingivitis (NUG) is a condition that has been recognized for many years. The name historically included the term "acute," however, most investigators have discontinued this because there is not a chronic form of the disease and it is unnecessary to consider it as anything other than necrotizing gingivitis. The organism *Fusobacterium nucleatum* has been implicated with several other organisms particularly Spirochetes in this condition. The infections seem to occur primarily following periods of psychological stress and this is the most common unifying factor in patients who suffer with NUG. In addition, immunosuppression, smoking, and local trauma have also been implicated. Generally, the classical appearance of NUG includes punched-out interdental papillae that are inflamed and appear blunted, somewhat necrotic at their tips. A pseudomembrane often is present and a strong fetor oris is usually present. The patient sometimes has fever and malaise as well. The treatment is generally conservative using gentle debridement. There is some benefit in using antibiotics such metronidazole, tetracycline, or amoxicillin. Historically, some clinicians have also chosen to add a vitamin supplement, generally a vitamin B complex with vitamin C, to help with the mucosal healing.

Another condition occasionally encountered is plasma cell gingivitis, a diffuse but intense erythema of the gingival complex, including a rapid onset and soreness to the oral gingival tissues. The implicated etiologies in plasma cell gingivitis include various chewing gums, toothpastes with herbal additives, as well as spicy candies, mints, peppers, and other potential allergens. The treatment of plasma cell gingivitis is local use of topical steroids; although by removing the dietary stimulant, generally the condition will resolve spontaneously. If plasma cell gingivitis is being considered as a diagnosis, the autoimmune desquamative gingival diseases must also be considered. A biopsy is usually necessary to determine a diagnosis.

MILD-TO-MODERATE FORMS OF ULCERATIONS AND EROSIONS

There are several over-the-counter preparations that may give the patient some or total relief, including Ulcerease®, BetaCell oral rinse®, Cankermelts-GX®, Gelclair® Bioadherent Oral Gel®, Orabase Sooth-N-Seal®, OraPatch®, Ricinol P.R.N.®, Zilactin® gel, Canker Cover®, and Orajel® Protective Mouth Sore Discs.

Aloclair (Ameseal™) is now available as a spray. It is marketed by OMNI Preventive Care as an oral lesion pain relief spray, useful for indications related to aphthous ulcerations and other mild-to-moderate oral erosions. Oralone® is a new formulation of triamcinolone acetonide dental paste which had previously been available as Kenalog in Orabase®.

SYMPTOMATIC GEOGRAPHIC TONGUE (BENIGN MIGRATORY GLOSSITIS, ERYTHEMA MIGRANS)

Geographic tongue is a localized, transitory loss of the tongue's filiform papillae. Although disconcerting in appearance, it usually is asymptomatic; however, occasionally patients will report a burning sensation. Fungal colonization has been implicated in symptomatic geographic tongue and this condition needs to be ruled out as a contributing factor (see Fungal Infections on page 1945).

After infection has been ruled out, palliation for symptomatic geographic tongue can sometimes be achieved with an approach similar to managing minor oral ulcerations. Benadryl® elixir, a potent antihistamine, is used in the oral cavity primarily as a mild topical anesthetic agent for the symptomatic relief of certain allergic deficiencies which should be ruled out as possible etiologies for the oral condition under treatment. It is often used alone as well as in 50:50 solutions with agents such as Kaopectate® or Maalox® to assist in coating the oral mucosa. Benadryl® can also be used systemically in capsule form although the elixir mixed with a coating agent as above provides excellent palliation prior to meals. Frequently, Benadryl® alone or in combination with the above agents will be very effective in the relief of symptomatic geographic tongue.

Amlexanox on page 112
Attapulgite on page 191
Chlorhexidine Gluconate on page 360
Clobetasol on page 408
Debacterol® on page 1563
Dexamethasone (Systemic) on page 492
DiphenhydrAMINE (Systemic) on page 540
Fluocinonide ointment with Orabase on page 751
Lactobacillus on page 976
MetroNIDAZOLE (Systemic) on page 1126
Mouthwash (Antiseptic) on page 1164

PredniSONE on page 1393
Sulfonated Phenolics in Aqueous Solution on page 1563
Tetracaine (Topical) on page 1610
Tetracycline on page 1611
Thalidomide on page 1615
Triamcinolone (Topical) on page 1672

EROSIVE LICHEN PLANUS AND OTHER VESICULOEROSIVE DISEASES

Lichen planus is a chronic dermatologic disease that often affects the oral tissues. The name was first selected in 1869 because of the flat appearance of the white lesions on the oral mucosa. Lichen planus ranges from being totally asymptomatic to severely painful when present in its erosive forms. Reticular forms of lichen planus with no erosions show a white lacy pattern that has become pathognomic for the condition. The lesions on the skin often have a purplish hue and form slightly raised papules, with an occasional white lacy or silvery appearance to the borders of the lesions. Patients do not need to have the skin lesions in order to suffer with oral lichen planus. The diagnosis of lichen planus is best performed by histopathology; however, often the pathognomic appearance and distribution of the lesions allows a presumptive diagnosis to be made from the clinical appearance. Generally the erosive forms of lichen planus require treatment based on the extent, severity, and pain level of the patient in question. Autoimmune desquamative gingival diseases, including pemphigoid and pemphigus, must also be considered. A biopsy is necessary to determine a diagnosis and systemic work-up for related disease effects must be completed in consultation with patient's physicians.

Elixir of dexamethasone, a potent anti-inflammatory agent, is used topically (as a 2-minute rinse and expectorate) in the management of acute episodes of erosive lichen planus and other vesiculo-erosive disease processes such as benign mucous membrane pemphigoid and pemphigus vulgaris. Some patients will not achieve relief from topical agents and systemic delivery either by swish and swallow or tablets may be necessary. Prednisone corticosteroid tablet is a popular and often effective starting point with a regimen consisting of burst therapy (eg, 6-80 mg) for several days followed by 7-10 days of a maintenance and tapering dose. Immunosuppressant agents such as tacrolimus (Protopic®) and pimecrolimus (Elidel®) have shown some efficacy in off-label applications for severe cases. Prolonged use should be carried out in consult with the patient's physician. Continued supervision of the patient during treatment is essential and the dentist must be aware that treatment of any secondary infections such as fungal overgrowth may be essential in gaining control of the erosive lesions. Also, patients should be counseled that maximum benefit of the medication will be achieved when oral hygiene is maintained at excellent levels.

For examples of sample prescriptions see Ulcerative and Erosive Disorders on page 1992

BURNING MOUTH SYNDROME

Burning mouth syndrome (BMS) is a relatively common condition, of unknown etiology, and is a significant problem when it occurs, both in diagnosis and in management. Individuals often experience a burning or a scalding pain on the lips, tongue, and sometimes other parts of the oral cavity. There are often no visible signs of irritation that the clinician can identify. The etiology of burning mouth syndrome remains unknown. The syndrome has been associated with everything ranging from vitamin deficiencies to the onset of menopause. It is estimated that nearly 5% of the population around the age of 60 may suffer with this condition. The symptoms often include burning mouth, dry mouth, a bitter or metallic taste, other taste alterations, changes in the patient's ability to eat, and onset of pain while attempting to sleep. Systemic conditions associated with BMS are abnormal hormonal fluctuations, diabetes, deficiencies in iron, zinc, and vitamins such as thiamine, B_{12}, niacin, complications associated with cancer therapy, and some patients report that the burning mouth syndrome symptoms occur after dental procedures.

The evaluation of a patient complaining of burning mouth begins with a detailed history/process of elimination and may lead to a biopsy to determine if any organic reason for the condition is identifiable. Dry mouth often accompanies burning mouth. The clinician should culture the tongue or oral mucosa to rule out oral fungal colonization. A normal hematologic work up will ensure that there is no developing diabetes, allergy, or abnormal liver or thyroid condition. The clinician should carefully examine all of the surfaces of the tissues to see if there are any abrasive components caused by rough teeth or prostheses. It is often necessary to have the patient evaluated by their primary care physician because of the common association of BMS with high stress situations, common in the process of aging. The condition has the features of a neuropathy and could be related to the production of toxic radicals that may be released at the cellular level during times of stress.

These widely divergent hypotheses related to the etiology of BMS have led to equally broad therapeutic suggestions. A variety of drugs have been suggested, including: Topical rinses and anesthetics for palliative management, clonazepam 0.25-3 mg/day, amitriptyline 25-100 mg/day, nortriptyline 10-50 mg/day, gabapentin 900-1500 mg/day, and doxepin cream, applied to the areas affected. Various studies indicate that alpha-lipoic acid in an initial dose of 600 mg may be used with a dose reduction to 200 mg after the initial 20 days. The rationale for attempting alpha-lipoic acid is the relationship between its antioxidant effects and the levels of glutathione and reduction of free radicals cellularly. In addition to alpha-lipoic acid, capsaicin has been used with some success. Capsaicin has been a prescription drug useful in arthritis care as a topical skin product. It has also been prescribed to assist with patients who have had shingles, post herpetic pain neuropathies associated with diabetes and other neuralgias. Its applications in oral use have been studied in very limited trials; however, it has recently been re-evaluated in a 0.75% topical application for use in BMS and oral mucositis. All of the medications suggested for managing burning mouth are off-label uses and there are limited data from placebo controlled clinical trials.

During a Cochrane analysis, nine clinical trials were reviewed. Of the nine trials, three interventions demonstrated reduction in BMS and all of these included varying effects of clonazepam and alpha-lipoic acid. Although the other trials considered randomized double-blind trials, study designs were small and lacked power to draw and define conclusions. There is little evidence to provide a clear standard of care for treating patients with burning mouth syndrome to date. The clinician must always be aware of this lack of conclusive evidence. These drugs should be selected and managed in collaboration with the patient's physician, particularly since many of these patients suffering with burning mouth syndrome have complicated medical histories including the use of additional medications that could be affected.

REFERENCES AND SELECTED READINGS

Basker RM, Sturdee DW, and Davenport JC, "Patients With Burning Mouths. A Clinical Investigation of Causative Factors, Including the Climacteric and Diabetes," *Br Dent J*, 1978, 145(1):9-16.

Beers MH and Berkow R, *The Merck Manual of Geriatrics*, 3rd ed, Whitehouse Station, NJ: Merck Research Laboratories, 2000.

Chakrabarty AK, Mraz S, Geisse JK, et al, "Aphthous Ulcers Associated With Imiquimod and the Treatment of Actinic Cheilitis," *J Am Acad Dermatol*, 2005, 52(2 Suppl 1):35-7.

Buchanan J and Zakrzewska J, "Burning Mouth Syndrome," *Clin Evid (online)*, March 14, 2008. Available at http://www.ncbi.nlm.nih.gov/pmc/articles/PMC2907957/pdf/2008-1301.pdf.

Donovan JC, Hayes RC, Burgess K, et al, "Refractory Erosive Oral Lichen Planus Associated With Hepatitis C: Response to Topical Tacrolimus Ointment," *J Cutan Med Surg*, 2005, 9(2):43-6.

Eisen D, "Hydroxychloroquine Sulfate (Plaquenil) Improves Oral Lichen Planus: An Open Trial," *J Am Acad Dermatol*, 1993, 28(4):609-12.

Epstein JB and Marcoe JH, "Topical Application of Capsaicin for Treatment of Oral Neuropathic Pain and Trigeminal Neuralgia," *Oral Surg Oral Med Oral Pathol*, 1994, 77(2):135-40.

Femiano F, "Burning Mouth Syndrome (BMS): An Open Trial of Comparative Efficacy of Alpha-Lipoic Acid (Thioctic Acid) With Other Therapies," *Minerva Stomatol*, 2002, 51(9):405-9.

Femiano F and Scully C, "Burning Mouth Syndrome (BMS): Double Blind Controlled Study of Alpha-Lipoic Acid (Thioctic Acid) Therapy," *J Oral Pathol Med*, 2002, 31(5):267-9.

Femiano F, Gombos F, Scully C, et al, "Burning Mouth Syndrome (BMS): Controlled Open Trial of the Efficacy of Alpha-Lipoic Acid (Thioctic Acid) On Symptomatology," *Oral Dis*, 2000, 6(5):274-7.

Femiano F, Gombos F, and Scully C, "Burning Mouth Syndrome: Open Trial of Psychotherapy Alone, Medication With Alpha-Lipoic Acid (Thioctic Acid), and Combination Therapy," *Med Oral*, 2004, 9(1):8-13.

Femiano F, Gombos F, and Scully C, "Burning Mouth Syndrome: The Efficacy of Lipoic Acid on Subgroups," *J Eur Acad Dermatol Venereol*, 2004, 18(6):676-8.

Femiano F, Scully C, and Gombos F, "Idiopathic Dysgeusia; An Open Trial of Alpha Lipoic Acid (ALA) Therapy," *Int J Oral Maxillofac Surg*, 2002, 31(6):625-8.

Gremeau-Richard C, Woda A, Navez ML, et al, "Topical Clonazepam in Stomatodynia: A Randomised Placebo-Controlled Study," *Pain*, 2004, 108(1-2):51-7.

Grushka M and Bartoshuk LM, "Burning Mouth Syndrome and Oral Dysesthesias," *Can J Diag*, 2000, 17:99-109.

Grushka M, Epstein JB, and Gorsky M, "Burning Mouth Syndrome," *Am Fam Physician*, 2002, 65(4):615-20.

Grushka M, Epstein J, and Mott A, "An Open-Label, Dose Escalation Pilot Study of the Effect of Clonazepam in Burning Mouth Syndrome," *Oral Surg Oral Med Oral Pathol Oral Radiol Endod*, 1998, 86(5):557-61.

Heckmann SM, Heckmann JG, Hilz MJ, et al, "Oral Mucosal Blood Flow in Patients With Burning Mouth Syndrome," *Pain*, 2001, 90(3):281-6.

Heckmann SM, Heckmann JG, Ungethüm A, et al, "Gabapentin has Little or no Effect in the Treatment of Burning Mouth Syndrome - Results of an Open-Label Pilot Study," *Eur J Neurol*, 2006, 13(7):e6-7.

Joint Formulary Committee, *British National Formulary*, 51st edition, London, England: Pharmaceutical Press, 2006.

Low PA and Dotson RM, "Symptomatic Treatment of Painful Neuropathy," *JAMA*, 280(21):1863-4.

Maina G, Vitalucci A, Gandolfo S, et al, "Comparative Efficacy of SSRIs and Amisulpride in Burning Mouth Syndrome: A Single-Blind Study," *J Clin Psychiatry*, 2002, 63(1):38-43.

Mínguez Serra MP, Salort Llorca C, Silvestre Donat FJ, "Pharmacological Treatment of Burning Mouth Syndrome: A Review and Update," *Med Oral Patol Oral Cir Bucal*, 2007, 12(4):E299-304.

Miyamoto SA and Ziccardi VB, "Burning Mouth Syndrome," *Mt Sinai J Med*, 1998, 65(5-6):343-7.

Olivier V, Lacour JP, Mousnier A, et al, "Treatment of Chronic Erosive Oral Lichen Planus With Low Concentrations of Topical Tacrolimus: An Open Prospective Study," *Arch Dermatol*, 2002, 138(10):1335-8.

Packer L and Colman C, *The Antioxidant Miracle: Your Complete Plan for Total Health and Healing*, 1st ed, New York, NY: John Wiley & Sons, 1999.

Patton LL, Siegel MA, Benoliel R, et al, "Management of Burning Mouth Syndrome: Systematic Review and Management Recommendations," *Oral Surg Oral Med Oral Pathol Oral Radiol Endod*, 2007, 103(Suppl S39):e1-13.

Petruzzi M, Lauritano D, De Benedittis M, et al, "Systemic Capsaicin for Burning Mouth Syndrome: Short-Term Results of a Pilot Study," *J Oral Pathol Med*, 2004, 33(2):111-4.

Reljanovic M, Reichel G, Rett K, et al, "Treatment of Diabetic Polyneuropathy With the Antioxidant Thioctic Acid (Alpha-Lipoic Acid): A Two Year Multicenter Randomized Double-Blind Placebo-Controlled Trial (ALADIN II). Alpha Lipoic Acid in Diabetic Neuropathy," *Free Radic Res*, 1999, 31(3):171-9.

Rhodus NL, Carlson CR, and Miller CS, "Burning Mouth (Syndrome) Disorder," *Quintessence Int*, 2003, 34(8):587-93.

Rhodus NL, Myers S, and Kaimal S, "Diagnosis and Management of Oral Lichen Planus," *Northwest Dent*, 2003, 82(2):17-9, 22-5.

Sardella A, Uglietti D, Demarosi F, et al, "Benzydamine Hydrochloride Oral Rinses in Management of Burning Mouth Syndrome. A Clinical Trial," *Oral Surg Oral Med Oral Pathol Oral Radiol Endod*, 1999, 88 (6):683-6.

Ship JA, Grushka M, Lipton JA, et al, "Burning Mouth Syndrome: An Update," *J Am Dent Assoc*, 1995, 126(7):842-53.

Spice R and Hagen NA, "Capsaicin in Burning Mouth Syndrome: Titration Strategies," *J Otolaryngol*, 2004, 33(1):53-4.

Tammiala-Salonen T and Forssell H, "Trazodone in Burning Mouth Pain: A Placebo-Controlled, Double-Blind Study," *J Orofac Pain*, 1999, 13(2):83-8.

Thomson MA, Hamburger J, Stewart DG, et al, "Treatment of Erosive Oral Lichen Planus With Topical Tacrolimus," *J Dermatolog Treat*, 2004, 15(5):308-14.

Vidal MA, Martinez-Fernandez E, Martinez-Vazquez de Castro J, et al, "Diabetic Neuropathy: Effectiveness of Amitriptyline and Gabapentin," *Rev Soc Esp Dolor*, 2004, 11(8):38-52.

White TL, Kent PF, Kurtz DB, et al, "Effectiveness of Gabapentin for Treatment of Burning Mouth Syndrome," *Arch Otolaryngol Head Neck Surg*, 2004, 130(6):786-8.

Woda A and Pionchon P, "A Unified Concept of Idiopathic Orofacial Pain: Clinical Features," *J Orofac Pain*, 1999, 13(3):172-84.

Woda A, Navez ML, Picard P, et al, "A Possible Therapeutic Solution for Stomatodynia (Burning Mouth Syndrome)," *J Orofac Pain*, 1998, 12(4):272-8.

Zakrzewska JM, Forssell H, and Glenny AM, "Interventions for the Treatment of Burning Mouth Syndrome," *Cochrane Database Syst Rev*, 2005.

Ziegler D, Hanefeld M, Ruhnau KJ, et al, "Treatment of Symptomatic Diabetic Polyneuropathy With the Antioxidant Alpha-Lipoic Acid: A 7-Month Multicenter Randomized Controlled Trial (ALADIN III Study). ALADIN III Study Group. Alpha-Lipoic Acid in Diabetic Neuropathy," *Diabetes Care*, 1999, 22 (8):1296-301.

Ziegler D, Reljanovic M, Mehnert H, et al, "Alpha-Lipoic Acid in the Treatment of Diabetic Polyneuropathy in Germany: Current Evidence From Clinical Trials," *Exp Clin Endocrinol Diabetes*, 1999, 107 (7):421-30.

DENTIN HYPERSENSITIVITY, ACID EROSION, HIGH CARIES INDEX, AND XEROSTOMIA

DENTIN HYPERSENSITIVITY

Suggested steps in resolving dentin hypersensitivity when a thorough exam has ruled-out any other source for the problem:

Treatment Steps

- Home treatment with a desensitizing toothpaste containing potassium nitrate (used to brush teeth as well as a thin layer applied, each night for 2 weeks)
- If needed, in office potassium oxalate (Protect® by Butler) and/or in office fluoride iontophoresis
- If sensitivity is still not tolerable to the patient, consider pumice then dentin adhesive and unfilled resin or composite restoration overlaying a glass ionomer base
- The use of 5% sodium fluoride varnishes (Duraflor® and Duraphat®) have been encouraged for the prevention of decay in persons of high-risk populations and also show some efficacy for reducing sensitivity following multiple applications.

Home Products (all contain nitrate as active ingredient):

Promise®
Denquel®
Sensodyne®
THERADENT™

Other major brand name companies have added ingredients to their dentifrice product lines that also make hypersensitivity claims.

ACID EROSION

Acid erosion is the loss of tooth enamel through prolonged exposure to acid rich foods, beverages, and even fruits. The problem has been raised primarily in pediatric patients and can be significant. Several oral care products claim surface remineralization efficacy and should be coupled with dietary counseling to achieve a desirable reduction in tooth damage.

ReNew® Remineralizing and Desensitizing Paste
Sensodyne® ProNamel™ for Children
Recaldent, found in GC America's Prospec™ MI Paste with Recaldent™ and Trident XTRA CARE™ chewing gum
Amorphous calcium phosphate (ACP) found in Arm & Hammer® Enamel Care® Toothpaste
Premier Dental's Enamel Pro™ polishing paste
SensiStat, found in Ortek Therapeutic's ProClude® and DenClude® products
NovaMin, a synthetic mineral composed of calcium, sodium, phosphorus, and silica

ANTICARIES AGENTS

Fluoride (Gel 0.4%, Rinse 0.05%) on page 752

New toothpastes with triclosan such as Colgate Total® show promise for combined treatment/prevention of caries, plaque, and gingivitis. The use of 5% sodium fluoride varnishes (Duraflor® and Duraphat®) have been encouraged for the prevention of decay in persons of high-risk populations.

FLUORIDES

Used for the prevention of demineralization of the tooth structure secondary to xerostomia. For patients with long-term or permanent xerostomia, daily application is accomplished using custom applicator trays, such as omnivac. Patients with porcelain crowns should use a neutral pH fluoride (see Fluoride monograph on page 752). Final selection of a fluoride product and/or saliva replacement/stimulant product must be based on patient comfort, taste, and ultimately, compliance. Experience has demonstrated that, often times, patients must try various combinations to achieve the greatest effect and their highest comfort levels. The presence of mucositis during cancer management complicates the clinician's selection of products.

OVER-THE-COUNTER (OTC) PRODUCTS

Form	Brand Name	Strength / Size
Gel, topical (stannous fluoride)	Gel-Kam® (cinnamon, fruit, mint flavors)	0.4% [0.1%] (65 g, 105 g, 122 g)
	Gel-Tin® (lime, grape, cinnamon, raspberry, mint, orange flavors)	0.4% [0.1%] (60 g, 120 g)
	Stop® (grape, cinnamon, bubblegum, piña colada, mint flavors)	0.4% [0.1%] (60 g, 120 g)
Rinse, topical (as sodium)	ACT®, Fluorigard®	0.05% [0.02%] (90 mL, 180 mL, 300 mL, 360 mL, 480 mL)
	Listermint® with Fluoride	0.02% [0.01%] (180 mL, 300 mL, 360 mL, 480 mL, 540 mL, 720 mL, 960 mL, 1740 mL)

PRESCRIPTION ONLY (Rx) PRODUCTS

Form	Brand Name	Strength / Size
Drops, oral (as sodium)		0.275 mg/drop [0.125 mg/drop]
	Fluoritab®, Flura-Drops®	0.55 mg/drop [0.25 mg/drop] (22.8 mL, 24 mL)
	Karidium®, Luride®	0.275 mg/drop [0.125 mg/drop] (30 mL, 60 mL)
	Pediaflor®	1.1 mg/mL [0.5 mg/mL] (50 mL)
Gel-Drops	Thera-Flur® (lime flavor), Thera-Flur-N®	1.1% [0.55%] (24 mL)
Gel, topical		
Acidulated phosphate fluoride	Minute-Gel® (spearmint, strawberry, grape, apple-cinnamon, cherry cola, bubblegum flavors)	1.23% (480 mL)
Sodium fluoride	Karigel® (orange flavor)	1.1% [0.5%]
	Karigel®-N	1.1% [0.5%]
	PreviDent® (mint, berry, cherry, fruit sherbet flavors)	1.1% [0.5%] (24 g, 30 g, 60 g, 120 g, 130 g, 250 g)
Lozenge (as sodium)	Flura-Loz® (raspberry flavor)	2.2 mg [1 mg]
Rinse, topical (as sodium)	Fluorinse®, Point-Two®	0.2% [0.09%] (240 mL, 480 mL, 3780 mL)
Solution, oral (as sodium)	Phos-Flur® (cherry, cinnamon, grape, wintergreen flavors)	0.44 mg/mL [0.2 mg/mL] (250 mL, 500 mL, 3780 mL)
Tablet (as sodium)		1.1 mg [0.5 mg]; 2.2 mg [1 mg]
Chewable	Fluor-A-Day®	0.55 mg [0.25 mg]
	Fluor-A-Day®, Fluoritab®, Luride® Lozi-Tab®, Pharmaflur®	1.1 mg [0.5 mg]
	Fluor-A-Day®, Fluoritab®, Karidium®, Luride® Lozi-Tab®, Luride®-SF Lozi-Tab®, Pharmaflur®	2.2 mg [1 mg]
Oral	Flura®, Karidium®	2.2 mg [1 mg]
Varnish	Duraflor®, Duraphat®	5% [50 mg/mL] (10 mL)

Tables copied from Newland, JR, Meiller, TF, Wynn, RL, et al, *Oral Soft Tissue Diseases,* 2nd ed, Hudson (Cleveland), OH: Lexi-Comp, Inc, 2002.

ANTIMICROBIAL ORAL RINSE

Chlorhexidine Gluconate (Peridex®) on page 360
Chlorhexidine Gluconate alcohol-free (CHX®) on page 360
Mouthwash (Antiseptic) (Listerine®) on page 1164

For examples of sample prescriptions see Antimicrobial Rinses on page 1987

MANAGEMENT OF SIALORRHEA

In patients suffering with medical conditions that result in hypersalivation, the dentist may determine that it is appropriate to use an atropine sulfate medication to achieve a dry field for dental procedures or to reduce excessive drooling. Currently there is one ADA approved medication sold under the name of Sal-Tropine™. Pro-Banthine® (propantheline bromide), an antimuscarinic used for excessive stomach acid production is advocated by some for off-label use. See Atropine on page 188

XEROSTOMIA

Xerostomia refers to the subjective sensation of a dry mouth while salivary gland hypofunction can be objectively measured. Numerous factors can play a role in the patient's perception of xerostomia. Changes in salivary function caused by drugs, surgical intervention, or treatment of cancer are among the leading causes of xerostomia. Other factors including aging, smoking, mouth breathing, and autoimmune disorders such as Sjögren's syndrome, can also be implicated in a patient's perception of xerostomia. Human immunodeficiency virus (HIV) may produce xerostomia when viral changes in salivary glands are present. Xerostomia often occurs in patients taking antianxiety and antidepressant medication and often accompanies burning mouth syndrome. Xerostomia affects women more frequently than men and is also more common in older individuals. Some alteration in salivary function naturally occurs with age, but it is extremely difficult to quantify the effects. Xerostomia and salivary gland hypofunction in the elderly population are contributory to deterioration in the quality of life.

Once a diagnosis of xerostomia or salivary gland hypofunction is made and possible causes confirmed, treatment for the condition usually involves management of the underlying disease and avoidance of unnecessary medications. In addition, good hydration is essential and water is the drink of choice. Also, the use of artificial saliva substitutes, selected chewing gums, and/or toothpastes formulated to treat xerostomia, is often warranted. In more difficult cases, such as patients receiving radiotherapy for cancer of the head and neck regions or patients with Sjögren's syndrome, systemic cholinergic stimulants may be administered if no contraindications exist. The clinician must also rule out and treat concomitant conditions such as fungal colonization and overgrowth which often occur subsequent to xerostomia.

CLINICAL PRODUCT USE

Because of the complex nature of xerostomia, management by the dental clinician is difficult. Treatment success is also difficult to assess and is often unsatisfactory. The salivary stimulants, pilocarpine and cevimeline, may aid in some conditions but are only approved for use as sialogogues in patients receiving radiotherapy and in Sjögren's patients, specifically as described above. Artificial salivas are available as over-the-counter products and represent the potential for continuous application by the patient to achieve comfort for their xerostomic condition.

The role of the clinician in attempting treatment of dry mouth is to first achieve a differential diagnosis and to ensure that other conditions are not simultaneously present. For example, many patients suffer burning mouth syndrome or painful oral tissues with no obvious etiology accompanying dry mouth. Also, higher caries incidence may be associated with changes in salivary flow. As previously mentioned, Sjögren's syndrome represents an immune complex of disorders that can affect the eyes, oral tissues, and other organ systems. The reader is referred to current oral pathology or oral medicine textbooks for review of signs and symptoms of Sjögren's syndrome.

Treatment of cancer often leads to dry mouth. Surgical intervention removing salivary tissue due to the presence of a salivary gland tumor results in loss of salivary function. Also, many of the chemotherapeutic agents produce transitory changes in salivary flow, such that the patient may perceive a dry mouth during chemotherapy. Most notably related to salivary dysfunction is the use of radiation regimens to head and neck tissues. Tumors in or about salivary gland tissue, the oral cavity, and oropharynx are most notably sensitive to radiation therapy and subsequent dry mouth. In the head and neck, therapeutic radiation is commonly used in treatment of squamous cell carcinomas and lymphomas. The radiation level necessary to destroy malignant cells ranges from 40-70 Gy. Salivary tissue is extremely sensitive to radiation changes. Radiation dosages >30 Gy are sufficient to permanently change salivary function. In addition to the mucositis and subsequent secondary infection by fungal colonization or viral exacerbation, oral tissues can become exceptionally dry due to the effects of radiation on salivary glands. In fact, permanent damage to salivary gland tissue within the beam path produces significant levels of xerostomia in most patients. Some recovery may be noted by the patient. Most often, the effects are permanent and even progressive as the radiation dosage increases.

Artificial salivas do not produce any protectant or stimulation of the salivary gland. The use of pilocarpine and cevimeline as salivary stimulants in pre-emptive treatment, as well as postradiation treatment, have been shown to have some efficacy in management of dry mouth. The success rate, however, still is often unsatisfactory and post-treatment management by the dentist usually requires fluoride supplements to prevent radiation-induced caries due to dry mouth. Also, management of dry mouth through patient use of the artificial salivary gel, solutions and sprays, or other over-the-counter products for dry mouth (eg, chewing gum, toothpaste, mouthwash, swabsticks, sugar-free candy) is highly recommended. The use of pilocarpine or cevimeline should only be considered by the dentist in consultation with the managing physician. The oftentimes severe and widespread cholinergic side effects of pilocarpine and cevimeline mandate close monitoring of the patient and certain medical conditions contraindicated their use.

The use of artificial salivary substitutes is less problematic for the dentist. The dentist should, in considering selection of a drug, base his or her decision on patient compliance and comfort. Salivary substitutes presently on the market may have some benefit in terms of electrolyte balance and salivary consistency. However, the ultimate decision needs to be based on patients' taste, their willingness to use the medication ad libitum, and improvement in their comfort related to dry mouth. Many of the drugs are pH balanced to reduce additional risk of dental demineralization or caries. Oftentimes, the dentist must try numerous medications, one at a time, prior to finding one which gives the patient some comfort. Another gauge of acceptability is to investigate whether the artificial saliva substitute has the American Dental Association's seal of approval. Most of the currently accepted saliva substitute products have been evaluated by the ADA.

In general, considerations that the clinician might use in a prescribed regimen would be that saliva substitutes are meant to be used regularly throughout the day by the patient to achieve comfort during meals, reduce tissue abrasion, and prevent salivary stagnation on teeth. Other than these, there are no specific recommendations for patients. Recommendations by the dentist need to be tailored to the patient's acceptance. Salivary substitutes may provide an allergic potential in patients who are sensitive to some of the preservatives present in artificial saliva products. In addition to this allergic potential, there is a risk of microbial contamination by placement of the salivary substitute container in close contact with the oral cavity.

Patient education regarding the use of saliva substitutes is also part of the clinical approach. The patient with chronic xerostomia should be educated about regular professional care, high performance in dental hygiene, the need to re-evaluate oral soft tissue pathology, and any changes that might occur long term. In patients with severe xerostomia, artificial salivary medications should be given in combination with topical fluoride treatment programs designed by the dentist to reduce caries.

PRODUCTS AND DRUGS TO TREAT DRY MOUTH

Medication	Manufacturer and Phone Number	Product Type	Manufacturer's Description	Indication	Ingredients	Directions for Use	Form and Availability
Artificial Salivas (OTC)							
Biotene® OralBalance® Mouth Moisturizing Gel	Laclede Professional Products, Inc (800) 922-5856	Gel	Sugar-free oral lubricant; relieves dry mouth symptoms up to 8 hours; soothes and protects oral tissue to promote healing; helps to inhibit harmful bacteria; improves retention under dentures	Relieves symptoms of dry mouth: burning, itching, cotton palate, sore tissue swallowing difficulties	Contains the "Biotene®" protective salivary enzyme system Active: Glucose oxidase (2000 units), lactoperoxidase (3000 units), lysozyme (5 mg), lactoferrin (5 mg) Other: Hydrogenated starch, xylitol, hydroxyethyl cellulose, glycerate polyhydrate, aloe vera	Using a clean fingertip, apply a 1" ribbon of gel on tongue; add additional amount of gel on other dry; use as needed	1.4 oz tube; available at mass merchandise stores, food stores, and drugstores
BreathTech™ Plaque Fighter Mouth Spray	Omnii Oral Pharmaceuticals (800) 445-3386	Pump dispenser	Plaque inhibitor in vanilla-mint flavor for breath malodor or reduced salivary flow	Treats the discomfort of oral dryness	Microdent® patented plaque-inhibitor formula	Spray directly into mouth; spread over teeth and tissue with tongue	18 mL pump dispenser; order directly from manufacturer
Moi-Stir® Moistening Solution	Kingswood Laboratories, Inc (800) 968-7772	Pump spray	Saliva supplement for moistening of mouth and mucosal area	Nontherapeutic treatment of dry mouth; intended for comfort only	Water, sorbitol, sodium carboxymethylcellulose, methylparaben, propylparaben, potassium chloride, sodium chloride, flavoring	Spray directly into mouth as necessary to treat drying conditions	4 oz spray bottle; order directly from manufacturer or various distributors
MouthKote® Oral Moisturizer	Parnell Pharmaceuticals, Inc (800) 457-4276	Aqueous solution	Pleasant lemon-lime-flavored oral moisturizer to lubricate and protect oral tissue	Treats the discomfort of oral dryness caused by medications, disease, surgery, irradiation, aging	Water, xylitol, sorbitol, yerba santa, citric acid, ascorbic acid, flavor, sodium benzoate, sodium saccharin	Swirl 1 or 2 teaspoonfuls in mouth for 8-10 seconds; swallow or spit out; shake well before using	2 oz and 8 oz bottles; available at drugstores or order directly from manufacturer
Oasis® Moisturizing Mouthwash	GlaxoSmithKline (800) 777-2500	Oral moisturizer, aqueous solution	Moisturizing mouthwash for a dry mouth indication	Moisturizes mouth and helps it from drying out	Active: Glycerin Other: Water, sorbitol, poloxamer 338, PEG-60 hydrogenated castor oil, cellulose gum, cetylpyridinium chloride, copovidone, disodium phosphate, flavor, methylparaben, propylparaben, sodium benzoate, sodium phosphate, sodium saccharin, xanthan gum, FD&C blue #1	Rinse for 30 seconds with 1 ounce of mouthwash first thing in the morning and before going to bed or as needed; do not swallow; use as part of an effective oral hygiene program	16 oz bottle
Optimoist™ Oral Moisturizer	Colgate Oral Pharmaceuticals (800) 225-3756	Oral moisturizer, aqueous solution	Pleasant tasting saliva substitute for instant relief of dry mouth and throat without demineralizing tooth enamel	Treats the discomfort of oral dryness	Deionized water, xylitol, calcium phosphate monobasic, citric acid, sodium hydroxide, sodium benzoate, flavoring, acesulfame potassium, hydroxyethylcellulose, polysorbate 20 and sodium monofluorophosphate (fluoride concentration is 2 parts per million)	Spray directly into mouth to relieve dry mouth discomfort; may be swallowed or expectorated; use as needed	2 oz and 12 oz bottles; available at mass merchandise stores, food stores, and drugstores

PRODUCTS AND DRUGS TO TREAT DRY MOUTH *continued*

Medication	Manufacturer and Phone Number	Product Type	Manufacturer's Description	Indication	Ingredients	Directions for Use	Form and Availability
Salivart® Synthetic Saliva, Aqueous Solution	Gebauer Co (800) 321-9348	Aerosol aqueous spray	Oral moisturizer for patients with reduced salivary flow	Replacement therapy for patients complaining of xerostomia	Sodium carboxymethylcellulose, sorbitol, sodium chloride, potassium chloride, calcium chloride dihydrate, magnesium chloride hexahydrate, potassium phosphate dibasic, purified water, nitrogen (propellant)	Spray directly into mouth or throat for 1-2 seconds; use as needed	2.48 fl oz (75 g); available at most drugstores or directly from manufacturer
Other Dry Mouth Products (OTC)							
Biotene® Dry Mouth Gum	Laclede Professional Products, Inc (800) 922-9348	Chewing gum	Sugar-free; helps stimulate saliva flow; fights cause/effect of bad breath; reduces plaque	Treats oral dryness	Active: Lactoperoxidase (0.11 Units), glucose oxidase (0.15 Units) Other: Sorbitol, gum base, xylitol, hydrogenated glucose, potassium thiocyanate	Chew 1 or 2 pieces; use as needed	Each package contains 17 pieces; available at drugstores or directly from manufacturer
Biotene® Dry Mouth Toothpaste	Laclede Professional Products, Inc (800) 922-9348	Toothpaste	Reduces harmful bacteria which cause cavities, periodontal disease, and oral infections	Use in place of regular toothpaste for dry mouth	Active: Lactoperoxidase (15,000 Units), glucose oxidase (10,000 Units), lysozyme (16 mg), sodium monofluorophosphate Other: Sorbitol, glycerin, calcium pyrophosphate, hydrated silica, xylitol, isoceteth-20, cellulose gum, flavoring, sodium benzoate, beta-d-glucose, potassium thiocyanate	Use in place of regular toothpaste; rinse toothbrush before applying; brush for 2 minutes; rinse lightly	4.5 oz tube; available at drugstores or directly from manufacturer
Biotene® Gentle Mouthwash	Laclede Professional Products, Inc (800) 922-9348	Mouthwash	Alcohol-free; strong antibacterial formula neutralizes mouth odors; soothes as it cleans to protect teeth and oral tissue	Treats dry mouth or oral irritations	Lysozyme, lactoferrin, glucose oxidase, lactoperoxidase	Use 15 mL (1 tablespoonful); swish thoroughly for 30 seconds and spit out; for dry throat, sip 1 tablespoonful of mouthwash 2-3 times/day	Available at drugstores or directly from manufacturer
Moi-Stir® Oral Swabsticks	Kingswood Laboratories, Inc (800) 968-7772	Swabsticks	Lubricates and moistens mouth and mucosal area	Lubricates and moistens mouth and mucosal area	Water, sorbitol, sodium carboxymethylcellulose, methylparaben, propylparaben, potassium chloride, sodium chloride, flavoring	Gently swab all intraoral surfaces of mouth, gums, tongue, palate, buccal mucosa, gingival, teeth, and lips where uncomfortable dryness exists	3 swabsticks/packet, 100 packets/case; order directly from manufacturer or from various distributors.
Oasis® Moisturizing Mouth Spray	GlaxoSmithKline (800) 777-2500	Oral moisturizer	Moisturizing mouth spray for a dry mouth indication	Moisturizes mouth and helps it from drying out	Active: Glycerin 35% (prediluted) Other: Cetylpyridinium chloride, copovidone, flavor, methylparaben, PEG-60 hydrogenated castor oil propylparaben, sodium benzoate, sodium saccharin, water, xanthan gum, xylitol	Use as required up to a maximum of 30 times or 60 sprays a day; spray 1-2 times into the affected area of mouth; do not rinse out	1 oz bottle

PRODUCTS AND DRUGS TO TREAT DRY MOUTH *continued*

Medication	Manufacturer and Phone Number	Product Type	Manufacturer's Description	Indication	Ingredients	Directions for Use	Form and Availability
Saliva Substitute (Rx)							
Aquoral™	Auriga Laboratories (877) 287-4428	Pump spray	Lipid-based solution designed to moisten and lubricate the oral cavity and oropharynx by formation of lipid film which limits loss of water and restores the viscoelasticity of the oral mucosa	Chronic and temporary xerostomia which may be the result of Sjögren's syndrome, oral inflammation, medication, chemo- or radiotherapy, and stress or aging. **Note:** Contraindicated if patient has a known history of hypersensitivity to any of its ingredients. No known interactions with medicinal or other products.	Oxidized glycerol triesters (TGO), silicon dioxide, aspartame, and artificial flavoring	Shake gently; 1 dose (2 sprays) into the mouth 3-4 times/day; spread product onto inflamed and/or dry areas of the mouth with the tongue.	1 bottle (40 mL = 400 sprays)
Cholinergic Salivary Stimulants (Rx)							
Cevimeline (Evoxac®)	Snow Brand Pharmaceuticals (800) 475-6473			Treats symptoms of dry mouth in patients with Sjögren's syndrome	Active: Cevimeline 30 mg Other: Lactose monohydrate, hydroxypropyl cellulose, magnesium stearate	1 capsule (30 mg) 3 times/day	30 mg capsules
Pilocarpine (Salagen®)	MGI Pharmaceuticals, Inc (800) 562-5580			Treats xerostomia caused by radiation therapy in patients with head/neck cancer, Sjögren's syndrome	Active: Pilocarpine 5 mg Other: Carnauba wax, hydroxypropyl methylcellulose, iron oxide, microcrystalline cellulose, stearic acid, titanium dioxide	1-2 tablets (5 mg) 3-4 times/day, not to exceed 30 mg/day	5 mg tablets

CHOLINERGIC SALIVARY STIMULANTS (PRESCRIPTION ONLY)

Pilocarpine (Systemic) (Salagen® on page 1346) and cevimeline (Evoxac® on page 355) are cholinergic drugs which stimulate salivary flow. They stimulate muscarinic-type acetylcholine receptors in salivary glands within the parasympathetic division of the autonomic nervous system, causing an increase in serous-type saliva. Thus, they are considered cholinergic, muscarinic-type (parasympathomimetic) drugs. Due to significant side effects caused by these drugs, they are available by prescription only.

Pilocarpine (Salagen®) is indicated for the treatment of xerostomia caused by radiation therapy in patients with head and neck cancer and xerostomia in patients suffering from Sjögren's syndrome. The usual adult dosage is 1-2 tablets (5 mg or 7.5 mg/tablet) 3-4 times/day, not to exceed 30 mg/day. Patients should be treated for a minimum of 90 days for optimum effect. The most frequent adverse side effect is perspiration, which occurs in about 30% of patients who use 5 mg 3 times/day. Other adverse effects (in about 10% of patients) are nausea, rhinitis, chills, frequent urination, dizziness, headache, lacrimation, and pharyngitis. Salagen® is contraindicated for patients with uncontrolled asthma and narrow-angle glaucoma.

Pilocarpine has been documented to overcome xerostomia from different causes. More recent studies confirm its effectiveness in improving salivary flow in patients undergoing irradiation therapy for head and neck cancer. A capstone study by Johnson, et al, reported the effects of pilocarpine in 208 irradiation patients at 39 different treatment sites. Salagen®, at a dose of 5 mg 3 times/day, improved salivation in 44% of patients, compared with 25% in the placebo group. They concluded that treatment with pilocarpine (Salagen®) produced the best overall outcome with respect to saliva production and relief of symptoms of xerostomia in patients undergoing irradiation therapy.

Additional studies have been published showing the effectiveness of pilocarpine (Salagen®) in stimulating salivary flow in patients suffering from Sjögren's syndrome and the FDA has approved the use of Salagen® for this indication.

Recent reports suggest that pre-emptive use of pilocarpine may be effective in protecting salivary glands during therapeutic irradiation; further studies are needed to confirm this. As of this publication date, the use of pilocarpine has not been approved to treat xerostomia induced by chronic medication. Pilocarpine could be used as a sialagogue for individuals with xerostomia induced by antidepressants and other medications. However, the potential for serious drug interactions is a concern and more studies are needed to clarify the safety and effectiveness of pilocarpine when given in the presence of other medications.

Cevimeline (Evoxac®) is indicated for treatment of symptoms of dry mouth in patients with Sjögren's syndrome. The usual dosage in adults is 1 capsule (30 mg) 3 times/day. Cevimeline (Evoxac®) is supplied in 30 mg capsules. Some adverse effects reported for Evoxac® include increased sweating (19%), nausea (14%), rhinitis (11%), sinusitis (12%), and upper respiratory infection (11%). Evoxac® is contraindicated for patients with uncontrolled asthma, narrow-angle glaucoma, acute iritis, and other conditions where miosis is undesirable. Cevimeline's half-life elimination is significantly slower than pilocarpine (0.76 hours versus 5 hours).

OTHER DRUGS IMPLICATED IN XEROSTOMIA

>10%	1% to 10%
ALPRAZolam	Acrivastine and Pseudoephedrine
Amitriptyline hydrochloride	Albuterol
Amoxapine	Amantadine hydrochloride
Anisotropine methylbromide	Amphetamine sulfate
Atropine sulfate	Astemizole (withdrawn from market)
Belladonna and Opium	Azatadine maleate
Benztropine mesylate	Beclomethasone dipropionate
BuPROPion	Bepridil hydrochloride
ChlordiazePOXIDE	Bitolterol mesylate
Clomipramine hydrochloride	Brompheniramine maleate
ClonazePAM	Carbinoxamine and Pseudoephedrine
CloNIDine	Chlorpheniramine maleate
Clorazepate dipotassium	Clemastine fumarate

OTHER DRUGS IMPLICATED IN XEROSTOMIA *(continued)*

>10%	1% to 10%
Cyclobenzaprine	CloZAPine
Desipramine hydrochloride	Cromolyn sodium
Diazepam	Cyproheptadine hydrochloride
Dicyclomine hydrochloride	Dexchlorpheniramine maleate
Diphenoxylate and Atropine	Dextroamphetamine sulfate
Doxepin hydrochloride	DimenhyDRINATE
Ergotamine	DiphenhydrAMINE hydrochloride
Estazolam	Disopyramide phosphate
FlavoxATE	Doxazosin
Flurazepam hydrochloride	Dronabinol
Glycopyrrolate	EPHEDrine sulfate
Guanabenz acetate	Flumazenil
GuanFACINE hydrochloride	FluvoxaMINE
Hyoscyamine sulfate	Gabapentin
Interferon alfa-2a	GuaiFENesin and Codeine
Interferon alfa-2b	Guanadrel sulfate
Interferon alfa-N3	Guanethidine sulfate
Ipratropium bromide	HydrOXYzine
Isoproterenol	Hyoscyamine, Atropine, Scopolamine, and Phenobarbital
ISOtretinoin	Imipramine
Loratadine	Isoetharine
LORazepam	Levocabastine hydrochloride
Loxapine	Levodopa
Maprotiline hydrochloride	Levodopa and Carbidopa
Methscopolamine bromide	Levorphanol tartrate
Molindone hydrochloride	Meclizine hydrochloride
Nabilone	Meperidine hydrochloride
Nefazodone	Methadone hydrochloride
Oxybutynin chloride	Methamphetamine hydrochloride
Oxazepam	Methyldopa
PARoxetine	Metoclopramide
Phenelzine sulfate	Morphine sulfate
Prochlorperazine	Nortriptyline hydrochloride
Propafenone hydrochloride	Ondansetron
Protriptyline hydrochloride	OxyCODONE and Acetaminophen
Quazepam	OxyCODONE and Aspirin
Reserpine	Pentazocine
Selegiline hydrochloride	Phenylpropanolamine hydrochloride
Temazepam	Prazosin hydrochloride
Thiethylperazine maleate	Promethazine hydrochloride
Trihexyphenidyl hydrochloride	Propoxyphene
Trimipramine maleate	Pseudoephedrine
Venlafaxine	RisperiDONE
	Sertraline hydrochloride
	Terazosin
	Terbutaline sulfate

TEMPOROMANDIBULAR DYSFUNCTION (TMD)

Temporomandibular dysfunction comprises a broad spectrum of signs and symptoms. Although TMD presents in patterns, diagnosis is often difficult. Evaluation and treatment is time-intensive and no single therapy or drug regimen has been shown to be universally beneficial.

The thorough diagnostician should perform a screening examination for temporomandibular dysfunction on all patients. Ideally, a baseline maximum mandibular opening along with lateral and protrusive movement evaluation should be performed. Secondly, the joint area should be palpated and an adequate exam of the muscles of mastication and the muscles of the neck and shoulders should be made. These muscle would include the elevators of the mandible (masseter, internal pterygoid, and temporalis); the depressors of the mandible (including the external pterygoid and digastric); extrusive muscles (including the temporalis and digastric), and protrusive muscles (including the external and internal pterygoids). These muscles also account for lateral movement of the mandible. The clinician should also be alert to indicators of dysfunction, primarily a history of pain with jaw function, chronic history of joint noise (although this can often be misinterpreted), pain in the muscles of the neck, limited jaw movement, pain in the actual muscles of mastication, and headache or even earache. The signs and symptoms are extremely variable and the clinician should be alert for any or all of these areas of interest. Because of the complexity of both evaluation and diagnosis, the general dentist often finds it too time consuming to spend the countless hours evaluating and treating the temporomandibular dysfunction patient. Therefore, oral medicine specialists trained in temporomandibular evaluation and treatment often accept referrals for the management of these complicated patients. TMD often accompanies other chronic pain conditions, such as fibromyalgia and chronic headache. Studies are currently being performed to determine the efficacy of chronic pain medications in the management of TMD.

The oral medicine specialist in TMD management, the physical therapist interested in head and neck pain, and the oral and maxillofacial surgeon will all work together with the referring general dentist to accomplish successful patient treatment. Table 1 lists the wide variety of treatment alternatives available to the team. Depending on the diagnosis, one or more of the therapies might be selected. For organic diseases of the joint not responding to nonsurgical approaches, a wide variety of surgical techniques are available (Table 2).

ACUTE TMD

Acute TMD oftentimes presents alone or as an episode during a chronic pattern of signs and symptoms. Trauma, such as a blow to the chin or the side of the face, can result in acute TMD. Occasionally, similar symptoms will follow a lengthy wide open mouth dental procedure.

The condition usually presents as continuous deep pain in the TMJ. If edema is present in the joint, the condyle sometimes can be displaced which will cause abnormal occlusion of the posterior teeth on the affected side. The diagnosis is usually based on the history and clinical presentation. Management of the patient includes:

1. Restriction of all mandibular movement to function in a pain-free range of motion
2. Soft diet
3. NSAIDs (eg, Anaprox® DS 1 tablet every 12 hours for 7-10 days)
4. Moist heat applications to the affected area for 15-20 minutes, 4-6 times/day
5. Consideration of a muscle relaxant, such as Methocarbamol (Robaxin®) on page 1096, adult patient of average height/weight, two (500 mg) tablets at bedtime; daytime dose can be tailored to patient

Additional therapies could include referral to a physical therapist for ultrasound therapy 2-4 times/week and a single injection of steroid in the joint space. A team approach with an oral maxillofacial surgeon for this procedure may be helpful.

CHRONIC TMD

Following diagnosis which is often problematic, the most common therapeutic modalities include:

- Explaining the problem to the patient
- Recommending a soft diet:
  - Diet should consist of soft foods (eg, eggs, yogurt, casseroles, soup, ground meat).
  - Avoid chewing gum, salads, large sandwiches, and hard fruit.
- Reducing stress; moist heat application 4-6 times/day for 15-20 minutes coupled with a monitored exercise program will be beneficial. Usually, working with a physical therapist is ideal.
- Medications include analgesics, anti-inflammatories, tranquilizers, and muscle relaxants

MEDICATION OPTIONS

Most commonly used medication (NSAIDs)

Choline Magnesium Trisalicylate on page 376
Diclofenac (Systemic) on page 513
Diflunisal on page 524
Etodolac on page 690
Fenoprofen on page 715
Flurbiprofen (Systemic) on page 763
Ibuprofen on page 884
Indomethacin on page 912
Ketoprofen on page 966
Ketorolac (Systemic) on page 969
Magnesium Salicylate on page 1051
Meclofenamate on page 1059
Mefenamic Acid on page 1062
Nabumetone on page 1172
Naproxen on page 1183
Oxaprozin on page 1262
Piroxicam on page 1360
Salsalate on page 1507
Sulindac on page 1564
Tolmetin on page 1645

Tranquilizers and muscle relaxants, when used appropriately, can provide excellent adjunctive therapy. These drugs should be primarily used for a short period of time to manage acute pain. In low dosages, amitriptyline is often used to treat chronic pain and occasionally migraine headache. Two drugs similar to the prototype drug, amitriptyline, have been approved for use in adults only, for treatment of acute migraine with or without aura: Almotriptan malate (Axert™ [tablets]; Pharmacia Corp) and frovatriptan succinate (Frova™ [tablets]; Endo Pharmaceuticals). Other approved abortive (but not preventative) antimigraine triptan drugs include eletriptan (Relpax®), naratriptan (Amerge®), rizatriptan (Maxalt®), sumatriptan (Imitrex®), and zolmitriptan (Zomig®). Selective serotonin reuptake inhibitors (SSRIs) are sometimes used in the management of chronic neuropathic pain, particularly in patients not responding to amitriptyline. Gabapentin (Neurontin®) has been approved for chronic pain. Problems of inducing bruxism with SSRIs, however, have been reported and may preclude their use. Clinicians attempting to evaluate any patient with bruxism or involuntary muscle movement, who is simultaneously being treated with an SSRI, should be aware of this potential association.

See individual monographs for dosing instructions.

Common minor tranquilizers include:

ALPRAZolam on page 85
Diazepam on page 509
LORazepam on page 1035

Chronic neuropathic pain management:

Amitriptyline on page 107
CarBAMazepine on page 301
Gabapentin on page 798

Acute migraine management:

Almotriptan on page 82
Eletriptan on page 593
Frovatriptan on page 793
Naratriptan on page 1188
Rizatriptan on page 1491
SUMAtriptan on page 1566
ZOLMitriptan on page 1751

Common muscle relaxants include:

Chlorzoxazone on page 374
Cyclobenzaprine on page 447
Methocarbamol on page 1096
Orphenadrine on page 1257

Note: Muscle relaxants and tranquilizers should generally be prescribed with an analgesic or NSAID to relieve pain as well.

Narcotic analgesics can be used on a short-term basis or intermittently in combination with non-narcotic therapy in the chronic pain patient. Judicious prescribing, monitoring, and maintenance by the practitioner is imperative whenever considering the use of narcotic analgesics due to the abuse and addiction liabilities.

Table 1. TMD - NONSURGICAL THERAPIES

1. Moist heat and cold spray
2. Injections in muscle trigger areas (procaine)
3. Exercises (passive, active)
4. Medications
   a. Muscle relaxants
   b. Minerals (magnesium, glucosamine, chondroitin)
   c. Multiple vitamins (Ca, B_6, B_{12})
   d. NSAIDs, opioid combinations, antidepressants
5. Orthopedic craniomandibular repositioning appliance (splints)
6. Biofeedback, acupuncture
7. Physiotherapy: TMJ muscle therapy
8. Myofunctional therapy (occasionally)
9. TENS (transcutaneous electrical neural stimulation), Myo-Monitor (occasionally)
10. Dental therapy
    a. Equilibration (coronoplasty) (occasionally)
    b. Restoring occlusion to proper vertical dimension of maxilla to mandible by orthodontics, dental restorative procedures, orthognathic surgery, permanent splint, or any combination of these

Table 2. TMD – SURGICAL THERAPIES

1. Cortisone injection into joint (with local anesthetic)
2. Bony and/or fibrous ankylosis: Requires surgery (osteoarthrotomy with prosthetic appliance)
3. Chronic subluxation: Requires surgery, depending on problem (possibly eminectomy and/or prosthetic implant)
4. Osteoarthritis: Requires surgery (arthroscopy), depending on problem
   a. Arthroplasty
   b. Meniscectomy
   c. Arthroplasty with repair of disc
   d. Arthrocentesis

5. Rheumatoid arthritis
   a. Arthroplasty
   b. "Total" TMJ replacement
6. Tumors: Require osteoarthrotomy – removal of tumor and restoring of joint when possible
7. Chronic disc displacement: Arthroscopy with arthrocentesis; possible removal of bone from condyle

MANAGEMENT OF THE PATIENT WITH ANXIETY OR DEPRESSION

ANXIETY AND DEPRESSION

Over the past two decades, there has been a gradual, but steady, increase in the number of patients who are taking antianxiety and antidepressant medications. Much of this is driven by the emergence of new medications for management of these conditions and an increasing awareness on the part of medical clinicians in recognizing signs and symptoms of depression and anxiety. In addition, society has now accepted that the quality of life for these patients can be improved on an outpatient basis.

The dentist often encounters patients taking medications that have the potential to induce mild-to-moderate adverse oral side effects and may create additional risk based on the types of medication used in the dental practice. In addition to a wide variety of depression-indicated signs and symptoms, antidepressant medications are prescribed for psychiatric disorders, pain control, sleep deprivation, smoking cessation, substance abuse, and eating disorders. The side effects of these drugs primarily fall into several categories. Xerostomia or altered salivary flow has long been known as a side effect of tricyclic antidepressants. Newer antidepressants, although the effects may be lessened, also have similar side effects. Coupled with xerostomia is an increased risk of fungal infections and a significant association with burning mouth syndrome (BMS). The reader is referred to Fungal Infections on page 1945 and Ulcerative, Erosive, and Painful Oral Mucosal Disorders on page 1950 for management if an infection is suspected. In addition, some drugs, including the selective serotonin reuptake inhibitors (SSRIs), have effects on orthostatic hypotension.

Another potential adverse reaction is cardiotoxicity associated with the use of combination drugs, including the antidepressant medication classes, and the use of a vasoconstrictor in local anesthetics. The reader is referred to Vasoconstrictor Interactions With Antidepressants on page 2026 in the appendix which discusses the classes of antidepressant and antianxiety medications and the potential risk of interactions with local anesthetics.

In reviewing the epidemiology of antidepressant and antianxiety medications, female subjects outnumber males by ~2.3:1 ratio with selective serotonin reuptake inhibitors being the most commonly prescribed medications. Tricyclic antidepressants, atypical third-generation antidepressants, and monoamine oxidase inhibitors are also used. Some of the drugs used for smoking cessation also fall into this atypical antidepressant class.

BIPOLAR DISORDER

Most people with bipolar disorder take combinations of lithium, valproate, and carbamazepine to manage symptoms and prevent recurrence of bipolar episodes. These medications are often called mood stabilizers, to even out emotional highs and lows. These patients may also be prescribed other medications to treat the agitation, anxiety, and sleep disturbances that may accompany their illness. In patients with concomitant depression, antidepressants can help manage the feelings of sadness, guilt, worthlessness, or hopelessness. Dry mouth, constipation, and nausea are the most common side effects.

SEDATION

Anxiety constitutes the most frequently found psychiatric problem in the general population. Anxiety can range from a simple phobia to a severe debilitating disorder. Functional results of this anxiety can, therefore, range from simple avoidance of dental procedures to panic attacks when confronting stressful situations, such as seen in some patients regarding dental visits. Many patients claim to be anxious over dental care, when in reality, they simply have not been managed with modern techniques of local anesthesia, the availability of sedation, or the caring dental practitioner.

The dentist may detect anxiety in patients during the treatment planning and evaluation phases of care. The anxious person may appear overly alert, may lean forward in the dental chair during conversation, or may appear concerned over time, possibly using this as a guise to cut short the dental visit. Anxious persons may also show signs of being nervous by demonstrating sweating; muscle tension, including their temporomandibular musculature; or they may complain of being tired due to an inability to obtain an adequate night's sleep.

The management of these patients requires a methodical approach to relaxation, discussing their dental needs, and then planning, along with the patient, the best way to accomplish dental treatment in the presence of their fears, either real or imagined. Consideration may be given to sedation. This sedation can be oral or parenteral, or inhalation in the case of nitrous oxide. The dentist must be adequately trained in administering the sedative of choice, as well as in monitoring the patient during the sedated procedures. Numerous medications are available to achieve the level of sedation usually necessary in the dental office: Valium®, Ativan®, Xanax®, Vistaril®, Serax®, and BuSpar® represent a few. These oral sedatives can be given prior to dental visits as outlined in the following prescriptions. They have the advantage of allowing the patient a good night's sleep prior to the day of the procedure and provide on-the-spot sedation during the procedure. Nitrous oxide is an in-the-office administered sedative that is relatively safe, but requires additional training and carefully planned monitoring protocols of auxiliary personnel during inhalation. Both oral and inhalation techniques can be used to manage the anxious patient in the dental office.

It is recommended that patients not drive themselves to or from dental appointments following use of these medications. Also, these medications should not be prescribed during pregnancy. For pediatric patients, oral preprocedural sedatives include primarily chloral hydrate, hydroxyzine, and liquid meperidine. Dosing suggestions are described in each of the respective monographs.

ALPRAZolam on page 85
BusPIRone on page 269
Chloral Hydrate on page 356
Diazepam on page 509
HydrOXYzine on page 877
LORazepam on page 1035
Meperidine on page 1073
Nitrous Oxide on page 1223
Prochlorperazine on page 1407
Triazolam on page 1674

Note: Although various antidepressants have been used for preprocedure sedation, no specific regimens or protocols have been established. Guidelines for use are still under study.

Doxepin (Systemic) on page 566
FLUoxetine on page 755
FluvoxaMINE on page 774
PARoxetine on page 1298
Sertraline on page 1518
TraZODone on page 1664

For examples of sample prescriptions see Sedation (Prior to Dental Treatment) on page 1995

REFERENCES

Brodine AH and Hartshorn MA, "Recognition and Management of Somatoform Disorders," *J Prosthet Dent*, 2004, 91(3):268-73.

Keene JJ Jr, Galasko GT, and Land MF, "Antidepressant Use in Psychiatry and Medicine: Importance for Dental Practice," *J Am Dent Assoc*, 2003, 134(1):71-9.

MANAGEMENT OF PATIENTS UNDERGOING CANCER THERAPY

CANCER PATIENT DENTAL PROTOCOL

The objective in treatment of a patient with cancer is eradication of the disease. Oral complications, such as mucosal ulceration, xerostomia, bleeding, and infections can cause significant morbidity and may compromise systemic treatment of the patient. With proper oral evaluation before systemic treatment, many of the complications can be minimized or prevented.

MUCOSITIS

Normal oral mucosa acts as a barrier against chemical and food irritants and oral microorganisms. Disruption of the mucosal barrier can lead to secondary infection, increased pain, delayed healing, and decreased nutritional intake.

Mucositis is inflammation of the mucous membranes. It is a common reaction to chemotherapy and radiation therapy. It is first seen as an erythematous patch. The mucosal epithelium becomes thin as a result of the killing of the rapidly dividing basal layer mucosal cells. Seven to ten days after cytoreduction chemotherapy and between 1000 cGy and 3000 cGy of radiation to the head and neck, mucosal tissues begin to desquamate and eventually develop into frank ulcerations. The mucosal integrity is broken and is secondarily infected by normal oral flora. The resultant ulcerations can also act as a portal of entry for pathogenic organisms into the patient's bloodstream and may lead to systemic infections. These ulcerations often force interruption of therapy.

Prevention of radiation mucositis is difficult. Stents can be constructed to prevent irradiation of uninvolved tissues. The use of multiple ports and fractionation of therapy into smaller doses over a longer period of time can reduce the severity. Fractured restorations, sharp teeth, and ill-fitted prostheses can damage soft tissues and lead to additional interruption of mucosal barriers. Correction of these problems before radiation therapy can diminish these complications.

CHEMOTHERAPY

Chemotherapy for neoplasia also frequently results in oral complications. Infections and mucositis are the most common complications seen in patients receiving chemotherapy. Also occurring frequently are pain, altered nutrition, and xerostomia, which can significantly affect the quality of life.

Certain chemotherapeutic agents, such as 5-fluorouracil, methotrexate, and doxorubicin, are more commonly associated with the development of oral mucositis. Treatment of oral mucositis is mainly palliative, but steps should be taken to minimize secondary pathogenic infections. Culture and sensitivity data should be obtained to select appropriate therapy for the bacterial, viral, or fungal organisms found.

RADIATION CARIES

Dental caries that sometimes follow radiation therapy is called radiation caries. It usually develops in the cervical smooth surface region of the teeth adjacent to the gingiva, often affecting many teeth. It is secondary to the irreversible damage done to the salivary glands and is initiated by dental plaque, but its rapid progress is due to changes in saliva. In addition to the diminution in the amount of saliva, both the salivary pH and buffering capacity are diminished, which decreases anticaries activity of saliva. Oral bacterial flora also change with xerostomia leading to the increase in caries activity. Typically patients that receive a cumulative radiation dose of 30 Gy or more will suffer significant loss of saliva production.

Osteonecrosis of the jaw (ONJ) is pertinent to cancer patient management and patients with osteoporosis (see Osteonecrosis of the Jaw on page 1894).

PERIORAL PREMALIGNANT LESIONS

Dentists are often the first to recognize changes in the skin, lips, or oral mucosal tissues that represent potential premalignancies. The general dentist may refer such patients or an oral and maxillofacial surgeon to a dermatologist for biopsy. There are numerous drugs under study to manage premalignancies by preventing the progression of lesions from dysplasia to frank cancer. On the skin, the condition actinic keratosis and on the lips, its perioral equivalent actinic cheilitis, create a diagnostic and management challenge for clinicians. Until now 5-fluorouracil preparations have been used with mixed success, but recently, Zyclara™ (imiquimod) has been approved for actinic keratosis.

SALIVARY CHANGES

Chemotherapy is not thought to directly alter salivary flow, but alterations in taste and subjective sensations of dry mouth are relatively common complaints. Patients with mucositis and graft-vs-host disease following bone marrow or stem cell transplantation often demonstrate signs and symptoms of xerostomia. Radiation does directly affect salivary production. Radiation to the salivary glands produces fibrosis and alters the production of saliva. If all the major salivary glands are in the field, the decrease in saliva can be dramatic and the serous portion of the glands seems to be most severely affected. The saliva produced is increased in viscosity, which contributes to food retention and increased plaque formation. These xerostomia patients have difficulty in managing a normal diet. Normal saliva also has bacteriostatic properties that are diminished in these patients.

The dental management recommendations for patients undergoing chemotherapy, bone marrow transplantation, and/or radiation therapy for the treatment of cancer are based primarily on clinical observations. The following protocols will provide a conservative, consistent approach to the dental management of patients undergoing chemotherapy or bone marrow transplantation. Many of the cancer chemotherapy drugs produce oral side effects including mucositis, oral ulceration, dry mouth, acute infections, and taste aberrations. Cancer drugs include antibiotics, alkylating agents, antimetabolites, DNA inhibitors, hormones, and cytokines.

All patients undergoing chemotherapy or bone marrow transplantation for malignant disease should have the following baseline:

A. Panoramic radiograph

B. Dental consultation and examination

C. Dental prophylaxis and cleaning (if the neutrophil count is >1500/mm^3 and the platelet count is >50,000/mm^3)

– Prophylaxis and cleaning will be deferred if the patient's neutrophil count is <1500 and the platelet count is <50,000. Oral hygiene recommendations will be made. These levels are arbitrary guidelines and the dentist should consider the patient's oral condition and planned procedure relative to hemorrhage and level of bacteremia.

D. Oral Hygiene: Patients should be encouraged to follow normal hygiene procedures. Addition of a chlorhexidine mouth rinse such as Peridex® or PerioGard® on page 360 is usually helpful. If the patient develops oral mucositis, tolerance of such alcohol-based products may be limited. Recently, a nonalcohol-containing chlorhexidine mouth rinse CHX® is also available.

PREVENTION AND TREATMENT OF MUCOSITIS

A. If the patient develops mucositis, bacterial, viral, and fungal cultures should be obtained. There are no standard of care recommendations for prevention of oral mucositis. The intravenous biologic product keratinocyte growth factor, palifermin (Kepivance®) is approved to help reduce the chance that certain cancer patients, those with blood cancers undergoing chemotherapy, would develop mucositis. Most therapies are palliative only or help in reducing secondary infection. Sucralfate suspension in a pharmacy-prepared form or Carafate® suspension, as well as Benadryl® on page 540 or Xylocaine® viscous on page 1010 can assist in helping the patient to tolerate food.

B. The oral barrier Gelclair® and the mucositis treatment aid Caphosol® are FDA approved for mucositis. Gargle and spit Gelclair® mixture of one single-use packet (15 mL) and water 3 times/day or as needed; follow mixing and administration instructions on packet.

C. Mix contents of 1 blue (A) and 1 clear (B) Caphosol® ampul in clean container, swish thoroughly with 1/2 of mixture (15 mL) for 1 minute and spit; repeat. Use immediately after mixing ampuls. Use 4 doses/day from the onset of high dose chemotherapy or radiation treatment. May use up to 10 doses/day if patient experiences pain from mucositis. Caphosol® may be used for duration of cancer treatment or as instructed by physician. Use Caphosol® 2-10 times/day for relief of dry mouth or as instructed by physician. Patients subjectively report some aid in swallowing and reduction of pain. Patients may also require systemic and topical analgesics for pain relief depending on the presence of mucositis. Positive fungal cultures may require a nystatin swish-and-swallow prescription or the selection of another antifungal agent (see Fungal Infections on page 1945).

D. The determination of performing dental procedures must be based on the goal of preventing infection during periods of neutropenia and reducing the risk of bleeding when platelet counts are low. Timing of procedures must be coordinated with the patient's hematologic status.

E. If oral surgery is required, at least 7-10 days of healing should be allowed before the anticipated date of bone marrow suppression (eg, ANC <1000/mm^3 and/or platelet count of ≥50,000/mm^3).

F. Daily use of topical fluorides is recommended for those who have received radiation therapy to the head and neck region involving salivary glands. Any patients with prolonged xerostomia subsequent to graft-vs-host disease and/or chemotherapy can also be considered for fluoride supplement. Use the fluoride-containing mouthwashes (Act®, Fluorigard®, etc) each night before going to sleep; swish, hold 1-2 minutes, spit out or use prescription fluorides (gels or rinses); apply daily for 1-4 minutes as directed; if mouth is sore (mucositis), use flavorless/colorless gels (Thera-Flur®, Gel-Kam®). Custom trays for fluoride applications can be produced by the clinician for the patient's home use using heat-formed materials such as omnivac. Improvement in salivary flow following radiation therapy to the head and neck has been noted with prescription sialogogue Salagen® on page 1346 or Evoxac® on page 355.

Benzonatate on page 222
Cevimeline on page 355
Chlorhexidine Gluconate on page 360
DiphenhydrAMINE (Systemic) on page 540
Gelclair® Bioadherent Oral Gel® on page 1168
Lidocaine (Topical) on page 1010
MuGard™
Pilocarpine (Systemic) on page 1346
Povidone-Iodine (Topical) on page 1382
Sucralfate on page 1554

ORAL CARE PRODUCTS

BACTERIAL PLAQUE CONTROL

Patients should use an extra soft bristle toothbrush and dental floss for removal of plaque. Sponge/foam sticks and lemon-glycerine swabs do not adequately remove bacterial plaque.

CHOLINERGIC AGENTS

See Products for Xerostomia on page 1955

Used for the treatment of xerostomia caused by radiation therapy in patients with head and neck cancer and from Sjögren's syndrome

Cevimeline on page 355
Pilocarpine (Systemic) on page 1346

FLUORIDES

See Fluorides in the Dentin Hypersensitivity, High Caries Index, and Xerostomia section.

Used for the prevention of demineralization of the tooth structure secondary to xerostomia. For patients with long-term or permanent xerostomia, daily application is accomplished using custom gel applicator trays, such as omnivac. Patients with porcelain crowns should use a neutral pH fluoride (see Fluoride monograph on page 752). Final selection of a fluoride product and/or saliva replacement/stimulant product must be based on patient comfort, taste, and ultimately, compliance. Experience has demonstrated that, often times, patients must try various combinations to achieve the greatest effect and their highest comfort levels. The presence of mucositis during cancer management complicates the clinician's selection of products.

SALIVA SUBSTITUTES

See Products for Xerostomia on page 1955

ORAL AND LIP MOISTURIZERS/LUBRICANTS

Note: Water-based gels should first be used to provide moisture to dry oral tissues.

Surgi-Lube®
K-Y Jelly®
Oral Balance®
Mouth Moisturizer®
Caphosol®

PALLIATION OF PAIN

Note: Palliative pain preparations should be monitored for efficacy.

- For relief of pain associated with isolated mucositis or ulcerations, topical anesthetic and protective preparations may be used.
  - Orabase-B® with 20% benzocaine on page 218
  - Zilactin-B® gel with 10% benzocaine
- For generalized oral pain:
  - Chloraseptic Spray® (OTC) anesthetic spray without alcohol on page 1336
  - Ulcer-Ease® anesthetic/analgesic mouthrinse
  - BetaCell® oral rinse
  - Xylocaine® 2% viscous on page 1010
    Note: May anesthetize swallowing mechanism and cause aspiration of food; caution patient against using too close to eating; lack of sensation may also allow patient to damage intact mucosa
  - Tantum Mouthrinse® (benzydamine hydrochloride); may be diluted as required
    Note: Available only in Canada and Europe

Patient-Prepared Palliative Mixtures

Coating agents:
Maalox® on page 93
Mylanta® on page 93
Kaopectate® on page 191

These products can be mixed with Benadryl® elixir (50:50):
DiphenhydrAMINE (Systemic) (Benadryl®) on page 540

Topical anesthetics (diphenhydramine chloride):
Benadryl® elixir or Benylin® cough syrup on page 540
Note: Choose product with lowest alcohol and sucrose content; ask pharmacist for assistance
Mucotrol gel wafer

Pharmacy Preparations

A pharmacist may also prepare the following solutions for relief of generalized oral pain:

Benadryl-Lidocaine Solution
Diphenhydramine injectable 1.5 mL (50 mg/mL) on page 540
Xylocaine viscous 2% (45 mL) on page 1010
Magnesium aluminum hydroxide solution (45 mL)
Swish and hold 1 teaspoonful in mouth for 30 seconds; do not use too close to eating

DENTIST'S ROLE IN RECOGNIZING DOMESTIC VIOLENCE, ABUSE, AND NEGLECT

Recognition of the signs and symptoms of domestic violence is an important topic for dental and medical professionals throughout the world. Unfortunately, statistics related to domestic abuse and/or neglect of women, children, and the elderly appear to be on the rise, perhaps, in part, due to increased recognition.

Statistics are indeed staggering. In the United States, a woman, child, or elder is physically abused every 5-15 seconds. In fact, violence is cited as one of the common causes of emergency room admissions for women 15-44 years of age. Furthermore, 50,000 deaths occur annually, which are attributable to violence in the form of homicide or suicide.

The dentist's responsibilities and professional role in this arena are not clear in all states. The literature, however, is clear regarding how each professional has the responsibility to understand current state laws regarding the reporting of domestic violence, abuse of children or the elderly, and/or neglect. Many states have existing codes defining the role of the professional in these regards. Many other states, such as Maryland, have adopted continuing education requirements specific to the subject. The overall problem of domestic violence, including child abuse, neglect, and other forms of abuse, are indeed public health issues. Likewise, the costs (eg, medical, dental, psychiatric, hospital, and emergency care fees) are borne to a great extent by the community as well as the individual.

Domestic abuse is defined as "controlling behavior." Neglect can take on a myriad of presentations. Although this often includes physical injury, the primary focus of domestic abuse is one person being in control of another person, making that person do something against his/her will. Women are often abused both physically and mentally in relationships that have existed for many years. Children are often the focus of domestic violence; however, the pattern for an entire family's abuse may be present. Abuse comes in many forms and many victims do not even realize that abuse is occurring. Some victims simply "chalk it up" to things that happen within families. Abuse may include battery and physical assault, such as throwing objects, pushing, hitting, slapping, kicking, or attacking with a weapon; sexual assault including the abuser forcing sexual activities upon another; and psychological abuse, such as forcing a victim to perform degrading or humiliating acts, threatening harm to a female or male partner or child, or destroying valued possessions of another. Verbal abuse can also be included; however, psychological forms of abuse are very difficult to ascertain and signs and symptoms may be difficult to separate from other psychological traits. Abuse tends to have a cyclic pattern, often where a partner or the controlling individual is extremely friendly, intimate, and a good household member; however, due to unknown reasons, as tension develops, family violence often erupts. Once battering has begun, it often increases in frequency and in severity with time. Early recognition can often prevent serious effects; however, until physical violence becomes part of the domestic abuse situation, recognition is usually difficult.

It is estimated that nearly 65% of abuse cases (where physical injury is involved) include injury to the head, neck, or mouth; therefore, dental professionals are in a unique position to detect and perhaps, if appropriate in that state, report suspected abuse. In children, these percentages are even higher. Being wards of adults, children are vulnerable. Child abuse includes any act that is not accidental, endangering or impairing a child's safety or emotional health. Types of child abuse may include physical abuse, emotional abuse and neglect, including neglect of proper healthcare. Any child suspected of suffering from an emotional injury, including sexual abuse or neglect, should be brought to the attention of the social welfare system. Occasionally, "Munchausen syndrome," which is defined as the guardians fabricating or inducing illness in the child, may be observed. Intentional poisoning and safety neglect are also included in this syndrome.

From a medical point-of-view, neglect is much more difficult to determine than abuse. The role of the dentist may be to define the state of normal and customary pediatric or elderly patient health within a locality; however, due to parents and families moving about the country, sometimes one standard may not be appropriate for all locations. Several key behavioral indicators:

- child, adult, or elderly patient:
  - avoids eye contact
  - is wary of a guardian or spouse

  - demonstrates fear when touched
  - exhibits dramatic mood changes (eg, hostile or aggressive behavior)
- history or reports of suicide attempts or running away
- unexplained injuries or injuries inconsistent with explanation or delay in seeking treatment
- inappropriate use of prescription drugs (ie, responsible adult controls compliance of a child or elderly patient)
- individual decides to change practitioner when questioned too intensely

For the dentist, head-neck examination is important and includes gathering an overall visual impression of general cleanliness, dress, and stature and examining for any specific physical indicators such as bruises, welts, bite marks, abrasions, lacerations, or other injuries to the head or neck. Contusions or bruises represent the highest percentage of abuse injuries to the young child. The extremely young child or infant often suffers fractures, which fall to second place in terms of incidence as the child matures. In the adult, fractures are much less common. The dentist needs to document the location since this often represents the characteristic that may be difficult for the person to explain. Common areas for injuries include the bony eminences over the knees, shins, and elbows but could also be on the face, including the zygomatic arch and the chin. Burns are rarer, but represent one of the most serious types of injuries. Intraoral injuries, including trauma to the oral mucosa, tooth fractures, palatal lesions, ecchymoses, and fractures, represent serious evidence of domestic or child abuse. Physical indicators of sexual abuse may not be obvious to the dentist; however, bruising of the hard palate or other evidence of sexual dysfunction may sometimes be found.

The dentist has the responsibility to document, from a forensic point-of-view, the characteristics of abuse that are observed. As with all diagnostic considerations, the dentist must form a differential diagnosis to rule in or out oral and dental pathologies before suspecting abuse or neglect. History and probability are key to making these determinations. If necessary, evidence including impressions for bite marks or photographs to document unexplained injuries to the head, neck, and face may be necessary. The legal liability for the dentist is determined by the state laws governing the dental practice. The dental practitioner's failure to diagnose child abuse and neglect is another consideration which goes along with ethical and legal considerations. States are generally much more clear in the area of child abuse than they are regarding spousal or elderly abuse or overall domestic violence. The dentist has a responsibility to refer a patient for a second opinion, such as to their primary care pediatrician or internist, if there are concerns of abuse.

Under the Federal Child Abuse Prevention and Treatment Act (CAPTA) passed in 1974, all 50 states have passed laws mandating the reporting of child abuse and neglect. CAPTA provides a foundation for states by identifying a minimum set of acts or behaviors that characterize physical abuse, neglect, and sexual abuse. These laws vary from state to state. Each states responsible for the following:

- providing its own definition of child abuse and neglect
- describing the circumstances and conditions that obligate mandated individuals to report known or suspected child abuse
- providing definitions for juvenile/family courts when to take custody of the child
- specifying the forms of maltreatment that are criminally punishable

Unfortunately, there is little uniformity in the state laws regarding either the responsibility for reporting adult domestic violence or abuse or in protecting the healthcare professional by reporting, in good faith, abuse situations. When spousal or elderly abuse or other domestic violence is suspected, the definitions become even less clear. They are very similar in ambiguity to those that are faced by the professional regarding neglect as opposed to direct physical or mental abuse. The American Dental Association code is clear on principles and ethics regarding professional conduct regarding the responsibility for recognition of child abuse. They are much less clear on spousal or other abuse and it is likely that in the future, as some consistency is noted between and among the various state laws, the ADA Council will undoubtedly take a stronger position.

It is clearly up to the individual states to take the lead in establishing strict guidelines for recognition and reporting of domestic abuse, including protection under the "good faith" statutes for the practitioner. Rules and regulations regarding malicious reporting should also be better defined. The national position is difficult to define because of the extreme variation among states. Dentists are encouraged to use their best judgment in proceeding in any situation of suspected domestic abuse or neglect. They should primarily know their state laws and join in the discussion of the topic so that appropriate state actions and formation of legal codes can be undertaken. The current move by some states toward requiring continuing education on these subjects is an excellent sign that there is movement in a constructive direction.

REFERENCES

American Academy of Pediatric Dentistry, "Clinical Guideline on Oral and Dental Aspects of Child Abuse and Neglect," *Pediatr Dent*, 2004, 26(7 Suppl):63-6.

Manea S, Favero GA, Stellini E, et al, "Dentists' Perceptions, Attitudes, Knowledge, and Experience About Child Abuse and Neglect in Northeast Italy," *J Clin Pediatr Dent*, 2007, 32(1):19-25.

"Oral and Dental Aspects of Child Abuse and Neglect. American Academy of Pediatrics. Committee on Child Abuse and Neglect. American Academy of Pediatric Dentistry. Ad Hoc Work Group on Child Abuse and Neglect," *Pediatrics*, 1999, 104(2 Pt 1):348-50.

Podnieks E, "Elder Abuse and Neglect: A Concern for the Dental Profession," *J Can Dent Assoc*, 1993, 9 (11):915-20.

Stechey F, "P.A.N.D.A. A Dentist's Introduction to Recognizing Child Abuse," *Dental Practice Management*, 2001. Available at: http://www.rcdso.org/life/ll_learning_pdf/DPM_PANDA.pdf

Tsang A and Sweet D, "Detecting Child Abuse and Neglect - Are Dentists Doing Enough?" *J Can Dent Assoc*, 1999, 65(7):387-91.

Wiseman M, "The Role of the Dentist in Recognizing Elder Abuse," *J Can Dent Assoc*, 2008, 74 (8):715-20.

ORAL MEDICINE TOPICS

PART III:

SAMPLE PRESCRIPTIONS

Drug prescriptions shown represent prototype drugs and popular prescriptions and are examples only. The pharmacologic category index is available for cross-referencing if alternatives and additional drugs are sought.

TABLE OF CONTENTS

INFECTIVE ENDOCARDITIS (PREVENTION)

General Prescription Comments

Prescriptions dispense amounts are for 3 visits. These numbers can be adjusted for each patient treatment plan.

Sample Prescriptions

Rx:

Amoxicillin 500 mg
Disp: 12 tablets
Sig: 4 tablets (2 g) 30-60 minutes prior to dental visit and repeat at each appointment

Rx:

Clindamycin (Systemic) 150 mg
Disp: 12 capsules
Sig: 4 capsules (600 mg) 30-60 minutes prior to dental visit and repeat at each appointment

Rx:

Cephalexin 500 mg
Disp: 12 tablets
Sig: 4 tablets (2 g) 30-60 minutes prior to dental visit and repeat at each appointment

Rx:

Azithromycin (Systemic) 500 mg
Disp: 3 tablets
Sig: 1 tablet 30-60 minutes prior to dental visit and repeat at each appointment

PROSTHETIC JOINT LATE INFECTIONS (PREVENTION)

General Prescription Comments

Prescriptions dispense amounts are for 3 visits. These numbers can be adjusted for each patient treatment plan.

Sample Prescriptions

Rx:

Amoxicillin 500 mg
Disp: 12 tablets
Sig: 4 tablets (2 g) 1 hour prior to dental visit and repeat at each appointment

Rx:

Clindamycin (Systemic) 150 mg
Disp: 12 capsules
Sig: 4 capsules (600 mg) 1 hour prior to dental visit and repeat at each appointment

Rx:

Cephalexin 500 mg
Disp: 12 tablets
Sig: 4 tablets (2 g) 1 hour prior to dental visit and repeat at each appointment

ORAL PAIN

Mild / Moderate Oral Pain

General Prescription Comments

Recently, the FDA has formally requested manufacturers to limit the amount of acetaminophen in prescription combination products (Vicodin®, Lortab®) to no more than 325 mg per dosage unit. The FDA is also requiring manufacturers to update labeling of all prescription combination acetaminophen products to warn of the potential risk for severe liver injury (see Oral Pain on page 1928 for more information).

Note: Numerous brand name products for infants and children that contain ibuprofen or acetaminophen have been voluntarily recalled by manufacturers due to investigation by the FDA.

Closely monitor and re-evaluate response at least every 2 weeks. If response is inadequate, re-evaluate diagnosis, medication choice, and dosage.

Sample Prescriptions

Rx:

Acetaminophen 325 mg tablets
Disp: To be determined by practitioner
Sig: Take 2-3 tablets every 4 hours

Note: Products include Tylenol® and others.
Note: Acetaminophen can be given if patient has allergies, bleeding problems, or stomach upset secondary to aspirin or NSAIDs.

Rx:

Ibuprofen 200 mg tablets
Disp: To be determined by practitioner
Sig: Take 1-2 tablets every 4 hours

Note: Ibuprofen is an available OTC as Advil®, Motrin® IB, Nuprin®, and many store brand generic names. NSAIDs should not be combined with aspirin. NSAIDs may increase post-treatment bleeding. Use with caution in patients receiving anticoagulants or antiplatelet drugs.

Rx:

Naproxen sodium 220 mg tablets
Disp: To be determined by practitioner
Sig: Take 1-2 tablets every 8 hours

Note: Naproxen sodium is an available OTC as Aleve® and many store brand generic names.

Rx:

Ibuprofen 400 mg tablets
Disp: 20 tablets
Sig: Take 1 tablet every 4-6 hours as needed for pain

Note: Prescription strength ibuprofen is available as the brand name Motrin®.

Rx:

Dolobid® 500 mg tablets
Disp: 16 tablets
Sig: Take 2 tablets initially, then 1 tablet every 8-12 hours as needed for pain

Ingredient: Diflunisal

Moderate / Moderately Severe Oral Pain

General Prescription Comments

Closely monitor and re-evaluate response at least every 2 weeks. If response is inadequate, re-evaluate diagnosis, medication choice, and dosage.

Sample Prescriptions

Rx:

Ibuprofen 800 mg tablets
Disp: 16 tablets
Sig: Take 1 tablet 3 times/day as needed for pain
Note: For severe pain can be given up to 4 times/day. Also available as 600 mg tablets.

Rx:

TraMADol 50 mg tablets
Disp: 36 tablets
Sig: Take 1-2 tablets every 4-6 hours as needed for pain

Note: Also available as the brand name Ultram®.

Rx:

Ultracet® tablets
Disp: 36 tablets
Sig: Take 2 tablets every 4-6 hours as needed for pain, not to exceed 8 tablets in 24 hours

Ingredients: Acetaminophen 325 mg and Tramadol 37.5 mg

Rx:

Vicoprofen® tablets
Disp: 16 tablets
Sig: Take 1-2 tablets every 4-6 hours as needed for pain

Note: Restrictions: C-III; no refills
Ingredients: Hydrocodone 7.5 mg and ibuprofen 200 mg; available as generic equivalent

Note: The following popular combination products, Vicodin® ES and Lortab®, contain more than 325 mg of acetaminophen; therefore, these products will be phased out over the next 3 years per the FDA request (see Oral Pain on page 1928 or the FDA website for more information).

Rx:

Vicodin® ES tablets
Disp: 16 tablets
Sig: Take 1 tablet every 4-6 hours as needed for pain

Note: Restrictions: C-III; no refills
Ingredients: Hydrocodone bitartrate 7.5 mg and acetaminophen 750 mg; available as generic equivalent. Also available as Vicodin® tablets: Ingredients: Hydrocodone bitartrate 5 mg and acetaminophen 500 mg; take 1 tablet every 4 hours as needed for pain.

Rx:

Lortab® 5 mg
Disp: 16 tablets
Sig: Take 1 or 2 tablets every 4 hours as needed for pain; not to exceed 8 tablets in 24 hours

Note: Restrictions: C-III; no refills
Ingredients: Hydrocodone 5 mg and acetaminophen 500 mg; available as generic equivalent

Rx:

Norco® 10 mg
Disp: 16 tablets
Sig: Take 1 or 2 tablets every 4 hours as needed for pain; not to exceed 8 tablets in 24 hours

Note: Restrictions: C-III; no refills
Ingredients: Hydrocodone 10 mg and acetaminophen 325 mg; available as generic equivalent

Rx:

Tylenol® #3
Disp: 16 tablets
Sig: Take 1 tablet every 4 hours as needed for pain

Note: Restrictions: C-III; no refills
Ingredients: Codeine 30 mg and acetaminophen 300 mg; available as generic equivalent

Rx:

Naproxen 275 mg tablets
Disp: 16 tablets
Sig: Take 2 tablets initially, then one tablet 3 times/day as needed for pain

Severe Oral Pain

General Prescription Comments

Closely monitor and re-evaluate response at least every 2 weeks. If response is inadequate, re-evaluate diagnosis, medication choice, and dosage.

Liquid volumes are suggested for a typical 2-week course. Check with pharmacist for available sizes.

Cream and ointment tube sizes may vary based on availability. Refer to individual monograph or check with pharmacist for available sizes.

Sample Prescriptions

Rx:

Percocet® tablets
Disp: 16 tablets or capsules
Sig: Take 1 tablet or capsule every 6 hours as needed for pain

Note: Restrictions: C-II; no refills
Ingredients: Oxycodone 5 mg and acetaminophen 325 mg; available as generic equivalent; triplicate prescription required in some states

Rx:

Oxycodone and Ibuprofen tablets
Disp: 16 tablets
Sig: Take 1 tablet every 6 hours as needed for pain

Note: Restrictions: C-II; no refills
Ingredients: Oxycodone 5 mg and ibuprofen 400 mg; triplicate prescription required in some states

Rx:

Demerol® 50 mg tablets
Disp: 16 tablets
Sig: Take 1 tablet every 4 hours as needed for pain

Note: Restrictions: C-II; no refills
Ingredients: Meperidine; triplicate prescription required in some states

BACTERIAL INFECTIONS AND PERIODONTAL DISEASES

General Prescription Comments

Closely monitor and re-evaluate response at least every 2 weeks. If response is inadequate, re-evaluate diagnosis, medication choice, and dosage.

Sample Prescriptions

Rx:

Penicillin V potassium 500 mg
Disp: 40 tablets
Sig: Take 1 tablet 4 times/day for 7-10 days (consider a loading dose of 1 g for acute infection)

Rx:

Clindamycin (Systemic) 150 mg
Disp: 40 capsules
Sig: Take 1 capsule 4 times/day for 7-10 days

Note: Prescription usually selected for patients allergic to penicillin; may be prescribed for 3 or 4 times/day

Rx:

Clindamycin (Systemic) 300 mg
Disp: 40 capsules
Sig: Take 1 capsule 4 times/day for 7-10 days

Note: Prescription usually selected for patients allergic to penicillin; may be prescribed for 3 or 4 times/day

Rx:

Azithromycin (Systemic) 250 mg
Disp: 1 Z-Pak®
Sig: 2 tablets day 1, then 1 tablet/day until gone

OTHER ANTIBIOTICS:

Rx:

Amoxicillin 250 mg
Disp: 30 capsules
Sig: Take 1 capsule 3 times/day for 7-10 days

Rx:

Amoxicillin 500 mg
Disp: 30 capsules or tablets
Sig: Take 1 capsule or tablet 3 times/day for 7-10 days

Rx:

Amoxicillin 875 mg
Disp: 20 tablets
Sig: Take 1 tablet twice daily

Rx:

Augmentin® 250 mg
Disp: 30 tablets
Sig: Take 1 tablet 3 times/day for 7-10 days

Rx:

Augmentin® 500 mg
Disp: 30 tablets
Sig: Take 1 tablet 3 times/day for 7-10 days

Rx:

Augmentin® 875 mg
Disp: 20 tablets
Sig: Take 1 tablet twice daily for 7-10 days

Rx:

Augmentin XR™ 1000 mg
Disp: 20 tablets
Sig: Take 2 tablets twice daily for 7-10 days

Rx:
Cephalexin 250 mg
Disp: 40 capsules
Sig: Take 1 capsule 4 times/day for 7-10 days

Rx:
MetroNIDAZOLE (Systemic) 500 mg
Disp: 40 tablets
Sig: Take 1 tablet 4 times/day for 7-10 days

Note: Usually used in combination with amoxicillin; may be prescribed for 3 or 4 times/day

Rx:
Erythromycin (Systemic) 250 mg
Disp: 40 tablets
Sig: Take 1 tablet 4 times/day for 7-10 days

Note: Prescription for patients allergic to penicillin

Rx:
Zithromax® TRI-PAK™ 500 mg
Disp: 1 PAK
Sig: Follow package insert directions until gone

Ingredient: Azithromycin (Systemic)

Rx:
Levaquin® 500 mg
Disp: 10 tablets
Sig: Take 1 tablet/day until gone

PERIODONTAL DISEASE:

Note: Sample prescriptions based on dosing suggestions from the American Academy of Periodontology

Rx:
Azithromycin (Systemic) 500 mg tablets
Disp: Dispense a dose pack
Sig: Take 1 tablet daily for 4-7 days as directed

Rx:
Ciprofloxacin (Systemic) 500 mg tablets
Disp: 16 tablets
Sig: Take 1 tablet 2 times/day for 8 days

Rx:
Clindamycin (Systemic) 300 mg tablets
Disp: 24 tablets
Sig: Take 1 tablet 3 times/day for 8 days

Rx:
Doxycycline or Minocycline 100-200 mg tablets
Disp: 21 tablets of selected dose
Sig: Take 1 tablet daily for 21 days

Rx:
MetroNIDAZOLE (Systemic) 500 mg
Disp: 24 tablets
Sig: Take 1 tablet 3 times/day for 8 days

Rx:
MetroNIDAZOLE (Systemic) and Amoxicillin 250 mg or 500 mg tablets
Disp: 24 tablets of each drug
Sig: Take 1 tablet of each drug 3 times/day for 8 days

Rx:
MetroNIDAZOLE (Systemic) and Ciprofloxacin (Systemic) 500 mg tablets
Disp: 16 tablets of each drug
Sig: Take 1 tablet of each drug 2 times/day for 8 days

SINUS INFECTION TREATMENT

General Prescription Comments

Closely monitor and re-evaluate response at least every 2 weeks. If response is inadequate, re-evaluate diagnosis, medication choice, and dosage.

Sinus infections represent a common condition which may present with confounding dental complaints. Treatment is sometimes instituted by the dentist, but due to the often chronic and recurrent nature of sinus infections, early involvement of an otolaryngologist is advised. These infections may require antibiotics of varying spectrum, as well as requiring the management of sinus congestion. Although amoxicillin is usually adequate, many otolaryngologists initially prescribe Augmentin®. Second generation cephalosporins, azithromycin and clarithromycin are sometimes used depending on the chronicity of the problem.

Sample Prescriptions

Rx:
Afrin® nasal spray [OTC]
Disp: 15 mg
Sig: Spray once in each nostril every 6-8 hours for no more than 3 days

Ingredient: Oxymetazoline (Nasal)

Rx:
Sudafed® 60 mg tablets [OTC]
Disp: 30 tablets
Sig: Take 1 tablet every 4-6 hours as needed for congestion

Ingredient: Pseudoephedrine

Rx:
Chlor-Trimeton® 4 mg [OTC]
Disp: 14 tablets
Sig: Take 1 tablet twice daily

Ingredient: Chlorpheniramine

Rx:
Azithromycin (Systemic) 250 mg
Disp: 1 Z-Pak®
Sig: 2 tablets day 1, then 1 tablet/day until gone

OTHER ANTIBIOTICS:

Rx:
Amoxicillin 250 mg
Disp: 30 capsules
Sig: Take 1 capsule 3 times/day for 7-10 days

Rx:
Amoxicillin 500 mg
Disp: 30 capsules or tablets
Sig: Take 1 capsule or tablet 3 times/day for 7-10 days

Rx:
Amoxicillin 875 mg
Disp: 20 tablets
Sig: Take 1 tablet twice daily

Rx:
Augmentin® 250 mg
Disp: 30 tablets
Sig: Take 1 tablet 3 times/day for 7-10 days

Rx:
Augmentin® 500 mg
Disp: 30 tablets
Sig: Take 1 tablet 3 times/day for 7-10 days

Rx:
Augmentin® 875 mg
Disp: 20 tablets
Sig: Take 1 tablet twice daily for 7-10 days

Rx:
Augmentin XR™ 1000 mg
Disp: 20 tablets
Sig: Take 2 tablets twice daily for 7-10 days

ANTIMICROBIAL ORAL RINSE

General Prescription Comments

Closely monitor and re-evaluate response at least every 2 weeks. If response is inadequate, re-evaluate diagnosis, medication choice, and dosage.

Liquid volumes for antimicrobial rinses are suggested for a typical 1 month course. Check with pharmacist for available sizes.

Sample Prescriptions

Rx:

Chlorhexidine gluconate 0.12% oral rinse
Disp: 32 oz bottle
Sig: Rinse with ½ oz twice daily for 30 seconds and expectorate

Note: Chlorhexidine gluconate available as the following brands: Peridex®, Perio-Gard®

Rx:

Listerine® antiseptic mouthwash [OTC]
Disp: Bottle
Sig: 20 mL, swish for 30 seconds twice daily

FUNGAL INFECTIONS

Topical Fungal Infections

General Prescription Comments

Closely monitor and re-evaluate response at least every 2 weeks. If response is inadequate, re-evaluate diagnosis, medication choice, and dosage.

Liquid volumes are suggested for a typical 2-week course. Check with pharmacist for available sizes.

Cream and ointment tube sizes may vary based on availability. Refer to individual monograph or check with pharmacist for available sizes.

Sample Prescriptions

Rx:
Nystatin (Oral) 100,000 units/mL oral suspension
Disp: 300 mL
Sig: Rinse with 1 teaspoon (5 mL) for 2 minutes 4-5 times/day and expectorate

Rx:
Nystatin (Topical) ointment
Disp: 15 g tube
Sig: Apply locally as directed with a thin coat to inner surface of denture and the affected area 4-5 times/day

Rx:
Mycelex® 10 mg troches
Disp: 70 troches
Sig: Dissolve 1 troche in mouth 5 times/day until gone; leave any prosthesis out during treatment and soak prosthesis in nystatin liquid suspension overnight

Ingredient: Clotrimazole (Oral)

Rx:
Nizoral® 2% cream
Disp: 15 g tube
Sig: Apply locally as directed with a thin coat to inner surface of denture and affected areas after meals

Ingredient: Ketoconazole (Topical)

Systemic Fungal Infections

General Prescription Comments

Note: Decision to use systemic antifungals should be based on diagnostic culture results or positive smear.

Closely monitor and re-evaluate response at least every 2 weeks. If response is inadequate, re-evaluate diagnosis, medication choice, and dosage.

Sample Prescriptions

Rx:
Nizoral® 200 mg tablets
Disp: 14 tablets
Sig: Take 1 tablet daily, with a meal for 2 weeks

Note: May cause irreversible liver damage; liver function should be monitored with long-term use (ie, >3 weeks)

Ingredient: Ketoconazole (Systemic)

Rx:
Diflucan® 100 mg tablets
Disp: 16 tablets
Sig: Take 2 tablets day 1, then 1 tablet/day until gone

Note: Sometimes a shorter course is adequate. However, oral infections commonly are more difficult to eradicate and often a 21-day course, or even a second course, may be necessary.
Ingredient: Fluconazole

Rx:

Posaconazole 100 mg tablets
Disp: 14 tablets
Sig: Take 2 tablets the first day, followed by 1 tablet each day for 13 days

Note: Posaconazole has been recently approved for use in patients refractory to itraconazole or fluconazole

Angular Cheilitis

General Prescription Comments

Closely monitor and re-evaluate response at least every 2 weeks. If response is inadequate, re-evaluate diagnosis, medication choice, and dosage.

Cream and ointment tube sizes may vary based on availability. Refer to individual monograph or check with pharmacist for available sizes.

Sample Prescriptions

Rx:

Iodoquinol and Hydrocortisone cream
Disp: 45 g tube
Sig: Apply locally as directed 3-4 times/day for 10 days to 2 weeks and then re-evaluate

Note: Available sizes may include 15 g, 30 g, and 45 g tubes. Other associated etiologies for angular cheilitis must also be considered such as loss of vertical dimension, trauma, and vitamin deficiencies.

Rx:

Nystatin and Triamcinolone acetonide ointment
Disp: 30 g tube
Sig: Apply locally as directed to affected area 4 times/day for 10 days to 2 weeks and then re-evaluate

Note: Available sizes may include 15 g, 30 g, and 60 g tubes. Other associated etiologies for angular cheilitis must also be considered such as loss of vertical dimension, trauma, and vitamin deficiencies.

VIRAL INFECTIONS

Herpes Simplex (Primary)

General Prescription Comments

Closely monitor and re-evaluate response at least every 2 weeks. If response is inadequate, re-evaluate diagnosis, medication choice, and dosage.

Sample Prescriptions

Rx:
Zovirax® 200 mg capsules
Disp: 50 or 60 capsules
Sig: Take 1 capsule 5 times/day for 10 days or 2 capsules 3 times/day for 10 days

Ingredient: Acyclovir (Systemic)

Rx:
Zovirax® ointment 5%
Disp: 15 g tube
Sig: Apply thin layer to lesions 6 times/day for 7 days.

Ingredient: Acyclovir (Topical)

Herpes Simplex (Recurrent)

General Prescription Comments

Closely monitor and re-evaluate response at least every 2 weeks. If response is inadequate, re-evaluate diagnosis, medication choice, and dosage.

Cream and ointment tube sizes may vary based on availability. Refer to individual monograph or check with pharmacist for available sizes.

Sample Prescriptions

Rx:
Denavir® topical cream 1%
Disp: 1.5 g tube
Sig: Apply locally as directed to lesion every 2 hours during waking hours (begin when symptoms first occur)

Ingredient: Penciclovir

Rx:
Famciclovir 500 mg tablets
Disp: 3 tablets
Sig: Take 3 tablets (1500 mg) as a singe dose; therapy should be initiated at the first sign of any prodrome such as tingling, burning, or itching

Note: Dispense in multiples of 3 so that patient has drug on hand for any recurrences; available as generic equivalent

Rx:
ValACYclovir 500 mg
Disp: 8 caplets
Sig: 4 caplets twice daily for 1 day (separate doses by 12 hours); therapy should be initiated at the first sign of any prodrome such as tingling, burning, or itching

Rx:
Abreva® cream [OTC]
Disp: 2 g tube
Sig: Apply to lesion 5 times/day during waking hours for 4 days (begin when symptoms first occur)

Ingredient: Docosanol

Rx:
Viroxyn® [OTC]
Disp: 1 pack of 3 individual swab kits
Sig: Apply locally as directed at first symptoms of recurrence

Ingredient: Benzalkonium 0.13% in isopropyl alcohol

Rx:

Zovirax® cream 5%
Disp: 2 g tube; 5 g tube
Sig: Apply 5 times/day for 4 days

Ingredient: Acyclovir (Topical)

Shingles (Varicella-Zoster Virus)

General Prescription Comments

Closely monitor and re-evaluate response at least every 2 weeks. If response is inadequate, re-evaluate diagnosis, medication choice, and dosage.

Sample Prescriptions

Rx:

Zovirax® 200 mg capsules
Disp: 200 capsules
Sig: Take 4 capsules 5 times/day for 10 days

Ingredient: Acyclovir (Systemic)

Rx:

Famciclovir 500 mg
Disp: 21 tablets
Sig: 1 tablet 3 times/day for 7 days

ULCERATIVE AND EROSIVE DISORDERS

Recurrent Aphthous Stomatitis

General Prescription Comments

Some intraoral uses are off-label. Write directions as "use locally as directed" and closely monitor and re-evaluate response at least every 2 weeks. If response is inadequate, re-evaluate diagnosis, medication choice, and dosage.

Liquid volumes are suggested for a typical 2-week course. Check with pharmacist for available sizes.

Cream and ointment tube sizes may vary based on availability. Refer to individual monograph or check with pharmacist for available sizes.

Sample Prescriptions

Palliative

Rx:
Amlexanox oral paste 5%
Disp: 5 g tube
Sig: Apply locally as directed, 4 times/day until area heals

Rx:
Orabase® Protective Barrier [OTC]
Disp: 1 package
Sig: Apply locally as directed, every 6 hours as needed

Rx:
Benadryl® liquid 12.5 mg/5 mL (mix 50/50) with Kaopectate®
Disp: 8 oz total
Sig: Rinse with 1-2 teaspoonfuls every 2 hours and expectorate

Note: Maalox® can be used in place of Kaopectate® if constipation is a problem. Benadryl® is available as a generic DiphenhydrAMINE liquid.

Rx:
Benadryl® liquid 12.5 mg/5mL / Kaopectate® / Lidocaine viscous (mix 1/3, 1/3, 1/3)
Disp: 8 oz total
Sig: Rinse with 1-2 teaspoonfuls every 2 hours and expectorate

Note: Maalox® can be used in place of Kaopectate® if constipation is a problem. Benadryl® is available as a generic DiphenhydrAMINE liquid. Lidocaine viscous is available as a prescription only.

Rx:
Benadryl® liquid 12.5 mg/5mL
Disp: 4 oz bottle
Sig: Rinse with 1-2 teaspoonfuls every 2 hours and expectorate

Note: Benadryl® is available as a generic DiphenhydrAMINE liquid.

Therapy Based (contain steroids)

Rx:
Oralone® 0.1%
Disp: 5 g tube
Sig: Apply locally as directed to the lesion after each meal and at bedtime

Ingredient: Triamcinolone (Topical)

Rx:
Fluocinonide 0.05% gel
Disp: 45 g tube
Sig: Apply locally as directed to lesion 4 times daily

Rx:
Temovate® 0.05%
Disp: 45 g tube
Sig: Apply locally as directed a small quantity with a Q-tip to affected area 3-4 times/day

Ingredient: Clobetasol propionate

Rx:

Betamethasone 0.1% ointment
Disp: 45 g tube
Sig: Apply locally as directed a small quantity with a Q-tip to affected area 3-4 times/day

Rx:

Decadron® elixir 0.5 mg/5 mL
Disp: 300 mL
Sig: Rinse with 1 teaspoon for 2 minutes 4 times/day and expectorate

Ingredient: Dexamethasone (Systemic)

Note: Depending on severity of ulceration, instructions can be tailored to include swallowing initial doses and then tapering to every other dose eventually over 4-7 days to no swallowing. See Erosive Lichen Planus, Other Biopsy-Proven Desquamative Oral Diseases, and Major Aphthae for more examples.

Mild Lichen Planus

General Prescription Comments

Some intraoral uses are off-label. Write directions as "use locally as directed" and closely monitor and re-evaluate response at least every 2 weeks. If response is inadequate, re-evaluate diagnosis, medication choice, and dosage.

Cream and ointment tube sizes may vary based on availability. Refer to individual monograph or check with pharmacist for available sizes.

Sample Prescriptions

Rx:

Oralone® 0.1%
Disp: 5 g tube
Sig: Apply locally as directed by coating the lesion with a thin film after each meal and at bedtime

Ingredient: Triamcinolone (Topical) 0.1%

Rx:

Fluocinonide 0.05% gel
Disp: 45 g tube
Sig: Apply locally as directed to lesion 4 times daily

Erosive Lichen Planus, Other Biopsy-Proven Desquamative Oral Diseases, and Major Aphthae

General Prescription Comments

Some intraoral uses are off-label. Write directions as "use locally as directed" and closely monitor and re-evaluate response at least every 2 weeks. If response is inadequate, re-evaluate diagnosis, medication choice, and dosage.

Liquid volumes are suggested for a typical 2-week course. Check with pharmacist for available sizes.

Cream and ointment tube sizes may vary based on availability. Refer to individual monograph or check with pharmacist for available sizes.

Note: Soft, thin, vacuum-formed trays can be made (similar to bleaching trays but extending slightly onto the gingiva) to deliver steroid ointments or creams to gingival lesions. Also, the pharmacist can compound potent steroids, such as clobetasol with Orabase®, to enhance adherence to oral tissues. For chronically recurring lesions, prednisone can be prescribed at 40 mg/day for week 1, 30 mg/day for week 2, continue tapering dose each week to 0. Occasionally, the clinician needs to tailor the regimen by using alternating doses every other day, such as 20 mg day 1, 10 mg day 2, then back to 20 mg. It is important to assess patient compliance when such a regimen is considered.

Sample Prescriptions

Rx:

Decadron® 0.5 mg/5 mL elixir
Disp: 400 mL bottle
Sig: For 3 days, rinse with 1 tablespoonful (15 mL) 4 times/day and swallow; then for 3 days, rinse with 1 teaspoonful (5 mL) 4 times/day and swallow; then for 3 days, rinse with 1 teaspoonful (5 mL) 4 times/day and swallow every other time. Then for 3 days rinse with 1 teaspoonful (5 mL) 4 times/day and expectorate. Continue the rinse and expectorate mode for 2 minutes but discontinue medication when mouth becomes completely comfortable.

Ingredient: Dexamethasone (Systemic); the practitioner can tailor this rinse, hold expectorate and/or swallow prescription to the severity and lesion location for each individual patient.

Rx:

Temovate® 0.05% cream
Disp: 15 g tube
Sig: Apply locally as directed 4-5 times/day

Ingredient: Clobetasol; high potency topical steroid

Rx:

PredniSONE 5 mg tablets
Disp: 40 tablets
Sig: Take 5 tablets in the morning for 5 days, then 5 tablets in the morning every other day until gone

Rx:

PredniSONE 10 mg tablets
Disp: 50 tablets
Sig: Take 4 tablets in the morning for 5 days, then decrease by 1 tablet on each successive series of 5 days

Rx:

Medrol® Dose Pak
Disp: 1 Pack
Sig: Follow package insert directions until gone

Ingredient: MethylPREDNISolone

SEDATION (PRIOR TO DENTAL TREATMENT)

General Prescription Comments

Sample prescription doses are for healthy adults. Use of these drugs and/or dosage may not be appropriate for children, elderly, and/or debilitated patients. Dental sedation should be used cautiously in these patients. Patients receiving sedative agents must be advised that they will need to have someone drive them to and from their appointment.

Sample Prescriptions for Adults

Rx:

Valium® 5 mg
Disp: 1 tablet
Sig: Take 1 tablet 1 hour before appointment

Note: Also available as 2 mg and 10 mg
Ingredient: Diazepam

Rx:

Ativan® 1 mg
Disp: 2 tablets
Sig: Take 2 tablets 1 hour before appointment

Note: Also available as 0.5 mg and 2 mg
Ingredient: LORazepam

Rx:

Xanax® 0.5 mg
Disp: 1 tablet
Sig: Take 1 tablet 1 hour before appointment

Ingredient: ALPRAZolam

Rx:

Vistaril® 25 mg
Disp: 2 capsules
Sig: Take 2 capsules 1 hour before appointment

Ingredient: HydrOXYzine

Rx:

Halcion® 0.25 mg
Disp: 1 tablet
Sig: Take 1 tablet 1 hour before appointment

Ingredient: Triazolam

APPENDIX TABLE OF CONTENTS

ABBREVIATIONS, ACRONYMS, AND SYMBOLS

Abbreviations Which May Be Used in This Reference

Abbreviation	Meaning
5-HT	5-hydroxytryptamine
AAP	American Academy of Pediatrics
ABG	arterial blood gases
ABW	adjusted body weight
AACT	American Academy of Clinical Toxicology
ACC	American College of Cardiology
ACE	angiotensin converting enzyme
ACLS	advanced cardiac life support
ACOG	American College of Obstetricians and Gynecologists
ACTH	adrenocorticotrophic hormone
ADH	alcohol dehydrogenase
ADHD	attention-deficit/hyperactivity disorder
ADLs	activities of daily living
AED	antiepileptic drug
AHA	American Heart Association
AIDS	acquired immune deficiency syndrome
AIMS	Abnormal Involuntary Movement Scale
ALS	amyotrophic lateral sclerosis
ALT	alanine aminotransferase
AMA	American Medical Association
ANC	absolute neutrophil count
aPTT	activated partial thromboplastin
ARB	angiotensin receptor blocker
ARDS	acute respiratory distress syndrome
AST	aspartate aminotransferase
AUC	area under the curve
BDI	Beck Depression Inventory
BEC	blood ethanol concentration
BLS	basic life support
BMI	body mass index
BMT	bone marrow transplant
BP	blood pressure
BPH	benign prostatic hyperplasia
BPRS	Brief Psychiatric Rating Scale
BSA	body surface area
BUN	blood urea nitrogen
CABG	coronary artery bypass graft
CAD	coronary artery disease
CAN	Canadian
CAPD	continuous ambulatory peritoneal dialysis
CAS	chemical abstract service
CBC	complete blood count
CBT	cognitive behavioral therapy
Cl_{cr}	creatinine clearance
CDC	Centers for Disease Control and Prevention
CF	cystic fibrosis
CGI	Clinical Global Impression

Abbreviations Which May Be Used in This Reference *(continued)*

Abbreviation	Meaning
CHD	coronary heart disease
CHF	congestive heart failure; chronic heart failure
CIE	chemotherapy-induced emesis
C-II	schedule two controlled substance
C-III	schedule three controlled substance
C-IV	schedule four controlled substance
C-V	schedule five controlled substance
CIV	continuous I.V. infusion
C_{max}	maximum plasma concentration
C_{min}	minimum plasma concentration
CMV	cytomegalovirus
CNS	central nervous system or coagulase negative staphylococcus
COLD	chronic obstructive lung disease
COPD	chronic obstructive pulmonary disease
COX	cyclooxygenase
CPK	creatine phosphokinase
CRF	chronic renal failure
CRP	C-reactive protein
CRRT	continuous renal replacement therapy
CSF	cerebrospinal fluid
CSII	continuous subcutaneous insulin infusion
CT	computed tomography
CVA	cerebrovascular accident
CVVH	continuous venovenous hemofiltration
CVVHD	continuous venovenous hemodialysis
CVVHDF	continuous venovenous hemodiafiltration
CYP	cytochrome
D_5W	dextrose 5% in water
DBP	diastolic blood pressure
DEHP	di(3-ethylhexyl)phthalate
DIC	disseminated intravascular coagulation
DM	diabetes mellitus
DMARD	disease modifying antirheumatic drug
DSC	discontinued
DSM-IV	Diagnostic and Statistical Manual
DVT	deep vein thrombosis
EBV	Epstein-Barr virus
ECG	electrocardiogram
ECMO	extracorporeal membrane oxygenation
ECT	electroconvulsive therapy
ED	emergency department
EEG	electroencephalogram
EF	ejection fraction
EG	ethylene glycol
EGA	estimated gestational age
EIA	enzyme immunoassay
ELISA	enzyme-linked immunosorbent assay
EPS	extrapyramidal side effects
ESR	erythrocyte sedimentation rate
ESRD	end stage renal disease
EtOH	alcohol
FDA	Food and Drug Administration

Abbreviations Which May Be Used in This Reference *(continued)*

Abbreviation	Meaning
FTT	failure to thrive
GABA	gamma-aminobutyric acid
GAD	generalized anxiety disorder
GERD	gastroesophageal reflux disease
GFR	glomerular filtration rate
GGT	gamma-glutamyltransferase
GI	gastrointestinal
GU	genitourinary
GVHD	graft versus host disease
HAM-A	Hamilton Anxiety Scale
HAM-D	Hamilton Depression Scale
HDL	high density lipoprotein
HF	heart failure
HFSA	Heart Failure Society of America
HIV	human immunodeficiency virus
HMG-CoA	3-hydroxy-3-methylglutaryl-coenzyme A
HOCM	hypertrophic obstructive cardiomyopathy
HPA	hypothalamic-pituitary-adrenal
HSV	herpes simplex virus
HTN	hypertension
HUS	hemolytic uremic syndrome
IBD	inflammatory bowel disease
IBS	irritable bowel syndrome
IBW	ideal body weight
ICD	implantable cardioverter defibrillator
ICH	intracranial hemorrhage
ICP	intracranial pressure
IDDM	insulin dependent diabetes mellitus
IDSA	Infectious Diseases Society of America
IHSS	idiopathic hypertrophic subaortic stenosis
I.M.	intramuscular
INR	international normalized ration
Int. unit	international unit
IOP	intraocular pressure
IUGR	intrauterine growth retardation
I.V.	intravenous
IVP	intravenous push
IVPB	intravenous piggyback
JIA	juvenile idiopathic arthritis
JNC	Joint National Committee
KIU	kallikrein inhibitor unit
LAMM	L-α-acetyl methadol
LDH	lactate dehydrogenase
LDL	low density lipoprotein
LFT	liver function test
LGA	large for gestational age
LR	lactated ringers
LVEF	left ventricular ejection fraction
LVH	left ventricular hypertrophy
MADRS	Montgomery Asbery Depression Rating Scale
MAOIs	monamine oxidase inhibitors
MDD	major depressive disorder

Abbreviations Which May Be Used in This Reference *(continued)*

Abbreviation	Meaning
MDRD	modification of diet in renal disease
MDRSP	multidrug resistant *streptococcus pneumoniae*
mEq	milliequivalent
mg	milligram
MI	myocardial infarction
mL	milliliter
mm	millimeter
mM	millimolar
mm Hg	millimeters of mercury
MMSE	mini mental status examination
M/P	milk to plasma ratio
MPS I	mucopolysaccharidosis I
MRHD	maximum recommended human dose
MRI	magnetic resonance imaging
MUGA	multiple gated acquisition scan
NAS	neonatal abstinence syndrome
NF	National Formulary
NFD	Nephrogenic fibrosing dermopathy
ng	nanogram
NIDDM	Noninsulin dependent diabetes mellitus
NKA	no known allergies
NKDA	No known drug allergies
NMDA	n-methyl-d-aspartic acid
NMS	neuroleptic malignant syndrome
NNRTI	non-nucleoside reverse transcriptase inhibitor
NRTI	nucleoside reverse transcriptase inhibitor
NS	normal saline
NSAID	nonsteroidal anti-inflammatory drug
NSF	nephrogenic systemic fibrosis
NSTEMI	Non-ST-elevation myocardial infarction
OA	osteoarthritis
OCD	obsessive-compulsive disorder
OHSS	ovarian hyperstimulation syndrome
OTC	over-the-counter
PAT	paroxysmal atrial tachycardia
PD	Parkinson's disease; peritoneal dialysis
PDA	patent ductus arteriosus
PDE-5	phosphodiesterase-5
PE	pulmonary embolus
PEG tube	percutaneous endoscopic gastrostomy tube
PHN	post-herpetic neuralgia
PID	pelvic inflammatory disease
PMDD	premenstrual dysphoric disorder
PONV	postoperative nausea and vomiting
PPN	peripheral parenteral nutrition
PROM	premature rupture of membranes
PSVT	paroxysmal supraventricular tachycardia
PT	prothrombin time
PTSD	post-traumatic stress disorder
PTT	partial thromboplastin time
PUD	peptic ulcer disease
PVD	peripheral vascular disease

Abbreviations Which May Be Used in This Reference *(continued)*

Abbreviation	Meaning
QT_c	corrected QT interval
QT_c-F	corrected QT interval by Fredricia's formula
RA	rheumatoid arthritis
REM	rapid eye movement
RPLS	reversible posterior leukoencephalopathy syndrome
SA	sinoatrial
SAD	seasonal affective disorder
SAH	subarachnoid hemorrhage
SBE	subacute bacterial endocarditis
SBP	systolic blood pressure
S_{Cr}	serum creatinine
SERM	selective estrogen receptor modulator
SGA	small for gestational age
SGOT	serum glutamic oxaloacetic aminotransferase
SGPT	serum glutamic pyruvate transaminase
SI	International System of Units or Systeme international d'Unites
SIADH	syndrome of inappropriate antidiuretic hormone secretion
SLE	systemic lupus erythematosus
SNRI	serotonin norepinephrine reuptake inhibitor
SSKI	saturated solution of potassium iodide
SSRIs	selective serotonin reuptake inhibitors
STD	sexually transmitted disease
STEM I	ST-elevation myocardial infarction
SubQ	subcutaneous
supp	suppository
SVT	supraventricular tachycardia
SWFI	sterile water for injection
syr	syrup
$T_{1/2}$	half-life
tab	tablet
TB	tuberculosis
TC	total cholesterol
TCA	tricyclic antidepressant
TD	tardive dyskinesia
TG	triglyceride
TIA	transient ischemic attack
TMA	thrombotic microangiopathy
T_{max}	time to maximum observed concentration, plasma
TNF	Tumor necrosis factor
TPN	total parenteral nutrition
tr, tinct	tincture
tsp	teaspoonful
UC	ulcerative colitis
ULN	upper limits of normal
URI	upper respiratory infection
USAN	United States Adopted Names
USP	United States Pharmacopeia
UTI	urinary tract infection
UV	ultraviolet
V_d	volume of distribution
VEGF	vascular endothelial growth factor
VF	ventricular fibrillation

Abbreviations Which May Be Used in This Reference *(continued)*

Abbreviation	Meaning
VT	ventricular tachycardia
VTE	venous thromboembolism
vWD	von Willebrand disease
VZV	varicella zoster virus
YBOC	Yale Brown Obsessive-Compulsive Scale
YMRS	Young Mania Rating Scale

Common Weights, Measures, or Apothecary Abbreviations

Abbreviation	Meaning
< [1]	less than
> [1]	greater than
≤	less than or equal to
≥	greater than or equal to
ac	before meals or food
ad	to, up to
ad lib	at pleasure
AM	morning
AMA	against medical advice
amp	ampul
amt	amount
aq	water
aq. dest.	distilled water
ASAP	as soon as possible
a.u.[1]	each ear
bid	twice daily
bm	bowel movement
C	Celsius, centigrade
cal	calorie
cap	capsule
cc[1]	cubic centimeter
cm	centimeter
comp	compound
cont	continue
d	day
d/c[1]	discharge
dil	dilute
disp	dispense
div	divide
dtd	give of such a dose
Dx	diagnosis
elix, el	elixir
emp	as directed
et	and
ex aq	in water
F	Fahrenheit
f, ft	make, let be made
g	gram
gr	grain
gtt	a drop
h	hour

Common Weights, Measures, or Apothecary Abbreviations *(continued)*

Abbreviation	Meaning
hs[1]	at bedtime
kcal	kilocalorie
kg	kilogram
L	liter
liq	a liquor, solution
M	molar
mcg	microgram
m. dict	as directed
mEq	milliequivalent
mg	milligram
microL	microliter
mL	milliliter
mm	millimeter
mM	millimolar
mm Hg	millimeters of mercury
ng	nanogram
no.	number
noc	in the night
non rep	do not repeat, no refills
NPO	nothing by mouth
NV	nausea and vomiting
O, Oct	a pint
o.d.[1]	right eye
o.l.	left eye
o.s.[1]	left eye
o.u.[1]	each eye
pc, post cib	after meals
PM	afternoon or evening
P.O.	by mouth
P.R.	rectally
prn	as needed
pulv	a powder
q	every
qad	every other day
qd[1,2]	every day, daily
qh	every hour
qid	four times a day
qod[1,2]	every other day
qs	a sufficient quantity
qs ad	a sufficient quantity to make
Rx	take, a recipe
SL	sublingual
stat	at once, immediately
SubQ	subcutaneous
supp	suppository
syr	syrup
tab	tablet
tal	such
tid	three times a day
tr, tinct	tincture
trit	triturate
tsp	teaspoon

Common Weights, Measures, or Apothecary Abbreviations *(continued)*

Abbreviation	Meaning
u.d.	as directed
ung	ointment
v.o.	verbal order
w.a.	while awake
x3	3 times
x4	4 times

[1]ISMP error-prone abbreviation.

[2]JCAHO Do Not Use list.

Additional abbreviations used and defined within a specific monograph or text piece may only apply to that text.

REFERENCES

The Institute for Safe Medication Practices (ISMP) list of Error-Prone Abbreviations, Symbols, and Dose Designations. Available at http://www.ismp.org/Tools/errorproneabbreviations.pdf

The Joint Commission Official "Do Not Use" list. Available at http://www.jointcommission.org/Do_Not_Use_List_of_Abbreviations/

STANDARD CONVERSIONS

APOTHECARY / METRIC EQUIVALENTS

Approximate Liquid Measures

Basic equivalent: 1 fluid ounce = 30 mL

Examples:

1 gallon	=	3800 mL	1 gallon	=	128 fluid ounces
1 quart	=	960 mL	1 quart	=	32 fluid ounces
1 pint	=	480 mL	1 pint	=	16 fluid ounces
8 fluid oz	=	240 mL	15 minims	=	1 mL
4 fluid oz	=	120 mL	10 minims	=	0.6 mL

Approximate Household Equivalents

1 teaspoonful	=	5 mL	1 tablespoonful	=	15 mL

Weights

Basic equivalents:

1 oz	=	30 g	15 gr	=	1 g

Examples:

4 oz	=	120 g	1 gr	=	60 mg
2 oz	=	60 g	1/100 gr	=	600 mcg
10 gr	=	600 mg	1/150 gr	=	400 mcg
7 1/2 gr	=	500 mg	1/200 gr	=	300 mcg
16 oz	=	1 lb			

Metric Conversions

Basic equivalents:

1 g	=	1000 mg	1 mg	=	1000 mcg

Examples:

5 g	=	5000 mg	5 mg	=	5000 mcg
0.5 g	=	500 mg	0.5 mg	=	500 mcg
0.05 g	=	50 mg	0.05 mg	=	50 mcg

Exact Equivalents

1 g	=	15.43 gr	0.1 mg	=	1/600 gr
1 mL	=	16.23 minims	0.12 mg	=	1/500 gr
1 minim	=	0.06 mL	0.15 mg	=	1/400 gr
1 gr	=	64.8 mg	0.2 mg	=	1/300 gr
1 pint (pt)	=	473.2 mL	0.3 mg	=	1/200 gr
1 oz	=	28.35 g	0.4 mg	=	1/150 gr
1 lb	=	453.6 g	0.5 mg	=	1/120 gr
1 kg	=	2.2 lb	0.6 mg	=	1/100 gr
1 qt	=	946.4 mL	0.8 mg	=	1/80 gr
			1 mg	=	1/65 gr

Solids[1]

1/4 grain	=	15 mg	1 1/2 grains	=	90 mg
1/2 grain	=	30 mg	5 grains	=	300 mg
1 grain	=	60 mg	10 grains	=	600 mg

[1]Use exact equivalents for compounding and calculations requiring a high degree of accuracy.

POUNDS / KILOGRAMS CONVERSION

1 pound = 0.45359 kilograms
1 kilogram = 2.2 pounds

lb	= kg	lb	= kg	lb	= kg
1	0.45	70	31.75	140	63.50
5	2.27	75	34.02	145	65.77
10	4.54	80	36.29	150	68.04
15	6.80	85	38.56	155	70.31
20	9.07	90	40.82	160	72.58
25	11.34	95	43.09	165	74.84
30	13.61	100	45.36	170	77.11
35	15.88	105	47.63	175	79.38
40	18.14	110	49.90	180	81.65
45	20.41	115	52.16	185	83.92
50	22.68	120	54.43	190	86.18
55	24.95	125	56.70	195	88.45
60	27.22	130	58.91	200	90.72
65	29.48	135	61.24		

DRUG INTERACTIONS: METABOLISM/ TRANSPORT EFFECTS

Most drugs are eliminated from the body, at least in part, by being chemically altered to less lipid-soluble products (ie, metabolized), and thus are more likely to be excreted via the kidneys or the bile. Phase I metabolism includes drug hydrolysis, oxidation, and reduction, and results in drugs that are more polar in their chemical structure, while Phase II metabolism involves the attachment of an additional molecule onto the drug (or partially metabolized drug) in order to create an inactive and/or more water soluble compound. Phase II processes include (primarily) glucuronidation, sulfation, glutathione conjugation, acetylation, and methylation.

Virtually any of the Phase I and II enzymes can be inhibited by some xenobiotic or drug. Some of the Phase I and II enzymes can be induced. Inhibition of the activity of metabolic enzymes will result in increased concentrations of the substrate (drug), whereas induction of the activity of metabolic enzymes will result in decreased concentrations of the substrate. For example, the well-documented enzyme-inducing effects of phenobarbital may include a combination of Phase I and II enzymes. Phase II glucuronidation may be increased via induced UDP-glucuronosyltransferase (UGT) activity, whereas Phase I oxidation may be increased via induced cytochrome P450 (CYP) activity. However, for most drugs, the primary route of metabolism (and the primary focus of drug-drug interaction) is Phase I oxidation, and specifically, metabolism.

CYP enzymes may be responsible for the metabolism (at least partial metabolism) of approximately 75% of all drugs, with the CYP3A subfamily responsible for nearly half of this activity. Found throughout plant, animal, and bacterial species, CYP enzymes represent a superfamily of xenobiotic metabolizing proteins. There have been several hundred CYP enzymes identified in nature, each of which has been assigned to a family (1, 2, 3, etc), subfamily (A, B, C, etc), and given a specific enzyme number (1, 2, 3, etc) according to the similarity in amino acid sequence that it shares with other enzymes. Of these many enzymes, only a few are found in humans, and even fewer appear to be involved in the metabolism of xenobiotics (eg, drugs). The key human enzyme subfamilies include CYP1A, CYP2A, CYP1B, CYP2B, CYP2C, CYP2D, CYP2E, and CYP3A.

CYP enzymes are found in the endoplasmic reticulum of cells in a variety of human tissues (eg, skin, kidneys, brain, lungs), but their predominant sites of concentration and activity are the liver and intestine. Though the abundance of CYP enzymes throughout the body is relatively equally distributed among the various subfamilies, the relative contribution to drug metabolism is (in decreasing order of magnitude) CYP3A4/5 (nearly 50%), CYP2D6 (nearly 25%), CYP2C8/9 (nearly 15%), then CYP1A1/2, CYP2C19, CYP2A6, CYP2E1, CYP1B1, and CYP2B6. Owing to their potential for numerous drug-drug interactions, those drugs that are identified in preclinical studies as substrates of CYP3A enzymes are often given a lower priority for continued research and development in favor of drugs that appear to be less affected by (or less likely to affect) this enzyme subfamily.

Each enzyme subfamily possesses unique selectivity toward potential substrates. For example, CYP1A1/2 preferentially binds medium-sized, planar, lipophilic molecules, while CYP2D6 preferentially binds molecules that possess a basic nitrogen atom. Some CYP subfamilies exhibit polymorphism (ie, multiple allelic variants that manifest differing catalytic properties). The best described polymorphisms involve CYP2C8/9, CYP2C19, and CYP2D6. Individuals possessing "wild type" gene alleles exhibit normal functioning CYP capacity. Others, however, possess allelic variants that leave the person with a subnormal level of catalytic potential (so called "poor metabolizers"). Poor metabolizers would be more likely to experience toxicity from drugs metabolized by the affected enzymes (or less effects if the enzyme is responsible for converting a prodrug to it's active form as in the case of codeine). The percentage of people classified as poor metabolizers varies by enzyme and population group. As an example, approximately 7% of Caucasians and only about 1% of Orientals appear to be CYP2D6 poor metabolizers.

CYP enzymes can be both inhibited and induced by other drugs, leading to increased or decreased serum concentrations (along with the associated effects), respectively. Induction occurs when a drug causes an increase in the amount of smooth endoplasmic reticulum, secondary to increasing the amount of the affected CYP enzymes in the tissues. This "revving up" of the CYP enzyme system may take several days to reach peak activity, and likewise, may take several days, even months, to return to normal following discontinuation of the inducing agent.

CYP inhibition occurs via several potential mechanisms. Most commonly, a CYP inhibitor competitively (and reversibly) binds to the active site on the enzyme, thus preventing the substrate from binding to the same site, and preventing the substrate from being metabolized. The affinity of an inhibitor for an enzyme may be expressed by an inhibition constant (Ki) or IC50 (defined as the concentration of the inhibitor required to cause 50% inhibition under a given set of conditions). In addition to reversible competition for an enzyme site, drugs may inhibit enzyme activity by binding to sites on the enzyme other than that to which the substrate would bind, and thereby cause a change in the functionality or physical structure of the enzyme. A drug may also bind to the enzyme in an irreversible (ie, "suicide") fashion. In such a case, it is not the concentration of drug at the enzyme site that is important (constantly binding and releasing), but the number of molecules available for binding (once bound, always bound).

Although an inhibitor or inducer may be known to affect a variety of CYP subfamilies, it may only inhibit one or two in a clinically important fashion. Likewise, although a substrate is known to be at least partially metabolized by a variety of CYP enzymes, only one or two enzymes may contribute significantly enough to its overall metabolism to warrant concern when used with potential inducers or inhibitors. Therefore, when attempting to predict the level of risk of using two drugs that may affect each other via altered CYP function, it is important to identify the relative effectiveness of the inhibiting/inducing drug on the CYP subfamilies that significantly contribute to the metabolism of the substrate. The contribution of a specific CYP pathway to substrate metabolism should be considered not only in light of other known CYP pathways, but also other nonoxidative pathways for substrate metabolism (eg, glucuronidation) and transporter proteins (eg, P-glycoprotein) that may affect the presentation of a substrate to a metabolic pathway.

SMOKING AND DRUG METABOLISM

A nonpharmaceutical interaction may be equally important because of its constant occurrence in users (tobacco). Smoking induces CYP1A2 activity, possibly causing a reduced effect of its substrates (eg, estradiol). Among postmenopausal women receiving 1 or 2 mg daily of oral estrogen, it has been found that the serum estradiol level in smokers was half that in nonsmokers. The effect was manifested by about a 50% reduction in breast tenderness in smokers. Thus, smoking may affect drugs metabolized by CYP1A2, with various consequences on target organs. A review of the literature suggests that at least a dozen drugs interact with cigarette smoke in a clinically significant manner. Polycyclic aromatic hydrocarbons (PAHs) are largely responsible for enhancing drug metabolism. Cigarette smoke induces an increase in the concentration of CYP1A2, the isoenzyme responsible for metabolism of theophylline. Theophylline is, therefore, eliminated more quickly in smokers than in nonsmokers. As a result of hepatic induction of CYP1A2, serum concentrations of theophylline have been shown to be reduced in smokers. Cigarette smoking may substantially reduce tacrine plasma concentrations. The manufacturer states that mean plasma tacrine concentrations in smokers are about one-third of the concentration in nonsmokers (presumably after multiple doses of tacrine).

Patients with insulin-dependent diabetes who smoke heavily may require a higher dosage of insulin than nonsmokers. Cigarette smoking may also reduce serum concentrations of flecainide. Although the mechanism of this interaction is unknown, enhanced hepatic metabolism is possible. Propoxyphene, a pain reliever, has been found to be less effective in smokers than in nonsmokers. The mechanism for the inefficacy of propoxyphene in smokers compared with nonsmokers may be enhanced biotransformation.

The norepinephrine and serotonin reuptake inhibitors, as a new class of smoking cessation drugs, have also received attention relative to metabolic interactions. *In vitro* studies indicate that bupropion (Zyban®) is primarily metabolized to hydroxybupropion by the CYP2B6 isoenzyme. Therefore, the potential exists for a drug interaction between Zyban® and drugs that affect the CYP2B6 isoenzyme metabolism [eg, orphenadrine (Norflex™) and cyclophosphamide (Cytoxan®)]. The hydroxybupropion metabolite of bupropion does not appear to be metabolized by the cytochrome P450 isoenzymes. No systemic data have been collected on the metabolism of Zyban® following concomitant administration with other drugs, or alternatively, the effect of concomitant administration of Zyban® on the metabolism of other drugs.

SUMMARY

Once a drug has been metabolized in the liver, it is eliminated through several different mechanisms. One is directly through bile, into the intestine, and eventually excreted in feces. More commonly, the metabolites and the original drug pass back into the liver from the general circulation and are carried to other organs and tissues. Eventually, these metabolites are excreted through the kidney. In the kidney, the drug and its metabolites may be filtered by the glomerulus or secreted by the renal tubules into the urine. From the kidney, some of the drug may be reabsorbed and pass back into the blood. The drug may also be carried to the lung. If the drug or its metabolite is volatile, it can pass from the blood into the alveolar air and be eliminated in the breath. To a minor extent, drugs and metabolites can be excreted by sweat and saliva. In nursing mothers, drugs are also excreted in mother's milk.

The clinical considerations of drug metabolism may affect which other drugs can and should be administered. Drug tolerance may be a consideration, in that larger doses of a drug may be necessary to obtain effect in patients in which the metabolism is extremely rapid. These interactions, via cytochrome P450 or its isoforms, can occasionally be used beneficially to increase/maintain blood levels of one drug by administering a second drug. Dental clinicians should attempt to stay current on this topic of drug interactions as knowledge evolves.

SELECTED READINGS

Bjarnason NH and Christiansen C, "The Influence of Thinness and Smoking on Bone Loss and Response to Hormone Replacement Therapy in Early Postmenopausal Women," *J Clin Endocrinol Metab*, 2000, 85(2):590-6.

Bjarnason NH, Jørgensen C, Kremmer H, et al, "Smoking Reduces Breast Tenderness During Oral Estrogen-Progestogen Therapy," *Climacteric*, 2004, 7(4):390-6.

Bjornsson TD, Callaghan JT, Einolf HJ, et al, "The Conduct of *in vitro* and *in vivo* Drug-Drug Interaction Studies: A PhRMA Perspective," *J Clin Pharmacol*, 2003, 43(5):443-69.

Drug-Drug Interactions, Rodrigues AD, ed, New York, NY: Marcel Dekker, Inc, 2002.

Hersh EV and Moore PA, "Drug Interactions in Dentistry: The Importance of Knowing Your CYP's," *J Am Dent Assoc*, 2004, 135(3):298-311.

Levy RH, Thummel KE, Trager WF, et al, eds, *Metabolic Drug Interactions*, Philadelphia, PA: Lippincott Williams & Wilkins, 2000.

Wilkinson GR, "Drug Metabolism and Variability Among Patients in Drug Response," *N Engl J Med*, 2005, 352(21):2211-21.

Wynn RL and Meiller TF, "CYP Enzymes and Adverse Drug Reactions," *Gen Dent*, 1998, 46(5):436-8.

Zhang Y and Benet LZ, "The Gut as a Barrier to Drug Absorption: Combined Role of Cytochrome P450 3A and P-Glycoprotein," *Clin Pharmacokinet*, 2001, 40(3):159-68.

SELECTED WEBSITES

http://www.gentest.com
http://www.imm.ki.se/CYPalleles
http://medicine.iupui.edu/flockhart
http://www.mhc.com/Cytochromes

NORMAL BLOOD VALUES

Test	Range of Normal Values
Complete Blood Count (CBC)	
White blood cells	4,500-11,000
Red blood cells (male)	4.6-6.2 x 10^6 µL
Red blood cells (female)	4.2-5.4 x 10^6 µL
Platelets	150,000-450,000
Hematocrit (male)	40% to 54%
Hematocrit (female)	38% to 47%
Hemoglobin (male)	13.5-18 g/dL
Hemoglobin (female)	12-16 g/dL
Mean corpuscular volume (MCV)	80-96 μm^3
Mean corpuscular hemoglobin (MCH)	27-31 pg
Mean corpuscular hemoglobin concentration (MCHC)	32% to 36%
Differential White Blood Cell Count (%)	
Segmented neutrophils	56
Bands	3.0
Eosinophils	2.7
Basophils	0.3
Lymphocytes	34.0
Monocytes	4.0
Hemostasis	
Bleeding time (BT)	2-8 minutes
Prothrombin time (PT)	10-13 seconds
Activated partial thromboplastin time (aPTT)	25-35 seconds
Serum Chemistry	
Glucose (fasting)	70-110 mg/dL
Blood urea nitrogen (BUN)	8-23 mg/dL
Creatinine (male)	0.1-0.4 mg/dL
Creatinine (female)	0.2-0.7 mg/dL
Bilirubin, indirect (unconjugated)	0.3 mg/dL
Bilirubin, direct (conjugated)	0.1-1 mg/dL
Calcium	9.2-11 mg/dL
Magnesium	1.8-3 mg/dL
Phosphorus	2.3-4.7 mg/dL
Serum Electrolytes	
Sodium (Na^+)	136-142 mEq/L
Potassium (K^+)	3.8-5 mEq/L
Chloride (Cl^-)	95-103 mEq/L
Bicarbonate (HCO_3^-)	21-28 mmol/L
Serum Enzymes	
Alkaline phosphatase	20-130 IU/L
Alanine aminotransferase (ALT) (formerly called SGPT)	4-36 units/L
Aspartate aminotransferase (AST) (formerly called SGOT)	8-33 units/L
Amylase	16-120 Somogyi units/dL
Creatine kinase (CK) (male)	55-170 units/L
Creatine kinase (CK) (female)	30-135 units/L

ANTIGINGIVITIS DENTIFRICES

Brand Name	Abrasive Ingredient	Therapeutic Ingredient	Foaming Agent
Colgate® Total® Advanced Clean Plus Whitening Gel[1]	Hydrated silica, mica	Sodium fluoride 0.24%, triclosan 0.3%	Sodium lauryl sulfate
	Other Ingredients: Water, glycerin, sorbitol, PVM/MA copolymer, flavor, cellulose gum, sodium hydroxide, propylene glycol, carrageenan, sodium saccharin, FD&C blue no. 1, D&C yellow no. 10		
Colgate® Total® Advanced Clean Plus Whitening Paste[1]	Hydrated silica	Sodium fluoride 0.24%, triclosan 0.3%	Sodium lauryl sulfate
	Other Ingredients: Water, glycerin, sorbitol, PVM/MA copolymer, flavor, cellulose gum, sodium hydroxide, propylene glycol, carrageenan, sodium saccharin, titanium dioxide		
Colgate® Total® Advanced Fresh Gel[1]	Hydrated silica	Sodium fluoride 0.24%, triclosan 0.3%	Sodium lauryl sulfate
	Other Ingredients: Water, glycerin, sorbitol, PVM/MA copolymer, flavor, cellulose gum, sodium hydroxide, propylene glycol, carrageenan, sodium saccharin, FD&C blue no. 1, D&C yellow no. 10		
Colgate® Total® Advanced Whitening Paste[1]	Hydrated silica	Sodium fluoride 0.24%, triclosan 0.3%	Sodium lauryl sulfate
	Other Ingredients: Water, glycerin, sorbitol, PVM/MA copolymer, flavor, cellulose gum, sodium hydroxide, propylene glycol, carrageenan, sodium saccharin, titanium dioxide		
Colgate® Total® Enamel Strength[1]	Hydrated silica, mica	Sodium fluoride 0.24%, triclosan 0.3%	Sodium lauryl sulfate
	Other Ingredients: Water, glycerin, sorbitol, PVM/MA copolymer, cellulose gum, flavor, sodium hydroxide, propylene glycol, carrageenan, sodium saccharin, titanium dioxide, FD&C blue no. 1, D&C yellow no. 10		
Colgate® Total® Clean Mint Paste[1]	Hydrated silica, mica	Sodium fluoride 0.24%, triclosan 0.3%	Sodium lauryl sulfate
	Other Ingredients: Water, glycerin, sorbitol, PVM/MA copolymer, cellulose gum, flavor, sodium hydroxide, propylene glycol, carrageenan, sodium saccharin, titanium dioxide, FD&C blue no. 1, D&C yellow no. 10		
Colgate® Total® Mint Stripe™ Gel[1]	Hydrated silica, mica	Sodium fluoride 0.24%, triclosan 0.3%	Sodium lauryl sulfate
	Other Ingredients: Water, glycerin, sorbitol, PVM/MA copolymer, cellulose gum, flavor, sodium hydroxide, propylene glycol, carrageenan, sodium saccharin, titanium dioxide, FD&C blue no. 1, D&C yellow no. 10		
Colgate® Total® Whitening Gel[1]	Hydrated silica, mica	Sodium fluoride 0.24%, triclosan 0.3%	Sodium lauryl sulfate
	Other Ingredients: Water, glycerin, sorbitol, PVM/MA copolymer, cellulose gum, flavor, sodium hydroxide, propylene glycol, carrageenan, sodium saccharin, titanium dioxide, FD&C blue no. 1		
Colgate® Total® Whitening Paste[1]	Hydrated silica	Sodium fluoride 0.24%, triclosan 0.3%	Sodium lauryl sulfate
	Other Ingredients: Water, glycerin, sorbitol, PVM/MA copolymer, cellulose gum, flavor, sodium hydroxide, propylene glycol, carrageenan, sodium saccharin, titanium dioxide		
Crest® Pro-Health Clean Mint[1]	Hydrated silica	Stannous fluoride 0.454%	Sodium lauryl sulfate
	Other Ingredients: Glycerin, sodium hexametaphosphate, propylene glycol, PEG-6, water, zinc lactate, trisodium phosphate, flavor, polyethylene, sodium gluconate, carrageenan, sodium saccharin, xanthan gum, titanium dioxide, blue no. 1		
Crest® Pro-Health Clean Cinnamon[1]	Hydrated silica	Stannous fluoride 0.454%	Sodium lauryl sulfate
	Other Ingredients: Glycerin, sodium hexametaphosphate, propylene glycol, PEG-6, water, zinc lactate, trisodium phosphate, flavor, polyethylene, sodium gluconate, carrageenan, sodium saccharin, xanthan gum, titanium dioxide, red no. 40 aluminum lake		

(continued)

Brand Name	Abrasive Ingredient	Therapeutic Ingredient	Foaming Agent
Crest® Pro-Health Clinical Gum Protection Invigorating Clean Mint	Hydrated silica	Stannous fluoride 0.454%	Sodium lauryl sulfate
	Other Ingredients: Glycerin, sodium hexametaphosphate, propylene glycol, PEG-6, water, zinc lactate, trisodium phosphate, flavor, polyethylene, sodium gluconate, stannous chloride, carrageenan, sodium saccharin, xanthan gum, titanium dioxide, blue no. 1 aluminum lake		
Crest® Pro-Health For Me Fluoride Anticavity Minty Breeze	Hydrated silica, mica	Stannous fluoride 0.454%	Sodium lauryl sulfate
	Other Ingredients: Water, disodium pyrophosphate, carbomer, sorbitol, flavor, polyethylene, sodium saccharin, xanthan gum, titanium dioxide, blue no. 1 aluminum lake, sodium hydroxide		
Crest® Pro-Health Night[1]	Hydrated silica	Stannous fluoride 0.454%	Sodium lauryl sulfate
	Other Ingredients: Glycerin, sodium hexametaphosphate, propylene glycol, PEG-6, water, zinc lactate, trisodium phosphate, flavor, polyethylene, sodium gluconate, carrageenan, sodium saccharin, xanthan gum, titanium dioxide, blue no. 1 aluminum lake		
Crest® Pro-Health Whitening[1]	Hydrated silica, mica	Stannous fluoride 0.454%	Sodium lauryl sulfate
	Other Ingredients: Glycerin, sodium hexametaphosphate, propylene glycol, PEG-6, water, zinc lactate, trisodium phosphate, flavor, polyethylene, sodium gluconate, carrageenan, sodium saccharin, xanthan gum, titanium dioxide, blue no. 1		
Crest® Pro-Health Enamel Shield	Hydrated silica	Stannous fluoride 0.454%	Sodium lauryl sulfate
	Other Ingredients: Glycerin, sodium hexametaphosphate, propylene glycol, PEG-6, water, zinc lactate, trisodium phosphate, flavor, polyethylene, sodium gluconate, carrageenan, sodium saccharin, xanthan gum, blue no. 1 aluminum lake		
Crest® Pro-Health Sensitive Shield	Hydrated silica	Stannous fluoride 0.454%	Sodium lauryl sulfate
	Other Ingredients: Glycerin, sodium hexametaphosphate, propylene glycol, PEG-6, water, zinc lactate, trisodium phosphate, flavor, polyethylene, sodium gluconate, carrageenan, sodium saccharin, xanthan gum, titanium dioxide, blue no. 1		
Listerine® Essential Care Toothpaste Mint Gel	Hydrated silica	Anticavity: Sodium monofluorophosphate 0.76% (0.13% W/V fluoride ion Antiplaque/ Antigingivitis: Eucalyptol 0.738%, menthol 0.340%, methyl salicylate 0.480%, thymol 0.511%	Sodium lauryl sulfate
	Other Ingredients: Water, sorbitol, glycerin, flavor, cellulose gum, sodium saccharin, phosphoric acid, FD&C blue no. 1, D&C yellow no. 10, sodium phosphate, benzoic acid, PEG-32, xanthan gum		

[1]Carries American Dental Association (ADA) seal indicating safety and efficacy.

Note: In addition to anticavity, these dentifrices have gained approval from the Food and Drug Administration to label the product as antigingivitis or prevention of gingivitis. The antigingivitis ingredient is either stannous fluoride, triclosan, or essential oils.

CALCIUM CHANNEL BLOCKERS AND GINGIVAL HYPERPLASIA

The last published report on calcium channel blocker-induced gingival hyperplasia (GH) by this author was in 1995 (Wynn, 1995). This present update reviews the reports up through 2008, relative to the incidence of GH in patients taking calcium channel blockers (CCBs) and the mechanisms by which these drugs cause GH.

The first reported cases of gingival hyperplasia induced by nifedipine were reported by Ramon et al, in 1984 (Ramon, 1984). Since that report, additional reports and case studies have been published describing gingival hyperplasia caused by nifedipine and other calcium channel blockers. The following table lists the number of reported cases up through the 1995 review, the specific drug involved, and the number of cases from 1995 to the present.

FDA Approval	General Preparation	Cases of Gingival Hyperplasia in Clinical Literature Through 1995	Cases Reported in Literature 1996-Present	Total Reported Cases
1982	Verapamil	7	9	16
1982	Diltiazem	20	32	52
1982	NIFEdipine	120	168	288
1989	NiCARdipine	0	0	0
1989	NiMODipine	0	0	0
1991	Isradipine	0	0	0
1992	AmLODIPine	0	26	26
1992	Felodipine	1	3	4
1993	Nisoldipine	0	0	0
2008	Nitrendipine[1]	1	0	1
	Clevidipine	0	0	0
	Pinaverium[1]	0	0	0

[1]Not approved in the United States

Calcium channel blockers are so named because of their effects on calcium at the cellular level. Contractile cells of the myocardium and smooth muscle cells of coronary and systemic arteries are influenced by the movement of calcium across their membranes. Part of this influence is in the regulation of contractile processes in these cells by way of movement of calcium ions through specific membrane channels. By blocking this channel movement of calcium, these drugs cause depression of the mechanical contraction of the myocardial cells, depression of electrical impulse formation and conduction velocity within the myocardium, and depression of smooth muscle contraction in coronary and systemic arteries. Thus, these drugs are useful in cardiovascular diseases, such as angina and hypertension, in which relaxation of these cells to cause vasodilatation is desired. These agents are sometimes referred to as calcium antagonists.

CLINICAL FINDINGS

Typical clinical findings of CCB-induced GH are hyperplastic gingiva around the maxillary and mandibular anterior teeth (Lederman, 1984). The hyperplastic gingiva usually originates in the interdental papilla, and in many areas, bleeding upon probing and small ulcerations are present. False periodontal pockets may be present with no evidence of bone loss. Histopathological analysis usually shows a thick layer of stratified squamous epithelium with parakeratosis and elongated rete pegs (Lederman, 1984; Lucas, 1985). In the submucosa, a proliferation of collagen fibers together with lymphocytic and plasma cell infiltration can be noticed (Lucas, 1985). The connective tissue usually shows large bundles of dense collagenous fibers with a moderate increase in fibroblasts. In addition, signs of inflammation are present with lymphocytes and plasma cells located perivascularly (Lucas, 1985).

MECHANISMS

Theories abound on the mechanism of CCB-induced gingival hyperplasia, but none have been proven. An early report using cell culture showed that the CCBs may lead to proliferation of selected fibroblasts, leading to an imbalance between regeneration and degeneration of those cells (Pernu, 1989). Brown et al, proposed that CCBs influence calcium/sodium flux in gingival fibroblast to result in decreased uptake of folic acid (Brown, 1990). The lack of intracellular folic acid then sets off a chain of events resulting in lack of production of active collagenases with no resultant catabolism of interstitial ground substance. The overabundance of ground substance manifests as gingival enlargement. Another theory suggests that these drugs elicit their effects indirectly through mediators which simulate proliferation and/or collagen synthesis by gingival fibroblasts (Giustiniani, 1987). Two of the mediators are reported to be Interleukin-2 from T cells and the testosterone metabolite 5-dihydrotestosterone (Nishikawa, 1991; Sooriyamoorthy, 1990). The report by Sooriyamoorthy et al, showed convincing evidence in controlled experiments that increased levels of 5-dihydrotestosterone occurred in gingival hyperplasia induced by nifedipine (Sooriyamoorthy, 1990). Their earlier work also showed that this testosterone metabolite had a stimulatory effect on the synthetic activity of fibroblasts (Sooriyamoorthy, 1988). In another theory, Nishikawa et al, suggests that alteration of the intracellular calcium level in gingival cells by nifedipine in combination with some local inflammatory factors is important in eliciting gingival hyperplasia (Nishikawa, 1991). Pre-existing gingival inflammation may be essential for onset of drug-induced gingival hyperplasia and that strict plaque control would be effective for preventing onset (Nishikawa, 1991). A more recent study using rats suggests that CCBs induce epithelial hyperplasia in gingival overgrowth not by an increase in keratinocyte proliferation, but by prolongation of cell life through reduction of apoptosis (controlled cell death) before epithelial hyperplasia is detected (Shimizu, 2002). Harel-Raviv et al, have argued that CCB-induced GH must be a calcium-dependent process because drugs, such as phenytoin and cyclosporin, which cause GH, also affect calcium ion cellular flux (Harel-Raviv, 1995). For example, phenytoin increases total intracellular calcium accumulation in gingival fibroblasts (Harel-Raviv, 1995).

INCIDENCE AND TREATMENT

The frequency and incidence of gingival hyperplasia caused by calcium channel blockers is difficult to assess. Literature numbers tell us that the effect by the calcium blockers is most prevalent with nifedipine (See table). The incidence of nifedipine-induced GH as currently reported are 28 cases out of 442 patients (6.3%), 11 cases out 29 patients (38%), and 79 cases out of 181 patients (44%) (Ellis, 1999; Nery, 1995; Steele, 1994). The other agents are diltiazem, 7 cases out of 33 patients (21%) and 4 cases out of 186 patients (2.2%), and amlodipine, 5 cases out of 150 patients (3.3%) and 3 cases out of 181 patients (1.7%) (Ellis, 1999; Jorgensen, 1997; Steele, 1994). For verapamil, the incidence has been reported as 5 cases out of 26 patients (19%) (Steele, 1994). A report from the Mayo clinic described the incidence of verapamil-induced GH as ranging between 4% to 19% (Meraw, 1998). Thus to summarize these values, nifedipine incidence ranged from 6.3% to 44%; diltiazem incidence ranged from 2.2% to 21%; amlodipine incidence ranged from 1.7% to 3.3%; and verapamil incidence ranged from 4% to 19%. In a more recent report, 20,636 patients taking a CCB or a non-CCB for treatment of various cardiovascular conditions were evaluated for incidence of gingival hyperplasia (Kaur, 2010). The report identified 103 patients with definite CCB-induced gingival hyperplasia. The number of CCB-identified cases included amlodipine (12), nifedipine (13), felodipine (1), verapamil (4), and diltiazem (8).

Treatment of CCB-induced GH includes the reinforcement and maintenance of good oral hygiene, along with frequent professional plaque removal (Camargo, 2000). The ideal treatment of choice; however, is the discontinuation of the suspected medication. Regression of GH has been demonstrated after discontinuation of the offending CCB (Meraw, 1998). In some situations, the use of another drug in the same class of medications has provided similar medical outcomes with reduced incidence of GH (Westbrook, 1997). If the nonsurgical approach is ineffective, then gingivectomy or periodontal flap procedures can reduce the enlarged gingival tissues (Camargo, 2000).

REFERENCES

Brown RS, Sein P, Corio R, et al, "Nitrendipine-Induced Gingival Hyperplasia. First Case Report," *Oral Surg Oral Med Oral Pathol*, 1990, 70(5):593-6.

Camargo PM, Melnick PR, Pirih FQ, et al, "Treatment of Drug-Induced Gingival Enlargement: Aesthetic and Functional Considerations," *Periodontol 2000*, 2001, 27:131-8.

Ellis JS, Seymour RA, Steele JG, et al, "Prevalence of Gingival Overgrowth Induced by Calcium Channel Blockers: A Community-Based Study," *J Periodontol*, 1999, 70(1):63-7.

Giustiniani S, Robustelli della Cuna F, and Marieni M, "Hyperplastic Gingivitis During Diltiazem Therapy," *Int J Cardiol*, 1987, 15(2):247-9.

Harel-Raviv M, Eckler M, Lalani K, et al, "Nifedipine-Induced Gingival Hyperplasia. A Comprehensive Review and Analysis," *Oral Surg Oral Med Oral Pathol Oral Radiol Endod*, 1995, 79(6):715-22.

Jorgensen MG, "Prevalence of Amlodipine-Related Gingival Hyperplasia," *J Periodontol*, 1997, 68 (7):676-8.

Kaur G, Verhamme KM, Dieleman JP, et al, "Association Between Calcium Channel Blockers and Gingival Hyperplasia, *J Clin Periodontol*, 2010, 37(7):625-30.

Lederman D, Lumerman H, Reuben S, et al, "Gingival Hyperplasia Associated With Nifedipine Therapy. Report of a Case," *Oral Surg Oral Med Oral Pathol*, 1984, 57(6):620-2.

Lucas RM, Howell LP, and Wall BA, "Nifedipine-Induced Gingival Hyperplasia. A Histochemical and Ultrastructural Study," *J Periodontol*, 1985, 56(4):211-5.

Meraw SJ and Sheridan PJ, "Medically Induced Gingival Hyperplasia," *Mayo Clin Proc*, 1998, 73 (12):1196-9.

Nery EB, Edson RG, Lee KK, et al, "Prevalence of Nifedipine-Induced Gingival Hyperplasia," *J Periodontol*, 1995, 66(7):572-8.
Nishikawa S, Tada H, Hamasaki A, et al, "Nifedipine-Induced Gingival Hyperplasia: A Clinical and *in vitro* Study," *J Periodontol*, 1991, 62(1):30-5.
Pernu HE, Oikarinen K, Hietanen J, et al, "Verapamil-Induced Gingival Overgrowth: A Clinical, Histologic, and Biochemic Approach," *J Oral Pathol Med*, 1989, 18(7):422-5.
Ramon Y, Behar S, Kishon Y, et al, "Gingival Hyperplasia Caused by Nifedipine - A Preliminary Report," *Int J Cardiol*, 1984, 5(2):195-206.
Shimizu Y, Kataoka M, Seto H, et al, "Nifedipine Induces Gingival Epithelial Hyperplasia in Rats Through Inhibition of Apoptosis," *J Periodontol*, 2002, 73(8):861-7.
Sooriyamoorthy M, Gower DB, and Eley BM, "Androgen Metabolism in Gingival Hyperplasia Induced by Nifedipine and Cyclosporin," *J Periodontal Res*, 1990, 25(1):25-30.
Sooriyamoorthy M, Harvey W, and Gower DB, "The Use of Human Gingival Fibroblasts in Culture for Studying the Effects of Phenytoin on Testosterone Metabolism," *Arch Oral Biol*, 1988, 33(5):353-9.
Steele RM, Schuna AA, and Schreiber RT, "Calcium Antagonist-Induced Gingival Hyperplasia," *Ann Intern Med*, 1994, 120(8):663-4.
Westbrook P, Bednarczyk EM, Carlson M, et al, "Regression of Nifedipine-Induced Gingival Hyperplasia Following Switch to a Same Class Calcium Channel Blocker, Isradipine," *J Periodontol*, 1997, 68 (7):645-50.
Wynn RL, "Update on Calcium Channel Blocker-Induced Gingival Hyperplasia," *Gen Dent*, 1995, 43 (3):218-20, 222.

CALCIUM PHOSPHATE PRODUCTS

Brand Name	Category	Formula	Availability
Arm & Hammer Age Defying™ Toothpaste	Remineralization	ACP Technology Sodium fluoride: 0.24%	OTC
Burt's Bees® Natural Toothpastes	Remineralization	Sodium monofluorophosphate: 0.77% Calcium sodium phosphosilicate: % not indicated	OTC
DayWhite® ACP Gel	Whitening Desensitization Remineralization	ACP: 0.5% Hydrogen peroxide: 7.5%, 9.5%	OD
MI Paste™	Desensitization Remineralization[1]	CPP-ACP (Recaldent™): 10%	OD
MI Paste Plus™	Desensitization Remineralization[1]	CPP-ACP (Recaldent™): 10% Sodium fluoride: 0.2%	OD
NiteWhite® ACP Gel	Whitening Desensitization Remineralization	ACP: 0.5% Carbamide peroxide: 10%, 16%, 22%	OD
Relief® ACP Oral Care Gel	Desensitization Remineralization	ACP: 0.375% Sodium fluoride: 0.22% Potassium nitrate: 5%	OD
		ACP: 0.75% Sodium fluoride: 0.22% Potassium nitrate: 5%	
Topex® ReNew™ Toothpaste	Desensitization Remineralization	Calcium sodium phosphosilicate (NovaMin®): 5% Neutral sodium fluoride: 1.1%	OD
Trident Xtra Care™ with Recaldent®	Remineralization	CPP-ACP (Recaldent™): 1%	OTC

CPP-ACP = casein phosphopeptide-amorphous calcium phosphate; ACP component may contain properties that rebuild enamel and remineralize teeth; **OD** = office dispensed; **OTC** = over-the-counter; **ACP** = amorphous calcium phosphate; **ACP technology** = calcium ions, phosphate ions

[1]Clinical cases available from GC America

DENTAL DRUG USE IN PREGNANCY AND BREAST-FEEDING[1]

Drug	FDA Pregnancy Category	Use During Pregnancy	Use During Breast-Feeding
Acetaminophen	B	Yes	Yes
Acetaminophen and codeine	C	Low dose for short duration	Yes (with caution)
Acetaminophen and tramadol	C	No information	No information
Acyclovir	B	No information	No information
Alclometasone	C	Yes	No information
ALPRAZolam	D	Avoid	Avoid
Amitriptyline	C	Yes	Avoid
Amlexanox	B	Yes	Yes
Ammonia spirit (aromatic)	C	No information	No information
Amoxicillin	B	Yes	Yes
Amoxicillin and clavulanate potassium	B	Yes	Yes
Ampicillin	B	Yes	Yes
Ampicillin and sulbactam	B	Yes	Yes
Articaine hydrochloride and epinephrine (U.S.)	C	Yes	Yes
Aspirin	C/D	Not in third trimester	Avoid
Aspirin and codeine	D	Not in third trimester	Avoid
Atropine sulfate (dental tablets)	C	Yes	Avoid
Azithromycin	B	Yes	Yes
Beclomethasone	C	Yes	Avoid
Benzocaine	C	Yes	Yes
Betamethasone and clotrimazole	C	Yes	No information
Bupivacaine	C	Yes	Yes
Bupivacaine and epinephrine	C	Yes	Yes
Butalbital, acetaminophen, caffeine, and codeine	C/D	Not in third trimester	Avoid
CarBAMazepine	D	Avoid	Avoid
Carbamide peroxide	C	Yes	Yes
Carisoprodol	C	Yes	Avoid
Carisoprodol and aspirin	C/D	Not in third trimester	Avoid
Carisoprodol, aspirin, and codeine	C/D	Not in third trimester	Avoid
Cefaclor	B	Yes	Yes
Cefadroxil	B	Yes	Yes
CeFAZolin	B	Yes	Yes
Cefditoren	B	Yes	Yes
Celecoxib[2]	C/D	No information	No information
Cephalexin	B	Yes	Yes
Cevimeline	C	No information	No information
Ciprofloxacin	C	Yes	Avoid
Clarithromycin	C	Yes	Yes
Clindamycin	B	Yes	Yes
Clobetasol	C	Yes	Yes
ClonazePAM	D	Avoid	Avoid
Clotrimazole	C (troches)	Yes	Yes
Cloxacillin	B	Yes	Yes
Codeine	C	Low dose for short duration	Yes (with caution)
Cyclobenzaprine	B	Yes	No information
Dexamethasone	C	Yes	No information

(continued)

Drug	FDA Pregnancy Category	Use During Pregnancy	Use During Breast-Feeding
Diazepam	D	Avoid	Avoid
Dibucaine	C	Yes	Yes
Diclofenac[2]	B/D	Not in third trimester	Yes
Dicloxacillin	B	Yes	Yes
Diflunisal	C/D	Not in third trimester	Yes
DiphenhydrAMINE	B	Yes	Yes
Doxycycline hyclate (periodontal)	D	Avoid	Avoid
Doxycycline (subantimicrobial)	D	Avoid	Avoid
EPINEPHrine	C	Yes	Yes
Erythromycin	B	Yes (avoid estolate)	Yes
Eszopiclone	C	Yes	No information
Etidocaine and epinephrine	B	Yes	Yes
Etodolac	C/D	Not in third trimester	Yes
Famciclovir	B	Yes	No information
FentaNYL	C/D	Yes (with caution)	Yes
Fluocinolone	C	Yes	No information
Fluocinonide	C	Yes	No information
Fluconazole	C	Yes	Yes
Flurbiprofen	C/D	Not in third trimester	Yes
Gabapentin	C	Yes	Avoid
Halobetasol	C	Yes (with caution)	Yes (with caution)
Hydrocodone and acetaminophen	C	Low dose for short duration	Yes (with caution)
Hydrocodone and aspirin	D	Not in third trimester	Avoid
Hydrocodone and ibuprofen	C/D	Not in third trimester	Yes (with caution)
Hydrocortisone	C	Yes	No information
Ibuprofen[2]	B/D	Not in third trimester	Yes
Iodoquinol and hydrocortisone	C	Yes	No information
Ketoconazole	C	Yes	Yes
Ketoprofen	B/D	Not in third trimester	Yes
Ketorolac	C/D	Not in third trimester	Yes
Lidocaine	B	Yes	Yes
Lidocaine and epinephrine	B	Yes	Yes
Lidocaine and prilocaine	B	Yes	Yes
LORazepam	D	Avoid	Avoid
Meperidine	B/D	Low dose for short duration	Yes (with caution)
Mepivacaine	C	Yes	Yes
Mepivacaine (dental anesthetic)	C	Yes	Yes
Mepivacaine and levonordefrin	C	Yes	Yes
Methocarbamol	C	Yes	No information
Methohexital	C	Yes	Yes
MethylPREDNISolone	C	Yes	No information
MetroNIDAZOLE	B	Yes (with caution)	Yes (with caution)
Midazolam	D	Avoid	Avoid
Minocycline	D	Avoid	Avoid
Minocycline hydrochloride (periodontal)	D	Avoid	Avoid
Naloxone	C	Yes	Yes

(continued)

Drug	FDA Pregnancy Category	Use During Pregnancy	Use During Breast-Feeding
Naproxen[2]	B/D	Not in third trimester	Yes
Nicotine	D	Avoid	Avoid
Nitrous oxide[3]	None reported	Acute use in patients: Yes (with caution)	Acute use in patients: Yes
Nortriptyline	D	Avoid	Avoid
Nystatin	B/C	Yes	Yes
Nystatin and triamcinolone	C	Yes	No information
OxyCODONE	B/D	Low dose for short duration	Yes
Oxycodone and acetaminophen	C/D	Low dose for short duration	Yes
Oxycodone and aspirin	D	Not in third trimester	Avoid
Oxycodone and ibuprofen	C/D	Not in third trimester	Yes (with caution)
Oxygen	None reported	Yes	Yes
Palifermin	C	Yes	No information
Penciclovir	B	Yes	Yes
Penicillin V potassium	B	Yes	Yes
Pentazocine and acetaminophen	C	Low dose for short duration	Yes (with caution)
Pilocarpine (dental)	C	Yes	Avoid
Pimecrolimus	C	Yes	No information
Posaconazole	C	Avoid	Yes (with caution)
PrednisoLONE	C	Yes	Yes (with caution)
PredniSONE	B	Yes	Yes
Prilocaine	B	Yes	Yes
Prilocaine and epinephrine	C	Yes	Yes
Propantheline	C	Yes	Yes
Propoxyphene and acetaminophen	C	Low dose for short duration	Yes (with caution)
Propoxyphene, aspirin, and caffeine	D	Not in third trimester	Avoid
Sulfonated phenolics in aqueous solution	C	Yes	Yes
Telithromycin	C	Yes	Yes (with caution)
Tetracaine	C	Yes	Yes
Tetracycline	D	Avoid	Avoid
Tetracycline (periodontal)	C	Avoid	Avoid
TraMADol	C	No (labor and delivery)	No
Triamcinolone acetonide paste	C	Yes	No information
Triazolam	X	Avoid	Avoid
ValACYclovir	B	Yes	Yes
Valdecoxib	C/D	No information	No information
Zaleplon	C	Yes	Avoid
Zolpidem	B	Yes	Yes (with caution)

[1]Pregnant or breast-feeding women should be encouraged to consult a physician prior to the use of any prescription or nonprescription medication. Additional information concerning other medications may be found in individual drug monographs.

[2]A study from Quebec Canada has shown that women who take prescribed nonsteroidal anti-inflammatory drugs (NSAIDs) in early pregnancy may increase their risk of giving birth to a child with congenital anomalies, especially cardiac septal anomalies, compared with women who do not take NSAIDs during this period. The NSAIDs involved included ibuprofen, naproxen, rofecoxib, diclofenac, and celecoxib. Of the 1056 women who took NSAIDs before giving birth, there were 93 (8.8%) live births of children with congenital anomalies. Of 35,331 women not taking any NSAID during pregnancy, there were 2478 (7%) live births of children with congenital anomalies. Further, the proportion of infants with one or more congenital defects who were born to women taking NSAIDs in the first trimester was 16.1% and the proportion of infants who were born to women not taking NSAIDs was 14.2%. Women who took NSAIDs during early pregnancy may be at greater risk of having children with congenital anomalies, specifically cardiac septal defects.

[3]Female dental personnel to avoid chronic exposure to unscavenged nitrous oxide.

REFERENCES

Della-Giustina K and Chow G, "Medications in Pregnancy and Lactation," *Emerg Med Clin North Am*, 2003, 21(3):585-613.

Drug Information for the Health Care Professional, 20th ed, Vol 1, Rockville, MD: Medical Economics Company, 2000.

Haas DA, Pynn BR, and Sands TD, "Drug Use for the Pregnant or Lactating Patient," *Gen Dent*, 2000, 48 (1):54-60.

Mariotti AJ, "Agents That Affect the Fetus and Nursing Infant," *ADA Guide to Dental Therapeutics*, 2nd ed, Chicago IL: ADA Publishing, 2000, 594-5.

Ofori B, Oraichi D, Blais L, et al, "Risk of Congenital Anomalies in Pregnant Users of Nonsteroidal Anti-Inflammatory Drugs: A Nested Case-Control Study," *Birth Defects Res B Dev Reprod Toxicol*, 2006, 77 (4):268-79.

TOOTHPASTES WITHOUT SODIUM LAURYL SULFATE (SLS) OR OTHER FOAMING AGENTS

Brand Name	Abrasive Ingredient	Therapeutic Ingredient
Arm & Hammer Advance White™ Toothpaste for Sensitive Teeth	Hydrated silica, sodium bicarbonate	Sodium fluoride 0.24%, triclosan 0.30%
	Other Ingredients: Cellulose gum, cocamidopropyl betaine, flavor, glycerin, sorbitol, titanium dioxide, water	
Baby Orajel® Tooth and Gum Cleanser (4-18 months of age)	None	None
	Other Ingredients: Purified water, sorbitol, propylene glycol, glycerin, cellulose gum, poloxamer 407, flavor, simethicone, methylparaben, potassium sorbate, sodium saccharin, propylparaben, citric acid	
Biotene® Sensitive	Hydrated silica, calcium pyrophosphate	Potassium nitrate 5% (antihypersensitivity), sodium monofluorophosphate 0.14% w/v fluoride ion (anticavity)
	Other Ingredients: Acesulfame K, calcium lactate, calcium pyrophosphate, cellulose gum, flavor, beta-d-glucose, glycerin, isoceteth-20, potassium thiocyanate, sodium benzoate, sorbitol, xylitol enzyme system (glucose oxidase, lactoferrin, lactoperoxidase, lysozyme)	
Oralgel® Toddler Training Toothpaste (≤4 years of age)	None	None
	Other Ingredients: Purified water, sorbitol, propylene glycol, glycerin, cellulose gum, poloxamer 407, flavor, simethicone, methylparaben, potassium sorbate, sodium saccharin, propylparaben, citric acid	
Rembrandt® Whitening Mint Toothpaste with FluorideSpecially Formulated for Canker Sores	Hydrated silica	Sodium fluoride 0.24%
	Other Ingredients: Water, glycerin, sorbitol, flavor, titanium dioxide, cellulose gum, polyvinylpyrrolidone (PVP), sodium saccharin, sucralose	
Sensodyne® Iso-Active® Toothpaste Multi Action	Hydrated silica	Potassium nitrate 5% (antihypersensitivity), sodium fluoride 0.15% w/v fluoride ion (anticavity)
	Other Ingredients: Carrageenan gum, Cocamidopropyl betaine, FD&C blue no. 1, flavor, glycerin, isopentane, PEG 6, sodium hydroxide, sodium methyl cocoyl taurate, sodium saccharin, sorbitol, water, xanthin gum	
Sensodyne® Iso-Active® Toothpaste Whitening	Hydrated silica	Potassium nitrate 5% (antihypersensitivity), sodium fluoride 0.15% w/v fluoride ion (anticavity)
	Other Ingredients: Blue no. 1, carrageenan gum, cocamidopropyl betaine, flavor, glycerin, isopentane, PEG 6, pentasodium triphosphate, sodium hydroxide, sodium methyl cocoyl taurate, sodium saccharin, sorbitol, water, xanthin gum	
Sensodyne® ProNamel™ Gentle Whitening	Hydrated silica	Potassium nitrate 5% (antihypersensitivity), sodium fluoride 0.15% w/v fluoride ion (anticavity)
	Other Ingredients: Cocamidopropyl betaine, flavor, glycerin, PEG 8, sodium hydroxide, sodium saccharin, sorbitol, titanium dioxide, water, xanthin gum	
Tom's™ of Maine Clean and Gentle with Fluoride	Hydrated silica	Sodium monofluorophosphate 0.13%
	Other Ingredients: Glycerin, water, calcium carbonate, aloe vera leaf juice (organic), xylitol, carrageenan, acacia gum, peppermint oil	
Tom's™ of Maine Fluoride-Free Clean & Gentle	Hydrated silica	None
	Other Ingredients: Glycerin, water, calcium carbonate, aloe vera leaf juice, xylitol, carrageenan, acacia gum, spearmint and peppermint oils	
Tom's™ of Maine Maximum Strength Sensitive Toothpaste for Sensitive Teeth and Cavity Protection with Fluoride	Hydrated silica	Potassium nitrate, sodium fluoride 0.243%
	Other Ingredients: Sorbitol, xylitol, water, glycerin, aloe vera leaf juice, natural flavor, cocamidopropyl betaine, xanthin gum, titanium dioxide	

Note: It is thought that patients suffering from canker sores benefit from using dentifrices without a foaming agent, such as SLS.

TOP 200 MOST PRESCRIBED DRUGS IN 2009

1. Hydrocodone and Acetaminophen
2. Lisinopril
3. Simvastatin
4. Levothyroxine
5. Amoxicillin
6. Azithromycin
7. Hydrochlorothiazide
8. AmLODIPine
9. ALPRAZolam
10. MetFORMIN
11. Lipitor®
12. Omeprazole
13. Atenolol
14. Furosemide (oral)
15. Metoprolol tartrate
16. Sertraline
17. Zolpidem
18. Metoprolol succinate
19. Oxycodone and Acetaminophen
20. NexIUM®
21. PredniSONE
22. Citalopram
23. Ibuprofen
24. Plavix®
25. Singulair®
26. Lexapro®
27. FLUoxetine
28. Gabapentin
29. Warfarin
30. TraMADol
31. ClonazePAM
32. Lisinopril and Hydrochlorothiazide
33. LORazepam
34. ProAir® HFA
35. Cephalexin
36. Cyclobenzaprine
37. Synthroid®
38. Amoxicillin and Clavulanate Potassium
39. Sulfamethoxazole and Trimethoprim
40. Ciprofloxacin
41. Fluticasone
42. Hydrochlorothiazide and Triamterene
43. Crestor®
44. Pravastatin
45. TraZODone
46. Propoxyphene and Acetaminophen
47. Alendronate
48. Advair Diskus®
49. Fexofenadine
50. Lovastatin
51. Carvedilol
52. PARoxetine
53. Diovan®
54. Cymbalta®
55. Meloxicam
56. Diazepam
57. Ranitidine
58. Effexor® XR
59. Fluconazole
60. Naproxen
61. Doxycycline
62. Klor-Con®
63. Prevacid®
64. Amitriptyline
65. MethylPREDNISolone
66. Allopurinol
67. Acetaminophen and Codeine
68. Diovan HCT®
69. Enalapril
70. Carisoprodol
71. CloNIDine
72. Actos®
73. Flomax®
74. SEROquel®
75. Levaquin®
76. AmLODIPine
77. Promethazine
78. Potassium chloride
79. Tricor®
80. Yaz®
81. Vytorin®
82. Viagra®
83. CeleBREX®
84. Lantus®

85. Nasonex®
86. Albuterol
87. OxyCODONE
88. Lyrica®
89. Glimepiride
90. Temazepam
91. Folic Acid
92. Spironolactone
93. Premarin®
94. Zetia®
95. Digoxin
96. Isosorbide mononitrate
97. Cefdinir
98. Ventolin® HFA
99. Ramipril
100. Triamcinolone
101. MetFORMIN
102. GlyBURIDE
103. Cozaar®
104. Concerta®
105. Valtrex®
106. Penicillin V Potassium
107. Benazepril
108. LamoTRIgine
109. Tamiflu®
110. RisperiDONE
111. Spiriva® HandiHaler®
112. GlipiZIDE
113. Amphetamine salt combination
114. Verapamil (sustained release)
115. Clindamycin
116. Benicar®
117. Ambien CR®
118. MetroNIDAZOLE
119. Ocella™
120. Potassium chloride (extended release)
121. Aricept®
122. Abilify®
123. Tri-Sprintec®
124. Cialis®
125. OxyCONTIN®
126. Estradiol (oral)
127. Levoxyl®
128. Phentermine
129. Benicar HCT®
130. HydrOXYzine
131. Diclofenac
132. Metoclopramide
133. Gemfibrozil
134. Diltiazem (extended release)
135. Divalproex
136. Nitrofurantoin
137. Mirtazapine
138. Xalatan®
139. Januvia™
140. Acyclovir
141. Proventil® HFA
142. Promethazine and Codeine
143. Doxazosin
144. Propranolol
145. Lunesta®
146. Budeprion XL®
147. Niaspan®
148. Guaifenesin and Codeine
149. Hyzaar®
150. Suboxone®
151. Topiramate
152. Adderall XR®
153. Detrol® LA
154. BusPIRone
155. Meclizine
156. Vyvanse®
157. BuPROPion
158. Quinapril
159. Pantoprazole
160. Toprol-XL®
161. Mupirocin
162. GlipiZIDE
163. Methotrexate
164. Polyethylene Glycol 3350
165. AcipHex®
166. NuvaRing®
167. FentaNYL
168. Benzonatate
169. Flovent® HFA
170. Avapro®
171. Combivent®
172. TriNessa®
173. Methadone
174. Betamethasone and Clotrimazole
175. SUMAtriptan
176. NIFEdipine

177. Famotidine
178. Butalbital, Acetaminophen, and Caffeine
179. Finasteride
180. Ferrous Sulfate
181. Boniva®
182. Terazosin
183. Glyburide and Metformin
184. Endocet®
185. Lovaza®
186. Actonel®
187. Namenda®
188. Loestrin®
189. TiZANidine
190. NovoLOG®
191. Methocarbamol
192. Clobetasol
193. Bisoprolol and Hydrochlorothiazide
194. Ortho Tri-Cyclen® Lo
195. Chantix®
196. Nitroglycerin
197. Evista®
198. Chlorhexidine Gluconate
199. Ondansetron
200. ROPINIRole

Based on units dispensed in U.S.

Source: SDI/Verispan, VONA, available at www.drugtopics.com

VASOCONSTRICTOR INTERACTIONS WITH ANTIDEPRESSANTS

Antidepressant	Effects with Epinephrine, Levonordefrin	Contraindicated	Recommendation
Tricyclics			
Amitriptyline (Elavil® [DSC])	Epinephrine (Systemic, Oral Inhalation) = increased pressor response; cardiac dysrhythmias Levonordefrin = increased pressor response	No	Potentially dangerous; use minimal amounts with caution in local anesthetics
Amitriptyline and Chlordiazepoxide			
Amitriptyline and Perphenazine			
Amoxapine			
Clomipramine (Anafranil®)			
Desipramine (Norpramin®)			
Doxepin (Systemic) (Prudoxin™, SINEquan®, Zonalon®)			
Imipramine (Tofranil-PM®, Tofranil®)			
Nortriptyline (Pamelor®)			
Protriptyline (Vivactil®)			
Trimipramine (Surmontil®)			
Serotonin / Norepinephrine Reuptake Inhibitor			
Desvenlafaxine (Pristiq™)	No adverse interactions reported	No	Suggest caution since serotonin/norepinephrine reuptake inhibitors block norepinephrine reuptake in CNS
Milnacipran (Savella™)			
Venlafaxine (Effexor® XR, Effexor®)			
Serotonin Only Reuptake Inhibitors			
Citalopram (CeleXA™)	No adverse interactions reported	No	No precautions appear to be necessary
Escitalopram (Lexapro™)			
FLUoxetine (PROzac® Weekly™, PROzac®, Sarafem™)			
FluvoxaMINE			
Olanzapine and Fluoxetine (Symbyax®)			
PARoxetine (Paxil CR™, Paxil®, Pexeva™)			
Sertraline (Zoloft®)			
Central Alpha-2 Antagonist			
Mirtazapine (Remeron SolTab®, Remeron®)	No adverse interactions reported	No	Suggest caution since mirtazapine increases release of norepinephrine
Dopamine Reuptake Inhibitor			
BuPROPion (Wellbutrin SR®, Wellbutrin XL™, Wellbutrin®, Zyban®)	No adverse interactions reported	No	Part of the mechanism of bupropion is to block norepinephrine reuptake within CNS; it has been suggested that vasoconstrictor be administered with caution

(continued)

Antidepressant	Effects with Epinephrine, Levonordefrin	Contraindicated	Recommendation
Others			
DULoxetine (Cymbalta®)	No adverse interactions reported	No	Part of the mechanism of duloxetine is to block norepinephrine reuptake within CNS; it has been suggested that vasoconstrictor be administered with caution
Maprotiline	Potential for increased pressor response	No	Potentially dangerous; use minimal amounts with caution in local anesthetics
MAO Inhibitors			
Isocarboxazid (Marplan®)	No effects on blood pressure or heart rate reported; however, potential exists for slight increase in pressor response	No	Use vasoconstrictor with caution
Moclobemide			
Phenelzine (Nardil®)			
Tranylcypromine (Parnate®)			
Serotonin Reuptake Inhibitor / Serotonin Antagonist			
Nefazodone (Serzone® [DSC])	No adverse interactions reported	No	No precautions appear to be necessary
TraZODone (Desyrel®)			
Serotonin Reuptake Inhibitor/5-HT_{1A} Receptor Partial Agonist			
Vilazodone (Viibryd™)	No adverse interactions reported	No	No precautions appear to be necessary

REFERENCES

Naftalin LW and Yagiela JA, "Vasoconstrictors: Indications and Precautions," *Dent Clin North Am*, 2002, 46(4):733-46.

Wynn RL, "Antidepressant Medications," *Gen Dent*, 1992, 40(3):192-7.

Yagiela JA, "Adverse Drug Interactions in Dental Practice: Interactions Associated With Vasoconstrictors. Part V of a Series," *J Am Dent Assoc*, 1999, 130(5):701-9.

Yagiela JA, "Injectable and Topical Local Anesthetics," *ADA Guide to Dental Therapeutics*, 2nd ed, Chicago, IL: ADA Publishing, 2000, 1-16.

PHARMACOLOGIC CATEGORY INDEX

Histamine H_1 Antagonist, First Generation

ALPHABETICAL INDEX

NOTES

NOTES

NOTES

NOTES

NOTES

NOTES

NOTES

NOTES

NOTES

NOTES

NOTES

NOTES

NOTES

NOTES

Other Products Offered by Lexicomp

Advanced Protocols for Medical Emergencies

by Donald P. Lewis, Jr, DDS and Ann Marie McMullin, MD

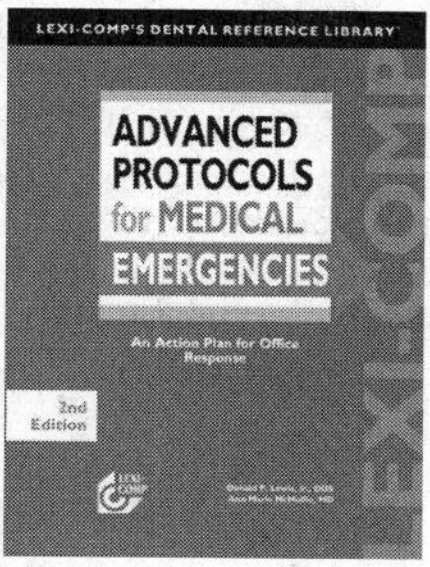

Advanced Protocols for Medical Emergencies is a must-have guide for offices that administer nitrous oxide, conscious sedation, and general anesthesia. This manual addresses specific medical emergency situations, which are presented in tabbed chapters for quick reference, to help ensure preparation for, and management of, office emergencies. Includes staff training guidelines.

Dental Office Medical Emergencies

by Timothy F. Meiller, DDS, PhD; Richard L. Wynn, BSPharm, PhD; Ann Marie McMullin, MD; Cynthia Biron, RDH, EMT, MA; Harold L. Crossley, DDS, PhD

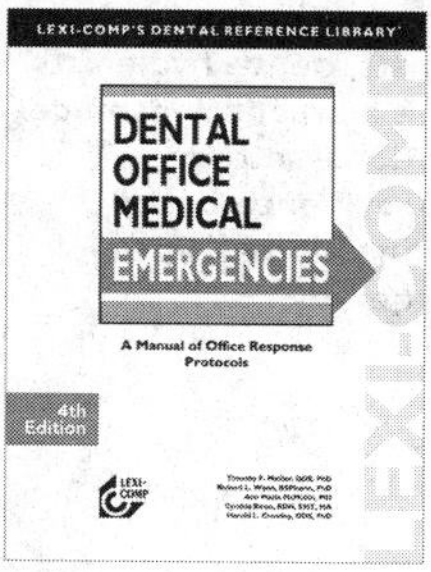

The *Dental Office Medical Emergencies* manual facilitates dental office emergency treatment and assists the dentist in addressing any developing situation by reinforcing basic life support techniques. This handy reference is intended for use by the entire dental office staff for preparedness training as well as during times of crisis.

Clinician's Endodontic Handbook

by Thom C. Dumsha, MS, DDS, MS and James L. Gutmann, DDS, FACD, FICD

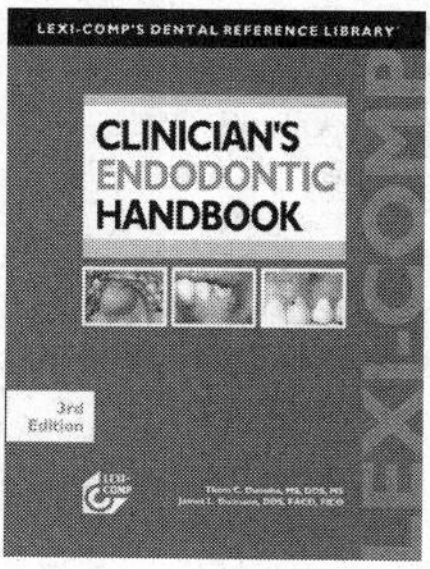

The *Clinician's Endodontic Handbook* is a fully-illustrated guide to current issues in endo-dontic therapy. Here, the latest techniques, procedures, and materials are presented, eliminating the need for multiple textbooks. This is a valuable reference for all dental practitioners with an interest in endodontics.

Other Products Offered by Lexicomp

Illustrated Handbook of Clinical Dentistry

by Richard A. Lehman, DMD, MPH and Michael A. Sullivan, DDS

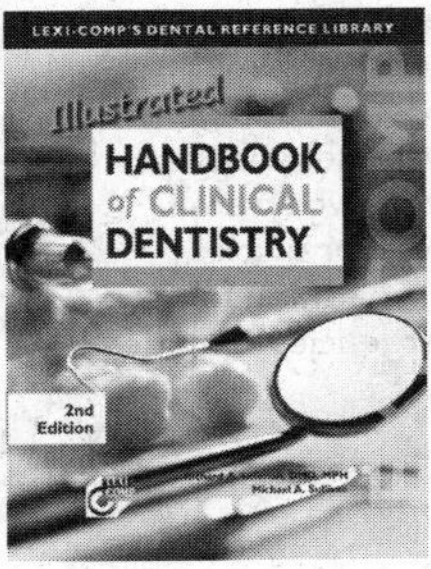

The *Illustrated Handbook of Clinical Dentistry* is a concise, yet comprehensive, resource for all dentists and dental students. This manual summarizes many basic dental principles and procedures and is designed to be used when transitioning into clinical practice or as a refresher for the seasoned dental professional.

Manual of Clinical Periodontics

by Francis G. Serio, DMD, MS, MBA and Charles E. Hawley, DDS, PhD

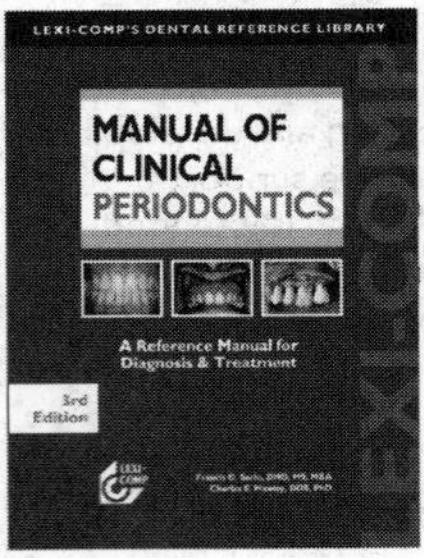

The *Manual of Clinical Periodontics* is a quick reference for general dentists, dental hygienists, and students. The manual is a practical resource for both clinical and educational settings, stressing patient-centered, evidence-based diagnosis, treatment planning, and accepted modalities of periodontic therapy.

Manual Of Dental Implants

by David P. Sarment, DDS, MS, Beth Peshman, RDH, and Robert F. Faulkner, DDS

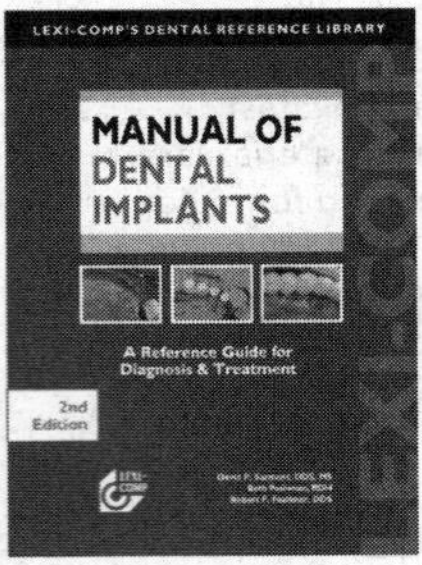

The *Manual of Dental Implants* introduces dental professionals to the world of restorative implant dentistry. Over 220 color photographs, plus diagrams and decision trees, help illustrate the diagnosis, treatment, and maintenance of implants. This reference is valuable at increasing levels of knowledge and training, so the user can continue to benefit as he or she gains implant experience.

www.lexi.com/dentistry • 1-866-397-3433

Other Products Offered by Lexicomp

Oral Hard Tissue Diseases

by J. Robert Newland, DDS, MS

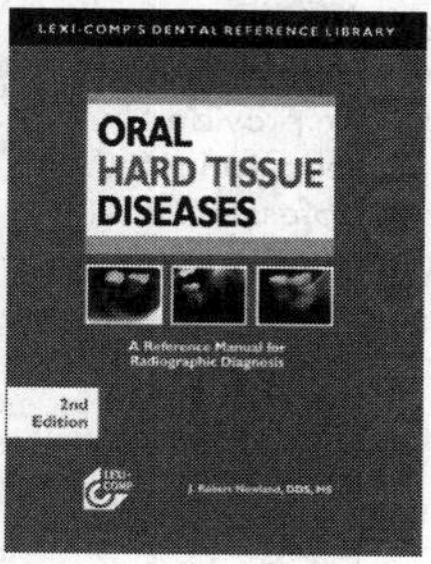

Oral Hard Tissue Diseases is a handy reference for visual recognition and diagnosis of common bone lesions. Each section of this manual is devoted to a specific diagnostic category and illustrated with high-quality black and white photographs. Recommendations for treatment and follow-up and an alphabetical index are included.

Oral Soft Tissue Diseases

by J. Robert Newland, DDS, MS; Timothy F. Meiller, DDS, PhD; Richard L. Wynn, BSPharm, PhD; Harold L.Crossley, DDS, Ph D

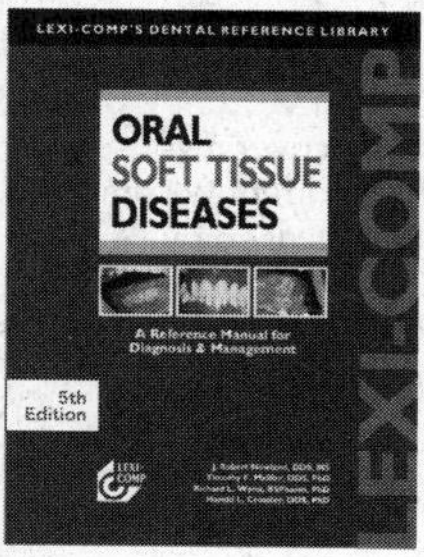

In this visually-cued manual, each lesion associated with soft tissue disease is illustrated by one or more color photographs depicting typical clinical features and common variations. Recommendations for treatment and follow-up, including sample prescriptions and concise drug monographs, are presented genomics knowledge into the management of drug therapy.

Oral Surgery for the General Dentist - Book and DVD Bundle

by Lawrence I. Gaum, DDS, FADSA, FICD

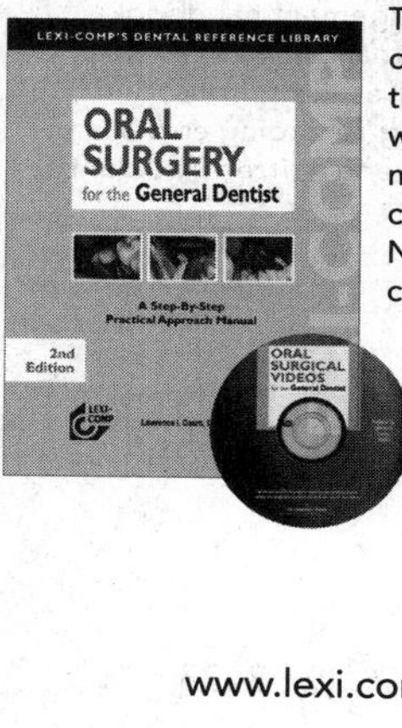

This clinical, step-by-step manual simplifies and demystifies everyday oral surgery and provides the knowledge needed to perform procedures with competency. The techniques detailed in this manual address commonly encountered dental conditions requiring surgical intervention. Numerous color photographs of actual surgical cases are included. Also available on DVD.

Own two valuable resources through t his unique bundled package. The *Oral Surgery for the General Dentist* manual will assist in viewing the 13 high-resolution videos available on the DVD.

www.lexi.com/dentistry • 1-866-397-3433

Other Products Offered by Lexicomp

The Little Dental Drug Booklet

by Peter L. Jacobsen, PhD, DDS

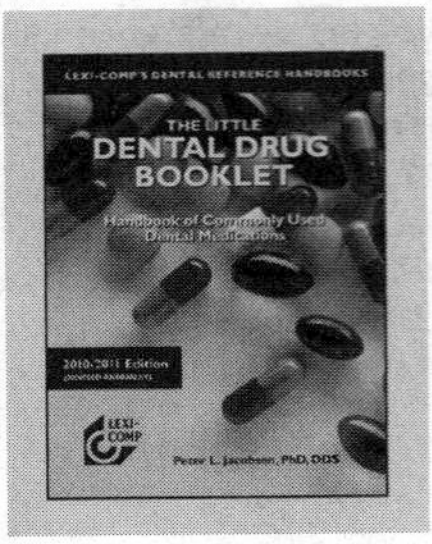

The Little Dental Drug Booklet is a pocket-sized reference to the drugs most commonly used in dental practice. The information provided in this booklet includes practical, practice-oriented suggestions made by dental professionals. A section on prescription writing and prescription requirements is included.

Employee Embezzlement and Fraud in the Dental Office

by Donald P Lewis, Jr., DDS, CFE

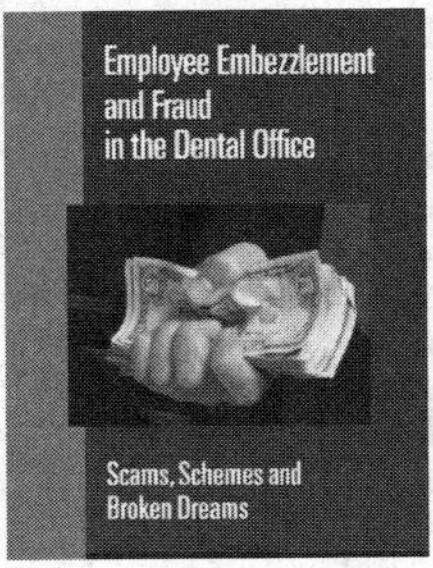

Incidents of fraud and embezzlement are on the rise, and dental offices are a particular target. This book, by a dentist in private practice, gives inside information on preventing fraud and embezzlement from occurring in your practice.

This book shows you how to discover if your practice is a target for theft and identify some of the common scams and schemes used by embezzlers in dentistry. With this book also learn how to establish internal controls to prevent thefts by enacting policies and procedures to protect your practice.

Your Roadmap to Financial Integrity in the Dental Practice

by Donald P. Lewis, Jr., DDS, CFE

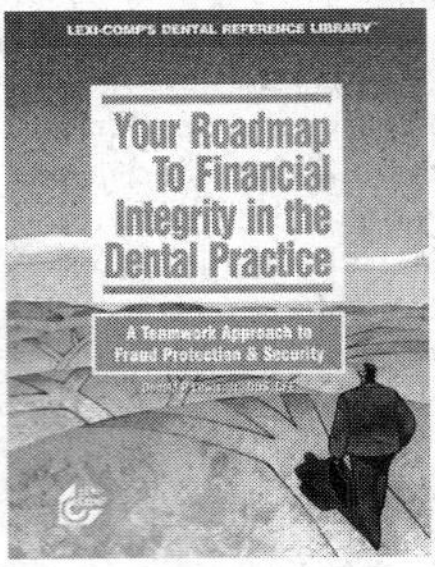

This ideal practice management handbook explains how good internal controls can help minimize problems such as theft, fraud, and unintentional accounting/recording errors in the dental office. Designed and written by a dentist in private practice.

www.lexi.com/dentistry • 1-866-397-3433

Other Products Offered by Lexicomp

A Patient Guide to Dental Implants

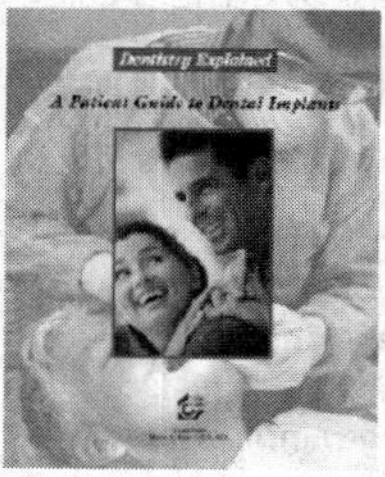

A highly illustrative description of the options available for various types of implants, including a frequently asked question-and-answer section. The flip-chart format allows for display on a desk, if required.

Tabbed sections include:
- Single Tooth Replacement
- Replacement of Several Teeth
- Four-Implant Retained Overdenture
- Two-Implant Retained Overdenture
- Screw-Retained Denture

Additional Features:
- Over 1600 bulleted points of interest
- Over 180 checklist options
- 13 real-life stories
- Over 80 boxed topics of special interest

A Patient Guide to Dental Implants Booklet

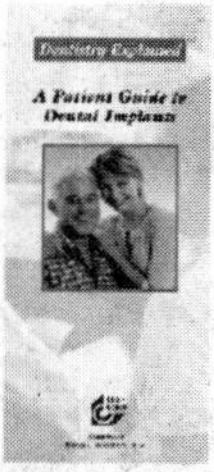

This simplified guide to dental implants will help your patients understand the different options for this procedure. Easy to read and illustrated in a non-frightening way, the diagrams show how single or multiple implants can be achieved. Useful for reception areas, these leaflets can be supplied in bulk quantities.

A Patient Guide to Periodontal Disease

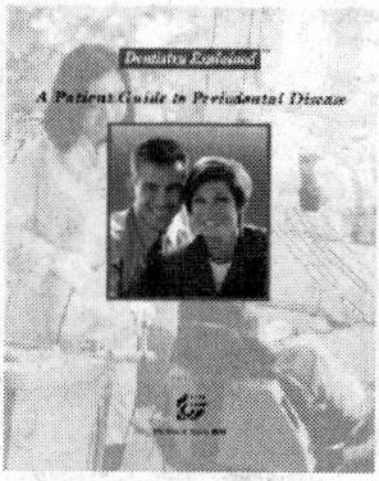

This informative patient guide provides a colorful visual overview of the procedures involved with the treatment of Periodontal Disease. The flip-chart format allows for display on a desk, if required.

Tabbed sections include:
- Healthy Gums
- Gingivitis
- Mild to Moderate Periodontitis
- Advanced Periodontitis
- Treatment Operations
- If Left Untreated
- Oral Hygiene Instruction
- Prevention

Patient Guide to Root Canal Therapy

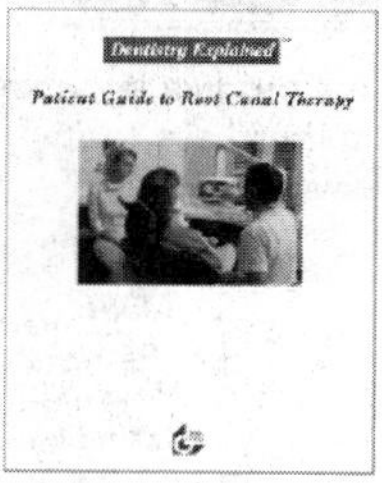

An illustrated, detailed explanation of Root Canal Therapy including a frequently asked question-and-answer section. The flip-chart format allows for display on a desk, if required.

Tabbed sections include:
- What is Root Canal Therapy?
- Access Opening
- Cleaning & Shaping the Root Canal System
- Filling the Root Canal System
- Temporary Restoration
- Permanent Restoration
- Crown Restoration

www.lexi.com/dentistry • 1-866-397-3433

Other Products Offered by Lexicomp

Lexicomp On-Hand for Dentistry

Lexicomp On-Hand for Dentistry provides instant access to point-of-care information on mobile/smartphone devices. Updates to our content are available on a daily basis, ensuring you always have the most timely clinical information at your fingertips.

Featuring Dental Lexi-Drugs, covering over 8000 drugs and herbal products with monographs containing up to 55 fields of information, including U.S. Brand Names, Special Alerts, Use, Local Anesthetic/Vasoconstrictor Precautions, Effects on Dental Treatment, Dental Dosing for Selected Drug Classifications, Adverse Effects, Contraindications, Warnings/Precautions, Drug Interactions and Dental Comment.

Lexicomp On-Hand for Mobile/Smartphone Devices

On-the-go access to Lexicomp's dental-specific drug information!

Available for smartphones and other mobile devices, Lexicomp's dental applications feature the full color images, charts and appendices from our trusted dental print manuals!

Available for the iPhone · Android · palm webOS · palm · Windows Mobile · BlackBerry

Available applications include:

☐ **Dental Lexi-Drugs *plus* Lexi-Interact**

☐ **Lexi-DENTAL SELECT**
Includes:

- Dental Lexi-Drugs
- Lexi-Interact
- Lexi-Drug ID
- Lexi-CALC
- Oral Soft Tissue Diseases
- Oral Hard Tissue Diseases
- Illustrated Handbook of Clinical Dentistry
- Dental Office Medical Emergencies
- The Little Dental Drug Booklet

☐ **Lexi-DENTAL COMPLETE**
Includes:

- Dental Lexi-Drugs
- Lexi-Interact
- Pediatric Lexi-Drugs
- Lexi-Drug ID
- Lexi-CALC
- Oral Soft Tissue Diseases
- Oral Hard Tissue Diseases
- Illustrated Handbook of Clinical Dentistry
- Dental Office Medical Emergencies
- The Little Dental Drug Booklet
- Clinician's Endodontic Handbook
- Manual of Clinical Periodontics
- Manual of Dental Implants
- Oral Surgery for the General Dentist
- Advanced Protocols for Medical Emergencies
- Harrison's Practice
- Stedman's Medical Dictionary for the Health Professions and Nursing

DAILY UPDATES

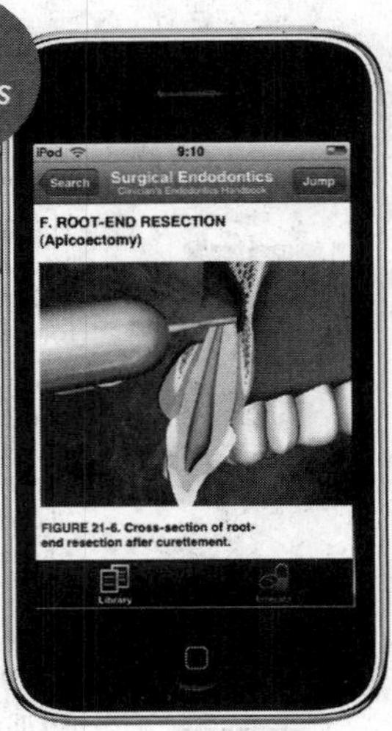

For complete product informatio[n]
and to purchase, visit:
www.lexi.com

Multi-year Subscription Discounts Available!

www.lexi.com/dentistry • 1-866-397-3433